W9-DCN-127

MEDICAL-SURGICAL NURSING:

Assessment and Management of Clinical Problems

MEDICAL-SURGICAL NURSING:
Assessment and Management of Clinical Problems

Sharon Mantik Lewis, R.N., M.S., CCRN

Assistant Professor
College of Nursing
University of New Mexico, Albuquerque
Doctoral Student
Department of Pathology
Medical Sciences
University of New Mexico, Albuquerque

Idolia Cox Collier, R.N., M.S.N.

Associate Professor
College of Nursing
University of New Mexico, Albuquerque
Doctoral Student
Department of Family Health Care Nursing
University of California, San Francisco

McGraw-Hill Book Company

New York St. Louis San Francisco Auckland Bogotá Hamburg
Johannesburg London Madrid Mexico Montreal New Delhi Panama
Paris São Paulo Singapore Sydney Tokyo Toronto

NOTICE
As new medical and nursing research and clinical experience broaden our knowledge, changes in treatment and drug therapy are required. The editors and the publisher of this work have made every effort to ensure that the drug dosage schedules herein are accurate and in accord with the standards accepted at the time of publication. Readers are advised, however, to check the product information sheet included in the package of each drug they plan to administer to be certain that changes have not been made in the recommended dose or in the contraindications for administration. This recommendation is of particular importance in regard to new or infrequently used drugs.

MEDICAL-SURGICAL NURSING:
Assessment and Management of Clinical Problems

2 3 4 5 6 7 8 9 0 VNHVNH 8 9 8 7 6 5 4 3

ISBN 0-07-037561-5

This book was set in Helvetica Light by Black Dot, Inc. (ECU).
The editors were David P. Carroll, Stuart D. Boynton, and James W. Bradley;
the designer was Merrill Haber;
the production supervisor was Dominick Petrellese.
Von Hoffmann Press, Inc., was printer and binder.

Illustration Credits

Mark Lefkowitz, M.A., *Medical Illustrator*
Marcia Williams, M.S., *Medical Illustrator*
JoEllen Murphy, B.F.A., *Instructional Illustrator*
Alice Vickery, *Graphic Illustrator*
Terry Buzzee, *Graphic Illustrator*

Educational Media Support Center
Boston University Medical Center

Library of Congress Cataloging in Publication Data

Lewis, Sharon Mantik.
Medical-surgical nursing.

Includes index.
1. Nursing. 2. Surgical nursing. I. Collier, Idolia Cox. II. Title. [DNLM: 1. Nursing care. 2. Nursing process. WY 100 L676m]
RT41.L68 1983 610.73 82-18673
ISBN 0-07-037561-5

To the Profession of Nursing

There comes a call and we answer
by learning,
caring,
sharing.

And we continue. . . .
Because we are a profession of dedication.

V. Lewis
1982

CONTENTS

Section 9 Problems Related to Regulatory Mechanisms

Section 10 Problems Related to Movement and Coordination

Section 11 Problems in Special Situations

Appendixes

LIST OF CONTRIBUTORS

Charlotte R. Abbink, R.N., M.S.N.
Associate Dean, Assistant Professor, College of Nursing, University of New Mexico, Albuquerque, New Mexico

Nancy R. Adams, R.N., M.S.N., CCRN
Major, U.S. Army Nurse Corps; *formerly Director,* Intensive Care Nursing Course, Fitzsimons Army Medical Center, Aurora, Colorado

Naomi R. Ballard, R.N., M.A.
Associate Professor, Medical-Surgical Nursing, School of Nursing, University of Oregon Health Sciences Center, Portland, Oregon

Audrey S. Bomberger, R.M., Ph.D.
Director of Education, St. Mary's Hospital, Reno, Nevada

Barbara J. Boss, R.N., Ph.D.
Associate Professor of Nursing, The University of Mississippi Medical Center, Jackson, Mississippi

Margaret Stapleton Brown, R.N., Ph.D.
Assistant Professor, College of Nursing, University of New Mexico, Albuquerque, New Mexico

Linda C. Carnago, R.N., M.S.N.
Instructor of Nursing, Henry Ford Community College, Dearborn, Michigan

Michael A. Carter, R.N., D.N.Sc.
Associate Professor, School of Nursing, University of Colorado, Denver, Colorado

Corina B. Casias, R.N., M.S.N., CFNP
Assistant Professor, College of Nursing, University of New Mexico, Albuquerque, New Mexico

Katherine L. Chipman, R.N., M.S.N.
Head Nurse—Obstetrics, University of Oregon Health Sciences Center, Portland, Oregon

Dorothy Hendel Clough, R.N., M.S.N.
Associate Professor, College of Nursing, University of New Mexico, Albuquerque, New Mexico

Idolia Cox Collier, R.N., M.S.N.
Associate Professor, College of Nursing, University of New Mexico, Albuquerque, New Mexico; *Doctoral Student,* Department of Family Health Care Nursing, University of California, San Francisco

JoAnn Ganje Congdon, R.N., M.S.
Assistant Professor, School of Nursing, University of Colorado, Denver, Colorado

Sandra Hower Currin, R.N., B.S.N.
Formerly Diabetes Nurse Specialist, Veteran's Administration Hospital, North Chicago, Illinois

Gladys Deters, R.N., M.S.
Assistant Professor, School of Nursing, University of Virginia, Charlottesville, Virginia

Linda Stevenson Dillion, R.N., M.S.
Renal Clinical Specialist, Methodist Hospitals of Dallas, Dallas, Texas

Patsy L. Orth Duphorne, R.N., M.N.
Assistant Professor, College of Nursing, University of New Mexico, Albuquerque, New Mexico

Barba Jean Edwards, R.N., M.A.
Director of Surgery, Archbishop Bergan Mercy Hospital, Omaha, Nebraska

Rachel E. Elrod, R.N., M.S.
Instructor, Community College of Denver, North Campus, Denver, Colorado

Sue E. Elster, R.N., M.N.
Research Associate, College of Nursing (Research Support Center), University of Utah, Salt Lake City, Utah

Marie E. Folk-Lighty, R.N., M.S.N., CCRN
Nurse Coordinator, Burn Center, Harborview Medical Center, Seattle, Washington; *Clinical Assistant Professor,* Department of Physiological Nursing, University of Washington, Seattle, Washington

Louise P. Gallagher, R.N., M.Ed.
Assistant Professor, Pace University, Pleasantville, New York

Anita Ann Wagner Garman, R.N., M.S.N.
Lieutenant Colonel, U.S. Army Nurse Corps; formerly, Academy of Health Sciences, Ft. Sam Houston, San Antonio, Texas

Diane Germain, R.N., B.S.
Instructor, Program of Practical Nursing, St. Mary's County Technical Center, Leonardtown, Maryland

Joan W. Goloskov, R.N., B.S.N., F.A.A.N.
Neurosurgical Nurse Associate, Wilmington, Delaware

Martha-Jane Greenberg, R.N., M.S.N.
Assistant Professor, Department of Nursing, Pace University, Pleasantville, New York

Patricia Robertson Hercules, R.N., M.S.
Assistant Director—Operating Rooms, The Methodist Hospital, Houston, Texas

Virginia M. Hunter, R.D.
Clinical Dietician, University of New Mexico Hospital, Albuquerque, New Mexico

Susan Searle Jackson, R.N., M.S.N.
Assistant Professor, School of Nursing, The Catholic University of America, Washington, D.C.

Bonnie Mowinski Jennings, R.N., M.S.
Major, U.S. Army Nurse Corps, Department of Nursing, Dwight David Eisenhower Army Medical Center, Fort Gordon, Georgia

Phyllis Gappa Jensen, R.N., M.S.N.
Instructor, Madison Area Technical College, Madison, Wisconsin

Carol Fair Keith, R.N., M.S.
Assistant Professor, School of Nursing, Ohio State University, Columbus, Ohio

Delores C. Lesher, R.N., B.S.
Director of Education, Lebanon Valley General Hospital, Lebanon, Pennsylvania

Sharon Mantik Lewis, R.N., M.S., CCRN
Assistant Professor, College of Nursing, University of New Mexico, Albuquerque, New Mexico; *Doctoral Student,* Department of Pathology, Medical Sciences, University of New Mexico, Albuquerque, New Mexico

Susan C. Littell, R.N., M.S., CCRN
Instructor, School of Nursing, University of Alaska, Anchorage, Alaska

Barbara J. Lockwood, R.N., M.S.
Systems Director of Nursing, St. Anthony Hospital Systems, Denver, Colorado

Karen H. May McArdle, R.N., M.A.
Coordinator, St. Therese Alternate Response Hospice, St. Therese Hospital, Waukegan, Illinois

Kathy Marquis, R.N., M.S.N., F.N.P.
Formerly Director of Women's Health Specialist Program, University of New Mexico, Albuquerque, New Mexico

Emilie Musci, R.N., M.S.N.
Associate Clinical Director, Post Master's Oncology Nursing Education Project, San Jose State University; *Doctoral Student,* University of California, San Francisco

Maureen Brady Nash, R.N., M.S.N., CPNP
School Nurse, Albuquerque Public School System, Albuquerque, New Mexico; *formerly Rehabilitation Nursing Specialist and Neurological Nursing Supervisor,* St. Joseph Hospital, Albuquerque, New Mexico

Sally J. Ness, R.N., M.S.N., CVNS, CCRN
Formerly Cardiovascular Clinical Nurse Specialist, Surgical Nursing Service, The Methodist Hospital, Houston, Texas

Judith M. Ozuna, R.N., M.N.
Assistant Professor, Department of Physiological Nursing, University of Washington, Seattle, Washington; *Clinical Nurse Specialist,* Epilepsy Center, Seattle, Washington

Donna J. Rodriguez, R.D.
Clinical Dietician, University of New Mexico Hospital, Albuquerque, New Mexico

Carol Cox Smith, B.S., M.A.
Formerly Instructor, Technical-Vocational Institute, Albuquerque, New Mexico

Carol E. Smith, R.N., M.S.N., Ph.D.
Assistant Professor of Nursing, Winona State University, Rochester Center, Rochester, Minnesota; Nurse Practitioner, Blooming Prairie, Minnesota

Roberta T. Spencer, R.N., M.S.
Associate Professor, Department of Nursing, State University of New York College at Plattsburgh, Plattsburgh, New York

Patricia Palmer Stephens, R.N., M.S., M.A.
Assistant Professor, College of Nursing, University of New Mexico, Albuquerque, New Mexico

Carol A. Stephenson, R.N., Ed.D., N.S.
Assistant Professor, Harris College of Nursing
Texas Christian University
Ft. Worth, Texas

Nancy Rojo Sypert, R.N., M.S.N.
Clinical Director for Surgery, Department of Nursing Services, Shands Teaching Hospital & Clinics, Inc., Gainesville, Florida; *Adjunct Assistant Professor,* College of Nursing, University of Florida, Gainesville, Florida

Patricia Van Sciver, R.N., M.S., CCRN
Critical Care Coordinator, Professional Nurse Associates, P.C.; *Visiting Instructor,* College of Nursing, University of New Mexico, Albuquerque, New Mexico

Sharon Wahl, R.N., M.S.N.
Formerly, School of Nursing, University of Oregon Health Sciences Center, Portland, Oregon

Susan N. Walker, R.N., Ed.D.
Associate Professor, School of Nursing, Northern Illinois University, De Kalb, Illinois

Kenneth J. Webb, R.N., OPA-C, M.S.
Orthopaedic Nursing Care Specialist, Coordinator and Instructor, Orthopaedic Allied Health Training Program, Department of Orthopaedic Surgery, Los Angeles County, University of Southern California Medical Center, Los Angeles, California

Earnestine Huffman White, R.N., M.S.N., M.A.
Professor, College of Lake County,
Grayslake, Illinois
Doctoral Candidate
Northern Illinois University

Joyce M. Yasko, R.N., Ph.D.
Assistant Professor—Graduate Program, Medical-Surgical Nursing, School of Nursing, University of Pittsburgh, Pittsburgh, Pennsylvania

Kathy Zarling, R.N., B.S.N.
Coronary Care Counselor and Coordinator, Cardiac Rehabilitation, Rochester Methodist Hospital, Rochester, Minnesota

Gayle L. Ziegler, R.N.
Rheumatology Research/Education, Division of Rheumatology and Clinical Immunology, School of Medicine, University of Pittsburgh, Pittsburgh, Pennsylvania

PREFACE

If nursing is to maintain and improve its position in the health care delivery system, nurses must continue to broaden the knowledge base upon which their decisions are made. *Medical-Surgical Nursing: Assessment and Management of Clinical Problems* has been written for this purpose and focuses on the nursing care of adult clients. The major strengths of this text are its use of the nursing process as an organizational thread as well as its commitment to the place of nursing in the health care team. The text is intended to have sufficient content flexibility to meet the needs of a variety of programs and learning styles.

The editors recognize that learning occurs in a variety of ways. This book intentionally addresses both the verbally oriented and the pictorially oriented learner. Accordingly, it utilizes both approaches, with many pictures, tables, and illustrations supplementing the text. Readability has been analyzed to keep content at the appropriate level.

Content is organized into two major divisions. The first division (Section 1: Chapters 1 through 5) discusses general nursing concepts related to adult clients. Basic nursing concepts such as death and dying, epidemiology, and health care systems, commonly found in medical-surgical texts, have been intentionally excluded to avoid overlap with material usually covered in fundamental nursing textbooks.

The second division (Sections 2 through 11: Chapters 6 through 60) presents both nursing assessment and nursing role in management of medical-surgical problems. The various body systems are grouped by section in a sequence that reflects their interrelated functions in order to promote the reader's understanding of the body as an integrated whole. Each section is organized around two main themes: assessment and management. Chapters dealing with the first theme, assessment of the body system, include a discussion of the following:

1. Anatomy and physiology in brief review, focusing on information that will promote understanding of nursing care
2. Health history and noninvasive physical assessment skills to expand the data base on which decisions are made
3. Common diagnostic studies, expected results, and related nursing care

The second theme is the nursing role in management of the various disorders of the body system. Chapters embracing this theme focus on the significance of the problem, pathogenesis and/or pathophysiology, clinical manifestations and complications with explanations of pathophysiological bases, and expected abnormalities of diagnostic studies. In addition, each chapter presents a concise discussion of medical management for major diseases and problems.

The nursing process is the basis for the organization of nursing management, and it enables the nurse to provide care in the following areas:

1. Health maintenance and promotion
2. Acute intervention
3. Rehabilitative or chronic management

Client education is a major concern in all areas of nursing care. Over 100 nursing care plans have been developed that include client problems, expected outcomes, and nursing interventions. For each major medical-surgical problem there is a specific discussion of pharmacological and nutritional intervention. Critical care content is included where appropriate. Appendix A deals with laboratory values and the significance of alterations. Appendix B includes samples of therapeutic diets based on cultural variations for traditional American, Spanish-American, and black-American populations.

Learning objectives precede each chapter to focus on essential content, and review questions follow each chapter to enable the reader to assess mastery of the content. (Appendix C lists answers to the review questions.) Each management chapter includes a case study with discussion questions. Sample charting for normal assessment of each body system is included in table form.

Although the basic content of the text was provided by multiple contributors, final rewriting and editing by the two editors achieves internal consistency. In addition, each chapter was thoroughly reviewed by one or more specialists in the subject area.

Note that to avoid the cumbersome repetition and alternation of the pronouns "he" and "she," the text consistently refers to the nurse as "she" and the client (with obvious exceptions) as "he." This usage of the traditional pronoun in referring to the nurse should not be interpreted as either an exclusion of the contributions of male nurses or a failure to acknowledge and support the increasing number of men who are entering the nursing profession.

The editors are especially grateful to many people at the McGraw-Hill Book Company who assisted with this major effort. In particular, we wish to thank

Laura Dysart Marcy, Former Nursing Editor
David P. Carroll, Former Nursing Editor
Stuart D. Boynton, Development Editor
James W. Bradley, Senior Editing Supervisor
Eileen Dowd, Editorial Assistant

Jerome Glickman and his artists at the Educational Media Support Center at Boston University are responsible for the fine art program. Carol Cox Smith has our special thanks for transferring our words into creative photographs to enhance the textual material. Shirley King is our perservering typist who typed all chapters prior to final submission as well as the instructor's manual.

And, of course, we wish to thank our contributors and reviewers, whose commitment to nursing excellence kept them at their tasks until the job was done. We sincerely hope that this book will assist both students and practitioners in practicing truly professional nursing.

Sharon Mantik Lewis
Idolia Cox Collier

MEDICAL-SURGICAL NURSING:

Assessment and Management of Clinical Problems

Section 1

General Concepts of Nursing Practice

Chapter 1

GENERAL CONCEPTS

Experience of Health and Illness

Patricia Palmer Stephens

Learning Objectives

1. Define health, wellness, and illness.
2. Describe modern theories of disease causation.
3. Differentiate among behaviors that promote health or result in illness.
4. Describe the behaviors characteristic of illness and sick role.
5. Differentiate between acute and chronic illness.
6. Explain the stages of acute illness.
7. Explain special concerns and tasks of the chronically ill.

INTRODUCTION

> The great secret known to internists, but still hidden from the general public, is that most things get better by themselves. Most things in fact are better by morning.[1]

> Life is a continual battle with the 'bugs.' In the end, however, the bugs will win out.[2]

There is an element of truth in both these contrasting views of health and illness. One view emphasizes the ability of the body to heal without medical intervention and the other view emphasizes that death comes to all.

The focus of this chapter is on the experience of health and illness. First, the meaning of health and illness will be addressed. Then, common role changes which may occur with illness will be discussed. In order to manage clients well, nurses must begin with an understanding of how health and illness may be defined and experienced. A general knowledge comes from health theorists and research studies, to which is added specific information gained from a client's nursing history. Thus, the general knowledge plus the specific information provide the data base for implementing the nursing process with an individual client (the nursing process is discussed in Chap. 2).

HEALTH AND ILLNESS

Conceptual Definitions of Health

A clear definition of health that can be easily understood and used is not easy to achieve. However, as a number of definitions are considered, a definition for this textbook will emerge. Sometimes the terms *health* and *wellness* are used interchangeably. However, there is an important difference. *Health* is often defined as merely the absence of illness. Also, the phrase "state of health" may be used to refer to excellent or poor health. However, *wellness* is often given a more positive connotation, suggesting that it involves more than absence of illness. The following paragraphs will demonstrate the differences in definition more clearly.

This chapter was reviewed by Chiyoko Furukawa, R.N., M.S., Assistant Professor, College of Nursing, University of New Mexico, Albuquerque, New Mexico.

WHO definition of health

Perhaps the most commonly quoted definition of health was stated in 1947 by the World Health Organization (WHO). It states that health is "a state of complete physical, mental, and social well-being and not merely the absence of disease or infirmity."[3] This means that to be healthy an individual must be in a state of well-being physically, mentally, and socially. Thus, according to the WHO definition, a person who is considered physically and mentally healthy is not truly healthy, if socially he is deprived access to basic education (this statement assumes that there is agreement that basic education is necessary for social health). The major problem with this definition is the difficulty health professionals have in agreeing to definitions of health in the physical, mental, and social dimensions.

High-level wellness

In the late 1950s, Halbert Dunn described the concept of high-level wellness.[4] It is based on a grid with two axes (Fig. 1-1). The health axis has death and peak wellness along it and the environmental axis has a very unfavorable environment and a very favorable environment along it. The health axis includes both physical and mental health. The environmental axis

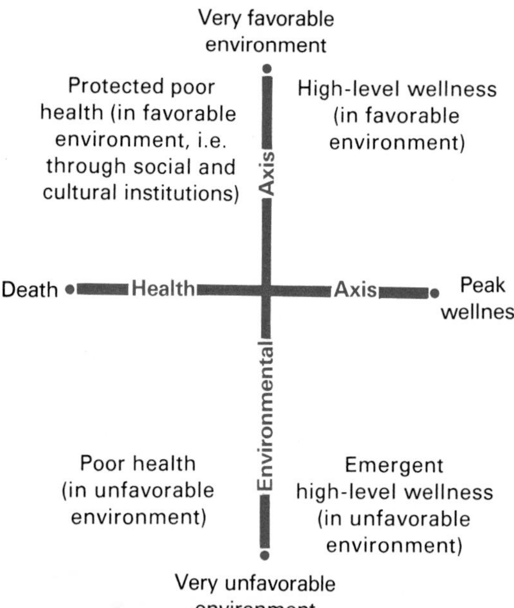

Figure 1-1 The health grid, its axes and quadrants. *(Source: U. S. Dept. of HEW, Public Health Service, National Office of Statistics.)*

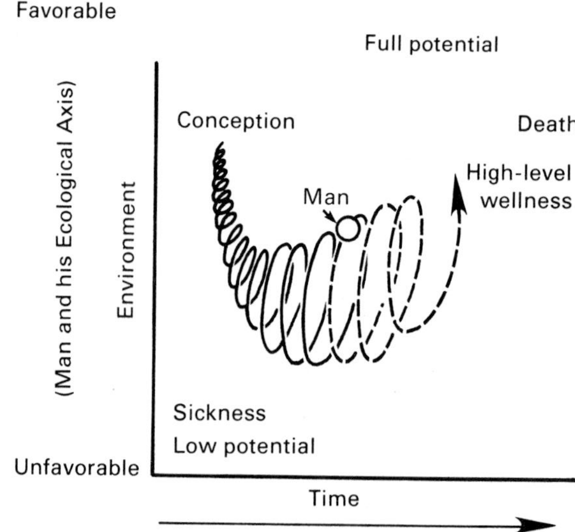

Figure 1-2 Spiral of Life. O-a person at a point in time. The spiral shows a person moving from conception to death. He or she "spirals" or moves from low potential or sickness to full potential or high-level wellness. *(Adapted from H. L. Dunn, High-Level Wellness, R. W. Beatty, Ltd., Arlington, Virginia, 1961, p. 240.)*

includes socioeconomic as well as biophysical factors in the environment which may affect health. Thus, high-level wellness refers to peak physical and mental health in a very favorable biophysical and socioeconomic environment.

Dunn further stated that "high-level wellness for the individual is *an integrated method of functioning which is oriented toward maximizing the potential of which the individual is capable, within the environment where he is functioning*."[5] He described wellness as a dynamic process which is moving toward a higher level of functioning. In contrast he described health as a passive state in which the individual is free from disease in a peaceful environment. Figure 1-2 uses a spiral to illustrate how an individual may move from conception to death between an unfavorable to favorable environment. An individual is considered to be body, mind, and spirit. At the bottom of the spiral an individual has low potential or energy. At the top of the spiral he has full potential or energy. Dunn's view of high-level wellness sees the body, mind, and spirit as interdependent and balanced. Ideally, during the life cycle the individual works to achieve this interdependence and balance as he progresses toward self-fulfillment and maturity.

An example of high-level wellness would be a 40-year-old college professor who is free of disease and jogs regularly. She is experiencing much personal satisfaction from her career and involvement in her church. She lives in a quiet town, relatively free from pollution and crime.

Developing wellness

Bruhn et al. in the mid-1970s stressed the *wellness process*.[6] They stated that *good health* is often described as a static position which is the consequence of avoiding those behaviors or circumstances which produce illness. However, *wellness* is a constantly evolving process in which the individual actively arranges his lifestyle and behavior. Figure 1-3 depicts the health continuum from illness to wellness. Note that good health, as frequently defined by health professionals, is in the middle of the continuum. Thus, the health continuum in Fig. 1-3 demonstrates that when a client has been rehabilitated from a specific illness, he is only halfway toward experiencing wellness. Table 1-1 further differentiates between the characteristics of wellness and good health. Bruhn et al. stress that wellness is always developing.

Sociological definition of health

Sociology is a source for a fourth possible definition of health. Sociologists see health as those bodily and emotional conditions which support or complement the pursuit and enjoyment of prized cultural values.[7] Thus, *illness* is any condition which interferes with the pursuit and enjoyment of desired cultural

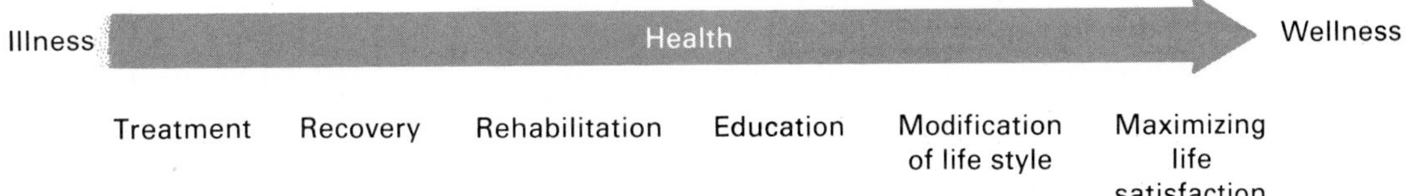

Figure 1-3 The linear health continuum. *[Source: J. G. Bruhn et al., "The Wellness Process," Journal of Community Health,* **2***(3):210 (Spring 1977).]*

values. This is similar to the results of several studies which find that laymen define good health as the ability to carry out normal activities. In addition, laymen see health as the absence of symptoms and a feeling of well-being.[8]

This latter definition of health moves from the view of the health professional to the view of the individual experiencing health or illness. Focus on the experience of the individual will be developed later in the chapter as theories of disease causation and sick role behavior are considered.

Definition for this textbook

Health, as used in this book, will be defined as high-level wellness. It is a dynamic condition in which a person is functioning at full energy levels in mind, body, and spirit to achieve his full potential. Wellness is the condition of a person which allows him to pursue desired goals with a sense of well-being. Events (physical, emotional, social, or environmental) which require adaptation by the individual will use energy and thus reduce the level of wellness experienced by him.

This textbook views nursing as having an important role in helping clients to develop wellness. In each of the management chapters those nursing measures which foster wellness will be called nursing management for *health promotion and maintenance.* Specific measures will be outlined which should assist the client in preventing or delaying the onset of certain diseases.

Holistic Health Care

Increased recognition that high-level wellness considers the needs of the whole person has led to the growth of holistic health (sometimes called holistic medicine). Holistic health practitioners focus on the promotion of health and prevention of illness as well as on the healing process. They emphasize the personal responsibility of the client in achieving high-level wellness. In addition, their care is focused on bringing the whole person (mind, body, and spirit) into harmony with the environment. Holistic health practitioners also see illness (a lack of harmony between the whole person and the environment) as an opportunity for personal growth. Health-promoting measures which are recommended by holistic care providers include such practices as meditation, prayer, massage, rolfing, nutrition, exercise, imagery, biofeedback, and therapeutic touch.[9]

When illness is present, holistic health measures may be used in addition to traditional western medical treatments. This may be done by one person or by a team made up of practitioners with different skills. An example of this approach is seen in the Medical Center Complex built in the early 1980s at Oral Roberts University in Oklahoma. Here, the physician, nurse, and spiritual counselor have equally important

Table 1-1
Difference Between Good Health and Wellness

Good Health	Wellness
1. State of being at one time. A stage on the health continuum. It can be lost.	1. A process that continues over time. Potential is not lost.
2. May exist without any effort by the individual.	2. Active utilization of all an individual's resources (biophysical, spiritual, sociocultural, psychological, and environmental).
3. An objective description of how an individual is doing at a point in time. It is lost when clinical signs of disease occur.	3. Part of the developmental tasks which the individual must meet. Cumulative learning. Delay in accomplishment of developmental tasks will decrease wellness potential.
4. State of being free from disease or clinical symptoms (Illness is the absence of wellness). Focus is on physical condition of a person.	4. Wellness and illness may exist together because a person may have a disease (headache) but experience wellness in the nonphysical areas of his life.

Compiled from J. G. Bruhn et al., "The Wellness Process," *Journal of Community Health,* **2**(3): 211–212 (Spring 1977).

roles in the treatment of illness. Each nursing unit has physical space allotted to each member of the team.

Sociocultural Considerations in Defining Health and Illness

There are variations in definitions of health and illness according to the social and cultural orientation of individuals. It is important for the nurse to recognize that these do exist and that nursing intervention be planned accordingly. Research has been conducted to determine if various socioeconomic groups within the majority American culture define health and illness in different terms. Little evidence has been found to support differences in definition among socioeconomic groups. However, there does seem to be a difference in help-seeking behavior. Generally, those from higher socioeconomic levels tend to seek help earlier when they suspect the presence of illness. However, other variables such as personal values and accessibility of health care (financially or geographically) affect this behavior.

There are more obvious variations in the definitions of health and illness by ethnic minority groups of color in the United States. Ethnic minority groups of color include Black Americans, Hispanic Americans, Native Americans (e.g., Eskimo, Iroquois, Seminole, Sioux, Navajo, Pueblo groups) and Asian-Americans. Those people who identify most closely with their ethnic group are called *traditional*. Those who identify most closely with the majority are called *acculturated*. The beliefs of many ethnic people are somewhere on a continuum between traditional beliefs and acculturated beliefs. Table 1-2 presents examples of the way three ethnic minority groups of color traditionally define health and describe causation of disease. It also describes traditional healers and methods of treatment.

Because dietary patterns are an important part of an individual's cultural practices, this textbook demonstrates, in Appendix B, how special diets may be modified. It is important when considering this table not to stereotype individuals but to use the information while implementing the nursing process (see Chaps. 2 and 3).

Theories of Illness Causation

Part of the science of medicine has been directed toward identifying the cause of disease. Great advances have been made in this area. Today we recognize that diseases may be caused by:

1. Inherited genetic defects
2. Developmental defects due to factors such as exposure to viral substances or certain chemicals or drugs during pregnancy
3. Biological agents or toxins
4. Physical agents such as temperature extremes, chemicals, or radiation
5. Generalized response of tissues to injury or irritation

Table 1-2
Variations in Defining and Treating Health and Disease Ethnic Groups

Ethnic Group	Definition of Health	Causation of Disease	Traditional Treatment Methods	Traditional Healers
Black Americans	Harmony with nature because all things influence each other. No separation between mind, body, and spirit.	Illness is disharmony due primarily to demons and evil spirits.	1. Voodoo—a belief system using white magic and black magic. Good *gris-gris* (pleasantly scented oils and powders) to prevent illness, cause success. Bad *grisgris* (vile-smelling oils and powders) used to cause illness, failure. Candles and Catholic relics are also used. 2. Many folk remedies. 3. Faith healers. Healing power of religion is stressed.	1. Women voodoo leaders who do *rooting* (determining source and treatment of a disease). 2. Faith healers (pray over the individual for healing; stress faith of the sick person).

Table 1-2 (Continued)

Ethnic Group	Definition of Health	Causation of Disease	Traditional Treatment Methods	Traditional Healers
Hispanic Americans A. Chicano (Mexican-American descent)	Balance or harmony in body due to either "luck," good behavior, or gift from God.	1. Imbalances of hot or cold, wet or dry in body due to punishment for wrongdoing. 2. Dislocation of body parts. 3. Magic causes outside of the body such as witchcraft or *malojo* (bad eye). 4. Strong emotions (e.g., *susto* from fright).	1. Use of certain religious rituals and artifacts such as confession, laying on of hands, lighting candles. 2. Massage. 3. *Cleanings,* or passing an unbroken egg or herbal bunch over the body. 4. Treatments are classified as hot or cold treatments and used for the opposite type of illness. 5. Magicoreligious practices such as pilgrimages, offering medals, lighting candles, making promises.	1. Curandero—a holistic faith healer. 2. Herbalist, skilled in using herbs for treatment.
B. Puerto Rican	Same	1. Similar to above. See illnesses as hot or cold. 2. Consider people who see visions as special people, not mentally ill.	1. Similar to Chicanos. Use of special herbs, foods, lotion. 2. Use of charms for prevention. 3. Treatments are classified as *frio* (cold), *fresco* (cool), or *caliente* (hot).	*Esperitista* or *curendera—a sophisticated folk practitioner. Santero*—treats mental illness.
Asian-Americans (e.g., Chinese)	Spiritual and physical harmony with nature. Balance maintained between *yin* (female, negative, cold, dark) and *yang* (male, positive, warm, light) by following *Tao*, the order or way of nature.	Upset in *yin* and *yang* balance.	1. Acupuncture (cold treatment), puncturing certain areas of the skin to cure disease or pain. 2. Moxibustion (hot treatment). Applying heated pulverized wormwood to specific areas of the skin to restore balance of *yin* and *yang*. 3. Wide variety of herbal remedies.	1. First-class physician—prevents occurrence of disease, plus treating disease. 2. Second-class physician—treats only those with disease.

Compiled from R. E. Spector, *Cultural Diversity in Health and Illness,* Appleton Century Crofts, New York, 1979, pp. 195–292.

6. Physiologic and psychological reactions to various stresses
7. Either an excessive or deficient production of various body secretions

It has also been found that many of these factors are interrelated.

However, there are still many unknowns about what causes disease. For many diseases there is not a direct cause-and-effect relationship between a specific disease-producing agent and the onset of disease. Theories of disease causation have been developed from research aimed at the discovery of the key to disease. The following theories are presented to demonstrate progress in determining the cause of diseases.

Historical theories of disease causation

Claude Bernard (a nineteenth-century physiologist) and Walter Cannon (an early-twentieth-century physician) described theories of disease causation that underlie modern theories. Bernard was the first to describe the internal environment of the body and the necessity for it to be maintained in a relatively constant state for health. He hypothesized that disease is the result of an upset in the internal environment, an interruption of the normal link between the internal and external environment of the body, and an overreaction of the body's attempt to adapt to the changes in the internal environment. Cannon was the first to use the term *homeostasis* when referring to the physiologic processes within the body. He defined homeostasis as dynamic equilibrium in which there is a constant change occurring in bodily processes which is so balanced that the end result is a constant environment. The support for his theory came from his study of self-regulating mechanisms in the body such as blood levels of oxygen and carbon dioxide, blood pressure, and body temperature.

General adaptation syndrome (GAS) or stress syndrome

Hans Selye, a physician, drawing from the work of Bernard on adaptive responses, published his early book on stress in 1950. He hypothesized that the stress syndrome was present in all diseases. His theory began with his observations as a young medical student of the "syndrome of being sick." He was struck more by the similarities of appearance and nonspecific symptoms of sick individuals than he was by their differences. He defines *stress* as "the state manifested by a specific syndrome which consists of all the non-specifically induced changes within a biologic system."[10] Stress is caused by a *stressor* which may be any agent such as physical exertion (swimming), emotional tension, or freezing temperatures which stresses the body. Selye calls the response the *General Adaptation Syndrome (GAS)* because it involves nonspecific changes, mediated by the sympathetic nervous system and adrenal cortices, which are directed toward adaptation of the body to the stressor. In his early work, Selye emphasized *acute* stressors and physiologic responses. In his recent work, Selye has put more emphasis on psychological stressors. A more detailed discussion of the syndrome follows later in Chap. 39.

Disease as maladaptation

In the 1950s and 1960s Harold Wolff, a psychiatrist, built on the work of Bernard and Selye. He emphasized psychological as well as physiologic responses to *chronic* stressors. Thus, he proposed that the entire life of the individual may be involved in disease causation. He noted that, because of a highly developed central nervous system, humans react not only to actual stressors but to symbols and threats of danger as if they were actual stressors. Therefore, reactions to symbolic danger may be inappropriate. In addition, he noted that certain organs may react inappropriately to stressors. Often, the organ which reacts inappropriately is specific to the individual.[11] For example, one person is more apt to have physiologic changes in the stomach when stressed, whereas another individual will have changes in the respiratory tract. He proposed that these individual, specific organ reactions are the cause of psychosomatic diseases. *Psychosomatic diseases* or disorders are ones with physiologic or structural changes thought to be at least partially due to psychological or mental influences. Psychosomatic medicine continues to look at the role emotions play in disease causation. Table 1-3 is a list of disorders thought to have psychological factors as part of their etiology.

Life changes and illness

The last theory of disease causation to be considered is life change units. Research has found that the number of life change units experienced by an individual has a positive correlation with the onset of disease. Much of the research in this area has been done by Rahe et al.[12,13] In one study Rahe and Holmes defined a *life change* as any positive or negative event in a person's life which requires that the person expend energy in order to adapt to it. The authors had various

Table 1-3
Possible Psychosomatic Disorders

Bronchial asthma
Dysmennorrhea
Hypertension
Hyperthyroidism
Migraine headache
Neurodermatitis
Paroxysmal tachycardia
Peptic ulcers
Raynaud's disease
Rheumatoid arthritis
Ulcerative colitis

All these disorders are thought to have psychological factors as part of their etiology.

Compiled from Raymond Adams, "Alteration in Nervous Function," in K. J. Isselbacher et al. (eds.), *Harrison's Principles of Internal Medicine*, 9th ed., McGraw-Hill Book Company, New York, 1980, p. 68.

Table 1-4
Social Readjustment Rating Scale

No.	Life Event Item	Mean Value
1.	Death of spouse	100
2.	Divorce	73
3.	Marital separation from mate	65
4.	Detention in jail or other institution	63
5.	Death of a close family member	63
6.	Major personal injury or illness	53
7.	Marriage	50
8.	Being fired from work	47
9.	Marital reconciliation	45
10.	Retirement	45
11.	Major change in health of a family member	44
12.	Pregnancy	40
13.	Sexual difficulties	39
14.	Gaining a new family member (e.g., birth or elderly parent)	39
15.	Major business readjustment	39
16.	Major change in financial state	38
17.	Death of a close friend	37
18.	Changing to different line of work	36
19.	Major change in number of arguments with spouse	35
20.	Taking on mortgage greater than $10,000	31
21.	Foreclosure of mortgage or loan	30
22.	Major change in responsibilities at work (e.g., promotion, demotion)	29
23.	Son or daughter leaving home	29
24.	In-law troubles	29
25.	Outstanding personal achievement	28
26.	Wife beginning or ending work outside the home	26
27.	Beginning or ending normal schooling	26
28.	Major change in living conditions (e.g., new home, remodeling)	25
29.	Revision of personal habits	24
30.	Trouble with boss	23
31.	Major change in working hours or conditions	20
32.	Change in residence	20
33.	Change in school	20
34.	Major change in type or amount of recreation	19
35.	Major change in church activities	19
36.	Major change in social activities (e.g., clubs, dancing, visiting)	18
37.	Taking on mortgage or loan less than $10,000	17
38.	Major change in sleeping habits	16
39.	Major change in number of family get-togethers	15
40.	Major change in eating habits	15
41.	Vacation	13
42.	Christmas	12
43.	Minor violation of law (e.g., traffic tickets)	11

Adapted from T. H. Holmes and R. H. Rahe, "Social Readjustment Rating Scale," *Psychosomatic Research*, **11:**216 (1967).

socioeconomic and cultural groups rank a number of life changes according to the amount of energy needed to adapt to the changes. The Social Readjustment Rating Scale (SRRS), Table 1-4, shows the results of this ranking plus the number of life change units associated with each event (marriage was given an arbitrary score of 50).

Additional research studies utilizing the SRRS have found a significant relationship between life changes and physical and mental illnesses. It is felt that the reason for the development of illness with life changes is that these changes require adaptive behavior. The adaptive behaviors then cause major alterations in the individual's psychophysiologic systems, thus lowering the resistance of the body to illness.[14] Table 1-5 describes the incidence of illness according to the number of life changes over a 1- to 2-year period. Other studies have shown that the higher the average number of life change units (LCU) over 2 years, the more serious is the illness. For example, the LCUs before developing bronchitis were around 320 whereas the LCUs before developing cancer were 780.[15]

Other factors such as health habits, social assets (family and financial security and academic achievement), and psychological well-being may be thought to have as much influence on health status as life change units. However, Pesznecker and McNeil found in their study that the number of life change units were the strongest variable predicting health status. However, all the variables were weakly associated with maintenance of health status.[16]

In conclusion, it is apparent that there are many factors involved in the causation of disease in a specific individual. These factors are found in both his external and internal environment. In addition, factors causing illness are both physical and psychological. Recent research findings regarding the stress of life changes are especially significant for health promo-

Table 1-5
Life Change Units and Incidence of Major Illness

Number of LCU	Amount of Change	Incidence of Major Illness
0–149	Insignificant	Minimal
150–199	Mild	33%
200–299	Moderate	50%
300+	Major	80%

This table describes the amount of stress as measured by life change units. This is followed by the statistical incidence of disease according to the number of LCUs. The chance of illness is based on the number of LCUs over a 1- to 2-year period.

Compiled from B. L. Pesznecker and J. McNeil, "Relationship Among Health Habits, Social Assets, Psychological Well-Being, Life Change, and Alterations in Health Status," *Nurs Res*, **24:**(6)443 (November–December 1975).

tion and maintenance in our rapidly changing society. This is especially true when the physiologic impact of stress is considered (see Chap. 39).

BEHAVIORS THAT PROMOTE HEALTH

Health Practices

The major focus of this chapter thus far has been on definitions of health and illness and factors which are likely to cause disease. There are, however, behaviors which seem to promote and maintain health. Certain health practices of the individual have been found to be positively correlated with health. These are:[17]

1. Sleeping regularly 7 to 8 hours per night
2. Eating breakfast
3. Eating regular meals with minimal or no snacking
4. Moderate eating to maintain ideal weight
5. Moderate exercising
6. Moderate drinking of alcohol
7. No smoking (best if have never smoked)

It has been found that the association of these behaviors with good health is independent of sex, age, and economic status. It has also been noted that they are cumulative; that is, the greater the number of these factors habitually practiced by the individual, the better his health.[18]

In addition to these primarily physical factors promoting health, good mental health practices are important for good health. These practices are primarily those which result in a realistic, positive self-concept and the ability to problem-solve.

Preventive Health Behavior

Preventive health behavior has been described as voluntary* action taken by an individual or group to decrease the potential threat of illness. This action is not curative or remedial because it is taken while the person is asymptomatic for a specific disease.[19] Preventive health behavior has both a decision-making phase and an action phase. The phases relate to both components of primary prevention and early detection. Primary prevention refers to those measures such as proper diet, proper exercise, and immunizations which may prevent the actual onset of a specific disease. Early detection refers to those measures such as blood pressure screening and breast self-examination which may detect the early onset of disease so early treatment may be instituted. This book includes both these components in the health promotion and maintenance sections of nursing care.

*Required school immunizations are the major exception to this definition.

Many times health care providers make the false assumption that a person will do what he knows is best for his health. Unfortunately, health care providers themselves disprove this assumption, as evidenced by the numbers who smoke, are overweight, underexercised, and overstressed! It is apparent that most human beings make choices about health practices which are the easiest, not necessarily the most healthy. Table 1-6 outlines the various factors affecting the decision-making process in preventive health behavior. Once a person has decided to carry out some preventive health behavior, he then needs cues to initiate action. These cues may be such things as a perception of aging, advertisements stressing healthy behavior, or a recent illness.

Nursing Management

The role of nursing in encouraging preventive behavior for better health can be identified when considering the decision-making factors. It is important that the nurse take steps to ensure that the client has the knowledge to select options. She may also need to help him find the resources needed to change his behavior. Table 1-7 further elaborates nursing measures which may be taken. Many of the disorders covered in this book could be prevented if an individual followed the seven health practices outlined earlier in this section. Thus, nursing care should begin by emphasizing these basic health habits.

TYPES OF ILLNESS

The two major categories of illness are generally classified as acute and chronic. *Acute illness* in this book refers to illness or disease (deviation from normal) of relatively rapid onset and short duration. It is usually self-limiting or responds readily to a specific treatment. Most acute illnesses allow the individual who develops no complications to return to his previous level of functioning after a period of recovery.

Chronic illness refers to those illnesses which lead to at least some of the following characteristics: (1) permanent impairments or deviations from normal, (2) nonreversible pathologic changes, (3) a residual disability, (4) special rehabilitation of the client, and (5) long-term medical and/or nursing management.[20] Chronic illnesses may have acute exacerbations in

Table 1-6
Decision-Making Phase Of Preventive Health Behavior

Factors	Motivating Perceptions	Basis
Personal determinants	Importance of health to the person	Activities it allows a person to do.
	Perceived vulnerability to a specific disease	Family history, present health status of the person, and incidence of the disease in the general population.
	Perceived value of early detection	Belief of the benefit of the specific technique for a specific illness, e.g., Pap smear for cervical cancer.
	Perceived seriousness of the disease	Degree of discomfort it threatens, degree of visibility, degree of disruption in family or occupational roles, and degree of communicability of the disease to others.
	Perceived efficacy of action	Choose those actions he perceives can lower threat of illness with least amount of risk and inconvenience.
	Perceived level of internal and external control	Those who feel powerless feel more vulnerable to illness because they have little control over their environment.
Interpersonal determinants	Concern of significant others	Family concern may cause a person to select healthy behavior to maintain family stability.
	Family patterns of utilization of health behavior	There is high maternal influence with a positive correlation between the level of education of the dominant female in the home and the level of preventive health behavior.
	Expectations of friends	Do what "good parents" should do.
	Expectations from professionals	The greater the credibility of the person giving the information, the greater the motivating factor.
Situational determinants	Cultural acceptance of health behaviors	Some cultures sanction the seeking of medical attention in presence of serious illness only. Preventive health behavior will follow when culture sanctions it as responsible action.
	Societal group norms and pressures	Complying with societal norms gives satisfaction.
	Information from nonpersonal sources	Use of mass media increases perceived vulnerability of individuals to disease.

Compiled from N. J. Pender, "A Conceptual Model for Preventive Health Behavior," *Nursing Outlook*, **23**(6):385–388 (June 1975).

which the client moves from a level of optimum functioning, with the illness in good control, to a period of physiologic instability where others may need to provide assistance.

Although both types of illnesses require nursing management, the specific nursing skills needed vary. In this book, nursing is divided into *health promotion and maintenance* (described earlier), *acute intervention,* and *chronic or rehabilitative management.* Nurses need to have the skills and knowledge base to meet the needs of a client within any of these categories. The specific skills for acute and chronic nursing intervention will be described with the particular problem where they are most applicable.

EXPERIENCE OF ILLNESS

Illness Behavior

The experience of illness as described by the terms *illness behavior* and *sick role* focuses attention on the individual rather than on the disease. An understanding of the various processes involved in the experience of illness will enable the nurse to provide care that considers the total person—in his biophysical, psychological, sociocultural, and environmental dimensions.

Illness behavior is the way a person deals with organic malfunctioning such as pain, discomfort, or

Table 1-7

Nursing Measures For Health Promotion

Nursing Measures	Example
Inform clients of the characteristics of at-risk disease.	Inform that a history of death of a parent at 40 years due to coronary artery disease is usually familial.
Explain the consequences of the disease to which the client is at risk.	Explain that because of family history, client may also have coronary artery disease at young age.
Give client specific information on how he may reduce his vulnerability to disease.	Counsel client on early detection measures by having lipid screening. Also counsel regarding moderate eating, regular exercise, and cessation of smoking.
Use nonhealth-related interpersonal determinants to encourage conformity.	For example, say: "I talked to your younger brother yesterday. He has cut down on desserts and started jogging every other day."

When carrying out these nursing measures, it is important to consider the whole person—the biophysical, psychological, sociocultural, and environmental dimensions.

Compiled from N. J. Pender, "A Conceptual Model for Preventive Health Behavior," *Nursing Outlook*, **23**(6):385–388 (June 1975).

fever. It includes the perception of symptoms, the evaluation of the significance (seriousness) of these symptoms, and the way the individual decides to respond to the symptoms and his evaluation of them. Each of these components of illness behavior are influenced by the severity of the symptoms and the individual's sociocultural environment.

An individual's response to illness will fall into three categories: (1) taking action, (2) taking no action, or (3) taking a counteraction.[21]

Taking action

Taking action to relieve symptoms may involve self-diagnosis and self-treatment, or seeking help from a health practitioner. Billions of dollars are spent annually by Americans on over-the-counter drugs (drugs not requiring a prescription) to alleviate symptoms which the ill person has diagnosed and decided to treat. This behavior is influenced by mass media advertising as well as the person's social grouping. Other ill persons may choose to self-treat using home or folk remedies. Other forms of self-treatment include such activities as rest, change in diet, or exercise.

If the self-treatment does not work, the individual who is taking action will probably seek out a health practitioner. The one he selects will depend primarily on his sociocultural background. One person may choose to go to a physician, whereas another may choose to go to such health practitioners as an herbalist, a chiropractor, or a spiritual healer. Sometimes the choice of health practitioner depends on the symptoms being experienced. For instance, an individual may go to a chiropractor for back problems or headache, but will go to a physician for a fever or abdominal pain.

Taking no action

Taking no action is another behavioral response to illness. It may be the result of a "wait-and-see" attitude or denial of the significance of the symptoms. The individual may be waiting to see if the symptoms will subside or worsen before he decides to take action. For example, he may say, "I will wait 2 or 3 days to see if my stomach pain will go away." On the other hand, the symptom may be so frightening that the individual denies it. He may completely ignore rectal bleeding although his father died of cancer of the colon. Some individuals delay action because they are unwilling to admit that they are sick or fear the consequences of their illness. Others may delay because they do not know which physician to see.

The individual's lack of action will be rewarded if the symptoms disappear. However, if the symptoms persist or worsen he will be forced to take action. This action may be taken because of pressure from family or friends, too much interference in his usual activities by the symptoms, or as a constructive response to a health-threatening symptom.

Taking counteraction

Taking counteraction refers to those behaviors which attempt to disprove the existence of symptoms. An example might be the man who decides to lift weights to work the "soreness" out of his left arm when the symptom suggests myocardial ischemia. Another example is an individual who has been diagnosed with a leukemia but who then shops around to find a health practitioner who will tell him that he does not have leukemia. Taking counteraction is an example of deviant illness behavior because the person wants to be defined as healthy when he is actually ill. He is not open to seeking help and thus is likely to have his condition worsen, possibly to the point of death.

Sick Role Behavior

Once the person defines himself as being ill, he enters the *sick role*. This means that he takes on the expected behaviors held by society of a sick person. Twaddle defines *sickness* as the judgment of health of

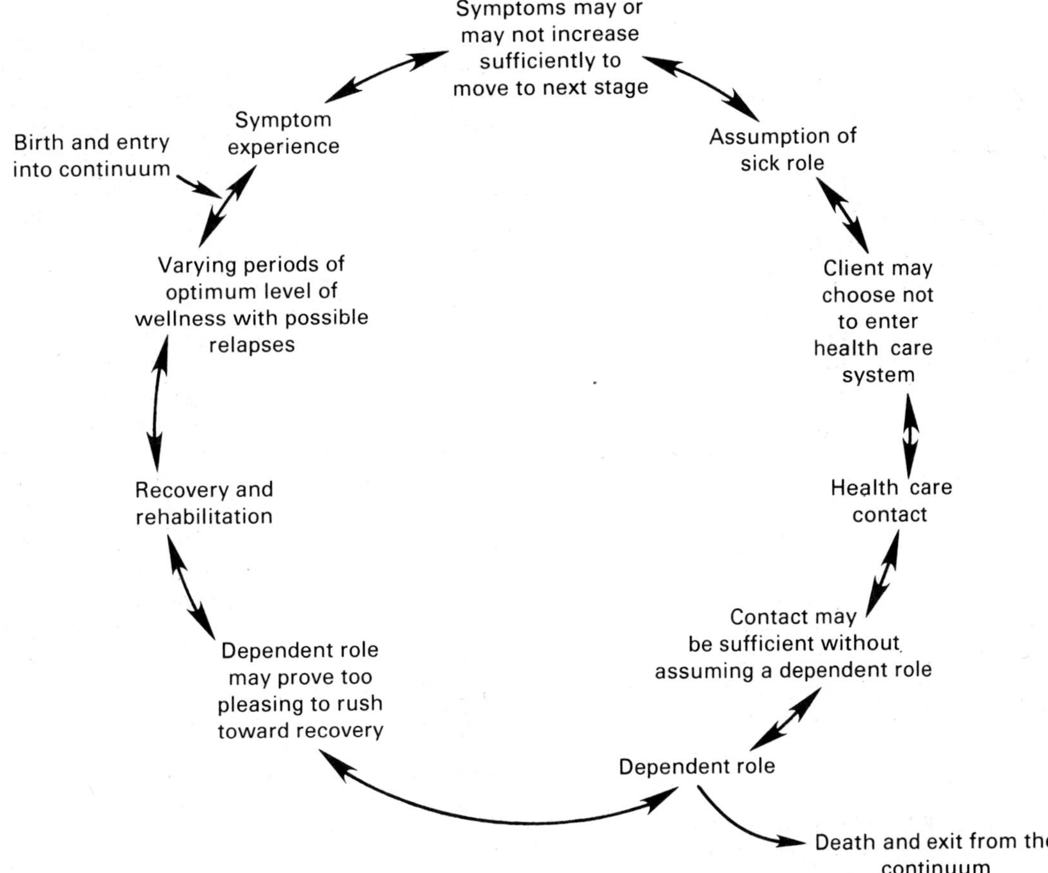

Figure 1-4 This circular health-illness continuum demonstrates the relationship between illness behavior and the sick role. Individuals may move around the circle many times during their lifetime. They may stop at the different places for varying times and may reverse their direction. *(Slightly modified from M. J. Fromer, Community Health Care and the Nursing Process, The C. V. Mosby Company, St. Louis, 1979, pp. 194–195.)*

one person by others. (He also sees *illness* as the symptoms the person experiences and disease as physical changes that either shorten life or reduce the individual's capacity to function).[22] This definition emphasizes that for someone to function in a sick role, those around him must perceive that he has a sickness.

The classic components of the sick role were defined by Parsons in the early 1950s. They are:[23]

1. The right of the individual to not be held responsible for his illness.
2. The right of the individual to be released from his usual responsibilities
3. The duty of the individual to try to get well and to see illness as undesirable
4. The duty of the individual to seek medically competent help and to cooperate with the treatment plan

These expectations of the sick role have been debated and analyzed over the last 30 years but have still been found to be an accurate description of the major components of sick role expectations.[24] This is especially true when applied to acute illness.

The relationship between illness behavior and the sick role are diagrammed in Fig. 1-4. It demonstrates that there is an overlap between seeking help (illness behavior) and assumption of the sick role. It also points out that a sick person needs to receive validation of his sick role from those around him and legitimization of it from a health care provider.

Stages of Acute Illness

An individual with an acute illness usually experiences a specific sequence of events from onset to recovery. The following sequence assumes that the individual is restored to health. He may even go on to a higher level of wellness than he had prior to his illness as a result of health teaching he received during his illness. The stages of acute illness combine illness behavior and sick role behavior.

Every person experiences forms of acute illness during their lives. Most people experience it many times between birth and death. Figure 1-4 demonstrates how the stages of acute illness fit into the health-illness continuum throughout life. It is based on Suchman's analysis of behavior patterns in illness.[25]

Symptom experience

The first stage is the experience of symptoms. As described under illness behavior, the individual recognizes he has sensations not compatible with his concept of health. If the symptoms subside while he is taking no action, he will skip the steps in the circle and return to his optimum level of wellness. The symptoms may also subside following his use of folk remedies or over-the-counter medications. However, if the symptoms persist or worsen, he will move on to the next stage. The most significant symptom suggesting illness is pain. Examples of other symptoms suggestive of illness are fever, chills, and shortness of breath. If these symptoms are severe, the person seeks professional health care more rapidly than if the symptoms are considered mild or moderate in degree. The person's emotional response to the symptom(s) is another factor in his total response to the symptoms.

Assumption of the sick role

When the individual perceives his symptoms as illness, he relinquishes his normal duties and activities. He seeks validation from family, friends, or work peers that he is sick. If they agree that he is ill, then he is allowed to enter the sick role. For many, this lay validation is only acceptable for a day or two. This is because American society requires professional validation of illness for the person to remain in the sick role (Fig. 1-5).

As the person takes on the sick role, he usually becomes preoccupied with his symptoms and other bodily functions. This is seen in his thoughts and conversations in which he focuses on minor variations in his pulse, elimination patterns, and temperature. His attention becomes inner-directed. Thus, if he goes to work when he feels he is sick, he is likely to do a poorer job because of this self-preoccupation.

Health care contact

Some people may choose not to seek professional health care. However, most people seek professional health care to legitimize their remaining in the sick role and because of the intensity and personal signifi-

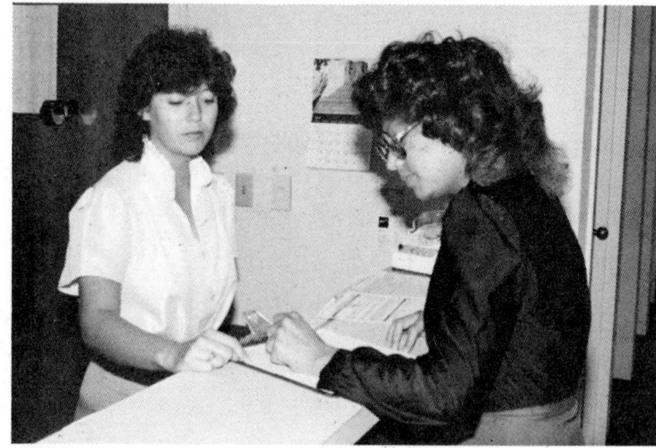

Figure 1-5 The ill person must seek professional validation if he or she remains in the sick role longer than 2 or 3 days.

cance of the symptoms. They make the medical contact (usually with a physician) for diagnosis, treatment, and prognosis of their illness. If their illness is validated, then they continue in the sick role. If it is not validated, they may decide to return to their normal role or they may decide to seek out another medical person who will validate their illness (called "shopping around"). Either response may be valid depending on the circumstances.

Dependent role

The person enters the dependent role stage when he decides to accept the diagnosis and treatment plan of his physician. For many persons with acute illnesses the physiologic effects of illness (fever, blurred vision, pain, cloudy thinking, etc.) allow less energy to be available for them to function independently, and thus they regress to dependency. The more severe the illness, the greater the dependency of the individual upon others. Thus, at this stage he may or may not be hospitalized.

Dependency falls into three categories:[26]

1. Compliance with or conformity to opinions and demands of others
2. The need for physical assistance in activities of daily living
3. The need for emotional support in the form of approval, reassurance, physical closeness, and protection

The person may initially be reluctant to enter this dependent role because it is usually viewed as undesirable. It may also be seen as the only means to the desired goal of restored health. Nurses often play an important part in helping sick individuals adapt to the dependent role. The acute nursing intervention described in the management chapters in this book focuses on assisting clients in this stage.

An important component of the dependent role is compliance. *Compliance* refers to the cooperation of the client with the treatment regimen prescribed. The term *adherence* is increasingly used instead of compliance because it stresses the active, knowledgeable cooperation of a client with the treatment regimen. The treatment may include a special diet, a modification in activity (change in type such as special exercises or an increase or decrease in level), or medications. Clinical experience as well as research have shown that there is rarely 100 percent adherence to a treatment regimen.

Several factors have been identified which have a positive correlation with a high level of adherence. Factors that are related to the client's relationship with medical providers are (1) perception of the care giver as friendly and understanding, (2) agreement with the care giver about the nature of the illness, and (3) perception of the treatment as appropriate to the illness. Psychological factors promoting adherence are the client's perception of (1) his personal susceptibility to a recurrence of the illness, (2) the seriousness of the illness, and (3) the effectiveness of the treatment in alleviating symptoms.[27] Thus, adherence involves good rapport between the health care giver and the client, an effective treatment plan, and knowledge of his illness by the client. The correlation between adherence and education points out why there is such a strong emphasis on client education in nursing care (see Chap. 5).

The individual may exit from the health-illness continuum at this point if death occurs. However, most people move on toward recovery. It is at this point of movement toward recovery that clients may experience some *secondary gain* or enjoyment of the dependency role. This is because they experience a release from their normal responsibilities and pressures of daily living and enjoy the attention they are receiving. Because of this secondary gain, recovery is often experienced physically before it is experienced emotionally. However, since part of the expectations of the sick role is that the individual perceives it as undesirable, health care providers and the client's family and friends encourage him to move on to recovery. If he does not move on to recovery, he is considered a *malingerer*—a deviant role in which a person pretends to be sick in order to avoid responsibilities.

Recovery and rehabilitation

The final stage of acute illness is that of recovery and rehabilitation. It may begin in the hospital but will conclude in the home. It requires that the individual chooses to give up his sick role and begin to resume his normal tasks and responsibilities. He may return to an even higher level of wellness than experienced before his illness. This may be due to the health education which he received, resulting in better health practices. Thus, it is essential that a person receive needed assistance with health promotion and maintenance practices as well as be treated to prevent recurrence of specific diseases. Nurses are in an ideal position to accomplish this task.

Special Tasks and Problems of the Chronically Ill

Chronic illness has been increasingly significant as medical care has advanced in the treatment of acute illness. Today the incidence of chronic illness is a major health problem (Table 1-8). When considering these figures it is also significant to note that there is an average of two chronic conditions per chronically ill individual. Some diseases are related, such as hypertension, congestive heart failure, and renal failure. Others may be unrelated, such as arthritis and emphysema.

Those who have chronic illnesses do not fit neatly into the five stages of acute illness just described. When a chronic illness such as diabetes mellitus is in good control, the person may experience no signs or symptoms of the disease. However, to remain symptom-free, the chronically ill individual needs to maintain contact with a medical care giver and to adhere to the treatment regimen (a degree of dependency found in the sick role). Depending on the disease and the stage it is in, there is a varying impact on the person's lifestyle. However, a chronic illness requires adaptation by the individual. Anselm L. Strauss, a medical sociologist, has identified the following seven tasks of those who are chronically ill:[28]

Table 1-8
Incidence of Chronic Illness

Age	Incidence Of Chronic Illness	Illness Limiting Major Activity
Under 17 years	23%	1%
17–44 years	54%	5%
45–64 years	71%	14%
65 years and above	84%	40%

These figures demonstrate that chronic illness affects all age groups, although it does increase with age. Comparison of incidence of chronic illness with limitation of activity suggests that many people with chronic illness live nearly normal lifestyles.

Adapted from A. L. Strauss, *Chronic Illness and The Quality of Life,* The C. V. Mosby Company, St. Louis, 1975, p. 2.

1. Preventing and managing crisis
2. Carrying out prescribed regimens
3. Controlling symptoms
4. Reordering of time
5. Adjusting to changes in the course of disease
6. Preventing social isolation
7. Attempting to normalize interactions with others

These tasks were identified as common themes in the lives of chronically ill persons who participated in several research studies conducted by Strauss et al.[29] The following is a summary of Strauss' work:

Preventing and managing medical crisis

Most chronic illnesses have the potential of an acute exacerbation of symptoms, which may result in increased disability or death. Examples include the client with cardiac disease who may have another myocardial infarction, or the client with asthma who may have a severe attack. Thus, a major task for the chronically ill person and his family is to learn to prevent or manage the crisis. First, this involves learning what the potential crisis is and ways to prevent it. The latter usually involves adherence to a prescribed medical regimen. Secondly, they need to know the clues or signs and symptoms of the onset of a crisis. These may occur rapidly, as with a seizure, or slowly, as with hyperglycemia in a diabetic.

A third step for learning to manage a crisis is making a plan of how one will deal with the crisis which is likely to occur. This may involve a diabetic carrying some candy with him for a sudden onset of hypoglycemia, or a plan to never leave an individual alone who is prone to sudden choking seizures. Factors affecting the organization of a plan to manage a crisis are the actual potential of the crisis occurring, association of a medical crisis with the original onset of disease, distance in time from an actual crisis, and the possibility of a breakdown in organization due to disruption in the lives of those who are to manage the crisis.

Managing regimens

Learning to live with a specific medical treatment regimen is the second major task of a chronically ill individual. Regimens vary in degree of difficulty and the impact they have on an individual's lifestyle. Each client evaluates his regimen and adapts it to some extent. Characteristics of regimens include:

1. *Degree of difficulty involved in learning the regimen.* This may range in difficulty from remembering to take a specific tablet once a day to learning to run a home hemodialysis unit.
2. *Amount of time required to implement the regimen.* Does it involve an activity lasting 1 minute three times a day, or 2 hours three times a day?
3. *Amount of discomfort and energy associated with the implementation of the regimen in its prescribed form.* Obviously, if it is uncomfortable and takes a considerable amount of energy, there is a decreased chance it will be carried out as prescribed. Thus, an insulin-dependent diabetic may decide to forgo an injection because "it hurts!" Another consideration affecting compliance is uncomfortable or undesirable side effects of the regimen, such as impotence from some antihypertensive drugs.
4. *Visibility of the regimen to other people and the social acceptability of the disease the regimen suggests.* For example, a Seeing Eye dog with a blind person in a restaurant is generally considered more socially acceptable than the frequent expectoration which occurs with chronic obstructive lung disease.
5. *Effectiveness and speed of the regimen in treating or preventing symptoms of the disease.* Some clients erroneously assume that if the signs or symptoms disappear they may stop taking their medication. A common example is the client with hypertension who stops his medicines "because my blood pressure is normal now."

Controlling symptoms

Learning to control symptoms so that desired activities may be continued is a third task of the chronically ill. Methods of managing the visibility of symptoms may also be included. Some individuals redesign their lifestyle by learning to plan ahead, such as the person with ulcerative colitis choosing to only go to events where there are restrooms near the seating area. Others may redesign their lifestyle by making changes in their environment or using special tools to assist them in daily activities. For example, a person with severe emphysema may need to adjust to the use of portable oxygen (Fig. 1-6). Another example is the person with arthritis who selects clothing having zippers with large pull tabs rather than small buttons. Some redesign their lifestyle by rearranging work schedules for times when their symptoms, such as coughing up a large amount of sputum, are less severe.

Important general considerations in symptom control is that the individual should learn about the pattern of his symptoms (typical onset, duration, severity) and if he can have an effect on their duration and intensity. The chronically ill person must also learn the limits of his own ability in controlling symptoms. Finally, he must learn to use his "good times," when symptoms are less severe, to do those things he cannot do when his symptoms are present. An example of the latter is the client with decreased levels of energy due to cardiac disease who elects to have sexual relations in the morning after a good night's sleep.

Reordering of time

The use of time is another problem area for the chronically ill. They may have too much or too little available time. For example, the individual who is forced to retire because of a chronic illness may find too much time on his hands and have to find activities which he enjoys doing to fill the empty hours. On the other hand, many regimens take tremendous amounts of time for the chronically ill and their helpers, thus presenting the opposite problem.

Adjusting to changes in the course of the disease

Learning to live with the usual course of a chronic illness is a fifth task for the chronically ill. Some diseases such as multiple sclerosis have unpredictable courses which make adjustments difficult. Other diseases are more predictable, such as controlled diabetes. Part of a person's task also involves developing a personal identity to include the chronic illness and the lifestyle changes it necessitates.

Preventing social isolation

As indicated earlier, social isolation may occur with chronic illness because the individual chooses to withdraw from previous activities or because others withdraw from the chronically ill person. An example of the former is the man who has been operated on for lung cancer, who avoids coffee breaks at work because everyone else smokes and he has stopped. An example of the latter would be the avoidance by his work peers of a person with partially controlled epilepsy.

Attempting to normalize interactions with others

A final related task is normalizing interactions with others. Most chronically ill individuals attempt to manage symptoms and to hide disabilities or disfigurement. This may involve wearing a prosthesis or demonstrating that they can function the same as a "normal" person, that is, one without the disability. A common example of this is the person with chronic lung problems who stops walking to catch his breath but who appears to be inspecting a plant or looking in a store window. Closely related to this is the desire of many dying individuals to be treated as being among the living, with normal interests and desires, and not as half-dead.

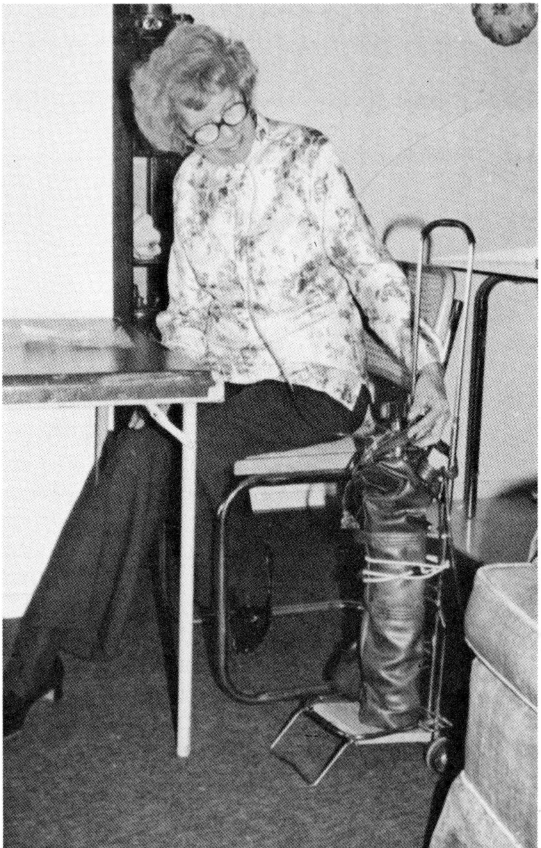

Figure 1-6 People with chronic illnesses may need to use special tools or equipment to assist them in daily activities.

Special Tasks and Problems of the Chronically Ill: Conclusions

These seven tasks of the chronically ill focus on managing disease and managing life. Nurses may use these tasks as important components in planning the management of chronically ill clients.

As the client and his family are assisted in achieving these various tasks, he will be moving toward his potential for high-level wellness. Many specific points of how to deal with a chronic illness will be covered in the management chapters. However, nurses may gain additional insights by asking their chronically ill clients how *they* deal with specific problems. Information gained in this manner may then be shared with other clients with similar problems.

This latter approach, gaining information from those with a specific chronic illness, has been formalized into a number of self-help groups. These groups, such as Alcoholics Anonymous, ostomy clubs, and Mended Heart clubs, are organized specifically to assist people with the same disorders in managing them. Such groups have the support of many health professionals and voluntary health agencies. Nurses may recommend these groups to their chronically ill clients or, if one is unavailable, assist in the organization of such groups.

SUMMARY

This chapter has presented a broad overview of the experience of health and illness. It has shown that, although health is defined in a variety of ways, there seems to be a consensus that it involves the whole person—mind, body, and spirit—functioning at full energy levels. Conversely, illness may be caused by physical, emotional, and spiritual factors. As factors associated with the onset of illness have been recognized, more measures which promote health have been recognized and communicated to the public. The important role of nursing related to health education is detailed in the various management chapters.

Generalities about the process people go through in deciding whether or not they are ill and the behaviors (role) typical of an acutely ill person are also discussed. These generalities present a framework which the nurse can use in understanding the unique experience of an individual with a specific illness. However, it is essential that the nurse not force an individual into a specific role pattern but recognize that illness will change the ability to function in various roles.

The chapter concludes with a focus on the special tasks of the chronically ill person. This is especially significant because of the increased incidence of chronic illness as the average age of the population increases. Nursing assists clients in learning to manage these tasks so that the chronically ill have time and energy for quality living.

In conclusion, the information in this chapter attempts to help the reader see the client as a unique person. This holistic attitude should form the framework on which the reader can learn the theory presented in this text.

REVIEW QUESTIONS

The number of the question corresponds to the same numbered objective at the beginning of the chapter.

1. Wellness is
   a. a dynamic condition in which a person is functioning in mind, body, and spirit to achieve his full potential
   b. a static condition which is the result of a person avoiding those factors which cause illness
   c. a state of complete physical, mental, and social well-being
   d. the absence of any symptoms of illness

2. Which one of the following individuals articulated the theory that disease is partially due to many changes in an individual's life?
   a. Cannon
   b. Selye
   c. Wolff
   d. Rahe

3. Factors which are positively correlated with preventive health behaviors include all the following *except*
   a. a mother with a college education as compared to a mother with a grade school education
   b. the belief that one is invulnerable to coronary artery disease despite a family history of it
   c. the use of mass media to highlight the risk of cancer, pulmonary, and heart disease due to smoking
   d. a perception that it is important to one's health to participate in activities such as skiing

4. Which of the following is an example of taking counteraction when symptoms of an illness exist?
   a. deciding to wait 2 or 3 days to see if the pain in his eye will disappear
   b. taking an over-the-counter medication for stomach pains
   c. changing dietary intake because "spices make me belch"
   d. increasing jogging "to work soreness out of my left leg and help decrease the swelling"

5. A characteristic of a chronic disease is
   a. it results in permanent deviation from normal
   b. it has a rapid onset
   c. it is self-limiting
   d. it has a short duration

6. An example of the dependent role in an acutely ill person is
   a. taking an antibiotic for his pharyngitis
   b. returning to work after appendicitis
   c. omitting morning dose of a diuretic
   d. seeing the physician because "I sprained my ankle"

7. All the following statements about living with chronic illness are true *except*
   a. chronically ill persons need to have a plan to deal with exacerbations of the acute stages of their illness
   b. chronically ill persons learn to control symptoms of their disease in order to minimize their social implications
   c. the major problem of chronically ill persons is extra time on their hands due to social isolation
   d. chronically ill persons attempt to normalize their interactions with others by disguising evidence of their illness

REFERENCES

1. L. Thomas, in *The Lives of a Cell* as quoted by Lawrence Cherry in "A Doctor Who Dispenses Joy," *Reader's Digest,* September 1980, p. 119.

2. D. E. Benson, Pastor of Agape Baptist Church, Albuquerque, N.M., sermon/conversation.
3. World Health Organization: *Constitution of the World Health Organization,* Chronicle of the World Health Organization 1, 1947, Geneva, Switzerland.
4. H. L. Dunn, "High-Level Wellness for Man and Society," *Am J Public Health and Nations Health,* **49:**786–792, (1959).
5. ———, "What High-Level Wellness Means," *Health Values,* **1**(1):9, (January/February, 1977).
6. J. G. Bruhn et al., "The Wellness Process," *J Community Health,* **2**(3):209–221, (Spring 1977).
7. B. L. Pesznecker and J. McNeil, "Relationship Among Health Habits, Social Assets, Psychological Well-Being, Life Change and Alterations in Health Status," *Nurs Res* **24:**297–298, (November–December, 1975).
8. Bruhn et al., op. cit., p. 210.
9. P. A. R. Flynn, *Holistic Health,* Robert J. Brady Co., Bowie, Maryland, 1980.
10. H. Selye, *The Stress of Life,* rev. ed., McGraw-Hill Book Company, New York, 1976, p. 64.
11. H. G. Wolff, *Stress and Disease,* 2d ed., Charles C Thomas, Springfield, Ill., 1968.
12. T. H. Holmes and R. H. Rahe, "Social Readjustment Rating Scale," *J Psychosomatic Res,* **II:**216 (1967).
13. E. K. Gunderson and R. H. Rahe (eds.), *Life Stress and Illness,* Charles C Thomas, Springfield, Ill. 1974.
14. L. O. Ruch, "A Multidimensional Analysis of the Concept of Life Change," *J Health and Social Behavior,* **18:**71 (March 1977).
15. D. L. Dudley and E. Welke, *How to Survive Being Alive,* Doubleday and Company, New York, 1977, p. 56.
16. Pesznecker and McNeil, op. cit., pp. 242–247.
17. N. B. Belloc and L. Breslow, "Relationship of Physical Health Status and Health Practices," *Preventive Medicine,* **1:**409–421 (1972).
18. Ibid.
19. N. J. Pender, "A Conceptual Model for Preventive Health Behavior," *Nursing Outlook,* **23:**386 (June 1975).
20. A. L. Strauss, *Chronic Illness and the Quality of Life,* The C. V. Mosby Company, St. Louis, 1975, p. 1.
21. R. Wu, *Behavior and Illness,* Prentice-Hall Inc., Englewood Cliffs, N.J. 1973, pp. 137–142.
22. A. C. Twaddle, "Sickness: A Sociological View," in J. R. Folta and E. S. Deck, *A Sociological Framework for Patient Care,* 2d ed., John Wiley & Sons, Inc., New York, 1979, pp. 315–316.
23. A. Arluke, L. Kennedy, and R. C. Kersler, "Re-examining the Sick Role Concept: An Empirical Assessment," *J Health and Social Behavior,* **20:**30 (March 1979.)
24. Ibid., pp. 30–36.
25. E. A. Suchman, "Stages of Illness and Medical Care," *J Health and Human Behavior,* **6**(3):114–128 (Fall 1965).
26. Wu, op. cit., p. 161.
27. J. Hover and N. Juelsgaard, "The Sick Role Reconceptualized," *Nursing Forum,* **17**(4):412 (1978).
28. Strauss, op. cit., pp. 7–8.
29. Ibid., pp. 13–65.

Chapter 2

GENERAL CONCEPTS

Nursing Process

Dorothy Hendel Clough

Learning Objectives

1. Describe commonalities of accepted definitions of nursing.
2. Describe the phases of the nursing process.
3. Differentiate between subjective and objective data.
4. Explain the components of a nursing diagnosis.
5. Differentiate between the roles of nursing and medicine.
6. Describe factors that affect information obtained during an interview.
7. Describe the progress note and its role in evaluation.
8. Describe rationale for components generally included in the nursing care plan.

The nursing process provides the foundation for professional nursing today. This chapter will present an overview of the nursing process as well as look at the place of nursing in the health care delivery system.

NURSING YESTERDAY AND TODAY

In primitive times there was no distinction between "nursing" and "medicine." The sick and injured were merely cared for by those with nurturant instincts.[1] In more recent times society has tried to differentiate between nursing and medical practice. However, even today there is not a clear delineation between nursing and medical practice.

Nursing's Territory

Many modern theorists such as Johnson, Orem, Rodgers, and Roy are presently attempting to define precisely nursing's territory.[2] Though such work is needed, it is interesting that many of the current issues in nursing were previously concerns of Florence Nightingale. In 1893 she addressed holistic health when she emphasized that one must nurse the whole person rather than the disease.[3] Health maintenance and promotion, health teaching, family and community nursing, establishing trust, use of good communication skills, and stress reduction techniques were all an integral part of nursing as defined by Florence Nightingale.[4]

In the 1960s the team concept became popular. Fragmentation of client care occurred as various nurses and health care workers descended upon the client to complete their designated tasks. The nursing profession was not satisfied with this system of care. Nursing roles are presently changing in response to client and nurse dissatisfaction as well as to technological advances, increased hospital costs, decreased hospital stay, changing societal attitudes toward the physician, changing needs of clients, a longer life span, and more leisure time. *Primary nursing care* is once again seen as a means to quality health care. Primary nursing care is a system where one nurse is responsible for ensuring that all the basic needs of her specific clients are met on a 24-hour basis, according to professional standards.

Expanded Roles

Today, those in the health care system are also talking of "expanded roles" for nurses. These roles emphasize health assessment, diagnosis, and treatment of conditions usually considered only within the physician's domain. Some nursing leaders dislike the term "expanded role." Mauksch states,[5]

> I do not believe there are expanded roles for nurses. I believe my role as a nurse clinician or practitioner is a new role because it encompasses new behaviors. These behaviors are risk taking, decision making, being accountable, and being assertive.

But are these expanded roles really new behaviors for nurses? Nursing leaders of the past such as Florence Nightingale, Esther Lucile Brown, and Margaret Sanger would not have made such strides for the profession lacking these assertive kinds of behaviors. A closer look at nursing history indicates that rather than expanding into totally new areas, nurses are merely reclaiming old territory once held.

Nurses have always assessed their clients' health

This chapter was reviewed by Joyce Van Landingham, Assistant Professor, Mount St. Mary's College, Los Angeles, California.

status. However, today, due to scientific and technological advances, there are new methods available requiring new equipment and skills. Nurses today are asserting that they have the right to learn and apply skills which enhance their ability to determine health status. By increasing their assessment skills, nurses increase their data base upon which to make sound judgments. It should be remembered that the thermometer was at one time the private domain of the chief physician. Today, no one questions whether the nurse should use this instrument to assess temperature.[6]

Scientific and technological advances have made an impact on health care and care of the sick. Nursing continues to be in a state of evolution in response to these advances. In its attempt to keep pace, nursing would do well to remember what the Queen in *Through the Looking Glass* said to Alice:[7]

> Now *here*, you see, it takes all the running *you* can do to keep in the same place. If you want to get somewhere else, you must run at least twice as fast as that.

Increasing emphasis on assertiveness, persistence, risk taking, and decision making are essential if nursing is to "get somewhere else."

Definition of Nursing

A basic question revolves around how the profession of nursing views itself. Several well-known definitions of nursing indicate that there exists a basic theme of health, illness, and caring, present since Florence Nightingale. Note the commonalities in the following definitions:

> The unique function of the nurse is to assist the individual, sick or well, in the performance of those activities contributing to health or its recovery (or to peaceful death) that he would perform unaided if he had the necessary strength, will or knowledge. And to do this in such a way as to help him gain independence as rapidly as possible.[8] (1969 International Council of Nurses, Geneva.)
>
> Nursing is putting the patient in the best condition for nature to act.[9]
>
> Nursing is a direct service, goal oriented, and adaptable to the needs of the individual, the family and community during health and illness.[10]

In this textbook nursing will be defined broadly as assisting the client in any setting, through the application of the nursing process, to maintain or attain a state of dynamic equilibrium at the highest possible level of wellness with the least possible expenditure of energy.[11]

In this definition the terms used are further defined as follows:

1. *Client*—Any individual, family, or group requiring nursing intervention.
2. *Nursing Process*—The systematic use of the steps of assessment, planning, intervention, and evaluation when providing nursing care.
3. *Dynamic equilibirum*—A relative state of balance, or homeostasis, where basic needs are met by minimal output of energy.
4. *Level of wellness*—The degree of physiologic and psychological adaptation.
5. *Assist*—Implies a doing with, not a doing for, to facilitate independence to the greatest degree possible.

Nursing's View of Humanity

Nursing's view of humanity must be considered when describing nursing. Although different terms have been used, there is widespread agreement among nursing theorists that an individual has *physiologic* (or biophysical), *psychological* (or emotional), *sociocultural* (or interpersonal), and *environmental* components or dimensions.[12] In this text the human individual will be considered "a biopsychosocial being in constant interaction with a changing environment."[13] The dimensions comprising the individual in actuality are not separate entities but interrelated. Thus, a problem in one dimension generally affects one or more of the other dimensions. Psychological anxiety, for instance, affects the autonomic nervous system, a part of the biophysical dimension.

Growth and development are influenced by an individual's interactions with others. No two individuals are ever exactly alike. No one individual remains the same from moment to moment. Each individual, therefore, has value as an irreplaceable member of humanity. Inherent in this individuality is the right to develop unique potentials according to a personal value system to the extent that the exercise of this right does not deny it to others.[14]

The individual's behavior is meaningful and oriented toward fulfilling needs and coping with environmental stresses. At times, however, the individual needs assistance in order to meet these needs and to cope successfully.

THE NURSING PROCESS

Nursing can best accomplish its goal of assisting others to maintain or attain optimal functioning by use of the *nursing process.* The nursing process is a problem-solving approach based on the scientific method. The use of this process enables the nurse to provide care in an organized and scientific manner in each of the following areas:

1. Health maintenance and promotion
2. Acute intervention
3. Rehabilitative or chronic management

Phases of the Nursing Process

The nursing process consists of four phases: assessment, planning, implementation, and evaluation (Fig. 2-1). There are, however, numerous other terms or phrases presently used in nursing to describe the steps of the nursing process. Table 2-1 lists other commonly used terms. The assessment phase is comprised of collecting information and drawing conclusions from the information. The planning phase consists of setting goals and determining strategies for accomplishing the goals. The implementation phase is the actual plan set in action. The evaluation phase is the analysis of the effectiveness of the assessment, planning, and implementation phases.

Interrelatedness of Phases

The four phases of the nursing process do not occur in isolation from each other. For example, the nurse can be gathering data about the wound condition (assessment) as she changes the soiled dressing (implementation). There is, however, a basic order to the nursing process, beginning at the assessment phase. This provides the data on which to base the plan. Implementation follows a careful plan. Once begun, the nursing process is continuous or cyclical in nature. There is no limit to the number of times the cycle can be reinitiated. Notice in Fig. 2-1 that evaluation is ongoing throughout the cycle. This continual evaluation provides feedback on the effectiveness of the plan or the need for revision. Revision may be needed in the data collection method, the diagnosis, the goals, the plan, or the implementation method.

Application of the nursing process requires sound knowledge of the physical and behavioral sciences

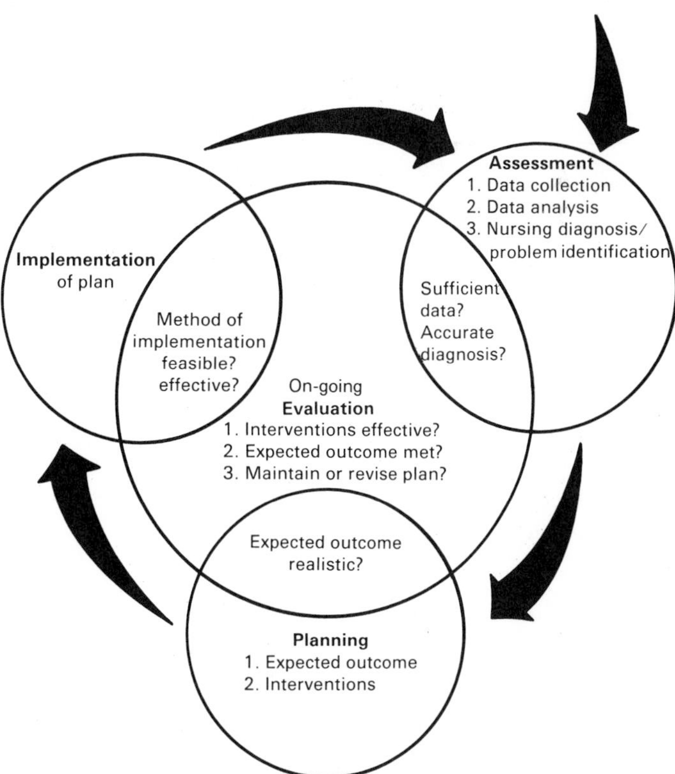

Figure 2-1 The nursing process.

Table 2-1
Commonly Used Terms Referring to Components of the Nursing Process

	Assessment Phase
Step I	Data Collection Data gathering Assessment Collection of information History and physical
Step II	Data Analysis Assessment Judgment Decision making Problem identification Determination of strength and weaknesses Determination of unmet needs Determination of assets and limitations
Step III	Nursing Diagnosis Assessment Problem identification Determining cause of problem Labeling the problem Classification of problem
	Planning Phase
Step I	Priority Setting
Step II	Expected Outcome Determined Goal setting Objective setting, subgoals Desired behaviors
Step III	Planning Interventions Planning nursing actions Nursing orders Planning strategies of care
	Implementation
	Application Intervention Nursing Care
	Evaluation
	Reassessment

and a repertoire of intellectual, interpersonal, and technical skills. Note the similarity of the nursing process and scientific method as compared in Table 2-2.

Both the nursing profession and the medical profession use a type of problem-solving process. The uniqueness of nursing's problem-solving approach stems from nursing's goals and its means of accomplishing these goals. This differs from medicine's format of examination-diagnosis-treatment.[15] The differences are compared in Table 2-3.

Independent and Dependent Functions

There is increasing overlap between nursing and medicine, particularly in the area of health maintenance and promotion. Nurses have both independent and dependent functions in relation to medicine. The nurse functions independently when she initiates *nursing* interventions such as health teaching, counseling, and other measures which assist clients to meet their basic needs. When the nurse assists in carrying out designated medical plans she functions dependently: Dependent functions include administering medications, performing or assisting with certain medical treatments, and assisting with diagnostic tests and procedures.

As mentioned earlier, the line between what comprises medical versus nursing interventions is vague. The exact lines are determined by individual state and agency policies. In general, the nurse is expected to have the following intellectual, interpersonal, and technical skills:

- Health assessment skills
  - Physical examination
  - Psychosocial assessment
- Analytical skills
- Decision-making skills
- Creativity and the ability to improvise
- Teaching skills
- Therapeutic skills
- Counseling and referral skills
- Technical skills
- Administrative skills
- Leadership and management skills
- Recording and reporting skills
- Research skills

Some or all of these skills are used during the various phases of the nursing process.

ASSESSMENT PHASE

Data Collection

A sound data base is the foundation for the entire nursing process. Collection of data is a prerequisite to making a diagnosis, to planning, and to intervening. A human being as a biopsychosocial being has needs and problems in all dimensions. A nursing diagnosis made without supporting data in all dimensions can lead to incorrect conclusions and depersonalized care. For example, a client who does not sleep all

Table 2-2
Similarities of the Nursing Process and the Scientific Method

	Scientific Method	Nursing Process
Defining a problem	Client identified	General problem areas are identified through health screening.
Collecting data	Assessment	Subjective and objective data are obtained in depth.
Forming the hypothesis	Planning	Data are analyzed. Diagnosis is made. Expected outcome is stated. Strategies are considered. Interventions are selected.
Testing the hypothesis	Implementation	Interventions are tried.
Forming conclusions	Evaluation	Results of the entire process are analyzed.

night may be mistakenly diagnosed as having insomnia. In fact he may have worked nights his entire adult life and is having trouble adjusting to the hospital routine. This information about his sleeping habits would be necessary to individualize his care so that he did not receive a sleep medication at 10 P.M.

Interventions implemented without careful prior assessment can be life-threatening. For example, if the nurse fails to assess head injury in a newly admitted client involved in an automobile accident, and subsequently intervenes to prevent shock by lowering the head and raising the feet, she could cause increased intracranial pressure which could result in permanent brain damage or death.

Subjective and objective data

A sound data base includes both subjective and objective data. *Subjective data* is what the client or family members state either spontaneously or by direct questioning. *Objective data* is what the nurse and other members of the health team gather by information, inspection, palpation, percussion, and auscultation. The client's chart, diagnostic tests, and other health team members also provide additional useful subjective and objective data. An easy way to remember the commonly used abbreviations "S" and "O" is:

S = Subjective statements
O = Objective observations

In the initial assessment phase, most of the subjective data are obtained through the health history. However, while interviewing, the nurse also observes the client's general appearance and nonverbal behavior. These observations provide some objective data. The majority of the objective data are obtained through physical examination of the client. Yet the nurse also obtains subjective data as the client makes statements during the examination procedures, especially in regard to pain during palpation. The history and physical examination are described in detail in Chap. 3.

Since nursing interventions are only as sound as the data base on which they are formulated, it is critical that the data base be accurate. Therefore, information gained from sources such as the chart, other health care workers, the client's family, and the nurse's observations should be validated with the client whenever possible. Likewise, questionable statements by the client should be validated by a knowledgeable other person when possible.

Table 2-3
Comparison of Primary Goals Nursing and Medicine

Nursing	Medicine
Determines level of wellness and need for assistance.	Determines illness or injury.
Provides physical care, emotional care, teaching, guidance, and counseling	Provides medical treatments, surgery.
Interventions aimed at assisting the client to meet his needs.	Interventions aimed at preventing and curing injury or illness.

Interviewing skills

There are several factors that affect success in obtaining information:

1. Rapport with the client
2. The timing of the interview
3. The surrounding environment
4. The amount of time available
5. Condition of the client

Each of these factors will be considered as basic generalizations related to interviewing techniques as presented. Since more in-depth discussion of communication is beyond the scope of this text the student is encouraged to refer to the bibliography for some excellent references in this area.

First, the nurse should identify herself and her role and inform the client what information is needed and why. Clients cannot be expected to discuss personal health concerns without a sound reason. Seemingly nonpersonal questions may be perceived by the client as very private information.

The time of the interview should be carefully selected. Pain, fear, fatigue, anxiety, and other common stressors associated with illness are examples of situations which should alert the nurse to defer an interview until a more appropriate time. A calm, comfortable client is much more likely to share information.

Careful attention should be directed to the surrounding environment. If necessary, the environment should be manipulated to make it more conducive to sharing information. Privacy for the client should be assured. Avoid backlighting since it limits good eye contact. The temperature of the room should be appropriate for the client's age and condition. Background noise should be minimal. The client's and nurse's full attention are required for an interaction to be successful.

The client should be informed of the approximate amount of time the interview will take. The amount of time should be realistic, considering the nurse's responsibilities and the client's condition. If additional time is required, the client should be consulted for a suitable time.

The client's condition must be a primary concern when planning a data-gathering session. If acutely ill, the client will be unable to expend energy on nonemergency questions. Other sources of information may need to be utilized such as old charts, family members, or friends in such a situation. The nurse must be attuned to the needs of the client when selecting an interview topic. For instance, the nurse may want to determine the learning needs of a preoperative client, while the client may only care to discuss what medication will be used postoperatively to control his pain.

Begin an interview with easily answered, impersonal questions. As rapport is established advance to the more personal questions. The nurse's comfort level with the topic, as well as a genuine concern for the client, promotes rapport. The nurse needs to know why certain information is necessary and must have insight into her own attitudes and feelings about asking personal questions.

Listen to, rather than anticipate, what the client has to say. If the nurse is mentally planning how to respond to the client, she cannot be listening to what is being said. While listening, closely observe the client, noting any incongruency between verbal and nonverbal behaviors. Before beginning a purposeful interview take time to hear the client's concerns. This not only helps to establish rapport, but can provide important additional information. It is neither necessary nor wise to strictly adhere to a rigid interviewing format, since much of the psychosocial data are obtained as the individual is allowed time to share his concerns. Open-ended rather than closed questions (closed questions can be answered by a yes or no or short statement) provide the most information. Give the client time to answer.

The number of questions asked during the history can give the client a sense of urgency which discourages communication. Select words carefully, based on the client's apparent ability to understand. Underestimating or overestimating a client's ability to comprehend can negatively affect communication. Remember the purpose is an interview, not an interrogation. It is important to use simple language. The author vividly remembers an English-speaking client who asked what a low hematocrit was. When the author explained that it meant the number of red blood cells were decreased, the client asked, "What's a cell?" Never assume you are being understood; look for nonverbal and verbal clues, and ask the client to request clarification of any unfamiliar terms.

Data Analysis

The second step of the assessment phase is the data analysis. The nurse mentally sorts through and organizes the information, determining unmet needs, strengths, and discrepancies between the two. The findings are then compared to documented norms to determine if there is anything which is interfering or could interfere with the client's needs or ability to maintain a state of dynamic equilibrium. Those things which can and do interfere are called potential problems and actual problems, respectively. The following list of human needs must be met to maintain wellness and can be used as a frame of reference for recognizing actual problems (or unmet needs) and potential problems (needs in jeopardy of not being met):

Oxygenation
Water
Food
Elimination
Temperature regulation
Rest
Activity
Cleanliness
Shelter
Clothing
Security
Affiliation
Esteem
Self-actualization

Nursing Diagnosis

After a thorough analysis of all available information, one of two possible conclusions results: (1) There are no problems which require intervention, or (2) the client needs assistance to solve a potential or actual problem. The final conclusions about the problems are the *nursing diagnosis*.

Nursing is moving toward standardized nomenclature for classifying client's unhealthy responses or problems. Until this time arrives the nurse must develop the nursing diagnosis. The nursing diagnosis should state a description of the problem (or *behavior* of concern) and a *cause*. Simply labeling a problem is not sufficient as individual interpretation can lead to confusion. For example, the term "anxiety" is too general and lacks specificity. A more descriptive nursing diagnosis would read:

> Calls the nurse every 10 minutes (behavior) due to fear of being alone when having dyspnea (cause).

The cause should be validated with the client whenever possible.

PLANNING PHASE

Priority Setting

After the problems are identified, the nurse must decide on the urgency of intervention which is needed. Problems of the highest priority require immediate intervention. Problems of lower priority can be dealt with at a later time.

One means of determining the urgency of the problem, and thus its priority, is to look at the impact it has on the individual:[16]

> *First priority*—Threats to life, dignity, and integrity of the client
>
> *Second priority*—Problems which destructively change the client
>
> *Third priority*—Problems that affect normal growth and development of the client

Maslow's hierarchy of needs also acts as a useful guide to determining priorities. These needs include physical needs, safety, love and belonging, esteem, and self-actualization.[17] As in climbing a mountain, the lower level must be reached before a higher level can be attained.

The nurse must be aware that the identified priorities change as the client's level of wellness fluctuates. For example, the client's highest priority in the morning may be a need for information about diabetes since she is going home and must care for herself. During the teaching session the client does not feel well and the nurse suspects a *potential* problem of insulin shock since the client has not eaten breakfast. The session is interrupted so that the nurse can get the client a glass of orange juice. Note that *impending (potential)* problems can be of higher priority than *existing (actual)* problems.

Setting Goals

After the priorities are established, *expected outcomes* or *goals* are mutually decided upon by the client and the nurse (Fig. 2-2). Both long-term and short-term goals need to be set.

Although the ultimate goal for the client is to maintain or attain a state of dynamic equilibrium at the highest possible level of wellness, the setting of more specific goals, both short- and long-term, is necessary for systematic evaluation of the client's progress.

Long-term goals

A client with a chronic illness who plans to return home from an acute-care setting would have long-term goals as follows:[18]

1. The client will be free from acute symptoms.
2. The client will show an adjustment to the impact of his illness on his life.
3. The client will follow home care regimens.

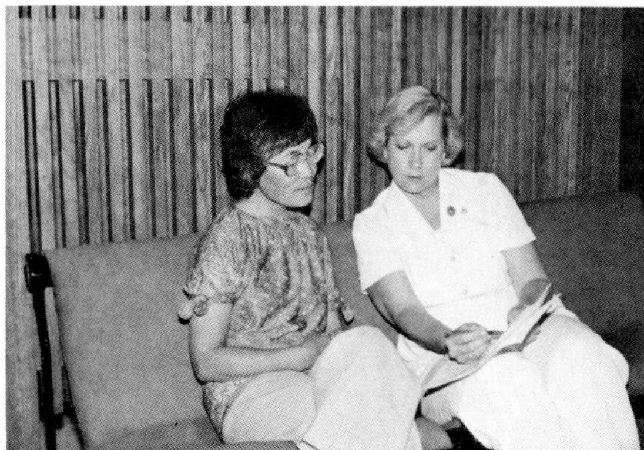

Figure 2-2 Cooperation between the client and the nurse is necessary in setting goals.

Short-term goals

Since these long-term goals are very broad, short-term goals which are easily measurable are also needed for evaluation purposes. They are the stepping stones to arrive at the long-term goal. Thus, goals must be worded as expected outcomes and worded specifically enough so that everyone caring for the client will be able to agree whether the goals have been achieved. Wording the goals in terms of desired, observable behaviors and specifying a date by when the expected outcome should be accomplished facilitates this process.

To be worthwhile, written short-term goals should

1. Be realistic and achievable
2. Be measurable, observable, behavioral
3. Be client-centered (the client's expected outcome)
4. Have a time designation (*Example*: The client will state he has no pain by 10-1-82.)

Short-term goals can serve as motivators for the client and nurse, especially when a goal takes a great deal of time and effort to reach. For example, if the long-term goal for the school child is to attain healthy gums and teeth, the short-term goals could be

1. That he brush his teeth after each meal
2. That he floss his teeth before going to bed at night
3. That he refrain from chewing gum containing sugar
4. That he visit the dentist by 11-9-82

Planning Intervention

Once the expected outcomes are determined, strategies to accomplish these desired behaviors should be developed. The nurse should use available resources when determining possible nursing interventions. The client often has a wealth of information about measures which were a success or a failure for him in the past. Much time and effort are saved by asking the client what has already been tried and discarded as worthless in the past. The client's family can also be consulted regarding the feasibility of a plan.

Other nurses and health care providers can be valuable sources for intervention ideas. Since members of the health team share common goals for the client, the sharing of ideas to reach these goals should be encouraged. A client-centered conference is a good way to foster such sharing of ideas.

Literature and research provide valuable suggestions and information which can facilitate the process of determining a means to accomplish the goals. Nurses need to foster the use of a research base approach to interventions. Intuition should no longer be the mainstay of intervention.

Sound knowledge, good judgment, and decision-making ability are required to effectively choose which methods the nurse will use to intervene. Interventions should be based on sound rationale from the behavioral and physical sciences. In addition, the nurse must also use her own ingenuity, creativity, and past experience to guide her in tailoring a plan to meet a client's individual needs. The benefits of the intervention must outweigh the disadvantages. Factors such as availability of help, equipment, time, money, and other resources must also be considered.[19] As in the case of goal determination, the final selection of which strategies are implemented remains the prerogative of the client.

When recording the plan on the chart or Kardex, the nurse needs to be very specific to enable everyone concerned with the client to understand precisely what is to be accomplished. The plan should be tailored to meet each particular client's individual needs and should note particulars such as how, when, how long, how often, where, by whom, and with what. For example, "Wound care qid" is not an adequate plan. The following plan communicates much more: "The nurse (*who*) is to irrigate the leg wound (*where*) with 200 mL $\frac{1}{2}$ H_2O_2 and $\frac{1}{2}$ NS (*with what*) @ 9-1-5-9 (*how often*)."

IMPLEMENTATION PHASE

The actual carrying out of a specific, individualized plan constitutes the implementation phase. The nurse may carry out the interventions herself or designate others who are qualified to intervene (Fig. 2-3).

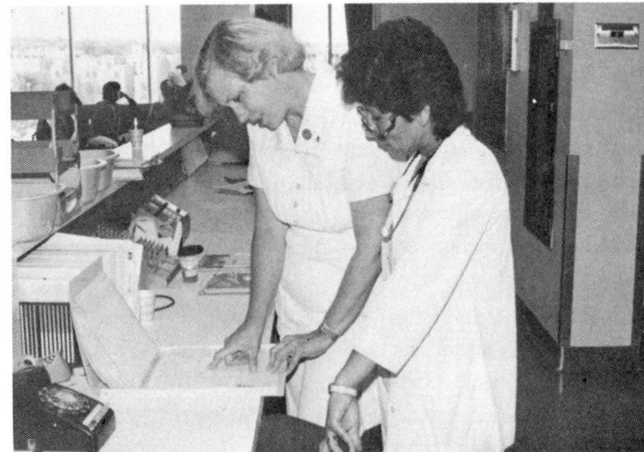

Figure 2-3 Even though the nurse may designate another to implement a nursing activity, the nurse maintains responsibility for the client's welfare.

Throughout this phase the nurse must evaluate the effectiveness of the particular method chosen to implement the plan. For example, she may determine that the nurse's assistant presently caring for a client with a mastectomy should not continue to be the person who implements the client's exercise plan. Perhaps the client is more depressed than anticipated and would benefit from contact with a nurse who is knowledgeable about changes in body image. The exercise plan might essentially remain the same, but the implementor of the plan would be different and would utilize different skills to carry out the plan. Referrals to other professionals may also be made when the nurse anticipates that expertise in specialized areas would be helpful to the client.

EVALUATION PHASE

A look at the diagram of the nursing process (Fig. 2-2) indicates that all phases must be evaluated. Note that evaluation not only occurs after implementation of the plan but is ongoing throughout the process.

The nurse evaluates whether or not sufficient assessment data have been obtained to allow a nursing diagnosis to be made. The diagnosis in turn is evaluated for its accuracy. For example, was the pain actually due to the wound itself or due to pressure from a constricting dressing?

Next, the nurse evaluates whether the expected outcomes and interventions as planned are realistic and achievable. If not, replanning must occur. This may involve revision of both goals and interventions. Consideration must be given to whether the plan should be maintained, modified, or totally revised in light of the client's present status.

The effectiveness of each individual intervention and its contribution to progress toward the goal is also evaluated. In addition, the nurse considers whether a different method of implementation of the same plan would provide better results.

Progress Notes

One systematic method of evaluating and recording client progress is the problem-oriented progress note, referred to as *SOAP*. This type of progress note is problem-specific and incorporates the components described in Table 2-4.

The SOAP term assessment has a more limited meaning than the term used to describe the first phase of the nursing process. With SOAP, assessment connotes data analysis and diagnosis.

The process of SOAP evaluation is as follows:

1. Additional subjective and objective data are gathered about the area of concern.
2. Based on old and new data an assessment of (*a*) the client's progress toward the goal and (*b*) the effectiveness of each intervention is made.
3. Based on the reassessment of the situation, the initial plan is maintained, revised, or discontinued.

   Example:

   Problem: Wound pain

   S. States wound is more painful today.

   O. Wound has moderate amount of yellow, foul-smelling drainage and is inflamed along the suture line.

   A. Postsurgical infection.

   P. 1. Notify physician.
   2. Take temperature q 2 hours.

Use of this SOAP format helps avoid conflict or duplication in services and allows all members of the health team to quickly evaluate the client's progress. This written evaluation should occur regardless of whether the client appears to be progressing satisfac-

Table 2-4
Components of a Problem-Oriented Progress Note

	Explanation
S = Subjective	Information supplied by client or knowledgeable other.
O = Objective	Information obtained by nurse directly, from client records, or diagnostic studies.
A = Assessment	Tentative conclusion based on subjective and objective data.
P = Plan	Specific interventions related to a problem considering diagnostic, therapeutic, and client education needs.

torily, appears unchanged, or appears to be regressing.

WRITTEN CARE PLANS

As mentioned earlier, the nursing care plan is recorded to facilitate continuity of care and help avoid duplication of services. When it is kept as a permanent part of the client's chart it can aid in the evaluation of nursing care. The term *care plan* can mean several different things. It is sometimes used to describe the planning portion of the SOAP progress notes. Most frequently, however, there is a care plan which is kept separate from the client's chart in a Kardex, and it serves as a quick reference on what nursing interventions should be implemented each shift.

Generally, only the more unusual or unexpected problems are addressed in the Kardex. Predictable routine difficulties that are experienced by many clients with the same diagnosis should be planned for but are not necessarily recorded on the Kardex. Both actual (or existing) and likely potential problems should be considered appropriate for the written care plan.

The Kardex care plan may be written in pencil so the outdated interventions can be erased. Then only the current plan remains, avoiding confusion. However, this method should not be used without some kind of permanent record of the plan, since the nurse also needs a source of information about which interventions were unsuccessful so they are not repeated. Table 2-5 presents a useful guideline for evaluating nursing care plans.

Institutions are continually experimenting with various methods of recording the care plan and there are many different formats available. An example of one format is shown in Fig. 2-4.

Some institutions write the care plan in ink and retain the entire plan as a part of the client's chart. This kind of care plan often has a fourth, *evaluation* column, where comments about the progress toward the expected outcome and the effectiveness of the interventions are recorded. The evaluation portion of the care plan is not generally necessary if the SOAP method of charting is used, since evaluation is ongoing with this system.

SUMMARY

Nursing roles are continually evolving as our society changes and we learn to apply new technology. Although nursing is defined in different ways by

Table 2-5
Guidelines for Evaluating Nursing Care Plans

Topic	Expectations *are met* if you answer yes to these questions:	Expectations *are not met*; you have made a common mistake if you answer yes to these questions:
Client problem Validation, cause	Is information included which tells how you knew this was a problem? Is the problem validated by subjective and/or objective data? *Example* *Problem: Overdependence on nurses for physical help as evidenced by* (validation) calling nurse to hand her items within her reach, possibly *due to* (cause) need for attention because of body image change (radical mastectomy). Are potential high-risk problems included as well as present problems? *Example* Possible R shoulder immobility due to pain upon movement and loss of muscle mass. Is your problem specific? (See examples above.) Is this the client's problem? What caused the problem? (Your assessment.)	Do you get another answer than what you have written down when you ask yourself how you knew this was a problem? If so, you have stated an inference or are too general. *Example* Problem: Demanding client Do you get other problems when you ask yourself what other problems does this problem cause? If so, your problem may be too general. *Example* Problem: Radical mastectomy Is this the nurse's problem? *Example* Problem: Time-consuming due to frequent requests. Is this an intervention? *Example* Problem: IV in left arm

Table 2-5 (Continued)

Topic	Expectations *are met* if you answer yes to these questions:	Expectations *are not met*; you have made a common mistake if you answer yes to these questions:
Expected outcome (client goal)	Is it stated in behavioral terms which are specific and measurable? Would everyone be able to agree when the expected outcome is accomplished? Is this the client's desired behavior? Is a deadline included? *Examples* Client *will* discuss her feelings or reaction to the surgery with the nurse before discharge. Client will not call the nurse to hand her items within reach.	Is it difficult to tell if the expected outcome is accomplished? *Example* Client will be less demanding. Is this the nurse's desired behavior or an intervention? If so, it does not belong under expected outcome. *Examples* The IV will not infiltrate The nurse will check the IV q 1 hour.
Plan of action	Are very *specific* steps given? Would a nurse new to the unit understand exactly how to do the activity? Did you note: how, when, how long, how often, where, by whom, with what, when appropriate? Were you specific for your client? Tailored to meet his particular problem? *Example* Spend 15 minutes per day sitting with a client to discuss *any* concerns she is having. Plan so that it can be an uninterrupted time. Tell her about any concerns *before* you begin.	Were you too general so different people might interpret the plan differently? *Example* Reassure the client bid. Did you use good-intention words such as: 1. support 2. encourage 3. teach 4. help 5. reassure 6. explain 7. explore with client If so, you are too general; these words may only be used when they are answered in the plan by "how," "when," "where," etc.
Evaluation	S. Did you gather subjective data to indicate the effectiveness of each intervention and movement toward the expected outcome? *Example* Client states she understands why she doesn't want to be alone. O. Did you gather objective data to indicate the effectiveness of each intervention and movement toward the expected outcome? *Example* called for nurse three times to hand her items within reach. A. Did you state whether your expected outcome was accomplished? *Example* Expected outcome accomplished: Client discussed horror at having only one breast; feels no one could like her this way. P. Did you assess the effectiveness of each intervention, and note whether to revise, continue, or discontinue interventions? *Example* Client needs a longer period of uninterrupted time before she expresses feelings. Spend 20 minutes per day instead of 15 with client.	Did you forget to mention that the expected outcome was: 1 accomplished? 2 not accomplished? Is the plan outdated?

Client Problem	Expected	Nursing Intervention
1. Dehydration due to nausea and vomiting	Drink 1,000cc fluid per shift.	a. Offer favorite drinks (apple juice, 7-Up) every 2h. b. Check water pitcher is full and within reach every 2h. c. Explain the reason why fluid intake must be increased d. Monitor I. and O. each shift.

Figure 2-4 Sample nursing care plan format. When possible, the client problem column should reflect a nursing diagnosis rather than a medical problem.

today's nursing theorists, the various definitions of nursing have commonalities of health, illness, and caring.

Nursing care is provided through the application of the steps of the nursing process: assessment, planning, implementation, and evaluation. There are three major steps to the assessment phase: data collection, data analysis, and nursing diagnosis. The nurse's skill at collecting both subjective and objective data affects the quality of the data base. Good interviewing skills are essential for obtaining this data. The planning phase also has three major steps: priority setting, goal formulation, and planning interventions. The plan of action must be founded on a sound data base. Implementation, the actual carrying out of the plan, may be done by the nurse or by someone the nurse designates. Evaluation is ongoing throughout the nursing process cycle.

There are several methods of record keeping used to promote continuity of client care and facilitate the nursing process. Two such methods are the SOAP progress notes and the written Kardex care plan.

The nursing process is a form of scientific method application, and it differs from medicine's problem-solving approach in its goals and means of accomplishing its goals. Knowledge from the physical and behavioral sciences and specific skills such as teaching, counseling, and technical skills are required to be able to apply the nursing process. Through the systematic use of the nursing process, nursing can best accomplish its goal of assisting others to maintain or attain optimal functioning.

REVIEW QUESTIONS

The number of the question corresponds to the same numbered objective at the beginning of the chapter.

1. A commonality in definitions of nursing is that nursing is
  a. client-centered
  b. an independent function
  c. a dependent function
  d. restorative in nature

2. The phases of the nursing process are
  a. assessment, problem solving, diagnosis, evaluation
  b. history and physical, diagnosis, treatment, evaluation
  c. assessment, planning, implementation, evaluation
  d. problem identification, goal setting, intervention, evaluation

3. Subjective data is
  a. what the nurse observes
  b. what the nurse states
  c. what the client exhibits
  d. what the client states

4. A nursing diagnosis consists of
  a. a subject, an action verb, and an explanation
  b. a stated behavior and cause
  c. a conclusion about a problem
  d. a label describing a behavior

5. A part of nursing's primary goal is to
  a. diagnose the illness or injury
  b. provide medical treatment
  c. assist the physician with the medical plan
  d. assist the client to meet his needs

6. Which of the following most affects one's success in obtaining an accurate, detailed nursing history?
  a. a cool, calm manner
  b. the ability to establish rapport
  c. self-confidence
  d. the client's age

7. A progress note should include
  a. a conclusion about the data
  b. a goal
  c. a summary of past treatment
  d. a medical diagnosis

8. In order to be useful, the nursing care plan should
  a. be general
  b. be specific
  c. be idealistic
  d. be a legal part of the chart

REFERENCES

1. M. Goodnow, *Outlines of Nursing History*, 6th ed., W. B. Saunders Company, Philadelphia, 1938, p. 25.
2. *Nursing Theories: The Base for Professional Nursing Practice*. The Nursing Theories Conference Group, Prentice-Hall, Inc., Englewood Cliffs, N.J., 1980.
3. F. Nightingale, *Notes on Nursing: What It Is and What It Is Not*, facsimile edition, J. B. Lippincott Company, Philadelphia, 1946.
4. F. L. Bower, and E. O. Bevis, *Fundamentals of Nursing Practice*, The C. V. Mosby Company, St. Louis, 1979, p. 13.
5. Ibid., p. 582.
6. Ibid., p. 582.
7. L. Carroll, *Alice's Adventures in Wonderland and Through the Looking Glass*, 8th printing, Collier Books, New York, 1973, p. 193.
8. V. Henderson, *The Nature of Nursing*, The Macmillan Company, New York, 1966, p. 3.
9. F. Nightingale, op. cit., p. 79.
10. American Nurses Association, Standards of Practice, 1973.
11. UNM Curriculum Overview, University of New Mexico, Albuquerque, New Mexico, June 1979, pp. 4–12.
12. Ibid.
13. Sr. C. Roy, *Introduction to Nursing: An Adaptation Model*, Prentice-Hall, Inc., Englewood Cliffs, N.J., 1976, pp. 11.
14. UNM Curriculum Overview, op. cit., p. 11.
15. S. Sundeen et al., *Nurse-Client Interaction: Implementing The Nursing Process*, The C. V. Mosby Company, St. Louis, 1976, p. 5.
16. Bowers, F. L., *The Process of Planning Nursing Care*, The C. V. Mosby Company, St. Louis, 1977, pp. 16–17.
17. A. Maslow, *Motivation and Personality*, Harper & Row Publishers, Incorporated, New York, 1954.
18. K. C. Sorenson, and J. Luckmann, *Basic Nursing: A Psychophysiologic Approach*, W. B. Saunders Company, Philadelphia, 1979, p. 302.
19. Sundeen et al., op. cit., p. 12.

Chapter 3

NURSING ASSESSMENT

Health History and Physical Examination

Corina B. Casias
Dorothy Hendel Clough

Learning Objectives

1. Explain the purpose, components, and techniques related to the health history and physical examination.
2. Describe the appropriate use and techniques of inspection, palpation, percussion, and auscultation.
3. Identify the equipment needed to perform a physical examination.
4. Describe the indications, purposes, and components of the branching or regional examination.
5. Describe a routine format for recording the health history and physical examination.
6. Describe a format for performing and recording a general survey.

The health history, general survey, and physical examination are part of the assessment phase of the nursing process. This information provides much of the data upon which the other phases of the nursing process are based. The *health history* provides subjective data. Subjective data are information supplied by the client either voluntarily or by direct questioning by the nurse. Knowledgeable others can contribute subjective data about the client. The *general survey* statement provides a descriptive statement about the client. The *physical examination* provides objective data related to the health status of the client. Objective data are gathered by the nurse through inspection, palpation, percussion, and auscultation. Additional sources of objective data include the findings of other health care providers and the results of diagnostic studies.

HEALTH HISTORY

The health history is the initial step in the assessment process. Collection of these data assists both the examiner and the client in identifying health problems as well as assets and resources. The nurse can use these data to identify areas where the client might be unable to meet personal needs and would require nursing assistance.

The health history is subjective data gathered about the client's present and past health status and lifestyle. The following areas are included in a comprehensive health history:

1. Demographic or identifying data
2. Chief complaint
3. History of present illness or problem
4. Past health history
5. Family health history
6. Social and personal history (client profile)
7. Review of systems

It generally takes 45 minutes to 1 hour to obtain a complete history. It may be completed in one or several sessions, depending upon the setting and the client. Allowing time for the client to volunteer information about his or her own particular areas of concern enables the nurse to work *with* the client to identify existing and potential health problems. When a client is unable to provide the necessary data (unconscious, aphasic) the nurse then asks the person who has assumed responsibility for the client's welfare to provide as much information as possible.

Before beginning the health history, the nurse should explain to the client that the purpose of a detailed history is to collect information that will provide the client with a comprehensive health supervision plan including health maintenance and promotion (Fig. 3-1). It should further be explained that the nurse needs to obtain personal and social data about the client in order to individualize the plan of care. This explanation is necessary as clients may not be accustomed to sharing personal information about themselves and need to know the purpose of such ques-

This chapter was reviewed by M. Carolyn Cecere, R.N., M.S.N., CPNA, Associate Professor, Indiana University School of Nursing Specialist Degree Program in Primary Health Care of Adults and Children.

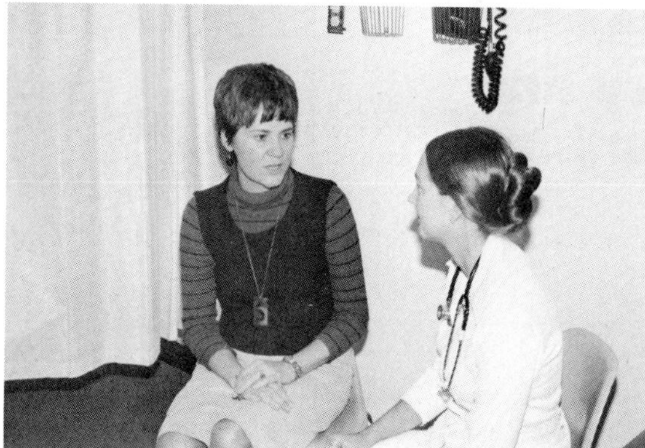

Figure 3-1 It is important that the nurse explain the purpose of the health history to the client.

tioning. The nurse should assure the client that all information will be kept confidential.

A variety of nursing history formats are available. Many of these forms are designed with a particular setting in mind. Both structured and unstructured forms are used. Some forms consist entirely of checklists which the client or the nurse completes. Other forms require an interview by the nurse. Regardless of the form used, the nurse must remember that the forms only assist in the assessment process. Completion of the form must be a means, not the end, in assessment.

The nurse must be flexible in the use of a health history form. For example, it may be more effective not to begin with the collection of demographic data. The use of such questions as "What brings you here today?" or "What seems to be the problem?" can be useful. It elicits the chief complaint and shows concern for what worries the client the most.[1] The nurse cannot assume the relative importance of a problem without validating this with the client.

The amount of information obtained at a first contact is a nursing judgment based on the client, the problem, and the setting. The nurse may ask only those questions which are pertinent to a specific problem, deferring the complete history until a more appropriate time.

The Format

The health history form presented in this text is a general screening assessment form for adults which could be used in a variety of settings (Table 3-1). The nurse should evaluate different forms until one is found which best suits her work situation and style.

The form presented here can assist the nurse to assess biophysical, psychological, sociocultural, and environmental dimensions of a client. Table 3-2 illustrates how all dimensions are assessed when this history format is used in conjunction with a physical examination.

There are often overlaps when viewing the dimensions which might be affected by a particular problem. For instance, occupational stress could result in problems in all dimensions. If categorization is necessary, it is usually done on the basis of the cause of the problem. Using this concept, occupational stress would be considered an environmental problem, as the work environment is the basic cause of the prob-

Table 3-1
Health History Form

I. **Demographic Data** (Identifying Data)
   1. Dates of assessment
   2. Client's name
   3. Parents' or guardian's name if a minor
   4. Address
   5. Age, birthdate
   6. Birthplace
   7. Sex, race, and ethnicity
   8. Primary language
   9. Marital status
   10. Occupation and place of employment
   11. Health coverage
   12. Informant/reliability

II. **CC** (Chief Complaint—problem and duration in client's own words) Reason for seeking health care

III. **HPI** (History of Present Illness—amplification of reason for entering the health care system)
Investigation of a symptom:
Bodily location, quality, quantity, chronology, setting, aggravating and alleviating factors, associated manifestations, meaning to individual. List significant positive and negative findings related to the chief complaint.

Table 3-1 (Continued)

IV. **Past Health History**

General health statement

Childhood illnesses: rubella, mumps, pertussis, scarlet fever, rheumatic fever, chickenpox, polio, measles, strep throat

Adult illnesses: rheumatic fever, hepatitis, cystitis, strep throat, pneumonia, anemia, tuberculosis

Immunizations: give type and dates

Injuries, hospitalization and operations

Therapeutic regimens: meds, diet, psychotherapy—past and present

Allergies: environmental, ingestion, drugs, other

Travel in last five years: dates, location, related illness

Habits: smoking, alcohol, caffeine, recreational drugs

Supportive devices: e.g., cane, walker, eyeglasses

V. **FH** (Family Health History)

Ask specifically about:

TB, diabetes, glaucoma, hypertension, heart disease, strokes, renal disease, alcoholism, VD, arthritis, gout, ulcers, cancer, epilepsy, depression, mental illness, other

Example: Genetic chart

Code: ○ = female, □ = male; ■, ● = deceased; × = client

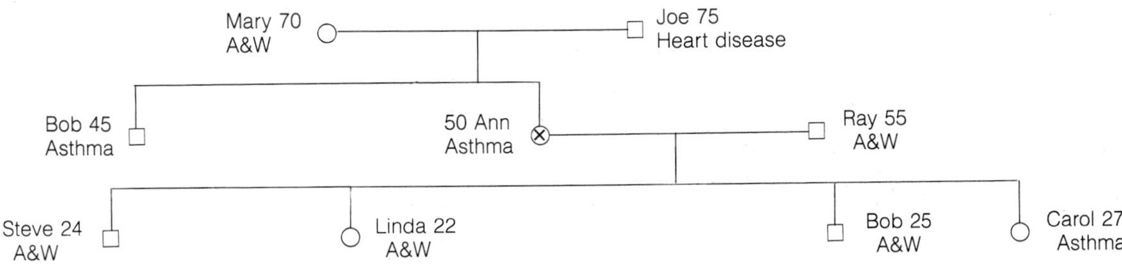

Record all significant positives and negatives including mental retardation, congenital abnormalities, hereditary diseases, and family allergies.

VI. **Social and Personal History** (Client Profile)

Typical day and typical weekend day

Diet habits with 24-hour recall—specifically, questions about intake of fluid, salt, artificial sweeteners, and sugar

Sleep patterns—number of hours, times awake, reason for awakening, how the client feels upon awakening in the morning

Exercise patterns—include exercise habits, duration, frequency

Recreation—include activities, frequency, individual or team sport

Occupation—include type, duration, satisfaction, stressors, time commitment

Safety practices—question specifically about safety practices related to exercise, recreation, or occupation

Education—highest grade achieved, future educational goals for self

Income—adequacy to meet needs, retirement planning, as a stressor

Family relationships—number of persons in household, ages, positive and negative relationships, expectations for children, significant others

Dependency/independency needs—need for privacy, need for others, available support systems

Client's perception of self-aspirations, hopes, disappointments, guilt, satisfactions

Spiritual needs—religious preference, strength of belief

Stressors—areas of life which cause concern to the client; all dimensions should be assessed as potential stressors

Coping patterns—ability to overcome obstacles

Ability to communicate—identify any problem areas, language barriers, attention span, memory

Sexual history—problems, satisfaction

Personal practices related to health promotion and maintenance—describe specific practices and duration

Client's perception of problem and expectation of the health care provider

VII. **Review of Systems**

General

Present weight (loss or gain of ± 10 lb) Weakness Fatigue Malaise Sleep patterns Fever Chills Sweats or night sweats Dizziness Fainting Headache

Vision and Hearing

Eyes: Pain Vision Glasses or contacts Spots or floaters Recent change in acuity Diplopia Infection Glaucoma Cataract Date of last examination

Ears: Earaches Hearing Tinnitus Discharge Infection Mastoiditis Ears pierced Vertigo Sensitivity to noise Date of audiometric testing, if ever

Table 3-1 (Continued)

Integumentary

Pruritus Pigmentary and other color changes Lesions/rashes Tendency to bruising Excessive dryness Texture or moisture Character of hair and nails Use of hair dyes or other possibly toxic agents

Respiratory

Nose: Sinus pain Nasal obstruction Rhinorrhea/discharge Postnasal drip Frequent colds sneezing

Mouth/Throat: Pain Difficulty chewing Hoarseness Expectoration Frequent sore throats Condition of teeth Voice changes

Lungs: Chest pain Pleurisy Cough Sputum Hemoptysis Dyspnea Wheezing Bronchitis Pneumonia Smoking Tuberculosis or contact with Exercise pattern Date of last chest x-ray TB skin test (date and results)

Hematological

Bleeding tendencies of skin or mucous membranes Anemia and treatment Blood transfusion and reaction Blood type Blood dyscrasia Exposure to toxic agents or radiation Lymph node enlargement

Cardiovascular

Chest pain or distress Palpitations Dyspnea on exertion Orthopnea Paroxysmal nocturnal dyspnea Nocturia (does it awaken you or do you awaken and then void?) Cyanosis History of heart murmur Rheumatic fever Hypertension Coronary artery disease Anemia Heart attack Date of last ECG Other cardiac W/U

Peripheral Vascular

Intermittent claudication Thrombophlebitis Varicose veins or complications Peripheral edema Raynaud's disease Cyanosis Hair loss Chronic coldness of extremities

Gastrointestinal

Appetite Food intolerances Dysphagia (solids, liquids) Heartburn Indigestion Postprandial pain or distress Use of antacids Other abdominal pain or distress Belching Nausea Vomiting Hematemesis Distension Flatulence Abdominal masses Use of laxatives Character of stool Melena Change in bowel habits Rectal conditions (pruritus, hemorrhoids, fissures, fistulas) Gallbladder disease Hepatitis Jaundice Appendicitis

Abdominal surgery Colitis Parasites Hernia Date of previous x-rays

Genitourinary

Renal colic/stones Frequency of urination Nocturia Polyuria Oliguria Dysuria Hematuria Albuminuria Pyuria Urination (hesitancy, urgency, narrow or weak stream, dribbling, incontinence) Kidney disease Facial edema Cystoscopy Infections Gonorrhea or syphilis (identify by common name and signs, note date, treatment, complications) Herpes simplex type 1 or type 2

Male: Prostatitis Hernia Testicular pain Discharge Change in size of scrotum

Reproductive/Sexual

Sexual: Drive Activity Pleasure Discomfort Impotence Frigidity Sterility Contraceptive methods (type, how long, methods, effectiveness)

Female: Menstrual history [last normal menstrual period (LNMP), menarche, cycle and duration, amount of flow, premenstrual tension/pain, dysmenorrhea, intermenstrual bleeding] Vaginal discharge Menopause and associated symptoms Vaginal or uterine surgery Date of last Pap smear and results Breast masses Breast self-exam (BSE)—Knows how? How often? Nipple discharge

Pregnancies: Gravida______Para______Abortions______Spontaneous or therapeutic______Stillbirths______Premature births______No. of living children______

Male: Impotence Premature ejaculation Prostate problems Rashes/lesions on penis or scrotum

Endocrine

Nutritional and growth history Thyroid function (tolerance to heat and cold, changes in skin, relationship between appetite and weight, nervousness, tremors, drowsiness, results of previous tests) Hair distribution/hirsutism Sexual vigor goiter Diabetes or its symptoms (polyuria, polydipsia, polyphagia) Sugar in blood or urine Excessive sweating Hormone therapy

Neurological

Headache Nervousness Sleep disturbance Vertigo Syncope Loss of consciousness Convulsions/fits Stroke Sensory or motor disturbance (speech disturbance, tremor, weakness, paralysis, clumsiness of movement) Paresthesia Memory loss Disorientation

Musculoskeletal

Muscle: Muscle weakness Pain Cramps Trauma Aches Atrophy Spasms

Joints: Pain Stiffness Swelling Rheumatoid arthritis Osteoarthritis Gout Bursitis Back (pain, stiffness, limitation of motion, sciatica, or disc disease)

Bones: Dislocation Fractures Osteomyelitis Flat feet

lem. The nurse should use a holistic approach, viewing all of an individual's dimensions in order to avoid only considering part of a problem.

It is important to note that the Health History Guidelines indicate what to ask, not how to ask it. Specific interviewing skills have been discussed in Chap. 2. In addition to understanding the principles of effective communication, each nurse must develop her own style of relating to clients. Although there is no single style that fits all people, the nurse will find that there are certain ways to word specific questions which elicit the needed information. Ease at asking questions, particularly those related to sensitive areas such as sexual functioning and income, comes with experience.

Table 3-2
Assessment in All Dimensions

Dimension	Assessment Area
Biophysical	Chief complaint (CC) History of present illness Past health history Family health history Review of systems (ROS) Physical examination
Psychological	Past health history Family history Social and personal history ROS (neurological, endocrine) Physical examination
Sociocultural	Demographic data Family history Social and personal history
Environmental	Past health history Family health history Social and personal history

Demographic Data

The first part of the health history, the demographic data, consists of identifying data such as name, date, age, etc. (See Table 3-1, Health History Guidelines.) When recording these data, mention should be made of who supplied the information (informant) and of how accurate the information is considered to be (reliability). Any discrepancies or inconsistencies should be noted.

Chief Complaint

In Part II, the *chief complaint* (CC) is the term used to describe what has motivated the client to seek health care. It should be recorded in the client's own words whenever possible. Quotation marks indicate that the client's words have been used. When a health problem is involved, the chief complaint should state the problem and its duration. For example, "Nausea for 36 hours" would be a properly recorded chief complaint. If the client does not have a health problem or chief complaint, the reason for entering the health care system at this time should be noted. For example, "I need an insurance physical," gives direction to the interview which follows.

It is important to deal initially with the client's perceived problems. Although the nurse may view other problems as more important, the client's concerns must be dealt with before progress can be made in other areas.

History of Present Illness or Problem

Part III is the history of present illness (HPI). The history of present illness provides detailed data about the chief complaint. The nurse should be quite directive in this phase. If the client has entered the health care system with a particular problem, the nurse then gathers very specific information about the client's symptoms. This is done in a systematic fashion and is referred to as the investigation of a symptom. The information obtained through this process helps to determine the cause of the problem. Table 3-3 lists the eight areas which must be investigated if a symptom is present.

For example, if the client stated that he had "pain in his leg at times," the nurse, in correctly exploring the symptom according to the above criteria, might obtain and record the following information:

Has right midcalf pain (*location*), described as "like being stabbed with a knife" (*quality*). Pain is so severe that it is not possible to continue walking (*quantity*). Onset is abrupt, lasting for 1 to 2 minutes; occurs once or twice daily; last occurred on 5/5/80 (*onset, duration, frequency*). Generally occurs at work when climbing stairs after lunch but last occurred when cutting lawn (*setting*). Pain is alleviated by rest for 2 to 3 minutes. The client has been salting his food "more heavily" than he used to, but "it doesn't help" (*alleviating factor*). Leg pain is sometimes accompanied by chest pain (*associated manifestations*). The client has not altered his lifestyle on account of the intermittent pain. He thinks it is caused "by muscle cramps from lack of salt" (*personal meaning*).

Throughout the health history, *any positive findings* are explored using the same criteria as the investigation of a symptom. A positive finding indicates that the client has had or does have a particular problem or symptom posed by the nurse. For example, if the client answers yes to the question of chest

Table 3-3

Investigation of a Symptom

The Location

Ask: "Where do you feel it?" "Where is it located?"
Record: Region of the body:
If local or radiating
If superficial or deep

The Quality

Ask: "What does it (feel, look) like?"
Record: The client's analogy (i.e., "Like being burned")

The Quantity

Ask: "How often do you have this feeling?" "How bad is it?" "How much is it?" or "How big is it?"
Record: Frequency, (mild, moderate, severe) volume, size, extent, or number

The Chronology

Ask: "When was the first time it occurred?" "Any particular time of day, week, month, or year?"
Record: Time of onset
The duration
Periodicity and frequency
Course of the symptoms

The Setting

Ask: "Where are you when this occurs?" "What were you doing?"
Record: Where the client is when the symptom occurs
What the client is doing
If the symptom is related to anything

The Aggravating or Alleviating Factors

Ask: "What makes it better? Worse?" "Is there any activity that seems to cause it?" "What have you done for it?" "Did it help?" "Was there some reason you didn't do anything about it?"
Record: The influence of physical and emotional activities
The client's attempts to alleviate (or treat) the symptom

The Associated Manifestations

Ask: "What other things do you see or feel when it occurs?"
Record: Other symptoms

The Meaning of the Symptom to the Client

Ask: "How has it affected you? Your life?" "Why have you sought care now?" "What do you think may be the cause?"
Record: Client's statements as to the effect of the symptom on himself and the cause of the symptom

pain, this indicates a positive finding. The nurse would then proceed to gather relevant information about this problem.

Negative findings may also be significant. A negative finding is lack of a symptom usually associated with a problem. It would be common to find peripheral edema in the client with congestive heart failure. If edema was not present in a client with congestive heart failure, it would be noted. Another type of negative finding includes the absence of usual health promotion practices. Lack of tetanus immunization is a negative finding and would be recorded.

Past Health History

Part IV of the health history is the past health history which provides information about the client's prior state of health and illness. The client is specifically questioned about major childhood and adult illnesses, immunizations, injuries, hospitalizations, operations, therapeutic regimens, allergies, travel, habits, and the use of supportive devices.

The nurse asks about specific childhood and adult illness as outlined in Table 3-1. This procedure is more effective than simply asking if the client has had any illnesses. Many illnesses are long forgotten or considered irrelevant. If there is a positive finding, the nurse needs to determine when the client had the problem, how it was treated, and if the client still experiences any health problems related to the illness. In some instances the client may not know about childhood illnesses. This should be indicated on the history.

The nurse also determines if the client's immunizations are current. A current immunization schedule from the local health department can serve as a checklist. Specific immunizations to ask about include polio, measles, mumps, tetanus, pertussis, rubella, and diphtheria.

All injuries, hospitalizations, and surgeries are recorded, along with a note of the date of the event, the treatment, and the outcome (whether or not the problem was completely resolved). Blood transfusions received by the client should be noted.

Specific details related to past or present therapeutic regimens should be obtained. This includes use of prescription or over-the-counter medications. Examples of specific medications to ask about include steroids, birth control pills, antibiotics, diuretics, aspirin, antacids, and laxatives. Data related to special diets, either prescribed or self-selected, should be obtained. Examples of common special diets to specifically ask about include restricted calorie, low salt, and low cholesterol diets.

The client needs to be questioned regarding allergies, including known allergens, specific reactions, and treatments. Information related to desensitization regimens should also be obtained. History of travel in the past 5 years is included in the questioning since different geographic locations may expose the client to new and different health hazards.

Habits related to smoking, alcohol intake, caffeine, and recreational drugs should be noted. The type, quantity, and duration of use should be specifically elicited and recorded.

Finally, the client needs to be questioned about the use of any supportive devices such as a cane, walker, eyeglasses, or hearing aid. The reason and duration of use should be included.

Family Health History

Part V of the health history is the family health history (FHH). A family health history is an inquiry about illnesses which have a genetic or familial tendency or which are communicable. The presence or absence of such conditions or problems listed in section V of Table 3-1 should be noted. Again, stating the most common diseases can help the client to remember what illnesses various family members have had.

A genetic chart of three generations should also be developed. The nurse notes the ages of family members and whether the family members are alive and well (A & W) or have a health problem. (See the example on the Health History Guidelines sheet.)

The genetic history can provide a wealth of information. It reveals: (1) a picture of the family composition, (2) information about the client's responses to health and illness of family members (i.e. grieving process), and (3) health trends and heredity and environmental predispositions.[2]

Social and Personal History (Client Profile)

Part VI of the health history is the social and personal history of the client. It presents a profile of the client in his social and personal world. These data gathered by the nurse allow problems to be assessed in a more individualized manner and is often unique to nursing. As mentioned in Chap. 2, the nurse is primarily concerned with the client's level of wellness. Assessment of the client profile assures that the client's sociocultural, environmental, and psychological status are considered in planning care. The review of systems, discussed later, assesses the client's biophysical status. Detailed information is needed in all these areas to accurately determine the client's health problems, coping ability, and assets. The specific areas to question the client about are detailed in the Health History Guidelines.

Gathering the personal and social history

Generally, this is the least structured portion of the health history and requires the most rapport with the client. Allow the client to tell his own story.[3] Obtaining the client's perspective is prerequisite to understanding his needs and concerns. Open-ended questions allow the client to discuss personal topics comfortably.

Attaching an explanation to the questions provides the client with a rationale for sometimes seemingly irrelevant questions. For example, "Knowing about your usual workday gives me some information about what stresses or health hazards you are exposed to. Please describe your typical workday for me." Another example is, "Relaxation is important to your health. What do you do to relax?" Informal teaching can be done when questions are posed in this manner.

In order to obtain accurate social and personal information, the nurse must communicate acceptance of the client as an individual. When asking sensitive questions, the nurse can communicate the acceptance or normalcy of behaviors by prefacing questions with "most people," or "frequently." For instance, stating "Most people have sexual concerns; are there any you would like to discuss?" shows the client his situation may not be unique. Another method of putting the client at ease is to word the question in such a way that an affirmative answer appears expected. An example of this technique would be to ask "What do you like to drink at a party?" instead of "Do you drink?" "How often do you drink alcohol?" is another way of obtaining this information. This is less likely to put the client on the defensive than "Do you ever drink?"[4]

From the social and personal history the nurse gains a view of the client as a unique individual. This perspective, along with the other parts of the health history, provides a firm foundation for assisting the client to set goals and develop a health care plan tailored to his own life situation.

Review of Systems

The review of systems (ROS) is the final portion of the health history. It is the systematic collection of specific information about the client's past and present health status related to common problems of body systems. It is considered subjective data since the information is supplied by the client. Leading, directed questions are posed to the client in an orderly manner using a systems approach.

In addition to questioning the client about current or past health problems, health promotion and maintenance practices are recorded with the appropriate system. Such practices include breast self-exam, eye exams, ECG testing, testicular exam, dental exams, tuberculin screening, and chest x-ray.

Before beginning the lengthy list of review of systems questions, the client should be told the importance of this information in planning health care. Generally, "yes" or "no" answers are satisfactory. If the client answers "yes" to a symptom or problem, it should be investigated using the criteria presented under history of present illness.

Responses that have already been elicited in previous portions of the health history need not be repeated. It is important to avoid asking repetitive questions. This can lead the client to believe that the nurse is not listening to what is being said. It is also important to use common, easily understood words to describe medical problems. Otherwise, the client may give inaccurate information due to lack of understanding.

Recording of responses should be standardized if a printed review of systems form is used. This assures that all care providers can understand the significance of the responses. For instance, all positive responses can be circled, all negative responses crossed out, and information not available responses underlined. The directions should clearly indicate the system used.

GENERAL SURVEY

Following the health history, the nurse makes a general survey statement. The general survey is a statement of the nurse's general impression of a client. This initial survey is considered a scanning procedure and begins with the nurse's first encounter with the client and continues during the health history.

Although the nurse may include other data which she feels are pertinent, the major areas generally included in the general survey statement include: (1) body features, (2) state of consciousness and arousal, (3) speech, (4) body movements, (5) physical signs, (6) nutritional status, and (7) stature. Vital signs, height, and weight are often included in the general survey statement. Observations of these areas provide the data for the general survey statement. The following is a sample of a general survey statement:

> This is a 34-year-old Mexican-American female. BP 130/84/80, P 88, R 18. No distinguishing body features. Alert but anxious. Speech rapid with trailing thoughts. Wringing hands and shuffling feet during interview. Skin flushed, hands clammy. Overweight in proportion to height. Sits with eyes downcast and shoulders slumped.

THE PHYSICAL EXAMINATION

The physical examination is the systematic assessment of the physical and mental status of a client and is considered objective data. During the physical examination additional subjective data may be obtained from the client. This may occur from direct questioning by the nurse regarding a finding or be coincidental to the client remembering a forgotten piece of information. It is not advisable to combine the review of systems with the physical examination. The review of systems gives valuable direction to the physical examination. Also, the two activities of questioning and examining can be confusing to both the client and the nurse. An exception to this might be in an emergency situation where time is a factor.

Types of Physical Examinations

There are two types of physical examinations, the branching or regional exam and the screening physical exam. The *screening physical examination* is performed for screening situations, health surveillance, and for health maintenance purposes. It is an organized superficial check of major body systems to detect any possible problems. If a problem is detected in the course of the screening physical, a more detailed branching examination of the involved system should be done.

A *branching or regional examination* is a more detailed assessment of a particular system such as the physical examination presented in the assessment chapters of this text. The client's clinical manifestations should alert the nurse to the appropriate branching exam. For instance, abdominal pain would indicate the need to do a branching exam of the abdomen. Some problems necessitate more than one branching exam. For example, a complaint of headache would indicate the need to do musculoskeletal, neurological, head and neck, and psychiatric exams.

Techniques of Physical Examination

There are four major techniques used in performing the physical examination. These are the techniques of inspection, palpation, percussion, and auscultation.

Inspection

Inspection is the visual examination of a part or region of the body to assess normal or deviations from normal. Inspection is more than just looking. This technique is deliberate, systematic, and focused. The nurse needs to compare what is seen with the known generally visible characteristics of the part being inspected. For instance, most 30-year-old women have hair on their legs. Absence of hair could indicate a vascular problem and would need to be investigated (Fig. 3-2). This same absence of hair in a 90-year-old man could represent a normal skin change of aging.

Palpation

Palpation is the examination of the body through the use of touch. The use of light and deep palpation can yield information related to masses, pulsatility, organ enlargement, tenderness or pain, swelling, muscular spasm or rigidity, elasticity, vibration of voice sounds, crepitus, moisture, and differences in texture.[5] The nurse will learn that different parts of the hand are more sensitive for specific assessments. For example, the tips of the fingers are used to palpate lymph nodes while the dorsa of hands and fingers would be used to assess temperatures (Fig. 3-3).

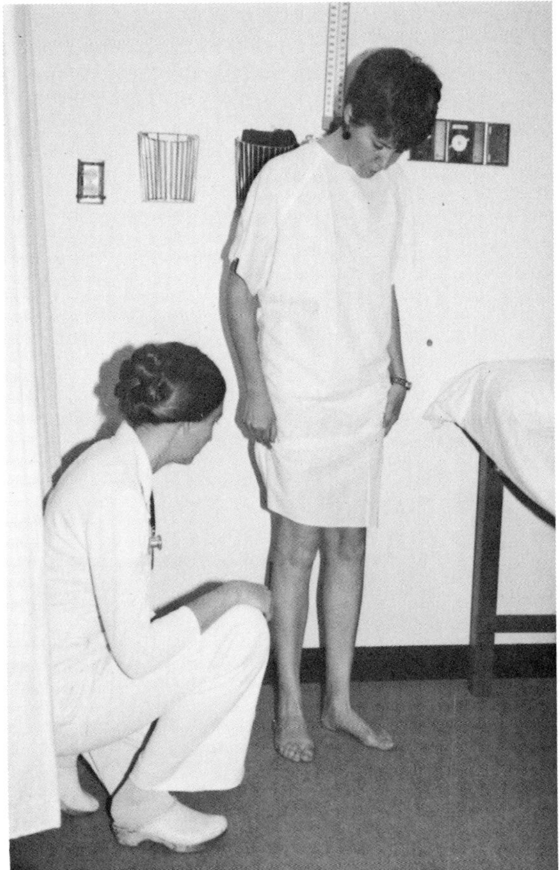

Figure 3-2 Inspection is the visual examination of a part or region of the body to assess normal or deviations from normal.

Percussion

Percussion is an assessment technique involving the production of sound to obtain information about the underlying area. The percussion sound may be produced directly or indirectly. Direct percussion is performed by directly tapping the body with one or two fingers to elicit a sound. Indirect or mediated percussion is the more common percussion technique. The middle finger (*pleximeter*) of the nondominant hand is placed firmly against the body surface (Fig. 3-4*a*). The tip of the middle finger of the dominant hand (*plexor*) strikes the distal phalanx of the pleximeter finger (Fig. 3-4*b*). A relaxed wrist and a rapid strike produce the best sounds. The sounds produced as well as the vibrations are evaluated relative to the underlying structures. Deviation from an expected sound could indicate a problem. For example, the usual percussion sound in the right lower quadrant of

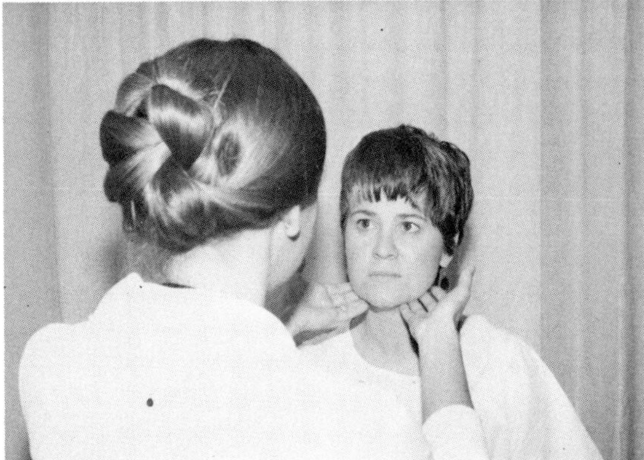

Figure 3-3 Palpation is the examination of the body through the use of touch.

the abdomen is tympany. Dullness in this area could indicate a problem and would need to be investigated. Specific percussion sounds of various body parts and regions are discussed in the appropriate assessment chapters.

Auscultation

Auscultation is the listening to sounds produced by the body to assess normal and deviations from normal. Auscultation is usually indirect, using a stethoscope to mediate the sounds (Fig. 3-5). The bell of the stethoscope is more sensitive to low-pitched sounds. The diaphragm of the stethoscope is more sensitive to high-pitched sounds. Auscultation is particularly useful in evaluating sounds from the heart, lungs, abdomen, bruits, and murmurs. Specific auscultatory sounds are discussed in the appropriate assessment chapters.

Not all assessment techniques are appropriate for all body parts and systems. The nurse will learn which technique to use to elicit the most information. The physical assessment techniques are usually performed in the sequence of inspection, palpation, percussion, and auscultation.

The only exception to this sequence is for the abdominal exam. In this situation, the sequence is inspection, auscultation, percussion, and palpation. Palpation and percussion of the abdomen before auscultation can alter bowel sounds and produce false findings.

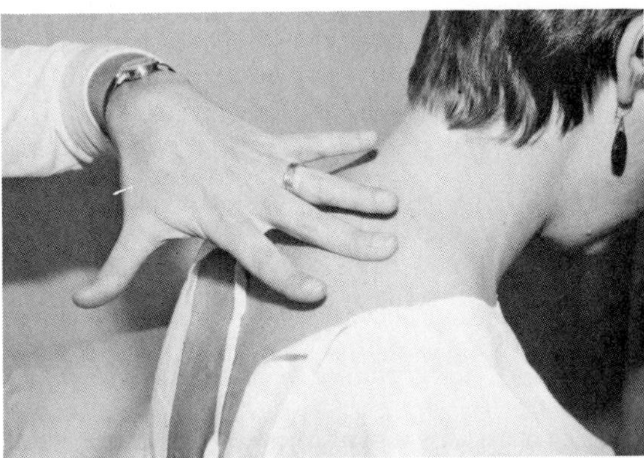

A

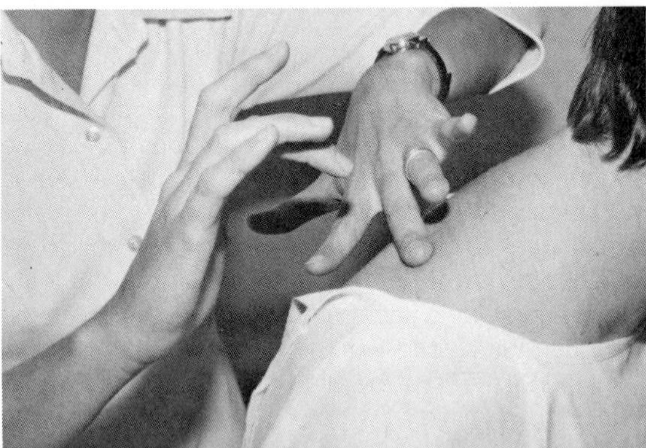

B

Figure 3-4 Percussion is an assessment technique involving the production of sound to obtain information about the underlying area. (*a*) Placement of the pleximeter finger. (*b*) Plexor finger striking the pleximeter finger to produce sound.

Equipment

It is important to have all equipment needed for the screening physical easily accessible during the

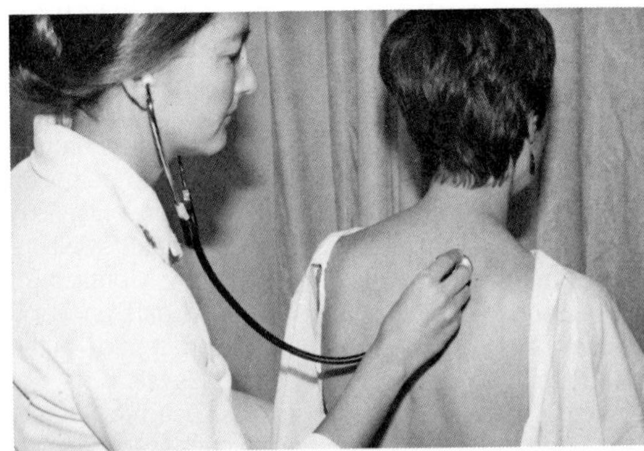

Figure 3-5 Auscultation is the listening to sounds produced by the body to assess normal and deviations from normal.

examination (Table 3-4). Organizing equipment before the exam saves the time and energy of both the client and the nurse. Lack of organization can discourage the client from the trust and confidence the nurse needs to collect the data base. The use of specific pieces of equipment are discussed in the appropriate assessment chapters.

Developing a System

The screening physical should be performed systematically and efficiently. Explanations should be given to the client as the examination proceeds. The factors considered should be for efficiency, client comfort, safety, and privacy. In developing a routine method, the examiner is less likely to forget a procedure, a step in the sequence, or a portion of the body if the same sequence is followed every time. Table 3-5 suggests an outline for the screening physical examination which is organized, logical, and complete.

Recording the screening physical examination

It is suggested that only abnormal findings be written down during the actual examination. This prevents needless interruptions in the examination to write lengthy normal findings. At the conclusion of the examination, the nurse can combine the normal and abnormal findings in a carefully recorded physical examination. Table 3-6 is an example of how to record a screening physical on a healthy adult.

Table 3-4

Equipment Necessary To Perform a Screening Physical Examination

Stethoscope (with bell and diaphragm, tubing 15–18" in length)
Wrist watch (with second hand)
Blood pressure cuff
Ophthalmoscope/otoscope set
Eye chart (either wall chart or Snellen pocket eye card)
Pocket flashlight
Tongue blades
Cotton balls
Percussion hammer
Tuning fork
Alcohol swabs
Client gown
Paper cup with water
Examining table or bed

Table 3-5

An Outline for the Screening Physical Examination

A. **General Survey:** Observe the client's general state of health including body features, state of consciousness and arousal, speech, body movements, physical signs, nutritional status, and stature. Vital signs, height, and weight are often included. *(Client usually remains seated until examination of the neck.)*
B. **Vital Signs:** Blood pressure, radial pulse, respiration, weight.
C. **Integumentary System:** Inspect and palpate for color, lesions, scars, bruises, edema, moisture, texture, temperature, turgor, vascularity. Nails for color, lesions, size, flexibility, shape, angle.
D. **Head and Neck**
   1. *Head:* Inspect and palpate for shape and symmetry of skull, masses, tenderness, hair, scalp, skin, temporal arteries, temporomandibular joint, sensory (CN V, light touch and pain), motor (CN VII, shows teeth, purses lips, raises eyebrows)
   2. *Eyes:* Inspect and palpate for visual acuity, eyebrows, position and movement of eyelids, visual fields, extraocular movements (CN III, IV, VI), cornea, sclera, and conjunctive, PERRLA, red reflex eyeball tension
   3. *Ears:* Inspect and palpate for placement, pinna, auditory acuity (Weber or Rinne, whispered voice, or ticking watch), mastoid process
   4. *Nose and sinuses:* Inspect and palpate external nose (shape, blockage, discharge) and internal (patency of nasal passages, shape, turbinates/polyps, discharge, frontal and maxillary sinuses)
   5. *Mouth:* Inspect and occasionally palpate lips (symmetry, lesions, color), buccal mucosa (Stensen's and Wharton's ducts), teeth (absent, state of repair, color), gums, tongue with strength (asymmetry, ability to stick out tongue, side to side, fasciculations), moisture, color, floor of mouth, palates, tonsils and pillars, uvular elevation (CN IX), posterior pharynx, gag reflex (CN X), jaw strength (CN XI), (Completion of cranial nerves) look up and wrinkle forehead (CN VII), raise shoulders against resistance (CM XI)
   6. *Neck:* Inspect and palpate (occasionally auscultate) skin (vascularity and visible pulsations), symmetry, postural alignment, range of motion, pulses (carotid). Midline structures of trachea and thyroid gland and cartilage, Lymph nodes (pre- and postauricular, occipital, mandibular, tonsillar, submental, anterior and posterior cervical, infra- and supraclavicular. (*Have client change to a standing position.*)
   7. *Neurological examination:* Motor status; walk, observe gait, toe walk, heel walk, assess drift; coordination; finger to nose, Romberg. Inspect and palpate spine; observe for scoliosis. (*Client returns to sitting position.*)

Table 3-5 (Continued)

E. Extremities: Gross observation for size and shape, symmetry and deformity, involuntary movements. (*Client in sitting position with examiner at the back.*)
1. Inspect and palpate arms, fingers, wrists, elbows, and shoulders for strength, range of motion, crepitus, joint pain, swelling, fluid.
2. Test reflexes, including biceps, triceps, bachioradialis, patellar, Achilles, plantar.
3. Inspect and palpate legs for strength of hips, edema, hair distribution, pulses (dorsalis pedis, posterior tibialis)

F. Thorax (Posterior): Inspect for muscular development, respiratory movement, approximation of A-P diameter; palpate for symmetry of respiratory movement, tenderness of CVA, spinous processes, tumors or swelling, tactile fremitus; Percuss for pulmonary resonance; auscultate for breath sounds.

G. Thorax (Anterior): Breasts: assess configuration, symmetry, skin for dimpling; nipples for rash, direction, inversion, retraction. Initiate teaching or review of breast self-exam, perform upright examination, palpate axilla. (*Client assumes supine position.*) Inspect, palpate, check breasts for discharge; complete teaching of breast self-exam.
1. *Chest:* Inspect for PMI and other precordial pulsations; palpate for thrills, lifts, heaves, tenderness over precordium; auscultate for rate and rhythm, character of S_1 and S_2; auscultate for S_1 and S_2 in the aortic, pulmonic, Erb's point, tricuspid and mitral areas, bruits at the carotid and epigastrium, breath sounds at RML.
2. *Neck:* Inspect for venous distension, pulsations and waves. (*Redrape chest and bare abdomen to symphysis pubis.*)

H. Abdomen: Inspect for scars, shape, symmetry, bulging, muscular development, position and condition of umbilicus, movements (respiratory, pulsations, presence of peristaltic waves); auscultate for peristalsis, femoral bruits; percuss the border of liver, all four quadrants; palpate to confirm positive findings, liver (size, surface contour, tenderness), spleen, kidney (size, contour, consistency, tenderness, mobility), urinary bladder (distension), femoral pulses, inguinofemoral nodes.

I. Completion of the Examination of the Extremities: Range of motion of hips, ankles, feet; crepitus, joint pain, swelling, fluid, muscle development, coordination (heel to shin), Homan's sign, proprioception (position sense of great toe)
[This examination(s) will have the female client supine for this portion. The male will be supine for a portion and upright for the remainder.]

J. Genitalia: Inspection and palpation.
It is not the objective of this book to have the nurse perform the speculum and bimanual examination of the female client, nor the digital examination of the male prostate gland. If the nurse had learned the above-mentioned procedures they would be conducted at this time. Otherwise, the nurse will perform the following:
1. *Male external genitalia:*
   Penis: Inspect for: Hair distribution, prepuce, glans, urethral meatus, scars, ulcers, eruptions, and structural alterations.
   Perineum: Inspect epidermis, rectum.
   Scrotum: Inspect skin. Palpate for both descended testes, masses, pain.
2. *Female external genitalia:*
   Inspect hair distribution, mons pubis, labia (minora and majora) urethral meatus, Bartholin, urethral and Skene's glands (may also be palpated, if necessary), introitus. Have client bear down to assess for presence of cystocele, rectocele or prolapse. Inspect perineum and rectum.

Table 3-6

Recording a Screening Physical Examination

Client's Name: ____________

Age: ____________

Date: ____________

Vital Signs: BP______ **P**______ **R**______

General: Well-nourished, well-hydrated, well-developed white ♀ (female) or ♂ (male) in NAD appears stated age, looks pleasant, smiles readily, speech clear and evenly paced, is alert and oriented ×3; cooperative, calm	**Skin:** Clear s̄ lesions, warm and dry, trunk warmer than extremities, turgor: returns quickly; no ↑ vascularity; no varicose veins **Hair:** Thick, brown, normal (♂, ♀) distribution **Nails:** Well-groomed, round 160° angle ō lesions; nail beds pink; nails flexible
Eyes: Visual fields intact on gross confront *V.A.:* OD 20/20 OS 20/20 OU 20/20 s̄ glasses *E.O.M.:* Intact on all gazes ō ptosis or nystagmus *Fundi:* Red reflex present bilat no opacities—fundi WNL's *Pupils:* PERRLA; cover/uncover test neg; Herschberge test neg	**Ears:** Pinna intact, in proper alignment, external canal patent, TM's intact, pearly gray LM & LR visible not bulging **Nose:** Patent bilaterally turbinates pink no swelling, smell intact bilaterally **Hearing:** Rinne—AC7BC; Weber—does not lateralize, whisper heard @ 4′ **Sinuses:** Nontender **Head:** Normocephalic

Table 3-6 (Continued)

Mouth: Moist, pink, soft and hard palates intact, uvula rises midline on "ahh" **Throat:** Tonsils surgically removed—no redness **Tongue:** Moist, pink, size appropriate for mouth **Teeth:** 24 present and in good repair, gums pink	**Neck:** Supple ō masses ō bruits, nontender *Thyroid:* Palpable, smooth, not enlarged *ROM:* Full, intact, strong *Trachea:* Midline, nontender
Lymph nodes *Supraclavicular:* Nonpalpable *Inguinal:* Nonpalpable *Cervical:* Nonpalpable *Axillary:* Nonpalpable	**Breasts:** Soft, nonpendulous, ō venous pattern; ō dimpling, puckering *Nipples:* ō inversion, point in same direction, areola dark and sizes sym., no discharge, no masses, nontender **Axilla:** Hair present, shaved, no lesions, nontender
Lungs: No increase in A-P diameter, resp rate 18, reg rhythm, no ↑ in tactile fremitus, no tenderness, lungs resonant throughout, diaphragmatic excursion 4 cm, lung fields clear throughout	**Heart:** Rate 82, reg rate and rhythm; no lifts or heaves *PMI:* c̄in MCL 5th ICS, L nonpalpable, nonpalpable thrills S_1, S_2 louder and softer in appropriate locations; no S_3, S_4, no murmurs, rubs, clicks *Carotid—femoral—pedis—radial:* all present equal and strong bilaterally
Abdomen: No pulsations visible, rounded; bowel sounds present and active; no bruits ō CVA tenderness **Liver:** Edge palpable, smooth, nontender, approx. 9 cm in size **Masses:** None palpable **Spleen:** Nonpalpable, nontender, no inguinal hernia palpable	**Female genitals** *External genitalia:* B. U. S. (glands) no swelling, redness, or tenderness; normal hair distribution, no cysts or rectocele *Vagina:* No lesions or discharge; pink *Cervix:* Os closed, no lesions or erosions, nontender *Uterus:* Small, firm, nontender, pink *Adnexa:* No enlargement, nontender *Rectovaginal:* Sphincter intact, confirms findings above
Neuro Cranial nerves I–XII intact Motor (drift, toe stand) intact Coord (FN, Romberg) intact Reflexes—see diagram Sensation (touch, vibration, prop) intact 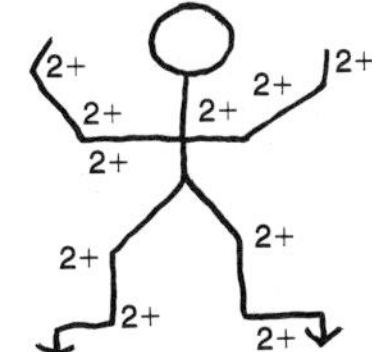 	**Male genitals** Normal male hair distribution *Penis:* Urethral opening patent; no redness, swelling, or discharge; no lesions or structural alterations *Scrotum:* Testes descended; no redness, masses, or tenderness *Rectal:* No lesions, redness; sphincter intact; prostate small, nontender
Psych.: Affect appropriate, eye contact *Orientation:* Oriented ×3—time, place, person *Mood:* Pleasant, appropriate *Thought content:* Intelligent, coherent *Memory:* Remote and recent intact *Serial sevens:* Not done or intact	**Musculoskeletal:** Well-developed, no muscle wasting; ō crepitus, nodules, or swelling *ROM:* Full, intact head to toe, no scoliosis *Strength:* Equal, strong bilaterally *Gait:* Walks erect 2′ steps, arms swinging @ side ō staggering

See problem list for summary of problems

____

Signature

PROBLEM IDENTIFICATION

Upon completion of the health history and physical examination, the nurse is ready to develop a problem list. Problems can be actual (currently present), potential (high probability of occurrence), or resolved (no longer needing intervention). Examples of actual problems include deviations from expected norms such as high blood pressure, diarrhea, shortness of breath, and depression.

Potential problems are problems which the nurse recognizes as high-risk areas for a client based on the assessment data. Such problems might include irregular practice of breast self-exam, family history of hypertension, unwilling to receive blood transfusion, or unable to pay for prophylactic dental care.

Resolved problems are problems which neither the client nor the nurse anticipate will need current intervention but which required intervention in the past. Examples of resolved problems include properly healed fractures, acute illnesses such as pneumonia, and many elective and emergency surgeries such as rhinoplasty and appendectomy. Following the identification of problems, the nurse is ready to proceed to the planning phase of the nursing process.

REVIEW QUESTIONS

The number of the question corresponds to the same numbered objective at the beginning of the chapter.

1. The health history is considered to be part of the
a. objective data
b. subjective data
c. general survey

2. Examination of the body through the use of touch is called
a. inspection
b. palpation
c. percussion
d. auscultation

3. The proper length for a stethoscope is
a. 10 inches
b. 15 inches
c. 20 inches
d. 25 inches

4. A branching examination is an examination of
a. a region of the body
b. the four extremities
c. mental status
d. a system of the body

5. In performing a screening history and physical, the first data to record is the
a. health history
b. problem list
c. general survey
d. physical examination

6. A general survey statement is recorded
a. after the physical examination
b. after the mental status examination
c. following collection of demographic data
d. before the physical examination

REFERENCES

1. E. T. Eggland, "How to Take a Meaningful Nursing History," *Nursing 77*, **7:**(7):28 (1977).
2. E. Baer, M.N. McGowan, and D.O. McGivern, "How to Take a Health History," *Nursing*, **77:**(7):1172 (1977).
3. Ibid., p. 1192.
4. Ibid.
5. J. M. Sana and R. Judge, *Physical Appraisal Methods in Nursing Practice*, Little, Brown and Company, Boston, 1975, p. 17.

Chapter 4

GENERAL CONCEPTS

Adult Development and the Impact of Disruption

Charlotte R. Abbink

Learning Objectives

1. Explain the major concepts in the adult developmental theories proposed by Erikson, Peck, Havighurst, and Levinson.
2. Contrast the Disengagement, Activity, and Identity Continuity psychosocial aging theories.
3. Describe the major psychodynamic concerns of young, middle, and elderly adults in terms of self-concept, intellectual processes, and sexuality.
4. List the major family developmental tasks for young, middle, and elderly adults.
5. Compare the community activities of young, middle, and elderly adults in terms of work, leisure, and civic participation.
6. Describe important health maintenance concerns for young, middle, and elderly adults related to changes due to the process of aging.
7. Describe the impact of illness on young, middle, and elderly adults related to their developmental status.

WHY CONSIDER DEVELOPMENTAL STAGES?

What picture flashes through your mind's eye when you read the words "developmental stages"? For many nurses and nursing students, the first, and sometimes only, mental picture is of children. However, we know that the entire human life span is a dynamic sequence of biological, psychological, and social changes which occur in predictable patterns. Adulthood, like childhood, can be divided into developmental stages, although adult stages have not been as comprehensively articulated as childhood stages.

The following discussion of adulthood will describe predictable patterns in adult growth and development. Understanding these patterns gives the nurse insight into what may be happening in a client's life at given points in the life cycle. Assessing growth and developmental status is just as crucial in planning appropriate nursing care for an adult as it is for a child. Nursing care is superficial and incomplete if it separates the experiences of illness from what the client is experiencing in all other areas of life. Although there are predictable developmental patterns, caution must be used in imposing these patterns upon a specific client before first validating the unique developmental processes this client is experiencing. For example, the nurse cannot determine that an unmarried young adult is not mastering the intimacy tasks until a complete developmental assessment is made and validated.

This chapter was reviewed by Joan B. Enggaard, B.S.N., M.S.N., Professor, College of Lake County, Grayslake, Illinois.

CONCEPTUAL APPROACHES TO ADULT DEVELOPMENT

Theorists have proposed models for understanding adult development based on the premises that:

1. Adult development continues to occur in definable, predictable, and sequential patterns.
2. Critical periods occur throughout the life span when one's physical and psychosocial growth undergo reorganization.
3. Within each stage of development, there are certain normative activities or tasks to be accomplished.
4. Mastering the tasks of preceding stages is foundational to transition and mastery of tasks in future stages.

The adult development models of Erikson, Peck, Levinson, and Havighurst all use this stage approach. Table 4-1 summarizes the adult developmental stages according to each of these theorists.

Erikson's Theory: Psychosocial Developmental Conflicts

Erikson[1] views personality development as resulting from the confrontations between one's ego and his social milieu. He identifies points in the life cycle where specific developmental conflicts become paramount because a person's capacities or experiences dictate that he must make a major adjustment to himself and his environment. In the process of making

Table 4-1
Adult Developmental Stage Theories

Theorist	Young Adulthood	Middle Adulthood	Elderly Adult
Erikson	Intimacy vs. isolation	Generativity vs. self-absorption	Ego-integrity vs. despair
Peck		Valuing wisdom vs. physical power Socializing vs. sexualizing relationships Emotional flexibility vs. emotional impoverishment Mental flexibility vs. mental rigidity	Ego differentiation vs. work role preoccupation Body transcendence vs. body preoccupation Ego transcendence vs. ego preoccupation
Havighurst	Mate selection and marriage adjustments Establishing family and child rearing Home management Occupation launching Beginning civic responsibility	Launching teenage children Maturing relationship with spouse Adjusting to aging parents Career/occupational maturity Adult social and civic responsibility Developing leisure activities Adjusting to physiologic changes	Adjusting to health decline Adjusting to retirement Adjusting to social role changes Establishing satisfactory living arrangements Adjusting to death of spouse
Levinson	Early Adult Transition Getting Into the Adult World 30s Transition Settling Down	Mid-life Transition Payoff years	

this adjustment, the individual moves toward one of two opposing positions, such as toward intimacy or toward isolation. When a person successfully masters a core conflict (such as intimacy) the negative sense (isolation) remains as a dynamic counterpart and may be demonstrated in new situations where this conflict needs to be mastered again at a higher level. Although there are critical times for mastery of each core conflict, all conflicts are present throughout the life span. For example, autonomy is especially important to a toddler; however, adolescents striving for identity need some independent space; and the elderly frequently suffer loss of autonomy when limitations are placed on their decision-making prerogatives.

Intimacy vs. isolation

In Erikson's model, the young adult task is *intimacy* (Fig. 4-1). This involves fusing self-identity with the identities of others in friendships, for causes or creative efforts, or in close personal relationships, including sexual union. Intimacy requires a degree of commitment which necessitates sacrifice, compromise, and self-abandonment for the benefit of others. If the young adult avoids making this type of commitment because of the fear of loss of identity, he will experience a sense of isolation and, consequently, self-absorption.

Generativity vs. stagnation

During middle adulthood, the primary task is *generativity*. The generative adult is concerned with establishing the next generation by nurturing and guiding either one's own children or other young people. A sense of productivity in the individual's work and creativity in living are also important components of this task. This core conflict probably arises out of an altruistic need to leave some mark which will make the world a better place in which to live. If generativity does not occur, the adult experiences a sense of *stagnation,* and turns inward, becoming self-preoccupied and overly concerned with physical and psychological health needs. The self-absorbed person's focus on middle-aged changes may result in his resorting either to invalidism or to inappropriate youthfulness in an attempt to stay young. There may be regression to an obsessive need for pseudointimacy, which may be expressed through affairs with younger members of the opposite sex.

Ego integrity vs. despair

Old age is a time for reviewing the past and rearranging the "photo album of life." This bringing together of all the previous life stages should result in a sense of wholeness, purpose, and a life well lived, or a sense of *ego integrity*, according to Erikson. As the individual reviews his history, he should accept and approve of his unique life. If a sense of *despair* arises, he only sees opportunities missed or wrong directions taken. He may wish to have the chance to correct failures, but knows the time is too short to start over. To the despairing, death is faced with fear because it robs him of the chance to make changes, whereas the ego-integrated individual accepts death as a meaningful stage of life. In this last stage of ego-integrity versus despair, each person must face his own adjustments and come to a final conflict resolution that is the product of all previous developmental conflict resolutions.

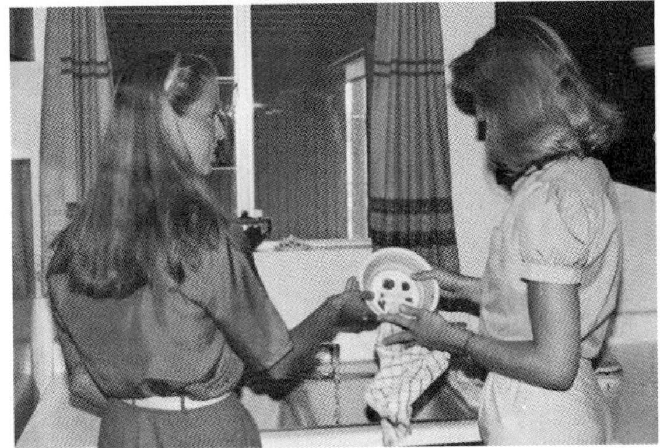

Figure 4-1 The sharing of everyday tasks by roommates can be an expression of intimacy for young adults.

Peck's Theory: Developmental Tasks

Building on Erikson's work, Robert Peck[2] has further defined psychosocial tasks of middle and old age.

Middle-adult tasks

Peck has identified four tasks relevant to middle adulthood. The first two tasks, *valuing wisdom versus physical power*, and *socializing versus sexualizing relationships*, reflect biological changes of middle age. With a general decline in physical and sexual functioning, the middle-aged adult's self-esteem can suffer if it is heavily based on these attributes. However, with experience, judgmental abilities tend to increase, so that valuing the use of one's "head" becomes a positive alternative for maintaining esteem. The progression to a socializing relationship is appropriate as sexual motivations decline. This allows a love relationship to focus on total personalities and companionship rather than sexual performance.

Tasks three and four, *emotional flexibility versus emotional impoverishment*, and *mental flexibility versus mental rigidity*, arise from the need for adjusting to life changes and new events which occur in the middle years. When children leave home, parents die, jobs change, and friends die or move away, the adult must be flexible enough to shift attachments and reinvest emotions in other people and pursuits. One also needs the mental flexibility to allow for new solutions to life problems, rather than being dogmatic and governed by past experiences or judgments.

Older-adult tasks

Peck delineated three tasks for old age. The first, *ego-differentiation versus work preoccupation*, is important for maintaining a sense of self-esteem after retirement. This is achieved by reassigning the value of the work role to other roles and dimensions of life. The task of *body transcendence versus body preoccupation* involves recognizing physical decline, but rising above aches and pains, so that happiness is not defined by physical well-being. This task is exemplified by the person who experiences suffering but retains a zest and pleasure in life. The final task of old age, *ego-transcendence versus ego-preoccupation*, is very similar to Erikson's ego-integrity task. It denotes an ability to accept one's personal death without fear. It is neither a denial nor passive resignation to death, but an acceptance which moves the individual to be actively and emotionally involved in a legacy that lives on. In contrast, the ego-preoccupied individual mires in the thought of personal death, being unable to let go of life and immediate gratification.

Havighurst's Theory: Developmental Tasks

Havighurst[3] has also proposed specific developmental tasks for each life stage. (See Table 4-1 for the list of tasks. The listed order does not imply hierarchical arrangement.) Like Erikson, he contends that there are optimal points in life to master these tasks, and that current mastery is contingent upon having successfully mastered the tasks of previous life stages. Unlike Erikson and Peck, who focused on individual developmental tasks, Havighurst also included family-oriented tasks which are significant to individual development.

Levinson's Theory: Evolution of Life Structures

Levinson's[4] basic concept, *individual life structure*, is the pattern of a given life at any point in time. Life structure is formed by the interactions of the individual's self-system (judgments, motives, values,

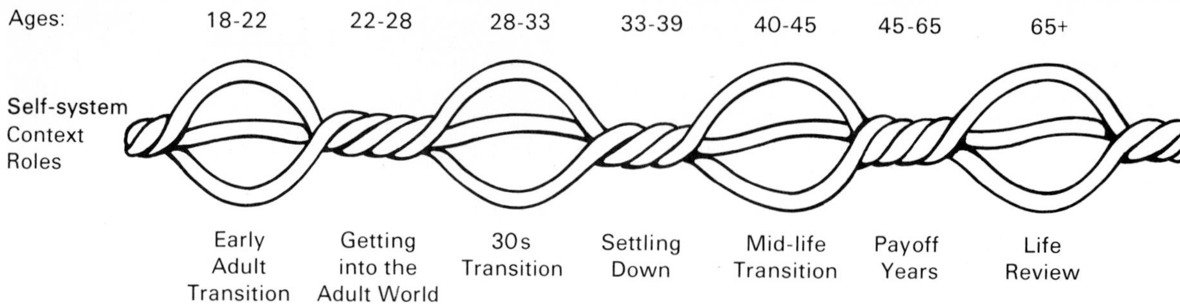

Figure 4-2 An individual's life structure. An individual is continually in the process of building and rebuilding his or her life structure, according to Levinson's theory. This may be seen as a "life rope" in which the interacting strands are taken apart during transition periods and rewoven in stable periods.

etc.), the social and cultural context of one's life (family, ethnicity, religion, occupation, social events such as war or inflation), and the particular set of roles in which he participates (husband/wife, worker, friend, etc.). When any of these components change, the life structure must reorganize (Fig. 4-2). Levinson considers some aspects of life structure, such as family and occupation as central, because they hold great significance to the individual; whereas other aspects are peripheral because they are less critical and more fluid.

Life structure is dynamic, with predictable changes occurring as the individual moves through life. There are four major periods in adult life, early adulthood from approximately age 20 to 40; middle adulthood, age 40 to 60; late adulthood, age 60 to 80; and late-late adulthood, beyond 80. Within each period, the individual experiences alternating times of transition and stability in life structure. *Transitions* are a time of evaluating and making changes which permit growth and redirection of life toward identified goals and values. *Stable times* are those times for building on changes while maintaining an intact life structure, in order to focus on the goals and values of that life period.

Early adult transition

The first transition is the *Early Adult Transition*, which occurs between the ages of 18 to 22. The major concerns of this time are to terminate or modify existing life structures and to make preliminary adult choices which move one toward new life structures that consolidate an initial adult identity. This transition includes breaking away from the family of origin, making an initial career choice, establishing new intimate relationships, and selecting personal goals, values, and lifestyle (Fig. 4-3).

Entering the adult world: The first stable period

From ages 22 to 28, the young adult is *Entering the Adult World*. This is a time for building on the tentative adult choices which were made during the previous transition. Concurrently, the young adult is

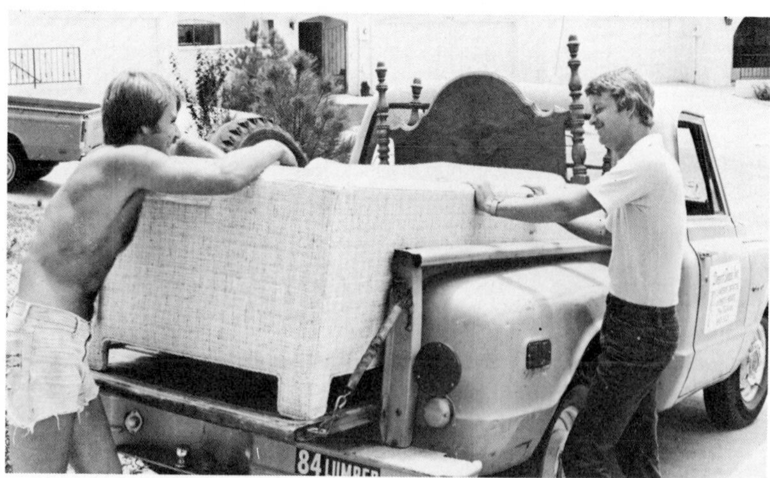

Figure 4-3 The move from home to an apartment is an external sign of early adult transition.

working out a balance between building on these choices and exploring alternative opportunities, so as to avoid cementing the future prematurely. Because of this exploring, there may be a transient quality to the occupational choices and relationships which are being established at this time.

The 30s transition

Another transition is experienced between ages 28 to 33. This may bring modifications and enrichment of the life built in the 20s, or it may be a time of dramatic change, depending on whether the individual reaffirms or discards previous commitments made to career, mate, values, goals, and friends. Single persons may consider marriage, unhappy marriages may terminate, childless couples may conceive or adopt, and careers may be left or reconfirmed with new vigor.

Settling down: A calm before the storm

During the 30s, there is a calm period referred to as *Settling Down*. This is a time of investing oneself into those areas of life which are of primary importance, be they family, work, friends, or community. It is now important to believe that one is establishing a place in society as a full-fledged adult, and that one can advance and attain whatever goals have been set. There is a striving toward exerting authority, and gaining status and recognition with respect and reward from others.

Mid-life transition

The *Mid-Life Transition*, from roughly 40 to 45, is the gateway into middle adulthood. This usually involves a profound reappraisal of life goals and values, with a concurrent emotional upheaval. Self-identity and authenticity are questioned and stripped of the illusions of young adulthood. All life structures are renegotiated, including marriage, friendships, occupation, and social roles. There is a realignment of time to the perspective of time left to live. For some individuals, this transition results in a continuance of the previous lifestyle, but with new confirmation and enthusiasm for the current life structure. For others, there are varying degrees of change and reorganization of life structures. For instance, a person may return to school to complete previously aborted educational plans.

The payoff years

As the middle adult emerges from the transitional stage, having reorganized or reaffirmed the direction of life, he enters into a time which may be very satisfying and creative. Ages 45 to 65 become the *Payoff Years* when one experiences a time of maximum influence, heightened self-perception, self-approval, and self-direction. Middle adults can demonstrate wisdom and sound judgment as well as vision and innovation. Levinson projects that beyond middle age there is a continued growth process which involves transition and stability and is based on previous life structures.

Psychosocial Aging Theories

Because developmental theories are least explicit about the later years of life, other theoretical approaches have been taken to explain the processes of aging. The *Disengagement Theory*[5] proposes that successful psychosocial aging is characterized by a reciprocal decline in the involvement of the individual with society, and society with the individual. The criticism of this theory has focused on the proposition that disengagement is intrinsic, and therefore a norm for successful aging. Disengagement will vary in old people, depending on factors such as health, abilities, previous lifestyle, and personality type. Contrasting with disengagement, the *Activity Theory*[6] maintains that continued productivity and social interaction are necessary for successful aging. Although forms of activity may need to change due to reductions in physical health and strength, the level of activity with society should be commensurate with lifelong patterns. The aging person, to remain engaged, will compensate for lost roles and activities by replacing them with new ones. The *Identity Continuity Theory*[7] assumes that adaptation to aging is correlated with the ability to maintain the same behavior patterns and lifestyle which existed prior to old age. This continuity is maintained by selectively attending to those things that fit previously established behavioral patterns. However, in our change-oriented society, it becomes increasingly difficult to maintain such consistencies in lifestyle.

PSYCHODYNAMIC ISSUES OF ADULTHOOD

Psychodynamic issues arise from confrontation between one's inner development and the demands of the social world. We continually try to find a comfortable fit between ourselves and our world, attempting to integrate our sense of who we are, and who we are becoming.

Self-Concept Throughout Adulthood

Self-concept and self-esteem are interdependent constructs. *Self-concept* may be defined as the totality of ideas one holds about oneself, and *self-esteem* is one's evaluation, that is, satisfaction or dissatisfaction with these ideas.

Young adult

During the young adult years, a strong theme in self-concept is "I can handle it." There is a sense of mastery and self-control over life events and the environment. The actions of young adults convey the attitude that self-will and boldness are the components of success. This confidence is a reflection of the high energy levels and the increasing power and control a young adult experiences over life, when moving out of adolescence.

Middle adult

During the middle-adult years, self-concept may vary greatly, depending on the perceived balance between positive and negative aspects of middle age. This perception is partially determined by culture, social class, personality, and health status. In some cultures, one is preprogrammed to consider oneself "old" at 40, whereas in others you have just "made it" at 40. It has been found that working-class men may consider themselves old at 40, whereas professionals perceive "old" as after 70. Some middle-agers have the time of their life, with an increased sense of self-approval because of peak family and career investments in terms of power, prestige, and income, and continued good health. On the other hand, if one experiences a decline in career or health, self-esteem may also decline.

The sense of self-control continues into middle age; however, during middle adulthood, one recognizes the finiteness of life and shifts to a more realistic appraisal of the limits of self-will. Recognizing that will-power alone does not overcome life circumstances, the individual becomes aware that help and advice from others can be valuable rather than allowing it to threaten his self-esteem. With this new insight regarding self-will, the middle-aged adult may also reevaluate his spiritual position. He may determine that placing trust in God is not a crutch for the weak personality, but a desire for living beyond his human finiteness (Fig. 4-4).

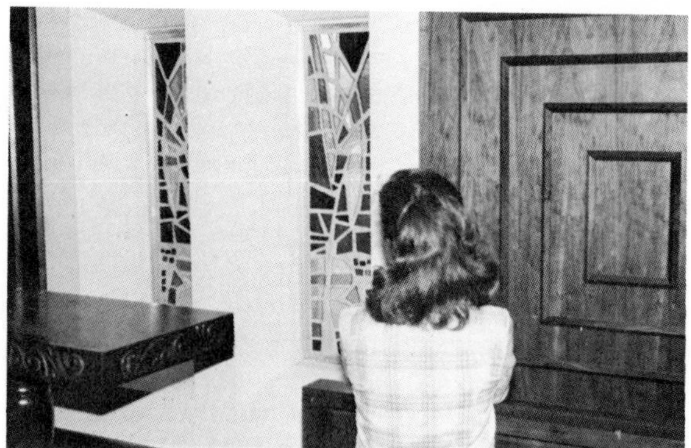

Figure 4-4 An increasing awareness of spiritual needs often occurs in the middle years.

Elderly adult

Although it is likely that self-concept is stable from middle age to old age, it is not static. Life events experienced with aging (poor health, loss of income, loss of roles, isolation, relocation, and institutionalization) all serve to decrease the elderly person's sense of control, and in turn may threaten self-esteem. However, it has been found that old people have compensatory mechanisms to offset some threats brought on by aging changes. A paradox exists in that age perception decreases with age. The elderly person may think of other cohorts as being "old" according to social stereotypes attributed to old people, but may not perceive oneself as old, and refuse to respond to others' suggestions that he is aging or needs help or care. Another compensatory mechanism is that many elderly retain their middle-age self-concepts by thinking of themselves in their former roles. A retired farmer still thinks of himself as a farmer, or a school teacher as a teacher. Being able to maintain a consistent sense of self, making decisions, and managing one's own life are clearly important to well-being at this stage of life. Autonomy and dignity are essential elements to an elderly person's positive self-esteem.

Mental Functioning: Intelligence and Memory

Intelligence

Traditionally it has been held that intelligence declines after age 30. However, recent longitudinal data indicate a gradual improvement in general intelligence until approximately age 50, and then stability until shortly before death.[8] In the months prior to death, an elderly person's intellectual abilities decrease sharply. This change is part of a complex phenomenon called *terminal decline*.

The patterns of change in adult intelligence vary with the specific mental abilities being measured. *Fluid intelligence* consists of those abilities which are related to neurologic development, and includes associative power, memory, figural relationships, and visual-motor flexibility. Because of degenerative neurologic changes, fluid intelligence may decline during middle age. *Crystallized intelligence* consists of those abilities which arise out of experience and the accumulation of learning, and includes verbal comprehension, formal reasoning, and general information. Crystallized intelligence improves with age.

A variety of environmental and individual variables such as education, social class, illness, personality, and motivation affect adult intelligence. Generally, individuals who have had above-average IQs as young adults, who have obtained more years of formal education, and have continued to use intellectual processes, demonstrate greater increases in intelligence throughout adulthood.[9]

It is very important for nurses to recognize that a major problem in mental functioning for older adults is the matter of speed. Because of central nervous system decline and sensory deficits such as poor eyesight, some older persons have trouble with quick thinking and performance (Fig. 4-5). It has been demonstrated that old people perform equally as well as young people when time is not a factor. Because of this, any teaching or skills practice should be carefully planned to allow the older client adequate time for comprehension and performance without the pressure of hurrying.

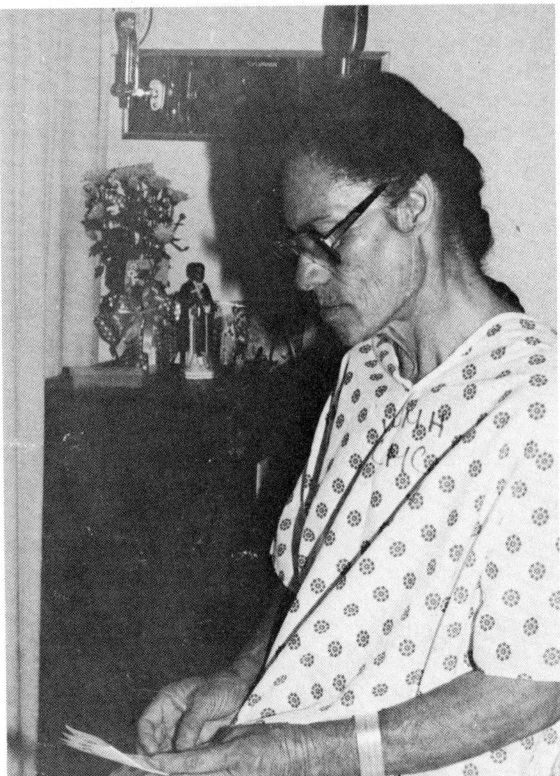

Figure 4-5 This client is compensating for failing vision and decreased speed of mental processes by the use of eyeglasses and solitary reading.

Memory

Although many middle adults fear becoming forgetful, no real decline in memory has been demonstrated until old age. *Short-term memory* deteriorates first. This refers to immediate recall which requires information retention for a few seconds to a few minutes. An example is remembering how to dial an unfamiliar phone number after having read it in the phone book. The decline in short-term memory may be related to neurotransmission interference or temporary storage integration problems. Because neurotransmission is slower, the elderly become vulnerable to interference from other stimuli, which impede acquisition and storage of information. Thus, information cannot be retrieved later because it was inadequately registered. This short-term memory problem can have significant effects on the learning process, because learning new material often requires speed in acquisition, comprehension, and registration.

Long-term memory seems quite resistant to aging. It is often noted that elderly persons can describe in minute detail past life events yet forget recent ones. This recall ability for past events may be attributed to the fact that once information is registered, people retain a sound memory for it. It is also likely that the memory for past events is firmly consolidated because the details have been previously recalled and rehearsed by the person.

Another memory difficulty in the elderly is the inability to recall specifics after recognizing a person or a place. For example, an elderly grandmother may recognize her grandchild, but call him by another family member's name. In this case, she has placed the child in the family, recognizing the person, but cannot recall the name. This problem seems to be in the retrieval process rather than in registration of information.

In addition to aging changes, the memory of an elderly adult is affected by health status, drugs, education, amount of stimulation, motivation, and the meaningfulness of the material. (See Table 4-2 for a summary of the effects of aging on mental functioning.)

Sexuality in Adulthood

Sexuality is a broad concept which incorporates physiologic characteristics, attitudes, values, and behaviors related to gender perceptions. The task of developing a compatibility between gender identity and one's expressions of sex-related roles is vital to self-concept integration during adulthood. This is an ongoing task which pervades practically all aspects of

Table 4-2
The Effects of Aging on Adult Mental Functioning

Function	Effect of Aging
1. Fluid intelligence	1. Declines during middle age
2. Crystallized intelligence	2. Improves
3. Vocabulary/verbal reasoning	3. Improves
4. Spatial perception	4. Constant or improves
5. Synthesis of new information	5. Declines during middle age
6. Mental performance speed	6. Declines during middle age
7. Short-term recall memory	7. Declines during old age
8. Long-term recall memory	8. Constant

adult life, including mate selection, career choices, friendships, and all forms of self-expression.

Young adult

For the young adult, gender identity and sexual relationships are primary concerns in achieving a sexual self-concept and sense of intimacy. Although intimacy transcends a sexual relationship to include affiliative sharing, for the sexually active young adult intimacy is usually established by commitment to a relationship which includes an expression of affection and physical sexuality. Sexual performance in a marriage relationship represents more than physical pleasure. It becomes an expression of caring and closeness, which helps the couple find satisfaction in sharing their work, play, childbearing, and child-rearing activities. It has been found that couples who are satisfied with their sexual relationship are most often satisfied with the overall marriage and vice versa.

Biologically, young adults are reproductively mature and in the prime of physical and reproductive performance. Many of their biosocial concerns center around sexual activity, including cyclic changes in sexual arousal and orgasm, use and selection of contraceptives, sexual changes with pregnancy and postpartum, abortion, infertility, and venereal disease. It has been found that in males, the peak sexual drive and responsiveness occurs during the late teens and early 20s; whereas this peak occurs between 30 to 45 in females. However, most healthy adults maintain a strong sex drive into their 60s and 70s.

Middle adult

During the middle years, both men and women experience hormonal declines which produce physiologic changes that affect sexual desire and responsiveness. However, more important than the physiologic changes are the psychological expectations related to these changes. It has been found that menopausal and postmenopausal women have fewer fears and negative feelings about the effects of menopause on their sexuality than do young adult women. Rather than experiencing a decline in sexual capacity, postmenopausal women frequently experience an increased libido and greater enjoyment. With the male climacteric, the decline in testosterone may result in a decreased libido and a slower sexual arousal and climax, but these changes do not necessarily lessen the pleasure in sexual intercourse.

Factors probably more important than hormonal changes which negatively affect sexual activity in the middle years include monotony in a repetitious sexual pattern, boredom with a relationship, career and economic preoccupation, mental and physical fatigue, excessive eating or drinking, fear of sexual failure, and becoming victim to the myth that a youthful body is equated with sexual desirability and potency. Middle-aged adults are also at risk for the potential onset of chronic illnesses, which could affect libido. Also, they may be taking a variety of prescribed drugs, which can reduce sexual responsiveness. Sexual activity continues to be a very important part of middle-adult life. Satisfaction with their sexual life is not so much related to frequency of intercourse as to vitality in the relationship and enjoyment derived from sexual experiences in younger years.

Elderly adult

Although our society attributes sexlessness to the elderly, people are sexual beings throughout their lives. Most studies attest to continued sexual activity well into the last decades of life for both men and women who have been sexually active as young and middle adults. Physical changes in the sexual organs should not be considered as biological limiters of sexual activity, nor should they reduce the satisfaction experienced by sexual partners. The most important criteria for remaining sexually active in old age are a receptive partner, reasonable physical health, and a positive attitude about regular sexual activity.

Because our society has been slow to recognize the sexual needs of the elderly, and most elderly have been socialized to not talk about sex, it becomes difficult for health care givers to identify and to intervene on sex-related problems. It has been suggested that sex education programs be developed for old people in order to inform them of normal changes and to help them cope with unmet sexual needs and social and familial attitudes about continued sexual activity.

Intimacy

In a broad context, *intimacy* incorporates the concept of attachment or seeking a relationship in which one can maintain contact or proximity to the object of attachment. From this perspective, intimacy is a need which is manifest from conception to death, and does not decrease in intensity or significance throughout adulthood. Intimacy is maintained *physically* by touching, stroking, patting, hugging, kissing, and sometimes through sexual intercourse; and *emotionally* by sharing joys, sorrows, affection, ideas, and values.

Throughout life touch plays an important role in receiving and expressing intimacy. However, as hearing and sight decline with age, reaching out to touch becomes an even more important way to make intimate physical contact. Old people often attempt to touch and be touched by others to experience some sense of physical closeness. The response to their touch communicates a message of acceptance or nonacceptance which might never have been expressed verbally.

The need for expressing physical intimacy in ways which have a sexual connotation is often disregarded for the elderly. Although these expressions are accepted as normal in younger adults, they may be viewed with disdain, disapproval, or as an amusing and childish behavior when expressed by old people. This disregard is seen in some institutional structures and policies. Many nursing homes provide little opportunity for expression of sexual needs. Private rooms and locked doors often are neither provided nor respected. Elderly couples may be segregated and placed on separate men's and women's units, or, if in the same room, may have single beds. Is it any wonder that an elderly person, who has for years shared a bed with a spouse, now becomes disoriented at night and wanders around or gets into bed with someone else? Our youth-oriented society has developed skewed ideas about appropriate sexual behavior in the elderly, and as a result has placed severe restrictions on intimate relationships during old age.

SOCIAL PROCESSES IN ADULTHOOD

Adulthood is lived out in a social context, with major developmental tasks being determined by the interaction of individuals with their social systems. Adult social concerns primarily involve family life, work and leisure, and community responsibilities.

The Family and Adult Development

Frequently the family is studied from the perspective of the child and his or her socialization. However, it is important to recognize that the family remains a major socializing agent for adults. The family is a focal source for adults in meeting their needs for emotional security, belonging, love, companionship, esteem, and approval from others. The process of family development reflects the developmental changes occurring in the adult members. (See Table 4-3 for a summary of family tasks during adulthood.)

Young adulthood

Emancipation from the family of origin is the first family task of young adulthood. This usually occurs as a gradual process which includes physical, economic, and emotional independence from one's parents. However, emancipation is not the end of a relationship with one's family, but rather the first step to establish-

Table 4-3
Family Tasks in Adult Development

Young Adulthood	Middle Adulthood	Elderly Adulthood
1. Emancipation from family of origin	1. Assisting teenage children to become responsible adults	1. Establishing satisfactory living arrangements with a limited income
2. Establishment of an interdependent adult relationship with one's parents	2. Restructuring the relationship with one's spouse as children leave home	2. Restructuring family roles and responsibilities following retirement
3. Selecting a mate and adjusting to an intimate relationship	3. Restructuring the relationship with aging parents	3. Adapting living arrangements to meet problems caused by physical decline
4. Adapting the family system to the demands of childbearing	4. Adjusting to death of parents	4. Adjusting to death of a spouse
5. Finding a balance to family, work, and social demands	5. Defining the roles and responsibilities of a grandparent	

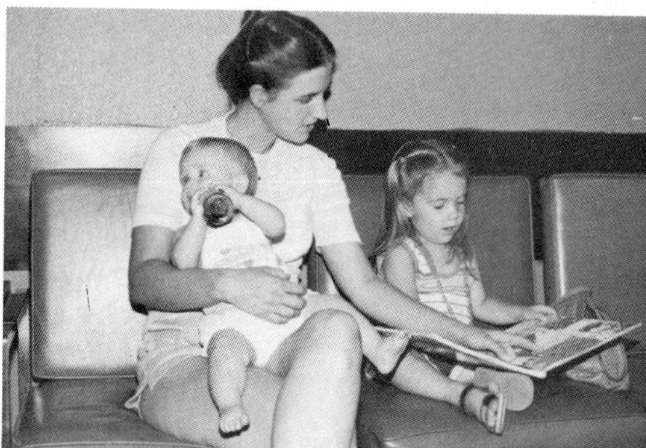

Figure 4-6 This young mother is communicating with her children through touch, reading, and sharing.

ing an interdependent adult relationship between the young adult and his parents.

Often concurrent with emancipation from the family of origin, the young adult is setting up a new family system in which roles, relationships, and expectations are being worked out. This usually includes adjusting to an intimate relationship requiring a high level of communication and compromise, and adapting to the predictable crises of childbearing (Fig. 4-6). Stress is frequently high in the emerging young adult family, because of the multiplicity of changing relationships and structures. Also, it is most often during this time that the work trajectory is launched, therefore placing new outside demands on the adult family members. Because of these changes, the emerging family may easily become dysfunctional. This is reflected in the fact that the highest divorce rate occurs during the first 3 to 5 years of marriage, involving young adults under age 30.

Following the initial family transition, young adults move into a more stable, comfortable family life period. Commitment to the success of the family is high and there is less turmoil with children, who are usually now in middle childhood. Couples without children also find this to be a time for strengthening relationships with each other and their social group.

Middle adulthood

Middle adults find themselves caught in the "family sandwich" between the needs of their children and their aging parents. Family life can be stressful because it is a complex chore to concurrently be working through one's own mid-life identity transition, the identity confusion of teenagers, and the redefinition of family roles and relationships in both the families of origin and procreation.

Disenchantment with the marital relationship is frequently experienced by middle-aged adults. Research has demonstrated that married couples are least satisfied with each other during the decade of the 40s. There are multiple contributing factors to this dissatisfaction. The husband may be preoccupied or confused about his occupational goals and blame his wife for his dissatisfaction with accusations that she has held him back or has not kept up with him intellectually and socially. At the same time, the wife may blame her husband for her lack of goals or skills now that the children are leaving home, believing that her self-development needs were sacrificed for his job and the family. Also, the financial and emotional strain of adolescent children may come between them. Although the divorce rate is not quite as high during middle adulthood as during early young adulthood, it does increase again during the years shortly after children leave home.

Middle-aged couples who recommit themselves to their spouses and a continuing marriage find marital satisfaction frequently hits a new high. Although there has been much discussion about the crisis of the "empty nest," many middle-aged men and women experience a new sense of self and unity as a couple after the children leave home. They again define their relationship as lovers and companions, rather than as parents. In many ways, the postparental years become the payoff for investing in a mutual relationship with shared problems and joys, if the couple survives the trials of the mid-life marriage.

During middle age, adults often come to appreciate their parents and understand the problems of old people in a new way. When the aging parent is in good health and basically self-reliant, the parent-child relationship is usually characterized by a friendship which is quite satisfactory to both. If aging parents are confronted with problems such as inadequate finances, ill health, or death of a spouse, making it impossible for them to remain independent, the parent-child relationship and roles may be restructured. A very difficult, and sometimes necessary, role reversal occurs when a middle-aged child must become the parent to his own parent. This requires giving up feelings of dependency on the parent, and often assuming an uncomfortable authority role, which the elderly parent may find difficult to relinquish. The manner in which the middle-aged adult responds to the parent's dependency needs will be determined by the previous relationship, available resources, and the other responsibilities of the middle-aged adult. Eventually, many middle-aged adults must deal with their feelings about the death of parents. Although little has been done to study the family changes at this time, certainly it must be an important phase in family life, when one becomes a member of the family's oldest generation due to death of parents.

Grandparenting Today an increasing number of adults become grandparents during middle adulthood (Fig. 4-7). This new social role may have positive or negative connotations for the grandparent's self-esteem. To some it is met with excitement and anticipation; for others it represents "growing old," which conflicts with how the grandparent wants to feel about himself.

Elder adulthood

The onset of this final period in family life is generally considered to be marked by retirement and poses new and unique developmental tasks for the aging family. The first task is to establish satisfactory living arrangements within a limited income, considering the role changes brought on by retirement and the physical incapacities of aging. In terms of living arrangements, most elderly adults live in their own households[10] (see Table 4-4). For the elderly who are in relatively good health and have an adequate income, living in their own homes, rather than with family members, allows them to maintain a sense of privacy, competency, and independence. The fact that now fewer old people live with their children than before should not be interpreted to mean that adult children have abandoned or neglected their aging parents. There is ample research evidence to demonstrate that family ties remain strong and contact is frequent.

Being able to adjust family responsibilities and routines becomes an important part of the adaptation a couple must make following retirement. Not only are schedules and activities readjusted, but frequently a retiree will turn to family members for meeting his self-esteem needs, which were previously met by the referent work group.

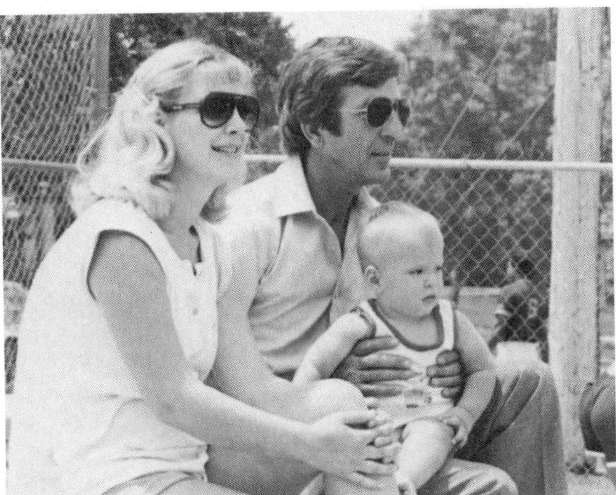

Figure 4-7 The active grandparent plays a positive role in the lives of both child and grandchild.

Table 4-4
Household Arrangements for Persons Over 65

Living with a spouse*	51%
Living with someone other than a spouse	18%
Living alone	26%
Living in a home or hospital for aged	5%

*80% of all men over 65 lived with a spouse whereas only 35% of all women over 65 were living with a spouse.

Adapted from U.S. Surgeon General's Report, *Healthy People,* Government Printing Office, Washington, D.C., 1979, p. 74.

Widowhood The loss of a spouse is a major crisis at any stage in life. The reaction to a spouse's death may vary, depending on how compatible the relationship was; the circumstances of the death; the available support systems, including family and religious beliefs; the physiologic independence of the survivor; and the adequacy of financial resources. Although the degree of marital happiness varies for old people, in general couples who have had a long marriage have established an interdependent symbiotic relationship that gives them a great deal of pleasure during their later years.

Developing a new social identity and adjusting living arrangements are major tasks of adjusting to widowhood. For many, widowhood is a time when they are socially marooned, unless they actively seek out activities they can participate in without a spouse. Some elderly people choose to move in with family members; others move to smaller apartments, trailers, or a community for the aged. In any case, relocation may be an additional trauma faced by the widowed.

Remarriage becomes an alternative to living alone, or to living with children or friends. Most elderly widowed remarry for companionship, and although there is the danger of idealizing the deceased mate and making unrealistic comparisons with the new spouse, most of these remarriages are happy.

Singlehood

Single adults include the never married, separated, divorced, and widowed. Singlehood is becoming increasingly common in America, partially because more people are marrying later for the first time and waiting longer to remarry. Factors related to not marrying include personal freedom and self-development; family responsibilities to parents or siblings; ill health, particularly having a genetically transmittable disease; concentration on a career; and simply not finding someone to marry. The healthy elderly single person who has never married or was divorced or widowed early in life usually has found ways to compensate for the lack of a nuclear family. However, problems may arise when the single elderly one becomes ill or frail and cannot care for himself without substantial assistance from those around him. Sometimes the most feasible living arrangement then becomes a nursing home.

Divorce

There are multiple social and individual factors which contribute to family dissolution, so the complexities of divorce will not be discussed here. Divorce is a source of personal crisis for all family members, and as such, affects their physical and mental health status. Developmentally, it requires that a reorientation process be started. Each family member must make adjustments in self-identity and establish new social roles. This process is harder for middle-aged and elderly adults, because life patterns and the incorporation of a spouse into one's own personal identity have become well established.

Community Life in Adulthood

Participating in community life is a major developmental task of adulthood. Personal and family well-being is strongly dependent on successful interactions with the community via work, leisure, and civic participation.

Work and young adulthood

Work provides more than just the financial means to support a standard of living. It becomes a salient feature of one's personal identity and self-concept. Launching a career is the first point in the work cycle and occurs in young adulthood for most men and women. This entry point confronts the young adult with many potentially stressful role adjustments, both on the job and within the family.

Work and the middle-aged career clock

The second major occupational crisis occurs during middle age when one assesses if he is "on time" or "behind time" according to one's personal career clock (Fig. 4-8). With the perspective of time until retirement, occupational goals often need to be revised toward more realistic expectations.

Frequently the middle-aged adult is at the peak of job performance, so work may become the pivot around which all relationships and activities are ordered. Because the job is so central, job stresses and dissatisfaction can have profound effects on physical and mental health. Also, the person who develops health problems which impede ability to work or threaten his career timing will experience less job satisfaction, thus producing a vicious, stressful cycle. Frequently, nurses must help middle-aged clients adjust to job restrictions created by hospitalization and medical regimens.

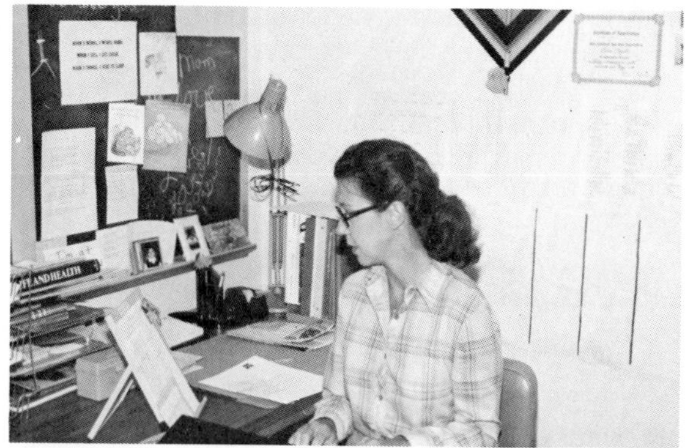

Figure 4-8 The middle-aged woman may experience the same career clock as a man due to economic concerns and greater life choices.

Retirement: Ending the work cycle

Retirement is the third major event in the occupation cycle. The significant issues adults must face with retirement include a lowered income, which can have profound effects on lifestyle; loss of work role and associated relationships, which are part of the individual's personal identity and social status; a readjustment of time and restructuring of daily activities; a change in family roles and arrangements; and the psychological mark of old age, which increases awareness of the aging process. However, with improved retirement benefits and better pension plans, more individuals are choosing to retire early. They view retirement as a reward for past productivity and an opportunity to satisfy previously unmet needs.

It is known that the transition from employed to retired is less stressful when the person has comprehensively planned for retirement. Gerontologic nurses should take significant roles in preparing clients for the predictable stresses that occur with retirement, and thus lessen some of the potential crises of this major life change. Table 4-5 further describes the work cycle.

Leisure During Adulthood

The concept of leisure is becoming more and more important in our society. It is not only of interest to the retiree, but also to young and middle-aged adults, who are experiencing more nonwork time and

Table 4-5
The Work Cycle

Work	Young Adulthood	Middle Adulthood	Elderly Adulthood
Focus	Career launch	Mid-life career crisis	Retirement
Expectations of each stage	Reorganization of time Job role adjustments Family role adjustments	Measuring accomplishments against goals Revising unrealistic career goals with the perspective of time until retirement If desired, changing jobs and/or careers before it is "too late"	Reorganization of time and daily activities Family role adjustments Establishing a referent group other than coworkers
Major Problems	Expectations for job not congruent with reality "Now is the time to make it" attitude with an imbalance between work, family, and personal development needs	A sense of occupational failure and frustration if unable to give up idealistic young adult goals and set realistic current goals Ego deflation with being at the "entry level" of a new career when changing careers at mid-life	Lowered income and standard of living Loss of self-esteem if unable to transfer status from the work role to other roles Psychological mark of old age

need to determine how to spend this in a satisfying manner. In general there is an increase in the amount of available leisure time as one moves from young adulthood to retirement (see Table 4-6). During any life stage, the occupational choice and leisure are interdependent. The job heavily influences the amount of leisure time available, the financial resources, and the physical and mental energy left for leisure activities.

Young adulthood

Young adults often have very busy schedules with little time for leisure. Attempts to balance work, school, family responsibilities and leisure often result in frustration. The forms of leisure they engage in are affected by personal interests and social factors including marriage and parenting roles, new friendships, occupational choices, and financial resources.

Table 4-6
Adult Leisure Time

	Young Adult	Middle Adult	Older Adult
Time factor	Minimal pure leisure time because of holding a second job or going to school and working full time	Increasing amounts of available time as there is usually greater occupational stability and less time spent on child-rearing activities.	May experience too much available time
Cost factor	Financial resources may limit time spent and type of leisure activities engaged in	More money available for leisure because of higher earning power	Reduced and fixed incomes may limit activities Government programs help reduce the cost of leisure activities for retired citizens
General types of leisure	Activities which sustain marital and family closeness such as family outings and home entertainment Activities with other young families Activities with same sex friends such as sports, arts and crafts	Less home-centered activities because of greater freedom; enjoy travel, going out with friends Activities which are less physically demanding and do not require quick reflexes Activities oriented toward health maintenance; swimming, jogging, exercising	Continue with those activities enjoyed during middle-adulthood if health and finances permit Creative arts and crafts and recreational activities such as cards and dancing Activities with family members and friends Volunteer services such as Foster Grandparents

Middle adulthood

The leisure patterns in middle adulthood change slightly from young adulthood because of physical and social changes in this stage of life. The use of leisure time is an important concern for middle-aged adults because they are beginning to prepare for retirement. It is now that they can develop interests which can be continued on into the retirement years and bridge the gap from the working life to full-time leisure. However, reseachers who sampled a population of middle-agers on their attitudes toward leisure time, found that 90 percent of the men and 80 percent of the women would want to continue working, even if they did not need to work, because they were gaining more satisfaction from work than from leisure.[11]

Elderly adults

Elderly adults tend to continue to fill their time with the leisure activities they enjoyed in middle age, as long as their health and finances remain adequate. However, as more elderly people have opportunities to participate in a variety of programs such as those provided by senior centers, they can increase their scope of activities and do the things they have never tried before. Government programs at federal, state, and local levels, as well as private enterprise, have joined to help provide and make leisure activities more accessible to old people. The Older American Act has established funds and programs such as multipurpose senior citizens' centers, which provide a variety of activities including classes, recreational activities, arrangements for discount tickets for entertainment programs and travel, and special education programs.

The elderly use their leisure time not only in self-oriented activities; they also contribute much to society through their volunteer services. Volunteering provides elderly people with an opportunity to share their expertise and to participate in meaningful activities which fill a need in our society.

With continued aging and decline in health, old people may engage in more home-bound solitary activities such as just relaxing in a rocking chair, thinking, daydreaming, people watching, and patting a pet. In general, the leisure activities of the elderly are determined by their health, previous activities, money, and current expectations about what they can do (Fig. 4-9).

Civic Participation

Participation in one's community through civic and governmental organizations, church groups, professional groups, and special interest groups begins in young adulthood, crescendos in middle adulthood, and generally declines during old age. Because young adults are very involved with the commitments of establishing an overall lifestyle, including a family, career, and friendships, their time and energy is limited for consistent participation in community activities.

Although we have a youth-oriented society, the control is held by middle adults. This becomes apparent when one looks at the ages of individuals who are in high decision-making positions at all levels of government and private enterprise. Not only do middle-aged adults participate in more community and professional activities, but they have developed the expertise and leadership qualities to participate at higher organizational levels. The increase in political

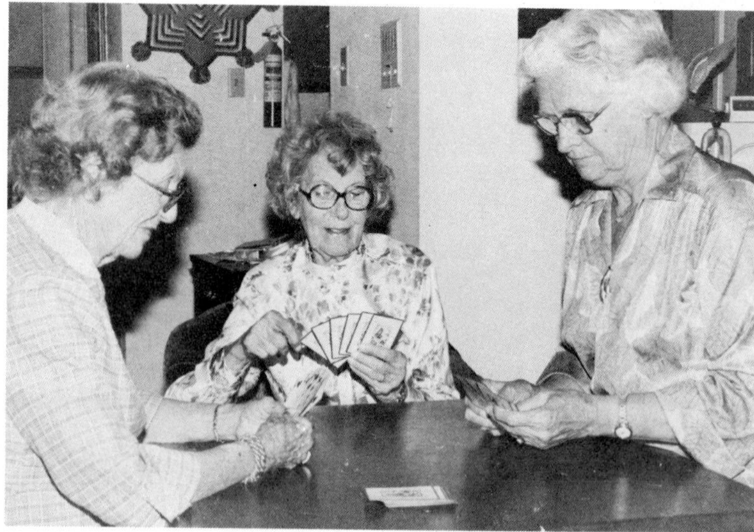

Figure 4-9 Good friends and pleasant activities help fill the lives of active older adults.

Table 4-7
Civic Participation in Adulthood

	Young Adulthood	Middle Adulthood	Elderly Adulthood
Factors encouraging/discouraging involvement	Time and energy for civic involvement is limited due to family and career commitments	Concern for future of society fosters civic participation as a priority	Available time, resources and special interest causes encourage civic participation Declining health reduces ability to participate
Type of participation	Activities perceived as having direct bearing on day-to-day lives, such as labor unions, PTA, church activities Usually participate at the local level	Increased political and professional activity Leadership and decision-making positions at all levels of government and private enterprise	Continue with civic involvements begun during the middle-adult years Retirement community activities Political involvement including political action groups which promote legislation for causes of special interest to the elderly

activism among middle-aged women has become especially prominent because of their successful election attempts. In general, middle-aged men and women are at the peak of their influence and responsibility for the affairs of our society in local, national, and international arenas.

Old people who have been active in their communities will probably remain active as long as their health and income permit. With the growing population of elderly, a new community focus has arisen; the retirement community. The elderly who live in these communities become very involved with all aspects of their community's life. Elderly people also remain politically active and organize for their own causes. Approximately 6 million elderly belong to local, state, and national political action groups for the elderly, such as the American Association of Retired Persons, National Council of Senior Citizens, and the Gray Panthers.[12] Most politicians recognize the political clout of the elderly as a group because of their organizations and the fact that the elderly do get out and vote. Table 4-7 further describes civic activities.

PHYSIOLOGIC PROCESSES IN ADULTHOOD

Having a healthy body is truly an asset and can be a major factor in the positive or negative feelings one has about himself.

Physiologic Changes During Adulthood

The *young adult* body is generally at its peak of health and performance. Although physical changes associated with aging are beginning at this time, the effects are not yet great enough to require attention. Extrinsic factors such as accidents and physical stressors such as lack of sleep and substance abuse are the most common source of disabling biophysical problems in young adults.

Structural and functional body changes which were unnoticed in young adulthood may begin to be apparent during *middle age*. One must remember that the rate and expressivity of physiologic aging changes are highly individual (Fig. 4-10). Frequently, changes in physical appearance, such as dry skin, wrinkles,

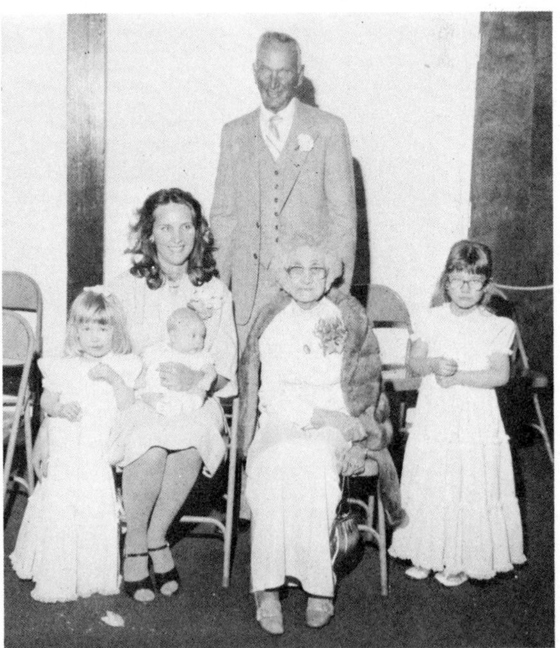

Figure 4-10 Intergenerational family.

thinning, graying hair, and inches on the waist and hips are the first noticeable clues of aging. Sometime during the middle years, most adults notice that muscle strength and agility are declining, but on a day-to-day basis most people make small compensations which minimize the effects of these changes. While the middle-ager is aware of these signs of aging, there are also changes in the vital organs which often are going on unnoticed. Table 4-8 describes physiologic changes resulting from the aging process. Because these changes involve aging rather than a pathologic process, they begin an insidious process, starting in young adulthood, becoming more manifest in middle adulthood, and culminating in death, when the body can no longer compensate for or adapt to the changes.

Although many *elderly* people remain vigorous beyond 80, the general decline in all systems and reduction of normally functioning cells caused by aging decreases the elderly person's overall ability to withstand and adapt to physical or emotional stress. When one system is placed under stress, there is a domino effect, in that without the ability to compensate, all systems may collapse. For example, the elderly person who breaks a hip and is immobilized is more vulnerable to urinary problems because of reduced renal function; to respiratory problems because of weakened muscles and rigid respiratory tissue; to circulatory problems because of decreased cardiac output; to skin problems because of thin skin and decreased peripheral circulation; to gastrointestinal problems because of decreased esophageal, stomach, and bowel motility; and to confusion because of decreased sensory input. Thus, maintaining physical and emotional integrity in the elderly person can be very precarious.

Considerations for Health Maintenance

Young adult

Although the young adult years are a time of generally good physical and emotional health, the young adult lifestyle may hold potential health hazards. Accidents, sleep deprivation, substance abuse, inactivity, obesity, exposure to environmental and occupational hazards, and stress-related illnesses

Table 4-8

Anatomic and Physiologic Changes With Aging

System	Normal Aging Changes	Outcomes
Cardiovascular		
Cardiac function	Decreased: Force of contraction Stroke volume Cardiac volume	Decreased: Cardiac output by 1% per year after 30 Peripheral circulation Blood flow to liver, GI tract, and kidneys; brain and heart receive maximum supply Physical endurance; increased fatigue
Cardiac rate	Resting state rate unchanged with age Exercise increases output, but to a reduced maximal rate Slowed response to stress with only slightly increased rate Slowed return to basal levels	Maximum attained rate 20-year-old 200/min 80-year-old 120/min Decreased ability to compensate for stress Absence of increased pulse rate may mask shock or infection.
Blood vessels	Elastic fibers straighten, fragment Accumulation of collagen and calcium	Decreased resilience, and distensibility Normal increase in BP 20-year-old 120/80 65-year-old 160/90
Respiratory	Alveolar wall thickens, decreased recoil Interalveolar septi lost, decreased number of alveoli/larger size Decreased vital capacity and tidal volume Increased residual air, and dead space Decreased ciliary movement Decreased strength of expiratory muscles Increased thoracic wall rigidity	Decreased endurance, fatigue easily Decreased capacity for deep breathing and coughing Increased potential for lower respiratory tract infection

Table 4-8 (Continued)

System	Normal Aging Changes	Outcomes
Cardiovascular		
Excretory		
Kidney	Kidney function declines 50% from age 20 to age 90. Decreased: Nephrons, 40% fewer by age 85 Renal plasma flow Glomerular filtration rate Age 40 normal GGR 120 mL/min Age 85 normal GFR 60–70 mL/min	Increased: Protein in urine BUN Drug toxicity Potential for electrolyte imbalance Potential for dehydration
Bladder	Decreased: Muscle tone Sphincter control Capacity	Urinary retention, dribbling Increased potential for infection
Gastrointestinal	Loss of teeth/dentures Decreased: Taste buds Saliva volume and salivary amylase Tone and motility of esophagus, stomach, and intestines Gastric acid production Decreased external intestinal sphincter reflex Increased biliary stones	Soft diet necessary Increased potential for: Hiatus hernia Difficulty swallowing, especially in supine position Aspiration Food intolerances, malnutrition Constipation Fecal incontinence
Endocrine		
Pancreas	Delayed insulin release Reduced peripheral sensitivity to insulin	Decreased glucose tolerance Slower return to fasting level
Gonads		
Male	Decreased testosterone production	Decreased libido, reproductive capacity remains
Female	Decreased estrogen/progesterone after menopause	No reproductive capacity Atrophy of reproductive structures
Musculoskeletal		
Muscles	Decreased mass, adipose replaces muscle cells Collagen fibers more rigid	Decreased strength, endurance, agility 10% decline age 30–60 Flabby appearance
Bones	Decreased mass, demineralization, and protein matrix loss (greatest in postmenopausal women)	Increased brittleness and fractures Potential osteoporosis
Joints	Cartilage erosion Increased calcium deposits Decreased water in cartilage	Painful articulation, crepitation Decreased range of motion Joint spaces narrowed Shortened vertebral column, decreased height Kyphosis
Integumentary		
Skin	Decreased: Subcutaneous fat Sweat glands Extracellular water Melanin Receptors Circulation to extremities	Wrinkles, bags under eyes Decreased homeostatic balance Thin, dry skin, easily bruised Liver spots Decreased pain sensitivity Nonhealing skin lesions
Hair	Thinning/loss Decreased pigment and oil	Aopecia Gray, dry hair
Nails	Decreased peripheral blood supply Increased keratin	Thickened, brittle nails Ridging, callus formation

Table 4-8 (Continued)

System	Normal Aging Changes	Outcomes
Cardiovascular		
Nervous		
Brain	Decreased: Number of cells Pyramidal tract function Blood flow and oxygen utilization Increased plaque/pigment accumulation	Reduced speed of mental processing Impaired proprioception Loss of balance/coordination Decreased CNS integration, more prolonged response to stress
Nerves	Decreased conduction velocity	Slower response/reaction time
Receptors	Decreased number/function	Decreased sensory input Potential depression
Sensory		
Vision	Decreased: Acuity/accommodation/visual fields Pupil size/dark adaptation Cones in retina Lens clarity, lens yellows with age Lacrimal secretion	Decreased: Visual input Binocular depth perception Color discrimination at blue spectrum Increased sensitivity to glare
Hearing	Decreased: Acuity/pitch discrimination Sensitivity to higher frequency Increased keratin/cerumen Tympanic membrane sclerosis Vestibular cone degeneration	Potential hearing loss, depression Impaired speech reception Diminished sound conduction Tinnitus Body sway/dizziness
Taste	Decreased number/function of taste buds	Increased taste threshold level
Smell	Fiber loss in olfactory bulb Cellular degeneration in parietal lobe	Diminished sense of smell, food not as pleasing
Touch	Decreased receptors	Less sensitive to tactile environment

Adapted from Ralph Goodman, "Aging Changes in Structure and Function," in D. L. Carnevali and M. Patrick (eds.), *Nursing Management for the Elderly*, J. B. Lippincott Company, Philadelphia, 1979, pp. 53–79; and Ann G. Yurick et al., *The Aged Person and the Nursing Process*, Appleton Century Crofts, New York, 1980, pp. 501–510.

such as ulcers, depression, and suicide are important health problems during this time of life. Chronic illnesses such as hypertension, coronary artery disease, and diabetes may have their onset in young adulthood without being known to the young adult, but become serious health threats later.

Middle adult

The middle-aged lifestyle should be assessed for areas which are detrimental to health. With a decline in strength and stamina, daily exercise is essential; however, sporadic weekend exercise or competitive physical overexertion can lead to injury (Fig. 4-11). Reducing caloric intake is often necessary to prevent weight gain. This may be particularly difficult for middle-aged adults whose social and business lifestyles encourage overindulgence at dinners and parties. Life pressures frequently mount during middle age, and in order to cope, a variety of substances may be used and overconsumed, including cigarettes, alcohol, and tranquilizers. Rather than relying on these, the individual may need assistance to deal with the sources of pressure.

Middle-aged adults need to be encouraged to seek routine medical and dental examinations directed toward disease prevention and early treatment of problems. The Surgeon General's Report recommends annual dental and biannual physical examinations for healthy middle-aged adults. It also recommends Pap smears every 3 years, unless estrogen therapy or oral contraceptives are being used, and periodic mammography after age 40 for women with a family history of breast cancer; otherwise, after age 50, when the personal and family history are negative for breast cancer.[13] Nurses have a fundamental role in health maintenance care by educating and promoting self-care responsibility among middle-aged adults.

Although a large number of middle-aged adults feel in the prime of their life, a rising incidence of chronic illnesses is associated with middle age. Some of the major health concerns, in addition to those which continue into middle age from young adulthood, include heart and vascular disease, cancer, liver cirrhosis, diabetes, and sexual dysfunctions.

Older adult

Eighty percent of the population over 65 have one or more chronic conditions with varying degrees of disability.[14] The health problems of older people reflect past health and lifestyle influences. The major problems include chronic or recurrent conditions from earlier adult stages, chronic brain syndrome, degenerative bone and joint diseases, malnutrition, acute and chronic respiratory diseases, renal diseases, drug-induced problems, and mental disorders.

The health of older adults is influenced not only by pathologic disease processes but also by the process of aging. Although the aging process cannot be stopped, the effects can be reduced by good health habits including proper nutrition, activity and rest, safety, and correct drug usage.

Nutrition Maintaining adequate nutrition can be a problem to the elderly for multiple physical and social reasons. Physiologically, with the decline in taste and smell, food may be less appealing; with dentures or loss of teeth, chewing is more difficult. Also, swallowing and digestive problems may accompany eating because of decreases in saliva, gastric motility and enzyme production. Socially, if a person eats alone, it becomes easier to snack on quick foods rather than prepare meals. Also, the lack of transportation or access to a grocery store, inability to see the merchandise, and financial poverty may be factors in poor nutrition. However, for some elderly, obesity is a problem. Usually this problem has arisen earlier in adulthood and continues because of difficulty in changing lifelong eating patterns.

Sleep Sleep is often a concern to the elderly because of changed sleep patterns. Old people lose the stage IV deep sleep and are easily aroused. As a result, they cannot maintain a prolonged night sleep. Even though the demand for sleep decreases with age, the elderly person may be disturbed by insomnia and complains that he spends more time in bed, but still feels tired. Frequently, elderly persons prefer to spread their sleep throughout the 24 hours, with short naps providing adequate rest.

Safety Environmental safety is crucial in health maintenance for old people. With normal sensory changes, slowed reaction time, decreased thermal and pain sensitivity, changes in gait and balance, and medication effects, the elderly are accident-prone.

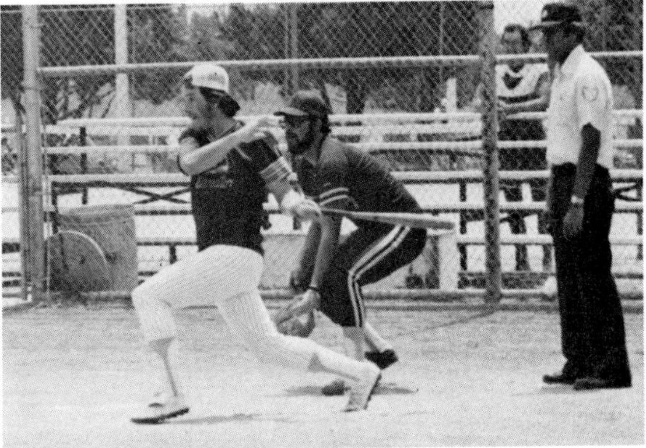

Figure 4-11 Both young and middle-aged adults are subject to injuries associated with sporadic activity.

Most accidents occur in or around the home. Falls, motor vehicle accidents, and fires are the common causes for accidental death in the elderly.[15] Another environmental problem for the elderly arises from an impaired thermoregulating system which cannot adapt to extremes in environmental temperatures. The elderly person's body can neither conserve nor dissipate heat efficiently, therefore, both hypothermia and heat prostration occur more readily. The elderly account for the majority of mortality statistics during severe cold spells and heat waves.

Medications Medication use poses a number of potential health problems for the elderly. With altered drug metabolism and excretion, individual sensitivities and side effects occur more readily. Drug interactions can occur because many elderly people take multiple prescription and nonprescription drugs. Self-medicating is often a hazard in that leftover drugs may be saved and used again after they are outdated, or may be shared with a friend or family member who reports similar symptoms. Dosages may be increased because if "a little does some good, more will do better," or dosages may be reduced so the medication will last longer if it is expensive. With memory changes, drugs may be taken sporadically, some doses being missed and others taken twice.

THE STRESS OF ILLNESS DURING ADULTHOOD

Illness is a situational crisis which can disrupt adult life at any time. The extent of the disruption may vary from a minor annoyance to a complete lifestyle change. The significance that "being ill" holds for an

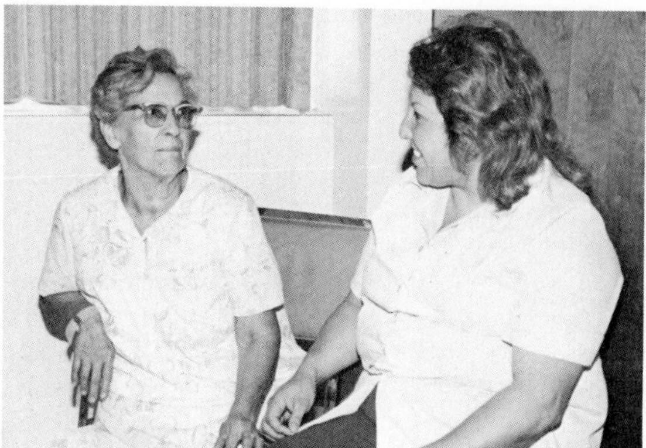

Figure 4-12 The mother's illness impacts on both her life and the life of her daughter.

individual is determined by multiple variables: the type of illness and its perceived threat, the personality type, socioeconomic resources, family or significant other support, and possible restrictions on current lifestyle or structure. Using Levinson's model, the impact of illness will differ, depending on whether the individual is in a transitional or stable period of his development. During stable periods, when life is generally going smoothly, one has more energy to cope with illness. On the other hand, with the changes being made in overall life structure during transitional periods, there is not only less energy to cope with illness, but illness and its potential effects add new variables to consider in the restructuring process. Because transitional stages represent a time of uncertainty, role changes, and anxiety, the individual is also more vulnerable to becoming ill. Conversely, the stable periods, which are typically times of commitment, confidence, and success, foster health. The presence of illness, either one's own or illness in a significant other, can also trigger movement from a stable period into a transitional stage (Fig. 4-12). This may be characteristically seen in the mid-life transition, when an illness can initiate the "time left" thinking which is fundamental to the profound reassessment of life during this transition.

Illness and Young Adults

The most frequent acute conditions in young adults are minor accidents, drug abuse, respiratory infections, influenza, gastroenteritis, urinary tract infections, and minor surgeries. These conditions may be developmentally significant to the young adult for several reasons. First, with the frequently hectic schedules of young adults, an acute minor illness is an annoyance factor because of disruption in life activities. With an acute disability, the young adult may know that the effects are short-term; however, he may become impatient with the healing process and be concerned that there will be long-term problems. Family rearrangements can be stressful, especially when hospitalization is required. Hospitalization also is frustrating because of forced dependency and limitations posed by treatment regimens. Maintaining control is very important for young adults, so they need to be informed and involved with decisions about care. Young adults are generally strongly motivated toward recuperation in order to resume life activities.

Although chronic conditions are not common in young adulthood, they can occur. Disabilities caused by accidents, multiple sclerosis, rheumatoid arthritis, and cancer are the common long-term conditions faced by young adults. Chronic illness and disability in young adulthood strikes at the very core of developmental tasks and can result in delayed development. With the onset of chronic illness or disability, the threat to the young adult's independence may precipitate multiple crises when there is a need to change personal, family, and career goals. It is essential for the nurse to identify and direct nursing intervention toward potential developmental problems in the areas of identity reorganization, establishment of independence, and reorganization of intimate relationships, family structure, and launching of a chosen career.

Illness and Middle Adults

The characteristics of acute illness are much the same in middle adulthood as in young adulthood. However, in middle adulthood there is a slowing in recuperative power, so that injuries and acute conditions, which rapidly resolved in young adulthood, may now have a longer recovery period and are more likely to become chronic problems.

Chronic conditions during middle age interfere with the individual's sense of generativity. This task requires outward-directed concerns and activities. Long-term recurrent illness often forces an interiority which can lead to physical and psychological self-absorption. When a middle-aged adult develops a chronic illness or disability, he may feel unable to influence his own destiny, let alone reach out and influence and provide for others. The impact on generativity includes changes in family, job, and community involvement.

With the onset of chronic illness in middle age, there is often a forced change in established family roles. The psychological trauma of these role changes is due to the fact that there is a strong emotional component to roles, which is based on how one values that role as a part of his identity and the vested power which the role holds. The nurse should be perceptive to the potential for family dysfunction, and should serve as a resource to the entire family, helping them to seek counseling and therapy as necessary.

Career or occupational orientation may need to change as a result of chronic illness. This is particularly stressful during the middle years, because it confounds the career timing and readjustment of goals which occurs with the mid-life occupational crisis. When the illness is severely disruptive, the person may need to change occupations or jobs, or may need to face an early forced retirement. Both these options may be a source of great stress and a threat to generativity because of occupational regression or being denied the gratification which comes from closing a career with the feeling of a job well done.

Illness and the Elderly

The distinction between acute and chronic illness in the aged adult is less precise, because acute conditions may become chronic or may be an exacerbation of chronic problems. However, there are acute problems such as gastroenteritis, primary pneumonia, removable tumors, and noncomplicated accidental injuries which can have a short course with complete recovery. The difficulties such illnesses pose for the elderly are that they add stress to a body system that physiologically and psychologically has a decreased ability to compensate for stress. The ability to care for oneself is an important problem for the elderly person when an acute illness occurs. If the person lives alone or with a frail spouse or housemate, and does not have adequate support systems, an acute illness can precipitate a life disorganization which results in a move out of one's own home and toward dependency.

When an elderly person is hospitalized, many situations occur which threaten ego-integrity and cause the hospitalization to be a very disorganizing experience. New situations and environments are often normally anxiety-producing for the elderly, and when combined with the stress of being sick, the unfamiliar becomes confusing. When giving care, the nurse needs to carefully orient and reorient the elderly person to the hospital environment. Allowing the elderly client to keep personal belongings within reach and visible will also help to maintain a sense of orientation, as well as to reduce the depersonalized feeling that accompanies hospitalization. Nursing care should be paced to allow the elderly client an opportunity to participate without hurrying, so that he can maintain control and has time to understand and cooperate with what is being done.

Family situations are an important concern in caring for the hospitalized elderly. It is essential for the nurse to recognize when role reversals are occurring between an elderly parent and the adult children. Children who have problems with this reversal may respond by withdrawing, or by becoming overprotective and smothering. In either case, the parent's self-worth will be threatened. The nurse should also be perceptive to other family concerns of the hospitalized elderly person, such as worry over a spouse being home alone, or concern for pets and plants or household maintenance if he was living alone.

Chronic conditions are very common deviances in health which the elderly learn to live with. Part of this process includes incorporating the accoutrements of aging such as canes, wheelchairs, dentures, and hearing aids into a healthy self-esteem. Chronic conditions also have social implications if the illness imposes an involuntary disengagement process. When this occurs, it becomes increasingly difficult to transcend the physical problems. The social isolation that is experienced may reduce self-esteem and the physical and emotional strength needed to cope with the stresses of disease and aging.

REVIEW QUESTIONS

The number of the question corresponds to the same numbered objective at the beginning of the chapter.

1. Erikson's developmental conflicts are based on
- **a.** biological changes during adulthood
- **b.** adjustments of self and social environment
- **c.** changes in the individual life structure
- **d.** instinctual energies and drives

2. Disengagement
- **a.** is a developmental stage theory
- **b.** occurs in all people over 65 years of age
- **c.** assumes that the elderly cannot adapt to aging
- **d.** varies according to health, abilities, and previous lifestyle

3. Significant changes in mental functioning during middle and older adulthood include
- **a.** improved fluid intelligence
- **b.** declining verbal comprehension and reasoning skill
- **c.** declining speed in mental performance
- **d.** improved synthesis of new information

4. Young adult family tasks involve
- **a.** establishing a new family system which focuses on internal structure and relationships
- **b.** adapting a family system to outside demands
- **c.** modifying the relationship with the families of origin
- **d.** all of the above

5. Select the *one correct* statement about work and adulthood.
   a. The only significance work has to an adult is as a means of financial support.
   b. The important role changes when launching a career are those related to the job.
   c. Resolution of the middle-aged occupational crisis requires self-evaluation of goals.
   d. Retirement is not stressful if the preretirement standard of living can be maintained.

6. Physical changes associated with aging in adulthood
   a. arise from extrinsic factors
   b. are pathologic in origin
   c. can be halted by proper health maintenance
   d. have an insidious beginning in young adults

7. Hospitalization can be a disorganizing experience for the elderly client because
   a. new environments are anxiety-producing and difficult to cope with
   b. disorientation may occur when personal belongings are out of sight and out of reach
   c. a hurried pace reduces the elderly person's ability to participate and maintain control
   d. all the above

REFERENCES

1. Erik Erikson, *Childhood and Society*, 2d rev. ed.; W. W. Norton & Company, Inc., New York, 1963, pp. 263–269.
2. Robert C. Peck, "Psychological Developments in the Second Half of Life," in B. L. Neugarten (ed.), *Middle-Age and Aging: A Reader in Social Psychology*, University of Chicago Press, Chicago, pp. 88–92.
3. Robert J. Havighurst, *Developmental Tasks and Education*, 3d ed., David McKay Company, Inc., New York, 1973, pp. 83–116.
4. Daniel J. Levinson et al., *The Seasons of a Man's Life*, Alfred A. Knopf, Inc., New York, 1978.
5. E. Cumming and W. E. Henry, *Growing Old: The Process of Disengagement*, Basic Books, Inc. Publishers, New York, 1961.
6. George L. Maddox, "Activity and Morale: A Longitudinal Study of Selected Elderly Subjects," *Social Forces*, **42** (2):195–204 (1963)
7. Bernice L. Neugarten, *Personality in Middle and Late Life*, Atherton Press, Inc., New York, 1964.
8. Douglas C. Kimmel, *Adulthood and Aging*, John Wiley & Sons, Inc., New York, 1974, p. 159.
9. K. W. Schaie, "Age Changes in Adult Intelligence," in D. S. Woodruf and J. E. Birren, (eds.), *Aging: Scientific Perspectives and Social Issues*, D. Van Nostrand Company, Inc., New York, 1975.
10. U. S. Surgeon General's Report, *Healthy People*, Government Printing Office, Washington, D.C., 1979, p. 74.
11. E. Pfeiffer and G. C. Davis, "The Use of Leisure Time in Middle-Life," *Gerontologist*, **11**:187–195 (1971).
12. Lewis Aiken, *Later Life*, W. B. Saunders Company, Philadelphia, 1978, p. 169.
13. U. S. Surgeon General's Report, 1979, p. 154.
14. Ibid., p. 155.
15. Ibid., p. 71.
16. Ralph Goodman, "Aging Changes in Structure and Function," in D. L. Carnevali and M. Patrick (eds.), *Nursing Management for the Elderly*, J. B. Lippincott Company, Philadelphia, 1979, pp. 53–79.
17. Ann G. Yurick et al., *The Aged Person and The Nursing Process*, Appleton Century Crofts, New York, 1980, pp. 501–510.

Chapter 5

GENERAL CONCEPTS

Client Education

Margaret Stapleton Brown
Carol Cox Smith

Learning Objectives

1. Identify four common characteristics of the adult learner.
2. Identify the factors contributing to successful learning for the adult client, including implications for nursing intervention.
3. Explain the basic steps in the teaching-learning process.
4. List and describe the four dimensions of assessment related to the teaching-learning process.
5. Explain the components of a correctly written learning objective.
6. Describe the seven basic teaching strategies.
7. Describe common methods of short-term and long-term evaluation.
8. Select appropriate teaching strategies based on assessment of learning styles.

Client education is an integral part of nursing intervention. Knowledge of the theory related to teaching-learning and the adult learner are prerequisite to developing effective teaching skills.

This chapter will present practical, useful teaching techniques that will help the nurse give clients the information they need to adjust to new skills and attitudes necessary for their total health care.

CHARACTERISTICS OF THE ADULT LEARNER

Common Characteristics

Why are adults more difficult to teach than children? There are four reasons, each one based on a basic principle of adult education.

First, as a person matures, he becomes increasingly *self-directed* regarding his educational needs and choices. If he wants to learn how to operate a computer, he may choose several books on the topic and from them figure out the process. He may choose to take a formal course of instruction or may simply visit several businesses and discuss the process with computer experts. He directs his own learning into channels that are best suited to his individual learning style.

However, the adult client in an acute-care setting is far from self-directed. If he loses control over the learning process, he can become frustrated and even hostile toward the very people who are trying to help him.

This chapter was reviewed by Joan B. Enggaard, B.S.N., M.S.N., Professor, College of Lake County, Grayslake, Illinois.

Second, the adult client has already accumulated a *lifetime of experiences*—good and bad—upon which he will base any new information received. If, for example, a diabetic client knows someone among his family or friends who is also diabetic and who is able to self-administer insulin, he will more likely have a positive attitude toward learning this skill.

Unfortunately, being in a hospital or other acute-care facility is often a totally new experience for the adult client. He has no previous positive experiences on which to base attitudes and feelings. Consequently, this client is fearful and suspicious, and the learning process cannot progress.

Third, an adult's *readiness to learn* depends on where he is on the continuum of adult developmental tasks (see Chap. 4 for a discussion of adult development). Whether or not he is ready to learn depends on his ability to identify a need to learn in relation to his development. For instance, if an adult client is experiencing Mid-Life Transition—a period of emotional upheaval, self-doubt, and reevaluation of life goals—he may not be ready to learn a new attitude or skill that is a threat to his identity. The nurse will need to be especially supportive and encouraging to this type of adult client and will need to show how new learning will adapt to his present lifestyle.

Fourth, the adult client's learning is based on *life problems* and on the ability to *apply learning immediately*.[1] The adult wants results *now*. This orientation makes the nurse's task particularly difficult in relation to chronic illnesses since they are long-term, lifetime experiences with no immediate solutions. To overcome the difficulties of this adult characteristic, the successful nurse-teacher should provide short-term, immediate, reachable goals that give the client a feeling of progress.

Effects of Illness on Adult Learning Characteristics

When an adult realizes that he is chronically ill, the psychological impact exaggerates already existing characteristics. In addition, the illness adds many stressors to an already stressful dilemma. The loss of control over one's destiny, the loss of strength and energy, the strain of financial and family pressures, worry over losing one's job, concern for the reactions of loved ones and friends—all these factors can make the adult client a very reluctant learner. There are several things the nurse-educator can do to help the adult client overcome these effects.

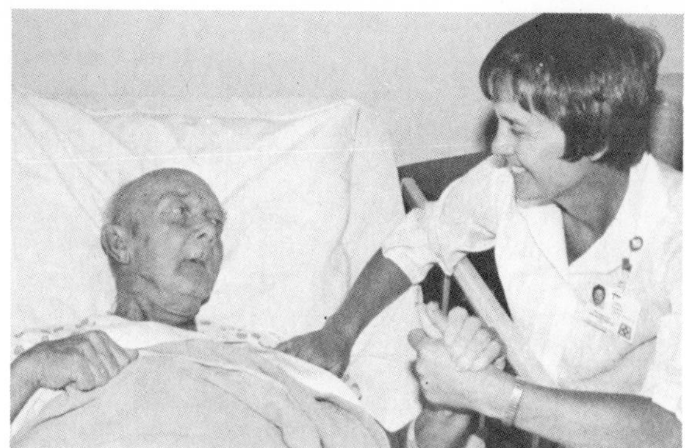

Figure 5-1 A touch and a smile are great motivators.

FACTORS CONTRIBUTING TO SUCCESSFUL TEACHING

Relevance

First, make sure that the material to be learned is *relevant* to the client's problem. The client is more likely to be motivated and cooperative when tasks are meaningful and of interest.[2] The nurse therefore should use only those printed or audiovisual materials which relate directly to the client's needs and should limit discussions and demonstrations to necessary content. In addition, the nurse should explain the learning objectives and should help the client understand the teaching strategies before implementing the teaching plan.

Motivation

Second, remember that the client will learn if he wants to. Wanting to learn is the greatest aid to learning, and this *motivation* can be enhanced in several ways. For instance, help the client to see the relationship of the new skill to his life. Give him short, reachable goals at which he can succeed immediately. Organize the material and present it in logical order from the simple to the complex. Give the client time to understand and practice each new task before proceeding to more advanced material. Always present a warm, caring, nonthreatening image to the client, using positive, supportive communications (Fig. 5-1). This is the time in the client's life when he needs every human relations skill the nurse can summon.

Active Participation

Next, the client should actively participate in the teaching-learning process. *Active participation* increases motivation and retention. For example, the nurse and client together should discuss and agree upon desired outcomes ("We agree that you need to be able to administer your own insulin injections" or "We want you to be able to successfully change your own colostomy bag"). The client may also participate in the selection of reading materials or audiovisual material ("Which pamphlet looks most interesting to you?" or "Do you prefer tapes or films?"). Remember that a characteristic of adult learning is the desire to be self-directed, to choose his own learning experiences. Building upon this fact is an important tool for the nurse-educator.

Along with active participation, the client needs frequent *measures of success*. A client who knows that he is learning and succeeding with each activity is strongly motivated to learn more. Support and encouragement are essential every step of the way. Immediate experiences of success in the learning process help to overcome the fear of failure which is a learning block for many adults.[3]

Practice and Review

Another factor that contributes to successful teaching is *practice and review*. Learning theory shows that repetition and practice of facts and skills increase memory. Frequency of repetition is important in acquiring and maintaining a skill. To help a client develop a skill or retain learning material, the nurse should incorporate spaced practice intervals in the teaching-learning plan. Also, a good practice is to briefly "quiz" the client verbally each time you see him ("Can you name the four basic food groups?" or "Tell me how to correctly measure an insulin injection" or, again, "Are you having any problems with your injections?"). Once the nurse is satisfied that previously given instruction is retained, she may confidently proceed with new content.

Expectations

What the nurse expects the client to learn and what the client expects to learn should be discussed and agreed upon. The client's expectations and the nurse's expectations should be the same. The nurse may develop a model of what the client should know or be able to do as a result of the learning experience. In some cases, a role model can be introduced to the client to help illustrate therapeutic expectations.

Time and Timing

Another factor is *time*. As people get older, their rate of learning declines.[4] Since it takes an older person longer to learn a new skill than a younger person, more time must be allowed. Time limits and pressures imposed upon the adult client may produce negative results. Best results usually occur when the adult client can proceed at his own rate. However, proceeding at one's own rate may not always be possible due to many factors such as early discharge. In this case, the nurse should plan to refer the client to a home care program, visiting nurse, or other follow-up agency.

Incorporated in the concept of time is *timing*: knowing when to teach and when not to teach. The nurse needs to be attuned to each client's needs as these needs change from hour to hour, day to day. Planning ahead and knowing the client's schedule is helpful. For example, if a client is being discharged but needs to know how to change his dressing, the nurse should plan to teach this skill as far ahead of discharge as possible. In this way, the client will have time to practice and review the skill so that he feels confident of this skill upon discharge.

Learning Environment

Another factor is the *learning environment*. From the moment the client enters the hospital until he is discharged—even before initial assessment is complete—the nurse must work to develop a feeling of trust, respect, and support. The client will learn best in an atmosphere of warmth, comfort, and caring. When the nurse and client establish rapport, the teaching-learning transaction will be more successful (see Chap. 2 for interviewing principles and developing rapport).

The learning environment is also a physical climate. Since distractions can reduce the efficiency of teaching and learning, the nurse should eliminate, rearrange, or control noise, lighting, ventilation, and odors. Close the window if too much traffic noise is coming from the street. Shut your office door and

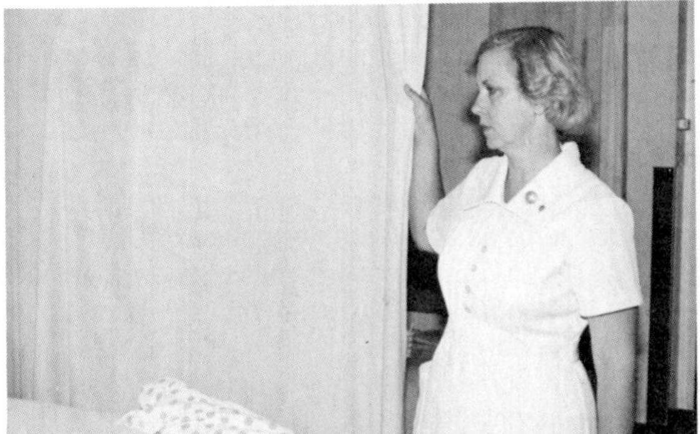

Figure 5-2 Closing the bedside curtain reduces distraction.

eliminate visual distractions from passersby. Turn off the television set or radio, or pull the privacy curtain (Fig. 5-2). Remembering that adult clients may have reduced visual or auditory ability, the nurse should provide clear visual cues (adequate illumination, larger print, reduced glare) and adequate auditory cues (speak clearly, face the client, slightly increase the volume of your speech).

With all these factors in mind, the nurse is prepared for a successful teaching-learning experience.

THE TEACHING-LEARNING PROCESS

The nurse-educator should be able to follow these basic steps in the teaching-learning process: (1) assessment, (2) determining objectives, (3) selecting teaching strategies, (4) implementation, and (5) evaluation.

Assessment

Assessment as a process may be defined as a systematic method of gathering relevant information about a particular client. Assessment for the purpose of developing a teaching plan encompasses collecting a complete data base, identifying the client's strengths and weaknesses, and determining personal characteristics, learning characteristics, and experiential characteristics of the client.

Biophysical dimension

Assessment begins when the nurse considers the client's biophysical dimension. How old is the client? His *age* will provide cues to the nurse concerning the rate of learning, past experiences, memory ability, mastery of developmental tasks, and possible impairments of vision, hearing, or reaction time.

The *physiologic condition* and *physical health* of an adult client can determine his readiness to learn. Sensory impairment, such as poor vision or hearing loss, can decrease ability to learn because of restricted sensory input. Learning requires an adequately functioning nervous system. Therefore, a client with such problems as a cerebral vascular accident, poor cardiac perfusion, or severe muscular or nervous system trauma may easily forget; and the nurse may need to repeat information frequently to facilitate learning. In some cases, the nurse may need to postpone teaching until the client is physiologically ready to learn: that is, until a certain amount of healing has taken place.[5]

Pain, fatigue, and *certain medications* will also influence a client's readiness to learn. No one can learn efficiently when he is in severe pain. To clients experiencing intense pain, the nurse should give only a brief explanation, then follow with more detailed instruction when pain has been managed.

The nurse must also be aware of the client's *energy level*. A tired or weak client cannot learn effectively because his concentration is low. The nurse should wait until the client is rested and has more energy before beginning instruction.

Medications may also influence a client's readiness to learn. Barbiturates, tranquilizers, and narcotic analgesics, for instance, can cause drowsiness, clouding of consciousness, and a general decrease in mental alertness. The nurse must continuously evaluate the client's physical condition, including his response to medications, and reassess readiness to learn.

Psychological dimension

A second aspect of assessment is the *psychological dimension*. Here, the nurse assesses the client's personal and social adjustment to his illness and the learning situation. Is the client anxious or afraid? Is he suspicious or defensive? Although mild anxiety increases the learner's perceptual and learning abilities, as anxiety increases, these abilities decrease. The nurse must lower anxiety before the client can learn efficiently.

Other psychological factors that can influence learning are the client's personality, the way he adapts to illness, and his outlook on life. If he is alienated, hopeless, or defensive, he may not want to learn.[6] Illness itself, or the threat of illness, can force the individual to reassess his goals and reevaluate his entire life.

In addition, if the client does not adapt well to his illness, he will not learn effectively. How well he adapts depends on his self-concept prior to the illness, the severity of illness, life changes due to illness, and the meaning the illness has to the client, and to his family, friends, and coworkers. Pertinent information can help the client adapt well if the nurse intervenes at the appropriate time.[7] (See Chap. 1 for factors related to appropriate time.)

Sociocultural dimension

The *sociocultural dimension* must also be assessed. Basically, this means that the nurse must examine the client's *lifestyle*. His lifestyle influences how he perceives the hospital setting and the entire learning experience. Lifestyle includes many elements: occupation, education, income, housing arrangement, living location (rural, urban, etc.), dietary pattern, sleep pattern, exercise, sexuality, coping mechanisms, and stressors. Also, the client's values and beliefs can influence how he views health and illness and therefore how he responds to the teaching-learning process.[8]

For example, a person who values a youthful figure can be taught to diet and exercise to retain that figure while at the same time bringing an ulcer under control. However, in many cultures, being fat is valued as a sign of financial success and sexuality. A client from such a culture would probably reject the concept of diet and exercise for weight control or any other reason.

Learning is closely related to the wider *culture* and the *subculture* to which the client belongs. Health beliefs and actions vary by religious belief, ethnic group, and family group. The nurse must assess and understand the client's cultural background, and must develop a teaching plan that takes this element into consideration.

For instance, a middle-aged, upper-income woman may belong to a subculture in which "popping pills" is widely accepted. She may therefore be willing to take prescribed pills but unwilling to learn to self-administer an injection. The nurse, in assessing the client's needs, must take a holistic approach and see the client as a total person within her subculture. The nurse's teaching plan must include ways to change the client's attitudes or show the client how her new skill will fit into her existing lifestyle.

An interesting element within the client's cultural group is the *leadership pattern*. Because people tend to follow the advice of their leaders, the nurse should try to identify and work with leaders or decision makers within the client's culture group. Their assistance may help the client accept new ideas and techniques.[9]

Environmental dimension

The environmental dimension is another part of assessment. A basic teaching motto is "Begin with what the learner knows." Previous life experiences ("what the learner knows") will determine where the nurse-educator should begin instruction. Since learning is a process by which individuals add to or modify their previously existing knowledge, skills, and attitudes, past experiences and types of informal and formal instruction should be determined. Ask questions related to previous hospital experiences, previous experiences with diet, medications, and other family illnesses. Has the client known anyone in the past with this illness? Has he read any material about the illness? Have previous hospital experiences been positive or negative? Have any previous treatments familiarized the client with similar equipment or processes? For example, previous experience with allergy immunizations will familiarize the client with syringes.

The nurse should also find out what educational experiences the client has had. If past educational situations have been negative (overly critical teachers, "waste of time" attitude, poor or failing grades, nonsupportive family or friends), the nurse-educator will need to provide continuous encouragement and the earliest possible experiences of success.

Learning styles

A related concept that the nurse should assess is the client's *learning style*. Everyone has a distinct style of learning, as individual as his personality. The three learning styles are (1) visual (reading), (2) aural (listening), and (3) physical (doing things) (Fig. 5-3). People often use more than one learning style. To determine the client's learning style, the nurse might ask the following questions:

1. In what kind of environment do you learn best? Formal classroom? Informal setting, such as home or office? Among a group of peers?
2. Do you learn best when you are alone or in a group?
3. Do you prefer to read information, hear it from a tape, listen to a lecture, watch a film or slide presentation? Or would you rather physically do something?
4. How do you feel that most of your learning has taken place? Have you learned primarily from classes, personal experience, discussion groups, personal reading, television?

Answers to questions such as these help both the nurse and the client focus on the most appropriate teaching strategies to fit the learning style.

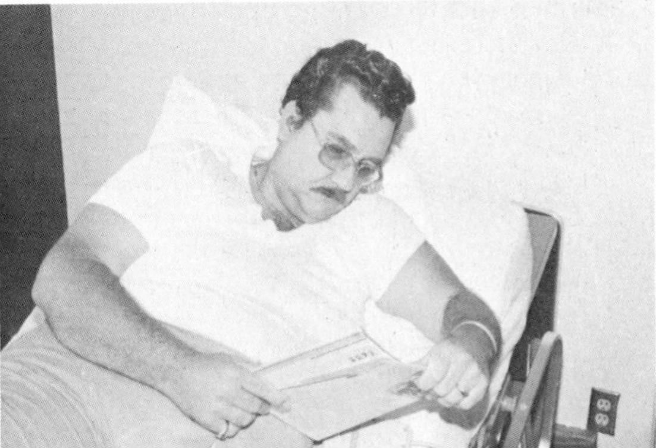

Figure 5-3 Written material is often the best technique for achieving a learning objective.

Determining Objectives

The second step in the teaching-learning process follows detailed assessment. In this step, the nurse involves the client in *determining objectives* and *planning the learning experience*.

Information obtained from the assessment (what the client knows, understands, believes, and is able to do) is compared with what the client should know, understand, and be able to do. Identifying the gap between the known and not known helps to motivate the client.

Mutual planning

Because individuals tend to feel more committed to a decision or activity when they participate in making or planning it, the client and the nurse should mutually agree upon learning objectives. If the physical or psychological condition of the client is such that he cannot actively participate, the nurse must assume the major role of designing the learning experience. The client's family or significant others can assist the nurse in this process, and the client can be involved as soon as he is able.

Learning objectives describe intended results of instruction, guide the selection of teaching strategies and materials, and help evaluate client and teacher progress. These objectives should be written down and made readily available to all members of the health care team. In order to communicate clearly to those who need to know, the nurse should acquire skill in writing clear, specific, measurable teaching objectives.

Writing specific learning objectives

Learning objectives are written statements that define exactly what learners are able to do to show that they have mastered the unit. They should contain the following four elements:

1. Who it is that will perform the activity or acquire the desired behavior.
   Example: The client will . . .
   . . . the client will . . .
   The client's family will . . .
2. The actual behavior that the learner will exhibit to demonstrate mastery of the objective.
   Example: . . . to list the symptoms . . .
   . . . to self-administer an insulin injection . . .
   . . . will identify from a hospital menu . . .
3. The conditions under which the behavior is to be demonstrated (how and where the learner will perform).
   Example: . . . in front of the nurse . . .
   . . . in his own home . . .
   . . . select from a random list . . .
   . . . will choose from a restaurant menu . . .
4. The specific criteria that will be used to measure the client's success, such as time and degree of accuracy.
   Example: . . . with 100 percent accuracy . . .
   . . . using correct technique . . .
   . . . within 3 minutes . . .

Note that well-written learning objectives contain very precise descriptions, using terms with few interpretations.[10] When writing objectives, use verbs such as "identify," "list," "describe," "demonstrate," "name," "recognize," or "compare and contrast." Avoid terms with vague, ambiguous meanings, such as "appreciate," "learn," "understand," "enjoy," "feel," or "value."

Examples of poorly written and well-written objectives

The following is an example of a poorly written learning objective:

> The client will appreciate the importance of proper foot care.

How will the client demonstrate that he "appreciates"? When and to whom will he demonstrate this behavior? What criteria will be used? In the above objective, these questions are not answered.

The following are examples of well-written learning objectives:

> The client will be able to demonstrate to the nurse the correct technique for changing his colostomy bag.
>
> The client will administer in front of the nurse a subcutaneous injection of insulin to herself using correct technique.
>
> The client will select a 1,000-mg Na diet from the hospital menu for breakfast, lunch, and dinner for 3 consecutive days with 100 percent accuracy.
>
> Given a list of symptoms of hyperglycemia and hypoglycemia, the client will be able to identify the early symptoms of hypoglycemia with 100 percent accuracy.

When learning objectives are clear and specific, and when they are written down and available in the client's record, all members of the health care team can work together to accomplish the same objectives. This type of communication will ensure good results.

Teaching Strategies

Once the objectives are clearly stated, the nurse and client (with input from other members of the health care team as available and appropriate) can develop the teaching plan. Together, they can select content and materials and decide on strategies and learning tasks. Selecting a particular strategy is determined by at least *three factors:* (1) the character of the learner (learning style, educational background, culture and subculture, etc.), (2) the subject matter, and (3) available facilities. The nurse and client must choose the strategy or strategies that can be used most effectively and from which the client can best benefit.

Types of strategies

There are *seven teaching strategies* which the nurse-educator can employ to achieve learning objectives. Each has advantages and disadvantages that make it more or less suitable to a particular learning situation.

Lecture For rapid learning when time is short, the *lecture* is an efficient, versatile, and economical teaching strategy. The nurse presents a series of related ideas or facts to one person or to a group (Fig. 5-4). Usually, the lecture is short, from 15 to 20 minutes, and some visual reinforcement, such as a diagram on a blackboard, emphasizes key points. Some disadvantages of the lecture are that it often has a negative "school learning" connotation, and individual learning is difficult to evaluate. In addition, the nurse-educator is active, but the clients are passive unless they are allowed to participate or ask questions.

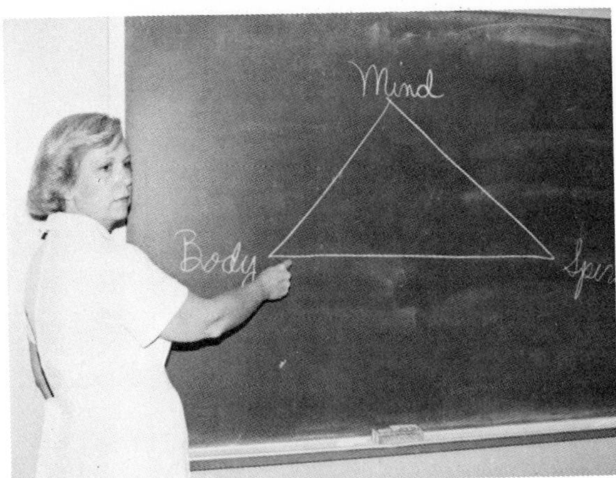

Figure 5-4 The lecture method lends itself to large group teaching situations.

Lecture-Discussion A second teaching strategy is the *lecture-discussion*, which can overcome some of the disadvantages of the straight lecture. With this strategy, the nurse presents specific information by using the lecture technique, followed by a period during which clients ask questions and exchange points of view with the nurse. This strategy assists the client to become an active participant in the learning process and creates a more informal give-and-take learning environment.

Discussion A third strategy is *discussion*, and its purpose may be to exchange points of view concerning a topic or question or to arrive at a decision or conclusion. The nurse can discuss content with an individual or with a group, keeping the specific learning objectives in mind and clarifying information as needed. This strategy is a good choice when the client or clients have previous experience with a subject and have information to share, such as stop smoking, postcoronary, or preoperative teaching classes. The discussion allows the client to actively participate and to apply his own experiences and observations to the learning process. However, one disadvantage must be remembered: The discussion will take longer to cover a given amount of material than some other methods. The informal sharing and nonthreatening environment of discussion are positive factors, but the time and difficulty of reaching desired objectives may present negatives.

Group Teaching *Group teaching* is a strategy in which the nurse acts as a facilitator of group discussion, not as a teacher (Fig. 5-5). The nurse introduces the client to an existing group or forms a group of persons with similar problems, such as women who have elderly parents living in their home. The group teaches itself; that is, the clients share knowledge of a subject. In this case, it is essential that all members of the group are at similar levels of learning and are prepared to teach each other; otherwise, there may be a great deal of repetition and discussion without real learning. However, this strategy does encourage peer teaching and self-help and does provide social support. Therefore, it is a good strategy for the client who needs encouragement and positive reinforcement. One caution: Avoid this strategy when any person or group is dysfunctional or when anxiety or stress is at a very high level.

Demonstration/Return Demonstration *Demonstration/return demonstration* is probably the most common strategy a nurse-educator uses. Its purpose may be to show how something works and the procedure to follow when doing it. Another purpose may be to illustrate to the client how a skill is performed, or to demonstrate ideas, problem solving, or motor skills. The focus is on correct procedure and application. To handle this strategy correctly, the nurse should tell the client the purpose of the demonstration and make sure that the client can see and hear clearly. Then the nurse presents the demonstration in an informal manner, defines unfamiliar terms, and watches for signs of confusion from the client. The nurse clarifies and repeats as needed, then the client returns the demonstration with the nurse as observer. The entire process should last no more than 15 to 20 minutes and should be briefly repeated during the nurse's next teaching session with the client.

Role Playing Another strategy that the nurse might employ, depending on teaching objectives, is *role playing*. When clients need to examine their attitudes and behaviors, when they need to under-

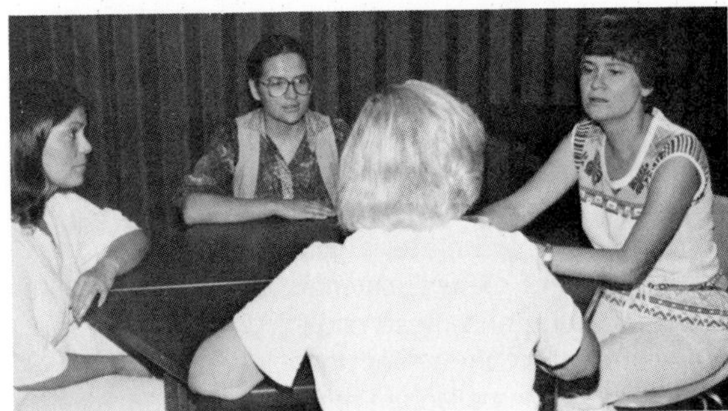

Figure 5-5 The nurse acts as facilitator in small group discussions.

stand viewpoints and attitudes of others, or when they need to practice carrying out thoughts, ideas, or decisions, this strategy may be effective. The nurse has a difficult and delicate position when employing this strategy: The nurse must define the problem, determine goals, set the climate, and determine the situation and roles to be played. She must then give information and instructions to role players and observers, and provide time for feedback and evaluation —all this while keeping the "play" from deteriorating into an emotional scene. Few clients are mature enough, confident enough, and flexible enough to role-play successfully. More often, clients feel uncomfortable and inhibited with this method. Again, time can be a negative factor, and results are difficult to evaluate. However, this strategy is ideal for some situations. For example, a wife may need to rehearse how to talk to her husband about his need to quit smoking. In this case, "play-acting" the discussion ahead of time will be a helpful strategy.

Audiovisual Material A final strategy for the nurse to consider is the use of *audiovisual materials*, including movies, film strips, slides, posters, charts, videotapes, audiotapes, or simple transparencies. This strategy can be used to present effectively most types of information in a more interesting manner than a lecture. The reason is that more than one sense is being used. To use this strategy, the nurse must know what materials are available within the care facility, from support agencies, and from professional groups (Fig. 5-6). These materials must be previewed and evaluated for accuracy, completeness, and appropriateness to the learning objectives before being shown to the client. Unfortunately, many audiovisual items are expensive, and viewing or listening space may be difficult to find. Additionally, audiovisual equipment, such as projectors or viewers, must be kept in good repair and available for the nurse's use. The nurse must also be able to operate the equipment alone.[11] However, in spite of these disadvantages, this strategy can be extremely beneficial, particularly when teaching content that is largely visual, such as teaching the steps, processes, or results of a surgical procedure. (See Fig. 5-7 for examples of selecting learning strategies.)

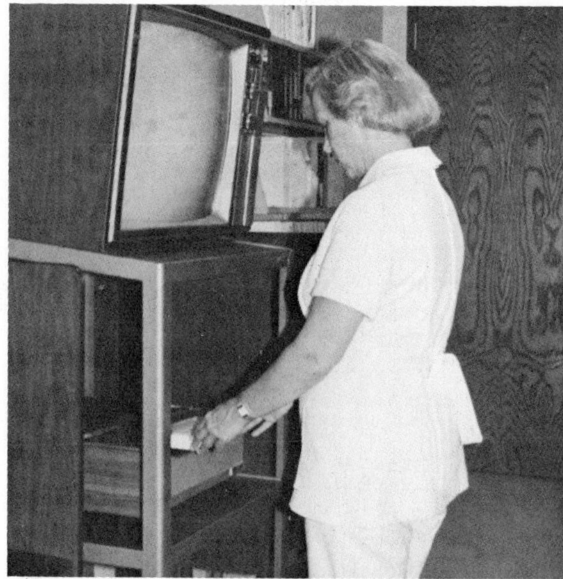

Figure 5-6 The nurse should be aware of audiovisual material available in a care facility.

Use of printed material with strategies

A wealth of *printed materials* is available for the nurse-educator, and these should be considered for use with each of the seven teaching strategies. For instance, following a lecture on the physiologic effects of smoking, the nurse could distribute a pamphlet from the American Cancer Society which reviews and reinforces the topic. Or, the nurse-educator might select a book or magazine article written by a woman who has had a mastectomy and instruct the client to read this material before viewing a film on the same topic.

Always keep in mind the learning style of the client. Many people prefer to read material in private at their own pace, before or after a learning experience. The care facility's library, the pharmacy, members of the health care team, the public library, federal and state agencies, universities, and research centers are some of the major resources for the nurse seeking relevant printed materials.

Barbara Klug Redman in *The Process of Patient Teaching in Nursing* presents an excellent section on the evaluation of printed materials for use with the adult client.[2] In brief, she suggests that the nurse evaluate the materials using nine criteria: (1) accuracy; (2) completeness; (3) whether or not the materials meet specific learning goals; (4) vocabulary and sentence length suitable to the client's educational level; (5) use of pictures of diagrams to stimulate interest; (6) use of one main idea or concept per pamphlet; (7) use of terminology that the client would understand, rather than use of undefined medical terminology; (8) whether or not the material contains information the client would like to know; and (9) whether or not the material is middle-class value-specific.[12]

Implementation

Implementation involves the actual presentation of learning material to the client. It requires the nurse to have an attitude of interest, enthusiasm, respect,

Client A

Learning Style:
Prefers direct, straightforward approach. Dislikes formal classroom environment. Task oriented. Good talker.

Educational Background:
High-school graduate. Took several vocational courses. Above average grades.

Subject matter:
Post-MI instruction.

Facilities:
A major urban hospital with extensive resources.

Client B

Learning Style:
Works well with other adults. Enjoys sharing ideas. Likes television talk shows.

Educational Background:
One year of college. Majored in elementary education.

Subject Matter:
Breast self-exam
Client fearful and depressed.

Facilities:
Meeting rooms in local women's resource center.

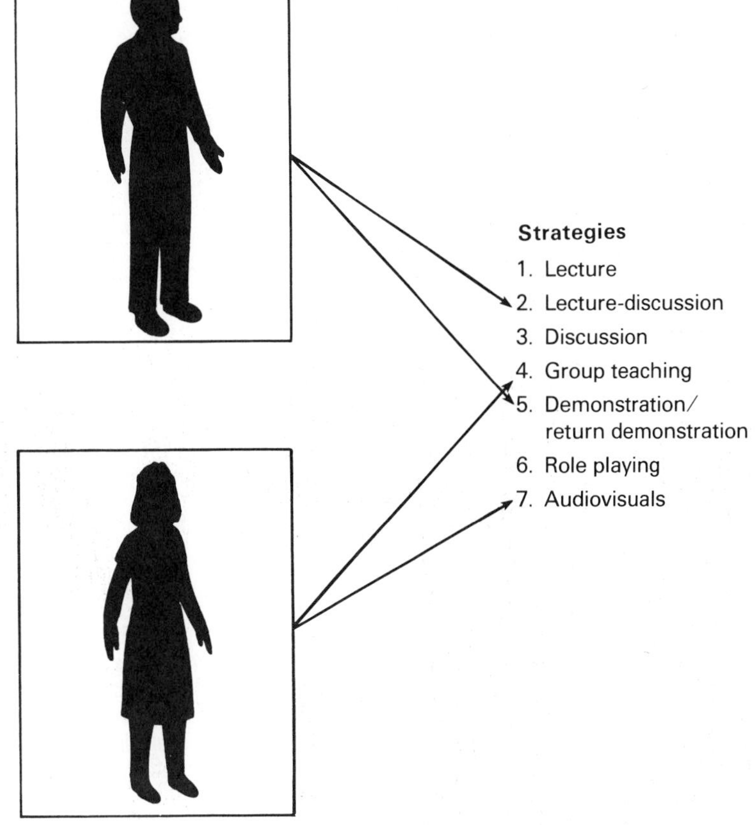

Figure 5-7 Selecting learning strategies.

and belief in the client's ability to learn. The client should not be placed in the position of passive recipient. Based on the assessment of the client's physical and psychological condition, the nurse should determine how much active participation the client can assume. The amount of time spent in the teaching-learning transaction should be based on the client's energy level. In most cases, short learning sessions are much more conducive to learning than are long learning sessions. The nurse should continuously reassess the client's condition so that the teaching situation can remain flexible and adaptable as the client's needs change.

In implementing the teaching plan, the nurse should remember the basic concepts for successful teaching:[13]

1. Keep the physical environment relaxed and nonthreatening.
2. Maintain a warm, enthusiastic, and respectful attitude.
3. Involve the client in the teaching-learning process as fully as possible. Emphasize active participation.
4. Utilize and build on the client's previous experiences.
5. Emphasize the practical application of the learned material to the client's lifestyle and immediate solution to problems.
6. When necessary, assist the client with unlearning poor habits or negative attitudes.
7. Time learning according to the client's needs.
8. Individualize the teaching-learning transaction, even if standardized teaching plans are used.
9. Identify what the client wants to learn first; this can then lead to additional learning.
10. Emphasize helping the client to learn, not just transmitting subject matter.
11. Allow the client to pace his own learning when possible.
12. Keep information relevant to the client's needs and goals.

Evaluation

Evaluation is the final step in the teaching-learning process, and is a measure of the degree to which the client has mastered the learning objectives. The nurse must be aware of the performance level of the client so that changes can be made as needed. The nurse may find that the client has achieved his goals; however, if certain goals were not reached, the nurse may need to develop a new teaching plan. If the client has developed *new needs*, the nurse will want to plan new goals, content, and strategies.

For example, recently an elderly male diabetic client entered the hospital with a blood sugar of 550 mg/dL. When the student nurse began to prepare his insulin injection, the head nurse asked, "Are you going to have him give his own insulin and observe his technique?" "Oh, no," replied the student nurse, "He has been a diabetic for 20 years!" The assumption was, of course, that a diabetic would certainly know how to perform this task correctly. The two nurses returned to the client's room and asked him to draw up his injection. They were astonished to see the client fill the syringe with 20 units of insulin and 20 units of air, instead of 40 units of insulin! After correcting the dosage and questioning the client more fully, the nurses concluded that the client could not accurately see the markings on the syringe; they believed that the client may have been administering insufficient insulin to himself for a long period of time. The client's vision was not as good as it had been 20 years ago—*his needs had changed*—and special equipment was now necessary for him to safely and accurately administer his insulin.

Short-term evaluation techniques

Evaluation techniques may be short-term or long-term. *Short-term evaluation techniques* may involve the client and nurse, the client's family, significant others, and/or members of the health care team. You may quickly evaluate the client's mastery of a skill or behavior change in one or more of the following ways:

1. Observing the client directly. "Show me how you will change your dressing." "Let me see how you administer your injection." By observation, the nurse determines if a task has been mastered, if further instruction is needed, or if the client is ready for new or additional content.
2. Observing verbal and nonverbal clues. If the client asks questions, asks you to repeat instructions, shakes his head, loses eye contact, slumps or droops in his chair or bed, becomes restless and fidgety, or otherwise expresses doubt about his understanding, he is indicating that further instruction is needed or a different approach should be taken. Be alert. Watch and listen to your client carefully for correct evaluation.
3. Asking the client direct questions. "What are the four major food groups?" "How often must you change your dressing?" "What are the warning signs of a heart attack?" Be sure to ask questions that require more than a "yes" or "no" answer.
4. Using a written measurement tool (a test, essay, or list) which can be graded for accuracy. Remember, however, that written tests tend to bring about or increase anxiety in adult clients and therefore may not produce accurate evaluation. Often, adult clients will "freeze" when given a test, or they "go blank" when asked to write something that they know will be graded. Assess the client's learning style before using this evaluation method.
5. Talking to the client's family, culture group members, group leaders, or other health professionals who are in contact with him (Fig. 5-8). "Is he eating regularly?" "How is he handling his walker?" "Did he participate in the group discussion?" Since the nurse cannot be with the client 24 hours a day, she must utilize other people who visit or assist the client.
6. Helping the client evaluate his own progress. What evidence does he have that he is reaching his objectives? How does he feel: confident or unsure? Apprehensive or ready to go forward with new material? The main thrust with this technique is to determine whether or not the client believes that he has control of the procedure.[14]

These short-term techniques should be used frequently and interchangeably to keep informed of the client's progress and his changing needs.

Long-term evaluation techniques

Long-term evaluation requires follow-up by the nurse, the care facility, or an outside agency. The nurse's role is to impress the client with the need for regular reevaluation by someone familiar with the client's needs. The nurse should set up a schedule of visits for the client before he leaves the hospital or clinic, or refer the client to the proper agencies. In addition, the nurse should keep accurate records for follow-up telephone calls or written reminders to urge the client to maintain his schedule. The client's family may also be familiarized with the follow-up procedures so that everyone is involved in the client's long-term progress.

The nurse must take the initiative in contacting persons or agencies involved in the client's follow-up. Telephone, visit, or write these health professionals and request updated information on the client's prog-

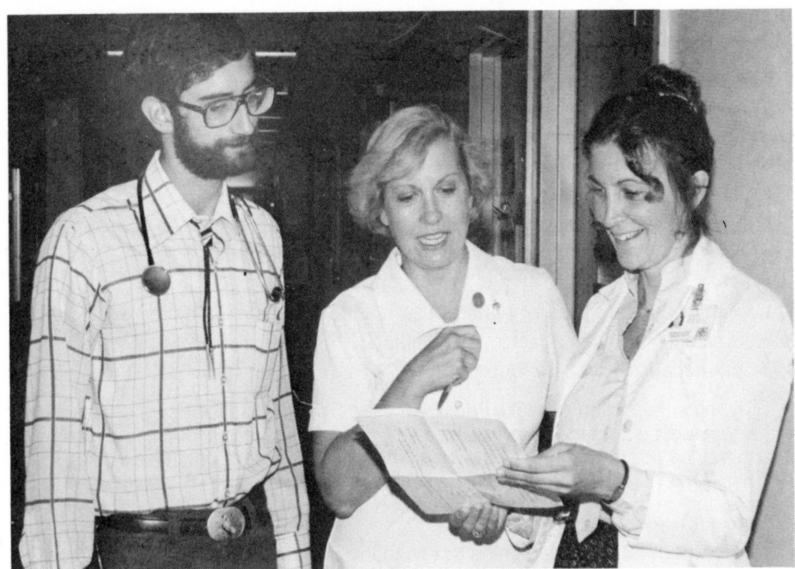

Figure 5-8 Health team members should cooperate in evaluating client progress.

ress. These data should be added to the client's records for future use.

Documentation is an essential component of the entire teaching-learning transaction. The nurse must record everything from the assessment through evaluation and must record each follow-up contact in detail. The documentation should be forwarded to the agency which will provide long-term follow-up for the client. Since many different members of the health care team will need to examine these records on many different shifts, in many different places, and for many different reasons, the teaching objectives, content, strategies, and evaluation results should be written as clearly and completely as possible. Health team members should be encouraged to add comments and observations to these records, and conferences should be held whenever possible to review the teaching-learning plan.

The use of *standardized teaching plans* for common major illnesses and surgeries has become an accepted method for developing a teaching plan. Standardized teaching plans contain widely accepted knowledges, understandings, and skills that a client needs to know concerning a specific medical illness or a surgical procedure. The nurse should, of course, individualize these plans to meet the specific client's needs.

Teaching the adult client in an acute-care setting is a challenging and rewarding experience for the nurse. It should be seen as a dynamic process that begins when you first see your client, continues with each contact day by day, and remains an integral part of the client's care over months and years. The following case study illustrates many of the principles related to client education discussed in this chapter.

Case Study / Example of the Teaching-Learning Process

Mr. B. was recently admitted to the hospital with a diagnosis of a gastric ulcer. Upon admission the nurse worked to develop a climate of trust with Mr. B. by answering his questions, making sure he felt as comfortable as possible in the environmental setting, ensuring his physical comfort, and maintaining an unhurried attitude.
Assessment revealed the following:

Age: 48
Occupation: Engineer, with Ph.D., recently promoted to department head.
Marital Status: Separated for last 6 months. In the process of filing for divorce.
Family: No history of ulcer; father recently diagnosed with cancer of the prostate, mother, healthy; sister is a radiologist; brother has a Ph. D. in counseling. States that family is close.
Diagnosis: Bleeding gastric ulcer

Treatment: Regular diet
Maalox 30 mL prn for gastric discomfort
Cimetidine (Tagamet) 300 mg qid with meals and at bedtime
Diazapan (Valium) 5 mg. qid
Resources: Daughter, 17 years old, who lives with Mr. B. One very close male friend who has been a support through the separation.
Learning Style: Learns best by personal reading followed by discussion. Enjoys informal learning rather than formal classroom experiences. Enjoys learning via television and in a one-to-one relationship.

Mr. B. states he is interested in learning and is assessed by the nurse as being physically and psychologically ready to participate in the learning process, e.g., alert, without pain, low anxiety at this time.

Mr. B. identified the following learning needs:

1. Causes of a gastric ulcer. He states that he already understands the anatomy and physiology of the GI tract.
2. How alcohol influences gastric secretions.
3. The therapeutic effects of Tagamet.

The nurse identified possible additional needs of Mr. B. as the need to discuss current stressors, methods to reduce stress, and side effects of Maalox, Tagamet, and Valium. Mr. B. agreed that these areas be included in the teaching plan. (*Note:* Many other areas could be included in the plan. The areas listed are only a sampling.)

Since Mr. B.'s daughter was a significant resource regarding meal planning, alcohol consumption, and possible stressors, her presence at some of the teaching-learning sessions was agreed upon.

Identified Learning Objectives:

Following the teaching-learning sessions I will be able to:

1. Describe to the nurse 3 causes of a gastric ulcer.
2. Discuss the major effects of alcohol on gastric secretions and the gastric mucosa with the nurse.
3. Describe the interactions of alcohol and Tagamet and Valium to the nurse with 90 percent accuracy.
4. Identify the therapeutic effects of Tagamet from a list with 90 percent accuracy.
5. Identify possible stressors in my life to Dr. M., a psychologist, after three consultations.
6. Discuss two ways to reduce stress in my life to Dr. M.
7. Demonstrate two relaxation techniques to the nurse.

Principles of the teaching-learning process implemented in the teaching-learning plan for this client (see table below) are as follows:

1. Motivation was enhanced by Mr. B identifying his needs, being actively involved in the teaching-learning plan, and by experiencing success in the learning process.
2. Mr. B. was able to review and practice the information by experiencing a variety of strategies for the presentation of material, e.g., pamphlet, video, discussion, return demonstration.
3. Lifestyle may need adaptation to incorporate good eating habits and elimination of alcohol. Follow-up is needed through the nurse practitioner in Mr. B.'s doctor's office.
4. Instructional periods need to be centered around adequate rest periods plus an assessment of any drowsiness, decreased mental orientation, or an increase in depression due to Valium.
5. Relaxation techniques need to be carried into the occupational setting, i.e., exercises that can be done while sitting at a desk or during lunch or coffee breaks.
6. Pamphlets—larger print for the middle-aged adult; reading level can be fairly advanced for Mr. B.
7. Slide-tape should be in a quiet, private setting, e.g., conference room or patient education room.

Sample Teaching Plan

Objectives	Content	Strategy	Evaluation
1. Describe to the nurse three causes of a gastric ulcer.	☐ Brief review of anatomy and physiology of the GI tract. ☐ Discussion of theories behind the development of a gastric ulcer. ☐ Discussion of psychogenic factors of a gastric ulcer.	☐ Pamphlet, "The Gastric Ulcer," developed by the hospital patient education department. ☐ Slide-tape, "Possible Causes of a Gastric Ulcer," developed by the hospital media center. ☐ Discussion with nurse to clarify information and answer questions related to pamphlet and slide-tape.	☐ Able to describe to nurse at least three theories related to the development of a gastric ulcer.

Sample Teaching Plan (Continued)

Objectives	Content	Strategy	Evaluation
2. Discuss the major effects of alcohol on gastric secretions and the gastric mucosa with the nurse.	☐ Physiologic effects of alcohol on gastric secretions.	☐ Slide-tape, "Possible Causes of a Gastric Ulcer." ☐ Discussion with the nurse over content.	☐ Able to describe the effects of alcohol on the gastric secretions and gastric mucosa.
3. Describe the interactions of alcohol, Tagamet, and Valium to the nurse with 90 percent accuracy.	☐ Specific potentiating effects of antihistamines, tranquilizers, and alcohol.	☐ One-on-one discussion with clinical pharmacist concerning interactions of alcohol and certain medication.	☐ Can state why alcohol should not be combined with tranquilizers and antihistamines.
4. Identify the therapeutic effects of Tagamet from a list with 90 percent accuracy.	☐ Therapeutic effects of Tagamet.	☐ Pamphlet on Tagamet developed by the hospital pharmacy. ☐ Article from the AJN on Tagamet. ☐ Discussion with the nurse on the therapeutic effects of Tagamet.	☐ From a list developed by the hospital pharmacy will be able to select the therapeutic effects of Tagamet.
5. Identify from a list the side effects of Tagamet, Valium, and Maalox.	☐ Side effects of Valium, Tagamet, and Maalox.	☐ Pamphlets on Tagamet, Valium, and Maalox developed by the hospital pharmacy. ☐ Discussion with the clinical pharmacist over these side effects. ☐ Follow-up discussion with the nurse.	☐ From a list developed by the hospital pharmacy will be able to select out the side effects of Tagamet, Valium, and Maalox.
6. Identify possible stressors in my life to Dr. M. after three consultations.	☐ Possible stressors in my life.	☐ Discussions with Dr. M. ☐ Follow-up discussions with the nurse if desired.	☐ Will be able to identify several causes of stress in my life.
7. Discuss two ways to reduce stress in my life to Dr. M.	☐ Alternatives for reducing stress in my life.	☐ Discussion with Dr. M. ☐ Follow-up discussion with the nurse.	☐ Identify and implement ways to reduce stress.
8. Demonstrate two relaxation techniques to nurse.	☐ Relaxation techniques and how they work. ☐ How to do relaxation exercises.	☐ Pamphlet on relaxation. ☐ Video-tape that illustrates relaxation techniques. ☐ Demonstration by nurse of relaxation techniques. ☐ Return demonstration by Mr. B. of relaxation techniques.	☐ Will be able to demonstrate two relaxation techniques to the nurse.

REVIEW QUESTIONS

The number of the question corresponds to the same numbered objectives at the beginning of the chapter.

1. Common characteristics of the adult learner include
  a. Learning is necessary for the development of the individual as an independent person.
  b. Readiness to learn is based on a need to learn.
  c. The adult learner is dependent on others in the learning process.
  d. The individual who is to learn is basically a passive recipient in the learning process.

2. Considering the factors contributing to successful teaching, which of the following statements is true?
  a. The nurse should decide what is relevant to the topic.
  b. Long-term goals should be accomplished within 7 days.
  c. Expectations are set when the learner's speed is determined.
  d. Privacy is important to a successful teaching plan.

3. The first step in the teaching-learning process is
  a. evaluation
  b. implementation
  c. assessment
  d. setting objectives

4. By identifying certain personality characteristics of the client, the nurse is incorporating principles from which dimension?

a. biophysical
b. psychological
c. sociocultural
d. environmental

5. Which learning objective listed below is properly written?
   a. The client will demonstrate ROM.
   b. The client will learn how to do a dressing change.
   c. The client will demonstrate to the nurse the correct technique for deep breathing and coughing.
   d. The client will be able to discriminate between foods high in sodium and foods low in sodium.

6. All the following are active learning strategies for the client except the
   a. lecture
   b. group discussion
   c. demonstration/return demonstration
   d. role playing

7. Methods of short-term evaluation include all the following except
   a. observing nonverbal cues during a demonstration
   b. asking a direct question
   c. questioning by the follow-up agency personnel
   d. talking to other staff members regarding client knowledge

8. An advantage of group teaching over individual teaching is
   a. it is useful for rapid learning
   b. it translates descriptive material into actual practice
   c. it allows practice in carrying out thoughts, ideas, or decisions
   d. it encourages peer teaching and self-help

REFERENCES

1. Malcolm Knowles, *Modern Practice of Adult Education*, Associated Press, New York, 1970, p. 39.
2. B. Redman, *The Process of Patient Teaching in Nursing*, The C. V. Mosby Company, St. Louis, 1976, pp. 138–143.
3. A. Knox, *Adult Development and Learning*, Jossey-Bass Publishers, San Francisco, 1978, p. 410.
4. Ibid., p. 410.
5. F. Storlie, *Patient Teaching in Critical Care*, Appleton Century Crofts, New York, 1975, p. 14.
6. Knox, op. cit., p. 423.
7. Redman, op. cit., p. 44.
8. J. R. Kidd, *How Adults Learn*, Follett Publishing Company, Chicago, 1973, p. 44.
9. R. Murray and J. Zentner, *Nursing Concepts for Health Promotion*, Prentice-Hall, Inc., Englewood Cliffs, N.J., 1975, pp. 123–124, 332, 343.
10. Robert F. Mager, *Preparing Instructional Objectives*, Pitman Learning, Inc., Belmont, Calif., 1975, 1962.
11. E. S. Popiel, *Nursing and the Process of Continuing Education*, The C. V. Mosby Company, St. Louis, 1976, pp. 100–107; B. K. Redman, *The Process of Patient Teaching in Nursing*, The C. V. Mosby Company, St. Louis, 1976, pp. 138–159; J.R. Verduin, Jr., et al., *Adults Teaching Adults*, Learning Concepts, Austin, Texas, 1977, pp. 125–130.
12. Redman, op. cit., pp. 138–143.
13. Knowles, op. cit., pp. 39–51.
14. M. Murray, *Fundamentals of Nursing*, Prentice-Hall, Inc., Englewood Cliffs, N.J., 1976, pp. 241–242.

BIBLIOGRAPHY FOR SECTION 1

Books

Bates, B.: *A Guide to Physical Examination*, 2d ed., J. B. Lippincott Company, Philadelphia, 1979.

Birmingham, J. J.: *The Problem-Oriented Record: A Self-Learning Module*, McGraw-Hill Book Company, New York, 1978.

Bower, F. L., and E. O. Bevis: *Fundamentals of Nursing Practice*, The C. V. Mosby Company, St. Louis, 1979.

———: *The Process of Planning Nursing Care: A Model for Practice,* 2d ed., The C. V. Mosby Company, St. Louis, 1977.

Brammer, L. M.: *The Helping Relationship: Process and Skills*, Prentice-Hall, Inc., Englewood Cliffs, N.J., 1979.

Burgess, A. W.: *Nursing: Levels of Health Intervention*, Prentice-Hall, Inc., Englewood Cliffs, N.J., 1978.

Burnside, I., et al.: *Psychosocial Caring Throughout the Life Span*, McGraw-Hill Book Company, New York, 1979.

Byrne, M. L., and L. F. Thompson: *Key Concepts for the Study and Practice of Nursing*, 2d ed., The C. V. Mosby Company, St. Louis, 1978.

Carroll, L.: *Alice's Adventures in Wonderland and Through the Looking Glass*, 8th printing; Collier Books, The Macmillan Company, New York, 1973.

Combs, A. W., E. L. Avila, and W. W. Purkey: *Helping Relationships*, 2d ed., Allyn and Bacon, Inc., Boston, 1978.

DeGowin, E., et al.: *Diagnostic Examination,* 3d ed., The Macmillan Company, New York, 1976.

Diekelmann, N.: *Primary Health Care of the Well Adult*, McGraw-Hill Book Company, New York, 1977.

Folta, J. R., and E. S. Deck: *A Sociological Framework for Patient Care*, 2d ed., John Wiley & Sons, Inc., New York, 1979.

Fromer, M. J.: *Community Health Care and the Nursing Process*, The C. V. Mosby Company, St. Louis, 1979.

Gillies, D., et al.: *Patient Assessment and Management by the Nurse Practitioner*, W. B. Saunders Company, Philadelphia, 1976.

Goodnow, M.: *Outlines of Nursing History*, 6th ed., W. B. Saunders Company, Philadelphia, 1938.

Gunderson, E. K., and R. H. Rahe (eds.): *Life Stress and Illness*, Charles C Thomas, Springfield, Il., 1974.

Henderson, V.: *The Nature of Nursing*, The Macmillan Company, New York, 1966.

Hengenhan, B. R.: *An Introduction to Theories of Learning*, Prentice-Hall, Inc., Englewood Cliffs, N.J. 1976.

ICN: *Basic Principles of Nursing Care*, Geneva, International Council of Nurses, 1972.

Jaco, E. G. (ed.): *Patients, Physicians and Illness*, 3d ed., The Free Press, New York, 1979.

Knowles, M.: *Informal Adult Education*, Associated Press, New York, 1961.

Malasanos, L., et al.: *Health Assessment*, The C. V. Mosby Company, St. Louis, 1977.

Marriner, A.: *The Nursing Process*, 2d ed., The C. V. Mosby Company, St. Louis, 1979.

Maslow, A.: *Motivation and Personality*, Harper & Row Publishers, Incorporated, New York, 1954.

Murray, M.: *Fundamentals of Nursing*, Prentice-Hall, Inc., Engelwood Cliffs, N.J., 1976.

Murray, R., and J. Zentner: *Nursing Assessment and Health Promotion Through the Life Span*, 2d ed., Prentice-Hall, Inc., Englewood Cliffs, N.J., 1979.

Mechanic, D.: *Medical Sociology*, 2d ed., The Free Press, New York, 1978.

Nightingale, F.: *Notes on Nursing: What it is and What it is Not*, facsimile edition, J. B. Lippincott Company, Philadelphia, 1946.

Rider, J., et al.: *Nursing: A Human Needs Approach*, Houghton Mifflin Company, Boston, 1977.

Rines, A. R., and M. L. Montag: *Nursing Concepts and Nursing Care*, John Wiley & Sons Inc., New York, 1976.

Rogers, C.: *Freedom to Learn*, Charles E. Merrill Publishing Company, Columbus, Ohio, 1969.

Rogers, D.: *The Adult Years: An Introduction to Aging*, Prentice-Hall, Inc., Englewood Cliffs, N.J., 1979.

Roy, Sr C.: *Introduction to Nursing: An Adaptation Model*, Prentice-Hall, Inc., Englewood Cliffs, N.J., 1976.

Sackett, D. L., and R. B. Haynes: *Compliance with Therapeutic Regimens*, The Johns Hopkins University Press, Baltimore, 1976.

Sana, J. M., et al.: *Physical Appraisal Methods in Nursing Practice*, Little, Brown and Company, Boston, 1975.

Schuster, C., and S. Ashburn (eds.): *The Process of Human Development: A Holistic Approach*, Little, Brown, and Company, Boston, 1980.

Selye, H.: *Stress Without Distress*, Signet Books, New York, 1974.

Sherman, J., et al.: *Guide to Patient Evaluation*, 2d ed., Medical Examination Publishing Co., Inc., New York, 1976.

Smith, D., et al.: *The Biological Ages of Man: From Conception through Old Age*, 2d ed., W. B. Saunders Company, Philadelphia, 1978.

Spector, R. E.: *Cultural Diversity in Health and Illness*, Appleton Century Crofts, New York, 1979.

Stevenson, J.: *Issues and Crises During Middlesence*, Appleton Century Crofts, New York, 1977.

Sundeen, S., et al.: *Nurse-Client Interaction: Implementing the Nursing Process*, The C. V. Mosby Company, St. Louis, 1976.

Tofler, A.: *Future Shock*, Bantam Books, New York, 1972.

Wu, R.: *Behavior and Illness*, Prentice-Hall, Inc., Englewood Cliffs, N.J., 1973.

Yura, H., and M. B. Walsh: *The Nursing Process: Assessing, Planning, Implementing, Evaluating*, Appleton Century Crofts, New York, 1978.

Periodicals

Baer, E., M. N. McGowan, and D. O. McGivern: "How to Take a Health History," *Am J Nurs*, **77**:7 (1977).

Becker, M. H.: "The Health Belief Model and Sick Role Behavior," *Nurs Digest*, 35–40, Spring 1978

Borland, D.: "Research on Middle Age: An Assessment," *The Gerontologist*, **18**(4):379 (1978).

Dayani, E.: "Concepts of Wellness," *Nurse Practitioner*, **4**(1):31 (January–February 1979).

Dunn, H. L.: "High-Level Wellness for Man and Society," *Am J Public Health Nation's Health*, **49**:786–792 (1959).

Eggland, E. T.: "How to Take a Meaningful Nursing History," *Nursing 77*, **7**:7 (1977).

Evans, S. K.: "Descriptive Criteria for the Concept of Depleted Health Potential," *Advances in Nursing Science*, **1**(4):67 74, (July 1979).

Falk, G., and U. Falk: "Sexuality and the Aged," *Nurs Outlook*, **28**(1):51 (1980).

Ford, L. C.: "Influencing Health Values," *Health Values*, **1**(1):17–22 (January–February 1977).

Gressow, Z., and G. S. Tracy: "The Role of Self-Help Clubs in Adaptation to Chronic Illness and Disability," *Nurs Digest*, 23–31 (Spring 1978).

Holmes, T. H., and R. H. Rahe: "Social Readjustment Rating Scale," *J Psychosomatic Res*, **II**:213–218 (1967).

Johnson, E., and B. Bursk: "Relationships Between the Elderly and Their Adult Children," *The Gerontologist*, **17**(1):90 (1977).

Lawerence, S. A., and R. M. Lawerence: "A Model of Adaptation to the Stress of Chronic Illness," *Nurs Forum*, **18**(1):33–42 (1979).

Lore, A.: "Supporting the Hospitalized Elderly Person," *Am J Nurs*, **79**(3):496 (1979).

McDaniels, C.: "Leisure and Career Development in Mid-Life: A Rationale," *The Vocational Guidance Quarterly*, **344**: 7 (June 1977).

Milco, N.: "A Framework for Prevention: Changing Health-Damaging to Health-Generating Life Patterns," *Am J Public Health*, **66**:(5) 435–439 (May 1976).

Tessler, R., and D. Mechanic: "Psychological Distress and Perceived Health Status," *J Health and Social Behavior*, **19**:254–262 (1978).

Treas, J.: "Family Support Systems for the Aged: Some Social and Demographic Considerations," *The Gerontologist*, **17**(6):486 (1977).

Weed, L.: "Medical Records, Medical Education and Patient Care, The Press of Case Western Reserve University, Cleveland, 1970.

Wiedenbach, E.: "The Helping Art of Nursing," *Am J Nurs*, **63**:54–57 (1963).

Organizations

Administration on Aging
U.S. Department of Health, Education and Welfare
Washington, D.C. 20201

American Association of Industrial Nurses (AAIN)-1942
79 Madison Avenue
New York, NY 10016
Official publication: *Occupational Health Nursing*

American Association of Nurse Anesthetists (AANA)-1931
111 East Wacker Drive
Chicago, IL 60601
Official publication: *The Journal of the American Association of Nurse Anesthetists*

American Association of Retired Persons
1909 K Street N.W.
Washington, D.C. 20049

American Nurses' Association (ANA)-1897
2420 Pershing Road
Kansas City, MO 64108
Official publication: *American Journal of Nursing*

Association of Operating Room Nurses (AORN)-1957
10170 East Mississippi Avenue
Denver, CO 80231
Official publication: *AORN Journal*

Concern for Dying
250 West 57 Street
New York, NY 10019

International Council of Nurses (ICN)
87 Rue de Vermont
1202 Geneva, Switzerland
Official publication: *International Nursing Review*

National Black Nurses' Association (NBNA)-1971
P.O. Box 8295
Canton, OH 44711

National Council on Aging
1828 L Street N.W.
Washington, D.C. 20036

National League for Nursing (NLN)-1952
10 Columbus Circle
New York, NY 10019

National Student Nurses Association (NSNA)-1953
10 Columbus Circle
New York, NY 10019
Official publication: *Imprint*

Nurses' Coalition for Political Action (N-Cap)-1974
2420 Pershing Road
Kansas City, MO 64108

Sigma Theta Tau - 1922
1232 West Michigan, Room 347
Indianapolis, IN 46202
Official publication: *Image*

The American Association for Nephrology Nurses and Technicians (AANNT)-1969
Middle City Station, P.O. Box 2368
Philadelphia, PA 19103

The American Association of Neurosurgical Nurses (AANN)-1968
428 East Preston Street
Baltimore, MD 21203
Official publication: *The Journal of Neurosurgical Nursing*

The American College of Nurse Midwives (ACNM)
50 East 92 Street
New York, NY 10028
Official publication: *The Journal of Nurse Midwifery*

The Nurses' Association of the American College of Obstetricians and Gynecologists (NAACOG)-1969
1 East Wacker Drive, Suite 2700
Chicago, IL 60601
Official publication: *Journal of Obstetric, Gynecologic and Neonatal Nursing*

Section 2

The Surgical Experience

Chapter 6

NURSING ROLE IN MANAGEMENT

Preoperative Client

Susan N. Walker

Learning Objectives

1. Identify common purposes and types of surgery.
2. Describe the psychosocial nursing assessment of the preoperative client.
3. Interpret the significance of data related to the preoperative client's health status and operative risk.
4. Identify the baseline nursing data to be recorded preoperatively as a basis for postoperative management.
5. Explain the characteristics of a voluntary and informed consent for surgery.
6. Describe the nursing role in the psychological and instructional preparation of the client for surgery.
7. Describe the nursing role in the physical preparation of the client for surgery.
8. Explain the rationale for preoperative medical and nursing management.

Surgery is any procedure that involves entry into the human body. It is usually performed with instruments. It is estimated that more than 15 million people undergo surgery in the United States each year.[1] Surgery may be done for any of the following reasons:

Diagnosis—Example: lymph node biopsy or exploratory incision (laparotomy)

Cure—Example: removal of diseased part or total hip replacement to restore function of lower limb

Palliation—Example: cutting a nerve root (rhizotomy) to remove symptoms of pain, or creating an artificial anus (colostomy) to alleviate bowel obstruction

Cosmetic improvement—Example: repairing a burn scar or changing breast shape (mammoplasty)

Specific suffixes are commonly used in combination with identifying a body part or organ in naming of surgical procedures (Table 6-1).

Surgery may be a carefully planned and anticipated event in the life of an individual. Sometimes, the need for surgery may arise with sudden and unanticipated urgency (Table 6-2). Both emergency and elective surgery may be performed in a hospital operating room, emergency room, doctor's office, or a clinic. The setting in which a surgical procedure may safely and effectively be done is influenced by the extent of the surgery, the possible complications, and the general condition of the client.

This chapter was reviewed by Patricia Robertson Hercules, R.N., M.S., Assistant Director—Operating Rooms, The Methodist Hospital, Houston, Texas.

The nurse plays a significant role in preparing the client for surgery, in maintaining surveillance of the client during surgery, and in preventing complications and facilitating recovery following surgery. To perform this role effectively, the nurse must have certain basic information. First, she must know the individual client's response to a stressful situation. Secondly, the nature of the disorder requiring surgery and of any coexisting disease processes must be established. Thirdly, results of appropriate diagnostic measures done preoperatively must be assessed. Lastly, the bodily alterations, risks, and possible complications associated with the surgical procedure must be considered.

The preoperative nursing measures included in this chapter are those which are applicable to any client in preparation for elective surgery. Specific measures in preparation for particular surgical procedures (such as intestinal, thoracic, or orthopedic surgery) are covered in other chapters. When a client

Table 6-1
Suffixes Describing Surgical Procedures

Suffix	Meaning	Example
-ectomy	Excision or removal of	Appendectomy
-lysis	Destruction of	Electrolysis
-orrhaphy	Repair or suture of	Herniorrhaphy
-oscopy	Looking into	Endoscopy
-ostomy	Creation of permanent opening into	Colostomy
-otomy	Cutting into or incision of	Tracheotomy
-plasty	Repair or reconstruction of	Mammoplasty

Table 6-2
Types of Surgery According to Need

Type	Example
Emergency	
1. Immediate (without delay)	Ruptured aortic aneurysm Gunshot wound Acute appendicitis Epidural hematoma
2. Urgent (within 24–48 hours)	Ureteral calculi Bleeding uterine fibroids Obstructed duodenal ulcer
Elective	
1. Required (within weeks or months)	Cataract extraction Benign prostatic hypertrophy Chronic cholecystitis
2. Recommended	Simple hemorrhoids Rectocele or cystocele Simple hernias
3. Optional or cosmetic	Facelift Rhinoplasty Breast plastic operations

Adapted from R. E. Rothenberg, *The Complete Surgical Guide*, Simon and Schuster, New York, 1974, pp. 6–7.

is to undergo emergency surgery, the nurse must establish priorities and include the essential preparation possible in the situation. While nursing assessment and intervention are discussed separately in this chapter, they are more realistically done simultaneously in practice.

ASSESSMENT OF THE PREOPERATIVE CLIENT

Psychosocial Assessment

Surgery, even when planned well in advance, is a physically traumatic experience which elicits the stress response. This is a desirable mechanism which enables the body to adapt and heal in the postoperative period.[2] However, fear and anxiety are also stressors. If they become excessive, they can magnify the stress response to such an extent that it becomes harmful and actually interferes with recovery. The nurse who is aware of a client's fears and anxieties will be able to provide support and information during the preoperative period so that stress will not become distress.

Common fears related to surgery

Fear of pain and discomfort is nearly universal. It includes concern about feeling pain during as well as after surgery. The nurse can reassure the client that surgery will not begin before anesthesia has taken effect and that adequate anesthesia will be maintained throughout the procedure. The nurse can encourage the client to talk with the anesthetist or anesthesiologist for further clarification. The nurse can help the client who fears postoperative pain by emphasizing the availability of drugs for pain relief. This is more effective than detailing the nature of the pain to be anticipated.

Fear of the unknown is also extremely common. It is based on lack of information about what to expect during the surgical experience as well as on the uncertainty about the outcome of surgery. The dread of cancer, so prevalent in our society, often contributes to this fear, both when the surgery is for diagnostic purposes as well as when the diagnosis is known. The client may have developed totally unrealistic expectations of what surgery will be like. This may be a result of his own past experience or the vicarious experiences provided by friends' stories and the mass media, especially television. The nurse can relieve the client's fear of the unknown by providing accurate, specific information about what to expect. The surgeon should be informed if the client requires any additional information.

Fear of mutilation or alteration of body image may be a factor, not only when radical surgery or amputation is to be performed, but also in much less extensive surgery. The prospect of one's blood being shed is anxiety-provoking to some persons. The presence of even a small scar on the body is abhorrent to others. An individual's body image and perception of a threat to it are unique. The nurse must listen to and assess the client's concern about this area with an open, nonjudgmental attitude.

Fear of death may be greater when the client knows that he or she has a malignancy or is a poor surgical risk. However, it may be experienced by others for even minor procedures. Surgery may be postponed if the client is convinced that he will not survive it. Attitude and emotional state are known to influence the surgical outcome.[3] The nurse should inform the surgeon if a client expresses such a fear.

Fear of anesthesia may include concern about an unpleasant induction or aftereffects, about hazards or complications (such as brain damage or paralysis), or about loss of control while under its influence. The nurse can reassure the client that anesthesia does not have the effect of "truth serum." The client also needs to know that it is not usual for persons to reveal their deepest secrets while under anesthesia. The anesthesiologist can provide detailed information about what the client can expect to experience with the particular agent(s) to be employed.

Fear of disruption of life pattern may be present in varying degrees. It may range from the person who fears permanent disability to the person who is concerned about not being able to play golf for a few weeks. Concerns about separation from family and about how spouse or children are managing are frequent. Financial concerns may be related either to an anticipated loss of income or to the costs of hospitalization.

Meaning of surgery to the client

Information about how each client perceives the surgical experience should be obtained. This information can be gathered by the nurse during the admission nursing interview as well as throughout the ongoing nurse-client relationship. Since the preoperative client is usually admitted to the hospital only 24 hours or less before surgery, it is essential that the initial nursing interview be purposeful and goal-directed. Areas to be covered include:

1. Previous experience with surgery or hospitalization
2. Client's knowledge of need for this surgery
3. Present symptoms or discomforts
4. Questions or concerns about planned surgery or recovery
5. Cultural (including religious) beliefs and practices which may affect surgery or nursing care
6. Occupation and nature of work and responsibilities
7. Health insurance coverage and other economic implications of surgery and recuperation
8. Usual means of dealing with stress (or crisis)
9. Sources of emotional support (including significant others)

Physiological Assessment

The preoperative period is used by both the physician and the nurse (1) to determine the adequacy of the client's health status to undergo the proposed surgery, (2) to identify and correct (if possible) any risk factors, and (3) to establish baseline data for comparison in the postoperative period. Table 6-3 shows the purpose of the diagnostic tests which are usually performed on preoperative clients. In some hospitals, the fasting blood sugar (FBS), blood urea nitrogen (BUN), and electrocardiogram (ECG) are only done when the client is over age 40. Additional tests may be done as indicated by the client's health status or for the planned surgical procedure.

Table 6-3
Routine Preoperative Diagnostic Tests

Diagnostic Test	To Detect
Urinalysis	Urinary tract infection Renal disease Diabetes
Chest x-ray	Pulmonary disease Cardiac enlargement
Blood studies	
RBC, Hb, Hct,	Anemia
WBC, Differential	Infection Reduced immune response
Prothrombin or partial thromboplastin time	Bleeding tendencies
Fasting blood sugar (FBS)	Diabetes
Blood urea nitrogen (BUN)	Renal disease
Electrocardiogram	Cardiac disease Electrolyte abnormalities

Health status and operative risk

The degree of operative risk may be affected by many psychological or physiological conditions of the client. However, it is particularly influenced by the factors of (1) age, (2) nutritional status, (3) respiratory status, (4) cardiovascular status, (5) renal and hepatic status, and (6) use of medication.

Age Advancing age may increase operative risk and the nurse must be particularly vigilant when caring for the elderly surgical client. Elderly clients are more likely to have multiple organ degenerative diseases, including many of the risks described below. They are also more apt to be dehydrated and thus have less reserve adaptation to fluid loss during surgery. The elderly are more sensitive to central nervous system depressants used during the surgical experience such as analgesics, sedatives, and anesthetics. They require a reduced dose of these drugs and should be observed for the untoward reaction of excitement when they are used. Despite these cautions, the healthy elderly client often tolerates even extensive surgery well when carefully managed.

Nutritional Status Assessment of nutritional status includes recognition of two problems which can increase operative risk: obesity and nutritional deficiencies. Obesity makes access to the surgical site more difficult and thus prolongs the surgery. It predisposes the client to wound dehiscence, wound infection, and incisional herniation. This occurs because adipose tissue impairs approximation of the wound edges and is less vascular than other tissues. Inhalation anesthetia is absorbed and stored by adipose tissue and then released postoperatively. Therefore, the obese client requires more anesthetic and recovers more slowly from its effects. Nutritional deficiencies of protein and vitamins C and B complex are particularly significant, since each of these substances is essential for wound healing. Surgery may be postponed until weight is reduced or deficiencies corrected.

Respiratory Status Assessment of respiratory status includes detection of both acute and chronic problems. The presence of an upper respiratory infection usually results in postponement of surgery. A history of respiratory allergy should be communicated to the anesthesiologist. It may increase the risks associated with inhalation anesthesia. Chronic obstructive lung disease impairs the client's gas exchange during and after surgery and also predisposes him to pulmonary infection and obstruction. The client who smokes should be encouraged to abstain preoperatively, but may find this difficult during a time of heightened anxiety. Both clients who smoke and those with chronic lung disease may receive pulmonary measures preoperatively, including intermittent positive pressure breathing (IPPB) and postural drainage in addition to the usual breathing and coughing instruction.

Cardiovascular Status Assessment of cardiovascular status is particularly focused on detection of angina, recent myocardial infarction, hypertension, or congestive heart failure. Each of these conditions may increase operative risk. Clients with recognized arrhythmias may be monitored electrocardiographically during and after surgery. Those on digitalis therapy will have serum potassium levels carefully watched to avoid toxicity. The presence of dehydration or anemia may require correction with fluid therapy or blood transfusion preoperatively. Blood typing and cross matching are done on many clients, so that compatible blood will be available for transfusion should this be necessary during or after surgery.

Renal and Hepatic Status Renal and hepatic status are of concern since many anesthetics and adjunctive drugs are detoxified by the liver and excreted by the kidneys. The kidneys also regulate fluid and electrolyte balance and eliminate metabolic wastes during the postoperative period. Chronic liver disease may be accompanied by bleeding tendencies as well as by poor wound healing and increased susceptibility to infection.

Use of Medications A careful history of medication use is essential to preoperative assessment. This should include drugs used for recreational as well as therapeutic purposes. Regular use of many prescription or nonprescription drugs may result in an increased operative risk:

1. *Steroids* may impair the body's ability to respond to the stress of anesthesia and surgery, and may mask symptoms of postoperative infection.
2. *Anticoagulants* and *salicylates* may increase bleeding during surgery.
3. *Antibiotics* may be incompatible with anesthetic agents.
4. *Tranquilizers* potentiate the effect of narcotics and barbiturates and cause hypotension.
5. *Antihypertensives* may predispose to shock by reducing blood pressure.
6. *Diuretics* may produce potassium deficiency which is also produced by the stress of surgery.

Chronic alcohol abuse also increases the operative risk (Chap. 60). It is often accompanied by impaired nutrition or liver disease, which are hazardous as described above. The alcoholic should also be observed for decreased effectiveness of pain medication and for delirium tremens during the postoperative period.

Clients using digitalis preparations or insulin may need their dosages individually adjusted during the operative period. Clients with diabetes mellitus are usually placed on sliding scale insulin in the immediate postoperative period (Chap. 41).

Recording of baseline nursing data

In addition to participating in the assessment of the client's health status and operative risk, the nurse records preoperative baseline data about the client to be used for comparison during the postoperative period. Observations may be recorded on a form designed for the purpose (Fig. 6-1) or in the nursing notes.

Such information, along with that obtained in the admission nursing interview, is extremely important for the nurses in the recovery room and on the postoperative nursing unit. It enables them to more accurately evaluate the client's postoperative status and to individualize postoperative care. Helpful data include a record of vital signs (including peripheral pulses),

PREOPERATIVE ASSESSMENT FORM TO PROVIDE BASELINE FOR POSTOPERATIVE EVALUATION

Directions: Complete this form 1-2 days before surgery. Circle appropriate words and fill in blanks. Comment when necessary. To go with patient to OR and to become part of bedside nursing record in postoperative unit.

Name: Doe Jane Hospital # 000 000 Age: 50 Date: 8-1-73

Preoperative Diagnosis: RHD c̄ MS, MI, AS, AI Angina Pectoris
post mitral commissurotomy (1966) venous ligation (1948)

VITAL SIGNS (indicate range): EKG: NSR c̄ 1° block

Blood Pressure	80/70 - 110/70		
Apical Pulse	60-80	(regular)	irregular 2 pillow
Respiration	18-24	normal	noisy (orthopneic) dyspneic irregular
Cough		(none)	occasional frequent dry productive
Temperature	97 (po) pr		
Weight	122 lbs		
SKIN: Color		(average) pale	dusky cyanotic (where) ______ jaundiced
Condition		(no problem)	bony areas redness decubitus rash (where) ______
NEUROLOGICAL STATUS:			
Consciousness		(conscious)	semi-conscious comatose
Orientation		(oriented)	disoriented to: time place person
Paralysis/Weakness		none	(present) (where) slight (L) eyelid ptosis
Pupils		equal (reactive)	(unequal) (R larger) L larger unreactive R L
Speech		(clear)	slurred
Handed		(right) left	
GENERAL INFORMATION:			
Emotional Status		normal anxiety	* (high anxiety) no apparent anxiety
Vision		(adequate)	decreased blind R L glasses contacts
Hearing		(adequate)	decreased R L deaf R L hearing aid
Dentures		none	upper lower (full) partial
Language		(speaks English)	speaks ______
Allergies		none	allergic to cardiac cath dye → V tach; adhesive tape → rash

COMMENTS (additional information, requests by patient, other prostheses, etc.):

* very anxious - seems hyper - c/o insomnia - says she feels "deathly afraid" - worried about blood clots and chest tube falling out
would like dentures when able
varicosities both legs
propensity → dig. toxicity

Completed by: E. Winslow M. Fuhs R.N.

Figure 6-1 Preoperative assessment for postoperative evaluation. *(E. H. Winslow and M. F. Fuhs, "Preoperative Assessment for Postoperative Evaluation," Am J Nurs,* ***73:****1373, August 1973.)*

allergies, nutritional and integumentary status, neurological status, vision and hearing, and speech and language.

NURSING MANAGEMENT OF THE PREOPERATIVE CLIENT

Legal Preparation: The Operative Permit

Before nonemergency surgery can be legally performed, the client must sign a *voluntary* and *informed consent* in the presence of a witness.[4] This document serves to protect not only the client but also the surgeon, the hospital, and its employees. While the responsibility for obtaining consent is ultimately the surgeon's, it is often the nurse who obtains and witnesses the client's signature on a permit such as the one in Fig. 6-2.

If consent is to be voluntary, the client must not be persuaded or coerced in any way in deciding to undergo the procedure. The nurse who stands at the bedside while the client reads the permit or who offers a pen along with the permit, may inadvertently be applying pressure for the client to hurry and sign it. A far better approach is to leave the client alone to read the permit in an unhurried atmosphere. Return after a

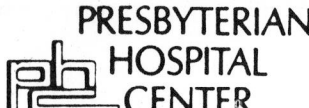

1. This check list shall be completed and placed in front of the chart for each patient, in-patient and out-patient, and shall accompany him/her to surgery.
2. Each item shall be checked and initialed by the person completing the step, when not applicable, dash and initial.
3. Final checking of the list is the responsibility of the charge nurse.
4. This form becomes a permanent part of the chart.

	✓	INITIAL
Identification Band Secured on Patient		
Check First and Last Name		
Check Birthdate		
Check Hospital Number		
Prep Done		
Time Voided or Catheterized — Charted		
Bathed and Charted		
Enema and/or Douche if Ordered — Given and Charted		
Mouth Care Given		
Pre-op TPR BP Time Charted		
Height and Weight — Out Patients Only		
Pre-Op Medication Given and Charted		
Allergies Determined, Charted and Taped to Face of Chart		
Clean Hospital Gown and Disposable Cap on All Underclothing Removed — Except on Children		

INSTRUCTIONS TO PATIENT AND FAMILY

	✓	INITIAL
NPO — Record Last Intake if Out-Patient		
Waiting Room		
Recovery Room		
Deep Breathing Exercises		
Side Rails Up		
Patient to Remain in Bed		
No Smoking		
Call Light in Reach		
Bed in Low Position		

INSTRUCTIONS TO PATIENT AND FAMILY (cont.)

	✓	INITIAL
Any Sign of Cold, Cough, Sore Throat Or Elevated Temperature		
Gum and/or Pacifiers Removed		
Surgical Stockings — Ace Bandage Applied		
Excess Eye Makeup Removed		
False Eyelashes Removed		

PROSTHESIS — NOTE ON FORM IF SENT HOME WITH FAMILY

	✓	INITIAL
Dentures in Patients Room — Labeled Container		
Upper Plate		
Lower Plate		
Partial Plate		
Fixed Bridge		
Contact Lenses Labeled Container — Patient's Own		
Glass Eye		
Artificial Limb(s)		
Other		

VALUABLES ENVELOPE

	✓	INITIAL
Rings and Watches Removed		
Release for Taping Signed (Release Form)		
Other (Wigs - Hearing Aid - Etc.) Itemize		
Money		
Billfold		
Credit Cards		
List if Out-Patient		
Checked by Name and Title		

THE FOLLOWING ARE TO BE IN THE PATIENTS' CHARTS

	✓	INITIAL
Laboratory and X-Ray Reports Including Routine Chest — If Indicated		
Routine Urinalysis		
Routine Hematology		
Proper Departments Notified if Test Not Completed		
Pathological Slips and Anesthesia Sheets Stamped		
Physician's Order Sheets with Adequate Space for Entries		
Progress Notes with Adequate Space for Entries		
Addressograph Plate Placed in Patient's Chart		
History and Physical for Oral Surgery		
Surgical Permits Signed		
Blood Typed and Crossmatched if Ordered		
Checked by		

This Equipment is to be in Patient's Room if Patient is not Sent to Recovery Room

Oral Suction Machine — I.V. Standard

B P Cuff and Stethoscope — Oxygen Mask and Gauge

PHC 040.4960

CHART

PREPARATION OF PATIENT FOR SURGERY - CHECK LIST

Figure 6-2 Operative permit. *(Courtesy of Presbyterian Hospital Center, Albuquerque, New Mexico.)*

brief time and ask if the client understands the permit or has any questions before signing. The client must also be mentally clear and competent at the time the consent is obtained. This includes freedom from the influence of any drugs which might affect rational thinking. Therefore, the permit should be signed before the client is given either analgesic or preanesthetic medication.

If consent is to be informed, two criteria must be met. First, the client must understand the nature of the surgery (including what, if any, organs are to be removed). Secondly, the client must be informed of the risks and benefits of the surgery (including possible complications as well as changes in body function). The client must be aware of available alternatives to the proposed surgery if a truly informed choice is to be made. Adequate time must be provided for the client to ask any questions before consenting. Even after signing the permit, the client must be made aware that permission may be withdrawn at any time. While the physician is responsible for providing the above explanations to the client, the nurse should determine that the client has received and understood them fully. If any confusion or doubt exists, the nurse should ask the physician to clarify further before having the client sign the permit.

The nurse plays a vital role as client advocate in ensuring that the consent for surgery is truly voluntary and informed. Fulfilling this role may present a difficult challenge. However, the extra effort is necessary and worthwhile.

Sometimes the client is a minor, unconscious, or mentally incapable of signing the written permit. In situations like this, the written permission may be signed by a responsible family member. In surgical procedures involving sterilization (e.g., vasectomy, tubal ligation) the spouse as well as the client may be required to sign the operative permit. Local hospital policies should be checked for further clarification on this matter.

Psychological Preparation

In preparing the client psychologically for surgery, the nurse must strike a balance between telling the client so little that he is unprepared and telling him so much that he is overwhelmed. The nurse who observes carefully and listens sensitively to the client will usually be able to determine how much information is enough in each instance.

A number of health team members participate in providing the client with information and instruction during the preoperative period. The admitting physician or surgeon is responsible for explaining the need for surgery and its nature during office visits prior to admission. In some instances, the client has not met the surgeon prior to hospitalization. The anesthesiologist or anesthetist visits the client on the day or evening before surgery. At this time, he writes the preanesthetic medication orders and explains plans for anesthesia to the client. In an increasing number of hospitals, the operating room nurse also makes a preoperative visit to offer information, assurance, and support in varying degrees. The operating room nurse may simply provide a face to be recognized when the client reaches the surgical suite or may participate extensively in the preoperative teaching detailed below. In addition, the client may be visited by a member of the clergy or by a spiritual counselor employed by the hospital.

The major responsibility for preparing the client for surgery generally falls to the staff nurse on the unit. It is this nurse who offers support and explanations, verifies that the client has understood information provided by other health team members, and instructs the client in specific activities to be done postoperatively.

Instructional Preparation

The positive values of preoperative teaching include reduction of (1) fear and anxiety, (2) postoperative vomiting, (3) use of pain medication, (4) number of complications, and (5) duration of hospitalization.[5-9] In addition, the client has a right to know what to expect and how to participate effectively during the surgical experience.

The principles of teaching and learning (Chap. 5) are applicable to the instruction of the preoperative client. The nurse should be particularly aware of the effect of anxiety upon learning and allow time for repetition and reinforcement, as well as for verification of the client's understanding. Preoperative instruction may be accomplished alone, in a group, or with a combination of these approaches. The nurse should consider choice of words carefully, stressing the positive whenever possible. The explanation that elastic stockings will be used to assist circulation during reduced activity is just as accurate and less alarming than saying that they are intended to prevent formation of blood clots. It is helpful to involve family members in teaching as well. This technique relieves their own concerns and engages their assistance in supporting and encouraging the client throughout the experience.

The areas to be covered in preoperative teaching are outlined in Table 6-4. In general, the client should be made aware of what will happen, when it will happen, why it is necessary, and how to participate

Table 6-4

Outline for Preoperative Teaching

About surgery and anesthesia
Nature and duration of surgery
Type of anesthesia
Time surgery scheduled
What to ask surgeon and anesthesiologist

What to expect the day before surgery
Skin prep
Enemas
Food and fluid restrictions
Bedtime sedation
Diagnostic measures (e.g., blood drawn, ECG)

What to expect on the day of surgery
Hygienic measures
Removal of cosmetics, dentures, etc.
Hospital attire
Care of possessions
Insertion of tubes (e.g., nasogastric, urinary)
Preoperative medications
Time to go to surgery
When family can visit
Where family can wait during surgery

What to expect after surgery
Recovery room stay (and intensive care unit if necessary)
Availability of analgesic
Equipment in use postoperatively (e.g., IV, oxygen, tubes and catheters, elastic stockings, dressings)

Postoperative preventive techniques
Deep breathing and coughing
Incisional splinting
Leg exercises
Turning in bed, getting out of bed, and ambulating

most therapeutically. When teaching the following postoperative preventive techniques, the nurse should first describe and demonstrate each technique. She then observes the client's return demonstration.

Deep breathing and coughing techniques

Deep breathing and coughing in the postoperative period help the client to eliminate inhalation anesthetics, to prevent alveolar collapse, and to move respiratory secretions to larger passages for expectoration. They should be done several times each hour during the immediate postoperative period.

The client should be instructed to practice deep breathing and coughing in a similar position (semi-Fowler's, flat in bed) that would be assumed after surgery. Because the sitting and standing positions allow maximum lung expansion, the client should also be encouraged to practice these breathing techniques when sitting at the side of the bed or ambulating.

Diaphragmatic or abdominal breathing is accomplished by inhaling slowly and deeply through the nose, holding the breath for a couple of seconds and then exhaling slowly but completely through the mouth. The client should place his hands lightly over the lower ribs and upper abdomen. This allows him to feel the abdomen rise during inspiration and fall during expiration.

Following four to six deep breaths, the client should cough deeply from the lungs rather than the throat. If secretions are present in the respiratory passages, deep breathing often will move them up to stimulate the cough reflex without any voluntary effort by the client and they can then be expectorated.

The client who is to have a thoracic or abdominal incision should also be shown how to splint it while deep breathing and coughing. This technique minimizes discomfort and increases willingness to carry out the respiratory exercises. Splinting may be accomplished in several ways by either the nurse or the client (Fig. 6-3).

Leg exercises

Leg exercises by the postoperative client help to facilitate venous return and prevent venous stasis. While any number of leg movements may be helpful, it is most important that the client rhythmically contract and relax the calf (gastrocnemius) and thigh (quadriceps) muscles to create a pumping action along the veins where thrombus formation is likely to occur. Gastrocnemius pumping is accomplished when the client alternately flexes and extends the ankle by pressing the feet against a footboard or the nurse's hands. Quadriceps setting is accomplished by pressing the back of the knee against the bed and then relaxing it. These should each be done about 10 to 12 times each hour.

Additional exercises which may be helpful, especially if the client is not allowed to ambulate immediately, are foot circles and hip and knee movements. The latter may prove too painful for the client who has an abdominal incision. These exercises are illustrated in Fig. 6-4.

Movement in bed and ambulation

The client will be expected to turn (usually from side to back to side) every hour postoperatively to prevent respiratory and circulatory complications. Preoperative practice using the side rails for assistance in turning is helpful. He should also practice getting out of bed to ambulate in a manner which minimizes strain on the incision and discomfort. One helpful technique is to turn on the side and then push up to a sitting position. Another technique is to raise

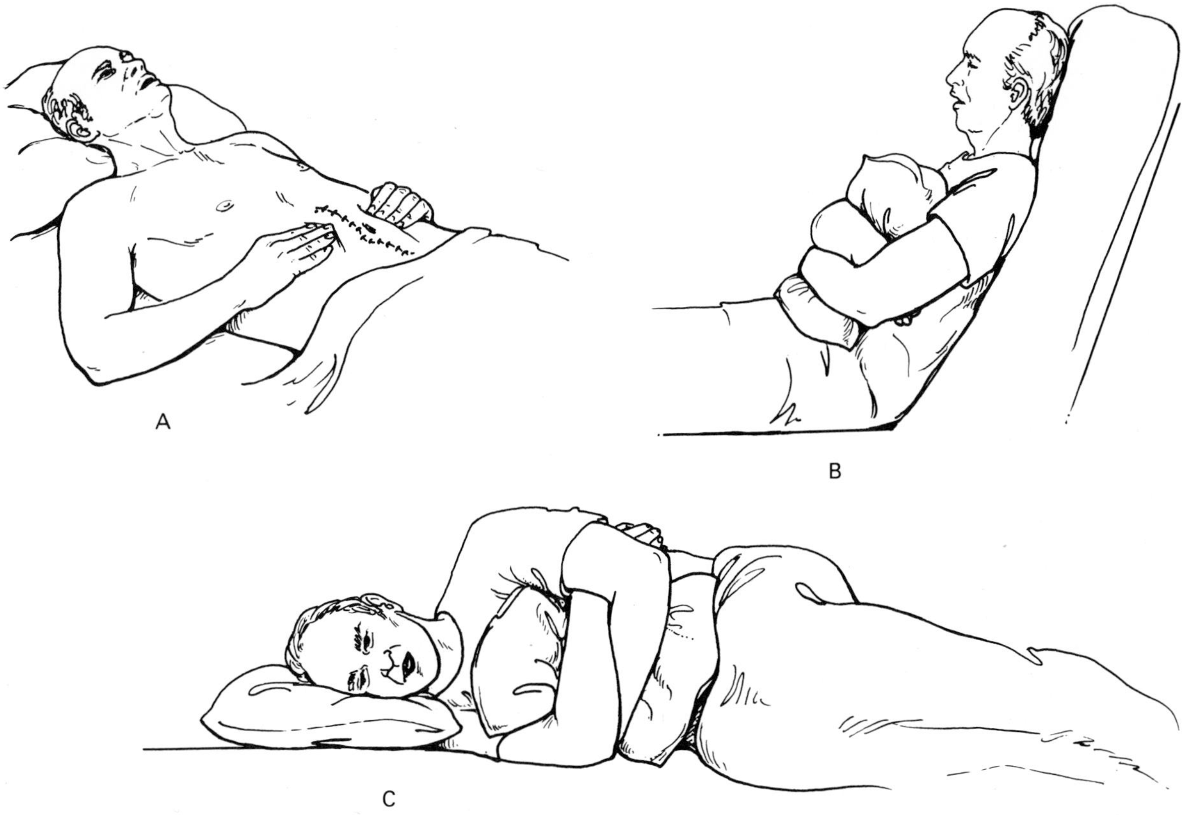

A

B

C

Figure 6-3 Techniques for splinting wound while coughing.

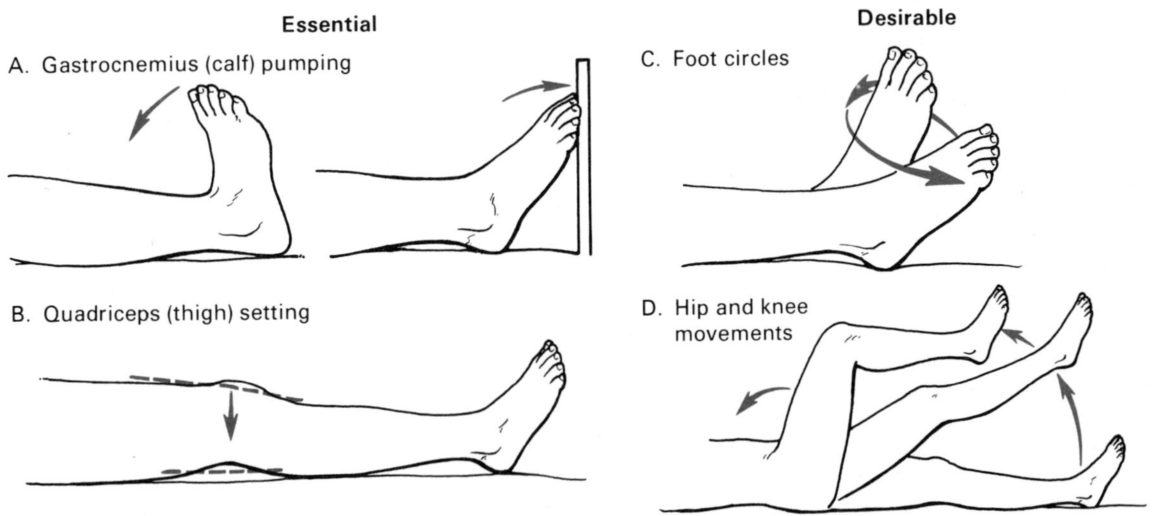

Figure 6-4 Postoperative leg exercises.

the head of the bed until sitting erect and then pivot the legs over the side of the bed.

The client should also be informed of his anticipated activity postoperatively. The trend is to ambulate clients on the day of surgery or the first postoperative day. If this will not be the plan, the client should know why.

Physical Preparation: The Evening Before Surgery

Physical preparation of the client for surgery is designed to minimize operative and postoperative risks and complications. Specific preoperative orders are written by the surgeon for each client. In many hospitals these orders automatically cancel any previous orders. The nurse needs to be alert for the inadvertent cancellation of therapies (e.g., drugs such as corticosteroids and antiarrhythmics) which should be continued throughout the surgical experience. If such an omission occurs, the physician should be notified.

Bowel elimination

A cleansing enema, small-volume hypertonic enema, or suppository may be ordered to empty the intestine before surgery. There are many reasons for emptying the bowel. It reduces the likelihood of involuntary defecation when sphincters relax under anesthesia. It collapses the bowel so that it will not obstruct access to abdominal organs or be nicked during abdominal surgery. It also prevents uncomfortable or even dangerous straining at stool during the first few days after certain operations (such as rectal, prostatic, or eye surgery). Bowel-elimination measures, if ordered, should be carried out well before bedtime so that they will not interfere with needed rest.

Skin preparation

Preparation of the skin at the surgical site is designed to reduce the number of microorganisms present as much as possible, while maintaining the skin in an intact and healthy condition to resist infection. These goals are usually accomplished by skin cleansing and hair removal over an extensive area surrounding the location of the planned incision (Fig. 6-5).

There is still considerable debate about how and when skin preparation is most effectively accomplished. Cleansing may involve simple washing with soap and water or more prolonged scrubbing with an antiseptic solution such as pHisoHex or Betadine. Hair removal is usually done by shaving with a safety razor. In some instances a depilatory cream may be used instead. Shaving is accompanied by the hazard of nicking the skin. Depilatories may produce skin irritation or rash, particularly when used in sensitive areas such as the groin or axilla. Any disruption of skin integrity is to be avoided. If a cut or skin irritation occurs, it should be recorded and reported.

When the skin prep is to be done the evening before surgery, it may be the responsibility of the staff nurse on the nursing unit or of a prep aide employed solely for that purpose. In some hospitals, the shave is delayed until the client is on the operating table. Lighting is best at this time and any nick incurred will not have the opportunity to harbor bacteria before surgery begins. In some instances, hair removal is omitted entirely in the belief that unshaven but clean skin is less likely to be associated with sepsis.

Hygienic measures

A bath or shower the evening before surgery not only cleanses the skin, but also may help the client to relax and sleep throughout the night. A shampoo is advisable at this time. It may be several days to a week before the client can again easily wash his hair. Depending upon the client's preference and the scheduled time of surgery, these activities may be deferred until morning.

Rest and sleep

A restful night's sleep before surgery is important so that the client will be in the best condition to withstand the surgical trauma and its aftermath. A hypnotic is usually given at bedtime to accomplish this goal. In addition, the nurse should employ all necessary comfort measures to ensure that the client falls asleep and stays asleep throughout the night.

Food and fluids

The client is usually kept NPO ("nothing by mouth") after midnight before surgery in order to ensure that the upper gastrointestinal tract will be empty. This reduces the possibility of vomiting and aspiration during anesthesia and postoperatively. Solid food must be withheld for a minimum of 6 hours before general anesthesia. Water is sometimes given up until 4 hours before surgery.

The client should be informed of these restrictions, encouraged to eat a nourishing supper, and to maintain a good fluid intake during the evening. Elderly or dehydrated clients may have an IV started to avoid a period without fluid intake. An NPO sign should be posted in a conspicuous place and all personnel informed of the restriction. Oral intake during the time of restriction could result in the delay of surgery.

Physical Preparation: The Day of Surgery

The nursing responsibility immediately before surgery includes final preparation of the client, as well as checking to determine that all orders have been carried out and that records are complete and ready to accompany the client to the operating room. The preoperative checklist (Fig. 6-6) provides an efficient and visible means for ensuring that no detail has been forgotten.

Hygiene and attire

The client should be awakened in time to complete morning care, including any hygienic measures not carried out the evening before. No cosmetics or nail polish should be worn. The color of skin, lips, and nail beds must be readily observable for indications of the adequacy of oxygenation during surgery. All prostheses, including dentures, wigs, and contact lenses, are generally removed to avoid loss or damage to them. Some anesthesiologists may prefer that dentures remain in place. Hairpins or clips are removed so that they will not accidentally injure the scalp or face. The client wears a hospital gown both for ease of access to the surgical site and to avoid staining or other damage to the client's own clothing. Caps and boots may also be required in some hospitals.

Care of valuables

All valuables, including jewelry and money, should be taken by the client's family or locked up securely according to agency policy. Their disposition should be recorded clearly.

If the client prefers not to remove a wedding ring, it may be securely tied with gauze which is then wrapped and fastened around the wrist. Adhesive or other tape is not used for this purpose since it may remove stones from their setting or be loosened by perspiration and slip off.

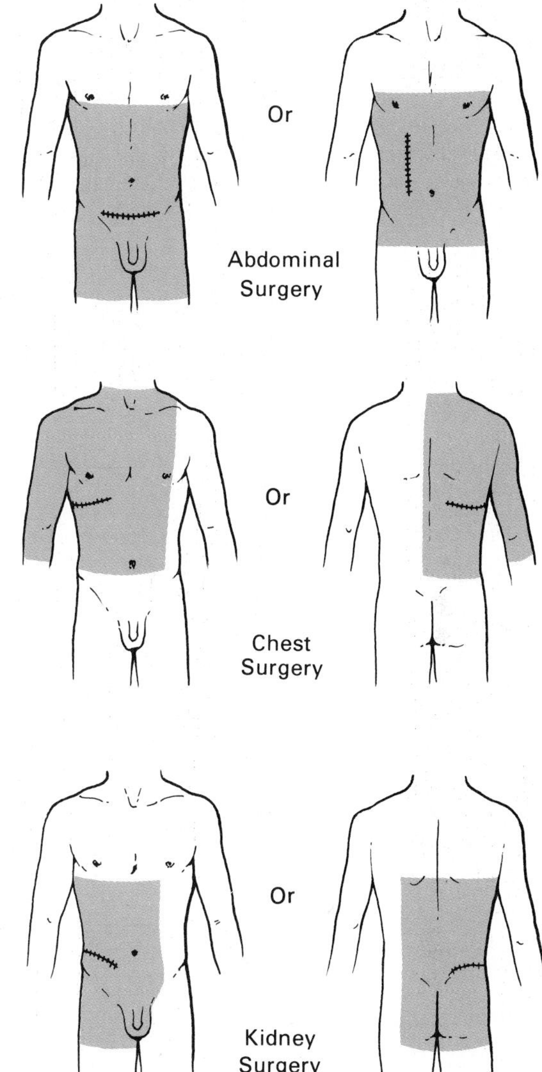

Figure 6-5 Areas for skin preparation in selected surgical procedures.

Completing the chart

The nurse should determine that all orders and procedures have been completed and recorded in the client's chart before giving the preanesthetic medication. This includes checking for the presence of a signed consent, a record of all consultations, baseline vital signs, diagnostic test results, and nurses' notes complete to that point.

Urinary elimination

The client should urinate immediately before being given preanesthetic medication. This prevents involuntary elimination under anesthesia, lessens the chance of accidental nicking of the bladder during surgery, and reduces the possibility of urinary retention during early postoperative recovery. When surgery is in the area of the bladder, as in gynecological procedures, an indwelling catheter may be inserted either preoperatively or in the operating room.

Preanesthetic medication

Preanesthetic medications are given either at a prescribed time 30 to 60 minutes before surgery, or "on call" when notified by the operating room. The on call procedure is used when many surgeries are planned in sequence in the same operating suite. The

CONSENT FOR MEDICAL PROCEDURE, FOR SURGERY
AND ACKNOWLEDGEMENT FOR RECEIPT
OF INFORMATION

Explanation

A physician obtains the patient's consent to surgery or medical procedure. You are asked to consent to an operation or a medical procedure and confirm that the operation or procedure has been explained to you, that you understand what is to be done, why it is necessary, and risks that may be involved. If you have any doubts or unanswered questions, do not sign this consent. The physician will be called.

Consent

The undersigned hereby requests and gives consent to Dr. ______________________
(Physician's name)

and assistants of his choice to perform or administer to ______________________
(Patient's name)

the following surgical or medical procedure for diagnosis or treatment: ______________________

____

____

and to do any procedure(s) that in the judgement of the above-named physician or his assistants may be deemed necessary or advisable on the basis of findings during the course of said operation or procedure. The consent also includes authority to administer any necessary medications or blood transfusions chosen by the physician or his assistants, and the disposal of any tissue removed.

Consent is also given for the administration of such anesthetics as are deemed necessary by the anesthetist as assigned.

The nature and purpose of this operation or medical procedure, possible alternative methods of treatment, the risks involved and the possibility of complications or unintended results have been explained. I acknowledge that no guarantee or assurance has been made as to the results that may be obtained.

I acknowledge that I have read and fully understand the above consent, the explanations referred to were made, and that all blanks or statements requiring insertion or completion were filled in before I affixed my signature.

Signature of Patient or
Patient's Representative ______________________

Witness ______________________

Date ______________________ Time ______________________ a.m./p.m.

Physician's Acknowledgement

I acknowledge that the medical procedure or surgery stated on this form was explained to the patient or his representative before the patient or his representative consented.

Physician's Signature ______________________

Patient Identification

PRESBYTERIAN HOSPITAL CENTER

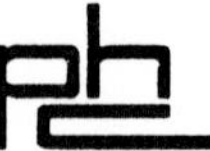

CONSENT FOR MEDICAL PROCEDURE, FOR SURGERY
AND ACKNOWLEDGEMENT FOR RECEIPT
OF INFORMATION

PHC 040.4950 (4-79)

Figure 6-6 Preoperative checklist. *(Courtesy of Presbyterian Hospital Center, Albuquerque, New Mexico.)*

operating room usually calls the unit about 30 to 60 minutes before the client's surgery is anticipated. The nurse needs to give the preanesthetic medication without delay as soon as she is notified so the medication can achieve its expected result. Preanesthetic drugs are designed to facilitate the administration of anesthesia and to reduce its risks (Table 6-5). The client usually receives an anticholinergic drug along with one or more central nervous system depressants (sedative, tranquilizer, or opiate).

These should be administered to the client in bed after all other preoperative preparation has been completed. The client should be told that they will help him to relax and feel drowsy without losing consciousness. He also needs to know that they will cause his mouth to feel dry. He should be instructed not to smoke or to get out of bed. Side rails should be raised. Family members may remain with the client until he is transferred to surgery. A quiet environment conducive to rest should be provided.

Transportation to the operating room

When operating room personnel arrive on the unit, the nurse assists in transfer of the client to a stretcher, covers him with a cotton blanket for modesty and warmth, raises the stretcher's side rails, and secures the safety belt(s). The nurse notes the time and mode of transfer in the chart and sends the chart, preoperative checklist, and any other required forms to the operating room with the client.

In many institutions, the family may accompany the client to the operating room suite. The nurse should make certain that any family members who are present at this time know where to wait during surgery and what to expect when the client returns.

During the client's absence, the nurse prepares

Table 6-5
Preoperative Medications (Anesthesia Adjunctive Drugs)

Drug Classification	Examples	Purpose and Effects
Sedatives		
Short-acting barbiturates	Sodium pentobarbital (Nembutal) Sodium secobarbital (Seconal)	Produces drowsiness and relaxation Facilitates anesthesia induction Permits less anesthesia to be used
Tranquilizers		
Phenothiazine-type (major tranquilizers)	Chlorpromazine (Thorazine) Prochlorperazine (Compazine)	Reduces anxiety and apprehension Smoother anesthesia induction Have antiemetic effect Potentiate action of narcotics and sedatives
Antianxiety agents (minor tranquilizers)	Diazepam (Valium) Hydroxyzine (Vistaril, Atarax)	
Opiates	Morphine Meperidine (Demerol) Levorphanol (Levo-Dromoran)	Induces euphoria Facilitates anesthesia induction Less anesthetic required
Anticholinergics		
Atropine-type drugs	Atropine Scopolamine	Reduces salivary and bronchial secretions Keeps respiratory passages clear and dry Makes inhalation of anesthesia easier Reduces hazard of atelectasis Blocks heart-slowing impulses from vagus nerve (atropine) Amnesic action blocks memory of pain or discomfort (scopolamine)

the room for his return by making up a surgical bed with a washable blanket for warmth. Additional plastic and cotton drawsheets are placed where drainage might occur. The nurse also brings any necessary additional equipment, such as an IV pole or suction machine, into the room. The furniture should be arranged so that the stretcher may easily be drawn alongside the bed when the client returns.

Case Study / Elective Surgery

Mrs. Gwendolyn Abbamonto, a 42-year-old elementary school teacher, is admitted to the hospital for an elective cholecystectomy. After several episodes of epigastric distress during the year, she consulted her family physician. X-rays revealed gallstones and she was referred to a surgeon who recommended surgery within a few months. She has chosen to have her surgery in June to allow time for full recuperation before returning to work in the fall. Her husband is taking 2 weeks' vacation to care for their children, ages 7 and 12.

Mrs. Abbamonto's previous hospitalizations were for a tonsillectomy at age 10 with open drip ether anesthesia and for delivery of her two children using the Lamaze psychoprophylactic method of childbirth. She smoked one pack of cigarettes a day until a year ago, when she stopped entirely.

Discussion Questions

1. What factors in Mrs. Abbamonto's background or personal situation may influence her emotional and physical reactions to this hospitalization and surgery?
2. What should she know if her consent to surgery is to be truly informed? How would you approach her to obtain her written consent?
3. In teaching her breathing exercises preoperatively what are the best techniques to use?
4. What measures would you expect to carry out on the evening before surgery? Why?
5. What measures would you expect to carry out on the morning of surgery? Why?

REVIEW QUESTIONS

The number of the question corresponds to the same numbered objective at the beginning of the chapter.

1. Which of these surgical procedures involves removal of a body organ?
   a. herniorrhaphy
   b. cholecystectomy
   c. mammoplasty
   d. colostomy

2. A nursing intervention to assist the client in coping with fear of pain would be to
   a. describe the degree of pain expected
   b. explain the availability of pain medication
   c. inform the client of the frequency of pain medication
   d. divert the client when talking about pain

3. More anesthesia may be required by the client who is
   a. dehydrated
   b. a smoker
   c. obese
   d. elderly

4. The range of preoperative vital signs should be recorded
   a. for all clients
   b. when general anesthesia is to be used
   c. if client has a history of cardiovascular disease
   d. when client is elderly

5. Mr. Jensen, an alert man of 75, is to undergo elective hip surgery. The operative permit must be signed in the presence of a witness by
   a. Mr. Jensen
   b. Mr. and Mrs. Jensen
   c. either Mr. or Mrs. Jensen
   d. Mr. Jensen and the surgeon

6. When teaching the preoperative client deep breathing techniques, the nurse should have him
   a. sit in a comfortable chair at the bedside
   b. keep abdominal muscles tight and flat while inhaling
   c. inhale through the nose and exhale through the mouth
   d. cough from the throat rather than from the lungs

7. Which measure should be done *last* on the morning of surgery?
   a. administer preanesthetic medication
   b. ask client to void in the bathroom
   c. remove jewelry and lock up securely
   d. check chart for signed consent form

8. The preoperative client is kept NPO after midnight in order to prevent
   a. overhydration or fluid overload postoperatively
   b. urinary incontinence in the operating room
   c. nicking of stomach or intestine during surgery
   d. vomiting and aspiration during anesthesia

REFERENCES

1. R. E. Rothenberg, *The Complete Surgical Guide,* Simon and Schuster, New York, 1974, p. 3.
2. M. B. Marcinek, "Stress in the Surgical Patient," *Am J Nurs,* **77:**1809–1811 (November 1977).

3. H. C. Polk, Jr., "Principles of Preoperative Preparation of the Surgical Patient," chap. 5 in *Davis-Christopher Textbook of Surgery,* D. C. Sabiston, Jr., W. B. Saunders Co., Philadelphia, 1977, p. 121.
4. L. B. Besch, "Informed Consent: A Patient's Right," *Nurs Outlook,* **27:**33 (January 1979).
5. R. G. Dumas and R. C. Leonard, "Effect of Nursing on the Incidence of Postoperative Vomiting," *Nurs Res,* **12:**12–15 (Winter 1963).
6. K. M. Healy, "Does Preoperative Instruction Make a Difference?" *Am J Nurs,* **68:**62–67 (January 1968).
7. C. A. Lindeman and B. VanAernam, "Nursing Intervention with the Presurgical Patient: Effects of Structured and Unstructured Preoperative Teaching," *Nurs Res,* **20:**319–332 (July–August 1971).
8. C. A. Lindeman, "Nursing Intervention with the Presurgical Patient: Effectiveness and Efficiency of Group and Individual Preoperative Teaching, Phase Two," *Nurs Res,* **21:** 196–209 (May–June 1972).
9. F. E. Schmitt and P. J. Wooldridge, "Psychological Preparation of Surgical Patients," *Nurs Res,* **22:**108–116 (March–April 1973).

Chapter 7

NURSING ROLE IN MANAGEMENT

Client During Surgery

Patricia Robertson Hercules
Barba Jean Edwards

Learning Objectives

1. Describe the physical environment of the operating room and the preoperative holding area.
2. Describe the functions of the members of the surgical team.
3. Explain activities of the operating room nurse in the preoperative and postoperative phases of the client's care.
4. Explain the nursing role during the intraoperative phase.
5. Describe basic principles of aseptic technique used in the operating room.
6. Differentiate between general and local anesthesia including methods, advantages and disadvantages, and rationale for administration.
7. Identify the basic characteristics of the methods and drugs used to achieve general anesthesia.
8. Discuss the various methods for administering local anesthesia.
9. Define the anesthetic mechanisms of controlled hypotension, hypothermia, cryoanesthesia, hypnoanesthesia, and acupuncture.

Nursing care of the surgical client requires understanding of the intraoperative phase of surgical care. This knowledge allows the nurse to monitor the client's response to the stressors related to the surgical experience. Utilization of the nursing process during the intraoperative phase is necessary as a framework for the delivery of care.

PHYSICAL ENVIRONMENT

Operating Room

The surgical environment is a unique acute-care setting removed from other hospital clinical units (Fig. 7-1). It is controlled geographically, environmentally, and bacteriologically and is restricted in terms of the inflow and outflow of personnel. Its physical location is preferably adjacent to the postanesthesia recovery area and surgical intensive care unit. This allows for close collaboration for postanesthesia recovery. Careful consideration of design, location, and control of the physical environment assists with the prevention of infection and provides physical safety and comfort for both the client and the operating room team.

Several methods are used to prevent the transmission of infection. Filters and controlled airflow in the ventilating systems provide dust control. Dust-collecting surfaces such as open shelves and ledges are omitted. Materials which are resistant to the corroding effects of strong disinfectants are used. The functional design lends ease to the practice of aseptic technique by the operating room team.

Physical safety and comfort are aided by the use of operating room furniture which is conductive, adjustable, easy to clean, and easy to move. Overhead and ancillary lighting and electrical plugs are explosion-proof. All equipment is checked frequently to ensure electrical safety. Humidity is regulated at 50 percent to prevent the accumulation of static electric sparks. The lighting is designed to provide a low- to high-intensity range for precise view of the surgical site. A communication system provides a means for the deliverance of routine and emergency messages.[1]

The temperature is controlled from 20 to 30°C (68 to 85°F) to ensure normothermia of the client. The higher ranges of temperature are used when large surgical areas are exposed (e.g., such as in abdominal or chest procedures). The lower ranges of temperature are used for most other types of procedures to ensure client comfort under the surgical drapes, team comfort during the procedure, and an environment which is unfavorable to bacterial incubation and growth.

The privacy of the client is achieved by a lack of windows and few doors to and from the room. The entire operating suite is restricted to the influx of hospital personnel and visitors. Special permission must be granted to enter during the surgical procedure.

This chapter was reviewed by Janice J. Arrott, CRNA, Supervisor, Department of Anesthesiology, University of New Mexico Hospital, Albuquerque, New Mexico.

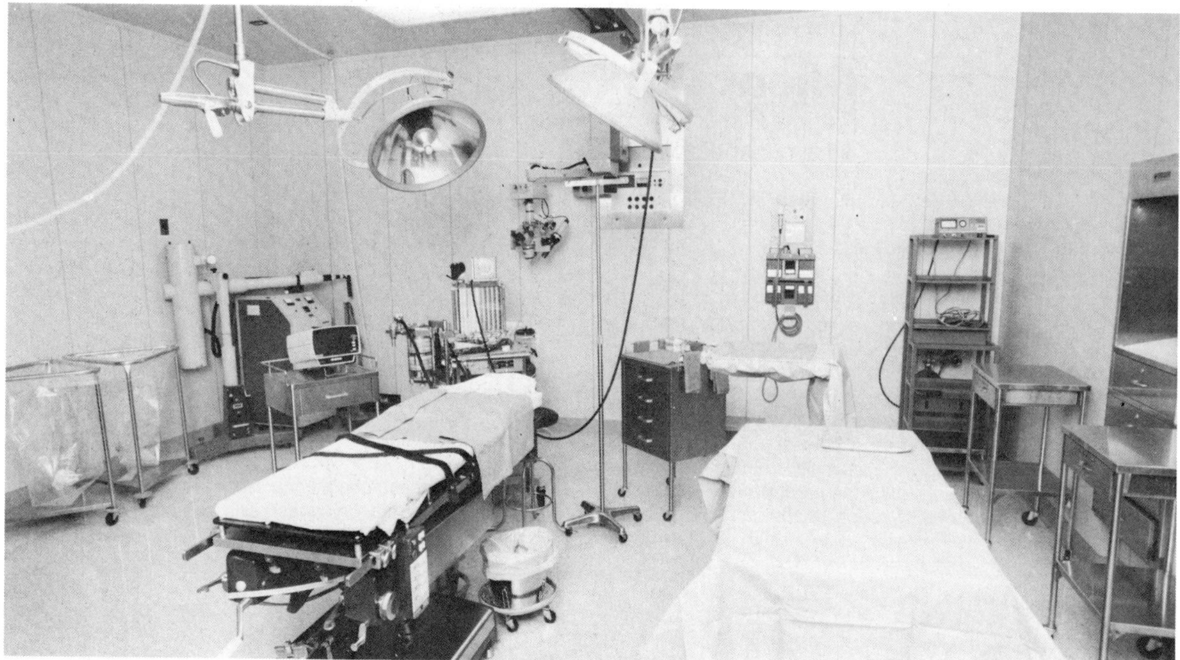

Figure 7-1 Physical environment of the operating room. *(Courtesy of The Methodist Hospital, Texas Medical Center, Houston, Texas.)*

Preoperative Holding Area

The preoperative holding area is a special waiting area outside the surgical suite. The size varies according to hospital design and can range from a centralized holding area to accommodate numerous clients to a small designated area immediately outside the actual room identified for the surgical procedure. In this area the operating room nurse makes the final identification and assessment before the client is transferred into the operating room for surgery.

Many institutions permit the family or a friend to accompany and wait with the client until it is time for him to be transferred to the operating room. Separation from loved ones at this time can be anxiety-producing.

HUMAN ENVIRONMENT: THE SURGICAL TEAM

When the client awaiting surgery is transported from the nonsurgical area to the preoperative holding area, usually the operating room nurse is the first member of the surgical team encountered. Along with the final assessment and necessary tasks prior to the surgery, this nurse provides physical comfort measures and assists in alleviating the client's anxiety.

Registered Nurse

The operating room nurse is a registered nurse who implements client care based on the nursing process. Two different roles may be assumed by the operating room nurse. Responsibilities of the nurse may involve either *sterile* or *nonsterile* activities depending on the role assumed for a particular surgery. If the nurse is not scrubbed, gowned, and gloved and remains in the unsterile field, the role of the *circulating nurse* is implemented. If the nurse follows the designated scrub procedure, gowns and gloves in sterile attire, and remains within the sterile field, the role of the *scrub nurse* is implemented. Specific task-oriented duties of each of these roles are outlined in Table 7-1.

However, the function of the operating room nurse is not limited to just these task-oriented duties. The operating room nurse actively implements nursing care in the preoperative, intraoperative, and postoperative phases of the surgical client's care. These three phases of client care are presented in the scope of practice developed by the Association of Operating Room Nurses as the Perioperative Role (Fig. 7-2). The nursing activities which characterize each of these phases are presented in Table 7-2. The *preoperative phase* begins with the decision to have surgery and ends when the client is transferred to the operating

Table 7-1
Duties of the Circulating Nurse and the Scrub Nurse

Circulating nurse
Reviews anatomy, physiology, and surgical procedures
Assists with preparing room
Practices aseptic technique
Monitors activities of others
Ensures that needed items are available and sterile (if required)
Checks mechanical and electrical equipment and environment factors
Arranges furniture in workable order
Identifies and assesses client
Checks chart and relates pertinent data
Admits client to operating room suite
Assists with transferring client to operating room bed
Protects client during induction with anesthesia
Positions client
Helps with insertion or application of monitoring devices
Preps client's skin for surgical incision
Monitors draping procedure and all activities requiring asepsis
Provides well-functioning suction
Completes intraoperative record
Records, labels, and sends to proper locations tissue specimens and cultures
Evaluates blood and fluid loss
Coordinates all activities in operating room between team members and other hospital departments
Counts sponges, needles, and instruments
Accompanies the client to postanesthesia recovery area
Reports pertinent information to recovery area nurses
Scrub nurse
Reviews anatomy, physiology, and surgical procedures
Assists with preparation of room
Scrubs, gowns, and gloves self and other members of surgical team
Prepares instrument table and organizes sterile equipment
Assists with draping procedure
Passes instruments to surgeon and assistants
Counts sponges, needles, and instruments
Monitors practices of aseptic technique
Keeps track of irrigation solution used for more accurate calculation of blood loss
Reports amount of local anesthetics and epinephrine solutions to anesthetist

room bed. The *intraoperative phase* begins with transference to the operating room bed and ends with admittance to the recovery area. The *postoperative phase* begins when the client is transferred to the recovery area and ends with a home or clinic evaluation.[2]

Licensed Vocational Nurse and Technician

In some institutions, the scrub nurse is a technically trained operating technician or a licensed practical nurse. Scrub nurses assist the surgeon by passing instruments during the surgical procedure. This role can also be assumed by a registered nurse.

Surgeon and Assistant(s)

The surgeon is the physician who assumes the responsibility for the surgical procedure. The surgeon may be the client's primary physician or one who was selected by the client's physician to collaborate with the primary physician. The surgeon is primarily responsible for:

1. Preoperative client assessment including need for surgical intervention, choice of surgical procedures, and management of preoperative workup.
2. Client safety and management in the operating room.
3. Postoperative management of the client.

The surgeon's assistant is a physician who functions in an assisting role during the surgical procedure. The assistant usually holds retractors to expose surgical areas and assists with hemostasis and suturing. In some instances, especially in educational settings, the assistant may perform some portions of the operative procedure under the direct supervision of the surgeon.

There are some institutions in which the surgeon's assistant is a nonphysician who is permitted to function in the role of the assistant. In these situations, role differentiation is defined according to hospital policy and physician responsibility.

Anesthesiologist and Nurse Anesthetist

The *anesthesiologist* is a medical doctor who has specialized in the field of anesthesia. The *nurse anesthetist* is a registered nurse who has also specialized in the field of anesthesia and has taken exams to become certified as a Certified Registered Nurse Anesthetist (CRNA). The anesthesiologist functions in the physician's role, whereas the CRNA functions within the realm of nursing. Both are qualified to administer anesthesia to the surgical client and assume the responsibility for the diminution of senses and cardiopulmonary homeostasis throughout the procedure.

Hospital policies vary regarding the responsibilities of the nurse anesthetist, depending on the availability of coverage by an anesthesiologist. Sometimes the surgeon assumes medical responsibility for the supervision of the nurse anesthetist. The responsibilities generally accepted for both the anesthesiologist and the CRNA are:

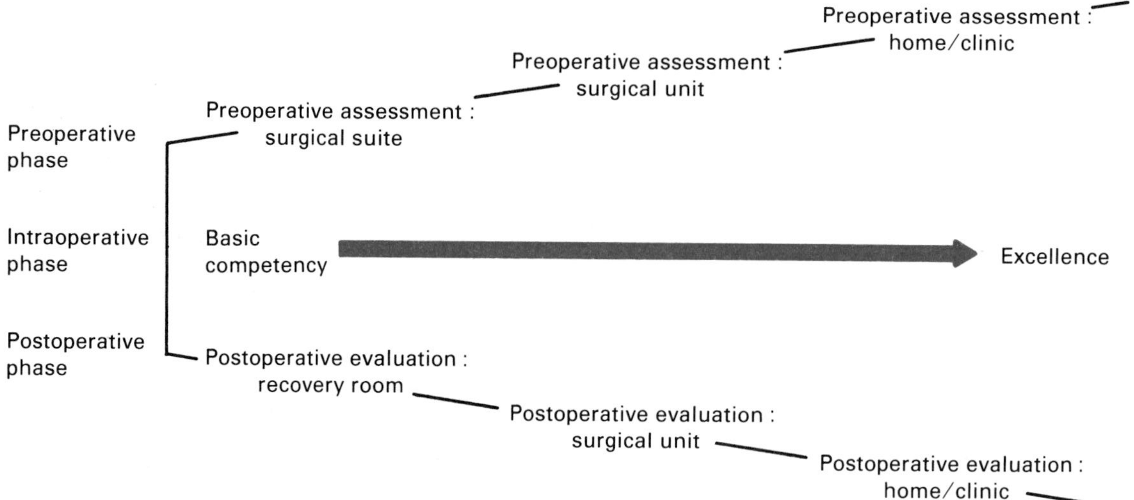

Figure 7-2 The perioperative role: A continuum. *(From "Perioperative Role," AORN J,* ***27:****1162–1165, 1978.)*

1. Assessing the client preoperatively to determine the safest anesthesia for the particular needs and operative procedure.
2. Administering the anesthesia during the surgical procedure and informing the surgeon if difficulties arise in the client's stability.
3. Administering fluids and electrolytes and medications throughout the surgical procedure.

The additional responsibilities of the anesthesiologist are generally:

1. Prescribing preoperative medications (Chap. 6).
2. Supervising the nurse anesthetist.
3. Supervising the postanesthesia recovery of the client.

In preparation for and carrying out the surgical procedure, each member of the surgical team (the circulating nurse, the scrub nurse, the surgeon, the assistant, and the anesthetist) collaborate to assure that the client is receiving the best possible care (Fig. 7-3).

NURSING INTERVENTIONS FOR THE SURGICAL CLIENT

Preoperative Phase

Assessment

The preoperative assessment of the surgical client establishes safe intraoperative and postoperative nursing care. Assessment data gathered by the nurse on the surgical unit were discussed in Chap. 6. The same information is pertinent to the nursing care implemented by the operating room nurse. Collaboration between the two nursing units is important so that continuity of client care will exist.

It is the responsibility of the operating room nurse to participate in the assessment process. When the data cannot be gathered on the surgical unit, they are acquired in the preoperative holding area of the surgical suite (Table 7-2). Components of information that specifically relate to intraoperative nursing care are explained in the next section.

Psychosocial Assessment The nurse who regularly implements nursing care in the operating room is knowledgeable about the activities which occur when the client is transferred into the surgical suite. This knowledge allows informative and reassuring explanations, especially to the fearful and frightened client.

Fear of the surgical procedure or anesthesia can be alleviated by the operating room nurse. Specific questions relating to details of the surgical procedure and anesthesia are referred to the surgeon or anesthetist. However, nondetailed questions regarding surgery or anesthesia should be answered by the operating room nurse. Examples of these questions might include: "When will I go to sleep?", "Who will be in the room?", "When will my doctor arrive?", "How much of my body will be exposed and to whom?", "Will I be cold?", and "When will I wake up?" Knowledge of hospital intraoperative routine is the data upon which to answer such general questions.

It is especially important that the operating room nurse have a knowledge of the client's spiritual and

Table 7-2
Examples of Nursing Activities in the Perioperative Role

Preoperative Phase	Intraoperative Phase	Postoperative Phase
Preoperative assessment Home/clinic 1. Initiates initial preoperative assessment 2. Plans teaching methods appropriate to client's needs 3. Involves family in interview Surgical unit 1. Completes preoperative assessment 2. Coordinates client teaching with other nursing staff 3. Explains phases in perioperative period and expectations 4. Develops a plan of care Surgical suite 1. Assesses client's level of consciousness 2. Reviews chart 3. Identifies client 4. Verifies surgical site **Planning** 1. Determines a plan of care **Psychological support** 1. Tells client what is happening 2. Determines psychological status 3. Gives prior warning of noxious stimuli 4. Stands near/touches client during procedures/induction 5. Communicates client's emotional status to other appropriate members of the health care team	**Maintenance of safety** 1. Assures that the sponge, needle, and instrument counts are correct 2. Positions the client a. Functional alignment b. Exposure of surgical site c. Maintenance of position throughout procedure 3. Applies grounding device to client 4. Provides physical support **Physiologic monitoring** 1. Calculates effects on client of excessive fluid loss 2. Distinguishes normal from abnormal cardiopulmonary data 3. Reports changes in client's pulse, respirations, temperature, and blood pressure **Psychological monitoring** (prior to induction and if client is conscious) 1. Provides emotional support to client 2. Continues to assess client's emotional status 3. Communicates client's emotional status to other appropriate members of the health care team **Nursing management** 1. Provides physical safety for the client 2. Maintains aseptic, controlled environment 3. Effectively manages human resources	**Communication of intraoperative information** 1. Gives client's name 2. States type of surgery performed 3. Provides contributing intraoperative factors, i.e., drain, catheters 4. States physical limitations 5. States impairments resulting from surgery 6. Reports client's preoperative level of consciousness 7. Communicates necessary equipment needs **Postoperative evaluation** Recovery area 1. Determines client's immediate response to surgical intervention Surgical unit 1. Evaluates effectiveness of nursing care in the OR 2. Determines client's level of satisfaction with care given during perioperative period 3. Evaluates products used on client in the OR 4. Determines client's psychological status 5. Assists with discharge planning Home/clinic 1. Seeks client's perception of surgery in terms of the effects of anesthetic agents, impact on body image, distortion, immobilization 2. Determines family's perceptions of surgery

Adapted from "Perioperative Role," *AORN J*, **27:**1165, 1978.

cultural habits and beliefs. Care must be taken that infringement upon the client's rights and privileges are not made without prior consent.

Physical Assessment Physical assessment data which are specifically important to intraoperative nursing care include baseline data such as vital signs, height, weight, age, allergic reactions, condition and cleanliness of skin, skeletal and muscle impairments, perceptual difficulties, level of consciousness, and any sources of pain or discomfort. Baseline vital signs are important when administrating drugs and anesthesia. These data provide a means to evaluate the effects of intraoperative medications. Height and weight guide the nurse regarding the width and length of the operating room bed. Age can indicate the need for extra warmth or cooling, as it can reflect the rate of basal metabolism. Allergic reactions can be avoided with such simple measures as a change in prepping solutions or the type of tape used with dressings. The condition and cleanliness of the skin guides the nurse in determining the amount and type of intraoperative skin prepping solutions, as well as alerting the team to the potential for infections due to open or closed skin lesions. A knowledge of skeletal and muscle impairments prevents injury to the client during positioning. Perception difficulty such as vision or hearing impairments will guide the nurse to alter communication techniques for adaptation to individual needs. Altered level of consciousness necessitates increased safety

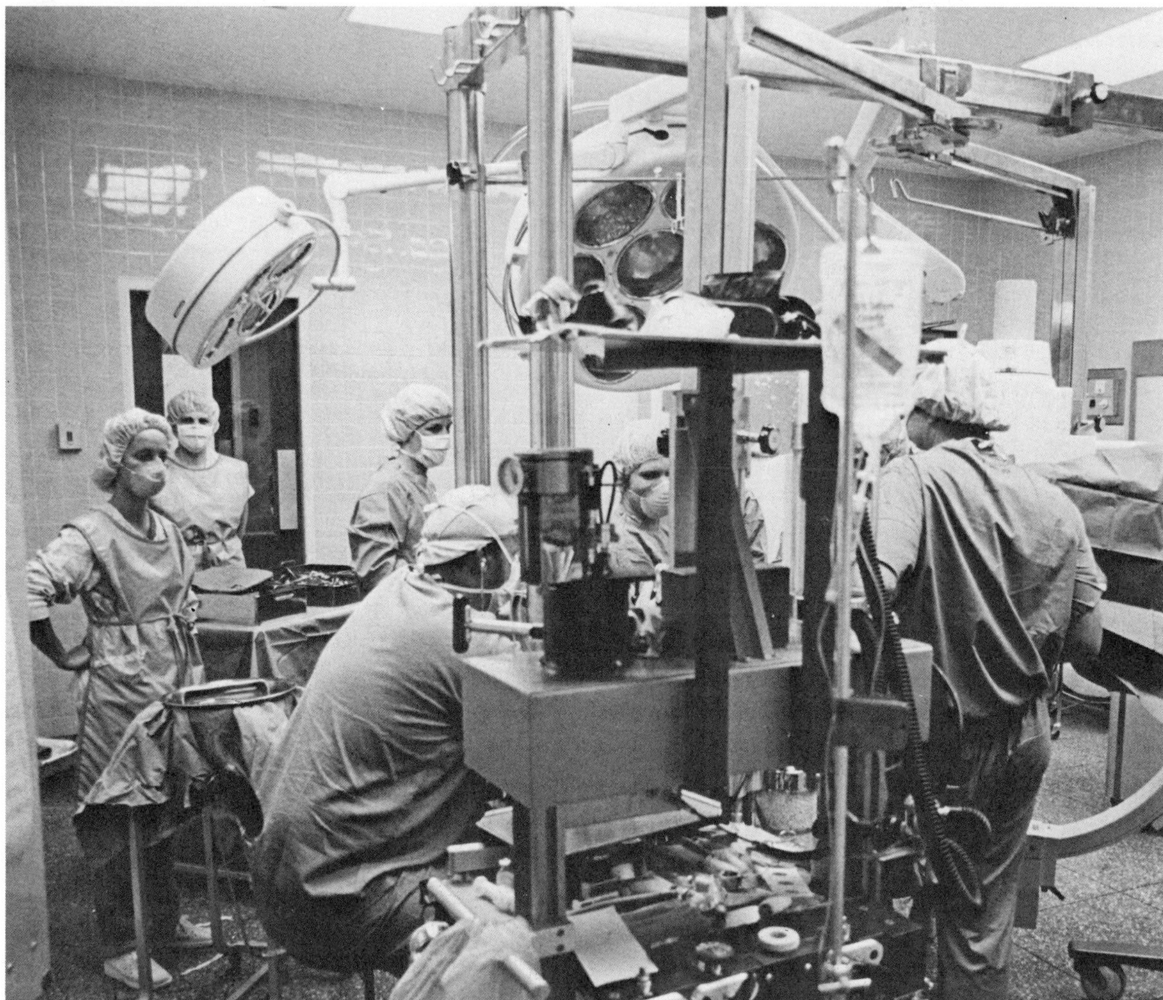

Figure 7-3 Operating room members during a surgical procedure.

and protection techniques. Communicating identified sources of pain to other health team members prevents subjecting the client to unnecessary discomfort.

Chart Assessment Chart data required vary with hospital policy and client condition. Chart data that should be gathered during the preoperative assessment include:

History and physical
Urinalysis
Complete blood count
Signed operative permit

Other information that may be required depending on hospital policy and client condition includes:

Serum electrolytes
Chest x-ray
Electrocardiogram
Special diagnostic tests

A knowledge of these chart data will contribute to an understanding of the client's past and present history, cardiopulmonary homeostasis, and potential for infection. The chart should be read carefully as other data pertinent for a particular client will be documented.

Admitting the client

Hospital policy designates the exact procedure which should be followed when admitting the client to the operating room suite. A general routine that is followed includes initial greeting, extension of human contact and warmth, and proper identification. The identification process includes asking the client to state his name, the surgeon's name, the operative procedure and location, and comparing the hospital identification numbers with the client's identification band and the chart. The client is further identified by the surgeon prior to the induction with anesthesia. In some institutions this is done in the holding area and in others in the operating room.

The admitting procedure is continued with reassessment of the client and time for last-minute questions. The nurse continues to review the chart for the previously mentioned data and notes any abnormalities. The client is questioned concerning valuables, prosthesis, and last intake of food and fluid. Validation is made that the preoperative medication was given as ordered and a warm blanket, pillow, or position adjustment is provided if the client is uncomfortable. Most hospitals require the client's hair to be covered just prior to transferring.

Intraoperative Phase

Transferring the client

Once the client has been properly identified and the operating room has been adequately prepared, the client is transferred into the room for the surgery. Anytime a client is transferred from one bed to another, the wheels of the stretcher should be locked, and a sufficient number of personnel available to lift, guide, and prevent accidental falling. Once on the operating room bed, a safety strap should be snugly tightened across the client's thighs. If monitor leads (e.g., electrocardiograph leads) or the intravenous catheter have not been inserted in the preoperative holding area, these are usually applied at this time.

Implementing aseptic technique

Prior to transferring the client into the specific operating room, the operating room nurses spend significant time preparing the room to ensure privacy, safety, and the prevention of infection. Surgical attire (specially designed pants or dresses, masks, caps or hoods, and shoe covers) is worn by all persons entering the operating room suite. All electrical and mechanical equipment is checked for proper functioning. Aseptic technique is practiced as each surgical item is opened and placed systematically on the instrument table for use. Sponges, needles, and instruments are counted to assure accurate retrieval at the close of the procedure.

During this time and during the procedure, the roles of the nurses are delineated. The scrub nurse scrubs her hands and arms, gowns and gloves in sterile surgical attire, and touches only those items within the sterile field. The circulating nurse remains in the unsterile field and implements those activities which permit touching all unsterile items and the client himself.

Scrubbing, Gowning, and Gloving All sterile members of the surgical team (scrub nurse, surgeon, and assistant) are required to mechanically cleanse their hands and arms with detergent prior to entering the sterile field. This is done to eliminate dirt and skin oil from the skin, and to decrease the microbial count as much as possible. The scrub helps prevent the growth of microbes beneath the surgical gown and gloves. The detergent used should be a broad-spectrum microbicidal agent. The procedure should involve a minimum of 5 minutes of mechanical friction with a specially designed sterile surgical brush.[3] During the actual procedure of scrubbing, the team member's fingers and hands should be scrubbed first and progression continued to the arms and elbows. The hands should be held higher than the elbows at all times to prevent detergent suds and water from draining from the unclean (above elbows) to the clean and previously scrubbed areas (hands and fingers) (Fig. 7-4).

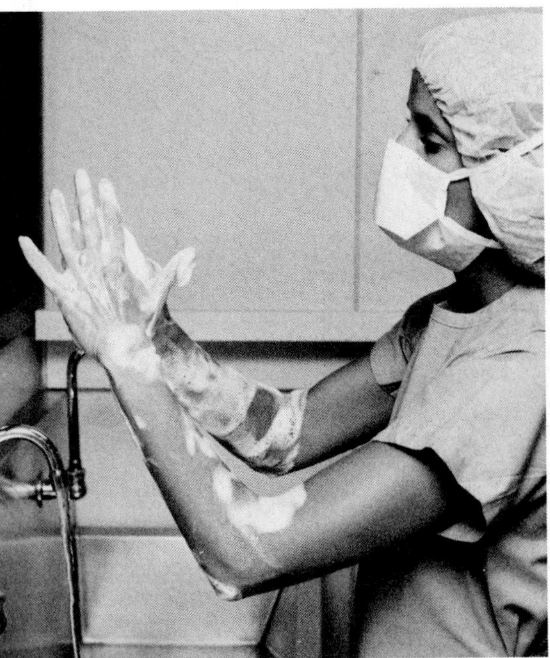

Figure 7-4 Surgical scrub. *(Courtesy of The Methodist Hospital, Texas Medical Center, Houston, Texas.)*

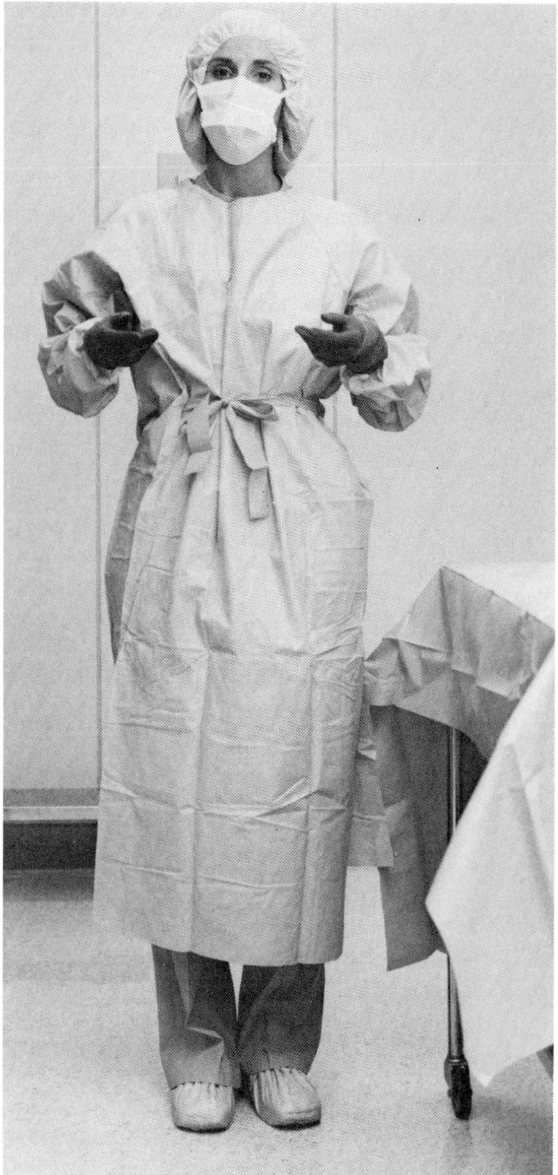

Figure 7-5 Sterile surgical attire. *(Courtesy of The Methodist Hospital, Texas Medical Center, Houston, Texas.)*

Once the scrub procedure is completed, the team members enter the room to clothe themselves in the surgical gowns and gloves (Fig. 7-5). Because the gowns and gloves are sterile, it is permissible for the scrubbed person to manipulate and organize all sterile items for use during the procedure.

Basic Aseptic Technique Aseptic technique is practiced in the operating room to prevent the entrance of microorganisms into the surgical wound and thus prevent infection. This is implemented through the creation and maintenance of a sterile field. The center of the sterile field is the site of the surgical incision. Its inanimate contents are surgical items and equipment which have been sterilized with appropriate sterilization methods.

There are specific principles which the team members should understand to practice aseptic technique. Unless these principles are followed, the safety of the client is compromised and the potential for postoperative infection is increased. Table 7-3 presents the principles of aseptic technique.[4,5]

Assisting the anesthesia team

During the time the nurse checks the operating room to finalize its preparation, the anesthesia team is preparing the client for the administration of anesthesia. It is essential that the nurse understand the mechanism of anesthesia administration as well as the pharmacologic effects of the agent(s). The nurse should know the location of all emergency drugs and equipment in the operating room area.

The circulating nurse is involved in establishing monitoring devices to be used during the surgical procedure (e.g., urinary catheter, ECG leads, etc.). She also assists in placement of the electrical grounding pad.

If the client is to have general anesthesia, the nurse remains at the client's side to ensure safety and assist the anesthetist if needed. These responsibilities may include obtaining blood pressure measurements, starting an intravenous line, and monitoring the client's level of consciousness and cardiorespiratory status during the procedure.

Positioning the client

Positioning the client usually follows administration of general anesthesia. At this time relaxation and surgical exposure can best be facilitated. When positioning for the surgical procedure, care must be instituted to (1) provide correct skeletal alignment, (2) prevent undue pressure on bony prominences and skin, (3) provide for adequate thoracic excursion, (4) prevent occlusion of arteries and veins, (5) avoid stretching and compression of nerve tissue, (6) provide modesty with exposure, and (7) recognize and respect individual needs such as previously assessed aches, pains, or deformities. It is a nursing responsibility to secure the extremities, provide adequate padding and support, and obtain sufficient physical or mechanical help to avoid unnecessary straining on self or the client.

Various positions in which the client may be positioned include supine, prone, Trendelenburg, lat-

Table 7-3
Principles of Aseptic Technique in the Operating Room

1. All materials that enter the sterile field must be sterile.
2. Sterilization is the only means by which an item can be considered sterile. If it comes in contact with an unsterile item, it becomes contaminated.
3. Contaminated items should be removed immediately from the sterile field.
4. Sterile team members must wear only sterile gowns. Once dressed for the procedure, they should recognize that all parts of the gown are considered *unsterile* except the front from chest to table level and the sleeves to 2 inches above the elbow (Fig. 7-5).
5. A wide margin of safety must be maintained between the sterile and unsterile field.
6. Team members' motions should be from sterile to sterile or from unsterile to unsterile.
7. Tables are considered sterile only at table top level and items extending beneath this level are considered contaminated.
8. The edges of a sterile package are considered contaminated once the package has been opened.
9. Bacteria travel on airborne particles and will enter the sterile field with excessive air movements and currents.
10. Bacteria travel with moisture and liquids by capillary action from surface to surface.
11. Bacteria harbor on the client's and the team members' hair, skin, and respiratory tract.

eral, kidney, lithotomy, jackknife (Kraske), and sitting (Fig. 7-6). The supine is the most common position used. It would be used for surgery involving the gastrointestinal tract, heart, breast, etc. The prone position allows easy access for back surgeries (e.g., laminectomies). The lithotomy position is used for some pelvic organ surgeries (e.g., vaginal hysterectomy). The sitting position is used for craniotomies.

Prepping the client

The goal of skin prepping is to reduce the number of organisms available to migrate to the surgical wound. The preoperative skin preparation discussed in Chap. 6 is vital. However, intraoperatively another skin preparation is done immediately prior to the incision. The task of prepping is often the responsibility of the circulating nurse.

The skin is prepared by mechanically scrubbing or cleansing with antimicrobial agents identified as being nonallergic to the client. The nurse first assures that excess hair has been shaved from the area around the surgical site. This area is then scrubbed in a circular motion. The principle of scrubbing from the clean area (site of the incision) to the dirty area (periphery) is observed at all times. A liberal area is cleansed to allow for extra protection and unexpected occurrences during the procedure.

Following the preparation of the client's skin, the sterile members of the surgical team drape the area. Only the site to be incised is left exposed.

Postoperative Phase

Toward the end of the surgical procedure the anesthetist begins to reverse the effects of the anesthetic agents so that the client will emerge more rapidly. This not only allows more physiological control of the client during the transfer to the postanesthesia area, but encourages more rapid and safer recovery. (Refer to the following sections on anesthesia.)

The anesthetist and surgeon or other member of the surgical team accompany the client to the recovery room. A report of the client's status and procedure is communicated (Chap. 8).

ANESTHESIA

Choice

Selection of the anesthetic method and agent is determined by the anesthetist* in collaboration with the surgeon and the client. Factors contributing to the decision include the client's current health status and history, emotional stability, and factors relating to the operative procedure (length, position, site, use of electrocautery.) The anesthesiologist* validates this information during the preoperative assessment, finalizes the decision, and writes the order for the preoperative medication.

Classification of Anesthesia

Anesthesia is classified according to the effect that it has on the client's sensorium (central nervous system) and pain perception. *General anesthesia* is defined as the loss of sensation with a loss of consciousness and reflexes. *Local anesthesia* is defined as the loss of sensation without a loss of consciousness. More specifically, general anesthesia has a direct effect on the central nervous system. In con-

*The terms anesthesiologist and anesthetist (certified registered nurse anesthetist or CRNA) are used interchangeably in this chapter.

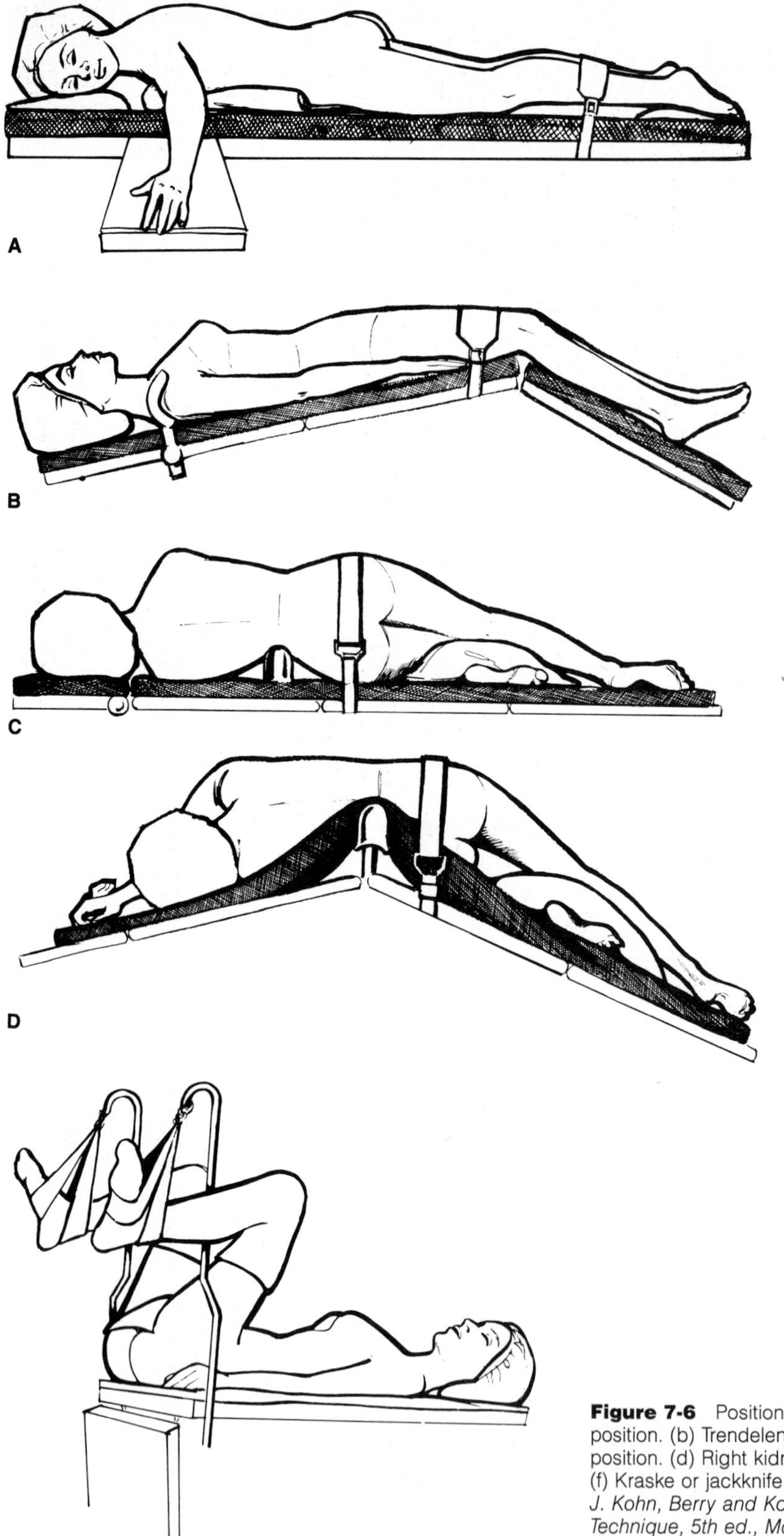

Figure 7-6 Positioning the client in surgery. (a) Prone position. (b) Trendelenburg's position. (c) Right lateral position. (d) Right kidney position. (e) Lithotomy position. (f) Kraske or jackknife position. *(From L. J. Atkinson and M. J. Kohn, Berry and Kohn's Introduction to Operating Room Technique, 5th ed., McGraw-Hill Book Company, New York, 1978, pp. 216, 217, 219, and 220.)*

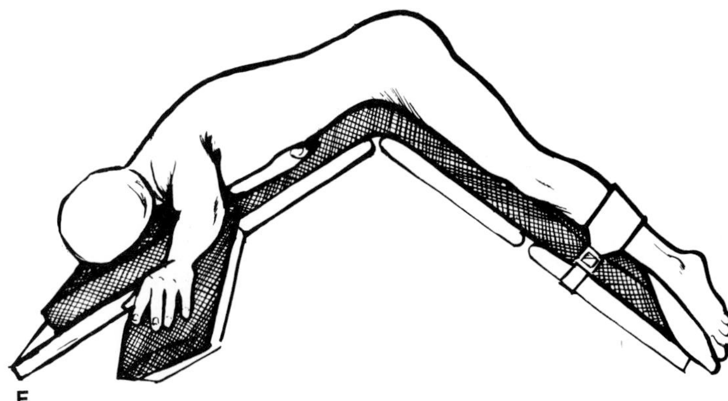

Figure 7-6 (continued)

trast, local anesthesia interrupts nerve impulses along the nerve cell fibers.

General Anesthesia

General anesthesia is usually the category of choice for clients who:

1. Are having surgical procedures requiring significant skeletal muscle relaxation, long period of time, and awkward positions due to the location of the incisional site.
2. Are extremely anxious.
3. Require the physiological monitoring that only general anesthesia will allow.

General anesthesia is administered by four different methods: inhalation, intravenously, rectally, and intramuscularly (Table 7-4).

Inhalation agents

The inhalation agents used for general anesthesia may be *volatile liquids* (liquid at room temperature) or *gases* (gas at room temperature). Volatile liquids are vaporized into a gaseous state together with a carrier gas such as oxygen. The oxygen and anesthetic agent are passed through a precalibrated vaporizer on the anesthesia machine. The gaseous agents are stored in pressurized tanks.

Inhalation agents enter the body through the respiratory tract to reach their desired effect in the brain. This characteristic makes them particularly desirable since they can be very easily controlled through the ventilatory process. However, the characteristic that makes them not so desirable is their irritating effect on the respiratory passages that can lead to respiratory obstruction and depression, cough, laryngospasms, and increased secretions. In addition, many of them stimulate the vomiting center of the brain, leading to the potential for postoperative aspiration of secretions.[6]

The face mask and intubation (nasotracheal, endotracheal, or tracheal tube) techniques of administration are the methods used to deliver inhalation agents. With the *mask induction,* the gas is inhaled through a face mask which is placed over the client's mouth and nose. It is attached to the anesthetic gas machine and gas is delivered through a mechanical system which allows for reabsorption of the exhaled carbon dioxide. This technique is more frequently used for surgical procedures which are shorter in length and require less muscular relaxation.

Inhalation of anesthetic gases through the cuffed *endotracheal tube* is considered the safest means of gas delivery, especially for lengthy procedures requiring deep muscle relaxation and sedation. The endotracheal tube with an inflated cuff permits mechanical ventilation, control of respiration with an open airway, easy access to the tracheobronchial tree for suctioning, and little possibility for regurgitation of stomach contents and aspirated secretions.

Complications or disadvantages of endotracheal intubation include those primarily associated with its insertion and removal. Irritation of the tracheobronchial tree at these times may cause laryngospasms (muscular spasms of the larynx), laryngeal edema (swelling of the laryngeal tissue), or hoarseness due to injury to the vocal cords. The nurse must be certain that suction is readily accessible to the anesthetist at the time of induction of anesthesia and throughout the intraoperative period.

After the tube is removed, the nurse should observe for respiratory complications. It is critical to have readily available oxygen, suction apparatus, emergency drugs to decrease the swelling, and equipment for reinsertion of the tube if necessary for airway maintenance.

Table 7-4

Drugs and Methods Used for General Anesthesia

Inhalation agents
- A. *Volatile liquids*
  - Chloroform*
  - Diethyl ether*†
  - Divinyl ether*†
  - Enflurance (Ethrane)
  - Halothane (Fluothane)
  - Isoflurane (Fourane)
  - Methoxyflurane (Penthrane)
  - Trichlorethylene (Trimar)*
- B. *Gaseous agents*
  - Cyclopropane*†
  - Ethylene*†
  - Nitrous oxide

Intravenous agents
- A. *Barbiturates* (short-acting)
  1. Thiopental Sodium (Pentothal)
  2. Sodium methohexitol (Brevital)
- B. *Narcotics*
  1. Meperidine hydrochloride (Demerol)
  2. Morphine sulfate
  3. Fentanyl (Sublimaze)
- C. *Neuroleptanesthesia + tranquilizers*
  1. Innovar
     - Fentanyl (Sublimaze)
     - Droperidol (Inapsine)
  2. Diazepam (Valium)
- D. *Dissociative anesthetics*
  - Ketamine hydrochloride (Ketalar)
- E. *Muscle relaxants*
  1. Depolarizing agents
     - Succinylcholine (Anectine)
  2. Nondepolarizing agents
     - Tubocurarine chloride (Curare)
     - Pancuronium bromide (Pavulon)
     - Gallamine triethiodide (Flaxedil)

Rectal agents
- A. *Barbiturates* (short-acting)
  1. Thiopental Sodium (Pentothal)
  2. Sodium methohexitol (Brevital)
  3. Tribromeothanol (Avertin)*

Intramuscular agents
- Innovar
- Ketamine hydrochloride (Ketalar)

*Historical significance only.
†Explosive.

Volatile Liquids *Diethyl ether* was introduced during the nineteenth century and was accepted as the first useful general anesthetic agent. With its frequent use, the signs and stages of anesthesia were clearly identified as the client passed from altered consciousness (stage 1) to excitement (stage 2) to surgical relaxation (stage 3) (Fig. 7-7). If an overdose had occurred, the client would have progressed to stage 4 (circulatory and respiratory failure). A variety of reflex reactions occur as the client passed through these stages. Since induction was prolonged with ether, these stages were readily documented. Today the client passes through the stages of anesthesia quite quickly, as induction with the newer agents is more rapid. Although the nurse should be aware that these stages do occur, priority is not placed on being able to identify them.[7]

Diethyl ether, cyclopropane, ethylene, and divinyl ether are considered obsolete because of their inflammable and explosive potential. The agents should only be used in operating rooms fulfilling all National Fire Protection Association recommendations.

Halothane (Fluothane) is a halogenated hydrocarbon which is nonexplosive and nonirritating. In appropriate doses it is a strong anesthetic and bronchodilator, and has a low incidence of postoperative nausea and vomiting. During its administration, cardiac depression and peripheral vasodilation resulting in hypotension may occur. The analgesic effects readily leave the client postoperatively. Because evidence of acute hepatic necrosis following the administration of halothane has been documented, each client is thoroughly evaluated for the potential of liver disease and recent exposure to the agent.

Halothane sensitizes the myocardium to the presence of epinephrine which increases the incidence of ventricular arrhythmias. The nurse should make careful calculations of the dosage of epinephrine injected during surgical procedures. The anesthetist needs to be informed of its use prior to injection.

When nursing the client postoperatively, blood pressure should be frequently assessed, fluid therapy evaluated, and complaints of pain recognized.[8, 9] Shivering is frequently present in emergence from anesthesia.

Enflurane (Ethrane) is a halogenated ether which is nonexplosive and rapid-acting. It allows ready management of cardiovascular status and produces little respiratory secretions. It is also a good muscle relaxant and provides for rapid postoperative recovery with minimal nausea and vomiting. Seizure activity has been seen during enflurane anesthesia. Because recovery is rapid and there is little residual analgesia, the nurse should realistically evaluate the occurrence of pain in the postoperative period. Enflurane is a highly accepted and much desired anesthetic agent.[10]

Isoflurane (Fourane) is a soon-to-be-released anesthetic agent. Its advantage over halothane and enflurane is the minimal degree to which it is metabolized. This would minimize untoward effects on the liver and kidney. One disadvantage of this drug may be its irritating effect on the respiratory system.

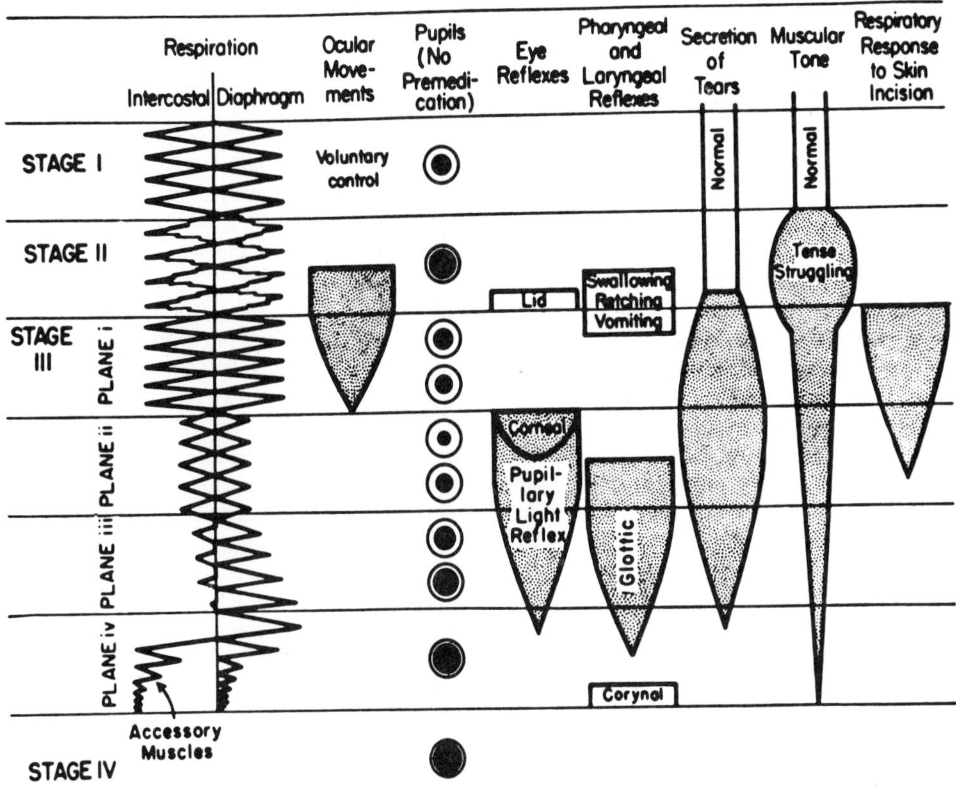

Figure 7-7 Signs and stages of anesthesia. The signs and reflex reactions of the stages of anesthesia. The wedge-shaped areas indicate not only client variability but the factor of variability in disappearance of the signs in the planes of anesthesia. Stage I, altered consciousness; stage II, excitement; stage III, surgical relaxation; and stage IV, circulatory and respiratory failure. *(From J. R. DiPalma, Basic Pharmacology in Medicine, McGraw-Hill Book Company, New York, 1976, p. 48.)*

Methoxyflurane (Penthrane), a nonexplosive agent, is the strongest of the volatile agents but least administered due to the occurrence of nephrotoxicity. The client's respiratory system is significantly depressed during its use. This situation frequently requires assisted ventilation to maintain the airway.

Postoperatively, the nurse should expect a lengthy recovery period and the potential for an artificial airway. She should specifically evaluate increased urinary output with a decreased specific gravity as evidence of possible early renal toxicity.[11]

Gaseous Agents *Nitrous oxide* is a gaseous agent providing more analgesia than unconsciousness. It is the most widely administered gas, alone or in combination, due to its numerous favorable qualities. Induction with nitrous oxide is rapid and recovery is rapid and void of hazardous occurrences. It is nonirritating and has a pleasant odor. Its effects are readily reversible. Although nitrous oxide is relatively innocuous, studies now show it does have some cardiac depressant effects.

Because it is a weak anesthetic, nitrous oxide is administered as a single agent only in minor procedures requiring little anesthesia and muscular relaxation. When it is administered in combination, its potentiating effects allow smaller amounts of the accompanying drugs. Its primary harmful effect would result from administration without a sufficient amount of oxygen. This can lead to varying degrees of hypoxia and respiratory depression.[12]

Primary nursing responsibilities for clients focus on assessment of respiratory status until adequate ventilation is assured. Oxygen should be routinely administered following nitrous oxide anesthesia until the nitrous oxide has been replaced in the client's alveoli by nitrogen in room air.

Intravenous agents

Induction with intravenous agents is rapid and pleasant. These are the primary characteristics for the client's preference for IV agents. Recovery is likewise rapid and lacks the unpleasantness of restlessness and gastrointestinal upset that frequently occurs with the inhalation agents.

Intravenous agents are rarely given alone. They are usually given in combination with two or more other drugs or inhalation agents. This is because even though they are depressants, they do not totally eliminate painful stimuli. In addition, once injected they are not as easily controlled as the inhalation agents and have a high potential for untoward drug interactions.[13]

Intravenous agents used alone or in combination to achieve the effects of general anesthesia include the barbiturates, tranquilizers, narcotics, disassociative agents, and muscle relaxants. It should be noted that each agent is not in itself a general anesthetic, but specific combinations achieve the desired effect.

Barbiturates The most frequently administered intravenous agents to achieve general anesthesia are the short-acting barbiturates. Of those available, the two most frequently used are thiopental sodium (Pentothal) and sodium methohexitol (Brevital).

Induction with both of these agents is rapid and smooth. However, these agents must be followed with a potent inhalation agent or muscle relaxant to achieve muscular relaxation. If a high concentration of the barbiturate is administered during induction, respiratory depression and apnea can occur, necessitating mechanical ventilation. Leakage of the barbiturates into the tissue surrounding the vein can cause severe pain and damage due to the alkalinity of the drugs. If injected into an artery, arterial spasms and thrombosis may occur.[14]

Narcotics Narcotics are not classified as anesthetics. Rather, they serve as adjuncts when used in combination with weak inhalation or IV barbiturates. Their primary disadvantage is slowing of the respiratory rate and the occurrence of respiratory depression. This effect and their analgesia effects in the postanesthesia period should alert the nurse to closely check the client's respiratory rate and depth and pain status.

Those narcotics most frequently administered to achieve anesthesia are meperidine hydrochloride (Demerol), morphine sulfate, and fentanyl (Sublimaze). Fentanyl, a synthetic opiate, is the most potent of this group. When used in combination with droperidol (Inapsine), it has a neuroleptanalgesia effect.

Neuroleptanesthesia This is the state in which there is a tranquilization with little cortical depression. The client has decreased motor activity, decreased anxiety, and a feeling of indifference. The ability to respond to commands remains.

The drug widely administered for neuroleptanesthesia is *Innovar*—a combination of the narcotic fentanyl (Sublimaze) and the tranquilizer droperidol (Inapsine). Innovar can be administered alone or in combination with other agents. Because of its pharmacological effect, the client recovering from Innovar should be assessed for extreme respiratory depression, prolonged analgesia, and tranquility. The client should be verbally stimulated to respond to commands of coughing and deep breathing, as prolonged sleepiness is likely to occur. Innovar may be administered IV or IM.[15]

Diazepam (Valium), given intravenously in combination with narcotics, is also used to achieve a neuroleptanesthesic effect.

Dissociative Anesthetics A dissociative drug is one that interrupts associative brain pathways while blocking sensory pathways. The client may appear awake but is actually asleep. The agent administered as a dissociative anesthetic is ketamine hydrochloride (Ketalar). It is particularly advantageous in that it does not relax upper airway muscles and tissues. Therefore, there is minimal probability of airway obstruction. In spite of this advantage, ketamine should never be administered without resuscitative equipment immediately available. Ketamine has no cardiac depressant effect so it is a suitable agent in poor surgical risk clients.

Ketamine's principal disadvantage is the hallucinogenic state it produces in the postoperative period. The likelihood of this is reduced by keeping the total dosage of the drug as low as possible and by using adjunct drugs such as Pentothal and diazepam. The nurse should approach the client slowly and quietly, as startling touch and loud sounds may elicit hallucinatory reactions.[16, 17] Ketamine may be administered IV or IM.

Muscle Relaxants–Neuromuscular Blocking Agents Use of the neuromuscular blocking agents allows deep muscle relaxation with relatively light levels of anesthesia. The hazards of deep anesthetic levels are significantly lessened as the stage of surgical relaxation is achieved. This is extremely important as adequate surgical exposure and relaxation is essential for the surgeon to operate. The nurse should know that client awareness occasionally occurs under deep relaxation, light anesthesia techniques. Therefore, care should be made to keep the operating room as quiet as possible.

The two categories of muscle relaxants or neuromuscular blocking agents are *depolarizing agents* and the *nondepolarizing agents.* Depolarizing agents such as succinylcholine (Anectine) interfere with depolarization of the motor end plate to prevent it from responding. The nondepolarizing agents such as tubocurarine chloride (Curare), pancuronium bromide (Pavulon), and gallamine triethiodide (Flaxedil) interfere with nerve impulse transmission at the myoneural junction by competing at the motor end plate with acetylcholine. Both types of relaxants achieve the same effect, muscular relaxation.[18]

Disadvantages involving the administration of muscle relaxants are of special concern to the postanesthesia nurse. The duration of their action may be longer than the surgical procedure or reversal agents may not have been effective in eliminating the residual effects. This requires that the client be carefully observed for airway patency and respiratory muscle movement. Lack of movement and return of reflexes and strength may indicate the need for an artificial airway and respirator. If intubated, the endotracheal tube should not be removed without careful assessment of return of muscular strength and tidal volume.

Rectal agents

Rectal administration of short-acting barbiturates is only occasionally used today due to individual differences in absorption rate in the colon (Table 7-4). This type of anesthesia is most frequently administered to children to produce a sleep state prior to the use of other anesthetics.[19]

Intramuscular agents

Drugs which have been administered intramuscularly to achieve general anesthesia are Innovar and ketamine hydrochloride (Ketalar). Although this method of administration is usually secondary to their administration by IV, the nurse should be aware of this choice of administration.

Local Anesthesia

Definition and examples

Local anesthetics allow for an operative procedure on a part of the body without loss of consciousness. Action of local anesthetics is by blocking the conduction of nerve impulses through altering nerve cell permeability to sodium and potassium ions.[20]

Local anesthetics frequently administered are cocaine, procaine hydrochloride, tetracaine hydrochloride (Pontocaine), dibucaine hydrochloride (Nupercaine), lidocaine hydrochloride (Xylocaine), mepivacaine hydrochloride (Carbocaine), and bupivacaine hydrochloride (Marcaine).

Advantages and disadvantages

Advantages of local anesthesia are numerous for the client assessed as a suitable recipient. A suitable client is one who is not allergic to the drug, is having a surgical procedure that lends itself to the technique, and anxiety or apprehension does not predominate the mental state. Because loss of consciousness does not occur, the induction and recovery hazards of a general anesthetic do not exist. Minimal equipment is needed and the cost is lower. Local anesthesia is especially beneficial for individuals who have not been kept NPO ("nothing by mouth") prior to surgery or are having minor procedures performed on an outpatient basis.

Disadvantages of local anesthesia include (1) lack of client acceptance due to awareness during the procedure, (2) lack of feasibility of localizing some anatomical sites, and (3) rapid absorption of the agent into the bloodstream in unsuspected circumstances.[21] Manifestations of overdose and/or rapid absorption include lightheadedness, dizziness, ringing in ears, loss of consciousness, and seizure activity.

Methods of administration

There are a variety of methods for administering local anesthesia (Table 7-5). *Topical application* is the application of the agent directly to the skin, mucous membrane, or open surface. *Local infiltration* is injection of the agent into the tissues through which the surgical incision will pass. *Regional application* is injection of the agent at some location along the conductive nerve pathway to and from the region selected to be anesthetized. Regional application is achieved away from the surgical field.

There are several types of regional anesthesia. The *nerve block* is the injection of a specific nerve at a given point, as an intercostal or median nerve block. The *intravenous regional block* with a tourniquet (Bier's block) is the injection of the agent intravenously into an extremity after a tourniquet has been applied and the extremity elevated to drain it of blood. The tourniquet should always remain inflated a minimum of 30 minutes. The nurse should observe the client when the tourniquet is released. It is possible to have

Table 7-5

Methods for Administering Local Anesthesia

I. Topical application
II. Local infiltration
III. Regional application—conduction block
  A. Nerve block
  B. Intravenous regional block—Bier's block
  C. Field block
  D. Central nerve blocks
    1. Spinal block
    2. Epidural block
      a. Lumbar-peridural block
      b. Caudal-sacral block

symptoms of local anesthetic overdose. The *field block* is a type of infiltration anesthesia in which the anesthesia surrounds the area of the surgical procedure by a series of injections. The *central nerve blocks* are those which anesthetize the spinal cord nerves (motor and sensory) near their origin. The *spinal block* affects the nerves in the subarachnoid space, and the *epidural block* affects those surrounding the dura mater. The epidural block may take a lumbar approach (*peridural block*) or the caudal approach (*sacral block*).[22, 23]

Epidural and spinal anesthesia

Epidural and spinal anesthesia are achieved by injection of a local anesthetic agent into the spinal cord between two lumbar vertebrae. Once injected, sensory and motor sympathetic routes of the nerve cell are anesthetized. Anesthesia spreads to the uppermost desired level as additional fibers are gradually affected. Epidural and spinal anesthesia is administered primarily for clients having surgery of the lower abdomen and lower extremities. The client can remain conscious during the surgical procedure or be sedated.

The onset of spinal anesthesia is faster than epidural because the spinal nerves are uncovered in the subarachnoid space and absorb the drug more rapidly. However, the effect of the two techniques are the same and the client must be closely observed for manifestations brought about by blockage of the sympathetic nervous system. These include hypotension, bradycardia, and nausea and vomiting. If the block extends upward, the client may experience respiratory depression. The level of the sensory and sympathetic block is controlled by the amount of drug used and the position of the operating room table.

An advantage of epidural over spinal anesthesia is lack of postanesthesia headache. The headache experienced after a spinal is thought to occur from a leakage of spinal fluid at the site of injection. All clients with spinal anesthesia should be encouraged to force fluids postoperatively to help prevent this complication.

Additional Anesthesia Mechanisms

Controlled hypotension is a technique used during the administration of anesthesia to decrease the amount of expected blood loss by lowering the blood pressure. *Hypothermia* is the deliberate lowering of the body temperature to decrease body metabolism and thus the need for oxygen. *Cryoanesthesia* involves cooling or freezing a localized area to block pain impulses of localized nerve impulses. *Hypnoanesthesia* utilizes hypnosis to produce an alteration in pain consciousness. *Acupuncture* achieves loss of sensation by the use of intense local stimulation with fine-gauge needles at meridian points throughout the body.[24]

REVIEW QUESTIONS

The number of the question corresponds to the same numbered objective at the beginning of the chapter.

1. Which of the following characteristics of the operating room environment facilitate the prevention of infection in the surgical client?
  a. conductive furniture
  b. filters in the ventilating system
  c. explosion-proof electrical plugs
  d. adjustable lighting

2. Select from the following the activity which is *not* a function of the registered nurse in the operating room.
  a. administering local anesthesia
  b. checking electrical equipment
  c. implementing the nursing process
  d. scrubbing for the surgical procedure

3. Preoperative assessment by the operating room nurse is initiated in a variety of settings. Select the *inappropriate* setting for preoperative client assessments.
  a. home or clinic setting
  b. clinical unit
  c. operating room
  d. preoperative holding area

4. After the client is transferred to the operating room bed, the nurse should place the safety strap across the client's
  a. abdomen
  b. thighs
  c. chest
  d. knees

5. Contaminated items in a sterile field should be
  a. covered
  b. pushed aside

c. washed off
d. removed immediately

6. A client is scheduled for an abdominal hysterectomy. She is extremely anxious and has the tendency to hyperventilate when upset. Which of the following types of anesthesia would be most appropriate for her?
a. general anesthesia
b. local anesthesia

7. Which of the following methods of achieving general anesthesia is considered to be the most desirable and controllable?
a. inhalation
b. intravenous
c. rectal
d. intramuscular

8. The injection of the local anesthetic into the tissues through which the surgical incision will pass is the technique of
a. topical application
b. nerve block
c. regional application
d. local infiltration

9. Cooling or freezing a localized area to block pain impulses of localized nerve impulses is known as
a. hypnoanesthesia
b. acupuncture
c. hypothermia
d. cryoanesthesia

REFERENCES

1. Marie J. Rhodes, Barbara J. Gruendemann, and Walter F. Ballinger, *Alexander's Care of the Patient in Surgery,* The C. V. Mosby Company, St. Louis, 1978, pp. 21–28.
2. Association of Operating Room Nurses, "Operating Room Nursing: Perioperative Role," *AORN J*, **27:**1170–1171 (1978).
3. Association of Operating Room Nurses, "Standards for Surgical Hand Scrubs," *AORN J,* **23:**976–977 (1976).
4. Rhodes, op. cit., p. 54.
5. Association of Operating Room Nurses, "Standards for Basic Aseptic Technique," in *AORN Standards of Practice,* Association of Operating Room Nurses, Denver, pp. 3–1 to 3–5.
6. Robert D. Dripps, James E. Eckenhoff, and Leroy D. Vandam, *Introduction to Anesthesia,* W. B. Saunders Company, Philadelphia, 1977, pp. 126–132.
7. Joseph R. Di Palma, *Basic Pharmacology in Medicine,* McGraw-Hill Book Company, New York, 1976, pp. 48–49.
8. Cecil B. Drain and Susan B. Shipley, *The Recovery Room,* W. B. Saunders Company, Philadelphia, 1979, pp. 138–139.
9. Di Palma, op. cit., pp. 50–52.
10. Dripps, op. cit., p. 159.
11. Drain, op. cit., pp. 139–140.
12. Nicholas M. Greene, "Anesthesia," in Seymour I. Schwartz et al. (eds.), *Principles of Surgery,* McGraw-Hill Book Company, New York, 1979, pp. 478–479.
13. Greene, op. cit., pp. 482–483.
14. Morton J. Rodman and Dorothy W. Smith, *Pharmacology and Drug Therapy in Nursing,* J. B. Lippincott Company, Philadelphia, 1979, pp. 292–293.
15. Drain, op. cit., pp. 157–160.
16. Rodman, op. cit., p. 293.
17. Greene, op. cit., p. 485.
18. Ibid., p. 486.
19. Rodman, op. cit., pp. 292–293.
20. Ibid., p. 303.
21. Dripps, op. cit., pp. 242–243.
22. Lucy Jo Atkinson and Mary Louise Kohn, *Berry and Kohn's Introduction to Operating Room Technique,* McGraw-Hill Book Company, New York, 1978, p. 170.
23. Rodman, op. cit., pp. 304–305.
24. Atkinson, op. cit., pp. 186–193.

Chapter 8

NURSING ROLE IN MANAGEMENT

Postoperative Client

Susan N. Walker

Learning Objectives

1. Identify the responsibilities of the nurse in admitting the postoperative client to the recovery room.
2. Explain the pathophysiology and nursing assessment and management for possible problems during the postanesthesia recovery period.
3. Describe the initial nursing assessment and management when receiving the client on the clinical unit from the recovery room.
4. Explain the pathophysiology and nursing assessment and management of possible problems during the postoperative period.
5. Identify the information needed by the postoperative client in preparation for discharge.

The postoperative period begins after surgery is over and continues until the client is discharged from medical care. This chapter focuses on the common features of postoperative nursing care for the client undergoing surgery. The unique problems and nursing care related to specific surgical procedures are discussed elsewhere in this text.

THE POSTOPERATIVE CLIENT IN THE RECOVERY ROOM

Receiving the Client from the Operating Room

The client's immediate recovery period is supervised by the recovery room nurse, a specially trained professional working in a specially equipped environment. The recovery room (RR) or postanesthesia recovery room (PAR) is located close to the operating suite. In the event of an emergency, the anesthesiologist and the surgeon are nearby.

The goal of the recovery room nurse is to provide the client with an uneventful recovery from anesthesia and the immediate effects of surgery. This requires that the nurse prevent complications when possible, recognize complications and intervene early when they do occur, and protect the client from injury during recovery.

The anesthesiologist* and operating room nurse (in some agencies) accompany the client to the recovery room and report to the recovery room nurse. This report should include the following information:

1. Client's name
2. Nature of surgery performed and findings
3. Type of anesthesia and agents used
4. Drugs administered during surgery
5. Special conditions (allergies, chronic illnesses) existing preoperatively
6. Complications (such as hemorrhage or cardiac arrhythmias) during surgery
7. Estimated blood loss and IV fluid and blood replacement
8. Amount of urine output during surgical procedure
9. Number and type of drains, tubes, or suction devices present
10. Overall evaluation of client's vital signs and general condition at conclusion of surgery

The initial nursing assessment of a client upon admission to the recovery room is listed in Table 8-1. The frequency of further observations and interventions is a nursing judgment. Factors involved include data obtained during this initial assessment, the client's preoperative status, the surgery performed, and the anesthetic and adjunct drugs used. Vital signs in the recovery room are usually monitored at least every 15 minutes until stable and then every 30 minutes.

A written record of all observations and treatment measures during the postanesthesia recovery period is essential. Many recovery rooms have special forms

*The terms anesthesiologist and anesthetist (certified registered nurse anesthetist or CRNA) are used interchangeably in this chapter.

This chapter was reviewed by Patricia Robertson Hercules, R.N., M.S., Assistant Director Operating Rooms, The Methodist Hospital, Houston, Texas.

Table 8-1
Client Assessment on Admission to Recovery Room

Time of arrival in recovery room
Patency of airway
Presence of artificial airway devices
 Pharyngeal airway
 Endotracheal tube
 Tracheostomy tube
Vital signs
 Temperature, pulse, and respirations
 Blood pressure
Color of skin, nail beds, and lips
Appearance of skin (moist or dry, warm or cool)
Level of consciousness
Presence or absence of reflexes
 Eyelid
 Pharyngeal
 Cough
 Gag and swallowing
Intravenous infusion
 Type of solution
 Amount in bottle or bag
 Flow rate
 Appearance and location of IV site
Dressings, drains, and tubes
 Intactness and function
 Connection to drainage
 Amount and character of drainage
Oxygen in use
 Mode of administration
 Flow rate
Presence or absence of urge to void
 Bladder distension

that are used for this purpose (Fig. 8-1). The frequency of recording is based on medical orders and nursing judgment.

Possible Problems During Postanesthesia Recovery

Respiratory problems

Nursing Assessment For an adequate respiratory assessment, the nurse needs to evaluate airway patency, chest symmetry, and depth, rate, and character of respirations. The nurse should place a cupped hand over the client's nose and mouth to evaluate the forcefulness of exhaled air.

The chest wall should be observed for symmetry of movement. Determine if abdominal and accessory muscles are being used for breathing. If they are moving excessively, it may indicate respiratory distress.

Breath sounds need to be auscultated. Decreased or absent breath sounds will be detected when airflow is diminished or obstructed. Coarse rales may indicate the need for suctioning of secretions.

Monitoring pulse and respirations at regular intervals permits the nurse to recognize early symptoms of respiratory distress. Hypoxia from any cause may be reflected by rapid breathing, gasping, apprehension, restlessness, or a rapid, thready pulse. Impaired ventilation may be first detected by observing a slowed breathing rate or diminished chest and abdominal movement during respiration.

The characteristics of sputum or mucus should be noted and recorded. Mucus from the trachea and throat is colorless and thin in consistency. Sputum from the lungs and bronchi is thick and yellow-tinged.

Pathophysiology Respiratory problems in the immediate postanesthesia period may be related to airway obstruction, hypoventilation, aspiration of vomitus, or a combination of these factors[1] (Table 8-2). These problems are more likely to develop in the client who smokes heavily or has chronic lung disease, but they may occur in any client who has been anesthetized.

Airway obstruction is most frequently produced by blockage of the oral airway by the client's own tongue.[2] The base of the tongue falls backward against the soft palate and occludes the pharynx. This is most pronounced in the supine position (Fig. 8-2).

Hypoventilation is inadequate ventilation resulting in elevated P_aCO_2 levels. Respirations are shallow and frequently show an altered pattern. Hypoventilation presents the immediate danger of hypoxia and asphyxia, as well as the later hazards of atelectasis and hypostatic pneumonia. The most frequent cause of hypoventilation is due to drugs for anesthesia and analgesia[3] (Table 8-2).

Aspiration of vomitus, that is, the intake of vomitus by the lungs, can asphyxiate the client. If not that, it may lead to the development of chemical pneumonitis, which responds poorly to treatment (Table 8-2).

Nursing Management During the postanesthesia recovery period, the nurse routinely carries out measures aimed at prevention or detection of possible respiratory problems.

Proper positioning to facilitate respiration is essential. Unless contraindicated by the surgical procedure, the unconscious or semiconscious client should be in a side-lying or semiprone position (Fig. 8-3). If the client must be supine, the head should be turned to the side to avoid aspiration. The client should be turned from side to side hourly to allow for bilateral lung expansion. The supine position should be avoid-

RECOVERY ROOM RECORD

PROCEDURE: Cholecystectomy

PRE-OP PROBLEMS: None

INTRA-OP PROBLEMS: None

ANTICIPATED POST-OP PROBLEMS: None

OR. INTAKE	
Fluids:	900
Blood Prod.:	None

TIME ADMITTED:	CONDITION ON ARRIVAL:	TIME RESPONDED:	EBL.:
2^{10} PM	good	3^{30} PM	300 ml

TIME	B/P	P	R	OBSERVATION & TREATMENTS
2^{10} PM	110/70	88	22	Dressing dry
2^{25} PM	112/72	90	20	
2^{30}	108/70	86	20	
3^{00}	108/72	84	22	
3^{30}	106/70	80	20	Responds to verbal stimuli

ANTICIPATED PARR PROBLEMS:

SURGEON:	TIME DISCH.:	SIGNATURE DISCH. RN:

INTAKE

TIME	IV FLUID & IV MEDICATION	AMOUNT INFUSED: CRYSTALOID	AMOUNT INFUSED: BLOOD PRODUCTS	P.O.	IRR.
2^{10} PM	5% D/W				
TOTALS					

TIME	URINE	EMESIS	IRRIG	CHEST TUBE	NG	OTHER
2^{10} PM						
3^{45} PM	200					
TOTALS						

ANESTHESIA: Nitrous oxide

PATIENT

Gwendolyn Abbamonto

DATE:

PL0065 (Rev. 10/77)

Figure 8-1 Recovery room record. *(Courtesy of University of New Mexico Hospital, Albuquerque, N.M.)*

ed until protective pharyngeal reflexes have returned. The client's uppermost arm should rest on a pillow rather than upon the chest wall to permit full chest movement. Dressings or binders on the chest or abdomen should be inspected to ensure that they are not constricting.

Patency of the airway is an ever-present concern in the unconscious client. If the upper respiratory tract appears to be obstructed, it may often be cleared simply by moving the client's lower jaw forward and upward (Fig. 8-2). If secretions are present, they may be removed by suctioning. Several mechanical devices are available to prevent airway obstruction in the anesthetized client (Fig. 8-4). *Pharyngeal airways* are usually removed by the client when he has recovered reflexes sufficiently either to gag or to push the device out with the tongue. *Endotracheal extubation* has traditionally been the responsibility of the anesthesiologist, but is beginning to be done by nurses in some areas.[4] Criteria for safe extubation include:

1. Adequate ventilation and movement of air evidenced by observation and auscultation.
2. Client can lift head off stretcher and hold it up for 30 seconds.

Deep breathing and coughing should be initiated as soon as the client enters the recovery room. Even while semiconscious, the client who has been instructed in these techniques preoperatively will respond to a verbal reminder. Deep breathing helps to clear inhalation anesthetic agents from the body and hasten recovery, prevent pooling of secretions, and decrease the tendency to hypoventilate. The client who is left alone tends to drift back to sleep and breathe shallowly or even become apneic. Verbal stimuli must be

Table 8-2
Respiratory Problems in the Postanesthesia Period

Problems and Causes	Mechanisms	Nursing Observations	Intervention
Airway obstruction			
Tongue falling back	Muscular flaccidity associated with ↓ consciousness and muscle relaxants	Snoring respirations Decreased air movement	Neck hyperextension Pull mandible forward Mechanical airway
Retained thick secretions	Secretion stimulation by anesthetic agents Dehydration of secretions from anticholinergic medication	Noisy respirations Rhonchi	Suctioning Deep breathing and coughing IV hydration IPPB with mucolytic agent Bronchoscopy
Laryngospasm	Irritation from endotracheal tube or anesthetic gases Most likely to occur following removal of endotracheal tube	Inspiratory stridor (crowing respiration) Sternal retraction	Oxygen Pull mandible forward IV atropine or muscle relaxant Intubation
Laryngeal edema	Allergic drug reaction Mechanical irritation from intubation Fluid overload	Similar to laryngospasm	Oxygen Antihistamines or steroids Sedatives Possible intubation
Bronchospasm	Preexisting asthma Irritation from anesthetic gases	Expiratory wheezing	IPPB IV bronchodilators (Isuprel or aminophylline)
Hypoventilation			
Drug-induced CNS depression	Prolonged effect of anesthesia and adjunct drugs Excessive pain medication	↓ respiratory rate Shallow respirations Apnea	Deep breathing and coughing Mechanical ventilation Narcotic antagonists
Drug-induced peripheral muscle paralysis	Excessive use of muscle relaxants	Similar to above	Deep breathing and coughing Mechanical ventilation Anticholinesterase drugs
Mechanical restriction	Tight casts or dressings Abdominal dissention Position preventing lung expansion	Shallow respirations	Deep breathing and coughing Repositioning Loosening of cast or dressing Nasogastric intubation
Pain	Shallow breathing to prevent incisional pain (especially with chest and abdominal surgery)	Similar to above	Analgesic in reduced dose
Aspiration of vomitus			
Retention of food or fluid in stomach	Gastric secretions may be accumulated even in fasting client	Vomitus may or may not be expelled via mouth	Turn on side or turn head to side Suctioning Nasogastric intubation Coughing
Delayed gastric emptying	Pain, fear, narcotics, anticholinergic medications delay gastric emptying		
Position change after narcotics	Narcotics stimulate chemoreceptor trigger zone (CTZ) in medulla Movement also stimulates CTZ		

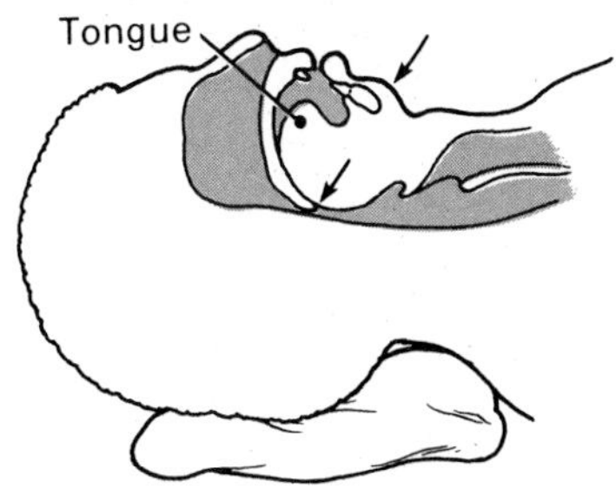

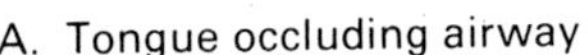

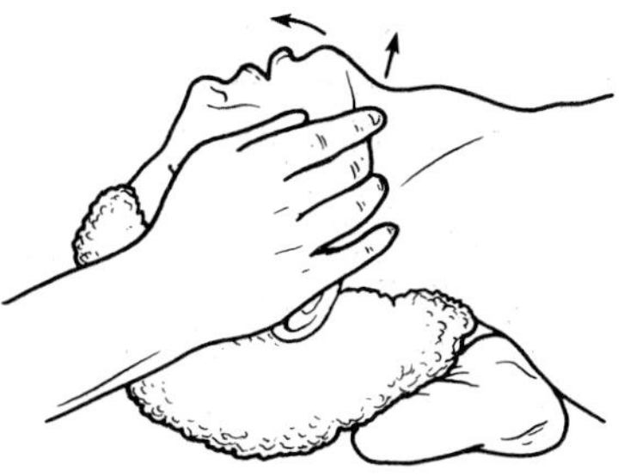

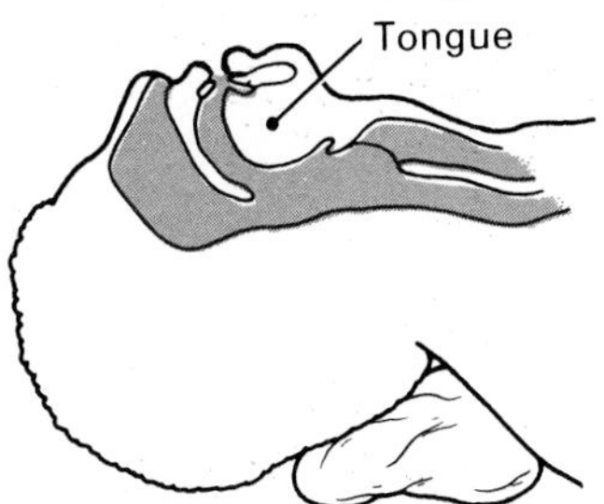

Figure 8-2 Etiology and relief of airway obstruction by client's tongue.

provided by the nurse until the respiratory center recovers sufficiently to respond to the usual stimulant of increased carbon dioxide concentration in the blood.[5]

Cardiovascular problems

Nursing Assessment The most important aspect of the cardiovascular assessment is frequent taking of *vital signs*. They are usually monitored every 15 minutes or more often until stabilized, and then at less frequent intervals. A common schedule is every 15 minutes × 4, every 30 minutes × 4, every 1 hour × 4, and then every 4 hours (the 4 × 4 rule). Postoperative vital signs should be compared with preoperative as well as with intraoperative readings to determine when they are stabilizing at a normal level for the client's situation. The anesthesiologist or surgeon should be notified if:

1. Systolic blood pressure is less than 90 mmHg or greater than 160 mmHg.
2. Pulse rate is less than 60 beats per minute (bpm) or greater than 120 bpm.
3. Blood pressure or pulse is markedly different from previous readings (e.g., 10 mmHg change in blood pressure, 10 bpm change in pulse).
4. Gradual decrease in blood pressure over several consecutive readings.
5. Development of irregular cardiac rhythm.

Assessment of skin color, temperature, and moisture provides valuable information in detecting cardiovascular problems. Hypotension accompanied by a normal pulse and warm, dry, pink skin usually represents the residual effects of anesthesia and suggests only a need for continued observation. Hypotension accompanied by a rapid pulse and cold, clammy, pale skin may be due to impending hypovolemic shock and requires immediate treatment.

Pathophysiology Transient hypotension is relatively common in the recovery room. However, if persistent and severe it may indicate shock. Hypotension and shock postoperatively are most commonly related to hypovolemia, residual effects of anesthesia, and severe pain. Other possible causes are adrenal insufficiency or cardiac failure (Table 8-3).

Hypovolemia results from inadequate fluid or

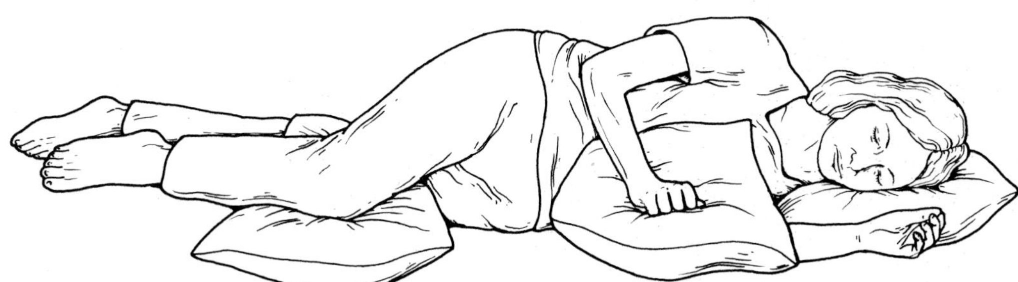

Figure 8-3 Positioning of client during recovery from general anesthesia.

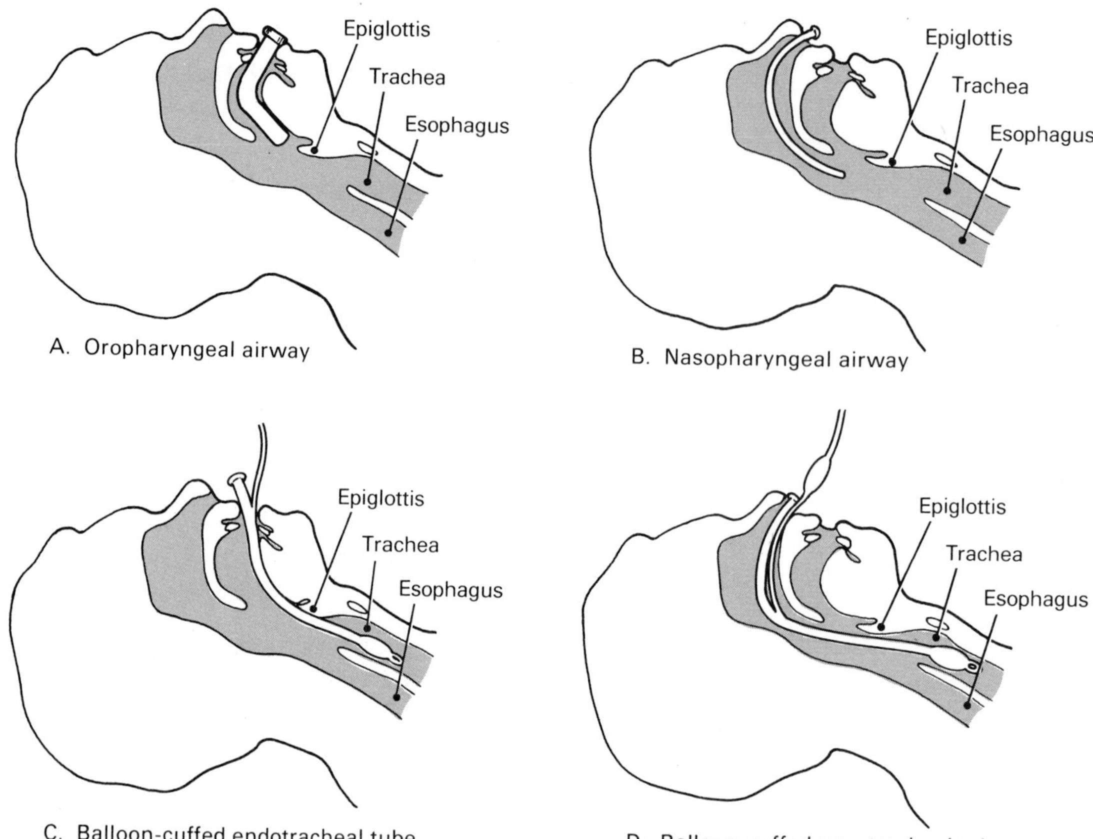

Figure 8-4 Mechanical devices to prevent airway obstruction during recovery from anesthesia.

blood replacement for dehydration, surgical losses, hemorrhage, and postoperative fluid losses. Blood loss during most surgical procedures ranges between 100 and 500 mL, but may be considerably greater if bleeding is difficult to control. Blood transfusions are generally given only if estimated blood loss exceeds 500 mL. Serious hypovolemic shock does not usually develop in the adult until 1.5 to 2 L of blood volume have been lost.[6]

Residual effects of anesthesia may produce mild hypotension during the recovery period from any general anesthetic.[7] A fall in blood pressure may also accompany the use of spinal or epidural anesthesia. This can be due to arteriolar dilatation due to paralysis of preganglionic sympathetic nerves and a fall in cardiac output due to reduced venous return.[8] As anesthesia wears off, the client's blood pressure usually returns to its preoperative level. Since narcotic analgesics may also lower blood pressure, their administration before the effects of anesthesia have dissipated may noticeably increase hypotension.

While moderate pain tends to produce an increase in blood pressure, more severe pain may cause hypotension as a result of autonomic reflexes mediated by norepinephrine release and result in a decrease in heart rate and cardiac output.[9] This response may be great enough to produce shock, particularly when pain occurs in combination with the residual effects of anesthesia and depleted fluid volume.

Nursing Management The nursing role in assessment and management of hypotension and shock is described in Chap. 26. During postanesthesia recovery, many of the nurse's actions are directed at prevention or early detection of hypotension, shock, and other cardiovascular problems (Table 8-3).

If shock develops, the client's legs should be elevated enough to maintain a downward slope toward the trunk of the body. The head should not be lowered. If a person has had spinal anesthesia, the legs should not be elevated because this position

Table 8-3
Hypotension and Shock in the Postanesthesia Period

Cause	Contributing Factors	Intervention
Hypovolemia	Blood loss Hemorrhage Preoperative dehydration Inadequate fluid or blood replacement GI drainage	Leg elevation Oxygen IV fluids or blood
Effects of anesthesia and drugs	Conduction anesthesia (vasomotor depression)	Leg elevation Oxygen IV fluids Vasopressors
	General anesthesia	Same as above Stimulate to regain consciousness
	Excessive narcotic dosage	Oxygen Narcotic antagonists (Nalline, Lorfan)
Pain	Withholding of narcotics	IV or IM analgesic in reduced dosage
Adrenal insufficiency	Chronic steroid use Prolonged or excessive stress	IV hydrocortisone IM cortisone or hydrocortisone
Cardiac failure	Preexisting cardiac disease Circulatory overload from excessive fluid replacement	Digitalization Diuretics

could cause impairment of the diaphragm. It is better to position that client with the head elevated 30° and a pillow under each leg.[10]

Pain and discomfort

Pathophysiology As the effects of anesthesia wear off, the client begins to perceive incisional pain as well as discomforts associated with the presence of dressings, drains, tubes, and other equipment. Pain or discomfort may also be associated with a distended bladder, uncomfortable positions during the operative procedure, or with a serious complication such as myocardial infarction.

Nursing Management Analgesic drugs are frequently administered in the recovery room for relief of pain. Sometimes the medical order is written that the dose may be reduced by one-third to one-half. A full dose of pain medication plus the residual effect of preanesthetic barbiturates or narcotics and of anesthetic agents can cause respiratory depression and decreased blood pressure. The hypotensive client is at particular risk from overdose. Hypotension in itself is not an indication to withhold pain medication. However, it does require nursing judgment when administering pain medication.

A client who has received a neuroleptic drug such as Innovar, which potentiates the action of narcotics, requires special caution and may have the dosage of narcotics and barbiturates reduced to one-half to one-fourth the usual dosage for up to 12 hours.[11,12]

Recovery From Anesthesia

Nursing assessment: Manifestations of recovery

General Anesthesia Recovery from general anesthesia occurs in the reverse sequence as described in Chap. 7. There is considerable variation in the mode of emergence experienced by clients, depending upon the nature and dosage of the anesthetic agent used and the client's idiosyncratic response to it. The nurse should always be alert to the possibility of unexpected deepening of anesthesia and reversal of recovery of consciousness and reflexes. This may occur as circulation increases and deposits of anesthesia are picked up from storage in various tissues. This change in level of consciousness presents a special danger to the client whose artificial airway already has been removed.

Regional Anesthesia Recovery from *regional anesthesia* (spinal and epidural) also occurs in a reverse sequence from induction. Position sense returns first, then motion, then sensation, and finally autonomic (sympathetic) vasomotor function.[13] The nurse should note the time of recovery of both motion and sensation. The client is considered recovered when he responds to a toe pinprick rather than when he can wiggle his toes.

Some clients develop a spinal headache when their head is raised after regional anesthesia.[14] This type of headache, involving severe constricting or throbbing occipital or sometimes frontal discomfort and some nuchal rigidity, may develop within an hour to 2 or 3 days after surgery. It may last from a day to a week or even longer. It is believed to be caused by a decrease in cerebrospinal fluid pressure due to leakage at the puncture site. This results in a "sagging" of the brain and tension on its pain-sensitive supporting structures. It is more frequent in young adults, in females during the preovulation phase of the menstrual cycle, and in those clients who expect it to happen. Spinal headache is less likely if a small size needle is used for spinal anesthesia and if postoperative hydration of the client is adequate. The practice of keeping the client flat for 12 to 24 hours to prevent a headache is generally considered outmoded but may still be employed in some instances.

Nursing management

Safety and Comfort The client must be turned and positioned carefully during recovery from anesthesia to avoid damage to eyes, skin, muscles, nerves, and blood vessels. Before lid reflexes return, the cornea may inadvertently be scratched by personnel or equipment, or the client. Before sensation and motion return, the client may remain in a position which places pressure on skin or nerves, or which obstructs circulation. Flaccid muscles may easily be overstretched and injured during turning if adequate support is not provided. The use of side rails and restraining straps on the recovery stretcher prevent injury during this period.

The client should be kept warm by receiving extra blankets. Anesthesia and many adjunctive drugs affect the body's temperature regulating mechanisms. The client may enter the recovery room with a body temperature as low as 36.5°C. The nurse must take appropriate measures to prevent chilling until the body temperature has stabilized.[15] The client with a low body temperature has slowed circulation and thus delayed elimination of the anesthetic, which prolongs recovery.

Communication Even the client who has been told what to expect in the recovery room may be frightened or confused as he awakens to the strange environment. Since hearing is the first sense to return in the unconscious client, the nurse should explain all actions from the moment of admission to the recovery room. Orientation includes telling the client that (1) the surgery is over, (2) he is in the RR, (3) his family knows he is there, (4) who the persons caring for him are and what they are doing, and (5) the time of day. Family members who are waiting should also be contacted by the recovery room nurse when possible.

Discharge from the Recovery Room

The surgeon or anesthesiologist will authorize the client's release from the recovery room and transfer to the clinical unit or intensive care unit. Recovery from anesthesia is usually judged to be sufficient when the following criteria are met:

1. Vital signs are stabilized.
2. Respirations and circulation are adequate.
3. Anesthetic effects have been reversed (usually requires 1 to 2 hours).
4. The client is awake or easily arousable.
5. Complications are not present or are under control.

The recovery room nurse accompanies the client to the clinical unit and assists in settling the client in bed. She gives a detailed report to the unit nurse related to the intraoperative and immediate postoperative period.

THE POSTOPERATIVE CLIENT ON THE CLINICAL UNIT

Receiving the Client from the Recovery Room

The nurse who receives the client on the clinical unit listens to the report from the recovery room nurse. She then completes and records an initial assessment and begins care (Table 8-4).

Possible Problems During the Postoperative Period

The nurse recognizes that problems of the immediate postanesthetic period continue into the early postoperative period. As recovery continues, these problems become less likely and are replaced by different problems during subsequent days (Fig. 8-5).

Nursing assessment and management are based upon knowledge of the possible symptoms and complications associated with surgery in general, as well as with the particular type of operation which the client has undergone.

Early ambulation is the most significant nursing measure to prevent postoperative complications. Since it was first advocated nearly four decades ago, experience has repeatedly shown the value of early ambulation.[16] The exercise associated with walking (1) increases smooth muscle tone; (2) improves gastrointestinal and urinary tract function; (3) stimulates circulation, which prevents venous stasis and speeds wound healing; and (4) increases vital capacity and maintains normal respiratory function.

Respiratory problems

Nursing assessment of respiratory problems has been discussed in the section on postanesthesia recovery.

Pathophysiology *Atelectasis and pneumonitis* (hypostatic pneumonia) are particularly common after abdominal and thoracic surgery.[17] *Atelectasis* (alveolar collapse) occurs when mucus blocks bronchioles and the air trapped beyond the block is gradually absorbed (Fig. 8-6). It may affect a portion of or an entire lobe of a lung. The primary reason that mucous plugs develop postoperatively is due to hypoventilation, a constant recumbent position, and ineffective coughing. Increased bronchial secretion occurs when respiratory passages are irritated by heavy smoking, acute or chronic pulmonary infection, inhalation anesthetics, or endotracheal intubation. Atelectasis can progress to *pneumonitis* when a secondary infection develops in the stagnant mucus.

Nursing Management The client should be assisted to breathe deeply several times every hour, as instructed preoperatively. Splinting the incision aids in coughing up any secretions which are present (Chap. 6). Position should be changed hourly to allow full expansion of both lungs, and ambulation (*not* just sitting in a chair) should be carried out aggressively. Adequate and regular analgesic medication should be provided, since incisional pain often is the greatest deterrent to adequate ventilation. The client should also be reassured that these activities present no danger to the incision. Adequate hydration, either parenteral or oral, is essential to keep secretions thin and loose so they can be raised with coughing. Nursing management of the client who develops atelectasis and pneumonitis is described in Chap. 20.

Table 8-4

Nursing Assessment and Care of Client on Admission to Clinical Unit

1. Record time of client's return to unit
2. Take baseline vital signs
3. Assess neurological status
   - Level of consciousness
   - Movement of extremities
4. Assess wound, dressing, and drainage tubing
   - Type and amount of drainage
   - Connect tubing to gravity or suction drainage
5. Assess color and appearance of skin
6. Assess urinary status
   - Time of voiding
   - Presence or absence of urge to void
   - Bladder distension
   - Urinary output (Report if <30 mL/h)
   - Presence of catheter
   - Patency of catheter
7. Assess pain and discomfort
8. Position for comfort and safety (usually on side with side rails up)
9. Intravenous Infusion
   - Type of solution
   - Amount remaining
   - Flow rate
   - Appearance and location of IV site
10. Attach call light within reach
11. Place emesis basin and tissues within reach
12. Check and carry out postoperative orders
13. Determine emotional condition and support

Cardiovascular problems

Nursing assessment of cardiovascular problems is discussed in the section on postanesthesia recovery.

Pathophysiology *Deep vein thrombosis* is a potentially life-threatening complication because it may lead to *pulmonary embolism*. Clotting tendencies are increased postoperatively as a result of the increased platelet production associated with glucocorticoid release in response to the stress of surgery. Blood clots may form in leg veins as a result of postoperative inactivity, position, and pressure which creates venous stasis. They may also form in pelvic veins following gynecologic surgery during which retractors or other instruments have injured the vein wall. If a piece of this clot becomes dislodged, it can cause a pulmonary infarction of a size proportionate to the vessel in which it lodges. *Superficial thrombophlebitis*, an uncomfortable but less ominous complication, may develop in the leg veins as a result of venous stasis, or in the arm veins as a result of irritation from IV needles or solutions.

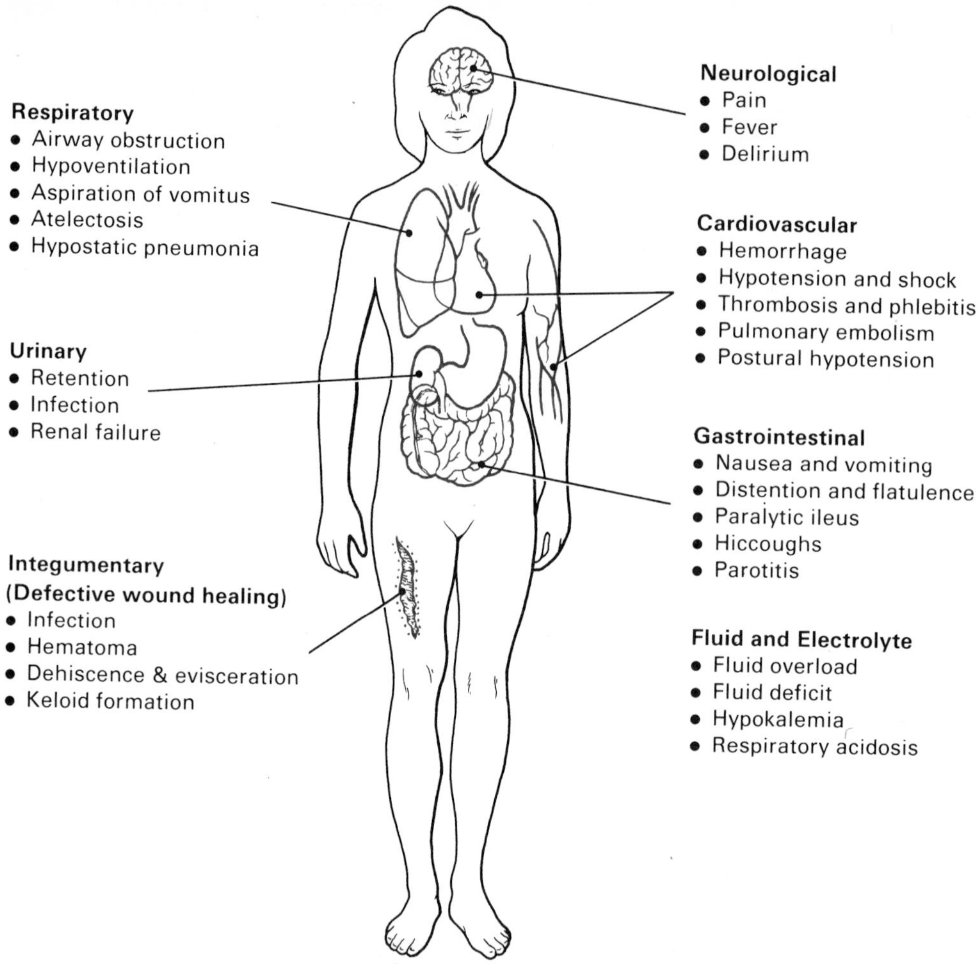

Respiratory
• Airway obstruction
• Hypoventilation
• Aspiration of vomitus
• Atelectosis
• Hypostatic pneumonia
Urinary
• Retention
• Infection
• Renal failure
Integumentary
(Defective wound healing)
• Infection
• Hematoma
• Dehiscence & evisceration
• Keloid formation
Neurological
• Pain
• Fever
• Delirium
Cardiovascular
• Hemorrhage
• Hypotension and shock
• Thrombosis and phlebitis
• Pulmonary embolism
• Postural hypotension
Gastrointestinal
• Nausea and vomiting
• Distention and flatulence
• Paralytic ileus
• Hiccoughs
• Parotitis
Fluid and Electrolyte
• Fluid overload
• Fluid deficit
• Hypokalemia
• Respiratory acidosis

Figure 8-5 Possible problems in the postoperative period.

Alveoli lined by flattened epithelium to allow gas exchange
Mucus plug accumulating
Mucus plug
Air absorbed from alveoli. Lung segment "collapses"
A
B
C

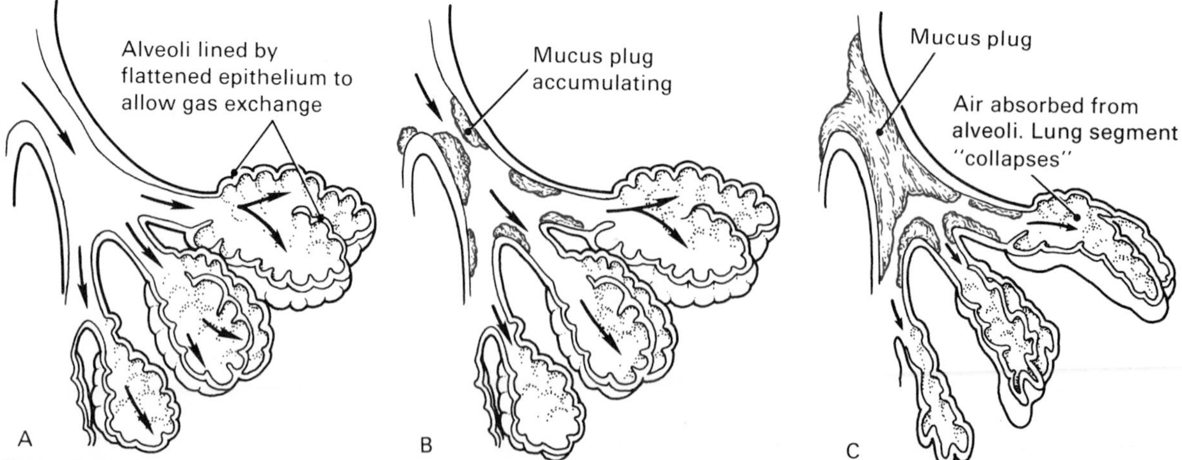

Figure 8-6 Postoperative atelectasis. (*a*) Normal bronchiole and alveoli. (*b*) Mucous plug in bronchiole. (*c*) Atelectactic collapse of alveoli.

Syncope may occur as a result of postural hypotension when the client ambulates. It is more common in the elderly and when surgery and recumbency have been prolonged. Normally, when the client comes quickly to a standing position, arterial pressoreceptors in the neck and thorax respond to the fall in blood pressure and cause sympathetic nervous stimulation which produces peripheral vasoconstriction. This causes a rise in blood pressure. After an extended time of recumbency or following the effects of anesthesia (which alters sympathetic and vasomotor function) this normal mechanism may be impaired. Consequently, syncope develops.

Nursing Management The client should be encouraged to exercise the legs 10 to 12 times each hour as instructed preoperatively (Chap. 6). The muscular contraction which these exercises (as well as that of walking) produces is effective in facilitating venous return from the lower extremities. When the client ambulates, he should pick up his feet sharply rather than shuffling them, so that muscular contraction is maximized. When sitting in a chair or lying in bed, there should be no pressure (from crossed legs, pillows behind the knee, or a raised knee gatch) to impede venous flow through the popliteal space.

Some surgeons routinely use elastic bandages or stockings to increase the massaging action which is transmitted to the veins when leg muscles contract. The nurse must remember that these are useless if the legs are not exercised, and may actually impair circulation if the legs remain inactive or if they are applied improperly. When used, elastic bandages and stockings should be removed and reapplied at least once on every shift.

The use of low-dose heparin therapy (5000 U subcutaneously every 8 to 12 hours) as a prophylactic measure against venous thrombosis and embolism is becoming increasingly common. It is begun 2 hours before surgery and continued for 7 days or until the client is fully ambulatory.[18] This low dose does not significantly increase the risk of bleeding during surgery or in the postoperative period.

Syncope may be prevented by raising the head of the client's bed for a minute or two before getting him out of bed. The nurse then has the client stand at the bedside while supporting him. If faintness occurs, the nurse can help the client sit on the edge of the bed. If the client faints during ambulation, he should be eased to the floor and allowed to lie there until recovery. Then the client can be assisted to walk back to bed. While perhaps frightening for the client (or the unprepared nurse), such syncope is of no real danger.

Nursing management of the client who develops thrombosis and embolism is described in Chap. 30.

Fluid and electrolyte imbalances

Pathophysiology Postoperative fluid and electrolyte imbalances may develop as a result of a combination of the body's normal response to the stress of surgery, excessive fluid losses, and improper intravenous replacement. The stress response (Fig. 12-9) results in fluid retention during the first 2 to 5 postoperative days. It is generally a useful mechanism to maintain blood volume and blood pressure. Fluid retention results from (1) increased adrenocorticotropic hormone (ACTH) secretion by the anterior pituitary, which leads to increased secretion of aldosterone and cortisol by the adrenal cortex, both of which produce sodium and water retention; and (2) increased antidiuretic hormone (ADH) secretion by the posterior pituitary, which leads to decreased urine output.

Fluid overload may develop during this period of fluid retention if intravenous fluids are administered too rapidly. Conversely, *fluid deficit* may be related to slow or inadequate fluid replacement for preoperative dehydration or intraoperative and postoperative losses from vomiting, bleeding, or drainage from various tubes. *Hypokalemia* may result from urinary and gastrointestinal losses if potassium is not replaced in intravenous fluids. Adequate replacement of potassium is 40 mEq/day. Potassium should not be given until adequate renal function has been established, which is generally considered to be at least 30 mL/hour.

Nursing Management *Thirst* is one of the most annoying discomforts with which the postoperative client must contend. It may be related to the drying effects of preoperative anticholinergic drugs, anesthetic gases, and a fluid deficit. Adequate and regular mouth care is helpful while the client is NPO. An increased rate of fluid replacement seems to relieve thirst. An accurate intake and output record should be kept during the postoperative period, and laboratory findings (electrolytes and hematocrit) should be monitored. Nursing responsibilities relative to IV management are critical during this period. In particular, the nurse should be alert for symptoms of too slow or too rapid a rate of fluid replacement, and for the possible infusion site discomfort and cardiac hazards associated with IV potassium administration (Chap. 12).

Urinary problems

Nursing Assessment The urine should be examined for color, amount, consistency, and odor. Retention catheters should be assessed for patency. Urine output should be at least 30 mL/hour if a client has an indwelling catheter. If a catheter is not present, the client should be able to void about 200 mL at the first voiding after surgery. Most people void within 6 to 8 hours after surgery.

If the client has not voided within 6 to 8 hours or bladder distension is suspected, the bladder should be palpated and percussed. These techniques are discussed in Chap. 36.

Pathophysiology Low urine output (800 to 1500 mL) in the first 24 hours may be expected regardless of fluid intake. This is due to increased ADH secretion following the stress of surgery, fluid restriction before surgery, loss of fluids due to evaporation during surgery, drainage, and diaphoresis. By the second or third day the client will have diuresis after fluid has been mobilized and the immediate stress reaction subsides.

Actual *urinary retention* can occur in the postoperative period for a variety of reasons. Anesthesia depresses the nervous system, including the micturition reflex arc and the higher centers which influence it. This allows the bladder to fill more completely than normal before the urge to void is felt. It also impedes voluntary micturition. Anticholinergic and narcotic drugs may interfere with the ability to initiate voiding or to empty the bladder completely. Retention is more likely to occur following lower abdominal or pelvic surgery because spasm or guarding of the abdominal and pelvic muscles interferes with their normal function in micturition. Pain may clutter perception centers and interfere with the client's awareness of the less intense and more familiar sensation arising as the bladder fills. Voiding ability is probably impaired to the greatest extent by immobility and the recumbent position in bed. Lack of skeletal muscle activity decreases smooth muscle (bladder detrusor) tone, and the supine position reduces the ability to relax the perineal muscles and external sphincter.

Oliguria associated with *acute renal failure* is a less common although more serious problem after surgery. It may result from renal ischemia from inadequate renal perfusion secondary to a hemolytic reaction due to the transfusion of incompatible blood or other causes. These prerenal causes of renal failure are described in Chap. 38.

Nursing Management The nurse may facilitate voiding by normal positioning (sitting for females, standing for males), reassuring the client of his or her ability to void, and techniques such as running water, drinking water, blowing bubbles through a straw, or heat application to relax the perineum. Ambulation (preferably to the bathroom) is the most helpful measure to facilitate voiding.

The surgeon often leaves an order to catheterize the client in 8 to 12 hours if he has not voided. Because of the hazard of infection associated with catheterization, the nurse should first try other measures to induce voiding and validate that the bladder is actually full. If the bladder becomes overdistended, it is traumatized and more susceptible to infection if catheterization becomes necessary. In assessing the need for catheterization, the nurse should consider fluid intake during and after surgery and evidence of bladder fullness (palpable fullness above the symphysis pubis, discomfort when pressure is applied over the bladder, or the presence of the urge to void).

Gastrointestinal problems

Nursing Assessment Bowel sounds should be assessed during the postanesthesia period and routinely thereafter. The abdomen should be auscultated in all four quadrants to determine the presence, frequency, and characteristics of the sounds.

Bowel sounds are frequently absent in the immediate postoperative period due to the effect of anesthesia and adjunct drugs which decrease peristalsis. In abdominal surgery, manual manipulation of the bowel causes temporary paralysis of the intestine, frequently called *paralytic ileus*.

Pathophysiology *Nausea and vomiting* are experienced by 10 to 30 percent of surgical clients.[19] These problems may be caused by the action of anesthetics or narcotics, by slowed peristalsis resulting from the handling of the bowel during surgery, and by resumption of oral intake too soon after surgery.

Abdominal distension is another common problem caused by decreased peristalsis due to handling of the intestine during surgery and to limited dietary intake after surgery. Motility of the large intestine may be reduced for 3 to 5 days, although motility in the small intestine resumes within 24 hours.[20] Swallowed air and gastrointestinal secretions may therefore accumulate in the colon, producing flatulence and gas pains.

Hiccoughs (singultus) are intermittent spasms of the diaphragm caused by irritation of the phrenic nerve which innervates the diaphragm. Postoperative sources of *direct irritation* of the phrenic nerve may be gastric distension, intestinal obstruction, intraabdominal bleeding, or a subphrenic abscess. *Indirect irritation* of the phrenic nerve may be produced by acid-base and electrolyte imbalances. *Reflex irritation* may come from drinking very hot or cold liquids or from the presence of a nasogastric tube. Hiccoughs usually last only a short time and subside spontaneously. Occasionally they may be persistent and debilitating.

Parotitis is an inflammation of the parotid glands which occurs when the normal stimulation of salivary secretion provided by eating is absent and the salivary ducts become blocked. It is uncomfortable for the client, producing considerable pain, swelling, and fever. It is also dangerous because a secondary staphylococcal infection can develop.

Nursing Management Depending upon the nature of surgery, the client may resume oral intake as soon as the gag reflex returns. Sometimes the client is kept NPO for several days until bowel sounds are heard. While the client is NPO, intravenous infusions are given to maintain fluid and electrolyte balance. A nasogastric tube may be used to decompress the stomach to prevent nausea, vomiting, and abdominal distension from developing. When oral intake is allowed after the return of bowel sounds, clear liquids are first given while the IV is still running. If these are well tolerated by the client, the IV is removed and the diet advanced until a regular diet is tolerated.

While the client is NPO, regular mouth care is essential for comfort and stimulation of salivary glands. Nausea and vomiting may be prevented or relieved by the administration of an antiemetic drug (usually of the phenothiazine type) intramuscularly. In some instances, a nasogastric tube may be inserted if symptoms persist.

Abdominal distension may be prevented or minimized by early and frequent ambulation and by resumption of a normal diet, both of which stimulate intestinal peristalsis. Although their efficacy in stimulating peristalsis is questionable, cholinergic drugs such as bethanechol (Urecholine), neostigmine (Prostigmin), or dexpanthenol (Ilopan) may be administered subcutaneously or intramuscularly. The nurse should assess the client regularly to detect the resumption of normal intestinal peristalsis, as evidenced by the return of bowel sounds and the passage of flatus.

The client may need to be encouraged to expel flatus and to be assured that this generally sociably unacceptable behavior is now highly desirable. *Gas pains*, which tend to become pronounced on the second or third postoperative day, may be relieved by ambulation, positioning, rectal tube placement or rectal lavage, and application of heat to the abdomen. These measures may be combined for effectiveness by positioning the client on the right side to permit gas to rise along the transverse colon, inserting a rectal tube attached to a container to collect any discharge, and applying heat to the abdomen. This treatment is most effective if maintained for about 20 minutes and repeated every 2 to 3 hours, and if the client ambulates between treatments. Some clients experience relief if a rectal lavage or Harris flush (the alternate instillation and siphonage of 200 to 300 mL of fluid) is used instead of the rectal tube placement. Bisacodyl (Dulcolax) suppositories may also be ordered to stimulate peristalsis and flatus expulsion.

The postoperative client who is *hiccoughing* should first be assessed in an attempt to determine the cause. In many instances, simply irrigating the nasogastric tube to restore patency will solve the problem. However, in other instances the cause is elusive, and trial and error must prevail. Techniques such as holding the breath while drinking water, swallowing 1 or 2 teaspoons of sugar, or rebreathing carbon dioxide from a paper bag may help. Drug therapy may include atropine or phenothiazine administration. For intractable cases, a phrenic nerve block or phrenic nerve crush may be employed.

Parotitis may be prevented primarily by meticulous mouth care. While chewing gum or sucking on hard candy are sometimes recommended to stimulate salivation, these activities may lead to increased air swallowing and distension in the postoperative client. If parotitis should develop, it is treated with antibiotics. Incision and drainage is sometimes necessary.

Integumentary problems

Pathophysiology Surgery involves an incision through skin and underlying tissues. Healing of the wound is one of the major concerns of the postoperative period. The surgical stress response includes protein catabolism which makes amino acids available for healing. A limited period of interrupted nutritional intake will not harm the adult who was well-nourished preoperatively. However, the poorly nourished client may have little reserve to draw upon and is considerably more prone to problems of wound healing.

Wound infection results from invasion of the wound by microbes from three major sources: exogenous flora (present in the environment and on the skin), oral flora, and intestinal flora.[21] The incidence of wound sepsis is higher among clients who are malnourished, and increases in proportion to the length of hospital stay and to the duration of time that the wound is open during surgery. Infection may involve the entire incision either superficially or deeply. Infection may form an abscess or it may involve body cavities, as in peritonitis. Evidence of wound infection usually does not become apparent before the third to fifth postoperative day. The signs include local manifestations of redness, swelling, and increasing pain and tenderness at the site. Systemic manifestations are fever and leukocytosis.

An accumulation of fluid within a wound may create pressure, impair circulation and wound healing, and predispose to infection. These are the reasons the surgeon may place a drain in the incision itself or a stab wound adjacent to the incision to allow for drainage. These drains may be soft rubber and drain into a dressing, or they may be firm catheters attached to a Hemovac or other source of gentle suction. Wound healing and complications are discussed in Chap. 9.

Nursing Assessment and Management Nursing assessment of the wound and dressing requires knowledge of the type of wound, drains inserted, and expected drainage related to the specific type of surgery. A small amount of serous drainage is common from any type of wound. If a Penrose drain is in the incision or close to it, a moderate to large amount of drainage may be expected. For example, a cholecystectomy incision with accompanying Penrose drain can be expected to drain a moderate amount of serosanguineous drainage with some bile drainage within the first 24 hours. In contrast, an inguinal herniorrhaphy should have only minimal serous drainage in the postoperative period.

In general, drainage should be expected to change from sanguineous (red) to serosanguineous (pink) to serous (straw-colored) over a period of hours and days. Bloody drainage may be normal after certain types of surgery (e.g., chest surgery). However, it should not last more than a few hours and should decrease in volume over time. Continuation of bleeding or an increase in drainage after it has once subsided often signals a problem. Wound infection may be accompanied by purulent drainage. Wound dehiscence (separation and disruption of previously joined wound edges) may be preceded by a sudden discharge of brown, pink, or clear drainage.

When drainage occurs on the dressing, it should be circled with a pen and marked with the date and time. The type, amount, color, consistency, and odor of drainage should be noted and recorded. The effect of position changes on drainage should also be assessed. The surgeon should be notified of any excessive or abnormal drainage and significant changes in vital signs indicating infection or hemorrhage.

The surgical incision may or may not be covered by a dressing after the first few hours. It is increasingly common to leave the incision open to the air after covering it with a waterproof spray. Hospital policy determines whether or not the nurse may change the initial operative dressing or simply reinforce it. Whether changing the first or a subsequent dressing, the nurse should always be aware of the number and type of drains present. Great care should be taken to avoid dislodging drains when removing the soiled dressing.

When the dressing is changed, the incision site should be examined carefully. The area around the sutures may be slightly reddened and swollen. But the skin around the incision should be of normal color and temperature. Abnormal findings include unusually warm skin around the incision, purple-appearing hard areas in the incision site (possibly from hemorrhage), and signs of infection as previously mentioned.

Neurological problems

Nursing Assessment The initial aspect of the neurological assessment is determination of the level of consciousness. Anesthetized clients resume consciousness in a predictable pattern. By the time the client returns to the clinical unit he is usually awake or easily arousable. The nurse always needs to be alert for possible deepening of anesthesia effects, especially when administering pain medication in the early postoperative period. (See section on recovery from anesthesia.)

Pain assessment may be difficult in the early postoperative period. The client may not be able to verbalize the presence or severity of pain. The nurse should observe for clues of pain such as wrinkling face or brow, clenched fist, moaning, diaphoresis, and increased pulse.

Pathophysiology Pain and fever are two symptoms mediated by the central nervous system which may be problems for the postoperative client. (The assessment and management of the client in pain are discussed in Chap. 49). *Postoperative pain* is produced by the interaction of a number of physiologic and psychological factors. The skin and underlying tissues have been traumatized by the incision and retraction during surgery. In addition, reflex muscle spasms around the incision may be present for several hours or days. Anxiety and fear, sometimes related to the anticipation of pain, create tension and further increase muscle tone and spasm. The effort and movement associated with deep breathing, coughing, or changing position may aggravate pain by creating tension or pull on the incisional area.

When the internal viscera are cut no pain is felt. However, pressure within the internal viscera elicits pain. Therefore, deep visceral pain may signal the presence of a complication, such as intestinal distension or bleeding or abscess formation.

Table 8-5
Significance of Postoperative Temperature Variations

Time After Surgery	Temperature	Possible Reasons
Up to 12 hours	Hypothermia To 34.5°C (94°F)	Effects of anesthesia (general or conduction) Body heat loss in OR
First 24–48 hours	Elevation To 38°C (100.4°F) Above 38°C (100.4°F)	Inflammatory response to surgical trauma Lung congestion, atelectasis Dehydration
Third and subsequent days	Elevation Above 37.7°C (100°F)	Wound infection Urinary infection Respiratory infection Phlebitis Parotitis (rare)

Postoperative pain is usually most severe within the first 48 hours and subsides thereafter. Variation is considerable according to the procedure performed and the client's individual pain tolerance or perception.

Temperature variation in the postoperative period provides valuable information about the client's status. Hypothermia may be present for a few hours while the client is recovering from the effects of anesthesia and body heat loss during surgery. *Fever* may occur at any time during the postoperative period (Table 8-5). A mild elevation (up to 38°C, 100.4°F) during the first 48 hours usually reflects the surgical stress response. A moderate elevation (above 38°C) is caused most frequently by respiratory congestion or atelectasis and less frequently by dehydration. After the first 48 hours, a moderate to marked elevation (above 37.7°C, 99.9°F) is usually caused by infection. Wound infection, particularly from aerobic organisms, is often accompanied by a fever which spikes in the afternoon or evening and returns near normal in the morning. The respiratory tract may be infected secondary to stasis of secretions in an atelectatic region. The urinary tract may be infected secondary to catheterization. Superficial thrombophlebitis may occur at the IV site or in the leg veins. The latter may produce a temperature elevation between 7 and 10 days after surgery. Intermittent high fever accompanied by shaking chills and diaphoresis suggests septicemia. This may occur at any time during the postoperative period because microorganisms may have been introduced into the bloodstream during surgery (especially in GI or GU procedures) or picked up later from the site of a wound, urinary, or vein infection.

Nursing Management Postoperative pain relief is essentially a nursing responsibility, since the surgeon's orders for analgesic medication and other comfort measures are usually written on a prn basis. During the first 48 hours or longer, narcotic analgesics (such as morphine or meperidine) are required to relieve the moderate to severe pain. After that time, nonnarcotic analgesics may be sufficient as pain intensity decreases. Too often nurses undermedicate their clients in an attempt to protect them from addiction, an imagined hazard which simply does not exist during the few days of extreme postoperative discomfort. During the first 24 to 48 hours, the client should be medicated freely every 3 to 4 hours if necessary because (1) the greatest relief is obtained when an analgesic is administered as pain is beginning, rather than when it has become more severe; and (2) relative freedom from pain is essential to gain the client's cooperation in activities of deep breathing, coughing, turning, and ambulation. When the client does request pain medication, it should be given promptly, for minutes can seem like hours to a person in pain.

Analgesic administration should be timed so that it is in effect during activities which may be painful for the client, such as ambulating. While narcotic analgesics are often essential for the postoperative client's well-being, they are not without undesirable side effects. These side effects (slowed intestinal peristalsis and bowel spasm, nausea and vomiting, respiratory and cough depression, and hypotension) are most pronounced with the opiates.

Before administering any analgesic, the nurse should first be sure of the nature of the client's pain. If it is incisional pain, the analgesic is appropriate. If it is remote chest or leg pain, medication may simply mask a complication. If it is gas pain, medication can aggravate it. The nurse should notify the physician and request a change in the order if the analgesic either fails to relieve the client's pain or if it makes him excessively lethargic or somnolent.

A number of other measures may be helpful in preventing or relieving postoperative pain. The client should be instructed to use his limbs rather than abdominal muscles in turning and getting out of bed after abdominal surgery. There is increasing interest in the application of controlled breathing and relaxation techniques used to obtain relief of postoperative pain. Both these measures have a similar rationale which includes anxiety reduction, attention distraction, muscle relaxation, and provision of a sense of control over the pain experience.[22,23]

The nurse's role related to postoperative fever may be preventive, diagnostic, and therapeutic. Nursing measures to prevent most sources of fever are described earlier in this chapter. In particular, meticulous asepsis should be maintained in regard to the wound and IV site, as well as frequent observation for early signs of inflammation.

The client's temperature is usually measured every 4 hours for the first 48 hours postoperatively and then less frequently if no problems develop. If fever develops, chest x-rays may be taken, along with cultures of the wound, urine, or blood, depending upon the suspected etiology. If infection is believed to be the cause, antibiotics are started IM or via IV piggyback as soon as cultures have been obtained. If the fever is extreme (>41°C, 105.8°F), antipyretic drugs and body cooling measures may be employed (Chap. 52).

Psychological problems

Pathophysiology Anxiety and depression may occur in the postoperative client for any of the reasons described in Chap. 6 (common fears related to surgery). They may be more pronounced in the client who has had radical surgery or amputation or whose findings suggest a poor prognosis. A prior history of a neurotic or psychotic disorder should alert the nurse to the possibility of postoperative anxiety and depression. However, they may develop in any client as part of the grief response to loss of a body organ or disturbance in body image, and may be exacerbated by a lowered response to stress.

Confusion or delirium may arise from a variety of psychological and physiologic sources, including fluid and electrolyte imbalance, hypoxia, drug toxicity, sleep deprivation, and sensory alteration, deprivation, or overload. Delirium tremens due to alcohol withdrawal may be responsible for as much as 25 percent of all postoperative delirium.[24] It is characterized by restlessness, insomnia and nightmares, tachycardia, apprehension, confusion and disorientation, irritability, and auditory or visual hallucinations, and may be treated by the administration of IV alcohol (Chap. 60).

Nursing Management The nurse attempts to prevent psychological problems in the postoperative period by providing adequate support for the client. Supportive measures include taking time to listen and talk with the client, offering explanations and genuine reassurance, and encouraging the presence and assistance of significant others. The nurse must observe and evaluate the client's behavior to distinguish a normal reaction to the stress situation from one which is becoming abnormal or excessive. The recognition of the alcohol withdrawal syndrome in a client not previously known to be an alcoholic presents a particular challenge. Any unusual or disturbed behavior should be reported immediately so that diagnosis and treatment may be instituted.

Planning for Discharge and Follow-up Care

Preparation for the client's discharge is actually an ongoing process throughout the surgical experience which begins during the preoperative period. The informed client is then prepared as events unfold, and gradually assumes greater responsibility for self-care during the postoperative period.

As the day of discharge approaches, the nurse should be certain that the client has the following information:

1. Care of wound site and any dressings
2. Action and possible side effects of any medications; when and how to take them
3. Activities allowed and prohibited; when various physical activities can be resumed safely (e.g., driving a car, going to work, sexual intercourse, playing golf, or jogging)
4. Dietary restrictions (if any)
5. Symptoms to be reported (e.g., development of incisional tenderness or increased drainage, discomfort in other parts of the body)
6. Where and when to return for follow-up care
7. Answers to any individual questions or concerns

If the physician has not provided information about particular diet or activity prescriptions or restrictions, the nurse should either obtain it or encourage the client to do so. Attention to fully informing the client before discharge may prevent needless distress or actual disruption of what was accomplished by surgical intervention. For the client, the surgical experience continues during the recuperative period after discharge.

Case Study / Elective Surgery

Mrs. Gwendolyn Abbamonto, a 42-year-old elementary school teacher who is married and the mother of two children, has undergone an elective cholecystectomy for gallstones. The surgery under general anesthesia was uncomplicated. A Penrose drain was placed in the gallbladder bed and brought out through a stab wound adjacent to the right upper quadrant abdominal incision. Her surgeon has written these postoperative orders:

Nasogastric tube to low intermittent suction; irrigate prn. IV Follow present 1000 mL 5% D/W with 1000 mL Ringer's lactate q 8 h and 1000 mL 5% D/W with 40 mEq KCl q 8 h

Turn, cough, and deep breathe q I h

Ambulate this P.M. and then qid

Vital signs per routine

Morphine sulfate 10 mg IM q 4 h prn

Change dressing over drain prn

Discussion Questions

What nursing measures should be taken in the recovery room to protect Mrs. Abbamonto from hazards during post-anesthesia recovery?

1. How would you determine that she was sufficiently recovered from general anesthesia to be transferred to her room?
2. What is the purpose of ambulating this client on the evening of surgery?
3. What factors may particularly predispose Mrs. Abbamonto to the following postoperative problems?
   - atelectasis
   - wound infection
   - abdominal distension
   - hyponatremia
4. What type of drainage would you expect from the incision and from the Penrose drain during the first three postoperative days?
5. What nursing observations would indicate to the surgeon that her Levine tube could be removed and oral intake resumed? Describe how you would implement the following doctor's orders:
   - remove nasogastric tube
   - sips of water to diet as tolerated
   - D/C IV
6. If Mrs. Abbamonto complains of cramping abdominal pain on the third postoperative day, what measures would you use to relieve it? Why?

REVIEW QUESTIONS

The number of the question corresponds to the same numbered objective at the beginning of the chapter.

1. As soon as the client enters the recovery room, the nurse routinely
   a. initiates ROM to extremities
   b. assesses level of consciousness and presence of reflexes
   c. starts a unit of whole blood
   d. removes the oropharyngeal airway

2. Which of these nursing actions would *not* be desirable during recovery from general anesthesia?
   a. encouraging deep breathing and coughing
   b. positioning the client supine
   c. suctioning to remove excess respiratory secretions
   d. auscultating the client's chest bilaterally

3. During the first 24 to 48 hours postoperatively, analgesic medication should be given
   a. every 3 hours even if pain is not present
   b. every 3 to 4 hours as soon as pain begins
   c. every 4 to 6 hours when pain becomes fairly severe
   d. as infrequently as possible to avoid addiction

4. A mild temperature elevation (up to 38°C) in the first 48 hours postoperatively usually reflects
   a. surgical stress response
   b. respiratory congestion
   c. wound infection
   d. urinary infection

5. Which of the following information should the client have in preparation for discharge?
   a. rationale for abstinence from sexual intercourse for 4 to 6 weeks
   b. calling hospital clinical unit to report any abnormal signs or symptoms
   c. when various physical activities can be resumed
   d. referral to nutritional center for management of dietary restrictions

REFERENCES

1. C. P. Artz and J. D. Hardy, *Management of Surgical Complications*, W. B. Saunders Company, Philadelphia, 1975, pp. 206–209.
2. R. H. Libman and J. Keithley, "Relieving Airway Obstruction in the Recovery Room," *Am J Nurs*, **75:**603 (April 1975).
3. J. D. Hardy, "Surgical Complications," chap. 20 in *Davis-Christopher Textbook of Surgery,* D. C. Sabiston, Jr., ed., W. B. Saunders Company, Philadelphia, 1977, p. 426.
4. M. Marcott, "There's More to Post-op Extubation Than Just Pulling Out a Tube," *RN*, **40:**43 (September 1977).
5. C. B. Drain, "Innovar, A Neuroleptic Drug," *Am J Nurs*, **74:**896 (May 1974).
6. Hardy, op. cit., p. 425.
7. M. B. Wiener et al., *Clinical Pharmacology and Therapeutics in Nursing*, McGraw-Hill Book Company, New York, 1979, pp. 758–759.
8. W. D. Wylie and H. C. Churchill-Davidson, *A Practice of Anaesthesia*, Year Book Medical Publishers, Inc., Chicago, 1972, pp. 1200–1202.
9. P. H. Mitchell, *Concepts Basic to Nursing*, McGraw-Hill Book Company, New York, 1977, p. 538.
10. T. Croushore, "Postoperative Recovery: Monitoring for Physiologic Equilibrium," *Nursing Critically Ill Patients Confidentially, Skillbook 79*, Horsham, Pennsylvania, 1979, p. 120.
11. Drain, op. cit.
12. Wiener et al., op. cit., p. 773.
13. Wylie and Churchill-Davidson, op. cit., pp. 1193–1194.
14. V. J. Collins, *Principles of Anesthesiology*, Lea & Febiger, Philadelphia, 1976, p. 690.
15. J. M. Ozuna and C. Foster, "Hypothermia and the Surgical Patient," *Am J Nurs*, **79:**646–648 (April 1979).
16. D. J. Leithauser, *Early Ambulation and Related Procedures in Surgical Management*, Charles C Thomas, Springfield, Ill, 1946.
17. M. Johnson, "Outcome Criteria to Evaluate Postoperative Respiratory Status," *Am J Nurs*, **75:**1474 (September 1975).
18. S. L. Chamberlain, "Low-Dose Heparin Therapy," *Am J Nurs*, **80:**1115 (June 1980).
19. Downs, op. cit.
20. M. Nachlas et al., "Gastrointestinal Motility Studies As a Guide to Postoperative Management," *Ann Surg*, **175** (4):510–522 (1972).
21. C. O'Byrne, "Clinical Detection and Management of Postoperative Wound Sepsis," *NCNA*, **14:**733–734 (December 1979).
22. S. Hudson, "Teach Breath Control to Ease Your Patients' Post-op Pains," *RN*, **40:**37–38 (January 1977).
23. G. G. Flaherty and J. J. Fitzpatrick, "Relaxation Technique to Increase Comfort Level of Postoperative Patients: A Preliminary Study," *Nurs Res*, **27:**352–355 (November–December 1978).
24. E. L. Hollan, "Alcohol Withdrawal: The Unexpected Post-op Syndrome," *RN*, **39:**42 (February 1976).

BIBLIOGRAPHY FOR SECTION 2

Books

Birch, A. A., and J. D. Tolmie: *Anesthesia for the Uninterested*, University Park Press, Baltimore, 1976.

Brand, Janet Coogan, and Stephen H. Tolins: *The Nursing Student's Guide to Surgery*, 1st ed., Little, Brown and Co., Boston, 1979.

Brooks, S. M.: *Fundamentals of Operating Room Nursing* 2d ed., The C. V. Mosby Company, St. Louis, 1979.

———: *Instrumentation for the Operating Room*, The C. V. Mosby Company, St. Louis, 1978.

Dunphy, J. E., et al.: *Current Surgical Diagnosis and Treatment*, 3d ed., Lange Medical Publications, Los Altos, California, 1977.

Gruendemann, Barbara J., et al.: *The Surgical Patient*, 2d ed., The C. V. Mosby Company, St. Louis, 1977.

Hardy, J. D.: *Rhoads Textbook of Surgery: Principles and Practice*, J. B. Lippincott Company, Philadelphia, 1977.

Kee, J.: "Abdominal Surgery, Fluid and Electrolyte Complications," in *Monitoring Fluid and Electrolytes Precisely*, Intermed Communications, Inc., Horsham, Pennsylvania, 1978, pp. 145–148.

LeMaitre, George D., and Janet A. Finnegan: *The Patient in Surgery: A Guide for Nurses*, 4th ed., W. B. Saunders Company, Philadelphia, 1980.

Liechty, R. D., and R. T. Soper (eds): *Synopsis of Surgery*, 3d ed., The C. V. Mosby Company, St. Louis, 1976.

Sabiston, D. C., Jr. (ed): *Davis-Christopher Textbook of Surgery*, W. B. Saunders Company, Philadelphia, 1977.

Periodicals

Aspinall, M. J.: "Scoring Against Nosocomial Infections," *Am J Nurs*, **78:**1704 (1978).

Baker, P. J.: "Postoperative Atelectasis," *Nurs Digest*, **5:**42 (1977).

Bastasaraswathi, K., and A. A. El-Etr: "Preoperative Evaluation of Drug History," *AORN J*, **23:**616–620 (1976).

Blackwell, A. K., and W. Blackwell: "Relieving Gas Pains," *Am J Nurs*, **75:**66 (1975).

Boore, J.: "Preoperative Care of Patients," *Nurs Times*, **73:**409 (1977).

Brandt, Raymond W.: "OR Safety for You—For Your Patients," *AORN Journal*, **17:**46 (1973).

Church, Russell, and William T. Hamlin: "Electrosurgery Demands OR Vigilance," *AORN Journal*, **22:**903 (1975).

Croushore, T. M.: "Postoperative Assessment: The Key to Avoiding the Most Common Nursing Mistakes," *Nurs 79*, **9:**47 (1979).

Cullen, D. J.: "Recovery Room Complications," *AORN J*, **26:**746 (1977).

Damsteegt, D.: "Pastoral Roles in Presurgical Visits," *Am J Nurs*, **75:**1336 (1975).

DeJong, Rudolph H.: "How Local Anesthetics Work," *AORN Journal*, **18:**286 (1973).

———: "Safer Local Anesthesia," *AORN Journal*, **18:**292 (1973).
Donn, M.: "Communication—The Key to Preparation for Surgery," *Nurs Mirror*, **143:**46 (1976).
Durham, N.: "Looking Out for Complications of Abdominal Surgery," *Nurs 75*, **5:**24 (1975).
Dziurbejko, M. M., and J. C. Larkin: "Including the Family in Preoperative Teaching," *Am J Nurs*, **78:**1892 (1978).
Esbach, D.: "Teaching Patients to Cough," *Nurs 78*, **8:**58 (1978).
Fay, M. R.: "Nursing Process in the Recovery Room," *AORN J*, **24:**1069 (1976).
Felton, C. L.: "Hypoxemia and Oral Temperatures," *Am J Nurs*, **78:**56 (1978).
Finn, K. L.: "How's Your Post-Op Ambulation Technique?" *RN*, **42:**69 (1979).
Fraser, I.: "Early Postoperative Bathing, Challenging Traditional Methods," *Nurs Times*, **72:**1844 (1976).
Fry, E. N. S.: "Postoperative Analgesia," *Nurs Times*, **73:**655 (1977).
Galloway, Albert L.: "Diverse Cultures in the OR," *AORN Journal*, **27:**1296 (1978).
Green, J. W., and R. P. Wenzel: "Postoperative Wound Infection," *Ann Surg*, **185:**264 (1977).
Gruendemann, B.: "The Impact of Surgery on Body Image," *NCNA*, **10:**635 (1975).
Harrington, J. D. (ed): "Symposium on Intensive Care of the Surgical Patient," *NCNA*, **10:**1 (1975).
Hewitt, D.: "Is that Pre-op Patient Terrified?" *RN*, **42:**44 (1979).
Holley, Steele H.: "Anesthesia, Methods to Recovery," *AORN Journal*, **21:**822 (1975).
Hoopes, N. M., et al.: "An Approach to Preoperative Visits," *AORN J*, **26:**1048 (1977).
Johnson, J. E., et al.: "A Better Way to Calm the Patient Who Fears the Worst," *RN*, **40:**47 (1977).
Karetzky, M. S., and A. U. Khan: "Review of Current Concepts in Aspiration Pneumonia," *Heart & Lung*, **6:**321 (1977).
Kelly, L. Y.: "The Patient's Right to Know," *Nurs Outlook*, **24:**26 (1976).
Kneedler, Julia A., et al.: "From Standards Into Practice," *AORN Journal*, **28:**603 (1978).
Laird, M.: "Techniques for Teaching Pre- and Postoperative Patients," *Am J Nurs*, **75:**1338 (1975).
Lewis, L.: "Confronting Alcoholism: How One Medical/Surgical Unit Faced the Problem," *Nurs 77*, **7:**56 (1977).
Lyons, M. L.: "What Priority Do You Give Preop Teaching?" *Nurs 77*, **7:**12 (1977).
MacClelland, D. C.: "Are Current Skin Preparations Valid?" *AORN J*, **21:**55 (1975).
McConnell, E. A.: "After Surgery," *Nurs 77*, **7:**32 (1977).
———: "Meeting the Special Needs of Diabetics Facing Surgery," *Nurs 76*, **6:**30 (1976).
———: "Nursing Care in the Surgical Reception Area," *AORN Journal*, **27:**1315 (1978).
Mehaffy, N. L.: "Assessment and Communication for Continuity of Care for the Surgical Patient," *NCNA*, **10:**625 (1975).
Metheney, N. A., and W. D. Snively: "Perioperative Fluids and Electrolytes," *Am J Nurs*, **78:**840 (1978).
Mezzanotte, E. J.: "Group Instruction in Preparation for Surgery," *Am J Nurs*, **70:**89 (1970).
Mitchell, M.: "An RR Experience: As Nurse and Patient Saw It," *RN*, **38:**46 (1975).
Myers, M. B.: "Sutures and Wound Healing", *Am J Nurs*, **71:**1725 (1971).
Paradis, Carol P.: "Nursing in the Recovery Room," *AORN Journal*, **18:**1117 (1973).
Parsons, M. C., and G. J. Stephens: "Postoperative Complications: Assessment and Intervention," *Am J Nurs*, **74:**240 (1974).
Pleitz, J. A.: "Psychological Complications of the Surgical Patient," *AORN J*, **16:**137 (August 1972).
Pomarski, M. E.: "The Alcoholic as a Surgical Patient," *AORN J*, **16:**137 (1972).
Regan, W. A.: "When it Comes to Consent, Empty Gestures Won't Do," *RN*, **42:**25 (1979).
Ridgeway, M.: "Preop Interviews Assure Quality Care," *AORN J*, **24:**1083 (1976).
Robertson, Patricia A.: "Respiratory Care in Local Anesthesia," *AORN Journal*, **21:**797 (1975).
Saylor, D.: "Understanding Presurgical Anxiety," *AORN J*, **22:**624 (1975).
Schumann, D. (ed): "Symposium on Wound Healing," *NCNA*, **14:**665 (1979).
Shafer, N.: "Preparing the Asthmatic Patient for Surgery," *Consultant*, **17:**84 (1977).
Silva, M. C.: "Preoperative Teaching for Spouses," *AORN J*, **27:**1081 (1978).
Skillings, I. L.: "Emotional Support for Surgery Patients," *AORN J*, **26:**263 (1977).
Smith, Betty J.: "After Anesthesia," *Nursing 74*, **4:**28, 1974.
———: "Safeguarding your Patient After Anesthesia," *Nurs 78*, **8:**53 (1978).
Smith, R. B., J. Petruscak, and D. Solosko: "In a Recovery Room," *Am J Nurs*, **73:**70 (1973).
Steele, B. G.: "Test Your Knowledge of Postoperative Pain Management," *Nurs 80*, **10:**76 (1980).
Strauss, R. J., et al.: "Operative Risks of Obese Patients: Nursing Care," *AORN J*, **25:**1053 (1977).
"Wound Suction: Better Drainage with Fewer Problems," *Nurs 75*, **5:**52 (1975).

Booklets

Association of Operating Room Nurses: *AORN Standards of Practice*, AORN Publishers, Denver, 1978.
Manuel, Bradley J.: *The Nursing Process Series-Mils*, AORN Publishers, Denver, 1978.

Organizations

American Association of Nurse Anesthetists (AANA), 111 East Wacker Drive, Chicago, IL 60601
Association of Operating Room Nurses (AORN), 10170 East Mississippi Avenue, Denver, CO 80231

Section 3

Problems of Altered Cell Structure

Chapter 9

NURSING ROLE IN MANAGEMENT

Cell Injury and Inflammation

Emilie Musci
Sharon Mantik Lewis

Learning Objectives

1. Describe the structures and functions of the normal cell.
2. Explain the cellular adaptive mechanisms to sublethal injury.
3. Describe the causes and mechanisms of lethal cell injury.
4. Differentiate among types of cell necrosis.
5. Describe the components and functions of the reticuloendothelial system.
6. Describe the inflammatory response including the vascular and cellular responses and exudate formation.
7. Explain local and systemic manifestations of inflammation and their physiological bases.
8. Differentiate among healing by primary, secondary, and tertiary intention.
9. Describe factors that delay wound healing and common complications of wound healing.
10. Describe the pharmacologic, dietary, and nursing management of a client with an inflammatory response.

The major work of the body goes on at the cellular level in the form of chemical reactions. Each cell has a specific function and, together with other cells, makes up body tissues, organs, and systems. Cellular reactions synthesize new products for growth and energy and break down used products.[1] It is necessary to understand the structure and function of an individual cell if the functioning of tissues, organs, and systems is to be understood.

The cell's response to adverse conditions depends on its ability to adapt to changing conditions. Adaptations include such responses as atrophy, hypertrophy, degeneration, inflammation, regeneration, and repair. When the cell fails to adapt, it undergoes a series of changes that can result in cell death (*necrosis*) and eventually tissue death.

THE HUMAN CELL

Cell Structure

The cell is the basic unit of structure in any living organism (Fig. 9-1). Each cell is surrounded by a semipermeable plasma membrane. The two basic parts of a cell are the cytoplasm and the nucleus.

Cytoplasm

Cytoplasm is composed of viscous protoplasm which is water, protein, lipid, carbohydrate, and inorganic solutes. Cytoplasm is organized into many subunits called *organelles* which carry out cellular functions (Table 9-1).

Nucleus

The nucleus, present in all cells that can divide, consists mostly of chromosomes. (The tangled threads of chromosomes found when the cell is not actively dividing are called chromatin.) There are 23 pairs of chromosomes in human somatic cells. The basic unit of the chromosome is the *gene*. *Deoxyribonucleic acid* (*DNA*) is the building block of the gene. The sequence of amino acids of the large complex DNA molecule is the genetic information, the heredity unit of the cell. Furthermore, DNA directs synthesis of specific proteins by the cell (Fig. 9-2), thus determining its special characteristics.

Ribonucleic acid (RNA), also found in the nucleus, transmits the information from DNA to ribosomes in the cytoplasm. Ribosomes are the site of protein synthesis of the cell. The protein products may be used for cellular metabolism (e.g., enzymes) or secreted for use in other parts of the body (e.g., insulin).

Basic Functions of Cells

The basic functions of cells include the following:

Transport of metabolites

Transport of metabolites is the movement of substances (e.g., electrolytes) across the cell membrane actively, passively, or with the assistance of a carrier.

This chapter was reviewed by Robin Meize-Grochowski, R.N., M.S.N., Instructor, College of Nursing, University of New Mexico, Albuquerque, New Mexico.

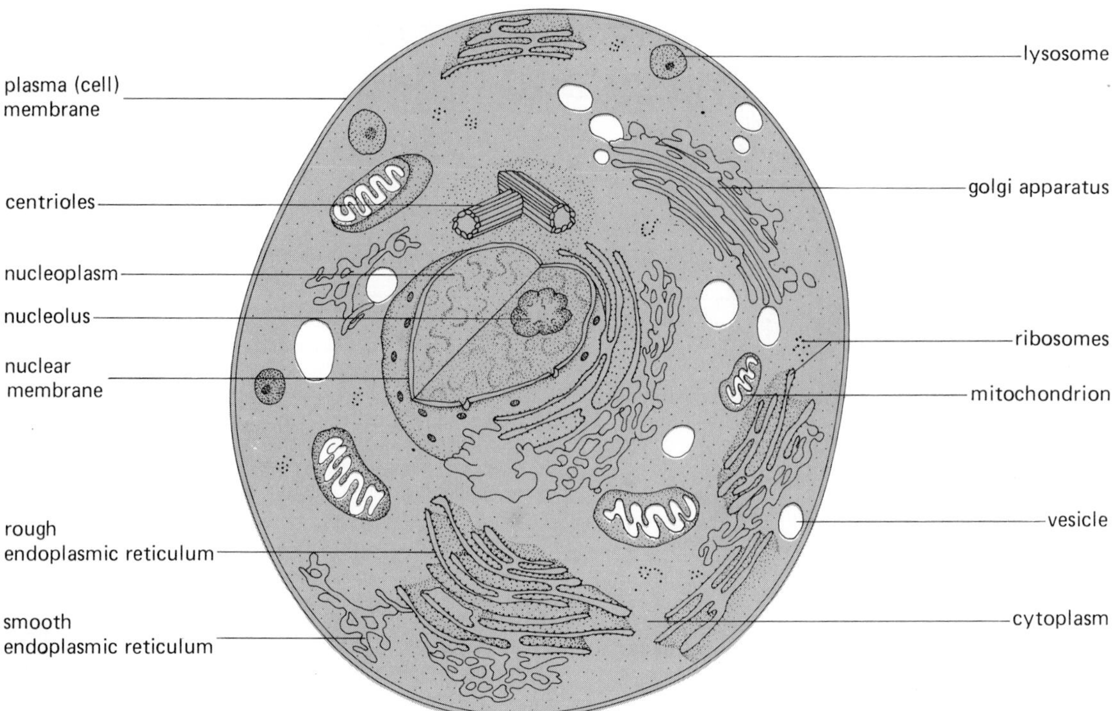

Figure 9-1 Human cell and organelles. *(From R. M. DeCoursey and J. L. Renfro, The Human Organism, 5th ed., McGraw-Hill Book Company, New York, 1980. Used by permission.)*

Table 9-1

Composition and Function of Cell Organelles

Organelle	Composition	Function
Nucleus	DNA (chromatin) RNA Nucleolus (contains RNA)	DNA: control system of cell; cellular reproduction RNA: transmits information to ribosomes Nucleolus: site for messenger-RNA synthesis
Endoplasmic reticulum Smooth (agranular or SER) Rough (granular or RER)	Network of tubular structures which provide communication between nucleus, cytoplasm, and cell membrane.	Lipid and steroid synthesis; bile conjugation; detoxification of unnecessary cell substances; protein synthesis
Ribosomes (found attached to RER or free in cytoplasm)	Granules of cytoplasmic RNA held together by protein May merge into clumps called polyribosomes	Protein synthesis
Golgi complex (or apparatus)	Flattened collection of tubules and vesicles	Packages proteins (hormones and enzymes) which are stored as secretion granules for later release from cell
Mitochondria	Layered cristae (folds) formed into small, oval bodies	Powerhouse of cell; production of ATP; cellular respiration
Lysosome	Membrane surrounded sac containing enzymes	Hydrolytic enzymes released on contact with phagocytized material and act to degrade it
Centrosome	Pair of centrioles	Spindle formation during cell division

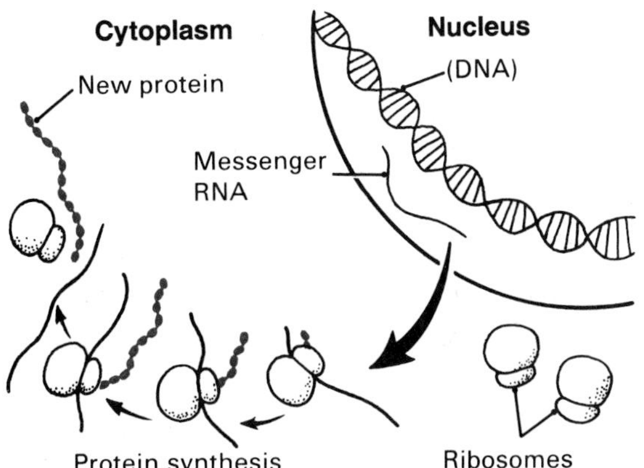

Figure 9-2 Protein synthesis directed by DNA.

Metabolism

The two phases of metabolism include *anabolism* and *catabolism*. Both take place within cells. The *anabolic phase* is concerned with conversion of simpler compounds into new, larger compounds (e.g., amino acids into proteins). In the *catabolic phase* these larger compounds are broken down into simpler compounds with the release of energy necessary for cell functioning.

Movement

Many body cells, especially muscle cells, band together in a coordinated manner to permit body movement.

Conduction

Conduction is transmission of a stimulus from one part of the body to another. Examples of conduction are transmission of a nerve impulse through nerve and muscle cells, and passage of heat and sound waves through various parts of the body.

Absorption

Absorption is the movement of a substance through a cell membrane. An example is glucose absorption by the lining cells of the gastrointestinal tract.

Body protection

Certain cells of the body, such as the epithelial cells of the epidermis, protect the body against injury from penetration or abrasion. Other cells, such as white blood cells, protect the body against invading agents by means of inflammation and the immune response.

Reproduction

New cells are necessary for replacement of aged cells and for growth of the body. *Mitosis*, or cell division, is the process by which cells replace themselves. Not all cells are capable of mitosis.

TISSUE TYPES

Cells similar in structure and function are organized to form tissues. The four types of tissue are epithelial, connective, muscular, and nervous. Table 9-2 discusses examples of the various tissue types and their regenerative ability.

CELL INJURY

Cell injury can be *sublethal* or *lethal*. *Sublethal* injury alters function without causing cell death. The changes caused by this type of injury are potentially reversible if the injurious stimulus is removed. *Lethal* injury is an irreversible process that causes cell death.

Table 9-2

Four Major Tissue Types

Tissue Type	Examples	Regenerative Ability
Epithelial	Skin Linings of blood vessels Mucous membranes	Cells readily divide and regenerate
Connective tissue	Bone	Active tissue that heals rapidly
	Cartilage	Regeneration possible but slow
	Tendons and ligaments	Regeneration possible but slow
	Blood	Cells actively regenerate
Muscle	Smooth	Regeneration usually possible (particularly in GI tract)
	Cardiac	Damaged muscle replaced by connective tissue
	Skeletal	Connective tissue replaces severely damaged muscle Some regeneration in moderately damaged muscle
Nerve	Neuron	Cells do not divide Regenerates only if cell body is not injured
	Glial	Regenerates Often forms scar tissue when neurons are damaged

Cell Adaptation to Sublethal Injury

Cell adaptations to sublethal injuries are common and part of many physiologic and disease processes.[2] Prolonged exposure to sunlight stimulates melanin production and thus protection of deeper skin layers by skin tanning. Lack of muscular activity can lead to decreased muscle tone. Adaptive processes of the cell include *hypertrophy hyperplasia*, *atrophy*, and *metaplasia*. Other adaptive responses that some consider maladaptive are *dysplasia* and *anaplasia*.

Hypertrophy

Hypertrophy refers to an increase in the size of cells without cell division. A pregnant uterus enlarges from hormonal stimulation. The heart of a person with severe hypertension enlarges to compensate for the increased resistance to its pumping action. Muscle hypertrophy results from an increase in size of muscle fibers.

Hyperplasia

Hyperplasia refers to the actual increase in number of cells. This process is reversible when the stimulus is removed. The female breast experiences hyperplasia during lactation. Hyperplasia of the liver may restore damaged liver tissue.

Atrophy

Atrophy refers to a decrease in the size of a tissue or organ due to the decreased number of cells or reduction in size of the individual cells. It frequently occurs as a result of disease (decreased muscle activity), lack of blood supply (thrombus formation), natural aging process (decreased breast size after menopause), and nutritional deficiency.

Metaplasia

Metaplasia is the transformation of one cell type into another. An example of physiologic metaplasia is when circulating monocytes change to macrophages in connective tissue. An example of pathologic metaplasia is when the normal pseudostratified columnar epithelium of the bronchi changes to stratified squamous epithelium in response to chronic cigarette smoking.

Dysplasia

Dysplasia is an abnormal differentiation of dividing cells resulting in changes in size, shape, and appearance of the cells. Minor dysplasia is found in some areas of inflammation. Dysplasia is potentially reversible if the stimulus is removed. Frequently, dysplasia is a precursor of malignancy.

Anaplasia

Anaplasia is cell differentiation to a more immature or embryonic form. Malignant tumors are often characterized by anaplastic cell growth.

Causes of Lethal Cell Injury

Many different agents and factors can cause lethal cell injury (Table 9-3). The mechanism of actual cell death varies. Examples include *pyknosis* (nuclear condensation and shrinking), *karyolysis* (dissolution of nucleus and contents), rupture of cell membrane, and alteration in cell metabolism.

Microbial invasion frequently, but not always, results in cell injury and death. Infection occurs when *pathogens* (microorganisms capable of producing disease) invade and multiply in body tissues. *Opportunistic* organisms are microorganisms which are not usually considered pathogens. However, they may cause injury if the resistance of the host is decreased from events such as trauma or illness.

Cell Necrosis

Necrosis is the death of cells within a living organism. The appearance of necrotic tissue varies, depending upon the results of lysosomal activity.[3]

Coagulative necrosis

Necrotic cells maintain their outline (lytic enzymes are somewhat inhibited). Proteins are denatured and enzymes lose their function. Coagulative necrosis is commonly due to lack of blood supply.

Liquefactive necrosis

Necrotic cells rapidly disappear as lytic enzymes digest tissues. Liquefactive necrosis commonly occurs in the brain where supply of lytic enzymes is abundant.

Caseous necrosis

Necrotic cells disintegrate but cell fragments remain for long periods of time. This type of necrosis is called *caseous* (cheeselike) because of its crumbly appearance. It is frequently found in tuberculosis of the lung.

Gangrenous necrosis

Gangrenous necrosis results from severe hypoxia and subsequent ischemic injury as is common after impaired circulation in the lower legs. "Dry" gangrene refers to the dry, shriveled, darkened area (Fig. 9-3) and "wet" gangrene to the liquefied underlying necrotic tissue.

Table 9-3
Causes of Lethal Cell Injury

Cause	Effect on Cell
Physical agents	
Heat	Denaturation of protein Acceleration of metabolic reactions
Cold	Vasoconstriction leads to decreased blood flow Slowed metabolic reactions Thrombosis of blood vessels Freezing of cell content which forms crystals and can burst cell
Radiation	Alteration of cell structure and activity Alteration of enzyme systems Mutations Destruction of cell
Electrothermal injury	Interruption of neural conduction Fibrillation of cardiac muscle Coagulative necrosis of skin and skeletal muscle
Mechanical trauma	Transfer of excess kinetic energy to cells causes rupture of cells, blood vessels, and tissue. Examples include: (*a*) Abrasion—scraping of skin or mucous membrane (*b*) Laceration—severing of vessels and tissue (*c*) Contusion (bruise)—crushing of tissue cells causing hemorrhage into skin (*d*) Puncture—piercing of a body structure or organ (*e*) Incision—surgical cutting
Chemical injury	Alteration of cell metabolism Interference with normal enzymatic action within cells
Microbial injury (about 1,000 different pathogens can produce disease)	
Viruses	Viral nucleic acid (either DNA or RNA) takes over cell metabolism and synthesizes new particles that may cause cell rupture
Bacteria	Destruction of cell membrane or cell nucleus Production of lethal toxins
Ischemic injury (lack of oxygen supply)	Compromised cell metabolism Acute or gradual cell death
Immunological (Chap. 10)	
Antigen-antibody response	Release of substances (histamine, complement) that can injure and damage cells
Autoimmune	Activation of complement destroys normal cells and produces inflammation
Neoplastic growth	Cell destruction from abnormal and uncontrolled cell growth
Normal substances	
E.g., digestive enzymes	Release into abdomen causes peritonitis
Uric Acid	Excess accumulation crystallizes in joints and renal tissue

DEFENSE AGAINST INJURY

In order to protect itself against injury, the body has various defense mechanisms. These defense mechanisms are (1) the skin and mucous membranes (first line of defense), (2) the reticuloendothelial system, (3) the inflammatory response, and (4) the immune system.

The function of the skin is discussed in Chap. 16. This chapter will cover the roles of the reticuloendothelial system and the inflammatory response in the immediate response to injury. The immune system, providing a secondary line of defense, is described in Chap. 10.

Reticuloendothelial System

The *reticuloendothelial system* (*RES*) is also called the *macrophage system*. It is not a body system

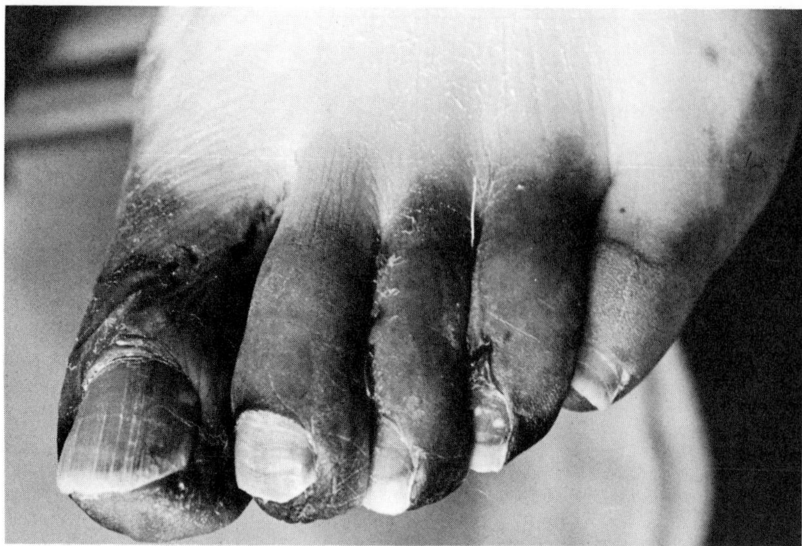

Figure 9-3 Gangrene of the toes. *(From S. Price and L. Wilson, Pathophysiology: Clinical Concepts of Disease Processes, 2d ed., McGraw-Hill Book Company, New York, 1982. Used by permission.)*

with distinctly defined tissues and organs. Rather, it consists of phagocytic cells located in various tissues and organs. The phagocytic cells are either *fixed* or *mobile* (Table 9-4). The macrophages of the liver, spleen, bone marrow, lungs, and lymph nodes are fixed phagocytes. The monocytes (in blood) and macrophages found in connective tissue, known as histiocytes, are mobile or wandering phagocytes.

Both monocytes and macrophages are derived from the bone marrow. Monocytes spend a few days in the blood and then enter tissues and change into macrophages. Tissue macrophages are larger and more phagocytic than monocytes.

The functions of the RES include:

Table 9-4

Location and Names of Macrophages*

Location	Name
Connective tissue	Histiocyte
Liver	Kupffer cell
Lung	Alveolar macrophage
Spleen and bone marrow	Sinusoidal lining macrophage
Bone tissue	Osteoclast
Nervous system	Microglial cell
Peritoneal cavity	Peritoneal macrophage

*In addition, monocytes become macrophages once they leave the blood and enter tissues.

1. Recognition and phagocytosis of foreign material such as microorganisms
2. Removal of old or damaged cells from circulation
3. Participation in the immune response (Chap. 10)

The specific function of macrophages in the inflammatory response is discussed in the next section.

Inflammatory Response

The inflammatory response is a sequential reaction to cell injury. It neutralizes the inflammatory agent, removes necrotic materials, and establishes an environment proper for healing and repair. *Inflammation* is often but incorrectly used as a synonym for *infection.* To simplify the difference, one can say that inflammation is always present in infection but infection is not always present with inflammation. An infection means invasion of tissues or cells by microorganisms such as bacteria, fungi, or viruses. Inflammation, on the other hand, can also be caused by nonliving agents such as heat, radiation, or trauma (Table 9-3). If, in addition, there is infection, it is from a superimposed invasion of microorganisms.

The mechanism of inflammation is basically the same regardless of the injuring agent. The intensity of the response depends on the extent and severity of injury and on the reactive capacity of the victim. The inflammatory response can be divided into a vascular response, cellular response, formation of exudate, and healing. A typical inflammatory response to bacterial infection will be described.

Vascular response

After the cell injury the capillaries of the area briefly undergo vasoconstriction. Next, following release of histamine and other chemicals by the injured cells, the vessels dilate (Fig. 9-4). This vasodilatation brings about *hyperemia* (increased blood supply) which raises filtration pressure. Vasodilatation along with the chemical mediators also make the capillaries more permeable. Movement of fluid from capillaries into tissue spaces is thus facilitated. Initially composed of serous fluid, this *inflammatory exudate* is later joined by plasma proteins, primarily albumin. The proteins exert oncotic pressure that further draws fluid from blood vessels. The tissue becomes edematous.

As the plasma protein fibrinogen leaves the blood it is activated to *fibrin* by the products of the injured cells. Fibrin strengthens a blood clot formed by platelets. The clot functions to trap bacteria, preventing their spread, and to serve as a framework for the healing process.

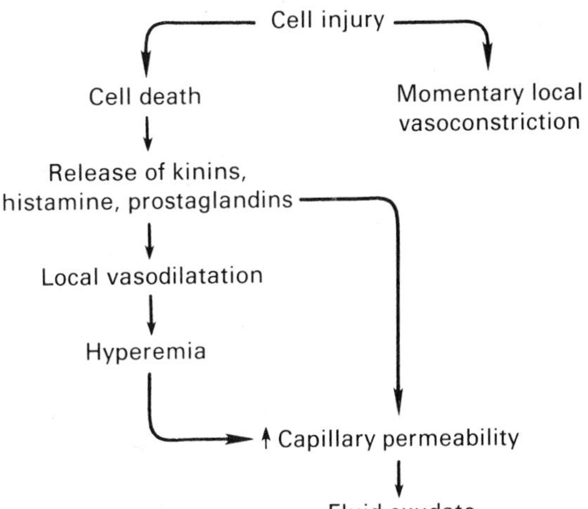

Figure 9-4 Vascular response in inflammation.

Cellular response (Fig. 9-5)

The blood flow through capillaries of the area slows as fluid is lost and viscosity rises. Certain leukocytes move to the inner surface of the capillaries (margination), then, in ameboid fashion, through the capillary wall (diapedesis) and to the site of injury (Fig. 9-6).

Chemicals released by injured cells exert an attractive force, called *chemotaxis*, on white blood cells in the circulation. The cells respond by moving to the site of injury.

Neutrophils Neutrophils are the first leukocytes to arrive. They phagocytize bacteria, other foreign material, and damaged cells. With their short life span dead neutrophils soon accumulate. In time the mixture of dead neutrophils, digested bacteria, and other cell debris builds to a creamy substance known as *pus*.

In order to keep up with the demand for neutrophils, the bone marrow releases more into circulation. This results in an elevated white blood cell count (especially the neutrophil count). Sometimes the demand for neutrophils increases so much that the bone marrow releases immature forms of neutrophils (*bands*) into circulation. (Mature neutrophils are called *segmented neutrophils*). The finding of increased numbers of band neutrophils in circulation is called a *shift to the left*.

Monocytes *Monocytes* are the second type of phagocytic cells that migrate from circulating blood. Upon entering the tissue spaces, the monocytes transform into macrophages. These macrophages, together with the tissue macrophages, assist in phagocytosis of the inflammatory debris. The macrophage role is very important in cleaning up the battlefield before healing can occur. Macrophages have a long life span. They can multiply and may stay in the damaged tissues for weeks.

In some cases macrophages perform tasks other than phagocytosis. They accumulate and fuse to form

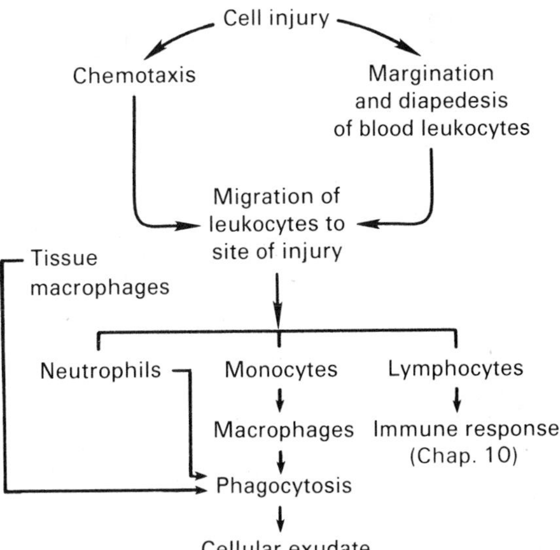

Figure 9-5 Cellular response in inflammation.

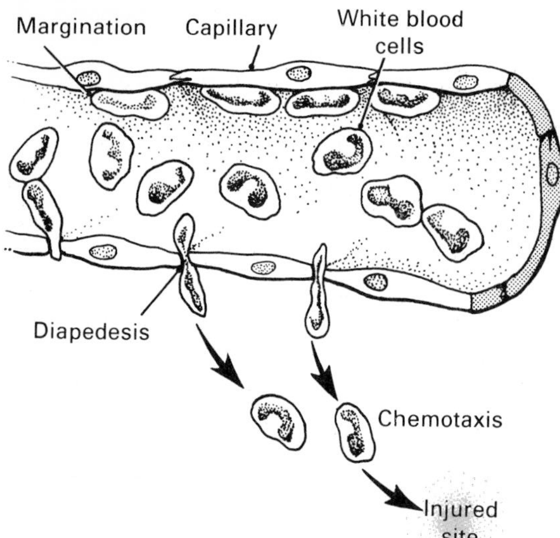

Figure 9-6 Margination, diapedesis, and chemotaxis of white blood cells.

a multinucleated *giant cell*. The giant cell serves to wall off the infection. The accumulation of the macrophages may lead to nodule formation (*granulomata*).[4] A classic example of this process occurs with the tubercle bacillus in the lung. A chronic state of inflammation exists as the bacillus is walled off. The granuloma formed is a cavity of necrotic tissue.

Lymphocytes Lymphocytes arrive later at the site of injury. Their primary role is related to immunity and the antigen-antibody response at the injured site (Chap. 10).

Eosinophils and Basophils Eosinophils and basophils are also phagocytic leukocytes but appear to have a more selective role in inflammation. Eosinophils are released in large quantities during an allergic reaction. They are involved in phagocytosis of the antigen-antibody complex. The histamine and heparin that basophils carry in granules are released during inflammation. Histamine is a potent vasodilator.

Exudate

Exudate is formed from both the fluid and the cells that move to the site as well as from the cellular debris. The nature and quantity of exudate depends on the type and severity of the injury and the tissues involved.

Serous Exudate Serous exudate results from the outpouring of fluid with few cells and low protein content. It is seen in the early stages of inflammation or when the injury is mild. Examples include skin blisters and pleural effusion.

Fibrinous Exudate This type of exudate occurs with increasing vascular permeability and fibrinogen leakage into the interstitial spaces. If fibrin is formed in excessive amounts, it may coat tissue surfaces and cause them to adhere. Adhesions may develop in the healing process and bind surfaces together (e.g., the pleura adhering together secondary to pneumonia).

Suppurative or Purulent Exudate Purulent exudate or pus consists of leukocytes, microorganisms (dead and alive), liquefied dead cells, and other debris. A *furuncle* (boil) and *abscess* are localized forms of purulent exudates. *Cellulitis* is a spreading form of the inflammatory process to the surrounding connective tissue.

Catarrhal Exudate Catarrhal exudate is found in tissues where cells have the ability to produce mucus. The inflammatory response accelerates mucus production. Catarrhal exudate occurs in the nasopharynx (e.g., the runny nose common with upper respiratory infection), lungs, and gastrointestinal tract.

Hemorrhagic Exudate This type of exudate occurs when there is rupture and/or necrosis of the blood vessel walls. It consists of erythrocytes that escape into the tissues.

Healing

Normally, inflammation is followed by healing (see ahead). If the cause of the inflammation is not effectively removed, the inflammation becomes chronic and persists.

Clinical Manifestations of Inflammation

The *local response* to inflammation includes the five manifestations of redness, heat, pain, swelling, and loss of function (Table 9-5).

Systemic manifestations of inflammation include (1) fever, (2) leukocytosis with a shift to the left, (3) malaise, (4) nausea and anorexia, (5) weight loss, and (6) increased pulse and respiratory rate.

Fever is due to pyrogens (protein substances) released from white blood cells which act on the hypothalamus to raise the core body temperature. *Leukocytosis* results from the increased release of leukocytes from the bone marrow. An increase in the circulating numbers of one or more types of leukocytes may be found. Inflammatory reactions are accompanied by vaguely defined constitutional symptoms of *malaise*, *nausea*, *anorexia*, and *fatigue*. The causes of these systemic changes are poorly understood. An increase in pulse and respiration follows the rise in metabolism due to an increase in body temperature.

Types of Inflammation

The basic types of inflammation are *acute*, *subacute*, and *chronic*. In *acute inflammation* the healing occurs within 2 to 3 weeks and usually leaves no residual damage. Neutrophils are the predominant cell type. A *subacute inflammation* has the features of the acute process but is extended in time. Examples include subacute bacterial endocarditis, a smoldering infection which has features of acute inflammation but persists over weeks or months.

Chronic inflammation lasts for weeks, months, and even years. The injurious agent persists or repeatedly injures tissue. The predominant cell types are lymphocytes, plasma cells, and macrophages. Examples of chronic inflammation include rheumatoid arthritis and tuberculosis. Tuberculosis is a type of chronic granulomatous inflammation.

A chronic inflammatory process is debilitating and over the long term can be devastating. It is proposed that the prolongation and chronicity of any inflammation is due to an alteration in the immune response.[5]

THE HEALING PROCESS

The final phase of the inflammatory response is healing. Healing includes the two major components of *regeneration* and *replacement*. *Regeneration* is the replacement of lost cells and tissues with cells of the same type. *Replacement* is healing as a result of lost cells being replaced by connective tissue. It is the more common type of healing and usually results in scar formation.[6]

Regeneration

The ability of cells to regenerate depends on the cell type (Table 9-2). *Labile cells* such as the skin, lymphoid, blood cells, and mucous membranes of the gastrointestinal, urinary, and reproductive tract divide constantly during their lifetime. Injury to these organs is followed by rapid regeneration.

Stable cells retain their ability to regenerate but do so only if the organ is injured. Examples of stable cells are the liver, pancreas, kidney, and bone cells.

Permanent cells do not regenerate. Examples of these cells are neurons of the central nervous system and cardiac muscle cells. Damage to heart muscle or central nervous system neurons leads to permanent loss. Healing will occur by repair with scar tissue.[7]

Table 9-5
Local Manifestations of Inflammation

Manifestations	Cause
Redness (rubor)	Hyperemia from vasodilatation
Heat (calor)	Increased metabolism at inflammatory site
Pain (dolor)	Change in pH Change in local ionic concentration Nerve stimulation by chemicals (e.g., histamine) Pressure from fluid exudate
Swelling (tumor)	Fluid shift to interstitial spaces Fluid exudate accumulation
Loss of function (functio laesa)	Swelling and pain

Replacement

Replacement is a more complex process than regeneration. Most injuries heal by this type of connective tissue repair. Replacement healing occurs by primary, secondary, or tertiary intention.

Primary (first) intention

Primary intention healing takes place when wound margins are neatly approximated such as in a surgical incision. There is a continuum of processes associated with primary healing (Fig. 9-7 and Table 9-6). These processes include three phases.

Initial Phase The initial phase lasts for 3 to 5 days. The edges of the incision are first aligned and sutured in place. The incision area fills with blood from the cut blood vessels and blood clots form. There is an acute inflammatory reaction because of the exudate and necrotic cells. As the wound debris is removed, the fibrin clot serves as a meshwork for future capillary growth and migration of epithelial cells.

Granulation Phase The granulation (or fibroplasia) phase is the second step and lasts from 5 days to 4 weeks. Fibroblasts are immature connective tissue cells that migrate into the healing site. (Histiocytes and some lymphocytes can change into fibroblasts.) Fibroblasts secrete collagen. Over a period of time the collagen is organized and restructured to strengthen the healing site. At this stage it is called *fibrous* or *scar tissue*.

During the granulation phase the wound is pink in appearance and very vascular. Numerous red gran-

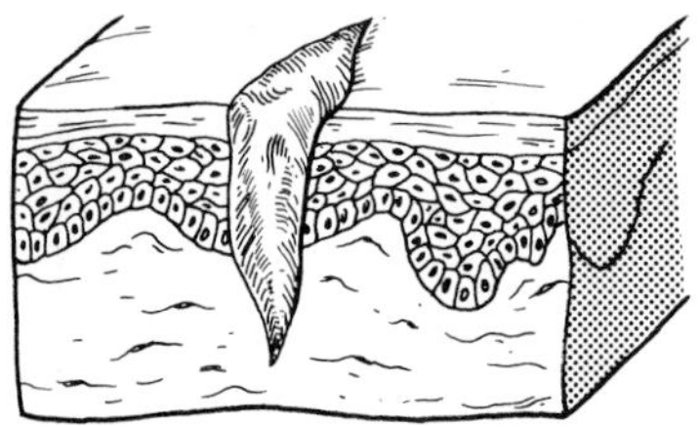
Incision with blood clot

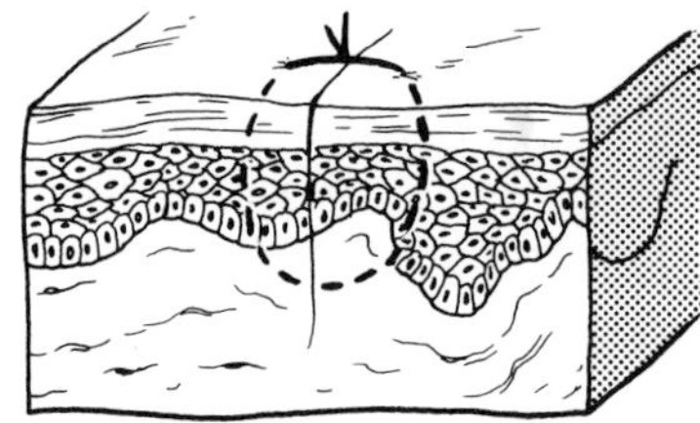
Edges approximated with suture

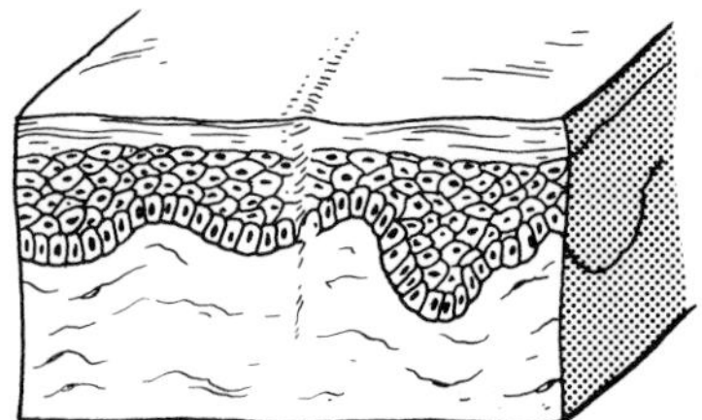
Fine scar

A. PRIMARY INTENTION

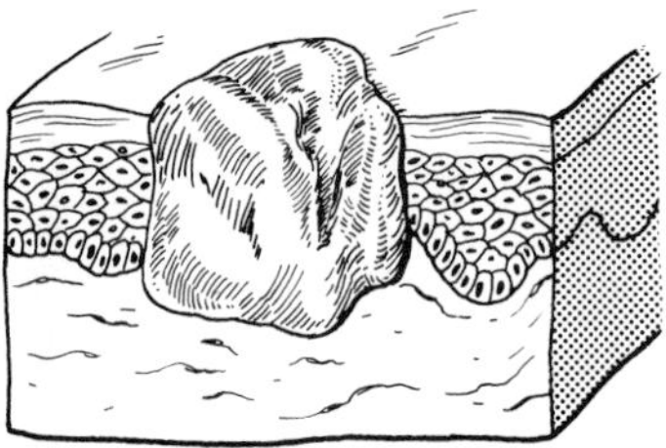
Irregular, large wound with blood clot

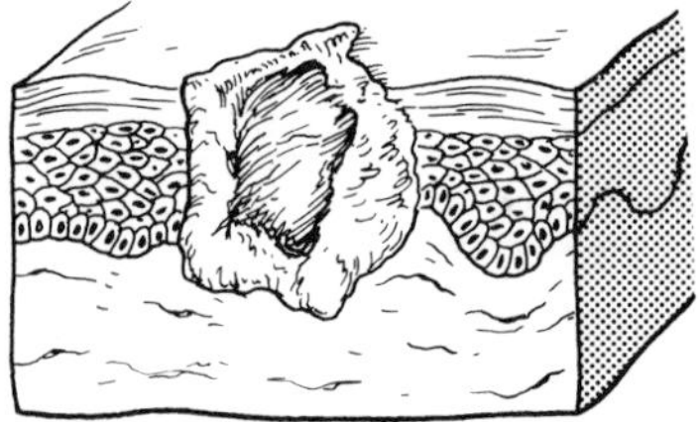
Granulation tissue fills in wound

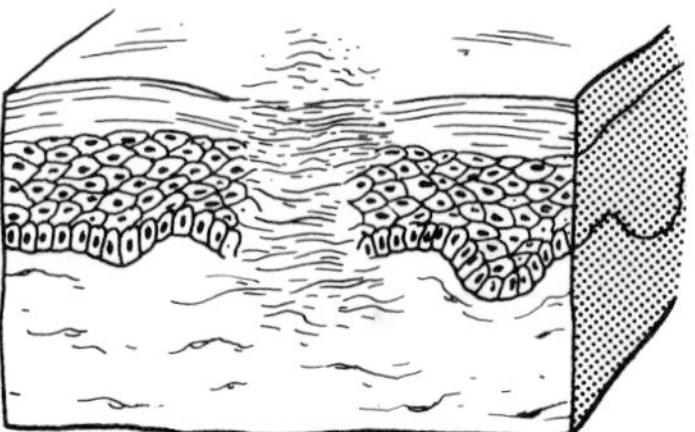
Large scar

B. SECONDARY INTENTION

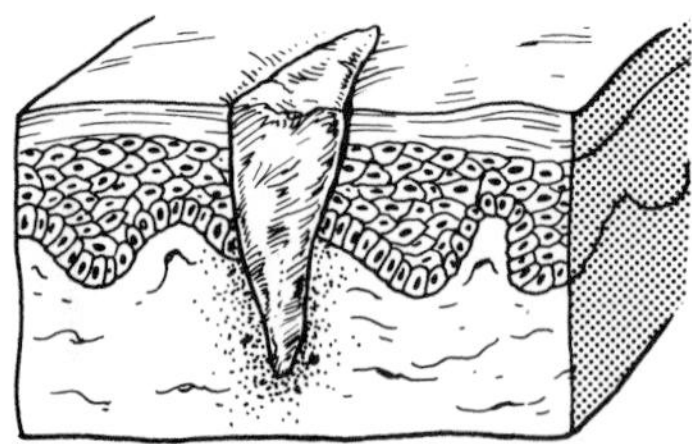
Contaminated wound

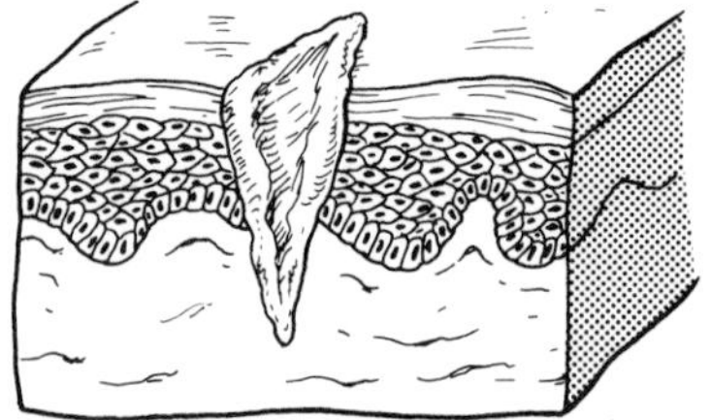
Granulation tissue

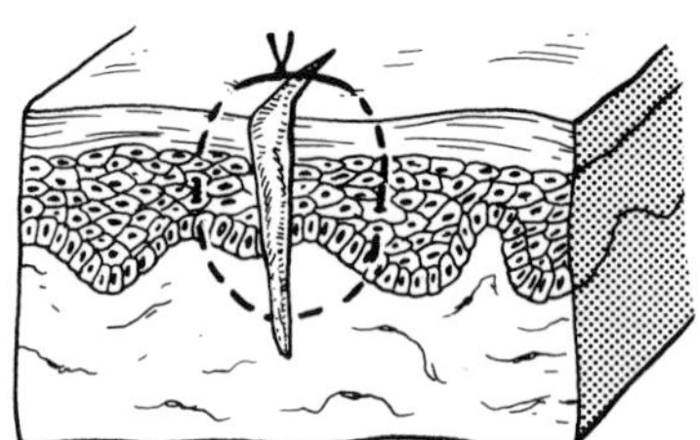
Delayed closure with suture

C. TERTIARY INTENTION

Figure 9-7 Types of wound healing.

ules (young budding capillaries) are present. At this point the wound is very friable, has an anesthetic quality, and is resistant to infection because of the increased leukocytes in the area.

Scar Contraction and Maturation Phase The scar contraction and maturation phase overlaps with the granulation phase. It may begin 7 days after the injury and continue for several months. Collagen fibers are further organized and the remodeling process occurs. Fibroblasts disappear as the wound becomes stronger. The active movement of the fibroblasts causes contraction of the healing area. This helps to close the defect and bring the skin edges closer together. A mature scar is then formed. In contrast to granulation tissue, a mature scar is virtually avascular, pale in color, and may be more painful than in the granulation phase.

Secondary intention

Wounds that occur from trauma, ulceration, infection, and other conditions and that have large amounts of exudate and wide irregular wound margins may not have edges that can be approximated. The inflammatory reaction may be greater than in primary healing. This results in more debris, cells, and exudate. The debris may have to be cleaned away (*debrided*) before healing can take place.

In some instances a primary incision may become infected, creating additional inflammation. The wound may reopen and healing by secondary intention would take place.

Table 9-6
Phases in Primary Intention Healing

Phase	Activity
Initial phase (3–5 days)	Incision edges approximated Migration of epithelial cells Clot serves as meshwork for starting capillary growth
Granulation (fibroplasia) (5 days–4 weeks)	Migration of fibroblasts Secretion of collagen Capillary buds abundant Wound is fragile
Scar contracture (maturation) (7 days–several months)	Remodeling of collagen Scar gains in strength

The process of healing by secondary intention is essentially the same as described in primary healing. The major differences are the greater defect and the gaping wound edges. Healing and granulation take place from the edges inward and from the bottom of the wound upward until the defect is filled. There is more granulation tissue and the result is a much larger scar.

Tertiary intention (delayed primary closure)

Tertiary intention occurs with delayed suturing of a wound when two layers of granulation tissue are sutured together. This would occur in situations where a contaminated wound was left open and later sutured together after the infection was removed. It would also occur in situations where a primary wound became infected, was opened, allowed to granulate, and then sutured. Tertiary intention results in a larger and deeper scar than primary intention.

Factors Which Delay Healing

In a healthy person, wounds heal at a normal, predictable rate. Little can be done to accelerate this process. However, there are factors which delay wound healing. These are summarized in Table 9-7.

Complications of Wound Healing

The shape and location of the wound determine how well the wound will heal. Complications result from interference with wound healing (e.g., poor nutrition and decreased blood supply). Some complications that could result are summarized.

Hypertrophic scars and keloids

Hypertrophic scars and keloids occur when the body produces an excess of collagen tissue. The scar

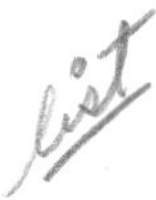

Table 9-7
Factors Which Delay Wound Healing

Factor	Effect on Wound Healing
Nutritional deficiencies	
Vitamin C (ascorbic acid)	Prevents formation of collagen fibers
Protein	Decreases supply of amino acids for tissue repair
Inadequate blood supply (from edema, vascular disease, etc.)	Decreases supply of nutrients to injured area Decreases removal of exudative debris
Corticosteroid drugs	Inhibits inflammatory response Depresses the formation of granulation tissue Inhibits wound contraction
Infection	Increases inflammatory response and tissue destruction
Mechanical friction on wound	Destroys granulation tissue Prevents apposition of wound edges
Advanced age	Slows the formation of collagen by fibroblasts Impairs circulation
Obesity	Decreased blood supply in fatty tissue
Poor general health	Generalized absence of factors necessary to promote wound healing

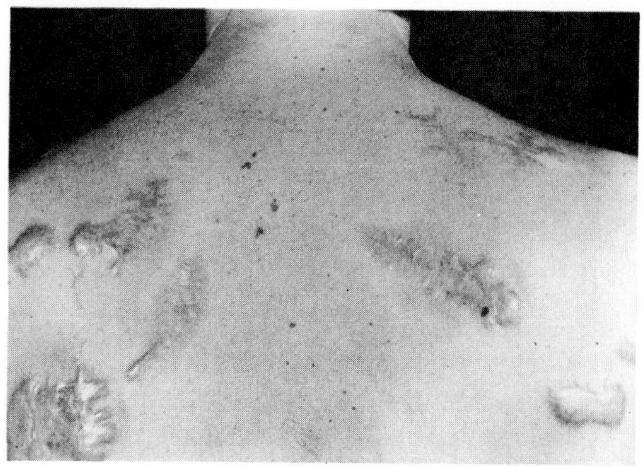

Figure 9-8 Keloid formation. [*From T. B. Fitzpatrick et al. (eds.) Dermatology in General Medicine, 2d ed., McGraw-Hill Book Company, New York, 1979. Used by permission.*]

enlarges and may protrude beyond the boundary of the incision. Hypertrophied scars are red, raised, and hard. Keloids are a greater protrusion of scar tissue and may assume tumorlike masses (Fig. 9-8). A predisposition to keloid formation is thought to be hereditary and occurs more often in dark-skinned people. Neither of these complications is life-threatening but can have serious cosmetic implications.

Contracture

A shortening of muscle or scar tissue results from excessive fibrous formation, especially if the wound is near a joint. Contracture frequently occurs in burns where there is great loss of skin and subcutaneous tissue (Chap. 13).

Dehiscence

Dehiscence is separation and disruption of previously joined wound edges. It usually occurs when a primary healing site bursts open. There are two possible causes of dehiscence. First, an infection may cause an inflammatory process. Second, the granulation tissue may not be strong enough to withstand the forces imposed on the wound.[8] *Evisceration* occurs when the wound edges separate to the extent that intestinal contents protrude through the wound.

Excess granulation tissue

Excess granulation tissue ("proud flesh") protrudes above the surface of the healing wound. If the granulation tissue is cauterized or cut off, healing normally continues.

Adhesions

Adhesions are bands of scar tissue between or around organs. Adhesions form as aging scar tissue shrinks. Adhesions may occur in the abdominal cavity or between the lungs and pleura. Adhesions in the abdomen may cause an intestinal obstruction. Adhesions between the lungs and pleura require *decortication* (stripping of pleura) to provide for normal ventilation.

Major organ dysfunction

Major organ dysfunction results when there is an acute inflammation of the heart, kidney, brain, etc. Alteration in physiologic functioning of the organ is due to the formation of scar tissue. The scar tissue "patch" will never function like the original tissue.

MEDICAL MANAGEMENT OF INFLAMMATION

The actual medical management of injury and inflammation is highly variable. It depends on the causative agent, degree of injury, and the client's condition. Superficial skin injuries may need only cleansing. Deeper skin wounds can be closed by suturing the edges together. Adhesive strips may be used instead of sutures. If the wound is contaminated, it needs to be converted into a clean wound before healing can adequately take place. It may be necessary to surgically debride a wound that has multiple fragments or devitalized tissue. Frequently, open, contaminated wounds are irrigated with nonabsorbable antibiotics like neomycin. If the source of injury or inflammation is an internal organ (e.g., appendix, ruptured spleen), surgical removal of the organ is the treatment of choice.

PHARMACOLOGIC MANAGEMENT OF INFLAMMATION

Pharmacologic agents are used in all types of inflammation. Drugs are used for the specific purpos-

Table 9-8
Pharmacologic Agents Used for Inflammation

Drug	Mechanism of Action
Antipyretic drugs	
Salicylates (aspirin)	Lowers body temperature by action on heat-regulating center in hypothalamus. This results in peripheral dilatation and heat loss Interference with formation and release of leukocyte pyrogens. Selective depression of central nervous system
Acetaminophen (Tylenol)	Action similar to aspirin but without CNS depression
Phenacetin	Action similar to aspirin (produces more central nervous system depression)
Antiinflammatory drugs	
Salicylates	Inhibits synthesis of prostaglandins Reduction of capillary permeability
Corticosteroids	Interferes with tissue granulation Immunosuppressive effects (decreased synthesis of lympocytes) Prevents liberation of lysosomes
Indomethacin (Indocin)	Inhibits synthesis of prostaglandins
Phenylbutazone (Butazolidin)	Inhibits synthesis of prostaglandins
Antibiotic and antimicrobial drugs	
Penicillin	Bacteriostatic and bactericidal Interferes with formation of bacteria cell wall
Cephalosporins	Bactericidal Interferes with formation of bacteria cell wall
Erythromycin	Bacteriostatic Inhibits synthesis of bacterial protein
Tetracycline	Bacteriostatic Inhibits synthesis of bacterial protein
Sulfonamides	Bacteriostatic Interferes with incorporation of para-aminobenzoic acid (PABA) into folic acid
Vitamins	
Vitamin A	Accelerates epithelialization
Vitamin B complex	Acts as coenzymes of metabolic reactions
Vitamin C	Needed for synthesis of collagen
Vitamin D	Needed for absorption of calcium

es of reducing fever (antipyretic agents), reducing the inflammatory response (antiinflammatory agents), and destroying the infectious agent (antibiotics) (Table 9-8). Antihistamine drugs may also be used to antagonize the action of histamine and prevent vasodilator effects. These drugs are discussed in Chap. 10.

DIETARY MEASURES TO PROMOTE WOUND HEALING

A high fluid intake is needed to replace perspiration and exudate losses. Water loss results from increased metabolic rate. There is a 7 percent increase in metabolism for every 0.3°C increase in temperature.

A diet high in protein, carbohydrate, and vitamins with moderate fat intake is necessary to promote healing. *Protein* is needed to correct the negative nitrogen balance resulting from the increased metabolic rate. Protein is also necessary for synthesis of immune factors, leukocytes, fibroblasts, and collagen. *Carbohydrate* is needed for the increased metabolic energy required in inflammation and healing. If there is a carbohydrate deficit, the body will break down protein for the needed energy. *Fats* are also a necessary component in the diet to help in the synthesis of fatty acids and triglycerides which are a part of the cellular membrane. *Vitamin C* is necessary to synthesize collagen. *The B-complex vitamins* are necessary as coenzymes for many metabolic reactions. If a vitamin B deficiency develops, there will be a disruption of protein, fat, and carbohydrate metabolism.

Vitamin A is also needed in healing because it aids in the process of epithelialization. It increases collagen synthesis and tensile strength of the healing wound.[9]

NURSING MANAGEMENT OF INFLAMMATION

Health Promotion and Maintenance

The best management of inflammation is the prevention of infection, trauma, surgery, and contact with potentially harmful agents. This is not always possible. A simple mosquito bite causes an inflammatory response. Since occasional injury is inevitable, concerted efforts to combat inflammation are needed. The following areas need to be considered to avoid serious illness from an inflammatory response.

Adequate nutrition

Adequate nutrition is essential so that the body has the necessary factors to promote healing when injury occurs.

Emotional and physical stress

Stress should be avoided or controlled. It suppresses immune factors and increases the body's susceptibility to inflammatory agents that cause disease.

Early recognition of inflammation

Early recognition of manifestations of inflammation is necessary so that appropriate treatment may be started. This treatment may be rest, pharmacologic, or specific treatment of the injured site. Immediate treatment may prevent the extension and complications of inflammation.

Acute Intervention

Observation and vital signs

The nurse's ability to recognize the clinical manifestations of inflammation is important. Observation and recording of wound healing is also very important. Any drainage (consistency, color, odor) should be recorded and reported if abnormal for the situation. *Staphylococcus* and *Pseudomonas* are common organisms that produce purulent draining wounds.

Vital signs are important to note with any inflammation and especially with an infectious process. When infection is present there may be a rise in temperature and an increase in pulse and respiration rates. If a wound infection develops in a postoperative client, vital signs will show a change 4 to 5 days after surgery.

Rest and immobilization

Rest and immobilization of the inflamed area will promote healing by decreasing the inflammatory process, assisting in the repair process, and decreasing metabolic needs. Immobilization with a cast, splint, or bandage will cause less wound debris and hemorrhage. The repair process is facilitated by allowing fibrin and collagen to form across the wound edges with little disruption. Rest helps the body better use its nutrients and oxygen for the healing process.

Elevation of inflamed area

Elevating the injured area (especially an extremity) will reduce the edema in the inflammatory site and increase venous return. This will help to reduce pain and improve circulation of blood which provides oxygen and nutrients needed for healing.

Oxygenation

Adequate oxygenation of the inflamed area is essential because oxygen promotes the differentiation of fibroblasts and collagen synthesis. Oxygen is also essential for cell growth and division. Moderate administration of oxygen can help protect the client against wound infection. People with arterial disease, hypovolemia, and hypotension are at greatest risk for infection and may benefit from oxygen administration.[10]

Heat and cold

Application of heat and cold are controversial interventions. Cold application is usually appropriate at the time of the initial trauma to cause vasoconstriction. This will decrease swelling, pain, and the congestion from increased metabolism in the area of inflammation. Heat may be used later to promote healing by increasing the circulation to the inflamed site and subsequent removal of debris. Heat is also used to localize the inflammatory agents. If necrotic material is present in the wound, warm, moist heat may help to debride the wound site.

Dressings

Dressings need to be applied properly. Unnecessary manipulation associated with dressing changes may destroy new granulation tissue and break down fibrin formation. Meticulous aseptic technique is essential in dressing and irrigating wounds. If a dressing does not adequately cover the entire wound, the parts exposed are subject to contamination. Dressings applied too tightly can cause pressure on the wound and interfere with normal blood supply. If a dressing (especially one with moist drainage) is changed infrequently, it may leave the wound more susceptible to infection. The frequency of dressing changes depends on the type, location, and drainage of wound.

Infection control

The nurse and the client must scrupulously follow aseptic procedures for keeping the wound free from infection. The client should not be allowed to touch a recently injured area. The client's environment should be as free as possible from contamination from items introduced by roommates and visitors. Antibiotics may be administered prophylactically to some clients. If an infection does develop, a culture and sensitivity test will be done to determine the antibiotic most effective against the specific organism.

If the client develops an infection that is considered a risk for others, *protective isolation* may be needed. He is placed in a private room which is kept closed. All persons entering must be gowned and masked and must wash hands on entering and leaving. Everyone who touches the client must be gloved.

A low white blood cell count and depressed immune responses (as during cancer chemotherapy) may indicate a need for another type of isolation called *reverse isolation.* The goal of reverse isolation is to protect the vulnerable client from environmental sources of infection. Institutional policies related to reverse isolation should be followed when the client's condition warrants this intervention.

Psychological implication

The client may be distressed at the thought or sight of an incision or wound. He may fear scarring or disfigurement. Drainage from a wound often causes increased alarm. The client needs to understand the healing process and the normal changes that occur as the wound heals. When a nurse is changing a dressing, facial expression can alert the client to problems with the wound or the nurse's ability to care for it. Wrinkling of the nose may convey disgust to the client. A nurse should also be careful not to focus on the wound to the exclusion of the client as a total person.

Chronic Management

The healing of wounds may not be complete for 4 to 6 weeks or longer. The measures of adequate rest, good nutrition, and limited physical and emotional stress need to be continued. Observing for wound complications such as contractures, adhesions, or secondary infection is important during the rehabilitative stage.

Medications will often be taken for a period of time after recovery from the acute infection. Awareness of the necessity to continue the drugs for the specified time is an important point to teach the client. For example, a client who is to take an antibiotic for 10 days may stop taking the medication after 5 days because he feels better. There is a possibility that the organism may not be entirely eliminated. In fact it could increase in number and virulence. Furthermore, the organism could become resistant to the antibiotic.

The client may also need teaching in some areas of personal care. He may need to be taught to change his own dressings and take care of his wound. He may need to take medication and observe for any adverse side effects. He needs to know about manifestations of abnormal wound healing so he can report any of these findings to his health care provider.

Case Study / Injury and Inflammation

Roger, 20 years old, was admitted to the hospital emergency room with burns estimated to be second degree that involved his face, neck, and upper trunk. He also had a lacerated right leg.

He was alert and his voice was slightly hoarse. An IV was started immediately and an indwelling catheter inserted into the bladder. His right leg was splinted and the lacerated wound cleaned and debrided.

By the third day post-burn Roger had marked edema throughout his body. He also developed a temperature of 39°C. On the sixth day post-burn his lacerated leg wound became infected and pus developed. His white blood cell count was 26,400 and a differential showed:

Neutrophils	75%	Basophils	0.5%	Monocytes	3%
Eosinophils	2%	Lymphocytes	20%		

By the third week, the burn sites and leg wound were healing well. When Roger complained of stiffness of his neck, the nurse noticed contractures developing in the neck area.

Discussion Questions

1. What clinical manifestations of inflammation did Roger exhibit? Explain the pathophysiologic mechanism for each manifestation.
2. What type of exudate formation did he develop?
3. What is the basis for the development of the temperature the third day post burn?

4. What is the significance of his white blood cell count and differential?
5. Because his wound was deep, primary tissue healing was not possible. How would you expect healing to take place?
6. What is the cause of the contracture development in the neck area?
7. What problems might Roger have with self-concept or body image? What concerns or problems might a nurse have in caring for Roger?

REVIEW QUESTIONS

The number of the question corresponds to the same numbered objective at the beginning of the chapter.

1. What is the function of deoxyribonucleic acid (DNA)?
   a. to transmit all genetic information
   b. to determine the occurrence of cell division
   c. to build ribonucleic acid (RNA)
   d. to regulate the sequence of genes on chromosomes

2. Physiologic hyperplasia is commonly found in
   a. the bronchi of a chronic cigarette smoker
   b. a distended urinary bladder
   c. the female breast during lactation
   d. an enlarged myocardium in congestive heart failure

3. Which of the following describes a mechanism of cell death?
   a. cytoplasm becoming more granular
   b. rupture of cell membrane
   c. increase in size of cell
   d. embryonic differentiation

4. Which of the following is a common cause of coagulation necrosis?
   a. autophagocytosis
   b. granulomatous inflammation
   c. lack of blood supply
   d. malignant brain tumor

5. A major function of the reticuloendothelial system (RES) is to
   a. stimulate fibrin formation
   b. synthesize neutrophils
   c. release histamine
   d. phagocytize foreign material

6. Which of the following phrases best describes inflammation?
   a. an antigen-antibody reaction
   b. sequential reaction to cell injury
   c. secondary defense mechanism
   d. detrimental defense mechanism of body

7. Which of the following are local manifestations of inflammation?
   a. contractures and adhesions
   b. pain and ulceration
   c. boil and cyanosis
   d. swelling and loss of function

8. Wound healing by primary intention involves all the following *except*
   a. abundant collagen formation
   b. an inflammatory reaction
   c. regenerating epithelium
   d. blood clot formation

9. Contractures frequently occur after burn healing due to
   a. weakness of connective tissue
   b. lack of adequate blood supply
   c. excess fibrous tissue formation
   d. secondary infection

10. Rest and immobilization are important measures of acute care for wound healing because
    a. the production of leukocytes will be decreased
    b. the inflammatory response will be decreased
    c. they are known mechanisms to increase the rate of healing
    d. they increase the body's production of corticosteroids

REFERENCES

1. J. Crouch and J. R. McClintic, *Human Anatomy and Physiology*, John Wiley & Sons, Inc., New York, 1976, pp. 23–33.
2. D. T. Purtilo, *A Survey of Human Diseases*, Addison-Wesley Publishing Company, Inc., 1978, p. 74.
3. S. Price and L. Wilson, *Pathophysiology: Clinical Concepts of Disease Processes*, 2d ed., McGraw-Hill Book Company, New York, 1982, p. 20.
4. C. E. Roesel, *Immunology: A Self-Instructional Approach,* McGraw-Hill Book Company, New York, 1978, p. 8.
5. M. Groër and M. Shekleton, *Basic Pathophysiology: A Conceptual Approach*, The C. V. Mosby Company, St. Louis, 1979, p. 101.
6. Ibid., p. 103.
7. J. Walter, *An Introduction to the Principles of Disease*, W. B. Saunders Company, Philadelphia, 1977, p. 107.
8. Ibid., p. 120.
9. S. Levenson and E. Seifter, "Dysnutrition, Wound Healing and Resistance to Infection," *Clinics in Plastic Surgery*, **4**:375–388, 1977.
10. J. Niinikoski, "Oxygen and Wound Healing," *Clinics in Plastic Surgery*, **4**:361–374, 1977.

Chapter 10

NURSING ROLE IN MANAGEMENT

Altered Immune Responses

Susan Searle Jackson

Learning Objectives

1. Describe the functions, properties, and components of the immune system.
2. Differentiate between natural and acquired immunity.
3. Compare and contrast humoral and cell-mediated immunity regarding lymphocytes involved, types of reactions, and effects on antigens.
4. Identify the five types of immunoglobulins and their characteristics.
5. Describe the purpose and mechanism of action of the complement system.
6. Differentiate between the four types of hypersensitivity reactions in terms of immunological mechanism, time sequence, and disease manifestations.
7. Identify the clinical manifestations and emergency treatment for a systemic anaphylactic reaction.
8. Describe the etiologic factors, clinical manifestations, and treatment modalities of autoimmune diseases.
9. Describe the etiologic factors, categories, and treatment for immunodeficiency disorders.
10. Explain the relationship between cancer and the immune system.
11. Describe the assessment and management of a client with chronic allergies.
12. Describe the pharmacologic intervention for the client with allergies.

Since the beginning, the human body has had to protect itself from invasion by microorganisms and tumor protein. A complex defense system has evolved to withstand these constant attacks. The defense system in humans consists of a nonspecific inflammatory response (including phagocytosis) and a specific immune response (humoral immunity and cell-mediated immunity). (The inflammatory response was discussed in Chap. 9.)

Immunocompetence exists when the body's immune system is able to identify and to inactivate or destroy foreign substances.[1] When the immune system is incompetent or underresponsive, autoimmune diseases, immunodeficiency diseases, and malignancies occur. When the immune system overreacts, hypersensitivity disorders occur.

NORMAL IMMUNE RESPONSE

Immunity

Immunity is a state of responsiveness to invading organisms and foreign or tumor protein. Immune responses serve three functions (Table 10-1):[2]

1. *Defense*—The body resists invasions of microorganisms and prevents infection from developing by attacking foreign pathogens.
2. *Homeostasis*—Damaged cellular substances that are constantly being catabolized in the body are removed. Through this mechanism the cell type remains uniform and unchanged.
3. *Surveillance*—Mutations continually arise in the body but are normally recognized as foreign cells and destroyed.

Properties of the Immune System

The immune system has three important properties that make its protection diverse and long-lasting. They are:

1. *Specificity*—When a foreign substance (antigen) enters the body, a series of cellular changes take place. These changes result in the formation of a specific antibody that attaches to the surface of the antigen.
2. *Memory*—The immune system has the unique ability to remember the antigen. Because of this property, a secondary immune response is more rapid and stronger.
3. *Self-recognition*—Since there frequently is little difference between the body's own proteins and foreign proteins, it is of utmost importance for the body to distinguish between the two. When the body fails to recognize self-proteins, autoantibodies develop, leading to tissue destruction.

Types of Immunity

Immunity is classified as *natural* or *acquired*. Natural immunity exists in a person without prior

This chapter was reviewed by Jacqueline M. Fritz, R.N., B.S.N., M.S.N., CCRN, Educational Coordinator, Advanced Nursing Service, Advanced Critical Care Nursing Service, Anaheim, California.

Table 10-1
Functions of the Immune System

Function	Adaptive Response	Maladaptive Response	
		Hyper	Hypo
Defense	Destruction of viruses, bacteria	Allergic disorders	Immunodeficiency disorders
Homeostasis	Removal of damaged cells	Autoimmune diseases	—
Surveillance	Removal of cell mutants	—	Malignant diseases

Adapted from J. A. Bellanti, *Immunology II,* W. B. Saunders Company, Philadelphia, 1979, p. 14.

contact with an antigen. It may be related to a species, race, or genetic tendency. Acquired immunity implies the development of immunity in man, either actively or passively (Table 10-2).

Active acquired immunity

Active acquired immunity results from invasion of the body by microorganisms and subsequent development of antibodies and sensitized lymphocytes. With each reinvasion of the microorganisms, the body responds more rapidly and vigorously to fight off the invader. Active acquired immunity may result naturally from a disease or artificially through inoculation of a less virulent antigen. Because antibodies are manufactured, immunity takes time to develop but it is long-lasting.

Passive acquired immunity

Passive acquired immunity implies that the host receives antibodies to an antigen rather than manu-

Table 10-2
Types of Acquired Specific Immunity

Type of Immunity	Acquisition of Immunity	Protection	Examples
Active: antibodies synthesized by body in response to antigenic stimulation	*Natural:* natural contact with antigen through clinical or subclinical case	*Development:* develops slowly; protective levels reached in a few weeks *Duration:* long-term; often lifetime *Spectrum:* specific to antigen contacted	Recovery from childhood diseases (e.g., chickenpox, measles, mumps)
	Artificial: immunization with antigen	*Development:* develops slowly; protective levels reached in a few weeks *Duration:* several years; extended protection with "booster" doses *Spectrum:* specific to antigen immunized against	Immunization with live or killed vaccines; toxoid immunization
Passive: antibodies produced in one individual are transferred to another	*Natural:* transplacental and colostrum transfer from mother to child	*Development:* immediate *Duration:* temporary; several months *Spectrum:* to all antigens that mother has immunity	Maternal immunoglobulins in neonate
	Artificial: injection of serum from immune human or animal	*Development:* immediate *Duration:* temporary; several weeks *Spectrum:* to all antigens that source has immunity	Injection of pooled human gammaglobulin; injection of animal hyperimmune sera

From W. J. Phipps, B. C. Long, and N. F. Woods, *Medical-Surgical Nursing: Concepts and Clinical Practice,* The C. V. Mosby Company, St. Louis, 1979, p. 171.

facturing them. This may take place naturally through the transfer of immunoglobulins across the placental membrane from mother to fetus. Artificial passive acquired immunity occurs through injection with gamma globulin or serum antibodies. The benefit of this immunity is its immediate effect. Unfortunately, the immunity is short-lived, since the host did not manufacture the antibodies and consequently does not retain memory cells for the antigen.

Antigens

An *antigen* is a foreign substance that elicits an immune response by the body. Most antigens are composed of protein. However, other substances such as large-size polysaccharides, lipoproteins, and nucleic acids can act as antigens. Of special significance are *haptens* (low molecular weight substances) that in themselves are harmless but when combined with high molecular weight carriers, form complexes that are antigenic. Common haptens include dust, animal danders, drugs, and industrial chemicals. Once antibodies are produced, future exposure to the hapten alone can elicit an immune response. Haptens are important in hypersensitivity reactions.

Most antigens are not chemically pure substances, but rather have multiple antigenic determinants on their surface with which antibodies can combine. Physical or chemical irritation may stimulate new antigenic determinants and this process results in hypersensitivity, autoimmunity, and neoplasia.[3]

Components of the Immune System

Lymphoid organs function in production of lymphocytes, one of the essential cells of the immune response.

Lymphoid organs

The lymph system is composed of both central and peripheral lymphoid organs. The *central lymphoid organs* are the thymus gland and the bone marrow. The *peripheral lymphoid organs* are the tonsils, gut-associated lymphoid tissues, lymph nodes, and spleen (Fig. 10-1).

Lymphocytes are synthesized in *bone marrow* and eventually migrate to the peripheral organs.

The *thymus* is important for the differentiation and maturation of *T lymphocytes*. The thymus is therefore essential for a cell-mediated immune response. In childhood the gland is large. However, the gland shrinks with age and can be removed in adults without causing a severe immunodeficient state.

Gut- and bronchial-associated lymphoid tissue is found in the submucosa of the respiratory, genitourinary, and gastrointestinal tracts. This tissue protects the body surface from external microorganisms. The tonsils are a typical example of such lymphoid tissue.

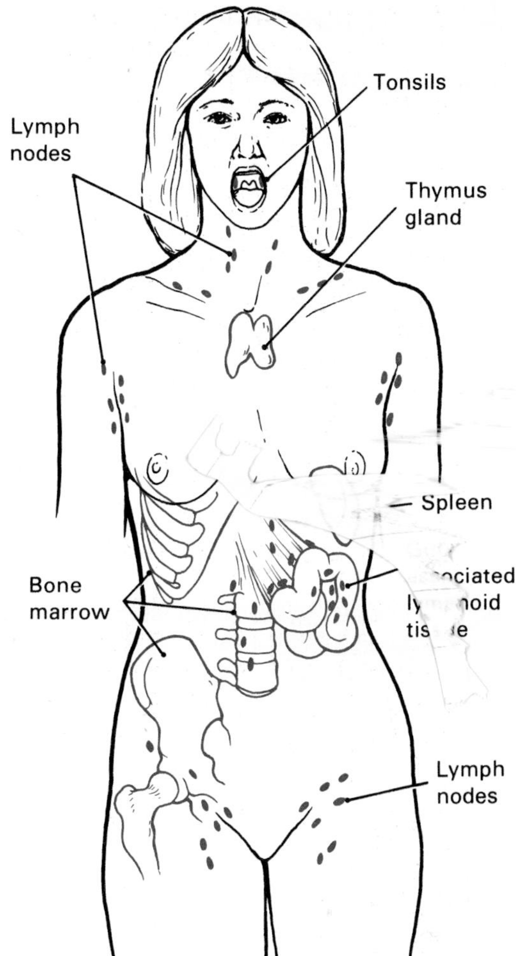

Figure 10-1 Organs of the immune system.

When antigens are introduced into the body, they may be carried via the blood stream or lymph channels to regional *lymph nodes*. The antigens interact with B and T lymphocytes and macrophages in the lymph node. The two important functions of lymph nodes are: (1) filtration of foreign material brought to the site, and (2) circulation of lymphocytes.

The *spleen* is important as the primary site for filtering foreign substances from the blood. It consists of two kinds of tissue: *white pulp* contains B lymphocytes and T lymphocytes; *red pulp* contains erythrocytes. If the spleen is removed in children, it can predispose to life-threatening septicemia.

Reticuloendothelial system (RES)

The reticuloendothelial system consists of macrophages found in lymphoid tissue. (See Chap. 9 for a more complete description of the RES and macrophages.) Macrophages have a critical role in the immune system. Macrophages are responsible for capturing, processing, and presenting the antigen to the lymphocytes. This stimulates a humoral or cell-mediated immune response. Capturing is accomplished through phagocytosis. The macrophage-bound antigen, which is highly immunogenic, is presented to circulating T lymphocytes or B lymphocytes, and thus triggers an immune response.[4]

Lymphocyte Production

Lymphocytes arise from undifferentiated stem cells in the fetal liver and later from the bone marrow (Fig. 10-2). Under the influence of a lymphoid structure, the lymphocytes differentiate into B lymphocytes and T lymphocytes.

B lymphocytes (bursa-equivalent or thymus-independent cells) mature under the influence of the bursa of Fabricius in birds. However, this lymphoid organ does not exist in man. The equivalent of the bursa has not yet been identified. Several sites have been suggested, including the bone marrow and gut-associated lymphoid tissue.

Cells that migrate from the bone marrow to the thymus differentiate into *T lymphocytes* (thymus-dependent cells). The thymus secretes thymosin hormone, which is believed to stimulate the maturation and differentiation of T lymphocytes. These cells compose 60 to 70 percent of the circulating lymphocytes and are primarily responsible for immunity to viruses, tumor cells, and fungi.

Humoral Immunity

A successful humoral immune response leads to humoral immunity. Production of antibodies (immunoglobulins) is an essential step in a humoral immune response. Immunoglobulins are composed of amino acids arranged on two light and two heavy polypeptide chains. Differences in the heavy chain configuration differentiates the five classes of immunoglobulins, which are IgG, IgA, IgM, IgD, and IgE. Each class of immunoglobulins has a special function (Table 10-3).

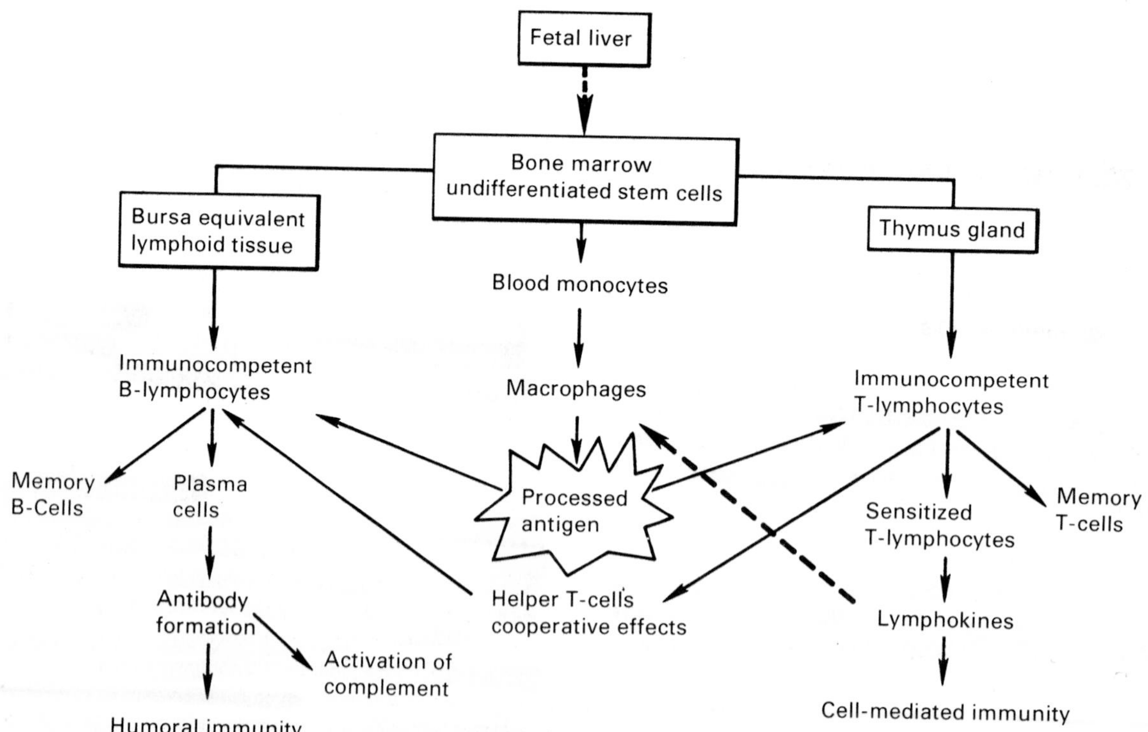

Figure 10-2 Relationships and functions of macrophages, B lymphocytes, and T lymphocytes in an immune response.

Table 10-3
Characteristics of Immunoglobulins

Class	Quantity	Location	Characteristics
IgG	76%	Plasma Interstitial fluid	Only Ig that crosses placenta Fixes complement Responsible for secondary immune response
IgA	15%	Body secretions tears, saliva, breast milk, colostrum	Lines mucous membranes and protects body surfaces
IgM	8%	Intravascular serum	Fixes complement Responsible for primary immune response With IgG has specific antitoxin action Forms antibodies to ABO blood antigens
IgD	1%	Serum	Present on lymphocyte surface Assist in the differentiation of B lymphocytes
IgE	0.002%	Serum, interstitial fluids, exocrine secretions	Responsible for symptoms of allergic reactions Antibody that fixes to mast cells Assist in defense against parasitic infections

Humoral immune response

When an antigen (especially bacteria) enters the body, it may encounter a B lymphocyte specific for that antigen. The B lymphocyte recognizes the antigen because it has cell surface receptors specific for the antigen. After contact with the antigen, most of the B lymphocytes differentiate into plasma cells (Figure 10-2). The mature plasma cell secretes immunoglobulins. Each plasma cell produces only one type of immunoglobulin. Some of the stimulated B lymphocytes remain as memory cells.

The *primary immune response* is evident 4 to 8 days after the initial exposure to the antigen. IgM is the first type of antibody formed. Because of the large size of the IgM molecule, this immunoglobulin is confined to the intravascular space. As the immune response progresses, IgG is produced and can move from the intravascular to the extravascular spaces.

When the individual is exposed to the antigen the second time, a *secondary antibody response* occurs. This response occurs faster (1 to 2 days), is stronger, and lasts for a longer time than a primary response. Memory cells account for the memory of the first exposure to the antigen and the more rapid production of antibodies. IgG is the primary antibody found in a secondary immune response.

During gestation, the fetus has some immunity to protect itself against in utero infections. However, the lymph nodes and spleen are underdeveloped at birth. Fortunately, IgG crosses the placental membrane and provides the newborn with passive acquired immunity for at least 3 months. Infants may also get some immunity from IgA concentrated in breast milk and colostrum. By 9 months of age, a baby's IgM level is at normal concentration and the lymph nodes and spleen are well developed.

Antigen-antibody interactions

Antigen-antibody interactions result in elimination or destruction of the antigen. The five kinds of interactions are:

1. *Precipitation*—Soluble antigens combine with antibodies to form a lattice formation of insoluble complexes which precipitate.
2. *Agglutination*—Antibodies may destroy antigen by forming clumps of the antigen (e.g., blood transfusion reactions).
3. *Opsonization*—Opsonins are immunoglobulins that make the antigen more likely to be phagocytized. Opsonization is the reaction of an antibody with highly resistant antigen (e.g., pneumococcus) in which a special chemical coating from opsonins provides a means for attachment of the antigen to the surface of phagocytes.
4. *Lysis*—Lysis occurs after complement acts on the antigen cell membrane to cause rupture and spillage of cell contents (see next section).
5. *Neutralization*—Antibodies neutralize some toxins released from bacteria. The RES system phagocyt-

izes the antigen-antibody complex and removes it from the body.

Complement System

The complement system consists of nine plasma proteins that interact to mediate and amplify the immune response. When activated, the components occur in the sequential order of: C1, C4, C2, C3, C5, C6, C7, C8, and C9 (Fig. 10-3). The numbering reflects the order of their discovery. Some components have subparts designated by lowercase letters (C3a, C3b, C5a, etc.). The primary pathway for activation of the complement system is through fixation of component C1 to an antigen-antibody complex. The immunoglobulins IgG and IgM are responsible for fixing complement. Each of the activated complexes is able to act on the next component, creating a cascade effect.

An alternate pathway (*properdin pathway*) exists, in which C3 is activated without prior antigen-antibody fixation. Bacteria products, lipopolysaccharides, and plasmin can stimulate the complement sequence at the C3 level with activation of C5 to C9.

Major functions of the complement system are enhanced phagocytosis, enhanced vascular permeability, and cellular lysis. All these activities are important to the inflammatory response.

Complement increases phagocytosis through opsonization and chemotaxis. Immune adherence and opsonization occur when antigen in combination with complement factor C3 and specific antibodies stick to the surface of phagocytic cells. This adherence leads to more rapid phagocytosis. In addition, complement component C5a promotes *chemotaxis*, which is the attraction of macrophages and granulocytes to the area of antigen-antibody reaction.

Both C3a and C5a generate anaphylatoxin factors which degrade mast cells and cause the release of histamine. Histamine causes smooth muscle contraction and an increase in vascular permeability.

The entire complement sequence C1 to C9 must be activated for cell lysis to occur. The final component C8,9 acts upon the cell surface causing rupture of the cell membrane and lysis. Bacteria, red blood cells, and nucleated cells are susceptible to the lysis.

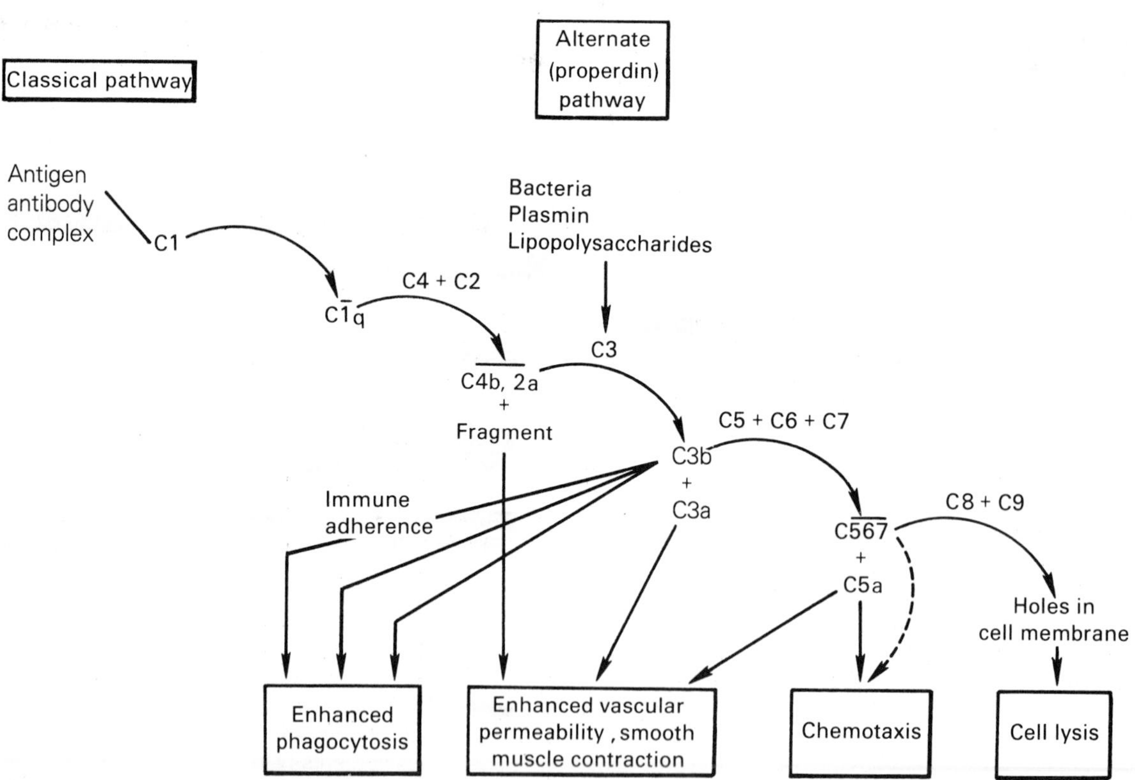

Figure 10-3 Sequential action and biologic effects of the complement system. *(Adapted from R. E. Stiehm and V. A. Fulginitti, Immunologic Disorders in Infants, W. B. Saunders Company, Philadelphia, 1973, p. 103.)*

Cell-Mediated Immunity

This type of immunity is achieved through production of a cell-mediated immune response. The first step is detection of antigen by T lymphocytes. They do not destroy the antigen by producing antibodies. Rather, their two methods of attack are (1) direct attack by the sensitized T lymphocytes (cytotoxic T cells), and (2) indirect attack by release of lymphokines. As with B lymphocytes, some sensitized T lymphocytes do not attack the antigen but remain as *memory T cells* in the lymphoid tissue. As in the humoral immune response, a second exposure to the antigen will result in a more intense and rapid cell-mediated immune response. Other sensitized T lymphocytes become *helper T cells* that assist B lymphocytes in the humoral immune response.

Cytotoxic T cells

After exposure to an antigen, some T lymphocytes transform into sensitized T cells known as cytotoxic T cells. Cytotoxic T cells attack the cell membrane and release cytolytic substances that destroy the antigen.

Lymphokines

Sensitized T lymphocytes release soluble chemical substances called *lymphokines*. Lymphokines attract, hold, and activate other uncommitted lymphocytes and macrophages to the affected area. The various kinds of lymphokines which act as mediators on the immune response are summarized in Table 10-4.

Summary of Immune Responses

Humans need both humoral and cell-mediated immunity to remain healthy. Each type of immunity has unique properties, different methods of action, and reacts against particular antigens. Table 10-5 is a comparison of humoral and cell-mediated immunity.

ALTERED IMMUNE RESPONSE

The immune system normally reacts protectively to invasion of antigens. However, sometimes the response is overreactive and results in tissue damage. This is called a *hypersensitivity reaction*. At other times the body fails to recognize self-proteins and reacts against its own protein. Tissue damage resulting from this mechanism is called autoimmunity. Finally, tissue damage may occur if the immune system is deficient. The *immunodeficiency state* may be primary or secondary to other diseases.

Table 10-4

Effects of Lymphokines on Body Cells

Lymphokine	Cell Involved	Effect
1. Lymphocyte-derived chemotactic factor (LDCF)	Macrophages, neutrophils	Attracts macrophages and neutrophils to area of antigen
2. Migration-inhibition factor (MIF) or macrophage activation factor (MAF)	Macrophages	Suppresses movement of macrophages so they remain in area of antigen, promotes adherence of macrophages to cell surface, activates macrophages metabolically
3. Transfer factor (TF)	Lymphocytes	Transforms nonsensitized T cells to sensitized T cells
4. Lymphotoxin (LT)	Tissue cells	Kills some antigens
5. Interferon	Tissue cells	Interferes with viral growth, stimulates phagocytic action of macrophages, and stimulates killing activity of sensitized lymphocytes and natural killer cells
6. Interleukin 2 (IL-2)	Lymphocytes	Promotes antibody production by B cells, stimulates thymocytes, and promotes the development of cytotoxic T cells

Table 10-5

Comparison of Humoral Immunity and Cell-Mediated Immunity

Characteristic	Humoral Immunity	Cell-Mediated Immunity
Cells involved	B lymphocytes	T lymphocytes
Products elaborated	Antibodies	Sensitized T cells Lymphokines
Memory cells	Present	Present
Reaction	Immediate	Delayed
Protection for	Bacteria Viruses Respiratory and gastrointestinal pathogens	Fungus Some viruses Chronic infectious agents Tumor cells
Examples	Anaphylactic shock Atopic diseases Transfusion reaction Neutralization of exotoxins	Tuberculosis Fungal infections Contact dermatitis Graft rejection Destruction of cancer cells

Hypersensitivity Reactions

Hypersensitivity implies an allergic condition in which the immune system plays an active role. The overreaction of the immune system to an antigen (*allergen*) may occur because of excessive amounts of antigen or antibody, inappropriate involvement of nonspecific tissue, and/or the response occurs in the wrong area of the body.

Classification of hypersensitivity reactions may be done according to the source of the allergen (exogenous, homologous, and autologous), time sequence (immediate or delayed), or according to the basic immunologic mechanisms causing the injury (Gell and Coombs classification). The Gell and Coombs classification is the most comprehensive and will be used in this chapter. Basically, there are four types of hypersensitivity reactions. Types I, II, and III are immediate and are examples of humoral immunity. Type IV is a delayed hypersensitivity reaction and related to cell-mediated immunity. See Table 10-6 for a summary of the four types of hypersensitivity reactions.

The manifestations of hypersensitivity reactions depend upon many etiologic factors. Among the most important are:

1. Degree of exposure to the allergen. The effect is more serious if the client ingested, inhaled, or touched a large amount of the allergen.
2. The type of antibody involved in the reaction determines the clinical manifestations.
3. Target organs and tissues affected by allergens. Especially vulnerable are the skin and gastrointestinal and respiratory tracts.
4. Release of chemical mediators on target organs.

Type I—Anaphylactoid reactions

Anaphylactoid reactions occur *only* in persons who are highly sensitized from *previous* exposure to low-dose allergens. Upon subsequent exposure to a challenge allergen, IgE (reaginic antibody) *immediately* reacts with the allergen and triggers the release of chemical mediators from mast cells. The mediators act upon target cells of the body, causing tissue damage. Common allergic reactions include anaphylactic shock (anaphylaxis), allergic asthma, allergic rhinitis, atopic dermatitis, urticaria, and angioedema.

The IgE immunoglobulins have a characteristic property of attaching to mast cells (Fig. 10-4). Within mast cells are granules containing potent chemical mediators (histamine, serotonin, SRS-A, ECF-A, acetylcholine, kinins, and bradykinin). When IgE-bound mast cells react with an allergen, the mast cell is *degranulated*, the mediators are released, and then attack target organs, causing clinical allergy symptoms. Fortunately, the mediators are short-acting and their effects are reversible.

Histamine, an important chemical mediator in humans, illustrates the effects on target organs. The release of histamine causes multifocal effects on the body. These effects include smooth muscle contraction, increased vascular permeability, vasodilation, hypotension, increased mucus secretion, and itching.

Table 10-6
Hypersensitivity Reactions

Type of Reaction	Antibody Involved	Complement Involved	Mediators of Injury	Clinical Examples	Skin Test
I. Anaphylactic	IgE	None	Histamine SRS-A	Allergic rhinitis Asthma	Wheal and flare
II. Cytotoxic	IgG or IgM	C1–9	Complement lysis, neutrophils	Transfusion reaction Goodpasture's syndrome	None
III. Immune-complex mediated	IgG or IgM	C1-9	Neutrophils Complement lysis	Serum sickness Systemic lupus erythematosus	Arthus reaction
IV. Delayed hypersensitivity (cell-mediated)	None	None	Lymphokines	Contact dermatitis Allograft or tumor rejection	Delayed reaction (TB test)

Adapted from H. B. Richerson, "Immunology of the Respiratory System," *Basics of RD*, American Thoracic Society, **2** (5):3, 1974.

Allergic Reactions The clinical manifestations of an anaphylactoid reaction depend upon whether the mediators remain local, become systemic, or affect particular organs. When the mediator remains *localized,* a cutaneous response called the *wheal* and *flare reaction* occurs. This reaction is characterized by a pale wheal containing edematous fluid surrounded by a red flare from the hyperemia. The reaction occurs in minutes or hours and is not usually dangerous. A classic example of a wheal and flare reaction is the mosquito bite. The wheal and flare reaction serves a positive purpose as a means of demonstrating allergic reactions to specific allergens during skin tests.

Anaphylactic shock (anaphylaxis) occurs when mediators are released *systemically* after injection of a drug or an insect sting. The reaction occurs within minutes and is life-threatening because of respiratory obstruction and vascular collapse. The *target organs* affected are seen in Fig. 10-5. Initial symptoms include edema and itching at the site of the allergen. Within minutes shock may occur, manifested by rapid, weak pulse, hypotension, dilated pupils, dyspnea, and cyanosis. This is compounded by bronchial edema and angioedema. Death will occur if emergency treatment is not initiated. Some of the important allergens leading to anaphylactic shock in hypersensitive persons are listed in Table 10-7.

Atopic Reactions A less severe type of anaphylactoid reaction occurs in persons who inherit a familial tendency to react to harmless environmental allergens (dust, animal danders, plant pollens, mole

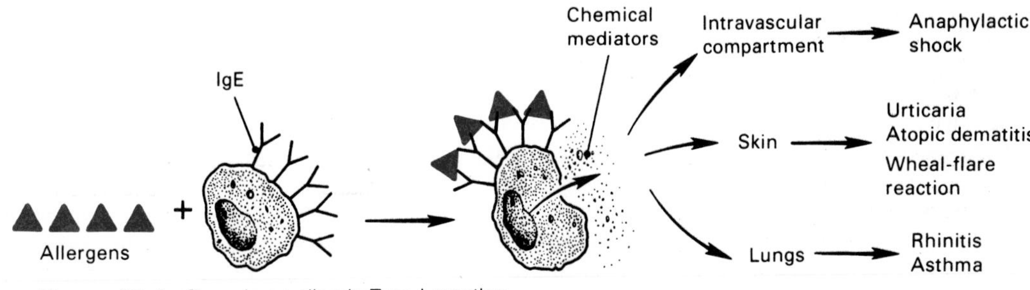

Figure 10-4 Steps in an allergic Type I reaction.

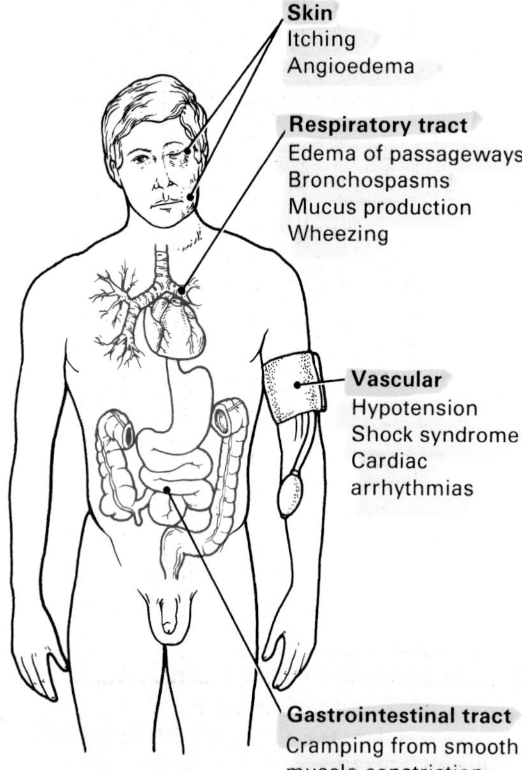

Figure 10-5 Clinical manifestations of a systemic anaphylactic reaction. (*Adapted from S. A. Price and L. M. Wilson, Pathophysiology: Clinical Concepts of Disease Processes, McGraw-Hill Book Company, New York, 1978, p. 110.*)

Table 10-7

Allergens That May Cause Anaphylactic Shock

Drugs
Penicillins
Insulin
Chemotherapy agents
Tetracycline
Insect venoms
Hymenoptera (wasps, hornets, yellow jackets, bumblebees, and ants)
Foods
Eggs
Nuts
Shellfish
Chocolate
Animal serums for antitoxins
Tetanus antitoxin
Diphtheria antitoxin
Rabies antitoxin
Snake venom antitoxin
Treatment measures
Blood products (whole blood and other particles)
Allergenic extracts in hyposensitization therapy
Iodine-contrast media dye for IVP or angiogram test

spores, cosmetics, and foods). Twenty percent of the population is believed to be *atopic* or have an inherited tendency to become sensitive to environmental allergens. The *atopic diseases* that can result are allergic rhinitis, allergic asthma, atopic dermatitis, urticaria, and angioedema.

Allergic rhinitis or *hay fever* is the most common Type I hypersensitivity reaction. It may occur year round (*perennial allergic rhinitis*) or be seasonal (*seasonal allergic rhinitis*). Persons afflicted with allergic rhinitis often have a sensitive nasal mucosa and are very susceptible to respiratory infections. Airborne substances (aeroallergens) are the primary cause of allergic rhinitis. The target areas affected are the conjunctiva of the eyes and the upper respiratory tract mucosa. Symptoms include nasal discharge, sneezing, lacrimation, mucosal swelling with airway obstruction, and pruritus around the eyes, nose, throat, and mouth. (Treatment of allergic rhinitis is discussed in Chap. 19.)

Fifty percent of asthmatics have *asthma* caused by hypersensitivity to allergens. The asthma may be *extrinsic* if caused by environmental allergens (foods, seasonal pollens, dust, and danders) or *intrinsic* if due to bacterial or viral infections of the respiratory tract. Most clients with extrinsic asthma present a past history of atopic disorders (infantile eczema, allergic rhinitis, or food intolerances). With intrinsic asthma there is no atopic history. Extrinsic asthma usually starts in people aged 5 to 30, while intrinsic asthma starts as an adult disorder.[5]

In allergic asthma, SRS-A (slow-reacting substance of anaphylaxis) and histamine are responsible for action on the bronchioles. These mediators produce bronchial smooth muscle constriction, excessive viscoid mucus secretion, edema of the mucous membranes of the bronchi, and decreased lung compliance. Because of these physiological alterations, clients manifest dyspnea, severe expiratory wheezing, coughing, tightness in the chest, thick sputum, and a fear of suffocation. (Treatment of asthma is discussed in Chap. 21.)

Atopic dermatitis is a chronic inherited skin disorder characterized by exacerbations and remissions. It is caused by a variety of environmental allergens that are difficult to identify. Frequently, children with infantile eczema have allergic respiratory disorders although the relationship between the two is not fully understood. Although clients with atopic dermatitis have elevated IgE levels and positive skin tests, the histopathologic features do not represent the typical localized wheal and flare Type I reactions. Rather, the skin lesions are more generalized and involve vasodilation of blood vessels, resulting in intracellular edema with vesicle formation (Fig. 10-6). (Dermatitis is discussed in Chap. 17.)

Urticaria or *hives* is a cutaneous lesion occurring in atopic persons. It is characterized by transient wheals (pink, raised, edematous, pruritic areas) that vary in size and shape and may occur throughout the body. Urticaria develops rapidly after exposure to an allergen and may last minutes or hours. Histamine causes (1) localized vasodilation (erythema), (2) transudation of fluid (wheal), and (3) stimulation of local axon reflexes (flaring).[6] Internal urticaria is characterized by edema in internal organs. Histamine also is responsible for the numbness and pruritus associated with the lesions. (Urticaria is discussed in Chap. 17.)

Angioedema is a localized cutaneous lesion similar to urticaria but involving deeper layers of the skin and the submucosa. The principal areas of involvement include the eyelids, lips, tongue, larynx, hands, feet, gastrointestinal tract, and genitalia. Usually, swelling occurs in only one area at a time. Dilation and engorgement of the capillaries secondary to release of histamine causes the diffuse swelling. Welts are not apparent as in urticaria. Rather, the outer skin appears normal or has a reddish hue. The lesions may burn, sting, or itch, cause no discomfort, or cause acute pain if in the gastrointestinal tract. The swelling may occur suddenly or over 2 hours and it usually lasts for 24 hours.

Type II—Cytotoxic and cytolytic reactions

Type II hypersensitivity reaction involves the direct binding of IgG or IgM antibodies to an antigen on the cell surface. IgG or IgM activates the complement system and helps mediate the reaction. Cellular tissue is destroyed in one of three ways: (1) activation of the complement cascade resulting in *cytolysis*, (2) enhanced phagocytosis from complement fixation, and (3) a *cytotoxic* reaction independent of complement involvement.

Target cells frequently destroyed in Type II reactions are erythrocytes, platelets, and leukocytes. Some of the antigens involved are the ABO blood group, Rh factor, and drug haptens such as chloramphenicol. Pathologic disorders characteristic of Type II reactions include ABO incompatibility transfusion reaction, Rh incompatibility transfusion reaction, autoimmune and drug-related hemolytic anemias, leukopenias, thrombocytopenias, erythroblastosis fetalis, and Goodpasture's syndrome. The tissue damage usually occurs rapidly.

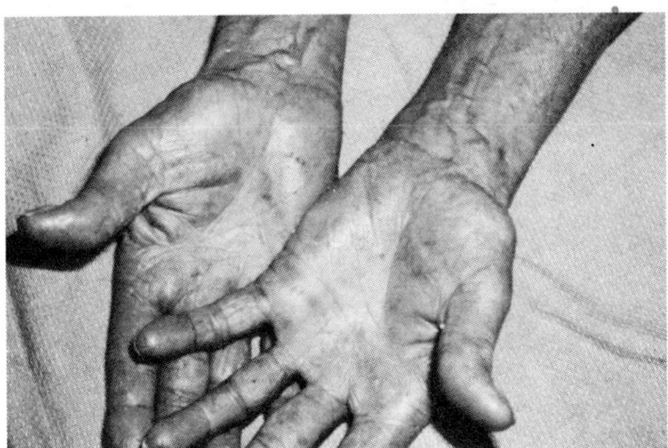

Figure 10-6 Chronic lesions of atopic dermatitis on the hands of a woman; erythema, crusts, cracks are evident. (*Film courtesy of Pad Meuron, M.D.*)

Hemolytic Transfusion Reactions A classicial Type II reaction occurs when a recipient receives ABO-incompatible blood from a donor. Within the recipient's serum are natural antibodies (agglutins) to antigens (agglutinogens) of the ABO blood group that are not present on his erythrocyte membranes (Table 23-7). For example, a person with type A blood has anti-B agglutinins, a person with type B blood has anti-A agglutinins, a person with type AB blood has no antiagglutinins, while a person with type O blood has both anti-A and anti-B agglutinins.

If the recipient is transfused with incompatible blood, agglutinins immediately coat the foreign erythrocytes, causing agglutination or clumping. The clumping of cells blocks all the small blood vessels in the body and also depletes the clotting factors, leading to bleeding. Within hours neutrophils and macrophages phagocytize the agglutinated cells. As complement is fixed to the antigen, cytolysis occurs. Cellular lysis causes the release of hemoglobin into the urine and plasma. In addition, a cytotoxic reaction causes vascular spasms in the kidney, which further block the renal tubules. Acute renal failure can result from the hemoglobinuria. (Blood transfusions are discussed in Chap. 26.)

Goodpasture's Syndrome This is a rare disorder involving the lungs and kidneys. An antibody-mediated autoimmune reaction occurs with the glomerular and alveolar basement membranes. The circulating antibodies combine with tissue antigen to activate complement, which causes deposits of IgG to form along the basement membranes of the lungs or kidney. This reaction may result in pulmonary hemorrhage and glomerulonephritis.

The disease is usually rapidly progressive and fatal. Corticosteroids may induce temporary remission but will not prevent death. Plasmapheresis transfusions offer the most hope.

Type III—Immune-complex reactions

Tissue damage in a Type III reaction occurs secondary to antigen-antibody complexes. Soluble antigens combine with immunoglobulins of the IgG and IgM classes to form complexes which are too small to be effectively removed by the reticuloendothelial system (RES). Therefore, the complexes deposit in tissue or small blood vessels. They cause the fixation of complement and the release of chemotactic factors which lead to inflammation and phagocytosis of the involved tissue.

Type III reactions may be local or systemic and immediate or delayed. The clinical manifestations depend upon the number of complexes and their location in the body. Common sites for deposit are the kidneys, skin, joints, and blood vessels. Severe Type III reactions are associated with some autoimmune disorders such as systemic lupus erythematosus (SLE), acute glomerulonephritis, and rheumatoid arthritis (RA). Two classic disorders that illustrate Type III reactions are *Arthus reaction* and *serum sickness*.

Arthus Reaction The Arthus reaction is a *localized* inflammatory response resulting from antigen-antibody complexes deposited in the small vessels of the skin. It may occur from inhalation of dust or spores, resulting in pneumonitis or farmer's lung.

The underlying defect that triggers an Arthus reaction appears to be the production of *excess IgG* to specific antigens. Upon subsequent exposure to soluble antigens, antigen-antibody complexes form, leading to a Type III reaction. Because of the chemotactic substances released by complement, neutrophils infiltrate to the site of the complex. The neutrophils which phagocytize the cells are the primary factor responsible for tissue damage.

Arthus reactions are manifested by edematous, hemorrhagic, and necrotic lesions that develop over 6 to 12 hours. Most classic Arthus reactions are not clinically significant because strong antigenic substances are not ordinarily given repeatedly to a hypersensitive individual. However, *allergic vasculitis* to drugs (penicillin, sulfonamides) resembles the Arthus reaction.

Serum Sickness Serum sickness is another Type III reaction that involves deposits of antigen-antibody complexes in blood vessel walls of the skin, joints, and especially in the renal glomeruli. In contrast to an Arthus reaction, this disorder is *systemic*. It develops slowly, 10 to 14 days after exposure to an antigen, and is self-limiting. Although the reaction is delayed, serum sickness is considered a humoral hypersensitivity reaction because of the presence of antibodies causing tissue damage.

The critical factor in serum sickness is the presence of *excess soluble antigen*. Common antigens triggering the reaction are horse antitoxin serums and certain drugs (penicillins, sulfonamides). Unlike a Type I reaction, the person does not need to be previously sensitized to react to the antigen. Rather, a single dose of the antigen that remains at high levels in the body for several days reacts with antibodies formed about 2 weeks after initial exposure to the antigen. The antigen-antibody complex then triggers complement to deposit in vessels resulting in an intravascular inflammation. The predominant signs and symptoms of serum sickness are urticaria, angioedema, fever, muscle soreness, malaise, lymphadenopathy, joint pain, polyarthritis, and nephritis.

Fortunately, with the use of human serums, serum sickness reactions can be avoided. However, it is still critical to watch for drug sensitivities. The actual treatment of serum sickness depends upon the severity of the reaction. For mild reactions, aspirin is prescribed for the fever and arthritis and antihistamines are given for urticaria and angioedema. Corticosteroids are prescribed for more severe reactions, especially when renal or neurologic changes are present.

Type IV—Delayed hypersensitivity reactions

A delayed hypersensitivity reaction is also called a cell-mediated immune response; however, a cell-mediated response is a protective mechanism while tissue damage occurs in delayed hypersensitivity reactions.

The tissue damage in a Type IV reaction does not occur in the presence of antibodies or complement. Rather, sensitized T lymphocytes may directly attack antigens or indirectly release lymphokines to interact with specific antigens. The process takes hours to days for a reaction to occur.

Clinical examples of a delayed hypersensitivity reaction include (1) contact dermatitis; (2) hypersensitivity reactions to bacterial, fungal, and viral infections; and (3) transplant rejections. Some drug sensitivity reactions also fall under this category.

Contact Dermatitis Allergic eczematous contact dermatitis (AECD) is an example of a delayed hypersensitivity reaction involving the skin. The reaction occurs when the skin is exposed to haptens. The haptens easily penetrate the skin to combine with epidermal proteins. The hapten-carrier substance then becomes antigenic. Over a period of 7 to 14 days memory cells form to the antigen. Upon subsequent exposure to the hapten, a sensitized person develops eczematous skin lesions within 48 hours.[7] The most common haptens encountered are: metal compounds (nickel, mercury); rubber compounds; catechols present in poison ivy, poison oak, and sumac; cosmetics; and some dyes.

In acute contact dermatitis, the skin lesions appear erythematous, edematous, and are covered with papules, vesicles, and bullae. The involved area is very pruritic but may also burn or sting. When contact dermatitis becomes chronic, the lesions resemble atopic dermatitis because they are thickened, scaly, and lichenified. The main difference between contact dermatitis and atopic dermatitis is the fact that contact dermatitis is localized and restricted to the area exposed to the allergens while atopic dermatitis is widespread (Fig. 10-7).

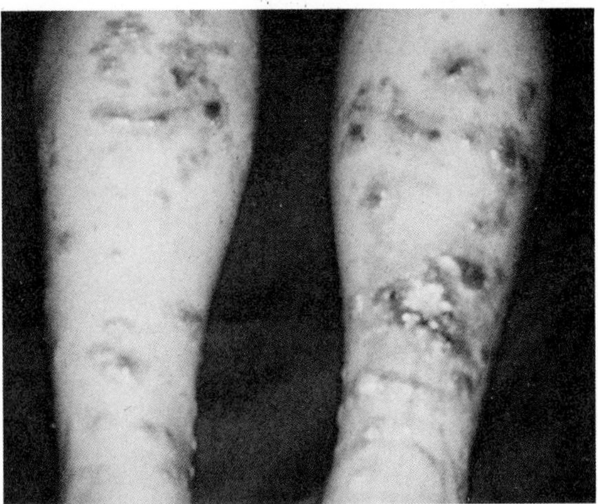

Figure 10-7 Acute chronic dermatitis on lower extremities. Note the edema, erythema, papules, bullae, and weeping vesicles. (*Film courtesy of Pad Meuron, M.D.*)

Microbial Hypersensitivity Reaction Although cell-mediated immunity plays an important defensive role in destroying viruses, bacteria, and fungi, delayed hypersensitivity reactions do occur as the surrounding tissue is damaged. Examples to illustrate infectious delayed hypersensitivity reactions include: skin rashes of measles and smallpox, lesions of leprosy and herpes simplex virus, and the generalized toxemia and caseous necrosis with tuberculosis.

The classic example of a bacterial cell-mediated immune reaction is the body's defense against *tubercle bacillus*. *Mycobacterium tuberculosis* results from invasion of lung tissue by highly resistant tubercle bacillus. The organism itself does not directly damage the lung tissue and may live in the host for some time before symptoms appear. However, over time antigenic material released from the tubercle bacillus reacts with T lymphocytes, initiating a cell-mediated response. The resulting lymphocytotoxicity causes extensive caseous necrosis of the lung.

After the initial cell-mediated reaction, memory cells persist so that subsequent contact with the tubercule bacillus or an extract of purified protein from the organism will cause a delayed hypersensitivity reaction. This is the basis for the PPD tuberculosis skin test read 48 to 72 hours after the injection. (Tuberculosis is discussed in Chap. 20.)

Transplant Rejection Rejection of organs occurs by cell-mediated immunity if the donor organ does not perfectly match the recipient's human leukocytic antigens (HLA), also called *histocompatibility antigens*. The rejection can be prevented by closely matching ABO, Rh, and HLA antigens between donor and recipient. Unfortunately, there are numerous different HLA antigens and a perfect match is nearly impossible unless the tissue is *autograftic* (self) or *isograftic* (identical twin). Once the major antigens are matched, minor histocompatibility antigens are attempted to be matched.

Graft rejection is a complicated process that involves sensitized T lymphocytes. If the tissue is mismatched, sensitized T lymphocytes arrive at regional lymph nodes within 6 to 10 days. The clinical signs of rejection appear in about 14 days when sensitized T lymphocytes attack the site. At this time the vascularization stops and the tissue becomes necrosed. Common manifestations of transplant rejection include fever, malaise, localized graft tenderness, hypertension, leukocytosis, elevated sedimentation rate, and elevated enzyme studies.

Drugs that interfere with cell-mediated immune responses are given to recipients of transplanted organs. Some of the agents used are summarized in Table 10-8. Unfortunately, the use of immunosuppressant drugs can result in major complications which are (1) increased susceptibility to infection, (2) increased risk of developing cancer, and (3) graft-versus-host disease.[8]

Autoimmune Phenomena

Autoimmunity is a state of responsiveness to certain self-proteins; the body no longer differentiates self from nonself with respect to these substances. For some unknown reason, cells that are normally unre-

Table 10-8

Immunosuppressive Agents Used In Organ Transplantations

Type of Agent	Mechanism
I. Anti-inflammatory	
Adrenocortical steroids: Prednisone, prednisolone, methylprednisolone	Stabilizes lysozomes, impairs antigen recognition and processing, lymphocytolysis, impairs antibody synthesis
II. Antimetabolites Azathioprine, 6-mercaptopurine	Impairs nucleic acid synthesis and pyrimidine ribonucleotide
III. Cytotoxic	
Alkylating agents: Cyclophosphamide, chlorambucil	Causes inter- and intrastrand DNA cross-linkage with alteration of DNA helix
X-irradiation	Karyorrhexis, destruction of DNA helix
Antilymphocyte globulin	Immune cytolysis

From J. A. Bellanti, *Immunology II*, W. B. Saunders Company, Philadelphia, 1979, p. 558.

sponsive (tolerant to self-antigens) are activated. Both T cells and B cells have the ability for tolerance to self-antigens. Therefore, an alteration in T cells alone or B cells and T cells can produce autoantibodies and autosensitized T cells to cause pathologic tissue damage. The various autoimmune diseases manifested depend upon which self-antigen is damaged.

Theories of causation

The cause of autoimmune diseases is still unknown. Age plays some role because it has been found that there are an increased number of circulating autoantibodies in persons over age 50.[9] It appears that no one theory is conclusive but rather a combination of etiological factors must be considered.

Forbidden-Clone Theory Through somatic mutation, a clone of mutant T cells or B cells could be allowed to survive. These new clone cells could become reactive against the body's own tissue, resulting in an autoimmune process.

Sequestered Antigen Theory Normally, during embryonic development (when immune tolerance develops) there are tissues that are separated or sequestered from the circulatory and lymph systems. These tissues include the lens of the eye, the thyroid, the testes, and the central nervous system. If later through trauma, infection, or chemical exposure, these cells are released into circulation, these cells will not be recognized as "self" and an autoimmune response occurs. An example of this reaction is Hashimoto's thyroiditis.

Immunologic Deficiency Theory Persons with a hypoactive immune system have a higher incidence of developing an autoimmune disease. In animal experiments, the tissue injury occurs because of autoreactive mutant lymphocytes or because of persistent antigens.

Viral Mutation of Cells Theory Viruses are believed to alter T cells and therefore prevent control of antibody production. There is evidence that hepatitis B virus is found in clients with polyarteritis nodosa, an autoimmune disease.

Tissue Injury Theory Sometimes, after severe trauma, necrosis, radiation, drugs, and infections the body tissue is altered such that the body no longer recognizes it as "self." An example is hemolytic anemia secondary to alpha-methyldopa (Aldomet) administration.

Cross-reacting Antigen Theory Autoimmunity sometimes develops because of the close structural resemblance between the body's own antigens and foreign antigens. The antibodies synthesized in response to the foreign invasion cross-react with healthy tissue. This appears to be the cause of rheumatic heart disease. Antibodies developed against group A beta-hemolytic streptococcus cross-react with heart muscle, heart valves, and synovial membrane, causing tissue damage.

Genetic Instruction Theory For some unknown reason the genetic instruction for antibody production is altered. There appears to be a genetic predisposition to develop autoimmune diseases within some families. Most of the research work in this area correlates certain HLA types with an autoimmune condition.[10]

Autoimmune diseases

Generally, autoimmune diseases are grouped according to *organ-specific* and *systemic* diseases. See Table 10-9 for a summary of autoimmune diseases. To illustrate these two types of diseases, autoimmune hemolytic anemia (AHA) and systemic lupus erythematosus (SLE) will briefly be described.

Autoimmune Hemolytic Anemia (AHA) AHA is a specific organ disease involving the erythrocytes. The autoimmune disease may be primary or secondary to other diseases such as SLE and lymphocytic leukemia. Regardless of the cause, the immune response is similar. The cause is unknown but it is believed that drugs and viruses may alter antigenic structure of the erythrocyte membrane, making it more susceptible to hemolysis. In addition, in some people there appears to be a genetically determined susceptibility to form autoantibodies.

Clients with AHA present signs and symptoms of

Table 10-9
Autoimmune Diseases

Disease	Autoantigen	Comments
	Systemic Diseases	
Systemic lupus erythematosus (SLE)	DNA, DNA proteins	Circulating-antinuclear antibodies attack DNA
Rheumatoid arthritis (RA)	IgG	Rheumatoid factor is an IgM that reacts with IgG
Progressive systemic sclerosis (PSS) Scleroderma	DNA proteins	
Mixed connective tissue disease (MCTD)	DNA proteins	
	Organ-Specific Diseases	
Blood		
Autoimmune hemolytic anemia (AHA)	RBC surface	Drugs and trauma may alter the RBC surface antigens
Idiopathic thrombocytopenic purpura	Platelet surface	
CNS		
Multiple sclerosis	Myelin sheath around nervous tissue	Possibly triggered by a viral infection. Helper T cells appear uncontrolled because of very reduced levels of suppressor T cells (see Chap. 51)
Guillain-Barré syndrome	Myelin sheath	Peripheral nerve damage
Muscle		
Myasthenia gravis	Muscle cells and thymus myoid cells	See Chap. 51
Heart		
Rheumatic fever	Cross-reactive streptococcal antigens	Occurs secondary to strep throat infection
Endocrine system		
Addison's disease	Adrenal cell	
Thyroiditis	Thyroid cell surface	See Chap. 42
Hypothyroidism	Thyroid globulin	
GI tract		
Pernicious anemia	Intrinsic factor of parietal cells	See Chap. 34
Ulcerative colitis	Colon cells	
Kidney		
Goodpasture's syndrome	Basement membrane	See Chap. 37
Glomerulonephritis	Cross-reactive streptococcal antigens	
Liver		
Primary biliary cirrhosis	Mitochondria	
Eye		
Uveitis	Uvea	See Chap. 17

pallor, fatigue, fever, jaundice, splenomegaly, and hepatomegaly. Diagnosis is based upon a positive Coomb's test and spherically shaped erythrocytes on a smear.

Systemic Lupus Erythematosus (SLE) SLE is a classic example of a systemic autoimmune disease characterized by vasculitic damage to multiple organs. It occurs most frequently in women aged 20 to 40 years. The etiology is unknown but there appears to be a loss of self-tolerance for the body's own DNA antigens. Viruses, drugs, and genetic factors are believed to affect the self-tolerance.

SLE meets the criteria of an autoimmune disease because laboratory analysis reveals: (1) elevated serum immunoglobulins present because of hyperactive humoral immunity, (2) defective T-cell function, (3) deposition of immune antigen-antibody complexes in small blood vessels of diseased organs, and (4) low serum complement levels.[11]

In SLE, tissue injury appears to be the result of the formation of antinuclear antibodies. For some reason (possibly a viral infection), the cell membrane is damaged and DNA is released into systemic circulation where it is viewed as "nonself." This DNA normally is sequestered inside the nucleus of cells. Upon release into circulation the DNA antigen reacts with an antibody. Some of these antibodies are involved in immune complex formation, and others may cause damage directly. Once the complexes are deposited, complement is activated and further damages the tissue, especially the renal glomerulus. (Systemic lupus erythematosus is discussed in Chap. 57.)

Plasmapheresis

Pheresis refers to a complicated laboratory procedure whereby selected blood components can be separated and removed from whole blood without damaging the other blood components. The four types of blood components are: platelets, white blood cells, red blood cells, and plasma. Pheresis is done to replace blood components that are defective or in inappropriate quantities. Of special significance to autoimmune diseases is the technique of removing large amounts of plasma from whole blood (*plasmapheresis*).

The procedure involves removal of whole blood through a needle inserted in one arm, circulation of the blood through a continuous-flow centrifuge machine to separate the components, and then reinsertion of the blood through a needle into the opposite arm. The plasma is generally replaced with an isooncotic fluid: fresh-frozen plasma, protein fractions, reconstituted dried plasma, or albumin. When blood is manually removed, only 500 mL may be taken at one time. However, with the use of a continuous-flow centrifuge machine (blood cell separator) up to 4 L of plasma can be removed in 2 hours.

Through removal of large quantities of plasma, investigators have been able to reduce the high levels of circulating antibody or antigen-antibody complexes that cause some autoimmune diseases. Plasmapheresis has proven somewhat successful in the treatment of Goodpasture's syndrome and SLE. In addition to removing antibodies and antigen-antibody complexes, plasmapheresis may also remove inflammatory mediators such as complement, C-reactive protein, and fibrinogen that are responsible for tissue damage. In the treatment of SLE, plasmapheresis is reserved for those clients in an acute attack who are unresponsive to steroids. Plasmapheresis seems to lower the level of DNA antibodies and immune complexes, allowing the RES system to take control of removing immune complexes.[12] Plasmapheresis is also being used to treat rheumatoid arthritis with vasculitis, idiopathic thrombocytopenia purpura, myasthenia gravis, and a variety of other autoimmune-related diseases.

As is true with administration of other blood products, nurses need to be aware of side effects associated with plasmapheresis. Because of the rapid depletion of plasma it is imperative to observe for development of edema secondary to loss of plasma albumin. Other complications that may arise are electrolyte imbalances, hypovolemia, hemorrhage, pyrogenic reaction, syncope, hyperventilation, nausea, and restlessness.

Immune Deficiency

When the immune system does not adequately protect the body, an *immunodeficient* state exists. The immunodeficiency disorders involve an impairment of one or more immune mechanisms which include (1) phagocytosis, (2) humoral response, (3) cell-mediated response, (4) complement, and (5) a combined humoral and cell-mediated deficiency. Immunodeficiency disorders may be *primary* if the immune cells are improperly developed or may be *secondary* to an interference with the immune system. Primary immunodeficiency disorders are rare and often serious whereas secondary disorders are more common and less severe.

Causative factors

Some of the important factors that may cause immunodeficiency disorders include stress, pregnancy, age, physical agents, nutrition, surgery, genetics, and other diseases. Stress suppresses the immune response by stimulating the release of cortisol which destroys lymphocytes. Normally, the immune response is suppressed during pregnancy to prevent rejection of the fetus.

A hypofunctional state of the immune system exists in young children and the elderly. Laboratory studies have demonstrated that the immunoglobulin levels decrease with age and therefore lead to a suppressed humoral immune response in the elderly.

Malnutrition has been found to impair cell-mediated immune responses. When protein is deficient over a prolonged period, there is atrophy of the thymus gland and a decrease in lymphoid tissue. In addition, there is always an increased susceptibility to infections. Studies of African children have shown that malnutrition at an early age may cause developmental failure of the immune system.[13]

Such physical agents as cigarettes and alcohol also exert a harmful effect on lymphocytes and can lead to immunodeficiency. Irradiation destroys lymphocytes either directly or through depletion of stem cells. As the radiation dose is increased, more bone marrow atrophies, leading to severe pancytopenia and severe suppression of immune function.

Surgical removal of lymph nodes, thymus, or spleen can suppress the immune response. Splenectomy in children is especially dangerous and may lead to septicemia from simple respiratory infections.

Some of the immunodeficiency disorders are the result of inheriting an autosomal recessive gene or sex-linked gene. For example, X-linked agammaglobulinemia (Bruton's disease) is a sex-linked recessive disorder that occurs only in male infants.

Hodgkin's disease greatly impairs the cell-mediated immune response and clients may die from severe viral or fungal infections. Viruses, especially rubella, may cause immunodeficiency by direct cytotoxic damage to lymphoid cells. Nephrotoxic syndrome, which is characterized by a tremendous loss of protein in the urine, leads to a suppressed humoral immune response.

Categories of immunodeficiency diseases

The four basic categories of primary immunodeficiency disorders include: (1) phagocytic defects, (2) B-cell deficiency, (3) T-cell deficiency, and (4) a combined B- and T-cell deficiency (Table 10-10). To illustrate these disorders, hypogammaglobulinemia, Di George's syndrome, and severe combined immunodeficiency disease will be described.

Hypogammaglobulinemia The defect in B cells can range from the complete absence of all immunoglobulin classes (*agammaglobulinemia*) to a defect in only one immunoglobulin class. *Hypogammaglobulinemia* refers to a decreased level of the circulating immunoglobulins. The disorder may be congenital or acquired. *Congenital hypogammaglobulinemia (Bruton's disease)* is a rare sex-linked recessive disorder that occurs only in males. It is characterized by a deficiency of B cells and immunoglobulins and an intact thymus gland and normal T-cell immune response. The disorder usually is first manifest around 3 months of age when the IgG antibody from mothers is depleted and the infant develops recurrent respiratory tract and pyrogenic bacterial infections.

Acquired hypogammaglobulinemia (common variable hypogammaglobulinemia) is a more common disorder that is characterized by the presence of T and B cells but no plasma cells. There appears to be a defect in differentiation of B cells to plasma cells. A possible cause of acquired hypogammaglobulinemia is an abundance of suppressor T cells that suppress B-cell maturation into plasma cells. The disorder resembles Bruton's disease except that the recurrent bacterial infections (primarily of the respiratory tract) do not occur until ages 15 to 35. The treatment

Table 10-10
Immunodeficiency Disorders

Disease or Syndrome	Defective Cells	Genetic Basis
Chronic granulomatous disease	PMN	Sex-linked
Job's syndrome	PMN	
Bruton's X-linked hypogammaglobulinemia	B	Sex-linked
Common variable hypogammaglobulinemia	B	
Selective IgA, IgM, or IgG deficiency	B	Some sex-linked
Di George's syndrome (thymic hypoplasia)	T	
Severe combined immunodeficiency disease (SCID)	Stem, B,T	Sex-linked
Ataxia-telangiectasia	B,T	Autosomal recessive
Wiskott-Aldrich syndrome	B,T	Sex-linked
Graft vs. host disease	B,T	

includes gamma globulin injections or transfusions of plasma.

Di George's Syndrome Di George's syndrome (also known as congenital thymic hypoplasia) is a condition in which neither the thymus nor parathyroid gland develop. B-cell function is normal but T-cell function is absent. The disorder is manifest by recurrent viral, fungal, and protozoan infections, inability to reject allografts, and inability to have a delayed skin test reaction. Symptoms of oral candidiasis and chronic diarrhea develop in the first year of life. Microscopically, there are no thymus-dependent areas in the spleen or lymph nodes. Because helper T cells are missing, the circulation levels of some antibodies may also be reduced. Hypocalcemic tetany is also present because of the absence of the parathyroid gland. Treatment consists of administration of calcium and a fetal thymus transplant. A fetal thymus gland (less than 14 weeks old) can be locally implanted intramuscularly or minced and injected intraperitoneally.[14] Once in place, mature T cells are produced.

Severe Combined Immunodeficiency Disease (SCID) This condition includes a group of inherited disorders in which both B- and T-cell functions are abnormal. The most common form of SCID is sex-linked *Swiss type agammaglobulinemia*. The etiology of the disorder is unknown but seems to represent a bone marrow stem defect or failure in normal development of thymus and bursa equivalent tissue. Microscopically the thymus gland is hypoplastic, and lymph nodes contain no B and T cells. The disorder is manifest by severe viral, bacterial, fungal, or protozoan infections that occur within the first 2 years of life. Treatment consists first of controlling the infection with antibiotics and placing the client in protective isolation. Histocompatible bone marrow transplants have been somewhat successful. Other treatments include thymus transplant, gamma globulin injections, fetal liver transplant, and administration of thymic epithelium. Even with treatment, the prognosis is guarded.

Relationship Between Cancer and the Immune System

Cancer cells are similar to other foreign proteins because they can trigger an immune response. If the tumor is slow-growing and small enough, the immune system may be able to destroy it. This property serves as the basis for immunotherapy treatment.

Immune response to cancer

Surveillance is one of the important functions of T lymphocytes. Many cancer cells are believed to carry tumor-specific antigens (TSA) on their surface. These antigens are thought to be synthesized within the cell and inserted into the cell membrane. Since tumor antigens differ from normal ones, they elicit a cell-mediated immune response.

Sometimes *enhancing antibodies* protect the tumor surface antigens from T lymphocytes. The enhancing antibodies combine with the surface antigens to form complexes which combine with T lymphocyte receptors to deactivate lymphocytes. It is believed that some tumors have weak surface antigens that are not easily recognized as foreign and therefore do not activate T lymphocytes. At other times the tumor cells reproduce too rapidly for the immune response to be effective. Cancer develops more frequently in the very young, elderly, immunodepressed, and clients on immunosuppressant therapy.

Role of immune tests in cancer

At times immunologic tests for tumor-specific antigens (TSA) have been used for the detection of cancer and for monitoring metastases. One such surface antigen is carcinoembryonic antigen (CEA), which is present during fetal growth but not normal adult life. In adults it is associated with colorectal and pancreatic carcinoma. Another surface antigen is alpha-fetoprotein (AFP), associated with testicular carcinoma and hepatocarcinoma. Unfortunately, both tests are not highly specific and may be elevated in clients with other types of conditions.

Skin testing with dinitrochlorobenzene (DNCB) is done to determine immunocompetence in a cancer client. A delayed hypersensitivity reaction occurring 7 to 14 days after exposure to DNCB indicates that a cancer client has intact sensitized lymphocytes. This is an important indicator for the effectiveness of nonspecific immunotherapy treatment. (Cancer is discussed in Chap. 11.).

Immunotherapy

Since the early 1970s research has been undertaken to determine the usefulness of immunotherapy as an adjunct to cancer treatment. In theory, three approaches are possible: (1) *active immunotherapy*, with injection of specific tumor antigens to produce specific tumor antibodies and sensitized T cells; (2) *passive immunotherapy*, with injection of antibodies from a donor immunized against the tumor antigens or in a remission state; and (3) *nonspecific active immunotherapy*, with injection of an antigen that will stimulate the client's immune response. Two nonspecific active immunotherapy agents are BCG (bacillus Calmette-Guérin) and thymosin.

BCG is believed to activate the macrophage system and gather lymphocytes at the tumor site. So far the best results with BCG have been achieved in clients with malignant melanoma who are immunocompetent to DNCB.

Thymosin factor V from bovine thymus has recently been used in clinical experiments with small-cell carcinomas of the lungs. Thymosin is believed to stimulate the maturation of T lymphocytes and maintain a high number of T lymphocytes in the bloodstream. This nonspecific immune treatment seems to benefit only those clients with decreased T-cell levels.

Another form of immunotherapy treatment involves the use of *interferon (IF)*, a natural protein substance with antiviral and antitumor properties. Interferon, which is species-specific, is produced by three sources in the body: (1) T lymphocytes, (2) fibroblasts, and (3) lymphoblasts. Because of the few side effects associated with its use, interferon is being investigated as a major therapeutic agent against cancer. Clinically promising results have been found with lymphoma, myeloma, and breast cancer.

Interferon does not directly inactivate viruses or tumor cells. Rather it is a lymphokine, a factor that mediates a reaction. In the case of viruses it acts upon an undamaged cell to stimulate DNA to produce antiviral proteins which inhibit viral multiplication. With malignant cells, interferon is believed to activate killer T cells, enhance phagocytosis by macrophages, and alter the cell surface. The cell-mediated response seems to be enhanced best when the tumor cell is in a resting state. (Immunotherapy is discussed in more detail in Chap. 11.)

Drug-Induced Immunosuppression

Immunosuppression is a state of decreased responsiveness by the immune system. It may occur naturally, secondary to pathologic diseases (e.g., leukemia), or be drug-induced. By far, drug-induced immunosuppression is the most common. It is prescribed for clients for treatment of autoimmune disorders and to prevent transplant rejection. In addition, immunosuppression is a serious side effect of cytotoxic drugs used in cancer chemotherapy. Generalized leukopenia often results, leading to a decreased humoral and cell-mediated response. Therefore, secondary infections are common in immunosuppressed clients. (Refer back to Table 10-8 for a summary of the specific action of the various drugs on the immune system.)

ALLERGIC RESPONSE

Although an alteration of the immune system may be manifested in many ways, allergies or hypersensitivity reactions are seen most frequently. Therefore, the remainder of this chapter will discuss the assessment, prevention, and treatment of allergic disorders.

Assessment

For a thorough assessment of a client with allergies, a complete data base must be obtained. This consists of a comprehensive client history, physical examination, diagnostic workup, and skin testing for allergens.

Client history

A comprehensive history that covers family allergies, past and present allergies, and social and environmental factors is essential. The information may be obtained from the client or the client's care giver.

Family history, including information about atopic reactions in relatives, is especially important in identifying high-risk clients. The specific disorder, clinical manifestations, and treatments prescribed should be assessed.

Past and present allergies must be noted. To control allergic reactions, it is essential to identify the allergens that may have triggered a reaction. Table 10-11 lists four major categories of allergens that should be evaluated. Determination of the time of year that an allergic reaction occurs can be a clue about a seasonal allergen (Table 10-12).

In addition to identification of the allergen, information about the clinical manifestations and course of allergic reaction should be obtained. If the client is a woman, assessment of symptoms during pregnancy, menstruation, or menopause may be important.

Social and environmental factors, especially the physical environment, are very important. Questions about pets, trees and plants on property, pollutants in the air, and cooling and heating systems in the home can provide valuable information about allergens. In

Table 10-11
Four Major Categories of Allergens

Inhalants	Contactants	Ingestants	Injectables
Pollens	Plants	Foods	Drugs
Molds	Drugs	Drugs	Vaccines
Spores	Metals		Animal saliva and venoms
Animal dander	Cosmetics		
House dust	Dyes		
	Fibers		
	Various chemicals		

From M. Lind, "The Immunologic Assessment: A Nursing Focus," *Heart Lung*, **9**(4):660 (July–August 1980).

Table 10-12
Seasonal Allergens In Various Regions of United States

Region	Winter	Spring	Summer	Autumn
Northeast	—	Elm, oak, maple	Grasses, ragweed, *Alternaria**	Ragweed, *Alternaria*
Southeast	Elm	Ash, oak, pecan, Bermuda grass	Bermuda grass, ragweed, *Alternaria*	Ragweed, *Alternaria*
North central	—	Elm, maple, oak	Grass, ragweed, *Alternaria*	Ragweed, *Alternaria*
South central	Elm	Oak, maple, sycamore, Bermuda grass, *Alternaria*	Bermuda grass, *Alternaria*	Ragweed
Plains	—	Maple, cottonwood	Grass, Russian thistle	Ragweed, sagebrush
Southwest	*Alternaria*	*Alternaria*, ash, Bermuda grass	Bermuda grass, Russian thistle	*Alternaria*
Intermountain basin	—	Elm, cottonwood, sycamore	Grass, Russian thistle	Sagebrush
Pacific coast north	—	Alder, oak, maple	Grass	—
Pacific coast south	*Alternaria*	Oak, walnut, olive	Bermuda grass	Elm, *Alternaria*

*A fungus species.

Adapted from *Asthma, A Practical Guide for Physicians*, American Lung Association in cooperation with the Allergy Foundation of America, 1973.

addition, a 24-hour or weekly food diary with a description of any untoward reaction is important. Of particular interest is a screening of any reaction to medication. Finally, questions about the client's lifestyle and stress level should be viewed in connection with the appearance of allergic symptoms.

Physical examination

A comprehensive head-to-toe physical exam should be given to each allergy client with particular attention focused on the site of the allergic symptom. A comprehensive assessment guide of body systems which includes objective and subjective data has been developed for assessing allergic reactions (Table 10-13).

Diagnostic studies

Many specialized immunologic techniques can be done to detect abnormalities of lymphocytes, eosinophils, and immunoglobulins. A complete blood count (CBC) and blood serology tests are commonly done.

A complete blood count (CBC) is required with a lab test to detect an *absolute lymphocyte count* and *eosinophil count*. Cellular immunodeficiency is diagnosed if the lymphocyte count is below 1200/uL. The eosinophil count is elevated with Type I hypersensitivity reactions involving IgE immunoglobulins.

Serum IgE level must be measured because it is generally elevated in Type I hypersensitivity reactions and serves as a diagnostic indicator of atopic diseases. It may be measured by radioimmunoassay or by radioallergosorbent test (RAST). RAST involves the measurement of IgE with a specific antigen. Although expensive, it is safer and more specific than skin tests for allergens.

An erythrocyte rosette test will detect adequate cell-mediated immunity. Normally, 60 percent of T lymphocytes aggregate around injected sheep red blood cells when they are mixed. Less than 60 percent indicates a cellular deficiency state.

Sputum, nasal, and bronchial secretions also may be tested for the presence of eosinophils. If asthma is suspected, pulmonary function tests for vital capacity, forced expiratory volume, and maximum midexpiratory flow rates are helpful.[15]

Skin tests

Once the other screening procedures are completed, skin testing is recommended to try to detect the specific allergen(s) causing the clinical manifestations. Skin testing may also be done to determine the initial titer concentration of the allergen extract used in immunotherapy treatment.

Procedure Skin testing may be done by one of two methods: (1) *a cutaneous scratch or prick*, or (2) *an intracutaneous injection*. The areas of the body involved in testing are the arms and back. Allergen extracts are applied to the skin in rows with a corresponding control site opposing the test site. Saline or another dilutant is applied to the control site. After the test is read, all allergen extracts are removed.

In the *scratch test*, the epidermis skin layer is scratched with a lancet and the allergen extract is applied at the site. The prick test involves placing a drop of allergen extract on the skin and then piercing the epidermis underneath with a needle.

In the *intracutaneous method* the allergen extract is injected intradermally in rows, usually on the arm. Since the allergic reaction is more severe, the test is used only for persons who do not react to cutaneous methods.

Findings If the person is hypersensitive to the allergen, a positive reaction will occur in 10 to 30 minutes after insertion in the skin and may last for 8 to 12 hours. A positive reaction is manifest by a local wheal and flare response. The size of the positive reaction does not always correlate with the severity of allergy symptoms. Sometimes the allergic reaction may be delayed and occur 24 to 48 hours after the administration of the test allergen. False-positive and false-negative results may occur. Negative results from skin testing do not necessarily mean the person does not have an allergic disorder. On the other hand, positive results do not necessarily mean that the allergen was causing the clinical manifestations. Positive results imply that the person is sensitized to that allergen. Therefore, it is very important to correlate skin test results with the client's history.

Precautions A highly sensitive person is always at risk for developing an anaphylactic reaction to skin tests. Therefore, a client should never be left alone during the testing period. Sometimes skin testing is completely contraindicated and the RAST test is used. If a severe reaction does occur with a cutaneous test, the extract is immediately removed and anti-inflammatory topical cream is applied to the site. For intracutaneous testing, the arm is used so that a tourniquet could be applied during a severe reaction. Subcutaneous epinephrine may also be necessary.

Table 10-13
Assessment Guide for Allergy

Objective Data Suggestive of Allergy	
Skin Dryness, scaliness Irritations, inflammations Pallor Rashes (note symmetry, location) Scratches Urticaria **Eyes** Allergic shiners Conjunctivitis Inflammation Lacrimation Long, silky eyelashes Rubbing or excessive blinking Styes **Nose** Allergic salute Nasal polyps Nasal voice Nose twitching Pale, boggy mucous membranes Rhinitis	**Nose** Sniffling, paroxysmal sneezing, snorting Swollen nasal passages Transverse nasal crease **Mouth and pharynx** Allergic gaping Continual throat clearing Geographic tongue Gingival hyperplasia Mouth wrinkling with facial grimaces Orofacial dental deformities Redness of throat Swollen lips or tongue **Ears** Decreased hearing Drainage Immobile or scarred tympanic membrane Absence of cone of light **Neck** Palpable lymph nodes
Subjective Data Suggestive of Allergy	
History of Failure to gain weight Tiring readily upon moderate exertion Wheezing or shortness of breath upon moderate exertion Food intolerances Colic, cramping, vomiting, diarrhea (in absence of general illness) Alterations in taste, smell, hearing	Unusual reactions to drugs, insect bites or stings, inhalants (odors and fumes) Recurrent respiratory problems Recurrent otitis media Specific problems, such as itching, rashes, hives, recurrent nosebleeds, headaches Seasonal exacerbations of any symptoms Behavior or learning problems

From S. C. Bridgewater, R. R. Voignier, and C. S. Smith, "Allergies in Children," *Am J Nurs*, **78**(4):616 (April 1978).

Therapeutic Management of Allergic Reactions

Once an allergic disorder is diagnosed, the therapeutic treatment is aimed at (1) reducing exposure to the offending allergen, (2) treating the symptoms, and (3) desensitizing the person through immunotherapy. All health care workers must be alert to the rare but life-threatening anaphylactic reaction that may occur and which requires immediate medical and nursing interventions.

Therapeutic management of anaphylaxis

Anaphylactic reactions occur suddenly following parenteral injection of drugs (especially antibiotics) and insect stings in hypersensitive clients. Therefore, the cardinal principle in therapeutic management is *speed* in (1) recognition of signs and symptoms of an anaphylactic reaction, (2) maintenance of a patient airway, (3) prevention of spread of the allergen by using a tourniquet, (4) administration of drugs, and (5) treatment for shock. Table 10-14 summarizes treatment of anaphylactic reaction.

The drug of choice is *epinephrine*, 1:1000 strength, administered in 0.01 mL/kg doses subcutaneously every 5 to 10 minutes according to the physician's orders or a hospital emergency drug protocol. The drug may be discontinued when anaphylactic signs and symptoms disappear. If the reaction is severe, then antihistamine drugs (e.g., diphenhydramine) are administered parenterally to counteract the effects of histamine on the body tissues. Theophylline ethylenediamine (Aminophylline) may be used to relax the bronchial smooth muscle spasms. Although not effective immediately, ACTH and corticosteroids may be used to suppress the immune and inflammatory response.

Hypovolemic shock may occur due to the loss of intravascular fluid into the interstitial spaces. To compensate for the fluid shift, peripheral vasoconstriction and stimulation of the sympathetic nervous system occur. However, unless shock is treated early, the body will no longer be able to compensate and irreversible tissue damage will occur, leading to death. Therefore, the following emergency measures should be undertaken immediately:

1. Intravenous administration of volume expanders (plasma, dextran, and normal saline) to correct the hypotension. Nurses must carefully monitor for signs of circulatory overload.
2. *Vasopressor* drugs are necessary to raise the blood pressure. However, these drugs are very dangerous when administered intravenously. Levarterenol bitartrate (Levophed) and metaraminol bitartrate (Aramine) may cause severe hypertension if the infusion rate is too rapid. Severe sloughing of tissue may occur if the IV infiltrates. Therefore, the nurse must continually monitor a client at the bedside during intravenous administration of a vasopressor. Vital signs should be monitored every 15 minutes and the IV flow rate adjusted to maintain a stable blood pressure as prescribed by the physician.

Table 10-14
Therapeutic Management of Anaphylactic Shock

Treatment	Rationale
I. Maintain an open airway (Initiate CPR as needed)	Bronchospasms and angioedema may be severe and block the airway. Unless oxygen exchange occurs, hypoxia will develop
II. Drug therapy	
A. Sympathomimetics (epinephrine)	Causes vasoconstriction of peripheral vessels and bronchodilation
B. Antihistamines (Benadryl)	Blocks histamine and thereby reduces urticaria and angioedema
C. Bronchodilators (Aminophylline)	Directly dilates the bronchial smooth muscle
D. Corticosteroids (Solu-Cortef)	Suppresses the immune and inflammatory responses
E. Vasopressors (Levophed)	Raises the blood pressure that is lowered in shock state
III. Administer oxygen as needed (monitor blood gases)	If bronchospasm is severe, give oxygen via nasal catheter. The amount of oxygen is determined by frequent blood gas analysis
IV. Start intravenous volume replacement (monitor CVP readings)	Since plasma shifts to the interstitial space, fluids are needed to increase the intravascular volume

General allergy management

Most allergic reactions are chronic and are characterized by remissions and exacerbations of symptoms. Treatment is focused upon identification and control of allergens, relief of symptoms through pharmacology interventions, and hyposensitization of a client to an offending allergen.

Allergen Recognition and Control First, the nurse plays an important role in helping a client adjust his lifestyle so that there is minimal exposure to offending allergens. Second, the nurse must reinforce the fact that even with drug therapy and immunotherapy, the client will never be desensitized or completely symptom-free. Third, the nurse can initiate various preventive measures that will help control the allergic symptoms.

Of primary importance is the need to identify the offending allergen. Sometimes this is done through skin testing. In the case of food allergies, an *elimina-*

tion diet is valuable. If an allergic reaction occurs, all food eaten should be eliminated and gradually added one at a time until the offending food is detected. In the case of infants with a strong family history of atopic disorders, new solid foods should be introduced one at a time for 3 consecutive days. The elimination system may also be used to detect fabric and cosmetic allergens.

Many allergic reactions, especially asthma and urticaria, are aggravated by fatigue and emotional stress. The nurse can be instrumental in initiating a stress management program with clients. Relaxation techniques can be practiced when clients come for frequent immunotherapy treatments.

Sometimes control of allergic symptoms requires *environmental control*, including such things as a change in occupation, a move to a different climate, or giving up a favorite pet. In the case of aeroallergens, sleeping in an air-conditioned room, damp dusting daily, and wearing a mask outdoors may be helpful.

If the allergen is a drug, the client should be instructed to avoid the drug. The client also has the responsibility to make his drug intolerance well known to all health care providers. The client should wear a medical-alert bracelet listing the particular drug allergy and have the offending drug listed on all medical and dental records.

For clients allergic to insect stings, commercial *bee-sting kits* containing preinjectable epinephrine and a tourniquet are available. The nurse has the responsibility to instruct the client about the technique of applying the tourniquet and self-injecting the subcutaneous epinephrine. These clients also should wear a medical-alert bracelet and carry the bee-sting kit with them whenever they go outdoors.

Pharmacologic intervention

The major categories of drugs used in symptomatic relief of chronic allergic disorders include: (1) sympathomimetic drugs, (2) antipruritic drugs, (3) bronchodilators, and (4) antihistamines. Many of these drugs may be obtained over the counter and are misused by clients. The drugs are summarized in Table 10-15.

Sympathomimetic Drugs The major sympathomimetic drug is epinephrine (Adrenalin) which is the drug of choice to treat an anaphylactic reaction. Epinephrine is a hormone produced by the adrenal medulla which stimulates both alpha and beta receptors. Stimulation of the alpha receptors causes vasoconstriction of peripheral blood vessels. Beta receptor stimulation relaxes bronchial smooth muscle spasms. The action of epinephrine lasts only a few minutes. The drug must be given parenterally or subcutaneously because it is digested in the gastrointestinal tract.

Table 10-15
Common Drugs Used For Treatment of Allergic Symptoms

Generic Name	Trade Name	Class	Prescription	Over-the-Counter
Theophylline	Aminophylline	Bronchodilator	×	
Contains $ZnCO_3$	Calamine lotion	Antipruritic		×
Methdilazine HCl	Tacaryl	Antipruritic	×	
Diphenhydramine HCl	Benadryl	Antihistamine	×	
Azatadine maleate	Optimine	Antihistamine	×	
Carbinoxamine maleate	Clistin	Antihistamine	×	
Methapyrilene HCl	Histadyl	Antihistamine	×	
Promethazine HCl	Phenergan	Antihistamine	×	
Tiprolidine	Actifed	Antihistamine	×	
Brompheniramine maleate	Dimetane	Antihistamine		×
Chlorpheniramine maleate	Coricidin, Chlor-Trimeton Teldrin	Antihistamine		×
Epinephrine	Adrenalin	Sympathomimetic	×	
Isoproterenol	Isuprel	Sympathomimetic	×	
Pseudoephedrine HCl	Sudafed, Isoephedrine	Sympathomimetic	×	
Phenylephrine HCl	Dristan, Demazine, Neo-Synephrine	Sympathomimetic		×
Propylhexedrine	Benzedrex	Sympathomimetic		×
Oxymetazoline	Alfin	Sympathomimetic		×

There are a variety of specific, minor sympathomimetic drugs which differ from epinephrine because they can be taken orally or nasally and last for several hours. Included in this category are isoproterenol (Isuprel), phenylephrine (Neo-Synephrine) and pseudoephedrine HCl (Sudafed, Isoephedrine). The minor sympathomimetic drugs are used primarily to treat chronic asthma and allergic rhinitis. The action of these drugs includes bronchodilation, nasal decongestion, reduction in nasal edema, elevation of blood pressure, and cardiac stimulation.

Of all the drugs used in the management of chronic allergy clients, ephedrine is abused most frequently. Since these drugs may be bought over the counter, there is a tendency for clients to overmedicate themselves. *Rhinitis medicamentosa*, a rebound effect in which nasal mucosa becomes more edematous and congested after medicating, may develop from the local overuse of nasal sprays containing ephedrine.

Antipruritic Drugs are most effective when the skin is not broken. These drugs protect the skin and provide relief from itching. Common over-the-counter drugs include calamine lotion, coal tar solution, and camphor. Menthol and phenol may be added to other lotions to produce an antipruritic effect. Some more potent drugs that require a prescription include methdilazine HCl (Tacaryl) and trimeprazine (Temaril). These drugs should be used with great caution because of the risk of agranulocytosis.

Bronchodilators The most common bronchodilator is theophylline (Aminophylline) which acts directly on bronchial smooth muscle to promote bronchodilatation. This drug may be given by mouth, intramuscularly, or intravenously. However, for an acute asthma attack the intravenous method is recommended. One of the side effects from theophylline preparations is myocardial stimulation. Therefore, vital signs should be frequently monitored by the nurse during intravenous administration and the IV drip rate slowed as necessary.

Antihistamines are the best drugs for treatment of allergic rhinitis and urticaria. They are less effective for severe allergic reactions. The drugs may be given intravenously or orally, applied topically, inhaled, or used as a nasal spray. Since the drugs inhibit further release of histamine from mast cells, best results are achieved if taken immediately after allergy signs and symptoms appear. With seasonal rhinitis, antihistamines should be taken during peak pollen seasons. A number of side effects are associated with antihistamines, especially drowsiness, sedation, and disturbed coordination. Therefore, clients should be cautioned about driving and operating machinery. Other side effects include dryness of mouth, gastrointestinal upset, blurred vision, and dizziness.

Hyposensitization (desensitization, immunotherapy program)

Immunotherapy is the recommended treatment for control of allergic symptoms when the allergen cannot be avoided. It involves administration of small titers of an allergen extract in increasing strengths until *hyposensitivity* to the specific allergen is achieved. Hyposensitization appears to be about 80 percent effective against allergic rhinitis. Less success has been achieved with allergic asthma and atopic dermatitis. For best results, the client should continue only limited exposure to the offending allergen because complete *desensitization* is impossible.

Mechanism of Action The IgE immunoglobulin level is elevated in atopic individuals. When IgE combines with an allergen in a hypersensitive person, a chemical reaction occurs, releasing histamine in various body tissues. It has been found that allergens more readily combine with IgG immunogobulin than with other immunoglobulins. Therefore, immunotherapy involves injecting allergen extracts that will stimulate increased IgG levels. The binding of IgG to allergen-reactive sites blocks IgE and reduces the number of chemical reactions that cause tissue damage. The goal of long-term immunotherapy is to keep IgG levels high and IgE levels low.

Method of Administration Immunotherapy involves the subcutaneous injection of titered amounts of allergen extracts biweekly or weekly. The dosage is small at first and is increased slowly until a maintenance dose is reached. The maintenance dose, which keeps the IgG level elevated, is given every 2 to 8 weeks for several years. For those clients with severe allergies and/or sensitivity to insect stings, maintenance therapy is continued indefinitely. Best results of immunotherapy are achieved when administered year round.[16] See Table 10-16 for a hypothetical immunotherapy schedule.

Nursing Management Nurses are primarily responsible for giving immunotherapy. To guarantee effectiveness, accuracy, and prevention of adverse reactions, the following steps should be taken:

1. Carefully keep the allergen vial in a refrigerator to prolong the shelf life. Be sure the vial is packed in

the labeled box in an *upright position* so that leakage and contamination do not occur.

2. Since the allergen extract is part protein, gently rotate the vial to mix the extract and warm the solution. *Without injecting air* into the vial, withdraw the extract into a tuberculin syringe using a 25 or 26 gauge needle. A tuberculin syringe is recommended for accuracy in measuring the amount of extract.
3. Immunotherapy always carries the risk of a severe anaphylactic reaction. Therefore, a physician, emergency equipment, and essential drugs should be available whenever injections are given. The important emergency equipment includes: oral pharyngeal airway, laryngeal scope and endotracheal tubes, oxygen, tourniquet, intravenous therapy equipment and fluids, and a cardiac monitor with a defibrillator. The essential drugs are epinephrine 1:1000 in an injectable syringe, antihistamines, corticosteroids, and vasopressor drugs.
4. *Record keeping* must be accurate and can be invaluable in preventing an adverse reaction to the allergen extract. Before giving an injection, the nurse should check the client's name with the name on the vial. Next the vial *strength, amount* of last dose, *date* of last dose, and any reaction information should be screened.
5. The physician should be consulted about the amount of allergen to administer whenever a previous severe reaction has occurred or the client has missed the previous appointment. The dosage will have to be adjusted before administering the next dose.
6. The nurse should always administer the allergen extract in an extremity away from a joint so that a tourniquet could be applied for a severe reaction. The site should be rotated for each injection. It is imperative that a nurse *aspirate* for blood before giving an injection to be sure the allergen extract is not in a blood vessel. An injection directly into the bloodstream could potentiate an anaphylactic reaction. After the injection is given, the client should be carefully observed for 20 minutes since systemic reactions are most likely to occur immediately. However, clients should be warned that a delayed reaction could occur as long as 24 hours later.
7. Adverse reactions should always be anticipated, especially when opening a new strength vial, after a previous reaction, or after a missed dose. Early signs and symptoms indicative of a systemic reaction include pruritus, urticaria, sneezing, laryngeal edema, and hypotension. Emergency measures for anaphylactic shock should be initiated immediately. A local reaction should be described according to the degree of redness and swelling at the injection site. If the area is greater than the size of a *nickel* in a child or a *fifty-cent piece* in an adult the reaction should be reported to the physician so that the allergen dosage may be decreased.[17]

Table 10-16

Schedule of Immunotherapy For a Client with Inhalant Allergies

Starting strength (1:1000,000), once weekly	Third strength (1:1,000), once weekly
.05 mL	.05 mL
.10 mL	.10 mL
.15 mL	.15 mL
.20 mL	.20 mL
.25 mL	.25 mL
.30 mL	.30 mL
.35 mL	.35 mL
.40 mL	.40 mL
.45 mL	.45 mL
.50 mL	.50 mL

Second strength (1:10,000), once weekly	Fourth strength (1:100), once weekly
.05 mL	.05 mL
.10 mL	.10 mL
.15 mL	.15 mL
.20 mL	.20 mL
.25 mL	.25 mL
.30 mL	.30 mL
.35 mL	.35 mL
.40 mL	.35 mL (becomes maintenance dose)
.45 mL	
.50 mL	

From R. R. Voignier and S. C. Bridgewater, "Allergies in Children: Testing and Treating," *Am J Nurs*, **78**(4):618 (April 1978).

REVIEW QUESTIONS

The number of the question corresponds to the same numbered objective at the beginning of the chapter.

1. Which of the following is not a component of the immune system?
   a. spleen
   b. thymus
   c. bone marrow
   d. connective tissue

2. Administration of the MMR (mumps, measles, rubella) vaccine is done to promote which type of immunity?
   a. active natural immunity
   b. passive natural immunity
   c. passive acquired immunity
   d. active acquired immunity

3. All the following statements are characteristic of cell-mediated immunity *except*
   a. effective in fighting fungal infections
   b. response occurs immediately within minutes

c. surveys the body for invasion by tumor cells
d. sensitized lymphocytes directly attack antigens

4. The reason newborns are protected for the first 6 months of life from bacterial infections is because of the maternal transmission of
   a. IgG
   b. IgA
   c. IgM
   d. IgE

5. Activation of the entire complement cascade is necessary for
   a. enhancement of phagocytosis
   b. stimulation of chemotactic factors
   c. destruction of the cell membrane
   d. enhancement of vascular permeability

6. In a Type I hypersensitivity reaction, the primary immunologic disorder appears to be
   a. binding of IgG to an antigen on a cell surface
   b. deposit of antigen-antibody complexes in small vessels
   c. release of lymphokines to interact with specific antigens
   d. release of chemical mediators from IgE-bound mast cells

7. The treatment of choice for an acute anaphylactic reaction is
   a. theophylline (Aminophylline)
   b. diphenhydramine (Bendaryl)
   c. epinephrine (Adrenalin)
   d. corticosteroids (Solu-Cortef)

8. Autoimmunity is defined as a phenomenon involving
   a. production of endotoxins that destroy B lymphocytes
   b. inability to differentiate self from nonself
   c. overproduction of reagin antibody
   d. depression of the immune response

9. Congenital hypogammaglobulinemia is characterized by all the following *except*
   a. deficiency of T lymphocytes
   b. recurrent otitis media infections
   c. symptoms manifest after age 3 months
   d. sex-linked recessive disorder

10. Administration of BCG as an adjunct to treat malignant melanoma is an example of
   a. active immunotherapy
   b. passive immunotherapy
   c. nonspecific passive immunotherapy
   d. nonspecific active immunotherapy

11. All the following are true about skin testing *except*
   a. a positive reaction is manifested by a wheal and flare reaction
   b. a highly sensitive person may develop an anaphylactic reaction
   c. the preferred site for intracutaneous testing is the back
   d. it may be done to determine initial titer of allergen extracts

12. Antihistamines are most effectively used in treating
   a. systemic lupus erythematosus
   b. intrinsic asthma
   c. allergic rhinitis
   d. anaphylactic shock

REFERENCES

1. D. A. Jones, C. F. Dunbar, and M. M. Jirovec, *Medical-Surgical Nursing: A Conceptual Approach*, 2d ed., McGraw-Hill Book Company, New York, 1982, p. 323.
2. J. A. Bellanti, *Immunology II*, W. B. Saunders Company, Philadelphia, 1979, p. 14.
3. Ibid., p. 101.
4. D. T. Purtilo, *A Survey of Human Diseases*, Addison-Wesley Publishing Company Inc., Reading, Mass., 1978, p. 106.
5. F. E. Hargreave and J. Dolovich, "Immunology of Pulmonary Disease," in Geoffrey Taylor (ed.), *Immunology in Medical Practice*, W. B. Saunders Company, Philadelphia, 1975.
6. Bellanti, op. cit., p. 486.
7. C. E. Roesel, *Immunology: A Self-Instructional Approach*, McGraw-Hill Book Company, New York, 1979, p. 148.
8. Bellanti, op. cit., p. 559.
9. Roesel, op. cit., p. 158.
10. A. N. Rana and A. Luskin, "Immunosuppression, Autoimmunity, and Hypersensitivity," *Heart Lung*, **9**:655 (July–August 1980).
11. N. Shahinpour, "The Patient with Systemic Lupus Erythematosus: Prototype of Autoimmunity," *Heart Lung*, **9**:682 (July–August 1980).
12. J. V. Jones, "Plasmapheresis: Current Research and Success," *Heart Lung*, **9**:671 (July–August 1980).
13. Bellanti, op. cit., p. 16.
14. R. M. Hyde and R. A. Patnode, *Immunology*, Prentice-Hall Company, Reston, Virginia, 1978, p. 183.
15. R. R. Voignier and S. C. Bridgewater, "Allergies in Children: Testing and Treating," *Am J Nurs*, **78**:617 (April 1978).
16. Ibid., p. 618.
17. Ibid., p. 619.

Chapter 11

NURSING ROLE IN MANAGEMENT

Problems with Abnormal Cell Growth

Joyce M. Yasko

Learning Objectives

1. Describe the prevalence and incidence of cancer in the United States.
2. Describe the pathophysiologic dysfunctions in cellular proliferation and differentiation in cancer.
3. Explain the stages in the development of cancer.
4. Describe the role of the immune system related to cancer.
5. Compare and contrast the classification systems for cancer.
6. Explain the role of the nurse in prevention and detection of cancer.
7. Explain the use of surgery, radiation therapy, chemotherapy, and immunotherapy in the treatment of cancer.
8. Differentiate between external and internal radiation.
9. Identify the classifications of chemotherapy drugs and methods of administration.
10. Describe the effects of radiation therapy and chemotherapy on normal tissues.
11. Describe the nursing management for the client receiving radiation therapy and chemotherapy.
12. Describe the types of immunotherapy and nursing management related to immunotherapy.
13. Describe the nutritional problems of the client with cancer and appropriate management.
14. Explain the role of the nurse related to unproven methods of cancer treatment.
15. Describe complications that can occur in advanced cancer.
16. Describe appropriate psychological support of the client with cancer and the family.

SIGNIFICANCE OF PROBLEM

It is believed that all multicellular organisms have the potential to develop cancer at some point in their lifetime. Hippocrates coined the word *carcinoma,* meaning a tumor that spread and destroyed the host. However, Galen was the first to describe cancer as being crablike in nature.

Cancer is a group of more than 100 diseases characterized by unregulated growth of cells. It can occur in people of all ages and all races and is a major health problem in the United States. It is estimated that one in four Americans will experience cancer at some point in their lifetime. The overall incidence of cancer has been steadily increasing since 1970. It is estimated that 805,000 people will be diagnosed as having cancer (excluding nonmelanoma skin cancer and cancer in situ) in 1981.[1] Some cancers such as cancer of the stomach, uterus, rectum, and esophagus have decreased in incidence in recent times, while other cancers such as cancer of the lung, colon, prostate, and bladder have increased in incidence. Differences are noted in the incidence of certain cancers in the male and female (Table 11-1).

Considerable progress has been made in controlling cancer for long periods of time. There are over 3 million Americans alive today who have had a history of cancer, 2 million of whom were initially diagnosed 5 or more years ago. Many of the 2 million show no evidence of disease (NED). *NED* usually means the person has remained disease-free and has the same life expectancy as a person who has never had cancer.[2] This term is frequently substituted for the term *cured,* which is used cautiously by oncologists due to the slow-developing nature of cancer.

Cancer is the second most common cause of death in the United States (heart disease is first). One out of every five deaths is due to cancer, with one-half of these deaths occurring before the age of 65. The death rate is leveling off or decreasing except for cancer of the lung, which is increasing (Table 11-2). In 1981 approximately 420,000 Americans died of cancer. The cancer incidence and death rate for blacks is higher than for whites. This is especially apparent for black males. Blacks also have a higher death rate than whites from cancer. Most of the differences in black and white cancer rates are attributed to environmental and social rather than biological factors.[3]

This chapter was reviewed by Joan A. Piemme, R.N., M.N.Ed., Assistant Professor of Nursing, George Mason University, Fairfax, Virginia; Marilyn Davis, R.N., B.S.N., Nurse Educator, Clinical Cancer Education Program, School of Medicine, University of New Mexico, Albuquerque, New Mexico; and William Black, M.D., Chief of Pathology, Cancer Research and Treatment Center, University of New Mexico, Albuquerque, New Mexico.

Table 11-1
Cancer Incidence by Site and Sex in 1981 (Excluding Nonmelanoma Skin Cancer and Cancer in Situ)

Male		Female	
Lung	22%	Breast	27%
Prostate	17%	Colon/rectum	15%
Colon/rectum	14%	Uterus	13%
Urinary Tract	9%	Lung	8%
Other	38%	Other	37%

From *Cancer Facts and Figures, 1981*, American Cancer Society, 1980.

Statistics do not reveal the physiologic, psychological, and sociologic impact of cancer. Cancer is known to be the most feared disease, greater by far than the fear of heart disease. The word cancer is synonymous with death, pain, disfigurement, and dependency. Attitudes toward cancer do not fit the present status of the treatment and control of cancer. Education of health professionals and the public is essential if current attitudes surrounding cancer and cancer care are to become more positive and realistic.

PATHOPHYSIOLOGY OF CANCER

Cancer is a group of many diseases of unknown and probably multiple causes that arise in any cell of the body capable of mitosis. Two major dysfunctions present in the process of cancer are: (1) dysfunction in cellular proliferation (growth), and (2) dysfunction in cellular differentiation (maturity) (Fig. 11-1). It is theorized that dysfunction in cellular proliferation has a genetic origin and dysfunction in cellular differentiation has a nongenetic origin.[4]

Table 11-2
Estimates of Cancer Deaths by Site and Sex in 1981 (Excluding Nonmelanoma Skin Cancer and Cancer in Situ)

Male		Female	
Lung	34%	Breast	19%
Colon/rectum	12%	Colon/rectum	15%
Prostate	10%	Lung	15%
Leukemia/lymphoma	9%	Leukemia/lymphoma	9%
Other	35%	Other	42%

From *Cancer Facts and Figures, 1981*, American Cancer Society, 1980.

Genetic—Genetic code (DNA) is altered; genetic information is added, substituted, or altered.

Nongenetic—Genetic code (DNA) is not altered but changes occur in cellular differentiation and function.

Existing knowledge cannot prove or disprove either of these theories. Both mechanisms may operate in the development of cancer.

Dysfunction in Cellular Proliferation

Normally, most tissues of the human adult contain a population of predetermined undifferentiated cells known as *stem cells. Predetermined* means that the stem cells of a particular tissue will ultimately differentiate and become mature functioning cells of that tissue and only that tissue.

Cell proliferation originates in the stem cell and begins when the stem cell enters the cell cycle (Fig. 11-2). The time from the birth of a new cell to the time the cell divides into two identical cells is called the *generation time* of a cell. A mature cell continues to function until it degenerates and dies. At any point in time, there are cells at various stages of the cell cycle in all body tissues.

All cells of a tissue are controlled by an intracellular mechanism that determines when cellular proliferation is necessary. Under normal conditions, a state of dynamic equilibrium is constantly maintained (i.e., cellular proliferation equals cellular degeneration/death). The process of cellular division and proliferation is activated only in the presence of cellular degeneration or death. Cellular proliferation will also occur if the body has a physiologic need for more cells. For example, there is a normal increase in white blood cells in the presence of infection.

Another explanation for the phenomenon of proliferation control of normal cells is *contact inhibition.* Normal cells respect the boundaries and the territory of the cells surrounding them. They will not invade a territory that is not their own. The neighboring cells are thought to inhibit cellular growth through the physical contact of the surrounding cell membranes.

The rate of normal cellular proliferation (from the time of cellular birth to the time of cellular death) differs in each body tissue. In some tissues such as bone marrow, hair follicle, and epithelial lining of the gastrointestinal tract, the rate of cellular proliferation is rapid. In other tissues such as the liver, myocardium, brain, and cartilage, the rate of cellular proliferation is much slower. In fact, in adult life, the proliferation rate of these cells is so slow that it is barely perceptible.

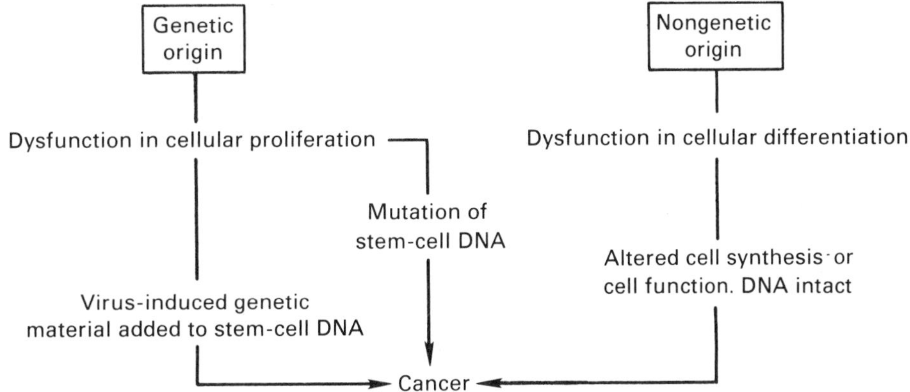

Figure 11-1 Theories of cancer formation.

Cancer cells usually proliferate in the manner and at the rate of the normal cells of the tissue from which they arise. However, cancer cells respond differently than normal cells to the intracellular signals that maintain the state of dynamic equilibrium. Cancer cells divide indiscriminately and haphazardly. Sometimes they produce more than two cells at the time of mitosis. Several authorities have postulated that the loss of intracellular control of proliferation occurs due to a mutation of the stem cells.[5] The stem cells are viewed as the target or the origin of cancer development. The DNA of the stem cell is substituted for or permanently rearranged. When this happens, the stem cell can mutate and has the potential to become a neoplastic cell (Fig. 11-1). It will usually proliferate at the rate of the tissue of origin and forms a malignant tumor that will closely resemble the tissue of origin. The stem cell theory of cancer development is not complete, since it has been noted that malignant stem cells can differentiate to form normal tissue cells.[6]

A common misconception regarding the characteristics of cancer cells is that their rate of proliferation is more rapid than that of any normal body cell. In most situations cancer cells proliferate at the same rate as the normal cells of the tissue from which they originate. The difference is that proliferation of the cancer cell is indiscriminate and continual. In this way, with each cell division creating two or more offspring cells, there is rapid growth of a tumor mass: 1→2→4→8→16, etc. The time required for a tumor mass to double in size is known as its *doubling time.*

Cancer cells are also characterized by *loss of contact inhibition.* They have no regard for cellular boundaries and will grow on top of one another and also on top of or between normal cells.

In addition, cancer cells are less cohesive than normal cells. This characteristic may explain their tendency to metastasize. Certain cancer cell surface characteristics such as low calcium content and a negatively charged surface may explain why these cells are less cohesive. It is also known that some types of cancer cells produce the enzyme hyaluronidase, which destroys intracellular cementing substances.

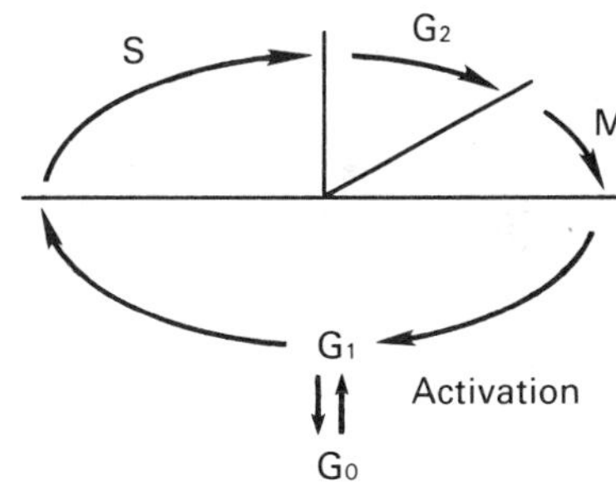

G = gap

G_0 = resting phase

G_1 = relatively dormant; some RNA and protein synthesized

G_2 = relatively dormant; some RNA synthesized

S = DNA is synthesized; RNA and protein synthesis continue

M = mitosis

Figure 11-2 Cell life cycle and metabolic activity. Generation time is the period from M phase to M phase. Cells not in the cycle, but capable of division, are in the resting phase (G_0).

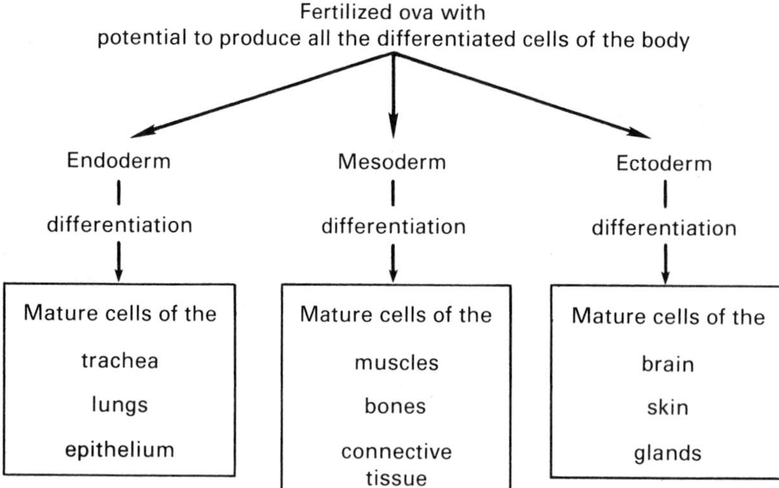

Figure 11-3 Normal cellular differentiation.

Dysfunction in Cellular Differentiation

Cellular differentiation is an orderly process that progresses from a state of immaturity to a state of maturity. Since all body cells are derived from the fertilized ova, all cells have the potential to perform all body functions. As cells differentiate, this potential is repressed and the mature cell is capable of performing only specific functions (Fig. 11-3).

With cellular differentiation there is a stable and orderly phasing out of cellular potential. Under normal conditions the differentiated cell is stable and will not dedifferentiate, that is, revert to a previous undifferentiated state. The exact mechanism controlling differentiation is presently unknown but is thought to be controlled by signals from the environment.[7]

Cancer cells are transformed cells which are morphologically different from the cells which gave rise to them. Some varieties resemble undifferentiated cells. The concept of dedifferentiation is sometimes used to explain the regression of these cells to a more immature state.

One theory for the transformation process in the development of cancer is that cells have undergone derepression of their genes; that is, all the potential functions and characteristics of the cell that have been repressed during normal development are allowed expression. The cell is transformed to a more embryonic or fetal appearance and function. For example, some cancer cells produce new proteins, such as those characteristic of the embryonic and fetal periods of life. These proteins include carcinoembryonic antigens and alpha-fetoprotein (see section on Role of the Immune System). Other cancer cells such as oat-cell carcinoma of the lung produce hormones (see section on complications of cancer).

Tumors can be classified as *benign* or *malignant.* In general, benign neoplasms are well differentiated and malignant neoplasms range from well differentiated to undifferentiated. The ability of malignant tumor cells to metastasize is the major difference between benign and malignant cells. Other differentiating characteristics are presented in Table 11-3.

Development of Cancer

The following presentation is a theoretical model of the development of cancer. It is important to remember that the basic cause of cancer is unknown. It is not known how many tumors have a chemical, environmental, genetic, immunologic, or viral etiology. It is possible that cancers arise spontaneously with no significant contributing cause.

Four stages in the development of cancer are initiation, latency, progression, and invasion. These stages occur over a period of time as altered cells proliferate and eventually produce evidence of clinical disease (Fig. 11-4).

Initiation

During the stage of initiation, a carcinogen acts on a target cell and causes changes in the genetic structure. A carcinogen produces an increased incidence of a specific cancer in people that are repeatedly exposed to the specific agent. Among carcinogens that have been identified are chemicals,

Table 11-3
Comparison of Benign and Malignant Growths

	Malignant Tumor	Benign Tumor
Encapsulated	Rarely	Usually
Differentiated	Poorly	Partially
Metastasis	Frequently present	Absent
Recurrence	Frequent	Rare
Vascularity	Moderate to marked	Slight
Mode of growth	Infiltrative and expansive	Expansive
Cell characteristics	Cells abnormal and become more unlike parent cell	Fairly normal and similar to parent cell

radiation, and viruses. Most authorities believe that the stage of initiation is irreversible.

Chemical Carcinogens Chemicals were identified as cancer-causing agents in the latter part of the eighteenth century when Percivall Pott noted that chimney sweeps, especially those with poor personal hygiene, had a higher incidence of cancer of the scrotum associated with exposure to soot residues in chimneys. As the years went on, more chemical agents were identified as actual and potential carcinogens by observing statistical evidence that showed that individuals exposed to certain chemicals over a period of time had a greater incidence of certain cancers than other individuals. The long latency period from the time of exposure to the development of cancer makes it difficult to identify cancer-causing chemicals. Also, those chemicals that cause cancer in animals may or may not cause that specific cancer in humans. Some chemicals are cancer causative in their environmental form, while others must first undergo certain metabolic changes. Chemical carcinogens thought to cause cancers in humans[8] are reviewed in Table 11-4.

Certain drugs have also been identified as carcinogens (Table 11-5). Drugs that are capable of interacting with DNA (e.g., alkylating agents) as well as immunosuppressive agents have the potential for causing neoplasms in humans. The use of alkylating agents (e.g., cyclophosphamide, nitrogen mustard) either alone or in combination with radiation therapy have been associated with increased incidence of acute myelogenous leukemia (incidence 1 to 5 percent) in individuals treated for Hodgkin's disease, non-Hodgkin's lymphomas, and multiple myeloma. These secondary leukemias are relatively refractory to an induction of remission with combination chemotherapy.[9]

It has already been mentioned that individuals on long-term immunosuppression therapy have an increased incidence of malignancy. (See section on Role of Immune System.) Kidney transplant recipients usually receive a combination of antilymphocytic serum, antimetabolites (e.g., azathioprine), and corticosteroids. At times cyclophosphamide (Cytoxan) is also used (see Chap. 38).

Radiation Since the turn of the century, it has been known that radiation can cause cancer in almost any human body tissue. At the present time, the dose of radiation that causes cancer is not known and there is considerable debate surrounding the effect of low-dose radiation exposure over a period of time.[10] When cells are exposed to a source of radiation, damage occurs to one or both strands of DNA (see section on radiation therapy and Chap. 59). Certain disorders have been correlated with radiation as a carcinogenic agent:

1. Leukemia, lymphoma, thyroid, and other cancers increased in incidence in the general population of Hiroshima and Nagasaki after the atomic bomb explosion.
2. A higher incidence of bone cancer occurs in persons exposed to radiation in certain occupational environments: radiologists, radiation chemists, uranium miners.
3. Thyroid cancer occurs at a higher incidence in those persons who received radiation to the head and neck area for a variety of reasons: acne, tonsillitis, sore throat, and an enlarged thyroid gland.
4. Persons exposed to direct sunlight over a period of time have a higher incidence of skin cancer: sailors, farmers, and construction workers.
5. A higher incidence of childhood cancers occur in children exposed to radiation during fetal life.

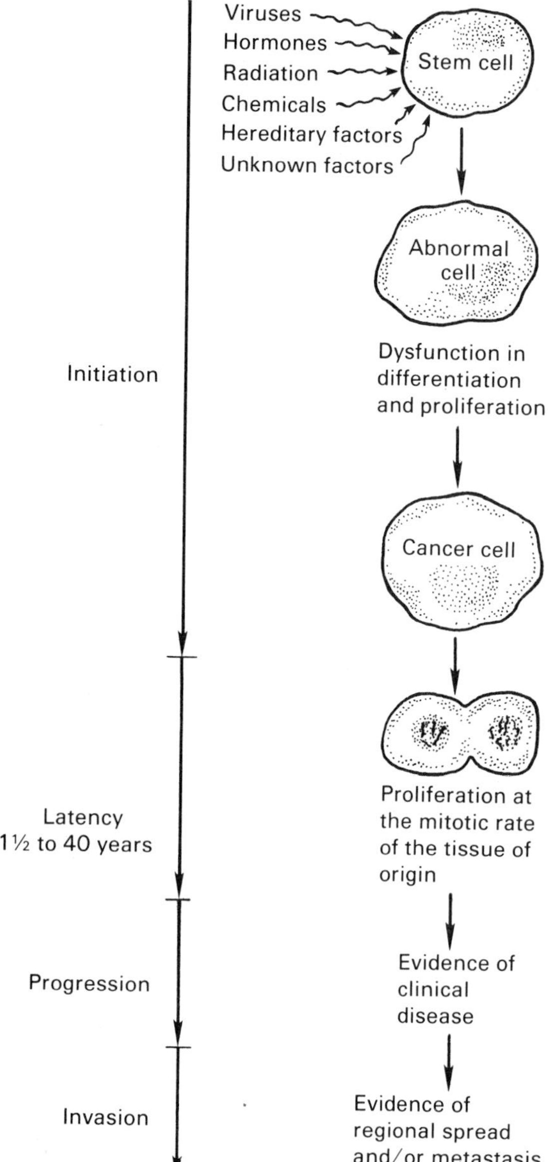

Figure 11-4 Process of cancer development.

6. A higher incidence of malignant melanoma in recent times is thought to be due to the decrease in the ozone layer, allowing more ultraviolet rays from the sun to enter the atmosphere.

Hormones Statistical evidence has become apparent in recent years indicating that diethylstilbestrol (DES), when given to a mother during the first trimester of pregnancy, may cause vaginal adenosis in female offspring. Some of these girls will also develop adenocarcinoma of the vagina or cervix (although the incidence is very low). Estrogens are also thought to be carcinogenic when administered to postmenopausal women for the relief of menopausal symptoms. These women have an increased incidence of endometrial cancer. When estrogens are administered to premenopausal women for the purpose of contraception, an increased incidence of adenomas of the liver and breast cancer has also been noted. Although the correlation between hormones and cancer has been statistically noted, the mechanics of carcinogenesis is not known. The evidence appears to be accumulating in favor of a dysfunction in cellular differentiation.

Table 11-4
Occupational and Environmental Carcinogens

Carcinogen	Associated Neoplasm
Cigarette smoke	Lung, upper respiratory tract, and other cancers
Asbestos	Mesothelioma, lung
Arsenic	Skin, lung
Cadmium	Prostate, kidney
Chromium	Lung .
Nickel	Lung, nasal sinuses
Uranium	Lung
Aflatoxin	Liver
Nitrites	Stomach
Chloramethyl ethers	Lung
Isopropyl oil	Nasal sinuses
Naphthalene dyes (aniline dyes)	Bladder
Vinyl chloride	Liver hemangiosarcoma
Benzene	Acute myelogenous leukemia
Schistosomiasis haematobia	Bladder

From K. Isselbacher et al. (eds.), *Harrison's Principles of Internal Medicine,* 9th ed., McGraw-Hill Book Company, New York, p. 1586. Used by permission of the publisher.

Hereditary Factors There are several genetic disorders that are associated with or identified as related to certain cancers. Familial polyposis of the colon is considered to be a premalignant lesion. It has been observed that after a period of time adenocarcinoma often occurs (see Chap. 34). Bilateral retinoblastoma is an inherited trait that has recently been associated with a chromosomal abnormality. Xeroderma pigmentosum is an inherited syndrome characterized by abnormal pigmentation of the skin that develops into cancer in areas exposed to the sun. "Cancer families" have also been identified in which several members of the family develop one or several specific cancers at a very early age. The specific cancers are usually cancer of the colon and cancer of the uterus. Multiple-site cancers or cancers that occur at an early age are thought to have a genetic link. Most authorities feel that the cause in these instances is due to inherited chromosomal abnormalities.

For many years, scientists have searched for genetic patterns in the most common cancer sites. A few patterns have emerged:

1. The incidence of postmenopausal breast cancer is three times higher and the incidence of premenopausal breast cancer is five times higher in the population of women with a family history of this disease. Breast cancer is rare in Oriental women and common in American women.
2. The incidence of lung cancer is greater in smokers with a family history of this disease than in smokers without a family history of the disease.
3. The incidence of leukemia is greater in an identical twin of a client with the disease.
4. The incidence of neuroblastomas has been found in increased frequency among siblings.

For a few specific cancers, the link between cancer and heredity is evident. However, most of the specific cancers do not have a hereditary link. Recent advances in the study of chromosomes may uncover some of the minor chromosomal alterations that may provide the missing information of the role of heredity in the development of cancer. At the present time, the evidence seems to indicate that cancer is an acquired disease and that certain genetic factors increase the risk of the development of cancer in a certain segment of the population.

Viruses Viruses have been identified as causative agents of cancer in animals. In humans this causative link has not been proven since ethics preclude the inoculation of humans with viruses that are thought to be causative agents for cancer. A cancer found in humans, Burkitt's lymphoma, has consistently shown evidence of the presence of the Epstein-Barr virus (EBV) in vitro. This virus is also present in infectious mononucleosis, but the answer to why some individuals develop an infectious disease and others a lymphoma is not known.[11]

At the present time, evidence is mounting that herpes virus type II is causative for cancer of the cervix (see Chap. 46). Viral causation has been suggested by many authorities for leukemia and cancer of the breast, lung, and brain. It is not known at the present time if the presence of viruses at the site of human cancer is evidence of a causative agent, or if the presence of the viruses is due to a favorable environment for viral proliferation that is provided by the presence of cancer.

Table 11-5

Cancers Related to Drug Exposures in Humans

Drug	Cancer
Radioisotopes:	
Phosphorus (^{32}P)	Acute leukemia
Radium, mesothorium	Osteosarcoma and sinus carcinoma
Thorotrast	Hemangioendothelioma of liver
Immunosuppressive agents (for renal transplantation):	
Antilymphocyte serum Antimetabolites Alkylating agents Corticosteroids	Reticulum-cell sarcoma, epithelial malignancies of skin and viscera
Cytotoxic drugs:	
Chlornaphazine Phenylalanine mustard Cyclophosphamide	Bladder cancer Acute myelogenous leukemia
Hormones:	
Synthetic estrogens:	
Prenatal	Vaginal and cervical adenocarcinoma (clear-cell type)
Postnatal	Endometrial carcinoma (adenosquamous type)
Androgenic-anabolic steroids	Hepatocellular carcinoma
Others:	
Arsenic	Skin cancer
Phenacetin-containing drugs	Renal pelvis carcinoma
Coal tar ointments	Skin cancer
?Diphenylhydantoin	Lymphoma
?Chloramphenicol	Leukemia
?Amphetamines	Hodgkin's disease

From K. Isselbacher et al. (eds.), *Harrison's Principles of Internal Medicine,* 9th ed., McGraw-Hill Book Company, New York, 1980. Used by permission of the publisher.

After R. Hoover and J. F. Froumeni, *J Clin Pharmacol,* **15**:16 (1975).

Latency

After the initiation phase, the environment plays a major role in the development of cancer. In order for the disease process to become clinically evident, the cells must reach a critical mass. A 1-cm tumor (the size usually detectable by palpation) contains 10^9 (1 billion) cancer cells. Depending on the environmental factors and the mitotic rate of the tissue of origin, it may take 1 ½ to 40 years before this critical mass is

Table 11-6
Examples of Factors that Promote Cancer Development

Promotion Factor	Effect on Cancer Development
1. Sex	↑ Incidence in the female.
2. Age	↑ Incidence in the very young and in persons over the age of 55 years.
3. Hormones	↑ Progression of breast cancer in the presence of estrogen.
	↓ Progression of certain cancers with removal of the thyroid, adrenal, ovaries, and/or pituitary gland.
4. Stress	↑ Progression of cancer in the presence of high levels of stress (not scientifically proven at the present time).
5. Diet	↑ Incidence and progression of cancer in persons who are 25% or more over their recommended weight.
	↑ Incidence and progression of breast and gallbladder cancers in the presence of a high-fat diet.
	↑ Incidence and progression of colon cancer in the presence of a low-fiber diet.
	↑ Progression of cancer in persons who are protein-deficient.
6. Chronic irritation	↑ Incidence and progression of cancer in the presence of chronic irritation.

reached. This period of time is called the latency period of cancer development.

Promotion Factors Factors in the environment may serve as promotion factors for cancer development. These promotion factors contribute to the growth of the cancer cells. Some of these factors include age, sex, level of stress, work environment, hormones, diet, chronic irritation (especially in the gastrointestinal tract), and the state of physical and emotional health (Table 11-6).

Some authorities believe that cancer will progress only in the presence of a *specific promotion factor.* An example of this phenomenon is the fact that saccharin increases the frequency of bladder cancer in the presence of *N*-methyl-*N*-nitrosurea (MNU). Without this additional substance, bladder cancer does not usually occur due to saccharin ingestion. This is the co-carcinogen theory of cancer development, which provides an explanation of why known carcinogens are not consistently seen in a cause-and-effect relationship.[12]

Progression

The key factor in the period of progression is the proliferation of the cancer cells in spite of controls of the host. The cancer cells at this point are said to be heterogeneous in nature. As the cancer cells attempt to survive in their environment, the cells lose or gain characteristics to facilitate their survival. In the progression phase, there is an increase in the rate of proliferation of those cancer cells that are best able to survive in the environment. The progression of cancer in situ of the cervix to invasive carcinoma of the cervix is an example of the progressive nature of cancer.

Another factor that must be present in order for tumor progression to occur is the development and maintenance of an independent blood supply. If a blood supply is not created, the cancer cells cannot grow beyond a diameter of 2 to 3 mm. A *tumor angiogenic factor* (TAF) has been identified, and it has been observed that the growth of capillaries into the mass of cancer cells can occur at a rapid rate (1 mm per day). Therefore, the blood vessels in a tumor are composed of normal tissue and the host supplies the blood to maintain the tumor.

Invasion

Cancer cells have the ability to invade surrounding tissue and organs *(regional invasion)* and to spread to distant body sites *(metastasis). Regional invasion* occurs by (1) cellular proliferation, (2) loss of contact inhibition, and (3) secretion of lytic substances. These lytic substances are usually cell surface proteases that can cause tissue destruction or reorganization or both. Cancer cells are known to grow in the path of least resistance and will grow over, under, and between normal cells.

Metastasis is a characteristic of cancer cells and is the major determining factor in the nature and prognosis of cancer. Metastasis can occur via the (1) vascular system, (2) lymphatic system, and (3) process of implantation (Fig. 11-5).

Vascular Spread Metastasis via the vascular system occurs in five steps:

1. Invasion of surrounding tissue from the primary site of the cancer cells. The cancer cells penetrate the blood and lymphatic vessels.
2. Cancer cells are released into the bloodstream. This environment is hostile to the cancer cells and the majority of the cells are quickly destroyed.
3. Circulatory emboli are trapped in the small capillaries of the tissues and/or organs.
4. Through the secretion of lytic substances (usually proteases) cancer cells penetrate the walls of the capillary and enter the adjacent tissue where they begin to proliferate.
5. A capillary bed is developed and the cancer cells in the metastatic site continue to proliferate.

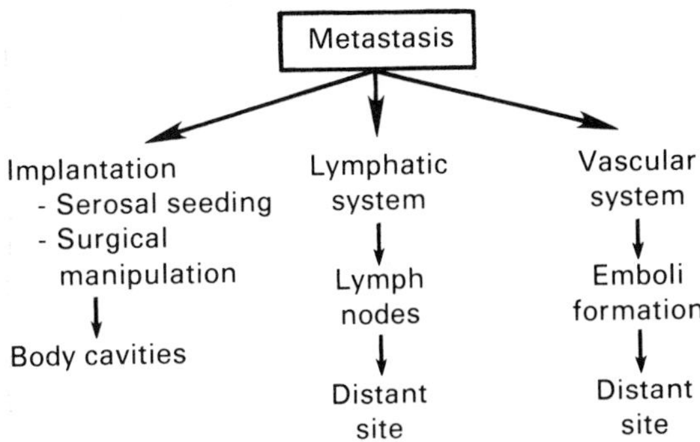

Figure 11-5 Routes of metastasis.

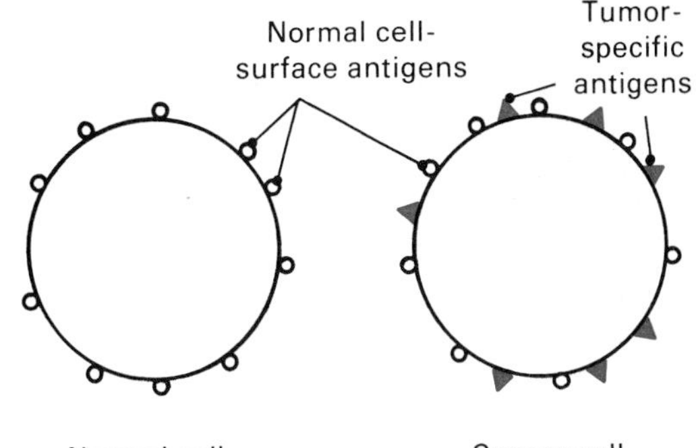

Figure 11-6 Tumor-specific antigens appear on the cell surface of malignant cells.

Lymphatic Spread Lymphatic spread occurs in a similar manner as vascular spread. It has been assumed for a long period of time that the lymph nodes serve as a barrier to metastatic spread. Clinically it has been observed that the prognosis of cancer is best when there is no detectable metastasis to the lymph nodes in the region of the primary tumor. The prognosis becomes worse the more lymph nodes that are involved. Some authorities feel that the lymph nodes may not provide as much of a barrier as was previously assumed.

Implantation Implantation occurs when cancer cells implant themselves in various body organs such as the peritoneal cavity or the pleural cavity. During surgical procedures, implantation may also occur in the primary organ or the regional area.

Some cancers metastasize early in the process of development (e.g., breast cancer) while others spread regionally and rarely metastasize (e.g., glioblastoma multiforme and basal cell carcinoma of the skin). Certain cancers seem to have an affinity for a particular tissue or organ as a site of metastasis while other cancers are unpredictable in their pattern of metastasis. It has been stated that certain cancers ("seed") require a particular site for proliferation ("soil"). The most frequent sites of metastasis are the lungs, brain, bone, and liver. Most metastatic lesions are multiple and widely disseminated, but a few cancers usually produce a single metastatic lesion.

Role of the Immune System

Both normal and abnormal cells have a complex array of antigenic determinants (markers) on the surface of their cell membrane as well as within the cell. The antigenic determinants differ from one cell type to another. When foreign cells are transplanted from one individual to another individual, these antigenic determinants elicit an immunologic response. This is the basis for rejection of a transplanted organ.

It is known that some cancer cells have changes in their cell surface antigens due to malignant transformation. These antigens are called tumor-specific antigens (TSA) (Fig. 11-6). It is believed that one of the functions of the immune system is to respond to these antigens. The response of the cellular immune system to antigens of the malignant cells is called *immunologic surveillance*. The T lymphocytes are continually checking cell surface antigens and are capable of detecting and destroying cells with abnormal or altered antigenic determinants. It has been proposed that malignant transformation occurs continuously and the malignant cells are destroyed by the cellular immune response (the cell-mediated response is discussed in Chap. 10). Three kinds of cells that are involved in cell-mediated immunity to tumors are:[13]

1. Cytotoxic T cells (T_c cells)
2. Antibody-dependent cell-mediated cytotoxic cells (ADCC cells)
3. Natural killer cells

In most cancers, the cytotoxic T cells are the dominant response. They can destroy cancer cells through direct contact. All cancers are susceptible to cellular immune mechanisms. Cancers of the hematolymphoid system are sensitive to both humoral and cellular mechanisms.[14]

Natural killer cells are not B or T lymphocytes but appear to be a type of lymphocyte. Natural killer cells do not need prior exposure to the antigen for activation. Their effect is immediate and is stimulated by several things such as viral infections, possibly through production of interferon.[15]

Certain groups of people have a higher incidence of malignancies than the general population. Nearly 10 percent of children with congenital immunodeficiencies develop cancer. These cancers are primarily derived from cells of the lymphoid system.

Individuals on high doses of immunosuppressive drugs have an eighty- to one-hundredfold increased risk of developing cancer. The types of malignancies found in immunosuppressed individuals are primarily epithelial in origin.[16] These findings are mostly reported from people treated with immunosuppressive agents for transplanted kidneys.

Other groups of people at an increased risk for malignancies are the very young and the elderly. In the very young, the immune system is immature. The incidence of malignancies increases dramatically in individuals over 40 to 50 years of age. The reasons for this are not known. It is possible that their immunologic surveillance system is working less effectively. It is known that the thymus undergoes involution and atrophy with aging. In addition, the functional efficiency of the T cells decrease with aging.

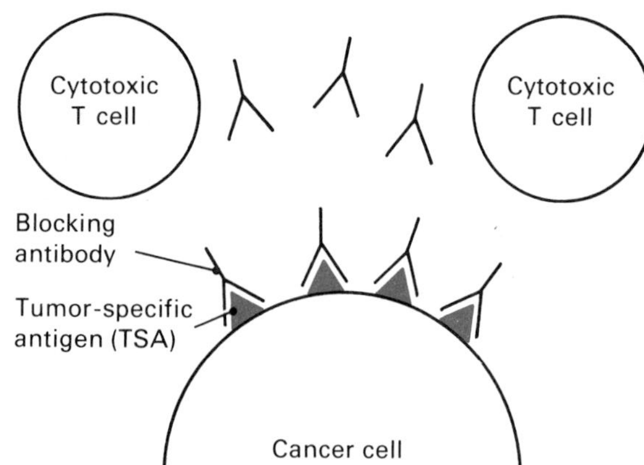

Figure 11-7 Blocking antibodies prevent the T cells from interacting with tumor-specific antigens and destroying the malignant cell.

Escape mechanisms from immunologic surveillance

Tumor development has often been referred to as *immunologic escape*. In many individuals with cancer there is evidence of an active immunologic response, yet the tumor survives. Some theoretical explanations for immunologic escape that have been proposed will be presented.

Sneaking Through This process is thought to occur when the cell surface antigens are weak in nature. Cancer cells in the early phase of growth may not excite an immunologic response. The transformed cell surface markers are of low antigenicity. By the time the immune system is altered, the cancer is well established and too large for the body to deal with.[17]

Antigenic Modulation The malignant cell has the ability to change or lose antigenic determinants during or after a response by the immune system. The cell may then express a new set of antigens. This process is known as *antigenic modulation*. The new set of antigens fails to adequately stimulate the immune system.

Overwhelming Antigen Exposure Cancers may escape attack by flooding the body with tumor antigen. The antigens bind to specific antibodies or to receptors on lymphocytes and prevent them from recognizing and destroying the cancer cells.[18] The excess of antigens paralyzes the host immune system. Therefore, tumor growth is enhanced.

Blocking Factors Blocking factors may prevent attack of the tumor-specific antigens by T lymphocytes. For example, blocking antibodies may bind with TSA and prevent their recognition by T cells (Fig. 11-7). Another possibility is that free antigen produced and released by the malignant cell may bind with the T cell and prevent it from recognizing the malignant cell. These blocking factors related to the immune system may actually enhance tumor growth. This is described by the term *immunologic enhancement*.

Oncofetal antigens

Oncofetal antigens, also carcinofetal antigens, are a type of tumor antigen. These antigens are found on the surfaces of cancer cells as well as cells found in the fetus. These antigens are an expression of the shift of cancerous cells to a more immature metabolic pathway, one usually associated with embryonic or fetal periods of life.[19] The reappearance of fetal antigens in malignant disease is not well understood.

Examples of oncofetal antigens are carcinoembryonic antigen (CEA) and alpha-fetoprotein (AFP). Carcinoembryonic antigen is found on the surfaces of cancer cells derived from the gastrointestinal system as well as normal cells from the fetal gut, liver, and pancreas. Normally, it disappears during the last 3 months of fetal life. CEA was originally isolated from colon cancer. However, in recent years elevated CEA levels have also been found in nonmalignant conditions (e.g., cirrhosis of the liver, ulcerative colitis, heavy smokers). The major value of CEA at this time is its use as an indicator of the success of the cancer treatment.[20] For example, if elevated preoperative CEA titers persist after surgery, it is an indication the tumor was not completely removed. A rise in CEA levels following chemotherapy or radiation therapy may indicate recurrence or spread of the malignancy.

Alpha-fetoprotein (AFP) is produced by malignant

liver cells as well as fetal liver cells. AFP levels have also been found to be elevated in testicular carcinoma, viral hepatitis, and other nonmalignant liver disorders. AFP has been found to be of diagnostic value in primary cancer of the liver (hepatoma) but is also produced when there is metastatic liver growth. The detection of AFP is of value in tumor detection and progression.

Other examples of oncofetal antigens currently being studied are fetal sulfoglycoprotein found in gastric carcinoma, pregnancy-specific β_1-glycoprotein (SP_1) found in testicular cancer, human chorionic gonadotropin (HCG), and pancreatic oncofetal antigen (POA) found in pancreatic and lung cancers.

Virus-induced antigens

Tumor-specific antigens may be induced by certain viruses. In experimental animals both DNA and RNA viruses have been found to induce unique nuclear and cell-surface antigens in cells. As mentioned earlier, it is difficult to establish these findings in humans. The DNA viruses include various herpesviruses and adenovirus. The three major candidates for human DNA virus-induced tumors are Burkitt's lymphoma, nasopharyngeal carcinoma, and cancer of the cervix.[21] RNA viruses have been correlated with leukemia in mice and other animals as well as in mouse mammary tumors.[22] At the present time, RNA viruses have not been linked to human cancers.[23]

CLASSIFICATION OF CANCER

Tumors can be classified according to:

Anatomic site
Histologic analysis (grading)
Extent of disease (staging)

Tumor classification systems are intended to provide a standardized way (1) to communicate the status of the cancer to all members of the health care professions, (2) to assist in decisions to determine the most effective treatment plan, (3) to evaluate the treatment plan, (4) to serve as a factor in determining the prognosis, and (5) as a way of comparing like groups for statistical purposes.

Anatomic Site Classification

In the anatomic classification of tumors, the tumor is identified by the tissue of origin, the anatomic site, and the behavior of the tumor (i.e., benign or malignant) (see Table 11-7). Carcinomas originate from embryonal ectoderm (skin and glands) and endoderm (mucous membrane linings of the respiratory tract, gastrointestinal tract, and genitourinary tract). Sarcomas originate from embryonal mesoderm (connective tissue, muscle, bone, and fat). Lymphomas and leukemias originate from the hematopoietic system.

Table 11-7
Anatomical Classification of Tumors

Site	Benign	Malignant
Epithelial tissue tumors: (body surfaces, lining of body cavities, and glandular structures)	*Oma*	*Carcinoma*
Surface epithelium	Papill*oma*	*Carcinoma*
Glandular eipthelium	Aden*oma*	Adeno*carcinoma*
Connective tissue tumors: (supporting tissue, fibrotic tissues, blood vessels)	*Oma*	*Sarcoma*
Fibrous tissue	Fibr*oma*	Fibro*sarcoma*
Cartilage	Chondr*oma*	Chondro*sarcoma*
Striated muscle	Rhabdomy*oma*	Rhabdomyo*sarcoma*
Bone	Oste*oma*	Osteo*sarcoma*
Nervous tissue tumors: (brain, nerves, retina)	*Oma* (Named according to cell type)	*Oma*
Meninges	Meningi*oma*	Meningeal *sarcoma*
Nerve cells	Ganglioneur*oma*	Neuroblast*oma*
Hematopoietic tissue tumors:	(No specific nomenclature)	
Lymphoid tissue		Malignant lymphoma
Plasma cells		Multiple myeloma
Bone marrow		Lymphocytic leukemia
		Myelogenous leukemia

Histologic Analysis Classification

In histologic grading of tumors the appearance of cells and their degree of differentiation are evaluated. For many tumor cells, four grades are used:

Grade I—Cells differ slightly from normal cells (mild dysplasia) and are well differentiated.

Grade II—Cells are more abnormal (moderate dysplasia) and moderately differentiated.

Grade III—Cells are very abnormal (severe dysplasia) and poorly differentiated.

Grade IV—Cells are immature and primitive (anaplasia) and undifferentiated; cell of origin is difficult to determine.

Extent of Disease Classification

The extent of disease classification is often called *staging*. This classification system is based on a description of the extent of the disease rather than on cell appearance. Although there are similarities in the staging of cancers, there are many differences based on a thorough knowledge of the natural history of each specific type of cancer. The following are two examples which illustrate the use of different staging classifications.

Clinical staging

This classification system determines the extent of the disease process of cancer.

Stage 0—Cancer in situ.

Stage I—Tumor is limited to the tissue of origin—localized tumor growth.

Stage II—Limited local spread.

Stage III—Extensive local spread and regional spread.

Stage IV—Metastasis.

This staging classification has been used in cancer of the cervix (see Chap. 46) and Hodgkin's disease (Table 24-26).

TNM classification system

The TNM classification system represents the standardization of the clinical staging of cancer by the International Union Against Cancer (UICC). This classification system (see Table 11-8) is used to determine the extent of the disease process of cancer utilizing three parameters: tumor size (T), degree of regional spread to the lymph nodes (N), and absence or presence of metastasis (M). This system has been applied to cancer of the breast in Chap. 44.

Staging of the disease can be done initially and at several intervals. *Clinical diagnostic staging* is done at the time of diagnosis to determine the most effective treatment plan. Examples of diagnostic studies that might be done to assess for spread of disease include bone and liver scans, ultrasonography, and computerized tomography (CT) scans.

Surgical evaluative staging is utilized to describe the extent of the disease process after biopsy or surgical exploration. For example, a laparotomy and splenectomy are frequently done in staging of Hodg-

Table 11-8
TNM Classification System

Primary Tumor (T)	
T_0	No evidence of primary tumor
T_{IS}	Carcinoma in situ
T_1, T_2, T_3, T_4	Ascending degrees of increase in tumor size and involvement
Regional Lymph Nodes (N)	
N_0	Regional nodes not demonstrable
N_{1a}, N_{2a}	Demonstrable regional lymph nodes; metastases not suspected
N_{1b}, N_{2b}, N_3	Demonstrable regional lymph nodes; metastases suspected
N_x	Regional lymph nodes cannot be assessed clinically
Distant Metastases (M)	
M_0	No evidence of distant metastases
M_1, M_2, M_3	Ascending degrees of metastatic involvement of the host, including distant nodes

From K. Isselbacher et al. (eds.), *Harrison's Principles of Internal Medicine*, 9th ed., McGraw-Hill Book Company, New York, 1980, p. 1593.

kin's disease. During a staging laparotomy, areas of lymph node biopsy and margins of any masses may be marked with metal clips. These clips are used as markers if radiotherapy is utilized as a treatment modality.

Postsurgical treatment pathologic staging is utilized after pathologic examination of the surgical specimen. The presence of residual tumor should be recorded at this time. The stages are R_0, no residual tumor; R_1, microscopic residual tumor; and R_2, macroscopic residual tumor.

Once the extent of disease is determined, the stage classification is not changed. The original description of the extent of the tumor remains part of the original record. If additional treatment is needed or if treatment fails, retreatment staging is done to determine the extent of the disease process at the time of retreatment.

Carcinoma in situ is a commonly used term in classification of malignancies. It is defined as a lesion with all the histologic features of malignancy except invasion. If left untreated, carcinoma in situ will eventually become invasive.

In addition to tumor classification systems, there are also classification systems used to describe the status of the client with cancer. The status of the client is recorded at the time of diagnosis, treatment, retreatment, and at each follow-up examination period. The Karnofsky performance scale is an example of a method used to evaluate the physical status of the client (see Table 11-9).

Table 11-9
Performance Status (Karnofsky Scale)

100	Normal; no complaints; no evidence of disease.
90	Able to carry on normal activity; minor signs or symptoms of disease.
80	Normal activity with effort; some signs or symptoms of disease.
70	Cares for self; unable to carry on normal activity or do active work.
60	Requires occasional assistance but is able to care for most of his needs.
50	Requires considerable assistance and frequent medical care.
40	Disabled; requires special care and assistance.
30	Severely disabled; hospitalization is indicated although death not imminent.
20	Very sick; hospitalization necessary; active supportive treatment is necessary.
10	Moribund, fatal processes progressing rapidly.
0	Dead.

PREVENTION AND DETECTION OF CANCER

Early detection and prompt treatment are directly responsible for increased survival rates in individuals with cancer. The nurse plays a major role in the prevention and detection of cancer. One important aspect is to educate the public to:

1. Reduce or avoid exposure to known or suspected carcinogens.
2. Eat a proper diet.
3. Get adequate, consistent exercise.
4. Reduce stress and/or increase the capacity to cope with stress.
5. Get consistent periods of relaxation and enjoyable use of leisure time.
6. Obtain adequate, consistent periods of rest (at least 6 to 8 hours per night).
7. Obtain health care on a consistent basis that includes a history, physical examination, and specific diagnostic parameters for common cancers according to guidelines specified by the American Cancer Society.
8. Know the seven warning signs of cancer as identified by the American Cancer Society (see Table 11-10).
9. Learn and practice self-examination (e.g., breast self-exam, testicular exam).
10. Seek immediate medical care if cancer is suspected. Early detection of cancer has a positive impact on the prognosis of cancer.

When educating the public regarding the disease process of cancer, care should be taken to minimize the fear that surrounds cancer. Tactics that increase fear should never be utilized. The facts should be taught in an accurate, low-key manner at the level of the learner. The goal of public education is to *motivate* the learner to change the pattern of behavior that is necessary to achieve and maintain an optimum state of health. The nurse can play a significant role in meeting this goal. Although the general public must

Table 11-10
Seven Warning Signs of Cancer

C hange in bowel or bladder habits
A sore that does not heal
U nusual bleeding or discharge from any body orifice
T hickening or a lump in the breast or elsewhere
I ndigestion or difficulty in swallowing
O bvious change in a wart or mole
N agging cough or hoarseness

be taught, those that are at high risk to develop cancer are the target population for effective cancer control (see Table 11-11). The nurse can have a definite impact on *convincing* people that change in habits will have a positive influence on health. If the nurse is to make any significant impact, the challenge needs to be recognized and strategies developed to teach effectively (see Chap. 5).

Diagnosis of the Client with Suspected Cancer

When a client is admitted to a health care agency with the possible diagnosis of cancer, it is a very stressful time for the client and family. The client typically undergoes several days of diagnostic studies. During this time the fear of the unknown is often more stressful than ultimately being told of a positive diagnosis of cancer.

During the time of waiting for the results of the diagnostic studies the nurse needs to be available to actively listen to the client's concerns. False reassurance that everything will be all right is inappropriate and is an effective way to shut off further communication with the client. During this time of high anxiety the client may need repeated explanations regarding the diagnostic workup. Explanations should be brief and reinforced as necessary.

The specifics of the health history and screening physical examination are presented in Chap. 3. A diagnostic plan for the client suspected of cancer includes a health history, physical examination, and specific diagnostic studies.

The health history includes particular emphasis on risk factors such as family history of cancer, exposure to or use of known carcinogens (e.g., cigarette smoking and occupational pollutants or chemicals), diseases characterized by chronic irritation (e.g., ulcerative colitis), and drug ingestion (e.g., hormone therapy). Other important information relates to dietary habits, ingestion of alcohol, and lifestyle.

The physical examination should be thorough and investigate for physical signs of suspected cancer. Particular attention should be focused on the lymph nodes, skin, liver, spleen, abdomen, and neurologic system. A thorough oral cavity examination, pelvic

Table 11-11
Screening for Specific Cancer Sites

Specific Cancer	High-Risk Profile	Screening	Medium and Low-Risk Profile	Screening
Lung cancer	History of 20 pack years of smoking (1 pack a day for 20 years) Exposure to airborne carcinogens, especially asbestos, uranium, hydrocarbons	Baseline chest x-ray with follow-up every 6 months to 1 year	History of less than 20 pack years of smoking Nonsmokers	Chest x-ray not recommended
	Age range 40–80 years Chronic lung disease	Client observes for a change in respiratory status: frequency of infections, change in cough, sputum, breathing		
Colon/rectal cancer	History of familial polyposis, ulcerative colitis, or Crohn's disease Diet with high fat, low fiber Age range 40–75 years	Guaiac test on stools every year after 50 Digital rectal examination every year Proctosigmoidoscopic examination every year Client observes for changes in bowel pattern: diarrhea, constipation, pain, flatus, black tarry stools and/or the presence of bleeding	Persons with no known risk factors	Guaiac test on stools every year after 50 Digital rectal exam every year Proctosigmoidoscopic exam as a baseline at age 50 years. After two normal examinations, repeat proctosigmoidoscopic examination every 3 to 5 years

Table 11-11 (Continued)

Specific Cancer	High-Risk Profile	Screening	Medium and Low-Risk Profile	Screening
Prostatic cancer	Presence of prostatic hypertrophy Presence of prostatic infection Blacks Risk increases with age	Rectal examination every year Client should observe for dysuria and/or difficulty in producing a stream of urine	The presence of one risk factor excluding age	Rectal examination every year after age 40
Cervical cancer	Early intercourse (prior to age 20) with multiple partners Noncircumcised partners Poor personal hygiene History of herpesvirus type II infection Cervical dysplasia	Pap test every year Pelvic examination every year Colposcopy if suspicious area is noted Client should observe for abnormal vaginal bleeding or discharge and/or the presence of pain or bleeding with sexual intercourse	No known risk factors	Pap test every year after age 18 for 2 years; if normal, every 3 years Pelvic examination every year for 2 years; if normal, every 3 years
Skin cancer	Prolonged exposure to sun Previous radiation Fair, thin skin	Physical examination every year Client observes for a sore that does not heal and/or a change in a wart or mole	Presence of one risk excluding prolonged exposure to the sun	Physical examination each year
Breast cancer	Caucasian Early menarche—late menopause Fibrocystic breast disease Infertility; over age 30 for first pregnancy; three or less children Mother or sister with a history of breast cancer Use of estrogen therapy (birth control pill, postmenopausal estrogen replacement) Age range 35–65 years	Monthly self-breast examination Breast examination by a health professional every year Baseline mammogram at age 35 and every year after that Client observes for a lump or thickening, discharge from the nipple and/or pain in the breast	Excluding family history of breast cancer, less than two risk factors	Monthly breast self-examination Breast examination by a health professional every 3 years Baseline mammogram
Endometrial cancer	Infertility Ovarian dysfunction Obesity Uterine bleeding Estrogen therapy over a long period of time Age range 30–80 years	Pap every year Pelvic examination every year Endometrial aspiration every year after menopause Client observes for abnormal uterine bleeding, pain, and/or a change in the menstrual pattern	The presence of one risk, excluding estrogen therapy, over a long period of time	Pap test every year for 2 years; if normal, every 3 years Pelvic examination every year for 2 years; if normal, every 3 years Endometrial aspiration is not recommended

Based on the American Cancer Society, 1980 Recommendations.

examination, and digital examination of the rectum should be included.

Diagnostic studies will be performed depending on the suspected primary or metastatic site(s) of the cancer. (Specific procedures as they relate to each body system are discussed in the respective assessment chapters.) Examples of diagnostic studies related to cancer detection include:

1. Cytology studies (e.g., Pap smear)
2. Chest x-ray
3. Complete blood count
4. Proctoscopic examination
5. Bone marrow examination (if a hematolymphoid malignancy is suspected)
6. Mammogram
7. Liver function studies
8. Lymphangiography
9. Presence of oncofetal antigens CEA, AFP, and POA (see section on Immunology)
10. Radioisotope scans (liver, brain, bone, lung)
11. Biopsy
12. Computerized tomography
13. Ultrasonography

Biopsy

The biopsy procedure is the definitive means of diagnosing cancer. It involves the histologic examination of a piece of tissue from the suspicious lesion by a pathologist. A biopsy is essential prior to planning a treatment regime for the client. A biopsy will determine (1) if the tissue is benign or malignant, (2) the anatomic tissue from which the tumor arises, and (3) the degree of cellular differentiation of the cancer cells present in the tumor.

Tissue biopsy can be obtained by *needle biopsy, incisional biopsy,* and *excisional biopsy.* Needle biopsy can be obtained by aspiration (e.g., bone marrow aspiration) or by the use of a large-bore needle. Large, long needles are used in obtaining samples of tissues such as prostate gland, breast, liver, and kidney.

Incisional biopsy performed by a scalpel or dermal punch technique is the most common technique used for making a diagnosis of cancer. The assumption that incisional biopsy may contribute to the spread of cancer has not been proven. Even if a minor risk is involved, the information gained by an incisional biopsy justifies the procedure.[24]

Excisional biopsy involves the removal of the entire tumor. It is usually used for small tumors such as skin lesions and intestinal polyps. This procedure can be considered a therapeutic as well as diagnostic approach. Often when a tumor is not easily accessible, a major surgical procedure is necessary (laparotomy, thoracotomy, craniotomy) to obtain a piece of the tumor tissue. Direct biopsies of the gastrointestinal, respiratory, and genitourinary tracts can be obtained by endoscopic procedures.

TREATMENT OF CANCER

Goals and Modalities

The goals of cancer treatment are *cure, control,* or *palliation* (Fig. 11-8). Factors that determine the treatment modality are the cell type of the cancer, the location and size of the tumor, and the extent of the disease. The physiologic and psychological status and expressed needs of the client also have an important part in determining the treatment plan. These factors influence the modalities chosen for treatment and the length of time the treatment plan is administered.

When caring for the client with cancer, it is important to know the goals of the treatment plan in order to appropriately communicate with and support the client. When *cure* is the goal, it is expected that after treatment the client will be disease-free and will live a normal life span. Many kinds of cancer have the potential to go into permanent remission with either an initial course of treatment or with treatment that extends for several weeks, months, or years. Basal cell carcinoma of the skin is usually cured by the surgical removal of the lesion or by a several-week course of radiation therapy. Acute lymphocytic leukemia (ALL) in children has the potential for cure. The treatment plan for ALL includes the administration of several chemotherapy drugs on a scheduled basis for a time span of 1 to several years.

Until a few years ago, a 5-year disease-free period was thought to be indicative of a cancer cure. It has been learned that this time span is not accurate for all cancers. Those clients who have been diagnosed as having a tumor with a rapid mitotic rate (e.g., rhabdomyosarcoma) are considered in remission if cancer is not detected in a 2-year time span. Clients with a tumor with a slow mitotic rate (e.g., postmenopausal breast cancer) need 20 or more disease-free years before being considered cured of cancer.

Control is the goal of the treatment plan for many cancers considered to be chronic. The client receives the initial course of therapy and is either continued on maintenance therapy for a period of time or is followed closely so that early signs and symptoms of returning

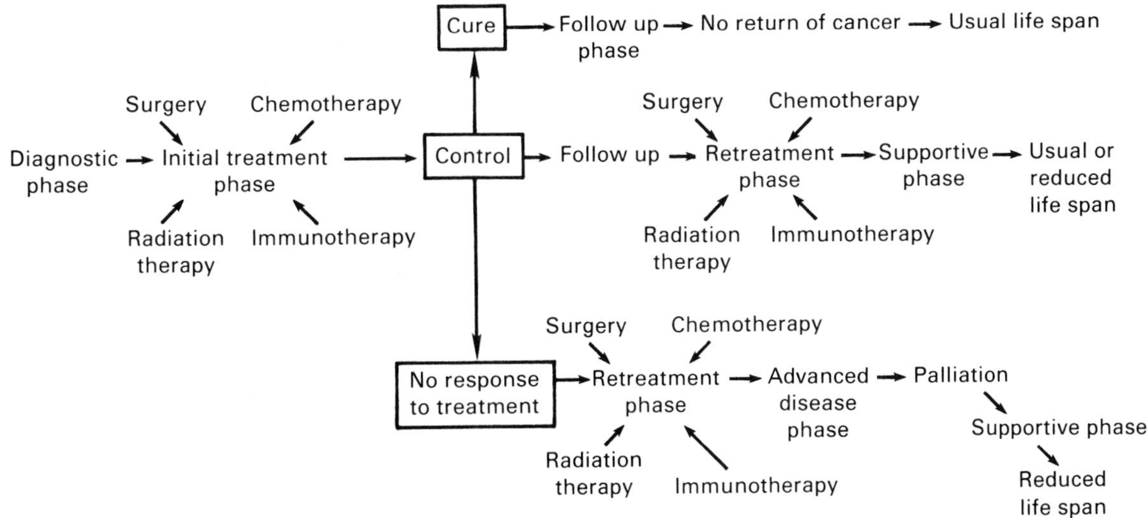

Figure 11-8 Goals of cancer treatment.

cancer can be detected. These cancers are never cured but they are controlled by therapy for long periods of time. They are controlled in a manner similar to other chronic illnesses, such as diabetes mellitus. An example of this type of cancer is chronic lymphocytic leukemia. (Chronic lymphocytic leukemia is discussed in Chap. 24.)

Palliation of symptoms can also be a goal of the treatment plan. With this treatment goal, relief of symptoms and the maintenance of a high quality of life are the primary goals rather than cure or control of the disease process. Radiation therapy given to relieve the pain of bone metastasis is an example of treatment with a goal of palliation.

The goals of cure, control, or palliation are achieved through the use of four treatment modalities for cancer: surgery, radiation therapy, chemotherapy, and immunotherapy. Since surgery was the first and only treatment for cancer for a long period of time, the other treatment modalities—radiation therapy, chemotherapy, and immunotherapy—are often said to be adjuvant to surgery. Surgery, radiation therapy, and chemotherapy can be used alone or in any combination as the treatment for cancer in the initial treatment phase as well as in the retreatment phase(s) of the process of cancer. Immunotherapy is not used alone in the treatment of cancer, but often is used with one, two, or all the other treatment modalities.

In many cancer sites, two or more of the treatment modalities are utilized to achieve the goal of cure or control for a long period of time. Table 11-12 gives examples of the use of the treatment modalities to achieve cure or control of the disease process of cancer.

Surgery

Surgery is the oldest form of cancer treatment and for many years was the only effective method of cancer diagnosis and treatment. The treatment of choice for many years was to remove the cancer and as much of the surrounding tissue as possible. Therefore, most of the surgical procedures utilized were considered radical in nature. In the mid-1950s, it was statistically observed that even though the radical procedures were technically sophisticated, the mortality rates associated with certain cancer sites were not improving (e.g., breast cancer). Many of the cancers that were thought to be local disease processes were found to be systemic diseases with metastatic lesions located in anatomic sites other than the site of the primary disease. By analyzing these statistics, it became obvious that surgery used alone, regardless of the extent of the surgical procedure, was not an effective treatment for every type of cancer.[25] At the present time, surgery plays several roles in the diagnosis and treatment of cancer (Fig. 11-9).

Surgery for cure and control

Several surgical principles are applicable when surgery is utilized to cure or control the disease process of cancer:

1. Cancer that arises from a tissue with a slow rate of

Table 11-12
Treatment Modalities Used in Cancer

Original Cancer	Surgery	Radiotherapy	Chemotherapy	Immunotherapy
Breast (stage I)	P	Alt	ND	ND
Ovary (stage I)	P	Adj, E	E	ND
Uterine cervix:				
In situ	P	P	NU	NU
Stage II	P	P	E	ND
Lung:				
Small (oat) cell	NU	Adj, E	P	E
Adenocarcinoma	P	Adj	E	E
Gastrointestinal:				
Colon	P	NU	E	E
Stomach	P	Adj	E	ND
Melanoma:				
Stage I	P	NU	NU	E
Head and Neck	P	P	E	E
Testes:				
Seminoma (stage I)	P	P	ND	ND
Prostate	P	Alt	E	ND
Kidney	P	Adj	ND	ND
Brain	P	Alt	E	E
Lymphomas:				
Hodgkin's disease:				
Stage I	NU	P	E	ND
Stage III	NU	Alt	P	ND

Note: **P** = Considered an integral part of standard primary treatment programs. **Alt** = An alternate, although less commonly used, method of primary treatment for which data are already available indicating results equivalent to more common approaches. **Adj** = Use an adjunctive therapy after localized tumor is treated by a primary method; routine use is not considered essential. **E** = Experimental; role in treatment is under examination in controlled clinical trials. Either a new approach to treatment or an older approach which, in the absence of sufficient data to support its frequent use, is being evaluated in controlled clinical trials. In the latter case, treatment is designated Alt, E. **NU** = Current information indicates no role in primary treatment program. Control rate of tumor in question may be sufficiently high with other forms of treatment to preclude testing of this modality. **ND** = No data available to evaluate this form of treatment.

Adapted from K. Isselbacher et al. (eds.), *Harrison's Principles of Internal Medicine,* 9th ed., McGraw-Hill Book Company, New York, 1980, p. 1612.

cellular proliferation/replication is most amenable to surgical treatment.

2. A margin of normal tissue must surround the tumor at the time of resection.
3. Only as much tissue as necessary is removed and adjuvant therapy is utilized. The trend at the present time is less radical surgery.
4. Preventive measures are utilized to reduce the occurrence of surgical "seeding" of cancer cells.
5. The usual sites of regional spread may be surgically removed.

Examples of surgical procedures utilized for cure or control of cancer include radical neck dissection, mastectomy, pneumonectomy, thyroidectomy, and bowel resection.

A *debulking procedure* may be utilized if the tumor is unable to be completely removed (e.g., is attached to a vital organ). When this occurs, as much as possible of the tumor is removed and the client is treated with chemotherapy, radiation therapy, and/or immunotherapy. This type of surgical procedure makes the adjuvant therapy more effective.

Supportive care

Surgical procedures can also be used to provide supportive care throughout the disease process of cancer. Examples of supportive surgical procedure include:

1. Insertion of feeding tubes in the esophagus or stomach
2. Creation of a colostomy to allow a rectal abcess to heal
3. Suprapubic catheter for client with advanced prostatic cancer

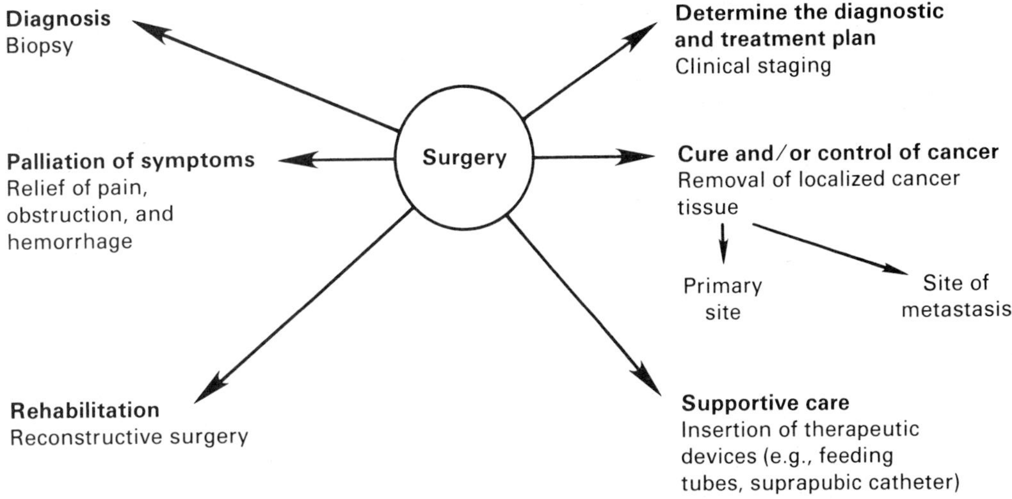

Figure 11-9 Role of surgery in the treatment of cancer.

Palliation of symptoms

When cure or control of cancer is no longer possible, the quality of life must be maintained at the highest possible level for the longest period of time. Examples of surgical procedure done for palliative care include:

1. Relief of pain by a cordotomy or rhizotomy (see Chap. 51)
2. Colostomy for the relief of a bowel obstruction (see Chap. 34)
3. Laminectomy for the relief of a spinal cord compression (see Chap. 53)

The reader should refer to the type of cancer in question to learn of specific operative procedures.

Rehabilitative management

Cancer surgery often mutilates and produces a change in the body image. This is often difficult for the client to cope with while attempting to maintain usual lifestyle patterns. As the treatment plans for certain cancers become more and more effective, the time the client must live with an alteration created by surgery will be increased. If quality of life is to be maintained, the body image must be one that the client is able to accept and cope with on a daily basis. To increase the quality of life, a greater emphasis has been placed in recent times on the rehabilitative role of surgery in cancer care. Mammoplasty following a mastectomy is an example of a rehabilitative surgical procedure (see Chap. 44). The new appliances and care of ostomies is another major focus of rehabilitative management (see Chap. 34).

A nursing challenge is to try to get the client to think of cancer as a *chronic* illness rather than a *terminal* illness. Many people with chronic illnesses such as arthritis and diabetes mellitus learn to cope and live a high quality of life.

Radiation Therapy*

Radiation therapy is a local treatment modality for cancer which can be administered externally *(teletherapy)* or internally *(brachytherapy)*. The route of administration depends on the cell type, location, size, and age of the cancer, the client being treated, and the current thinking regarding the most effective treatment plan for the specific cancer. Radiation therapy is a frequently used treatment modality. It is estimated that over 50 percent of clients diagnosed as having cancer will be treated with radiation therapy at some point in the course of their illness.

Radiation is the emission of tiny particles or waves of energy from radioactive sources (see Chap. 59). Radiation from these sources has the ability to release electrons from the outer shell of an atom. This process changes the atom to an ionized state. When living cells become ionized, physical and chemical changes occur within the cells.

Types of radiation

Radiation therapy is the clinical use of various forms of ionizing radiation. Two types of radiation

*This section was adapted from Yasko, J., *Care of the Client Receiving External Radiation Therapy,* Reston Publishing Co., Inc., Reston, Va., 1982.

utilized in the treatment of cancer are (1) *electromagnetic radiation* (gamma rays and x-rays), and (2) *particulate radiation* (alpha particles, beta particles, protons, neutrons, and pi mesons). *Gamma rays and x-rays,* which have similar properties, are produced when electrons are liberated from their orbits in an x-ray vacuum tube or during nuclear disintegration (e.g., cobalt 60 and radium). Radium is an example of naturally occurring radiation. Artificial radioactive isotopes such as cobalt 60 are produced in a nuclear reactor. The range and penetration of gamma rays and x-rays is great and dense material such as lead or concrete is necessary to shield tissue from this type of radiation (Fig. 59-2). Electromagnetic radiation is used extensively in radiation therapy.[26]

Particulate radiation has characteristics that are different from electromagnetic radiation. The depth to which these particles can penetrate depends on the energy with which they are propelled and the density of the substance to be penetrated. A thin sheet of paper or a piece of cloth will stop all alpha rays and a piece of wood or plastic will stop beta rays. The other particulates are stopped by substances of a higher density such as lead or concrete. Protons and negative pi mesons produce denser ionizing beams, transfer energy to a smaller area, and produce a greater effect on tumor and normal tissue.

Measurement of radiation

There are several units used to measure radiation (see Table 11-13).

Detection of radiation

Special machines are available to detect the presence of radiation. The *film badge* is the most familiar device to detect radiation and is widely used to monitor the exposure of health care personnel to radiation in the work setting. Radiation causes a change in the density of the film which is detected when the film is processed. The film is then compared to film of known radiation exposure to determine the amount of radiation exposure experienced by the person wearing the badge. Nurses who are exposed to sources of radiation in the work setting must:

1. Wear the film badge at all times during the time of potential or actual exposure to a source of radiation.
2. Keep the badge away from sources of heat or moisture as these substances will alter the validity of the film reading.
3. Wear *only* the film badge that has been assigned to you. Personnel must not interchange film badges as the film badge provides the only record of the individual's exposure to radiation over a period of time.

The film badge is a monitoring device and offers no protection from radiation for the individual wearing the badge.

An instrument utilized to measure the amount of ionizing radiation present in the environment is the Geiger-Müller detector. This instrument is used to determine the presence of a source of radiation and to measure the levels of radiation. When an internal source of radiation is utilized in the treatment plan, a Geiger detector is always utilized to determine if the radiation source has been dislodged or if the entire source of radiation has been removed at the completion of the treatment plan.

Table 11-13
Measurement of Radiation

Unit	Definition
Curie (Ci)	Measures the number of atoms of a particular radioisotope that disintegrate in one second.
Roentgen (R)	A measure of the radiation required to produce a standard number of ions in air; therefore, a unit of exposure to radiation.
Rad	Measurement of radiation dosage absorbed by the tissues.
Rem	Measurement of the biological effectiveness of various forms of radiation on the human cell (1 rem = 1 rad).

Effect of radiation on cells

The interaction of radiation with human cells results in a variety of biological effects. Radiation interacts with the molecules of the tissues and produces activated molecules through the processes of excitation and ionization. The unstable activated molecules undergo secondary reactions to produce chemically active free radicals. These free radicals such as OH^-, H^+, and H_3O^+ form from the water molecule and are powerful reducing or oxidizing agents that will go on to cause further chemical reactions within the cell. The cellular changes that occur primarily involve the interaction of these free radicals with the DNA, RNA, and enzymes of the cell.

The DNA of the cell is seen as the target of the radiation effect and it is now known that the chemically active hydroxyl radical (OH^-) causes most of the DNA alterations. The principal lesion produced by radiation is a single chromosomal strand break (Fig. 11-10). This lesion becomes lethal when it combines with another single strand break of a cell that has also been exposed to radiation. In normal cells a single chromosomal strand break is usually reparable. However, in

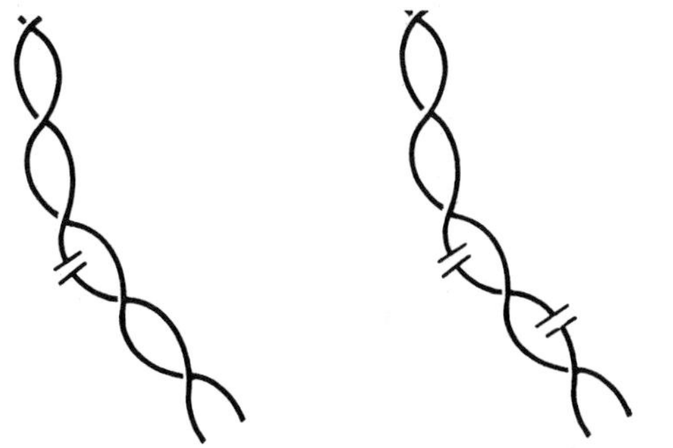

Figure 11-10 Lesions produced in cells by radiation.

cancer cells repair of this alteration is at best difficult. Often, radiation produces a double chromosomal strand break which is lethal to both normal cells and cancer cells.

The amount and degree of DNA damage is greatly influenced by the amount of oxygen available in the cellular environment. The greater the amount of oxygen, the greater the amount of damage to DNA. Studies are being conducted to determine the effectiveness of radiosensitizers [e.g., drugs such as nitroimidazole (Misonidazole)] that are thought to biochemically mimic the action of oxygen. Other studies are being conducted to determine if hyperbaric oxygenation and/or hyperthermia prior to or during the time of the radiation treatment will increase the cellular effect of radiation.

The effect of radiation on the tissues represents a summation of the effect of radiation on the cells forming the tissue. The cells of any given tissue depend on the cellular arrangement of that tissue for their life, replication, and functioning. Therefore, cellular damage or death in a critical area may result in the death of the entire tissue. In addition to the effect on the cells of a given tissue, the capillaries supplying the tissues with blood are also sensitive to the effects of radiation. The cellular destruction of a tissue that occurs from a decreased blood supply may be greater than the cellular destruction that occurs from exposure to radiation.

External radiation: Treatment plan

Radiation therapy is the delivery of radiation to a small amount of tissue at a high dose in a short period of time. The radiation dose is determined by the *radiosensitivity of the tumor cells, therapeutic ratio,* and *volume of tissue.*

Radiosensitivity The clinical definition of a radiosensitive tumor is one that is eradicated by radiation in a dose that is well tolerated by the surrounding normal tissues. Cells with a rapid generation time such as those of the bone marrow, ovaries, testes, epithelial cells of the lining of the gastrointestinal and genitourinary tract, the hair follicle, and the lymphatic tissue are said to be radiosensitive (Table 11-14). The effect of the radiation on these tissues is dramatic. Cells are destroyed and an inflammatory response occurs. As more and more cells are destroyed, cells may slough off, causing the tissue to become thin, denuded, or ulcerated. This process causes side effects such as mucositis, nausea, vomiting, diarrhea, and cystitis. Alopecia, leukopenia, thrombocytopenia, and sterility will also occur when a sufficient number of normal cells of these tissues begin to repair the cellular damage. However, the tissues may never return to their original state. This is due to the formation of fibrosis, which is a normal consequence of cellular repair (see Chap. 9). These changes in the tissue structure continue to occur for several months or even years after the exposure to radiation.

In tissues that have a slow generation time such as the muscles, tendons, and nerves, the response to radiation is less dramatic. Little if any cellular destruction occurs in these tissues since few cells are in the process of cellular division at any one point in time. These cells are said to be *radioresistant*. Even though little cellular destruction occurs when radioresistant tissues are exposed to radiation, the capillaries of these tissues will be destroyed, with resulting edema and inflammation of the surrounding tissue. The degree of atrophy, fibrosis, and necrosis of the tissues will depend on the adequacy of the blood supply to these tissues.

Therapeutic Ratio The second determining factor of radiation dose, the *therapeutic ratio,* is defined

Table 11-14
Tumor Radiosensitivity

High radiosensitivity	Moderate radiosensitivity
Ovarian dysgerminoma	Skin carcinoma
Testicular seminoma	Oropharyngeal carcinoma
Hodgkin's disease	Esophageal carcinoma
Non-Hodgkin's lymphoma	Breast adenocarcinoma
Wilms' tumor	Uterine and cervical carcinoma
Neuroblastoma	Prostate carcinoma
	Bladder carcinoma
Mild radiosensitivity	**Poor radiosensitivity (radioresistant)**
Soft tissue sarcomas (e.g., chondrosarcoma)	Osteosarcoma
Gastric adenocarcinoma	Malignant melanoma
Renal adenocarcinoma	Malignant gliomas
Colon adenocarcinoma	

as the relationship between the radiation dose that normal tissues in the area of the tumor can tolerate and the radiation dose necessary to destroy the tumor cells:

$$\text{Therapeutic ratio} = \frac{\text{normal tissue tolerance dose}}{\text{tumor lethal dose}}$$

If the therapeutic ratio is greater than 1 (> 1), it is likely that the tumor can be successfully eradicated. If the therapeutic ratio is less than 1 (< 1), radiation therapy will not be an effective treatment. It must be remembered that radiation will affect the normal cells as well as the cancer cells in the treatment field.

If the entire tumor lethal dose of radiation was given in one treatment, the exposure would be classified as an acute radiation exposure similar to that of an atomic bomb blast or a nuclear power plant accident (Chap. 59). To avoid radiation exposure that would be detrimental to the health of a client, the total tumor lethal radiation dose is divided into smaller doses (called *fractionation*) given on a daily basis until the total tumor lethal dose is reached.

The usual time schedule for the course of treatment with external radiation therapy is a series of treatments given over a period of 2 to 8 weeks on a 5-day-a-week schedule. Since most tumors require a radiation dose of between 4500 and 7500 rads, most clients receive a daily fractionated radiation dose of 200 ± 50 rads and a weekly radiation dose of 1000 ± 250 rads.

The immediate effect of radiation therapy occurs within the first 2 hours after exposure to a source of radiation. After this period of time, the normal cells as well as the tumor cells in the treatment field will attempt to repair themselves. The repair process will continue during the 24-hour time period from one radiation treatment to the next. The normal cells in the treatment field have a greater capacity for cellular repair, both in the rate and quality of the repair. Cancer cells can repair themselves, but the rate and quality of repair is slower and less accurate than normal cells.

To further enhance the repair of normal tissues, radiation therapy is sometimes given as a *split course* of therapy. In this treatment plan, the treatments are given for a period of 2 to 4 weeks, discontinued for several weeks so that the normal cells can repair themselves, and resumed for another 2-to-4-week period of time. It is important that the client receive each of the scheduled radiation treatments. If for some reason a treatment is omitted, the radiation therapist may add another treatment to the end of the treatment plan or increase the daily dose of each remaining radiation treatment. The client is usually reevaluated during and near the end of the course of treatment. Depending on the tumor response to radiation or the side effects of radiation therapy experienced by the client, the number of treatments may be increased or decreased and/or the daily dose of radiation may be altered.

Volume of Tissue The third factor that must be considered in radiation therapy is the *volume* of tissue exposed to the source of radiation. The volume of tissues radiated is known as the *treatment field* and it includes the tumor and the smallest possible amount of normal tissue. The tumor lethal dose delivered to the treatment field must be a dose that is high enough to destroy the cancer cells but one that will not have a highly detrimental effect on the normal cells present in the field. If the volume of tissue radiated is small, the tumor lethal dose of radiation can be increased, the rate of tumor cell destruction will be greater, and the side effects experienced by the client will be fewer and less severe.

Goals of treatment

The treatment goals of radiation therapy are cure, control, or palliation. In order to accomplish these treatment goals, radiation therapy can be used alone as a treatment modality or as an adjuvant treatment modality in combination with surgery, chemotherapy, and/or immunotherapy.

Cure is the goal when radiation therapy is used alone as a curative treatment modality for treating clients with:

1. Basal cell carcinoma of the skin
2. Tumors confined to the vocal cords
3. Stage I or IIA Hodgkin's disease

Radiation therapy can be combined with surgery, chemotherapy, and immunotherapy to cure certain cancers such as:

1. Stage IIB, IIIA, and IIIB Hodgkin's disease in combination with chemotherapy
2. Wilms' tumor in combination with surgery and/or chemotherapy
3. Ewing's sarcoma in combination with chemotherapy
4. Head and neck cancer in combination with surgery and/or chemotherapy

Control of the disease process of cancer for a period of time is considered a reasonable goal in some situations. Initial treatment is offered at the time of diagnosis and additional treatment is instituted each time symptoms of disease recur. Most clients enjoy a high quality of life during the symptom-free period. Radiation therapy can be combined with surgery to further enhance the local control of cancer. It can be given preoperatively to reduce the size of the tumor so that it can be more easily resected, or postoperatively to destroy any remaining tumor cells.

Inoperable tumors can be treated with radiation therapy. These tumors are large and have extended regionally. An example of an inoperable cancer treated for control with radiation therapy is oat-cell cancer of the lung.

Palliation is often the goal of radiation therapy. The client can be treated to control the distressing symptoms that are occurring as a result of the disease process. Tumors can be reduced in size to relieve symptoms such as pain and obstruction. Examples of the use of radiation therapy for palliation include the relief of:

1. Pain associated with bone metastasis
2. Pain and neurologic symptoms associated with brain metastasis
3. Spinal cord compression
4. Intestinal obstruction
5. Superior vena cava obstruction
6. Bronchial and/or tracheal obstruction

Types of radiation therapy machines

The *kilovoltage machine,* the first available radiation therapy machine, delivers x-rays at a low energy level and is similar to machines used for diagnostic x-rays. The depth of the maximum delivered dose of radiation is on the skin surface. A problem experienced when this machine is used is that the radiation scatters when it strikes the skin surface, causing the skin surrounding the treatment field to experience radiation exposure. At the present time, the kilovoltage machine is rarely used.

The cobalt 60 machine is a *megavoltage machine* which emits high-energy gamma rays as the source of radiation (Fig. 11-11). Because radioactive cobalt is a high energy source of radiation, the penetration of the radiation is greater and the maximum radiation dose occurs below the surface of the skin. Therefore, this machine is used to treat tumors located below the skin surface with minimal radiation exposure of the skin surface and less radiation scatter. Although this machine is gradually being replaced by higher voltage

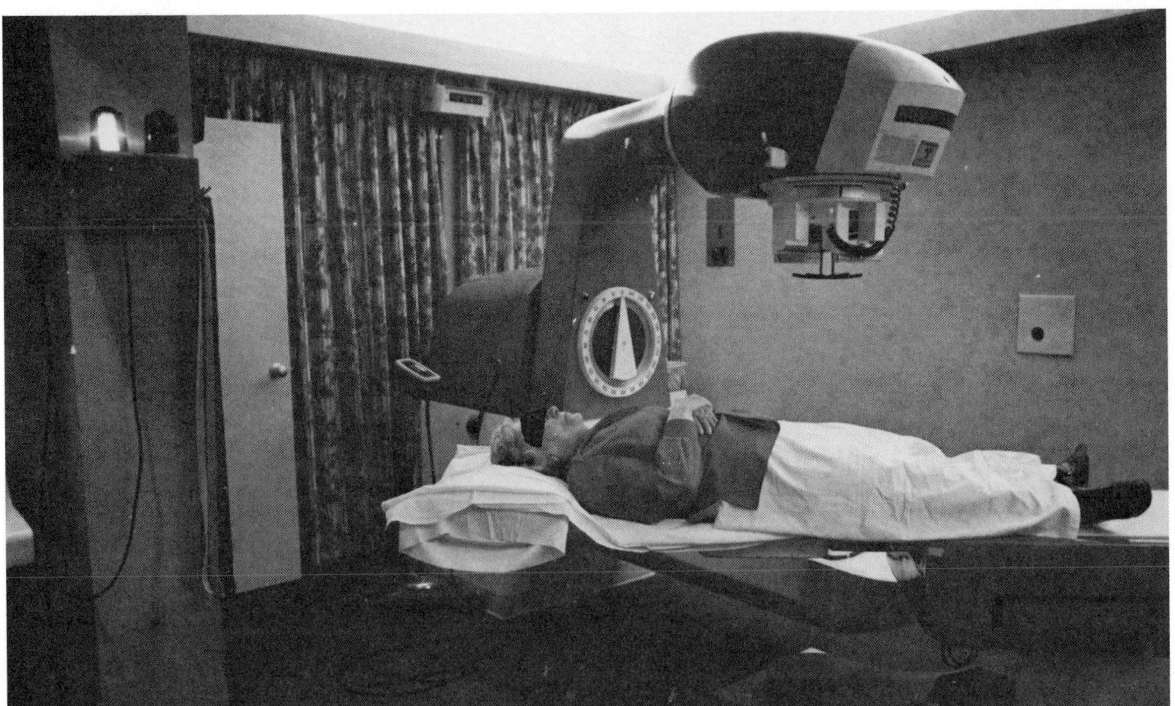

Figure 11-11 Cobalt 60 radiation therapy machine. *(From J. Yasko, Care of the Client Receiving External Radiation Therapy—A Self-Learning Module For the Nurse, American Cancer Society, Pennsylvania Division, Inc., 1980.)*

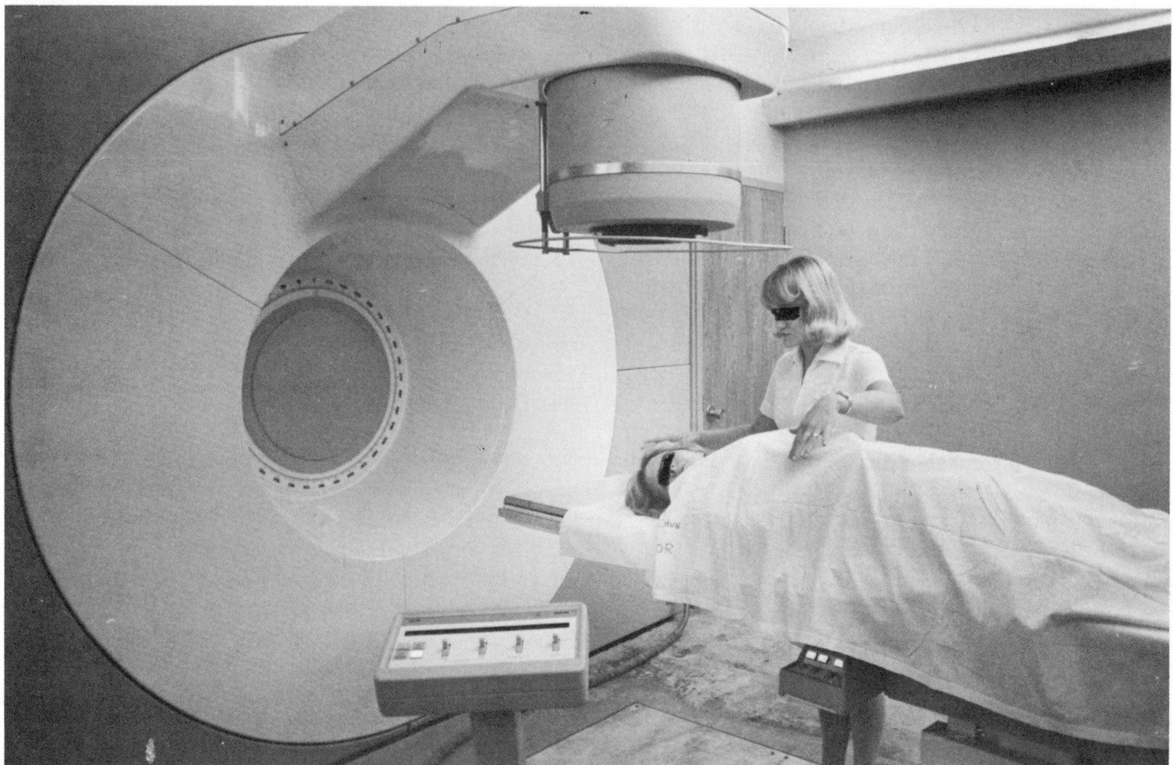

Figure 11-12 Linear accelerator. *(From J. Yasko, Care of the Client Receiving External Radiation Therapy—A Self-Learning Module For the Nurse Caring For the Client With Cancer, American Cancer Society, Pennsylvania Division, Inc., 1980.)*

machines, its widespread use continues at the present time.

The large, high-energy *supervoltage machine* is the *linear accelerator.* It utilizes x-rays or electrons as a source of radiation to the treatment fields (Fig. 11-12). Since the penetration of the source of radiation from this machine is great and the radiation scatter is minimal, tumors located several centimeters below the skin surface can be effectively treated. These machines are currently popular and are supplementing and/or replacing the cobalt 60 machine.

Cyclotrons and betatrons are other examples of supervoltage machines. The betatron machine utilizes electrons while the cyclotron utilizes protons, neutrons, or electrons as a source of radiation. These machines are being utilized in several cancer centers.

Effects of radiation therapy on normal tissues

Side effects of radiation therapy are common. They are caused by destruction of irradiated normal tissues in the area of the tumor. All clients receiving radiation in a particular anatomic site will not experience the same side effects, nor will the side effects be experienced to the same degree. In some clients, the side effects will be so slight that they will hardly be noticed, while in other clients the side effects will seriously alter the usual lifestyle patterns.[27]

Many side effects are dependent on the site being radiated. For example, a client who had radiation therapy to the scalp will usually develop alopecia. Some side effects are more general in nature and common to clients receiving radiation regardless of the area being radiated. These include skin reactions, fatigue, and anorexia.

Skin Reactions During each treatment, radiation will pass through the skin. Since megavoltage or supravoltage machines are presently used to deliver the source of radiation to the treatment field, the maximum effect of radiation therapy occurs below the skin surface and the skin is said to be spared. However, the epithelial cells of the skin have a rapid rate of cellular division so that some epithelial cells of the skin will be destroyed as the radiation enters the treatment field. The greater the dose of radiation used in therapy, the more likely the skin reaction. Fair-skinned persons are usually more sensitive than darker-skinned individuals.

There are four degrees or levels of the skin reaction. Most clients will remain at level I or II throughout the course of the treatment plan (Table 11-15). The skin reaction must not be referred to as a radiation burn. A skin reaction is usually expected. When the word "burn" is used, it suggests that a mistake has been made resulting in a burn.

Level I—Erythema of the skin in the treatment field. The skin in this area will be pink to red in color and will resemble a first-degree reaction of the skin to the sun.

Level II—Dry desquamation of the skin in the treatment field. The skin will become dry and scaly and the client may complain of itching.

Level III—Wet desquamation of the skin in the treatment field. The skin may become blistered and the superficial layers may be lost through peeling. This reaction resembles a second-degree reaction of the skin to the sun. The damage to the skin is reversible but it may be necessary to discontinue the treatment plan until healing occurs.

Level IV—Loss of hair on the skin in the treatment field. Permanent loss of hair in the treatment field as well as suppression of sweat glands occurs with high doses of radiation therapy. Late side effects may occur 6 months to 5 years following the completion of the treatment plan. These include:

1. Fibrosis of the skin and telangiectasis due to dilatation of capillaries in the treatment field.
2. Impairment of the lymphatic drainage in the treatment field and the development of lymphedema due to fibrosis of the lymph glands.

Side effects of radiation therapy are presented in Table 11-16.

Nursing management related to external radiation

In order to effectively care for the client receiving external radiation therapy, the nurse must be aware of what the client will experience while being treated with radiation therapy.

Once the preliminary examinations (e.g., history and physical examination, review of medical records) are completed, the client is prepared for radiation

Table 11-15
Nursing Management of Radiation Skin Reactions

1. If necessary, gently cleanse the skin in the treatment field using a mild soap, tepid water, a soft cloth, and a gentle patting motion. Rinse the area thoroughly and pat dry.
2. In the presence of a level II skin reaction, apply A & D ointment or baby oil to alleviate the dry skin. This substance must be gently cleansed from the treatment field prior to each treatment and reapplied. (Note: Care differs from institution to institution.)
3. If a level III skin reaction is present, cleanse the area involved with half-strength hydrogen peroxide and normal saline. The solution is best applied with an irrigating syringe to avoid friction. Rinse the area with saline. Expose the area to air as often as possible. If copious drainage is present, nonadhesive absorbent dressings are warranted and they must be changed as soon as they become wet. Observe the area on a daily basis for signs of infection.
4. Avoid wearing tight-fitting clothing over the treatment field, such as bras, girdles, and belts.
5. Avoid wearing harsh fabrics such as wool and corduroy. A light-weight cotton garment is best. If possible, expose the treatment field to the air.
6. Utilize gentle detergents such as Dreft® and Ivory Snow® to wash the clothing that will come in contact with the treatment field.
7. Avoid direct exposure to the sun. If the treatment field is in an area that is exposed to the sun, wear protective clothing, such as a wide-brimmed hat, when exposed to the sun.
8. Avoid all sources of heat on the treatment field (hot water bottles, heating pads, and sun lamps).
9. Avoid exposing the treatment field to cold temperatures (ice bags or cold weather).
10. Avoid swimming in salt water or in chlorinated swimming pools during the time of treatment.
11. Avoid the use of all medications, deodorants, perfumes, powders, or cosmetics on the skin in the treatment field. Tape, dressings, and adhesive bandages should also be avoided unless permitted by the radiation therapist. Avoid shaving the hair in the treatment field.
12. Sensitive skin must continue to be protected after the treatment plan is completed. Teach the client to:
    a. Avoid direct exposure to the sun. A sunscreening agent containing PABA and/or protective clothing must be worn if the potential of exposure to the sun is present.
    b. Use an electric razor if shaving is necessary in the treatment field.

J. Yasko, *Care of the Client Receiving External Radiation Therapy—A Self-Learning Module for the Nurse Caring for the Client With Cancer*, The Reston Publishing Co., Reston, Va., 1982.

Table 11-16
Problems Caused by Radiation Therapy and Chemotherapy

Problem	Etiology and Comments
Gastrointestinal	
1. Dryness of the mucous membranes of the mouth	When salivary glands are located in the radiation treatment field, they are frequently damaged. This side effect is often a permanent side effect of radiation therapy. It can be quite disturbing to the client since it is difficult to eat, swallow, and/or talk when the mucous membranes are dry.
2. Stomatitis and mucositis	Occurs when epithelial cells are destroyed by chemotherapy and/or radiation therapy. These cells are extremely sensitive because of their normal high cell turnover rate. Mucositis can precipitate complications of infection and hemorrhage.
3. Esophagitis	Inflammation and ulceration of mucous membranes of esophagus due to rapid cell destruction. Occurs as a side effect of chemotherapy and radiation therapy to the area of the neck, chest, and/or back.
4. Nausea and vomiting	Stimulation of the vomiting center in the medulla of the brain by products of cellular breakdown that occurs in response to chemotherapy and radiation therapy. The drugs used in chemotherapy also stimulate the vomiting center. Destruction of the epithelial lining of the gastrointestinal tract in response to chemotherapy and radiation therapy to chest, abdomen, and back. Strong psychological impact associated with nausea and vomiting and the high stress level associated with cancer and cancer treatment.
5. Anorexia	*Site specific* side effects of radiation therapy—dry mouth, mucositis, esophagitis, nausea, vomiting, and diarrhea. Presence of fatigue, pain, infection. Alteration in the sensation of taste which occurs when tumors release waste products into the bloodstream. Psychological and social impact of cancer and cancer therapy resulting in an increased level of stress and changes in the usual lifestyle pattern.
6. Altered taste sensation	The destruction of the taste buds in the treatment field with radiation therapy. The amount of taste alteration or loss depends on the radiation dosage and the extent of the treatment field. Complete loss of taste often occurs. Often taste changes may be a permanent outcome of therapy. Waste products that occur in response to cellular destruction from radiation therapy and chemotherapy. These waste products are thought to be responsible for alterations in the sensation. The reduction in the amount of saliva due to the location of the salivary glands in the treatment field. Food must be in solution to be tasted.
7. Diarrhea	Denuding of the epithelial lining of the small intestines as a side effect of chemotherapy and as a side effect of radiation therapy to the abdomen and/or lower back.
8. Constipation	Related to dysfunction of autonomic nervous system caused by neurotoxic effects of plant alkaloids (vincristine, vinblastine).
9. Hepatotoxicity	Due to toxic effects of certain chemotherapy drugs such as methotrexate, mithramycin, 6-MP, Cytosar.
Hematopoietic system	
1. Anemia	Depressant effect on bone marrow function due to chemotherapy and radiation therapy. Malignant infiltration of bone marrow by cancer. Ulceration, necrosis, and bleeding of neoplastic growth.
2. Leukopenia	Depressant effect on bone marrow activity due to chemotherapy and radiation therapy. Especially significant because of the short life span of WBC. Infection is the most frequent cause of morbidity and mortality in the cancer client. Usual sites of infection are the respiratory and genitourinary systems.
3. Thrombocytopenia	Depressant effect on bone marrow function due to chemotherapy and radiation therapy. Malignant infiltration of the bone marrow. Abnormal destruction of circulating platelets. When the platelet count is less than 20,000/mL, spontaneous bleeding can occur.
Integumentary	
1. Alopecia	Alopecia occurs as a side effect of chemotherapy and radiation therapy to the skull. The hair loss that occurs in response to chemotherapy is usually temporary and the hair loss that occurs in response to radiation therapy is usually permanent. The hair begins to fall out during the first week of therapy and may progress to complete hair loss. Many emotions are expressed when hair loss occurs: anger, grief, embarrassment, and fear. Loss of hair may be the most stressful event that is experienced during the course of their illness.
2. Skin reactions	(See text for causes of radiation skin reactions.) Extravasation of certain chemotherapeutic drugs (e.g., Adriamycin) given intravenously cause severe necrosis.

Table 11-16 (Continued)

Problem	Etiology and Comments
Genitourinary	
1. Cystitis	Occurs when the epithelial lining of the bladder is destroyed as a side effect of chemotherapy (e.g., cyclophosphamide) and as a side effect of radiation therapy when the bladder is located in the treatment field. Clinical manifestations of urgency, frequency, and hematuria.
2. Sexual dysfunction	Effect of chemotherapy on the cells of the testes or the ova. Effect of radiation therapy when the cells of the testes or ova are located in the treatment field. Symptoms of cancer and cancer therapy: fatigue, diarrhea, nausea, vomiting, anxiety, fear, and pain.
3. Nephrotoxicity	Necrosis of proximal renal tubules due to an accumulation of drugs (e.g., Cis-Platinum) in the kidney.
Nervous system	
1. Increased intracranial pressure	May result from radiation edema in the central nervous system. This phenomenon is not well understood. Easily controlled with steroids and pain medication.
2. Peripheral neuropathy	Paresthesias, areflexia, skeletal muscle weakness, and smooth muscle dysfunction (e.g., paralytic ileus, constipation) can occur as a side effect of chemotherapy, especially from plant alkaloids (e.g., vinblastine, vincristine,) and Cis-Platinum.
Respiratory system	
1. Pneumonitis	When the lungs are located in the treatment field, radiation pneumonitis may develop 2 to 3 months after the start of the treatment plan. It is characterized by a dry, hacking cough, fever, and exertional dyspnea. After 6 to 12 months, fibrosis will occur which will be persistently evident on x-ray. The client with fibrosis is more susceptible to respiratory infection. Can also occur as a result of chemotherapy (e.g., bleomycin, busulfan).
Cardiovascular	
1. Pericarditis and myocarditis	Infrequent complications when chest wall is irradiated. May occur up to 1 year after treatment.
2. Cardiotoxicity	Chemotherapeutic agents such as Adriamycin and Daunomycin can cause nonspecific electrical changes (i.e., low voltage) and rapidly progressive heart failure. The drug therapy needs to be modified if these effects occur.
Biochemical	
1. Hyperuricemia	Increase in uric acid levels due to cell destruction by chemotherapy. Can cause a secondary form of gout.
2. Hypomagnesemia	Occurs with Cis-Platinum therapy.
Psychoemotional	
1. Fatigue	Increase in the metabolic rate that occurs when cancer is present, with the resultant increase in the amount of energy utilized. Destruction of cancer cells and normal cells by chemotherapy and radiation therapy with the release of waste products into the bloodstream. Increase in anabolic processes of cellular proliferation and differentiation that are necessary to repair the normal cells and tissues destroyed by chemotherapy and radiation therapy.
2. Pain	Compression or infiltration of the blood vessels, lymphatic vessels, and the nerves. Obstruction of the gastrointestinal and/or genitourinary system. Inflammation, ulceration, or necrosis of the tissues and/or organs. Fear, anxiety, and depression experienced in response to the diagnosis of cancer.

therapy. This preparation is known as *treatment simulation.* The client is placed in the anticipated treatment position on a treatment table under a machine called the *simulator.* The simulator is a diagnostic x-ray machine that can mimic the treatment capabilities of the radiation therapy machine. The client will be asked to lie very still while a series of measurements and x-rays are performed. In order to maintain the exact position the client must assume during treatment, various immobilization devices are utilized. Immobilization devices can be in the form of clamps, or plaster of paris molds or casts. The measurements and x-rays are necessary to determine the dose of radiation, the volume of tissue to be radiated, and the length, number, and frequency of the radiation therapy treatments. All these computations are done with the assistance of a computer.

When the treatment field is determined, the area will be outlined using indelible dye or ink such as felt-tip ped markers, gentian violet, or india ink. Dye or ink which is visible only under black light is also used and is particularly beneficial for clients who have tumors in exposed areas of the body, such as in the region of the head or neck.

Another method used to determine the treatment field is the use of lead blocks that are placed over the radiation source within the machine. The client is placed in exactly the same position for each treatment and the lead blocks permit radiation exposure only to the treatment field. The lead blocks are said to shield the vital organs from exposure to radiation. The skin markings and/or lead blocks are necessary to assure that during each radiation treatment the source of radiation is directed to exactly the same area of the body.

The skin markings must not be washed off or removed in any way. If they are accidentally removed, the client must be cautioned not to attempt to redraw the skin markings. The radiation technician should be notified that the skin markings have been removed and they will be redrawn according to the original treatment plan. Many times the skin markings are a source of stress for the client. If they are visible with the naked eye, they become a constant reminder to the client that the client has and is being treated for cancer.

Prior to the start of the treatment plan, it is helpful to allow the client to see either the actual machine that will be used in the treatment plan or a picture of the machine so that many of the fears of the unknown will be minimized. These strange-looking machines are often associated with many client fears, concerns, and misconceptions.

Receiving a radiation treatment is very similar to having an x-ray taken. Although the client is alone in the room during the treatment, visual and auditory communication is provided via a television monitor and an intercom system. The client should be made aware that radiation is invisible, silent, and painless. Sometimes machines do make unusual whirring or clicking sounds. The client should be informed that it is the machine and not the source of radiation that causes these sounds to occur.

The client should also be informed that lying immobile on the hard, flat treatment table may cause discomfort or pain. If the client is experiencing pain, pain medications should be administered 1 hour prior to the time of treatment to assure comfort.

Clients will often ask if they are radioactive and a danger to others or if their clothing is radioactive. Clients must be assured that once the radiation therapy machine is turned off, radiation is no longer emitted.

Periodically throughout the course of the treatment the client will be evaluated by the radiation therapist and nurse. The effect as well as the side effects of radiation therapy will be assessed. Interventions to prevent or minimize the side effects of radiation therapy will be planned and implemented (see Table 11-17). Adjustments of the original treatment plan will occur if warranted. The client should be aware that it is expected that changes in the original treatment plan may be necessary.

Clients treated with radiation therapy should receive regularly scheduled follow-up care for the rest of their lives. The client should understand that follow-up care is an essential part of the treatment plan. Initially, after the completion of the treatment plan, the radiation therapist will examine the client every 4 to 6 weeks. If the cancer appears to be cured or controlled, the time period for follow-up care is extended to every 6 months to 1 year. Consistent long-term follow-up care is also necessary to evaluate the late side effects of radiation therapy, some of which will not be evident for 5 to 10 years after the completion of the course of treatment.

Internal radiation*

Internal radiation therapy (brachytherapy) is the placement of a source of radiation in a specific area within or on the body. The source of radiation utilized in internal radiation therapy is either a *mechanically positioned* (sealed radiation source) or an *unsealed radiation* source. The selection of the type of internal radiation therapy used in the treatment plan is determined by the size, cell type, and location of the cancer. Table 11-18 lists the characteristics of the various sources of radiation utilized in internal radiation therapy.

Mechanically Placed Internal Radiation *Mechanically placed internal radiation therapy* or *sealed internal therapy* is the placement of a source of radiation in (1) an externally placed mold, (2) interstitially (directly into the tissues of a tumor), or (3) intracavitary (within a body cavity). When a mold containing a source of radiation is *externally placed,* it is made to fit a particular anatomic site and the source of radiation is embedded within the mold. The mold is then applied directly over the skin or mucous membranes covering the tumor. The sources of radiation usually in this form of internal radiation therapy include cobalt 60, tantalum 182, and strontium 90. The usual anatomic sites of treatment are the nostrils, lips, ears, scalp, mouth, larynx, skin, and penis.[28]

In the *interstitial placement of a radiation source,*

*This section was adapted from Yasko, J., "Internal Radiation," in M. L. Donovan, *Cancer Care: A Guide to Patient Education,* Appleton Century Crofts, New York, 1981.

Table 11-17
Nursing Care Plan for the Client with Cancer*

Client Problem	Expected Outcome	Nursing Intervention
Nausea and vomiting	Decreased symptoms of nausea and vomiting. Normal nutritional intake.	Administer antiemetics as ordered and evaluate efficacy of drug, dose, and time administered (e.g., prns vs. routine, around-the-clock administration). Administer sedatives and tranquilizers as ordered to augment the effect of antiemetics when indicated. Maintain a quiet, restful environment. Modify diet to include bland, lukewarm, high-caloric, high-protein foods. Try small, frequent feedings vs. fewer large meals. Teach client to eat and drink slowly. Offer client chewing gum, warm lemon-lime soda pop, Coke syrup, soda crackers, tepid tea, or anything the client knows to work for him. Remove all sights, sounds, or smells which have the potential for initiating nausea, such as emesis basin, unpleasant odors. If these procedures do not work, tetrahydrocannabinol (THC), also known as marijuana, may be considered for treatment.
Stomatitis, mucositis, and dry mouth	Normal integrity of mucous membranes. Absence of oral infections.	Assess oral mucosa every day. Teach client to inspect oral cavity. Remember to remove dentures. Observe for dryness, redness, and white or yellow membrane and the presence of any breaks in the integrity of the tissues. If the client wears dentures, assess to determine if the dentures fit properly. Distinguish stomatitis from candidiasis (presents as soft white patches on mucous membranes.) Maintain good oral hygiene. Use mouth washes of baking soda, H_2O_2, normal saline, or elixir of Benadryl every 2 hours. Use soft bristle toothbrushes, toothettes, or an irrigation syringe as a cleansing agent. Avoid the use of lemon and glycerine swabs for mouth care. Apply topical anesthetics such as viscous xylocaine, chlorseptic, or oxethazaine. Modify diet to avoid hot, spicy, acidic foods. Discourage the use of irritants such as tobacco and alcohol. Encourage water or other liquids at frequent intervals throughout the day or utilize artificial saliva to keep mucous membranes moist. Moisten lips with a small amount of petroleum jelly, baby oil, or cocoa butter.
Anorexia and weight loss	Maintenance or improvement in nutritional intake. Normal body weight.	Provide a well-balanced diet including the basic four with increased protein-calorie intake. Provide a small amount of food every few hours. The client should be gently encouraged to eat but nagging must be avoided at mealtime. Teach the client what to eat rather than stressing the fact that more food should be eaten. (Home-prepared items are often more appealing.) Set realistic goals. Gradually increase the food served at each meal. (A full plate can be overwhelming to the client with anorexia.) Eat primarily high-protein, high-caloric foods. Avoid foods that are filling or gas-forming such as salads, the gas-forming vegetables (cabbage, broccoli), fruits, or beer. Serve all foods attractively and in a pleasant environment. Soft music and a glass of wine will relax the client and stimulate the appetite. Remove all unpleasant sensory stimuli (emesis basin, bed pan, loud noises.) Augment dietary intake with nutritional supplements. Serve them cold in another container other than the can. Teach the client to sip the nutritional supplement slowly between meals.
Diarrhea	Normal bowel elimination pattern.	See Table 34-2.

Table 11-17 (Continued)

Client Problem	Expected Outcome	Nursing Intervention
Alopecia	Cope with loss of hair. Maintain usual lifestyle pattern.	Provide psychological support and inform client as soon as possible of the expected hair loss. Encourage client to select a wig prior to time of hair loss. Begin to wear a wig prior to the time of hair loss. Wear a scarf and/or turban to conceal hair loss. Utilize a mild, protein-based shampoo, cream rinse, and hair conditioner every 4 to 7 days. Excessive shampooing should be avoided. Wash hair with dry shampoo rather than liquid shampoo. Avoid excessive brushing and combing of the hair. Avoid the use of electric hair dryers, curlers, curling rods, and hair spray. When administering drugs which induce alopecia reduce or occlude blood flow to hair follicles by using icepacks, scalp tourniquets, or scalp sphygmomanometers (see text).
Fatigue	Understand the causes of fatigue. Adjust the usual lifestyle pattern to obtain the needed rest.	Inform the client that fatigue is occurring as an expected side effect of therapy and that it usually begins during the first week of therapy, reaches its peak in 2 weeks, continues, and then gradually disappears 2 to 4 weeks after the treatment plan has ended. Encourage the client to rest when fatigue is experienced, and maintain as closely as possible usual lifestyle patterns and pace activities in accordance with the energy level. Force fluid to 3000 mL a day unless contraindicated. Maintain an optimal nutritional status (refer to the nursing interventions for anorexia).
Anemia	Feeling of being rested.	See Table 24-4.
Leukopenia	No signs of infection.	See Table 24-21.
Thrombocytopenia	No bleeding.	See Table 24-13.
Cystitis	No hematuria. No signs of bladder infection.	Drink 3000 mL of fluid a day. A rate of 1000 mL every 8 hours is an effective schedule to follow. Avoid foods, liquids, and substances that may be irritating to the epithelial lining of the bladder, such as coffee and tea; alcoholic beverages; foods containing spices (e.g., pepper and curry); tobacco. Encourage client to void frequently. Maintain the pH of the urine at 7.0 or lower to avoid the development of infection. Ascorbic acid, taken each day, is the most effective way to maintain acidic urine.
Hyperuricemia	Uric acid levels within normal range.	Monitor uric acid levels. Record intake and output every shift. Force fluids to prevent uric acid crystals from causing obstruction. Evaluate urine pH (alkaline urine enhances uric acid excretion). Administer allopurinol (Zyloprim) as ordered. Observe for rash development as an indication of significant drug reaction.
Neurotoxicity (Peripheral neuropathy, ataxia, paresthesias, autonomic nervous system alterations)	No symptoms of peripheral or autonomic nervous system neuropathy.	Evaluate gait for slapping and staggering. Evaluate deep tendon reflexes. Assess fine grasp and coordination. Assist client with hygiene, eating, moving as needed. Maintain a safe environment as extremities may be weak. Encourage use of footboard and active range of motion to extremities. Assess number and character of bowel movements, complaints of gas and abdominal pain, and bowel sounds. Evaluate for urinary incontinence as a sign of bladder atony.
Chronic pain	Maintain maximal level of mental and physical functioning. Gain control of pain.	See Chap. 50.

*This nursing care plan is applicable to the client being treated with radiation therapy and/or chemotherapy. Not all problems apply to every client.

Table 11-18
Sources of Radiation Utilized in Internal Radiation Therapy

Isotope	Emission	Half-Life	External Hazard	Use	Administration
^{131}I (iodine)	Gamma rays	8.05 days	Yes	Thyroid cancer	Systemically by mouth
^{32}P (phosphorous)	Beta particles	14.3 days	No	Malignant pleural or peritoneal effusion	Intracavitary in colloidal form
^{226}Ra (radium)	Alpha particles Beta particles Gamma rays	1,602 years	Yes	Cancer of the uterus, cervix, nasopharynx, bladder	Intracavitary in an applicator
^{192}Ir (iridium)	Beta particles Gamma rays	74.4 days	Yes	Cancers of head and neck Breast cancer	Interstitially Intracavitary in an applicator
^{125}I (iodine)	Gamma rays	60.2 days	Yes	Cancer of neck, tongue, bladder, muscle	Interstitially
^{222}Rn (radon)	Alpha particles Beta particles Gamma rays	3.82 days	Yes	Gynecological cancer	Intracavitary in an applicator
^{137}Cs (cesium)	Beta particles Gamma rays	30.0 years	Yes	Gynecological cancer	Intracavitary in an applicator

Kathleen Gillick, "Radiation Therapy: Internal Radiation," *Cancer Nursing,* **II**(4):314–25 (August 1979).

the source of radiation is in the form of a seed, needle, wire, or tube that is implanted within the tissues of the tumor. The interstitial placement of a radiation source is usually done by the radiation therapist in the operating room. Cobalt 60, cesium 137, iridium 192, gold 198, iodine 125, radon 222, and tantalum 182 are the sources of radiation utilized in this placement technique[29] (Table 11-18). All these radiation sources emit gamma rays. The *half-life* of the particular isotope utilized in the treatment plan determines if the interstitial placement will be temporary (remaining in place for 24 to 72 hours) or permanent. (*Half-life* is used to indicate the rate of decay. It is defined as the amount of time needed for a radioisotope to decay to half its original radioactivity.) The permanent interstitial radiation sources have a short half-life, which results in an inert substance in a short period of time. Radon, gold, and iodine seeds are the radiation sources generally utilized in permanent implants.

Intracavitary placement of a radiation source is the placement of a source of radiation within a particular body cavity by either preloading or afterloading placement. In *preloading placement,* the radiation source is placed within a capsule or applicator and the capsule or applicator is then placed within a particular body cavity. This is done in the operating room. In *afterloading placement,* the empty capsule or applicator is placed in the particular body cavity in the operating room and the client returns to his room for placement of the radiation source within the capsule or applicator. The advantage of the afterloading placement is that it minimizes the number of persons exposed to the radiation source during the time of placement. In both forms of intracavitary placement, an x-ray is taken to determine if the applicator is in the correct position for the treatment plan. The usual sources of radiation for this placement technique are cesium, cobalt, and radon, all of which emit gamma rays. This form of internal radiation therapy is used in the treatment plan of cancer of the uterus, cervix, or vagina (see Fig. 11-13). The intracavitary placement of a source of radiation is always temporary and usually remains in place for 24 to 72 hours.

Safety Precautions for Internal Radiation Specific safety precautions *must* be observed to assure that persons coming in contact with the client being treated with an internal source of radiation emitting gamma rays are exposed to a *minimum* amount of radiation. These safety precautions include:

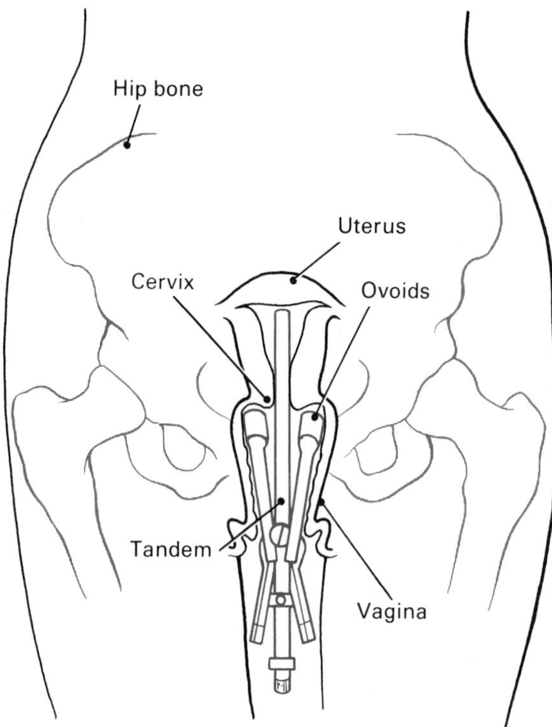

Figure 11-13 Placement of tandem and ovoids into vagina for internal radiation therapy.

1. Admitting the client to a private room (preferably lead-lined) that is fully equipped with everything (including bathroom facilities) the client will need during the period of time the source of radiation remains in place. The client will remain confined to the room until the source of radiation is removed.
2. Informing all persons coming in contact with the client that an internal source of radiation is being used in the treatment plan and that certain specific safety precautions will be necessary.
3. Placing a "Caution—Radiation Area" sign with the radiation symbol (Fig. 11-14) on the door of the client's room and on the client's chart. These yellow and magenta signs and tags are standard and are utilized by all health care agencies that treat clients with internal radiation therapy.
4. Placing in the chart by the radiation safety officer a written list of instructions and precautionary measures. The list includes the type of radiation, time inserted, removal time, as well as name and phone number of radiation safety officer and any special precautions.
5. Restricting persons under the age of 18 and pregnant women from visiting or caring for the client with internal radiation.
6. Utilizing radiation monitors or film badges for caretakers who will come in contact with clients with internal radiation therapy.

Time, Distance, and Shielding All persons coming in contact with the client must utilize the principles of *time, distance,* and *shielding* (see Fig. 59-4). The principle of *time* refers to the amount of time that a person can safely spend in the same room with the client. All client contacts should be arranged so that the greatest amount of care can be accomplished in the shortest period of time. The greatest amount of radiation exposure will occur over the anatomic area of the body that contains the source of radiation. All persons should limit contact with this anatomic site.

The *distance,* or the amount of space between the client and person, has the greatest influence on the maximum exposure time each person can remain in contact with the client. A source of radiation is known to lose its intensity according to the inverse square law. This means that if one remains twice as far from the source of radiation, one will receive one-fourth the amount of radiation exposure. For example, if the maximum exposure time is 6 hours and 40 minutes at a distance of 3 feet from a particular source of radiation, the maximum exposure time will increase to 42 hours and 30 minutes when the distance from the source is increased to 6 feet. The only time any person should be at a distance of 3 feet or less from the source of radiation is when direct care is being given. At all other times the person in the room must remain at a distance of 6 *feet* or greater from the source of radiation.

A few health-care agencies use the principle of *shielding.* Shielding refers to the placement of a thick lead shield between the care givers and the source of radiation. The shield can be a portable or permanent shield. Shielding equipment is very heavy and difficult to manage. It is felt that no practical amount of shielding will completely protect from the penetrating gamma rays. It is felt that if the principles of time and distance are followed exactly and consistently, the additional burden of shielding is not necessary.

The body excreta (urine, feces, perspiration) and soiled linen and dressings are not radioactive. In some health agencies they are collected in the client's room until it can be determined via monitoring that they do not contain a source of radiation that has become dislodged from the site of placement. A sealed lead-lined container should be present in the client's room at all times for immediate use if a dislodgement should occur. When a dislodgement is noted, the source of radiation must be picked up with a pair of long-handled forceps or tongs and placed in the lead container. The radiation source must *never* be picked up with the bare hands and the radiation source must *never* be placed in the sewage system via the sink or toilet. The radiation safety officer and/or the radiation therapist must be notified *immediately* if dislodgement occurs.

The removal of a radiation source must occur at the exact time designated in the treatment plan. The radiation source is gently removed and placed in the sealed lead container that is present in the client's room. The radiation source is then taken to the radiation therapy department and the client and room are monitored to make certain that all the radiation source has been removed. Once the radiation source is removed, all the safety precautions are discontinued, since the client is no longer radioactive.

Unsealed Internal Radiation Unsealed internal radiation therapy is the use of a liquid source of radiation which is administered orally, intravenously, or via instillation into a specific body cavity. This form of internal radiation therapy is metabolized and absorbed by the body and then concentrated in a specific body organ often referred to as the *target organ.* Because the source of radiation is absorbed systemically in the body and metabolized, all body fluids and excreta are considered contaminated by the source of radiation utilized.

Iodine 131 is the most commonly encountered and most widely used absorbed radiation source. It is used to treat thyroid cancer as well as the benign diseases of hyperthyroidism and Graves' disease. This isotope is administered orally and the client is asked to sip the liquid containing iodine 131 through a straw. Gamma rays with a half-life of 8 days are emitted. The same precautions used to avoid radiation exposure for mechanically placed internal radiation therapy are utilized. The body fluids and excreta containing the greatest amount of contamination from the radiation source are the saliva, perspiration, blood, vomitus, and urine. Considering the half-life of the isotope, the excretion rate of 50 percent in the first 24 hours, and the fact that it takes 3 to 5 days before the isotope concentrates in the thyroid gland (target organ), the time of greatest danger from radiation contamination of the body fluids is the first 24 to 96 hours after the administration of the isotope. During this period of time, special precautions must be taken when other persons, equipment, and supplies come in contact with the radioactive body fluids and excreta of the treated client. After 96 hours, it can be assumed that the greatest portion of the radioactivity will be concentrated in the thyroid gland, so special precautions will not be necessary for the remainder of the time the isotope remains radioactive. Since the major portion of the isotope will be excreted by the kidneys, kidney function must be monitored prior to, during, and after the isotope administration. If the kidneys are not functioning within normal limits, it may take a longer period of time to rid the body of the isotope than what the half-life predicts. Care of the client with unsealed radioactive iodine is presented in Table 11-19.

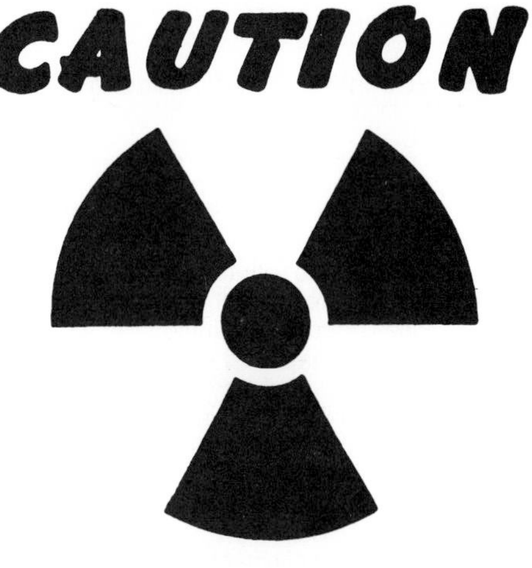

RADIATION AREA

Figure 11-14 Caution: Radiation area warning sign.

Radioactive phosphorus (phosphorus 32) is an isotope which emits beta particles and has a half-life of 14 days. Beta particles present no external hazard to persons coming in contact with the client as long as the isotope is contained within the client. Even though beta particles can penetrate several layers of skin, the particles are shielded by the body fluids and tissues. Phosphorus is administered orally or intravenously in multiple doses over a period of several weeks and is usually used in the treatment of the metastatic lesions of primary breast and prostatic cancer. Soluble phosphorus 32 is given in multiple doses over a period of several weeks. A frequently occurring side effect of soluble phosphorus is leukopenia. Phosphorus 32 in the soluble form is present in all body fluids and is excreted by the kidneys in the urine. All precautions associated with body fluids and urine that were utilized for iodine 131 are to be utilized when soluble phosphorus 32 is administered.

Chemotherapy

Chemotherapy is the systemic treatment of cancer with chemicals (drugs). In the 1940s, chemothera-

Table 11-19
Care of the Client Treated with Radioactive Iodine

During the First 4 Days
1. Utilize the safety measures discussed for sealed mechanically placed radiation (see text).
2. If vomiting occurs, the vomitus will be highly contaminated with gamma radiation. All persons coming in contact with the vomitus are considered contaminated.
3. Take precautionary measures with the urine in accordance with the standards of the health care agency.
4. If the urine is to be deposited directly into the sewage system, the client must flush the toilet three times after each use, making sure no urine is deposited on the toilet seat.
5. If the urine is to be decontaminated prior to disposal in the sewage system, the client utilizes a bedpan and the urine is collected in lead containers and stored for 10 to 40 days prior to placement in the sewage system.
6. Thoroughly wash the hands or anything contaminated with urine with soap, water, and friction for 5 minutes or longer. Use rubber gloves and effective handwashing techniques when coming in contact with the client's urine.
7. Utilize paper plates and plastic eating utensils and discard after meals.
8. Wear hospital gown and store all soiled linen in tightly closed plastic bags. The linen is stored for 10 to 40 days prior to washing.
9. Monitor all articles coming in contact with the client. If contamination is present, all articles must be stored for 10 to 40 days and then checked again for contamination before being used or discarded.
Days 5 through 14
1. Continue to flush the toilet three times after voiding, and utilize effective handwashing techniques.
2. Instruct the client to sleep alone.

Adapted from J. Yasko, "Radiotherapy: A Patient/Significant Other Teaching Plan," in M. L. Donovan (ed.), *A Guide to Patient Education*, Appleton Century Crofts, New York, 1981, pp. 101–102.

py was in the infancy stages. Nitrogen mustard, a chemical warfare agent in World War II, was used in the treatment of acute leukemia and a folic acid antimetabolite (5-FU) was found to have antitumor activity. In the 1950s considerable experimentation with single drug therapy was begun and in the 1960s the emphasis was on the development and use of combination chemotherapy. By the 1970s chemotherapy was established as an effective treatment modality for cancer. It is now used as the treatment of many solid tumors. Chemotherapy has gone from a palliative, "last-ditch effort" treatment modality to a treatment modality that can cure certain cancers, control other cancers for long periods of time, and offer palliative symptom relief when cure or control no longer is possible (Fig. 11-15).

Effect of chemotherapy on cells

The effect of chemotherapy is at the cellular level. As discussed earlier, all cells (cancer cells and normal cells) enter the cell cycle for replication and proliferation (Fig. 11-1). The effects of the chemotherapeutic

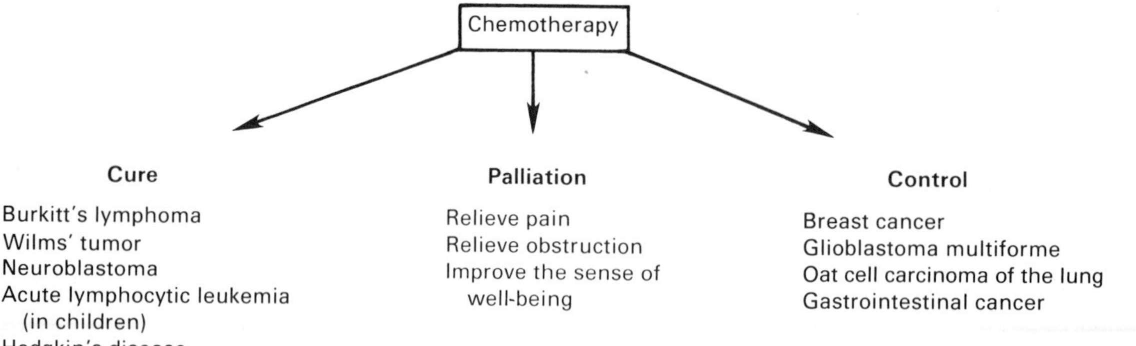

Figure 11-15 Goals of chemotherapy.

agents are described in relationship to the cell cycle. The two major categories of chemotherapeutic drugs are cell cycle nonspecific and cell cycle specific.

Cell Cycle Nonspecific Chemotherapeutic Drugs These drugs have their effect on the cells that are in the process of cellular replication and proliferation as well as on the cells that are in the resting phase (G_0).

Cell Cycle Specific Chemotherapeutic Drugs These drugs have their effect on cells that are in the process of cellular replication/proliferation (G_1, S_1, G_2 or M). The cell cycle specific chemotherapeutic drugs can be categorized more specifically into *phase-specific chemotherapeutic agents.* These drugs are only effective at one specific phase of the cell cycle.

The goal of chemotherapy is to reduce the number of cancer cells present in the primary tumor site(s) and the cancer cells present in metastatic tumor sites. Several factors will determine the response of cancer cells to chemotherapy. These include:

1. *Mitotic rate of the tissue from which the tumor arises.* The more rapid the mitotic rate, the greater the response to chemotherapy. Chemotherapy is the treatment of choice in acute leukemia, choriocarcinoma of the placenta, Wilms' tumor (used in conjunction with surgery), and neuroblastoma. These cancer cells have a rapid rate of cellular proliferation.
2. *Size of the tumor.* The smaller the number of cancer cells, the greater the response to chemotherapy.
3. *Age of the tumor.* The younger the tumor, the greater the response to chemotherapy. Young tumors have a greater percentage of proliferating cells.
4. *Location of the tumor.* Certain anatomic sites provide a protected environment from the effects of chemotherapy. For example, only a few drugs cross the blood/brain barrier (nitrosureas and bleomycin).
5. *Physiologic and psychological status of the host.* A state of optimum health and a positive attitude will allow the client to better withstand aggressive treatment with chemotherapy.

When the cancer first begins to grow, most of the cells are actively dividing. As the tumor increases in size, more and more cells become inactive and convert to a resting state (G_0). Since most chemotherapeutic agents are most effective against dividing cells, cells can escape death by staying in the G_0 phase.[30] The main problem in cancer chemotherapy is the presence of drug-resistant resting and noncycling cells.[31]

Classification of chemotherapy

Chemotherapy drugs are categorized or classified according to their structure and mechanisms of action (see Table 11-20 and Fig. 11-16). Each of the drugs in a particular drug classification has many similarities, but major differences in the drugs are also evident.

Methods of administration

Chemotherapy can be administered via a variety of routes (see Table 11-21). The oral and intravenous routes are the most common. Some guidelines for intravenous administration are:

1. Start an intravenous infusion of normal saline or 5% dextrose in water or saline with a small lumen, short needle, or catheter.
2. Select a vein that is large enough to promote infusion without irritating the intima of the vein. When a vesicant is administered, avoid the veins located in the hand, wrist, and antecubital area.
3. Check for a blood return prior to infusing the chemotherapy drug, especially if the drug is a vesicant.
4. Slowly push those drugs that are to be given via the push or bolus method. Pause 30 to 60 seconds and allow the intravenous infusion to flush the vein and again gently push $\frac{1}{2}$ to 1 mL of the medication. Repeat until the medication has been given and allow the intravenous infusion to flush the vein for several minutes.
5. Stop the intravenous infusion *immediately* if the client complains of a burning or stinging pain, especially if a vesicant is being administered. Under these circumstances, the infusion should be discontinued even in the presence of a good blood return.

If extravasation occurs, (1) stop the intravenous infusion immediately; (2) notify the physician; (3) pack the involved area in ice for 30 minutes, remove, and apply warm soaks for 30 minutes. Alternate cold and warm soaks every 30 minutes for 48 hours. (4) Follow other established protocols (some centers treat extravasation by injecting sodium bicarbonate and hydrocortisone into the area of infiltration and then applying hydrocortisone cream).

Pain is the cardinal symptom of extravasation, although it has been known to occur without causing pain. Swelling, redness, and the presence of vesicles on the skin are other early signs of the presence of

Table 11-20
Classification of Chemotherapy Drugs

Mechanisms of Action	Examples
Alkylating Agents	
Cycle nonspecific Damage DNA by causing breaks in the double strand helix (similar to the effect of radiation therapy). If repair does not occur, the cells will die immediately (cytocidal) or when they attempt to divide (cytostatic).	Mechlorethamine (Nitrogen Mustard) Cyclophosphamide (Cytoxan) Chlorambucil (Leukeran) Melphalan (Alkeran) Triethylene thiophosphoramide (Thiotepa) Busulfan (Myleran)
Antimetabolites	
Cycle specific Interfere with the synthesis of DNA by mimicking certain essential cellular metabolites which the cell incorporates into the synthesis of DNA. The cells will die immediately (cytocidal).	Methotrexate (Amethopterin) Cytosine arabinoside (Ara-C, Cytosar) 5-Fluorouracil (5-FU) 6-Mercaptopurine (6-MP) Thioguanine (6-TG)
Antitumor Antibiotics	
Cycle nonspecific Modify the function of DNA and interfere with the transcription of RNA. The cells will die immediately (cytocidal) or when they attempt to divide (cytostatic).	Doxorubicin (Adriamycin) Bleomycin (Blenoxane) Mitomycin (Mutamycin) Daunorubicin (Daunomycin)
Plant Alkaloids	
Cycle specific Interrupt cellular replication in mitosis at metaphase. The cells will die immediately (cytocidal).	Vinblastine (Velban) Vincristine (Oncovin)
Nitrosureas	
Cycle nonspecific Effect similar to the alkylating agents and also blocks specific enzymes needed for the synthesis of purine. The cells will die immediately (cytocidal) or when they attempt to divide (cytostatic).	Carmustine (BCNU) Lomustine (CCNU) Semustine (Methyl CCNU) Streptozotocin (STZ)
Corticosteroids	
Cycle nonspecific Disruption of the cell membrane and the inhibition of the synthesis of RNA to protein. Lysis of the circulating lymphocytes. Inhibit mitosis. Depression of the immune system. Increase the feeling of well-being.	Meticorten (Prednisone) Dexamethasone (Decadron)
Hormones	
Cycle nonspecific Stimulate the process of cellular differentiation; metastatic lesions are less able to survive in the unfavorable environment. Decrease the process of cellular proliferation.	Androgens [Testosterone, Fluoxymesterone (Halotestin)] Estrogens [Diethylstilbestrol (DES)] Progestins (Provera, Delalutin)
Miscellaneous	
Heavy metal—effect on DNA is similar to the alkylating agents.	Cis-Platinum diammine dichloride (Cis-Platinum, Platinol)
Destroys the exogenous supply of L-asparagine, which is needed for cellular proliferation. Normal cells can synthesize, but cannot be synthesized by cancer cells.	L-Asparaginase (Elspar)
Effect on DNA similar to alkylating agents. Also blocks the incorporation of thymidine into DNA.	Hydroxyurea (Hydrea)
Suppresses mitosis at interphase; also has an effect similar to the alkylating agents.	Procarbazine (Matulane, Natulan)
Nonsteroidal antihormones that are used in breast cancer.	Nafoxidine, Tamoxifen (Nolvadex)
Alkylating activity. Inhibition of DNA synthesis. Purine synthesis blocking.	Imidazole (DTIC)

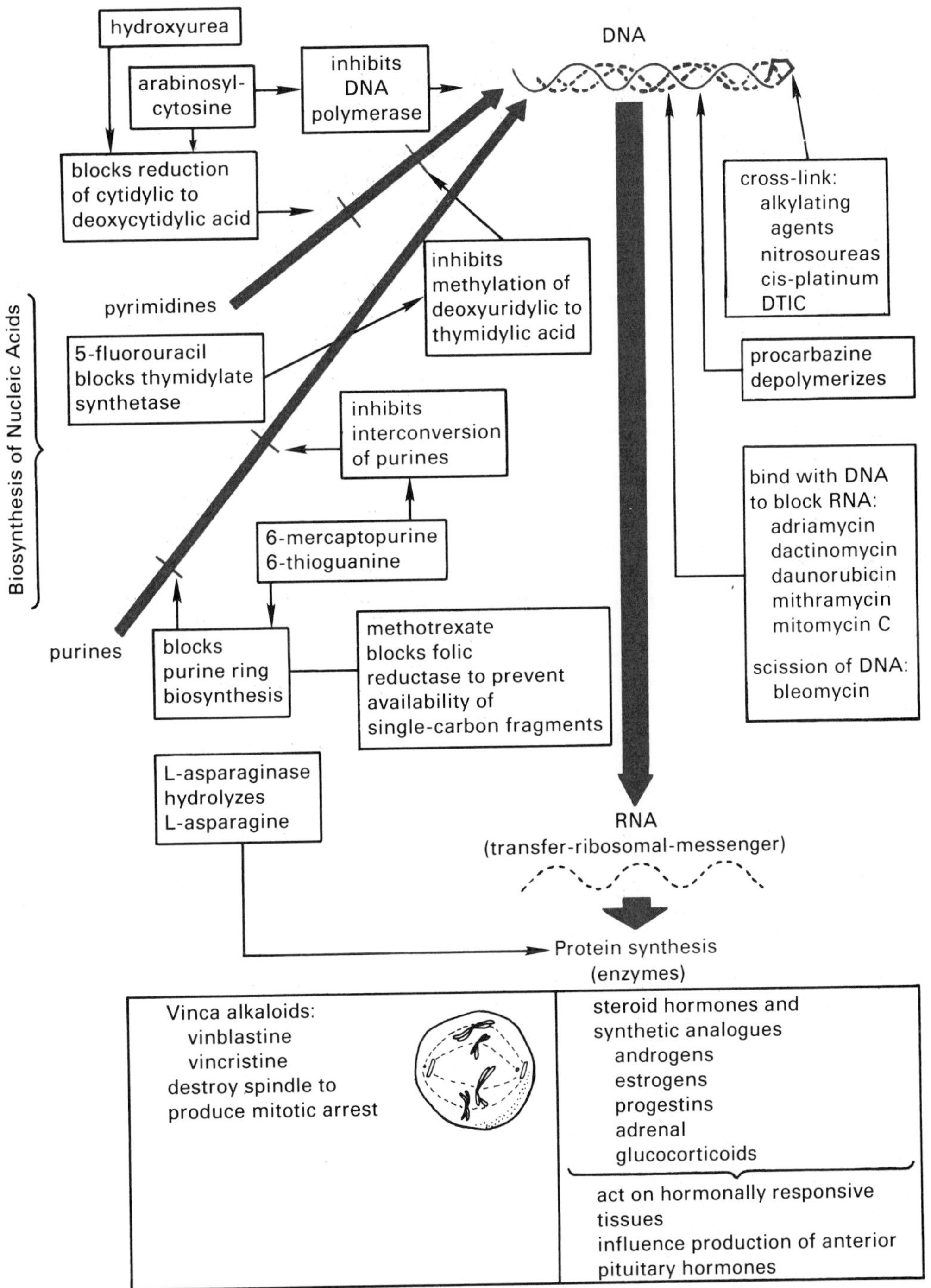

Figure 11-16 Actions of chemotherapeutic drugs. [*Adapted from I. Krakoff, Ca-ACJClin,* **27:**130 (1977).]

Table 11-21
Methods of Chemotherapy Administration

Method	Examples
Oral	Cyclophosphamide (Cytoxan)
Intramuscular	Bleomycin
Intravenous	Adriamycin, vincristine
Intracavitary (pleural, peritoneal)	Radioisotopes, alkylating agents
Intrathecal (meningeal leukemia)	Methotrexate, cytosine arabinoside
Intraarterial	DTIC, 5-FU, methotrexate
Perfusion	Alkylating agents
Continuous infusion	5-FU, methotrexate, cytosine arabinoside
Subcutaneous	Cytosine arabinoside
Topical	5-FU cream
Intraperitoneal	Methotrexate, 5-FU

extravasation. After a few days, the tissue will begin to ulcerate and necrosis will be evident. The process has the potential to progress to a deep, wide crater that often warrants closure with skin grafts. This is a very serious problem that may be life-threatening if infection occurs.

Intracavitary therapy is used primarily to treat ascites and pleural effusions. *Perfusion* therapy attempts to isolate an extremity using tourniquets to obstruct venous return. This approach is used to treat malignant melanoma. Hepatic artery infusion has been used in hepatoma and liver metastases. *Continuous infusion* has been used for cancer of the head and neck, liver, pelvis, and acute myelocytic leukemia.

Effects of chemotherapy on normal tissues

Chemotherapeutic agents are unable to selectively distinguish between normal cells and cancer cells. When normal cells are destroyed, the client experiences certain signs and symptoms that are the expected side effects or toxic effects of chemotherapy. Effects of chemotherapy are due to (1) destruction of cells with a rapid rate of cellular proliferation (see Table 11-22), (2) response of the body to the products of cellular destruction (cellular waste products in circulation may cause fatigue, anorexia, and taste alterations), and (3) specific drug toxicities (Table 11-23). Some drugs possess an affinity for a particular tissue due to the processes of metabolism or excretion (see Table 11-17 for examples).

Chemotherapy treatment plan

When chemotherapy is used in the treatment of cancer, several drugs are usually given in combination. Single drug chemotherapy is rarely chosen for a treatment plan today. The drugs given are carefully selected to most effectively kill the cancer cells while allowing the normal cells to repair themselves and proliferate. The dosage of each drug is carefully calculated according to the body weight or the body surface area of the client being treated. The choice of the drugs selected to be given together to treat a particular cancer is based on the following principles of combination chemotherapy:

Table 11-22
Cells with Rapid Rate of Proliferation

Cells and Generation Time	Effect of Cell Destruction
Bone marrow stem cell, 6–24 h	Myelosuppression: infection/bleeding/anemia
Neutrophils, 12 h	Leukopenia, infection
Epithelial cells lining the gastrointestinal tract, 12–24 h	Anorexia, stomatitis, esophagitis, nausea/vomiting, diarrhea
Cells of the hair follicle, 24 h	Alopecia
Ova/testes, 24–36 h	Sexual dysfunction

1. The drugs utilized in the treatment plan are effective against the cancer being treated.
2. When drugs are given in combination, a synergistic effect occurs.
3. The drug combination includes drugs that are cycle specific and cycle nonspecific and which have different mechanisms of action.
4. The drugs combined include drugs that have different toxic side effects.
5. The drug combination includes drugs whose nadir occurs at different time intervals. A *nadir* of a particular drug is the point in time when the effect and toxic side effects of the drug are at the greatest degree possible. The nadir of most chemotherapeutic agents ranges from 5 to 28 days.

Combination chemotherapy can only reduce tumor cell mass to numbers ranging from 10^3 to 10^5 cells. Natural immunity is capable of destroying 10^3 to 10^5 cancer cells. Because chemotherapeutic agents are immunosuppressive, the client's immune system can handle less than 10^5 cancer cells.[32]

The MOPP protocol, utilized extensively in the treatment of Hodgkin's disease, is an example of a combination chemotherapy treatment regimen.

M=Nitrogen mustard:
- cycle nonspecific
- alkylating agent
- toxic side effects—myelosuppression, nausea, vomiting, alopecia
- nadir—7 to 14 days

Table 11-23
Toxic Side Effects of Chemotherapy

	Myelo-suppression	Stomatitis	Nausea and Vomiting	Alopecia	Vesicant	Allergic Reaction	Other Specific Toxicities
Actinomycin D (Cosmegen)	+	+	+	+	+	0	Diarrhea
5-Azacytidine	+	+	+	0	0	0	Hepatotoxicity
Bleomycin (Blenoxane)	±	±	0	+	0	+	Pulmonary toxicity Skin Rash
Busulfan (Myleran)	+	0	±	0	0	0	Pulmonary fibrosis
Carmustine (BCNU)	+	0	+	0	+	0	Hepatotoxicity
Chlorambucil (Leukeran)	+	0	±	0	0	0	
Cis-Platinum (Platinol)	+	0	+	0	0	+	Nephrotoxicity Peripheral neuropathy Ototoxicity
Cyclophosphamide (Cytoxan)	+	±	+	+	0	0	Sterile hemorrhagic cystitis
Cytosine arabinoside (Cytosar, Ara-C)	+	0	+	+	0	0	Hepatotoxicity
Dacarbazine (DTIC)	+	0	+	0	+	0	Hypotension
Daunorubicin (Daunomycin)	+	+	+	+	+	0	Cardiotoxicity
Dianhydrogalact-itol (Galactitol)	+	0	+	0	+	0	
Dibromomannitol (DMB)	+	0	±	0	0	0	
Diethylstilbestrol (DES)	0	0	+	0	0	0	CHF
Doxorubicin (Adriamycin)	+	+	+	+	+	0	Cardiotoxicity, diarrhea
5-Fluorouracil	+	+	±	0	0	0	Diarrhea
Fluoxymesterone (Halotestin)	0	0	+	0	0	0	Masculinization
Hexamethylmelamine (HXM)	+	0	+	+	0	0	Peripheral neuropathy
Hydroxyurea (Hydrea)	+	+	+	+	0	0	
L-Asparaginase (Elspar)	0	0	+	0	0	+	Major organ failure
Lomustine (CCNU)	+	+	+	±	0	0	Hepatotoxicity
Megestrol acetate (Megace)	0	0	0	0	0	0	
L-Phenylalanine Mustard (Melphalan, L-Pam)	+	0	+	0	0	0	
6-Mercaptopurine (6 MP)	+	+	+	0	0	0	Decrease dose if on allopurinol
Methotrexate (MTX, Amethopterin)	+	+	±	±	0	0	Nephrotoxicity
Mithramycin (Mithracin)	+	+	+	0	+	0	Hemorrhagic tendency
Mitomycin (Mutamycin)	+	+	+	+	+	0	Nephrotoxicity
Neocarzinostatin	+	0	+	+	+	+	
Mechlorethamine (Nitrogen Mustard)	+	0	+	+	+	0	
Oxymethalone (Androl-50)	0	0	+	0	0	0	Masculinization

Table 11-23 (Continued)

	Myelo-suppression	Stomatitis	Nausea and Vomiting	Alopecia	Vesicant	Allergic Reaction	Other Specific Toxicities
Piperazinedione	+	0	+	0	+	0	
Prednisolone	0	0	0	0	0	0	Steroid side effects
Prednisone	0	0	0	0	0	0	Steroid side effects
Procarbazine hydrochloride (Matulane)	+	±	+	0	0	0	Monoamine oxidase inhibitor
Semustine (Methyl CCNU)	+	+	+	0	0	0	
Streptonigrin	+	0	+	0	0	0	
Streptozotocin (STZ)	+	0	+	±	+	0	Nephrotoxicity
6-Thioguanine (6-TG)	+	±	±	0	0	0	
Uracil mustard	+	0	+	0	0	0	
Vinblastine (Velban)	+	+	±	±	+	0	Neurotoxicity
Vincristine (Oncovin)	0	0	0	+	+	0	Neurotoxicity
Vindesine (DVA)	+	+	+	+	+	0	Neurotoxicity
VP-16	+	0	+	+	0	+	

Adapted from Cheryl Lane, *Cancer Chemotherapy Guidelines*, Oncology Research Center, Bowman Gray School of Medicine, Wake Forest University, Winston-Salem, N.C. 1980.

O=Oncovin (vincristine):
- phase specific
- plant alkaloid
- toxic side effects—neurotoxicity, alopecia
- nadir—not known

P=Procarbazine:
- cycle specific
- MAO inhibitor
- toxic side effects—myelosuppression, nausea, vomiting
- nadir—2 to 8 weeks

P=Prednisone:
- hormone
- toxic side effects—steroid effects
- nadir—not known

The agents in this drug protocol differ in mechanisms of action, toxic side effects, and nadir, but the combination is synergistic in nature and effectively destroys the cancer cells present in the early stages of Hodgkin's disease.

The drugs are given according to a specific schedule that includes a time of drug administration and a time of rest from drug administration. The rest period is necessary to allow the normal body cells that have been destroyed to proliferate and repair the damaged tissue. The example in Table 11-24 describes a typical drug schedule. This drug schedule is repeated a specific number of times. Most chemotherapy treatment plans extend for 6 months to 2 years or more. The client is evaluated prior to the administration of each course of chemotherapy to determine if the normal cells have proliferated to a sufficient degree.

Often, the most difficult decision to make is when to stop the administration of chemotherapy. The client is evaluated according to the following criteria:

Complete remission—Complete absence of all evidence of cancer and a return to the usual performance status. The duration of a complete remission must exceed 1 month.

Partial remission—Regression of 50 percent or more of the disease process without evidence of progression and with subjective improvement. The duration of a partial remission is usually several months.

Improvement—Regression of 25 to 50 percent of the disease process with subjective improvement.

No Response—Regression of 25 percent or less of the disease with no subjective improvement.

Progression—Progression of the disease process.

Table 11-24
MOPP Chemotherapeutic Drug Schedule

	Days														
Drug	1	2	3	4	5	6	7	8	9	10	11	12	13	14	15 — 28
Nitrogen Mustard (intravenous administration)	↔							↔							No drugs given
Oncovin (intravenous administration)	↔							↔							
Procarbazine (oral administration)	←													→	
Prednisone (oral administration)	←													→	

In the presence of a complete remission that has extended for a period of time, the chemotherapy is usually discontinued and the client is evaluated at frequent intervals. When partial remission or improvement occurs, the same treatment plan or a revised treatment plan is administered over a long period of time (several years) and the client is evaluated at frequent intervals. No response or progression of disease warrants a change in the treatment plan or a decision to utilize treatment for palliation.

Marijuana to control nausea and vomiting

Research has indicated that tetrahydrocannabinol (THC), an ingredient in marijuana, is effective in preventing and/or minimizing the nausea and vomiting that occur in certain individuals as a side effect of radiation therapy or chemotherapy. In addition to controlling nausea and vomiting, marijuana also produces an elevation of mood, a tranquilizing effect, an enhancement of appetite, and a reduction in the sensation of pain. All these effects of marijuana can be of benefit to the client being treated for cancer. However, the individual response to marijuana is variable.[33]

The nurse must be aware that unless marijuana is being utilized as part of a research study, its use is *illegal* in most states. In a few states, marijuana has been legalized for medical purposes. At the present time, bills are before other state legislatures to legalize marijuana for medical use.

Clients who have chosen to use marijuana should be taught to:[34]

Avoid the use of other antiemetics during the time when marijuana is being utilized.

Begin using marijuana 1 to 2 hours prior to receiving radiation therapy and chemotherapy and continue to use it for 2 to 4 hours after the treatment.

Avoid the use of antihistamines when using marijuana.

Use small amounts of marijuana and gradually increase the amount for an increased effect.

When marijuana is inhaled in smoking, three to five puffs will begin to control nausea and vomiting in 5 to 10 minutes and the effect will last approximately 2 hours.

When marijuana is ingested in food such as brownies, cookies, or tea or taken in capsule form, the nausea-controlling effect begins in 45 to 120 minutes and lasts 2 to 6 hours.

When marijuana is used in suppository form, the nausea control begins in 30 minutes and lasts 2 to 6 hours.

Nursing management related to chemotherapy

The role of the nurse in cancer chemotherapy has greatly expanded during the past decade. Regardless of the health care agency setting, the nurse will meet individuals who are receiving or have received chemotherapy. One of the most important responsibilities of the nurse is differentiating between toxic effects of the drug and progression of the malignant process. The nurse also needs to be able to differentiate between tolerable side effects and acute toxic effects of chemotherapeutic agents. For example, nausea and vomiting are expected side effects of many drugs. However, if paresthesia presents with the use of vincristine, or signs of heart failure present with the use of Adriamycin, these need to be reported to the physician so the drug dosages can be modified or discontinued. Specific nursing measures related to problems associated with chemotherapy are presented in the nursing care plan for the cancer client (Table 11-17).

It is important to monitor results of laboratory studies for the client receiving chemotherapy. Particular attention should be given to the white blood cell, platelet, and red blood cell counts. If the white blood cell count falls to less than 1 to 2000/μL, the client may need to be put in reverse isolation or the drug dosage may need to be modified or discontinued. Granulocyte transfusions may be indicated if the white blood cell count falls to less than 500/μL. Every measure possible needs to be taken to prevent infections in a client with leukopenia (Table 24-21). If the platelet count falls to less than 50,000/μL, the client must be assessed for any signs of bleeding and measures should be taken to prevent bleeding (Table 24-13). The administration of platelet transfusions may be necessary. Red blood cell transfusions may also be indicated for symptomatic anemia.

Uric acid and creatinine levels are usually monitored weekly. Optimal hydration is important to prevent uric acid crystals from causing obstructive uropathy and allopurinol is often administered as a prophylactic measure. Other diagnostic monitoring depends on the type of drug. For example, an ECG is performed and cardiac ejection fractions are measured to monitor potential cardiotoxic effects of Adriamycin and Daunomycin.

Client Education Client education is an extremely important part of the nursing role related to the use of chemotherapy. To decrease the fear and anxiety often associated with chemotherapy, the client must be taught what to expect during a course of treatment. The client's attitude toward treatment should be explored so any misconceptions or fears can be discussed. The client needs to be told that some of the effects of chemotherapy will make him feel sick, perhaps sicker. This is a discouraging realization. Therefore, the client must be reassured that this is a temporary situation and the client should be feeling better within a few weeks after chemotherapy is discontinued. The client should also be informed that supportive care (e.g., antiemetics, antidiarrheals) will be provided as needed.

Prevention of Hair Loss Alopecia due to the administration of chemotherapeutic agents is usually reversible. The degree and duration of the hair loss depends on the dose of the chemotherapeutic agent, the duration of the treatment, and the nutritional status of the client. At times, the hair will begin to grow back while the client is receiving chemotherapeutic agents, but generally, the hair cells grow back when the agents are discontinued. Often, the new hair growth will be of a different color and texture than the hair that was lost.

Often, hair loss caused by certain chemotherapeutic drugs (e.g., cyclophosphamide, Adriamycin) administered via the bolus intravenous route, can be minimized or prevented by using a scalp sphygmomanometer, tourniquet, and/or hypothermia.[35] The scalp tourniquet/sphygmomanometer is applied around the hairline to decrease the blood flow through the superficial scalp arteries prior to, during, and for 20 minutes after the drug has been infused. (This technique protects hair follicles from high concentrations of cytotoxic drugs.) To prevent tissue damage when the sphygmomanometer is utilized, the cuff should never be more than 70 mmHg above the normal systolic blood pressure. When hypothermia is utilized, the hypothermic agent is applied at least 10 minutes prior to, during, and for 20 to 30 minutes after the chemotherapeutic agent has been infused.

Scalp tourniquets and hypothermia should not be used for clients undergoing chemotherapy for hematopoietic malignancies. When these devices are used, chemotherapeutic agents may be prevented from reaching the cancer cells circulating in the vascular system of the scalp. Therefore, these cancer cells would be protected from the effects of the chemotherapeutic agents.

Counseling Regarding Sex and Sexuality Sexual dysfunction may be manifested as temporary or permanent sterility, disruption in the menstrual cycle (for the female), temporary or permanent impotence (for the male), or chromosomal damage leading to possible genetic mutation.

The client (either male or female) should be instructed to use an effective means of birth control during the time of treatment with chemotherapy and/or radiation and for 1 to 2 years after treatment. This is necessary to avoid birth defects due to chromosomal damage, to allow the sperm count to return to normal, and to determine the expected prognosis of the client. Sexual or genetic counseling is necessary prior to the conception of a child to determine the risk of chromosomal damage.

Sexual relations can be continued in the usual patterns during and after the treatment plan if an effective method of birth control is utilized. It may be necessary to alter the time of day chosen for sexual relations if fatigue is present. Early morning may be the time of day the client feels most rested.

Denuding of the epithelial lining of the vagina may result in inflammation, edema, and ulceration. Sexual intercourse should be avoided if mucositis or ulceration are present. Sitz baths or sitting in a tub of warm water will provide some degree of comfort. A steroid-based cream ordered by the physician may also provide comfort. A water-based lubrication may be used during the time of intercourse to increase vaginal lubrication. Lubrication is necessary to prevent trauma to the vaginal lining and to prevent discomfort or pain.

The client should be encouraged to use other forms of physical contact to obtain sexual pleasure during the period of time when there is disruption in sexual functioning. Hugging, caressing, touching, and quiet talking can provide sexual pleasure when sexual intercourse is not possible. The client's partner must be included in all teaching and counseling sessions to be fully informed of the temporary or permanent changes in the client's sexual functioning. Both client and partner must understand that adjustments in sexual functioning patterns will take time, patience, and understanding.

Immunotherapy

Immunotherapy as a treatment modality is based on the ability of certain substances to stimulate the immune system. The object is to direct the response against cancer cells. Immunotherapy is most effectively used against a small tumor mass. This is why it is used as adjuvant therapy with surgery, radiation, or chemotherapy to assist the body in destroying any remaining cancer cells.

Immunotherapy has been effective when used in the treatment plan for bronchogenic carcinoma, malignant melanoma, acute leukemia, bladder carcinoma, head and neck tumors, colon carcinoma, osteogenic sarcoma, Hodgkin's disease, and various skin cancers.[36] For immunotherapy to be most effective, the tumor bulk or load should be small, individuals should have optimal nutritional status, and the immune system should not be severely depressed by other therapy.

Evaluation of the immune response

Several parameters are utilized to evaluate the status of the immune response, including the number of circulating lymphocytes (normal level is 15 to 40 percent of the total white blood cells), and response to skin testing.

Several common antigens can be used for skin testing. They are injected intradermally and are used to assess the cellular immune response (delayed hypersensitivity). Several antigens that can be used are:

1. Mumps virus
2. Purified protein derivative (PPD)
3. Streptokinase/streptodornase (SKSD)
4. Dinitrochlorobenzene (DNCB)
5. *Candida*

The inner aspect of the forearm is the usual intradermal injection site. The injection site should be marked with ink and the client instructed not to remove the markings. The injection site is evaluated at the end of 24 hours and again at the end of 48 hours. The presence of a raised erythematous wheal with induration (hardened area) indicates that the cellular immune system is intact and functioning properly. The size of induration determines the degree of cellular immune system competence. To measure the size of induration, draw a line with a pen from the top to the bottom and from one side to the other side of the wheal. The indurated area of the wheal will not absorb the ink and it is this area that is measured. Depleted capacity to mount a cellular immune response is indicated by an induration of less than 15 mm. From 10 to 15 mm the depletion is considered mild; from 5 to 10 mm, moderate; and if 5 mm or less, severe.

A positive response to one or more of the antigens indicates a normal cellular immune response. Immunotherapy is most effective in the client with a competent functioning immune system. When induration is 5 mm or less for all antigens, the client is said to be *anergic*. This means that the client's cellular immune system is not functioning adequately or actively. It has been determined that clients who are anergic have a poorer prognosis than clients who are immunocompetent.

Types of immunotherapy

The two basic types of immunotherapy are *passive* and *active*. *Passive* immunotherapy involves the administration of antibody, usually in the form of plasma. *Active* immunotherapy is the injection of antigen to stimulate the body's natural immune response against cancer cells. Active immunotherapy may be further divided into *specific* or *nonspecific*. *Specific* immunotherapy involves the use of inactivated tumor cells or their derivatives. *Nonspecific* immunotherapy involves the use of nontumor antigens such as vaccines.

Passive Immunotherapy This method involves collecting antibodies or lymphocytes from clients who have or have had certain cancers and are thought to be immune to these specific cancers. After the serum (containing antibodies) or lymphocytes is collected, it can be injected directly into the recipient with the same type of cancer. Another technique of administration is to treat the collected material in a manner to extract the material that is responsible for the immunity and injecting this substance *(transfer factor).* A major problem with this form of immunotherapy is the recipient's rejection of the foreign cells. Passive immunotherapy has a very limited role in the treatment of cancer at this time.[37]

Active Specific Immunotherapy This procedure is largely experimental and involves the injection of a vaccine produced from the client's cancer cells or from donor cells which closely resemble the client's cancer cells. These vaccines are usually administered intradermally and the client may experience pruritus, inflammation, and pain at the injection site as well as fever, chills, and general malaise.

Active Nonspecific Immunotherapy This method is the most commonly used form of immunotherapy. This approach uses vaccines, usually BCG (bacillus Calmette-Guérin), to stimulate the immune response. BCG is a weakened derivative of the bacteria which causes tuberculosis in cattle. This substance was utilized for many years to vaccinate humans against tuberculosis. The exact mechanisms by which BCG stimulates the immune system is not well understood. It seems to be effective in promoting both cell-mediated immunity and antibody production. It may be effective in partially reversing the immunosuppressant effects of radiation and chemotherapy as well as that due to the malignant process.

Other active nonspecific immunotherapy agents include (1) *Corynebacterium parvum,* a killed suspension of bacteria; (2) *methanol extracted residue* (MER), an insoluble residue of BCG vaccine; and (3) *levamisole,* an antihelminthic that is not an immunostimulant but which has the capacity to restore an impaired immune status to normal.[38] These agents are still under investigation and as yet have not been shown to have a substantial impact on human cancer.

Administration of BCG

BCG can be administered in many different ways: orally, intradermally, scarification (using multiple etched scratches), multiple puncture (prong) technique, intralesional injection, inhalation, and intracavitary injection. BCG can be given in any area of the body, depending on the site of the primary tumor. Optimal results may be obtained when the vaccine is deposited in the immediate vicinity of the tumor. For example, a client with a melanoma on the upper back may receive BCG in that region or the BCG may be injected into the lesion. When injected into a lesion, BCG has been shown effective in causing regression of malignant melanoma.[39]

Most clients tolerate therapy well but several reactions usually occur when BCG is administered. *Local reactions* include pruritus, erythema, pustule formation, and pain at the injection site. If the immune response is present, these reactions will increase in severity with each subsequent injection of BCG. *Systemic reactions* include fever, chills, malaise, myalgia, and enlargement of regional lymph nodes. The client should be instructed about the lymphadenopathy so that this finding is not misinterpreted as an extension of the disease process. Occasionally the lymph nodes become pustular. Liver dysfunction with elevated enzyme levels and granulomatous hepatitis have also been reported. The client must keep the injection site dry and not use ointment, lotions, or dressings on the site. Even though pruritus may be present, to prevent infection and scarring, the site should not be scratched. The site should not be exposed to the sun.

Interferon

Interferon can be considered a form of active nonspecific immunotherapy. It is a naturally occurring protein that is produced by cells in response to a viral infection and other immune stimuli. The protein is released from cells that have been infected by a virus and taken up by neighboring noninfected cells (Fig. 11-17). Interferon is thought to protect these neighboring cells from viral invasion and replication.[40]

Interferon has also been found to have an antitumor effect. It inhibits cellular growth, has a selective effect on cellular protein synthesis, and activates the natural killer cells.[41]

The three sources of interferon are from leukocytes, fibroblasts (cells that form connective tissue), and T lymphocytes (called immune interferon). Since interferon is species-specific, it is effective only in the cells of the same species in which it was produced. Interferon is not virus-specific and has been shown to be active against a wide variety of viruses. This discovery was made when the original researchers tried unsuccessfully to induce a second viral infection in an animal already infected with a virus.

Interferon has been used clinically against hepatitis B, upper respiratory infections, and some forms of cancer. One of the main problems with its use is obtaining sufficient quantities because it is produced in minute quantities in living cells and extracting it is difficult and costly. Another problem with interferon's clinical use is its relatively short life span when in circulation. Because of this characteristic, a person needs repeated injections every 12 to 24 hours to maintain effective blood levels.

Interferon is administered intramuscularly daily for a specified period that may range from 1 to 2 months. The most common side effects are local erythema and discomfort at the injection site. There may be an initial rise in temperature, especially with high doses. Systemic reactions include malaise, fatigue, nausea, anorexia, reversible leukopenia, and thrombocytopenia.

Clients or a family member are often taught how to administer the substance intramuscularly. Acetaminophen (Tylenol) is the drug of choice to treat elevated temperatures that occur with interferon therapy. Aspirin should be avoided because of its anticoagulant effect. Small, frequent meals and preparation of favorite foods may be helpful for the anorexic client.

Thymosin

Thymosin, a purified fraction of bovine thymus, can also be considered a form of active nonspecific immunotherapy. It acts to stimulate the maturation of T-lymphocyte precursors. Thymosin has been shown to be effective in increasing the number of T cells in circulation in persons with initially low T-cell numbers. Individuals with normal T-cell levels are not likely to benefit from thymosin therapy.[42]

Thymosin is administered subcutaneously two times a week for a period of about 6 weeks. Local reactions may include local irritation, erythema, urticaria, and swelling. Systemic reactions that may occur include fever, chills, myalgia, and hypersensitivity reactions to bovine extract.

Nursing management related to immunotherapy

The client who receives immunotherapy has usually experienced multiple diagnostic and treatment regimens prior to being considered for immunotherapy. The client needs to be honestly told that immunotherapy is at the present time still in the early stages of development and its effectiveness is still being studied. Usually immunotherapy is not debilitating and the client experiences very little discomfort or only for a short period of time. This knowledge might be a welcome relief to some individuals who have experienced multiple side effects from radiation therapy and chemotherapy.

The client needs to seek medical care if the temperature exceeds 38°C, if he experiences severe malaise, or if he develops a fine rash, blistering, or pain over and/or around the administration site. It is important to encourage the client to return for follow-up visits to assess the effectiveness of immunotherapy.

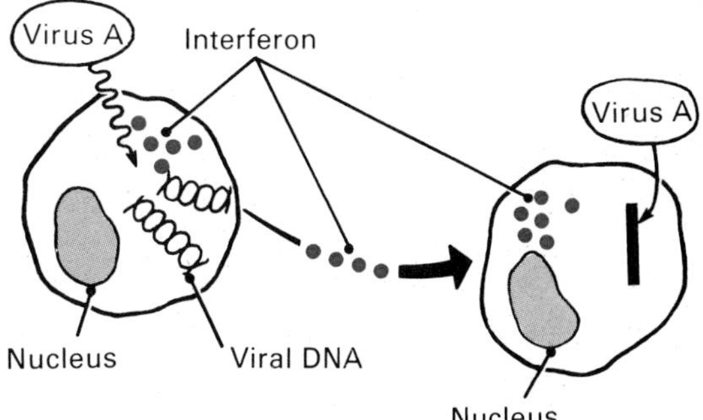

Figure 11-17 Mechanism of action of interferon. Virus A attacks a cell. The cell begins to synthesize viral DNA and interferon. Interferon serves as an intercellular messenger. Interferon induces the production of antiviral proteins. Virus A is not able to replicate in the cell.

In considering the effectiveness of any immunotherapy treatment, it is important to remember that these treatments are not miracle cures for cancer. Immunotherapy at best is a form of adjunct therapy along with surgery, radiation, and chemotherapy in an attempt to actively destroy cancer cells. Until more definitive answers can be found regarding the cause of cancer, the selective use of one or any combination of these approaches is probably the best treatment regimen available.

Nutritional Management of the Client with Cancer

Nutritional problems that most frequently occur in clients with cancer are malnutrition, anorexia, and altered taste sensation. These problems can be caused by a combination of many factors: drug toxicity, effects of radiation therapy, tumor involvement, recent surgery, emotional distress, or difficulty with ingestion or digestion of food. If the client is inadequately nourished, the normal cells will not be able to recover from the effects of therapy and the immune system will be depressed due to depletion of protein stores.

Malnutrition

The client with cancer usually experiences calorie and protein malnutrition characterized by fat and muscle depletion. Assessment of the degree of malnutrition is discussed in Chap. 33. Food suggestions to increase the protein intake to facilitate repair and regeneration of cells are presented in Table 11-25. High-calorie foods for energy and to minimize weight

Table 11-25

Protein Foods with High Biological Value

Milk

One cup of whole milk = 9 g protein
Double-strength milk—1 quart of whole milk plus 1 cup of dried skim milk blended and chilled:
1 cup = 14 g protein
Milkshake—1 cup of ice cream plus 1 cup of milk = 15 g protein, 416 calories
Use evaporated milk, double-strength milk, or half-and-half to make casseroles, hot cereals, sauces, gravies, puddings, milkshakes, and soups.
Yogurt (regular and frozen)—check labels and purchase the brand with the highest protein content: 1 cup = 10 g protein

Eggs

Egg = 6 g protein
Eggnog (1 cup) = 15.5 g protein
Add eggs to salads, casseroles, and sauces. Deviled eggs are especially well tolerated.
Desserts that contain eggs include angel food cake, sponge cake, custard, and cheesecake.

Cheese

Cottage	$\frac{1}{2}$ cup	15 g protein
American	1 slice	3 g protein
Cheddar	1 slice	6 g protein
Cream	1 tbsp	1 g protein

Use cheese on a sandwich or as a snack.
Add cheese to salads, casseroles, sauces, and baked potatoes.
Cheesecake is usually a welcome treat.
Cheese spread with crackers is a wholesome snack that can be made and stored in the refrigerator for easy accessibility.

Meat/Poultry/Fish

Beef	3 oz	Approx. 21 g protein
Pork	3 oz	Approx. 19 g protein
Chicken	$\frac{1}{2}$ Breast	Approx. 26 g protein
Fish	3 oz	Approx. 30 g protein
Tunafish	$6\frac{1}{2}$ oz	Approx. 44.5 g protein

Add meat, poultry, and fish to salads, casseroles, and sandwiches.
Add strained and junior baby meats to soups and casseroles.
Cocktail weiners or deviled ham on crackers are wholesome snacks. These snacks can be made and stored in the refrigerator for easy accessibility.

Adapted from J. Yasko, *Care of the Client Receiving External Radiation Therapy—A Self-Learning Module for the Nurse Caring for the Client with Cancer,* The Reston Publishing Co., Reston, Va., 1982; and C. Donoghue Nunnally and J. Yasko, *Nutritional Aspects of Cancer—A Self-Learning Module for the Nurse Caring for the Client with Cancer,* The Reston Publishing Co., Reston, Va., 1982.

loss are presented in Table 11-26. A sample high-calorie, high-protein diet is presented in Appendix B, Table 1.

The nurse should suggest the need for a nutritional supplement to the physician as soon as a 5 percent weight loss is noted or if the client has the potential to develop protein and calorie malnutrition. Once a 10-pound weight loss occurs, it is very difficult to maintain the nutritional status. The client can be taught to use nutritional supplements in place of milk when cooking and/or baking. Foods to which nutritional supplements can be easily added include scrambled eggs, pudding, custard, mashed potatoes, cereal, and cream sauces. Instant Breakfast ® can be sprinkled on cereals, desserts, and casseroles.

If the malnutrition cannot be treated with dietary intake, it may be necessary to use total parenteral nutrition (TPN) as an adjunct nutritional measure.[43] (TPN is discussed in Chap. 33.)

Anorexia

It is important to realize that anorexia experienced by the client with cancer is a challenging problem. An intervention may be effective one day and ineffective the next. Continual assessment and intervention are necessary to successfully manage this problem. The nurse must develop the philosophy that something can be done to prevent or minimize anorexia. Evaluate each intervention and continue to use those that have been successful in the past. Some suggestions are presented in the nursing care plan for the client with cancer (Table 11-18).

Altered taste sensation

It is theorized that cancer cells release substances that resemble amino acids and stimulate the bitter taste buds. Clients have also experienced an alteration in the sweet taste sensation as well as the sour and salty taste sensations. The physiologic basis of these varied taste alterations at this point in time is unknown. Other causes for altered taste sensation are presented in Table 11-17.

To assist the client with this problem, the client should be instructed to avoid foods for which he has a strong dislike. Frequently a client may feel compelled to eat certain foods because he believes they are good for him. He can be taught to experiment with spices and other seasoning agents in an attempt to mask the taste alterations that are occurring. Lemon juice, onion, mint, basil, and fruit juice marinades may improve the taste of certain meats and fish. Bacon bits, onion, or pieces of ham may enhance the taste of vegetables. Adding an additional amount of a spice or a seasoning agent is usually not effective.

Table 11-26
High Calorie Foods

Food	Amount
Mayonnaise	1 tbsp = 101 cal
Butter/margarine	1 tsp = 35 cal
Sour cream	1 tbsp = 72 cal
Peanut butter	1 tbsp = 94 cal
Whipped cream	1 tbsp = 53 cal
Corn oil	1 tbsp = 119 cal
Jelly	1 tbsp = 49 cal
Ice cream	1 cup = 256 cal
Honey	1 tbsp = 64 cal

Unproven Methods of Cancer Treatment

Unproven methods of cancer treatment, sometimes referred to as cancer quackery, are as old as the disease itself. Cancer quackery is defined as the intentional misrepresentation and/or misapplication of measures that delay or impede the entry of the client into the health care system for treatment. At the present time cancer quackery is a multimillion-dollar business in the United States. Fear appears to be the major factor that motivates clients to seek "miracle cures." Other reasons include (1) impatience with the progress of their present cancer treatment, (2) the need to exercise control over their daily lives, (3) impersonal approach of health care workers, (4) a need for hope when terminal illness is a reality, (5) lack of information on methods that are proven versus those that are not, and (6) suspicion that the health care system is not providing the client with the most effective treatment plan available.[44]

The major hazard of cancer quackery is that it delays or prevents the client from receiving proven methods of cancer diagnosis and treatment. The delay may make the difference between cancer cure or control and terminal illness. The nurse can play a very significant role in preventing or minimizing the use of cancer quackery. This role includes:

1. Providing the client with accurate information concerning the benefits of the proven methods of cancer treatment.
2. Informing the American Cancer Society, the Medical Association, the health department, and the local consumer's protection office when it is learned that clients are being approached by persons promoting unproven methods of cancer treatment.
3. Discussing the fallacies of the unproven methods of cancer treatment with the client and family. The current methods of cancer quackery include chemicals and drugs, dietary alterations, occult techniques, and mechanical devices.

Chemicals and drugs

The two drugs that have been most associated with cancer quackery are Krebiozin (the wonder drug of the 1950s and 1960s) and Laetrile (the wonder drug of the 1970s and 1980s). A National Cancer Institute study on a large number of clients who used Krebiozin failed to demonstrate any anticancer effects of this drug. Chemical analysis revealed that the major ingredient of Krebiozin is mineral oil with minute amounts of creatine and amyl alcohol.

Laetrile, also known as vitamin B-17 and Cyto H-3, has been actively used as a treatment for cancer for the past 25 to 30 years. The active ingredient of Laetrile is hydrogen cyanide and it is derived from apricot or peach pits. It is available in parenteral and tablet form and the parenteral form contains 30 to 40 times as much cyanide as the oral form. Several studies have been conducted by some of the major cancer centers and all have failed to show evidence of an anticancer effect of this drug.

Since Laetrile is frequently used by clients with cancer, and has until recently been thought a harmless drug, the nurse must be aware of the possible toxic effects that may be experienced. The cyanide content of Laetrile is released in the presence of hydrolyzine β-glucosidase enzymes. These enzymes are present in raw fruits and vegetables such as lettuce, mushrooms, green peppers, celery, and sweet almonds. When these foods are eaten after the ingestion of Laetrile, cyanide intoxication may occur. The bacteria of the intestinal tract are also thought to contain this enzyme. When the cyanide is released, it inhibits cellular respiration and the resulting hypoxia produces symptoms such as dizziness, nausea/vomiting, hypotension, and shock. Because the drug is not controlled by the FDA, many impurities may exist which have the potential for causing systemic bacterial, viral, and fungal infections. When the nurse is aware that the client is interested in taking Laetrile, the client should be taught to:

1. Observe for signs and symptoms of cyanide intoxication and maintain the respiratory status
2. Observe for signs and symptoms of infection

3. Avoid fresh fruits and vegetables that contain the enzyme hydrolyzine β-glucosidase
4. Avoid taking the parenteral medication orally

Dietary alterations

Books proposing a cure for cancer are sold which enumerate the foods to eat and avoid, offer special recipes, and usually recommend the use of an expensive blender to assure the proper potency of the food mixture. Examples of nutritional alterations that have been used are eating raw foods, fasting for long periods of time, the grape diet, the carrot juice diet, the coffee and Coke diet, and the use of coffee, buttermilk, and/or yogurt enemas during the time of a special diet. None of these diets has been found effective in treating cancer. Nutritional alterations can have a profound effect on the client with cancer, since a great amount of protein and calories is needed to maintain weight and prevent a negative nitrogen balance.

Occult techniques

The most commonly used occult form of cancer quackery is "psychic surgery." This surgery is performed by a healer without an incision. The client presents the problem, has the healing surgery, and leaves believing that the tumor has been removed. During the surgery, the area where the problem exists is massaged and rubbed with animal blood. At some point, the client is shown a piece of animal tissue and told that it is the diseased tissue or organ. This tissue is thrown away and the massage with blood continues and then the client is told his tumor is gone and the cancer is cured.

Mechanical devices

Mechanical devices are an old form of cancer quackery that have lost their popularity in recent times. These devices are usually nothing more than light bulbs, vibrators, a low-voltage generator, dials, and knobs. The client is told to place the device on or in front of the area of cancer for a certain period of time each day and the device will destroy the cancer present.

Supportive care

One of the cancer quack's greatest assets is the emotional support he gives to the client and family. This should be a message to the nurse for the need to provide psychological support, caring, and active listening to the cancer client. The nurse needs to be available, listen, and counsel the client during times when side effects are being experienced, the treatment is not effective, or when the client is experiencing fear, anger and depression.

If the client chooses an unproven method of cancer treatment, the nurse needs to support the client and assume a nonjudgmental attitude. The nurse should attempt to convince the client to continue the proven treatment plan and to maintain the nutritional status while using an unproven method of cancer treatment. Belief in the treatment may provide a placebo effect that may offer some benefits. It is important that all doors remain open to clients so that they can return to the health care system without feelings of fear and/or guilt.

COMPLICATIONS RESULTING FROM CANCER

If the client fails to respond to the treatment plan and the disease process of cancer progresses, the client is said to be in the advanced phase of cancer. In this phase the client may develop complications related to the continual growth of the malignancy.

Infection

Infection is the most frequent cause of death in the client with cancer. The usual sites of infection include the lung, genitourinary system, mouth, rectum, peritoneal cavity, and the blood (septicemia). Infection occurs due to ulceration and necrosis of the tumor, compression of the tumor on vital organs, and the state of neutropenia due to the disease process or the treatment of cancer. Fungi and gram-negative bacteria are the usual causative organisms.

Paraneoplastic Syndrome

Paraneoplastic syndrome includes all the physiologic effects that occur due to the release of certain hormones by cancer cells in the primary and/or metastatic site(s). Hormone secretion from cancer cells that arise from tissues that do not normally release this hormone is due to the process of derepression. This process allows the stored potential of all cells to become evident. Paraneoplastic syndrome can occur during all phases of the process of cancer, but is commonly associated with the advanced illness phase. The most common paraneoplastic syndromes include:

1. Hypercalcemia, which occurs when a parathormone-like substance and/or calcitonin is secreted by the cancer cells. Hypercalcemia oc-

curs most frequently in clients with lung, breast, kidney, colon, or thyroid cancer.

2. Inappropriate ADH syndrome (SIADH), due to secretion of antidiuretic hormone by cancer cells located in the lung, pancreas, or prostate gland.
3. Secretion of ACTH by a tumor of the lung, thymus, pancreas, thyroid, stomach, or ovary.
4. Secretion of insulin by a tumor of the pancreas, liver, adrenal glands, stomach, or ovary.

Hypercalcemia

Hypercalcemia is a serious electrolyte disorder that occurs in cancer. Serum levels of calcium in excess of 15 mg/dL can be life-threatening. Hypercalcemia can be associated with the paraneoplastic syndrome as described. In addition, it can be caused by extensive bone involvement in clients with multiple myeloma and bony metastasis. Chronic hypercalcemia can result in nephrocalcinosis and irreversible renal failure. The long-term treatment of hypercalcemia is to treat the primary disease. Acute hypercalcemia is treated by hydration (3 L/day), diuretic administration, and mithramycin if the client is severely symptomatic.

Superior Vena Cava Syndrome

Superior vena cava syndrome results from obstruction of the superior vena cava by a tumor. The clinical manifestations include facial edema, distension of veins of the neck and chest, headache, and convulsions. Often, the presence of a mediastinal mass is visible on a chest x-ray. The most common causes are Hodgkin's disease, non-Hodgkin's lymphomas, and lung cancer. Superior vena cava syndrome is considered a serious medical problem and treatment is usually radiation therapy to the site of obstruction.

Hemorrhage

Hemorrhage can occur due to the presence of thrombocytopenia, tumor invasion of a blood vessel causing the vessel to rupture, or the development of an ulcer. Petechiae, epistaxis, hematuria, or melena may be signs of the possibility of an impending major hemorrhage. The usual sites of massive hemorrhage are the brain, gastrointestinal tract, the major vessels of the neck, the lungs, and the peritoneal cavity. Disseminated intravascular coagulation (DIC) can also occur in cancer clients. It is due to the release of thromboplastic substances from cancer cells. DIC is described in Chap. 24.

Infarction and Organ Failure

Infarction occurs due to the formation of thrombi composed of tumor cells. When the thrombi occlude vessels in major body organs they cause necrosis of vital organ tissue. The major sites of infarction are the lungs, heart, and brain. Organ failure is the result of primary or metastatic disease involvement of the vital organ: brain, liver, kidney, and lung. The involvement is sufficient to cause physiologic dysfunction, failure, and/or death.

PSYCHOLOGICAL SUPPORT OF THE CLIENT WITH CANCER

Psychological support of the client with cancer is an important aspect of cancer care. Due to the effectiveness of cancer treatment, many clients with cancer are cured or their disease process is controlled for long periods of time. Because of this trend in cancer treatment, an emphasis must be placed on maintaining an optimum quality of life after the diagnosis of cancer. It has been observed that a positive attitude of the client, family, and care givers toward cancer has a significant positive impact on the quality of life the client experiences. Some authorities have stated that a positive attitude may also influence the prognosis of the client with cancer.[45]

The diagnosis of cancer is viewed by most individuals as a crisis. The most common fears experienced by clients with cancer include:

Disfigurement
Dependency
Pain
Emaciation
Financial depletion
Death
Abandonment

In order to cope with these fears, the client with cancer will utilize different behavioral patterns: shock, anger, denial, bargaining, depression, helplessness, hopelessness, rationalization, acceptance, and intellectualization. These behavioral patterns may occur at any time during the process of cancer. However, some patterns appear to occur more frequently or at a greater intensity at certain specific stages of the disease process. Several factors may determine how the client will cope with the diagnosis of cancer:

1. *Ability to cope with stressful events in the past*

(e.g., loss of job, major disappointment). By simply asking how the client has coped with stressful events, the nurse can gain an understanding of the client's coping patterns, the effectiveness of the usual coping patterns, and the usual coping time framework.

2. *Availability of significant others.* It has been observed that those clients with effective support systems tend to cope more effectively than those clients without a meaningful, available support system.
3. *Ability to express feelings and concerns.* Those clients who are able to express their feelings and needs and to seek and ask for help appear to cope more effectively than those clients who internalize their feelings and needs.
4. *Age at the time of diagnosis.* This determines the coping strategies to a great degree. A young mother with cancer will have concerns that differ from a 70-year-old woman with cancer.
5. *Extent of disease.* Cure or control of the disease process is usually easier to cope with than the reality of terminal illness.
6. *Disruption of body image.* Disruption of the body image (radical neck dissection, alopecia, mastectomy) may intensify psychological impact of cancer.
7. *Presence of symptoms.* Symptoms such as fatigue, nausea, diarrhea, and pain may intensify the psychological impact of cancer.
8. *Past experience with cancer.* If past experience with cancer has been negative, it is likely that the client will view his own status as negative.
9. *Attitude associated with the cancer.* A client who feels in control and has a positive attitude about cancer and cancer treatment is better able to cope with the diagnosis and treatment of cancer than the client who feels hopeless, helpless, and out of control.

In order to facilitate the development of a hopeful attitude toward cancer and to support the client and family during the various stages of the process of cancer, the nurse should:

1. Be available and continue to be available, especially during difficult times.
2. Exhibit a caring attitude.
3. *Listen actively* to fears and concerns.
4. Provide relief of distressing symptoms.
5. Provide essential information regarding cancer and cancer care.
6. Maintain a relationship based on trust and confidence. Be open, honest, and caring in your approach.
7. Utilize touch to exhibit caring. A squeeze of the hand or hug may at times be more effective than words.
8. Assist client in setting realistic, reachable short- and long-term goals.
9. Maintain *hope,* the key to effective cancer care. Hope varies, depending on the status of the client; hope that the symptoms are not serious, hope that the treatment is curative, hope for independence, hope for relief of pain, hope for a longer life or hope for a peaceful death. Hope provides control over what is occurring and is the basis of a positive attitude toward cancer and cancer care.
10. Assist the client in maintaining usual lifestyle patterns.

Hospice Care*

Hospice is not a place but a concept of care that provides compassion, concern, support, and skilled professional care for the dying. Hospice care seeks to enhance the remaining time for those persons who are living with a dying body. The term *hospice* is derived from a medieval word that means a place of shelter for people on a difficult journey. The hospice concept of care has existed in England for many years. During the 1970s the idea took hold in the United States and by the end of the decade every state had existing hospice programs.

The National Hospice Organization has defined hospice as a centrally administered program of palliative and supportive services which provide physical, psychological, social, and spiritual care for dying persons and their families. Services are provided by a medically supervised interdisciplinary team of professionals and volunteers.

Admission to a hospice program is on the basis of client and family need. Hospice services are available in both the home and the inpatient setting. Home care is provided on a part-time, intermittent, regularly scheduled, or around-the-clock on-call basis. Hospice services are available on a 7-day-a-week, 24-hour basis to provide help to clients and families in their homes. Some hospice programs also have an inpatient unit in a hospital. Usually, the in-hospital units have been deinstitutionalized to make the atmosphere as free and homelike as possible. Staff and volunteers are available to the client and family. A multidisciplinary team approach provides holistic personal care.

Philosophy of hospice care

There is often a point in terminal disease when curative treatment is no longer appropriate. It is at this

*This section was written by Karen May McArdle.

time that the hospice philosophy of promoting the quality of life and providing palliative care is appropriate. Palliative care controls symptoms and provides comfort but does not cure. Palliative care does not prolong life but provides comfort.

Hospice care is a return to previous times where the dying were helped to remain at home and to die at home, if possible, surrounded by familiar sights, sounds, and smells, and by the love of those who care. Hospice exists to provide support and care for persons in the last phases of incurable diseases so that they might live as fully and comfortably as possible.

Differences between traditional and hospice care

Hospice care differs from traditional care in a number of ways. The goals of traditional hospital and medical care are to (1) treat and cure disease, (2) prolong life, (3) utilize all appropriate technology, and (4) treat pain with limited, well-defined amounts of medication. Traditional medical care views death as a treatment failure.

In hospice care, the client and family are the focus of care. Preparation for dying is a task with which the family as well as the client must deal. Hospice provides a milieu where this is more easily accomplished. Hospice recognizes dying as a normal process. It neither hastens nor postpones death. Hospice exists in the hope and belief that, through appropriate care and the promotion of a caring community sensitive to their needs, clients and families may be free to attain a degree of mental and spiritual preparation for death that is satisfactory to them.

Hospice care is not technology oriented. Rather, it is intensive personal care that provides skilled bedside nursing and focuses attention on the emotional, social, spiritual, and familial aspects of the client. Hospice offers little opportunity to do things *to* clients but offers great opportunity to do things *with* clients and families.

Pain is a common concern among terminally ill cancer clients. In hospice, pain is considered as a total experience rather than a physiologic event. Adequate medication (usually narcotics) is used to provide relief. The prn order for pain is not found in hospice. Analgesia is routinely given in an attempt to eliminate the pain and, more important, to prevent its recurrence and to erase the memory of pain. Attention is also given to all the other factors that contribute to pain or to its increasing intensity: fear, loneliness, anxiety, insomnia, spiritual doubts or concerns, financial concerns, and depression.

When the client dies, the hospice team continues to follow the family and significant others through the bereavement period. The hospice team makes itself available to aid survivors through the grief period.

Support groups are available to hospice staff and volunteers. Crises and grief result in varying forms of stress for care givers. In order to give to clients and families, the staff and volunteers must also have a means to be nourished and refreshed. Various means of stress relief are utilized by different hospices. Professionally assisted groups, informal rap sessions, flexible time schedules, and additional time off are a few ways to decrease stress. The needs of the care giver must be considered important or the care receiver will find he is getting less and less of what he requires.

REVIEW QUESTIONS

The number of the question corresponds to the same numbered objective at the beginning of the chapter.

1. Which type of cancer is increasing in incidence?
 a. uterine cancer
 b. esophageal cancer
 c. stomach cancer
 d. lung cancer

2. Cancer is a name for a large group of diseases, all of which are characterized by
 a. cell growth which escapes normal control
 b. rapid, explosive proliferation of cells
 c. production of toxins which alter cells
 d. long and painful course

3. A characteristic of the stage of progression in the development of cancer is
 a. mutation of stem cell
 b. continual steady growth facilitated by promoting factors
 c. proliferation of cancer cells in spite of host control mechanisms
 d. invasion of surrounding tissues

4. The primary protective role of the immune system related to malignant cells is
 a. immunologic surveillance
 b. immunologic enhancement
 c. antigenic blindfolding
 d. antigenic modulation

5. The primary difference between benign and malignant neoplasms is
 a. rate of cell proliferation
 b. requirements for cellular nutrients
 c. characteristic of tissue invasiveness
 d. site of malignant tumor

6. Important nursing roles related to prevention and detection of cancer include all the following *except*
 a. teaching people self-examination of breast and testicles

b. instructing people to eat low-fiber, refined carbohydrate diets
c. instructing individuals on ways to increase capacity to cope with stress
d. teaching people to obtain regular health care

7. The only definitive means of diagnosing cancer is by
a. radiologic study
b. culture
c. chemical testing
d. biopsy

8. Which of the following is a radiation hazard when a client has radium needles implanted in a tongue lesion?
a. saliva
b. bed linen
c. urine
d. displaced needle

9. Which of the following sets of drug classifications and examples are incorrect?
a. alkylating agent—nitrogen mustard
b. antibiotic—actinomycin D
c. antimetabolite—5-fluorouracil
d. plant alkaloid—L-asparaginase

10. Stomatitis, a common side effect of chemotherapeutic agents, occurs because the
a. general health of the client with cancer is poor
b. rapidly dividing cells of the mucous membranes of the mouth are being destroyed
c. chemotherapeutic drugs have an external, local, and irritating effect
d. site of the malignancy is near the oral cavity

11. Radiation precautions on the clinical unit must be observed by the nurse caring for a client
a. receiving supervoltage radiation therapy for lung cancer
b. who has ingested radioactive iodine for diagnostic brain scan
c. having cobalt teletherapy for esophageal cancer
d. who has implanted radium needles in her breast

12. A client with cancer receives a vaccine containing tumor cells from another client that are similar to the cells of the client's tumor. This is an example of
a. active specific immunotherapy
b. active nonspecific immunotherapy
c. passive specific immunotherapy
d. passive nonspecific immunotherapy

13. The most common nutritional problems found in cancer clients include all the following *except*
a. malnutrition
b. anorexia
c. altered taste sensation
d. hypernatremia

14. If a client decides to take Laetrile the nurse should inform him that he
a. should avoid foods with hydrolyzine β-glucosidase enzymes
b. should not take chemotherapy and Laetrile simultaneously
c. will probably develop a pulmonary fungal infection
d. should simultaneously drink buttermilk to avoid toxic effects

15. Paraneoplastic syndrome that occurs in certain types of malignancies is primarily due to
a. invasiveness of cancer cells
b. gram-negative septicemia
c. ectopic hormonal production
d. autoimmune reaction

REFERENCES

1. Cancer Facts and Figures, 1981, American Cancer Society, 1980, p. 3.
2. Ibid.
3. Ibid, p. 5.
4. Richard La Fond, *Cancer—The Outlaw Cell,* American Clinical Society, Washington, D.C., 1978, p. 4.
5. Ibid., p. 47.
6. Pierce G. Barry et al., *Cancer—A Problem of Developmental Biology,* Prentice-Hall Inc., Englewood Cliffs, New Jersey, 1978, p. 48.
7. Ibid., p. 130.
8. G. P. Marginson, *Carcinogenesis,* Pergamon Press, New York, 1978.
9. J. E. Ultmann and H. M. Golumb, "Neoplasia," in Isselbacher, *Harrison's Principles of Internal Medicine,* 9th ed., McGraw-Hill Book Company, New York, p. 1587.
10. Barry, op. cit., p. 119.
11. J. T. Barrett, *Basic Immunology and Its Medical Application,* 2d ed., The C. V. Mosby Company, St. Louis, 1980, p. 253.
12. H. Pinot, *Fundamentals of Oncology,* Marcel Dekker, Inc., New York, 1978, p. 20.
13. L. E. Hood et al., *Immunology,* Benjamin Cummings, Menlo Park, Calif., 1978, p. 428.
14. Ibid.
15. C. McKhann, "Cancer Immunotherapy: A Realistic Appraisal," *Ca-ACJ Clin,* **30:**286–287 (1980).
16. Ibid., p. 429.
17. L. J. Old, "Cancer Immunology," *Sci Am,* **236:**62–79 (1977).
18. Ibid.
19. Barrett, op. cit., p. 249.
20. Ibid.
21. Hood, op. cit., p. 426–427.
22. Barrett, op. cit., p. 248.
23. M. A. Litchman et al., *Hematology and Oncology,* Grune and Stratton, New York, 1980, p. 246.
24. J. Rosai and L. V. Ackerman, "The Pathology of Tumors, Part II: Diagnostic Techniques," *Ca-ACJClin,* **29:**66–77 (1979).
25. O. T. Pace and B. Cady, "Overall Principles of Cancer Management," in *Cancer: A Manual for Practitioners,* American Cancer Society, Massachusetts Division, Boston, 1978, pp. 43–48.
26. C. G. Varrichio, "The Patient on Radiation Therapy," *Am J Nurs,* **81:**334–337 (1981).
27. P. P. Kelly and C. Tinsley, "Planning Care for the Patient Receiving External Radiation," *Am J Nurs,* **81:**338–342 (1981).
28. S. S. Ogi, "Radiotherapy, Cancer, and the Nurse," in P.

K. Burkhalter and D. L. Donley, *Dynamics of Oncology Nursing,* McGraw-Hill Book Company, New York, 1978, pp. 155–158.

29. Varrichio, op. cit., pp. 336–337.

30. P. C. Hetzel et al., "Overall Principles of Cancer Management: IV. Chemotherapy," in *Cancer: A Manual for Practitioners,* American Cancer Society, Massachusetts Division, Boston, 1978, pp. 59–61.

31. C. A. Bingham, "The Cell Cycle and Cancer Chemotherapy," *Am J Nurs,* **78:**1201–1205 (1978).

32. D. R. Toal, "Tumor Cell Kinetics and Cancer Chemotherapy," *Am J Nurs,* **80:**1802–1804 (1980).

33. "Using Marijuana in the Reduction of Nausea Associated with Chemotherapy," Murray Publishing Company, Inc., 1979.

34. T. Andrysiak, "Marijuana for the Oncology Patient," *Am J Nurs,* **79:**1396–1398 (1979).

35. M. B. Maxwell, "Scalp Tourniquets for Chemotherapy-Induced Alopecia," *Am J Nurs,* **80:**900–903 (1980).

36. M. E. Koren and C. S. Herrmann, "Cancer Immunotherapy," *Nursing 81,* **11:**36–39 (1981).

37. B. M. Morrin, "Cancer Immunology," *Heart Lung,* **9:**686–688 (1980).

38. Ibid.

39. Ibid.

40. C. W. McAdams, "Interferon: The Penicillin of the Future?" *Am J Nurs,* **80:**714–718 (1980).

41. B. M. Morrin, op. cit., pp. 688–689.

42. Ibid.

43. E. M. Copeland, "Intravenous Hyperalimentation as an Adjunct to Cancer Patient Management," *The Cancer Bulletin,* **30:**102–108 (1978).

44. *Unproven Methods of Cancer Management—1979,* American Cancer Society Inc., 1979.

45. C. Simonton et al., *Getting Well Again,* J. P. Tanker Inc., Los Angeles, 1978.

BIBLIOGRAPHY FOR SECTION THREE

Books

Alexander, W., and Good, R.: *Fundamentals of Clinical Immunology,* W. B. Saunders Co., Philadelphia, 1977.

Bayly, Joseph: *The View from a Hearse,* Cook Publishing Co., Elgin, 1973.

Bellaniti, Joseph: *Immunology II,* W. B. Saunders Co., Philadelphia, 1978.

Boldonada, Ardeline, and Dulalina A. Stabb: *Cancer Nursing,* Medical Examination Publishing Company, Inc., Garden City, New York, 1978.

Cochran, Alistair: *Man, Cancer and Immunity,* Academic Press, New York, 1978.

Cohen, Kenneth P.: *Hospice,* Aspen Systems Corp., Germantown, Md., 1979.

Davidson, Glen W.: *The Hospice,* Hemisphere Publishing Corp., Washington/London, 1978.

Durland, Frances C.: *Coping with Widowhood,* Liguori Publications, Liguori Missouri, 1978.

Eys, Jan: *Nutrition and Cancer,* S. P. Medical and Scientific Books, New York, 1977.

Frazier, C. A.: *Psychosomatic Aspects of Allergy,* Van Nostrand Reinhold, New York, 1977.

Fudenberg, H. H., Stites, D. P., Caldwell, J. L., and J. V. Wells: *Basic and Clinical Immunology,* 2d ed., Lange Medical Pub., Los Angeles, 1980.

Han, S. S., and J. O. Holmsteat: *Cell Biology,* McGraw-Hill Book Company, New York, 1979.

Hyde, R. M., and R. A. Patnode: *Immunology,* Prentice-Hall, Reston, Virginia, 1978.

Kruse, Louise C., et al.: *Cancer: Pathophysiology, Etiology and Management,* The C. V. Mosby Co., St. Louis, 1979.

Kübler-Ross, Elisabeth: *On Death and Dying,* Macmillan, New York, 1973.

———: *Questions and Answers on Death & Dying,* Collier, New York, 1974.

Lack, S. A., and R. W. Buckingham: *The First American Hospice—Three Years of Home Care,* Conn. Hospice, Inc., New Haven, 1978.

LaFond, Richard, ed.: *Cancer—The Outlaw Cell,* American Clinical Society, Washington, D.C., 1978.

Leahy, Irene, Jean M. St. Germain, and Claudette G. Varricchio: *The Nurse and Radiotherapy,* The C. V. Mosby Co., St. Louis, 1979.

Lessner, Howard: *Medical Oncology,* Elsevier, New York, 1978.

Marino, L. B.: *Cancer Nursing,* The C. V. Mosby Co., St. Louis, 1981.

McCaffery, Margo: *Nursing Management of the Patient with Pain,* J. B. Lippincott Company, New York, 1979.

Middleton, E., et al.: *Allergy, Principles and Practice,* The C. V. Mosby Co., St. Louis, 1978.

Parkes, C. M.: *Bereavement: Studies of Grief in Adult Life,* International, New York, 1979.

Pierce, G. Barry, et al.: *Cancer—A Problem of Developmental Biology,* Prentice-Hall Inc., Englewood Cliffs, N.J., 1978.

Pinot, Henry: *Fundamentals of Oncology,* Marcel Dekker, New York, 1978.

Rubin, Philip, ed.: *Clinical Oncology,* 5th ed., The American Cancer Society, New York, 1978.

Stoddard, Sandol: *The Hospice Movement,* Vintage Books, Random House, New York, 1978.

Temes, Roberta: *Living with an Empty Chair,* Mandala, Amherst, Mass., 1977.

Tripp, A.: *Basic Pathophysiologic Mechanisms of Inflammation,* McGraw-Hill Book Company, New York, 1979.

Windle, W. F.: *Textbook of Histology,* 5th ed., McGraw-Hill Book Company, New York, 1976.

Periodicals

Baker, S.: "Late Onset Systemic Lupus Erythematosus," *Am J Med,* **66:**727–730 (1979).

Breeding, Mary Anne: "Working Safely Around Implanted Radiation," *Nursing 76* (May 1976).

Bridgewater, S. C., and Voignier, R. R.: "Allergies in Children: Teaching," *Am J Nurs,* **78:**620–621 (1978).

——— and C. S. Smith: "Allergies in Children: Recognition," *Am J Nurs,* **78:**614–616 (1978).

Costa, Giovanni: "Cachexia, the Metabolic Component of Neoplastic Disease," *Cancer Res,* **37:**235–237 (1977).

Cove-Smith, J. R., et al.: "Transplantation, Immunosuppression, and Plasmapheresis in Goodpasture's Syndrome," *Clin Nephrol,* **9:**125–129 (1978).

Croft, C. L.: "BCG Administration and Nursing Implications," *Am J Nurs,* **79:**315–319 (1979).

DeWys, William: "Anorexia in Cancer Patients," *Cancer Res,* **37:**2354–2348 (1977).

——— and Karen Walters: "Abnormalities of Taste Sensation in Cancer Patients," *Cancer,* **39:**1888–1896 (1975).

Dharan, M.: "Immunoglobulin Abnormalities," *Am J Nurs,* **76:**1626–1628 (1976).
Dodd, M. J.: "Theoretical Bases of Immunotherapy," *Am J Nurs,* **79:**310–314 (1979).
Donley, D. L.: "Nursing the Patient Who Is Immunosuppressed," *Am J Nurs,* **76:**1619–1625 (1976).
Elpern, E. H.: "Asthma Update: Pathophysiology and Treatment," *Heart Lung,* **9:**665–670 (1980).
Faulk, W. P., et al.: "Some Effects of Malnutrition on Immune Response in Man," *Am J Clin Nutr,* **27:**638 (1974).
Fruth, R.: "Anaphylaxis and Drug Reactions: Guidelines for Detection and Care," *Heart Lung,* **9:**662–664 (1980).
Glasser, Ronald J.: "How the Body Works Against Itself . . . Autoimmune Diseases," *Nurs 77,* **7:**38–43 (1977).
Goel, J.: "Cancer Cachexia and Gluconeogenesis," *Ann New York Acad Sci,* **230:**103–110 (1974).
Gold, W. N.: "Asthma," *Basics Respir Dis,* **4:**1 (1976).
Groenwald, S. L.: "Physiology of the Immune System," *Heart Lung,* **9:**645–650, (1980).
Haylock, Pamela, and Laura Hart: "Fatigue in Patients Receiving Localized Radiation," *Cancer Nursing,* 461–467 (1979).
Hill, J. S.: "Urticaria and Angioedema: Common Clinical Problems," *Postgraduate Med,* **65:**83 (1979).
Holland, Jimmie, Julia, Rowland, and Marjorie Plumb: "Psychological Aspects of Anorexia in Cancer Patients," *Cancer Res,* **37:**2455–2428 (1977).
Jones, J. V.: "Plasmapheresis: Current Research and Success," *Heart Lung,* **9:**671–674 (1980).
Kotwas, Letty: "Pheresis Donor Reactions and Complications: Prevention, Recognition and Management," in American Association of Blood Banks, Fundamentals of a Pheresis Program, New York, 1979, pp. 63–77.
Lawrence, W.: "Effects of Cancer on Nutrition: Impaired Organ System Effects," *Cancer,* **43:**2020–2029 (1979).
Lind, M.: "The Immunologic Assessment: A Nursing Focus," *Heart Lung,* **9:**658–661 (1980).
Lister, J.: "Nursing Intervention in Anaphylactic Shock," *Am J Nurs,* **72:**720–721 (1972).
Mandell, G. L.: "When to Suspect Immune Defects," *Consultant,* **19:**83 (1979).
Mayer, M. M.: "The Complement System," *Sci Am,* 54–56 (1973).
McAdams, C. W.: "Interferon: The Penicillin of the Future?" *Am J Nurs,* **80:**714–718 (1980).
McColla, J.: "Immunotherapy: Concepts and Nursing Implications," *Nurs Clin North Am,* **11:**59–74 (1976).
McLeod, B. C.: "Immunologic Factors in Reactions to Blood Transfusions," *Heart Lung,* **9:**675–681 (1980).
Morrin, B. M.: "Cancer Immunology," *Heart Lung,* **9:**686–689 (1980).
Munroe, H. N.: "Tumor/Host Competition for Nutrients in the Cancer Patient," *J Am Dietetic Assoc,* **71:**380–84 (1977).
Nizami, R. H., et al.: "Hyposensitization Therapy in Allergic Disease," *Ann Allergy,* **53:**296 (1975).
Nysather, J. O., A. E. Katz, and J. L. Length: "The Immune System: Its Development and Functions," *Am J Nurs,* **76:**1614–1618 (1976).
Rana, A. N., and A. Luskin: "Immunosuppression, Autoimmunity, and Hypersensitivity," *Heart Lung,* **9:**651–657 (1980).
Richardson, H. B.: "Immunology of the Respiratory System," *Basics Respir Dis,* **5:**1–6 (1974).
Rossman, M., R. Slavin, and E. G. Taft: "Pheresis Therapy: Patient Care," *Am J Nurs,* **77:**1135–1141 (1977).
Samter, M., (ed.): "Symposium on Immunotherapy in Malignant Disease," *Med Clin North Am,* **60:**1–618 (1976).
Schien, P. S., and S. H. Winokur: "Immunosuppressive and Cytotoxic Chemotherapy, Long Term Complication," *Ann Intern Med,* **82:**84 (1975).
Shahinpoir, N.: "The Patient with Systemic Lupus Erythematosus: Prototype of Autoimmunity," *Heart Lung,* **9:**682–685 (1980).
Slavin, R. G.: "Immunotherapy: A Safe and Effective Way to Treat Allergies," *Consultant,* **19:**117 (1979).
Sophie, L. R.: "Meeting the Immunologic Challenge of Transplant Nursing," *Heart Lung,* **9:**690–694 (1980).
Tenozynski, J.: "Leukapheresis: The Process," *Am J Nurs,* **77:**1133–1134 (1977).
Theologides, A.: "Cancer and Anorexia," *J Med Soc New Jersey,* 785–786 (1979).
———: "Cancer Cachexia," *Cancer,* **43:**2004–2012 (1979).
Torbett, H. P., and J. Ervin: "The Patient with Systemic Lupus Erythematosus," *Am J Nurs,* **9:**1299 (1977).
Voignier, R. R., and S. C. Bridgewater: "Allergies in Children: Testing and Treating," *Am J Nurs,* **78:**617–619 (1978).
White, J. F.: "Teaching Patients to Manage Systemic Lupus Erythematosus," *Nurs 78,* **8:**26–35 (1978).

Booklets

A Guide to Proper Nutrition for the Patient Undergoing Cancer Therapy, Mead Johnson and Company, Evansville, Ind., 47721, 1979.
Cancer Facts and Figures—1981, The American Cancer Society, New York, 1980.
Manual for Staging of Cancer, 1978, American Joint Committee for Cancer Staging and End-Results Reporting, Chicago, Ill., 1978.
Nutrition—A Helpful Ally in Cancer Therapy, Ross Laboratories, Division of Abbott Laboratories, Columbus, Oh., 43216, 1979.
Unproven Methods of Cancer Management—1979, The American Cancer Society, New York, 1979.
Using Marijuana in the Reduction of Nausea Association with Chemotherapy, Murray Publishing Company, Inc., 1979.

Organizations

Allergy Foundation of America, 801 Second Avenue, New York, NY 10017
American Cancer Society, 219 East 42 Street, New York, NY 10017
Concern for Dying, 250 West 57 Street, New York, N.Y. 10019
National Hospice Organization,1311 A Dolly Madison Blvd., McLean, VA 22101

Section 4

Problems with Fluid and Electrolyte Balance

Chapter 12

NURSING ROLE IN MANAGEMENT

Fluid and Electrolyte Imbalances

Nancy R. Adams
Sharon Mantik Lewis

Learning Objectives

1. Identify the major fluid compartments and the electrolytes in each compartment.
2. Describe the mechanisms controlling fluid and electrolyte movement.
3. Describe the mechanisms and causes of extracellular fluid shifts.
4. Explain the physiologic mechanisms which regulate fluid and electrolyte balance.
5. Describe the common causes, clinical manifestations, and medical and nursing management of fluid and electrolyte imbalances.
6. Describe pH and the mechanisms that regulate acid-base balance.
7. Describe the common causes, pathophysiology, compensatory mechanisms, and clinical manifestations of respiratory and metabolic acidosis and alkalosis.
8. Identify the significant assessment data and common abnormal assessment findings related to fluid and electrolyte imbalances.
9. Compare and contrast the types of solutions available for fluid and electrolyte therapy, including osmolarity and indications for use.

HOMEOSTASIS

The cells that make up body tissue exist in a chemically constant but physiologically dynamic internal environment. Physiologic processes function to regulate this environment so that responses to stimuli minimally affect the body. The chemical consistency achieved through fluid, electrolyte, and acid-base balance is essential to the maintenance of *homeostasis*. *Homeostasis* is the term used to describe the stable state produced by physiologic processes which interact "to keep a physical or chemical parameter in the body relatively constant."[1]

As long as life exists, the body is affected by stressors. Stressors such as disease and injury alter the normal balance. A stress state is produced by failure to satisfy a psychological or physiologic need. Homeostatic mechanisms participate in the adjustment to stressors so that the body efficiently and effectively reestablishes a steady state.

The homeostatic mechanisms that regulate fluid and electrolye balance represent an interaction between chemical and physiologic processes. The chemical composition of fluid and electrolytes is not difficult to understand. However, understanding the many shifts in maintaining a stable chemical composition may be difficult.

Note: The opinions or assertions in this article are the views of the author and are not to be construed as official or as reflecting the views of the Department of the Army or the Department of Defense.

This chapter was reviewed by Carolyn Baratta Yucha, R.N., M.S., Instructor, School of Nursing, Syracuse University, Syracuse, New York.

WATER CONTENT OF THE BODY

Water is the primary body fluid. It is the solvent utilized to transport nutrients to cells and to remove waste products produced by cellular metabolism. Temperature regulation is assisted by evaporation of water on the body's surface.

Variations in Water Content

The adult human body is composed of about 60 percent water. The water content varies with sex, lean body mass, and age. Males generally have a larger amount of water content due to more lean body mass than females. Adipose tissue contains less water than an equivalent amount of muscle tissue. Age also influences the body's water content (Fig. 12-1). In the elderly, body water content averages 45 to 55 percent of body weight. For an infant, water content is 70 to 80 percent of the infant's weight.[2] Therefore, the young are at risk for fluid problems because of the large

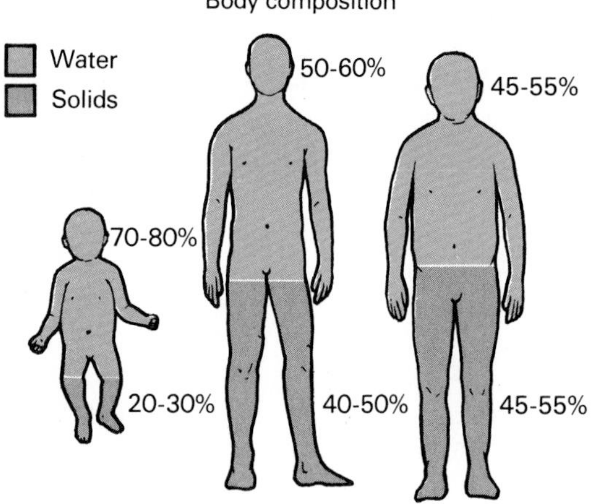

Figure 12-1 Changes in body water content correlated with age.

percentage of their body weight that is water. The elderly are at risk because they have less fluid reserve.

Body Fluid Compartments

The two main fluid compartments in the body are *intracellular* and *extracellular* (Fig. 12-2). The intracellular fluid (ICF), located within cells, constitutes about 40 percent of body weight or 70 percent of the total body water. The extracellular fluid (ECF) constitutes about 20 percent of body weight or 30 percent of total body water.

The extracellular fluid consists of interstitital (fluid between cells), intravascular (plasma), cerebrospinal, and intraocular fluid, and secretions of the gastrointestinal tract. Sometimes the term *transcellular* (a product of secretion and diffusion from cells) is used to refer to cerebrospinal fluid, intraocular fluid, and gastrointestinal secretions together.

Fluid spacing is a term used to classify the distribution of body water. First spacing means that there is a normal distribution of fluid in both the extracellular and intracellular compartments. Second spacing refers to an excess accumulation of interstitial fluid (edema). Third spacing is fluid accumulation in areas that normally have no fluid or a minimum amount of fluid. Some examples of third spacing are ascites, sequestration of fluid in the bowel with peritonitis, and edema associated with burns. Third spacing is a concern because it takes away fluid from the normal fluid compartments and may produce hypovolemia.

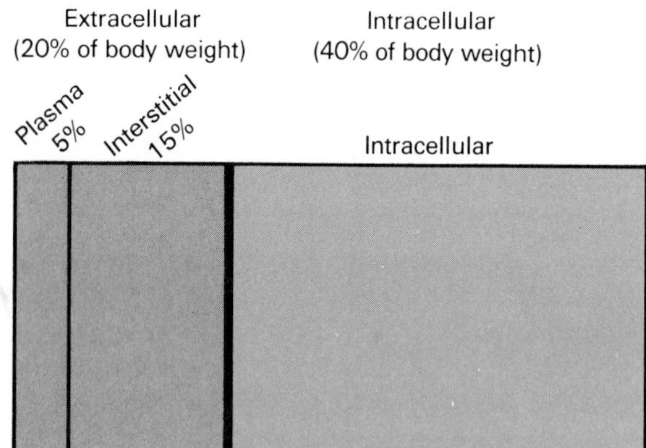

Figure 12-2 Fluid compartments within the body. Water is 60 percent of the body weight. Water is contained in two main compartments: the intracellular and extracellular. The extracellular fluid is divided into interstitial and intravascular (plasma).

Calculating Fluid Gain or Loss

One L of water weighs 1 kg (2.2 pounds). If a client drank 240 mL of fluid, his weight gain would be 0.24 kg (0.5 pound). A client on diuretic therapy and no dietary changes who loses 2 kg in 24 hours has experienced a fluid loss of about 2 L. A sudden weight change is the best indicator of fluid volume deficit or excess.

ELECTROLYTES

Definition

Electrolytes are substances whose molecules dissociate or split into ions when placed in water. Ions are electrically charged particles. *Cations* are positively charged ions. Examples include sodium (Na^+), potassium (K^+), calcium (Ca^{2+}) and magnesium (Mg^{2+}). *Anions* are negatively charged ions. Examples include bicarbonate (HCO_3^-), chloride (Cl^-) and phosphate (PO_4^{2-}). (Terminology related to body fluid chemistry is presented in Table 12-1.)

Measurement of Electrolytes

Electrolytes can be measured by weight or combining power. The unit of weight is milligrams per deciliter (mg/dL) and combining power is milliequivalents per liter (mEq/L). Milliequivalents equal molecular weight (in milligrams) divided by the valence of the ion:

$$\text{mEq} = \frac{\text{molecular weight (in mg)}}{\text{valence}}$$

Table 12-1
Terminology Related to Body Fluid Chemistry

Anion	Electrolyte that carries a negative charge.
Cation	Electrolyte that carries a positive charge.
Electrolyte	Substance which exists in solution as dissociated molecules, each with an electrical charge. A molecule of sodium chloride (NaCl) in solution becomes Na^+ and Cl^-.
Nonelectrolyte	Substance which in solution does not dissociate into its component molecules. Examples include glucose and urea.
Osmolality	A measure of the total solute concentration per kilogram of solution.
Osmolarity	A measure of the total solute concentration per liter of solution.
Solute	Substance that is dissolved in a solvent.
Solution	A homogeneous mixture of solutes dissolved in a solvent.
Solvent	Substance that is capable of dissolving a solute (liquid or gas).

The weight of an electrolyte gives no direct information regarding the number of ions or number of charges carried by an electrolyte. Milliequivalents expresses the chemical activity of an electrolyte. For example, 1 mEq of sodium combines with 1 mEq of chloride, whereas 1 mEq of calcium combines with 2 mEq of chloride.

Electrolyte Composition of Fluid Compartments

The electrolytes found in the ECF and ICF are essentially the same. However, their concentrations vary somewhat between the compartments (Fig. 12-3). The primary intracellular cation is potassium while the primary extracellular cation is sodium. The primary intracellular anion is phosphate while the primary extracellular anion is chloride. The main difference between plasma fluid and interstitial fluid is a higher concentration of protein in the plasma. Calcium is found only in ECF.

Electrolyte Functions

The roles of electrolytes in cellular function include

1. Regulation of water distribution
2. Transmission of nerve impulses
3. Clotting of blood
4. Generation of adenosine triphosphate (ATP)
5. Regulation of acid-base balance

The specific function of electrolytes will be discussed in the section on electrolyte imbalances.

MECHANISMS CONTROLLING FLUID AND ELECTROLYTE MOVEMENT

There are many different processes that control movement of fluid between the various compartments. These include diffusion, osmosis, active transport, hydrostatic pressure, and oncotic pressure.

Diffusion

Diffusion is a movement of molecules from an area of higher concentration to an area of lower concentration (Fig. 12-4). It occurs in liquids, gases, and solids. Diffusion stops when the concentrations are the same in both areas. It does not require active energy to carry out the transport system. Diffusion is an efficient and effective way for movement of substances in and out of the cell to maintain a chemically stable environment. This process is a prerequisite for normal cell function.

Osmosis

Osmosis is a special type of diffusion. It is the flow of water between two compartments separated by a membrane permeable to water but not to a solute. Water moves through the membrane from an area of low solute concentration to an area of high solute concentration (Fig. 12-5). Another way of saying this is that water moves from the compartment that is more dilute (has more water) to the side that is more concentrated (has less water). The semipermeable membrane prevents movement of larger solute particles. Osmosis requires no outside energy sources and stops when concentration differences disappear. In addition to diffusion, osmosis is very important for maintaining the chemical stability of body cells.

Osmotic pressure or force is a term used to describe the movement of water by the process of osmosis. *Osmolarity* and *osmolality* are both measurements of osmotic pressure. Osmolality measures the osmotic force of solute per unit of weight of solvent (mOsm/kg). Osmotic force is in units of milliosmols. Osmolarity measures the total milliosmoles of solute per unit of total *volume* of solution (mOsm/L).

For body fluids the acceptable term is *osmolality* because it allows for the comparison of fluids such as plasma and urine, which do not have the same weight

Electrolyte composition of serum in intravascular compartment (mEq/L)

Intravascular (Plasma)

Cations | Anions

Na^+ 142
K^+ 4
Ca^{2+} 5
Mg^{2+} 3
154

103 Cl^-
27 HCO_3^-
2 HPO_4^-
1 SO_4^{2-}
5 Organic acids
16 Protein
154

Totals

Electrolyte composition of interstitial fluid (mEq/L)

Interstitial

Cations | Anions

Na^+ 145
K^+ 4
Ca^{2+} 3
Mg^{2+} 2
154

115 Cl^-
30 HCO_3^-
2 HPO_4^{2-}
1 SO_4^{2-}
5 Organic acids
1 Protein
154

Totals

Electrolyte composition of intracellular fluid (mEq/L)

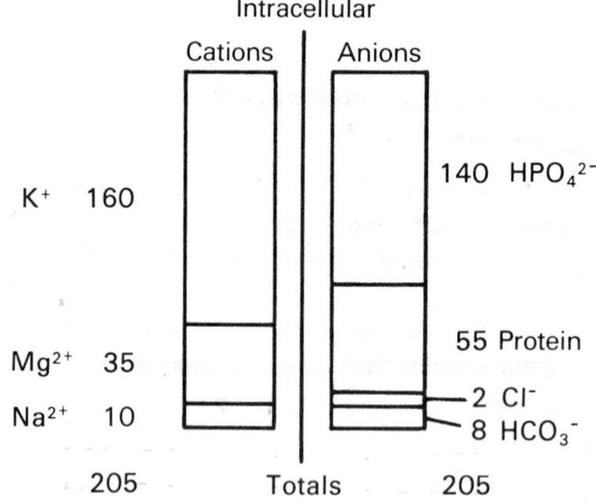

Figure 12-3 Electrolyte content of fluid compartments.

for an equal volume.[3] Osmolarity is used to compare solutions of equal weight and volume, such as plasma with an intravenous solution.

Measurement of osmolality

Osmolality is measured in milliosmoles per kilogram of water (mOsm/kg). Normal osmolality of body fluids is 275 to 295 mOsm. A high serum glucose increases the osmolality of extracellular fluid. This elevation of osmolality explains the increased requirement for fluids in the treatment of diabetic ketoacidosis.

The kidneys are responsible for keeping the concentration of body fluids constant at 275 to 295 mOsm. The normal range for urine osmolality is 300 to 1090 mOsm/kg.

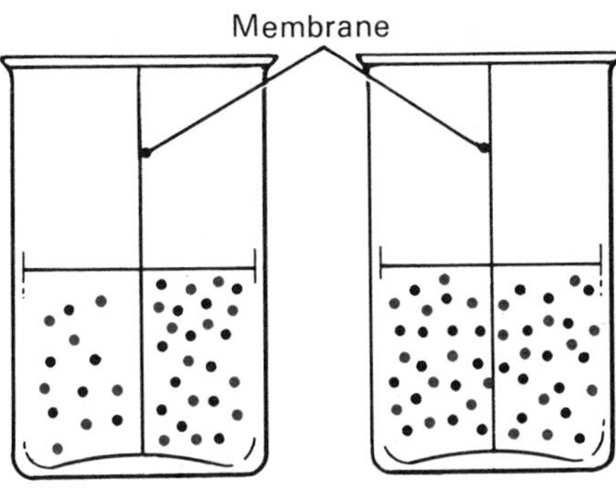

Figure 12-4 Diffusion is the movement of molecules from an area of higher concentration to an area of lower concentration.

Osmotic movement of fluids

Cells are affected by the osmolality of the fluid which surrounds them. When fluids are added to the body, those having the same osmolality as the cell interior are called *isotonic*. Solutions which contain more water than the cell are *hypotonic* and those with less water than the cell are *hypertonic* (Table 12-2).

Normally, the ECF and ICF are *isotonic* to one another; hence no net movement of water occurs. Of course, in the metabolically active cell, there is constant exchange of substances between the compartments, but no net gain or loss of water occurs.

If a cell is surrounded by *hypo*tonic fluid, water moves into the cell, causing it to swell and possibly to burst. If a cell is surrounded by *hyper*tonic fluid, water leaves the cell to dilute the ECF. The cell shrinks and may eventually die.

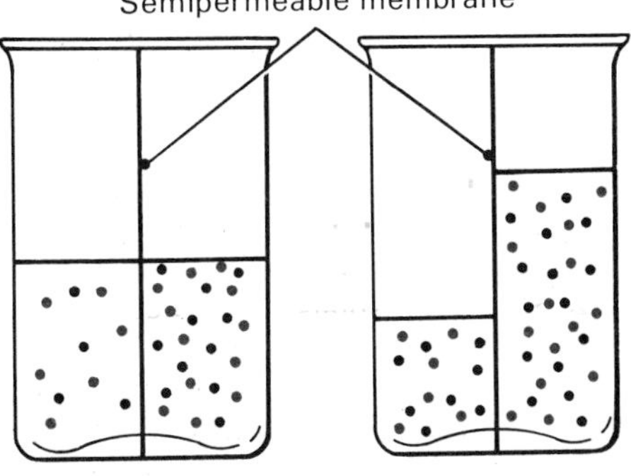

Figure 12-5 Osmosis is the process of water movement through a semipermeable membrane from an area of low solute concentration to an area of high solute concentration.

Table 12-2
Definitions of Tonicity

Tonicity	Osmolality	Effects on Cell Size
Hypotonic	Less than 270 mOsm	Swelling
Isotonic	275–295 mOsm	None
Hypertonic	More than 300 mOsm	Shrinking

Active Transport

Active transport is an energy-using process in which electrolytes are pumped into and out of cells. One type of active transport is the *sodium-potassium pump* and like all biological pumps, it works against normal pressure gradients (Fig. 12-6). The energy source for the pump is adenosine triphosphate (ATP) produced in the mitochondria.

Hydrostatic Pressure

Hydrostatic pressure is the force generated by the column of blood contained within a blood vessel. At the arterial end of the capillary system, hydrostatic pressure moves fluid into the interstitial spaces (Fig. 12-7). At the arterial end, the hydrostatic pressure is 32 mmHg. The hydrostatic pressure decreases to 12 mmHg on the venous side because of the fluid movement from the capillary to the interstitium.

Oncotic Pressure

Oncotic pressure (colloidal osmotic pressure) is osmotic pressure created by plasma proteins. Their large size compels plasma proteins to remain within the vascular system. They attract water and contribute to the osmotic pressure within the vascular system. Other particles in solution (both electrolyte and nonelectrolyte substances) also exert osmotic pressure, but the term *oncotic pressure* specifically refers to the osmotic pressure of plasma proteins.

Since plasma proteins are normally found only within the vascular system, there is a significant difference between the vascular system and interstitium. Figure 12-7 illustrates the effect of hydrostatic and oncotic pressure at the capillary level.

FLUID SHIFTS

When the equilibrium of the body is altered, shifts of fluid may occur from one fluid compartment to another. The two shifts of fluid seen most frequently

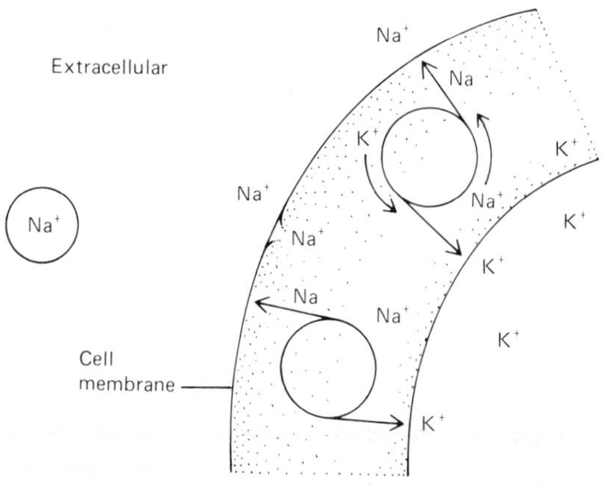

Figure 12-6 Sodium-potassium pump. As sodium diffuses into the cell and potassium out of the cell, an active transport system supplied with energy delivers sodium back to the extracellular compartment and potassium to the intracellular compartment. (*Taken from J. Barry, Emergency Nursing, McGraw-Hill Book Company, New York, 1978, p. 13.)*

occur in the extracellular fluid. They are (1) plasmato-interstitial, and (2) interstitial-to-plasma.

Plasma-to-Interstitial Fluid Shift

Two types of plasma-to-interstitial shift are edema and hypovolemic changes.

Edema

Edema is the accumulation of fluid in the interstitial spaces. It can be due to (1) increased hydrostatic pressure, (2) decreased oncotic pressure, (3) breaks in the integrity of vessel walls, and (4) obstructed lymph drainage.

Increased hydrostatic pressure can occur in clients with fluid overload (e.g., congestive heart failure). Decreased oncotic pressure can occur in situations of excess protein loss (nephrotic syndrome) or deficient protein synthesis (liver disease). Blood vessel wall integrity can be damaged by trauma, burns, or inflammatory reactions. If lymphatics are obstructed, their

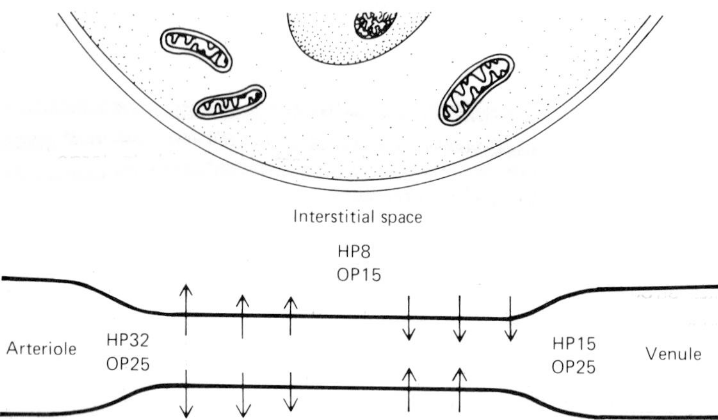

Figure 12-7 Dynamics of fluid exchange between the vascular volume and the interstitial space. The arrow indicates direction of filtration flow. HP is hydrostatic pressure: OP is oncotic pressure. At the arteriolar end an HP of 32 mmHg is forcing outward filtration while an OP of 25 mmHg resists this flow. The result is a 7-mmHg filtration gradient. The tissue resists this capillary flow with an HP of 8 mmHg but enhances the filtration with 15 mmHg OP, resulting in a 7-mmHg drawing force. The net arteriolar filtration gradient is 14 mmHg. At the venule end, HP decreases to 15 mmHg, but the OP remains the same, and so there is an inward capillary pull of 10 mmHg. The tissue pressures remain the same with 7 mmHg resistance. Therefore, fuild is reabsorbed into the capillary pressure gradient of 3 mmHg. (*Taken from J. Barry, Emergency Nursing, McGraw-Hill Book Company, New York, 1978, p. 12.)*

normal function in removing excess fluid from the interstitium and returning it to the venous system is impaired.

Hypovolemia

Hypovolemia may result from massive fluid loss into the interstitial spaces. Clinical causes of this shift include traumatic injuries that disrupt the integrity of capillary walls. Examples include:

- Massive burns
- Peritonitis
- Pleural effusion
- Intestinal obstruction
- Fractures (especially femur and pelvis)
- Occlusion of large arteries, producing ischemia

Interstitial-to-Plasma Fluid Shift

Interstitial-to-plasma fluid shift may occur with remobilization of edema fluid following a plasma-to-interstitial shift. This usually occurs in severe burns about the third day. This shift can also occur due to excessive IV administration of plasma, dextran, and other hypertonic solutions. The concentrations of these solutions are so great that interstitial water is drawn back into the plasma.

Another type of interstitial-to-plasma fluid shift is a compensatory response to blood loss. In both internal and external blood loss, there is an acute shift of fluids from the interstitium to plasma.

REGULATION OF FLUID AND ELECTROLYTES

Cerebral Regulation

Water intake is equal to water excretion when the client is not exposed to any environmental stresses and has access to water. Water ingestion in the conscious client is regulated by the thirst center in the hypothalamus. Factors which signal a need to drink water include a decreased cardiac output and extracellular and intracellular dehydration. A dry mouth will cause the client to drink even when there is no measurable body water deficit.

Pituitary Regulation

The thirst center in the hypothalamus regulates water ingestion. The adjacent posterior pituitary secretes antidiuretic hormone (ADH) which regulates water retention by the kidneys. The distal tubules and collecting ducts in the kidney respond to ADH by becoming more permeable to water so that water is reabsorbed into the blood, leaving a more concentrated urine to be excreted.

Normally an increase in plasma osmolality or a decrease in circulating volume will stimulate ADH secretion. If ADH secretion occurs when there is a normal plasma osmolality and normal circulating plasma volume, this is called *syndrome of inappropriate antidiuretic hormone* (SIADH) (Chap. 42.) Causes of SIADH secretion include stress, trauma, tumors, surgery, ventilation with a positive-pressure respirator, and certain drugs. The inappropriate ADH causes water retention, which produces a decrease in plasma osmolality below the normal value and an increase in urine osmolality.

Absence of antidiuretic hormone produces diabetes insipidus (Chap. 42). A copious amount of dilute urine is excreted because the renal tubules and collecting ducts do not reabsorb water. If the water losses are not replaced, the client will become dehydrated and hypernatremic.

Adrenal Cortical Regulation

Extracellular fluid volume is maintained by a combination of hormonal influences. ADH affects only water reabsorption. The adrenal cortex secretes two groups of hormones: glucocorticoids and mineralocorticoids. The glucocorticoids have an anti-inflammatory effect while the mineralocorticoids are known for their enhancement of sodium retention and potassium excretion (Fig. 12-8). When sodium is reabsorbed, some water is also reabsorbed because of the osmotic effect of sodium.

Cortisol is the most common example of a naturally occurring adrenocortical steroid. In large doses

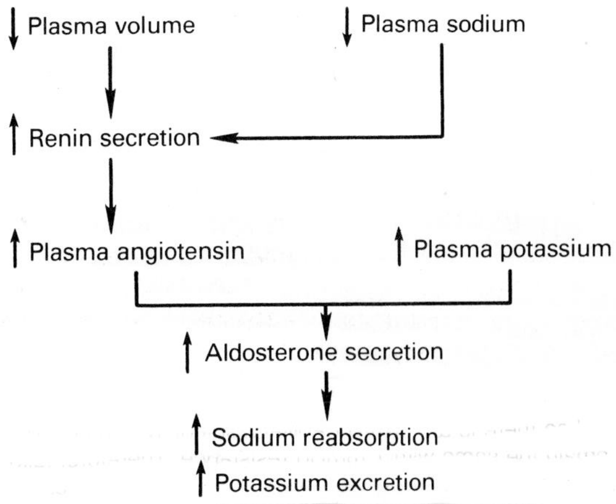

Figure 12-8 Influences of aldosterone secretion.

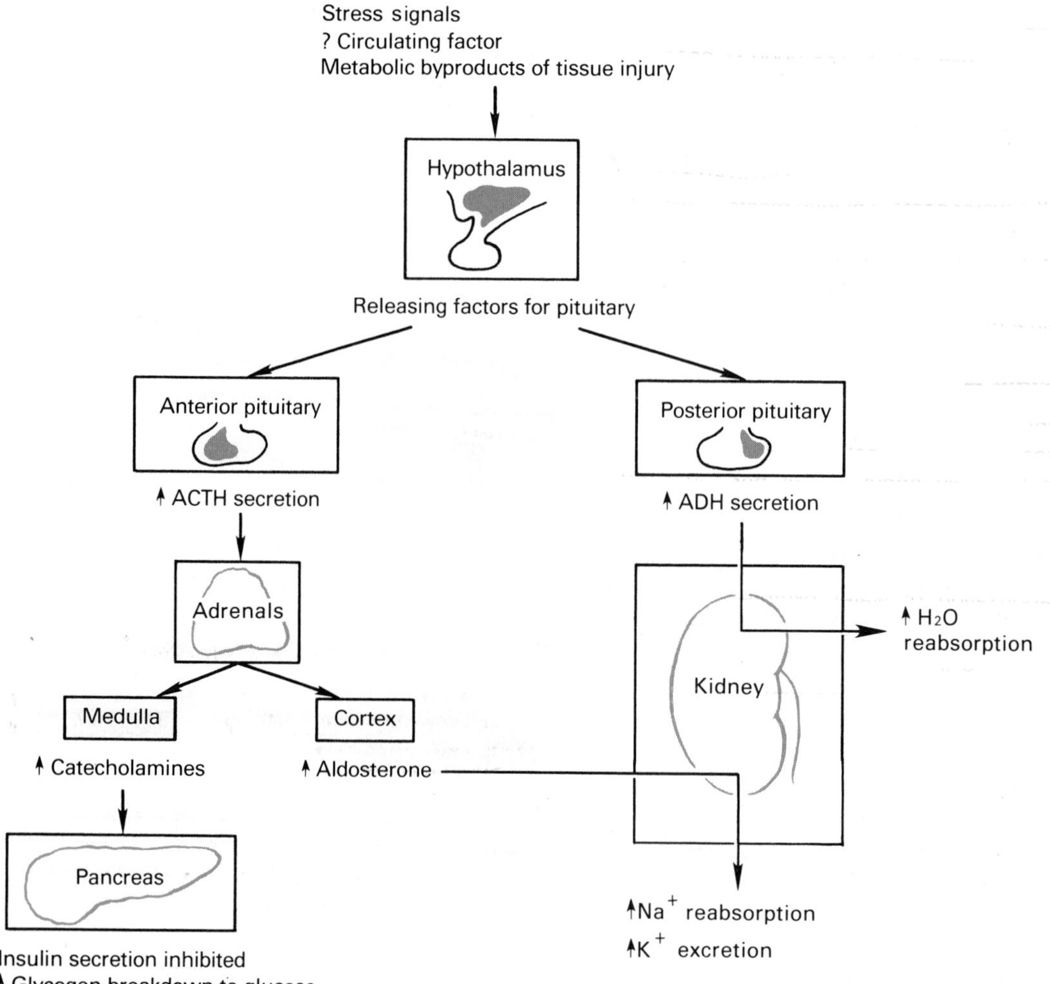

Figure 12-9 Effects of stress on fluid and electrolyte balance.

cortisol has both glucocorticoid (anti-inflammatory) and mineralocorticoid (sodium retention) properties. The adrenocortical hormone cortisol is secreted whenever the body experiences stress. Many body systems including fluid and electrolyte balance are affected by stress (Fig. 12-9).

Aldosterone is the naturally occurring mineralocorticoid with the most potent sodium retention and potassium excreting capability. The secretion of aldosterone is raised by a decrease in plasma volume and decreased serum sodium. The kidney responds by secreting renin into the plasma. Angiotensinogen produced in the liver is acted on by the renin to form angiotensin, which stimulates the adrenal cortex to secrete aldosterone (Fig. 12-8).

Renal Regulation

The primary organ for regulation of fluid and electrolyte balance is the kidney (Chap. 36). Normally the kidney reabsorbs 99 percent of the glomerular filtrate. Selective reabsorption and secretion of fluid and electrolytes function to maintain normal plasma osmolality and blood volume. The renal tubules are the site for the hormonal action of ADH and aldosterone.

With impaired renal function, the kidneys are not able to maintain fluid and electrolyte balance. This results in edema, potassium retention, impaired bicarbonate reabsorption, and many other problems (Chap. 38).

Gastrointestinal Regulation

Our daily water intake is between 2000 to 3000 mL (Table 12-3). The gastrointestinal tract accounts for most of the water intake. Water intake includes fluids, water from food metabolism, and the water present in solid foods. Fruits and vegetables are 50 to 60 percent water while the water content of lean meats approaches 70 percent.[4]

Most of the water excreted is eliminated by the kidneys. A small amount of water is eliminated by the gastrointestinal tract in feces.

Insensible Water Loss

Insensible water loss is unavoidable vaporization from the lungs and skin. It functions in regulating body temperature. Normally, about 900 mL per day is lost. The amount of water loss is increased by accelerated body metabolism.

Insensible perspiration should not be confused with the vaporization of water excreted by sweat glands. Only water is lost by insensible perspiration. Excessive sweating (perspiration) caused by fever or high environmental temperatures may lead to large losses of water and sodium chloride.

FLUID AND ELECTROLYTE IMBALANCES

Fluid and electrolyte imbalances occur to some degree in most clients with a major illness or injury. This is because illness disrupts the normal homeostatic mechanism. Some fluid and electrolyte imbalances are directly caused by the illness or disease (e.g., burns, congestive heart failure). At other times therapeutic measures (e.g., IV fluid replacement, diuretics) cause or contribute to a fluid and electrolyte imbalance.

Table 12-3

Normal Fluid Balance in the Adult

Intake	
Fluids	1200mL
Solid food	1000mL
Water from oxidation	300mL
	2500mL
Output	
Insensible loss (skin and lungs)	900mL
In feces	100mL
Urine	1500mL
	2500mL

Table 12-4

Normal Serum Electrolyte Values

Bicarbonate (HCO_3^-)	20–30 mEq/L
Calcium (Ca^{2+})	9–11 mg/dL 4.5–5.5 mEq/L
Chloride (Cl^-)	96–106 mEq/L
Potassium (K^+)	3.5–5.5 mEq/L
Magnesium (Mg^{2+})	1.5–2.5 mEq/L
Sodium (Na^+)	135–145 mEq/L
Phosphate (PO_4^{2-})	2.8–4.5 mg/dL
Protein	6.0–8.0 g/dL

The imbalances are commonly classified as deficits or excesses. Each imbalance is discussed separately (for normal values, see Table 12-4). In actual clinical situations it is common to find two or more imbalances in the same client. For instance, a client with prolonged nasogastric suction may lose Na^+, K^+, and HCl. This could result in both a sodium and potassium deficiency as well as metabolic alkalosis.

Water and Sodium Imbalances

Sodium is the major cation in ECF. It participates in the generation and transmission of nerve impulses, is an essential electrolyte in the sodium-potassium pump, regulates osmotic pressure, and controls distribution of water throughout the body.

A frequent saying is "where sodium goes, water goes." For this reason, sodium and water problems are often not differentiated. This can be very confusing because primary water problems require significantly different treatment than primary sodium problems. For example, a pure water gain produces a decreased serum sodium because the added water dilutes the sodium. Treatment with a normal saline solution would overload the client with both sodium and water. The appropriate treatment for a low serum sodium (hyponatremia) caused by an excess of water is restriction of fluid.

Sodium and water alterations can be classified into *primary water imbalances, primary sodium imbalances*, and *extracellular imbalances.*

Primary water imbalances

Common causes of primary water imbalances are listed in Table 12-5.

Water Deficit (Dehydration) *Water deficit* is not a problem in an alert person who has access to water

Table 12-5
Primary Water Imbalances: Causes and Clinical Manifestations

Primary Water Deficiency	Primary Water Excess
Causes	
Impaired thirst mechanism (injury) Swallowing problems Diabetes insipidus Decreased water intake Coma Debility Decreased availability Watery diarrhea	Psychiatric disorder of large amounts of H_2O ingestion Renal disease Excess administration of hypotonic fluids Excess tap water enemas Inappropriate secretion of ADH
Appearance	
Decreased skin turgor Dehydrated Dry, sticky mucous membranes Rough, dry tongue Weight loss Fever	Weight gain Edema Good skin turgor
Behavior	
Agitation Restlessness Weakness	Confusion Lethargy Weakness Seizures
Cardiovascular	
Orthostatic hypotension ↓ CVP Rapid, weak pulse	Full, bounding pulse ↑ CVP Jugular venous distension
Gastrointestinal	
Hard stools	Nausea Vomiting Liquid stools
Urinary Findings	
Urine volume ↓ Specific gravity >1.030	Urinary volume ↑ Specific gravity <1.010
Serum Values	
Na ↑ Protein ↑ Hematocrit ↑ Serum osmolality ↑ Urine osmolality ↑	Na ↓ Protein ↓ Hematocrit ↓ Serum osmolality ↓ Urine osmolality ↓

and is able to swallow. Primary water deficiency is often the result of impaired level of consciousness and/or inability to ingest oral fluids. Clients who receive only high-protein tube feedings will become water-deficient. Often, elderly people, especially if they are ill, do not drink enough fluids.

The clinical manifestations of primary water deficiency are listed in Table 12-5. The client appears dehydrated. A deficiency of water concentrates the serum sodium, increases the serum sodium, and decreases the ECF volume.

Water Excess (Overhydration) A *water excess* in a healthy individual will not occur unless the fluid intake exceeds 20 L over a day[5] Problems with water excess are most frequently associated with impaired renal function.

In primary water excess (Table 12-5) the client will appear hydrated and may have edema. The changes in the ECF volume are reflected in decreases in hematocrit and serum sodium and increases in urine volume and central venous pressure (CVP).

Medical Management of Primary Water Imbalances The goal of treatment in both types of water imbalances is to treat the underlying cause. In primary water deficit, the continued water loss must be prevented and water replacement provided. If oral fluids cannot be administered, intravenous solutions of 5% dextrose in water are given initially. If adequate renal function is present, electrolytes can be added to the IV solution.

In primary water excess, fluid restriction is often all that is needed to treat the problem. If severe symptoms (e.g., convulsions) develop, small amounts of hypertonic saline may be given to restore the serum sodium while the body is returning to a normal water balance.

Sodium imbalances

The common causes of sodium imbalances are presented in Table 12-6. Sodium imbalances are usually directly related to water imbalances. Hyponatremia (low serum sodium level) may result from sodium loss or water excess. Hypernatremia (increased serum sodium levels) may result from excess sodium, water loss, or insufficient water intake. The clinical manifestations of sodium imbalances are similar to those of water imbalances (Table 12-6).

Medical Management of Sodium Imbalances Treatment of sodium imbalances needs to be directed at the underlying cause. Differential assessment of ECF volume is helpful (Fig. 12-10). The goal of treatment for sodium deficit is to restore sodium level without causing fluid volume excess. If the client also has a fluid excess (dilutional hyponatremia), therapy is aimed at restricting fluids. If there is a fluid deficit or normal fluid balance associated with the hyponatremia, usually intravenous isotonic saline (0.9% NaCl) is given. Occasionally, 3% NaCl is given.

The goal of treatment for sodium excess is to dilute the sodium concentration and promote excretion of the excess sodium. Intravenous solutions of 5 percent dextrose in water are usually given. Diuretics may be used to remove excess sodium.

Extracellular fluid volume imbalances

The terms *extracellular fluid volume deficit* (hypovolemia) and *extracellular fluid volume excess* (hypervolemia) are commonly used in describing fluid imbalances (Table 12-7). These terms refer to a deficit or excess not just of water, but of both water and electrolytes (primarily sodium) in approximately the same proportion. ECF deficit could result from severe diarrhea or fistula drainage where both water and electrolytes are lost. ECF excess would result from excessive infusion of isotonic fluids. The clinical manifestations of ECF imbalances are similar to those of both water and sodium imbalances.

Medical Management of Fluid Volume Imbalances The goal of treatment for fluid volume deficit is to correct the underlying cause (e.g., hemorrhage, diarrhea) and to replace both water and electrolytes, especially if the problem has existed for several days. Balanced intravenous solutions such as lactated Ringer's solution are usually given.

The goal of treatment for fluid volume excess is removal of sodium and water without producing abnormal changes in electrolyte osmolality or composition of ECF. The primary cause needs to be identified and treated. Intravenous therapy is usually not indicated for this type of fluid imbalance. Usually diuretic therapy is indicated. Reducing oral sodium intake may also be indicated. If the fluid excess leads to problems of ascites or pleural effusion, an abdominal paracentesis or thoracentesis might be indicated.

Nursing management of sodium and water imbalances

Intake and Output Twenty-four-hour intake and output records give valuable information regarding fluid and electrolyte problems. Sources of excessive intake or fluid losses can be identified on a properly recorded intake and output flowsheet. Intake should include oral, intravenous, and tube feedings. Output includes urine, excess perspiration, wound or tube drainage, vomitus, and diarrhea. Estimated fluid losses should be made on wound and perspiration losses.

Table 12-6
Sodium Imbalances: Causes and Clinical Manifestations

Hyponatremia (Na^+<135mEq/L)	Hypernatremia (Na^+>145 mEq/L)
Causes	
Excess sweating plus drinking water Diuretic excess Adrenal insufficiency Gastrointestinal suction with H_2O irrigations Edema (water retention exceeds sodium retention) Cirrhosis Congestive heart failure Excess IV administration of D5/water Fresh water drowning	Decreased water intake Excess intake of saline or salt tablets Adrenal hyperfunction Heatstroke High fever Salt water drowning Rapid breathing with H_2O vapor loss Excess IV administration of 0.9% NaCl Watery, profuse diarrhea
Appearance	
Clammy skin Dehydrated Shocky Weakness	Edema Weight gain
Behavior	
Anxiety Lethargy Stupor→coma	Weakness Lethargy Restlessness
Cardiovascular	
Rapid, thready pulse Postural hypotension ↓ CVP Decreased jugular venous filling	Normal vital signs (can deteriorate into congestive heart failure) ↑ CVP Distended veins
Gastrointestinal	
Anorexia, nausea Vomiting Abdominal pain	No specific findings
Neuromuscular	
Muscle weakness Lower extremity muscle cramps	Depressed reflexes
Urinary Findings	
Urinary output ↓ Specific gravity ↑	Urinary output ↓ Specific gravity ↑
Serum Values	
Serum Na ↓ Hematocrit ↑ Serum protein ↑ Urine osmolality ↑	Serum Na ↑ Hematocrit ↓ Serum protein ↓

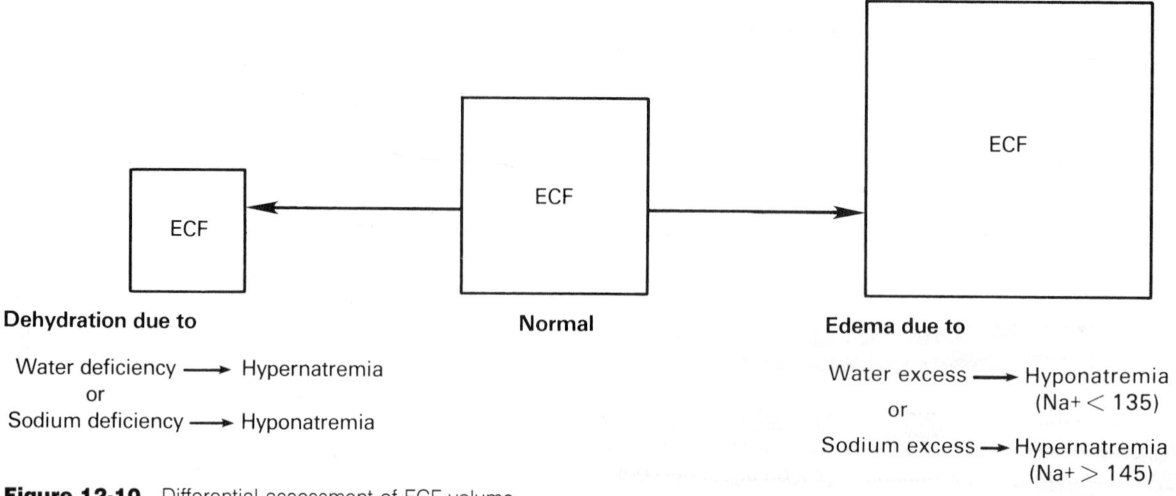

Figure 12-10 Differential assessment of ECF volume.

Table 12-7
Causes of Extracellular Fluid Volume Imbalances

Extracellular Fluid Volume Deficit	Extracellular Fluid Volume Excess
Decreased water intake	Congestive heart failure
Vomiting and diarrhea	Hyperaldosteronism
Fistula drainage	Chronic liver disease with portal hypertension
Intestinal obstruction	Long-term use of corticosteroids
Systemic infection	Renal diseases
	Excessive IV administration of isotonic fluids

Daily Weights Accurate daily weights are known to provide the best bedside measurement of hydration status.[6] A rapid increase of 1 kg (2.2 pounds) is equal to 1000 mL fluid retention (providing the person has maintained usual dietary intake or been NPO). However, weights are often not relied upon because they are not properly obtained.[7] An accurate weight requires the client to be weighed at the same time every day and on the same scale. Excess clothing and bedding should be removed, and all drainage bags emptied prior to the weighing. If there are bulky dressings present or tubes which may not necessarily be present day to day, a notation regarding these variables should be recorded on the flowsheet or nursing notes.

Skin Assessment and Care Dehydration and overhydration can be detected by inspection of the skin. Skin should be examined for turgor and mobility. Normally, a fold of skin when pinched will readily move and upon release snap back into its former condition. Skin over the sternum, abdomen, and anterior forearm are the usual sites for evaluation of tissue turgor (Fig. 12-11).

In dehydration, skin turgor is diminished so that there is a lag in the pinched skin fold returning to its original state. The skin may be cool and moist if there is sympathetic vasoconstriction to compensate for the decreased fluid volume. Mild dehydration usually does not stimulate this compensatory response so the skin will be warm and dry. Dehydration may also cause the skin to appear dry and wrinkled. This sign may be difficult to evaluate in the elderly because their skin may be normally dry, wrinkled, and nonelastic.

Skin that is edematous may feel cool due to fluid accumulation and a decrease in blood flow secondary to the pressure of the fluid. The fluid can also stretch the skin so that it feels taut and hard. *Pitting edema* is the term used to describe edema when the examiner's thumb leaves an indentation over the edematous area. The areas to be evaluated for pitting edema are those where soft tissues overlay a bone. Skin over the tibia, fibula, and sacrum are the preferred sites.

Good skin care for both the overhydrated and dehydrated person is very important. Edematous tissues need to be protected from extremes of heat and cold, prolonged pressure, and trauma. Frequent skin care and position changes will prevent edematous tissues from skin breakdown. Elevating edematous extremities helps to promote venous return. Dehydrated skin needs frequent skin care without soap application. The application of moisturizing creams or oils will increase moisture retention and stimulate circulation.

Other Nursing Measures The infusion rates of intravenous fluid solutions should be carefully monitored. Attempts to "catch up" should be considered carefully. This is especially true for clients with heart, renal, or neurologic problems. The nurse needs to encourage and often assist the elderly or debilitated client to maintain an adequate oral intake. Clients on tube feedings may need to have supplementary water added to their regular tube feedings.

Clients with nasogastric suction should not be allowed to drink water because it will be suctioned out along with electrolytes. Occasionally, limited ice chips are allowed for the client to suck on. A nasogastric tube should always be irrigated with isotonic saline and not water.

Potassium Imbalances

Potassium is the major cation in ICF. Its functions include maintenance of the regular cardiac rhythm, transmission and conduction of nerve impulses, and utilization of glucose by cells. Furthermore, K^+ is part of the enzyme system necessary for cell energy production.

The kidneys play the primary role in K^+ excretion. If the kidney function is impaired, toxic levels of K^+ may result. However, the kidneys are unable to conserve potassium, which may be flushed out by diuresis even in the presence of a body deficit.

The laboratory measurement of potassium measures the amount in ECF. This is only an indirect determination of potassium found intracellularly. Causes of potassium imbalance are presented in Table 12-8.

Hypokalemia

Hypokalemia (low serum potassium) can result from loss of potassium in intestinal tract fluids, excretion in urine, or from a shift of potassium from the ECF to the ICF. Metabolic alkalosis will cause potassium to move intracellularly in exchange for hydrogen ions. This type of hypokalemia will usually correct itself with treatment of the alkalosis.

Hypokalemia may be associated with the treatment of diabetic ketoacidosis. When glucose and insulin move intracellularly they take potassium with them and decrease the ECF potassium. Other causes of hypokalemia (reflecting a decrease in total body potassium) include diuretic therapy, increased aldosterone secretion, and gastrointestinal losses in diarrhea, vomiting, and ileostomy drainage.

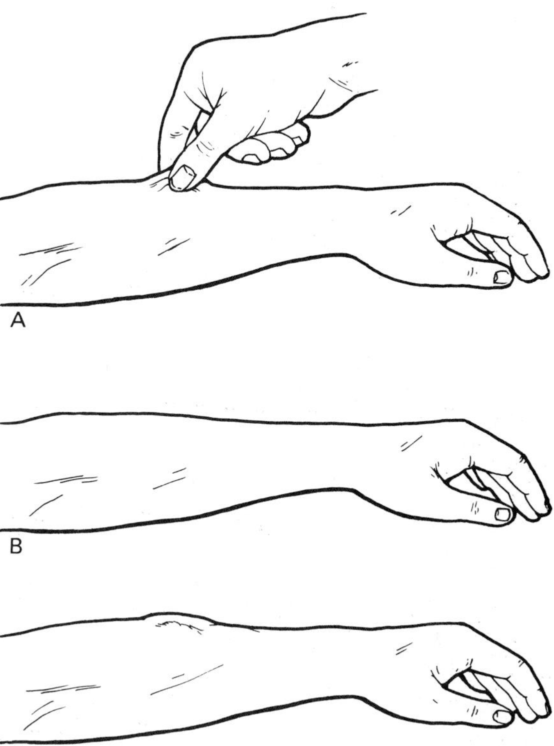

Figure 12-11 Assessment of skin turgor. When normal skin is pinched (*a*), it resumes shape within seconds (*b*). If the skin remains wrinkled for 20 to 30 seconds, the client has poor skin turgor (*c*).

Clinical manifestations of hypokalemia are listed in Table 12-8. Hypokalemia decreases cell excitability but produces a stronger contraction. Hyperkalemia (high serum potassium) increases cell excitability but produces a weaker contraction. Cardiac cells demonstrate the most clinically significant changes with potassium imbalance (Fig. 12-12).

Hyperkalemia

Hyperkalemia occurs following a shift of potassium from the ICF to the ECF from massive cell destruction (e.g., burns or a crush injury) or with an excessive intake and resultant increase in total body potassium as in renal failure. Metabolic acidosis causes a shift of potassium from ICF to ECF. Correction of the acidosis causes a shift of potassium from ICF to ECF. Correction of the acidosis will usually correct the hyperkalemia except when renal function is impaired.

Table 12-8

Potassium Imbalances: Causes and Clinical Manifestations

Hypokalemia ($K^+<3.5$ mEq/L)	Hyperkalemia ($K^+>5.5$mEq/L)
Causes	
Vomiting Diarrhea Potent diuretics Aldosterone-producing tumor Potassium-free IV solutions Recovery phase of diabetic acidosis Fistulas Metabolic alkalosis	Renal failure Early stage of burns Adrenal insufficiency Massive crushing injury Excess IV administration of K^+ Metabolic acidosis
Appearance	
Drowsy	No specific findings
Behavior	
Confusion Irritability	No alteration in mentation
Cardiovascular	
ECG Changes ST depression T wave inversion or flattening U waves Bradycardia, 1st and 2d degree heart block, atrial arrhythmias PVCs, especially for clients on digitalis Postural hypotension	ECG Changes Peaked T waves PR interval prolonged P wave disappears QRS widens Complete heart block, ectopic beats Ventricular fibrillation → ventricular standstill
Gastrointestinal	
Anorexia, nausea, vomiting Paralytic ileus	No specific findings
Neuromuscular	
Hyporeflexia Muscle weakness→paralysis Muscle cramps and paresthesias	Decreased deep tendon reflexes Ascending paralysis Paresthesias
Urinary Findings	
Urinary output ↑ Specific gravity ↓ May have decreased output because of urinary retention	Urine potassium ↑
Serum Values	
Serum potassium ↓ pH ↑	Serum potassium ↑ pH ↓

Medical and nursing management of potassium imbalances

Treatment of hyperkalemia consists of:

1. Decreasing dietary sources of potassium (Appendix B, Table 11)
2. Administering sodium bicarbonate intravenously
3. Administering calcium gluconate
4. Infusing glucose and insulin intravenously
5. Use of cation exchange resins (Kayexalate)
6. Dialysis

Sodium bicarbonate corrects acidosis and facilitates potassium movement to the ICF. Calcium antagonizes the effect of potassium on the heart. Glucose and insulin infusion is used in the acute management of hyperkalemia because potassium moves to the ECF when glucose is metabolized. Kayexalate binds potassium in exchange for sodium and the resin is excreted in feces (Chap. 38).

Hypokalemia is treated by giving potassium chloride supplements and increasing dietary intake of potassium. Potassium chloride (KCl) supplements can be given orally or intravenously. KCl should never be given unless there is urine output of at least 30 mL/hr. KCl supplements added to intravenous solutions should never exceed 80 mEq/L. The preferred is 40 mEq/L. The rate of IV administration of KCl should never exceed 30 mEq/hour. When potassium is given IV, it may cause pain in the area of the vein where it is entering.

Clients taking diuretics (especially thiazide and loop diuretics) need to be aware of the need to increase dietary potassium intake (Appendix B, Table 11). It may be necessary for them to take oral KCl supplements. These people should be instructed to recognize clinical manifestations of hypokalemia and report them to their health care provider. If this client is also on digitalis preparations, serum potassium must be closely monitored because hypokalemia enhances the action of digitalis.

Calcium Imbalances

Calcium is only found in ECF. Its functions include transmission of nerve impulse, blood clotting, formation of teeth and bone, and muscular contraction. Normally, the amount of calcium and phosphorus found in the body is in an inverse relationship. Calcium is usually present in the body either in an ionized form or bound to protein. The ionized form is the biologically active form.

Calcium balance depends on the proper functioning of three hormones: vitamin D, parathormone, and calcitonin. *Vitamin D* is formed through the action of

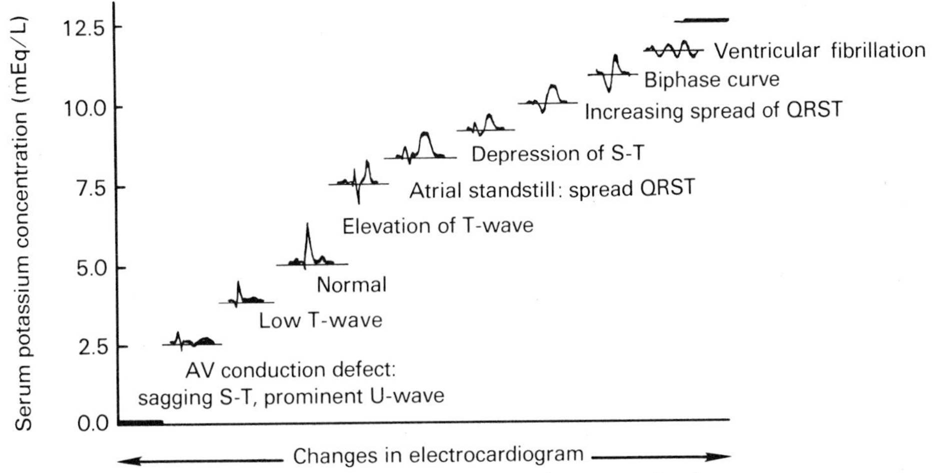

Figure 12-12 ECG changes associated with changes in serum potassium.

ultraviolet rays on a precursor found in the skin, or is ingested in the diet. Vitamin D is essential for absorption of calcium from the gastrointestinal tract.

Parathormone is produced by the parathyroid gland. Its production and release is stimulated by low serum calcium levels. Parathormone increases bone resorption (movement of calcium out of bones), increases gastrointestinal absorption of calcium, increases renal reabsorption of calcium, and decreases phosphate reabsorption.

Calcitonin is produced by the thyroid gland and is stimulated by high serum calcium levels. It opposes the action of parathormone and thus lowers the serum calcium level.

Causes of calcium imbalance are listed in Table 12-9.

Hypocalcemia

Hypocalcemia is commonly associated with hypoparathyroidism caused by surgical removal of the parathyroids. Surgical removal of the parathyroids may be done primarily for treatment of tumors or occur inadvertently with thyroid surgery. Acute pancreatitis is another common cause of hypocalcemia. Clients who receive multiple blood transfusions can become hypocalcemic because the citrate used to anticoagulate the blood binds with the calcium. Clinical manifestations of hypocalcemia are listed in Table 12-9.

Since calcium is essential for conduction of nerve impulses and muscle contraction, procedures which evaluate neuromuscular irritability are useful for assessing a low serum calcium. Trousseau's sign refers to carpopedal spasms induced by inflating a blood pressure cuff on the arm (Fig. 12-13). The blood pressure cuff is inflated above the systolic pressure. Carpopedal spasms are evident within 3 minutes if hypocalcemia is present.[8] Chvostek's sign is contraction of facial muscles in response to a tap over the facial nerve in front of the ear (Fig. 12-13).

Tetany refers to the increased neuroexcitability and sustained muscle contraction associated with hypocalcemia. Manifestations of tetany include wrist and carpopedal spasms (Fig. 12-13), laryngeal stridor, dysphagia, dysarthria, cardiac arrhythmias, and convulsions.

Hypercalcemia

Excess serum calcium (hypercalcemia) also affects muscle tone and strength because neural excitability is depressed (Table 12-9). Hypercalcemia is most commonly associated with malignancy with skeletal metastasis, multiple myeloma, and hyperparathyroidism.

Medical and nursing management of calcium imbalances

The primary goal in treatment of calcium imbalance is aimed at treating the cause. Hypocalcemia can be treated with oral or intravenous calcium supplements. Calcium lactate (oral) and calcium gluconate (intravenous) are commonly used supplements. Any client who has had thyroid surgery must be observed closely for symptoms of hypocalcemia.

The basic treatment of hypercalcemia is to promote excretion of calcium in urine by administering a loop diuretic (furosemide or ethacrynic acid) and hydrating the client with normal saline. In chronic hypercalcemia the client needs to drink 3000 to 4000 mL of fluid daily to decrease the possibility of renal calculi formation.

Table 12-9
Calcium Imbalances: Causes and Clinical manifestations

4.5 -> 5.5 mEq/L

Hypocalcemia (<8.6 mg/dL)	Hypercalcemia (>10.5 mg/dL)
Causes	
Acute pancreatitis Primary hypoparathyroidism Steatorrhea Generalized peritonitis Chronic renal failure Vitamin D deficiency Surgical removal of parathyroids Excess administration of citrated blood	√Excess milk-product ingestion Hyperparathyroidism Prolonged immobilization √Multiple myeloma Pathologic fracture Thyrotoxicosis
Appearance	
Tonic and clonic convulsions	Lethargic Weight Loss Dehydrated
Behavior	
Personality changes Depression Irritability Easy fatigability	Decreased intellectual function Malaise Confusion Coma Increased thirst
Cardiovascular	
ECG changes QT-prolonged	ECG changes Broadened T waves Shortened QT then lengthened QT with severe elevation Hypertension
Gastrointestinal	
Colicky discomfort	Anorexia Nausea Constipation
Neuromuscular	
Hyperreflexia Muscle cramps Numbness and tingling in extremities Carpopedal spasms Chvostek's sign Trousseau's sign	Decreased muscle strength Depressed reflexes
Urinary Findings	
No specific findings	Increased urinary output
Serum Values	
Correction of acid pH may precipitate symptomatic hypocalcemia	Serum albumin increased —client may not be symptomatic despite increased Ca^{2+}

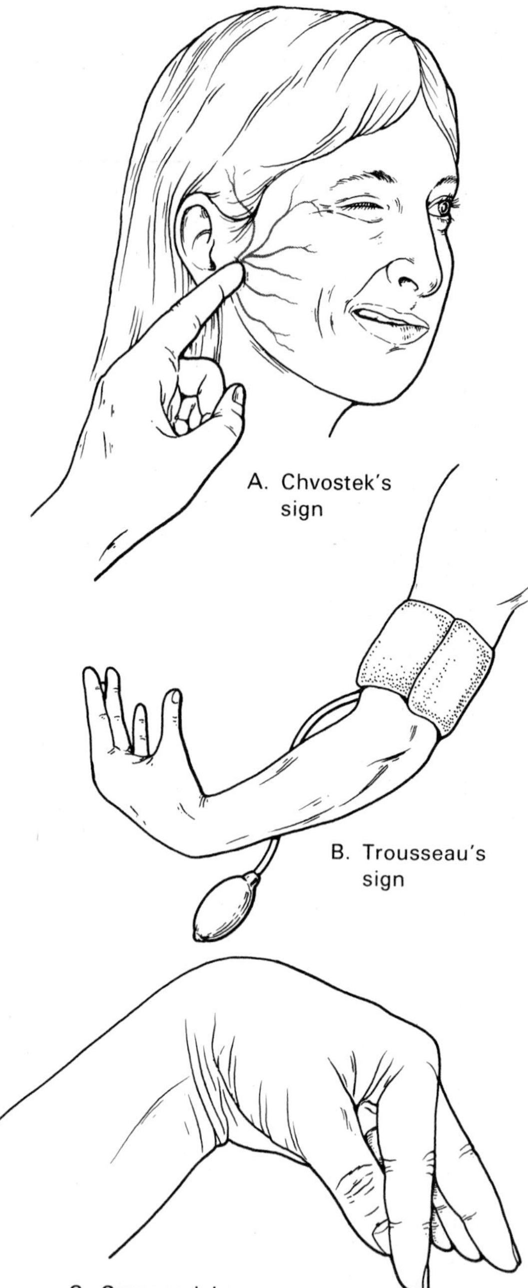

Figure 12-13 (*a*)Chvostek's sign is a contraction of facial muscles in response to a light tap over the facial nerve in front of the ear. (*b*) Trousseau's sign is a carpopedal spasm (*c*) induced by inflating a blood pressure cuff above the systolic pressure.

Phosphate Imbalances

An imbalance in phosphate often occurs with calcium problems because a high serum calcium level promotes phosphate excretion while a low serum calcium causes phosphate reabsorption. *Hyperphosphatemia* (elevated serum phosphate) occurs with chronic renal failure. Dialysis clients require phosphate binders in the form of aluminum hydroxide (Amphogel, Alternagel, Basaljel) to decrease their serum phosphate. Phosphate dialyzes poorly and is present in all foods. Ordinarily, calcium and phosphate are deposited only in bone. However, an increased serum phosphate along with an increased serum calcium precipitates readily and calcified deposits can occur in soft tissue.

Hypophosphatemia (low serum phosphate) is seen most frequently in malnourished clients. Hypophosphatemia produces a variety of nonspecific clinical manifestations including paresthesias, diminished reflexes, stupor, coma, and seizures. The most specific findings are those affecting the blood. Hypophosphatemia causes alterations in the shape and stability of the red blood cell, impairs white blood cell functioning, and decreases the number and effectiveness of platelets.[9] A low serum phosphate is treated by administering potassium or sodium phosphate in intravenous fluids.

Magnesium Imbalances

Magnesium functions as a coenzyme in the metabolism of both carbohydrates and protein. It is also involved in metabolism of cellular nucleic acid and proteins.[10] Causes of magnesium imbalance are listed in Table 12-10.

Neuromuscular excitability is profoundly affected by alterations in serum magnesium. *Hypomagnesemia* (a low serum magnesium) produces neuromuscular and central nervous system hyperirritability. A high serum magnesium (*hypermagnesemia*) depresses neuromuscular and central nervous system functions.

Hypomagnesemia

Hypomagnesemia develops gradually. Prolonged intravenous feeding without magnesium supplementation or excessive losses of fluids from the gastrointestinal tract are the common causes. The significant clinical manifestations are hyperactive deep tendon reflexes, tremors, and convulsions. Clinically, hypomagnesemia resembles hypocalcemia.

Hypermagnesemia

Hypermagnesemia usually occurs only with an increase in magnesium intake accompanied by renal insufficiency. Chronic renal failure clients who ingest products containing magnesium (e.g., Maalox, milk of magnesia) will have a problem with excess magnesium. The pregnant female who receives magnesium sulfate for the management of eclampsia could develop magnesium excess. Initial effects of increased magnesium are diminished deep tendon reflexes, followed by somnolence, then respiratory and ultimately cardiac arrest. Respiratory and cardiac arrest can occur when serum magnesium values approach 15 mEq/L.[11]

Table 12-10
Causes of Magnesium Imbalances

Hypomagnesemia	Hypermagnesemia
Diarrhea	Renal failure (if client given magnesium products)
Vomiting	
Chronic alcoholism	
Impaired GI absorption	
Malabsorption syndrome	

Medical management of magnesium imbalances

The treatment of hypomagnesemia is intravenous or intramuscular administration of magnesium sulfate. The emergency treatment of hypermagnesemia is administration of calcium chloride intravenously to physiologically oppose the effects of the magnesium on cardiac muscle. Promoting urinary excretion will decrease serum magnesium. Clients with impaired renal function will require dialysis since the kidney is the only route of excretion for magnesium.

Protein Imbalances

Plasma proteins are a significant determinant of ECF content. Due to their large molecular size they attract water and contribute to the osmotic pressure within the vascular system. Causes of protein imbalance are listed in Table 12-11.

Clinical manifestations of protein deficit include edema (from decreased oncotic pressure), slow healing, anorexia, fatigue, anemia, and muscle loss resulting from the breakdown of body tissue to meet the body's need for protein.

Management of protein deficit includes providing a high-carbohydrate, high-protein diet, and dietary protein supplements. If the client cannot meet his

Table 12-11
Causes of Protein Imbalances

Hypoproteinemia	Hyperproteinemia
Decreased food intake	Dehydration
Starvation	Hemoconcentration
Diseased liver	
Massive burns	
Loss of albumin in renal disease	
Major infection	

needs for protein orally, hyperalimentation may be used (Chap. 33).

ACID-BASE IMBALANCES

Hydrogen Ion Concentration

The acidity or alkalinity of a solution depends on its hydrogen ion (H^+) concentration. An increase in H^+ concentration leads to acidity, a decrease to alkalinity. (Definitions related to acid-base balance are presented in Table 12-12).

The weight of ionized hydrogen in water is about 0.0000001 g/L. This quantity may be expressed as 10^{-7}. Hydrogen ion concentration (symbolized as pH) is usually written as a negative logarithm. The pH may range from 1 to 14. The use of the negative logarithm means the lower the pH, the higher the hydrogen ion concentration. In contrast, to a pH of 7, a pH of 8 represents a tenfold decrease in hydrogen ion concentration.

A solution with a pH of 7 is considered neutral. An acid solution has a pH less than 7 and an alkaline solution has a pH greater than 7. Blood is slightly alkaline (pH 7.35 to 7.45), yet if it drops below 7.35, one can say the person has *acidosis*, even though it may never become truly acidic. If the blood pH is greater than 7.45, the person has *alkalosis* (Fig. 12-14). The pH of blood is computed through the use of the Henderson-Hasselbalch equation (Table 12-13).

Table 12-12
Terms Used in Acid-Base Physiology

Acid	Donor of hydrogen ions (H^+). In solution an acid separates into hydrogen and its accompanying anion.
Acidemia	Signifies an arterial blood pH of less than 7.35.
Acidosis	Process which adds acid or eliminates base from body fluids.
Alkalemia	Signifies an arterial blood pH of more than 7.45.
Alkalosis	Process which adds base or eliminates acid from body fluids.
Base	Acceptor of hydrogen ions. When hydrogen ions are added to a solution containing a base, the acid and base chemically combine. Bicarbonate (HCO_3^-) is the most abundant base in body fluids.
Buffer	Substance that reacts with an acid or base to prevent a large change in pH.
pH	Negative logarithm of the hydrogen ion concentration. A pH of 7 signifies 10^{-7} or 0.0000001 g/L of hydrogen ion.

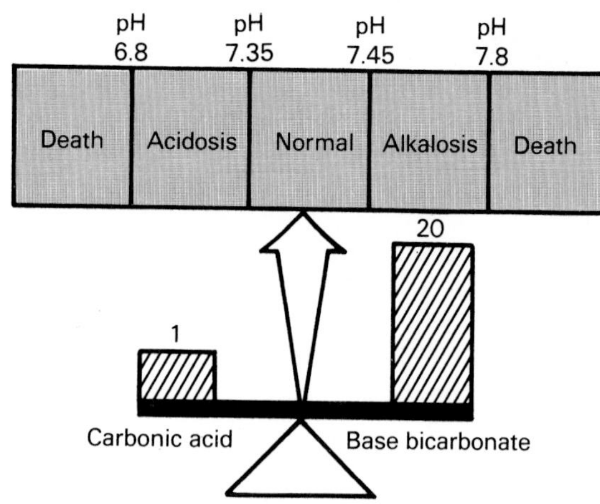

Figure 12-14 The normal range of plasma pH is 7.35–7.45. A normal pH is maintained by a ratio of one part carbonic acid to 20 parts base bicarbonate.

Acid-Base Regulation

Normally, the body has three mechanisms by which it regulates acid-base balance of extracellular fluid to maintain it between 7.35 and 7.45. These mechanisms are (1) the buffer systems, (2) the respiratory system, and (3) the renal system.

The regulatory mechanisms react at different speeds. Buffers react immediately. The respiratory system takes a few minutes to respond and reaches maximum effectiveness in about 1 hour. The renal response takes 2 to 3 days to respond maximally, but the kidneys can maintain balance for a long period of time.

Buffer system

The buffer system is the fastest-acting system and the primary regulator of acid-base balance. The buffers in the body are:

1. Carbonic acid-bicarbonate
2. Disodium-monosodium phosphate
3. Hemoglobin
4. Intracellular and plasma proteins

A buffer consists of a weakly ionized acid or base and its salt. The most important buffer system in the body is the carbonic acid-bicarbonate system. Normally, a ratio of 20 parts bicarbonate to 1 part carbonic acid is present in extracellular fluid (Fig. 12-14). Addition of hydrochloric acid (HCl) will result in more carbonic acid (H_2CO_3) in the following way:

$$\underset{\text{strong acid}}{H^+Cl^-} + \underset{\text{strong base}}{Na^+HCO_3^-} \rightarrow \underset{\text{salt}}{Na^+Cl^-} + \underset{\text{weak acid}}{H_2CO_3}$$

Table 12-13
Calculation of pH (Henderson-Hasselbalch Equation)

$$pH = pK\ (\text{constant}) + \log \frac{\text{base}}{\text{acid}}$$

$$pH = 6.1 + \log \frac{HCO_3^-\ (\text{renal})}{H_2CO_3\ (\text{lung})}$$

$$pH = 6.1 + \log \frac{25.4\ \text{mEq}}{1.27}$$

$$pH = 6.1 + \log \frac{20}{1}$$

$$pH = 6.1 + 1.3$$

$$pH = 7.4$$

In this way hydrochloric acid is prevented from making a large change in the solution's pH and more H_2CO_3 is formed. The carbonic acid, in turn, is broken down to H_2O and CO_2. The CO_2 is excreted by the lungs. In this process the buffer system maintains the 20:1 ratio between bicarbonate and carbonic acid and the normal pH.

The body buffers an acid load better than it neutralizes base excess. Buffers cannot maintain pH without the adequate functioning of the respiratory and renal systems.

Respiratory system

The lungs excrete carbon dioxide and water, which are by-products of cell metabolism. When released into the circulation, CO_2 and H_2O combine to form H_2CO_3, which then dissociates into hydrogen and bicarbonate. This process is reversed in the lung. Carbon dioxide is formed and exhaled from the lung. The overall reversible reaction is expressed as:

$$CO_2 + H_2O \rightleftharpoons H_2CO_3 \rightleftharpoons H^+ + HCO_3^-$$

The amount of CO_2 in the blood is directly related to carbonic acid concentration and subsequently to hydrogen ion concentration. With increased respirations, less CO_2 remains in the blood. This leads to less carbonic acid and fewer H^+ ions.

With decreased respirations, more CO_2 remains in the blood. This leads to increased carbonic acid and more hydrogen ions.

Renal system

The kidneys reabsorb and conserve most of the bicarbonate. In addition, the kidney can eliminate excess hydrogen. The three mechanisms of acid elimination include (1) secretion of small amounts of free hydrogen into the renal tubule, (2) combining hydrogen with ammonia (NH_3) to form ammonium (NH_4^+), and (3) excreting weak acids.

The kidneys normally excrete an acidic urine (average pH = 6). The kidneys have the ability to decrease or increase bicarbonate reabsorption. In renal failure metabolic acidosis is the usual finding.

Alterations in Acid-Base Balance

An acid-base imbalance is produced when the ratio between acid and base content is altered (Table 12-14). A primary disease or process may alter one side of the ratio (e.g., CO_2 retention in pulmonary disease). The compensatory process attempts to maintain the other side of the ratio (e.g., increased renal bicarbonate reabsorption). When the compensatory mechanism fails, an acid-base imbalance results. The compensatory process may be inadequate, either because the pathologic process is overwhelming or there is insufficient time for the compensatory process to function.

Acid-base imbalances are classified as *respiratory* and *metabolic*. Respiratory imbalances affect carbonic acid concentrations. Metabolic imbalances affect the base bicarbonate. Therefore, acidosis can be caused by an increase in carbonic acid (respiratory acidosis) or a decrease in bicarbonate (metabolic acidosis), and alkalosis can be caused by a decrease in carbonic acid (respiratory alkalosis) or an increase in bicarbonate (metabolic alkalosis).

Respiratory acidosis (carbonic acid excess)

Respiratory acidosis occurs whenever there is hypoventilation (Table 12-14). Carbon dioxide and subsequently carbonic acid accumulate in the blood. Carbonic acid dissociates, liberating H^+, and there is a decrease in pH. If carbon dioxide is not eliminated from the blood, acidosis results from the accumulation of carbonic acid (Fig. 12-15a).

The renal compensatory mechanism may operate if the problem has been present for several days. The kidneys conserve bicarbonate. The kidneys also secrete increased concentrations of hydrogen ion. In acute respiratory acidosis the renal compensatory mechanisms are not yet functioning and a low or normal serum bicarbonate level is usually found.

Respiratory alkalosis (carbonic acid deficit)

Respiratory alkalosis occurs with hyperventilation (Table 12-14). Anxiety, central nervous system disease, and mechanical overventilation all increase ventilation and decrease the PCO_2. This leads to decreased carbonic acid and alkalosis (Fig. 12-15a).

Table 12-14
Acid-Base Imbalances

Imbalance	Common Etiologies	Pathophysiology	Laboratory Findings
Respiratory acidosis (carbonic acid excess)	Chronic obstructive pulmonary disease Barbiturate or sedative overdose Guillain-Barré syndrome Pneumonia Atelectasis	CO_2 retention from hypoventilation. Impaired respiratory efforts due to airway obstruction, weakened respiratory muscles, or depressed respiratory center. Compensatory response by kidney is HCO_3^- retention.	Plasma pH ↓ PCO_2 ↑ HCO_3^- normal (uncompensated) ↑ (compensated) Urine pH <6
Respiratory alkalosis (carbonic acid deficit)	Mechanical overventilation Hyperventilation due to anxiety Encephalitis Fever	Increased CO_2 excretion from hyperventilation. Compensatory response by kidney is HCO_3^- excretion.	Plasma pH ↑ PCO_2 ↓ HCO_3 normal (uncompensated) ↓ (compensated) Urine pH >7
Metabolic acidosis (base bicarbonate deficit)	Diabetic ketoacidosis Uremia Lactic acidosis Starvation Severe diarrhea Renal tubular acidosis	Gain of fixed acid, inability to excrete acid, or loss of base. Compensatory response by lungs is CO_2 excretion.	Plasma pH ↓ PCO_2 ↓ (compensated) HCO_3 ↓ Urine pH <6 (compensated)
Metabolic alkalosis (base bicarbonate excess)	Severe vomiting Excess gastric suctioning Diuretic therapy Potassium deficit Excess $NaHCO_3$ intake	Loss of strong acid or gain of base. Compensatory response by lungs is CO_2 retention	Plasma pH ↑ PCO_2 ↑ (compensated) HCO_3 ↑ Urine pH >7 (compensated)

Compensated respiratory alkalosis is not usually seen unless the client has been maintained on a ventilator or has a CNS problem. The decreased bicarbonate level differentiates compensated respiratory alkalosis from acute or uncompensated respiratory alkalosis.

Metabolic acidosis (base bicarbonate deficit)

Metabolic acidosis occurs when an acid other than carbonic acid accumulates in the body or when bicarbonate is lost from body fluids (Table 12-14 and Fig. 12-15b). In both cases there is a bicarbonate deficit. Acetoacetic acid accumulation in diabetic ketoacidosis and lactic acid accumulation with shock are examples of accumulation of acids. Severe diarrhea results in loss of bicarbonate. In renal disease the kidneys lose their ability to reabsorb bicarbonate and secrete hydrogen ions.

The compensatory response is to increase CO_2 excretion by the lungs. The client often develops Kussmaul's breathing (deep, rapid breathing). In addition, the kidneys attempt to excrete additional acid.

Metabolic alkalosis (base bicarbonate excess)

Metabolic alkalosis occurs when there is loss of acid (HCl from prolonged vomiting or gastric suction) or gain in bicarbonate (e.g., self-ingestion of baking soda) (Table 12-14 and Fig. 12-15b). Compensatory mechanisms include a decreased respiratory rate to increase CO_2 and renal excretion of bicarbonate.

Clinical Manifestations of Acid-Base Imbalance

Clinical manifestations of acidosis and alkalosis are summarized in Table 12-15 and Table 12-16. Because a normal pH is vital to all cellular reactions, the clinical manifestations of acid-base imbalances are generalized and nonspecific. The actual compensatory mechanisms also produce some of the clinical manifestations.

Interpretation of Blood Gases

Blood gas values provide information essential for evaluation of acid-base problems. These include pH,

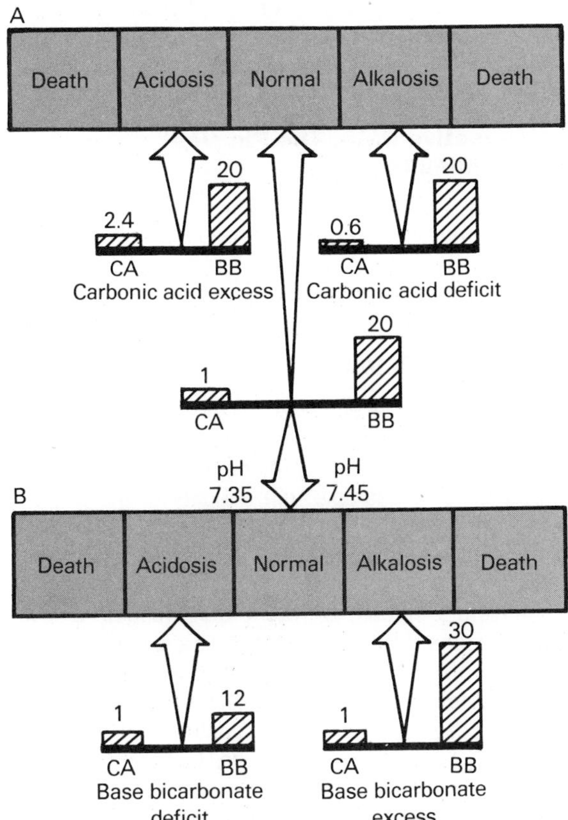

Figure 12-15 Kinds of acid-base imbalances. (*a*) Respiratory imbalances due to carbonic acid excess and carbonic acid deficit. (*b*) Metabolic imbalances due to base bicarbonate deficit and base bicarbonate excess.

PCO_2, and PO_2. The pH determines the acidosis or alkalosis of the blood. A normal pH can signify no problem or a mixed imbalance that results from metabolic and respiratory problems occurring simultaneously. With a compensated problem, the pH will approach normal with the direction of deviation from normal identifying the primary problem.

Also commonly included in blood gas determinations are bicarbonate levels, base excess levels, and oxygen saturation. Base excess indicates the excess or deficit of either alkali or acid. Positive values indicate alkalinity and negative values indicate acidity. Oxygen saturation can be calculated from PO_2, pH, and hemoglobin.

Either arterial or venous blood can be used as long as one is consistently used for comparison. The arterial method is usually preferred. (For arterial puncture technique see Chap. 18.) The values of blood gases differ slightly between arterial and venous samples (Table 12-17).

Table 12-15

Clinical Manifestations of Acidosis

Respiratory (↑ PCO_2)	**Metabolic (↓ HCO_3)**
Appearance	
Drowsy Coma	Coma Dehydration
Behavior	
Disoriented	Disoriented—weak
Cardiovascular	
Decreased BP Tachycardia	No significant findings
Gastrointestinal	
No significant findings	Nausea, vomiting, diarrhea, abdominal pain
Neuromuscular	
Asterixis	Asterixis
Respiratory	
Rapid, shallow breaths or hypoventilation with hypoxia	Hyperventilation

Table 12-16

Clinical Manifestations of Alkalosis

Respiratory (↓ PCO_2)	**Metabolic (↑ HCO_3)**
Appearance	
Lethargic	Stupor Coma
Behavior	
Confusion	Confusion
Gastrointestinal	
No significant findings	Anorexia Nausea Vomiting
Neuromuscular	
Tetany Numbness Tingling of Extremities Hyperreflexia	Tremors Hypertonic muscles Muscle cramps Tetany
Respiratory	
Hyperventilation	Hypoventilation

Table 12-17
Comparison of Values between Arterial and Venous Blood

	Arterial	Venous
pH	7.35–7.45	7.35–7.45
PCO_2	35–45 mmHg	40–45 mmHg
Bicarbonate	20–30 mEq/L	20–30 mEq/L
PO_2*	80–100 mmHg	40–50 mmHg†
Oxygen saturation	96–100%	40–70%
Base excess	±2.0	±2.0

*Decreases above sea level and with increasing age.
†Oxygen tension is defined as the significant difference between the PO_2 of arterial and venous blood.

Use of a nomogram

A *nomogram* is a graph that facilitates interpretation of acid-base imbalances with the known values for pH and PCO_2 (Fig. 12-16). To use a nomogram, the value of the PCO_2 is located first. Then the value of the pH is located. The area in which the values for PCO_2 and pH intersect is the acid-base status. For example, if the PCO_2 is 40 mmHg and the pH is 7.36, acid-base balance is normal. If the PCO_2 is 70 mmHg and the pH is 7.2, acute respiratory acidosis is possible. If the values intersect in a white area, a combination of the two types of imbalances which border it are present.

ASSESSMENT OF FLUID AND ELECTROLYTE IMBALANCES

Subjective Data: The History

Past medical history

An assessment of the client's current and past use of medications is very important. The ingredients in many drugs (especially over-the-counter drugs) are often overlooked as sources of sodium, potassium, calcium, magnesium, and other electrolytes. There are many prescription drugs that could cause fluid and electrolyte problems. Examples include diuretics, corticosteroids, and electrolyte supplements. The client should be questioned about any primary disease or condition that could cause fluid and electrolyte imbalances, such as renal disease, diabetes mellitus, ulcerative colitis, and respiratory disease.

Social and personal history

Extremes of climate and activity markedly alter the fluid requirement. Clients who live alone may not satisfy their need for balanced fluid and electrolytes because they may not adequately prepare their meals. The client needs to be questioned regarding his diet, especially if he has been on a special diet (reducing, low-sodium, or fad diet).

Objective Data: The Physical Examination

There is no unique physical examination for fluid and electrolytes. Common abnormal assessment findings of major body systems give clues to possible fluid and electrolyte imbalances (Table 12-18).

Laboratory Values

Normal serum electrolyte values are a good starting point for identifying fluid and electrolyte imbalance (Table 12-4). However, they often provide only cursory information. For example, the majority of the potassium in the body is found intracellularly. Serum potassium values only indirectly reflect the total body potassium.

A serum sodium of 120 mEq/L reflects a low serum sodium. Does the value indicate a total body sodium depletion as occurs when sodium losses exceed water loss, or does the client have a low serum sodium because normal sodium content is diluted with an excess of water? A reduced hematocrit could indicate an anemia or it could be caused by fluid volume excess.

INTRAVENOUS FLUID AND ELECTROLYTE REPLACEMENT

Intravenous (IV) therapy is used to replace fluid and electrolytes if the problem requires immediate correction of the fluid and electrolyte imbalance. Intravenous therapy is also used in clients who are NPO because of paralytic ileus, gastrointestinal fistulas, swallowing problems, unconsciousness, etc. The amount and type of solution will be determined by the normal daily maintenance requirements and by imbalances identified by laboratory results. The normal daily requirement for fluids and electrolytes is

Electrolytes
Na^+ and Cl^-: 70 mEq
K^+: 40 to 60 mEq
Glucose
150 to 200 g (1 g equals 4 kcal)
Water
3000 mL

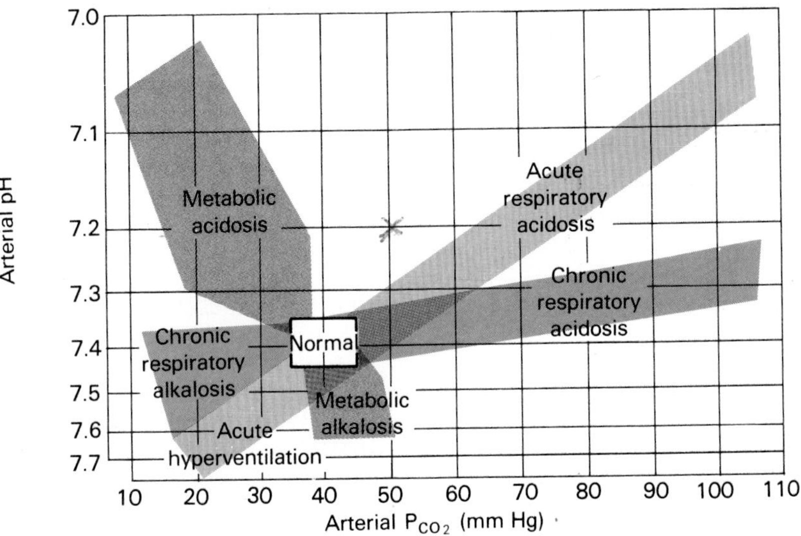

Figure 12-16 Nomogram used for blood gas interpretation. (*Taken from M. Groer and M. Shekleton, Basic Pathophysiology: A Conceptual Approach, The C. V. Mosby Co., St. Louis, 1979, p. 278.*)

Table 12-18
Common Abnormal Assessment Findings of Fluid and Electrolyte Imbalances

Finding	Possible Etiology
Skin	
Poor skin turgor	Fluid volume deficit
Cold, clammy skin	Sodium deficit Plasma-to-interstitial fluid shift
Pitting edema	Fluid volume excess
Flushed, dry skin	Sodium excess
Pulse	
Bounding pulse	Fluid volume excess Interstitial-to-plasma fluid shift
Rapid, weak, thready pulse	Plasma-to-interstitial fluid shift Sodium deficit Fluid volume deficit
Weak, irregular, rapid pulse	Severe potassium deficit
Weak, irregular, slow pulse	Severe potassium excess
Blood Pressure	
Hypotension	Fluid volume deficit Plasma-to-interstitial fluid shift Sodium deficit
Hypertension	Fluid volume excess Interstitial-to-plasma fluid shift
Respirations	
Deep, rapid breathing	Metabolic acidosis
Shallow, slow, irregular breathing	Metabolic alkalosis
Shortness of breath	Fluid volume excess
Moist rales	Fluid volume excess Interstitial-to-plasma fluid shift
Skeletal Muscle	
Cramping of exercised muscle	Calcium deficit
Carpopedal spasm (Trousseau's sign)	Calcium deficit
Flabby muscles	Potassium deficit
Positive Chvostek's sign	Calcium deficit
Behavior or Mental	
Picking at bedclothes	Potassium deficit Magnesium deficit
Indifference	Fluid volume deficit Sodium deficit
Apprehension	Plasma-to-interstitial fluid shift
Extreme restlessness	Potassium excess Fluid volume deficit
Confusion and irritability	Potassium deficit Fluid volume excess

Table 12-19
Normal Daily Maintenance Requirements for Fluids and Electrolytes

Maintenance IVs	Volume	NaCl/L	K^+/L	Glucose/L
D5/$\frac{1}{2}$ NS with 20 mEq KCl	2000 mL	77 mEq	20 mEq	50 g
D10/water	1000 mL			100
	3000 mL	144 mEq	40 mEq	200 g

Maintenance IVs are described in Table 12-19. Intravenous solutions vary not only in amount of electrolytes but also in osmolarity (Table 12-20).

Types of Solutions

Hypotonic

A hypotonic solution dilutes the ECF. Osmosis then produces a movement of water from the ECF to the ICF. After osmotic equilibrium has been achieved, the ICF and the ECF have the same osmolality. Total body water is increased by the amount of fluid infused or ingested. Examples of hypotonic solutions are 0.45‘ NaCl, 0.2‘ NaCl, and 5‘ dextrose.

Isotonic

Administration of an isotonic solution produces no net movement between the ICF and the ECF. An isotonic fluid is ideal fluid replacement for a client with extracellular fluid volume deficit. Examples of isotonic solutions are lactated Ringer's, Normosol, and 0.9‘ NaCl. Lactated Ringer's (Hartmann's) solution contains sodium potassium, chloride, calcium, and lactate (precursor of bicarbonate) in the same concentrations as those of the ECF.

Hypertonic

A hypertonic solution initially raises the osmolality of ECF. Total body water is increased. In addition, the higher osmotic pressure draws water out of the cell into the ECF.

Examples include 5% dextrose/0.9% NaCl, 5% dextrose/0.45% NaCl, and 10% dextrose/0.9% NaCl.

Intravenous additives

In addition to the basic solutions which provide water and a minimum amount of calories and electrolytes, there are additives to replace specific losses. These have been previously mentioned during the discussion of the particular electrolyte deficiency. Potassium chloride, calcium chloride, magnesium sulfate, and bicarbonate are the common additives which are added to the basic intravenous solutions.

Plasma expanders

Plasma expanders stay within the vascular space and increase the oncotic pressure. Plasma expanders include colloids and dextran. Colloids are protein solutions such as plasma, albumin, and commercial plasmas (Plasmanate). Dextran is a complex synthetic sugar. It is metabolized slowly so it remains in the vascular system for a prolonged period but not as long as the colloids.

If the client has lost blood, whole blood or packed red blood cells will be necessary to restore the hemoglobin. Packed red blood cells have the advantage of giving the client primarily red blood cells; the blood bank can use the plasma for blood components. Also, packed cells have a decreased plasma volume which may be a significant consideration in a client who has received plasma expanders as emergency treatment

Table 12-20
Osmolarity and Use of Common Intravenous Solutions

Solution	Osmolarity	Indications for Use
5% dextrose in water (D5/W)	253	Insensible water loss
Normal saline (0.9% NaCl)	308	Hyponatremia
5% dextrose and 0.45% saline (D5/$\frac{1}{2}$ NS)	406	Maintenance fluid
5% dextrose and normal saline (D5/NS)	561	Maintenance fluid
3% normal saline	1026	Symptomatic hyponatremia
Lactated Ringer's	273	ECF volume deficit

of blood loss. Whole blood with its additional fluid volume could cause circulatory overload.

REVIEW QUESTIONS

The number of the question corresponds to the same numbered objective at the beginning of the chapter.

1. The major intracellular cation is
a. sodium
b. magnesium
c. potassium
d. calcium

2. Diffusion can best be defined as
a. movement of molecules from an area of lesser concentration to an area of greater concentration
b. movement of molecules from an area of greater concentration to an area of lesser concentration
c. movement of water from an area of lesser concentration to an area of greater concentration
d. movement of water from an area of greater concentration to an area of lesser concentration

3. A client is admitted to the hospital in congestive heart failure. His severe generalized edema can be explained by
a. interstitial-fluid-to-plasma shift
b. plasma-to-interstitial fluid shift
c. extracellular-to-intracellular fluid shift
d. interstitial-to-intracellular fluid shift

4. Body water loss from the skin and lungs is known as
a. obligatory loss
b. insensible water loss
c. partial water loss
d. essential water loss

5. Three days post-burn, a client started to have diuresis and his urinary output was 6000 mL in 2 days. The next day the nurse found him picking his bedclothes. His grasp was weak and reflexes were absent. What electrolyte imbalance might these symptoms suggest?
a. potassium deficit
b. potassium excess
c. sodium excess
d. sodium deficit

6. To maintain a normal pH, it is necessary for the body to keep a ratio of
a. 10 parts of bicarbonate to 1 part carbonic acid
b. 15 parts bicarbonate to 1 part carbonic acid
c. 20 parts bicarbonate to 1 part carbonic acid
d. 20 parts carbonic acid to 1 part bicarbonate

7. Hyperventilation causes an acid-base imbalance. The body compensates for this respiratory alkalosis primarily by
a. lungs retaining CO_2
b. kidneys retaining bicarbonate
c. lungs eliminating CO_2
d. kidneys eliminating bicarbonate

8. What is the possible etiology of a bounding pulse that is not easily obliterated?
a. sodium deficit
b. potassium deficit
c. fluid volume deficit
d. fluid volume excess

9. If hypertonic saline is injected intravenously, in which of the following ways will body water shift?
a. intracellular to intravascular
b. interstitial to intracellular
c. intravascular to interstitial
d. intravascular to intracellular

REFERENCES

1. A. J. Vander, J. H. Sherman, and D. S. Luciano, *Human Physiology: The Mechanisms of Body Function*, McGraw-Hill Book Company, New York, 1980, p. 161.
2. A. Burgess, *The Nurse's Guide to Fluid and Electrolyte Balance*, 2d ed., McGraw-Hill Book Company, New York, 1979, p. 9.
3. Ibid., p. 29.
4. A. J. Vander et al., op. cit., p. 367.
5. I. F. Maher and F. C. Bartter, "Maintenance of Dynamic Equilibrium of Body Fluids Electrolytes," in E. D. Frohlich (ed.), *Pathophysiology*, 2d ed., J. B. Lippincott Company, Philadelphia, 1976, chap. 11, p. 254.
6. M. M. Grant and W. M. Kubo, "Assessing a Patient's Hydration Status," *Am J Nurs*, **75:**1310 (1975).
7. S. S. Pflaum, "Investigation of Intake Output as a Means of Assessing Body Fluid Balance," *Heart Lung*, **8:**498 (1979).
8. R. R. Recker and P. D. Saville, "Hypercalcemia and Hypocalcemia in Clinical Practice," *Hospital Practice*, **15:**83 (September 1979).
9. G. W. Zeluff, W. N. Suki, and D. Jackson, "Depletion of Body Phosphate—Ubiquitous, Subtle, Dangerous," *Heart Lung*, **6:**523 (1977).
10. N. Elbaum, "Magnesium the Forgotten Electrolyte," in H. Hamilton (ed.), *Monitoring Fluids and Electrolytes*, InterMed Communications, Horsham, Pa., 1978, p. 108.
11. Ibid.

Chapter 13

NURSING ROLE IN MANAGEMENT

Burn Client

Sue E. Elster

Learning Objectives

1. Describe types and prevention of burn injuries.
2. Describe burn injury in terms of involved structures and clinical appearance of full- and partial-thickness burns.
3. Identify the parameters used to determine the severity of burns.
4. Describe the pathophysiologic changes, clinical manifestations, and medical and nursing management occurring in each burn phase.
5. Explain fluid and electrolyte shifts during the emergent and acute phases.
6. Differentiate among the nutritional needs of the burn client during the three burn phases.
7. Explain the physiologic and psychosocial aspects of burn rehabilitation.
8. Describe medical and nursing management of the emotional needs of the burn client and family.
9. Describe special needs of nursing staff caring for the burn client and possible ways to meet those needs.

SIGNIFICANCE OF PROBLEM

An estimated 2 million Americans seek medical care each year for burns. Approximately 130,000 are hospitalized and 70,000 require intensive care services at a cost of over $300 million dollars per year.[1] An estimated 12,000 to 15,000 of these people die annually as a direct result of their burns.[2] Children (especially preschoolers) and elderly persons account for over two-thirds of all burn fatalities.[3]

Cigarette smoking is the main cause of deaths from fires in the home. Other major causes of burns include hot water heaters set above 55°C (131°F), cooking accidents, space heaters, combustibles such as gasoline and charcoal lighter fluid, steam from radiators, and chemicals.[4] Currently, there are over 40 major burn centers in the United States and well over 70 additional burn specialty units providing highly skilled, specialized care to burn victims.

PROBLEM IDENTIFICATION

Definition of Burn Injury

Burn injury involves the destruction of the integumentary system (Chap. 16). The skin is divided into three layers (Fig. 13-1). The *epidermis*, or nonvascular outer layer of the skin, is about the thickness of a sheet of paper. It is composed of many layers of nonliving epithelial cells that provide a protective barrier to the skin, hold in fluids and electrolytes, regulate heat, and keep harmful agents in the external environment from injuring or invading the body. The *dermis*, lying below the epidermis, is about 30 to 45 times thicker than the epidermis. The dermis contains connective tissues with blood vessels and highly specialized structures consisting of hair follicles, nerve endings, sweat glands, and sebaceous glands. Under the dermis lies the *subcutaneous tissue* containing major vascular networks, nerves, and lymphatics. The subcutaneous tissue acts as shock absorber and heat insulator for the underlying structures: muscles, tendons, bones, internal organs, etc.

In the past, burns were defined by degrees: first degree (1°), second degree (2°), and third degree (3°). The American Burn Association currently advocates a more explicit definition categorizing the burn according to depth: partial- and full-thickness. Table 13-1 reflects the comparison of the classification system.

Types of Burn Injury

Thermal Injury

The most common type of burn is thermal injury, which can be caused by flame, flash, scald, and contact burns (Table 13-2 and Fig. 13-2).

Smoke and inhalation injury

Smoke and inhalation injury occurs when heat or noxious chemicals cause respiratory tissue damage. Although breathing very hot, dry air can burn respiratory mucosa, it rarely happens because the vocal

This chapter was reviewed by Melva Kravitz, R.N., M.S., Associate Director, Intermountain Burn Center, University of Utah Medical Center, and Clinical Instructor, University of Utah College of Nursing, Salt Lake City, Utah.

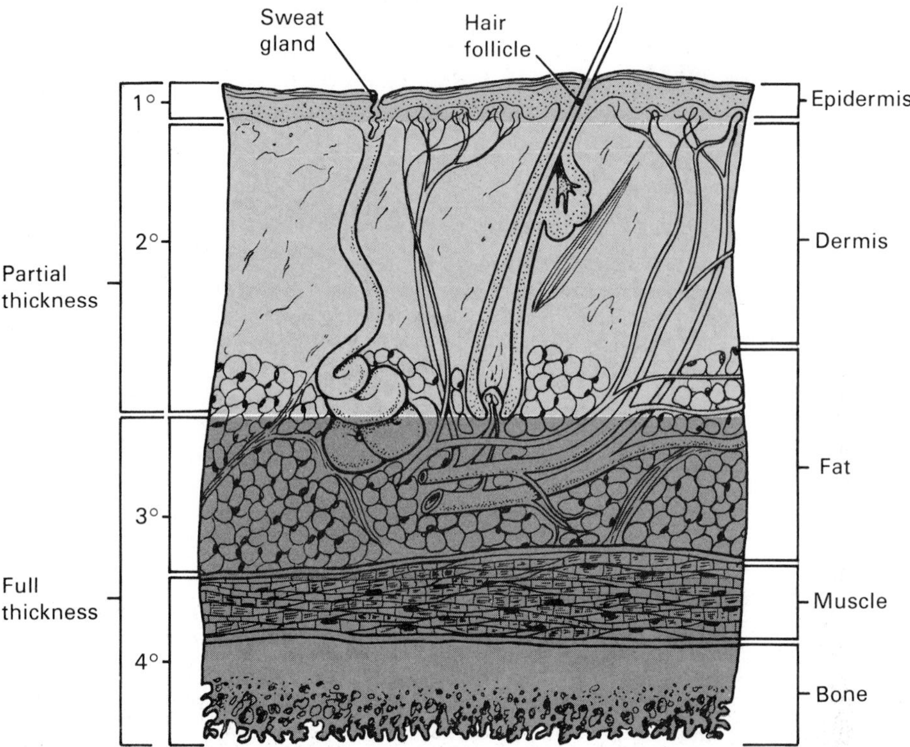

Figure 13-1 Cross-section of skin indicating burn and structures involved.

cords and glottis close as a protective mechanism. Thermal burn of the respiratory tract will usually be limited to the oropharynx. However, smoke inhalation injury of the lower respiratory tract is a more common injury and a frequent cause of death in burn clients. If a victim with flame burns was also trapped in a closed space or near an explosion, it must be assumed that an inhalation injury also occurred until proven other-

Table 13-1
Classification of Burns

Classification	Clinical Appearance and Cause	Morphology (Fig. 13-1)
Partial-thickness		
1° (Superficial)	Characterized by erythema. Blanches on pressure. Pain and mild swelling present. No vesicles or blisters (although after 24 hours skin may blister and peel). Caused by superficial sunburn or quick heat flash.	Only superficial devitalization with local hyperemia.
2° (Deep)	Fluid-filled vesicles. Red, shiny, wet (if vesicles have ruptured). Very painful due to nerve injury. Mild to moderate edema. Caused by flash, scald, or flame burn.	Involves both epidermis and dermis to varying depth. Some skin elements remain viable from which epithelial regeneration occurs.
Full-thickness		
3° and 4°	Dry, waxy white, leathery, or hard. Thrombosed vessels often visible. Insensitive to pain and pressure due to nerve destruction. Can involve muscles, tendons, and bones. Caused by flame, scald, chemicals, tar, or electric current.	All skin elements destroyed as well as nerve endings. Coagulation necrosis present.

Table 13-2
Causes of Thermal Burn Injury

Cause	Examples
Flame	Clothing ignited with fire
Flash	Flame burn associated with explosion (combustible fuels)
Scald	Too-hot bath water Spilled hot beverages Steam burns (pressure cookers, automobile radiators)
Contact	Hot metal (outdoor grill) Hot, sticky tar Hot grease or liquids from cooking

wise. It is estimated that 30 to 40 percent of major burn injuries are accompanied by inhalation injuries.

Although the corneal reflex generally protects the eye from burn injury, corneal burns and abrasions can occur under circumstances similar to inhalation injuries. Intense heat or noxious chemical by-products damage delicate corneal tissue. When corneal burns are suspected, an ophthamologist should see the client as soon as possible. Because of rapid facial edema that can occur with burns, a rapid nursing assessment is needed because the eyelids may become swollen shut within the first few hours after injury.

Chemical injury

Chemical injuries are the result of tissue contact and destruction from necrotizing substances. In chemical injuries it is important to remove the person from the burning agent, or vice versa. The latter is accomplished by lavaging the affected area with copious amounts of water. Any clothing containing the chemical should be removed. Otherwise, the burning process would continue while the chemical is in contact with the skin.[5]

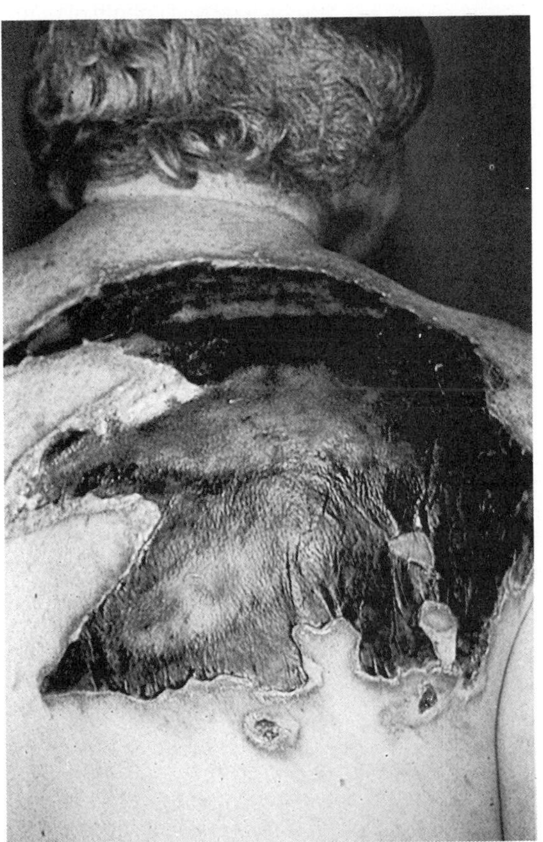

A

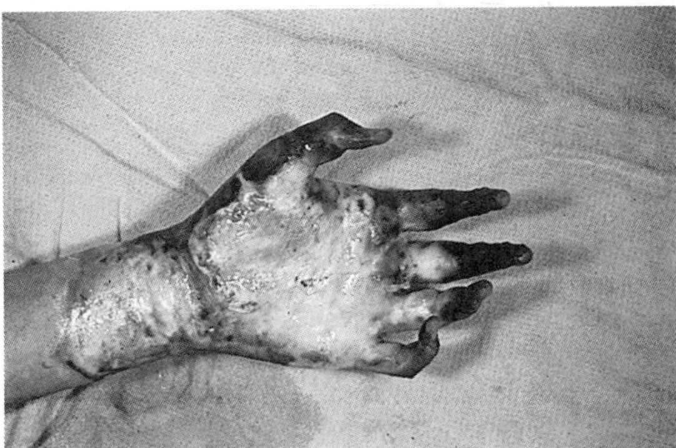

B

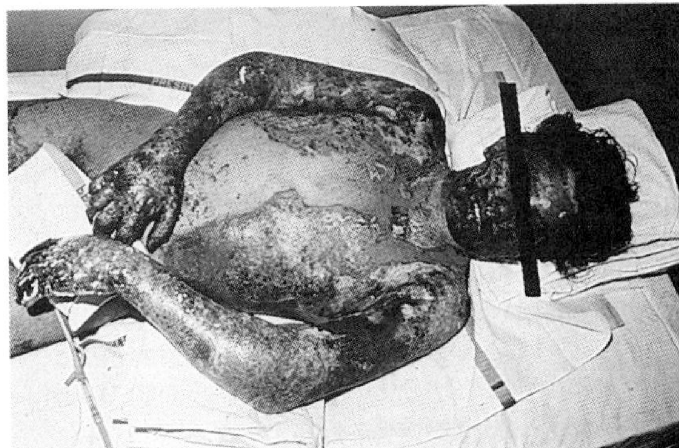

C

Figure 13-2 Types of burn injury. *a.* Elderly client who fell against a hot radiator. *b.* Full thickness burn of hand. Blackened fingertips are burned to the bone. *c.* Full thickness burns with massive edema. Accident occurred from a firecracker factory explosion. *(Courtesy of MEDCOM.)*

Chemicals can produce respiratory injury as well as skin or eye injury. When chlorine is inhaled, the toxic gas produces respiratory distress. By-products of burning substances (e.g., carbon) are toxic to the sensitive respiratory mucosa. The extent of this type of injury may not become evident until up to 72 hours post insult.

Chemical burns are most commonly caused by acids. However, alkali burns also occur and they are more difficult to manage than acid burns. Alkaline substances are not neutralized by tissue fluids as readily as acid substances are. Alkalies adhere to tissue, causing protein hydrolysis with liquefaction. This damage continues even when the alkali is neutralized.[6] Examples of alkalies that cause burn injury are phenols, sodium metals, calcium hydroxide, and lyes.

Electrical injury

Electrical injury occurs from coagulation necrosis due to intense heat that is generated from an electric current. It can also occur from direct damage to nerves and vessels causing tissue anoxia and death. The severity of the electrical injury depends on the amount of voltage, tissue resistance, current pathways, surface area in contact with the current, and the length of time current flow was sustained. Tissue densities offer various amounts of resistance to electric current. For example, fat and bone offer the most resistance while nerves and blood vessels offer the least resistance. Current that passes through vital organs (brain, heart, kidneys) will produce more profound damage than current passing through muscle tissue. A person submerged in water sustaining an electric shock has more surface area in contact with electricity than one out of water touching a live wire.

Nursing assessment of the client with electrical injury should be thorough. Often the wounds of electric current entry and exit are all that are visible, masking the possibility of extensive, underlying tissue damage. Noting the client's position when the injury was sustained in conjunction with identifying the entry and exit wounds can assist in the assessment of which underlying organ structures may have been affected.

Myoglobinuria from extensive muscle damage can produce acute tubular necrosis, and eventual renal failure if not treated aggressively with fluids and diuretics (Chap. 38). Adults who sustain high-voltage electrical burns frequently have varying degrees of cardiac muscle damage. This can result in arrhythmias, infarction, or sudden death.

Health Promotion and Maintenance

Most burns can be prevented. The nurse as a citizen and health care provider is in a good position to do home safety assessment and client education before accidents occur.

Home safety measures include the use of smoke alarms and fire extinguishers. Families should have fire drills with each family member knowing where to go and what to do in case of fire. Local fire departments are willing to inform the public of regional fire codes as well as performing home safety checks.

Knowledge of potential sources for burn injury allows problem solving for burn prevention (Table 13-3). Teaching people proper use of appliances such as space heaters, electric cords, wiring, outlets, outdoor grills, and hot water heaters can do much to prevent burn injury. Nurses can be instrumental in teaching minor burn home care to the public. Industrial nurses should teach burn prevention in the work setting.

Severity of Burn Injury

The treatment of burns is related to the severity of the injury. Severity is determined by (1) depth of burn, (2) extent of burn calculated in percent of body surface area (BSA), (3) location of burn, (4) age of victim, and (5) past medical history indicating poor risk factors.

Depth

Determination of partial- and full-thickness injuries was previously discussed (Table 13-1).

Extent

Two commonly used guides for determining the extent of a burn wound are the Lund and Browder chart (Fig. 13-3) and the Rule of Nines chart (Fig. 13-4). The Lund and Browder chart is considered to be more accurate because the client's age in proportion to relative body-part size is taken into account.[7] The Rule of Nines is easy to remember and is considered very adequate for initial assessments. For irregular or odd-shaped burns, the palmar surface of the hand is considered to be about 1 percent of the BSA.[8] The extent of a burn is often revised after edema has subsided and demarcations of zones of injury are more clear.

Location

Not all body parts deserve equal consideration in determining the severity of a burn. Burns involving the hands, face, neck, eyes, ears, feet, joints, or genitalia, or any circumferential burn deserve special attention. Edema in the face or neck can mechanically obstruct the airway. The hands and feet have an abundant vascular and nerve supply and are a major concern

Table 13-3
Common Places and Causes of Burn Injury

Occupational Hazards	Home and Recreational Hazards
Steam pipes	Hot water heaters set greater than 55°C (131°F)
Chemicals	Multiple extension cords per outlet
Hot metals	Frazzled or defective wiring
Tar	Pressure cookers
Electricity from power lines	Radiators
Combustible fuels	Open space heaters
	Carelessness with cigarets or matches
	Excessive exposure to sunlight
	Electrical storms
	Improper use of outdoor grills
	Improper use of flammables (e.g., starter fluid, gasoline, kerosene)
	Hot grease or liquids from cooking

when burned. The ears, composed mainly of cartilage, are highly susceptible to infection because of their poor blood supply. Edema causing stricture of the urethra can be a serious problem for the burn client.

Age

Because of an immature immune system and generally poor body defense mechanisms, infants are less able to cope with burn injury. The elderly heal more slowly and have more difficulty with rehabilitation than do children or younger adults. Infection of the burn wound and pneumonia are common complications in elderly burn clients.

Poor risk factors

Any person having preexisting cardiovascular, pulmonary, or renal disease has a poorer prognosis for recovery because of the tremendous demands put on the body from a burn injury. Clients with diabetes or peripheral vascular disease are at high risk for gangrene and poor healing, especially with foot and leg burns. General physical debilitation from any chronic disease, including alcoholism, drug abuse, and malnutrition renders the client less physiologically competent to deal with a burn injury. In addition, clients who have concurrently sustained fractures, blunt trauma, or head injuries have a poorer prognosis for recovery from burn injury.

Major versus minor burns

The American Burn Association categorizes burns into major, moderate, and minor injuries using depth, extent, location, and poor risk factors (Table 13-4). The American Burn Association recommends that major burn injuries be triaged to burn centers or burn units which have optimum facilities and personnel for handling such severe trauma.[9]

PHASES OF BURN MANAGEMENT

Discussion of burn management can be classified into three phases: *emergent, acute,* and *rehabilitative*. These phases are the focus of the remainder of the chapter. Prehospital care will briefly be considered. Emergency care of the burn victim is discussed in Chap. 58.

Prehospital Care

The initial consideration for the burn victim is to remove the person from the source of burn. If the burn is small, it may be covered with a clean, cool, tap-water dampened towel for the client's comfort and protection until medical care is instituted. It is thought that cooling of the injured area (if small) within 1 minute minimizes the depth of injury. Tap water for flushing is acceptable. Time should not be wasted trying to find sterile water or saline solution.

If the burn is large, primary consideration is focused on the "ABCs" (Chap. 28):

Airway—Check for patency, smoke around nares, or singed nasal hair.

Breathing—Check for adequacy of ventilation.

Circulation—Check for presence and regularity of pulses.

If the burn is large, it is not advisable to immerse the burned body part in cool water due to heat and electrolyte loss. The burn should never be packed in ice. As much clothing as possible should be removed. The victim should be wrapped in a dry, clean sheet or blanket to prevent further contamination of the wound and to provide warmth.

It must be remembered that the burn client may also be a trauma client. Often the burn is accompanied by other life-threatening injuries that may demand priority over the burn wound.

Emergent Phase (Initial or Critical Phase)

Definition

The emergent phase is the period of time required to resolve the immediate problems resulting from burn injury.[10] This time period may last from burn onset to 5 or more days, but usually lasts 24 to 48 hours. This

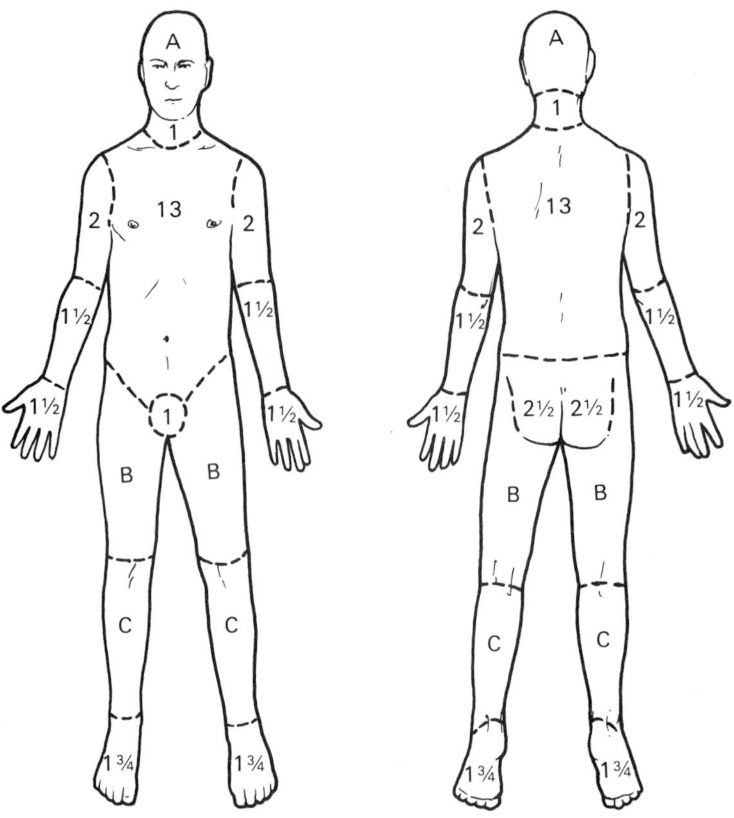

Relative Percentage of Areas Affected by Growth

	Age in Years					
	0	1	5	10	15	Adult
A—½ of head	9½	8½	6½	5½	4½	3½
B—½ of one thigh	2¾	3¼	4	4¼	4½	4¾
C—½ of one leg	2½	2½	2¾	3	3¼	3½

Figure 13-3 Lund and Browder chart.

phase begins with fluid loss and edema formation and continues until fluid mobilization and diuresis occur.

Pathophysiologic Changes

Fluid and Electrolyte Shifts The greatest initial threat to a major burn victim is hypovolemic shock. It is caused by a massive shift of fluids out of blood vessels. This shift is primarily caused by increased capillary permeability resulting from histamine release from injured cells, as well as by direct injury. Histamine, a potent vasodilator, promotes increased blood supply to an injured area but also causes loss of capillary integrity. As the capillary walls become more permeable, water, sodium, and later plasma proteins (especially albumin) move into the interstitial spaces and other surrounding tissue (Fig. 13-5).

The colloidal osmotic pressure decreases with progressive loss of protein from the vascular space. This results in more fluid shift out of the vascular space into the interstitial spaces. (Fluid accumulation in the interstitium is called *second-spacing*.) Fluid also moves to areas that normally have minimal to no fluid, a phenomenon called *third-spacing*. Examples of third-spacing in burn injury are exudate and blister formation.

The net result of the fluid shift is volume depletion within the vasculature. Edema, decreased blood pressure, increased pulse, and other manifestations of hypovolemic shock are clinically detectable manifestations (Chap. 26). If not corrected, these events can lead to cardiac arrest.

Another source of fluid loss is from increased

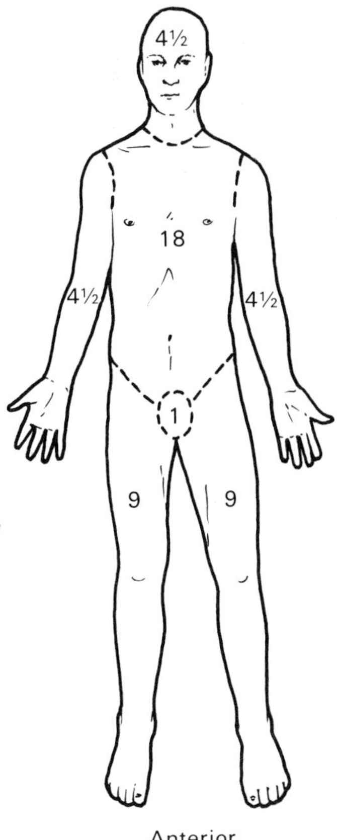

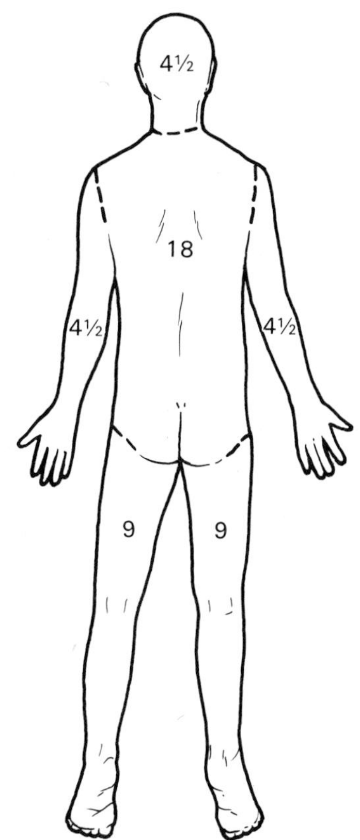

Figure 13-4 Rule of Nines chart.

insensible loss via evaporation from large, denuded body surfaces. The normal insensible loss of 30 to 50 mL/hour may increase to as much as 500 to 700 mL/hour in the severely burned client.

The circulatory status is also impaired due to hemolysis of red blood cells. The red blood cells are hemolyzed from the direct insult of the burn injury. Thrombosis in the capillaries of burned tissue causes an additional loss of red blood cells. An elevated hematocrit is common due to hemoconcentration. After fluid balance has been restored, lowered hematocrit levels are found and the anemic state is more readily detectable.

Sodium and potassium are involved in electrolyte shifts. Sodium is rapidly shifted to the interstitial space and remains there until edema formation ceases (Fig. 13-5). A potassium shift develops in the first 24 to 48 hours because injured cells and hemolyzed red blood cells release potassium into the extracellular spaces.

Toward the end of the emergent phase, if fluid

Table 13-4
American Burn Assocation Burn Classification: Major vs. Minor Burns*

Magnitude of Burn Injury	Partial Thickness (Second Degree)	Full Thickness (Third Degree)	Areas of Special Concern	Poor Risk Factors
Major	>25%	≥10%	Face, eyes, ears, hands, feet, and genitalia	Preexisting cardiovascular, renal, pulmonary disease
Moderate	15–25%	<10%		
Minor	<15%	< 2%		

*Percentage figures indicate % of total body surface area (BSA)

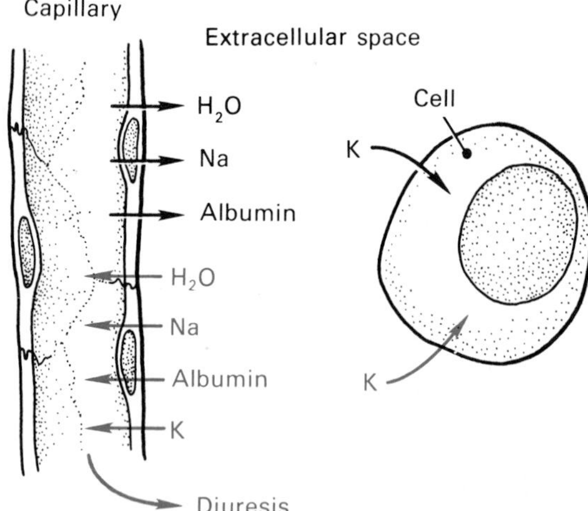

Figure 13-5 Fluid and electrolyte shifts in the emergent phase. (1) In the early stage of the emergent phase, water, sodium, and albumin leak into the interstitial space due to increased capillary permeability. Injured cells release potassium into the extracellular space. (2) In the later stage of the emergent phase (arrows in color), fluid mobilization occurs with reabsorption of water, sodium, albumin, and potassium. Potassium also moves back into the cell. Massive diuresis results in loss of fluid accompanied by sodium and potassium.

replacement is adequate, capillary membrane permeability will be restored. Fluid loss and edema formation cease. Interstitial fluid will gradually return to the vascular space (Fig. 13-5). Clinically, massive diuresis will be seen with very low urine specific gravities. Serum potassium will be markedly elevated initially as fluid mobilization brings potassium from the interstitium to the vascular space (Fig. 13-6). Hypokalemia may result at this time or in a few days due to the loss of potassium in diuresis and potassium movement back into cells. Serum sodium will increase as sodium returns to the vascular space. Later, normal serum sodium values are found with loss of sodium in urine.

Inflammation and Healing Burn injury causes coagulation necrosis whereby tissue and vessels are disrupted or destroyed. Interstitial fluid, cellular elements, and connective tissue interact to bring leukocytes to adhere to vascular epithelium. Polymorphonuclear leukocytes and monocytes accumulate at the site of injury. Fibroblasts and newly formed collagen fibrils appear to begin wound repair within the first 6 to 12 hours after injury. (The inflammatory response is discussed in Chap. 9.)

Clinical manifestations

The client may be in shock from pain and hypovolemia. Large areas of full-thickness and deep partial-thickness burns will be anesthetic. Denuded areas will be very painful. Blisters filled with fluid and protein will occur in partial-thickness burns. The client will experience an intense thirst due to the relative fluid loss. The fluid is not actually lost from the body as much as it is sequestered in the interstitial spaces and third spaces. It is hard to visualize severe dehydration in someone who is obviously edematous.

The client may be disoriented and have difficulty recalling the sequence of events that led up to the burn injury. The client will have minimal urine output and may begin to have signs of paralytic ileus due to the body's response to massive trauma and potassium shifts. Shivering may be present from chilling due to heat loss, anxiety, and pain.

Complications

The three major organ systems most susceptible to complications during the emergent phase of burn injury are the cardiovascular, respiratory, and renal systems.

Cardiovascular System Cardiovascular system complications include hypovolemic shock, arrhythmias, and cardiac arrest. Circulation to extremities can

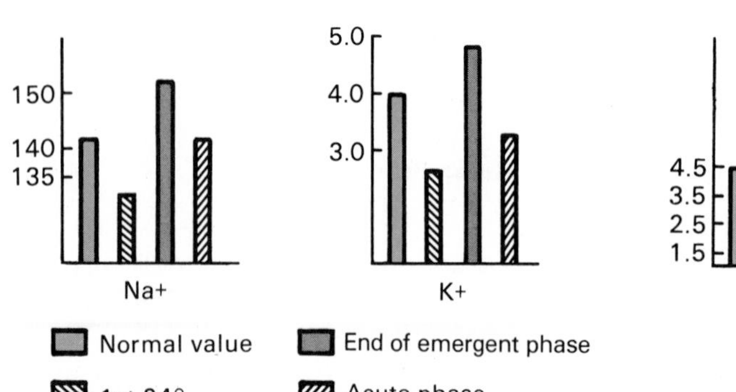

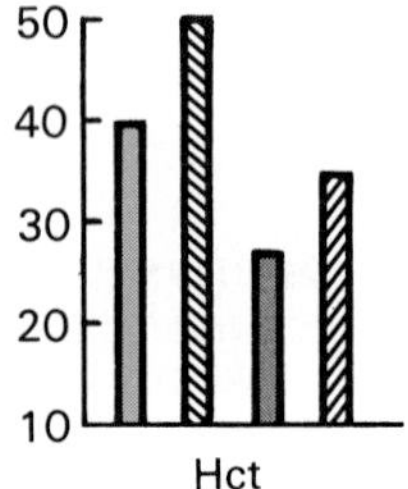

Figure 13-6 Laboratory value changes during emergent and acute phases of burn.

be severely impaired by circumferential burns and edema formation. These processes occlude the blood supply causing ischemia, necrosis, and eventually gangrene. *Escharotomies*, incisions through the eschar, are frequently done to restore circulation to compromised extremities (Fig. 13-7). Because of increased blood viscosity due to fluid loss, microcirculation is impaired resulting in a phenomenon called *sludging*. This can be corrected by adequate fluid replacement.

Respiratory System The respiratory system is especially vulnerable to two types of respiratory injury: (1) upper airway burns causing edema formation and obstruction of the airway, and (2) inhalation injury causing adult respiratory distress syndrome (see Chap. 22). Thermal burns to the head and neck can occlude the airway by edema formation compressing the trachea (Fig. 13-8). Circumferential burns of the thorax prevent lung expansion and necessitate an escharotomy.

The need for a tracheostomy is, in itself, a complication because of alteration of the natural airway and easy access of pathogens into the respiratory system. If the client has preexisting pulmonary problems (e.g., chronic obstructive pulmonary disease) he is more likely to sustain a respiratory infection. Pneumonia is a common complication of major burns due to debilitation, abundant microbial flora, and relative immobility of the client. If fluid replacement is too vigorous, the client can succumb to pulmonary edema.

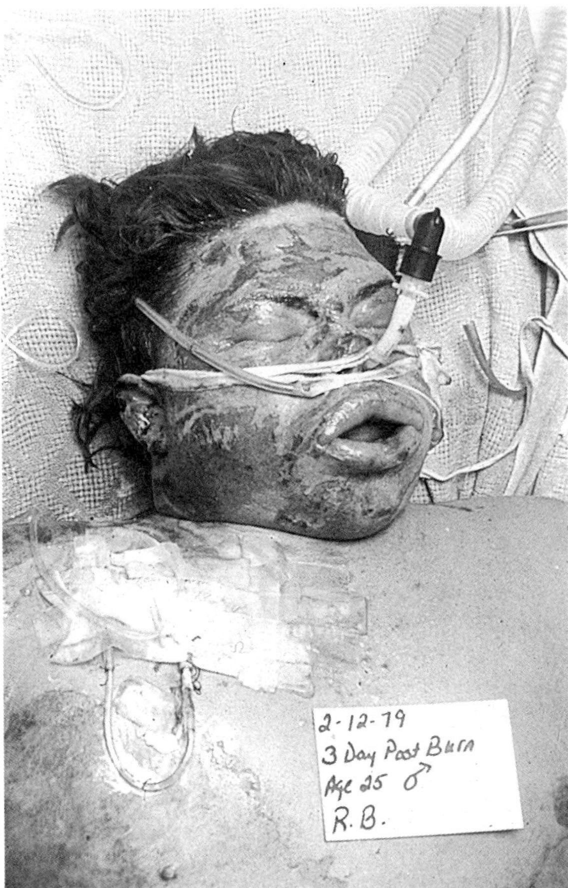

Figure 13-8 Massive facial edema in the emergent phase. *(Courtesy of University of Utah Medical Center.)*

Renal System The most common renal complication is acute tubular necrosis (ATN). Because of the hypovolemic state, blood flow to the kidneys is decreased, causing renal ischemia. If this continues, acute renal failure may develop.

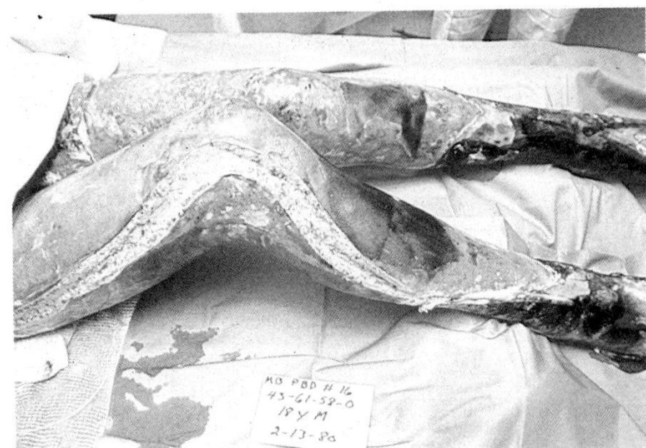

Figure 13-7 Circumferential leg burn necessitating escharotomy. *(Courtesy of University of Utah Medical Center.)*

With full-thickness and electrical burns, myoglobin (from muscle cell breakdown) is released into the bloodstream and occludes renal tubules. Adequate fluid replacement and diuretics can counteract myoglobin obstruction of the tubules.

Medical management

From onset of the burn event until the client is stabilized, medical therapy predominantly consists of fluid therapy and wound care (Table 13-5). Upon arrival at a health care facility, a fluid replacement line is secured in a large vein, preferably by percutaneous puncture. If this is not feasible, a jugular or subclavian line is inserted through unburned or even burned tissue. A cutdown is a final measure, rarely used because of high incidence of infection and sepsis. It is critical to establish access to a large vein that can

Table 13-5

Medical Management of the Burn Client

Emergent Phase

1. Fluid therapy
   a. Assess fluid needs (Table 13-6)
   b. Intravenous fluid replacement
   c. Indwelling catheter
   d. Monitor urine output
2. Wound Care
   a. Tub and debridement
   b. Assess extent and depth of burns
   c. Topical antibiotic therapy
   d. Systemic antibiotics for 5–7 days
   e. Tetanus toxoid or tetanus antitoxin

Acute Phase

1. Fluid therapy
   a. Replacement depends on individual client needs
   b. Administer RBC
2. Wound Care
   a. Assess wound daily
   b. Observe for complications
   c. Continue tubbing and debridement
3. Early excision and grafting
   a. Homografts
   b. Autografts
   c. Donor site care

Rehabilitation Phase

1. Counsel and teach client and family
2. Encourage and assist client in resuming self-care
3. Physical therapy for maintenance and rehabilitation of motion
4. Correct contractures and scarring (surgery, physical therapy, or splinting)
5. Possible cosmetic or reconstructive surgery

accommodate large volumes of fluid. Peripheral veins, especially those in the feet or legs, are not generally used.

Fluid Therapy Fluid therapy is usually instituted in clients with burns greater than 20 percent BSA. The type of fluid replacement is determined by size and depth of burn, age, and any individual considerations such as dehydration in the preburn state or preexisting congestive heart failure. Three types of fluid replacement are:

1. Crystalloids—physiologic saline, lactated Ringer's solution, dextrose, and saline
2. Colloids—blood dextran, plasma
3. Water—dextrose 5% in water

Of the many formulas that are used for fluid replacement, the Evans formula, the Brooke formula, the hypertonic saline formula, and the Baxter (Parkland) formula are most commonly employed[11,12] (Table 13-6). All formulas are estimates. The Baxter formula has received wide use because it is easy to calculate and monitor, and provides a reliable method of fluid resuscitation in most clients.

As noted in Table 13-6, the Baxter formula gives fluid in the following manner: 4 mL lactated Ringer's/kg of body wt/% BSA. This quantity is calculated for the first 24 hours with one-half of the total quantity given in the first 8 hours after injury because it is during that period that the fluid loss is greatest. (*Note*: this 24 hours is not calculated from time of arrival to hospital, but from the time of injury.) One-quarter of

Table 13-6

Formulas for Estimating Fluid Replacement of an Adult Burned Client

	First 24 Hours			Second 24 Hours		
	Electrolytes	**Colloid**	**Glucose in Water**	**Electrolytes**	**Colloid**	**Glucose in Water**
Evans	Normal saline 1.0 mL/kg/% burn	1.0 mL/kg/% burn	2000 mL	$\frac{1}{2}$ of 1st 24-hour requirement	$\frac{1}{2}$ of 1st 24-hour requirement	2000 mL
Brooke	Lactated Ringer's 1.5 mL/kg/% burn	0.5 mL/kg/% burn	2000 mL	$\frac{1}{2}$ to $\frac{3}{4}$ of 1st 24-hour requirement	$\frac{1}{2}$ to $\frac{3}{4}$ of 1st 24-hour requirement	2000 mL
Baxter-Parkland	Lactated Ringer's 4 mL/kg/% burn				20%–60% of calculated plasma volume	

Adapted with permission from B. A. Pruitt, "Fluid and Electrolyte Replacement," *Surg Clin North Am*, **58:**1293 (1978).

the total quantity is then given in the second 8-hour period, and the final one-quarter given in the last 8-hour period.

The second 24 hours of fluid replacement consists of ensuring adequate dextrose in water replacement to maintain serum sodium below 140 mEq/L. Potassium and plasma are also given. In burns greater than 30 percent, approximately 250 mL of plasma is required for each 20 percent of burn.[13] Plasma is not replaced until the second 24 hours, when capillary permeability begins to return to normal. Infusion of plasma during the first 24 hours would cause it to leak out of the vascular space. After this time, plasma remains in the vascular space and expands the circulating volume.

Assessment of the adequacy of fluid replacement is best made by using more than one parameter, with urinary output being the most commonly used. Assessment parameters include:

1. Hemodynamic factors
   Blood pressure* (systolic≥ 90 to 100 mmHg)
   Pulse rate (≤100)
   Pulmonary wedge pressure (PWP) (≤ 18 mmHg)
2. Urine production
   30 to 70 mL/hour
3. Sensorium
   Clear (in absence of narcotics or concomitant head injury)
4. Gastrointestinal function
   Absence of ileus or nausea

Wound Care Wound care may be delayed until a patent airway, adequate circulation, and adequate fluid replacement have been established. Goals of wound care are to:

1. Cleanse and debride the area of necrotic tissue and debris that would promote bacterial growth
2. Minimize further destruction to viable skin
3. Promote client comfort[14]

Cleansing and debridement are usually accomplished in a Hubbard tank in which the entire body can be immersed comfortably (Fig. 13-9). While the person is in the tub, loose, necrotic skin is removed. Large blisters are opened to eliminate a media for bacterial growth. All burned areas with hair (except eyebrows) should be shaved, including the head and perineum. Care should be taken to accomplish this procedure as quickly and deftly as possible. Immersion for longer than 20 to 30 minutes can cause electrolyte loss from open burned areas. Prolonged immersion can lead to chilling following the bath. The water does not need to be sterile. Tap water not exceeding 40°C (104°F) is acceptable. Because pathogenic organisms are normally present on the skin, clean technique is adequate.

*Blood pressure is most appropriately measured by an arterial line. Peripheral measurement is often invalid due to early vasoconstriction and edema.

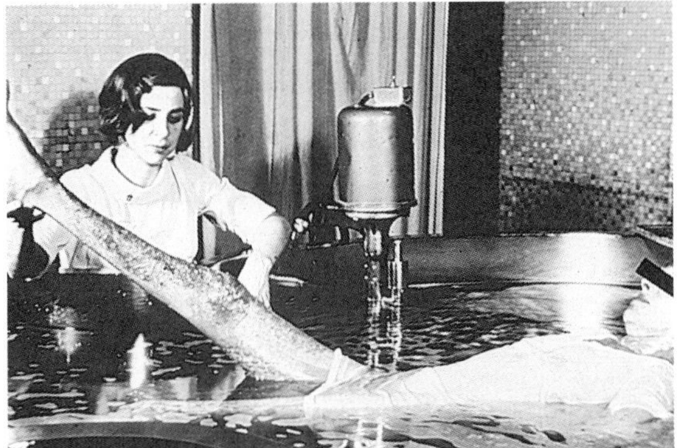

Figure 13-9 Hubbard tank (tub) for hydrotherapy. *(Courtesy of MEDCOM.)*

Infection is the most serious threat to further tissue injury and possible sepsis. Two methods of wound treatment used to control infection are the *open* and *closed method*. In the *open method* the client's burn is covered with a topical antibiotic and has no dressing (Fig. 13-10). The *closed method* employs sterile gauze dressings impregnated with or laid over a topic antibiotic. These dressings are changed two to three times every 24 hours.

Other Measures Tetanus toxoid is given routinely to all burn victims because of the likelihood of burn wound contamination. Routine lab tests are performed initially and serially to monitor electrolyte balance.

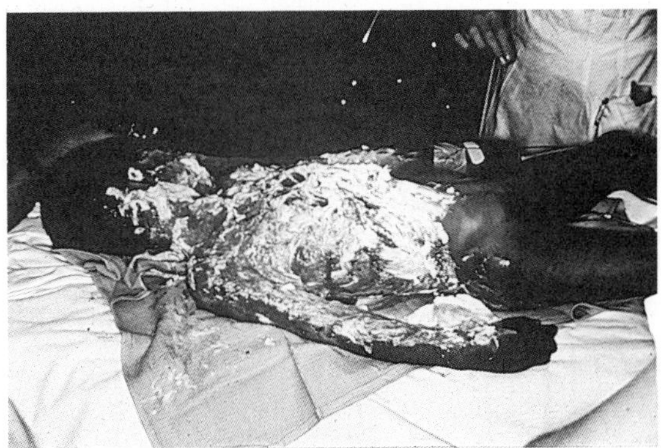

Figure 13-10 Silver sulfadiazine topical application to burn wound. *(Courtesy of MEDCOM.)*

Arterial blood gases may be drawn to determine adequacy of ventilation and perfusion. Physical therapy is begun immediately, sometimes in the Hubbard tank. Early range of motion is necessary in order to facilitate mobilization of the extravasated fluid back to the vascular bed. Exercise of body parts also maintains function and reassures the client that movement is still possible.

To promote client comfort, analgesics are ordered. Early in the post burn period, pain medications should be given intravenously because (1) gastrointestinal function is slowed or impaired due to shock or paralytic ileus, and (2) intramuscular injections will not be absorbed adequately in burned areas or edematous areas. Pooling of medications will occur in the tissues because of poor circulation. When fluid mobilization begins, the client can be overdosed from the interstitial accumulation of previous IM medications.

Pharmacologic intervention

The use of topical and systemic antibiotics early in burn treatment controls bacterial growth and prevents sepsis. Burns are initially sterile unless contaminated by the environment. However, within 24 hours, endogenous organisms (staphylococci and streptococci) that reside in hair follicles and sweat glands proliferate and produce dense colonization. Systemic antibiotics in conjunction with topical antibiotics are used to control infection and minimize further tissue damage (Table 13-7). It is recommended that systemic antibiotic therapy supplement topical therapy for the first 5 to 7 days.

Narcotics used for pain control are listed in Table 13-7. The need for analgesia should be evaluated early relative to the burn injury. The drug of choice for pain control is morphine sulfate. Meperidine may also be used. These drugs provide adequate pain control and a sedative effect. The client is in great pain with large burns (especially those that are predominantly partial-thickness). Withholding pain medication in the early phases of burn recuperation is not only inhumane but unethical as well.

For large full- and partial-thickness burns, wound coverage is the primary goal. Survival is directly related to the amount of time required for burn wound closure.[15] Since there is rarely enough available unburned skin in the major burn victim for skin grafting, other temporary wound closure is used. *Allograft* or

Table 13-7
Common Drugs Used in Burn Therapy

Antibiotics	**Examples**	**Indications for Use**
Topical	Silver sulfadiazene Mafenide (Sulfamylon) Silver nitrate Furazoleum Neomycin sulfate Cerium nitrate	While burn wound is open
Systemic	Penicillin Erythromycin Polymyxin-B Carbenicillin Gentamicin Amikacin	First 5–7 days or in presence of sepsis
Narcotics	Morphine sulfate Meperidine Codeine Dilaudid	Acute pain control
	Codeine (p.o.) Tylenol with codeine (p. o.)	When healing has progressed
Immunosuppressives	Antithymocyte globulin Azathioprine (Imuran)	Before primary excision and temporary allograft, continuing for 40–50 days
Miscellaneous	Ophthalmic ointments and drops	Corneal injury
	Lactinex Mycostatin mouthwash	Prophylaxis
	Vitamins Iron	Supplementary

Modified from D. R. Haburchak and B. A. Pruitt, "Use of Systemic Antibiotics in the Burned Patient," *Surg Clin North,* Am, **58:**1125 (1978).

homograft (usually from cadavers) is commonly used for wound closure (Table 13-9). However, rejection takes place within 12 to 20 days by the host's immune system. Because it may take up to 3 months to cover the full-thickness burned areas with the client's own skin, immunosuppression must be used.[16] Antithymocyte globulin is preferred (where possible) to azathioprine for immunosuppression. Strict environmental control is imperative with clients on immunosuppression because of their decreased ability to fight infection.

A variety of miscellaneous drugs may be administered to the burn client (Table 13-8). Frequently, superinfections develop in the client's mucous membranes (mouth and genitalia) due to antibiotic therapy and low host resistance. The offending organism is usually *Candida albicans*. This is treated with nystatin (Mycostatin) mouthwash. When the diet is resumed, *Lactobacillus* (Lactinex) may be given by mouth to maintain normal intestinal flora that has been destroyed by antibiotic therapy. Supplemental vitamins and iron may be initiated as early as the emergent phase. However, the need for these supplements usually does not occur until the acute phase.

Nutritional intervention

Fluid replacement takes priority over nutritional needs in the initial emergent phase. Clients with large burns frequently develop ileus within a few hours due to the body's response to major trauma and altered potassium metabolism. A nasogastric tube is inserted and connected to low intermittent suction for decompression. When bowel sounds return 48 to 72 hours after injury, alimentation can be initiated beginning

Table 13-8
Initial Nursing Care Plan for The Burn Client

Client Problem	Expected Outcome	Nursing Intervention
Fluid and electrolyte shifts	Urine output of $\leq$30 mL/hour Stable vital signs Clear sensorium	Give fluids according to client needs. Assess pulses, blood pressure, circulation, and sensation to all extremities every 1–2 hours. Assess mental status. Hourly intake and output. Daily weights. Assess pulmonary function. Have client cough and deep breathe every hour. Monitor serial laboratory tests.
Generalized discomfort and pain	Decreased anxiety Rest in comfort	Give analgesia if needed (morphine IV). Keep client warm. Elevate burned arms on pillows. Ambulate (if possible) qid.
Potential wound infection	Wound will be free of debris and loose necrotic tissue	Hydrotherapy and debridement for not greater than 30 minutes. Shave appropriate areas. Evacuate blisters, remove devitalized tissue. Cleanse area around eyes with normal saline (if burned). Perineal care every 2 hours (while catheterized). Apply topical antibiotic or sterile dressings as indicated. Systemic antibiotics IV. Give tetanus if necessary. Observe wound daily for separation of eschar and wound margins for cellulitis.
Decreased peristalsis	Positive nitrogen balance within 72 hours after burn	Place client NPO. Insert nasogastric tube. Assess for return of bowel sounds. Hyperalimentation and intravenous fluid replacement. Institute progressive diet to meet nutritional needs after bowel sounds return.
Potential contractures	Full ROM of all extremities and joints	Passive and active ROM during hydrotherapy and during waking hours. Maintain neck, arms, legs in extension positions. Hands in functional position. Have client assume facets of self-care as soon as possible.
Anxious client and family	Verbalize expected course of treatment Ask questions of nursing personnel	Allow opportunities to verbalize fears and concerns. Explain course of therapy and rationale to client and family. Give them frequent progress reports. Allow family to assume as much of client care as they desire.

with clear liquids and progressing to a diet high in protein and calories.

A hypermetabolic response proportional to the size of the wound is observed. Resting metabolic expenditure may be increased by 50 to 100 percent over normal for major burns. Temperature is elevated. Plasma catecholamines that stimulate heat production and substrate mobilization are increased. Massive catabolism is seen characterized by protein mobilization and increased gluconeogenesis. Caloric needs are often in the 5000 kcal/day range. Failure to supply adequate calories and protein actually causes starvation.[17]

Nursing management

In the emergent phase, client survival depends on quick and thorough nursing assessment and intervention. It is frequently the nurse who makes the initial assessment of depth, degree, and percent of burn, and who coordinates the actions of the burn team. The nurse assesses the adequacy of fluid replacement, provides wound care, and offers support to the client and family (Table 13-8).

Care of special areas is nursing initiated. The face is very vascular and subject to a greater amount of edema. The face is treated by open method because dressings would be difficult to maintain. Eye care for corneal burns or edema is done with slightly warmed normal saline as often as every hour. Periorbital edema can prevent opening of the eyes. This can be very frightening to the client and requires that the nurse assure the client that the swelling is not permanent and vision will soon be restored. An ophthalmic antibiotic ointment may be ordered. Instillation of methylcellulose drops into eyes for moisture provides additional client comfort.

Hands and arms should be elevated on pillows to minimize edema. Ears should be kept free of pressure due to poor vascularization and predisposition to infection.

The perineum must be kept clean and as dry as possible. In addition to providing hourly urine outputs, an indwelling catheter prevents urine contamination of the perineal area. Good perineal and catheter care is essential.

Acute Phase (Intermediate Phase)

Defintion

The acute phase begins when diuresis is complete and wound healing and coverage are under way. The acute phase is concluded when all burned areas are healed or grafted.

Pathophysiologic changes

Burn injury involves pathophysiologic changes in many body systems. Massive diuresis from fluid mobilization has just occurred at the end of the emergent phase and the client is no longer grossly edematous. It is more evident which areas of burn are full- or partial-thickness. Bowel sounds have returned. The client is aware of the enormity of body changes and the presence of pain. Healing begins when white blood cells have surrounded the burn wound and phagocytosis begins. Necrotic tissue begins to slough. Fibroblasts begin to lay down matrices of the collagen precursors which eventually form granulation tissue. Kept free from infection, a partial-thickness burn wound will heal from the edges and from below. However, with full-thickness burns, normal healing needs to be assisted with skin grafting.

Clinical manifestations

The wound will be dry, waxy white to dark brown in full-thickness areas and wet and shiny with serous exudate in partial-thickness areas. *Epithelialization* will begin, usually at burn margins, appearing as a bright red, granular surface. The granulations are called epithelial buds (Fig. 13-11). The margins of thick eschar will begin to separate, leaving a creamy yellow color. Areas of facial burns may show signs of healing very quickly because of the rich vascularization.

Laboratory values

Because the body is attempting to reestablish fluid and electrolyte homeostasis in the initial acute phase, it is important to follow serum values closely.

Sodium *Hyponatremia* can occur with silver nitrate topical antibiotic therapy due to sodium loss through the eschar. If hydrotherapy is too lengthy (usually greater than 20 to 30 minutes) the hypotonicity of the bath water pulls sodium from the open burn areas. Other causes of hyponatremia include excessive gastrointestinal drainage and diarrhea. Symptoms of hyponatremia include weakness, dizziness, muscle cramps, fatigue, headache, tachycardia, and confusion. Burn clients may also develop a dilutional hyponatremia referred to as *water intoxication*. To avoid this compulsion, the client should take ice chips sparingly and drink fluids other than water, such as juices or soft drinks.

Hypernatremia may be seen following successful fluid replacement if copious amounts of Ringer's lactate were required (each liter contains 130 mEq of sodium). Other causes of hypernatremia include improper tube feeding therapy or improper fluid administration. Manifestations of hypernatremia include thirst, dry, furry tongue, lethargy, confusion, and possibly convulsions.[18]

Potassium *Hyperkalemia* will be seen if the client has renal failure, adrenocortical insufficiency, or massive deep muscle injury with large amounts of potassium released from damaged cells. Cardiac arrhythmias and ventricular failure can occur with excessive elevations (K > 7 mEq/L). Muscle weakness and ECG changes will be seen clinically (Chap. 12).

Hypokalemia is seen with silver nitrate therapy and lengthy hydrotherapy. Other causes of this deficit include digitalization therapy, vomiting, diarrhea, prolonged gastrointestinal suction, and prolonged intravenous therapy without potassium supplement. Use of thiazide diuretics may also cause excessive amounts of potassium to be excreted. Constant potassium losses occur through the burn wound and from hemolysis of cells caused by debridement.

Complications

Infection The course of recovery from major burn injury is never smooth. The body's first line of defense, the skin, has been destroyed by burn injury. Pathogens often proliferate before phagocytosis has begun. The media for pathogenic growth is quite favorable. When organisms reach 100,000 (10^5)/μL the client is said to have a wound infection. In the presence of an infection, localized inflammation and suppuration will be seen at burn wound margins. Partial-thickness burns can convert to full-thickness burns in the presence of infection.

Wound infection may progress to transient bacteremia from wound manipulation (i.e., after debridement and hydrotherapy). The client may develop an invasive infection or sepsis. Manifestations of sepsis include an elevated temperature, increased pulse and respiratory rate, decreased blood pressure, and decreased urine output. There may be mild confusion, chills, malaise, and loss of appetite. The white blood cell count will usually be between 10,000 and 20,000/μL. The causative organisms of sepsis are usually gram negative (e.g., *Pseudomonas, Proteus*), putting the client in further jeopardy of possible septic shock (Chap. 26).

When sepsis is suspected, cultures should be obtained immediately from all possible sources: urine, oropharynx, IV site, and wound. However, treatment should not be delayed pending results of the culture and sensitivity studies. Usual therapy will begin with carbenicillin and gentamicin intravenously. Topical antibiotics may be continued. Steroids may be given immediately to stabilize the cell membrane and minimize endotoxin release. At this stage the client's condition is critical, requiring very close monitoring of vital signs.

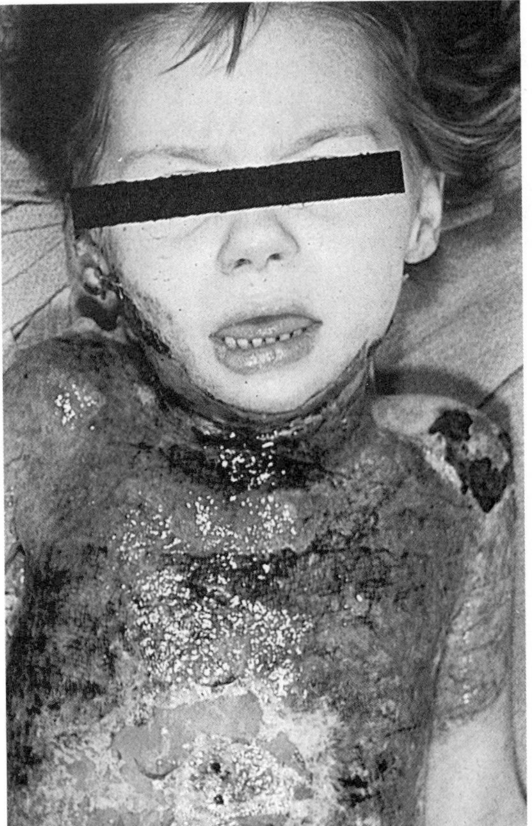

Figure 13-11 Epithelialization of burn wound. *(Courtesy of MEDCOM.)*

Cardiovascular and Respiratory Systems The same cardiovascular and respiratory system complications may be present in the acute phase as were discussed in the emergent phase.

Neurologic System Neurologically, the client usually has no physically based problems. However, a poorly understood phenomenon is likely to be seen. The client becomes extremely disoriented, may withdraw or become combative, and has hallucinations and frequent nightmarelike episodes. Delirium is more acute at night and occurs more often in older patients. This is a transient state lasting from a day or two to several weeks. Various causes have been considered, including electrolyte imbalance, massive stress, cerebral edema, sepsis, and ICU psychosis syndrome.

Musculoskeletal System The *musculoskeletal system* takes center stage for complications during the acute phase. As the burns begin to heal and scar tissue forms, the skin is less supple and pliant. Range of motion can be limited and contractures result (Fig. 13-12). Rigorous physical therapy is imperative to maintain optimal joint function. A good time for exercise is right after hydrotherapy when the skin is softer. Passive and active range of motion should be done to all joints. Clients with neck burns should sleep without pillows or with their heads hanging slightly over the head of the mattress to encourage hyperextension. Splints may be applied to keep joints in functional positions.

Gastrointestinal System The *gastrointestinal system* also exhibits complications. Paralytic ileus results from potassium alterations or sepsis. Diarrhea is more commonly found than ileus. It is due to the use of antibiotics and rich supplemental feedings. Constipation can occur as a side effect from narcotic analgesics and decreased mobility. *Curling's ulcer* is due to a generalized stress response resulting in decreased mucus production and increased gastric acid secretion. It is estimated that over half of all major burn clients have occult blood in their stools during the acute phase. The best treatment of Curling's ulcer is the prophylactic use of antacids and cimetidine which prevents histamine stimulation.

Endocrine System *Stress diabetes* may be seen transiently due to increased mobilization of glycogen stores and conversion to glucose. There is also an increase in insulin production and release. However, insulin's effectiveness is decreased, leading to an elevated blood sugar. As the client's metabolic demands are met and less stress is placed on the entire system, this process reverses. Adrenocortical insufficiency may occur, although this is rare. This is seen when the body's systems are so severely stressed that they can no longer withstand the metabolic demands placed on them. Symptoms include a sustained hyperthermia (>39.4°C; 103°F) or hypothermia (<37.2°C; 99°F), leukopenia, anorexia, weakness, hypotension, decreased urine potassium, and increased urine sodium. Hydrocortisone is given intravenously to reverse adrenocortical crisis.[19]

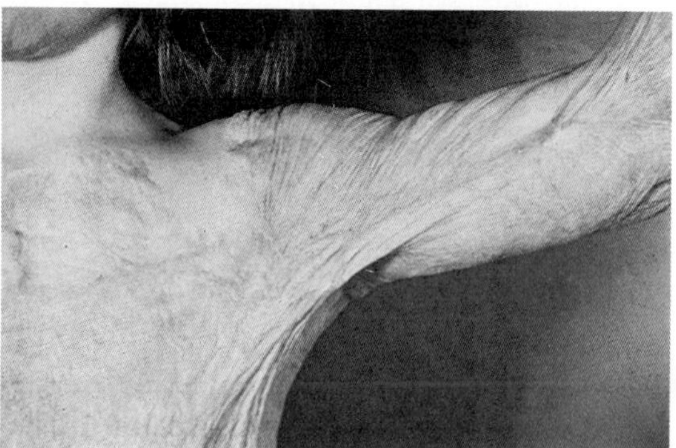

Figure 13-12 Contracture of axilla. *(Courtesy of MEDCOM.)*

Medical management

The three predominant medical interventions in the acute phase are (1) fluid replacement, (2) wound care, and (3) early excision and grafting (Table 13-5).

Fluid Replacement *Fluid replacement* continues from the emergent phase into the acute phase, based on client needs. Intravenous therapy is given to replace fluid losses, administer medications, administer transfusions of plasma or blood products, and to maintain nutrition. The type of fluid replacement depends on the client's specific needs. Common types of replacement are normal saline, Ringer's lactate, and various concentrations of glucose in saline or water. Packed red blood cells are also commonly given at this time.

Wound Care *Wound care* consists of daily observation and assessment, debridement, and perhaps *grid escharotomy*. This procedure involves cross-hatching through the eschar with a scalpel. This is a painless procedure for the client and allows more of the burn surface to be an edge, thus promoting eschar separation from viable tissue.

Excision and Grafting The most remarkable medical therapy which has changed the management of burn care in the last 10 years is *early excision and grafting*. In the past, major burn clients had low rates of survival because healing and wound coverage took so long that the client usually first succumbed to infection or starvation. Now, mortality can be greatly reduced and morbidity decreased by this type of intervention. Candidates for early excision and grafting are those with uninfected wounds and no preexisting complications.

Two types of excision are (1) tangential excision for partial-thickness burns, and (2) full-thickness excision for full-thickness burns. *Tangential excision* is best done 3 to 7 days post burn or when edema is beginning to subside and before infection has had an opportunity to develop. Devitalized tissue is removed as far down as viable deep dermis and covered with *autograft* or *allograft* (Table 13-9). Function is restored

Table 13-9
Sources of Grafts

Source	Graft Name	Coverage
Client's own skin	Autograft	Permanent
Cadaveric skin	Homograft or allograft (same species)	Temporary
Porcine skin	Heterograft (different species)	Temporary

Table 13-10
Types of Autografts

Sheet Graft	Mesh Graft	Postage Stamp Graft
Used for covering joints or areas of high stress (neck, axilla) or the face	Used to cover larger, flatter areas (back, arms, buttocks, legs.) Maximizes skin coverage with small amount of graft	Used when there is only a small amount of skin to cover a large area

and scar tissue formation is lessened. A disadvantage of tangential excision is the problem of hemostasis. Since the dead tissue is planed off until viable tissue is reached, much bleeding is expected to occur. Excessive bleeding poses a problem when grafting is performed. Clots between the graft and the wound keep the graft from adhering to the wound. One method of managing the clotting problem is to excise the wound one day and graft the next day, making sure that the excised areas are soaked every 4 hours with an antibiotic solution.

Full-thickness excision is done for the same reasons as tangential excision. However, in large burns it is not possible to accomplish excision for all burned areas at one time due to bleeding, surgical stress, and lack of sufficient autograft harvesting sites. Therefore, sequential excision may be done on full- and partial-thickness burns, allowing the client time between surgeries to recover and grow more skin.

Skin is taken from the client for *grafting* by using a dermatome that takes a very thin element of skin, called *split-thickness* (Table 13-10). A split-thickness graft can then be *meshed* to allow stretching for greater wound coverage, or cut into small squares for a *postage stamp* graft (Fig. 13-13).

The graft must be placed onto clean, viable tissue in order for the graft to take. Fresh granulation is usually seen 14 to 21 days post burn for partial-thickness injury and longer for full-thickness injury. Grafting, especially autografting, is done in the operating room under sterile conditions with the client under general anesthesia.

Nutritional intervention

The goals of nutritional management of the burn client during the acute phase are to (1) minimize energy demands, and (2) provide adequate exogenous calories to promote healing.

The burn client is in a hypermetabolic and highly catabolic state as a result of the burn injury. Decreasing catecholamine release by minimizing pain, fear, anxiety, and cold can maximize client comfort and conserve energy. Infection is also highly energy-consuming.

Daily caloric intake is crucial. Adult needs for burns greater than 20 percent BSA can be estimated:[21]

25 kcal/kg of body weight + 40 kcal/% burn

Caloric needs are often 5000 kcal/day. By the end of the first postburn week, the client's caloric and nutritional requirements should be met. Encourage high-protein, high-carbohydrate foods to meet increased caloric needs (Appendix B, Table 1). Ideally, the client should not lose greater than 10 percent of his preburn weight.

Optimally, the client should take a normal diet by mouth as soon as bowel function returns. If this is not possible, a small silastic feeding tube can be placed nasogastrically and a complete liquid diet administered. Diet supplements can be given by mouth or intravenously in the form of fat emulsions (Intralipid) or total parenteral nutrition (see Chap. 33).

If family members wish to bring in the client's favorite foods, this should be encouraged. Calories and protein are desired in high quantities. Adequate nutritional intake can decrease the recovery time.

Nursing management

During this phase wound care consumes most of the nursing care hours. Yet this should not negate the importance of supportive care, comfort and hygiene measures, and physical therapy.

Pain Assessment and Management One of the most critical functions a nurse performs during this phase is pain assessment and management. It becomes very difficult in burn nursing to separate empathy from sympathy and act appropriately when clients are so vulnerable and ill. Almost every intervention

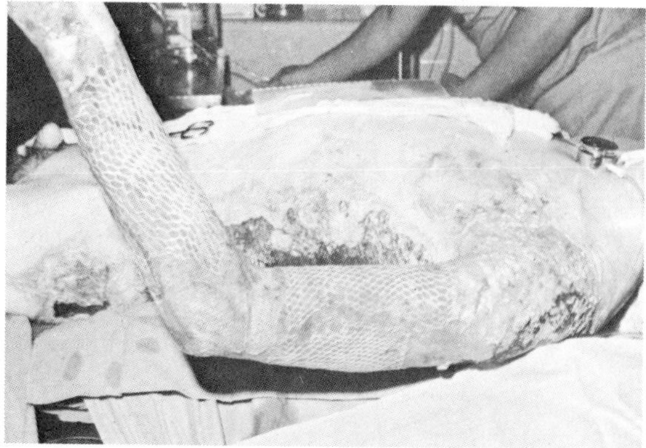

A

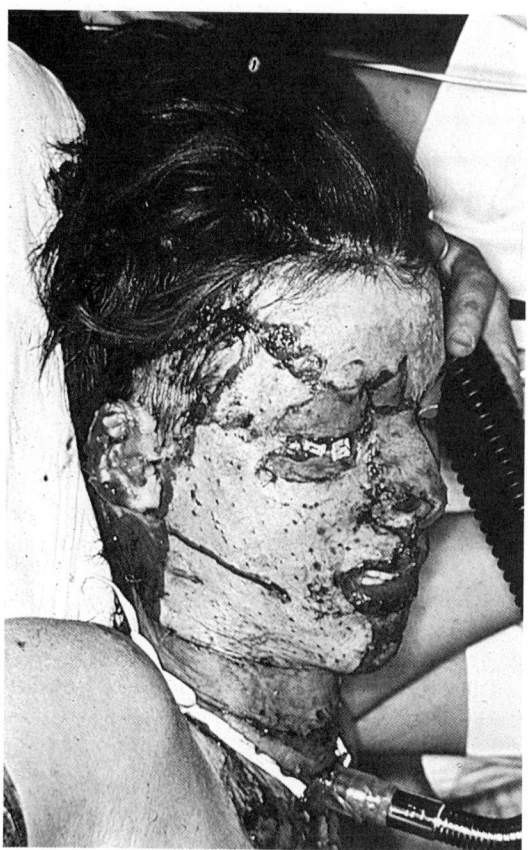

B

Figure 13-13 Types of grafts. *(a.)* Autograft using mesh graft. *(Courtesy of D. Jones et al., Medical-Surgical Nursing: A Conceptual Approach, McGraw-Hill Book Company, New York, 1982, p. 540.)* *(b.)* Sheet grafts used to cover entire side of face. *(Courtesy of MEDCOM.)*

done for the client causes pain in spite of the fact that helping to cure is the goal (Fig. 13-14). The client may find rare times of relative comfort, but knows they will not last. The nurse must understand physiologic as well as psychological bases of pain (Chap. 50). Allowing the client to ventilate feelings of anger, hostility, and frustration serve to assist the client in pain expression.

Wound Care Debridement, dressing changes, topical antibiotic therapy, graft care, and donor site care are done daily. Appropriate coverage of the graft (if it is not kept open to air) should include fine-mesh gauze in closest proximity to the graft before other dressings are applied. Grafts must be free of serous blebs. Blebs prevent the graft from interfacing and growing to the wound itself. Evacuation of blebs is done by aspiration with a tuberculin syringe or by pricking or cutting the peripheral margin of the bleb and rolling (with a sterile swab) the fluid from the center of the bleb to the exit site. Never roll the bleb to the edge of the graft. This only serves to separate adherent graft from the wound. Donor sites must be kept dry for optimal healing. Heat lamps serve to dry the gauze over the donor site and initiate scab formation. Epithelialization soon follows and healing is complete in 10 to 14 days.

Emotional Support Since the nurse has the most prolonged contact with the client and family, it is natural for them to see the nurse as their source of emotional support. The nurse must assist the client in maintaining personal worth and reestablishing a satisfactory body image. The nurse must have an almost unlimited supply of patience and understanding. Often health care personnel are the targets for anger and hostility from clients who have no other way to express these feelings.

Working with the family is a challenge for the nurse. Loved ones need to see the importance of reestablishment of a client's independence. Family members will be confused by all the changes they see in the various burn phases. It is helpful for the family to view the burned areas frequently so they can see the progress of healing.

Rehabilitation Phase

Definition

The rehabilitation phase is defined as beginning when the client's burn is "reduced to less than 20% BSA and the client is capable of assuming some self-care activity."[22] This can be as soon as 2 weeks to as long as 2 months. Goals for this period are to assist

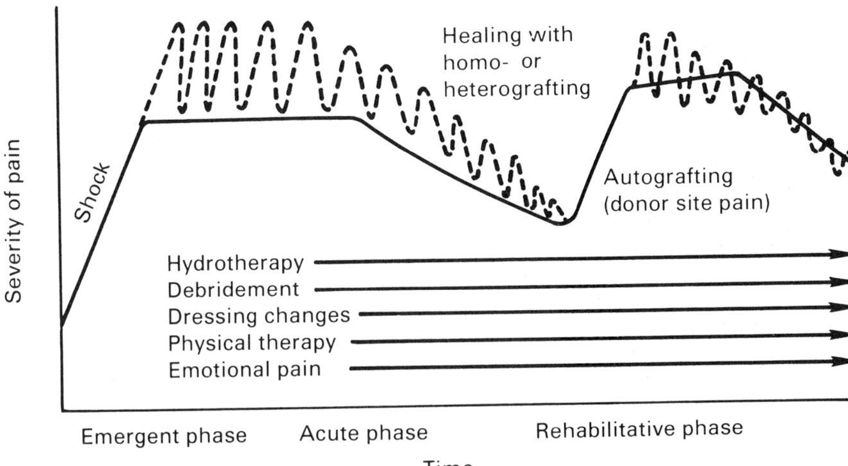

Figure 13-14 Pain trajectory for burns.

the client in resuming a functional role in society and to accomplish functional and cosmetic reconstruction.[23]

Pathophysiologic changes and clinical manifestations

The burn wound heals either by primary intention or by grafting. Layers of epithelialization begin building back the tissue structure destroyed by the burn injury. Collagen fibers present in the new scar tissue help healing, weakened areas to be stronger. After healing the new skin appears flat and pink. In approximately 4 to 6 weeks the area becomes raised and hyperemic. If adequate range of motion is not instituted, the new tissue will shorten, causing contracture. Mature healing is reached in 6 months to a year when suppleness has returned and the pink or red color has faded to a slightly lighter color than the surrounding unburned tissue. In blacks, since many of the melanocytes are destroyed, it takes longer for black skin to regain its dark color. Often the skin never regains its original color.

The client will experience discomfort from itching where healing is occurring. Nivea cream and diphenhydramine (Benadryl) serve to ease the itching. As "old" epithelium is replaced by new cells, flaking will occur. The newly formed skin is extremely sensitive to trauma. Blisters are likely to form from very slight pressure or friction. Additionally, these newly healed areas can be hyper- or hyposensitive to cold, heat, or touch. Grafted areas are more likely to be hyposensitive until peripheral nerve regeneration occurs.

Complications

The most common complications are skin and joint contractures and hypertrophic scarring. Due to pain the client will prefer to assume a flexed position for comfort. This position predisposes to contracture formation. To minimize this complication, positioning, splinting, and exercise should be instituted very early in the course of recovery. These procedures should be continued until the skin matures.

Areas that are most subject to contracture formation include the anterior and lateral neck areas, axillae, antecubital fossae, fingers, groin areas, popliteal fossae, and ankles. These areas encompass major joints. Not only does the skin develop contractures, but also the underlying tissues such as the ligaments and tendons suffer shortening. Therapy is aimed at extension of body parts because the flexors are stronger than the extensors.

Medical and nursing management

Members of the health care team share responsibilities for assisting the client in returning to optimal function during the rehabilitation phase. Because of the severe psychological impact of burn injury, health care providers must be sensitive and attuned to the client's feelings. The client is assisted with emotional adjustments by ventilation of fears such as loss of function, deformity, disfigurement, and financial burdens. Clients can then be assisted in realistic appraisal of their particular situation and emphasis is placed on what they can do, not what they cannot do. Self-esteem is usually low for burn injury victims. Allowing them appropriate independence and encouraging them to assist with the care of other burn clients involves them in activities that help to restore self-esteem. Counseling continues when the client goes home. They need reassurance that their adjustment feelings are normal and that frustration is common as they resume their normal lifestyles.[24]

During the rehabilitation phase the client and family are actively learning how to care for the healed and healing wounds. Since the client may go home with unhealed open areas, instruction will be needed in dressing changes and wound care. To keep the skin supple and decrease itching and flaking, an emollient cream (e.g., Nivea) should be used routinely on healed areas. The client and family will need anticipatory guidance in order to know what to expect physiologically as well as psychologically during recovery.

Cosmetic or reconstructive surgery is often needed for major burns. It is important that the client understand the need or possibility of reconstructive surgery before leaving the hospital.

The role of exercise and appropriate physical therapy cannot be overemphasized. The progression of physical therapy from hydrotherapy to passive range of motion, to active range of motion, to stretching, ambulation and ultimate restoration of function is a lengthy and painful process. Constant encouragement and reassurance are necessary to maintain the client's spirits and morale. Clients soon regard physical therapy as an integral part of their treatment.[25]

Nutritional intervention

By this time in the client's recovery, the negative nitrogen balance has been corrected. However, it is still important to maintain a high-calorie, high-protein diet. There is usually no problem with anorexia at this time. The client with a functional problem in eating can get assistance from occupational therapy in use of a device to correct or ameliorate the problem. Often, all that is necessary is padding the handle of a fork or spoon with several layers of gauze so that grip is better established. Toward the end of hospitalization clients occasionally need assistance from a dietitian. Because they have been encouraged to *eat, eat, eat* for such a long period of time while their burn wounds were acute, it becomes very difficult to gear the body's appetite down as healing approaches completion and to avoid an unwanted weight gain.

EMOTIONAL NEEDS OF THE CLIENT AND FAMILY

Because of the suddenness and severity of burn trauma, the client and family are plunged into physical and emotional crises. Health care providers must be prepared to assess psychoemotional cues from the client and family and provide appropriate intervention throughout the client's course of recovery.

The client will be experiencing thoughts and feelings that are very frightening and disturbing to him such as guilt over the burn accident, reliving the experience, fear of death, and concern about future therapy and the concomitant pain. The family may share any or all of these feelings. They will feel helpless to assist their loved one. The nurse should provide time for the client and family to be alone. Allow family members (if they indicate a desire) to assist the client with position changes and eating. It is important that the family be kept informed of the client's progress.

In order for nursing to adequately deal with the enormous range of emotional response that the burn client may exhibit, it is important to have an understanding of the circumstances of the burn, past family interactions, and past coping experiences with stressful stimuli. At any time the various emotional responses of fear, anxiety, anger, guilt, and depression may be experienced (Table 13-11). Another commonly seen emotional response is *regression*. Clients will revert to behavior that helped them cope with stressful past situations. Frank psychosis can also be seen. Unless the client had a psychiatric condition prior to the burn injury, this psychosis is usually transient.

Therapeutic intervention for the client at this point does not necessarily indicate the use of a psychiatrist. Nurses, physicians, social workers, or anyone else having a rapport with the client and a good understanding of their own feelings in such situations can be therapeutic. The client can best convey some of these negative, but normal, emotions to a health care provider who can interact without the client sensing retaliation. Acknowledgment that the feelings are real and valid does much to help the client. The nurse should not belittle or scorn a client's regression, but be firm and consistent in assisting the client to cope.

Major emotional tasks confront the client and family. As more and more independence is expected from the client, he must confront new fears: "Can I *do* it?" "What will people think when they see me?" "Will I be a burden?" "Am I a desirable partner, father, etc.?" Open communication needs to exist in the client's environment during this phase of recovery.

The difficult issue of sexuality must be met with honesty. Physical attractiveness will be altered in the major burn client. Acceptance of this alteration is very difficult at first for the client and family. The nature of skin injury in itself causes modifications in processing sexual stimuli. Since touch is such an important part of sexuality, the client's need for this may be altered.

Immature scar tissue may make touch unpleasant or dulled. The normal pleasure response is altered and the client's sexuality is affected. This is usually transient, but the client and family need to know that it is normal and thus receive anticipatory guidance from health care personnel to avoid undue emotional strain.

Table 13-11
Emotional Responses of Burn Clients

Emotion	Possible Verbal Expression
Fear	Will I die? What will happen next? Will I be disfigured?
Anxiety	I feel out of control. What's happening to me?
Anger	Why did this happen to me? Those doctors enjoy hurting me.
Guilt	If only I'd been more careful. I was punished because I was bad.
Depression	It's no use going on like this. I don't care what happens to me. I wish people would leave me alone.

SPECIAL NEEDS OF THE NURSING STAFF

Psychoemotionally Demanding Role

From the discussion in previous sections about the emotional trauma of the client, a logical extension includes the emotional trauma of the nurse. The nurse must deal with unpleasant, rejective, hostile clients and the idea that the burn therapy is almost always painful. The nurse will see many hours of client care suddenly obliterated by sepsis and death. Because of long hospitalizations and intense contact, clients and their care providers often form dependency bonds. Although these bonds at times are unavoidable, they sometimes make therapy difficult. Burn clients can develop demanding or punitive attitudes which cause the nurse to be reluctant to care for the client. The frequency of family contact can be rewarding as well as draining to nursing personnel. Newcomers to burn nursing often find it difficult to deal with the deformities caused by burn injury.

Intensive Care Milieu

Most major burn victims are cared for in an intensive care unit. This means critical and frequent assessments, as well as frequent changes in therapy as the client's condition changes. Highly stressful environments tend to result in a rapid staff turnover. Thus, new personnel are continuously being trained to function in this complex environment. Concern over whether or not to resuscitate a severely burned victim causes much internal stress. The assortment of sophisticated equipment can in itself be overwhelming. Tension and intense emotions are ever-present in this intensive care environment.

Support services for burn nurses in the form of group meetings led by a psychiatrist, psychologist, or social worker are often organized. Such meetings help the nursing staff deal with difficult feelings they experience in caring for the burn client. Nurses need the opportunity to ventilate their feelings of anger and hostility to a non-retaliatory listener. This therapeutic communication process often distinguishes truly fine burn nursing from custodial burn nursing.

Case Study / Severe Burn Client

Mac, a 57-year-old male, was admitted to the emergency room via ambulance with severe burns, full- and partial-thickness, over his body (Fig. 13-15). He had good health prior to an explosion from a gas heater in his apartment. His injury was sustained 3 hours ago.

A physical examination reveals a 70-kg male in acute distress. His pulse is 128 and slightly irregular. His blood pressure is 106/80. An IV was started and an indwelling catheter inserted into his bladder.

Discussion Questions

1. Estimate from the Lund and Browder diagram the client's percentage of burn. Is the client critical? Why?
2. How would you expect the burn injuries to appear?
3. What fluid and electrolyte changes would Mac encounter during the first 48 hours? Explain their pathophysiologic bases.
4. What is the rationale for ordering a tracheostomy set to be kept at Mac's bedside?
5. After fluid replacement is started, Mac's urine output increased to 80 mL/hour. What is the significance of this finding?
6. What physical changes that will occur in the first few days after his burn injury does the nurse need to inform Mac about?

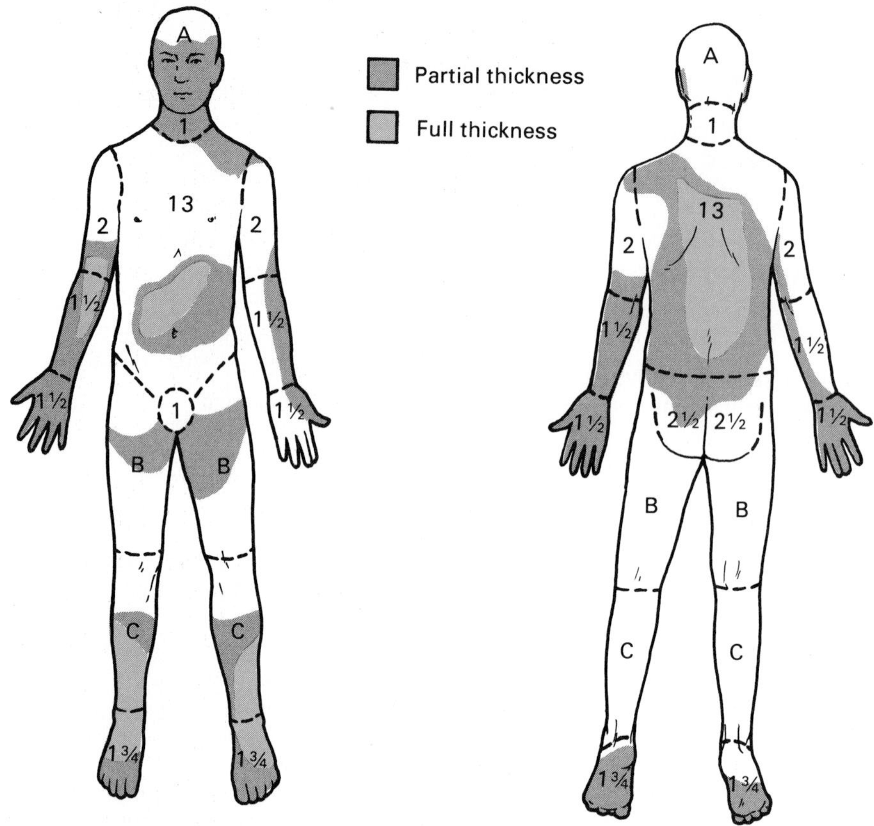

Relative Percentage of Areas Affected by Growth

	Age in Years					
	0	1	5	10	15	Adult
A—½ of head	9½	8½	6½	5½	4½	3½
B—½ of one thigh	2¾	3¼	4	4¼	4½	4¾
C—½ of one leg	2½	2½	2¾	3	3¼	3½

Figure 13-15 Case Study—Estimation of Mac's burns.

REVIEW QUESTIONS

The number of the question corresponds to the same numbered objective at the beginning of the chapter.

1. Extent of electrical injury can be difficult to assess because
   a. victims are often in shock
   b. the entry and exit wounds are very deep
   c. internal damage is not readily apparent
   d. electrical injury is usually smaller than thermal injury

2. A partial-thickness burn would have which of the following characteristics?
   a. red, shiny, wet appearance
   b. generalized erythema with no vesicles
   c. exposed fascia
   d. dry, waxy white appearance

3. The extent of burns is assessed by
   a. looking at which body parts are involved
   b. determining preexisting risk factors
   c. using guides to indicate burn location relative to total body surface
   d. estimating what is a full- vs a partial-thickness burn

4. Silver sufadiazine is the topical antibiotic of choice because it
   a. is rapidly absorbed by blood
   b. is effective against bacterial growth with few side effects
   c. is a carbonic anhydrase inhibitor
   d. maintains adequate pH of the newly forming skin buds

5. Which of the following events occurs during the early emergent phase?
   a. large proteins adhere to vascular walls
   b. potassium moves into the cell

c. sodium and water are sequestered in interstitial fluid
d. red blood cells hemolyze from large volumes of rapidly administered fluid

6. In order to maintain a positive nitrogen balance in a major burn, the client must
a. eat at least 500 calories three times per day
b. eat rice and whole wheat for the chemical effect on nitrogen balance
c. increase normal adult caloric intake by three times
d. eat a high-protein, carbohydrate diet

7. A burn client is said to be in the rehabilitative phase when
a. less than 20 percent of the burn is ungrafted or unhealed
b. physical therapy is no longer needed
c. scars have faded and skin looks normal
d. the client can return to work

8. It is important for the burn client and family to
a. see the burn wound three times per day
b. talk frequently with the nurse about the client's progress
c. allow nurses to do total care for the client to prevent infection
d. avoid discussion of the client's progress to minimize false hopes

9. The burn nurse needs
a. special psychological training
b. to be sensitive to the needs of the client and family
c. much physical strength due to the client's debilitation
d. to hide all personal feelings for the client and family

REFERENCES

1. B. J. Montgomery, "Consensus for the Sickest Patients You'll Ever See," *JAMA*, **241**:345 (1979).
2. Robert T. Fitzgerald, "Prehospital Care of Burn Patients," *Crit Care Q*, **1**(3):13 (1978).
3. Accident Facts (1977), National Safety Council, Chicago, Ill., 1978.
4. Andrew McGuire, "Prevention of Burns," *Crit Care Q*, **1**(3):2–10 (1978).
5. Fitzgerald, op. cit., pp. 13–24.
6. Ibid., p. 23.
7. C. C. Lund and N. C. Browder, "The Estimation of Areas of Burns," *Surg, Gynecol, Obstet*, **79**:352 (1944).
8. C. P. Artz and J. A. Moncrief, "The Treatment of Burns," W. B. Saunders Company, Philadelphia, 1969, p. 2.
9. Fitzgerald, op. cit., pp. 13–24.
10. Irving Feller and Claudella Archambeault-Jones, *Nursing the Burn Patient*, Institute for Burn Medicine, Ann Arbor, Michigan, 1973, p. 35.
11. Basil Pruitt, Fluid and Electrolyte Replacement in the Burned Patient, *Surg Clin North Am*, **58**(6):1291–1309 (1978).
12. Janet Marvin, "Acute Care of the Burn Patient," *Crit Care Q*, **1**(3):30 (1978).
13. Ibid., p. 30.
14. Feller, op. cit., p. 62.
15. John F. Burke, William Quinby, and Conrado Bondoc, "Early Excision and Prompt Wound Closure Supplemented with Immunosuppression," *Surg Clin North Am*, **58**(6):1141–1150 (1978).
16. Ibid., p. 1145.
17. William Curreri and Arnold Luterman, "Nutritional Support of the Burned Patient," *Surg Clin North Am*, **58** (6):1151–1156 (1978).
18. Feller, op. cit., p. 267.
19. Ibid., p. 286.
20. Ronald Sato, David Beesinger, John Hunt, and Charles Baxter, "Early Excision and Closure of the Burn Wound," *Crit Care Q*, **1**(3):51–62 (p. 60) (1978).
21. Curreri and Luterman, op. cit., p. 1153.
22. Feller, op. cit., p. 320.
23. Ibid.
24. N. J. Andreason, A. S. Norris, and C. E. Hartford, "Incidence of Long-Term Psychiatric Complications in Severely Burned Adults," *Ann Surg*, **174**(5):785–793 (1971).
25. Phala Helm, Marjorie Head, Gerry Pullium, Maureen O'Brien, and G. Fred Cromes, Jr., "Burn Rehabilitation—A Team Approach," *Surg Clin North Am*, **58**(6):1263–1278 (1978).

BIBLIOGRAPHY

Books

Bricker, N. S.: *The Sea Within Us: A Clinical Guide to Fluid and Electrolyte Balances*, Science and Publishing Company, New York, 1975.

Burgess, A.: *The Nurse's Guide to Fluid and Electrolyte Balance*, 2d ed., McGraw-Hill Book Company, New York, 1979.

Collins, R. D.: *Illustrated Manual of Fluid and Electrolyte Disorders*, J. B. Lippincott Company, Philadelphia, 1976.

Feller, Irving: *International Bibliography on Burns*, National Institute for Burn Medicine, Ann Arbor, Mich., 1978.

Hamilton, Helen (ed.): *Monitoring Fluid and Electrolyte Precisely*, Nursing '79 Skillbook Series, InterMed Communications, Inc., Horsham, Pa, 1978.

Jacoby, Florence: *Nursing Care of the Patient with Burns*, The C. V. Mosby Company, St. Louis, 1972.

Metheny, N. M., and W. D. Snively: *Nurses' Handbook of Fluid Balance*, 3d ed., J. B. Lippincott Company, Philadelphia, 1979.

Periodicals

Adlard, J. M., and J. M. George, "Hyponatremia," *Heart Lung*, **7**:587 (1978).

Andreason, N. J., et al: "Management of Emotional Reactions in Seriously Burned Adults," *N Engl J Med*, **268**:65–69 (1972).

Fagerhaugh, Shizuko: "Pain Expression and Control on a Burn Care Unit," *Nurs Outlook*, **22**:645–650 (1974).

Felver, L: "Understanding the Electrolyte Maze," *Am J Nurs*, **80**:1591–1595 (1980).

Fox, C. L., and John Stanford, "Comparative Efficacy of Hypo-, Iso-, and Hypertonic Sodium Solutions in Experimental Burn Shock," *Surgery*, **75**:71–79 (1974).

Gelin, Lars-Erik: "Reaction of the Body as a Whole to Injury," *J Trauma*, **10**:932–939 (1970).

Hayter, Jean: "Emergency Nursing Care of the Burned Patient," *NCNA*, **13**:223–234 (1978).

Humes, H. D., Narins, R. G., and B. M. Brenner: "Disorders of Water Balance," *Hosp Pract*, **14**:133 (1979).

Kleeman, C. R.: "CNS Manifestations of Disordered Salt and Water Balance," *Hosp Pract*, **14**:59 (1979).

Kosman, M. E.: "Management of Potassium Problems During Long-Term Diuretic Therapy," *JAMA*, **230**:743 (1974).

Kubo, W. M., and M. M. Grant, "The Syndrome of Inappropriate Secretion of Antidiuretic Hormone," *Heart Lung*, **7**:469 (1978).

Monafo, William, and Vatche H. Ayvazian: "Topical Therapy," *Surg Clin North Am*, **58**:1157–1172 (1978).

Moylan, Joseph, et al.: "Resuscitation with Hypertonic Lactate Saline in Thermal Injury," *Am J Surg*, **125**:580–584 (1973).

O'Dorisio, T. M.: "Hypercalcemic Crisis," *Heart Lung*, **7**:425 (1978).

Ricci, M. M.: "Water and Electrolyte Metabolism in Patients with Intracranial Lesions," *J Neurosurg Nurs*, **9**:165 (1977).

Shoemaker, W. C., et al.: "Burn Pathophysiology in Man—Part I, Sequential Hemodynamic Alterations," *J Surg Res*, **14**:64–73 (1973).

Trunkey, D. D.: "Review of Current Concepts in Fluid and Electrolyte Management," *Heart Lung*, **4**:115 (1975).

Zeluff, G. W., W. N. Suki, and D. Jackson: "Depletion of Body Phosphate—Ubiquitous, Subtle, Dangerous," *Heart Lung*, **6**:519 (1977).

———, ———, and ———: "Hypokalemia—Cause and Treatment," *Heart Lung*, **7**:854 (1978).

Section 5

Problems with Sensory Input

Chapter 14

NURSING ASSESSMENT

Vision and Hearing

Carol Fair Keith

Learning Objectives

1. Describe the structures and functions of the visual and auditory systems.
2. Describe the physiologic processes involved in normal vision and hearing.
3. Identify the significant subjective and objective data related to the visual and auditory systems that should be obtained from a client.
4. Describe the appropriate techniques used in the physical assessment of the visual and auditory systems.
5. Differentiate normal and abnormal findings of a physical assessment of the visual and auditory systems.
6. Describe the purpose and significance of results of diagnostic studies used to assess problems of the visual and auditory systems.

The importance of vision and hearing to well-being and communication cannot be overestimated. Not only do the eyes and ears sense nearby stimuli, they also provide information about the world away from the immediate environment of the client. Impairment of either the visual or auditory systems causes many changes in the client's mobility and interaction with others.

The visual system consists of both internal and external parts. The external parts are the lids, lashes, conjunctiva, cornea, sclera, and extraocular muscles. The internal parts are the iris, lens, ciliary body, choroid, and retina.

VISUAL SYSTEM: STRUCTURES AND FUNCTIONS

Ocular Structures

External structures and functions

The external structures of the eye serve a very important role in protecting the eye. The eyelids or *palpebrae* and eyelashes protect the eye from dust and foreign particles. The eye is further protected by the surrounding bony orbit and fat pads inferiorly (below) and posteriorly (behind) to the eyeball. The upper palpebrae blink spontaneously approximately 15 times per minute, distributing tears over the anterior eyeball.

The palpebrae open and close by the action of muscles innervated by the third (oculomotor) and seventh (facial) cranial nerves respectively. Muscular action also helps hold the lids against the eyeball, and along with the *tarsal plate*, a tough sheet of connective tissue within the lids, maintains the shape of the eyelids.

The space between the opened eyelids is called the *palpebral fissure*. When open, the upper lid margin is just below the *limbus* (Fig. 14-1). The inner surface of the lids is covered by a transparent mucous membrane, the *palpebral conjunctiva*, which takes on the pink color of the underlying tissue. This continuous membrane forms a pocket and covers the anterior sclera and joins the cornea at the *limbus*. This membrane, or *bulbar conjunctiva*, appears white with tiny vessels visible, especially in the periphery.

Many glands provide secretions to make up the tear film that covers the surface of the anterior eyeball. The tear film moistens the cornea and provides nourishment, especially oxygen. Tears, moved over the eye by blinking and eye movements, are drained via the *lacrimal punctum*, *lacrimal sac*, and *duct* into the nose (Fig. 14-1). The amount of tears produced decreases with sleeping, some diseases, and with aging. Increased production of tears occurs with trauma, foreign body, and diseases of the conjunctiva, cornea, eyelids, and nasal mucosa.

Each eye is moved by six extraocular muscles (four rectus or straight and two oblique) that are innervated by cranial nerves III (oculomotor), IV (trochlear), and VI (abducens). Neuromuscular coordination produces simultaneous movement of the eyes in the same direction. This is called *conjugate* movement.

The eyeball: Internal structures and functions

The eyeball is composed of three layers or tunics and is filled with fluid (Fig. 14-2). The tough *outer layer* is composed of the white *sclera* and the transparent

This chapter was reviewed by Tana Durnbaugh, R.N., B.S.N., M.S., Assistant Professor, College of Lake County, Grayslake, Illinois.

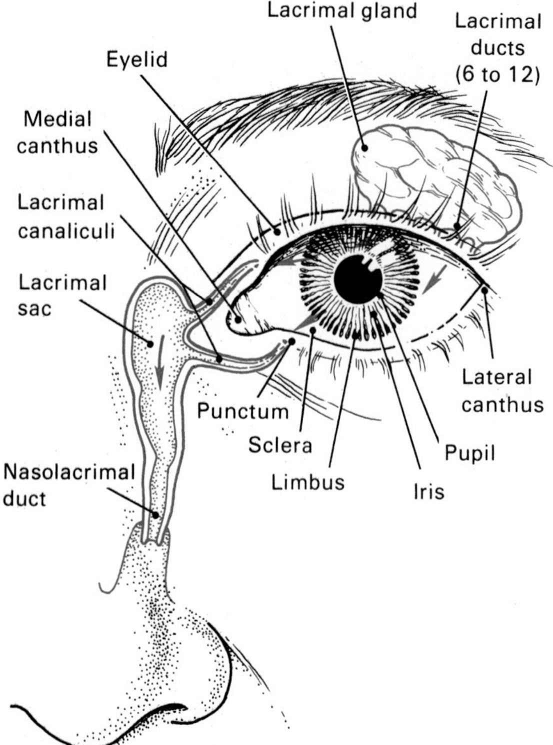

Figure 14-1 Anterior section of the eye and lacrimal apparatus. (*From L. L. Langley et al., Dynamic Anatomy and Physiology, 5th ed., McGraw-Hill Book Company, New York, 1980. Used with permission of McGraw-Hill Book Company.*)

cornea. The *middle layer* or *uveal tract* includes the *choroid*, *ciliary body*, and the *iris*. The *innermost sensory layer* lines the posterior cavity only. The lens is suspended behind the iris by zonule fibers. The pupil appears black and is the opening that varies in size by the action of muscles within the iris.

The white, tough *sclera* encircles the eyeball and joins the cornea at the *limbus*. The avascular clear *cornea* is one of the most sensitive tissues in the body and is innervated by cranial nerve V (trigeminal). Composed of five layers, the cornea maintains its transparency by obtaining oxygen via the top epithelial layer and also by a pump mechanism in the innermost layer, the endothelium, which maintains the corneal layers free of excess fluid. When the cornea receives decreased oxygen supply or is affected by trauma or disease, it becomes swollen and cloudy. This prevents transmission of light and is very painful. The cornea also has important refractive powers. The curvature of the cornea bends the light rays or *refracts* to help bring the light rays into focus on the retina.

The highly vascular choroid of the middle layer nourishes the retina in the posterior cavity. In the anterior part of the eye, the *uveal tract* continues as the ciliary body whose muscles cause the lens to change in convexity and aids in accommodation. *Accommodation* is changing of the lens to view both near and far. Loss of accommodation results in the inability to change focus from far to near. The ciliary body also secretes *aqueous humor*, the clear fluid in

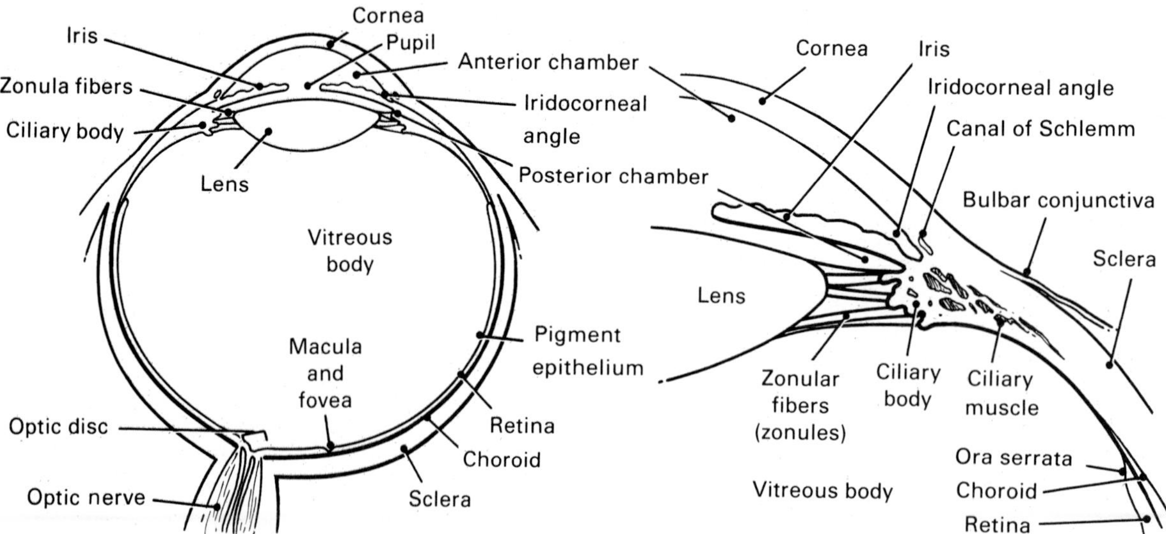

Figure 14-2 Diagram of horizontal section of the eye. (*From C. R. Noback and R. Demarest, The Human Nervous System: Basic Principles of Neurobiology, 2d ed., McGraw-Hill Book Company, New York, 1975. Used with permission of McGraw-Hill Book Company.*)

the anterior and posterior chambers in the anterior part of the eye. The iris, which provides color to the eyes, changes the size of the pupil by two muscles. The iris sphincter, innervated by the parasympathetic nervous system, causes the pupil to become smaller by contraction. The iris sphincter action can be blocked by cycloplegic drugs such as atropine. A cycloplegic drug causes paralysis of the ciliary muscles, resulting in dilation of the pupil and loss of accommodation. The dilator muscle of the iris causes the pupil to dilate. Drugs such as Neo-Synephrine 10% applied topically also produce pupillary dilation. Mydriatic drugs dilate the pupils but do not result in loss of accommodation.

The *retina*, the light-sensitive layer, is composed of two types of visual cells, the *rods* and the *cones*. The rods are stimulated in dim or darkened environments and the cones are receptive to bright environments and colors. The *macula*, a centrally located area free of vessels, has a high concentration of cones, which provides central or sharp and color vision. Within the macula is the *fovea centralis*, a pinpoint depression composed of cones only. This is the area of sharpest vision and central focusing point. Nourishment to the macula is from the underlying *pigment epithelium*, the lowermost layer of the retina, and the choroid.

With the exception of the macular area, the retina is nourished by four sets of retinal arterioles and veins entering from the optic disk. These vessels are very important as they can be easily inspected with an opthalmoscope. The condition of the retinal arteries is a good indicator of the vascular system in general.

The *optic disk* is located nasally from the macula, and has a depression within called the *physiological cup*. The optic disk is the optic nerve (cranial nerve II) and carries the visual impulses to the brain (Fig. 14-3).

Fluids of the eye

The posterior cavity, located in front of the retina, is filled with clear gelatinous material called the *vitreous humor* (Fig. 14-2). The vitreous humor helps to hold the retina in place. With aging, it becomes more liquid.[1] The lens also contains a thick gelatinous material enclosed in a clear capsule. Degenerative changes and disease cause the lens to become thicker and cloudy or opaque. This condition is called a *cataract*.

The fluid in the anterior portion of the eye is the *aqueous humor*, a clear, crystalline, watery fluid produced by the ciliary body. The route of flow is from behind the iris through the pupil and into the anterior chamber. It is absorbed by the trabecular meshwork in the iridocorneal angle into the *canal of Schlemm*, a

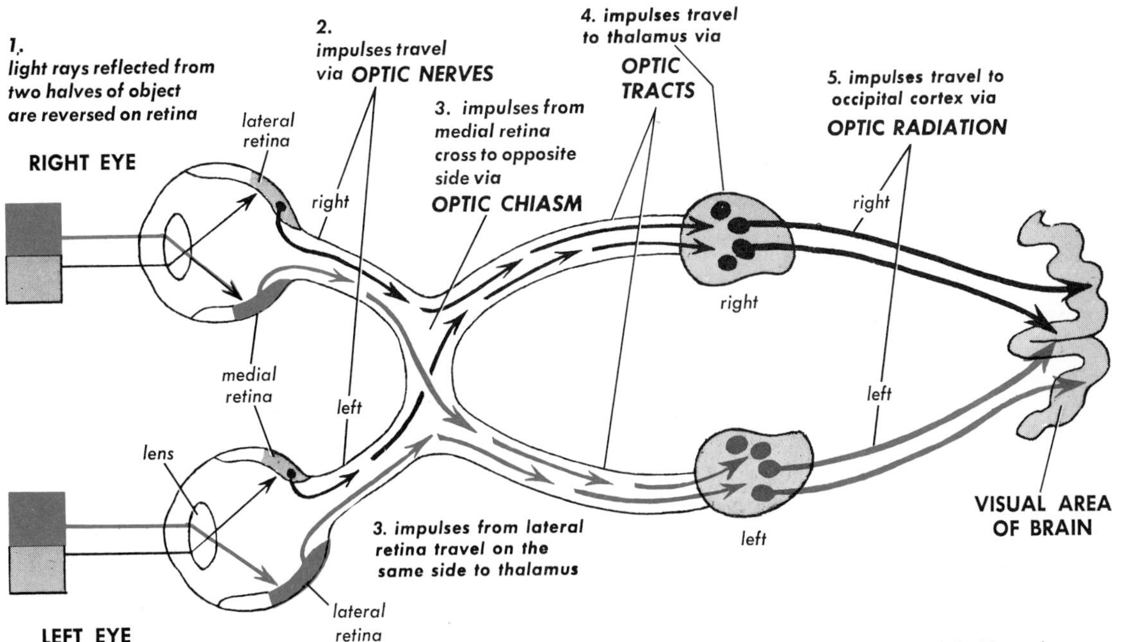

Figure 14-3 Visual pathways. Note how objects are reversed right to left on the retina. (*From E. J. Reith et al., Textbook of Anatomy and Physiology, 2d ed., McGraw-Hill Book Company, New York, 1978. Used with permission of McGraw-Hill Book Company.*)

circular canal that conveys the fluid into scleral veins and into the circulation of the body. Most cases of glaucoma are caused by a block of this meshwork. The aqueous humor bathes and nourishes the lens and the endothelium of the cornea (Fig. 14-2).

Vision: Visual Fields

Visual pathways

Vision occurs when the eye is focused upon an object in a lighted environment. The light waves reflected from the object travel through the cornea, the aqueous humor, the lens, and the vitreous humor and are then focused upon the retina. Objects are formed upside down and reversed right to left on the retina. For instance, if the object is seen in the left upper temporal field, it will be focused on the retina upside-down and in the lower nasal area of the retina of the left eye. From here the impulses travel back to the optic chiasm where the fibers from the left field of both eyes form the left optic tract and travel to the left occipital cortex. The fibers from the right field of both eyes form the right optic tract and travel to the right occipital cortex (Fig. 14-3).

In order for a near object to be focused upon the retina of an *emmetropic eye* (an eye with no refractive error) the lens must accommodate. This is accomplished by the ciliary muscle which contracts and causes the lens to become more convex or thicker. Distance vision does not require the lens to change in the emmetropic eye (Fig. 14-4). For the eye with a refractive error, the lens thickens or flattens to focus near and distant objects. As the lens ages, it becomes less elastic and cannot be focused for near vision, resulting in a need for convex lenses for reading and near vision (presbycusis). In Table 15-2 refractive errors are described as well as the correction possible by glasses and contact lenses.

ASSESSMENT OF THE VISUAL SYSTEM

Subjective Data: The Health History

Past medical history

The eye not only reflects diseases of the eye, but often indicates other systemic diseases. In addition to asking about specific diseases known to cause visual problems, it is important to ask the client about the following:

1. Pediatric and adult illnesses
   Diabetes
   Hypertension
   Hyperthyroidism, hypothyroidism
   Rheumatism, arthritis
   Syphilis
   Specific eye problems
   a. Childhood
      Strabismus, amblyopia (lazy eye), use of eyeglasses, refractive error
   b. Adult
      Glaucoma
      Cataract
      Refractive error—last exam and change of glasses
2. Immunizations
   Measles (especially women of childbearing age)
3. Hospitalizations, trauma, medications

Questions should be asked regarding hospitalizations, especially surgery involving the eye or brain, and injuries such as automobile accidents and blows to the head or eye. It is important to ask about current prescription drugs the client is taking such as cortisone preparations, diabetic and thyroid medications, and any eye medications such as pilocarpine. Cortisone preparations may contribute to the formation of glaucoma and cataracts. Questions regarding allergies and related eye problems are included. The nurse also needs to determine if the client has any allergies related to eye medications or which result in eye symptoms such as itching or tearing.

Family history

Refractive errors and many eye problems are hereditary and a careful family history is necessary. Questions regarding the following problems should be included:

1. Systemic diseases
   Arteriosclerosis
   Diabetes
   Thyroid disease
   Arthritis
2. Eye disease
   Cataracts
   Eye tumors
   Glaucoma
   Refractive errors, especially myopia and hyperopia
   Retinal degenerative changes, e.g., retinal detachment, macular degeneration, retinitis pigmentosa
   Congenital corneal problems

Social and personal history

Background Information The client should be asked if he is employed where fumes, smoke, or eye irritants are present. Information is obtained regarding

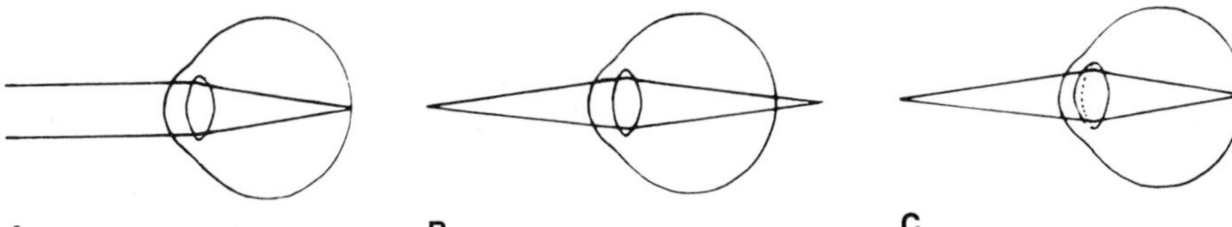

Figure 14-4 Emmetropia and accommodation. (*a*) Parallel rays from a distant object focus on the retina. (*b*) No adjustment has been made to accommodate for near vision. (*c*) The lens thickens increasing its refractive power and the light rays focus upon the retina. (*From W. DeMyer et al., Technique of the Neurologic Examination, 3d ed., McGraw-Hill Book Company, New York. Used with permission of McGraw-Hill Book Company.*)

the use of eye safety practices such as wearing protective glasses in occupations involving welding and shop work where the possibility of flying objects or molten metals exists.

Lifestyle Information regarding lifestyle is important, especially if the client wears contact lenses. Questions regarding health practices, care of lenses, and dexterity to insert contacts is of concern. Type of contacts used and wearing time may provide information for health teaching. Obtain information regarding the use of sunglasses for bright sunlight only or if used more frequently due to photophobia and light sensitivity.

If the client is a diabetic, it is important to determine adherence to a diabetic regimen and amount of control achieved. Increased blood sugars may cause the lens to absorb more fluid and the client to become myopic.[2] Determine if eye problems keep the client from engaging in any favorite activity or occupation.

Review of systems

Symptoms related to other systems can mimic eye problems. It is necessary to ask questions regarding possible sinusitis and neurologic problems such as headaches and migraine. Clinical manifestations related to the visual system include:

1. Pain or discomfort in one or both eyes
   - Foreign body sensation—lessened with lid closure?
   - Photophobia (increased sensitivity to light)
   - Irritation/itching
   - Severe, sharp, throbbing
2. Changes in vision
   - One or both eyes—time and rate of onset
   - Blurred
   - Diplopia (double vision)
   - Blind spot (scotoma)
   - Spots or floaters
   - Curtain or veil over visual field
   - Loss of parts or all of vision
   - Tunnel vision, decreased peripheral vision
   - Decreased color perception
   - Halos around lights
   - Flashes of light within eye
3. Redness
   - Eyelids, parts of eyelids
   - Conjunctiva
4. Swelling, if present throughout the day
   - Circumscribed areas of lid
   - Periorbital edema
5. Drainage
   - Increased tearing
   - Decreased tearing
   - Purulent drainage
   - Crusting of eyelid, eyelashes

Objective Data: The Physical Examination

Most of the objective data regarding the eyes are obtained by inspection. Since there are many parts of the visual system available for inspection, it is important that the nurse have a good understanding of the anatomy of the eye. A normal physical assessment is recorded as shown in Table 14-1.

Visual acuity and functions of the eye tests

Visual acuity and functions of the eye are usually tested prior to physical inspection of the eye.

Visual Acuity The client is seated or standing 20 feet from the Snellen chart (Fig. 14-5). Glasses or contact lenses should be left in place unless they are used only for reading. The client is asked to read the 40-foot line. If this can be done, the examiner instructs the client to read the next lowest line. If the client cannot read the 40-foot line, the examiner instructs him to start at the 200-foot line. The client reads the lowest line possible with no more than two mistakes. The standard of 20 feet is recorded, then the distance in feet on the line of the Snellen chart that the client read successfully. If the client were able to read down to the 30 foot line, it would be recorded 20/30. It is also recorded if the left eye (oculus sinister, or O.S.), right

Table 14-1

Recording Normal Physical Assessment of the Visual System

Eyes bilaterally symmetrical; eyebrows, lids, and lashes intact without deformity; conjunctiva, cornea, and sclera clear
Visual acuity 20/20 O.U., without glasses
E.O.M. intact without nystagmus, ptosis, or lid lag
PERRLA
Parallel corneal light reflex
Able to read newsprint at 35 cm (14 inches) with corrective lenses

eye (oculus dexter, or O.D.) or both eyes (oculus uterque, or O.U.) were tested, e.g., 20/30 O.D. This means that the client reads at 20 feet what the normal visioned person can read at 30 in the right eye.

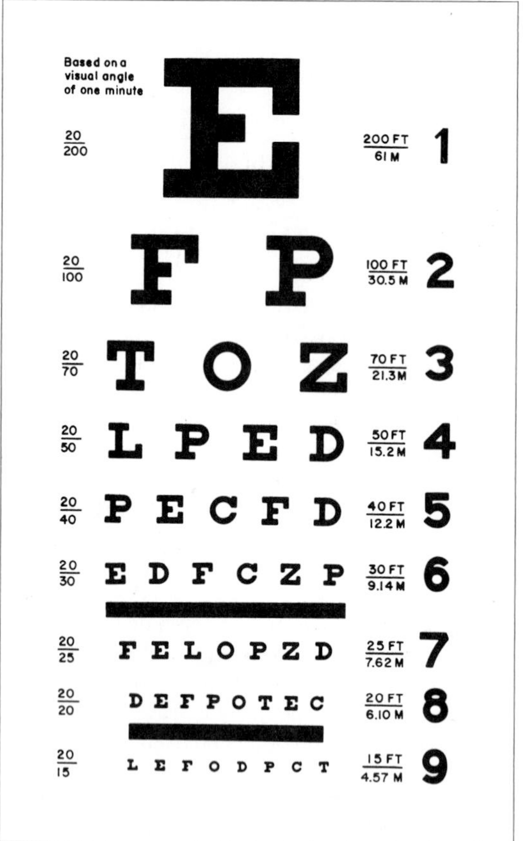

Figure 14-5 Snellen chart. The subject with normal visual acuity who stands 6.10 m (20 ft) from the full-sized chart can read line 8, marked 20/20. *(From L. L. Langley et al., Dynamic Anatomy and Physiology, 5th ed., McGraw-Hill Book Company, New York, 1980. Used with permission of McGraw-Hill Book Company.)*

Visual Fields Peripheral vision is assessed by testing visual fields. A simple although gross method of determining visual fields is the *confrontation test.* The client and examiner are seated, facing each other 60 to 90 cm (2 to 3 feet) apart. The client and examiner each cover opposite eyes. The examiner holds a pencil equidistant and without moving their eyes, both report when unable to view the pencil when moved peripherally to left upward, downward, and to the right upward and downward.[3] Any difference from the examiner's field (assuming it is normal) is recorded. The other eye is tested similarly. *Perimetry*, employing a semicircular instrument marked in degrees, is a more precise method of recording the visual fields of each eye and can be diagnostic of eye and neurologic problems.

Extraocular Muscle Functions The *corneal light reflex* is used to grossly evaluate the position of the eyes. In a darkened room, the client is asked to look straight ahead and a penlight is shone directly on the cornea. The light reflection should be located in the center of both corneas if the client looks directly at the light source.

The *cover-uncover test* will also detect faulty alignment of the eyes. While the client looks at an object held by the examiner, one eye is covered. The examiner observes for movement of the uncovered eye. If the uncovered eye moves to look at the object, then it was deviating before the straight eye was covered. Both eyes are tested. Movement of the uncovered eye indicates strabismus (crossing of the eye). If no movement of the uncovered eye occurs, the eyes must be straight.

The *extraocular movements* of the eyes are tested to determine neuromuscular balance. The client is asked to follow the examiner's index finger through the cardinal gazes (Fig. 14-6). Starting in front of the eyes, the finger is moved slowly through the positions of cardinal gaze. The eyes should follow equally with parallel and coordinated movements. Inability to move the eyes into a specific position indicates paralysis of the corresponding extraocular muscles.

Corneal Reflex The corneal reflex tests the functioning of the fifth cranial nerve (trigeminal). To test this reflex, the client is asked to keep both eyes open and look up. A wisp of cotton is brought in laterally and touched to the cornea. The client should blink with both eyelids when touched.

Inspection of extraocular structures

Inspection of the external ocular structures includes *observation* of both eyes. The physical charac-

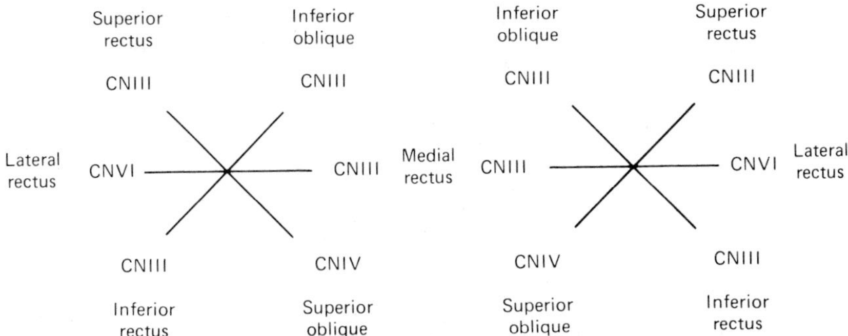

Figure 14-6 The six cardinal gazes used to test extraocular movement. Inability to move the eye into a specific position indicates pathology of the controlling extraocular muscle (LR–lateral rectus, cranial nerve VI; SR–superior rectus, cranial nerve III; IO–inferior oblique, cranial nerve III; MR–medial rectus, cranial nerve III; SO–superior oblique, cranial nerve IV; IR–inferior rectus, cranial nerve III).

teristics should be *similar* unless one eye has had previous surgery or problems. The client is seated and at eye level with the examiner. The nurse should assess the following extraocular structures.

Lids and Lashes The lids are the same color as the face and have a fold in the upper lid that disappears when the client looks up. Edema may be present immediately after arising but should subside rapidly. With age, the lids exhibit redundant tissue. The lashes are equally distributed and without crusting. Note also the condition of the eyebrows. The hair of the eyebrows should be of equal distribution without crusting. The openings of the lids (*palpebral fissures*) are equal. The upper lid should cover the superior limbus by 1 to 3 mm and the lower lid should be below the inferior limbus margin. The lids should close at the same rate and smoothness when the client is asked to follow an object in a downward gaze. The position of the lower lid should be against the eyeball with the lashes not touching the conjunctiva (entropion) or turned out from the eyeball (ectropion).

Conjunctiva and sclera

It is necessary to further expose the conjunctiva. It is *very important that your hands have been washed and that no pressure is applied to the eyeball* to prevent irritation or damage to the eye. To examine the lower lid the examiner should place a forefinger over the cheekbone and gently pull down. The client is asked to look up, down, and to both sides. The upper lid is not usually everted unless a problem is suspected. To evert the upper lid, the examiner places an applicator tip on the lid at the crease. With the client looking down, the lashes are grasped and the lid is turned over the applicator. The client should look up to reposition the lid. If the upper lid is everted, examine for any raised or reddened areas. The bulbar conjunctiva is clear, with fine vessels visible, especially in the periphery. The palpebral conjunctiva is pink. The sclera is white and may have a slight yellowish cast in dark-pigmented individuals.

Cornea A light is shone obliquely on the cornea. The surface should be smooth and without irregularities. The cornea is clear, transparent, and shiny. In an older client a white ring at the limbus (arcus senilis) is not abnormal. An additional test which can determine corneal trauma is the fluorescein strip test. A fluorescein strip is touched to the lower conjunctival sac. Any irregularities of the cornea will stain a brilliant green.

Anterior Chamber Using the oblique light the anterior chamber is inspected. The iris should appear flat and not bulging toward the cornea. The area between the cornea and iris should be clear and without particles.

Iris Both irides should be of equal color and shape. However, a color difference between the irides occurs in 5 percent of the population. The iris should be inspected with the upper lid raised for any "v" or notch-shaped black areas due to surgery for cataract or glaucoma.

Pupils The pupils are examined for shape and size. Approximately 5 percent of the population have unequal size of the pupil, which is considered a normal variation.[4] The pupil size varies by age. The infant and elderly have a miotic or small pupil; also, those with hyperopia (farsightedness) may have a miotic pupil. Pupils are larger in childhood and less large during adulthood. Normal diameter range of the pupil is 3 to 7 mm.

The pupils are tested for *pupillary response*. The client is asked to focus on a distant object straight ahead. The examiner places an object (e.g., finger) 10 to 12 cm in the client's central vision. The client is asked to focus on the near object. The normal response is for the pupils to converge and constrict symmetrically. The response is slower in older persons.

To check *consensual pupillary response* the room is darkened. A penlight is brought in laterally and shone on one pupil. The opposite eye is tested similarly. The examined pupil constricts (direct response) and the other pupil constricts simultaneously (indirect response). Normal characteristics and response of the pupil are charted as PERRLA—pupils equal, round, reactive to light and accommodation.[5]

Palpation

The eyelids are gently palpated to detect irregularities, nodules, and discomfort. Intraocular pressure can be roughly estimated by gently placing the index finger and second fingertips over the closed lid with the client looking down. With experience, the examiner will be able to detect an increase or decrease in the intraocular pressure. This test should not be done when injury to the eye is suspected or when ocular surgery has been done recently.

Finally, the *lacrimal sac* is palpated. The index finger is pressed below the inner canthus against the orbital rim to detect the presence of nodules, swelling, drainage, or pain.

An experienced examiner would proceed with an ophthalmoscopic examination to view the internal eye. The reader is referred to an assessment text for details of this examination.

Table 14-2 summarizes common assessment abnormalities of the visual system.

DIAGNOSTIC STUDIES OF THE VISUAL SYSTEM

Other diagnostic tests are available which provide specific information about the internal parts of the eye, especially the anterior chamber and vessels. Many are done in the doctor's office and outpatient clinic with special equipment (Table 14-3). There are often similar tests ordered for eye and neurologic problems.

One of the most frequent diagnostic tests done is the *tonometry test* using the Schoitz tonometer (Fig. 14-7). The intraocular pressure of the eye is measured by resting the tonometer on the anesthetized cornea. The client, lying flat or seated with the head turned upward, is directed to look at a spot overhead and to hold both eyes wide open. The tonometer is brought in from the side and the footplate is placed on the cornea in a perpendicular position. The tonometer is stabilized and the pressure read and converted in terms of the weight used.[6] A chart is available for this conversion. Normal intraocular pressure is 12 to 22 mmHg. An *applanation tonometer* applied to the cornea during examination with a biomicroscope provides a more accurate reading of intraocular pressure (Fig. 14-8). The client must be cautioned not to rub his eyes for 15 minutes as he can scratch the anesthetized cornea. Elevations of intraocular pressure may indicate glaucoma. Other tests are used to confirm the diagnosis.

THE AUDITORY SYSTEM: STRUCTURES AND FUNCTIONS

The auditory system is composed of the external ear, middle ear, inner ear, cranial nerve VIII (acoustic), cochlear nuclei, and cortex of the brain. It contains the smallest bone in the body, the stapes. Parts of the auditory system are surrounded by the temporal bone, one of the hardest bones in the body. The mastoid bone with its honeycomblike air cells is part of the temporal bone.

External Ear

The external ear is composed of the *auricle* or *pinna* and the auditory canal. The auricle is composed of cartilage and connective tissue covered by epithelium which also lines the external auditory canal (Fig. 14-9). The external auditory canal in the adult is approximately 2.5 cm long and has a slight S shape. Sebaceous and other glands in the outer half of the canal secrete *cerumen* or wax. Cerumen is moist and sticky in Caucasians and blacks, dry or hard in the Mongoloid race and American Indians. The color of cerumen ranges from a creamy pink through brown and black.[7] Cerumen has a protective function.

Hair is present in the outer half of the canal. This hair may be profuse and coarse, especially in the older male client. The inner half of the ear canal is quite sensitive. The function of the external ear and canal is to collect and transmit sound waves to the eardrum or *tympanic membrane*. This shiny, translucent membrane of pearl-gray coloration, is composed of skin, connective tissue, and mucous membrane. It is obliquely positioned at the medial end of the canal.

Table 14-2
Common Assessment Abnormalities of the Eye

Findings	Description/Definition	Possible Etiology/Significance
	Subjective Symptoms	
Pain	Foreign body sensation	Superficial corneal erosions from wearing contact lenses (hard); foreign body on conjunctiva, cornea
	Lessened with lid closure	Corneal abrasion
	Severe, deep, throbbing	Iritis, acute glaucoma, infection of the eye
Photophobia, sudden and persistent	Abnormal intolerance to light	Inflammation of cornea, iris, conjunctiva
Blurred vision	Gradual or sudden inability to see clearly	Many possibilities: refractive errors, corneal opacities, cataract, retinal changes as detachment, macular degeneration; optic neuritis or atrophy, central retinal vein or artery thrombosis, changes related to diabetic control
Scotoma	Blind spot or loss of vision within visual field	Glaucoma, chorioretinitis, injury, migraine headache
(central)	Blind spot involving central vision	Macular degeneration, occlusion of vessels of eye or brain
Spots or floaters (sudden appearance)	Sudden appearance of spots or floaters within field of vision	Hemorrhage into the vitreous humor, impending retinal detachment, intraocular hemorrhage, chorioretinitis
Dryness of eyes	Decreased tear formation or changes in tear composition. Decrease in amount of fluid bathing the eye	Can cause changes in cornea. Sleep, age, certain diseases
Halo around lights	Presence of halo when looking at lights	Glaucoma, acute
Excessive glare	Light reflects onto retina periphery	Cataract formation and aging
Diplopia	Double vision	Involvement of cranial nerves, extraocular muscles
	Objective Observations	
Eyelids		
Allergies	Redness with watering and itching along lashes	Multiple possible allergens. Itching can result in eye trauma
Hordeolum or stye	Small abscesses along lid edge	Bacterial invasion of lids and glands of eyelids
Chalazion	Infection of Meibomian glands within the tarsal framework of the lids	Bacterial invasion of sebaceous glands (Meibomian) of the eyelid
Marginal blepharitis	Reddened lid margins, crusting of lashes	Requires instruction in care of eyelids to prevent spread of infection
Dacrocystitis	Inflammation of lacrimal sac resulting in raised area near nose and medial lower lid.	Blockage of the nasolacrimal duct and subsequent infection
Xanthelasma	Raised, yellowish plaques that are circumscribed along nasal portion of each lid	May accompany lipid disorders or may be normal
Conjunctiva		
Conjunctivitis	Reddened, swollen mucous membrane	Conjunctivitis (pinkeye), trauma, edema, iritis, bacterial infection
Sclera jaundiced	Yellow color to all of sclera	Jaundice
Cornea		
Corneal abrasion	Irregularity of epithelium of cornea, usually causing much pain	Trauma, overwearing of contact lens, improper fit of contact lens

Table 14-2 (Continued)

Findings	Description/Definition	Possible Etiology Significance
Corneal opacity	Whitish color of part or all of normally transparent cornea	Scar tissue formation due to inflammation, infection. Blocks visual stimuli causing blindness, requires referral if recent
Pterygium	Triangular thickening of bulbar conjunctiva that grows over the cornea	Distorts vision, must be surgically removed if progressing to central cornea
Lid position		
Ptosis	Upper lid margin over pupil when eyes are open, may be unilateral or bilateral	Cranial nerve III involvement, myasthenia gravis, congenital, trauma
Ectropion	Outward turning of lower lid and lashes	Relaxation of framework of eyelid associated with aging, paralysis of facial nerve; edema of palpebral conjunctiva may cause maceration of skin
Entropion	Inward turning of lower lid and lashes	Contraction of scar on conjunctiva or tarsus, muscle contraction. Eyelashes may rub conjunctiva, cornea, causing irritation of conjunctiva, cornea
Lid lag	Lid closes more slowly than other lid and/or with jerky movements	Possible involvement of cranial nerve VII
Blepharospasm	Inability to open lids	Inflammation, involvement of cranial nerves V, VII
Decreased blinking		
Monocular, bilateral	Decreased closure of upper palpebral fissure	Possible involvement of cranial nerve VII; causes dryness and damage to cornea
Exophthalmos		
Monocular, bilateral	Protrusion of eyeball, lids may not close over eyes; white sclera seen above iris when eyelids open	Possible thyroid disease, tumor behind eye, possible frontal sinus enlargement. Unable to close lids causing dryness of cornea
Pupils		
Irregular, square		Intraocular lens that clips onto iris, normal
Asymmetrical in reaction to light and accommodation		Involvement of cranial nerves or extraocular muscles
Constricted	Smaller than 3 mm, miosis	Miotic medication for glaucoma, normal for elderly. Damage to sympathetic nerve supply; narcotic use
Asymmetrical corneal light reflex		Weakness of intraocular muscles, strabismus; involvement of extraocular muscles, cranial nerves III, IV, VI
Cloudiness/gray color		Formation of cataract
Iris		
Change in color		Iritis, uveitis
Extraocular muscles		
Strabismus	Extraocular movements deviate in one or more positions	Neuromuscular involvement; involvement of cranial nerves III, IV, VI
Visual field defect		
Peripheral	Partial or complete loss of peripheral vision	Glaucoma, complete or partial interruption along the vision pathway
Central	Loss of central vision	Macular disease, possible nuclear cataract
Lens		
Cataract	Opacification of the lens leading to progressive loss of vision	Diabetes, aging, congenital, trauma

Middle Ear

Mucous membrane lines the middle ear and is continuous from the nasal pharynx via the *auditory*, or *eustachian*, *tube*. The middle ear cavity contains the *malleus*, *incus*, and *stapes bones* (collectively called the *ossicular chain*). The malleus articulates with the incus, which articulates with the head of the stapes. These articulations are freely movable synovial joints. The footplate of the stapes vibrates and causes the fluid in the inner ear to be disturbed or to be set in motion. The round window covered with mucous membrane also opens into the inner ear and allows for dissipation of the fluid disturbances. The superior part of the middle ear is called the *epitympanum* or the attic and also communicates with air cells within the mastoid bone. The air cells are lined with the same mucous membrane as the middle ear.

Table 14-3
Diagnostic Studies of the Visual System

Study	Description and Purpose	Nursing Responsibility
Perimetry	Semicircular instrument marked in degrees. Accurate map of peripheral vision, visual fields. Noninvasive. Painless.	Explain procedure to client.
Refraction	A. Refractor containing a large number of lenses mounted on rotating wheels is used with the client in a sitting position. Client identifies lens that increases visual acuity. Cycloplegic drugs are usually used to block accommodation. Determines refractive error and aids in prescription of eye glasses, contact lenses.	Explain procedure to client. Administer ordered cycloplegic in correct eye or eyes. Assess dilation of pupil. Protect from light while dilated; inform client to wear sunglasses. Explain temporary difficulty in reading due to dilation.
	B. Retinoscope—held by the physician at a distance of 2 feet—directs focused light into the eye. A specific refractive error will distort the focused light, aiding the identification of refractive error. Can be easily used on infants.	Explain procedure to client. If cycloplegics used, same nurse actions as above.
Ophthalmoscopy fundoscopy	An ophthalmoscope magnifies and lights the fundus (inner layer) of the eye, thus allowing visualization of optic disk, four main pairs of vessels, and macular area.	Explain procedure to client. Darken room.
1. Direct	Used for diagnosis of abnormalities of the above parts. Requires dilated pupil to examine peripheral retina.	Administer ordered cycloplegic.
2. Indirect	An indirect ophthalmoscope is worn on the head of the physician and a hand-held magnifying lens is used to observe the retina for holes or detachment. The stereoscopic view is larger and has more illumination. Peripheral retina can be better observed.	Place client in a seated or supine position.
Biomicroscopy (Slit lamp exam—see Fig. 14-8)	A binocular microscope is capable of ×50 magnification. Assessment of anterior eye for abnormalities of the cornea, iris, lens, and depth of anterior chamber angle.	Position client in chair, chin on chin rest.
Tonometry		
1. Schiotz	Indentation or flattening of cornea by slight pressure to measure intraocular pressure.	Position in chair, head back, or in the supine position with the head facing upward. Cornea is anesthesized with one drop of 0.5% proparacaine. *Caution not to rub* eyes for 15 minutes after drops are instilled.
2. Applanation with biomicroscope	Measures the force required to flatten lens. No anesthetic medication needed.	Seated as for biomicroscopy.

Table 14-3 (Continued)

Study	Description and Purpose	Nursing Responsibility
Gonioscopy 1. Direct 2. Indirect	Special lens and instruments used to observe anterior chamber of eye, especially in glaucoma, and inflammation of anterior eye.	Explain procedure to client.
Ultrasonography	Used to determine the tissue masses when unable to view the fundus due to hemorrhage; to determine tumor within eye or orbit. Done prior to vitrectomy for diabetic retinopathy to determine status of retina.	Explain procedure to client.
Fluorescein angiography	Fluorescein 5 mL given IV in hand or arm. Serial pictures are made at time of injection, 5 minutes, and 20 minutes. Allows microscopic visualization and slides of the flow of blood through the vessels of the pigment epithelium and the retina for diagnosis of abnormalities of vessels and retina.	Administer cycloplegics for dilation of pupil. Seat client in front of camera with chin on chin rest. The flashing bright blue light used for the camera may cause client discomfort, blinking, and difficulty seeing 1–2 minutes after test. Use caution if client epileptic. Explain that client may notice yellow coloration of face for 6–24 hours, urine will be greenish-yellow for 24–36 hours. Observe for extravasculation at IV site, and manifestations of allergy to dye.

The middle ear cavity is air-filled and equalization of atmospheric air pressure is accomplished by the auditory tube. This tube is opened when yawning or swallowing. Blockage of the tube can occur with allergies, nasopharyngeal infections, and enlarged adenoids. Of clinical significance is the fact that cranial nerve VII (facial) traverses above the oval window of the middle ear. The thin bony covering of the cranial (facial) nerve VII can become eroded or traumatized by chronic ear infection and/or trauma due to ear surgery.

In summary, the external and middle portions of the ear function to conduct and magnify sound waves picked up from the environment. This is called *air conduction*. Problems in these two parts of the ear may cause *conductive hearing* loss, causing the client not to hear loud sounds as well as normal.

Inner Ear

The inner ear, composed of the bony labyrinth and the membranous labyrinth, houses the end organ receptors for hearing and balance. The receptor organ for hearing is the *cochlea*, a coiled structure. It contains the *organ of Corti*, whose tiny hair cells are bathed in endolymph which transmits the sound waves from the oval window. The mechanical stimulus is converted into an electric chemical impulse and then transmitted via cranial nerve VIII to the brain.

The *vestibular apparatus*, the organ of balance, is composed of the three semicircular canals and the utricle. The vestibular apparatus is bathed by the same endolymph fluid. Surrounding the endolymph is the perilymph fluid which cushions these two sensitive organs and communicates with the brain and subarachnoid spaces of the brain. The nervous stimuli are communicated via the vestibular portion of cranial nerve VIII.

Pathology of the inner ear or along the nerve pathway from the inner ear to the brain can result in *sensorineural hearing loss*. This causes the client to hear high-pitched tones as muffled and distorted, but not necessarily decreased in loudness. Problems within the brain auditory system from the auditory nuclei to the cortex cause *central* hearing loss. Types of hearing loss will be discussed in Chap. 15.

Transmission of Sound

Sound waves are conducted by air and picked up by the auricles and auditory canal. The taut tympanic membrane is struck by the sound waves, causing it to vibrate. The ossicular chain is set in motion and conducts the waves by vibration to the footplate of the stapes in the oval window. The much smaller size of the oval window compared to the tympanic membrane results in a much greater force being exerted by the sound waves on the oval window. The energy to set the perilymph in motion is provided by the force advantage due to this difference in size.[8]

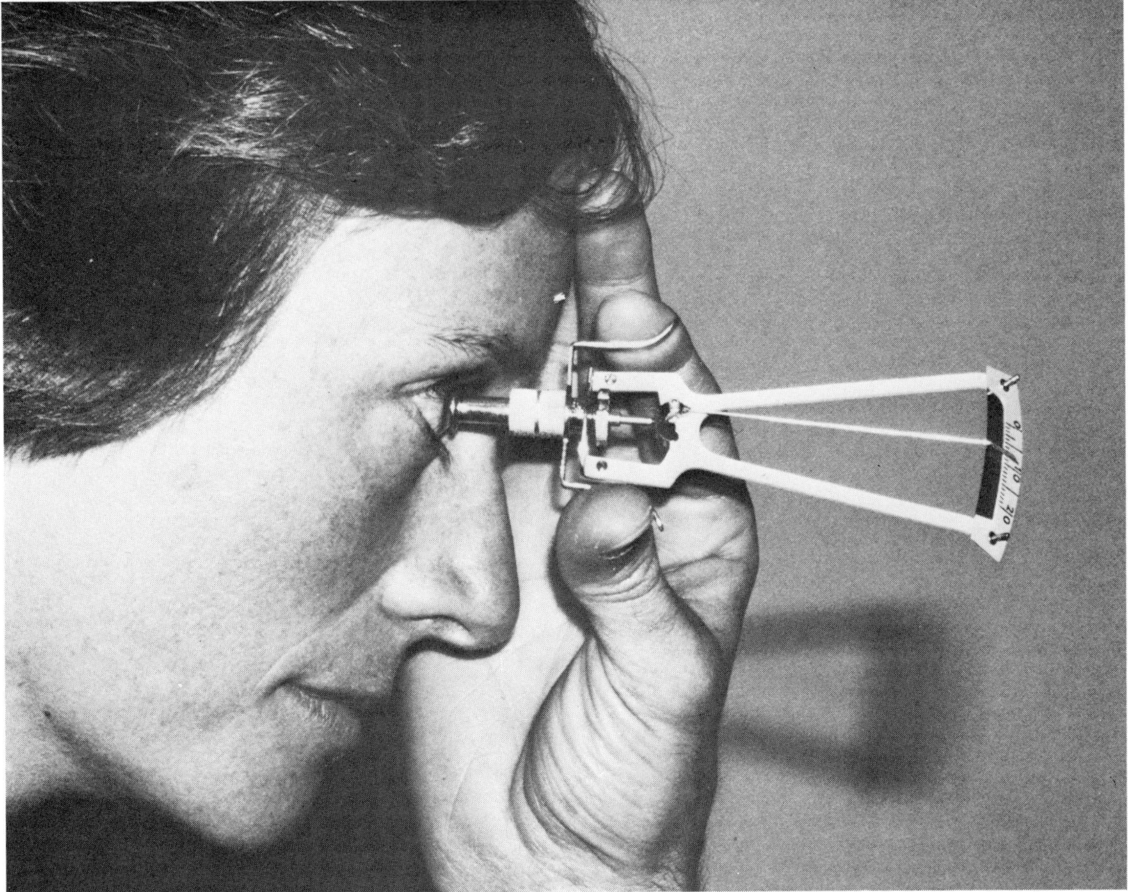

Figure 14-7 Schiotz tonometer. The sterile footplate is resting on the anesthetized cornea. One hand of the examiner is stabilizing the manometer. Although not shown the lids can be held apart with the other hand.

Once sound has been transmitted to the liquid medium of the inner ear the disturbance is picked up by the tiny sensory hair cells of the cochlea which initiate nerve impulses. These impulses are carried by nerve fibers to the main branch of the acoustic portion of cranial nerve VIII (acoustic). From here, it goes to the brain. Problems occurring in the auditory nuclei and cortex cause difficulty understanding the meaning of the words heard. This is referred to as *central* loss.

ASSESSMENT OF THE AUDITORY SYSTEM

Subjective Data: The Health History

Many problems related to the ear are sequelae of childhood illnesses or result from problems of adjacent organs. Consequently, a careful assessment of past medical problems is important.

Past medical history

Pediatric and Adult Illnesses The client needs to be questioned regarding previous problems regarding the left and right ears, especially those problems experienced during childhood. The frequency of acute middle ear infections (otitis media), perforations of the eardrum, drainage, complications, and history of mumps and measles need to be recorded. Residual or chronic otitis media, perforation of the eardrum, pain, and amounts and frequency of drainage are data that are also obtained. Problems such as dizziness and hearing loss are recorded in the client's words. It is important to ask the client to describe a complaint of dizziness in detail.

Immunizations Congenital hearing losses can result from rubella or influenza in the first trimester of pregnancy. Therefore, young women of childbearing age and those who are pregnant are questioned

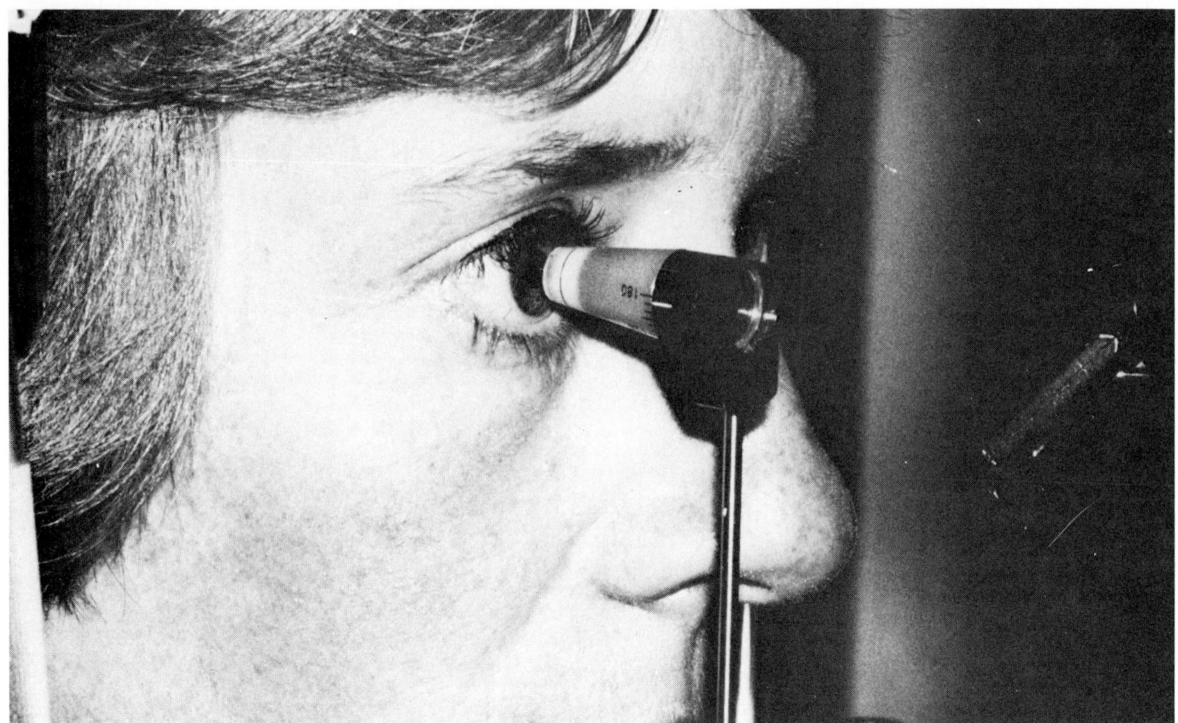

Figure 14-8 Applanation tonometry with biomicroscopy.

regarding whether they were vaccinated against rubella or ever had rubella.

Hospitalizations, Trauma, and Medication Information regarding previous hospitalizations for ear surgery as well as tonsillectomy and adenoidectomy (T & A) is obtained. Information regarding current or past medications that are ototoxic (cause damage to cranial nerve VIII) and can produce hearing loss and/or tinnitus (ringing) and dizziness is obtained (Table 14-4). The amount and frequency of aspirin used is important as tinnitus can result from high aspirin intake. Tinnitus is reversible if aspirin is discontinued. Information regarding allergies is important as the eustachian tube can become edematous and prevent aeration of the middle ear. This occurs more frequently in children.

Since prematurity can cause hearing problems, information about the client's birth is important. Head injury is a frequent cause of decreased or lost hearing and should be investigated.

Family history

Information regarding family members with hearing loss and type of hearing loss is important, especially in congenital and sensorineural hearing loss with the aging client (presbycusis).

Social and personal history

The client should be questioned regarding employment or contact with environments with excessive noise levels such as work with jet engines and machinery, contact with the firing of firearms, and electromagnified music. Use of preventive devices worn in noisy environments is also recorded. Information regarding swimming habits, especially in contaminated waters, is also obtained.

Review of systems

Symptoms related to the auditory system are similar to many of the symptoms of the upper respiratory and neurologic systems. Information to be obtained regarding each ear and its function includes the following:

Hearing loss—Sudden, gradual over hours or months; type, can hear certain words, sounds, muffled sounds; effect of environmental noise on hearing

Pain—Discomfort, fullness, increased on movement of auricle, sharp (referred from throat—determine if there are problems in throat)

Drainage from external ear—Serosanguineous, bloody, purulent, clear, odor (putrid)

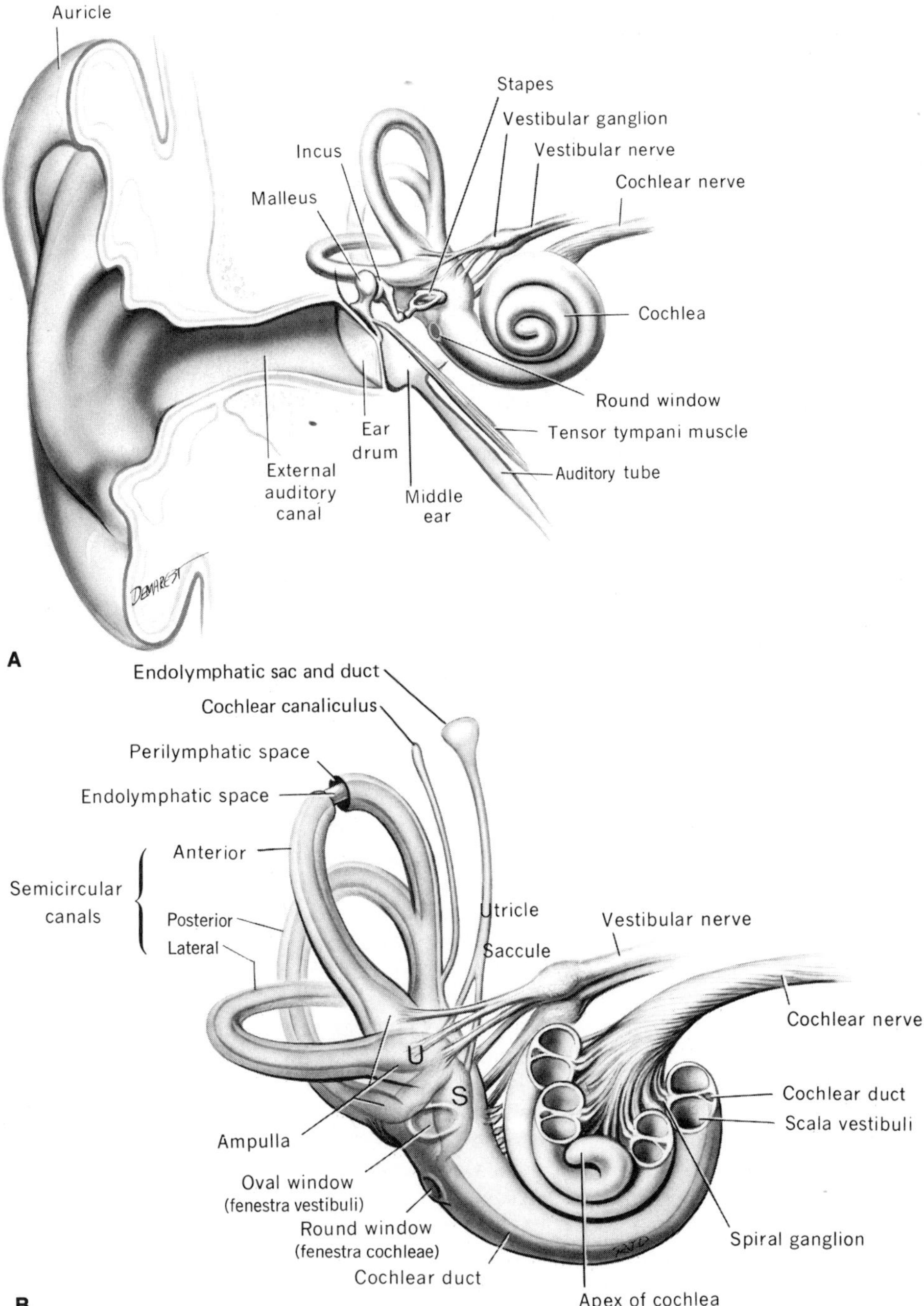

Figure 14-9 (*a*) External ear, middle ear, and inner ear, (*b*) The labyrinth. (*From C. R. Noback and R. Demarest, The Human Nervous System: Basic Principles of Neurobiology, 2d ed., McGraw-Hill Book Company, New York, 1975. Used with permission of McGraw-Hill Book Company.*)

Tinnitus (ringing in ear)—Type and pitch (low, high); roaring, humming, hissing, time of day
Dizziness—Vertigo, lightheadedness, environment whirling with eyes open, client whirling with eyes closed, relationship to activity
Nausea/vomiting—Along with dizziness, vertigo

Table 14-4

Ototoxic Drugs

Toxic to cochlea and/or labyrinth:

Severely ototoxic
- Aminoglycosides
  - Amikacin
  - Dihydrostreptomycin
  - Gentamicin
  - Kanamycin
  - Neomycin
  - Tobramycin
  - Vancomycin
- Chemotherapeutics
  - Cis-Platinum (platinol)
  - Mechlorethiamine (Mustargen, nitrogen mustard)

Moderately ototoxic
- Chloroquine (Aralen)
- Ethacrynic acid (Edecrin)
- Furosemide (Lasix)
- Quinidine gluconate
- Quinine sulfate, Polygalacturonate (Quinaglute, Cardioguin Cen-Quin, Quinidex, Quinora)
- Salicylates
- Chloramphenicol (topical) (Amphicol, Chloromycetin, Mychel)
- Oral contraceptives
- Streptomycin sulfate (causes vestibular toxicity first)

Cause/dizziness
- Antihypertensives
- Barbiturates
- Central nervous system depressants
- Estrogens
- Phenothiazines
- Phenylbutazone

Adapted from W. H. Saunders, and R. W. Gardier, *Pharmacotherapy in Otolaryngology,* The C. V. Mosby Company, St. Louis, 1976, p. 38.

Objective Data: The Physical Examination

The nurse can collect valuable objective data regarding the client's ability to hear during the health history interview. Clues such as posturing of the head and appropriateness of responses should be noted. Does the client ask to have certain words repeated? Does he intently watch the examiner but miss comments when not looking at the examiner? Such observations are significant and should be recorded. This is also important because the client often is not aware of hearing losses or does not admit to decreases until moderate losses have occurred. A normal assessment of the ear is recorded as shown in Table 14-5.

The external ear

The external ear is observed and palpated prior to inspection of the external canal and tympanum.

Table 14-5

Recording Normal Physical Assessment of the Auditory System

Ears symmetrical in location and shape
Auricles without lesions or discharge
Canal clear; T. M. intact. Landmarks and light reflex intact.
Able to hear low whisper at 30 cm; Rinne—AC > BC;
Weber—lateralization equal

The auricle, preauricular area, and mastoid area are inspected for equality of conformation of both ears, the color of skin, nodules, swelling, redness, and lesions. The auricle and mastoid areas are then palpated for tenderness and nodules. Grasping the auricle may elicit pain, especially if inflammation of the external ear and/or canal is present.

The external auditory canal and tympanum

After inspecting the canal opening for patency, an otoscopic exam is done. A speculum slightly smaller than the size of the canal is selected. The client's head is tipped to the opposite shoulder. To straighten the canal in the adult client, the top of the auricle is grasped and gently pulled up and back. The otoscope, held in the examiner's right hand and stabilized on the client's head by his fingers, is inserted slowly (Fig. 14-10). Observe for the color and amount of cerumen. If a large amount of cerumen is present the tympanum may not be visible. The tympanum is observed for color, landmarks, and intactness (Fig. 14-11).

The tympanic membrane separates the external ear from the middle ear. It is pearl-gray, shiny, and translucent. The anterioinferior quadrant is situated obliquely in the ear canal and is furthest from the examiner. The major landmarks are formed by the *short process of the malleus* superiorly, the handle or *manubrium*, and the *umbo*. From the innermost part of the tympanum a light reflex or *cone of light* is formed with the point directed toward the umbo. The circumference of the tympanum is surrounded by a dense, whitish, fibrous ring or *annulus* with the exception of the superior area. The tympanum within the annulus is taut and referred to as the *pars tensa*. Superior to the short process of the malleus is the pars flaccida or flaccid part of the tympanum. The malleolar folds are both anterior and posterior to the short process of the malleus. Changes of the tympanum to observe include color, landmarks, and effect of light. Table 14-6 summarizes common assessment abnormalities of the auditory system. The inner ear cannot be examined directly with the otoscope because of the tympanic membrane.

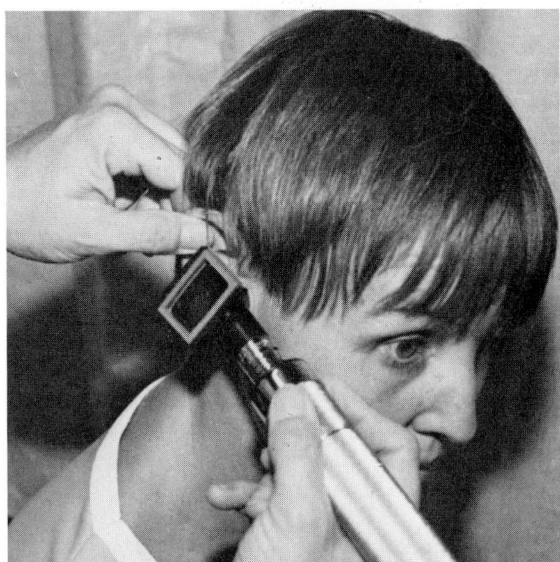

Figure 14-10 Proper technique for otoscopic examination of the adult ear. Note position of left hand to pull auricle up and back. The right hand stabilizes otoscope with fingers on client's face.

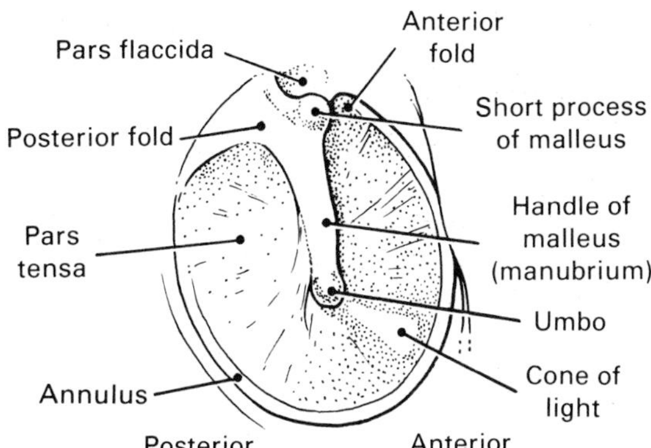

Figure 14-11 Normal landmarks of the right tympanic membrane.

Tests for hearing acuity

Whispered and Spoken Voice Tests These tests can provide gross screening information about the client's ability to hear. Audiometry provides more specific information which can be used for diagnosis and treatment.

Whispered test

The examiner stands 30 to 60 cm to the side of the client and, after exhaling, speaks using a low whisper. A louder whisper is used if the client does not respond correctly. Spoken voice, increasing in loudness, is similarly used. The client is asked to repeat numbers, words, or answer questions. Each ear is tested. Masking of the ear not being tested is done with the client occluding the ear, or examiner or client moving his finger rapidly close to the ear canal.

Ticking watch

A watch is placed 2 to 5 cm from the ear being tested and the opposite ear is masked. The client with normal hearing should be able to hear the ticking. However, the variations among watches makes this test a very gross one for assessing hearing acuity. Clients with sensorineural loss cannot hear the high-pitched tones of a ticking watch.

Tuning Fork Tests Tuning fork tests aid in differentiating between conductive and sensorineural hearing loss. Tuning forks of 500 and 1000 cycles per second are used. Both skill and experience are necessary to assure accurate results. If a problem is suspected, further evaluation by pure tone audiometry is essential. The most common tuning fork tests are the Rinne and the Weber.

The Rinne test

The test is conducted by holding the base of an activated tuning fork on the mastoid bone until the client signals he can no longer hear it. It is then moved to 2.5 cm from the ear canal. The client reports if the sound can be heard and for how long. The examiner times each. The Rinne is positive when the client reports air conduction (AC) is heard longer than bone conduction (BC). This can indicate normal hearing or a sensorineural loss. If the client hears the tuning fork better by bone conduction, the Rinne test is negative and indicates that a conductive hearing loss is present.

The Weber test

The test is conducted by placing an activated tuning fork on the midline of the skull, the forehead, or the teeth. The client is asked to identify where the sound is heard best. Normal response is equal loudness bilaterally. If a client has a conductive hearing loss of one ear, sound is heard louder (lateralizes) in that ear. If a sensorineural loss is present, sound will be louder in the good ear. It must be noted that hearing losses may be mixed and further diagnostic testing is required.[9]

Vestibular system

Nystagmus, an abnormal rhythmic jerking motion of the eyes within the field of binocular vision, can be caused by disturbances in the endolymph fluid. The movement of the endolymph fluid stimulates receptor

Table 14-6
Common Assessment Abnormalities of the Auditory System

Findings	Definition/Description	Etiology/Significance
	External Ear and Canal	
Sebaceous cyst behind ear	Usually within the skin, may have black dot which is opening to sebaceous gland	Requires removal and/or incision and drainage if painful
Tophi	Hard nodules in the helix or antihelix consisting of uric acid crystals	Associated with gout, metabolic disorder; further diagnosis needed
Impacted cerumen (wax)	Wax that has not normally been excreted from the ear. Eardrum cannot be visualized.	May cause decreased hearing; sensation of fullness in auditory canal; requires removal before otoscopic exam
Discharge in canal	Infection of external ear, usually painful	Swimmer's ear, infection of external ear; may be due to ruptured eardrum and otitis media
Swelling of pinna, pain	Infection of glands of skin; hematoma due to trauma	Requires aspiration
Changes in skin; scaling, lesions	Change in usual appearance of skin due to scaling or lesions.	Seborrheic dermatitis; squamous cell carcinoma
Exostosis	Bony growth extending into canal causing narrowing of canal	May interfere with visualization of tympanum; usually asymptomatic
	Tympanum	
Retracted eardrum	Malleus appears shorter, more horizontal; cone of light bent, absent	Air absorbed from middle ear and eustachian tube blocked; negative pressure in middle ear
Hairline fluid level Bubbles above fluid level, yellow amber color	Due to transudate of blood and serum; meniscus of fluid produces the hairline appearance	Serous otitis media
Bulging red or blue eardrum, lack of landmarks	Middle ear filled with fluid; pus, blood	Acute otitis media, may perforate
Early stage hyperemic vessels	Complaint of pain, severe	Usually in children
Perforation of the eardrum (central or marginal)	In adult, usually previous perforations of the eardrum that have failed to heal. May be covered by a thin, transparent layer of epithelium	Chronic otitis media; needs referral
Recruitment	Malfunction of inner ear which causes sound to be heard disproportionately loud	May make hearing aid difficult to use

cells and causes nystagmus. Lesions in the central nervous system and drug toxicity can also cause nystagmus. To test for nystagmus, have the client look straight ahead and then follow the examiner's finger to an extreme lateral gaze. Quick jerking movement along the way, except on extreme lateral gaze, is considered abnormal. Nystagmus can also be caused by a central nervous system lesion. Caloric testing and electronystagmography also test the function of the vestibular system.

DIAGNOSTIC STUDIES OF THE AUDITORY SYSTEM

Audiometry

Audiometry is useful both as a screening test for hearing acuity as well as a diagnostic test for determining the degree and type of hearing loss. The audiometer produces pure tone of simple sound waves. Sound is described according to how many vibrations take place each second. Cycles per second (cps) or more recently Hz (Hertz) will follow the number representing the vibrations such as 2000 cps or Hz.

The *frequency* of sound is determined by how fast a sound source vibrates. The higher the frequency, the higher the pitch. Hearing loss can affect specific sound frequencies and influences the success of a hearing aid. The intensity or strength of a sound wave is expressed in terms of decibels (dB) ranging from 0 dB to 140 dB, with 0 being the softest. Zero decibels represents the intensity of a sound required to make any frequency barely audible to the average normal ear. *Threshold level* refers to the lowest level of intensity at which pure tones are heard correctly by a particular client in one ear at least 50 percent of the time.

Normal speech presented comfortably loud is approximately 40 to 65 dB; a soft whisper is 20 dB. Normally, a child and young adult can hear frequencies of 20 to 20,000 Hz, but hearing is most sensitive from 500 to 4000 Hz. This is similar to the frequencies used in speech. A 40 to 45 dB loss in all frequencies would cause the client moderate difficulty in hearing normal speech. A hearing aid would be helpful, since it magnifies sound. A client with a 15 to 20 dB loss in only the higher frequencies such as 4000 Hz would have difficulty hearing the high-pitched consonants. Words such as cheese, thin, and fin would not be perceived accurately. They would sound muffled or distorted. A hearing aid will not be as helpful, as it would only cause the sound to be louder but not clearer. Table 14-7 presents frequently heard sounds and their decibel intensity.

Table 14-7
Frequently Heard Sounds and Their Decibel Intensities

Sound	Decibels
Air raid siren (painful to ear)	140
Jet engine	130
Rock band	
Loud shout (1 ft away)	120
Thunder	
Motorcycle	110
Aircraft engine (propeller)	
Power mower (discomfort for pure tones)	100
Electric food blender	90
Train	
Pneumatic jackhammer	80
Heavy traffic (outside)	70
Average conversation	60
Vacuum cleaner	50
Automobile	40
A quiet room	30
Soft whisper	20
Breathing	10
Hearing threshold	0

From D. A. Jones et al., *Medical-Surgical Nursing,* 2d ed., McGraw-Hill Book Company, 1982, p. 1423. Used with permission of McGraw-Hill Book Company.

Screening Audiometry

Screening audiometry is the testing of large numbers of people using a fast, simple test to detect possible hearing problems. A pass/fail criterion is used to screen out people who will or will not be given additional diagnostic testing. Although many tests are used, the most common is the pure-tone "sweep" frequency test. In this test, a 20 dB tone is presented, usually at 500, 1000, 2000; and a 25 dB tone at 4000 Hz.

The sweep test is simple to administer. The subject is instructed to raise a hand when a sound is heard. The audiometer is set at the appropriate hearing level, and the tester sweeps through the test tones. Each ear is tested separately.

The person passes the sweep test if sound is heard at all the test frequencies in both ears. If the test is failed, further evaluation is indicated. Many older adults will have difficulty passing the sweep test due to hearing losses associated with aging. They should be referred for threshold audiometry to determine if the hearing loss is sensorineural or conductive.

Pure-Tone Threshold Test

Nurses often have the opportunity to perform pure-tone threshold audiometry. The test setting does not always provide the quiet atmosphere required for accurate testing. The results of the test are recorded on an audiogram (Fig. 14-2) with the right ear represented by a red circle and the left ear represented by a blue X. The following suggestions will produce more reliable audiograms:[10]

1. Select a quiet setting.
2. Develop rapport with the client.
3. Seat the client so he cannot see you or the audiometer.
4. Avoid repetitive patterns of tone selection.
5. Get as much information as quickly as possible.

Directions for performing the pure-tone audiometric threshold test (air conduction) are presented in Table 14-8. Specific criteria for referring children with hearing losses detected by audiometry are available.

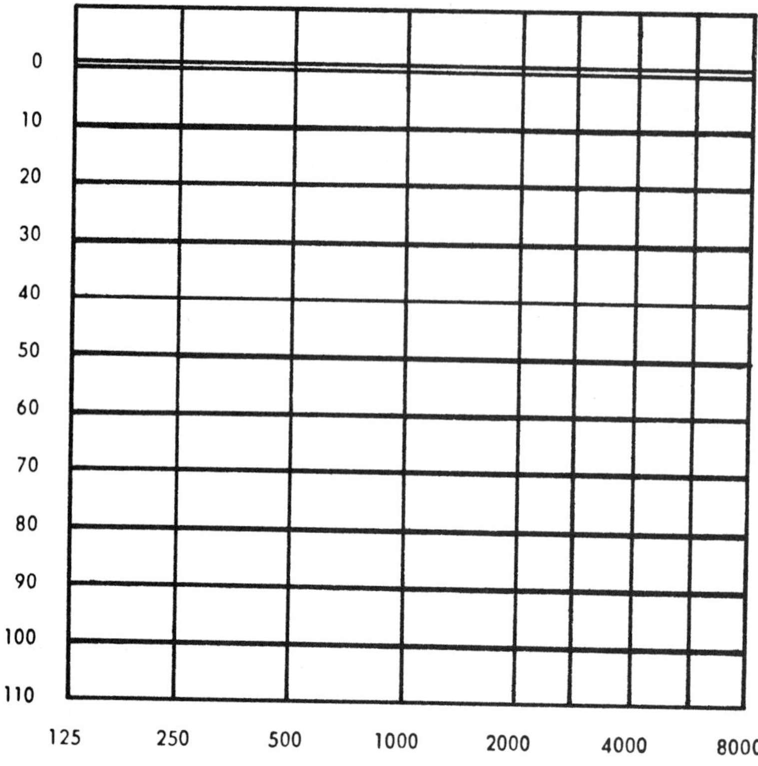

Figure 14-12 The client's hearing level is plotted on the audiogram. Each ear is tested separately. (*Courtesy Estelle Rosenblum.*)

Table 14-8
Pure-Tone Audiometric Threshold Testing: Air Conduction

1. Set the frequency control at 1000 Hz and the hearing level control at 40 dB.
2. Seat the person to be tested in such a position that he cannot see the controls.
3. Give instructions before putting on the earphones. Be sure to emphasize that some of the sounds may be very soft and far away but that he should respond even to these faint tones.
4. Be sure that hats, glasses, etc., are removed.
5. Place the earphones properly on the person's head with the right earphone on the right ear.
6. Begin by testing the better ear first, if the person reports that there is a difference between ears. If not, the right ear should be tested first as a matter of routine.
7. The first tone presentation will be at 1000 Hz at an intensity of 40 dB. (Tone presentations should be no longer than two to three seconds.)
8. If there is a response, descend in intensity in 10 dB steps until the patient no longer responds.
9. Starting at the first level at which there was no response, ascend in intensity in 5 dB steps until there is a response.
10. Descend by 10 dB and present a tone at that level and at levels in ascending 5 dB steps until another response is obtained.
11. Continue this procedure—descending in 10 dB steps and ascending in 5 dB steps—until you have obtained two responses at one level. This is the hearing threshold for that frequency. (For audiometric purposes, *threshold* is defined as the lowest level to which a person responds correctly to the presence of a tone at least 50 percent of the time.)
12. Continue in the same manner and establish thresholds at all frequencies to be tested, recording the result in the appropriate place on the audiogram.
13. If there is no response at the 40 dB hearing level, ascend in 10 dB steps until you obtain a response, then continue in the manner described earlier to establish the hearing threshold.
14. The order in which the frequencies are tested is usually as follows: 1000 Hz, 2000 Hz, 4000 Hz, 8000 Hz, 1000 Hz, 500 Hz.
15. When there is no response at a test frequency, this should be indicated on the audiogram (Fig. 14-12). This is commonly done by writing the symbol on the audiogram at the maximum level which can be tested at that frequency, with an arrow attached to the symbol and pointing downward.

From Estelle Rosenblum, *Fundamentals of Hearing for Health Professionals,* Little, Brown and Co., Boston, 1979, pp. 111–112.

Reasonable guidelines for referral of adults are failure to hear two frequencies in one ear at 25 dB or failure to hear the 500 frequency in one ear at 25 dB.[11] In addition, the client who complains of hearing loss but has a normal audiogram should be referred for further evaluation.

Specialized Tests

The audiologist can perform many additional tests as a result of newer audiometers and computers that record pressures of electric impulses from the middle ear, inner ear, and brain. Some of these tests are described in Table 14-9. The most common test performed by the audiologist is pure-tone audiometry done under ideal testing conditions. A soundproof room is used for greater accuracy of results. The audiologist can also test bone conduction by audiometry to diagnose conductive hearing loss. The more specialized tests of the auditory system are most often performed in an outpatient setting by an audiologist. There is seldom any nursing responsibility involved.

Test for Vestibular Function

The *caloric test* is done to determine the function of the vestibular system. The external ear is irrigated with cold or warm water, which causes disturbances in the endolymph. The client's reaction is observed for type of eye movements (opposite to ear stimulated),

Table 14-9
Diagnostic Studies of the Auditory System

Study	Description and Purpose	Nursing Responsibility
Auditory		
Audiometry Pure tone	An audiometer is an electroacoustic instrument that produces pure tone frequencies of 125 to 8000 cps or Hz, at intensities of low to excessively loud dB (decibels). Sounds are presented through earphones in a soundproof room. Client responds nonverbally when sound is heard. Response is recorded on an audiogram. Purpose is to determine hearing range of client in terms of dB and Hz for diagnosing conductive and sensorineural hearing loss.	Nurse does not usually participate in this examination.
Bone conduction	Vibrator placed on mastoid process and hearing by bone conduction is recorded. Necessary to diagnose conductive hearing loss.	
Spoken voice, word lists, one-and-two-syllable words, high-frequency words	Presented by microphone, recorded or spoken voice used at comfortable level of hearing, lower and higher dB used.	
Pure tone decay; threshold pure tone	Normally a client can hear a pure tone for 1 min. Those with pressure on cranial nerve VIII cannot hear 1 tone for 1 min. Levels of intensity increased which client cannot hear.	
High-frequency pure tones of 12,000 to 15,000 cps, Hz	Similar pure tone but higher frequencies used. If used prior to ototoxic drug administration, decrease at this level during drug administration indicative of cochlear damage and need to discontinue use of drug.	Same as for pure tone audiometry.
Bebesky audiometry	Self-recording audiogram—the client listens to tones and increases or decreases intensity. Responses are recorded automatically on paper. Differentiates between cochlear and cranial nerve VIII disease, conductive and sensorineural hearing losses.	Explain use of instrument to client.
Evoked response audiometry or audiometric brainstem response (ERA or ABR)	Similar to electroencephalogram (EEG). Electrodes are attached to client in a darkened room. A computer is used to isolate the auditory from other electrical activity of the brain. Useful for uncooperative client or those clients who cannot volunteer useful information.	Explain procedure to client. Do not leave client alone in darkened room.
1. Cortical (stimulus, pure tone, or broadband)	Focuses on electrical activity at cerebral cortex level.	
2. Brainstem (stimulus, pure tone, or broadband stimulus)	Measures electrical peaks along auditory pathway of the inner ear to brain. Possible diagnosis of acoustical neuromas, brainstem problems, or a vascular accident.	

Table 14-9 (Continued)

Vestibular	Description and Purpose	Nursing Responsibility
Caloric test stimulus; cold water (20°C; 68°F), warm water (36°C; 96.8°F)	The endolymph of the semicircular canals can be stimulated by cold (20°C) or warm (36°C) solution irrigated into ear. Client is seated or in supine position. Observation of type of nystagmus, nausea and vomiting, falling and vertigo produced is helpful in diagnosing disease of the labyrinth. Decreased function is indicated by decreased response and indicates disease of vestibular system. Other ear tested similarly and results compared.	Observe client for vomiting. Assist if necessary. Ensure client safety.
Electronystagmography	Electrodes are placed near client's eyes and movement of eyes (nystagmus) is recorded on a graph when ear is irrigated. Diagnoses disease of vestibular system.	

past pointing with eyes closed, and falling toward the ear stimulated. Drugs that may affect the test include alcohol, CNS depressants, and barbiturates, and should be known to the physician prior to testing.

REVIEW QUESTIONS

The number of the question corresponds to the same numbered objective at the beginning of the chapter.

1. The third, fourth, and sixth cranial nerves control
a. visual fields
b. extraocular movement
c. nystagmus
d. pupil size

2. The parts of the eye that refract light rays are the
a. anterior and posterior chambers
b. cornea and pupil
c. bulbar conjunctiva and lens
d. cornea and lens

3. A history of a high intake of aspirin could result in
a. tinnitus
b. vertigo
c. sensorineural hearing loss
d. conductive hearing loss

4. The abbreviation used to designate both eyes is
a. O.U.
b. O.D.
c. O.S.

5. Which of the following is a normal finding in assessing the ear?
a. absent cone of light
b. dry, brown cerumen
c. BC > AC
d. retracted tympanum

6. The purpose of tonometry is to determine
a. refractive error
b. corneal curvature
c. intracular pressure
d. sensitivity of the cornea

REFERENCES

1. D. Vaughan and T. Asbury, *General Ophthalmology*, 9th ed., Lange, Los Latos, 1980, p. 13.
2. M. Yanoff, "Diabetes Mellitus," chapter 5 in *Ocular Pathology Update*, D. H. Nicholson (ed.), Masson Publishing Press, New York, 1980, p. 94.
3. Lois Malasanos et al., *Health Assessment*, The C. V. Mosby Company, St. Louis, 1977, pp. 150–151.
4. W. H. Saunders et al., *Nursing Care in Eye, Ear, Nose and Throat Disorders*, 4th ed., The C. V. Mosby Company, St. Louis, 1978, p. 57.
5. L. Malasanos, *Health Assessment*, The C. V. Mosby Company, St. Louis, 1977, pp. 155–156.
6. W. H. Havener, *Synopsis of Ophthalmology*, 5th ed., The C. V. Mosby Company, St. Louis, 1979, pp. 406–408.
7. J. M. Thompson et al., *Clinical Manual of Health Assessment*, The C. V. Mosby Company, St. Louis, 1980, pp. 117
8. W. H. Saunders et al., *Nursing Care in Eye, Ear, Nose, and Throat Disorders*, 4th ed., The C. V. Mosby Company, St. Louis, 1978, p. 381.
9. J. Sataloff et al., *Hearing Loss*, 2d ed., J. B. Lippincott Company, Philadelphia, 1980, p. 27.
10. E. Rosenblum, *Fundamentals of Hearing for Health Professions*, Little, Brown and Company, Boston, 1979, p. 109.
11. Ibid., p. 105.

Chapter 15

NURSING ROLE IN MANAGEMENT

Problems of Vision and Hearing

Carol Fair Keith

Learning Objectives

1. Describe the types of refractive errors and appropriate corrections.
2. Describe the etiology and management of external ocular disorders.
3. Explain the pathophysiology, clinical manifestations, and medical and nursing management for the client with selected intraocular disorders.
4. Describe nursing measures to promote health maintenance and promotion of the eyes and ears.
5. Explain the general preoperative and postoperative care of the client undergoing surgery of the eye or ear.
6. Describe the action and uses of common pharmacologic agents used in treating problems of the eyes and ears.
7. Explain the pathophysiology, clinical manifestations, and medical and nursing management of common ear problems.
8. Compare conductive and sensorineural hearing loss as to cause, management, and rehabilitative potential.
9. Explain the use, care, and client education related to assistive devices for eye and ear problems.
10. Describe the common causes and assistive measures for blindness and deafness.

VISUAL PROBLEMS

Health Promotion and Maintenance

The nurse must be aware of the great potential for preventing problems of vision by appropriate nursing intervention. Early recognition of conditions that can cause blindness is a major nursing responsibility. Conditions or situations which should alert the nurse to potential visual problems follow.

1. Congenital blindness can be due to a rubella infection in the mother in the first trimester of pregnancy. This condition could be prevented by the use of rubella (German measles) vaccine to maintain normal rubella titers in women of childbearing age. Those who come in contact with this group of women, especially those who work in health care agencies, should also be immunized.
2. Monitoring the levels of oxygen delivered to premature and newborn infants and arterial blood gas levels to prevent development of retrolental fibroplasia is very important. Excessive oxygen given to newborn infants results in fibrovascular growths within the eye, causing blindness.
3. Community education is an important nursing responsibility. Teaching the need for eye examinations, especially for adults over 40, is essential. Glaucoma can cause blindness if not treated. Open-angle glaucoma is often first identified by measurement of intraocular pressure by tonometry. The nurse can also support and assist with community glaucoma screening programs. Clients with diabetes should have yearly ophthalmic examinations to assure early treatment of retinopathy.[1] It is also essential that children who have strabismus or suppression amblyopia be identified early.
4. Eye injuries can lead to blindness. It is estimated that 90 percent of eye injuries can be prevented.[2] Potential sources of eye injuries need to be identified and corrected. Many eye injuries are caused by flying metal pieces in home workshops and in the use of welding equipment.[3] Use of safety glasses would greatly reduce these injuries.
5. Incorrect wearing of contact lenses is also an important source of trauma to the eye.[4] Correct wearing and proper cleaning techniques would reduce many of the problems that can potentially cause impaired vision or blindness.
6. The correct use of safety equipment such as the wearing of seat belts and shoulder harnesses in cars and the use of goggles and helmets when riding motorcycles needs to be encouraged.
7. Correct handling of cleaning solutions containing alkali or acid that can cause chemical burns needs to be emphasized. Many home products contain lye, which, if splashed in the eye, can cause blindness. It is important to teach that the immediate and prolonged irrigation of the eye prior to seeking medical attention is critical emergency treatment.
8. As more information becomes known about the causes of congenital blindness and inherited eye problems, genetic counseling would be helpful in reducing visual problems.

This chapter was reviewed by Tana Hinson Durnbaugh, R.N., B.S.N., M.S., Assistant Professor, College of Lake County, Grayslake, Illinois.

Refractive Error

The most common visual problem is refractive error.[5] This is a defect of the refracting media of the eye, preventing light rays from converging into a single focus on the retina. Defects are due to irregularities of the corneal curvature, the focusing power of the lens, and the length of the eye. The major symptoms are blurred vision and discomfort. Corrective lenses are used to better focus the light rays upon the retina (Fig. 15-1). Approximately one-half, or 115 million, of the U.S. population requires some form of visual correction. One-third of the adult population, or 70 million persons, are nearsighted or *myopic,* requiring corrective lenses for distant vision.[6]

Types of refractive error

Myopia The myopic eye causes light rays to focus anterior to the retina when focused on a distant object. Light rays from near objects focus upon the retina. Myopia requires fairly frequent changes of glasses during childhood and especially during adolescence when the eyeball lengthens excessively. This excessive lengthening is generally attributed to genetic factors. A few authorities, however, support the theory that excessive use of the eyes for near vision early in life contributes to myopia.[7] Other causes of myopia are due to the excessive bending of light rays by the cornea and the lens. A minus lens (concave) is required for better focus.

Hyperopia Hyperopia or farsightedness causes the light rays to focus behind the retina and requires the use of accommodation to focus the light rays on the retina for near and far objects. The treatment of excessive hyperopia is a convex or plus lens which is used to facilitate focusing.

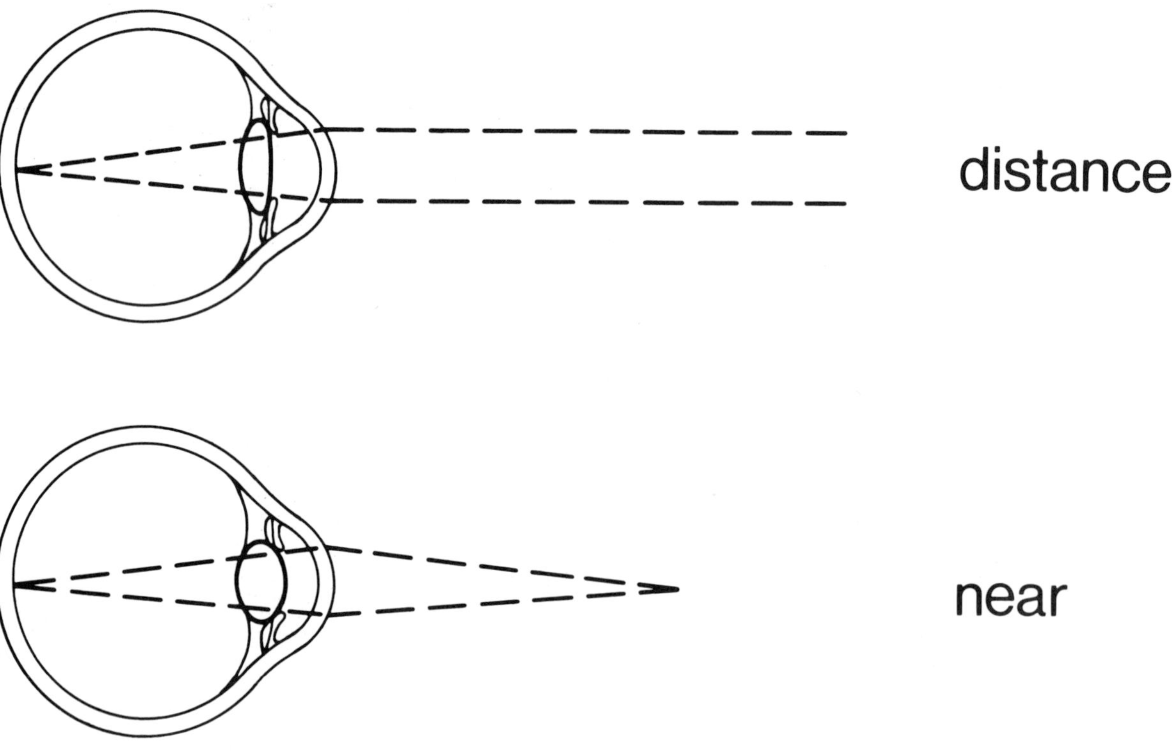

Figure 15-1 Comparison of emmetropic eye with corrected and uncorrected vision. (*From Ohio State University, College of Optometry, Instructional Media Center. Drawings by Wendy Clark.*)

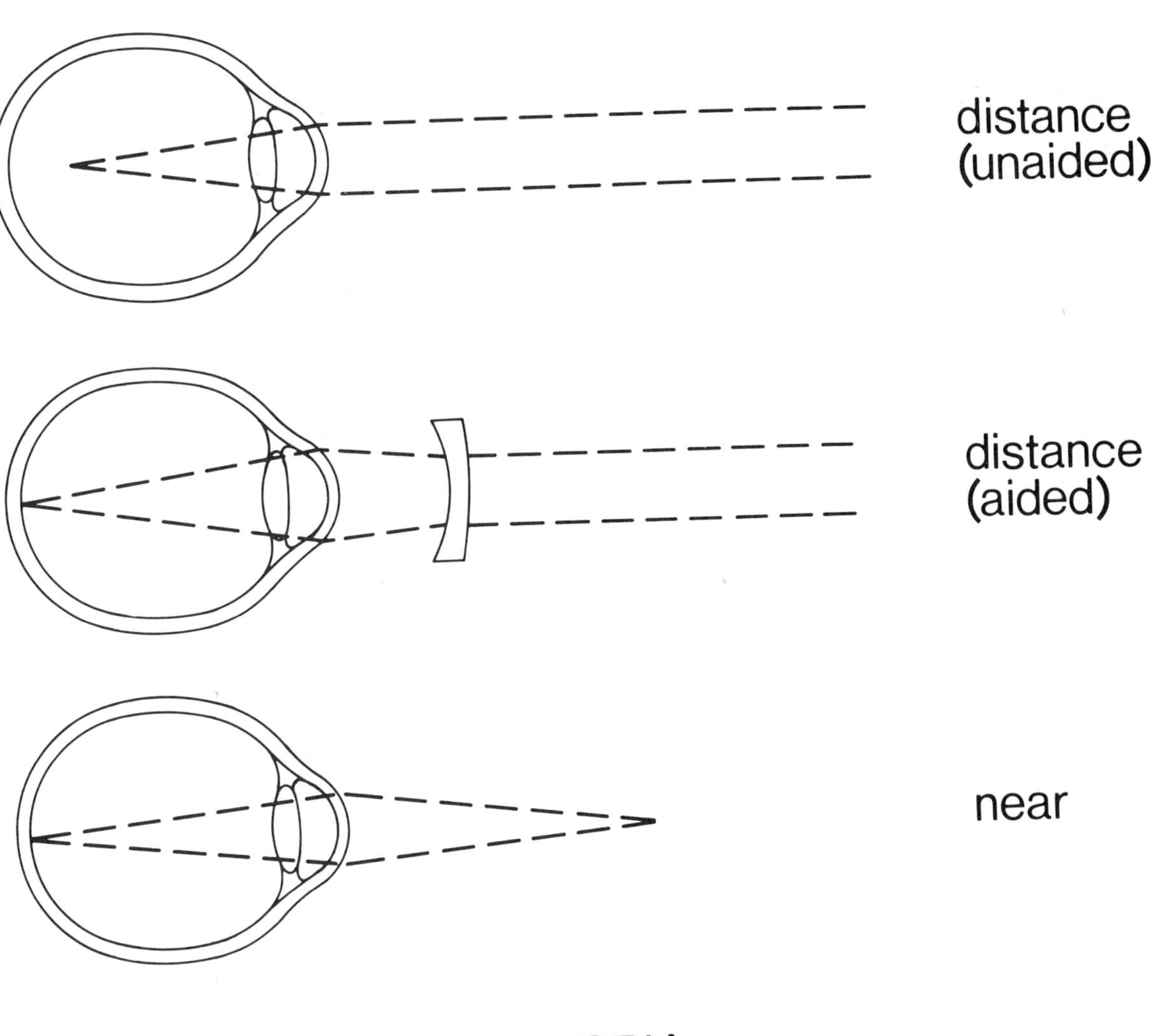

Figure 15-1 (continued)

Astigmatism Astigmatism is due to the unequal curvature of the cornea and causes the light rays to be bent unequally and not come to a single focus on the retina. Correction of the unequal curvature of the cornea is by use of a cylinder lens. Myopia or hyperopia can coexist with astigmatism.

Presbyopia Presbyopia is the loss of accommodation due to age. As the eye ages, the ocular lens becomes less elastic, larger, and firmer, and the accommodative ability decreases. After the age of 60 the lens has become so inelastic that accommodation is not possible.[8] Initially, the client experiences difficulty in reading newsprint unless held at arm's length. Visual correction is by reading glasses if no other refractive error is present. Bifocal glasses are prescribed for those with other refractive errors. Trifocals are prescribed when the client requires correction for middistance of 68 to 137 cm (27 to 50 inches).

Types of correction

Glasses or contact lenses are used to correct refractive errors (Table 15-1). The contact lens, riding on the tear film of the cornea, usually provides better vision without the distortion of glasses and their frames. The contact lens is held in place by surface tension. Blinking causes the tear film to move under and over the contact lens. The tear film is very

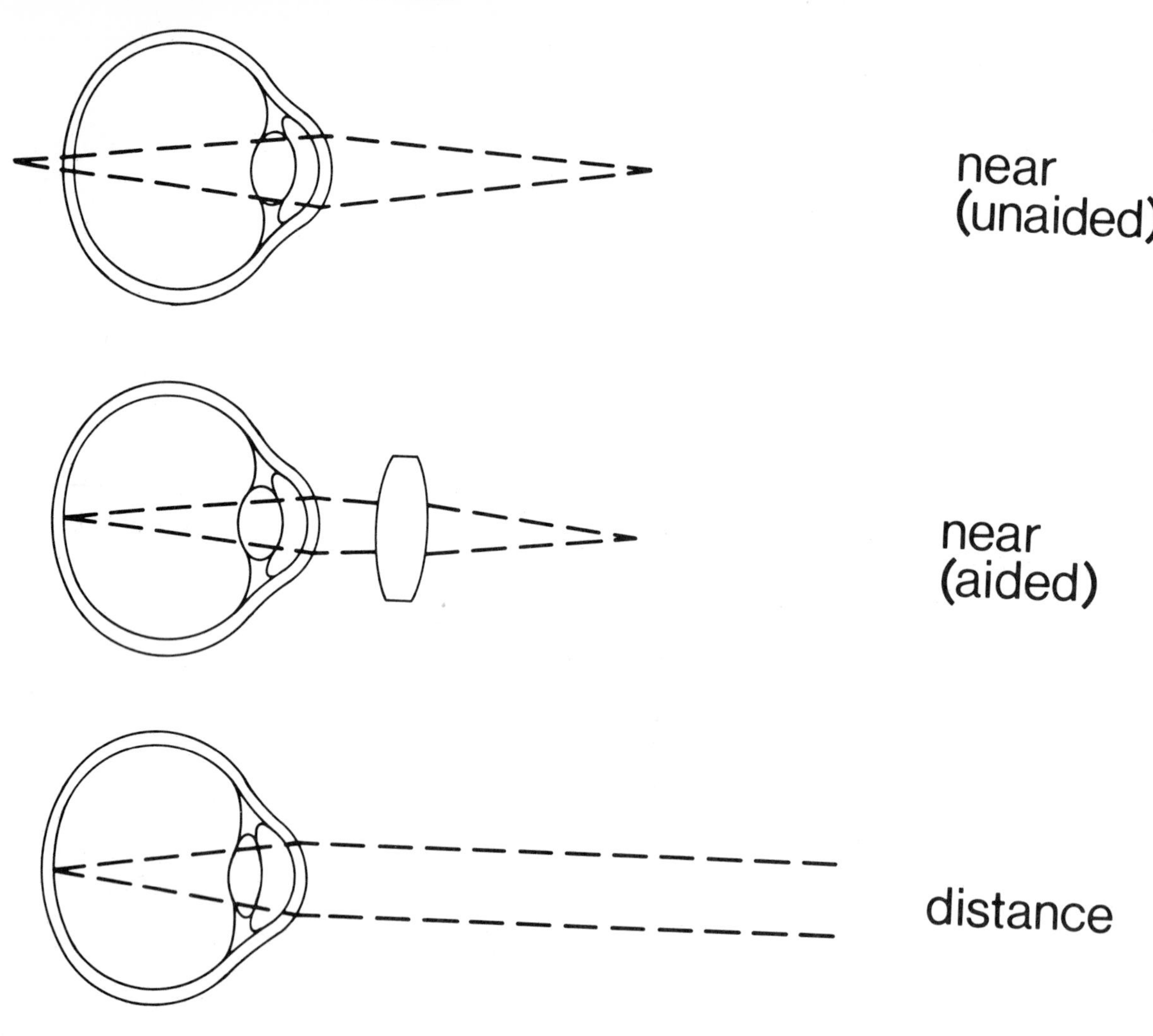

Figure 15-1 (continued)

important as it provides oxygen for the cornea. Should the oxygen become depleted, the corneal epithelium becomes swollen, visual acuity decreases, and the client experiences severe discomfort.[9]

Altered or decreased tear formation can make the wearing of contact lenses difficult. Drugs that can disturb tear production include antihistamines, decongestants, diuretics, birth control pills, and the hormones produced by pregnancy. Conjunctivitis caused by allergies also can affect the wearing of contact lenses.[10]

The types of contact lenses, their advantages, and disadvantages are presented in Table 15-2. In general, the nurse needs to know if the client wears contact lenses, the type, frequency of medical supervision, and care practices (Fig. 15-2). The nurse must be able to identify the presence of contacts and know how to remove them in an emergency situation. Shining a light obliquely on the eyeball can help identify a contact lens. If the client is unable to remove the contact lenses, a small suction cup can be used to lift the lens off the cornea. The client needs to be instructed on the signs and symptoms of possible contact lens problems that indicate the need for medical

Table 15-1
Refraction and Visual Condition—Type of Correction Possible

Refraction/ Condition	Description	Symptoms	Type of Spectacle Correction	Type of Contact Lenses
Emmetropia	Light is focused on the retina; distance vision without accommodation, near vision with accommodation.	Normal vision.	Not indicated.	Not indicated.
Myopia (nearsighted)	Elongated eyeball or excessive refractive power of cornea and lens. When viewing a distant object, light rays are focused in front of the retina; a near object causes light rays to be focused on the retina, accommodation is used for closer objects.	Blurred distance vision, evident in early school years, squinting to narrow amount of light entering eye and improve focus.	Biconcave lens (plus). Requires new glasses every one or two years in adolescence. Stabilizes during adulthood.	Hard, soft, gas-permeable.
Hyperopia (farsighted)	Short eyeball with insufficient refractive power to focus light rays on the retina without accommodation, e.g., when viewing a near object, light rays are focused behind the retina. Light is focused on retina for far and near vision by accommodation. May experience presbyopia earlier than emmetropic eye.	Ocular fatigue.	Convex lens (Minus).	Hard, soft, gas-permeable.
Astigmatism	Unequal curvature of cornea causing light to focus at no clear point. Associated with any of the above refractions.	Blurred vision, ocular fatigue.	Cylinder lens.	Hard lens can correct unequal curvature. Soft lens will not correct unless special Toric* lens (two lenses in one: cylinder) for moderate astigmatism.
Presbyopia (inability to change focus)	Aging lens becomes larger and harder and cannot flatten or accommodate for near vision.	Blurred near vision, holding fine point further away from eye than 10 inches.	Reading glasses, bifocals, convex for near vision.	Monovision* (one eye with distance correction; other eye with near vision correction); loses depth perception; hard and soft lenses.
Aphakia	Without lens; congenital, due to trauma or surgery (cataract extraction).	Near vision impossible. If only one eye involved, image on retina will be $\frac{1}{3}$ larger than normal eye.	Thick, concave glasses can decrease image difference to 20–25%. Difficulty with restriction of visual field. Asperial lens causes less distortions.	Soft extended wear can reduce difference to 9%. [Intraocular lens (surgical implant) eliminates image size difference].

**Consumer Reports*, May 1980, pp. 288–292.

Table 15-2
Comparison of Types of Contact Lenses

Type	Description	Advantages	Disadvantages
Hard			
Polymethylmethacrylate (PMMA)	Rigid plastic, 8–10 mm in diameter (do not completely cover cornea). Requires specific wetting, cleansing, and soaking solutions.	Can be tinted, polished, and reground. Last 4–7 years. Least expensive in terms of cost, equipment, follow-up care.	Requires gradually increased wearing time up to 14 hours. If wearing schedule disrupted, restart wearing schedule. Dust particles under lens cause discomfort. Painful corneal edema with overwearing. "Spectacle blur" (hazy vision) when using glasses following contact use.
Gas-permeable			
Cellulose acetate butyrate (CAB) or 65% PMMA with silicone	Rigid plastic that allows oxygen and other gases to pass through and nourish cornea. Same size as hard contacts.	More comfortable than hard contact lenses. Requires less adaptation time and less problem with corneal edema.	More expensive than hard contact lenses.
Soft			
Hydrophilic plastic (many products); 30–40% water	Consistency of cornflake until immersed in sterile water or normal saline when becomes soft, gelatinlike. Larger than hard lenses. 12.5–16 mm in diameter (completely cover the cornea and a small portion of sclera). Requires conscientious cleaning (see Fig. 15-2). Enzymatic cleaner used weekly.	Fits snugly on cornea, prevents particles entering under lens. Little adaptation. Can be worn intermittently and up to 18 hours per day.	Fragile, lasts approximately 2 years. Cannot be tinted. Can shrink in dry environments or deficient tear film (tighten and blur vision). Visual acuity less than with hard contacts. Easily absorbs dust, smoke, protein from tears, aerosol sprays, oil from makeup, and microorganisms.
Extended wear			
Hydrophilic plastic 60–80% water Approved by FDA, 1979	Similar to soft lens.	Can be worn for several weeks without removal. Used after cataract extraction; reduces distortion of cataract glasses and image size difference if only one cataract removed. Useful for clients with decreased manual dexterity.	More fragile than soft lenses, splits easily. Requires close medical supervision. Most expensive. Complications of infections and vascularization of cornea.

consultation. These include: (1) red and painful eye; (2) a sudden change in vision; (3) repeated irritation of the eye; (4) excess secretions from the eye; and (5) "spectacle blur" (hazy vision), that lasts more than 24 hours after wearing hard contact lenses.

Strabismus

The deviation of one eye from the other in an outward, inward, upward, or downward manner when the client is fixing on an object is called strabismus. In children, strabismus requires medical intervention early to prevent development of *suppression amblyopia*. Suppression amblyopia is reduced vision in an eye caused by cerebral blockage of the visual stimulus although the eye is normal by examination.

Should strabismus develop in the adult client, *diplopia* or double vision is the chief complaint. Causes of strabismus in the adult may be due to thyroid disease, neuromuscular problems of eye muscles, and cerebral lesions.[11]

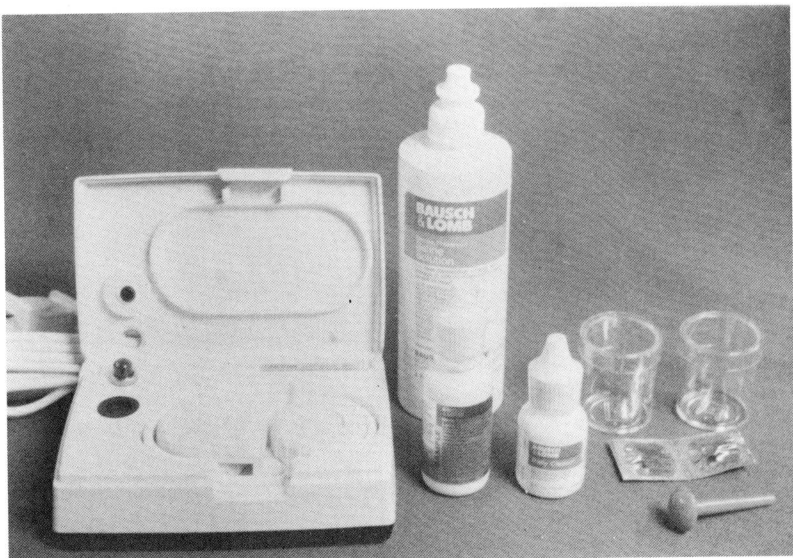

Figure 15-2 Equipment required for care of soft contact lenses. Heat sterilizer used once a day is to the right. Solutions for storage, sterilizing, and wetting the lenses are in the center. On the right are enzymatic tablets and equipment used for weekly cleaning to remove protein deposits.

External Ocular Disease

Infections

One of the most common conditions encountered by the ophthalmologist is infection of the external eye. Many microorganisms affect the lids and conjunctiva and can involve the avascular cornea. Conditions that predispose to infection of the cornea are irritation of the cornea, decreased tear film, or decreased blinking. The client who has decreased resistance or is immunosuppressed is more prone to ocular infections. Infection of the cornea can cause corneal ulceration with a potential for perforation and/or scarring and blindness. Common ocular problems due to infections will be presented related to the part of the eye affected and the type of microorganisms involved. Many eye infections are treated on an outpatient basis. It is a nursing responsibility to teach the client appropriate interventions related to the specific infection.

Lids *Hordeolum* or "stye," a staphylococcal infection of the lid margin, is fairly common. A red, swollen, circumscribed, and acutely tender area develops rapidly. If there is a tendency for recurrence, appropriate antibiotic ointments are indicated. A search for other possible sources of staphylococcal infection elsewhere on the body is indicated. Warm, moist compresses are applied at least three to four times a day.

Chalazion, an inflammation of the Meibomian glands within the lids, usually develops slowly over a period of weeks. The blocked gland enlarges and becomes tender. Redness of the palpebral conjunctiva may be noted when the eyelid is everted. Management includes warm compresses and antibiotics if infected. If the chalazion becomes chronic, excision of the gland may be necessary.

Marginal blepharitis is a common chronic bilateral inflammation of the lid margins. The lids are red-rimmed with many scales or crusts on the lid margins and lashes (Fig. 15-3). The client complains of burning, itching, irritation, and photophobia. Small ulcers may occur at the lid margins.

If caused by a *Staphylococcus* infection, medical management includes the use of an appropriate ophthalmic antibiotic ointment. Seborrheic blepharitis related to seborrhea of the scalp and eyebrows is treated with an antiseborrheic shampoo for the scalp and eyebrows. Often blepharitis is due to both staphylococcal and seborrheal microorganisms and the treatment must be more vigorous to avoid hordeola, keratitis (inflammation of the cornea), and other eye infections.[12] Good hygienic practices involving skin and scalp need to be emphasized. Gentle cleansing of the lid margins with baby shampoo, olive oil, or hydrogen peroxide can effectively soften and remove crusting.

Conjunctiva: Bacterial Infections Acute conjunctivitis or "pinkeye" is a common bacterial infection in children and is often epidemic. If caused by *Pneumococcus* or *Hemophilus* microorganisms, the

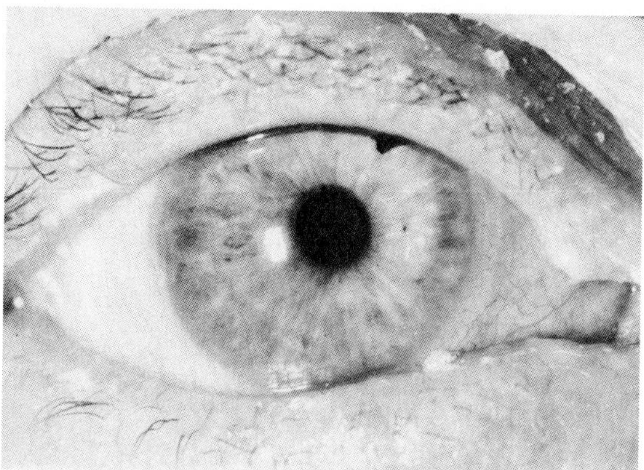

Figure 15-3 Marginal blepharitis: Note crust on lids. The client has had a peripheral iridectomy when a cataract was removed. The dark "v" area just below the upper lid is the part of the iris that was removed. *(Courtesy of Department of Ophthalmology, The Ohio State University.)*

conjunctiva rapidly becomes red and a mucopurulent drainage develops. The client complains of mild irritation. The condition is usually self-limiting but prevention of spread is important by careful handwashing and use of individual or disposable towels and washcloths. Topical antibiotics are prescribed.

Conjunctiva: Viral Infections Viral infections are caused by herpesvirus type I, herpes zoster, and adenoviruses. Viral infections of the conjunctiva produce redness, a watery discharge, and usually follicles of the conjunctiva. Follicles are avascular white or gray, round, raised areas. Viral infections produce a mild self-limiting to a severe debilitating disease.

Herpesvirus type I Herpesvirus type I is one of the most common severe ocular infections in the United States.[13] It is a growing problem, especially with immunosuppressed clients such as those receiving chemotherapy and corticosteroids. Small, clear vesicles surrounded by erythema appear on the palpebral conjunctiva and spread to the cornea. The *corneal ulcer* has a characteristic zigzag appearance. Pain and photophobia are common. Usually self-limiting, the disease may last for 2 to 3 weeks. Medical management is with idoxuridine ointment (Stoxil, IDU). *Corticosteroids are contraindicated* as they contribute to a longer course, possible deeper ulceration of the cornea, and systemic complications. If not responsive to IDU after 7 to 10 days, vidarabine adenine arabinoside, (Ara-A), or trifluorothymidine are prescribed for topical administration.[14]

Herpes zoster or varicella-zoster (V-Z virus) occurs in clients with lymphomas and chronic lymphocytic leukemia, and in those over 80 years of age.[15] The V-Z virus spreads by dorsal root or cranial nerve ganglion. Involvement of superficial branches of the ophthalmic division of the trigeminal nerve (cranial nerve V) involves the forehead, eyelid, and eyes. The first symptom is pain in the ocular area followed by a fine, fluid-filled papular rash. The papules become turbid and yellow, break open, and form crusts with eventual scarring. In 40 percent of clients with ocular V-Z virus, the cornea will develop lesions and will eventually lose its sensation. Involvement of the inner eye also occurs. The disease process lasts 5 to 6 weeks or longer. *Medical management* includes analgesia for the pain, topical corticosteroids to reduce the inflammatory process, mydriatics to dilate the pupil and relieve pain, and topical antibiotics.[16] Careful diagnosis is important because the lesions may be similar to herpesvirus type I, but the medical management is quite different.

The adenoviruses are the most frequent cause of epidemic ocular disease. Several of the adenoviruses are resistant to chlorine and are spread during the swimming season. They are also spread by hands and ophthalmic equipment such as tonometers.

Chlamydial Infections Although rare in the United States, the chlamydial infection *trachoma* is the leading cause of blindness in the world. It is especially prevalent in the Middle East, Africa, and South America. Trachoma affects only isolated groups in the southwestern United States.[17] Progressing through several stages, trachoma eventually causes blindness due to corneal scarring. The World Health Organization advocates treatment with systemic and topical antibiotics. A preventable cause of blindness, trachoma control requires better health delivery systems, sanitation, and education of the underdeveloped populations affected.

Fungal Infections Fungal infections are on the increase in developed countries and are more prevalent in the temperate zone. Ocular fungal infections are more common in southern and southwestern parts of the United States.[18] Fungal organisms attacking the lids, conjunctiva, and cornea include *Candida albicans, Fusarium,* and *Aspergillus* species. Fungal infections are often associated with corneal abrasions caused by vegetable matter. No characteristic corneal lesion occurs. At first, the lesion may resemble a staphylococcal infection. *Medical management* for fungal infections includes amphotericin B (Fungizone), flucytosine (Ancobon) and natamycin (Pimercin).[19] Fungal infections within the eye, involving the uveal tract and retina, are common in certain areas. *Histoplasmosis* is endemic in the Ohio River valley and eastern United States and produces a chorioretinitis resulting in decreased vision and retinal detachment.

Allergies and irritants

Common manifestations of allergic reactions include a milky, edematous (chemosis) appearance to the conjunctiva, tearing, stringy secretions, and complaints of itchiness. Although there are limitless possibilities for allergens to the eyes, grasses, pollens, and animal dander are common offenders. Antihistamines may be useful.

Contact allergies caused by topical medication such as atropine, neomycin, contact lens solutions, and broad-spectrum antibiotics produce hyperemia and irritation. Management is removal of the offending agent. Topical corticosteroids provide relief, but should not be continued over a long period of time.

Common irritants to the eye causing redness, swelling of the conjunctiva, tearing, and irritation include smoke, smog, chemicals, makeup (mascara), and silver nitrate ophthalmic drops (administered at birth). *Medical management* includes elimination of the source. Redness and discomfort may continue for a period of time after removal of the offending agents.

Nursing management of extraocular problems

Careful medical asepsis and frequent, thorough handwashing are essential to prevent spread of organisms from one eye to the other, to other clients, and to the nurse. Specific procedures including isolation must be carried out conscientiously. Warm compresses may be ordered. The material used for the compress should be disposed of appropriately to prevent cross-contamination.

The medication regimen may be complicated and involve the use of several eye medications at frequent intervals. Careful administration and recording of medications is essential. If eye medications are to be used at home, the nurse should instruct the client on proper administration as well as on the importance of handwashing.

The nurse must assess and record changes in the eye such as edema, redness, decreasing visual acuity, and increasing discomfort. Analgesia may need to be given based on this assessment. Often, a darkened room may increase client comfort. If vision is decreased, the nurse should attempt to provide stability in the environment.

Trauma

Although well protected by the bony orbit and the fat pads, many sources of trauma to the eye are encountered associated with everyday activities. Emergency treatment of a laceration, penetrating foreign body, corneal foreign body, and chemical burns of the eye are covered in Table 58-6.

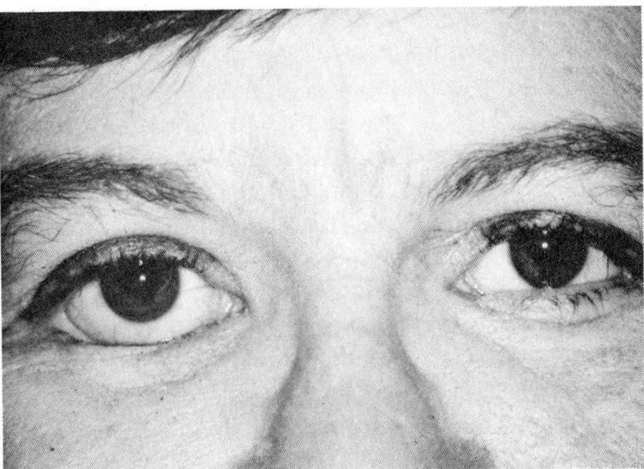

Figure 15-4 Entropion of right lower lid: Note the amount of sclera below the limbus and increased vessels in the conjunctiva due to the lower lid and lashes rubbing the conjunctiva. The cornea could also become irritated if not treated. *(Courtesy of Department of Ophthalmology, The Ohio State University.)*

Entropion, the turning in of the lower lid margin, can easily traumatize the cornea by movement of the eye against the lid and lashes (Fig. 15-4). The client will complain of pain and irritation. Temporary management includes taping the lower lid to the face or pulling the lid away from the globe, but surgical correction is necessary.

Alteration in the corneal tear film

Decrease or alteration in the tear film can cause drying and/or irritation of the cornea. Decreased tear formation and lack of the mucoid layer occur with aging, with arthritis, and other connective tissue diseases.[20] Other frequent causes of dry eye follow.

Ectropion Ectropion is the turning out and sagging of the lower lid due to aging. Tears spill out onto the cheeks. Irritation and drying of the conjunctiva and cornea can occur. Plastic surgery is necessary to correct the lid position.

Decreased Blinking or Closure of the Eyelid These conditions allow for drying of the cornea. Injury to cranial nerve VII (facial) prevents closure of the eyelid on the affected side. Clients with *exophthalmus* (abnormal forward displacement of the eye usually associated with hyperthyroidism) may be unable to completely close their lids.

Medical Management Management to prevent drying of the cornea is aimed at treatment of the cause. Application of topical lubricants such as methylcellulose (Ultra Tears) every 1 to 2 hours provides symptomatic relief. Lacri-Lube, a bland ointment, can be used when drops cannot be applied frequently. If topical medication fails to relieve the irritation, an eyepad taped with enough pressure to keep the lid closed can be used. This can also be used during sleep. A plastic shield without holes or Saran wrap can provide increased humidity and moisture. Surgical treatment to suture the lids together, a *tarsorraphy*, may be necessary to protect the cornea, especially for unconscious clients.

Acute nursing management Nurses play an important role in observing the affected eye or eyes, noting the client's complaints, and reporting changes. Administration of eye medications at the frequency needed is especially important. If plastic tape or pressure eyepads are used, the lids must remain closed so no further irritation of the cornea can occur. Increasing the humidity of the environment may decrease the discomfort of the nonblinking eye. If able, clients may manually close the lid to moisten the cornea and to decrease discomfort.

Cornea

There are many problems that affect the cornea. Over 2 million persons in the United States experience corneal disorders each year. Corneal disease accounts for only 6 percent of legal blindness in the United States.[21] This low percentage is probably due to the fact that most corneal problems cause severe pain, requiring the client to seek early medical treatment. Early treatment is essential in treating inflammations and infections of the cornea (keratitis).

Keratitis is caused by bacterial, viral, and fungal microorganisms as well as chemical and mechanical injuries to the epithelium of the cornea. Keratitis is very painful and reduces visual acuity. Once the epithelium is denuded, the area is open to the possibility of infection. Clients with decreased resistance, lack of vitamin A, malnutrition, diabetes, and those on systemic corticosteroids are more susceptible to a variety of microorganisms. Infection of the cornea will not produce drainage because the cornea is avascular. The inflammatory reaction can extend to the iris and ciliary body and pus or a *hypopyon* can form in the anterior chamber. Depending on the depth of the corneal ulcer and virulence of the disease, corneal perforation can occur with loss of eye contents if the eye is rubbed. After many infections, scarring and opacities result, causing decreased visual acuity.

The affecting agent is diagnosed by scrapings of the corneal layer, which are sent for cultures and sensitivity studies. Biomicroscopy and ophthalmoscopic examinations aid in diagnosis. *Medical management* includes immediate topical antibiotics administered every 1 to 2 hours. Parenteral antibiotics are administered after sensitivity studies are done. However, systemic administration of antibiotics does not reach high levels in the anterior chamber and cornea. Deep ulcerations can be treated by subconjunctival daily injections of antibiotic. Specific antibiotics injected under the bulbar conjunctiva can maintain therapeutic levels of the cornea for 24 hours.[22] Corticosteroids are not advocated systemically but are used topically to decrease the inflammatory response and scarring of the cornea. Topical anesthetics are also avoided as they can result in further corneal damage secondary to rubbing. *Eyepads are also contraindicated as organism growth is increased in dark environments.*

Corneal Scarring and Opacities If corneal scarring occurs, causing opacities of the cornea and decreased visual acuity, a corneal transplant or *keratoplasty* can be done to replace the cloudy cornea.

Keratoconus is a bilateral degenerative disease inherited as an autosomal recessive trait. The anterior cornea thins and becomes cone-shaped. Keratoconus appears during adolescence and is slowly progressive between 20 through 60 years of age. The only symptom is blurred vision. Hard contact lenses are used to correct the refractive error as well as decrease the pointedness of the cornea early in the process. The cornea can perforate as the thinning of the central cornea progresses. Keratoplasty is indicated prior to perforation.

Medical Management: Corneal Transplant Surgery (Keratoplasty) Keratoplasty is indicated for clients who experience corneal degeneration and dystrophies, scarring, opacities, chemical burns, and trauma. Although corneal problems are not common, a corneal transplant can provide vision that otherwise would be impossible. The clients may be young, including infants, and many are in their productive years when a corneal transplant is performed. Approximately 10,000 transplants are performed a year. The success rate has increased and is currently about 85 percent.[23] A second transplant can be performed should rejection occur. Healthy donor eyes are obtained as soon as possible after death, and placed in a specially nutritive solution and refrigerated or cryopreserved until used. Tissue typing, better instru-

Table 15-3
Types of Corneal Grafts (Keratoplasty)

Type	Descriptions	Use
Penetrating	All five layers of cornea removed. Circular, 7–8 mm in diameter.	Total corneal layers involved. Keratoconus. Most frequently used.
Lamellar	Epithelial and subepithelial layers removed; endothelial layer of client left intact. Circular.	Superficial corneal opacities (herpesvirus scars). Infants, children.
Keyhole lamellar	Section of cornea, ephithelial, and underlying layer removed.	Opacity or a section of cornea. Extraocular growths involving cornea (pterygium).

ments, finer sutures, use of topical corticosteroids postoperatively, and careful follow-up has decreased rejection of the donor graft.

The types of corneal grafts are listed in Table 15-3. The most commonly used corneal transplant is the *penetrating keratoplasty*. It is sometimes necessary to also remove the lens of the affected eye as it becomes opaque (cataract) with the disease process of the cornea, especially with chemical burns of the cornea and penetrating eye injuries. A cataract extraction can also be performed with this type of corneal transplant.[24]

The client may be "on call" for a donor graft for days, months, or longer. Surgery is performed as soon as possible or up to 48 hours after obtaining a donor cornea unless the cornea has been cryopreserved. The surgery is usually performed under local anesthesia. Besides the routine preoperative preparation for a penetrating keratoplasty, specific medications may be ordered. The client's eyes may be treated with a miotic to constrict the pupil to prevent trauma to the lens. A mydriatic (Table 15-4) may be used if the lens is to be removed due to cataract. To assure a "soft eye" during surgery and prevent a possible evisceration of the vitreous humor, the surgeon may massage the eyeball prior to the incision and/or order hyperosmotic agents prior to surgery to reduce intraocular fluid (see Table 15-12).

The donor cornea is prepared after ascertaining the correct size required. The host cornea is removed by a disposable trephine, a round cutting instrument. The donor cornea or "button" is sutured in place by a continuous 10-0 nylon suture and the anterior chamber is reformed with a balanced saline solution. An eyepad and metal shield are applied to the operative eye. An eyepad may be applied to the opposite eye to reduce quick eye movement of the operative eye.

The main concerns after surgery are that the corneal grafts remain intact, that rejection is minimal or recognized early, and complications such as infection do not occur. Healing will be prolonged because the avascular cornea and the corticosteroids used will reduce the inflammatory process. The sutures will remain in place 5 to 6 months or longer. Progress of the eye will be monitored by biomicroscopic examination and tonometry. Topical medications are ordered accordingly. Clients usually are discharged with corticosteroids, an antibiotic, and a mydriatic topical medication. The nursing care postoperatively is similar to the care of the client after cataract extraction. The client must be kept comfortable and the incision protected from external pressure. An increase in intraocular pressure is to be avoided.

Intraocular Diseases

Cataract

Cataract formation is the development of opacities of the ocular lens. It usually occurs in both eyes, but at different rates in each eye. It is not a "growth over the eye" as many people describe cataract formation.

Significance Opacities of the lens cause one-sixth of all visual impairment. The incidence increases with age. Of persons 85 years of age or older, 95 percent have developed lens opacities. Cataract surgery is the most common eye surgery. Of clients hospitalized for eye problems, approximately one-half have cataract as the main diagnosis and 300,000 to 400,000 operations are performed each year to remove the ocular lens. Yet over 1.6 million Americans of all ages have difficulty seeing with one or both eyes even with glasses because of developing cataracts.[25]

Etiology The lens enlarges with age and cataracts develop due to alterations of metabolism and transport of nutrients within the lens. The most com-

Table 15-4
Common Eye Medications for Dilating the Pupil

Drug	Action	Uses	Implications
Mydriatics and Cycloplegics	Mydriatics dilate pupil by contracting radial muscle or iris, constrict conjunctival blood vessels.	Pupil dilation.	Systemic tachycardia and ↑ BP, trembling, sweating, pallor.
Sympathomimetics			
Phenylephrine HCl (Neo-Synephrine HCl)	One of the most potent mydriatics without cycloplegic action.	Often used with cycloplegics. Given preoperatively.	Given cautiously to clients with hypertensive cardiovascular disease.
Parasympatholytics			
Cycloplegics	1. Blocks acetycholine and radial muscles of iris → dilatation → mydriasis. 2. Paralyzes ciliary muscle and blocks accommodation for near vision cycloplegic.	Mydriatics and cycloplegics used to treat inflammation (uveitis and keratitis) by relaxing intraocular muscles.	Contraindicated in glaucoma, causes narrowing of iridocorneal angle.
Atropine sulfate (Atropisol, Isopto Atropine)	Most potent cycloplegic, long duration. Produces mydriasis in 30 min. Lasts 2–4 weeks.	Permits examination of inner parts of the eye. Used pre- and postoperatively in intraocular surgery.	Side effects—dryness of mouth. Sensitivity to light—wear sunglasses. Will have difficulty focusing. In infants, children: hot, flushed, dry skin; fever, ↑ pulse. Store out of reach of children.
Scopolamine hydrobromide (Isopto Hyoscine)	Faster action than atropine; shorter duration.		
Homatropine hydrobromide (Isopto Homatropine)			
Cyclopentolate hydrochloride (Cyclogyl)		Used solely as mydriatic.	Lesser response in heavily pigmented (dark brown or black) irises. Assess effectiveness of drug; report if pupil not dilated.
Tropicamide (Mydriacyl)	Fast onset, short duration.	Used in examination but not inflammatory conditions.	

mon type of cataract is degenerative or "senile." Degenerative cataracts develop over a period of 3 to 20 years. Ten to 15 percent of clients with senile cataract have diabetes or blood sugar alterations. Clients with diabetes tend to be younger than other clients when cataracts develop. Accumulation of sorbitol from sustained high levels of glucose leads to a high osmotic gradient within the lens fibers.[26] Other etiologic factors in the development of opacities of the lens are presented in Table 15-5.

Clinical Manifestations The clinical manifestations of cataracts include gradual decrease in vision, blurry vision, glare caused by the scattering of light by the opacities, and decreased perception of colors. If only one lens is involved, the client may be unaware of the changes until the good eye is accidently covered and he experiences "sudden" loss of vision. One type of senile cataract in which there is rapid enlargement of the lens causes the client to become more myopic. This condition requires frequent spectacle correction prior to surgery. Presently, no treatment for cataracts is available other than surgical removal. If the cataract is not removed, the client will become blind. Secondary glaucoma can also occur if the enlarging lens causes increased intraocular pressure.

Table 15-5
Etiologic Factors of Cataract Formation

1. Degenerative (senile)
2. Trauma
   Penetrating injury
3. Congenital
   Maternal rubella
   Inborn errors of metabolism
   Chromosomal defects
4. Radiation-induced
   Environmental
   Therapeutic
5. Drug-induced
   Systemic corticosteroids
   Prolonged use of topical corticosteroids
   Triparanol (MER/29)
   Echothiophate (miotic)
   Chlorpromazine (Thorazine)
6. Secondary
   Ocular infections (uveitis)

Diagnostic Study Abnormalities Diagnosis is based on decreased visual acuity. Examination by ophthalmoscope and biomicroscope demonstrates the presence of the opacity. Excessive enlargement of the lens can also be detected by these methods. Tonometry may indicate increased intraocular pressure due to the enlarged lens.

Medical Management Most surgery is performed when the client's vision causes difficulty in normal activity. Preoperative preparation will be similar to the preparation of the client for corneal transplant (see Table 15-6). The client is usually older than the client who has a corneal transplant. Chronic diseases will need to be assessed and controlled. The pupil will be dilated by mydriatic and cycloplegic medications (Table 15-4). Some clients may require a reduction of intraocular pressure by hyperosmolar drugs. Most cataract extractions are performed under local anesthesia.

Intraoperative phase

Surgical removal of the lens is an intraocular procedure. If the whole lens is removed, it is an *intracapsular extraction.* If the lens material is removed without the lens capsule, it is an *extracapsular extraction.* In the intracapsular cataract extraction, a cryoprobe freezes and adheres to the lens and with the use of alpha-chymotrypsin, an enzyme, the zonule fibers are softened and break as the frozen lens is removed by withdrawing the cryoprobe. A *peripheral iridectomy* is performed by cutting a "V" shape opening at the iris' periphery to prevent pupil block. Without the lens in the eye, the vitreous humor can block the flow of aqueous humor through the pupil and cause secondary glaucoma; however, the iridectomy allows aqueous humor to flow into the anterior chamber via this new route. The extracapsular cataract extraction procedure allows placement of certain types of intraocular lens in the posterior chamber between the iris and the remaining posterior lens capsule. A much smaller incision is made when the newer technique of *phacoemulsification* is used. A special instrument inserted into the anterior chamber delivers ultrasonic vibrations and breaks up the lens content. The lens particles are then irrigated and aspirated by this same instrument.

Table 15-6
Medical Management: Cataract*

Diagnostic
1. Measurement of visual acuity
2. Ophthalmoscopy, direct
3. Biomicroscopy
4. Tonometry

Therapeutic
1. Preoperative
   a. Mydriatic, cycloplegic
   b. Antibiotic, topical
   c. Osmotic diuretics
2. Surgery
   a. Removal of lens
      (1) Intracapsular extraction
      (2) Extracapsular extraction
      (3) Phacoemulsification
   b. Peripheral iridectomy
   c. Other—insertion of intraocular lens
3. Postoperative
   a. Analgesia
   b. Mydriatic
   c. Corticosteroids, topical
   d. Antibiotic, topical
   e. Eye shield
   f. Compresses

*Reviewed by Robert A. Bruce, Jr., M.D., Assistant Professor, Department of Ophthalmology, The Ohio State University.

Intraocular lens insertion

Intraocular lenses are tiny plastic lenses that are inserted into the anterior or posterior chamber, in front of or behind the iris. One type of intraocular lens may be clipped onto the iris. The choice of lens depends upon the type of cataract extraction performed, the size of the eye, and the ophthalmologist's preference. Clients considered for an intraocular lens are usually over 60 years of age. The older person has more difficulty adjusting to the thick glasses or contact lenses required after cataract surgery. More complications do occur after lens implantation. In 1979, a panel of ophthalmologists investigated and reported to the National Eye Institute that the risk of complication after intraocular lens insertion is small but significant. These complications include vitreous loss, intraocular infection, and postoperative inflammation. Most complications are temporary and can be treated successfully.[27]

Postoperative phase

The client is usually hospitalized for 1 to 3 days after surgery. The day of surgery, the client is out of bed with assistance. The surgeon will carefully check the anterior chamber for depth. A flat chamber may cause adhesions of the iris and cornea. Atropine 1% is administered daily to decrease spasms of the ciliary body and to relieve pain. Warm or cold compresses may be ordered to decrease the conjunctival and lid edema and to remove secretions from the lid and lashes. The eye shield must be worn during sleep for 1 month or more to prevent inadvertently rubbing and causing damage to the operated eye. The eye shield may be removed during the day if the client needs to wear glasses for serviceable vision with the unoperated eye. The lower layer of the cornea heals over in 48 hours, but it will take approximately 6 weeks for all layers of the corneal incision to heal.

Nursing Management

Acute intervention (Table 15-7)

Preoperatively, the nurse must assess the client's visual acuity, especially in the unoperated eye. With the operated eye patched after surgery, the client will need special consideration if blind in the unoperated eye. Clients are fearful of eye surgery and need an opportunity to voice their fears. *Postoperatively,* the nurse's main concerns are the comfort and safety of the client, the avoidance of external pressure to and increased intraocular pressure within the eye, and the preventions of complications. The client usually experiences minimal pain and scratchiness of the eye. Mild analgesics are usually sufficient to relieve these problems. Atropine eyedrops and compresses will also decrease the pain. If pain increases, the surgeon should be notified as it may indicate complications of hemorrhage and secondary glaucoma.

Ophthalmologists differ in the amount of activity and restrictions allowed postoperatively. Avoidance of activity that increases intraocular pressure such as squeezing the eyelids, bending over to put on slippers, and straining for lifting or defecating is usually requested. Usually a laxative of the client's choice is allowed. Vomiting also increases intraocular pressure and is to be prevented whenever possible. The nurse must maintain a safe environment to avoid trauma to the client from falling or bumping the eye.

Rehabilitative management

The client must be instructed in care of his eye prior to discharge. The client's family should be included in the instruction since many clients will be unable to administer their own medications due to poor vision. Opportunity for return demonstration of eye medication administration should be planned. Written directions and schedules are valuable teaching aids related to medication and activity restrictions.

The client's aphakic eye (without lens) after surgery will require correction. If only one cataract has been removed, images will be 33 percent larger than the vision perceived by the normal eye. Glasses reduce the difference to 20 to 25 percent but the brain may not fuse this difference.[28] Glasses can provide good central vision, but distort peripheral vision. Objects suddenly pop into view. Walls and steps are curved and distorted, and the client will under-reach for objects. The newer aspheric plastic lenses decrease some of the peripheral distortion and are lighter, but the cost is greater. A hard contact lens can be fitted at 1 month (see Tables 15-2 and 15-3).

Most clients can wear an extended wear lens for at least 90 days. If the lens becomes uncomfortable, or if tearing, redness, or decreased vision develops, the ophthalmologist should be contacted. If discomfort develops, the lens should be removed and examined for coating, deposit, and damage. Abrasions, ulceration, infection, or irritation should also be reported. The wearer of an extended-wear lens should avoid swimming and irritating or noxious fumes.

Retinal tear and detachment

Retinal detachment is a separation of the two layers of the retina, the neural retina and the underlying pigment epithelium. Once separated, fluid can enter between these layers and cause permanent loss of vision unless corrected surgically. Of the 25,000 clients diagnosed yearly as having a retinal detachment, 6000 lose vision in at least one eye.[29]

Etiology There are many causes of retinal detachment. The most common cause of separation is formation of a *hole* or *tear* in the retina, called a *rhegmatogenous* retinal detachment. Retinal tears can be caused by vitreous traction as the vitreous humor shrinks with age. The liquid vitreous humor enters the hole and separates the retina layers. As the eye moves, more separation can occur in minutes or over a period of years. As the retina separates, the corresponding field of vision becomes distorted. Contributing factors of rhegmatogenous retinal detachment include the myopic and aphakic eye that has a larger posterior cavity. This causes more force to be exerted on the retina as the eye moves. Degenerative disease,

Table 15-7

Nursing Care Plan for the Client Undergoing Eye Surgery

Client Problem	Expected Outcome	Nursing Intervention
		Preoperative Phase
Potential for infection	No postoperative infection.	Clip lashes according to established procedure. Cleanse lids from inner to outer canthus. Instill eyedrops as ordered without contaminating eyedropper. Maintain container for individual client.
Adequate pupil dilation	Mydriasis adequate for surgery.	Give ordered medication. Observe for mydriasis (very dark brown eyes may require more medication. Notify MD). Give correct medication in correct eye at ordered times. Place drop in lower conjunctival sac without contamination of dropper tip. Allow time for absorption before next drop. Blot excess with clean tissue.
Possible increased intraocular pressure	Soft eyeball during surgery.	Administer glycerin PO, mannitol, or urea IV as ordered. Monitor output. If general anesthesia used, Foley catheter may be inserted prior to surgery.
Anxiety over possible loss of vision	Relaxed, well-prepared client.	Answer questions. Provide psychological and physical support as appropriate.
		Postoperative Phase
Stress response of surgery, anesthesia	Safe postoperative course: vital signs within normal limits.	Monitor vital signs, IV rates, recovery from general anesthesia. Note progress of urine checks, blood sugar, vital signs, etc.
Nausea and vomiting especially if extraocular muscle manipulation or general anesthesia	Minimal nausea and no vomiting.	Administer antiemetics as ordered (vomiting increases intraocular pressure). Start with clear liquids, increase diet as tolerated.
Moderate pain, scratching sensation	Minimal discomfort.	Administer analgesics as ordered; monitor effects. If severe pain, call MD. Administer atropine ophthalmic drops as ordered (relaxes ciliary body and decreases pain).
Local eye reaction; edema and redness	Minimal edema and redness.	Monitor drainage on eyepad. Administer warm compresses using clean washcloth or established procedure; check temperature to avoid burning. Avoid pressure to eyeball. Change compresses when cold. Teach client to apply compresses.
Potential for complications; intraocular bleeding	Absence of complications.	Monitor for increasing complaints of pain. Do not change initial eyepad unless ordered.
Impaired vision and safety	Safe environment; movement within environment without trauma.	Side rails until recovered and/or allowed up. Assess vision acuity of unoperative eye. Keep environment stable. Assist out of bed, and with activities of daily living. Keep call button in place. Keep eye shield over pad for intraocular surgery (cataract, corneal transplant).
		Rehabilitative Phase
Potential for inappropriate self-administration of medications	Client and/or significant other will demonstrate safe skill in administering eye medications. States name and time of administration of eye medications.	Teach client specific medications to take. Provide demonstration and return demonstration.
Possible activity restriction	Performs appropriate activities.	Assess home situation and employment. Assist with alternative plans.
Inadequate follow-up care	Explain date and time of follow-up care.	Assess client's understanding of need and arrangements for follow-up care.
Development of complications	Describe signs and symptoms indicating eye problem.	Instruct client/significant other to recognize signs of eye problem such as pain, purulent drainage, decreasing vision.

such as lattice degeneration which develops a firm vitreoretinal adhesion, causes approximately one-third of tear-induced detachments. Severe diabetic retinopathy can cause shrinkage of the vitreous humor due to retinal vessel hemorrhage into it. Trauma to the head or eye, although a less common cause, may precipitate a detachment, especially in an eye, with degenerative changes. The majority of retinal tears, however, do not develop into detachments. It is difficult to determine which tears will eventually detach. Both eyes can be involved. *Nonrhegmatogenous* retinal detachments are caused by fluid accumulating between the choroid and retinal layers due to tumor or an inflammatory disease of these layers.

Table 15-8
Medical Management: Detached Retina*

Diagnostic
1. Measurement of visual acuity
2. Ophthalmoscopy, direct
3. Ophthalmoscopy, indirect
4. Biomicroscopy

Therapeutic
1. Eye pads O.U.
2. Position client with retinal hole area lowermost
3. Photocoagulation
4. Surgery

Procedure	Purpose
a. Cryotherapy (Cryoretinopexy) b. Diathermy	Stimulation of scar
c. Silicone explant d. Encircling procedure fascia silicone e. Release of subretinal fluid f. Intraocular air/gas	Approximation of retinal layers against choroid

Postoperative
1. Analgesia
2. Position as ordered
3. Eyepads
4. Mydriatics
5. Compresses

*Reviewed by Robert A. Bruce, Jr., M.D., Assistant Professor, Department of Ophthalmology, The Ohio State University.

Clinical Manifestations and Complications A common symptom of retinal detachment is the appearance of flashing lights lasting only a few seconds, followed by the sudden presence of many moving spots or "floaters." Retinal detachment causes the release of blood cells that become suspended in the vitreous humor and can be seen by the client. Another manifestation is a visual field loss which is often described as a curtain coming across the field of vision. The visual field loss will be reversed from the area of retinal involvement. A visual field loss in the inferior temporal area of the left eye will be due to a detachment in the superior nasal retina of the left eye. On ophthalmoscopy, the retina will appear pale, translucent, in folds, and tremulous as the eye moves.

Retinal detachment can result in the loss of vision in the area of detachment. If the detachment involves the macular area, permanent loss of central vision occurs, resulting in less than 20/200 vision. However, some peripheral vision can be restored if treated early.

Medical Management Direct and indirect ophthalmoscopy is used to identify the site of the tear or detachment (Table 15-8). Once diagnosed, the client will usually be referred to an ophthalmologist who specializes in retinal surgery. The client may need to be transported with his head down and/or bilaterally patched to avoid further detachment. The principles of treatment include sealing the hole by creation of an inflammatory reaction that will cause a chorioretinal adhesion or scar and approximation of the detached retina against the underlying layer.

Photocoagulation is the use of an intense, precisely focused light beam such as the argon laser or a xenon light to create an inflammatory reaction. The light is directed at the area of retinal tear with the client awake. Photocoagulation is used when there is only a retinal tear. After the treatment, the client will experience marked blurring of vision due to the flashing bright lights, but vision should return to the previous level within 12 hours.

Cryotherapy or diathermy is the application of extreme cold or heat to create an inflammatory reaction and produce a scar. A cryoprobe or diathermy instrument is applied to the external globe over the tear during surgery. Cryotherapy is used more frequently today because less tissue reaction occurs. Approximation of the detached retina is accomplished by indenting the eyeball, causing the pigment epithelium, choroid, and sclera to move toward the detached retina. This is accomplished by several procedures. A silicone explant can be sutured against the sclera for localized detachments. A scleral buckling procedure using an encircling band with the knot over the area of the retinal tear is used for larger detachments (Fig. 15-5). A tuck can also be taken in the sclera. Materials used are silicone, Teflon, or fascia from the client or a cadaver. A large accumulation of fluid between the retinal layers is released by inserting a needle and performing a subretinal tap to facilitate approximation of the retinal layers. General anesthesia is usually used, although local anesthesia can be used when there is minimal detachment.

Surgical treatment is 80 to 90 percent success-

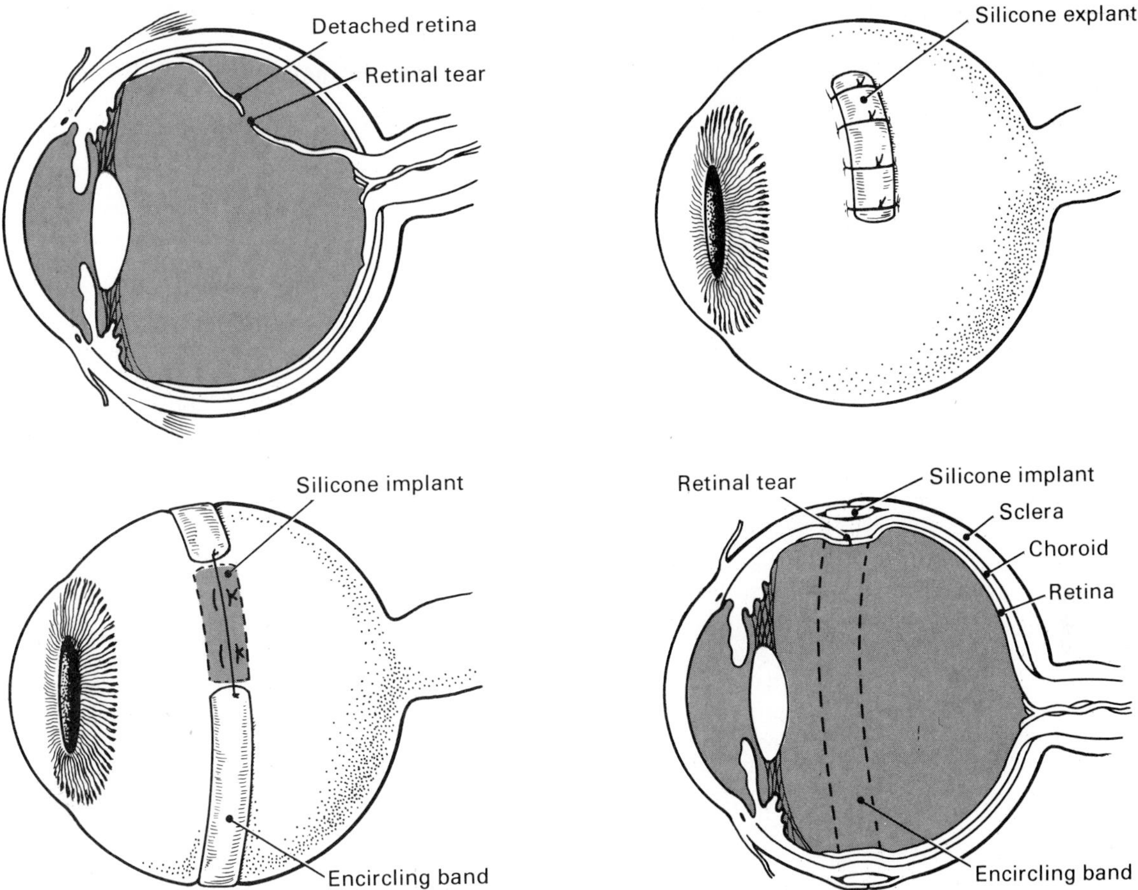

Figure 15-5 Diagram of retinal detachment and surgical treatment.

ful.[30] Additional procedures may be necessary for some clients. Retinal attachment can involve one or both eyes. Other areas of detachment can occur later. The treated eye may not regain maximal vision for 3 months.

Preoperatively, the client is often on bedrest and restricted position with possible bilateral eyepads. The rationale for positioning a retinal detachment preoperatively or immediately postoperatively is to keep the *retinal tear lowermost* (dependent position) within the eye, allowing the retina to fall back against the pigment epithelium. Preoperatively, this position is used to prevent further detachment, especially if the macular area is endangered. Bilateral patches are used to reduce quick eye movements that could facilitate further detachment. Not all ophthalmologists patch both eyes.

Postoperatively, the client may be on bed rest for 1 to 2 days or up and about depending on the position of the repair and the surgeon's preference. A position with the detachment area lowermost may be indicated to assist in approximation of the two layers, allowing the adhesion scar to form. Mydriatics, analgesics, and compresses will be ordered. The conjunctiva and lids will be red and swollen.

Nursing Management (Table 15-9)

Acute intervention

Since retinal detachment is an emergency situation, the client is often extremely anxious. Emotional needs and fear of blindness must not be overlooked as preparations for surgery progress. Information regarding past experience with retinal surgery will be helpful in planning care. Specific nursing interventions are detailed in Table 15-9.

The client is usually hospitalized for 2 to 5 days following surgical repair. Ambulation is permitted on the first or second day. Discharge planning should be started as soon as possible to allow for supervised practice of eyedrop instillation and compress application.

Table 15-9

Nursing Care Plan for Client with Rhegmatogenous Retinal Detachment

Problem	Expected Outcome	Nursing Intervention
Potential extension of tear or detachment	Macula intact and/or no further retinal detachment	Maintain ordered position with retinal tear (hole) lowermost in relation to eye 1. Client flat in bed and lying on left side 2. Client flat in bed and lying on right side Restrict activities. Bilateral eye patches as ordered. No reading if unpatched; may look at TV.
	Retinal tear will be flat and against choroid	Maintain ordered position as above. Bilateral patches 24 hours or longer, as ordered. Avoid jerking movement of head, e.g., combing hair, possibly shaving, brushing teeth, coughing, vomiting. Administer appropriate medications to prevent nausea, coughing.
Restricted activity	No complications of bed rest, e.g., thrombophlebitis	Encourage isometric exercises, range of motion exercises without head movement. Back care as needed. Encourage deep breathing.
Decreased sensory input	Free of signs of sensory restriction/deprivation, e.g., boredom, withdrawal, noncompliant behavior	Provide meaningful stimulation via other senses; use radio, read to client, identify self before touching.
Potential for trauma	Free of trauma	Stabilize environment, use of side rails, assist with ambulation and activities of daily living. Test temperature of water before applying warm compress to sensitive lids.
Edema of lids and redness of conjunctiva	Minimal redness and edema of conjunctiva, lids	Apply warm compresses as ordered; use clean washcloth. Teach client to do after thorough handwashing.
Fear of blindness	Optimistic attitude toward positive outcome	Encourage verbalization. Give careful explanations of all treatments and activities. Include family in planning and teaching.
Self-care following discharge	States signs and symptoms of retinal detachment, restrictions and follow-up care	Review written directions with client/family. Return demonstration on compresses, instillation of eyedrops, and eyepads.

Rehabilitative

Reading is restricted for a period of 3 weeks or more. This is because the rapid eye movements used in reading may cause further detachment. Watching TV is allowed. An eyepad is worn for comfort as needed. Some clients may be restricted from certain activities such as combing or shampooing hair and shaving. Resumption of light activities such as secretarial duties may be allowed in 3 weeks. No heavy work or lifting is allowed for 6 weeks or more. In preparing for discharge, it is imperative that the client be able to identify the signs of retinal detachment and the action to take should this occur again. The client will be seen by his ophthalmologist 10 to 14 days post discharge.

Diabetic retinopathy

Diabetic retinopathy is a complication of diabetes mellitus that affects the arterioles and capillaries within the eye (see Chap. 41). It is the most rapidly increasing visual problem in the United States. About one-sixth of newly diagnosed cases of blindness are due to the effect of diabetes on the retina.[31] Nevertheless, the actual risk of legal blindness in someone who has been diabetic for 20 to 30 years is only 7 to 9 percent.[32] Yet most diabetic clients develop some retinopathy over a period of 10 to 15 years.

The two types of vessel changes are *nonproliferative* and *proliferative retinopathy.* The nonproliferative type causes dilatation and microaneurysms of the retinal vessels which can rupture, causing hemorrhage into the retinal layers. Proliferative retinopathy refers to formation of many new vessels *(neovascularization)* that are weak and bleed into the vitreous humor, causing blood staining of the vitreous humor. The bloody vitreous humor develops adhesions and contracts, causing retinal tears and retinal detachment. The client may experience glare as light hits the edematous retina. Floaters due to red blood cells in the vitreous humor are seen. Visual acuity decreases as the hemorrhage clouds the vitreous humor.

Diagnostic Study Abnormalities The changes in vessels are visible on ophthalmoscopic examination unless the vitreous humor is opaque. Fluorescein angiography readily identifies the vascular changes in the subretinal and retinal areas by leakage of dye into the vitreous humor. Ultrasonography will help identify detached retinal areas, especially if the vitreous humor is opaque. Electroretinography is used to elicit retinal response by use of a very bright light transmitted through the opaque vitreous humor.

Medical Management Until recently, little could be done to treat diabetic retinopathy. Currently, photocoagulation is used early in the disease process (Table 15-10). If bleeding into the vitreous humor occurs, a vitrectomy can be performed.

Photocoagulation with the argon laser or xenon light is used to coagulate the microaneurysms and new growth of vessels in and on the retina. This procedure may require several treatments. There is evidence that photocoagulation will prevent severe bleeding within the eye (see section on photocoagulation under Retinal Detachment).

Since 1970, surgery involving the removal of the vitreous humor by entering the posterior cavity of the eye (vitrectomy) has been developed. *Vitrectomy* has provided a means of removing the blood-stained vitreous humor and allows for return of vision in clients who previously had no hope of visual improvement. The eye should be "quiet" or should have had no bleeding 6 months prior to the surgery (see Chap. 41 for description of vitrectomy and related nursing care).

Complications of a vitrectomy include further bleeding of the vessels during surgery. If bleeding occurs after surgery, the blood is no longer trapped in the vitreous humor to block vision, but will be absorbed over a period of a week or more. Secondary glaucoma due to bleeding can occur. Severe infection within the eye (endophthalmitis) can occur and requires immediate treatment. The vision of the client who has had a vitrectomy will not clear immediately and may be poorer for a short time after surgery than preoperatively. It may take up to 6 months for vision to reach its maximum.[33] Approximately 75 percent of clients undergoing vitrectomy experience increased vision.[34] These procedures only treat the manifestations of diabetic retinopathy. They do not halt either the disease or the progress of the retinopathy.

Table 15-10

Medical Management: Diabetic Retinopathy*

Diagnostic

1. Measurement of visual acuity
2. Ophthalmoscopy
3. Biomicroscopy
4. Tonometry
5. Fluorescein angiography
6. Ultrasonography
7. Electroretinopathy (ERG)

Therapeutic

1. Photocoagulation
2. Surgery
   Vitrectory
   Repair of retinal detachment (see Table 15-10)

*Reviewed by Robert A. Bruce, Jr., M.D., Assistant Professor, Department of Ophthalmology, The Ohio State University.

Nursing Management

Acute intervention

Preoperatively, the client should understand the purpose of the surgery and expected results. The diabetes should be well controlled. Postoperatively, the vital signs are monitored closely as an elevation of blood pressure may cause hemorrhage within the eye. Increased or sharp pain in the eye is significant and must be reported. Sleeping with the head of the bed elevated can decrease pressures in the retinal capillaries. The client should be instructed not to bend over or perform activities which increase intraocular pressure. The client's understanding of diabetes should be assessed during the hospitalization. A teaching plan should be initiated should lack of knowledge be determined.

Intraocular hemorrhage

Retinal Hemorrhage Arteries or arterioles are present throughout the retina and choroid in addition to those that are visible on the surface of the retina on ophthalmoscopic examination. Bleeding from any of these vessels can occur in the choroid, between the choroid and pigment epithelium of the retina, in the subretinal layers, and on the surface of the retina. These hemorrhages may be small to large, staining a large area of tissue. Fluorescein angiography is used to diagnose the source of bleeding.

Vitreous Hemorrhage Vitreous hemorrhage refers to a small amount of red blood cells within the vitreous humor (floaters) to a mass of blood within the vitreous gel that blocks perception of light. The blood is usually from the superficial vessels of the retina.

Etiology of the hemorrhage includes changes within the arterial walls due to hypertension, arteriosclerosis, and diabetes. Blood disorders such as leukemia can also cause bleeding of the retinal and choroidal vessels. Vitreous hemorrhage is often caused by traction upon the retina by vitreous contraction (see retinal detachment) and changes due to diabetes.

Treatment is according to the cause. Photocoagulation can be used to stop bleeding vessels early in the disease process.

Anterior Chamber Hemorrhage (Hyphema) Blood in the anterior chamber can occur as a result of trauma to the eye or, rarely, iridocyclitis (inflammation of the iris and the ciliary body) associated with rheumatoid arthritis, especially in the young. The blood is visible in the anterior chamber. If the hemorrhage is due to trauma, the client's eye will need to be immobilized using bedrest and bilateral eye patches until the bleeding stops.

Glaucoma

Glaucoma comprises a number of problems within the eye that are characterized by *increased intraocular pressure.* Increased intraocular pressure initially causes damage to the optic disk and nerve cells of the retina. At this point the client has no signs of symptoms. If not recognized and treated, glaucoma causes blindness that could have been prevented in most clients.

Significance Two percent or more than 1 million of those over 40 years of age in the United States have increased intraocular pressure requiring medical treatment. Many are not aware they have glaucoma. More women than men are afflicted; 200,000 have visual impairment and 56,000 are legally blind, attributable to glaucoma.[35]

Pathophysiology Although the visual problem occurs at the optic disk and retina of the eye, the mechanism causing increased intraocular pressure is in the anterior part of the eye. The ciliary body secretes approximately 4 to 5 mL of aqueous humor per day which bathes the lens with nutrients. It then flows through the pupil and is absorbed by the trabecular meshwork and the canal of Schlemm in the iridocorneal angle of the anterior chamber (Fig. 14-2). The outflow of aqueous humor is decreased by several mechanisms.

Primary open-angle glaucoma (chronic simple glaucoma) is the most common form of glaucoma. Approximately 90 percent of clients with glaucoma have primary open-angle glaucoma.[36] It is hereditary and is due to degenerative changes in the trabecular meshwork or aqueous outflow. Some authorities feel that the disease process also involves degenerative changes in the optic nerve and its vascular supply. Because the aqueous humor cannot leave the eye at the same rate it is produced, increased aqueous humor remains in the eye, increasing the pressure. This increased pressure is reflected first in the optic nerve and eventually in all parts of the eye if not controlled. The sensitive nervous tissue becomes ischemic and dies first.

Primary angle-closure glaucoma (acute glaucoma) is due to blockage of the trabecular meshwork. Although rare, it occurs suddenly and is an emergency. The iris in an eye with a flat anterior chamber is pushed forward, blocking the outflow channels and increasing pressure. This may be precipitated by several conditions: (1) The lens blocks the flow of aqueous humor into the anterior chamber and increased pressure quickly builds up in the posterior eye, causing the iris to fall forward and block outflow channels; (2) narrowing of the peripheral angle of the anterior chamber secondary to aging. Dilatation of the pupil pushes the iris forward and blocks the outflow mechanism. Dilatation of the pupil can be caused by a mydriatic drug, excitement, or darkness. *Mydriatic ophthalmic medications should not be given to a person with a narrow angle of the anterior chamber. Subacute or chronic angle-closure glaucoma* is a condition similar to the above which has the potential for an acute attack.

Secondary glaucoma is caused by other ocular diseases that block the outflow channels, cause a narrow angle, or increase the volume of fluid within the eye. Increased cells produced by hemorrhage in the eye, inflammatory processes such as uveitis, and trauma can block the outflow channels. Poor wound healing after cataract surgery with aqueous loss can cause a flat anterior chamber. Tumors within the eye increase the volume and intraocular pressure rises.

Clinical Manifestations and Complications Primary open-angle glaucoma develops slowly and without symptoms. The gradual visual field defects are usually not identified by the client until much peripheral vision is lost (tunnel vision). Vague signs may include headaches without cause or frequent change of glasses in the client over 40 years of age.

Acute angle-closure glaucoma causes definite symptoms including sudden, excruciating pain about the eyes, and/or headache. The associated nausea, vomiting, and abdominal pain may cause the clinician to suspect an abdominal problem. Colored haloes about lights and sudden blurred vision with decreased light perception are other symptoms. The eye may be reddened and the cornea appear steamy.

Subacute or chronic angle-closure glaucoma manifestations appear gradually and include transient blurred vision, haloes about lights, and slight pain about the eyes. Manifestations of secondary glaucoma include increasing pain, increased intraocular pressure, and other specific symptoms depending on the causative ocular disease.

Depending upon the type of glaucoma, the result is decreased visual fields due to the pressure and resultant ischemia of the nervous tissue. If not treated, blindness can occur slowly or rapidly.

Diagnostic Study Abnormalities Intraocular pressure as measured by tonometry will be elevated in glaucoma. If the client has an elevated reading, several readings need to be taken over a period of time and at various times of the day to determine a pattern. In open-angle glaucoma, the tonometry reading will be between 22 to 32 mmHg (normal readings are 12 to 20/22 mmHg). In acute angle-closure glaucoma, the tonometry reading may be 50 mmHg or higher. Biomicroscopy will demonstrate a normal angle for open-angle glaucoma, but a markedly narrow or flat anterior chamber angle, an edematous cornea, a fixed and moderately dilated pupil, and ciliary injection in acute glaucoma. Gonioscopy examination will reveal specifics of the iridocorneal angle. The visual fields will initially show a small football-shaped defect gradually progressing to a nasal and superior field defect in chronic open-angle glaucoma. In acute angle-closure glaucoma, the visual fields will be markedly decreased. Central vision may be 20/20. The optic disk becomes wider, deeper, and paler (light gray or white). This may be one of the first signs of chronic open-angle glaucoma. Photographs over time will demonstrate changes. Secondary glaucoma would reveal causative factors on examination such as inflammation, tumor, and hemorrhage.

Medical Management (Table 15-11)

Medical

Initially, the treatment of chronic open-angle glaucoma is pharmacologic (Table 15-12). Surgery is performed if control of intraocular pressure cannot be achieved. Miotic medications which increase the outflow of aqueous humor and constrict the pupil are used. A carbonic anhydrase inhibitor and a beta-adrenergic blocking agent may also be used to reduce the secretion of aqueous humor.

Table 15-11

Medical Management: Glaucoma*

Diagnostic

1. Visual acuity
2. Tonometry
3. Biomicroscopy
4. Ophthalmoscopy
5. Perimetry
6. Gonioscopy

Therapeutic

A. Chronic open-angle
   1. Cholinergic agents (miotics), topical
   2. Adrenergic agent (epinephrine), topical
   3. Carbonic anhydrase inhibitors
   4. Beta-adrenergic blocker, topical
   5. Surgery
      a. Filtering procedures
         (1) Trabeculectomy
         (2) Argon laser trabeculotomy
             Trephination, iridencleisis
         (3) Others: sclerectomy, thermal sclerotomy
      b. Reduction of aqueous production by cyclotherapy
         (1) Cyclodiatherapy
         (2) Cyclocryotherapy
         (3) Laser cyclocoagulation
   6. Avoidance of corticosteroids, topical, systemic
B. Acute angle-closure
   1. Cholinergic, topical (pilocarpine 4%)
   2. Hyperosmotic agents, PO or IV
   3. Analgesia—narcotic
   4. Surgery (may be ophthalmic emergency)
      Peripheral iridectomy

*Reviewed by Frederick M. Kapetansky, M.D., Associate Professor, Department of Ophthalmology, The Ohio State University.

Surgical

If pharmacologic control of intraocular pressure is not successful, a filtering procedure to create a bypass of the trabecular meshwork and the canal of Schlemm is performed. Currently, the trabeculectomy procedure (which causes fewer complications) is used. A channel is made by an incision into the conjunctiva and sclera for the creation of a scleral flap and removal of part of the iris and trabecular meshwork. The scleral flap is closed loosely, but the conjunctival incision is tightly sutured. Aqueous humor then drains under the conjunctiva. Success rate with these procedures is 80 to 90 percent.[37] If the filtering procedure is not effective, *cyclocryotherapy* is used. A cryoprobe is touched to the sclera external to the ciliary body, freezing parts of the ciliary body. Freezing causes local destruction of the ciliary tissue and

Table 15-12

Common Medications Used for Glaucoma

Types and Examples	Mechanism of Action	Implications and Use
Miotics		
A. Cholinergic action (Parasympathomimetics)	Direct acting. Lowers intraocular pressure. Causes contraction of iris sphincter muscle → pupil constriction (miosis); causes dilatation of vessels where aqueous humor leaves eye; increases outflow of aqueous humor.	Toxicity; headache; salivation, sweating, nausea and vomiting, diarrhea, bronchial spasm. May take 6 months to develop.
1. Carbachol (Miostat, IsoptoCarbachol)	Longer duration of action than pilocarpine.	Open-angle or closed-angle glaucoma.
2. Philocarpine (Isopto-Carpine, Pilocar)	Safest and most widely used miotic; causes miosis in 15 min and reaches maximum effect in 30–60 min. Causes spasms of accommodation with fixation of lens for near vision for 2 hours.	↓ Visual acuity. Requires administration 3–4 times daily. Stings on administration. May become resistant to action. Dosage must be titered to client. Neutralizes mydriatics used for eye exams. Used in Ocusert-reservoir placed in upper or lower conjunctival cul-de-sac for continuous delivery.
B. Anticholinesterase agents	Indirect acting. Inhibit the destruction of acetylcholine and allow iris sphincter to constrict pupil and ciliary muscle to be in spasm.	Side effects of headache, eye pain, blurred vision, dilated vessels of conjunctiva.
1. Isoflurophate (Diisopropyl)	Powerful miotic lasts up to 2 weeks. Used every 12–72 hours.	Systemic effects: hypotension, sweating, vomiting and diarrhea, abdominal pain, bronchial constriction. Used in accommodative esotropia, glaucoma.
2. Physostigmine (Eserine)	Moderate action.	Oxidizes and turns pink or brown—discard.
3. Neostigmine bromide (Prostigmin)		Open-angle glaucoma. Conjunctivitis, allergic reaction can occur.
4. Demecarium bromide (Humorsol)		
5. Echothiophate iodide (Phospholine Iodide)		Open-angle glaucoma, aphakic glaucoma, and congenital glaucoma. Loses potency at room temperature; store in refrigerator.
Adrenergic agent		
(Sympathomimetics, mydriatics)	↓ Formation of aqueous and ↑ outflow → ↓ intraocular pressure (IOP). Constriction of conjuctival blood vessels.	Treat wide-angle glaucoma and glaucoma secondary to uveitis. Can precipitate attack of acute glaucoma. Local reactions of hyperemia, corneal edema, allergic reaction, brow ache. Stings on administration. Systemic tachycardia and ↑ BP.
1. Epinephrine HCl (Epifrin, Glaucon, Epitrate, Epinal, Eppy)		
2. Dipivefrin (Propine)	Converted to epinephrine upon entering the eye.	Less frequent administration; can be used with other antiglaucoma drugs. Less systemic side effects.
Beta-adrenoreceptor blocking agent		
Timolol maleate (Timoptic)	Reduces IOP by unknown mechanisms.	Open-angle glaucoma. Used with miotics and carbonic anhydrase inhibitors if necessary. May slow pulse rate; may have additive effect with systemic beta-blocking agents [e.g., propranolol (Inderal) or metoprolol (Lopressor)]. Long duration, given once or twice daily.

Table 15-12 (Continued)

Types and Examples	Mechanism of Action	Implications and Use
Carbonic anhydrase inhibitors		
1. Acetzaolamide (Diamox) 2. Ethoxzolamide (Cardrase, Ethamide)	Slows production of aqueous humor by inhibiting the enzyme carbonic anhydrase.	May result in K^+ depletion and side effects of lethargy, anorexia, numbness and tingling of face and extremities.
Hyperosmotic agents		
1. Glycerin (Glyceral, Glysol, Glycerol) 50%, 75% solutions for oral use only. 2. Mannitol (Osmitrol) IV solution for IV use only, 5%, 25%. 3. Urea (Urevert, Ureaphil) IV—for IV use only.	Elevate osmotic pressure of the plasma, reduce the volume of intraocular fluid → ↓ IOP rapidly.	Used preoperatively to reduce IOP (cataract extraction, iridectomy, keratoplasty, etc). Used in acute and hemorrhagic glaucoma. Observe diabetics for hyperglycemia. Use cautiously with cardiovascular and pulmonary disease. Monitor intake and output, vital signs, electrolytes.

decreased production of aqueous humor. The procedure may be repeated. It can also be used in the treatment of acute glaucoma. Photocoagulation is also used instead of a cryoprobe.

Acute angle-closure glaucoma

This is treated as an emergency. Immediate intervention to lower intraocular pressure with miotics and oral glycerin (glycerol) is initiated. If this is not successful, intravenous mannitol or urea is used. Meperidine or other narcotics are given for pain. If the pressure has not been reduced, emergency surgery is done. A peripheral iridectomy as discussed with cataract extraction is performed, allowing the aqueous humor to flow through this opening into normal outflow channels. This same operation may be performed on the other eye as a large number of clients have an acute attack in the other eye.[38] Miotics may be used for individuals predisposed to narrow iridocorneal angle glaucoma, but an acute attack can still occur. The surgical procedure of peripheral iridectomy is considered curative for acute angle glaucoma unless complications occur.

Secondary glaucoma

This is managed by treating the underlying problem and by using antiglaucoma drugs. Should treatment fail or not be followed, glaucoma can progress to absolute glaucoma, resulting in a hard, sightless, and usually painful eye requiring enucleation (surgical removal of the eye).

Pharmacologic Management The most common miotic used is pilocarpine 1 to 4%. Carbachol may be used if pilocarpine is not effective. Epinephrine, 0.5 to 2% instilled 1 to 2 times a day, decreases formation of aqueous humor and increases aqueous humor outflow. This drug may be prescribed by some ophthalmologists prior to a miotic medication. A carbonic anhydrase inhibitor such as acetazolamide (Diamox) may be used to reduce production of aqueous humor and maintain a low intraocular pressure. Recently, a beta-adrenergic blocking agent has been approved for use. Timolol maleate (Timoptic) reduces aqueous humor secretions without pupil constriction. It can be used in combinations with the above drugs. The client requires continued supervision as these drugs control but do not cure glaucoma. By maintaining normal intraocular pressures, the optic nerve theoretically receives a better blood supply and oxygen. Table 15-12 lists common medications used in the treatment of glaucoma.

Corticosteroids may be used postoperatively with the filtering procedure to delay healing of the scleral flap and keep the fistula open. A possible side effect of corticosteroids is increased intraocular pressure.

Nursing Management

Open-angle glaucoma

Acute nursing intervention for the client with primary open-angle glaucoma primarily involves preoperative and postoperative care. The procedure to be done should be explained to the client. Appropriate medications should be administered and recorded. Time should be spent to allow the client to verbalize fears and clarify information before surgery. The client's fear of blindness should be recognized by the nurse.

Postoperatively, meticulous attention to accurate administration of eye medication is critical. The operative eye may be receiving a mydriatic, an antibiotic, and corticosteroids. The unoperative eye may be receiving a miotic and a beta-blocking agent. Error in drug administration would result in serious consequences.

Planning for discharge needs to be very specific in terms of medications, their purpose and frequency, and the eye each medication is to be used in. Vague symptoms indicating increased intraocular pressure such as aching around the eye and change in vision need to be reported and follow-up care sought. Compliance of medication for chronic conditions is known to be as low as 50 percent.[39] Therefore, every effort must be made to make sure the client continues with antiglaucoma medications. A client with open-angle glaucoma must always take medication. The nurse must stress the need for supervised follow-up care.

Acute angle-closure glaucoma

Because of the suddenness of symptoms and presence of pain the client with acute-angle closure glaucoma will usually be very frightened. Every effort should be made to reduce stress and provide a quiet, dark environment. The need for frequent administration of pilocarpine drops and tonometry readings should be explained. Administration of osmotic diuretics requires keeping accurate intake and output records and monitoring the cardiovascular system. Since surgery is usually necessary, explanations and preparations need to be made to the client and significant others. Postoperatively, the client should experience relief of the severe pain. Plans for similar surgery in the other eye are usually made. Preparation for use of postoperative eye medications at home should be included. This client will not usually need antiglaucoma medications, but the need for follow-up care should be stressed.

Macular degeneration

Macular degeneration is one of the most common causes of legal blindness. Currently, there is very little medically that can stop the progress of this degenerative process. The most common form, *senile macular degeneration,* occurs in about 30 percent of the older age group.[40] Due to decreased nourishment of the macular area by the choroid, new vessels develop which hemorrhage easily under the neural retina and cause detachment of the macular area. Once the macula is detached, the light-sensitive cones lose their function. The client experiences blurry vision which may partially resolve, only to occur again. Laser photocoagulation may decrease the bleeding and slow the process. The client eventually loses his central vision, but peripheral vision remains. Mobility without assistance is usually possible, but the client is unable to read. This results in a very frustrating handicap (see Nursing Management of the Blind Client).

Intraocular inflammation

Uveitis includes a variety of diseases that affect part or all of the uveal layer and the adjacent retina. Besides microorganisms, the uveal tract is affected by collagen diseases such as arthritis (with accompanying iritis and sclero-uveitis) and autoimmune reactions such as sympathetic uveitis. Pain and photophobia are the common symptoms. Medical management is determined by the causative agent and tissue affected and often requires extended treatment.

Endophthalmitis is an extensive intraocular infection involving the posterior cavity or the anterior parts of the eye. Although rare, it can be a complication of intraocular surgery and penetrating eye injuries. Causative organisms include fungi and gram-positive and gram-negative bacteria with an increasing incidence of the latter group of organisms. Symptoms include ocular pain, photophobia, decreased visual acuity, headaches, upper lid edema, reddened and swollen conjunctiva, and corneal edema.

Panophthalmitis is extension of the infectious process to the extraocular muscles and the orbit. There is pain on movement of the eye and involvement of cranial nerve V (trigeminal) which can cause exquisite but diffuse pain such as on combing the hair. Medical management includes appropriate antibiotics systemically, subconjunctivally, and/or intravitreally (into the vitreous humor). Corticosteroids may be given to decrease the inflammatory reaction and destruction of tissue. If the infection is not controlled, enucleation may be necessary.

Enucleation

Enucleation is the removal of the eye as a result of injury, infection, absolute glaucoma, pain, sympathetic ophthalmia, and malignancy of the eye. Fewer enucleations are being done for malignancy of the eye due to current management with cryotherapy, radiation, and chemotherapy. Surgery includes severing the extraocular muscles close to the globe and suturing the muscles over a round plastic or Teflon globe. The sutured muscles over the globe provide some movement to the prosthesis and help fill the cavity. The conjunctiva is then closed, forming a mucous membrane-lined socket. A plastic shell or conformer is placed over the tissue until the prosthesis is fitted. A pressure dressing is applied for 48 hours.

Nursing observations to be made postoperatively

that indicate development of complications include excessive bleeding on the dressing, increased pain, and temperature elevation. Instruction in care of the eye includes instilling topical antibiotics, ointment or drops; compresses; and cleansing of the wound.

The prosthesis is fitted by the optician in approximately 1 month. The client is taught how to insert, remove, and cleanse the prosthesis. Special polishing, usually done by the optician, is periodically required to remove dried protein secretions. The nurse may need to remove the prosthesis when the client is unconscious or unable to do it. The procedure is as follows: After thorough handwashing, the lower lid is pulled down and depressed. The prosthesis usually will slip out. A special small suction tip can also be used (Fig. 15-6). After washing and scrubbing the prosthesis with fingers under running water, the upper lid is opened by pressure on the upper bony orbit, the top of the prosthesis (usually marked) is placed under the upper lid, and the lower lid is then pulled down. The lower edge of the prosthesis slips under the lid with a little pressure on the prosthesis (Fig. 15-7). If the prosthesis is to be stored when a client is going into surgery, it should be placed in a normal saline or water solution.

Blindness

Blindness does not necessarily imply total inability to see. Many people are classified as legally blind (Table 15-13) who have some light perception present. Those persons legally blind are eligible for federal and state aid to the blind, income tax exemptions, and state service programs for rehabilitation. Another group defined as *visually impaired* includes those with monocular vision and some who cannot read newsprint, but have better than 20/200 vision. This group also qualifies for some state aid.

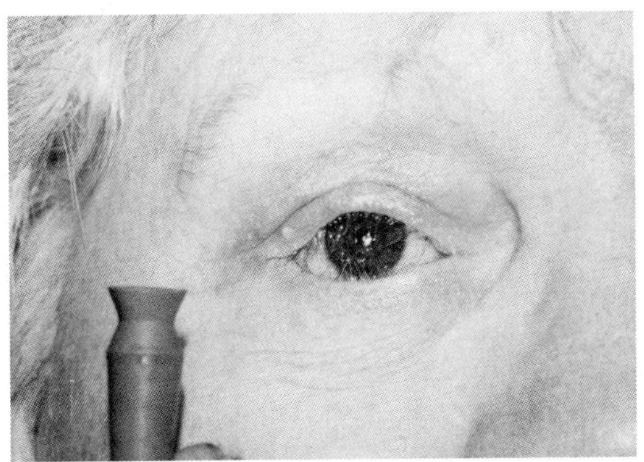

A

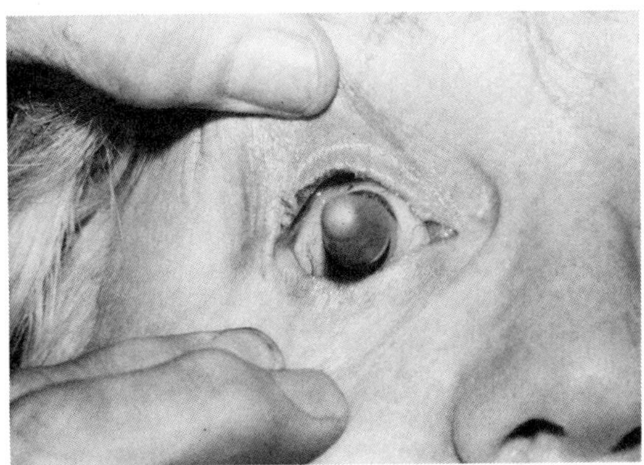

B

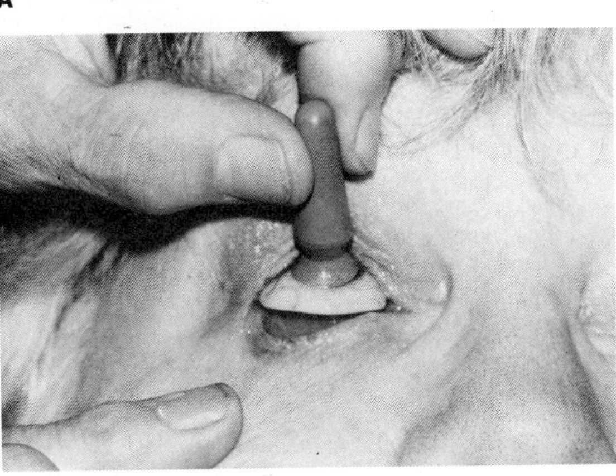

C

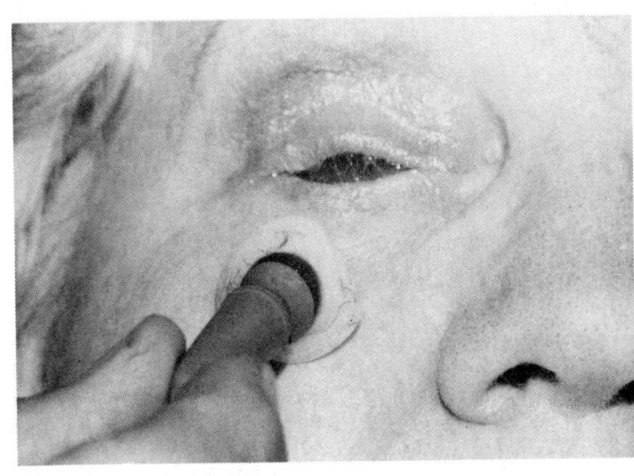

D

Figure 15-6 Removal of eye prosthesis. *(a)* Suction tip. *(b)* Suction tip in place. *(c)* Removal of prosthesis. *(d)* Prosthesis removed.

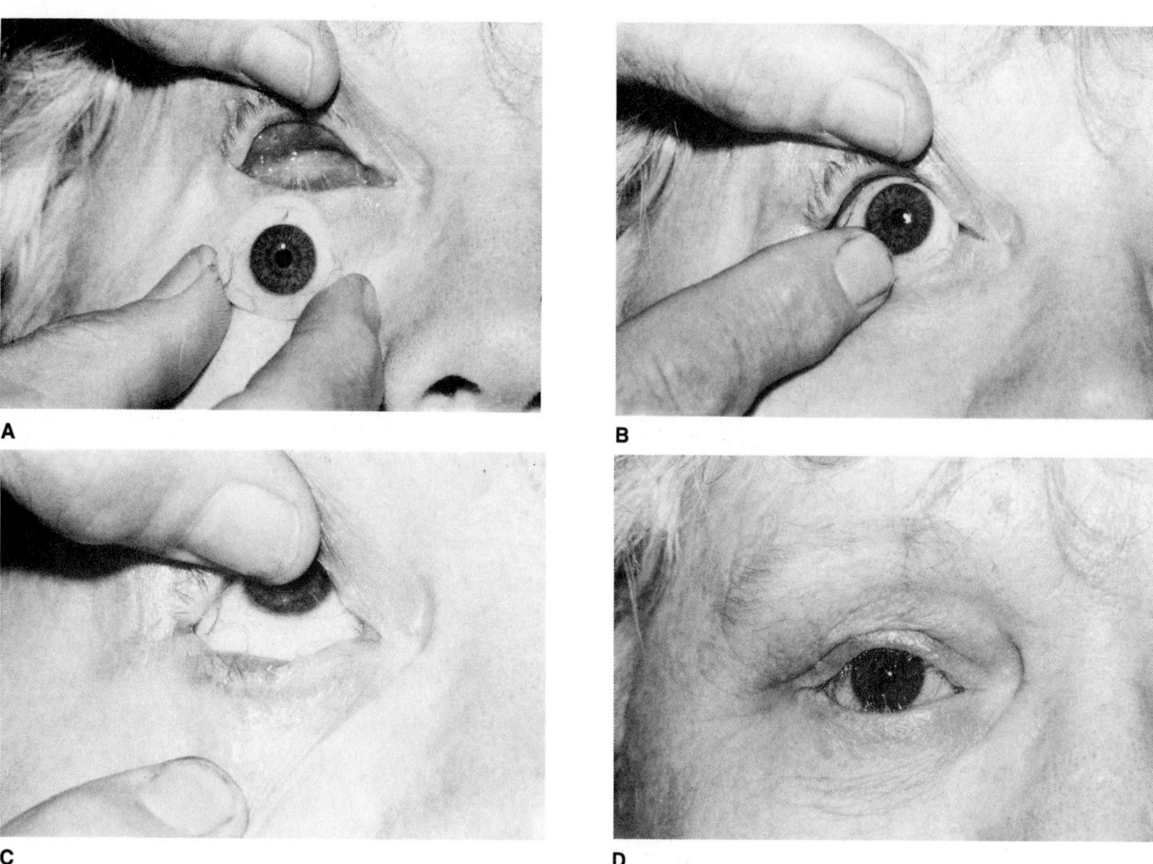

Figure 15-7 Insertion of eye prosthesis. *(a)* Lifting upper lid. *(b)* Top of prosthesis in place. *(c)* Lower lid pulled down. *(d)* Prosthesis in place.

Incidence and etiology

In the United States, it is estimated that there are 11 million persons who are *visually impaired,* one-third of whom have monocular vision only. Most persons who have vision impairment are between 25 and 64 and are male, while the majority of persons legally blind are elderly and female[41](Fig. 15-8).

Table 15-13

Definition of Legal Blindness in the United States

Persons who have a central visual acuity for distance of 20/200 or poorer in the better eye, with correction; or a visual acuity of better than 20/200, but with a field of vision no greater than 20° in its widest diameter.*

*Operational Research Department, National Society to Prevent Blindness, *Data Analysis, Vision Problems in The U.S.,* National Society for Prevention of Blindness, 1980, p.3.

Nursing management

Acute Intervention Emotional support of the client depends upon the time frame associated with the blindness. Sudden blindness allows no time to arrive at acceptance or learn compensatory skills. If vision fails gradually the client and nurse have an opportunity to plan and work through many of the emotional aspects of this situation. Both the nurse and the client need to reflect on their attitude toward this catastrophic occurrence. The client must be allowed to express anger and depression and work through the grieving process. The nurse must know when teaching can be best implemented. The client's family needs to be included in discussions and allowed to express concern.

In caring for the blind in the hospital or health care agencies, the nurse needs to be aware of certain factors to facilitate communication and provide a safe environment for the blind client. In approaching the

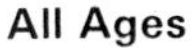

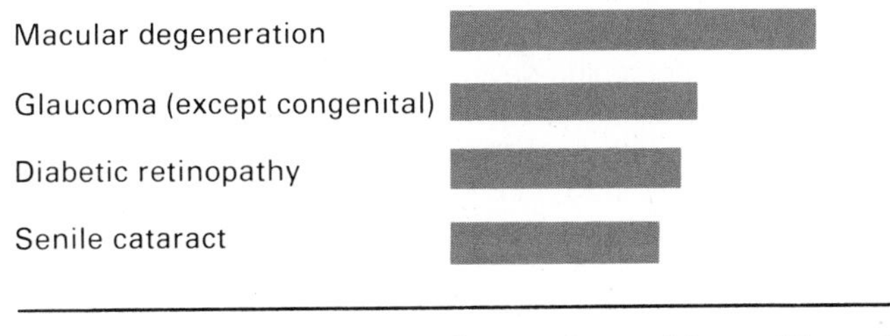

Figure 15-8 Leading causes of new cases of legal blindness—all ages, 1978. *(Reproduced from Vision Problems in the U.S., National Society to Prevent Blindness, 1980.)*

client, the nurse should call the client's name before touching him, introduce herself, and provide information regarding the purpose of the interaction. The client should be informed when the nurse leaves the room so he is not left talking to himself. The family should not be questioned about the client if the client is present. Activity and noise about the client should be described to assist the client in orientation and validation of the environment. The nurse should talk normally and not be hesitant about such words as "see." Often people raise their voices when talking to the visually impaired or blind, which does not help the communication.

The client should be encouraged to be as independent as possible. Independence is facilitated by a stable environment. Once the visually impaired or blind person has placed an object such as clothing or furniture in a certain position, it should not be rearranged. Doors should be fully open or shut but never left half open. Items on a meal tray can be described in terms of a clock superimposed over the plate, such as eggs are at 6:00 o'clock and bacon is at 12:00 o'clock. When uncertain if help is needed, the client should be consulted. Such openness is usually appreciated by the blind person and avoids misunderstanding and dependency.

When ambulating in an unfamiliar place the blind client usually appreciates assistance. The client should place his hand on the assistant's arm. The assistant should walk one-half step ahead of the blind person, describing objects that are approaching as "on your left is an open door" (Fig. 15-9). The blind person should never be pushed ahead of the assistant.

Other senses of the blind person should be stimulated in meaningful ways. A radio and/or television may be quite relaxing to some while others would prefer someone to read or talk with them. The use of touch can be a means of security and comfort to the blind when in an unfamiliar environment.

Rehabilitative Management Those clients legally blind are eligible for mobility training, braille, and rehabilitative training funded by state and federal agencies. Specific nursing skills associated with these activities are not within the scope of this book. The client or family should contact Services for the Blind, Welfare Department, of their state. Pilot dogs are

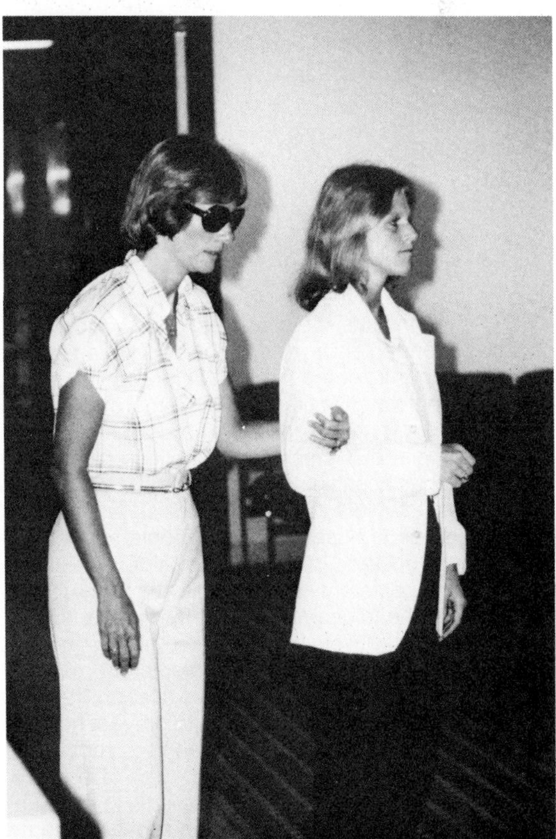

Figure 15-9 Assisting a visually impaired person to walk by allowing client to grasp arm and follow one-half step behind the nurse.

available to a certain group of clients who can care for them and need assistance with travel. Often, young blind persons prefer a dog. Although costly, a variety of electronic and computer devices are available. Talking books are available through some libraries. A list of agencies servicing the blind can be obtained from the American Foundation for the Blind, Incorporated (15 West 16th Street, New York, New York, 10011). Many of these agencies are listed after the bibliography.

For those with impaired vision, a large number of low-vision aids are available, ranging from magnifying glasses to small cameras incorporated into eyeglasses. Clients should be encouraged to seek help and information about available aids. Specific devices are available to help in measuring and injecting insulin for the visually impaired or blind diabetic client.

HEARING PROBLEMS

Health Promotion and Maintenance

The nurse has an important role in the preservation of hearing. In order to fulfill this role, the nurse should:

1. Instruct clients to keep objects out of the ear. Ears should be cleaned only with a washcloth and finger. Bobby pins and cotton-tipped applicators should especially be avoided. A quick movement can cause a perforated eardrum.
2. Support environmental noise control. It is known that sensorineural hearing loss due to increased and prolonged environmental noise such as amplified sound is occurring in young adults at an increasing rate. Health teaching regarding avoidance of continued exposure to noise levels of 85 to 90 decibels (dB) is essential. Continued exposure to noise has been shown to cause some persons to be more irritable and tense. Nurses should monitor noise levels in hospitals and at home to promote rest and recovery from illness. Interventions such as seeking different and less noisy equipment or a different time to use noisy equipment are possible solutions. In work environments known to have high noise levels (over 90 dB), ear protectors must be worn. A variety of protectors are available. They are worn over the ears or in the ears to prevent hearing loss. Periodic audiometric screening should be part of the health maintenance policies of industry. This provides baseline data on hearing to measure subsequent hearing loss. Ear protectors should be worn during skeet shooting and other recreational pursuits with high noise levels. Hearing loss due to noise is not medically correctable.
3. Promote use of childhood immunization, including MMR (measles, mumps, rubella). Rubella has been identified as a cause of deafness, especially if it occurs during the first trimester of pregnancy. High fever has been the cause of inner ear damage in many documented cases of sensorineural deafness.[42]
4. Monitor the client's reaction to drugs that cause ototoxicity. Clients who are receiving ototoxic drugs such as aspirin should be assessed for tinnitus and decreased hearing. When these symptoms develop, immediate withdrawal of the offending drug may prevent further damage and/or the symptoms may disappear.
5. Identify clients who have potential for hearing loss. Children who are chronic mouth breathers need referral. Enlarged adenoids can block the nasal passages as well as the eustachian tube, preventing aeration of the middle ear. This also predisposes to serous otitis media. Children who have acute otitis media frequently need to be followed for possible signs of chronic otitis media. It is important that children receive the full course of antibiotics prescribed.
6. Be observant of symptoms that indicate hearing loss in all ages. These symptoms include asking others to speak up, answering questions inappropriately, not responding when not observing the speaker, straining to hear, cupping hands around ear, showing irritability with others who do not speak up, and increasing sensitivity to slight increases in noise level. Often the client is not aware of minimal hearing loss or may compensate by the above-mentioned mannerisms. Children will often be inattentive, bored, or uncooperative when they have decreased hearing due to a middle ear infection (conductive type loss) or an inner ear problem (sensorineural loss).

External Ear and Canal

Trauma

Trauma to the ear can cause injury to the subcutaneous tissue that may result in a hematoma. If not aspirated, an inflammation of membranes of the ear cartilage (perichondritis) can result. Antibiotics are given to prevent infection. Blows to the ear also cause hearing loss if there is dislocation of the ossicles of the middle ear. It is important to obtain a very careful history of the accident and to assess the hearing of a client who has had a blow to the ear.

External otitis

External otitis involves the inflammation or infection of the epithelium of the ear canal. It is more common in the summer. Swimming in contaminated waters is frequently implicated and is called "swimmer's ear." Trauma caused by picking the ear and/or use of sharp objects such as hairpins frequently causes the initial break in the skin.

Etiology The most common causes of external otitis are the gram-positive organisms, staphylococci and streptococci. However, there is increasing incidence of gram-negative infections caused by organisms such as *Pseudomonas.* Fungi are often the causative agent of external otitis, especially in warm, moist climates. The warm, dark environment of the ear canal provides a good media for microorganisms to grow in.

Clinical Manifestations and Complications Pain is one of the first signs of external otitis. It is due to stretching of the tight epithelium of the ear canal by the inflammatory process. Pain is especially noted on movement of the auricle or pressure applied to the tragus (directly in front of the ear). Drainage from the ear may be serosanguineous or purulent. If it is due to a *Pseudomonas* infection, the drainage will be green and musty-smelling. Temperature elevations occur when there is extensive involvement of the tissue. The swelling of the ear canal can block hearing and cause dizziness.

Medical and Nursing Management Diagnosis is made by observation using the otoscope light and the largest speculum the ear will accommodate. The eardrum may be normal if it can be visualized. Culture and sensitivity studies of the drainage may be done. Aspirin or codeine usually control the pain. After the ear canal is cleansed, a wick of cotton is placed in the ear canal to help deliver the antibiotic ear drops. Wicking should be used with caution in a client who might push it further into the ear, such as the very young and confused or psychotic clients. Antibiotics include polymyxin B, colistin, neomycin, and chloromycetin. Nystatin is used for fungal infections. Corticosteroids may also be used.[43] If the surrounding tissue is involved, systemic antibiotics are prescribed. Warm, moist compresses or heat may be prescribed. Improvement should occur in 48 hours, but time is required for resolution (Table 15-14).

Careful handling and disposal of material saturated with drainage is important. Otic (ear) drops should be administered at room temperature. If stored in a refrigerator, only the dropper is warmed under running water. The tip of the dropper should not touch the auricle during administration. The ear is positioned so that the drops can run down the canal. This position should be maintained for several minutes to allow absorption of drops.

Table 15-14
Medical Management: External Otitis*

Diagnostic
1. Otoscopic examination
2. Culture and sensitivity

Therapeutic
1. Analgesics
2. Warm compresses
3. Cleansing canal
4. Ear wick
5. Antibiotic otic drops
6. Systemic antibiotics

*Reviewed by David R. Kelly, M.D., Assistant Professor, Department of Otolaryngology, The Ohio State University.

Cerumen (impacted), foreign bodies in the external ear canal

Impacted cerumen can cause discomfort and decreased hearing, which is often described as a hollow sensation. In older persons, the earwax becomes drier and is not easily removed from the canal. Water which enters the canal during a shower or swimming may cause expansion of the cerumen, causing blockage of the canal. Management is by irrigation of the canal with body temperature solutions. Special syringes can be used and vary from the simple bulb syringe to special irrigating equipment used in the doctor's office or clinic (Fig. 15-10). The client is placed in a sitting position with an emesis basin under the ear. The auricle is pulled up and back. The flow of solution is directed to the top of the canal. It is important that the ear canal not be completely

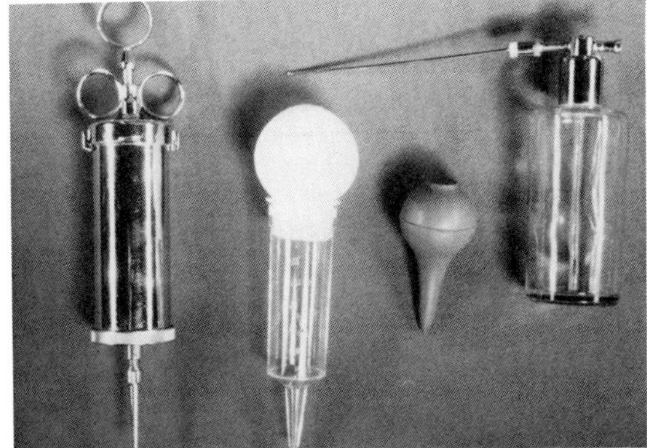

Figure 15-10 Types of equipment used to irrigate the ear: On the left is the metal Pomeroy syringe, a bulb syringe, an ear syringe as an irrigating tip, and a bottle used with a positive-pressure machine. The latter equipment is often used in doctors' offices and clinics.

occluded with the syringe tip. If this irrigation does not remove the wax, a special cerumen spoon can be used. Mild lubricant drops may be used to soften the earwax and irrigation may then be effective in removing the impacted cerumen. Some clinicians suggest the use of a Water Pik set at the lowest setting to remove impacted cerumen.[44]

Foreign Bodies Should an insect enter the ear canal, the best action is to drown it with mineral oil or alcohol, then flush it out. If a wood tick has become attached to the tissue, it is removed with an ear forcep.

Malignancy

Malignancy of the external ear and canal is not uncommon. The most common signs include a chronic ulcer of the auricle or persistent drainage from the canal. This drainage is blood-tinged and does not diminish with treatment. Medical management includes biopsy and other diagnostic studies to determine invasion of underlying tissue and bone. Treatment is by surgery. If the malignancy involves the ear canal and temporal bone, radical surgery of the middle and inner ear with resection of the facial nerve (cranial nerve VII) and auditory nerve (cranial nerve VIII) may be necessary.

Middle Ear and Mastoid

The most common problem of the middle ear is *acute otitis media,* usually a childhood disease associated with colds, sore throats, and blockage of the eustachian tube. Pain, fever, malaise, headache, and reduced hearing are clinical manifestations of acute otitis media. Medical management is with antibiotics and, if necessary, a *myringotomy.* This surgery involves an incision in the tympanum to release the increased pressure and exudate in the ear. Since treatment with antibiotics, the incidence of severe and prolonged ear infections of the middle ear and mastoid have been greatly reduced except in areas where there is inadequate health care.

Chronic otitis media and mastoiditis

Significance and Etiology In the adult, the most common infection of the middle ear is chronic otitis media. It is usually related to previous episodes of acute otitis media that did not completely resolve. Organisms involved in chronic otitis media include *Staphylococcus, Streptococcus, Proteus,* and *Pseudomonas.* The latter two organisms are more commonly cultured. Because the mucous membrane is continuous, both the middle ear and the air cells of the mastoid are usually involved in the chronic infectious process.

Clinical Manifestations In chronic otitis media, there is a continuous or intermittent ear drainage that may be thin and mucoid or thick, white, yellow, or green with a foul odor. The main client complaint is hearing loss due to destruction of the ossicles from the purulent discharge. Occasionally, a facial palsy or attack of vertigo may alert one to this condition. Chronic otitis media is usually painless. If pain is present, it indicates drainage under pressure and possible extension of the infection to the brain.

The eardrum is usually perforated. If the perforation is marginal, the epithelium of the external ear can grow into the middle ear. The skin sheds, and debris and drainage form a ball or growth called a *cholesteatoma.* This can cause pressure and erode the thin bony covering over the facial nerves (cranial nerve VII) resulting in decreased motor function of the same side of the face. A labyrinth fistula can also result, causing vertigo.

Diagnostic Study Abnormalities Otoscopic examination reveals a marginal or central perforation of the eardrum (Fig. 15-11). A central perforation has tympanum remaining around all points of the circumference. Some eardrums may be healed, but have an area that is more flaccid and thinner, indicating a previous perforation. Cultures and sensitivity tests are necessary to identify the organisms involved and the appropriate antibiotic to use. The audiogram may demonstrate no loss in hearing or a loss as great as 50 to 60 dB if the ossicles have been partially destroyed or disarticulated (separated). The x-rays may demonstrate a small, poorly pneumatized bone due to early acute otitis media.

Medical Management The aim of treatment is to rid the middle ear of infection. Systemic antibiotic therapy based on the sensitivity study is initiated. In addition, ear irrigations with otic solutions of 2% acetic acid or an aqueous merthiolate are used often to remove the drainage and debris. Antibiotic eardrops and/or powder are also used to reduce infection. If there is a recurrence, the client may need to be hospitalized for parenteral antibiotics such as the cephalosporins (gentamicin, carbenicillin) if the offending organisms are gram-negative (Table 15-15).

Often, the perforation will not heal by conservative treatment and surgery is necessary. Surgery to restore the conductive hearing loss by reconstruction of the middle ear is called a *tympanoplasty.* Diseased

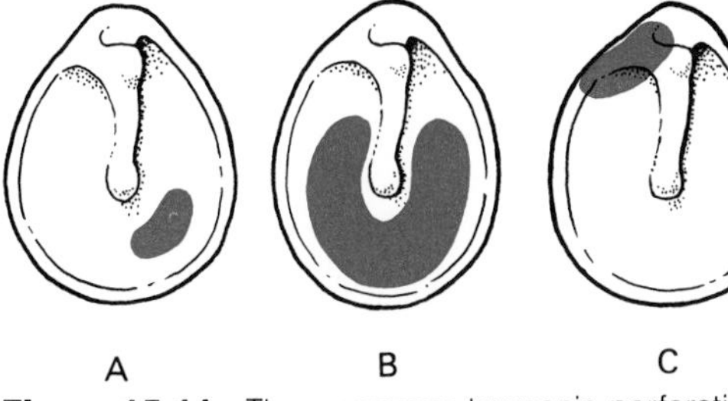

Figure 15-11 Three common tympanic perforations. 1. Small central perforation (hearing is usually good). 2. Large central perforation around the handle of the malleus (hearing is usually poor). 3. Marginal perforation of Shrapnell's membrane (hearing is usually good). *(From D. D. DeWeese and W. H. Saunders, Textbook of Otolaryngology, The C. V. Mosby Company, St. Louis, 1977.)*

tissue and ossicles are removed and a graft is used to make an intact tympanum. The graft is either tissue from the external canal or fascia (usually from the temporalis muscle). The graft is placed over the tympanum; Gelfoam (which is absorbed) is placed in the middle ear and a cotton ball holds the graft in place in the external ear canal. The incision may be endaural (incision around the tympanum) or postauricular (behind the auricle or ear). The type of tympanoplasty depends upon the amount of involvement (Table 15-16). Less hearing would be restored with types IV and V.

A mastoidectomy is often done concurrently with tympanoplasty to remove diseased tissue and the source of infection. A *modified mastoidectomy* aims at preserving function by removing as little tissue as possible. Removal of tissue stops short of the middle ear structures which appear capable of survival. A *radical mastoidectomy* is required when disease is extensive, requiring complete removal of all middle ear structures (except the stapes) or when complete exposure is necessary. No attempt is made to restore conductive hearing. The middle ear and mastoid become one large cavity. This surgery is rarely done

Table 15-15

Medical Management: Chronic Otitis Media*

Diagnostic

1. Otoscopic examination
2. Culture and sensitivity
3. Mastoid x-rays

Therapeutic

1. Ear irrigations
   Acetic acid
   Aqueous merthiolate
2. Otic drops, powders
3. Antibiotics, systemic
4. Surgery
   Tympanoplasty (see Table 15-18)
   Mastoidectomy—modified
   Analgesic
   Antiemetic

*Reviewed by David R. Kelly, M.D., Assistant Professor, Department of Otolaryngology, The Ohio State University.

Table 15-16

Tympanoplastic Procedures

Type	Middle Ear Problem	Description of Surgery
I	Perforation of tympanum; ossicular chain normal	Closure of tympanum with Gelfoam, fascia graft
II	Perforation of tympanum; erosion of malleus	Removal of all or parts of malleus. Closure with graft over remaining malleus
III	Destruction of tympanum, malleus, and incus; intact and mobile stapes remain	Removal of necrosed malleus and incus. Closure with graft over mobile stapes
IV	Destruction of tympanum, malleus, incus and *most* of stapes; footplate of stapes *mobile*	Removal of remaining malleus, incus, and stapes, except footplate. Closure with graft over footplate of stapes
V	Same as IV above except footplate of tapes *fixed*	(a) Fenestration (window) into horizontal semicircular canal; provides sound protection to round window. Closure with graft sealing off middle ear (b) Stapes footplate removed. Closure with graft over oval window

Adapted from W. H. Saunders, W. H. Havener, C. F. Keith, and G. Havener, *Nursing Care of Eye, Ear, Nose and Throat Disorders*, 4th ed., The C. V. Mosby Company, St. Louis, 1978, p. 421.

Table 15-17
Nursing Care Plan for the Client Following Middle Ear Surgery

Client Problem	Expected Outcome	Nursing Intervention
Bleeding from operative site	Minimal or no bleeding	Assess dressing frequently, chart. Do not remove initial dressing or cotton ball in external ear canal by tympanum. Position as ordered postoperatively.
Surgical disruption of tympanum	No fluctuation of air pressure in middle ear	Instruct client not to blow nose or cough. Sneeze with mouth open.
Possible facial nerve trauma	Intact facial nerve	Assess facial nerve function, e.g., client able to wrinkle eyebrows, close lids, wrinkle nose, smile, bare teeth symmetrically.
Nausea and vomiting	Minimal nausea; no vomiting	Administer antiemetics prn. Order appropriate diet.
Dizziness	Absence of dizziness Safe ambulation	Assist when getting up. Monitor ability to ambulate.
Discomfort	Minimal or no discomfort	Administer pain medication. Plan periods of rest. Keep room dark and monitor environmental noise.
Potential for infection, extending to brain	No temperature elevation	Monitor vital signs, temperature, headache. Give antibiotics as ordered. Instruct client not to get ear wet in shower or to shampoo.

today but was used prior to treatment of ear infections with antibiotics.

Nursing Management Routine care is provided, including teaching postoperative expectations (Table 15-17). Postoperatively, concerns are the avoidance of complications and of increased pressure in the middle ear. The client is instructed to avoid blowing his nose. This causes increased pressure in the eustachian tube and the middle ear cavity and could dislodge the fascia graft to the tympanum. Coughing and sneezing can cause similar disruption and are to be avoided if possible. If the client must cough or sneeze, leaving the mouth open will reduce the pressure increase. It is essential that the client be helped when getting up the first time as he may feel dizzy, lose his balance, and fall. Depending on the type of surgery, the client remains in the hospital from 1 to 4 days after surgery.

An eyepad or small dressing is used for an endaural incision. If a postauricular incision is used and a drain is in place, a *mastoid* dressing is used. A 4 × 4 dressing is cut to fit behind the ear and fluffs applied over the ear to prevent the outer circular head dressing from placing pressure on the auricle. It is necessary to monitor the tightness of the dressing and the amount of drainage postoperatively.

Serous otitis media (effusion of the middle ear)

Serous otitis media is an accumulation of sterile fluid (serous or mucoid) in the middle ear. The middle ear fluid may be very thick (called "glue" ear) and may be bloody. It may occur at any age, but is more frequent in children. Causes of serous otitis media include an obstruction of the eustachian tube or failure of the eustachian tube to open. Failure to open can occur during rapid descent in an airplane or during underwater diving (barotrauma or aerotitis). If the eustachian tube does not open and allow equalization of atmospheric pressure, negative pressure within the middle ear pulls (effuses) fluid from the tissues and capillaries. Allergic reaction of the mucosa can also cause blockage of the eustachian tube and/or cause fluid within the ear.

Complaints include a feeling of fullness of the ear, decreased hearing, and pain. Otoscopic examination reveals a retracted eardrum with the cone of light bent or broken. A hairline fluid line may be evident. Medical management utilizes decongestants and antihistamine medication, decongestant nasal spray, and exercises such as swallowing and gum chewing to open the eustachian tube. If not relieved in a few days or a week, a *myringotomy* is performed or the fluid is aspirated with a needle. A ventilating tube is frequently used for children who have recurrent serous otitis media or others with dysfunction of the eustachian tube. The client who has a ventilating tube in the eardrum must be instructed not to swim or get water in the ear.

Otosclerosis

Otosclerosis, an autosomal dominant disease, is the fixation of the footplate of the stapes in the oval window by a bony growth. It is a common cause of conductive hearing loss in young adults, especially women, and may be accelerated during pregnancy. It involves both ears, but at different rates. This condition is rare in blacks. Spongy bone develops from the bony labyrinth, causing immobilization of the footplate of the stapes. Approximately 10 percent of the population has this condition, but not all develop symptoms.[45] The client complains of a progressive hearing loss. If bilateral, the client speaks softly. Symptoms develop in one ear first.

Otoscopic examination may reveal a pinkish-orange discoloration of the tympanum (Schwartz's sign) due to the vascular and bony changes within the middle ear. The Rinne test, using the 512 tuning fork, favors bone conduction. Bone conduction is equal to or greater than air conduction (BC ≥ AC). This is a negative Rinne test. The Weber test lateralizes to the poor ear or to the ear with the greatest conductive hearing loss. An audiogram will demonstrate good hearing by bone conduction, but poor hearing by air conduction or an "air-bone" gap audiogram. Usually a 20 to 25 dB difference between air-conduction and bone-conduction levels of hearing is seen.

Medical Management The stapedectomy surgical procedure is the operation of choice today and is usually done under local anesthesia (Table 15-18). The poorer ear is done first and the other ear is operated on later. An endaural incision is made and, using the operating microscope, the stapes bone is broken and removed, including the footplate seated in the oval window. The oval window is covered with Gelfoam or a fascia graft and a prosthesis is attached to the incus. The prosthesis completes the ossicular chain and movement initiated by sound waves can now occur and be transmitted to the perilymph (Fig. 15-12). The tympanum is replaced and packing placed in the external ear canal. An eyepad dressing is placed over the auricle. During surgery, the client will often report the increased ability to hear in the operative ear. Due to blood and fluid accumulation in the middle ear, the hearing level decreases but does return to near-normal levels in 1 to 2 weeks in 90 to 95 percent of the clients.[46]

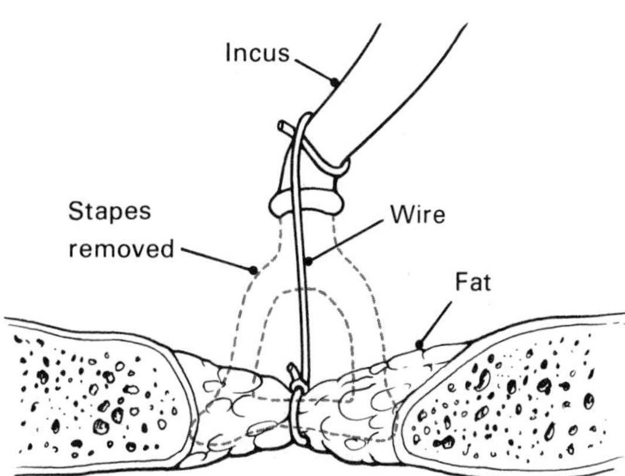

Figure 15-12 A commonly used stapedectomy technique. A wire-fat prosthesis replaces the stapes (Schukneekt). The graft thins out and becomes contiguous with the adjacent mucoperiosteum.

Table 15-18
Medical Management: Otosclerosis

Diagnostic
1. Otoscopic examination
2. Rinne test (512 Hz tuning fork)
3. Weber test
4. Audiometry

Therapeutic
1. Hearing aid
2. Surgery—Stapedectomy
   - Analgesia
   - Antiemetic
   - Antibiotic
   - Antimotion drugs

A perilymph fistula can occur with symptoms of widely fluctuating hearing levels, tinnitus, and dizziness. A few clients (2 to 3 percent) may develop a sensorineural hearing loss.[47] An audiogram is repeated when the ear is healed.

Nursing Management Similar care is provided for the client after a stapedectomy as for the client who had a tympanoplasty. Postoperatively, this client may experience dizziness and nausea and vomiting due to the proximity of the surgery to the labyrinth. Some clients will demonstrate nystagmus on lateral gaze because of disturbance of the perilymph.

Inner Ear Problems

Three symptoms which indicate disease of the inner ear include *vertigo* (whirling), *sensorineural hearing loss,* and *tinnitus* (ringing). Vertigo arises from the vestibular labyrinth while hearing loss and tinnitus arise from the auditory labyrinth. There is much overlap between manifestations of inner ear problems and central nervous system disorders.

Ménière's disease or syndrome

Ménière's disease is characterized by the triad of symptoms caused by inner ear disease—vertigo, tinnitus, and hearing loss. It incapacitates clients because of sudden, severe attacks of vertigo. Symptoms begin between the ages of 20 and 60. Usually one ear is involved; however, 20 to 30 percent of clients have bilateral involvement.[48]

The etiology of the disease is unknown but hydrops (dilatation) of the endolymphatic system occurs. The client's attacks of vertigo are sudden and without warning, possibly caused by autonomic nervous system dysfunction and vascular constriction. The client complains that the environment is whirling wildly about him and he must lie down or fall. Some clients report that they are whirling in space. The duration may be hours or days and attacks occur several times a year. Nausea and vomiting accompany the vertigo.

Tinnitus of a low pitch is present in the affected ear all the time and worsens during an attack. Hearing loss fluctuates, but over a period of years worsens until no functional hearing remains.

Medical management (Table 15-19) includes diagnostic tests to rule out central nervous system disease. The audiogram demonstrates a hearing loss in the low tones. Vestibular tests indicate decreased function. Nystagmus is present during an attack. During the acute attack, atropine may be given to decrease the autonomic nervous system function. Diazepam (Valium), Innovar, or droperidol are often used instead of atropine. Management between attacks may include vasodilation, diuretics, Diazepam, antihistamines, a low-sodium diet, and other medications. Over a period of time, most clients respond to the medications prescribed but must learn to live with the unpredictability of the attacks. Approximately 20 percent of clients have symptoms that become incapacitating in terms of frequency and severity and loss of useful hearing. When involvement is unilateral, surgical destruction of the labyrinth, causing loss of the vestibular and cochlear function, is performed. Shunting or drainage procedures are done for those with some hearing. Careful medical management can decrease the possibility of progressive sensorineural loss in many patients.

During the acute attack, the client is kept in a quiet, darkened room in a position that is of his choosing. Since motion aggravates the whirling and roaring sensations, the client is only moved for essential care; bathing may not be essential. An emesis basin should be available as vomiting is common. Medications and fluids are administered parenterally and intake and output monitored. When the attack subsides, the client is assisted with ambulation since unsteadiness may remain. Similar care is provided after surgical destruction of the labyrinth as the client will have severe tinnitus and vertigo which decreases over a period of days.

Table 15-19
Medical Management: Ménière's Disease*

Diagnostic

1. Audiometric studies; speech discrimination, tone decay, loudness balance, etc.
2. Vestibular tests: caloric test, positional tests
3. Electronystagmography
4. Neurologic exam
5. Polytomes (x-ray) of internal auditory canal

Therapeutic

1. Acute (one or more)
   Atropine
   Diazepam (Valium)
   Diphenhydramine (Benadryl)
   Fentanyl and droperidol (Innovar)
   Droperidol
2. Chronic (one or more)
   Diuretics
   Antihistamines
   Vasodilators
   Vitamins
   Diazepam (Valium)
   Low-salt diet

*Reviewed by David R. Kelly, M.D., Assistant Professor, Department of Otolaryngology, The Ohio State University.

Labyrinthitis

Infection or inflammation of the inner ear may affect the cochlear or vestibular portion of the labyrinth or both. Infection can enter from the meninges, the middle ear, or the bloodstream. Symptoms of vertigo, tinnitus, and sensorineural hearing loss are due to problems in the labyrinth. Nystagmus, an abnormal rhythmic, jerking movement of the eye, accompanies the vertigo and has a horizontal beat. Nystagmus is caused by abnormal currents in the endolymph fluid causing the eyes to have a rhythmic jerking movement with a quick and a slow component. Nystagmus is also caused by dysfunction of the cerebellar system. Vertical nystagmus is indicative of brainstem disease rather than labyrinthine disease.[49]

Suppurative labyrinthitis due to infection causes severe vertigo similar to a Ménière's attack. It lasts for a week or more progressing until the vestibular function is destroyed. Complete destruction of the cochlear portion occurs, causing deafness. Eventually the client learns to walk without support. *Vestibular neuronitis* causes only symptoms of vertigo with nystagmus, the quick component toward the normal ear. A viral infection may be the etiologic factor. The client recovers after a week or more. No hearing loss occurs. *Toxic labyrinthitis* is caused by ototoxic drugs that may cause vertigo. However, most ototoxic drugs affect the ear, resulting in tinnitus and eventually hearing loss.

Acoustic neuroma

An acoustic neuroma is a benign tumor which occurs as cranial nerve VIII (acoustic) enters the internal auditory canal or the temporal bone from the brain. It is important that early diagnosis be made as the neuroma can compress the facial nerve and arteries within the internal auditory canal. It can expand into the cerebellopontine angle and involve other cranial nerves and the brain by compression.

Early symptoms are unilateral progressive sensorineural hearing loss, unilateral tinnitus, and intermittent vertigo (unsteadiness). Diagnostic tests include neurologic, audiometric, and vestibular tests.

Surgery to remove the tumor is performed through a postauricular incision through the labyrinth, which is destroyed. A permanent hearing loss results in the affected ear, but the facial nerve is preserved. If the tumor is larger, a cranial approach is used.

Hearing Impairment and Deafness

Incidence

Hearing impairment is the second most common physical disability in the United States. In the United States, more than 15 million persons have impaired hearing in one or both ears. Over one-half have a bilateral hearing loss and the majority of these are 65 years or older. Males have a higher incidence of hearing loss than do females.[50]

Etiology and types of hearing loss

The types of hearing loss and pertinent characteristics follow (Table 15-20):

Conductive loss occurs in the outer and middle ear and impairs the sound being conducted from the outer to the inner ear. It is caused by interference of air conduction such as impacted cerumen, middle ear disease, and otosclerosis. Antibiotics, tubes in the eardrum, and surgery usually correct the problem. The audiogram will demonstrate an air-bone gap of at least 15 dB. The voice may be soft because the client hears his own voice conducted by bone as loud. This client hears better in a noisy environment. A hearing aid is quite helpful for a client with a 40 to 50 dB loss or more, although often is not necessary due to the excellent results of treatment.

Sensorineural hearing loss is caused by impairment of function of the organ of Corti or its central connections. Congenital and hereditary factors, noise trauma over a period of time, aging (presbycusis), Ménière's disease, and ototoxicity can all cause sensorineural hearing loss. Systemic diseases such as certain collagen diseases, diabetes, syphilis, and Paget's disease can also cause sensorineural deaf-

Table 15-20
Comparison of Types of Hearing Loss

	Air Conduction Pattern	Bone Conduction Pattern	Air-Bone Gap	(Weber) Lateralization of 500 Hz Fork	Discrimination	Voice	Other Findings
Conductive	Greater low tone loss—maximum is 70 dB	Normal or almost normal	At least 15 dB	To worse ear	Good	Soft or normal	Hears better in noisy environment
Sensorineural	Greater high tone loss or flat loss	BC = AC	None	To better ear	Reduced	Louder	Hears worse in noisy environment
Mixed	Components of both the above	Normal or almost normal	At least 15 dB	Variable	Reduced	Variable	Hears worse in noisy environment
Central	Variable or normal	BC = AC or absent BC	No gap	None	Reduced	Normal	Hears poorly in noisy environment, poor integration of complex stimuli

Adapted from Joseph Sataloff et al., *Hearing Loss*, 2d ed., J. B. Lippincott Company, Philadelphia, 1980, pp. 290–291.

ness. The two main problems associated with sensorineural loss are ability to hear sound but not understand speech and other's lack of understanding of the problem. Ability to hear high-pitched sounds diminishes. The consonants are high-pitched sounds and give intelligibility to speech. Words are difficult to distinguish and sound muffled. An audiogram demonstrates a loss in dB levels of the 4000 Hz range which can progress to the 2000 Hz range. A hearing aid may help some who have a 30 dB loss or more by reducing the strain of trying to hear, but the sounds will still be muffled.

Presbycusis, degenerative change in the ear, is a major cause of sensorineural hearing loss, especially in the elderly. It is a progressive problem which results in many social and emotional problems for the elderly. The control of inner ear diseases such as Ménière's disease can prevent further hearing loss. If the sensorineural loss is due to an ototoxic drug, further loss should not occur if the drug is discontinued.

Mixed hearing loss is caused by a combination of conductive and sensorineural losses. Careful evaluation is needed before corrective surgery for conductive loss is planned as the cause of the sensorineural loss will still remain.

Central hearing loss is caused by problems in the central nervous system from the auditory nucleus to the cortex. The client is unable to understand or put meaning to the incoming sound.

Functional hearing loss may be due to an emotional or psychological cause. The client does not seem to hear or respond to pure tone hearing tests but no organic cause can be identified. A careful history is helpful as there is usually a reference to deafness within the family. Psychological counseling may help. Referral to qualified hearing and speech services is indicated.

Levels of Hearing Loss Hearing loss can also be classfied by the decibel (dB) level or loss as recorded on the audiogram. Normal hearing is in the 0 to 25 decibel range. A *mild impairment* is in the range of 30 to 40 dB hearing level. A *moderate impairment* is in the 40 to 60 dB range. The *severely impaired* have a loss in the 60 to 80 dB range. The *profoundly* deaf have a loss greater than 80 dB. Many in this latter group are the congenitally deaf.

Manifestations of hearing loss

If the hearing loss is congenital and profound, the great difficulty in learning speech and conceptual thinking is quite evident. Rehabilitation must be started early. Those who develop hearing loss vary in the amount of loss and the reactions to it. The variables which affect the results of hearing loss include age at which the loss occurred, extent of loss, type of loss, frequencies affected, and communicative demand on the hearing system.[51] Interference in communication and interaction with others can be the source of many problems for both client and family. Often, the client refuses to admit or may be unaware of his impaired hearing. Irritability is common because of the difficulty in understanding speech. The loss of clarity of speech in clients with sensorineural hearing loss is most frustrating. The client may hear what is said but cannot understand it. Withdrawal, suspicion, loss of self-

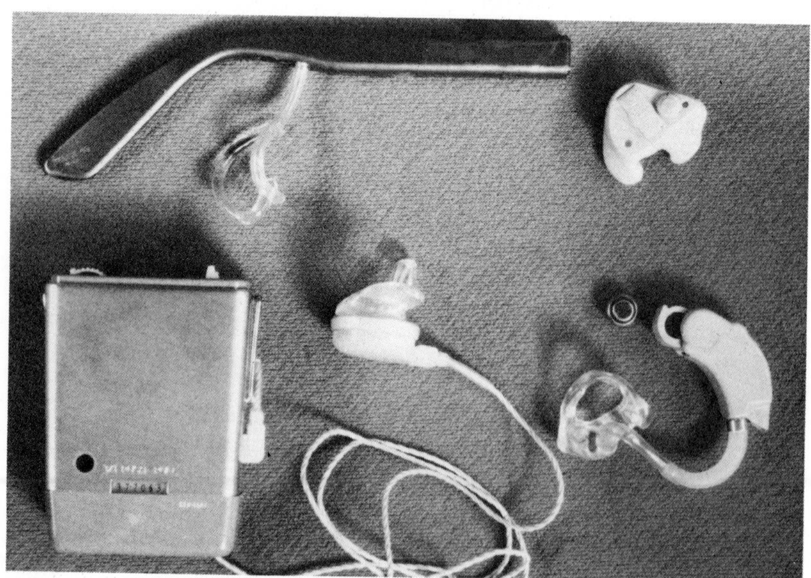

Figure 15-13 Types of hearing aids. At the top is the earpiece of glasses with battery and clear plastic mold, that fits the external auditory meatus. On the left is the battery pack worn on the body. The behind-the-ear model and in-the-auditory-meatus model are to the right.

Table 15-21

Care of a Hearing Aid

1. The hearing aid should be stored in a dry, cool place when not being used.
2. The battery should be disconnected or removed when the hearing aid is not in use.
3. Only a month's supply of batteries should be purchased at one time. (Battery life averages one week in average use.)
4. The earmold should be cleaned at least once a week.
5. A clogged eartip can be cleaned with a toothpick or pipe cleaner.

From Christina C. Clark and Gretchen C. Mills, "Communicating with Hearing Impaired Elderly Adults," *Gerontological Nurse,* **5**(3) (May/June 1979).

Table 15-22

Communicating with the Client Who Has Impaired Hearing

Nonverbal aids

Draw attention by hand movements
Have light on face
Avoid covering mouth or face with hands
Avoid chewing, eating, smoking while talking
Maintain eye contact
Avoid distracting environments
Avoid careless expression that the client may misinterpret
Use touch
Move close to better ear
Avoid light behind speaker

Verbal aids

Speak normally, slowly
Do not overexaggerate facial expression
Do not overenunciate
Use simple sentences
Rephrase sentence, use different words
Write name or difficult words
Avoid shouting

Observe client for understanding by

Attention, facial expression
Appropriate response
Accurately repeating information

esteem, and insecurity are common reactions to hearing loss. Irritability is common because of the intenseness with which the client must listen to hear others. Withdrawal, loss of self-esteem, and insecurity are common reactions.

Rehabilitation of the client with impaired hearing

It is important that the client with a suspected hearing loss have a hearing assessment by a qualified audiologist. If a hearing aid is indicated, it should be fitted by an audiologist or a speech and hearing specialist. There are four types of aids available—the body-worn aid, the eyeglasses style, the behind-the-ear style, and an in-the-ear style—each with advantages and disadvantages (Fig. 15-13). Client acceptance of a hearing aid may present a real problem. The nurse needs to be prepared to give careful instruction on its use and maintenance and to assist the client during the period of adjustment.

Initially, the hearing aid should be worn for short periods of time (15 to 30 minutes). This time can be gradually increased as the client adjusts to the increase in sound and learns to filter out environmental noise.[52] The nurse should assure the client and family that nervousness is not unusual during the period of adjustment. Table 15-21 summarizes care of a hearing aid.

Speech reading can be helpful in increasing communication. It allows for approximately 40 percent understanding of the spoken word. In speech reading, many words will look alike to the client; for example, "rabbit" and "woman." If the client wears glasses, they should be used to facilitate speech reading. The nurse can help the client by using and teaching verbal and nonverbal communication techniques (Table 15-22). The hearing aid should go with the client if he goes to other departments in the hospital or to surgery.

Case Study / Cataract extraction

Mr. O., a 62-year-old lawyer, has been admitted to the hospital for cataract extraction O.S. He noticed a gradual decrease in visual acuity O.S. and complained of glare, especially when in bright lights.

Visual acuity O.S. 20/80, O.D. 20/40 with correction (bifocal lens). Biomicroscopic examination revealed a nuclear cataract O.S. Small cataract O.D.

Preoperative orders included: Atropine 1% gtts ṫ O.S., h.s. and in a.m.
Neosporin ophthalmic gtts ṫ O.S., h.s. and in a.m.
Phenylephrine 10% gtts ṫ O.S. Cyclopentolate 2% gtts T O.S. The preop gtts ÷ q 15 min x 4 or 3
Valium 10 mgm PO with small amount of water on call to surgery
NPO after midnight

The surgery was performed under local anesthesia. The lens was removed intact (intracapsular). A peripheral iridectomy was also performed. Mr. O. returned to his room with an eyepad and a metal shield O.S.

Discussion Questions:

1. Explain the reasons for Mr. O.'s symptoms.
2. Why were the above preoperative eye medications given? What are the actions of each?
3. Why was a peripheral iridectomy performed?
4. Would Mr. O. be able to fill out his menu after surgery without his glasses? He will not use glasses until shield is removed.
5. What precautions would need to be taken with the operative eye?
6. What will vision of O.S. be when the patch is removed?
7. Once the eye is healed, Mr. O. may have glasses or an extended wear contact lens. Which will provide the best vision for him?
8. What signs should the client be aware of indicating complications?

REVIEW QUESTIONS

The number of the question corresponds to the same numbered objective at the beginning of the chapter.

1. Causes of myopia include
   a. short eyeball
   b. flat cornea
   c. excessive refractive power of lens
   d. increased intraocular pressure

2. All the following actions may be helpful for the client who has decreased blinking because of nonfunction of a facial nerve (cranial nerve VII) *except*
   a. bilateral patches
   b. lubricant eyedrops instilled frequently
   c. increased moisture in the environment
   d. securely placed eyepad to close eyelid during sleep
   e. closing lid manually when eye feels dry

3. The client who is experiencing a retinal detachment (rhegmatogenous) may complain of all the following *except*
   a. curtain over part of field
   b. increase of floaters
   c. halo around bright lights
   d. flashing lights for a short period of time
   e. unable to wipe dark spots in visual field away

4. Health maintenance and promotion of the ear include all *except*
   a. obtaining rubella titers on all women of childbearing age
   b. wearing ear protectors with noise levels above 70 dB
   c. monitoring environmental noise levels
   d. monitoring hearing on clients receiving ototoxic drugs

5. Postoperatively, the client who has had cataract extraction will need to
   a. stay in bed for several days
   b. wear an eye shield for 1 month, especially at night
   c. receive narcotics for 24 to 48 hours for pain
   d. have an immediate fitting with prescription glasses

6. Pilocarpine eyedrops
   a. dilate the pupil
   b. constrict the pupil
   c. decrease the flow of aqueous humor
   d. relax iris sphincter muscle

7. Characteristics of serous otitis media include
   a. purulent drainage
   b. dilation of eustachian tube
   c. perforated eardrum
   d. retracted eardrum

8. The client who has a sensorineural hearing loss will
   a. hear words as muffled
   b. hear better in a noisy environment
   c. speak softly
   d. have better bone conduction than air conduction

9. The least expensive contact lens as far as cost, equipment, and follow-up care is the
   a. soft lens
   b. hard lens
   c. gas-permeable lens
   d. extended wear lens

10. When communicating with a hearing-impaired client, it is helpful to
    a. increase voice pitch
    b. have light behind the speaker
    c. increase enunciation
    d. avoid hands to face

REFERENCES

1. Operational Research Department, National Society to Prevent Blindness, *Vision Problems in the U.S., Facts and Figures, Diabetic Retinopathy,* National Society to Prevent Blindness, 1980.
2. Operational Research Department, National Society to Prevent Blindness, *Vision Problems in the U.S., Highlights,* National Society to Prevent Blindness, p. 8, 1980.
3. Ibid., p. 11.
4. Ibid., p. 10.
5. Ibid., p. 14.
6. The 1977 Report of the National Advisory Eye Council, *Vision Research: A National Plan, 1978–1982,* vol. 1, Summary, U.S. Department of Health, Education and Welfare, Public Health Service, National Institutes of Health, DHEW Publication No. (NIH) 78–1258, p. 53.
7. Ibid., p. 53.
8. R. A. Moses, "Accommodation," chap. 11 in *Adler's Physiology of the Eye: Clinical Application,* 7th ed., R. A. Moses (ed.), The C. V. Mosby Company, St. Louis, 1981, p. 328.

9. *Contact Lenses,* part one, *Consumer Reports* **45**(5):289 (1980).
10. Ibid., p. 288.
11. W. H. Saunders, W. H. Havener, C. F. Keith, and G. Havener, *Nursing Care in Eye, Ear, Nose and Throat Disorders,* 4th ed., The C. V. Mosby Company, St. Louis, pp. 101–103, 1978.
12. D. Vaughn and T. Asbury, *General Ophthalmology,* 9th ed., Lange Medical Publications, Los Altos, 1980, p. 47.
13. The 1977 Report of the National Advisory Eye Council, vol. I, op. cit., p. 71.
14. M. Grayson, *Diseases of the Cornea,* The C. V. Mosby Company, St. Louis, 1979, pp. 142–146.
15. Ibid., pp. 148–149.
16. Ibid., pp. 150–160.
17. Vaughn, op. cit., pp. 65–66.
18. Grayson, op. cit., p. 60.
19. Vaughn, op. cit., p. 94.
20. Ibid., p. 55.
21. Grayson, op. cit., p. 60.
22. G. A. Peyman, D. R. Sanders, and M. F. Golberg, *Advances in Uveal Surgery, Vitreous Surgery and the Treatment of Endophthalmitis,* Appleton-Century-Crofts, New York, 1975, pp. 218–219.
23. The 1977 Report of The National Advisory Council, vol. I, op. cit., p. 70.
24. J. H. King and J. A. C. Wadsworth, *An Atlas of Ophthalmic Surgery,* 3d ed., J. B. Lippincott Company, Philadelphia, 1981, p. 274.
25. The 1977 Report of the National Advisory Committee, vol. I, op. cit., pp. 84–85.
26. Ibid., pp. 90–91.
27. *Contact Lenses,* part two, *Consumer Reports* **45**(5):288 (1980).
28. The 1977 Report of the National Advisory Committee, vol. I, op. cit., p. 95.
29. Ibid., p. 58.
30. W. H. Havener, *Synopsis of Ophthalmology,* 5th ed., The C. V. Mosby Company, St. Louis, 1979, p. 463.
31. The 1977 Report of the National Advisory Council, vol. I, op. cit., p. 51.
32. M. Yanoff, "Diabetes Mellitus," chap. 5 in *Ocular Pathology Update,* D. H. Nicholson (ed.), Masson Publishing U.S.A. Inc., New York, 1980, p. 93.
33. R. Machemer and T. M. Aabery, *Vitrectomy,* 2d ed., Grune and Stratton, New York, 1979, pp. 16–18.
34. Vaughn, op. cit., p. 150.
35. The 1977 Report of the National Advisory Council, vol. I, op. cit., p. 97.
36. J. T. Wilensky, "Glaucoma: The Scope of the Problem," chap. I in *Glaucoma: Contemporary International Concepts,* J. G. Bellows (ed.), Masson Publishing U.S.A. Inc., New York, 1979, pp. 1–2.
37. J. E. Cairns, "Trabeculectomy," chap. 24 in *Glaucoma: Contemporary International Concepts,* J. G. Bellows (ed.), Masson Publishing U.S.A. Inc., New York, 1979, p. 376.
38. S. A. Obstbaum and M. A. Galin, "Primary Angle Closure Glaucoma," chap. 14 in *Glaucoma: Contemporary International Concepts,* J. G. Bellows (ed.), Masson Publishing U.S.A. Inc., New York, 1979, p. 208.
39. D. A. Sackett, "The Magnitude of Compliance and Noncompliance," chap. 2 in *Compliance with Therapeutic Regimens*, D. L. Sackett and R. B. Haynes (eds.), Johns Hopkins University Press, Baltimore, 1976, pp. 16–17.
40. Operational Research Department, National Society to Prevent Blindness, *Vision Problems in the U.S.: Highlights,* pp. 4–6.
41. Ibid., p. 7.
42. W. W. Deatsch, "Ear, Nose and Throat," chap. 5 in *Current Medical Diagnosis and Treatment*, M. A. Krupp and M. J. Chatton (eds.), Lange Publishing Co., Los Altos, Ca., 1980, p. 97.
43. Saunders et al., op. cit., pp. 385–388.
44. G. Larsen, "Removing Cerumen with a Water Pik," *Am J Nurs,* **76**:264–265 (February 1976).
45. G. L. Adams, L. R. Boies, Jr., and M. M. Paparella, *Boies' Fundamentals of Otolaryngology,* 5th ed., W. B. Saunders Company, Philadelphia, 1978, p. 224.
46. D. D. DeWeese and W. H. Saunders, *Textbook of Otolaryngology,* 5th ed., The C. V. Mosby Company, St. Louis, 1977, p. 385.
47. J. Sataloff, R. T. Sataloff, and L. A. Vassallo, *Hearing Loss,* 2d ed., J. B. Lippincott Company, Philadelphia, 1980, p. 252.
48. L. A. Harker and B. F. McCabe, "Ménière's Disease and Other Peripheral Labyrinthine Disorders," chap. 41 in *Otolaryngology,* vol. 2, 2d ed., M. M. Paparella, and D. A. Shumriek (eds.), W. B. Saunders Company, Philadelphia, 1980, p. 1878.
49. Saunders et al., op. cit., p. 477.
50. J. F. Mauer and R. R. Rupp, *Hearing and Aging: Tactics for Prevention,* Grune and Stratton, New York, 1979, p. 17.
51. J. H. McCartney and G. Nadler, "How to Help Your Patient Cope with Hearing Loss," *Geriatrics,* **69,** March 1979.
52. C. C. Clark and G. C. Mills, "Communicating with Hearing Impaired Elderly Adults," *J Gerontological Nurs,* **5**(3) (May/June 1979).

Chapter 16

NURSING ASSESSMENT
Integumentary System

Idolia Cox Collier

Learning Objectives

1. Describe the structures and functions of the integumentary system.
2. Describe the significant subjective and objective data related to the integumentary system that should be obtained from a client.
3. Describe specific assessments to be made during the physical examination of the skin and appendages.
4. Explain the critical components for describing a lesion.
5. Describe the appropriate techniques used in the physical assessment of the integumentary system.
6. Explain the normal variants of aging and black skin.
7. Differentiate normal from common abnormal findings of a physical assessment of the integumentary system.
8. Describe the purpose, significance of results, and nursing responsibilities of diagnostic studies of the integumentary system.

The integumentary system is composed of the skin, hair, nails, and glands (sebaceous, apocrine, and eccrine). The skin is further divided into three layers: the epidermis, dermis, and subcutaneous layers (Fig. 16-1).

STRUCTURES OF THE SKIN AND APPENDAGES

Epidermis

The *epidermis* is the thin, avascular outermost layer of the skin. It is nourished by diffusion from blood vessels in the dermis and returns waste products in this same manner. The two main types of cells of the epidermis are melanocytes and keratinocytes.

Melanocytes are scattered throughout the basal layer of the epidermis. They produce melanin, a pigment which shields the deeper structures of the skin from sunlight. All races have basically the same number of melanocytes. The wide range of skin colors is due to the size and distribution of the melanosomes produced by the melanocytes.

Keratinocytes develop from cells in the basal layer of the epidermis. As the keratinocytes mature and make their way to the skin surface (stratum corneum of the epidermis), they flatten, dehydrate, and become keratinized. The upward movement of keratinocytes from the basement membrane to the stratum corneum takes about 14 days. The sloughing of the stratum corneum takes an additional 14 to 30 days. If dead cells fall off too rapidly, the skin will appear thin, eroded, or atrophic. If new cells are forming faster than old cells are shed, the skin becomes scaly and thickened. Deviations in this cycle account for many dermatologic problems.

This chapter was reviewed by Bernadette M. Forget, Clinical Nurse Specialist, Department of Dermatology, Yale University School of Medicine, New Haven, Connecticut.

Dermis

The dermis is the layer beneath the epidermis. It is primarily composed of fibrils of collagen. In addition, there are blood vessels, nerves, lymphatics, hair follicles, and sebaceous and sweat glands. Collagen, water, and a gellike ground substance serve to support the structures of the epidermis and dermis. Collagen is responsible for the mechanical strength of the skin.

Subcutaneous Layer

The *subcutaneous layer,* or hypodermis, is constructed of loose connective tissue and fat cells. This layer gives substance to the skin and is like the dermis except for the presence of fat cells. The anatomic distribution of the subcutaneous layer is a secondary sex characteristic. The subcutaneous layer acts as absorber and insulator for the body.

Epidermal Appendages

Appendages of the skin include the hair, nails, and glands (apocrine, eccrine, and sebaceous). These originate from the epidermal layer although they are anatomically located in both the epidermis and dermis. Hair and nails are specialized keratin that becomes dry and firm. The growth of *hair* (Fig. 16-1)

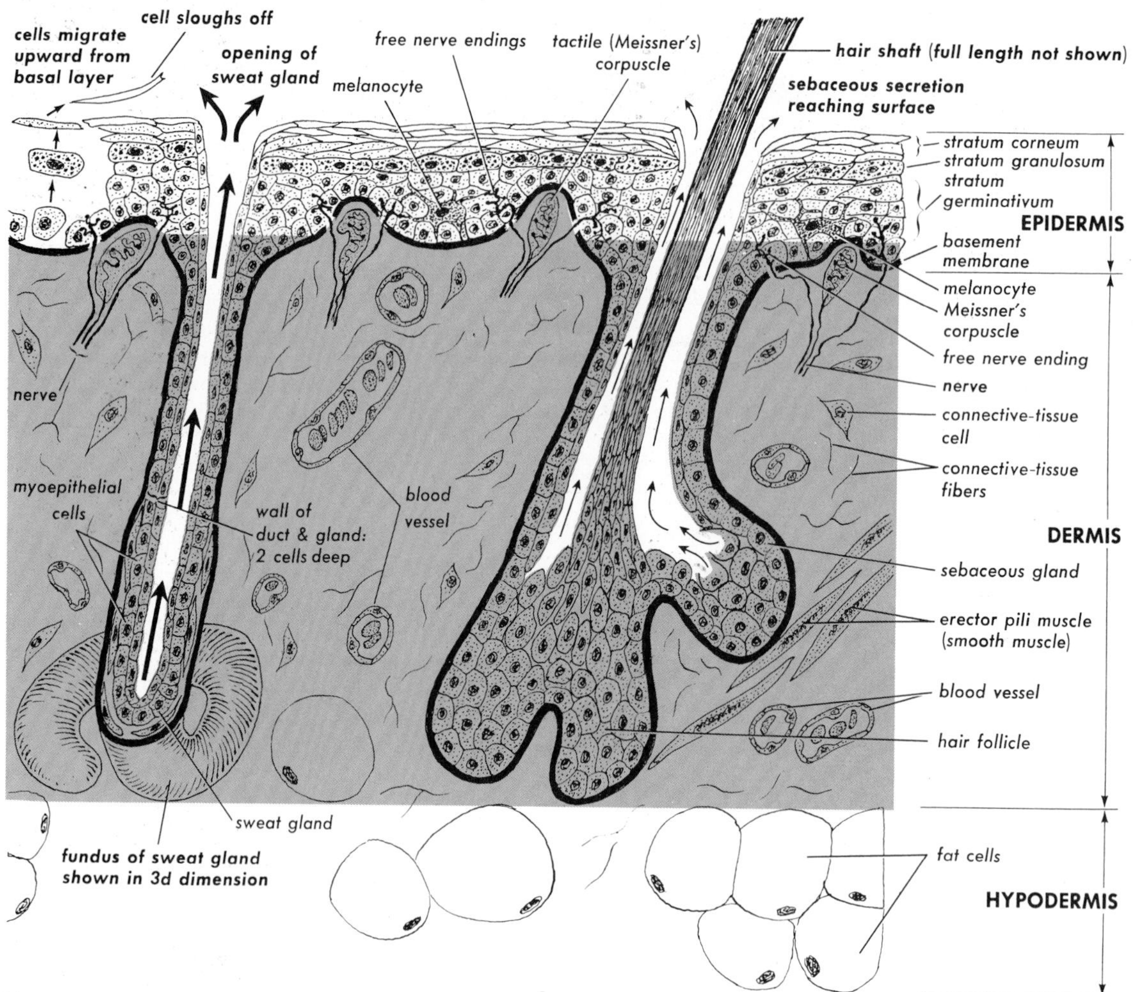

Figure 16-1 Cross section of the skin (diagrammatic). *(From E. Reith, B. Breidenbach, and M. Lorenc, Textbook of Anatomy and Physiology, 2d ed. New York, McGraw-Hill Book Company, 1978. Used by permission of the publisher.)*

occurs in several phases. Each hair goes through a resting (telogen), growth (anagen), and an atrophy (catagen) phase. A scattered pattern of phases keeps the numbers of hairs relatively constant. Chemical, mechanical, or psychological factors can convert all hair to the atrophy phase, resulting in baldness. There are no hair follicles on the palms or soles. No new hair-producing structures develop after birth. Scalp hair grows about 1 cm per month.

Nails grow from the nail matrix which is usually hidden by skin at the base of the nail (Fig. 16-2). Nails can be injured by direct trauma and are subject to the same problems as the skin.

Glands—sebaceous, apocrine, and eccrine glands—complete the epidermal or accessory appendages. The *sebaceous glands* secrete sebum, a complex lipid mixture which is emptied into the hair shaft. These glands are dependent on the male hormone, androgen, to initiate and continue production. Sebaceous glands are present on all areas of the skin except the palms, soles, and dorsa of the feet. They are most numerous and largest on the face, scalp, upper chest, and back.

Apocrine glands secrete an odorless fluid from the hair shaft which produces a distinctive body odor when acted upon by bacteria normally present on the skin. These glands are found in the axillae, anogenital area, nipples, and periumbilical areas. There is no known useful purpose for these glands. Apocrine glands become functional at puberty, atrophy with

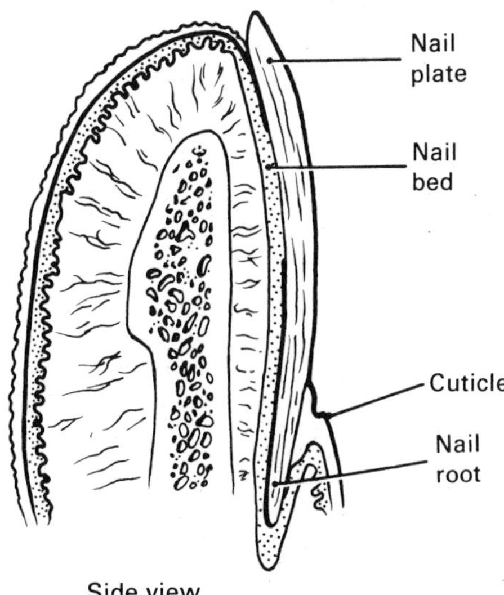

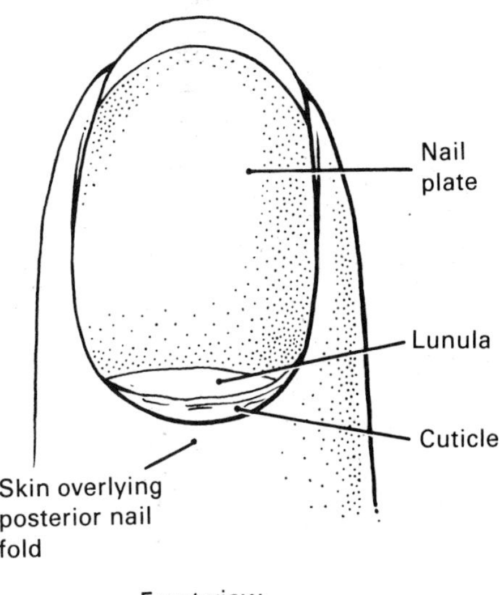

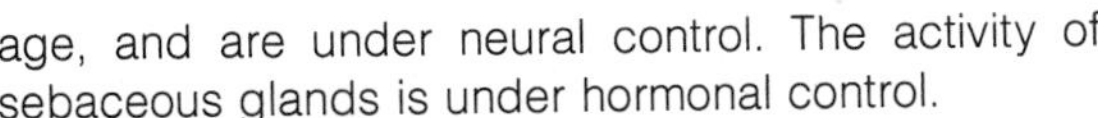
Figure 16-2 Structure of a nail.

age, and are under neural control. The activity of sebaceous glands is under hormonal control.

Eccrine (sweat) *glands* are stimulated by heat and emotional stress. They are located all over the body, especially on the forehead, palms, and soles. Eccrine glands secrete sweat to the surface of the body via the sweat duct. They function in the heat-regulating activities of the skin.

FUNCTIONS OF THE SKIN

The primary function of the skin is *protection* of the underlying tissue by acting as a surface barrier to the external environment. The skin also protects by preventing excessive loss of water, preventing mechanical trauma, and inhibiting bacterial invasion.

The skin is the major receptor for general *sensation.* The nerve endings within the skin supply information related to pain, touch, pressure, and temperature to the brain. The skin controls *heat regulation* by its ability to respond to internal and external temperature variations by vasoconstriction or vasodilation. Coincidental to heat regulation is the skin's function of *excretion.* Between 600 to 900 mL of water is lost daily through insensible perspiration.

The fat of the subcutaneous layer *insulates* the body as well as functions in the *activation of vitamin D.* The *esthetic* functions of the skin include the mirroring of emotions as well as displaying the individual identity of a person. Since it is almost a complete barrier, the skin plays a minimal role in absorption.

ASSESSMENT OF THE INTEGUMENTARY SYSTEM

The assessment of the skin begins at the initial contact with the client and continues throughout the examination. Specific areas of the skin are examined while examining other areas of the body unless the chief complaint is a dermatologic problem. A general statement about the skin would be recorded (Table 16-1) and specific problems would be noted under the appropriate system. In addition to investigating a problem according to criteria presented in Chap. 3, several specific questions are important to ask if a skin problem is present:[1]

1. How long have you had this problem?
2. Does it itch or bother you?
3. How does it bother you?

Subjective Data: The History

Past medical history

Past medical history would indicate the reasons for scars related to trauma or surgery. Specific major illnesses which could have dermatologic implications include collagen, renal, and hepatic diseases. A careful medication history is important, especially in relation to vitamins, steroids, hormones, and antimetabolites. Any food, drug, or contact allergy and the specific pattern of allergic reaction would be recorded.

Table 16-1
Recording the Normal Physical Assessment of the Integumentary System

Skin pink and warm; good turgor; no petechiae, purpura, lesions, or excoriations.
Nails pink, round, and mobile with 160 angle.
Hair shiny and full.
Amount and distribution of hair appropriate for age and sex.
No flaking of the scalp.

Family history

The client should be questioned about a family history of diabetes, blood dyscrasias, allergic disorders, cancer, or specific dermatologic problems. Many congenital or familial problems such as sickle-cell anemia have skin manifestations as the primary or secondary problem. Often, these conditions are rare. Ask the client if such problems are present in any member of the family. It is often helpful to ask, "Has anyone in your family ever had this same problem with their skin?"

Social and personal history

The unique identity and lifestyle of a client often affect the skin. Advancing *age* brings anticipated changes to the skin. Wrinkling and coolness result from a loss of subcutaneous fat. Decreased blood flow to the skin produces a thickening of fingernails and toenails and a loss of hair.

Hygiene practices and use of cosmetics should be investigated carefully. Specific brand names that are used should be recorded. A *diet history* would reveal the adequacy of nutrients essential to healthy skin such as vitamins A, D, E, C, dietary fat, and protein. Food allergies should be elicited. The client should be questioned regarding exposure to irritants, the sun, unusual cold, or unhygienic conditions related to his recreation or occupation. Exercise and sleep practices should be investigated. The client should be encouraged to express the personal and emotional implication of a dermatologic problem.

Review of systems

The client would be specifically questioned about any past problems such as rashes, lumps, itching, dryness, lesions, ecchymoses, masses, or specific changes in the hair or nails. If the client admits to any of these problems, specific characteristics of the symptom would need to be obtained.

Objective Data: The Physical Examination

General principles of the assessment of the skin are:[2]

1. Have a good source of light, preferably daylight.
2. Be systematic and proceed from head to toe.
3. Compare symmetrical parts.
4. Examine lesions individually.
5. Use the metric system for measurements.
6. Use appropriate terminology and nomenclature when reporting or recording.

Inspection (Table 16-2)

Color The skin is inspected for color, vascularity, and the presence of lesions. The critical factor when assessing skin color is change. Many skin colors which are normal for a particular client would be pathologic in another client. The color of the skin is dependent on the amount of melanin (brown), carotene (yellow), oxyhemoglobin (red), and reduced hemoglobin (bluish red) present at a particular time. The most reliable areas in which to assess color are the areas of least pigmentation such as the sclera, conjunctiva, nail beds, lips, and buccal mucosa. Activity, emotions, cigarette smoking, and edema as well as respiratory, cardiovascular, and hepatic problems can all directly affect the color of the skin.

Vascularity The skin is examined for problems related to *vascularity* such as areas of bruising, and vascular and purpuric lesions such as angioma, petechiae, or purpura. Reaction to direct pressure should be noted. If a lesion blanches on direct pressure, the redness was due to a dilated blood vessel. If the discoloration remains, it is the result of subcutaneous or intradermal bleeding which may be due to vasculitis.

Lesions If a *lesion* is found on inspection of the skin, a detailed examination must follow. *Type, color, size, distribution and grouping, location,* and *consistency* should be recorded. Characteristics of common skin lesions are described in Fig. 16-3. Measure lesions with a transparent ruler. If more than one lesion is present, record the range of sizes. *Distribution* refers to the localized or generalized occurrence of the lesion. *Grouping* or *configuration* is identified as annular (circular), linear (in a line), or clustered (a group of lesions located close together). The *location* of the lesion should be carefully described. A full-body diagram is often useful for this purpose. Accurate description is the key. Use of the appropriate terms to describe the lesion should give a mental picture of the characteristics of the lesion.

Palpation

Palpation of the skin provides information about temperature, turgor and mobility, moisture, and tex-

Table 16-2
Common Assessment Abnormalities of the Skin

Finding	Definition/Description	Possible Etiology
Alopecia	Loss of hair, may be localized or general.	Heredity, friction, rubbing, traction, trauma, infection, inflammation, chemotherapy, pregnancy, stress, emotional shock, tinea capitis.
Angioma	A form of tumor consisting of blood or lymph vessels.	Normal increase with aging, liver disease, vitamin B deficiency, pregnancy, varicose veins.
Comedo (blackheads and whiteheads)	Keratin, sebum, microorganism, and epithelial debris within a dilated follicular opening.	Acne vulgaris.
Cyanosis	Slightly bluish-gray or dark purple discoloration of the skin and mucous membranes due to presence of excessive amounts of reduced hemoglobin in capillaries.	Cardiorespiratory problems; vasoconstriction, asphyxiation, anemia, leukemia, and malignancies.
Cyst	A sac containing fluid or semisolid material.	Obstruction of a duct or gland, parasitic infection.
Ecchymosis	A large bruiselike lesion caused by collection of extravascular blood in dermis and subcutaneous tissue.	Trauma, bleeding disorders.
Erythema	Redness occurring in patches of variable size and shape.	Heat, certain drugs, alcohol, ultraviolet rays, any problem which causes dilatation of the skin.
Excoriation	Superficial excavations of epidermis.	Pruritus, trauma.
Hematoma	An extravasation of blood of sufficient size to cause a visible swelling.	Trauma, bleeding disorders.
Hirsutism	Male distribution of hair in women and children.	Abnormality of gonads or adrenal glands, decrease in estrogen levels, familial trait.
Intertrigo	Dermatitis of apposing surfaces of the skin.	Moisture, obesity, *Monilia* infections.
Jaundice	Yellow (Caucasian) or yellowish brown (black) discoloration of the skin best observed in the sclera secondary to increased bilirubin in the blood.	Liver disease, red blood cell hemolysis, pancreatic cancer, common duct obstruction.
Keloid	Hypertrophied scar beyond margin of incision or trauma.	Genetic predisposition more common in blacks.
Lichenification	Thickening of the skin with accentuated skin markings.	Repeated scratching and irritation.
Mole (melanocytic nevus)	Benign overgrowth of melanocytes.	Defects of development. Excessive numbers tend to be familial.
Petechiae	Smaller than 1 cm discrete deposit of blood in the extravascular tissues and visible through the skin or mucous membrane.	Inflammation, marked dilatation, blood vessel trauma, blood dyscrasias which result in bleeding tendencies (e g., thrombocytopenia).
Telangiectasia	Visibly dilated superficial cutaneous small blood vessels commonly found on face and thighs.	Aging, acne, sun exposure, alcohol, liver failure, steroid medication, irradiation, certain systemic diseases, and skin tumors. Normal variant.
Tenting	Failure of skin to immediately return to normal position following gentle pinching.	Aging, dehydration, cachexia.
Varicosity	Increased prominence of superficial veins.	Interruption of venous return (e g., tumor, incompetent valves, inflammation).
Vitiligo	Acquired loss of melanin resulting in white, depigmented areas.	Genetic disease of unknown etiology. Occasionally from chemical agents.

Primary

Macule

A flat, circumscribed area of color change in the skin without surface elevation
Size: 1 mm to 2 cm

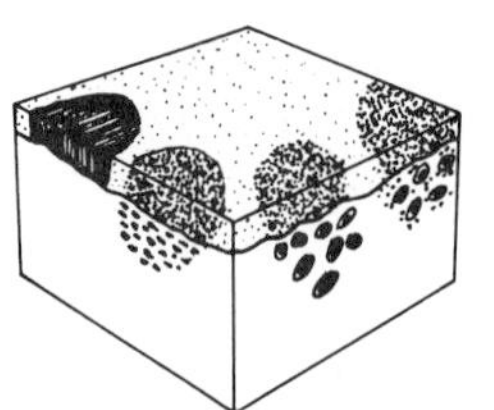

Papule

A circumscribed solid and elevated lesion
Size: 1 mm to 1 cm

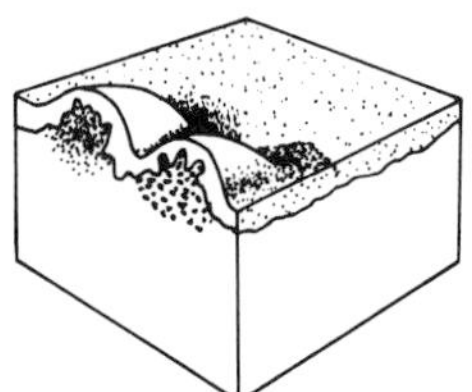

Nodule

A solid, elevated lesion extending deeper in the dermis
Size: 1 to 2cm

Tumor

A solid mass larger than a nodule
Size: Larger than 2 cm

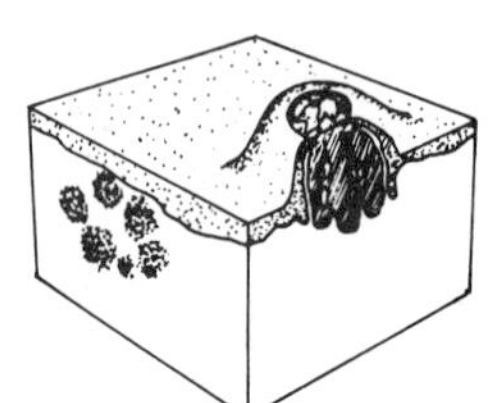

Cyst

A papule or nodule containing fluid or viscous material
Size: 1 mm or larger

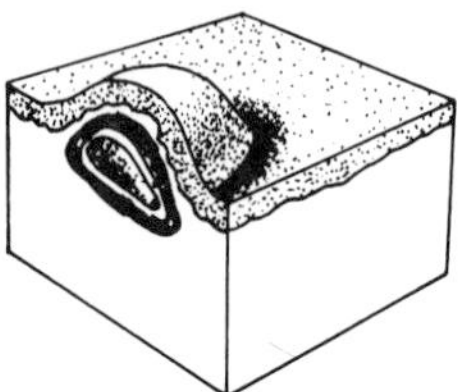

Wheal

A clustering of papular-type lesions creating an edematous plaque
Size: 1 mm to several cm

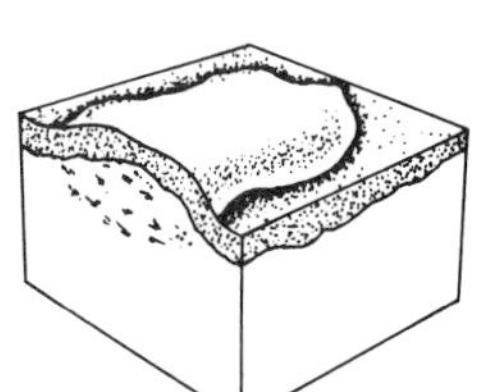

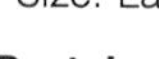

Vesicle

A bulging, small, sharply defined lesion filled with serous fluid or blood
Size: Smaller than 1 cm

Bulla

Larger than a vesicle
Size: Larger than 1 cm

Pustule

A vesicle or bulla filled with pus
Size: 1 mm to 1 cm

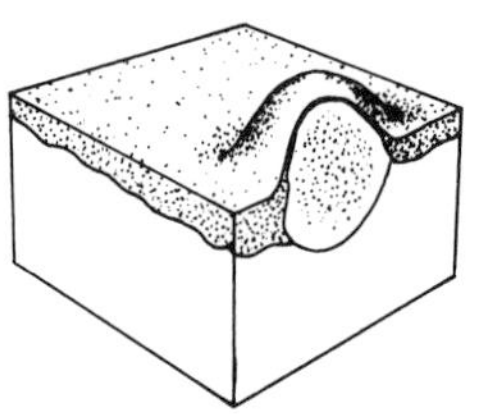

Secondary

Crust

Dried serum, blood, pus, or sebum which forms on the surface of any vesicle or pustule lesion when it ruptures

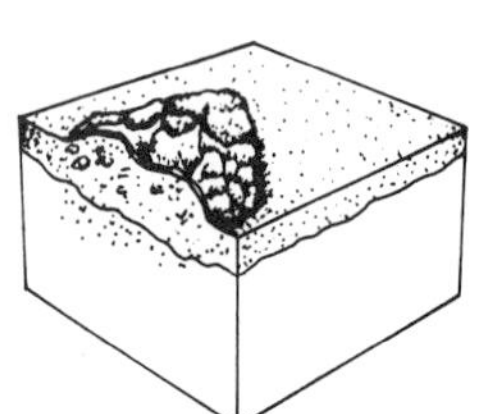

Scale

Dried fragments of sloughed, dead epidermis

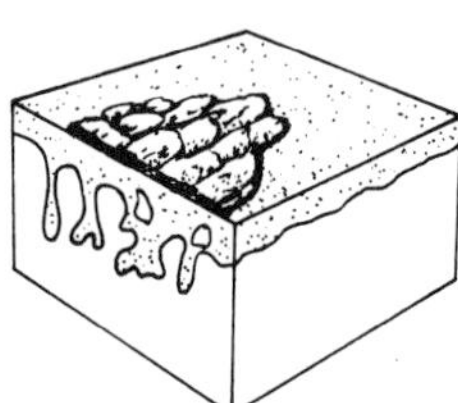

Excoriation

Scratch or scrape of original lesion

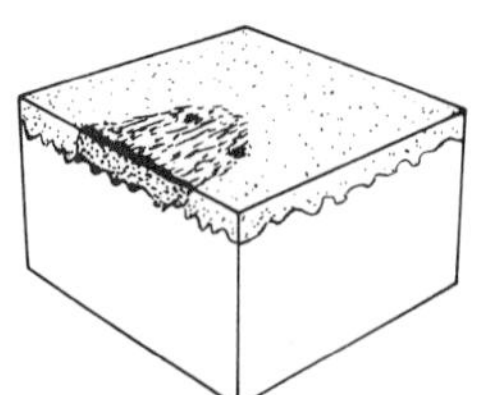

Fissure

A crack in the skin, usually through the dermis

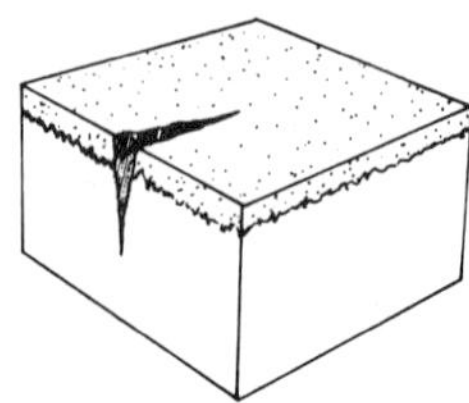

Figure 16-3 Characteristics of common skin lesions. *(Adapted from M. Kinney et al., AACN's Clinical Reference for Critical Care Nursing, McGraw-Hill Book Company, New York, 1981. Used by permission of the publisher.)*

Secondary (continued)

Ulcer	**Scar**
A depressed lesion resulting from loss of epidermis and the papillary layer of the dermis 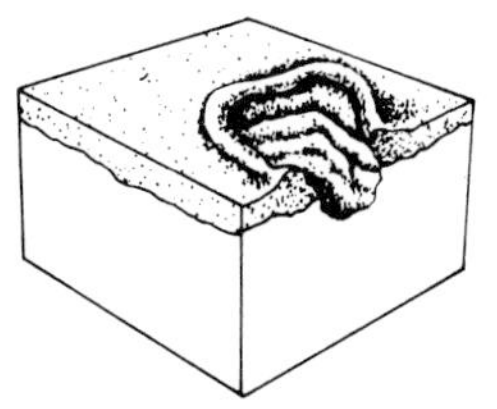	Replacement of destroyed tissue by fibrous tissue or excessive collagen 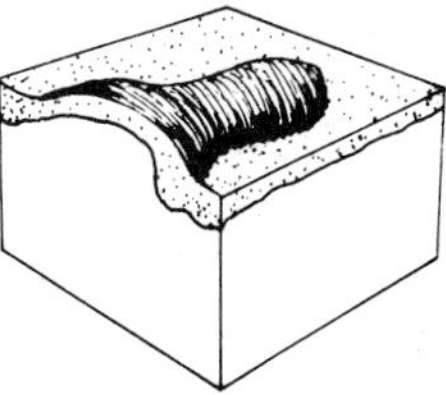

Figure 16-3 (Continued)

ture. *Temperature* of the skin is best assessed by palpating the upper lip, palms, and forehead with the back of the hands. The temperature of the skin increases when blood flow to the dermis is increased. There will be a localized increase with burns and local inflammation. A generalized increase in temperature will result from fever. A decreased body temperature will be noted due to shock, chilling, and emotional trauma.

Turgor and mobility refer to the elasticity of the skin. There is a loss of turgor with dehydration and aging. Emotional tension increases turgor. The examiner assesses turgor by gently pinching an area of skin together. The best area to use for assessing turgor is the skin over the sternum. Skin with good turgor will immediately return to its original position.

Moisture of the skin is the dampness or dryness of the skin. Moisture increases in intertriginous (two surfaces approximate) areas. The amount of moisture present on the skin varies with the temperature of the environment, with muscular activity, and body temperature. Skin dries with age due to a decrease in the activity of the sebaceous glands. Decreased humidity also causes dry skin.

Texture refers to the fineness or coarseness of the skin. Extremes of either type of texture can reflect local trauma or systemic disease. Increased coarseness is often work-related and should not be mistaken for pathology.

Normal Variants of Physical Assessment of the Skin

Aging skin

The rate of age-related skin changes is influenced by the person's history of sun exposure, hygiene practices, heredity, nutrition, and general state of health. Exposure to ultraviolet rays hastens skin aging. In addition, a decrease in the level of sex hormones and atrophy of the skin and epidermal appendages correlate with the look of aging.

Dry, thin skin, increased capillary permeability, the presence of lentigines (brown spots), and seborrheic keratoses all confirm advancing age. Poor nutrition is a contributing factor due to a decrease in protein, calories, and vitamins. The collagen stiffens, elastic fibers degenerate, and the amount of subcutaneous tissue decreases. The end result is wrinkling (Fig. 16-4). Blood vessels close to the skin give a ruddy appearance. Sweating diminishes as eccrine glands become less active. The rate of hair and nail

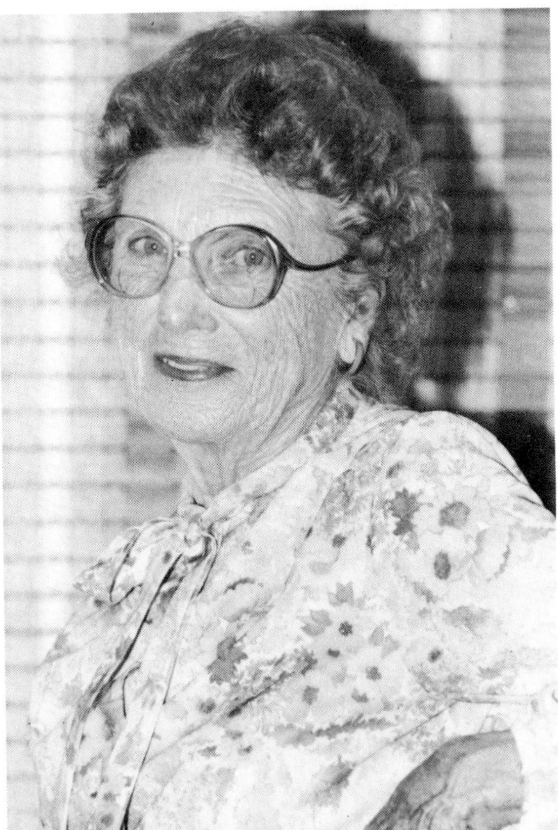

Figure 16-4 A person with wrinkled skin.

Table 16-3
Diagnostic Studies of the Integumentary System

Study	Description and Purpose	Nursing Responsibility
Biopsy Punch Excisional or incisional Shave	Removal of a small sample of skin for microscopic examination to determine diagnosis of a specific problem.	Obtain consent form. Inform client local anesthetic will be used. Instruct client to keep biopsied area dry until healed. Instruct client to contact physician for biopsy results.
Microscopic tests		
Potassium hydroxide (KOH)	Examination of hair, scales, or nails for hyphae of fungus infection. Put on glass slide and 10–40% concentration of KOH added.	Client instruction regarding purpose of test. Preparation of slide.
Tzanck test (Wright's, Giemsa's, and Papanicolaou stain)	Examination of fluid and cells from vesicles or bullae to diagnose herpes virus, herpes zoster, and chicken pox. Specimen put on slide, stained and examined microscopically for multinucleated giant cells.	Inform client of purpose of test. Sterile collection of fluid for examination.
Miscellaneous Wood's light	Examination of skin with long-wave ultraviolet light causes specific substances to fluoresce (e.g., *Pseudomonas,* erythrasma, fungus infections, vitiligo.	Inform client of purpose of exam. Inform client it is not painful.

production decreases due to atrophy of the involved structures. Vitamin deficiencies can cause dry, thin hair that has a tendency to fall out.

Black skin

The degree of color of black-skinned people is genetically determined. The dark skin color results from the reflection of light as it strikes the underlying skin pigment. Increased activity of melanocytes resulting in large amounts of melanin production accounts for the darker skin color. This increased melanin forms a natural sun shield for black skin.

The structures and functions of black skin are basically no different than Caucasian skin. However, they are more difficult to assess. Practice and comparison are necessary. Less pigmented areas such as the buccal mucosa, tongue, lips, and nail beds are areas which best indicate color changes such as cyanosis or pallor. Rashes are often difficult to observe and may need to be palpated.[3]

Black skin is predisposed to certain skin conditions. These include pseudofolliculitis, keloids, and Mongolian spots. Because of the darkness of the skin of blacks, it often cannot be used as an indicator for systemic conditions (e.g., flushed skin with fever).

DIAGNOSTIC STUDIES OF THE INTEGUMENTARY SYSTEM

The main diagnostic technique related to skin problems is inspection of an individual lesion and a careful history related to the problem. If a definitive diagnosis cannot be made by inspection alone, other tests may be indicated (Table 16-3).

A biopsy of a characteristic skin lesion is a common diagnostic aid. Early lesions are usually selected for biopsy since they are most typical. A biopsy is indicated in all conditions where a malignancy is suspected or a specific diagnosis is questionable.

Incisional, excisional, and scrape or shave biopsies can be both therapeutic and diagnostic. A punch biopsy is done using a small tubular knife that looks much like a cookie cutter. This tool cuts out a small piece of tissue for microscopic examination. The size of the biopsy specimen is determined by the location of the biopsy. If the site would normally be visible, such as on the face, the smallest possible piece of tissue which would still yield accurate diagnosis is taken. Immunofluorescence, a special technique performed on the biopsy specimen, may be indicated in certain conditions such as bullous diseases or lupus erythematosus.

REVIEW QUESTIONS

The number of the question corresponds to the same numbered objective at the beginning of the chapter.

1. Melanocytes are located in the
- **a.** epidermis
- **b.** dermis
- **c.** subcutaneous layer

2. The best area to assess skin color is the
a. sternum
b. feet
c. nail beds
d. abdomen

3. Increased vascularity of the skin results in
a. blanching
b. coolness
c. erythema
d. purpura

4. Localized or generalized occurrence of a lesion refers to
a. distribution
b. configuration
c. location
d. type

5. The most important assessment technique related to the skin is
a. inspection
b. palpation
c. percussion
d. auscultation

6. Black skin is less susceptible to sunburn than lighter skin due to the presence of increased amounts of
a. melanin
b. keratin
c. stratum corneum
d. follicles

7. The most common cause of an excoriation is
a. vasoconstriction
b. pruritus
c. moisture
d. hemolysis

8. Fungal infections are diagnosed by the use of
a. Papanicolaou test
b. fluorescence
c. Giemsa's stain
d. potassium hydroxide

REFERENCES

1. T. F. Fitzpatrick et al. (eds.), *Dermatology in General Medicine,* McGraw-Hill Book Company, New York, 1979, p. 11.
2. R. D. Judge et al., *Methods of Clinical Examination: A Physiologic Approach,* 3d ed., Little, Brown and Company, Boston, 1974, p.
3. Lora Roach, "Color Changes in Dark Skin," *Nursing 77,* January 1977, p. 49.

Chapter 17

NURSING ROLE IN MANAGEMENT

Problems of the Integumentary System

Idolia Cox Collier

Learning Objectives

1. Describe health promotion and maintenance practices related to the skin.
2. Explain the etiology, clinical manifestations, and medical and nursing management of common acute dermatologic problems.
3. Describe the psychological and physiologic effects of chronic dermatologic conditions.
4. Explain the etiology, clinical manifestations, and management of malignant dermatologic disorders.
5. Explain the etiology, clinical manifestations, and management of bacterial, viral, and fungal infections of the integument.
6. Explain the etiology, clinical manifestations, and management of infestations and bites.
7. Explain the etiology, clinical manifestations, and management of dermatologic disorders related to allergies.
8. Explain the etiology, clinical manifestations, and management related to benign dermatologic disorders.
9. Describe the dermatologic manifestations of common systemic diseases.
10. Explain the indications and nursing management related to plastic surgery and skin grafts.

Problems of the skin are often difficult to manage due to the visibility of this organ. Although clothing and cosmetics can disguise or cover some skin problems, many problems cannot be hidden so easily. The emotional impact of skin problems often is more serious than the skin problem itself. For instance, acne is little more than a nuisance disease in relation to systemic health. However, to the adolescent attempting to establish his own identity, it can be a barrier to establishing a peer group and pleasant social outlets.

A dichotomy often exists between the actual seriousness of a skin problem and the emotional impact of the problem. The medical and nursing management of integumentary problems is presented before specific problems are discussed. These general considerations common to many dermatologic problems apply to many specific diseases as well.

MEDICAL AND NURSING MANAGEMENT

Health Promotion and Maintenance

Health promotion and maintenance practices related to problems of the skin often parallel health practices appropriate for general good health. The skin reflects both physical and psychological well-being. Specific health promotion and maintenance areas appropriate to good skin health include avoidance of environmental hazards, adequate rest and exercise, proper hygiene and nutrition, and cautious use of self-treatment.

Environmental hazards

Sun Many people are unaware that the cumulative effects of years of sun exposure are irreversible. The ultraviolet rays of the sun cause degenerative changes in the dermis which result in premature aging due to loss of elasticity, and thinning, wrinkling, and drying of the skin. Prolonged and repeated sun exposure is a major factor in precancerous and cancerous lesions.

Nurses should be strong advocates of moderation in sun exposure. Vitamin D_3 is produced in the skin and is necessary for vitamin D synthesis. However, only a few minutes of sun on small areas of the body is adequate to meet this need.[1] Specific wavelengths of the sun (Table 17-1) stimulate epithelial turnover. Tanning is the body's defense against further sunburn and is caused by increased production of melanin. The turnover time of the skin is shortened and results in peeling. Fair-skinned people should be especially cautious about excessive sun exposure since they have smaller amounts of the natural protection afforded by melanin.

Sunscreens block out UV-B wavelengths. The most effective sunscreens contain para-aminobenzoic acid (PABA). The Food and Drug Administration has rated popular sunscreen products. The higher the sun

This chapter was reviewed by Bernadette M. Forget, Clinical Nurse Specialist, Department of Dermatology, Yale University School of Medicine, New Haven, Connecticut.

Table 17-1
Wavelengths of the Sun and Effect on Skin

Wavelength	Nanometer Rating	Effect
Short (UV-C)	Below 290	Does not reach earth Blocked by atmosphere
Middle (UV-B)	280–315	Causes sunburn and cumulative effect of sun damage
Long (UV-A)	315–400	Undetermined effect on skin except for photosensitive client where sunburn results

protective factor (SPF), the greater the screening effect. Consumers need to select the sunscreen most appropriate for their needs. Reapplication is necessary after swimming and every 1 to 2 hours if exercising or perspiring. Directions accompanying specific products should be read as application time prior to exposure varies according to the product.

The nurse can also inform the client about other means of protection from the damaging effects of the sun such as wearing a large-brimmed hat, longsleeved shirts, and carrying an umbrella. Clients need to know that the rays of the sun are most dangerous between 10 A.M. and 2 P.M. standard time or 11 A.M. and 3 P.M. daylight time regardless of the latitude. Even on overcast days a serious sunburn can occur.

Certain medications potentiate the effect of the sun, even with brief exposure. These photosensitizing medications include tetracyclines, some diuretics or hypoglycemic agents, sulfonamides, phenothiazines, barbiturates, certain topical anesthetics, perfume, and psoralens.[2] The chemicals in these medications absorb light and release intense heat and fluorescence that harm cells and tissues.

Irritants and Allergens The nurse needs to reinforce the need to avoid exposure to known irritants (e.g., ammonia, harsh detergents). In addition, allergens which have troubled the client in the past or are known to produce problems upon exposure (e.g., poison ivy) should be avoided. Many irritants and allergens have a cumulative effect, producing more serious dermatoses upon repeated exposure. Aside from costly and time-consuming desensitization, the most obvious strategy is avoidance.

Radiation Although most radiology departments are extremely cautious in protecting both themselves and clients from the effects of excessive radiation, the nurse should help the client make intelligent decisions about radiologic procedures. X-rays can be invaluable in both diagnosis and therapy, but indiscriminate use can cause serious side effects to the skin as well as other body processes.

Rest and Sleep

Rest and sleep are important health promotion considerations in relation to the skin. Although the exact effects of sleep are not known, it is thought to be restorative.[3] Slow-wave sleep is believed to have physically restorative functions.[4] Rest reduces the threshold of itching and protects the skin from the effects of scratching.[5]

Exercise

Exercise increases circulation and dilates the blood vessels. In addition to the healthy glow produced by exercise, the psychological effects can also improve one's appearance and mental outlook. However, caution needs to be used to avoid overexposure to heat, cold, and sun during outdoor exercise.

Hygiene

Hygienic practices should match the skin type, lifestyle, and culture of the client. The person with oily skin will need to cleanse the skin more often with a drying agent than will the person with dry skin. Dry skin might benefit from superfatted soaps and measures to increase moisture such as moisturizers applied to the skin.

The normally acidic skin (pH 4.2 to 5.6) and perspiration protect against bacterial overgrowth. Most soaps are alkaline with degreasing power and cause a neutralization of the skin surface and loss of protection. More neutral soaps and the avoidance of very hot water and vigorous rubbing can noticeably decrease local irritation and inflammation.

In general, the skin and hair should be washed often enough to remove excess oil and excretions as well as to prevent odor. Older people should avoid the use of harsh soaps and shampoos and decrease the frequency of bathing.

Nutrition

A well-balanced diet adequate in the basic four food groups can produce healthy skin, hair, and nails. Certain elements are particulary essential to good skin health, however. These include:

1. *Vitamin A*—essential for maintenance of normal cell structure in epithelial surfaces.
2. *Vitamin B complex*—essential to complex metabolic functions. Deficiencies of niacin and pyridoxine

manifest with dermatologic symptoms such as erythema, bullae, and seborrhea-like lesions.

3. *Vitamin C (ascorbic acid)*—essential for connective tissue formation and normal wound healing. Absence causes damage to the dermis.
4. *Vitamin K*—deficiency interferes with normal prothrombin synthesis in the liver which can lead to cutaneous purpura.
5. *Protein*—adequate supply of protein is necessary for cell synthesis.
6. *Unsaturated fatty acids*—specifically linoleic and arachidonic acids. Necessary to maintain the function and integrity of cellular and subcellular membranes in tissue metabolism.

Obesity has an adverse effect on the skin. The increased subcutaneous fat deposits can lead to stretching and overheating. Overheating causes an increase in sweating which has an adverse effect on normal or inflamed skin. Obesity also has an influence on the development of type II diabetes with its concomitant skin complications (see Chap. 41).

Self-treatment

The nurse needs to increase client awareness of the dangers of self-diagnosis and treatment. The wide variety of over-the-counter skin preparations can indeed confuse the consumer. General instructions which the nurse can discuss with the client would stress the duration of the treatment and the need to follow package directions closely. Skin problems are generally slow to develop symptoms and slow to resolve. If the package insert of an over-the-counter drug says its use should not exceed 7 days, this warning should be heeded. If the directions say to apply twice daily, the urge to double the dose and hasten the cure must be avoided. If any systemic signs of inflammation or extension of the skin problem develop, such as increased number of lesions or increased erythema or swelling, self-care should be stopped and the help of a professional enlisted.

General Measures to Treat Acute Dermatologic Problems

Diagnostic

A careful history is of prime importance in diagnosing skin problems. The clinician must be skilled at detecting any evidence which could lead to the cause of the extraordinary number of skin problems. Following a careful history and examination, individual lesions are inspected. Based on the history, physical examination, and appropriate diagnostic tests, either a medical, surgical, or combination therapy will be planned.

Medical and pharmacologic management

There are many treatment methods used in dermatology. Some are disease-specific, while others work for unknown reasons. Advances in this field have brought relief to many previously chronic, untreatable conditions. Many of the specific medical treatments require specialized equipment and are usually reserved for use by the dermatologist. Pharmacologic treatments are prescribed by many clinicians. Their effectiveness can often be related to the base (or vehicle) in which the medication is prepared. Table 17-2 summarizes the common agents used as bases for topical preparations and their therapeutic considerations.

Phototherapy The use of the sun as a source of ultraviolet wavelengths (UVL) causes erythema, desquamation, and pigmentation. It also has bactericidal effects. Ultraviolet light causes a temporary suppression of basal cell mitosis followed by a rebound increase in cell turnover.[6] Certain photosensitizing drugs such as psoralens enhance the effect of ultraviolet light in the UV-A spectrum (Table 17-1). Conditions which are responsive to effective wavelengths with or without drugs include acne vulgaris, psoriasis, and vitiligo.[7]

Ultraviolet light in the specific wavelengths can be produced artificially. Therapeutic doses of UV-A and UV-B can be measured and used to treat spectrum-specific diseases (Fig. 17-1). Prolonged exposure to UVL can result in basal or squamous cell carcinoma.

Table 17-2
Common Bases for Topical Medications

Agent	Therapeutic Considerations
Powder	Promotes dryness. Increases evaporation. Area may absorb moisture. Common base for antifungal preparations.
Lotion	Suspension of insoluble powders in water. When water evaporates it cools, dries, and leaves film of powder. Useful in subacute pruritic eruptions.
Cream	Emulsions of oil and water. Most common base for topical medications. Lubricates and protects.
Ointment	Oil with differing amounts of water added in suspension. Lubricates and protects. Petrolatum most common.
Paste	Mixture of powder and ointment. Not occlusive. Absorbs moisture, so use is limited to where some drying effect is needed.

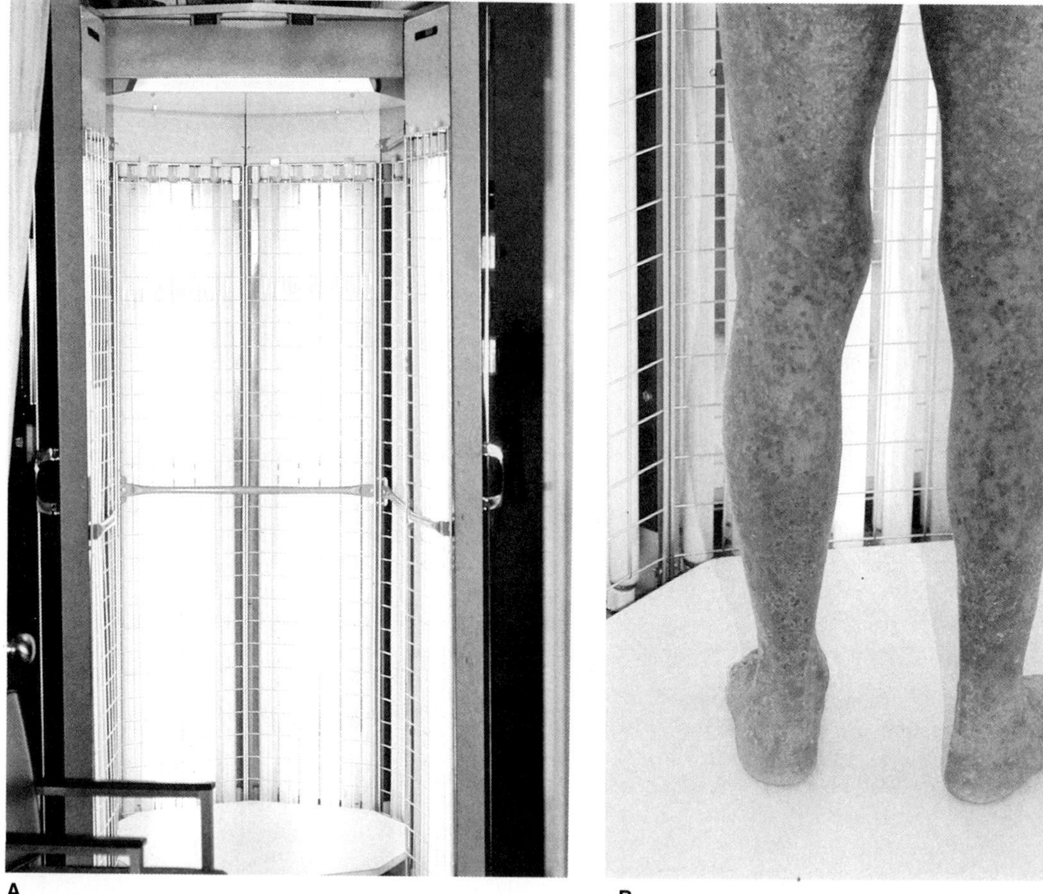

Figure 17-1 Phototherapy is a method for treating spectrum-specific diseases. The client's eyes must be protected during the phototherapy session. (*a*) PUVA unit. (*b*) Client with psoriasis undergoing PUVA therapy. *(Courtesy of William Chapman, M.D.)*

Radiation The use of radiation for the treatment of dermatologic conditions has decreased since the Second World War. Better treatments are now available for most benign conditions. However, radiation is useful in the treatment of cutaneous malignancies, especially basal cell carcinomas.

Radiation to cutaneous malignancies is a painless, relatively inexpensive treatment which produces minimal damage to surrounding tissue. It is a particularly effective treatment for the aged, the debilitated, and for areas such as the nose, eyelids, and canthal areas. Careful shielding is necessary to prevent ocular lens damage if the irradiated area is around the eyes.

Radiation therapy usually requires multiple visits. It is most effective on lesions above the neck. It produces permanent alopecia of the irradiated areas. Adverse effects include telangiectasia, atrophy, hyperpigmentation, depigmentation, ulceration, chronic radiodermatitis, and squamous cell carcinoma (see Chap. 11).

Antibiotics Antibiotics are used both topically and systemically to treat dermatologic problems. The use of topical antibiotics is controversial and reflects the philosophy of the care provider as to their efficacy. If used, topical antibiotics should be applied to clean debrided skin. Occlusive dressings should not be used. Common topical antibiotics include bacitracin (used with gram-positive organisms), and neomycin and gentamicin (used with *Staphylococcus* and most gram-negative organisms).

If signs of systemic infection are present, a systemic antibiotic should be used. Systemic antibiotics (most often synthetic penicillins and erythromycin) are useful in bacterial infections and acne vulgaris. They are particularly useful in erysipelas, cellulitis, carbuncles, and severe infected eczema. Culture of the lesion should guide the choice of antibiotic. Many of the more popular systemic antibiotics are not used topically due to the danger of allergic contact dermatitis.

Corticosteroids Over one-half of the prescriptions written by dermatologists are for glucocorticoids. Glucocorticoids are amazingly effective in treating a wide variety of dermatologic conditions and can be used topically, intralesionally, or systemically.

Topical glucocorticoids are used for their local anti-inflammatory action as well as for their antipruritic effects. Attempts to diagnose a lesion should be made before a steroid preparation is applied, since steroids will mask the clinical picture. Steroids are useful in the treatment of atopic eczema, seborrheic dermatitis, and psoriasis. With prolonged use the more potent steroid formulations such as Halog® cream, Lidex® cream, and other fluoridated steroid creams can cause adrenal suppression, especially if occlusion is used.

Fluoridated corticosteroids are more effective than nonfluoridated corticosteroids. However, fluoridated corticosteroids produce side effects including atrophy of the skin, rosacea eruptions, striae, severe exacerbations of acne vulgaris, and dermatophyte infections when their use is prolonged. Rebound dermatitis is not uncommon when therapy is ceased. Nonfluoridated corticosteroids such as hydrocortisone and triamcinolone act more slowly, but can be used for a longer period of time without producing serious side effects. Nonfluoridated corticosteroids are used on the face and intertriginous areas.

Intralesional glucocorticoids are injected directly into or just beneath the lesion. This method provides a reservoir of medication whose effect will last several weeks to months. Intralesional injection is particularly useful in psoriasis, lupus erythematosus, cystic acne, and eczema. A 2.5 mg/mL suspension of triamcinolone acetonide (Kenalog) is the most common dose for intralesional injection. A small amount is injected into the site of each lesion.

Systemic glucocorticoids can have remarkable results in treating dermatologic conditions. However, they often have undesirable systemic effects (Chap. 42). Steroids can be administered as short-term therapy for acute conditions such as poison ivy. They may also be used for life-threatening situations such as anaphylaxis. Long-term steroid therapy for dermatologic conditions is reserved for chronic bullous diseases, severe systemic effects of collagen and immunologic responses, and as a last resort when other therapies have failed.

Antihistamines Use should be limited to conditions which exhibit urticaria, angioedema, nocturnal pruritus associated with drug reactions, and other allergic cutaneous reactions. Antihistamines block the action of histamine. Several different antihistamines may need to be tried before the satisfactory therapeutic effect is achieved. A major side effect of histamine use is sedation. The client must be warned about sedative effects, particularly when driving or operating heavy machinery.

Topical Fluorouracil (5-FU) This is a topical cytotoxic agent with selective toxicity for sun-damaged cells. It does not damage normal tissue. 5-FU is very effective in treating actinic (sun-damaged) areas on the face, but is less effective on the hands and treatment must be modified. It is not an adequate treatment for diagnosed skin cancers. If treatment is not effective, the suspicious areas should be biopsied.

Client compliance is the major problem with the use of 5-FU. The medication produces painful, ulcerated areas over the damaged skin in 4 days to 3 weeks (Fig. 17-2). Fluorouracil is a photosensitizing drug so the client must be instructed to avoid sunlight during treatment.

Disease-Specific Drugs Many dermatologic conditions are treated by specific drug preparations.

Surgical management

Certain dermatologic conditions are best treated by surgical methods. Common surgical procedures are discussed below.

Electrodesiccation and Electrocoagulation These procedures convert electrical energy to heat via the tip of an electrode. This results in tissue being destroyed by burning. The major uses of this type of therapy is point coagulation of bleeding vessels and destroying small telangiectasia. Electrodesiccation usually refers to more superficial destruction. Electrocoagulation refers to a deeper effect with better hemostasis and an increased possibility of scarring.

The major disadvantages to electrodesiccation and electrocoagulation are scarring, inability to control depth of burning, and lack of a specimen to biopsy.

Curettage Curettage refers to the removal of tissue using an instrument with a circular cutting edge attached to a handle. The tissue is scooped away. Although the curette is not strong enough to cut normal skin, it is very useful in removing many types of small skin tumors such as warts, keratoses, and small

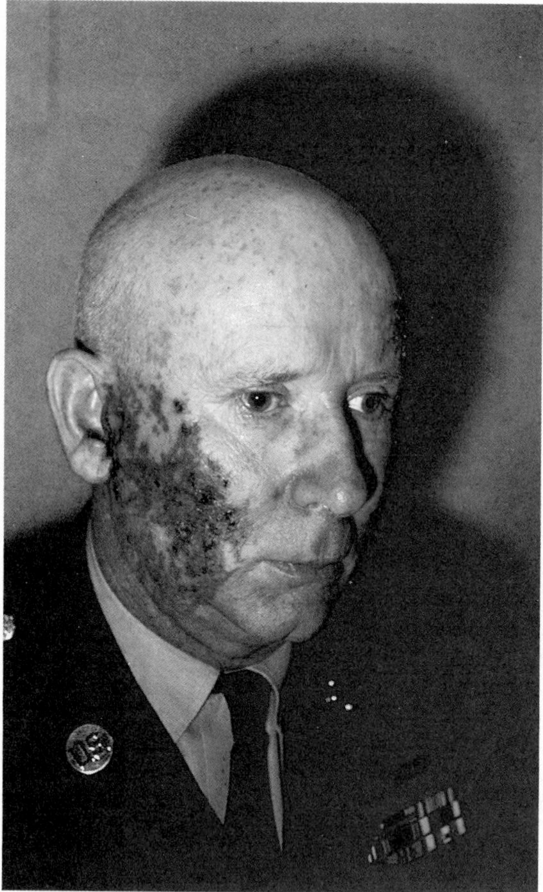

Figure 17-2 Client being treated with 5-FU. *(Courtesy of Larry Becker, M.D.)*

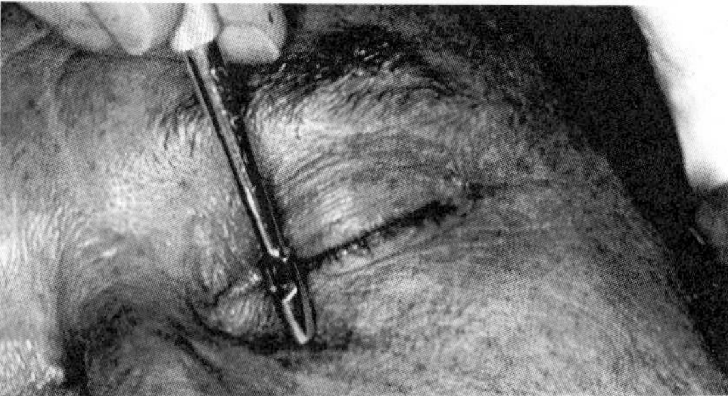

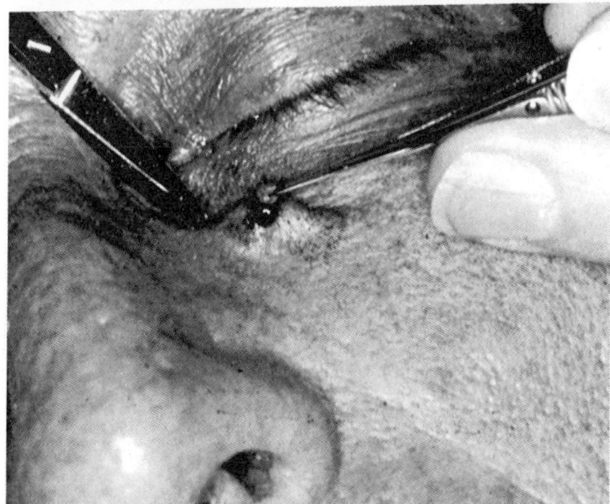

Figure 17-3 Punch biopsy for pathology specimen. *(G. D. Weinstein, Skin Cancer, Recognition and Treatment, Famous Teachings in Modern Medicine, Medcom, Inc., New York, 1973.)*

basal and squamous cell cancers. The area to be curetted is anesthetized before the treatment. Hemostasis is obtained by using ferric tincture chloride, Monsel's solution, or gelatin foam.

Punch biopsy This is a very common dermatologic procedure used to obtain a tissue sample for histologic study or to remove small lesions. Its use is generally reserved for lesions under 0.5 cm. Prior to local anesthesia, the area to be biopsied is outlined so landmarks will not be obscured. The biopsy punch cores out a small cylinder of skin when its sharp edge is twirled between the fingers. The core of skin is snipped from the subcutaneous fat and appropriately preserved for examination (Fig. 17-3). Hemostasis is usually by gelatin foam packing to reduce scarring. Suturing is generally not required. Multiple small biopsies can help delineate the borders of a basal cell carcinoma.

Cryosurgery Skin lesions are destroyed by freezing. Topical or intralesional liquid nitrogen is the most common agent used for cryosurgery. Although the exact mechanism is not clearly understood, the use of liquid nitrogen causes death or destruction of the treated skin.

Liquid nitrogen is a cold, liquefied gas with a temperature of −196°C (−320.8°F). In order for cells to be destroyed, the agent used must go to at least −20°C (−4°F). Liquid nitrogen can explode if kept in an air-tight container.

Liquid nitrogen can be applied topically by direct application or with the appropriate container directly onto the benign or precancerous lesion. The lesion will first become swollen and red. It may blister. Next, a scab forms and falls off in 1 to 3 weeks. The skin lesion will be sloughed along with the scar. Growth of new skin follows. It is a useful treatment for acne, warts, cutaneous tags, keloids, seborrheic keratoses, actinic keratoses, and many other less common skin conditions.

When used for a neoplasm, a microthermocouple needle is inserted to measure tissue temperature at placed depth. Liquid nitrogen is then applied topically until the desired temperature is measured. Local anesthesia is usually required. Cryosurgery is inexpensive, rapid, and leaves minimal scarring. The major disadvantage to this treatment is lack of a tissue specimen.

Excision This procedure should be considered if the lesion involves the dermis. Complete closure of the excised area usually results in good cosmetic results. Fair cosmetic results can be obtained by partial closure, but cosmetic reconstruction may be required. This method is particularly suited to problems on the face. To minimize scarring, hemostasis can be obtained by direct pressure or by packing with absorbable material.

Acute nursing intervention

Dermatologic conditions are not common reasons for hospitalizations. Although it may not be the primary reason for hospitalization, many clients will exhibit concurrent skin problems while hospitalized which warrant nursing intervention and client education.

If the nursing care is in an acute-care setting, the nurse will be both doing and teaching the appropriate therapeutic treatments. If the client is in an outpatient setting, the nursing focus would be on client education with opportunities provided for demonstration and redemonstration. Subsequent visits would provide the opportunity to evaluate client understanding and treatment effectiveness.

Nursing interventions related to dermatologic conditions fall into broad categories. They are applicable to many skin problems in both inpatient and outpatient settings. Table 17-3 discusses nursing care for a client with open lesions.

Wet Dressings The use of wet dressings is a common dermatologic procedure used to dry exudative lesions, relieve itching, and reduce erythema. In addition, wet dressings will increase penetration of topical medications, promote sleep by relieving discomfort, and enhance removal of scales, crusts, and exudate.[8] Materials such as thin sheeting or gauze sponges can be used for dressings. Ingenuity is sometimes necessary to cover odd-shaped parts of the body.

The prescribed dressing is put in fresh solution, held until it is no longer dripping, and applied to the affected area (Fig. 17-4). Occlusion of the dressing with plastic or additional material is rarely done due to maceration (wrinkling) of the skin. The dressing may be rewet and reapplied every 5 minutes, moistened regularly with a syringe, or applied thickly enough to keep it wet for up to 6 hours. Most commonly, the wet dressings are applied for 15 minutes four to six times per day. If the skin appears macerated, the dressings should be discontinued for 2 to 3 hours. The client should be protected from discomfort and chilling by protecting linens and bedclothes with protective pads or plastic.

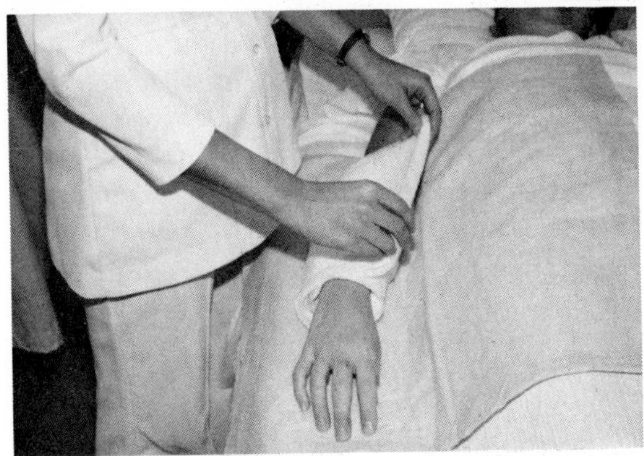

Figure 17-4 Wet dressings are a common dermatologic procedure. They are particularly effective in drying moist, oozing wounds.

Common solutions used for wet dressings are Burow's solution (aluminum sulfate and calcium acetate) and potassium permanganate. Potassium permanganate must be completely dissolved before use since the crystals may burn the skin. This solution must be freshly prepared in order to maintain its oxidative properties. If potassium permanganate solution turns brown, it should be discarded and fresh solution made. The best solution to use on the eyes is plain cool water.

Wet dressings do not need to be sterile. The best temperature to use is tepid to cool to cause vasoconstriction and decrease itching. These treatments are excellent ways to remove the scabs left by the collection of debris at a wound site. Although the scab initially is protective, it later retards healing and feeds bacteria.

Baths Baths are appropriate when large body areas need to be treated. They also have sedative and antipruritic effects. Some medications such as oilated oatmeal, potassium permanganate, and sodium bicarbonate can be added directly to the bath water. The tub should be half full of water. Both the bath water and the prescribed solution should be at a comfortable temperature for the client. The client can soak for 15 to 20 minutes 3 to 4 times a day, depending on the

Table 17-3

Nursing Care Plan for a Client with Open Lesions

Client Problem	Expected Outcome	Nursing Intervention
Exudate	Drying and healing of lesion.	Apply wet dressings to dry, clean skin to collect exudate and debride. Avoid maceration of skin by removing dressings at intervals. Keep lesions exposed to air when wet dressings not used.
Pruritus	Minimal to no pruritus.	Decrease environmental irritants (e.g., heat, scratchy covering). Use topical, systemic, or local anti-inflammatory medications. Provide a cool environment. Use cool, wet dressings, soaks, and baths. Administer sedatives and tranquilizer as necessary. Keep client's nails trimmed short.
Secondary infection	No evidence of secondary infection.	Teach client measures to prevent scratching. Give good skin hygiene. Use of careful handwashing by care givers.
Dry skin	Moist, well-lubricated skin.	Use of nonirritating moisturizing agents. Give adequate fluid (2000–3000 mL/day) and fat intake. Avoid frequent bathing.
Poor self-image	Realistic hope for resolution of open lesions.	Discuss situation with client in open, accepting manner. Do not show shock or disgust at the site of the lesions. Touch the client as would be appropriate to the situation.
Inappropriate use of self-medication	Seek medical help if self-medication ineffective or condition worsens.	Question client's knowledge of cause of lesion and knowledge of medication being used. Advise client to carefully follow guidelines for over-the-counter medication. Inform client of signs indicating a worsening of condition such as increase in number of lesions, increase in erythema and swelling, and fever.
Scarring and lichenification	Minimal scarring. No lichenification.	Prevent secondary infections by careful handwashing and good hygiene. Instruct client in care of lesions and medication regimen. Advise client on interventions possible to remove or minimize scarring such as dermabrasion and chemical peel. Continue measures to prevent itching.
Frustration over chronicity of problem	Remain hopeful regarding cessation of new lesions.	Encourage client to continue with medical regimen. Counsel client regarding healthy life practices. Advise client on skillful use of cosmetics.
Social isolation	Seek outside activities and friends.	Encourage socialization in client's interest areas. Arrange psychiatric referral if indicated. Teach skillful use of cosmetics, cover-up agents, and clothing.

severity of the dermatitis and the client's discomfort. It is important to stress to the client that the skin not be towel dried but allowed to air dry when possible. If this is too chilling for the client, the skin should be gently patted to prevent increasing irritation and inflammation. The addition of oils makes the bathtub extremely slippery and should be avoided. If oils are used in the tub, the utmost caution must be used in transferring clients to prevent disastrous accidents. An equally effective means of lubricating the skin is to apply a moisturizer to gently dried skin directly after the bath. This helps to retain the moisture in the hydrated cells.

Topical Medications These medications are generally best applied with the ungloved hand. This method allows the nurse to palpate the lesion and assess progress of the treatment. A thin layer of ointment and cream should be applied to clean skin and spread evenly. An alternate method is to apply the medication directly onto the dressings. However, pastes are designed to protect the affected area. They should be applied thickly using a tongue blade or gloved hand. Draining lesions and lesions with greasy medication can be covered with a light dressing to prevent soiling clothes.

Control of Pruritus Pruritus (itching) can be caused by almost any physical or chemical stimulus to the skin such as drugs, insects, and dry skin. The annoying sensation of itching is probably an automatic attempt to remove the offending agent from the skin and thus relieve the itch. The itch sensation is carried by the same nonmyelinated nerve fibers as pain. If the epidermis is damaged or absent, the sensation will be felt as pain rather than an itch.

The itch-scratch-itch cycle needs to be broken to prevent excoriation and eventual lichenification. Certain circumstances make itching worse. Anything that causes vasodilation such as heat or rubbing should be avoided. Dryness of the skin lowers the itch threshold and increases the itch sensation. Any internal or external factors which decrease blood flow to an area increase itching.

Measures which the nurse can do or teach the client to perform to break the itch cycle should be attempted. A cool to cold environment or dressings cause vasoconstriction and decrease itching. The use of topical corticosteroids reduces inflammation and causes vasoconstriction. The itch receptors can be numbed with menthol, camphor, or phenol. Systemic use of antihistamines, tranquilizers, and sedatives can be used if necessary to provide relief to a miserable client while the underlying cause of the pruritus can be diagnosed and treated.

When wet dressings are used to relieve pruritus, they should be used in the following way. Thin, old sheets are placed in very warm water, wrung out, and placed over the pruritic area. After 10 to 15 minutes the dressing is removed and the skin allowed to air dry. A lubricant is then applied to the skin. This procedure can be repeated as necessary for comfort. Topical antipruritic medications should be applied as directed by the physician.

Preventing Spread Most skin problems are not contagious. The unnecessary use of gloves can be demoralizing to an already sensitive client. However, if in doubt, the nurse should wear gloves until a definite diagnosis has been established. The most common contagious lesions which should be easily recognized by nurses include impetigo, staphylococcus pyoderms, primary chancre and secondary syphilis lesions, scabies, and pediculosis. Careful handwashing and safe disposal of soiled dressings are the best prevention of spread of skin problems.

Preventing Secondary Infections Open lesions on the skin are susceptible to invasion by other organisms. Meticulous hygiene, handwashing, and dressing changes are important to prevent secondary infections. Also, the client should be warned about scratching lesions which can cause excoriations and an entry for pathogens. The client's nails should be trimmed short to minimize trauma from scratching. Measures to decrease pruritus previously mentioned should be employed.

Specific Skin Care Nurses are often in a position to advise clients regarding care of the skin following simple dermatologic surgical procedures such as freezing and cryosurgery. In general, the healing process would include care of oozing wounds, scabs, and stitched wounds.

Oozing wounds are best treated with wet to dry dressings for debridement and an antibiotic ointment such as polymyxin B (Polysporin) or bacitracin. The ointment will inhibit infection and keep the bandage from sticking. If the bandage gets wet, simply reapply both ointment and bandage.

Initially, a *scab* should be left alone to be the protective coating for the damaged skin beneath it. Scabs should be kept dry. They can be covered during the day for cosmetic purposes, but should be exposed at night. If a scab gets wet, it should be dried gently. After a while, the scab should be removed gently after soaking to encourage healing and remove a site for bacterial growth.

A wound which required stitches is handled much like an oozing wound. The area should be covered with an adhesive bandage and an antibiotic ointment used. Stitches will generally be removed in 2 to 10 days. The client can expect some swelling and discomfort in the first 24 hours. Mild analgesics such as aspirin or acetiminophen (Tylenol) should control the discomfort. The client needs to know the manifestations of inflammation such as redness, fever, or increased pain or swelling so that he can seek professional help.

Management of chronic disorders

Psychological Effects of Chronic Dermatologic Problems The emotional toll is indeed heavy for persons who suffer from chronic skin problems such as eczema, psoriasis, and seborrheic dermatitis. The sequelae of chronic skin problems could result in employment problems with subsequent financial implication, a frail and easily damaged body image, problems with sexuality, and increasing and progressive frustration. The usual lack of systemic overt illness coupled with the visibility of the skin lesions presents a real problem to the client.

The nurse must continue to be optimistic and help

the client comply with the prescribed regimen. The client must be allowed to verbalize the "Why me?" question, even though there is no ready answer. Reinforcement of the prescribed hygiene and treatment measures is an important part of the nursing management.

Most lesions will not be harmed by the skillful use of cosmetic cover. Individual sensitivity to product ingredients must always be considered when selecting a cosmetic product.

In addition to specific skin conditions which tend to chronicity, other factors affecting the outcome of long-term dermatologic problems include skin type, history of previous attacks, family history, complications, intolerance to therapy, environmental factors, lack of adherence to the prescribed regimen, endocrine factors, and psychological factors.[9] Lesions which follow a chronic pattern often are associated with lichenification and scarring.

Physiologic Effects of Chronic Dermatologic Problems *Scarring* of old lesions may take place concurrently with continuing exudation in a chronic skin condition. When a lesion is large and deep, the edges cannot approximate and excessive amounts of keratinocytes are destroyed. The defect is filled with granulation tissue which is replaced with dense bundles of collagen. The resulting scar is permanent with loss of hair or sweat glands and decreased innervation.

Scars are pink and vascular at first. As they age they become avascular and white with increasing strength. An old scar will have 85 percent of the strength of the undamaged skin.[10] Different parts of the body scar differently. Other than the face and neck which heal fairly well due to a good blood supply, scars usually remain conspicuous.

Although there are methods to reduce or remove scars, these are usually not practical for use with chronic skin conditions. Since acute lesions are often present concurrently with the chronic lesions, the scarring would simply repeat itself. Obviously, the location of the scar is the determining factor as to its cosmetic implications. Facial scars are the most damaging psychologically since they are so visible. Again, creative use of cosmetics can do much to mask the scarring of chronic skin conditions. The best treatment is prevention of scarring by control of the problem in the acute phase.

Lichenification is another consequence of chronic skin problems. It is the thickening of skin due to proliferation of keratinocytes with accentuation of the normal markings of the skin. The resulting plaque may be uniform or irregular. The cause of lichenification is scratching or rubbing of the skin and is often associated with atopic dermatoses and pruritic conditions. Although any area of the body may be affected, the hands and forearms are common sites. Treatment of the cause of the itching is the key to prevention of lichenification. Excoriations are often evident in the thickened skin as a result of the pruritus.

The side effects of both topical and systemic long-term steroid therapy must always be considered when used to treat chronic skin conditions. The dangers of prolonged use of topical glucocorticoids are discussed earlier in this chapter. Systemic steroid therapy is discussed in Chap. 42.

SPECIFIC DERMATOLOGIC DISORDERS

Malignant Conditions of the Skin

Malignant neoplasms of the skin exhibit the characteristics of all malignant conditions (Chap. 11). However, skin malignancies are generally slow-growing. Adequate and early treatment can lead to complete cure. The visibility of skin lesions increases the likelihood of early detection and diagnosis. The presence of a lesion that persists and does not heal is highly suspicious. Evidence from the client's history related to race, chronic sun exposure, and exposure to tar and systemic arsenicals in addition to the persistent lesion is an indication for a biopsy of the lesion. A biopsy should be done before specific treatment is started to confirm the diagnosis.

Many types of skin cancer are preventable. The most common etiologic factor, chronic sun exposure, should be consciously avoided by the use of sunscreens and protective clothing. The incidence of skin cancer increases with age. Dark-skinned people are less susceptible to skin cancers due to the naturally occurring increase in melanin. Melanin is the most effective sunscreen and increases due to increased activity of melanocytes.

Basal cell epithelioma (BCE) is probably the most common human malignancy[11] (Fig. 17-5). Table 17-4 compares the most common types of skin cancers.

Infections of the Skin

Bacterial infections

The skin is covered with great numbers of microorganisms, especially bacteria. *Staphylococcus epidermidis* and diphtheroids are the most common bacteria present on the skin. The skin provides the ideal environment for bacterial growth with abundant supplies of warmth, food, and water.

Bacterial infection *(pyoderma)* occurs when the balance between the host and the microorganisms is

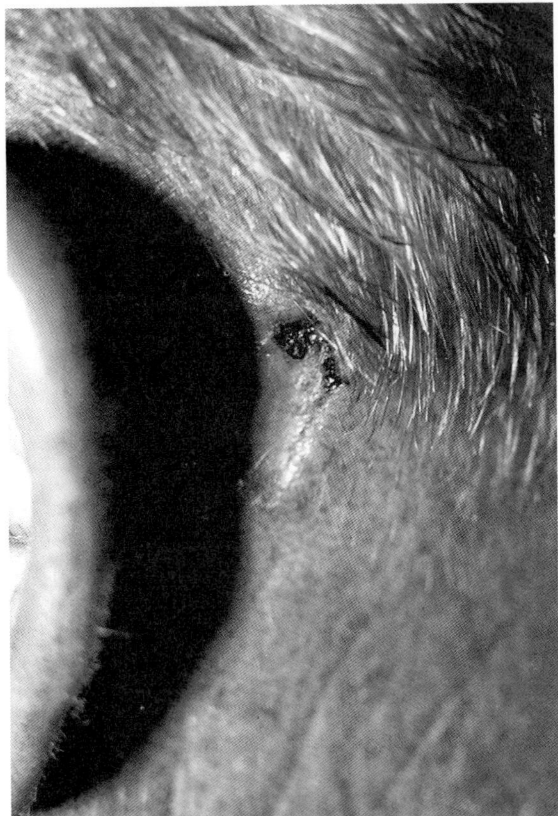

Figure 17-5 Basal cell epithelioma. Note the typical pearly border. *(Courtesy of Larry Becker, M.D.)*

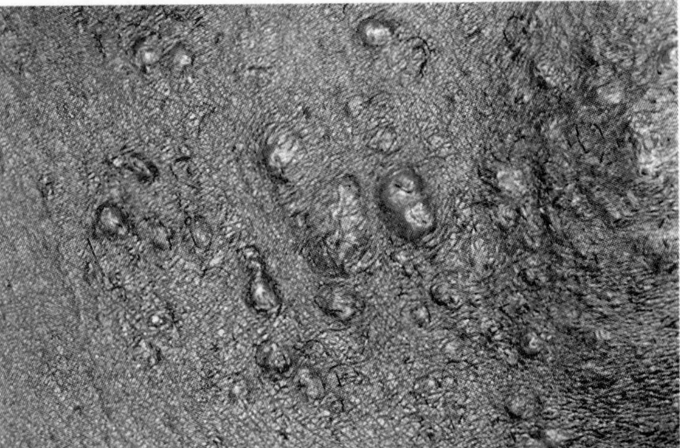

Figure 17-6 Pseudofolliculitis barbae on a black client. *(Courtesy of Larry Becker, M.D.)*

upset (Table 17-5 and Fig. 17-6). This can occur as a primary infection following a break in the skin. It can also occur as a secondary infection to already damaged skin or as a sign of a systemic disease.

Healthy people can develop bacterial skin infections. Predisposing factors such as moisture, obesity, skin disease, systemic steroids and antibiotics, chronic disease, and diabetes mellitus all increase the likelihood of infection. Good hygiene practices and general good health inhibit bacterial infections. If an infection is present, drainage is infectious. Meticulous skin hygiene is necessary to prevent spread of infection.

Viral infections

Viral infections of the skin are as difficult to treat as viral infections anywhere in the body. A virus is an ultramicroscopic organism which is an obligatory parasite. That is, it requires living cells. Viruses must go to the lower layers of the epidermis in order to replicate since the outer layers are dead cells. The stratum corneum, hair, and nails cannot be affected by viruses.

The body attempts to destroy the protein coat surrounding the core of the genetic material of the virus. The affected cell can become injured in this attempt and a lesion can result (Fig. 17-7). Lesions can also result from an inflammatory response to the viral interference with cell function and morphology (Table 17-6).

Fungal infections

Due to the huge number of identified fungi, it is almost impossible to avoid exposure to some pathologic varieties. Many fungi have valuable functions in modern society, such as in food preparation (e.g., molds, cheese) and drug synthesis (e.g., penicillin). Many fungi have serious deleterious effects as well.

The clinical characteristics of fungal infections are easily recognized (Table 17-7). Microscopic examination of the scraping of suspicious lesions in 10 to 20% KOH is an easy, inexpensive diagnostic aid. The appearance of hyphae (threadlike structures) is indicative of a fungal infection (Fig. 17-8*a* and *b*).

Dermatophytes are those fungi which cause ring-

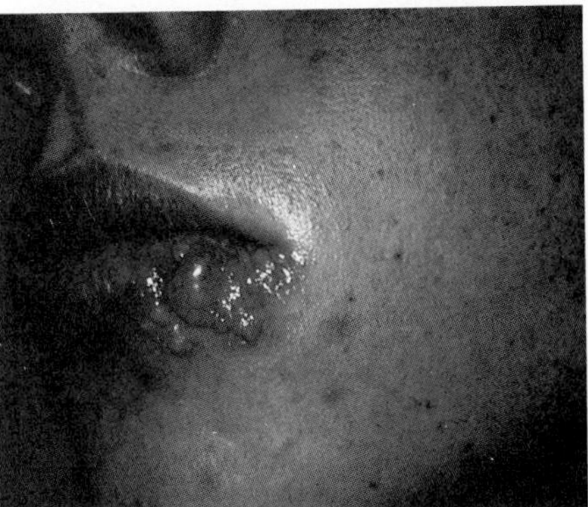

Figure 17-7 Herpesvirus on the lips. *(Courtesy of Larry Becker, M.D.)*

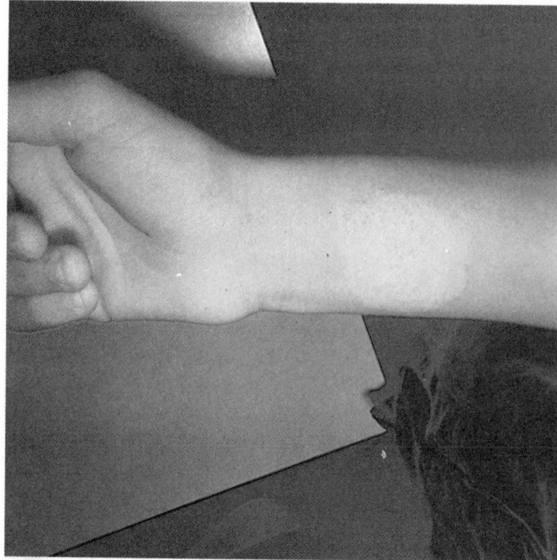

A

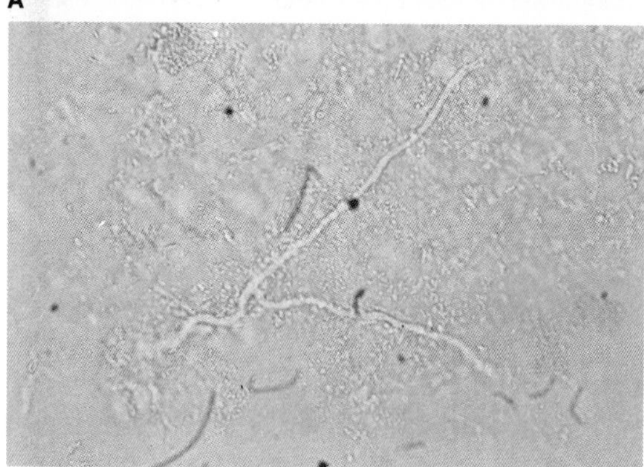

B

Figure 17-8 (*a*) Tinea corporis (ringworm). (*b*) Hyphae on slide prepared with KOH. *(Courtesy of Larry Becker, M.D.)*

worm. These are referred to as tinea. This word is followed by a word designating the location of the lesion (e.g., tinea capitis occurs on the head).

Infestations and Insect Bites

The possibilities of exposure related to insect bites and infestations is almost limitless (Table 17-8). In many instances, an allergy to the venom plays a major role in the reaction. In other cases, the clinical manifestations are due to a reaction to the eggs, feces, or body part of the invaders (Fig. 17-9). Certain individuals will react with a severe hypersensitivity (anaphylaxis) which can be life-threatening (Chap. 10).

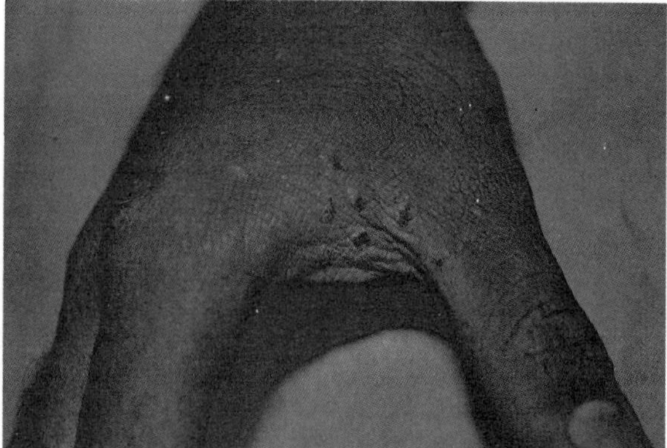

Figure 17-9 Scabies on a hand. *(Courtesy of Larry Becker, M.D.)*

Prevention of insect bites by avoidance or the use of repellants is somewhat effective. Meticulous hygiene related to personal articles, clothing, and bedding, as well as careful selection of sexual partners, can reduce the incidence of infestations.

Allergic Dermatologic Problems

Dermatologic problems associated with allergies and hypersensitivity reactions present a real challenge to the clinician. The pathophysiology related to allergic and contact dermatitis is covered in Chap. 10. Often only the most careful family history and discussion of possible offending agents will yield valuable data. The best treatment of allergic dermatitis is avoidance. The extreme pruritus of atopic dermatitis as well as its chronicity make it a frustrating problem for the client, the nurse, and the dermatologist. Table 17-9 summarizes common allergic conditions of the skin.

Benign Dermatologic Problems

Although the list of benign dermatoses is extensive, some of the most commonly seen and distressing problems have been summarized in Table 17-10.

DERMATOLOGIC MANIFESTATIONS OF SYSTEMIC DISEASES

Dermatologic manifestations of systemic disease may be either specific or nonspecific. Specific conditions display the same pathologic process in relation to the skin as the internal disease process. Nonspecific conditions do not resemble the internal problem but are helpful in establishing a diagnosis. The skilled clinician should always consider the possibility that a

Table 17-4
Malignant Conditions of the Skin

Name	Etiology and Pathogenesis	Clinical Characteristics	Treatment and Prognosis
Actinic keratoses (premalignant)	Caused by actinic (sun) damage.	Flat or slightly elevated, dry, hyperkeratotic scaly papule. Can be flat, rough, or verrucous. Adherent scale which returns when removed. Often multiple. Rough scale on red base. Often on erythematous sun-exposed areas. Increase in number with age.	Curettage, electrosurgery, cryosurgery, chemical caustics, topical application of 5-fluorouracil applied over entire area for 7–10 days. Healthy skin and other lesions not affected. No recurrence with adequate treatment. If untreated, can lead to squamous cell carcinoma.
Basal cell epithelioma	Change in basal cell. Does not mature and keratinize normally. Continues to divide as basal cells and form enlarging mass. Predisposing factors are excessive sun exposure, genetic tendency, arsenicals, x-ray irradiation, scars, and some types of nevi. Basal cells can be pigmented but do not arise in nevi.	*Nodular/ulcerative:* Small, slowly enlarging papule. Borders semitranslucent or "pearly," with overlying telangiectasia. Center erodes, ulcerates, and becomes depressed. Normal skin markings lost. *Superficial:* Erythematous, sharply defined, barely elevated multinodular plaques with varying scaling and crusting. Looks like eczema.	Excisional surgery, chemosurgery, electrosurgery, cryosurgery, x-ray therapy. 95% cure rate. Slow-growing tumor that invades local tissue. Metastasis very rare.
Squamous cell carcinoma (epidermoid carcinoma)	Occurs frequently on previously damaged skin (e.g., sun, irradiation, scar). Malignant tumor of squamous (prickle) cell of epidermis. Invades dermis, surrounding skin. May metastasize.	*Early:* Firm nodules with indistinct borders with scaling and ulceration, opaque. *Later:* Keratinization results in lesion being covered with sclae or horn. Most common on sun-exposed areas like face and hands.	Surgical removal, radiation therapy, or chemosurgery, electrodesiccation and curettage. If untreated, can metastasize to regional lymph nodes.
Malignant melanoma	Neoplastic growth of melanocytes anywhere on skin, eye, or mucous membrane. Classified according to major histologic mode of spread. Has potential for invasion and widespread metastases.	Irregular color, irregular surface, irregular border. Variegated color including red, white, blue, black, gray, brown. May be flat or elevated, eroded or ulcerated. Often under 2.5 cm in size. Most common sites: males—back, females—legs, but can occur anywhere.	Wide excision, full-thickness surgical removal. Survival rate correlates with depth of invasion. Poor prognosis unless diagnosed and treated early. Spreads by local extension, regional lymphatics, and bloodstream. Adjuvant therapy may be used following surgery if lesions greater than 0.76 mm in depth.

particular dermatosis is a clue to an internal, less obvious problem.

Certain life changes have recognized associated dermatoses. At *puberty,* male or female pattern hair growth will be evident as secondary sex characteristics. Increased apocrine gland activity can lead to body odor. The increased sebaceous gland activity stimulated by androgens can result in seborrhea and acne.

Pregnancy is characterized by physiologic skin changes including hyperpigmentation and increased perspiration. *Menopause* is often accompanied by hot flashes, increased perspiration, facial hair growth, and varying degrees of scalp hair loss. Old age often presents skin problems related to dryness, wrinkling, hyperpigmentation, and actinic changes. System-specific dermatologic manifestations of internal disorders are presented in Table 17-11.

Table 17-5
Common Bacterial Infections of the Skin

Name	Etiology and Pathogenesis	Clinical Characteristics	Treatment and Prognosis
Impetigo	Group A beta-hemolytic streptococci. Associated with poor hygiene and low socioeconomic status. May be primary or secondary infection. Contagious.	Vesiculopustular lesions which develop thick, honey-colored crust surrounded by erythema. Pruritic. Most common on face.	Systemic antibiotics 400,000 units oral penicillin qid × 10 days or 600,000 units of benzathine penicillin IM in single injection. Client allergic to penicillin—250 mg erythromycin qid × 10 days. Local—Warm saline or aluminum acetate soaks followed by soap and water removal of crusts. Topical antibiotic cream. If untreated, glomerulonephritis can occur when streptococcal strain is nephritogenic. Meticulous hygiene essential.
Folliculitis	Usually staphylococci. Found in areas subjected to friction, moisture, oil, or grease.	Small pustule at hair follicle opening with minimal erythema. Crusting develops. Most common on scalp, beard, and extremities in men. Tender to touch.	Soap and water cleansing. Warm compresses of water or aluminum acetate solution. Usually heals without scarring. If extensive and deep, may lead to scarring and loss of involved hair follicles.
Furuncle (boil)	Deep infection with *Staphylococcus* around a hair follicle. Often associated with severe acne or seborrheic dermatitis.	Tender erythematous area around a hair follicle. Upon rupture, drains pus and a core of necrotic debris. Most common on face, back of neck, axillae, breasts, buttocks, perineum, or thighs. Painful.	Incision and drainage. Occasionally antibiotics. Meticulous care of involved skin.
Furunculosis (multiple or recurrent)	Increased incidence in clients who are obese, chronically ill, regularly exposed to grease or oils, or who have diabetes mellitus.	Lesions as above. Malaise, regional adenopathy, elevated temperature.	Warm compresses. Systemic antibiotic after culture and sensitivity study of drainage (usually semisynthetic, penicillinase-resistant, oral penicillin such as cloxacillin and oxacillin). Measures to reduce surface staphylococci include antimicrobial cream to nares, armpits, and groin; antiseptic to entire skin. Often recurrent with scarring. Incision and drainage of soft lesions. Prevent or correct predisposing factors. Meticulous personal hygiene.
Carbuncle	Multiple, interconnecting furuncles.	Many pustules appearing in an erythematous area. Most common on nape of neck.	Treatment same as furuncles. Often recurrent despite production of antibodies. Heals slowly with scar formation.
Cellulitis	Inflammation of subcutaneous tissues. May arise as secondary complication or be primary infection. Often follows break in skin. Most often caused by *S. aureus* and streptococci. Bacteria produce enzymes which results in deep inflammation of subcutaneous tissue.	Hot, tender, erythematous, and edematous area with diffuse borders. Malaise and fever.	Moist heat. Immobilization and elevation. Systemic antibiotic therapy. Hospitalization if severe. Can progress to gangrene if untreated.

Table 17-5 (Continued)

Name	Etiology and Pathogenesis	Clinical Characteristics	Treatment and Prognosis
Erysipelas	Superficial cellulitis primarily involving the dermis. Group A beta-hemolytic streptococcus.	Red, hot, sharply demarcated plaque which is indurated and painful. Bacteremia may develop. Most common on face and extremities. Toxic signs such as fever, elevated WBC, headache, malaise.	Systemic antibiotics—usually penicillin. Hospitalization often required.

Table 17-6
Common Viral Infections

Name	Etiology and Pathogenesis	Clinical Characteristics	Treatment and Prognosis
Herpesvirus (fever blister, cold sore)	Extragenital infections usually caused by herpesvirus type I. Virus stays in nerve root ganglion and may return to skin to produce recurrence when exacerbated by sunlight, trauma, menses, stress, and systemic infection. Contagious to those not infected.	*First episode:* Painful local reaction. Grouped vesicles on an erythematous base. May have systemic symptoms as fever and malaise or be asymptomatic. *Recurrent:* Small and recur in similar spot. Characteristic grouped vesicles on an erythematous base.	Symptomatic medication. Soothing, moist compresses. Petrolatum to the lesions. Scarring does not usually result. Antiviral agents.
Herpes zoster (shingles)	Activation of the zoster varicella virus in the hypoimmune host. Frequently occurs in immunosuppressed clients. Potentially contagious to anyone who has not had varicella or who is immunosuppressed.	Linear patches along dermatome of grouped vesicles on an erythematous base. Usually unilateral and on trunk. Burning, pain, and neuralgia precede outbreak. Mild to severe pain during outbreak.	Symptomatic. Acetic acid compresses, white petrolatum to fissures. Analgesia. Mild sedation at bedtime. Systemic corticosteroids to shorten course and likelihood of postherpetic neuralgia. Usually heals without complications but may scar. May develop postherpetic neuralgia.
Verruca vulgaris (warts)	Caused by human papova virus. May disappear spontaneously in 1–2 years. Mildly contagious by autoinoculation. Specific response depends on body part affected.	Circumscribed hypertrophic, flesh-colored papule limited to epidermis. Painful on lateral compression.	Multiple treatments: Surgery—scoop removal using scissors and currette. Liquid nitrogen therapy. Blistering agents—cantharidin. Keratolytic agents—salicylic acid. If scarring occurs, due to the treatment rather than the primary lesion.
Plantar warts	Caused by human papova virus.	Wart on bottom surface of foot which grows inward due to pressure of walking or standing. Painful when pressure is applied. Skin markings interrupted. Cone shaped with black dots (thrombosed vessels) when pared down.	Padding the affected area. Chemical destruction: Salicylic acid; Formalin. Overaggressive destruction can result in a painful, hypertrophic scar.

Table 17-7
Common Fungal Infections of the Skin and Mucous Membrane

Name	Etiology and Pathogenesis	Clinical Characteristics	Treatment and Prognosis
Candidiasis (moniliasis)	Caused by yeast-like fungus of *Candida albicans*. 50% of adults are asymptomatic carriers. Presents in warm, moist areas as the crural area, oral mucosa, and submammary folds. Vaginal candida (vulvo vaginitis) occurs often in pregnant or diabetic women on steroid therapy, birth control pills, or antibiotics. Symptoms produced by imbalance between host and normal inhabitant of gastrointestinal tract, the mouth, and vagina.	*Mouth:* White, cheese-like patches which leave erosions when removed (thrush). *Vagina:* Vaginitis—red, edematous, painful vaginal wall, white patches. Vaginal discharge. Pruritus. Pain on urination and intercourse.	Microscopic examination and culture. Nystatin or other specific medication as vaginal suppository or oral lozenge. Abstinence or use of condom. Infection can be eradicated with appropriate medication.
Tinea corporis (ringworm)	Various dermatophytes.	Typical annular appearance, well-defined margins with fine cigarette paper scale. Erythematous.	Cool compresses. Topical antifungals for isolated patches. Clotrimazole, miconazole, tolnaftate, and haloprogin creams or solutions.
Tinea cruris ("jock itch")	Various dermatophytes.	Well-defined border in groin area.	Topical antifungals—clotrimazole, miconazole, tolnaftate, and haloprogin cream or solution.
Tinea unguium (onychomycosis)	Various dermatophytes.	Affects only a few nails on one hand. May affect nails on toes. Fungal scale is close to outer margin of lesion. Brittle, thickened, broken nails with white or yellow discoloration.	Topical antifungals—clotrimazole, miconazole, tolnaftate, and haloprogin cream or solution. Griseofulvin is moderately successful on fingernails. 25% of toenails will respond. Debride toenails to normal contour if problematic.
Tinea pedis (athlete's foot)	Various dermatophytes.	Interdigital scaling and maceration. Erythema and blistering. Pruritus. Painful.	Topical antifungals—clotrimazole, miconazole, tolnaftate, and haloprogin cream or solution.

Table 17-8
Common Infestations and Insect Bites

Name	Etiology and Pathogenesis	Clinical Characteristics	Treatment and Prognosis
Bees and wasps	Hymenoptera.	Intense, burning, local pain. Swelling and itching. Severe hypersensitivity can lead to anaphylaxis. See Chap. 10 for treatment of anaphylaxis.	Cool compresses. Local application of antipruritic lotion. Antihistamines if indicated. Usually uneventful recovery.
Bedbugs	Cimicidae. Feed periodically, usually at night. Live in furniture, walls, etc., during day.	Wheal surrounded by vivid flare. Firm urticaria transforms into persistent lesion. Severe pruritus. Often grouped by three appearing on noncovered parts of body.	Bedbug controlled by chlorocyclohexane. Lesions usually require no treatment. Severe itching may necessitate use of antihistamines or steroids.

Table 17-8 (Continued)

Name	Etiology and Pathogenesis	Clinical Characteristics	Treatment and Prognosis
Pediculosis			
Head lice	*Pediculus humanus* var. *capitis.*	Minute, red, noninflammatory. Points flush with skin. Progress to papular wheallike lesions. Pruritus. Secondary excoriation, especially parallel linear excoriations in intrascapular region. With hand lens oval eggs (nits) can be seen firmly attached to hair shaft in head and body lice.	Gamma benzene hexachloride or pyrethrins to treat various parts of the body. Apply as directed.
Body lice	*Pediculus humanus* var. *corporis.*		
Pubic lice	*Phthirius pubis* The above three lice are obligate parasites that suck blood, leave eggs and excrement on skin. Reaction due to delayed hypersensitivity to saliva and feces acting on antigen. Pubic lice often spread by sexual contact.		
Scabies (mites)	*Sarcoptes scabiei* Stratum corneum penetrated. Eggs deposited. Allergic reaction develops due to presence of eggs, feces, and mite parts. Spread by direct physical contact; only occasionally by shared personal items.	Severe itching, especially at night, usually not on face. Presence of burrows especially in interdigital webs, flexor surface of wrists, and anterior axillary folds. Redness, swelling, and vesiculation.	10% crotamiton, gamma benzene hexachloride, benzyl benzoate 12–25%. Directions for specific drug should be followed. Can be completely eradicated. Recurrence is possible. Treatment of sexual partner in positively diagnosed scabies. Antibiotics may be prescribed if dermatitis and secondary infections are present.

Table 17-9
Common Allergic Conditions of the Skin

Name	Etiology and Pathogenesis	Clinical Manifestations	Treatment and Prognosis
Contact dermatitis	Manifestation of delayed hypersensitivity. The absorbed agent acts as antigen. After several exposures, sensitization occurs. Lesions appear 12–48 hours after contact with allergen.	Red, hivelike papules and plaques. Sharply circumscribed with occasional vesicles. Exposed areas more common. Usually pruritic. Area of dermatitis related to causative agent (e.g., metal allergy and dermatitis on ring finger.)	Topical corticosteroids. Skin lubrication. Eliminating contact allergen. Avoid irritating affected area. Systemic steroids if sensitivity severe.
Urticaria	Usually results from allergic phenomena. Caused by presence of edema in upper dermis due to local increase in permeability of capillaries. Usually caused by histamine.	Spontaneously occurring and rounded elevations. Size may vary. Usually multiple.	Removal of source. Antihistamine therapy.
Drug reaction	Can be caused by any drug which acts as antigen and causes hypersensitive reaction. Certain drugs more prone to reactions (e.g., penicillin, mediated by circulating antibodies).	Rash of any morphology. Often appears as red, macular and papular, semiconfluent, generalized rash with abrupt onset. May present as late as 14 days after cessation of drug. May be pruritic.	Withdrawal of drug if possible. Antihistamines. Local or systemic corticosteroids may be required.

Table 17-9 (Continued)

Name	Etiology and Pathogenesis	Clinical Manifestations	Treatment and Prognosis
Atopic dermatitis (eczema)	Exact etiology unknown. Often starts in infancy and clears with age. Associated with allergic conditions. Many have elevated IgE levels. Genetically determined. Often family history. Clients have decreased itch threshold.	Scaly, red to red-brown, circumscribed lesions. Accentuation of skin markings. Pruritic. Adult—symmetrical eruptions common in antecubital and popliteal space.	Topical corticosteroids. Coal tar therapy. Intralesional steroids. Lubrication of dry skin. Systemic steroids if severe. Reduce stress.

Table 17-10

Common Benign Conditions of the Skin

Name	Etiology and Pathogenesis	Clinical Manifestions	Treatment and Prognosis
Acne	Inflammatory disorder of sebaceous glands. More common in teenagers. May persist into adulthood. May result secondary to iodides, bromides, corticosteroids, androgen-dominant birth control pills.	Noninflammatory lesions: comedones (blackheads) and closed comedones (whiteheads). Inflammatory lesions: papules and pustules. Most common on face, neck, and upper back.	Multiple lesions can be mechanically removed with comedon extractor after comedon opened with fine needle or blade. Benzoyl peroxide used topically as antibacterial and peeling agent. Peeling and irritating agents such as retinoic acid used. Long-term antibiotic therapy—topical or systemic. Phototherapy. Treatment is aimed at suppressing new lesions. Can undergo spontaneous remission. Often improves with summer sun exposure.
Moles (nevi)	Grouping of normal cells derived from melanocytelike precursor cells. May have hereditary determination.	Hyperpigmented areas which vary in form and color. May be flat, slightly elevated, haloid, verrucoid, polypoid, dome-shaped, sessile, and papillomatous. Normal skin markings preserved. Hair may grow in around nevus.	No treatment necessary except for cosmetic reasons. Excisional biopsy for diagnostic decisions.
Psoriasis	Chronic dermatitis which involves excessively rapid turnover of epidermal cells. Strong family predisposition.	Sharply demarcated scaling plaques of the scalp, elbows, and knees. Can affect palms, soles, and fingernails. May be localized or general, intermittent or continuous.	Aimed at retarding growth of epidermal cells. Difficult to medicate. Usually topical corticosteroids, tar, anthralin. Intralesional injection of corticosteroids. Sunlight. Ultraviolet light; alone, with topical or systemic potentiation. Cannot be cured. Can be controlled. Wrapping of affected areas is often indicated. Antimetabolites (esp. methotrexate) used in difficult cases.
Seborrheic keratoses	Benign, genetically determined growths. Found in increasing number with age. Not associated with sun exposure.	Irregularly round or oval, flat-topped papules or plaques. Surface often warty. Appear stuck on. Pigmentation increases with age of lesion. Usually are multiple.	Removal by curettage or liquid nitrogen freezing if diagnosis is in question or for cosmetic reasons. Minimal scarring results.

Table 17-10 (Continued)

Name	Etiology and Pathogenesis	Clinical Manifestions	Treatment and Prognosis
Skin tags (acrochordon)	Common after midlife. Appear on neck, axillae, and upper trunk.	Small, skin-colored, soft, pedunculated papules.	No treatment required unless for cosmetic reasons or repeated trauma. If requested, can be removed surgically.
Lipoma	Benign tumor of adipose tissue. Often encapsulated. Most common in 40–60-year-old age group.	Rubbery, compressible, round mass of adipose tissue. Single or multiple. Variable in size. Occur most often on trunk, back of neck, and forearms.	Usually no treatment. Biopsy to differentiate from liposarcoma. Excision is usual treatment when indicated.
Vitiligo	Unknown etiology. Genetically influenced, most noticeable in dark-skinned people and with summer tan. Complete absence of melanocytes. Noncontagious.	Focal amelanosis (complete loss of pigment). Macular. Varies in size and location. Usually symmetrical and permanent.	Attempts at repigmentation with sunlight and psoralens. Depigmentation of pigmented skin with extensive disease. (>50% of body involved). Cosmetics and stains used for camouflage and to deemphasize vitiliginous areas.
Lentigo	Increased number of normal melanocytes in basal layer of epidermis. Senile lentigos (liver "spots") related to aging and sun exposure.	Hyperpigmented, brown to black, flat lesion. Usually occurring on sun-exposed areas.	Only treated for cosmetic purposes. Medicate with liquid nitrogen. May recur in 1–2 years.

Table 17-11

Dermatologic Manifestations of Systemic Problems*

System	Systemic Problem	Dermatologic Manifestation
Endocrine	Increased growth hormone	Hyperplasia and thickening of dermis, hair, nails.
	Hyperthyroidism	Increased sweating; skin warm with persistent flush; thin nails; vitiligo and alopecia; fine, soft hair.
	Hypothyroidism	Cold, dry, pale to yellow skin; slightly hyperkeratotic epidermis with follicular plugging; generalized nonpitting edema; dry, coarse, brittle hair; brittle, slow-growing nails.
	Glucocorticoid excess (Cushing's syndrome) induced endogenously or exogenously	Atrophy; striae; epidermal thinning; telangiectasia; acne; decreased subcutaneous fat over extremities; thin, loose dermis; impaired wound healing; increased vascular fragility; mild hirsutism; excessive collection of fat over clavicles, back of neck, abdomen, and face; increased incidence of pyodermas.
	Addison's disease	Loss of body hair (especially axillary) generalized hyperpigmentation.
	Androgen excess	Enlarged facial pores; male sex characteristic; acne; acceleration of coarse hair growth.
	Androgen deficiency—post-puberty	Hair becomes sparse; marked reduction in sebum production.
	Hypoparathyroidism	Opaque, brittle nails with transverse ridges; coarse, sparse hair with patchy alopecia; eczematous and exfoliative dermatitis; hyperkeratotic and maculopapular eruptions.
	Hyperpituitarism (acromegaly)	Coarsened skin, deepened lines; increased oiliness and sweating; acne; increased number of nevi, hyperpigmentation; hypertrichosis.
	Hypopituitarism (Froelich's syndrome)	Smooth skin; scant hair growth; obesity; small, thin fingernails.
	Diabetes mellitus	Increased xanthomas and carotene; skin spots; necrobiosis lipoidica diabeticorum.

Table 17-11 (Continued)

System	Systemic Problem	Dermatologic Manifestation
Gastrointestinal	Ulcerative colitis; Crohn's disease	Pyoderma gangrenosum; mouth ulcers.
	Liver disease Biliary tract obstruction	Jaundice; itching; pigmentary abnormalities; alterations in nails and hair; spider angiomas, telangiectasia.
	Deficiency of essential fatty acids (EFA)	Scaly skin.
	Malabsorption syndrome	Acquired ichthyosis.
	Fibrocystic disease	Abnormal sweat gland function resulting in failure to conserve sodium.
Musculoskeletal and connective tissue	Systemic lupus erythematosis	Maculopapular semiconfluent rash (butterfly rash).
	Scleroderma	Leathery hardening and stiffness of skin.
	Dermatomyositis	Edema; purplish-red color to upper eyelids; butterfly rash; scaly, macular erythema over knuckles; linear telangiectasia of posterior nail fold.
Metabolic	Lipidoses	Xanthomas.
	Vitamin A deficiency	Generalized dry hyperkeratoses (phrynoderma).
	Hypervitaminosis A	Hair loss; dry skin.
	Vitamin B_1 (thiamine) deficiency	Edema; redness of soles of feet.
	Vitamin B_2 (riboflavin) deficiency	Red fissures at corner of mouth; glossitis.
	Nicotinic acid deficiency (niacin)	Causes pellagra; redness of exposed areas of hand /feet, face/neck. Results in infected dermatitis.
Immune	Drug sensitivity	Rash of any morphology.
	Serum sickness	Pruritus.
	Cancer of breast, stomach, lung, uterus, kidney, ovary, colon, bladder	Metastasis to skin.
	Hodgkin's disease	Pruritus and nonspecific erythemas.
	Lymphomas	Papules, nodules, plaques, pruritus.
Cardiovascular	Arteriosclerosis	Venous thrombosis, decreased oxygenation leading to gangrene.
	Rheumatic heart disease	Petechiae, urticaria, rheumatic nodules, erythema nodosum and multiforme.
	Periarteritis nodosa	Periarteritis nodules.
	Thromboangiitis obliterans (Buerger's disease)	Superficial migrating thrombophlebitis, pallor or cyanosis, gangrene, ulceration.
Respiratory	Inadequate oxygenation secondary to respiratory pathology	Cyanosis.
Hematologic	Anemia	Pallor, hyperpigmentation, pale mucous membrane, hair loss, nail dystrophy.
	Clotting disorders	Purpura, petechiae, ecchymosis.
Renal	Chronic renal failure	Dry skin, pruritus, uremic frost, pallor, dry skin, bruises, petechiae.
Reproductive	Primary syphilis	Chancre.
	Secondary syphilis	Generalized skin lesions.
	Late benign syphilis	Gummas.
Neurologic	Syringomyelia; chronic sensory polyneuropathies; spinal cord trauma	Trophic changes in skin due to sensory denervation, decubitus ulcers, anesthesia, paresthesias.

*Refer to the systemic disease for specific information.

PLASTIC SURGERY

Elective Cosmetic Surgery

The possible cosmetic changes that can be made surgically are almost limitless. Cosmetic surgery includes such techniques as breast enlargement; breast reduction; chemical, mechanical, and surgical face-lift; eyelid lift; hair transplant; nose corrections; removal of double chin; correction of receding or prominent chin; abdomen lift; buttocks reduction;

thigh lift; and correction of elephant ears. You can even get dimples!

The reasons for the surgery are as varied as the techniques. The most common reasons for people to suffer the pain and financial expense (most are not covered by insurance) of cosmetic surgery is to improve their body image. People project their personal image of themselves. If they feel better about themselves as a result of cosmetic surgery, they will often act more confident and self-assured. Often social position and economic considerations are part of the decision. Our youth-oriented society often feels uncomfortable doing business with someone who appears to be aging. Also, increased longevity provides a larger population to whom cosmetic surgery is especially appealing.

Regardless of the reason for electing to have cosmetic surgery, the nurse should maintain a supportive, nonjudgmental attitude. If the client wishes to change a body feature perceived as unattractive, then it is his decision to undergo cosmetic surgery and the nurse should uphold this decision.

Chemical face-lift or peel

A *chemical face peel* utilizes a cauterant to the skin to cause a controlled burn. This results in superficial destruction of the upper layers of the skin and a tightening of the deep layers. The most common indications for a chemical peel include pigmentation problems, skin damage due to radiation, removal of freckles, and superficial acne scarring.

After the client is sedated a solution (buffered phenol) is painted on the skin, avoiding the eyes. The treated areas may be covered with waterproof tape (except the mouth, nose, and eyes) and left on for 24 to 48 hours. During this time, the client refrains from talking and eats only liquids through a straw. When the tape is removed there is moderate swelling and crusting for a week. Redness will persist for 6 to 8 weeks. A pink tone will be apparent for several months. Once healing is complete, the skin will have a more youthful appearance due to a new superficial layer of skin.

Since there is a reduction of melanin due to the procedure, the client must be instructed to absolutely avoid the sun for 6 months to avoid unsightly hyperpigmentation. Aside from the fact that it is relatively painful, chemical peeling results in the new skin being lighter than the old skin. This can cause a disparity in the color between the treated and untreated areas. There is a possibility that this procedure can cause scarring. Chemical peeling is considered the better treatment for wrinkles and certain types of hyperpigmentation.

Dermabrasion

Dermabrasion is the removal of epidermis and a portion of the superficial layer of the dermis with preservation of sufficient epidermal adnexa to allow for spontaneous reepithelialization of the abraded surface.[12] Dermabrasion is considered the better treatment for acne and other depressed scars.

There has been marked improvement in the tools used for this procedure. Dermabrasion uses an electrically driven waterproof carbide abrasive paper cylinder and diamond-impregnated burrs. The client may or may not be hospitalized, depending on the preference of the surgeon and the client.

Following the formation of a coagulum from the serum, there is a proliferation of squamous epithelium from the adnexal elements. By the third to fourth postoperative day, a thin epidermis begins to regenerate and collagen is laid down. Pigmentation does not begin until 3 to 4 weeks post abrasion. Exposure to the sun must be strictly avoided for 2 to 4 months to prevent hyperpigmentation.

The important consideration post abrasion is to keep the abraded areas dry for the first week. A hairdryer is handy for this purpose. After 1 week, cold cream or vegetable oil is applied to soften the area and keep the skin supple. Sunscreens should be used if the client is outdoors.

Face-lift (rhytidectomy)

A *face-lift* is the redistribution of facial skin and excision of excess soft tissue (Fig. 17-10). Indications for this procedure include:[13]

1. Redundant soft tissue resulting from dermatitis (e.g., smallpox or acne scarring)
2. Asymmetric redundancy of soft tissues (e.g., facial palsy)
3. Redundant soft tissues resulting from trauma
4. Preauricular lesions
5. Redundant soft tissues resulting from solar elastosis, changes in body weight, and gravitation
6. Restoration of body image

The surgical approach and lines of incisions vary according to the nature of the deformity and the position of the hairline. Prevention of hematoma formation is the most important postoperative consideration. A pressure dressing is usually used the first 24 to 48 hours to reduce the possibility of hematoma formation. Once the dressing is removed, there is little pain. The sutures are removed from the fifth to the tenth postoperative day. Antibiotics are used at the discretion of the surgeon. Infection is not a common problem.

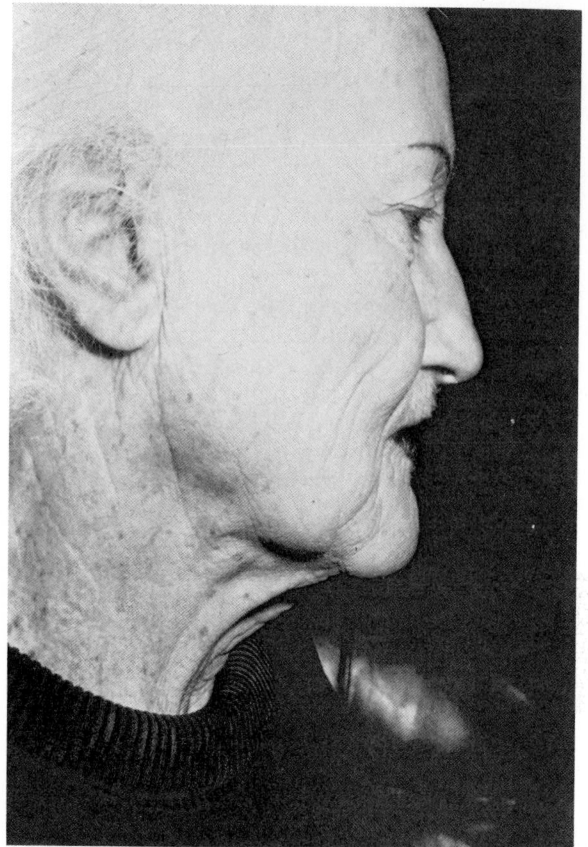
A

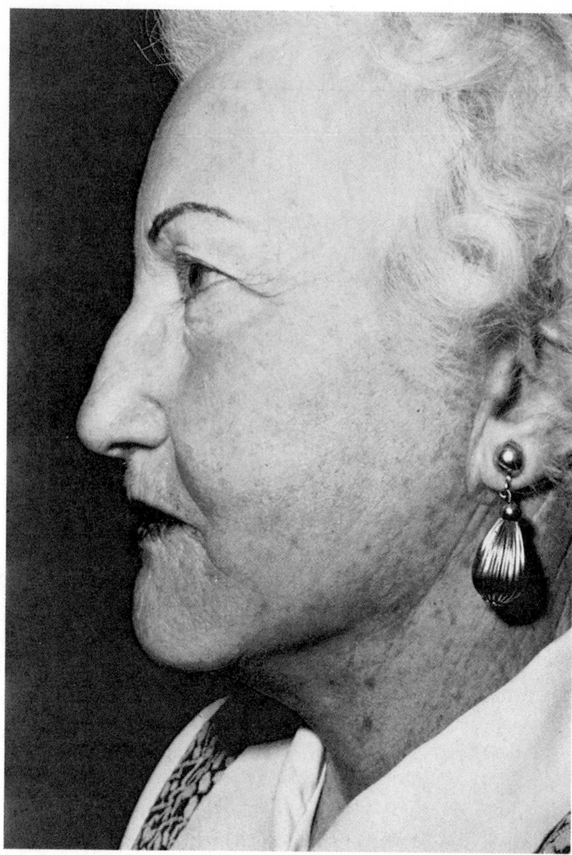
B

Figure 17-10 (*a*) Before face-lift. (*b*) After face-lift. (*Courtesy of Richard Gooding, M.D.*)

Nursing Management of Cosmetic Surgery

Many cosmetic surgeries are being performed in well-equipped day surgeries or in plastic surgeons' office surgery suites. Several interventions related to cosmetic surgery are appropriate, regardless of where or how the nurse-client relationship develops.

Preoperative management

A major consideration relates to informed consent and realistic expectations of what cosmetic surgery can accomplish. Although this information is usually provided by the surgeon, the nurse can and should reinforce this dialogue and answer questions and concerns. For instance, face-lifting has little or no effect on deep wrinkling of the forehead and temples, deep nasolabial grooves, or vertical lip wrinkles. Before and after pictures are often helpful in aiding the client to set realistic expectations.

The client also needs to understand the time frame for healing. The fullest results cannot, in some instances, be expected for as long as 1 year after the procedure. The oozing, crusting phase of the abrasive procedures must be explained so the client can plan time off from work if this seems necessary. The final results of the cosmetic procedures is affected by age, general state of health, and general skin type. Should a health problem be apparent, efforts should be made to correct or control the problem prior to the procedure.

Postoperative management

Most of the cosmetic surgeries are not exceptionally painful. Usually, mild analgesics are sufficient to keep the patient comfortable.

Even though infection is not a common problem following cosmetic surgery, the nurse needs to assess the surgical sites for signs of infection. Systemic signs such as temperature and respirations should also be carefully monitored. The client should be aware of signs of infection and told to report any such signs immediately so appropriate antibiotic intervention can be started.

If the surgery involved alteration in the circulation to the skin such as the undermining done in a face-lift, a careful monitoring of adequate circulation is necessary. Warm, pink skin that blanches with pressure indicates adequate circulation is present in the surgical area.

Skin Grafts

Uses of skin grafting

Skin grafts may be necessary to provide protection to underlying structures or to reconstruct areas for cosmetic or functional purposes. Ideally, wounds heal by primary intention. However, large, surgically created wounds, trauma, and chronic wounds can cause extensive tissue destruction, making primary intention healing impossible. In these cases, skin grafting may be necessary. Improved surgical techniques make it possible to graft skin, bone, cartilage, fat, fascia, muscles, and nerves.

Types of grafts

The two types of skin grafts are *free grafts* and *skin flaps*. Free grafts are further differentiated, based on the method of providing blood supply to the grafted skin. One method is to transfer the graft (epidermis and part or all of the dermis) to the recipient site from the donor site. If the graft is an autograft (from the client's own body) or an isograft (from an identical twin), it will revascularize and become fixed to the new site. Chapter 13 discusses full and split skin grafts in detail.

Another method for free skin grafting is by reconstructive microsurgery. Using an operating microscope, circulation is immediately established in the free flap by anastomosis of the blood vessels from the skin flap to the vessels in the recipient site. This highly technical and time-consuming surgery is being used in many situations which were previously treated by the use of skin flaps.[14]

Skin flaps involve moving a section of skin and subcutaneous tissue from one part of the body to another without terminating the vascular attachment (Fig. 17-11). The vascular attachment is called a pedicle. Skin flaps are used to cover wounds with a poor vascular bed, when padding is needed, and to cover wounds over cartilage and bone. There may be the need for intermediate flap placement if the recipient site is far removed from the donor.

The flap is advanced to the recipient site when circulation is well established at the intermediate site. The type of flap and route of transfer is individually determined, based on the needs of the client and the nature of the defect to be repaired.

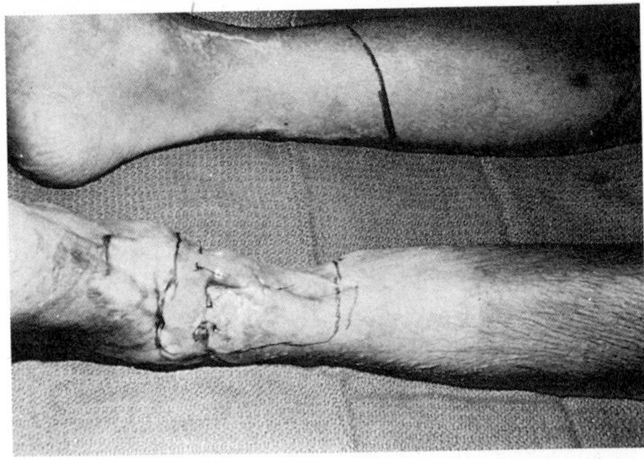

A

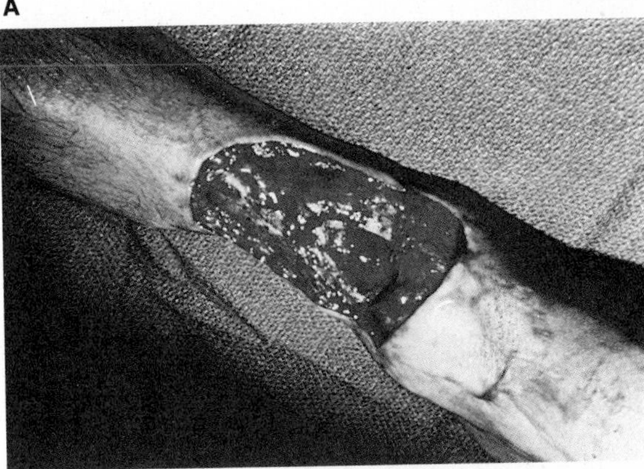

B

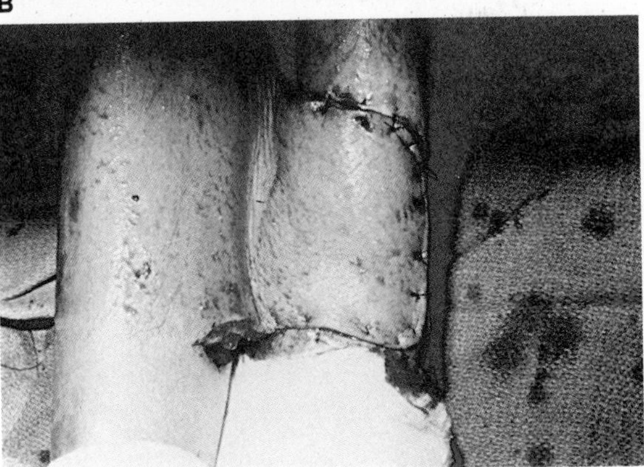

C

Figure 17-11 Skin flap being progressed. (*a*) Area of excision of damaged skin marked on right leg and flap marked on left leg. (*b*) Excised wound. (*c*) Cross-legged flap in place. *(W. Nickell and K. Salver, Plastic Surgery, part 1, Basic Plastic Surgery, Famous Teachings in Modern Medicine, Medcom, Inc., New York, 1973.)*

Nursing care following skin grafts

Following a skin graft, several areas need to be assessed. The most critical assessment is related to the vascular supply to the grafted site. If the area is not dressed, it should be regularly assessed for color, warmth, capillary refill, and turgor. If the grafted area has a dressing, it is usually left in place until removed by the surgeon. Systemic signs of infection such as fever and pain must be monitored.

The client may often have to assume unnatural positions which lead to pain, stiffness, and frustration. The nurse is challenged to assist the client to divert attention from this awkward situation. Often, tranquilizers or sedatives are necessary to assist the client through this period. Appropriate nursing intervention related to altered mobility must also be considered.

Although pain is not usually a major problem, the nurse should provide pain relief when necessary. Conversation, diversion, and massage, as well as medication, should be used to maintain client comfort. The immobility enforced by certain grafting procedures presents the expected potential complication of pneumonia, pulmonary emboli, and decubiti. Aggressive measures by the nursing staff should be instituted to prevent such complications.

Skin grafting often involves long periods of hospitalization with the constant threat of graft death. Since this is a particularly difficult time emotionally for the client, the nurse needs to be supportive and understanding. Expectations of the results of the graft must be realistic if the client is not to suffer depression as the result of unfulfilled expectations. The family and friends of the client need consideration and explanation of procedures and restrictions imposed by the grafting procedures.

Case Study / Basal Cell Epithelioma

John Martin, 67, is a fair-skinned, balding, retired construction worker. He presents at dermatology clinic with a papule of 6 months' duration behind his right ear. He states that a scab forms, falls off, and reforms. On inspection, the lesion has semitranslucent borders with absence of normal skin marking. A diagnosis of basal cell epithelioma is made on biopsy.

Discussion Questions

1. What facts about this client support the diagnosis?
2. What are the usual clinical characteristics of a basal cell carcinoma?
3. How was a definitive diagnosis made?
4. What treatment options are available for a basal cell epithelioma?
5. What is the likelihood of metastatic spread with this lesion?
6. What are the nursing responsibilities related to client education for Mr. Martin?

REVIEW QUESTIONS

The number of the question corresponds to the same numbered objective at the beginning of the chapter.

1. Sunscreens primarily block out
   a. UV-A wavelengths
   b. UV-B wavelengths
   c. UV-C wavelengths

2. The most common medications used to treat dermatologic problems are
   a. corticosteroids
   b. antibiotics
   c. keratolytics
   d. antipruritics

3. Scars that result from chronic skin conditions have
   a. increased innervation
   b. increased sweating
   c. decreased collagen
   d. loss of hair

4. The most common etiologic factor related to skin cancer is
   a. chronic sun exposure
   b. hereditary predisposition
   c. prolonged irritation
   d. inadequate vitamin C intake

5. The pathogen involved in impetigo is
   a. *Escherichia coli*
   b. *Pseudomonas aeruginosa*
   c. *Proteus*
   d. group A beta-hemolytic streptococci

6. Scabies is spread by
   a. systemic involvement
   b. contaminated articles
   c. direct physical contact
   d. airborne transfer

7. A common site for the lesions associated with atopic dermatitis is the
   a. palmar surface of the feet
   b. antecubital space
   c. temporal area
   d. buttocks

8. A common benign skin problem associated with aging is
   a. psoriasis

b. skin tags
c. vitiligo
d. lipomas

9. A systemic respiratory problem would most commonly affect the skin by
a. increase in pruritus
b. pallor
c. changes in color
d. increased perspiration

10. An important client instruction following a chemical peel or dermabrasion is
a. increased fatty acids in the diet
b. use of superfatted soaps
c. avoidance of sun exposure
d. keep the treated areas moist

REFERENCES

1. Gail McBride, "What Sunlight Does to Your Skin," *Family Health,* January 1978, p. 39.
2. Ibid., p. 38.
3. Wilse B. Webb, "Theories of Sleep Functions and Some Clinical Implications," Rene Drucker-Colin (ed.), *The Function of Sleep,* Academic Press, Inc., New York, 1979, p. 21.
4. Ernest L. Hartmann, *The Functions of Sleep,* Yale University Press, New Haven, Conn., 1973, p. 145.
5. D. S. Wilkinson, *The Nurse and Management of Skin Disease,* Faber and Faber, Ltd., London, 1977, p. 85.
6. John A. Parrish, *Dermatology and Skin Care,* McGraw-Hill Book Company, New York, 1975, p. 107.
7. Herbert Goldschmidt (ed.), *Physical Modalities in Dermatologic Therapy,* Springer-Verlag New York, Inc., New York, 1978, p. 223.
8. Kathy Hawkins, "Wet Dressings—Putting the Damper on Dermatitis," *Nursing 78,* February 1978, p. 64.
9. D. S. Wilkinson, *The Nurse and Management of Skin Diseases,* Faber and Faber Ltd., London, 1977, p. 58.
10. Harmon C. Bickley, *Practical Concepts in Human Disease,* The Williams & Wilkins Company, Baltimore, 1975, p. 49.
11. John A. Parrish, *Dermatology and Skin Care,* McGraw-Hill Book Company, New York, 1975, p. 206.
12. Thomas D. Rees et al., *Cosmetic Facial Surgery,* W. B. Saunders Company, Philadelphia, 1973, p. 218.
13. Frank W. Masters (ed.), *Symposium on Aesthetic Surgery of the Face, Eyelid and Breast,* vol. 4, The C. V. Mosby Company, St. Louis, 1972, p. 33.
14. Ian A. McGregor, *Fundamental Techniques of Plastic Surgery and their Surgical Applications,* 7th ed., Churchill Livingstone, Edinburgh, 1980, p. 59.

BIBLIOGRAPHY FOR SECTION 5

Books

Adams, G. I., L. R. Boies, and M. M. Paparella: *Boies's Fundamentals of Otolaryngology*, 5th ed., W. B. Saunders Company, Philadelphia, 1978.

Alford, B. R.: *Complications of Suppurative Otitis Media and Mastoiditis*, chap. 11 in *Otolaryngology*, vol. 2, *The Ear*, M. M. Paparella and D. A. Shumrick, W. B. Saunders Company, Philadelphia, 1980.

Ballantyne, D. L.: *Experimental Skin Grafts and Transplantation Immunity*, Springer-Verlag New York Inc., New York, 1979.

Bates, B.: *A Guide to Physical Examination*, 2d ed., J. B. Lippincott Company, Philadelphia, 1979.

Bellows, J. G. (ed.): *Glaucoma Contemporary International Concepts*, Masson Publishing U.S.A. Inc., New York, 1979.

Burton, B. T.: *Human Nutrition*, 3d ed., McGraw-Hill Book Company, New York, 1976.

Canada, W.: *Beauty Surgery*, copyrighted by William H. Canada, M.D., Houston, Texas, 1976.

Conn, H. F.: *Current Therapy*, W. B. Saunders Company, Philadelphia, 1979.

DeWeese, D. D. and W. H. Saunders: *Textbook of Otolaryngology*, 5th ed., The C. V. Mosby Company, St. Louis, 1977.

Ellis, P. P.: *Ocular Therapeutics and Pharmacology*, 5th ed., The C. V. Mosby Company, St. Louis, 1977.

Emery, J. M., and J. H. Little: *Phacoemulsification and Aspiration of Cataracts*, The C. V. Mosby Company, St. Louis, 1979.

Epstein, E.: *Common Skin Disorders: A Manual for Physicians and Patients*, Medical Economics Company, Oradell, N.J., 1979.

Fitzpatrick, T. B., et al.: *Dermatology in General Medicine*, 2d ed., McGraw-Hill Book Company, New York, 1979.

Fraunfelder, T., and F. Roy: *Current Ocular Therapy*, W. B. Saunders Company, Philadelphia, 1980.

Frost, P., et al. (ed.): *Recent Advances in Dermatopharmacology*, Spectrum Publications, New York, 1978.

Glickman, F. S.: *Dermatology in General Medicine*, PSG Publishing Company, Inc., Littleton, Mass., 1979.

Grayson, M.: *Diseases of the Cornea*, The C. V. Mosby Company, St. Louis, 1979.

Havener, W. H.: *Ocular Pharmacology*, 4th ed., The C. V. Mosby Company, St. Louis, 1978.

———: *Synopsis of Ophthalmology*, 5th ed., The C. V. Mosby Company, St. Louis, 1979.

Hoehne, C. N., et al.: *Ophthalmological Considerations in the Rehabilitation of the Blind*, Charles C Thomas, Publisher, Springfield, Ill., 1980.

Judge, R. D., et al.: *Methods of Clinical Examination: A Physiologic Approach*, 3d ed., Little, Brown and Company, Boston, 1974.

Kart, C. S., et al.: *Aging and Health: Biologic and Social Perspectives*, Addison-Wesley Publishing Company, Inc., Reading, Mass., 1978.

King, J. H., Jr., and J. A. C. Wadsworth: *An Atlas of Ophthalmic Surgery*, 3d ed., J. B. Lippincott Company, Philadelphia, 1981.

Krizek, T. J., et al. (eds.): *Symposium on Basic Science in Plastic Surgery*, vol. 15, The C. V. Mosby Company, St. Louis, 1976.

Krupp, M. C., and M. J. McChatton: *Current Medical Diagnosis and Treatment*, Lange Medical Publications, Los Altos, Calif., 1980.

Lazarus, G. S., et al.: *Diagnosis of Skin Disease*, F. A. Davis Company, Philadelphia, 1980.

Loebl, S., G. Spratto, and E. Heckheimer: *The Nurses' Drug Handbook*, 2d ed., John Wiley & Sons, Inc., New York, 1980.

Luciano, D. S., et al.: *Human Function and Structure*, McGraw-Hill Book Company, New York, 1978.

Machemer, R., and T. M. Aaberg: *Vitrectomy*, 2d ed., Grune & Stratton, Inc., New York, 1979.

Maurer, J. F., and R. R. Rupp: *Hearing and Aging: Tactics for Prevention*, Grune & Stratton, Inc., New York, 1979.

McGregor, I. A.: *Fundamental Techniques of Plastic Surgery*, Churchill Livingstone, Edinburgh, 1980.

Moses, R. A. (ed.): *Adler's Physiology of the Eye: Clinical Application*, 7th ed., The C. V. Mosby Company, St. Louis, 1981.

Northern, J. L., and M. R. Downs: *Hearing in Children*, 2d ed., The Williams & Wilkins Company, Baltimore, 1978.

Paparella, M. M., and D. A. Shumrick (eds.): *Otolaryngology*, 2d ed., vol. 2, *The Ear*, W. B. Saunders Company, Philadelphia, 1980.

Parrish, J. A.: *Dermatology and Skin Care*, McGraw-Hill Book Company, New York, 1975.

Purtilo, D.: *A Survey of Human Diseases*, Addison-Wesley Publishing Company, Reading, Mass., 1978.

Reith, E. J., et al.: *Textbook of Anatomy and Physiology*, 2d ed., McGraw-Hill Book Company, New York, 1978.

Robinson, C., et al.: *Normal and Therapeutic Nutrition*, 15th ed., The Macmillan Company, New York, 1977.

Sataloff, J., R. T. Sataloff, and I. A. Vassallo: *Hearing Loss*, 2d ed., J. B. Lippincott Company, Philadelphia, 1980.

Saunders, W. H., W. H. Havener, C. F. Keith, and G. Havener: *Nursing Care in Eye, Ear, Nose and Throat Disorders*, 4th ed., The C. V. Mosby Company, St. Louis, 1978.

———, Paparella, M. M., and A. W. Miglets: *Atlas of Ear Surgery*, 3d ed., The C. V. Mosby Company, St. Louis, 1980.

Schachar, R. A.: *Intraocular Lenses*, Charles C Thomas, Publisher, Springfield, Ill., 1979.

Schaie, H. G., and D. M. Albert: *Textbook of Ophthalmology*, 9th ed., W. B. Saunders Company, Philadelphia, 1977.

Simmons, R. E., and D. A. Keller: *One Pair for a Lifetime*, Keller Publishing, Columbus, Ohio, 1979.

Smith, J. F., and D. P. Nachazel: *Ophthalmologic Nursing*, Little, Brown and Company, Boston, 1980.

Vander, J. A., et al.: *Human Physiology: The Mechanism of Body Function*, 3d ed., McGraw-Hill Book Company, New York, 1980.

Vaughan, D., and T. Asbury: *General Ophthalmology*, 9th ed., Lange Medical Publications, Los Altos, Calif., 1980.

Yanoff, M.: "Diabetes Mellitus," chap. 5 in *Ocular Pathology Update*, ed. by D. H. Nicholson, Masson Publishing U.S.A. Inc., New York, 1980

Periodicals

Bielan, B.: "If It's Wet, Dry It; If It's Dry, Wet It," *Occupational Health*, **47:**32–34, September/October (1978).

"Black Skin Problems," *Am J Nurs*, **79**(6):1092–1094, June (1979).

Boger, W. L.: "Treatment of Glaucoma: Role of β-Blocking Agents," *Drugs*, **18:**25–32 (1979).

Boyd-Monk, H.: "Examining the External Eye: Part I," *Nursing 80*,**5:**58 (1980).

———: "Examining the External Eye: Part 2," *Nursing 80*,**6:**58 (1980).

———: "Screening for Glaucoma," *Nursing 79*, **8:**42 (1979).

Boyles, V. A.: "Injection Aids for Blind Diabetics," *Am J Nurs*, **77**(9):1456–1458 (1977).

Bozian, M. W., and H. M. Clark: "Counteracting Sensory Changes in the Aging," *Am J Nurs*, **80**(3):473–476 (1980).

Choulinard, F.: "Vigilant Nursing Care After Reconstructive Surgery," *Nursing 79*, **9:**18–25, June (1979).

Clark, C. C., and G. C. Mills: "Communicating with Hearing Impaired Elderly Adults," *J Gerontol Nurs*, **5**(3) (1979).

Contact Lenses: part 1, *Consumer Reports*, **45:**288–292, May (1980).

Contact Lenses: part 2, *Consumer Reports*, **45:**383–386, June (1980).

Coskey, R. J.: "Dermatologic Therapy," *Cutis*, **19**(6):807–839, June (1977).

———: "Dermatologic Therapy," *Cutis*, **24:**78–85, July (1979).

——— and R. B. Rees: "Dermatologic Therapy," *Cutis*, **24**(91)78–83, July (1977).

Dupont, J.: "EENT Emergencies," *Nursing 79*, **11**:65–70 (1979).

———: "What to Do For Common Eye Emergencies," *Nursing 76*, **11:**65 (1976).

Durkee, D. R., and B. G. Bryant: "Drug Therapy Review: Drug Therapy of Glaucoma," *Am J Hosp Pharm*, **35**(6):682–690 (1978).

Eddy, D. M.: "Vitrectomy," *Am J Nurs*, **78**(4):608–609 (1978).

Farah, A.: "The Skin Game: New Rules for the 80's," *Family Health*, **12:**27–28, February (1980).

Finn, K.: "Rebuilding Skin—Meeting the Challenge of Skin Care," part 1, *RN*, **39:**41–45, October (1977).

———: "Rebuilding Skin—Meeting the Challenge of Skin Care," part 2, *RN*, **40:**47–52, November (1977).

Gates, N.: "The Elderly Deaf," *Nursing Mirror*, **144**(3):67–68, January (1977).

Herman, R., et al.: "Cutaneous Reaction Rates to Penicillins—Oral Versus Parenteral," *Cutis*, **24**(2):232–233, August (1979).

Jolly, H. W.: "Superficial X-ray Therapy in Dermatology—1978," *Int J Dermatol*, **17**(9):691–697, November (1978).

Kass, M., et al.: "Dipivefrin and Epinephrine Treatment of Elevated Intraocular Pressure: A Comparative Study," *Arch Ophthalmol*, **97**(10):1865–1866 (1979).

Levenson, L., and J. Levenson: "Corneal Transplantation," *Am J Nurs*, **77**(7):1160–1163 (1977).

MacFadgen, J. S.: "Caring for the Patient with a Primary Retinal Detachment," *Am J Nurs*, **80**(5):920–921 (1980).

Marritt, E.: "The Hair Transplant Model: A Three Dimensional Approach to the Patient Consultations," *Cutis*, **24** (2):153–164, August (1979).

Maters, N. R.: "Topical Therapy: Choosing and Using the Proper Vehicle," *Nursing 77*, **7:**8 (November 1977).

McCartney, J. H., and G. Nadler: "How to Help Your Patient Cope with Hearing Loss," *Geriatrics*, **34**(3):69–76 (1979).

McFadden, J. W.: "Burn and Sunburn Products," *Handbook of Nonprescription Drugs*, 6th ed., American Pharmaceutical Association (1979).

McNamee, C.: "Communicating with the Lord of Hearing," *Canadian Nurse 74*, **3:**27–29 (1978).

National Institute of Health, Public Health Service: The 1977 Report of the Advisory Eye Council, Vision Research, A National Plan. 1978–1982, vol. 1: Summary U.S. Department of Health, Education and Welfare, DHEW Pub. No. (NIH) 78–1258, 1978.

National Institute of Health, Public Health Service: The 1977

Report of the Advisory Eye Council Vision Research: A National Plan: 1978–1982, vol. II: Panel Reports. U.S. Dept. of Health, Education and Welfare, DHEW. Pub. No. (NIH) 78–1258, 1978.

Orem, S. E.: "A Time for Trust," *Nursing 77*, **2:**120 (1977).

Perks, J.: "Nursing a Blind Patient," *Nursing Times*, **44:**1728–1729 (October 1975).

Perron, D. M.: "Deprived of Sound," *Am J Nurs*, **74**(6):1057–1059 (1974).

Proctor, C.: "Diagnosis, Prevention and Treatment of Hereditary Sensoreneural Loss," *Larynoscope* (supplemental, no. 7), LXXVII, **2**(10):1–54 (1977).

Rees, R. B.: "Current Dermatologic Treatment," *Cutis*, **18** (4):568–574 (October 1976).

Reynolds, B. J.: "Suddenly Blind at 80," *Nursing 79*, (7):46–49 (1979).

Roach, L.: "Color Changes in Dark Skin," *Nursing 77*, **7**(1):48 (January 1977).

Roberts, S. L.: "Skin Assessment for Color and Temperature," *Am J Nurs*, **75**(4):610–613 (April 1975).

Rubin, B. A.: "Black Skin: Here's How to Adjust Your Assessment and Care," *RN*, **42**:31–35 (March 1979).

Sataloff, R. T., and C. M. Colton: "Otitis Media: A Common Childhood Disease," *Am J Nurs*, **81**(8):1480–1483 (1981).

Schrader, E. S.: "Perioperative Nurses Reassure Ophthalmic Patients," *AORN J*, **30**(12):1066–1077 (1979).

Shelby, J. P.: "Sensory Deprivation," *Image*, **10**(6):49–55 (1978).

Smith, J.: "Focusing Your Care for the Patient with an Intraocular Lens Implant," *RN*, **41**(3):46–50 (1978).

Smith, J. G.: "Skin Problems of Blacks," *JAMA*, **236**(3)(July 1976).

Stough, D. B.: "Innovative Adjuncts in Hair Transplantation," *Cutis*, **24**(2) (August 1979).

Torosian, G., et al.: "Sunscreen and Suntan Products," *Handbook of Nonprescription Drugs*, 6th ed., American Pharmaceutical Association (1979).

Uhler, D. M.: "Common Skin Change in the Elderly," *Am J Nurs*, **8**(8):1342 (August 1978).

Wiley, L.: "The Defeated Patient: Her Worries Come First," *Nursing 77*, **7:**28–33 (April 1977).

———: "Trauma Care: Don't Forget the Patient," *Nursing 79*, **9:**46–51 (August 1979).

Wong, E. K., Jr., S. Wong, and I. H. Leopold: "How Ophthalmic Drugs Can Fool You," *RN*, **43**(3):37–44 (1980).

Yeacoumettis, A. M., et al.: "Better Results from Delayed Primary Skin Grafting," *Nursing Mirror*, **147:**28–30 (August 24 1978).

Zigmore, J.: "For the New Year: Clearer, Cleaner Skin," *Family Health*, **10:**14–15 (January 1978).

Organizations

American Foundation for the Blind, Inc.
15 West 16 Street
New York, NY 10011
A national research and service agency concerned with all aspects of work for the blind. Publishes books, pamphlets, monographs, and reports of a professional nature, including the *Directory of Agencies Serving Blind Persons in the United States* and *The New Outlook for the Blind*. Sells special appliances for the blind.

American Speech and Hearing Association (ASHA)
9030 Old Georgetown Road
Washington, D.C. 20014
ASHA is a scientific and professional organization with approximately 15,000 members. Members must have a master's degree or equivalent in the field of human communication. The purposes of the organization are to encourage basic scientific study of the processes of human communication, with special reference to speech, hearing, and language; to promote investigation of disorders of human communication; and to foster improvement of clinical procedures with such disorders. Official communications include *The Journal of Speech and Hearing Disorders* and *The Journal of Speech and Hearing Research. The Annual Directory*, published yearly, lists all members and their qualifications, and recognized state associations.

American Academy of Facial, Plastic and Reconstructive Surgery, Inc.
1110 West Main Street
Durham, NC 27701

Division for the Blind and Physically Handicapped
Library of Congress
Washington, D.C. 20542

Fight for Sight, Inc.
41 West 57 Street
New York, NY 10019

Guide Dogs for the Blind, Inc.
San Rafael, California 94902

National Psoriasis Foundation
Suite 250
6415 S.W. Canyon Court
Portland, OR 97221

National Society to Prevent Blindness, Inc.
79 Madison Avenue
New York, NY 10016
Engages in a nationwide program to eliminate preventable blindness in both children and adults through field consultation and publications

Recording for the Blind, Inc.
121 East 58 Street
New York, NY 10022
Provides free records and tapes of textbooks and other educational material for individuals unable to read the printed word because of visual or other physical limitations. Will record books at the specific request of borrowers.

Rehabilitation Services Administration
Division of Services to the Blind
U.S. Department of Health, Education and Welfare
Washington, D.C. 20201
Provides national leadership, technical and consultative assistance, and financial support to the federal-state programs of vocational rehabilitation. Each state administers its own program and provides complete rehabilitation services to eligible blind persons. Vocational guidance, training, placement, and follow-up are available. Information on local services can be obtained at individual state offices of vocational rehabilitation.

The American Foundation for the Blind
15 West 16 Street
New York, N.Y. 10011

The National Association for the Deaf
814 Thayer Avenue
Silver Springs, Maryland 20910

National Association for the Deaf
814 Thayer Avenue
Silver Springs, MD 20910
This organization has done much to eliminate unjust traffic and liability laws and to promote the welfare of the deaf in education, legislation, and employment. *The Silent Worker* is the official monthly publication.

National Association for Visually Handicapped
305 East 24 Street
New York, NY 10010

The Seeing Eye, Inc.
P.O. Box 375
Morristown, NJ 07960
Serves the United States, Canada, and Puerto Rico. Qualified blind persons spend 1 month learning to use and control guide dogs. Maintains a follow-up service for graduates. Conducts an extensive program of public education.

Veterans Administration
810 Vermont Avenue, N.W.
Washington, D.C. 20005
An intensive and comprehensive program of basic reorganization to blindness is provided at the Blind Rehabilitation Center, Hines, Illinois. Prosthetic and sensory aids are provided to help overcome the handicap of blindness for veterans who meet specific eligibility requirements.

Section 6

Problems of Oxygenation

Chapter 18

NURSING ASSESSMENT

Respiratory System

Carol A. Stephenson

Learning Objectives

1. Describe the structures and functions of the respiratory system.
2. Describe the process and control mechanisms for inspiration and expiration.
3. Describe the process of gaseous diffusion within the lungs.
4. Describe the structures and functions of the respiratory defense mechanisms.
5. Describe the significance of arterial blood gas values and the oxyhemoglobin dissociation curve in relationship to respiratory function.
6. Identify the significant subjective and objective data related to the respiratory system that should be obtained from a client.
7. Describe the appropriate techniques used in the physical assessment of the respiratory system.
8. Differentiate normal from common abnormal findings on physical assessment of the respiratory system.
9. Describe the purpose, significance of results, and nursing responsibilities related to diagnostic studies of the respiratory system.
10. Identify the common pulmonary function studies and what they measure.

The respiratory system includes the respiratory tract, lungs, and supporting structures. Its primary purpose is to obtain oxygen from atmospheric air. Oxygen is necessary for normal cellular function within the body. The respiratory system also performs an excretory function by ridding the body of some of the end products of metabolism (e.g., carbon dioxide).

RESPIRATORY SYSTEM: STRUCTURES AND FUNCTIONS

The respiratory system is continuous but is often divided into two portions for discussion and study. These portions are the *upper respiratory tract,* or upper airway, and the *lower respiratory tract,* or lower airway (see Fig. 18-1). The upper airway structures are the *nose, tonsils, adenoids, pharynx, epiglottis, larynx,* and *trachea.* The lower airway structures are the *bronchi, bronchioles, alveolar ducts,* and *alveoli.* Except for the primary bronchi, the lower airway structures are contained within the *lungs.* The lungs are divided into three lobes on the right (upper, middle, and lower lobes) and two lobes on the left (upper and lower lobes) (Fig. 18-2). The *chest wall structures* are also essential to respiration. These include the *rib cage, pleura,* and *muscles of respiration.*

This chapter was reviewed by Leslie Kirilloff, R.N., Ph.D., Assistant Professor, Graduate Program, Medical-Surgical Nursing, University of Pittsburgh, Pittsburgh, Pennsylvania.

Upper Respiratory Tract

The *nose* is made of bone and cartilage. Internally, the nose is divided into two passages, or *nares,* by the *septum.* The interior of the nose is shaped into many rolling projections called *turbinates.* These increase the surface area for warming and moistening air. The nose, like the rest of the respiratory tract, is lined with *mucous membrane.* It is also lined with very small hairs. The internal nose is in open communication with the various sinuses.

As air enters the nose, it is conditioned for use in the lower airway by being warmed, moistened, and filtered. This conditioning serves a protective function. In addition, most of the large foreign particles which are inhaled are removed in the nose or pharynx. This occurs as they are either caught by the nasal hairs or strike the nasal mucosa. The large number of angular projections in the nasopharynx facilitate particle impaction.

The *olfactory nerve endings,* receptors for the sense of smell, are located in the roof of the nose. The adenoids and tonsils, which are small, paired lymphatic structures, are found in the posterior nose and pharynx, respectively.

Air passes through the nose to the pharynx. Air may also enter the pharynx via the mouth. However, the mouth breather loses the protective and conditioning functions of the nose. The epiglottis is a small flap at the base of the tongue. During swallowing, the larynx elevates so that a small cartilage tips against the epiglottis. This movement serves a protective function and prevents the entrance of food into the

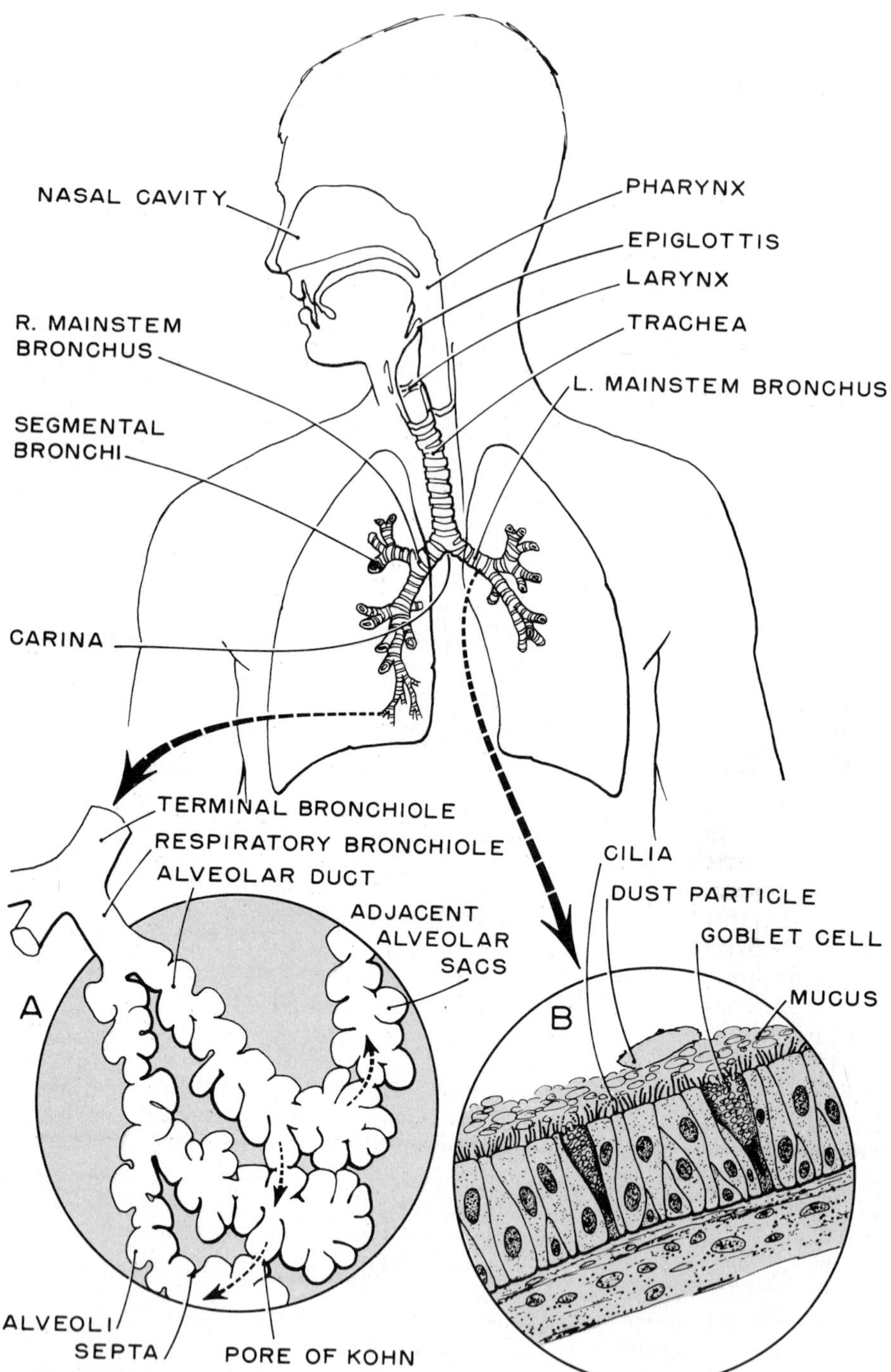

Figure 18-1 Structures of the respiratory tract. *(a)* Pulmonary function unit *(b)* Ciliated mucous membrane. *(From S. Price and L. Wilson, Pathophysiology: Clinical Concepts of Disease Processes, McGraw-Hill Book Company, New York, 1978, p. 385.)*

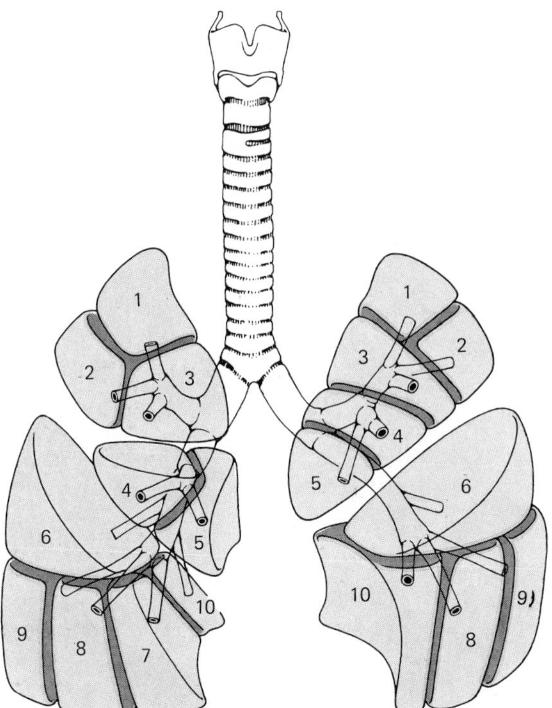

Figure 18-2 Bronchopulmonary segments of human lung. Left and right upper lobes: (1) apical, (2) posterior, (3) anterior, (4) superior lingular, and (5) inferior lingular segments. Right middle lobe: (4) lateral and (5) medial segments. Lower lobes: (6) superior (apical), (7) medial-basal, (8) anterior-basal, (9) lateral-basal, and (10) posterior-basal segments. The medial-basal segment (7) is absent in the left lung. *(From A. P. Fishman, Pulmonary Diseases and Disorders, McGraw-Hill Book Company, New York, 1980, p. 225.)*

larynx, which could result in severe coughing or aspiration.

Air moves from the pharynx to the larynx, where the vocal cords are located, and then down into the trachea. The trachea is a cylindrical tube about 10 to 15 cm long and 1.5 cm in diameter in the adult. It is supported by C-shaped cartilages which are incomplete at the posterior surface. The cartilage keeps the trachea open. The opening of the C is bridged by connective tissue and smooth muscle. This design permits expansion of the esophagus when a bolus of food is swallowed. Each cartilage is connected by elastic ligaments. The trachea bifurcates into the *right* and *left mainstem bronchi* at a point called the *carina.* The carina is located at the level of the manubriosternal junction. The manubriosternal junction is sometimes called the *angle of Louis.*

Lower Respiratory Tract

Once air passes the carina, it is in the lower respiratory tract. The right mainstem bronchus is shorter, wider, and straighter than the left mainstem bronchus. Because of these characteristics, aspiration of foreign objects is more likely to occur in the right lung than in the left lung.

The mainstem bronchi subdivide several times to form the *lobar, segmental,* and *subsegmental bronchi.* Further divisions form the bronchioles. The most distant bronchioles are called the *terminal* and *respiratory bronchioles.* Beyond these lie the alveolar ducts and sacs. This configuration of branching airways looks like an upside-down tree and hence is termed the *respiratory tree.* This method of branching allows the surface area of each smaller type of tube to be greater than the surface area of the larger tubes preceding it.

Up to the point of the respiratory bronchioles, no gaseous exchange takes place. The area of the respiratory tract from the nose to the respiratory bronchioles serves only as a conducting pathway and is therefore *anatomical dead space* (V_D). This dead space must be filled with every breath, but the air that fills it is not available for gaseous exchange. A normal adult has about 1 mL per pound of body weight of anatomical dead space.

After moving through the conducting zone, air reaches the respiratory zone, composed of the respiratory bronchioles and alveoli (Fig. 18-3). Although most gas exchange occurs in the alveoli, some gas exchange also occurs in the respiratory bronchioles. Respiratory bronchioles have alveoli that open directly into the lumen of the bronchioles.

Alveoli are small compartments that form the air cells and functional units of the lungs. The alveoli are interconnected by *pores of Kohn,* which allow for collateral movement of air from alveoli to alveoli (Fig. 18-1). The 300 million alveoli in the adult have a total volume of about 2500 mL and a surface area for diffusing about the size of a tennis court. The alveoli are in intimate contact with the capillary network. This alveolar-capillary membrane is very thin (less than 0.5 hm) and is the site of gas exchange.[1]

Surfactant

The structure of alveoli is inherently unstable. The natural tendency for alveoli is to collapse. *Surfactant,* a phospholipid secreted by type II alveolar cells, decreases the alveolar surface tension as the diameter of the alveoli becomes smaller. This increases the stability of the alveoli and prevents their collapse. The

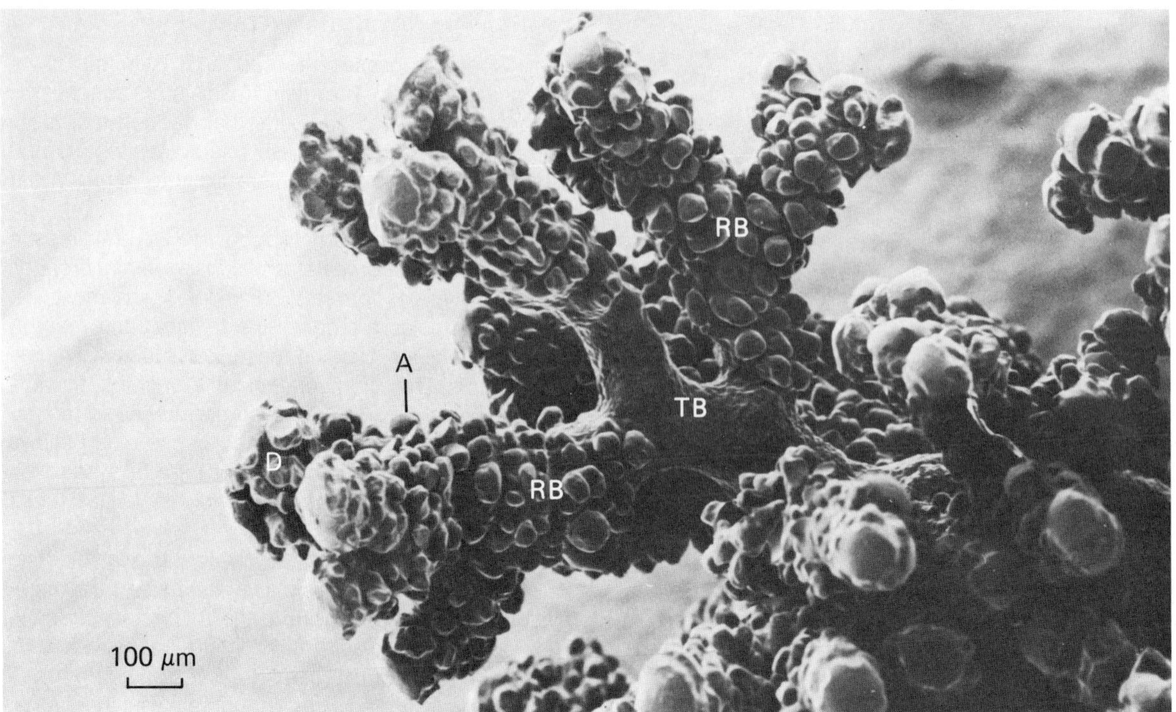

Figure 18-3 Scanning electron micrographs of airway branches peripheral to the terminal bronchiole. *(From A. P. Fishman, Pulmonary Diseases and Disorders, McGraw-Hill Book Company, New York, 1980, p. 229.)*

presence of surfactant also decreases the amount of pressure needed to inflate the alveoli. Therefore, the physiological advantages of surfactant are:[2]

1. They promote alveoli stability.
2. They increase lung compliance and decrease the work of breathing.

When there is a deficiency of surfactant in the alveolar lining, the lungs become stiff due to decreased compliance and there is widespread *atelectasis* (collapsed, airless alveoli). This condition is referred to as the *respiratory distress syndrome* and is discussed in Chap. 22.

Blood supply to the lungs

The lungs have two different types of circulation, pulmonary and bronchial. The *pulmonary* circulation provides the lungs with blood for gas exchange. It begins with the pulmonary artery from the right ventricle of the heart and branches so that each alveolus is in direct communication with a pulmonary capillary. It is at this point that oxygen and carbon dioxide exchange occurs. The pulmonary venous system returns oxygenated blood to the left atrium of the heart.

The *bronchial* circulation starts with the bronchial arteries, which arise from the thoracic aorta. It functions to meet the metabolic needs of the airways and other pulmonary tissues. Most of this blood is carried away from the lungs by the pulmonary veins.

Chest Wall

The chest wall structures include the rib cage, intercostal muscles, and diaphragm (Fig. 18-4). The chest cavity is lined with a membrane called the *parietal pleura,* and the lungs are covered with a membrane called the *visceral pleura*. The parietal and visceral pleurae are joined and form a closed, double-walled sac. The pleura secretes small amounts of fluid into the intrapleural space (potential space between the visceral and parietal pleurae) for the purpose of lubrication, which allows the layers of pleura to slide over each other during breathing. This fluid film serves to hold the lung and chest wall together as a single unit while allowing them to move separately.

The chest is shaped, supported, and protected by 24 ribs (12 on each side). The ribs and sternum make up the thorax. The ribs have several muscles attached to them. The *external intercostal muscles*

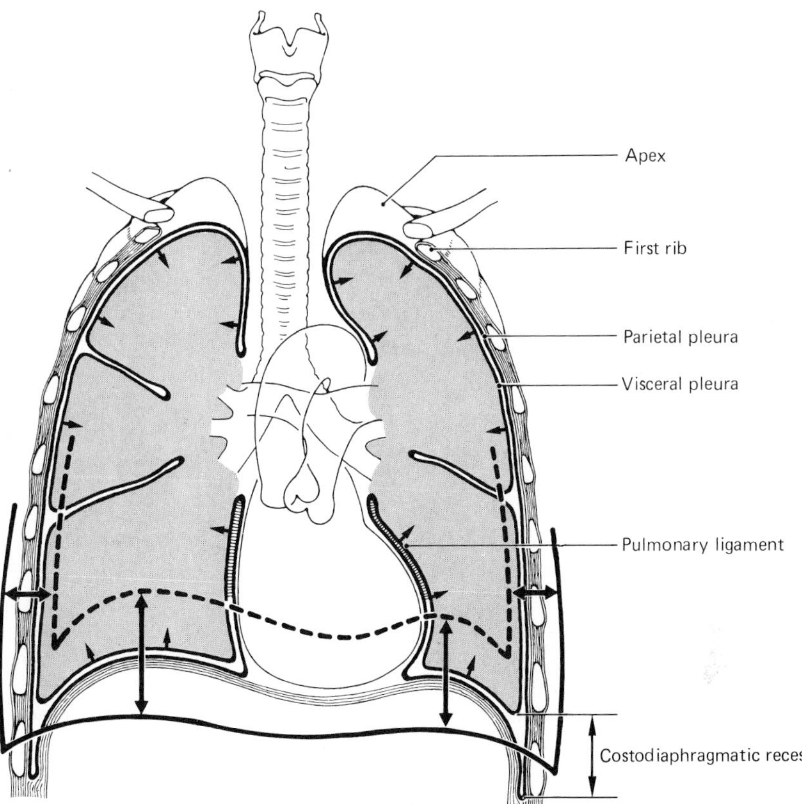

Figure 18-4 Frontal section of chest and lung showing pleural space. Single arrows indicate the retractive force; double arrows show the excursion of the lung bases and periphery between deep inspiration and expiration. *(From A. P. Fishman, Pulmonary Diseases and Disorders, McGraw-Hill Book Company, New York, 1980, p. 225.)*

and *parasternal muscles* function in normal inspiration to raise the rib cage and thereby help to increase the size of the thoracic cavity. The *scalene muscles* and *sternocleidomastoid muscles* function similarly in forced inspiration. However, the major muscle of respiration is the *diaphragm,* a dome-shaped muscle separating the chest from the abdomen. When the diaphragm contracts, it descends, increasing the size of the thoracic cavity. The abdominal contents move downward with the diaphragm and may limit its movement in conditions such as obesity or abdominal distension.

The intercostal muscles are innervated by nerves coming from the spinal cord between T1 and T11. The diaphragm is innervated by the phrenic nerve, which comes from the spinal cord between C3 and C5. All the nerves are linked to the respiratory center in the medulla via the spinal cord. This pattern of innervation is significant when considering the effect of brainstem or high spinal cord injuries. Persons who no longer have functional intercostal muscles may still be able to breathe by using their diaphragm. Other persons may be assisted in their breathing by implanting a phrenic nerve stimulator (see Chap. 53).

Physiology of Respiration

Ventilation

Ventilation involves *inspiration* (movement of air into the lungs) and *expiration* (movement of air out of the lungs). The physical process of ventilation is accomplished by the changing intrathoracic pressures in relation to atmospheric pressure so that air will move into or out of the lungs. The pressure within the lungs and thorax must be less than atmospheric pressure for inspiration to occur. This is because gases flow from an area of greater pressure to one of lesser pressure. The intrathoracic pressure is lowered by enlarging the thoracic cavity. This is accomplished by contraction of the diaphragm and intercostal muscles (see Fig. 18-5). As the thoracic cavity enlarges, the intrathoracic pressure becomes less than the atmospheric pressure, and air moves into the lungs. In quiet respiration, the diaphragm moves only about 1 cm, but it may move up to 10 cm on forced inspiration. Diaphragmatic movement temporarily compresses the abdominal contents. Consequently, this movement can be impeded by changes in abdominal size or pressure such as those resulting from obesity, preg-

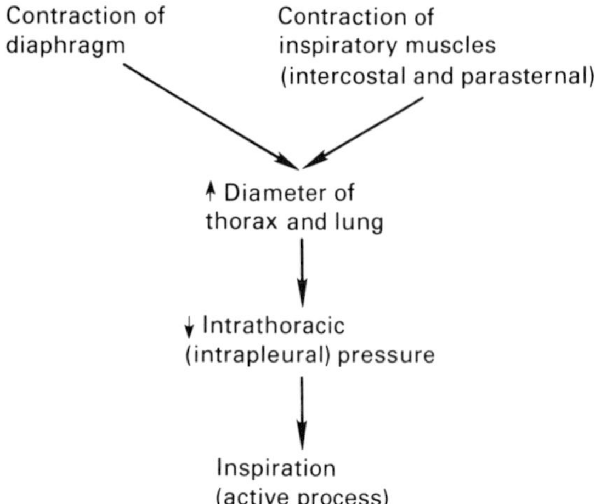

Figure 18-5 Inspiratory process.

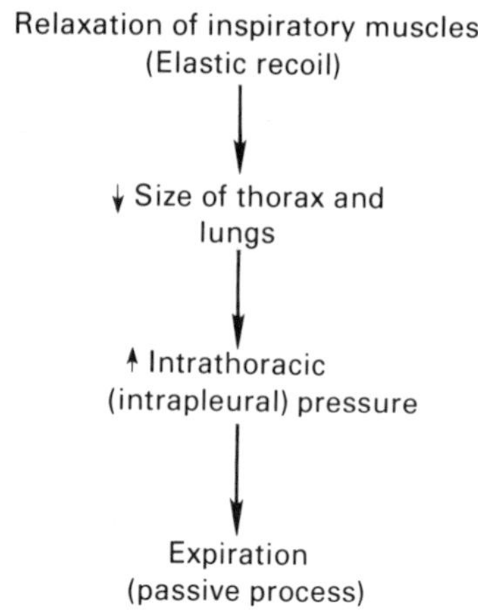

Figure 18-6 Expiratory process.

nancy, overeating, or abdominal pathological conditions.

In contrast to the active efforts of inspiration, expiration is passive. As the muscles relax, the thoracic cavity becomes smaller by elastic recoil. Intrathoracic pressure rises, and air moves out of the lungs into the atmosphere (see Fig. 18-6). Expiration can become an active process by increasing the intraabdominal pressure.

Compliance and elastic recoil

Compliance (or distensibility) is a measure of expansibility or elasticity of the lungs and thorax. Compliance is decreased in restrictive lung diseases such as diffuse fibrosis and pleural effusion. Compliance is also decreased when there is a deficiency of surfactant. Increased compliance is found in obstructive lung diseases such as pulmonary emphysema.

Elastic recoil is the tendency for the lungs to recoil after being stretched or expanded. The elasticity of lung tissue is due to the elastin fibers found in the alveolar walls and surrounding the bronchioles and capillaries.

Diffusion

When a person inhales normally, the alveoli fill with air. This causes the alveolar oxygen concentration to become higher than the concentration of oxygen in the blood. At the same time, the alveolar concentration of carbon dioxide is less than the carbon dioxide concentration of the blood in the pulmonary capillary. Therefore, oxygen diffuses across the alveolar-capillary membrane into the blood, and carbon dioxide diffuses into the alveoli until equilibrium is reached (Fig. 18-7).

Dalton's law is basic to understanding the process of gas diffusion. It states that in a mixture of gases found in an enclosed space, each gas exerts a pressure independent of those of the other gases present. The total pressure in the container is the sum of the partial pressures exerted by each gas. This means that the action of oxygen and carbon dioxide can be considered independently of the actions of other gases. Each gas occupies a fixed percentage of the air, regardless of the distance above sea level. However, even though the percentage of each gas remains constant, its partial pressure is reduced because the total barometric pressure is reduced. This is because the partial pressure, or tension of a given gas in the air, is a function of barometric pressure. Table 18-1 is based on typical barometric pressures at sea level and at an altitude of 1 mile.

As the oxygen in the air moves through each stage of transport from the atmosphere to the arterial blood and then to the tissues, some of its tension or partial pressure is lost. The partial pressure of a gas can be increased by therapeutic interventions such as oxygen therapy.

Arterial Blood Gases *Arterial blood gases* (ABGs) measure the partial pressures of gases in the arteries. The partial pressures of oxygen and carbon dioxide in arterial blood are recorded as P_aO_2 and P_aCO_2 and are frequently abbreviated as PO_2 and PCO_2. Bicarbonate (HCO_3), acidity (pH), and oxygen saturation of the hemoglobin are also measured by ABGs. This is a critical measurement for the assessment of oxygenation, ventilatory status, heart function, and metabolic status. The ABG measurements provide important data for making clinical decisions. For

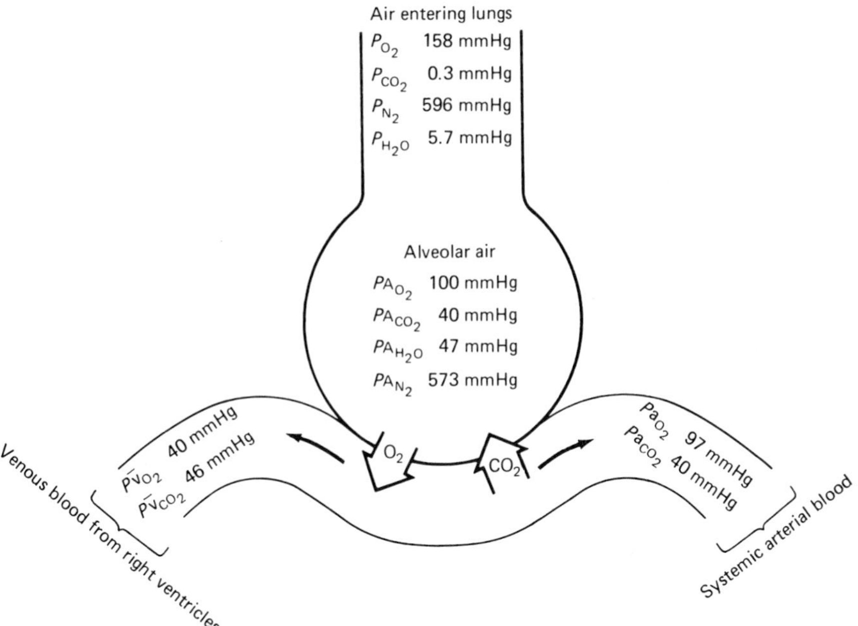

Figure 18-7 Partial pressures of respiratory gases in normal respiration. $P\bar{v}$ refers to mixed venous blood (combining blood from inferior and superior venae cavae). *(From M. R. Kinney et al., AACN's Clinical Reference for Critical Care Nursing, McGraw-Hill Book Company, New York, 1981, p. 19.)*

a detailed discussion on ABGs and acid-base balance, see Chap. 12.

Oxygen saturation is also part of ABG studies. Only a small percentage (about 3 percent) of the total oxygen in the blood is carried as dissolved oxygen. Most of it is carried in chemical combination with hemoglobin.

$$\text{Oxygen saturation} = \frac{\text{amount of oxygen being carried by hemoglobin}}{\text{amount of oxygen hemoglobin could carry}}$$

For example, if the oxygen saturation is 90 percent, then 90 percent of the hemoglobin attachments for oxygen have oxygen attached to them.

Normal values for ABG measurements vary according to whether a person is at sea level or at a higher altitude, and whether the blood is drawn from a peripheral artery or the pulmonary artery (mixed venous blood) (see Table 18-2). Blood in the pulmonary artery has not yet passed through the pulmonary capillary bed, so it will be lower in oxygen and higher in carbon dioxide than blood which has just left the lungs and entered the arterial system. The normal value of the PO_2 also decreases with age. Arterial blood compared with venous blood is a better reflection of the ventilatory status of the client because it has just gone through the pulmonary capillary beds. Nursing responsibilities for ABGs are discussed later in this chapter.

ABG results for PCO_2 are also used as a measure of whether ventilation is normal or whether the client is hyperventilating or hypoventilating. Carbon dioxide

Table 18-1
Partial Pressures of Gases in the Air*

Component of Air	%	Pressure at Sea Level, mmHg	Pressure at 1 Mile High, mmHg
Nitrogen	78.62	597.0	491.37
Oxygen	20.84	159.0	130.26
Carbon dioxide	0.04	0.3	0.25
Water vapor	0.50	3.7	3.12
Total	100.00	760.0	625.00

*The partial pressure of each gas in the air is independent of the partial pressures of the other gases and is dependent on the barometric pressure. Average barometric pressures for altitudes at sea level and at 1 mile high are given above. The partial pressure of a specific gas is determined by multiplying the percentage of that gas in air by the atmospheric pressure at a particular altitude. For example, the partial pressure of oxygen at sea level = 20.8% × 760 = 159 mmHg.

Table 18-2
Normal ABG Values

Laboratory Value	Arterial Blood at Sea Level	Arterial Blood at 1 Mile High	Mixed Venous Blood
pH	7.35–7.45	7.35–7.45	7.31–7.41
PO_2	80–100 mmHg*	65–75 mmHg*	35–40 mmHg*
O_2 saturation	95% or more	92–94%	70–75%
PCO_2	35–45 mmHg	35–45 mmHg	41–51 mmHg
HCO_3	22–28 mEq/L	22–28 mEq/L	22–28 mEq/L

*Value decreases with age.
Adapted with permission from Carolyn M. Hudak, Thelma Lohr, and Barbara M. Gallow, *Critical Care Nursing,* 2d ed., J.B. Lippincott Company, Philadelphia, 1977, p. 273.

diffuses more readily than oxygen across the alveolar-capillary membrane. Therefore, it is more readily given up when it is carried to the lungs. Since it is so exchangeable, PCO_2 is used as a measure of how well a person is exchanging air. *Hyperventilation* results in exhalation of greater than normal amounts of carbon dioxide, while *hypoventilation* results in retention of carbon dioxide. Hyperventilation or hypoventilation should not be used as a label for how a person looks when he is breathing. He may be in distress and may appear to be working very hard to breathe, while at the same time actually exchanging very little carbon dioxide or oxygen. The states of hyperventilation and hypoventilation can be determined only by the measurement of ABGs.

Oxygen-Hemoglobin Dissociation Curve[3] The affinity of hemoglobin for oxygen is described by the *oxygen-hemoglobin dissociation curve* (Fig. 18-8). This curve reflects the ease with which hemoglobin gives up or takes on oxygen. Oxygen delivery to the tissues depends greatly on the ease with which hemoglobin will give up oxygen once it reaches the tissues. In the upper flat portion of the curve, fairly large changes in the PO_2 cause a small change in hemoglobin saturation. For this reason, if the oxygen tension drops from 100 to 60 mmHg, the saturation of hemoglobin changes by only 7 percent (from the normal of 97 to 90 percent). Thus, the hemoglobin remains 90 percent saturated despite a 40 mmHg drop in the PO_2. This portion of the curve also explains why increased administration of high levels of oxygen does little good if the hemoglobin has already been fully saturated.

The lower portion of the curve indicates a different type of protection. Here, as the hemoglobin becomes further desaturated, larger amounts of oxygen are released for tissue use. This is an important method of maintaining the pressure gradient between the blood and tissues. It also assures an adequate oxygen supply to peripheral tissues even when the decrease in capillary PO_2 is small.

Many factors alter the affinity of hemoglobin for oxygen. An increase in hemoglobin affinity for oxygen causes the curve to shift to the left. This is seen in alkalosis, decreased PCO_2, and decreased temperature.

A decrease in the hemoglobin affinity for oxygen causes the curve to shift to the right. This is seen in acidosis, increased PCO_2, and increased temperature. A shift to the right favors release of oxygen to the tissues. An increase in 2,3-diphosphoglycerate (2,3-DPG) is associated with chronic hypoxia and causes a shift to the right. (This is explained in the section on anemia in Chap. 24.)

Control of Respiration

Respirations are controlled very precisely in order to supply adequate amounts of oxygen to the body and rid the body of carbon dioxide. The respiratory rate changes in response to a variety of metabolic needs.

The *respiratory center* is composed of cell clusters in both the *medulla* and *pons* in the brain. These cells respond to both chemical and mechanical signals from the body. Impulses are sent from the respiratory center to the body via the spinal cord and the phrenic nerves.[4] Respirations are controlled by both chemical chemoreceptors and mechanical sensors.

Chemical chemoreceptors

A *chemoreceptor* is a receptor that responds to a change in the chemical composition (especially blood gases and pH) of the fluid around it. The *central chemoreceptors* are located in the medulla and respond to changes in the H^+ ion concentration. An increase in the H^+ ion concentration stimulates ventilation, while a decrease inhibits it. The carbon dioxide level in blood regulates ventilation primarily by its effect on the pH of the cerebrospinal fluid.

Peripheral chemoreceptors are located in the carotid bodies at the bifurcation of the common carotid arteries and in the aortic bodies located above and below the aortic arch. The peripheral chemoreceptors respond to decreases in arterial PO_2 and pH and to increases in arterial PCO_2. These changes will cause stimulation of the respiratory center.

In a healthy individual an increase in PCO_2 and a decrease in pH cause an immediate increase in the respiratory rate. Alveolar ventilation is increased and excess carbon dioxide removed. A decrease in PO_2 will also stimulate respiration, but this mechanism is less important. When pulmonary disease prevents efficient removal of carbon dioxide by increasing the respiratory rate, a decrease in the PO_2 (or hypoxic drive) becomes the more important mechanism to stimulate the respiratory center. This is seen in a person with chronic obstructive lung disease (Chap. 21).

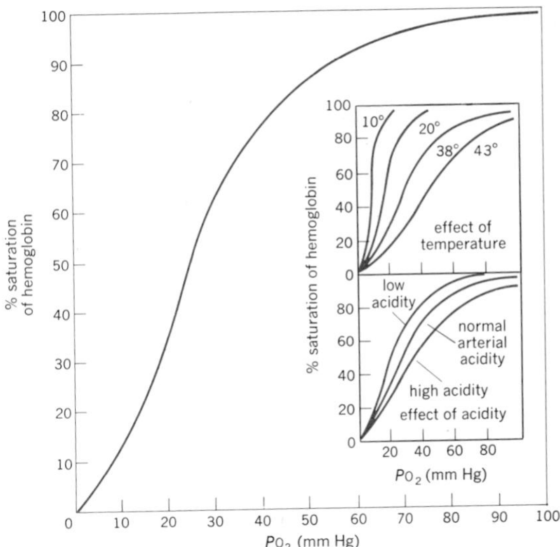

Figure 18-8 Oxygen-hemoglobin dissociation curve. The insets show the effects of acidity changes and temperature changes. *(From E. J. Reith et al., Textbook of Anatomy and Physiology 2d ed., McGraw-Hill Book Company, New York, 1978, p. 364.)*

Mechanical sensors

Mechanical sensors are located in the lungs, upper airways, chest wall, and diaphragm. They are stimulated by a variety of physical factors such as airway obstruction, irritants, muscle stretching, and alveolar wall distortion. Signals from the stretch receptors aid in the control of respiration. As the lungs inflate, pulmonary stretch receptors aid in the control of respiration. As the lungs inflate, pulmonary stretch receptors activate the inspiratory center to inhibit further lung expansion. This is called the *Hering-Breuer reflex.* It prevents overdistension of the lungs. Impulses from the mechanical sensors are sent via the vagus nerve to the brain.

Respiratory Defense Mechanisms

Respiratory defense mechanisms are very efficient in protecting the lungs from inhaled particles, microorganisms, and toxic gases. The defense mechanisms include (1) filtration of air, (2) the mucociliary clearance system, (3) the cough reflex, (4) reflex bronchoconstriction, and (5) the alveolar macrophage.

Filtration of air

Nasal hairs *filter* the inspired air. In addition, the sharp angulation of airflow which occurs as air moves over the nasal pharynx, the tongue, and the larynx increases air turbulence. This results in the impaction of particles and bacteria on the mucosal lining of these structures. Most particles over 10 μm in diameter are removed in this manner.

The airflow slows greatly after it passes the larynx, facilitating the deposition of smaller particles (1 to 10 μm). They are deposited on the mucosa by sedimentation. Particles less than 1 μm are deposited and removed by diffusion.

Mucociliary clearance system

Below the larynx, mucus movement is accomplished by the *mucociliary clearance system.* This term is used to indicate the interrelationship between mucus secretion and ciliary activity. Mucus is continually secreted at a rate of about 100 mL/day by goblet cells and submucosal glands. It forms a mucus blanket which contains the impacted particles and debris from distal lung areas (Fig. 18-1). Secretory immunoglobulin A in the mucus contributes to protection against bacteria and viruses.

Most of the lower airway cells are equipped with cilia (Fig. 18-9). Each ciliated cell contains about 200 cilia. These beat rhythmically about 1200 times per minute in order to move the upper layer of the mucus blanket toward the mouth.[5] Ciliary action is reduced by increased mucus viscosity, dehydration, smoking, inhalation of high oxygen concentrations, infection, and ingestion of drugs such as atropine, alcohol, or anesthetics.

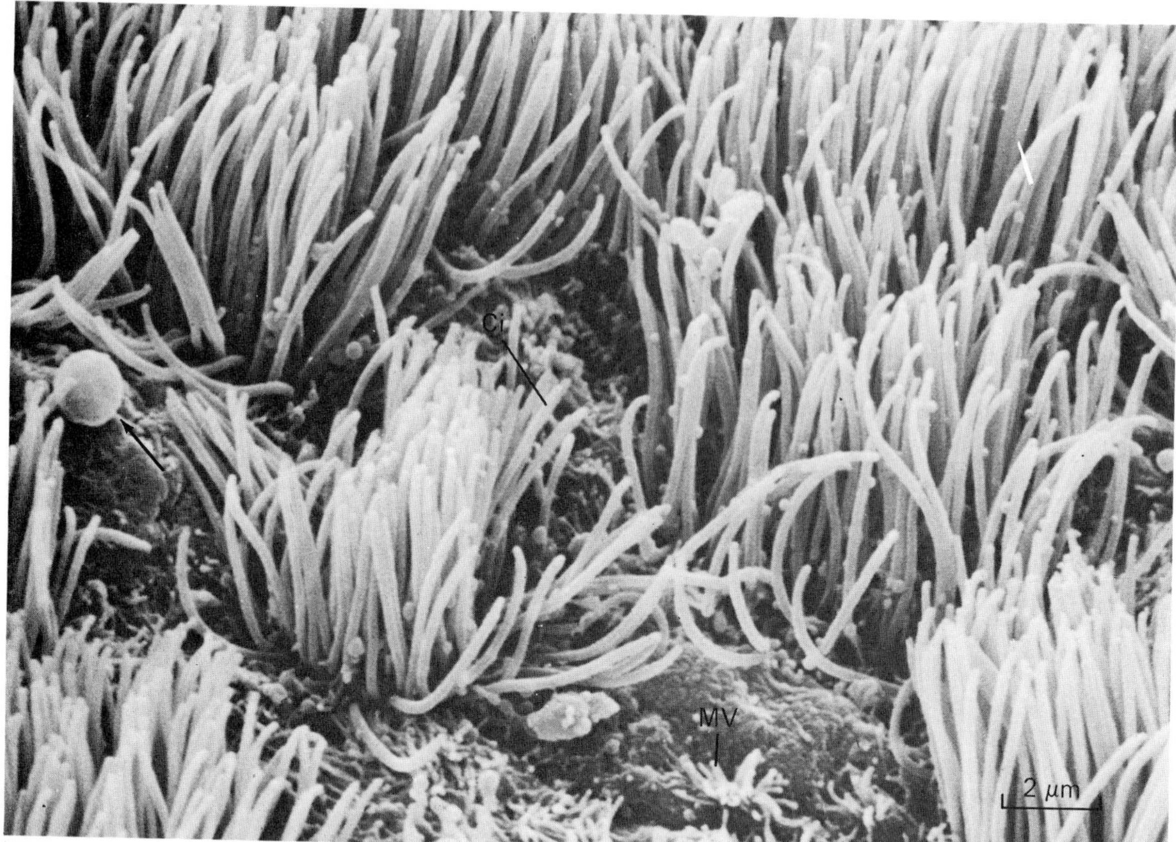

Figure 18-9 Surface view of bronchiolar epithelium showing tufts of cilia (Ci) and microvilli (MV). Note droplet secretion (arrow). *(From A. P. Fishman, Pulmonary Diseases and Disorders, McGraw-Hill Book Company, New York, 1980, p. 247.)*

Cough reflex

The *cough* is a protective reflex action which clears the airway by a high-pressure, high-velocity flow of air. It is a backup mechanism for the mucociliary clearance mechanism. This is especially true when the mucociliary clearance mechanism is overwhelmed or ineffective. Coughing is usually more effective in clearing the larger airways than the smaller ones. The most effective method of coughing is first to take several deep breaths and then on the last breath to generate a series of smaller or staged coughs during expiration. The deep breaths and smaller coughs help to move mucus up the airway. The person with severe lung or neuromuscular disease may have a greatly impaired cough (see Chap. 21).

Reflex bronchoconstriction

Another defense mechanism is *reflex bronchoconstriction.* In response to the inhalation of large amounts of irritant substances (e.g., dusts, aerosols), the bronchi constrict reflexly in an effort to prevent entry of the irritants. This may protect the distal lung tissues to some extent. Some individuals, such as asthmatics, have hyperractive airways and experience bronchoconstriction after inhalation of dust or cold air.

Alveolar macrophage

The mucociliary clearance system does not extend into the alveoli. The primary defense mechanism at this level is the *alveolar macrophage.* (Macrophages are discussed in Chap. 10.) These macrophages rapidly phagocytize inhaled foreign particles such as bacteria. The debris is moved to small airways for removal by the mucociliary system, or it is removed from the lungs by the lymphatic system. Normal macrophage activity can be impaired by cigarette and marijuana smoking, pollutants, ingestion of alcohol, and administration of corticosteroids.[6]

Particles which cannot be adequately phagocytized tend to remain in the lungs for indefinite periods and can stimulate *inflammatory* or *fibrogenic* responses. Coal dust and silica can stimulate a fibrous reaction (see Chap. 20).

ASSESSMENT OF THE RESPIRATION SYSTEM

Subjective Data: The History

Past medical history

Pediatric and Adult Illnesses The upper and lower respiratory systems are common sites of both minor and major health problems. The client should be specifically asked about a history of lower respiratory problems such as pneumonia, tuberculosis, asthma, emphysema, or bronchitis. The frequency of upper respiratory problems (colds, sore throats, sinus problems) should be determined. Problems related to other systems that affect the respiratory system should also be investigated. For example, cardiac and peripheral vascular problems can adversely affect the respiratory status, as can severe neurological problems.

Immunizations Question the client about the frequency and results of tuberculin skin testing. The date of the last test should be recorded. The status of immunization related to pertussis and polio should also be recorded.

Hospitalizations Determine if the client has ever been hospitalized for a respiratory problem. If the response is positive, the dates, chief complaint, therapy (including surgery), and current status of the problem should be recorded. If the client mentions hospitalization for any other reason, ask if a chest x-ray was taken at that time. This x-ray could provide valuable baseline data should a respiratory problem be identified. Since tonsillectomy and adenoidectomy are usually pediatric procedures, specifically ask your adult client if he had these surgeries. Past events are easily forgotten. For this reason, specific questions must be asked.

Injuries Ask whether the client has ever sustained trauma to structures of the respiratory system, such as a broken nose, fractured ribs, or pneumothorax (collapsed lung).

Medication History It is important to record a medication history with particular reference to antituberculosis drugs, antibiotics prescribed for respiratory problems, bronchodilators, steroids, cardiotonics, diuretics, and anticoagulants. Include over-the-counter drugs as well as prescription drugs. Past and present usage should be determined. The reason for taking the medication, the name, dose, and frequency, duration of use, effect, and side effects of the medication should be obtained.

The client should also be questioned about drugs which have adverse effects on respiration. Such drugs include sedatives, narcotics, heroin, and alcohol (depress respiratory function), aspirin (causes severe allergic hypersensitivity in some asthmatics), beta blockers such as propanolol (causes bronchoconstriction) and oil-based nasal products (cause lipoid aspiration pneumonia).

Many pulmonary clients use equipment at home to alleviate their breathing problem. Inquire if they use IPPB (intermittent positive-pressure breathing) machines, nebulization, mist, or other equipment. If they do, determine the type of equipment used, how and when it is employed, and what solutions are used with it. Also inquire about the use of home oxygen and such treatments as postural drainage and percussion.

Allergies Many clients with allergies also have respiratory problems. Carefully inquire about food, drug, contact, or inhalant allergens which might cause an allergic reaction. Have the client describe the specific reaction and precipitating factors such as runny nose, wheezing, scratchy throat, or tightness in the chest. Determine if the client has ever had an anaphylactic reaction. Inquire about any past or ongoing desensitization therapy. Ask the client if he has ever been told about the presence of nasal polyps or was ever treated for them.

Family history

The client needs to be questioned about a family history of such problems as tuberculosis, heart disease, alcoholism, hypertension, cancer, anemia, asthma, allergies, eczema or hives, bronchitis, or emphysema which can affect the respiratory system either directly or indirectly. These problems in parents, spouse, children, and siblings should be noted.

Personal and social history

Almost all components of a person's life can influence his respiratory status. The following areas are of particular importance.

Occupation Obtain specific data related to the job history. Where does the client work, what are his responsibilities, and is he exposed to any dusts, fumes, toxins, asbestos, coal dust, or silica? If exposed, what safety equipment does he use to decrease the potential lung damage? Determine if a past job entailed exposure to respiratory irritants.

Geographic Locations Ask where the client has lived and traveled. Coccidioidomycosis (valley fever) is a special problem for persons who have lived in the Arizona desert and in the San Joaquin valley of California. Histoplasmosis is prevalent in the Ohio valley. Other fungal lung infections and their common geographic locations are presented in Table 20-10.

Exercise and Recreation Lack of exercise is detrimental to respiratory health. Inquire about the client's type and frequency of exercise. Ask the client to compare his activity level within the last 5 to 10 years. Also, ask the client how strenuous exercise or recreation affects his breathing now as compared to the past.

Diet Obtain data to determine the adequacy of fluid intake during a 24-hour period. Inadequate fluid intake can alter respiratory secretions, making them thicker, more tenacious, and more difficult to expectorate. Also, note if the diet is balanced according to the basic four food groups. Adequate vitamin A intake is necessary to maintain soft, moist tissues of the respiratory tract and to increase resistance to infective organisms. Vitamin C, iron, and protein are also important to maintain the health of the respiratory tract.

Habits

Smoking

A careful smoking history is a critical part of the health history because smoke is known to increase mucus production and decrease ciliary action. Ask the client if he now smokes or has ever smoked cigarettes, pipes, or cigars. If the answer is positive, determine the number of pack-years by multiplying the number of packs smoked per day by the number of years smoked. For example, a person who smoked $1\frac{1}{2}$ packs per day for 10 years would have a 15-year pack history. It is generally believed that a person with a 20-year pack history cannot escape having some small airway changes. However, this person may not exhibit any respiratory symptoms. If the client has stopped smoking, find out if he did so because of respiratory problems.

Alcohol

There is a high correlation between alcoholism and heavy smoking, although the converse is not necessarily true. The client should be questioned about the pattern of drinking. Alcohol decreases ciliary action, which in turn reduces the movement of mucus from the lungs. Alcohol also reduces the rate of respiration and the cough reflex. In addition, many alcoholics do not eat adequately. If a problem is suspected, a detailed drinking history should be elicited (see Chap. 60).

Activity Obtain information related to the lifelong activity pattern of your client. As a child, did he miss school frequently because of colds and respiratory problems? Could he keep up with his peers and participate in physical education? As an adult, can he keep up with his peers in their activities? Although some lessening of activities is expected with aging, it should not occur as a result of breathing problems associated with activity. If this has occurred, carefully document these changes.

Current Stresses and Coping Mechanisms Tactfully elicit a history of current problems and stresses. The usual and current methods of coping with stress should be obtained. Does stress cause any change in the respiratory pattern such as sighing, shallow breathing, or hyperventilation? When under stress, does the client often come down with a cold or sore throat? Determine who and what the client views as available resources and support systems.

Review of systems

While the nurse is directly questioning the client regarding symptoms which could indicate a respiratory problem, she should also be making pertinent observations. Does the client speak comfortably in complete sentences, or is he limited to phrases or even single words with a breath in between? Is any hoarseness noted? Does the client swallow frequently or sniff as if his nose were full?

Specifically question the client about past or current problems of the upper and lower respiratory systems. Inquire about problems of the nose and sinuses, such as colds, discharge, epistaxis, sinus pain, or swelling. Problems of the throat can include sore throats, hoarseness, difficulty in swallowing, and occurrence of strep throat. Ask about the presence of a cough, sputum, dyspnea, orthopnea (the need to sit up in order to breathe), wheezing, chest pain, hemoptysis (coughing up blood), fever, shaking chills, or night sweats. Record the date of the last chest examination. If the client responds positively to any of the problems asked in the review of systems, obtain detailed information according to the criteria outlined in Chap. 3.

Since respiratory problems often affect other systems, the client should be questioned specifically about anxiety, personality changes, disorientation, poor judgment, irritability, and headache which could indicate a neurological problem secondary to oxygen deficit or increased carbon dioxide. Cardiac symptoms such as tachycardia, paroxysmal nocturnal dyspnea (PND), hypertension, angina or other chest pain, and palpitations on exertion could result from a respiratory problem.

Objective Data: The Physical Examination

Vital signs including temperature, pulse, respirations, and blood pressure, as well as weight, are important data to collect prior to examination of the respiratory system.

Nose

Inspect the external shape of the nose for inflammation, form, and symmetry. Then, utilizing a nasal speculum and a good light, inspect the interior of the nose (Fig. 18-10). The mucous membrane should be observed for color, edema (bogginess), exudate, and bleeding. It should be pink and moist, with no evidence of edema, exudate, or bleeding. The nasal septum should be observed for deviation, perforations, or bleeding. The turbinates should be observed for *polyps,* fingerlike projections of swollen nasal mucosa. Polyps are abnormal and usually associated with long-term irritation of the mucosa, often secondary to allergies.

Mouth and pharynx

Using a good light source, inspect the interior of the mouth. The presence, symmetry, and condition of the tonsils should be noted. They should have the same pink color as the oral mucosa (lighter in color than the nasal mucosa), moist, and with no exudate or ulcerations. In order to visualize the pharynx, press a tongue blade against the middle of the back of the tongue. The pharynx should be smooth, moist, and pink, with no evidence of exudate, ulcerations, or swelling (Fig. 18-11). (Further descriptions of the mouth examination for conditions that may affect the gastrointestinal system are provided in Chap. 31.)

Neck

Inspect the neck for symmetry and swollen areas. Also, inspect the trachea to see if it is in the midline. Palpate the lymph nodes with the client sitting erect and with the neck slightly flexed. Progress from the nodes around the ears (front to back) to the nodes at the base of the skull and then to those located under the angles of the mandible (jaw) to the midline. Small, mobile, nontender individual nodes (shotty nodes) may be felt normally. However, tender, hard, or fixed nodes are indicative of pathology. Describe the location and characteristics of any nodes that are palpated (lymph node palpation is described in more detail in Chap. 23). Palpate the trachea to see that it is in the midline above the sternal notch.

Heart

Cardiac assessment is discussed in Chap. 25. Findings that reflect respiratory health include heart

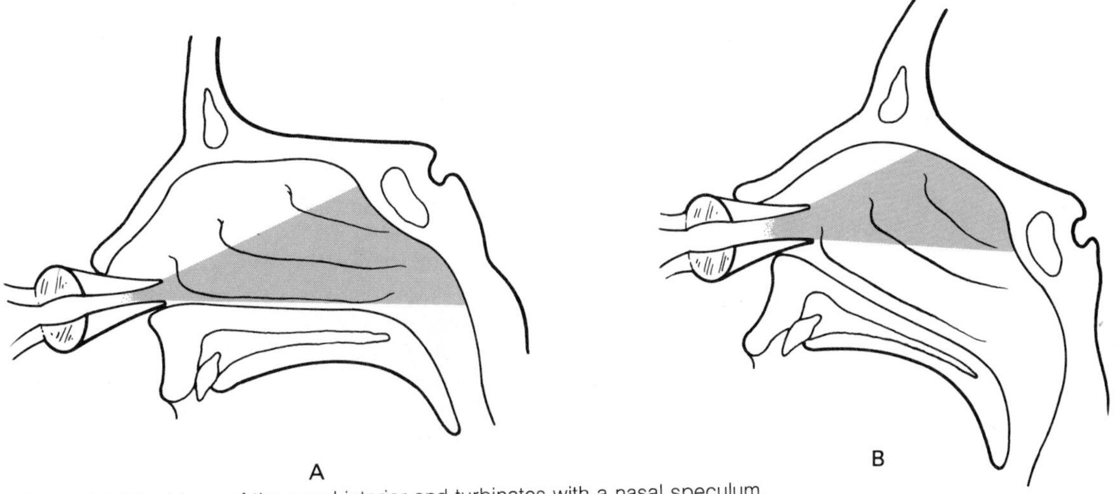

Figure 18-10 Views of the nasal interior and turbinates with a nasal speculum.

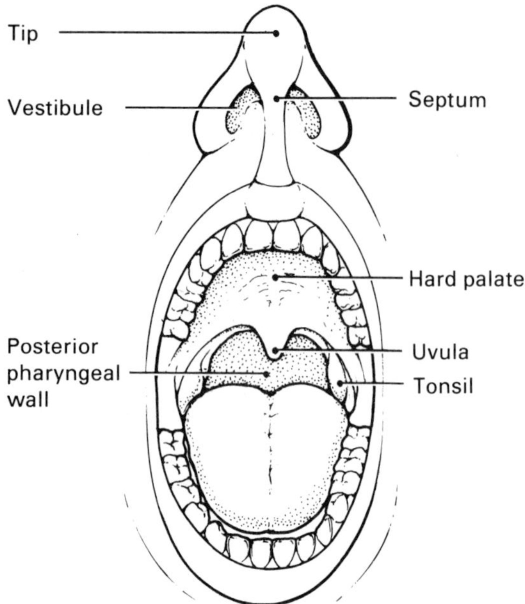

Figure 18-11 Structures of the nose and mouth.

sounds (also covered in Chap. 28), heart rate, location of the point of maximal impulse (PMI), jugular venous distension (JVD), and dependent edema.

Thorax and lungs

Inspection If possible, the client should be sitting in an upright position for a respiratory examination. Have the client undress down to the waist. Compare one side of the chest with the other side and work from the top down. The posterior chest is usually examined before the anterior chest. Observe the respirations for rate, depth, and rhythm. Note whether the respirations are costal (from the ribs) or abdominal. Note the posture and the use of accessory muscles in breathing.

Also, note whether the respirations appear very shallow or if there is intercostal bulging or *retraction* (outward or inward movement of the interspaces between the ribs on expiration or inspiration). In addition, watch for *splinting* of the chest during breathing (decreased movement of an area of the chest). Note the presence of diaphoresis on the skin. In addition, inspect the skin for any evidence of chest trauma, such as bruising or lacerations.

When inspecting anteriorly, watch for pursing of the client's lips on exhalation, flaring of the nares, and cyanosis of the lips. The client's fingers should be inspected for evidence of clubbing (the angle between the base of the nail and the fingernail is greater than 180°).

Inspect for symmetry and shape of the chest. Both sides should appear alike. Measure the distance between the anterior and posterior axillary lines and the posterior axillary line on each side and compare the ratio (transverse). The anterior-posterior (AP) diameter should range from a ratio of 1:2 to 5:7 in relation to the transverse measurement. Alterations in the shape of the thorax which can restrict ventilation include such conditions as kyphoscoliosis and are discussed in Chap. 21.

Palpation Palpation is done to assess symmetry of motion, tactile fremitus, and the presence of tenderness or masses. It is helpful for the nurse to visualize mentally the underlying structures during the examination.

Symmetry of motion or *excursion* should be checked on both the front and back of the chest. The examiner places both hands against the lower part of the posterior chest, as shown in Fig. 18-12. To check the symmetry of the anterior chest, the examiner places both hands over the lower anterior thorax, thumbs along the coastal margin pointing toward the neck. As the client takes a deep breath, the examiner watches the movement of her hands. Having the hands on the chest makes it possible to detect asymmetry of motion, as evidenced by unequal movement of the thumbs away from each other. Normal chest motion is symmetrical.

Tactile fremitus reflects the transmission of the vibration of air resulting from phonation. These vibrations are transmitted to the chest wall. It is important to compare the same location on both sides of the chest for findings to be accurate. Tactile fremitus is elicited by placing the palms or the ulnar surfaces of the examiner's hands against the client's chest. The client is asked to repeat a phrase, such as "ninety-nine." The examiner moves the hands to a lower spot and repeats the process. This should be continued all the way down the back, comparing the sides symmetrically. A soft, buzzing sensation decreasing in intensity should be felt at each site and should be symmetrical at each level.

Increased, decreased, or absent fremitus should be noted. Problems such as pneumonia and tumors increase the density of lung tissue and increase palpable fremitus. Air, upper airway blockage, or obstruction of a major airway interferes with the transmission of sounds and decreases fremitus. The anterior chest is more difficult to palpate for fremitus due to the presence of large muscles and breast tissue.

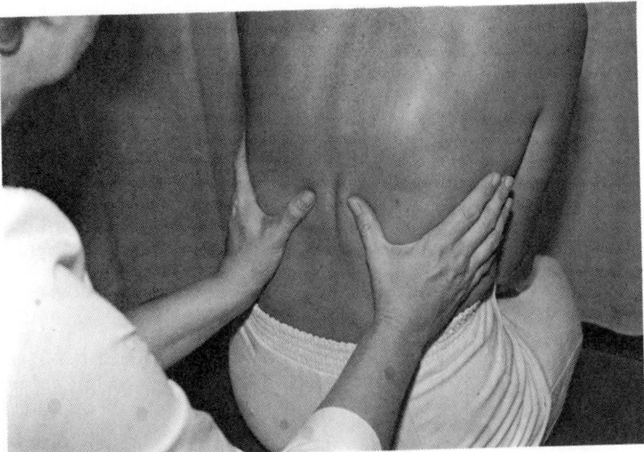

Figure 18-12 Evaluating respiratory excursion.

Percussion Percussion is done to assess the density or aeration in the lungs. The technique for percussion is described in Chap. 3. The usual percussion sounds are presented in Table 18-3.

The client should sit with his arms folded in order to pull the scapulas apart so that more area may be percussed. Percussion should begin across the top of the shoulder to identify the apices of the lungs. There should be a resonant area about 5 cm long. Then continue down, interspace by interspace (Fig. 18-13). Many examiners alternate sides to compare findings. Normally, there will be the same sound and less resonance as the examiner approaches the base of the lungs. An alternate technique is to progress down one side, then down the other side, and finally to compare notes on alternate sides if any changes are found.

The anterior chest is usually percussed with the client in a supine position. Starting below the clavicles, percuss downward, interspace by interspace. The entire thorax should be resonant, with the exception of the area of cardiac dullness.

Diaphragmatic excursion (amount of downward movement of the diaphragm with a full inspiration following a full expiration, normally 4 to 6 cm) may be assessed by percussion, although it is usually evaluated by chest x-ray. To percuss for diaphragmatic excursion, the examiner should have the client breathe normally while the examiner percusses down the back. When the percussion note changes from resonance to dullness, note the location. Ask the client to inspire and hold his breath. Starting at the previous area of dullness, percuss down until dullness is again noted. The difference between the two areas of dullness is the diaphragmatic excursion.

Auscultation The diaphragm of the stethoscope is used for auscultation of the lungs because it transmits the higher-pitched sounds. The stethoscope should be pressed tightly against the body surface. The examiner should ask the client to take repeated slow, deep breaths through his mouth during auscultation. The examiner should begin auscultating at the *posterior* base of the lungs and work from side to side

Table 18-3
Percussion Sounds

Sound	**Description**
Tympany	Drumlike, loud, empty quality. May be elicited over gas-filled stomach or intestine, or pneumothorax.
Resonance	Sound elicited over normal lungs. Low-pitched.
Hyperresonance	Louder, low-pitched sounds. This term often used to describe hyperinflated lungs, such as in chronic obstructive lung disease or acute asthma.
Dull	Medium-intensity pitch and duration. Elicited over areas of "mixed" solid and lung tissue, as over the top area of the liver or partially consolidated lung tissue (pneumonia), or the fluid-filled pleural space.
Flat	Soft, high-pitched sound of short duration. Heard over very dense tissue where air is not present.

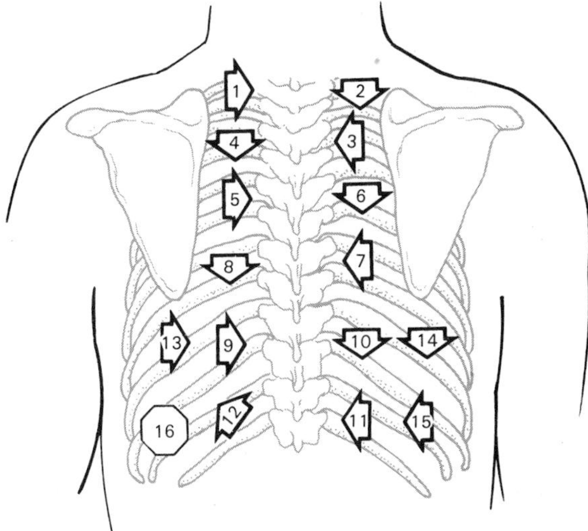

Figure 18-13 Diagram of percussion areas on the posterior chest wall. Percussion should progress symmetrically, as shown in the numbered sequence. *(From D. A. Jones et al., Medical-Surgical Nursing: A Conceptual Approach, McGraw-Hill Book Company, New York, 1978, p. 772.)*

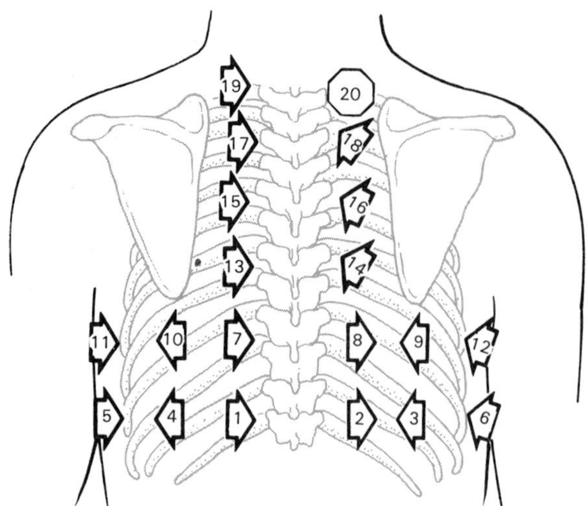

Figure 18-14 Diagram of auscultation of the posterior chest. Auscultation should proceed symmetrically, beginning at the posterior bases so that atelectatic rales are not overlooked.

and upward until reaching the apices (Fig. 18-14). This allows the examiner to note any atelectatic rales, which can disappear with deep breathing. The *front* of the chest wall is auscultated from top to bottom. The findings should be described by both character and exact location.

At each location in the auscultatory process, the examiner should listen to a full cycle of breath sounds (inspiration and expiration). She should listen for three qualities: character and intensity of breath sounds, the presence of adventitious (abnormal) sounds, and the transmission of voice sounds.

There are three normal breath sounds: vesicular, bronchial, and bronchovesicular (Fig. 18-15). *Vesicular* breath sounds are normal in the adult. The inspiratory phase is longer and stronger than the expiratory phase. The sound is soft and low-pitched.

Bronchial breath sounds are normal in the child because there is less tissue between the alveoli and the stethoscope. In the adult, they are generally associated with lung consolidation. The expiratory phase is longer than the inspiratory phase. The quality is tubular, harsh, loud, and high-pitched.

Bronchovesicular breath sounds are intermediate between the other two types. They are of medium intensity and pitch and are normally heard anteriorly and posteriorly in the area of the bronchi. The duration of inspiration and expiration is equal.

Adventitious breath sounds are abnormal sounds which may be heard on auscultation. Table 18-3 describes them and gives possible etiologies.

A record of the normal physical assessment of the respiratory system is shown in Table 18-4. Common assessment abnormalities are presented in Table 18-5.

DIAGNOSTIC STUDIES OF THE RESPIRATORY SYSTEM

Blood Studies

Common blood studies used to assess the respiratory system are the hemoglobin (Hb or Hbg), hematocrit (Hct), and ABG (see Table 18-6). Others that may be done include electrolyte and enzyme studies. Analysis of ABGs is the most important test for determining the adequacy of ventilation. Table 18-6 describes the nursing responsibility associated with this test. To obtain accurate findings:

1. Maintain the client at room air or prescribed supplemental oxygen for at least 20 minutes (this is

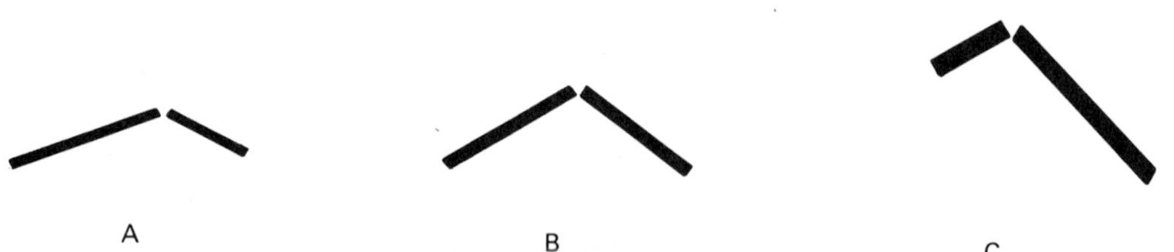

Figure 18-15 A diagrammatic model of breath sounds. Normal vesicular sounds have a longer inspiratory phase. Bronchovesicular breath sounds have approximately equal inspiratory and expiratory phases. Bronchial breath sounds have a longer and louder expiratory phase.

especially critical when a client's oxygen therapy or ventilator is being manipulated).

2. Maintain the client at complete physical and emotional rest as much as possible in order to decrease the metabolic rate.
3. Prevent the mixing of air with the blood sample, which would affect both oxygen and carbon dioxide findings. Do this by expelling all air bubbles prior to puncture and covering the tip of the needle.
4. Slow the chemical activity in the blood sample by surrounding the syringe with ice in a tray.

Sputum Studies

Single sputum specimens are examined for cellular and bacterial components. In diagnosing infections

Table 18-4
Recording the Normal Physical Assessment of the Respiratory System

Nose is symmetrical, with no deformities. Nasal mucosa is pink and moist with no edema, exudate, or blood. Nasal septum is straight, without perforations. No polyps are evident. Oral mucosa is light pink and moist, with no exudate or ulcerations. Tonsils are present. Pharynx is smooth, moist, and pink. Neck is symmetrical and trachea is in the midline. No nodes are palpable. Chest has a normal configuration, without evidence of injury. Respirations are normal, at the rate of 14/min. Excursion is equal bilaterally, with no increase in tactile fremitus. Percussion is resonant throughout. Breath sounds are normal throughout without rales, ronchi, or wheezes. No axillary nodes are palpable.

Table 18-5
Common Assessment Abnormalities of the Thorax and Lungs

Finding	Definition/Description	Possible Etiology*
	Inspection	
Use of accessory muscles; tripod position	Client leans forward on arms and elbows and actively uses neck and shoulder muscles to enlarge thorax.	Respiratory distress due to air trapping (COPD, asthma)
Increased AP diameter (barrel chest)	Chest abnormally wide from front to back. Ribs nearly horizontal rather than having normal 45° slope.	Chronic air trapping Aging COPD Some skeletal diseases
Kyphosis	Convex curvature of spine.	Trauma Musculoskeletal disease Vertebral tuberculosis (Pott's disease) Long-term steroid administration
Scoliosis	Lateral curvature of spine.	Poor posture Rickets Uneven leg length Idiopathic
Lordosis	Concave curvature of spine.	Poor posture Musculoskeletal disease Idiopathic
Pectus excavatum (funnel chest)	Depressed lower sternum with reduced AP diameter.	Congenital
Pectus carinatum (pigeon chest)	Forward projection of sternum with increased AP diameter and narrow thoracic width.	Congenital
Pursed lips on exhalation	Client exhales with lips pursed together in order to slow exhalation.	Asthma COPD Cystic fibrosis
Inspiratory flaring of nares	Nares flare on inspiration in an effort to increase air intake.	Respiratory distress
Splinting	Client holds chest rigid in order to avoid increasing pain with respiratory movement.	Recent thoracic and abdominal incisions Chest trauma Musculoskeletal problems

Table 18-5 (Continued)

Finding	Definition/Description	Possible Etiology
	Inspection	
Intercostal retractions	Intercostal muscles between ribs pull in with respiration, markedly increasing the work of breathing.	COPD Asthma Pulmonary fibrosis If sudden, may be airway obstruction
Intercostal bulging	Intercostal spaces (usually in a localized area) bulge out between ribs.	Aneurysm Cardiac enlargement Pleural effusion
	Palpation	
Uneven chest excursion	Two sides of chest do not move symmetrically with respirations.	Chest trauma Splinting Pneumothorax Hemothorax Pleural effusion
Altered tactile fremitus	Change from normal decrease of vibrations.	Reduced: Pleural effusion Pneumothorax Increased: Atelectasis
	Percussion	
Hyperresonance	Abnormally loud resonance (usually generalized).	Air trapping: COPD Asthma Pneumothorax
Dullness	Abnormal dullness (usually localized).	Consolidation Pleural effusion Hemothorax
	Auscultation	
Rales	Crackling, bubbling sounds secondary to fluid film in small airways and alveoli. Usually occur on inspiration and may or may not clear with coughing. Rales sound similar to soda fizzing, cellophane crinkling, or rolling hair between fingers just behind the ear.	Atelectasis Emphysema Bronchitis Pneumonia Pulmonary fibrosis Congestive heart failure
Atelectatic rales	Crackling sounds indicating slight fluid accumulation due to shallow breathing. Clear with a few deep breaths.	Atelectasis
Rhonchi	Rumbling, snoring, or rattling sounds due to obstruction of large airways with secretions. Most prominent on expiration. Often change with coughing or suctioning.	Bronchitis Cystic fibrosis Pneumonia
Wheezing	High-pitched musical whistling sounds due to air rushing over narrowed small airways. Heard with stethoscope first on expiration, but may be heard on inspiration as obstruction of the airway increases. May be audible without stethoscope.	Bronchospasm: Asthma Pneumonia Airway obstruction: Foreign body Tumor

Table 18-5 (Continued)

Finding	Definition/Description	Possible Etiology
Pleural friction rub	Localized click or grating due to decrease or absence of pleural fluid which causes the pleura to rub together. It is heard during inspiration and expiration and does not clear with coughing. Area is usually uncomfortable on inspiration.	Postpleural effusion removal Myocardial infarction Pericarditis Pneumonia
Bronchophony, whispered pectoriloquy	Spoken or whispered syllable heard more distinctly than normal on auscultation.	Pneumonia Pleural effusion
Egophony ("e" to "a" change)	Due to altered transmission of voice sounds, the spoken "e" sounds like "a" on auscultation.	Pneumonia

*Limited to common etiologies. (Further discussion of conditions listed may be found in Chaps. 19 to 21.)

of the lung, a smear and stain of the sputum followed by appropriate culture techniques are needed to diagnose the type of infection. In addition, 24-hour specimens may be collected to determine the quantity, color, tenaciousness, and amount of solids present. The nursing responsibilities for collection of these specimens are given in Table 18-6. It is important that the nurse observe the sputum for color, presence of blood, volume, and viscosity.

Skin Testing

Persons who have suspected or diagnosed respiratory disease may be skin tested for allergies (Chap. 10) or for an immune reaction to a bacterial, fungal, or viral disease. Skin tests involve the intradermal injection of an antigen. Positive reactions are an inflammatory response consisting of redness and *induration* (a raised, hardened area). Table 18-7 describes commonly used skin tests.

Table 18-6
Diagnostic Studies of the Respiratory System

Study	Description and Purpose	Nursing Responsibility
Blood studies		
1. Hemoglobin (Hbg, Hb)	Reflects amount of hemoglobin available for combination with oxygen. Venous blood is used. Normal adult male: 13–16 g/dL Normal adult female: 12–14 g/dL	Nonfasting. No specific responsibilities.*
2. Hematocrit (Hct)	Ratio of red blood cells to plasma. Increased hematocrit (polycythemia) found in chronic hypoxia. Venous blood is used. Normal adult male: 42–50% Normal adult female: 40–48%	No specific responsibilities.* Nonfasting.
3. ABG studies	Done to determine oxygenation, ventilation, and metabolic status. Arterial blood is obtained through arterial puncture of the radial, brachial, or femoral artery. It may also be obtained through an arterial line. Normal persons: see Table 18-3.	Mark request with time to be done and flow of supplemental oxygen. Stabilize client for 20 min prior to procedure on ordered oxygen flow and by maintaining bed rest. Blood is collected in a heparinized syringe. No air should remain in the syringe, and the tip of the needle should be occluded with a cap or cork. Place specimen on ice immediately after it is withdrawn and send to the lab for analysis. After procedure, apply pressure to puncture site by hand for 5–10 min. This is especially important because an arterial puncture is involved.

Table 18-6 (Continued)

Study	Description and Purpose	Nursing Responsibility
Sputum studies		
1. Culture and sensitivity	Single sputum specimen is collected in a sterile container. Purpose is to diagnose bacterial infection and to select an effective antibiotic. Specimen may also be collected to evaluate treatment.	For all sputum specimens, collect specimen to be cultured prior to giving antibiotics unless the purpose is evaluation of treatments. Be sure to obtain sputum (mucoid-like), not saliva. Give the sputum container with its cover to the client at night. Instruct him to expectorate sputum into the container after coughing deeply, when he first awakens. Ideally, this should be done before the client swallows the sputum which has collected in the back of his throat overnight. If a specimen has not been obtained successfully, the following steps may be taken: 1. Increase oral fluid intake (unless fluid restriction is indicated). 2. Use ultrasonic nebulizer to liquefy secretions. 3. Administer aerosol bronchodilator treatment or IPPB treatment. 4. Suction trachea and use a sputum trap to collect specimen.
2. Gram stain	Staining of sputum permits classification of bacteria into gram-negative and gram-positive types. Guides therapy until culture and sensitivity results are obtained.	
3. Acid-fast stain	Single sputum specimen is collected to diagnose infection by acid-fast bacilli (tuberculosis). It is collected early in the morning for 3 consecutive days. Specimen may also be collected to evaluate treatment.	Cover all sputum specimens. Remove containers when specimen is obtained or container is full. Replace with fresh container to decrease spread of infection as well as to maintain aesthetics. It is especially important to transport the specimen to the lab quickly.
4. Cytology	Single sputum specimen is collected in a special container with fixative solution. Purpose is to determine the presence of abnormal cells that may indicate a malignancy.	
Radiology		
1. Chest x-ray	For screening, diagnosis, and evaluation of change. Most common views are PA and lateral.	Client should undress to waist and put on a gown. There should be no metal between the neck and the waist. Nurse should be out of range of or shielded from radiation.
2. Bronchogram	Used to diagnose abnormality of airway structures. Dye is introduced into the trachea, and the client is tilted to various positions for x-rays.	Ask client if he has any iodine or dye allergies and obtain signed permit. Client should be NPO prior to the procedure for 6–12 h. Oral hygiene should be given and dentures removed immediately before procedure. Also, note permanent bridges. Administer premedication as ordered. *During procedure,* monitor pulse and report changes. Also, observe for reaction to local anesthetic and dye. *After procedure,* position client on side and keep NPO until gag reflex returns. Observe for respiratory distress and signs of bleeding.
3. Lung scan	Used to diagnose pathology in ventilation-perfusion status, especially pulmonary embolus. A radionuclide is injected intravenously, and a radioactive gas is inspired by the client. A gamma-detecting device records the radioactivity within the lungs.	Preparation is same as for chest x-ray. Also, check for dye allergy.

Table 18-6 (Continued)

Study	Description and Purpose	Nursing Responsibility
4. Pulmonary angiogram	Used to visualize pulmonary vasculature and locate obstruction or pathology such as pulmonary embolus. A radiopaque dye is injected, usually through a catheter into the pulmonary artery or right heart.	Prepare as for chest x-ray. Dye injection may cause flushing, warm sensation, and cough. *After procedure,* pressure dressing is applied to injection site. Monitor blood pressure, pulse rate, and circulation distal to injection site closely. Report and record significant changes.
Bronchoscopy	Use of flexible fiberoptic scope for diagnosis, biopsy, specimen collection, or assessment of changes. May also be done to suction out mucus plugs or remove foreign objects. Sometimes done in radiology department using fluoroscopy.	Prepare as for bronchogram. *During procedure,* cover the client's eyes with a towel to protect against droplets of solution. Monitor pulse and encourage client to relax and not talk or cough. *After procedure,* provide care as for bronchogram. Sputum may be slightly blood-tinged for a few hours if biopsy specimen has been taken. Report frank bleeding. Ice bags applied to throat may promote comfort. Discourage talking, coughing, smoking, and clearing of throat for a few hours to decrease throat irritation. After return of gag reflex, throat lozenges may be ordered for sore throat.
Thoracentesis (Fig. 18-18)	Used to obtain specimen of pleural fluid for diagnosis, to remove pleural fluid, or to instill medication. The physician inserts a large-bore needle through the chest wall into the pleural space. A chest x-ray is usually done after the procedure to check for pneumothorax and other changes. Abnormal findings discussed in Chap. 21.	*Before procedure,* explain procedure to client and obtain signed permit. *During procedure,* position client upright. Instruct him not to talk or cough. Assist the physician and monitor client's pulse. Small dressing usually applied postprocedure. *After procedure,* assist the client to bed and observe for possible complications: signs of shock, pneumothorax, or infection and leakage at the puncture site. Send labeled specimens to laboratory.
Pulmonary function studies (PFT)	To evaluate lung function. Involves use of a spirometer to diagram air movement as client performs prescribed respiratory maneuvers. Normal persons: see Tables 18-8, 18-9.	Avoid scheduling immediately after mealtime. Explain procedure to client. Give much verbal encouragement and support during procedure. Monitor client's pulse. Terminate test early if client experiences difficulty or extreme fatigue. Provide rest after the procedure.
Lung biopsy	Biopsy specimens may be obtained of any tracheobronchial structures via a bronchoscope. Needle biopsy specimens can also be obtained of lung or pleural tissue. These biopsies are most often done to detect malignant growths.	Same as for thoracentesis.

*For all studies, the nurse should explain the procedure and its purpose. In addition, procedures requiring penetration of the skin should be carried out with aseptic technique.

Nursing responsibilities are similar for all skin tests. First, the nurse should be sure that the injection is intradermal and not subcutaneous to prevent a false-negative reaction. After the injection, the sites should be circled and the client instructed not to remove the marks. When charting administration of the antigen, the nurse should draw a diagram of the forearm and hand and label the injection sites. The diagram is especially helpful when more than one test is administered.

When reading the test results, the nurse should use a good light. If induration is present, a marking pen should be brought in from the periphery on all four sides of the induration. As the pen touches the raised

Table 18-7
Skin Tests Used in Respiratory Disorders

Test	Purpose and Description
Mantoux	Positive result indicates that a client's immune system has reacted to the tubercle bacillus. Does *not* differentiate between active and dormant infection. The test involves the intradermal injection of 0.1 mL of intermediate strength purified protein derivative (PPD) into the inner aspect of the forearm. The test is read 48–72 h after injection. Results are interpreted as follows: *Positive reaction* = 10 mm or more of induration. Interpreted as positive for past or present infection with *Mycobacterium tuberculosis*. *Doubtful reaction* = 5–9 mm of induration. A person who is known to have been in close contact with an infectious person, i.e., a subject with infectious sputum, or a person having radiographic or clinical evidence of disease compatible with tuberculosis, should be regarded as probably infected with *M. tuberculosis*. *Negative reaction* = 0–4 mm of induration. No repeat test necessary unless there is evidence of clinical tuberculosis.
Multiple puncture test (Heaf, Tine, Mono-Vacc)	Positive results indicate that a client's immune status has reacted to the tubercle bacillus. In determining the size of the induration, measure the diameter of the largest single reaction. If the reaction consists of discrete papules, the diameters of separate areas of induration should not be added. For screening tests, the following interpretation is suggested:[7] *Positive reaction* = Vesiculation. If vesiculation is present, the test may be interpreted as positive, in which case the management of the subject is the same as that for one classified as positive to the Mantoux test. *Doubtful reaction* = 2 mm or more of induration. Even though such reactions may be due to *M. tuberculosis*, a significant proportion of them may not be confirmed by a positive standard Mantoux test. This is particularly true of smaller reactions. Therefore, a standard Mantoux test should be done on all subjects in this group, and management should be based on the reaction to the Mantoux test or on the results of dual testing using PPD-tuberculin and PPD-B. *Negative reaction* = Less than 2 mm of induration. There is no need for retesting unless the individual is in contact with someone who has tuberculosis or there is clinical evidence suggestive of the disease.
Coccidioidomycosis test	Positive results indicate an active or previous coccidioidomycosis infection. The test involves the intradermal injection of coccidioidin or spherulin. It is read at 24–72 h. Positive findings are a reddened area and induration of 5 mm or more. The immediate reaction is nonspecific.
Histoplasmosis test	Positive results indicate an active or previous histoplasmosis infection. The test involves the intradermal injection of histoplasmin. It is read at 24–48 h. Positive findings are a reddened area and induration of 5 mm or more. Previous histoplasmosis tests may also cause a positive reaction.
Shick test	Measure of a person's immunity to diphtheria. Positive results indicate that a client lacks immunity to diphtheria. The test involves the intradermal injection of 0.1 mL purified diphtheria *toxin* into the inner aspect of the forearm. In addition, 0.1 mL of inactivated purified diphtheria *toxoid* is injected into the other arm as a control. The test is read at 24 and 48 h and between the fourth and seventh days after the injection. Results are negative if there is no inflammation at either site (client has immunity). A false-positive reaction may occur at both sites within 12–72 h and then fade away in a few days. Positive results begin within 24 h at the site where the toxin was injected, and the lesion may become larger than 2 cm (no reaction at the site of toxoid injection).

area, a mark should be made. The nurse then determines the diameter of the induration in millimeters. The reddened, flat areas should not be measured.

When mass screening is done for tuberculosis, the Heaf, Tine, or Mono-Vacc tests are used. These tests rely on pushing a drop of liquid antigen through the skin with a small object that causes multiple punctures. Since the amount of solution delivered this way is unpredictable, positive reactions should be checked with a Mantoux test or a chest x-ray.

Radiology

Chest x-ray

Chest x-rays are probably the most common test used for respiratory screening and diagnosis. They are also used for assessment of changes showing the progression of disease or the response to treatment. The most common views used are the posterior-anterior (PA) views and lateral. An anterior-posterior (AP) view is used when a portable bedside chest x-ray is necessary. In a PA view the ray passes from back to front, and in an AP view it passes from front to back. The results of the final product are slightly different. The heart size appears larger in the AP view. See Table 18-6 for nursing responsibilities related to chest x-rays.

Bronchography

Bronchography involves the instillation of an iodine radiopaque dye into the lungs, one lung at a time (Fig. 18-16). This permits the airways to be clearly outlined for x-ray so that airway abnormalities may be seen. To promote the client's comfort and cooperation, he is usually premedicated with meperidine, atropine, and a sedative. In addition, a local anesthetic is applied to the oropharynx. Then the dye is instilled into the trachea with a catheter or fiberoptic bronchoscope (a flexible tube with a light on it). The client is tilted to various positions to promote the flow of the dye and thus better visualization of the airways by x-ray. After the x-rays have been taken, the dye is removed by postural drainage.

Throughout the procedure, the client needs to be watched closely for a reaction to the local anesthetic or dye. Following the procedure, the client needs to be protected from aspiration of secretions or fluids until the gag reflex returns, usually within 2 to 4 hours. If an oil-based dye is used, the client needs to be observed for the development of pneumonia. Other nursing responsibilities are discussed in Table 18-6.

Lung scan

A *lung scan* is used primarily to check for the presence of a pulmonary embolus. There is no specific preparation or aftercare for the procedure. An intravenous radionuclide dye is given, and the pulmonary vasculature is outlined and photographed. Then, the client inhales a radioactive gas which outlines the alveoli. The two photographs of the lung in each position are compared. They should look the same. If there are areas which are ventilated but not perfused, the presence of an embolus is suspected.

Bronchoscopy

Bronchoscopy is a procedure in which the bronchi are visualized through a fiberoptic tube (Fig.

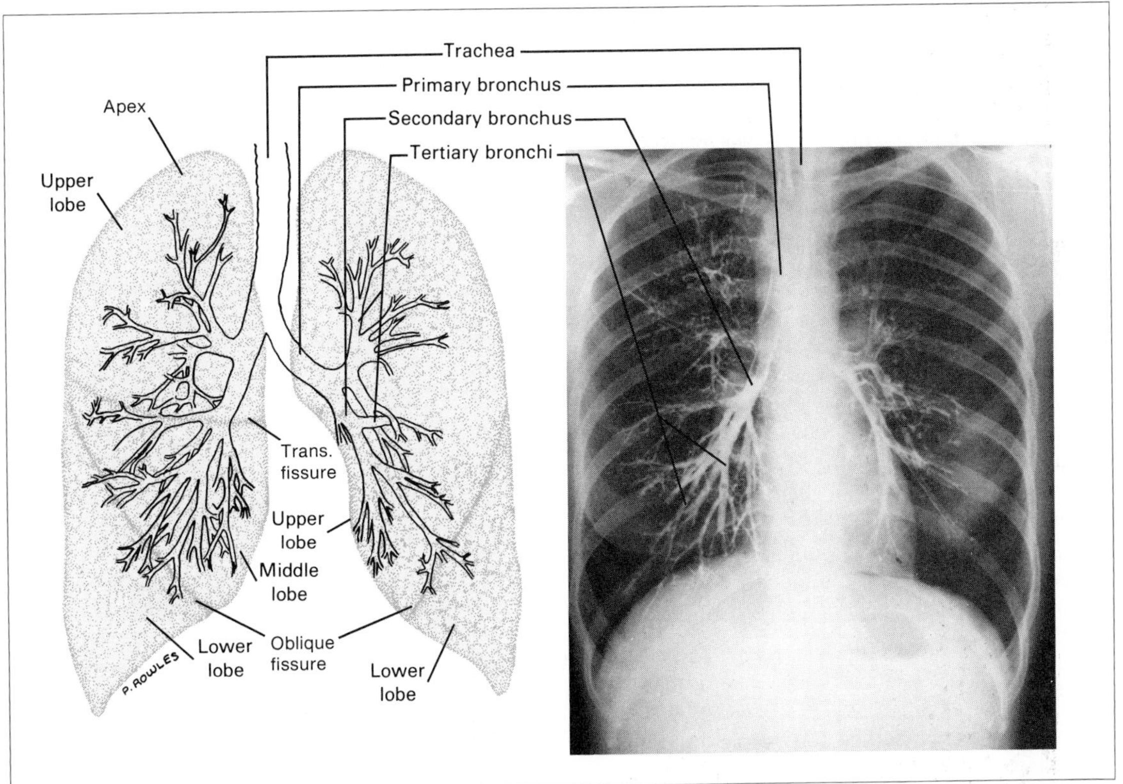

Figure 18-16 Schematic drawing of lungs compared with a bronchogram. *(From L. L. Langley et al., Dynamic Anatomy and Physiology, 5th ed., McGraw-Hill Book Company, New York, 1980, p. 518.)*

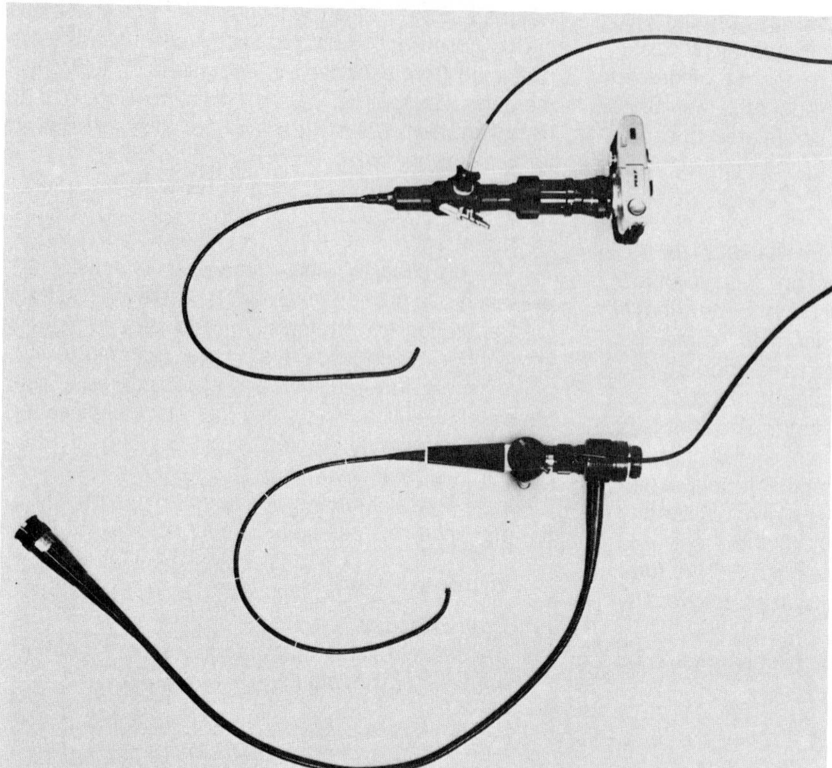

Figure 18-17 Bronchofiberscopes. One is manufactured by the Machida Company and the other by Olympus. A 35-mm camera is attached to the Machida bronchofiberscope. A teaching attachment to permit an observer to view the endoscopy is shown with the Olympus bronchofiberscope. The cables to the light source pass to the right of the instruments. *(From A. P. Fishman, Pulmonary Diseases and Disorders, McGraw-Hill Book Company, New York, 1980, p. 123.)*

18-17). It may be used for (1) diagnosis, (2) specimen collection or biopsy, (3) assessment of changes due to treatment, or (4) to remove mucus plugs or foreign bodies. Preparation is the same as for bronchography. A signed permit is required. Diazepam is often given intravenously during the procedure to aid relaxation.

The procedure is done in a darkened room with the client either lying down or seated, depending on the physician's preference. Once the nasal pharynx and oral pharynx have been anesthetized with local anesthetic, a flexible fiberoptic bronchoscope is inserted, usually via the nose, and threaded down into the airways. The nursing care for the procedure is described in Table 18-6.

Thoracentesis

Thoracentesis is the insertion of a needle through the chest wall into the pleural space (Fig. 18-18). It is done to obtain specimens for diagnostic evaluation, to

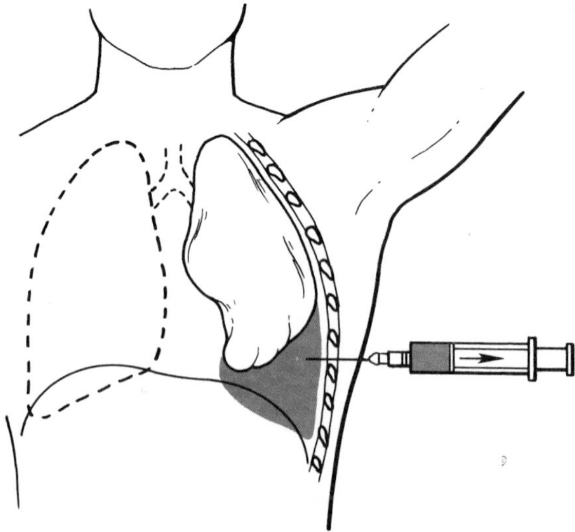

Figure 18-18 Thoracentesis. The needle has penetrated into the fluid-filled pleural space to remove fluid.

remove pleural fluid accumulation, and to instill medication into the pleural space. A signed permit is necessary in most agencies.

For a thoracentesis, the client is positioned upright, usually sitting on a chair and leaning on his elbows on the bed or the over-bed table. His feet and legs should be well supported. The back and lateral areas of his chest are exposed. The physician cleanses the skin at the site of choice and uses a local anesthetic such as 1% Xylocaine prior to insertion of the thoracentesis needle. The nursing care is described in Table 18-6.

Pulmonary Function Tests

Pulmonary function tests (PFTs) measure lung volumes and capacities (Tables 18-8, 18-9). The results of PFTs are important in the diagnosis and evaluation of pulmonary status. PFTs involve the use of a *spirometer,* an instrument that measures and diagrams the movement of air volume across time; it can measure the volume of air exhaled at 1-second intervals. When a client is having a PFT he is instructed in a variety of respiratory maneuvers which are performed while he is in a sitting position. The client is instructed to breathe into a mouthpiece attached to the spirometer. A nose clamp is used to ensure that no air will escape through the nose.

Accurate measurements depend on the client's ability to cooperate and follow the given directions. Thus it is important that the procedure be carefully explained by the nurse prior to the test. In addition, the technician will give further directions and encourage the client throughout the test. It will also be easier for the client if the test is not scheduled immediately after a meal, when the stomach causes pressure against the diaphragm. The test can be very tiring for persons with pulmonary disorders, so the client should be allowed to rest afterward.

In order to understand PFTs, it is helpful to look at the way the lungs' contents can be measured and classified. The contents can be divided into four lung capacities (compartments), each of which is made up

Table 18-8
Lung Volumes and Capacities

Term	Abbrev.	Definition	Typical Values
		Lung Volumes	
Tidal volume	V_T	Volume of air inhaled and exhaled with each breath. Is only a small proportion of the total capacity of the lungs for air.	0.5 L
Expiratory reserve volume	ERV	The additional air that can be forcefully exhaled after a normal exhalation (V_T) is complete. Does not completely empty the lungs.	1.5 L
Residual volume	RV	The amount of air remaining in the lungs after a forced expiration. Allows air to be available in the lungs for gas exchange between breaths.	1.5 L
Inspiratory reserve volume	IRV	Maximum volume of air that can be inhaled forcefully after normal inhalation (V_T).	2.5 L
		Lung Capacities	
Total lung capacity	TLC	Maximum volume of air that the lungs can contain. $TLC = IRV + V_T + ERV + RV$.	6.0 L
Functional residual capacity	FRC	Volume of air remaining in lungs at end of normal exhalation (at V_T). $FRC = ERV + RV$. May increase or decrease with lung pathology.	3.0 L
Vital capacity	VC	Can be measured as either expiratory VC or inspiratory VC. Is the maximum volume of gas that can be forcefully exhaled or inhaled. Usually expiratory VC equals inspiratory VC. $VC = IRV + V_T + ERV$. Males generally have a higher VC than do females.	4.5 L
Inspiratory capacity	IC	Maximum volume of air that can be inhaled after a normal expiration. $IC = V_T + IRV$.	3.0 L

*Twenty-year-old male: weight = 70 kg, height = 165 cm.
Adapted from A. P. Fishman, *Pulmonary Disease and Disorders*, McGraw-Hill Book Company, New York, 1980, p. 1832.

Table 18-9

Common Measures of Pulmonary Functions*

Term	Abbrev.	Description	Normal Value†
Forced expiratory volume in first second of expiration	$FEV_{1.0}$	Amount of air exhaled in first second of forced expiration. Valuable clue to severity of airway obstruction.	About 83%
Ratio of $FEV_{1.0}$ to forced vital capacity	$FEV_{1.0}$/FVC	Over 80% of the total air moved during the exhalation should be exhaled in the first second of that breath. Useful in assessing airway obstruction.	Over 80%
Maximal expiratory flow rate	MEFR	Measure of the flow rate of the first 1000 mL of air exhaled in the forced expiration. Rarely used.	250–450/4 min
Forced midexpiratory flow rate	FEV 25–75%	Measures airflow rate in middle half of the forced expiration. Is more accurate than MEFR because it is less dependent on client effort.	Smaller than MEFR
Maximal voluntary ventilation	MVV	Client breathes as deeply and rapidly as possible for a specified period. The amount of air moved is reported in liters per minute. Tests airflow, muscle strength, coordination, and airway resistance. An important factor in exercise tolerance.	About 170 L/min for adult male. Decreases in women and with age
Peak flow rate	PFR	Maximum airflow rate during the forced expiration.	Up to 600 L/min in young men
Inspiratory force	IF	Amount of negative pressure generated on inspiration. Gives some idea of ability to breathe and cough.	−25 cmH_2O minimum

*Pulmonary function studies also include those described in Table 18-8.
†Normal values must be computed for each individual and are variable.

of two or more volumes. These are illustrated and defined in Fig. 18-19 and Table 18-8.

Tables of norms of pulmonary function based on age, sex, weight, and height are used by physicians to predict norms for the client. However, these norms are not totally reliable. One reason is that separate tables are not available for smokers and nonsmokers. A second reason is that some persons have a vital capacity (VC) which is greater than the predicted normal vital capacity. This occurs because predicted values are based on averages, and the range of normal is quite wide. For example, a person's predicted VC may be 5 L. In reality, when he was healthy, his VC was 7 L. Now, in the early stages of disease, his VC has decreased to 5 L, which is the normal value predicted for him. In reality, he has lost about 28 percent of his VC while still remaining within the normal VC predicted for him. Since the VC is variable, it is not considered abnormal until it is less than 80 percent of the predicted norm. Although the range of normal is wide, measurements can be reproduced in the same individual that are within very close limits. Thus, PFTs can be used to monitor individual progress, to make a prognosis, and to detect early evidence of pulmonary disease if done repeatedly.

Since complete PFTs are both costly and fatiguing, it is impractical to perform them frequently. However, the simple screening test of measuring a single forced expiration can yield important information. The client is given a mouthpiece which is attached to a recording or measuring machine. He is asked to put the mouthpiece in his mouth, to take as deep a breath as possible, and to blow out as hard, as fast, and as long as possible. Much verbal encouragement must be given to him to continue blowing out even after he feels that the exhalation is complete. Fig. 18-20 is an example of the curve that might be produced by a normal person.

The shape of the curve produced by a single forced expiration is important in detecting abnormalities. It is measured to determine the $FEV_{1.0}$ (Table 18-9). This is the volume of air expired in the first

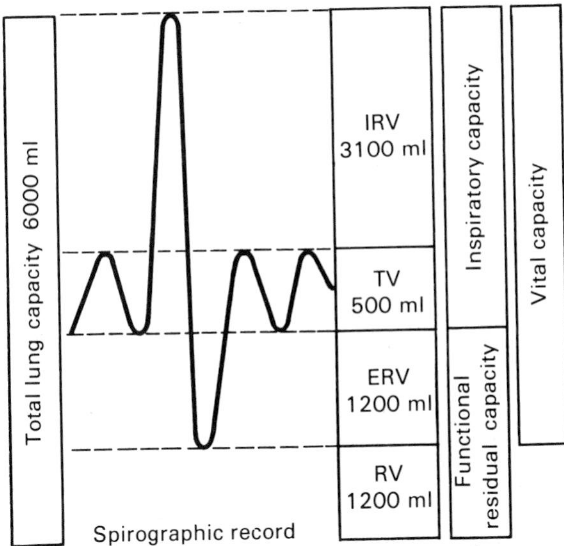

Figure 18-19 Relationship of lung volumes and capacities. *(From S. Price and L. Wilson, Pathophysiology: Clinical Concepts of Disease Processes, McGraw-Hill Book Company, New York, 1978, p. 404.)*

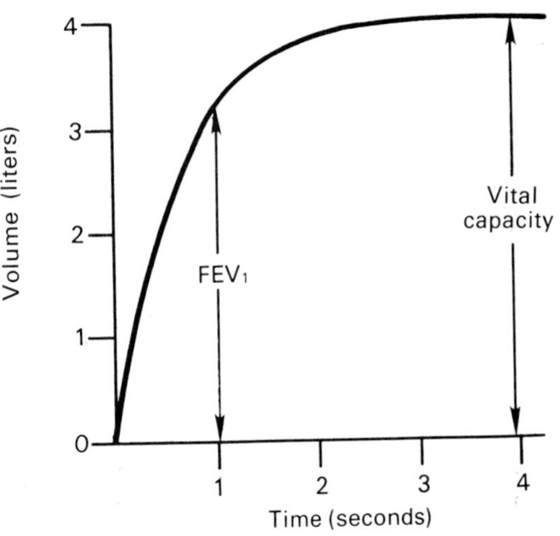

Figure 18-20 The normal forced expirogram. Volume in the spirometer is plotted against time. The vital capacity (VC) is represented by the total volume expired. One-second forced expiratory volume ($FEV_{1.0}$) is the volume expired during the first second.

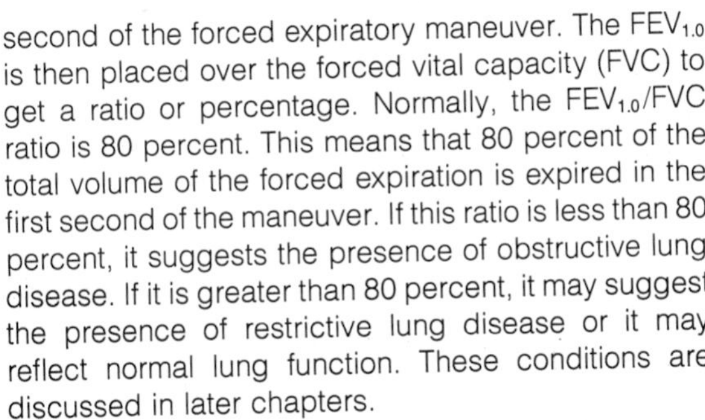
second of the forced expiratory maneuver. The $FEV_{1.0}$ is then placed over the forced vital capacity (FVC) to get a ratio or percentage. Normally, the $FEV_{1.0}$/FVC ratio is 80 percent. This means that 80 percent of the total volume of the forced expiration is expired in the first second of the maneuver. If this ratio is less than 80 percent, it suggests the presence of obstructive lung disease. If it is greater than 80 percent, it may suggest the presence of restrictive lung disease or it may reflect normal lung function. These conditions are discussed in later chapters.

REVIEW QUESTIONS

The number of the question corresponds to the same numbered objective at the beginning of the chapter.

1. What is the function of surfactant?
- **a.** It facilitates oxygen transport across the alveolar membrane.
- **b.** It provides a continuous nutrient supply to the alveoli.
- **c.** It decreases resistance to expansion and prevents collapse of the alveoli.
- **d.** It allows air exchange between alveolar sacs.

2. The primary regulators of respirations are
- **a.** decreased carbon dioxide and increased pH
- **b.** decreased pH and increased carbon dioxide
- **c.** decreased oxygen and increased pH
- **d.** increased oxygen and increased carbon dioxide

3. The partial pressure of oxygen in the atmosphere is dependent on the
- **a.** partial pressure of carbon dioxide
- **b.** barometric pressure
- **c.** pressures of other gases in the air
- **d.** moisture in the air

4. The most important respiratory defense mechanism distal to the respiratory bronchioles is the
- **a.** alveolar macrophage
- **b.** reflex bronchoconstriction
- **c.** mucociliary clearance mechanism
- **d.** impaction of particles

5. A rightward shift of the oxyhemoglobin dissociation curve
- **a.** interferes with release of oxygen at the tissue level
- **b.** causes oxygen to have a greater affinity for hemoglobin
- **c.** facilitates release of oxygen at the tissue level
- **d.** is caused by metabolic alkalosis

6. Which of the following drugs is usually not significant as related to a history of the respiratory system?
- **a.** corticosteroids
- **b.** antihistamines
- **c.** sedatives
- **d.** insulin

7. When auscultating the chest, the nurse should use which part of the stethoscope?
- **a.** diaphragm

b. bell
c. both diaphragm and bell
d. whatever part the examiner prefers

8. Which of the following is the normal percussion sound for examination of the lungs?
a. dull
b. flat
c. resonant
d. tympany

9. Which of the following nursing measures related to ABG collection is not accurate?
a. Stabilize the client for 20 minutes prior to the procedure on the ordered oxygen flow.
b. Collect blood in a heparinized syringe.
c. Place the specimen immediately on ice after it is withdrawn.
d. Apply pressure to the puncture site for 1 minute.

10. The amount of air left in the lungs after a forced exhalation is called the
a. dead space volume
b. function residual volume
c. residual volume
d. expiratory reserve volume

REFERENCES

1. J. B. West, *Respiratory Physiology: The Essentials,* 2d ed., The Williams & Wilkins Company, Baltimore, 1979, p. 3.
2. Ibid., pp. 94–95.
3. A. P. Fishman, *Assessment of Pulmonary Function,* McGraw-Hill Book Company, New York, 1980, pp. 187–188.
4. E. G. Pavlin and T. F. Hornbein, "The Control of Breathing," *Basics Resp Dis,* **7:**1–2 (1978).
5. D. L. Sexton, *Chronic Obstructive Pulmonary Disease: Care of the Child and Adult,* The C. V. Mosby Company, St. Louis, 1980, p. 11.
6. Ibid., p. 142.
7. *Diagnostic Standards and Classification of Tuberculosis and Other Mycobacterial Diseases,* American Lung Association, New York, 1974, pp. 18–19.

Chapter 19

NURSING ROLE IN MANAGEMENT

Upper Respiratory Problems

Martha-Jane Greenberg

Learning Objectives

1. Describe the pathophysiology, clinical manifestations, and medical and nursing management of problems of the nose.
2. Describe the pathophysiology, clinical manifestations, and medical and nursing management of problems of the paranasal sinuses.
3. Describe the pathophysiology, clinical manifestations, and medical and nursing management of inflammatory problems of the pharynx and larynx.
4. Compare and contrast the physiological effects, purposes, and indications for and complications of tracheostomy and endotracheal intubation.
5. Describe the nursing care of clients with a tracheostomy or endotracheal intubation.
6. Describe the significance, types, and clinical manifestations of cancer of the larynx.
7. Explain the medical, surgical, and nursing management of the client with cancer of the larynx.
8. Describe the nursing management of clients with temporary or permanent loss of speech.

The structures that make up the upper respiratory tract are the nose, the paranasal sinuses located in the frontal, sphenoid, ethmoid, and maxillary bones, the pharynx, the larynx, and the trachea. These structures are subject to repeated exposure of disease-producing microorganisms, carcinogens, and noxious elements during the process of breathing. Disorders involving the upper respiratory tract, especially viral infections, are very common in humans.

STRUCTURAL AND TRAUMATIC DISORDERS OF THE NOSE

Deviated Septum

Deviated septum occurs as a result of trauma or factors related to the growth process. The nasal septum is usually straight at birth unless bending occurs as a result of birth trauma. As persons grow older, there is a tendency for the septum to deviate to one side.[1] Injury may also cause the septum to deviate. Symptoms of a deviated septum are nasal obstruction with or without accompanying breathing distress, headache, sinusitis, and nosebleeds. On inspection, the septum is seen to be bent to one side, with the airway greatly reduced. The obstruction may be anterior (cartilaginous) or posterior (bony).

Submucous resection (SMR) is nasal septal reconstruction which straightens and thins the nasal septum. This reconstruction is indicated to relieve nasal obstruction. The major complications of this surgery are tearing of the septum and saddle deformity. Saddle deformity occurs as a result of the bridge of the nose being pulled downward by a scar contracture or falling after excess cartilaginous or bony support is removed.

Nursing care related to SMR is similar to that of rhinoplasty, which is described later. Health promotion is aimed at preventing precipitating factors such as accidental falls sustained in childhood.

Nasal Fracture

Nasal fracture is most often caused by trauma sustained as a result of athletic injury and accidents (automobile accidents and miscellaneous causes). Complications of the fracture are airway obstruction and cosmetic deformity, with a resultant change in body image. Most nasal fractures are simple or comminuted, and are rarely compound. The type of fracture is determined by the direction of the blow and the intensity of the force. The nose is more resistant to fracture from direct frontal blows than it is from lateral blows.

On inspection, the fractured nose is noted to be deviated to one side or depressed frontally, with misalignment of the septum. Crepitation, edema, ecchymosis, and difficulty in breathing may be present. The client will complain of pain. The diagnosis of nasal fracture is based on the client's history and direct observation of the internal and external nasal structures. X-ray findings are not always accurate.

Upon examination, it is crucial to determine the client's ability to breathe through each side of the nose and whether there is evidence of hemorrhage, leak-

This chapter was reviewed by Leslie Kirilloff, R.N., Ph.D., Assistant Professor, Graduate Program, Medical-Surgical Nursing, University of Pittsburgh, Pittsburgh, Pennsylvania.

age of cerebrospinal fluid, and/or a pronounced change in the shape of the nose. A positive reaction for glucose indicates that the nasal discharge is cerebrospinal fluid.

Management

The goal of nasal fracture management is to reduce the fracture via open or closed reduction. This will reestablish the cosmetic appearance and proper function of the nose and provide an adequate airway. Lateral fractures are usually reduced without anesthesia by using simple thumb pressure on the convex side. Depressed fractures require surgery using anesthesia.

The major goals of nursing care are edema reduction, observation for and prevention of complications, client education, and emotional support (see Rhinoplasty).

Rhinoplasty

Rhinoplasty is surgical reconstruction of the nose performed for cosmetic or physiologic reasons (e.g., septum deviation). Many individuals have a grossly deformed nose as a result of trauma or the growth process. This deformity affects each person differently with some suffering psychologically. A person's perception of his body is difficult to assess, owing to the highly personal and complex nature of this phenomenon. Body image is multidimensional, including the perception of one's body as a psychological, social, and physical entity. For this reason, any physical alteration such as a deformed or enlarged nose can influence the individual's environmental interactions.[2] The client may feel ugly, act embarrassed, or joke about his appearance. The client who undergoes rhinoplasty for cosmetic reasons needs the same emotional reassurance as the client who has this operation because of trauma. Each must incorporate the bodily change into his perceptions of self.

Surgical procedure

Rhinoplasty is most often performed under local anesthesia. Topical anesthesia of the nose is achieved by the insertion of cocaine-impregnated applicators or by spraying Pontocaine into each nostril. Procaine is injected externally near the infratrochlear and infraorbital nerves. Incisions are made both internally and externally. Tissue may be added or removed and the nose lengthened or shortened. A variety of plastic prosthetic implants may be utilized for both the nose and the chin. The nose is often augmented at the time of rhinoplasty to achieve overall balance. Postoperatively, nasal packing is placed in the nasal vestibule, a nasal splint may cover the nose, and a "mustache dressing" covers the nasal tip. Packing and splinting help to maintain the proper position of the nasal structures and prevent postoperative edema, bleeding, and further injury. The nasal packing is generally removed within 24 to 48 hours.

Nasal Packing Nasal packing is utilized following rhinoplasty, SMR, sinus surgery, and for epistaxis control. The goal when using nasal packing is to control bleeding by direct pressure. Packing can be local or postnasal. *Local packing* consists of a small piece of petroleum gauze or a cotton ball wedged firmly in the desired location. *Postnasal packing* is large and made of gauze or a tampon to which strings are attached. The strings are brought to the outside and taped to the cheek. Large postnasal packs may compress the eustachian tube. A reminder that packing is in place should be given in an obvious place in the client's record. Nasal packing is usually removed within 24 to 48 hours. Following the removal of the nasal packing, the nares may be gently cleaned and lubricated with petroleum jelly.[3]

Nursing management

Photographs are usually taken for preoperative and postoperative comparison. The client should be instructed to refrain from taking aspirin for 2 weeks prior to surgery to prevent postoperative bleeding. Explain the procedures that the client can expect following the surgery (Table 19-1).

Nursing intervention during the acute postoperative period includes frequent assessment of vital signs. The surgical site should also be observed for hemorrhage, edema, and discoloration. Nursing interventions are directed toward pain control, reduction of edema, and prevention of infection. Infection and hemorrhage are rare, but not unanticipated complications of rhinoplasty. The client should be told that edema can persist for weeks or months but will subside over time.

The outcome of rhinoplasty is most often satisfactory and pleasant to the client. The client's self-esteem and self-perception may increase as a result of a positive mind-body interaction and an altered physical image following the surgery.

Epistaxis (Nosebleeds)

Epistaxis occurs as a result of bleeding from a rich network of veins in the anterior nares. Ten percent of all nosebleeds do not stop spontaneously and require treatment. For these clients, epistaxis is a serious, though rarely fatal problem. Epistaxis occurs

Table 19-1
Nursing Care Plan for the Client with a Rhinoplasty

Client Problem	Expected Outcome	Nursing Intervention
Inability to breathe through nose	No respiratory distress. Successful adaptation to mouth breathing.	Check rate and character of the respirations q 2 h for 12 h. Maintain bed rest in semi-Fowler's position for 8–12 h with back of head flat against bed. Turn and deep breathe q 2 h–q 4 h. NPO for 6–8 h. Observe nasal packing placement. Check back of throat q 1 h. Observe for bleeding, difficulty in breathing, choking. Inquire about any earaches. Offer oral hygiene frequently.
Bleeding and potential hemorrhage	No bleeding. Normal hemoglobin and hematocrit.	Check BP, P, R q 2 h for 12 h, then q 4 h for 24 h. Give no aspirin. Observe the client for frequent swallowing, hematemesis, melena, or tarry stool, which may indicate hemorrhage. Warn client that stool may be tarry due to swallowed blood. Observe the nasal packing and mustache dressing qh for 12 h. Using a flashlight, check posterior packing in the throat q 2 h. Note the correct placement of exterior dressing, interior nasal packing, and the character and amount of drainage. Change the mustache dressing prn. Apply ice packs to nose. Inform client that nose blowing is contraindicated. Report any fresh or frank bleeding to the physician.
Nasal edema and discoloration	Minimal to no swelling.	If present, observe nasal splint for pressure and alignment. Elevate head of bed. Apply ice packs to nose prn. Inform client that edema and discoloration will subside over time. Cosmetic effect of rhinoplasty cannot be judged until several weeks after surgery.
Pain	Minimal to no pain.	Describe to client the amount of pain expected. Include client in planning the rest periods. Administer analgesics and ice packs prn.
Disruption in eating habits	Resumption of normal food and bowel habits.	Check gag reflex. Add clear liquids to diet as tolerated when gag reflex is present. Administer laxative as ordered if constipation develops.
Potential delayed hemorrhage	State ways to prevent hemorrhage. No signs of hemorrhage.	Teach client gentle cleaning technique and lubrication with a water-soluble jelly following removal of the packing. Avoid nose blowing for 3–4 days. Teach open-mouth method of nose blowing. Explain signs of hemorrhage (tachycardia, hypotension, bright red drainage). Instruct client to contact physician immediately if signs of bleeding occur.
Potential infection	Normal temperature. No manifestations of infection.	Explain signs of inflammation to client (fever, increased pain and swelling at site, malaise). Instruct client to notify physician if these occur. Teach importance of correct hand-washing techniques, clean nasal care, rest, activity limitations, adequate fluid intake, and good nutrition.

as a result of nasal picking (the most common cause), vitamin C and K deficiency, tumor growth, blood dyscrasia, hypertension, blowing the nose too hard, acute sinusitis, or toxic metal ingestion.

Management involves accurate localization of the bleeding site and cauterization or ligation of the problem vessel. In addition, the nose may be packed. The nurse should observe the client for any signs of acute blood loss, monitor vital signs, advise the client to keep the head elevated, restore fluid balance, and monitor hemoglobin levels.

Facial Trauma

Fractures of the maxilla, zygoma, mandible, and nose usually result from severe direct trauma such as a blow with a fist, a fall, or an automobile accident. Diagnosis is based on the history, physical examination, and x-ray. In cases of severe facial injury, intracranial or cervical damage must be determined prior to correction. Fractures are most often reduced using various techniques of open reduction.

Facial injury rarely threatens life but requires immediate assessment since airway obstruction and hemorrhage may occur. Any obstruction by dentures, vomitus, or broken teeth must be removed promptly. Hemorrhage in the facial area (e.g., the cheek) is usually treated with direct pressure. Impaled foreign bodies should not be removed until medical assistance is present. Removal of the foreign body may cause hemorrhage of an otherwise tamponaded vessel.[4]

INFLAMMATION AND INFECTION OF THE NOSE AND PARANASAL SINUSES

Rhinitis

Rhinitis is an acute or chronic inflammation of the nasal mucous membrane. It may be caused by allergic reactions, nonallergic reactions, or infection. The most common allergic reaction is allergic rhinitis. Infections are most commonly caused by viruses (acute viral rhinitis). Causes of nonallergic reactions are nasal polyps, hypertrophied and inflamed turbinates, and deviated septum. (These disorders are discussed under separate headings.)

Allergic rhinitis (hay fever)

Allergic rhinitis is the reaction of the nasal mucosa to a specific antigen (allergen). Manifestations of allergic rhinitis are nasal obstruction, sneezing, headache, itching and tearing of the eyes, and increased mucus secretion. *Acute* attacks are usually seasonal and caused by allergy to pollens from trees, flowers, and grasses. The typical acute attack lasts for several weeks (most commonly during the hay fever season), disappears, and recurs at the same time the following year. *Chronic* or *perennial* rhinitis is present intermittently or constantly. Usually the client is allergic to environmental contacts such as house dust, wool, feathers, or food. The client may complain of frequent "colds." Physical examination of the nose will show edematous mucous membranes, a smooth, glistening nasopharynx, and enlarged posterior turbinates. There may also be (especially in chronic rhinitis) abnormal amounts of connective tissue, hypertrophy of the nasal septum, and atrophy of the mucous membranes and cartilage.

Allergic rhinitis is a significant medical problem because of its incidence (at least 10 percent of the population may be involved) and its duration (since symptoms may last for months or for the entire year). The disease may begin in early childhood and persist for most of the client's life.

Allergic rhinitis results from the reaction of IgE antibody fixed to the surface of mast cells in the tissues lining the respiratory tract. When an allergen diffuses across the mucous membrane, there is a resultant release of vasoactive mediators. Histamine and other vasoactive mediators (bradykinin, serotonin, prostaglandins, and eosinophil chemotactic factor) released in the nose induce vasodilatation and increased capillary permeability. Swelling of the nasal mucosa and edema occur due to leakage of intravascular fluid into the tissues following increased capillary permeability. (See Chap. 10 for a further discussion regarding the antigen-antibody response.)

Clinical Manifestations In addition to coldlike symptoms, the nasal turbinates will appear pale and boggy. If they are infected, they will appear red and edematous, with a smooth, glistening surface mucosa. The turbinates fill the air space and press against the nasal septum. The posterior ends of the turbinates may become so enlarged that they protrude into the nasopharynx.

Microscopic examination of the thin, clear nasal discharge reveals large numbers (as high as 90 percent) of eosinophils where normally there are none or few. IgE antibodies will be present in the serum.

Management Therapy includes avoidance of the antigen, altering the immune response (desensitization; see Chap. 10), and symptomatic treatment (Table 19-2). Antihistamines are used for the management of rhinorrhea, while sympathomimetic amines are prescribed for nasal congestion (see Table 10-15). Antihistamines block histamine effects at the receptor site, causing vasoconstriction and decreased capillary permeability. Antihistamines are not without side effects, and careful instructions should be given to the client regarding their use (Table 19-3).

Oral and nasal sympathomimetic amine preparations treat nasal congestion by stimulating receptors of the adrenergic nervous system. This results in marked vasoconstriction of the arterioles of the nasal mucosa. Blood flow and edema are reduced, and stuffiness is relieved. The sympathomimetic amines provide symptomatic relief of nasal congestion whether due to allergy, trauma, or infection. These drugs are contraindicated in persons with hypertension, thyroid disease, diabetes mellitus, and those taking MAO (monoamine oxidase) inhibitors. Such drugs may produce a severe hypertensive reaction when taken in combination with sympathetic amine preparations. The client should be advised of the adverse effects and the proper use of these preparations (Table 19-3).

Rhinitis medicamentosa or rebound nasal congestion is a phenomenon that often results from prolonged use of vasoconstrictors in excessive amounts.

Table 19-2
Medical Management: Allergic Rhinitis and Acute Viral Rhinitis

	Allergic Rhinitis	Acute Viral Rhinitis
Diagnostic	Inspection of turbinates during attack Stain of nasal discharge for eosinophil count	Viral isolation and assay History of recent exposure to current contaminant Microscopic evaluation of nasal discharge for desquamated cells, lymphocytes, and large numbers of polymorphonuclear leukocytes
Therapeutic	Avoid exposure to or eliminate allergen (if possible) Desensitization Antihistamines Decongestants	Bed rest Force fluids (2–3 L/day) Isolation Antipyretics Antitussives Antihistamines Decongestants Vitamin C Nutritious diet

Such use results in chronic reactive hyperemia.[5] Initial vasoconstriction is followed by a secondary vasodilatation and chronic nasal obstruction.

Nursing management for acute and chronic rhinitis is directed toward client education. Instructions can be given regarding the reduction of the occurrence of allergy symptoms and the use of pharmacologic preparations to alleviate symptoms. The nurse may also refer the client to resources that may assist in determining the allergen and desensitizing the client (see Chap. 10).

Acute viral rhinitis (common cold)

The *common cold* (acute coryza) is caused by various viruses that invade the upper respiratory tract. It is the most prevalent infectious disease among

Table 19-3
Antihistamine and Sympathomimetic Preparations

Preparation	Mechanisms of Action	Side Effects	Nursing Concerns
Antihistamines (e.g., Benadryl, Dimetane, Chlor-Trimeton)	Blocks histamine at receptor sites, causing vasoconstriction and decreased capillary permeability.	Anticholinergic properties of dry mouth, decreased secretions, drowsiness, sedation.	Warn client that operating machinery and driving may be dangerous due to sedative effect. CNS effect can be potentiated by use of depressants, alcohol, hypnotics, and antianxiety agents.
Sympathomimetic amines Phenylephrine hydrochloride (Neo-Synephrine) Oxymetazoline hydrochloride (Afrin) Hydroxyamphetamine hydrobromide (Paredrine) Tetrahydrozoline hydrochloride (Tyzine)	Stimulates alpha (α) receptors of the adrenergic nervous system, causing vasoconstriction of nasal arterioles. Produces shrinking of mucous membranes and opening of nasal passages.	Rhinitis medicamentosa (rebound nasal congestion). Severe hypertensive reaction when used in combination with MAO inhibitors.	Advise client of adverse reactions. These preparations should be used for only 3–5 days and not more than three to four times per day. Discard bottles, sprays, inhalers when no longer needed. Never allow another person to use the same applicator. Contraindicated for persons with hypertension, diabetes mellitus, or thyroid disease.

people of all ages. The most common causative agents are rhinoviruses, respiratory syncytial virus, and coronaviruses. The organisms are spread by airborne droplet sprays emitted during respiration, talking, sneezing, and coughing. The virus may also be spread by direct hand contact. The frequency of common colds is due to multiple infections with multiple antigenically unrelated viruses.

The number and frequency of colds increase in the winter months, when staying indoors and overcrowding are more common. In addition, other factors such as chilling, fatigue, and physical and emotional stress may increase a person's susceptibility. Host susceptibility or resistance to infection is determined by the immunologic status of the client. The potential for catching a cold is increased by the time spent in the presence of a person with a cold, by the severity of the symptoms, and by the amount of virus shed into the surrounding atmosphere.

With the common cold, it is unlikely that antibody formation per se is the immediate mechanism of recovery. It takes 5 to 7 days for adequate antibody production. Interferon, a nonspecific, nontoxic product of virus-infected cells, is more closely related to the decline of viruses in tissues and to recovery from infection.[6] (See Chaps. 10 and 11 for discussions of interferon.)

Clinical Manifestations The client with acute viral rhinitis complains of cough, malaise, headache, low-grade fever, sneezing, nasal obstruction, and copious nasal discharge. The client is contagious between the first and third days. The cold is self-limiting within 2 to 7 days. Sore throat is an unusual symptom.[7]

Knowledge of the current viruses that are "going around" and the client's history of recent exposure to the contaminant are the usual methods of diagnosis. Viral isolation and assay for serum neutralization antibody and microscopic examination of the nasal discharge for desquamated cells, lymphocytes, and large numbers of polymorphonuclear leukocytes can also be done.

Medical Management Rest, fluids, proper diet, isolation, antipyretics, and analgesics are recommended. A viral disease causes cell death. These necrotic cells form an excellent culture medium for secondary bacterial infection. Bacterial infection is indicated by fever and a purulent nasal discharge. If the client's complaints are *not* severe, antibiotic therapy is contraindicated. Antibiotics have no effect on viruses and, if taken injudiciously, may produce resistant organisms. A culture and sensitivity study of the throat or nasal discharge may be indicated if severe secondary bacterial invasion is present.

Nursing Management During the cold season, the client should be advised to avoid crowded, close situations and people with obvious cold symptoms. The nurse may recommend that the client increase the vitamin C intake, obtain adequate rest, and avoid situations which are stress-producing. If the client is exposed to a cold virus, frequent hand washing may prevent contamination through direct spread.

Nursing intervention is directed toward relieving annoying symptoms, promoting comfort, instructing the client, and preventing secondary bacterial invasion (Table 19-4). In addition, the client should be encouraged to take increased amounts of fluids, which serve to liquefy secretions in the lungs, ensure hydration, and compensate for evaporative loss due to fever. Vitamin C taken during the acute period may be beneficial in reducing the severity of the cold and the length of time the symptoms persist.

The client should be taught to recognize the symptoms of the *uncommon* cold such as a temperature higher than 38°C (100.4°F), exudate on the tongue, tender glands, a severly red throat, and petechiae in the throat. If these symptoms appear, the client should seek immediate medical attention.

Influenza (Flu)

Influenza is an acute, contagious respiratory disease characterized by sudden onset of headache, fever, and prostration. Influenza reaches epidemic to pandemic proportions and is responsible for thousands of deaths each year. Respiratory viruses called influenza *types A, B,* and *C* cause a wide variety of upper respiratory tract diseases (acute bronchitis, croup, pneumonia) and influenza (the "flu"). Influenza viruses undergo antigenic shifts or changes over time, making immunization difficult.

The primary lesion of influenza is a necrosis of the ciliated epithelium of the respiratory tract. In an uncomplicated infection, epithelial damage is confined to the upper and middle portions of the respiratory tract.

Clinical manifestations and complications

Influenza is spread by direct or indirect airborne droplets. The client typically complains of respiratory tract involvement with symptoms of coryza, cough (often productive), sore throat, headache, high fever, chest pain, malaise, apathy, myalgia, anorexia, nausea and vomiting, and prostration. Influenza is most contagious in the first 3 days and lasts for 1 week to 10 days, with prolonged convalescence.

Table 19-4

Nursing Care Plan for the Client with Upper Respiratory Infections (Cold or Influenza)

Client Problem	Expected Outcome	Nursing Intervention
Fever	Absence of diaphoresis and chills. Normal body temperature.	Isolate client. Give antipyretic medications as ordered. Use cooling sponge bath or alcohol as indicated. Check T q 4 h. Encourage frequent intake of fluids. Reduce room temperature. Monitor I & O. Encourage small, frequent feedings, progressing to usual diet.
Malaise	Absence of aches and pains.	Encourage bed rest and reduction of physical activity. Apply hot packs or rubs if not contraindicated. Give analgesics (aspirin) prn.
Rhinitis	Absence of nasal obstruction and discharge.	Humidify room air. Encourage intake of fluids. Administer antihistamines and decongestants prn.
Cough	Relief of throat discomfort. Absence of cough.	Encourage frequent oral hygiene. Use warm saline throat gargles. Increase humidity in room air. Administer antitussives prn.
Recurrence of infection	No manifestations of cold or influenza.	Instruct client to avoid overcrowded situations during cold/influenza seasons and to avoid contact with persons known to have viral infections. Employ frequent hand washing. Recommend increase in vitamin C intake. Encourage client to seek influenza immunization prior to flu season (refer to Table 19-5).
Potential secondary bacterial infection	Normal WBC. No infection.	(Measures included above.) Instruct in proper diet, rest, activity. Teach differentiation between cold symptoms and bacterial infection (refer to Table 19-8).

Viral pneumonia is one of the main complications of flu. Persons who have chronic rheumatic heart disease with mitral stenosis are particularly predisposed. Influenzal pneumonia develops rapidly and progresses to pulmonary involvement and vascular collapse. Bacterial pneumonia most often affects persons with preexisting pulmonary disease, pregnant women, and the elderly. Other groups at risk for developing complications of flu are infants and clients on immunosuppressive drugs.

Factors that are important in making a diagnosis are the client's history, clinical findings, knowledge of the current prevalent virus, and recovery of the virus from nasopharyngeal specimens. In uncomplicated cases, lymphocytopenia and an elevated or normal erythrocyte sedimentation rate may be present.

Management

The primary goals of treatment are (1) supportive measures directed toward symptomatic relief and (2) prevention of secondary infection. Prophylactic vaccination of the currently prevalent live attenuated and formalin-inactivated influenza strains is recommended for high-risk groups by the Atlanta Center for Disease Control[8] (Table 19-5).

The objectives of vaccination differ in epidemic and pandemic years. The increased morbidity associated with pandemics has been used to justify the consideration of mass immunoprophylaxis. Mass immunization may also lead to problems, as evidenced by the development of increased number of cases of Guillain-Barré syndrome following mass immunization for swine flu virus. Although immunity of varying degrees follows the disease or vaccination, further booster shots are required for a sustained effect. To be effective, the vaccine must be given before the flu

Table 19-5

Indications for Influenza Immunizations*

The following groups should be immunized against influenza:

1. Persons over age 65
2. Persons with a history of:
   - Heart disease
   - Diabetes mellitus
   - Chronic renal disease
   - Chronic anemia
   - Chronic pulmonary disorders
3. Persons who have immune problems or are taking immunosuppressive drugs
4. Pregnant women—should be evaluated using above criteria 2 and 3

*Recommended by the Public Health Service Advisory Committee on Immunization Practices, Center for Disease Control, Atlanta.

virus is contracted. Vaccination should be performed with caution in infants, young children, pregnant women, and those persons who are hypersensitive to egg proteins.

Amantadine hydrochloride has been demonstrated to have the chemoprophylactic effect of producing lower infection rates and less severe illness in those who receive the drug before exposure to influenza virus. The drug is presumed to act by inhibiting virus penetration. However, central nervous system toxicity may limit the use of the drug in the elderly. The nursing management of influenza is described in Table 19-4.

Sinusitis

Acute sinusitis

Acute sinusitis is an inflammation of one or more of the sinus cavities (Fig. 19-1). It may accompany or follow rhinitis (allergic or viral) or occur as a result of a deviated nasal septum and nasal polyps. Because the nasal and sinus mucous membranes are continuous, infections spread rapidly from the nasal passages to the sinuses. Gram-positive cocci (*Streptococcus pneumoniae, Staphylococcus pyogenes, S. aureus,* and *Haemophilus influenzae*) are the most common causative organisms of acute sinusitis.

Clinical Manifestations and Complications The client with acute sinusitis has nasal blockage and stuffiness, a nasal discharge that may be blood-tinged or purulent, a slightly elevated temperature, pressure over the involved sinus which slowly becomes more severe, and malaise. The client looks and feels sick. Sinus pain is due to the accumulation of pus and absorption of air behind a blocked ostium. In most instances, the location of the pain marks the site of infection. Pain over the cheek and upper teeth indicates *maxillary* involvement; pain over the forehead above the eye indicates *frontal* involvement; and pain medial and deep to the eye indicates *ethmoid* involvement. The manifestations of *sphenoid* involvement are tenderness and pain over the vertex of the skull, the mastoid bones, and the occipital portion of the head. When all of the sinuses are infected, *pansinusitis* exists. Typically, the pain of frontal and maxillary sinus inflammation appears 1 to 2 hours after arising from sleep, peaks within 3 to 4 hours, and then becomes less severe in the late afternoon. Unilateral sore throat is often present on the affected side.

Complications of acute sinusitis occur when the infection extends beyond the limits of the sinuses. Epidural abscess, meningitis, frontal lobe abscess, blocking of the natural ostium of the involved sinus, osteomyelitis, mucocele, and orbital cellulitis may occur because of the close proximity of the sinus cavities to the eyes and the brain. Signs of increased intracranial pressure such as changes in behavior, headache, blurred vision, vomiting, high fever, chills, convulsions, or edema should be reported to the physician *immediately.*

Diagnostic Study Abnormalities Direct observation of the nasal mucosa, palpation of the sinus points for pain, x-ray of the sinus, and *transillumination*

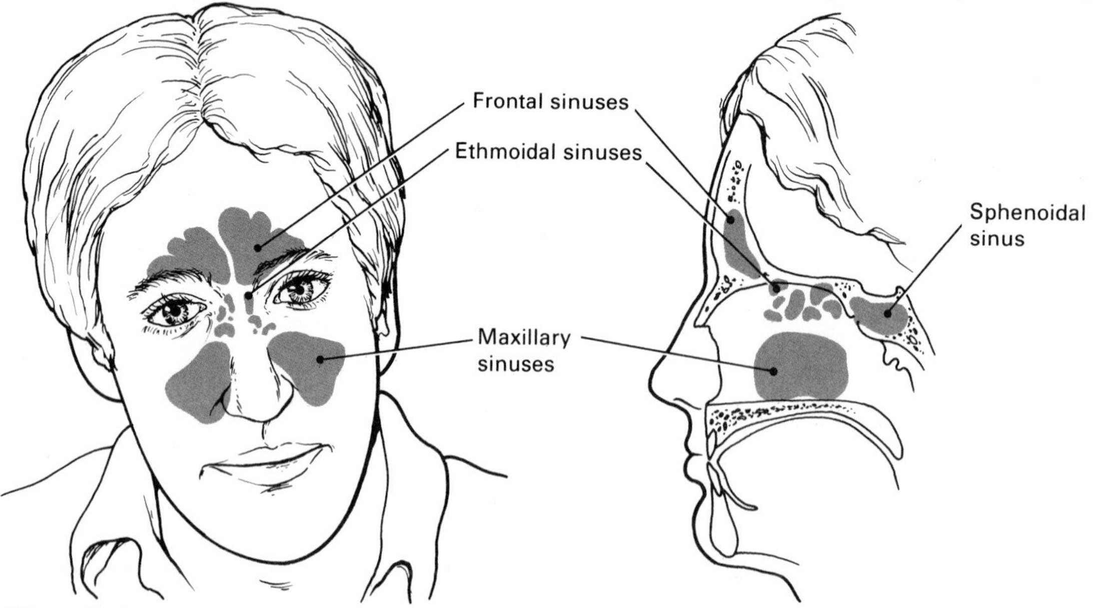

Figure 19-1 Locations of the sinuses.

(shining of a bright light in the client's mouth with the mouth closed to light the sinus) provide diagnostic information. Physical examination findings indicative of acute sinusitis include a hyperemic and edematous mucosa on the involved side and enlarged turbinates which press against the septum and fill the air space. The maxillary and frontal sinuses will be dark to transillumination and appear cloudy, with a visible fluid level on x-ray.

Since antibiotics are highly effective for bacterial infections, culture and sensitivity tests of the drainage material are indicated. The white blood cell (WBC) count usually remains normal.

Medical and Nursing Management Therapeutic goals for acute sinusitis are pain relief, infection control, and promotion of sinus drainage (Table 19-6). Analgesics and application of heat (hot wet packs) give symptomatic relief. Nose drops with vasoconstrictor action help to keep the nose open (Tables 10-15 and 19-3). Antibiotics may be prescribed. In some clients, the condition persists as a subacute infection. When there is severe pain and pus fails to drain, more vigorous methods may be employed. Drainage of the sinuses may be accomplished by irrigation of the maxillary sinus through the natural ostium in the middle meatus or through the thin bone of the medial wall of the sinus under the inferior turbinate.

Surgical intervention employs *antral puncture* or *antrostomy,* which is the insertion of a large-gauge (16 to 18) needle under the inferior turbinate through the medial wall of the antrum and into the sinus cavity. The presence of purulent material or air signals entry of the needle into the antral cavity. Following proper placement of the needle, the sinus cavity can be irrigated with normal saline. Drainage of the sinuses is *contraindicated* during active infection since osteomyelitis can occur. The nursing intervention is described in Table 19-7.

Table 19-6
Medical Management: Acute and Chronic Sinusitis

Diagnostic
1. Inspection of the nose and throat
2. Palpation of sinuses
3. Transillumination
4. Sinus x-ray
5. Culture and sensitivity of nasal discharge
6. Antral puncture

Therapeutic
1. Heat application/inhalation
2. Antibiotics
3. Sympathomimetic (vasoconstrictor) sprays
4. Analgesics
5. Irrigation (chronic)
6. Antral puncture (incision and drainage)
7. Radical antrum surgery

Chronic sinusitis

Sinusitis becomes a chronic problem when no or inadequate treatment is received in the acute or subacute stage or when recurrent bacterial attacks damage the sinus mucosa, causing irreversible tissue damage. The primary clinical manifestations are a purulent nasal discharge and symptoms of allergy.

Diagnosis is based on the history. The client usually has a history of repeated sinus infections. Transillumination, x-ray, and antral puncture are utilized.

When the infection becomes prolonged or complications develop, therapeutic surgical intervention is indicated to (1) eradicate the infection, (2) remove all diseased tissue and bone, (3) restore adjacent postoperative drainage, and (4) obliterate the preexisting sinus cavity when possible.

Types of Surgery The *antral window* is an operative procedure done under local anesthesia as a means of providing sinus drainage in chronic maxillary sinusitis. The inferior turbinate of the nose is fractured medially and the bony wall between the nose and the antrum is removed, producing a permanent window. The window allows pus to drain into the nose.

The *Caldwell-Luc radical antrum procedure* is a more radical type of surgery performed under local or general anesthesia. An incision is made under the upper lip above the roots of the teeth to enter the maxillary sinus. Following removal of part of the anterior wall of the antrum (which creates a window), the diseased mucosa and periosteum are also removed. Packing may be inserted into the antrum to control hemorrhage. However, bleeding is usually very slight.

Ethmoidectomy or exenteration of the ethmoid air cells can be accomplished either through the nose (intranasally) or around the inner canthus of the eye (externally).

The nursing management of clients with chronic sinusitis is described in Table 19-7.

Obstructions of the Nose and Paranasal Sinuses

Polyps

Polyps are benign, recurring focal accumulations of tissue filled with edema fluid. The edema is accom-

Table 19-7
Nursing Care Plan for the Client with Acute and Chronic Sinusitis

Client Problem	Expected Outcome	Nursing Intervention
	Acute Management	
Pain and severe headache	Comfort. Nontender sinus points.	Give steam inhalations and encourage fluid intake to liquefy secretions. Utilize heat lamp. Apply warm compresses to sinus points. Maintain a constant room temperature. Administer analgesics and vasoconstrictors prn. Teach client proper use of vasoconstrictor medication. Raise head of bed. Discourage smoking.
Infected nasal discharge	Normal nasal secretions. Normal temperature.	Encourage frequent oral hygiene. Administer antibiotics as indicated. Give warm gargles. Encourage fluids intake, proper diet, and rest.
Anorexia	Usual appetite.	Encourage frequent oral hygiene. Promote rest. Provide nutritious, attractive foods.
	Surgical Management	
Anxiety	Remain calm.	Give general preoperative instructions. Include teaching the client to mouth-breathe. Advise client that nose blowing is contraindicated. Explain equipment for and methods of pain relief such as warm or cool vapor inhalations, frequent oral hygiene, ice bags to the operative site, analgesics. Teach deep breathing and relaxation techniques.
Hemorrhage	Stable vital signs. No bleeding.	Take vital signs q 2 h for 24 h. Observe client for excessive swallowing. Check nasal packing for dislodgement. Change mustache dressing. Administer ice bags to the operative site. Instruct client to avoid nose blowing.
Infection	No signs of inflammation. Normal temperature and WBC.	Administer antibiotics as ordered. Encourage generous fluid intake. Provide rest. Administer oral hygiene before and after meals if there is an oral incision. Check T q 4 h, Report any signs of inflammation and infection to physician.
Diplopia	Normal visual acuity.	Assess optic nerve status. Report any deviations to the physician.
Postoperative pain	Minimal to no pain.	Reinforce preoperative learning and relaxation techniques. Place ice bag on the operative site. Raise head of bed. Administer analgesics prn. Report severe pain to physician since it may indicate infection or inadequate drainage.
	Chronic Management	
Chronic cough, headache, purulent nasal discharge	Minimal to absent cough, headache, nasal discharge.	Teach client to avoid factors that lead to exacerbations such as cold, damp places, and air conditioning. Discourage smoking. If allergy is the cause, follow directions regarding the type of allergen responsible for condition.

panied by hyperplasia of submucosal connective tissue. Polyps occur in both the nose and sinuses as a result of infection, trauma, allergy, or thermal changes. They can cause great anxiety for the client who fears they are malignant. Allergic rhinitis is the most common predisposing factor. Polyps tend to recur if the underlying allergy is not well controlled.

Polyps are classified as *edematous* (a glistening, gray-white, grapelike lesion filled with edema fluid) or *fibrous* (a firm growth of fibrous tissue) and vascular (pink in color). They are noted when they protrude into the airway or occlude the nose. Clinical manifestations are nasal obstruction, nasal discharge (usually clear mucus), and speech distortion.

Nasal polyps are removed surgically under local anesthesia with a wire snare or forceps. Small polyps may be injected with long-acting steroids to reduce edema. However, they often return to their previous size when the drug is discontinued.

Foreign bodies

Foreign bodies are any objects or substances located in any tissue or body cavity that are foreign to the location in which they are found. Foreign bodies in the nose are most often removed by sneezing. However, if they are not removed, they may result in infection and obstruction. Nearly all nasal foreign bodies result from accidents. Regardless of the cause, the usual outcome is local obstruction with mucosal edema and swelling. A seropurulent discharge and a putrid odor often occur concurrently. A unilateral, foul-smelling discharge should alert the nurse or physician to this problem. The client may have no pain.

All foreign bodies should be removed from the nose through the route of entry. Irrigation of the nose or pushing the object backward should *not* be attempted. Either intervention could force the object into the laryngotracheal tree, causing airway obstruction and death. The object should be removed with a forceps following shrinkage of the nasal mucosa with a vasoconstrictor.[9] A calcium deposit called a *rhinolith* may form around an object that is left in the nose for many years.

PROBLEMS RELATED TO THE PHARYNX

Pharyngitis

Acute pharyngitis (viral)

The most common throat inflammation in adults is *acute viral or bacterial pharyngitis*. The viruses responsible are primarily adenovirus type 4 or 7, Coxsackie group A virus, and ECHOviruses. A viral causative agent is suggested by the occurrence of infection during summer, winter, and spring epidemics. Viral causation is further confirmed by exclusion of a bacterial etiology on throat culture.

The inflammation usually causes a mild, sore, red throat, slight fever, and difficulty in swallowing. A dry, raspy cough and hoarseness may be present. The tonsils, palatine arches, and soft palate will have a dusky or bright red appearance with marked edema. Acute viral pharyngitis is best treated by rest, warm saline gargles, and aspirin.

Acute follicular pharyngitis (streptococcal sore throat)

Acute follicular pharyngitis (strep throat) results from bacterial invasion by group A beta-hemolytic streptococci. The problem is endemic during the winter months because people stay indoors more frequently and are in close contact. The organism is transmitted by moist droplets expelled from the respiratory tract by coughing and sneezing.

Clinical Manifestations The clinical manifestations of strep throat are sore throat (ranging from a scratchy throat to difficulty in swallowing), dysphagia, fever, malaise, loss of appetite, earache, and headache. Physical examination shows a markedly elevated temperature and cervical adenopathy. The pharynx will be hyperemic and edematous. The tonsils, if present, will be reddened and swollen and often covered with a removable white or yellow patchy exudate. The WBC will be elevated, with marked neutrophil leukocytosis.

Complications are peritonsillar abscess, otitis media, scarlet fever, rheumatic fever, and glomerulonephritis. Rheumatic fever and glomerulonephritis occur as a result of the formation of antibodies against streptococcal bacteria which then combine with heart or kidney tissue to cause local tissue damage. (Rheumatic heart disease is discussed in Chap. 29 and glomerulonephritis in Chap. 37.)

Management The physician will usually order benzathine penicillin G intramuscularly (IM) or oral phenoxynethyl penicillin. If the client is allergic to penicillin, erythromycin is substituted.

The client should be instructed in methods to prevent contamination and infection, such as washing hands frequently and avoiding exposure to known carriers. The client should also be told about the difference between streptococcal and viral pharyngitis and the common cold (Table 19-8).

Nursing management includes encouraging bed rest with modified activities, alleviation of the sore throat with warm saline gargles and an ice collar, steam vaporization to soothe inflamed mucous membranes, and administration of analgesics for pain and antipyretics to reduce fever. The client's temperature should be checked frequently and antibiotics administered as ordered. The client should be encouraged to increase fluid intake and to take cool, bland liquids and gelatin that will not irritate the pharynx. Citrus juices should be avoided since they irritate the mucous membrane.

Tonsillitis

Acute follicular tonsillitis (palatine)

Acute follicular tonsillitis, a problem common to adolescents and young adults, is most commonly

Table 19-8
Comparison of Common Upper Respiratory Problems

Problem	Pathogenic Organism	Local Manifestations	Systemic Manifestations
Acute follicular tonsillitis	Group A beta-hemolytic streptococci	Tonsillar cover of white, patchy, non-adherent exudate	Fever, chills, sore throat, headache, and malaise
Diphtheria	*Cornyebacterium diphtheriae*	Tonsillar and oropharyngeal cover of firm, gray, leathery, adherent membrane	Toxicity (related to exotoxin production), fever, late myocarditis, and perineuropathy
Acute viral pharyngitis	Adenoviruses 4 and 7 Coxsackie virus group A ECHOviruses	Hyperemic throat	Slight fever

caused by bacterial invasion of the tonsils by group A beta-hemolytic streptococci. Other causative agents may be pneumococci, staphylococci, and *H. influenzae*. Predisposing factors are preexisting upper respiratory infections, exposure to temperature extremes, and fatigue.

Clinical Manifestations The onset of acute follicular tonsillitis may be sudden, with chills, high fever, dysphagia due to a sore throat, headache, malaise, and joint pains. On examination of the throat, the tongue is found to be coated with a grayish material and thick, tenacious mucus in the oral cavity. The tonsils will be large, edematous, and covered with small patches of a nonadherable, soft, friable, whitish exudate. The mucosa underlying the exudate will be inflamed. The WBC count will be elevated and a culture of tonsil tissue will be positive for bacteria. A major complication of tonsillitis is peritonsillar abscess (quinsy), which is described later.

Management After the history and physical examination, a culture of tonsillar exudate is obtained. Systemic antibiotics (e.g., penicillin) are given for 7 to 10 days to eradicate the organism and reduce the risk of producing antibiotic-resistant bacteria. The client needs to understand the importance of taking all the medication.

Supportive nursing intervention is directed toward assisting the client with an adequate fluid intake, hygienic measures, rest, warmth, oral gargles with warm saline, analgesics, and antipyretics. Lozenges with topical anesthesia may decrease the dysphagia. Soft foods should be provided.

Chronic tonsillitis

Chronic tonsillitis occurs when there is recurrent infection. The invading viral or bacterial pathogens produce tonsillar enlargement through hyperplasia or fibrous obstruction of the tonsillar crypts.

Clinical manifestations are frequent upper respiratory and systemic infections, chronic recurrent sore throats, fever, malaise, cervical adenopathy, foul breath, and small (or enlarged) tonsils. Medical treatment is supportive unless surgical removal is indicated. See Table 19-9 for nursing care of the client.

Acute Adenoiditis (Pharyngeal Tonsillitis)

Acute adenoiditis occurs as a result of inflammation involving the pharynx and tonsils. On examination, erythema and edema of adenoidal tissue are present concurrently with localized pustules and cervical adenopathy. The client typically has dysphagia, malaise, fever, headache, sore throat, sinusitis, decreased hearing, and otalgia due to eustachian tube obstruction.

Supportive therapy as described for acute follicular tonsillitis is tried initially. If chronic inflammation persists, surgical removal, which is described later, is indicated.

Peritonsillar Abscess (Quinsy)

Quinsy occurs when a suppurative inflammation of the tonsils results in a localized accumulation of pus within the peritonsillar tissue. It is usually a complication of acute pharyngitis. The most common causative organisms are *S. pyogenes* and *S. aureus.* The client recalls having a lingering sore throat which worsens and localizes to one side. This is accompanied by high-grade fever, chills, malaise, local pain, dysphagia, tender cervical adenopathy, drooling followed by rancid breath, *trismus* (spasms of the jaw), difficulty in speaking, and a thickened, nasal voice.

Physical examination shows infection and edema

Table 19-9
Nursing Care Plan for the Client with Tonsillectomy and Adenoidectomy

Client Problem	Expected Outcome	Nursing Intervention
	Preoperative Management	
Inadequate knowledge of impending surgery	Increased knowledge of surgical and postoperative procedures.	Give client brief explanation of surgical procedures, hospital routine, and expected postoperative course. Instruct client to turn and deep-breathe (*coughing is contraindicated*), to expectorate rather than swallow drainage, and to avoid using a straw. Pain relief measures should be discussed (see below) and questions answered.
	Postoperative Management	
Potential respiratory distress	Normal respiratory rate. Patent airway.	In the recovery room, place client in modified Trendelenburg position to facilitate removal of secretions and prevent aspiration. Observe for respiratory distress (e.g., crowing, chest retraction). Check for tonsillar packing. Exercise extreme caution if oropharyngeal suctioning is necessary.
Potential hemorrhage	Normal vital signs. No excessive bleeding.	Monitor vital signs hourly for 12 h and pulse q h while client is asleep. Check the back of the throat with a flashlight for excess bleeding q 1 h to q 2 h. Report tachycardia, bright red drainage, hypotension, increased swallowing to physician. Tell client to avoid coughing, clearing throat, and using a straw.
Pain	Minimal to no pain.	Instruct client in proper and frequent oral hygiene. Administer an ice collar. Give nonaspirin analgesics prn as ordered. Client should gargle with warm saline q 2 h. Client should also chew Aspergum before and between meals for soreness and avoid smoking. Advise client that pain in ears is usual after T and A. Give mild analgesic as needed.
Dehydration	Normal intake and output.	Give oral fluids (ice chips, ice cream, gelatin) when client is alert and responsive. Encourage a generous intake (see below).
Delayed wound healing, weight loss	Good nutritional intake.	Emphasize the importance of good nutrition for wound healing. Instruct the client to eat soft foods (e.g., custard, strained vegetables, gelatins, broths) and to drink warm liquids, which are less irritating than cold ones. Client should avoid drinking citrus and tomato juices, which cause throat to burn. Gradually, add foods such as ground meat, mashed potatoes, bread without crusts.
Potential infection	No signs of inflammation. Normal temperature.	Instruct the client to drink fluids and eat well. Instruct in and institute frequent oral hygiene using warm saline or a mild mouthwash. *Avoid* persons with an infectious process.
Delayed hemorrhage	Normal vital signs.	Instruct client regarding the signs of hemorrhage and advise client to call physician immediately if they appear. If mild bleeding occurs, instruct client to spit out blood and gargle gently with ice water. Notify physician if bleeding does not stop promptly. Client should limit activity, rest frequently, avoid heavy lifting and vigorous exercise for at least 2 weeks. Advise the client that white patches will form where the tonsils were removed.

of the involved peritonsillar tissue, bulging and redness of the soft palate or tonsillar pillars, and lateral deviation of the uvula.

Following culture and sensitivity testing, early treatment consists of antibiotic therapy. If pus forms, incision and drainage are indicated. Once the abscess has subsided, the nurse should teach the client careful oral hygiene and give instructions regarding upper respiratory problems that require medical intervention.

Complications of recurrent peritonsillar abscess can be life-threatening. These include supraglottic edema with airway obstruction, sepsis, phlebitis, endocarditis, nephritis, hemorrhage, and brain abscess. Because of the possibility of serious complications, a tonsillectomy is often advocated as the treatment of choice of peritonsillar abscess.

Tonsillectomy and Adenoidectomy (T and A)

Removal of the tonsils is indicated when the client experiences recurrent, incapacitating episodes of acute or chronic tonsillitis. These attacks often number two or more per year and result in time lost from school or work. Tonsillectomy is also required for clients who have tonsillar or adenoidal hypertrophy which obstructs the airway, peritonsillar abscess (quinsy), recurrent middle ear disease secondary to eustachian tube obstruction, hearing loss related to enlargement of the tonsils and adenoids, or complications of ethmoid sinusitis. Tonsillectomy is also indicated for the client who is a diphtheria carrier since the tonsils function to seed infection. Adults who have recurrent sore throats, earaches, or problems with snoring are also candidates for this procedure.

Tonsillectomy is most often performed during childhood since developing immunity renders the tonsillar lymphoid tissue the most frequent site of repeated bacterial invasion and hypertrophy. Adenoidal tissue usually atrophies by adulthood, necessitating removal of only tonsillar tissue. Combination surgery is more frequent in childhood. The surgery should not be done when acute infection is present, during the active stage of tuberculosis or polio epidemics, or when the client has a blood dyscrasia such as purpura or hemophilia.[10]

Preoperative management

Preoperative management begins with a history, which includes careful questioning about bleeding disorders and any prior medical problems. A complete blood count (CBC) is obtained. Prothrombin time, partial thromboplastin time, and the platelet count are determined to assess bleeding or clotting problems. Prophylactic antibiotics may be ordered to prevent transitory bacteremias. Other preparations are similar to those used in all preoperative regimes (see Chap. 6).

Surgical management

T and A may be performed under general or local anesthesia. Local anesthesia is preferred for adults. The tonsils are removed by dissection and a snare. Hemostasis is achieved through local pressure with a gauze sponge, ligation of vessels, or electrocoagulation. The alternative to the use of dissection and a snare is the guillotine method of tonsillectomy. This method is less effective when the tonsils are located deep in the throat. Adenoidectomy is accomplished by use of an *adenotome* or adenoid curette.

Healing by granulation begins within 24 hours and is usually complete by 3 weeks. A membrane of white patches forms where the tonsils were removed. The client should be told that the membrane may separate and bleed between the fifth and tenth postoperative days. If this bleeding does not stop spontaneously, hemostasis can be achieved by the local application of epinephrine or pressure. Complications of T and A are infrequent but may include an adverse reaction to anesthesia (e.g., cardiac arrest), hemorrhage, infection, tissue trauma, delayed healing, and regrowth of tissue.

A relatively new method involving the use of *cryosurgical technique* in tonsillectomy may also be selected. This technique is of great benefit for clients with blood dyscrasias. The cryosurgical procedure may not destroy all of the lymphoid tissue, but the tissue that remains appears to be somewhat more resistant to infection. Edema is a major problem postoperatively, but hemorrhage is uncommon since necrosis is gradual.[11]

Nursing management in the pre- and postoperative periods is described further in Table 19-9.

Diphtheria

Diphtheria is a localized infection of the upper respiratory tract resulting from invasion by *Corynebacterium diphtheriae,* a gram-positive, aerobic bacterium. Delayed systemic manifestations of myocarditis and perineuropathy may follow local invasion. These complications occur as a result of excretion of a potent soluble exotoxin by the microorganisms. This exotoxin is absorbed systemically.

The incidence of diphtheria has been extremely

low for the last 4 decades. However, it is again increasing due to lack of immunization in childhood. Diphtheria most often occurs in temperate climates, in inadequately immunized hosts, and with overcrowding. Infection is most prevalent during the fall and winter.

The incubation period is from 1 to 7 days. Clinical manifestations include elevated temperature, an increased, thready pulse, and the appearance of a characteristic gray-white pseudomembrane covering the oropharynx, nasopharynx, and laryngopharynx which sometimes extends to the trachea. The membrane is adherent to the underlying ulcerated mucosa. Diphtheria should be managed as an *acute emergency* since death may ensue as a result of airway obstruction.

Diagnosis is based on the history, physical examination of the throat, and a culture of pharyngeal scrapings. Medical management should begin immediately. Administration of antitoxin and antimicrobials (e.g., penicillin) should *not* be delayed until the microscopic diagnosis is made. Isolation, rest, and hydration are utilized as supportive medical and nursing measures.

Diphtheria can be prevented by administration of a toxoid which produces active immunity. In emergencies such as exposure to the infection with no prior immunization, passive immunity of 3 weeks' duration can be attained by use of diphtheria antitoxin. The nurse can aid in preventing this sometimes fatal disease by giving instruction to adults and children regarding immunization.

PROBLEMS RELATED TO THE TRACHEA AND LARYNX

Tracheostomy

Tracheotomy is a surgical incision into the trachea for the purpose of establishing an airway. *Tracheostomy* is the tracheal stoma or opening that results from tracheotomy (Fig. 19-2). Tracheostomy is a procedure that is over 2000 years old and has evolved as a planned rather than an emergency procedure. The frequent use and efficacy of nonirritating oral and nasal endotracheal tubes has reduced the incidence of tracheostomy.

Indications for tracheostomy

There are four basic indications for tracheostomy:[12]

1. To bypass upper airway obstruction (e.g., tumors, laryngeal edema, facial injuries)
2. To prevent aspiration of secretions (requires a cuffed tube)
3. To assist or control breathing when mechanical ventilation is used for a prolonged period
4. To facilitate the removal of respiratory tract secretions

Tracheostomy has decided advantages over endotracheal intubation (discussed below). These advantages include increased comfort for the client (since no tube will be present in the mouth), less chance of tube displacement (since the tracheotomy tube is shorter than the endotracheal tube and cannot enter the right mainstem bronchus), and the ability to swallow and eat with the tube in place.

Surgical procedure

Tracheostomy can be performed at the bedside but is most frequently done in an operating room. Following local anesthetization with the client's head down and the neck hyperextended, a horizontal incision is made midway between the cricoid cartilage and the suprasternal notch. The trachea is incised between the second and third tracheal rings. The tracheostomy tube is inserted, hemostasis is provided, and the wound is easily closed. Chest x-ray confirms the placement of the tube.

During insertion of a double-cannula tracheostomy tube, an obturator is placed in the outer cannula (Fig. 19-3). After insertion, it is immediately removed and replaced by the inner cannula, which is then secured by locking it to the outer cannula. The obturator should always be placed in a conspicuous place at the bedside so that it is available if the tracheostomy tube is accidentally removed.

Tracheostomy tubes and cuffs

Tracheostomy tubes can be made of synthetic material (e.g., plastic, nylon) or metal. They can be single or double (inner and outer) cannula. Tracheal tubes can be cuffed or uncuffed. *Cuffs* are plastic balloons encircling the tube that are inflated to form a seal between the tube and the trachea.

Single-cannula tracheostomy tubes (e.g., Portex) have a low-pressure cuff which is bonded to the cannula (Fig. 19-4). A single-cannula tracheostomy tube has no inner cannula, and encrusted secretions may occlude the tube if no additional source of humidification is used. Ambulatory clients with tracheostomies may not continuously receive additional hu-

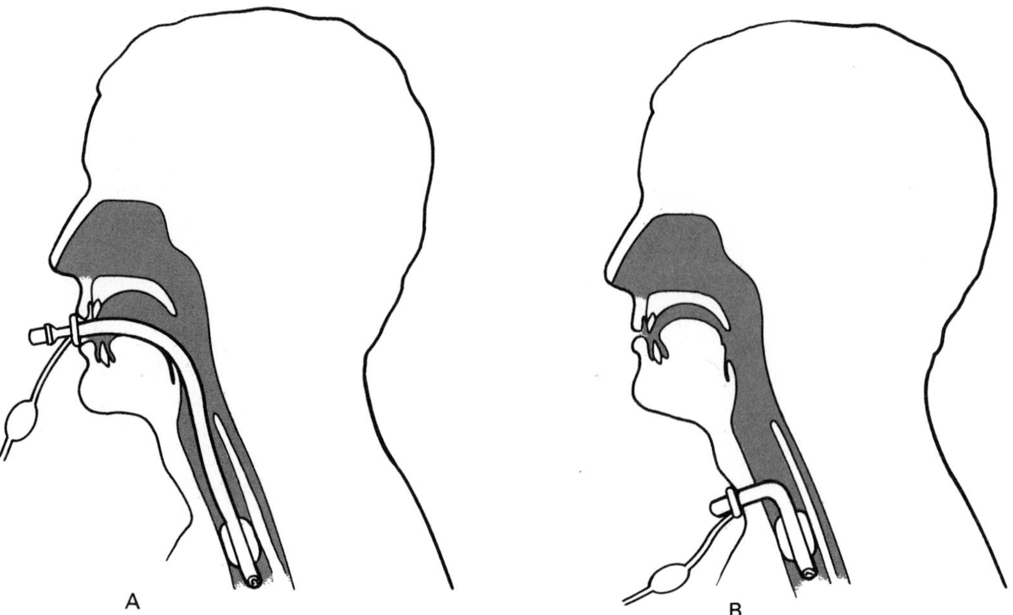

Figure 19-2 *(a)* Placement of the endotrachael tube. *(b)* Placement of tracheostomy tube. (Both tubes have inflated cuffs.)

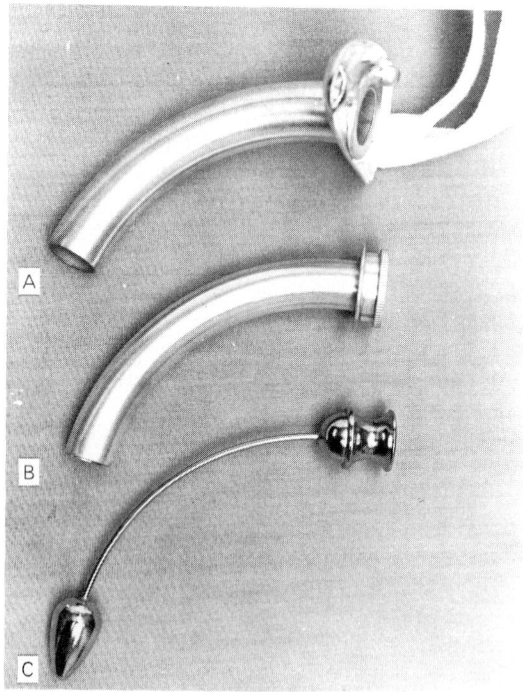

Figure 19-3 Metal tracheostomy tube set. (*a*) Outer cannula. (*b*) Inner cannula. (*c*) Obturator. *(From H. Moidel et al., Nursing Care of the Patient with Medical-Surgical Disorders, 2d ed., McGraw-Hill Book Company, New York, 1976, p. 499.)*

midification, and therefore, secretions may crust inside the tube. Some plastic cannulas are now supplied with an inner cannula (e.g., Lanz, Shiley) which can be removed for cleaning. Single-cannula tubes are not removed for cleaning.

When a metal tracheostomy tube is used, a rubber cuff may be attached to the outside of the outer tube. Such cuffs often achieve very high pressures on inflation. Other disadvantages of metal tubes are the rigidity and expense of the metal and potential slippage of the cuff over the end of the tube. Slippage will not occur with cuffs on plastic tubes because the plastic is bonded to the plastic tube.

Tracheostomy cuffs should be soft to permit tube movement without movement of the cuff against the tracheal membrane. A pliable, soft cuff reduces friction between the cuff and the wall of the trachea and permits an airtight seal. Low-pressure, high-volume cuffs reduce the hazards of tracheal necrosis and anatomic distortion. The cuffed tracheostomy cannula should meet a number of requirements which are described in Table 19-10.

Cuff Inflation The cuff should be inflated when the client is eating or drinking, when the swallowing reflex is absent, or when the client is attached to a mechanical ventilator. A cuff is inflated by injecting air into the fine-bore tubing leading to the balloon. The

Cuff Inflation The cuff should be inflated when the client is eating or drinking, when the swallowing reflex is absent, or when the client is attached to a mechanical ventilator. A cuff is inflated by injecting air into the fine-bore tubing leading to the balloon. The cuff should be inflated with the least amount of air that will adequately seal the trachea. The amount of air needed to inflate the cuff varies depending on the size of the tracheostomy tube and the client's trachea. An adequate seal has been made when the nurse cannot hear or feel air escaping from the client's mouth or nose and the client cannot speak. If the client is on a mechanical ventilator, the leak is detectable by a harsh sound heard during the inspiratory phase.

Rupture of the cuff will be apparent when large amounts of air will not inflate the balloon, when the client is able to speak, when more air can be removed from the cuff than was injected originally, or when the positive-pressure respirator cannot maintain adequate respiratory movement.

To reduce the possibility of tracheal ischemia and necrosis, always monitor cuff pressures. The volume of air instilled should not exceed 20 mmHg or 25 cm H_2O. Shiley, Lanz, and Portex have systems which allow such monitoring. When low-pressure cuffs are not used, deflate the cuff for 1 minute each hour. The recommended procedure for minimizing cuff damage to the trachea when low-pressure cuffs are used is to (1) inflate the cuff to the *minimal* occluding pressure or allow a slight leak, (2) make sure that the intracuff pressure is less than 25 cmH_2O during exhalation, and (3) allow the cuff to remain deflated except when the airway needs to be sealed[13] (e.g., when there is a risk of aspiration or when mechanical ventilation is required).

Fenestrated Cannula The *fenestrated cannula* is a double cannula with openings cut into the curvatures of the outer cannula. The fenestrated tube is usually inserted during weaning procedures. When the inner cannula is in place, the tube functions as a normal double cannula. When it is removed, the openings in the outer cannula permit air to rise over the vocal cords. The fenestrated cannula permits the client to speak since inspired air passes through the

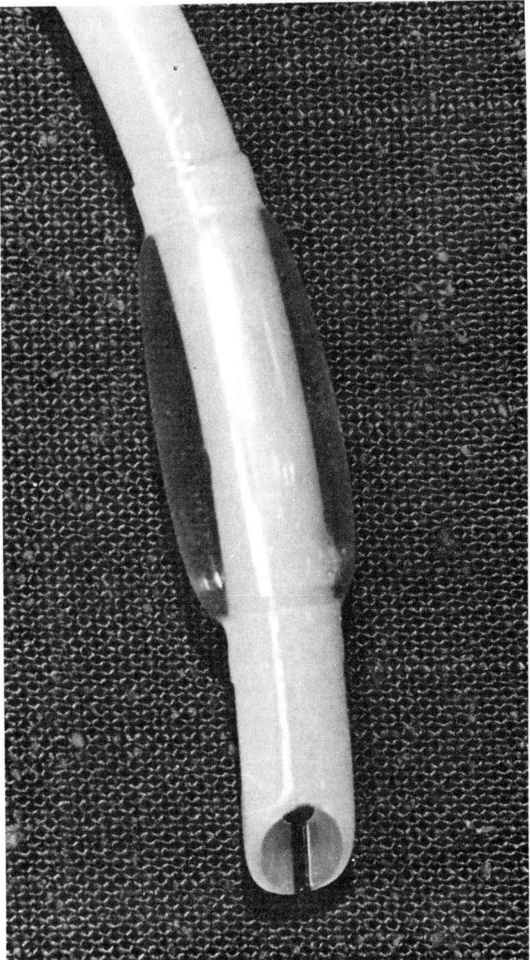

Figure 19-4 Distal tip of a cuffed tracheostomy tube with the cuff inflated. *(From H. Moidel et al., Nursing Care of the Patient with Medical-Surgical Disorders, 2d ed., McGraw-Hill Book Company, New York, 1976, p. 498.)*

Table 19-10
Requirements for Cuffed Tracheostomy Cannulas

1. The cuff should be:
   - Bonded to the cannula
   - Smooth and evenly inflatable
   - Low pressure, high volume
   - Comformable to the trachea
2. The cannula should:
   - Have a smooth lumen with a wide diameter
   - Not be long enough to cause endobronchial intubation or pressure on the carina
   - Not be rigid
   - Be made of inexpensive, nontoxic, tissue-compatible materials
   - Be comfortable to the client

larynx. The client's ability to breathe spontaneously through the larynx and cough up tracheobronchial secretions may be evaluated when this cannula is used.

Tracheostomy Button (Kischner) The *tracheostomy button* is a short outer tube that fits into the stoma. This device contains a one-way valve that permits the client to speak, but its presence prevents closing of the tracheostomy opening. The button helps to wean the client from the tracheostomy tube. If the tracheostomy must be maintained, a tracheostomy tube can easily be reinserted.

Complications of tracheostomy

The operative procedure may cause the following complications: (1) bleeding because of inadequate hemostasis, (2) subcutaneous emphysema, (3) posterior tracheal penetration, or (4) left recurrent laryngeal nerve damage. Most of these complications are avoidable if the procedure is elective and is performed in a controlled environment.

Complications following the operative procedure are postoperative hemorrhage, airway obstruction secondary to cannula occlusion, kinking, or displacement of the tube, and infection.

Problems increase over the period that the tracheostomy tube is in place. Late complications include tracheal stenosis, tracheal esophageal fistula, tracheal necrosis or ulceration, and tracheomalacia (the loss of cartilaginous support of the tracheal wall). Potential causes of tracheal damage may be excessive cuff pressure, high ventilatory pressures, or a large cannula diameter relative to the diameter of the trachea.

Nursing management

Prior to the tracheostomy, the nurse should explain to the client and family the purpose of the surgery and state that the client will not be able to speak. However, the client will be provided with a pad and pencil, and a means for contacting the nurse (bell, light) will be available. The client's hearing, language, and writing ability should be assessed. The client should be given adequate information to reduce anxiety.

Care of the tracheotomized client is challenging and utilizes the full realm of nursing skills and knowledge. The nursing care of this client is described in Table 19-11.

A replacement tracheostomy tube, an obturator, and a hemostat should be kept at the bedside, where they are readily available for emergency use. If a tracheostomy tube is accidentally removed, the stoma wound should be separated with a hemostat and the replacement tube inserted.

Decannulation

Decannulation of the tracheotomized client is similar to that of the client with endotracheal intubation. When the client no longer needs mechanical ventilation to assist breathing, blood gases are satisfactory, and the client can adequately clear the secretions, decannulation will begin. The procedure may be initiated with a methylene blue dye test to assess the client's gag and swallow reflexes. In this test, the cuff is first deflated and then the client swallows 30 mL of water colored with methylene blue dye. The trachea is next suctioned to check for the presence of blue-colored secretions. If there is no indication of dye in the secretions, the client is judged to have competent epiglottal function.[14] A fenestrated tube or tracheal button may then be employed.

The client needs to relearn to breathe through the nose. This can be facilitated by reducing the lumen of the tube for a day or two and then corking or taping the tube closed. If this procedure is well tolerated, the tube can be removed. The stoma is covered with a dressing and taped. It will begin to form epithelial tissue within 24 to 48 hours and close on its own. No surgery is required. The stoma may also be closed with Steristrips and covered with a dry sterile dressing.[15]

Endotracheal Intubation

Endotracheal intubation is the insertion and placement of a tube into the trachea via the mouth (*orotracheal*) or nose (nasotracheal) to ensure a patent airway (Fig. 19-2). Tubes may be cuffed or uncuffed (Fig. 19-6).

Orotracheal intubation

Orotracheal intubation is indicated in emergencies since it can be accomplished quickly and atraumatically in most clients. The orotracheal route is used to (1) maintain a patent airway in clients who develop an obstruction, (2) remove secretions from the tracheobronchial tree, (3) provide deep breaths with a self-inflating bag, (4) deliver oxygen or general anesthetics, and (5) control or facilitate ventilation for short time periods.[16]

Orotracheal tubes are inserted via a laryngoscope. The client's airway is suctioned, and the lungs are hyperventilated with oxygen. Topical anesthesia may be applied to the larynx and trachea. If the client is conscious, a muscle relaxant and morphine sulfate may be administered. The client is placed in a supine position with the head in moderate dorsiflexion and

Table 19-11
Nursing Care Plan for a Client with a Tracheostomy

Client Problem	Expected Outcome	Nursing Intervention
Moist rales	Chest clear to auscultation.	Suction client (see Table 19-12).
Dry mucous membranes of respiratory tract	Moist, intact mucous membranes.	Add moisture to inspired air via oral intake, humidifiers, nebulization, or tracheal instillation of normal saline. Assess client for signs of fluid overload. Assess mucous membranes of mouth and pharynx.
Potential infection	Normal WBC and temperature. No sign of inflammation.	Utilize strict aseptic technique for tracheostomy care (see Table 19-13). Wash hands frequently. Avoid cross-contamination. Change all oxygen and humidification tubing at least daily.
Potential hemorrhage	Stable vital signs.	Monitor P, R, and BP as ordered. Observe client for restlessness and hematoma formation. Do not administer heated, humidified air if client is bleeding. Inflate tracheostomy cuff to prevent aspiration of blood. Notify physician.
Airway obstruction	Normal respiratory rate. No hypoxia. Patent airway.	Observe the client for restlessness, hypoxia, and dyspnea. Kinking or displacement of the cannula and impingement of the cannula tip on the carina may occur.
Accidental extubation	Successful reintubation with minimal trauma.	Always maintain an extra tracheostomy tube, obturator, and hemostat at the bedside. If the tube is coughed out (e.g., while changing tracheostomy tapes), spread the opening with a hemostat. Insert the sterile replacement tube with the obturator at an angle. Straighten and remove the obturator. Act quickly!
Communication impairment	Able to communicate needs.	Reassure client that assistance is available. Provide a magic slate, writing materials, call bell, or light.
Complications of tracheal ischemia, fistula, stenosis	No complications.	Observe for complications. Prevent overinflation of cuff (if present). Use caution when suctioning. Prevent trauma to the trachea.
Nutritional imbalance	No weight loss. No aspiration.	Assist client in modifying the diet (if necessary). Inflate the tracheal cuff when eating or swallowing fluids to prevent aspiration. Assist the client in holding the head flexed with the chin down to open the esophagus and narrow the airway.

elevated 2 or 3 inches above the bed. The orotracheal tube is then inserted. If the tube has a cuff, it is inflated to prevent aspiration of mouth or stomach contents into the lungs. Another reason to inflate the cuff is to prevent air leakage around the tube if the person is attached to a mechanical ventilator.

Following intubation, the client is oxygenated and suctioned (Table 19-12). The client may be placed on mechanical ventilation. A chest x-ray should be taken to confirm the placement of the tube. Additional signs of correct intubation are auscultation of breath sounds in both lungs, movement of the chest wall, and warm exhaled air felt at the end of the tube if the client is breathing spontaneously. After placement is confirmed, a mark should be placed at the point where the endotracheal tube emerges from the mouth. The tube is then taped securely to the face at the side of the mouth. An oral airway or bite block is placed in the mouth to stabilize the tube and prevent the client from biting down on it. Pressure areas may form at the side of the client's mouth if the tube is not repositioned daily. It should be alternated from side to side on a daily basis. When the tube is retaped, it is important to ensure adequate fixation to prevent extubation and loss of a patent airway. The presence of breath sounds in both lungs should be noted on auscultation if the tube is correctly positioned.

Oral endotracheal tubes are uncomfortable for conscious clients and may induce coughing and retching. Vocal cord damage may develop following prolonged use (more than 10 days).

The nurse who manages the care of the client with

Table 19-12

Suctioning Procedure

1. Explain procedure to the client.
2. Auscultate lungs and suction when respirations sound moist.
3. Collect necessary sterile equipment (usually available in sterile disposable set).
   a. Suction catheter (should be no larger than half the diameter of the endotracheal or tracheostomy tube)
   b. Cup or basin
   c. Towel
   d. Sterile water
   e. Sterile gloves
4. Wash hands.
5. Utilizing sterile technique, unwrap sterile equipment and fill cup (or basin) with water.
6. Preoxygenate with 100% O_2 using ventilating bag or by increasing the inspired O_2 concentration for a few breaths.
7. Often, it is helpful to instill 2–5 mL of normal saline into tube before suctioning.
8. Insert catheter into suction outlet, put on sterile gloves, and pick up sterile suction catheter with one hand.
9. Lubricate catheter tip with water and insert catheter about 6 inches (for tracheostomy tube) or full length (for endotracheal tube) with Y connector or thumb valve open (finger off).
10. After catheter is fully inserted, apply suction while withdrawing in a rotating manner.
11. Occlude Y side or thumb valve intermittently while withdrawing catheter.
12. Do not suction longer than 15 seconds at one time.
13. Reoxygenate manually or with O_2 mask between suctioning periods.
14. Rinse catheter with sterile water between insertions.
15. When finished with suctioning, auscultate lungs to assess lung sounds.

orotracheal intubation must be aware of the immediate complications that may occur. These complications include bronchospasm, aspiration during the intubation procedure, apnea secondary to respiratory inhibition, injury to the teeth, and lacerations of the oral mucosa. Failure to intubate immediately creates an emergency situation because of the muscle relaxants used with the procedure. A manual resuscitation bag

Table 19-13

Tracheostomy Care

1. Explain procedure to client.
2. Gather necessary sterile equipment (often available as a prepackaged tracheostomy kit).
   a. Basins
   b. Towel
   c. Forceps
   d. Pipe cleaners
   e. Tracheostomy ties
   f. Brush
   g. Hydrogen peroxide (3% solution)
   h. Sterile saline or water
   i. Suction catheter
   j. Bib
3. Suction and oxygenate client (see Table 19-12).
4. Using aseptic technique, unlock and remove inner cannula.*
5. Immerse inner cannula in hydrogen peroxide (H_2O_2) and clean inside with brush.
6. Drain H_2O_2 off the cannula and then immerse it in sterile water or saline. (Do not dry it, just shake off excess fluid.)
7. Insert the inner cannula into the outer cannula with the curved part down and lock in place.
8. Clean around the tracheostomy opening with H_2O_2 using applicators or 4× 4 dressings. Then apply antiseptic solution (e.g., Betadine).
9. Change the tracheostomy bib or especially slit 4 × 4 dressing underneath the tracheostomy. (Regular 4 × 4 dressing should not be cut to achieve this purpose because frayed threads will be created.)
10. Change the tracheostomy ties.† Two twill tapes (about 41 cm or 16 inches in length) should have slits cut in one end (Fig. 19-5) about 1 inch from the end. The slit end is put into the opening of the outer cannula and a loop is made with the other end of the tape. The tapes are tied together with a double knot on the side of the neck. The tie should be loose enough to allow fingertips to be inserted under the tapes.

*Many synthetic tubes do not have inner cannulas. Tracheostomy care for these tubes includes everything mentioned in the table except for inner cannula care.

†The tapes should not be changed in the first 24 h postoperatively.

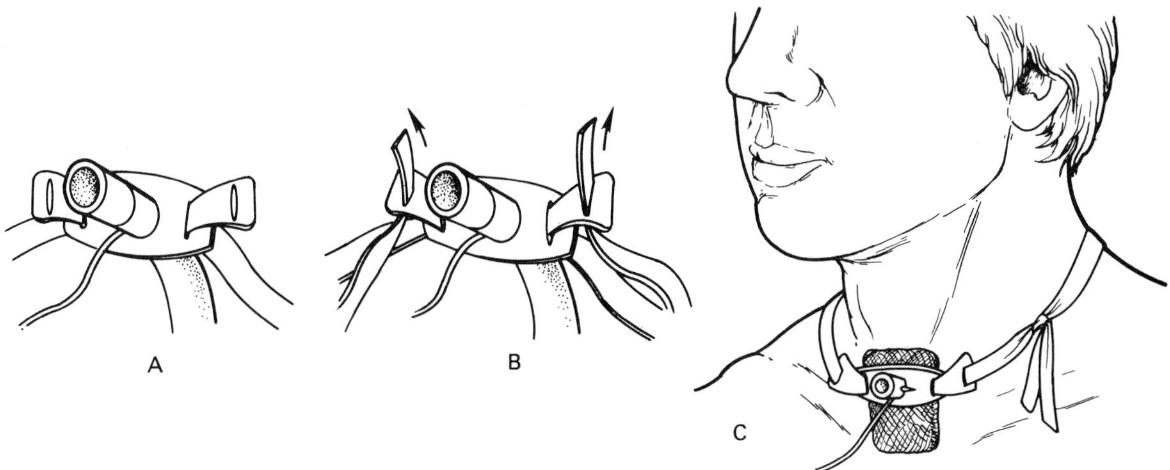

Figure 19-5 Changing tracheostomy ties. *(a)* A slit should be cut about 1 inch from the end. The slit end is put into the opening of the cannula. *(b)* A loop is made with the other end of the tape. *(c)* The tapes are tied together with a double knot on the side of the neck.

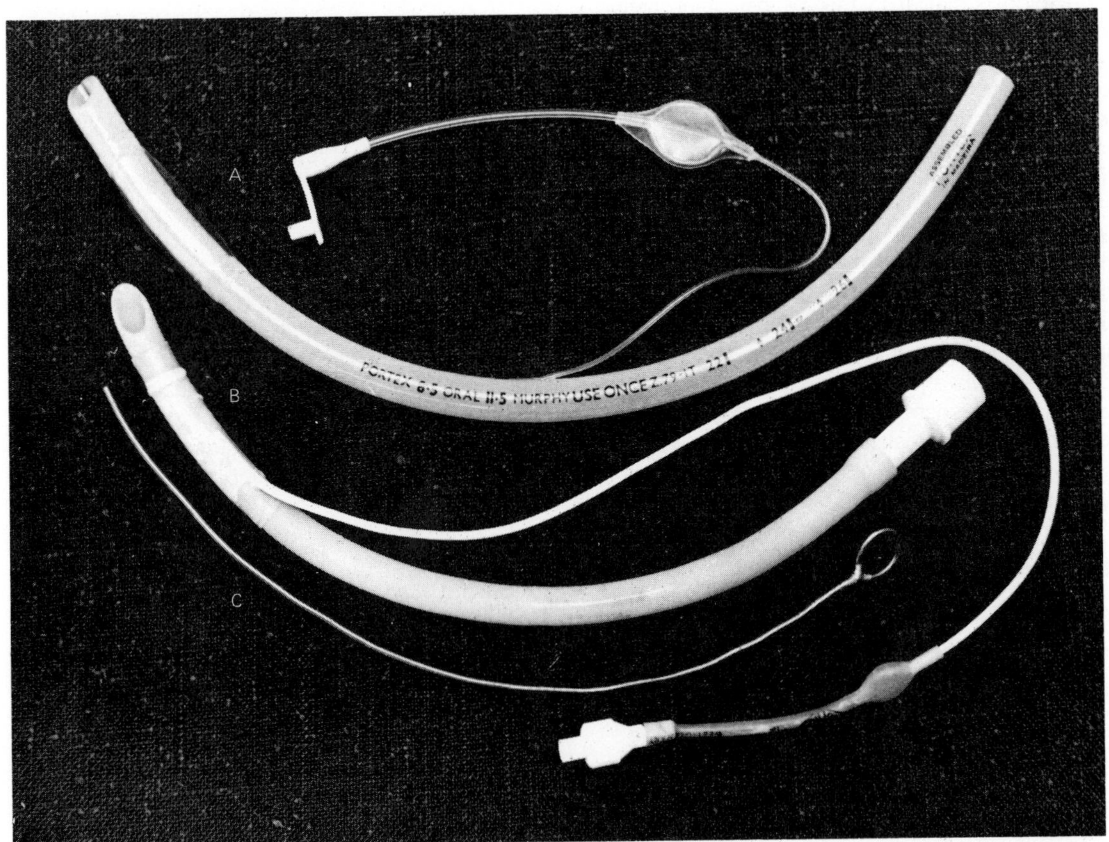

Figure 19-6 Endotrachael tubes. Note the two types of cuffs, (*a*) and (*b*), and the obturator (*c*). *(From H. Moidel et al., Nursing Care of the Patient with Medical-Surgical Disorders, 2d ed., McGraw-Hill Book Company, New York, 1976, p. 497.)*

and mask connected to 100% oxygen should be available for use in the event of an emergency.

Nasotracheal intubation

Some clinicians advocate *nasotracheal intubation* (1) when long-term intubation is necessary, (2) for those clients who cannot tolerate an oral tube, and (3) when jaw fracture or trismus are present. Nasal tubes are contraindicated when clients have sinusitis or a nasal obstruction such as a fractured nose.

Disadvantages of nasotracheal intubation include (1) bleeding following removal of the tube, (2) development of pressure necrosis of the nasal mucosa, (3) maxillary sinusitis, (4) difficulty in weaning from a mechanical ventilator, and (5) difficulty in suctioning since the nasotracheal tube has a smaller lumen than the orotracheal tube. Nasotracheal intubation may be more traumatic than orotracheal intubation and is not commonly used.

Nursing management

The nursing management of clients with endotracheal intubation is similar to that of the client with tracheotomy, which is described in Table 19-11. Special instructions include (1) auscultation for bilateral breath sounds, (2) alternating the placement of the oral tube from side to side to prevent pressure necrosis, and (3) careful observation for extubation.

The client is extubated when ventilation measurements, arterial blood gases, and clinical judgment indicate that the client can maintain a patent airway. After the procedure is explained to the client, the endotracheal tube is suctioned. The client is placed in a sitting position, and the cuff is deflated. Oxygen is administered and the tube is withdrawn. Oxygen is then administered via a face mask. The nurse should observe for laryngospasm, hemorrhage, and signs of laryngeal edema. If extubation is not possible within 10–14 days of endotracheal intubation, a tracheostomy is often performed.

Cancer of the Larynx

Oral cancer strikes approximately 26,000 persons in the United States each year and accounts for about 3 percent of all cancers that occur annually in the nation. About 28 percent of oral cancers are pharyngeal in origin. Over 9000 new cases of cancer of the larynx occurred in 1980 with an estimated 4000 deaths.[17] Early detection of laryngeal cancer is essential to increase cure rates, enhance the quality of survival, diminish complications, reduce functional disabilities, and simplify rehabilitation.[18]

Cancer of the larynx is closely related to the personal habits of our society, primarily alcohol consumption and cigarette smoking. Males in middle or later life are most commonly affected. Other factors increasing the risk are heavy use of tobacco and alcohol and frequent exposure to pollutants and irritants. Since cigarette smoking has increased in women, it is likely that there will also be an increased incidence of laryngeal cancer in women.

The majority of laryngeal malignancies (95 percent) are squamous cell carcinomas. Adenocarcinoma and sarcoma also occur. Squamous cell carcinomas are usually well differentiated and grow slowly. They remain superficial for prolonged periods, but when they infiltrate, extension is rapid. While there is no evidence that alcohol per se is carcinogenic, it has been suggested that alcohol may aid in the absorption of tobacco carcinogens, irritate tissues, or make squamous cells more susceptible to conversion to cancer cells.[19] Heavy alcohol intake may also contribute to nutritional deficiencies. Other agents such as heavy metals irritate the larynx and may lead to histologic changes.

Types of cancers and clinical manifestations

Supraglottic Cancer Supraglottic, or extrinsic laryngeal cancer, is a serious threat to both voice and life. Supraglottic structures include the epiglottis, false cords, and medial aryepiglottic fold. This cancer is likely to be subtle in symptomatology and is often in the advanced stage when first recognized. There is often no warning since the cancer does not impinge on the true vocal cords and cause voice changes. Since the epiglottis is in the midline and the lymphatic drainage is rich, both sides of the neck are threatened with metastasis. There may be *no early warning* symptoms. Early clinical manifestations may include localized throat pain, vague neck and throat discomfort, or a lump in the neck. Late manifestations include glottic hoarseness, vocal cord fixation by extension of the tumor, pain, blood-tinged sputum, or frank hemoptysis.

Glottic Cancer Glottic (intrinsic or true vocal cord) cancer is the most frequently occurring laryngeal cancer. Since this cancer impinges on the true vocal cords, hoarseness is an early symptom. Unfortunately, many clients do not consult physicians early enough, and the diagnosis is delayed. Hoarseness lasting in excess of 2 weeks should be evaluated by a physician. Dyspnea is a late symptom.

Subglottic Cancer Subglottic cancers are tumors that arise in the area that extends from below the vocal cords to the lower border of the cricoid cartilage. Less than 2 percent of cancers of the larynx originate below the vocal cords.

The TNM (Tumor, Nodes, Metastasis) system recommended by the American Joint Committee on Cancer Staging and End Results Reporting is most often utilized for the classification and staging of laryngeal cancer (the TNM system is explained in Chap. 11). This is important for both choice of treatment and accurate prognostic predictions.[20]

Diagnostic study abnormalities

Diagnosis is based on the client's history, physical examination, direct or indirect laryngoscopy, and biopsy of the laryngeal mass. Radiologic examination of the lesion is a valuable adjunct to clinical and endoscopic examinations. Currently employed methods are lateral soft tissue films of the neck, frontal tomography of the larynx, barium swallow, and contrast laryngography. Evidence of a tumor mass includes thickening or deformity of the involved structures, irregularity of the mucous membrane, and fixation of normally mobile laryngeal structures. Computerized tomography (CT) offers a quick, noninvasive, three-dimensional display of the larynx. CT provides information that augments or reinforces the clinical examination. Neoplastic tissue is identifiable because it contains tissue of greater density and/or because it distorts, displaces, or destroys normal anatomic structures.[21]

Medical management

Treatment of laryngeal cancer is accomplished through surgical removal of the tumor, irradiation, and chemotherapy. In many cases, treatments may be only palliative (Table 19-14).

Surgery *Partial laryngectomy* or *laryngofissure* is performed when the client has an early lesion confined to one cord or to the anterior part of the larynx. The amount of tissue removed depends on the extent of the disease. Usually, one true vocal cord is removed. The client retains his voice and normal airway capacities. There is usually no swallowing problem. If the client is a candidate for this procedure, a high cure rate is expected.

Supraglottic laryngectomy, used in certain extrinsic tumors, involves removal of the hyoid bone, epiglottis, and false vocal cords. The true vocal cords and trachea are left intact. Usually, a radical neck dissection is done on the involved side. The great advantage of this procedure is that it preserves the voice.

Hemilaryngectomy (or vertical laryngectomy) involves removal of one true vocal cord, one false cord, and one-half of the thyroid cartilage. The person has a hoarse but usable voice and a normal airway.

Table 19-14
Medical Management: Cancer of the Larynx

Diagnostic
1. History and physical examination
2. Indirect laryngoscopy
3. Direct laryngoscopy
4. Biopsy
5. Contrast laryngography
6. Computerized tomography

Therapeutic
1. Laryngectomy: partial or complete
2. Irradiation
3. Chemotherapy
4. Speech rehabilitation

Total laryngectomy is done when the client has far advanced lesions. It is contraindicated in clients who have nonresectable local tumors and/or distant metastasis. The entire larynx is removed along with the hyoid bone, preepiglottic space, strap muscles, and one or two tracheal rings (Fig. 19-7). The client is left with a permanent tracheostomy and without a normal voice.

Radical neck dissection frequently accompanies supraglottic and total laryngectomy. Radical neck dissection removes nonvital neck structures, cervical lymph nodes on the side of the tumor, and muscle and vessels that may contain tumor tissue. See Chap. 32 for a further discussion of this procedure and related nursing management.

The *carbon dioxide laser* is becoming an instrument commonly used in laryngeal surgery. It has the advantages of accuracy, cost effectiveness, and minimal morbidity. The laser has been used for diagnosis, tumor reduction prior to definitive treatment, and as a curative tool in supraglottic laryngectomy.[22]

Complications of total or conservative laryngectomy may be severe and often life-threatening. The client is subjected to further complications when radical neck dissection is performed concurrently (Table 19-15).

Irradiation Irradiation therapy is effective in certain cases. However, there is only a narrow dose range that will offer a good cure rate and little tissue damage. The best results occur in clients with early carcinomas involving one cord, without cord fixation, or with extralaryngeal extension. The advantage of irradiation therapy is the retention of the voice. The major problem associated with radiotherapy is the destruction of healthy as well as tumor tissue.

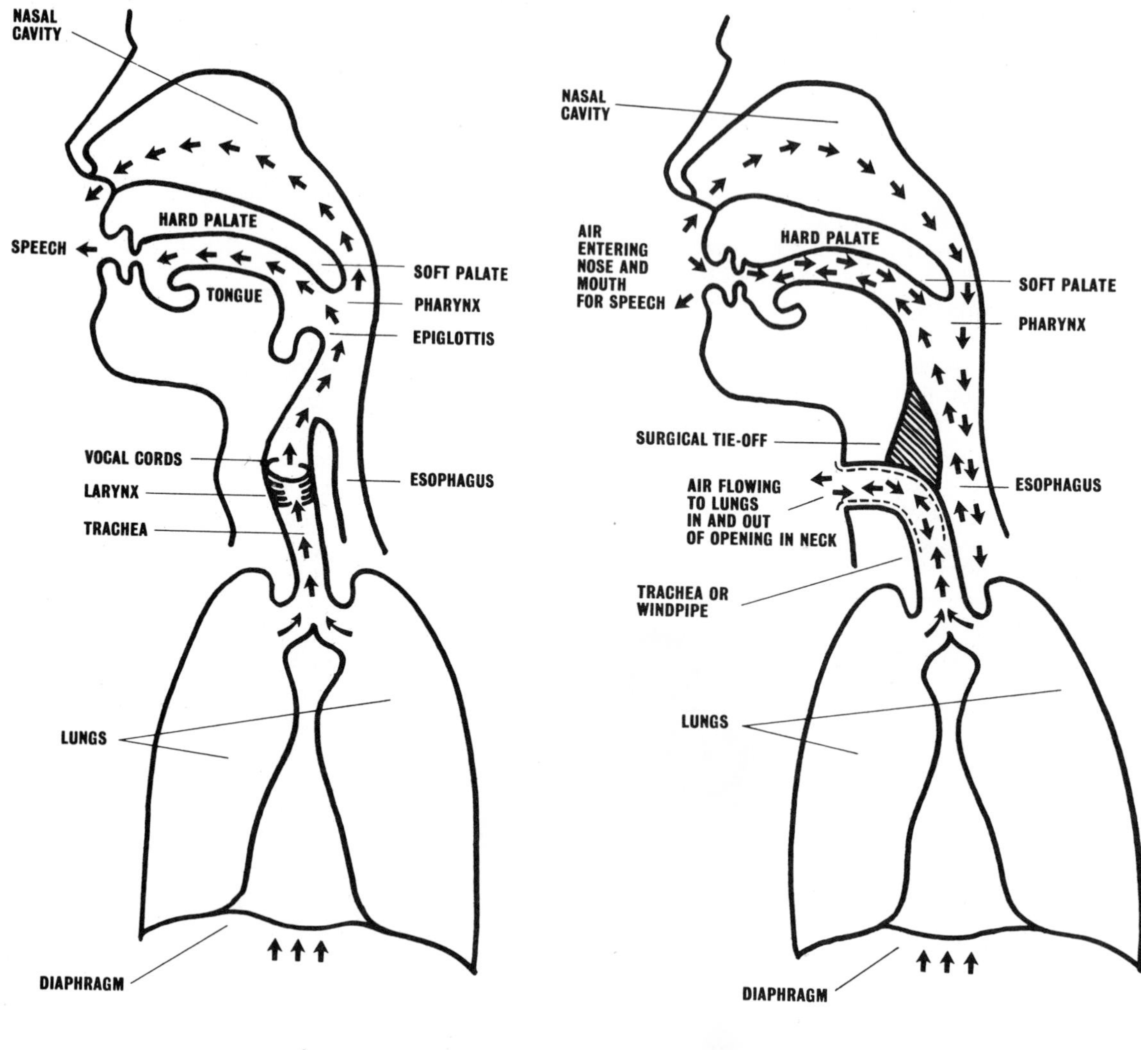

Figure 19-7 (*a*) Physiology of the head and neck before total laryngectomy. (*b*) Physiology of the head and neck after total laryngectomy. *(From the American Cancer Society.)*

Combination of Surgery and Irradiation When used in combination with surgery, irradiation can be given either before or after the operation. The advantages of preoperative irradiation are that it decreases tumor volume, eradicates unsuspected microscopic mucosal extensions of the tumor, reduces iatrogenic dissemination of tumor cells during surgery, and helps to abolish tumor recurrences since viable cells will not seed into the surgical wounds. The disadvantages of preoperative irradiation are primarily time related. Surgery must be delayed for 6 weeks following irradiation. Surgery on an irradiated area also increases operative complications and morbidity. When preoperative irradiation is performed, the client is more prone to postoperative complications of fistula formation, dehiscence, and carotid artery necrosis. The disadvantages of postoperative irradiation include a decreased vascular supply in the area (resulting from surgery) and the need to irradiate a large field due to tissue manipulation during the operative procedure.

Table 19-15
Complications of Laryngectomy and Radical Neck Dissection

Procedure	Complication	Rationale
Laryngectomy	Carotid artery rupture	Occurs due to preoperative irradiation and fistula formation.
	Fistula formation	Occurs when hypopharynx is reconstructed to the skin and lymph channels are interrupted. Healing is delayed.
	Tracheostomy stenosis	Occurs when tracheostomy becomes too small to function.
Radical neck dissection	Pneumothorax	Occurs due to injury to the apex of the pleural reflection at the root of the neck.
	Facial edema	Occurs due to interruption of the lymphatic vessels, surgical trauma, and excision of the jugular system of veins.
	Iatrogenic nerve injury	Occurs due to surgical incising of hypoglossal, glossopharyngeal, phrenic, vagus, and spinal accessory nerves.
	Infection	Occurs due to entering of oral cavity and postoperative hematoma or seroma formation under skin flap.
	Skin flap necrosis	Occurs due to decreased blood supply and irradiation.

Palliative Treatment Uncontrolled metastatic cancer of the larynx is often painful, leaving the individual in a severely debilitated state. When a lesion with disabling metastasis becomes ulcerated, fungated, or infected, the ulcer will be removed surgically. If there is no fungation, chemotherapeutic drugs and palliative radiotherapy may be employed.

Rehabilitative Surgery One of the major problems that the client must cope with is voice loss following total laryngectomy. A number of surgical reconstructive procedures have been developed and are being refined. One such procedure provides serviceable speech through the construction of a subcutaneous skin-lined tube sutured to the hypopharynx and trachea. The client occludes the tracheostomy with the thumb, directs air upward through the subcutaneous tube into the pharynx, and speaks. Retrograde aspiration of liquids may be a problem following this procedure.[23]

Nursing management

Health Promotion and Maintenance One of the nursing responsibilities is identification of groups at risk for developing laryngeal cancer. Smokers, persons who consume large amounts of alcohol, and particularly middle-aged males who both smoke and drink may be referred to "I Quit Smoking" clinics, Alcoholics Anonymous, dental clinics, and family physicians. As a health educator, the nurse should instruct clients in the warning signs of cancer (see Chap. 11) and in methods of early detection such as oral screening programs or routine physical examination. As a counselor, the nurse should understand the reluctance of some individuals to seek health care. Stimulating the client's accountability and motivation to practice preventive health care is often challenging for the nurse.

Preoperative Management Head and neck cancer surgery is anxiety-provoking, traumatizing, and frightening to the client and his family. The client and family need to deal with the psychological impact of the diagnosis of cancer in addition to possible altered modes of communication and changes in body image. It is vital to implement a consistent team approach as well as to include the client and family in all aspects of care. The physician, nurse, speech pathologist, social worker, and clergy should be aware of the psychological ramifications of the voice impairment or loss, potential disfigurement, and distorted body image that the client and family will face. Assessment of the client's past coping mechanisms as well as his knowledge and understanding of the surgery are integral to the plan of care.

The client should be thoroughly prepared in the following areas prior to surgery:[24]

1. What to expect immediately after surgery

2. Physical changes that will occur (e.g., tracheostomy)
3. Surgical procedure
4. Causes, nature, and treatment of laryngeal cancer
5. Methods of laryngeal speech and speech pathology
6. Sources of community help
7. Changes in lifestyle
8. Emotional adjustments to be anticipated by the client and family

The client should be acquainted with equipment that will likely be used, such as the tracheostomy tube, nasogastric tube, laryngectomy tube, and suction apparatus. The nurse should encourage the client to ask questions and express anxieties. It may be beneficial to the client if alternate methods of communication, such as writing and a communication board, are discussed prior to the surgery.

Laryngectomized clients experience high degrees of depression, frustration, and suicide. A large number (15 to 50 percent) fail to develop alaryngeal speech or never return to full-time employment postoperatively.[25] When asked, many clients and families state that they were inadequately prepared prior to the operative experience. The nurse should work to ensure that the client and family take an active role in preoperative and postoperative planning.

The client may benefit from the preoperative visit of a laryngectomized volunteer from the Lost Chord Club. The nurse must assess the client's ability to discuss with another laryngectomee the changes that will soon take place.

Postoperative Management (Table 19-16)

When *laryngofissure* has been performed, a temporary tracheostomy tube will be in place. Nasogastric tube feedings and intravenous therapy will be instituted. (The nasogastric tube is usually inserted at the time of surgery.) Oral feedings are usually started on the first postoperative day if tolerated by the client. Whispering is permitted about the third or fourth postoperative day, followed by gradual use of the voice.

When *total laryngectomy* is performed, the client will have a laryngectomy tube in place (Fig. 19-8). The laryngectomy tube functions as a tracheostomy tube but is wider and shorter. The nurse must ensure tube

Table 19-16
Nursing Care Plan for a Client with a Laryngectomy

Client Problem	Expected Outcome	Nursing Intervention
	Preoperative Management	
Impending surgery **Fear of the unknown**	Successful adaptation following surgical procedure. Alleviation of fears.	Explain policies and expected procedures following surgery: recovery room, suctioning, humidification, coughing and deep breathing, intravenous fluids, tube feedings. Answer questions. Encourage client to talk of fears and hopes following surgery. Prepare client for probable change in appearance.
Change in oral communication pattern	Successful modification of communication pattern.	Assess client's hearing and writing ability. Orient the client to anticipated change in the mode of communication when indicated. Demonstrate use of magic slate or communication board. Arrange for interpreters if client is non-English-speaking. Demonstrate use of artificial larynx and laryngeal speech.
	Postoperative Management	
Altered communication pattern **Inability to speak**	Adaptation to altered communication pattern.	Provide client with paper and pencil or magic slate. Destroy written notes to protect client's privacy. Observe client's nonverbal behavior. Provide a call bell or light. Allow client to ask questions. Do not anticipate answers. Avoid starting intravenous infusion in client's writing arm. Arrange for a volunteer laryngectomee to meet with client to demonstrate esophageal or artificial speech. Provide client with information regarding the Lost Chord Club and IAL.

Table 19-16 (Contined)

Potential obstructed airway	No cyanosis. Normal respiratory rate.	Observe for patent airway. Maintain head of bed in semi-Fowler's position unless contraindicated. Instruct client to cough and deep-breathe. Suction and clean tracheostomy tubes prn. Assess lungs through percussion and aucultation q 4 h. Provide humidification. Assess functioning of tracheostomy-laryngectomy tube and seal. Increase hydration to liquefy secretions. Suction the nose with a nasal catheter since laryngectomee is unable to blow nose.
Pain	Minimal or no pain.	Elevate head of bed. Teach client to move head by supporting back of neck with hands each time it is necessary to lift or turn head. Administer analgesics as needed.
Potential hemorrhage	Stable vital signs.	Assess vital signs. Observe for signs of excess bleeding (amount and character of Hemovac secretions, edema at surgical site, tachycardia, hypotension, restlessness). Notify physician if evident. Client should be placed on hemorrhage precautions if local radiation has preceded the surgery.
Potential infection	Normal WBC. Normal body temperature.	Monitor T q 4 h. Encourage fluid intake via tube feedings or orally if indicated. Maintain aseptic technique when suctioning. Clean tracheostomy tube q 8 h with peroxide and saline. Change tube tapes prn. Use aseptic technique when changing dressing at suture line. Observe for signs of inflammation. Monitor Hemovac for color and character of drainage. Administer antibiotics as ordered. Provide frequent oral hygiene through irrigation and power spray.
Inability to swallow **Poor nutritional state**	Successful adaptation to temporary tube feedings. Nutritional balance.	Institute tube feedings as ordered. Progress from water to formula as ordered. Encourage additional liquids such as coffee, tea, and carbonated beverages to increase client's morale and improve hydration. Encourage client to feed himself. (Tube feeding is discussed in Chap. 33.)
Fear of injuring stoma	Confidence in ability to care for self.	See Table 19-17.
Difficulty in communicating	Successful adaptation to alternate methods of speech.	The client should be referred to a speech therapy center where training will begin when the operative area is healed. Esophageal speech or artificial devices may be demonstrated by the therapist or a volunteer member of the Lost Chord Club.
Depression and embarrassment regarding altered appearance	Recognition that feelings are normal.	Refer the client and significant others to support services available following discharge, e.g., social services, clinics, speech therapists, volunteer organizations such as IAL. Encourage grooming, personal hygiene, and wearing of attractive clothing.

patency in much the same way as with a tracheostomy tube. The permanent laryngectomy fistula forms within 3 to 6 weeks. Liquid feedings are given via a nasogastric tube on the first postoperative day. Oral feedings may begin around the eighth postoperative day, when the suture line has healed. The client should be instructed to burp following feedings. The burping mechanism paves the way for esophageal speech.

When a *radical neck dissection* accompanies laryngectomy, the client will have wound suction (e.g., via Hemovac) and/or a pressure dressing. The head of the bed should be elevated since the bulky dressing may interfere with respirations. The client should be observed for any manifestations of hemorrhage. Carotid artery rupture is an uncommon complication following irradiation and radical neck dissection.

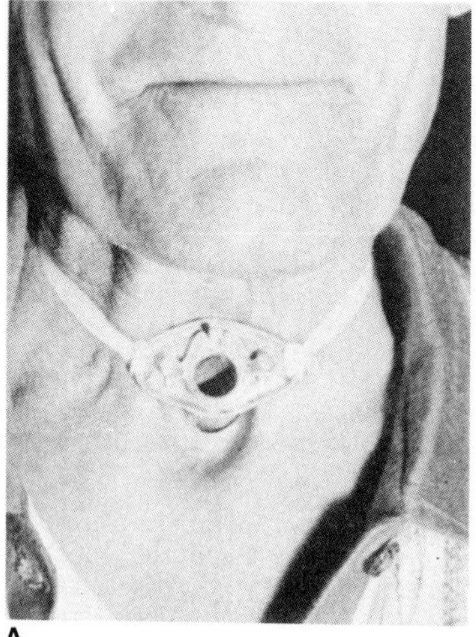
A

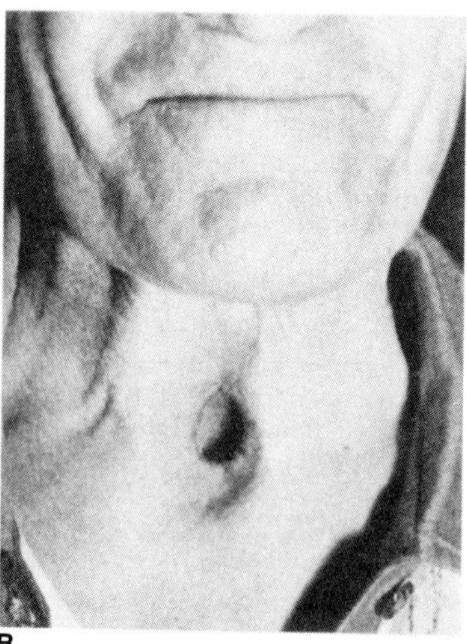
B

Figure 19-8 (*a*) Client with a laryngectomy tube in place. (*b*) Client with a permanent stoma. *(From First Aid for Laryngectomees, American Cancer Society, New York.)*

Many laryngectomees are elderly and debilitated, with a history of tobacco and alcohol abuse. Preoperative nutritional deficiency and stress lead to generalized catabolism postoperatively. Therefore, parenteral hyperalimentation may be utilized for a period of time postoperatively. The nutritional status generally improves within 14 to 21 days with this therapy.[26]

Rehabilitative management

Rehabilitation begins as soon as the client is admitted to the hospital. A speech therapist or speech pathologist should meet with the client to discuss alaryngeal speech. A laryngectomee volunteer should visit with the client either preoperatively or postoperatively to demonstrate esophageal speech or speech with the artificial larynx. Esophageal speech training is available through speech clinics and therapists. Esophageal speech utilizes burping that exerts pressure against the folds of the esophagus and produces a vibration. For those clients who cannot master this form of speech, an artificial larynx is available through the American Cancer Society or the telephone company.

Prior to discharge, the client should be instructed in the care of the laryngectomy stoma. The area around the stoma should be washed daily with a moist cloth and kept moist with petroleum jelly. If dried secretions form around the stoma, they may be removed with tweezers. To shield and filter the stoma, a metal, crocheted, or plastic stoma shield can be applied. The client should cover the stoma with a loose dressing or the hand when coughing, since mucus will be expectorated. Suggest to the client alternate methods of humidifying the air, such as placing pans of water around the house, using a humidifier, running a hot shower, or simply growing houseplants. Decrease clients' self-consciousness about their physical appearance by advising the use of a shirt, tie, or scarf or the wearing of jewelry. The client should be informed of the importance of wearing an emblem or tag such as Medic-Alert jewelry that can alert others in an emergency situation of his status as a neck breather (Table 19-17, Fig. 19-9).

Advise the client that swimming is no longer possible. When the client showers or bathes, the stoma should be protected by a shield or wash cloth. The stream of water should be directed below the stoma.

Since the client no longer breathes through his nose, the ability to smell smoke and food may be absent. Advise the client to install smoke detectors in the home. It is important for food to be colorful, prepared attractively, and nutritious since taste may also be diminished.

The client can resume exercise, recreation, and sex when he is able. Most laryngectomized clients can return to work 1 to 2 months following surgery. However, as many as 50 percent never return to full-time employment. The changes that follow laryngectomy are upsetting. Loss of speech, loss of the ability to taste and smell, the inability to produce audible sounds including laughing and weeping, and the presence of a permanent tracheal stoma that produces undesirable mucus are often overwhelming to the client and family. It is essential for the nurse to support the client's coping mechanisms and provide information regarding community resources. Organizations such as the New Voice Club and the Lost Chord Club of the International Association of Laryngectomees (IAL) provide vital support, counseling, and assistance in locating needed supplies.

Table 19-17
Teaching Self-Care to the Client with a Laryngectomy

	Client Education
Stoma guards	Demonstrate types of guards available, e.g., metal, plastic, nylon bibs. The stoma may also be covered with a light scarf, blouse, or shirt for cosmetic purposes and to prevent foreign bodies from entering.
Stoma care	Instruct the client to prevent cracking of the skin around the stoma by applying water-soluble lubricants or mineral or baby oil for 10 min daily.
Mouth care	Crusting of the tongue and halitosis can be controlled by brushing the tongue with a soft toothbrush and using oral astringents.
Humidification	Provide a vaporizer or room humidifier. Taking a tub bath or shower will increase the humidity. Instruct client to protect the stoma with a towel or shield to prevent water from entering the stoma while bathing. The shower nozzle should be directed well below the level of the stoma.
Precautions	Laryngectomized men should be cautioned about the use of razors when shaving since the area will be numb for approximately 6 mo. Guard against having shaving cream enter the stoma by recommending a nonaerosal type of cream. The client should be warned not to swim.
Emergency care	The client should be instructed to wear a Medic-Alert tag stating that he is a neck breather (Fig. 19-9).
Coughing	Instruct the client to lean forward to expel secretions and to cover the stoma when sneezing or coughing.

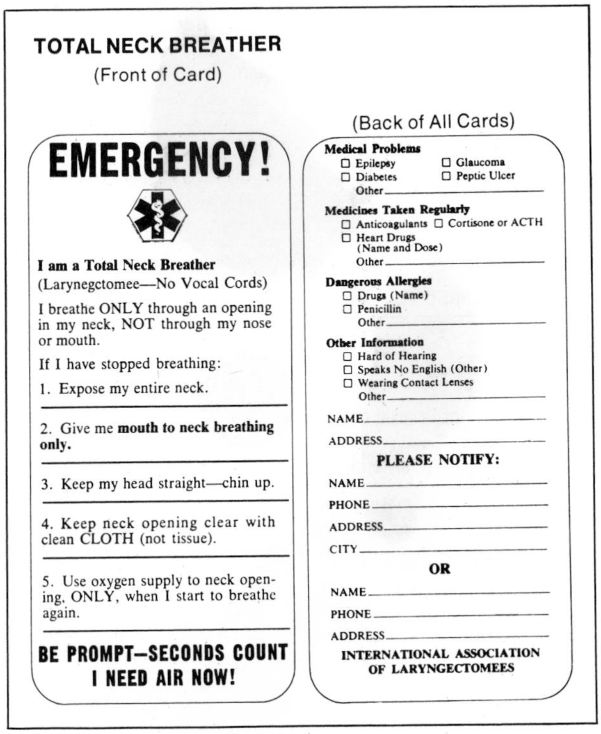

TOTAL NECK BREATHER
(Front of Card)

EMERGENCY!

I am a Total Neck Breather
(Larynegctomee—No Vocal Cords)

I breathe ONLY through an opening in my neck, NOT through my nose or mouth.

If I have stopped breathing:

1. Expose my entire neck.
2. Give me **mouth to neck breathing only.**
3. Keep my head straight—chin up.
4. Keep neck opening clear with clean CLOTH (not tissue).
5. Use oxygen supply to neck opening, ONLY, when I start to breathe again.

BE PROMPT—SECONDS COUNT
I NEED AIR NOW!

(Back of All Cards)

Medical Problems
☐ Epilepsy ☐ Glaucoma
☐ Diabetes ☐ Peptic Ulcer
Other ____

Medicines Taken Regularly
☐ Anticoagulants ☐ Cortisone or ACTH
☐ Heart Drugs (Name and Dose)
Other ____

Dangerous Allergies
☐ Drugs (Name)
☐ Penicillin
Other ____

Other Information
☐ Hard of Hearing
☐ Speaks No English (Other)
☐ Wearing Contact Lenses
Other ____

NAME ____
ADDRESS ____

PLEASE NOTIFY:

NAME ____
PHONE ____
ADDRESS ____
CITY ____

OR

NAME ____
PHONE ____
ADDRESS ____

INTERNATIONAL ASSOCIATION OF LARYNGECTOMEES

Figure 19-9 Emergency identification of a neck breather.

Laryngeal Edema

Acute laryngeal edema may occur as a result of anaphylaxis, inflammation, or injury. Hoarseness and dyspnea are the major symptoms. Dyspnea is ominous. The airway must be immediately restored by endotracheal intubation or tracheostomy. When anaphylaxis is the cause, epinephrine 1:1000 subcutaneously, adrenal corticosteroids, and ice collars may be used.

Chronic laryngeal edema may result from tumors of the neck and infections that obstruct lymph drainage. Intubation or tracheostomy may be necessary to restore a patent airway.

Laryngeal Spasm

Laryngeal spasm of muscle tissue may occur following the use of some general anesthetics. Tetany, occurring in clients with low blood calcium levels, also causes laryngeal spasm. Calcium chloride or calcium gluconate is given intravenously to elevate calcium levels and relieve tetany-induced laryngeal spasm.

Acute Laryngitis

Acute laryngitis is inflammation of the larynx due to a number of causes. The disorder most often occurs due to local infection of parainfluenza virus. Other etiologic factors are overuse of the voice and exposure to irritating inhalants and combustion products from fire. A serious complication of laryngitis is subglottic edema.

The primary clinical manifestations are acute hoarseness, dysphagia, dry cough, pain aggravated by talking, and tenacious sputum. Complete loss of voice may occur. The diagnosis is determined by the laryngeal examination, which should differentiate between tumor growth and laryngitis. An x-ray of the neck may be done to detect subglottic edema.

Supportive medical and nursing interventions include steam inhalations, topical anesthetic throat lozenges for the cough, voice rest, and discontinuance of smoking. Bronchodilators and antibiotic therapy may be indicated in some cases. In severe cases of accompanying glottic edema, tracheostomy may be indicated.[27]

Case Study / Cancer of the Larynx

Mr. W., an outgoing 64-year-old widower, had been complaining of sore throats with persistent hoarseness for the last 2 months. Following consultation with his primary physician, he was admitted to the hospital for laryngoscopy. The biopsy report revealed squamous cell carcinoma involving both vocal cords. He agreed to have a total laryngectomy performed.

Following total laryngectomy, Mr. W. returned to his room with a Hemovac in place, a laryngectomy tube, and a nasogastric tube. His vital signs were stable. The head of the bed was elevated, and he complained of little pain.

Discussion Questions

1. What are the etiologic factors related to cancer of the larynx?
2. What are the clinical manifestations of laryngeal cancer? What causes the hoarseness?
3. What preoperative needs should the nurse be aware of?
4. What are the nursing interventions in the immediate postoperative period?
5. When is the ideal time to begin vocal rehabilitation? How is it done?
6. Describe the predischarge rehabilitative teaching that the nurse does. What precautions should the laryngectomee take?

REVIEW QUESTIONS

The number of the question corresponds to the same numbered objective at the beginning of the chapter.

1. "Rebound nasal congestion" or rhinitis medicamentosa is the result of
   a. antigen-antibody interaction
   b. prolonged overuse of vasoconstrictor agents
   c. frequent nasal infections
   d. resistant sinusitis

2. A severe complication of acute sinusitis which necessitates immediate reporting to the physician is
   a. adenoiditis
   b. increased intracranial pressure
   c. pain
   d. purulent nasal discharge

3. Influenza vaccination may *not* be recommended when the client is
   a. a diabetic
   b. elderly
   c. sensitive to egg proteins
   d. taking immunosuppressive drugs

4. Tracheal-esophageal fistula, tracheal stenosis, and ulceration are most likely to occur as a complication of
   a. orotracheal intubation
   b. laryngectomy
   c. tracheostomy
   d. nasotracheal intubation

5. Suctioning the client with an endotracheal tube is most often performed
   a. every 30 minutes
   b. when the lungs sound moist to auscultation
   c. utilizing a clean technique
   d. when the cuff is deflated

6. Which of the following would not be a clinical manifestation of laryngeal cancer?
   a. hoarseness
   b. dyspnea
   c. dysphagia
   d. fever

7. Which of the following alterations would be caused by a laryngofissure (partial laryngectomy)?
   a. no significant alterations would be anticipated
   b. loss of neck muscle tissue
   c. permanent hoarse, low voice
   d. difficulty in swallowing

8. Which of the following nursing interventions is inappropriate when managing a client with speech loss following laryngectomy?
   a. providing the client with writing implements
   b. providing a light or call bell
   c. introducing the client to a Lost Chord Club member
   d. anticipating answers to decrease the client's need to communicate

REFERENCES

1. D. D. DeWeese and W. H. Saunders, *Textbook of Otolaryngology,* The C. V. Mosby Company, St. Louis, 1977, p. 210.
2. M. J. Dropkin, "Compliance in Post Operative Head and Neck Patients," *Cancer Nurs,* **10:**379 (1979).
3. DeWeese and Saunders, op. cit., p. 205.
4. D. L. D'Acuti, "Eyes, Ears, Nose Emergencies," *J Emerg Nurs,* **1:**24 (1975).
5. M. Wiener et al., *Clinical Pharmacology and Therapeutics in Nursing,* McGraw-Hill Book Company, New York, 1979, p. 197.
6. P. Beeson et al., *Cecil Textbook of Medicine,* W. B. Saunders Company, Philadelphia, 1979, p. 229.
7. R. Hutchinson, "The Common Cold Primer," *Nurs 79,* **9:**58 (1979).
8. "Influenza Vaccine," *Ann Intern Med,* **89:**657 (1978).
9. V. Passey et al., "Foreign Bodies in the Throat, Nose and Ear," *Hosp Med,* **13:**17 (1977).
10. DeWeese and Saunders, op. cit., p. 71.
11. S. T. Westerman, "Clinical Experience with Cryosurgical Tonsillectomy," *EENT* **59:**48 (1980).
12. P. A. Selecky, "Tracheostomy: A Review of Present Day Indications," *Heart Lung,* **3:**272 (1974).
13. P. A. Selecky, "Tracheal Damage and Prolonged Intubation with a Cuffed Endotracheal or Tracheostomy Tube," *Heart Lung,* **5:**733 (1976).
14. M. Morrison et al., *Respiratory Intensive Care Nursing,* Little, Brown and Company, Boston, 1979, p. 198.
15. Morrison, op. cit., p. 93.
16. D. Greenbaum, "Decannulation of the Tracheotomized Patient," *Heart Lung,* **5:**122 (1976).
17. "Cancer Facts and Figures 1980," American Cancer Society, New York, 1979, p. 19.
18. *Nursing Inservice Education Programs on Cancer of the Head and Neck,* American Cancer Society, New York, 1979, p. 3.
19. P. Rubin et al., *Current Concepts in Cancer Multidisciplinary Views,* American Cancer Society, New York, 1972, p. 3.
20. G. M. English, *Otolaryngology,* Harper & Row, Publishers, Incorporated, Hagerstown, Md., 1976, p. 533.
21. S. Sagel et al., "High Resolution Computed Tomography in the Staging of Carcinoma of the Larynx," *Laryngoscope,* **91:**292 (1981).
22. C. W. Vaugh et al., "Laryngeal Carcinoma: Transoral Treatment Utilizing the Transoral Laser," *Am J Surg,* **136:**490 (1978).
23. DeWeese and Saunders, op. cit., p. 136.
24. R. Keith et al., "Presurgical Counseling Needs of Laryngectomees: A Survey of 78 Patients," *Laryngoscope,* **88:**1660 (1978).
25. J. Johnson et al., "Toward the Total Rehabilitation of the Alaryngeal Patient," *Laryngoscope,* **89:**1813 (1979).
26. S. Sobol et al., "Enteral and Parenteral Nutrition in Patients with Head and Neck Cancer," *Ann Otol,* **88:**495 (1979).
27. H. A. Lyons, "Guide to Acute Upper Airway Infections," *Hosp Med,* **12:**99 (1976).

Chapter 20

NURSING ROLE IN MANAGEMENT

Lower Respiratory Problems

Sharon Mantik Lewis

Learning Objectives

1. Describe the pathogenesis, types, clinical manifestations, and medical and pharmacological management of pneumonia.
2. Explain the nursing role in management of the client with penumonia.
3. Describe the pathogenesis, classification, clinical manifestations, complications, diagnostic abnormalities, and medical, pharmacological, and nursing management of tuberculosis.
4. Identify the causes of pulmonary fungal infections.
5. Explain the pathophysiology, clinical manifestations, and medical and nursing management of bronchiectasis and lung abscess.
6. Identify the indications for oxygen therapy, methods of delivery, and complications of oxygen administration.
7. Identify the clinical features and management of occupational lung diseases.
8. Describe the etiology, risk factors, pathogenesis, clinical manifestations, and medical and nursing management of lung cancer.
9. Identify the mechanisms involved and the clinical manifestations of pneumothorax, fractured ribs, and flail chest.
10. Describe the purpose, methods, and nursing responsibilities related to chest tubes.
11. Explain the types of chest surgery and appropriate pre- and postoperative care.
12. Compare and contrast extrapulmonary and intrapulmonary restrictive lung disorders in terms of causes, clinical manifestations, and management.
13. Describe the pathophysiology, clinical manifestations, and management of pulmonary hypertension and cor pulmonale.

There is a wide variety of problems affecting the lower respiratory system. Lung diseases which are characterized primarily by an obstructive disorder such as asthma, emphysema, chronic bronchitis, and cystic fibrosis are discussed in Chap. 21. All other lower respiratory problems will be discussed in this chapter.

PULMONARY INFECTIONS

Pulmonary infections annually rank among the top 10 causes of death in the United States. Bacterial pneumonias remain the leading infectious cause of death in spite of the availability of antimicrobial agents.[1] Tuberculosis, although potentially curable and preventable, is still an important public health problem in the United States and worldwide.

Pneumonia

Significance of the problem

Pneumonia, or *pneumonitis,* is an acute inflammation of the lung parenchyma. Until 1936, pneumonia was the leading cause of death in the United States. Then sulfa drugs and penicillin were discovered and used in the treatment of pneumonia. However, in spite of antibiotics, pneumonia is still quite common, and some types of the disease have a very high mortality rate. About 1 percent of the American population develop pneumonia at some time in their lives, and there is about a 10 percent mortality rate.

This chapter was reviewed by Mary V. Hanley, R.N., M.A., CCRN, Assistant Professor, Graduate Medical-Surgical Program, School of Nursing, Boston University, Boston, Massachusetts; and Lela Lottermoser, CRTT, RRT, B.A., formerly Director of Pulmonary Services, University of New Mexico Hospital, Albuquerque, New Mexico.

Pathogenesis of pneumonia

Normal Defense Mechanisms Normally, the airway distal to the larynx is sterile because of protective defense mechanisms. These mechanisms, described in Chap. 18, include:

1. Filtration and humidification of air
2. Warming of inspired air
3. Epiglottis closure over the trachea
4. Cough reflex
5. Mucociliary escalator
6. Secretory immunoglobulin A
7. Alveolar macrophage
8. Serum immunoglobulin G

Factors Predisposing to Pneumonia Pneumonia is more likely to result when the defense mechanisms become incompetent or are overwhelmed by

Table 20-1
Factors Predisposing to Pneumonia

1. Smoking
2. Air pollution
3. Altered consciousness
   - Alcoholism
   - Head injury
   - Seizures
   - Anesthesia
   - Drug overdose
4. Tracheal intubation (endotracheal, tracheotomy)
5. URI infection
6. Chronic diseases
   - Chronic lung disease
   - Diabetes mellitus
   - Heart disease
   - Uremia
   - Cancer
7. Immunosuppressive drugs
   - Corticosteroids
   - Cancer chemotherapy
8. Malnutrition
9. Inhalation or aspiration of noxious substances
10. Debilitating illness
11. Bed rest and prolonged immobility
12. Altered oropharyngeal flora

the virulence or quantity of infectious agents. Factors that may impair defense mechanisms are listed in Table 20-1. Altered consciousness depresses the cough and epiglottis reflexes, which may allow aspiration of oropharyngeal contents into the lungs. Tracheal intubation interferes with the normal cough reflex and the mucociliary escalator mechanism. It also bypasses the upper airways, where filtration and humidification of air normally take place. The mucociliary escalator mechanism is impaired by air pollution, cigarette smoking, viral upper respiratory tract infections (URI), and normal changes of aging. In malnutrition, the formation and activity of lymphocytes and polymorphonuclear leukocytes are altered. Certain diseases, such as leukemia, alcoholism, and diabetes mellitus, are associated with an increased frequency of gram-negative bacilli in the oropharynx.[2] (These organisms are not normal flora.) Altered oropharyngeal flora can also occur secondary to antibiotic therapy given for an infection elsewhere in the body.

Acquisition of Organisms Organisms that cause pneumonia reach the lung by:

1. Aspiration from the nasopharynx or oropharynx. Many of the organisms that cause pneumonia are normal inhabitants of the pharynx in healthy adults.
2. Inhalation of microbes present in the air. Examples include *Mycoplasma pneumoniae* and fungal pneumonias.
3. Hematogenous spread from a primary infection elsewhere in the body.

Types of pneumonia

Pneumonia can be caused by bacteria, viruses, *Mycoplasma,* fungi, *Pneumocystis carinii,* chemicals, dust, gases, and a variety of other factors (Table 20-2).

Gram-Positive Bacterial Pneumonias Gram-positive bacteria (*Streptococcus pneumoniae, Staphylococcus aureus,* and group A beta-hemolytic streptococci) account for most bacterial pneumonias acquired in the community. Recently, *S. aureus* has become an increasingly common cause of nosocomial pneumonia. The most common type of pneumonia is pneumococcal pneumonia caused by *S. pneumoniae.*

Gram-Negative Bacterial Pneumonias There has been an increasing incidence of aerobic gram-negative bacterial pneumonias. They account for 20 percent of community-acquired pneumonias and 40 to 60 percent of hospital-acquired pneumonias.[3] Organisms causing gram-negative pneumonias include *Klebsiella, Pseudomonas, Hemophilus, Serratia, Escherichia coli,* and *Proteus.* Most of these organisms enter the lung following aspiration of particles from the client's own pharynx. Immunosuppressive therapy, general debility, endotracheal intubation, and prolonged antibiotic therapy may be predisposing factors. Respiratory therapy equipment that is not appropriately cleaned is a potential source of infection.

Anaerobic Bacterial Pneumonias Most anaerobic pneumonias are caused by aspiration of oropharyngeal secretions. Infections usually involve multiple organisms, with aerobic organisms found concurrently in many cases of anaerobic pneumonia.

Mycoplasma Pneumonia. Mycoplasma pneumonia is transmitted from person to person by respiratory droplets. Intrafamily or intragroup (e.g., military) spread is common. Mycoplasma pneumonia is usually treated with antibiotics.

Viral Pneumonias About one-half of all pneumonias are caused by viruses, primarily influenza viruses and adenoviruses. The initial manifestations of viral pneumonia are highly variable but are usually similar to those of influenza, including fever, myalgia, headache, and dry cough. On chest x-ray there is usually an interstitial pattern of lung involvement. The x-ray may demonstrate extensive pulmonary involvement, with minimal physical findings on examination. These

Table 20-2
Comparison of Types of Pneumonia

Causative Agent	Characteristics	Clinical Manifestations and Complications
	Gram-Positive Bacterial Pneumonias	
Pneumococcal pneumonia (*Streptococcus pneumoniae*)	Usually preceded by URI Usually involves one or more lobes Incubation period is 1 to 3 days Peak incidence in winter and spring Damages host by overwhelming growth of the organism Does not usually cause necrosis of lung tissue Chest x-ray shows lobar infiltration (Fig. 20-1) Nasopharyngeal carriers Herpes labialis frequently found in association with pneumonia Individuals at risk include those with chronic heart or lung disease, diabetes mellitus, and cirrhosis	Abrupt onset of manifestations Elevated temperature Tachypnea Chills Productive cough (often bloody, rusty, or green) Nausea Vomiting Malaise Myalgia Weakness Pleuritic chest pain Atelectasis Lung abscess (rare) Pleural effusions (frequent) Empyema
Staphylococcal pneumonia (*Staphylococcus aureus*)	Acquired via the hematogenous route or aspiration into the lungs Nasopharyngeal carriers (35–50% of population) Necrotizing infection causing destruction of lung tissue Chest x-ray shows bronchopneumonia (Fig. 20-1) Risk factors include chronic lung disease, leukemia, and other debilitating diseases Often preceded by influenza infection 10–14 days earlier Individuals at risk as carriers include drug abusers, diabetics, and clients on chronic hemodialysis Occurs more frequently in hospitalized clients than in people in the community Usually requires prolonged antibiotic therapy Associated with a high mortality rate in chronically debilitated clients and newborns	Abrupt onset of manifestations Multiple chills High fever Productive cough with sputum (often bloody and purulent) Tachypnea Progressive dyspnea Pleuritic chest pain Empyema Pleural effusions Lung abscess
Streptococcal pneumonia (*Streptococcus pyogenes*)	Rare in adults Occurs in military populations, after influenza epidemics, and sporadically in the community Often associated with strep throat Occurs most frequently in winter Enters the lung by inhalation or aspiration Lung tissue is destroyed Chest x-ray shows bronchopneumonia (Fig. 20-1)	Temperature usually > 39°C (102.2°F) Chills Cough Pharyngitis Hemoptysis Pleuritic chest pain Dyspnea Myalgia Empyema (common) Pleural effusion Bacteremia Mediastinitis Pneumothorax Bronchiectasis
Bacillus pneumonia (*Bacillus anthracis*)	Associated with agricultural or industrial exposure (e.g., individuals working with animal hair or contaminated animal hides or bones) Acquired via inhalation Spore-forming Alveolar macrophages ingest spores and carry them to hilar lymph nodes, where multiplication of bacillus occurs Hemorrhagic pneumonitis can occur	Early manifestations Insidious onset (2–4 days) Mild fever Myalgia Malaise Fatigue Nonproductive cough Later manifestations Dyspnea Profuse diaphoresis Cyanosis

Table 20-2 (Continued)

Causative Agent	Characteristics	Clinical Manifestations and Complications
	Gram-Negative Bacterial Pneumonias	
Klebsiella pneumonia (*Klebsiella pneumoniae;* also called *Friedländer's bacillus*)	Most common gram-negative pneumonias acquired outside the hospital Individuals at high risk include alcoholics, diabetics, people with chronic lung disease, and postoperative clients Acquired via aspiration of oropharyngeal organisms into the lungs Chest x-ray shows lobar consolidation (Fig. 20-1) Can rapidly progress to lung abscess Often associated with high mortality and morbidity rates	Sudden onset Fever Cough Purulent sputum Hemoptysis Malaise Pleuritic chest pain Extensive lung necrosis Lung abscess Empyema Pericarditis Meningitis
Pseudomonas pneumonia (*Pseudomonas aeruginosa*)	Most common gram-negative hospital-acquired pneumonia Predisposing conditions include endotracheal intubation, IPPB treatments, suctioning, respiratory therapy equipment High mortality rate in critically ill clients Chest x-ray shows nodular bronchopneumonia (Fig. 20-1) Individuals at risk include those with chronic lung disease, debilitating diseases, tracheostomies, cancer, and kidney transplants or those taking immunosuppressive therapy or broad-spectrum antibiotics High mortality rate	High fever Cough Copious sputum Hypoxia Cyanosis Lung abscess
Hemophilus influenza pneumonia (*Hemophilus influenzae*)	Increasing in incidence Acquired via endogenous aspiration Chest x-rays show bronchopneumonia in multiple lobes or lobar consolidation Individuals at risk include those with alcoholism, chronic lung disease, recent viral infections, and immune deficiencies Mortality rate is high, especially in elderly clients	Onset may be abrupt, but is usually gradual Fever Chills Cough Purulent sputum Hemoptysis Sore throat Dyspnea Nausea and vomiting Pleuritic chest pain Pleural effusions Lung abscess (common) Empyema (common)
Legionnaires' disease (*Legionella pneumophila*)	Named when major outbreak occurred in 1976 at American Legion Convention in Philadelphia May occur in outbreaks or sporadically Caused by gram-negative bacteria Acquired from airborne organisms Organisms proliferate in water reservoirs (e.g., air-conditioning cooling towers) Individuals at increased risk include cigarette smokers and those with serious underlying diseases (e.g., chronic lung or heart conditions) Erythromycin effective as a treatment measure	Myalgia (initially) Headache (initially) Fever Chills Nonproductive cough Pleuritic chest pain Nausea and vomiting Diarrhea Mental confusion Respiratory failure (major complication)
	Anaerobic Bacterial Pneumonias	
Common causative agents: **Anaerobic streptococci** **Fusobacteria** ***Bacteroides* species**	Most types of pneumonia caused by aspiration of oropharyngeal secretions but occasionally via blood from GI or GU tract or wound infections Infections usually are caused by three or four anaerobes Clients often have poor dental hygiene, periodontal disease, and a history of altered consciousness Chest x-ray often shows lung abscess, empyema, and necrotizing pneumonia	Similar to pneumococcal pneumonia, except for insidious onset Foul-smelling sputum Necrotizing pneumonitis (aspiration-induced) Lung abscess Empyema

Table 20-2 (Continued)

Causative Agent	Characteristics	Clinical Manifestations and Complications
	Mycoplasma Pneumonia (*Mycoplasma pneumoniae*)	
Organism has characteristics of both bacteria and viruses	Transmitted from person to person by respiratory droplets Incubation period of 9–21 days Organisms attack epithelial lining of respiratory system Common in children, military populations, and college-age groups Increase in cold agglutin titer in serum or complement fixation with negative bacterial culture Chest x-ray shows interstitial pneumonia, often bilaterally (Fig. 20-1)	Gradual onset URI Fever (low-grade) Nasal congestion Pharyngitis Lower respiratory tract involvement (bronchitis, bronchiolitis) Headache Malaise Cough (initially usually nonproductive of sputum) Maculopapular rashes
	Viral Pneumonia	
Common causative agents: **Influenza viruses** **Adenovirus** **Parainfluenza viruses**	Accounts for about one-half of all pneumonias Quite common in adults Transmitted from person to person by respiratory droplets Usually self-limiting and treated symptomatically Adversely affects many respiratory defense mechanisms, predisposing to secondary bacterial pneumonia Chest x-ray shows interstitial pneumonia (Fig. 20-1)	Fever Chills Headache Myalgia Anorexia Sneezing Nasal congestion Cough (initially nonproductive)

types of pneumonias are typically mild and self-limiting, and result in no permanent lung damage in previously healthy individuals. Treatment is usually symptomatic, as antibiotics are not effective. Occasionally, viral pneumonias set the stage for bacterial involvement. The client may have concurrent viral and bacterial pneumonia.[4]

Primary influenza viral pneumonia syndrome, although rare, is severe and may be fatal. It occurs primarily in clients who are elderly or debilitated or who have chronic lung or heart disease. The alveoli fill with fibrin, fluid, RBCs, and macrophages. These individuals have severe hypoxemia, tachycardia, and tachypnea. The mortality rate is extremely high in spite of ventilatory support.[5] If the individual survives, pulmonary fibrosis is a common complication.

Viral pneumonia is also found in association with systemic viral diseases such as measles, herpes varicella-zoster virus, and herpes simplex. Varicella pneumonia is more common in adults with chicken pox than in children.

Vaccines against adenovirus and influenza are currently available. Since adenovirus pneumonia is not common in the general population, the use of adenovirus vaccine has been limited to high-risk groups such as military recruits. Influenza vaccine is considered a mainstay of prevention and is recommended annually for use in individuals considered to be at high risk of serious influenza (see Table 19-5).[6]

Amantadine (an antiviral drug) has been used as a chemoprophylactic agent against influenza A virus infections. It acts by preventing the penetration of the virus into the host cell. It is used primarily in outbreaks of the virus and in high-risk individuals. It needs to be given daily throughout the period of influenza exposure. Side effects are uncommon and consist primarily of reversible minor central nervous system effects.

Fungal Pneumonia Fungi may also be a cause of pneumonia and are discussed in a later section on Pulmonary Fungal Infections.

Aspiration Pneumonia Aspiration pneumonia is frequently called *necrotizing pneumonia* because of the pathological changes in the lungs. It usually follows aspiration of material in the mouth into the trachea and subsequently the lungs. The aspirated material—food, water, vomitus—is the triggering mechanism for the pathogenesis of pneumonia. Multiple organisms, including both aerobes and anaerobes, are isolated from the sputum of these individuals.

Persons who develop aspiration pneumonia usually have a history of loss of consciousness (e.g., seizure, anesthesia, head injury, alcohol-induced). With loss of consciousness, the gag and cough re-

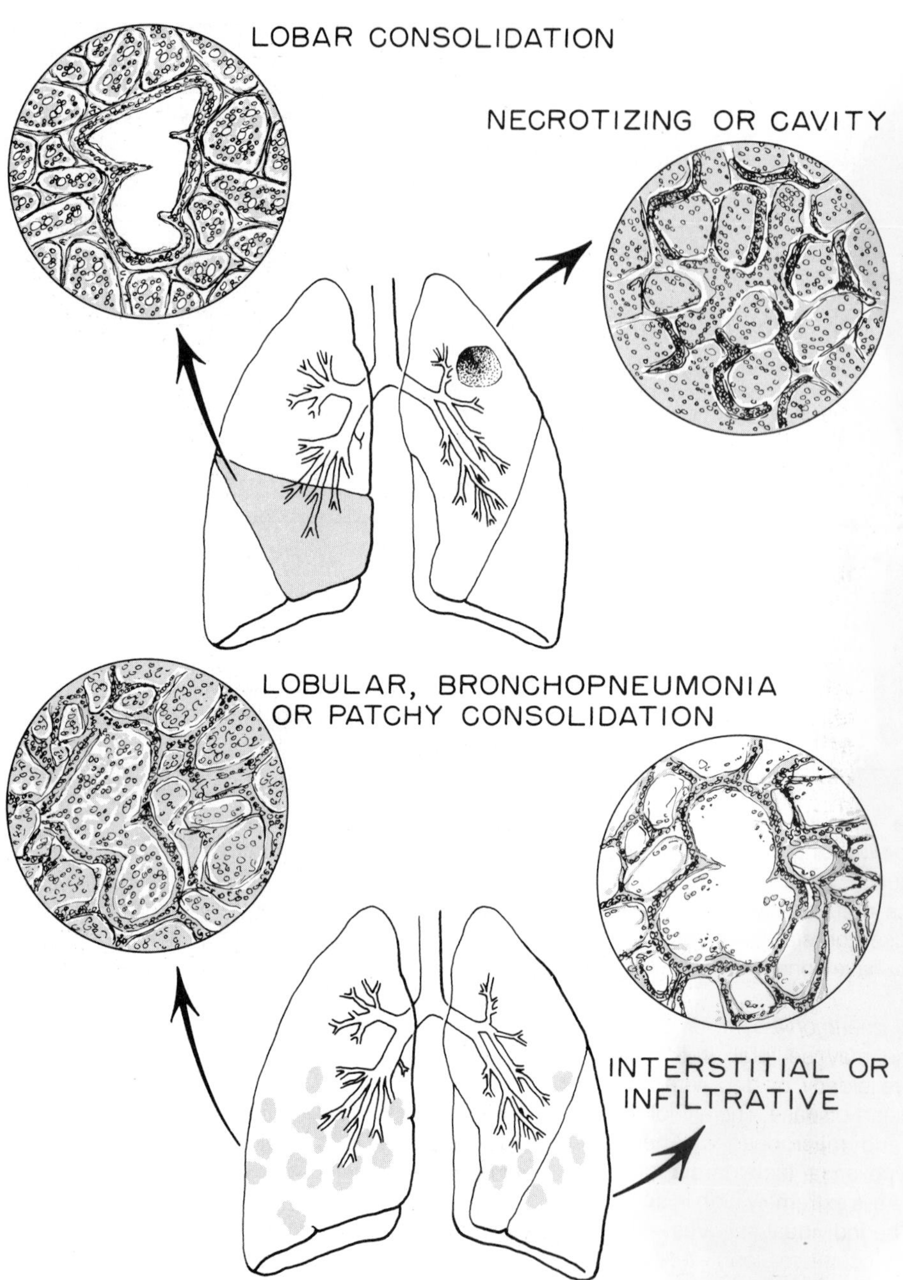

Figure 20-1 Forms of pneumonia: *Lobar*—entire lobe consolidated; exudate chiefly intra-alveolar (inset); *Pneumococcus* and *Klebsiella* are common infecting organisms. *Necrotizing*—granuloma may undergo caseous necrosis and form a cavity; fungi and tubercle bacillus are common infecting organisms. *Lobular*—patchy distribution; fibrinous exudate chiefly in bronchioles; *Staphylococcus* and *Streptococcus* are common infecting organisms. *Interstitial*—perivascular exudate and edema between the alveoli, caused by virus or mycoplasmal infection. *(From S. Price and L. Wilson, Pathophysiology: Clinical Concepts of Disease Processes, 2d ed., McGraw-Hill Book Company, New York, 1982, p. 452.)*

flexes are depressed, and aspiration is more likely to occur.

Pneumonias in the Compromised Host Certain clients with an altered immune response are highly susceptible to respiratory infections. Individuals considered at high risk are those with severe protein-calorie malnutrition, immune deficiencies, post-transplant clients, and clients being treated with radiation therapy, cancer chemotherapy drugs, and corticosteroids (especially for a prolonged period). These individuals have a variety of altered conditions, including suppressed B and T lymphocyte function, depressed bone marrow function, and decreased levels of neutrophils and macrophages. In addition to the causative agents (especially gram-negative bacteria) previously discussed, other agents causing pneumonia in immunosuppressed clients are *Pneumocystis carinii* (a protozoan), cytomegalovirus, and fungi (see the section on Pulmonary Fungal Infections).

Pneumocystis carinii rarely causes pneumonia in healthy individuals. In widespread disease the lungs are massively consolidated. Clinical manifestations are insidious and include fever, tachypnea, tachycardia, dyspnea, nonproductive cough, and hypoxemia. Pulmonary physical findings are minimal in proportion to the serious nature of the disease. Treatment consists of trimethoprim and sulfamethoxazole (Bactrim) as the primary agents and pentamidine isethionate as a secondary one. The mortality rate is about 50 percent. Untreated, the mortality rate may reach 100 percent.

Cytomegalovirus, also called *cytomegalic inclusion virus,* is the most important type of viral pneumonia in immunocompromised clients. Cytomegalovirus, a type of herpesvirus, gives rise to latent infections and reactivation with shedding of infectious virus. This type of interstitial pneumonia can be a mild disease, or it can be fulminant and produce pulmonary insufficiency and death. Often, cytomegalovirus coexists with other opportunistic bacterial, fungal, or protozoan agents in causing pneumonia. There is no specific therapy available for this type of pneumonia.[7]

Pneumococcal pneumonia

Because pneumococcal pneumonia is the most common cause of bacterial pneumonia, it will be the primary focus of this section.

Pathogenesis There are four characteristic stages of the disease process:

1. *Congestion.* After the pneumococcus reaches the alveoli via droplets or saliva, there is an outpouring of edema fluid into the alveoli. The organisms multiply in the serous fluid, and the infection is spread. The pneumococci damage the host by overwhelming growth and interfering with lung functions.
2. *Red hepatization.* There is massive dilatation of the capillaries, and alveoli are filled with organisms, neutrophils, RBCs, and fibrin. The lung appears red and granular, or liverlike, which is why the process is called hepatization.
3. *Gray hepatization.* Blood flow decreases, and leukocytes and fibrin consolidate in the affected part of the lung.
4. *Resolution.* Complete resolution and healing occur if there are no complications. The exudate becomes lysed and is processed by the macrophages. The normal lung tissue is restored, and the person's gas-exchange ability returns to normal.

Clinical Manifestations A preceding URI is typically found in cases of pneumococcal pneumonia. The incubation period is 1 to 14 days. Presenting manifestations include an acute onset of fever, chills, productive cough with greenish, bloody, or rusty sputum, and pleuritic chest pain. Nausea and vomiting are also seen, and systemic manifestations such as malaise, myalgia, and weakness are common. Tachycardia, tachypnea, and chest splinting are commonly found. Findings on physical examination of the chest may include dullness to percussion, diminished breath sounds in the affected part of the lung, rales, and a pleural friction rub. The client's skin may have a dusky appearance because of hypoxemia. If the lower lobes are involved, the client may experience mild to severe abdominal pain.

Complications Pneumococcal pneumonia generally runs an uncomplicated course. The associated mortality rate is about 10 percent. Complications are not common and develop more frequently in individuals with underlying chronic diseases. Complications may include the following:

1. *Pleurisy* (inflammation of the pleura) is a relatively common accompanying problem of pneumonia. Pain develops when the parietal and visceral pleurae rub together.
2. *Pleural effusion* occurs in about 5 percent of clients. Usually, the effusion is sterile and is reabsorbed in 1 to 2 weeks. Occasionally, it requires aspiration via a thoracentesis.
3. *Atelectasis* (collapsed, airless alveoli) of one or part of one lobe may occur. These areas usually clear with effective coughing and deep breathing or vigorous tracheal suctioning.
4. *Delayed resolution* results from persistence of the infection and is seen on x-ray as residual consoli-

dation. Usually, the physical findings return to normal within 2 to 4 weeks.

5. *Lung abscess* is *not* a common complication of pneumococcal pneumonia. It is seen more frequently with other types of pneumonia, such as staphylococcal and gram-negative pneumonias. Lung abscess is discussed in a later section of this chapter.
6. *Empyema* (accumulation of purulent exudate in the pleural cavity) is relatively infrequent but requires antibiotic therapy and drainage of the exudate by a chest tube or open surgical drainage.
7. *Pericarditis* results from spread of the infecting organism from an infected pleura or via a hematogenous route.
8. *Arthritis* results from systemic spread of the organism. The affected joint is swollen, red, and painful, and a purulent exudate can be aspirated.
9. *Meningitis* caused by pneumococcus is second only to meningococcus as a cause of purulent meningitis. Any client with pneumococcal pneumonia who is disoriented, confused, or somnolent should have a lumbar puncture to evaluate the possibility of pneumococcal meningitis.
10. *Endocarditis* can develop when the organisms attack the endocardium and the valves of the heart. The clinical manifestations are similar to those of acute bacterial endocarditis (see Chap. 29).

Medical management of pneumonia

Diagnostic The common diagnostic measures for pneumonia are presented in Table 20-3. Immediate identification of the organism is critical in order to institute appropriate antimicrobial therapy. Blood and sputum cultures may take 24 to 72 hours. Therefore, a Gram stain of the sputum provides the information on which the initial therapy is based. Usually, the predominant organism can be identified on a Gram stain. If the client cannot voluntarily produce a sputum specimen after trying the techniques suggested in Table 18-6, procedures such as transtracheal aspiration and fiberoptic bronchoscopy may be used. Transtracheal aspiration involves inserting a catheter into the trachea through the cricothyroid membrane.

Chest x-rays often show a typical pattern characteristic of the infecting organism. Arterial blood gases, if obtained, usually reveal hypoxemia. Leukocytosis is found in about 80 percent of clients with pneumonia.

Table 20-3

Medical Management: Bacterial Pneumonia

Diagnostic

1. History and physical examination
2. Gram stain of sputum
3. Sputum culture and sensitivity
4. Chest x-ray
5. Arterial blood gases (if indicated)
6. Complete blood count
7. Blood cultures

Therapeutic

1. Appropriate antibiotic therapy (see Table 20-4)
2. Increased fluid intake (at least 3 L/24 h)
3. Limited activity or bed rest
4. Antipyretics
5. Analgesics
6. Oxygen therapy (if indicated)
7. Aerosol therapy

Therapeutic Prompt treatment with the appropriate antibiotic almost always cures bacterial and mycoplasma pneumonia. Currently, there is no effective treatment for viral pneumonia. The specific types of antibiotics are discussed under Pharmacological Management. In uncomplicated cases, the client responds to drug therapy within 1 to 2 days. Indications of improvement include decreased temperature, improved breathing, and reduced chest pain.

In addition to antibiotic therapy, supportive measures may be used, including oxygen therapy to treat hypoxemia, chest physiotherapy to mobilize secretions, analgesics such as codeine to relieve the chest pain, and antipyretics such as aspirin or acetominophen to decrease the temperature. During the acute febrile phase, clients' activity should be restricted, and rest should be encouraged and planned.

Most individuals with mild to moderate illness who have no other underlying disease process can be treated on an outpatient basis. If there is a serious underlying disease or the pneumonia is accompanied by severe dyspnea, hypoxemia, or other complications, the client should be hospitalized.

Pneumococcal Vaccine Pneumococcal vaccine has been developed, and its use is indicated primarily for those individuals considered at high risk who:[8]

Have chronic illnesses such as lung and heart disease and diabetes mellitus

Are recovering from a severe illness

Are age 50 or older

Are in nursing homes or other long-term care facilities

The vaccine is not recommended for pregnant women, children under 2 years of age, or those with febrile disease. Usually 0.5 mL is given intramuscularly or subcutaneously. The vaccine offers protection for at least 3 years, and booster injections should be given every 3 years. Influenza vaccine was previously discussed under Viral Pneumonias.

Pharmacological management

The introduction of sulfonamides in the 1930s and penicillin in the 1940s revolutionized the treatment of pneumonia. Today penicillin is still the drug of choice for a great number of bacterial pneumonias. The main problems with the use of antibiotics in pneumonia are (1) the development of resistant strains of organisms and (2) the client's hypersensitivity or allergic reaction to certain antibiotics.[9] Table 20-4 outlines the major antimicrobial agents used in the treatment of pneumonia and respiratory infections. It is extremely important to identify accurately the infecting organism so that the appropriate drug therapy can be instituted. Initial

Table 20-4
Antibiotic Drug Therapy Used for Pneumonia

Drug	Common Side Effects	Comments
Penicillins		
Penicillin G Penicillin G with procaine Penicillin V Ampicillin Amoxicillin Carbenicillin Methicillin Nafcillin Oxacillin Cloxacillin Dicloxacillin	Low incidence of side effects Hypersensitivity reactions (1–10%) Neurotoxicity (from procaine penicillin) Hepatotoxicity Neutropenia Interstitial nephritis (especially from methicillin)	Frequently the drug of choice in treating bacterial and anaerobic pneumonias Broad-spectrum activity Observe for superinfection
Cephalosporins		
Cephalothin (Keflin) Cephapirin (Cefadyl) Cephaloridine (Lorridine) Cefazolin (Ancef, Kefsol) Cephradine (Anspor) Cephalexin (Keflex) Cephaloglycin (Kafocin)	GI disturbance Phlebitis (from IV administration) Nephrotoxicity Hypersensitivity reactions (2–5%)	Indicated as primary therapy in *Klebsiella* pneumonia, along with an aminoglycoside Useful for therapy when mixed infection is present Broad-spectrum activity Often used when client has known hypersensitivity to penicillins
Aminoglycosides		
Kanamycin (Kantrex) Gentamicin (Garamycin) Tobramycin (Nebcin) Amikacin (Amikin)	Nephrotoxicity Audiotoxicity Hypersensitivity reactions Neuromuscular blockade	Particularly valuable against gram-negative bacilli Poorly absorbed after oral administration Monitor BUN and serum creatinine Assess hearing before and during therapy
Miscellaneous Drugs		
Erythromycin	GI disturbances Infrequent hypersensitivity reactions Reversible hepatotoxicity Phlebitis (with IV administration)	Considered primary therapy for Legionnaires' disease
Tetracycline	GI disturbances Photosensitivity Hypersensitivity	Primarily effective against gram-positive bacilli GI absorption altered with antacid or milk ingestion
Clindamycin	GI disturbances Hypersensitivity reactions	Particularly effective against anaerobic bacteria Also effective against gram-positive bacteria
Chloramphenicol	Bone marrow suppression Optic neuritis	Broad-spectrum antibiotic
Vancomycin	Nephrotoxicity Audiotoxicity Phlebitis	Requires IV administration Infrequently used for pulmonary infections Effective against gram-positive organisms

antimicrobial therapy is based in large part on the results of the Gram stain smear analysis. More definitive information may later be obtained from the sputum culture and sensitivity, and the antibiotic can be changed if indicated.

In acute cases, antibiotics are usually given parenterally for the first few days and then administered orally. In mild cases, oral administration is adequate for the duration of the illness. It is extremely important that the client continue taking the antibiotics for the prescribed period (usually at least 10 days) to prevent a relapse of pneumonia and the development of resistant strains of the organism. Before antibiotics are given, it is necessary to obtain the client's history regarding possible drug allergies.

Nutritional measures

Fluid intake of at least 3 L/day is very important in the supportive treatment of pneumonia. If oral intake cannot be maintained, intravenous administration of fluids and electrolytes may be necessary for the acutely ill client. A liquid blenderized or processed liquid diet may be tolerated better than solid food in the acute phase of pneumonia. An intake of at least 1500 calories daily should be maintained to provide energy for the increased metabolic processes in the client. Small, frequent meals are tolerated better by the dyspneic client. Oral hygiene prior to eating is very important to improve the person's appetite. Expectoration of sputum often decreases the client's taste sensation and contributes to anorexia.

Nursing management

Health Promotion and Maintenance There are many nursing interventions to help prevent the occurrence as well as the morbidity associated with pneumonia. Teaching individuals to practice good health habits such as proper diet and hygiene, adequate rest, and regular exercise can maintain their natural resistance to infecting organisms. If possible, exposure to URIs should be avoided. If a URI occurs, it should be treated promptly with supportive measures (e.g., rest, fluids, antipyretics). If symptoms persist for more than 3 or 4 days, the person should obtain medical care. Individuals at high risk for pneumonia (e.g., the chronically ill and the elderly) should be encouraged to obtain both influenza and pneumococcal vaccines.

In the hospital, the nursing role involves identifying clients at risk (Table 20-1) and taking measures to prevent the development of pneumonia. Clients with altered consciousness should be placed in positions (e.g., side-lying, upright) that will prevent them from aspirating. They should be turned and repositioned at least every 2 hours to facilitate adequate lung expansion and to discourage pooling of secretions. Clients who have difficulty swallowing (e.g., stroke clients) need assistance in eating, drinking, and taking medication to prevent aspiration. Postoperative clients and others who are immobile need assistance with turning, coughing, and deep-breathing measures at frequent intervals (see Chap. 8). The nurse must be careful to avoid overmedication with narcotics or sedatives, which can cause a depressed cough reflex and accumulation of fluid in the lungs. The gag reflex should be present in individuals who have had local anesthesia to the throat prior to the administration of fluids or food.

Strict medical asepsis should be practiced by the nurse to reduce the incidence of nosocomial infections. The client with an infection should not be placed in the same room with a postoperative client or one with chronic lung disease. Respiratory therapy equipment should be properly cleaned and changed, and disposable equipment used as much as possible. Strict sterile aseptic technique should be used when suctioning a client.

Acute Intervention Although many clients with pneumonia are treated on an outpatient basis, the nursing care plan presented in Table 20-5 is applicable to both these individuals and the in-hospital client. It is important for the nurse to remember that pneumonia is an acute, infectious disease. Although most cases of pneumonia are potentially completely curable, complications can result. Nurses must be aware of these complications and of the manifestations of their occurrence.

Chronic Management The client needs to be reassured that complete recovery from pneumonia is possible. It is extremely important to emphasize the need to take all the prescribed medication and to return for follow-up medical care and evaluation. Adequate rest is needed to maintain progress toward recovery and to prevent a relapse. Clients need to be told that it may be weeks before they feel their usual vigor and sense of well-being. A prolonged period of convalescence may be necessary for the elderly or chronically ill client.

Those clients considered to be at high risk for pneumonia should be told about available vaccines and should discuss them with the health care provider. Deep-breathing and coughing exercises should be practiced for 6 to 8 weeks after the client is discharged from the hospital.

Table 20-5
Nursing Care Plan for the Client with Pneumonia

Client Problem	Expected Outcome	Nursing Intervention
Shallow, rapid respirations with dyspnea	Respiratory rate of 12–18/min.	Assess degree of pain and anxiety. Take vital signs and auscultate lungs every 2–4 h. Monitor arterial blood gases if ordered. Administer oxygen as indicated. Assess its effectiveness. Decrease anxiety (e.g., with relaxational techniques, diversion) and provide a quiet, restful environment. Position client in semi-Fowler's or other comfortable position for breathing (may use reclining chairs).
Productive cough	Lungs clear to auscultation. Normal chest x-ray finding. Client will observe changes in sputum.	Assist client to cough by splinting chest and teaching how to cough effectively. (Inhale slowly through nose, exhale, and cough; see Table 21–9.) Provide receptacle and tissues for disposal of sputum. Provide oral hygiene after production of sputum. Give expectorants and cough suppressants as ordered. Provide humidification of inhaled air. Maintain fluid intake of 3 L daily. Use chest physiotherapy if indicated to mobilize secretions. Observe characteristics of sputum and report any significant changes (e.g., from mucoid to grossly purulent).
Chest pain	Alleviation of chest pain. Normal lung excursion.	Administer analgesics as ordered. Position client comfortably. Premedicate with analgesics before uncomfortable therapies are given. Assist with intercostal nerve block if necessary. Observe for possible complications if pain persists (e.g., pleural effusion, empyema, etc.).
Fever and chills	Normal body temperature (≤37°C, ≤98.6°F).	Administer antibiotics as prescribed. Observe for side effects and toxicity associated with antibiotic therapy. Administer antipyretics as ordered. Take temperature every 2–4 h. Observe for continuing or recurring fever and report finding to physician. Provide fluid intake (at least 3 L/day). Provide frequent clothing and linen changes if diaphoresis occurs. Keep client comfortable and dry.
Fatigue	Feeling of being rested.	Provide bed rest and limited physical activity. Assess response to activity and plan changes accordingly. Limit visitors and long conversations. Plan nursing care in blocks to ensure periods of rest. Maintain a pleasant, calm environment. Place needed items (e.g., tissues, call bell) within easy reach. Plan for uninterrupted sleep periods.
Anorexia, nausea, or vomiting	Normal nutritional intake.	See Table 33–19.
Possible spread of infection	No spread of infection.	Teach client to use tissues when coughing and expectorating sputum. Place used tissues in wax-lined paper bag and dispose of properly. Wash hands thoroughly after contact with infected client. Teach client to practice these techniques at home as well as in hospital. Do not put infectious client in same room with client at high risk for pneumonia (e.g., postoperative, with chronic lung disease, immunosuppressed, elderly).
Possible relapse and recurring pneumonia	No evidence of pneumonia. Client will follow prescribed regimen, including: Medications Fluid therapy Activity schedule	Assess ability to continue self-care at home. Encourage client to continue on full course of antibiotic therapy. Instruct client on the importance of rest and limited activity. Encourage client to obtain adequate rest, good nutrition, and fresh air. If indicated, encourage client to stop or decrease cigarette smoking. Teach client to continue coughing and deep-breathing exercises. Teach client the importance of follow-up care and the need to seek medical attention for symptoms related to respiratory infections. Encourage client to obtain vaccinations (pneumococcal and influenza) if at high risk for pneumonia.

Tuberculosis

Tuberculosis (TB) is a bacterial infectious disease transmitted by *Mycobacterium tuberculosis.* It usually involves the lungs, but it also occurs in the kidneys, bones, lymph nodes, and meninges, and can be disseminated throughout the body.

Significance of the problem

Since the introduction of chemotherapy in the late 1940s and early 1950s, there has been a dramatic decrease in the prevalence of TB. About 15 million people are infected with or harbor the tubercle bacillus. The majority of these individuals have healed or dormant TB. It is estimated that about 30,000 cases of active TB will be reported each year. About 10 percent of these cases represent relapse.[10] These statistics indicate that TB, in spite of being potentially curable and preventable, is still a major public health problem in the United States.

The tubercle bacillus may remain dormant for many years, and then reactivate and produce clinical TB. Infection with *M. tuberculosis* involves a lifelong relationship between humans and the tubercle bacillus; dormant organisms may remain alive in the host for life. The infected host has been referred to as a "walking time bomb" in whom TB may develop and serve as a source of infection for others.

High-risk individuals for TB include residents of inner-city neighborhoods, foreign-born persons, the elderly, and the socioeconomically disadvantaged of all races. TB is found in high incidence in a few areas of the United States where there is a large population of American Indians, such as Arizona and New Mexico, and in counties near the Mexican border. Hawaii has had the highest rate of new cases in the past few years.

Etiology and pathogenesis

Mycobacterium tuberculosis, a gram-positive, acid-fast bacillus, is usually spread via airborne droplet nuclei which are produced when infected individuals cough, sneeze, or speak. Once released into a room, the organisms are dispersed and can be inhaled by a susceptible host. Brief exposure to a few tubercle bacilli rarely causes an infection. Rather, it is more commonly spread to individuals who have had repeated close contact with an infected person. TB is not highly infectious, and transmission usually requires close, frequent, or prolonged exposure.[11] The disease cannot be spread by hands, books, glasses, dishes, or fomites.

When the bacilli are inhaled, they pass down the bronchial system and implant on the respiratory bronchioles or alveoli. The lower parts of the lungs are usually the site of initial bacterial implantation. After implantation, they multiply, with no initial resistance from the host. The organisms are engulfed by phagocytes (initially neutrophils and later macrophages) and may continue to multiply within the phagocyte.

While a cellular immune response is being activated, the bacilli can be spread through the lymphatic channels to regional lymph nodes and via the thoracic duct to the circulating blood. Thus, organisms may be spread throughout the body before sufficient activation of the cell-mediated immune response is available to bring the infection under control. The organisms find favorable environments for growth primarily in the upper lobes of the lungs, kidneys, epiphyseal lines of the bone, and cerebral cortex.

Eventually, the acquired cellular immunity limits further multiplication and spread of the infection. A characteristic tissue reaction called an *epithelioid cell granuloma* results after the cellular immune system is activated. This granuloma (also called an *epithelioid cell tubercle*) is due to fusion of the infiltrating macrophages. The granuloma is surrounded by lymphocytes. This reaction usually takes 10 to 20 days.

The central portion of the lesion (called a *Ghon tubercle*) undergoes necrosis characterized by a cheesy appearance and hence is named *caseous necrosis.* The lesion may also undergo liquefactive necrosis, with the liquid sloughing into connecting bronchi and producing a cavity. Therefore, tubercular material may enter the tracheobronchial system,[12] allowing airborne transmission of infectious particles.

Healing of the primary lesion usually takes place by resolution, fibrosis, and calcification. The granulation tissue surrounding the lesion may become more fibrous and form a collagenous scar around the tubercle. A *Ghon complex* is formed consisting of the Ghon tubercle and regional lymph nodes. Calcified Ghon complexes may be seen on chest x-rays.

When a tuberculous lesion regresses and heals, the infection enters a latent period in which it may persist without producing a clinical illness. The infection may remain dormant for life, or it may develop into clinical disease if the persisting organisms begin to multiply rapidly.[13]

If the initial immune response is not adequate, control of the organisms is not maintained and clinical disease results. Certain individuals are at a higher risk for clinical disease, including those who are immunosuppressed, have diabetes mellitus, are less than 2 years old, and are adolescents.

About 5 percent of individuals are incapable of containing the initial infective process. An additional 5 percent of those who do produce an effective immune response later lose this capability; dormant bacilli then begin to multiply, and the disease is reactivated. The reasons for reactivation are not well understood, but they are related to decreased resistance found in the elderly, individuals with concomitant diseases, and those taking immunosuppressive therapy.

Classification of TB

In 1974 the American Thoracic Association and American Lung Association adopted a classification system that covers the entire population (Table 20-6).

Table 20-6

Classification of TB

Class O: No TB exposure, not infected (no history of exposure, negative tuberculin skin test)

Class I: TB exposure, no evidence of infection (history of exposure, negative tuberculin skin test)

Class II: TB infection without disease (positive tuberculin skin test, negative bacteriological studies, no roentgenographic findings compatible with tuberculosis, no symptoms caused by tuberculosis)

Class III: TB infection with disease (positive bacteriological studies, abnormal roentgenographic findings, positive tuberculin skin tests, symptomatic)

Adapted from *Diagnostic Standards and Classification of Tuberculosis and Other Mycobacterial Diseases,* American Lung Association, New York, 1974.

Clinical manifestations

In the early stages of TB, the person is usually asymptomatic. Many cases are found incidentally when routine chest x-rays are done, especially with the elderly.

Systemic manifestations initially may consist of fatigue, malaise, anorexia, weight loss, low-grade fevers (especially in the late afternoon), and night sweats. These manifestations are related to the lymphokine production stimulated by the hypersensitivity immune response to the tubercle bacilli. The weight loss may not be excessive until late in the disease and is often attributed to overwork or other factors. Irregular menses may also be present in premenopausal females.

A characteristic pulmonary manifestation is a cough which progresses to become frequent and productive of mucoid or mucopurulent sputum. Chest pain characterized as dull or tight may also be present. Hemoptysis is not a common finding and is usually associated with more advanced cases. Sometimes TB has more acute, sudden manifestations, and the client presents with high fever, chills, generalized flulike symptoms, pleuritic pain, and a productive cough.

Complications

Miliary (Hematogenous) TB If a necrotic Ghon focus erodes through a blood vessel, large numbers of organisms invade the bloodstream and are spread to all body organs. This is called *miliary or hematogenous TB.* The person may either be acutely ill with fever, dyspnea, and cyanosis or chronically ill with systemic manifestations of weight loss, fever, and gastrointestinal (GI) disturbance. Hepatomegaly, splenomegaly, and generalized lymphadenopathy may be present.

Pleural Effusion A pleural effusion is caused by the release of caseous material into the pleural space. The bacteria-containing material triggers an inflammatory reaction and a pleural exudate of protein-rich fluid.

A form of pleurisy called "dry" pleurisy may result from a superficial tuberculous lesion involving the pleura. It appears as localized pleuritic pain on deep inspiration.

Tuberculous Pneumonia Acute pneumonia may result when large amounts of tubercle bacilli are discharged from the liquefied necrotic lesion into the lung or lymph nodes. The clinical manifestations are similar to those of bacterial pneumonia, including chills, fever, productive cough, pleuritic pain, and leukocytosis.

Other Organ Involvement Although the lungs are the primary site of tuberculosis, other body organs may also be involved. The meninges may become infected following rupture of a caseous tubercle into the subarachnoid space. Bone and joint tissue may be involved in the infectious disease process. The kidneys, lymph nodes, and both female and male genital tracts may also be infected.

Diagnostic study abnormalities

Tuberculin Skin Testing The body's immune response can be demonstrated by testing for hypersensitivity to a tuberculin skin test. A positive reaction develops 3 to 10 weeks after the initial infection, corresponding to the time needed to mount an immune response.

Purified protein derivative (PPD) of tuberculin is used primarily to detect the delayed hypersensitivity response. (The procedure for doing the tuberculin skin test is described in Chap. 18.) Once acquired, sensitivity to tuberculin tends to persist throughout life. A positive reaction indicates the presence of a tuberculous infection, but it does not show whether the infection is dormant or causing a clinical illness.

Chest X-Ray Although the findings on chest x-rays are extremely important, it is not possible to make a diagnosis of TB based solely on this examination. This is because other diseases can mimic the appearance of TB.

The abnormality most commonly found in TB is multinodular lymph node involvement with cavitation in the upper lobes of the lungs. This is often referred to as the *parenchymal lymph node complex*. Calcification of the lung lesions generally occurs within several years of the infection.

Bacteriological Studies The demonstration of tubercle bacilli bacteriologically is essential for establishing a diagnosis. Microscopic examination of stained *sputum smears* for acid-fast bacilli is usually the first bacteriological evidence of the presence of tubercle bacilli. It is a quick, easy examination and provides the physician with valuable information. A major disadvantage is that over 10,000 bacteria per milliliter of specimen are required to produce a positive smear. In addition to sputum, material for examination can be obtained from gastric washings, cerebrospinal fluid, or pus from an abscess.

The most accurate means of diagnosis is a *culture technique*. The major disadvantage of this method is that it takes 2 weeks or more for the mycobacterium to grow. The advantage is that it can detect small quantities (10 bacteria per milliliter of specimen).

Medical management

The treatment of TB rarely requires in-hospital treatment. Most clients are treated on an outpatient basis, and many can continue working or maintain their lifestyle with few changes (Table 20-7). Hospitalization may be used for diagnostic evaluation, for the severely ill or debilitated, and for those with adverse drug reactions or treatment failures.

The mainstay of TB treatment is pharmacological. Drug therapy is used to treat individuals with clinical disease as well as to prevent disease in an infected person. Drugs are usually administered as a single dose before breakfast to ensure adequate GI absorption.

Table 20-7
Medical Management: TB

Diagnostic
1. History and physical examination
2. Tuberculin skin test
3. Chest x-ray
4. Bacteriological studies
   a. Sputum
   b. Culture

Therapeutic
1. Long-term antimicrobial drugs (Table 20-8)
2. Follow-up bacteriological studies

Pharmacological management

Active Disease The main form of treatment of TB is pharmacological. Treatment of TB usually consists of a combination of at least two drugs. The reason for combination therapy is to increase the therapeutic effectiveness and decrease the development of resistant strains of *M. tuberculosis*. It has been shown that single-drug therapy can result in rapid development of resistant strains.

The four primary drugs used are isoniazid, rifampin, streptomycin, and ethambutol (see Table 20-8). Other drugs are primarily used for treatment of resistant strains or if the client develops toxicity to the primary drugs.

A problem with anti-TB therapy is the length of time medication must be taken. In the past, 18 to 24 months was the usual period of time required for individuals to adhere to the medical regimen. Recent studies have indicated that a shorter course of therapy may be effective. Although there are variations, protocol consists of using isoniazid and rifampin for a minimum of 9 months. After a period of time (2 weeks to 2 months), daily administration may be changed to twice weekly.[14]

The recommendation of the American Thoracic Society is that treatment continue for at least 9 months, and longer if necessary (until at least 6 months have elapsed from conversion of a positive sputum to negative).[15] If the case of TB is complicated, these guidelines need to be individualized.

Follow-up care for clients on long-term therapy is very important to monitor for (1) effectiveness of drugs and (2) development of toxic side effects. Usually, sputum specimens are initially obtained on a weekly basis and then monthly to assess the effectiveness of the medication. The regimen is considered effective if the client converts to a negative sputum status. (Over 90 percent of persons convert to negative sputum status within 3 months.)[15]

An important reason for follow-up care is to ensure adherence to the treatment regimen. About 35 percent of individuals do not adhere to the treatment program in spite of understanding the disease process and the value of treatment.[16] Methods to improve

Table 20-8
Drug Therapy Used in TB

Drug	Mechanism of Action	Side Effects	Comments
		First-Line Drugs	
Isoniazid (INH)	Interferes with DNA metabolism of tubercle bacillus	Peripheral neuritis Hepatotoxicity Hypersensitivity (skin rash, arthralgia, fever) Optic neuritis Vitamin B_6 neuritis	Drug is metabolized primarily by the liver and excreted by the kidney. Pyridoxine (vitamin B_6) should be administered during high-dose therapy as a prophylactic measure. Used as a single prophylactic agent for active TB in individuals whose PPD converts to positive. Can cross the blood-brain barrier.
Rifampin	Broad-spectrum antibiotic. Inhibits RNA polymerase of tubercle bacillus	Hepatitis Febrile reaction GI upset Peripheral neuropathy Hypersensitivity	Most commonly used with isoniazid. Incidence of side effects is low. Negates the effect of birth control pills. Urine may turn orange.
Ethambutol (Myambutol)	Inhibits RNA synthesis and is bacteriostatic for the tubercle bacillus	Skin rash GI upset Malaise Peripheral neuritis Optic neuritis	Side effects are uncommon and are reversible with discontinuation of the drug. Its most common use is as a substitute drug when toxicity occurs with isoniazid or rifampin.
Streptomycin	Inhibits protein synthesis and is bactericidal	Audiotoxicity (VIIIth cranial nerve) Nephrotoxicity Hypersensitivity	Should be used with caution in older clients, those with renal disease, and pregnant women.
		Second-Line Drugs	
Ethionamide	Inhibits protein synthesis	GI upset Hepatotoxicity Hypersensitivity	Valuable for retreatment of resistant organisms. Contraindicated in pregnancy.
Capreomycin	Inhibits protein synthesis and is bactericidal	Audiotoxicity Nephrotoxicity	Should be used with caution in older clients.
Kanamycin	Interferes with protein synthesis	Audiotoxicity (VIIIth cranial nerve) Nephrotoxicity	Used in selected cases for retreatment of resistant strains.
Pyrazinamide	Bactericidal. Exact mechanism unknown	Jaundice (rare) Fever Skin rash Hyperuricemia	Very effective when used with streptomycin or capreomycin.
Para-aminosalicylic acid (PAS)	Interferes with metabolism of tubercle bacillus	GI upset (frequent) Hypersensitivity Hepatotoxicity	Interferes with absorption of rifampin. Not frequently used.
Cycloserine	Inhibits cell wall synthesis	Personality changes Psychosis Rash	Should not be used in individuals with a history of psychosis. Used in retreatment of resistant strains.

client adherence are discussed in the section on Nursing Management.

The client needs to be followed for 12 months after completion of therapy to check for the development of resistant strains. The major causes of treatment failure are poor client adherence and an inappropriately prescribed drug regimen. Retreatment regimens are more complicated, require the use of completely new drugs, and are more expensive.

Preventive Treatment (Chemoprophylaxis) Pharmacological management can be used to prevent a TB infection from developing into a clinical disease. The indications for preventive therapy are presented in Table 20-9. Close contacts of individuals with infectious clinical TB should be examined with tuberculin skin tests. Close contacts who are less than 4 years of age should be given treatment even if the tuberculin skin test is negative.

Some individuals carry dormant TB infections that may develop into active disease in some situations. Examples of this include positive reactors who (1) are on prolonged steroid therapy, (2) have a malignancy such as Hodgkin's disease, and (3) develop diabetes mellitus. These individuals would benefit from prophylactic treatment of TB.[17]

The drug generally used in prophylactic chemotherapy is isoniazid. It is effective and inexpensive and can be administered orally. It is usually administered once daily for a period of 12 months.

BCG Vaccine Bacillus Calmette-Guérin (BCG) is a live attenuated vaccine which has limited usefulness in the United States because of the low rate of infection. It is recommended for people who have negative tuberculin skin tests but who are repeatedly exposed to pulmonary tuberculosis (e.g., individuals assigned to work in countries with a high prevalence rate). It is used for young children in countries with a high rate of TB. The vaccine does not reduce the chance of natural infection but does decrease the seriousness of clinical TB when it occurs. BCG is being used as a form of immunotherapy in the treatment of cancer (see Chap. 11).

Nursing management

Health Promotion and Maintenance The ultimate goal related to TB in the United States is eradication. The public health nurse and clinic nurse have especially important responsibilities. Selective screening programs in known high-risk groups may be of value in detecting individuals with TB. Persons with positive tuberculin skin tests should have chest x-rays to assess for the presence of TB. Another important measure is to identify the contacts of individuals who develop TB. These contacts need to be assessed for the possibility of infection and perhaps given chemoprophylactic treatment.

When an individual has respiratory symptoms such as cough, dyspnea, or productive sputum, the nurse should assess for the presence of TB even if the suspected respiratory problem is something else, such as emphysema, pneumonia, or lung cancer. It is possible that the client may also have TB.

Acute Intervention Acute in-hospital care is seldom required for clients with TB. If hospitalization is needed, it is usually for a brief period of time. Respiratory isolation is generally indicated until the client responds to chemotherapy (usually within days to a few weeks). Clients who are unlikely to transmit tubercle bacilli do not need to be placed in respiratory isolation. Masks are of limited value unless they are made of fabric designed to filter out droplet nuclei. They also need to be molded to fit tightly around the nose and mouth. Adequate ventilation of room air is important. Ultraviolet radiation in client rooms or air ducts enhances the effect of normal ventilation. From 1 to 2 hours of direct sunlight may kill the bacillus.

The client should be taught to cover his nose and mouth with paper tissue every time he coughs, sneezes, or produces sputum. The tissues should be thrown into a paper bag and disposed of with the trash, burned, or flushed down the toilet. The client should also be taught careful handwashing techniques after handling sputum and soiled tissues.

As discussed in the section on Pharmacological Management, most treatment failures are due to the client's neglecting to take the medication, discontinuing it prematurely, or taking it irregularly. It is important for the nurse to develop a therapeutic, consistent relationship with the client. The nurse needs to understand the client's lifestyle and to provide flexibility in planning a program that facilitates the client's participation in and completion of therapy. The nurse should educate the client so that he fully understands the need for dedication to the prescribed regimen. Ongoing reassurance helps the client understand that faithfulness can mean cure. If the client cannot or will not adhere to a self-administered medication regimen, medication may have to be given directly on a daily or intermittent basis.

Table 20-9
Indications for Preventive TB Therapy

1. Household members and other close associates of newly diagnosed client.
2. Newly infected client.
3. Positive tuberculin skin test reactors with abnormal chest x-ray.
4. Positive tuberculin skin test reactors in special clinical situations (taking steroids, having diabetes mellitus, silicosis, gastrectomy).
5. Other positive tuberculin skin test reactors up to age 35.
6. Other positive tuberculin skin test reactors over age 35 only in special epidemiological situations.

Adapted from L.S. Farer, "All about TB," *Clinical Notes on Respiratory Diseases,* American Lung Association, New York, 1978.

Some clients may feel that there is a social stigma attached to TB. These feelings need to be discussed and the client reassured that individuals with TB can be cured if they follow the prescribed regimen. Many people still remember when TB victims were sent away to TB sanitoriums and isolated from society. The health professional's attitude toward individuals with TB should be no different from the attitude toward those with pneumonia. Both diseases are infectious and potentially curable. The American Lung Association provides excellent literature related to teaching as well as providing emotional support to the client and family.

Chronic Management When the chemotherapy regimen has been completed, most individuals can be considered adequately treated. Follow-up care may be indicated during the subsequent 12 months, including bacteriological studies and chest x-rays. Because about 5 percent of individuals experience relapse, clients should be taught to recognize the symptoms that indicate recurrence of TB. If these symptoms occur, they should seek immediate medical attention.

The client needs to be instructed about certain factors which could reactivate TB, such as immunosuppressive therapy, malignancy, and prolonged debilitating illness. If the client experiences any of these events, he needs to tell his health-care provider so he can be closely monitored for reactivation of TB. In some situations, it may be necessary to put the person on anti-TB chemotherapy.

Atypical mycobacteria

Pulmonary disease closely resembling TB may be caused by atypical acid-fast mycobacteria. This type of pulmonary disease is indistinguishable from TB clinically and radiologically but can be differentiated by bacteriological culture. These organisms are not believed to be airborne and thus are not transmitted by droplet nuclei.

Atypical mycobacteria that affect the lung include *Mycobacterium kansasii, M. scrofulaceum, M. intracellularis,* and *M. xenopi.* These bacteria (especially *M. intracellularis* and *M. scrofulaceum*) may also invade the cervical lymph nodes, causing lymphadenitis. This type of pulmonary disease typically occurs in white males with a history of chronic obstructive lung disease or silicosis.

Treatment depends on identification of the causative agent and determination of drug sensitivity. Many of the drugs used in treating TB are employed in combating infections from atypical mycobacteria.

Pulmonary Fungal Infections

Pulmonary fungal infections are increasing in incidence. They are found most frequently in seriously ill clients being treated with corticosteroids, antineoplastic and immunosuppressive drugs, and multiple antibiotics.[18] Types of fungal infections are presented in Table 20-10. These infections are not transmitted from person to person, and the client does not have to be placed in isolation. The clinical manifestations are similar to those of bacterial pneumonia. Skin and serology tests are available to assist in identifying the infecting organism. However, identification of the organism in a sputum specimen or other body fluids is the best diagnostic indicator.

Amphotericin B is the drug most widely used in treating systemic fungal infections. It must be given intravenously to achieve adequate blood and tissue levels because it is poorly absorbed from the GI tract. Amphotericin B is considered an α-toxic drug with many possible side effects, including hypersensitivity reactions, fever, chills, malaise, nausea and vomiting, thrombophlebitis at the injection site, and abnormal renal function. Monitoring of renal function is critical while a person is receiving this drug. Renal changes are at least partially reversible. Amphotericin infusions are incompatible with most other drugs. Therapy is frequently administered every other day after an initial period of several weeks of daily therapy. Total treatment with the drug may range from 4 to 10 weeks.[19]

5-Fluorocytosine has also been used in selected types of pulmonary fungal infections. It is given orally and becomes widely distributed in the body. Adverse reactions include abdominal discomfort, diarrhea, hepatotoxicity, and bone marrow suppression.

Bronchiectasis

Pathophysiology

Bronchiectasis is a disorder characterized by permanent, abnormal dilatation of one or more large bronchi. The pathological change resulting in dilatation is destruction of the elastic and muscular structures of the bronchial wall. There are two types of bronchiectasis, saccular and cylindrical (Fig. 20-2). *Saccular* bronchiectasis occurs mainly in large bronchi and is characterized by cavitylike dilatations. The affected bronchi end in large sacs. *Cylindrical* bronchiectasis involves medium-sized bronchi which are mildly to moderately dilated.

The most common cause of bronchiectasis is usually a bacterial infection, but other conditions such as congenital factors and obstruction predispose to the development of infection. *Congenital* factors include altered bronchial structures such as cysts and

Table 20-10
Fungal Infections of the Lung

Type	Organism	Characteristics
Histoplasmosis	*Histoplasma capsulatum*	Found in soil of North American river valleys Mycelia inhaled into the lungs Many infected individuals are asymptomatic Generally self-limiting disease Chronic disease resembles TB
Coccidioidomycosis	*Coccidioides immitis*	Found in semiarid regions of the southwestern United States Arthrospores inhaled into the lungs Causes suppurative and granulomatous reaction in the lungs One-third have symptomatic infection
Blastomycosis	*Blastomyces dermatitidis*	Found in the southeastern and midwestern United States Inhalation of fungus into lungs Disease often progresses insidiously May also involve the skin
Cryptococcosis	*Crytococcus histolyticus*	True yeast found in soil and pigeon excreta Inhalation of fungus into lungs May also cause meningitis
Aspergillosis	*Aspergillus niger or Aspergillus fumigatus*	True mold that inhabits the mouth Widely distributed in nature May invade lung tissue and cause necrotizing pneumonia In asthmatics, allergic bronchopulmonary aspergillosis may occur, requiring corticosteroid therapy
Actinomycosis	*Actinomyces bovi*	Not a true fungus, but has pseudohyphae Organisms are anaerobic, gram-positive, higher bacteria with branching hyphae Found as commensals in mouth and GI tract Necrotizing pneumonia produced after aspiration
Nocardiosis	*Nocardia asteroids*	Not a true fungus Organisms are aerobic, higher bacteria with branching hyphae Soil saprophyte widely distributed in nature Infection acquired from nature

cul-de-sacs which lead to pooling of secretions. In cystic fibrosis, there is retention and thickening of mucus that may plug the airways. A variety of immunodeficiency diseases are associated with recurrent bacterial pneumonias.

Obstructive processes of any kind can predispose to bronchiectasis. Examples include lung tumors, tumor masses in the chest cavity, aspirated foreign objects, and thick, tenacious secretions such as those found in chronic bronchitis. The obstruction causes the bronchi and bronchioles to distend and balloon out below the level of obstruction. This provides a good place for organisms to proliferate.

Almost all forms of bronchiectasis are associated with bacterial infections. Infections cause the bronchial walls to weaken, and pockets of infection begin to form. When the walls of the bronchial system are injured, the mucociliary mechanism is damaged, allowing bacteria, mucus, and dust to accumulate within the pockets. The infection becomes worse and results in bronchiectasis.

The disease process is often thought to start in childhood as an acquired disorder, beginning with respiratory complications secondary to influenza, measles, or whooping cough. Recurring lower respiratory tract infections are another pattern of disease in childhood that may predispose to bronchiectasis. This pattern typically is seen in individuals with cystic fibrosis, asthma, and immune-deficiency diseases.[20]

Clinical manifestations

The primary manifestations of bronchiectasis vary considerably depending on the extent and location of the disease process. They include chronic cough with production of mucopurulent sputum, hemoptysis, and recurrent pneumonia. The cough is paroxysmal and is often stimulated with position changes. Other manifestations include exertional dyspnea, fatigue, weight loss, anorexia, and fetid breath. Sinusitis frequently

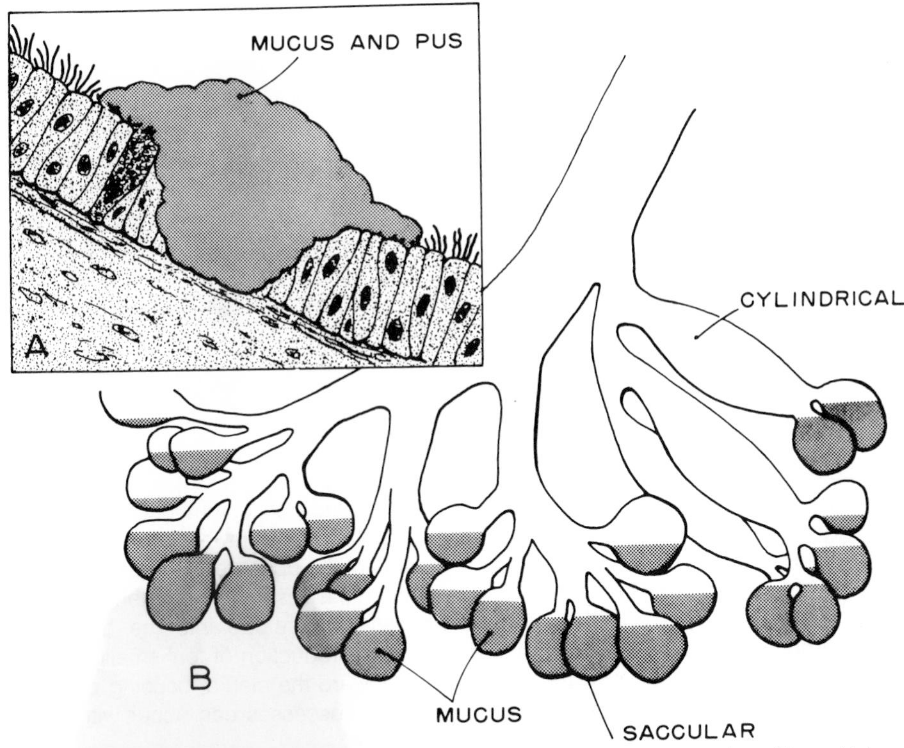

Figure 20-2 Pathological changes in bronchiectasis. *(a)* Longitudinal section of bronchial wall, where chronic infection has caused damage; *(b)* collection of purulent material in dilated bronchioles, leading to persistent infection. *(From S. Price and L. Wilson, Pathophysiology: Clinical Concepts of Disease Processes, 2d ed., McGraw-Hill Book Company, New York, 1982, p. 439.)*

accompanies diffuse bronchiectasis. The manifestations of advanced, widespread bronchiectasis are generalized wheezing, digital clubbing, and cor pulmonale.

Medical management

Diagnostic An individual with a chronic productive cough with increased sputum (that may be blood-streaked) should be suspected of having bronchiectasis. Characteristic findings in the health history such as childhood diseases complicated by respiratory infections or chronic bronchitis are very significant. Chest x-rays are usually done and may show streaky infiltrates. *Bronchography* involves instilling radiopaque material into the bronchial system via a catheter or bronchoscope and is useful in evaluating individuals with moderate to severe cases of bronchiectasis. *Bronchoscopy* may be useful in identifying the source of secretions or sites of hemoptysis in individuals with chronic productive cough.

Collection of sputum to evaluate its quantity, characteristics, and microbial content may provide additional information regarding the severity of impairment and the presence of active infection. Pulmonary function studies may be abnormal in advanced bronchiectasis. A complete blood count may be normal or show evidence of anemia and leukocytosis.

Therapeutic Bronchiectasis is difficult to treat. Antibiotics are the major form of treatment and should be given based on sputum culture results. Other forms of drug therapy may include bronchodilators, mucolytic agents, and expectorants. Maintaining good hydration is very important to liquefy secretions. Postural drainage is vital to facilitate expectoration of sputum. (Postural drainage is discussed in Chap. 21, in the section on Chest Physiotherapy in clients with chronic obstructive pulmonary disease [COPD].) The individual should reduce exposure to excessive air pollutants and irritants, avoid cigarette smoking, and obtain pneumococcal and influenza vaccines.

Surgical resection of parts of the lungs, although not used as often as previously, may be done if medical treatment is not effective. Surgical resection of an affected lobe or segment may be indicated for the client with repeated bouts of pneumonia and hemoptysis and disabling complications. Surgery is not advisable when there is diffuse or widespread involvement. (The surgical approaches are discussed in the section on Chest Trauma and Surgery later in this chapter.)

Nursing management

Health Promotion and Maintenance Bronchiectasis has shown a decline in recent years. This is partially due to the administration of measles and pertussis vaccines, which decreases the incidence of bronchiectasis from these diseases. Early detection and treatment of lower respiratory tract infections prevent them from developing into complications such as bronchiectasis. Any obstructing lesion or foreign body should be removed promptly. Other measures to decrease the occurrence or progression of bronchiectasis include avoiding cigarette smoking and decreasing exposure to pollution. Children with persistent coughs should receive a medical evaluation to determine the source of the problem.

Acute and Chronic Intervention An important nursing goal is to promote drainage and removal of bronchial mucus. The client should be taught effective deep-breathing exercises and how to cough effectively (Table 21-10). Postural drainage should be done on affected parts of the lung (see Fig. 21-9). Some individuals require elevation of the foot of the bed by 4 to 6 inches to facilitate drainage. Pillows may be used in the hospital as well as the home to help the client assume postural drainage positions. Administration of the prescribed antibiotics, bronchodilators, or expectorants is important. The client needs to understand the importance of taking the prescribed regimen of drugs to obtain maximum effectiveness. The client should be aware of possible side or adverse effects that must be reported to the physician.

Rest is important to prevent overexertion. Bed rest may be indicated during the acute phase of the illness. Chilling and excess fatigue should be avoided.

Good nutrition is important and may be difficult to maintain because the client is often anorexic. Oral hygiene to cleanse the mouth and remove dried sputum crusts may improve the person's appetite. Offering foods that are appealing may also increase the client's desire to eat.

The client and family should be taught to recognize significant manifestations to be reported to the health care provider. These manifestations include increased sputum production, grossly bloody sputum, increasing dyspnea, fever, chills, and chest pain.

Lung Abscess

Pathophysiology

Lung abscess is a pus-containing lesion of the lung parenchyma which gives rise to a cavity. The cavity is formed by necrosis of the lung tissue. In many cases, the etiology and pathogenesis of lung abscess are similar to those of pneumonia. The most common etiological factor is aspiration of material into the lungs (Table 20-11). In addition to producing infection, the organisms involved cause necrosis of the lung tissue. Examples include enteric gram-negative organisms such as *Klebsiella, S. aureus,* and anaerobic bacilli. Lung abscess can also result from hematogenously spread lung infarct secondary to pulmonary embolus, malignant growth, TB, and various parasitic and fungal diseases of the lung.

The areas of the lung most commonly affected are the apical segments of the lower lobes and the posterior segments of the upper lobes. Fibrous tissue usually forms around the abscess in an attempt to wall it off. The abscess may erode into the bronchial system, causing the production of foul-smelling sputum. It may grow toward the pleura, causing pleuritic pain. Multiple small abscesses can occur within the lung.

Clinical manifestations and complications

The onset of a lung abscess is usually insidious, especially if anaerobic organisms are the primary cause. A more acute onset occurs with aerobic organisms. The most common manifestation is cough productive of purulent sputum (often dark brown) that is foul smelling and foul tasting. Hemoptysis is common, especially at the time an abscess ruptures into a bronchus. Other common manifestations are fever, chills, prostration, pleuritic pain, dyspnea, cough, and weight loss. The history may reveal a predisposing condition such as alcoholism, pneumonia, or oral infection.

Physical examination of the lungs indicates dullness to percussion and decreased breath sounds on auscultation. Rales may also be present in the later stages as the abscess drains. Oral examination often reveals dental caries, gingivitis, and periodontal infection.

Complications that can result include chronic pulmonary abscess, hemorrhage from abscess erosion into blood vessels, brain abscess due to the spread of infection, bronchopleural fistula, and empyema from abscess perforation into the pleural cavity.

Medical management

Diagnostic A chest x-ray before emptying of the abscess reveals a circumscribed area of infiltration.

After the abscess is drained, a chest x-ray will show an area of consolidation with a wall around a lucent zone. Sputum culture and Gram stain are necessary to identify the infecting organism. Bronchoscopy may be used to locate the site of the abscess. Leukocytosis is usually present.

Therapeutic Antibiotics given for a prolonged period (up to 6 weeks) are usually the primary method of treatment. Penicillin is generally the drug of choice because of the frequent presence of anaerobic organisms. Chest physiotherapy and postural drainage are sometimes used to drain abscesses located in the lower or posterior portions of the lung. Surgery is rarely indicated. The use of bronchoscopy for drainage of an abscess is controversial. Some clinicians feel that this procedure may spread the infection to other parts of the lung. If used, bronchoscopy should be done 24 to 48 hours after initiation of antimicrobial therapy.

Nursing management

Drainage of the abscess and treatment of the infection are the primary goals. The client should be taught how to cough effectively. Chest physiotherapy will help to loosen secretions. Postural drainage according to the lung area involved will aid the removal of secretions (see Fig. 21-9). Frequent (every 2 to 3 hours) mouth care is needed to relieve the putrid odor from the foul-smelling sputum. Diluted hydrogen peroxide and mouthwash are often effective.

Because of the need for prolonged antibiotic therapy, the client must be aware of the need to continue taking medication for the prescribed period. The client needs to know about untoward side effects to be reported to the health care provider. Sometimes the client is asked to return periodically during the course of antibiotic therapy for repeat cultures and sensitivity tests to ensure that the organism is not becoming resistant to the antibiotic. When antibiotic therapy is completed, the client is reevaluated.

Rest, good nutrition, and adequate fluid intake are all supportive measures to facilitate recovery. If dentition is poor and dental hygiene is not adequate, the client should be encouraged to obtain dental care.

Table 20-11
Common Causes of Lung Abscess

Type of Abscess	Cause
Aspiration abscess	Alcoholism Postanesthesia Oversedation Coma (e.g., diabetic, epileptic, drug overdose, cerebrovascular accident) Oral infection Food or foreign body Laryngeal palsy Carcinoma of esophagus ("spillover" aspiration)
Malignant abscess	Necrotic bronchial carcinoma Secondary to bronchial obstruction and stasis of secretions Head and neck malignancies
Pulmonary embolus	Pulmonary infarct infection Septic emboli Fragments from bacterial endarteritis
Infection	Pneumonia Pyogenic bacteria (notably *Staphylococcus aureus*) Defective ciliary action Ineffective expectoration Infected cysts Necrotic lesions Subdiaphragmatic infections (usually liver) Open chest wounds

M. Kinney et al., *AACN's Clinical Reference for Critical-Care Nursing,* McGraw-Hill Book Company, New York, 1981, p. 506.

OXYGEN THERAPY

Oxygen therapy will be discussed in this section since it is frequently used in the treatment of respiratory problems. Oxygen (O_2) is a colorless, odorless, tasteless gas that constitutes 20.95 percent of the atmosphere. Used clinically it is considered a drug. Administering supplemental oxygen raises the partial pressure of oxygen (PO_2) in inspired air.

Indications for Oxygen Administration

Oxygen is usually administered to treat hypoxemia caused by:

1. *Respiratory disorders* such as COPD, pneumonia, lung cancer, and pulmonary emboli
2. *Cardiovascular disorders* such as myocardial infarction, arrhythmias, and cardiogenic shock
3. *Central nervous system disorders* such as overdose of narcotics, anesthesia, and head injury

Methods of Oxygen Administration

The goal of oxygen administration is to supply the client with adequate oxygen to maximize the oxygen-carrying ability of the blood. There are various methods of oxygen administration (Table 20-12 and Figs. 20-3 and 20-4). The method selected depends on factors such as the forced inspiratory oxygen (FIO_2)

Table 20-12
Methods of Oxygen Administration

Method	Advantages	Disadvantages	Comments
Nasal catheter	Allows continuous, uninterrupted O_2 therapy. Client will receive O_2 even if a mouth breather. Does not interfere with client care.	Must be inserted into nasopharynx through a nostril. Can produce excoriation of the nares. High flow rates (>6 L/min) can cause drying of nasal membranes. Inadvertent gas flow distends into stomach. Does not permit a high degree of humidification. Must be taped to client's face.	Catheter should be changed every 8 h. Alternate the nostrils. Distance catheter is to be inserted is measured from distance between tip of nose and earlobe. A flow rate of 5–6 L/min gives an oxygen concentration of about 30%. Best used for short-term therapy.
Nasal cannula (nasal prongs)	May be used by a restless client. Safe and simple method. Relatively comfortable and acceptable. Useful for clients requiring low O_2 concentrations (e.g., COPD). Allows client to move about in bed. Client can eat, talk, or cough while wearing device.	Difficult to maintain in position and can be easily dislodged. Client must be alert and cooperative to keep cannula in proper place. High flow rates (>5 L/min) dry the nasal membranes and may cause pain in frontal sinuses.	Nasal cannula should be stabilized when caring for a restless client. A flow rate of 2 L/min gives an oxygen concentration of about 24%. Amount of O_2 inhaled depends on room air and client's own breathing. Most clients with COPD can tolerate 2 L/min via cannula.
Simple face mask	Oxygen can be given quickly for short periods of time. With flow rates of 6–12 L/min, O_2 concentrations of 35–60% can be achieved. Provides for adequate humidification of inspired air.	Lack of client tolerance results in inadequate therapy. May be uncomfortable since a tight seal must be maintained between face and mask. Mask may produce a pressure necrosis of the skin. Confines heat radiating from the face about the nose and mouth. Must be removed to eat or drink.	Wash, dry, and powder under mask every 2 h. Mask needs to fit tightly. Nasal cannula may be provided while eating. Watch for pressure necrosis at the top of ears from elastic straps.
Venturi mask	Can deliver precise, high-flow rates of O_2. Lightweight plastic, cone-shaped, fitted to face. Masks are available for delivery of 24, 28, 31, 35, and 40% O_2. Adaptors can be applied to increase humidification.	Mask is uncomfortable. Must be removed when client eats. Client can talk, but voice may be muffled.	Mask must be changed to deliver higher concentrations of O_2. Especially helpful for administering low, constant O_2 concentrations to clients with COPD. Air entrainment ports must not be occluded.
Partial rebreathing mask	Lightweight and easy to use. Reservoir bag conserves O_2. Concentrations of 35–90% can be achieved using flow rates of 6–10 L/min.	Cannot be used with a high degree of humidity.	Useful when the blood O_2 concentrations must be raised. Not recommended for client with COPD. Should never be used with a nebulizer. Bag should not be allowed to deflate.
Nonrebreathing mask	High concentrations of O_2 can be delivered accurately. Oxygen flows into bag and mask during inhalation. Valve prevents expired air from flowing back into bag. Concentrations of 95–100% can be achieved.	Cannot be used with a high degree of humidity.	Mask should fit snugly. Flow rate must be sufficient to keep bag from collapsing.

Table 20-12 (Continued)

Method	Advantages	Disadvantages	Comments
Face tent (face hood)	Ideal for providing moderate to high-density aerosol. Oxygen concentration administered varies with oxygen flow rate.	Less reliable than face mask for maintaining high inspiration of O_2 concentration.	Open plastic mask that fits under the chin. Temperature of aerosol needs to be checked to prevent burning the client.
Tent	Able to control temperature and humidity.	Limited usefulness. Difficult to maintain adequate concentrations of O_2. Isolates client from environment.	Tent should be flushed with O_2 every time it is opened. Assess for leaks around canopy.
Tracheostomy collar	Can deliver high humidity and O_2 via tracheostomy.	Condensed fluid in tubing may drain into tracheostomy. Secretions collect inside collar and around tracheostomy. Oxygen concentration lost into atmosphere because collar does not fit tightly.	Attaches to neck with elastic strap. Should be removed and cleaned at least every 4 h to prevent aspiration of fluid and infection.
Tracheostomy T bar (T tube, Brigg's adaptor)	Tight fit allows better O_2 and humidity delivery than tracheostomy collar.	Condensed fluid in tubing may drain into tracheostomy. Empty as necessary.	Needs to be removed for suctioning. May use norche swivel and eliminate the need for removal.

and humidification required, client cooperation, and comfort.

Most methods of oxygen administration are low-flow devices which deliver O_2 in concentrations that vary with the person's breathing. In contrast, the Venturi mask is a high-flow device that delivers fixed concentrations of oxygen.[21] With the Venturi mask, O_2 is delivered to a small jet (Venturi device) in the center of a wide-based cone (Fig. 20-5). Air is *entrained* (pulled through) openings in the cone as oxygen flows through the small jet. The mask has large vents through which exhaled air can escape. The degree of restriction or narrowness of the jet determines the amount of entrainment and dilution of pure O_2 with room air, and thus the concentration of oxygen.

Humidification and Nebulizers

Oxygen obtained from cylinders or wall systems (Fig. 20-6) is dry. Dry oxygen has an irritating effect on mucous membranes and dries up secretions. Therefore, it is important that O_2 be humidified when administered, either by humidification or nebulization. A common device used for humidification when the client has a catheter, cannula, or low-flow mask is a *bubble humidifier*. It is a small plastic jar filled with sterile distilled water. It is attached to the oxygen source by means of a flowmeter. Oxygen passes into the jar, bubbles through the water, and then goes through tubing to the client's catheter, cannula, or mask. The purpose of the bubble humidifier is to restore the humidity conditions of room air.

Another means of administering humidified oxygen is via a *nebulizer*. It delivers particulate water mist (aerosols) with a high humidity. The humidity can be raised by heating the water and thus increases the ability of the gas to hold moisture. Heated (37°C, 98.6°F) and humidified (100%) gas is required when the upper airway is bypassed. When nebulizers are

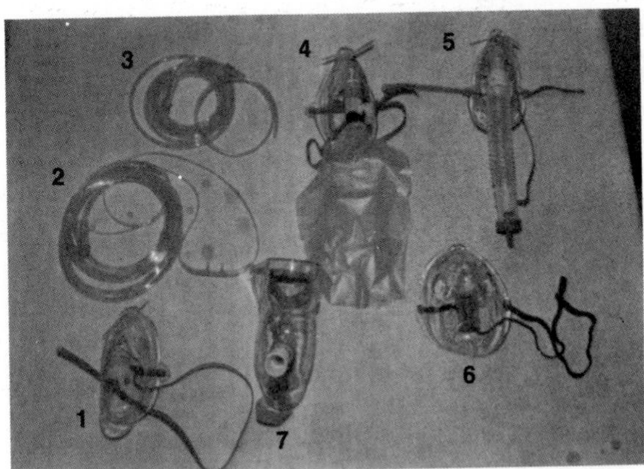

Figure 20-3 Methods of oxygen administration. Shown are (reading clockwise from lower left): (1) aerosol mask; (2) nasal cannula (prongs); (3) nasal catheter; (4) rebreathing mask; (5) Venturi mask; (6) face tent; and (7) simple face mask.

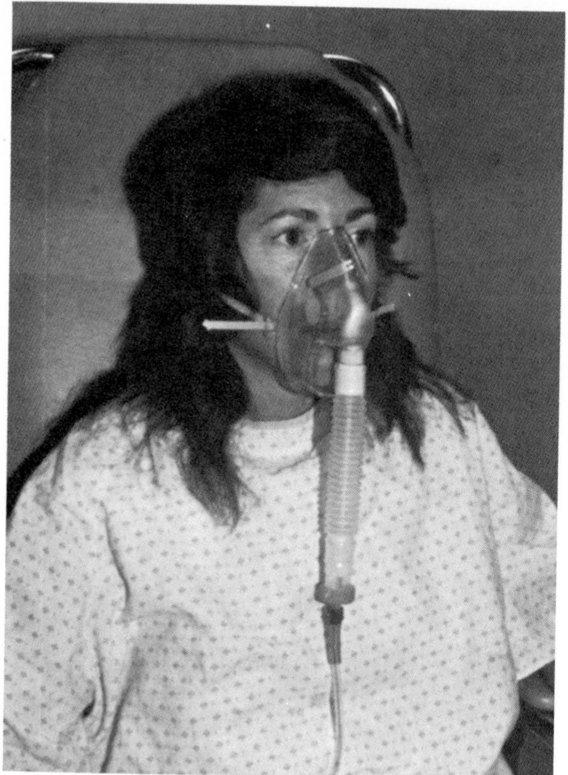
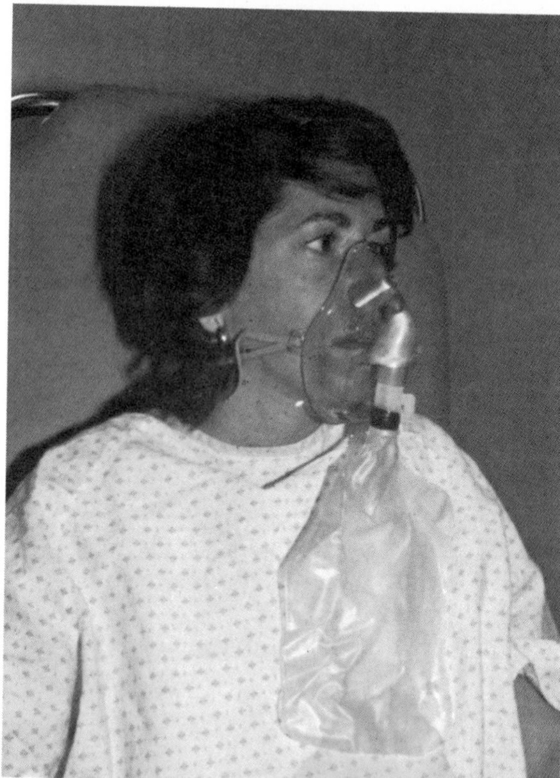

Figure 20-4 *(a)* Venturi mask in place. *(b)* Rebreathing mask in place.

used, large-size tubing should be employed to connect the device to a face mask or T bar. If small-size tubing is used, condensation can occlude the flow of oxygen.

Complications of Oxygen Therapy

Combustion

Oxygen supports combustion and increases the rate of burning. This is why it is so important that smoking be prohibited in the area where oxygen is being used. A "No Smoking" sign should be prominently displayed on the client's door. The client should also be cautioned against smoking cigarettes with O_2 prongs or a catheter in place.

CO_2 narcosis

It is important to remember that in some cases of respiratory distress, increasing the oxygen flow rate may be quite harmful. Normally, carbon dioxide (CO_2) accumulation is a major stimulant of the respiratory center. However, individuals with a long-standing history of COPD or who are heavily sedated develop a tendency to hypoventilate and to retain carbon dioxide. Gradually, the respiratory center loses its sensitivity to the elevated carbon dioxide level. For these individuals, the major stimulant of respiration is hypoxemia. When oxygen is administered in high concentrations, the hypoxic stimulus is eliminated and the rate and depth of ventilation will decrease. The client will subsequently develop hypercapnia and eventually CO_2 narcosis.

It is critical to start oxygen at low flows until arterial blood gases can be obtained. Arterial blood gases are used as a guide to determine what FIO_2 level is sufficient and can be tolerated. The client's mental status and vital signs should be assessed before starting O_2 therapy and frequently thereafter.

Oxygen toxicity

Pulmonary oxygen toxicity may result from prolonged exposure to a high P_aO_2. The development of O_2 toxicity is determined by client tolerance, exposure time, and effective dose. It is thought that high concentrations of oxygen may inactivate pulmonary surfactant and lead to the development of the adult respiratory distress syndrome (ARDS). The lungs from individuals who die after prolonged administration of

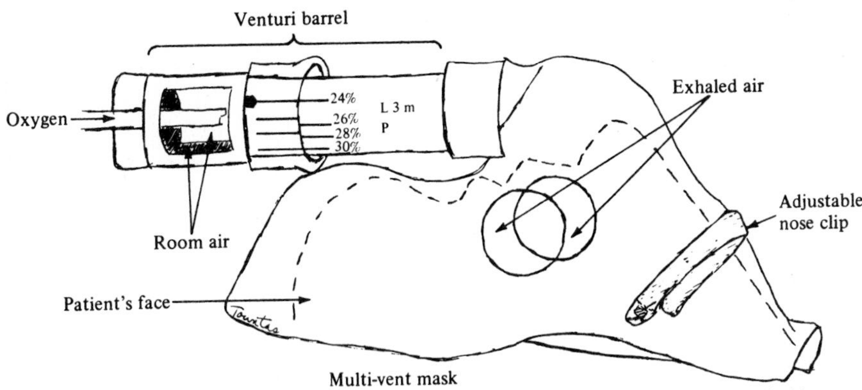

Figure 20-5 Venturi mask mixes room air with oxygen at present ratios. *(From L. M. Shortridge and E. J. Lee, Introductory Skills for Nursing Practice, McGraw-Hill Book Company, New York, 1980, p. 311.)*

100% O_2 show some or all of the following abnormalities on autopsy:[22]

1. Lungs are heavy, "beefy," and edematous.
2. Hyaline membranes cover many alveoli, alveolar ducts, and respiratory bronchioles.
3. Many alveoli are filled with hemorrhagic exudate.
4. Alveolar septa are markedly increased.

Early manifestations of oxygen toxicity are a reduced vital capacity, cough, substernal chest pain, nausea and vomiting, paresthesia, nasal stuffiness, sore throat, and malaise. The later stages of oxygen toxicity affect the alveolar-capillary gas exchange unit, causing edema and production of copious sputum. The end stage of oxygen toxicity is progressive fibrosis of the lung.

Prevention of oxygen toxicity is very important for the client receiving O_2. The amount of O_2 administered should be just enough to maintain the arterial oxygen pressure (P_aO_2) within a normal or acceptable range for the client. Arterial blood gases should be monitored frequently to evaluate the effectiveness of therapy as well as to guide the tapering of supplemental O_2. A safe limit of O_2 concentrations has not yet been established. All levels above 50 to 60% should be considered potentially toxic. Levels of 40% and below may be regarded as relatively nontoxic.

Absorption atelectasis

Normally nitrogen, which constitutes 79 percent of the air we breathe, is not absorbed into the bloodstream, and it prevents alveolar collapse. When high concentrations of oxygen are given, nitrogen is washed out of the alveoli and replaced with O_2. If airway obstruction occurs, the oxygen is absorbed into the bloodstream and the alveoli collapse. This process is called *absorption atelectasis.*

Infection

Infection can be a major hazard of oxygen administration. Heated nebulizers present the highest risk. The constant use of humidity supports bacterial growth; the most common infecting organism is *Pseudomonas.* To prevent infection, disposable equipment should be used and changed every 24 hours. A hospital policy of frequent changes of disposable equipment should be instituted. Both equipment and respiratory secretions should be Gram-stained and cultured frequently. (Nursing care of the client receiving oxygen therapy is presented in Table 20-13.)

Oxygen supply at home

Some individuals who are disabled with severe chronic lung disease benefit considerably by having an oxygen supply in their home. Nasal prongs are used to deliver O_2 from a central source which can be

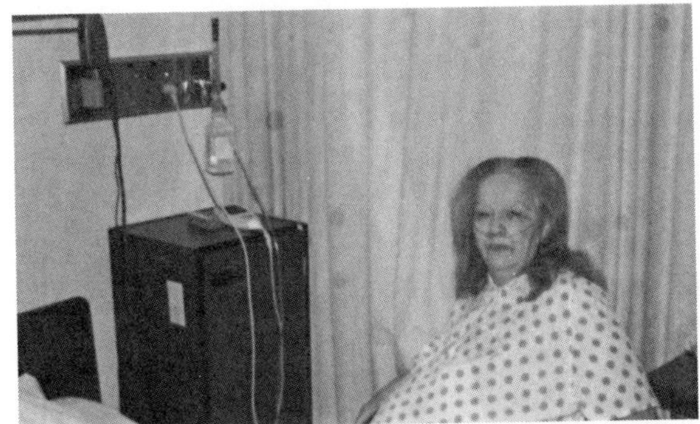

Figure 20-6 Oxygen wall unit with nasal prongs used for oxygen administration.

Table 20-13

Nursing Care Plan for the Client Receiving Oxygen Therapy

Client Problem	Expected Outcome	Nursing Intervention
Hypoxemia (inadequate arterial oxygenation)	Client's P_aO_2 will be appropriate. No manifestations of hypoxia.	Monitor arterial blood gases (ABGs) before starting oxygen if possible, after 20–30 min of receiving oxygen, and with every change in oxygen administration. Assess client for signs of inadequate oxygenation (e.g., tachycardia, restlessness). Device should fit snugly. Assess client's comfort with device in place.
Potential skin breakdown	No skin breakdown under delivery device or strap.	Do not fit strap too tightly. If mask is used, remove it every 2 h and wash and dry skin. Pad any pressure points. Observe tops of ears for skin breakdown at pressure points.
Potential mucosal drying	No evidence or complaints of mucosal discomfort.	If needed, water-based jelly may be used on lips and nasal mucosa. Do not obstruct cannula outlets with jelly. Provide frequent oral hygiene. Provide humidification via humidifier or nebulizing device.
Potential bacterial contamination of equipment	No evidence of infection.	Remove mask or collar and cleanse with water every 4–8 h. Cleanse skin carefully at this time and prn. Regularly obtain Gram stains and culture of secretions. Disposable equipment should be changed frequently. Remove secretions that are coughed out. Empty container by flushing down the toilet.
Potential fire from O_2-enriched environment	No spark or other hazard will exist.	Post "No Smoking" warning sign prominently. Do not use electric razors, portable radios, open flames, wool blankets, or mineral oils. No smoking in the room. Teach client about precautions related to home O_2 therapy.
Potential CO_2 narcosis in client with chronic COPD	No CO_2 narcosis as evidenced by rising PCO_2 and/or decreased level of consciousness.	Identify clients at risk for CO_2 narcosis. Administer oxygen at ordered level only. Monitor results with ABGs. Do not increase the oxygen flow to treat respiratory distress. Start oxygen at low flow rates (1–3 L/min) until ABGs can be obtained. Assess baseline level of consciousness, respiratory rate, and pulse rate and monitor frequently.
Potential oxygen toxicity	Client will receive minimal O_2 therapy to maintain adequate P_aO_2.	Administer oxygen at the lowest level which produces acceptable ABGs. Monitor ABGs frequently. Monitor client for manifestations of substernal discomfort, cough, nasal congestion, sore throat, and confusion. Do not attempt to use FIO_2 over 60% for more than 24 h unless specifically indicated.
Rapid fall in P_aO_2 when O_2 is discontinued	Maintain adequate arterial oxygenation.	Administer oxygen continuously unless it is specifically ordered only for exercise or sleep. Encourage client to wear the oxygen-delivery device properly. If a mask is used, provide a nasal cannula during meals. Take rectal temperature if mask is being used. Provide enough tubing to reach from oxygen source to bathroom if client is ambulatory or to move around house if client is at home. Provide portable oxygen for ambulation outside hospital room or home. Client should be weaned from O_2 in increments.

a liquid oxygen storage system, a gas cylinder storage bank, or a machine that makes O_2. Long tubing can be used to increase the client's mobility around the home (e.g., climbing stairs). A small, portable O_2 tank on a special cart can be used away from home for shopping or traveling. Portable oxygen can greatly increase the client's level of activity and provide more mobility.

Home oxygen systems are usually rented from a company which sends a respiratory therapist or pulmonary nurse specialist to the client's home. The therapist will teach the client how to use the system, care for it, and recognize when the oxygen supply is running low and should be reordered.

The client who uses home oxygen therapy should be encouraged to travel normally. If he is traveling by car, he can make arrangements for oxygen to be available when he makes motel reservations in advance. If a client flies, he should know that he must use the plane's oxygen system while in flight. Most portable oxygen systems are not properly pressurized for use during flight. In general, the client should also be encouraged to plan his travels so as to avoid areas of high elevation.

OCCUPATIONAL LUNG DISEASES

Occupational lung diseases result from inhaled dust or chemicals.[23] The duration of exposure and the amount of inhalant have a major influence on whether exposed individuals will develop lung damage. Another factor is the susceptibility of the host.

Pneumoconiosis is a general term for lung diseases caused by inhalation and retention of dust particles. The literal meaning of pneumoconiosis is "dust in the lungs." Examples of this condition include silicosis, asbestosis, and berylliosis. The classic response to the inhaled substance is diffuse parenchymal infiltration with phagocytic cells. This results eventually in *diffuse pulmonary fibrosis* (excess connective tissue). Fibrosis is the result of tissue repair following inflammation. Pneumoconiosis and other types of occupational lung diseases are presented in Table 20-14.

Clinical Features

Symptoms of occupational lung disease usually do not occur until at least 10 to 15 years after the initial exposure to the inhaled irritant. Dyspnea and cough are often the earliest manifestations. Chest pain and productive sputum usually occur later. Complications that often result are pneumonia, chronic bronchitis, emphysema, and lung cancer. Manifestations of these diseases can be presenting symptoms.

Pulmonary function studies show reduced vital capacity. A chest x-ray will often reveal lung involvement specific to the primary problem. Cor pulmonale is a late complication, especially in conditions characterized by diffuse pulmonary fibrosis.

Management

The best approach to management is to try to prevent or decrease occupational risks. Well-designed, effective ventilation systems can reduce exposure to irritants. Wearing masks is appropriate in some occupations. Mining and industrial commissions are planning ways to decrease exposure to dusts and other irritants. New materials that are developed need to be studied in terms of their potential risks. Cigarette smoking adds increased insult to the lungs, and persons at risk for occupational lung disease should not smoke.

Early diagnosis is essential if the disease process is to be halted. The best treatment is to decrease or stop exposure to the harmful agent. Some places of employment where there is a known risk of lung disease may require periodic chest x-rays and pulmonary function studies. These measures can detect pulmonary changes before symptoms develop.

There is no specific treatment for occupational lung diseases. Treatment is directed toward providing symptomatic relief. If there are coexisting problems such as pneumonia, chronic bronchitis, or emphysema, they are appropriately treated.

LUNG CANCER

Significance of the Problem

Primary lung cancer is the leading cause of death in men who die of malignant disease in the United States. The incidence of lung cancer in women is also rapidly rising. In 1981 there were an estimated 122,000 new cases of lung cancer. The incidence of this disease has doubled every 10 years in the past few decades.[24]

In 1981 there were an estimated 105,000 deaths due to lung cancer. The mortality rate is high, with only about 10 percent of lung cancer victims living for 5 years or more after diagnosis.[25]

Lung cancer occurs most commonly in an individual more than 50 years old with a long history of cigarette smoking. The disease is found most frequently in persons 40 to 75 years of age. Until recently, more cases of lung cancer were found in men than in women. That situation is changing, probably due to the fact that since the 1930s and 1940s cigarette smoking became socially acceptable for women.

Etiology and Risk Factors

Cigarette smoking is by far the major risk factor in the development of lung cancer. Smoking is responsible for more than 75 percent of all lung cancers.[26] About 1 out of every 10 heavy smokers eventually develops lung cancer. Cigarette smoking causes a change in the bronchial epithelium, which usually returns to normal when smoking is discontinued. The risk of lung cancer is gradually lowered to that of a nonsmoker after 10 to 13 years of nonsmoking.[27]

Studies are also beginning to show that there may be a risk from secondhand smoke; that is, the nonsmoking spouse of a smoker has a higher risk of developing lung cancer than the nonsmoking spouse of a nonsmoker. Heredity may play a role in both the tendency to smoke and the predisposition to develop

Table 20-14
Occupational Lung Diseases

Disease	Agents/Industries	Description	Complications
Asbestosis	Asbestos fibers found in: Insulation Construction (roof tiling, cement products) Shipyards Textiles (fireproofing) Automobile clutch and brake linings	Disease appears 15–35 yr after first exposure. Interstitial fibrosis develops. Pleural plaques, which are calcified lesions, develop on pleura. Dyspnea, basal rales, and decreased vital capacity are early manifestations.	Lung cancer, especially in cigarette smokers. Mesothelioma (rare type of cancer affecting pleura and peritoneal membrane).
Berylliosis	Beryllium dust found in: Aircraft manufacturing Metallurgy Rocket fuels	Formation of noncaseating granulomas. Acute pneumonitis occurs after heavy exposure. Interstitial fibrosis can also occur.	Disease can progress after removal of stimulating inhalant.
Byssinosis	Cotton, flax, and hemp dust. Textile industry.	Airway obstruction caused by contraction of smooth muscles. Chronic disease results from severe airway obstruction and decreased elastic recoil.	Chronic disease progresses after dust exposure ceases.
Coal worker's pneumoconiosis (black lung)	Coal dust.	Incidence is high (20–30%) in coal workers. Deposits of carbon dust cause lesions to develop along respiratory bronchioles. Dilatation of bronchioles due to loss of wall structure. Development of chronic airway obstruction and bronchitis. Dyspnea and cough are common early symptoms.	Progressive, massive lung fibrosis. Smoking increases risk of chronic bronchitis and emphysema.
Farmer's lung	Inhalation of airborne material from moldy hay or similar matter.	Hypersensitivity pneumonitis. The *acute* form is similar to pneumonia, with manifestation of chills, fever, malaise, etc. The *chronic*, insidious form is a type of pulmonary fibrosis.	Progressive fibrosis of the lung.
Siderosis	Iron oxide found in: Welding Foundries Iron ore mining	Dust deposits found in lung.	
Silicosis	Silica (SiO_2) dust found in quartz rock in mining of gold, copper, tin, coal, and lead. Also present in sandblasting, foundries, quarries, pottery making, and masonry.	In *chronic disease*, dust is engulfed by macrophages and may be destroyed, resulting in fibrotic nodules. *Acute disease* results from intense exposure in a short time period. Within 5 yr, it progresses to severe disability from lung fibrosis.	Lungs more susceptible to TB. Progressive, massive fibrosis. High incidence of chronic bronchitis.
Silo filler's disease	Nitrogen oxides from fermentation of vegetation in freshly filled silo.	Chemical pneumonitis.	Progressive bronchiolitis obliterans.

lung cancer. Since only a few persons (1 out of 10) who are at high risk actually develop lung cancer, there must be a difference in the host's ability to deal with the repeated insult of smoking.

Another major risk factor in the etiology of lung cancer is inhaled carcinogens. These include asbestos, nickel, iron and iron oxides, uranium, chromates, arsenic, and air pollution. The cigarette smoker who is also exposed to one or more of these chemicals or to high amounts of air pollution significantly increases the risk of lung cancer.

Lung cancer does occur in individuals who have never smoked or worked with carcinogens. The reasons for this are not known, but heredity may play a part. As previously mentioned, the host's response to environmental insults is important. It is also possible that the susceptibility to lung cancer is inherited, as family correlations have been found.[28]

Another possible risk factor is preexisting pulmonary diseases such as TB, pulmonary fibrosis, bronchiectasis, and COPD. It has been shown that chronic inflammatory conditions often precede cancer. The incidence of lung cancer correlates with the degree of urbanization and population density. The reason for this may be increased exposure to irritants and pollutants.

Pathogenesis

The pathogenesis of primary lung cancer is not well understood. Over 90 percent of cancers originate from the epithelium of the bronchus (bronchogenic). They grow slowly; it takes 8 to 10 years for a tumor to reach 1 cm in size. Lung cancers occur primarily in the segmental bronchi or beyond and have a preference for the upper lobes of the lungs. Pathological changes in the bronchial system show nonspecific inflammatory changes with hypersecretion of mucus, desquamation of cells, reactive hyperplasia of the basal cells, and metaplasia of normal respiratory epithelium to stratified squamous cells.

Primary lung cancers are often categorized into histological types (Table 20-15). They metastasize primarily by direct extension and via the blood circulation and the lymph system. The common sites for metastatic growth are the scalene lymph nodes, liver, brain, adrenal glands, and bones.

Paraneoplastic syndrome

Certain lung cancers cause the *paraneoplastic syndrome,* which is characterized by various manifestations caused by certain substances (hormones, enzymes, antigens) produced by the tumor cells. Oat-cell (small cell) carcinomas are most commonly associated with the paraneoplastic syndrome. The systemic manifestations are:[29]

1. *Hormonal*—See Table 20-16
2. *Dermatologic*—Including dermatomyositis and acanthosis nigricans
3. *Neuromuscular*—Including peripheral neuropathy, cortical cerebellar degeneration, and a myasthenialike syndrome
4. *Vascular and hematologic*—Including thrombocytopenic purpura, anemia, leukemoid reaction, thrombophlebitis, and nonbacterial endocarditis
5. *Connective tissue*—Including nonspecific arthralgias, hypertrophic pulmonary osteoarthropathy, and digital clubbing

Clinical Manifestations

The clinical manifestations of lung cancer are usually nonspecific and present late in the disease process. Manifestations depend upon the type of primary lung cancer. Often there is extensive metastasis before symptoms become apparent. Persistent pneumonitis due to obstructed bronchi may be one of the earliest manifestations, causing fever, chills, and cough.

One of the most significant symptoms, and often the one reported first, is a persistent cough that may be productive of sputum. Blood-tinged sputum may be produced due to bleeding of the malignancy but hemoptysis is not a common early presenting symptom. Chest pain may be present; it may be localized or unilateral, mild to severe. Dyspnea and an auscultatory wheeze may be present if there is bronchial obstruction.

Later manifestations may include nonspecific systemic symptoms such as anorexia, fatigue, weight loss, and nausea and vomiting. Hoarseness may be present due to involvement of the recurrent laryngeal nerve. Unilateral paralysis of the diaphragm, dysphagia, and superior vena cava obstruction may occur due to intrathoracic spread of the malignancy. There may be palpable lymph nodes in the neck or axilla. Mediastinal involvement may lead to pericardial effusion, cardiac tamponade, and arrhythmias.

Medical Management

Diagnostic

Chest x-rays are widely used in the diagnosis of lung cancer (Table 20-17). Anyone who has had a cough or a change in a cough for more than 2 to 3

Table 20-15
Comparison of the Types of Primary Lung Cancer

Cell Type	Risk Factors	Characteristics	Response to Therapy
Squamous cell (epidermoid) carcinoma	Almost always associated with cigarette smoking. Exposure to environmental carcinogens (e.g., uranium, asbestos)	Accounts for 60% of lung cancers More common in men Arises from the bronchial epithelium (Fig. 20-7) Produces earlier symptoms because of bronchial obstructive characteristics Does not have a strong tendency to metastasize Metastasizes locally by direct extension Causes cavitating pulmonary lesions	Surgical resection is often attempted Life expectancy better than for undifferentiated (anaplastic) carcinoma
Undifferentiated or anaplastic carcinoma (includes large-cell and oat-cell types)	High correlation with cigarette smoking and exposure to environmental carcinogens	Accounts for 20% of lung cancers Highly metastatic Metastases primarily via lymphatics Found in younger age groups than other cell types Occurs primarily in males	Prognosis is usually poor. Often fatal within 1 yr Surgery is not usually attempted because of high rate of metastases Tumor is usually radiosensitive and responds well to radiation therapy, but often recurs
Adenocarcinoma	Has been associated with lung scarring and chronic interstitial fibrosis Not related to cigarette smoking	Accounts for 15% of lung cancers Occurs about equally in men and women Often presents no clinical manifestations until there is widespread metastasis. Metastasis via bloodstream Most commonly located in peripheral portions of the lungs (Fig. 20-7)	Surgical resection is often attempted Does not respond well to chemotherapy
Bronchioalveolar cell (alveolar cell) carcinoma	Does not seem to be related to cigarette smoking	Accounts for 2% of lung cancers Located in peripheral portions of the lungs (Fig. 20-7) Originates in alveoli or bronchioles Onset insidious and resembles pneumonia Abundant expectoration of mucoid sputum	Prognosis poor unless affected lobe can be surgically resected at an early stage

weeks should be evaluated by chest x-ray. The findings may show the presence of the tumor and/or abnormalities related to the obstructive features of the tumor, such as atelectasis and pneumonitis. The x-ray can also show evidence of metastasis to the ribs or vertebrae and the presence of pleural effusion.

A definitive diagnosis of lung cancer is made by identifying malignant cells. Sputum specimens may be obtained for cytology studies. An early-morning specimen that has been obtained by coughing deeply provides the most accurate results. However, malignant cells may not be obtained even in the presence of a lung cancer.

The use of the fiberoptic bronchoscope is very important in the diagnosis of lung cancer. It provides direct visualization and allows biopsy specimens to be obtained. A biopsy is usually the best method for establishing the presence of a malignant tumor.

Mediastinoscopy involves the insertion of a scope via a small anterior chest incision into the mediastinum to examine for metastasis in the anterior mediastinum or hilum, or extrapleurally in the chest. It is also used to stage the lung cancer, which is important in determining the treatment plan.

Other diagnostic procedures include a scalene lymph node biopsy to determine metastatic spread, pulmonary angiography, and lung scans to assess the overall pulmonary status. If a thoracentesis is performed to relieve a pleural effusion, the fluid should be analyzed for malignant cells.

Therapeutic

Surgical Resection Surgical resection is usually the only hope for cure in lung cancer (Table 20-17). Unfortunately, detection is often so late that the tumor is no longer localized and is not amenable to resection. Resectability of the tumor is a major consideration in planning the surgical intervention. Oat-cell (small-cell) carcinomas usually have widespread metastasis at the time of diagnosis. Therefore, surgery is usually contraindicated. In contrast, squamous-cell carcinomas are more likely to be treated with surgery because they remain localized or, if they metastasize, it is primarily by local spread.

When the tumor is considered operable with a potential for cure, the client's cardiopulmonary status must be evaluated to determine his ability to withstand surgery. This is done by clinical studies of pulmonary function, arterial blood gases, and others, as indicated by the individual's status. Contraindications for thoracotomy include hypercapnia, pulmonary hypertension, cor pulmonale, and markedly reduced lung function. Coexisting conditions such as cardiac, renal, and liver diseases are also contraindications for surgery.

A tumor may be potentially resectable, but because it is located in a critical area such as the trachea or is too close to the heart, it is considered inoperable. The type of surgery performed is usually a *lobectomy* (removal of one or more lobes of the lung) and less often a *pneumonectomy* (removal of the entire lung).

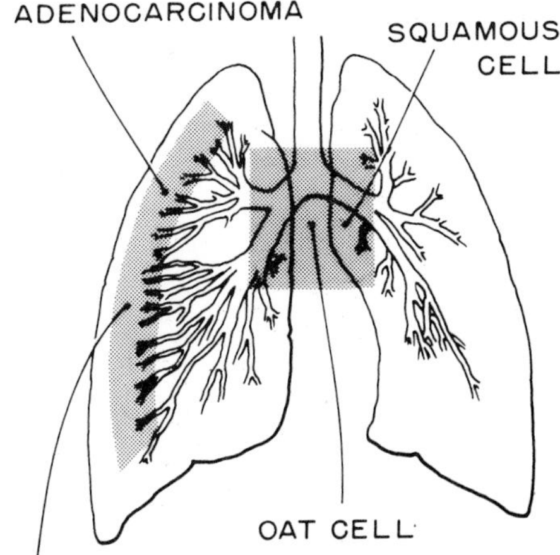

Figure 20-7 Anatomic distribution of lung cancer. *(From S. Price and L. Wilson, Pathophysiology: Clinical Concepts of Disease Processes, 2d ed., McGraw-Hill Book Company, New York, 1982, p. 470.)*

Surgical procedures related to the lung and thorax are discussed in the section on Chest Surgery.

Radiation Therapy Radiation therapy is used as a curative approach in individuals who have resectable tumors but are considered poor surgical risks. It is also done as a palliative procedure to reduce distressing symptoms such as cough, hemoptysis, and bronchial obstruction. It can be employed to treat pain due to metastatic bone lesions or cerebral metastasis. Radiation used as a preoperative or postoperative adjunctive measure has not been found to increase survival in the client with lung cancer.

Chemotherapy Chemotherapy is used in the treatment of nonresectable tumors. Multiple drug regimens (protocols including combination chemothera-

Table 20-16
Ectopic Hormone Syndromes of Lung Cancer

Syndrome	Ectopic Hormone	Most Common Cell Type
Cushing's syndrome	ACTH	Oat cell
Inappropriate secretion of antidiuretic hormone (ADH)	ADH	Oat cell
Hypercalcemia	Parathyroid hormone	Squamous cell
Gynecomastia	Follicle-stimulating hormone (FSH)	Large cell
Carcinoid syndrome	5-Hydroxyacetic acid from serotonin breakdown	Oat-cell Bronchial adenoma

Table 20-17

Medical Management: Lung Cancer

Diagnostic

1. History and physical examination
2. Chest x-ray
3. Sputum for cytology
4. Bronchoscopy
5. Mediastinoscopy
6. Scalene node biopsy
7. Pulmonary angiography
8. Lung scan
9. CT scan

Therapeutic

1. Surgery
2. Radiation therapy
3. Chemotherapy
4. Immunotherapy

py) using cyclophosphamide, methotrexate, methyl-CCNU, and vincristine have increased the survival rate in oat-cell carcinomas. Chemotherapy has not shown any significant results when used with squamous cell carcinoma and adenocarcinoma.[30] Symptomatic improvement and tumor regression will usually last for only a period of months.

Immunotherapy Immunotherapy as adjuvant therapy has been used in individuals with cancer, including malignant lung tumors. BCG and *Corynebacterium parvum* are nonspecific immunostimulants and may increase the immune system's ability to destroy tumor cells. (Immunotherapy is discussed in Chap. 11.)

Nursing Management

Health promotion and maintenance

The best way to halt the epidemic of lung cancer is for cigarette smoking to stop. An important nursing role is to disseminate information related to the dangers of cigarette smoking. Assistance should be provided to individuals who want to stop smoking (Chap. 60). Nurses should be familiar with antismoking resources in their communities so that they can provide this information to their clients.

The American Cancer Society has a campaign called "Smoking Stinks," reflecting the idea that smoking is not socially appropriate. It is especially important to promote antismoking programs for youth to prevent them from acquiring the smoking habit.

Those individuals who cannot or will not quit smoking should be urged to alter their habit by smoking (1) cigarettes with tar yields of less than 10 mg, (2) filtered cigarettes, (3) fewer cigarettes per day, and (4) only half of each cigarette.[31] These persons should understand that, at best, these measures only slightly reduce the risk of lung cancer.

Nurses who smoke are in a difficult position to help clients change their smoking habits. Nurses as role models can do much to facilitate or harm their educational attempts with people in the community as well as in the hospital. Therefore, if a nurse smokes, she must try to stop before she can serve as a role model for her clients. A smoker turned nonsmoker may be in a good position to suggest strategies for success.

Screening chest x-rays every 6 to 12 months may be of value for individuals who are considered at high risk for lung cancer. This consideration applies to persons employed in uranium mining, asbestos-related industries, iron foundries, and other industries with known respiratory carcinogens, as well as for those who are heavy cigarette smokers.

When a nurse is obtaining a history from a client (even one with nonrespiratory problems), it is important to get information related to respiratory carcinogens. The client should be asked about occupational exposure to asbestos, uranium, arsenic, nickel, iron and iron oxides, and excessive exposure to air pollution. In addition, a detailed history of cigarette smoking should be obtained. This information should be used to evaluate the client's risk of developing lung cancer and also to teach the client about early recognition of symptoms. Anyone with a history of exposure to respiratory carcinogens who has pneumonitis that persists for longer than 2 weeks in spite of antibiotic therapy should be evaluated for the possibility of lung cancer.[32]

Individuals with a chronic cough or a change in the character of a cough should be encouraged to obtain medical care. In addition, persons with chronic or recurring respiratory infections should be carefully evaluated, especially if they are cigarette smokers.

Acute intervention

Care of the client with lung cancer will initially involve support and reassurance during the diagnostic evaluation. Specific nursing measures related to the diagnostic studies are outlined in Chap. 18.

Another major responsibility of the nurse is to help the client and his family deal with the diagnosis of lung cancer. The client may feel guilty about his cigarette smoking having caused the cancer and needs to discuss this feeling with someone who has a nonjudgmental attitude. Questions regarding his condition should be answered honestly. Additional counseling from a social worker, psychologist, or member of the clergy may be needed.

Specific care of the client will depend on the treatment plan. Surgical care related to thoracotomy is discussed in the section on Chest Surgery. Care of the client undergoing radiation therapy and chemotherapy is discussed in Chap. 11. The nurse has a major role in providing client comfort, teaching methods to reduce pain, and assessing indications for hospitalization (Chap. 11).

Chronic management

The client who has had a surgical resection with intent to cure should be followed carefully for manifestations of metastasis. The client and family should be told to contact the physician if symptoms such as hemoptysis, dysphagia, chest pain, and hoarseness develop.

For many individuals who have lung cancer, very little can be done medically to significantly prolong their lives. Radiation therapy and chemotherapy can be used to provide palliative relief from distressing symptoms. Constant pain becomes a major problem. (Measures used to relieve pain are discussed in Chap. 50.) Care of the client with cancer is discussed in Chap. 11.

Other Types of Lung Tumors

Other types of primary lung tumors include sarcomas, lymphomas, and bronchial adenomas. *Bronchial adenomas* are small tumors that arise from the lower trachea or major bronchi and are considered malignant because they are locally invasive and frequently metastasize. Clinical manifestations of bronchial adenomas include hemoptysis, persistent cough, localized obstructive wheezing, and purulent bronchitis. There may be secondary bronchiectasis in long-standing cases. Bronchial adenomas frequently cause endocrine paraneoplastic manifestations. They can usually be treated successfully with surgical resection.

The lung is a common site for secondary metastases and is more often affected by metastatic growth than by primary lung tumors. The pulmonary capillaries, with their extensive network, are ideal sites for tumor emobli. In addition, the lung has an extensive lymphatic network. The primary malignancies that spread to the lung often originate in the GI and genitourinary (GU) tracts and breast. General symptoms of lung metastases are chest pain and nonproductive cough.

Benign tumors of the lung are generally classified as mesenchymal. Their occurrence is rare, and they have the potential to become malignant. The most common mesenchymal tumors are *chondromas,* which arise in the bronchial cartilage, and *leiomyomas,* which are myomas of smooth, nonstriated muscle fibers.

Hamartomas of the lung are mixtures of fibrous tissue, fat, and blood vessels. They are congenital malformations of the connective tissue of the bronchiolar walls.

CHEST TRAUMA AND SURGERY

Chest Trauma

Emergency treatment of chest trauma is discussed in Chap. 58. The most common thoracic injuries are presented in Table 58-7. The most frequent types of chest trauma will be reviewed in this section.

Pneumothorax

A *pneumothorax* is a complete or partial collapse of a lung due to an accumulation of air in the intrapleural space. A pneumothorax may be closed or open.

Closed Pneumothorax Closed pneumothorax has no associated external wound. The most common form of closed pneumothorax is a *spontaneous pneumothorax,* which is caused by rupture of small blebs on the visceral pleural space. The cause of the blebs is unknown. This condition occurs most commonly in otherwise healthy individuals between 20 and 40 years of age, usually in male cigarette smokers. There is a tendency for pneumothoraces to recur.

Other causes of closed pneumothorax include:

1. Injury to the lung from mechanical ventilation
2. Injury to the lung from insertion of a subclavian catheter
3. Perforation of the esophagus
4. Injury to the lungs from broken ribs
5. Ruptured blebs or bullae in a client with COPD

Open Pneumothorax Open pneumothorax occurs when air enters the pleural space through an opening in the chest wall (Fig. 20-8). Examples include stabbing or gunshot wounds and surgical thoracotomies. A penetrating chest wound is often referred to as a *sucking chest wound.* Emergency treatment of these wounds is described in Chap. 58.

Tension Pneumothorax Tension pneumothorax may result from either an open or a closed pneumothorax. In an open chest wound, a flap may act as a one-way valve. Therefore, air can enter on inspiration but cannot escape. Intrathoracic pressure increases,

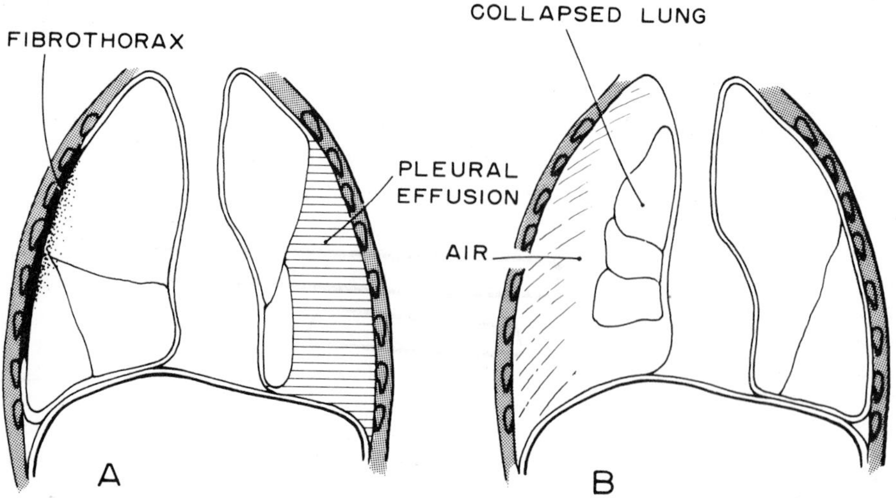

Figure 20-8 Disorders of the pleura. *(a)* Fibrothorax resulting from an organization of inflammatory exudate and pleural effusion; *(b)* collapse of lung due to an open pneumothorax. *(From S. Price and L. Wilson, Pathophysiology: Clinical Concepts of Disease Processes, 2d ed., McGraw-Hill Book Company, New York, 1982, p. 448.)*

the lung collapses, and the mediastinum is shifted toward the unaffected side, which is subsequently compressed. As the intrathoracic pressure increases, cardiac output is altered because there is decreased venous return and compression of the great vessels. Tension pneumothorax is a medical emergency because both the respiratory and circulatory systems are affected. Tension pneumothorax may also occur when chest tubes are clamped or become blocked in a client after insertion for treatment of pneumothorax.

Hemothorax Hemothorax is an accumulation of blood in the intrapleural space. It is frequently found in association with open pneumothorax and is then called a *hemopneumothorax.* Causes of hemothorax include chest trauma, lung malignancy, complication of anticoagulant therapy, pulmonary embolus, and tearing of pleural adhesions.

Clinical Manifestations The client with a pneumothorax has respiratory distress, including shallow, rapid respirations, dyspnea, and air hunger. Chest pain and a cough with or without hemoptysis may be present. On auscultation there are no breath sounds over the affected area, and hyperresonance may be heard. A chest x-ray shows the presence of pneumothorax.

If a tension pneumothorax develops, severe respiratory distress, tachycardia, and cyanosis occur. The trachea and point of maximal impulse (PMI) shift to the unaffected side.

Management Emergency care of pneumothorax is discussed in Chap. 58. If the amount of air or fluid accumulated in the intrapleural space is small, no treatment is needed because it will gradually be absorbed. If the amount of air or fluid is minimal, the pleural space can be aspirated with a large-bore needle. Needle aspiration is often a lifesaving measure. The most definitive and common form of treatment of pneumothorax and hemothorax is to insert a chest tube and connect it to water-seal drainage (discussed later in the chapter). Repeated spontaneous pneumothorax may have to be treated surgically by a partial pleurectomy or application of irritants to the pleural surfaces to promote adherence.

Fractured ribs

Rib fractures are the most common chest injuries resulting from trauma. Ribs 4 to 9 are most commonly fractured because they are least protected by chest muscles. If the fractured rib is splintered or displaced, it may damage the pleura and lungs.

Clinical manifestations of fractured ribs include pain (especially on inspiration) at the site of injury. The individual splints the affected area and takes shallow breaths to try to decrease the pain. Because the individual is reluctant to take deep breaths and cough, atelectasis may develop because of decreased ventilation.

The main goal in treatment is to decrease pain so that the client can breathe adequately to promote good chest expansion. *Intercostal nerve blocks* using local anesthesia are most frequently employed to provide pain relief. The nerve(s) of the affected rib(s) and the two intercostal nerves above and below the injured rib(s) are also blocked. The effect of the anesthesia lasts for a period of hours to days. It needs to be repeated as necessary to provide pain relief. Strapping the chest with tape or using a binder is not common practice. Most physicians feel that these measures should be avoided because they reduce lung expansion and predispose the individual to atelectasis. Narcotic drug therapy must be individualized and used with caution because these drugs can depress respirations.

Flail chest

Flail chest results from multiple rib fractures, causing instability of the chest wall (Fig. 58-7). The chest wall cannot provide the bony structure necessary to maintain bellow action and ventilation. The affected (flail) area will move paradoxically to the intact portion of the chest during respiration. During inspiration the affected portion is sucked in, and during expiration it bulges out. This *paradoxical chest movement* prevents adequate ventilation of the lung in the injured area. Inadequate ventilation results in retained secretions, atelectasis, hypoxia, and hypercapnia. The client manifests rapid, shallow respirations, cyanosis, and tachycardia. On inspection, the paradoxical chest movement is apparent.

Emergency management of a flail chest is discussed in Chap. 58. Basically, it involves stabilizing the chest by applying pressure, such as by strapping a pillow over the affected area.

Definitive treatment of flail chest involves internal stabilization using tracheal intubation and controlled mechanical ventilation. Positive end-expiratory pressure (PEEP) used with mechanical ventilation to improve oxygenation will maintain positive pressure in the lungs throughout the respiratory cycle. (Mechanical ventilation is discussed in Chap. 22.) The lung parenchyma and fractured ribs will heal with time. Mechanical ventilation will be necessary for 1 to 2 weeks.

Chest Tubes and Water-Seal Drainage

Intrapleural pressure and the intrapleural space were described in Chap. 18. Under normal conditions, intrapleural pressure is below atmospheric pressure (about 4 to 5 cmH_2O below atmospheric pressure during expiration and about 8 to 10 cmH_2O below atmospheric pressure during inspiration). If intrapleural pressure becomes equal to atmospheric pressure, the lungs will collapse (pneumothorax). Air and fluid can enter the intrapleural space by a variety of mechanisms, including traumatic chest injury (e.g., gunshot wound, fractured rib), thoracotomy, and spontaneous pneumothorax (see the section on Pneumothorax). The purpose of chest tubes and water-seal drainage is to remove the air and fluid and restore normal intrapleural pressure so that the lungs can reexpand.

Chest tube insertion

A physician can insert a chest tube in the emergency room, at the client's bedside, or in the operating room, depending on the situation. In the operating room, the chest tubes will be inserted using the thoracotomy incision. In the emergency room or at the bedside, the client is placed in a sitting position or lying down with the affected side elevated. The area is prepared with antiseptic solution, and the site is infiltrated with a local anesthetic agent. After a small incision is made, one or two chest tubes are inserted into the pleural space. One catheter is placed anteriorly through the second intercostal space to remove air (Fig. 20-9). The other is placed posteriorly through the 8th or 9th intercostal space to drain fluid and blood. The tubes are sutured to the chest wall, and the puncture wound is covered with an airtight dressing. During insertion, the tubes are kept clamped. After the tubes are in place in the pleural space, they are connected to drainage tubing and water-seal drainage. Each tube may be connected to a separate drainage system and suction. More commonly, a Y connector is used to attach both chest tubes to the same drainage system.

Water-seal drainage

The chest tube is connected to a glass connecting tube that is placed inside a bottle containing water. The tube is placed below the water level (hence the name *water-seal*). The water-seal drainage acts as a one-way valve. On inspiration, air and fluid from the intrapleural space enter the drainage system. Atmospheric air cannot enter the tubing because of the water barrier, and water is too heavy to be pulled up into the tubing. A water-seal drainage system can be set up using one, two, or three bottles or commercial disposable plastic units.

One-Bottle Water-Seal Drainage The chest tube is connected to a glass tube that is submerged 2 cm below the water level in a capped, covered bottle (Fig. 20-10). An air vent in the top of the bottle allows air to escape. This system does not use suction. Gravity drainage is facilitated by the client's inspiratory effort. Inspiration, especially when deep, forces air and fluid through the chest tube. Bubbles are seen coming up

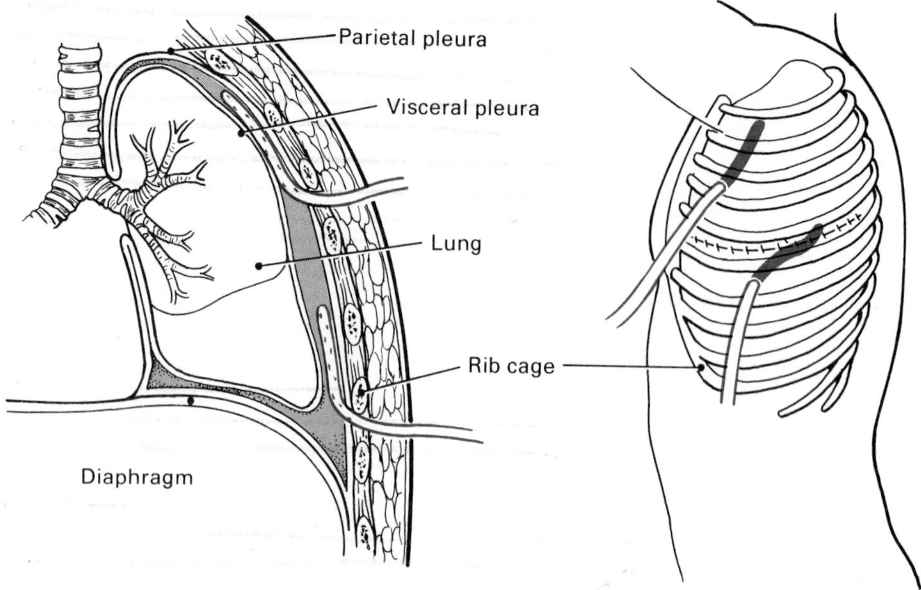

Figure 20-9 Placement of chest tubes.

through the water, and air escapes via the vent. Water can be seen to oscillate during a respiratory cycle. On inspiration, the water level should rise in the connecting tube, and on expiration it should fall. The drainage bottle should be well secured below the level of the client's chest.

Drainage Systems with Suction In most situations, gravity drainage with a one-bottle setup does not provide adequate lung reexpansion. Suction is required to remove larger amounts of air and blood. In a *two-bottle drainage system,* the water-seal bottle is set up like the first bottle (Fig. 20-11). The second bottle is attached to a suction source. If wall suction is used, the degree of suction may be too great; control is achieved by the depth of submersion of the glass tube. If the tube is submerged 10 cm below the water and suction is turned on, a negative pressure will result equal to 10 cm of suction applied to the pleural space. The greater the depth of the tube in the water, the greater the amount of suction delivered. An Emerson pump can also be used as the source of suction. The amount of suction desired (usually between −10 and −20 cmH_2O) is set on the pump.

In a *three-bottle drainage system,* there is a bottle for drainage collection, a water-seal bottle, and a suction control bottle (Fig. 20-12). Commercial disposable plastic units such as Pleur-evac are designed to be used as three-bottle systems (Fig. 20-13). This unit has chambers for collection, water-seal, and suction control. The unit can also be used only for collection or collection and water-seal. The manufacturer's suggestions for use are included with the equipment. The plastic units allow the client mobility and decrease the risk of breaking or spilling the drainage system.

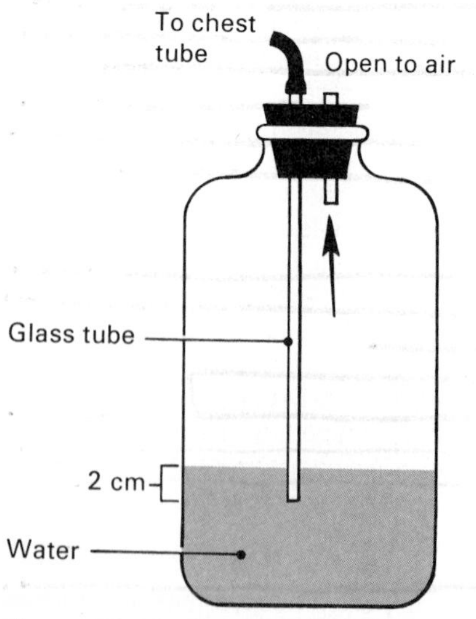

Figure 20-10 One-bottle water-seal drainage.

Chest tube removal

Clients with chest tubes usually have daily chest x-rays to follow the course of lung reexpansion. The chest tubes are removed when the lungs are reexpan-

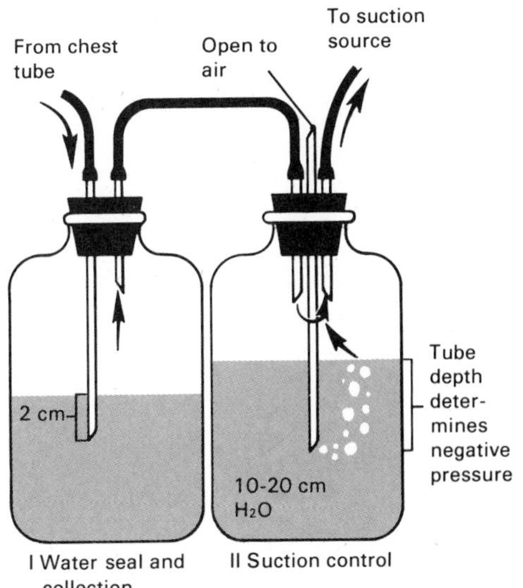

Figure 20-11 Two-bottle water-seal suction. Bottle I is the water seal, and bottle II is the suction control bottle.

ded and fluid drainage has ceased. Sometimes the amount of suction is decreased or the tubes are clamped off for a period of time before being removed. The tube is removed by cutting the sutures, applying a sterile Vaseline gauze dressing, having the client take a deep breath, exhale, and bear down (Valsalva maneuver), and then removing the tube. The site is covered with an airtight dressing, the pleura seals itself off, and in a few days the wound is healed. The wound should be observed for drainage and reinforced if necessary. The client should be observed for any manifestations of respiratory distress.

Nursing responsibilities related to chest tubes

Some general guidelines for nursing care of clients with chest tubes and water-seal drainage systems include the following:

1. Keep all tubing as straight as possible, coiled loosely, and do not let the client lie on it.
2. All connections between chest tubes, drainage tubing, and the drainage collector should be tight. Taping at connections and at the top of the bottle will help prevent air leaks.
3. A piece of tape should be placed on the outside of the drainage bottle. The time of measurement and the fluid level should be marked according to the prescribed orders. Marking intervals may range from once per hour to every 8 hours. Any change in the quantity or characteristics of drainage (e.g., clear yellow to bloody) should be recorded and reported to the physician.
4. The chest tubes and drainage tubing should be "milked" or stripped every 1 to 2 hours to dislodge mucus or blood clots. Special mechanical strippers are available to do this. Otherwise, stripping can be done manually by holding the proximal part of the tubing with one hand and squeezing

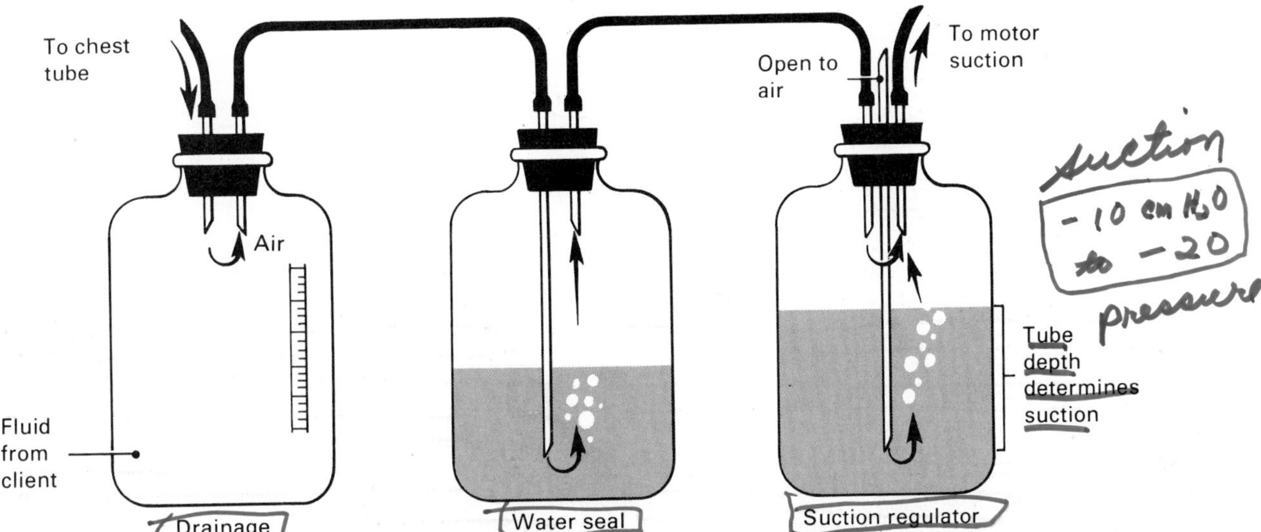

Figure 20-12 Three-bottle water-seal suction. Bottle I is the drainage bottle. A verticle piece of tape should be applied to the outer surface of the drainage bottle. The time of measurement and the fluid level should be marked hourly on the tape. Bottle II is the water-seal bottle. Bottle III is the suction-control bottle. The length of glass tube below the water surface determines the amount of suction.

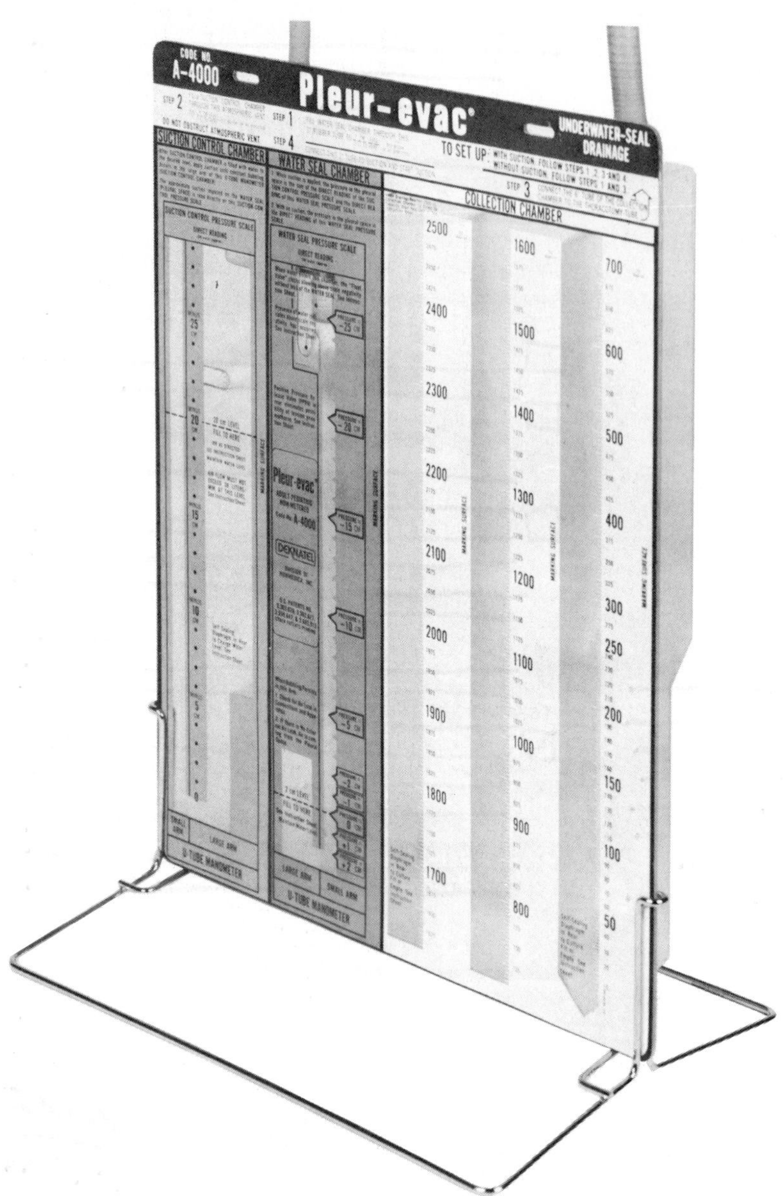

Figure 20-13 Pleur-evac, a modern, disposable, lightweight chest suction unit. *(Courtesy of DeKnatel, Inc.)*

the distal portion in a downward direction. Lotion applied to the hands may facilitate milking.

5. Observe for air bubbles in the water-seal chamber and fluctuations in the glass tube or chest tubes. Air should be bubbling out from the glass tube. If no fluctuations (rising with inspiration and falling with expiration) are observed, the drainage system is blocked or the lungs are reexpanded. If bubbling increases, there may be an air leak in the system.

6. The client's clinical status should be monitored. Vital signs should be taken frequently, lungs auscultated, and the chest wall observed for any abnormal chest movements.

7. Never elevate the drainage system to the level of the client's chest. Secure the bottles to the metal drainage stand or racks. The drainage bottles should not be emptied unless they are in danger of overflowing.

8. Kelly clamps should be available at the bedside at all times in case the tube becomes disconnected or the bottle breaks. If either of these things

happens, the chest tube should be clamped as close to the skin as possible and the physician notified immediately.

9. The client should be encouraged to cough and deep-breathe periodically to facilitate lung expansion.

10. If the bottle is overturned and the water seal is disrupted, return the bottle to an upright position and encourage the client to take a few deep breaths.

Chest Surgery

Chest surgery is done for a variety of reasons, some unrelated to primary lung problems. For example, a thoracotomy is done for heart and esophageal surgery. The types of chest surgeries are compared in Table 20-18.

Preoperative care

General preoperative care is discussed in Chap. 6. Prior to chest surgery, baseline data are obtained on both the respiratory and cardiovascular systems. Diagnostic studies usually performed are pulmonary function studies, chest x-ray, lung scans, electrocardiograph (ECG), arterial blood gases, blood urea nitrogen (BUN), serum creatinine, blood glucose, serum electrolytes, and complete blood count. Additional studies of cardiac functioning such as cardiac catheterization may be done for the client undergoing a pneumonectomy.

A careful physical assessment of the lungs, including percussion and auscultation should be done. This will allow the nurse to compare preoperative and postoperative findings.

The client should be encouraged to stop smoking preoperatively to decrease secretions and increase oxygen saturation. In the anxious period before surgery, this is not an easy thing for the habitual smoker to do.

Postural drainage may be indicated to help drain the lungs of accumulated secretions. This is indicated especially for the client with a lung abscess or bronchiectasis.

Preoperative teaching was discussed in Chap. 6. One aspect to focus on is effective deep breathing and coughing (see also Table 21-9). If the client practices these techniques before surgery, they will be easier to perform postoperatively. The client should be told that adequate medication will be given to reduce the pain, and the client will be helped to splint the incision with a pillow to facilitate deep breathing and coughing.

For most types of chest surgery, chest tubes are inserted and connected to water-sealed drainage. The purpose of these tubes should be explained to the client. In addition, oxygen is frequently given the first day postoperatively. Range-of-motion exercises on the operative side similar to those for the mastectomy client (see Chap. 44) should be taught to the client.

The thought of losing part of a vital organ is frequently frightening. The client should be reassured that the lungs have a large degree of functional reserve. Even after the removal of one lung, there is enough lung tissue to maintain adequate oxygenation.[33]

The nurse should be available to deal with the questions asked by the client and the family. Questions should be answered honestly. The nurse should try to facilitate the expression of concerns, feelings, and questions.

Surgical procedure

Thoracotomy surgery is considered major surgery because the incision is large, cutting into bone, muscle, and cartilage. The two types of thoracic incisions are (1) *median sternotomy*, performed by splitting the sternum, and (2) *lateral thoracotomy*. The median sternotomy is primarily used for surgery involving the heart.

The two types of lateral thoracotomy are posterolateral and anterolateral. The *posterolateral* thoracotomy is used for most surgeries involving the lung. The incision is made from the anterior axillary line below the nipple level posteriorly at the 4th, 5th, or 6th intercostal space. It is rarely necessary to remove the ribs. Strong mechanical retractors are used to gain access to the lung. The *anterolateral* incision is made in the 4th or 5th intercostal space from the sternal border to the midaxillary line. This procedure is commonly used for trauma victims, mediastinal operations, and wedge resections of the upper and middle lobes of the lung.

The extensiveness of the thoracotomy incision often results in severe pain for the client postoperatively. Because muscles have been severed, the client is reluctant to move the shoulder and arm on the operative side. Chest tubes are placed in the pleural space except in pneumonectomy surgery. In a pneumonectomy, the space where the lung was removed gradually fills with serosanguineous fluid.

Postoperative care

General postoperative care is discussed in Chap. 8. Specific measures related to the care following a thoracotomy are presented in Table 20-19. The specif-

Table 20-18
Chest Surgeries

Type of Surgery	Description	Indication	Comments
Lobectomy	Removal of one lobe of the lung	Lung cancer Bronchiectasis TB Emphysematous bullae Benign lung tumors Fungal infections	Most common lung surgery. Two chest tubes inserted postoperatively. Remaining lung tissue expands to fill up space.
Pneumonectomy	Removal of entire lung	Lung cancer (most common) Extensive TB Bronchiectasis Lung abscess	Done only when lobectomy or segmental resection will not remove all diseased lung. Drainage tubes are not generally used. Fluid gradually fills space where lung has been removed. Client should not be turned to unaffected side postoperatively.
Segmental resection	Removal of one or more lung segments	Bronchiectasis TB	Technically difficult surgery done to remove lung segment. Chest tubes inserted. Remaining lung tissue expands to fill space.
Wedge resection	Removal of small, localized lesion that occupies only part of a segment	Lung biopsy Excision of small nodules	Chest tubes needed postoperatively.
Decortication	Removal or "stripping" of thick, fibrous membrane from visceral pleura	Empyema	Chest tubes and drainage used postoperatively.
Exploratory thoracotomy	Incision into thorax to look for injured or bleeding tissues	Chest trauma	Chest tubes and drainage used postoperatively.
Thoracotomy not involving the lungs	Incision into thorax for surgery on other organs	Hiatal hernia repair Open heart surgery Esophageal surgery Tracheal resection Aortic aneurysm repair	See discussion of individual diseases in text.
Thoracoplasty	Removal of ribs without entering pleura	Reduced size of chest cavity	Historically important in treating TB. May be used to decrease lung size in area of chronic empyema. On rare occasions, may be performed prior to resectional surgery.

ic follow-up care depends on the type of surgical procedure.

RESTRICTIVE RESPIRATORY DISORDERS

Restrictive respiratory disorders are characterized by decreased compliance of the lungs or chest wall or both. This is in contrast to obstructive disorders, which are characterized by increased resistance to airflow. Pulmonary function tests are the best measurement to use in differentiating between restrictive and obstructive respiratory disorders (Table 20-20). Restrictive disorders are characterized by reduced vital capacity (VC), and reduced total lung capacity, with a normal or reduced functional residual capacity (FRC) and residual volume (RV). Obstructive disorders are characterized by normal or decreased vital capacity, increased total lung capacity, reduced ratio of forced air expiration volume in the first second of expiration to functional vital capacity ($FEV_{1.0}$/FVC), increased FRC, and increased RV. Mixed obstructive

Table 20-19
Nursing Care Plan for the Client Following Thoracotomy

Client Problem	Expected Outcome	Nursing Intervention
Accumulation of lung secretions	Lungs clear to auscultation. Client able to clear secretions	Place client in semi-Fowler's position. Assist client to turn, deep-breathe, and cough every 1–2 h initially. Splint chest incision when breathing exercises and coughing are performed. Plan coughing exercises after pain relief is obtained. Auscultate lungs before and after deep-breathing and coughing regimens. If secretions are not being removed, suctioning may be necessary. Observe the color and characteristics of sputum.
Air and fluid collections in intrapleural space	Chest x-ray shows lungs fully expanded. Increased breath sounds at involved site	Monitor chest drainage system. (See section on Nursing Responsibilities Related to Chest Tubes.)
Pain	Client free from pain Able to cough effectively	Administer analgesics every 3–4 h (if needed) for 1–2 days postoperatively. Assist client with deep breathing and coughing after pain relief is obtained. Position client to prevent client's lying on tubes or occluding drainage. Assist physician with intercostal nerve block if indicated.
Dyspnea	Respiratory rate 12–18/min	Administer O_2 via nasal prongs or mask (if ordered). Assess respiratory rate every 1–2 h. Auscultate lungs every 2–3 h. Monitor the results of ABGs. Observe for manifestations of complications such as pneumothorax or hemothorax. Assist client with deep breathing. Position for comfort and ease of breathing.
Restricted motion of upper extremities on affected side	Has full, active range of motion in shoulder on operative side	Begin passive range-of-motion exercises evening and first postoperative day. Then active range of motion should be practiced 2 to 3 times per day. (Exercises similar to those for postmastectomy can be performed; See Chap. 41.) Assist with ambulation 3 to 4 times per day.
Inadequate nutritional and fluid intake	Maintenance of normal weight	Provide fluid intake of at least 3 L/day. Assess client's ability to tolerate gradual progression to a general diet. Weigh client daily.
Postoperative complications	Client will practice activities to promote recovery	Instruct client to: 1. Continue deep-breathing exercises 2. Practice shoulder range-of-motion exercises 3. Avoid people with URI 4. Try to stop or cut back on cigarette smoking 5. Obtain adequate rest and nutrition 6. Know clinical manifestations of infection 7. Know when to call the physician

and restrictive disorders are often manifested. For example, a client may have both chronic bronchitis (an obstructive problem) and pulmonary fibrosis (a restrictive problem). Restrictive problems are generally categorized into extrapulmonary and intrapulmonary disorders.

Extrapulmonary Restrictive Disorders

Extrapulmonary causes of restrictive lung disease include disorders involving the central nervous system, neuromuscular system, and chest wall (Table 20-21). In these disorders, the lung tissue is normal. Most of these conditions are discussed in detail in other chapters.

Intrapulmonary Restrictive Disorders

Intrapulmonary causes of restrictive lung disease involve the pleura or the lung tissue (Table 20-22).

Pleural effusion

Types of Pleural Effusions Pleural effusion is a collection of fluid in the pleural space (Fig. 20-8). It is not a disease, but rather a sign of a serious disease. It is frequently classified as transudative or exudative according to whether the protein content of the effusion is low or high, respectively. A transudate occurs primarily in noninflammatory conditions and is an accumulation of protein-poor, cell-poor fluid. *Transudative pleural effusions* (also called *hydrothorax*) are

Table 20-20

Relationship of Lung Volumes to Type of Ventilatory Impairment

Interpretation	FVC	$FEV_{1.0}$	$FEV_{1.0}/FVC\%$	RV	TLC
Normal	Normal	Normal	Normal	Normal	Normal
Airway obstruction	Normal or low	Low	Low	High	High
Lung restriction	Low	Normal or low	Normal or high	Normal or low	Low
Both obstruction and restriction	Low	Low	Low	Variable	Variable

Chronic Obstructive Pulmonary Disease, 5th ed., American Lung Association, New York, 1977.

Table 20-21

Extrapulmonary Causes of Restrictive Lung Disease

Disease or Alteration	Description	Comments
	Central Nervous System	
Head injury, CNS lesion (e.g., tumor, CVA)	Injury to or impingement on respiratory center. Causes hypo- or hyperventilation. Manifestations related to increased intracranial pressure (see Chap. 54).	Management is directed at treating the underlying cause, maintaining the airway, using mechanical ventilation for supportive care, and assessing for manifestations of increased intracranial pressure.
Narcotics and barbiturates	Depression of the respiratory center. Causes respiratory rate of <12/min.	Caused by drug overdose or inadvertent administration of drugs to a person with respiratory difficulty. These drugs should not be administered to a person with a respiratory rate of <12/min.
	Neuromuscular System	
Guillain-Barré syndrome	Acute inflammation of peripheral nerves and ganglia. Paralysis of intercostal nerves leads to diaphragmatic breathing. Paralysis of the vagal preganglionic and postganglionic fibers leads to reduced ability of bronchioles to constrict, dilate, and respond to irritants.	See Chap. 53 for clinical manifestations and management. Client often has to be put on mechanical ventilation for supportive care.
Amyotrophic lateral sclerosis	Progressive degenerative disorder of the motor neurons in the spinal cord, brainstem, and motor cortex. Respiratory system becomes involved due to interruption of nerve transmission to respiratory muscles, especially diaphragm.	See Chap. 51 for clinical manifestations and management.
Myasthenia gravis	Disease caused by defect in neuromuscular junction. Respiratory system becomes involved due to interruption of nerve transmission to respiratory muscles.	See Chap. 51 for clinical manifestations and management.
Muscular dystrophy	In this hereditary disease, all skeletal muscles eventually become involved. Paralysis of the respiratory muscles, including intercostals, diaphragm, and accessory muscles.	Pulmonary problems develop late in disease process.

Table 20-21 (Continued)

Disease or Alteration	Description	Comments
	Chest Wall	
Chest wall trauma (e.g., flail chest, fractured rib)	Rib fracture causes inspiratory pain. The person voluntarily splints the chest, resulting in shallow, rapid breathing. A person with a flail chest has impaired ventilatory ability due to paradoxical breathing (air shunted back and forth in pendulum fashion between lungs during respiratory cycle; see Fig. 58-7).	These conditions discussed in the section on Chest Trauma.
Pickwickian syndrome (extreme obesity)	Excess adipose tissue interferes with chest wall and diaphragmatic excursion. Characterized by somnolence due to hypoxemia and CO_2 retention and polycythemia due to chronic hypoxia. Disease named after the sleepy fat boy in Charles Dickens' *Pickwick Papers*.	Weight loss generally causes a reversal of symptoms. Prevention and prompt treatment of respiratory infections are important. Condition is worsened in the supine position.
Kyphoscoliosis	Posterior and lateral angulation of the spine. Restricts ventilation due to alteration in thoracic excursion. The work of breathing is increased. Person develops a pattern of rapid, shallow breathing. Lung volume is reduced, and both alveoli and blood vessels are compressed.	Only a small number of people with the condition develop severe respiratory problems.

Table 20-22
Intrapulmonary Causes of Restrictive Lung Disease

Disease or Alteration	Description
	Pleural Disorders
Pleural effusion	Accumulation of fluid in pleural space secondary to altered hydrostatic or oncotic pressure. If fluid collection is greater than 250 mL, it usually shows up on chest x-ray.
Pleurisy (pleuritis)	Inflammation of the pleura. Can be classified as fibrinous (dry) or serofibrinous (wet). Wet pleurisy is accompanied by an increase in pleural fluid and can result in a pleural effusion.
Pneumothorax	Accumulation of air in pleural space with accompanying lung collapse.
	Parenchymal Disorders
Atelectasis	Condition of lung characterized by collapsed, airless alveoli. Can be acute (e.g., in the postoperative client) or chronic (e.g., in the client with a malignant tumor).
Pneumonia	Acute inflammation of the lung tissue caused by bacteria, viruses, fungi, chemicals, dusts, and other factors.
Pulmonary fibrosis	Excessive connective tissue in the lungs resulting from healing and tissue repair following an inflammation. Fibrosis can be localized (e.g., from lung abscess, TB, pneumonia) or diffuse (e.g., from pneumoconiosis, sarcoidosis, cystic fibrosis, Hamman-Rich syndrome). Condition characterized by progressive dyspnea on exertion due to decreased compliance of the lungs and increased work of breathing. Diffuse pulmonary fibrosis is progressively disabling and frequently fatal.
Adult respiratory distress syndrome (ARDS)	Characterized by atelectasis, pulmonary edema, congestion, and hyaline membrane lining the alveolar wall. Can be caused by a variety of conditions, including shock lung, oxygen toxicity, gram-negative sepsis, cardiopulmonary bypass, and aspiration pneumonia. See Chap. 22 for clinical manifestations and management.

caused by (1) increased hydrostatic pressure found in congestive heart failure or (2) decreased oncotic pressure (from hypoalbuminemia) found in chronic liver or renal disease. In these situations, fluid movement is facilitated out of the capillaries and into the pleura space.

An exudate is an accumulation of fluid and cells in an area of inflammation. An *exudative pleural effusion* results from increased capillary permeability characteristic of the inflammatory reaction. Examples of this type of effusion occur secondary to pulmonary inflammations or malignancies.

The type of pleural effusion can be determined by a sample of pleural fluid obtained via thoracentesis (a procedure done to remove fluid from the pleural space). Exudates have a specific gravity above 1.015 and a high protein content, and the fluid is clear or pale yellow in appearance. Transudates have a lower specific gravity and low to no protein content. The fluid is dark yellow or amber in color. The fluid can also be analyzed for red and white blood cells, malignant cells, bacteria, glucose, pH, and lactic dehydrogenase.

An *empyema* is a pleural effusion that contains pus. It is caused by conditions such as pneumonia, TB, and lung abscess. A complication of empyema is *fibrothorax,* in which there is fibrous fusion of the visceral and parietal pleurae.

Clinical Manifestations Common clinical manifestations of pleural effusion are progressive dyspnea and decreased movement of the chest wall on the affected side. There may be pleuritic pain from the underlying disease. Physical examination of the chest will indicate dullness to percussion and absent or decreased breath sounds over the affected area. The chest x-ray will indicate an abnormality if the effusion is greater than 250 mL.

Manifestations of empyema include those mentioned for pleural effusion, as well as fever, night sweats, cough, and weight loss. A thoracentesis will reveal an exudate containing thick, purulent material.

Thoracentesis If the cause of the pleural effusion is not known, a diagnostic thoracentesis is needed to obtain pleural fluid for analysis (Fig. 18-18). If the degree of pleural effusion is severe enough to impair breathing, a therapeutic thoracentesis is done to remove fluid.

A thoracentesis is performed by having the client sit on the edge of a bed and lean forward over a bedside table. The puncture site is determined by chest x-ray and percussion of the chest to determine the maximum degree of dullness. The skin is cleaned with an antiseptic solution and anesthetized locally. The physician inserts the thoracentesis needle into the intercostal space. Fluid can be aspirated using a syringe, or tubing can be connected to allow fluid to drain into a sterile collecting bottle. After the fluid is removed, the needle is withdrawn and a bandage applied over the insertion site.

Usually only 1000 to 1200 mL of pleural fluid is removed at one time to prevent mediastinal shift and compromised venous return. A follow-up chest x-ray should be done to detect a possible pneumothorax that could have been induced by perforation of the pleura. Following the procedure, the client should be observed for any manifestations of respiratory distress.

Management The main goal of management of pleural effusions is to treat the underlying cause. For example, adequate treatment of congestive heart failure with diuretics and sodium restriction will result in a decreased pleural effusion. The treatment of pleural effusions secondary to malignant disease represents a more difficult problem. These types of pleural effusions are frequently recurrent and accumulate quickly following thoracentesis. Infusions of cancer chemotherapeutic agents directly into the pleural space are attempted to decrease the number of recurrent effusions.

Treatment of empyema is directed at drainage of the pleural space via thoracentesis or a closed thoracotomy tube. Appropriate antibiotic therapy is also needed to eradicate the causative organism. If a fibrothorax results from the empyema and causes severe pulmonary restriction, a *decortication* surgical procedure is done in which the pleural membranes are separated.

Pleurisy

Pleurisy (also called *pleuritis*) is an inflammation of the pleura. The most common causes are pneumonia, TB, chest trauma, pulmonary infarctions, and neoplasms. The inflammation usually subsides with adequate treatment of the primary disease. Pleurisy can be classified as *fibrinous* (dry), with fibrinous deposits on the pleural surface, or *serófibrinous* (wet), with increased production of pleural fluid that may result in pleural effusion.

The pain of pleurisy is typically abrupt and sharp in onset and is aggravated by inspiration. The client's breathing is shallow and rapid to avoid unnecessary movement of the pleura and chest wall. A pleural friction rub may be heard 1 to 2 days after the onset of symptoms.

Treatment of pleurisy is aimed at treating the

underlying disease and providing pain relief. Analgesics as well as lying on or splinting the affected side may provide some relief. The client should be taught to splint the rib cage when coughing. Intercostal nerve blocks may be done if the pain is severe.

Atelectasis

Atelectasis is a condition of the lungs characterized by collapsed, airless alveoli. The most common cause of atelectasis is airway obstruction due to retained exudates and secretions. This is frequently seen in the postoperative client. Normally, the pores of Kohn provide for collateral passage of air from one alveolus to another. Deep inspiration is necessary to open the pores effectively. For this reason, coughing and deep-breathing exercises are important in preventing atelectasis in high-risk clients (e.g., postoperative, immobilized clients). Pulmonary fibrosis can occur as a complication of chronic atelectasis. The prevention and treatment of atelectasis are discussed in Chap. 8.

Pulmonary fibrosis

A common cause of diffuse pulmonary fibrosis is organic and inorganic occupational inhalants (see the section on Occupational Lung Diseases). Other causes of diffuse pulmonary fibrosis include the Hamman-Rich syndrome, which is an unusual form of interstitial pneumonia, and sarcoidosis.

Sarcoidosis is the presence of granulomatous lesions and proliferation of lymph tissue that can involve any body organ, including the lungs. The disease is most common in American blacks. The clinical course of the disease varies from self-limiting to progressive, widespread granulomatous inflammation and fibrosis. There can be marked pulmonary fibrosis with severe restrictive lung disease. Cor pulmonale can develop in the advanced stages. There is no specific treatment for sarcoidosis. Often the disease is self-limiting, and the client gets well without treatment. Corticosteroids have been used to relieve symptoms and suppress the acute inflammation.[34]

VASCULAR LUNG DISORDERS

Pulmonary Edema

Pulmonary edema is an abnormal accumulation of fluid in the alveoli and interstitial spaces of the lung. It is a complication of various heart and lung diseases (Table 20-23). It is considered a medical emergency and may be life-threatening.

Normally, there is a balance between the hydrostatic and oncotic pressures in the pulmonary capillaries. If the hydrostatic pressure increases or the colloid oncotic pressure decreases, the net effect will be fluid leaving the pulmonary capillaries and entering the interstial space. This stage is referred to as *interstitial edema*. At this stage, the lymphatics can usually drain away the excess fluid. If fluid continues to leak from the pulmonary capillaries, it will enter the alveoli. This stage is referred to as *alveolar edema.* Pulmonary edema interferes with gas exchange by causing an alteration in the diffusing pathway between the alveoli and the pulmonary capillaries.

The most common cause of pulmonary edema is left-sided congestive heart failure. The clinical manifestations and management of pulmonary edema are described in Chap. 28.

Chronic forms of pulmonary edema are not common. This condition can be asymptomatic for a long period of time while structural changes such as pulmonary fibrosis result. An early manifestation of this condition may be *paroxysmal nocturnal dyspnea* due to increased hydrostatic pressure in the lungs in the recumbent position.

Pulmonary Embolism

Pulmonary embolism is the most frequently encountered pulmonary illness in a general hospital and is responsible for more than 50,000 deaths annually in the United States.[35] A pulmonary embolism is caused by thrombotic occlusion of the pulmonary arterial system. The most common source of the thrombus is the deep veins of the legs. The thrombus breaks loose

Table 20-23
Causes of Pulmonary Edema

1. Congestive heart failure
2. Overhydration with IV fluids
3. Hypoalbuminemia
   a. Nephrotic syndrome
   b. Hepatic disease
   c. Nutritional disorders
4. Altered capillary permeability of the lungs
   a. Inhaled toxins
   b. Inflammation (e.g., pneumonia)
   c. Severe hypoxia
   d. Near-drowning
5. Mechanical ventilation
6. Lymph malignancies
7. Respiratory distress syndrome (e.g., oxygen toxicity)
8. Unknown etiology
   a. Neurogenic
   b. Narcotic overdose
   c. High altitude

and travels as an embolus until it lodges in the pulmonary vasculature.

The result of the thromboembolic occlusion is complete or partial occlusion of the pulmonary arterial blood flow to parts of the lung. Therefore, the lung is ventilated but not perfused. As the pressure increases in the pulmonary vasculature, pulmonary hypertension may result. Pulmonary embolism is described in detail in Chap. 30.

Pulmonary Hypertension

Pathophysiology

Normally, the pulmonary circulation is characterized by low resistance and low pressure. Cardiac output can increase significantly with no increase in the pressure in the pulmonary vasculature. In pulmonary hypertension, the pulmonary pressure is elevated due to an increase in pulmonary vascular resistance to blood flow through small arteries and arterioles.

A 60 to 70 percent reduction in the vascular bed is required before pulmonary hypertension develops. The increase in vascular resistance may be anatomic or vasomotor in origin.

The reasons for *anatomic increase* in vascular resistance include:

1. Loss of capillaries due to alveolar wall damage as found in chronic obstructive lung disease
2. Stiffening of the pulmonary vasculature, as found in pulmonary fibrosis
3. Obstruction of blood flow, as found in pulmonary emboli

Vasomotor increase in pulmonary vascular resistance is found in conditions characterized by alveolar hypoxia and hypercapnia. These conditions cause localized vasoconstriction and shunting of blood away from poorly ventilated alveoli. Alveolar hypoxia and hypercapnia can be caused by a wide variety of conditions, including the Pickwickian syndrome, kyphoscoliosis, neuromuscular diseases, and other conditions characterized by alveolar hypoventilation with normal lungs.

It is possible to have a combination of anatomic restriction and vasomotor constriction. This is found in the client with long-standing chronic bronchitis who has chronic hypoxia in addition to loss of lung tissue.

Pulmonary hypertension is almost always caused by pulmonary or cardiac disorders. One type, called *primary pulmonary hypertension,* is not associated with either pulmonary or cardiac disease. The person with this disorder is typically a female between the ages of 20 and 40. The basic cause of the problem is unknown. No definitive therapy is available, and the course is often one of slow downhill progression.

Clinical course

The most common manifestations of pulmonary hypertension are dyspnea and weakness. These symptoms initially present only when there is an increased cardiac output (e.g., during exercise or with fever) or during hypoxia (e.g., pulmonary infection). Eventually, the condition occurs even during rest. Pulmonary hypertension increases the work load of the right ventricle and causes right ventricular hypertrophy, a condition called *cor pulmonale.*

Cor Pulmonale

Cor pulmonale is characterized by hypertrophy of the right ventricle secondary to a respiratory disorder. Pulmonary hypertension is usually a preexisting condition in individuals with this condition. Cor pulmonale may be present with or without overt cardiac failure.

The most common cause of acute cor pulmonale is a massive pulmonary embolism. In general, however, cor pulmonale is chronic, resulting from alveolar hypoxia in COPD. Almost any disorder that affects the respiratory system can cause cor pulmonale. The etiology and pathogenesis of cor pulmonale are outlined in Fig. 20-14.

Clinical manifestations

Clinical manifestations of cor pulmonale include dyspnea, cough, retrosternal or substernal pain, and fatigue. Chronic hypoxia leads to polycythemia and increased total blood volume and viscosity of the blood. Thus, compensatory mechanisms due to hypoxemia can aggravate the pulmonary hypertension. Attacks of cor pulmonale in a person with underlying chronic respiratory problems are frequently triggered by an acute respiratory tract infection.

If heart failure accompanies cor pulmonale, additional manifestations such as peripheral edema, weight gain, distended neck veins, full, bounding pulse, and enlarged liver will also be found. (Heart failure is discussed in Chap. 27.) A chest x-ray will show the presence of an enlarged right ventricle and pulmonary artery.

Management

The primary treatment of cor pulmonale is directed at treating the underlying pulmonary problem which precipitated the heart problem (Table 20-24). Low-flow oxygen therapy is used to correct the hypoxemia and reduce vasoconstriction in chronic states of

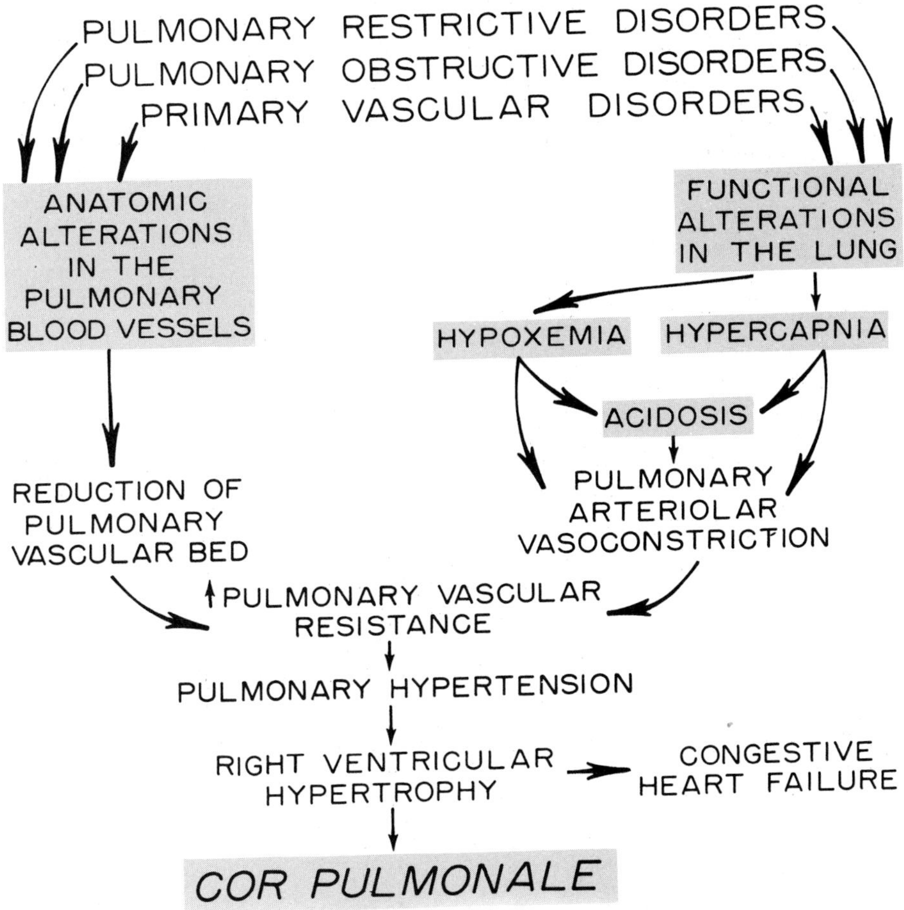

Figure 20-14 Etiology and pathogenesis of cor pulmonale. *(From S. Price and L. Wilson, Pathophysiology: Clinical Concepts of Disease Processes, 2d ed., McGraw-Hill Book Company New York, 1982, p. 467.)*

respiratory disorders. In acute states (e.g., due to pulmonary emboli), higher concentrations of oxygen may be required. If fluid and electrolyte and acid-base imbalances are present, they need to be corrected. Diuretics and a low sodium diet will help to decrease the plasma volume and the load on the heart. Bronchodilator therapy is indicated if the underlying respiratory problem is due to an obstructive disorder. Antibiotic therapy is indicated if the cor pulmonale was precipitated by an infection. The use of digitalis may be necessary to treat the accompanying heart failure. If used, smaller doses than usual are recommended because hypoxemia predisposes to digitalis toxicity. Antiarrhythmic drugs are given if indicated. Phlebotomies may be needed in clients with hematocrits over 60 g/dL to reduce the hematocrit and blood volume.

Long-term management of cor pulmonale due to COPD is similar to that described for COPD in Chap. 21. Continuous low-flow oxygen during sleep, exercise, and eating may allow the client to feel better and be more active. (See the section on Oxygen Therapy.)

Table 20-24
Medical Management: Cor Pulmonale

Diagnostic
1. History and physical examination
2. Arterial blood gases
3. Serum and urine electrolytes
4. Continual monitoring with ECG

Therapeutic
1. Bed rest
2. Oxygen therapy
3. Bronchodilators
4. Diuretics (e.g., furosemide)
5. Low sodium diet
6. Fluid restriction
7. Antibiotics
8. Digitalis

LUNG TRANSPLANTATION

In 1963 the first clinical lung transplant was performed in the United States. Since that time, about 40 additional lung transplants have been performed in human beings. The recipient with the longest survival time lived for 10 months after the surgery. At the present time, there is a virtual moratorium on lung transplants due to the poor results that have been obtained thus far. The infection and rejection that occur in the recipient presently preclude long-term success.[36]

One reason for the poor results is that the clients who receive lung transplants are at high risk. They usually have severe chronic lung disease and have not responded to other forms of treatment. In addition, they usually have a lung infection at the time of the lung transplant, and the effectiveness of antibiotics may well have been exhausted.

Case Study / Bacterial Pneumonia

Greg, a 31-year-old construction worker, was admitted to the hospital with cold sweats, chills, a deep productive cough with thick, rust-colored sputum, and generalized muscle and joint pain. For the past week, he stated, he had had a "chest cold" and was taking various antihistamines and decongestants that brought no relief. That morning, he had experienced increased difficulty in breathing and developed intermittent chills.

Results of a physical examination included dusky nail beds and mucous membranes and shallow respirations. Greg's vital signs showed a temperature of 40°C (104°F), pulse 114, respiration 28, and blood pressure 140/88. Lung sounds were barely audible in the lower lobes of the lungs, and rales were heard. A chest x-ray showed bilateral lobar pneumonia of the lower lobes.

Laboratory Results

White blood cell count	28,000/μL
Differential	76% segmented neutrophils, 6% band neutrophils
Culture of sputum	*S. pneumoniae*

Medical Treatment

Diagnosis: Acute bacterial pneumonia, pneumococcal origin
Procaine penicillin 600,000 units intramuscular (IM) immediately and every 12 h
Force fluids to 3 L/24 h
Repeat chest x-ray every other day
O_2 administration at 4 L/min (as needed)

Discussion Questions

1. What are the main classifications of pneumonia and their characteristics? What is the most common type of pneumonia?
2. What predisposing factors contribute to the development of pneumonia?
3. What are the typical manifestations of acute bacterial pneumonia? Which ones did Greg exhibit? What are the pathophysiological bases for the various clinical manifestations?
4. Explain the bases for each of the medical treatments that were prescribed for Greg.
5. What complications may result from bacterial pneumonia? Compare these complications to those characteristic of viral pneumonia.
6. Explain the results of the chest x-ray and the laboratory studies.

REVIEW QUESTIONS

The number of the question corresponds to the same numbered objective at the beginning of the chapter.

1. Which of the following statements characterize pneumococcal pnuemonia?
   - **a.** generally causes an interstitial type of pneumonia
   - **b.** usually self-limiting and treated symptomatically
   - **c.** characterized by productive cough with rust-colored sputum
   - **d.** most common complication is pneumothorax

2. Which of the following would not be considered an appropriate nursing intervention for the client with pneumonia?
   - **a.** assisting with postural drainage every 2 to 3 hours
   - **b.** teaching the client proper disposal of soiled tissues
   - **c.** allowing the client to sleep in the semi-Fowler's position
   - **d.** administering analgesics for chest pain

3. Clinical manifestations of TB include
   - **a.** chest pain and morning sweats
   - **b.** productive cough and high-grade fevers
   - **c.** night sweats and cough
   - **d.** hemoptysis and rust-colored sputum

4. All the following are types of fungal infections *except*

a. histoplasmosis
b. coccidioidomycosis
c. aspergillosis
d. mycoplasmosis

5. Bronchiectasis is characterized by
a. bronchoconstriction and mucosal edema
b. hypersensitivity of small bronchioles
c. chronic dilatation of the bronchi
d. rupture of bronchi secondary to fibrosis

6. The major advantage of a Venturi mask is that it can
a. deliver precise, high-flow rates of O_2
b. provide continuous 100% humidity
c. be used while a client eats and sleeps
d. deliver up to 80% oxygen

7. A common pathological characteristic of many types of pneumoconiosis is
a. diffuse airway obstruction
b. diffuse pulmonary fibrosis
c. benign tumor growth
d. liquefactive necrosis

8. The type of lung cancer generally associated with the best prognosis because it is potentially surgical resectable is
a. squamous-cell carcinoma
b. anaplastic carcinoma
c. adenocarcinoma
d. bronchioalveolar carcinoma

9. A common cause of flail chest is
a. multiple rib fractures
b. spontaneous pneumothorax
c. kyphoscoliosis
d. atelectasis

10. The purpose of closed chest-tube drainage is to
a. prevent the escape of air from the pleural space
b. produce additional negative alveolar pressure
c. equalize the pressure in the chest cavity
d. remove air and fluid from the pleural space

11. Nursing measures that should be instituted following a thoracotomy include all the following except
a. range-of-motion exercises on the affected upper extremity
b. keeping the client off the unaffected side following a pneumonectomy
c. monitoring chest tube drainage and functioning
d. using a shoulder sling to immobilize the affected upper extremity

12. The Guillain-Barre syndrome causes respiratory problems primarily by
a. depressing the central nervous sustem
b. paralyzing the diaphragm secondary to trauma
c. interrupting nerve transmission to respiratory muscles
d. deforming chest wall muscles

13. Which of the following descriptions best characterizes cor pulmonale?
a. right ventricular hypertrophy secondary to increased pulmonary vascular resistance?
b. right ventricular hypertrophy secondary to congenital heart disease
c. pulmonary congestion secondary to left ventricular failure
d. excess serous fluid collection in the alveoli secondary to heart failure

REFERENCES

1. D. D. Briggs, "Pulmonary Infections," *Med Clin North Am*, **61:**1163–1180, (1977).
2. J. V. Hirschmann, "Pneumonia and Lung Abscess," in K. Isselbacher et al. (eds.), *Harrison's Principles of Internal Medicine* 9th ed., McGraw-Hill Book Company, New York, 1980, pp. 1223–1229.
3. M. P. Reyes, "The Aerobic Gram-Negative Bacillary Pneumonias," *Med Clin North Am*, **64:**363–382 (1980).
4. R. C. Reichman and R. Dolin, "Viral Pneumonias," *Med Clin North Am*, **64:**491–503 (1980).
5. Briggs, op. cit., p. 1174.
6. Reichman and Dolin, op. cit., p. 500.
7. Ibid., p. 498.
8. *Pneumonia,* American Lung Association, New York, 1979.
9. B. E. Murray and R.C. Moellering, "Antimicrobial Agents in Pulmonary Infections," *Med Clin North Am*, **64:**319–340 (1980).
10. L. S. Farer, "All about TB," in *Clinical Notes on Respiratory Diseases,* American Lung Association, New York, 1978.
11. Ibid.
12. S. Price and L. Wilson, *Pathophysiology: Clinical Concepts of Disease Processes,* 2d ed., McGraw-Hill Book Company, New York, 1982, p. 476.
13. Isselbacher et al., op. cit., p. 702.
14. J. A. Sbarbaro, "Tuberculosis," *Med Clin North Am*, **64:**417–429 (1980).
15. "Guidelines for Short-Course Tuberculosis Chemotherapy," *Am Rev Respir Dis*, **121:**1–4 (1980).
16. Ibid.
17. Sbarbaro, op. cit., p. 428.
18. Briggs, op. cit., p. 1175.
19. Ibid.
20. J. F. Murray, "Bronchiectasis and Broncholithiasis," in Isselbacher et al., op. cit., pp. 1229–1233.
21. P. L. Fuchs, "Getting the Best Out of Oxygen Delivery Systems," *Nursing 80*, **10:**34–43 (1980).
22. H. M. Sweetwood, *Nursing in the Intensive Respiratory Care Unit,* 2d ed., Springer Publishing Co., New York, 1979, pp. 237–238.
23. J. M. Anderson, *Occupational Lung Diseases: An Introduction,* American Lung Association, New York, 1979.
24. *Cancer 1981 Facts and Figures,* American Cancer Society, New York, 1980.
25. Ibid.
26. D. Rodescu, "Lung Cancer," *Med Clin North Am*, **61:**1205–1215 (1977).
27. Ibid.
28. G. M. Tisi, "Neoplasms of the Lung," in Isselbacher et al., op. cit., pp. 1260–1265.
29. Ibid.
30. Ibid.

31. L. Begg Marino, *Cancer Nursing,* The C. V. Mosby Company, St. Louis, 1981, p. 197.
32. Ibid., p. 195.
33. M. Cameron, "Before and after Thoracotomy," *Nursing,* **8:**28–36 (1978).
34. C. J. Johns, "Sarcoidosis," in Isselbacher et al., op. cit., pp. 928–929.
35. K. M. Moser, "Pulmonary Thromboembolism," in Isselbacher et al., op. cit., pp. 1249–1251.
36. J. D. Hardy, "Lung Transplantation," in A. P. Fishman, *Pulmonary Diseases and Disorders,* McGraw-Hill Book Company, New York, 1980, pp. 1739–1747.

Chapter 21

NURSING ROLE IN MANAGEMENT

Obstructive Pulmonary Diseases

Sharon Mantik Lewis

Learning Objectives

1. Describe the effects of cigarette and marijuana smoking on the lungs.
2. Describe the types, pathophysiology, clinical manifestations, and medical and pharmacological management of asthma.
3. Describe the nursing role in management of the client with asthma.
4. Differentiate among the etiology, pathogenesis, clinical manifestations, complications, and medical management of chronic bronchitis and pulmonary emphysema.
5. Explain the respiratory therapy and nursing management of the client with chronic bronchitis and pulmonary emphysema.
6. Describe the pathophysiology, clinical manifestations, and medical and nursing management of the client with cystic fibrosis.

Chronic obstructive airway disease is a descriptive term for diseases characterized by obstruction of the small airways (Fig. 21-1). Included in this grouping are asthma (usually reversible), pulmonary emphysema (usually irreversible), and chronic bronchitis (usually irreversible or only partially reversible). The client with a diagnosis of chronic obstructive pulmonary disease (COPD) may have distinguishing features of two or even all three diseases. Asthma will be discussed as a separate entity. Emphysema and chronic bronchitis will be considered together, and their differences will be indicated where appropriate.

Cystic fibrosis is another type of obstructive aiway disease. Although it resembles chronic bronchitis, its pathogenesis is different. The effects of smoking will be considered intially. Smoking, especially of cigarettes, is an important etiological factor and contributes to the progression of many forms of obstructive airway disease.

EFFECTS OF SMOKING

Cigarette Smoking

In 1979 the *U.S. Surgeon General's Report* stated that cigarette smoking is the single most important environmental factor contributing to premature mortality in the United States. About 325,000 premature deaths each year are related to cigarette smoking. In addition to being responsible for more than 75 percent of all lung cancers, it has been implicated in cancers of the mouth, pharynx, larynx, esophagus, pancreas, and bladder. An American Cancer Society study showed that smokers of low-tar and low-nicotine cigarettes had lower death rates than those who smoked brands with higher levels, although these cigarettes were clearly more dangerous than not smoking at all.[1]

There are hundreds of chemicals and gases in cigarettes that are inhaled into the lungs in smoking. Although many carcinogens have been isolated from cigarette smoke, 3,4-benzpyrine has been shown to be the most dangerous. Nicotine is probably not a carcinogen, but it has other important effects. It acts by stimulating the sympathetic nervous system, resulting in increased heart rate, increased peripheral vasoconstriction, increased blood pressure, and increased cardiac work load. These effects of nicotine compound the problems in a person with coronary artery disease (see Chap. 27). Other effects of nicotine are discussed in Chap. 60.

Cigarette smoke has a number of direct effects on lung tissue. The irritating effect of the smoke causes hyperplasia of cells, including goblet cells, which subsequently results in increased mucus production. Hyperplasia reduces airway diameter and increases the difficulty of clearing secretions. Smoking reduces the ciliary activity and may cause actual loss of ciliated cells. Many cells develop large, atypical nuclei, which is considered a precancerous condition. Lung tissue can be destroyed, possibly as a result of severe coughing efforts to clear the airways. There is fibrous thickening of the alveolar and capillary walls which lead to decreased diffusion of oxygen and subsequent hypoxemia.

Carbon monoxide is a component of tobacco smoke. Carbon monoxide has a high affinity for hemo-

This chapter was reviewed by Mary V. Hanley R.N., M.A., CCRN, Assistant Professor, Graduate Medical-Surgical Program, School of Nursing, Boston University, Boston, Massachusetts; and Lela Lottermoser CRTT, RRT, B.A., formerly Director of Pulmonary Services, University of New Mexico Hospital, Albuquerque, New Mexico.

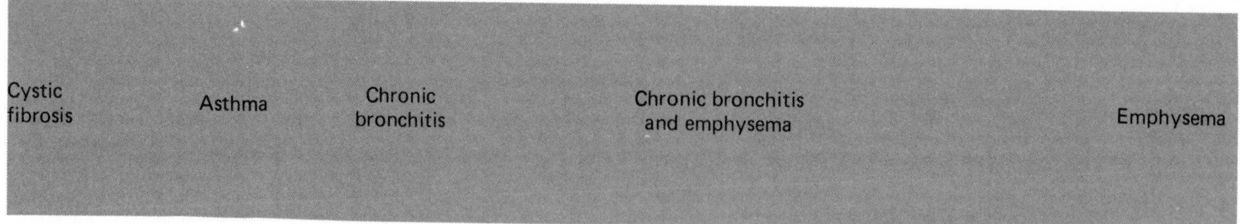

Figure 21-1 Spectrum of obstructive disease of the airways. Pure forms of either end are uncommon. Especially for the middle of the spectrum (chronic bronchitis and emphysema), mixtures are the rule. *(From A. P. Fishman, Pulmonary Diseases and Disorders, McGraw-Hill Book Company, New York, 1980, p. 459.)*

globin and combines with it more readily than does oxygen. Therefore, the smoker's oxygen-carrying capacity is reduced. In addition, when inhaling the smoke, the smoker is inhaling a lower percentage of oxygen than normal. Therefore, there is less oxygen available at the alveolar level. The heart's need for oxygen is increased due to the sympathetic stimulation of nicotine. Since the blood's oxygen-carrying capacity is reduced, the heart must pump more rapidly to supply tissues adequately with oxygen. Carbon monoxide also seems to impair psychomotor performance and judgment and may cause psychological stress. Children who live in a home with smoking parents have an increased incidence of respiratory illnesses.

Marijuana Smoking

Marijuana is the most widely used illicit drug and constitutes the greatest single new threat to the lungs of people in the United States. Although the research findings are still not conclusive, marijuana may be more dangerous to the lungs than cigarette smoking. An estimated 16 million Americans use marijuana regularly, and 44 million have smoked it at least once. In the late 1960s marijuana started to come into vogue, and by the mid-1970s, smoking it became commonplace.[2]

Over 400 chemicals are contained in marijuana, 60 of them known as *cannabinoids*, which are specifically found only in the cannabis plant (from which marijuana and hashish are prepared). The principal psychoactive ingredient is the chemical constituent Δ^9-tetrahydrocannabinol (THC). Ten years ago, the average THC content in a marijuana cigarette was 0.2 percent. Today the THC content is 4 to 6 percent.

In contrast to the cigarette smoker, the marijuana smoker inhales deeply and holds the breath to maximize absorption. Within seconds after it is inhaled, THC enters circulation and stimulates the heart rate dramatically. After 5 to 7 days, half the original THC is still in the body.[3]

Marijuana smoke contains 50 percent more carcinogens than tobacco smoke, so its potential for causing lung cancer is high. Marijuana smoke is a respiratory irritant and causes inflammatory changes in the epithelium which may be precancerous.[4]

Marijuana smoke interferes with the ability of the alveolar macrophages to fight off invading organisms. This alteration contributes to a higher incidence of respiratory infections in the chronic marijuana smoker. In addition, marijuana may suppress the immune system, especially the T lymphocytes.

Habitual marijuana smoking causes manifestations of early COPD. In addition, there is a rise in carbon monoxide in the blood when marijuana is smoked. The altered effect created by marijuana may be a contributing factor in car accidents when a person combines marijuana smoking and driving. (Other effects of marijuana are discussed in Chap. 60.)

OBSTRUCTIVE DISORDERS OF THE LUNGS

Asthma

Asthma is an intermittent, reversible, obstructive airway disease characterized by hyperirritability of the airways. Its clinical course is unpredictable, and it varies from person to person. It is characterized by periodic exacerbations. Between attacks, the person is usually clinically asymptomatic. In some persons, spontaneous remissions occur. Asthma differs from other obstructive disorders such as emphysema and chronic bronchitis, which are chronic, progressive, and irreversible or only partially reversible conditions.

Significance of the problem

A study by the National Institute of Allergy and Infectious Disease found that 8.9 million Americans are presently affected by asthma. Five percent of children less than 15 years of age have asthma.

Approximately 17 percent of all Americans have had asthma at some time in their life.[5]

The morbidity associated with the disease is dramatic. It affects school attendance, occupational choices, physical activity, and many other aspects of life. The mortality rate is relatively low, at about 2000 persons per year.[6]

Types of asthma

Asthma is often categorized as (1) extrinsic (allergic), (2) intrinsic (idiopathic or nonallergic), or (3) mixed asthma (both allergic and nonallergic factors). (See Table 21-1.)

Extrinsic Asthma Extrinsic asthma is caused by a known allergen or allergens (Fig. 21-2). Individuals with extrinsic asthma usually have a family history of allergies and a past medical history of infantile eczema or allergic rhinitis. Exposure to allergens such as inhaled pollen, animal dander, mold spore, or certain foods (e.g., milk or chocolate) triggers an asthmatic attack. Pure extrinsic asthma is found in only a minority of individuals with asthma.

Intrinsic Asthma Intrinsic asthma is not related to specific precipitating allergens, and there is usually

Table 21-1
Comparison of Intrinsic and Extrinsic Asthma

Intrinsic	Extrinsic
Onset after 35 years of age	Onset in childhood or adolescence
Incidence of atopic family history same as in the general population	Positive family history for atopic illnesses
Course is unpredictable, often chronic and severe	Seasonal course associated with environmental changes; symptoms often clear entirely after childhood
Attacks precipitated by inhaled irritants, weather changes, infection, aspirin, drugs, emotion, and exercise	Attacks precipitated by exposure to certain allergens, such as pollen, danders, feathers, mold, dusts, and some foods
Skin tests usually negative	Skin tests generally positive
Normal serum IgE	Elevated serum IgE

From E. H. Elpern, "Asthma Update: Pathophysiology and Treatment," *Heart Lung* **9**:666 (1980).

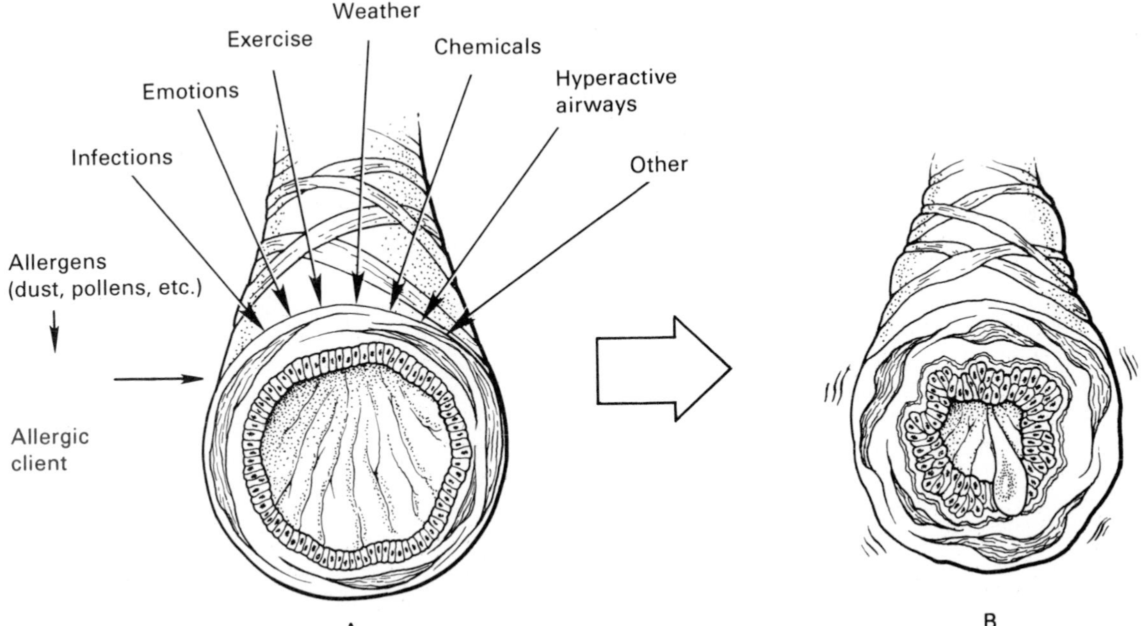

Figure 21-2 (*a*) Normal respiratory bronchiole and provoking factors that may trigger an asthma attack. (*b*) In asthma, the changes in the respiratory bronchiole include spasm from smooth muscle contraction, mucosal edema, and excess mucus production. (*Adapted from D. L. Sexton, Chronic Obstructive Pulmonary Disease, The C. V. Mosby Company, St. Louis, 1981, p. 90.*)

no family history of asthma. Nonspecific factors such as a common cold, respiratory tract infections, exercise, emotions, and environmental pollutants may trigger an attack (Fig. 21-2). Aspirin and nonsteroidal anti-inflammatory drugs may also be precipitating factors. The attacks become more severe and frequent with time, and the condition can progress to chronic bronchitis or emphysema.[7] Most individuals with chronic bronchitis and emphysema have bronchospastic aspects of the disease which may be considered as asthma.

Mixed Asthma Mixed asthma is the type of asthma that affects most individuals with this condition. It has characteristics of both extrinsic and intrinsic asthma. Children with extrinsic asthma often outgrow the condition by adolescence. Some individuals with intrinsic asthma develop mixed asthma. Mixed asthma will be the focus of this discussion.

Pathophysiology of asthma

The prominent feature of bronchial asthma is reversible, diffuse airway obstruction. Three processes involved in airway obstruction are (1) constriction of bronchial smooth muscles, (2) excess mucus production, and (3) mucosal edema (Fig. 21-3). Accompanying these changes are bronchial muscle hypertrophy, mucous gland hypertrophy, thick, tenacious sputum, and hyperinflation and air trapping in the alveoli.

The exact mechanism responsible for these changes is not known. Etiological evidence centers on alterations involving the immunological system and the autonomic nervous system.

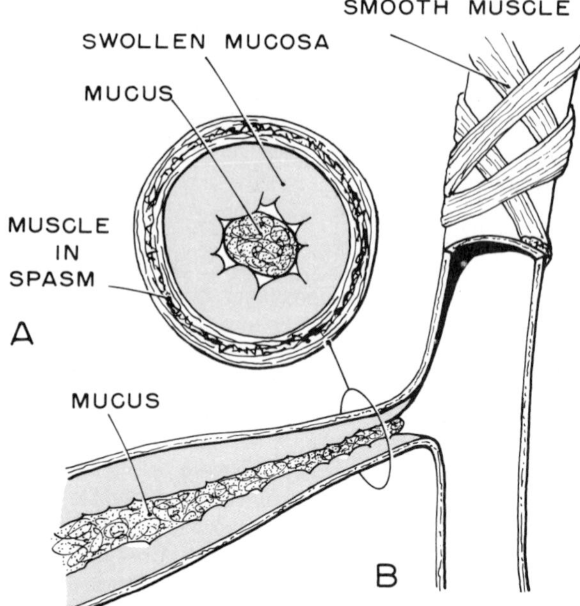

Figure 21-3 Factors causing expiratory obstruction in bronchial asthma. (*a*) Cross section of a bronchiole occluded by muscle spasm, swollen mucosa, and mucus in the lumen; (*b*) longitudinal section of a bronchiole. *(From S. Price and L. Wilson, Pathophysiology: Clinical Concepts of Disease Processes, 2d ed., McGraw-Hill Book Company, New York, 1982, p. 434.)*

Immunological Alterations Asthma is an example of a Type I hypersensitivity reaction (Chap. 10). Some asthmatics develop exaggerated immunoglobin E (IgE) responses to their environment. It has been shown that abnormally large amounts of IgE are produced in response to certain antigens or allergens (e.g., dust, pollen, drugs, grasses, microorganisms). IgE antibodies attach to mast cells (Fig. 21-4). Reexposure to even minute amounts of the antigen results in antigen binding to the antibody. This event triggers the release of mast cell products such as histamine which acts locally and systemically. The IgE–mast cell complexes remain for long periods of time, so that the second exposure will trigger mast cell release even years after the initial exposure to the antigen.

An interesting observation regarding inhaled antigens is their need to pass through the respiratory mucosa into the bloodstream to make contact with mast cells. Normally, secretory immunoglobulin A (IgA) found in secretions such as mucus, saliva, and sweat protects against invasion of foreign substances into underlying tissue. In asthma there is a possible deficiency in secretory IgA which may be one factor contributing to the disease.[8] It is also known that some mast cells are located in the mucosa. Interaction with the antigen there can facilitate penetration of the antigen into the submucosa and, thus, the bloodstream.[9]

When mast cells degranulate, they release chemical mediators which cause a variety of biological activities (Table 21-2). The effects of these mediators may result from direct contact with the bronchial mucosa. They also result from the effects of reflex vagal nerve stimulation by irritant receptors in the mucosa. The chemical mediators consist of all the factors needed for a locally controlled inflammatory reaction. The end results of the action of these mediators are bronchial smooth muscle contraction, increased secretion of mucus, and dilatation and increased permeability of small blood vessels (primarily venules).

Autonomic Nervous System Alterations The autonomic nervous system, consisting of the parasympathetic and sympathetic systems, innervates the

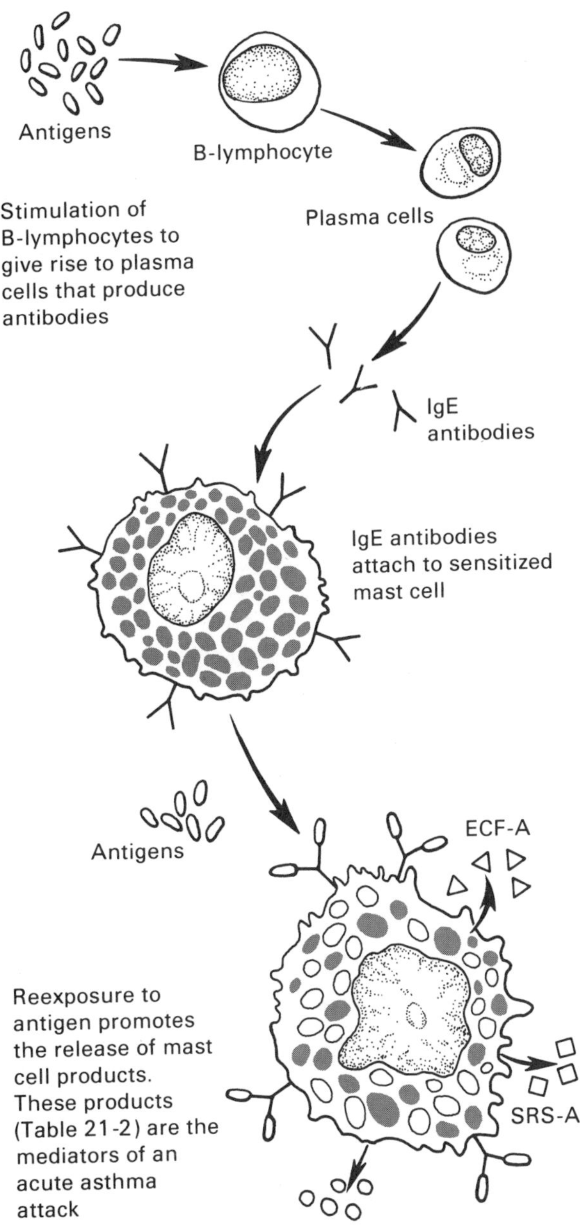
Antigens
B-lymphocyte
Plasma cells
Stimulation of B-lymphocytes to give rise to plasma cells that produce antibodies
IgE antibodies
IgE antibodies attach to sensitized mast cell
Antigens
ECF-A
Reexposure to antigen promotes the release of mast cell products. These products (Table 21-2) are the mediators of an acute asthma attack
SRS-A
Histamine
Figure 21-4 Mechanism of mediator release in an asthma attack.

lungs. Bronchial muscle tone is regulated by vagal nerve impulses via the parasympathetic system. Afferent and efferent impulses are conducted via the vagus nerve to the medulla and back to the lungs. When airway nerve endings are stimulated by mechanical or chemical stimuli (e.g., air pollution, cold air, dust), increased release of acetylcholine causes reflex bronchoconstriction as well as increased production of chemical mediators, as described in the preceding section.[10] These chemical mediators also produce bronchoconstriction. Therefore, parasympathetic stimulation results in bronchoconstriction and release of chemical mediators. A proposed theory is that asthmatics have a low threshold for parasympathetic responses. This may explain why the airways of asthmatics are sensitive to nonspecific irritants.[11]

Both alpha- (α-) and beta- (β-) adrenergic receptors of the sympathetic nervous system are located in the bronchi. When the α receptors are stimulated, bronchoconstriction occurs. When the β receptors (primarily β_2 receptors are located in the bronchi) are stimulated, bronchodilatation occurs.

The balance between alpha and beta receptors is mediated primarily by cyclic adenosine monophosphate (c-AMP). Alpha-adrenergic stimulation results in decreased levels of c-AMP, leading to (1) increased mast cell release of chemical mediators and (2) bronchoconstriction. Beta-adrenergic stimulation results in increased levels of c-AMP, which (1) inhibits release of chemical mediators and (2) promotes bronchodilatation. Epinephrine acts primarily on beta receptors.

A proposed theory is that there is a beta-adrenergic blockade in asthmatics. Therefore, their beta-adrenergic response is altered, and they are prone to increased release of chemical mediators and constriction of bronchial smooth muscle.[12] Broncho-

Table 21-2
Chemical Mediators Involved in Type I Hypersensitivity Reactions

Mediator	Biological Activity
Histamine	Constricts bronchial smooth muscle. Dilates capillaries and venules. Stimulates irritant receptors in the mucosa. Increases mucus production.
Slow reacting substance of anaphylaxis (SRS-A)	Causes prolonged smooth muscle spasm. Dilates and increases venule permeability.
Eosinophil chemotactic factor of anaphylaxis (ECF-A)	Attracts eosinophils.
Serotonin	Causes contraction of smooth muscle. Increases vascular permeability.
Neutrophil chemotactic factor (NCF-A)	Causes migration of neutrophils.
Bradykinin (made from blood proteins known as *kininogens*)	Constricts bronchial smooth muscle. Increases blood vessel permeability. Stimulates irritant receptors in the mucosa.

constriction is the predominant response mediated by cholinergic receptors (parasympathetic system) and alpha-adrenergic receptors.

Other Factors Related to Asthma Another factor often discussed in relationship to the etiology of asthma is psychological or emotional stimuli. Rarely are these factors the sole cause of asthma. Contrary to the thinking of some persons, asthma is not a psychosomatic disease. Psychological or emotional factors may aggravate symptoms of asthma and on occasion initiate an asthma attack. Having an asthma attack is a very frightening experience. It is possible that the emotional components develop as a result of the client's feelings and reactions to his diagnosis of asthma. Therefore, it is difficult to assess whether the observed emotional reaction is part of the etiological mechanism or a consequence of the disorder.

Viral and, to a less extent, bacterial infections are common precipitating factors in an asthma attack. These infections cause inflammatory changes in the tracheobronchial system and alter the mucociliary mechanism. Therefore, they increase the hyperresponsiveness of the bronchial system.

Exercise-induced asthma (EIA) may be the only form of asthma in some individuals, especially children. Typically, it occurs after several minutes of vigorous exercise (e.g., jogging) and is characterized by bronchospasm. Cromolyn sodium may be of value in helping these individuals to maintain bronchodilatation during exercise (see the section on Pharmacological Management for a discussion of this drug). Physical exertion, by causing obligatory mouth breathing of cold, dry air, may induce bronchospasm. This is probably why physical exertion is a contributing factor to an attack in many asthmatics.

Clinical manifestations

Asthma is characterized by an unpredictable and variable course. An attack of asthma may have an abrupt onset but is usually more gradual. Attacks often occur at night. Most of them last for a few minutes to several hours, and then the client recovers. Between attacks, the client may be asymptomatic, with normal pulmonary function. However, in some individuals, compromised pulmonary function may result in a state of continuous asthma and chronic debilitation.

The characteristic clinical manifestations of asthma are wheezing, coughing, and dyspnea following exposure to the causative allergen or precipitating factor. Expiration is more difficult than inspiration. Normally, the bronchioles constrict during expiration. However, expiration becomes more difficult when the bronchioles are constricted, edematous, and filled with mucus. Prolonged, wheezing expirations are characteristic. The cough may be nonproductive or produce thick, tenacious, white, gelatinous mucus. The attack usually ends with the client producing large quantities of thick, stringy mucus.

Asthmatics feel as though they are suffocating because they have difficulty moving air in and out of the lungs. The asthmatic sits upright and uses the accessory muscles of respiration during an acute attack to try to get enough air. The more difficult breathing becomes, the more anxious the client feels.

Findings of physical examination of the client during an acute attack may include transient cyanosis, increased pulse and respiratory rate, use of accessory muscles, and observable dyspnea—especially on prolonged expiration. Auscultation of the chest may indicate the presence of rhonchi. Wheezing, both on inspiration and on expiration, is usually present.

Chronic asthma can result in complications such as pulmonary emphysema, chronic bronchitis, and bronchiectasis. Status asthmaticus is another possible complication and is described in the next section.

Status asthmaticus

Status asthmaticus is severe asthma that persists for longer than 24 hours and does not respond to conventional therapy such as epinephrine, terbutaline, and aminophylline. The condition is potentially life-threatening and requires constant monitoring in a hospital setting. Causes of status asthmaticus may include abrupt discontinuation of drug therapy (especially corticosteroids), respiratory infection, abuse of aerosol medications, massive exposure to allergens, and ingesting β-adrenergic blocking drugs (e.g., propanolol).

The client has clinical manifestations similar to those mentioned in the previous section, but they are more severe and more prolonged. Hypoxemia with hypocapnia is usually detected initially in arterial blood gases. As the severity of the attacks increases, hypoxemia with hypercapnia may develop.

Treatment consists of establishing an intravenous (IV) line for administration of drugs and IV fluids. Aminophylline is given intravenously as a loading dose and is then followed with a continuous IV drip for maintenance therapy. Supplementary oxygen is usually best given via nasal prongs or a Venturi mask (see the section on Oxygen Therapy in Chap. 20). Arterial blood gases are tested at frequent intervals to monitor the acid-base balance of the client. Mechanically assisted ventilation may be necessary if the blood gases indicate respiratory failure (see Chap. 22). IV administration of corticosteroids (e.g., Solu-Cortef) is usually begun if the above measures do not result in significant improvement. Sodium bicarbonate will be given intravenously to correct respiratory acidosis.

Continuous monitoring of the client is critical. Knowing that someone is observing will help decrease the client's anxiety. It will also ensure prompt recognition of changes in the client's status and provide the basis for possible changes in therapy. A bronchoscopy may be necessary to remove thick mucus plugs.

Repeated attacks of status asthmaticus can lead to irreversible emphysema. Cor pulmonale may occur late in the course of severe status asthmaticus. Death from status asthmaticus is usually due to respiratory arrest or cardiac failure.

Diagnostic study abnormalities

Wheezing and respiratory distress characterize a variety of disorders, including chronic bronchitis and emphysema, cystic fibrosis, pulmonary edema, bronchial obstruction, and bronchial asthma. It is necessary to perform certain diagnostic studies to determine if these symptoms are caused primarily by asthma. The client's history may indicate previous attacks of a similar nature, often precipitated by a known cause. A chest x-ray obtained during an acute asthma attack may show findings resembling emphysema, with the presence of hyperinflation. Small areas of atelectasis may also be found. After the attack, the x-ray findings are often normal.[13]

Pulmonary function studies are valuable diagnostic tools and often show early evidence of increased airway resistance. Typical findings are decreases in forced expired volume in one second ($FEV_{1.0}$), peak expiratory flow rate (PEFR), and forced expiratory flow rate during the middle of forced vital capacity ($FEF_{25-75\%}$). The functional residual capacity (FRC) is increased, reflecting increased air trapping in the distal airways.[14] An improvement in abnormal values is usually obtained after inhalation of a bronchodilator drug.

Arterial blood gas monitoring is essential to assess the client during an asthmatic attack. It provides information on the severity of the attack as well as on the response to therapy. Characteristically, there is decreased arterial oxygen pressure (P_aO_2) throughout the attack. The level of arterial carbon dioxide pressure (P_aCO_2) is usually low or normal, and respiratory alkalosis is present. A rise in P_aCO_2 indicates increasing severity of the airway obstruction.

Allergy skin testing may be of some value in trying to determine the sensitivity to a specific antigen. However, a positive skin test does not necessarily mean that the allergen is causing the asthma attack. On the other hand, a negative allergy test does not mean that the asthma is not allergy-related.

A sputum specimen for Gram stain and culture is often obtained to detect the presence of a bacterial infection. A sputum specimen can also be analyzed for the presence of eosinophils. Blood levels of eosinophils are often elevated in asthma.

Medical management

Acute Asthma A client frequently comes to the emergency room or a physician's office in acute respiratory distress (Table 21-3). The objectives of management at this stage are to:[15]

1. Restore and maintain ventilation
2. Relieve bronchospasm and decrease mucosal edema
3. Facilitate secretion removal

Oxygen therapy should be started immediately and its administration should be monitored by arterial blood gases. The drugs used are described in the section on Pharmacological Management. Aminophylline is considered essential to treatment. A loading dose is usually administered and is then followed by continuous infusion. Terbutaline or epinephrine given subcutaneously can be repeated 2 to 3 times within a 30-minute period.

Table 21-3
Medical Management: Asthma

Diagnostic
1. History and physical examination
2. *Pulmonary function studies,* including the response to bronchodilator therapy
3. Chest x-ray
4. Arterial blood gases
5. Allergy skin testing
6. Sputum specimen for eosinophils, Gram stain, and culture
7. Blood level of eosinophils

Therapeutic for acute asthma
1. Nasal oxygen
2. Aminophylline intravenously
3. Terbutaline or epinephrine subQ
4. Corticosteroids intravenously
5. Chest physiotherapy and postural drainage
6. Fluid intake of 3 L/day

Therapeutic for chronic asthma
1. Elimination of causative agents
2. Desensitization (immunotherapy) if indicated
3. Stepwise addition of medication
   a. Theophylline compound (oral)
   b. Beta-adrenergic (inhalant)
   c. Cromolyn sodium (inhalant)
   d. Beclomethasone (inhalant)
   e. Beta-adrenergic (oral)
   f. Corticosteroids (oral)
4. Chest physiotherapy and postural drainage

Corticosteroids do not have an immediate effect. They are usually effective 4 to 8 hours after administration.[16] Adequate fluid intake is necessary to replace the fluid lost because of hyperventilation and diaphoresis. It will also help to liquefy tenacious sputum. If postural drainage is indicated, it should focus on the affected areas as identified on chest x-ray or by physical examination (e.g., auscultation).

Therapy should be continued until the client is breathing comfortably, wheezing has disappeared, and pulmonary function study results are near the client's normal values. If the attack subsides, the client often returns home. If recovery is incomplete, the client will be hospitalized for further observation and treatment.

Chronic Asthma Chronic asthma is characterized by a previous diagnosis of asthma as well as frequent, severe, episodic dyspnea. The chronic asthmatic needs a bronchodilatation program to prevent periodic attacks and to improve the pulmonary reserve.[17]

In one therapeutic approach, the client attempts to avoid or control environmental irritants, allergens, and precipitating factors. A program of desensitization (immunotherapy) may be of value for the individual with a well-demonstrated sensitivity to an allergen, especially if the asthma is related to a seasonal allergen. (Desensitization is described in Chap. 10.)

Bronchodilator drug therapy is usually begun as a prophylactic measure. These drugs are outlined in Table 21-4 and discussed in the section on Pharmacological Management. If satisfactory control cannot be obtained with one agent, then other drugs are added to the client's regimen.

Ongoing chest physiotherapy and postural drainage may be of value in some clients to mobilize secretions. These procedures are discussed later in the chapter. Before asthmatics undergo these procedures, they should be given a bronchodilator.

Pharmacological management

Methylxanthine Derivatives Methylxanthine derivatives (theophylline preparations) are the mainstay of pharmacological management of asthma. Methylxanthine may be the only drug required to treat mild attacks.[18] The main therapeutic action of methylxanthine derivatives on the respiratory system is bronchodilatation. Theophylline inhibits the breakdown of c-AMP, which is needed for bronchodilatation (Fig. 21-5). These drugs are especially effective in relieving bronchospasm. They are readily absorbed orally, parenterally (excluding the intramuscular [IM] route), and rectally. Absorption by the rectal route is not reliable or predictable and is not frequently used. IM injections can cause tissue irritation.

Theophylline preparations stimulate the heart and production of gastric hydrochloric acid (HCl) and act as a diuretic. They can also stimulate the central nervous system. Specific side effects are listed in Table 21-4.

Theophylline levels of 10 to 20 μg/mL are considered to be therapeutic.[19] This is a narrow margin of safety, and toxicity can easily occur. Aminophylline (a theophylline derivative) is usually used initially in the treatment of an acute asthmatic attack. Then a continuous IV infusion at a prescribed rate is given. There are many theophylline preparations, some of which are listed in Table 21-4.

Adrenergic Stimulants Sympathomimetic adrenergic drugs can be classified according to their receptor activity. The receptors on cells are alpha (α), beta$_1$ (β_1), and beta$_2$ (β_2). The alpha and beta$_1$ receptors are discussed in Chap. 26 and Table 26-7. The beta$_2$ receptors located in the smooth muscle of the bronchi and pulmonary blood vessels are of particular importance in understanding the action of sympathomimetic drugs on the respiratory system. Sympathomimetic stimulation of the β_2 receptors results in bronchodilatation by increasing the level of c-AMP (Fig. 21-5). Drugs producing this effect are classified as sympathomimetic bronchodilators and are presented in Table 21-4. These drugs can be administered orally, parenterally, or by inhalation using a metered-dose aerosol or a hand nebulizer.

In acute asthmatic attacks, terbutaline or epinephrine is given subcutaneously. Many adrenergic drugs are available as aerosol inhalants. The main problem with this method of administration is the potential for abuse, which can lead to serious and potentially lethal cardiovascular toxicity. These agents

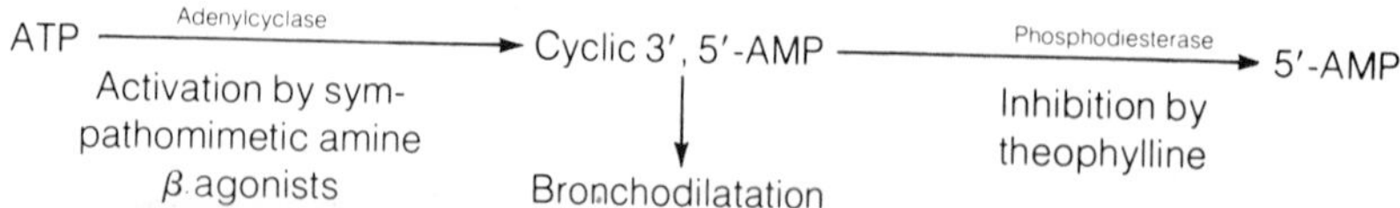

Figure 21-5 Theoretical mechanism of bronchodilatation for sympathomimetic β_2 agonists and theophyline. *(From M. Wiener et al., Clinical Pharmacology and Therapeutics in Nursing, McGraw-Hill Book Company, New York, 1979, p. 358.)*

should be prescribed only for those clients who are not likely to overuse them.

Chromones Cromolyn sodium (Aarane, Intal) stabilizes the mast cell and prevents its degranulation, thus inhibiting antigen-induced bronchospasm.[20] It is available as gelatinous capsules which are placed in a special inhaler. It is a relatively safe drug. A common side effect is irritation of the upper airway. Cromolyn sodium has been shown effective in preventing exercise-induced asthma if administered prior to the start of exercise. Unfortunately, there is poor compliance with cromolyn sodium because the client does not feel any immediate effect.

Corticosteroids Corticosteroids are used primarily when other therapy has failed to work. In acute asthma attacks, they are used to relieve symptoms of bronchospasm. Initially, hydrocortisone (Solu-Cortef) is given intravenously. The onset of action occurs about 4 to 6 hours after steroids are started. When the client improves clinically, oral corticosteroids should be substituted and the dosage tapered quickly. If continued steroid therapy is necessary, an alternate-day schedule of administration may minimize the side effects.

Inhaled steroids such as beclomethasone (Vanceril) have been used in the management of asthmatics. This drug acts directly on the bronchial mucosa with a minimum of systemic absorption.

Antibiotics The prophylactic use of antibiotics in asthma is not indicated. If they are used in this manner, they encourage the growth of resistant strains of bacteria. Therefore, the client with asthma who develops respiratory infections may be resistant to commonly used antibiotics and may subsequently die.

The organisms that cause pneumonia most frequently are *Streptococcus pneumoniae, Haemophilus influenzae*, and viruses. Appropriate antibiotic therapy should be based on Gram stain and sputum culture and sensitivity.

Antihistamines Antihistamines are of little value in the management of asthma. One reason for this is that histamine is only one of the mediators involved in the asthmatic process. Antihistamines do not affect such substances as slow reacting substance of anaphylaxis (SRS-A). Antihistamines cause drying of the respiratory mucosa, which can thicken the mucus, an undesired effect in asthmatics.

Nonprescription Combination Drugs Several combination products are available as over-the-counter drugs. They are usually combinations of a bronchodilator, an expectorant, and a sedative. (Some of these combination drugs are listed in Table 21-5.) These agents are advertised as drugs to relieve bronchospasm. In general, they should be avoided by individuals with obstructive lung disease. Many persons consider these drugs safe because they can be obtained without a prescription.

Some of the dangers of these drugs are as follows:[21]

1. Epinephrine acts for only a short period of time, and rebound bronchospasm may occur.
2. Clients seeking relief have a tendency to overuse the agent.
3. A combination of ephedrine and theophylline can enhance toxicity.
4. Guaifenesin, an expectorant, can increase secretions from mucous glands (salivary, nasal, lacrimal).
5. Phenobarbital interferes with the action of steroids and thus is contraindicated in asthmatics receiving steroid therapy.
6. Freon is a gas used to propel some inhalant medications. It can cause bronchospasm and possibly cardiac arrhythmias.

An important teaching responsibility of health professionals is to warn clients about the dangers associated with nonprescription combination drugs. These drugs are especially dangerous to clients with underlying cardiac problems. If a client insists on or persists in taking one of these medications, then he should be cautioned to read and follow the accompanying directions on the label. Another way of discouraging the use of these drugs is to monitor carefully and reevaluate the effectiveness of the prescribed drug therapy. The drug regimen may have to be adjusted to help the client obtain maximum relief from bronchospasm. An attitude of understanding and caring will often reassure the client that the medical and nursing professions are concerned. This may prevent the client from attempting to find relief at the local drugstore.

Therapy Plan The pharmacological treatment plan depends on the severity of the disease and the individual's response to treatment. Mild asthma can usually be controlled with the prophylactic use of a single oral agent, usually a theophylline preparation or a β_2-specific sympathomimetic drug. If this plan is not effective and asthma attacks continue, then a theophylline preparation and a sympathomimetic drug are used together. A more vigorous regimen requires aerosol bronchodilators, cromolyn sodium, or beclomethasone. In moderately severe to severe asthma,

Table 21-4
Drugs Used in the Treatment of COPD

Drug	Route of Administration	Mechanism of Action	Side Effects	Comments
		Sympathomimetic Bronchodilators		
Epinephrine (Adrenalin)	Subcutaneous (1:100 solution Aerosol (Medihaler-Epi)	β-adrenergic stimulant. Relaxes bronchial smooth muscle. Constricts blood vessels in bronchial mucosa due to its β_1 and α activity. (Cardiac stimulant effects are discussed in Chaps. 26 and 28.)	Headache Dizziness Palpitations Tremors Restlessness Hypertension	Used primarily to treat bronchial asthma attacks. Should not be used in clients with arrhythmias or hypertension. Paradoxical fall in PO_2 due to vasodilation.
Isoproterenol (Isuprel)	Parenteral Aerosol (Medihaler-Iso)	β-adrenergic stimulant. Primarily affects β_2 receptors. Quick-acting bronchodilator. Does not cause decongestion because it causes vasodilatation.	Tachycardia Headache Nausea Palpitations Tremor Insomnia	Instruct client regarding self-administration of inhalants. Abuse can lead to excessive cardiac side effects.
Metaproterenol (Alupent, Metaprel)	Aerosol Oral tablets Elixir	Similar to above. Has a longer duration than isoproterenol.	Tachycardia Hypertension Nervousness Palpitations	Should not be used in clients with angina or other cardiac disorders.
Ephedrine	Oral tablets Elixir	Stimulates both α and β_2 receptors. Causes bronchodilatation. Action is more prolonged, although less effective, than that of epinephrine. α-stimulant effect results in vasoconstriction.	Same as those of epinephrine	
Isoetharine (Bronkometer, Bronkosol)	Aerosol	Stimulates β_2-adrenergic receptors, producing bronchodilatation.	Tachycardia Hypertension Nervousness Palpitations	
Terbutaline (Bricanyl)	Oral tablets Aerosol* Parenteral	Stimulates β_2-adrenergic receptors, producing bronchodilatation. Also stimulates β_1 and receptors. Has long-acting effects.	Nervousness Tachycardia Palpitations Resting tremor	Relatively few side effects when used as prescribed. Has fewer cardiotoxic effects than other sympathomimetic bronchodilators.
Salbutamol	Aerosol	Same as that of terbutaline.	Same as those of terbutaline	Same as above.

		Methylxanthine Derivative Bronchodilators		
Theophylline preparations **Aminophylline** **Slophyllin, Quibron (theophylline and guaifenesin)** **Choledyl (oxtriphylline)** **Brophylline** **Quadrinal**	Oral tablets Elixir Rectal Parenteral	Produce relaxation of the bronchial smooth muscles.	Tachycardia Hypertension Arrhythmias Anorexia Nausea Vomiting Nervousness Irritability Headache	Wide variety in response to drug metabolism. Half-life decreased by smoking and increased by congestive heart failure and liver disease. GI side effects may be alleviated by taking drug with food. Client should be instructed to lie down if dizziness is experienced.
		Chromones		
Chromolyn sodium (Aarane, Intal)	Aerosol	Inhibits the release of histamine and SRS-A by acting directly on the mast cell.	Irritation of the throat Relatively nontoxic	Not a bronchodilator and should not be used in an acute asthmatic attack. Used for asthma (e.g., before exercise) prophylactically if an allergen is a causative agent.
		Mucolytics		
Acetylcysteine (Mucomyst)	Aerosol	Enzyme that breaks down mucoproteins. Decreases mucus viscosity and enhances mobilization of secretions.	Bronchospasm Hemoptysis Nausea Vomiting	After administration of mucolytics, secretions may become very profuse. Use of mucolytic agents may not be necessary if client is kept well hydrated and humidified.
		Corticosteroids		
Hydrocortisone (Solu-Cortef) **Methylprednisolone (Medrol)** **Prednisone**	IV Oral Oral	Anti-inflammatory and immunosuppressive effects. Decreases edema in bronchial airways.	Cushingoid appearance Skin changes (acne, striae, bruising) Osteoporosis Increased appetite Obesity Peptic ulcer Hypertension Hypokalemia Cataracts Menstrual irregularities Muscle weakness	Alternate-day therapy minimizes the side effects. Tapering of dose needs to be done slowly to prevent adrenal insufficiency.
Beclomethasone (Vanceril)	Aerosol	Same as above. Acts locally in respiratory tract with relatively little absorption.	Oral thrush infections. Few systemic effects.	Not recommended for an acute attack of asthma. Rinse mouth after use.

*Not currently FDA approved.

Table 21-5
Nonprescription Combination Asthma Drugs

Drug Product	Ingredients		
	Sympathomimetic	Xanthine	Other
Amodrine	Ephedrine	Aminophylline	Phenobarbital
Asthma Nefrin inhalant	Epinephrine		Chlorobutanol
Bronkaid tablets	Ephedrine	Theophylline	Guaifenesin
Bronkaid mist	Epinephrine		Ascorbic acid Alcohol
Bronkotabs	Ephedrine	Theophylline	Guaifenesin Phenobarbital
Primatene M tablets	Ephedrine	Theophylline	Pyrilamine
Primatene P tablets	Ephedrine	Theophylline	Phenobarbital
Primatene Mist	Epinephrine		Ascorbic acid Alcohol
Tedral	Ephedrine	Theophylline	Phenobarbital
Vaponefrin inhalant	Epinephrine		Chlorobutanol

oral prednisone is added to regular doses of bronchodilators.[22]

Acute severe asthma attacks are treated with IV aminophylline, subcutaneous (SC) terbutaline or epinephrine, and a nebulizer administration of sympathomimetic bronchodilators.

Nursing management

Health Promotion and Maintenance The nursing role in preventing asthma attacks or decreasing their severity focuses primarily on teaching the client and family. The client should be taught to avoid, if possible, known potential allergens (e.g., cigarette smoke) and precipitating factors (e.g., excess exercise, cold air, aspirin). Staying indoors when there is a high degree of air pollution may be helpful. If cold air cannot be avoided, dressing properly with scarves or using a mask may prevent an asthma attack. Aspirin and nonsteroidal anti-inflammatory drugs such as indomethacin should be avoided if they are known to precipitate an attack. Many over-the-counter drugs contain aspirin, and the client should be instructed to read the labels carefully. Desensitization (immunotherapy) may be partially effective in decreasing the individual's sensitivity to known allergens (see Chap. 10).

Prompt diagnosis and treatment of upper respiratory tract infections may prevent an exacerbation of asthma. If occupational irritants are involved as etiological factors, the individual may need to consider changing jobs. Beta-blocking agents, such as propanolol, are contraindicated. (These drugs and their indications for use are discussed in Chap. 27.)

The client should be encouraged to maintain a fluid intake of 2 to 3 L/day, good nutrition, and adequate rest. If exercise is planned, administering cromolyn sodium 15 to 30 minutes beforehand should prevent bronchospasm.

Acute Intervention An important nursing goal during an acute attack is to decrease the sense of panic experienced by the client (Table 21-6). A calm, quiet, reassuring attitude may help the client to relax. He should be positioned comfortably (usually sitting). Staying with the client and being available provide additional comfort. It is important to monitor the client's respiratory and cardiovascular systems. This includes auscultating lung sounds, observing for cyanosis, and taking the pulse rate, respiratory rate, and blood pressure.

When the acute attack subsides, the nurse should provide rest and a quiet environment for the client. When the client has recovered from exhaustion, the nurse should attempt to obtain information about the

Table 21-6
Nursing Care Plan for the Client with Asthma

Client Problem	Expected Outcome	Nursing Intervention
	Acute Management	
Dyspnea	Absence of wheezing and chest tightness. Respiratory rate of 12–18/min. Arterial blood gases within normal limits.	Provide comfortable position (e.g., bed rest in high Fowler's position or recliner chair). Administer bronchodilators as ordered (e.g., IV aminophylline, subQ terbutaline). Administer humidified O_2 (see Table 20-13). Auscultate breath sounds every 1–2 h. Monitor arterial blood gases. Assess BP, HR, RR, and level of consciousness every 15 min until stable and then every 2–4 h. Premedicate with bronchodilators before doing deep-breathing and coughing exercises or chest physiotherapy. Teach client pursed-lip and diaphragmatic breathing.
Dehydration	Moist mucous membranes and thin sputum.	Administer IV fluids as ordered. Later, force oral fluids to 3000 mL/day. Provide for oral hygiene. Monitor intake and output and body weight. Use *humidified* oxygen equipment.
Apprehension, anxiety	Calm feeling. Reduced anxiety over asthma.	Do *not* oversedate. Stay with client. Encourage slow, deep breathing. Promptly treat any exacerbations of an attack. Anticipate client's needs. Provide anticipatory guidance for client to prevent exacerbations.
Fatigue	Feeling of being rested. Increased energy to do self-care activities.	Plan 90–120-min rest periods. Provide total care for client at onset with progressive self-care as tolerated. Provide small amounts of liquid, progressing to a soft diet. Provide for good-quality sleep.
Inflammation	No bronchospasm or coughing.	Monitor and control environment for possible allergens (e.g., dust, smoke, flowers). Administer IV or po steroids as ordered. Administer inhalant medication via hand nubulizer (e.g., metaproterenol sulfate).
Infection	No sputum or clear to white sputum. Normal temperature.	Obtain sputum for Gram stain and culture and sensitivity. Then, give antibiotic as ordered. Assess rectal or axillary temperature every 4 h. Monitor changes in color, viscosity, and volume or sputum. Provide mouth care every 2–4 h and prn. Provide deep-breathing and coughing exercises.
	Long-Term Management	
Wheezing	Eliminate symptoms of bronchospasm. Respiratory rate of 12–16/min. Explain home management program: 1. Describe purpose and show how to take medications 2. Develop schedule of self-medication 3. Demonstrate use of hand nebulizer 4. Describe prophylactic measures to prevent an attack	Administer bronchodilators as prescribed. Increase activity as tolerated. Assess client's response to bronchodilators, hydration, and increased activity. Assess client's understanding and develop a teaching plan for home care, including proper balance of rest and activity; the names, actions, side effects, frequency, and dose of prescribed medications; the use of a hand nebulizer; utilization of an inhaled bronchodilator prior to strenuous activity; and the avoidance of allergens and irritants.
Dehydration	State the importance of adequate fluid intake. Describe a plan for implementation of the desired volume.	Explain the effect of dehydration on sputum production and the consequent effect on bronchospasm. Assist in planning the client's self-administered adequate fluid intake, excluding milk.
Respiratory infection	State ways to avoid infection. Describe evidence of possible infection. State appropriate action to take if infection is suspected.	Explain factors that may contribute to infections and assist in planning preventive measures. Explain a method to evaluate the color, character, and amount of sputum on a regular basis. Review the physician's orders in regard to infection (take medications as ordered or seek medical attention).
Anxiety over possible attack	State factors which may precipitate an attack (emotional stress, infections) and appropriate action to take if attack occurs.	Assist in identifying factors that have precipitated attacks and develop plans to prevent them. Stress importance of taking medications regularly as ordered. Teach client to seek medical attention if medicine does not relieve the attack or dyspnea occurs at night. Tell client about the American Lung Association and its services and literature, such as *Living with Asthma*.

Prepared by Carol Stephenson, R.N., M.S.N., N.S., Assistant Professor of Nursing, Baylor University, Dallas, Texas.

client's history and pattern of asthma. Questions to ask include: When do attacks occur? What are the exacerbating factors? How does the client respond to the first clues of an exacerbation? Any history of allergies? What medications are used? Is there any indication of abuse of prescription or nonprescription drugs? Is there any evidence of aggravating psychological factors? This information is important in planning an individualized nursing care plan for the client.

Chronic Management It is important to remember that asthma is potentially controllable, and every effort should be made to keep the client asymptomatic. The client and the health professionals need to monitor the client's responsiveness to medication. It is very easy to under- or overmedicate an asthmatic unless careful monitoring is ongoing. Some clients may benefit from keeping a diary to record the medication used, the presence of wheezing or coughing, the drug's side effects, and the activity level. This information will be valuable in helping the physician adjust the medication. The client needs to understand the importance of continuing the medication even when symptoms are not present. If worsening bronchospasm or severe side effects of the drugs occur, the client needs to seek medical attention.

The client should be taught to maintain a fluid intake of 2 to 3 L/day. Good nutrition and avoidance of overeating are other important measures. Physical exercise (e.g., swimming) within the client's limit of toleration is also beneficial. If dyspnea on exertion is experienced, it can be prevented with cromolyn sodium.

Psychotherapy may be indicated to help clients and their families resolve personal, family, social, or occupational problems that have resulted from asthma. Relaxation therapies (e.g., yoga, meditation) may be of value in helping some clients relax their respiratory muscles and decrease their respiratory rate. A healthy emotional outlook can also be very important in preventing future asthmatic attacks.

Pulmonary Emphysema and Chronic Bronchitis

The clinical use of the terms *chronic obstructive pulmonary disease (COPD)* and *chronic obstructive lung disease (COLD)* is common. These expressions are generally used to describe the clinical picture of chronic bronchitis and/or pulmonary emphysema. Although the preferred term is *predominant emphysema* or *predominant chronic bronchitis*, in actuality there is usually some overlap between them. This section will consider the two conditions together as COPD, with discussions of their differences where appropriate.

Significance of the problem

At least 13 million Americans suffer from emphysema and chronic bronchitis. The prevalence and death rate have increased dramatically in recent years. The death rate is more than 40,000 per year, making COPD the sixth leading cause of death. White males account for more than three-fourths of the deaths.[23]

The increase in COPD is related primarily to cigarette smoking. There seems to be a 30- to 35-year lag between taking up smoking and developing the disease.[24] Currently, COPD is found primarily in men over 45 years of age. However, the incidence in women is now steadily increasing. (Women began smoking in large numbers in the 1930s and 1940s.) Disability allowances paid by Social Security for COPD rank second after heart disease.

Etiology

Chronic irritation of the lungs is the primary etiological mechanisms in COPD. Three irritants, cigarette smoking, infection, and inhaled irritants, will be considered. Heredity and aging are also possible etiological factors.

Cigarette Smoking Cigarette smoking is the most common cause of COPD in the United States. The effects of smoking on the respiratory tract were described earlier in this chapter. Cigarette smoke alters the mucociliary mechanisms, increases airway resistance by reflex bronchoconstriction, and alters the activity of alveolar macrophages. Cigarette smokers have more sputum production, coughing, and wheezing than nonsmokers. Respiratory infections are more common and severe among cigarette smokers.

Infection No viral or bacterial agent has been identified as the sole cause of COPD. However, recurring respiratory tract infections are a major contributing factor to the aggravation and perpetuation of COPD. Recurring infections impair normal defense mechanisms, making the bronchioles and alveoli more susceptible to injury. In addition, individuals with COPD are more prone to develop respiratory infections, which subsequently intensify the pathological destruction of lung tissue and the progression of COPD. The most common causative organisms are *H. influenzae* and *S. pneumoniae*. Retained secretions provide a good medium for the proliferation of these organisms.

Inhaled Irritants The incidence of COPD is higher in urban than in rural areas. This may partially be explained by the air pollution and occupational irritants to which individuals are exposed. Inhaled irritants cause a nonspecific inflammatory response. More macrophages and leukocytes are found in the lungs. Proteases in these cells can destroy alveoli, and this process has been implicated in the pathogenesis of COPD.

Exposure to occupational gases and dusts can cause lung fibrosis and focal areas of emphysema. Exposure to air pollution and occupational irritants worsens the dyspnea of COPD by causing bronchospasm and mucosal edema.

Heredity A form of familial primary emphysema is related to a deficiency of alpha$_1$-antitrypsin (AAT), a glycoprotein that normally has an inhibitory effect on proteolytic enzymes. The level of AAT is controlled by a pair of autosomal codominant genes. Low levels of AAT are related to homozygosity for the deficiency gene (ZZ), intermediate levels to heterozygosity (MZ), and normal values to homozygosity for the normal gene (MM). About 0.1 percent of the population is homozygous, and 5 to 10 percent are heterozygous.[25] In the homozygous group, onset of symptoms often occurs before age 40 and as frequently in women as in men. Although somewhat controversial, some evidence suggests that individuals with the heterozygous condition may also be predisposed to develop emphysema.

Emphysema results when AAT deficiency causes lysis of lung tisues by proteolytic enzymes from leukocytes and macrophages. Normally, AAT inhibits the action of these enzymes. Therefore, lower levels of AAT result in insufficient inactivation and subsequent destruction of lung tissue.

Aging Some degree of emphysema is common in the lungs of older persons, even nonsmokers, and is often referred to as *senile emphysema*. With aging there is dilatation of the air spaces, decreasing elasticity of lung tissue, and increasing rigidity of the chest wall. However, clinically significant emphysema is usually not caused by aging alone.

Pathogenesis of COPD

It is very common clinically to find in the same person a mixture of emphysema and chronic bronchitis, often with one condition predominating. The pathogensis of these diseases will be considered here separately.

Pulmonary Emphysema Pulmonary emphysema is abnormal enlargement of the air spaces distal to the terminal nonrespiratory bronchioles, with destruction of their walls. Structural changes include (1) hyperinflation of alveoli, (2) destruction of alveolar walls, (3) destruction of alveolar capillary walls, (4) narrowed, tortuous, small airways, and (5) loss of lung elasticity.

There are two major types of emphysema, *centrilobular* and *panlobular* (Fig. 21-6). In centrilobular emphysema the primary area of involvement is the central part of the lobule. Respiratory bronchioles enlarge, the walls are destroyed, and the bronchioles become confluent. Chronic bronchitis is often associated with centrilobular emphysema. It is more common than panlobular emphysema.

In contrast, panlobular emphysema involves distension and destruction of the whole lobule. Respiratory bronchioles, alveolar ducts and sacs, and alveoli are all affected. There is progressive loss of lung tissue and a decreased alveolar-capillary surface area. Severe panlobular emphysema is usually found in individuals with alpha$_1$-antitrypsin deficiency. In some clients with emphysema, bullae (large cystic areas) develop. When emphysema is severe, it is difficult to distinguish the two types, which may coexist in the same lung.

The pathophysiological mechanisms involved in emphysema are not totally understood. Small bronchioles become obstructed due to mucus, smooth muscle spasm, the inflammatory process, collapse of bronchiolar walls, and other causes. Recurrent infectious processes lead to increased leukocytes and macrophages. These cells release proteolytic enzymes which can destroy alveolar tissue. This process results in more inflammation, more edema, exudate formation, etc. With severely constricted bronchioles, air is trapped in the distal alveoli, resulting in hyperinflation and overdistension of the alveoli. As more alveoli are destroyed and alveoli coalesce, larger air spaces called *blebs* (in the visceral pleura) and *bullae* (in the lung parenchyma) develop (Fig. 21-7). The loss of alveolar-capillary surface area decreases the diffusing capacity of the lungs. Hypoxemia eventually develops due to ventilation-perfusion mismatch. Hypercapnia and respiratory acidosis do not develop until late in the disease process.

Chronic Bronchitis Chronic bronchitis is excessive production of mucus in the bronchi accompanied by a recurrent cough that persists for at least 3 months of the year during at least 2 successive years. Pathological changes in the lung consist of (1) hypertrophy and hyperplasia or mucus-secreting glands in the bronchi, (2) increase in goblet cells, (3) disappearance of cilia, and (4) chronic inflammatory changes and narrowing of small airways. Frequently, an infection is present. Excess amounts of mucus are found in the airways and sometimes may occlude small bronchioles. Eventually,

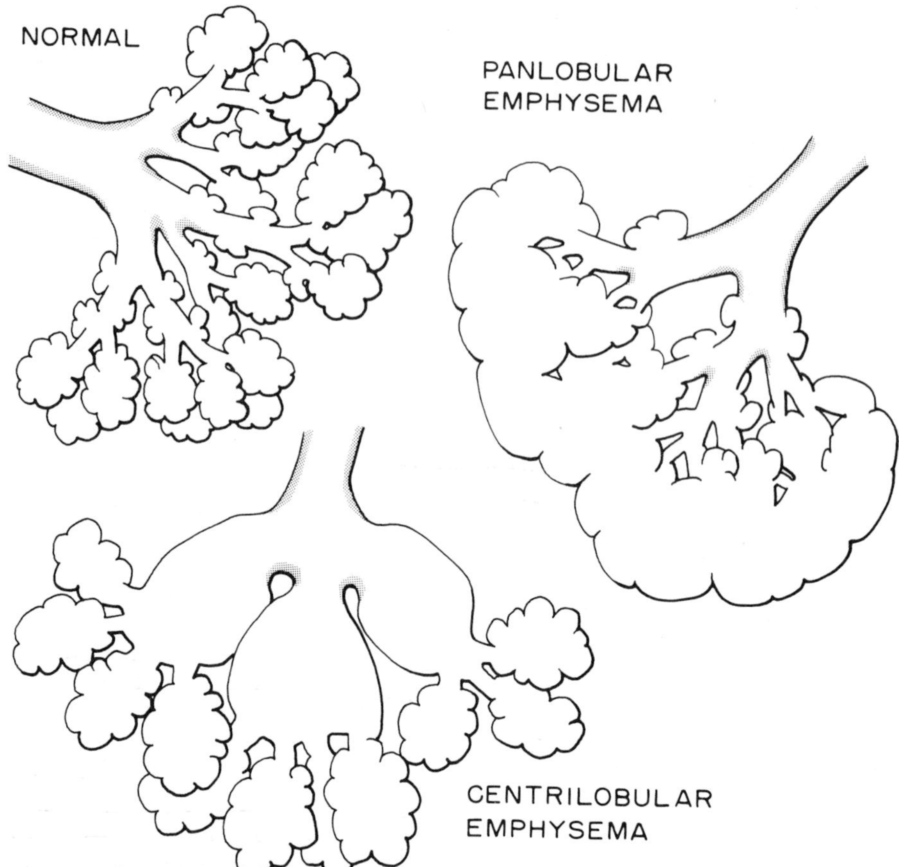

Figure 21-6 Morphological types of emphysema. Panlobular entire primary lobule involved with destruction and distension distal to the respiratory bronchioles. Centrilobular destruction is central involving primarily the respiratory bronchioles. *(From S. Price and L. Wilson, Pathophysiology: Clinical Concepts of Disease Processes, 2d ed., McGraw-Hill Book Company, New York, 1982, p. 435.)*

there may be scarring of the bronchial wall. In contrast to emphysema, the alveolar structure and capillaries are normal.

Chronic inflammation is the primary pathophysiological mechanisms involved in causing the pathological changes characteristic of chronic bronchitis. The inflammatory response causes vasodilatation, congestion, and mucosal edema. The mucous glands are stimulated to hypertrophy and become hyperplastic. This hyperplasia, inflammatory swelling, and excess, thick mucus cause narrowing of the airway lumen and result in diminished airflow.[26] Greater resistance to airflow increases the work of breathing. Hypoxemia and, later, hypercapnia develop. Peribronchial fibrosis may also result from the healing process secondary to inflammatory changes.

Coughing is stimulated by retained mucus which cannot adequately be removed due to decreased cilia and lessened mucociliary activity. The cough is often ineffective to remove secretions adequately because the person cannot inspire deeply enough to cause air to flow distal to retained secretions. The chronic cough may dilate and even destroy susceptible bronchioles weakened by inflammatory changes.

Bronchospasm found in COPD may result from asthma. However, it can also be stimulated by inhaled irritants. Bronchospasm results in greater work of breathing and impaired alveolar-gas exchange.

Clinical manifestations

The clinical manifestations of COPD vary from those of pure emphysema ("pink puffers") to those of pure chronic bronchitis ("blue bloaters"). Most clients with COPD have features of both (Table 21-7).

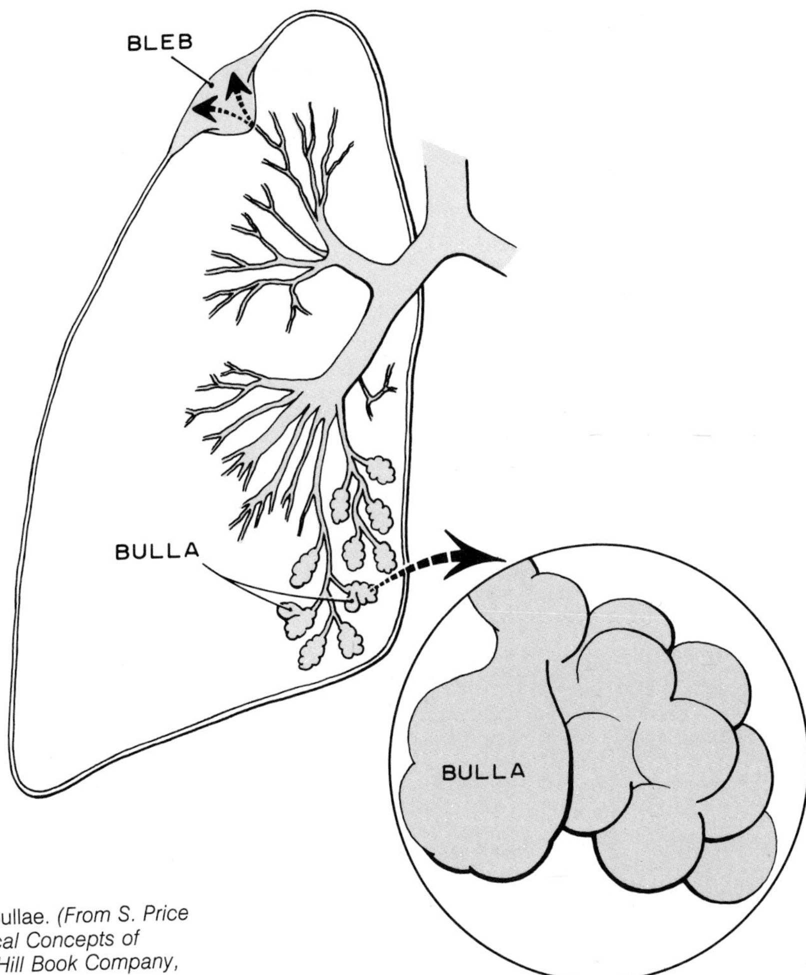

Figure 21-7 Pulmonary bleb and bullae. *(From S. Price and L. Wilson, Pathophysiology: Clinical Concepts of Disease Processes, 2d ed., McGraw-Hill Book Company, New York, 1982, p. 436.)*

Emphysema In emphysema, an early symptom is dyspnea beginning at 30 to 40 years of age and becoming progressively more severe. Minimal coughing is present, with no sputum or small amounts of mucoid sputum. As more alveoli become overdistended, increasing amounts of air are trapped. This causes a flattened diaphragm and an increased anterior-posterior diameter of the chest, forming the typical barrel chest. Effective abdominal breathing is decreased due to the flattened diaphragm from the overdistended lungs. The person becomes more of a chest breather, relying on the intercostal muscles. However, this type of breathing is not very effective because the ribs become fixed in an inspiratory position.

Hypoxemia may be present, but hypercapnia does not develop until late in the disease. The term *pink puffer* is used because there is adequate oxygenation of tissues and no cyanosis is present. The person is characteristically thin due to the (1) extra energy required for eating, (2) increased physical effort required to eat, and (3) full stomach which presses on the diaphragm and contributes to dyspnea. There is frequently muscle wasting and recent weight loss. Later in the course of the disease, secondary chronic bronchitis may develop. In advanced stages, finger clubbing may be present in both emphysema and chronic bronchitis. Other characteristics are presented in Table 21-7.

Chronic Bronchitis In chronic bronchitis the earliest symptom is usually a frequent, productive cough. It is often exacerbated by respiratory irritants and cold, damp air. Frequent respiratory infections are

Table 21-7
Comparison of Pulmonary Emphysema and Chronic Bronchitis*

	Pulmonary Emphysema	Chronic Bronchitis
	Clinical Features	
Age	60–70 years (disabling) 30–40 years (onset)	40–50 years (disabling) 20–30 years (onset)
Body build	Thin	Tendency toward obesity
Past medical history	Generally healthy Occasional insidious dyspnea	Recurrent respiratory tract infections
General appearance	Pink puffer	Blue bloater Cyanosis
Weight loss	Often marked	Absent or slight
Dyspnea	Slowly progressive	Variable, relatively late
Sputum	Scanty, mucoid	Copious, mucopurulent
Cough	Negligible	Considerable
Chest examination	Marked overdistension, quiet breath sounds, chest expansion less than 3 cm	Slight to marked overdistension, scattered rales, rhonchi, and wheezing
Cor pulmonale	Infrequent	Common
	Diagnostic Study Results	
Arterial blood gases	Near normal, mild ↓ P_aO_2	↓ P_aO_2, ↑ P_aCO_2
Chest x-ray	Hyperinflation, flat diaphragm, attenuated peripheral vessels, small or normal heart, widened intercostal margins	Cardiac enlargement, normal or flattened diaphragm, evidence of chronic inflammation, congested lung fields
Lung volumes		
TLC	Increased	Normal or slightly increased
RV	Increased	Increased
VC	Decreased	Decreased
$FEV_{1.0}$	Decreased	Decreased
Hematocrit and hemoglobin	Normal until late in disease	Increased
	Pathology	
	Widespread emphysema, usually panlobular type	May have some centrilobular emphysema

*Most individuals with COPD have features of both pulmonary emphysema and chronic bronchitis.

another common manifestation. Somewhat later, dyspnea on exertion may develop. A history of cigarette smoking for many years is almost always present. Unfortunately, clients often attribute their chronic cough to smoking.

Hypoxemia and hypercapnia result from hypoventilation due to increased airway resistance. These individuals are referred to as *blue bloaters* because their skin is often a reddish-blue color. This color results from polycythemia and cyanosis. Polycythemia develops as a result of increased production of red blood cells secondary to the body's attempt to compensate for chronic hypoxemia. Hemoglobin concentrations may reach 20 g/dL or more. Cyanosis develops because there is at least 5 g/dL of unoxygenated hemoglobin.

These individuals are usually of normal weight or heavyset, with a robust appearance. Emphysema of the centrilobular type frequently develops.

Complications

Cor Pulmonale Cor pulmonale is hypertrophy of the right side of the heart, with or without heart failure, due to pulmonary hypertension. In COPD, pulmonary hypertension is caused primarily by (1) loss of the total cross-sectional area of the pulmonary vasculature and (2) constriction of pulmonary vessels in response to hypoxia. The loss of surface area is due to destruction of alveolar septa with loss of capillaries. Chronic alveolar hypoxia causes constriction of pulmonary vessels. This constriction is reversible if the alveolar PO_2 is increased. Chronic hypoxia also stimulates erythropoiesis, which increases the viscosity of the blood. This change contributes in a small way to the pulmonary hypertension. Pulmonary hypertension results in hypertrophy of the right ventricle and eventually in heart failure.

Clinical manifestations of cor pulmonale include splitting of the pulmonic second sound, a right-sided diastolic gallop, and an early systolic pulmonary ejection click. If right-sided failure results from cor pulmonale, the client will have distended neck veins, hepatomegaly, and peripheral edema.

Acute Respiratory Failure Sedatives and narcotics may precipitate respiratory failure by depressing the respiratory center. Infection of the tracheobronchial tree is the most common cause of acute respiratory failure in COPD. The added inflammation and increased secretion formation lead to worsening hypoxemia and increasing CO_2 retention.[27] The hypercapnia (elevated CO_2) presents a serious problem when oxygen therapy is being given. Due to the persistent elevation of CO_2, the respiratory center no longer responds to increases in CO_2. Therefore, hypoxemia is the primary respiratory stimulant. If too much oxygen is administered, the hypoxic drive is removed and breathing slows or stops. These individuals should be treated with low flow rates of oxygen, with careful monitoring of arterial blood gases. (Respiratory failure is discussed in detail in Chap. 22.)

Peptic Ulcer The incidence of peptic ulcer disease is increased in individuals with COPD. It has been estimated that as many as 25 percent of individuals with COPD develop peptic ulcers.[28] The reason for this occurrence is not known. Possibly it is due to side effects from chronic use of a bronchodilator or steroid drugs. Another factor may be the stressful nature of the disease. It is important to test gastric aspirates and feces for occult blood.

Pneumonia *Pneumonia* is a frequent complication of COPD. As previously mentioned, the most common causative agents are *S. pneumoniae, H. influenzae, Mycoplasma,* and viruses. The most common manifestation is purulent sputum. Systemic manifestations such as fever, chills, and leukocytosis may not be present. The treatment of pneumonia was discussed in Chap. 20.

Diagnostic study abnormalities

An important goal of the diagnostic workup is to determine the major disease component of COPD (e.g., emphysema, asthma, or bronchitis) and the severity of progression. This enables the physician to design an individualized treatment plan.

Chest x-rays taken early in the disease may show no abnormalities. Later in the disease the findings presented in Table 21-7 may be present.

Pulmonary function studies are very useful in diagnosing and assessing the severity of COPD. The most significant findings are related to increased resistance to expiratory airflow. Typical findings are:

Reduced forced expiratory volume in one second ($FEV_{1.0}$)
Reduced forced midexpiratory flow ($FEF_{25-75\%}$)
Reduced maximum voluntary ventilation (MVV)
Reduced vital capacity (VC)
Increased residual volume (RV)
Increased total lung capacity (TLC)
Increased functional residual capacity (FRC)

Arterial blood gases are usually monitored. In the later stages of COPD, typical findings are low P_aO_2, elevated P_aCO_2, decreased pH, and increased bicarbonate. In the early stages, there may be a normal or only slightly decreased P_aO_2 and a normal P_aCO_2.

The Reid Index is the ratio of bronchial gland thickness to bronchial wall thickness. Normally, the ratio is small. In chronic bronchitis, when the bronchial mucosal glands enlarge, the Reid index becomes larger. In order to determine the Reid index, a specimen of bronchus is obtained by bronchoscopy. An electrocardiogram (ECG) may be normal or show signs indicative of right ventricular failure (e.g., low voltage, right axis deviation, P-pulmonale).

Medical management

In general COPD is an irreversible process. In the early stages, it may be partially reversible. The primary goals of medical management are to (1) improve ventilation, (2) promote secretion removal, (3) prevent complications and progression of symptoms, and (4) promote client comfort and participation in care (Table 21-8). The majority of these clients are treated on an outpatient basis. They will be hospitalized for acute

Table 21-8
Medical Management: COPD

Diagnostic
1. History and physical examination
2. Chest x-ray
3. Pulmonary function studies
4. Sputum culture
5. Arterial blood gases
6. Reid index
7. ECG

Therapeutic
1. Treatment of respiratory infections
2. Maintenance of bronchodilator therapy
3. Chest physiotherapy and postural drainage
4. Breathing exercises
5. Low flow rate of oxygen (1–3 L/min)
6. Hydration of 3 L/day
7. Cessation of cigarette smoking
8. Appropriate rest periods

exacerbations and complications such as respiratory failure, pneumonia, and congestive heart failure.

Cessation of cigarette smoking in the early stages is probably the most significant factor in halting the progression of the disease. Other environmental or occupational irritants should be evaluated for their possible effect, and ways to control or avoid them should be determined. For example, aerosol hair sprays and smoked-filled rooms can be avoided.

Respiratory infections should be treated as soon as possible. Often, the best indication of their presence is the increasing purulence, viscosity, or quantity of sputum. Clients are sometimes given a 7- to 10-day supply of antibiotics and told to begin taking them at the first signs of change in sputum.

Bronchodilator drug therapy is often helpful in relieving symptoms. These drugs were discussed in the section on Pharmacological Management of asthma. Theophylline is commonly used for maintenance therapy. Orally administered expectorants and aerosol-delivered mucolytic agents have not been shown to be any more effective than maintaining good hydration. Chest physiotherapy is discussed in a later section.

Pharmacological management

The general classes of drugs used for clients with COPD are presented in Table 21-4 and discussed in the section on Pharmacological Management of asthma. This section will focus on how these drugs are used in the treatment plan for clients with chronic bronchitis and emphysema.

Bronchodilators Bronchodilators are effective for clients whose airway obstruction is partially reversible. This partial reversibility is usually shown by improved pulmonary function studies following the use of an aerosol bronchodilator. Even if there is not significant improvement using this diagnostic approach, bronchodilatation is often tried in clients with COPD. Follow-up pulmonary studies may indicate improvement. If the bronchial obstruction is irreversible, improvement with bronchodilator therapy is negligible.

Corticosteroids Corticosteroids are generally effective in asthma, ineffective in emphysema, and occasionally effective in chronic bronchitis. In general, they should not be used unless other measures have proved ineffective.

Depressant Drugs The use of narcotics, sedatives, and tranquilizers for clients with COPD has to be monitored carefully. Inappropriate or injudicious use of these agents is one of the most frequent causes of acute respiratory failure in clients with COPD.[29] If these individuals are anxious, restless, or irritable, they should first be evaluated for hypoxemia and treated accordingly.

Expectorants The use of expectorants in facilitating removal of secretions is not uniformly recommended for clients with COPD. In many clients, adequate hydration and aerosol humidification are quite effective in loosening secretions. In some individuals, expectorant drugs may be used to stimulate secretion of mucus and thus facilitate the clearing of thick, tenacious sputum from the bronchial system. The most commonly used expectorants are glyceryl guaiacolate (Guaifenesin) and saturated solution of potassium iodide (SSKI).

Respiratory therapy

Respiratory care is a collaborative effort involving respiratory therapists and nurses.

Breathing Exercises The client with COPD develops a rapid respiratory rate to try to compensate for dyspnea. In addition, the accessory muscles of breathing in the neck and upper chest are used excessively to promote chest wall movement. Breathing exercises can assist the client during rest and activity (e.g., lifting, walking, stair climbing). The main types of breathing exercises are (1) pursed-lip breathing and (2) diaphragmatic breathing.

The purpose of using *pursed-lip breathing* is to prolong exhalation and thereby prevent bronchiolar collapse and air trapping. Clients are taught to inhale slowly through the nose and then exhale slowly through pursed lips almost as if they wanted to whistle.

Exhalation should be twice as long as inhalation. Various techniques can be used to teach pursed lip breathing, such as:

1. Blowing through a straw in a glass of water with the intent of forming small bubbles
2. Blowing at a lit candle enough to bend the flame without blowing it out
3. Blowing a table tennis ball across a table at a steady pace

Diaphragmatic breathing focuses on using the diaphragm instead of accessory muscles to achieve maximum inhalation and to slow the respiratory rate. The client should be made aware of the difference between chest breathing and abdominal breathing. This can be done by having the client lie down or assume a semi-Fowler's position, placing one hand on the chest and the other on the abdomen. The client should observe which hand moves during inspiration. The abdomen should protrude on inhalation with diaphragmatic breathing. The value of diaphragmatic movement in increasing lung expansion should be stressed by the nurse.

To practice abdominal or diaphragmatic breathing, the client should keep the hand on the abdomen and concentrate on filling up the abdomen by inhaling slowly through the nose. Another technique is to wrap a towel gently around the abdomen and during exhalation to pull it tight. The client then attempts to stretch the towel with slow inhalation using diaphragmatic breathing. On exhalation, the client uses pursed-lip breathing and draws the towel tighter to promote effective expiration.

Another technique to assist in diaphragmatic breathing is to place a small pillow, magazine, or book on the abdomen. This provides tactile stimulation and visual feedback. If the object rises on inspiration, the individual is given positive feedback that diaphragmatic breathing is taking place.

Pursed-lip breathing and diaphragmatic breathing should be practiced together for 8 to 10 repetitions 3 or 4 times per day. These techniques give the client more control over breathing, especially when experiencing dyspnea.

Effective Coughing Many individuals with COPD have developed ineffective coughing patterns that cannot clear their airways adequately or raise sputum. In addition, they fear that they may develop spastic coughing resulting in dyspnea. Guidelines for effective coughing are presented in Table 21-9. The main goals of effective coughing are to conserve energy, reduce fatigue, and facilitate removal of secretions.

Chest Physiotherapy Chest physiotherapy consisting of percussion, virbration, and postural drainage is an important measure used to treat pulmonary problems (Table 21-10). Percussion and vibration are manual techniques used to augment postural drainage. Postural drainage uses the principle of gravity to assist in bronchial drainage. Percussion and vibration are used after the person has assumed a postural drainage position to assist in loosening the mobilizing secretions. It is very important that these procedures be performed by a trained person.

Postural drainage

The lungs are divided into five lobes, three on the right side and two on the left. There are 18 segments in the lungs (see Fig. 18-2). The purpose of various positions in postural drainage is to drain each segment toward the larger airways, from which sputum can be coughed up. The postural drainage positions are determined by the areas of involved lung, which are assessed by chest x-ray, percussion, palpation, or auscultation (Fig. 21-8). Bronchodilator aerosol drug and/or hydration therapy is frequently administered prior to postural drainage. The chosen postural drainage position is maintained for a designated period of time (usually 5 to 15 minutes). The degree of slope can

Table 21-9

Guidelines for Effective Coughing

1. Have client assume a sitting position with head slightly flexed, shoulders relaxed, knees flexed, and forearms supported by pillow.
2. Client then drops his head and bends forward while using slow, pursed-lip breathing to exhale.
3. Sitting up again, client now uses diaphragmatic breathing to inhale slowly and deeply.
4. Steps 2 and 3 are repeated 3–4 times to facilitate mobilization of secretions.
5. Before initiating a cough, client should take a deep abdominal breath, bend slightly forward, and then huff cough (cough 3–4 times on exhalation). It may be necessary to support or splint the thorax or abdomen to achieve a maximum cough.

Table 21-10

Steps in Chest Physiotherapy

1. Perform procedure before meals or 2–3 h following meals.
2. Administer bronchodilator (if ordered) about 15 min before procedure.
3. Collect needed equipment, such as tissues, emesis basin, paper bag, and pillows.
4. Help client assume correct position for postural drainage based on findings from x-ray, auscultation, palpation, and percussion of chest. The position should be maintained for 5–15 min to mobilize secretions via gravity.
5. Have client take several deep abdominal breaths.
6. Percuss the appropriate area for 1–2 min.
7. Vibrate the same area while the client exhales 4–5 deep breaths.
8. Assist client to cough while assuming the same position. Splinting with towel or hands may be necessary to aid in effective coughing. Client may have to assume a sitting position to generate enough airflow to expel secretions. (Coughing productively may be a long waiting process which may occur 30 min after the procedure.) Suction may be necessary if coughing is not effective.
9. Repeat percussion, vibration, and coughing until client no longer expectorates mucus.
10. Repeat same procedure in all necessary positions.
11. After procedure, help client assume a comfortable position, assist with oral hygiene, and discard used tissues.

be obtained using pillows, blocks, books, or a tilt-board.

The frequency of postural drainage depends on the client's condition. A common order is for 2 to 4 times per day. In acute situations, postural drainage may be done as frequently as every 1 to 2 hours. The procedure should be planned to occur at least 45 minutes before meals.

If a client experiences difficulty in assuming various positions, adaptations will need to be made. The angle can be reduced or the time decreased. A side-lying position can be used for those individuals who cannot tolerate a head-down position.Some positions for postural drainage (e.g., Trendelenburg) should not be performed on clients with chest trauma, hemoptysis, heart disease, or head injury and in other situations where the client's condition is not stable.

Percussion

Percussion is done with the hands in a cuplike position (Fig. 21-9). The hands are cupped and the fingers and thumbs closed. The cupped hand should create an air pocket between the client's chest and the hand. Both hands may be cupped and used in an alternating rhythmic fashion. Percussion is done with flexion and extension of the wrists. A hollow sound should be heard if it is done correctly. The air-cushion impact facilitates the movement of thick mucus. A thin towel may be placed over the area to be percussed, or the client may choose to wear a T-shirt or hospital gown. Percussion should not be performed over the kidneys, sternum, spinal cord, or any tender or painful area. Other contraindications to percussion include hemoptysis, carcinoma, and induced bronchospasm.

Vibration

Vibration is done by tensing the hand and arm muscles and pressing mildly with the flat of the hand on the affected area (Fig. 21-10). It is done while the client slowly exhales a deep breath. The vibrations facilitate movement of secretions to larger airways. Mild vibration is tolerated better than percussion and can be used in situations where percussion may be contraindicated (as discussed above). Commercial vibrators are available for the client to use at home.

Intermittent Positive-Pressure Breathing (IPPB)

IPPB is the use of a pressure-limited respirator to deliver gas with humidity and/or aerosol on an intermittent basis. It can be done in 10 to 20 minutes and used several times a day. The machine applies positive pressure, and the client inspires passively. IPPB can transiently decrease the work of breathing and improve ventilation. The use of IPPB for clients with COPD is controversial. Its value has probably been overrated, and its long-term beneficial effects have not been demonstrated. Aerosol medication may be administered just as effectively with simpler devices.

Indications for the use of IPPB include the following:[30]

1. *Provide large inspiratory volumes*. May be effective in inflating lungs to a larger volume than can be achieved by voluntary effort. This is beneficial in treating atelectasis.

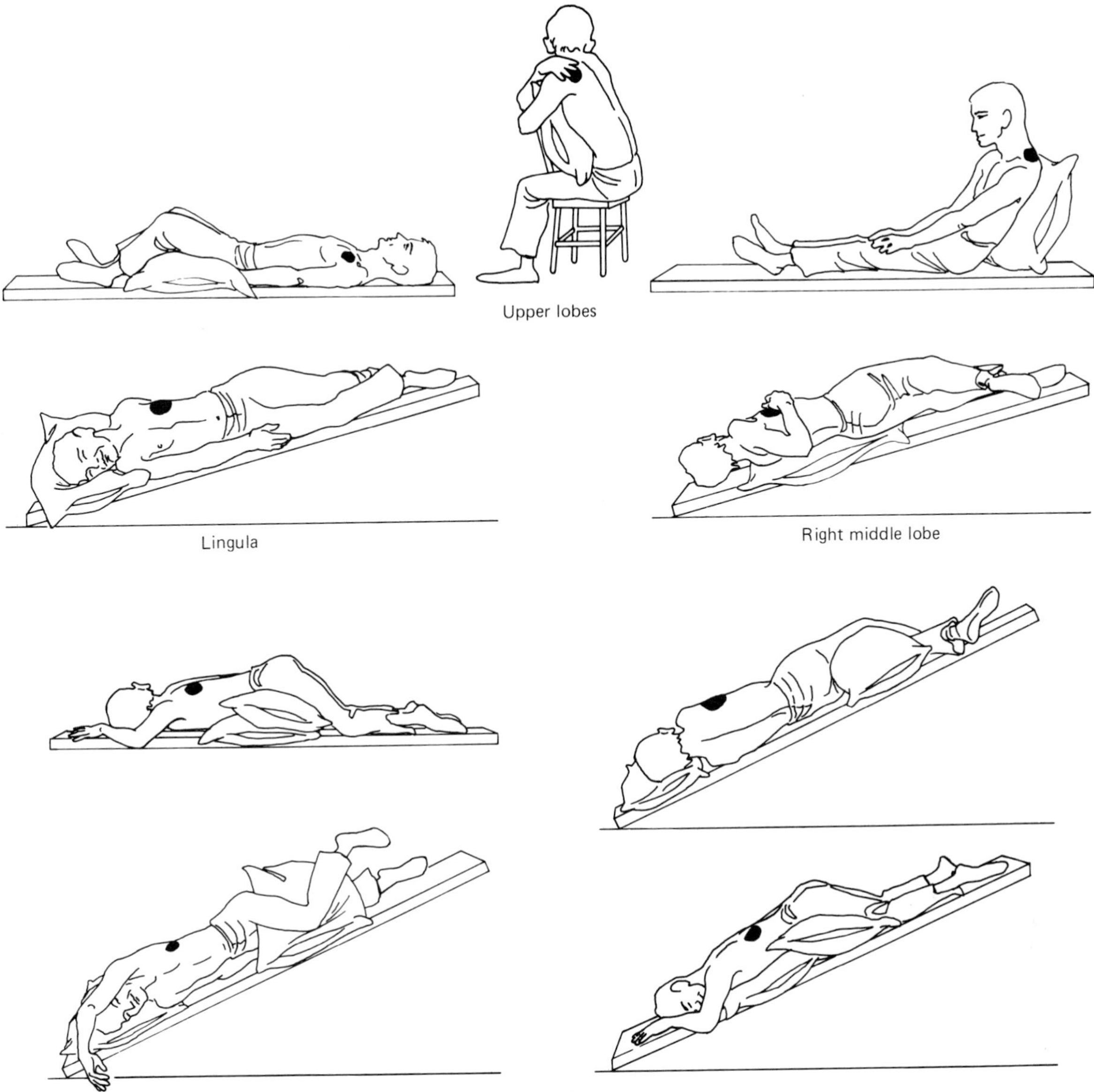

Figure 21-8 Representative positions for postural drainage. The shaded area in each drawing indicates the portion of the lung in which drainage is to be promoted. *(Adapted from A. P. Fishman, Pulmonary Diseases and Disorders, McGraw-Hill Book Company, New York 1980, p. 1624.)*

2. *Improve delivery of medications.* Aerosol medications may be more effectively delivered to areas of the lungs, especially if simple aerosol devices are not effective.
3. *Improve coughing and expectoration.* Aerosol medication and increased inspiratory volumes may help stimulate productive coughing.
4. *Decrease P_aCO_2 and increase P_aO_2.* Better ventilation of lungs may promote increased removal of CO_2 and increased delivery of O_2.

Disadvantages of the use of IPPB include the following:

1. The possibility of inducing a pneumothorax
2. The possibility that the machinery will serve as a source of respiratory infection
3. Aggravation of bronchopulmonary bleeding
4. Hyperventilation with a rapid decrease in elevated P_aCO_2 leading to respiratory alkalosis

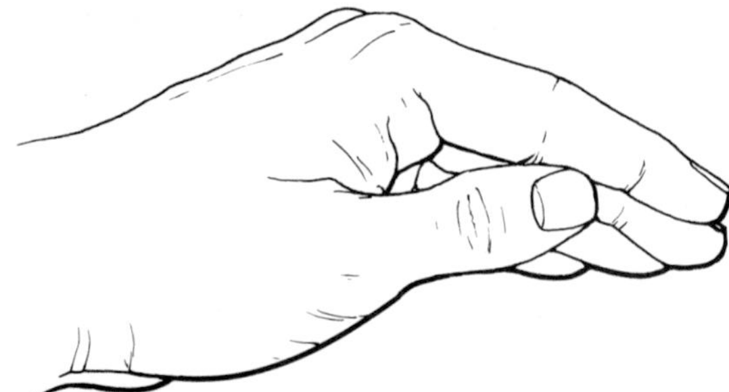

Figure 21-9 Cupped-hand position for percussion. The hand should be cupped as though to scoop up water.

5. Reduction in cardiac output by impeding the return of blood to the right side of the heart
6. Gastric dilatation

The client and a family member should be instructed in the proper use and maintenance of IPPB equipment. If bronchodilator medication is being administered, the client should be told to breathe as deeply and slowly as possible to facilitate distribution of the medication throughout the lungs. The client must learn to initiate inspiration and then allow the machine to fill the lungs. The client should be able to perform the therapy effectively before professional supervision is discontinued at home.

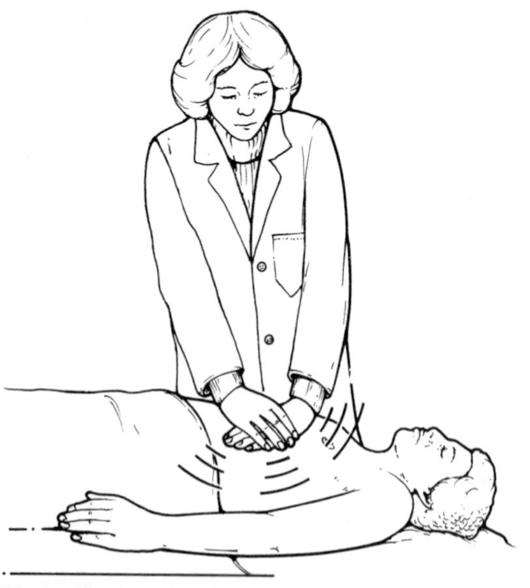

Figure 21-10 Vibration is rhythmic massage with the flat of the hand during a long exhalation.

The client's condition and response to therapy should be evaluated periodically. Pulmonary function studies, arterial blood gases, and subjective improvement are indicators of the value of IPPB. It is possible that the client can change to a simpler or less costly treatment modality.

Nutritional measures

The client with COPD should try to keep body weight at or a little below the ideal weight. Eating becomes a real effort, especially in the later stages of COPD. It is difficult for some clients to hold their breath while swallowing, and therefore, inadequate amounts of food are eaten. The physical activity involved in the preparation and eating of food is often very fatiguing. A full stomach puts pressure on the diaphragm and decreases lung movement. Liquid blenderized or commercial diets may be helpful.

The general diet recommended for a client with COPD is a high calorie diet with five to six small meals per day. The high calorie diet may counteract the weight loss. Gas-forming foods should be avoided. Use of supplemental O_2 via nasal prongs while eating may also be beneficial. Fluid intake should be at least 3 L/day unless contraindicated for other medical conditions such as heart failure. Sodium restriction may be indicated if there is accompanying heart failure.

Nursing management

Health Promotion and Maintenance The incidence of COPD could be decreased if more individuals chose not to start smoking cigarettes or stopped smoking. Avoiding or controlling exposure to occupational and environmental pollutants is another preventive measure to maintain healthy lungs. These factors are discussed in the section on Nursing Management of lung cancer in Chap. 20.

Early detection of small-airway disease is important. Individuals who have smoked for only a few years may have early evidence of obstructive airways. Often, these changes cannot be detected from pulmonary function studies until extensive damage is present. It is extremely important for these individuals to stop smoking and avoid inhaling irritants while their disease is still reversible. Failure to follow this advice will inevitably lead to irreversible COPD.

Early diagnosis and treatment of respiratory tract infections are another way to decrease the incidence of COPD. Avoiding exposure to large crowds in the peak periods for influenza may be necessary, especially for the elderly and those with a history of respiratory problems.

Families with a history of alpha$_1$-antitrypsin deficiency need to be aware of the genetic nature of the disease. Genetic counseling may be appropriate for those clients who are planning to have children.

Acute Intervention Clients with COPD will require acute intervention for complications such as pneumonia, cor pulmonale, and acute respiratory failure. The nursing care for these conditions are discussed in Chaps. 20 and 22. Once the crisis in these situations has been resolved, the nurse can assess the degree and severity of the underlying respiratory problem. The section on Assessment in Chap. 18 provides a beginning tool to use in obtaining information from the client. The information obtained will help to plan the nursing care (Table 21-11).

When an individual with COPD is first diagnosed, or has complications that require hospitalization, the nurse should expect a variety of responses ranging from guilt to depression. Guilt may be experienced due to the individual's realization that the disease was caused largely by cigarette smoking. Depression may be experienced as the severity and chronicity of the disease are realized. The nurse needs to convey a sense of understanding and caring to the client.

Chronic Management The nurse should help the client understand that it is possible to plan treatment aimed at preserving lung function and slowing the progression of the disease. Client and family participation in the treatment plan is essential. Respiratory care will be ongoing, as well as the approaches outlined in Table 21-11.

The client should be encouraged to engage in physical activities within the limits of his capacity. Mild exercise such as walking may improve the physical health and mental outlook. The client may need to walk at a slower pace or to rest more frequently. It is important to encourage continuation of occupational or recreational activities to prevent the client from becoming a physical and psychological invalid. Exercise tolerance is often increased through gradual physical conditioning activities. The client should be assisted with energy conservation techniques such as using elevators.

Clients frequently ask if moving to a warmer or drier climate will help. In general, such a move is not significantly beneficial. Moving to places with an elevation of 4000 feet or more should be discouraged because of the lower P_aO_2 found there. A disadvantage of moving may be that persons leave their occupation, friends, and familiar environment, which could be psychologically stressful. Any advantage gained from a different climate may be outweighed by the psychological effects of the move.

Long-term use of oxygen therapy has improved the quality of life for many clients with COPD. The use of controlled, low-flow oxygen at home can improve the client's exercise tolerance and appetite and alleviate pulmonary hypertension. (Increased pulmonary vascular resistance is associated with alveolar hypoxia.) If pulmonary hypertension is reduced, the risk of cor pulmonale decreases. In addition, chronic hypoxia is partially corrected, and secondary polycythemia is less likely to develop. One of the major reasons that physicians are recommending oxygen use at home is that clients experience a sense of well-being and gain more freedom in their choice of activities. Since hypoxemia worsens during sleep in clients with severe hypoxemic COPD, supplemental O_2 during the night is definitely indicated for them. (Oxygen therapy is discussed in Chap. 20.)

Cystic Fibrosis

Cystic fibrosis is discussed primarily in pediatric texts because it is a relatively common disease among white American children. With better treatment, more affected children are living to young adulthood. Therefore, this disease will be discussed briefly in this section. Cystic fibrosis is an autosomal recessive disease characterized by altered function of the exocrine glands involving primarily the lungs, pancreas, and sweat glands. Abnormally thick, abundant secretions from mucous glands can lead to a chronic, diffuse, obstructive pulmonary disorder. Exocrine pancreatic insufficiency causes about 80 percent of the cases of cystic fibrosis. Sweat glands excrete increased amounts of sodium and chloride.

Significance of the problem

The disease occurs primarily in Caucasians, with a frequency of 1 in 1600 births. Both sexes are equally affected. The life expectancy has increased from 2 years in 1948 to 19 years at present.[31] The primary cause of death is respiratory failure.

Pathophysiology

The etiology of the disease is not really known. No biochemical or structural alteration has been clearly defined. Cystic fibrosis is transmitted as an autosomal recessive trait. The carrier rate in the Caucasian population is 1 in 20. There is no diagnostic method currently available to detect carriers. The basic pathological mechanism is obstruction of exocrine gland ducts with thick, viscous secretions which adhere to the lumen of the ducts. The glands distal to the duct eventually undergo fibrosis.

In the lungs, thick secretions obstruct bronchioles and lead to air trapping and hyperinflation of the

Table 21-11
Nursing Care Plan for the Client with Emphysema or Chronic Bronchitis

Client Problem	Expected Outcome	Nursing Intervention
Dyspnea	Respiratory rate of 12–18/min. Client feels in control of breathing.	Teach client pursed-lip and diaphragmatic breathing. Instruct client to use these techniques during physical exertion and at times of breathlessness. Teach client to avoid activities that cause excess dyspnea. Provide humidified O_2 at 1–3 L/min. Instruct client in the use of home O_2. Administer bronchodilators by aerosol before physical activity. Encourage client to plan rest periods during times of physical activity. Teach client to avoid or try to control situations that precipitate emotional stress. Include family in teaching.
Chronic cough	Production of sputum from coughing. No development of spastic coughing.	Teach client to use effective coughing technique (Table 21-9). If the cough is productive, instruct client to avoid cough suppressant medications and antihistamines. Splint abdomen with pillow or towels if additional support is needed to help client produce a more expulsive cough.
Difficulty in removing secretions	Lungs clear to auscultation. Client or family member can demonstrate chest physiotherapy techniques.	Encourage client to maintain fluid intake at a minimum of 3 L/day. Teach client and family member chest physiotherapy (Table 21-10). Provide oral hygiene after expectoration of sputum. Provide tissues, emesis basin, paper bags, etc., needed to collect expectorated sputum. Remove all equipment before meals.
Weight loss and poor nutrition	Maintenance of normal body weight.	Place client in a comfortable position. Plan rest periods before meals. Perform postural drainage at least 45 min before meals, followed by oral hygiene. Provide small, frequent feedings with foods high in calories. Avoid gas-forming foods. Give liquid refreshments high in calories (e.g., milk shakes). Assist client to plan and eat a nutritionally balanced diet.
Fatigue	Feeling of being rested.	Assess client's sleep patterns. Plan rest periods before and after activities, such as bathing, eating, and postural drainage. Have client use breathing techniques during activities to control breathing. Plan activities that require low amounts of energy. Assist client with graduated-exercise reconditioning program. Use low-flow oxygen (if indicated) to assist in activities of daily living.
Chronic illness	Client verbalizes willingness to participate in self-care related to disease.	Allow client and family to verbalize feelings about disease. Discuss possible changes in lifestyle that will be needed. Instruct client about community resources such as the American Lung Association, Better Breathing Clubs, and smoking cessation groups. Arrange for follow-up counseling visits.
Progression of disease and increased potential for infection	Client able to perform activities of daily living. Client identifies early manifestations of infection.	Teach client to: 1. Avoid excess air pollution and environmental irritants (fumes, dust, chemicals) 2. Stop smoking or decrease amount of smoking 3. Avoid extremely cold weather 4. Wear scarf over face if cold weather cannot be avoided 5. Avoid temperature extremes 6. Recognize side effects of prescribed medications Instruct client to seek medical attention for manifestations such as changes in sputum characteristics, chest pain, excessive fatigue, increased cough, hemoptysis, peripheral edema, increased breathlessness. Discuss the use of home humidifier systems and electronic air filters. Teach client to seek early treatment of respiratory tract infections. Avoid contact (if possible) with individuals who have such infections. Encourage client to obtain vaccines for influenza and pneumococcal pneumonia.

lungs. The stasis of mucus provides a growth medium for bacteria. In infancy or young childhood, the initial infecting agent is *Staphyloccoccus aureus*. Sometime later, *Pseudomonas aeruginosa* colonizes and becomes the predominant infecting agent. Lung disorders that can result include pneumonia, bronchiolitis, bronchitis, bronchiectasis, atelectasis, and emphysema. There is progressive loss of lung tissue from inflammation and scarring. Death is usually due to extensive respiratory infection. Cor pulmonale is a common late complication due to extensive loss of lung tissue and chronic hypoxia.

Pancreatic insufficiency is due primarily to mucus plugging the pancreatic duct and its branches, which results in fibrosis of the acinar glands of the pancreas. The exocrine function of the pancreas is altered and may completely stop. Pancreatic enzymes such as trypsinogen, lipase, and amylase do not reach the intestine to digest ingested nutrients. There is malabsorption of fat, protein, and fat-soluble vitamins (A, D, E, K). Fat malabsorption results in steatorrhea, and protein malabsorption results in failure to grow and gain weight. In advanced pancreatic insufficiency, diabetes mellitus may occur if the islets of Langerhans become fibrotic.

The sweat glands excrete 4 times the normal amount of sodium and chloride. This abnormality does not seem to affect the general health of the person. However, this finding is useful as a diagnostic indicator.

The liver may become involved. Biliary cirrhosis may not be recognized until late in the disease. Complications of cirrhosis such as portal hypertension and hypersplenism are not commonly found.

The reproductive system's function is altered. This finding is important, since more individuals with cystic fibrosis are living to adulthood. The adult male is usually sterile due to structural changes in the vas deferens, seminal vesicles, and epididymis. The female usually has delayed menarche and may develop secondary amenorrhea. She may be unable to become pregnant because of the increased viscosity of the cervical mucus. However, females do become pregnant, but the fertility rate is lower than in healthy women. The baby is heterozygous (and hence a carrier) for cystic fibrosis if the father is not a carrier. If the father is a carrier, there is 1 in 2 chance that the baby will have cystic fibrosis.

Clinical manifestations and complications

The clinical manifestations of cystic fibrosis vary depending on the severity of the disease. An initial finding of meconium ileus in the newborn is present in 10 percent of individuals with cystic fibrosis. Early manifestations in childhood are failure to grow, dyspnea on exertion, persistent cough with mucus production, tachypnea, and large, frequent bowel movements. A large, protuberant abdomen may develop with an emaciated appearance of the extremities. Other respiratory problems that may be indicative of cystic fibrosis are recurring lung infections such as bronchiolitis, bronchitis, or pneumonia.

The severity and progression of the disease vary from one person to another. In the past decade, it has been shown that with early diagnosis and immediate institution of intensive care, the prognosis can be significantly improved. As previously mentioned, respiratory complications are the main cause of debilitation and death.

Medical management

Diagnostic The main diagnostic test for cystic fibrosis is the sweat chloride test using the pilocarpine iontophoresis method. Pilocarpine carried by a small electric current is used to stimulate sweat production. The sweat is collected on filter paper or gauze and then analyzed for sodium and chloride concentrations. The test takes about 40 minutes. Values greater than 65 mEq/L for both sodium and chloride are suggestive of cystic fibrosis, especially in a person who has other clincial features of the disease. The degree of sodium and chloride elevation does not necessarily correlate with the severity of the disease.[32]

Other diagnostic studies that may be done include chest x-ray, fecal analysis for fat, and duodenoscopy for quantitative determination of enzymes.

Therapeutic The management of pulmonary problems in cystic fibrosis includes postural drainage and the use of antibiotics when pulmonary infections occur. Bronchodilatation may be indicated if bronchospasm is present.

The management of pancreatic insufficiency includes a drug preparation of pancreatic enzymes such as pancreatin (Viokase) or pancrelipase (Cotazym), high calorie intake, reduction of dietary fat, and multivitamins. Added dietary salt is indicated whenever sweating is excessive, such as during hot weather, when a fever is present, or from intense physical activity.

Nursing management

The family or person with cystic fibrosis has a great financial and emotional burden. The cost of drugs, special equipment, and continual medical care is often a great financial hardship. Emotionally, the burden of living with a chronic disease at a young age can be overwhelming. Community resources are often available to help the family. In addition, in many areas the Cystic Fibrosis Foundation can be of assistance.[33]

The nurse can assist young adults to gain independence by helping them assume responsibility for their medical care as well as their vocational or school goals. A major problem that needs to be discussed at this time is sexuality. Delayed or irregular menstruation is not uncommon. There may be delayed development of secondary sex characteristics such as breasts in girls or prolonged short stature in boys. The person may use the illness to avoid certain events or relationships. On the other hand, healthy individuals may be hesitant to make friends with someone who is sick.

The issue of marrying and having children is difficult. Most males with cystic fibrosis are sterile. Females with the disease may have difficulty becoming pregnant, as previously mentioned. The additional factor here is that any child produced will either be a carrier of cystic fibrosis or will have the disease. Genetic counseling may be an appropriate suggestion for the couple planning to have children.

Regardless of how well the individual is coping with living with the disease, a normal life span is not possible. As the person continues toward and into adulthood, the nurse needs to be available to help the client and family cope with complications resulting from the disease and to prepare for dying.

Case Study / Acute Asthmatic Attack

Fred, 20 years old, was seen in the emergency room for an asthma attack. He stated that he had had a history of asthma since childhood and had positive reactions to various allergens, including house dust and grasses. He was not aware of what precipitated his current attack, but it occurred while he was trying out for the college football team.

Fred takes aminophylline and uses an Alupent inhaler at home. During the past 24 hours, he has increased his Alupent inhalations every 2 hours without relief. At present, he is not on steroid therapy.

On physical examination, he was in acute respiratory distress. Vital signs revealed a temperature of 39°C (102.2°F), pulse 126, respirations 32, and blood pressure 140/88. He was sitting upright using his accessory muscles for ventilation, audibly wheezing, and diaphoretic. Auscultation of the chest revealed diffuse expiratory and inspiratory wheezing.

Discussion Questions

1. Explain the pathophysiology of asthma.
2. How does asthma differ from chronic bronchitis and pulmonary emphysema?
3. What could be precipitating factors in Fred's asthma attack?
4. What are the clinical manifestations of an asthma attack? Which of these did Fred manifest?
5. What can a nurse do to alleviate his acute respiratory distress?

REVIEW QUESTIONS

The number of the question corresponds to the same numbered objective at the beginning of the chapter.

1. Which of the following effects does cigarette smoking have on the respiratory system?
   a. hyperplasia of goblet cells and increased mucus production
   b. increased proliferation of ciliated cells
   c. hypertrophy of the alveolar membrane
   d. destruction of all alveolar macrophages

2. Bronchial asthma is best characterized by which description?
   a. partially reversible, obstructive disease of the bronchioles
   b. intermittent, reversible, obstructive airway disease
   c. obstructive disease with loss of alveolar walls
   d. steady progression of bronchoconstriction

3. The teaching plan for the asthmatic client would include all the following *except*
   a. preventing or limiting exposure of the client to antigens
   b. placing the client in isolation to prevent respiratory infections
   c. preventing psychological invalidism
   d. deep-breathing and coughing exercises to clear the airway

4. Chronic obstructive pulmonary disease is characterized by all the following *except*
   a. increased airway resistance on expiration
   b. fibrosis of the alveolar capillary surface
   c. an excessive amount and retention of secretions
   d. decreased residual volume

5. One of the most important things a nurse can teach a client with COPD is to
   a. obtain adequate rest in the supine position
   b. move to a hot, dry climate

c. practice pursed-lip expiratory breathing
d. practice chest inspiratory breathing

6. Diagnostic studies that would probably be abnormal in a person with cystic fibrosis are
a. pancreatic enzymes and hormones
b. pulmonary function study and sweat test
c. sweat test and vitamin B tolerance test
d. insulin tolerance and blood sugars

REFERENCES

1. *Cancer 1981 Facts and Figures*, American Cancer Society, New York, 1980, p. 14.
2. R. L. DuPont, "Marijunana Smoking: A National Epidemic," *Am Lung Assoc Bull* (September 1980).
3. N. C. Doyle, "Marijuana and the Lungs," *Am Lung Assoc Bull* (November 1979).
4. Ibid.
5. "Asthma and the Other Allergic Diseases," *Niaid Task Force Report,* NIH Publication No. 79, U.S. Dept. of Health, Education, and Welfare, May 1979, p. 387.
6. N. T. Feldman and E. R. McFadden, "Asthma: Therapy Old and New," *Med Clin North Am,* **61**:1239–1249 (1977).
7. S. Price and L. Wilson, *Pathophysiology: Clinical Concepts of Disease Processes*, 2d ed., McGraw-Hill Book Company, New York, 1982, p. 434.
8. E. H. Elpern, "Asthma Update: Pathophysiology and Treatment," *Heart Lung,* **9**:665–670 (1980).
9. E. R. McFadden and K. F. Austen, "Asthma," in K. Isselbacher et al. (eds.), *Harrison's Principles of Internal Medicine*, McGraw Hill Book Company, New York, 1980, pp. 1204–1205.
10. D. L. Sexton, *Chronic Obstructive Pulmonary Disease: Care of the Child and Adult*, The C. V. Mosby Company, St. Louis, 1981, p. 85.
11. J. B. West, *Pulmonary Pathophysiology: The Essentials*, The Williams & Wilkins Company, Baltimore, 1977, p. 83.
12. Price and Wilson, op. cit., p. 122.
13. H. M. Sweetwood, *Nursing in the Intensive Respiratory Care Unit*, 2d ed., Springer Publishing Co., Inc., New York, 1979, p. 382.
14. Sexton, op. cit., p. 91.
15. Ibid., p. 96.
16. D. W. Hudgel and L. A. Madsen, "Acute and Chronic Asthma: A Guide to Intervention," *Am J Nurs,* **80**:1791–1795 (1980).
17. Ibid.
18. Feldman and McFadden, op. cit., p. 1239.
19. M. Wiener et al., *Clinical Pharmacology and Therapeutics in Nursing,* McGraw-Hill Book Company, New York, 1979, p. 362.
20. Feldman and McFadden, op. cit., p. 1246.
21. J. E. Webber-Jones and M. K. Bryant, "Over-the-Counter Bronchodilators," *Nursing 80,* **10**:34–39 (1980).
22. Feldman and McFadden, op. cit., pp. 1248–1249.
23. *Chronic Obstructive Pulmonary Disease*, 5th ed, American Lung Association, New York, 1977.
24. M. F. Fuhs and A. M. Stern, "Better Ways to Cope with COPD," *Nursing 76,* **6**:29–38 (1976).
25. *Chronic Obstructive Pulmonary Disease*, 5th ed., American Lung Association, New York, 1977, p. 26.
26. Sexton, op. cit., p. 112.
27. R. H. Ingram, "Chronic Bronchitis, Emphysema, and Chronic Airways Obstruction," in Isselbacher et al., op. cit., pp. 1235–1241.
28. Sweetwood, op. cit., p. 49.
29. W. F. Miller and A. M. Geumei, "Respiratory and Pharmacologic Therapy in COPD," in T. L. Petty (ed.), *Chronic Obstructive Pulmonary Disease*, Marcel Dekker, New York, 1978.
30. "Intermittent Positive Pressure Breathing," in *Clinical Notes on Respiratory Diseases*, American Lung Association, New York, 1979.
31. H. L. Schwachman, "Cystic Fibrosis," in Isselbacher et al., op. cit., pp. 1233–1234.
32. N. Larter, "Cystic Fibrosis," *Am J Nurs,* **81**:527–532 (1981).
33. *Living with Cystic Fibrosis: A Guide for the Young Adult*, Cystic Fibrosis Foundation, Atlanta.

Chapter 22

NURSING ROLE IN MANAGEMENT

Critical Care of the Respiratory Client

Patricia Van Sciver
Carol Stephenson

Learning Objectives

1. Describe the types, mechanisms, etiology, and clinical manifestations of acute respiratory failure.
2. Describe the medical and nursing management of the client in acute respiratory failure.
3. Describe the etiology, pathophysiology, and clinical manifestations of adult respiratory distress syndrome.
4. Explain the medical and nursing management of the client with adult respiratory distress syndrome.
5. Describe the types of artificial airways, including their hazards and the interventions utilized to prevent them.
6. Explain the various modes of mechanical ventilation and their indications.
7. Describe the nursing management of the client on a mechanical ventilator.

Respiratory intensive care may be administered in a specialized respiratory intensive care unit or in a medical, surgical, coronary, or trauma unit. Respiratory intensive care of the critically ill client with a respiratory problem requires an organized team approach to provide a continuous, well-defined management program. The intensive care nurse is an integral member of this health team. Respiratory intensive care nursing is based on understanding cardiopulmonary anatomy and physiology and the pathophysiology of acute respiratory failure. Essential nursing skills include the ability to monitor clients closely, with an understanding of physiological parameters, and to anticipate and detect complications and initiate measures to correct them immediately. Adept performance of technical skills involved in airway care and respiratory management of the client is essential. The nurse is also responsible for the regulation and coordination of the emotional and physical aspects of care for the totally dependent client.

Nurses working in specialized respiratory intensive care units may share with the respiratory therapist a variety of skills unique to this setting, including such things as intubation, extubation, changing of tracheostomy tubes, performance of pulmonary function tests, use of the ear oximeter for weaning clients from mechanical ventilation, administration of aerosolized bronchodilators and mucolytic agents, and use of long-term arterial blood gas monitoring equipment.

The goal of this chapter is to provide an introduction to the knowledge and skills involved in the care of the client with acute respiratory failure. Four general areas discussed are:

1. Pathophysiology of acute respiratory failure and related medical-surgical management
2. Adult respiratory distress syndrome (ARDS), a type of acute respiratory failure
3. Care of the artificial airway
4. Physiological principles, types, modes, hazards, and nursing care of mechanical ventilation

Psychological support measures for the client and the family in acute respiratory distress are discussed throughout the chapter.

ACUTE RESPIRATORY FAILURE

Acute respiratory failure is present in a client with "normal" lungs when alveolar ventilation is inadequate to meet the body's needs. The lungs can no longer adequately oxygenate the blood. It is commonly accepted that acute respiratory failure exists in a client with supposedly normal lungs when arterial blood gas levels demonstrate an arterial oxygen pressure (P_aO_2) of $<$ 50 to 60 mmHg (hypoxemic failure) and/or an

This chapter was reviewed by Joyce C. Tremper, R.N., M.S., N.S., Pulmonary Clinical Nurse Specialist, Veteran's Administration Medical Center, Tucson, Arizona, and Nursing Associate, College of Nursing, University of Arizona, Tucson, Arizona; and Major Bettye Ball, R.N., A.N.S., Fitzsimmons Army Medical Center, Aurora, Colorado.

arterial carbon dioxide pressure (P_aCO_2) of > 50 mmHg, and a pH of < 7.35 (hypercapnic or ventilatory failure).

Acute respiratory failure in a client with chronic restrictive or obstructive lung disease cannot be defined according to the criteria used for the client with normal lungs. Clients with chronic pulmonary diseases are able to tolerate and compensate for a significant degree of hypoxemia and/or hypercapnia. Many stable, ambulatory chronic pulmonary disease clients maintain P_aO_2 levels of ≤ 50 to 60 mmHg and/or P_aCO_2 levels of ≥ 50 mmHg with a normal pH. In chronic lung disease, acute respiratory failure can be defined as alveolar ventilation inadequate to oxygenate the blood sufficiently, as evidenced by an acute decrease in P_aO_2 and/or an increase in P_aCO_2 (with an acidic pH) from the individual's baseline parameters.

Risk Factors

All critically ill clients are at risk for developing respiratory distress and/or acute respiratory failure. These clients have already sustained significant injury to one or more body organ systems. Since there are so many functional systemic interrelationships in the body, disequilibrium in one body system frequently leads to disequilibrium in other systems.

Clients who have undergone recent abdominal or thoracic surgery are at risk for developing respiratory failure due to splinting of their incision and reduced ventilation due to pain. Comatose clients or those with decreased levels of consciousness (e.g., post anesthesia with head injury) are prone to aspiration pneumonia and respiratory failure. Clients who have sustained thoracic or spinal injuries are predisposed to ineffective ventilation. Because of a loss of normal respiratory or protective mechanisms and decreased ventilatory reserve, clients who show evidence of lung disease or are heavy smokers are at high risk for developing acute respiratory failure. These clients are especially vulnerable when they develop an infection, have surgery, or develop other diseases.

Prevention of Acute Respiratory Failure

Measures to help prevent respiratory failure include preoperative screening and evaluation of all high-risk clients. Pulmonary function tests should be performed and arterial blood gas levels assessed preoperatively to determine the operative risk and to establish baseline parameters for postoperative care. Measures to optimize ventilation such as the use of parenteral and aerosolized bronchodilators, incentive spirometry, and teaching effective coughing and deep-breathing techniques are important to prepare the client for surgery. Preoperative teaching of all surgical clients is essential, especially for clients preparing for thoracic or abdominal surgery, so that they will be familiar with what is necessary and expected postoperatively.

Frequent monitoring of the respiratory status of clients who are critically ill or comatose is imperative. Arterial blood gas analysis is often an initial part of the workup during admission to the intensive care unit. Astute observation and measurement of the client's respiratory status will assist in early detection of respiratory problems. These measurements include the breathing rate, pattern, and depth; vital signs and level of consciousness; and arterial blood gases. Subjective client evaluation is also important. Early recognition of the clinical symptoms of respiratory distress and immediate implementation of corrective measures may prevent further deterioration and failure of the client's respiratory mechanisms.

Pathophysiology of Acute Respiratory Failure

The mechanisms involved in acute respiratory failure result in an increase of CO_2 and/or a decrease of O_2 in the blood. Mechanisms which contribute to or cause the development of *hypercapnic ventilatory failure* (↑ P_aCO_2) are alveolar hypoventilation and ventilation-perfusion mismatch. These are listed in Table 22-1. Mechanisms which contribute to or cause

Table 22-1

Causes of Hypercapnic Ventilatory Failure

1. Alveolar hypoventilation
   A. Decreased ventilatory drive
      (1) Sedative and narcotic overdosage
      (2) Excessive oxygen tensions (especially in the presence of chronic hypercarbia)
   B. Decreased ventilatory response
      (1) Neuromuscular diseases
         Guillain-Barré syndrome
         Myasthenia gravis
         Bulbar poliomyelitis
      (2) Chest wall deformity
         Kyphoscoliosis
      (3) Muscle splinting or spasm
         Postoperative pain
         Pleurisy
         Rib fracture
      (4) Airway obstruction
      (5) Sleep apnea
   C. Increased CO_2 production
      (1) Increased work of breathing
      (2) Anxiety
      (3) Fever, infection
2. Ventilation-perfusion mismatch (see Table 22-2)

the development of *hypoxemic respiratory failure* ($\downarrow P_aO_2$) are alveolar hypoventilation, ventilation-perfusion mismatch, shunts, and diffusion abnormalities. These are listed in Table 22-2.

Mechanisms of hypercapnic ventilatory failure

Alveolar Hypoventilation ($\uparrow P_aCO_2$) Alveolar or effective ventilation is the volume of gas per breath which is available for gas exchange in functioning alveoli or terminal respiratory units. When an adult takes a normal breath (tidal volume, or V_T) of 500 mL, approximately 150 mL of this gas never reaches the alveoli to be involved in gas exchange. This 150 mL is called the *anatomical dead space* (V_D) and is approximately equal to a person's weight in pounds (a 150-lb person has approximately 150 mL of anatomical dead space). The remaining 350 mL is the gas available for alveolar ventilation per breath.

Adequate alveolar ventilation is necessary to exchange O_2 for CO_2 in the alveoli. The amount of CO_2 in the arterial blood (P_aCO_2) is related directly to the amount of CO_2 produced metabolically and inversely to the effective alveolar ventilation. Therefore, increased P_aCO_2 indicates decreased alveolar ventilation (hypoventilation) and increased CO_2 produced metabolically. Decreased P_aCO_2 indicates increased alveolar ventilation (hyperventilation). In order for the P_aCO_2 to remain constant, alveolar ventilation must increase or decrease in proportion to the CO_2 produced metabolically.

Alveolar hypoventilation exists when effective ventilation of the alveoli is no longer adequate for the body's metabolic rate. Less O_2 is supplied, and less CO_2 is removed. Consequently, alveolar and arterial CO_2 levels increase and O_2 levels decrease. Alveolar hypoventilation is commonly caused by diseases outside of the lungs, and very often the lungs are normal (Table 22-1).

Physiological effects of hypoventilation

The main physiological feature of hypoventilation is elevated P_aCO_2 (>50 mmHg). A subsequent physiological effect of increased P_aCO_2 is a decrease in P_aO_2. In the lungs, the blood extracts more O_2 from the alveolar gas for delivery to the tissues than it gives up CO_2 to the lungs, so a one-to-one relationship does not exist for exchange of O_2 and CO_2 in the blood. When the P_aCO_2 increases by 8 mmHg, the P_aO_2 falls by about 10 mmHg in the presence of pure hypoventilation. As the level of CO_2 increases in the blood (P_aCO_2), the level of CO_2 in the alveoli also increases. Less space is left in the alveoli for oxygen. This results in a decrease in P_aO_2 that is proportional to the rise in P_aCO_2. Arterial PO_2 cannot fall to very low levels from pure hypoventilation since even if P_aCO_2 increases from 35 to 75 mmHg, P_aO_2 decreases from 100 to 50 mmHg. If hypoxemia exists prior to the hypoventilation, P_aO_2 may be decreased significantly (i.e., a client with a P_aO_2 of 60 mmHg would drop to 50 mmHg with a P_aCO_2 increase of 10 mmHg).

A second physiological effect of increased P_aCO_2 is decreased pH. Respiratory acidemia results as CO_2 accumulates in the plasma ($CO_2 + H_2O \rightleftharpoons H_2CO_3 \rightleftharpoons H^+ + HCO_3^-$). There is no significant increase in plasma bicarbonate in acute hypercapnia since it takes the kidney 48 to 72 hours to retain enough bicarbonate to compensate for the acidemia. In contrast, in chronic hypercapnia the plasma bicarbonate is elevated enough to bring the pH of the blood within the normal range. In chronic hypercapnia, metabolic alkalosis compensates for the respiratory acidosis.

A low serum chloride level occurs in acute respiratory failure. The mechanism for this is as follows: As bicarbonate ions (HCO_3^-) move from the cells to the plasma to buffer the H_2CO_3, the chloride ions move into the cell to maintain electroneutrality. This is called the *chloride shift.* As the CO_2 accumulates, and with it hydrogen ions (H^+), the serum becomes more acidic. H^+ enters the cells and potassium (K^+) flows from the cells to the plasma in an attempt to achieve electroneutrality. Initially, serum K^+ may be increased, but as the acidemia becomes prolonged or more pro-

Table 22-2
Causes of Hypoxemic Respiratory Failure

1. Alveolar hypoventilation (see Table 22-1)
2. Ventilation-perfusion mismatch
   - A. Decreased ventilation
     - (1) Pneumonia
     - (2) Atelectasis
     - (3) Asthma
     - (4) Chronic and acute bronchitis
     - (5) Emphysema
   - B. Decreased perfusion
     - (1) Severe emphysema
     - (2) Pulmonary embolus
3. Diffusion abnormalities
   - A. Diffuse interstitial fibrosis
   - B. Collagen diseases of the lung
     - (1) Scleroderma
     - (2) Systemic lupus erythematosus
     - (3) Rheumatoid lung
   - C. Asbestosis
   - D. Sarcoidosis
   - E. Interstitial pneumonia
4. Shunts
   - A. Consolidated pneumonias
   - B. ARDS

nounced, total body K^+ (both intracellular and extracellular) will be depleted as the excess K^+ is excreted by the kidneys. Thus, the client can demonstrate both hypokalemia and hypochloremia as a result of respiratory failure.

Hypoxemia alone can cause vasoconstriction of the pulmonary circulation, resulting in pulmonary hypertension. Respiratory acidemia seems to potentiate this effect. Therefore, as CO_2 rises, with the subsequent development of acidosis, the elevation of the pulmonary artery pressure increases relative to the level of hypoxemia.

Central nervous system alterations may occur secondary to the combination of hypoxemia, increased P_aCO_2, and acidemia. The client may complain of a headache, since increased CO_2 causes vasodilatation of cerebral blood vessels and increased cerebral blood flow. Cerebrospinal pressure may be elevated, and the client may exhibit papilledema, drowsiness, convulsions, tremors, confusion, slurred speech, restlessness, decreased deep tendon reflexes, fluctuations of mood, and asterixis (flapping tremor).

Ventilation-Perfusion Mismatch Ventilation-perfusion mismatch can cause an elevated P_aCO_2 as well as a decreased P_aO_2. This will be discussed in detail following the next two paragraphs.

Mechanisms of hypoxemic respiratory failure

Hypoxemia, or *low oxygen tension* in the arterial blood (P_aO_2 <50 to 60 mmHg), can contribute to the development of hypoxia, or lack of tissue oxygen, and acute respiratory failure. Arterial oxygen levels are not solely responsible for effective tissue oxygenation. The hemoglobin level, hemoglobin oxygen-carrying capacity, cardiac output, and distribution of blood flow to the tissues are all involved in the delivery of O_2 to the tissues and thus determine the state of tissue oxygenation. Respiratory mechanisms which may cause hypoxemia and subsequent acute hypoxemic respiratory failure are (1) alveolar hypoventilation, (2) ventilation-perfusion mismatch, (3) shunts, and (4) diffusion abnormalities.

Alveolar Hypoventilation Alveolar hypoventilation, although manifested predominantly by increased CO_2, also causes hypoxemia for reasons discussed in the previous section.

Ventilation-Perfusion Mismatch Altered ventilation-perfusion relationships in the lungs, or ventilation-perfusion mismatch, is the most common cause of hypoxemia. The concept of ventilation-perfusion relationships means that where there is ventilation or oxygen in the lung, there must be matching blood perfusion to that area for efficient gas exchange to occur (Fig. 22-1). In the normal lung, the ratio of ventilation to perfusion ($\dot{V}/\dot{Q}$) is 0.8. Normal resting alveolar ventilation is approximately 4 L/minute, and cardiac output is approximately 5 L/minute in an adult. Therefore, the ratio of ventilation to perfusion is 4:5 or 0.8. An alteration or mismatch will occur if there is blood flow to underventilated areas or ventilation to areas where blood flow is decreased or absent (Fig. 22-2).

Hypoventilation (generalized decreased alveolar ventilation) is usually not classified as $\dot{V}/\dot{Q}$ mismatch. CO_2 retention and subsequent hypoventilation may occur as a result of $\dot{V}/\dot{Q}$ mismatch if a client is unable to compensate by increasing the ventilation in the presence of airway obstruction. Regional alterations in ventilation and perfusion are more frequently classified as $\dot{V}/\dot{Q}$ mismatch.

Examples of processes which cause ventilation-perfusion mismatch are pneumonia, atelectasis, chronic and acute bronchitis, severe emphysema, asthma, and pulmonary embolism. In pulmonary embolism (depending upon the size of the vessel blocked), there is sustained ventilation to an area that is perfused either poorly or not at all. The other examples are processes in which there is sustained perfusion of poorly ventilated zones of the lung.

Sometimes ventilation-perfusion mismatch or imbalance is referred to as *physiological shunting*. This term implies that blood does not become well oxygenated despite contact with alveoli.

Shunts Shunting is also a cause of hypoxemia (Fig. 22-3). A shunt can be viewed as an extreme ventilation-perfusion disturbance, one in which there is perfusion but no ventilation at all or ventilation in the

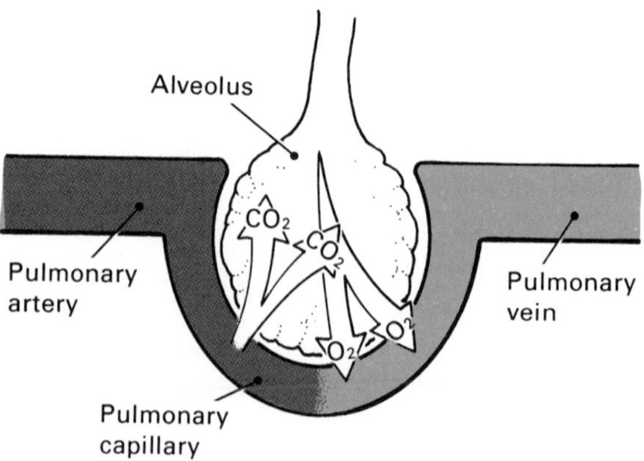

Figure 22-1 Normal gas exchange unit in the lung.

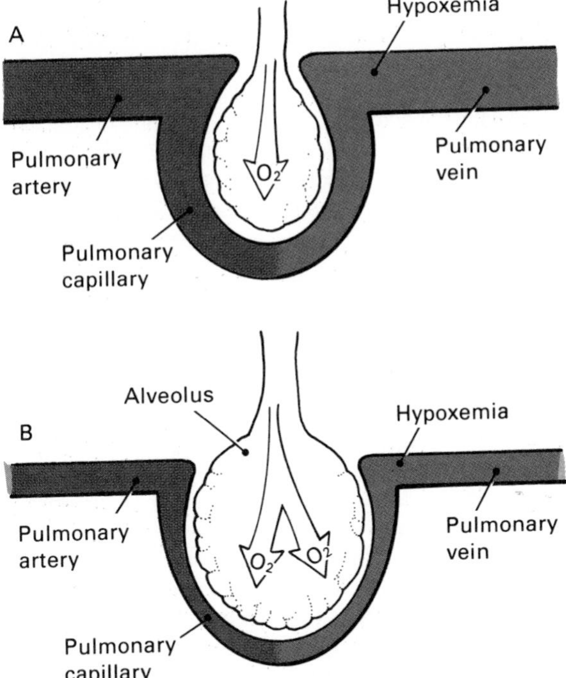

Figure 22-2 Gas exchange unit illustrating ventilation-perfusion ($\dot{V}/\dot{Q}$) mismatch. *(a)* $\dot{V}/\dot{Q}$ mismatch with decreased ventilation and normal perfusion. *(b)* $\dot{V}/\dot{Q}$ mismatch with normal ventilation and decreased perfusion. Note the narrowing of the blood vessel.

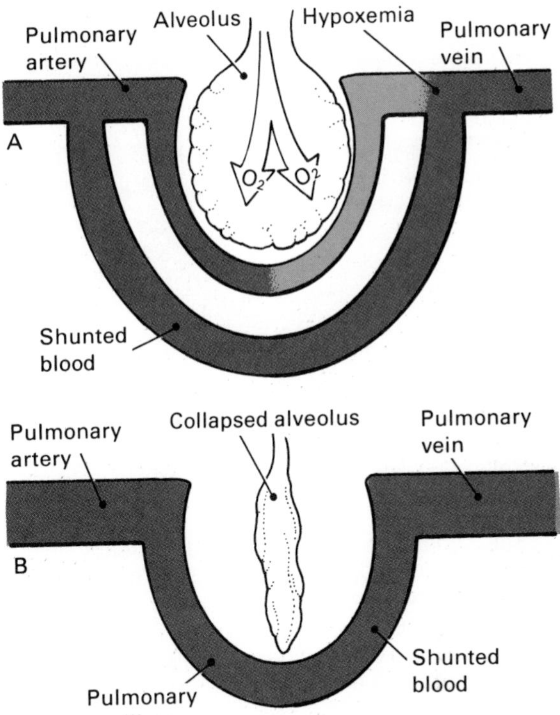

Figure 22-3 Schematic illustration of two types of shunts. *(a)* Anatomic shunt. The vessel which receives no ventilation has shunted blood that mixes with oxygenated blood. *(b)* Anatomic-like shunt. Perfusion continues in the absence of ventilation, and blood cannot become oxygenated.

absence of perfusion. The most common shunts are extrapulmonary and include those which occur in congenital heart disease through atrial or septal defects or a patent ductus arteriosus. These represent an anatomic shunt of blood from the right to the left side of the heart, bypassing gas exchange in the lung.

Intrapulmonary anatomic shunts are associated with arteriovenous fistulas in congenital defects and in hepatic cirrhosis. Anatomiclike shunts exist when there is obstruction to the flow of gas to lobes or segments of the lung, as in pneumonia with consolidation.

The classic difference between $\dot{V}/\dot{Q}$ mismatch and anatomiclike shunts is demonstrated by having the client breathe 100% oxygen for about 15 to 30 minutes. The client with $\dot{V}/\dot{Q}$ mismatch will increase the P_aO_2 to >400 mmHg, whereas the client with a shunt cannot increase the P_aO_2 to approximately the level seen in normal individuals or those with a $\dot{V}/\dot{Q}$ mismatch. In $\dot{V}/\dot{Q}$ mismatch, the increased FIO_2 (the fraction of inspired oxygen or the fractional concentration of oxygen delivered to the client) in poorly or intermittently ventilated areas provides enough oxygen to correct the ventilation problem by increasing the P_aO_2 and saturating the hemoglobin. However, in a client with shunting, the increased FIO_2 does not correct the oxygenation problem because mixed venous blood continues to flow through the "shunted" area and mixes with blood that has perfused normal alveoli. The poorly oxygenated blood from the shunt area lowers the P_aO_2 of the blood with which it is mixed, resulting in no increase or a limited increase in P_aO_2.

ARDS is a common clinical entity which is characterized by shunting. It is discussed in detail later in the chapter.

Diffusion Abnormalities Diffusion abnormalities are also a cause of hypoxemia. These abnormalities indicate an impairment in the equilibration between the PO_2 in the alveoli and in the pulmonary capillaries (Fig. 22-4). Diffusion does not occur normally for the following reasons:

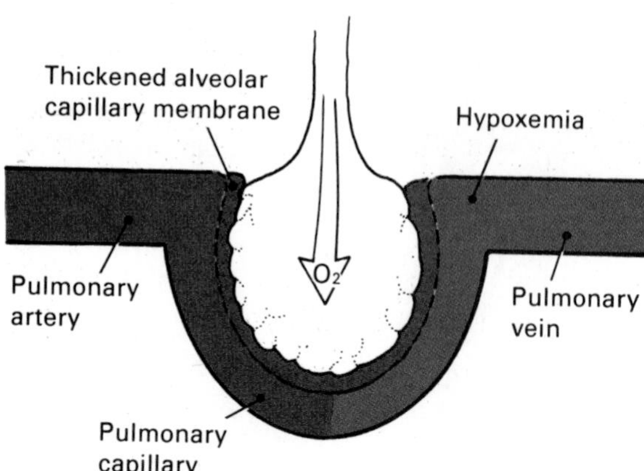

Figure 22-4 Diffusion abnormality. Exchange of CO_2 and O_2 cannot occur because of the thickened alveolar-capillary membrane.

1. The contact time for the red blood cells at the capillary membrane is decreased (e.g., intense physical exercise increases blood flow).
2. There is a reduction of pulmonary capillary blood secondary to obstruction or destruction of vessels (e.g., in severe emphysema).
3. There is a thickened blood-gas membrane, also classified as alveolar-capillary block (e.g., in fibrosis, pulmonary edema).

There may also be a combination of these effects to disrupt diffusion.

Hypoxemia caused by diffusion impairment can be corrected by the administration of 100% oxygen. This is not usually done in the client who has chronic CO_2 retention, such as in chronic obstructive pulmonary disease (COPD), because CO_2 narcosis may develop (see Chap. 21).

Severe diffusion problems must be present to cause a clinical decrease in the P_aO_2. Usually, clients have concurrent $\dot{V}/\dot{Q}$ abnormalities or shunt problems. Diseases in which a diffusion abnormality may contribute to hypoxemia include diffuse interstitial fibrosis, collagen-vascular disease of the lung (e.g., scleroderma, systemic lupus erythematosus), asbestosis, sarcoidosis, and interstitial pneumonia.

Interrelationship of Mechanisms Frequently, hypoxemic respiratory failure is caused by a combination of hypoventilation, diffusion impairment, shunting, and/or ventilation-perfusion mismatch. The client with acute respiratory failure secondary to acute pneumonia has a $\dot{V}/\dot{Q}$ imbalance because the inflammation, edema, and hypersecretion of exudate within the bronchioles and terminal respiratory units obstruct airways and impair ventilation in the alveoli. Hypoventilation can occur secondary to pain from pleuritic inflammation and subsequent shallow breathing. Interstitial edema due to secretion and fluid accumulation can cause diffusion abnormalities. Consolidation of lung lobules secondary to secretion accumulation and alveolar collapse can cause shuntlike effects.

Physiological effects of severe hypoxemia (P_aO_2 <40 to 50 mmHg) are manifested by altered function of the vital organs. The oxygen supply fails to support adequate tissue oxygen tension, and hypoxia develops. If oxygen insufficiency persists, the cells shift to anaerobic metabolism, which can lead to metabolic acidosis and cell death. Various organ systems are affected. The central nervous system is particularly vulnerable to hypoxia, and the client may manifest headache, restlessness, somnolence or clouding of consciousness, poor concentration, Cheyne-Stokes respirations, lethargy, and electroencephalogram (EEG) abnormalities. Frequently, the initial clinical symptoms of decreased O_2 are subtle changes in mental status. As hypoxemia progresses and becomes more severe, convulsions, retinal hemorrhages, and permanent brain damage may occur.

Clinical manifestations related to the cardiovascular system include tachycardia, mild hypertension (due partly to the release of catecholamines), increased cardiac output, cardiac arrhythmias, and deleterious effects on cardiac function with subsequent failure. These manifestations are especially true in the presence of coronary artery disease and pulmonary hypertension (secondary to alveolar hypoxia) and is further aggravated by respiratory acidosis (if present). With very severe, prolonged hypoxemia, bradycardia and hypotension may result. Renal function is impaired and sodium retention, proteinuria, edema formation, tubular necrosis, and uremia may occur. Gastrointestinal function alterations include abnormal liver function, abdominal pain, and bowel infarction.

Clinical Manifestations

Clinical manifestations of respiratory failure are related either to the accumulation of CO_2 and/or to the decrease in O_2 in the bloodstream. The rapid onset of symptoms is related to the rate of buildup of CO_2, the loss of O_2, and the ability of the client's compensatory mechanisms to overcome these changes. When the client's compensatory mechanisms fail to facilitate removal of CO_2 and the conservation of O_2, symptoms of tissue hypoxia and/or hypercapnia in the vital organs appear. The client may have rapid, shallow respirations because the lungs contain fluid and are noncompliant and stiff. The client may increase the respiratory rate in an effort to blow off accumulated CO_2. As CO_2 continues to increase, a slower respiratory rate may indicate that the client is no longer able to eliminate accumulated CO_2.

Acceptable arterial blood gas values may be present, but the client may be working extremely hard to attain them. Accessory muscles may be utilized during inspiration and/or expiration. During normal tidal breathing, the diaphragm moves about 1 cm. However, with forced inspiration or expiration, diaphragmatic excursion may be as much as 10 cm. Accessory muscles of inspiration that may be used are the scalene muscles, which elevate the first two ribs, and the sternocleidomastoids, which raise the sternum. Small muscles of the neck, hand, and face play a minor role as accessory inspiratory muscles. Normally, expiration is passive. When expiration becomes active during distress or increased exercise, the abdominal muscles and internal intercostals are used. Intercostal and supraclavicular retractions are an indication that these muscles are working hard to aid in ventilation.

The length of inspiration compared to that of expiration (I/E ratio), which is normally $1:1\frac{1}{2}$ or 1:2, may be decreased. The expiratory time is usually prolonged in airway obstruction. The pattern of respiratory response to activity may be altered. The client may use few accessory muscles at rest but may activate more muscle groups with increased activity.

The position the client assumes is also a clue to the effort associated with breathing. The client may prefer to sit straight up or lean forward, resting on the elbows, or to lie partially on one side or the other depending upon the location of the pulmonary pathology. Asymmetrical chest expansion may occur from (1) splinting an incision or trauma site, (2) pleural effusion, (3) pneumothorax, or (4) a paralyzed hemidiaphragm. Pursed-lip or open-mouth breathing may be utilized. The client who is working hard to breathe may become extremely diaphoretic. He may be able to speak only two to three words at a time between breaths.

As the level of P_aO_2 decreases, the mucous membranes, lips, tongue, and earlobes become a dusky grayish color. Cyanosis occurs when there is more than 5 g of unsaturated hemoglobin per deciliter of blood. If vasoconstriction occurs, the skin will become pale, cool, and clammy.

Clinical manifestations of tissue hypoxia to the vital organs may occur. The central nervous system is particularly prone to low O_2 and high CO_2 levels. The cardiovascular, renal, and gastrointestinal systems are also affected. These effects were discussed in the previous section, Interrelationship of Mechanisms.

Clients with chronic pulmonary disease may be able to tolerate a significant degree of hypoxemia and hypercarbia. Clinical signs of hypercapnia (tachycardia, papilledema, decreased deep tendon reflexes, confusion, etc.) may be apparent if the CO_2 retention is of rapid onset. However, these clinical signs are often absent or very subtle if chronic hypercapnia has been a feature of the client's disease. Only when the condition progresses to coma, with slow or gasping respirations or even apnea, may the diagnosis of respiratory failure be clinically obvious. For this reason, it is important to observe the client with chronic pulmonary disease very closely for subtle changes in respiratory pattern or mental status, and for overall clinical appearance.

Diagnostic Study Abnormalities

The most specific diagnostic study used to determine respiratory failure is assessment of arterial blood gases. Arterial blood gases are monitored as indicated by the client's respiratory status to detect changes, trends, and response to therapy. Other routine studies performed are chest x-ray, complete blood count, serum electrolytes, urinalysis, and electrocardiogram (ECG). Cultures of the sputum and blood are obtained as necessary to determine sources of possible infection. If pulmonary embolus is suspected, a ventilation-perfusion lung scan or pulmonary angiography may be done. Pulmonary function tests may be used to determine respiratory function.

In severe respiratory failure, measurement of cardiac output and mixed-venous blood gases via a thermodilution Swan-Ganz catheter (see Chap. 28) is an important aid in determining the amount of blood flow to tissues and the response to treatment. Monitoring of pulmonary artery, pulmonary wedge, and left atrial pressures is done to determine if the etiology of lung fluid accumulation is cardiac or pulmonary. These parameters are also monitored to determine the response of the lung and heart to hypoxemia, their state of compliance, and the client's response to therapeutic regimens. Swan-Ganz catheters and monitoring are discussed in detail in Chap. 28.

Blood from the pulmonary artery port (mixed-venous blood) of the Swan-Ganz catheter can be sampled. Mixed venous-blood oxygen tension ($P_{\bar{v}}O_2$) is an indication of the state of tissue oxygenation. The normal PO_2 of mixed-venous blood is 35 to 40 mmHg with an O_2 saturation of 75%. An increase in $P_{\bar{v}}O_2$ of >60 mmHg indicates that the tissues are not extracting and utilizing oxygen or are not being perfused (e.g., in cyanide poisoning). A decrease in $P_{\bar{v}}O_2$ (<35 mmHg) indicates that the tissues are utilizing more oxygen than they would normally. Clinically, a decreased $P_{\bar{v}}O_2$ is evident in severe hypoxemia due to decreased P_aO_2, decreased O_2-carrying capacity of hemoglobin, or decreased cardiac output.[1]

Calculation of the shunt fraction ($\dot{Q}S/\dot{Q}T$) utilizing $P_{\bar{v}}O_2$ in the client receiving 100% oxygen is useful in diagnosing the presence and degree of intrapulmonary shunt. The shunt fraction is expressed as a fraction or percentage of the cardiac output which does not become oxygenated in the lungs. A $\dot{Q}S/\dot{Q}T$ of >30 percent of the cardiac output is an ominous sign and signifies significant cardiopulmonary deterioration and hypoxemia.[2]

Calculation of the difference between the alveolar and arterial tensions [$D(A - a)O_2$ or $P(A - a)O_2$] is an aid in determining whether the cause of hypoxemia is secondary to hypoventilation. $D(A - a)O_2$ also assesses the difficulty with which oxygen moves from the alveolus across the alveolar-capillary membrane and into the arterial blood.

When one breathes room air, the normal $D(A - a)O_2$ is approximately 10 mmHg. In the presence of alveolar hypoventilation when an extrapulmonary factor affects the lungs (e.g., central nervous system depression secondary to drugs or paralysis of respiratory muscles), the alveolar ventilation rate decreases. Consequently, the amount of oxygen reaching the alveolus will decrease ($\downarrow P_AO_2$), with a subsequent but proportional decrease in P_aO_2. Thus, the $D(A-a)O_2$ will remain constant. However, if an intrapulmonary defect is present (for example, $\dot{V}/\dot{Q}$ mismatch, shunt), the alveolar ventilation rate is not usually effected adversely until the later stages of the disease, and the P_AO_2 remains contant or slightly increases. The amount of oxygen reaching the alveolus from the air is not effected. However, the P_aO_2 will decrease disproportionately, depending upon the exchange defect at the alveolar-capillary membrane. Consequently, the $D(A - a)O_2$ will be widened.

To calculate $D(A - a)O_2$, one must first calculate the partial pressure of oxygen in the alveolus (P_AO_2), and then subtract the P_aO_2 which is given in the arterial blood gas. The following equation, known as the alveolar air equation, is utilized to calculate P_AO_2:

$$P_AO_2 = FIO_2 \times (P_B - 47\text{ mmHg}) - \frac{P_aCO_2}{R}$$

In this equation, P_B is the barometeric pressure (i.e., at sea level $P_B = 760$ mmHg) and 47 mmHg is the partial pressure of water vapor in the trachea. Thus $FIO_2 \times (P_B - 47)$ is equal to the partial pressure of inspired oxygen (PIO_2). One must then subtract the carbon dioxide gas. The amount of CO_2 will depend upon *R*, the respiratory exchange ratio of CO_2 produced to O_2 consumed. For most calculations, *R* is assumed to be 0.8, the respiratory quotient at rest. Therefore, the partial pressure of oxygen in the alveolus is:

$$P_AO_2 = PIO_2 - \frac{P_aCO_2}{0.8}$$

Calculation of the $D(A - a)O_2$ at an FIO_2 greater than 0.21 may also be performed but requires different guidelines. Calculation of the $D(A - a)O_2$ at which the client is breathing 100% oxygen will also give an indication of the extent of the shunt. $D(A - a)O_2$ determination is also helpful in assessing the effects of positive end-expiratory pressure (PEEP), chest physiotherapy, fluid administration, diuretics, and dialysis.

Medical and Nursing Management of Acute Respiratory Failure

Management of acute respiratory failure depends on the underlying disease process (Table 22-3). However, several aspects of management are common to many types of respiratory failure, and these will be discussed. Because the medical and nursing management of acute respiratory failure are strongly interdependent and contiguous, the overall management of the client is presented in this section.

Maintenance of adequate oxygenation

Oxygen Administration If hypoxemia is secondary to hypoventilation, then provision and maintenance of adequate ventilation will usually overcome the problem of gas exchange. Hypoxemia secondary to $\dot{V}/\dot{Q}$ mismatch usually responds favorably to the lowest concentration of oxygen necessary to maintain the arterial PO_2 at ≥50 to 60 mmHg administered via mask or cannula. Hypoxemia secondary to shunting is usually refractory (refractory hypoxemia) to the administration of high concentrations of oxygen via mask and ultimately requires mechanical ventilation. The client with chronic pulmonary disease requiring oxygen should receive low-flow oxygen (1 to 3 L/minute) via a nasal cannula or Venturi mask. The Venturi mask provides an exact concentration of oxygen. In contrast, low flow via a nasal cannula delivers O_2 concentrations which vary with the client's minute ventilation. Both low-flow O_2 and the Venturi mask generally correct severe arterial hypoxemia in chronically ill clients without unduly suppressing respiration by reducing the hypoxic drive.

Maintenance of Hemoglobin Concentration and Cardiac Output In order to ensure adequate oxygen delivery to the tissues, adequate hemoglobin

Table 22-3
Management of Acute Respiratory Failure

1. Maintenance of adequate oxygenation
   A. Oxygen administration to keep P_aO_2 >60 mmHg
   B. Maintenance of adequate hemoglobin concentration
   C. Maintenance of adequate cardiac output
   D. Prevention and assessment of tissue hypoxia
   E. Measures to decrease stress and anxiety and promote comfort
2. Improvement of alveolar ventilation
   A. Maintenance of a patent airway
      (1) Effective coughing
      (2) Suctioning
      (3) Positioning
   B Measures to assist in liquefaction and movement of secretions
      (1) Humidification
      (2) Adequate hydration
      (3) Chest physiotherapy
      (4) Bland aerosols and ultrasonic nebulization
   C. Relief of bronchospasm
      (1) Bronchodilators
      (2) Aerosolized bronchodilators
   D. Reduction of pulmonary congestion
      (1) Diuretics
   E. Mechanical ventilation
3. Treatment of the underlying cause of failure
4. Continuous monitoring and evaluation of treatment

saturation can be provided by keeping the client's P_aO_2 above 60 mmHg. Recall from the oxyhemoglobin dissociation curve (Fig. 18-8) that when the P_aO_2 is 60 mmHg or greater, the hemoglobin is 90% saturated. An adequate hemoglobin concentration of 10 g/dL or greater and maintenance of an adequate cardiac output are also important in ensuring adequate oxygen delivery.

Blood pressure (BP) should be maintained at the most efficient level for each client. Usually, a systolic BP of ≥90 mmHg is adequate to maintain perfusion to the vital organs. A urine output of ≥30 mL/hour is an indication of adequate renal perfusion. If the systolic BP is maintained at ≥90 mmHg, then changes in mental status may be attributed to the levels of O_2 and CO_2 in the blood rather than to decreased perfusion to the brain.

Prevention and Assessment of Tissue Hypoxia Close observation for clinical manifestations of vital organ hypoxia is necessary. This includes frequent assessment of the client's mental and neurological status for cloudiness of sensorium, poor concentration, restlessness, stupor, lethargy, somnolence, tremors, slurred speech, depressed tendon reflexes, and asterixis. Cardiovascular status assessment includes direct or indirect BP monitoring; monitoring of cardiac output, pulmonary artery and wedge pressures, and cardiac rate and rhythm; and assessment for symptoms of right- and left-sided heart failure. Older clients and clients with coronary artery disease are very susceptible to the effects of decreased tissue oxygen upon the myocardium. Fluid and electrolyte levels should be carefully assessed in relation to renal and cardiac response. Serial evaluations of serum electrolytes are made to determine the existence of anion or cation excesses or deficiencies. Incremental replacement of potassium and bicarbonate may be indicated in the presence of hypokalemia and severe acidemia.

Measures to Decrease Stress and Promote Comfort The client should be maintained in an atmosphere as quiet and relaxed as possible. Rising levels of stress and anxiety can further increase oxygen demands. The respiratory rate can also be increased. In clients with COPD, this results in decreased time for exhalation, increased air trapping, and therefore an enhanced sensation of dyspnea. Fear of suffocation or death is not uncommon, and the client must be supported emotionally as well as physically at this time. Providing reassurance, spending as much time as possible with the client at the bedside, and ensuring that he can get help immediately (e.g., by making a call light readily available) may help to decrease his anxiety level. Frequently, a family member or friend may have a soothing effect on the client. It is important to evaluate the effect of visitors on his anxiety level.

Often, clients in respiratory distress (especially those with chronic lung disease) prefer to be in an open area without curtains or with a door or window open. Activity should be kept to a minimum within reason. Positioning the client for comfort and for the most efficient ventilation is important. Frequent rest periods need to be provided, and efficient scheduling of care, treatments, assessments, and diagnostic studies is important.

The client who has pronounced acute hypercarbia is often sleepy. In this case, it is very important to keep the client awake and breathing at regular intervals, since sleeping will result in further hypoventilation. Patting him on the back, keeping the lights on, and giving frequent reminders to breathe can all help. Interpreting facial expressions and body language, using questions that require short yes and no answers or head nodding, or using a word board for communication will help to limit the amount of energy the client utilizes for communication.

Measures to increase physical comfort are also important. A cool cloth placed on the forehead to remove perspiration and to refresh the face is usually appreciated. Sips of cool water or ice chips (if tolerated) can also be offered with assistance. Mouth care is especially important for the client who is a mouth breather because of the drying effects of inspired air upon the mucous membranes. Removing a perspiration-soaked gown, lightly sponging the client's upper torso, and helping him into a dry gown will often suffice for a daily bath.

Improvement of alveolar ventilation

In respiratory failure, the work of breathing is increased, and often the CO_2 production may be excessive in relation to the amount of alveolar ventilation that is occurring. Reduction of both CO_2 production and the work of breathing, with subsequent improvement in alveolar ventilation, can be accomplished by instituting therapy to relieve airway obstruction or pulmonary congestion. If all these intensive measures fail, mechanical ventilation may be required to assist or control the ventilation.

Maintenance of a Patent Airway Maintenance of a patent airway is essential. Obstruction of the airway due to the accumulation of secretions and/or bronchospasm occurs frequently. If secretions are obstructing the airway, the client should be encouraged to cough if possible. Effective coughing requires a deep inhalation, effective glottic closure, and high expiratory flows (see Table 21-9). These abilities need to be evaluated in the client to determine if the cough is effective.

Clients with neuromuscular weakness may have a flow limitation due to decreased volume and an inability to produce high enough pleural pressures. Augmented coughing may be helpful in these clients or in an exhausted client. Augmented coughing is performed by placing the flat palm of your hand or hands on the thorax (rib springing) in the area where the presence of secretions has been detected by auscultation or upon the abdominal musculature below the xiphoid process. As the client ends the deep inspiration and begins expiration, the hands should be moved forcefully downward, facilitating chest compression or increased abdominal pressure. This measure helps to produce muscle movement, increases pleural pressure and expiratory flows, and augments or assists the cough. Coughing at the end of expiration is helpful in clients with severe airway obstruction because it can cause compression of the more distal or peripheral airways and may help to "milk" or move secretions into the proximal airways. Frequently, having the client breathe as deeply as possible (if he is able) may stimulate the cough. "Huff" coughing with the glottis open may be used for clients who have problems with glottic closure, such as those with endotracheal or tracheal tubes in place.

Positioning the client either by elevating the head of the bed to 90° (if tolerated) or by using a reclining chair bed may maximize thoracic expansion. The client should be placed on the side if there is any possibility that the tongue will obstruct the airway or that aspiration may occur. An oral or nasal airway should be kept at the bedside and utilized when necessary.

If the client's cough is ineffective in removing secretions, nasopharyngeal or nasotracheal suctioning is indicated. Adequate oxygenation and monitoring of the client are essential during these procedures. Although rarely indicated, bronchoscopy may be employed to remove secretions, especially if they are extremely thick and tenacious.

Measures to Liquefy and Mobilize Secretions If bronchial secretions are thick, viscid, and difficult to raise, efforts to thin them should be made. Adequate hydration is necessary to keep secretions thin and easy to remove. All inspired oxygen should be well humidified to avoid dehydration and thickening of secretions.

Bland aerosols utilizing normal saline solutions or water administered via a nebulizer may be used to liquefy secretions. Occasionally, ultrasonic nebulization treatments of water or saline may be used. The client's response to aerosol therapy must be assessed. Aerosol therapy may induce bronchospasm, severe bouts of coughing, and decreased P_aO_2. Nebulized acetylcystine (Mucomyst) or other mucolytic agents have been used to thin secretions. However, the value of these agents is questionable, and they are often very irritating. In some clients, they induce bronchospasm. They have not proved to be more effective than bland mists or adequate hydration.

Chest physiotherapy in certain situations can be an effective means of improving the removal of retained secretions (see Fig. 21-9). If tolerated, postural drainage, percussion, and vibration performed manually or via a mechanical vibrator to the affected lung segments may assist in moving secretions to larger airways, where they can be removed by effective coughing or suctioning. If nasotracheal suctioning and other measures to liquefy and mobilize secretions are ineffective, it may become necessary to insert an endotracheal or tracheotomy tube to facilitate suctioning of secretions.

Relief of Bronchospasm Relief of bronchospasm (if present) will aid in maximal bronchodilatation and increase effective alveolar ventilation. An intravenous loading dose of aminophylline is infused initially in an acute attack of bronchospasm. The loading dose is followed by a continuous infusion sufficient to maintain theophylline blood levels of 10 to

20 μg/mL. Aerosolized bronchodilators such as isoproterenol (Isuprel), metaproterenol (Alupent), and isoetharine (Bronkosol) (see Table 21-4) diluted with sterile water or normal saline solutions may also be administered at regular intervals depending upon the client's response. Subcutaneous injections of terbutaline (Brethine) given at regular intervals can also reduce bronchospasm.

The client's response to the effects of these beta-adrenergic bronchodilators should be monitored. In some clients, bronchodilator administration results in an initial worsening of arterial hypoxemia. This is due to redistribution of the inspired gas away from areas which continue to be perfused to areas with decreased perfusion due to localized hypoxia. Administration of an oxygen-enriched gas mixture simultaneously with the bronchodilator may help to alleviate the subsequent hypoxemia. Side effects and nursing management related to bronchodilators are discussed in Chap. 21 and Table 21-4.

Reduction of Pulmonary Congestion A previously healthy person who goes into shock is given intravenous (IV) fluids to maintain the BP and contribute to extracellular volume. Pulmonary congestion and alveolar-capillary damage may result as a complication of this fluid administration. Lung water accumulation may also develop in an acute exacerbation of respiratory failure in a client with chronic lung disease or coronary artery and left ventricular disease. The accumulation of lung water can further aggravate and inhibit alveolar ventilation.

Diuretics may be used to treat pulmonary congestion. Digitalization is not usually recommended. If digitalis is used, arterial blood gases, ECG, and serum electrolytes are monitored closely since digitalis in the presence of hypoxemia, hypokalemia, and acidemia can increase cardiac irritability.

Mechanical Ventilation If all of the previously discussed procedures fail to improve alveolar ventilation and the client continues to deteriorate clinically, mechanical ventilation may be instituted to assist or control ventilation. Guidelines for determining the need for mechanical ventilation for clients without chronic lung disease are listed in Table 22-9. It is necessary to remember that these are only numbers; clinical observation of the client is equally important in making a decision to institute mechanical ventilation.

The client with chronic lung disease needs to be evaluated based upon his own limited pulmonary function. Baseline values for the client with chronic disease obtained when respiratory distress is not present often meet the criteria for mechanical ventilation. The client needs to be evaluated relative to the clinical manifestations and the response to therapy. For example, the client who is experiencing an acute exacerbation of asthma usually demonstrates hypocapnia and respiratory alkalemia with hypoxemia in the early stages rather than hypercapnia and respiratory acidemia with hypoxemia. In these clients, a rise in P_aCO_2, even into the normal range, is an ominous sign since it signifies exhaustion and impending respiratory failure. Ventilatory support is imperative. The types of mechanical ventilation and management of the client on a mechanical ventilator are discussed later in this chapter.

Treatment of the underlying cause of respiratory failure

In clients with absolute hypoventilation, the primary problem can usually be diagnosed rapidly and appropriate therapy initiated. When the problem is drug overdose, dialysis or other methods to promote excretion of the drug are undertaken. Specific measures are available for clients with myasthenia gravis, whereas clients with Guillain-Barré syndrome often require long-term ventilatory support until the disease process runs its course. Infection is often the primary cause of acute respiratory failure in the immunosuppressed client. Appropriate cultures must be obtained and antibiotic therapy begun as soon as possible. Bronchoscopy or lung biopsy may need to be performed to obtain specimens for determining the underlying respiratory pathology. Specific therapies for various diseases and problems are discussed in other chapters.

Continuous monitoring of the effects of treatment

A flowchart which shows the client's arterial blood gases and other laboratory and clinical studies, including vital signs, pulmonary artery and wedge pressures, weights, intake and output, medications and dosage, electrolytes, complete blood count, and respiratory parameters, is extremely helpful. Accurate, clear documentation of objective and subjective assessments on the client's flowchart is an important aspect of care. Management of the client should be evaluated continuously and the therapeutic regimen altered as indicated by the client's response.

ADULT RESPIRATORY DISTRESS SYNDROME

Adult respiratory distress syndrome (ARDS) is a descriptive term that has been applied to a variety of acute and diffuse infiltrative lung lesions which cause severe refractory arterial hypoxemia and life-

Table 22-4

Common Terms Synonymous with Adult Respiratory Distress Syndrome

ARDS
Shock lung
Traumatic wet lung
Wet lung
Septic lung
Congestive atelectasis
Hemorrhagic atelectasis
Capillary leak syndrome
Postperfusion (pump) lung
Posttraumatic pulmonary insufficiency
Acute respiratory failure (ARF)
Low-flow lung syndrome
Noncardiogenic pulmonary edema
Adult hyaline membrane disease
White lung
Progressive pulmonary consolidation
Da Nang lung

Table 22-5

Conditions Predisposing to ARDS

Sepsis
Shock
Generalized trauma
Fluid overload
Massive blood transfusions
Aspiration
Postcardiopulmonary resuscitation
Pancreatitis
Oxygen toxicity
Fat embolism
Massive smoke inhalation
Pneumonia
Inhaled or circulating toxins
DIC
Immunologic reactions (drug allergy, anaphylaxis)
Neurologic injuries
Drug overdose

threatening respiratory distress. This syndrome is more commonly encountered in adults with previously normal lungs than in those with preexisting lung disease. ARDS is known by a variety of clinical terms (Table 22-4). Frequently, the general term *adult respiratory distress syndrome* is utilized with reference to the suspected etiology, such as ARDS secondary to pancreatitis.

The prevalence of ARDS is not known. In 1972 an estimated 150,000 cases were treated, and it appears that this number is increasing.[3] The mortality rate (50 to 60 percent) of ARDS is still quite high.[4] This represents an improvement in survival from the mortality rate of almost 100 percent a few years ago and is a result of improved recognition and modern treatment techniques.

Pathophysiology

The initial insult to the lungs in ARDS can be caused by a variety of clinical disorders (Table 22-5, Fig. 22-5). Since all clients with these types of clinical disorders do not develop ARDS, it is assumed that there is a disturbance in normal protective pulmonary mechanisms. Despite the heterogeneity of the disorders which may cause ARDS, the common abnormal finding is diffuse alveolar-capillary membrane injury, which leads to the subsequent leakage of fluid and cellular components from the vascular space into the interstitium and alveoli (Fig. 22-6).

In most cases of ARDS, the initial alveolar-capillary membrane insult is thought to be due to a period of pulmonary hypoperfusion. The pulmonary hypoperfusion is thought to occur because of intravascular coagulation with subsequent thromboembolism within the pulmonary microvasculature. Thromboemboli cause release of potent broncho- and vasoconstrictors and mechanical obstruction of the pulmonary blood flow. The vasoconstriction and stagnation of blood flow in the pulmonary circulation lead to hypoxia, acidosis, and intravascular clotting.[5] Ultimately, the capillary membrane is damaged by these insults and the permeability is increased, allowing leakage of fluids and cellular components into the interstitial spaces. As the disease progresses, the fluid also moves into the alveoli. Normally, fluid moves from the pulmonary vessels into the interstitial space, but equilibrium is maintained by lymphatic removal of excess fluid. However, lymph channels become compressed by the extravasated fluid, and fluid accumulates in the interstitium (Fig. 22-6).

As endothelial cells are damaged and capillary membrane permeability increases, interstitial edema is intensified. This leads to an increase in the distance between alveoli and capillaries, with consequent reduced oxygen diffusion from the alveoli to the capillaries. Congestive atelectasis begins to develop at this point. The pulmonary capillaries are progressively dilated and filled with red blood cells. An increasingly diffuse microatelectasis develops as the pulmonary capillary endothelium is disrupted, and red blood cells migrate into the interstitium. Peribronchial hemorrhage may occur. The first clinical symptoms of ARDS are evident at this point.[6]

As interstitial edema increases, fluid moves from the interstitium into the alveoli. The alveolar type II cells are damaged, impairing their ability to make surfactant (see Chap. 18). Surfactant normally lowers

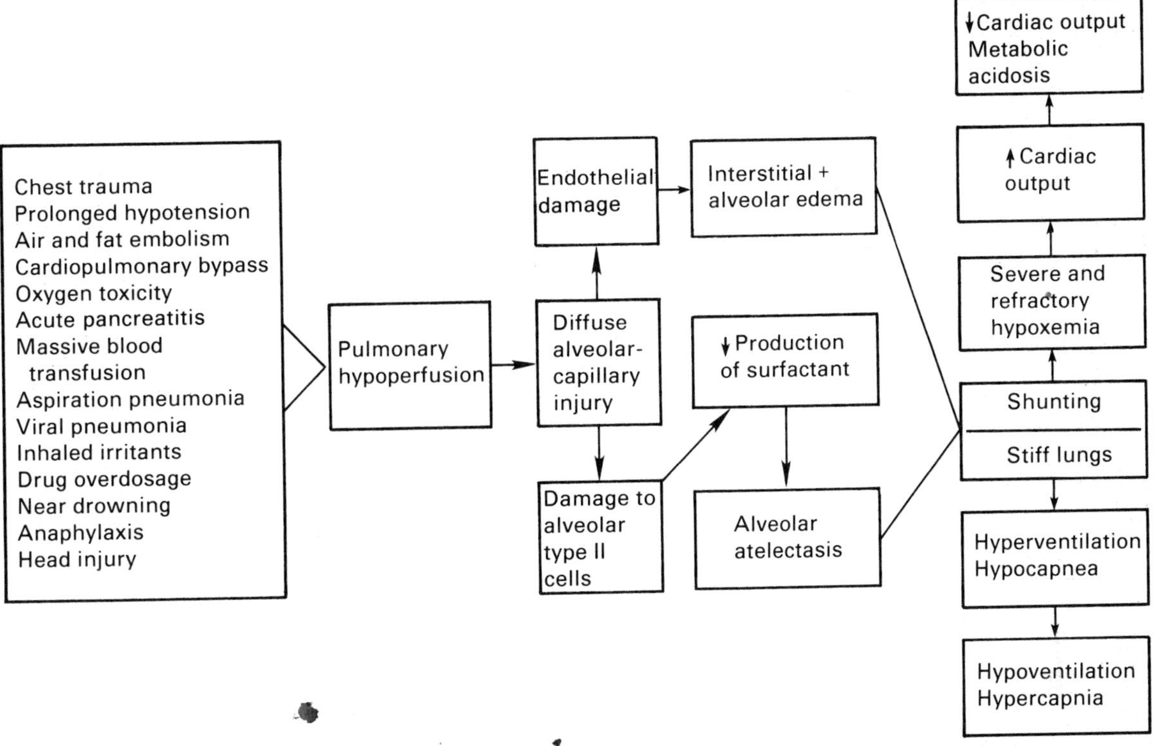

Figure 22-5 Pathogenesis of ARDS. *(Adapted from A. Fishman, Pulmonary Diseases and Disorders, McGraw-Hill Book Company, New York, 1980, p. 1676.)*

the surface tension of the alveolar lining fluid. Usually, surfactant maintains alveolar stability by preventing alveolar collapse, increases lung compliance, and reduces the work of expanding the lung with each breath. When alveolar type II cells are damaged, not only is the production of surfactant decreased, but the effectiveness of the existing surfactant is reduced by the alveolar fluid and its inactivation by fibrin. The alveoli become increasingly unstable and tend to collapse unless filled with fluid from the interstitium.

The essential disturbances which characterize ARDS are interstitial and alveolar edema (noncardiogenic pulmonary edema) and atelectasis. Severe ventilation-perfusion mismatch and shunting of blood occur as blood flows through alveoli which are collapsed or filled with fluid. Diffusion limitations and impairment may occur because of thickening of alveolar-capillary interfaces due to progressive interstitial fibrosis. Hypoxia and subsequent severe hypoxemia which is refractory to increasing concentrations of oxygen (refractory hypoxemia) develop.

The lungs become stiff and less compliant because of the loss of surfactant, interstitial edema, and alveolar collapse. Large inspiratory pressures must be generated by the respiratory muscles to inflate the noncompliant lungs. Therefore, the work of breathing is greatly increased. In addition, the functional residual capacity (FRC) is decreased due to alveolar collapse, alveolar filling, and interstitial thickening.

Both hypoxemia and the stimulation of juxtacapillary receptors in the stiff lung parenchyma (J reflex) cause an increase in respiratory frequency and decreased tidal volume. This results in alveolar hyperventilation due to increased removal of CO_2. The alveolar hyperventilation and a reflexive increase in cardiac output attempt to compensate for the severe hypoxemia. However, as alveoli collapse and fill with fluid, increased shunting of blood occurs, and alveolar hypoventilation and symptoms of decreased cardiac output and decreased tissue perfusion develop. The pathogenesis of ARDS is summarized in Fig. 22-5.

Clinical Manifestations

At the time of the initial injury and for several hours to 1 to 2 days afterward, the client may have no

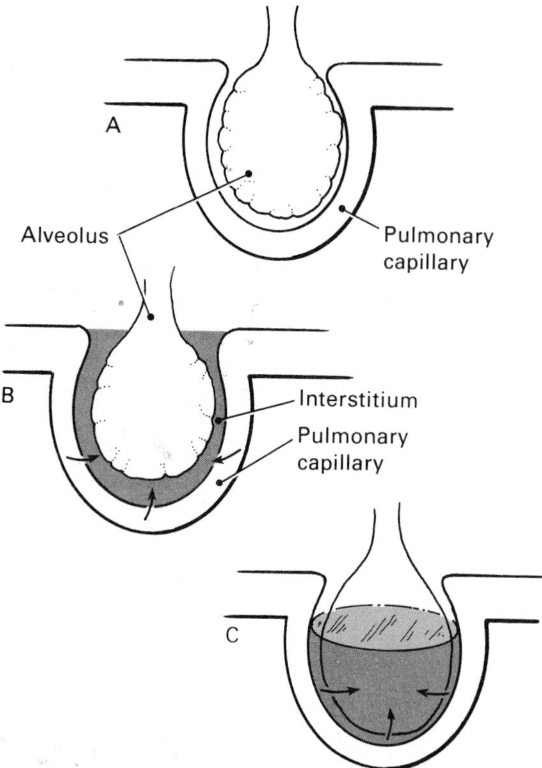

Figure 22-6 Stages of edema formation in ARDS. (*a*) Normal alveolus and pulmonary capillary. (*b*) Interstitial edema occurs with increased flow of fluid into the interstitial space. (c) Alveolar edema occurs when fluid crosses the blood-gas barrier.

respiratory symptoms. The initial phase of ARDS is often insidious. The client may exhibit dyspnea, tachypnea, cough, and restlessness. Chest auscultation may be normal or reveal fine, scattered rales (crackles). Arterial blood gas analyses usually demonstrate mild hypoxemia and respiratory alkalosis. The alkalosis is due to the compensatory increase in alveolar ventilation. The chest x-ray may be normal, or there may be evidence of minimal scattered interstitial infiltrates. There must be a large increase in lung congestion before the chest x-ray becomes abnormal.[7]

In the second phase of ARDS, symptomatology is related to increased lung water accumulation and decreased lung compliance. Respiratory discomfort becomes evident as the work of breathing increases. Noisy tachypneic and hyperpneic respirations as well as intercostal and suprasternal retractions may be present. Pulmonary function tests reveal decreased static and effective compliance and decreased lung volumes, particularly FRC (although it is not measured). Tachycardia, diaphoresis, changes in sensorium with decreased mentation, cyanosis, and pallor may be present. Chest auscultation usually reveals scattered to diffuse rales and rhonchi. The chest x-ray usually demonstrates diffuse and extensive bilateral interstitial and alveolar infiltrates.

Progressive arterial hypoxemia in spite of the increased oxygen tension of air inspired via mask, cannula, or endotracheal tube is a *hallmark* of ARDS. This is referred to as *refractory hypoxemia.* $D(A - a)O_2$, or the difference between alveolar and arterial PO_2, can be as high as 200 to 500 mmHg when breathing room air (normal <15 to 20 mmHg). A calculated shunt fraction ($\dot{Q}S/\dot{Q}T$) of >30 percent of the cardiac output is generally considered incompatible with prolonged spontaneous ventilation.[8] Arterial blood gas values may demonstrate a normal P_aCO_2 in spite of severe dyspnea and hypoxemia. A normal P_aCO_2 signifies that the client is no longer able to compensate and is increasing the alveolar ventilation in response to hypoxemia and other stimuli.

The final stage of ARDS is associated with profound respiratory distress requiring endotracheal intubation and assisted ventilation. Bronchial breath sounds are frequently associated with this stage. The chest x-ray is often termed "white out" or "white lung" as consolidation and coalescing infiltrates pervade the lungs, leaving few recognizable air spaces.[9] Severe hypoxemia, hypercarbia, and metabolic acidosis with symptoms of end organ or tissue hypoxia may ensue if prompt therapy is not instituted.

Complications

Complications may develop as a result either of ARDS itself or of treatment. *Disturbances in heart rhythm* may occur secondary to hypoxia and/or alkalosis. Cardiac monitoring as well as monitoring of electrolytes and the acid-base status is imperative to prevent or immediately treat arrhythmias.

Secondary bacterial infections may occur in the client with ARDS. Frequent monitoring of sputum smears and cultures and assessment of the quality, quantity, and consistency of sputum should be done. The presence of fever warrants a workup to determine the source of infection. Serial chests x-rays and blood counts with a white blood cell differential must be closely monitored.

Sepsis may occur since the client usually has numerous cannulas and tubes inserted directly into the venous or arterial system. Observing and changing cannula sites as necessary may prevent sepsis. All stopcocks should be capped or covered and old blood flushed from them to prevent bacterial contamination and growth.

Stress ulcers are not uncommon and prophylactic

use of antiacids every 1 to 2 hours (to keep the gastric pH >5) and/or IV cimetidine (Tagamet) may prevent gastrointestinal hemorrhage. Guaiac testing of stools and emesis and monitoring of hematocrit values are important to detect occult bleeding.

Disseminated intravascular coagulation (DIC) may occur with ARDS. (The pathophysiology of DIC is discussed in Chap. 24.) Frequent monitoring of platelet counts, fibrinogen level, and partial thromboplastin and prothrombin times is helpful in the early detection of DIC. Observation and assessment of bleeding from venipuncture sites and mucous membranes and during endotracheal suction are important. The client should also be observed for the presence of bruises and petechiae.

Medical and Nursing Management

Preventive measures for ARDS include those for acute respiratory failure. Astute observation of the respiratory status of high-risk clients is especially important. Judicious fluid administration and monitoring of the fluid status via intake and output records, weights, clinical manifestations of increased lung water (e.g., rales, deteriorating arterial blood gases, increased work of breathing), and body fluid accumulation (e.g., jugular venous distension, sacral, periorbital, or peripheral edema, hepatomegaly, splenomegaly) are important. Expeditious treatment of the initial disorder (e.g., prompt treatment with antibiotics or surgery to remove the source of infection in sepsis and maintenance of BP and urine flow in shock) is necessary and may prevent further deterioration of the client and the development of ARDS.

At the time of the initial lung injury and for as long as 12 to 48 hours thereafter, the client may be free of respiratory symptoms or signs of distress. Usually, abnormal findings on physical examination are indications that ARDS has progressed beyond the initial stages. Prompt recognition of clinical manifestations and treatment may help to prevent the development of severe forms of ARDS.

Management of ARDS includes many of the medical and nursing regimens used in acute respiratory failure. Measures to improve alveolar ventilation and maintain adequate oxygen discussed in the section on Medical and Nursing Management of Acute Respiratory Failure also apply to ARDS. However, there are many medical and nursing therapies unique to ARDS which are described in this section.

Treatment of the underlying disorder

Sepsis is often an initiating mechanism of ARDS. Prompt culturing of exudates and secretions and surgical debridement (if indicated) of an infected area are necessary. Antibiotic therapy should be instituted as soon as possible.

If severe arterial hypotension and shock are the initiating factors, restoration of adequate BP is essential. Not infrequently, overzealous administration of fluids in the attempt to restore BP leads to circulatory overload and pulmonary edema. Other conditions contributing to ARDS are presented in Table 22-5, and their treatment is discussed in other chapters.

Maintenance of adequate oxygenation

Oxygen administration via a face mask or cannula (prongs) is usually inadequate to treat the refractory hypoxemia of ARDS. The rule of thumb for oxygen administration is to give the client the lowest concentration of oxygen in inspired air that suffices to maintain a P_aO_2 of approximately 60 mmHg. When the FIO_2 concentration exceeds 0.5 for more than a few days, O_2 toxicity is virtually inevitable.

Endotracheal intubation with subsequent mechanical ventilation is almost always required. The indications for mechanical ventilation are discussed later in the chapter. When the client is placed on the mechanical ventilator, large tidal volumes (10 to 15 mL/kg) are utilized to reverse microatelectasis and shunting. The respiratory rate of the ventilator is set to keep the pH at 7.35 to 7.45 and to prevent alkalosis which may impair oxygen unloading at the tissue level, depress cardiac output, and initiate arrhythmias.

When adequate oxygenation is not achieved by mechanical ventilation of the client at high lung volumes, or when the P_aO_2 remains less than 60 mmHg with an FIO_2 of >0.5 to 0.6, the use of PEEP is indicated. PEEP is a ventilatory maneuver which applies positive pressure to the airway and lungs at the end of exhalation. Expiration normally occurs when the pressure in the chest becomes equal to atmospheric pressure or zero. When positive pressure is applied to the lung at the end of expiration, the lung is kept partially expanded and the alveoli are prevented from totally collapsing. The mechanism of action of PEEP is related to its ability to recruit or open up collapsed alveoli and increase the FRC. It also acts in this way to decrease shunting and improve oxygenation and lung compliance. PEEP is discussed in more detail in the section on Mechanical Ventilation.

Extracorporeal Membrane Oxygenation (ECMO) When acute pulmonary disease becomes severe and prolonged enough to carry a high mortality risk with continued therapy, ECMO can sustain life support for all organs while maintenance or new treatment is pursued. The concept of ECMO is similar to that of kidney dialysis or cardiopulmonary bypass. Blood which cannot be oxygenated by the lungs is removed from the body, passed through a membrane oxygenator where it undergoes gas exchange, and returned to the circulation. These are several cannulation sites and perfusion routes which may be chosen. Venoarterial (VA) bypass, which is accomplished by cannulation of the femoral artery and vein, is currently the most popular method. ECMO is indicated for clients with severe, reversible respiratory failure unresponsive to conventional treatment methods. Mechanical ventilation of the lungs must be continued to prevent deflation and atelectasis. Because the client must be anticoagulated during ECMO, strict anticoagulant precautions must be enforced. Special attention to the circulatory status of the area or extremity distal to the cannulation site is also important. Measures to promote secretion removal and lung clearance are also part of the management program. The use of ECMO for desperately ill clients with acute respiratory insufficiency has been associated with a 10 to 20 percent survival rate.[10] Further studies are needed to determine the effectiveness and indications for the use of ECMO.

Maintenance of cardiac output and hemoglobin concentration

There is a need for continuous hemodynamic monitoring of the client with ARDS who is receiving PEEP therapy. An arterial line should be inserted to obtain continuous recording of blood pressure and to make it easier to obtain frequent arterial blood gas measurements. Specific nursing measures for the client with an indwelling arterial cannula are discussed in Chap. 28.

Cardiac output can be assessed via the thermodilution port of the Swan-Ganz catheter. Mixed venous-oxygen samples can also be obtained from the pulmonary artery (distal) part of the catheter. Calculation of the arterial-venous oxygen $(A - V)O_2$ difference can be performed utilizing $P_{\bar{v}}O_2$. The arterial-venous oxygen difference is the difference in the oxygen content of arterial and mixed venous blood. This value gives an indication of cardiac output if thermodilution is not available. The normal $(A - V)O_2$ difference is 4 to 5 vol%, and an $(A - V)O_2$ difference of >5 vol% suggests impaired cardiac output.[11] It is very important to be able to assess cardiac output accurately utilizing one of these methods in order to determine the effects of PEEP and other therapies on the client's cardiopulmonary status.

If cardiac output falls, it may be necessary to administer fluids or colloid solutions or to lower PEEP. Use of inotropic drugs such as dopamine (Intropin) or dobutamine (Dobutrex) may also be necessary.

Hemoglobin is usually kept at levels of >10 g/dL with an adequate saturation of >90% (when P_aO_2 is >50 to 60 mmHg). Packed red blood cells may be administered to increase the oxygen-carrying capacity of the blood.

Maintenance of fluid balance

Maintenance of fluid balance is precarious in the client with ARDS. On the one hand, leaky capillaries increase lung water and cause pulmonary edema; on the other hand, the client may be volume-depleted and prone to hypotension and decreased cardiac output from mechanical ventilation and PEEP.

Generally, the client is kept "dry." The pulmonary capillary wedge pressure (which indicates the fluid status of the left side of the heart) is kept as low as possible without impairing cardiac output. The client is usually placed on mild fluid restriction and diuretics are used as necessary. The client is maintained on strict intake and output and daily weights. Electrolytes and the fluid status are monitored.

Other management considerations

The use of corticosteroids in the management of ARDS is controversial. There is no clear experimental evidence which substantiates or disproves the proposed effects of steroids. Steroid effects are believed to result mainly from decreasing pulmonary edema by stabilizing the lysosomal membranes and decreasing the amount of fibrosis after the acute phase of the illness.

Sedation is often utilized in clients with ARDS who are restless and tachypneic and who become overventilated and breathe out of phase with the ventilator. Morphine and diazepam (Valium) are frequently used. If sedatives are not sufficient to allay restlessness, paralysis of the client may be necessary. If curare or pancuronium (Pavulon) is used, small doses of opiates should be given in conjunction with the neuromuscular blocking agents. Administering opiates with the paralyzing agents will facilitate body paralysis. Providing for both mental and physical rest promotes optimal oxygenation.

ARTIFICIAL AIRWAY

An artificial airway is created by inserting a tube into the trachea which bypasses the upper airway and laryngeal structures. *Intubation* is the process of tube insertion, and *extubation* is the process of its removal. Artificial airways are required for individuals receiving mechanical ventilation. Other indications for their use include relief of airway obstruction, airway protection (e.g., after general anesthesia until the cough and other protective mechanisms return), and facilitation of secretion removal.

There are two basic types of artificial airways, *endotracheal (ET) tube* and *tracheostomy*. An ET tube may be inserted into the mouth (orotracheal) or nose (nasotracheal). The types of tubes and indications for use are discussed in Chap. 19.

Complications of Endotracheal Intubation

The major complications of endotracheal intubation are related to the pressure exerted on upper airway structures by the tube and cuff. Improper tube placement, aspiration, oral and nasal pressure sores, and accidental extubation are also potential problems. These complications will be discussed, along with preventive nursing measures.

Oral, nasal, and pharyngeal damage

Nasotracheal intubation may cause erosion and necrosis of the nasal septum and turbinates, and sinusitis by blockage of the ostia. Injury to the lips, teeth, tongue, and posterior pharynx may occur when the oral intubation route is used. Measures to prevent these complications include proper positioning and stabilization of the endotracheal tube so that it does not put pressure on the sides of the nose or mouth, as well as daily changes in the position of the oral endotracheal tube from one side of the mouth to the other. The mouth and nose should be inspected frequently for evidence of pressure areas and ulceration.

Laryngeal and tracheal damage

Laryngeal injury from endotracheal tubes and cuffs is common. Movement of the client and the tube during the ventilatory cycle contributes to laryngeal and tracheal injury. Almost half of all clients develop vocal cord congestion or a membranous glottis even when intubated for less than 24 hours.[12] The incidence of more serious laryngeal and tracheal damage increases with the duration of intubation. Ulceration of the tracheal mucosa and problems with tracheal stenosis, tracheomalacia, tracheoesophageal fistulas, and trachea-innominate bleeding have greatly decreased in incidence and severity with the use of low-pressure cuffs.

Tracheal stenosis is a stricture or narrowing of the airway caused by the healing process, resulting in scarring of the trachea. *Tracheomalacia,* a destruction or softening of the tracheal cartilages, results in collapse of the trachea during inspiration. Stenosis may occur alone, although malacia and stenosis often occur together.

Tracheomalacia may be present when increasing volumes of air are required to seal the cuff, or if there is a persistent air leak around the cuff. An increase in the cuff/tube width ratio seen on chest x-ray may also be a clue to the presence of tracheomalacia. Tracheal stenosis should be suspected if decreasing volumes of air are required to seal the endotracheal tube cuff. Tracheoesophageal fistulas may be detected or tested for by adding food coloring to tube feeding and observing for the coloring in suctioned secretions. Suctioned secretions can be tested with a dipstick for the presence of glucose. Normally, tracheal secretions should be negative for glucose.

If symptoms of laryngeal and tracheal problems occur, they usually become evident after extubation. Clients need to be observed closely for manifestations of airway obstruction after extubation, including hoarseness, cough, aspiration, swallowing difficulties, sore throat, inspiratory stridor, and respiratory distress. Usually, hoarseness, cough, and sore throat end after a period of time. If these manifestations persist, they must be investigated. An intubation tray should be kept near the client's bedside in case reintubation becomes necessary.

Laryngeal and tracheal injuries may be minimized by the following procedures:

1. Use of the smallest-diameter endotracheal tube which permits efficient ventilation
2. Use of swivel connectors and flexible tubing to connect the client's tube to the ventilator (which minimizes traction on the airway)
3. Stabilization of the airway
4. Support of the client's head and tubes when turning and avoiding undue head motion
5. Use of proper cuff inflation and low pressure cuffs

Improper tube placement and accidental extubation

Improper tube placement is another potential hazard of endotracheal intubation. It is possible for the tube to be inserted or to slip so that it extends into the right mainstem bronchus and ventilates only the right lung. Positioning of the distal tube orifice against the carina or tracheal wall may cause airway obstruction. Kinking of the endotracheal tube when the client moves the head may occur and cause airway obstruction. The use of a bite block or placement of an oral airway will prevent the client from biting on the endotracheal tube. There are also ready-made orotracheal tube holders which help to stabilize the tube.

Chest x-ray should be performed immediately after intubation or at any time if there is ever a question of tube placement so that the tube may be repositioned as needed. Chest auscultation should also be done immediately after intubation and prior to securing the tube to determine the presence of bilateral equal breath sounds. Auscultation of breath sounds is performed on a regular basis at least every 4 hours. The tube must be well secured to prevent slipping or accidental extubation. Accidental extubation can be prevented in the client who is not fully mentally alert (e.g., post anesthesia, heavily sedated) by the use of soft wrist restraints. It is wise to mark the tube with India ink at the lip or nose level, or to note the centimeter mark closest to the lip or nose level and chart it on the Kardex or flowchart. This mark provides a quick reference point to check proper tube placement.

Aspiration

Aspiration is a potential hazard since oral secretions can accumulate above the cuff; then, when the cuff is deflated, the secretions may move into the lungs. For this reason, the posterior pharynx should be suctioned prior to cuff deflation. Oral intubation increases salivation, so the mouth should be suctioned frequently. Clients themselves can use a Yankauer or tonsil suction. Other factors which may cause aspiration include cuff leak, tracheal distension, and tracheoesophageal fistula.

Tracheostomy tubes

Tracheostomy tubes are currently the preferred artificial airway for long-term intubation[*] (see Chap. 19). Upper airway damage is minimized and the client's comfort maximized. However, a recent study has shown that tracheostomy was associated with a higher incidence of complications. Problems with tracheostomy included stomal infection, stomal hemorrhage, excessive cuff pressure requirements, and subcutaneous emphysema. Follow-up studies revealed a higher prevalence of tracheal stenosis after tracheotomy than after endotracheal intubation.[13]

There is much debate on the subject of when to perform a tracheotomy in the client with an oral or nasotracheal endotracheal tube. The situation varies with the client, physician, and institution. The span of time ranges from 72 hours to 2 to 3 weeks; some institutions use endotracheal intubation in clients for up to 6 weeks without harmful sequelae. Nasotracheal intubation can usually be tolerated by the client for longer periods of time than oral intubation.

Care of the Artificial Airway

Types of cuffs

Endotracheal and tracheostomy tubes may have either hard (high-pressure, low-volume) or soft (low-pressure, high-volume) cuffs. The purpose of the cuff is to create a seal between the airway and the tube so that gas from the ventilator will go into the lung instead of escaping around the tube. A secondary purpose of the cuff is to minimize aspiration of gastric contents into the lungs.

Hard cuffs have high intracuff pressures and a narrow area of tracheal wall contact. These are used mostly for short-term intubation, usually in the operating room. Soft cuffs are made of soft, pliable material which tends to inflate evenly and conforms to the tracheal contour. Soft cuffs are also known as *low-pressure cuffs*. Lower cuff pressures are diffused over a wider area of the trachea, minimizing tracheal and laryngeal damage. Soft cuffs are preferred and are used almost exclusively today.

There are several different types of low-pressure cuffs, varying in composition and in the inflation methods used. The Kamen-Willanson foam cuff, the Lanz tube, and the Shiley PRV tubes are examples of the many types of cuffed tracheal tubes available.[14]

Cuff problems

A common problem which may occur in all cuffs inflated with air is the phenomenon of "chasing the trachea," which is seen with positive-pressure, no-leak ventilation.[15] A cuff inflated to seal during the peak inspiratory phase is overinflated during the exhalation phase. This overinflation of the cuff results in tracheal dilatation. To ensure no-leak ventilation, the cuff is reinflated with additional air, and the cycle is repeated as tracheal dilatation progresses. Tracheal dilatation may lead to esophageal compression, causing aspiration and difficulty in swallowing. This problem is prevented by the minimal occlusive volume or the minimal leak technique of cuff inflation and maintenance of intracuff pressures at <25 cmH_2O.

Another rare problem peculiar to some low-pressure cuffs is ballooning of the cuff over the tube lumen, resulting in airway obstruction. This can occur if the cuff is overinflated. If this problem is suspected, the cuff should be totally deflated, the airway patency checked, and the cuff slowly reinflated.

Cuff care

Three popular techniques recommended for cuff inflation and maintenance are (1) the minimal leak technique, (2) minimal occlusive volume, and (3) intracuff pressure measurement. The minimal leak technique and intracuff pressure measurement are frequently used in conjunction. Minimal occlusive volume and intracuff pressure measurement should be used together.

In the *minimal leak technique,* a minimal leak should be present in the cuff at the moment in the ventilatory cycle when the tracheal diameter is maximal (peak inspiration). To do this, the back of the oropharynx is first suctioned to prevent aspiration of secretions that may lodge on top of the cuff. Next, the cuff is deflated totally to prevent accidental overinflation. With the diaphragm of the stethoscope placed in the neck area (approximately where the cuff is situated), air is slowly injected into the cuff via a syringe at end-inspiration on a ventilator-delivered breath until no gurgling sounds are heard. Then enough air is withdrawn into the syringe until a slight leak is auscultated at the peak of inspiration on a ventilator-delivered breath. The nurse should record the amount of air necessary for the minimal leak and the amount of air in milliliters on the flowchart or nurse's notes at least once a day and as needed (some hospitals perform this every shift).

To obtain a *minimal occlusive volume* (MOV) in the cuff, the same procedure as above is followed except that the minimal leak procedure is left out. Air should be injected into the cuff until no gurgling is auscultated at the neck. To *measure the intracuff pressure,* the cuff port is connected via a three- or four-way stopcock to an anaeroid pressure gauge, and the pressure is read at the end of expiration. The cuff pressure should not exceed 25 cmH_2O or 18 to 20 mmHg. This is considered the maximal amount of pressure which will permit maximal capillary flow under normal blood pressure conditions.[16] The volume of air in the cuff and the intracuff pressure should be checked every day or every shift, depending upon hospital policy, and recorded on the flowchart or nurse's notes. When MOV is used, it is essential to check cuff pressures to ensure that the cuff is not overinflated, thus increasing pressure on the tracheal wall. Intracuff pressures may also be utilized to check the pressure attained in the cuff when the minimal leak technique is utilized. This ensures double protection for the airway structures.

When PEEP is utilized, MOV and intracuff pressure measurements are necessary since use of a minimal leak may allow air to escape from the lungs during end-exhalation. In addition, PEEP may be slightly decreased. Changes in head and neck position can also cause pressure and volume variations in the cuff. For these reasons, cuff pressure and volume measurements should be obtained with the client in a consistent position, preferably with the head of the bed elevated to 30°. Adjustments in cuff volume and/or pressure may have to be made with changes in the client's position.

Suctioning

Suctioning of the client's endotracheal or tracheotomy tube should be performed as needed and not just routinely (Fig. 22-7). Signs which may indicate the presence of secretions in the airways include dyspnea, increased ventilator peak inspiratory pressures, activation of the ventilator pressure alarm, noisy or gurgling respirations, coarse rales, and rhonchi. The recommended procedure for suctioning is presented in Table 22-6.

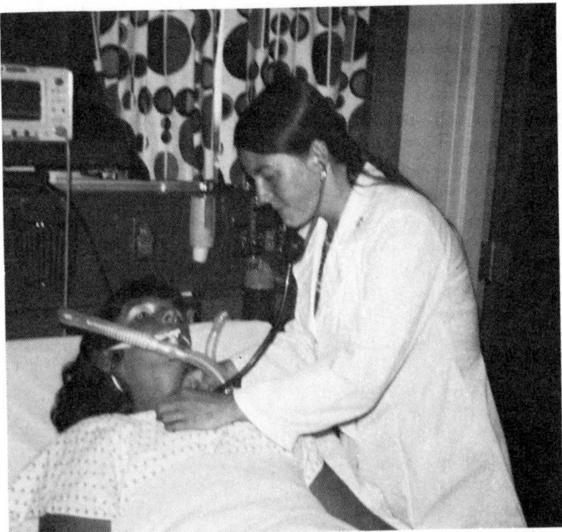

Figure 22-7 Auscultation of the lungs to detect the presence of rhonchi.

Complications associated with suctioning include hypoxemia, cardiac arrhythmias, damage to the mucosal membrane, pneumothorax, contamination and infection, retained secretions, and anxiety. Hypoxemia occurs when oxygen-enriched gas is sucked out of the lungs with the secretions and replaced by room air that enters around the catheter. Other causes of hypoxemia may be bronchospasm due to airway irritation and microatelectasis secondary to aspiration of intrapulmonary air. After 15 seconds of suctioning, P_aO_2 may be reduced by an average of 33 mmHg at 30 seconds after withdrawal of the suction catheter.[17]

Measures to prevent hypoxemia include preoxygenation and hyperinflation of the client's lungs with 100% oxygen via a bag ventilator for three to five breaths (Fig. 22-8), limiting each suction pass to 10 to 15 seconds, and returning the client to the ventilator or continuing to use the bag ventilator at the client's own respiratory rate between suctioning passes. Spontaneously breathing clients with chronic hypercarbia (e.g., COPD) should not be bag-ventilated with 100% oxygen. Instead, bag ventilators with 35 to 60% oxygen should be used, and the client should be assessed for spontaneous ventilatory activity after the suctioning procedure.

If possible, two persons should perform the suctioning procedure so that one person can use both hands to bag-ventilate the client. This is important

Table 22-6

Suctioning Procedure for a Client on a Mechanical Ventilator

1. Wash hands
2. Explain procedure, purpose, and sensations to client
3. Prepare all equipment
   A. Check negative suction pressure (usual range is between −80 and −120 mmHg)
   B. Pour sterile normal saline solution (NSS) into sterile container
   C. Turn on oxygen flow to bag ventilator to 15 L.
   D. Place bag ventilator on bed
   E. Open suction catheter and glove packages. Suction catheter should be no wider than one-half the diameter of the artificial airway

One-person method

4. Disconnect client from ventilator (instill 5–10 mL sterile NSS via needleless syringe into artificial airway during inspiration *if secretions are thick*)
5. Preoxygenate with 100% oxygen* and hyperventilate client with bag ventilator 3–5 times (this procedure should be done before and after suctioning)
6. Connect client to ventilator
7. Put on sterile glove and pick up catheter with sterile hand
8. Connect catheter to suction tubing, using sterile hand for catheter and nonsterile hand for suction tubing
9. Disconnect client from ventilator
10. Using nonsterile hand, stabilize the artificial airway and hold catheter suction regulator (at this point, client may turn head to right with chin up to attempt to place catheter in left mainstem bronchus)
11. Insert catheter gently with sterile hand, swiftly and without suction
12. When resistance is met, pull back catheter 1–2 cm without suction
13. Begin depressing suction vacuum regulator in an on-off (intermittent) fashion with nonsterile hand while rotating catheter in sterile hand between thumb and forefinger
14. Swiftly remove catheter. Each suctioning pass should not exceed 15 s
15. Rinse catheter in sterile saline between suctioning passes as necessary.
16. With nonsterile hand, reconnect client to ventilator
17. Depress manual breath or sigh button (if activated) on ventilator to hyperventilate or ventilate client†
18. Let client equilibrate for 30 s to 1 min or as needed
19. Rinse catheter with sterile NSS
20. Repeat procedure as needed
21. Place client back on ventilator
22. Suction oropharynx
23. Discard catheter
24. Hyperventilate and oxygenate for three to five breaths
25. Assess client's tolerance to suctioning

Two-person method

26. First person: Instills NSS as necessary; hyperventilates and preoxygenates before, between, and after suctions; stabilizes airway
27. Second person: Suctions as above

*Use an O_2 concentration of 60% or less for clients with chronic hypercarbia who are breathing spontaneously.

†As the nurse becomes more adept at suctioning, bag ventilation may be done with the nonsterile hand between suctioning passes. Ideally, it would be better for two persons to hyperventilate with two hands, but ideal situations do not always exist. (One nurse with one hand on the bag ventilator can generate up to 800 mL, and with two hands up to 1000 mL.)

because hyperinflation with volumes $1\frac{1}{2}$ times the tidal volume have been demonstrated to cause less hypoxemia.[18] One-handed bagging may not ensure this volume. Also, it is not satisfactory to turn the FIO_2 on the ventilator up to 1.0 (100% O_2) during the suctioning procedure, since there is a delay of 1 to 2 minutes before the ventilator actually delivers the increased concentration of 95 to 100% O_2.

During the suctioning procedure, the client must be observed for tachycardia, arrhythmias, hypertension, diaphoresis, and pallor or graying of mucous membranes. If any of these manifestations occur, the client should be bag-ventilated or placed back on the ventilator until equilibration occurs before another suction pass is attempted.

Three causes of cardiac arrhythmias during suctioning are arterial hypoxemia producing myocardial hypoxia, vagal stimulation secondary to tracheal irritation, and sympathetic nervous system stimulation due to anxiety. Specific arrhythmias that may occur include tachycardia; premature atrial, junctional, and ventricular beats; bradycardia; and possibly asystole.

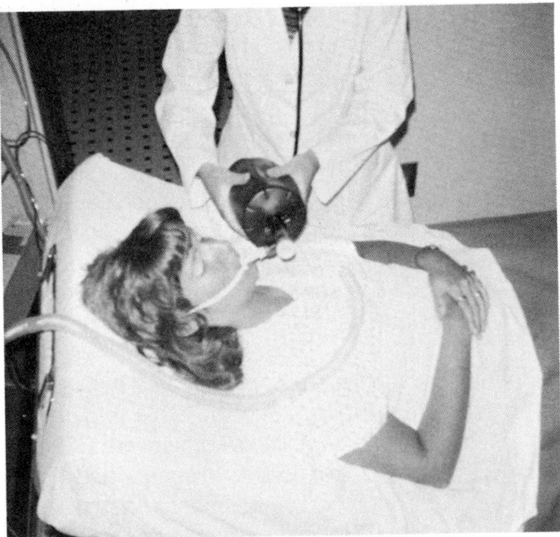

Figure 22-8 Ambu bag.

A suctioning pass should be limited to 5 to 10 seconds in clients with hypoxemia or bradycardia. Suctioning should be terminated if serious arrhythmias develop, and the client should be bag-ventilated slowly with 100% oxygen until they subside. Excessive suctioning should be avoided in clients with hypoxemia or bradycardia.

Mucosal damage to tracheal structures may occur because of excessive negative suction pressures, too vigorous insertion of the catheter, and the characteristics of the suction catheter itself. The presence of blood streaks and/or tissue shreds in aspirated mucus indicates that mucosal damage has occurred. Trauma to the mucosa can be prevented by:

1. The use of blunt or ring-tipped catheters with side holes
2. Limiting negative suction pressure to −80 to −120 mmHg
3. Insertion of the catheter without suction
4. Withdrawal of the catheter 1 to 2 cm before applying suction to prevent the catheter from adhering to the mucosa
5. Lubrication of the catheter tip with sterile saline
6. Application of intermittent suction as the catheter is removed
7. Insertion of the catheter as gently and quickly as possible
8. Stabilizing the endotracheal tube
9. Gently rotating the catheter and removing it swiftly

The client is prone to infection for a variety of reasons, including loss of upper airway protective mechanisms, disease, poor host defenses, and cross-contamination. Specific measures involved with suctioning that may help to prevent infection are frequent handwashing, use of disposable one-time fluid reservoirs and catheters, covering the end of the T piece or ventilator tubing in a catheter wrapper to limit contamination from bedclothes, use of meticulous sterile technique, and never suctioning the trachea with a catheter contaminated from the pharynx.

Pneumothorax, although rare, may occur when a client is suctioned with a large catheter inserted into a small-diameter artificial airway. There is inadequate space for air to move in or out around the catheter so that when a vacuum is applied, the lung may collapse (microatelectasis may also occur). To prevent lung collapse, the suction catheter should not occupy more than one-half of the internal diameter of the tube being suctioned, negative suction pressures should be maintained at −80 to −120 mmHg, and on-off suction pressure should be used when removing the catheter to prevent excessive buildup of negative pressure.

Secretions may be thick and difficult to suction due to inadequate hydration, inadequate humidification, or inaccessibility of the left mainstem bronchus or lower airways. Chest physiotherapy and having the client turn and cough before suctioning may help to move secretions into larger airways. Instillation of 5 to 10 mL of sterile saline into the artificial airway during inspiration will both cleanse the tube and stimulate coughing and the removal of thick secretions. Using angle-tipped or coude catheters while tilting the client's head up and to the right may increase the possibility of entering the left mainstem bronchus. Turning the client's head to the right *may* make access to the left mainstem bronchus easier if angle-tipped or coude catheters are not available.

Feelings of anxiety may arise in the client during suctioning because he feels he is unable to breathe or is choking, or because he has never been suctioned before and does not know what to expect. A simple explanation should precede each suctioning procedure. The client should be made aware that he will not be able to breathe for a short period but that he will soon be connected to O_2 and ventilated.

The client should also know that suctioning often stimulates coughing. If the client has a severe coughing spell during suctioning, bag ventilation with slow, small-volume breaths may help to alleviate his cough. Large volumes of air are not recommended because they may distend the lungs and reflexly stimulate further coughing episodes. The nurse should assume a calm, assured manner and allow the client to participate by bag-ventilating himself if possible. The client who has been placed immediately on a ventilator may need to be disconnected and bagged until the coughing spell diminishes.

Suctioning a client on PEEP greater than 10 cm H_2O must be carefully performed utilizing the hyperventilation and preoxygenation procedure which is best tolerated by the client. Hyperventilation and preoxygenation may be performed using special ventilator bags with PEEP attachments. These bags are somewhat difficult to maneuver and may require the two-person suctioning method. A special popoff port between ventilator and the artificial airway used in some institutions allows suctioning through the port. Immediate closure of the port after each suctioning pass may help to maintain PEEP and oxygenation. In the latter case, the FIO_2 may be increased to 1.0 for 2 minutes prior to suctioning if time is available. If a PEEP bag ventilator or a popoff port is not available, turning up the FIO_2 to 1.0 as mentioned previously and reconnecting the client to the ventilator (without sighing) between suctioning passes is superior to bag-ventilating the client with a non-PEEP bag. Nursing care of the client with an artificial airway is summarized in Table 22-7.

MECHANICAL VENTILATION

Mechanical ventilation is the process in which ventilation (the movement of air or oxygen-enriched air into and out of the lungs) is performed by a mechanical ventilator (Fig. 22-9). Mechanical ventilation is not a curative measure. It is a supportive technique that assists in ventilating the client while medical and nursing treatments enable recovery of the underlying disease process. For a summary of general guidelines on the need for mechanical ventilation, refer to Table 22-9.

Mechanical ventilation is not indicated in cases in which disease reversibility is not possible (e.g., end-stage respiratory failure in clients with severe COPD). Clients with chronic pulmonary disease and their families who are managed by pulmonary health care specialists on a continuous, long-term basis frequently have the opportunity to decide the issue of mechanical ventilation long before terminal respiratory disease develops. Other clients with chronic disease never discuss the subject, and the decision to use mechanical ventilation must be made by the physician and

Table 22-7

Nursing Care Plan for the Client with an Artificial Airway*

Client Problem	Expected Outcome	Nursing Intervention
Increased accumulation of secretions in the lungs	Lungs clear to auscultation. Secretions thin and easily removed.	Use effective suctioning technique (Table 22-6). Observe for blood streaks or tissue particles in suctioning aspirate. Suction only as needed, not routinely. Use blunt ring-tipped catheters. Use catheter with a diameter less than one-half of the tube diameter. Use negative suction pressure of −80 to −120 mmHg. Use modified postural drainage, vibration, and percussion maneuvers (when not contraindicated), concentrating on lung areas with evidence of infiltration or atelectasis (see Chap. 21). Change the client's position every 2 h as tolerated. Suction prior to position change if clinical signs warrant. Keep ventilator tubing cleared of all H_2O that condenses. Empty ventilator tubings prior to client position changes and prn. (Assess need for other measures to facilitate secretion mobilization.) Instill 5–10 mL sterile saline via needleless syringe if secretions are thick. Administer ultrasonic nebulization and aerosolized bronchodilators (if indicated).
Increased risk of respiratory infection	No evidence of infection. Negative sputum cultures.	Observe sputum for viscosity, quantity, color, and odor. Obtain sputum culture and do sensitivity test if secretions become purulent or tenacious, change color, or become odorous. Make sure that ventilator tubing is changed at least every 24–48 h. Periodically clean and change bedside bag ventilator and tubing. Observe for clinical signs of acute infection (such as fever, tachycardia, flushing of skin, elevated WBC, worsening of arterial blood gases, chest x-ray evidence of infection, increased rales or rhonchi, and decreased lung compliance.)
Drying of respiratory mucous membranes	Intact, moist mucous membranes.	Check temperature on the ventilator thermostat or feel the temperature of the ventilator gas with the hand to ensure that adequate humidity and warmth are being applied via a mechanical ventilator or O_2 source. Check cascade H_2O level on ventilator. Discard water in cascade prior to refilling with distilled H_2O.

Table 22-7 (Continued)

Client Problem	Expected Outcome	Nursing Intervention
Possible aspiration of gastric secretions	No aspiration. No evidence of gastric contents in tracheal aspirate.	Suction posterior pharynx and mouth prior to cuff deflation. Elevate head of bed and inflate cuff during tube feedings. Check for aspiration of tube feeding by observing consistency of suctioned tracheal aspirate. Add food coloring to feedings to make identification easier. Test secretions with dipstick for glucose. If positive, aspiration or regurgitation may have occurred. If client is eating, encourage anteflexion of the head to open the esophagus wide. Keep cuff inflated and elevate head of bed while client is eating. Insert nasogastric tube if client feels nauseated and is apt to vomit. Position client in side-lying position (never flat on back) if danger of aspiration is high.
Possible upper airway damage secondary to cuffed tube	Maintenance of normal integrity of upper airway structures.	Use smallest-diameter endotracheal tube that will support effective ventilation. Use only low-pressure cuffs for intubation. Use minimal leak or MOV technique and cuff pressures of <15–18 mmHg (or <25 cmH_2O). Stabilize tube, tubing, and client's head when turning. Limit client's head movements. Use a swivel adapter connection between client and ventilator. Provide frequent care of mouth and nares. Inspect nares with flashlight and sides of mouth around oral endotracheal tube for areas of pressure or ulceration. Change positions of oral endotracheal tube at least once a day. Secure tube firmly with tape, tube holder, or umbilical tape. Monitor chest x-ray results by assessing for tracheal size and relationship to tube. Observe for clinical signs of aspiration. Record the amount of air and pressure in the cuff every 8–24 h. Assess for cuff leak (e.g., hissing or gurgling sounds at mouth, decreased tidal volume). Immediately after extubation, monitor client closely for signs of respiratory distress secondary to laryngeal edema (e.g., inspiratory stridor). Assess client for hoarseness, sore throat, cough, and swallowing difficulties post extubation.
Tube position problems Right mainstem intubation Accidental extubation Mechanical obstruction	Proper alignment of tube. No accidental extubation.	Use a bite block or oral airway if client bites on tube. Stabilize and secure tube. Move client with care if connected to ventilator. Support client's head and airway. Mark the tube with India ink or indelible marker at lip or nose insertion point. Support long tube that protrudes from insertion point. Use rolled towel or sheet. Cut off excess endotracheal tube once tube is in correct position. Make sure to note on chart that tube has been cut. Auscultate breath sounds immediately after intubation and every 4 h. Make sure that chest x-ray is done immediately after intubation and whenever there is a serious question of tube position. If there is any question of mechanical obstruction, place client in sniffing position (hyperextend the head) and attempt to pass catheter. If catheter will not pass, deflate cuff totally and try again. Oxygenate and ventilate client after cuff has been slowly reinflated.
Inability to speak	Effective method of communication.	Provide client with paper and pencil, magic slate, alphabet board, or talking tracheotomy tubes. Use therapeutic touch. Learn to read client's body language, facial expression, and signals. Attempt to anticipate client's needs. Provide call light or bell that is easily accessible. Explain the temporary nature of this problem.
Inability to eat (client with oral or nasopharyngeal tube)	Maintenance of optimal nutrition.	Consult with physician regarding dietary needs if client has been without food for 3–5 days and is expected to remain intubated. Weigh client daily. Remember that fever, work of breathing, pain, and anxiety increase caloric needs. Institute total parenteral nutrition (Chap. 33) or tube feedings as ordered. Clients with tracheostomy can eat. Clients with nasotracheal tube may take liquid and semiliquid feedings with care but usually need more complete nutrition. Monitor client's response to feedings. Monitor serum albumin, hemoglobin, and daily weights.

*The nursing care for a client with a tracheostomy is presented in Table 19-11.

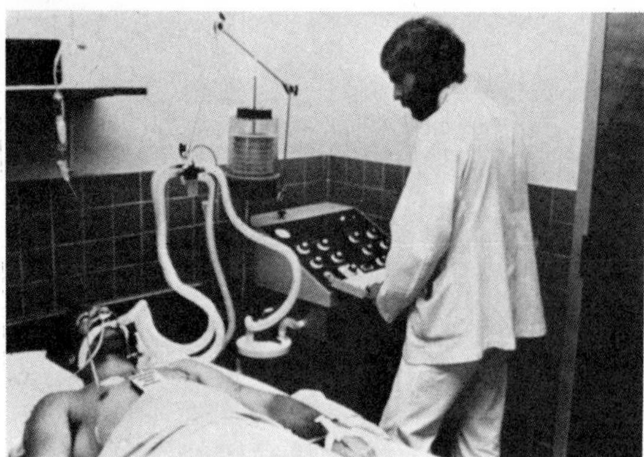

Figure 22-9 Client being ventilated using a Bennett MA ventilator.

family at the onset of clinical deterioration. It is much easier for the physician and family to decide not to institute ventilatory support initially than it is to remove the support system once it has been initiated. Therefore, the decision to use mechanical ventilation must be made very carefully.

Types of Mechanical Ventilators

Mechanical ventilators are divided into two major categories: negative- and positive-pressure ventilators.

Negative-pressure ventilators

Negative-pressure ventilators are chambers that encase the chest or body and produce a subatmospheric or negative pressure around it. The negative pressure surrounding the chest wall causes the chest wall to be pulled outward. This reduces intrathoracic pressure and causes air to rush in through the upper airway, which is outside the sealed chamber. Expiration is passive, since the machine cycles off and allows the chest to relax. This type of ventilation is similar to the normal mode of ventilation, since inspiration is normally produced by decreasing the pleural and intrathoracic pressures and since expiration is normally passive.

The iron lung formerly used in some persons with poliomyelitis is an example of a negative-pressure ventilator. A newer type of negative-pressure ventilator is the *chest cuirass.* It is more portable than the iron lung and is used today for long-term ventilatory support of some clients with neuromuscular disease. Negative-pressure ventilators are not satisfactory for use in acutely ill clients. The ventilators are bulky, observation of the client is limited, and the negative intrapleural pressure must not be interrupted.

Positive-pressure ventilators

Positive-pressure ventilation is the primary method of mechanical ventilation used in acutely ill clients. The inspiratory cycle of ventilation is accomplished when the ventilator forces air into the lungs under positive pressure. Intrathoracic pressure is raised by the inflation of the lungs with positive pressure rather than lowered, as it is normally on inspiration. Expiration occurs by passive relaxation of the diaphragm, just as in normal expiration. Positive pressure can also be added to the lungs during expiration. This is discussed in detail later.

The three types of positive-pressure ventilators are (1) time-cycled or -limited, (2) pressure-cycled or -limited, and (3) volume-cycled or -limited. Each type is classified by the physical parameter that ends the inspiratory cycle.

Time-Cycled or -Limited Ventilators Time-cycled or -limited ventilators terminate inspiration and switch to expiration at a definite preset time. The tidal volume is regulated by adjusting the length of inspiration and the flow rate of the pressurized gas. The tidal volume and inspiratory pressure delivered to the client may vary somewhat from one breath to the next. Time-cycled ventilators such as the Baby Bird, Air Shields, and Veriflo CV 200 are used primarily for neonates and infants. The Emerson postoperative ventilator, Emerson IMV, Engstrom ER 500, Engstrom ECS 2000, and Veriflo CV 2000 are time-cycled ventilators used for adults. Time-cycled ventilators also have fail-safe pressure limits beyond which the ventilator ceases to push gas into the lungs.

Pressure-Cycled or -Limited Ventilators Pressure-cycled or -limited ventilators terminate the inspiratory phase or the tidal volume delivered to the client when a preselected airway pressure is achieved. The volume of gas delivered to the client and the duration of delivery will vary according to airway resistance, pulmonary compliance, and integrity of the ventilator circuit. For instance, increased resistance (pressure) in the airway secondary to secretions or decreased chest compliance will cause the pressure-limited ventilator to cease delivering gas before an adequate volume is reached. In addition, unless each breath delivered to the client is measured, there is no way to know the exact gas volume delivered.

Pressure-limited ventilators usually lack a system to deliver precisely controlled levels of oxygen and a means for administering PEEP. Pressure-cycled ventilators are not utilized as frequently as time- or volume-cycled ventilators for acutely ill clients. They are used predominantly for intermittent positive-pressure breathing (IPPB) treatments, home therapy, short-term ventilation, or in a client whose lungs are relatively free of resistance and compliance disease. Examples of pressure-cycled ventilators are the Bennett PR-1 and PR-2 and the Bird Mark 7. These may be used with a mask, mouthpiece, or artificial airway.

Volume-Cycled or -Limited Ventilators The most popular mechanical ventilators for intubated adults and older children are the volume-cycled or -limited ventilators. Volume-cycled ventilators terminate the inspiratory phase or flow of gas into the lung when a designated, preset volume of gas is delivered into the ventilator circuit (e.g., after the client has received the inspiratory gas). Volume-cycled ventilators also have built-in pressure-limiting valves which prevent excessive pressure from building up in the lung so that the preset volume is achieved. Once the pressure limit is reached, the remainder of the tidal volume is vented to the air.

The major advantages of volume-cycled ventilators are that a readily measurable volume of gas is delivered to the client, volume delivery remains constant despite resistance and compliance changes in the lung (unlike the situation with pressure-cycled ventilators), and a consistent inspired oxygen concentration can easily be maintained. The disadvantages are that these ventilators are often bulky and expensive and may provide excessive intrathoracic and airway pressures. Examples of volume-cycled ventilators are the Bennett MA I, Bennett MA II, Bournes Bear I, Ohio 560, Monaghan 225, Foregger 210 (Fig. 22-10), Searle, and Sieman Servo 900. Some ventilators, such as the Monoghan 225, can be adapted to function as pressure-, time-, or volume-cycled.

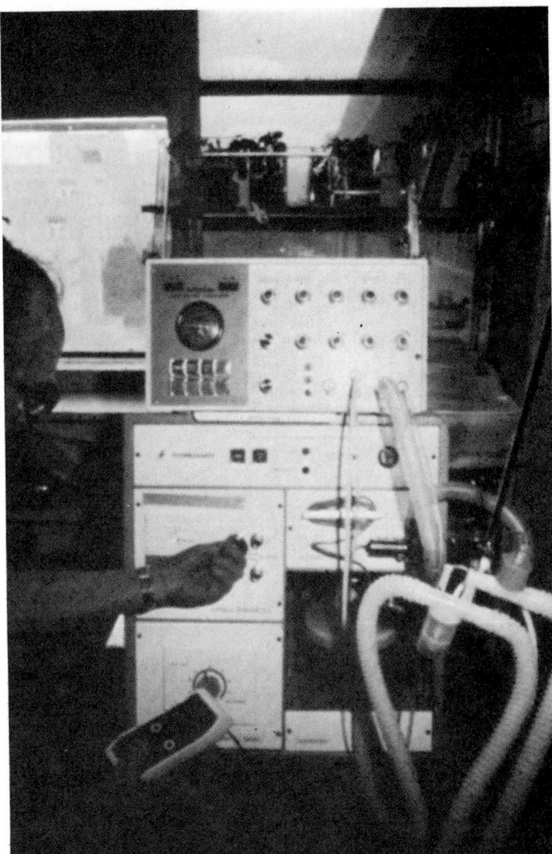

Figure 22-10 Foregger volume ventilator.

Settings of Mechanical Ventilators

The various functions and settings of the mechanical ventilator are discussed in this section. These settings are chosen by the physician after carefully evaluating the client's status (e.g., arterial blood gases, body weight, level of consciousness) and after consulting with the respiratory therapist and nurse who are caring for the client. The mechanical ventilator must be as finely tuned as possible to the client's ventilatory pattern. Therefore, the settings must be frequently evaluated and adjusted until the client achieves optimal ventilation.

Tidal volume

The *tidal volume* is the amount of air exchanged with each ventilator-delivered breath. The amount of tidal volume delivered to the client varies with the institution and the physician. Generally, the appropriate tidal volume is estimated as 10 to 15 mL per kilogram of the client's body weight. For clients of average weight, the tidal volume is usually 500 to 1000 mL.

Respiratory rate

The *respiratory rate* is the number of breaths per minute the ventilator delivers to the client. This depends upon the mode of ventilation [e.g., control, assist-control, or intermittent mandatory ventilation, (IMV)]. Usually, the rate is set in the different modes to keep the client's pH and P_aCO_2 within the normal range. The respiratory rate can vary from as low as 1 breath per minute (when the client is on IMV) to 20 to 30 breaths per minute.

Inspiratory expiratory ratio

The *inspiratory-expiratory (I/E) ratio* is the ratio of the time involved in inspiration to the time in expiration.

Normally, during spontaneous breathing, expiration takes about twice as long as inspiration. Ventilators can be set to maintain this ratio by controlling the rate of gas flow into the lungs during inspiration. The I/E ratio on the ventilator is usually set at $1\frac{1}{2}$ or 1:2.

Fraction of inspired oxygen

The *fraction of inspired oxygen* (FIO_2) will vary with the client's arterial blood gases. It can range from 0.21 (ambient air) to 1.00 (100% oxygen). The FIO_2 is analyzed frequently by the respiratory therapist to determine if the ventilator is acutally delivering the FIO_2 at which it is set. Many new ventilators have on-line oxygen analyzers with a digital display.

System pressure gauge

The volume-cycled ventilator also has a *system pressure gauge*. This is a dial which fluctuates with the pressure in the client's airway during the ventilatory cycle. The dial is similar to a clock; it is round and has increments of pressure measured in centimeters of water. The zero point corresponds to atmospheric pressure in the airways. During a ventilator inspiration, a stylus moves to the positive or left side of the dial, indicating the pressure at which the preset volume of gas is delivered. This is the amount of positive pressure in the airways at maximal inspiration (maximal inspiratory pressure or peak airway pressure). During exhalation, the stylus returns to zero if no positive pressure is applied to the airway at end-exhalation (PEEP). If positive pressure is applied during end-exhalation, the stylus falls only to that point above zero. For example, with 10-cm PEEP, the stylus falls to 10 cm above the zero point, but as inspiration begins, the stylus may dip down 1 or 2 cm as the client initiates his next inspiration. When the client attempts to breathe spontaneously without PEEP, his negative inspiratory effort registers as a swing of the stylus past zero to the negative side of the dial.

The system pressure gauge is important because it reflects the pressure and volume characteristics of the lung. If during peak inspiration the pressure stylus is 40 cmH_2O or greater, this indicates that a lot of pressure is required to push gas into the lungs. Therefore, the lungs have decreased compliance or are stiff, such as in ARDS or acute asthma. If the pressure stylus reaches only 5 to 10 cm on peak inspiration, this indicates that it is relatively easy for the lungs to become inflated and the lungs are probably very compliant, such as in emphysema. In other words, lung compliance is inversely related to peak inspiratory pressures. As lung compliance decreases, peak inspiratory pressures increase; as lung compliance increases, peak inspiratory pressures decrease.

Pressure limit dial

Volume-cycled ventilators also have a *pressure limit dial* which is separate from the system pressure gauge. The pressure limit dial is set at about 10 cm of H_2O pressure above the pressure needed to deliver the desired tidal volume. The pressure alarm will be activated if this pressure is reached. Conditions which may cause the pressure alarm to sound include resisting the machine, coughing, secretion accumulation, occlusion of the endotracheal or tracheotomy tube, decreased lung compliance, and/or the development of a pneumothorax. The low-pressure alarm sounds if pressure in the system drops. This may occur with disconnection from the client or gas source or disconnection of tubing within the machine.

Sighs

Because *sighs* are larger than normal breaths, they inflate more alveoli and help to prevent atelectasis. Normally, we all sigh periodically. Most volume-cycled ventilators can be set to deliver sighs at a preset rate and volume (usually 200 to 300 mL greater than the tidal volume). Sighing is generally not used when large tidal volumes or PEEP are utilized since these maneuvers also serve to increase lung inflation and prevent atelectasis.

Spirometer

The *spirometer* is an instrument which measures the expired tidal volume. Some ventilators have spirometers which are readily visible as a bellowlike container (e.g., MA I), whereas others are built within the machine (Foregger, Bournes Bear I). Tidal volume and/or minute volume can be easily read from the spirometer. When the client receives a ventilator breath, it is important to check whether the exhaled tidal volume is equal to the amount set on the ventilator. Usually, there is some small loss of volume with each breath due to dissipation in the tubing.

A spirometer alarm sounds when the exhaled tidal volume is less than the volume present on the spirometer. Conditions which can cause the spirometer alarm to be activated are (1) spirometer malfunction, such as sticking of the bellows or blockage of movement of the bellows by pushing against the volume stick (particularly in the MA I), (2) disconnection or leakage of tubing within the ventilator system, and (3) disconnection of the ventilator from the client. A large air leak in the cuff of the endotracheal or tracheostomy tube can allow gas to escape into the upper airway, causing a decrease in the tidal volume of gas returned to the spirometer. It is especially important to ensure that all ventilator alarms are turned on at all times. Alarms can alert the nurse and respiratory therapist to potentially dangerous situations of mechanical malfunction or client asynchrony with the ventilator. On many ventilators, the alarms can be temporarily bypassed or silenced for up to 2 minutes for suctioning. After that period of time, the alarm system automatically becomes functional again.

Sensitivity

Sensitivity is also a setting on most ventilators. It is discussed in the section on Assist-Control Ventilation.

Modes of Volume-Cycled Ventilation

There are a number of modes in which the volume-cycled ventilator may be set to operate (Fig. 22-11). *Mode* refers to the manner in which the ventilator delivers breaths to the client. The mode chosen usually depends upon current institutional practice. Another factor influencing the choice of mode is the ventilatory status of the client, as evidenced by his respiratory drive and pattern and arterial blood gas analysis. The three basic modes of mechanical ventilation are (1) controlled ventilation, (2) assist-control ventilation, and (3) IMV.

Controlled mechanical ventilation

In *controlled ventilation,* the client has no active role in the ventilatory cycle. The machine initiates inspiration, provides the power for it, and determines the rate of ventilation and the depth of the tidal volume. The client is totally passive and does none of the work of breathing. The mechanical ventilator's sensitivity is not tuned to the client's respiratory effort. Controlled ventilation is used in clients who are unable to breathe for themselves, such as those with neuromuscular disease or high cervical-spinal cord injuries, and in clients who are heavily sedated or have been paralyzed with drugs such as pancuronium (Pavulon) or tubocurarine (curare) in order to help them tolerate mechanical ventilation.

The major disadvantages of controlled ventilation are that it does not allow the client to initiate any breaths, does not allow the respiratory rate to change with changing client needs, and prevents respiratory system compensation for metabolic pH imbalances. Clients on controlled ventilation who are not apneic usually require some type of sedation or paralyzing agent. In addition, because the airway pressure is always positive during inspiration, the effects of positive intrathoracic pressure must be assessed in relation to compromising venous return and decreasing cardiac output.

Assist-control ventilation

In the *assist-control* mode of ventilation, both the mechanical ventilator and the client play an active role. The sensitivity dial of the mechanical ventilator is set so that the machine is sensitive to the negative pressure pull or inspiratory efforts of the client. This contrasts to controlled ventilation, in which the sensitivity dial is turned almost completely off. The client on assist-control ventilation is able to initiate active breathing. Once breathing begins, the ventilator cycles in and provides the preset flow and tidal volume of gas to complete inspiration. Should the client fail to initiate active breathing, the ventilator cycles in as it would in controlled ventilation.

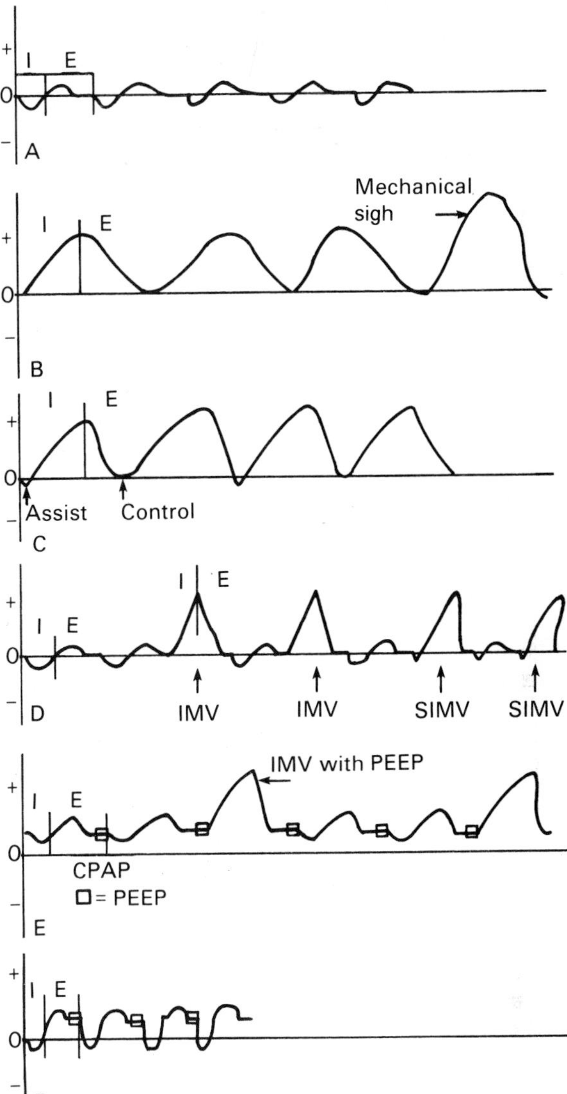

Figure 22-11 Airway pressures with the use of different ventilatory modes.

The sensitivity of the machine can be regulated so that the client can initiate active breathing. A high sensitivity setting indicates that the machine is extremely sensitive to any attempt by the client to inspire, and the client can initiate inspiration with a minimal amount of effort. If the sensitivity setting is too high, the client can easily be overventilated and become alkalotic. A low sensitivity setting means that the machine is not as sensitive to the client's inspiratory effort, and the client must work harder (i.e., pull more negative pressure) to "trigger" the machine. The sensitivity must be carefully calibrated to the client's level of inspiratory pull and drive to prevent problems of over- and underventilation. Usually, the sensitivity should be set so that if the client exerts approximately 2 cm of negative inspiratory pressure, the machine will deliver a breath.

The advantages of assist-control ventilation are that the client can initiate his own breathing and thereby use his own inspiratory muscles. In addition, the client can alter his ventilations according to need. Because the client initiates the ventilatory cycle, intrathoracic pressure decreases transiently prior to the mechanical inspiratory phase so that venous return and cardiac output are enhanced.

The disadvantages of assist-control ventilation are the problems of over and underventilation. These effects occur primarily in extremely anxious clients or clients with low lung compliance.

Intermittent mandatory ventilation (IMV)

When the *IMV* mode is used, the client breathes spontaneously at his own tidal volume and rate for the majority of the time. At a preset frequency, the ventilator will deliver a specific volume under positive pressure. On IMV, the ventilator breaths are not synchronized to the client's own respiratory pattern. A machine breath can be given during the client's exhalation or peak inhalation.

Synchronized IMV (SIMV) or intermittent demand ventilation (IDV) is available on some recently manufactured ventilators. On SIMV or IDV, the ventilator is synchronized to the client's own ventilatory rate. The machine is set to give a certain number of breaths and is triggered by the client's inspiration so that the breath is delivered as the client is normally inhaling. SIMV is theoretically safer since it eliminates the possibility that the ventilator could initiate a mandatory inspiration just at the peak of spontaneous inspiration and overdistend the lung as well as disrupt the regularity and ease of breathing. The major difference between IMV and assisted ventilation is that with assisted ventilation the client only starts the breath and the ventilator then delivers the tidal volume. With IMV, the client independently determines the tidal volume of each spontaneous breath.

IMV is now the primary mode of ventilatory support in most centers. It is utilized both to provide continuous ventilation and to wean the client from the ventilator. The advantages of IMV are numerous. It allows the maintenance of even minor spontaneous respiratory excursions. The client's ventilatory muscles remain in use. However, since his efforts may be inadequate for efficient alveolar ventilation, the ventilator breaths provide it. The client is not forced to submit to a pattern of ventilation controlled by the ventilator. Instead, the ventilator augments the client's own ventilatory effort to the degree necessary. Ventilator breaths can be titrated to adjust alveolar minute ventilation levels to normal and thereby decrease the incidence of respiratory alkalosis. Because of the spontaneous breaths during IMV, it is possible to achieve normal alveolar ventilation, avoid respiratory alkalemia, and maintain normal arterial pH more easily than with controlled or assisted ventilation.[19]

There are major differences between the cardiopulmonary effects of IMV and those of controlled or assisted ventilation. Spontaneous inspiration decreases intrathoracic pressure, reduces mean intrathoracic pressure, and enhances venous return. Cardiac output and venous return are more normal than with the other modes of mechanical ventilation. Therefore, higher levels of PEEP may be utilized than with assisted or controlled ventilation.[20]

Weaning the client from the ventilator can be accomplished in a way that seems more physiologically sound. Instead of abruptly removing the client from the ventilator and letting him breathe totally on his own, IMV may be utilized. IMV allows a smooth transition from controlled to spontaneous ventilation by gradually decreasing the IMV or ventilator rate as the client assumes an increasing percentage of the total work of breathing.

The disadvantages of IMV are not as great as the advantages. One disadvantage occurs when the client on a very low IMV rate (receiving one to four breaths per minute) ceases active, spontaneous breathing. In this situation, ventilation will not be adequately supported. IMV at low rates should be utilized only in clients who have regular, spontaneous breathing. Weaning with or without IMV demands close clinical assessment of the client. Weaning with IMV may take a longer time as each IMV breath is gradually removed. Another disadvantage of IMV is that during weaning from mechanical ventilation, clients are often left at low IMV rates rather than being rested, and they often become overly fatigued. (This is a concern for the client especially during the night.)

Some mechanical ventilators are not equipped to deliver IMV. Often, parallel circuits and other "homemade" devices are utilized. However, improper assembly of the circuitry is possible. Reservoir bags providing gas for the client's spontaneous ventilation must be fully inflated and remain inflated despite the client's inspiratory flow rates. The concentration of oxygen in the ventilator and the circuitry from which the client takes his spontaneous breaths should be the same. As more and more ventilators have IMV systems incorporated into them this problem will decline.

The delivery of an IMV breath from the ventilator just as the client finishes spontaneous inspiration may lead to overdistension of the lung. It is debatable whether this concern is justified in light of the sigh mechanism on many mechanical ventilators, which attempts to achieve this purpose. SIMV or IDV eliminates this problem.

Other Ventilatory Maneuvers

Positive end-expiratory pressure (PEEP)

PEEP is a ventilatory maneuver in which positive pressure is applied to the client's airway at end-exhalation. Normally, expiration is passive, and the airway pressure on the ventilator system pressure dial would drop to zero. With PEEP, the pressure falls only to the level of positive pressure which is left to expand the lungs at end-exhalation.

The lungs are partially inflated even during end-exhalation. Therefore, PEEP increases the functional residual capacity (FRC), or the amount of gas in the lung after normal exhalation, helps reinflate collapsed alveoli, and consequently improves oxygenation of the client. PEEP allows the FIO_2 to be reduced to less than 0.50, which prevents the hazard of oxygen toxicity. As an example of how PEEP works, a client may need an FIO_2 of 0.7 to maintain a P_aO_2 of 60 mmHg. With a PEEP of 5 to 10 cmH_2O, the FIO_2 can be reduced to 0.5 while a P_aO_2 of 60 mmHg is maintained.

Since PEEP is a unit of pressure, it is measured in centimeters of water. PEEP is prescribed in increments of 2.5 to 5.0 cmH_2O. Levels as high as 60 cm of PEEP have been used. PEEP greater than 20 cm is frequently called *Super-PEEP*, Currently, 5 cm of PEEP is often used prophylactically in many critically ill clients on ventilators to prevent atelectasis. The term *physiologic PEEP* is currently in vogue. According to this concept, 5 cm of PEEP in the intubated client will replace the glottic mechanism and help to maintain a normal FRC. Clinical studies vary as to the benefits of physiologic PEEP.

PEEP of 5 cmH_2O is also utilized for clients who have a history of alveolar collapse during weaning. PEEP has demonstrated an improvement in gas exchange, vital capacity, and inspiratory force when used during weaning.[21]

When PEEP is used during mechanical ventilation, the maximal inspiratory pressure increases in relation to the amount of PEEP added. For example, if a client is receiving a ventilator breath, and his maximal inspiratory pressure recorded on the ventilator pressure gauge is 30 cmH_2O and the expiratory pressure is zero, then when 10 cm of PEEP is added, the client's maximal inspiratory pressure will be 40 cm H_2O and his end-expiratory pressure will be 10 cm H_2O. Thus, the level of positive pressure achieved during mechanical ventilation with PEEP is often quite high. When PEEP is applied during controlled or assist-control ventilation, the term *continuous positive-pressure ventilation (CPPV)* may be utilized. Ventilator terminology is confusing and usually varies from institution to institution. If one understands the basic concepts of the different modes and maneuvers of ventilatory assistance, then it becomes easy to apply the terms used by the individual institution.

The use of IMV with PEEP is now the preferred method to administer PEEP. The decreased mean airway pressure which occurs during spontaneous breathing is enough to prevent some of the adverse effects produced by the increased pressures.

In general, it is believed that the major purpose of PEEP is to maintain adequate tissue oxygenation and gas exchange while trying to prevent oxygen toxicity. Its secondary role in the prevention of atelectasis is also important. Some practitioners think that PEEP may assist in healing damaged lungs by maintaining airway stability and accelerating the production of surfactant. This belief is not yet supported in clinical studies.

PEEP is indicated in lungs which are characterized by diffuse disease, severe hypoxemia unresponsive to FIO_2 greater than 0.5, and loss of compliance or stiffness. The classic example of indications for PEEP therapy is in ARDS. (This syndrome was discussed earlier in the chapter.)

PEEP is generally contraindicated or must be used with extreme caution in clients with highly compliant lungs, unilateral or nonuniform disease, hypovolemia, and low cardiac output. In these situations, the adverse effects of PEEP may outweigh any benefits obtained.

Continuous Positive Airway Pressure (CPAP)

CPAP is the use of PEEP in a client who is breathing spontaneously. With CPAP, there is a constant flow of gas at a rate that is greater than the client's spontaneous inspiratory flow rate. Therefore, the client's airway pressure never falls to zero, and there is always some degree of positive pressure (perhaps 1 to 2 cm during inspiration) on the airway at all times. For example, if CPAP of 5 cm is applied to the client's airway at end-exhalation, when the client inspires, he pulls 1 to 2 cmH_2O down from the 5 cm CPAP to inhale. At exhalation, the airway pressure is 5 cmH_2O. The client who is receiving IMV with PEEP receives CPAP when breathing spontaneously. In the past, the client receiving CPAP was usually an infant, but currently CPAP is being utilized more and more in adults. CPAP can be administered via a tight-fitting mask, or an endotracheal or tracheal tube. The latter two methods are preferred. One problem associated with CPAP in adults is that unless the person can cooperate (and not fight and attempt to exhale his air down to atmospheric pressure), the work of breathing may be increased.[22]

Expiratory Positive Airway Pressure (EPAP) EPAP is PEEP applied during spontaneous ventilation without the high flow of gas that occurs during the entire cycle. Airway pressures are required to fall below atmospheric pressure before inspiratory gas flow can occur. EPAP is not used as frequently as CPAP. One reason may be the increased work of breathing (greater than with CPAP) that occurs. Clients who have excellent ventilatory reserve but who also have hypovolemia seem to tolerate EPAP better than CPAP. This increased toleration of EPAP is due to the absence of positive airway pressure during inspiration, which leaves venous return uncompromised.[23]

Adverse Effects of Mechanical Ventilation

Although mechanical ventilation may improve the client's alveolar ventilation and oxygenation, it can also cause adverse effects. In this section, these effects are summarized according to the body system involved. Other general effects of mechanical ventilation are also discussed. The nursing measures related to these problems are presented in Table 22-8.

Table 22-8
Nursing Care Plan for the Client on Mechanical Ventilation*

Client Problem†	Expected Outcome	Nursing Intervention
Decreased cardiac output	Blood pressure and cardiac output within client's normal range.	Monitor vital signs every 2–4 h. Observe for clinical manifestations of decreased cardiac output (e.g., restlessness, decreasing levels of consciousness, low urine output, weak peripheral pulses, narrowed pulse pressure, slow capillary refill, pallor, fatigue, and chest pain). Monitor direct measurement of cardiac output via thermodilution, $P_{\bar{v}}O_2$, or $(A-V)O_2$ difference when >10 cm PEEP is utilized. Administer plasma expanders and vasopressors as ordered.
Fluid overload	No signs of peripheral or pulmonary edema.	Maintain strict intake and output. Take into account the blockage of insensible H_2O loss via respiration and the closed humidification system of the mechanical ventilator when considering accurate intake and output. Weigh client daily. Observe for clinical manifestations of fluid overload (such as weight gain or failure to lose weight if the only nutrition is maintenance intravenous solutions), hemodilution (low hematocrit, low serum sodium), edema, and rales. Take readings of PCWP, PAS, and PAD at end-exhalation while client is on the ventilator, preferably via a strip chart recorder or from the waveform.
Pneumothorax or pneumomediastinum	Normal breath sounds auscultated for both lungs.	Observe for manifestations of pneumothorax (see text). If not already done, an upright chest x-ray should be performed. Observe for symptoms of tension pneumothorax (see text). Bag-ventilate with O_2 source or use lower tidal volume. Notify physician and set up for chest tube insertion as soon as possible. Check ventilator settings at every shift. Record the level of peak inspiratory pressure to establish a baseline from which to tell if changes in lung compliance are occurring. (This assessment is especially important in clients on PEEP, since they are more prone to pneumothorax.)

Table 22-8 (Continued)

Client Problem	Expected Outcome	Nursing Intervention
Mechanical underventilation (alveolar hypoventilation)	Arterial blood gases within normal range for client. Breath sounds normal in both lungs.	Use large tidal volumes (15 mL/kg). Change client's position every 2 h. Client with unilateral lung disease should be positioned for only a limited amount of time with the diseased side down. Rotate frequently from good side to back. Suction as indicated. Use chest physiotherapy to areas of the lung with increased secretions. Have client cough and deep-breathe every 2 h. Monitor arterial blood gases. Check cuff for leaks. Auscultate breath sounds every 2–4 h. Monitor weaning of client carefully. Observe for symptoms of increased P_aCO_2 (e.g., somnolence, lethargy, tachycardia, confusion, headache).
Mechanical overventilation (alveolar hyperventilation)	Arterial blood gases within normal range for client. Maintenance of pH in the range 7.35–7.45.	Begin mechanical ventilation slowly (especially in clients with COPD) so that drastic falls in P_aCO_2 causing alkalemia do not occur. P_aCO_2 should be lowered only to client's baseline level. Monitor acid-base status, arterial blood gases, $P_{\bar{v}}O_2$, and $D(A-a)O_2$. Arterial blood gases should be drawn approximately 20 min after each ventilator setting change, serially thereafter, and whenever there are changes in client's clinical status. Assess client for other possible causes of hyperventilation (e.g., retained secretions, hypoxemia, pain, fear, and anxiety). Check tidal volume (may be too high), O_2 flow rate (may be too low), respiratory rate (may be too high), and I/E ratio. Clients who are fighting the ventilator may be slowly bag-ventilated for three to six breaths to help synchronize them with the ventilator. Determine cause of asynchrony. Try verbally coaching the client to breathe with the ventilator. Sedation (with morphine or diazepam) may be necessary if pain or anxiety is identified as the cause. Observe client for complications of alkalemia (e.g., hypokalemia, cardiac arrhythmias, poor tissue oxygenation, neuromuscular irritability, seizures, and coma). Administer potassium and bicarbonate supplements as ordered. Client on PEEP should not be pulling subatmospheric or negative airway pressures on inspiration. Sedate as tolerated and ordered.
Pulmonary infection	See Tables 20-2 and 22-6.	
Gastrointestinal problems Stress ulcer Gastric distension Gastrointestinal bleeding Ileus	Maintenance of gastrointestinal integrity. Normal bowel sounds. No evidence of gastrointestinal bleeding.	Take daily measurements of abdominal girth at the umbilicus. Assess for abdominal distension, tympany, and bowel sounds. Test stools and gastric drainage for occult blood. Assess client's complaints of pain, fullness, bloated feeling, or need for a laxative. Maintain adequate bowel evacuation program. Monitor hematocrit. Check for gastric air on chest x-ray. Administer antacids, cimetidine, and tube feedings as ordered. If abdominal distension is present, elevate head of bed to allow for optimal diaphragm excursion. Provide privacy for client to have a bowel movement.
Immobility	Normal range of motion of joints. No evidence of thromboemboli.	Assess client's ventilatory muscle pattern. Encourage client to breathe with the ventilator if on assist-control ventilation. If on IMV, encourage deep breaths (if client can tolerate) between IMV breaths. Encourage coughing. Provide adequate analgesia for pain if present. Provide progressive ambulation for long-term ventilator clients. Walk client while pushing ventilator or bag client with O_2 periodically. Perform active and passive range-of-motion exercises (e.g., leg lifts, knee bends, quadriceps setting, arm circles). Prevent contractures and external rotation of hips by proper positioning. Observe for pressure areas. Prevent decubitus ulcers by frequent turning, massaging pressure points, maintaining good nutrition, and use of air-pressure or egg-crate mattress. Prevent foot drop with use of foot board, high-top sneakers, having client flex the foot several times. Elevate head of bed as much as possible, especially during weaning. As soon as medically stable, the client should sit in a chair. Use elastic stockings and prophylactic heparin as ordered.

Table 22-8 (Continued)

Client Problem	Expected Outcome	Nursing Intervention
Psychological stress	Client and family communicate feelings and anxieties.	Assess client's behavior for clues of effectiveness of coping mechanisms. Make yourself available to family and offer support and help. Give simple, honest explanations regarding care and progress of the client. Offer positive reinforcement for client behaviors which demonstrate improvement. Allow client to make decisions regarding care (e.g., which side to turn on, when to bathe, when to eat). Provide periods of privacy for client and significant others. Converse with client and family members about client and family interests. Provide for diversion and occupational therapy as needed. Schedule care to allow for frequent rest periods. Encourage family to bring client's personal items to bedside. Provide a calendar and clock. Close off lights at night, perform bedtime preparations (e.g., wash face and hands, rub back, provide oral care). Sedate client as necessary. Move client to room with window (if available). Relaxation techniques and tapes may promote relaxation. Encourage and help family to participate directly in client's care. Encourage other members of health team to promote client's and family's well-being.
Machine malfunction	Early detection, correction, or prevention of complications associated with mechanical malfunction.	Turn all alarms on. If audible alarms are turned off during suctioning, turn them on immediately after. Check ventilator settings, FIO_2, respiratory rate, tidal volume, PEEP, airway pressure, thermister temperature. Keep bag ventilator connected to oxygen source at bedside of every ventilator client. Respond immediately to alarm. One person should bag-ventilate client while another person checks ventilator tubings for disconnections, leaks, sticky bellows, etc.

*The nursing care for a client with an artificial airway is presented in Table 22-7.
†All problems are listed as potential problems.

Cardiovascular system

Decreased Cardiac Output Circulatory problems can result from positive-pressure mechanical ventilation due to transmission of the increased mean airway pressure to the thoracic vessels, causing their compression during inspiration. This results in a decreased venous return to the heart, decreased cardiac output, and lowered blood pressure. Mean airway pressure may be further increased with higher and higher increments of PEEP. Maintenance of an I/E ratio of 1:1½ or 1:2 allows a longer period of time in the low-pressure exhalation cycle. This measure enhances venous return.

If the lungs are stiff and noncompliant (as in ARDS), airway pressures will not be easily transmitted to the heart and blood vessels. Therefore, the effects of mechanical ventilation on cardiac output are reduced accordingly. However, the danger of transmission of high airway pressures with very compliant lungs (e.g., in emphysema) is increased, and cardiac output may decrease.

The hemodynamic complications induced by positive-pressure ventilation are exaggerated by hypovolemia, sustained high airway pressures, prolonged inspiration, neurologic disease, and pharmacological depression. As mentioned previously, IMV reduces the cardio vascular effects of mechanical ventilation.

Cardiac output must be monitored carefully. Direct measurement via Swan-Ganz thermodilution, measurement of P_aO_2, or calculation of the $(A - V)O_2$ difference is extremely important in clients receiving 10 cm of PEEP or more. If cardiac output does fall, vasopressors, plasma expanders, and increased intravenous fluids may be required. Also, clients who are hypovolemic or who have decreased cardiac output may be volume-loaded prior to the institution of increased levels of PEEP. This decreases the problems associated with a drop in cardiac output. As positive airway pressure is removed and venous return increased, the client must be observed for symptoms of cardiac overload and pulmonary edema.

Positive Water Balance After 48 to 72 hours of mechanical ventilation, progressive fluid retention often occurs. This fluid retention can lead to pulmonary edema without evidence of cardiac failure, particularly when the level of mean airway pressure on the ventilator is increased (e.g., in PEEP therapy). Although several explanations have been proposed, the exact mechanism for the development of fluid retention is not clear. One popular theory is that the secretion of antidiuretic hormone (ADH) is increased. This may be due to vagal stretch receptors in the left atrium sensing the decreased venous return associated with positive-pressure ventilation, interpreting this as hypovolemia, and stimulating the neurohypophysis to secrete ADH.[24]

Another mechanism contributing to fluid retention is the prevention of the normal insensible loss of water (300 to 500 mL/day) from the client's respiratory system by the closed humidification system on the ventilator. In addition, the inspired air is saturated with humidity before the client inhales it. A net water gain of 300 to 500 mL or more per day may occur. Fluid restriction and diuretic therapy may be needed to promote water loss.

Pulmonary system

Barotrauma As higher and higher inflation pressures are required to inflate the lungs, there is an increased risk of pneumothorax, pneumomediastinum, and subcutaneous emphysema. Clients with highly compliant or floppy lungs (e.g., in emphysema) are at greater risk since the increased airway pressure readily distends the lungs and may rupture alveoli or emphysematous blebs.

Air can escape from the alveoli or interstitium into the pleural space, accumulate, and become trapped. This buildup of air increases pleural pressure and collapses the lung under it. This condition is called *pneumothorax* (see Fig. 20-8). "Ball-valving" is a common cause of pneumothorax. This phenomenon occurs in an area of the lung that can accept air during inspiration but cannot expel it during expiration. Because respiratory bronchioles are larger on inspiration than on expiration, they may close on expiration, thus contributing to the buildup of gas in the lung.[25] Some pneumothoraxes may be small (10 to 15 percent) and may not require a chest tube to evacuate the air and promote lung expansion, whereas larger pneumothoraxes (30 percent or greater) do require a chest tube. A chest tube may be inserted in a client on PEEP even with a small pneumothorax because of the possibility of increasing the pneumothorax.

A *tension pneumothorax* may occur if the pneumothorax expands rapidly, causing the mediastinum and its contents to be pushed to the opposite side of the pneumothorax. Cardiac output is extremely compromised, and a medical emergency exists. Fortunately, this is a rare occurrence. If a tension pneumothorax develops, the client should be removed from the ventilator and put on a bag ventilator connected to an O_2 source, or the tidal volume on the ventilator can be decreased to reduce airway pressures until a chest tube can be inserted.

Pneumomediastinum usually begins with the rupture of alveoli into the interstitium of the lung, followed by progressive movement of air into the mediastinum and the subcutaneous tissues of the neck. This is commonly followed by the development of a pneumothorax. The presence of new, unexplained subcutaneous air should indicate the need for immediate chest x-ray. Frequently, pneumomediastinum and subcutaneous emphysema in the neck are too small to be detected radiographically or clinically prior to the development of a pneumothorax.

Subcutaneous emphysema may occur after a tracheotomy due to leakage of air from the surgical site. Or it may occur around the site and area of the chest where a chest tube has been placed for a pneumothorax. In this latter instance, subcutaneous emphysema is usually due to the passage of gas from the pleural space into the tube wound, indicating that the space is not being adequately drained. The patency of the chest tube must be determined to prevent a further increase in the pneumothorax.

Clinical manifestations which may indicate the development or presence of a pneumothorax include tachypnea, asymmetrical chest expansion, decreased or absent breath sounds and/or hyperresonance to percussion on the affected side, subcutaneous emphysema with crepitus (crackly edema), particularly in the neck area, sharply increased peak inspiratory pressures on the system pressure gauge, and absence of lung markings at affected sites demonstrated on chest x-ray. The client may complain of not getting enough air or of having chest pain on the affected side.

Clinical manifestations of tension pneumothorax are more severe and may include all of the above signs plus tracheal deviation to the unaffected side, neck vein distension, thready pulse, hypotension, and mediastinal shift visualized on chest x-ray.

Alveolar Hypoventilation or Mechanical Underventilation The pressurized gas of the mechanical ventilator tends to flow to the areas of least resistance and high compliance. Therefore, some of the alveoli which are collapsed may not be ventilated, producing hypoventilated lung areas and atelectasis. The use of large tidal volumes, small increments of PEEP, and/or sighing of the client lessens the likelihood of the development of atelectasis. Frequent position changes and suctioning also help. The major clinical indicators of atelectasis are decreased breath sounds over the area and a drop in the P_aO_2. Increased secretions in the lungs can also cause hypoventilation. This can be prevented by turning the client every 1 to 2 hours, providing chest physiotherapy to areas of the lung with increased secretions, encouraging deep breathing and coughing, and performing suctioning as needed.

A tidal volume or respiratory rate set too low on the ventilator can decrease minute ventilation and lead to hypoventilation. A cuff that leaks or tubings which are not securely attached may cause leakage of air and may lower the delivered tidal volume. Too low an IMV rate in a client who is unable to produce adequate spontaneous ventilation can also lead to hypoventilation.

Alveolar Hyperventilation or Mechanical Overventilation Respiratory alkalosis occurs most often in clients with chronic respiratory acidosis (chronic alveolar hypoventilation and CO_2 retention, such as found in clients with COPD) in whom compensatory renal retention of bicarbonate has restored the pH toward normal. The mechanical ventilator removes CO_2, whereas the serum bicarbonate level stays elevated. (Normally, the kidneys require 2 to 3 days to alter the bicarbonate level.) Therefore, the ventilator can move the client from a state of compensated acidosis to one of severe alkalosis.

Alkalemia, especially if induced abruptly, can have serious consequences. As the bicarbonate level increases in the blood, H^+ and K^+ decrease. The resulting hypokalemia predisposes the client with oxygenation or cardiac problems to arrhythmias. Alkalemia also shifts the oxyhemoglobin dissociation curve to the left, making oxygen release to the tissues more difficult (see Fig. 18-8). Neuromuscular irritability, seizures, coma, and even death can also occur.

To prevent the occurrence of alkalosis in the client with compensated respiratory acidosis, mechanical ventilation should begin slowly and remain at a level that will not dramatically lower the arterial P_aCO_2. The client's arterial blood gases must be assessed 15 to 30 minutes after mechanical ventilation begins and after each ventilator change, serially thereafter, and whenever changes in the client's clinical status occur. The P_aCO_2 should be lowered only to the individual's baseline (pre-acute illness) level.

Respiratory alkalosis can also occur if the rate or tidal volume is set too high (mechanical overventilation) or if the client on assisted ventilation with IMV is hyperventilating. Hyperventilation means that the client's P_aCO_2 is less than 35 because he or the ventilator is blowing off CO_2 too rapidly. Decreasing the respiratory rate or tidal volume can help correct the respiratory alkalosis. However, if the current rate and volume are necessary to provide adequate ventilation and prevent atelectasis, mechanical dead space may be added.

Mechanical dead space is created by extending the client's anatomical dead space. Recall that anatomical dead space is that volume of gas not involved in gas exchange (see Chap. 18). Extra tubing, the amount of which is measured in inches or cubic centimeters (determined by the amount of water needed to fill the tubing), is connected from the client's artificial airway to the ventilator. This causes more of each breath to be rebreathed, and therefore less CO_2 is blown off. Arterial blood gases must be obtained to assess the effect of the added dead space. Mechanical dead space is rarely used with IMV since the IMV supplements the client's ventilatory status and overventilation is rarely a problem. (If overventilation is a problem, the IMV rate or volume can be decreased or adjusted accordingly.)

It is important to determine the cause of the hyperventilation or decreased P_aCO_2. Hyperventilation can be caused by retained secretions, hypoxemia, pain, fear, and anxiety, or it can be a compensatory mechanism for metabolic acidosis. The arterial blood gas levels need to be analyzed to determine if the respiratory alkalosis or hyperventilation is compensating for a primary problem of metabolic acidosis (e.g., diabetic acidosis). In the client with diabetic acidosis as an underlying problem, the diabetes must be controlled (see Chap. 41). Sedation and the addition of dead space as treatments for this problem can block the client's one available compensatory mechanism.

Clients who fight the ventilator or breathe out of synchrony with it may be very anxious and/or in pain. Secretion accumulation and movement or kinking of the endotracheal tube in the airway may also cause this problem. If the client is anxious and fearful, sitting with him and providing body contact by touching his hand or arm and verbally coaching him to breathe with the ventilator will help. If these measures fail, manually bagging the client slowly with the bag ventilator connected to an oxygen source may help to slow down the breathing enough to bring it in synchrony with the ventilator. The client may require morphine, diazepam, or other prescribed sedatives if pain or extreme anxiety occur. However, sedation must be administered with extreme caution in clients on IMV at low rates since the respiratory drive may be significantly depressed.

Pulmonary Infection Pulmonary infection is a common complication of mechanical ventilation. Because the normal defenses of the upper airway have been bypassed by the endotracheal or tracheal tube, the client is at increased risk of infection. In addition, the client's poor nutritional state, immobility, and the underlying disease process make him more prone to infections.

In clients on prolonged mechanical ventilation, sputum cultures invariably grow organisms which are usually gram-negative.[26] Gram-negative bacteria such as *Pseudomonas, Serratia,* and *Klebsiella* are abundant in both the hospital environment and the client's digestive tract. *Pseudomonas* has been found in handwashing sinks, suction apparatus, ice machines, distilled water, and water traps of ventilators.[27] Colonization of the upper respiratory tract by aspiration of gram-negative organisms is a predisposing factor in the development of gram-negative pneumonia.[28] (Gram-negative pneumonia is discussed in Chap. 20.)

The risk of infection can be minimized by using strict aseptic technique while suctioning or handling the artificial airway. Frequent handwashing is imperative. The humidifier and tubing on the ventilator provide a warm, moist environment conducive to the growth of organisms. Ventilator tubing is changed at least every 24 to 48 hours. When water has condensed in the tubing, it should be drained out of the system, especially prior to turning or repositioning the client. This measure will prevent the client from aspirating the water. Corrugated ventilator tubings must be pulled gently to remove H_2O that has condensed in the folds. Chest physiotherapy, adequate humidification of inspired gases, and sterile suctioning all may help to prevent infection by eliminating secretion accumulation. The manual ventilator bag (e.g., Ambu bag) and oxygen tubing kept at the client's bedside also need to be replaced and cleaned periodically (at least every 24 to 48 hours).

Clinical evidence suggesting pulmonary infection includes fever, an elevated white blood cell count, increasing purulence of sputum, sputum odor, auscultation which reveals rales or rhonchi, and chest x-ray evidence of pulmonary infection. The client is treated with antibiotics only after appropriate cultures are taken and when there is evidence of infection. Antibiotics should not be utilized prophylactically.[29]

Gastrointestinal system

The process of mechanical ventilation is stressful and increases the client's risk of developing *stress ulcers* and *gastrointestinal bleeding.* Clients who have a preexisting ulcer or who are on corticosteroid therapy are at an especially increased risk. Gastroscopy evidence exists which demonstrates that gastric mucosal changes occur in many critically ill clients.[30] It is also believed that PEEP may contribute to ischemia of the gastric mucosa by increasing resistance in splanchnic blood vessels.[31]

Prophylactic administration of antacids to maintain a gastric pH of greater than 5 has dramatically reduced the occurrence of gastrointestinal bleeding.[32] Early and frequent nasogastric feedings have also been successfully used to decrease gastric ulcers and bleeding. Prophylactic use of cimetidine (Tagamet), administered intravenously or orally, decreases the acidity of gastric secretions and prevents stress ulcer formation and hemorrhage. Cimetidine has been used alone or in combination with antacid therapy.

Gastric dilatation, although rare, may occur due to the accumulation of gas in the stomach. Gas may escape from around the cuff of the endotracheal tube and may be swallowed or aspirated into the stomach. The irritation of an artificial airway may cause excessive air swallowing and subsequent gastric dilatation. Gastric dilatation may put pressure on the vena cava, decrease cardiac output, and prohibit adequate diaphragmatic excursion during spontaneous breathing. Decompression of the stomach can be accomplished by the insertion of a nasogastric tube. Some physicians still routinely insert nasogastric tubes prophylactically when mechanical ventilation is initiated. It is especially important to insert a nasogastric tube to prevent aspiration if the client is in danger of vomiting.

Immobility, sedation, and stress contribute to decreased peristalsis. The inability to exhale against a closed glottis may make defecation difficult. Therefore, the client is predisposed to the development of paralytic ileus and constipation.

Inadequate nutrition

Mechanical ventilation, immobility, and the physical and emotional stresses associated with critical illness contribute to the poor nutritional status of the client. The presence of an endotracheal tube eliminates the normal route for eating. Clients with a nasotracheal tube have been allowed to have liquid and semiliquid feedings orally if test feedings indicate lack of aspiration. It is difficult for the client to swallow and to ingest sufficient calories, protein, and fat. A client with a tracheostomy can eat normally once the wound has healed. When eating with a tracheotomy or nasotracheal tube, the cuff should be inflated and the client should tilt his head slightly forward to facilitate swallowing and to prevent aspiration. Often, soft foods (e.g., puddings, ice cream) are more easily swallowed than liquids.

Clients who have been without food for 3 to 5 days and who are unlikely to eat within a week should have some type of nutritional program initiated. Inadequate nutrition makes the client on prolonged mechanical ventilation more prone to poor oxygen transport secondary to anemia and to poor tolerance of minimal exercise. Disuse of respiratory muscles, as well as poor nutrition, can result in decreased respiratory muscle strength. In addition, caloric expenditure is elevated in the presence of fever, anxiety, pain, and the increased work of breathing. Serum albumin and transferrin levels are usually decreased. Inadequate nutrition can delay weaning and decrease the speed of recovery from illness.

Total parenteral nutrition (TPN) supplemented with intralipids fulfills the nutritional requirements for many clients. Nasogastric or gastric feedings of high protein liquids (Ensure, Ensure Plus, Isocal, Vivonex) are another method of attaining adequate nutrition. Vitamin and mineral replacements, as well as water, are also important. A dietitian must be involved in this aspect of the client's care. (These nutritional measures are discussed in Chap. 33.)

The intubated client receiving nasogastric feedings should have the endotracheal cuff inflated and the head of his bed elevated. Tube feedings are given as a slow, continous drip, since rapid infusion can cause diarrhea and absorption problems. Problems with malabsorption and decreased gastric emptying can be assessed by discontinuing the tube feeding for 30 to 60 minutes and checking for the amount of residual tube feeding in the stomach by aspirating with an asepto syringe. Small feeding tubes must be aspirated gently with smaller syringes to prevent clogging.

If more than half the amount of the tube feeding given per hour is aspirated, the aspirate should be reintroduced slowly into the stomach, and the tube should be clamped for another 30 minutes to 1 hour and rechecked for residual. The gastric emptying time varies from person to person. The feedings should be administered in an amount and at an infusion rate best tolerated by the client.

Tube feedings should be temporarily stopped if the client is in a head-down postural drainage position (for at least 30 minutes prior to treatment), if bowel sounds are absent, or if regurgitation occurs. The client must be observed closely for signs of hypoglycemia if the tube feedings are rapidly discontinued for long periods of time. Food coloring placed in the feedings can help to identify the presence of feedings in material suctioned from the trachea. The presence of a positive glucose reaction on a dipstick of tracheal secretions may indicate insufflation of feedings into the trachea. If there is evidence that aspiration may have occurred, the tube feeding should be discontinued immediately and the physician notified. Nursing care related to tube feedings is discussed in Table 33-10.

Musculoskeletal system

Improvement or maintenance of muscle strength and prevention of the problems of immobility are important. Exercise tolerance is enhanced by adequate analgesia for pain and adequate nutritional intake. Progressive ambulation of long-term ventilator clients can be attained while the client is on the ventilator. This is done by pushing the ventilator with the client or by ambulating with an oxygenized bag ventilator (e.g., Ambu bag) while giving periodic hyperinflations. Passive and active exercises, consisting of movements to maintain muscle tone in the upper and lower extremities, should be done in bed. Simple maneuvers such as leg lifts, knee bends, quadriceps setting, or arm circles are always possible and appropriate. Prevention of contractures, pressure areas, decubitus ulcers, foot drop, external rotation of the hip and legs, and other deformities by proper positioning is also important.

Psychological effects

The client who is receiving mechanical ventilation is often under a great deal of physical and emotional stress. His vital functions have been altered. He is unable to speak, eat, or breathe normally. He is restricted in his activity. Often the client is in the center of a maze of tubes and machines whose presence creates fear and anxiety. Ordinary functions such as having a bowel movement or coughing are complicated. Death may seem inevitable, or the condition may be considered a punishment from God. The client's productive role in society and in his family is temporarily suspended. Being unable to participate fully in family matters may cause feelings of inadequacy, overwhelming helplessness, and frustration.

These problems are further compounded by the sensory overload and deprivation experienced in the intensive care unit. Ringing alarms, flickering lights, frequent interruptions by personnel (often without warning), and lack of meaningful input are examples of such experiences. The passage of time loses its meaning when lights are on constantly or when noises prevent sleep. Sleep and waking cycles are disturbed. Problems caused by sleep deprivation add to the client's stress.

It is the responsibility of the nurse to ensure that the client's needs are met. The nurse should be able to pick up behavioral clues to determine if the client is coping effectively with the stressful situation. If coping is not effective, the health team needs to be alerted, and supportive measures must be sought. For example, the client may be distressed because of a family problem that can be solved through consultation with family members and the health team. Effective coping mechanisms require positive reinforcement and sustained strengthening. The need for psychological support cannot be overemphasized.

The client must be given a means to communicate. Signals, paper and pencil, alphabet boards, word boards, magic slates, and in some instances talking trach tubes can be used. Touching the client's arm or hand and being able to read his body language and facial expressions are also important.

Measures to make the client's environment more restful include (1) efficient scheduling of care to reduce interruptions, (2) simulation of a night-day environment by turning the lights off at night, (3) a calendar and clock near his bed, (4) personal articles and pictures of loved ones, and (5) a calm, reassuring approach. Tape-recorded relaxation tapes or soothing music may also help the client to relax. Sedation may be required to enhance sleep. The long-term ventilator client should be moved to an area where there is a window in order to appreciate better both night and day and the outside world. Even though the client is unable to converse, he will still appreciate being spoken to. Talk to him about his interests and, most of all, explain in simple terms what the different tubes and equipment are and what progress is being made. Reassuring the client honestly about his progress and allowing him as much control as possible over his care may ease the frustration of dependence. Deciding when he wants to bathe, have his hair washed, which direction to turn, or what to eat may be the client's only way of maintaining control in an overwhelming situation.

The client's family needs emotional support as well. The first time a family member visits the client, it may be important for the nurse to go with them. The family should be told briefly what the tubes are for, and they should be encouraged to touch, hug, and speak to the client. A chair should be provided and the siderail lowered so that they can have contact with their loved one. Privacy should be provided as much as possible. The effect of the client's visitor should be assessed. Ocassionally, significant others have a difficult time dealing with a sick loved one and may need help and support. The family should be included in the plan of care. If a family member expresses a wish to participate in physical care such as shaving or oral hygiene, the nurse should encourage such activity.

Many institutions have family support systems available. Chaplains, social workers, and psychologists are often members of the health team. These support personnel may assist the family and client to adjust to problems resulting from the client's hospitalization.

Machine malfunction

It is possible for mechanical ventilators to malfunction or for a temporary pause to occur in the delivery of electric current. Alarm systems, when turned on and operative, can alert the nurse and respiratory therapist to problems. Alarms should be turned on if there is no silencer button to press during suctioning. If the alarms are temporarily turned off, they must be turned on again immediately after suctioning. Some of the most serious ventilator malfunctions include mechanical breakdown, overheating of inspired air, inadequate nebulization, and alarm failure. The sounding of an alarm does not identify the problem. It is merely a signal that a problem exists. The respiratory therapist or nurse must determine the cause of the problem and correct it. The client should be immediately ventilated with an oxygenized manual resuscitation bag until the machine is fixed. If the client can be ventilated without resistance, the problem is located within the ventilator system.

The Manual Resuscitation Bag Although the Ambu (air mask bag unit) is not the only example of a manual resuscitation bag or bag ventilator, it is the one best known. This unit consists of a bag which is fitted to either a face mask or an attachment that fits the client's tracheotomy or endotracheal tube. There are basically two types of bags, the *anesthesia bag* and the *self-inflatable bag*. The anesthesia bag is used by the anesthesiologist in surgery to ventilate the client; with its oxygen source, it delivers 100% oxygen. Adaptations of this bag have been made to produce PEEP bags for clients on PEEP greater than 10 cm H_2O.

Several kinds of self-inflatable bags are used for resuscitation and kept at the bedside for clients on mechanical ventilators. If a mask is used in resuscitation, it is important first to insert an oral or nasopharyngeal airway to maintain airway patency. The mask must then be tightly fitted to the face (first placed on the chin and then over the nose) and the neck hyperextended to keep the airway patent. The nurse should use a regular rate of about 10 breaths per minute and watch the rise and fall of the client's chest for confirmation that ventilation is adequate.

Self-inflatable bags vary in the concentration of oxygen delivered. All bags require liter flows of 15 L/minute. Bags which usually contain reservoir tubings and other devices to entrain oxygen deliver oxygen concentrations of 90 to 95%. The slower the bag is deflated and inflated, the higher the O_2 concentration which will be delivered. An example of the Hope II bag is seen in Fig. 22-12. Both the Hope II and old Hope bag with reservoir tubing and adaptor

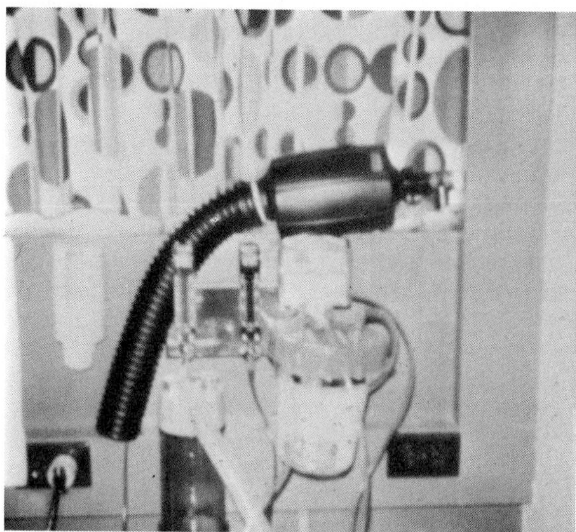

Figure 22-12 Hope II manual resuscitation bag.

deliver an FIO_2 of 0.90 to 0.95. The Laerdal bag (clear green) delivers an FIO_2 of 0.5 to 0.6 and with reservoir tubing, 0.75 to 0.8. The Bennett Puritan bag (brown) delivers an FIO_2 of 0.35 to 0.40.[33]

Weaning from Mechanical Ventilation

Weaning is the process of gradually reducing ventilator support until the client is able to perform self-ventilation. Clients who require mechanical ventilation will either be weaned from the ventilator and the endotracheal tube promptly (e.g., in drug overdose and postoperative open heart surgery without complications) or will require prolonged ventilatory assistance via a tracheostomy or endotracheal tube (e.g., in ARDS or COPD). Clients likely to require prolonged mechanical ventilation can generally be identified as those who have underlying lung disease and then because of surgical procedures, trauma, or infection develop respiratory failure. Preparations for the weaning process begin when the client is initially placed on the ventilator. These preparations include the optimization of nutritional status, exercise tolerance, fluid electrolyte and acid-base balance, cardiac output and status, level of consciousness, and pulmonary status.

Data to determine the weaning ability of clients should be compiled from many sources (Table 22-9). Criteria also vary from client to client depending upon previous lung status and ventilatory reserve. For weaning to be successful, the client should be as clinically stable as possible. It is hoped that the event(s) or condition which necessitated mechanical ventilation will have been reversed. Respiratory parameters should demonstrate that the client has a patent effective airway, adequate ventilatory muscle strength, and an effective cough. The lung's ability to oxygenate the arterial blood adequately is evident when stable arterial blood gases (with a P_aO_2 of 60 mmHg or greater) can be achieved on an FIO_2 of less than 0.5. The lungs should be reasonably clear on chest x-ray and to auscultation. It is important to have an alert, well-rested client relatively free from pain who will readily take deep breaths to obtain optimal alveolar ventilation and prevent atelectasis. This does not mean complete withdrawal from sedatives or analgesics, as is often thought when one speaks of avoiding central nervous system depression of the respiratory center. Instead, an intelligent approach to titration of medications to achieve pain relief and decreased anxiety without excessive drowsiness is indicated.

Basically, two weaning methods are in clinical use. The most common method is to place the client on IMV and gradually reduce the frequency of ventilation breaths as the client's ventilatory status permits. In another method, the client is transferred from assisted or IMV mechanical ventilation to humidified oxygen via a T piece of Brigg's adaptor. Clients usually require an FIO_2 of 10 percent higher off the ventilator to maintain adequate P_aO_2 and saturation levels, since the tidal volume usually drops with spontaneous respiration and there is an increase in P_aCO_2. The time off the ventilator is usually limited to 5 to 10 minutes/hour, increasing by increments of 5 to 10 minutes/hour if tolerated. The weaning procedure is carried out during the day, and the client is placed back on the ventilator at night until he is able to breathe all day with only periodic sighing. Allowing the client to rest at night is important regardless of the weaning technique employed.

Prior to weaning, the client should be prepared psychologically, and continued psychological support should be maintained. The nurse should explain the weaning process and report the client's progress. The client should be placed in a sitting or semirecumbent position and should be as comfortable as possible. Prior to weaning, respiratory parameters are measured (see Table 22-9) to provide a baseline with which frequent serial determinations can be compared. The tidal volume, inspiratory force, and vital capacity are most frequently measured. Arterial blood gases are drawn at specified periods during the weaning procedure. The cuff may be deflated totally or partially during weaning unless it is needed to prevent aspiration, since tracheal tubes add to airway resistance.

The client must be monitored closely for signs of respiratory distress, restlessness, tiring, somnolence,

Table 22-9
Indications for Mechanical Ventilation and Weaning[34–36]

	Measurement and Significance	Normal Values*	Mechanical Ventilation Indicated*	Weaning Feasible*
	Tests of Ventilatory Reserve or Mechanical Ability			
Tidal volume	Amount of air exchanged during normal breathing at rest.	6–7 mL/kg	<5 mL/kg	>5 mL/kg
Respiratory rate per minute		12–20	<10 or> 35	12–20
Forced vital capacity	Maximal inspiration and then measurement of air during maximal forced expiration. Determines if client can sigh deeply enough to avoid atelectasis. Best indicator of ventilatory reserve. Requires client's cooperation	65-75 mL/kg	<10–15 mL/kg	>10–15 mL/kg
Peak inspiratory pressure or negative inspiratory force	Aneroid manometer attached to airway or mouth is completely occluded for 10–20 s while negative inspiratory efforts of client are noted. Useful index of neuromuscular strength. Requires less client cooperation than forced vital capacity.	75–100 cm H_2O	<25 cm H_2O	>20 cm H_2O
Forced expiratory volume in 1 s ($FEV_{1.0}$)	Volume of air measured in the first second of exhalation of a forced vital capacity maneuver. Used in clients with COPD to determine whether adequate ventilation exists.	50–60 mL/kg	<10 mL/kg	>16 mL/kg
Resting minute ventilation	Tidal volume multiplied by respiratory rate. Gives a general indication of the client's total mechanical ventilation.	5–10 L/min	>10 L/min	<10 L/min
	If the client can double the minute ventilation with a *maximal voluntary ventilation* maneuver (exertion of maximum breathing effort for 10–15 s and comparing this to effort for 1 min), the ability to sustain the muscular effort necessary for normal gas exchange is shown.	>10–20 L/min	<20 L/min	>20 L/min
Dead space to tidal volume ratio (V_D/V_T)	Can be estimated from tidal volume (anatomical dead space equals 1 mL per pound of body weight). Accurate calculation requires P_aCO_2 and partial pressure of CO_2 in mixed expired gas. Measures portion of each breath that actually does not participate in gas exchange. Indicates lung's efficiency in removing CO_2.	0.25–0.40	>0.6	<0.5–0.6
Arterial P_aCO_2	Indicates lung's efficiency in removing CO_2 and reflects body's acid-base status.	35–45 mmHg	>55 mmHg	<45 mmHg
	Tests of Oxygenation Capability			
$\dot{Q}_S/\dot{Q}_T$(shunt fraction)	Calculated by formula which determines the amount of cardiac output shunted ($\dot{Q}_S$) in relation to the amount of total cardiac output ($\dot{Q}_T$). Indicates the extent of shunt, expressed as a percentage of cardiac output.	<5%	>20%	<15%
$D(A-a)O_2$ or $P(A-a)O_2$	Calculated from P_aO_2, P_AO_2, and respiratory quotient on FIO_2 of 1.0. Indicates the lung's ability to oxygenate blood. Gives an index of the extent of $\dot{V}/\dot{Q}$ mismatch, diffusion defect, or shunt.	25-65 mmHg	>450 mmHg	<300-350 mmHg
Arterial PO_2	Provides evidence of lung's ability to oxygenate arterial blood. P_aO_2 of 60 mmHg is required to saturate the hemoglobin by 90%. This is necessary for adequate tissue oxygenation.	80–110 mmHg (altitude dependent)	<60 mmHg with FIO_2 >0.6	>70–80 mmHg with FIO_2 ≤0.5

*These parameters are only guidelines and must be related to the individual client's status (e.g., clients with severe COPD may have a normal P_aCO_2 of 60 and values lower than normal for FEV, VC, MV, and MVV).

shallow breathing, use of accessory muscles of ventilation, tachycardia, decrease or increase in BP, tachypnea or bradypnea, ECG changes, pallor or graying of mucous membranes, and excessive secretion buildup with a need for frequent suctioning. Statements from the client regarding his weaning tolerance must also be considered.

When the client is to be extubated, the airway should be thoroughly suctioned and the cuff deflated. An oxygen mask or cannula should be set up at the bedside and be ready for use. Care of the mouth or nares is also given after extubation once the client has been stabilized on O_2 delivered by mask or cannula. Arterial blood gases are obtained 20 to 30 minutes after extubation. The client must be monitored continuously for the presence of respiratory distress, not only because of previous lung problems but also because laryngeal and/or tracheal edema may develop and symptoms of acute upper airway obstruction may occur. Measures to ensure pulmonary toilet, coughing, deep breathing, turning, and suctioning (if necessary) must be continued.

REVIEW QUESTIONS

The number of the question corresponds to the same numbered objective at the beginning of the chapter.

1. Which of the following is *not* a cause of hypoxemic respiratory failure?
 a. ventilation-perfusion mismatch
 b. shunting
 c. diffusion abnormalities
 d. alveolar hyperventilation

2. Which of the following may enhance ventilation in the client with expiratory wheezing and prolonged exhalation?
 a. bronchodilator administration (intravenous, subcutaneous, aerosol)
 b. ultrasonic nebulization with normal saline
 c. aerosolized Mucomyst
 d. administration of a large volume of intravenous fluids

3. The most common early manifestations of ARDS which the nurse may observe are
 a. cyanosis and apprehension
 b. dyspnea and tachypnea
 c. respiratory distress and frothy sputum
 d. hypotension and tachycardia

4. Which of the following is *true* concerning fluid management in the stable ARDS client?
 a. Pulmonary capillary wedge pressure is maintained at high levels (>10 mmHg).
 b. Pulmonary capillary wedge pressure is kept as low as possible without impairing cardiac output.
 c. Diuretics and fluid restriction are rarely used.
 d. Frequent and vigorous administration of salt-poor albumin is used.

5. The nurse can reduce the danger of hypoxemia induced by suctioning the ventilated client by
 a. preoxygenating and hyperventilating the client before and after suctioning
 b. suctioning only once per hour
 c. asking the client to take deep breaths before and after suctioning
 d. asking the client to cough during suctioning

6. A volume-cycled ventilator does which of the following?
 a. delivers gas flow for a preset period of time
 b. delivers gas flow until a preset pressure is reached
 c. delivers gas flow until a preset volume is reached
 d. any of the above depending on the settings used

7. Maintenance of client safety is extremely important for the client receiving mechanical ventilation. Which of the following is imperative to ensure this?.
 a. Maintain an oral airway in place on all intubated clients.
 b. Restrain all clients who are mechanically ventilated.
 c. Decrease the sound of ventilator alarms to avoid startling the client.
 d. Keep a bag ventilator with an O_2 source at the bedside at all times

REFERENCES

1. S. Nadel, "Adequate Oxygenation," in M. R. Kinney (ed.), *AACN's Clinical Reference for Critical Care Nursing,* McGraw-Hill Book Company, New York, 1981, pp. 366–367.
2. B. Shapiro, R. Harrison, and C. Trout, *Clinical Application of Respiratory Care,* 2d ed., Year Book Medical Publishers, Inc., Chicago, 1979, pp. 420–422.
3. Respiratory Diseases Task Force, *Report on Problems, Research Approaches and Needs,* Pub. No. NIH 73-432, Department of Health, Education and Welfare, Washington, D.C., 1972.
4. R. Ingram, "Adult Respiratory Distress Syndrome," in K. Isselbacher et al. (eds.), *Harrison's Principles of Internal Medicine,* 9th ed., McGraw-Hill Book Company, New York, 1980.
5. G. Burton, G. Gee, and J. Hodgkin, *Respiratory Care: A Guide to Clinical Practice,* J. B. Lippincott Company, Philadelphia, 1977, pp. 766–767.
6. R. Wilson and W. Sibball, "Acute Respiratory Failure," *Crit Care Med,* **4:**78–79 (1976).
7. Burton et al., op. cit., p. 772.
8. Shapiro et al., op cit., pp. 420–423.
9. Burton et al., op. cit., p. 773.
10. Respiratory Diseases Task Force, op. cit., p. 243.
11. Shapiro et al., op. cit., pp. 423–424.
12. J. Hedley-Whyte, G. Burgess, T. Feeley, and M. Miller, *Applied Physiology of Respiratory Care,* Little, Brown and Company Boston, 1976, p. 3.
13. J. L. Stauffer et al., "Complications and Consequences of Endotracheal Intubation and Tracheostomy: A Prospective Study of 150 Critically Ill Patients," *Am J Med,* **70:**65–76 (1981).
14. Shapiro et al., op. cit., p. 293.
15. Ibid., pp. 293–294.
16. N. Ching and T. F. Nealon, "Cuff Pressure Measurements," *Chest,* **66:**604 (1974).

17. G. Skelley, S. Deeren, and M. Powaser, "The Effectiveness of Two Pre-Oxygenation Methods to Prevent Endotracheal Suction Induced Hypoxemia," *Heart Lung,* **9**(2):320 (1980).
18. Ibid., p. 323.
19. M. Douglas and J. Downs, "Cardiopulmonary Effects of Intermittent Mandatory Ventilation," *Int Anesthesiol Clin,* **18**(2):103 (1980).
20. Hedley-Whyte et al., op. cit., p. 140.
21. S. Gherine, R. Peters, and R. Virgilo, "Mechanical Work on the Lungs and Work of Breathing with Positive End Expiratory Pressure and Continued Positive Airway Pressure," *Chest,* **76**(3):251 (1981).
22. Douglas and Downs, op. cit., pp. 113, 116.
23. Hedley-Whyte et. al., op. cit., p. 70.
24. J. Lagerson, "Mechanical Support of Ventilation," in Kinney, op. cit., p. 968.
25. R. Geer, "Mechanical Ventilation," in A. P. Fishman, *Pulmonary Diseases and Disorders,* McGraw-Hill Book Company, New York, 1980, p. 1616.
26. Hedley-Whyte et al., op. cit., p. 38.
27. Ibid., p. 41.
28. Geer, op. cit., p. 1616.
29. C. E. Lucas et al., "Natural History and Surgical Dilemma of Stress Gastric Bleeding," *Arch Surg,* **102**:266–272 (1971).
30. Hedley-Whyte et al., op. cit., p. 32.
31. Ibid., p. 35.
32. S. K. Harris et al., "Gastrointestinal Hemorrhage in Patients in a Respiratory Intensive Care Unit," *Chest,* **72**:301 (1977).
33. Burton et al., op. cit., p. 772.
34. Ibid.
35. Geer, op. cit., p. 1618.
36. S. Sahn et al., "Weaning from Mechanical Ventilation," *JAMA*:, 2200–2212 (1976).

Chapter 23

NURSING ASSESSMENT

Hematologic System

Bonnie Mowinski Jennings

Learning Objectives

1. Describe the structures and functions of the hematologic system.
2. Differentiate among the types of blood cells and their functions.
3. Explain the normal clotting mechanism.
4. Identify the significant subjective and objective assessment data related to the hematologic system that should be obtained from a client.
5. Describe the appropriate techniques used in the physical assessment of the lymphatic system.
6. Differentiate normal from common abnormal findings of a physical assessment of the hematologic system.
7. Describe the purpose, significance of results, and nursing responsibilities related to diagnostic studies of the hematologic system.

Hematology is the study of the blood and blood-forming tissues. This includes the blood cells, bone marrow, spleen, and lymph system. A basic knowledge of hematology is used in clinical settings to evaluate the client's ability to transport oxygen and carbon dioxide, coagulate blood, and combat infections. The study of the blood often includes the reticuloendothelial (macrophage) system. The macrophage cells are involved in phagocytosis and the immune response (Chaps. 9 and 10).

HEMATOLOGIC SYSTEM: STRUCTURES AND FUNCTIONS

Bone Marrow

Bone marrow is the soft material that fills the central core of bones. It produces the three major cell components of the blood: *erythrocytes* (red blood cells), *leukocytes* (white blood cells), and *platelets*. In the fetus, most of the bone marrow is actively producing blood cells. However, in the adult, actively producing marrow is generally limited to the ends of long bones, vertebrae, flat cranial bones, sternum, and ribs.[1] The blood components develop from a common stem cell (Fig. 23-1).

The opinions or assertions expressed in this chapter are the views of the author and are not to be construed as official or as reflecting the views of the Department of the Army or the Department of Defense.

This chapter was reviewed by Bonnie L. Luhmann, R.N., B.S.N., Assistant Director, Medical-Surgical Nursing, St. Mary's Hospital, Rochester, Minnesota.

Blood Cells

Erythrocytes

Several distinct cell types evolve during erythrocyte maturation (Fig. 23-1). The *reticulocyte* is an immature erythrocyte. Assessing the number of reticulocytes is a useful means of evaluating the adequacy of erythrocyte production. The reticulocyte count measures the rate at which new red cells appear in the circulation. Normally, after erythrocytes mature in the marrow, they enter the circulation. The functions of erythrocytes include transport of gases (both oxygen and carbon dioxide) and assistance in maintaining the acid-base balance through the buffering capability of hemoglobin.

Hemoglobin is found within the erythrocytes and gives them their characteristic red color. Iron and protein form the molecular structure of hemoglobin. The function of hemoglobin is to transport oxygen. Therefore, although adequate oxygen may be inspired into the lungs, it may not reach the tissues unless there is an adequate amount of hemoglobin to carry it.

Erythropoiesis (the production of erythrocytes) is regulated largely by cellular oxygen requirements and general metabolic activity. *Hemolysis* (destruction of erythrocytes) by the macrophage system removes abnormal, defective, damaged, and old red cells from circulation.

Leukocytes

Leukocytes also develop in a series of cell types varying in maturity (Fig. 23-1). The three kinds of mature leukocytes are *granulocytes*, *lymphocytes*, and *monocytes*. The main function of the granulocytes

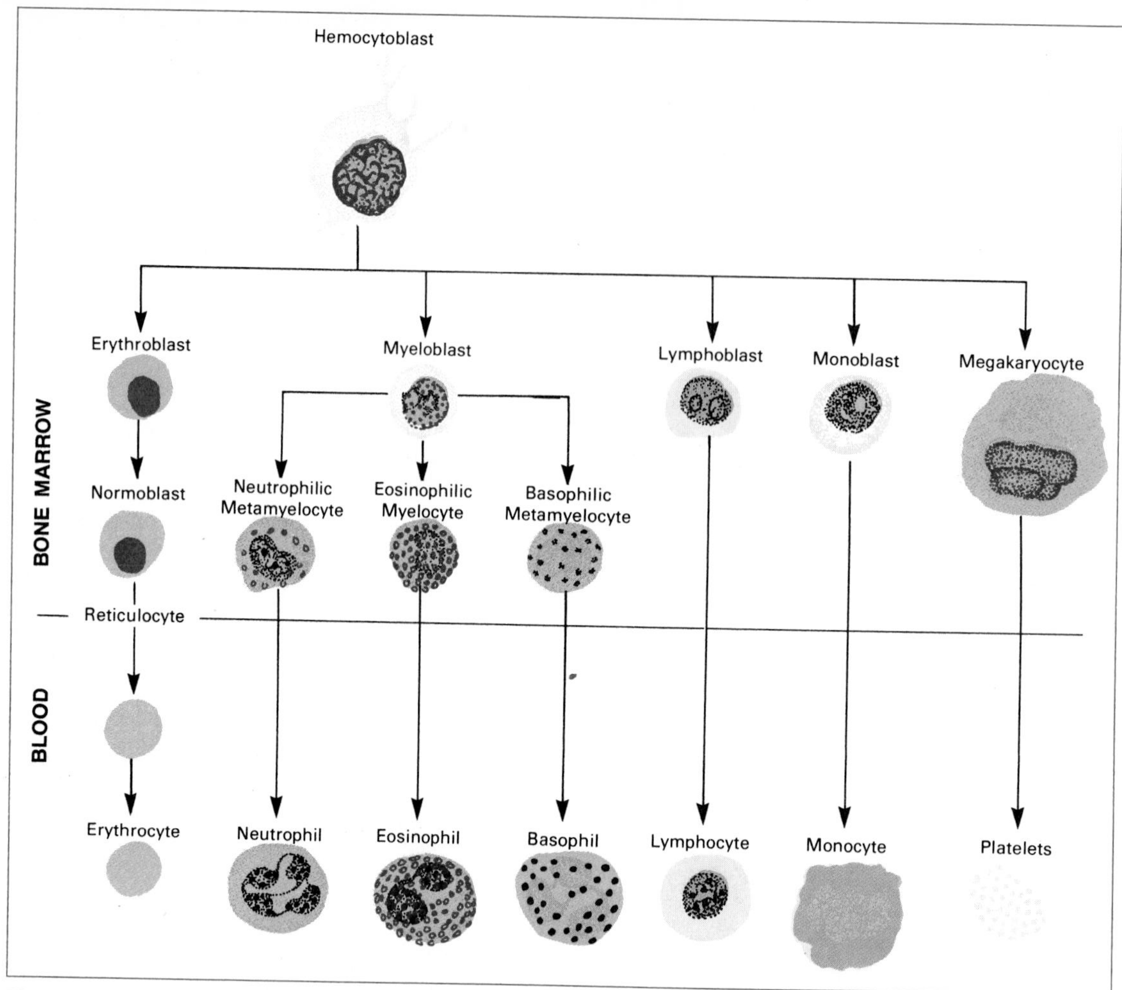

Figure 23-1 Development of blood cells. *(Modified from L. L. Langley et al., Dynamic Anatomy and Physiology, 5th ed., McGraw-Hill Book Company, New York, 1980, p. 385. Used by permission of the publisher.)*

and monocytes is *phagocytosis* of bacteria and foreign particles which invade the body. Phagocytosis is a process by which cells ingest or engulf any unwanted organism and then digest or kill it. The main function of lymphocytes is related to the immune response (Chap. 10).

Granulocytes Granulocytes are so named because they contain granules in their cytoplasm. The granulocytes (also known as *polymorphonuclear leukocytes*, or *PMNs*) consist of *neutrophils*, *eosinophils*, and *basophils*.

Neutrophils, also called *polys* or *segs*, have strong phagocytic activity. They are the primary phagocytic cell type during an acute inflammatory response. They are a major source of endogenous pyrogen that causes fever. Neutrophils are responsible for the inflammation following an antigen-antibody reaction.[2]

Eosinophils have a similar but reduced ability for phagocytosis. They are concerned mainly with phagocytosis of antigen-antibody complexes during an immune response (especially an allergic response). Basophils have a limited role in phagocytosis. Their granules in the cytoplasm contain heparin and histamine. If a basophil is stimulated by either an antigen or tissue injury, it will respond by releasing histamine. This is part of the response seen in allergic reactions.

Lymphocytes Lymphocytes are produced in the lymph system, bone marrow, and spleen. The two lymphocyte cell types are *B cells* and *T cells*. B cells, produced in the bone marrow, mediate the humoral immune response. When B cells are stimulated by antigens, they are activated to *plasma cells*. Plasma cells produce antibodies, also known as *immunoglobulins*.

T cells are produced by the thymus gland. They mediate cellular immunity. T cells are involved in the cellular immune response against some viruses, tuberculosis, contact irritants (e.g., poison ivy), cancer, parasites, fungus, and transplant antigens. The details of lymphocyte function are presented in Chap. 10.

Monocytes Monocytes are produced in the bone marrow and circulate briefly in the blood. They are large, slow-moving, potent phagocytic cells which can ingest small or large masses of matter such as bacteria, dead cells, or tissue debris. Monocytes are the second type of white blood cell that arrives at the scene of an injury (neutrophils are the first). When attracted to sites of injury, monocytes differentiate into *macrophages*. Macrophages may be either mobile (circulate in the blood) or fixed (present in tissue) (Chap. 9). They are more phagocytic than monocytes. In addition, macrophages facilitate lymphocytes in producing antibodies.

Platelets

Platelets, or *thrombocytes*, are derived from megakaryocytes (Fig. 23-1). The primary function of platelets is to participate in blood clotting. Platelets must be available in sufficient numbers and must be structurally sound in order to work properly. Platelets are also involved in maintaining capillary integrity by working as "plugs" to close any openings in the capillary wall. They are also important to the process of clot shrinkage and retraction. More specific functions of platelets will be discussed in the section on Normal Clotting Mechanisms.

Spleen

Another component of the hematologic system is the spleen, which is located in the upper left quadrant of the abdomen.

The five basic functions of the spleen include:

1. Production of red cells during fetal development
2. Production of lymphocytes and antibodies
3. Removal from the circulation of old and defective erythrocytes by the macrophage system
4. Catabolism of hemoglobin released by hemolysis, and return of the iron component of the hemoglobin to the bone marrow for reuse
5. Storage of 1 to 2 percent of the red cell mass, which can be released as needed

Lymph System

The *lymph system* carries fluid from the interstitial spaces to the blood. It is by means of the lymph that proteins, fat from the gastrointestinal tract, and certain hormones are able to return to the blood. The lymph system also returns excess interstitial fluid to the blood, which is important in preventing the development of edema.

Lymph fluid is pale yellow and circulates through a special vasculature, much as blood moves through blood vessels. Lymph fluid is interstitial fluid which has flowed into the lymphatics. The formation of lymph fluid increases when interstitial fluid pressure rises, and therefore more fluid enters the lymph system. When too much interstitial pressure develops, or when something interferes with the flow of lymph, *lymphedema* develops. The lymphedema that may occur as a complication of a radical mastectomy is often due to the obstruction of lymph flow caused by the removal of nodes.

The lymphatic capillaries are thin-walled, endothelial-lined vessels which have an irregular diameter. They are somewhat larger than blood capillaries and do not contain valves. Lymphatic capillaries unite to form lymphatic vessels which carry all lymph to either the right lymphatic duct or the thoracic duct. These large lymphatic ducts drain into subclavian veins in the neck.

The lymph nodes are also a part of the lymphatic system. Structurally, the nodes are small and round to bean-shaped organs of varying sizes. Two functions of lymph nodes are (1) production of lymphocytes and plasma cells, and (2) filtering of bacteria and foreign particles carried by lymph. Lymph nodes are distributed throughout the body. They are situated both superficially and deep. The superficial nodes can be palpated, but the deep nodes must be visualized radiographically (refer to Fig. 23-5).

Normal Clotting Mechanisms

Blood clotting maintains the integrity of the body when various body structures are injured. Three components which contribute to normal clotting are a *vascular response*, *platelets*, and *plasma proteins*. A countermechanism to lyse the clot, the *fibrinolytic system*, maintains blood in its fluid form.

Vascular response

When a blood vessel is injured, an immediate local vasoconstrictive response occurs (Fig. 23-2). Vasoconstriction reduces the leakage of blood from the vessel not only by restricting the vessel size but also by pressing the endothelial surfaces together. The latter reaction enhances vessel wall stickiness and maintains closure of the vessel even after the vasoconstriction subsides.

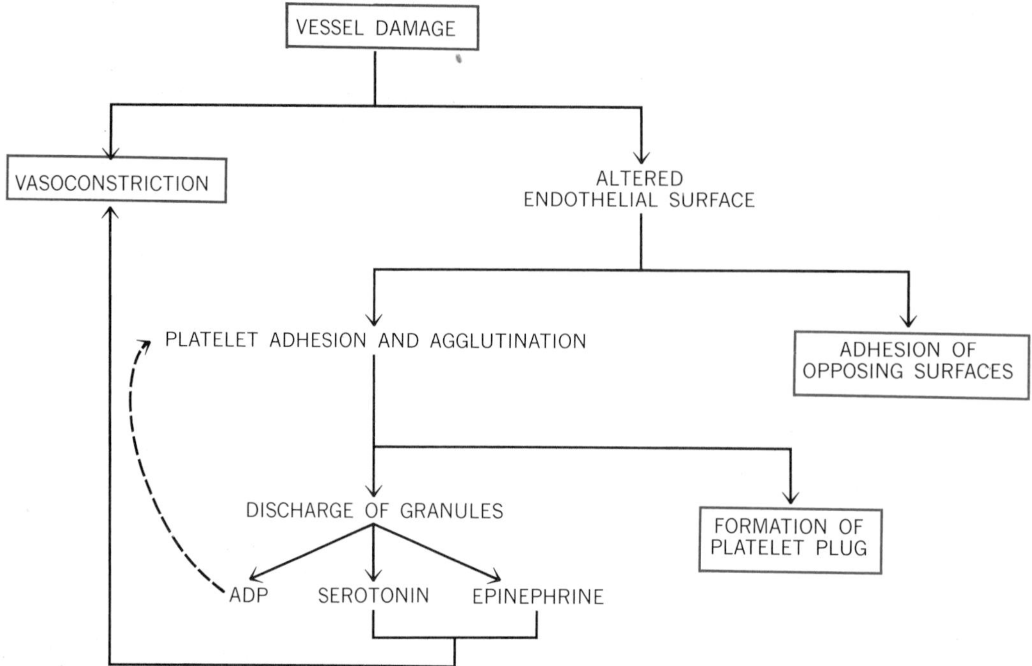

Figure 23-2 Hemostatic mechanisms involved in clotting. (*From D. Luciano, A. J. Vander, and J. H. Sherman, Human Function and Structure, McGraw-Hill Book Company, New York, 1978, p. 369. Used by permission of the publisher.*)

Platelet response

Platelets are activated when they are exposed to interstitial collagen from an injured blood vessel. Platelets stick to one another and form clumps. The stickiness is known as *adhesion*, and the formation of clumps is called *aggregation* or *agglutination*. When a blood vessel is injured, the circulating platelets are exposed to the collagen from the inner lining of the vessel. This interaction causes the platelets to release their substances, such as platelet factor three (PF3), serotonin, and epinephrine, which facilitate coagulation (Fig. 23-2). At the same time, platelets release adenosine diphosphate (ADP), which increases platelet adhesivity and aggregation, thereby enhancing the formation of a platelet plug.

Plasma proteins

The plasma proteins are known as *factors*, which are labeled in various ways to include the use of both names and Roman numerals (Table 23-1). Plasma proteins circulate in inactive forms until stimulated to initiate clotting through one of two pathways, *intrinsic* or *extrinsic*. The intrinsic pathway is activated by endothelial injury or blood vessel damage, whereas the extrinsic pathway is initiated when tissue thromboplastin is released extravascularly from injured tissues.

Regardless of whether clotting is initiated by substances internal or external to the blood vessel, coagulation follows the common pathway of the clotting cascade. It is important to understand that the *thrombin* in the common pathway is the most powerful enzyme in the coagulation process (Fig. 23-3).

Fibrinolysis

The *fibrinolytic* system is the countermechanism to blood clotting. It provides clot-lysing activities to maintain blood in a fluid state. The fibrinolytic system begins when plasminogen is activated to plasmin (Fig. 23-4). The plasmin attacks either fibrin or fibrinogen by splitting the molecules into smaller elements known as *fibrin split products* (*FSPs*) or *fibrin degradation products* (*FDPs*).

If fibrinolysis is excessive, clients will be predisposed to bleeding. In such a situation, bleeding results from the destruction of fibrin in platelet plugs or the effects of increased FSPs, which include impaired platelet aggregation, reduced prothrombin, and an inability to stabilize fibrin.

ASSESSMENT OF THE HEMATOLOGIC SYSTEM

Subjective Data: The History

Much of the evaluation of the hematologic system is based on a thorough history. Consequently, the nurse must be knowledgeable about what items to include in the nursing history so that questions may be phrased in a manner which will produce the most information related to the hematologic problem.

Past medical history

It is important to learn if the client has had prior hematologic problems. A previous laboratory determination of anemia must be explored, as should diagnoses of mononucleosis and malabsorption. Specific past surgeries to ask about include splenectomy, tumor removal, prosthetic heart valve placement, and surgical excision of the duodenum, which is responsible for iron absorption. The nurse should also ascertain how wound healing progressed postoperatively and if and when any bleeding problems occurred in relation to the surgery. Wound healing and bleeding

Table 23-1
Coagulation Factors

Factor	Name or Synonym
I	Fibrinogen
II	Prothrombin
III	Thromboplastin Tissue factor
IV	Calcium
V	Proaccelerin Labile factor Ac globulin
VI	Not assigned
VII	Stable factor Convertin Serum prothrombin conversion accelerator (SPCA)
VIII	Antihemophilic globulin (AHG) Antihemophilic factor (AHF)
IX	Plasma thromboplastin component (PTC) Antihemophilic factor B
X	Stuart-Prower factor Stuart factor
XI	Plasma thromboplastin antecedent (PTA) Antihemophilic factor C
XII	Hageman factor Antihemophilic factor D
XIII	Fibrin-stabilizing factor (FSF)

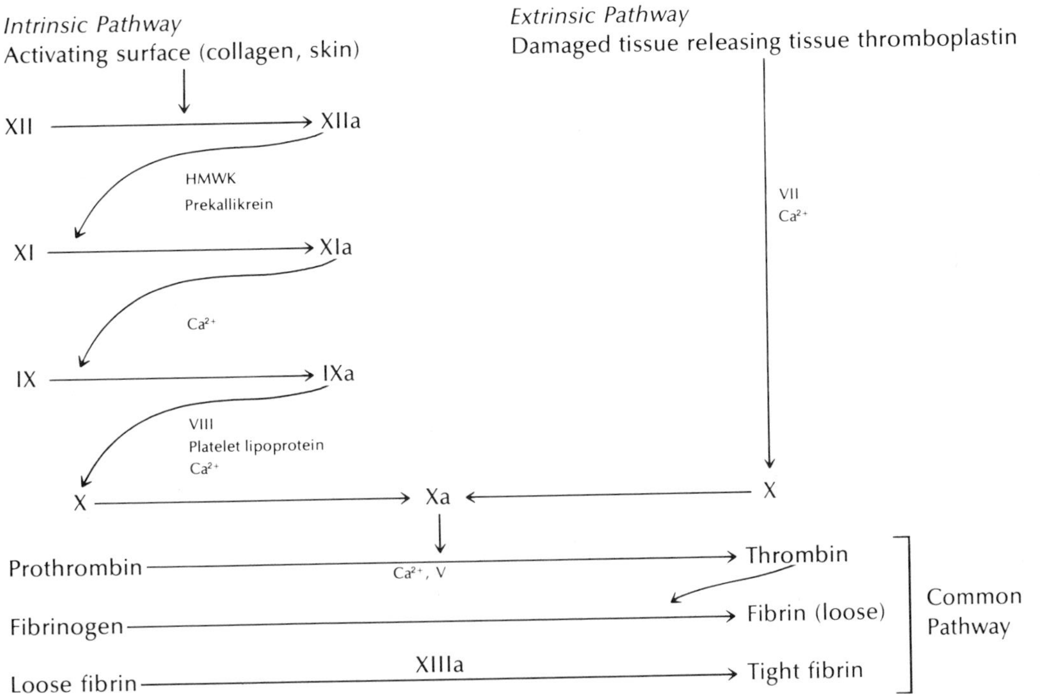

Figure 23-3 Pathways to coagulation. [*From S. Price and L. Wilson (eds.), Pathophysiology, Clinical Concepts of Disease Processes, 2d ed., McGraw-Hill Book Company, New York, 1982, p. 192. Used by permission of the publisher.*]

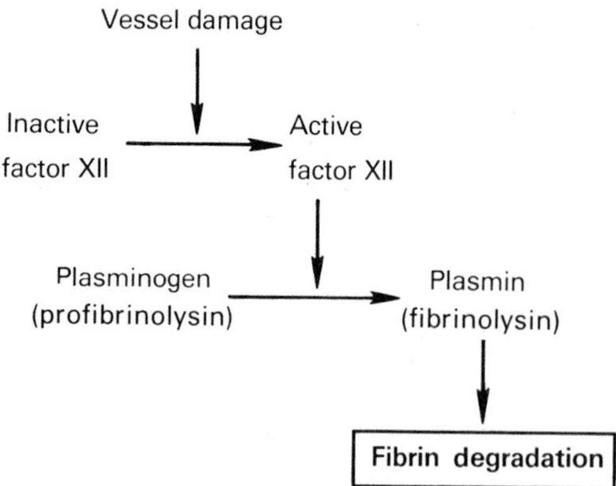

Figure 23-4 Fibrinolytic system.

should also be discussed as responses to other past injuries and to dental extractions. The nurse should also ask about any recurring infections and problems with blood clotting.

Known allergies and allergic reactions, including anaphylaxis, must be addressed. The number of previous blood transfusions and possible complications during the blood administration must also be evaluated. The nurse should ask if the client has had any abnormal bleeding or bruising in the past. Prior diagnosis of liver problems such as hepatitis or cirrhosis must also be noted.

Current medications

There are many drugs which may interfere with normal hematologic function (Table 23-2). In addition to these drugs, many antineoplastic agents used to treat malignant disorders cause depression of the bone marrow (Chap. 11).

Family history

There is a known genetic influence in certain hematologic conditions, as well as other blood diseases which follow familial patterns. When taking a family history, be sure to explore the following: jaundice, anemia, malignancies, congenital red blood cell dyscrasias such as sickle cell disease, and bleeding disorders (the predisposition both to bleed, as in hemophilia, and to clot, as in polycythemia).

Social and personal history

The significant sources of data related to social and personal history are exposure to radiation, exposure to chemicals, and dietary history. It is known that individuals who have been exposed to radiation, as a treatment modality or by accident, have a higher incidence of certain hematologic problems. The same is true for individuals who are exposed to chemicals (e.g., benzene, lead, naphthalene, and phenylbutazone).

A dietary history may provide clues to the cause of erythrocyte deficiencies. Iron, vitamin B_{12}, and folic acid are necessary for the development of red cells. Iron and folic acid deficiencies may be prevented by adequate intake of such foodstuffs as liver, meat, eggs, whole-grain and enriched breads and cereals, potatoes, leafy green vegetables, dried fruits, legumes, and citrus fruits. Inadequate vitamin B_{12} ingestion may be due to poor dietary intake (especially lack of liver, milk, and eggs). Folic acid deficiencies may be offset by a diet including foods which are also high in iron.

Alcohol abuse must be tactfully explored because the calories from the ethanol suppress the appetite for more nutritious foods. Chronic alcohol abusers frequently have vitamin deficiencies. Alcohol also exerts a damaging effect on the liver, where several clotting factors are produced. Consequently, bleeding problems can develop.

Review of systems

Many of the symptoms related to hematologic dysfunction are more generalized than specific. General complaints which should alert the nurse to the possibility of a hematologic disorder include fatigue, apathy, lethargy, malaise, weakness, chills, fever, night sweats, weight loss, heat intolerance, and poor wound healing. Specifics of the chief complaint should be evaluated and a methodical review of systems completed. A general complaint (e.g., a bruise on the thigh) indicates a need to assess the skin and musculoskeletal system of the involved area.

The client should be questioned about anemia, unusual or excessive bleeding or bruising, and lymph node swelling as well as poor wound healing. Past blood transfusions and possible reactions should be recorded. If there is a positive response, a review of systems of the involved area should be obtained.

Bleeding and bruising are significant findings. To avoid missing critical information about these problems, specific questions such as the following can be asked:[3]

How often do you notice a new bruise on your body?

What is the largest bruise that you have developed following injury so minor that you did not recall it until after you saw the bruise?

Do you develop bruises at sites of immunization or parenteral injections of drugs?

Table 23-2
Drugs Which May Affect Hematologic Function

Drug	Clinical Use	Hematologic Effect
Aminosalicylic acid (Pamisyl, PAS)	Antituberculin	Leukocytosis secondary to hypersensitivity
Amphotericin B (Fungilin, Fungizone)	Antifungal	Anemia
Acetylsalicylic acid (aspirin)	Analgesic, antipyretic, anti-inflammatory	Reduced platelet aggregation Prolonged bleeding time
Azathioprine (Imuran)	Immunosuppression	Anemia Leukopenia
Carbamazepine (Tegretol)	Pain of trigeminal neuralgia	Anemia Leukopenia Thrombocytopenia
Chloramphenicol (Chloromycetin)	Antibiotic	Anemia Neutropenia Thrombocytopenia
Chlorothiazide (Diuril)	Diuretic	Occasional thrombocytopenia
Oral contraceptives and diethylstilbestrol	Birth control Menopausal symptoms Functional uterine bleeding Cancer of prostate Postmenopausal cancer of the breast	Increase factors II, V, VII, VIII, IX, X; increase fibrinogen; increase thrombin; decreases prothrombin and partial thromboplastin times. Overall effect is to increase coagulation and thromboemboli formation
Diphenylhydantoin (Dilantin)	Anticonvulsant	Anemia
Epinephrine (Adrenalin)	Sympathomimetic	Leukocytosis
Glucocorticoids (ACTH, prednisone, etc.)	Anti-inflammatory	Lymphopenia Neutrophilia
Isoniazid (INH)	Antituberculin	Neutropenia
Methyldopa (Aldomet)	Antihypertensive	Hemolytic anemia
Phenacetin (APC, Empirin compound)	Analgesic antipyretic	Anemia
Phenylbutazone (Butazolidin)	Anti-inflammatory	Anemia Leukopenia Neutropenia Thrombocytopenia
Trimethoprim-sulfamethoxazole (Bactrim, Septrin)	Antibacterial	Anemia Leukopenia Neutropenia Thrombocytopenia

Objective Data: The Physical Examination

In order to examine accurately all systems which affect or are affected by the hematologic system, a complete physical examination is necessary (see Chap. 3). For instance, a decreasing level of consciousness may be due to an intracranial hemorrhage and indicates the need for a neurologic examination. Absent bowel sounds may be due to abdominal hemorrhage and indicate the need for a complete gastrointestinal examination. The nurse must keep in mind that signs and symptoms can be due to hematologic problems even though these are not the obvious cause (Table 23-3).

Table 23-3
Common Assessment Abnormalities of the Hematologic System

System	Manifestation	Possible Etiology/Significance
Skin	Pallor	Decreased quantity of hemoglobin (anemia)
	Flushing	Increased hemoglobin (polycythemia)
	Jaundice	Accumulation of bile pigment due to rapid or excessive hemolysis
	Purpura, petechiae, and ecchymoses	Hemostatic deficiency resulting in hemorrhage into the skin
	Excoriation and pruritus	Scratching from intense pruritus secondary to disorders such as Hodgkin's disease
	Leg ulcers	Common in sickle cell disease; especially prominent on the malleoli
	Brownish discoloration	Hemosiderin and melanin from the breakdown of erythrocytes
	Cyanosis	Increased amounts of reduced hemoglobin (secondary polycythemia)
Eyes	Jaundiced sclera	Accumulation of bile pigment due to rapid or excessive homolysis
	Conjunctival pallor	Reduced quantity of hemoglobin (anemia)
	Retinal hemorrhages	Seen more frequently in concurrent states of thrombocytopenia and anemia than with thrombocytopenia alone
Mouth	Pallor	Reduced quantity of hemoglobin (anemia)
	Gingival and mucosal ulceration	Neutropenia
	Gum infiltration (swelling, reddening, bleeding)	Leukemia either because of impeded movement of granulocytes and monocytes through the gingival-tooth attachment into the mucous membrane or because of inability of impaired leukocytes to combat oral infections
	Mucosal bleeding	Hemorrhagic diseases, thrombocytopenia
	Smooth tongue texture	Pernicious and iron deficiency anemia
Lymph nodes	Lymphadenopathy, tenderness	Hyperplasia of lymphatic tissue: a normal response to infection in infants and children; in adults, is caused by cancerous invasion, enlargement due to infection, foreign infiltrates, or metabolic disturbances, especially with lipids
Chest	Widened mediastinum	Enlarged lymph nodes
	Sternal tenderness:	
	Generalized	Leukemia resulting from increased bone marrow cellularity, which causes increased pressure and bone erosion
	Localized	Multiple myeloma due to stretching of the periosteum
	Tachycardia	Compensatory mechanism in anemia to increase cardiac output
	Widened pulse pressure	Compensatory mechanism in anemia to increase cardiac output by increasing stroke volume
	Murmurs	Usually a systolic murmur in anemia due to increased quantity and speed of low-viscosity blood going through the pulmonic valve
	Bruits (especially carotid bruits)	In anemia, due to increased flow of low-viscosity blood swirling through the blood vessels
Abdomen	Hepatomegaly	Leukemia
	Splenomegaly	Leukemia, lymphomas, mononucleosis
	Splenic bruits and rubs	Splenic infarction
Nervous system	Pain and touch, position and vibratory sensation, tendon reflexes	Impaired nervous system function due to vitamin B_{12} deficiency or compression of the nerves by masses

Table 23-3 (Continued)

System	Manifestation	Possible Etiology/Significance
Back and extremities	Back pain	Acute hemolytic reaction from flank pain due to renal involvement with hemolysis; multiple myeloma from enlarged tumors which stretch the periosteum or weaken supportive tissue, causing ligament strain and muscle spasm
	Arthralgia	Leukemia due to aching in bones which contain marrow; sickle cell disease from hemarthrosis
	Bone pain	Bone invasion by leukemia cells

Since specific system examinations are covered in other assessment chapters, the evaluation of the hematologic system will focus on examination of the lymph nodes.

Lymph nodes are distributed throughout the body. The superficial nodes can be evaluated by light palpation (Fig. 23-5). Deep nodes are detected radiographically. Lymph nodes should be assessed symmetrically in regard to five characteristics:

1. Location
2. Size in centimeters
3. Degree of fixation (e.g., movable, fixed)
4. Tenderness
5. Texture

The examiner should lightly palpate lymph nodes over the appropriate areas. The pads of the index and third fingers are most often used. The examiner should gently roll the skin over the area and concentrate on feeling for possible lymph node enlargement. When not specifically examined for their status, lymph nodes are usually palpated during the examination of the region where the nodes are located. For example, the axillary lymph nodes are examined at the completion of the breast examination.

It is important to develop a sequence when examining the lymph nodes. The lymph nodes of the head and neck drain areas of the mouth, throat, abdomen, breast, thorax, and arm. A convenient sequence for examination is preauricular, posterior auricular, occipital, tonsillar, submaxillary, submental, superficial cervical, posterior cervical chain, deep cervical chain, and supraclavicular (Fig. 23-5). This portion of the lymph node examination is usually done while the examiner is standing behind the client.

The axillary lymph nodes drain lymph from the chest wall, breasts, arms, and hands. The pectoral, subscapular, and lateral groups of nodes are next palpated. The epitrochlear nodes, located in the antecubital fossa between the biceps and triceps muscles, are then examined. These nodes drain specific areas of the forearm and hand. The inguinal lymph nodes are palpated last. These nodes drain the lower extremities.

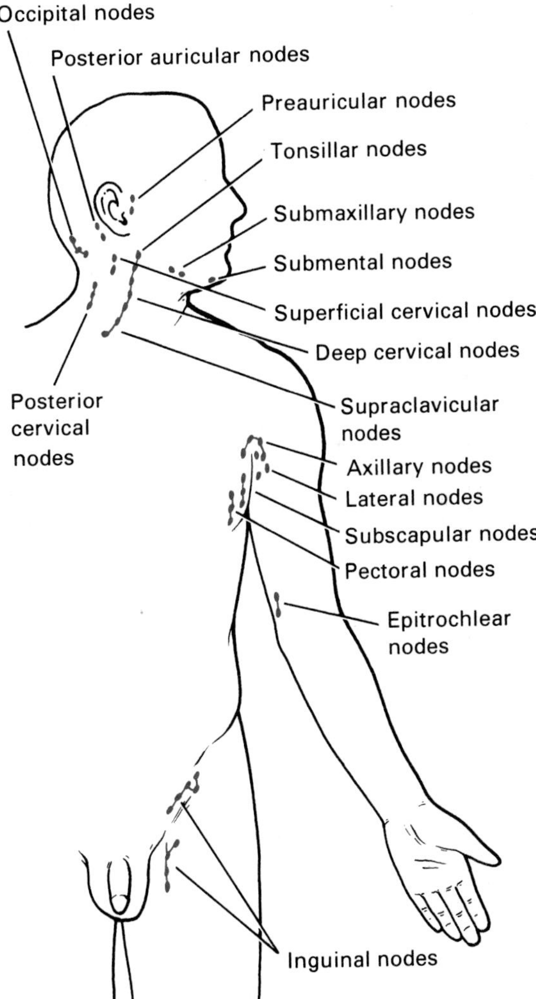

Figure 23-5 Palpable superficial lymph nodes.

Lymph nodes are generally not palpable unless there is residual enlargement from a previous or current infection. It may be normal to find small (0.5 to 1.0 cm), mobile, discrete, firm, nontender nodes, known as *shotty nodes*. Tender nodes are usually due to inflammation, whereas hard or fixed nodes are suggestive of malignancy.

Additional hematologic data can also be acquired from other body systems. Careful inspection of the skin (Chap. 16) and palpation of the liver and spleen (Chap. 31) are important examinations to include in a hematologic assessment. The most direct means of evaluating the hematologic system is through laboratory analysis and other diagnostic studies.

DIAGNOSTIC STUDIES OF THE HEMATOLOGIC SYSTEM

The nurse should recognize the need to explain thoroughly any diagnostic procedures to the client. It is not uncommon for clients to be anxious when faced with illness. Therefore, instructions must be simple, clear, and repeated when necessary to decrease anxiety and ensure client compliance with preparatory protocols. Whether studies are performed on an outpatient or inpatient basis, written instructions regarding the procedures may facilitate compliance.

It must also be recognized that the repeated acquisition of blood specimens may be very disconcerting for the client. Some clients, as well as staff, may become concerned that the amount of blood withdrawn for tests could lead to adverse effects. Although multiple blood studies may be uncomfortable, research has shown that only in rare situations does diagnostic blood withdrawal predispose clients to significant volume loss.[4]

Laboratory Studies

Complete blood count

The *complete blood count* (*CBC*) involves several laboratory tests (Table 23-4).

Red Blood Cells Normal values of some red blood cell tests are reported separately for men and women because normal values are based on body mass, and men usually have a larger body mass than women.

Hemoglobin (*Hb*) will be reduced in cases of anemia, hemorrhage, or states of hemodilution such as those that occur when the fluid volume is excessive. Increases in hemoglobin are found in polycythemia or in states of hemoconcentration which can develop from volume depletion.

The *hematocrit* (*Hct*) is done by spinning blood in a centrifuge, which causes erythrocytes and plasma to separate. The erythrocytes, being the heavier elements, settle to the bottom. Reductions and elevations of hematocrit are seen in the same conditions which raise and lower the hemoglobin. The hematocrit generally equals three times the hemoglobin.

The *total red blood cell* (*RBC*) *count* is reported on a laboratory slip as RBCs $\times 10^6$ (million). However, total RBC count is not always reliable in determining the adequacy of red cell function. Consequently, other data such as hemoglobin, hematocrit, and red cell indices must also be evaluated. The RBC count is altered by the same conditions which raise and lower the hemoglobin and hematocrit.

Red cell indices are special indicators which reflect red cell volume, color, and saturation. These parameters may provide insight into the cause of anemia. The significance of these parameters is discussed further in Chap. 24.

White Blood Cells The *white blood cell* (*WBC*) *differential* is of considerable significance because it is possible for the total WBC count to remain essentially normal despite a marked change in one type of leukocyte. For example, a client may have a normal WBC count of 8800/μL. The differential count may show a relative proportion of lymphocytes to be 10 percent. This is an abnormal finding which warrants further investigation.[5]

An important concept related to neutrophil counts is the *shift to the left*. When infections are severe, more granulocytes are released from the bone marrow as a compensatory mechanism. In order to meet the increased demand, many young, immature PMNs or *bands* are seen. The usual laboratory procedure is to report the white blood cells in order of maturity, with the less mature forms on the left side of the written report. Consequently, the existence of many immature cells is referred to as a *shift to the left*.

Platelet Count Bleeding may occur when *platelet counts* are depressed, a condition known as *thrombocytopenia*. If platelets are functioning properly, most hematologists believe that clients can undergo necessary surgery with platelet counts as low as 50,000/μL (the normal count is 150,000 to 400,000/μL). Once platelet counts drop to between 30,000 and 20,000/μL, spontaneous hemorrhage is probable. When platelets are depressed to 10,000/μL, the possibility of intracerebral hemorrhage is significantly increased. Clotting studies are presented in Table 23-5.

Table 23-4
CBC Studies

Study	Description and Purpose	Normal Values
Hb	Measures the gas-carrying capacity of the red cell. Gives red cells their color.	Female: 12–16 g/dL Male: 13.5–18 g/dL
Hct	Compares volume of RBCs to volume of plasma. Measured as a percent of total blood volume (%).	Female: 38–47% Male: 40–54%
Total RBC count	Count of the number of RBCs.	Female: 4.2–5.4 × $10^6/\mu L$ Male: 4.6–6.2 × $10^6/\mu L$
Red cell indices		
Mean corpuscular volume (MCV) $= \frac{Hct \times 10}{RBC \times 10^6}$	Determines relative size of the RBCs. Low MCV reflects microcytosis. High MCV reflects macrocytosis.	82–98 fl
Mean corpuscular hemoglobin (MCH) $= \frac{Hb \times 10}{RBC \times 10^6}$	Measures the amount of Hb/RBCs. Low MCH indicates microcytosis or hypochromia. High MCH indicates macrocytosis.	27–31 pg
Mean corpuscular hemoglobin concentration (MCHC) $= \frac{Hb}{HcT} \times 100$	Evaluates RBC saturation with Hb. Low MCHC indicates hypochromia. High MCHC seen in spherocytosis.	32–36%
WBC count	Measures total number of leukocytes.	5000–10,000/μL
WBC differential (neutrophils, eosinophils, basophils, lymphocytes, monocytes)	Determines if each kind of WBC is present in the proper proportion. Absolute values are determined by multiplying the percentage of the cell type by the total WBC count and dividing by 100.	Neutrophils:40–70% Eosinophils:2–4% Basophils:<1% Lymphocytes:20–40% Monocytes:4–8%
Platelet count	Measures the number of platelets available to maintain platelet clotting functions (Does not measure the quality of platelet function.)	150,000–400,000/μL

Erythrocyte sedimentation rate (ESR, or sed rate)

Increased sedimentation rates are common during acute and chronic inflammatory reactions when cell destruction is increased. They are also found in malignancy, myocardial infarction, and end-stage renal disease. Although the sed rate is a very nonspecific test, it is often used as a routine screening procedure.

Blood typing and Rh factor

Blood group antigens (A and B) are found on red cell membranes and form the basis for the ABO blood typing system. The presence or absence of one or both of the two inherited antigens is the basis for the four blood groups: A, B, AB, and O. Blood group A has A antigens, group B has B antigens, group AB has both antigens, and group O has neither A nor B. Each person has antibodies in the serum called *anti-A* and *anti-B* that react with A or B antigens. These antibodies are found when the corresponding antigen is absent from the red cell surface. For example, B antibodies are found in individuals with A blood (Table 23-6).

Blood reactions based on ABO incompatibilities result from intravascular hemolysis of the red blood cells. Erythrocytes agglutinate when a serum antibody is present to react with the antigens on the red cell membrane. Therefore, agglutination occurs in group A blood when B antigens are introduced. The anti-B antibodies will react with the B antigen, thus initiating the process which results in red cell hemolysis.

The Rh system is based on a third antigen, D, which is also found on the red cell membrane. Rh-positive individuals have the D antigen, whereas Rh-negative individuals do not. About 85 percent of

Table 23-5

Clotting (Coagulation) Studies

Study	Description and Purpose	Normal Values
Prothrombin time (PT)	Assesses extrinsic coagulation by measuring factors II, VII, IX, and X. These vitamin K–dependent factors are depressed by coumarin derivatives.	12–15 s
Partial thromboplastin time (PTT)	Assesses intrinsic coagulation by measuring factors I, II, V, VIII, IX, X, XI, XII. Prolonged by use of heparin.	30–60 s
Bleeding time	Measures the length of time a small skin incision bleeds. Reflects the ability of small blood vessels to constrict.	1–6 min
Activated clotting time (ACT)	Evaluates the ability of the blood to clot. Nonspecific, since a deficiency of any clotting factor will prolong the clotting time.	92–128 s
Thrombin time (TT)	Reflects adequacy of thrombin. A prolonged TT indicates that coagulation is inadequate secondary to decreased thrombin activity.	8–12 s
Fibrinogen	Reflects level of fibrinogen. Increased fibrinogen indicates enhancement of fibrin formation, making the client hypercoagulable. Decreased fibrinogen suggests that the client may be predisposed to bleeding.	200–400 mg/dL
Fibrin split products (FSPs). (Also known as fibrin degradation products, or FDPs)	Reflects the degree of fibrinolysis. Presence of FSPs reflects excessive fibrinolysis, and clients will be predisposed to bleed. May also indicate disseminated intravascular coagulation (DIC) (Chap. 24).	None, although 1–10 may occur without the development of bleeding
Protamine sulfate tests	Reflects the presence of fibrin monomer, the portion of fibrin remaining after the elements which polymerize and stabilize the clot are detached. A positive test indicates that the client is predisposed to bleed and may have DIC.	Negative

Table 23-6

ABO Blood Group Names and Compatibilities*

Blood Group or Type	Red Blood Cell Agglutinogen(s)	Serum Agglutinin(s)	Compatible Donor Blood Groups or Types	Incompatible Donor Blood Groups or Types
A	A	Anti-B	A and O	B and AB
B	B	Anti-A	B and O	A and AB
AB	A and B	Neither (universal recipient)	A, B, AB, and O	None
O	Neither (universal donor)	Anti-A and Anti-B	O	A, B, and AB

*ABO blood groups are named for the antigen (agglutinogen) found in the red blood cells. Compatibility is based on the antibodies (agglutinins) present in the serum.

D. A. Jones et al., *Medical-Surgical Nursing: A Conceptual Approach*, 2d ed., McGraw-Hill Book Company, New York, 1982, p. 401.

persons are Rh positive and 15 percent are Rh negative. As a result of transfusion therapy or during childbirth, an Rh-negative person may be exposed to Rh-positive blood. Such exposure results in that person's formation of an antibody, anti-D, which acts against Rh antigens. (Rh-positive persons normally have no anti-D.) The person is then said to be sensitized to Rh-positive blood, and a second exposure to Rh-positive blood will cause a severe hemolytic reaction. A Coombs' test can be used to evaluate the Rh status (Table 23-7).

Radiologic Studies

Lymphangiography is radiologic visualization of the lymph system after the injection of dye. The purpose of this procedure is assessment of the deep lymph nodes. It is particularly useful in detecting lymph node involvement in malignant conditions.

The procedure begins with the injection of a blue dye intracutaneously into the webs of the toes. (It is less commonly done through the hands.) The dye is absorbed by the lymph vessels, making them visible through the skin on the dorsum of the foot. Once visible, the dorsum of each foot is injected with a local anesthetic agent, and a small superficial incision is made over the lymph vessels. The lymph vessel is then cannulated with a very small needle. Once the needle is inserted, it is important that the client not move his feet to avoid the possibility of dislodging the needles. When the lymph vessels are cannulated, a radiopaque oil is injected very slowly by an automated pump. The usual dose of oil for adults is 7 mL in each foot administered over 45 to 60 minutes. Fluoroscopy may be used during the injection to watch the filling of the lymph vessels. Immediately after the dye has been injected, several radiographs will be done from various angles. A second set of radiographs will be done the next day when the lymph channels are emptied. The incisions on the feet are sutured closed when the procedure is complete. Nursing responsibilities related to lymphangiography and other common studies of the hematological system are presented in Table 23-8.

Biopsies

Biopsy procedures specific to hematologic assessment are *bone marrow examination* and *lymph node biopsy*.

Bone marrow examination

Bone marrow examination is important in the evaluation of many hematologic disorders. It involves

Table 23-7
Miscellaneous Laboratory Blood Studies

Study	Description and Purpose	Normal Values
ESR or sed rate	Measures the rate at which RBCs settle to the bottom of a test tube in 1 h. Affected by certain blood elements, especially protein.	Female: 1–20 mm in 1 h Male: 1–15 mm in 1 h
Reticulocyte count	Immature RBCs. Reflects bone marrow activity in producing RBCs.	0.5–1.5% of RBC count
Bilirubin Total Direct Indirect	Measures degree of RBC hemolysis or the liver's inability to excrete normal quantities of bilirubin. Indirect bilirubin rises when hemolytic problems occur.	Total: 0.3–1.3 mg/dL Direct: 0.1–0.3 mg/dL Indirect: 0.1–1.0 mg/dL
Iron		
Serum iron	Reflects the amount of iron combined with proteins in the serum. Accurately indicates the status of iron storage and use.	50–150 μg/dL
Total iron-binding capacity (TIBC)	Measures the percentage of saturation of transferrin, a protein which binds iron. Evaluates the amount of extra iron which could be carried.	250–410 μg/dL
Coombs' test	Purpose is to differentiate among types of hemolytic anemias and to detect immune antibodies.	
Direct	Detects antibodies (IgG) which are attached to RBCs.	Negative
Indirect	Detects antibodies (IgG) in the serum.	Negative

Table 23-8
Diagnostic Studies of the Hematologic System

Study	Description and Purpose	Nursing Responsibility
Blood studies (see Tables 23-4, 23-5, and 23-7)		
Urine studies		
Bence-Jones protein	An electrophoretic measurement used to detect the presence of the Bence-Jones protein, which is found in most cases of multiple myeloma (Chap. 24). Negative finding indicates that the client is normal.	No specific role other than to acquire a random urine specimen.
Radioisotope studies		
Spleen scan	Radioactive isotope is injected intravenously. Images from the radioactive emissions are used to evaluate the structure of the spleen.	No dietary preparation. Isotope administered in nuclear medicine. Client is not a source of radioactivity.
Bone scan	Same as for the spleen scan, except for the purpose of evaluating the structure of the bones.	Same as for the spleen.
Radiologic studies		
Lymphangiography	Purpose is to evaluate deep lymph nodes. Radiopaque oil-based dye is infused slowly into the lymph vessels via small needles in the dorsum of each foot. Radiographs are done immediately and on the next day.	*Before procedure*: Teach the client about what to anticipate. Consent form required. Assess for iodine sensitivity. Preop sedation often given. *After procedure*: Instruct client that urine will be blue from the dye excretion for 1–2 days. Client may experience transient fever, general malaise, and diffuse muscle aches for 12–24 h. Watch for signs of oil embolus to lungs (hacking cough, dyspnea, pleuritic pain, and hemoptysis).
Biopsies		
Bone marrow	Removal of bone marrow through a locally anesthetized site to evaluate the status of the blood-forming tissue. Indicated in diagnosing multiple myeloma, all types of leukemia, and some lymphomas. Also done to assess the efficacy of leukemic therapy (Chap. 24).	Explain procedure to client. Obtain signed consent form. Apply pressure dressing after procedure. Assess biopsy site for bleeding.
Lymph node biopsy	Purpose is to obtain lymph tissue for histologic examination to determine the diagnosis and therapy.	Explain procedure to client. Obtain signed consent form. Employ sterile technique in dressing changes after the procedure. Carefully evaluate the wound for healing. Assess the client for complications, especially bleeding.
1. Open	Done in surgery with direct visualization of the area.	
2. Closed (needle)	Done at the bedside.	

the aspiration of bone marrow with a syringe and needle.

The site of bone marrow aspiration is determined by the age of the client and the skill of the physician or specially credentialed nurse. In adults, the sites most easily biopsied are the sternum and anterior or posterior iliac crests. The tibia may provide an additional site in young children. Although hazards of bone marrow aspiration are minimal, there is the possibility of penetrating the bone and damaging underlying structures.

The skin over the puncture site is cleansed with a bactericidal agent. The skin, subcutaneous tissue, and periosteum are infiltrated with a local anesthetic agent. The client will be uncomfortable when the periosteum is infiltrated. Once the area is anesthetized, the special marrow needle is inserted through the cortex of the bone. The stylet of the needle is then removed, the hub is attached to a 10-mL syringe, and 0.2 to 0.5 mL of the fluid marrow is aspirated. The aspiration is experienced by the client as a suction pain which may be quite uncomfortable but lasts for only a few seconds.

After the marrow aspiration, the needle is removed. Pressure is applied over the aspiration site to ensure hemostasis. If the client is thrombocytopenic, pressure may be required for 5 to 10 minutes or longer.

If a bone biopsy is required, the preparatory procedure remains the same, but a different needle is used. The needle has a cutting blade which allows a specimen of the bone to be removed. When either a marrow aspirate or biopsy is acquired, a glass slide is carefully prepared with a thin film of the marrow. Laboratory personnel should be available at the bedside to perform this essential part of the procedure.

Lymph node biopsy

Lymph node biopsy involves obtaining lymph tissue for histologic examination to determine the diagnosis and therapy. This may be accomplished by either an *open biopsy* or a *needle* (*closed*) *biopsy*. In the open biopsy, an incision is made and the lymph node and surrounding tissue will be dissected whenever possible. Neoplastic cells can be disseminated during the biopsy if the knife passes through tissues containing cancerous cells. An open biopsy may be done with local or general anesthesia in the operating room.

A needle or closed biopsy may also be done to analyze lymph tissue. This bedside technique is done by a skilled physician. Sterile technique is essential throughout the procedure. Nursing personnel must recognize the possibility of insidious bleeding, and direct pressure should be applied after the biopsy to achieve hemostasis. Personnel should continue to observe the site for bleeding, and vital signs should be monitored. The sterile dressing should be changed as ordered and the wound inspected for healing. It is important to recognize that if a needle biopsy is negative, it may signify only that the cancer cells were not a part of the tissue in the biopsy specimen. However, a positive finding is sufficient evidence for confirming a diagnosis.

REVIEW QUESTIONS

The number of the objective corresponds to the same numbered objective at the beginning of the chapter.

1. An important function of the spleen in the adult is
  a. red blood cell production
  b. monocyte production
  c. removal of defective erythrocytes
  d. platelet production

2. Which of the following are both types of granulocytes?
  a. basophils and neutrophils
  b. monocytes and eosinophils
  c. thrombocytes and lymphocytes
  d. erythrocytes and eosinophils

3. Which of the following substances are necessary for converting prothrombin to thrombin?
  a. fibrinogen and factor IX
  b. thromboplastin and calcium
  c. platelet factor III and factor V
  d. fibrin-stabilizing factor and sodium

4. Which of the following data obtained from the health history has a significant relationship to the hematologic system?
  a. multiple pregnancies
  b. early menopause
  c. jaundice
  d. bladder surgery

5. Which of the following statements accurately describes the technique to palpate lymph nodes?
  a. Gentle, firm pressure should be applied to deep lymph nodes.
  b. Normally, superficial lymph nodes are not palpable.
  c. The index and third fingers should lightly palpate superficial lymph nodes.
  d. The tips of the second, third, and fourth fingers should apply firm pressure for palpation.

6. Which of the following is considered a normal finding of the lymph node examination?
  a. shotty nodes
  b. firm, tender nodes
  c. hard, fixed nodes
  d. mobile, hard nodes

7. Which of the following is an important nursing responsibility following lymphangiography?
  a. Apply pressure dressing to biopsy site.
  b. Take precautions for isotope elimination.
  c. Immobilize lower extremities for 24 hours.
  d. Instruct client that urine may be blue.

REFERENCES

1. W. J. Williams, "Examination of the Bone Marrow," in W. J. Williams, E. Beutler, A. J. Erslev, and R. W. Rundles (eds.), *Hematology*, McGraw-Hill Book Company, New York, 1977, p. 25.
2. T. P. Stossel, "Functions of Granulocytes," in Williams et al., op. cit., pp. 691–693.
3. S. I. Rapaport, *Introduction to Hematology*, Harper & Row Publishers, Incorporated, New York, 1971, p. 305.
4. D. M. Lanuza and J. A. Jennrich, "The Amount of Blood Withdrawn for Diagnostic Tests in Critically Ill Patients," *Heart Lung*, **5**(5):933–938 (1976).
5. D. A. Nelson, "Leukocyte Disorders," in J. B. Henry (ed.), *Todd-Sanford-Davidsohn Clinical Diagnosis and Management by Laboratory Methods*, 16th ed., vol. I, W. B. Saunders Company, Philadelphia, 1979, pp. 1036–1037.

Chapter 24

NURSING ROLE IN MANAGEMENT

Hematologic Problems

Bonnie Mowinski Jennings

Learning Objectives

1. Describe the general clinical manifestations and complications of anemia.
2. Differentiate between the etiological and morphological classifications of anemia.
3. Describe the causes, specific clinical manifestations, diagnostic findings, and medical and pharmacological management of iron-deficiency anemia, pernicious anemia, and sickle cell anemia.
4. Explain the nursing management of anemia.
5. Describe the pathophysiology, clinical manifestations, and medical and nursing management of polycythemia vera.
6. Compare and contrast the pathophysiology, clinical manifestations, and medical management for idiopathic thrombocytopenic purpura (ITP) and acquired thrombocytopenia.
7. Explain the nursing management of thrombocytopenia.
8. Describe the types, clinical manifestations, diagnostic findings, and medical and nursing management of hemophilia.
9. Explain the pathophysiology, diagnostic findings, and medical and nursing management of disseminated intravascular coagulation (DIC).
10. Describe the common causes, clinical manifestations, and medical and nursing management of granulocytopenia.
11. Compare and contrast the major types of leukemia in regard to age at onset and distinguishing clinical and laboratory findings.
12. Explain the rationales for induction and maintenance chemotherapy and combination chemotherapy.
13. Describe the nursing management of the client with leukemia.
14. Differentiate between Hodgkin's and non-Hodgkin's lymphomas in terms of clinical manifestations, staging, and medical and nursing management.
15. Describe the pathophysiology, clinical manifestations, and medical and nursing management of multiple myeloma and mononucleosis.
16. Differentiate between splenomegaly and hypersplenism in terms of etiology and medical management.

The purpose of this chapter is to provide information on red cell abnormalities, clotting disorders, white cell abnormalities, lymph system disturbances, and spleen disorders.

ANEMIA

Definition and Classification

Anemia is a reduction below normal in the number of erythrocytes, the quantity of hemoglobin, and the volume of packed red cells (hematocrit).[1] Because red blood cells transport oxygen, a deficit in erythrocytes leads to tissue hypoxia. This hypoxia accounts for most of the clinical manifestations of anemia. Anemia is not a specific disease but a symptom of a pathological process. Anemia is identified by laboratory evaluation. In addition, further investigation must be done to determine its cause.

The opinions or assertions in this article are the views of the author and are not to be construed as official or as reflecting the views of the Department of the Army or the Department of Defense.

This chapter was reviewed by Bonnie Luhmann, R.N., B.S.N., Assistant Director, Medical-Surgical Nursing, St. Mary's Hospital, Rochester, Minnesota.

Anemia may result from primary hematologic problems or may develop as a secondary consequence of defects in other body systems. The many kinds of anemia can be grouped according to either a *morphological* or an *etiological classification*. Morphological classification is based on descriptive, objective laboratory information about erythrocyte size and color. The terms used in this classification system were explained in Chap. 23. Etiological classification is related to the clinical conditions causing the anemia, such as decreased erythrocyte production, blood loss, and increased erythrocyte destruction (Table 24-1). While the morphological system is the most accurate means of classifying anemias, it is easier to discuss client care by focusing on the etiological problem. Table 24-2 relates morphological classifications to various etiologies. The etiological classification will be used in this chapter to discuss anemia.

Mechanisms to Compensate for Hypoxia

Regardless of the source of anemia, the deficit in erythrocytes reduces the blood's oxygen-carrying capacity, which leads to tissue hypoxia. Both tissue

Table 24-1
Etiological Classification of Anemia

Decreased erythrocyte production
- Decreased hemoglobin synthesis
  - Iron deficiency
  - Thalassemias (decreased globin synthesis)
- Nuclear cytoplasmic defects (DNA)
  - Vitamin B_{12} deficiency (pernicious anemia)
  - Folic acid deficiency
- Decreased number of erythrocyte precursors
  - Hypoplastic anemia
  - Marrow infiltration (leukemia, lymphoma, myelofibrosis)
  - Chronic disease

Blood loss
- Acute
  - Trauma
  - Blood vessel rupture
- Chronic
  - GI
  - Menstrual flow

Increased erythrocyte destruction (hemolytic anemias)
- Intrinsic
  - Abnormal hemoglobin (HbS—sickle cell anemia)
  - Defective glycolysis with enzyme involvement (G6PD deficiency)
  - Membrane abnormalities (paroxysmal nocturnal hemoglobinuria)
- Extrinsic
  - Physical trauma
  - Antibodies (isoimmune and autoimmune)
  - Infectious agents and toxins

Table 24-2
Relationship of Morphological Classification and Etiologies of Anemia

Morphology	Etiology
Normocytic, normochromic	Hypoplastic anemia, chronic renal disease, acute blood loss, pregnancy, diseases of endocrine deficiency, hemolytic anemias
Macrocytic, normochromic	Pernicious anemia, folic acid deficiency, chronic liver disease
Microcytic, normochromic	Chronic illness (e.g., infection, malignancy)
Microcytic, hypochromic	Iron-deficiency anemia, thalassemia

hypoxia and activation of physiological compensatory mechanisms attempt to meet cellular oxygen needs that stimulate the pathophysiological effects of anemia.

The four major compensatory responses are as follows:

1. Shift of the oxyhemoglobin dissociation curve to the right, thereby facilitating removal of more oxygen by the tissues at the same partial pressure of oxygen (Fig. 24-1)
2. Redistribution of blood by an automatic physiological process that diverts the blood away from tissues which have an abundant blood supply but a low oxygen requirement (e.g., skin) to tissues which have higher oxygen needs (e.g., brain, muscle, myocardium)
3. Increased cardiac output achieved by increased heart rate or increased stroke volume to meet oxygen demands of the tissues as the severity of the anemia increases
4. Increased rate of erythrocyte production within 4 to 5 days after erythropoietin production has increased in response to tissue hypoxia[2]

Clinical Manifestations

The clinical manifestations of anemia are primarily due to the body's response to hypoxia. The intensity of the manifestations will vary depending upon the severity of the anemia and the presence of coexisting diseases. The severity of anemia may be determined by the hemoglobin levels. *Mild* states of anemia (Hb 10–14 g/dL) may exist without causing symptoms. If symptoms do develop, they are usually attributed to either an underlying disease or a compensatory response to heavy exercise. Cardiopulmonary adaptations to exercise include palpitations, dyspnea, and excessive diaphoresis. In cases of *moderate* anemia

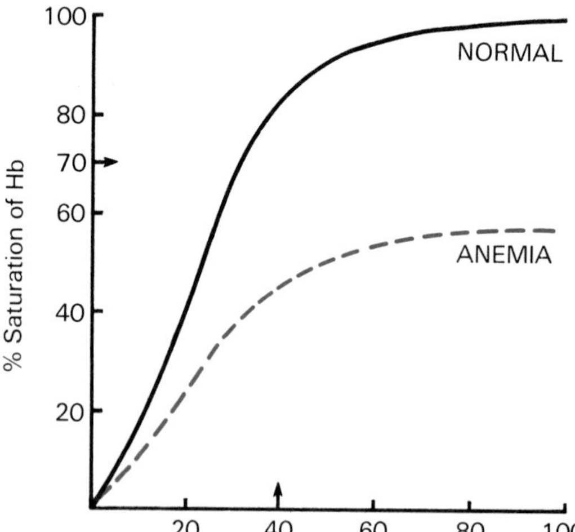

Figure 24-1 Oxyhemoglobin dissociation curve. The oxyhemoglobin curve of a normal person (bold line) with Hb of 15 g/dL compared to that of a person with anemia (dotted line) with Hb of 6 g/dL. The shift to the right seen with the anemic person is a compensatory mechanism. While the oxygen transport capability of hemoglobin is decreased with the shift to the right, hemoglobin release of oxygen to the tissues is facilitated.

Table 24-3
Clinical Manifestations of Anemia

Body System	Severity of Anemia		
	Mild (Hb 10–14 g/dL)	**Moderate (Hb 6–10 g/dL)**	**Severe (Hb < 6g/dL)**
Integument	None	None	Pallor, jaundice, pruritus
Eyes	None	None	Icteric conjunctivae and sclera, retinal hemorrhage, blurred vision
Mouth	None	None	Glossitis, smooth tongue
Cardiovascular	Palpitations	Increased palpitations	Tachycardia, increased pulse pressure, systolic murmurs, intermittent claudication, angina, congestive heart failure
Pulmonary	Exertional dyspnea	Dyspnea	Tachypnea, orthopnea
Neurological	None	None	Headache, vertigo, irritability, depression, impaired thought processes
GI	None	None	Nausea, vomiting, anorexia, hepatomegaly, splenomegaly
Skeletal	None	None	Bone pain
General	None	Fatigue	Sensitivity to cold, weight loss, lethargy

(Hb 6–10 g/dL), the cardiopulmonary symptoms are increased. Also, chronic fatigue will present during rest as well as activity.

Severe anemia

Clients with *severe* anemia (Hb less than 6 g/dL) will display many manifestations in multiple body systems (Table 24-3).

Integumentary Changes Integumentary changes may be reflected as pallor, jaundice, and pruritus. The pallor results from reduced amounts of hemoglobin and reduced blood flow to the skin. Jaundice occurs when the skin is stained by bile pigment, which increases from hemolysis of red blood cells. Pruritus occurs due to increased serum and skin bile salt concentrations. In addition to the skin, the eyes and mucous membranes should be evaluated because they reflect the integumentary changes more accurately.

Cardiopulmonary Manifestations Cardiopulmonary manifestations of severe anemia result from additional attempts by the heart and lungs to bring adequate amounts of oxygen to the tissues. Cardiac output is maintained by tachycardia. A widened pulse pressure reflects an increased stroke volume. The low viscosity of the blood contributes to the development of systolic murmurs and bruits. In extreme cases or when concomitant heart disease is present, angina pectoris and high output failure may occur if myocardial oxygen needs cannot be met. Cardiomegaly, pulmonary congestion, ascites, and peripheral edema may develop as the heart is overworked. The dyspnea of severe anemia, demonstrated by the presence of orthopnea and tachypnea, is an inappropriate response of the body to hypoxia or hypercapnia. It is inappropriate because the available hemoglobin is already fully saturated with oxygen.

Nursing Management

The many causes of anemia necessitate different nursing interventions specific to the needs of the client. Nevertheless, there are certain general components of care which may be required by all clients with anemia. These are given in the nursing care plan presented in Table 24-4. Nursing management for the specific causes of anemia is presented under the appropriate discussion on etiology.

ETIOLOGICAL CLASSIFICATIONS OF ANEMIA

Anemia Due to Decreased Erythrocyte Production

Normally, red cell production is in equilibrium with red cell destruction and loss. This balance is necessary to ensure that adequate numbers of erythrocytes are available. Red cells must be replenished, as they

Table 24-4
Nursing Care Plan for the Client with Anemia

Client Problem	Expected Outcome	Nursing Intervention
Fatigue	Feeling of being rested.	Plan care to alternate rest periods with activity periods (e.g., $\frac{1}{2}$ h activity, $1\frac{1}{2}$ h rest). Help client with bathing, eating, turning, hair brushing, oral hygiene. Reduce number of visitors, phone calls, and repeated unplanned interruptions by hospital staff (e.g., radiology, laboratory staffs). Assess BP, P, R as ordered or at least every 2–4 h.
Hypoxia	Heart rate less than 20 bpm above normal for the client. Respiratory rate 12–18/min.	(All of the interventions mentioned above.) Administer supplemental oxygen as ordered. Transfuse with blood products. Change client's position slowly and evaluate dizziness resulting from cerebral hypoxia.
Reduced blood volume	Blood pressure approximates pre-illness values.	(All of the inverventions mentioned for fatigue and hypoxia.) Administer parenteral fluids as ordered. Monitor urine output to maintain output to 30–50 mL/h. Evaluate body excreta for gross or occult blood.
Anorexia, weight loss, nausea, vomiting	Cessation of weight loss. Normal nutritional intake.	Small, frequent feedings of foods which require minimal chewing. Serve soft, bland, cool or minimally spicy foods. Offer foods which are nutritionally adequate but also appealing to the client. Assess the need for temporary use of antiemetics.
Predisposition to decubital ulcer formation and poor wound healing	No decubital ulcers or injuries secondary to trauma or pressure.	Turn client at least every 2 h during the day and every 4 h at night. Post a schedule and be specific. Use protective devices on the bed mattress (sheepskin, eggshell mattress, alternating air-pressure mattress). Assess the skin for redness when turning, especially over bony prominences and pressure areas. Ambulate client as soon as possible. Protect client from injury.
Mouth and tongue sores	Resolution of sores.	Use soft-bristle toothbrush or cotton swabs for mouth care. Plan the use of soothing mouthwashes every 2–4 h. Use low-flow Water Pik for cleansing.
Anxiety	Relaxed feeling.	Explain slowly and in a soothing tone the reasons for symptoms and treatment. Use understandable terms. Correct client's misconceptions. Employ imagery and relaxation techniques. Assess the need for sedatives or tranquilizers.
Predisposition to infection	Normal temperature. No signs of infection.	Assess oral temperature every 4 h. Use good handwashing techniques for self and client. Use isolation technique if ordered. Prevent contact with individuals known to be infected. Help client turn, cough, and deep-breathe to maintain respiratory function.
Predisposition to thermal injury	No thermal injuries.	For complaints of cold or chilling, *do not* use hot water bottles or mechanical heating devices. Provide warmth with extra clothing and blankets.
Dietary deficiency of needed erythropoietic elements	Understanding of adequate dietary intake of missing nutrients.	Initiate teaching with client and family regarding diet complete with deficient nutrients. Provide time for feedback and questions from client and family.
Need for supplemental drugs or blood products	Adequate intake of pharmacological agents or blood products.	Teach client the rationale behind using various pharmacological agents or blood products. Know usual doses, amounts, and times of administration and side effects for drugs and blood products.

are viable for only 120 days. Three significant alterations in erythropoiesis may occur which decrease red cell production:

1. Decreased hemoglobin synthesis may lead to iron-deficiency anemia and thalassemia.
2. Defective nuclear cytoplasm of the red cells may lead to pernicious anemia and folic acid deficiency.
3. Diminished availability of erythrocyte precursors may result in hypoplastic anemias and chronic disease anemias (Table 24-1).

Iron-deficiency anemia

Iron-deficiency anemia is one of the most common chronic disorders found in humans. It is present in 10 to 30 percent of the United States' population. This type of anemia is prevalent among the poor and in areas of the world where dietary intake of iron is inadequate. Regardless of economics or geography, iron-deficiency anemia is also common in infants, children, and women who are premenopausal or pregnant.

Iron is present in the body as heme in hemoglobin and in a stored form. The heme in hemoglobin accounts for two-thirds of the iron. The other one-third of iron is stored as ferritin and hemosiderin in the bone marrow, spleen, and liver. Normally, 1 mg of iron is lost daily through the gastrointestinal (GI) tract, sweat, and urine. When the stored supplies of iron are depleted, hemoglobin production is reduced.

Causes Iron deficiency may develop from inadequate dietary intake, malabsorption, blood loss, or hemolysis. Iron is obtained from foods in our diet. Approximately 1 mg of iron is absorbed from every 10 to 20 mg of iron ingested. Therefore, only about 5 to 10 percent of the ingested iron is absorbed. This amount of iron is adequate to meet the needs of men and older women, but it is inadequate for those individuals who have higher iron needs (e.g., pregnant females). Table 24-5 lists nutrients needed for erythropoiesis.

Malabsorption of iron is common after certain forms of GI surgery and in malabsorption syndromes. Surgical procedures such as subtotal gastric resection often involve the removal of the duodenum. Most of the iron absorption primarily occurs in the duodenum. Malabsorption syndromes commonly involve disease of the upper small intestine. The absorption of iron is impeded in malabsorption states because the absorption surface is lost.

Blood loss is a major cause of iron deficiency in adults, as 2 mL of blood contains 1 mg of iron. The three major sources of chronic blood loss are GI, genitourinary (GU), and respiratory. GI bleeds are often occult and therefore may exist for a considerable time before the diagnosis is made. From 50 to 75 mL of blood from the upper GI tract is required to cause stools to appear as *melena*. The black color of melena results from the action of intestinal enzymes on the blood. This condition must be differentiated from other causes of black stools, such as excessive iron intake. Common causes of GI blood loss in the adult are peptic ulcer, hiatal hernia, neoplasia, and gastritis. GU blood loss occurs primarily from menstrual bleeding. The average monthly menstrual blood loss is about 45 mL and therefore causes the loss of about 22 mg of iron. Hemoptysis may account for significant blood loss from the respiratory tract. While the hemoptysis may be overt, clients can swallow the bloody sputum in quantities large enough to show up as occult blood in stools.

Pregnancy contributes to iron deficiency because of the extra need for iron by the fetus.[3] Iron-deficiency anemia may also develop from intravascular hemolysis of red cells which may develop from the mechanical trauma of prosthetic heart valves.

Clinical Manifestations In the early course of iron-deficiency anemia, the client may be asymptomatic. As the disease becomes chronic, any of the

Table 24-5
Nutrients Needed for Erythropoiesis

Nutrient	Role in Erythropoiesis	Food Sources
Vitamin B_{12}	RBC maturation	Organ and muscle meats, especially liver
Folic acid	RBC maturation	Green leafy vegetables, liver, meat, fish, legumes, whole grains
Iron	Hemoglobin synthesis	Liver and muscle meats, eggs, dried fruits, legumes, dark green leafy vegetables, whole-grain and enriched bread and cereals, potatoes
Vitamin B_6	Hemoglobin synthesis	Meats (especially pork and liver), wheat germ, legumes, potatoes, cornmeal, bananas
Amino acids	Synthesis of nucleoproteins	Eggs, meat, milk and milk products (cheese, ice cream), poultry, fish, legumes, nuts
Vitamin C	Conversion of folic acid to its active form; aids in iron absorption	Citrus fruits, leafy green vegetables, strawberries, cantaloupe

general manifestations of anemia may be displayed (Table 24-3). There are also some specific clinical symptoms which typify iron-deficiency anemia. While pallor is the most common finding, *glossitis* (inflammation of the tongue) is the second most general feature in iron-deficiency anemia. Other findings include *cheilitis* (inflammation of the lips) and splenomegaly. In addition, the client may report headache, paresthesias, and a burning sensation of the tongue, all of which are caused by lack of iron in the tissues.

Diagnostic Study Abnormalities Laboratory abnormalities characteristic of iron-deficiency anemia are presented in Table 24-6. Other diagnostic studies will be done to determine the cause of the iron deficiency. For example, endoscopy and radiography may be used to detect GI bleeding.

Medical Management The goal of medical treatment for iron-deficiency anemia is to replace iron (Table 24-7). This may be done through increasing intake. If nutrition is adequate, increasing iron intake by dietary means may not be reasonable, as severe anemia might necessitate ingesting 10 lb of steak a day.[4] Consequently, oral or parenteral iron supplements are generally used. If the iron deficiency is caused by significant acute blood loss, transfusion of blood products may be required. (Blood transfusions are discussed in Chap. 26.)

Pharmacological Management Oral iron should be used whenever possible, as it is inexpensive and convenient. Innumerable iron preparations are available. Four factors that should be considered in the administration of iron are as follows:

1. About 300 mg of ferrous sulfate should be administered in the form of three to four tablets per day. (A 300-mg tablet of ferrous sulfate contains 65 mg of elemental iron.)
2. Iron is best absorbed in an acidic environment. For this reason, and to avoid binding the iron with food, iron should be given about an hour before meals, when the duodenal mucosa is most acidic. (Taking iron with orange juice, a form of ascorbic acid, also enhances iron absorption.) Enteric coated iron may prove ineffective, as the iron may not be released in an area in the intestine which facilitates absorption.
3. Undiluted liquid iron may stain the client's teeth. Therefore, it should be diluted and ingested through a straw.
4. Mild GI side effects of iron administration may occur. These include pyrosis (heartburn), constipation, and diarrhea. If side effects develop, the dose and type of iron supplement may be adjusted. All clients should know that the use of iron preparations will cause their stools to become black, as excess iron is excreted via the GI tract.

In some situations, it may be necessary to administer iron parenterally. Parenteral use of iron is indicated for malabsorption, intolerance of oral iron, a need for iron beyond oral limits, or poor client compliance in taking the iron.

Because intramuscular (IM) iron solutions may stain the skin, separate needles should be used for withdrawing the solution and for injecting the medication. About 0.4 to 0.5 mL of air should be left in the syringe to clear the iron completely from the syringe.

Iron should be given deep intramuscularly in the upper outer quadrant of the buttocks. A 2- to 3-inch needle with a 19 to 20 gauge should be used. Preferably, no more than 2 mL of iron is given in a single injection. To prevent leakage of the iron solution from the IM to the subcutaneous (SC) tissue, a Z-track technique should be used for injection. The site should not be massaged after the injection is given.

Dietary Management The client should be told which foods are good sources of iron (Table 24-5).

Nursing Management It is important to recognize groups of individuals who are at an increased risk to become iron deficient. These include infants, teenage girls, premenopausal and pregnant females, persons from low socioeconomic backgrounds, and individuals suffering from blood loss. Diet teaching, with an emphasis on foods high in iron, is very important for these groups. Supplemental iron is especially important for the pregnant female.

If anemia is present, it is important to discuss with the client the need for diagnostic studies to identify the cause. Appropriate nursing measures for the anemic client are presented in Table 24-4. Compliance with dietary and drug therapy needs to be emphasized. The hemoglobin level and red blood count should be reassessed to evaluate the response to therapy. The client should be encouraged to take iron therapy for 2 to 3 months after the hemoglobin returns to normal. This is necessary to replenish the iron stores within the body. If the hemoglobin remains low, the client should be reevaluated for the cause of anemia.

Thalassemia

Another cause of decreased erythrocyte production is known as *thalassemia*. Like iron deficiency, it is a disease of inadequate production of normal hemoglobin. (Hemolysis also occurs in thalassemia, but

Table 24-6

Laboratory Studies Correlated with Various Types of Anemias

	Fe Deficiency	Thalas-semia Major	Pernicious Anemia	Folic Acid Deficiency	Hypo-prolifer-ative Anemia	Chronic Disease	Acute Blood Loss	Chronic Blood Loss	Sickle Cell Anemia	G6PD Deficiency	Hemolyt Anemia
Hb	↓	↓	↓	↓	↓	↓	↓	↓	↓	↓	↓
Hct	↓	↓	↓	↓	↓	↓	↓	↓	↓	↓	↓
RBC	↓	↓	↓	↓	↓	↓	↓	↓	↓	↓	↓
MCV	↓	N	↑	↑	N		N	↓	N	N	N
MCH	↓	N	N or slight ↓	N or slight ↓	N	↓	N		N	N	N
MCHC	↓	N	↑	↑	N		N	↓	N	N	N
Retic	N or ↓	↑	↓	N	↓	N	N	N or ↓	↑	↑	↑
Serum Fe	↓	↑	N	N	± N	↓	N	↓	N to ↑	N to ↑	↑
TIBC	↓	↑	N	N	± N	↓	N	↓	N to ↓	N to ↓	↓
Bilirubin	N to ↓	↑	N	N	N	± N	N	N to ↓	↑	N to ↑	N to ↑
Sed rate	N or slight ↑					↑		N or slight ↑	Very ↓		
Platelets	↑		↓		↓	↑		↑	↑		
Other findings			↓ Vitamin B_{12} + Schilling achlorhydria	↓ Folate	↓ WBC				See Table 24-9		

Table 24-7
Medical Management: Iron Deficiency Anemia

Diagnostic
1. History and physical examination
2. RBC count
3. Reticulocyte count
4. Hematocrit and hemoglobin
5. Serum iron
6. TIBC
7. Fecal examination for occult blood

Therapeutic
1. Identify and treat underlying cause
2. Ferrous sulfate 300 mg three to four times per day
3. Iron dextran IM or IV
4. Diet rich in iron-containing foods
5. Transfusion of blood products

insufficient production of normal hemoglobin is the predominant problem.) In contrast to iron-deficiency anemia, in which heme synthesis is the problem, thalassemia involves a problem with globin protein. Therefore, the basic defect of thalassemia is abnormal hemoglobin synthesis.

Etiology Thalassemias are a group of *autosomal recessive genetic disorders* commonly found in members of ethnic groups originating near the Mediterranean Sea. Individuals may be heterozygous or homozygous. Persons who are *heterozygous* have one thalassemic gene and one normal gene. They are said to have *thalassemia minor* or the *thalassemic trait*, which is a mild form of the disease. *Homozygous* individuals have two thalassemic genes, causing a severe condition known as *thalassemia major*.

Clinical Manifestations Clients with thalassemia minor are frequently asymptomatic because they adjust to their gradually acquired chronic state of anemia. Occasionally, these individuals may develop splenomegaly, and mild jaundice may be manifested if malformed erythrocytes are rapidly hemolyzed. Individuals who have thalassemia major are pale and display other general symptoms of anemia (Table 24-3). In addition, they have marked splenomegaly and hepatomegaly. Jaundice from red cell hemolysis is prominent. Chronic bone marrow hypertrophy may cause thickening of the cranium, leading to an appearance resembling that of Down's syndrome. Thalassemia major is such a life-threatening disease that growth, both physically and mentally, is often retarded.

Medical Management The diagnostic findings of thalassemia major are summarized in Table 24-6. Thalassemia minor requires no treatment because the body adapts to the reduction of normal hemoglobin. Thalassemia major is usually treated with blood transfusions. There is no medication or diet therapy to treat thalassemia. Transfusions are administered often enough to keep the hemoglobin at about 10 g/dL. This level is low enough to foster the client's own erythropoiesis without enlarging the spleen. Because red blood cells are sequestered in the enlarged spleen, thalassemia may be treated by splenectomy. However, even with medical management, thalassemia major will gradually progress to a fatal outcome.

Pernicious anemia

The most common cause of vitamin B_{12} deficiency is *pernicious anemia*, in which intrinsic factor secretion ceases. Normally, a protein known as *intrinsic factor* is secreted by the parietal cells of the gastric mucosa. Intrinsic factor is required for vitamin B_{12} (extrinsic factor) absorption. Therefore, if intrinsic factor is not secreted, vitamin B_{12} cannot be absorbed. (Vitamin B_{12} is normally absorbed in the distal ileum.)

One of the functions of vitamin B_{12} is related to deoxyribonucleic acid (DNA) synthesis and erythrocyte production. When DNA synthesis is impaired, defective red blood cell maturation results. The red cells are large (macrocytic) and abnormal, and are referred to as *megaloblasts*. These red cells are easily destroyed because of their fragile membranes. Another common cause of megaloblastic anemia is folic acid deficiency (see Folic Acid Deficiency).

Etiology Pernicious anemia is predominantly manifested in persons over 60 years of age. This condition is always seen in clients who have undergone either total gastrectomy or small bowel resection involving the ileum. This is due to the loss of the mucosal surface which secretes intrinsic factor, either by surgery or because of malabsorption syndromes. Individuals who develop pernicious anemia were once believed to be genetically predisposed. Currently, the mechanism of disease transference is unknown. An autoimmune reaction against gastric parietal cells has been suggested to account for the gastric atrophy which leads to the development of pernicious anemia.[5] Relatives of persons with pernicious disease show an increased incidence of the disease.

Clinical Manifestations General symptoms of anemia develop because of tissue hypoxia (Table 24-3). A megaloblastic anemia is seen. GI manifestations occur as a result of gastric mucosal changes. These include a sore tongue, anorexia, nausea, vomiting, and abdominal pain. Neurological symptoms may present when the nervous system needs more vitamin

B_{12} to function properly. Typical neurological manifestations of the disease involve paresthesias of the feet and hands, reduced vibratory and position senses, muscle weakness, and impaired thought processes. Because pernicious anemia has an insidious onset, it may take several months for these manifestations to develop.

Diagnostic Study Abnormalities Laboratory assessment will yield data reflective of megaloblastic anemia (Table 24-6). The erythrocytes will appear large (macrocytic) and abnormally shaped. This structure contributes to the ease of erythrocyte destruction, as the cell membrane is very fragile.

When pernicious anemia is suspected, several additional studies will be conducted. *Serum vitamin B_{12}* levels will be reduced below 100 μg. To ascertain the cause of the vitamin B_{12} deficiency, a *gastric analysis* will be done. In this study, a nasogastric tube is inserted, the client is injected with histamine to stimulate gastric juice secretion, and the gastric juice is aspirated via the nasogastric tube over a given period of time. If analysis of the gastric juice reveals *achlorhydria* (an absence of free hydrochloric acid in a pH never less than 3.5), depressed parietal cell function can be determined. This feature is diagnostic of pernicious anemia.

Another means of assessing parietal cell function is by doing a *Schilling's test*. After radioactive vitamin B_{12} is administered to the client, the amount excreted in the urine is measured. Individuals who cannot absorb vitamin B_{12} will excrete only a small amount of the radioactive form. The same procedure may be followed with the addition of intrinsic factor parenterally. Absorption of vitamin B_{12} when intrinsic factor is added is diagnostic of pernicious anemia.

Medical and Pharmacological Management In addition to specific identification and treatment of the underlying disorder, the treatment of pernicious anemia is based on replacement of vitamin B_{12}. Without vitamin B_{12} administration, these individuals will die in 1 to 3 years. However, as long as supplemental vitamin B_{12} is used, pernicious anemia will remain in remission.

Parenteral use of vitamin B_{12} (cyanocobalamin or hydroxycobalamin) is the treatment of choice for pernicious anemia. The efficacy of Vitamin B_{12} injections in altering the otherwise fatal course of pernicious anemia cannot be overemphasized. The dosage and frequency of vitamin B_{12} administration may vary. A typical administration pattern might be as follows: 100 μg IM daily for 2 weeks; 100 μg IM twice a week for 4 weeks, and then 100 to 250 μg IM monthly for life.

Dietary Management Regardless of how much vitamin B_{12} is ingested, the client will not be able to absorb it due to the lack of intrinsic factor. Therefore, dietary management is not a reasonable approach for vitamin B_{12} replacement in pernicious anemia. However, the client should be instructed on adequate dietary intake to maintain good nutrition (Table 24-5).

Nursing Management Due to the familial predisposition involved in pernicious anemia, clients who have a positive family history should be evaluated for symptoms of anemia. Although disease development cannot be prevented, early detection and treatment can lead to reversal of symptoms.

The nursing measures presented in Table 24-4 are appropriate for the client with pernicious anemia. In addition to these measures, the nurse should make sure that injuries are not sustained due to the diminished sensations to heat and pain resulting from the neurological impairment. The client must be protected from burns and trauma. If heat therapy is required, the client's skin must be evaluated at frequent intervals to detect reddening. Irritation from nasogastric tubes and restrictive clothing may not be perceived by the client due to reduced pain sensations.

Ongoing care for the person with pernicious anemia is primarily related to ensuring good client compliance in returning for monthly vitamin B_{12} injections. There must also be careful follow-up to assess for neurological problems. Neurological problems may not be fully corrected even by adequate therapy. Because the potential for gastric carcinoma is increased in pernicious anemia, clients should have frequent and careful medical follow-up care.

Folic acid deficiency

Folic acid deficiency also causes megaloblastic anemia. Folic acid is required for DNA synthesis leading to red cell formation and maturation. Three common causes of folic acid deficiency are as follows:

1. Poor nutrition, especially a lack of leafy green vegetables, liver, citrus fruits, yeast, dried beans, nuts, and grains. The inadequate diet seen in chronic alcohol abusers frequently leads to folic acid deficiency.
2. Malabsorption syndromes.
3. Drugs which impede the absorption and use of folic acid, such as methotrexate and oral contraceptives, and anticonvulsants such as phenobarbital and diphenylhydantoin.

The *clinical manifestations* of folic acid deficiency are similar to those of pernicious anemia. The disease develops insidiously, and the client's symptoms may be attributed to other coexisting problems, such as cirrhosis or esophageal varices. GI disturbances include dyspepsia and a smooth, beefy red tongue. Of diagnostic significance is the *absence* of neurological problems. This lack of neurological involvement differentiates folic acid deficiency from pernicious anemia.

The diagnostic analysis for folic acid deficiency will reveal the laboratory data reflective of megaloblastic anemia. In addition, the *serum folate level* will be less than 4 ng (normal is 7 to 20 ng), the serum vitamin B_{12} level will be normal, and the gastric analysis will be positive for hydrochloric acid (Table 24-6).

Folic acid deficiency is treated by replacement therapy. The usual dose is 1 mg/day by mouth. In malabsorption states, up to 5 mg/day may be required. The duration of treatment depends on the reason for the deficiency. The client should be encouraged to eat foods containing large amounts of folic acid.

Hypoplastic (aplastic) anemia

When bone marrow fails to produce adequate numbers of erythrocytes, a condition known as *hypoplastic* or *aplastic anemia* exists. This term is somewhat of a misnomer in that all marrow elements—erythrocytes, leukocytes, and platelets—are quantitatively decreased, although they are qualitatively normal. The etiology of hypoplastic anemia is somewhat unclear, but there are three contributing factors:

1. Congenital origin due to chromosomal alterations
2. Toxic substances to the bone marrow, such as radiation, alkylating, and antimetabolite drugs used to treat various forms of cancer, and idiosyncratic reactions to drugs such as chloramphenicol, benzene, diphenylhydantoin, and phenylbutazone
3. Idiopathic or unknown reasons for development which account for about half the cases of hypoplastic anemia

Clinical Manifestations Clinically, the client may present with symptoms caused by suppression of any or all bone marrow elements. General symptoms of anemia, as well as cardiovascular and cerebral responses, may be seen (Table 24-3). Granulocytopenia may be reflected by fever and susceptibility to infection. Thrombocytopenia will be manifested by a predisposition to bleed (petechiae, ecchymoses, or nosebleeds).

Diagnostic Study Abnormalities Confirmation of the diagnosis is done by laboratory studies. The client will be pancytopenic (Table 24-6). Since the red cell indices are normal, the condition is classified as a normocytic, normochromic anemia. The reticulocyte count will be low. Other tests of platelet function, such as the bleeding time, will be prolonged.

Hypoplastic anemia can be further evaluated by assessing various iron studies. The serum iron and total iron-binding capacity (TIBC) will be elevated as initial signs of erythroid suppression. Bone marrow examination may be done for any anemic state. However, the findings are especially important in hypoplastic anemia, as the marrow will be hypocellular with increased yellow marrow (fat content).

Medical and Nursing Management Management of hypoplastic anemia is based on identifying and removing the causative agent (when possible) and offering supportive care until the pancytopenia can be treated. Nursing interventions appropriate for the anemic client are presented in Table 24-4. Nursing care plans for thrombocytopenic and neutropenic clients are presented in Tables 24-13 and 24-21, respectively. Generally, every effort must be made to prevent complications from infection and hemorrhage. Until bone marrow production is restored, blood products such as red cells, white cells, and platelets may be administered. Antibiotics are usually not given prophylactically, but they will be used to treat infections. Corticosteroids may be employed both to reduce capillary fragility and to decrease antibiotic-resistant idiopathic fevers. However, the long-term use of steroids may increase clients' susceptibility to infections. Oral androgens, such as synthetic testosterone, may be used to stimulate bone marrow production. Bone marrow transplantation may be attempted if a suitable donor can be found.

Unfortunately, regardless of the diagnosis and management, hypoplastic anemia is ultimately fatal in about 75 percent of clients. The disease may be controlled for months or years until such time as the marrow failure can no longer be offset. Recently, good success has been achieved using marrow transplants in children with hypoplastic anemia.

Anemia of chronic disease

Anemia may develop in several chronic conditions. In *renal disease* there is a relationship between the degree of anemia and the severity of uremia. Although several mechanisms may be involved in the development of anemia with renal disease, the primary factor is decreased erythropoietin, which is a hormone made in the kidneys that is necessary for erythropoiesis. With decreased renal function, decreased levels of erythropoietin are produced (Chap. 38).

Chronic liver disease may also contribute to the

development of anemia. Anemia may be from the folic acid deficiencies caused by inadequate nutrition in alcohol abusers or from blood loss due to chronic gastritis. The use of alcohol itself may reduce erythropoiesis. Anemia may also result from splenomegaly, which is commonly found in advanced stages of cirrhosis (Chap. 35).

Chronic inflammations and *malignancies* are other conditions in which anemia may be present. The mechanisms involved include increased red blood cell destruction from unidentified causes accompanied by a failure to augment erythropoiesis to compensate for the rise in destruction.

Chronic endocrine diseases may also lead to anemia. *Hypopituitary* and *hypothyroid* states both lead to reduced tissue metabolism. Therefore, tissue oxygen needs are diminished, leading to a reduced production of erythropoietin by the kidneys. *Adrenal hypofunction* caused by either *adrenalectomy* or *Addison's disease* will also evoke an anemic response. This, too, is believed to result from lowered metabolic requirements and decreased oxygen needs.

Anemia Due to Blood Loss

Anemia resulting from blood loss may be caused by either acute or chronic problems.

Acute blood loss

Acute blood loss occurs when there is sudden hemorrhage. Causes of acute blood loss include trauma, complications of surgery, and diseases which disrupt vascular integrity. The major clinical concerns in such situations are two. First, there is a sudden reduction in the total blood volume that may lead to hypovolemic shock. Second, if the acute loss is more gradual, the body maintains its blood volume by slowly increasing the plasma volume. Consequently, the circulating fluid volume is preserved, but the number of erythrocytes available to carry oxygen is significantly diminished. For example, there will be loss of 25 percent of the blood volume before the hematocrit drops below 30.

Clinical Manifestations The clinical manifestations of anemia from acute blood loss are caused by the body's attempts to maintain an adequate blood volume and meet oxygen requirements. Table 24-8 summarizes the clinical manifestations of clients with varying degrees of blood volume loss. It is essential to understand that clinical symptoms are valuable indicators of the degree of blood loss, as laboratory data may not accurately reflect the severity of hemorrhage for 2 to 3 days.

Table 24-8
Clinical Manifestations of Acute Blood Loss

Total Body Volume Lost	Clinical Manifestations
10%	None.
20%	At rest, no detectable signs or symptoms. With exercise, tachycardia and slight postural hypotension.
30%	At rest, normal supine blood pressure and pulse. With exercise, postural hypotension and tachycardia.
40%	Blood pressure below normal at rest. Rapid, thready pulse and cold, clammy skin.
50%	Shock and potential death.

The nurse should be alert to the client's expression (verbal or nonverbal) of pain. Internal hemorrhage may cause pain because of tissue distension, organ displacement, and nerve compression. Pain may be localized or referred. In the case of retroperitoneal bleeding, the client may not experience abdominal pain. Instead, he may present with numbness and pain in a lower extremity secondary to compression of the lateral cutaneous nerve, which is located in the region of the first to third lumbar vertebrae. The main complication of acute blood loss is irreversible shock (see Chap. 26).

Diagnostic Study Abnormalities When blood volume is lost suddenly, the body reacts by constricting the vascular space. Also, plasma volume has not yet had a chance to increase, so the loss of red cell mass is not perceived. These mechanisms will skew laboratory data, and the results may seem normal or high for 2 to 3 days. However, once the plasma is replaced by both endogenous and exogenous means, the red cell mass is less concentrated. At this time, erythrocytes, hemoglobin, and hematocrit levels are usually low and reflect the blood loss.

Medical Management Medical management is initially concerned with (1) replacing blood volume to prevent the development of shock and (2) identifying the source of the hemorrhage and stopping the blood loss.[6] IV fluids used in emergencies may be plasma proteins, dextran, or noncolloidal electrolyte solutions such as Ringer's lactate. The amount of infusion will vary with the solution used.

Once volume replacement is established, then attention can be directed to correcting red cell loss. The body needs 2 to 5 days to manufacture more red cells in response to increased erythropoietin. Consequently, blood transfusions may be necessary to achieve an immediate effect. While whole blood replaces blood volume at the rate of 500 mL/U, 12 to 24 hours must elapse before hemoglobin and hematocrit changes are seen. Packed red cells provide half the volume of whole blood and replace about 2 times as much hemoglobin as 1 U of whole blood.

Another component of medical management may be to provide the client with supplemental iron, as the iron supply affects the marrow production of erythrocytes. When anemia exists after acute blood loss, dietary sources of iron will probably not be adequate to maintain iron pools. Remember that for every 2 mL of blood lost, 1 mg of iron is also lost. Therefore, either oral or parenteral iron preparations will be administered.

Nursing Management In the case of trauma, it may be impossible to prevent the situation leading to the blood loss. For postoperative cases, exact evaluation of blood loss via various drainage tubes and dressings will facilitate early intervention to find the source of hemorrhage and treat it.

The nursing care plan in Table 24-4 is relevant to the anemia resulting from acute blood loss. In this situation, blood product replacement will almost certainly be necessary. Therefore, the techniques for proper transfusion therapy discussed in Chap. 26 should be followed.

Once the source of hemorrhage is identified, blood loss is controlled, and fluid and blood volume are replaced, the anemia should begin to correct itself. There should be no need for long-term treatment of the anemia.

Chronic blood loss

Only a brief summary of chronic blood loss is necessary, as the sources of chronic blood loss are similar to those of iron-deficiency anemia (bleeding ulcer, hemorrhoids, menstrual blood loss, etc.) The effects of chronic blood loss are usually related to the depletion of iron stores and therefore are usually considered as iron-deficiency anemia.

Management of chronic blood loss anemia involves identifying the source and stopping the bleeding. Supplemental iron may be required. The nursing measures correlate with those presented in Table 24-4 depending on the severity of the anemia.

Anemia Due to Increased Erythrocyte Destruction (Hemolysis)

The third major cause of anemia is the destruction or *hemolysis* of red cells at a rate higher than the rate of production. Hemolysis may occur because of problems intrinsic or extrinsic to the red blood cells. *Intrinsic hemolytic anemias* result from defects in the red blood cells themselves due to abnormal hemoglobin (e.g., sickle cells), enzyme deficiencies which alter glycolysis (glucose-6-phosphate dehydrogenase deficiency), or red cell membrane abnormalities. Intrinsic hemolytic anemias are usually hereditary. Because defective red blood cells are hemolyzed, these clients may benefit from the administration of normal erythrocytes. *Extrinsic hemolytic anemias* are acquired. The client's red cells are normal, but damage is caused by external factors, such as antibodies, toxins, or mechanical injury (e.g., prosthetic heart valves).

The two sites of hemolysis are classified as *intravascular* or *extravascular*. Intravascular destruction occurs within the circulation, while extravascular hemolysis takes place in the reticuloendothelial cells of the spleen, liver, and bone marrow. The spleen is the primary site of destruction of red blood cells which are moderately damaged. Figure 24-2 indicates the sequence of events involved in extravascular hemolysis.

The client with hemolytic anemia will manifest the general symptoms of anemia (Table 24-6) as well as others. Jaundice is a likely occurrence, as the increased destruction of red blood cells causes an elevation in bilirubin. The spleen and liver may enlarge because of their hyperactivity, which is needed to phagocytize the defective erythrocytes. Also, cholelithiasis may develop because the excessive bilirubin forms pigmented stones in the gallbladder.

In all causes of hemolysis, one of the main concerns of treatment is to maintain renal function. When a red cell is hemolyzed, the hemoglobin molecule is released and cleared by the kidneys. The hemoglobin molecule can obstruct the renal tubule and lead to acute tubular necrosis (Chap. 38). In addition, excessive amounts of urobilinogen develop from the red cell breakdown and must be cleared by the kidneys.

The three types of hemolytic anemias that will be discussed are sickle cell anemia, glucose-6-phosphate dehydrogenase deficiency, and acquired hemolytic anemias.

Sickle cell anemia

Sickle cell disease occurs when an abnormal hemoglobin, known as S, develops in place of the normal A hemoglobin. For unknown reasons, the disease is predominant in blacks, affecting 1 person in 10. The difficulty with sickle cell anemia is that when deprived of oxygen, the hemoglobin S (HbS) assumes various crescent or sickle shapes. Erythrostasis develops when sickled red cells are trapped in small blood

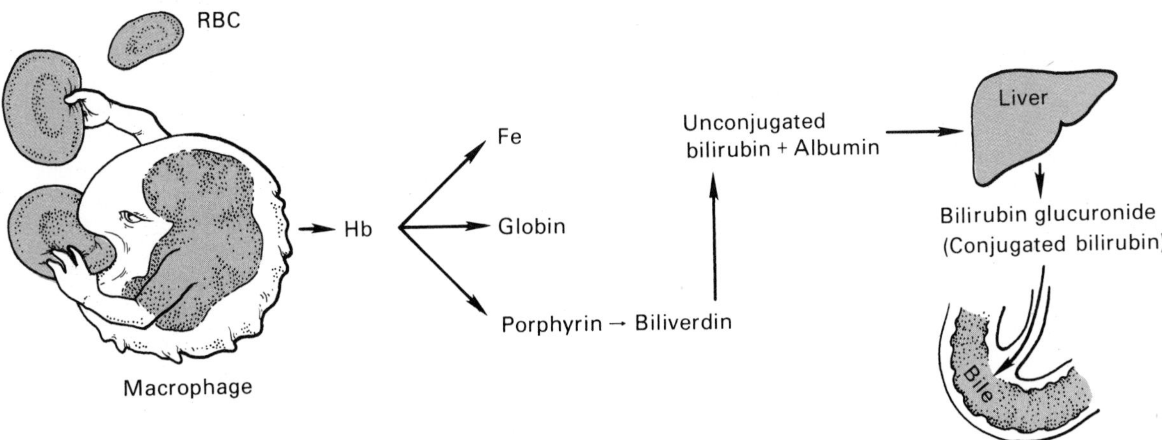

Figure 24-2 Sequence of events in extravascular hemolysis.

vessels. The erythrostasis causes further oxygen deprivation which potentiates more sickling. The increased concentration of sickle cells makes the circulation more sluggish. The abnormal shape of the hemoglobin is recognized by the body, and therefore the cell is hemolyzed.

Etiology Sickle cell anemia is an autosomal recessive genetic disorder in which the person is homozygous for HbS. Some individuals may have *sickle cell trait*, a mild condition which may be asymptomatic. Persons with sickle cell trait are heterozygous, with about one-fourth of their hemoglobin in the abnormal S form and three-fourths as normal A (Fig. 24-3). They develop *sickle cell crises* (exacerbations of sickling) only if they become extremely hypoxic.

The mutation which causes HbS to develop involves only one amino acid. One valine amino acid is

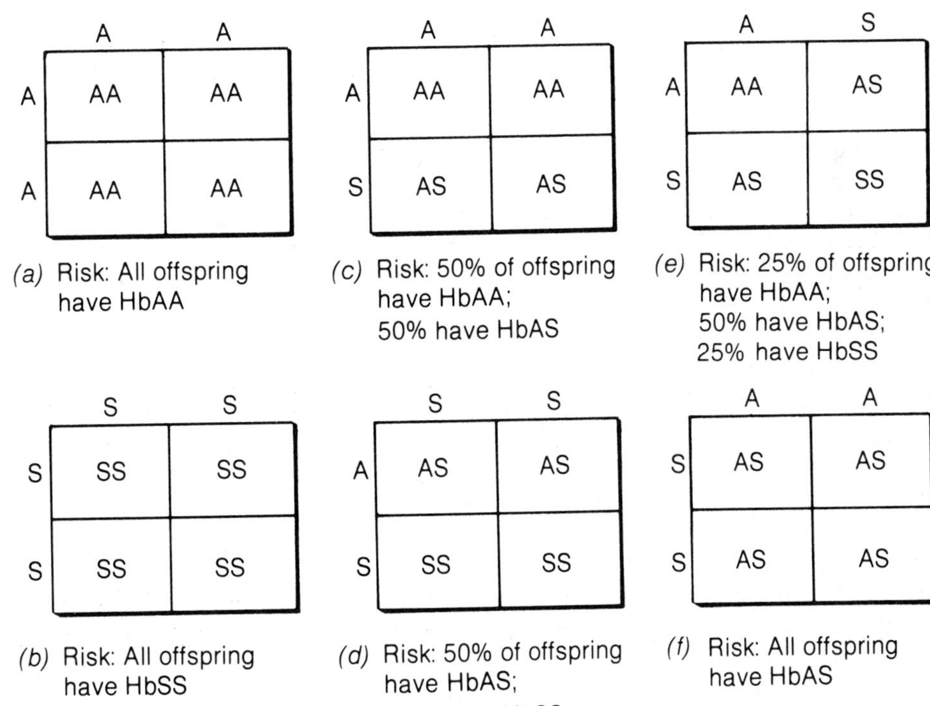

Figure 24-3 Inheritance patterns of sickle cell disease. *[From M. Smith et al. (eds.), Child and Family, Concepts of Nursing Practice, McGraw-Hill Book Company, New York, 1982, p. 721.]*

substituted for a glutamic acid. This substitution leads to an abnormal linking reaction which causes the development of deformed crescent-shaped cells when oxygen tension is lowered (Fig. 24-4).

Clinical Manifestations Children do not manifest symptoms until after the sixth month, at which time most of the fetal hemoglobin (HbF) has been replaced by HbS. Children manifest a general impairment of growth and development and a failure to thrive. In general, they have an increased susceptibility to infection. One reason for this increased susceptibility is the failure of the spleen to phagocytize foreign substances due to marked impairment of splenic function from fibrosis.

Individuals with sickle cell anemia have a severe form of hemolytic anemia. The mean red blood cell survival time is 10 to 15 days. As a result of the accelerated red blood cell breakdown, the client has characteristic clinical findings of hemolysis (jaundice, elevated serum bilirubin, hepatomegaly) and laboratory test results (Table 24-6).

Sickle Cell Crisis Sickle cell crisis refers to a syndrome that develops rapidly and results in exacerbated sickling. The painful crisis is due to intertwining of the sickle cells. Upon deoxygenation, the red blood cell containing HbS changes from a biconcave disc to an elongated, crescent-shaped or sickle-shaped cell. These sickling cells clog the small capillaries. As blood vessels become occluded, they can thrombose. This can ultimately lead to necrosis of the infarcted tissue from lack of oxygen.

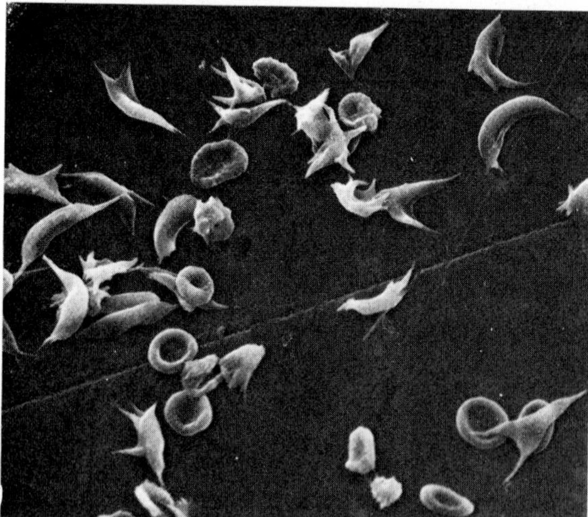

Figure 24-4 Comparison of a normal red blood cell with sickled red cells. *[From M. Smith et al. (eds.), Child and Family, Concepts of Nursing Practice, McGraw-Hill Book Company, New York, 1982, p. 722.]*

Precipitating factors include anything that causes hypoxia or deoxygenation of the red blood cell, including viral or bacterial infections, high altitudes, emotional or physical stress, and blood loss. Sometimes the crisis occurs spontaneously, with no apparent precipitating event. The frequency of sickle cell crisis is variable. Crises may occur frequently and then may not recur for months or years. The attack may last for 4 to 6 days.

These attacks may appear suddenly and affect various parts of the body, especially the abdomen, chest, and joints. Organs which have a high need for oxygen are most immediately affected. The heart may become ischemic and enlarged, leading to electrocardiographic changes. Pulmonary infarctions may cause chest pain and ultimately lead to cor pulmonale. The kidneys may be injured from the increased blood viscosity as well as the lack of oxygen. Spleen enlargement is not common in adults because the spleen is usually fibrosed from prior episodes of thrombosis. However, hepatomegaly is a frequent finding. Bone changes may include osteoporosis and, after infarction, osteosclerosis. Aching in the joints, especially those of the hands and feet, is a common complaint. Chronic leg ulcers may result from the hypoxia and are especially prevalent around the ankles.

Sickle cell crises may occasionally involve the central nervous system. Clients may present with seizures or impaired consciousness. Although these crises may be fatal, they usually are reversible.

Additional symptoms may develop during the crises which complicate sickle cell anemia. These symptoms are related to pain and aplasia. The pain may occur spontaneously or may be precipitated by infection, cold intolerance, etc. The pain usually begins in the extremities and lasts for 4 to 6 days. Aplastic crises occur when a stressor significantly decreases erythropoiesis. The anemia will therefore be exacerbated as hemolysis continues.

Shock is also a possible development in sickle cell crisis. Capillary hypoxia may result in changes in membrane permeability, leading to plasma loss, hemoconcentration, and further circulatory stagnation which causes an increased reduction of the circulating fluid volume.

Diagnostic Study Abnormalities Differentiating sickle cell trait from sickle cell anemia is essential during the diagnostic workup. Table 24-9 indicates the significant distinguishing laboratory features. In addition, an intravenous pyelogram may be done to evaluate the kidneys, and radiographs of the bones may show skeletal changes.

Table 24-9
Laboratory Assessment of Sickle Cell Trait and Sickle Cell Anemia

Study	Sickle Cell Trait	Sickle Cell Anemia
Peripheral smear	Normal	Partially or completely sickled cells seen
Sickle cell preparation (observe blood specimen reaction in hypoxic setting)	Sickle cells seen	Sickle cells seen
Sickledex (blood is mixed with a solution which deoxygenates HbS. This becomes insoluble and causes turbidity. Development of cloudiness is positive for presence of HbS)	Positive	Positive
Hemoglobin electropheresis (types of hemoglobin are separated when blood specimen is exposed to an electric field)	Both HbS and HbA	HbS

Medical Management Medical care for clients with sickle cell anemia is essentially supportive. There is no treatment specific for the disease. Therapy is usually directed toward alleviating the symptoms due to complications of the disease. For example, chronic leg ulcers may be treated with bed rest, antibiotics, warm saline soaks, mechanical or enzyme debridement, and sterile dressings.

Sickle cell crises usually require hospitalization. Oxygen may be administered to alter hypoxia and control sickling. Rest is instituted to reduce metabolic requirements, and fluids and electrolytes are administered to reduce blood viscosity and maintain renal function. Sedatives and analgesics are used to treat pain. Transfusion therapy is indicated when an aplastic crisis occurs.

Because these clients have increased needs for folic acid, it is important for them to obtain daily supplements. Blood transfusions should be used judiciously to treat a crisis. They have little, if any, role in the treatment between crises. In general, iron therapy is not indicated.

Nursing Management Because of the hereditary nature of sickle cell disease, sexual counseling is the only form of prevention. For sexual counseling to be effective, screening must be done to detect those individuals who have sickle cell trait. Otherwise, its mild effects may go unrecognized.

The basic care for clients with sickle cell anemia is discussed in Table 24-4. Long-term care for these clients is also of great importance. Chronic management is based mostly on client education. Individuals and their families must understand the basis of the disease and the reasons for supportive care. Clients must be taught ways to avoid crises. These include taking steps to reduce the chance of developing hypoxia, such as avoiding high altitudes, and seeking medical attention quickly to counteract problems such as upper respiratory tract infections.

Glucose-6-phosphate dehydrogenase (G6PD) deficiency

G6PD is a red cell enzyme that acts as the initial catalyst in glycolysis. G6PD is a sex-linked disorder and directly affects the erythrocyte's ability to resist oxidative damage. Consequently, when G6PD is reduced, there is a decrease in glucose utilization by the red blood cell. If erythrocytes are exposed to oxidative foods and drugs, the red cell's metabolic needs increase. However, the G6PD deficiency interferes with glucose metabolism and leads to damage of older red cells. The damaged red cells are then destroyed by hemolysis over a period of 7 to 12 days.

G6PD deficiency is relatively common, especially in blacks and individuals with a Mediterranean heritage. Hemolytic episodes are triggered by viral and bacterial infections. Drugs and toxins also cause hemolysis in individuals deficient in G6PD. Drugs that may cause oxidative problems are antimalarial drugs, sulfonamides, nitrofurantoins, analgesics (e.g., phenacetin), and chloramphenicol.

Generally, the only clinical manifestation and laboratory reflection of G6PD dificiency is hemolytic anemia (Table 24-6). A definitive diagnosis can be made by doing serum assays of the G6PD level.

Managing the hemolysis seen in G6PD deficiency is relatively easy. Because only older red cells are destroyed by the oxidative agent, the younger cells will survive. The cause of the hemolytic reaction must be removed. During the period of acute hemolysis, the client will require rest, adequate hydration, and assessment of kidney function. Attention should be focused on preventing the hemolytic disorders by treating infections promptly and screening black clients for G6PD deficiency before giving an oxidant drug.

Acquired hemolytic anemia

Extrinsic causes of hemolysis can be separated into the three categories: (1) *physical factors*, (2) *antibodies*, and (3) *infectious agents and toxins*. Physical destruction of red cells results from the exertion of extreme force on the cells. Traumatic events causing disruption of the red cell membrane include the use of extracorporeal circulation used in heart-lung bypass and prosthetic heart valves. In addition, the force needed to push blood through abnormal vessels, such as those that have been burned or affected by angiopathic disease (e.g., diabetes mellitus), may also physically damage the red cell.

Antibodies may destroy red blood cells by the mechanisms involved in antigen-antibody reactions. The reactions may be of an *isoimmune* or *autoimmune* type. Isoimmune reactions occur when antibodies develop against antigens from another person of the same species. Blood transfusion reactions typify this response, especially when donor cells are hemolyzed by the recipient's antibodies due to an ABO mismatch.

Autoimmune reactions result when individuals develop antibodies against their own erythrocytes. Autoimmune hemolytic reactions may be *idiopathic*, developing with no prior hemolytic history as a result of the immunoglobulin IgG covering the red cells, or *secondary* to other autoimmune diseases (systemic lupus erythematosus, leukemia, lymphoma) or drugs (penicillin, indomethacin, phenylbutazone, phenacetin, quinidine, quinine, and methyldopa).

The third category of acquired hemolytic disorders is caused by infectious agents and toxins. Infectious agents may foster hemolysis in four ways:

1. By invading the red cell and destroying its contents (e.g., parasites such as malaria)
2. By releasing hemolytic substances (e.g., *Clostridium perfringens*)
3. By generating an antigen-antibody reaction
4. By contributing to splenic hypertrophy as a means of increasing the removal of damaged erythrocytes from the circulation

Various agents may be toxic to the red cells and cause hemolysis. These *hemolytic toxins* involve chemicals such as the oxidative drugs (see Glucose-6-Phosphate Dehydrogenase Deficiency), arsenic, lead, copper, and snake venom.

Treatment and management of acquired hemolytic anemias involve general supportive care until the causative element can be eliminated or at least rendered less injurious to the erythrocytes. To compare and contrast the laboratory findings in the various types of anemia, refer to Table 24-6.

POLYCYTHEMIA

Polycythemia involves the production and presence of increased numbers of circulating erythrocytes. There is usually an associated increase in the blood's hemoglobin concentration. The increase in erythrocytes is so great that blood circulation is impaired due to the increased blood viscosity and volume.

Etiology

The two types of polycythemia are *polycythemia vera* and *secondary polycythemia*. They have different etiologies and pathogenesis, although their complications and clinical manifestations are similar. Polycythemia vera, also known as *primary polycythemia*, has an unknown etiology, although it is postulated that an intrinsic cell defect may be the cause. The disease develops insidiously and follows a chronic, vacillating course. Clients who develop it are usually over 50 years of age. This myeloproliferative disorder causes an increase not only in erythrocytes but also in leukocytes and thrombocytes. The client experiences enhanced blood viscosity and blood volume, as well as congestion of organs and tissues with blood.

The other main type of polycythemia, *secondary polycythemia*, is caused by hypoxia rather than a defect in the red cell itself. Hypoxia stimulates erythropoietin production in the kidney to stimulate erythrocyte production. The need for oxygen may be due to high altitude, pulmonary disease, cardiovascular disease, alveolar hypoventilation, defective oxygen transport, or tissue hypoxia. Consequently, secondary polycythemia is a physiological response that tries to compensate for a problem rather than a pathological response. (The discussion of polycythemia in this section will focus on polycythemia vera. Secondary polycythemia is discussed in Chap. 21.)

Clinical Manifestations and Complications

Circulatory manifestations of polycythemia vera are due to the hypertension caused by the increased blood volume and viscosity. They are often the first symptoms and include subjective complaints of headache, vertigo, dizziness, tinnitus, and visual disturbances. In addition, the client may experience angina, congestive heart failure, intermittent claudication, and thrombophlebitis which may be complicated by embolization. These manifestations are caused by blood vessel distension, impaired blood flow, circulatory stasis, and tissue hypoxia caused by the hypervolemia and hyperviscosity.

Hemorrhagic phenomena caused by either vessel rupture from overdistension or inadequate platelet function may be displayed by petechiae, ecchymoses, epistaxis, or GI bleeding. Hemorrhage can be acute and catastrophic.

Hepatomegaly and *splenomegaly*, which develop from organ engorgement, may contribute to client complaints of satiety and fullness. The client may also experience *pain* due to peptic ulcer caused by the increased gastric secretions or the liver and spleen engorgement. *Skin* manifestations include severe pruritus, which is believed to be due to altered histamine metabolism, and plethora (ruddy complexion).

Hyperuricemia is caused by the increase in cell destruction which accompanies the excessive cell production. Uric acid is one of the products of cell destruction. As cell destruction increases, uric acid production also increases, thus leading to hyperuricemia.

Abnormal Diagnostic Findings

The following laboratory manifestations will be seen in clients with polycythemia vera:

1. Elevated hemoglobin and red blood cell count
2. Elevated white blood cell count
3. Elevated platelets
4. Elevated leukocyte alkaline phosphates, uric acid, and vitamin B_{12}

If a bone marrow examination is used in establishing the diagnosis, it will show a hypercellularity of red cells, white cells, and platelets. Splenomegaly will be found in 75 percent of the clients with polycythemia.

Medical Management

Once polycythemia vera is diagnosed, its treatment will be directed toward reducing blood volume and viscosity as well as bone marrow activity. *Phlebotomy* may be done to diminish blood volume until the desired hematocrit is achieved. *Hydration* therapy will be used to reduce the blood's viscosity. *Myelosuppressive drugs* such as melphalan, busulfan, and chlorambucil may be given to inhibit bone marrow activity. Allopurinol may reduce the number of acute gouty attacks.

Nursing Management

Since the etiology of polycythemia vera is unclear, preventing it may not be possible. However, because secondary polycythemia is generated by any source of hypoxia, it can be prevented from causing problems by maintaining adequate oxygenation. Therefore, controlling chronic pulmonary disease and avoiding high altitudes may be important.

When acute exacerbations of polycythemia vera develop, the nurse has several responsibilities. Depending on the institution's policies, the nurse may either assist with or perform the phlebotomy. Fluid intake and output must be judiciously evaluated during hydration therapy to avoid both fluid overload (which would further complicate the circulatory congestion) and underhydration (which could cause the blood to become even more viscous). If myelosuppressive agents are used, the nurse must administer the drugs as ordered and observe the client for side effects.

Assessment of the client's nutritional status and collaboration with the dietitian may be necessary to offset the inadequate food intake which could result from GI symptoms of fullness, pain, and dyspepsia. Activities must be instituted to decrease thrombus formation. The immobility normally imposed by hospitalization may rapidly compromise the client. Active or passive leg exercises, and ambulation when possible, should be initiated.

Due to its chronic nature, polycythemia vera requires ongoing evaluation. Phlebotomy may be done every 2 to 3 months, reducing the blood volume by about 500 mL each time. The nurse must evaluate the client for the development of complications. Although the incidence is small, some clients with polycythemia develop leukemia and lymphomas. These occurrences may be due to the chemotherapeutic drugs used to treat the disease. However, some clients with polycythemia have developed these malignant disorders without chemotherapy treatment.

CLOTTING PROBLEMS

Clotting disorders may be caused by a disturbance in any component of the hemostatic process. Three major clotting problems are (1) thrombocytopenia (platelet deficiency), (2) hemophilia (a particular clotting factor deficiency), and (3) disseminated intravascular coagulation (a syndrome that affects both platelets and clotting factors).

Thrombocytopenia

Etiology

Thrombocytopenia is a reduction of platelets below the normal range of 150,000 to 400,000/μL. The two primary etiological types are idiopathic and acquired. *Idiopathic thrombocytopenic purpura (ITP)* is so named because its cause is unknown. However, various autoimmune mechanisms are being investigated as a possible cause. It is believed that in ITP, platelets are coated with antibodies. Nevertheless, these platelets function normally. However, when these platelets reach the spleen, macrophages sequester and destroy them because of their altered structure.[7] This platelet destruction results in the extravasation of small amounts of blood into tissues and mucous membranes, forming bruises. Acute ITP is seen predominantly in children following a viral illness. Chronic ITP occurs most commonly in women between 20 and 40 years of age. Chronic ITP has a gradual onset, and transient remissions occur.

Whereas ITP is the result of increased platelet destruction, *acquired thrombocytopenia* is due to diminished or defective platelet production. Acquired thrombocytopenia may result from many conditions (Tables 24-10 and 24-11). It is important for the nurse to become aware of the numerous conditions which may affect platelet production and destruction.

Clinical manifestations

Thrombocytopenia may be manifested by the appearance of bruises known as *purpura*. Small, pinpoint red or reddish-brown purpura are known as *petechiae*, while larger purplish lesions caused by hemorrhage are called *ecchymoses* (Fig. 24-5). Either type of purpura results from blood loss into the tissues. Petechiae result from intradermal bleeding due to vascular or platelet abnormalities. Ecchymoses develop from subcutaneous bleeding caused by trauma or clotting disorders.[8]

Prolonged bleeding after routine procedures such as excessive bleeding after venipuncture or prolonged oozing of blood following an intramuscular injection may also indicate thrombocytopenia. Because the bleeding may be internal, the nurse must also be aware of manifestations which reflect this type of blood loss. Internal bleeding may be manifested as weakness, fainting, dizziness, tachycardia, abdominal pain, and hypotension.

The major complication of thrombocytopenia is *hemorrhage*. The hemorrhage may be insidious or acute, internal or external. It may occur in any area of the body, including bleeding into joints, the retina, and the brain. Insidious hemorrhage may first be detected by discovering the anemia which accompanies blood loss.

Table 24-10
Causes of Acquired Thrombocytopenia

Acquired aplastic anemia
Bone marrow infiltration from carcinoma, lymphoma, leukemia
Exposure to ionizing radiation
Exposure to myelosuppressive drugs
Drugs which suppress platelet production (see Table 24-11)
Deficiencies of vitamin B_{12}, folic acid, and iron
Immunological platelet destruction (see Table 24-11)
Viral infections
Paroxysmal nocturnal hemoglobinuria
DIC

Table 24-11
Drugs that Can Cause Thrombocytopenia

Suppression of platelet production
- Thiazide diuretics
- Alcohol
- Estrogen hormones

Immune-mediated platelet destruction
- Analgesics
  - Acetaminophen
  - Aspirin
  - Phenylbutazone
- Antibiotics
  - Cephalothin
  - Penicillin
  - Streptomycin
  - Sulfa drugs
  - Para-aminosalicylate
- Cinchona alkaloids
  - Quinidine
  - Quinine
- Sedatives, hypnotics, anticonvulsants
  - Diphenylhydantoin (Dilantin)
  - Phenobarbital
  - Meprobamate

Diagnostic study abnormalities

The *platelet count* will definitely be decreased in cases of thrombocytopenia. Any reduction below 150,000/μL may be termed thrombocytopenia. However, bleeding does not usually occur until platelet counts are less than 50,000/μL. When the count drops below 20,000/μL, a serious bleeding tendency exists.[9,10]

The *bleeding time*, a reflection of platelet function,

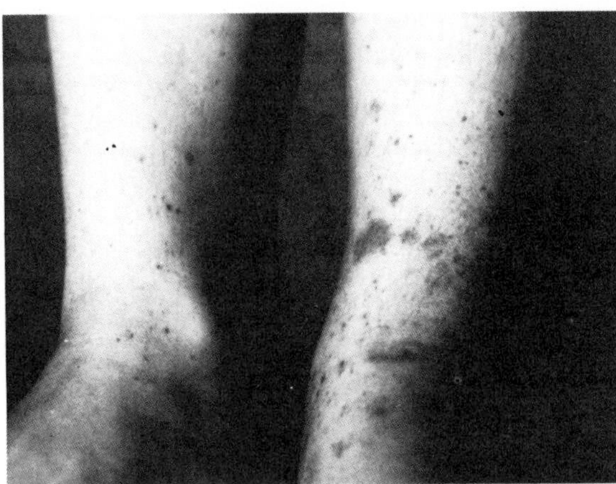

A

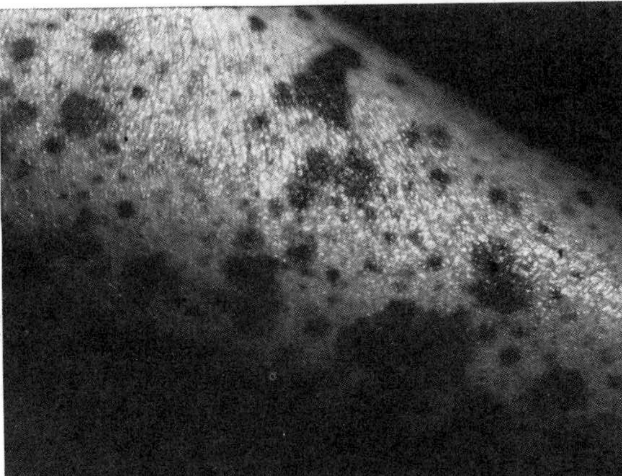

B

Figure 24-5 Examples of ecchymoses.

will be prolonged. Tests which assess other clotting mechanisms, such as the clotting time, prothrombin time, and partial thromboplastin time, will be normal. Bone marrow analysis will show megakaryocytes (precursors of platelets) to be normal or increased, but platelets will be reduced. Bone marrow examination is done to rule out possible causes, such as leukemia and other myeloproliferative disorders.

Anemia will be present in proportion to the amount of blood lost. Therefore, it is important to monitor hemoglobin and hematocrit values as well as to observe the patient for cardiopulmonary distress and other manifestations of anemia.

Medical management

Medical management of thrombocytopenia is based on differentiating the etiology of ITP from that of acquired thrombocytopenia, as each requires a different treatment plan (Table 24-12).

Table 24-12
Medical Management: Thrombocytopenia

Diagnostic
1. History and physical examination
2. Platelet count
3. Bleeding time
4. Bone marrow biopsy
5. Hematocrit and hemoglobin

Therapeutic
- A. Idiopathic
    1. Corticosteroids
    2. Platelet transfusion
    3. Immunosuppressives (cyclophosphamide, azathioprine)
    4. Splenectomy
- B. Acquired
    1. Identify and treat cause
    2. Corticosteroids
    3. Platelet transfusions

Idiopathic Thrombocytopenic Purpura The three main therapies used to manage the client with ITP are *corticosteroids, platelet transfusions*, and *splenectomy*.[11]

Adrenal corticosteroids are used to treat ITP because of their ability to suppress the phagocytic response of splenic macrophage cells. This alters the spleen's recognition of platelets and increases their life span. In addition, corticosteroids depress antibody formation. They also reduce capillary fragility and bleeding time. The mechanism that causes these latter events is poorly understood. The steroid usually administered is prednisone, and the doses vary with the severity of the ITP.

Platelet transfusions may be employed as a means of elevating platelet counts in cases of life-threatening hemorrhage (platelet count less than 20,000/μL). Platelets should not be administered prophylactically because of the possibility of antibody formation. ABO compatibility is not a necessary prerequisite for platelet transfusions. However, it was discovered that after multiple platelet transfusions from more than 20 donors, isoimmunization develops. The immunity is caused by the presence of human leukocyte antigens (HLA) on the platelet membrane. Therefore, by using lymphocyte typing to determine that the HLA types of the donor and the recipient are identical, multiple platelet transfusions can be used more effectively. Compatible donors are most often siblings or parents.[12,13]

The spleen is removed if the client does not respond to steroids. A splenectomy removes the major site of platelet destruction and the source of platelet antibody synthesis. While there is no clear understanding of why splenectomy works, 70 to 90 percent of the clients with ITP improve following spleen removal. Platelet levels increase following surgery because normally about one-third of the platelets are maintained in the spleen's reservoir.

Acquired Thrombocytopenia The medical management of acquired thrombocytopenia is based upon identifying and removing the causative agent. While the precipitating factor is being investigated, the client may receive *corticosteroids* to enhance capillary integrity and *platelet transfusions* if life-threatening hemorrhage develops. Splenectomy is not used because the spleen is not contributing to the thrombocytopenia.

In some situations, acquired thrombocytopenia may be caused by the medical therapy. For example, in leukemia the client may receive certain chemotherapeutic drugs that will cause bone marrow suppression. Therefore, the client must be supported throughout the course of thrombocytopenia in order to give the chemotherapy medication an opportunity to be effective.

Nursing management

Health Promotion and Maintenance It is very important for the nurse to discourage abuse of over-the-counter medications known to be possible causes of acquired thrombocytopenia. Many medications contain aspirin as an ingredient, especially those used to treat upper respiratory infections.

It is also important for the nurse to encourage individuals to have a complete medical evaluation if they develop manifestations of bleeding tendencies (e.g., prolonged epistaxis, petechiae). In addition, the nurse must be observant for early signs of thrombocytopenia in clients taking cancer chemotherapy drugs.

Acute Intervention The goal during acute episodes of thrombocytopenia is to prevent or control hemorrhage (Table 24-13). In thrombocytopenic clients, bleeding is usually from superficial sites, while deep bleeding (into muscles, joints, abdomen) occurs only when clotting factors are diminished. It is important to emphasize that a seemingly minor nosebleed may lead to hemorrhage in a severely thrombocytopenic client. Bleeds from the posterior nasopharynx may

Table 24-13

Nursing Care Plan for the Client with Thrombocytopenia

Client Problem	Expected Outcome	Nursing Intervention
Predisposition to hemorrhage	No evidence of bleeding.	Assess for blood loss via mucous membranes (e.g., epistaxis) and skin (e.g., petechiae, ecchymoses). Test all body excreta for occult blood and observe for overt bleeding in emesis, sputum, feces, urine, wound drainage, NG secretions. Evaluate CBC and platelet counts. Measure blood loss via any route. Weigh blood-soaked linen and dressings. Count sanitary napkins used during menstruation. Evaluate client for blurred or impaired vision (suggestive of retinal hemorrhage). Do not administer aspirin or aspirin-containing products. Use ice and direct pressure or packing to control active bleeding. Administer platelets as ordered, using correct technique (see text).
Fragile mucous membranes and skin	Intact mucous membranes and skin.	Avoid irritating and injuring mucous membranes. Provide oral hygiene with little friction by using soft-bristle toothbrush, cotton swabs, mild mouthwash, or Water Pik. Evaluate integrity of nares, especially if NG tube, NT tube, or nasal oxygen is in use. Use an electric razor for shaving. Avoid IM and SC injections if possible. If used, apply local pressure with a dry, sterile 2 × 2 for 5–10 min after needle is removed.
Possible injury from trauma	Client experiences no trauma or injuries.	Protect client from trauma. Reduce frequency of BP monitoring and alternate extremities used for readings. Pad side rails and other firm or sharp surfaces. Be very gentle when turning client, changing dressings, etc.
Possible bleeding into CNS	No bleeding into CNS.	Prevent rise in intracranial pressure. Teach client to avoid Valsalva maneuver (e.g., straining at stool). Administer stool softeners as ordered. Teach client to cough, sneeze, and blow nose gently. Prevent shivering. Evaluate mental status (headaches, vertigo, irritability, confusion).

be difficult to detect, as the blood may be swallowed. If an intramuscular or subcutaneous injection is unavoidable, use a small-gauge needle and apply direct pressure for at least 5 to 10 minutes afterward.

In the thrombocytopenic female, menstrual blood loss may exceed the usual amount and duration. Counting sanitary napkins used during menses is another important intervention to detect excess blood loss. It takes 50 mL of blood to soak a sanitary napkin completely.

An important nursing role is the proper administration of platelets. Platelet concentrate is administered because it is not practical to give the client the amount of fresh blood needed to increase the platelet level effectively. Platelet concentrate is a yellow-appearing liquid which contains only plasma and platelets. It contains 30 to 50 mL per unit of platelets. One unit of platelets can be derived by centrifuging 500 mL of whole blood.

One unit of platelets will increase the platelet count by about 10,000/μL. Therefore, several units of platelets are usually transfused. Once acquired from a donor, platelets are stored at room temperature for up to 3 days. Therefore, when platelets are received from the blood bank, they will not be cold, and they should be kept at room temperature until they are given. Gentle agitation of the bag is useful to prevent the platelets from adhering to the plastic.

The actual infusion procedure may vary among institutions. A filter tubing is always used. Platelets may be given by intravenous drip infusion or by a direct-push method at a steady rate of 20 to 50 mL/minute. If platelets are given by direct push, a sterile system must be established and maintained. This can be done by attaching a 50-mL syringe to the special platelet transfusion tubing and drawing the platelets into the syringe. Then, without disconnecting the syringe, the platelet tubing can be clamped while the platelets are pushed directly into the vein. This method is repeated until all the platelets are infused (Fig. 24-6).

Chronic Management Clients with ITP who are taking glucocorticosteroids should be monitored frequently for their response to therapy. If the ITP is treated by splenectomy, there is usually no recurrence. Persons with acquired thrombocytopenia must be educated to avoid causative agents when possible (Table 24-11). If the causative agents cannot be avoided, clients must be taught to detect the development of thrombocytopenic problems.

For clients with either ITP or acquired thrombocytopenia, there should be planned periodic medical evaluations to assess the client's status and to intercede in situations in which exacerbations and bleeding are likely to occur. The client must be cautioned to avoid trauma if platelet counts are below normal. Contact sports such as football should be avoided.

Hemophilias

Hemophilias are hereditary bleeding disorders caused by reduced clotting activity of specific coagulation factors. The three major forms of hemophilia are

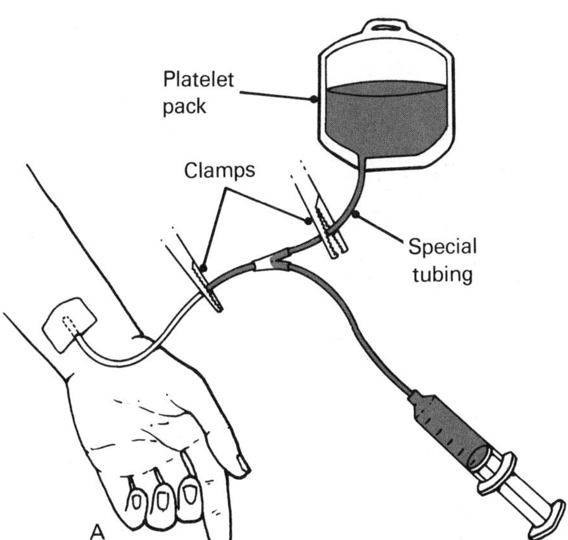

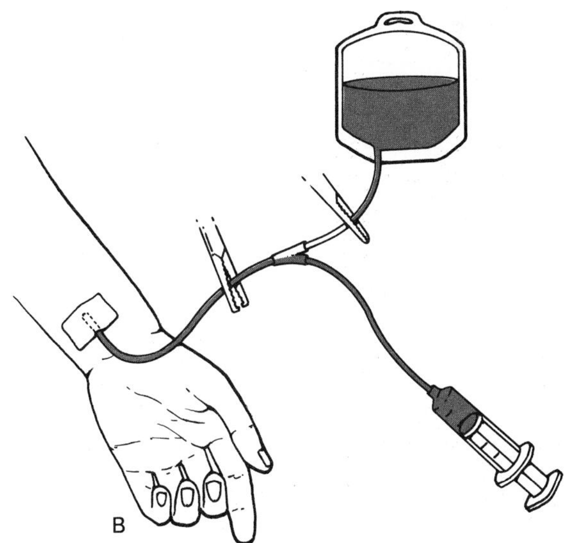

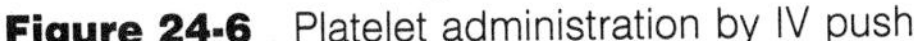
Figure 24-6 Platelet administration by IV push.

hemophilia A (classic hemophilia), *hemophilia B* (Christmas disease), and *von Willebrand's disease*. Hemophilia A is the most common form of hemophilia, comprising about 80 percent of all cases. The incidence of hemophilia A is about 1 in 10,000 males, while hemophilia B is seen in 1 in 100,000 males. The deficiency and inheritance patterns of the three forms of hemophilia are compared in Table 24-14.

Clinical manifestations and complications

There are significant clinical manifestations suggestive of the presence of hemophilia. These include the following:

1. Slow, persistent, prolonged bleeding from minor trauma and small cuts
2. Delayed bleeding after minor injuries (the delay may be several hours or days)
3. Uncontrollable hemorrhage following dental extractions or irritation of the gums with a hard-bristle toothbrush (Fig. 24-7)
4. Epistaxis, especially following a facial blow
5. GI bleeding from ulcers and gastritis
6. Hematuria from GU trauma and splenic rupture resulting from falls or abdominal trauma
7. Ecchymoses and subcutaneous hematomas (these are common; petechiae are rare)
8. Neurological signs such as pain, anesthesia, and paralysis, which may develop from nerve compression caused by hematoma formation
9. *Hemarthrosis* (bleeding into the joints), which may lead to joint deformity severe enough to cause unresolvable crippling (occurs most commonly in the knees, elbow, and ankles)

These manifestations are especially important when seen in children, as the disease may not yet be diagnosed. In adults, these developments are also significant, as they suggest that the hemophilia is poorly controlled. All of the clinical manifestations relate to bleeding, and any bleeding episode in hemophiliacs may result in death from hemorrhage.

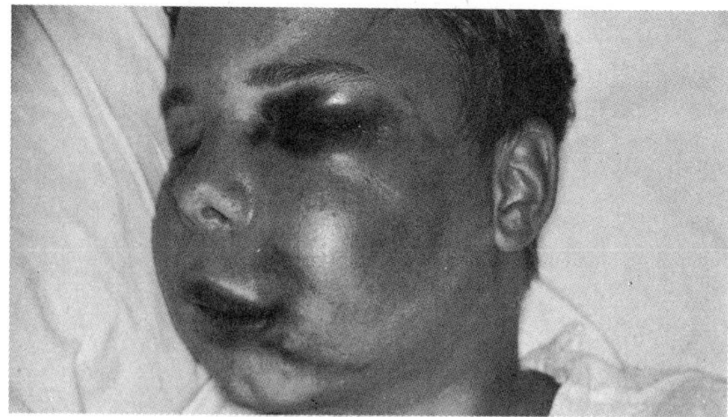

Figure 24-7 Hematoma that developed in a hemophiliac after dental treatment. *[From W. J. Williams et al. (eds.), Hematology, 2d ed., McGraw-Hill Book Company, New York, 1977, plate 12-10.]*

Table 24-14
Comparison of Hemophilic States

Problem	Deficiency	Inheritance pattern
Hemophilia A	Factor VIII	Recessive sex-linked (transmitted by female carriers; displayed almost exclusively in males)
Hemophilia B	Factor IX	Recessive sex-linked (transmitted by female carriers; displayed almost exclusively in males)
von Willebrand's disease	Factor VIII and platelet dysfunction	Autosomal dominant; seen in both sexes

Hemophilia had been considered primarily a disease of childhood because of early death from the complications. Advances in its treatment now enable hemophiliacs to live into adulthood. Although it is now possible to control the complications, hemarthroses and severe hemorrhage are the most common difficulties to be managed. In addition, due to the repeated use of blood components, the development of hepatitis is common.

Medical and pharmacological management

Laboratory studies are used to determine the type of hemophilia present. Any factor deficiency within the intrinsic system (factors VIII, IX, XI, or XII) will yield the laboratory results given in Table 24-15.

The goals of medical management are to prevent and treat bleeding. The medical regimen for a person with hemophilia will be focused on maintaining adequate blood levels of the deficient clotting factors. This goal is achieved by assessing clinical manifestations, determining blood levels of the factors concerned, and then administering the necessary blood component. Factors may be provided via fresh frozen plasma (FFP) or fresh whole blood (Table 24-16).

A more specific component is cryoprecipitate, which contains primarily factor VIII and fibrinogen. Cryoprecipitate is prepared from plasma, frozen rapidly and kept frozen until used. Prior to administration, the cryoprecipitate is thawed slowly and must then be used within 6 hours.

Frequently, commercially prepared antihemophilic factors (AHF) are given (Table 24-16). The commer-

Table 24-15
Laboratory Results Found in Hemophilia

Test	Comments
Prothrombin time (PT)	Extrinsic system is not involved
Thrombin time (TT)	Thrombin-fibrinogen reaction is not impaired
Platelet count	Platelet production is adequate
Partial thromboplastin time (PTT)	Prolonged due to a deficiency in any of the intrinsic clotting system factors
Bleeding time	Prolonged in von Willebrand's disease because of structually defective platelets Normal in hemophilia A and B because platelets are not affected
Factor assays	Reduced factor VIII in hemophilia A and von Willebrand's disease, and reduced factor IX in hemophilia B

cially prepared forms of AHF are known as lyophilized AHF. They represent pooled human donor AHF from which the liquid has been removed. The lyophilized AHF powder must be reconstituted properly and used within 12 hours due to the short life span of the clotting factors. Lyophilized AHF is easy to handle, store, and administer. Unlike cryoprecipitate, commercially prepared AHF provides a predictable, standardized amount of AHF. The disadvantage of commercial AHF is that it poses a higher risk of hepatitis because each vial is produced from multiple donors. Another complication of repeated AHF use is the development of autoimmune inhibitors (anti-AHF factor) which inactivate the AHF and complicate the treatment of bleeding episodes.[14]

Replacement of the deficient clotting factor is the primary means of supporting clients with hemophilia. A factor level of at least 5 percent of normal is usually adequate to prevent spontaneous bleeding, whereas normal hemostasis is possible with 25 percent of normal levels. Surgical procedures necessitate preoperative factor levels of 50 percent of normal, with postoperative levels at 25 percent for about 10 days. In addition to treating acute crises, the commercial AHF may be given to clients prior to surgery and dental care as a prophylaxis against bleeding.

The most common difficulties with medical management are starting AHF therapy too late and stopping it too soon. Generally, minor bleeding episodes should be treated with AHF for at least 72 hours, while surgery and traumatic injuries may dictate support with AHF for 10 to 14 days.[15]

Nursing management

Health Promotion and Maintenance Because of the hereditary nature of hemophilia, referral for genetic counseling is essential when considering preventive measures. This is especially important today, since hemophiliacs are living longer and reaching an age when reproduction is likely.

Acute Management Nursing intervention is related primarily to controlling bleeding and includes the following:

1. Stopping the topical bleeding as quickly as possible by applying direct pressure or ice, packing the area with Gelfoam or fibrin foam, and applying topical hemostatic agents such as thrombin.
2. Administering the blood component ordered to raise the client's level of the deficient coagulation factor.
3. Preventing crippling deformities from hemarthrosis. When joint bleeding occurs, it is important to rest

Table 24-16
Antihemophilic Factor Preparations

Name	Factor Replacement		Source
Fresh frozen plasma (FFP)	Replaces all clotting factors except platelets. Frequently used until the diagnosis is confirmed, as it replaces both factor VIII and factor IX.		Blood bank
Cryoprecipitate	Replaces factor VIII and fibrinogen.		Blood bank
Factorate	VIII	*Note*: None of these preparations can be used to treat von Willebrand's disease, as the factor for platelet adhesion is removed during the manufacturing process.	Lyophilized (commercially prepared dried concentrate)
Hemophil	VIII		
Humafac	VIII		
Koate	VIII		
Profilate	VIII		
Konyne	IX		
Proplex	IX		

the involved joint totally, in addition to administering AHF. The joint may be packed in ice. Analgesics will be needed to reduce the severe pain. As soon as bleeding has ceased, it is important to encourage mobilization of the affected area through range-of-motion exercises and physical therapy. Actual weight bearing should be avoided until all swelling has resolved and muscle strength has returned.

4. Managing any life-threatening complication which may develop as a result of hemorrhage. Examples include nursing interventions to prevent or treat airway obstruction from hemorrhage into the neck and pharynx, as well as early assessment and treatment of intracranial bleeding.

Chronic Management Chronic management is a primary consideration for hemophiliacs because the disease follows an incurable, chronic course. The quality as well as the length of life may be significantly affected by the client's knowledge of the illness and how to live with it. The client and family can be referred to the local chapter of the National Hemophilia Society to encourage association with other individuals who are dealing with the problems of hemophilia. The nurse must provide ongoing assessment of the client's adaptation to the illness. Psychosocial support and assistance should be readily available as needed.

Most of the chronic care measures are related to client education. Hemophiliacs must be taught to recognize disease-related problems and to learn which can be resolved at home and which require hospitalization. Immediate medical attention is required for severe pain or swelling of a muscle or joint which restricts movement or inhibits sleep, head injury, a swelling in the neck or mouth, abdominal pain, hematuria, melena, and skin wounds in need of suturing.

Daily oral hygiene must be done atraumatically, which may require knowledge of the techniques mentioned in Table 24-13. Understanding how to prevent injuries is another consideration. This is no easy task when one considers all the potential sources of trauma. Clients can learn to participate in noncontact sports (e.g., golf) and wear gloves when doing household chores to prevent cuts or abrasions from knives, hammers, and other tools. The client should wear a Medic-Alert tag to ensure that health care providers know about the hemophilia in case of an accident.

Clients need information about routine follow-up care and their compliance with scheduled visits must be assessed. Reliable individuals can be taught to administer AHF at home. This requires instruction regarding venipuncture and infusion techniques.

Disseminated Intravascular Coagulation (DIC)

DIC is a serious bleeding disorder resulting from acceleration of normal clotting with a subsequent decrease in clotting factors and platelets. These changes may lead to uncontrollable hemorrhage. The name of the problem may be misleading because it suggests that the blood is clotting, which is only partially true.

Etiology

DIC is not a disease but rather an abnormal *syndrome* caused by another process. The disorders known to predispose clients to DIC are listed in Table 24-17.

Initially in DIC, the normal coagulation mechanisms are enhanced. Abundant intravascular thrombin, the most powerful coagulant, is produced (Fig. 24-8). It catalyzes the conversion of fibrinogen to fibrin and enhances platelet aggregation. There is widespread fibrin deposition in capillaries and arterioles. Excessive clotting activates the fibrinolytic system to produce fibrin-splint products. These products inhibit the clotting of normal blood by acting as anticoagulants. Ultimately, with clots being lysed and clotting factors being depleted, the blood loses its ability to clot. Therefore, a stable clot cannot be formed at injury sites. This situation predisposes the client to hemorrhage.

Clinical manifestations

The manifestations of DIC are related to indications that the client's coagulation system is impaired. The following are likely findings:

1. Bleeding occurs in clients who have no history of bleeding problems.
2. The severity of bleeding may vary from mild oozing at venipuncture sites to hemorrhage from all orifices.
3. Any of the manifestations of anemia may be indicative of blood loss.
4. The clinical manifestations of thrombocytopenia are also present as platelets are destroyed.

Consequently, uncontrollable, life-threatening hemorrhage is the major complication of DIC.[16]

Diagnostic study abnormalities

There are five tests which may be employed to screen clients for DIC and three laboratory assessments which are diagnostic for the condition. These studies and their findings are listed in Table 24-18.

Table 24-17
Conditions which Predispose to DIC Development

Conditions in which DIC may be stimulated by thromboplastic substances (extrinsic system activity)
Obstetrical
Abruptio placentae
Retained dead fetus
Amniotic fluid embolus
Neoplasia
Prostate cancer
Acute leukemias
Giant cavernous hemangioma
Bronchogenic cancer
Conditions in which DIC may be stimulated by activation of factor XII (intrinsic system activity)
Hemolytic processes
Transfusion of mismatched blood
Acute hemolysis from infection or immunological disorders
Tissue damage
Extensive burns and trauma
Heat stroke
Transplant rejections
Postoperatively, especially following extracorporeal membrane oxygenation
Fat emboli
Snake bites
Conditions in which DIC is stimulated by poorly defined mechanisms
Acute bacterial infections, especially leading to septicemia
Glomerulonephritis
Thrombotic thrombocytopenic purpura
Cirrhosis
Acute fulminant hepatitis
Shock

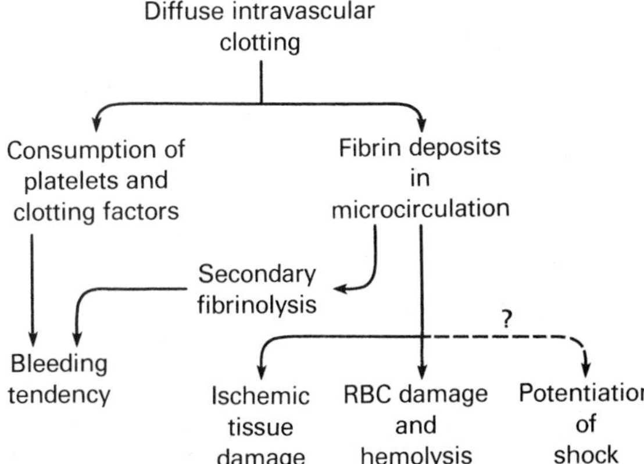

Figure 24-8 Mechanisms involved in disseminated intravascular coagulation. *[From W. J. Williams et al. (eds.), Hematology, 2d ed., McGraw-Hill Book Company, New York, 1977, p. 1455.]*

Table 24-18
Laboratory Abnormalities Found in DIC

Screening Tests	Findings in DIC
Prothrombin time (PT)	Prolonged
Partial thromboplastin time (PTT)	Prolonged
Thrombin time (TT)	Prolonged
Fibrinogen	Reduced
Platelets	Reduced
Special Tests	
FSP	Elevated
Protamine sulfate	Strongly positive
Factor assays (for factors V, VII, VIII, X, XIII)	Reduced

It is important to understand why the three special tests are diagnostic for DIC. As more clots are made in the body, more breakdown products from fibrinogen and fibrin are also formed. These are called *fibrin-split products (FSP)*, and they work in three ways to interfere with blood coagulation. First, they coat the platelets and interfere with platelet function. Second, they interfere with thrombin and thereby disrupt coagulation. Third, the FSPs attach to fibrinogen, which interferes with the polymerization process necessary to form a stable clot.

The *protamine sulfate test* may be the most sensitive diagnostic test of active DIC. Protamine sulfate can bind with fibrin split products and free the fibrin monomer so that it can be polymerized and form a stable clot. A weakly positive test may occur after surgery, with liver disease, or with thrombosis. A strongly positive protamine sulfate test is highly significant for DIC.

The last special test involves assessing the client's plasma for particular plasma protein factors which are suspected to be deficient. Factor assays may be performed to determine the exact amounts of the different plasma proteins.

Medical management

It is important to diagnose DIC quickly, institute therapy which will resolve the underlying causative disease, and then to treat the DIC itself. Establishing that DIC is occurring and investigating potential causes are considerably easier than knowing what therapy should be employed to counteract the condition. The treatment of DIC is currently under continual investigation as researchers attempt to validate the most suitable means of managing this dangerous syndrome. Consequently, it is imperative that the nurse maintain an ongoing awareness of current modes of therapy. What is suggested as the best approach for treatment at present may be revised in the future.

Treating the disease which causes DIC might entail supportive measures for those entities which are self-limiting. Other causes of DIC may require highly specific therapeutic intervention. Regardless of the etiology, treating the primary disease process is essential to the resolution of DIC.

Depending upon its severity, DIC may be treated by one of the following methods. First, if DIC is diagnosed in a client who is not bleeding, no therapy for this condition is necessary. Treatment of the underlying disease may be sufficient to reverse the DIC. Second, when the client is bleeding, therapy is directed toward providing support with necessary blood products while treating the primary disorder. The blood products are administered based on specific component deficiencies. Platelets will be given to correct thrombocytopenia, cryoprecipitate will replace factor VIII and fibrinogen, and FFP will replace all clotting factors except platelets as well as providing a source of antithrombin.

While the use of heparin in DIC is controversial, its proponents believe that the antithrombin activity of heparin interrupts the DIC process by preventing activation of the clotting mechanism. The important consideration is that if heparin is used to treat DIC, it *must* be used in conjunction with blood product support.

Another treatment has been employed, but its usefulness is extremely speculative. Epsilon aminocaproic acid (EACA, Amicar) has been tried as therapy for DIC because of its ability to inhibit fibrinolysis. The fibrinolysis offers protection against the thrombosis common to DIC. Therefore, EACA may potentiate the syndrome.[17]

Nursing management

The main consideration for nurses is always to be alert for the development of DIC. It is important to recognize which illnesses predispose clients to this potentially lethal problem. Early detection of the manifestations of bleeding is essential in the treatment of DIC.

The acute care required by a client with DIC is based on four principles:

1. Fulfill the nursing responsibilities related to resolving the cause of the DIC.
2. Administer blood products properly (if ordered).
3. Implement nursing measures related to anemia which is caused by blood loss and hemolysis (Table 24-4).
4. Protect the client from additional foci of bleeding (Table 24-13).

The administration of platelets has already been discussed. Infusing cryoprecipitate or FFP is similar to giving any other blood product (Chap. 26). Cryoprecipitate comes in bags of 10 to 20 mL each. When it is used to treat DIC, up to 30 bags of cryoprecipitate may be required to support the client. FFP is also frozen to preserve factors V and VIII. It takes about 20 minutes to thaw a unit which contains 200 to 250 mL.

NEUTROPENIA, GRANULOCYTOPENIA, AND AGRANULOCYTOSIS

Leukopenia refers to a decrease in the total white blood cell count (granulocytes, lymphocytes, and monocytes). *Granulocytopenia* is a deficiency of granulocytic white cells, including neutrophils, eosinophils, and basophils. However, traditionally granulocytopenia actually refers to *neutropenia* (an insufficient amount of neutrophils). Neutropenia is defined as a neutrophil count of less than 2,000/μL. The term *agranulocytosis* is actually a synonym for *neutropenia*, but it has come to imply a more serious problem.[18] Regardless of the terminology, it is important to recognize that a leukopenic state can develop in many diseases, but it itself is not a disease. Neutropenia is of concern because of the neutrophil's role in phagocytosis. The major causes of granulocytopenia or neutropenia are summarized in Table 24-19.

Clinical Manifestations

Clients who are granulocytopenic will be predisposed to infection. When the white count is depressed or immature white cells are present, the usual phagocytic mechanisms are impaired. As a consequence of the diminished phagocytic response, the classic signs of infection, redness, heat, and swelling, are not manifested. Therefore, the presence of fever is of great significance.

When fever is associated with granulocytopenia, it is generally assumed to be due to infection.[19,20] Other manifestations of granulocytopenia may include symptoms of fatigue and weakness. The mucous membranes of the throat and mouth are particularly susceptible to bacterial invasion. If an infection develops in these areas, the client may complain of sore throat and dysphagia. Other manifestations of granulocytopenia may include ulcerative lesions of the pharyngeal and buccal mucosa, tachycardia, and severe chills.

Medical Management

Diagnostic

The main methods for assessing granulocytopenia are peripheral blood and bone marrow examinations (Table 24-20). A total white blood cell count of less than 5000/μL reflects leukopenia. Only a differential count can confirm the presence of neutropenia (neutrophil count <2000/μL). If the differential white blood cell count reflects an absolute neutropenia of 500 to 1000/μL, the client is at moderate risk for a bacterial infection, while an absolute neutropenia of less than 500/μL places the client at severe risk. If the monocyte count is 400 to 600/μL or greater, the neutropenic client is afforded some intrinsic resistance to infection.

A peripheral blood smear is used to assess for immature forms of granulocytes. The hematocrit, reticulocyte count, and platelet count are done to evaluate general bone marrow function. Bone marrow biopsies and smears are done to examine cellularity, megakaryocytes, and malignant cells. Additional studies may be done as indicated to assess spleen and liver function.

Therapeutic

The factors involved in medical management for neutropenia include (1) determining the etiology of the neutropenia, (2) identifying the offending organisms if infection has developed, (3) instituting antibiotic therapy, (4) determining the need for granulocyte transfusions, and (5) assessing the usefulness of laminar air flow isolation (Table 24-20).

The cause of the granulocytopenia may be easily removed (e.g., by termination of phenothiazines), or it may be recognized but not altered (e.g., the need to continue chemotherapy to treat leukemia). In some situations, the neutropenia will resolve if the primary disease is treated (e.g., folic acid deficiency).

Systemic infections caused by both bacterial and fungal septicemia are common in granulocytopenic clients. Pneumonias of both bacterial and fungal origin are also prevalent. *Pneumocystis carinii* is an especially severe cause of pneumonia. Organisms that are known to be common sources of infection include *Staphylococcus aureus* and gram-negative organisms such as *Escherichia coli*, *Pseudomonas aeruginosa*, and *Klebsiella pneumoniae*. Fungi and the client's own bacteria have been identified as contributing significantly to life-threatening infection. The fungi which are involved include *Candida* (usually *C. albicans*) and *Aspergillus*. Viral infections caused by *varicella-zoster* and *herpes simplex* may also prove difficult to treat.[21]

The medical approach to *identifying the infective organism* is dependent upon acquiring cultures from various sites. Serial blood cultures (at least two) are essential, along with cultures of sputum, the throat, lesions, wounds, urine, and feces. It may also be necessary to do a tracheal aspiration, bronchoscopy with bronchial brushings, or lung biopsy to diagnose the cause of pneumonic infiltrates.

Once cultures are acquired, *antibiotic therapy* must be initiated if fever is present. The use of antibiotics prophylactically is not recommended. The life-threatening nature of granulocytopenia necessitates the institution of broad-spectrum antibiotics until

Table 24-19

Clinical Conditions Associated with Granulocytopenia (Neutropenia)

Hematological
- Idiopathic neutropenias
- Leukemia
- Aplastic anemia

Nutritional deficiences
- Vitamin B_{12}
- Folic acid

Drug-induced
- Alkylating agents (e.g., chlorambucil, cyclophosphamide)
- Antimetabolites (e.g., methotrexate, 6-mercaptopurine)
- Phenothiazine* (e.g., chlorpromazine)
- Anticonvulsants* (e.g., diphenylhydantoin)
- Antimicrobials* (e.g., chloramphenicol, penicillin, sulfonamides)

Secondary to other diseases
- Severe sepsis
- Malignancies with bone marrow infiltration
- Diseases with splenomegaly

*Infrequently causes neutropenia.

Table 24-20

Medical Management: Neutropenia

Diagnostic
1. History and physical examination
2. WBC count with differential count
3. Peripheral blood smear
4. Hematocrit and hemoglobin
5. Reticulocyte and platelet count
6. Bone marrow biopsy

Therapeutic
1. Identify the cause
2. Identify the source of infection (if present)
3. Antibiotic therapy
4. Granulocyte transfusions
5. Reverse isolation
6. Laminar airflow isolation

culture results return. Administration of antibiotics must be via the intravenous route due to the rapidly lethal effects of infection. Oral antibiotics are not sufficiently potent and do not act as rapidly.

Granulocyte transfusions may be used when the granulocytopenic client remains febrile in spite of antibiotic therapy.[22-24] Just as red cell and platelet transfusions are used to treat anemia and thrombocytopenia, respectively, granulocyte transfusions in conjunction with antibiotics improve survival for severely granulocytopenic clients.

Not all health care facilities have the capability to prepare granulocyte transfusions, as a technique known as *leukapheresis* is required. White cells may be obtained by cell separation. Donors are connected to the leukapheresis machine, and the white cells are separated from other blood elements. The remaining blood elements are returned to the donor.

Once the decision is made to administer granulocytes, one or two donors should be obtained. The donor needs to be someone who is ABO and Rh compatible with the client because some red cells will be present in the white cell concentrate. Donor HB_sAg (hepatitis B surface antigen) testing must be done, but HLA typing is not necessary. The donor must be counseled about the leukapheresis procedure and the time involved (generally 5 to 6 hours several times a week).

A final medical consideration is to assess the usefulness of *reverse isolation* and *laminar airflow isolation*. It is known that measures must be instituted to protect the granulocytopenic client from other persons who are infected. There is agreement that it is important to place the client in a private room with an attached bathroom and that everyone in contact with the client should use good handwashing procedures. However, the need for complete reverse isolation is controversial. Opponents of reverse isolation base their beliefs on the fact that this procedure has not substantially reduced infections in granulocytopenic clients. Reverse isolation probably only protects against transmission of organisms by direct physical contact. Therefore, the client is still exposed to contaminates from bathrubs, sinks, air ducts, and even hospital food.[25]

Laminar airflow rooms (LAFRs) are useful in preventing infection in clients whose treatment will lead to granulocytopenia (e.g., leukemics receiving chemotherapy or waiting for bone marrow recovery). These rooms provide a virtually sterile environment by filtering the air through extremely efficient air filters and employing a blower system which provides a laminar flow of air free from convection and conduction currents (Fig. 24-9). There are two reasons for using LAFRs for granulocytopenic clients. First, they reduce the incidence of hospital-acquired infections in these individuals. Second, they provide an environment in which the client's own flora, also a potential source of infection, may be reduced to a minimum through the use of prophylactic topical and oral antibiotics.

Prior to being placed in a LAFR, the client receives topical sterilization by being bathed and shampooed with antiseptic solution. In addition, topical antimicrobial ointments are applied to the ears, nose, rectum, and umbilicus. Oral nonabsorbable antibiotics are given to sterilize the GI tract.

Any personnel who enter the LAFR must be masked, capped, and gowned and must wear sterile covers over their shoes. The oral and topical antibiotic regimens continue while the client is in the LAFR.

Nursing Management

The nursing measures presented in Table 24-21 are critical to the survival of neutropenic clients. The value of good nursing care in reducing the development of infection or limiting its extent cannot be overemphasized.

The nurse is usually responsible for giving granulocyte transfusions if they are ordered. Granulocytes are given through standard blood filter tubing with normal saline to minimize cell lysis. Microaggregate filters are not employed, as they would eliminate infusion of platelets present in the granulocyte suspension.

Granulocytes are usually administered over a 2- to 4-hour period. There are usually 200 to 300 mL per granulocyte suspension. Granulocytes can be stored for only 48 hours. Remember that red cells, platelets, and other white cells may also be in the suspension. Consequently, transfusion reactions may occur. Therefore, the initial 50 to 75 mL of the granulocyte infusion should be administered over about 1 hour and the client monitored closely for any manifestations of a reaction.

The nurse must also monitor the client for untoward developments during granulocyte transfusion. These include fever and shaking chills, allergic reactions, hypotension, respiratory changes, hemolytic reactions, and graft-versus-host reaction.

Fever and *shaking chills* occur commonly. In fact, these responses occur more frequently if the client is febrile at the time the transfusion begins. Therefore, transfusion may be postponed until the client's temperature is less than 38.7°C (101.7°F). The source of this febrile response is not clear, but prophylactic premedication with steroids and antihistamines has proved to reduce the febrile episode.[26]

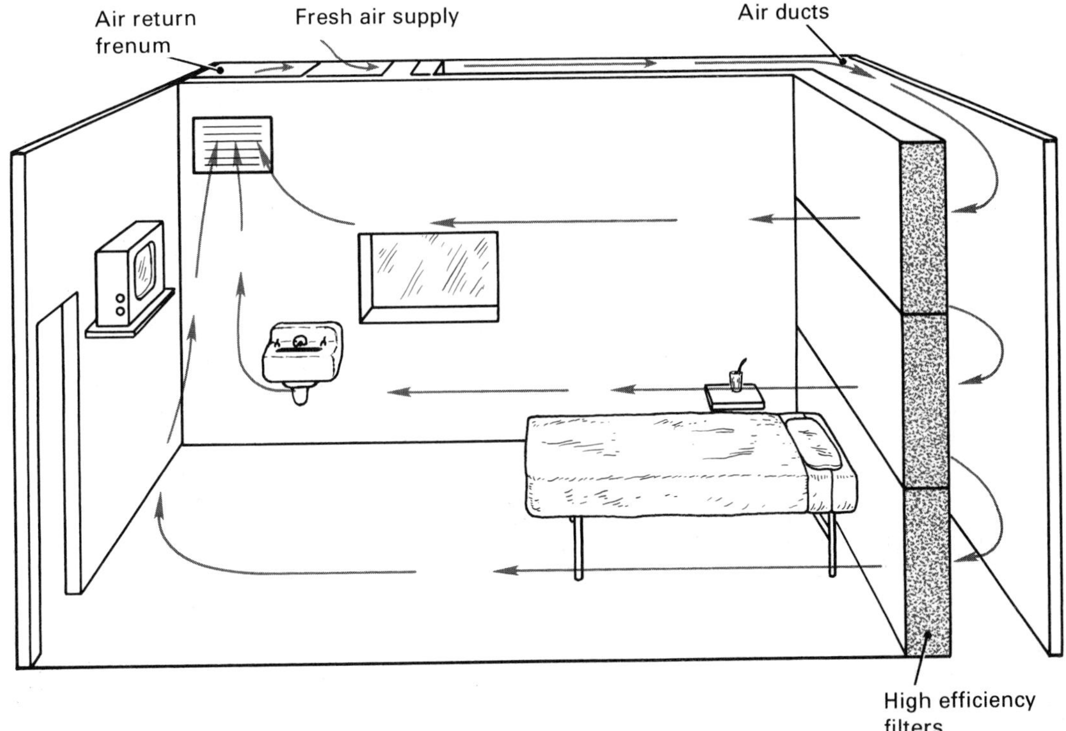

Figure 24-9 Laminar airflow room. Air filtration is combined with horizontal airflow across the room. In this way, a sterile environment can be achieved.

The nursing role in dealing with the febrile state is important. There is no need to stop the granulocyte transfusion, but the reaction may be minimized by slowing the infusion so that it takes 4 hours.

With *allergic reactions* manifested by urticaria, hives, wheezing, or hypotension, the transfusion should be stopped and the physician notified. As with reactions to other blood products, the IV line should be kept open with normal saline. The physician will determine whether the granulocyte transfusion can proceed.

Two situations which require the discontinuation of the granulocyte infusion are *hypotensive responses* and *respiratory reactions*. Hypotensive responses occur infrequently. A moderate reaction will reduce blood pressure by 10 mmHg, while more severe reactions may involve symptoms of shock. With moderate reactions, the transfusion can continue, but severe hypotension dictates discontinuing the transfusion, keeping the IV site open with normal saline, and notifying the physician. Respiratory reactions manifested by dyspnea and cyanosis are rare. The occurrence of these reactions is more frequent when pulmonary infections exist. It is believed that the reaction results from the migration of the leukocytes to the pulmonary microvasculature. In this situation, intervention follows the pattern used with severe hypotension.

Hemolytic reactions may occur due to the presence of erythrocytes in the granulocyte suspension. These may be immediate or delayed for up to 3 days. *Graft-versus-host reactions* may develop from lymphocytes in the granulocyte suspension if the client is immunosuppressed. In this type of reaction, the donated transfused lymphocytes mount an immune response against the recipient's cells.

LEUKEMIA

Leukemia is the general term used to describe a malignant disorder affecting the blood-forming tissues of the bone marrow, lymph system, and spleen. It is a disease which, in differing forms, may affect all age groups. Leukemia follows a progressive course that is eventually fatal if untreated. Leukemias comprise 6 percent of all cancers. All types of leukemia are slightly more common in males than females.

Table 24-21

Nursing Care Plan for the Client with Neutropenia

Client Problem	Expected Outcome	Nursing Intervention
Potential infection from pathogenic organisms	Limited exposure to potential pathogens. No fever or other signs of infection.	Reduce client exposure to pathogens in the hospital environment. Place client in private room. Limit number of visitors. Hospital staff with colds or other potentially communicable illnesses must not be assigned to work with the client. Institute good handwashing technique with antiseptic solution for all individuals who contact the client. Serve cooked, pasteurized, or sterilized food. Client should use sterile water for drinking and bathing. Conduct routine culturing of common sources of contamination (e.g., bathtub, sitz baths, respiratory therapy equipment).
Interruption of skin surface	Maintenance of skin integrity.	Reduce the number of venipunctures. Avoid the use of IV catheters and other invasive procedures except when absolutely necessary. Use an iodophor sponge for skin decontamination before venipuncture. Change IV sites every 24–48 h (ensure that a new IV is established before the old one is discontinued). If IVs are necessary, change IV tubing, dressings, and bottles every 24 h. Observe the insertion site for signs of infection. Use new tubing with the administration of each blood product. Ambulate client to reduce decubitus ulcer formation. If client is on bed rest, change position every 1–2 h by a predetermined schedule posted by the client's bed. Use measures to reduce pressure over bony prominences (alternating-pressure mattress, eggshell mattress, sheepskin, foam pads, etc.). Provide meticulous perianal care. Assess the character and number of bowel movements, as both diarrhea and constipation can irritate the bowel mucosa. Avoid taking T and administering medication by rectum. Avoid rectal enemas. Institute nonsurgical management of anorectal lesions, including sitz baths, topical anesthetic ointments, and analgesics to control the pain. Prevent breaks in skin integrity by using techniques discussed with thrombocytopenia (Table 24-13).
Potential infection from endogenous organisms	Reduction of normal endogenous organisms. No fever or other signs of infection.	Avoid using urinary catheters. Provide good personal hygiene for the client. Teach proper handwashing techniques especially before meals and after micturition or bowel movements. Provide and/or teach proper techniques of hair washing, bathing, grooming of fingernails and toenails, and oral hygiene. Teach pulmonary hygiene techniques such as turning, coughing and deep breathing every 2 h.
Developing or existing infection	Normal temperature and negative cultures. No other signs of infection.	Recognize signs of developing infection (especially fever). Be alert for abnormal complaints (chills or complaints of being cold in a warm environment, sore throat, persistent cough, chest pain, burning on urination, rectal pain). Routinely assess the oral mucosa for the development of candidiasis so that treatment can be instituted. Administer nystatin (Mycostatin), an antifungal, as ordered. Monitor vital signs every 2–3 h. Report a temperature of >38°C (100.4°F) to the physician. Administer acetaminophen, if ordered, as an antipyretic. Do not administer aspirin. Encourage increased intake of fluids during febrile episodes. Evaluate intake and output, along with fluid loss via perspiration. Assess skin turgor and mucous membranes. Recognize that increased metabolism during febrile states requires increased caloric ingestion to prevent weight loss. Have dietitian consult with client to ascertain food likes and desires. Monitor weight. Recognize that mouth sores may limit number of tolerable foods. Institute antibiotic therapy as ordered. Dilute medication sufficiently to reduce vein irritation. Administer all antibiotics separately. Devise a timing schedule so that drug interaction is minimized while desired physiological effects are maximized. Evaluate the client for side effects of antibiotic therapy. Be alert for superinfections which may develop with long-term antibiotic therapy.

Pathophysiology

Regardless of the specific type of leukemia involved, the etiology is unknown. However, several predisposing factors have been identified, including various chemical agents such as benzol, genetic factors such as chromosomal alterations, viral factors such as the Epstein-Barr virus, immunological deficiencies, and the prior use of certain antineoplastic drugs. Exposure to large doses of radiation is another predisposing cause of leukemia. There is an increased incidence of leukemia in radiologists, persons living near areas where radiation testing is conducted, persons treated with radiotherapy, and survivors of the bombing of Nagasaki and Hiroshima.

Leukemia is characterized by a disorderly, unregulated proliferation of white blood cells. The cellular defect involves proliferation of abnormal immature white blood cells or increased production of mature-appearing white cells. As leukemia progresses, fewer normal blood cells are produced. The abnormal leukocytes continue to multiply. They infiltrate and damage the bone marrow, lymph nodes, spleen, and other organs, including the central nervous system. Due to crowding of the bone marrow by leukemic cells, there is bone marrow suppression. The client is predisposed to anemia from the lack of red cells, thrombocytopenia from reduced platelets, and granulocytopenia from the deficiency of functional white cells.

Classification of Leukemia

The two major categories of leukemia are acute and chronic. In the past, these designations had significant prognostic implications related to the duration of the illness. However, current therapeutic measures have increased the survival of clients with certain forms of acute leukemia beyond that of clients with certain forms of chronic leukemia. While the terms *acute* and *chronic* are still used, they refer primarily to cell maturity and the nature of the disease onset. In *acute leukemia*, the bone marrow is infiltrated with young, undifferentiated, immature cells, often referred to as *blasts*. The disease has a rapid onset and requires immediate and aggressive intervention. The bone marrow in individuals with *chronic leukemia* consists primarily of differentiated mature white cells, and the disease onset is more gradual.[27]

Additional classification of leukemia is done by identifying the type of leukocyte involved, whether a *granulocyte (myelocyte)* or a *lymphocyte*. By combining the acute and chronic categories with the cell type involved, specific types of leukemia can be identified. Four major kinds of leukemia are acute myeloblastic (granuloblastic) leukemia, chronic granulocytic (myelocytic) leukemia, acute lymphoblastic leukemia, and chronic lymphocytic leukemia. These forms of leukemia are compared in Table 24-22.

Acute myeloblastic (granulocytic) leukemia (AML, AGL)

AML is characterized by uncontrolled proliferation of myeloblasts, the precursors of granulocytes. There is hyperplasia of the bone marrow and spleen. The clinical manifestations are usually related to replacement of normal hematopoietic cells in the marrow by leukemic cells and, to a lesser extent, to infiltration of other organs (Table 24-22).

Acute lymphoblastic leukemia (ALL)

In ALL, immature lymphocytes proliferate in the bone marrow. Fever is present in the majority of clients at the time of diagnosis. Symptoms may appear abruptly with bleeding or fever, or they may be insidious with progressive weakness, fatigue, and bleeding tendencies. Central nervous system manifestations are especially common in ALL and represent a serious problem. Leukemic meningitis due to arachnoid infiltration occurs in many clients with ALL. While ALL is primarily a disease of children, adults may also develop it.

Chronic granulocytic leukemia (CGL)

CGL is caused by an excessive development of neoplastic granulocytes in the bone marrow. The excess granulocytes move into the peripheral blood in massive numbers and ultimately infiltrate the liver and spleen. Immature and mature granulocytes are found in the bone marrow and peripheral blood, but mature cells are dominant peripherally. Complications of CGL are related to *blastic crises* which change chronic leukemia to acute disease (infiltration of more immature cells). Increased numbers of myeloblasts are found in both bone marrow and blood. The chronic phase of CGL usually can be well controlled by treatment and persists for 2 to 4 years. The blastic phase of CGL is refractory to therapy, and the client lives for only a few months.

Chronic lymphocytic leukemia (CLL)

CLL is characterized by the production and accumulation of functionally inactive but long-lived, mature-appearing lymphocytes. Eventually, the lymphocytes infiltrate the bone marrow, spleen, and liver. Lymph node enlargement throughout the body is commonly found (Fig. 24-10). There is an increased incidence of infection. Complications from CLL are uncommon initially but may develop as the disease advances. Pressure on nerves from enlarged lymph nodes can

Table 24-22
Comparison of Various Types of Leukemia

	AML	ALL	CGL	CLL
Age at onset	Increasing incidence with advancing age	Before age 14; peak incidence 2–4 yr	30–50 yr old	50–70 yr old (rare below age 45)
Clinical manifestations	Fatigue and weakness Headache Mouth sores Minimal hepatosplenomegaly and lymphadenopathy Anemia Bleeding Fever Infection Sternal tenderness	Fatigue and weakness Headache Mouth sores Hepatosplenomegaly Generalized lymphadenopathy Anemia Bleeding Fever Neurological manifestations (CNS metastases, increased intracranial pressure secondary to meningeal infiltration) Bone and joint pain	Asymptomatic early in disease Fatigue and weakness Fever Sternal tenderness Weight loss Bone pain Massive splenomegaly	Usually asymptomatic; often found during an examination for an unrelated disease Chronic fatigue Anorexia Splenomegaly and lymphadenopathy Hepatomegaly
Diagnostic study abnormalities	RBC, Hb, Hct: low Platelets: very low WBC: low or normal Bone marrow: markly hypercellular with myeloblasts	RBC, Hb, Hct: low Platelets: low WBC: low, normal, or high Long-bone x-rays show transverse lines of rarefaction at the ends of the metaphysis	RBC, Hb, Hct: low Platelets: elevated early, reduced later WBC: PMNs increased, lymphs normal, monocytes normal or low Leukocyte alkaline phosphatase: low Philadelphia chromosome present in 90% of clients (only disease in which Philadelphia chromosome is found)	Mild anemia as disease progresses Mild thrombocytopenia as the disease progresses WBC: increased lymphocytes Bone marrow: increased presence of lymphocytes
Prognosis	Poor. High mortality from infection and hemorrhage	Good response to treatment (95% initial remission), 50–60% of clients under age 15 achieve 5-year survival	Clients survive for 2–4 yr after diagnosis, with death usually resulting from infection and hemorrhage	Clients live well with this type of leukemia. Prognosis is related to extent of organ infiltration. Survival ranges from 2 to 10 yr

cause pain and even paralysis. Mediastinal node enlargement can lead to pulmonary symptoms.

Rare forms of leukemia

In addition to the four types of leukemia just discussed, there are two kinds of leukemia which are seen infrequently. One of these affects the monocytes and therefore is known as *monocytic leukemia*. Acute monocytic leukemia presents with weakness and fatigue progressing to exhaustion, anorexia, pallor, chills, and fever. Chronic monocytic leukemia is typified by a more insidious onset. In both types of monocytic leukemia, common findings are gum hyperplasia, inflammation, bleeding, and infection. The second rare form of leukemia affects red blood cells and is known as *erythroleukemia or DiGugliemo's syndrome*. It is considered a white cell disorder because ultimately the disease progresses to affect granulocytes.

Clinical Manifestations

As indicated in Table 24-22, the manifestations of leukemia are varied. Essentially, they relate to prob-

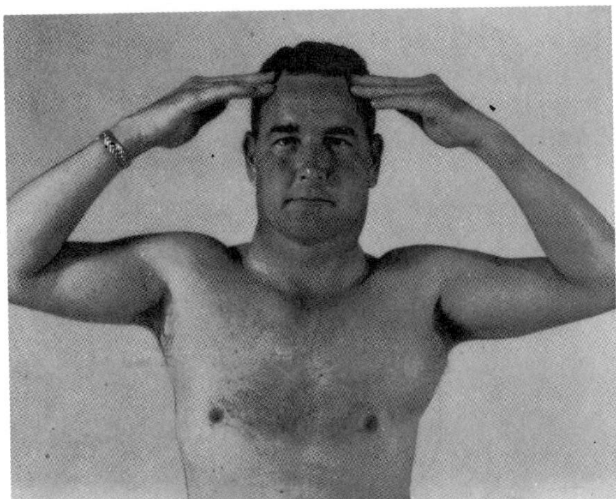

Figure 24-10 Axillary and cervical lymph node enlargement in a person with chronic lymphocytic leukemia. *[From Hematology, 2d ed., W. J. Williams et al. (eds.), McGraw-Hill Book Company, New York, 1977, plate 8-1.]*

lems caused by bone marrow failure and the formation of masses composed of leukemic infiltrates. *Bone marrow failure* results from a lack of production of normal marrow elements. Therefore, clinical manifestations of anemia, thrombocytopenia, and neutropenia will be found. *Leukemic infiltration* will lead to such findings as splenomegaly, hepatomegaly, lymphadenopathy, bone pain, meningeal irritation, and oral lesions.

Diagnostic Study Abnormalities

Peripheral blood evaluation and bone marrow examination are the primary methods of diagnosing leukemia. See Table 24-22 for the usual findings. It is often current practice to identify acute leukemia as ALL or acute nonlymphoblastic leukemia (ANLL), the latter possibly being a single disease with several forms of morphological expression.[28,29]

Medical and Pharmacological Management

Once leukemia has been diagnosed, medical management consists of ordering chemotherapeutic drugs, examining the client on an ongoing basis to evaluate his progress, and intervening to prevent complications of the disease and the therapy (e.g., hemorrhage and infection). In order to understand better the aggressive medical approach needed by the leukemic client, it is necessary to know the principles of cancer chemotherapy, including cellular kinetics, the use of multiple drugs rather than single agents, and the cell cycle. This information is presented in Chap. 11.

An important treatment consideration in regard to chemotherapy is the concept of *remission*. Remission is the goal of treatment for leukemia. Although the disease cannot be cured at this time, in remission it is under maximum control. In *complete remission* there is no evidence of overt disease on physical examination, and both the bone marrow and peripheral blood appear normal. A lesser state of control is known as *partial remission*. Partial remission is characterized by no overt clinical disease and a normal peripheral blood smear, but the disease remains in the bone marrow.

While curing leukemia is not currently possible, the survival period after diagnosis is increasing as a result of attaining and maintaining remissions. However, each time a client relapses, the succeeding remission will be much more difficult to achieve. Consequently, client compliance during maintenance therapy and evaluation of its efficacy are of paramount importance. (Maintenance therapy is usually done on an outpatient basis.)

Another important aspect of chemotherapy is the use of *induction therapy* and *maintenance therapy*. Induction therapy is the attempt to induce or bring about a remission, while maintenance therapy is the effort to maintain the remission once it is achieved. Induction is exceedingly aggressive treatment which seeks to destroy leukemic cells in the tissues, peripheral blood, and bone marrow. It is during induction therapy that a client may become devastatingly ill and predisposed to complications, as the bone marrow is severely depressed by the drugs in an attempt to allow normal cells to regenerate. Throughout induction, medical and nursing interventions to combat anemia, thrombocytopenia, and leukopenia may significantly affect the client's survival. Maintenance therapy is less potent ongoing therapy that strives to keep the body disease-free. Consequently, it is better tolerated by most clients and leads to fewer complications. Chemotherapy may also be used when remission is not a realistic goal to help with disease *palliation*, or the relief of symptoms to enhance the quality of life.

In addition to chemotherapy, radiotherapy may be ordered for clients with chronic leukemia. Total body radiation may be used, or fields may be restricted to the liver and spleen or other organs affected by infiltrates. For CML, radioactive phosporus (^{32}P) may be used instead of radiotherapy. In acute leukemia, cranial irradiation and intrathecal methotrexate are used prophylactically or in the treatment of central nervous system involvement. The use of immunotherapy in the treatment of leukemia is being investigated (Chap. 11). Bone marrow transplants are also under investigational use in the treatment of acute leukemias.

Chemotherapy regimens

The chemotherapeutic agents used in treating leukemia vary. The choice of drugs and the sequence of therapy depend on the preference of the cancer specialist as well as on current research findings. Therefore, it is impossble to present definitive protocols of treatment for the various types of leukemias. Table 24-23 lists chemotherapeutic agents used to treat leukemia. Table 24-24 gives examples of treatment regimens used in various types of leukemia.

Combination chemotherapy is the mainstay of treatment for leukemia. The three purposes for using multiple drugs are to (1) decrease drug resistance, (2) minimize the toxicity of high doses of single agents by using multiple drugs with varying toxicities, and (3) interrupt cell growth at multiple points in the cell cycle.

Acronyms made from the letters of the drugs used in the combination may be used to identify the regimen. For example COAP stands for the following drugs: cyclophosphamide, oncovin, arabinoside, and prednisone. This combination of drugs is used in the treatment of acute leukemia. These drugs are given in a sequential fashion following a predetermined format. Table 24-25 presents a normal 14-day cycle of COAP therapy. After a cycle, the client receives no antileukemic medications for a specified period of time (2 weeks for COAP), and then another cycle is started if peripheral blood counts are adequate.

Table 24-23
Chemotherapeutic Agents Used to Treat Leukemia

Drug Classification	Drug Name
Alkylating agent	Busulfan (Myleran) Chlorambucil (Leukeran) Cyclophosphamide (Cytoxan/Endoxan) Triethylenemelamine (TEM)
Antibiotic	Daunorubicin (Daunomycin/Rubidomycin) Doxorubicin (Adriamycin)
Antimetabolite	Cytarabrine/ Cytosine arabinoside (Cytosar/Ara-C) 6-Mercaptopurine (Purinethol) Methotrexate (Amethopterin) 6-Thioguanine (6-TG)
Corticosteroid	Prednisone
Miscellaneous	L-Asperaginase (Elspar) Hydroxyurea (Hydrea)
Nitrosureas	Carmustine (BCNU)
Plant alkaloid	Vincristine (Oncovin) Vinblastine (Velban)

Nursing management

Acute Intervention The nursing role during acute phases of leukemia is extremely challenging, as the client will have many physical and psychosocial needs. The diagnosis of leukemia, a form of cancer, often evokes great fear. It may be viewed as a hopeless, horrible disease with many painful and undesirable consequences. Leukemia is often equated with death. The diagnosis of leukemia elicits many emotional responses, with the realization that life is finite. The nurse has a special responsibility in helping clients and families deal with these feelings. The nurse must help clients realize that, although their future may be uncertain, they must learn to live in spite of their illness. Families may need help in adjusting to the chronic effects of illness (e.g., dependence, withdrawal, and changes in role responsibilities and body image) and the losses imposed by the sick role.

The nurse must develop skills to help the clients resolve their problems. A positive outlook by the client may increase the efficacy of therapy and will certainly affect the quality of the client's life. It must also be recognized that, at a time when human compassion is most needed, it is often least available, as chronically ill clients are often deserted and isolated. Because nurses have contact with clients 24 hours a day, nurses can help to reverse feelings of abandonment and loneliness. However, more technical needs usually take priority over talking with clients. Therefore, nurses face a special challenge in learning how to meet the intense psychosocial needs of clients with leukemia while continuing to offer the complex physical care which is usually required. Consulting with other health professionals (e.g., psychiatric clinical specialists, oncology clinical specialists, social workers) may help the nurse develop the skills required to meet the broad spectrum of needs manifested by leukemic clients.

From a physical care perspective, the nurse will be challenged to make astute assessments and plan care to help the client survive the severe side effects of chemotherapy. The life-threatening results of bone marrow suppression (anemia, thrombocytopenia, neutropenia) require aggressive nursing interventions, such as those recommended in Tables 24-4, 24-13, and 24-21. Additional complications of chemotherapy may affect the client's GI tract, nutritional status, skin

Table 24-24
Examples of Drug Regimens Used in the Treatment of Leukemia*

Type of Leukemia	Drug Regimens
AML	Cytosine arabinoside + 6-thioguanine + daunorubicin + prednisone
	Cytosine arabinoside + adriamycin + vincristine + prednisone
	COAP (cyclophosphamide, + Oncovin + arabinoside + prednisone)
	ADOP (Ara-C + adriamycin + Oncovin + prednisone)
ALL	Vincristine + prednisone + L-Asparaginase
	COAP (same as under AML)
	ADOP (same as under AML)
	Methotrexate given intrathecally to prevent CNS involvement
	Methotrexate (given in maintenance therapy)
CGL	Alkylating agents (busufan most commonly)
	For blastic crises, treatment similar to that of AML
CLL	Alkylating agents (e.g., chlorambucil, cyclophosphamide)
	Prednisone
	Irradiation (total body or spleen)

*Treatment protocols vary. See explanation in text.

and mucosa, cardiopulmonary status, hepatorenal system, and neuromuscular system. Nursing interventions to reduce discomfort related to these problems are discussed in Chap. 11.

The nurse needs to be knowledgeable about all drugs being administered. This includes the mechanism of action, purpose, routes of administration, usual doses, potential side effects, and toxic effects of the drugs. In addition, the nurse must know how to assess laboratory data reflecting the effects of the drugs. Client survival and comfort during aggressive chemotherapy are significantly affected by astute, innovative, knowledgeable nursing care.

Chronic management

Ongoing care for the client with leukemia is necessary in order to ensure that the disease remains in remission or under control. As stated previously, client compliance with maintenance chemotherapy regimens is very important. Therefore, the client and his significant others must be educated to understand the nature of leukemia and the rationale for treatment. They must also be taught about the drugs and when to seek medical attention.

Rehabilitation must also seek to provide psychological support to the client and family as they deal with the negative connotations of the diagnosis of leukemia. Assistance may be needed to reestablish the various relationships which are a part of the client's life. Friends and family may not know how to interact with the client. All the individuals involved may need help to focus on reality and living as opposed to being obsessed with death. Involving the client in groups such as Can Surmount and Make Today Count may help the client adapt to living with illness by learning from others with similar problems. Exploring resources in the community (e.g., American Cancer Society, Meals-on-Wheels, wheelchair taxis) may reduce the financial burden and the feelings of dependence. Spiritual support may give the client inner strength and peace.

It is expected that the client will need support in adapting to any physical limitations or changes imposed by the illness. The client may feel more positive

Table 24-25
Administration of Drugs for One Cycle of COAP Therapy

Drug	Day													
	1	2	3	4	5	6	7	8	9	10	11	12	13	14
Cyclophosphamide	×	×	×	×	×	×	×	×	×	×	×	×	×	×
Oncovin	×							×						
Ara-C	×							×						
Prednisone	×	×	×	×	×	×	×	×	×	×	×	×	×	×

if emphasis is placed on what he can do rather than on the restrictions that now exist. The nurse may involve other health care providers in meeting the client's needs, but the nurse must recognize the obligation at least to identify these needs and initiate a referral or consultation. For example, physical therapy personnel may be asked to develop an exercise program to prevent posttreatment deficits caused by drug-induced peripheral neuropathy.

It is evident that the nurse's approach to the chronic management of leukemia will affect the quality of the client's life. It is a responsibility which cannot be minimized. This is especially true because leukemia is marked by a cyclical course of remissions and exacerbations which constantly impinges on and affects the client's relationships and ability to function.

LYMPHOMAS

Lymphomas are malignant neoplasms of the reticuloendothelial system. They affect lymphatic structures and involve proliferation of histiocytes and lymphocytes. The two major types of lymphoma, Hodgkin's disease and non-Hodgkin's lymphoma, will be discussed separately.

Hodgkin's Disease

Hodgkin's disease is a malignant condition characterized by proliferation of abnormal histiocytes called *Reed-Sternberg cells*. The disease has a bimodal age-specific incidence, occurring most frequently in persons from ages 15 to 35 and above age 50. In adults, it is twice as prevalent in men as in women.

Pathophysiology

The cause of Hodgkin's disease remains unknown. It is possible that genetic, immunological, and viral factors interact to cause it.

Normally, the lymph nodes are composed of connective tissues which surround a fine mesh of reticular fibers and cells. In Hodgkin's disease the normal structure of lymph nodes is destroyed by hyperplasia of the reticuloendothelial system. It is believed that the disease arises in a single location (it originates in lymph nodes in 90 percent of clients) and then spreads along adjacent lymphatics. It eventually infiltrates other organs, especially the lungs, spleen, and liver. In about two-thirds of clients, the cervical lymph nodes are the first to be affected. When the disease begins above the diaphragm, it remains confined to lymph nodes for a variable period of time. Disease originating below the diaphragm frequently spreads to extralymphoid sites such as the liver.

A diagnostic feature of Hodgkin's disease is the presence of Reed-Sternberg cells. They are malignant histiocytes with large, multinucleated cells. These cells are often seen in lymph node biopsy material before they appear in the bone marrow or peripheral blood.

Clinical manifestations

The onset of symptoms in Hodgkin's disease is usually insidious. The initial development is usually an enlargement of cervical, axillary, or inguinal lymph nodes. This *lymphadenopathy* affects discrete nodes which remain movable and nontender. The enlarged nodes will not be painful unless nerves are involved.

Client complaints may include weight loss, fatigue, weakness, fever, chills, tachycardia, and night sweats. The findings of fever, night sweats, and weight loss (referred to as *B symptoms*) correlate with a poor prognosis. After the ingestion of even small amounts of alcohol, individuals with Hodgkin's disease will complain of rapid onset of pain at the site of disease. The cause for the alcohol-induced pain is unknown. Generalized pruritus without skin lesions may develop. Cough, dyspnea, stridor, and dysphagia may all be reflective of mediastinal node involvement.

Other physical findings may include hepatomegaly and splenomegaly, but they are usually not present unless the disease is advanced. Anemia results from increased destruction as well as decreased production of erythrocytes. Other physical signs vary depending on where the disease has spread. For example, intrathoracic involvement may lead to superior vena cava syndrome, enlarged retroperitoneal nodes may cause palpable abdominal masses, jaundice may occur from liver involvement, and spinal cord compression leading to paraplegia may occur with extradural involvement. Bone pain occurs due to osteoblastic bone lesions.

Diagnostic study abnormalities

Peripheral blood analysis, lymph node biopsy, bone marrow examination, and *radiological evaluation* are all important means of evaluating Hodgkin's disease. Peripheral blood analysis will often reveal a hypochromic microcytic anemia, neutrophilic leukocytosis (15,000 to 25,000/μL which may be associated with lymphopenia, and an increased platelet count Leukopenia and thrombocytopenia may develop, but they are usually a consequence of either treatment or superimposed hypersplenism. In addition to evaluating marrow elements, other blood studies may show hypoferremia due to excessive iron uptake by the liver and spleen, elevated leukocyte alkaline phosphatase from liver and bone involvement, hypercalcemia from bone involvement, and hypoalbuminemia.

Excisional lymph node biopsy offers a definitive means of diagnosis. An enlarged peripheral lymph node, if removed, can be examined histologically for the presence of the diagnostic Reed-Sternberg cells.

Bone marrow biopsy is rarely helpful, as there are no characteristic findings. In Hodgkin's disease there may be indications of granulocytic and megakaryocytic hyperplasia, but these findings are not unique to Hodgkin's disease. Reed-Sternberg cells may be found in the bone marrow of clients with advanced disease.

Radiological evaluation can help to localize the disease. Chest radiographs may show mediastinal adenopathy, and an intravenous pyelogram may show renal displacement due to retroperitoneal node enlargement. Lymphangiography is especially useful, as it allows for assessment of lymph nodes and lymph vessels, especially the retroperitoneal structures, which are difficult to visualize.

Medical management

In order for treatment to be as precise as possible, Hodgkin's disease needs to be staged. Staging involves determining the extent and involvement of the disease. This is important because Hodgkin's disease may be very localized or very diffuse. Treatment depends on the nature of the disease. The nomenclature used in staging will involve an A or B classification, depending upon whether symptoms are present when the disease is found, and a roman numeral (I to IV) which reflects the location and extent of the disease (Table 24-26).

Diagnostic studies, as already mentioned, will be conducted to assess the stage of Hodgkin's disease. However, there is also a need to demonstrate the actual extent of abdominal involvement. Some individuals believe that this is best accomplished by using peritonoscopy to obtain spleen, liver, and retroperitoneal node biopsies.[30] The other option for intraabdominal evaluation is to perform an exploratory laparotomy. The proponents of this approach believe that it is the most accurate way to detect intraabdominal disease. However, even they emphasize that laparotomy should be used not as a routine means of establishing the numerical stage but rather to help establish the best management regimen. Laparotomy offers the advantages of allowing performance of splenectomy which may be a foci of disease. In addition, radiopaque clips can be placed in the abdomen to serve as guides in planning future radiotherapy.[31]

Once the stage of Hodgkin's disease is established, medical management will focus on selecting a treatment plan. Radiation therapy can cure 95 percent of clients with stage I and stage II disease. Radiation

Table 24-26
Staging Classification for Lymphomas

Stage	Definition
I	Involvement of a single lymph node region (I) or of a single extra-lymphatic organ or site (I_E).
II	Involvement of two or more lymph node regions on the same side of the diaphragm (II), or localized involvement of an extra-lymphatic organ or site and of one or more lymph node regions on the same side of the diaphragm (II_E).
III	Involvement of lymph node regions on both sides of the diaphragm (III), which may also be accompanied by involvement of the spleen (III_s) or by localized involvement of an extra-lymphatic organ, or site (III_E), or both (III_{sE}).
IV	Diffuse or disseminated involvement of one or more extra-lymphatic organs or tissues, with or without associated lymph node involvement.
Symptoms	
A	No general symptoms.
B	Presence of one of the following symptoms: (1) unexplained weight loss of more than 10% of the body weight in the 6 months before admission, (2) unexplained fever with temperatures above 38°C (100.4°F), (3) night sweats.

Note: Biopsy-documented involvement of stage IV sites is also denoted by letter suffixes: marrow = M+; lung = L+; liver = H+; pleura = P+; bone = O+; skin and subcutaneous tissue = D+.

Adopted at the workshop on the Staging of Hodgkin's Disease held at Ann Arbor, Mich., April 1971. Adapted from K. Isselbacher et al. (eds.), *Harrison's Principles of Internal Medicine,* 9th ed., McGraw-Hill Book Company, New York, 1980, p. 1637.

given over 4 to 6 weeks may permanently cure Hodgkin's disease. Stage IIIA disease will be treated with both radiotherapy and chemotherapy. The role of radiation as a supplement to chemotherapy in Stages III and IV is controversial.[32] Advances in treatment now enable even some stage IIIB and stage IV diseases to be cured with chemotherapy. (Cure is defined as an absence of disease for more than 5 years.) Refer to Chap. 11 to review the principles of radiotherapy and chemotherapy.

Pharmacological management

Chemotherapy is the treatment of choice for disseminated Hodgkin's disease (stages IIIB and IV). Combination chemotherapy works well because, just as in leukemia, drugs are used which have an additive antitumor effect without increasing the side effects. As with leukemia, therapy must be aggressive. Therefore, potentially life-threatening problems are encountered in an attempt to achieve a remission.

The most widely known chemotherapy regimen is known as MOPP, which stands for the four drugs comprising it: M—nitrogen mustard, O—Oncovin (vinblastine), P—procarbazine (Matulane), and P—prednisone. One cycle of MOPP requires drugs to be given at various times over a 14-day period followed by a 14-day period without drugs (Table 24-27). At least six cycles are given with modifications in dosage based on white blood cell values. Other drug combinations which may be less toxic than MOPP are being studied. Bleomycin and adriamycin are used in various combinations with the drugs mentioned in the MOPP protocol. MOPP plus bleomycin has demonstrated an 84 percent remission rate, compared to 64 percent for MOPP.[33]

Maintenance chemotherapy does not contribute to increased survival once a complete remission is achieved. Occasionally, single drugs may be administered palliatively to clients who cannot tolerate intensive combination therapy. These include nitrogen mustard, cyclophosphamide, chlorambucil, vinblastine, procarbazine, adriamycin, and bleomycin.

Nursing management

The nursing care for Hodgkin's disease is largely based on dealing with pancytopenia and other side effects of therapy. Because the survival of clients with Hodgkin's disease is based on their response to treatment, supporting the client through the myelosuppressive state is extremely important (see Tables 24-4, 24-13, and 24-21). Psychosocial considerations are just as important as they are with leukemia (see Nursing Management, under Leukemia). In fact, because the prognosis for Hodgkin's disease is better than that for many forms of leukemia, the client must be helped to deal with his disease in a realistic manner even though he knows that it is a malignant disorder.

The client undergoing radiotherapy will need special nursing consideration. In addition to the side effects, which are similar to those of chemotherapy, the skin in the radiation field will require special attention. Also, the nurse must understand the concepts related to administration of radiotherapy. These are explained in Chap. 11.

Once the client is in remission, ongoing maintenance treatment is not needed. However, it is imperative that the client learn the importance of returning for subsequent examinations as scheduled.

Non-Hodgkin's Lymphoma

Non-Hodgkin's lymphomas are malignant neoplasms of the reticuloendothelial system. They are identified by both the cell type involved (lymphocyte or histiocyte) and the pattern of lymph node involvement. The node patterns are either nodular or diffuse.

Table 24-27
Administration of Drugs for One Cycle of MOPP Therapy

Drug	Days													
Drug	**1**	**2**	**3**	**4**	**5**	**6**	**7**	**8**	**9**	**10**	**11**	**12**	**13**	**14**
Nitrogen mustard (Mustargen)	×							×						×
Vinblastine (Oncovin)	×							×						×
Procarbazine	×	×	×	×	×	×	×	×	×	×				
Prednisone	×	×	×	×	×	×	×	×	×	×	×	×	×	×

Note: Followed by 14 days of rest before the second cycle is started.

Common names for different types of non-Hodgkin's lymphoma include *Burkitt's lymphoma*, *reticulum cell sarcoma*, and *lymphosarcoma*. There is no hallmark feature in non-Hodgkin's lymphomas that parallels the Reed-Sternberg cell of Hodgkin's disease.

Non-Hodgkin's lymphomas usually originate outside the lymph nodes, the method of spread cannot be anticipated, and the majority of clients have widely disseminated disease at the time of diagnosis. The primary clinical manifestation is painless lymph node enlargement. Because the disease is usually disseminated when it is diagnosed, other symptoms will be present depending upon where the disease has spread (e.g., hepatomegaly with liver involvement).

Diagnostic studies used for non-Hodgkin's lymphoma resemble those used for Hodgkin's disease. Lymph node biopsy will establish the cell type and pattern. While the prognosis for non-Hodgkin's lymphoma is not as good as that for Hodgkin's disease because of its diffuse nature, staging will nevertheless be conducted as a means of guiding therapy. Treatment for non-Hodgkin's lymphoma involves both radiotherapy and chemotherapy. Radiotherapy by itself may be effective for palliation with stage I disease, but combination radiation therapy and chemotherapy are used for other stages.

MULTIPLE MYELOMA

Multiple myeloma is a condition in which neoplastic plasma cells infiltrate bone marrow and destroy bone. Clients usually live for about 2 years following diagnosis if left untreated. The incidence of multiple myeloma approximates that of Hodgkin's disease. The disease is twice as common in males as in females and usually develops after age 40, with a peak incidence around age 55.

Pathophysiology

There are many hypotheses regarding the etiology of multiple myeloma (e.g., chronic inflammation, chronic hypersensitivity reactions, viral influences), but no actual cause has been identified. The disease process involves excessive production of neoplastic plasma cells. The plasma cells infiltrate the bone marrow and develop into tumors. Ultimately, the plasma cells destroy bone and invade the lymph nodes, liver, spleen, and kidneys. The neoplastic plasma cells produce an abnormal immunoglobulin which cannot develop into antibodies. This abnormal immunoglobulin is known as a *myeloma protein*. As myeloma protein increases, normal plasma cells are reduced in number, which further compromises the body's normal immune response.

Clinical Manifestations

Multiple myeloma is characterized by slow and insidious development. Clients will remain relatively asymptomatic until the disease is advanced, at which time *skeletal pain* is the major manifestation. Pain in the pelvis, spine, and ribs is particularly common. Diffuse osteoporosis develops as the myeloma protein destroys more bone. Osteolytic lesions are seen in the skull, vertebrae, and ribs. *Vertebral destruction* can lead to collapse of vertebrae with ensuing compression of the spinal cord, requiring emergency laminectomy to prevent paraplegia. Loss of bone integrity can lead to the development of pathological fractures. Also, bony degeneration causes calcium to be lost from the bones. It enters the serum, causing hypercalcemia.

Hypercalcemia may be reflected by renal, GI, or neurological changes. These include polyuria, anorexia, and confusion. In addition, cell destruction contributes to the development of *hyperuricemia*, which, along with the high protein levels caused by the presence of the myeloma protein, can result in renal failure due to renal tubular obstruction as well as interstitial nephritis from the uric acid precipitates. The client may display symptoms of *anemia*, *thrombocytopenia*, and *granulocytopenia*, all of which are related to the replacement of normal bone marrow elements with plasma cells.

Diagnostic Study Abnormalities

Evaluation of multiple myeloma will involve laboratory, radiological, and bone marrow examination. *Pancytopenia* may be found on laboratory assessment. *High serum protein* may be present. *Hyperuricemia*, *hypercalcemia*, and *elevated creatinine* can also be determined by laboratory tests. In addition to serum tests, a special urine study can be done. An abnormal globulin in the urine, known as *Bence-Jones protein*, is found only in cases of multiple myeloma.

Radiological studies will involve normal radiographs and isotope scans to establish the degree of bone involvement. The studies document the presence of diffuse bony lesions, demineralization, and osteoporosis in areas of the affected skeleton.

Bone marrow analysis will show significantly increased numbers of plasma cells in the bone marrow. Other components of the marrow will be normal.

Medical Management

The medical approach involves managing both the disease and its symptoms. *Ambulation* and *adequate hydration* will be ordered to offset hypercalcemia, hyperuricemia, and dehydration. Weight bearing helps the bones reabsorb some calcium, while fluids dilute the calcium load and prevent protein precipitates from causing renal tubular obstruction.

Pain control is another goal of medical therapy. Analgesics, orthopedic supports, and localized radiation all help to reduce the skeletal pain. *Chemotherapy* will be used to reduce the number of plasma cells. The agents most frequently used are melphalan (Alkeran) and cyclophosphamide (Cytoxan). Adrenocorticosteroids may be added, as they exert an antitumor effect in some clients. The combination of melphalan and predisone has been particularly effective.

Drugs may also be used to counteract complications. For example, allopurinol (Zyloprim) may be given to reduce hyperuricemia, while IV sodium chloride and furosemide will help to promote renal excretion of calcium.

Nursing Management

Dealing with the hypercalcemia and its resulting renal complications requires an understanding of what constitutes adequate hydration. Fluids will be administered to attain an output of $1\frac{1}{2}$ to 2 L per day. This may require an intake of 3 to 4 L. In addition, weight bearing helps the bones to reabsorb some of the calcium, while steroids may augment the excretion of calcium. Once chemotherapy is initiated, the uric acid levels will rise because of the increased cell destruction. Hyperuricemia must be resolved by hydration together with the use of allopurinol.

Because of the potential for pathological fractures, the nurse must use careful planning and methods to move and ambulate clients. A slight twist or strain in the wrong area (e.g., a weak area in the client's bones) may be sufficient to cause fracture.

Pain control requires innovative and knowledgeable nursing intervention. If radiotherapy is used to diminish pain from localized myeloma lesions, then appropriate skin care techniques must be employed. The nurse must understand that mild analgesics such as aspirin or aspirin and codeine may be more effective than potent analgesics in diminishing bone pain. Braces, especially for the spine, may also help control pain. As in any pain management situation, the nurse is responsible for assessing the client wisely and for implementing innovative, necessary nursing measures to reduce if not alleviate the pain (see Chap. 50).

Chemotherapy, as already noted, must be given properly, with attention to the client's development of side effects. Pancytopenia, in particular, requires nursing intervention.

The client's psychosocial needs will require sensitive, skilled management. As with leukemia, it is important to help the client and significant others adapt to changes fostered by chronic sickness, to deal with reality rather than create fantasies, to adjust to losses of various magnitudes, and to recognize the need to live and enjoy life while dying (see Nursing Management, under Leukemia). The symptoms of multiple myeloma will resolve and exacerbate. Consequently, hospital care will be needed at various times during the course of the illness.

MONONUCLEOSIS

Mononucleosis, often referred to as "mono" or the "kissing disease," is a benign, self-limiting disease characterized by lymph node enlargement, lymphocytosis, and elevated temperature. It occurs most commonly among children of ages 3 to 5 and adolescents and young adults of ages 15 to 25. It may occur in isolated cases or epidemics.

Etiology

Mononucleosis is caused by the Epstein-Barr virus, a type of herpesvirus. The exact mode of transmission is not known, but secretions from mucous membranes of the mouth and GI tract are believed to be involved. Persons who have antibodies to the Epstein-Barr virus do not develop mononucleosis; those who are deficient in these antibodies acquire the disease when infected by the Epstein-Barr virus. Once exposed, susceptible clients will manifest symptoms of disease after a 30- to 40-day incubation period. Symptoms will evolve gradually, intensifying as the disease becomes apparent. After causing mononucleosis, the Epstein-Barr virus may lie dormant in lymphocytes and other lymphatic tissue, thus contributing to the development of immunity.

Clinical Manifestations

General complaints prior to the actual onset of mononucleosis are rather nebulous. A severe headache, fatigue, malaise, chills, puffy eyelids, anorexia, and a distaste for smoking cigarettes may develop early in the illness. As the disease becomes more acute, more than 80 percent of clients will present a triad of symptoms including fever, painful lymph node enlargement (especially cervical, axillary, and groin nodes), and sore throat. The sore throat may be severe enough to cause dysphagia. If the spleen is enlarged by massive lymphocyte infiltration, left upper quadrant pain will occur.

It is rare for significant complications to develop from mononucleosis. The problems which may occur include pneumonia, neurological changes, splenic rupture, thrombocytopenia, hemolytic anemia, airway obstruction, and cardiac involvement.

Diagnostic Study Abnormalities

Initially, the white blood cell and differential cell counts will be normal, but within a week a leukocytosis (WBC> 20,000/μL) will occur. There will be a rise in lymphocytes and monocytes to over 50 percent, with 10 to 20 percent atypical lymphocytes. Another laboratory study evaluates the presence of heterophil antibody. Still another test measures the Epstein-Barr virus antibody. When positive, this test is absolute confirmation of the presence of mononucleosis. Because the viral level fluctuates, a negative finding does not totally rule out the presence of mononucleosis. Liver function studies may be used to ascertain if any liver involvement exists. And finally, throat cultures may be positive for beta-hemolytic streptococci in one-third of the clients.

Medical and Nursing Management

There is no specific medical protocol for clients with mononucleosis. Because the disease is often seen in college students and military personnel, clients may need to be hospitalized for 2 to 3 weeks to ensure that they get adequate rest, nutrition, fluids, and management of fever. Isolation procedures are not required, as mononucleosis is minimally contagious in adults. Antibiotics have not proved useful unless the throat culture is positive for beta-hemolytic streptococci. Analgesics may alleviate discomfort, and steroids may reduce pharyngeal swelling and fever.

Most nursing interventions will occur when the disease is actually present. Helping the client to comply with the physician's orders, especially bed rest, may prove challenging. The nurse may suggest the use of a saline gargle to ease sore throat pain. The nurse must also detect the development of complications. For the client with splenomegaly, the nurse must emphasize the need to avoid any possible activities which could lead to splenic rupture. For example, the client should avoid the Valsalva maneuver with bowel movements, and abdominal trauma from lifting or sports must be avoided until the splenic enlargement resolves.

The need for ongoing care after mononucleosis is uncommon. After 2 to 3 weeks, the client can usually return to a normal lifestyle. If the mononucleosis is seen in older adults, complications may be more prevalent and complete disease resolution may take longer.

DISORDERS OF THE SPLEEN

The spleen performs many functions, as discussed in Chap. 23. The spleen is affected by many illnesses. *Splenomegaly* occurs in neoplastic diseases such as lymphoma and leukemia, as well as in nonneoplastic disorders such as infections, collagen vascular diseases, anemias, thrombocytopenic purpura, hypersensitivity reactions, and cirrhosis. When the spleen enlarges, its normal filtering capacity increases. Consequently, there is often a reduction in the number of circulating blood cells.

Hypersplenism is a spleen disorder in which destructive spleen functions are exaggerated, leading to decreased peripheral blood elements and increased bone marrow cellularity. Splenomegaly usually develops, but it is not an absolute occurrence. Hypersplenism may be a primary condition, such as with ITP, or it may develop secondary to another illness, such as with lymphomas, leukemia, or any problem leading to portal hypertension.

Splenectomy is a treatment of choice for primary hypersplenism, as it will remove the problem. Spleen removal may be done in cases of secondary hypersplenism, but only as a palliative intervention. Another major indication for splenectomy is splenic rupture. The spleen may rupture from trauma, inadvertent tearing during other surgical procedures, and diseases such as mononucleosis.

Nursing responsibilities for clients with spleen disorders will vary depending on the nature of the problem. Splenomegaly may be painful and may require analgesic administration, care in moving, turning, and positioning, and evaluation of lung expansion, as spleen enlargement may impair diaphragmatic excursion. If anemia, thrombocytopenia, or leukopenia develops from splenomegaly or hypersplenism, nursing measures must be instituted to support the client and prevent life-threatening complications. If splenectomy is performed, the nurse must provide the meticulous care warranted following any surgery. In addition, there must be special observation for hemorrhage which could lead to shock, fever, and abdominal distension.

Splenectomy in young children requires special consideration. While an adult can live quite well without a spleen, this organ plays a major role in antibody development in children. Therefore, splenectomy is not done routinely in children. Should it be necessary for a child, the compromised immune system must be supported by prophylactic antibiotic administration.

Case Study / Anemia

Clare, a 20-year-old black bookkeeper who lives in New York City, was brought to a Denver emergency room with severe joint and abdominal pain. She complained of frequent urination during the past 2 nights and knee joint swelling. Two days ago, she had gone hiking in the Rocky Mountains with her brother, whom she had come to visit in Denver.

Clare's history included one other similar episode when she had acute pneumonia at age 11. She stated that she usually felt fatigued but thought it was due to her active social life. Physical assessment demonstrated the presence of splenomegaly and an enlarged, inflamed knee joint. Laboratory results included the following:

Hct 30%
Hb 10 g/dL
WBC 20,000/μL

Discussion Questions

1. What components of the laboratory results suggest anemia?
2. What is the pathophysiological basis of Clare's anemia? Why might symptoms have developed in Denver?
3. What precipitates a crisis of this type of anemia?
4. How is an anemic crisis with this etiology treated?
5. How is pain related to this type of anemia?
6. What measures should Clare take to prevent further crises?

REVIEW QUESTIONS

The number of the question corresponds to the same numbered objective at the beginning of the chapter.

1. Which of the following are both clinical manifestations of anemia?
   a. muscle twitching and petechiae
   b. pallor and bleeding tendencies
   c. headaches and tachycardia
   d. polyphagia and purpura

2. A normocytic, normochromic anemia may be caused by
   a. bone marrow suppression
   b. folic acid deficiency
   c. vitamin B_{12} deficiency
   d. chronic infection

3. The clinical manifestations of sickle cell crisis develop primarily as a result of
   a. capillary permeability
   b. erythrostasis
   c. hemorrhage
   d. transfusions

4. Which of the following is an important nursing intervention to provide warmth for an anemic client who complains of being cold?
   a. hot water bottle
   b. hyperthermia blanket
   c. heating pad
   d. socks and blankets

5. The vascular problems in polycythemia result from
   a. hyperviscosity and hypovolemia
   b. hypoviscosity and hypervolemia
   c. hyperviscosity and hypervolemia
   d. hypoviscosity and hypovolemia

6. The etiologies of ITP and acquired thrombocytopenia, respectively, are
   a. increased platelet destruction for both
   b. decreased platelet production for both
   c. increased platelet destruction; decreased platelet production
   d. decreased platelet production; increased platelet destruction

7. When providing care for a thrombocytopenic client, the nurse must avoid administering aspirin or aspirin-containing products because they
   a. disguise fevers
   b. destroy red blood cells
   c. increase intracranial pressure
   d. interfere with platelet aggregation

8. Which blood elements do the three major types of hemophilia affect?
   a. factor VIII, factor IX, platelets
   b. factor VII, factor IX, red cells
   c. factor VI, factor X, fibrinogen
   d. factor VIII, factor IX, thrombin

9. DIC is
   a. a hereditary disorder which may lead to diffuse hemorrhage

b. an acquired disorder which may lead to diffuse hemorrhage
c. a hereditary disorder which may lead to localized hemorrhage
d. an acquired disorder which may lead to localized hemorrhage

10. Which signs of infection is the clients with granulocytopenia most likely to display?
   a. redness
   b. pus
   c. heat
   d. fever

11. A 65-year-old female presents with enlarged cervical lymph nodes, an elevated lymphocyte count, and severe anemia. Which of the following types of leukemia does this description most likely characterize?
   a. acute lymphocytic leukemia
   b. acute myelocyte leukemia
   c. chronic lymphocytic leukemia
   d. chronic granulocytic leukemia

12. Multiple drugs are used in predetermined combinations to treat leukemia and lymphomas because
   a. The chance that one drug will be effective is increased.
   b. They are more effective without having exacerbating side effects.
   c. No one knows what drugs help clients with lymphoma.
   d. They can interrupt cell growth at multiple points in the cell cycle.

13. An important nursing measure in the management of a client with chronic leukemia is to
   a. reassure the client that most chemotherapy agents induce remission
   b. tell the client that induction chemotherapy is less toxic than maintenance chemotherapy
   c. discuss the client's feelings about the disease
   d. discuss with the family the client's need to maintain a dependent role

14. Stage IA Hodgkin's disease means that the
   a. disease is on one side of the diaphragm, and symptoms are present
   b. disease is on one side of the diaphragm, and symptoms are absent
   c. disease is on both sides of the diaphragm, and symptoms are present
   d. disease is on both sides of the diaphragm, and symptoms are absent

15. As mononucleosis becomes more acute, a common triad of symptoms develops, including
   a. fatigue, cough, and headache
   b. chills, anorexia, and vomiting
   c. fever, painful lymphadenopathy, and sore throat
   d. weight loss, night sweats, and splenomegaly

16. Clients with mononucleosis who have splenomegaly are at risk for
   a. infection
   b. red cell abnormalities
   c. splenic rupture
   d. renal failure

REFERENCES

1. R. Refkind et al., *Fundamentals of Hematology*, Year Book Medical Publishers, Inc., Chicago, 1976.
2. A. J. Erslev, "General Effects of Anemia," in W. J. Williams et al. (eds.), *Hematology*, 2d ed., McGraw Hill Book Company, New York, 1977, pp. 251–254.
3. V. F. Fairbanks and E. Beutler "Iron Deficiency," in Williams et al., op. cit., pp. 363–370.
4. Ibid.
5. Ibid.
6. R. S. Hillman, "Acute Blood Loss Anemia," in Williams et al., op. cit., pp. 618–623.
7. G. W. Zeluff, E. A. Natelson, and D. Jackson, "Thrombocytopenic Purpura—Idiopathic and Thrombotic," *Heart and Lung*, **7**:327–333 (1978).
8. S. L. Moschella, D. M. Pillsbury, and H. J. Hurley, *Dermatology*, vol. I, W. B. Saunders Company, Philadelphia, 1975, p. 859.
9. S. I. Rapaport, *Introduction to Hematoloy*, Harper & Row, Publishers, Incorporated, 1971, pp. 320–321.
10. W. J. Williams, "General Effects of Disorders of Hemostasis," in Williams et al., op. cit., pp. 1313–1316.
11. R. H. Aster, "Thrombocytopenia Due to Enhanced Platelet Destruction," in Williams et al., op. cit., pp. 1326–1340.
12. F. H. Gardner, "Preservation and Clinical Use of Platelet Preparations," in Williams et al., op. cit., pp. 1553–1560.
13. B. A. Myhre (ed.), *Blood Component Therapy: A Physician's Handbook*, American Association of Blood Banks, Chicago, 1975, pp. 16–17.
14. *AMA Drug Evaluation*, American Medical Association, Chicago, 1980.
15. T. C. Bithell and M. M. Wintrobe, "Disorders of Blood Coagulation," in M. M. Wintrobe et al. (eds.), *Harrison's Principles of Internal Medicine*, McGraw-Hill Book Company, New York, 1974.
16. H. C. Kwaan, "Disseminated Intravascular Coagulation,66 *Med Clin North Am*, **56**:177–191 (1972).
17. S. I. Rapaport, , "Defibrination Syndromes," in Williams et al., op. cit., pp. 1454–1458.
18. S. C. Finch, "Granulocyte Disorders—Benign, Quantitative Abnormalities of Granulocytes," in Williams et al., op. cit., pp. 717–730.
19. J. A. Dilworth and G. L. Mandell, "Infections in Patients with Cancer," *Semin Oncol*, **2**:349–359 (1975).
20. V. Rodriguez, M. Burgess, and G. P. Bodey, "Management of Fever of Unknown Origin in Patients with Neoplasma and Neutropenia," *Cancer*, **32**:1007–1012 (1973).
21. A. S. Levine, "Protected Environment—Prophylactic Antibiotic Programmes: Clinical Studies," *Clin Hematol*, **5** :409–424 (1976).
22. R. H. Herzig et al., "Successful Granulocyte Transfusion Therapy for Gram-Negative Septicemia," *N Engl J Med*, **296**:701–705 (1977).
23. J. B. Alavi et al., "A Randomized Clinical Trial of Granulocyte Transfusions for Infection in Acute Leukemia," *N Engl J Med*, **296**:706–711 (1977).
24. V. Graham and B. J. Rubal, "Recipient and Donor

Response to Granulocyte Transfusion and Leukapheresis," *Cancer Nurs*, **3**:97–100 (1980).

25. G. Bodey and G. P. Rodman, "Protected Environment—Prophylactic Antibiotic Programmes: Microbiological Studies," *Clin Hematol*, **5**:395–408 (1976).

26. I. Djerassi and J. S. Kim, "Problems and Solutions with Filtration Leukapheresis," *Progr Clin Biol Res*, **13**:395–313 (1977).

27. K. Isselbacher et al. (eds.), *Harrison's Principles of Internal Medicine*, 9th ed., McGraw Hill Book Company, New York, 1980, pp. 1630–1633.

28. M. Beard and G. Fairley, "Acute Leukemia in Adults," *Semin Hematol*, **9**:5–24 (1974).

29. M. Lichtman and M. Klemperer, "The Leukemias," in P. Rubin (ed.), *Clinical Oncology for Medical Students and Physicians*, American Cancer Society, New York, 1978, p. 246.

30. V. T. DeVita et al., "Peritonoscopy in the Staging of Hodgkin's Disease," *Cancer Res*, **31**:1746–1750 (1971).

31. S. B. Sutcliffe, A. R. Timoth, and T. A. Lister, "Staging in Hodgkin's Disease," *Clin Hematol*, **8**:593–609 (1979).

32. J. S. Greenberger, S. E. Come, and R. R. Weichselbaum, "Issues of Controversy in Radiation Therapy and Combined Modality Approaches to Hodgkin's Disease," *Clin Hematol*, **8**:611–624 (1979).

33. R. C. Young and V. T. DeVita, "Chemotherapy of Hodgkin's Disease," *Clin Hematol*, **8**:625–644 (1979).

Chapter 25

NURSING ASSESSMENT

Cardiovascular System

Carol E. Smith

Learning Objectives

1. Describe the anatomical location and function of the following cardiac structures: pericardial layers, atria, ventricles, semilunar valves, and atrioventricular valves.
2. Describe coronary circulation and the areas of heart muscle supplied by each blood vessel.
3. Explain the normal sequence of events involved in the conduction pathway of the heart.
4. Describe the structure and function of arteries, capillaries, and veins.
5. Define blood pressure and the mechanisms involved in its regulation.
6. Identify the significant subjective and objective assessment data related to the cardiovascular system that should be obtained from a client.
7. Describe the appropriate techniques used in the physical assessment of the cardiovascular system.
8. Differentiate normal from common abnormal findings of a physical assessment of the cardiovascular system.
9. Describe the purpose, significance of results, and nursing responsibilities of invasive and noninvasive diagnostic studies of the cardiovascular system.
10. Identify waveforms of a normal electrocardiogram and components of the normal sinus rhythm.

The cardiovascular system consists of the heart, arteries, veins, and capillaries. The function of this system is to circulate the blood, enabling oxygen, nutrients, and hormones to reach cells of the body and waste products of cells to be eliminated.

CARDIOVASCULAR SYSTEM: STRUCTURES AND FUNCTIONS

Heart

Structure

The heart is a four-chambered muscular organ about the size of a fist. It is the pump of the cardiovascular system. The heart lies within the thorax between the lungs. Its beating is sometimes visible on the body surface at the fifth intercostal space about 2 inches left of the midline (Fig. 25-1). This pulsation, arising at the apex of the heart, is known as the *apex beat.*

The heart wall is composed of three layers. *Endocardium* is the thin inner lining, *myocardium* is the middle muscular layer, and *epicardium* is the outer serous membrane. Around the heart is the *pericardial sac,* enclosing it the way a glove encloses a fist. This sac consists of a visceral (inner) layer and a parietal (outer) layer. The visceral layer is in contact with the epicardium. Between the visceral and parietal layers is *pericardial space.* In it is a small amount of fluid that acts as a lubricant for the movement of the layers with each heartbeat.

The heart's four chambers are separated by a septum, with two chambers on the right side and two on the left. The upper chamber on each side is the *atrium,* and the lower chamber is the *ventricle.* (Fig. 25-2). The atrial myocardium is thinner than that of the ventricles, and the left ventricular wall is much thicker than the right ventricular wall. Its added thickness is needed to allow the chamber to pump blood into the systemic circulation.

This chapter was reviewed by Carol Rehtmeyer, R.N., M.S.N., Coordinator, Medical-Surgical Nursing, College of Saint Mary, Omaha, Nebraska.

Blood flow through the heart

Cardiac Valves The right atrium receives venous blood from the inferior and superior venae cavae. The blood then passes through the *tricuspid valve* into the right ventricle. With each contraction, the right ventricle pumps blood into the pulmonary artery. At the entrance to the pulmonary artery is the *pulmonic valve,* which prevents the regurgitation of blood into the ventricle.

Blood from the lungs flows into the left atrium by way of the pulmonary veins. It then passes through the *mitral valve* and into the left ventricle. As the heart contracts, blood is ejected through the aortic valve into the aorta and thus enters the systemic circulation.

The four valves of the heart serve to keep blood flowing in one direction. The atrioventricular valves (tricuspid and mitral) prevent backflow into the atria at the start of each contraction of the ventricles. The cusps of the valves are attached to thin strands of fibrous tissue called *chordae tendineae* (Fig. 25-3).

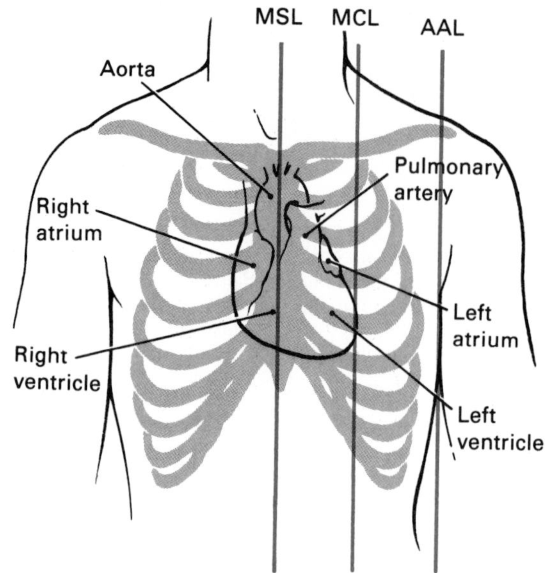

Figure 25-1 Orientation of the heart within the thorax. The red lines indicate the midsternal line (MSL), midclavicular line (MCL), and anterior axillary line (AAL). *(Adapted from S. Price and L. Wilson, Pathophysiology: Clinical Concepts of Disease Processes, 2d ed., McGraw-Hill Book Company, New York, 1982, p. 300.)*

These are anchored in papillary muscles projecting from the walls of the ventricles. The pulmonic and aortic valves prevent blood from regurgitating into the ventricles at the end of each ventricular contraction. These valves have three cusps. They are also known as *semilunar valves*.

Blood supply to the myocardium

The myocardium must be constantly nourished by blood so that contraction can continue. Immediately above the cusps of the aortic valve are the *sinuses of Valsalva*, with openings to the right and left coronary arteries. Each coronary artery has two main branches which carry blood to different areas of the myocardium (Fig. 25-4). The right coronary artery and its branches usually supply the right atrium, the right ventricle, and a portion of the posterior wall of the left ventricle. The left coronary artery and its branches supply the left atrium and the massive walls of the left ventricle.[1] In 90 percent of individuals, the atrioventricular node, part of the cardiac conduction system (see Cardiac Conduction System), receives its nourishment from the right coronary artery. For this reason, obstruction of this artery often causes serious defects in cardiac functioning.

If blood flow through any part of the coronary arterial system is interrupted, some myocardium will lose its ability to function. The effect on the heart as a whole depends on the size of the area deprived of oxygen. If blood flow is reduced gradually, alternate routes may develop in time to nourish the endangered myocardium. These alternate routes are called *collateral circulation* and may be compared to a detour for a road blocked with traffic.

The three divisions of coronary veins essentially

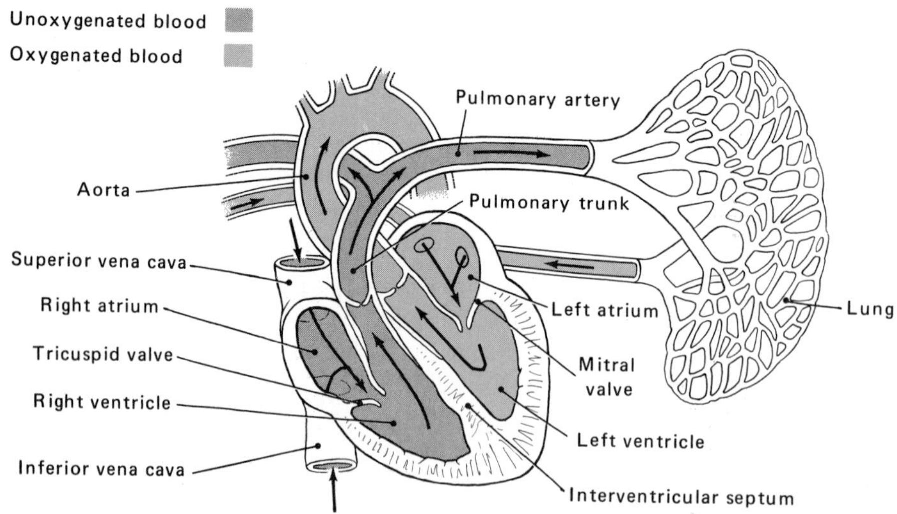

Figure 25-2 Schematic representation of blood flow through the heart. Arrows indicate the direction of flow. *(From L. L. Langley et al., Dynamic Anatomy and Physiology, 5th ed., McGraw-Hill Book Company, New York, 1980, p. 420.)*

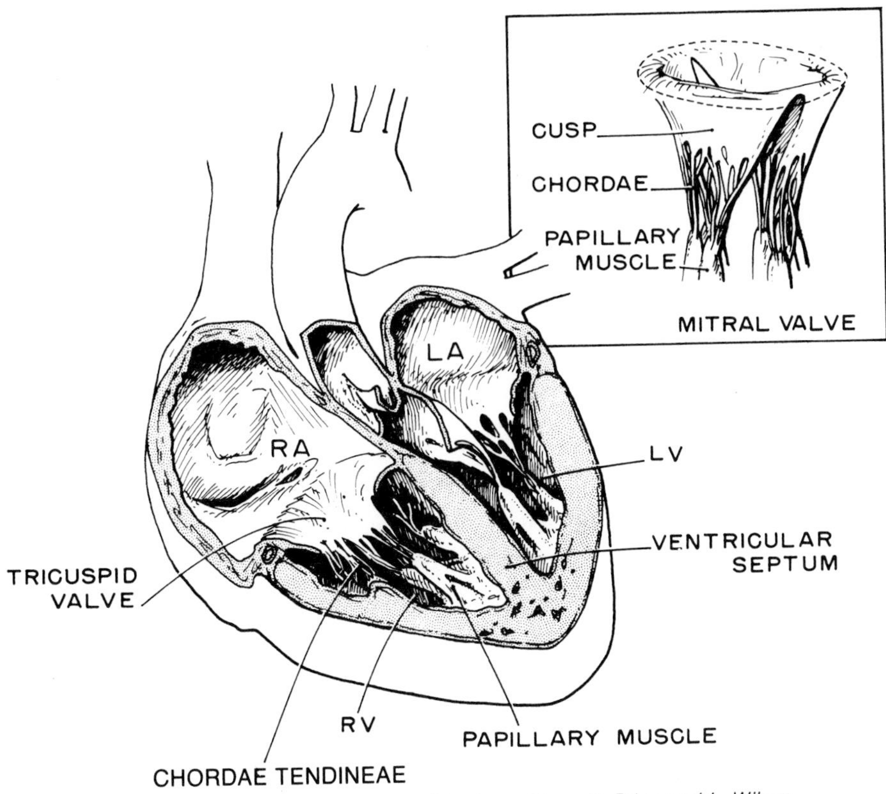

Figure 25-3 Anatomical structures of the AV valves. *(From S. Price and L. Wilson, Pathophysiology: Clinical Concepts of Disease Processes, 2d ed., McGraw-Hill Book Company, New York, 1982, p. 302.)*

parallel the coronary arteries. Most of the blood from the coronary system drains into the coronary sinus, which empties into the right atrium near the entrance to the inferior vena cava.

Conduction system

In the heart wall are pathways of special myocardial tissue for the wave of excitation, or action potential, that triggers each contraction of the heart muscle. This conduction system starts at the *sinoatrial (SA) node,* a tiny knob of tissue in the wall of the right atrium near the entrance of the superior vena cava (Fig. 25-5).

Because the normal heartbeat begins as an action potential generated in the SA node, this node is called the *pacemaker* of the heart. The action potential is the consequence of a sudden change in the membranes of node cells. This change abolishes the polarized condition which exists when node cells are at rest (electrically negative inside, positive outside); the cell membranes become *depolarized.* The action potential created at that instant moves in concentric waves through ordinary muscle fibers of the atria. These also depolarize and carry out their specialized function, contraction. As the muscle fibers are in communication with one another, the walls of the atria contract almost as one fiber.[2]

The action potential simultaneously travels along the internodal tracts to the *atrioventricular (AV) node,* located in the right atrium near the ventricle. The action potential pauses briefly in the AV node, which allows contraction and emptying of the atria to proceed before contraction of the ventricles begins. The excitation then moves through the *bundle of His* and, by way of the *left* and *right bundle branches,* along the interventricular septum. From there, the action potential diffuses widely through the walls of both ventricles by means of *Purkinje fibers.* The conduction system allows coordinated contraction of the heart chambers.

The cardiac cycle starts with depolarization of the SA node. Its climax is ejection of blood into the pulmonary and systemic circulations. It ends with *repolarization,* when the contractile fiber cells and the conduction pathway cells regain their resting polarized condition. Between depolarization and repolarization, the cells are responsive to a new stimulus in

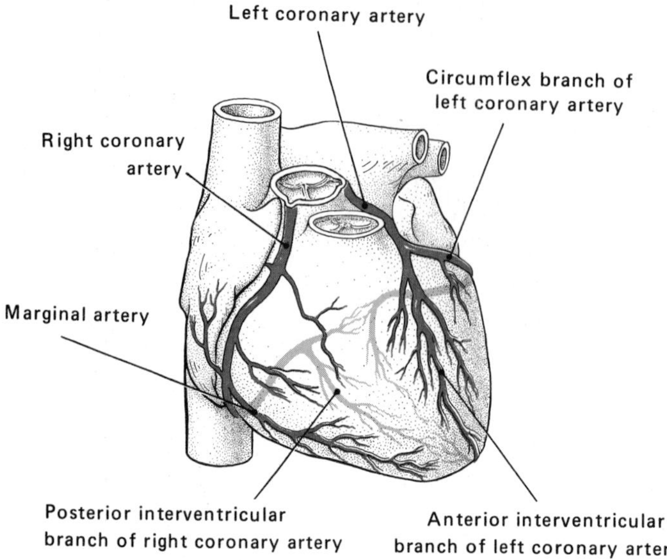

Figure 25-4 Coronary arteries. *(From L. L. Langley et al., Dynamic Anatomy and Physiology, 5th ed., McGraw-Hill Book Company, New York, 1980, p. 423.)*

various degrees. However, immediately after depolarization, they are not. This period is called the *absolute refractory period.*

Electrocardiogram The action potential can be detected on the body surface and recorded as an *electrocardiogram (ECG).* The letters P, QRS, and T are used to identify the separate waveforms (Fig. 25-6). The first wave, P, begins with the firing of the SA node and represents depolarization of the fibers of the atria. The QRS wave represents depolarization from the AV node throughout the ventricles. The last component of the cardiac cycle, the T wave, represents repolarization of the ventricles.

Intervals between these waves reflect the length of time it takes for the impulse to travel from one area of the heart to the other. These time intervals can be measured (Table 25-1). Deviations from these time references can indicate pathology.

Cardiac output

Cardiac output (CO) is the amount of blood pumped by each ventricle in 1 minute. It is calculated by multiplying the *stroke volume (SV)* (the amount of blood ejected from one ventricle with one heartbeat) by the *heart rate per minute (HR):*

$$CO = SV \times HR$$

For the normal adult at rest, cardiac output is maintained at around 5 L/min.[3]

Factors Affecting Cardiac Output There are numerous factors which can affect either the heart rate or the stroke volume. The heart rate is regulated primarily by the autonomic nervous system (see Regulation of the Cardiovascular System). The factors affecting the stroke volume are *preload, contractility,* and *afterload.*

Preload refers to the fact that the more fibers are stretched, the greater is their force of contraction. The volume of blood entering the ventricles determines fiber stretch, that is, the preload. Up to a point, therefore, venous return determines the stroke volume. Another factor is the contractility of heart muscle. This can be influenced by the sympathetic nervous system as well as by epinephrine, whether produced by the body or administered. Increasing contractility raises the stroke volume by increasing ventricular emptying.

Afterload is the amount of force the ventricle must exert to open the semilunar valves and eject blood. Afterload is affected by both the size of the ventricles and the arterial pressure. If the arterial pressure is elevated, the ventricles will meet increased resistance to ejection of blood. Eventually, this can result in ventricular hypertrophy. Thus, increased afterload results from either increased arterial pressure or ventricular hypertrophy. Certain drugs, such as hydralazine (Apresoline), decrease afterload by dilating arterioles. Such drugs are used in the treatment of conditions in which afterload is increased (e.g., congestive heart failure).

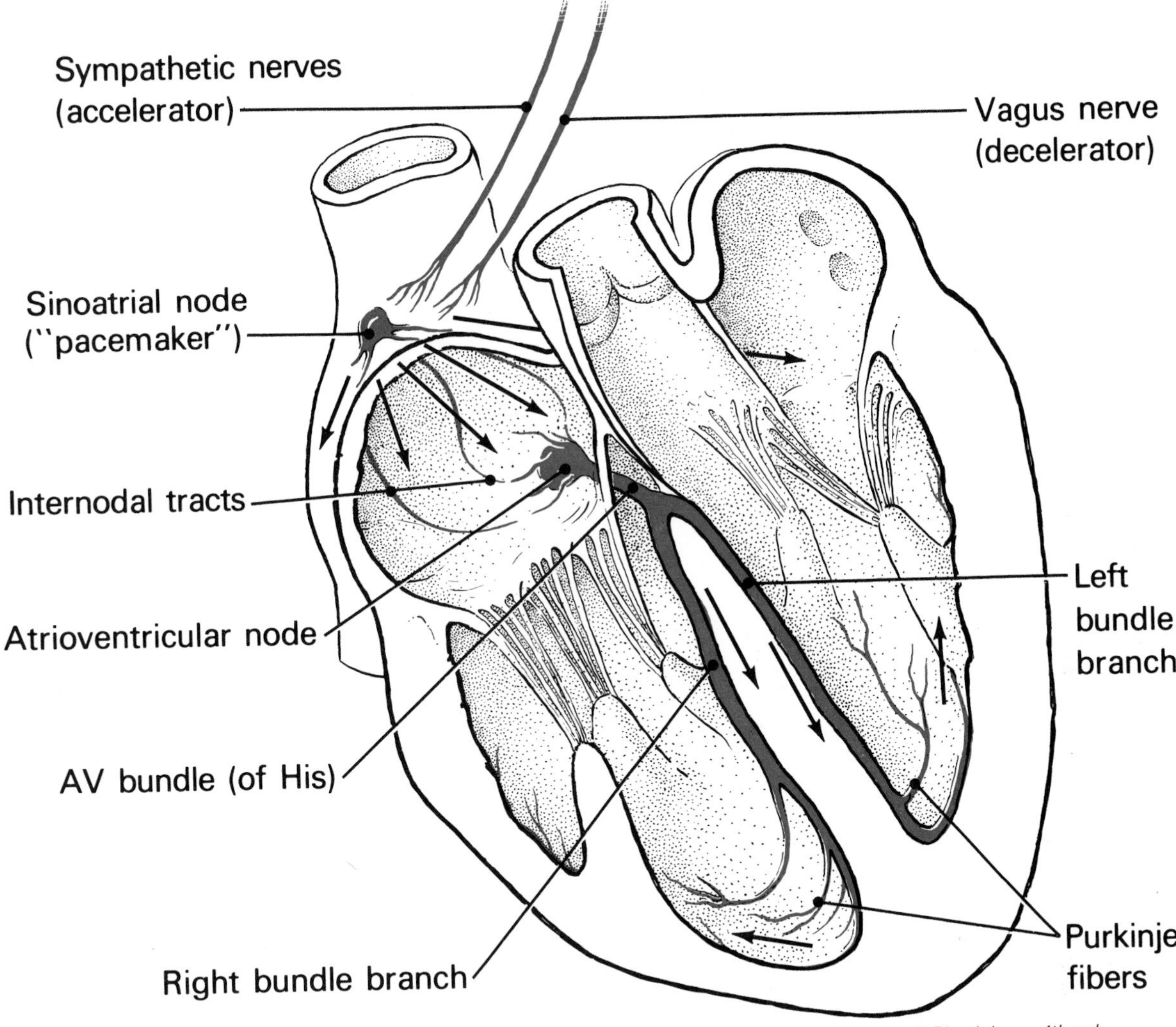

Figure 25-5 Conduction system of the heart. *(From L. L. Langley et al., Dynamic Anatomy and Physiology, 4th ed., McGraw-Hill Book Company, New York, 1974, p. 406.)*

Cardiac reserve

Considering the numerous factors affecting cardiac output, the fact that the cardiovascular system is able to adjust to the body's demands is a marvel. For example, the demand for increased output occurs with hypovolemia, exercise, or stress. The ability to respond to these demands and increase cardiac output three- or fourfold is referred to as *cardiac reserve.*

The increase in cardiac output results from an increase in heart rate or stroke volume. The heart rate can increase to as high as 180 beats per minute (bpm) for short periods without deleterious effects. The stroke volume can be increased by increasing either preload or contractility.

Vascular System

Blood vessels

The three major types of blood vessels of the vascular system are the *arteries, veins,* and *capillaries.* Arteries travel away from the heart and, except for the pulmonary artery, carry oxygenated blood. Veins travel toward the heart and, except for the pulmonary veins, carry deoxygenated blood. Small arteries are called *arterioles,* and small veins

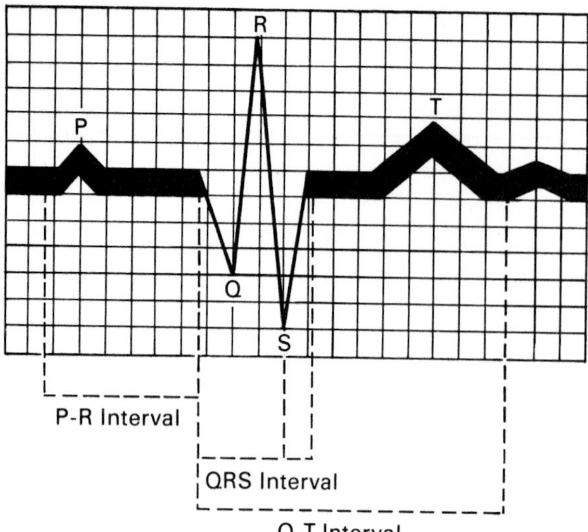

Figure 25-6 The normal ECG pattern. The P wave represents depolarization of the atria. The QRS complex indicates depolarization of the ventricles. The T wave represents repolarization of the ventricles. The P-R interval is a measure of the time required for the impulse to spread from the SA node to the ventricles.

are called *venules*. Blood circulates in the following sequence: from the heart into arteries, arterioles, capillaries, venules, veins, and back to the heart.

Arteries and Arterioles The arterial system differs from the venous system by the amount or type of tissue which makes up arterial walls (Fig. 25-7). The large arteries have thick walls that are composed mainly of elastic tissue. This elastic property creates a low-resistance reservoir for blood as well as a recoil which propels blood forward into the circulation. Large arteries also contain some smooth muscle. Examples of large arteries are the aorta and the pulmonary artery.

Arterioles have relatively little elastic tissue but much smooth muscle. They respond readily to autonomic nervous control by dilating or constricting. The amount of blood flow to each organ and various tissues is directly related to the degree of constriction of the arteriole lumen.[4] Arterioles serve as the major control of arterial blood pressure and distribution of blood flow.

Capillaries The thin *capillary wall* is made up of endothelial cells, with no elastic or muscle tissue present (Fig. 25-7). The capillary network is so extensive that each cell is no more than 0.0127 mm (0.0005 inch) from a capillary.[5] It is through these many thin-walled vessels that the exchange of cellular nutrients and metabolic end products takes place.

Veins and Venules Veins are large-diameter, thin-walled vessels which return blood to the right atrium (Fig. 25-7). The larger veins contain semilunar valves at intervals to maintain the blood flow toward the heart and to prevent backward flow. The amount of blood in the venous system is affected by a number of factors, including arterial flow, compression of veins by skeletal muscles, alterations in thoracic and abdominal pressures, and right atrial pressure.

The largest veins are the *superior vena cava,* which returns blood to the heart from the head, neck, and arms, and the *inferior vena cava,* which returns

Table 25-1
Assessment Guide for Electrocardiographic Waves

Normal Waveforms and Intervals	Normal Timing	Normal Sinus Rhythm (60–100 bpm)
P	0.06–0.12 s	Precedes QRS-T waves
QRS	0.06–0.10 s	Follows each P wave
T	0.16 s	Follows each QRS wave
P-R interval	0.12–0.20 s	Should not vary from one complex to another
Q-T interval	Timing varies with the pulse rate (0.31–0.38 s at a heart rate of 72 bpm)	Should not vary from one complex to another
R-R interval	Timing varies with the pulse rate	Should be equidistant, with slight variations on respiration

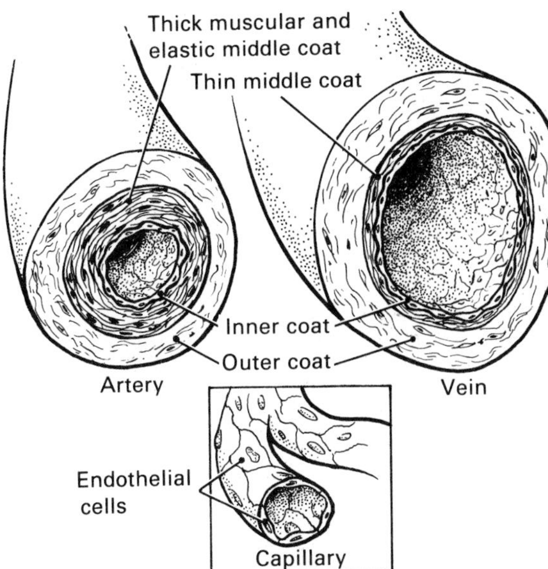

Figure 25-7 Comparative thickness of layers of the artery, vein, and capillary.

blood to the heart from the lower part of the body. These large-caliber vessels are affected by the pressure in the right side of the heart. Elevated right atrial pressure can cause distended neck veins or liver engorgement due to resistance of blood flow.

Venules are relatively small tubules made up of a small amount of muscle and connective tissue. Venules serve to collect blood from various capillary beds and channel it to the larger veins.

Regulation of the Cardiovascular System

Autonomic nervous system

The autonomic nervous system consists of the *sympathetic system* and the *parasympathetic system.*

Effect on the Heart Stimulation of the sympathetic system increases the heart rate, the speed of impulse conduction through the AV node, and the force of atrial and ventricular contractions. This effect is mediated by specific sites in the heart called *beta receptors,* which respond to sympathetic release of norepinephrine.[6]

In contrast, stimulating the parasympathetic system (mediated by the vagus nerve) causes a decrease in heart rate by the action on the SA node. Other factors affecting the heart, such as exercise, emotion, temperature, and medications, may also be mediated through this autonomic receptor system.

Effect on Blood Vessels The source of neural control of blood vessels is also the autonomic nervous system. Sympathetic fibers extend to the peripheral vasculature. It has been postulated that vessels contain two types of receptors in the smooth muscle which respond differently to sympathetic nerve stimulation. These are the *alpha* and *beta receptors.* When the alpha receptors are stimulated, vasoconstriction occurs. When the beta receptors are stimulated, vasodilatation occurs. The parasympathetic system does not have a major influence on the peripheral vasculature.

Baroreceptors

Baroreceptors in the aortic arch and carotid sinus (at the origin of the internal carotid artery) are sensitive to stretch or pressure within the arterial system. Stimulation of these receptors sends information to the vasomotor center in the brainstem. This results in inhibition of the sympathetic nervous system and enhancement of the parasympathetic influence, causing a decreased heart rate and peripheral vasodilatation.[7]

Decreased arterial pressure causes the opposite effect. Baroreceptors control only temporary changes, such as changes in position.

Chemoreceptors

Chemoreceptors are located in the aortic arch and carotid body. They are capable of initiating changes in heart rate and arterial pressure in response to chemical stimulation. They are stimulated by decreased PO_2, increased PCO_2, and decreased plasma pH. When the chemoreceptor reflexes are stimulated, they subsequently stimulate the vasomotor center to increase cardiac activity.

Blood Pressure

The arterial blood pressure is a measure of the pressure exerted by blood against the walls of the arterial system. The *systolic* pressure is the peak pressure exerted against the arteries when the heart contracts. The *diastolic* pressure is the residual pressure of the arterial system during cardiac relaxation. Blood pressure is usually expressed as the ratio of systolic to diastolic pressure.

The two main factors influencing blood pressure are *cardiac output (CO)* and *peripheral vascular resistance (PR):*

$$BP = CO \times PR$$

Peripheral resistance is the force opposing the movement of blood. This force is created primarily in small arteries and arterioles.

The arterial blood pressure is influenced by changes in either cardiac output or peripheral resistance. These factors are discussed in Chap. 26.

Measurement of arterial blood pressure

Blood pressure can be measured by both invasive and noninvasive techniques. The invasive technique consists of catheter insertion into an artery. The catheter is attached to a recording device, and the pressure is measured directly (Chap. 28).

However, the easiest technique is the noninvasive, indirect measurement of blood pressure using a sphygmomanometer and a stethoscope. The sphygmomanometer consists of an inflatable cuff and a pressure gauge. The blood pressure is measured externally by listening for sounds, called *Korotkoff sounds,* produced over an artery when it is constricted. The brachial artery is the common site for taking blood pressure.

The balloon cuff is inflated to a pressure in excess of the systolic pressure. This causes blood flow in the artery to cease. As the pressure in the cuff is lowered, Korotkoff sounds are heard. The Korotkoff sounds are divided into five phases. The *first* phase is a tapping sound caused by the spurt of blood into the constricted artery as the pressure in the cuff is gradually deflated. This sound is considered the systolic measurement. The *second* phase begins with a murmur, usually 10 to 15 mmHg below the systolic tap. The *third* phase begins 14 to 20 mmHg below the second phase and begins when the murmur changes again to a tapping sound. The *fourth* phase begins when this tapping sound becomes muffled and less intense. The *fifth* phase occurs when the sound disappears.

The true diastolic pressure lies between the fourth and fifth phases. For greatest accuracy, the diastolic pressure should be recorded as both the muffled sound and the disappearance of sound (e.g., 120/84/80).[8] Occasionally, the sounds will be heard all the way to zero. In this case, the blood pressure should be recorded as 120/80/0. In actual practice, the blood pressure is often recorded as two numbers. The first number indicates the appearance of sound, and the second number represents the cessation of sound.

Pulse pressure and mean arterial pressure

Pulse pressure is the difference between the systolic and diastolic pressures. It is normally about one-third of the systolic pressure. If the blood pressure is 120/80, the pulse pressure would be 40. An increased pulse pressure may occur in exercise or in arteriosclerosis of the larger arteries. A decreased pulse pressure may be found in cardiac failure or hypovolemia.

Another measurement related to blood pressure is *mean arterial pressure.* This is not simply the average of the diastolic and systolic pressures because the duration of diastole exceeds that of systole at normal heart rates. Consequently, mean arterial pressure is calculated by adding the diastolic pressure to one-third of the pulse pressure:

$$\text{Mean arterial pressure} = \text{diastolic pressure} + \tfrac{1}{3}\ \text{pulse pressure}$$

A person with a blood pressure of 120/60/0 would have a mean arterial pressure of 80.

ASSESSMENT OF THE CARDIOVASCULAR SYSTEM

Subjective Data: The History

A careful health history and physical examination of the cardiovascular system provide critical assessment data. Common chief complaints which should alert the nurse to the possibility of underlying cardiac or vascular pathology must be explored and documented (Table 25-2).

Past medical history

Pediatric and Adult Illnesses The client should be questioned about the existence or history of the following conditions, which may have an influence on his current cardiovascular status:

- Alcoholism or excessive drinking
- Anemia
- Asthma
- Bleeding disorders
- Bronchitis
- Collagen diseases
- Diabetes mellitus
- Gout
- Hypertension
- Influenza
- Intermittent claudication
- Kidney disease
- Pneumonia
- Rheumatic fever
- Rubella
- Scarlet fever
- Stroke
- Thrombophlebitis
- Varicosities

Hospitalizations The client should also be asked about specific treatments or hospitalizations he may have experienced in the past. Any hospitalizations for diagnostic workups or cardiovascular symptoms should be explored. It should be noted if an ECG or chest x-ray was taken for baseline data.

Current Medications An assessment of the client's current and past use of medication should be done. This includes over-the-counter drugs as well as prescription drugs. For example, aspirin, which prolongs the blood-clotting time, is contained in many drugs used for alleviation of cold symptoms.

A medication assessment should list the name of the drug and the client's understanding of its purpose, side effects, and self-administration. Specific categories of drugs frequently used in clients with cardiovascular problems include antihypertensives, anticoagulants, diuretics, glycosides, and nitrates. Drugs which may adversely affect the cardiovascular system should also be assessed. Some of these, and examples of their effect on the cardiovascular system, are as follows:

Tricyclic antidepressants—arrhythmias
Phenothiazines—arrhythmias and hypotension
Oral contraceptives—thrombophlebitis
Doxorubicin (Adriamycin)—cardiomyopathy
Lithium—arrhythmias
Corticosteroids—sodium and fluid retention

Allergies A question about the client's allergies is appropriate. If the client has been treated for allergies, his understanding of this therapy should be ascertained. He should also be asked if he has ever had an anaphylactic reaction.

Obstetrical and Gynecological Problems The obstetrical or gynecological background, such as water weight gain, use of oral contraceptives, or venereal disease, should be noted.

Family history

Confirmed illnesses of blood relatives can highlight any hereditary or familial tendencies toward hypertension, bleeding, cardiac disorders, diabetes mellitus, atherosclerosis, or stroke. In addition, disorders affecting the vascular system, such as anemia, intermittent claudication, or varicosities, may be familial. Lastly, a family history of noncardiac conditions, such as asthma, renal disease, or obesity, should be assessed.

Social and personal history

Background Information The client's sex, race, and age are all related to his cardiovascular health. Discussing the client's marital status, role in the household, age and number of children, living environment, significant others, spiritual orientation, and coping mechanisms may assist the nurse in identifying stressors or strengths and support systems in the client's life.

Table 25-2
Cues to Cardiovascular Problems

Symptom	Description
Fatigue	Has no energy Requires more rest than normal Cannot engage in normal activities without tiring
Fluid retention	Weight gain, bloated feeling Reports swelling; clothing seems tight, and shoes no longer fit comfortably Reports marks or indentations left from constricting garments
Irregular heartbeat	Reports sensation of heart in the throat or skipped beats, racing heart, and dizziness
Dyspnea	Reports air hunger, especially after exertion Requires pillows for sleep or must sleep in a chair
Pain	Reports indigestion, burning, numbness, or tightness in midchest Pain may be in neck or left arm
Tenderness in calf of leg	Inability to bear weight, swelling of the involved extremity, inflamed, warm skin over a vein
Aching in calves	Distended, discolored, tortuous veins in calves of legs Reports ache in lower extremities after standing for short periods

Lifestyle The strong correlation between components of a client's lifestyle and cardiovascular health support the need for a careful scrutiny of stressors, exercise, diet, sleep, and habits.

Stressors

The client should be asked to identify areas of his life that cause him stress or anxiety. Potentially stressful areas include marital relationships, family, job, church, friends, finances, and housing. Although many people enjoy certain activities, they can be stressful at the same time as they are rewarding. The usual methods of coping with stress should be investigated.

Exercise

The benefit of exercise to cardiovascular health is indisputable. Sustained aerobic exercise is the most beneficial. Carefully inquire about the types of exercise done, the duration and frequency of each, and the occurrence of any untoward effects. The length of time the exercise program has been practiced should be recorded. Participation in individual or group sports should also be noted, along with its frequency and duration. Any symptoms indicative of cardiovascular problems while engaging in exercise should be recorded.

Diet

The client's weight in relation to his height and build should be determined. Problems of underweight or overweight should be noted. The amount of salt, saturated fats, and triglycerides in the diet should be determined. A typical day's diet should be examined for its adequacy in relation to the client's lifestyle. In addition to actual food habits, the client's attitudes and plans in relation to diet should be investigated. Food intake and exercise patterns should be complementary. The big eater should be the disciplined exerciser. Conversely, the sedentary person should adjust his caloric intake accordingly to avoid overtaxing the heart by increasing the work load due to excessive weight.

Sleep

The client should be asked specific questions related to sleep habits. How many pillows does the client use to sleep on at night? How big are the pillows? How many times a night does he awaken to urinate? Does he ever wake up suddenly and feel as if he cannot catch his breath? What does he do when this happens? A healthy, content person should fall asleep easily, sleep soundly without awakening, and wake up feeling refreshed and ready to face the day. Although there are many possible causes, cardiovascular problems are often to blame for interrupted sleep patterns.

Habits

The most critical question to ask about habits is, does the client smoke? The number of pack-years of smoking (number of packs per day times the number of years the client has smoked) should be computed. The client's attitude toward smoking, as well as his attempts to stop, should be discussed. Alcohol use should also be recorded. This information should include the type of beverage, amount, frequency, and any changes in the reaction to it. The use of habit-forming drugs should also be noted.

Review of systems

The client should be questioned about his past problems with the cardiovascular system. Specific inquiry should be made about the following conditions:

Hypertension	Chest pain
Rheumatic fever	Palpitations
Murmurs	Wheezing
Weight gain	Fainting
Shortness of breath	Leg cramps
Orthopnea	Claudication
Edema	Varicose veins
Fatigue	Cold or blue feet

When a cardiovascular problem is present, it affects other body systems, especially the pulmonary, renal, and neurological systems. Questions should be asked about these systems. This includes an appraisal of manifestations such as the following:

Wheezing	Dark, concentrated urine
Productive cough	Leg edema or numbness
Shortness of breath	Loss of memory
Asymmetrical weakness	

Objective Data: The Physical Examination

Blood pressure

After the client's general appearance has been observed, vital signs including blood pressure, heart and respiratory rate, and temperature are taken. The blood pressure should be measured while the client is sitting, lying, and standing. An appropriate cuff size should be used for accurate readings. Normally, there is a reduction of up to 15 mmHg in the systolic blood pressure and 3 to 5 mmHg in the diastolic blood pressure in the standing position. Blood pressure measurements should be taken in both arms. These readings may vary from 5 to 15 mmHg. A greater variance indicates pathology. Blood pressure in the lower extremities is expected to be 10 mmHg higher than in the upper extremities.[9]

Physical examination of the peripheral vascular system

Inspection Inspection of the skin color, hair distribution, and venous blood flow provides information about arterial blood flow and venous return.

The extremities should also be inspected for conditions such as edema, thrombophlebitis, varicose veins, and lesions such as stasis ulcers. Edema in the extremities can be caused by gravity, interruption of venous return, or elevation of right atrial pressure.

A measure used for assessing arterial flow to the extremities is the *capillary filling time*. The client's nail beds are squeezed to produce blanching and observed for the return of color. With normal arterial capillary perfusion, the color will return within 6 seconds.

The large veins in the neck (*internal* and *external jugulars*) should be inspected while the client is gradually elevated to an upright position. Distension and prominent pulsations of these neck veins can be caused by right atrial pressure elevation.

Palpation Palpation of the pulses in the neck and extremities also provides information on arterial blood flow. The pulses should be palpated to assess the volume or pressure within each vessel, as well as the condition of the arterial walls. Then, characteristics of the arteries on the right and left sides of the body are compared. It is important to palpate each carotid pulse separately in order to avoid vagal stimulation and subsequent arrhythmias.

When palpating the arteries identified in Fig. 25-8, the assessor should note the pressure of the pulse wave or how far the vessel wall distends when the pulse occurs. This judgment of the pulsation volume is recorded as *normal, bounding, thready,* or *absent.* The *rigidity* (hardness) of the vessel should also be noted. The normal pulse will feel like a tap, whereas a vessel wall which is narrowed or bulging will vibrate. The medical term for a palpable vibration is *thrill.*

Auscultation An artery which has a narrowed or bulging wall may also create an abnormal buzzing or humming sound called a *bruit.* It can be heard through a stethoscope placed over the vessel. Auscultation of major arteries, such as the abdominal aorta, carotids, and femorals, should be part of the initial cardiovascular assessment. Abnormalities of the vascular system are described in Table 25-3.

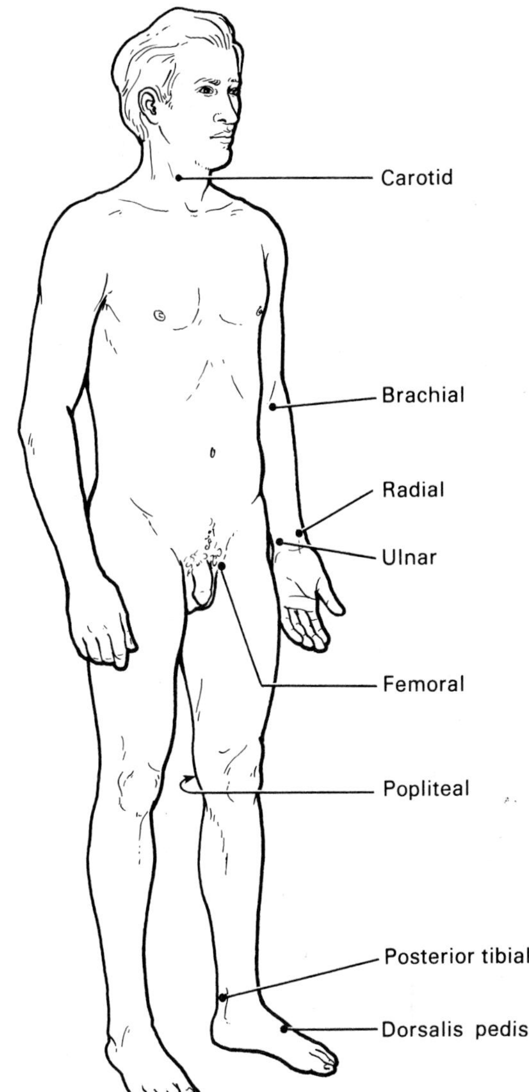

Figure 25-8 Common sites for palpating arteries.

Physical examination of the thorax

Inspection and Palpation An overall inspection of the bony structures of the thorax, such as the sternoclavicular joints, the manubrium, and the upper part of the sternum, is the initial step in the examination. Pulsations of the aortic arch or the innominate arteries may be observed or palpated in this area in some normal individuals. *Thrills* caused by abnormalities of these vessels may also be detected.

The next step in examining the thorax is to inspect the areas where the cardiac valves project their sounds by identifying the *intercostal spaces (ICSs).* The raised notch *(angle of Louis)* which is created where the manubrium and body of the sternum are joined is readily palpable in the midline of the sternum. The angle of Louis is at the level of the second rib and can therefore be used to distinguish the ICSs.

The following auscultatory areas can be located (Fig. 25-9): the *aortic area* in the second right ICS near the sternum, the *pulmonic area* in the second left ICS near the sternum, the *tricuspid area* in the fifth left ICS close to the sternum, and the *mitral area* in the left midclavicular line at the level of the fifth ICS. A fifth auscultatory area is *Erb's point,* located at the third left ICS near the sternum.

Normally, no pulsations are found in these areas unless the client has a very thin chest wall. Valvular disorder may be suspected if abnormal pulsations or

Table 25-3
Common Assessment Abnormalities of the Cardiovascular System

Finding	Description/Definition	Possible Etiology
	Pulse	
Pulse volume		
Bounding	Sharp, brisk, rapidly rising pulse.	Bradycardia, anemia, aortic valve incompetency.
Thready	Weak, slowly rising pulse.	Blood loss, mitral stenosis.
Absent	Lack of pulse.	Atherosclerosis, thrombus, trauma.
Thrill	Vibration of vessel or chest wall.	Aneurysms, aortic regurgitation.
Rigidity	Stiffness or inflexibility of vessel wall.	Hardening or thickening of wall, atherosclerosis.
Bruit	Humming heard through stethoscope held over vessel.	Narrowing of vessel, atherosclerosis, or aneurysms.
Tachycardia	Heart rate over 100 bpm.	Exercise, anxiety, shock, need for increased cardiac output.
Bradycardia	Heart rate less than 60 bpm.	Rest, SA node (pacemaker) damage, athletic conditioning.
Arrhythmia	Irregular heart rate, skipped heartbeats.	Damage to cardiac conduction pathway, ischemia, or side effect of drugs.
	Venous Abnormalities	
Distended neck veins	Present when the vertical distance is greater than 3 cm between the intersection of the angle of Louis and the level of jugular distension with the client sitting at a 45° angle.	Elevated right atrial pressure.
Pitting edema of lower extremities or sacral area	Finger indentation of imprint visible after firm pressure is applied.	Interruption of venous return to the heart, fluid in the tissues.
Thrombophlebitis	Red, warm, tender, hard vein. Edema, pain, and tenderness of extremity.	Venous stasis, damage to the endothelial layer of the vein, hypercoagulability of blood.
Positive Homan's sign	Calf pain which occurs during sharp dorsiflexion of the foot.	Thrombophlebitis.
	Skin	
Unusually warm hands or feet	Warmer than normal.	May occur with thyrotoxicosis or severe anemia.
Cold hands or feet	Cold to touch. Client requires external covering for comfort.	Intermittent claudication, peripheral arterial obstruction, low cardiac output.
Central cyanosis	Bluish or purplish color seen in central areas, such as the tongue, conjunctiva, or inner surface of the lips.	Arterial blood is not fully saturated with oxygen due to pulmonary or cardiac disorders (eg., congenital defects).
Peripheral cyanosis	Bluish or purplish color seen in exremities or in nose and ears.	Reduced blood flow to these areas due to heart failure, vasoconstriction, or cold environment.

Table 25-3 (Continued)

Finding	Description/Defination	Possible Etiology
Color changes in extremities with postural change	Pallor, cyanosis, or mottling of skin after limb has been elevated. Glossy appearance of skin.	Chronic decreased arterial perfusion.
Stasis ulcers	Darkly pigmented, edematous areas of the skin. May be open or oozing fluid.	Poor venous return, varicose veins, incompetent venous valves.
	Extremities	
Clubbing of nail beds	Obliteration of normal angle between base of nail and skin.	Endocarditis, congenital defects, prolonged O_2 deficiency.
Splinter hemorrhages	Small red to black streaks under fingernails.	Infective endocarditis (infection of endocardium, usually in area of the cardiac valves).
Abnormal capillary filling time	Blanching of nail bed for more than 6 s after pressure is released.	Reduced arterial capillary perfusion, anemia.
Varicose veins	Dilated, tortuous vessels visible in lower extremities.	Incompetent valves in the vein.
Asymmetry in limb circumference	Swelling of involved limb may not be observable, but differences in circumference can be measured.	Thrombophlebitis, varicose veins.
	Cardiac Ausculatory Abnormalities	
Third heart sound (S_3)	Extra heart sound, low-pitched, therefore heard best with bell of the stethoscope in the apical area. Falls in early diastole. Sounds like a gallop.	Usually indicates left ventricular failure.
Fourth heart sound (S_4)	Extra heart sound, low-pitched, therefore heard best with bell of the stethoscope along the left sternal border. Falls in late systole. Sounds like a gallop.	Usually indicates atrial failure.
Cardiac murmurs	A swishing noise heard between normal heart sounds that can be characterized by loudness, pitch, shape, quality, duration, and timing.	Usually indicates cardiac valve disorder.

thrills are felt. Next, the *epigastic area,* which lies on either side of the midline just below the xyphoid process, is inspected and palpated. The pulsation of the abdominal aorta may be visible and can normally be palpated here. Next, the *precordium,* which is located between the apex and sternum, is inspected for *heaves.*[10] Heaves are sustained lifts of the chest wall in the precordial area that can be seen or palpated. They may be caused by left ventricular enlargement. Normally, no pulsations are seen or felt here.

The *mitral area* is inspected for the point of maximum impulse (PMI) when the client is recumbent. This pulsation or ventricular thrust normally has a short duration and lies within the midclavicular line in the fifth ICS (apex). If the PMI is not visible, the area should be palpated by placing the palm of the right hand in the apical area and feeling for the thrust. If the PMI is palpable, its position is recorded in relation to the midclavicular line and ICSs. When the PMI is left of the midclavicular line, the heart may be enlarged.

Percussion The right and left heart borders can be estimated by percussion. The examiner stands to

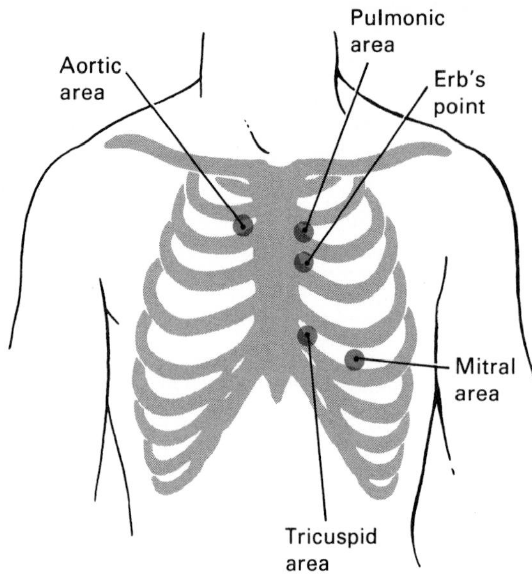

Figure 25-9 Cardiac auscultatory areas. *(Adapted from L. Shortridge and E. Lee, Introductory Skills for Nursing Practice, McGraw-Hill Book Company, New York, 1980, p. 126. Used with permission of McGraw-Hill Book Company.)*

Pulmonic and aortic areas

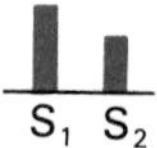

Tricuspid and mitral areas

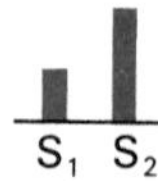

Normal physiological splitting of S_2 (best heard at pulmonic area)

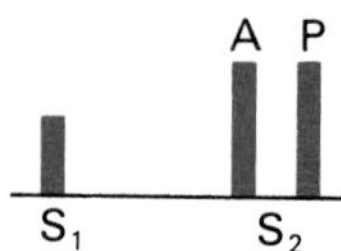

Legend:
A = Aortic
P = Pulmonic

Figure 25-10 Heart sounds.

the right of the recumbent client and percusses along the curve of the rib in the fourth and fifth ICSs, starting at the *midaxillary line*. The percussion note over the heart will be dull (in comparison to the resonance over the lung) and is recorded in relation to the midclavicular line.

Auscultation The movement of the cardiac valves creates some turbulence in the blood flow. The vibration of the blood causes normal heart sounds. These sounds can be heard through a stethoscope placed on the chest wall (Fig. 25-10). The first heart sound (S_1), which is associated with the closure of the aortic and pulmonic (AV) valves, has a soft *lub* sound. The second heart sound (S_2), which is associated with the closure of the tricuspid and mitral (semilunar) valves, has a sharp *dub* sound. S_1 signals the beginning of systole, the period of ventricular contraction. S_2 signals the beginning of diastole, the period of ventricular relaxation (Fig. 25-11). The examiner should listen to the auscultatory areas in sequence with both the diaphragm and bell of the stethoscope.

The first and second heart sounds are heard best with the diaphragm of the stethoscope because they are high-pitched. *Extra heart sounds* (S_3 or S_4), if present, are heard best with the bell of the stethoscope because they are low-pitched. It is important to explain to the client that the nurse will be listening while he is sitting leaning forward and in the *left lateral decubitus position.* Leaning forward while sitting accentuates sounds from the second ICSs (aortic and pulmonic areas). The left lateral decubitus position accentuates sounds produced at the mitral area.[11]

Initially, the nurse will listen at the apical area with the diaphragm of the stethoscope while simultaneously palpating the radial pulse. If fewer radial than apical pulses are counted, a *pulse deficit* is present. A client with a pulse deficit should have his apical/radial pulse taken often to monitor this abnormality. A judgment about the rhythm (regular or irregular) is also made when listening at the apex.

Palpating the carotid artery while auscultating is also important, as it allows differentiation of S_1 from S_2 and systole from diastole. Because S_1 (lub) occurs almost simultaneously with ventricular ejection, it is heard when the carotid pulse is felt. When listening at the other valvular areas, the examiner should always concentrate on the periods of systole and diastole, as well as on the first and second heart sounds.

Normally, no sound is heard between S_1 and S_2 during the periods of systole and diastole. Sounds that are heard during these periods probably represent abnormalities and should be described. An exception to this is a normal splitting of S_2, which is best heard at the pulmonic area.

If an abnormal sound is heard, it should be recorded. This description should include the timing (during systole or diastole), location (the site on the

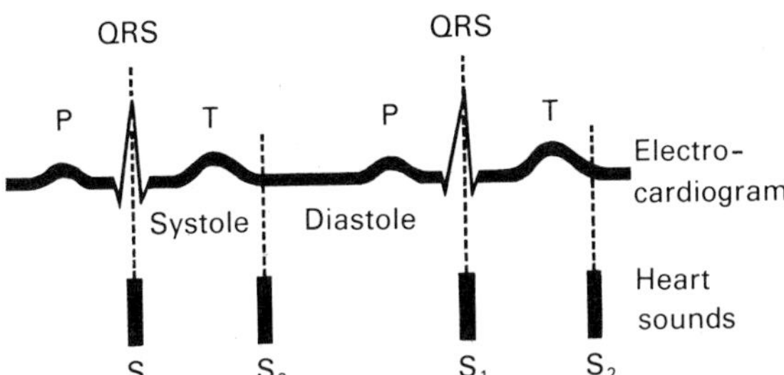

Figure 25-11 Relationship of ECG, cardiac cycle, and heart sounds.

chest where it is heard the loudest), pitch (heard best with the diaphragm or bell of the stethoscope), position (heard best when client is recumbent, sitting and leaning forward, or in the left lateral decubitus position), characteristic (harsh, musical, soft, short, long, etc.), and any other abnormal findings (irregular cardiac rhythms or palpable chest wall heaves) associated with the sound.

The abnormal sounds occurring during systole and diastole are classified as either murmurs or extra sounds. The most common abnormal sounds are described in Table 25-3. The data from inspection, palpation, percussion, and auscultation are presented in Table 25-4.

DIAGNOSTIC STUDIES OF THE CARDIOVASCULAR SYSTEM

There are numerous diagnostic techniques which add to the information obtained from the history and physical examination of the cardiovascular system. These procedures are usually classified as noninvasive or invasive. If only needle insertion for withdrawal of blood or injection of dye is used, these studies are usually considered noninvasive. Catheter insertion for angiography is considered an invasive procedure. The most common studies done to assess the cardiovascular system are presented in Table 25-5.

The responsibilities of the nurse remain the same whether the client is to undergo an invasive or a noninvasive procedure. First, the nurse must see that the procedure is scheduled and that any necessary preliminaries (e.g., special diets or changes in medication) are carried out. Appropriate safety measures, such as use of bedside rails following administration of pre-procedure medications or identification of client allergies, should be instituted. Comfort measures, such as oral care prior to the procedure, are important. The nurse must also check to see that the client's permission for the procedure has been obtained if it is required. It is important that the client understand the procedure to be done. Many times the client may have inaccurate information that causes unnecessary anxiety regarding the diagnostic study.

Table 25-4
Recording the Normal Physical Assessment of the Cardiovascular System

Inspection	Normal skin color and capillary filling time. Thorax symmetrical. PMI not visible.
Palpation	PMI palpable in the fifth ICS at the midclavicular line. No forceful pulsations, thrills, or heaves noted. Slight, palpable pulsations of abdominal aorta noted in epigastric area. Carotid pulses equal bilaterally. No jugular-venous distension with client sitting at a 45° angle.
Percussion	Dull to percussion 10 cm to the left on the midsternal line. Right heart border cannot be distinguished by percussion.
Auscultation	Heart sounds readily heard across the four valvular areas. Heart rate regular at 72 bpm. No murmurs or extra heart sounds. Apical pulse louder when patient is in left lateral decubitus position. All pulses of the extremities equal bilaterally. No evidence of impaired arterial flow or venous return noted in lower extremities.

Noninvasive Studies

Chest x-ray

A radiographic picture can depict cardiac contours, heart size and configuration, and anatomical changes in individual chambers (Fig. 25-12). The radiographic image records any displacement or enlargement of the heart. It is more accurate than percussion in determining the size of the heart.

Electrocardiogram

The normal ECG and the meaning of the waveforms were discussed in the first section of this chapter. The basic P, QRS, and T waveforms are used to assess cardiac function. Deviations from the normal sinus rhythm can indicate abnormalities in heart function.

There are numerous types of electrographic monitoring, including *continuous monitoring, telemetry,* in which waveforms are sent across telephone lines, and *stress testing,* in which the ECG of an exercising individual is recorded.

Table 25-5
Diagnostic Studies of the Cardiovascular System

Study	Description and Purpose	Nursing Responsibility
	Noninvasive	
Radiological Chest x-ray	The client is placed in three or four upright positions so that the size of the heart and any calcifications can be noted. *Normal:* heart size and contour for the individual's age, sex and size. No calcifications seen in coronary arteries or valves.	Inquire about the frequency of recent x-rays and the possibility of pregnancy. Provide lead shield for unexposed areas.
ECG	Small electrodes are placed on the surface of the chest and extremities while leads are changed to detect conduct patterns as the direction of current varies. ECG can detect rhythm of heart, site of pacemaker, position of heart, size of ventricles, and presence of injury. (For normal findings see Table 25-1.)	Observe for electrical safety hazards. Tell client that no discomfort is involved.
Echocardiogram	Small transducer which emits ultrasonic sound waves is moved across the client's chest wall above the heart. Transducer records sound waves that are bounced off the heart.	Instruct the client and his family about the procedure and sensations (pressure and rubbing from the movement of the transducer across the chest). No contraindication to the procedure since there is no risk to the client.
Phonocardiogram	Graphic recording of heart sounds done by placing a microphone on the surface of the body. Better than stethoscope for recording low-frequency sounds (gallop sounds). Provides information on murmurs and the timing of various sounds.	Explain procedure to client.
Nuclear cardiology	Involves intravenous injection of radioactive isotope. Radioactive uptake is counted over the heart by a gamma radiation camera. Supplies information about myocardial contractility, myocardial perfusion, and acute cell injury.	Explain procedure to client. Explain that radioactive isotope used is a small, diagnostic amount.
Blood studies: **Serum enzymes** CPK	Within 6 h of a myocardial infarction, the CPK will be elevated. It will return to normal within 48–72 h. *Normal:* 5–55 mU/mL (male) 5–35 mU/mL (female)	CPK enzymes are found in heart, skeletal muscle, and brain cells. It is important to avoid CPK elevation created by IM injections which damage muscle cells.
CPK-MB fraction	CPK isoenzyme that is cardiospecific.	
SGOT or AST	Six to eight hours following cardiac infarction, the SGOT (AST) rises. It will peak within 24–48 h and return to normal in 4–8 days. *Normal:* 15–45 mU/mL	Because the SGOT (AST) can be elevated by other disorders, such as liver damage, thorough history taking is important.
LDH	Has five different isoenzymes. Pattern of elevation is similar to that of SGOT following cardiac infarction, except that LDH remains elevated for 5–7 days. *Normal:* 80–120 Wacker units	When drawing blood ensure that it is not hemolyzed, as hemolysis will falsely raise the LDH level.
LDH_1	LDH isoenzyme subgroup contained in heart muscle.	
Serum lipids Cholesterol	Cholesterol is a blood lipid. Elevated cholesterol is considered a risk factor for developing atherosclerotic heart disease. *Normal:* 150–270 mg/dL (varies with age and sex)	Client must be fasting to obtain useful information. For all fasting blood studies, the nurse must be sure that the client understands that he is to limit his diet to noncalorie fluid intake for 12 h prior to the examination.

Table 25-5 (Continued)

Study	Description and Purpose	Nursing Responsibility
	Noninvasive	
Triglycerides	Triglycerides are mixtures of two or three fatty acids. Elevations are associated with cardiovascular disease. *Normal:* 40–150 mg/dL	
Lipoproteins	When elevated (especially in younger individuals), they can predict the development of cardiac disease. *Normal:* Lipoprotein electrophoresis 40–50 mb/dL	There are marked day-to-day fluctuations in serum lipid levels. More than one determination is needed for accurate diagnosis and treatment.
Total lipids	*Normal:* 400–850 mg/dL	
Drug levels Digitoxin Digoxin	Blood tests done to determine therapeutic and toxic levels of drugs in the body. *Digitoxin:* Therapeutic: 14–30 ng/mL Toxic: >30 ng/mL *Digoxin:* Therapeutic: 1–2 ng/mL Toxic: >3 ng/mL	Appropriate timing of test with medication schedule.
	Invasive	
Cardiac catheterization	Involves insertion of a catheter into the heart. Information can be obtained about the oxygen saturation and pressure readings within the chambers. Dye can be injected to assist in examining the structure and motion of the heart. The procedure is done by inserting a catheter into a vein (for the right side of the heart), or an artery (for the left side of the heart). For details of the procedure, see text.	*Before procedure:* Written permission required. Withhold food and fluids for 6–18 h prior to procedure. Sedative often given. Inform client about use of local anesthesia, insertion of catheter, and feeling of warmth and fluttering sensation of heart as catheter is passed. Client may cough when catheter is inserted into the pulmonary artery. Will be monitored by ECG throughout procedure. *After procedure:* assessment of circulation to extremity used for catheter insertion. Check peripheral pulses, color, and sensation of extremity every 15 min for 4 h and then with decreasing frequency. Observe injection site for swelling and bleeding. Sandbag often placed over arterial site. Vital signs monitored. Assessment for abnormal heart rates and arrhythmias and signs of pulmonary emboli (respiratory difficulty).
Coronary Angiography (arteriography)	Injection of radiopaque dye directly into coronary arteries using the same procedure as for cardiac catheterization. Used to evaluate the patency of coronary arteries and the collateral circulation.	Same as for cardiac catheterization.
Peripheral arteriography (angiography) and **venography** (phlebography)	Involves injection of radiopaque dye into either arteries or veins. Serial x-rays are taken to detect and visualize any atherosclerotic plaques, occlusions, aneurysms, or traumatic injury.	*Before procedure:* Carefully explain procedure to client. A mild sedative may be given. *After procedure:* check extremity with puncture site for pulsation, warmth, color, and motion. Inspect insertion site for bleeding or swelling. Observe client for allergic reactions to dye.

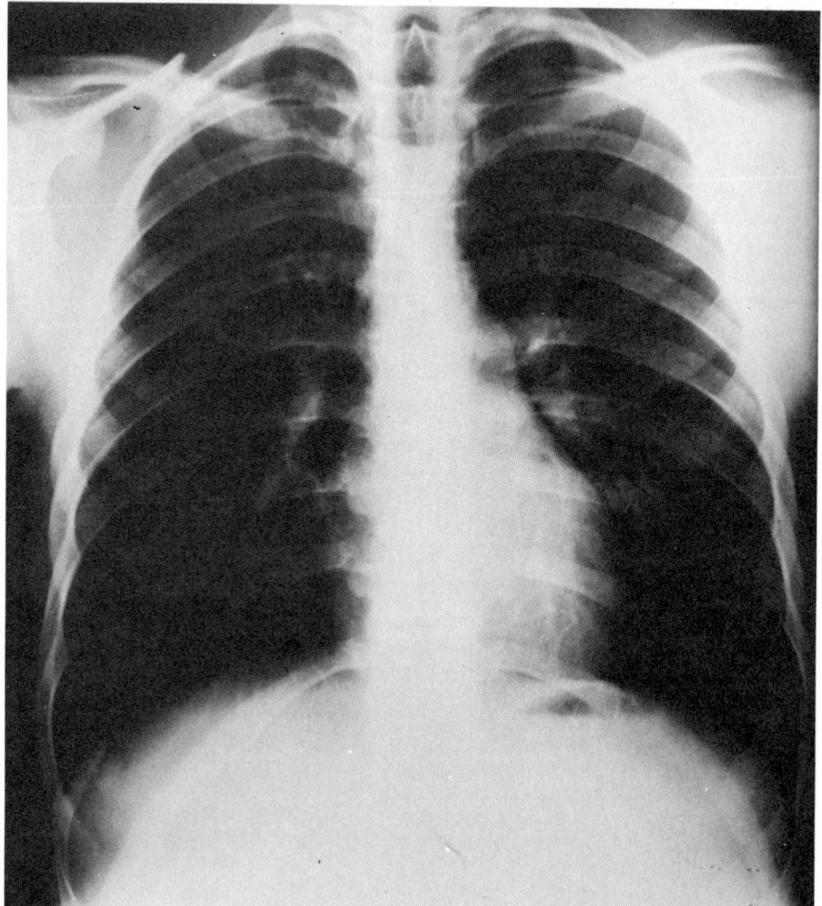

Figure 25-12 Chest x-ray showing outline of the heart. *(From N. K. Wenger et al., Cardiology for Nurses, McGraw-Hill Book Company, New York, 1980, p. 20. Used with permission of McGraw-Hill Book Company.)*

ECG Leads Recording of an ECG involves the use of five electrodes. An electrode is placed on each of the four limbs. The right-leg electrode is used as an inactive ground electrode. The fifth electrode is used for various placements on the precordium.

Electrical impulses generated by the heart are picked up by the electrodes, magnified by an amplifier, and recorded. The recording is done by machines which produce a direct tracing by a stylus on paper. The paper contains a graphic background which permits rapid interpretation of the waveforms.

Each combination of electrodes used in standard electrocardiography is called a *lead*. Each lead gives a continuous recording of changes in potential (or voltage) during the cardiac cycle between any two of the electrodes or between one electrode and a combination of others.[12]

The three standard leads are I, II, and III (Fig. 25-13). Lead I records the difference detected by the right- and left-arm electrodes. Lead II is a right-arm, and left-leg combination. Lead III records the electrical activity between the left arm and left leg.

The precordial leads are six standard positions over the heart (Fig. 25-14). The fifth electrode is placed in various locations, starting at the right sternal border in the fourth ICS (V_1) and moving across the chest, as indicated in Fig. 25-14.

Echocardiogram (ultrasound cardiogram)

The echocardiogram uses ultrasound waves (high-frequency sound waves) to record the movement of the structures of the heart. In the normal heart, ultrasonic sound waves directed at the heart will be reflected back in typical configurations. The echocardiogram provides information about abnormalities of valvular structure and motion, cardiac chamber size

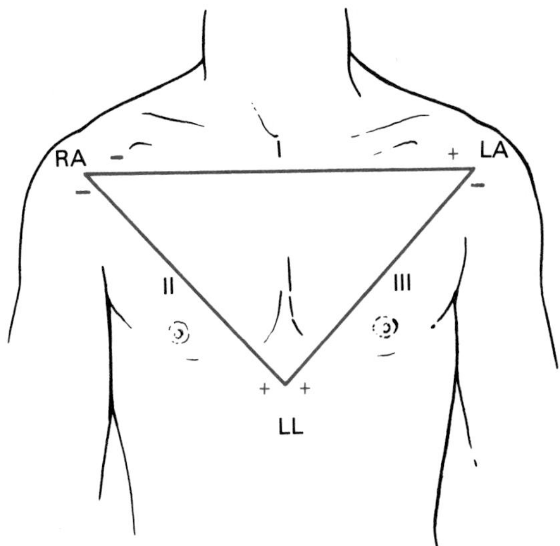

Figure 25-13 Conventional polarity of the three standard leads is indicated by + and −. *(From S. Price and L. Wilson, Pathophysiology: Clinical Concepts of Disease Processes, 2d ed., McGraw-Hill Book Company, New York, 1982, p. 329. Used with permission of McGraw-Hill Book Company.)*

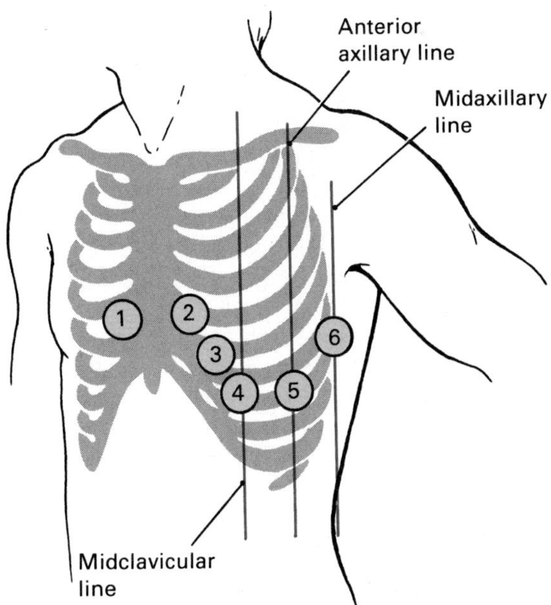

Figure 25-14 Placement of chest leads for a 12-lead ECG.

and contents, and ventricular muscle and septal motion and thickness.

Nuclear cardiology

Radioactive tracer studies are being used with increasing frequency to diagnose cardiovascular problems. Radioactive isotopes are injected into a vein, and recordings are made of the radioactivity emitted over a specific area. The circulation of this tagged material can be used to detect coronary artery blood flow, intracardiac shunts, motion of ventricles, and size of the heart chambers. This procedure is also used in evaluating the site and extent of myocardial ischemia or infarction.

Blood tests

There are numerous blood studies which contribute information about the cardiovascular system. For example, studies of the blood itself reflect the oxygen-carrying capacity (red blood cell count and hemoglobin), and coagulation properties (clotting times). See Chap. 23 for hematology studies.

Enzymes Enzymes are found in all cells, with each cell type having its own specific enzymes. When cells are injured, they release their enzymes into the circulation. The enzymes characteristic of cardiac injury are creatine phosphokinase (CPK), serum glutamic-oxaloacetic acid (SGOT)—also called serum aspartate aminotransferase (AST)— and lactic dehydrogenase (LDH) (Table 25-5).

Because these enzymes are found in a variety of body tissues, they can be elevated as a result of injury to the muscles, liver, and other organs. For example, an elevation of LDH could mean heart, liver, or skeletal muscle damage. *Isoenzymes* can be identified by electrophoresis and can indicate more clearly which tissue is actually damaged. The isoenzymes CPK-MB and LDH_1 are found primarily in heart muscle. Therefore, their determination is a better indicator of cardiac injury than the assessment of the total enzymes.

Blood Lipids Blood lipids consist of cholesterol, triglycerides, and phospholipids. They circulate in the blood bound to protein. Thus, they are often referred to as *lipoproteins*. Electrophoresis techniques are available to separate the lipoproteins. Abnormalities of blood lipids vary in such a way that several classifications of hyperlipoproteinemias have been developed (Chap. 27). The correlation between hyperlipidemia and coronary artery disease is well established.

Invasive Studies

Cardiac catheterization

Cardiac catheterization is a definitive means of obtaining information about cardiac disorders. This procedure can be used to measure intracardiac pressures and oxygen levels in various parts of the heart, as well as cardiac output. With injection of dye and x-ray visualization, the chambers of the heart can be outlined.

Cardiac catheterization is performed by inserting a radiopaque catheter into the right or left side of the heart. For the right side of the heart, a catheter is inserted via an arm vein (basilic or cephalic) or a femoral leg vein. The catheter is advanced into the vena cava, the right atrium, and the right ventricle. The catheter is further inserted into the pulmonary artery, where it can be wedged or lodged in position. This position is called the *pulmonary capillary wedge* position and can be used to measure pressures reflecting the function of the left side of the heart.

The left-sided approach is performed by inserting a catheter into the brachial artery or femoral artery. The catheter is passed in a retrograde manner up the aorta, across the aortic valve, and into the left ventricle.

Blood is taken from various chambers and analyzed for its oxygen content. Pressures in the various chambers are recorded. With the use of dye injections, the structures of the heart can be visualized and the size of the chambers determined.

Complications of cardiac catheterization include looping, kinking, or breaking off of the catheter, blood loss, allergic reaction to the dye, air or blood embolism, arrhythmias, and puncture of the ventricles, cardiac septum, or lung tissue. The procedure has a 1 percent mortality risk.[13]

Nurses have both pre-procedure and post-procedure responsibilities for clients undergoing cardiac catheterization. The client should be told how long (2 to 3 hours) the catheterization procedure will take, as well as where it will take place. Most hospitals have a cardiac catheterization laboratory specifically designed to perform the procedure. See Table 25-5 for the nursing responsibilities related to cardiac catheterization.

Coronary angiography (arteriography)

The coronary angiography is a modification of the cardiac catheterization. The left-sided catheter approach is modified so that the catheters are inserted up the aorta and into the openings of the coronary arteries. Dye is injected, and x-ray films are taken. This procedure is useful in identifying any lesions, obstructions, and collateral circulation of the coronary arteries.

Coronary angiography is used to obtain information about the presence and severity of coronary artery disease. This is needed to confirm the diagnosis and to determine the therapy. The nursing responsibilities for this procedure are similar to those for a client with a cardiac catheterization.

Blood flow and pressure measurements

Peripheral Vessel Blood Flow Peripheral vessel blood flow can be assessed by injection of radiopaque material (arteriography and venography). With these tests, arterial occlusions and venous abnormalities can be located.

Pressure Measurements Bedside measurements of pressures in the cardiovascular system are frequently used to assess cardiac output and the appropriate fluid management of the hospitalized client. One such measurement is the *central venous pressure (CVP).*

To obtain a CVP reading, a catheter is threaded through the jugular or subclavian vein into the superior vena cava to the right atrium. The end of the catheter is connected to a three-way stopcock, a fluid system, and a water manometer (Fig. 25-15). An intravenous solution is maintained at a slow drip rate into the vein. To take a reading, the stopcock is opened to the manometer which is then filled with intravenous solution. The stopcock is then turned to allow the fluid in the manometer to flow through to the client.

When the fluid level stabilizes, a reading is taken. Then the stopcock is returned to the original position so that the intravenous solution can flow to the client.

For an accurate reading, the base of the manometer should be at the level of the right atrium. The pressure readings directly reflect the right ventricular filling and diastolic pressure. The CVP reading is influenced by the function of the left side of the heart, pressures in the pulmonary vessels, venous return to the heart, and the position of the client when the reading is taken. The last factor must be kept in mind if an accurate reading is to be obtained. The CVP reading is now used less frequently since the introduction of pulmonary artery pressures.

Other pressure readings taken at the bedside include the *mean arterial pressure, pulmonary artery pressure,* and *pulmonary wedge pressure* (Chap. 28).

REVIEW QUESTIONS

The number of the question corresponds with the same numbered objective at the beginning of the chapter.

1. A semilunar valve is located between the
   a. vena cava and right atrium
   b. right atrium and right ventricle

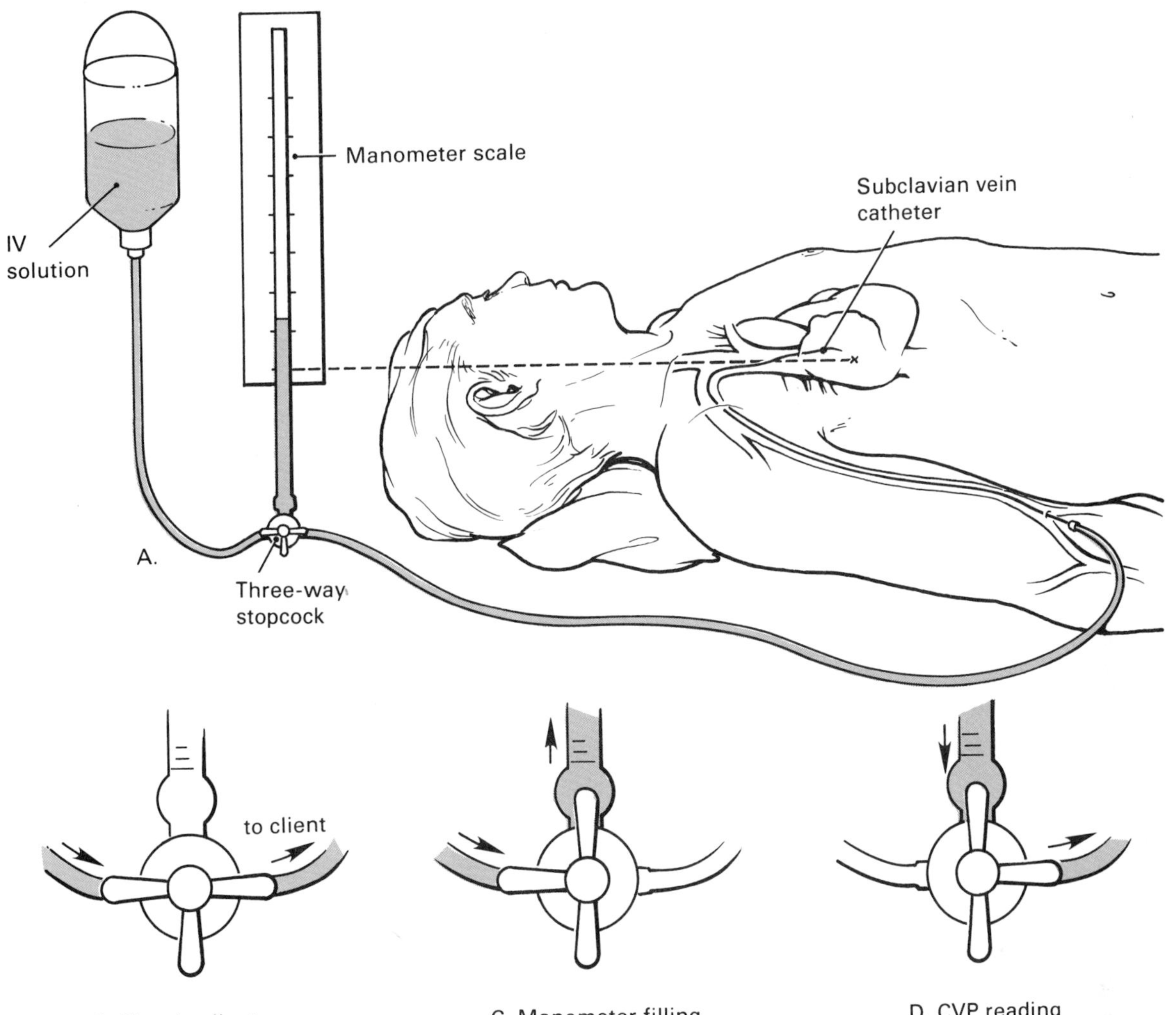

Figure 25-15 CVP measurement. *(a)* Placement of the manometer in relationship to the client. *(b)* Stopcock is turned for intravenous flow to the client. *(c)* Stopcock is turned so that manometer fills with fluid. *(d)* Stopcock is turned so that fluid in manometer flows to the client. A CVP reading is obtained when the fluid level stabilizes.

c. right ventricle and pulmonary artery
d. left atrium and left ventricle

2. If a person had a myocardial infarction of the anterior wall of the left ventricle, which of the following arteries is most likely occluded?
a. left circumflex artery
b. left anterior descending artery
c. right marginal artery
d. right anterior descending artery

3. Which of the following structures is not involved in the conduction pathway of the heart?
a. sinuses of Valsalva
b. Purkinje fibers
c. bundle branches
d. bundle of His

4. Which of the following blood vessels has the primary function of diffusing nutrients and metabolites?
a. venules
b. arterioles
c. arteries
d. capillaries

5. Chemoreceptors in the arch of the aorta and carotid body are stimulated by
a. decreased PCO_2
b. increased pH
c. decreased PO_2
d. increased arterial pressure

6. The purpose of testing for capillary filling time is to assess
a. arterial flow to the extremities

b. venous circulation to the hands
c. lymphatic obstruction of venous return
d. thrombus formation in veins

7. The auscultatory area in the left midclavicular line at the level of the fifth ICS is the
   a. tricuspid area
   b. mitral area
   c. aortic area
   d. pulmonic area

8. Palpable precordial thrills may be caused by
   a. heart murmurs
   b. pulmonary edema
   c. gallop rhythms
   d. right ventricular hypertrophy

9. Which one of the following is an important nursing responsibility for a client having an invasive cardiovascular diagnostic study?
   a. Tell him that he will have general anesthesia.
   b. Instruct the client to do a surgical scrub of the insertion site.
   c. Check the peripheral pulses and cutdown site.
   d. Instruct the client about radioactive isotope injection.

10. A P wave on an ECG represents an impulse
   a. arising at the AV node and spreading to the bundle of His
   b. arising at the AV node and depolarizing the atria
   c. arising at the SA node and repolarizing the atria
   d. arising at the SA node and depolarizing the atria

REFERENCES

1. C. D. Clemente et al., *Anatomy—A Regional Atlas of the Human Body,* Lea & Febiger, Philadelphia, 1975, pp. 126–145.
2. S. A. Price and L. M. Wilson, *Pathophysiology: Clinical Concepts of Disease Processes,* 2d ed., 1982 McGraw-Hill Book Company, New York, 1978, pp. 301–302.
3. A. J. Vander et al., *Human Physiology—The Mechanisms of Body Function,* McGraw-Hill Book Company, New York, 1980, p. 275.
4. Ibid., pp. 282–287.
5. Ibid., p. 289.
6. V. B. Montcastle, *Medical Physiology,* 13th ed., The C. V. Mosby Company, St. Louis, 1974, pp. 953–954.
7. N. K. Wenger et al., *Cardiology for Nurses,* McGraw-Hill Book Company, New York, 1980, pp. 44–45.
8. A. Ravin, *The Clinical Significance of the Sounds of Korotkoff,* Merck, Sharp and Dohme, West Point, Pa., pp. 1–29.
9. D. A. Jones et al., *Medical-Surgical Nursing,* McGraw-Hill Book Company, New York, 1978, p. 776.
10. W. Hurst, R. B. Logue, and R. Bruce, *The Heart, Arteries and Veins,* McGraw-Hill Book Company, New York, 1974, p. 196.
11. J. L. Sherman et al., *Guide to Patient Evaluation,* Medical Examination Publishing Company, Garden City, N.Y., pp. 180–195.
12. Wenger et al., op. cit., pp. 115–117.
13. A. Selzer, *Principles of Clinical Cardiology,* W. B. Saunders Company, Philadelphia, 1975, pp. 18–254, 326–626.

Chapter 26

NURSING ROLE IN MANAGEMENT

Blood Pressure Disturbances

Nancy Rojo Sypert
Louise P. Gallagher

Learning Objectives

1. Describe the mechanisms involved in the regulation of normal blood pressure.
2. Define the shock syndrome.
3. Differentiate among the three classifications of the causes and mechanisms of shock.
4. Describe the pathophysiology and clinical manifestations of the three stages of the shock syndrome.
5. Describe the medical and pharmacological management for the client with the shock syndrome.
6. Discuss the nursing management for the client in shock.
7. Explain the mechanisms and clinical manifestations of blood transfusion reactions.
8. Describe the nursing management for the client receiving blood transfusions.
9. Differentiate between the pathophysiological mechanisms of essential and secondary hypertension.
10. Identify the risk factors associated with essential hypertension.
11. Describe the clinical manifestations and complications of hypertension.
12. Describe the medical, pharmacological, and dietary management of hypertension.
13. Describe the nursing management for the client with hypertension, emphasizing client education.
14. Explain the clinical manifestations and management of hypertensive crisis.

Adequate systemic arterial blood pressure is essential for circulation of blood to all body tissues. This chapter discusses the regulation of blood pressure and then focuses on two disturbances in blood pressure, shock and hypertension.

REGULATION OF SYSTEMIC ARTERIAL PRESSURE

When reviewing the regulatory mechanisms of systemic arterial pressure, it is important to consider the following equation:

$$\text{Arterial blood pressure (BP)} = \text{cardiac output (CO)} \times \text{total peripheral resistance (TPR)}$$

Cardiac output is defined as the *stroke volume* (amount of blood pumped from one ventricle per beat, approximately 70 mL) times the heart rate (HR) for 1 minute. *Total peripheral resistance* (TPR) or *peripheral vascular resistance* (PVR) refers primarily to the amount of vasomotor tone of the blood vessels in the peripheral vascular system. Peripheral resistance is the force opposing the movement of blood. This force is created primarily in the small arteries and arterioles. If peripheral resistance is increased, a greater amount of pressure will be required to force the blood around the circulatory pathways.

The mechanisms that regulate blood pressure have an effect on either cardiac output or peripheral resistance. Regulation of normal systemic arterial pressure is a complex process involving the nervous, renal, and endocrine systems (Fig. 26-1).

Nervous System

Sympathetic nervous system

The nervous system, which reacts quickly to alterations in BP, increases arterial pressure primarily by activation of the sympathetic nervous system. When blood pressure falls to below-normal levels, the sympathetic nervous system is activated. Activation results in secretion of epinephrine and norepinephrine from sympathetic nerve endings and the adrenal medulla. Sympathetic stimulation accelerates the heart rate and the force of myocardial contraction. This results in increased cardiac output.

When the sympathetic nervous system is stimulated, it, in turn, stimulates the peripheral vasculature to constrict. This vasoconstriction causes an increase in peripheral resistance. Sympathetic control is the most important factor related to increasing peripheral resistance.

The sympathetic vasomotor center is located in the medulla of the brain. During exercise, the motor

This chapter was reviewed by Marlene McGann-Gilliland, R.N., M.S., M.S.N., Certified Adult Nurse Practitioner, Director of Wellness Center, Sioux Valley Hospital, Sioux Falls, South Dakota, and Adjunct Associate Professor, South Dakota State University, Brookings, South Dakota.

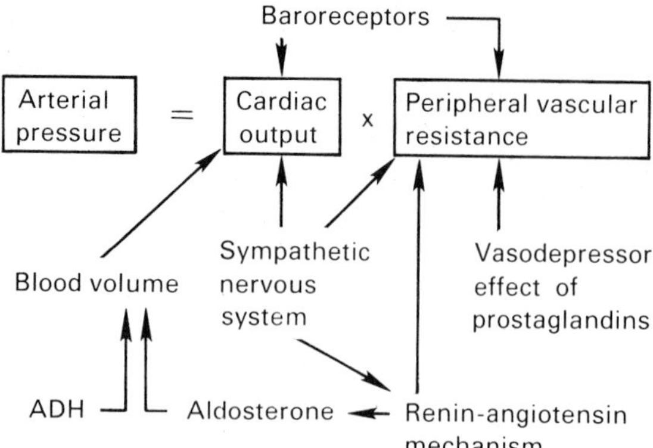

Figure 26-1 Mechanisms involved in regulation of blood pressure.

area of the cortex is activated, which in turn activates the vasomotor center and therefore the sympathetic nervous system. During postural changes from lying to standing, the vasomotor center is stimulated to activate the sympathetic nervous system. If this did not happen, there would be inadequate blood flow to the brain. Blood pressure may be reduced by stimulation of the parasympathetic system, which decreases the heart rate (via the vagus nerve) and thereby decreases cardiac output.

Baroreceptors (pressoreceptors)

Baroreceptors are specialized nerve receptors in the carotid arteries and arch of the aorta. When blood pressure rises to above-normal levels, the baroreceptors are stimulated. They are sensitive to stretch and, when stimulated by increased pressure, they send inhibitory impulses to the sympathetic vasomotor center and stimulate the vagus nerve. This results in dilatation of peripheral arterioles, a slowed heart rate, and decreased contractility of the heart.

A fall in blood pressure leads to activation of the sympathetic system because the inhibitory effect of the baroreceptors has been removed. The baroreceptors control only temporary changes in blood pressure. In the presence of long-standing hypertension, the baroreceptors become adjusted to elevated levels of blood pressure and recognize this level as "normal."

Renal System

The kidneys assist in regulating blood pressure by controlling sodium and extracellular fluid (ECF) volume (see Chap. 36). The retention of sodium results in increased water retention, which causes an increased ECF volume. This increased ECF volume will increase the venous return to the heart and therefore elevate the stroke volume which elevates the BP.

Another important mechanism related to the renal system is the renin-angiotensin mechanism. In response to sympathetic stimulation or decreased blood flow through the kidneys, renin is secreted from the juxtaglomerular apparatus in the afferent arterioles of the kidney. Renin activates angiotensinogen to angiotensin I, which, in turn, activates angiotensin II and III (Fig. 36-6). Angiotensin stimulates the adrenal cortex to secrete aldosterone. Increased aldosterone levels eventually result in increased blood volume and increased cardiac output (Fig. 26-2). Angiotensin is also a potent vasoconstrictor, thus increasing peripheral resistance.

The types of prostaglandins secreted by the renal medulla have a vasopressor effect on the systemic circulation. This results in decreased peripheral resistance and lowering of blood pressure. One type of prostaglandin increases renal blood flow and promotes sodium excretion, which also helps to maintain blood pressure within normal limits. (Prostaglandins are discussed in Chap. 40.)

Endocrine System

When the sympathetic nervous system is stimulated, it, in turn, stimulates the adrenal medulla to release epinephrine and norepinephrine. These hormones increase blood pressure by causing vasoconstriction, which increases total peripheral resistance. They also increase cardiac output by increasing heart rate and myocardial contractility.

The adrenal cortex is stimulated by angiotensin to release aldosterone. (Release of aldosterone is also regulated by other factors, such as low sodium levels; see Chaps. 12 and 40.) Aldosterone stimulates the kidneys to retain sodium and therefore water. This increases blood pressure by increasing cardiac output (Fig. 26-2).

The increased sodium in the blood stimulates the release of antidiuretic hormone (ADH) by the pituitary

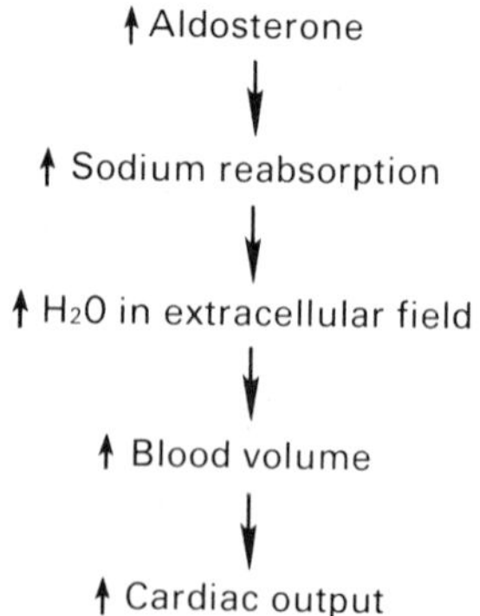

Figure 26-2 Mechanism of aldosterone.

gland. ADH increases the ECF volume by stimulating the kidneys to retain water. Therefore, blood pressure is increased by increasing blood volume and thus cardiac output.

In the healthy person, these regulatory mechanisms function in response to the demands of the body. When the person develops either shock or hypertension, the blood pressure-regulating mechanisms become defective. Medical and nursing management is directed toward changing the cardiac output or peripheral resistance of the client so that his blood pressure will return to normal.

THE SHOCK SYNDROME

Shock is a clinical syndrome of relatively rapid onset characterized by inadequate tissue perfusion. As a result, the metabolic needs of cells are not met.[1,2] Shock is a complex group of signs and symptoms that may be precipitated by a variety of etiological factors. It is important to note that shock cannot be defined in terms of hypotension since the shock syndrome may be manifested in the absence of hypotension. Conversely, hypotension may occur in the absence of shock.

Significance of the Problem

The morbidity and mortality associated with shock are extremely difficult to determine. Some estimates have been reported. For example, cardiogenic shock occurs in approximately 10 to 15 percent of clients hospitalized with acute myocardial infarction and has an estimated mortality of more than 80 percent.[3,4] About 40 percent of hospitalized clients with gram-negative bacteremia will develop some degree of septic shock.[5] Mortality from septic shock may approach 30 to 40 percent.[6] In addition, fatalities in the United States occurring as a result of anaphylactic reactions to penicillin alone have been estimated at as many as 300 per year.[7] Death in trauma victims is often due to complications of shock.

Etiology and Pathogenesis of the Shock Syndrome

There have been many attempts to classify shock. None have been totally satisfactory. Table 26-1 presents one classification system listing common types of shock and possible causes. This classification is based on a consideration of defects in the three primary mechanisms responsible for adequate circulation: (1) vascular tone (*relative hypovolemia*), (2) blood volume (*actual hypovolemia*), and (3) the ability of the heart to act as a pump (*pump failure*). Table 26-2 compares the cardiovascular effects of the three types of shock.

Table 26-1
Classification of the Shock Syndrome

Relative hypovolemia

1. Neurogenic shock
   - Spinal anesthesia or deep general anesthesia
   - Hyperinsulinism (insulin shock)
   - Spinal cord injury (spinal shock)
   - Barbiturate overdose
   - Extreme emotional stress, fear, or anxiety
   - Severe pain
2. Vasogenic shock
   - Hypersensitivity
   - Septicemia (toxic or septic shock)

Actual hypovolemia (hypovolemic shock)

- Hemorrhage (hemorrhagic shock)
- Burns (cutaneous or burn shock)
- Diabetes insipidus
- Ketoacidosis (diabetic shock)
- Gastrointestinal fluid loss (vomiting and diarrhea)
- Excessive use of diuretics
- Internal sequestration of fluid (ascites, peritonitis)

Pump failure (cardiogenic shock)

- Myocardial infarction
- Cardiac arrhythmias
- Congestive heart failure

Relative hypovolemia

Relative hypovolemia occurs when the size of the vascular space increases due to vasodilatation. The usual blood volume cannot adequately fill the expanded capillary bed. In this situation, there is no change in the ability of the heart to pump blood or in the blood volume. Relative hypovolemia can occur secondary to either neurogenic or vasogenic causes.

Neurogenic Shock In neurogenic shock, there is a decrease in efferent impulses from the sympathetic nervous system to the vascular smooth muscle. This results in vasodilatation due to a decrease in the ability of the vessels to constrict. This causes pooling of blood, decreased venous return to the heart, decreased cardiac output, and eventually inadequate tissue perfusion.

Vasogenic Shock Vasogenic shock occurs because the peripheral vessels are unable to respond to sympathetic impulses due to hypersensitivity reactions or bacterial toxins.[8] Hypersensitivity reactions result when substances such as histamine or bradykinin act directly on blood vessels to cause vasodilatation. This is most commonly found in anaphylactic shock (Chap. 10).

Table 26-2
Cardiovascular Effects of Shock

Type of Shock	Cardiac Output	Central Venous Pressure	Peripheral Resistance	Pulmonary Artery Pressure*	Pulmonary Artery Wedge Pressure*
Relative hypovolemia	↑ or ↓	↑ or ↓	↓	↑ or ↓	↑ or ↓
Actual hypovolemia	↓	↓	↑	↓	↓
Pump failure	↓	↑	↑	↑	↑

*Pulmonary artery pressures are explained in Chap. 28.

Bacterial endotoxins released from gram-negative bacteria are the primary cause of death from septicemia. Septic shock can also occur secondary to staphylococcal and streptococcal infections. In the early stages of septic shock, the toxins released into the blood may cause intense vasoconstriction, which may result in normal and greater than normal venous return and cardiac output. In the more advanced stages of septic shock, the same process occurs as in neurogenic shock, resulting in vasodilatation, decreased venous return, decreased cardiac output, and inadequate tissue perfusion.

Actual hypovolemia

Actual hypovolemia occurs when there is a loss of intravascular fluid volume. This loss results in decreased venous return to the heart, decreased cardiac output, circulatory insufficiency, and eventually inadequate tissue perfusion. In this situation, there is no change in the pumping ability of the heart or in the size of the vascular space. The fluid that is lost may be either whole blood, plasma, or water and electrolytes. Common causes of actual hypovolemia include hemorrhage, burns, and gastrointestinal fluid losses. Other causes are listed in Table 26-1.

Hemorrhage Hemorrhage refers to an excess loss of whole blood. The amount of blood loss that will result in the shock syndrome is dependent upon the efficiency of the individual's compensatory mechanisms. In general, a loss of 15 to 25 percent of the circulatory blood volume can result in shock, and a loss of 45 percent or more is often fatal.[9] Hemorrhagic shock frequently occurs following trauma and is secondary to such problems as bleeding esophageal varices or ruptured aortic aneurysms.

Burns Plasma is the primary fluid lost from the vascular space in burn injuries (Chap. 13). This loss results from a rapid shift of plasma from the vascular space to the interstitial space. The greater the burn area, the greater the quantity of plasma lost. This loss of plasma from the intravascular space causes increased viscosity of the blood and sludging of blood components. The latter also contributes to decreased tissue perfusion.

Gastrointestinal Fluid Losses Gastrointestinal fluid losses usually occur secondary to severe vomiting or diarrhea and result in a loss of water and electrolytes. Susceptibility to shock due to these causes is generally age-related. Infants and the elderly are at highest risk because of the decreased efficiency of their physiological compensatory mechanisms.

Pump failure

Pump failure (cardiogenic shock) occurs when the heart can no longer pump blood efficiently to all parts of the body and cardiac output is decreased. There is no decreased intravascular volume or increased vascular space. The major cause of this type of shock is extensive loss of myocardium due to myocardial infarction.[10] Other causes of pump failure include cardiac arrhythmias, which impair the efficiency of myocardial contractions, and end-stage congestive heart failure (see Chaps. 27 and 28).

Clinical Manifestations of the Shock Syndrome

Clinical manifestations of the shock syndrome are directly related to the pathophysiological mechanisms involved. Shock is a dynamic process in which several different events may be occurring at any one point in time. In addition, a client may progress toward death or toward normal homeostatic functioning over widely varying time periods. The shock syndrome can be divided into three stages: (1) *early* or *compensatory shock,* (2) *intermediate* or *progressive shock,* and (3) *late* or *irreversible shock.*

Early or compensatory shock

Early or compensatory shock is the initial, reversible stage in which compensatory mechanisms are effective in maintaining a normal or near-normal blood pressure. In this stage, most of the metabolic needs of the body continue to be met. The pathophysiological sequence of events occurring during this stage is detailed in Fig. 26-3.

Pathophysiology Regardless of the cause, the body attempts to compensate for the decreased arterial pressure in a variety of ways. First, a decrease in arterial pressure causes a similar decrease in capillary hydrostatic pressure. When the hydrostatic pressure no longer exceeds the colloidal osmotic pressure, fluid moves from the interstitial space to the intravascular space. This process is sometimes called *autotransfusion.* It may add sufficient volume to the vascular space to maintain normal arterial pressure without the aid of other compensatory mechanisms.

In addition to autotransfusion, baroreceptors sense a fall in arterial pressure. This results in increased sympathetic nervous system activity in the form of alpha- and beta-adrenergic receptor stimulation (see Table 26-6). Stimulation of alpha-adrenergic receptors causes selective peripheral vasoconstriction. Blood flow to the heart and brain is maintained, while blood flow to the kidneys and skin is decreased. Venous return of blood to the heart is increased by cutaneous and renal vasoconstriction.

The decreased blood flow to the kidneys stimulates the adrenal cortex to release aldosterone, which stimulates the kidneys to reabsorb sodium (Fig. 26-2). The increased sodium reabsorption raises the osmolarity of the blood and stimulates the release of ADH. This results in increased water reabsorption by the kidneys, increased blood volume, and increased venous return to the heart. Thus, venous return is increased by the combination of autotransfusion, vasoconstriction, and hormonal changes. Increased venous return, as well as the increased heart rate and myocardial contractility caused by beta-adrenergic receptor stimulation, result in increased cardiac output and maintenance of blood pressure.

Clinical Manifestations The clinical manifestations of early or compensatory shock are subtle and often overlooked (Table 26-3). During this stage, the resting supine blood pressure may be slightly elevated, slightly decreased, or normal for the client. For example, a hypertensive person may be in shock, with a blood pressure of 110/60. Resting supine blood pressure is not, therefore, a reliable indicator of early shock. On the other hand, *orthostatic hypotension* (a decrease in systolic blood pressure of at least 15 mmHg when a client is raised from a flat position to an elevation of 45 °) is significant and indicates the need for very careful assessment.[11]

The heart rate in early shock is slightly increased. The pulse may be either bounding or thready, depending on the stroke volume and the degree of peripheral vasoconstriction. The respiratory rate is generally normal or only slightly elevated. However, in early septic shock, hyperpnea is seen and is believed to be due to the effect of bacterial endotoxins. Urine output in early shock may decrease somewhat but usually remains within normal limits. Because of extravascular volume depletion, the client may complain of thirst. In addition, thirst may be due to decreased secretion of saliva secondary to peripheral vasoconstriction. The skin may feel cool, though not cold or clammy. An exception is septic shock, in which the skin will feel warm and dry. The temperature at this stage will be slightly decreased, except in septic shock.

One of the most reliable signs of early or compensatory shock is the client's level of consciousness. Subtle changes in sensorium, usually in the form of restlessness, irritability, or apprehension, are frequently observed and are believed to be due to sympathetic nervous system activity or hypoxia of brain cells. If the nurse misinterprets these signs and administers sedation, not only will an important assessment parameter be eliminated but the client will be predisposed to respiratory depression.[12]

Intermediate or progressive shock

Intermediate or progressive shock is the stage during which compensatory mechanisms are becoming ineffective and may even be detrimental to the client. The pathophysiological sequence of events occurring during this stage is outlined in Fig. 26-4.

Pathophysiology When shock is not detected and the precipitating cause is not corrected during the early stage, a massive sympathetic nervous system response occurs. Alpha- and beta-adrenergic responses continue, causing profound constriction of most vascular beds. Renal ischemia leads to activation of the renin-angiotensin mechanism, causing even more pronounced vasoconstriction (see Fig. 36-6). Despite the attempt of the body to increase cardiac output by increasing the heart rate and myocardial contractility, there is a net decrease in cardiac output. This is largely due to release of a myocardial depressant factor from the pancreas. This decreased output and profound peripheral vasoconstriction lead to tissue hypoxia, which causes the cells to undergo

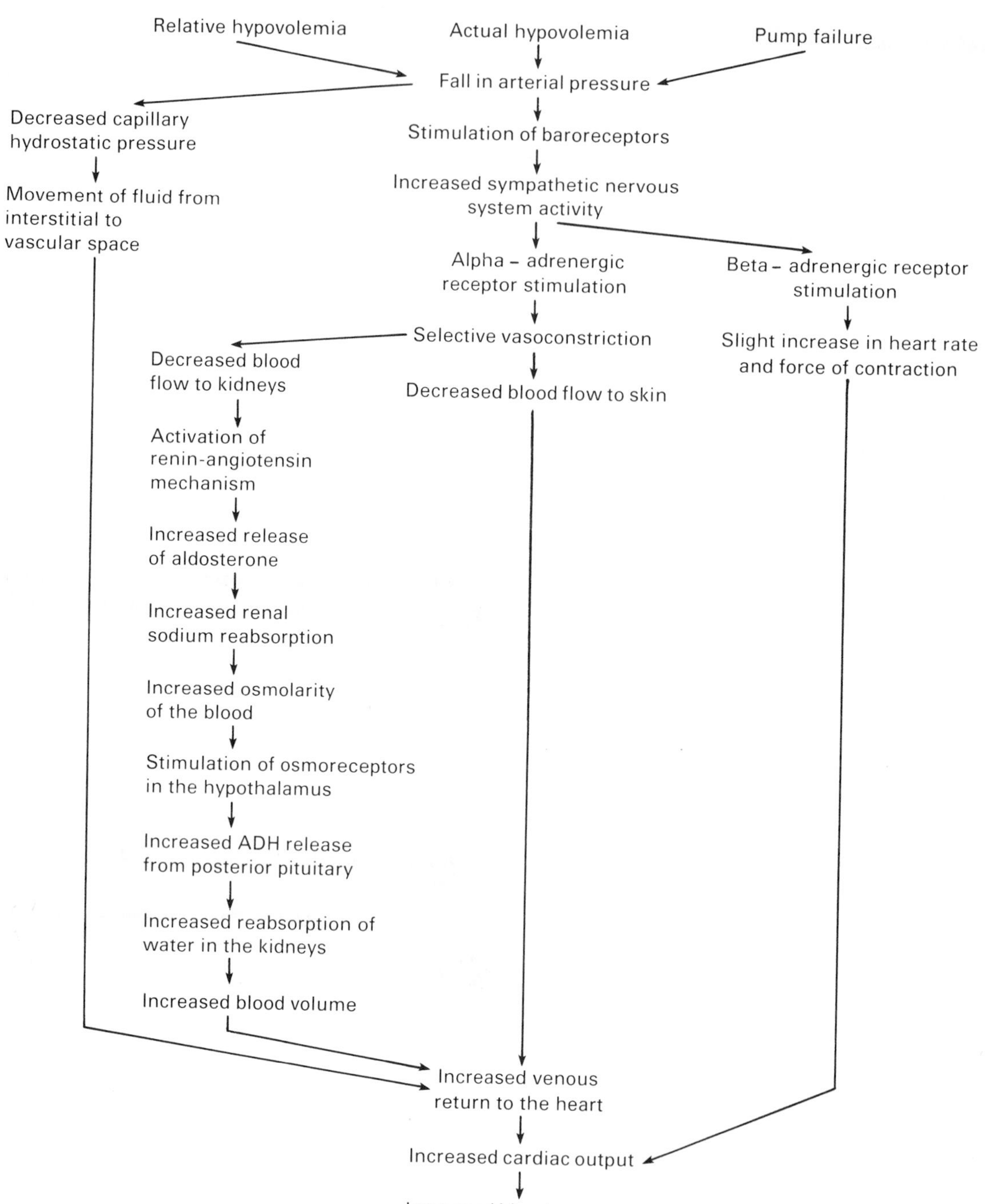

Figure 26-3 Early or compensatory shock: initial reversible stage when compensatory mechanisms are effective.

anaerobic metabolism. A by-product of anaerobic cellular metabolism is lactic acid production. The accumulation of lactic acid leads to metabolic acidosis.

Associated with the sympathetic response is the secretion of large amounts of catecholamines from the adrenal medulla. These augment the alpha- and beta-receptor effects. In addition, catecholamines facilitate

Table 26-3
Clinical Manifestations Correlated with Severity of Shock

Clinical Manifestation	Early Compensatory Shock	Intermediate or Progressive Shock	Late or Irreversible Shock
Neurological status			
Orientation	Oriented; a few slightly slurred words but normal sentences.	Fairly well oriented; slowed speech.	May be confused and disoriented; slurred speech, incoherent.
Pupils	Normal size (2–4 mm).	Normal size.	Normal to dilating to dilated, slowly constricting or nonreactive.
Level of consciousness	Restlessness, irritability, and apprehension.	Listlessness, apathy, and confusion.	Unconscious; reflexes may be absent.
Heart rate			
Rate	Slight increase.	Tachycardia.	Slowed and irregular.
Amplitude	Bounding or thready.	Weak and thready.	Thready—often a pulse deficit.
Blood pressure (mmHg)			
Systolic	Normal or slightly elevated or decreased.	Decreased—usually 25% below usual blood pressure.	Continues to fall.
Diastolic	Normal or slightly lowered.	Decreased, but less so than the systolic pressure.	Approaches zero.
Urinary output via catheter (mL/h)	Slight decrease, but within normal limits.	Oliguria (<20 mL/h). Increased specific gravity.	18 mL/h or less. Anuria, proteinuria.
Assessment for orthostatic hypotension			
Blood pressure	15- to 25-mmHg decrease.	25- to 50-mmHg decrease.	Marked decrease to unobtainable.
Symptoms	No light-headedness.	Light-headedness.	Unable to sit up.
Appearance of skin*	Pale and cool.	Cold and clammy. Cyanosis may be present.	Cold and clammy, Cyanotic.
Respiratory rate*	Normal or slightly increased.	Rapid and shallow.	Slow and shallow, with an irregular rhythm. Cheyne-Stokes respirations or sighing.
Thirst (degree)*	Normal or slightly increased.	Marked increase.	Severely increased.
Body temperature (°)*	Decreased.	Decreased.	Significantly decreased.

*These changes are found primarily in hypovolemic shock.

the cellular metabolism of the brain and heart. They cause the release of lipids which can be readily metabolized by the heart. Catecholamines also cause the liver to release its glycogen stores in the form of glucose. In addition, the pancreatic release of insulin is suppressed. Therefore, the brain, which does not require insulin for glucose utilization, has large quantities of glucose available for metabolism.

Clinical Manifestations The manifestations of the intermediate or progressive stage of shock are presented in Table 26-3. The sign mentioned most often is *hypotension*. While hypotension is frequently defined as a systolic pressure under 90 mmHg and/or a diastolic pressure under 70 mmHg, these guidelines can be used only in a client whose usual blood pressure is within the normal range for his age. A good

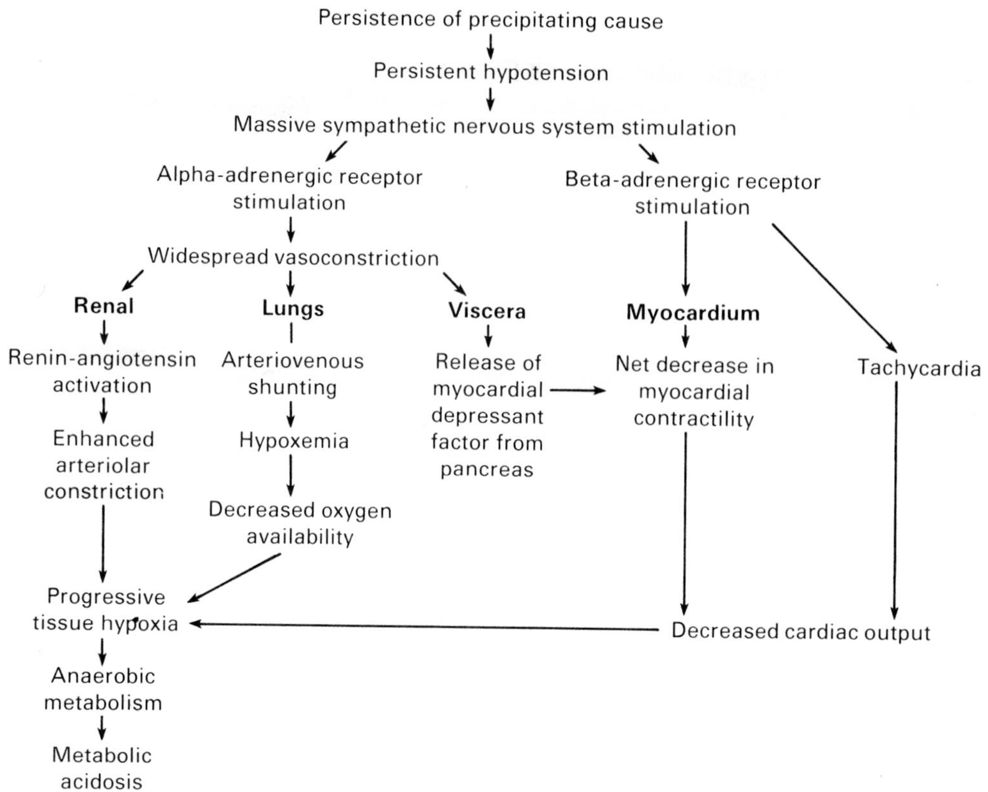

Figure 26-4 Intermediate or progressive shock: compensatory mechanisms are becoming ineffective.

guide for determining hypotension is a reduction in blood pressure greater than 25 percent of the baseline level for the client. Since cuff pressures may be inaccurate during this stage of shock due to the peripheral vasoconstriction, intraarterial monitoring or the use of a Doppler apparatus will provide more reliable pressure readings (Chap. 28). If this equipment is unavailable, it may be necessary to take a palpated blood pressure. This is done by palpating the brachial or radial pulse rather than listening for the first Korotkoff sound. The point at which the pulse is first felt is the systolic reading. It is not possible to obtain a diastolic reading with this procedure. In addition to hypotension, a narrowed pulse pressure may be present. This finding is indicative of decreased stroke volume.

Tachycardia is evident during this stage of shock, and the pulse is weak and thready. Elderly clients may be an exception and show little change in their heart rates. Other cardiovascular effects of shock during the intermediate or progressive stage are shown in Table 26-3.

Respirations increase in rate and depth in an attempt to compensate for tissue hypoxia and metabolic acidosis. Clients in anaphylactic shock will usually demonstrate stridor and wheezing. Urine output decreases and may fall below 20 mL/hour, indicating inadequate renal perfusion which can lead to renal failure. The lips and mucosa will be dry, and the client may continue to complain of thirst. The skin will be cold, pale, and clammy, with slow capillary refill. Cyanosis may be present due to tissue hypoxia. Body temperature will usually be subnormal. However, clients in septic shock will have warm, pink, dry skin and will usually have an elevated body temperature. The client will demonstrate listlessness, apathy, and confusion.

Late or irreversible shock

Late or irreversible shock is the stage during which compensatory mechanisms are either nonfunctioning or totally ineffective.

Pathophysiology As shock progresses, there is little or no evidence of sympathetic nervous system discharge. Thus, one of the major compensatory

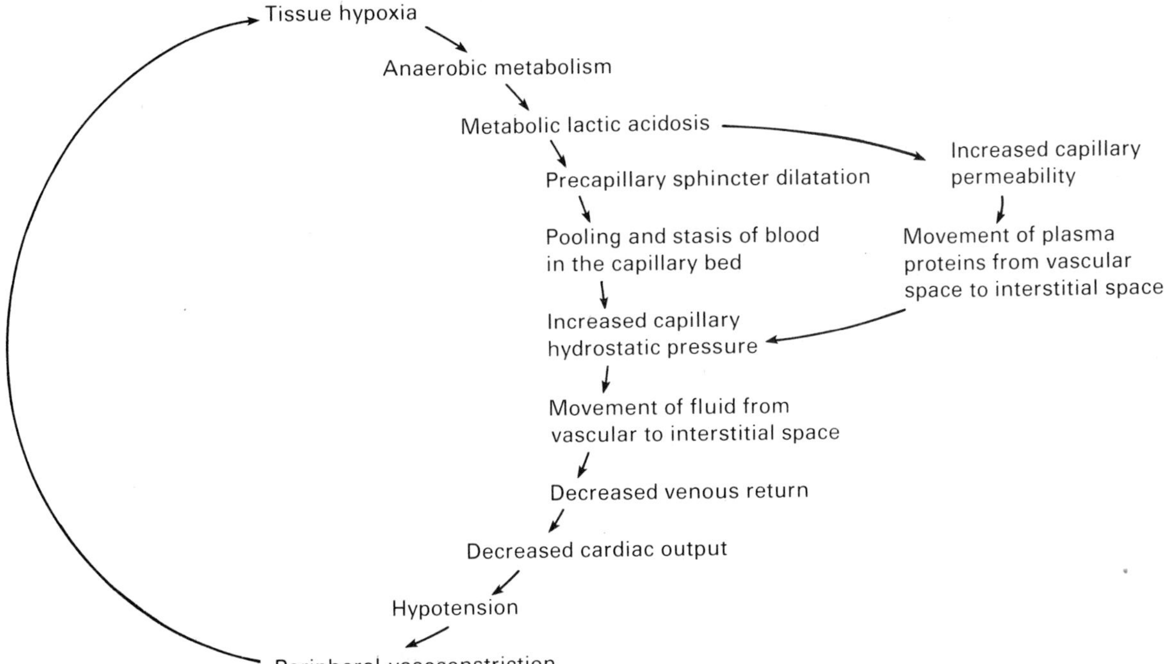

Figure 26-5 Late or irreversible shock: compensatory mechanisms are not functioning or are totally ineffective.

mechanisms has failed. There is much pooling and sludging of blood due to lack of vasomotor tone. Thrombosis of the small blood vessels also occurs.

As previously stated, tissue hypoxia resulting from peripheral vasoconstriction and decreased cardiac output makes it necessary for cells to metabolize anaerobically (Fig. 26-5). The accumulation of lactic acid and other acid metabolites in the body's tissues contributes to cell death. The acid environment also causes increased capillary permeability and dilatation of the precapillary sphincters. Increased capillary permeability allows fluid and plasma proteins to leave the vascular space. Because the venous end of the capillaries remains constricted while the arterial end is dilated, blood pools in the capillary bed. This also causes fluid to move out of the vascular space. The loss of fluid from the vascular space leads to hypotension, which causes peripheral vasoconstriction, and a vicious cycle of decompensation ensues. The brain and heart rapidly consume liberated lipid and glucose stores. After these are depleted, the brain and heart also begin to manifest the adverse effects of shock.

Clinical Manifestations During the late or irreversible stage of shock, all body systems, especially the cardiovascular system, show evidence of decompensation. The systolic blood pressure continues to fall and may not respond to therapeutic measures to raise it. The diastolic blood pressure falls toward zero. The heart rate usually becomes progressively slower. Cardiac arrhythmias may develop due to (1) ischemic myocardium and (2) increased potassium levels resulting from the release of intracellular potassium from dead cells. The pulse is weak, and the client may have a pulse deficit.

Due to respiratory center depression, there may be slow, shallow respirations with an irregular rhythm and sometimes Cheyne-Stokes respirations. The client is usually unconscious and may be unresponsive to all stimuli. Reflex responses may also be absent. Cyanosis may be present and is usually observed in the lips and nail beds. However, it may be more obvious in the palms, soles, and palpebral conjunctiva (inside the eyelid) of dark-skinned clients. There may be a progressive rise in serum creatinine and blood urea nitrogen (BUN), indicating some degree of renal failure.

Complications of Shock

Infection may be a complication of shock as well as a potential cause of the shock syndrome. The shunting of blood to the vital organs results in a decreased supply to the various parts of the reticuloendothelial system (RES). This may severely depress the RES and thus decrease the body's ability to remove bacteria and their endotoxins from the blood. The vascular changes resulting in hypoxia to the intestine, in combination with the depressed RES, cause clients to be particularly susceptible to septicemia due to *Escherichia coli.*

A variety of complications may result from prolonged and/or severe shock. Acute tubular necrosis may occur when impaired renal perfusion causes destruction of tubular epithelial cells (see Chap. 38). *Adult respiratory distress syndrome (ARDS, shock lung)* is frequently associated with shock syndrome. Although many factors have been implicated in the etiology of ARDS, no one specific cause is known (see Chap. 22). Finally, stasis of blood in capillary beds, as well as other factors present during shock, predispose to a disorder called *disseminated intravascular coagulation (DIC),* particularly in clients with septic shock (see Chap. 24). Finally, shock may end in death.

Diagnostic Study Abnormalities

While no single laboratory test can diagnose the presence of the shock syndrome, a variety of diagnostic studies may assist in monitoring the progression and severity of shock. These studies are detailed in Table 26-4. Abnormalities of diagnostic studies which are characteristic of DIC, acute tubular necrosis, and myocardial infarction are discussed elsewhere in this text.

Medical Management of the Shock Syndrome

For both the physician and the nurse, the critical factor in the management of the shock syndrome is early recognition and treatment before irreversible cell damage occurs. Successful management of shock is dependent upon the ability to:

1. Identify clients at high risk for shock
2. Diagnose the shock syndrome swiftly and accurately
3. Control or alleviate the primary etiology
4. Apply appropriate therapeutic measures to correct pathophysiological changes and enhance tissue perfusion

Diagnostic

The history and physical examination provide initial clues leading to a diagnosis of shock as well as identifying individuals at high risk for shock (Table 26-5). A history of a recent event which may be associated with shock (i.e., trauma, infection, crushing chest pain) is significant. Changes in sensorium and decreased levels of consciousness reported by others are also important considerations.

During the physical examination, it is important to observe for the clinical manifestations of shock discussed earlier in this chapter. Of particular importance is the immediate overall impression of central nervous system function, which is a measure of cerebral perfusion. Also, the status of the cutaneous vascular bed is noted because it may be indicative of impaired peripheral tissue perfusion.

In addition to the history and physical examination, various diagnostic studies will be ordered to corroborate the diagnosis and assist in identifying the etiology of the shock. A central venous pressure (CVP) catheter (see Chap. 12) and/or a Swan-Ganz catheter (Chap. 28) will be placed for accurate, ongoing hemodynamic monitoring. A chest x-ray may reveal thoracic trauma or pulmonary changes consistent with shock. A 12-lead electrocardiogram or cardiac monitor may indicate alterations in cardiac electrical activity which can be an effect of the shock syndrome. Arterial blood gases may be ordered to detect any acid-base abnormalities and to assess the oxygenation status of the client. An indwelling catheter is placed in the bladder to measure urine output, an indicator of renal perfusion.

Therapeutic

Oxygen and Ventilatory Assistance Medical therapy for shock begins with ensuring that the client has an adequate airway. This is accomplished by hyperextension of the neck (unless contraindicated), placement of an oral airway, or endotracheal intubation. Clients who are not breathing spontaneously require mechanical ventilatory assistance. In addition, all clients in shock must receive sufficient supplemental oxygen (usually via nasal prongs or a mask) to maintain a P_aO_2 of 60 mmHg or higher to avoid hypoxemia.

Fluid Resuscitation Since shock almost always involves a decreased effective circulating blood volume, the cornerstone of shock therapy is expansion of that volume by the intravenous administration of appropriate fluids. The choice of fluid for volume expansion remains controversial. However, it is generally accepted that balanced electrolyte solutions (e.g., lactated Ringer's solution) are used in the initial resuscitation from shock due to hemorrhage. Such solutions are not sufficient by themselves because 75 percent of their volume will diffuse out of the vascular system. Whole blood or packed cells are administered as soon as they are available after typing and cross-matching. The client's hematocrit can be used as a guide for

Table 26-4
Diagnostic Study Abnormalities in Shock Syndrome

Diagnostic Study	Abnormal Finding	Significance of Abnormality
	Blood	
RBCs hematocrit, hemoblogin	Normal	Remains within normal limits in shock due to relative hypovolemia and pump failure and in hemorrhagic shock prior to fluid resuscitation.
	Decreased	Decreased in hemorrhagic shock following fluid resuscitation when fluids other than blood are used.
	Increased	Increased in nonhemorrhagic shock due to actual hypovolemia since the fluid lost does not contain erythrocytes.
WBC with differential	Leukopenia	Occurs in severe shock, especially when it is due to gram-negative sepsis.
	Leukocytosis with increased neutrophils	Common in all forms of shock, especially hemorrhagic shock. Neutrophils increase in response to tissue injury.
Erythrocyte sedimentation rate	Increased	Nonspecific; increases in response to tissue injury.
BUN	Increased	Usually indicates impaired kidney function due to hypoperfusion.
Serum creatinine	Increased	Usually indicates impaired kidney function due to hypoperfusion. A more sensitive indicator of renal function than BUN.
Blood sugar	Increased	Occurs in early shock due to release of liver glycogen stores in response to catecholamines.
	Decreased	As shock progresses, glycogen stores are depleted and hepatocellular dysfunction may occur.
Serum electrolytes		
Sodium	Increased	Occurs when shock is due to gastrointestinal fluid loss or diabetes insipidus. Also occurs during the diuretic phase of acute tubular necrosis.
	Decreased	May occur iatrogenically when excess hypotonic fluid is administered following a fluid loss.
Potassium	Increased	Occurs when cellular death liberates intracellular potassium. Also occurs in acute renal failure, following RBC hemolysis in transfusion reactions, and when acidosis is present.
	Decreased	May occur when vomiting or excessive gastric suctioning is the cause of shock.
Calcium	Decreased	Sometimes occurs following rapid infusion of large amounts of citrated blood. Also occurs secondary to the respiratory alkalosis of early shock.
	Increased	Occurs secondary to lactic acidosis, which permits increased ionization of calcium.
Arterial blood gases	Respiratory alkalosis	Occurs early in shock secondary to hyperventilation.
	Metabolic acidosis	Occurs when organic acids, such as lactic acid, accumulate in the blood from anaerobic metabolism.
Blood cultures	Growth of one organism (usually)	Gram-negative organisms are most frequently seen in patients who are in septic shock.
	Urine	
Specific gravity	Increased	Occurs secondary to the action of ADH.
	Fixed at 1.010	Occurs in acute tubular necrosis.

Table 26-5

Medical Management: Shock Syndrome

Diagnostic

1. History and physical examination
2. Diagnostic studies (see Table 26-4)
3. Placement of CVP and/or Swan-Ganz catheters
4. Chest x-ray
5. Twelve-lead electrocardiogram or cardiac monitor

Therapeutic

1. Oxygen and/or ventilatory assistance with endotracheal entubation
2. Control of hemorrhage, if necessary
3. Fluid resuscitation
   a. Typing and cross-matching for whole blood or packed cells
   b. Placement of at least one large (16-to-18-gauge) peripheral intravenous line
   c. Crystalloids (balanced electrolyte solutions)
   d. Plasma volume expanders
4. Correction of acid-base imbalance as indicated by arterial blood gases
5. Pharmacological therapy (see Table 26-8)
6. Treatment of cardiac arrhythmias
7. Placement of indwelling urinary catheter

blood administration, since 1 unit of whole blood or packed cells will raise the hematocrit 2 to 4 points. (Blood transfusions are discussed later in this chapter.)

Balanced electrolyte solutions may be the only fluid used in volume replacement when neither blood nor serum proteins have been lost, such as in shock due to gastrointestinal fluid loss or cardiogenic shock. Plasma volume expanders (fluids with large molecules that can be retained in the blood vessels) are used in the treatment of shock when plasma protein loss is excessive, such as in burn shock and peritonitis (see Volume Expanders in Table 26-8).

The amount and type of fluid given depend on the client's need. This can be assessed by observing the blood pressure, pulse rate, urine output, skin perfusion, and the presence and location of rales. The most widely used and accurate guides to fluid therapy are the responses of the CVP and pulmonary artery wedge pressure (PAWP) to a fluid challenge of 200 mL of a balanced electrolyte solution over 10 minutes.[13] If the CVP and PAWP remain low or normal during fluid challenge, the need for more fluid is indicated.

Acid-Base Imbalance Frequent monitoring of arterial blood gases allows the physician to prescribe therapy to correct acid-base imbalances. This may be accomplished through the intravenous infusion of sodium bicarbonate or through the use of ventilatory assistance. When a mechanical ventilator is used to correct acid-base imbalances, it is usually necessary to administer a paralyzing drug (e.g., succinylcholine) to suppress the client's own respiratory effort. This allows control of the rate and depth of respirations by the ventilator.

Cardiac Arrhythmias Methods of treating cardiac arrhythmias are detailed in Chap. 28.

Pharmacological Management of Shock

Many of the drugs used in the treatment of shock have an effect on the sympathetic nervous system. Drugs which mimic the action of the sympathetic nervous system are called *adrenergic stimulants.* Sympathetic nervous system receptors are classified as alpha (α) and beta (β) receptors. Beta receptors in the heart respond to sympathetic stimulation with increased heart rate, increased force of contraction, and increased speed of contraction. The smooth muscle of the blood vessels have both α and β receptors (Tables 26-6 and 26-7).

The primary purpose of drugs used in the treatment of shock is correction of the poor tissue perfusion. These drugs are usually administered intravenously. Drugs used in the treatment of shock are presented in Table 26-8.

Vasopressor drugs

Vasopressor drugs were once thought to be of great value in the treatment of shock, but their use is being critically evaluated at this time. This is because these drugs cause peripheral vasoconstriction and

Table 26-6

Sympathetic Nervous System Receptors

Beta receptors in the heart

When stimulated:
↑ heart rate (+ chronotropic effect)
↑ force of contraction (+ inotropic effect)

When inhibited:
↓ heart rate (− chronotropic effect)
↓ force of contraction (− inotropic effect)

Beta receptors in the smooth muscles of blood vessels

When stimulated: mild vasodilatation
When inhibited: mild vasoconstriction

Alpha receptors in the smooth muscles of blood vessles

When stimulated: vasoconstriction or increased peripheral resistance
When inhibited: vasodilatation or decreased peripheral resistance

Note: The receptors in the lungs are discussed in Chap. 21.
Adapted from J. Barry, *Emergency Nursing,* McGraw-Hill Book Company, New York, 1978, p. 219.

Table 26-7
Drugs Which Affect Sympathetic Nervous System Receptors*

Alpha-adrenergic Methoxamine (Vasoxyl)	**Alpha blocker** Phentolamine (Regitine) Phenoxybenzamine (Dibenzyline) Tolazoline (Priscoline) Chlorpromazine (Thorazine) Prazosin (Minipress)
Beta-adrenergic Isoproterenol (Isuprel)	
Alpha- and beta-adrenergic Levarterenol (Levophed) Metaraminol (Aramine) Epinephrine (Adrenalin)	**Beta blocker** Propranolol (Inderal) Metoprolol (Lopressor) Nadolol (Corgard) Atenolol (Tenormin) Timolol (Blocadren)

*Some of these drugs are discussed in the section on Hypertension.

may therefore further jeopardize tissue perfusion either directly or indirectly.

These drugs often have an effect on the myocardium. A positive *inotropic* effect occurs when the force of the contraction is strengthened. A *chronotropic* effect occurs when the rate or timing of the contractions is affected.

It is generally agreed that vasopressors can be used as a temporary adjunctive measure to increase cerebral and coronary blood flow. This is especially true in elderly clients, who may not be able to tolerate prolonged, profound hypotension because of arteriosclerotic narrowing of coronary and cerebral arteries.[14] The goal of vasopressor therapy in this instance is to achieve and maintain a *mean* arterial blood pressure of 70 to 80 mmHg and improved tissue perfusion. This would ensure adequate blood flow to the heart and brain to prevent a myocardial infarction

Table 26-8
Drugs Used in the Treatment of Shock

Drug	Effect	Type of Shock	Nursing Implications
		Vasopressors	
Levarterenol (Levophed)	Stimulates both α- and β-adrenergic receptors. Causes marked vasoconstriction, as well as inotropic and chronotropic effects.	All types, especially neurogenic shock.	Sometimes given with phentolamine to prevent excessive vasoconstriction. Tissue sloughing if IV infiltration occurs. Best adminstered through a central venous line. Rapid fluctuations in BP.
Metaraminol (Aramine)	Stimulates both α- and β-adrenergic receptors. Causes marked vasoconstriction; inotropic effects in some clients.	Shock due to relative or actual hypovolemia.	Observe for bradycardia, oliguria, and decreased level of consciousness.
Dopamine (Intropin)	Precursor of epinephrine and norepinephrine. Stimulates both α- and β-adrenergic receptors. Causes peripheral vasoconstriction and has a positive inotropic effect. Causes renal and splanchnic vasodilatation.	All types, especially cardiogenic shock.	Monitor fluid intake and output. May be given through a large peripheral vein. Do not give with $NaHCO_3$. Observe for hypotension and tachycardia.
Dobutamine (Inotrex)	Similar to dopamine, except that it stimulates primarily β-receptors of heart. Minimal α- adrenergic effect.	Cardiogenic shock.	Increases myocardial contractility without inducing marked tachycardia. Do not give with $NaHCO_3$.
Epinephrine (Adrenalin)	Causes vasoconstriction as well as inotropic and chronotropic effects.	Anaphylactic shock. Cardiac arrest.	Observe for cardiac arrhythmias. Do not administer to clients taking digitalis. Observe for dyspnea, pulmonary edema, and severe headache.
Methoxamine (Vasoxyl)	Stimulates α-adrenergic receptors. Causes vasoconstriction.	Shock due to relative hypovolemia and cardiogenic shock.	Observe for cardiac arrhythmias, especially bradycardia.

Table 26-8 (Continued)

Drug	Effect	Type of Shock	Nursing Implications
		Vasodilators	
Isoproterenol (Isuprel)	Stimulates β-adrenergic receptors. Causes vasodilatation and marked inotropic and chronotropic effects.	Shock due to actual hypovolemia.	Observe for ventricular arrhythmias.
Nitroprusside (Nipride)	Causes vasodilatation (both venous and arterial) from relaxation of vascular smooth muscle. Decreased peripheral resistance. Increased cardiac output.	Cardiogenic shock.	Administer via a peripheral line. Use only D_5W to reconstitute; do not mix with other drugs; protect solution from light and discard after 4 h.
Phentolamine (Regitine)	α-adrenergic blocker. Causes vasodilatation.	Shock due to actual hypovolemia.	Observe for cardiac arrhythmias. Commonly given with levarterenol (Levophed).
Phenoxybenzamine (Dibenzyline)	α-adrenergic blocker. Causes vasodilatation.	Shock due to actual hypovolemia.	Observe for tachycardia; keep client flat. Give adequate fluid replacement to fill expanded vascular spaces.
Chlorpromazine (Thorazine)	α-adrenergic blocker. Causes vasodilatation.	Shock due to actual hypovolemia.	Ensure that adequate blood volume exists before administering.
		Corticosteroids	
Hydrocortisone (Solu-Cortef) **Methylprednisolone (Solu-Medrol)** **Dexamethasone (Decadron Hexadrol)**	Decreased peripheral resistance, gluconeogenesis, "antitoxic" effect, lysosomal membrane stabilization, sodium retention, possible inotropic effect. Improved cell metabolism.	Primarily septic shock, but sometimes other types occur.	Observe for GI bleeding. May make control of diabetes mellitus difficult.
		Miscellaneous Drugs	
Calcium chloride	Corrects hypocalcemia secondary to infusion of citrated blood.	Hemorrhagic shock.	Monitor use of the drug by observing for signs of hypocalcemia and hypercalcemia. Give slowly, as it is irritating.
Glucose-insulin-potassium (GIK) infusion	Theoretically, stimulates anaerobic glycolysis to maintain minimally adequate levels of high-energy phosphate compounds.	All types.	Monitor serum electrolyte and blood sugar levels.
		Volume Expanders	
Dextran (Expandex)	Expansion of plasma volume to slightly more than the volume infused.	All types of shock. Used in hemorrhagic shock only if client's religious beliefs forbid the use of blood.	Do not administer more than 1.5 L/24 h. Observe for anaphylactoid allergic reactions. Observe for prolonged bleeding time.
Dextran 40 (Rheomacrodex)	Expansion of plasma volume to almost twice the volume infused, but expansion dissipates over 3–4 h.	As above.	As above.

(or extension of an infarction in cardiogenic shock) or a cerebral vascular accident. Vasopressors may also be useful in treating some kinds of neurogenic shock, such as that which may occur secondary to spinal anesthesia. However, these drugs are used as briefly as possible because clients often develop a tolerance for them (increasingly higher doses are required to prevent hypotension). In addition, withdrawal after prolonged use may be extremely difficult.

Vasodilator drugs

The use of vasodilator drugs in shock therapy has recently achieved popularity. These drugs are administered on the assumption that inhibiting peripheral vasoconstriction will allow redistribution of pooled blood so that capillary flow and tissue perfusion, especially of the kidneys and splanchnic area, will improve. The major need in using vasodilators is ensuring adequate plasma volume and myocardial tone to fill the dilated vessels. Therefore, they are often used in conjunction with plasma volume expanders and inotropic drugs. The goal in vasodilator therapy, as in vasopressor therapy, is to maintain a mean blood pressure of 70 to 80 mmHg. It is also important to closely monitor CVP and arterial pressure so that fluid administration can be increased if a precipitous fall in pressure occurs.

Corticosteroids

There have been conflicting claims regarding the usefulness of corticosteroids in treating shock. Many investigators recommend the administration of relatively large doses of adrenocorticoids early in the course of the shock syndrome, especially in septic shock.

Experimental evidence indicates that adrenocorticosteroids may have an inotropic effect on the heart and may significantly decrease peripheral resistance. These drugs are also used to normalize cell and capillary membrane permeability. In addition, steroids promote gluconeogenesis (synthesis of glucose from amino acids and fatty acids). Furthermore, immunological studies on endotoxemia have shown that steroids exert an "antitoxic" effect by either fixing complement or preventing complement production. This anticomplement activity has also been postulated to protect the integrity of the lysosomal membrane.[15] Finally, corticosteroids can potentially increase blood volume by increasing sodium retention.

When steroids are administered in the high-dose ranges used in shock, they may cause a variety of problems for the client. The most serious of these is acute gastrointestinal bleeding. Therefore, feces, emesis, and contents of gastric suction should be examined for both occult and frank blood in all clients receiving steroids.

Antibiotics

Susceptibility to infection is increased in all clients with prolonged shock of nonseptic etiology. Broad-spectrum prophylactic antibiotic therapy may be indicated. Antibiotics are always used in the treatment of septic shock.

Before antibiotic therapy is begun, specimens of blood, urine, wound exudate, and sputum should be obtained for bacteriological culture and sensitivity studies. The anatomical sites of origin of the infection should be identified, if possible, so that the most likely etiological agent can be predicted. The organisms which most frequently cause septic shock are gram-negative.

Factors to consider in the initial selection of antibiotics for the client are as follows:

1. A broad-spectrum antibiotic may be needed because culture and sensitivity study reports are not yet available.
2. The serum half-life of drugs may be increased due to renal or hepatic insufficiency.
3. Some antibiotics are nephrotoxic or hepatotoxic.

Glucose and insulin

Since the availability of an energy source for cells is decreased in all types of shock, the use of hypertonic (50 percent glucose) has recently received considerable attention. It is generally administered with insulin and potassium to aid glucose utilization. However, hypertonic glucose therapy does not have widespread use in the treatment of shock, except for insulin shock. This is because it has not been demonstrated to have a significant impact on decreasing client mortality.

Dietary Considerations

During the acute phase of the shock syndrome, the client will receive nothing by mouth. As recovery begins, nutrition plays an important role in limiting morbidity. Since anorexia is almost universally present, parenteral or enteral feeding is often utilized.

Low complication rate, low cost, and ease of management make continuous enteral tube feeding via a pump the preferred method.[16] Contraindications include absence of bowel sounds, peritonitis, and intestinal anastomosis. Parenteral feeding, on the other hand, is generally adopted only if tube feeding fails to meet the client's caloric requirements. Total parenteral nutrition (TPN) and enteral tube feeding are discussed in Chap. 33.

Nursing Management of Shock

Health promotion and maintenance

To prevent shock, the nurse must first identify those persons who are at risk. In general terms, the very old, the very young, and those persons who have chronic, debilitating diseases have increased susceptibility to shock. More specifically, any person who sustains either surgical or accidental trauma is at high risk of shock due to hemorrhage, spinal cord injury, burn injuries, and the conditions listed in Table 26-1. Elderly persons who take barbiturates, as well as diabetics whose disease is not well controlled or who do not adhere to medical therapy may develop shock. Individuals who experience angina or who have a history of myocardial infarction are potential candidates for cardiogenic shock. Persons with a severe allergy to such substances as drugs, shellfish, and insect bites, and individuals who use diuretics or who have diabetes insipidus, may also develop shock.

After identifying susceptible individuals, the nurse may attempt to prevent the development of shock by controlling risk factors. Immediate first aid administered when trauma occurs outside the hospital may prevent shock from occurring (see Chap. 58). Vital signs and wound sites of postoperative and other clients should be observed for changes which might indicate hemorrhage. Clients who have severe allergies should be cautioned to wear a Medic-Alert tag and to report their allergies to health care providers. These clients may also be instructed that special kits are available which contain equipment and medication for the treatment of acute hypersensitivity reactions. In addition, health education is often provided to prevent the onset of disease that may result in shock, such as advice to stop smoking and to exercise regularly in order to decrease the risk of myocardial infarction.

Acute intervention

As care is begun, it is essential for the nurse to obtain the following brief history from the client or another knowledgeable person:[17]

1. Description of the events leading to the shock condition
2. Time of onset and duration of symptoms
3. Past medical history, especially medications and allergies
4. Care received prior to hospital admission
5. Date of last tetanus immunization if shock is due to trauma
6. Client's religious faith
7. Presence of Medic-Alert jewelry

The nurse's role primarily involves monitoring the client's ongoing physical and emotional status, carrying out specific medical therapy, and providing emotional support to both the client and significant others. Nursing care during the acute phase of shock also includes judging when it is necessary to alert other health team members to changes in the client's status which may warrant reevaluation of treatment.

Cardiovascular Status Much of the medical therapy for shock is based on information about the client's cardiovascular status. Initially, blood pressure, CVP, pulmonary artery pressure, and PAWP should be ascertained every 5 minutes. The client's electrocardiogram should be monitored continuously to detect arrhythmias which may result secondary to the shock itself or to medications used in treatment. Peripheral and apical pulses should be compared as to rate and quality every 5 to 10 minutes, and heart sounds should be assessed for quality and the presence of gallops or murmurs. The latter may indicate early heart failure. The frequency of this monitoring is decreased as the client's condition improves.

In addition to carrying out the above measures, which are necessary to monitor the client's cardiovascular status, the nurse must administer the prescribed therapy, which is designed to correct the client's impaired cardiovascular status.

In terms of the client's cardiovascular status, the recommended position for the treatment of shock is supine, with the legs elevated to an angle of 45°. The trunk should be horizontal, the head at the level of the chest, and the knees straight. The Trendelenburg (head-down) position should be avoided because it:

1. May initiate aortic and carotid sinus reflexes, causing impaired cerebral blood flow
2. May cause the abdominal organs to press against the diaphragm, thus limiting respiratory excursion
3. May decrease filling of the coronary arteries, causing myocardial ischemia
4. May cause an increase in intracranial pressure in the presence of a head injury

Respiratory Status The respiratory status of the client in shock must be frequently assessed to ensure adequate oxygenation and early detection of respiratory complications, as well as to provide data regarding the client's acid-base status. The rate, depth, and rhythm of respirations are initially monitored every 10 minutes. Increased rate and depth provide information regarding the client's attempts to correct metabolic acidosis. Alterations in respiratory rhythm may indicate cerebral complications. Chest sounds should be assessed every hour for the development of rales from fluid in the lungs.

Arterial blood gases are often measured as frequently as every 30 minutes. The nurse generally withdraws the blood specimen with a heparinized syringe from an arterial line. Initial interpretation of blood gases is often the responsibility of the nurse. A P_aO_2 below 60 mmHg indicates the presence of hypoxemia and the need for administration of higher oxygen concentrations or for a different method of oxygen administration. A low P_aCO_2 in the presence of a low pH and a low or normal bicarbonate level indicates that the client's hyperventilation is compensating for the metabolic acidosis. On the other hand, a rising P_aCO_2 in the presence of a persistently low pH indicates the need for intubation and ventilatory assistance.

Renal Status Hourly measurements of urinary output are essential in assessing the adequacy of renal perfusion. Urine output less than 20 mL/hour indicates inadequate perfusion of the kidneys. To facilitate measurements, an indwelling catheter is inserted. Measurement of urinary specific gravity every hour is also important to detect the onset of acute tubular necrosis. Specific gravity changes may also be indicative of the actions of aldosterone and ADH (see Table 26-3). The nurse should be sure that blood is drawn daily for serum BUN and creatinine and should alert the physician if elevations occur in these values.

Body Temperature and Skin Changes Rectal temperatures should be obtained hourly. The client should be kept comfortably warm by the use of light covers and the control of environmental temperature. If the client's temperature rises, this condition may be treated with medication such as acetaminophen suppositories, tepid sponge baths, removal of some covers, or a hypothermia blanket. It is important to avoid extremes of temperature since they cause an increased metabolic need for oxygen and increased carbon dioxide production.

Skin color should be assessed for pallor, flushing, and cyanosis. Diaphoresis or piloerection should be noted. In addition, the rapidity of capillary refill should be assessed as an indicator of peripheral vasoconstriction.

Neurological Status Neurological checks, including pupillary response, orientation, and level of consciousness, should be performed at least every hour. The client's neurological status is the best indicator of his cerebral blood flow. The nurse should be alert to clinical manifestations that may indicate neurological involvement, such as blurred vision, agitation, confusion, overalertness, or paresthesias.

Attempts should be made to orient the client to time, place, and person. If the client is in an intensive care unit, orientation to the environment is particularly important. Measures should be taken to control sensory input, such as minimizing noise and light levels. A day-night cycle of activity and rest should be maintained as much as possible. Sensory overload and disruption of the client's diurnal cycle may contribute to an altered neurological status.

Nutritional Status Clients in shock should be weighed daily to determine whether their caloric needs are being met. If the client experiences a significant weight loss, dehydration should be ruled out before additional calories are provided parenterally. Measurements of serum BUN also provide pertinent data since falling levels may indicate overhydration.

Since clients in shock usually receive nothing by mouth, oral care is essential. A water-soluble lubricant applied to the lips will prevent drying and cracking. Moist swabbing of the tongue and oral mucosa with saline, diluted mouthwash, or half-strength peroxide is also helpful. Lemon and glycerine swabs should not be used because they can cause drying of the mucosa.

Gastrointestinal Status Bowel sounds should be auscultated every 8 hours, and abdominal distension should be assessed through percussion and serial measurements of abdominal girth. If bowel sounds are not present, a nasogastric tube may need to be inserted. Decompression via suction should continue until bowel sounds return. The nasogastric aspirate should be measured as part of the fluid output and tested for occult blood. If the client has a bowel movement, the stool should also be checked for occult blood.

Personal Hygiene Hygiene is especially important to clients in shock since their impaired tissue perfusion predisposes to infection and skin breakdown. Oral and perineal hygiene, as well as a complete bath, should be done when necessary and not according to a schedule. If the client is able to perform some self-care, the nurse should allow independent action and assist only when necessary. The use of an alternating-pressure or egg-crate mattress, turning the client every 1 to 2 hours, and positioning the client in good body alignment will help to prevent decubitus ulcer formation.

Emotional Support The effects of the client's anxiety and fear in the face of this critical, life-threatening situation are frequently overlooked or underestimated. Anxiety and fear may aggravate respiratory distress and increase cathecholamine secretion. It is important for the nurse to remember that compassionate understanding is as essential as scientific and technical expertise in the total care of a client in shock.

In planning and implementing the nursing care of the client in shock, the nurse should assess the client's anxiety. While medication to decrease anxiety may seem to be the simplest mode of therapy, much more can be accomplished by nonpharmacological intervention. In many shock situations, sedation is contraindicated.

The nurse should always talk to the client, even though he is intubated or appears comatose. If the intubated client is capable of writing, a magic slate or pencil and paper should be provided. The client should also receive simple explanations of procedures *before* they are carried out, as well as information regarding his current plan of care and its rationale. If the client asks questions about his progress and prognosis, simple and honest answers should be given.

Privacy should be provided as much as possible, but the client should be assured that assistance is readily available should he require it. The call bell should be within reach. In addition, joking, teasing, and "kidding around" among health care personnel should be kept to a minimum or carried out where the client cannot hear it. This sort of behavior can often lead the client to believe that staff members are having too much fun to be able to care for him adequately. Furthermore, conversations about the client should not take place where the client can overhear them. Such conversations can constitute a violation of the client's confidence or may be misinterpreted in a way that causes the client unnecessary distress.

Finally, many clients desire the comfort of their priest, rabbi, or minister at this time. The nurse should offer to call a clergyman rather than wait for the client or his family to express a wish for spiritual comfort.

The client's family and significant others also need support and comfort at this time. They should be kept informed of the client's status and prognosis, and of the current plan of care and its rationale. The liaison nurse should be kept as consistent as possible to decrease anxiety and avoid confusing contradictions. Family members and friends should be shown where they can wait and where a telephone can be found. Directions to the bathrooms and the hospital cafeteria are also appropriate.

Visits with the client should be facilitated rather than hindered. The nurse should explain in simple terms the purpose of the tubes and machines surrounding the client, and the family should be informed of what they may and may not touch. Privacy should be ensured as much as possible. The family should also be instructed to avoid tiring the client.

Chronic management

Rehabilitation of the client in shock necessitates prevention or early treatment of complications and correction of the precipitating cause. The nurse should continue to assess the client for indications of complications throughout the recovery period. Health teaching and other measures discussed earlier, which are designed to correct or prevent the precipitating cause, should be implemented.

The potential complications of shock will need to be managed. These include such problems as chronic renal failure or fibrotic lung following acute tubular necrosis or ARDS (see Chaps. 38 and 22).

BLOOD TRANSFUSIONS*

Blood transfusions are discussed in this chapter because they are frequently used in the management of shock. Traditionally, the term *blood transfusion* meant the administration of whole blood. Blood transfusion now has a broader meaning, including whole blood as well as blood components such as platelets, red blood cells, and plasma (Table 26-9). Blood component therapy allows a single unit of donated whole blood to be given to three or four recipients. Whole blood is most frequently used in the treatment of hypovolemic shock due to hemorrhage.

Administration Procedure

An intravenous line using an 18-gauge needle should be started. (Smaller-size needles may be used for platelets, albumin, and cryoprecipitates.) The blood administration tubing with a filter should have a Y connector, one side for the blood and the other side for the isotonic saline solution. Glucose solutions should not be used because they induce red blood

*This section was written by Sharon Mantik Lewis.

Table 26-9
Comparison of Various Blood Products

Blood Product	Description	Special Considerations	Indications for Use
Whole blood	Contains normal constituents of whole blood. Coagulation is prevented by collecting blood with citrate-phosphate-dextrose or acid-citrate-dextrose. (Citrate complexes the calcium. Dextrose provides an energy source for RBCs.) Donor unit contains 450 mL of whole blood and 60 mL of preservative.	Should not be stored for more than 21 days, at which time 70–80% of RBCs are viable. WBCs and platelets are nonviable. Hyperkalemia develops when in storage due to death of RBCs.	Acute, rapid bleeding. Hypovolemia due to hemorrhage.
Fresh whole blood	Whole blood used less than 12 h after donation.	The use of fresh blood has been replaced by component therapy.	Rarely indicated unless RBCs, platelets, factors V and VIII are required (e.g., in a client who requires massive transfusion).
Packed RBCs	Prepared from whole blood by sedimentation or centrifugation. Have hematocrit of about 80%. One unit contains 250–300 mL.	Use of RBCs for treatment allows remaining components of blood (e.g., platelets, albumin, plasma) to be used for other purposes. Fresh packed cells needed if hyperkalemia is a consideration.	Anemia. Client with high risk of fluid overload (e.g., renal and cardiac disease). Acute bleeding.
Frozen RBCs	Prepared from RBCs using glycerol for protection and then frozen. Can be stored for 3 yr at −87°C (−188.6° F).	Must be used 24 h after thawing. During thawing process, successive washings with saline remove majority of WBCs and plasma proteins.	Autotransfusion—donate own blood and use it later. Useful in client with previous febrile reactions to transfusions.
Platelets	Prepared from fresh white blood within 4 h after collection. One unit contains 20–30 mL of platelet concentrate.	Multiple units of platelets can be obtained from one donor by platelet pheresis. Can be kept at room temperature for 3 days. Best used within 24 h of donation.	Bleeding due to thrombocytopenia (see Chap. 24).
Fresh frozen plasma	Liquid portion of whole blood. Separated from cells and then frozen. One unit contains 200–250 mL. Plasma is rich in clotting factors but contains no platelets. May be stored for 1 yr. Must be used within 2 h after thawing.	The use of plasma in treating hypovolemic shock is being replaced by pure preparations, such as albumin, and by plasma expanders.	Bleeding due to liver disease. Hypovolemia due to burns. Multiple transfusions. Clotting defects.
Albumin	Prepared from plasma. Can be stored for 5 yr. Available in 5% or 25% solution. Does not transmit hepatitis.	Osmotically, albumin 25 g/100 mL is equal to 500 mL of plasma.	Hypovolemic shock. Liver failure. Excessive albuminuria.
Cryoprecipitates and commercial concentrates	Cryoprecipitate is prepared from fresh frozen plasma. Can be stored for 1 yr. Once thawed, needs to be used.	See Table 24-16.	Bleeding due to hemophilia.
WBCs	Prepared by continous-flow centrifugation or filtration leukopheresis. Investigation is needed on best ways to collect and store WBCs.	Neutrophils have a very short life span in circulation. Administered slowly over 2–4 h.	Neutropenia (e.g., in clients with bone marrow transplants, chemotherapy with resultant bone marrow suppression) (see Chap. 24).

cell aggregation, which can cause plugging of the filter and tubing. Glucose also causes hemolysis of the red blood cells. The tubing should be flushed with isotonic saline before as well as after the administration of blood.

When the blood or blood components have been obtained from the blood bank, positive identification of the donor blood and recipient must be made. (Check the local hospital policy for the exact procedure.) The blood bank is responsible for typing and crossmatching of the donor blood with the recipient's blood. (These procedures are discussed in Chap. 23.)

The blood should be administered as soon as it is brought to the client. It should not be refrigerated on the unit because the refrigeration will not be controlled. If the blood is not used right away, it should be returned to the blood bank.

During the first 15 minutes of blood infusion, the nurse should stay with the client. If there are any untoward reactions, they are most likely to occur at this time. The rate of infusion during this period should be about 5 mL/minute. Blood should not be quickly infused unless an emergency exists. Rapid infusion of cold blood causes the client to chill. If rapid replacement is necessary, a blood-warming device should be used.

After the first 15 minutes, the rate of infusion is governed by the state of the client. If the person is not in shock or is not predisposed to circulatory overload, a rate of 10 to 20 mL/minute is satisfactory. Another guideline is that 1 unit of blood should not take more than 4 hours to administer. Usually 1 unit of blood can be administered in 2 hours.

If a transfusion reaction occurs, the following steps should be taken:

1. Discontinue the transfusion.
2. Maintain a patent intravenous line with dextrose or saline solution.
3. Notify the physician.
4. Save the blood bag and tubing and send them to the blood bank for examination.
5. Obtain urine samples for free hemoglobin.
6. Obtain serum samples for free hemoglobin.

The blood bank or laboratory will try to identify the cause of the reaction by repeating the type and cross match or by doing a direct and an indirect Coombs' test or other studies.

Autotransfusion

Autotransfusion, or autologous transfusion, consists of removing whole blood from a person and transfusing that blood into the same person. The problems of incompatibility, allergic reactions, and transmission of disease can be avoided. There are various methods of autotransfusion. These include:

1. *Elective phlebotomy,* in which a person donates blood prior to a planned surgical procedure. The blood can be frozen and stored for up to 3 years. Usually the blood is stored without being frozen and is given to the person within a few weeks of donation. This technique is especially beneficial to the client with a rare blood type.
2. Autotransfusion after collection of blood lost during major surgical procedures or traumatic injury. The blood is collected and filtered. Anticoagulants are added, and the blood is reinfused into the person. There are now commercially available autotransfusion systems, such as the Sorenson autotransfusion system and the Haemonetic Cell Saver, which prepare the blood for reinfusion.

Blood Transfusion Reactions

Blood transfusion reactions can be classified as immunological and nonimmunological (Table 26-10).

Immunological

Hemolytic Reactions The most common cause of hemolytic reactions is transfusion of ABO-incompatible blood. This is an example of a type II cytotoxic hypersensitivity reaction (Chap. 10). Severe hemolytic reactions are rare. Most mistakes are due to mislabeling of specimens and administration of blood to the wrong individual.

When a hemolytic reaction occurs, antibodies in the recipient's serum react with antigens on the donor's red blood cells. This results in agglutination of cells, which can cause obstruction of capillaries and blockage of blood flow. Hemolysis of the red blood cells releases free hemoglobin into the plasma. The hemoglobin is filtered by the kidney and is found in the urine (hemoglobinuria). Hemoglobin may obstruct the renal tubules, leading to acute renal failure (Chap. 38).

The clinical manifestations of the hemolytic reaction may be mild or severe and usually develop within the first 15 minutes of transfusion. Infrequently, delayed transfusion reactions occur 2 to 14 days after the administration of blood. The clinical manifestations and nursing management for the client with a hemolytic reaction are presented in Table 26-10.

Allergic Reaction Allergic reactions are due to the recipient's sensitivity to a component of the donor's blood. These reactions are more common in atopic individuals with a history of allergies. Antihista-

Table 26-10
Transfusion Reactions

Type of Reaction	Prevention	Clinical Manifestation	Nursing Management
Hemolytic transfusion reaction	Identify client and blood product to ensure proper match. Double-check all blood products with another nurse or health professional. Begin infusion at a slow rate, and remain with client for first 15 min. Severe reactions tend to begin soon after initiation of transfusion.	Usually immediate onset. Delayed onset may be observed when an Rh incompatibility is involved. Burning sensation along the vein. Facial flushing. Fever, chills. Temperature may be 40°C (104°F) or higher. Chest pain; rapid, labored respirations. Headache. Low back pain. Shock.	Stop transfusion immediately to reduce further risk. Severity of reaction is related to amount transfused. Treat shock if present. Administer oxygen, fluids, epinephrine as ordered by physician. Recheck blood slip with unit of blood and client's blood to determine if error was made. Obtain two blood samples from a vein distant from the infusion site. One specimen is sent for centrifugation (pink or red plasma indicates hemolysis); the other specimen is sent to the blood bank with the remainder of the transfusion. Obtain first voided urine to test for hemoglobinuria. Specimen may be red or black, indicating potential renal damage. With suspected renal involvement, prompt treatment with mannitol is ordered to promote diuresis and prevent renal tubular damage. Monitor fluid and electrolyte balance as soon as diuresis begins.
Allergic reaction	Determine whether client has a history of allergy, particularly a previous allergic reaction to transfused blood products. Administer antihistamine [e.g., diphenhydramine (Benadryl)] orally or parenterally 15–20 min. before starting infusion.	Urticaria (hives), pruritus. Facial and/or glottal edema (rare). Asthma (rare). Pulmonary edema with infiltrates (rare). Anaphylaxis.	Stop transfusion immediately. Treat life-threatening reactions (edema, anaphylaxis) immediately. Administer antihistamine parenterally.
Febrile reaction	Keep client covered and warm during transfusion. Administer antipyretic medication to persons known to have this reaction. Transfusion with leukocyte-poor RBCs or frozen washed packed cells may prevent this reaction in persons susceptible to it.	Chills and fever, usually beginning about 1 h after start of infusion. Headache, flushing, tachycardia, and general discomfort may be present. Symptoms may persist for 8–10 h; most are more transient.	Stop transfusion immediately. Treat symptomatically.
Bacterial reaction	Maintain aseptic collection techniques. Change transfusion equipment frequently. Do not allow blood to stand at room temperature unnecessarily, even while infusing. Do not use blood that has been heated to above room temperature. Do not prewarm infusions. Inspect all blood for evidence of hemolysis.	Shaking fever. Severe hypotension. Dry, flushed skin. Pain in abdomen and extremities. Vomiting and bloody diarrhea.	Stop transfusion immediately. Administer broad-spectrum antibiotics, as ordered immediately, by the most rapid route. Treat shock aggressively. Monitor vital signs, fluid, and electrolyte balance.

Table 26-10 (Continued)

Type of Reaction	Prevention	Clinical Manifestation	Nursing Management
Circulatory overload	Give packed cells to clients susceptible to circulatory overload (elderly, infants, persons with cardiac or respiratory disorders). Administer infusion slowly, with client in a sitting position.	Tightness in chest, labored breathing. Dry cough. Rales at base of lungs. Pulmonary edema.	Stop or slow the transfusion, depending on the severity of symptoms. Have client sit up. Monitor vital signs. Treat severe overload with rotating tourniquets or phlebotomy. Administer diuretics as ordered.
Air embolism	Avoid introducing air into system. If air is introduced, stop the infusion.	Cyanosis. Dyspnea. Shock. Cardiac arrest.	Lower client's head and turn client on left side. Air will collect in right atrium, where it can be released gradually to the lungs. Treat shock and/or cardiac arrest immediately if these conditions should occur.

Adapted from L. C. Cullins, "Preventing and Treating Transfusion Reactions," *Am J Nurs*, **79**:936 (1979).

mines may be used to prevent allergic reactions. Epinephrine or corticosteroids may be used to treat a severe reaction. Clients who develop allergic reactions often have fewer problems with washed or leukocyte-depleted red blood cells.

Febrile Reactions Febrile reactions are most commonly due to the presence of leukocyte or thrombocyte incompatibility (e.g., the donor's platelets vs. the recipient's antibodies) induced by previous transfusions. Many individuals who receive five or more transfusions develop circulating antibodies to white blood cells. Febrile reactions are less likely to occur due to contaminated tubing or equipment. These reactions can often be prevented by using washed red blood cells from which the white blood cells and plasma proteins have been removed.

Nonimmunological

Nonimmunological reactions include circulatory overload, infections, adverse effects of massive blood transfusion, and air embolism.

Circulatory Overload Individuals with cardiac or renal insufficiency are at risk for the development of congestive heart failure due to circulatory overload. This is especially true if a large quantity of blood is infused in a short period of time. When possible, these individuals should be given packed red blood cells instead of whole blood. When blood is needed, it should be infused as slowly as possible and monitored with CVP readings. CVP readings above 15 cm usually indicate circulatory overload.

Infection Many infections can be transmitted by blood transfusion, including hepatitis, malaria, and cytomegalovirus. In addition, blood can become infected from improper handling and storage. In spite of careful handling, bacterial contamination and growth occasionally occur.

Hepatitis is the most common infection transmitted, although its incidence has been decreasing. Hepatitis B virus can be detected in the blood by the presence of hepatitis B surface antigen (HB_sAg). It is now becoming more apparent that hepatitis non-A, non-B viruses are responsible for a large number of hepatitis cases (see Chap. 35). There is no screening test available to detect these viruses.

Massive Blood Transfusion Massive blood transfusion is defined as replacement that exceeds the total blood volume within 24 hours. Some problems that can result from this process, with possible solutions, are presented.

Hypothermia with cardiac arrhythmias can result from rapid infusion of large quantities of cold blood. Therefore, blood-warming equipment should be used to prevent this problem.

In stored whole blood, platelets deteriorate, clotting factors become deficient, and hyperkalemia and acidosis develop. To avert problems from excessive use of stored whole blood, 1 unit of fresh blood should be used for every 5 to 6 units of stored whole blood. If fresh blood is not available, platelet concentrate, fresh frozen plasma, or packed red blood cells can also be used.

Hypocalcemia can occur from the use of large

quantities of citrated blood (calcium binds to the citrate). To prevent this problem, calcium gluconate should be administered intravenously after the infusion of every 2 units of blood. (Calcium should never be added to the blood.)

Air Embolism The incidence of air embolism has been decreased by the use of plastic bags. Air may be introduced if the tubing is changed during the transfusion procedure.

HYPERTENSION

(*Hypertension,* commonly called *high blood pressure,* is sustained high arterial pressure. Since blood pressure varies among individuals, it is difficult to define high blood pressure as a specific number of units greater than normal. Generally, individuals less than 50 years old are considered to be hypertensive if their sustained arterial pressure is greater than 140/90.) Individuals more than 50 years old are considered to be hypertensive if their sustained arterial pressure is greater than 160/95.

The classification of hypertension as a disease is a very recent development. Hypertension was not an area of medical concern before 1930, and even then, many thought that the blood pressure should not be lowered because inadequate tissue perfusion might result. They were particularly concerned that decreased perfusion to the brain would lead to decreased intelligence.[18]

In the late 1920s, research on the mechanisms of hypertension began. Since that time, there have obviously been many advances. Yet today, for the majority of persons with hypertension, the exact cause of their elevated blood pressure cannot be determined.

Significance of the Problem

High blood pressure is often asymptomatic, which is the crux of the problem. Many times there are no symptoms to motivate individuals to seek treatment. When symptoms do occur, they are often ignored by the individual, who feels that they are probably insignificant. The majority of persons with hypertension are initially diagnosed during an incidental military, life insurance, or other periodic examination.[19]

Approximately one-sixth of all Americans, or more than 35 million persons, have hypertension, and one-half of them are unaware of their illness. In 1 year, at least 250,000 Americans will die from complications.[20] Untreated hypertension can reduce the average life expectancy by 20 years.[21]

Classification of Hypertension

The common classifications for hypertension include primary, secondary, benign, and malignant. Primary and secondary classifications refer to the etiology, while benign and malignant classifications refer to the course of the disease.

Essential (primary, idiopathic) hypertension

Essential hypertension accounts for 85 to 90 percent of all hypertension. The onset of essential hypertension is usually between the ages of 30 and 50 years. The exact cause remains unknown. The term *essential* was used because there was no readily available explanation; hence, it was considered an "essential" part of the person's makeup (see Table 26-11).

Secondary hypertension

Secondary hypertension, which accounts for 10 to 15 percent of hypertension, is an elevation of blood pressure due to an underlying primary disease. In contrast to essential hypertension, secondary hypertension often develops before age 30 or after age 50.

Table 26-11
Risk Factors in Essential Hypertension

Age	Develops between 30 and 50 yr of age. Peak incidence is 35 yr of age.
Sex	Primarily affects men over 35 yr and women over 45 yr.
Race	Blacks have twice the incidence of hypertension of whites.
Family history	Multifactorial genetic factors account for an estimated one-third of the cases of essential hypertension.
Obesity	Weight gain is associated with increased frequency of hypertension. High correlation of obesity and physical inactivity with hypertension.
Stress	Stress results in increased sympathetic nervous system activity.
Cigarette smoking	Nicotine in cigarettes causes vasoconstriction and increased catecholamine release, resulting in increased heart rate.
Excess sodium intake	Relationship between high sodium intake and hypertension, especially in obese individuals.
Elevated serum lipids	Elevated levels of cholesterol and triglycerides are primary risk factors in atherosclerosis, which is a contributing factor to hypertension.

Treatment of the primary cause can reduce the elevated blood pressure.

Secondary hypertension occurs most often in children, but it can occur in adults as well. The most common causes of secondary hypertension in adults are coarctation of the aorta, renal disease, endocrine disorders, hormonal therapy, and pregnancy (Table 26-12).

Benign hypertension

Benign hypertension refers to a moderate rise in blood pressure which occurs over a long period of time. It generally runs a slow, progressive course over a period of 20 to 30 years. It has been suggested that the term *benign* be abandoned because hypertension in any form can lead to death due to strokes, myocardial infarction, and renal failure.

Malignant hypertension

Malignant hypertension, also called *accelerated hypertension,* is characterized by an abrupt, severe rise in blood pressure associated with a diastolic pressure above 130 mmHg and papilledema. Males and blacks are particularly prone to this type of hypertension. Malignant hypertension can occur without any evidence of preexisting benign hypertension.

Pathophysiology of Essential Hypertension

As described earlier, arterial blood pressure is the product of cardiac output and the total peripheral resistance (BP = CO × TPR). The total peripheral resistance is the force, primarily created in the small arteries and arterioles, opposing the movement of blood. For arterial pressure to rise, there must be an

Table 26-12
Secondary Hypertension

Etiology	Pathophysiology of Hypertension	Clinical Features	Treatment
Coarctation of the aorta	Congenital heart disease resulting in narrowing of the aortic lumen due to a localized deformity of the vascular media.	Presents with various degrees of constriction. If sufficiently severe in an infant, surgery is indicated. If the person is asymptomatic and not hypertensive, surgery is generally postponed. The chief complaint of adult-type coarctation is leg pain on exertion. A chest x-ray will show notching of the ribs. A diagnosis is positive for coarctation if the following conditions are found: *Lower extremities* Pulse: Absent or weak BP: Lower in legs than arms *Upper extremities* Pulse: Bounding BP: Above normal	Surgical correction of the coarction
Renal disease Parenchymal disease	Mechanism not always clear. Factors may involve fluid retention, altered renin/angiotensin/aldosterone system, and decreased prostaglandin synthesis.	Any condition that decreases the overall activity of the kidney can cause hypertension. Examples include acute and chronic glomerulonephritis, polycystic kidneys, chrònic pyelonephritis, and renal artery stenosis. (These diseases are discussed in Chaps. 37 and 38).	Depends upon the cause. Antihypertensive medication. Dialysis treatment for renal failure.
Renal artery stenosis	Causes renovascular hypertension due to increased renin secretion.		Surgery indicated in renal artery stenosis.

Table 26-12 (Continued)

Etiology	Pathophysiology of Hypertension	Clinical Features	Treatment
Endocrine disorders			
Pheochromocytoma (see Chap. 42)	Catecholamine-producing tumor of the adrenal medulla or ganglia, resulting in excess secretion of epinephrine and norepinephrine.	Clinical manifestations are related to increased secretions of epinephrine and norepinephrine. May develop spontaneously or be precipitated by emotional or physical stress. Manifestations include paroxysmal hypertension, pounding headache, sympathetic overactivity (sweating, palpitations, apprehension), elevated fasting blood sugar, excessive catecholamines in the urine.	Surgical excision of the tumor.
Cushing's syndrome (see Chap. 42)	Neoplasia or hyperplasia of the adrenal cortex, resulting in excess secretion of glucocorticoids.	Large amounts of glucocorticoids have a sodium-returning effect. Some individuals with Cushing's syndrome also have increased production of mineralocorticoids. In some cases, renin production is increased by glucocorticoids. Excess secretion of 17-hydroxycorticoids and 17-ketosteroids in the urine.	Surgical excision of the tumor.
Primary aldosteronism (see Chap. 42)	Neoplasia of adrenals, resulting in excess secretion of aldosterone.	Moderate hypertension, hypokalemia, muscle weakness, fatigue, polyuria. Clinical finding of both hypertension and hypokalemia is highly suggestive of primary aldosteronism.	Medication (spironolactone or triamterene). Surgical resection of the adrenal gland.
(Hormone therapy oral contraceptives, estrogen preparations)	Unclear pathogenesis. Possible activation of renin-angiotensin mechanism, resulting in increased production of angiotensin and aldosterone.	Slight increase in blood pressure. From 5% to 7% develop hypertension.	Discontinuation of oral contraceptive therapy and estrogen preparations. Usually normotensive within 6 mo following discontinuation of the drug.
Toxemia of pregnancy	Unclear pathogenesis. Some indication of altered renin/angiotensin system.	Moderate to severe hypertension. Headaches, visual disturbances, epigastric distress, edema, proteinuria, convulsions.	Medication therapy if severe. (See section on hypertensive crisis.)
Combination of drugs containing monoamine oxidase (MAO) inhibitors and tyramine (vasopressor agent)	Certain cheeses, such as cheddar, camembert, and Stilton, beer, and pickles contain tyramine, which is capable of liberating stored catecholamines when ingested with MAO inhibitors.	Can produce a hypertensive crisis. Visual disturbances, papilledema, vomiting, coma, and death.	Discontinue medication or instruct client to avoid ingesting tyramine-containing substances.

increase in either cardiac output or peripheral resistance. If peripheral resistance is increased, a greater amount of pressure is required to pump blood throughout the body. The concept of peripheral resistance is so important in understanding arterial blood pressure that some have defined hypertension as increased peripheral resistance. Most individuals with hypertension have a normal cardiac output.

Although the cause of essential hypertension is not known, several factors have been identified as contributory mechanisms. Whether these factors and alterations are the cause or the result of hypertension is not always clear.[22]

Risk factors

There are certain risk factors known to be related to essential hypertension or suspected of being independent and additive predictors of the disease. These are presented in Table 26-11.

Retention of sodium and water

Excessive salt intake is considered responsible for initiation of hypertension in some individuals. Studies done on populations with a high salt intake in their diets (e.g., blacks who eat many foods that are high in sodium and island natives who cook fish in ocean water) develop hypertension at an extremely early age. In early essential hypertension, the kidney is unable to excrete sodium and water at a normal rate.[23] Consequently, the abnormal sodium metabolism leads to increased sodium and water retention, expanding the ECF volume and increasing cardiac output.

In addition, an excessive amount of sodium has been found in the arteriolar walls of some hypertensive individuals. The pressure of sodium causes the walls to swell, with resulting constriction of the lumen and increased peripheral resistance. Therefore, both actions (increased cardiac output and increased peripheral resistance) may result in increased blood pressure.

Altered renin-angiotensin mechanism

In some individuals with essential hypertension, excess quantities of renin are secreted by the kidney. This results in the conversion of angiotensinogen to angiotensin (Fig. 36-6). The angiotensin causes direct arteriolar constriction and a secondary increase in aldosterone. This is followed by retention of water and electrolytes, with resultant hypertension. In most clients with essential hypertension, the plasma renin level is normal. But in 10 to 17 percent of clients, the plasma level has been found to be elevated. These clients are referred to as *high-renin essential hypertensives.*

Excessive mineralocorticoids

In the presence of elevated renin levels, aldosterone will be increased. However, hypertensive clients with normal or low renin levels have also been found with elevated aldosterone levels. Some of these clients also have an elevation of other mineralocorticoids.

Stress and increased sympathetic activity

It has long been recognized that arterial pressure is influenced by factors such as anger, fear, pain, and exercise. Physiological responses to stress which are normally protective may persist to a pathological degree, resulting in increased sympathetic nervous activity. Increased sympathetic stimulation results in increased peripheral vasoconstriction and an increased heart rate. Renin release is stimulated by increased sympathetic nervous activity. This results in activation of the angiotensin mechanism and increased aldosterone secretion, both leading to elevated blood pressure.

Decreased prostaglandin activity

Prostaglandins synthesized by the renal medulla have a role in dilating peripheral blood vessels, increasing sodium and water excretion, and reducing blood pressure.[24] One proposed theory for hypertension is that there is decreased synthesis of renal prostaglandins. In the absence of prostaglandins, vasoconstriction with increased peripheral resistance and blood pressure occurs.

Hypertension in the Elderly

Atherosclerotic changes in the elderly cause increasing rigidity of the aortic wall and peripheral arteries. These changes result in decreased vascular compliance. Elderly persons usually develop systolic hypertension with a wide pulse pressure because the diastolic pressure remains relatively normal. Treatment is usually reserved for those elderly persons with elevations of both systolic and diastolic pressures. A general guideline for treatment is to lower the blood pressure slowly. The purpose of therapy is to reduce the blood pressure to about 160/95 rather than 140/90, which is the goal for individuals under age 50.

Clinical Manifestations

Hypertension is often called the "silent killer" because symptoms do not usually develop until the disease is advanced. If symptoms do develop as a late manifestation, they are usually secondary to effects on blood vessels in the various organs and tissues or to the increased work load of the heart. The most common complaint is a headache, which occurs frequently in the morning and disappears as the day goes on. It is usually in the occipital region and may be no more than a feeling of stiffness or tightness. Headache is characteristic of severe hypertension and is thought to be due to changes in cerebrospinal fluid (CSF). In the supine position, CSF pressure increases, resulting in headache. After the person stands upright, the CSF pressure decreases and headache disappears.

Other possible manifestations are easy fatiguability, dizziness, and palpitations. Blurring of vision and epistaxis (nosebleed) may also occur as a result of vascular disease. Epistaxis is not a common manifestation and is associated with severe hypertension.

Complications

The most common complications are target organ damage occurring in the heart (hypertensive heart disease), brain (cerebrovascular disease), kidney (nephrosclerosis), and eyes (retinal damage).

Heart (hypertensive heart disease)

Coronary Artery Disease Cardiac disease is the leading cause of death in individuals with hypertension. Hypertensives develop coronary artery disease two to three times more frequently than normotensives.[25] Hypertension is a major risk factor in accelerated atherosclerosis and coronary artery disease (see Chap. 27).

In addition to increasing the rate of atherosclerosis, elevated blood pressure causes the entire inner lining of the arteriole to become thickened as a reaction to the high pressure. This characteristic change results from hyperplasia of connective tissues in the intima of the arteriole. These arteriolar changes account for a high incidence of coronary artery disease and the resulting problems of angina pectoris and myocardial infarction.

Congestive Heart Failure Congestive heart failure occurs when the heart can no longer pump effectively against the increasing resistance. The increased resistance to blood flow increases the cardiac work load. To generate greater pressure, the myocardium of the left ventricle hypertrophies. If this is not effective, then the left ventricle dilates. Heart failure can result from excess dilatation (Chap. 27). The client may complain of shortness of breath on exertion and paroxysmal nocturnal dyspnea. A chest x-ray will show an enlarged heart, and an ECG will show left ventricular hypertrophy.

Brain (cerebrovascular disease)

As a result of hypertension, the blood vessels become more rigid due to thickening of vessels walls and replacement of smooth muscle tissue with fibrous tissue. The vessel is weakened by this process and tends to rupture more easily. Because of these abnormal processes, changes in cerebral circulation include:

1. Intense constriction of cerebral arterioles
2. Microaneurysms of small cerebral arteries
3. Progressive atherosclerotic changes
4. Increasing intracranial pressure

As a result of these changes, the client may experience transient ischemic attacks (TIA) or a cerebral vascular accident (CVA) due to thrombosis of cerebral vessels, intracerebral hemorrhage, or emboli. The Framingham study found that hypertensives have seven times as many CVAs as the general population.[26]

Hypertensive encephalopathy may occur following a marked rise in blood pressure if the cerebral blood flow is not decreased by autoregulation. With the increase in blood pressure, the cerebral vessels dilate, and cerebral edema develops and produces a rise in intracranial pressure. The increased intracranial pressure may be sufficient to decrease or halt blood flow to the brain. Clinical manifestations of hypertensive encephalopathy are discussed under Hypertensive Crisis or Emergency.

Kidneys (nephrosclerosis)

In the kidney, nephrosclerosis results from longstanding hypertension. This disorder is the direct result of ischemia due to the narrowed lumen of the intrarenal blood vessels. Gradual closure of the arteries and arterioles leads to destruction of the glomeruli and atrophy of the tubules and eventual death of nephrons. These changes eventually lead to renal failure. Common laboratory abnormalities are proteinuria, elevated BUN and serum creatinine, and microscopic hematuria.

Renal complications are much more prevalent and severe in malignant hypertension than in benign hypertension. In malignant hypertension, there is rapid deterioration in renal function due to necrotizing arteriolitis.

Eyes (retinal damage)

An ophthalmoscope is used to visualize the blood vessels of the eye. The appearance of the retina provides important information about the severity and prognosis of the hypertensive process. The retina is the only place in the body where the blood vessels can be directly visualized. Therefore, retinal damage provides an indication of vessel damage in the heart, brain, and kidney. Manifestations of retinal damage include blurring of vision, retinal hemorrhage, and loss of vision.

Retinal changes are graded according to severity of damage. The Keith-Wagener classification of retinal

Table 26-13
Keith-Wagener Classification of Retinal Changes

Grade I	Vascular spasm and arteriolar narrowing in terminal branches of vessels.
Grade II	Definite arteriovenous nicking (arterioles cross a vein and compress it).
Grade III	Flame-shaped hemorrhages and fluffy cotton-wool exudates.
Grade IV	Any of the above plus papilledema (swelling of the optic disk).

changes is presented in Table 26-13. Grade IV findings of papilledema are characteristic of malignant hypertension.

Medical Management

Diagnostic

In order to detect hypertension, the client's blood pressure measurements should be carefully evaluated (Table 26-14). Initially, when the blood pressure is taken, it should be taken two or three times, at least 1 or 2 minutes apart and the average pressure recorded as the value for that visit. Waiting for 1 or 2 minutes between readings allows the venous blood to drain from the arm and prevents inaccurate readings. Measurements should be taken in the supine, standing, and sitting positions. A rise in diastolic pressure when the person goes from the supine to the standing position suggests essential hypertension. A fall in pressure suggests secondary hypertension.[27] Usually, the diagnosis of hypertension is not made solely on the basis of an elevated reading on one occasion. The client is usually asked to return for subsequent reevaluation.

Controversy exists regarding the extensive diagnostic studies that should be performed in a person with hypertension. The main question is: Because most hypertension is essential, how much testing should be done to detect secondary hypertension?

Included in Table 26-14 are basic laboratory studies that are performed in individuals with sustained hypertension. Routine urinalysis, BUN, and serum creatinine tests are used to screen for renal involvement. Measurement of serum electrolytes, especially potassium levels, is important to detect aldosteronism. Blood glucose levels are important because they can assist in identifying endocrine causes of hypertension, such as diabetes mellitus, Cushing's syndrome, and pheochromocytoma. Serum cholesterol and triglyceride levels may provide an indication of risk factors that predispose to atherogenesis. Uric acid levels are determined to establish a baseline, as the levels often rise with diuretic therapy. A chest x-ray provides baseline information regarding heart size, as well as aortic dilatation and rib notching, which occur in coarctation of the aorta. An ECG provides baseline information regarding the cardiac status.

Table 26-14
Medical Management: Hypertension

Diagnostic
1. History and physical examination
2. Routine urinalysis
3. Serum electrolytes and uric acid
4. BUN and serum creatinine
5. Blood glucose (preferably 2 h postprandial)
6. Complete blood count
7. Serum cholesterol and triglycerides
8. Chest x-ray
9. ECG

Therapeutic
1. Diet
   a. Restrict sodium
   b. Restrict calories
   c. Restrict cholesterol and saturated fats
2. Exercise program
3. Relief of stress
4. Antihypertensive drugs (Table 26-15)
5. Periodic monitoring of BP
   a. Weekly if diastolic BP > 105 mmHg
   b. Every 4 mo if client is symptom-free and has stable diastolic BP <105 mmHg

Therapeutic

Treatment is individualized and depends on the degree of hypertension (Table 26-14). Decisions about treatment are usually based on blood pressure measurements taken over two to three visits. If the diastolic blood pressure is consistently greater than 105 mmHg, antihypertensive drug therapy is indicated if other measures (e.g., diet, exercise) have not worked to reduce the blood pressure. In clients with diastolic pressures between 90 and 105 mmHg, other factors, such as age, sex, race, and other risk factors, are taken into consideration before drug therapy is begun. (Pharmacological management is discussed in the next section.)

Follow-up monitoring of the blood pressure is very important. Weekly recordings are indicated for clients with a diastolic blood pressure above 105 mmHg. After the blood pressure has stabilized, it should be monitored every 4 months to ensure control and to assess for target organ damage.

Nondrug therapeutic interventions are indicated in all individuals with either borderline or sustained hypertension. These measures include diet management, regular exercise, stress relief, and control of modifiable risk factors contributing to hypertension. Dietary measures are discussed in a subsequent section. Management of risk factors is discussed in Chap. 27 and Table 27-4.

Regular Exercise Regular exercise can help to control blood pressure, promote relaxation, and control body weight. A moderate amount of exercise at regular intervals is better than vigorous exercise at irregular intervals. The type of exercise that is done is very important. *Isometric* exercises, such as pushing heavy weights or tightening muscles against fixed objects, can raise the blood pressure significantly and should be avoided in known hypertensives. On the other hand, *isotonic* exercises, such as swimming, bicycling, or rhythmic calisthenics, cause no significant change in blood pressure and promote aerobic metabolism (Chap. 27).

Stress Reduction and Management Stress reduction and management will not only help reduce blood pressure but will help control other aspects of the client's life. The individual should learn to identify the events and agents that act as stressors in his life and develop and implement methods to cope with them. *Relaxation techniques* are one means of dealing with stress. They include yoga, transcendental meditation, and physical relaxation. Relaxation techniques have been used successfully in mitigating stress and decreasing sympathetic activity, thereby lowering blood pressure, especially in clients with mild hypertension.

One simple relaxation exercise is walking. Another is to stand still and breathe slowly through the nose, let the breath rise from the diaphragm (not the stomach), and concentrate on exhalation.

Psychotherapy has been used as a method of lowering blood pressure, with successful results reported. It can help clients deal with anxiety and with hostile and aggressive impulses. Counseling has always been advocated as a method of increasing client adherence to the medical regimen.

Biofeedback is still in the experimental stages in treatment of hypertension. It employs equipment which gives the client continuous feedback so that bodily processes that are regulated by the autonomic nervous system (but not consciously perceived and controlled) can be self-regulated. Decreases in blood pressure as the result of biofeedback have been reported, although there are no data that demonstrate its long-term effectiveness.

Pharmacological Management

The general goals of pharmacological management of hypertension are to (1) reduce and maintain the diastolic blood pressure at less than 90 mmHg (95 mmHg if over age 50) and (2) keep uncomfortable or disabling side effects to a minimum. The drugs currently available for treating hypertension have two main actions: (1) reducing peripheral resistance and/or (2) decreasing the volume of circulating blood. The drugs used in the treatment of hypertension include diuretics, sympathetic nervous system inhibitors (sympatholytics), and vasodilators (Table 26-15). Although the precise action of diuretics in the reduction of blood pressure is unclear, they do produce a negative sodium balance in the arteriolar walls, release water for excretion and reduce plasma volume, and reduce the vascular response to catecholamines. Sympatholytics act by diminishing the sympathetic reflexes that increase blood pressure. Vasodilators decrease the blood pressure by dilating the arterioles.

The stepped-care approach to treatment is based on stepwise additions of various antihypertensive drugs until adequate control is achieved.[28] In this approach, therapy is usually started with a diuretic (Fig. 26-6). Diuretics are effective in controlling at least 30 to 40 percent of individuals with mild to moderate hypertension. If adequate control is not achieved with diuretics, a different diuretic agent may be prescribed.

In step two, sympathetic nervous system inhibitor agents are used. If used alone, they would cause sodium and water retention. The use of these drugs with the previously prescribed diuretic therapy prevents sodium and water retention.

If step two drugs are inadequate or produce undesirable side effects, step three drugs are added. Vasodilator drugs such as hydralazine (Apresoline), when used in combination with sympathetic inhibitors, are very effective. Vasodilator drugs cause a compensatory increase in sympathetic nervous activity, resulting in tachycardia and increased cardiac output. If vasodilators are used with sympathetic inhibitors, reflex activation of the sympathetic nervous system does not occur.

In step four, guanethidine is added for those individuals who are resistant to other drugs. In addition, minoxidil (Loniten) may be substituted for hydralazine.

Dietary Management

Dietary management of hypertension consists of sodium restriction, caloric restriction if the individual is overweight, and cholesterol and fat restriction.

Sodium restriction

For clients with very mild hypertension, a low-sodium diet may be the only treatment necessary. The mechanism by which the blood pressure is lowered by

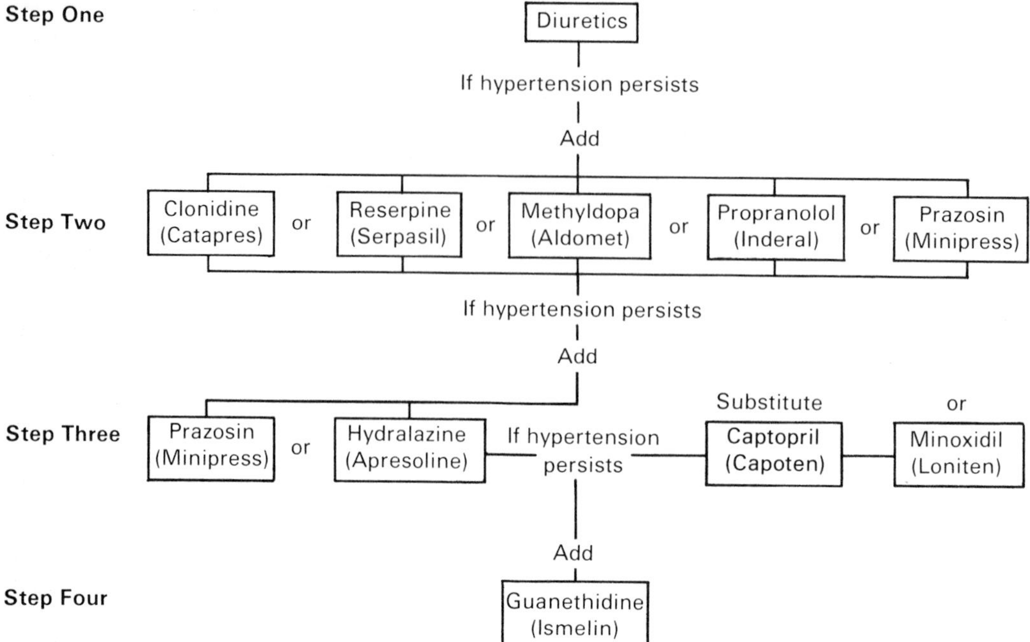

Figure 26-6 Stepped-care program for antihypertensive therapy.

restricting sodium is not fully understood. However, it is known that restricting sodium reduces the ECF volume and the circulating plasma volume, and thus the work of the heart.

The introduction of diuretic agents for hypertension has decreased the need for rigid sodium-restricted diets except in the most severe hypertensive states. A common recommended dietary restriction is 3 to 4 g of sodium per day. This involves not adding salt in the preparation of foods or at meals and avoiding foods known to be high in sodium (Appendix B, Table 12).

Caloric restriction

Obesity has been found to have a high correlation with hypertension. It has been shown that weight reduction has a significant effect on lowering blood pressure in many individuals. The amount of caloric restriction depends on the degree of obesity. When a person decreases caloric intake, sodium intake is also reduced. Therefore, an additional benefit is achieved with a weight-reduction diet.

Lipid restriction

Lipid restriction should include limiting the intake of cholesterol as well as saturated fats. This practice may retard the progress of atherosclerosis (see Chap. 27).

Alcohol consumption needs to be assessed in clients with hypertension. The exact mechanism by which alcohol raises blood pressure is not known. It is possible that alcohol increases renin or aldosterone. Chronic alcohol abuse elevates cortisol.

A study by Kaiser-Permanente has determined that three or more drinks daily is a definite risk factor in hypertension.[29] Therefore, alcohol consumption needs to be evaluated, and the client should be advised to reduce his intake if he is a heavy drinker. Moderate use of alcohol (2 ounces/day) usually should have no adverse effect on the client with mild to moderate hypertension.

Nursing Management

Health promotion and maintenance

Individual Screening The majority of cases of hypertension are identified through routine screening procedures such as insurance, preemployment, and military physical examinations. Nurses in these settings, as well as most other practice settings, are in an ideal position to (1) assess hypertension, (2) identify the risk factors, and (3) educate clients regarding this disease. In addition to blood pressure determination, a complete health assessment should include factors such as age, sex, race, diet history including sodium and alcohol intake, weight patterns, and identification of physical and psychosocial stressors. Other factors

Table 26-15
Antihypertensive Drug Therapy

Agent	Mechanism of Action	Side Effects and Adverse Effects	Special Considerations
		Diuretics	
Thiazide and thiazide derivatives Bendroflumethiazide (Naturetin) Benzthiazide (Aguatag, Exna) Chlorothiazide (Diuril) Chlorthalidone (Hygroton) Cyclothiazide (Anhydron) Hydrochlorothiazide (Esidrix, HydroDiuril, Oretic) Hydroflumethiazide (Saluron) Metolazone (Zaroxolyn) Methyclothiazide (Enduron) Polythiazide (Renese) Quinethazone (Hydromox) Trichlormethiazide (Metahydrin, Nagua)	Act on the distal ascending loop of Henle and distal tubule. Prevent reabsorption of sodium and chloride. Initial effect is due to reduced ECF and cardiac output. Long-term effect is due to reduced peripheral vascular resistance. Thiazide drugs are relatively inexpensive, effective orally, and relatively innocuous.	Electrolyte imbalances Hypokalemia (10–40% incidence) Hypercalcemia Hypochloremia Orthostatic Hypotension Hyperglycemia (1–2% incidence) Hyperuricemia (3–4% incidence) GI Anorexia Vomiting Diarrhea Central nervous system Dizziness Vertigo Headache Hematological Leukopenia Agranulocytosis Thrombocytopenia Hypersensitivity Photosensitivity Purpura Rash	Monitor for hypokalemia, alkalosis. Advise client to supplement diet with potassium-rich foods (see Appendix B, Table 11). If a potassium chloride solution supplement is needed, advise client to drink it with fruit juice or water in order to minimize unpleasant taste. Thiazides potentiate cardiotoxicity of digitalis by producing hypokalemia.
Loop diuretics Ethacrynic acid (Edecrin) Furosemide (Lasix)	Act on the ascending loop of Henle. Prevent reabsorption of chloride and sodium.	Same as thiazides. Fluid and electrolyte depletion. Reversible hearing loss. GI upset (most common with ethacrynic acid).	Monitor for hypokalemia, alkalosis. Measure fluid intake and output. Weigh client daily. Effect of drug increases with dose.
Potassium-sparing diuretics Spironolactone (Aldactone) Triamterene (Dyrenium)	Spironolactone competes with and blocks the effect of aldosterone on the kidney tubule. Mechanism of action of triamterene is unknown. Both drugs block the sodium-potassium exchange mechanism in the distal portion of the tubule. Prevent sodium from being reabsorbed and retain potassium.	Renal insufficiency. Hyperkalemia. Gynecomastia in males. Menstrual irregularities in females. Inability to achieve or maintain erection. Cramping. Skin eruptions. Hirsutism. Headache. Urticaria. Drug fever. Ataxia with spironolactone. Photosensitivity. Blood dyscrasias (with triamterene).	Monitor for hyperkalemia. Do not use potassium supplements.
		Vasodilators	
Minoxidil (Loniten)	As a class of drugs with similar actions, vasodilators act primarily on smooth muscle of arterioles to cause vasodilatation and to reduce peripheral resistance. Minoxidil produces arterial vasodilatation with no venous effect.	Reflex tachycardia. Sodium and water retention. Hypertrichosis. Congestive heart failure. Weakness.	Major disadvantage is reflex increased sympathetic activity.

Table 26-15 (Continued)

Agent	Mechanism of Action	Side Effects and Adverse Effects	Special Considerations
Hydralazine (Apresoline)	Direct relaxant effect on arterial smooth muscle. Arterioles affected more than veins. Less potent than minoxidil.	Tachycardia. Flushing. Headache. Palpitations. GI symptoms. Congestive heart failure. Angina exacerbation. Lupus-like syndrome.	Headaches sometimes occur when drug is started or when dosage is increased. Drug should be discontinued if lupus-like syndrome occurs.
Nitroprusside (Nipride)*	Direct-acting vasodilator. Administered by continuous IV infusion. Used in hypertensive emergencies.	Nausea. Sweating. Headache. Restlessness. Confusion. Muscle twitching.	Dosage titrated to client's response. Light-sensitive, short stability (4 h).
Trimethaphan (Arfonad)*	Blocks neural transmission at autonomic ganglia. Administration. Used in hypertensive emergencies.	Dry mouth. Urinary retention. Constipation.	Rapid onset of action. Should be given using constant monitoring.
Diazoxide (Hyperstat)*	Direct-acting vasodilator. Injected via IV push. Used only in hypertensive emergencies.	Sodium and water retention. Hyperglycemia. Postural hypertension. Skin rash. Fever. Arrhythmias. GI distress.	Decrease of BP seen in 1–5 min. Needs to be injected within 10 s.
	Sympathetic Nervous System Inhibitors		
Central sympathetic effect Clonidine (Catapres)	Inhibits impulse transmission through sympathetic nerve pathways. Causes central alphareceptor stimulation, which decreases sympathetic tone peripherally. Results in dilatation of both arterioles and veins.	Dry mouth. Sedation. Impotence. Constipation. Allergic rash. Dizziness. Headache. Fatigue. Anxiety.	Suggest chewing gum or hard candy to relieve dry mouth. Withdrawal syndrome of hypertensive crisis in 12–48 h if drug abruptly discontinued. Alcohol and sedatives increase central nervous system depression.
Methyldopa (Aldomet)	Same as clonidine.	Sedation. Drowsiness. Fatigue. Postural hypotension. Decreased libido. Impotence. Dry mouth. Hemolytic anemias. Hepatotoxicity. GI symptoms.	Client should be instructed about daytime sedation. Hazardous activities should be avoided. Activities requiring mental work may be an indication not to use drug.
Peripheral sympathetic effect Guanethidine (Ismelin)	Generally used for severe or refracting hypertension. Prevents the release of norepinephrine. Produces greatest effects in the standing position.	Orthostatic hypotension. Diarrhea. Cramps. Bradycardia. GI distress. Retrograde ejaculation.	Hypotensive effect delayed for 2–3 days and persists for 7–10 days after withdrawal. To prevent orthostatic hypotension, discuss with client the necessity of sitting or squatting at the first sign of dizziness and exercising the lower legs when standing for long periods of time. Toe-to-thigh bandages or support hose may be helpful.

Table 26-15 (Continued)

Agent	Mechanism of Action	Side Effects and Adverse Effects	Special Considerations
Reserpine (Serpasil)	Produces depletion of catecholamines from peripheral sympathetic system; endings may produce this effect centrally.	Nasal congestion. Drowsiness. GI distress. Mental depression. Bradycardia. Impotence. Bizarre dreams. Syncope. Breast cancer.	Monitor for depression (e.g., early-morning awakenings, with fatigue and inability to return to sleep, lack of interest in food) and personality changes. Advise client to eliminate barbiturates, alcohol, and narcotics.
Alpha blocker			
Prazosin (Minipress)	Blocks postsynaptic alpha receptors in peripheral vasculature. Results in dilatation of both arterioles and veins.	Postural hypotension. Syncope. Dizziness. Headache. Drowsiness. Paresthesias. Blurred vision. Impotence. Frequent urination.	Produces very little reflex tachycardia.
Phentolamine (Regitine)	Blocks alpha-adrenergic receptors.	Acute, prolonged hypotension. Cardiac arrhythmias. Tachycardia. Weakness. Flushing.	Primarily used in pheochromocytoma.
Beta blockers Propranolol (Inderal) Metoprolol (Lopressor) Nadolol (Corgard) Atenolol (Tenormin) Timolol (Blocadren)	Reduce blood pressure by decreasing cardiac output, decreasing sympathetic stimulation, and decreasing renin secretion by the kidney. With long-term use, beta blockers reduce peripheral resistance.	Asthma attacks (precipitate or aggravate). Heart failure. Bradycardia. AV conduction block. Impaired peripheral circulation. Nightmares. Depression. Weakness. GI symptoms.	Assess client for manifestations of heart failure and heart block. Check pulse regularly. Propranolol is contraindicated in individuals with a known history of congestive heart failure, asthma, or diabetes mellitus.
Miscellaneous			
Investigational drug			
Captopril	Inhibitor of angiotensin-converting enzyme. Lowers total peripheral resistance.	Loss of taste. Transient maculopapular rash.	
Combination therapy			
Aldochlor	Combination of methyldopa and hydrochlorothiazide.		
Aldactazide	Combination of aldactone and hydroclorothiazide.		
Dyazide	Combination of hydrochlorothiazide and triamterene.		
Ser-Ap-Es	Combination of reserpine, hydralazine, and hydrochlorothiazide.		
Combipress	Combination of chlorthalidone and clonidine.		
Apresazide	Combination of hydralazine and hydrochlorothiazide.		

*Used in hypertensive emergencies.

to include in the health history are a family history of heart disease, stroke, renal disease, and diabetes mellitus. Medications taken, both prescribed and over-the-counter, should be noted. The client should be asked about any previous documentation of high blood pressure and the results of treatment (if any).

Blood pressure measurements should be done under standardized conditions and with accurate equipment. The client's arm should be suitably uncovered. The blood pressure is assessed most accurately if readings are taken in three positions: sitting, supine, and standing. Usually the systolic pressure decreases upon standing, while the diastolic pressure increases. Both systolic and diastolic pressures should be recorded for each position.

The cuff should be inflated at least 20 mmHg above the systolic pressure to ensure vascular occlusion. In obese individuals, a cuff larger than the normal 12- to 14-cm cuff should be used to obtain an accurate reading.

To establish a baseline blood pressure level, blood pressure measurements should be taken on at least two visits, and the average pressure should be recorded based on the values of those visits. Common sources of error in measuring blood pressure are presented in Table 26-16.

Screening Programs The detection and control of hypertension in the community are important. Large numbers of screening programs have been established by state and local agencies to identify individuals with high blood pressure and refer them for treatment. It is particularly important to screen blacks since the prevalence of hypertension is much greater in this group. Nurses involved in screening programs should be aware of general guidelines for blood pressure detection and evaluation (Table 26-17). At the time of the blood pressure measurement, each client should be informed in writing of the numerical value of his blood pressure and, if necessary, why further evaluation is important.

Risk Factors Client education regarding risk factors is appropriate for both individual and mass screening programs. Risk factors can easily be identified and their modification discussed with the client. Health-promoting behaviors for risk factors related to coronary artery disease are discussed in Table 27-4. These same approaches are applicable to the client with hypertension.

Acute intervention

Clients with severe hypertension, either newly diagnosed or uncontrolled, are frequently hospitalized. The purpose of hospitalization is to lower the blood pressure, determine the cause, and treat the cause if it is due to secondary hypertension. The majority of individuals with mild to moderate hypertension are managed on an outpatient basis. The primary goal of the nurse at this stage of intervention is to assist in reducing blood pressure and to begin client education.

Severe Hypertension For the client with severe hypertension, the nurse needs to monitor the blood pressure every 1 to 2 hours and then with decreasing frequency as the pressure stabilizes. Antihypertensive drug therapy at this time is often given parenterally. Careful monitoring of vital signs provides information regarding the effectiveness of these drugs.

If the client has headaches, the nurse should assess when they occur and what the precipitating factors are. Nursing interventions for headaches include modification of factors which may cause stress, elimination of excess noise in the client's environment, administration of analgesics, and lowering the blood pressure.

For the client with fatigue and anxiety, a schedule should be provided that alternates long rest periods with periods of activity. It is important to plan for emotional as well as physical rest. The nurse should discuss with the client measures to reduce stress and decrease tension. In some situations, it may be appropriate to administer tranquilizers if ordered.

Mild to Moderate Hypertension Education is a primary goal for clients initially diagnosed with mild to moderate hypertension and for those clients who stabilize after treatment for severe hypertension.

Diet therapy

Dietary measures were previously discussed. The client and family need education about sodium-restricted diets. The client needs to be instructed on reading the labels of over-the-counter drugs as well as packaged foods to identify "hidden" sources of sodium. Sometimes it is helpful to review the client's normal diet and have the client identify foods high in sodium. Weight-reduction diets are discussed in Chap. 33, and diets low in cholesterol and saturated fat are discussed in Chap. 27.

Drug therapy

Antihypertensive drugs have varied mechanisms to lower the blood pressure (Table 26-15). A common side effect of some of these drugs is orthostatic (postural) hypotension. The drugs alter the nervous system mechanisms regulating pressure that are re-

Table 26-16
Common Sources of Errors in Measuring Blood Pressure

Environmental factors

Noise When measuring blood pressure inside, close doors, turn off radios or televisions, and stop conversation. For outdoor settings, avoid locations near music and heavy vehicular and pedestrian traffic.

Artifacts Arrange furniture and equipment so tubing from stethoscope and blood pressure cuff hangs free.

Temperature Avoid chilly environments. The ambient temperature can affect dilation and constriction of small arterioles.

Biological factors

Activity Clients should rest 5 minutes to minimize the effects of recent physical exertion on the cardiac output.

Position Avoid isometric muscle contractions, which can elevate blood pressure, by comfortably supporting the client's arm.

Stress Anxiety about the blood pressure reading or a procedure that is about to be done in a clinic or physician's office can affect the reading. Other biological factors, such as pain or discomfort from a distended bladder, should be corrected and the blood pressure repeated after the client has had an opportunity to rest. If these things cannot be corrected, note their presence with the blood pressure recording.

Equipment

Sphygmomanometer A mercury manometer in which the mercury level is not at zero or an uncalibrated aneroid instrument can give erroneous readings. Calibrate equipment and check frequently for leaks and smooth functioning. Mercury and aneroid manometers are endorsed by the American Heart Association and Joint National Committee on Detection, Evaluation, and Treatment of High Blood Pressure. While the aneroid type is more convenient, the mercury manometer is considered more accurate and durable.

Cuff The most common error is using a cuff that is too small for a large or obese adult or child. A cuff that is too narrow will give a false high reading. A false low reading will be obtained if the cuff is too wide.

Tears or cracks in the rubber bladder or tubing or faulty connectors will cause air leaks in the system and make it difficult to regulate the rate of deflation.

Ripped fabric on the cuff will allow bulging during inflation. This causes an uneven distribution of pressure and inaccurate readings.

Stethoscope Cracked or kinked tubing will not transmit sound well. Any stethoscope should be in good condition. Ear pieces should be clean and fit snugly in the ears.

Technique

Poor technique is usually due to inadequate training and/or the development of poor habits. Selection of incorrect cuff size, improper placement of the stethoscope, and excessively rapid deflation of the cuff are common sources of inaccurate readings.

Clients, lay volunteers, and health professionals who will be measuring blood pressures should be properly trained and periodically reevaluated. They should possess the following characteristics:

Hearing acuity	sufficient to identify and interpret Korotkoff's sounds
Visual acuity	sufficient to read a moving column of mercury and distinguish 2-mm markings
Manual dexterity	sufficient to wrap cuff and control air valve
Concentration and coordination	eye, hand, and ear coordination adequate to control the rate of inflation and deflation and not confuse auditory and visual cues

Interpretation

Digit preference Individuals have a preference for rounding to certain numbers. This practice has been documented as being common because the incidence of recorded readings ending in zero (130/80, 120/70) is greater than the expected incidence by change. Some people seem to cluster to the mean within a 10-mm range, preferring figures that end in 5 (135/85, 125/75).

Observer bias People measuring blood pressure can have an unconscious prejudice about what reading they expect to hear. This may be influenced by knowledge of the client's sex, race, age, weight, and prior readings. For example, one might expect to hear higher Korotkoff's sounds in a middle-aged, obese, black female than in a young, thin, white female, or one might expect to hear sounds lower than prior readings in a client who has begun drug therapy.

From Martha N. Hill, "What Can Go Wrong When You Measure BP," *AJN*, **80**:946 (May 1980).

quired for positional changes. Consequently, the client may feel dizzy, weak, and faint when assuming an erect position after sitting or lying down. Specific measures to control or decrease orthostatic hypotension are presented in Table 26-18.

Side effects of drug therapy are common. Sometimes the number or degree of side effects decreases with long-term use of the drug. In certain cases, it is necessary to change the drug or decrease the dosage. With some drugs, side effects can be alleviated by arranging a convenient schedule. For example, diuretics work best if taken early in the morning. Side effects of vasodilators and sympatholytics decrease if the drugs are given in the evening. With some drugs, side effects can be decreased if the drugs are given with meals. Dry mouth and frequent voiding are com-

Table 26-17
Procedure for Monitoring Blood Pressure

Client	Blood Pressure	Recommended Action
All adults	Diastolic 120 or higher	Prompt evaluation and treatment
All adults	160/95 or higher	Check BP within 1 mo
Younger than 50 yr	Between 140/90 and 160/95	Check BP every 2–3 mo
Older than 50 yr	Between 140/90 and 160/95	Check BP every 6–9 mo
All adults	Diastolic below 90	Check BP every year

The Joint National Committee on Detection, Evaluation, and Treatment of High Blood Pressure.

mon side effects of diuretics. Chewing sugarless gum or candy can relieve the dry mouth.

Stress modification

The first approach is to identify areas or factors that produce stress. The client needs to be told the relationship between stress and hypertension. The nurse and client together should plan ways for the client to handle stress more effectively (Chap. 39).

Exercise

The client needs assistance in developing a graduated exercise plan. Isometric exercises should be discouraged. An isotonic exercise program can be planned based on the client's current exercise activities (Table 27-11).

Chronic management

In most individuals, hypertension is a chronic problem. It usually cannot be cured, but it can be controlled. The client needs to understand that hypertension is a long-term condition which will require regular treatment. Education is one of the most impor-

Table 26-18
Teaching Plan Related to Antihypertensive Therapy

1. Learn the names, actions, dosages, and side effects of prescribed medications.
2. Take drugs at a regular and convenient time.
3. Do not discontinue drugs, or decrease the dosage if side effects develop. Consult first with the health care provider.
4. Do not abruptly discontinue drugs, as withdrawal may cause a severe hypertensive reaction.
5. Do not make up missed drug dosages.
6. If impotency or sexual problems develop, consult with the health care provider about changing drugs or dosages.
7. Side effects often diminish with time.
8. Do not take a medication belonging to someone else.
9. Do not take an increased dosage if BP increases before consulting with the health care provider.
10. Supplement diet with foods high in potassium (e.g., citrus fruits, green leafy vegetables) if taking potassium-losing diuretics.
11. Avoid hot baths, excessive amounts of alcohol, strenuous exercise within 3 h of taking medications which promote vasodilatation.
12. To decrease orthostatic hypotension:
    Arise slowly from bed.
    Sit on side of bed for a few minutes.
    Stand slowly.
    Do not stand still for prolonged periods of time.
    Do leg exercises to increase venous return.
    Wear support stockings.
    Sleep with head of bed raised or on pillows.
    Lie down or sit down when dizziness occurs.

tant ways to assist the client in controlling his blood pressure and adhering to his therapeutic regimen.

The biggest problem at this stage is *poor client adherence.* For some reason, many clients stop taking their medication and become indifferent about their diet. The reasons for poor adherence are many: (1) inadequate client instruction, (2) discomforting side effects of drugs (3) subsiding of symptoms, so that the client feels cured, (4) lack of motivation, (5) high cost of drugs and (6) lack of a trusting relationship between the client and the health care provider.

Careful planning of measures to help the hypertensive client follow the prescribed regimen is necessary to increase adherence to the therapeutic regimen. Careful planning includes complete assessment of those factors that will influence implementation of the therapeutic plan. A regimen needs to be designed that is compatible with the client's personality, habits, and lifestyle. It is important to help the client and his family understand that hypertension is a chronic condition that cannot be cured but can be controlled by drug therapy, diet therapy, reduction of stress, exercise programs, periodic evaluation, and possibly other lifestyle changes.

Another measure that may be used is teaching the client to take his blood pressure at home. Clients should be assessed individually as to the feasibility of this measure. For most clients, home blood pressure measurement gives a more valid indication of the blood pressure since the client is more relaxed at home. It is important to emphasize to the client that a single reading is not as important as a series of readings over a period of time. The client should be instructed to take his blood pressure weekly (unless otherwise instructed) after the blood pressure has stabilized.

Hypertensive Crisis or Emergency

Hypertensive crisis is an emergency situation in which the degree of hypertension creates a life-threatening situation. Severe hypertension (usually a diastolic pressure above 130 mmHg) can cause irreversible injury to the brain, heart, or kidneys and can progress rapidly to death. In individuals with a previously compromised cardiovascular status (e.g., congestive heart failure, myocardial infarction), a diastolic pressure greater than 110 mmHg may be life-threatening. Hypertensive emergencies can be a complication of essential hypertension or may be due to chronic renal disease, acute glomerulonephritis, acute toxemia of pregnancy, pheochromocytoma, Cushing's syndrome, or adrenocorticotropic hormone toxicity.

Clinical manifestations

Hypertensive crisis is often manifested as *hypertensive encephalopathy,* a syndrome in which severe hypertension is associated with headache, nausea, vomiting, convulsions, confusion, stupor, and coma. Other common manifestations are blurred vision and transient blindness. The manifestations of encephalopathy are probably due to cerebral edema and spasms of cerebral vessels.

Renal insufficiency ranging from minor impairment to complete renal shutdown may take place. Rapid cardiac decompensation with developing pulmonary edema can also occur.

Management

Treatment of the hypertensive crisis depends upon the nature of the underlying disorder and how rapidly the blood pressure needs to be reduced. The management of hypertensive crisis usually requires parenteral administration of antihypertensives. The drugs used in the treatment are:

1. Vasodilators—diazoxide (Hyperstat) and nitroprusside (Nipride)
2. Ganglionic blocker—trimethaphan (Arfonad)
3. Diuretic—furosemide (Lasix)

The mechanisms of action and the side effects of these drugs are presented in Table 26-15. The drugs are administered intravenously and have a rapid (within minutes) onset of action. The client's blood pressure and pulse should be taken every 5 to 10 minutes during the administration of these drugs. Monitoring of arterial blood pressure can be done using an intraarterial line (Chap. 28). The rate of administration is titrated based on the level of blood pressure. It is important to prevent hypotension and its effects in a person whose body has adjusted to hypertension. Continual ECG monitoring is frequently done to observe for cardiac arrhythmias. Hourly urinary output should be measured to assess for adequacy of cardiac output.

Lowering the blood pressure with the antihypertensive drugs may reverse the crisis in a day or two. If the hypertension cannot be controlled, the prognosis is very poor.

Once the hypertensive crisis is resolved, it is important to determine the cause of the hypertension. Then the client will need appropriate management and teaching to avoid future crises.

Case Study / Essential Hypertension

Mr. K. is a 49-year-old black male. For the last 3 years, he had been unable to work because of hypertension. He has a strong family history of hypertension.

Mr. K. was first admitted to the hospital in June with gross hematuria of unknown etiology and hypertension with retinopathy. On admission, his blood pressure was 234/134. His physical examination revealed no abnormalities. A laboratory workup was within normal limits except for a urinalysis, which revealed occult blood and proteinuria.

He was placed on a low-sodium diet, methyldopa (Aldomet), and chlorothiazide (Diuril). His hematuria cleared up in 1 week, and he was discharged with instructions to continue with his medications.

One year later, in July, he was readmitted to the hospital with a blood pressure of 170/120. He complained of severe chest pains with syncope, sharp occipital headaches, and dyspnea. His ECG showed an inferior wall myocardial infarction with ischemic S-T changes. His eye examination revealed grade II retinopathy in the left eye and grade I retinopathy in the right eye.

Discussion Questions

1. What risk factors related to hypertension were present in Mr. K's situation? What are other possible risk factors?
2. What evidence of target organ damage was present?
3. Explain the rationale for his medical therapy.
4. What client teaching measures should have been included in Mr. K's nursing care on his first admission?
5. What are the possible explanations for the finding of hypertension on the second admission after he demonstrated a good response to treatment?

REVIEW QUESTIONS

The number of the question corresponds to the same numbered objective at the beginning of the chapter.

1. Mechanisms which regulate normal blood pressure include all the following *except*
 a. parathormone feedback
 b. cardiac output
 c. peripheral vascular resistance
 d. renin-angiotensin mechanism

2. Shock is best defined as
 a. cardiovascular collapse
 b. vasodilatation
 c. inadequate tissue perfusion
 d. acute pump failure

3. The type of shock which results from vasodilatation is
 a. diabetic shock
 b. neurogenic shock
 c. cutaneous shock
 d. hemorrhagic shock

4. Which of the following events occurs during intermediate or progressive shock?
 a. activation of the renin-angiotensin mechanism
 b. stimulation of aortic and carotid sinus baroreceptors
 c. movement of plasma proteins into the interstitial space
 d. movement of fluid into the intravascular space

5. Which of the following fluids is generally used in the initial resuscitation of hemorrhagic shock?
 a. Ringer's lactate
 b. packed red cells
 c. dextran
 d. plasma

6. The appropriate position for the client in shock is
 a. Trendelenburg
 b. high Fowler's
 c. reverse Trendelenburg
 d. supine with legs elevated

7. Clinical manifestations of a hemolytic transfusion reaction include
 a. chills and low back pain
 b. vomiting and urticaria
 c. tachycardia and asthmatic attack
 d. severe hypotension and petechiae

8. Which of the following nursing measures is appropriate following a blood transfusion reaction?
 a. Discontinue the intravenous line and force fluids.
 b. Lower the client's head and turn the body to the left side.
 c. Stop the transfusion and maintain the intravenous line.with normal saline.
 d. Slow the transfusion and monitor vital signs.

9. Which of the following include causes of secondary hypertension?
 a. pheochromocytoma and Stokes-Adams syndrome
 b. birth control pills and renal vascular disease
 c. aldosteronism and coumadin therapy
 d. coarctation of the aorta and tetralogy of Fallot

10. Which of the following would not be considered a risk factor in hypertension?
 a. rural living
 b. family history of hypertension
 c. being a black male
 d. increasing age

11. Complications of hypertension include
 a. rheumatic heart disease and renal disease
 b. retinal damage and myocardial infarction

c. congestive heart failure and diabetes
d. stroke and pheochromocytoma

12. What is the most common problem in the management of hypertension?
    a. The disease is too complicated to treat adequately.
    b. Clients fail to adhere to the treatment regime.
    c. Hypertensive drugs are seldom effective.
    d. There is a sudden onset of retinal complications.

13. In preparing your teaching plans for a client with essential hypertension, which of the following would you include?
    a. elimination of all dietary sodium
    b. instructions regarding a low-residue diet
    c. awareness of common side effects of drugs
    d. explanation of myocardial infarction

14. Clinical manifestations of hypertensive encephalopathy include
    a. halo vision and paresthesias
    b. vomiting and headache
    c. seizures and hyperventilation
    d. irritability and blindness

REFERENCES

1. J. A. Jahre et al., "Medical Approach to the Hypotensive Patient and the Patient in Shock," *Heart Lung,* **4:**577 (1975).
2. J. Barry, *Emergency Nursing,* McGraw-Hill Book Company, New York, 1978, p. 199.
3. G. D. Park, "Cardiogenic Shock," *Crit Care Q,* **2:**43 (1980).
4. C. E. Rackley et al., "Cardiogenic Shock," *Res Staff Physician,* **26:**35 (1980).
5. R. A. Eskridge, "Septic Shock," *Crit Care Q,* **2:**55 (1980).
6. Barry, op. cit., p. 200.
7. N. F. Adkinson, "Drug Hypersensitivity—Prevention, Diagnosis and Management," *Del Med J,* **47:**645 (1975).
8. M. A. Thompson, *Shock Syndrome,* Addison-Wesley Publishing Company, Inc., Menlo Park, Calif., 1978, p. 18.
9. R.F. Wilson, "Diagnosis and Treatment of Shock," *Consultant,* **18:**109 (1978).
10. Rackley et al., op. cit.
11. Barry, op. cit., p. 204.
12. Ibid., p. 205.
13. Wilson, op. cit., p. 114.
14. R. F. Wilson, "The Diagnosis and Management of Severe Sepsis and Septic Shock," *Heart Lung,* **5:**422–427 (1976).
15. B. J. Guglielmo, "Evaluation of the Use of Corticosteroids," *Crit Care Q,* **2:**37–38 (1980).
16. T. F. O'Donnell and S. C. Belkin, "The Pathophysiology, Monitoring, and Treatment of Shock," *Orthop Clin North Am,* **9:**589–604 (1978).
17. A. Oakes and M. de Give, "Traumatic Injuries," M. E. Armstrong et al. (eds.), *McGraw-Hill Handbook of Clinical Nursing,* McGraw-Hill Book Company, New York, 1979, p. 1342.
18. H. Dustan, *Clinician: Hypertension,* Searle & Company, New York, 1973, pp. 8, 9.
19. K. Isselbacher et al. (eds.), *Harrison's Principles of Internal Medicine,* 9th ed., McGraw-Hill Book Company, New York, 1980, p. 179.
20. National High Blood Pressure Education Program, High Blood Pressure Coordinating Committee, *New Hypertension Prevalence Data and Recommended Public Statements,* Bethesda, Md., 1978.
21. *Hypertension Handbook,* Merck, Sharp, and Dohme, West Point, Pa., p. 21.
22. M. Kochar and L. Daniels, *Hypertension Control for Nurses and Other Health Professionals,* The C. V. Mosby Company, St. Louis, 1979, pp. 17–19.
23. Arthur Guyton, *Textbook of Medical Physiology,* 5th ed., W. B. Saunders Company, Philadelphia, 1976, pp. 286–290.
24. R. B. Zurier, "Prostaglandins: Their Potential in Clinical Medicine," *Postgrad Med,* **68:**70–77 (1980).
25. M. B. Marcinek, "Hypertension: What Does It Do to the Body?" *AJN,* **80:**931 (1980).
26. W. B. Kannel et al., "Epidemiologic Assessment of the Role of Blood Pressure in Stroke," *JAMA,* **214:**301 (1970).
27. Isselbacher et al., op. cit., p. 1170.
28. N. Wenger et al., *Cardiology for Nurses,* McGraw-Hill Book Company, New York, 1980, p. 338.
29. A. K. Klatsky et al., "Alcohol Consumption and Blood Pressure: Kaiser-Permanente Multiphasic Health Examination Data," *N Engl J Med,* **296:**1194 (1977).

Chapter 27

NURSING ROLE IN MANAGEMENT

Coronary Artery Disease and Congestive Heart Failure

Sue Elster
Kathy Zarling

Learning Objectives

1. Describe the etiology and pathogenesis of coronary artery disease.
2. Explain the nursing role in health promotion and maintenance related to risk factors in coronary artery disease.
3. Describe the precipitating factors, types, clinical manifestations, and medical and pharmacological management of angina pectoris.
4. Explain the nursing role in the management of the client with angina pectoris.
5. Describe the pathophysiology of myocardial infarction from the onset of injury through the healing process.
6. Describe the clinical manifestations, complications, diagnostic study abnormalities, and medical management of myocardial infarction.
7. Describe the nursing role in the rehabilitative management of the client following myocardial infarction.
8. Identify the emotional and behavioral reactions to myocardial infarction.
9. Explain the significance of an exercise program following myocardial infarction.
10. Differentiate between the pathophysiology and clinical manifestations of right-sided and left-sided congestive heart failure.
11. Describe the medical, pharmacological, dietary, and nursing management of the client with congestive heart failure.
12. Describe the actions and nursing implications of the following drugs used in the treatment of coronary artery disease and congestive heart failure: lipid-lowering agents, vasodilators, sedatives, digitalis, beta-adrenergic blockers, and diuretics.

SIGNIFICANCE OF THE PROBLEM

Coronary artery disease (CAD) is a type of blood vessel disorder that is included in the general category of *atherosclerosis*. Atherosclerosis is derived from two Greek words: *athere*, meaning fatty mush, and *skleros*, meaning hard. This word combination indicates that atherosclerosis begins as soft deposits of fat that harden with age. Atherosclerosis is often referred to as "hardening of the arteries." Although this condition can occur in any artery in the body, the *atheromas* (fatty deposits) have a preference for the coronary arteries. *Arteriosclerotic heart disease (ASHD), cardiovascular heart disease (CVHD), ischemic heart disease (IHD), coronary heart disease (CHD)*, and *coronary artery disease (CAD)* are all synonymous terms used to describe the disease process. Other terms used to describe the disease mechanisms involved in CAD are *plaque formation, atheromatous deposits*, and *coronary occlusions*.

CAD is the major cause of death in the United States (Fig. 27-1). The American Heart Association reports that over 640,000 people die yearly from heart attacks. An estimated 4,330,000 people have had a heart attack and/or have angina pectoris. The estimated prevalence of the major cardiovascular diseases is presented in Fig. 27-2.

Consumer costs related to heart disease are great and often exceed insurance compensation. In 1980 transportation costs of ambulance and paramedic services for a heart attack victim were approximately \$120 to \$150. Hospitalization may last for as

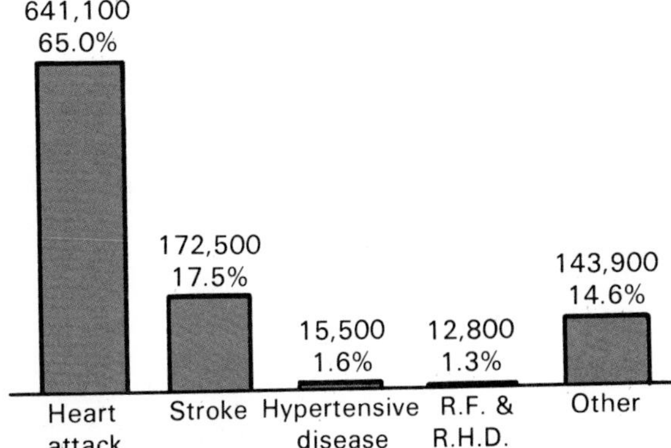

Figure 27-1 Deaths due to cardiovascular diseases. *(American Heart Association, Heart Facts, 1981, National Center, Dallas, 1980.)*

This chapter was reviewed by Beverly Hydo, R.N., M.S.N., Coordinator, Inpatient Cardiac Rehabilitation, William Beaumont Hospital, Royal Oak, Michigan.

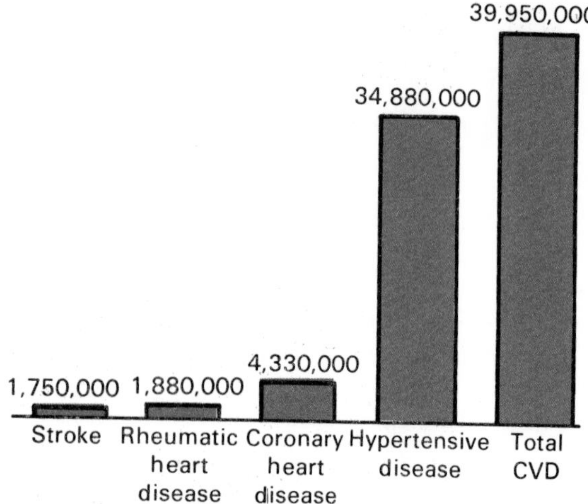

Figure 27-2 Estimated prevalence of the major cardiovascular diseases. *(American Heart Association.)*

long as 2 to 3 weeks. Coronary care unit (CCU) costs range from $600 to $700 per day, depending on the type and number of support systems required. General unit care amounts to approximately $350 per day. Follow-up visits to a clinic or physician may be as high as $50 per visit. Medications to be taken after discharge may average $30 per month. If there are indications for further studies, such as a treadmill exercise-tolerance test, echocardiography, or arteriography, the client can add several hundred dollars more to his health care bill. If the client is unable to return to work, he may be paid disability. The American Heart Association has estimated that cardiovascular disease cost the United States *$46.2 billion* in 1981. The costs in terms of personal tragedy are very difficult to measure.

ETIOLOGY AND PATHOGENESIS OF CORONARY ARTERY DISEASE

Atherosclerosis is the major cause of CAD. It is characterized by a focal deposit of cholesterol and lipids primarily within the intimal wall of the artery. The condition occurs most often in medium- to large-size vessels. Growth of smooth muscle cells and other arterial wall changes take place, leading to obstruction or occlusion of the arteries.

The exact mechanisms which allow for the multifocal deposition of fatty materials in the vessel wall are unclear. Atherosclerosis was once thought to be a disease of old age. However, current data suggest that the disease process can begin in youth.

Theories of Atherogenesis

Several theories exist to explain the process of atherogenesis (Table 27-1). None are conclusive or entirely explain the cause of atherogenesis. But whether occlusion is caused by thrombus formation, stenosis (narrowing), or arterial spasm from an irritation or a lack of O_2, the result is a decreased flow of blood to the myocardium. This produces either ischemia or necrosis, which is manifested as angina, infarction, or death.

Development Stages of Atherosclerosis

CAD takes many years to develop. When it becomes symptomatic, the disease process is usually well advanced. The stages of development in atherosclerosis are (1) *fatty streak*, (2) *raised fibrous plaque*, and (3) *complicated lesion* (Fig. 27-3).

Table 27-1
Theories of Atherogenesis

Theory	Mechanism
Lipid infiltration theory	Lipids from the circulation enter the endothelium and accumulate in smooth muscle in response to mechanical or inflammatory trauma. Lipoproteins become trapped, and damage occurs. Endothelial permeability is altered.
Thrombogenic theory	RBCs, platelets, and lipids accumulate along the intima of arteries. Microthrombi are formed. Platelets aggregate, releasing substances that alter endothelial permeability. The thrombus extends and reactivates the cycle.
Vascular dynamics theory	Mechanical factors (e.g., hypertension) increase intraluminal pressure, which leads to altered membrane permeability, resulting in increased lipid infiltration.
Capillary hemorrhage theory	Lipids accumulate in plaques as a result of capillary hemorrhage.
Lipid metabolic theory	LDL migrate into the arterial wall, accumulating in the intimal and medial layers of the artery. Since LDL are responsible for transporting cholesterol, cholesterol is also deposited at the same time.
Aging theory	Atherosclerotic changes occur in everyone and become more evident as aging progresses.

Fatty streak

Fatty streaks are the earliest lesions of atherosclerosis and are characterized by lipid-filled smooth muscle cells. As streaks of fat develop within the smooth muscle cells, a yellow color appears. Fatty streaks are usually observed in the coronary arteries by age 15 and involve an increasing amount of surface area as the client ages. It is generally believed that fatty streaks are reversible, but the evidence is inconclusive.[1]

Raised fibrous plaque

This stage is the beginning of progressive changes in the arterial wall. These changes appear in the coronary arteries by age 30 and increase with age. The arterial wall changes are initiated by chronic endothelial injury which results from many factors, including elevated blood pressure, high blood cholesterol, heredity, carbon monoxide produced by smoking, and possibly toxic substances within the blood. Once endothelial injury has occurred, lipoproteins (the carrier substances within the bloodstream) transport cholesterol and other lipids into the arterial intima. With endothelial injury, overgrowth and migration of smooth muscle cells occur (Fig. 27-3). This proliferation leads to thickening of the intima and causes a growing lesion. Lipids may cause smooth muscle damage as well as contribute to plaque thickening and instability. As these lipids and other substances pass through the vessels, they adhere to the roughened, damaged wall, thereby causing the lesion buildup or structural abnormality. Collagen tissue, elastic fibers, and smooth cells filled with fat cover the lesion. The fibrous plaque is grayish or whitish in appearance.

Platelets also play a part in the overgrowth of smooth muscle cells. Once the artery's inner wall has become damaged, platelets may accumulate in large numbers, leading to a thrombus. The thrombus may adhere to the wall of the artery, leading to narrowing and total occlusion of the artery. The thrombus may also break loose, causing an embolus to the heart, lungs, or other vital organs.

Complicated lesion

The final stage in the development of the atherosclerotic lesion is the most dangerous. The plaque consists of a core of lipid materials (mainly cholesterol) within an area of dead tissue. With the incorporation of lipids, thrombi, damaged tissue, and some accumulation of calcium, the growing lesion becomes complex. As the lesion continues to grow and becomes complex, dark, hardened, necrotic tissue appears within the arteries, causing rigidity and hardening.

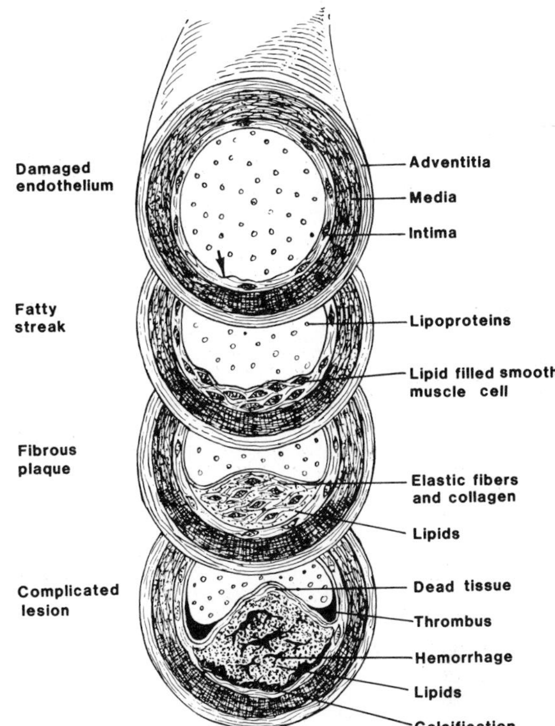

Figure 27-3 The stages of development in the progression of atherosclerosis include *(a)* fatty streaks, *(b)* raised fibrous plaque, and *(c)* complicated lesion. *(After Herb Smith.)*

Collateral Circulation

Normally, some arterial branching (called *collateral circulation*) exists within the coronary circulation. When an atherosclerotic plaque occludes the normal flow of blood through a coronary artery, increased collateral circulation develops (Fig. 27-4). When occlusion of the coronary arteries happens slowly over a long period of time, the myocardium may still receive an adequate amount of oxygen through the collateral circulation. Thus, the client may not develop symptomatic heart disease until a severe strain is placed on the heart.

RISK FACTORS IN CAD

Risk factors are characteristics or conditions which are statistically associated with a high incidence of a disease. Many risk factors have been associated with atherosclerosis but the three most

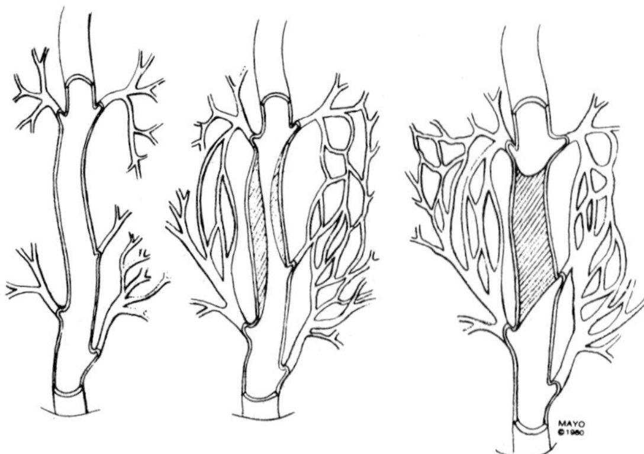

Figure 27-4 Vessel occlusion with collateral circulation. *(a)* Open, functioning coronary artery. *(b)* Partial coronary artery closure with collateral circulation being established. *(c)* Total coronary artery occlusion with collateral circulation bypassing the occlusion to supply the myocardium. *(Mayo Clinic.)*

significant ones are elevated serum lipids, hypertension, and cigarette smoking.[2]

These correlations are derived from studies using very large populations. Risk factors in different populations may vary in prominence. For example, glucose intolerance has been found to be a major risk factor in European populations but only a minor one in U.S. populations. Major risk factors in the United States, such as high serum cholesterol and hypertension, are less prevalent in Japanese, Puerto Rican, and Hawaiian populations.[3]

Risk factors can be categorized as unmodifiable and modifiable (Table 27-2). Unmodifiable risk factors are age, sex, race, genetic inheritance, and diabetes mellitus. Modifiable risk factors include elevated serum lipids, hypertension, smoking, obesity, sedentary lifestyle, and stress in daily living. Diabetes mellitus can be either modifiable by weight reduction and dietary regulation or unmodifiable through inheritance.

Table 27-2
Risk Factors in Coronary Artery Disease

Unmodifiable	Modifiable
Age	*Major*
Sex (males > females until 60 yr of age)	Elevated serum lipids
Race (blacks < whites)	Hypertension
Genetic predisposition and family history of heart disease	Cigarette smoking
	Diabetes mellitus*
	Minor
	Obesity
	Sedentary lifestyle
	Stressful lifestyle

*May be hereditary.

Adapted from the American Heart Association, *Heartbook*, E. P. Dutton & Co., Inc., New York, 1980, and J. W. Hurst et al., *The Heart*, 4th ed., McGraw-Hill Book Company, New York, 1980.

Data on risk factors have been obtained in several major studies. In the Framingham study, one of the most widely known, 5209 men and women were observed for 20 years. Over time, it was noted that elevated serum cholesterol (>250 mg/dL), elevated systolic blood pressure (≥160 mmHg), and cigaret smoking (one or more packs per day) were correlated with an increased incidence of CAD. The younger the subject at the time of induction to the study, the more predictive were the values. Other implicated risk factors and indicators included altered carbohydrate tolerance, sedentary lifestyle, electrocardiographic abnormalities, and reduced lung vital capacity.[4,5]

The Evans County, Georgia, longitudinal study looked at differences in risk factors between blacks and whites. Blacks manifested a lower incidence of risk in all categories. Occupation seemed to be the only clue to the differences. Blacks engaged in more activity and physical labor than did the more sedentary whites.[6] Blacks are known to be at higher risk for hypertension. This is discussed in Chap. 26.

The Western Collaborative Group longitudinal study addressed psychosocial issues of behavior in relation to risk factors.[7] Personal characteristics, such as competitiveness, high achievement orientation, impatience, time urgency, excessive drive and hostility, and abrupt speech and gestures, are described as type A behaviors. These characteristics are discussed further under Stress and Behavior Patterns.

Unmodifiable Risk Factors

Age, sex, and race

These factors were mentioned earlier in the discussion of some major epidemiological studies. The incidence of the first myocardial infarction (MI) is greater for the white, middle-aged male. After the age of 60, the incidence in males and females equalizes, although there is early evidence to suggest that more women are presenting with CAD earlier due to increased stress, increased cigaret smoking, and use of birth control pills. Blacks, although more prone to hypertension, are at less risk than whites of the same age for CAD. Myocardial infarctions in the oriental population in the United States are less frequent than in whites, but the rates are higher than in the countries of origin.

Family history and heredity

Genetic predisposition is an important factor in the occurrence of CAD, although the exact mechanism of inheritance is not fully understood. Some congenital defects in coronary artery walls predispose to the formation of plaques. Familial hyperlipoproteinemia, an autosomal dominant trait, has been strongly associated with CAD at early ages. In most cases of angina or MI, the client can name a close family member who has died either suddenly from an unknown cause or from a documented heart attack.

Diabetes mellitus

The incidence of CAD is greater for diabetic persons, even those with well-controlled blood sugar, than for the general population. Diabetics manifest CAD not only more frequently but also at earlier ages. There is no age difference between diabetic males and females for the onset of manifestations of CAD. Diabetes virtually eliminates the lower incidence of cardiovascular disease in females. Latent diabetes is frequently diagnosed at the time of infarction. Because diabetics have an increased tendency to develop connective tissue degeneration, it is thought that this condition may account for the tendency toward atheroma development seen in the diabetic population.

Modifiable Risk Factors

Elevated serum lipids

An elevated serum lipid level is one of the three most firmly established risk factors in CAD. More specifically, the risk of CAD is especially associated with a serum cholesterol level of more than 250 mg/dL or a fasting triglyceride level of more than 150 mg/dL. The liver is capable of producing cholesterol from saturated fats even when the dietary intake of fats is severely limited. A high correlation between cholesterol and triglyceride levels has been found. Elevated triglyceride levels are correlated with obesity and a sedentary lifestyle.

In order for lipids to be used and transported by the body, they need to become soluble in blood by combining with proteins. Lipids combine with protein to form macromolecules called *lipoproteins*. Lipoproteins are vehicles for fat mobilization and transport. The different types of lipoproteins vary in composition and are classified as high-density lipoproteins (HDL), low-density lipoproteins (LDL), and very low density lipoproteins (VLDL) (Fig. 27-5).

HDL contain more protein by weight and less lipid than any other lipoprotein. HDL may carry lipids away from arteries and to the liver for metabolism. This process prevents lipid accumulation within the arterial walls. The higher the HDL levels in the blood, the lower the risk of CAD. HDL levels are generally higher in women than in men and are increased by physical activity. Individuals who have had an MI have lower concentrations of HDL than matched controls.[8] In general, HDL are high in children and women, decrease with age, and are lowest in individuals with CAD.[9] Current research on drug and dietary therapy is concentrating on ways to elevate HDL levels.

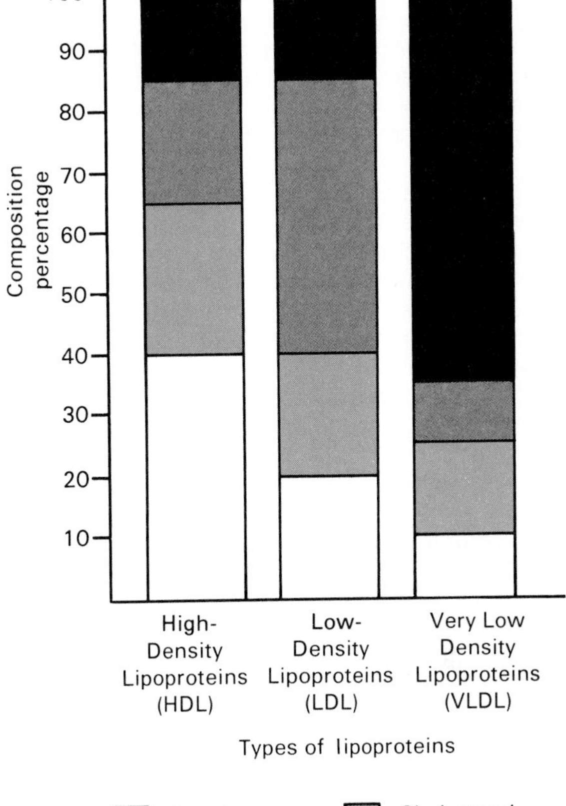

Figure 27-5 Composition of various types of lipoproteins.

LDL contain more cholesterol than any of the other lipoproteins and have an affinity for arterial walls. Elevated LDL correlates most closely with an increased incidence of atherosclerosis.

VLDL contain most of the triglycerides. The direct correlation of VLDL with heart disease is uncertain. High VLDL may increase the risk of premature atherosclerosis when associated with other risk factors, such as diabetes, hypertension, and cigarette smoking.[10]

Hypertension

The second primary risk factor is hypertension, which is defined as a blood pressure greater than or equal to 140/90 mmHg. In the Framingham study, a threefold increase in the incidence of CAD was reported for middle-aged males with arterial pressures exceeding 160/95 mmHg compared with those having blood pressures of 140/90 mmHg or less.[11] The cause of hypertension in 90 percent of those affected is unknown, but it is usually controllable with diet or medication.[12]

The stress of a constantly elevated blood pressure increases the rate of atherosclerotic development. Atherosclerosis, in turn, causes narrowed, thickened arterial walls and decreases the distensibility and elasticity of vessels. More force is required to pump blood through diseased arterial vasculature, and this increased force is reflected in a higher blood pressure. This increased work load is also manifested by an enlarged heart (cardiac hypertrophy) and/or a loss of efficiency with each contraction. Salt intake is positively correlated with elevated blood pressure due to fluid retention, adding volume and increasing peripheral resistance to the cardiac work load.

Smoking

The third primary risk factor in CAD is cigarette smoking. Pipe and cigar smokers are not at increased risk because they do not usually inhale. The risk of developing CAD is two to six times higher in smokers than in nonsmokers.[13] Risk is proportional to the number of cigarettes smoked. Cessation of smoking has been shown to reduce the risk to nonsmoker levels.

Nicotine in the cigarette smoke causes catecholamine (epinephrine, norepinephrine) release. These hormones cause an increased heart rate, increased blood pressure, and peripheral vasoconstriction. These changes increase the cardiac work load, necessitating greater myocardial oxygen consumption.

Carbon monoxide, a by-product of combustion, affects the oxygen-carrying capacity of hemoglobin by reducing the sites available for oxygen transport. Thus, the effects of an increased cardiac work load, combined with the oxygen-depleting effect of carbon monoxide from smoking, significantly decrease the oxygen available to the myocardium.

Obesity

Obesity is defined as a weight 30 percent or more than that considered standard for an individual's height and body build. The mortality from CAD is statistically higher in obese persons than in those of normal weight. The increased risk is proportional to the degree of obesity. However, obesity in the absence of other high-risk factors probably subjects a person to only a modest increase in risk.[14] Obesity is often associated with hypertension. The risk of developing hypertension is three times greater in obese individuals than in those with normal weight. Obesity does not lead to hypertension, but hypertension is present in 60 percent of obese clients.[15] As obesity increases, the heart size grows, causing increased myocardial oxygen consumption. In addition, obesity increases the work load of the heart because of the greater peripheral vascular resistance.

Sedentary lifestyle

A sedentary lifestyle implies a lack of adequate physical exercise on a regular basis. Some practitioners define regular physical exercise as exercise that occurs at least 3 times per week for at least 30 minutes, causing perspiration and an increase in the heart rate by 30 to 50 beats per minute (bpm). The role of physical activity, or the lack of it, as a cardiac risk factor is complex, and the study of this factor is only beginning. There is evidence to suggest that physically inactive persons are more prone to develop CAD. Some occupational studies have indicated that jobs involving heavy physical activity are associated with a lower risk than sedentary jobs, but a confounding variable is socioeconomic status, which may be responsible for some of the risk association.[16]

The mechanism by which a sedentary lifestyle predisposes to CAD is still unknown. It is possible that (1) physically active people have increased HDL levels and that (2) exercise enhances fibrinolytic activity, thus reducing the risk of clot formation. The theory that exercise encourages the development of collateral circulation has not been effectively demonstrated in humans.

Exercise training for those who are physically inactive is thought to minimize the risk of CAD through more efficient lipid metabolism and more efficient oxygen extraction from the working muscle groups, thereby decreasing the cardiac work load. It may be observed that physically active people are seldom obese, thus diminishing two risk factors in CAD.

Stress and behavior patterns

The Framingham study provides evidence that certain behaviors and lifestyles are conducive to the development of CAD.[17] Type A and type B behaviors were described by Friedman and Rosenman in the 1960s and were further elaborated in the 1970s by Jenkins and Zyzanski. Type A behaviors include perfectionism and a hard-working, driving personality. Type A people suppress anger and hostility, have a sense of time urgency, are impatient, and create stress and tension within themselves, often when a situation does not warrant it (Table 27-3). They are more prone to heart attacks than type B people. Type B people are more easygoing; they take upsets in stride, know their limitations, take time to relax, are not overachievers, and are able to keep priorities in perspective. Although not all characteristics are present in one person all the time, people *tend* to be type A or type B.

In the Framingham study, type A women manifested twice the incidence of CAD and three times the incidence of angina of type B women. Among type A men, there was a twofold risk of angina, MI, and CAD compared to type B men.[18]

Sympathetic stimulation and its effect on the heart is generally considered to be the physiological mechanism by which stress predisposes to the development of CAD. Sympathetic stimulation causes an increased release of epinephrine and norepinephrine from the adrenal medulla. This stimulation influences the heart by increasing the heart rate and intensifying the force of myocardial contraction. Therefore, the demand for oxygen consumption greatly increases.

Table 27-3
Type A Personality Characteristics

Perfectionistic
Competitive
Aggressive
Constantly time-oriented
Has hurry sickness
Can never say "no"
Compulsive
Impatient
Always tense
Unduly irritable
Obsessed with number of:
- Sales made
- Articles written
- Clients seen
- Forms completed

Holds feelings in
Never has leisure time
Rarely takes a relaxing vacation or any vacation

Adapted from Meyer Friedman and Ray H. Roseman, *Type A Behavior and Your Heart*, Fawcett Publications, Inc., Greenwich, Conn. 1974.

Health Promotion and Maintenance Related to Risk Factors

The appropriate management of risk factors in CAD may prevent, modify, or retard the progression of the disease. In the United States during the past 20 to 30 years, there has been a gradual and persistent decline in coronary deaths.

Identification of high-risk individuals

In both the acute-care setting and the community, the nurse needs to identify individuals at high risk for CAD. Screening for high risk involves obtaining personal and family histories. Clients are questioned about a family history of heart disease in parents, grandparents, or siblings. The presence of any cardiovascular symptoms should be noted. Environmental factors such as eating habits, type of diet, and level of exercise are assessed to elicit lifestyle patterns. A psychosocial history is included to determine smoking habits, alcohol ingestion, type A behaviors, recent life stresses (events), sleeping habits, and the presence of anxiety and/or depression. The place of work and type of work can yield important information on the kind of activity performed, exposure to pollutants, allergens, or noxious chemicals, and the degree of emotional stress associated with employment.

The interviewer seeks to identify the client's attitudes and beliefs about health and illness. This information can give some indication of how disease and lifestyle changes may affect the client and can reveal the client's misconceptions about heart disease. Knowledge of the client's educational background is frequently helpful in deciding at what level to begin teaching. If the client is on medications, it is important to know what they are, when they are taken, and what the client's attitude is regarding taking medications.

Management of high-risk individuals

Once high-risk persons are identified, preventive measures can be taken. Risk factors such as age, sex, and genetic inheritance cannot be modified. However, the individual with any of these risk factors can modify the risk of CAD by controlling or changing the additive effects of modifiable risk factors. For example, a young male with a family history of heart disease can decrease the risk of an MI by maintaining an ideal weight, getting adequate physical exercise, and reducing his intake of saturated fats.

Individuals who have modifiable risk factors need to be encouraged and motivated to make changes in their lifestyle to reduce the risk of heart disease. The nurse can play a major role in teaching health-promoting behaviors to individuals at risk for CAD (Table 27-4). For highly motivated people, knowing *how* to reduce this risk may be the only information needed to make changes.

For those who are less motivated to assume responsibility for their health, the idea of risk factor reduction may be so remote that they are unable to bring the threat of CAD into their real world. Especially in the absence of symptoms, few people desire to make lifestyle changes. The nurse should first assist these people in clarifying their personal values. Then, by explaining the risk factors and having them identify

Table 27-4
Management of Risk Factors in Coronary Artery Disease

Risk Factor	Health-Promoting Behaviors
Hypertension	Have regular blood pressure checkups Take prescribed medications for blood pressure control Reduce salt intake Stop smoking Control or reduce weight
Smoking	Enroll in a structured program to stop smoking if a support system is needed Change daily routines associated with smoking to reduce the desire to smoke Substitute other activities for smoking Ask family members to support efforts to stop smoking
Obesity	Change eating patterns and habits (See Chap. 60) Reduce calorie intake Exercise regularly to increase calorie expenditure Avoid fad and crash diets, which are not effective in the long run Avoid large, heavy meals
Diabetes mellitus	Follow the recommended diet Weight reduction and/or diet control often control the disease Test urine glucose regularly to ensure control of disease See Chap. 41
Elevated serum lipids	Reduce animal (saturated) fat intake Reduce total fat intake Adjust total calorie intake to achieve and maintain ideal body weight Increase amount of complex carbohydrates and vegetable proteins in diet
Sedentary lifestyle	Develop and maintain a routine for physical activity that is done at least 3 times per week Increase activities to a fitness level (see Table 27-14 for the relative merit of various exercises)
Stressful lifestyle	Increase awareness of behaviors that are detrimental to health Alter patterns that are conducive to stress and rushing (e.g., get up 30 min earlier so that breakfast is not eaten in transit to work, take 20 min/day to meditate) Set realistic goals for self and others Reassess priorities in light of health needs Learn to cope with unavoidable stress Avoid excessive and/or prolonged stress Plan time for adequate rest and sleep

their own vulnerability to various risks, the nurse may help them to recognize their susceptibility to CAD. Some people will prove recalcitrant until they begin to manifest overt symptoms or actually suffer an infarction. Other individuals, having suffered a heart attack, find the idea of changing lifelong habits totally unacceptable. The nurse must be able to identify such attitudes and respect them as human rights.

Physical fitness in the community

The last two decades have seen a surge of interest in attaining and maintaining health. Physical fitness has become a field of major importance. Communities are developing exercise programs for persons of all ages and with all health needs, ranging from "slimnastic" classes to cardiac walking-jogging programs. Local YMCAs often sponsor exercise classes, jogging courses, bicycling courses, and related events. Jogging has become almost a science. The American Heart Association takes pride in its annual "Run for Your Life" race as well as other events dramatizing the need for physical activity to promote health. Many large corporations provide gyms where their employees can exercise.

Health education in schools

The recent awareness of the body and physical health is also seen in school systems. School nurses have a receptive and captive audience to whom they teach health practices. Besides teaching physical fitness topics, the school nurse can inform students on how the body functions and responds to daily living. Lifestyle habits can be positively influenced at early ages to decrease the need for drastic changes later in life that confront the student's parents. The school nurse must take advantage of the social climate that promotes health and health practices and find innovative ways to present these values to a receptive, youthful audience before their habits become inflexible.

Pharmacological Management of Risk Factors

Various pharmacological agents are available to treat hyperlipidemia. Lipid-lowering drugs are usually reserved for clients in whom diet control, weight control, and cessation of smoking have not been effective. Lipid-lowering agents can be classified as (1) drugs that restrict lipoprotein production and (2) drugs that increase lipoprotein removal.

Drugs that restrict lipoprotein production

Drugs that restrict lipoprotein production include nicotinic acid (Niacin) and clofibrate (Atromid). Nicotinic acid is effective in lowering both cholesterol and triglycerides by interfering with their synthesis. Many clients refuse to take it because it can cause severe flushing, pruritus, and gastrointestinal (GI) distress. Clofibrate is effective primarily in lowering serum triglyceride levels and has some cholesterol-lowering activity as well. It appears to act by decreasing the synthesis of lipids. Side effects include malaise, nausea, diarrhea, and occasional increases in liver enzymes.

Drugs that increase lipoprotein removal

Drugs that increase lipoprotein removal include cholestyramine (Questran) and colestipol (Colestid). Cholestyramine is a bile-acid binding resin which lowers cholesterol in the GI tract and prevents its absorption into the blood. The drug has an offensive taste and smell. It also interferes with the absorption of many other drugs, such as digoxin, antibiotics, and diuretics. Colestipol is similar to cholestyramine but is tasteless and odorless.

Dextrothyroxine (Choloxin) has also been used to treat hyperlipidemia. It increases the metabolism of cholesterol and its excretion via the biliary tract.

Dietary Management of Risk Factors

Clients with elevated serum cholesterol and triglyceride levels should first achieve a normal weight if they exceed it. Then they should be maintained on a diet emphasizing a decreased intake of saturated fat and cholesterol (see Appendix B, Table 3). Meats, eggs, and milk products are major sources of saturated fat and cholesterol. If the serum triglyceride level is elevated, alcohol intake should be reduced or eliminated. Although there is no conclusive relationship between sodium intake and hypertension, the client at risk for CAD should avoid excessive sodium intake.

The role of dietary management is not yet well defined. None of the current dietary regimens used to treat hyperlipidemia have demonstrated a significant reduction in morbidity and mortality from CAD.

ANGINA PECTORIS

Angina pectoris is literally translated as pain (angina) in the chest (pectoris). More specifically, angina pectoris is transient chest pain due to myocardial ischemia. It usually lasts for only a few (3 to 5) minutes and commonly subsides when the precipitating factor (usually exertion) is relieved.

Pathophysiology

Myocardial ischemia develops when the demand for myocardial oxygen exceeds the ability of the coronary arteries to supply it (Table 27-5). The primary reason for insufficient flow is coronary artery narrowing by atherosclerosis. Normally, the myocardium extracts about 75 percent of the available oxygen from the coronary circulation. If myocardial oxygen needs are not met from this near-maximal extraction, then coronary blood flow can be increased through vasodilatation.

In persons with CAD, the coronary arteries are unable to dilate in order to meet metabolic needs. This creates an oxygen deficit. In addition to atherosclerotic stenosis, oxygen deficit is caused by coronary artery spasm and coronary thrombosis. In coronary artery spasm, the constriction is transient and revers-

Table 27-5
Factors Determining Myocardial Oxygen Needs

Decreased Oxygen Supply	Increased Oxygen Demand or Consumption
1. ↓ Hematocrit	1. ↑ Heart rate
2. ↓ Hemoglobin-binding capacity	2. ↑ Contractility
3. ↓ Coronary blood flow	3. ↑ Wall tension (left ventricular wall)
a. ↑ Diastolic pressure, filling time	a. ↑ Systolic BP
b. ↑ Coronary vascular resistance	b. ↑ Ventricular volume
c. Coronary spasm	c. ↑ Myocardial wall thickness
d. ↓ Blood volume (low-flow state)	

ible, and causes either subtotal or total narrowing of the coronary artery. The duration of the spasm determines whether the myocardium will sustain ischemia (not resulting in cell death) or actual infarction (resulting in cell death).[19]

Coronary thrombosis resulting from ulceration of a plaque, with subsequent fibrin and platelet aggregation leading to clot formation, was formerly thought to be the cause of coronary occlusion. It is now known that thrombosis, stenosis, and spasm are all causes of coronary occlusion and the resulting angina pectoris.

Other factors responsible for a discrepancy between myocardial oxygen needs and oxygen supply include low blood pressure, low blood volume, drugs causing vasoconstriction, valvular disorders, and aortic stenosis. Anemia, oxyhemoglobin disorders, and chronic lung disease may also contribute to myocardial ischemia.[20]

Ischemia causes transient left ventricular dysfunction, resulting in an increased left ventricular diastolic pressure. Ischemia also causes elevated pulmonary capillary wedge pressure and elevated right heart pressure. These three factors eventually increase the oxygen deficit of the myocardium. Arrhythmias may occur in the presence of myocardial ischemia due to cellular irritability. Arrhythmias decrease the efficiency of the cardiac pump and thereby increase the need for myocardial oxygen while decreasing the available supply.

On the cellular level, the myocardium becomes cyanotic within the first 10 seconds of coronary occlusion. Electrocardiographic changes will appear. With total occlusion of the coronary arteries, contractility ceases after several minutes, depriving the myocardial cells of glucose for aerobic metabolism. Anaerobic metabolism begins, and lactic acid accumulates. Myocardial nerve fibers are irritated by the increased lactic acid and transmit a pain message to the cardiac nerves and upper thoracic posterior roots (the reason for referred cardiac pain to the left shoulder and arm). Under ischemic conditions, cardiac cells are viable for about 20 minutes. With restoration of blood flow, aerobic metabolism resumes and contractility is restored. Cellular repair also begins.

Precipitating factors

Extracardiac factors may precipitate myocardial ischemia and anginal pain. These including the following:

1. *Physical exertion*, which increases the heart rate. Increasing the heart rate decreases the time the heart spends in diastole, which is the time of greatest coronary blood flow. Walking outdoors is the most common form of exertion which produces an attack.
2. *Strong emotions*, which stimulate the sympathetic nervous system and increase the work of the heart by increasing the heart rate, blood pressure, and myocardial contractility.
3. *Consumption of a heavy meal* (especially if the person exerts himself afterward), which can increase the work of the heart. During the digestive process, blood is diverted to the GI system, causing a low flow rate in the coronary arteries.
4. *Cold weather*, which increases the work load of the heart due to the growing peripheral vascular resistance (blood vessels constrict in response to a cold stimulus). Cold weather also causes increased metabolism to maintain internal temperature regulation.
5. *Cigarette smoking*, which causes vasoconstriction and an increased heart rate due to nicotine's stimulation of catecholamine release. It also diminishes available oxygen by increasing the level of carbon monoxide.
6. *Sexual activity*, which increases the cardiac work load and sympathetic stimulation. In a person with severe CAD, the resulting extra work load of the heart may precipitate angina.

Types of Angina

Stable angina

Stable angina (classic) refers to chest pain occurring intermittently over a long period of time with the same pattern of onset, duration, and intensity of symptoms. The discomfort may be mild or severe and disabling, but it is usually infrequent because the person restricts his activities so as not to precipitate pain.

Unstable angina

Unstable angina (progressive or *crescendo angina)* is different from stable angina. Its frequency, duration, and intensity of symptoms increase dramatically (usually over a 3-month period) as the disease in the vessels rapidly progresses, culminating in infarction within 18 months after its onset. Prolonged bouts of chest pain (lasting for 20 minutes or longer) are considered unstable angina and treated as such.

Prinzmetal's angina

Prinzmetal's angina (variant angina) occurs at rest, usually due to spasm of a major coronary artery which causes pain and a marked transient ST-segment elevation. (This contrasts to the characteristic ST-segment depression of the typical effort angina syndrome.) The pain may occur during rapid eye movement (REM) sleep when myocardial oxygen consumption increases; it may be relieved by some form of exercise or may disappear spontaneously. Cyclical, short bursts of pain at a usual time each day may also occur with this type of angina.[21]

Nocturnal angina and angina decubitus

Nocturnal angina occurs only at night, but not necessarily in the recumbent position or during sleep. *Angina decubitus* is chest pain that occurs only while lying down and is usually relieved by standing or sitting.

Clinical Manifestations

The most common initial symptom of a client with angina is chest pain or discomfort. The exact cause of the pain is unknown, but neurogenic pain at the site of ischemia is most likely. On direct questioning, some clients may deny feeling pain but will refer to a vague sensation, strange feeling, pressure, or ache in the chest. It is an unpleasant feeling often described as a constrictive, squeezing, heavy, choking, or suffocating sensation. Many people complain of severe indigestion or burning. Although most of the discomfort experienced by people with angina appears substernally, the sensation may occur in the neck or radiate to the shoulders and down the arms (Fig. 27-6). Often, people will complain of pain between the shoulder blades and dismiss it as not being heart pain. Depending on the severity of the anginal attack, the person may remain motionless or may clench a fist over the sternal area. Persons experiencing angina often refer to a feeling of anxiety and impending doom. Relief of classic angina pectoris is usually obtained with rest or cessation of activity.

Complications

Arrhythmias, such as premature contractions or fibrillations, may occur in a person with angina. The cells deprived of oxygen and nutrients may become irritable and develop into sites for ectopic pacemaker cells.

Because some anginal pains may be vague, the client may not perceive it as important, dismiss its occurrence, proceed with an activity, and sustain an MI. (If ischemia persists in the presence of an increased myocardial oxygen demand, then MI will occur.) When chest pain is reported to a health care provider, the diagnosis of angina may not be the first consideration since many problems can mimic midthoracic discomfort (Table 27-6).

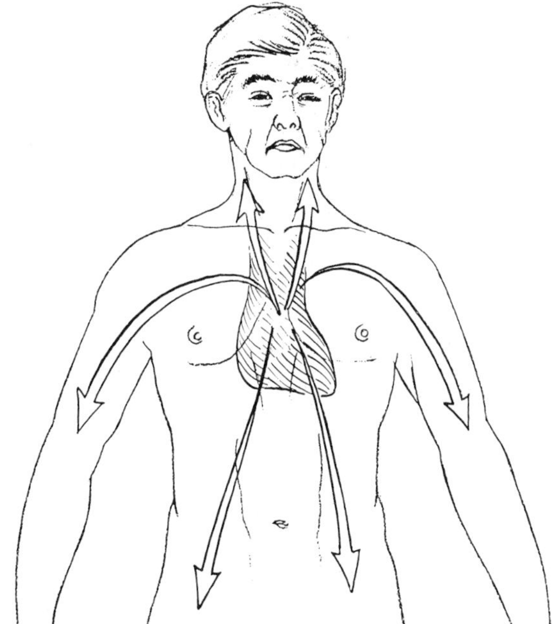

Figure 27-6 Location of chest pain and other symptoms during angina or MI. *(Mayo Clinic.)*

Medical Management

Diagnostic

When a client presents with a history indicating CAD, the physician may take several courses of action (Table 27-7). After a detailed history and physical examination are done, a chest x-ray is usually taken to look for cardiac enlargement, cardiac calcifications, and pulmonary congestion. Laboratory tests may be done to ascertain serum lipid and enzyme values. Serum lipid levels are assessed to screen for positive risk factors, and enzyme levels are checked to rule out the occurrence of infarction. An electrocardiogram (ECG) may be done and compared to an earlier tracing when possible.

More frequently now, treadmill exercise testing is done for clients with stable angina to examine ST-segment changes during exercise as an indirect assessment of coronary artery obstruction. Severely abnormal ECGs on exercise testing, indicating gross disease processes, may show the need for angiography. Unfortunately, the ECG stress test is not always conclusive for CAD. A false-positive reaction may be found (especially in women), and a false-negative reaction may be seen if the client is exercised submaximally.

If the client is not elderly and if there are no other significant health problems, the physician may propose coronary angiography. This study allows visuali-

Table 27-6
Comparison of the Pain of Angina Pectoris and Myocardial Infarction

Angina	Myocardial Infarction
Precipitating Factors	
Stress, either physiological (exertion) or psychological Digestion of a heavy meal Valsalva maneuvers during micturition or defecation Extremes of weather Hot baths or showers Sexual excitation	May occur with exertion or at rest May be precipitated by physical or emotional stress Often there are no precipitating factors
Location	
Midanterior chest Substernal Abdominal with radiation to neck, back, arms, fingers Diffuse, not easily located	Midanterior chest Substernal Subscapular Midscapular Radiation to neck and jaw or down arm(s) to fingers
Description	
Deep sensation of tightness or a squeezing feeling Mild to moderate in severity or pressure Attacks are usually similar each time	Severe pressure, squeezing, or heaviness with a crushing, oppressive quality Clients report that they would rather die than have such a pain again
Onset and Duration	
Onset can be either gradual or sudden Pain usually lasts for 15 min or less (usually no more than 30 min) Sometimes reported as "twinges"	Onset is sudden May last for 30 min to 2 h Not relieved by rest or nitroglycerin Client may report residual "soreness" for several days following MI
Associated Clinical Manifestations	
Apprehension Dyspnea Diaphoresis Nausea Desire to void Belching	Apprehension Nausea and vomiting Dyspnea Diaphoresis Extreme fatigue Once pain abates, dizziness or faintness occurs

zation of the coronary arteries for obstruction and helps to determine the prognosis.

Therapeutic

The most common initial medical intervention for angina is the use of nitrate therapy for enhancing coronary blood flow (Table 27-7). This is discussed under Pharmacological Intervention.

Generally, coronary artery bypass surgery is recommended if the client is under the age of 65 and has (1) significant left main coronary artery obstruction, (2) double- or triple-vessel disease, or (3) single-vessel disease involving the proximal left anterior descending coronary artery. Bypass surgery is usually recommended for those persons with unstable angina who demonstrate a poor response to medical therapy.[22] The success of such treatment varies. (Coronary bypass surgery is discussed in Chap. 28.)

Pharmacological Intervention

Nitrates

The first line of pharmacological intervention for angina consists of the *nitrates*, which are commonly classified as vasodilators. Nitrates produce their principal effects by:

1. Dilating peripheral blood vessels, which results in decreased peripheral resistance, venous pooling, and decreased venous blood return to the heart. Therefore, myocardial oxygen requirements are lessened due to the reduced cardiac work load.
2. Dilating coronary arteries and/or collateral vessels. This may increase blood flow to the ischemic areas of the heart. However, when the coronary arteries are severely atherosclerotic, the mechanism of coronary dilatation is difficult to demonstrate.

Nitroglycerin Nitroglycerin given sublingually will usually relieve pain in about 3 minutes but has a duration of approximately 45 minutes. The usual recommended dosage is one tablet taken sublingually, which can be followed at 5-minute intervals with two more doses. If nitroglycerin tablets have been necessary and relief from anginal pain has not been obtained, the client should be instructed to seek medical attention.

Nitroglycerin can be used prophylactically prior to undertaking an activity which the client knows may precipitate an anginal attack. In these instances, the client can take a tablet 5 to 10 minutes before beginning the activity.

Nitroglycerin tables are marketed in light-resistant bottles closed with metal caps. Since they tend to lose potency, the client should be advised to purchase a new supply every 6 to 9 months.

Nitroglycerin Ointment (Nitrol, Nitropaste) A 2% nitroglycerin topical ointment is dosed by the inch. It is placed on the skin (preferably the chest), where it is absorbed slowly, producing anginal prophylaxis for 3 to 6 hours. It has been found especially useful for nocturnal and unstable angina because it acts for a longer period of time than sublingual nitroglycerin.

Long-Acting Nitrates Long-acting nitrates, such as isosorbide dinitrate (Isordil, Sorbitrate), are longer-acting than nitroglycerin and, when used in adequate doses, are effective in reducing the incidence of anginal attacks. Their mechanisms of action and side effects are similar to those of nitroglycerin. The effects of oral isosorbide dinitrate may last for up to 8 hours.

Because of the vasodilating properties of nitrates, the predominant side effect of nitrate drugs is headache from the vasodilatation of cerebral blood vessels. This problem can be alleviated by reducing the dosage. Sometimes the body can build up a tolerance for the drug, so that the headache abates but the principal antianginal effect is still present. Other complications of the vasodilator drugs are orthostatic hypotension (nitrate syncope) and an aggravation of cerebral vascular insufficiency.

Table 27-7
Medical Management: Angina Pectoris

Diagnostic
1. History and physical examination
2. Chest x-ray
3. ECG
4. Serum enzyme level tests (CPK, SGOT, LDH)
5. Serum lipid level tests
6. Exercise stress tests
7. Angiography studies

Therapeutic
For acute angina attacks:
1. Nitroglycerin

For chronic anginal prophylaxis:
1. Nitroglycerin ointment (e.g., Nitrol)
2. Long-acting nitrates (Isordil, Sorbitrate)
3. Beta-adrenergic blocking agents
4. Calcium-blocking agents

Beta-adrenergic blocking agents

Beta-blocking agents available for the prophylaxis of angina are *propranolol (Inderal), metoprolol (Lopressor), nadolol (Corgard), atenolol (Tenormin), and timolol (Blocadren)*. These drugs produce a direct decrease in myocardial contractility, heart rate, peripheral resistance, and blood pressure, all of which reduce the myocardial oxygen demand. Side effects of the beta blockers include bradycardia, hypotension, wheezing, and GI complaints. The beta blockers should not be discontinued abruptly without medical supervision.

Calcium-blocking agents

Calcium-blocking agents such as nifedipine (Procardia) and verapamil (Calan, Isopin) have been recently used in the treatment of angina. These agents act at the cellular level by selectively blocking calcium access to the contractile force in the arterial cell. Through this action coronary artery spasm can be prevented, myocardial O_2 supply is increased, and peripheral arteries are dilated, resulting in reduced afterload and decreased myocardial O_2 demand.

Nursing Management

Acute intervention

Some of the main nursing objectives for the client with angina are pain assessment, evaluation of treatment, and reinforcement of appropriate therapy. Because chest pain can be due to many factors other than ischemia (e.g., pericarditis, valvular disease, pulmonary artery stenosis, MI, and congestive cardiomyopathy), it is important to have a clear understanding of the client's chest pain. By the questions a nurse asks, a history of anginal pain may be revealed. The nurse should determine if breathing in or out or changing positions makes the client's chest pain better or worse. Anginal pain does not vary with body position or respirations. In contrast, the pain of pericarditis does. It should be ascertained if the pain is deep or superficial, mild or intense. Cardiac pain is usually described as deep and intense, but occasionally it may be characterized as a dull ache. Very few people can successfully ignore cardiac pain. The client should be asked if the pain is diffuse or well localized. Cardiac pain is usually diffuse. The client may rub the entire chest to explain where the pain is occurring.

If a nurse is present during an anginal attack, the following measures are instituted: (1) administration of oxygen, (2) prompt pain relief with a nitrate or narcotic analgesic, (3) determination of vital signs, (4) ECG, (5) physical assessment of the chest, and (6) comfortable positioning of the client. The client will most likely appear distressed and have pale, cool, clammy skin. The blood pressure and pulse will probably be elevated, and an atrial gallop (S_4) sound may be heard. If a ventricular gallop (S_3) is heard, it may indicate transient left ventricular decompensation. Supportive and realistic assurance, as well as a calm, soothing manner will help to reduce the client's anxiety.

The client needs to be instructed in the proper use of nitroglycerin. It should be easily accessible to the client at all times. For protection from degradation, it should be kept in a tightly closed dark glass bottle. The client should be instructed to place a nitroglycerin tablet beneath the tongue and allow it to dissolve. This may cause a fizzing or slightly warm feeling locally. The client should be warned that the heart rate may increase and a pounding headache, dizziness, or flushing may occur. The client should be cautioned against rising to a standing position quickly because postural hypotension after nitroglycerin ingestion is not uncommon. If the pain has not been relieved after 5 minutes, the client should be told to take another nitroglycerin tablet. This procedure may be repeated for pain relief every 5 minutes, not to exceed the ingestion of three tablets. If pain persists after three doses, the client should seek immediate medical attention.

Rehabilitative management

The client needs to be reassured that a long, productive life is possible even though he has angina. Prevention of angina is preferable to its treatment, and this is where instruction is important. The client needs to be educated regarding coronary artery disease and angina, precipitating factors, risk factors, and medications.

Client teaching can be handled in a variety of ways. One-to-one contact between nurse and client is often the most effective procedure. The time spent in providing daily care is often an ideal teaching period. Teaching tools such as pamphlets, films used at the bedside, a heart model, and especially written information are all necessary components of client and family education (see Chap. 5).

Clients need to be assisted in identifying factors that precipitate angina (see the section on Precipitating Factors). They should be given instruction on how to avoid or control precipitating factors. For example, they should be cautioned to avoid exposures to extremes of weather. They should be taught not to eat large, heavy meals. If a heavy meal is ingested, adequate rest should be planned for 1 to 2 hours after eating.

The client needs to be assisted in identifying personal risk factors in CAD. Once these risk factors are known, various methods of decreasing them should be discussed (Table 27-4).

Educating the client and family about diets that are low in sodium and reduced in saturated fats may be appropriate. Maintaining ideal body weight is most important in controlling angina, as weight above this level increases the myocardial work load and may cause pain. Eating large meals also contributes to angina, and clients may need to eat several small meals in place of three moderate to large meals each day.

Adhering to a regular, individualized exercise program which conditions the heart rather than overstressing the myocardium is most important. Nurses should consult with a physician or physical therapist in instructing the client regarding an exercise program. (This is discussed in the section on Rehabilitative Management of the client with MI.)

It is important to educate both the client and the family in the use of nitroglycerin. Nitroglycerin tablets or ointments may be used prophylactically, such as prior to an emotionally stressful situation, before sexual intercourse, or before physical exertion (e.g., climbing a long flight of stairs).

Counseling should be provided to assess the psychological adjustment of the client and family to the diagnosis of CAD and the resulting angina pectoris. Many clients feel stripped of their identity and self-esteem and unable to fulfill their role in society. These emotions are normal and very real.

MYOCARDIAL INFARCTION

MI occurs when ischemic intracellular changes become irreversible and necrosis results. As described earlier, angina due to ischemia causes reversible cellular injury. Infarction is the result of sustained ischemia, causing irreversible cellular death (Fig. 27-7).

Mortality among clients with acute MI is approximately 30 to 40 percent. A substantial number of these deaths occur prior to hospitalization. Mortality among clients who reach the hospital is about 20 percent. Most of these deaths occur within the first 3 to 4 days.[23]

Pathophysiology

Cardiac cells can withstand ischemic conditions for about 20 minutes before cellular death (necrosis) takes place. Contractile function of the heart stops in the areas of myocardial necrosis. The degree of altered function depends on the area of the heart involved and the size of the infarct. Most infarcts involve the left ventricle. A *transmural MI* occurs when the entire thickness of the myocardium in a region is involved (Fig. 27-8). A *subendocardial MI* exists when the damage has not penetrated through the entire thickness of the myocardial wall.

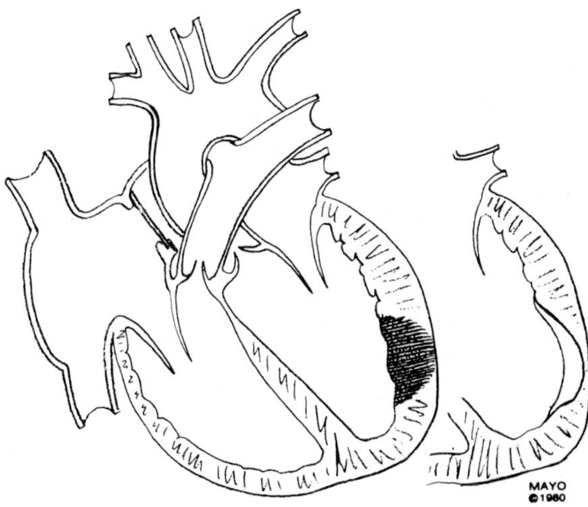

Figure 27-8 Transmural MI involving the thickness of the total wall. *(Mayo Clinic.)*

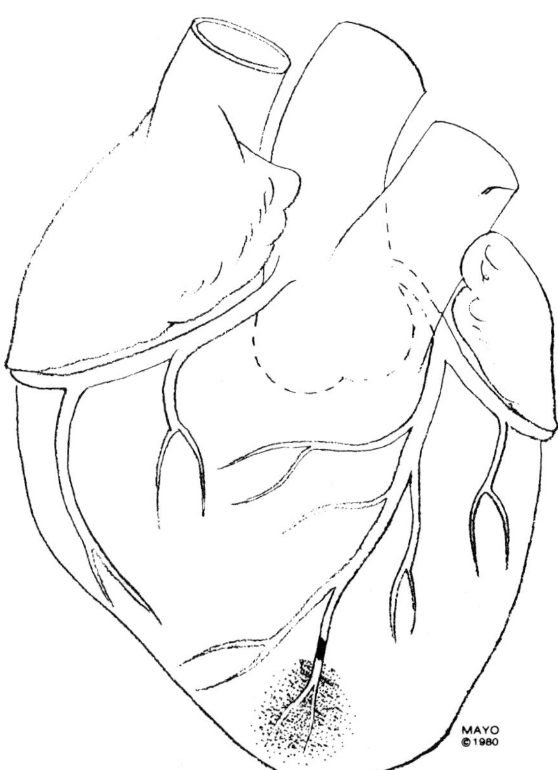

Figure 27-7 Occlusion of coronary artery, causing MI. *(Mayo Clinic.)*

Common areas of infarction are described as anterior, inferior, lateral, or posterior wall infarctions. Common combinations of areas are the anterior-lateral or anterior-septal MI. An inferior MI is also called a *diaphragmatic MI (DMI)* (Fig. 27-9).

The location and area of the infarct correlate with the part of the coronary circulation involved (Fig. 25-4). For example, inferior wall infarctions are usually due to right coronary artery lesions. Anterior wall infarctions are usually due to lesions in the left anterior ascending artery.

The degree of preestablished collateral circulation will also determine the severity of infarction. In individuals with a history of heart disease, adequate collateral channels may have been established which provide the area surrounding the infarction with some blood supply and oxygen. This is one explanation of why younger individuals who have a severe MI are often more likely to have a more serious impairment than an older individual with the same degree of infarction.

Healing process

As described in Chap. 9, the body's response to cell death is the inflammatory process. Within 24 hours, leukocytes infiltrate the area. Enzymes are released from the dead cardiac cells and are important diagnostic indicators (see Clinical Manifestations). The proteolytic enzymes of the neutrophils remove all necrotic tissue by the second or third day.

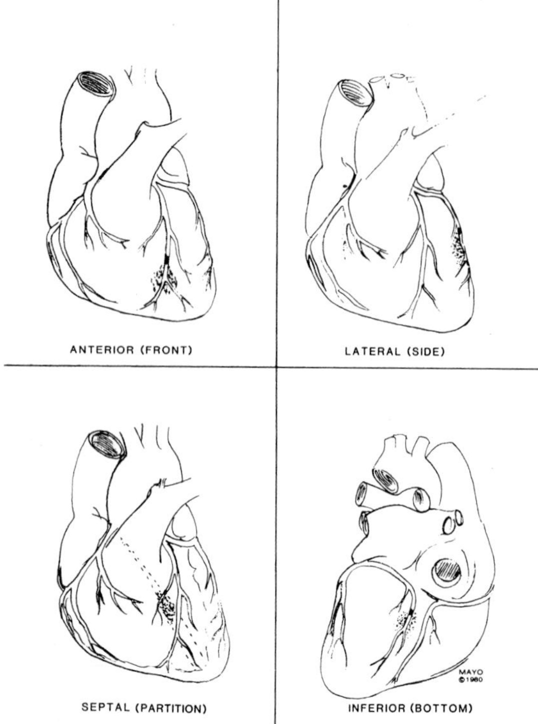

Figure 27-9 Four common locations where MI occurs. *(Mayo Clinic.)*

During this time, the necrotic muscle wall is thin. The development of collateral circulation will improve areas of poor perfusion and may limit the zones of injury and infarction. Once infarction takes place, cate cholamine-mediated lipolysis and glycogenolysis occur. These processes allow the increased plasma glucose and free fatty acids to be utilized by the oxygen-depleted myocardium for anaerobic metabolism. For this reason, serum glucose levels are frequently elevated post-MI and may be reponsible for a pseudodiabetic state.

Within 4 to 10 days, the necrotic zone is clearly identifiable by electrocardiographic changes or radionuclide imaging. At this point, the phagocytes (neutrophils and monocytes) have cleared the necrotic debris from the injured area, and the collagen matrix is laid down that will eventually form scar tissue.

At 10 to 14 days post-MI, the beginning scar tissue is still weak. The myocardium is considered to be especially vulnerable to increased stress because of the "mushy" state of the healing heart wall. (It is also at this time that the client may be increasing his activity level, so that special caution and assessment will be necessary.) By 6 weeks post-MI, scar tissue has replaced necrotic tissue. At this time, the injured area is said to be healed. The scarred area is often less compliant than the surrounding fibers. This condition may be manifested by uncoordinated wall motion, ventricular dysfunction, and/or pump failure.[24]

Clinical Manifestations

Pain

Severe, immobilizing chest pain is the hallmark of MI (Table 27-6). The pain is due to the inadequate oxygen supply to the myocardium. Persistent and unlike any other pain, it is usually described as a heaviness, tightness, or constriction. Common locations are substernal or retrosternal, radiating to the neck and arms or to the back. It may occur while the client is active or at rest, asleep or awake. It usually lasts for 20 minutes or more and is described as more severe than anginal pain.

The pain may be located atypically in the epigastric area. The client will take antacids without relief. Also infrequent is the atypical (or asymptomatic) MI. The client without a typical MI may not experience pain but may have profound weakness due to low cardiac output or syncope from severe bradycardia or tachycardia.

Nausea and vomiting

The client may be nauseated and vomit. Nausea and vomiting can result from reflex stimulation of the vomiting center by the severe pain (see Chap. 33). These symptoms can also result from vasovagal reflexes from the area of the infarcted myocardium which affect the GI tract.

Sympathetic stimulation

During the initial phases of MI, increased catecholamines (norepinephrine and epinephrine) are released. The increased sympathetic response results in diaphoresis and vasoconstriction of peripheral blood vessels. On physical examination, the client's skin will be ashen, clammy, and cool. This condition is often referred to as a "cold sweat."

Fever

The temperature may increase within the first 24 hours up to 38°C (100.4°F), and occasionally to 39°C (102.2°F). The temperature elevation may last for as long as 1 week. This increase in temperature is a systemic manifestation of the inflammatory process due to the infarcted myocardium.

Cardiovascular manifestations

The blood pressure and pulse will be elevated initially. Later, the blood pressure will drop due to decreased cardiac output. Urine output may be decreased. Rales may be noted in the lungs, persisting for several hours to several days. Hepatic engorgement and peripheral edema may indicate overt cardiac failure. Jugular neck veins may be distended and may have obvious pulsations, indicating early right ventricular dysfunction and pulmonary congestion.

Cardiac examination may reveal abnormal precordial movements suggestive of ventricular aneurysm. Heart sounds may seem distant, but close auscultation may reveal splitting of heart sounds, indicating left ventricular dysfunction. Other abnormal sounds suggesting ventricular dysfunction are S_4 (atrial gallop) and S_3 (ventricular gallop). In addition, the presence of murmurs indicates valve incompetency. A loud holosystolic apical murmur is due to papillary muscle rupture.

Complications

Arrhythmias

The most common complications post-MI are arrhythmias, found in 80 percent of MI clients. Arrhythmias are caused by any condition that affects the myocardial cell's sensitivity to nerve impulses, such as ischemia, electrolyte imbalances, and/or sympathetic nervous system stimulation. The intrinsic rhythm of the heartbeat is disrupted, causing either a very fast heart rate (tachycardia) or a very slow heart rate (bradycardia), both of which adversely affect the ischemic myocardium.

Life-threatening arrhythmias occur most often with anterior wall infarction, pump failure, and shock. Complete heart block is seen in massive infarction. Ventricular fibrillation, a common cause of sudden death, is a lethal arrhythmia. Premature ventricular contractions (PVCs) may precede ventricular tachycardia and fibrillation. Ventricular arrhythmias need immediate treatment. (See Chap. 28 for a detailed description of arrhythmias and their management.)

Heart failure

Heart failure is a complication that occurs when the pumping power of the left ventricle has diminished due to massive injury. It is common to see some degree of left ventricular dysfunction in the client with an acute MI in the first 24 hours. Depending on the severity and extent of the injury, heart failure will occur initially with subtle signs such as slight dyspnea, restlessness, agitation, or slight tachycardia. Jugular vein distension from right-sided heart failure, rales heard in the lungs, distension of upper lobe veins on an upright chest x-ray, and the presence of an S_3 or S_4 heart sound may indicate the onset of heart failure. (The treatment of acute heart failure is discussed in Chap. 28.)

Cardiogenic shock

Cardiogenic shock occurs when inadequate oxygen and nutrients are supplied to the tissues due to heart failure. It appears when there is dysfunction of much of the left ventricle due to infarction. Cardiogenic shock occurs in 10 to 15 percent of clients hospitalized with acute MI. (The treatment of cardiogenic shock is described in Chap. 28.)

Papillary muscle dysfunction

Papillary muscle dysfunction may occur if the infarcted area includes or is adjacent to these structures. Papillary muscle dysfunction causes mitral regurgitation, which increases the volume of blood in the left ventricle. This condition aggravates an already compromised left ventricle. It is detected by a systolic murmur at the cardiac apex radiating toward the axilla. *Papillary muscle rupture* is a severe complication causing massive mitral regurgitation, which results in dyspnea, gross pulmonary edema, and decreased cardiac output. Treatment consists of (1) rapid afterload reduction with nitroprusside and (2) immediate open heart surgery with mitral valve replacement.

Ventricular aneurysm

Ventricular aneurysm results when the infarcted myocardial wall becomes thinned and bulges out during contraction (Fig. 27-10). In the acute stage post-MI, this is called an *ischemic bulge*. If the aneurysm still exists after scar tissue is laid down, then it is called a *ventricular aneurysm*. Ventricular aneurysms are identified by palpation of ectopic impulses, bulges seen on x-ray or fluoroscopy, or persistent, long-term ST-segment changes on an ECG. Ventricular angiography can definitively diagnose ventricular aneurysm.

The client with a ventricular aneurysm may experience intractable failure, arrhythmias, and angina. Besides ventricular rupture, which is fatal, ventricular aneurysms harbor thrombi, cause arrhythmias, and promote left ventricular dysfunction. Surgical excision is the treatment for ventricular aneurysms severe enough to cause dysfunction.

Pericarditis

Pericarditis, an inflammation of the pericardium, is a common complication occurring 2 to 3 days after infarction. Pain is localized and is quite alarming to the client, who fears reinfarction. It is usually located in the precardial area and is accompanied by a friction rub. (This is different from infarction pain.) The pain is relieved by sitting up and is aggravated by deep

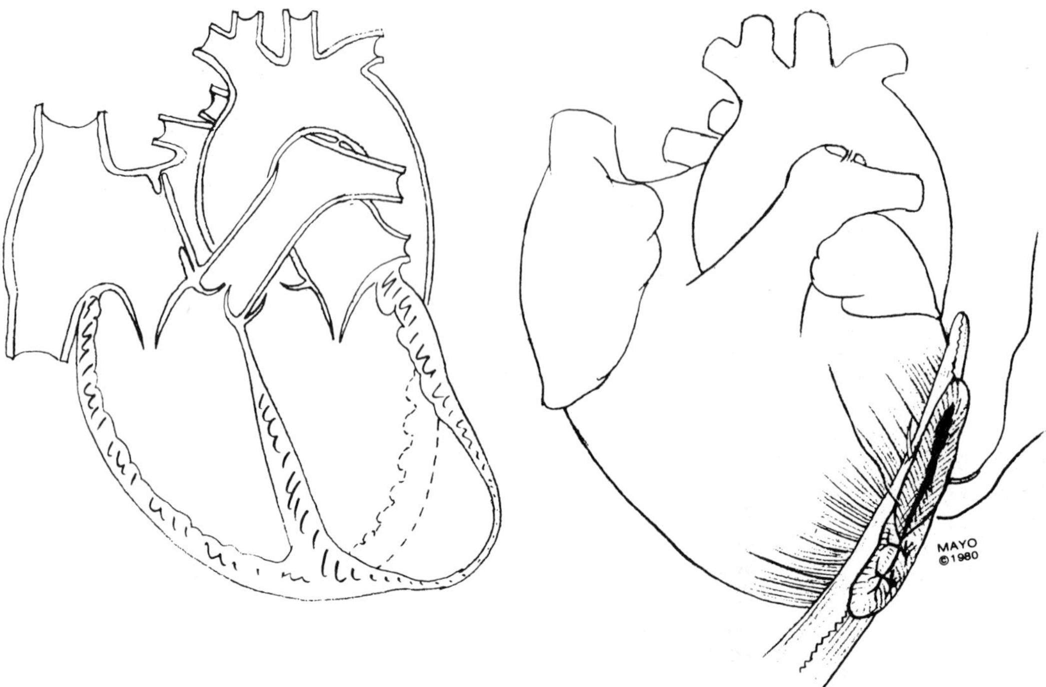

Figure 27-10 Ventricular aneurysm and surgical repair. *(Mayo Clinic.)*

inspiration. Aspirin, steroids, or indomethacin (Indocin) relieve the pain. Anticoagulants are usually discontinued to prevent pericardial bleeding.

Pulmonary embolism

Pulmonary embolism may be seen in the client with acute MI who has had bouts of congestive heart failure or has been extremely immobile because of prolonged bed rest. The source of the thrombus may be the roughened endocardium or leg veins. Early detection of emboli is accomplished by observing for pallor or cyanosis, heart failure unresponsive to treatment, and an unexplained pleural effusion. Acute massive pulmonary embolism causes sudden, severe dyspnea and is usually fatal. (Pulmonary emboli are discussed in more detail in Chap. 30.)

Dressler syndrome

Dressler syndrome (post-MI syndrome) is pericarditis with effusion and fever that develops 1 to 4 weeks post-MI. It is thought to be due to an antigen-antibody reaction to the necrotic myocardium. The client experiences pericardial pain, fever, a friction rub, left pleural effusion, and arthralgia. Laboratory findings include an elevated white blood cell (WBC) count and an elevated sedimentation rate. Steroids are used to treat this condition.

Abnormal Diagnostic Findings

The most important diagnostic laboratory measurement is that of the serum enzymes, especially lactic dehydrogenase (LDH), serum glutamic-oxaloacetic transaminase (SGOT), and creatine phosphokinase (CPK). When cardiac cells die, their cellular enzymes are released. The increase in these enzymes over their normal levels can demonstrate if cardiac damage has occurred and indicate the approximate extent or severity of the damage. (Figure 27-11 indicates the peak level and duration of these enzymes in the presence of MI.) These enzyme values must be interpreted with great care since other associated conditions can cause increased enzyme levels (e.g., hepatic congestion, pulmonary embolism, and intramuscular injections).

CPK begins to rise at about 6 hours post-MI and returns to normal 2 to 3 days thereafter. This enzyme is a more specific diagnostic indicator than LDH or SGOT because it comes primarily from the heart, skeletal muscle, and brain. (SGOT and LDH are found in large quantities in liver cells.) The MB fractions of CPK are found only in the myocardium. When they are elevated, the information obtained from CPK is even more specific. Similarly, cardiac muscle has an LDH isoenzyme composition distinctly different from that of other tissues and contains predominantly isomer LDH.

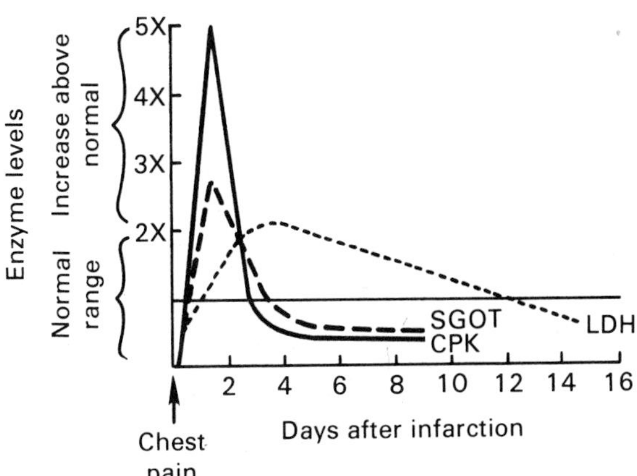

Figure 27-11 Heart muscle enzyme levels in the blood after MI.

Although serial ECGs are only about 80 percent accurate in diagnosing acute MI, these tests are important. Arrhythmias can be detected, and indications of the area of injury can be obtained from electrical alterations on the tracing. Since these changes are specific, they can be used as "road maps" for those trained in ECG interpretation (Table 27-8).

For assessment of cardiac size and pulmonary congestion, an initial chest x-ray is helpful. The appearance of distended upper-lobe veins may indicate early left ventricular dysfunction. The WBC count may rise to 12,000 to 14,000/μL or higher. The fasting glucose level increases to 300 mg/dL. (This finding makes the diagnosis of latent diabetes difficult because of the intense sympathetic reaction associated with MI.)

Radionuclide imaging has become increasingly important in establishing the diagnosis of MI. This technique uses radioactive isotope technetium pyrophosphate. (See Chap. 25 for an explanation of the technique.) The isotope concentrates in necrotic myocardial cells, and with scanning, the "hot spot" can be identified. Nuclear imaging is considered a very sensitive indicator of myocardial damage.

Medical Management

This section presents an overview of the medical management of acute MI (Table 27-9). Chap. 28 provides an in-depth discussion of the management of acute MI, cardiogenic shock, arrhythmias, pacemakers, and pulmonary edema.

Management of the client with MI is best accomplished in a CCU, where constant monitoring is available. Continuous electrocardiographic monitoring detects arrhythmias for prompt treatment. An intravenous route is established to provide an accessible means for emergency drug therapy. Morphine sulfate or meperidine is given intravenously for prompt pain relief.

A continuous intravenous infusion of lidocaine is given to prevent ventricular fibrillation, the greatest threat to life immediately post-MI. In many individuals, episodes of fibrillation are preceded by premature ventricular contractions.

Oxygen is usually administered via nasal cannula at a rate of 3 to 6 L/minute. Heparin may be given prophylactically to decrease the risk of thromboembolic complications. Its use is somewhat controversial because its effectiveness does not seem to be statistically significant.[25] If anticoagulants are selected by the physician, oral anticoagulants are given in place of heparin when the client is out of the intensive care unit.

Vital signs are taken frequently during the first few hours after admission and monitored closely thereafter. Bed rest and activity limitation are usual initially, with a gradual increase in activity later on.

A Swan-Ganz catheter and intraarterial line may be used to accurately monitor intracardiac, pulmonary artery, and systolic arterial pressures in order to determine the most effective mode of treatment in the acute phase. In the presence of severe left ventricular dysfunction, an intraaortic balloon pump may be used

Table 27-8
Electrocardiographic Changes Due to Myocardial Infarction

Phase I	Phase II	Phase III	Phase IV
Abnormal Q waves Elevated ST segment Inverted T waves	Gradual return of ST segment to baseline	T waves return to normal or near-normal configuration	Remnant Q wave

Inferior wall infarction: ST elevation, T inversion, pathological Q wave in leads II, III, and a VF
Inferior-lateral and posterior-lateral wall infarction: reduced R, T inversion, ± ST elevation in V_5, V_6, and aVL
Posterior wall infarction: mirror image of normal ECG
Anterior wall infarction: typical infarction pattern in leads I, aVL, V_2–V_6

Table 27-9
Medical Management: Myocardial Infarction

Diagnostic
1. History and physical examination
2. Serum enzyme level tests (CPK, SGOT, LDH)
3. ECG
4. Chest x-ray
5. CBC
6. Radionuclide imaging

Therapeutic
1. IV therapy
2. Continual electrocardiographic monitoring
3. Morphine sulfate IV every 2–4 h prn (meperidine if client is allergic to morphine)
4. Oxygen therapy
5. Vital signs every 1–4 h
6. Lidocaine IV drip infusion
7. Bed rest with progressive activity
8. Intake and output every shift
9. Heparin IV or SC (depending on physician's preference)

to assist ventricular ejection and promote coronary artery perfusion. (These procedures are explained in Chap. 28.)

Pharmacological Intervention

Morphine

Morphine sulfate is most commonly given for acute cardiac pain relief because it reduces anxiety and decreases the cardiac work load by lowering myocardial oxygen consumption, reducing contractility, lowering the blood pressure, and slowing the heart rate. Morphine is given intravenously because (1) after infarction there may be poor peripheral perfusion which may cause medication pooling, rendering the medication ineffective until the circulation is restored, when drug overdose might occur; and (2) serum enzymes would be affected by an intramuscular injection.

Meperidine (Demerol) is also given, but less frequently than morphine because it is more apt to induce vomiting and to initiate a vasovagal response. Both drugs can depress respirations, which could cause hypoxia, a condition to be avoided in infarction.

Stool softeners

The client post-MI is predisposed to constipation as a result of bed rest and narcotic administration. Stool softeners, such as dioctyl sodium sulfosuccinate (Colace), are given to facilitate and promote the comfort of bowel elimination. This prevents straining and the resultant vagal stimulation and Valsalva maneuver. (The Valsalva maneuver is explained in Chap. 34.) Vagal stimulation produces bradycardia and can provoke arrhythmias. Another real danger of straining is that when the action is stopped, venous return to the heart is suddenly increased. This may result in overloading of a weakened heart.

Antiarrhythmic drugs

Arrhythmias are the most common complication following an MI. The drugs used in the treatment of arrhythmias are discussed in Chap. 28.

Sedatives

Manifestations of anxiety post-MI may be related to the realization of the illness as well as the forced inactivity. Often the anxiety decreases with reassurance, education, and support. If drug therapy is indicated, the most commonly used antianxiety agents are diazepam (Valium) and chlordiazepoxide (Librium).

Digitalis

The use of digitalis preparations following an acute MI is controversial since these drugs increase myocardial oxygen requirements.[26]

Dietary Measures

During the first 5 days post-MI, a soft, bland diet is usually given in multiple feedings. Because an increased cardiac output is needed for digestion, this type of diet decreases energy expenditures. The diet may be restricted in saturated fats or cholesterol and is usually low in sodium.

Nursing Management

Acute intervention

Acute nursing intervention for the client with MI is best done in a specialized care unit such as a CCU, where monitoring and emergency equipment is available (Table 27-10). Since the advent of CCUs in the early 1960s, medical and nursing care has improved dramatically and countless lives have been saved.

An overview of the nursing intervention in acute MI is presented here. Chap. 28 discusses the specific nursing care related to acute MI, arrhythmias, cardiogenic shock, and pacemakers. Priorities for client care in the initial phase of recovery after MI include (1) pain assessment and relief, (2) physiological monitoring, (3) promotion of rest and comfort, (4) alleviation of stress and anxiety, and (5) understanding of the client's emotional and behavioral reactions. Proper management of these priorities will decrease the need for oxygen delivery to a compromised myocardium.

Table 27-10

Nursing Care Plan for the Client with Myocardial Infarction

Client Problem	Expected Outcome	Nursing Intervention
Pain	Free from pain. Comfortable and able to rest.	Administer O_2 per nasal cannula. Administer morphine sulfate IV as needed. Monitor vital signs every 1–2 h. Assess mental status frequently. Continue to evaluate client's level of comfort. Explain to client the importance of reporting any pain so that it can be evaluated and treated.
Altered oxygenation	Blood pressure and pulse within normal limits for individual. Respiratory rate 12–18/min.	Minimize cardiac work load during healing. Explain necessity for bed rest and decreased activity. Allow rest periods between concentrated nursing-care times. Provide for long, uninterrupted rest periods. Monitor O_2 administration. Assess comfort level (try to keep client pain-free). Assess urine output to determine adequacy of renal blood flow. Assess vital signs every 1–2 h. Auscultate heart and lung sounds every 2–3 h.
Anxiety	Physical and emotional comfort. A sense of well-being.	Assess anxiety with regard to the stressors affecting the client. Determine the client's past coping style and assess its effectiveness. Provide support and facilitate the client's coping mechanisms. If client needs information, provide it clearly and simply at client's level of understanding. Administer diazepam (Valium) prn. Allow support systems to operate (i.e., family may be most effective in reducing client's stress).
Fatigue	Minimal expenditure of energy in the first few days post-MI.	Monitor flow of people into client's room. Plan nursing care to provide optimal rest. Have articles client may need or want (tissues, glasses, water) within easy reach. If client's condition is stable, postpone taking vital signs until client awakens. Give care in a calm, quiet, efficient manner.
Altered self-concept	Client will see recovery from MI as a time-limited curtailment of his normal activities. Client will understand the importance of limited activity at this time and will see the future realistically.	Allow client as much autonomy as possible by giving him necessary information that will provide a feeling of control. Allow client to assist in planning his own care. Inform client of what to expect in the hospital routine. Teach client to take his own pulse so that he can determine what his own limits are during recovery.
Possible constipation	Normal bowel elimination pattern.	Administer stool softeners as ordered. Provide bedside commode for client to sit on. Instruct client to avoid straining. Provide foods high in bulk. If client is unsuccessful, laxative order may need to be obtained from physician.
Lack of information	Client will feel informed about: 1. What caused the heart attack 2. What to do for possible future symptoms 3. Changes that are recommended in lifestyle 4. Immediate plan of care 5. What to expect on homecoming 6. Activity guidelines	Teach at client's level of understanding. Provide guidelines with a rationale for recommended actions to be taken. Make sure that recommendations are presented to client in a realistic manner so that the client can see himself carrying them out. Include family when information is given, especially regarding homecoming. Be specific when giving discharge instructions. Write them down for the client to take home.
Preparation for uncertain future	Client will know the range of normal regarding recovery from MI.	Anticipate what recovery might be like for the client and discuss what the client may expect in future. This helps client gain perceived control and promotes a sense of well-being which aids recovery. Make sure that guidelines are specific and individualized.
Change in lifestyle	Client will be able to talk about anticipated changes in lifestyle.	Ensure that client understands which changes will be temporary (until healing is complete) and which ones should be permanent. Ensure that changes are realistic in relation to the severity of cardiac disease. Ensure that client and family have similar expectations and understandings of client's new lifestyle. Let client discuss how some of the changes are to be made.

Pain Morphine should be given as needed to eliminate or reduce chest pain. In addition to relieving pain, morphine acts as a sedative to relieve anxiety. Since clients do not always verbalize their pain, the nurse must be attuned to other manifestations of pain, such as restlessness, elevated pulse or blood pressure, clutching of the bedclothes, or other nonverbal cues. Once pain is relieved, the nurse may have to deal with denial in a client who interprets the absence of pain as an absence of cardiac damage. For some clients, nitroglycerin may have to be kept at the bedside so that pain relief is as prompt as possible. After the pain medication has been administered, the efficacy of the drug and the client's response should be assessed.

Monitoring The client will have continuous electrocardiographic monitoring while in the CCU and usually after transfer to a step-down or general unit. The nurse should be trained in ECG interpretation so that she will be able to identify and eliminate arrhythmias that can cause further deterioration of the cardiovascular status. During the initial post-MI period, ventricular fibrillation is the most common arrhythmia. In many clients, this arrhythmia is preceded by premature ventricular contractions.

Besides frequent vital signs, intake and output should be evaluated at least once a shift, and physical assessment should be carried out to detect deviations from the client's baseline parameters. Included is the assessment of lung sounds and heart sounds and inspection for evidence of fluid retention (distended neck veins, hepatic engorgement, presacral or anterior tibial edema). Since clients are frequently on strict bed rest initially, dorsiflexion of the feet (Homan's sign) to elicit deep calf pain should also be done to evaluate the presence of deep-vein thrombosis.

Assessment of the client's oxygenation status is helpful, especially if the client is receiving oxygen. Also, the nares should be checked for irritation or dryness, which can cause considerable discomfort.

Rest and Comfort With a severe insult to the myocardium, as in the case of infarction, it is important for the nurse to promote rest and comfort. Bed rest may be ordered for the first 3 to 5 days in a severe MI. Clients with an uncomplicated MI may rest for part of the time in a chair.

When sleeping or resting, the body requires less work from the heart than it does when aroused. It is important to plan nursing and medical actions to ensure adequate rest periods free from interruption. Comfort measures that can promote rest are smooth bedclothes, frequent oral care, adequate warmth, dim lighting, a quiet atmosphere, and assurance that personnel are nearby and responsive to the client's needs.

It is important that the client understand *why* his activity is limited. In spite of this limitation, however, the client is not immobilized. Probably the most comprehensive model for resumption of activity after MI is described by Wenger (see Table 27-11). This program, like many others, includes self-care, use of bedside commode or nearby toilet, and passive and active range-of-motion exercises while lying and sitting in bed or in a chair during the first few days of hospitalization. Gradually, the cardiac work load is increased through more demanding physical tasks so that the client can achieve a discharge activity level for home care.

Anxiety Anxiety is present in all clients in various degrees. The nurse's role is to identify the source of anxiety and assist the client in reducing it. If the client is afraid of being alone, a family member should be allowed either to sit quietly by the bedside or to check in with the client frequently. If a source of anxiety is fear of the unknown, the nurse should explore these concerns with the client and assist him with appropriate reality testing.

If anxiety is due to lack of information, the nurse should provide teaching appropriate to the client's stated need and level. This does not mean that the nurse initiates the cardiac education protocol. Instead, she answers the client's questions with clear, simple explanations sufficient to reduce the client's anxiety.

It is very important to start teaching at the client's level rather than to present a prepackaged protocol. Usually, clients are not yet ready to hear about the pathophysiology of heart disease. The earliest questions usually relate to how the disease affects their perceived control and independence. These questions usually include the following:

When will I leave the CCU?
When can I be out of bed?
When will I be discharged?
When can I return to work?
How much change will I have to make in my life?
Will this happen again?

The client should be advised that when he is feeling stronger, a more complete teaching program will be available. If the client experiences anxiety and is unable to identify the source, a mild tranquilizer may help to promote a sense of calmness.

Table 27-11
Fourteen-Step Myocardial Infarction Rehabilitation Program

Step	Exercise	Ward Activity	Educational and Craft Activity
1	Passive ROM* to all extremities (5× ea); client to do *active* plantar and dorsiflexion of ankles several times/day.	Feeding self, sitting with bed rolled up to 45°, trunk and arms supported by over-bed table.	Initial interview and brief orientation to program.
2	Repeat exercises of Step 1.	1. Feed self. 2. Partial A.M. care (wash hands, face, brush teeth) in bed. 3. Dangle legs on side of bed (1×).	Light recreational activity, such as reading.
3	Active assistive exercise in shoulder flexion; elbow flexion and extension; hip flexion, extension, and rotation: knee flexion and extension: rotation of feet (4× ea).	1. Begin sitting in chair for short periods as tolerated, 2×/day. 2. Bathing whole body. 3. Use of bedside commode.	More detailed explanation of program. Continue light recreation.
4	Minimal resistance, lying in bed in above ROM, 5× ea. Stiffen all muscles to the count of 2 (3×).	1. Increase sitting 3×/day. 2. Change gown.	Begin explanation of what is an MI.* Give client pamphlets to read. Begin craft activity: 1. Leather lacing. 2. Link belt. 3. Hand sewing, embroidery. 4. Copper tooling.
5	Moderate resistance in bed at 45° in above ROM exercises; hand on shoulder, elbow circling (5× ea arm).	1. Sitting ad lib. 2. Sitting in chair at bedside for meals. 3. Dressing, shaving, combing hair—*sitting down*. 4. Walking in room, 2×/day.	Continue education about healing of heart, reasons for early restrictions in activity.
6	1. Further resistive exercises sitting on side of bed, manual resistance of knee extension and flexion (7× ea). 2. Walk to bathroom and back (note if client needs help).	1. Walk to bathroom, ad lib if client can tolerate. 2. Stand at sink to shave.	Continue craft activity or supply client with another one. Client may attend group meetings in a wheelchair for no more than 1 h.
7	1. Standing warm-up exercises: a. Arms in extension and shoulder abduction, rotate arms together in circles (circumduction), 5× ea arm. b. Stand on toes, 10×. c. May substitute abduction, 5× ea leg. 2. Walk length of hall (50 ft) and back at average pace.	1. Bathe in tub. 2. Walk to telephone or sit in waiting room (1×/day).	May walk to group meetings on the same floor.
8	1. Warm-up exercises: a. Lateral side bending 5× ea side. b. Trunk twisting, 5× ea side. 2. Walk $1\frac{1}{2}$ lengths of hall, down 1 fl stairs, elevator up.	1. Walk to waiting room, 2×/day. 2. Stay sitting up most of the day.	Continue all previous craft and educational activities.
9	1. Warm-up exercises: a. Lateral side bending, 10× ea side. b. Slight knee bends, 10× with hands on hips. 2. Increase walking distance, walk down one flight of stairs.	Continue above activities.	Discussion of work simplification techniques and pacing of activities.
10	1. Warm-up exercises: a. Lateral side bending with 1-lb weight (10×). b. Standing—leg raising leaning against wall, 5× ea. 2. Walk two lengths of hall and downstairs, take elevator up.	Continue all previous ward activities.	1. Client may walk to OT* clinic and work on craft project for $\frac{1}{2}$ h. a. Copper tooling; b. woodworking; c. ceramics; d. small weaving project e. metal hammering; f. mosaic tile. 2. Discussion of client's home exercises.

Table 27-11 (Continued)

Step	Exercise	Ward Activity	Educational and Craft Activity
11	1. Warm-up exercises: a. Lateral side bending with 1-lb weight, leaning against wall, 10× ea side. b. Standing, leg raising, 5× ea. c. Trunk twisting with 1-lb weight, 5× ea. side. 2. Repeat part 2 of Step 10.	Continue all previous ward activities.	Increase time in OT clinic to 1 h.
12	1. Warm-up exercises: a. Lateral side bending with 2-lb weight, 10×. b. Standing—leg raising, leaning against wall, 10× ea. c. Trunk twisting with 2-lb weight, 10×. 2. Walk down two flights of stairs.	Continue all previous ward activities.	Continue craft activity with increased resistance.
13	Repeat all exercises of Step 12.	Continue all previous ward activities.	Complete all projects.
14	1. Warm-up exercises: a. Lateral side bending with 2-lb weight, 10× ea. side. b. Trunk twisting with 2-lb weight, 10× ea. side. c. Touch toes from sitting position, 10×. 2. Walk up flight of 10 stairs and down.	Continue all previous ward activities.	Final instructions about home procedures and activities.

*ROM = range of motion, MI = myocardial infarction, OT = occupational therapy.

Reproduced from N. K. Wenger and C. A. Gilbert, "Rehabilitation of the Myocardial Infarction Patient," in J. W. Hurst, R. B. Logue, R. C. Schlant, and N. K. Wenger (eds.), *The Heart*, 4th ed., McGraw-Hill Book Company, New York, 1978.

Emotional and Behavioral Reactions The emotional and behavioral reactions of a client are varied and frequently follow a predictable response pattern (Table 27-12). The role of the nurse in intervention is to understand what the client is currently experiencing, to assist the client in testing reality, and to support the use of constructive coping styles. Denial may be a positive coping style in the early phase of recovery from MI. Lazarus has identified situations in which denial and illusion may be the healthiest strategies available when the client is under stress.[27]

The nurse has an obligation to maximize and enhance the client's support systems. This entails assessing the support structure of the client and family and allowing it to function. Often clients are separated from their most significant support systems at the time of hospitalization. The nurse's role can include talking with the family, informing them of the client's progress, allowing the client and family to interact as necessary, and supporting the family members who will be able to provide the necessary support to the client.

Rehabilitative management

Rehabilitation may be defined as the process of helping the client adjust to a disability by teaching him to integrate all of his resources and to concentrate more on *existing abilities* than on permanent disabilities. Cardiac rehabilitation is the restoration of an individual to an optimal state of function in six areas: physiological, psychological, mental, spiritual, economic, and vocational. Many people recover from an MI attack physically, yet may never attain psychological well-being due to misconceptions about their illness or a need to practice illness behaviors. Returning to work or resuming all activities have long been outcome measures of cardiac rehabilitation and are important in terms of the cost effectiveness of cardiac care and rehabilitation. Wenger has described rehabilitation goals in terms of phases (Table 27-13).

In considering rehabilitation, nurses and clients must recognize that CAD is a chronic disease. It will not be cured, nor will it disappear by itself. Therefore, basic changes in lifestyle must be made in order to promote recovery and health. These changes must frequently be made at a time when a person is middle aged, and is already dealing with aging and all its associated stresses. The client must also realize that recovery takes time. Resumption of physical activity after MI is a slow, gradual process. For type A personalities, who have always had difficulty in being patient, this is an extra stress. With appropriate and

Table 27-12
Emotional and Behavioral Responses Following an Acute Myocardial Infarction

Denial
May have a history of ignoring symptoms related to heart disease
Minimizes the severity of the medical condition
Ignores activity restrictions
Avoids discussing MI or its significance.

Anger
Commonly expressed as "why did this happen to me?"
May be directed at family, staff, or medical regimen

Anxiety and fear
Fear of death and long-term disability
Overtly manifests apprehension, restlessness, insomnia, tachycardia
Less overtly manifests increased verbalization, projection of feelings to others, hypochondriasis
Fear of activity, recurrent heart attacks, or sudden death

Dependency
Totally reliant on staff
Unwilling to perform tasks or activities unless approved by physician
Wants to be monitored by ECG at all times
Hesitant to leave CCU or, later, to leave the hospital

Depression
Mourning period over loss of health, altered body function, and changes in lifestyle
Realizes the seriousness of the situation
Begins to worry about future implications of the health problem
Manifested by withdrawal, crying, anorexia, apathy
May be more evident after discharge

Realistic acceptance
Focuses on optimum rehabilitation
Plans changes compatible with altered cardiac function

Table 27-13
Phases of Rehabilitation

Phase I. Time when client is in the CCU (usually 3–5 days):
Activity level depends on severity of MI; client may rest in bed or chair
Attention focused on management of pain, arrhythmias, and cardiogenic shock

Phase II. Time from transfer from the CCU to discharge from the hospital:
Gradual resumption of activities to the point of self-care at the time of discharge
Information giving and teaching appropriate at this time

Phase III. Time of convalescence at home:
Client and family examine and possibly restructure their lifestyles and roles
Exercise program started, commonly a walking program, which progresses daily during the first week and then weekly
Client undergoes exercise treadmill test at about 8 wk to determine the work load of the recovering myocardium

Phase IV. Time of recovery and maintenance:
Involvement with the community rehabilitation program for physical training and fitness

Adapted from N. K. Wenger et al. (eds.), *Cardiology for Nurses*, McGraw-Hill Book Company, New York, 1980, pp. 310–312.

adequate supportive care, however, recovery will most likely occur.

Client Education Once the acute stage of MI has passed, the client is transferred to a step-down, intermediate care, or regular hospital unit. The goals of nursing care discussed in the section on Acute Intervention are ongoing. In addition, a very important nursing goal now becomes client and family education. This teaching begins in the CCU nurse and progresses through the staff nurse to the community health nurse. The purpose of education is to give the client and family the tools they need to make informed decisions about attainment of health. In order for teaching to be meaningful, the client must have a need to learn. Careful assessment of the client's learning needs helps the nurse to set goals and objectives that are realistic and can be met. (Guidelines for client teaching are discussed in Chap. 5.)

The timing of the teaching is important. When clients or families are in crisis (either physiological or psychological), they may or may not have learning needs. It is important to remember that (1) early questions should be answered initially in simple, brief terms, without detailed elaboration, and that (2) the answers to these questions will require repetition and follow-up (elaboration) as the shock and disbelief accompanying a crisis subside.

In addition to teaching the client and family what they wish to know, there are several types of information that are considered necessary in achieving health. A teaching plan for the client with MI should include the following:

1. Anatomy and physiology of the heart and vessels
2. Cause and effect of atherosclerosis
3. Definition of terms (CAD, angina, MI, congestive heart failure, etc.)
4. Signs and symptoms of angina, MI, and why they occur
5. Healing after infarction
6. Identification of risk factors
7. Rationale for tests and treatment, including ECG,

blood tests, angiography; and monitoring, rest, diet, and medications

8. What to expect in terms of recovery and rehabilitation (anticipatory guidance)
9. Measures to take to promote recovery and health
10. Importance of the gradual, progressive resumption of activity

When medical terminology is used, its meaning should be explained in lay terms. For example, it can be explained that (1) the heart is a four-chambered pump; it is a muscle that needs oxygen, like all other muscles; (2) when vessels become narrowed by atherosclerosis, the process is similar to a build up of mineral deposits inside water pipes, causing less water to flow through at a higher pressure. It is a good idea for the nurse to have a model of the heart or to use a pad and pencil to sketch what she is explaining. Literature written for a lay audience is available through the American Heart Association.

Anticipatory guidance involves preparing the client and family for what to expect in the course of recovery and rehabilitation. By learning what to expect during treatment and recovery, the client gains a sense of control over his life. This sense of *perceived control* allows the client to consciously consider stressors and thus possibly to promote his recovery.[28] The idea of perceived control is operationalized as the process by which the client exercises choice and makes decisions by *cutting back*. Cutting back is one way of minimizing the psychophysiological losses after MI (or any other life-changing event).[29] The client considers what he is told *must* be cut back (changed), weighs this against what *should* be cut back, and finally determines what he is *willing* to cut back. For instance, a middle-aged male who smokes two packs of cigarettes per day, is 20 lb overweight, and gets no physical exercise has a seemingly overwhelming task. He may decide that he *can* live with a weight-reduction diet and will get more exercise (although perhaps not daily), but to quit smoking is not possible for him. So, he reasons that since he is modifying two of the three risk factors, he will be safe if he cuts back on smoking.

Physical Exercise Exercise is an integral part of the rehabilitation program. It has a direct, positive effect on maximal oxygen uptake, increasing cardiac output, decreasing blood lipids, decreasing blood pressure, and increasing blood flow through the coronary arteries. A regular schedule of moderate exercise, even after many years of sedentary living, has been shown to be very beneficial.

One method used to identify levels of physical activities is through metabolic equivalent (MET) units. One MET is the amount of oxygen needed at rest, or 3.5 mL of oxygen/kg per minute, or 1.4 calories/kg of body weight per minute. The MET is used to determine the energy costs of various exercises (Table 27-14).

In the hospital, a client's activity level will be gradually increased so that by the time of discharge he will be able to tolerate moderate-energy activities of 3 to 5 METs. Usually, a stress exercise test is carried out 1 to 2 months post-MI,. This is done with a controlled rate of energy expenditure while the client's ECG and vital signs are being monitored. The client's exercise is increased until his heart rate reaches the safe maximum level. This test identifies the client's tolerance of activities so that the physician is able to develop an individualized exercise regimen. He can individualized exercise regimen. He can equate this exercise program to MET units. The client can then be started on a conditioning program consisting of planned exercises.

The nurse's role is to teach clients to check their own pulse. They should then be taught the parameters within which to exercise. They will be told the maximum heart rate that they should have at any point. If their heart rate exceeds this level or does not return to the rate of the resting pulse, they should stop. Clients should be instructed to stop exercising if pain or dyspnea occurs.

The basic categories of exercise are static (*isometric*) and dynamic (*isotonic*). Most daily activities are a mixture of the two. Static exercise involves the development of tension during muscular contraction but produces little or no change in muscle length or joint movement. Lifting, carrying, and pushing heavy objects are primarily isometric activities. Since the heart rate and blood pressure increase very rapidly during isometric-type work, exercise programs involving isometric exercises should be avoided.

Isotonic exercises involve changes in muscle length and joint movement with rhythmic contractions at relatively low muscular tension. Walking, jogging, swimming, bicycling, and jumping rope are examples of activities that are predominantly isotonic. Isotonic exercise can put a safe, steady load on the heart and lungs and may also improve the circulation in many organs.

Resumption of Sexual Activity It is important to include sexual counseling for both male and female cardiac clients and their partners. This often neglected area of discussion may be difficult for both clients and health care providers. Yet the cardiac client's concern about resumption of sexual activity after MI

Table 27-14
Energy Expenditure in METs for Various Activities

Equivalents
1 MET = oxygen needed at rest
or 3.5 mL of oxygen/kg of body weight per minute
or 1 cal = 200 mL of oxygen consumed

Activity	METs
Low-energy activities (less than 3 METs or less than 4 cal/min)	
Activities in hospital	
Rest, supine	1.0
Sitting	1.2
Eating	1.4
Conversation	1.4
Washing hands, face	2.5
Activities outside of hospital	
Sewing by hand	1.4
Sweeping floor	1.7
Painting, sitting	2.5
Driving car	2.8
Assembling radio	2.7
Sewing by machine	2.9
Moderate-energy activities (3–5 METs or 4–6 cal/min)	
Activities in hospital	
Sitting on bedside commode	3.6
Walking at 2.5 mph	3.6
Showering	4.2
Using bedpan	4.7
Walking at 3.75 mph	5.6
Activities outside of hospital	
Bricklaying	4.0
Tractor plowing	4.2
Ironing, standing	4.2
Mopping	4.2
Bowling	4.4
Cycling at 5.5 mph on level ground	4.5
Golfing	5.0
Dancing	5.5
High-energy activities (5–7 METs or 6–8 cal/min)	
Ambulation with braces and crutches	8.0
Carpentry	6.8
Mowing lawn by hand	7.7
Singles tennis playing	7.1
Trotting horse	8.0
Walking at 5 mph	6.5
Ascending stairs	7.0
Very-high-energy activities (7–9 METs or 8–10 cal/min)	
Skiing	9.9
Jogging at 5 mph	8.0
Shoveling snow	8.5
Ascending stairs with a 17-lb load	9.0
Extremely high-energy activities (more than 10 METs or more than 11 cal/min)	
Handball playing	
Cycling at 13 mph	
Ascending stairs with a 22-lb load	

often produces more stress than the physiological act itself.

It is reported that most cardiac clients do not resume sexual activity after MI.[30,31] The majority of these clients changed their sexual behavior *not* because of cardiac inability but because they were frequently concerned about sexual inadequacy, death during coitus, and impotence. The misconceptions held by these people could have been clarified with specific counseling by a concerned health care provider.

Before providing guidelines on resumption of sexual activity, it is important to know the physiological status of the client, the physiological effects of sexual activity, and the psychological effects of having a heart attack. One study concluded that sexual activity for middle-aged men with their usual partners is no more strenuous than climbing two flights of stairs.[32]

Most nurses are unsure of how and when to begin counseling about resumption of sex. It is helpful to consider sex as a physical activity and to discuss or explore feelings in this area when other physical activities are discussed. One helpful approach is: "Many people who have had a heart attack wonder when they will be able to resume sexual activity. Has this been of concern to you?" This type of nonthreatening statement (1) brings up the topic, (2) allows the client to explore his own feelings, and (3) gives the client an opportunity to raise questions with the nurse or another health care provider. Common guidelines are presented in Table 27-15.

Clients need to know that the inability to perform sexually after MI is not uncommon and that impotence usually disappears after several attempts. The nurse should reinforce the idea that patience and understanding usually solve the problem. Clients may assume the position of choice.[33]

It is not uncommon for clients who experience chest pain on physical exertion to have some angina during sexual stimulation or intercourse. Clients should be instructed to take nitroglycerin prophylactically. It is also helpful to have clients avoid sex soon after a heavy meal or after excessive ingestion of alcohol, when extremely tired or stressed, or with unfamiliar partners. Anal intercourse is to be avoided because of the likelihood of eliciting a vasovagal response.

Clients should be counseled that resumption of sex depends on their own desires and on the physician's assessment of the extent of recovery. It is usually recommended that clients refrain from sex until 4 to 8 weeks post-MI. Some physicians believe that the client should decide when he is ready to resume sex. Others say that the client must be able to climb

Table 27-15
Guidelines for Resumption of Sexual Activity After Myocardial Infarction

Plan resumption of sexual activity corresponding to sexual activity *before* the heart attack.
Physical training (exercise) seems to improve the physiological response to coitus, so encourage daily exercise during recovery.
Reduce consumption of food and alcohol before intercourse is anticipated (i.e., wait 3–4 h after ingesting a large meal before engaging in sexual activity).
Familiar surroundings and a familiar partner reduce anxiety.
Masturbation may be a useful sexual outlet and may reassure the client that sexual activity is still possible.
Temperature should be comfortable, not extreme. (Hot or cold showers should be avoided just before and just after intercourse.)
Foreplay is desirable in that it allows a *gradual* increase in heart rate prior to orgasm.
Positions during intercourse are a matter of individual choice.
Oral-genital sex places no undue strain on the heart. This form of sexual expression depends entirely on the individuals involved.
A relaxed atmosphere free of fatigue is optimal.
Prophylactic use of nitrates is effective in decreasing angina during sexual activity.
Anal intercourse may cause undue cardiac stress because of the possibility of inducing a vasovagal response.

two flights of stairs briskly without dyspnea or angina before sexual activity can be resumed.

CHRONIC CONGESTIVE HEART FAILURE

Congestive heart failure (CHF) is a cardiovascular state in which the heart is unable to pump an adequate amount of blood to meet the metabolic needs of the tissues. CHF is not a disease but a syndrome caused by a variety of pathophysiological processes (Table 27-16). This section will focus on chronic CHF. Acute CHF and pulmonary edema are discussed in Chap. 28.

Pathophysiology

Chronic CHF may include dysfunction in one or both ventricles. Normally, the pumping actions of the left and right sides of the heart complement each other, producing a continuous flow of blood. However, due to pathological conditions, one side may fail while the other side continues to function normally for a period of time. Due to the prolonged strain, the functioning side of the heart will eventually fail, resulting in total heart failure.

The most common form of initial heart failure is left-sided failure. This will usually lead to and is the main cause of right-sided failure. The majority of individuals with cardiac disease will eventually develop CHF.

Table 27-16
Causes of Congestive Heart Failure

Coronary artery disease
Hypertensive heart disease
Rheumatic heart disease
Congenital heart disease
Cor pulmonale

Left-sided failure

Left-sided failure results from left ventricular dysfunction, which causes blood to back up through the left atrium and into the pulmonary veins. The increased pressure causes fluid extravasation from the pulmonary capillary bed which is manifested as pulmonary congestion and edema. The most common causes are diseases of the coronary arteries, hypertension, and rheumatic heart disease.

When MI occurs, myocardial tissue is damaged and replaced by scar tissue. The scar tissue is less elastic and has poorer contractility than undamaged myocardium. The loss of myocardial mass increases the work load on the remaining functional tissue. If the functioning myocardium cannot compensate for this loss, the volume of blood ejected from the ventricle is decreased and heart failure results.

When hypertension is present, the heart must pump blood against a high arterial pressure. Eventually, this can lead to left ventricular hypertrophy.

In aortic valvular heart disease, the left ventricle must contract forcefully to pump blood through the stenotic aortic valve. This requires an increased amount of pressure that must be generated by the left ventricle. In addition, the valve often fails to close completely, and blood is regurgitated into the left ventricle. In mitral valve disease, a similar process involving the left atria occurs.

Right-sided failure

Right-sided failure from a weakened right ventricle causes venous congestion in the systemic circulation and results in peripheral edema. The primary cause of right-sided failure is left-sided failure. In this situation, left-sided failure results in pulmonary congestion and increased pressure in the blood vessels of the lung *(pulmonary hypertension)*. Eventually, pulmonary hypertension results in right-sided failure. Cor pulmonale (right ventricular dilatation and hypertrophy due to pulmonary pathophysiology) can also cause right-sided failure. Causes of cor pulmonale include chronic obstructive pulmonary disease and pulmonary emboli. Distended neck veins can be seen when a client with right-sided failure is in a semirecumbent position. This is due to increased pressure in the right atria.

Factors that precipitate heart failure

There are certain factors that can precipitate heart failure in an individual with heart disease (Table 27-17). Examples include (1) arrhythmias, which lead to ineffective mechanical pumping, (2) anemia, which causes an increased heart rate as a compensatory mechanism to maintain tissue oxygenation, and (3) thyrotoxicosis, which causes an increased heart rate.

Compensatory mechanisms

CHF is an insidious process and the result of slow, progressive changes. The chronically overloaded heart resorts to certain compensatory mechanisms to try to maintain adequate cardiac output. These are described below.

Hypertrophy Hypertrophy is an increase in the muscle mass and the cardiac wall thickness due to strain. It occurs slowly because it takes time for muscle tissue to develop. As myocardial mass increases, the need for additional blood and oxygen grows. This additional demand cannot always be met in the client with heart disease.

Dilatation Dilatation is an enlargement of the chambers of the heart. It occurs when pressure in the heart chambers (usually the left ventricle) is elevated over time. The muscle fibers of the heart stretch and thereby increase their contractile force. However, this increased contractility produces greater wall tension, and more myocardial oxygen is required for contraction. Therefore, dilatation is a mechanism developed to cope with increasing blood volume. Eventually, dilatation gradually becomes inadequate as the elastic elements of the muscle fibers are overstrained. Dilatation can progress to mitral valve incompetence and regurgitation, which further increase the cardiac work load.

Sympathetic Nervous System Activation Because there is inadequate stroke volume and cardiac output, baroreceptor reflexes cause sympathetic nervous system activation, which increases the release of epinephrine and norepinephrine. This results in an increased heart rate and myocardial contractility in order to raise cardiac output. This response also increases myocardial oxygen demands.

Table 27-17
Factors that Precipitate Heart Failure

Factors
Common
Acute myocardial infarction
Iatrogenic (including client noncompliance)
Pulmonary emboli
Pulmonary infection
Ectopic rhythm
Less common
Thyrotoxicosis
Anemia
Bacterial endocarditis
Prostatic hypertrophy with urine retention

Renal response to heart failure

As cardiac output falls, blood flow to the kidneys decreases, causing decreased glomerular filtration. This is interpreted by the juxtaglomerular apparatus in the kidneys as *decreased volume*. A complex reaction begins: The kidneys release renin, which reacts with angiotensinogen to form angiotensin (Fig. 36-6). Angiotensin causes (1) the adrenal cortex to release aldosterone, which causes sodium retention, and (2) increased vasoconstriction, which increases the arterial pressure.

The posterior pituitary senses the increased osmotic pressure due to sodium retention and secretes antidiuretic hormone (ADH). ADH increases water reabsorption in the renal tubules, causing water retention. The decreased renal blood flow also stimulates the secretion of ADH.

Clinical Manifestations

The clinical manifestations of chronic CHF are dependent on age, on the underlying type and extent of heart disease, and on which ventricle is failing to pump effectively. These manifestations include fatigue, dyspnea, tachycardia, edema, nocturia, skin changes, behavioral changes, and chest pain.

Fatigue

Fatigue is one of the earliest symptoms of chronic CHF. The client notices fatigue following activities that normally are not tiring. The fatigue is due to impaired circulation and oxygenation of the tissues. It is sometimes described as "sick fatigue" because of the decreased amounts of blood reaching the musculoskeletal system.[34]

Dyspnea

Dyspnea is a common sign of chronic CHF. It is caused by poor gas exchange due to fluid in the alveoli. The shortness of breath makes the client conscious of air hunger which prompts rapid, shallow respirations. Dyspnea can occur with mild exertion or at rest. Orthopnea is shortness of breath that occurs when the client is in a recumbent position.

Paroxysmal nocturnal dyspnea (PND) occurs when the client is asleep. It is probably caused by the reabsorption of fluid from dependent body areas when the person lies down. The client awakens in a panic, feels that he is suffocating, and has a strong desire to sit up to seek respiratory relief. Careful questioning of the client will reveal adaptive behavior such as sleeping with two or more pillows to aid breathing.

Tachycardia

Because cardiac output is diminished, there is an increased sympathetic nervous system stimulation to compensate for low output. (Remember: cardiac output = stroke volume × heart rate.) If the stroke volume decreases, the heart rate increases to maintain the cardiac output.

Edema

Edema is a common sign of CHF. It may occur in the legs (peripheral edema), liver (hepatomegaly), abdominal cavity (ascites), lungs (pulmonary edema and pleural effusion), and other parts of the body. Pressing the edematous skin with the finger may leave a transient indentation (pitting edema). The development of dependent edema and/or a sudden weight gain of 2 kg or more is often indicative of exacerbated CHF.

Nocturia

A person with chronic CHF will have decreased cardiac output, impaired renal perfusion, and decreased urinary output during the day. However, when the person lies down at night, fluid movement from interstitial spaces back into the circulatory system is enchanced. This causes increased renal blood flow and diuresis. The client may complain of having to void six or seven times during the night.

Skin changes

Because tissue capillary oxygen extraction is increased in a person with chronic CHF, the skin appears dusky. It is also cold and diaphoretic to the touch. The peripheral vasoconstriction that occurs to shunt blood to vital organs and the heart is a minor compensatory mechanism in chronic CHF.

Behavioral changes

Cerebral circulation may be impaired with chronic CHF, especially in the presence of more pervasive atherosclerosis. The client or family may report unusual behavior, including restlessness, confusion, and decreased attention span or memory. These behavioral changes seem to occur at night, possibly because the client is experiencing less stimulation than during the day.

Chest pain

In the presence of atherosclerosis, chronic CHF can precipitate chest pain due to decreased coronary perfusion from decreased cardiac output.

The determination of which side of the heart is in failure can be made only in early dysfunction. The circulatory system is a closed circuit, and the inefficiency of one part of the heart will eventually affect other parts as well, resulting in ventricular failure of both sides. Table 27-18 lists the physical manifestations of left and right ventricular failure. It should be kept in mind that the client with chronic CHF will probably have manifestations of biventricular failure.

Complications

Pulmonary edema and pleural effusion

As pulmonary congestion increases, the distended capillaries leak fluid into the alveoli (discussed in Chap. 28). Pleural effusion results from increasing pressure in the pleural capillaries. A transudation of fluid occurs from these capillaries into the pleural space. (Pleural effusion is discussed in Chap. 20.)

Table 27-18
Clinical Manifestations of Heart Failure

Right Heart Failure	Left Heart Failure
Peripheral edema	Left ventricular hypertrophy (PMI displaced inferiorly and posteriorly)
Weight gain	Poor oxygen exchange (arterial blood gases: ↓ P_aO_2, slight ↑ $P_a CO_2$)
Edema of dependent body parts (sacrum, anterior tibias, pedal edema)	Pulmonary edema (rales)
Anasarca (massive generalized body edema)	Unproductive cough
Jugular vein distension	Dyspnea (shallow respirations up to 32–40/min)
Liver engorgement (hepatomegaly)	Orthopnea, paroxysmal nocturnal dyspnea
	Cough (dry hacking caused by alveolar irritation from fluid accumulation)
	S_3 heart sound (from vibrations of ventricle wall due to resistance to ventricular filling)

Cirrhosis of the liver

CHF can lead to severe hepatomegaly. The liver lobules become congested with venous blood. The hepatic congestion leads to impaired liver function. Eventually, liver cells die, fibrosis occurs, and cirrhosis can develop (see Chap. 35).

Weight loss

There are many factors that contribute to weight loss. The client with CHF has an increased metabolic rate. At the same time, decreased oxygen and nutrients are transported to the tissues. Often, the client is too sick to eat. Abdominal fullness from ascites and hepatomegaly frequently causes anorexia and nausea. In many cases, the weight loss is masked by the client's edematous condition.

Decompensated heart failure

The compensatory mechanisms of dilatation, hypertrophy, and tachycardia were discussed earlier. When they function to provide adequate cardiac output to maintain tissue oxygenation, the client has *compensated heart failure*. When these mechanisms can no longer assist the heart in providing cardiac output, the client has *decompensated heart failure*. Without treatment, this state is fatal. Even with treatment, the prognosis is not good.

Medical Management

Diagnostic (Table 27-19)

The primary goal in diagnosis is to determine the underlying cause of heart failure. Diagnostic measures to assess the degree of heart failure include chest x-ray, ECG, stress testing, and echocardiography.

The chest x-ray is the most important diagnostic measure for assessing and monitoring heart failure. Initial abnormalities in CHF, such as prominent, congested upper lobe pulmonary veins, can be seen on x-rays. Later changes, such as interstitial pulmonary edema and pulmonary effusion, can also be visualized. The degree of cardiac enlargement is also readily observed.

An ECG is of no value in detecting heart failure. However, it can be used to detect cardiac arrhythmias and changes due to myocardial ischemia or MI. Exercise stress testing may provide more valuable information than an ECG taken at rest.

Echocardiography can be used to measure the size of the cardiac chambers and to assess ventricular function. Cardiac catheterization and angiocardiography are useful in detecting underlying heart disease.

Table 27-19

Medical Management: Congestive Heart Failure

Diagnostic

1. History and physical examination
2. Determine the underlying cause
3. Chest x-ray
4. ECG
5. Exercise-stress testing
6. Echocardiography

Therapeutic

1. Treat the underlying cause
2. Oxygen therapy at 2–6 L/min
3. Rest
4. Digitalis preparations
5. Diuretics
6. Vasodilator drugs
7. Daily weights
8. Sodium-restricted diet

The New York Heart Association has developed functional guidelines for classifying individuals with CHF. The classification is based on the individual's tolerance to physical activity (Table 27-20).

Therapeutic (Table 27-19)

Treatment of the Underlying Cause One of the most important goals of medical treatment for CHF is to treat the underlying cause. If arrhythmias have precipitated the failure, then they should be treated accordingly. If the underlying cause is hypertension, then antihypertensives should be of help (Chap. 26). Valvular defects can be treated with surgery (Chap. 29).

Table 27-20

New York Heart Association Functional Classification of Persons with Congestive Heart Failure

Class 1
No limitation on physical activity. Ordinary physical activity does not result in symptoms.

Class 2
Slight limitation on physical activity. No symptoms at rest, but symptoms may be produced with ordinary physical activity.

Class 3
More severe limitations. Client is usually comfortable at rest. Symptoms are manifested with many unusual physical activities.

Class 4
Inability to carry on any physical activity without producing symptoms. Symptoms may be present at rest.

Oxygen Therapy In a person with CHF, oxygen saturation of the blood is reduced because the blood is not adequately oxygenated in the lungs. Administration of oxygen improves oxygen saturation and assists greatly in meeting tissue oxygen needs. Thus, oxygen therapy helps to relieve dyspnea and fatigue.

Physical and Emotional Rest Physical and emotional rest allows the client to conserve energy and decreases the need for additional oxygen. The degree of rest recommended depends on the severity of heart failure. A client with severe CHF needs to be on bed rest with limited activity. A person with mild CHF can be ambulatory with a restriction of strenuous activity.

Pharmacological Management

Pharmacological therapy for CHF includes the use of digitalis preparations, diuretics, and vasodilator drugs.

Digitalis preparations (cardiac glycosides)

Digitalis preparations are very effective in increasing the force or strength of cardiac contraction (*inotropic* action). They also decrease the conduction speed within the myocardium and slow the heart rate (*chronotropic* action). This action provides more complete emptying of the ventricles, thus diminishing the volume remaining in the ventricles during diastole. Cardiac output increases because of an increased stroke volume from improved contractility.

Digitalis promotes diuresis by improving the efficiency of the cardiac pump. The stroke volume and glomerular filtration increase. Thus, more urine is excreted via the kidneys.

Many digitalis preparations are available (Table 27-21). The main differences between them relate to the onset and duration of action and the primary mechanism of elimination. With all digitalis preparations, a digitalizing dose much higher than the maintenance dose is given to achieve adequate blood levels rapidly. The maintenance dosage varies from individual to individual. Digoxin and digitoxin are the most commonly used drugs for maintenance therapy.

The range between therapeutic and toxic effects is narrow and can be affected by other drugs or concurrent disease processes. Monitoring the blood levels of digoxin and digitoxin is becoming common practice. The normal therapeutic range for digoxin is 1 to 2 ng/mL, and for digitoxin it is 14 to 30 ng/mL.

All persons receiving digitalis preparations are subject to digitalis toxicity (Table 27-22). Some of the earliest symptoms of toxicity are anorexia, nausea, and vomiting. Arrhythmias are a common indication of digitalis toxicity. Although almost any arrhythmia can occur, the types most frequently found are premature beats, atrial fibrillation, and first-degree heart block.

Hypokalemia is one of the most common causes of digitalis toxicity, resulting in arrhythmias because low serum potassium levels enhance ectopic pacemaker activity. It is very important to monitor the serum potassium levels of clients receiving both digitalis preparations and potassium-losing diuretics (thiazides, loop diuretics). Other electrolyte imbalances, such as hypercalcemia and hypomagnesemia, can also precipitate toxicity.

Diseases of the kidney and liver cause susceptibility to toxicity because most of the preparations are metabolized and eliminated by these organs. Elderly people are prone to digitalis toxicity because digitalis has more time to accumulate since body metabolism is slowed by aging.

Table 27-21
Digitalis Preparations Used in Congestive Heart Failure

Name	Digitalizing Dose	Maintenance Dose (Daily)	Onset of Action	Peak Effect	Average Half-Life	Primary Route of Elimination
Ouabain	0.3–0.5 mg IV	—	5–10 min	30 min–2 h	21 h	Kidney
Deslanoside (Cedilanid-D)	0.8 mg IV	—	10–30 min	1–2 h	33 h	Kidney
Digoxin (Lanoxin)	1.25–1.5 mg po 0.75–1.0 mg IV	0.125–0.5 mg	15–30 min	1–5 h	36 h	Kidney
Digitoxin (Crystodigin, Purodigin)	0.7–1.2 mg po 0.2–1.0 mg IV	0.1–0.2 mg	30 min–2 h	4–12 h	4–6 days	Liver
Digitalis (Digifortis)	—	0.1 g	—	—	4–6 days	Liver

The treatment of toxicity consists of withholding the drug until the symptoms abate. The treatment of life-threatening arrhythmias is instituted as needed (see Chap. 28.)

Diuretics

Diuretics are used in heart failure to mobilize edematous fluid and reduce pulmonary venous pressure (Table 27-23). If excess vascular volume is excreted, blood volume returning to the heart can be reduced and cardiac function improved.

Diuretics act on the kidney by promoting excretion of sodium and water. Many varieties of diuretics are available, and some have specific indications for use. Thiazide diuretics are usually the first choice because of their convenience, safety, and effectiveness. They are particularly useful in treating edema secondary to CHF as well as in controlling hypertension. The thiazides inhibit sodium reabsorption in the distal tubule, thus promoting excretion of sodium and water.

Two potent diuretics are furosemide (Lasix) and ethacrynic acid (Edecrin). These drugs act powerfully on the ascending loop of Henle to promote sodium and water excretion. Furosemide is more commonly used because it is slightly more predictable in its response.

Spironolactone (Aldactone) and triamterene (Dyrenium) are potassium-sparing diuretics that promote sodium and water excretion but block potassium excretion. These are milder diurectics because of their potassium-sparing property.

Vasodilator drugs

The use of vasodilator drugs such as nitrates, sodium nitroprusside (Nipride), and hydralazine (Apresoline) has been particularly important in treating CHF refractory to digitalis and diuretics. These drugs reduce peripheral resistance and pulmonary venous pressure. Reducing peripheral resistance increases left ventricular stroke volume and cardiac output. Reducing pulmonary venous pressure causes a reduction in left ventricular preload. Thus, myocardial function is enhanced and myocardial oxygen demand lessened. Morphine sulfate, used primarily in acute CHF, decreases afterload by causing peripheral pooling of blood, which decreases the cardiac work load. (Vasodilator drugs are discussed in more detail in Chap. 28.)

Table 27-22
Manifestations of Digitalis Toxicity

Cardiovascular	Bradycardia Tachycardia Pulse deficit Arrhythmias Premature ventricular contractions First-degree AV blocks Atrial fibrillation
Gastrointestinal	Anorexia Nausea Vomiting Diarrhea Abdominal pain
Neurological	Headache Drowsiness Confusion Insomnia Muscle weakness
Visual	Double vision Blurred vision Colored vision (usually green or yellow) Visual halos

Dietary Management

The edema of congestive heart failure is often treated by dietary restriction of sodium. The degree of sodium restriction depends on the severity of the heart failure and the effectiveness of diuretic therapy. Diets that are severely restricted in sodium are rarely prescribed because they are unpalatable and client compliance is very low.

The normal daily dietary intake of sodium ranges from 3000 to 7000 mg. A commonly prescribed diet for a client with mild CHF is a 2-g sodium diet (Appendix B, Table 2). All foods high in sodium should be eliminated (Appendix B, Table 12). For more severe CHF, sodium intake is restricted to 500 to 1000 mg. On this diet, milk, cheese, bread, cereals, and canned soups and vegetables must be eliminated.

Fluid restrictions are not commonly prescribed for individuals with mild to moderate CHF. Diuretic therapy and digitalis preparations act as effective diuretics to promote fluid excretion.

The client and family need to be told which foods are high in sodium. Salt substitutes frequently contain potassium, and their use should be verified by the physician. The client needs to be instructed on how to read labels to look for sodium as an ingredient.

Nursing Management

Health promotion and maintenance

An important measure used to prevent heart failure is the treatment or control of the underlying heart disease. In rheumatic valvular disease, valve replacement should be planned before the client develops lung congestion. Prophylactic antibiotics

Table 27-23
Diuretic Therapy Used in Congestive Heart Failure*

Drugs	Mechanism of Action	Side Effects and Adverse Effects
	Thiazides	
Chlorothiazide (Diuril) **Hydrochlorothiazide (HydroDiuril, Oretic, Esidrix)** **Chlorthalidone (Hygroton)**	Increase sodium, chloride, and H_2O excretion by inhibiting reabsorption of sodium and chloride in the distal tubule. K is excreted in conjunction with Na.	Hypokalemia Increased uric acid Hypercalcemia Hyperglycemia Dermatological reactions
	Loop Diuretics	
Furosemide (Lasix) **Ethacrynic acid (Edecrin)**	Very potent diuretics which increase urine output by preventing sodium and water reabsorption in the loop of Henle and distal tubule	Hypokalemia Hyperglycemia Hyperuricemia
	Potassium-Sparing Products	
Spironolactone (Aldactone)	Antagonizes the action of aldosterone in the distal tubule. Results in increased sodium excretion and potassium retention.	Hyperkalemia Gynecomastia Amenorrhea GI disturbances
Triamterene (Dyrenium)	Mechanism of action unknown. Acts on distal tubule to cause sodium excretion and potassium retention.	Hyperkalemia Nausea and vomiting Leg cramps
	Combination Products	
Aldactazide (spironolactone + hydrochlorothiazide) **Dyazide (triamterene + hydrochlorothiazide)**	Has more potent diuretic effect than single agents alone. Advantage of potassium-sparing effects.	

*For more information on diuretic therapy, see Table 26-15.

should be given to individuals with a known history of rheumatic heart disease when they undergo surgery or procedures involving instrumentation (e.g., cystoscopy, tooth extraction).

Another important preventive measure concerns early and continued treatment of hypertension. Hyperlipidemic states in individuals with CAD need to be managed with diet, exercise, and medication. The use of antiarrhythmic agents or pacemakers is indicated for individuals with serious arrhythmias or conduction disturbances.

Acute intervention

Many individuals with CHF do not experience an acute episode. If they do, they are usually initially managed in a CCU or critical care unit and later transferred to a general unit when their condition has stabilized. The nursing care plan in Table 27-24 applies to the client with stabilized acute or chronic CHF. The nursing management of acute CHF is discussed in Chap. 28.

Chronic management

It is important to realize that CHF will be a chronic illness for most individuals. Important nursing responsibilities are (1) educating the client about the physiological changes that have occurred and (2) assisting the client to adapt to both the physiological and psychological changes. It must be emphasized to the client that it is possible to live productively with this health problem.

Diet and Weight Management Diet education and weight management are critical to the client's control of chronic CHF. The nurse or dietitian should take a detailed diet history, determining not only what foods the client eats and when but also the sociocultural value of food. The nurse can use this data base to assist the client in solving problems. The client should be taught not only what foods are low and high in sodium but also ways to enhance food flavors without the use of salt (e.g., substituting lemon juice and various spices). Low-sodium, potassium-rich diets are

Table 27-24
Nursing Care Plan for the Client with Congestive Heart Failure

Client Problem	Expected Outcome	Nursing Intervention
Fatigue	Reduction in physical activity. Feeling of being rested.	Have client rest in bed or chair when tired. Provide emotional as well as physical rest. If client is in bed, teach leg exercises to prevent phlebothrombosis. Assess client daily for dyspnea, fatigue, and pulse rate to determine the level of activity that can be performed. Provide frequent small feedings instead of three large meals per day. Teach client about expenditure of energy on various activities (Table 27-14).
Edema	Reduction or elimination of edema.	Evaluate degree of peripheral edema and measure abdominal girth daily. Give good skin care to edematous areas. Administer digitalis agents and diuretics as prescribed. Assess intake and output every 8 h. Weigh client daily. Observe for manifestations of hypokalemia. Provide sodium-restricted diet as ordered. Teach client about sodium content of various foods (Appendix B, Table 12). Encourage eating of foods high in potassium (Appendix B, Table 11).
Dyspnea	Respiratory rate of 12–18/min.	Elevate head of bed to Fowler's position. Support arms with pillows. Use footboard. Administer oxygen via nasal cannula. Auscultate for lung and heart sounds every 4 h.
Predisposition to constipation	Normal elimination pattern.	Teach client to avoid straining at defecation. Administer stool softeners or laxatives as ordered. Provide bedside commode if indicated. Create relaxed environment.
Altered lifestyle	Rehabilitated to maximum capacity.	Teach client about the disease process and altered physiological function. Instruct client regarding medications and dietary restrictions. Encourage client to adopt a lifestyle compatible with the degree of heart impairment. Assist client and family in planning necessary changes. Encourage the client who seems discouraged or hopeless.
Recurring or decompensated CHF	Report symptoms to health care provider.	Teach client manifestations to report, including: Shortness of breath at rest Swelling of ankles, feet, or abdomen Loss of appetite; nausea or vomiting Weight gain of 1–2 kg in a 2-day period Frequent urination Persistent cough Changes in heart rate ± 20 beats different than usual

usually prescribed for chronic CHF clients. However, low sodium diets are not palatable and require a strong dedication on the part of the client and family in order to make necessary changes.

Where weight reduction is indicated to decrease the cardiac work load, the nurse and dietitian can assist the client and family in menu planning. Instructing the client to weigh himself daily is important for monitoring fluid retention as well as weight reduction. The client should be instructed to weigh himself at the same time each day, preferably before breakfast, with the same type of clothing. This helps to ensure valid comparisons from day to day and to identify early signs of fluid retention.

Drug Therapy The client with CHF is usually required to take medication for the rest of his life. This often becomes difficult because the client may be asymptomatic when CHF is under control. It must be stressed to the client that the disease is chronic and that medication must be continued to keep the heart failure under control. The client needs to understand the importance of maintaining adequate drugs levels as well as the danger of omitting or making up missed doses. In some situations, it is helpful to work out a system that helps the client to remember to take the medication.

The client needs to evaluate the action of the prescribed medication. He should be taught to recognize the manifestations of digitalis toxicity (Table 27-22). The client should also be taught how to take his pulse and to know under what circumstances drugs, especially digitalis preparations, should be held and a physician consulted. The pulse should always be taken for a full minute. A pulse lower than 60 bpm may be a contraindication to taking a digitalis preparation unless specified otherwise by the physician. A slow pulse may indicate a need to alter the digitalis therapy. However, in the absence of primary heart block or the development of ventricular ectopy, a pulse of 60 bpm or less is not a contraindication to taking digitalis. A pulse of 50 bpm (especially in a client who is also taking beta-blocking drugs) may be acceptable.

Clients should also be taught the symptoms of hypokalemia if they are taking diuretics that cause potassium excretion. (Manifestations of hypokalemia are discussed in Chap. 12.) Hypokalemia sensitizes the myocardium to digitalis. Consequently, the client may develop toxicity from an ordinary dosage of digitalis. Frequently, clients who are taking thiazide or loop diuretics are given supplemental potassium.

Rest The nurse can instruct the client in energy-saving and energy-efficient behaviors after an evaluation of daily activities has been done. For instance, once the nurse understands the client's daily routine, suggestions can be made for simplification of work or modification of an activity. Sometimes, an activity that the client enjoys may need to be eliminated. In such cases, the client should be helped to explore alternative activities that cause less physical and cardiac stress. The physical environment may require modification in situations where there is an increased cardiac work load demand (e.g., frequent climbing of stairs, inaccessibility to shopping areas). The nurse can help the client identify areas where outside assistance can be obtained.

Nurses are also responsible for encouraging clients who are discouraged and for motivating those who feel that their situation is unmanageable. This may require that the nurse assist the client and family in making lifestyle changes that they can accept and comply with. Often, the nurse can begin this process by establishing small, *achievable* goals with the client. Continuous support by the family and health care providers is important. If the client does not adhere to the prescribed regimen, it is important to determine the reasons. After this evaluation process, it may be necessary to plan an alternative therapeutic regimen that is more compatible with the client's lifestyle.

Case Study / Myocardial Infarction

Chester T., a 47-year-old successful businessman, was rushed to the hospital by a rescue squad after experiencing crushing substernal pain radiating down his left arm. He also had dizziness, nausea, diaphoresis, and shortness of breath.

He revealed a history of angina pectoris, hypertension, and obesity (although he had just lost 10 lb). He has three teenage children who were causing problems for him, and his business partner had just died of cancer.

After an ECG was taken, a diagnosis of inferior-lateral wall MI was made. His ECG also showed premature ventricular contractions and tachycardia.

Laboratory results indicated that all of the following were significantly elevated:

Triglycerides	220 mg/dL
Cholesterol	350 mg/dL
CPK	730 units/L

Medical treatment:

Hydrochlorothiazide 50 mg twice a day
Oxygen at 3 L/minute
Bed rest
Vital signs every hour
1500-calorie, 3-g sodium, low cholesterol diet
IV at keep-open rate
Lidocaine drip for PVCs
Morphine prn

Discussion Questions

Which coronary artery was most likely occluded in Chester's coronary circulation?

1. Explain the pathogenesis of CAD. What risk factors may contribute to its development? What risk factors were present in Chester's life?
2. What is angina pectoris? How does angina differ from MI?
3. What happens to the infarcted muscle of the heart after the initial injury?
4. List the clinical manifestations that Chester exhibited and explain the pathophysiological bases.
5. Explain the significance of the results of the ECG and the laboratory tests.
6. For each treatment measure Chester received, explain the physiological bases for its use.
7. What complications may result from an MI?

REVIEW QUESTIONS

The number of the question corresponds to the same numbered objective at the beginning of the chapter.

1. Which of the following changes occurs in the development of CAD?
   a. formation of fibrous tissue around coronary artery orifices
   b. accumulation of lipid and fibrous tissue within the coronary arteries
   c. diffuse involvement of plaque formation in coronary arteries and veins
   d. chronic vasoconstriction of coronary arteries leading to permanent vasopasm

2. Which of the following measures is not appropriate to include in a teaching plan to decrease risk factors for CAD?
   a. modification of a stressful lifestyle
   b. weight reduction and decreased dietary intake of saturated fats
   c. reduction and control of hypertension
   d. weight lifting to increase cardiac output

3. Which of the following describes the pain associated with angina pectoris?
   a. pain that is not relieved by nitroglycerin or rest
   b. substernal chest pain precipitated by activity
   c. crushing, heavy pain lasting for 15 to 20 minutes
   d. substernal pain penetrating to and radiating down the back

4. Which of the following should be included in a teaching plan for a client with angina?
   a. prophylactic use of nitroglycerin
   b. behavior modification to prevent recurrent MI
   c. symptoms of digitalis toxicity
   d. knowledge of foods that are high in potassium

5. Healing following MI is well established
   a. within 3 weeks after the infarction
   b. when chest pain and dyspnea are not present
   c. in about 6 to 8 weeks after the infarction
   d. at 4 to 6 days after the infarction

6. The most common complication in the first week post-MI is
   a. ventricular rupture
   b. Dressler syndrome
   c. cardiogenic shock
   d. arrhythmias

7. A client 5 days post-MI is very restless and apprehensive. The nurse can help him by
   a. structuring his environment and routine so that he can rest
   b. encouraging the family to provide for his physical care and emotional support
   c. allowing him to participate in planning and carrying out his activities
   d. providing all care by doing everything for him

8. Three days post-MI, a client states that he does not understand what the alarm is about because his problem is just bad indigestion. His reaction is an example of
   a. anger
   b. projection
   c. depression
   d. denial

9. When a client post-MI is being prepared for discharge, he should be instructed to
   a. take it easy until his healing is complete
   b. stay at home and avoid exposure to the environment
   c. begin a graduated, progressive exercise program
   d. do isometric exercises in a relaxed environment

10. Manifestations of left-sided heart failure include
   a. peripheral edema, jugular vein distension, and varicose veins
   b. dyspnea on exertion, rales, and an S_3 heart sound
   c. fatigue, cyanosis, and hepatomegaly
   d. substernal soreness, hypertension, and diplopia

11. The dietary management of a client with CHF emphasizes primarily a
   a. reduction in dietary sodium
   b. decreased fluid intake
   c. low cholesterol, low saturated fat diet
   d. reduction in dietary potassium

12. Manifestations of digitalis toxicity include
   a. rapid pulse, nausea, and cyanosis
   b. nausea, headache, and visual disturbances
   c. constipation, bradycardia, and polyuria
   d. arrhythmias, urinary retention, and diaphoresis

REFERENCES

1. K. Isselbacher et al. (eds.), *Harrison's Principles of Internal Medicine*, 4th ed., McGraw-Hill Book Company, New York, 1980, p. 1158.
2. M. J. Karvonen, "Epidemiology of Atherosclerosis and Risk Factor Identification in the Asymptomatic Population," in W. E. James and E. R. Amsterdam (eds.), *Coronary Heart Disease: Exercise Testing and Cardiac Rehabilitation*, Symposia Specialists, Miami, 1977, p. 14.
3. T. Gordon et al., "Differences in Coronary Heart Disease in Framingham, Honolulu, and Puerto Rico," *J Chronic Dis*, **27:**329–344 (1974).
4. W. B. Kannel and T. R. Dawber, "Contributors to Coronary Risk—Implications for Prevention and Public Health: The Framingham Study," *Heart and Lung*, **1**:797–809 (1972).
5. W. B. Kannel et al., "Electrocardiographic Left Ventricular Hypertrophy and Risk of Coronary Artery Disease: The Framingham Study," *Ann Intern Med*, **72:**813–822 (1970).
6. J. C. Cassel, "Summary of Major Findings of the Evans County Cardiovascular Studies," *Arch Intern Med*, **128:** 887–889 (1971).
7. C. D. Jenkins et al., "Prediction of Clinical Coronary Heart Disease by a Test for Coronary-Prone Behavior Pattern," *N Engl J Med*, **290:**1271–1275 (1974).
8. Gordon et al., op. cit., p. 707.
9. K. T. Francis, "High Density Lipoprotein Cholesterol and Coronary Heart Disease," *South Med J*, **73**(2):169–173 (1980).
10. Isselbacher et al., op. cit., p. 1162.

11. N. K. Wenger et al. (eds.), *Cardiology for Nurses*, McGraw-Hill Book Company, New York, 1980, p. 268.
12. American Heart Association, *Heart Facts—1981*, National Center, Dallas, 1980, p. 24.
13. American Heart Association, *Heartbook*, E. P. Dutton Co., Inc., New York, 1980.
14. Wenger et al., op. cit., p. 269.
15. K. G. Andreoli et al., *Comprehensive Cardiac Care*, 4th ed., The C. V. Mosby Company, St. Louis, 1979, p. 28.
16. Karvonen, op. cit., p. 18.
17. S. G. Haynes et al., "The Relationship of Psychosocial Factors to Coronary Heart Disease in the Framingham Study," *Am J Epidemiol*, **111:**37–58 (1980).
18. Ibid.
19. C. R. Conti and R. C. Curry, Jr., "Coronary Artery Spasm and Myocardial Ischemia," *Mod Concepts Cardiovasc Dis*, **49**(1):1–6 (1980).
20. D. A. Jones, C. F. Dunbar, and M. M. Jirovec, *Medical-Surgical Nursing: A Conceptual Approach*, 2d ed., McGraw-Hill Book Company, New York, 1982, p. 1027.
21. R. S. Cain, R. M. Ferguson, and J. H. Tillisch, "Variant Angina: A Nursing Approach," *Heart Lung*, **8**(6):1122–1125 (1979).
22. Wenger, et al., op. cit., p. 281.
23. Andreoli et al., op. cit., p. 70.
24. Jones, Dunbar, and Jirovec, op. cit., p. 1030.
25. Isselbacher et al., op. cit., p. 1129.
26. M. B. Wiener et al., *Clinical Pharmacology and Therapeutics in Nursing*, McGraw-Hill Book Company, New York, 1979, p. 673.
27. R. S. Lazarus, "Positive Denial: The Case for Not Facing Reality," *Psychology Today*, **13:**44–60 (1979).
28. D. S. Krantz, "Cognitive Processes and Recovery from Heart Attack: A Review and Theoretical Analysis," *J Human Stress*, **6:**27–38 (1980).
29. P. R. Mullen, "Cutting Back after a Heart Attack: An Overview," *Health Educ Monogr*, **6**(3):295–311 (1978).
30. W. B. Tuttle and W. L. Cook, "Sexual Behavior in Post-Myocardial Infarction Patients," *Am J Cardiol*, **13:**140 (1964).
31. H. K. Hellerstein and E. H. Friedman, "Sexual Activity and the Post-Coronary Patient," *Arch Intern Med*, **125:** 992 (1970).
32. Ibid., pp. 987–999.
33. E. Nemec et al., "Heart Rate and Blood Pressure Responses During Sexual Activity in Normal Males," *Am Heart J*, **92:**276 (1976).
34. R. Pineo, *Congestive Heart Failure*, Appleton Century Crofts, New York, 1978, p. 26.

Chapter 28

NURSING ROLE IN MANAGEMENT

Critical Care of the Coronary Client

Patricia Palmer Stephens
Susan C. Littell

Learning Objectives

1. Explain the purpose and essential elements of a coronary care unit.
2. Differentiate between common life-threatening and non-life-threatening arrhythmias.
3. Describe the medical and nursing management of common arrhythmias.
4. Explain the essential elements of Basic Cardiac Life Support and Advanced Cardiac Life Support.
5. Describe the principles of hemodynamic monitoring and related nursing management.
6. Describe the purpose and function of the intraaortic balloon pump.
7. Describe the early management of a client with an acute myocardial infarction.
8. Describe the management of a client with acute pulmonary edema.
9. Describe the management of cardiogenic shock.
10. Describe the preoperative and postoperative care of the client who has cardiac surgery.
11. Describe the management of clients with pacemakers, differentiating between temporary and permanent placement.

CORONARY CARE UNIT (CCU) ENVIRONMENT

Purpose and History

The coronary or cardiac care unit (CCU) is a highly specialized unit for the care of clients who are critically ill or suspected of having a critical illness due to cardiac malfunction. The purpose of a CCU is to reduce the mortality and morbidity of cardiac clients. To achieve this purpose, a CCU contains specialized equipment for assessing and treating the cardiac client. However, the most important factor determining the effectiveness of a CCU is a well-educated, highly motivated nursing staff. The most sophisticated instrumentation is useless without the presence of competent nursing personnel to interpret data and to give the needed care.

The first CCU was established in 1962 to respond to life-threatening cardiac disturbances. This was possible because of advances in continuous cardiac-monitoring techniques, closed-chest cardiac resuscitation, and the development of defibrillation and cardioversion techniques. However, mortality rates did not decrease significantly until nursing personnel were educated in the early detection of abnormal rhythms.[1] Today, mortality rates of clients with acute myocardial infarction (MI) who reach the hospital are 20 percent, compared with 35 percent in earlier days.[2] Deaths today occur largely from massive MI resulting in severe cardiac dysfunction or from persistent arrhythmias. The decrease in mortality is due primarily to the greater emphasis on preventing catastrophic events, such as cardiac arrest, by early detection of arrhythmias or other changes indicating that a catastrophic event is likely to occur.

Physical Factors

Equipment

The uniqueness of a CCU is due, in part, to the type and variety of equipment available to help in the ongoing assessment and management of the cardiac client. Fig. 28-1 illustrates equipment that may be found in the client's room. Some equipment, such as the crash cart and the intraaortic balloon pump, is brought into the room when needed, whereas other equipment is standard for each room. Specific nursing responsibilities for the use of this equipment are described later in this chapter.

Bed Special beds which are electronically grounded are generally used. These beds have removable headboards and footboards for client acces-

*This chapter was reviewed by Mary Ann Cammarano, R.N., M.S.N., CCRN, Research Nurse, Southwest Cardiology Research Conference, Albuquerque, New Mexico, and former Head Nurse, Adult Intensive Care Unit, Parkway General, North Miami, Florida; Julie M. Dax, R.N., B.S.N., CCRN, Trauma Coordinator, former Assistant Head Nurse, Surgical Intensive and Coronary Care Units, University of New Mexico Hospital, Albuquerque, New Mexico; and Gertrude E. Marquis, R.N., B.S., CCRN, Staff Nurse ICU/CCU, Anna Kaseman Hospital, Albuquerque, New Mexico.

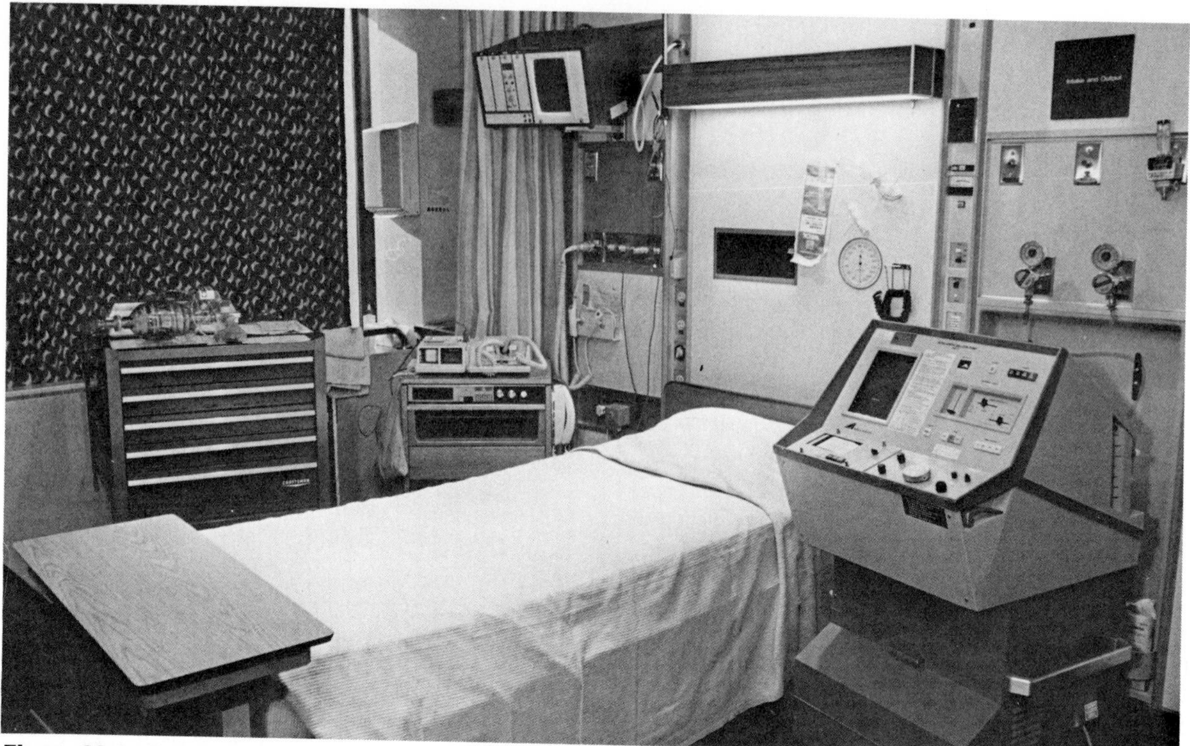

Figure 28-1 Equipment in a CCU.

sibility and use in cardiopulmonary resuscitation. They are narrower than standard hospital beds because of smaller rooms and have hard mattresses. In addition, some beds are radiographically transparent for use with fluoroscopy.

Monitors Bedside monitors for assessing the client's electrophysiological and hemodynamic status are available. Monitoring equipment varies in sophistication from simple portable bedside monitors to computerized wall banks capable of continuously reporting rhythm abnormalities and arterial and venous pressures, as well as other hemodynamic parameters, such as cardiac output, blood chemistries, and oxygen concentrations.

Most CCUs have the capability for continuous electrocardiogram (ECG) monitoring to determine arrhythmias, especially life-threatening ventricular arrhythmias. In addition, most CCUs have the capability of continuously monitoring arterial and venous pressures.

The typical CCU has a central monitoring station which displays information from each client's bedside monitor. This central unit should be observed continuously by a nurse or technician trained in the detection of rhythm disturbances. Many of these central units are equipped with automatic recorders, a memory loop, and freeze displays which aid in the detection and documentation as well as the diagnosis of arrhythmias.

Defibrillators Defibrillators, first developed in 1960,[3] are used to deliver direct electrical current via special paddles to the heart in order to interrupt fibrillation, or chaotic electrical activity in the conduction system of the heart. Some defibrillators are built in with a central console at the nursing station, but the activator and paddles are at the bedside. Many models are battery-powered and portable (see Fig. 28-20). It is essential that every CCU have at least one defibrillator available at all times. Defibrillators need to be checked regularly to determine if they are delivering the desired level of electrical current.

Emergency Cart Emergency or crash carts are specialized carts containing equipment and medications which are most often needed for treating cardiovascular or respiratory emergencies. Table 28-1 lists the contents of a typical emergency cart. These carts must be clearly labeled, readily accessible, and easily movable to the client's location. Each CCU needs to follow a systematic, regular process of checking the contents of the emergency cart for missing, outdated, or nonworking items.

Intraaortic Balloon Pump (IABP) Developed in the late 1960s, the IABP is used to decrease the work load of the left ventricle, lower the myocardial oxygen consumption, increase cardiac output, and enhance perfusion of the coronary arteries and vital organs. The IABP consists of a polyurethane balloon mounted on the end of a vascular catheter which is externally connected to a control console. This portable console houses controls and alarms, monitoring equipment, and gas tanks. The nursing management of the client with an IABP is discussed later in this chapter.

Doppler Flowmeters Doppler flowmeters are special devices which amplify the sound of blood flow. They are used to verify the presence of nonpalpable pulses and to determine inaudible blood pressures when the client does not have an arterial line for recording arterial pressures.

Rotating Tourniquets Rotating tourniquet machines are sometimes used in place of manually applied tourniquets to reduce venous return to the heart in pulmonary edema. The machine has four cuffs (similar to those on a sphygmomanometer) which are applied to all four extremities. Automatically, it then alternately inflates and deflates the cuffs in a set time and order.

Electrical hazards

Electrical hazards are a major factor to consider in the CCU environment. This is especially true when multiple pieces of electrical equipment are used for a single client. Some clients are electrically sensitive because of their body's lowered electrical resistance (e.g., clients with wet skin or skin that has been disrupted by punctures or abrasions). Thus, they may receive a *microshock,* electrical injury from current not sensed by a healthy individual. Currents of 180 microamperes (180/1,000,000 ampere) have been known to cause ventricular fibrillation. A *macroshock* is that current sensed by a healthy individual at 1 milliampere (1/1000 ampere).

Electrical hazards are due to (1) mechanical defect or malfunction (a common hazard for everyone) and (2) low-level leakage current found in all electrical circuits (a hazard for only electrically sensitive clients).

Table 28-1
Common Emergency Cart Contents

Alcohol or betadine wipes
Blood gas equipment
Blood pump
Cardiac arrest tray
Cardic board
CVP tray
Cutdown tray
Emergency drugs (see Table 28-15)
Endotracheal tubes with stylets
Examination and sterile gloves
IV solutions and administration sets
Laryngoscopes with extra batteries and lamps
Lubricant
Medication labels and IV flowmeter tapes
Needles and syringes
Nasogastric tubes and irrigating syringe
Oral airways
Oxygen bottle and flowmeter
Oxygen masks and cannulas with tubing
Pacemaker tray
Self-inflating resuscitation bag with masks (Ambu bag)
Suction catheters
Suction machine and tubing
Tape
Tourniquets
Tracheostomy tray and tubes with ties

There is special equipment that can be used to measure the amount of leakage, as well as other electrical conditions. These measurements are usually made by the hospital engineer. The procedures that nurses may use to reduce electrical hazards are outlined in Table 28-2.

Personnel Factors (Staff)

Personnel factors are the most critical factors in the environment of a CCU. Ideally, the nursing staff in a CCU should consist of well-educated, skilled practitioners who are highly motivated and assertive. They work very closely with their physician colleagues in giving care. The staff in a CCU should have completed a coronary care or critical care course prior to assuming full responsibilities in the unit. A typical course outline is found in Table 28-3. This content goes beyond that found in a basic nursing curriculum. It provides the framework for the daily nursing care of cardiac clients in a specialized unit.

In addition to the basic knowledge of coronary care, the CCU nursing staff requires regular continuing education programs to stay up-to-date on changes in diagnosis and treatment, to remedy problems in nursing practice, and to improve the level of care.

Table 28-2

Ways to Reduce Electrical Hazards[4,5]

1. Heed early warnings of circuit overload, such as dimming of lights or blowing of fuses, to prevent electrical fires.
2. Inspect all electrical plugs and cords for damaged prongs and frayed wiring. Do not use them if any defect is noted to prevent shocks.
3. Use electrically operated equipment only with an independent conductive ground wire (have three-wire line cords).
4. Never use any form of three-prong to two-prong adaptor ("cheater") because they remove the ground.
5. Do not use two-wire line cords (found in television sets and beauty aids) in electrically sensitive areas (e.g., near dialysis machines) or with electrically sensitive clients since they have no ground.
6. Use relatively short electrical cords because the amount of electrical leakage is related to the length of the cord.
7. Unplug all equipment which is not in use.
8. Plug all pieces of electrical equipment used for one client into the same cluster of wall outlets to maintain minimal ground resistance.
9. If a cord or plug is warm to the touch, replace the equipment and send it for repairs.
10. Insert and *remove* all line cords from wall sockets by grasping the plug, not the cord, to prevent damaging of the wiring.
11. Do not touch the client and the electrical equipment at the same time. Send any equipment that produces a tingling sensation for repairs.
12. Be sure that insertion of an electrical plug into an outlet requires some force and that the socket holds the plug securely to ensure proper grounding.
13. Check with the hospital engineer if you are unsure about any potential electrical problems.

Table 28-3

Coronary Care Course Outline

Anatomy and physiology of the heart
Mechanical physiology
Electrophysiology
Monitoring and arrhythmias
Twelve-lead ECGs and vectors
Examination of the cardiovascular system
Pathophysiology of atherosclerosis
Acute phase of MI
Nursing care of the client with an acute MI
Heart sounds
Digitalis and diuretics
Drugs, oxygen, and other measures used in MI
Interaction skills
CHF and nursing care
CPR
Drugs used in CPR
Cardiogenic shock
Swan-Ganz catheter
Intraaortic balloon pump
Antiarrhythmic drugs
Cardiac surgery and nursing care
Pacemakers
Pericarditis
Cardiac catheterization and nursing care
Pressure monitoring
Cardiac rehabilitation
Acid-base balance and blood gases
Respiratory assessment

Formal and informal classes and skill demonstrations and practice are utilized to keep nurses up-to-date on critical care content.

The goal of this preparation and continuing education is to assist the nursing staff in meeting the standards for nursing performance published by the American Nurses' Association[6] and the American Association of Critical Care Nurses (AACN).[7] The standards need to be individualized for each unit and then used in client care audits to ascertain their effectiveness. In addition, individual nurses may take an examination administered by the AACN to become certified in critical care nursing (CCRN).

The stress level of the nursing staff in CCUs is well documented, and examples of professional burnout are common.[8] There are several approaches which may be used to help the nursing staff cope with stress. Of critical importance is the maintenance of a good physician-nurse relationship through regular, frequent meetings.[9] A second means of helping the staff is to increase their ability to communicate. Thirdly, the enforcement of break times away from the unit helps to reduce stress. Adequate staffing and ongoing continuing education also help to lower stress by decreasing anxiety. Some hospitals also provide new patterns in staffing instead of the traditional 8-hour-day, 5-day-week schedules.

Clients

Types of clients admitted to a CCU

The purpose of highly skilled nurses and sophisticated equipment in CCUs is to decrease mortality and morbidity from critical cardiac problems. This is accomplished primarily by constant observation and monitoring of clients. The key is to detect complications early and to institute treatment immediately in order to prevent catastrophic events, such as cardiac arrest. Table 28-4 lists common diagnoses and problems for which clients are admitted to a CCU.

General nursing management

Whatever the suspected or actual diagnosis or problem, the care of clients admitted to a CCU has a basic structure. All clients need continual monitoring

Table 28-4
Reasons for Admission to a CCU

Angina
Congestive heart failure
Arrhythmias
Acute MI
Pulmonary embolus
Cardiac arrest
Conduction disturbances
Digitalis intoxication
Cardiac and vascular surgeries
Chest pain of undetermined origin
Stokes-Adams syndrome

of (1) vital signs and neurological status, (2) heart rhythm, (3) signs and symptoms of disease or potential complications, and (4) responses to treatment and medication. In addition, these clients need emotional support and teaching as an aid in coping with their illness. In meeting these needs, nurses and physicians work closely together, with much overlap in their responsibilities. Because of this close working relationship and the specialized skills of the CCU nurse, the management of clients will not be separated into medical and nursing components but will be discussed as a single entity.

Monitoring As indicated, close monitoring of the CCU client is imperative. Regularly ordered vital signs, including heart rate and the observation of heart rhythm, blood pressure, respiratory rate and rhythm, and temperature, bring the nurse in close contact with the client. This contact provides for inspection of the client's skin color, temperature, turgor, moistness or dryness, and the presence and quality of peripheral pulses.

Other parameters will also be closely monitored, such as intake and output and pulmonary artery and wedge pressures. The frequency of these measurements will depend on the client's condition. Equipment for making various observations may range from the simple stethoscope and sphygomomanometer to sophisticated arterial lines attached to oscilloscopes and computer banks. The various machines used to extend the nurse's observation are never a substitute for actual physical observation by the nurse because machines may malfunction. Some changes in vital signs and their implications are outlined in Table 28-5. The level of consciousness should be noted on an ongoing basis since inadequate perfusion of oxygenated blood will affect the sensorium. Clients also need to be observed for their level of activity. For example, restlessness can be caused by pain, anxiety, impending shock, and inadequate brain perfusion.

Table 28-5
Possible Implications of Changing Vital Signs

↑ temperature	Inflammation Infection Atelectasis
↓ temperature	Sepsis Therapeutic hypothermia Shock
↑ pulse	Anxiety Hemorrhage ↑ temperature Arrhythmias
↓ pulse	Heart block ↑ vagus tone Head injury
↑ respirations	Metabolic acidosis Pain Anoxia
↓ respirations	Pain Metabolic alkalosis
↑ blood pressure	Pain Hypertension Activity Hypervolemia
↓ blood pressure	Hemorrhage Cardiac tamponade Arrhythmias Hypovolemia Orthostatic changes Shock

The nurse should assess the client for pain, as described in Chap. 50. Table 27-6 compares the pain of MI and angina. Respiratory problems, such as pleurisy, that may cause chest pain are described in Chap. 20.

The nurse also needs to observe the client's level of anxiety. Table 28-6 outlines some physical and psychological manifestations of anxiety. The more anxious the client, the more manifestations will be noted.

Treatment The client will also be receiving various medications and treatments to aid in his recovery. Many of these require special skill in their administration and evaluation of their effects.

Rest and energy conservation are also important parts of the treatment. Providing for adequate rest is often difficult because of the frequent treatments and assessments of the client. However, the low nurse/client ratio should make it possible for the nurse to assist the client in all of his activities.

Table 28-6
Manifestations of Anxiety[10]

Physical	Psychological
Heart rate 10 bpm or more over baseline	Avoiding looking at nurse when speaking
Systolic blood pressure 10 mmHg over baseline	Nail or lip biting
Dry mouth	Verbal expressions of fear
Rapid, darting eye movement	Rapid, abrupt speech in a high, loud-pitched voice
Excessive perspiration	Constant talking
Generalized trembling or tremor of the hands	Shift of focus of conversation from illness
Strained facial muscles	Hesitation in answering questions, stammering, difficulty in concentrating on simple questions, and makes repetitive statements
Marked pallor or flushing of the face	Preoccupation with conceptions of dying
Sitting in a rigid posture with arms folded across chest	Evidence of crying
Clenching fists	

Psychological Support The CCU nurse has an extremely important function in supporting the client and his family during this crisis period. CCU clients frequently experience claustrophobia, loss of control, hopelessness, and depression.[11] Anger and denial are commonly used coping mechanisms. Others include distortion, repression, suppression, dissociation, rationalization, identification, projection, displacement, and intellectualization. (Table 27-12 presents emotional and behavioral responses following an acute MI.)

Nurses need to be aware of the possible presence of these coping mechanisms. However, nurses should not eliminate them, leaving the client defenseless against the stress of his illness and hospitalization. Some basic principles of crisis intervention are as follows:

1. Assist the client and his family to talk about the problem that confronts them.
2. Present facts about the situation in manageable increments (e.g., do not tell them everything they need to know about an MI in one sitting).
3. Encourage the client and his family to accept help from outside sources (e.g., a religious adviser, friends, extended family).
4. Assist the client and his family in identifying their own strengths or those to which they have access in helping them cope with the situation.

An important nursing measure is listening to the client and allowing him to set the pace and discuss his feelings. Both clients and their families need understandable, consistent answers to the numerous questions about unit routines, as well as the diagnosis, treatment, and prognosis. Television viewing sometimes provides diversion for clients who cannot or do not wish to read or do handiwork.

A supportive family also helps the client. The family should be present when explanations and teaching are offered to the client. This ensures that everyone is receiving the same information. The client should have the authority to decide which visitors (including family members) he will receive and how much information they are given. Rules and regulations regarding visiting are very rigid in some institutions. These should be enforced when necessary, but the client's condition and desires should dictate the visiting policy. For example, if a man wishes his wife to stay in the room, and if his condition is stable and she does not upset him, she should be allowed to stay. On the other hand, families often begin to offer advice to the client when he is still in the CCU, such as, "You'll stop smoking now" or "No more eggs for you." Such advice often takes the form of nagging that may be due to family anxiety. The nurse needs to be aware that this may occur and to inform the family that nagging may place undesirable stress on the client.

Teaching Teaching CCU clients and their families is another important function of the nurse. Chap. 5 outlines the basic principles of client education. An important factor is the client's readiness to learn. Since many clients are admitted to a CCU on an emergency basis, there is no opportunity for preparatory teaching. Thus, teaching begins with brief explanations of the care being given. Much teaching is done on this informal basis. However, retention of information and comprehension of what is taught may be hindered by the degree of illness, the medications given, and the anxiety level of the client. It is recommended that standard teaching plans be developed and individualized for use in teaching clients. The nurse must recognize that content supposedly learned in the CCU may need to be repeated several times before the client is able to retain it.

Formal teaching in a CCU should be done in very short, structured segments, and the statements must be direct, brief, clear, and simple.[12] In dealing with the CCU client, it is important to avoid subjects of no interest or great complexity. In addition, the nurse who is instructing a CCU client should stop the teaching session if the client exhibits any of the following: tachycardia or ectopic beats, increased respiratory rate, diaphoresis or flushing, chest pain, dyspnea, and withdrawal by closing of the eyes. Clients who have open heart surgery are usually admitted to the hospital soon enough before surgery to allow time for preoperative teaching. The teaching plan for these clients is described later in this chapter.

Response to the environment

A common response to the environment of the CCU is sensory disturbances. These may take the form of *sensory overload* or *sensory deprivation.* Sensory overload refers to the situation in which a client experiences an increase in the quality and quantity of stimuli. This may be due to the continuous use of bright lights, the ongoing noise of monitors, respirators, and suctioning apparatus, and so on. This sensory overload may result in sleep deprivation. Symptoms of sensory overload include agitation, restlessness, slowness in thinking, thought disorganization, severe anxiety, and hallucinations.

Sensory deprivation refers to the situation in which a client experiences a decrease in the quality and quantity of meaningful stimuli. This may be due to decreased stimuli in an unfamiliar environment, sensory loss, and continuous low murmuring sounds of equipment in the CCU. Symptoms of sensory deprivation include alternating periods of irritability and amusement, disorientation in space and time, physical discomfort, inability to concentrate, distorted sensations, and hallucinations.[13]

Nursing measures to help decrease sensory disturbances include the following:

1. Introduce oneself to the client and orient the client to time and place.
2. Decrease noise by *(a)* talking only when necessary when near the client's bedside, *(b)* turning off suction equipment when not in use, and *(c)* placing monitors so that audible sounds are not heard by the client.[14]
3. Dim the lights, especially at night, to help provide daytime/nighttime orientation.
4. Do not awaken the client when he is sleeping if monitoring information indicates that he is stable.
5. Give nursing care in blocks of time to allow the client to rest.
6. Provide meaningful stimuli for the clients by *(a)* using touch as appropriate, *(b)* conversing with the client, and *(c)* allowing the client to have a few visitors.

Table 28-7

Properties of Cardiac Tissue

Automaticity: Ability to initiate an impulse spontaneously and continuously
Contractility: Ability to respond mechanically to an impulse
Conductivity: Ability to transmit an impulse along a membrane in an orderly manner
Excitability: Ability to be eledtrically stimulated

SPECIAL SKILLS AND PROCEDURES COMMON TO A CCU

Arrhythmia Identification and Treatment

As mentioned earlier, the ability to recognize *arrhythmias (dysrhythmias)* is a critical skill for a CCU nurse. This section will explain common arrhythmias and describe basic principles in arrhythmia interpretation. (The reader is referred to books on interpreting ECGs for more detailed information.) To understand arrhythmias (abnormal cardiac rhythms) and their effect on the heart, it is important to know the normal function of the electrical system of the heart. (See Fig. 25-5 and Chap. 25 for an introductory presentation.)

Conduction system

The conduction system consists of neuromuscular tissue embedded in the heart muscle, arranged as shown in Fig. 25-5. Each cell in this tissue has the properties described in Table 28-7. Automaticity is normally greatest in the sinoatrial (SA) node. The SA node normally sends out an impulse 60 to 100 times per minute. This electrical stimulus then travels throughout the conduction system and results in muscle excitation, or contraction.

Because every part of the conduction system possesses automaticity, if one part fails for some reason, a lower portion of the conduction system can institute an impulse. The inherent conduction rates of various structures are listed in Table 28-8. For example, if the SA node is diseased and does not initiate an impulse, the atrioventricular (AV) junction will send out an impulse 40 to 60 times per minute. This arrange-

Table 28-8

Rates of the Conduction System

SA node	60–100 times per min
AV junction	40–60 times per min
Purkinje fibers	20–40 times per min

ment attempts to ensure regular electrical stimulation of cardiac muscle.

ECG monitoring

Chap. 25 describes the mechanism and process of recording an ECG (Figs. 25-6 and 25-14). This chapter will focus on continuous monitoring of one lead of an ECG. As described earlier, each client in a CCU is attached to a bedside monitor which is also attached to a central console. The lead used varies from institution to institution. It also varies according to the client's problems since different leads reflect different areas of the heart. The most common leads for continuous monitoring are leads II and MCL_1 (similar to V_1 of the standard 12-lead ECG).

The electrical activity is displayed on an oscilloscope on a bedside monitor and may also be printed on ECG paper. "Running a strip" refers to recording on ECG paper what is visible on the monitor oscilloscope. A strip is run every time there is an arrhythmia that requires documentation. It is also important to run a baseline strip every 4 to 8 hours. In addition, any time there is a change in rhythm or a significant change in the rate or shape of the complexes, strips are run for documentation and analysis. These ECG strips are usually placed in the client's chart.

For more detailed analysis, a 12-lead ECG will be done on the client (Fig. 25-14). This allows for 12 different electrical views of the conduction system of the heart and may demonstrate such morphological changes as heart damage due to ischemia, enlarged chambers due to abnormal pressures, or valvular damage. The results of a normal 12-lead ECG are illustrated in Fig. 28-2.

In order to interpret the ECG strip, it is essential to know how to measure time and voltage on the ECG paper. ECG paper is a grid consisting of large (heavy lines) and small (light lines) squares (Fig. 28-3). Each large square contains five small squares, horizontally and vertically. Each small square represents 0.04 second horizontally and 0.1 millivolt (mV) vertically. This means that one large square equals 0.20 second and that it takes 300 large (1500 small) squares to equal 1.0 minute. These squares are used in calculating the heart rate and the intervals between different ECG complexes.

There are a variety of ways to calculate the heart rate. One method is to count the number of small boxes between two QRS complexes (RR interval) and then divide that number into 1500 to obtain the heart rate per minute. There are tables which show these calculations (Fig. 28-4). An estimate of the heart rate may be quickly obtained if the nurse memorizes the landmarks (at increments of the large squares).

A second method used for determining the heart rate involves counting the number of the vertical lines imprinted above the ECG grid at 3-second intervals. The number of QRS complexes occurring in 6 seconds can be multiplied by 10 for an estimate of the heart rate. This method is helpful when the heart rhythm is irregular.

A third way to measure distances on the ECG grid is to use calipers (Fig. 28-5). Calipers are used for fine measurements, especially of components of a specific wave. Many times a P or R wave will not fall directly on a light or heavy line. The fine points of the calipers can be placed exactly on the components to be measured and then moved to another part of the grid for time measurement accurate to 0.04 second.

Leads are usually attached to the client's chest wall, with electrical conductive paste between the chest wall and the electrode. Wires leading away from the electrode are then connected to a cable, which in turn is attached to the monitor. If leads are not attached properly, then *artifacts* (distortions in the baseline or waves of the ECG due to electrical or physical interference) may occur. Since muscle activity generates electrical activity, electrodes should be placed over bone rather than muscle mass. Because hair may prevent good contact, the nurse needs to shave the chest of a client with a lot of hair. When a client is moving or dyspneic, the baseline of the ECG will wander. In this case, the nurse needs to do a bedside assessment of the client.

Assessment of cardiac rhythm

Normal sinus rhythm (NSR) refers to the normal conduction pattern of the cardiac cycle which originates in the SA node. Fig. 28-6 illustrates the normal cardiac cycle and the normal time periods for the various waveforms and intervals. Fig. 28-7 is a strip of an NSR. The P wave represents the depolarization of the atrium, the passing of the electrical impulse through the atrial muscle. The QRS complex represents depolarization of the ventricles. The T wave shows the resting phase, or repolarization, when the muscle returns to its prestimulated state. The PR interval represents the period during which the electrical impulse passes through the AV junctional tissue, and the QT interval represents the time needed for ventricular depolarization and repolarization. (Table 25-1 presents an assessment guide for ECG waves.)

Normally, the SA node initiates the impulse and gives the P wave a rounded shape. If another area in the heart is more irritable, it may initiate the impulse before the SA node. This is called an *ectopic focus* or a *premature beat.* Because the contraction does not originate in the SA node, the waveform will be shaped

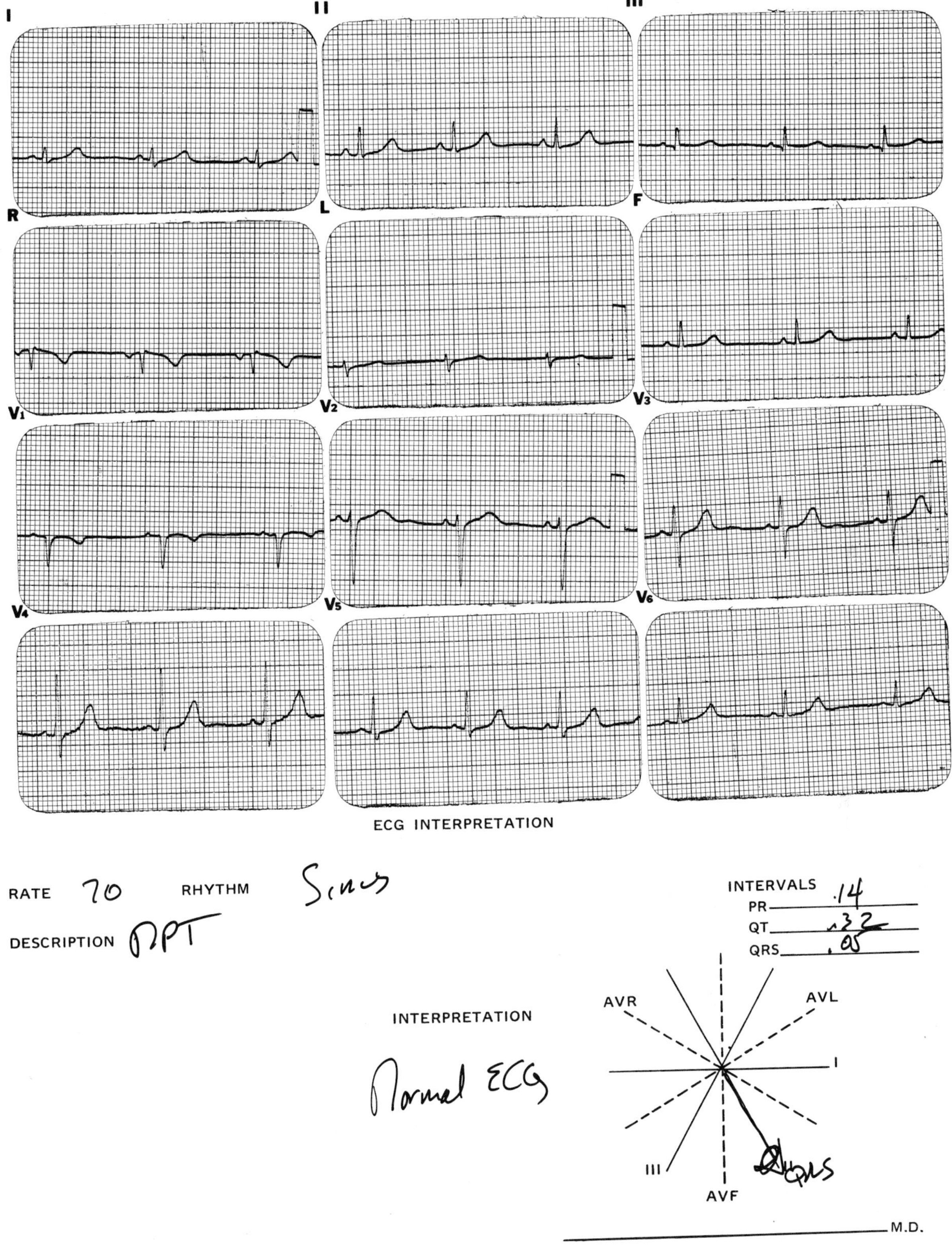

Figure 28-2 Twelve-lead ECG showing an NSR.

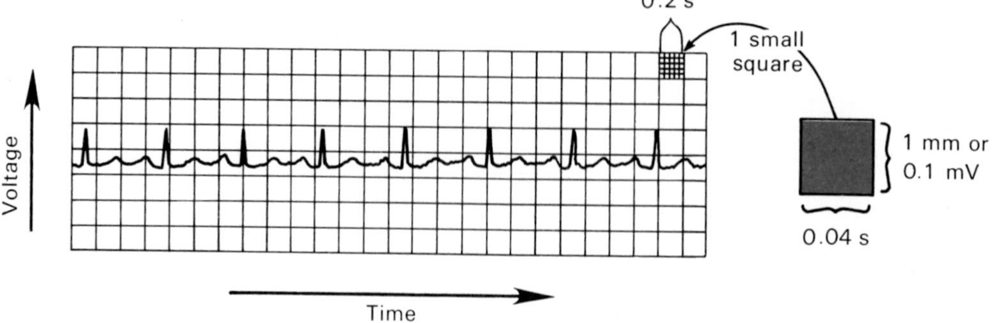

Figure 28-3 Time and voltage on the ECG.

differently from normal waves. This means that if it originates in the atrium, the P wave will have a different shape than normal, and if the ectopic beat originates in the ventricles, there will not usually be a P wave. These arrhythmias will be discussed later.

The interval between the P wave and the QRS complex is affected by the health of the AV junctional tissue. The timing is significant for arrhythmia identification. The length and shape of the QRS waveform are also affected by the health of the conduction system within the ventricles. Changes in the normal QRS configuration indicate that the electrical impulse does not follow the normal conduction pathway. The change may be temporary or permanent.

It is important for the nurse to note the T wave in relation to the rest of the cycle. This is because the T wave represents the resting phase in the cardiac cycle during which the cardiac cells are repolarizing, or restoring their electrical charge. During repolarization, there is a period in which no transmission of an electrical impulse can occur, called the *absolute refractory period.* This period is followed by the *rela-*

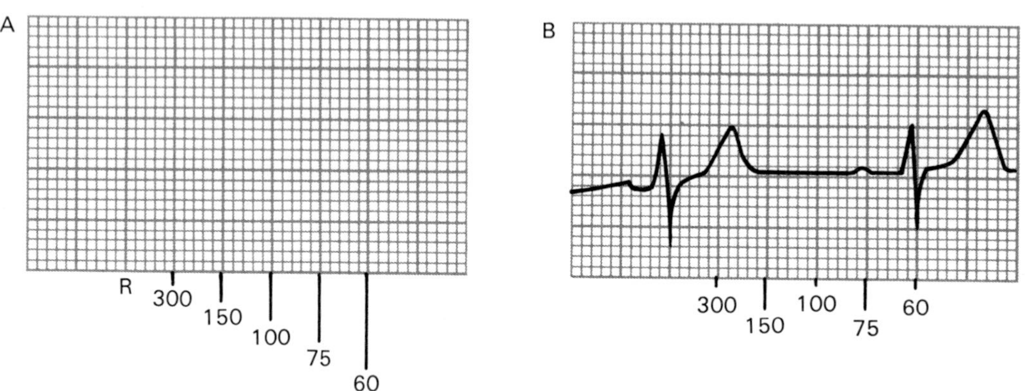

Figure 28-4 *(a)* The R represents the first QRS complex. The lines represent the location of the second QRS complex (RR interval), and the number indicates the heart rate.

5 small squares = 300	11 small squares = 136
6 small squares = 250	12 small squares = 125
7 small squares = 214	13 small squares = 115
8 small squares = 187	14 small squares = 107
9 small squares = 167	15 small squares = 100
10 small squares = 150	20 small squares = 75

(b) A rate of 60 cycles per minute, determined with the estimated rate scale: 300–150–100–75–60–50. The scale always starts with the first heavy, dark line to the right of the R or S wave, *not* the heavy, dark line on which the R or S wave is located. *(From J. Passman and C. D. Drummond, The EKG: Basic Techniques for Interpretation, McGraw-Hill Book Company, New York, 1976, p. 119.)*

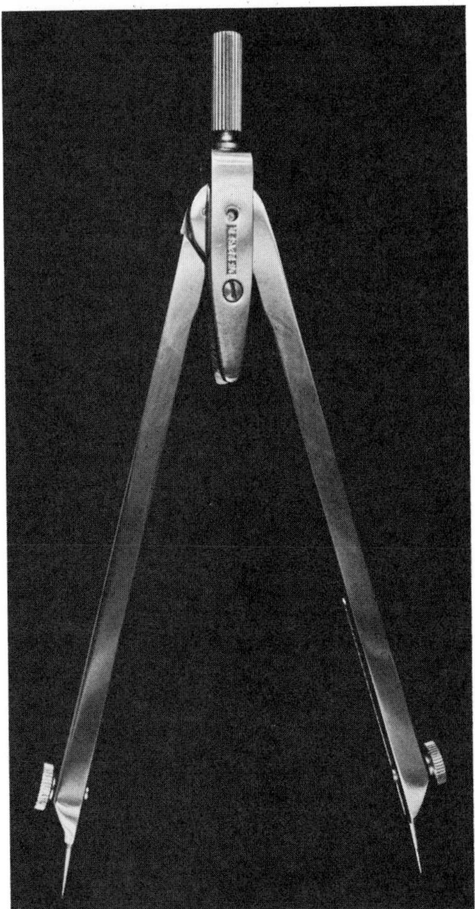

Figure 28-5 Calipers used to help make wave and baseline measurements. *(From J. Passman and C. D. Drummond, The EKG: Basic Techniques for Interpretation, McGraw-Hill Book Company, New York, 1976, p. 49.)*

tive refractory period, during which electrical impulses may be transmitted, but at a slower rate than normal because the cells have only partially recovered. The refractory period is the time needed for the cells to return to normal, i.e., when they can transmit impulses at a normal rate. Diseased cardiac cells usually have longer relative and absolute refractory periods than normal cells.

When analyzing an ECG, it is important to use a systematic approach. A recommended procedure is to note rate, rhythm, P wave, PR interval, QRS complex, ST segment, and T wave. All of the arrhythmias will be described in relation to the NSR.

Table 28-9 outlines some of the major causes of arrhythmias. Common arrhythmias will be discussed in two basic categories: life-threatening and non-life-threatening. Both types can affect adequate cardiac

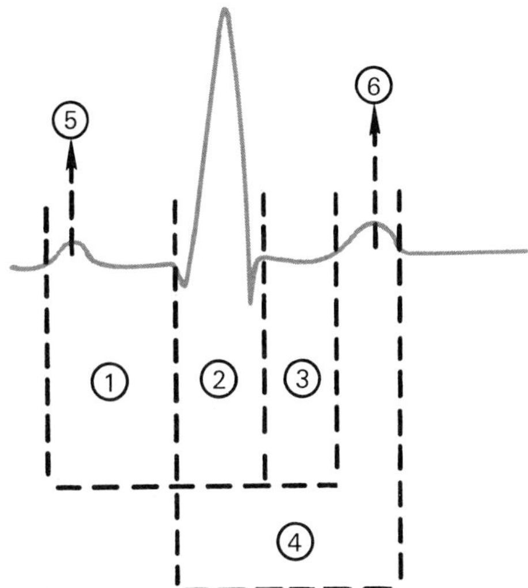

Figure 28-6 The ECG complex as seen in an NSR.

1 = PR interval	Normal is 0.12–0.20 second
2 = QRS complex	Normal is 0.06–0.10 second
3 = ST segment	Normal is 0.12 second
4 = QT interval	Normal is 0.34–0.43 second
5 = P wave	Normal is 0.06–0.12 second
6 = T wave	Normal is 0.16 second

functioning in time, but the life-threatening arrhythmias may result in death in a few minutes if they are not reversed.

Common life-threatening arrhythmias

Premature Ventricular Contractions (PVCs)

PVCs are contractions that originate somewhere in the ventricles rather than in the SA node (Fig. 28-8). They are potentially serious because they may precede life-threatening arrhythmias in the diseased heart.

Clinical associations: Stimulants such as caffeine, fever, aminophylline, epinephrine, and isoproterenol (Isuprel); digitalis drugs; hypokalemia; hypox-

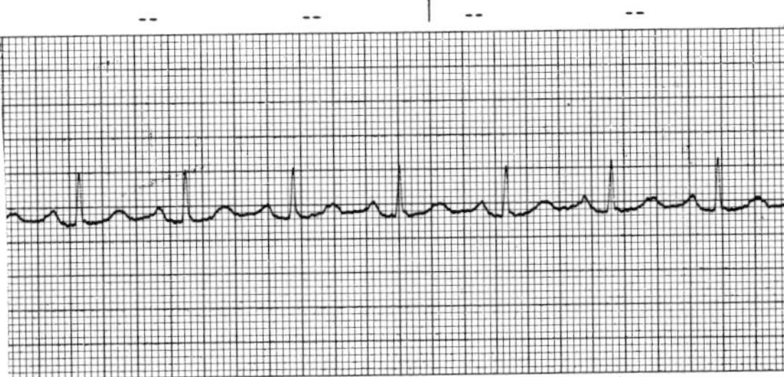

Figure 28-7 NSR.

Table 28-9
Common Causes of Arrhythmias

Common Causes of Arrhythmias
Electrolyte imbalance
Cellular hypoxia
Stretched cardiac tissue
Edema
Acid-base imbalances
Myocardial ischemia
Degeneration of the conduction system
Drug effects or toxicity
Myocardial cell degeneration
Hypertrophy of cardiac muscle with strain
Emotional crisis
Connective tissue disorders
Alcohol
Coffee, tea, tobacco

ia; emotional stress; MI, mitral valve prolapse, arteriosclerotic heart disease, and congestive heart failure (CHF).

Rate: Varies according to the underlying ventricular rate and the number of PVCs.

Rhythm: Irregular because of the PVCs.

P wave: Rarely visible because it is lost in the QRS complex of the PVC.

PR interval: Not measurable.

QRS complex: Wide and distorted in shape, and greater than 0.10 second.

T wave: Usually in the opposite direction from the QRS complex of the PVC.

Sequence: An irritable focus in one of the ventricles discharges before the SA node initiates the next regular impulse. This ectopic focus stimulates the ventricles directly to contract, causing the abnormal QRS shape. This abnormal beat occurs before the next expected normal beat (premature). The time between the beats preceding and following the PVC is equal to the time needed for three normal beats. This is because there is a compensatory pause after a PVC. Most PVCs are followed by a compensatory pause which aids in differentiating a PVC from a premature atrial contraction. *Multifocal* PVCs may arise from more than one irritable focus, as evidenced by their various shapes. When every other beat is a PVC, it is called *ventricular bigeminy;* when every third beat is a PVC, it is called *ventricular trigeminy,* etc. Two consecutive PVCs are called *coupled PVCs.* The rate at which PVCs follow each other is significant and should be measured. The *R on T phenomenon* occurs when a PVC comes so quickly in the cardiac cycle that it falls on the T wave of the preceding beat.

Significance: In a healthy person, PVCs are usually not considered a threat to health. In a setting of ischemic heart disease or an acute MI, PVCs reflect myocardial irritability. The danger signs requiring immediate treatment and reporting are (1) frequent PVCs (more than five per minute), (2) coupled PVCs, (3) multifocal PVCs, and (4) the R on T phenomenon. If these are not treated immediately, ventricular tachycardia or ventricular fibrillation may occur.

Treatment: Intravenous (IV) push of lidocaine 50 to 100mg, followed by an IV infusion of lidocaine at a rate of 1 to 4 mg/minute. This is followed by treatment of the underlying cause, if possible.

Ventricular Tachycardia (V tach) V tach is a run of three or more consecutive PVCs. This occurs when repetitive firing of an ectopic focus in the ventricles acts as the pacemaker rather than the SA node (Fig. 28-9). V tach is very dangerous because it severely reduces cardiac output and can be a precursor to a lethal arrhythmia, ventricular fibrillation. V tach may end spontaneously and abruptly without treatment.

Clinical associations: Any cardiac disease, especially MI, respiratory acidosis or alkalosis, hypokalemia, digitalis intoxication, and irritation by intracardiac catheters.

Rate: Ventricular rate is 100 to 250 beats per minute (bpm).

Rhythm: Usually regular, but occasionally may be irregular.

P wave: Not usually visible; occasionally seen with slower rates, with which the QRS complex is not very wide.

PR interval: Not measurable.

QRS complex: Greater than 0.10 second. Has a wide, distorted shape that is repeated with each contraction (same etopic focus).

Sequence: The contraction is initiated by an ectopic focus in the ventricles. The impulse travels from that point throughout the ventricles and atria. This impulse takes longer and follows a different route from that of the impulses initiated by the SA node. Consequently, the QRS complex is wider and bizarre-appearing.

Significance: V tach is very dangerous because it causes a severe decrease in cardiac output due to inadequate time for filling of the atria and ventricles and inefficient contraction (ventricles before atria) of the heart muscle. This may result in the rapid development of CHF, shock, and cerebral insufficiency. Sudden death may also occur. Also, at any time during the course of V tach, the arrhythmia may change abruptly to ventricular fibrillation. Thus, it is essential that treatment be vigorous and immediate. Even if V

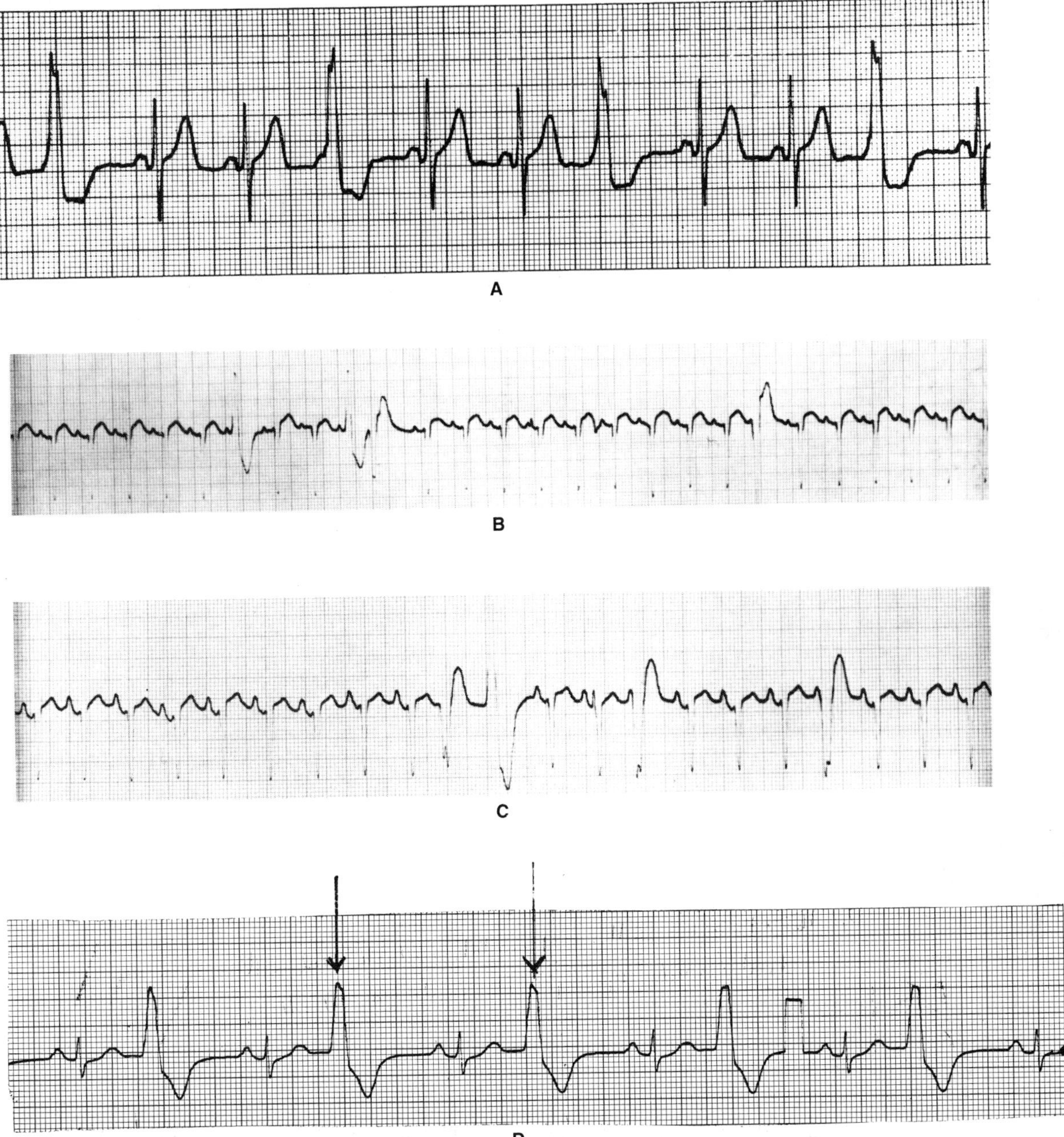

Figure 28-8 PVCs. *(a)* Ventricular trigeminy. *(b)* Multifocal PVC. *(c)* Fusion PVCs. *(d)* Ventricular bigeminy. *(b, c, and d from M. Kinney et al., AACN's Clinical Reference for Critical Care Nursing, McGraw-Hill Book Company, New York, 1981, p. 1124.)*

tach occurs briefly and stops spontaneously, it must be treated because there is a high risk of further episodes of V tachcardia or the onset of ventricular fibrillation.

Treatment: If the client is fairly stable, he should be treated with an IV push of lidocaine 50 to 100 mg and then started on a lidocaine IV infusion at a rate of 1 to 4 mg/minute. If there is no response to the lidocaine or other drugs, such as Procainamide or bretylium, or if the client is unstable (e.g., has loss of consciousness or hypotension), the treatment is *cardioversion.*

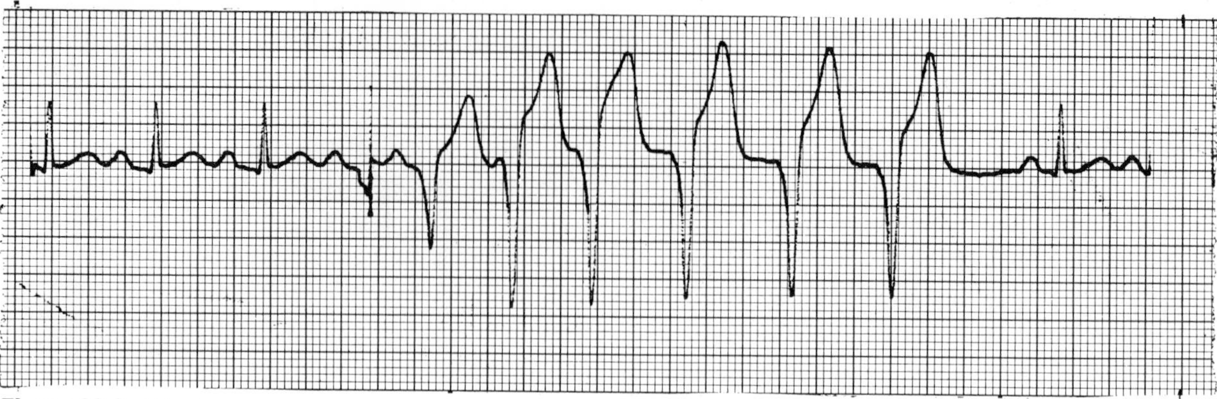

Figure 28-9 V tach.

Cardioversion is the administration of an electrical charge of 200 to 400 watt-seconds to the client's chest in an attempt to convert him to a NSR. A defibrillator is used to do emergency cardioversion when its synchronization mechanism is set to discharge the electrical shock on the R wave and not the T wave. If the shock is administered on the T wave, it may cause ventricular fibrillation. The procedure is similar to that used for defibrillation, described later. If the client is awake before cardioversion, he is usually given a minor tranquilizer, such as diazepam, via IV push just prior to the cardioversion.

If the cause of the V tach is digitalis intoxication, the treatment is slow IV administration of a potassium solution while closely monitoring the client.

Ventricular Fibrillation (V fib) V fib is a lethal arrhythmia in which there are multiple ventricular ectopic foci stimulating the heart to contract (Fig. 28-10). These contractions are very rapid and weak. The fibrillating heart looks like a rapidly quivering bowl of Jello. There is no measurable cardiac output and therefore no blood circulation.

Clinical associations: Various cardiac diseases, especially acute MI, electrocution, and hyperkalemia.

Rate: Not measurable.

Rhythm: Irregular and chaotic because uncoordinated.

P Wave: Not visible.

PR interval: Not measurable.

QRS complex: Wide (greater than 0.10 second), sloppy waves of varying contour.

Sequence: Many ectopic foci in the ventricles initiate a weak impulse. These impulses travel throughout the heart, resulting in a chaotic, disorganized wave pattern due to the uncoordinated twitching of heart.

Significance: V fib results in biological death if an effective rhythm is not reestablished within 3 to 4 minutes. This is because there is no cardiac output and therefore no circulation to any of the vital organs. This state is called *cardiac arrest.*

Treatment: Immediate initiation of cardiopulmonary resuscitation (Basic Cardiac Life Support) and definitive treatment with defibrillation and drugs (Advanced Cardiac Life Support). These are described in more detail later.

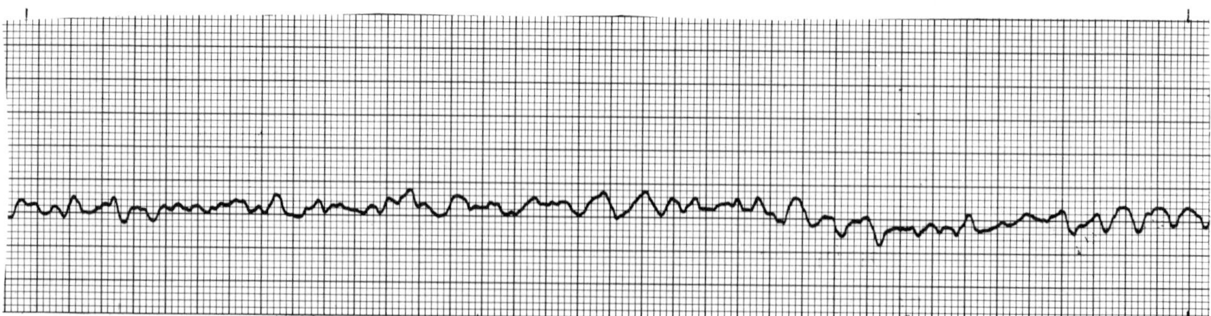

Figure 28-10 V fib.

Asystole Asystole is the cessation of any electrical activity in the heart muscle. It is lethal and requires immediate treatment. The prognosis is very poor.

Clinical associations: Usually due to advanced cardiac disease, as with end-stage CHF, ischemic heart disease, or advanced disease of the induction system.

Rhythm and significance: There are no identifiable waveforms on the monitor. The waveform is essentially flat because there is no electrical activity. No blood is being circulated.

Treatment: Cardiopulmonary resuscitation. Epinephrine is given IV or into the trachea through the endotracheal tube in an attempt to stimulate the heart into V fib. Then it is treated as V fib. Other drugs to stimulate cardiac muscle activity include isoproterenol and calcium chloride.

Electromechanical Dissociation (EMD) EMD refers to situations where impulses are being transmitted by the conduction system of the heart but the muscles (mechanical part) are not contracting. Therefore, no blood is circulating even though there is a pattern on the monitor. The client will have no pulse or blood pressure. EMD is most often associated with cardiac tamponade or hypovolemia. Treatment is the same as for asystole. If the underlying cause is known, it needs to be treated.

Common non-life-threatening arrhythmias

Sinus Bradycardia Sinus bradycardia is a slowed heart rate initiated by the SA node (Fig. 28-11).

Clinical associations: Normal variation of the heart rate in well-trained athletes, in sleep, and with extreme fear. It also occurs in conjunction with carotid sinus massage, ocular pressure, increased vagal influence, Valsalva maneuvers, and hypothermia. Disease conditions with which it is associated are myxedema, increased intracranial pressure, obstructive jaundice, and MI of the inferior surface.

Rate: Less than 60 bpm.

Rhythm: Regular.

P wave: Precedes each QRS complex and has a normal contour.

PR interval: Normal.

QRS complex: Normal in contour.

Sequence: The SA node, as the pacemaker, fires less frequently than normal. However, the impulse moves through the conduction system normally.

Significance: Varies with the cause of the bradycardia and the client's tolerance of it. In a client with an acute MI, the low rate predisposes him to PVCs or decreased cardiac output and thus to hypotension.

Treatment: Symptomatic clients may be treated with atropine and isoproterenol (Isuprel). If these drugs are not effective, a pacemaker may need to be inserted.

Sinus Tachycardia Sinus tachycardia is a heart rate greater than 100 bpm originating in the SA node.

Clinical associations: Common causes are fever, exercise, anxiety, pain, and shock. Others include hypoxia, CHF, anemia, thyrotoxicosis, and drugs (e.g., epinephrine, norepinephrine, caffeine, atropine, and theophylline).

Rate: More than 100 bpm.

Rhythm: Regular.

P wave: Precedes each QRS complex and has a normal contour.

PR interval: Normal.

Sequence: The SA node, as the pacemaker, fires more frequently than normal. However, the im-

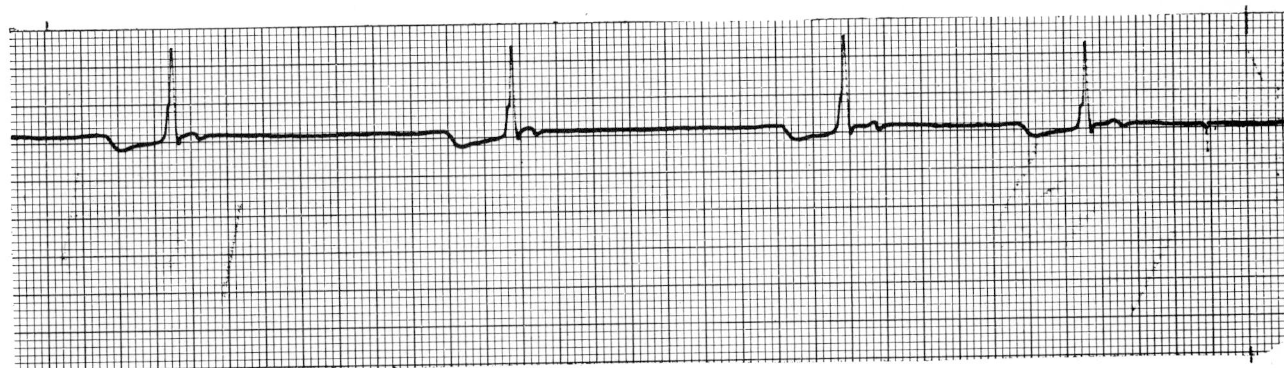

Figure 28-11 Sinus bradycardia.

pulse moves throughout the conduction system normally.

Significance: Depends on the client's tolerance. If it is prolonged, fatigue may occur.

Treatment: The underlying cause is treated.

Premature Atrial Contractions (PAC) A PAC is a contraction that originates in the atrium in a location other than the SA node (Fig. 28-12).

Clinical associations: In a normal heart, it occurs with emotional stress and anxiety, caffeine, tobacco, and alcohol. In disease states, it occurs with thyrotoxicosis, arteriosclerotic heart disease (especially with diseased or enlarged atria), and rheumatic heart disease.

Rate: Varies with the underlying rate and frequency of PACs.

Rhythm: Irregular.

P wave: The early P wave has a different contour from the normal P wave. It may be seen as a notch on the T wave preceding it. Occasionally, it is hidden in the preceding T wave.

PR interval: The time interval is within normal limits, but it may be shorter or longer than the PR interval with the client's normal contractions.

QRS complex: Usually normal. If it is 0.10 second or longer, abnormal conduction through the ventricles is indicated.

Sequence: An ectopic focus in either the right or left atrium initiates an electrical impulse before the next normal beat from the SA node occurs. This impulse travels across the atria by an abnormal path, thereby creating the distorted P wave. When the impulse reaches the AV node, it is stopped (nonconducted PAC), delayed (longer PR interval than normal), or conducted normally. The way the AV node reacts to the impulse depends on how early in the previous cycle the PAC occurs and if the AV node is still refractory. Once the impulse moves through the AV node, it travels normally throughout the ventricles (normal QRS) unless aberrancy occurs. Usually, there is no compensatory pause with PACs.

Significance: May be a prelude to atrial tachyarrhythmias.

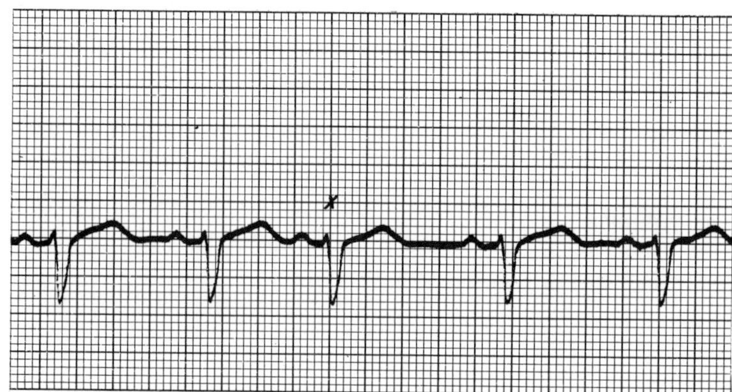

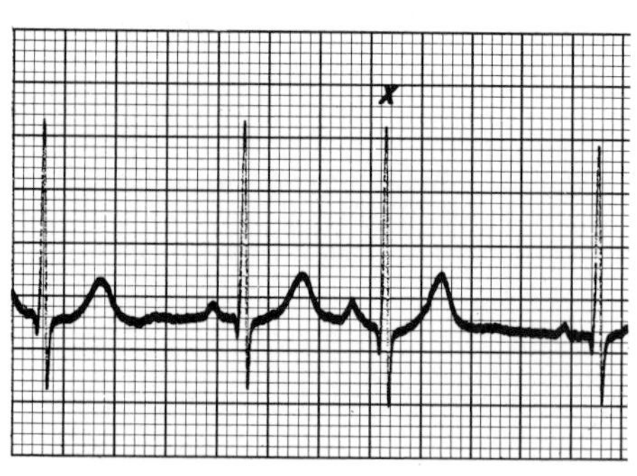

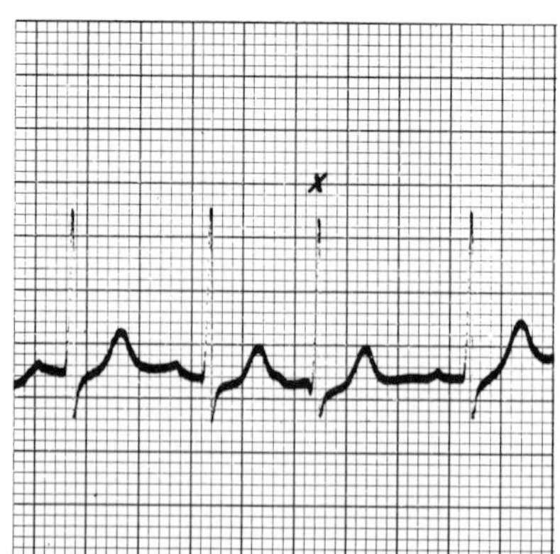

Figure 28-12 Several examples of PACs. *(From J. Passman and C. D. Drummond, The EKG: Basic Techniques for interpretation, McGraw-Hill Book Company, New York, 1976, p. 95.)*

Treatment: Required only if the client is symptomatic. If stimulants or other drugs are the cause, then they should be omitted. Drugs that are used include digitalis, quinidine, propranolol, and procainamide.

Paroxysmal Supraventricular Tachycardia Paroxysmal supraventricular tachycardias are tachycardias with an abrupt onset and termination and a regular rate (Fig. 28-13). They originate in an ectopic focus anywhere above the bifurcation of the bundle of His. They may be AV junctional rhythms or atrial rhythms. It is difficult to identify the site of origin.

Clinical associations: Common in normal hearts and associated with overexertion, emotional stress, deep inspiration, ingestion of heavy meals, changes in position, and stimulants such as coffee and tobacco. In diseased hearts, it is commonly found with rheumatic heart disease, Wolff-Parkinson-White syndrome, digitalis intoxication, arteriosclerotic heart disease, and pulmonary emboli.

Rate: 100 to 300 bpm (commonly about 200 bpm).

Rhythm: Regular.

P wave: If seen, it has an abnormal contour. It is often hidden in the preceding T wave.

PR interval: Prolonged at the initiation of the paroxysmal supraventricular tachycardia, then normal.

Sequence; An ectopic focus above the bifurcation of the bundle of His or the *reentry phenomenon* (reexcitation of the atria when there is a sufficient one-way AV nodal block) suddenly initiates a run of repeated premature beats. Its onset is usually heralded by a PAC. Abrupt termination of the tachycardia may be followed by a brief period of asystole.

Significance: Varies with the cause and the client's tolerance. Usually is not of concern except in clients with underlying heart disease or prolonged periods of tachycardia with a heart rate greater than 200 bpm.

Treatment: Rest and reassurance is the treatment of choice for those who have symptoms of palpitations and anxiety. For those with more severe symptoms, treatment includes vagal stimulation by carotid sinus massage or the Valsalva maneuver. Use of a calcium channel blocker such as verapamil is the treatment of choice. If hypotension is symptomatic, vasopressors such as dobutamine are used. If these do not work, then digitalis or propranolol may be used. If the SV tachycardia is complicated by angina or hypotension, then cardioversion is done.

Atrial Flutter Atrial flutter is a form of rapid atrial contraction usually associated with a slower ventricular contraction (Fig. 28-14*a*). The P waves may be counted and have a typical sawtooth pattern.

Clinical associations: Associated with arteriosclerotic heart disease, hypertension, pulmonary embolism, mitral valve disorders, and drugs such as digitalis, quinidine, and epinephrine. Not usually present in healthy people.

Rate: The atrial rate is 250 to 350 bpm (usually 300 bpm). The ventricular rate will vary with the degree of block (e.g., 2:1, 3:1, or 4:1)

Rhythm: The atrial rhythm is regular. The ventricular rhythm is usually regular.

P wave: Sawtooth waves called *F waves* (for "flutter").

PR interval: Varies.

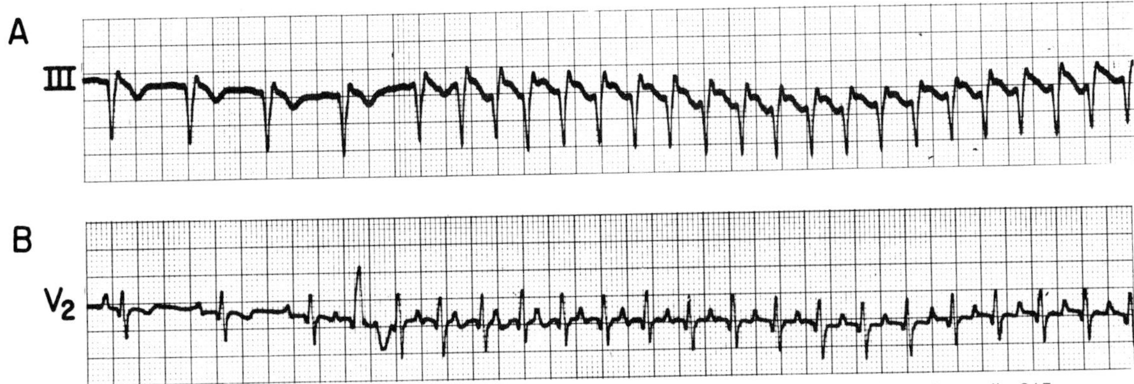

Figure 28-13 Paroxysmal supraventricular tachycardia. *(a)* Sudden onset of supraventricular tachycardia 215 ppm). The P waves cannot be identified. *(b)* Supraventricular tachycardia (172 bpm) initiated by a PAC. The first beat of the tachycardia indicates aberration; subsequent beats show normal conduction. *[From N. Wenger, J. W. Hurst, and M. C. McIntyre (eds.), Cardiology for Nurses, McGraw-Hill book Company, New York, 1980 p. 235.]*

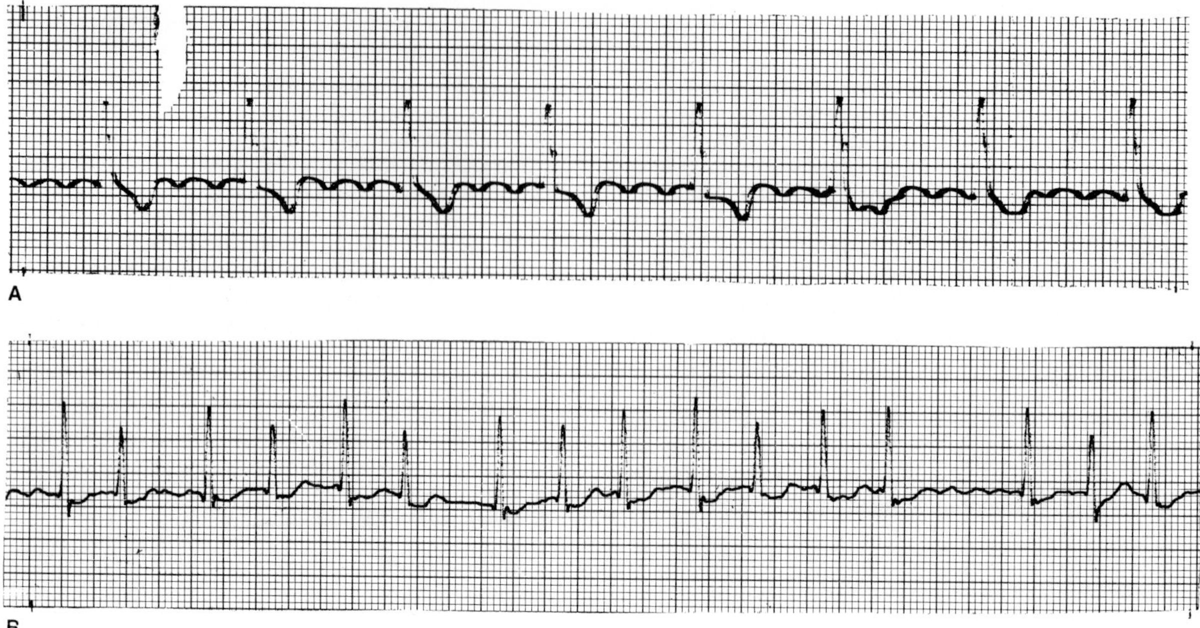

Figure 28-15 *(a)* Accelerated junction rhythm (88 bpm), *(b)* Junctional tachycardia (100 bpm). Inverted P waves occur on the ST segment and are produced by a 1:1 retrograde atial activation. *[From N. Wenger, J. W. Hurst, and M. C. McIntyre (eds.), Cardiology for Nurses, McGraw-Hill Book Company, New York, 1980, p. 241.]*

QRS complex: Normal in contour.

Sequence: Ectopic atrial focus rapidly fires an impulse about 300 times per minute. The rapid and abnormal path of depolarization of the atria results in a sawtooth configuration. The ventricles do not usually respond to each atrial beat because of the refractoriness of the AV node. Therefore, there is usually a fixed conduction ratio of 2:1 or 4:1 F waves to QRS responses.

Significance: If the client has an underlying disease, such as MI, atrial flutter is very serious. The situation may also be urgent if there is a high ventricular rate.

Treatment: The purpose is to slow the ventricular rate, often by increasing the AV block. This may be dangerous when the ratio goes from 2:1 to 4:1 or higher because the ventricular rate may suddenly go from 150 to 75 bpm or lower. In urgent situations, such as with acute MI, when the client is not tolerating the fast ventricular rate, reduction of the ventricular rate is temporarily accomplished with IV verapamil. This drug therapy is often followed by IV digitalis in an attempt to convert the atrial fibrillation to an NSR. If the client continues to have a rapid (or uncontrolled) ventricular rate, cardioversion may be done.

Atrial Fibrillation Atrial fibrillation is an arrhythmia in which ectopic foci cause rapid, irregular contractions of the atria (Fig. 28-14*b*). These are seen on the ECG as *fibrillatory waves* (a wavy line). There is an irregular ventricular response. Atrial fibrillation is the most common supraventricular tachyarrhythmia.[15]

Clinical association: Usually occurs in clients with different types of organic heart disease, such as rheumatic heart disease with mitral valve involvement, atrial septal defect, coronary artery disease, heart failure, pericarditis, hypertensive heart disease, chronic lung disease, and heart or chest trauma. It is also associated with thyrotoxicosis, gastroenteritis, stress, coughing, nausea, pain, infection, and a large intake of alcohol.

Rate: The atrial rate may be as high as 350 to 600 bpm. The ventricular rate varies but is usually 110 to 180 bpm.

Rhythm: Ventricular rhythm is sometimes irregular.

P wave: No definite P wave seen. Baseline is a wavy, "squiggly" line that may be very fine or very coarse. The coarse lines resemble those of atrial flutter.

PR interval: Not measurable.

QRS complex: Usually has a normal contour, but the amplitude may vary.

Sequence: Ectopic atrial foci fire rapidly and irregularly. Thus, the depolarization of the atria is totally disorganized and is seen on the ECG as fibrillatory waves. Sometimes there is no sign of atrial activity on certain ECG leads. The ventricular response to impulses from the atria is totally irregular and may be slow or quite rapid. When an arrhythmia has a grossly irregular ventricular rate without definite P waves, it is considered atrial fibrillation until proven otherwise.

Significance: Atrial fibrillation can result in a significant decrease in cardiac output due to inefficient atrial contractions and a rapid, irregular ventricular rate. In addition, thrombi may form in the atria and send out emboli throughout the arterial system. Some clients can tolerate atrial fibrillation for a long time, but especially with a sudden onset there may be significant changes in cardiac output.

Treatment: The goal of treatment is to decrease the ventricular rate. This is usually done with a digitalis preparation. Sometimes propranolol is used with digitalis. For rapid, temporary slowing of the ventricular response, verapamil may be given in conjunction with digitalis. Occasionally, in the presence of hypotension and severe CHF, direct current (DC) countershock is used to return the heart to the NSR.

Junctional Arrhythmias A junctional rhythm refers to an arrhythmia that originates in the tissue surrounding the AV node, i.e., the tissue above the AV node through the bundle of His (the AV node does not polarize spontaneously) (Fig. 28-15). There may be premature junctional contractions (PJCs) which are treated similarly to PACs. In addition, there are other arrhythmias which are at least partially defined by their rate and by evidence of their origin in the AV node. These are described below.

Clinical associations: In the well-trained athlete with sinus bradycardia, the junctional escape rhythm is normal. Otherwise, the junctional escape rhythm may occur with acute MI, any degenerative disease of the SA node, or increased vagal tone. Accelerated junctional rhythm and junctional tachycardia are also seen with acute

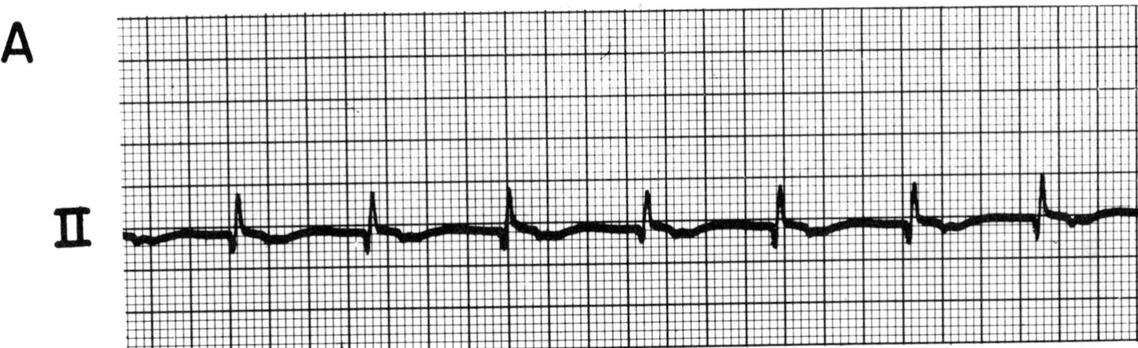

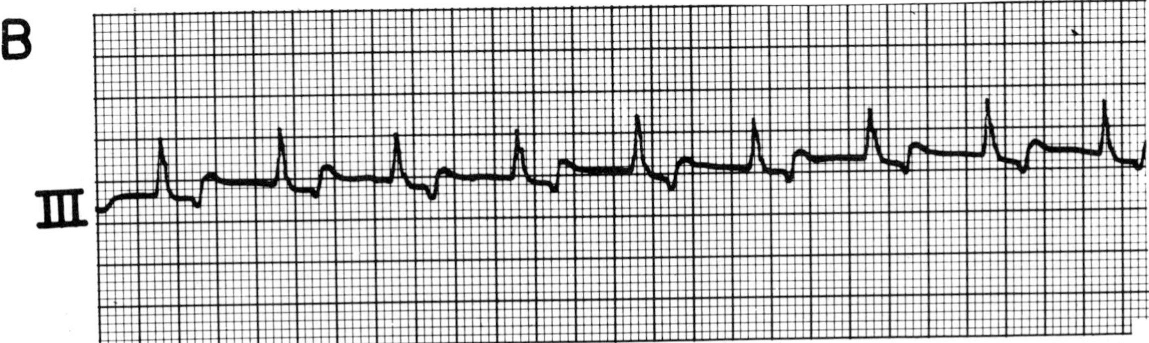

Figure 28-14 *(a)* Atrial flutter with two to three P waves before the QRS complex. *(b)* Atrial fibrillation. Note the jagged, irregular baseline between the QRS complexes.

inferior MI, as well as with digitalis toxicity, acute rheumatic fever, and open heart surgery.[16]

Rate: In junctional escape rhythm, the rate is 40 to 60 bpm; in accelerated junctional rhythm, it is 60 to 100 bpm; and in junctional tachycardia, it is 100 to 140 bpm.

Rhythm: Regular.

P wave: Abnormal in contour. Is usually inverted and closely precedes or follows the QRS complex (may be hidden in the QRS complex).

PR interval: When the P wave precedes the QRS complex, the interval is less than 0.12 second.

QRS complex: Normal.

Sequence: AV junctional tissue serves as the pacemaker in initiating the impulse. The impulse may then move in a retrograde manner up through the atrium, resulting in an abnormal P wave just before, during, or after the QRS complex representing depolarization of the ventricles. The impulse moves through the ventricles, normally resulting in a normal QRS complex.

Significance: The junctional escape rhythm is a defense mechanism when the SA node or atria do not initiate a beat. Therefore, escape rhythms should not be suppressed. The accelerated junctional rhythm and junctional tachycardia indicate that there may be something seriously wrong with the SA node. Also, if they are prolonged, there may be a decrease in cardiac output.

Treatment: Based on the underlying cause. If it is due to digitalis toxicity, then this drug should be discontinued. If digitalis is not involved, then the accelerated junctional rhythm is treated like other supraventricular arrhythmias. In junctional tachycardia, phenytoin and propranolol may be used.

First-Degree AV Block First-degree AV block is a type of *AV block. AV block* refers to various degrees of slowing or actual stopping of the conduction of the electrical impulse from the SA node as it passes through the AV node and down the ventricular conduction system. First-degree AV block involves only a slowing of the impulse (Fig. 28-16*a*).

Clinical associations: Rheumatic fever, chronic ischemic heart disease, acute MI, hyperthyroidism, vagal stimulation, and drugs such as digitalis and propranolol.

Rate: Normal.

Rhythm: Normal.

P wave: Precedes each QRS complex and has a normal contour.

PR interval: Prolonged; is greater than 0.20 second. The interval is the same for each beat.

QRS complex: Normal and follows every P wave.

Sequence: The impulse initiated by the SA node moves normally through the atrium but is slowed when going through the AV node. After the impulse goes through the AV node, it moves through the ventricles normally.

Significance: May be a precursor of higher degrees of block.

Treatment: None.

Second-Degree Heart Block, Type I (Mobitz I, Wenckebach) Second-degree heart block is a type of AV block in which the SA node impulse has increasing difficulty in going through the AV node until one impulse is stopped. The impulse then starts the conduction process again (Fig. 28-16*b*).

Clinical associations: Any disease or drug which slows AV conduction. Most common causes are digitalis toxicity and acute inferior MI.

Rate: Atrial rate is normal. Ventricular rate is slower than atrial rate because of some dropped QRS complexes.

Rhythm: Ventricular rhythm is irregular. The PR interval shortens progressively before the nonconducted P wave.

P wave: Normal in contour.

PR interval: Lengthens progressively until a QRS complex is dropped.

QRS complex: Normal in contour.

Sequence: The impulse from the SA node moves normally to the AV node, where it is slowed. Each successive impulse from the SA node arrives earlier and earlier in the relative refractory period of the AV node until an impulse finally fails to move through. Once a ventricular beat is dropped, the cycle repeats itself with progressively lengthening PR intervals until a QRS complex is dropped again.

Significance: Usually this condition is transient in acute MI. However, it may warn of impending higher degrees of block.

Treatment: None, unless cardiac output is decreased significantly. Atropine will increase the heart rate. In the setting of an acute MI, a temporary transvenous pacemaker may be inserted if the client is symptomatic.

Second-Degree Heart Block, Type II (Mobitz II) Second-degree heart block is a more serious form of heart block in which a certain number of SA node impulses are not transmitted to the ventricles. This occurs in a ratio of 2:1, 3:1, 4:1, etc., where there are two, three, four, or more atrial contractions (P waves) for a ventricular contraction (QRS complex) (Fig. 28-16*c*).

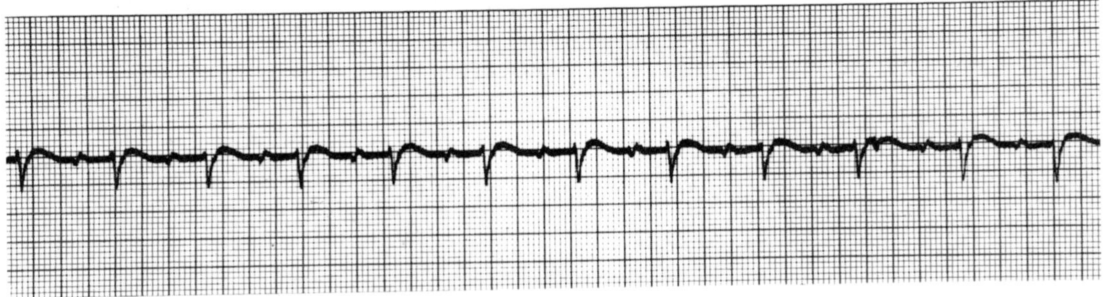

A

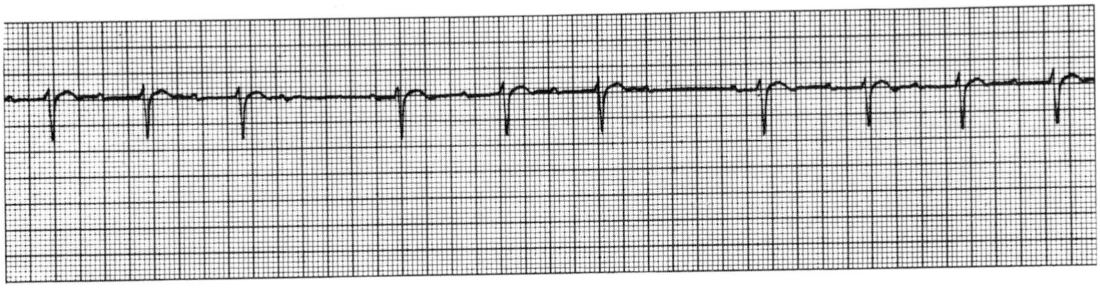

B

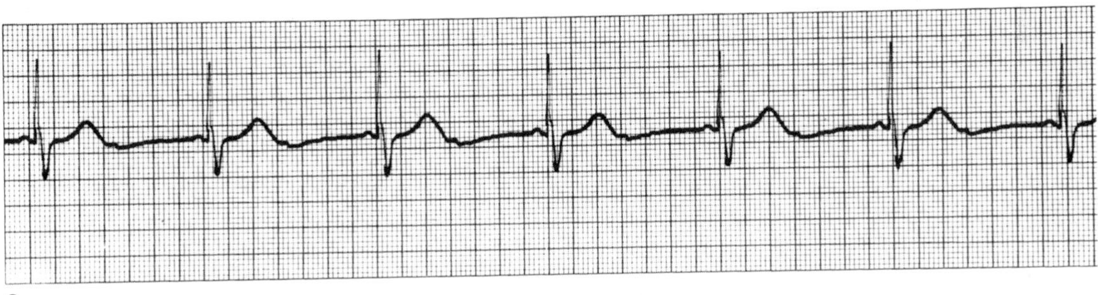

C

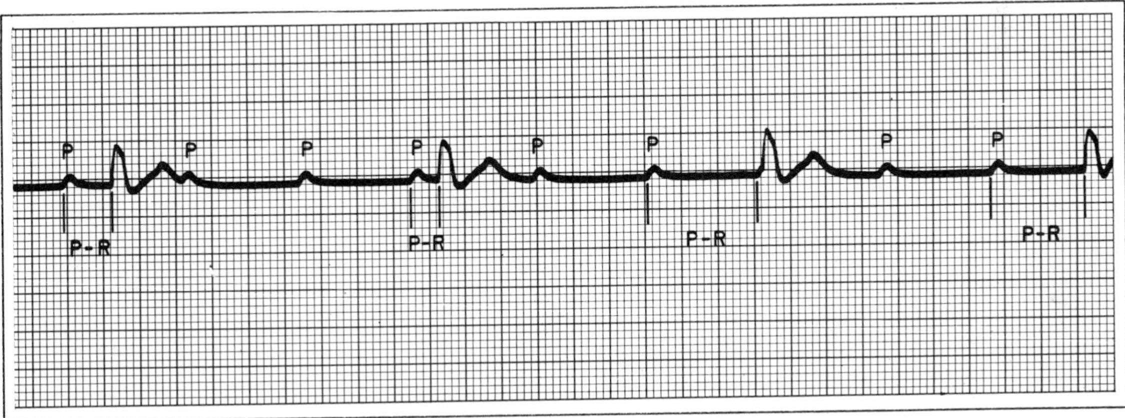

D

Figure 28-16 Heart block. *(a)* First-degree heart block. Note the delayed PR interval. *(b)* Second-degree heart block, type I (Mobitz 1, Wenckebach). *(c)* Second-degree heart block, type II (Mobitz II). *(d)* Complete heart block (third degree). The irregular PR intervals indicate the presence of a complete heart block. *(a, b, and c from M. Kinney et al., AACN's Clinical Reference for Critical Care Nursing, McGraw-Hill Book Company, New York, 1981, pp. 1129–1131; d from J. Passman and D. C. Drummond, The EKG: Basic Techniques to Interpretation, McGraw-Hill Book Company, New York, 1976, p. 135.)*

Clinical associations: Rheumatic and atherosclerotic heart disease, acute anterior wall MI, digitalis toxicity, and Lenegre's disease and Lev's disease.

Rate: The atrial (sinus) rate is normal. The ventricular rate depends on the sinus rate and the amount of block, but it is usually less than 60 bpm.

Rhythm: The sinus rhythm is regular. The ventricular rhythm may be slightly irregular.

P wave: Normal in contour.

PR interval: May be normal or prolonged on conducted beats.

QRS complex: Abnormally widened because there is a bundle branch block associated with the AV block.

Sequence: The SA node fires normally, and the impulse travels normally through the AV node tissue. It is blocked intermittently by the ventricular conduction system below the bundle of His. On conducted beats, the PR interval is constant.

Significance: This is a serious arrhythmia because it usually progresses to complete heart block. In addition, depending on the ventricular rate, it may severely limit cardiac output. Exercise, in the presence of Mobitz II, *slows* the heart rate.

Treatment: Insertion of a temporary or permanent pacemaker depending on the cause. If the client is severely symptomatic, an isoproterenol drip may be used to increase the ventricular rate until a pacemaker is inserted.

Third-Degree AV Heart Block (Complete Heart Block) Third-degree AV block refers to the situation in which no impulses from the atria are transmitted to the ventricles (Fig. 28-16*d*). Thus, the atria and ventricles contract independently of each other because of a block in the AV node or ventricular specialized conduction system (Purkinje system). The ventricular contractions are called *escape beats* because they occur without an SA node impulse.

Clinical associations: Acute MI, rheumatic heart disease, Lenegre's disease, Lev's disease, and atherosclerotic heart disease.

Rate: The atrial rate is dependent on the sinus rate, which is usually 60 to 100 bpm. The ventricular rate is 40 to 60 bpm if the block is located in the AV node and is 20 to 40 bpm if the block is located in the Purkinje system.

Rhythm: Both atrial and ventricular rates are regular, but not synchronized.

P wave: Normal in contour.

PR interval: Varies, with no set pattern.

QRS complex: Normal if the escape beat is initiated in the bundle of His or above; widened if the escape beat is initiated in lower areas.

Sequence: The SA node fires normally and moves normally through the atria but is blocked from moving through the ventricles. When complete heart block occurs, either the ventricles remain inactive (ventricular standstill) or, more likely, an independent ventricular pacemaker takes over and initiates ventricular contraction.

Significance: This is a serious arrhythmia because of significantly decreased cardiac output. Many clients develop syncope (Stokes-Adams attack) because of the decreased cardiac output, especially if the block is sudden. They may also develop angina and CHF. The ventricular rhythm does not increase with exercise. In addition, the ventricular escape beats may suddenly stop in ventricular standstill or may be replaced by V fib when ectopic foci become irritable.

Treatment: Temporary treatment is the use of drugs, such as atropine and isoproterenol or epinephrine. The treatment of choice is insertion of a pacemaker.

Table 28-10 summarizes some key characteristics of the common arrhythmias described here. The reader is referred to more specialized books for further detail on these and other arrhythmias.

Cardiopulmonary Resuscitation (CPR)

Every nurse and physician should be skilled in *CPR* because *cardiac arrest,* the sudden, unexpected cessation of breathing and adequate circulation of blood by the heart, may occur at any time or in any setting. *CPR* is the process of externally supporting the circulation and respiration of a person who has cardiac arrest. Resuscitation measures are divided into two components, *Basic Cardiac Life Support (BCLS)* and *Advanced Cardiac Life Support (ACLS).* The American Red Cross is actively involved in training lay people in BCLS. The American Heart Association establishes the standards for CPR and is actively involved in teaching both BCLS and ACLS to health professionals. The American Heart Association recommends that nurses and physicians working with CCU clients be certified in both BCLS and ACLS. Certification involves attending formal classes and passing cognitive and skill tests.

BCLS

BCLS involves the ABCs of CPR: *airway, breathing,* and *circulation.* This section will deal with CPR in any setting. Artificial respiration (mouth-to-mouth, mouth-to-mask, mouth-to-nose, or mouth-to-

Table 28-10
Summary of Characteristics of Common Arrhythmias

Pattern	Rate and Rhythm	P wave	PR Interval	QRS complex
		NSR		
NSR	60–100 bpm and regular	Present	Normal	Normal
		Life-Threatening		
PVC	60–100 bpm and irregular	Not usually present	Normal	Wide, sloppy
V tach	100–250 bpm and regular	Not usually present	Not measurable	Wide, sloppy
V fib	Not measurable and irregular	Not visible	Not measurable	Wide, sloppy Various shapes
		Non-Life-Threatening		
Sinus bradycardia	<60 bpm and regular	Normal	Normal	Normal
Sinus tachycardia	>100 bpm and regular	Normal	Normal	Normal
PAC	Usually 60–100 bpm and irregular	Abnormal shape	Normal or variable	Normal
Paroxysmal supraventricular tachycardia	100–300 bpm and regular	Abnormal shape	Normal	Normal (usually)
Atrial flutter	Atrial: 250–350 bpm and regular Ventricular: >100 bpm and irregular	Sawtooth	Variable	Normal
Atrial fibrillation	Atrial: 350–600 bpm and irregular Ventricular: >100 bpm and irregular or could be any rate	Squiggly line	Not measurable	Normal
Junctional rhythms	40–140 bpm and regular	Abnormal	Variable	Normal
First-degree heart block	Normal and regular	Normal	>0.20	Normal
Mobitz I	Low normal and irregular	Normal	Progressively lengthens	Normal
Mobitz II	Usually 60 bpm and either regular or irregular	Normal	Normal or prolonged	Normal or preceded by a widened wave; two or more P waves
Third-degree heart block	Ventricular rate is 20–40 bpm and regular	Normal, but no connection with QRS	Variable	Normal or widened; no connection with P waves

stoma) and external chest compression substitute for spontaneous breathing and circulation. BCLS or CPR must be initiated within 4 to 6 minutes of cardiac arrest in order to prevent *biological death* or death of brain cells. Brain cells start to die with 6 minutes of anoxia. A person who has no pulse or respirations and whose pupils are dilated is considered *clinically dead* if more than 4 to 6 minutes have elapsed since the onset of the cardiac arrest.

When giving CPR, it is critical that oxygenated blood be circulated. Brain cells are the first cells to die from anoxia. (This occurrence led to the term *brain death.*) CPR that is performed perfectly will result in a cardiac output that is 25 to 30 percent of normal. In

BCLS courses, potential rescuers are not certified unless they meet national standards in both knowledge and skills.

Patent Airway When administering BCLS, the first step is to establish a patent airway. Table 28-11 outlines the sequence of steps involved in managing a victim with an obstructed airway. An adult victim's airway may be opened by hyperextending his head. This is done by tilting the head back with one hand and lifting the neck slightly with the other hand (Fig. 28-17). If no respirations are noted, the rescuer attempts to ventilate the victim by mouth-to-mouth resuscitation. Breaths should be given with the nostrils pinched shut and the rescuer's mouth making a tight seal around the victim's mouth. In each ventilation, there should be a volume of 800 mL of air, which can be seen by the chest's rising 1 to 2 inches. (If the victim has a tracheostomy, ventilations should be given through the stoma.)

If there is an obstruction to ventilation, the rescuer should reposition the victim's head and then again attempt to provide ventilation. If an obstruction still exists, the rescuer should assume that it is caused by a foreign body. To remove the object, the rescuer turns the victim on his thighs and gives four rapid, forceful blows to the back between the scapulae. The rescuer then turns the victim on his back so that the rescuer's knees are close to the victim's hips. Having turned the victim's head to one side, the rescuer then gives four quick abdominal thrusts by placing the heel of one hand between the lower sternum and the navel and the second hand on top of the first (see Fig. 58-4). Thrusts are given upward in an attempt to dislodge the foreign object. The rescuer then examines the victim's mouth to see if the obstructing object can be reached by the fingers. If it is visible, the rescuer attempts to carefully remove it. If the object is not visible, the rescuer then attempts to ventilate the victim. If the obstruction remains, then the procedure is repeated until the victim can be ventilated. Even if the victim's heart has stopped, cardiac compressions are not started until the client can be ventilated.

With certain conditions, such as advanced preg-

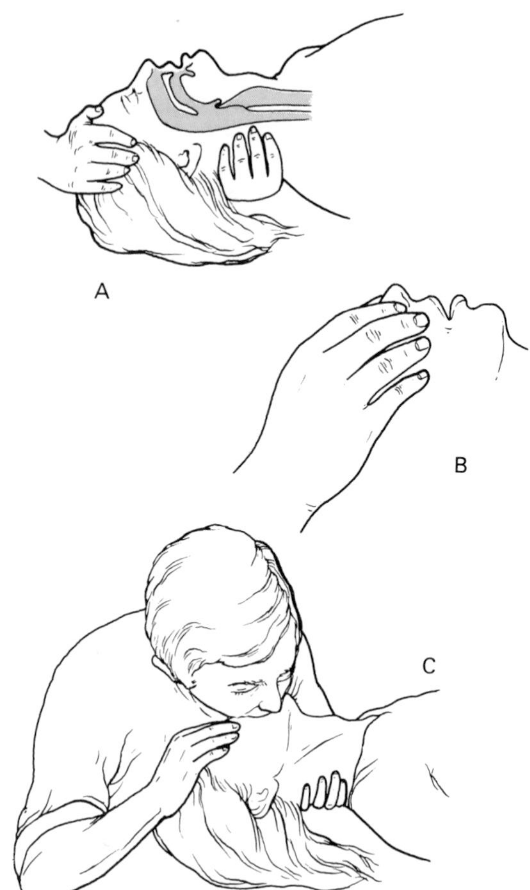

Figure 28-17 Opening the airway to give mouth-to-mouth resuscitation. This is done by tilting the head back with one hand and lifting the neck slightly with the other hand.

Table 28-11

Sequence for Managing an Obstructed Airway

1. Ascertain that the victim is unresponsive by shaking and shouting at him. Call out for help as you position him on his back.
2. Open the victim's airway by hyperextending his head.
3. Ascertain that the victim is breathless by taking 3–5 s to look, listen, and feel for respirations.
4. Attempt to ventilate the victim. If unsuccessful, then reposition the victim's head.
5. If still unable to ventilate the victim, roll him toward you, using your thighs for support.
6. Rapidly give four forceful blows to the victim's back between his shoulder blades.
7. Roll the victim onto his back and quickly give four abdominal thrusts or four chest thrusts.
8. Turn the victim's head to the side, open his jaw, and sweep deeply to remove any foreign body.
9. Attempt to ventilate the victim by hyperextending his head.
10. If the airway remains obstructed, then repeat the above sequence until the obstruction is removed.
11. If the airway is patent but the victim is still breathless, give ventilations once every 5 s. If there is no pulse, proceed with the steps given in Table 28-12.

Adapted from American Heart Association, *Standards of the American Heart Association for Cardiopulmonary Resuscitation and Emergency Cardiac Care.*

nancy or extreme obesity, and with infants, chest thrusts are used in place of abdominal thrusts. The hands are positioned as for giving cardiac compressions, and four quick downward thrusts are given.

Once the victim can be ventilated, he is given four quick breaths before his pulse is checked. These breaths bring oxygen into the lungs preparatory to circulating blood.

External Cardiac Massage Table 28-12 outlines the sequence of steps for CPR. It is critical to remember that although a person may be given mouth-to-mouth resuscitation in almost any position, he must be lying flat on his back on a firm surface for cardiac compression. The headboards and footboards of many CCU beds come off and may be used to provide a firm surface under a client. In other areas of the hospital, meal trays may also be used if a cardiac board is not available. The important point is to be sure that the victim is lying on a hard surface that reaches from his shoulders to his hips. Pulling the victim off the bed and onto the floor should be done only as a last resort because that position makes it more difficult to carry out definitive treatment (described later). However, outside of the hospital setting, the victim is usually placed on the ground or floor.

A patent airway is established as outlined in Table 28-11. The next step is to palpate for a carotid pulse. This can be done by placing the pads of the rescuer's fingers on the trachea and then sliding to the groove on the side (not both sides) closest to him. Palpating the carotid keeps the rescuer close to the victim's head and reduces unnecessary movement. If no pulse is palpated, then chest compressions are initiated. Figure 28-18 illustrates the important points in giving cardiac compressions.

The rescuer positions himself close to the side of the victim's chest. Using the middle and index fingers of the hand closest to the victim's feet, the rescuer locates the lower margin of the victim's rib cage on the side next to the rescuer. The fingers are then run along the rib cage to the notch where the ribs meet the sternum. One finger is placed on the notch, and the other finger is placed next to the first one on the lower sternum. (Because direct pressure on the xiphoid process may lacerate the liver, this technique ensures

Table 28-12
Sequence of Steps for CPR

I. Unwitnessed arrest
   A. Ascertain that the victim is unresponsive by shaking and shouting at him. If there is no response, call for help as you position him flat on his back.
   B. Open the victim's airway by hyperextending his neck.
   C. Ascertain that the victim is breathless by taking 3–5 s to look, listen, and feel for respirations.
   D. If there are no respirations, rapidly give the victim four mouth-to-mouth (or mouth-to-nose or -stoma) breaths without allowing for exhalations between breaths.
   E. Ascertain that the victim is pulseless by taking 5–10 s to palpate for a carotid pulse.
   F. If there is no pulse, immediately begin chest compressions at a rate of 80 per minute if you are alone. When you are alone, give 15 compressions followed by two breaths. If a second rescuer is available, then give 60 compressions per minute, with the second rescuer interspersing breaths between every fifth breath.
   G. Check for the return of the pulse or respirations every few minutes during a switch of the two rescuers. (If the victim is on a cardiac monitor, you can observe the return of an effective heart beat.)
II. Witnessed arrest
   A. Ascertain that there is no pulse by tilting the victim's head back and palpating the carotid artery.
   B. Visually note the presence of respirations. If there are none, proceed with steps C–E.
   C. Give four quick breaths.
   D. Ascertain the victim's continued lack of pulse and breath by checking for pulse and respiration.
   E. Begin as outlined in steps A–D.

Adapted from American Heart Association, *Standards of the American Heart Association for Cardiopulmonary Resuscitation and Emergency Cardiac Care.*

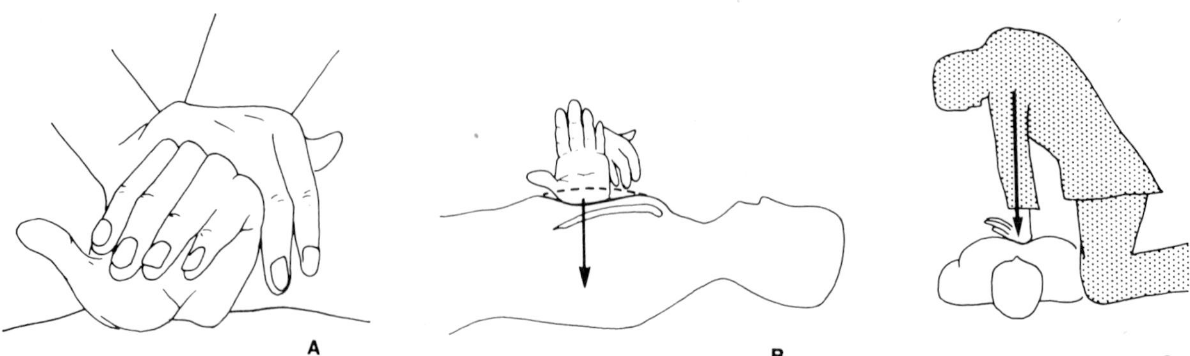

Figure 28-18 CPR or external cardiac massage. *(a)* Position of the hands during application of external cardiac massage. *(b)* When pressure is applied, the lower portion of the sternum is displaced posteriorily with the palm of the hand. *(c)* In order to apply maximal downward pressure, the resuscitator leans forward so that both arms are at right angles to the client's sternum. *[From K. Isselbacher et al. (eds.), Harrison's Principles of Internal Medicine, 9th ed., McGraw-Hill Book Company, New York, 1980, p. 186.]*

hand placement above the xiphoid.) The heel of the hand closest to the head is placed on the lower half of the sternum next to the index finger of the first hand that located the notch. The heel of the rescuer's hand should be placed on the long axis of the breastbone.[17] The other hand is placed on top of it. The fingers are kept off the chest.

The heart is compressed between the sternum and spine when 80 to 100 lb of pressure is applied. To apply pressure, the rescuer should have his shoulders directly over the sternum, keep his arm straight, maintain the hand position on the sternum at all times, and slightly rock back and forth from the hip joints. The sternum should be compressed smoothly $1\frac{1}{2}$ to 2 inches in a rhythmic manner. It has been found that if the downstroke is 50 percent of the cycle, there is better circulation of blood.

When there are two rescuers, the cardiac compressions, along with ventilations, need to be performed at a rate of 60 compressions per minute with a ventilation interspersed between every fifth compression. When there is one rescuer, the rate of compression should be 80 per minute, with a ratio of 15 compressions to 2 ventilations. The effectiveness of CPR is assessed by another person, who palpates a pulse in the victim during compression to ensure adequate force of compression and observes for decreased pupil dilatation and improvement in skin color as blood is circulated. The return of a spontaneous pulse and respirations is the goal, but it is rarely achieved without definitive therapy, described in the next section.

The precordial thump is recommended for use exclusively in the setting of an ECG-monitored client. (It is no longer recommended for use as a BCLS maneuver.) A precordial thump may be administered immediately after the monitor recognizes ventricular tachycardia or ventricular fibrillation. A blow to the heart within 1 minute of the onset of ventricular fibrillation or tachycardia may be sufficient to defibrillate the heart and restore an NSR. The precordial thump is delivered as a sharp, quick, single blow over the midportion of the sternum, hitting with the bottom fleshy portion of the fist from about 20 to 30 cm (8 to 12 inches) over the chest. BCLS should be instituted immediately if it is not apparent that cardiac output is being maintained.[18]

ACLS or definitive therapy

ACLS is a formal program developed by the American Heart Association for certification of nurses and physicians in the "D" (ABCD) of CPR. The "D" stands for definitive therapy, which was established in 1974. Table 28-13 outlines the major units covered in

Table 28-13
ACLS Course Content

Adjuncts for airway and breathing
Adjuncts for artificial circulation
Monitoring and dysrhythmia recognition
Defibrillation and synchronized cardioversion
IV techniques
Essential drugs in emergency cardiac care
Useful drugs
Acid-base balance
Stabilization and transportation

"Standards for Cardiopulmonary Resuscitation (CPR) and Emergency Cardiac Care (ECC)," *JAMA* **227**(suppl.):883–868 (1974).

this course. This section will deal with emergency cardiac drugs and defibrillation. BCLS must be continued during ACLS until breathing and circulation are restored.

Emergency Cardiac Drugs Table 28-14 lists the objectives of drug therapy. In order to administer emergency cardiac drugs, the CCU nurse needs to be skilled in various ways of administering oxygen (Chap. 20) and in the initiation and maintenance of IV therapy. Clients admitted to a CCU should have an IV line inserted to provide a pathway for emergency drugs that may be needed. Table 28-15 describes drugs commonly used in cardiac emergencies. The table is divided into drugs *essential* for cardiac emergencies and those *useful* for cardiac emergencies and less urgent cardiac stiuations. In addition to the drugs listed, two diuretics, furosemide and ethacrynic acid, are frequently used in acute CHF to prevent pulmonary edema and cerebral edema after a cardiac arrest. Corticosteroids are sometimes used with cardiogenic shock or shock lung following cardiac arrest. Figure 28-19 contains a decision tree for the treatment of serious arrhythmias.

Defibrillation Defibrillation is the treatment of choice for ventricular fibrillation. There are many types of defibrillators (Fig. 28-20). Nurses should familiarize themselves with the controls on the ones they will be using. Commonly used defibrillators are DC machines which give a monophasic discharge of several thousand volts lasting for only a few milliseconds when the discharge button is pushed. This discharge causes simultaneous contraction (depolarization) of all the myocardial cells. The repolarization of the cells frequently allows the SA node to resume as the pacemaker. Electrical defibrillation is most effective when the cells are *not* anoxic or acidotic. Therefore, it should ideally be done within 15 to 20 seconds of the onset of ventricular fibrillation. The amount of electricity given is usually 400 watt-seconds, but it may vary from 200 to 400 watt-seconds (joules). Controversy exists about whether or not some defibrillators should deliver more than 400 joules for use with large clients.[19] V tach has been terminated by as little as 100 joules.[20]

The procedure for defibrillation, once it is considered necessary, is as follows. In the presence of cardiac arrest, it is critical that CPR (BCLS) be carried out continuously while the nurse is preparing to defibrillate the victim. (In continuously monitored clients who go into V fib, defibrillation is attempted prior to CPR.) The machine must be turned on with the plug in the electrical outlet (if it is not battery operated). The desired amount of energy, as indicated by standing orders, should be selected. The nurse should be sure that the synchronization button is off. (This technique is used in cardioversion and requires an R wave to discharge. V fib does not have an R wave.)

Saline pads, electrode paste, or defibrillator gel pads are placed on the skin where the paddles will go to decrease skin resistance and prevent burns. Excess amounts of paste or saline can cause electrical "bridging," resulting in burns and decreased energy for defibrillation. Alcohol sponges should *never* be used because of the danger of fire. The paddles are placed on the chest wall (Fig. 28-21), one in the right second interspace and one to the left of the precordium. The operator calls, "Stand back," and *everyone* who is nearby breaks contact with the client or his bed. The operator applies 20 to 25 lb of pressure to the paddles, makes sure that he is not touching the client or the bed, and then simultaneously pushes the buttons on both paddles. CPR should be reinstituted immediately if no carotid pulse is felt, even if the monitor shows a regular pattern. This is because of the possibility of electromechanical dissociation.

If the first defibrillation attempt is unsuccessful, a second one should be made immediately using 200 to 300 joules of energy. If a second defibrillation attempt is unsuccessful, it is recommended that BCLS be continued with supplemental O_2. Epinephrine and sodium bicarbonate ($NaHCO_3$) may be given during the continuing CPR. The specifics of drugs, dosages, and procedures are outlined in the standing orders for each CCU.

In contrast to emergency defibrillation, cardioversion (the conversion of an arrhythmia back to an NSR using DC) may be a nonemergency, elective procedure. Clients to be cardioverted receive nothing by mouth and are sedated with diazepam or anesthetized with a short-acting barbiturate prior to the procedure.

Table 28-14
Objectives of Drug Therapy in Cardiac Emergencies

Correct hypoxia due to inadequate ventilation and circulation
Correct metabolic acidosis due to inadequate ventilation and circulation
Increase perfusion pressure during cardiac compression
Stimulate spontaneous and more forceful myocardial contraction
Accelerate the heart rate
Suppress ectopic activity in the ventricles
Relieve pain
Treat pulmonary edema

Adapted from American Heart Association, *Advanced Cardiac Life Support Textbook*, 1975, p. vii.

Table 28-15
Drugs Commonly Used in Cardiac Emergencies

Drug	Indications	Routine of Administration	Major Effect or Pharmacological Effect	Adverse Effects	Nursing Considerations
Oxygen*	Hypoxia	Nasal cannula, face mask, mask device, ventilators (refer to Table 20-12)	Used by all body cells for aerobic metabolism	Oxygen toxicity	In emergency situations, such as cardiac arrest, give without fear of toxicity.
Sodium bicarbonate*	Metabolic and respiratory acidosis	IV bolus	Corrects metabolic acidosis by the following simple formula: $HCO_3^- + H^+ \leftrightharpoons H_2CO_2 \leftrightharpoons CO_2 + H_2O \leftrightharpoons H_2CO_3$	Metabolic alkalosis, Hypernatremia Water overload	In cardiac arrest, be sure to ventilate victim well to aid in the removal of CO_2 gas. Acidosis increases chance for V fib and decreases contractile force of the ventricles and decreases the myocardial response to epinephrine. Do not mix it with any drug.
Epinephrine (Adrenalin)*	Asystole Electromechanical dissociation Bronchospasm Anaphylaxis	IV bolus Nebulization into endotracheal tube IM IV drip	Sympathomimetic drug that stimulates both α- and β-receptor sites, resulting in: ↑ heart rate ↑ myocardial contractile force ↑ systemic vascular resistance ↑ arterial blood pressure ↑ myocardial O_2 consumption ↑ automaticity ↓ blood flow to kidneys and skin	Transient anxiety Palpitations Headache Necrosis of tissue from local injections ↑ blood glucose ↑ O_2 consumption of heart	It is preferable to correct acidosis before using IV administration.
Atropine*†	Symptomatic sinus bradycardia Mobitz I heart block Complete heart block	IV, IM	Parasympatholytic drug ↑ discharge rate of the SA node (vagolytic action) ↓ refractory period and ↑ speed of conduction through AV node	Dry mouth Pupil dilation Difficulty in voiding ↓ bronchial secretions PVCs, V tach, or V fib (especially in acute MI client)	May also be given with morphine to counteract its vagomimetic effect.
Lidocaine (Xylocaine)*	PVCs V tach V fib	IV	↓ automaticity of Purkinje fibers ↑ threshold for V fib ↓ conduction velocity and refractory period of Purkinje fibers	Lethargy Confusion Slurred speech Tingling lips and tongue Disorientation Hypotension Convulsions SA arrest Heart block Bradycardia	Seldom used in clients with slow heart rates or heart block. Need to continuously monitor ECG of clients receiving this drug. Has slower detoxification in clients with liver disorder.

Morphine*	Pain with acute MI or acute pulmonary edema	IV	Analgesic and sedative effects ↑ venous pooling and therefore venous return ↓ left ventricular end diastolic pressure ↓ myocardial O_2 consumption ↓ left ventricular afterload	Respiratory depression Hypotension Confusion	Give in small increments carefully titrated to the response of the client.
Calcium chloride*	Asystole Electromechanical dissociation	IV	↑ myocardial contractility ↑ ventricular excitability	Moderate decrease in blood pressure Hypercalcemia Local necrosis if extravasation occurs	Do not mix with $NaHCO_3$. Give slowly if heart is beating (can cause severe bradycardia or sinus arrest). Use cautiously with digitalized client (can enhance toxicity).
Levarterenol (Levophed)	Peripheral vascular collapse (hypotension without significant peripheral vasodilatation)	IV	Directly stimulates both α- and β-receptors ↑ peripheral vasoconstriction (resistance) ↑ dilatation of coronary arteries ↑ myocardial contractility ↓ blood flow to kidneys	Bradycardia Headache Hypertensive response	Titrate dose according to arterial blood pressure. Taper slowly when discontinuing. Avoid extravasation.
Metaraminol (Aramine)	Peripheral vascular collapse (hypotension without significant peripheral vasodilatation) Supraventricular tachycardias	IV, IM	Indirectly stimulates both α- and β-receptors ↑ peripheral vasoconstriction (resistance) ↑ cardiac output ↑ systolic and diastolic blood pressure Reflex vagal stimulation	Hypertensive response Ventricular arrhythmias Reflex bradycardia	Same as with levarterenol.
Isoproterenol (Isuprel)	Complete heart block Asystole Electromechanical dissociation	SL, po, IV, inhalant	Stimulates β-receptor sites (β_1 and β_2) ↑ myocardial contractility ↑ heart rate ↑ myocardial O_2 consumption ↓ peripheral vascular resistance ↓ diastolic pressure (may reduce mean arterial pressure) Relaxes smooth muscle in bronchitis, GI tract	Sinus tachycardia PVCs V tach, V fib Hypotensions in presence of hypovolemia, headache, flushing of skin, angina, nausea, tremor, dizziness, weakness, and sweating	Isoproterenol is contraindicated in the presence of digitalis-induced tachycardias. Use very cautiously in presence of hypokalemia (↑ arrhythmias). If ventricular irritability occurs, decrease IV infusion rate. Titrate IV dose to achieve heart rate of 60 bpm.
Dopamine (Intropin)	Cardiac decompensation, as with CHF or cardiogenic shock Mainly used for hypotension Open heart surgery	IV	Stimulates β_1-receptor sites ↑ myocardial contractility but not heart rate Mild vasoconstriction in skeletal muscles ↑ cardiac output and stroke volume Dilates renal and mesenteric vessels in doses of 1–2 mg/kg/min to 10 mg/kg/min (> 10 mg/kg/min causes vasoconstriction)	Ectopic arrythmias Nausea and vomiting Angina Dyspnea Headache Hypotension Palpitations Vasoconstriction PVCs	Prevent extravasation by infusing into large vein. Do not mix with alkaline substance. Titrate dose to desired hemodynamic or renal response. Slow rate if an increased diastolic pressure results in a decreased pulse pressure. Continuously monitor ECG and blood pressure.

Table 28-15 (Continued)

Drug	Indications	Routine of Administration	Major Effect or Pharmacological Effect	Adverse Effects	Nursing Considerations
Dobutamine (Dobutrex)	Cardiac decompensation, especially with CHF and cardiogenic shock	IV	Stimulates β_1-receptor sites ↑ myocardial contractility but not heart rate Slightly stimulates α and β_2 vascular receptor (does *not* dilate renal and mesenteric arteries nor have vasoconstrictive activity at higher doses)	Marked elevation in heart rate (30 bpm or more) Marked elevation in blood pressure (50 mmHg) Ventricular ectopic arrhythmias Nausea Headache Chest pain Palpitations Shortness of breath	Client should have continuous monitoring of EGG, blood pressure, pulmonary wedge pressure, and cardiac output. Do not mix with alkaline substance.
Propranolol (Inderal)	Tachyarrythmias due to digitalis toxicity Recurrent V tach and V. fib Atrial flutter Atrial fibrillation Sinus tachycardia Paroxysmal supraventricular tachycardia	IV, po	β- adrenergic receptor blocking agent ↓ heart rate and myocardial contractility ↓ myocardial O_2 consumption Depresses automaticity of pacemakers and suppresses ectopic beats Prolongs AV conduction time and refractory period	Bradycardia, hypotension, heart block, fatigue, dizziness, blood sugar disturbances, insomnia, GI distress	Do not use in presence of CHF, bradycardia, heart block, and bronchospasm.
Procainamide (Pronestyl)	PVCs V tach Supraventricular tachycardia	IV, po	↑ refractory period in atrium ↓ excitability in atria and ventricles ↓ automaticity of pacemaker cells ↑ threshold to fibrillation ↑ conduction time	GI distress: anorexia, nausea, vomiting, diarrhea CNS: depression and hallucinations Systemic lupus-like syndrome: arthralgia, fever, skin rash, etc. Hypotension, convulsions, AV block, PVCs, V fib, agranulocytosis	Do not give to client with complete heart block. When giving IV, monitor ECG and blood pressure of client. Stop drug if QRS complex widens or PR or ST intervals become prolonged.
Digitalis (Ouabain, digoxin, digitoxin); see Table 27-21	Atrial flutter Atrial fibrillation Paroxysmal supraventricular tachycardia Junctional tachycardia CHF	IV, po	↑ myocardial contractility ↑ rate at which force is developed ↑ refractory period of AV node ↓ left ventricular end diastolic volume and pressure ↑ ventricular automaticity ↓ atrial automaticity	See Table 27-22 Cardiac: PVCs, junctional rhythms, AV block, V tach or V fib, sinus arrest	Always assess pulse before giving the drug because many arrhythmias are caused by digitalis. Monitor ECG when using IV administration. Poor renal function. Hypercalcemia and hypokalemia predispose client to digitalis toxicity. When given with quinidine, dose may need to be decreased because quinidine reduces renal clearance of digoxin

Quinidine	Premature contractions Paroxysmal supraventricular tachycardia V tach Atrial fibrillation Atrial flutter	po	↑ refractory period of atrial and ventricular muscle ↑ conduction time in myocardium, Purkinje fibers, and AV node ↓ excitability ↓ myocardial contractility ↓ automaticity of pacemaker cells	Hypersensitivity (hypotension, convulsions, thrombocytopenia) Cinchonism (nausea, vomiting, tinnitus, vertigo, blurred vision) Cardiac: SA node block, AV node block sinus arrest, V tach or V fib Asystole	Give test dose to check for hypersensitivity. In presence of atrial fibrillation or atrial flutter, client must receive digitalis *prior* to quinidine. IV administration has high incidence of toxicity.
Phenytoin (Dilantin)	Digitalis-induced arrhythmias, especially: Paroxysmal supraventricular tachycardia PVCs V tach	po, IV	↓ automaticity of pacemaker cells ↓ contractility ↑ AV node conduction	Ataxia, vertigo, nystagmus, seizures, confusion, hypertrophy of gums, nausea and vomiting V fib Asystole	If giving IV, dilute well and administer slowly. Oral anticoagulants slow metabolism of phenytoin; therefore, watch for toxicity. Do not give in presence of sinus bradycardia or SA or AV block
Bretylium (Bretylol)	Recurrent V tach not responsive to lidocaine, procainamide, etc.	IV, IM, po	Transient (increase in blood pressure and arrhythmias followed by a decrease) in blood pressure and arrhythmias due to sympatholytic action ↑ myocardial contractility ↑ V fib threshold ↑ refractory period of Purkinje fibers and ventricular muscle	Postural hypotension, nausea and vomiting ↑ sensitivity to catecholamines Aggravates existing angina pectoris	Watch client closely for hypersensitivity reaction if he is receiving catecholamine drugs concurrently. In clients with renal failure, watch closely for toxicity.
Disopyramide (Norpace, Rhythmodan)	PVCs V tach Supraventricular arrhythmias	po	↓ automaticity ↓ conductivity ↑ AV node conduction ↓ excitability	Anticholinergic side effects: dry mouth, urinary hesitancy and retention, constipation, blurred vision GI distress Headache and fatigue Heart block Syncope ("Norpace syncope") Prolonged OT interval; then paroxysmal ventricular tachycardia	Similar in action to quinidine but has greater negative inotropic action. Therefore, clients with preexisting CHF may experience hypotension and worsening of failure. Clients with atrial tachyarrhythmias should receive digitalis concurrently.
Nitroprusside (Nipride)	Severe or malignant hypertension Heart failure and other low output states (as with cardiac surgery, MI)	IV	Vasodilates both arterioles and venules In clients with elevated left ventricular filling pressure, causes increased cardiac output Also causes decreased ventricular filling pressure, mean PAP, peripheral vascular resistance, and mean arterial pressure. Increased cardiac output is due more to decreased afterload than decreased preload.	Acute: hypotension, tachycardia, increased intracranial pressure. Chronic: fatigue, nausea and anorexia, disorientation, psychotic behavior, muscle spasm	Drug needs to be infused continuously because its effect takes 3–5 min. Slow infusion rate if there is excessive increase in heart rate or lowering of blood pressure. When used for low output states, nurse should monitor ECG, intraarterial pressure, PCWP, and cardiac output.

*These drugs are considered essential for use in cardiac emergencies.
†Has many uses. Only those related to cardiac disorders are described.

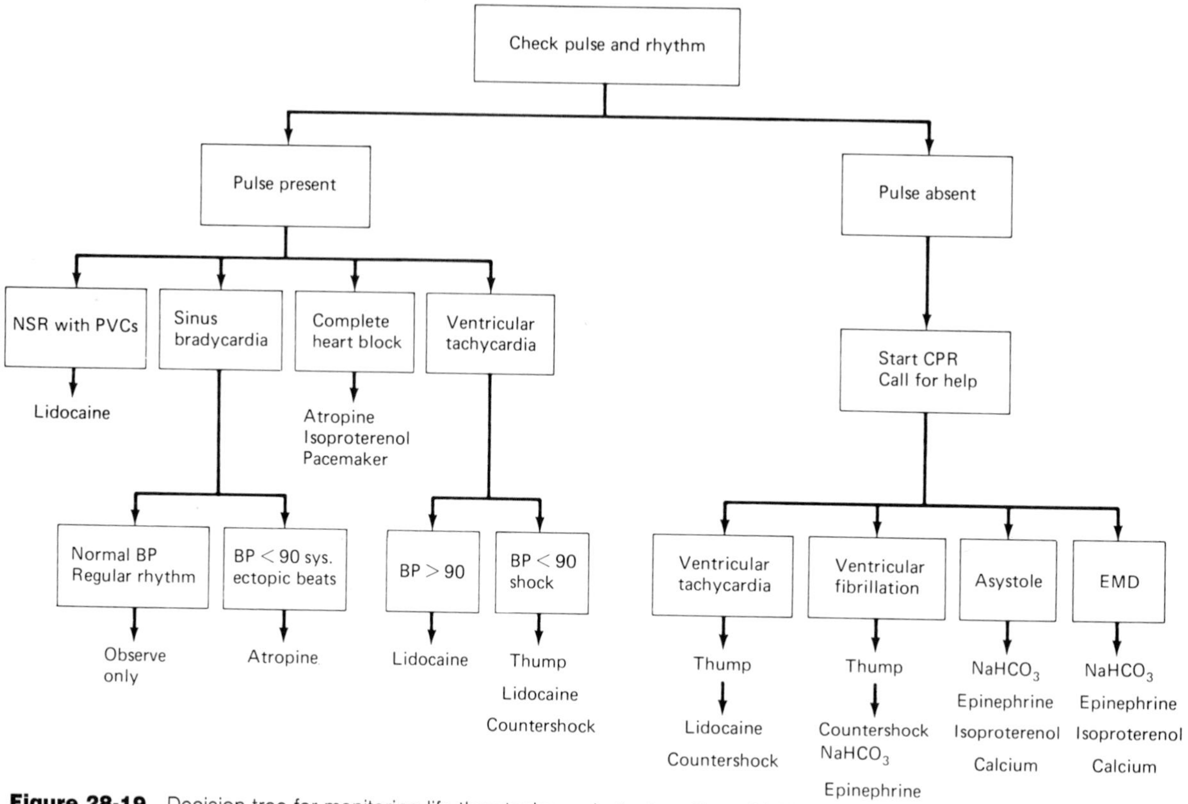

- Check pulse and rhythm
  - Pulse present
    - NSR with PVCs → Lidocaine
    - Sinus bradycardia
      - Normal BP, Regular rhythm → Observe only
      - BP < 90 sys., ectopic beats → Atropine
    - Complete heart block → Atropine, Isoproterenol, Pacemaker
    - Ventricular tachycardia
      - BP > 90 → Lidocaine
      - BP < 90 shock → Thump, Lidocaine, Countershock
  - Pulse absent
    - Start CPR, Call for help
      - Ventricular tachycardia → Thump → Lidocaine, Countershock
      - Ventricular fibrillation → Thump → Countershock, $NaHCO_3$, Epinephrine
      - Asystole → $NaHCO_3$, Epinephrine, Isoproterenol, Calcium
      - EMD → $NaHCO_3$, Epinephrine, Isoproterenol, Calcium

Figure 28-19 Decision tree for monitoring life-threatening arrhythmias. *(From M. Kinney et al., AACN's Clinical Reference for Critical Care Nursing, McGraw-Hill Book Company, New York, 1981, p. 919.)*

The synchronization button on the defibrillator is pushed so that the machine will discharge on the downward slope of the R wave. Both discharge buttons are held down until the machine discharges on the R wave. The purpose of synchronizing the electrical discharge with the client's rhythm is to avoid the period of electrical vulnerability during recovery (T wave).

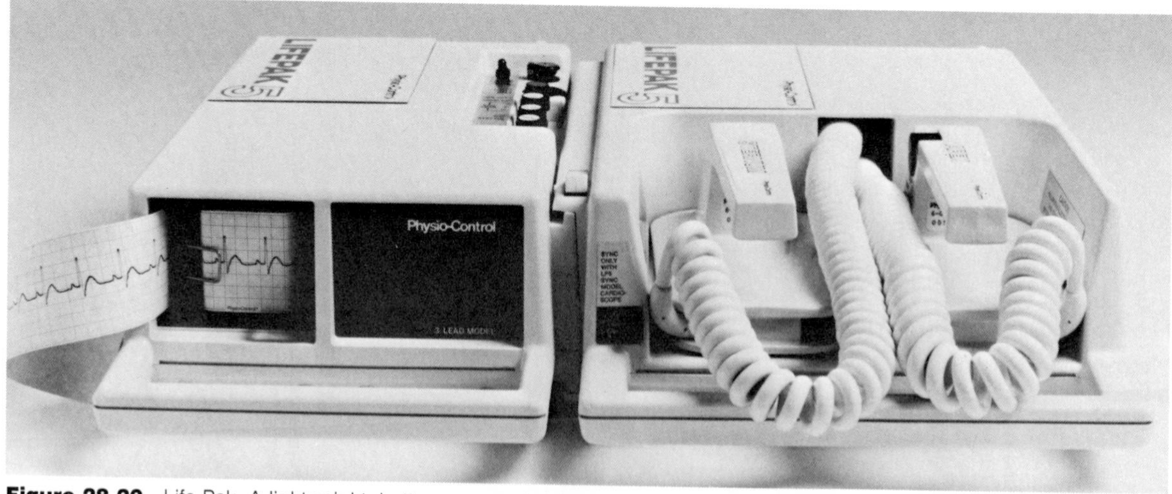

Figure 28-20 Life-Pak. A lightweight, battery-powered defibrillator with monitoring capabilities.

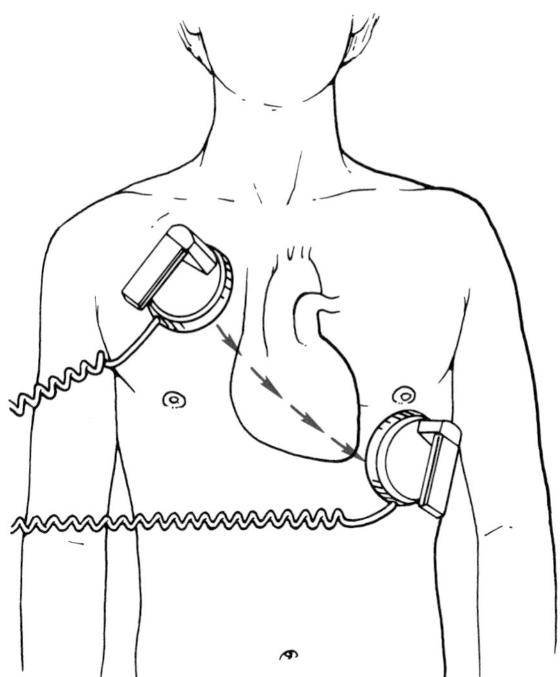

Figure 28-21 Paddle placement and current flow in defibrillation.

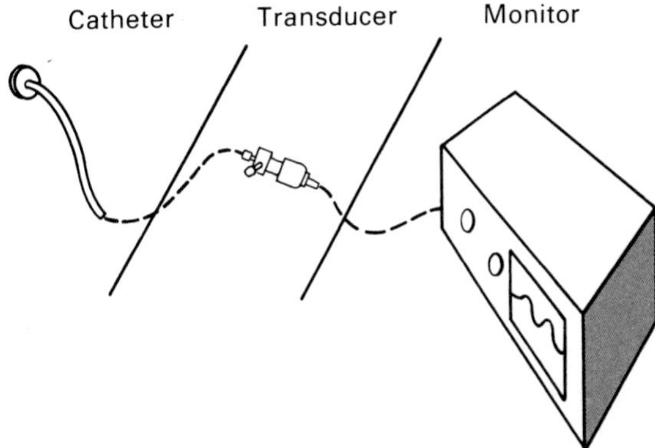

Figure 28-22 Hemodynamic monitoring systems consist of a fluid-filled catheter, a transducer, and a monitor.

Hemodynamic Monitoring

Hemodynamic monitoring refers to the monitoring of blood flow and pressure. *Indirect monitoring* involves a noninvasive procedure. A common example is taking an arterial blood pressure with a syphgmomanometer and stethoscope. The steps involved in taking an accurate blood pressure reading are presented in Chap. 25.

Direct or *invasive monitoring* allows for the ongoing assessment of critical blood pressures in and around the heart. It is commonly used in critical care areas because direct monitoring provides the quickest and most accurate physiological data.

Basic pressure system

In direct monitoring, physiological pressures in the heart chambers or blood vessels (measured in millimeters of mercury) must be converted into electrical current that varies with the change in pressures. Figure 28-22 illustrates the three basic components for pressure monitoring: a *catheter,* a *transducer,* and a *monitor.* A specialized catheter or line (depending on the purpose) is inserted into the area where pressure is to be measured. The catheter is filled with an IV solution, such as dextrose and water and heparin, to help maintain the patency of the catheter. A special flush device allows continual movement of the solution at a rate of 3 to 5 mL/hour.

Pressure measurement requires the transformation of a biological event into an electrical event that can be displayed, recorded, and quantified. This transformation is accomplished with a transducer. The transducer is the device that converts physiological (or mechanical) energy to electrical energy. It is attached to the catheter by a series of tubes and stopcocks. The fluid against the diaphragm of the transducer exerts pressure equal to that in the catheter and transforms this pressure to an oscilloscope for evaluation and documentation.

Nursing management of pressure lines

There are certain basic principles of nursing care in clients with pressure lines. Each CCU will have a specific protocol to follow. Nurses should familiarize themselves with the procedures designed to reduce the three major risks: (1) *hemorrhage,* (2) *thrombosis with emboli,* and (3) *infection.*

To prevent hemorrhage, or bleeding back into the line, the flush solution is kept in a closed system under a pressure greater than the client's systolic pressure. This is done by using a blood pump on the IV solution bag. It is important to tape all connections to maintain a closed system. Pressure on the flush bag must be kept at a preset level to prevent backup of blood into the tubing.

To prevent thrombus formation, a solution with heparin is continuously flushed through the line. If a thrombus should begin to form, this is indicated by a dampening of the waveform. In such cases, the line should be flushed with the fast flush valve found on the tubing. If the wave is still dampened, the nurse should attempt to aspirate the clot with a syringe. Any aspirated blood should not be injected back into the client because it may be clotted.

To prevent infections, careful technique for both

insertion and maintenance of the line is mandatory. Lines are inserted under aseptic conditions whenever possible since they are potential direct routes by which bacteria can enter the vascular system. The skin is cleaned according to hospital procedure, usually with an iodine preparation. A cutdown or percutaneous stick is performed under local anesthesia. All lines are sutured to the skin and covered with an occlusive dressing. Insertion sites should be dressed daily with an iodine-based ointment that is applied to the site and covered with an occlusive dressing. The line should be removed if there is any sign of infection at the insertion site. Lines should not be left in any longer than necessary because of their susceptibility to infection.

Another important nursing procedure is balancing and calibration of the transducers. Since physiological pressures are related to atmospheric pressures, the transducer must be balanced at atmospheric pressure. Once the transducer is balanced, the monitor is then calibrated to show the desired pressure. The procedures for balancing and calibrating the transducer are specified by the type of equipment used and the unit protocol. After calibration is completed, pressure tracing readings are taken with the client in the same position (flat or with the head of the bed elevated) used when the transducer was calibrated. This ensures accurate pressure readings.

Arterial blood pressure

Continuous monitoring of the arterial blood pressure is indicated for critically ill clients who (1) have hypotension with peripheral vasoconstriction, (2) are receiving potent vasoactive drugs, such as nitroprusside or dopamine, (3) require frequent blood samples, such as arterial blood gases, and (4) have increased intracranial pressure.

An arterial line is commonly inserted in the radial or brachial artery. It is important that the site of insertion be stabilized so that the line is not being moved back and forth. This may be done by using an arm board.

Figure 28-23 illustrates a typical arterial waveform for a normal blood pressure. Note the sharp ascent during systole, which is correlated with the depolarization and contraction of the ventricles. Diastole is represented by a slower descent starting with the *dicrotic notch,* which indicates the closing of the aortic valve.

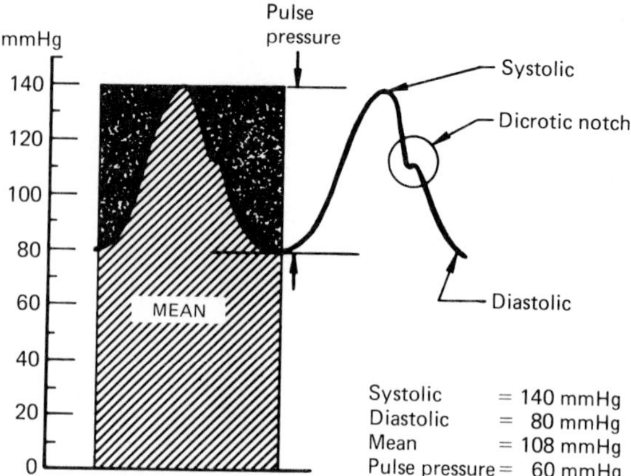

Figure 28-23 Typical arterial pressure waveform. *(From M. Kinney et al., AACN's Clinical Reference for Critical Care Nursing, McGraw-Hill Book Company, New York, 1981, p. 1010.)*

Swan-Ganz flow-directed catheter

The Swan-Ganz flow-directed catheter is used for measuring the pulmonary artery pressure (PA or PAP) and the mean pulmonary capillary wedge pressure (PCW or PCWP). These pressures are an indirect reflection of the left ventricular end diastolic pressure (LVEDP). In the absence of acute mitral valve incompetence (insufficiency), the PAP and PCWP are good indicators of left ventricular function.

The original Swan-Ganz catheters had a double lumen, with one lumen terminating at the tip of the catheter and the other, smaller one in the balloon near the tip. The balloon can be inflated near the tip without occluding it. Newer triple-lumen Swan-Ganz catheters have a third lumen for measuring the right atrial pressure and a thermister tip for measuring blood temperature, which is used in determining cardiac output. These catheters are also equipped with an atrial electrode or pacing wire. The electrode may be used to record atrial electrograms and to pace the atrium, as well as to perform the functions of any other triple-lumen catheter. This arrangement is of great benefit to the client since only one catheter is passed to serve multiple functions.

After the catheter is attached to the transducer (set up similarly to an arterial line), it is inserted via the internal or external jugular, subclavian, antecubital, or femoral vein and advanced into the right atrium. In the right atrium or ventricle, the balloon is fully inflated and allowed to float into the pulmonary artery until it wedges in a pulmonary arteriole (Fig. 28-24). During the insertion procedure, the monitor is observed for changes in pressure waves, which aids in determining the location of the catheter tip (Fig. 28-25). Once the catheter is in place, as evidenced by the characteristic wedge wave, an x-ray is taken to confirm the proper placement and the catheter is sutured in place.

When the balloon is inflated, pressures from the

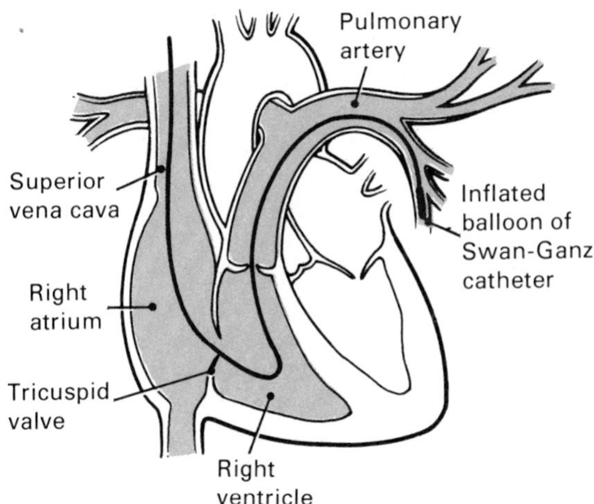

Figure 28-24 Insertion of a Swan-Ganz catheter through the right side of the heart to the pulmonary artery. *(From M. Armstrong et al., McGraw-Hill's Handbook of Nursing, McGraw-Hill Book Company, New York, 1979, p. 787.)*

right side of the heart are blocked so that the catheter tip measures pressure in the pulmonary capillaries. The normal PCWP reading is 4 to 12 mmHg. As soon as the PCWP reading is taken, the balloon must be deflated to prevent pulmonary infarction. Another potential risk associated with taking the PCWP reading is rupture of the pulmonary capillary due to overinflation.

The PAP is normally 25/10. The PA systolic pressure (top of the wave) represents contraction of the right ventricles. The PA end diastolic pressure (bottom of the wave) represents the pressure in the pulmonary arterioles and capillaries to the flow of blood. If there is a difference of more than 6 mmHg between the PCW and PA end diastolic pressures, this is an indication of obstructive vascular pathology in the lungs.[21]

There are other hazards associated with the Swan-Ganz catheter that are not found with arterial lines. In addition to thrombosis and embolus formation, there may be *air emboli* due to the injection of air into the ports or to rupture of the balloon. Fragments from balloon rupture may embolize. The longer the catheter is in place, the higher the possibility of rupture.

The Swan-Ganz catheter may also *advance into a wedge position* on its own. This can be seen by the change in waveform, underlining the need for continuous monitoring. If the catheter is left in a wedge position, a small pulmonary infarction may occur.

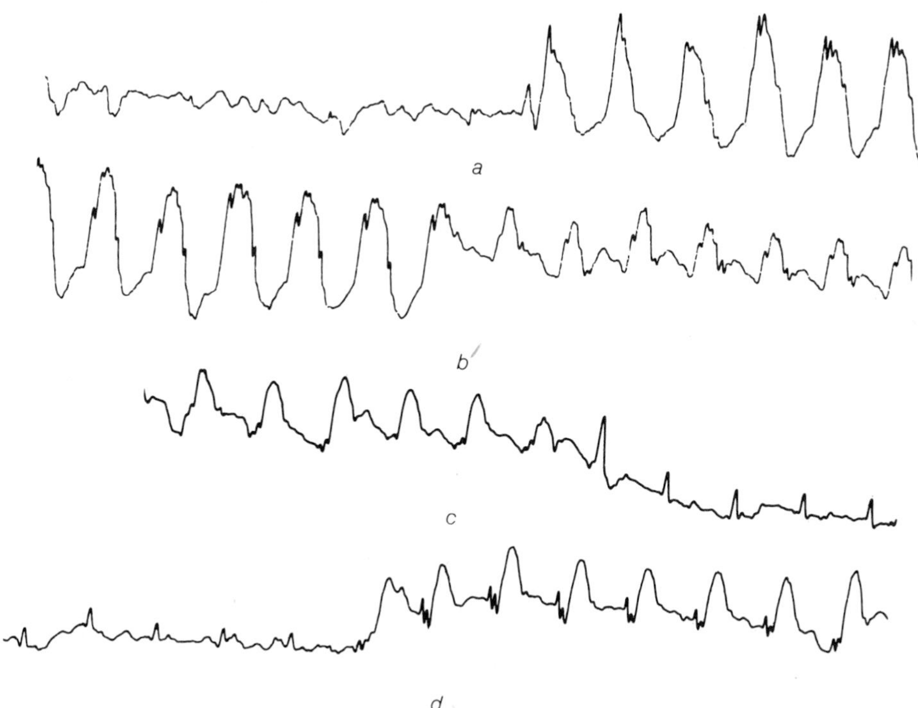

Figure 28-25 Changing pulmonary artery waveforms during insertion of the Swan-Ganz catheter. *(a)* Right atrium to right ventricle. *(b)* Right ventricle to PA. *(c)* PA to PCW. *(d)* PCW to PA. *(From M. Kinney et al., AACN's Clinical Reference for Critical Care Nursing, McGraw-Hill Book Company, New York, 1981, p. 1015.)*

Table 28-16
Determinants of Cardiac Output

Cardiac output =	stroke volume	× heart rate
4–8 L/min	60–130 mL/beat	60–80 bpm

Factors affecting stroke volume:
- Afterload
- Preload
- Contractility of left ventricle
- End diastolic volume of left ventricle

Factors affecting heart rate:
- Autonomic nervous system
- Effects of exercise

Changing a client's position or withdrawing the catheter 1 to 2 cm should alleviate the problem.

Ventricular arrhythmias may occur on insertion or removal or if the catheter falls back into the ventricle. This may be noted by changes in the pressure waveform (Fig. 28-25) as well as on the ECG. The physician should be notified if this occurs.

Cardiac output

Cardiac output (stroke volume × heart rate) is another measure of cardiac function. Table 28-16 summarizes the determinants of cardiac output. To maintain cardiac output, any change in the stroke volume or heart rate must be balanced by a change in the other value. If the stroke volume is decreased because a massive hemorrhage has reduced the circulating blood volume, the heart rate will increase to compensate. If the heart rate increases, the stroke volume decreases (e.g., in fast cardiac rhythms the heart does not fill well).

Most types of Swan-Ganz catheters allow direct cardiac output determinations. The catheter allows iced solution to be injected at a specified rate into the proximal port of the catheter or into the right atrium. A thermistor in the tip of the catheter senses the temperature of the blood as it passes, and a special computer (Fig. 28-26) calculates the cardiac output based on

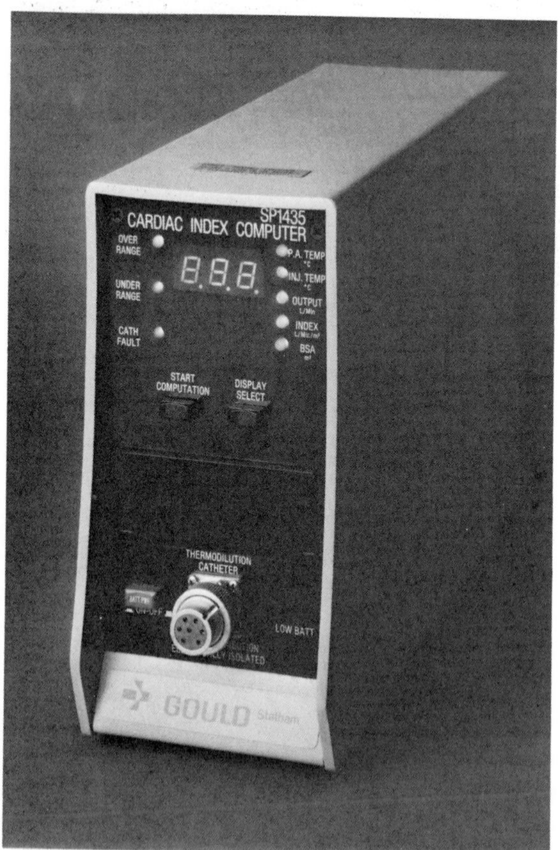

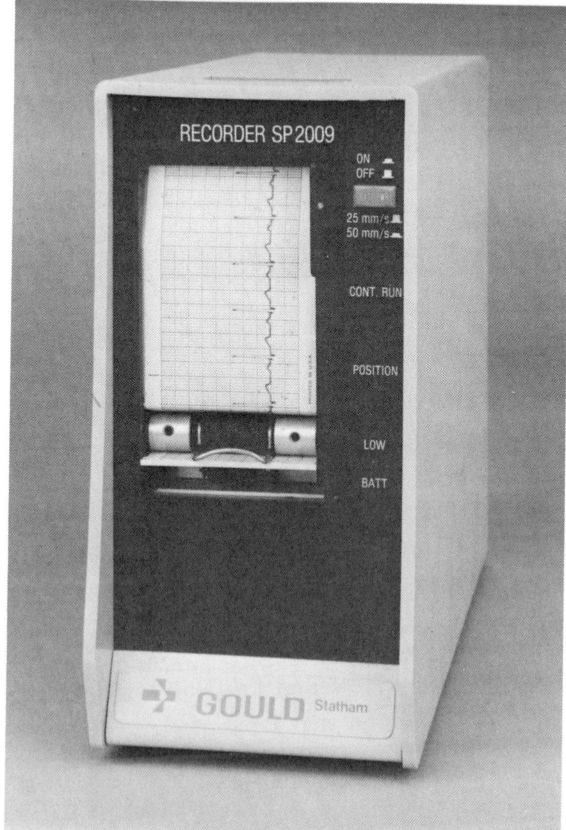

Figure 28-28 Cardiac output computer with recorder. *(Gould, Inc., Oxnard, Calif.)*

time and on changes in the temperature of the blood. Normal cardiac output is 3 to 5 L/minute. Although cardiac output gives information regarding left ventricular function, it varies from individual to individual according to one's size. A more accurate indicator of left ventricular function is the cardiac index. Cardiac output divided by body surface area yields the cardiac index. The normal cardiac index is 2.4 to 4.8 L/minute/m^2.

Other pressures

Two other pressures that are monitored are central venous pressure (CVP), described in Chap. 25, and left atrial pressure (LAP). LAP measurement requires that a catheter be inserted directly into the left atrium during a surgical procedure. Thus, it is associated with cardiovascular surgery. This pressure is used in determining the LVEDP. It is especially critical in preventing the entrance of air into this line because of the high risk of an air embolus to the coronary arteries or brain.

IABP

Description

The IABP is a mechanical device that provides circulatory assistance to the compromised heart by reducing *afterload* (the amount of tension the ventricle must develop during contraction to eject blood) and augmenting the diastolic pressure. Table 28-17 lists the various clinical conditions for which an IABP is used.

The sausage-shaped balloon is inserted into the common femoral artery under local anesthesia and advanced upward until it is in the descending thoracic aorta just below the left subclavian artery and above the renal arteries. The balloon is timed to inflate and deflate in synchrony with the client's heart action. Usually, the ECG is used initially to time deflation of the balloon on the R wave and inflation on the T wave. The arterial wave is used to adjust the timing precisely so that balloon inflation occurs at the dicrotic notch on the arterial tracing and deflation occurs just before systole. The balloon pump console contains the controls and alarms for inflation and deflation of the balloon. The balloon action is referred to as *counterpulsation* because the timing of the balloon inflations is the opposite of the ventricular contractions.

Effects of counterpulsation

The effects of counterpulsation are seen with both inflation and deflation of the balloon. The balloon is rapidly inflated at the beginning of diastole immediately after the aortic valve has closed, partially occluding the aorta (Fig. 28-27). Displaced blood is forced downward into the extremities and upward into the coronary arteries and the main branches of the aortic arch. The diastolic arterial pressure rises (diastolic augmentation), increasing perfusion of the vital organs and the perfusion pressure for the coronary

Table 28-17

Uses for the IABP

Indications

1. Preinfarction, accelerating or crescendo angina (when conventional modes of therapy, such as bed rest, nitrates, and propranolol, have failed)
2. Unstable angina; client is undergoing cardiac catherization
3. Severe cardiac disease; client is undergoing cardiac catherization or noncardiac surgery
4. Acute MI followed by:
    a. Ventricular aneurysm accompanied by ventricular arrhythmia
    b. Acute ventricular septal defect
    c. Acute mitral regurgitation
    d. Cardiogenic shock
    e. Continuing chest pain

    } Allows time for emergency angiography and corrective cardiac surgery to be performed
5. Preoperative, intraoperative, and postoperative open heart surgery (e.g., aneurysectomy, revascularization, or valve replacement)
    Cardiogenic shock associated with any of the above conditions

Contraindications

1. Irreversible brain damage
2. Terminal or untreatable disease of any major organ system
3. Ruptured or dissecting aortic or thoracic aneurysm
4. Generalized peripheral vascular disease (may prevent placement of balloon)
5. Insufficient aortic valve (considered an *absolute* contraindication)

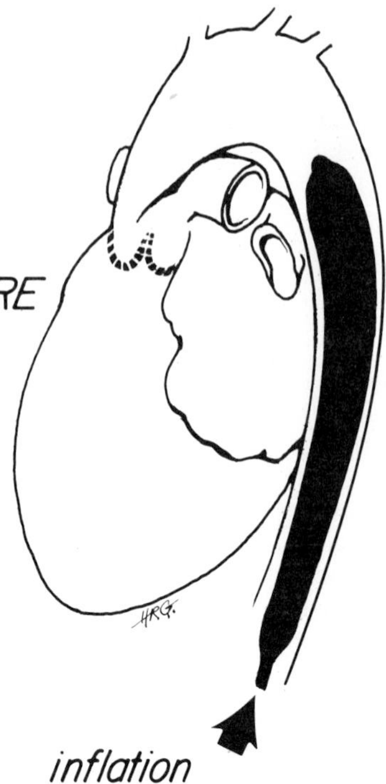

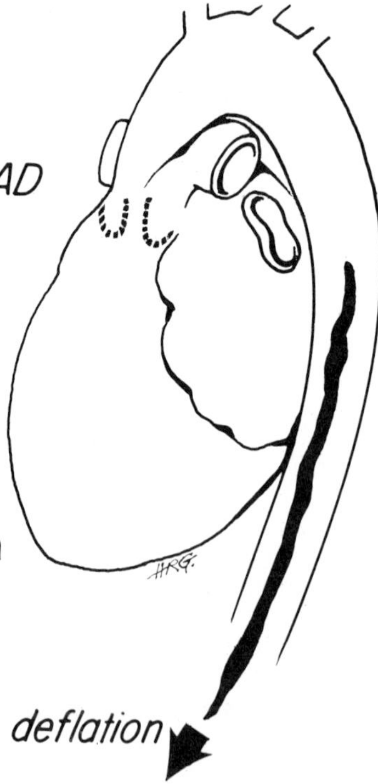

Figure 28-27 Effects of the IABP. *(a)* Inflation. *(b)* Deflation. *(From S. Price and L. Wilson, Pathophysiology: Clinical Concepts of Disease Processes, McGraw-Hill Book Company, New York, 2d ed., 1982, p. 361.)*

arteries. The rise in coronary artery perfusion pressure usually causes an increase in the total blood flow to the myocardium and may also increase the development of coronary artery collateral circulation.[22]

The balloon is rapidly deflated just before systole (Fig. 28-27). The suddenly created void causes the pressure in the aorta to drop below the pressure that would exist if no balloon were in place. With the aortic resistance to left ventricular ejection reduced (reduced afterload), the left ventricle empties more easily and completely. As a result, the oxygen consumption of the myocardium decreases.

Management of the IABP

Beginning, maintaining, and terminating the IABP require nurses who are highly skilled and who work closely with skilled physicians. The procedures involved are beyond the scope of this book. Clients on the IABP are prone to infections and to arterial, thromboembolic, and hematological complications. Complications are rarely due to malfunction of the balloon or console because the fail-safe alarm systems and automatic unit shut down if an unsafe pumping condition develops. Nursing management of the complications is briefly covered in Table 28-18. In addition, the nurse will be monitoring the ECG, hemodynamic parameters, and clinical condition of the client every 15 to 60 minutes to determine the effectiveness of the balloon pump.

Assessment of the CCU client

Prior to or shortly after the CCU client is admitted, a thorough history is taken and a physical examination is performed by a physician. This usually results in a tentative diagnosis. Since a thorough nursing history is usually difficult to obtain at the time of admission, an abbreviated history should be taken. The essential components of this assessment are listed in Table

Table 28-18
Nursing Management of Potential Complications of the IABP

Potential Complication	Nursing Management
Wound Infection Due to multiple lines into the cardiovascular system	Use strict aseptic technique for the insertion and dressing changes for all lines. Apply iodine ointment to all insertion sites and cover with occlusive dressings. Administer prescribed prophylactic antibiotic for entire course of therapy.
Respiratory Infection Due to immobilization	Reposition client every 2 h, being careful not to displace the balloon. Avoid causing ECG artifact during chest physical therapy.
Arterial trauma Due to insertion or displacement of the balloon	Evaluate and mark peripheral pulses prior to insertion of the balloon to use as baseline for assessing pulses after insertion. After insertion of the balloon, evaluate perfusion to both extremities every 1 h. Measure urine output every 1 h (occlusion of renal arteries causes severe decrease). Observe arterial waveforms for sudden changes. Restrain cannulated leg to prevent flexion. Do not elevate head of bed higher than 30° or flex the cannulated leg at the hip.
Thromboembolism Due to trauma, balloon obstruction of flow distal to the catheter	Administer prophylactic heparin if ordered. Evaluate pulses, urine output every 1 h. Evaluate level of consciousness every 1 h. Do not allow balloon to be deflated for more than 30 min. Manually inflate and deflate balloon if console malfunctions.
Hematological Due to platelet aggregation along the balloon (may cause decrease in platelets)	Administer prescribed Rheomacrodex (low molecular weight dextran). Monitor anticoagulation status and hematocrit.

Compiled from M. R. Kinney et al., *AACN's Clinical Reference for Critical Care Nursing*, McGraw-Hill Book Company, New York, 1981, pp. 938–943.

Table 28-19

Assessment of the CCU Client

Admission assessment
- Document symptoms and response to treatment
- Ascertain any allergies to medications or food
- Weigh client (if possible)
- Determine drugs being taken, dosage, schedule, and if any were taken on the day of admission
- Time of last meal
- Name and phone number of significant others

Ongoing assessment
- Cardiovascular system (see Chap. 25)
  - Symptoms
  - Observation of precordium
  - Palpation of precordium
  - Auscultation (S_1, S_2, S_3, S_4 heart sounds)
  - ECG monitoring
  - Peripheral pulses
  - Neck veins
- Respiratory system (see Chap. 18)
  - Respiratory pattern
  - Chest configuration and accessory muscles
  - Percussion
  - Auscultation
- Neurological/musculoskeletal (see Chaps. 49, 55)
  - Level of consciousness
  - Pupillary response
  - Range of motion
- Integumentary (see Chap. 16)
  - Intactness
  - Color
  - Temperature
  - Dryness
- Genitourinary-gastrointestinal systems (see Chaps. 31, 36)
  - Urinary difficulties/distended bladder
  - Abdominal distension

28-19. The techniques for examining each body system are described in the various chapters of this text. Assessments should be done quickly and thoroughly on admission and then at least once every 2 to 4 hours depending on the client's condition. The findings should be documented on the client's chart. This ongoing assessment is essential because subtle changes may be the first indication of developing complications, disease processes, or adverse responses to medications or other treatments. Observation and physical assessment are the CCU nurse's chief responsibilities since critically ill clients need constant monitoring and evaluation.

EARLY MANAGEMENT OF THE CLIENT WITH AN ACUTE MI

The management of acute MI was covered in detail in Chap. 27. Since clients who have had this condition spend the critical phase of their disease, usually the first 3 to 5 days, in a CCU, this chapter will focus briefly on their initial management. The typical client with an acute MI is admitted to the CCU with symptoms of substernal pain; pressure or tightness which may radiate to the arms, back, or jaws; shortness of breath; cold perspiration; nausea or vomiting; faintness, dizziness, and weakness; and feelings of impending doom.

Nurses and physicians work together closely in managing the client since both are proficient in the special skills and procedures common to a CCU. During the admission process, the aim is to deal with the client's anxiety and pain while observing and diagnosing his condition.

Chest pain, or pain associated with MI, indicates decreased coronary blood flow with ischemia and impending infarction, or the infarction may have already occurred. A vicious cycle exists whereby more pain causes more anxiety, which causes more pain, etc. This cycle must be broken. A combination of IV pain medication, usually morphine, and a confident, competent nurse answering questions honestly and explaining equipment and procedures as they are instituted will provide relief from pain and anxiety. Vital signs and the essentials of the nursing history and assessment should be obtained while the client is being admitted and made comfortable. The client must be instructed to notify the nurses if any discomfort returns. Pain relief is essential to prevent extention of the infarction.

Typical admitting orders (Fig. 28-28) contain elements of diagnosis and treatment. It may take several days to confirm a diagnosis. However, the client needs to be treated as if he has had an acute MI until proven otherwise, especially since arrhythmias are the most common complication of acute MI. V fib is especially likely to occur within the first 4 hours after the onset of pain.

The diagnosis is established with a combination of the history, the ECG, and enzyme changes. Strong indications for admitting a client to a CCU are a history of prior cardiovascular disease, the presence of cardiovascular risk factors, and pain suggestive of ischemic cardiovascular disease.

The 12-lead ECG may be normal when the client presents to an emergency room with a complaint of pain typical of ischemic chest pain, but within a few hours it may have changed to show the infarction process. These changes take place when cellular damage has occurred, interrupting the normal electrical depolarization. Fig. 28-29 correlates the anatomy with areas of infarction and with changes that occur on the ECG. Changes which are present in the leads that

CCU ADMISSION ORDERS

I. Admission

a. Continuous monitor, rhythm strips and arrhythmia analysis by nurses or monitor technicians.
b. Vital signs (TPR, BP, CVP) q 2 h for first 8 h, then q 4 h from 0600 to 2400.
c. Intake and output per shift.
d. IV of 500cc 5% Dextrose and water started with a plastic needle.
e. Diet: Soft diet for 12 h if client ill, otherwise regular diet - or - 2 Gm Na
f. Weigh daily ✓
(must be checked if wish to have done)
g. Oxygen 3 L/min per cannula or 5-8 L/min per mask.
h. Absolute bedrest with bedside commode for 48 h, Bedbath.
i. Heparin 1 unit/cc to main I.V. solution.
j. Routine lidocaine prophylaxis.

II. C.P.R.: (By certified personnel)

a. Defibrillation with 400 watt-seconds for V.F.
b. $NaHCO_3$ .5 meq/kg I.V. push; then repeat q 5 min.
c. Adrenalin 1 mg. I.V. push.
d. Type of resuscitation
DNR ______ EPS (treatment of arrhythmias and defibrillation only — no CPR to be done) ______ Dr. Heart Stat ✓ Open Chest ______
(if none of above checked, open chest massage will be performed).

III. Arrhythmias:

a. Lidocaine 75-100 mg bolus, then IV drip of 2-4 mg/min for PVC's more than 6/min, R-on-T, multifocal or sequential. (Drip=500cc 5% Dextrose in water with 2 g Lidocaine).
b. Atropine 0.4 - .6 mg IV may be given for a ventricular rate. 50 with B/P < 90 and/or symptoms of poor cerebral perfusion. Legs should be elevated before giving Atropine.

IV. Medication

a. Pain: 1. Severe M.S. 3 mg IVP every 5 min. until relief
2. Mild Acetominophen 600 mg po q 3-4 hrs
b. Sedation: Diazepam 5 mg po qid
c. Hypnotic: Dalmane 15 mg po hs MR × 1
d. Laxative: MOM 30 cc q hs prn
e. Stool softener: Colace 100 mg po bid
f. Antiemetic: ——

IV. Laboratory: (Circle desired tests by letter).

a. Cardiac Profile first morning after admission. (includes enzymes)
b. ECG: Dates 4/5, 4/6, 4/7
c. Serum K+ q.o.d. while in CCU.
d. Routine Lab: U.A., CBC, VDRL
e. Other ______

Figure 28-28 Typical standing orders.

examine infarcted areas of the heart are called *indicative* changes, i.e., they are indicative of infarction. Changes in the leads opposite infarcted areas are called *reciprocal* changes. Table 27-8 presents ECG changes due to MI.

In general, the area of infarction correlates more closely with side effects and complications than with mortality rates. In inferior damage, because the AV node is fed from the right coronary artery in 80 to 90 percent of persons, AV blocks are commonly seen. CHF, left ventricular aneurysms, cardiogenic shock, and complete heart block are more frequently seen with anterior MI because the front surface of the left ventricle and part of the septum are damaged. Acute MI occasionally occurs in the right ventricle. It presents with a picture of pain, signs of increased venous

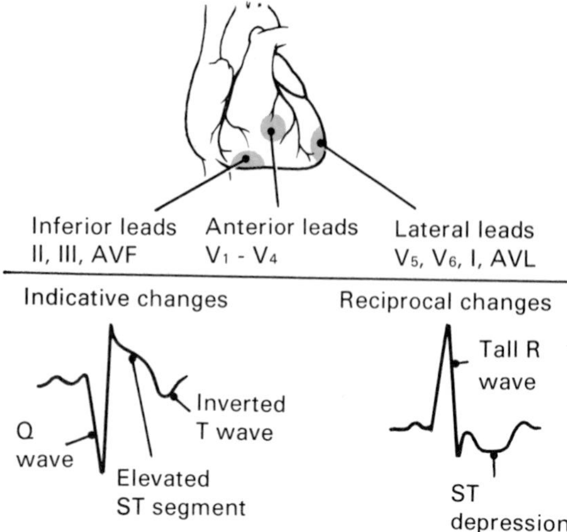

Figure 28-29 Indicative changes occur in leads that examine the area of infarction. Reciprocal changes occur in leads opposite the area of infarction.

pressure (distended neck veins, low PCWP but high CVP), and low cardiac output.

The heart muscle contains many enzymes, but three which are specifically released into the bloodstream when cells are infarcted are creatinine phosphokinase (CPK), serum glutamic-oxaloacetic transaminase (SGOT), and lactic dehydrogenase (LDH). Diagnostic levels of these enzymes and their pattern of rising and falling in the setting of an acute MI are seen in Fig. 27-11. The extent of myocardial damage correlates roughly with the degree of elevation of the enzymes (e.g., a CPK level of 1000 IU/L indicates the presence of more infarcted tissue than a level of 250 IU/L).

Sometimes one parameter points to an acute MI but another does not. Enzyme elevation may occur with or without ECG changes. A diagnosis of acute MI can be made with any two of the following three diagnostic findings: ECG changes, serum enzyme elevation, and/or pain indicative of myocardial ischemia. Myocardial scans, done by injecting IV radioactive isotopes, can help make the diagnosis of acute MI when other data are inconclusive. Following an IV injection of thallium, the amount of thallium present in each myocardial region is determined by two factors: the amount of coronary blood flow to that region and the degree of viable myocardium. Ischemia or infarcted myocardial regions receiving little or no coronary blood flow accumulate little or no IV thallium. Such regions appear as "cold spots" on the scan and thus indicate an area of ischemia or infarct.[23]

The acute nursing care of the client with an MI is described in Table 27-10. In addition to the responsibilities covered there, the nurse needs to institute measures to avoid the various hazards of immobility while encouraging rest. It is hoped that the client who is admitted with an acute MI has no complications and can be transferred out of the CCU in a few days. However, if complications are present, the nursing staff should be prepared to initiate treatment immediately. Two serious complications, pulmonary edema and cardiogenic shock, will be discussed in this chapter. Other complications are discussed in Chap. 27.

Experimental treatment of acute MI

Intracoronary Streptokinase The cause of acute transmural MI is unknown. However, the presence of intracoronary thrombus is directly associated with transmural infarction. If the MI is caused by a thrombus, then its lysis would reopen the coronary artery and restore the blood supply. The intracoronary infusion of streptokinase is a new approach to decreasing myocardial damage during the acute phase of MI.

Streptokinase is an enzyme that initiates the lysis of fibrin clots. The overall effect of streptokinase is thrombus degradation and improved microcirculation, contributing to improved oxygen delivery and the prevention of new thrombus formation.

Recently, clinical trials of intracoronary streptokinase instillation have documented clot lysis with minimal side effects. Studies have shown that instillation of streptokinase into coronary arteries within 3 to 5 hours after the onset of pain has reduced the thrombus and improved the coronary circulation.

Percutaneous Transluminal Coronary Angioplasty (PTCA) Although still in the investigative stage, PTCA is an innovative, nonoperative alternative to surgery for patients who have coronary artery occlusion. Transluminal dilatation can increase the diameter of the artery with the use of percutaneous, fluoroscopically guided catheters to relieve stenotic or occlusive lesions of the cardiovascular system. The techniques is similar to that of cardiac catheterization. A double-lumen polyvinyl balloon catheter is guided into the coronary artery where the occlusion occurs. The balloon is then inflated at the site of stenosis or occlusion, thereby directly increasing the diameter of the artery. After PTCA, regional coronary blood flow is increased and myocardial metabolism is restored.

MANAGEMENT OF THE CLIENT WITH PULMONARY EDEMA

Pulmonary edema is a term used to refer to an acute, life-threatening situation in which the lung alveoli become filled with serous or serosanguineous fluid. The most common factor in the onset of pulmonary edema is left ventricular failure due to coronary artery disease. Other etiological factors are listed in Table 20-23. Distinctive histories will aid in differentiating pulmonary edema from adult respiratory distress syndrome (Chap. 22).

Pathogenesis and Clinical Manifestations

The mechanisms of all the conditions resulting in pulmonary edema are not fully understood. This discussion will focus on the mechanism that occurs in the presence of left ventricular failure. Chap. 27 discusses the mechanisms involved in the development of CHF and the compensatory mechanisms of the heart. Pulmonary edema may occur when these compensatory mechanisms fail to effectively handle additional stress.

In most cases of left-sided heart failure, there is an increase in the pulmonary venous pressure due to decreased efficiency of the left ventricle. This results in engorgement of the pulmonary vascular system (veins, capillaries, and arteries). As a result, the lungs become less compliant (stiff), and there is increased resistance in the small airways. In addition, the lymphatic system increases its flow to help maintain a constant volume of the pulmonary extravascular fluid. This stage is associated with a mild increase in the respiratory rate and a decrease in both arterial P_aO_2 and P_aCO_2.

If pulmonary venous pressure continues to increase, the increase in intravascular pressure causes more fluid to move into the interstitial space than the lymphatics can handle. The edema is interstitial at this point. At this stage, there is more severe tachypnea, the blood gases worsen, and radiographic changes can be noted. If the pulmonary venous pressure further increases, the tight alveoli lining cells are disrupted, and fluid containing red blood cells and large molecules moves into the alveoli (*alveolar edema*) because the pulmonary hydrostatic pressure exceeds 20 mmHg (normal is 7 mmHg). As the disruption becomes worse due to further increases in the pulmonary venous pressure, the alveoli and airways are flooded with fluid (see Fig. 22-6). This is accompanied by a worsening of the blood gases (i.e., lower P_aO_2 and possible increased P_aCO_2 and progressive acidemia). The tissue hypoxia due to impaired perfusion also contributes to the worsening of the edema.

Clinical manifestations of pulmonary edema are unmistakable. The client is terrified that he is going to die. He is either sitting or standing and appears very agitated, pale, and cyanotic. His skin is clammy and cold. He has severe dyspnea, as evidenced by flaring of the nares, obvious use of accessory muscles of respiration (retractions in the intercostal spaces and supraclavicular area), and a respiratory rate of 30 to 40 per minute. He may be wheezing and coughing up frothy, blood-tinged sputum. Auscultation of the lungs may reveal bubbling rales, wheezes, and rhonchi throughout the lungs. The client's heart rate will be rapid, but his blood pressure may be elevated or at shock levels depending on the severity of the edema. In addition, the PCWP will be elevated.

Management

Diagnostic

The diagnosis of pulmonary edema is based primarily on a typical history and the clinical manifestations described above (Table 28-20). The classic diagnostic findings include:

1. Metabolic acidosis with decreased P_aO_2
2. Chest x-ray findings of alveolar edema
3. Clinical findings of tachycardia, tachypnea, rales,

Table 28-20
Medical Management: Pulmonary Edema

Diagnostic
1. History and physical examination
2. Arterial blood gases
3. Chest x-ray
4. Insert Swan-Ganz catheter and peripheral arterial line
5. Twelve-lead ECG and monitor

Therapeutic
1. Maintain in high-Fowler's position
2. O_2 by mask or nasal catheter
3. Morphine IV
4. Ethacrynic acid or furosemide IV
5. Digitalis IV
6. Nitroprusside IV
7. Aminophylline IV (if wheezing)
8. Rotating tourniquets
9. IPPB (if indicated)
10. BP, HR, RR, PCWP, urinary output at least every 1 h
11. Weigh client daily
12. Possible cardioversion

shortness of breath, orthopnea, and an S_3 heart sound

Therapeutic

Since the nurse and physician will be working closely together to care for the client with pulmonary edema because of its emergency nature, the medical and nursing management will be described together. Table 28-20 lists the major components of the therapeutic approach. Therapy is directed toward reducing anxiety, improving gaseous exchange and oxygenation, decreasing venous return, improving cardiac function, and decreasing the intravascular volume if indicated.[24] Many of the measures may be done simultaneously.

Reducing Anxiety Reduction of anxiety is facilitated by the sedative action of morphine administered intravenously. When morphine is used, the client needs to be watched closely for respiratory depression. In addition, a calm approach in providing care conveys to the client the idea that he is in good hands.

Improving Gaseous Exchange and Oxygenation Gaseous exchange may be improved by several measures. IV morphine helps to decrease oxygen demands which may be raised secondary to anxiety and the subsequent increased musculoskeletal and respiratory activity. Administration of O_2 helps increase the percentage of O_2 in inspired air (oxygen therapy is discussed in Chap. 20). Sometimes intermittent positive-pressure breathing (IPPB) is ordered because it decreases alveolar fluid, facilitates ventilation of the entire lung, increases arterial oxygen, and slows the respiratory rate. IPPB may cause a severe decrease in cardiac output due to decreased venous return. This may result in hypotension. Aminophylline may be ordered to dilate the bronchioles and stop wheezing. In addition, an arterial line is used to assess arterial pressure as well as to provide a site for withdrawal of specimens for blood gases. In severe pulmonary edema, the client may need to be intubated and placed on a mechanical ventilator.

Decreasing Venous Return Decreasing venous return may involve reducing preload, afterload, or both. Placing the client in a high Fowler's position helps to decrease venous return because of pooling of the blood in the extremities. It also helps to increase the thoracic capacity. The client should be positioned with his arms resting on pillows. IPPB also decreases venous return due to its effects on increasing intrathoracic pressures.

Medications that are used to decrease venous return affect *preload* and *afterload.* Preload is related to ventricular filling pressure, and left ventricular preload may be estimated by measuring the PCWP. The preload is directly related to the amount of fluid in pulmonary veins. Afterload is the wall tension the left ventricle must develop during systole and is primarily a function of systemic peripheral vascular resistance.[25]

Drugs which decrease preload will improve the mechanical efficiency of the heart and thus increase cardiac output. Nitrates such as nitroglycerin and isosorbide dinitrate reduce preload.

If afterload is reduced, the cardiac output from the left ventricle usually improves and there is less pulmonary congestion. Hydralazine is primarily a vasodilator and thus decreases afterload.

Drugs which decrease both preload and afterload are often the medications of choice. IV nitroprusside is usually administered in acute pulmonary edema (Table 27-15). It reduces both preload and afterload. Morphine, which is often considered the most important medication used to treat pulmonary edema, decreases both preload and afterload. It dilates both pulmonary and systemic blood vessels and thus decreases venous return. Another drug that decreases both preload and afterload is prazosin (Minipress).

Rotating tourniquets have long been used and are still occasionally used to decrease venous return. Tourniquets are placed on all four extremities, with three tightened sufficiently to prevent venous return while allowing arterial flow. The pulse distal to the tourniquets must be palpable. Every 15 minutes, working in a clockwise pattern, one tourniquet should be tightened and the next one loosened. The rotating tourniquets are discontinued by releasing one every 15 minutes. Rotating tourniquet machines are available that automatically perform the same procedures.

Improving Cardiac Function Cardiac function is enhanced by the measures already mentioned. In addition, if the client is not already on digitalis, he should be given it. The client needs to be closely monitored for arrhythmias while receiving digitalis (see Table 28-15). Cardioversion may also be used to convert serious supraventricular tachycardias or V tach in the presence of pulmonary edema. Reverting to an NSR will greatly improve cardiac function.

Decreasing Intravascular Volume Decreasing the intravascular volume will help the client who has pulmonary edema resulting from an excess of intravascular fluid, such as is found with CHF. However, in clients who have a normal vascular volume, it may precipitate serious hypotension and arrhythmias.[26] Potent diuretics, ethacrynic acid and furosemide, are the drugs of choice for decreasing the intravascular volume. They also decrease cardiac output and the cardiac work load by decreasing both preload and afterload. This is thought to help in moving fluids from the lungs, thus increasing gaseous exchange.

A second method of decreasing intravascular volume (although seldom used today) is *phlebotomy,* which involves the removal of 300 to 500 mL of whole blood. Rotating tourniquets are a form of phlebotomy and are usually tried before a phlebotomy is done.

MANAGEMENT OF THE CLIENT WITH CARDIOGENIC SHOCK

Cardiogenic shock is the shock syndrome due to primary cardiac dysfunction. It is also called *pump failure* and has replaced arrhythmias as the most frequent fatal complication of MI. It occurs in approximately 20 percent of clients with acute MI and is responsible for 70 percent of the deaths in the hospitals following acute MI. The mortality rate from cardiogenic shock following acute MI in any setting is as high as 85 to 95 percent.[27] The cause of cardiogenic shock is acute MI resulting in destruction of a large portion of the left ventricle. It is more likely to occur when there has been previous infarction or when the current infarction is so massive that at least 50 percent of the myocardium is destroyed.

Pathophysiology and Clinical Manifestations

The primary mechanism of cardiogenic shock (pump failure) is a significant reduction in the size of the contracting myocardium due to acute MI. Pump failure causes a decrease in tissue perfusion and eventually involves all body organs. Figure 28-30 illustrates the sequence of events involved.

The process is initiated by an obstruction of a major coronary artery which results in myocardial ischemia and infarction. With the infarction, there is a decrease in the amount of myocardial contraction. Thus, decreased functioning of the left ventricle occurs, as evidenced by a decreased cardiac output and blood pressure. There is then less arterial pressure to perfuse the coronary arteries. This continued decrease in coronary perfusion may increase the size of the infarction and cause arrhythmias and metabolic acidosis. These conditions further reduce the effective functioning of the left ventricle.

Hemodynamic studies done in clients with cardiogenic shock demonstrate a high LVEDP, a high PWCP, low cardiac output, a low cardiac index, severe hypotension, and no evidence of hypovolemia. The cycle continues to repeat itself until it is reversed or death occurs. This process may be enhanced by production of a *myocardial depressant factor (MDF).* A severe decrease in cardiac output is thought to stimulate production of MDF by activating splanchnic lysosomes.[28]

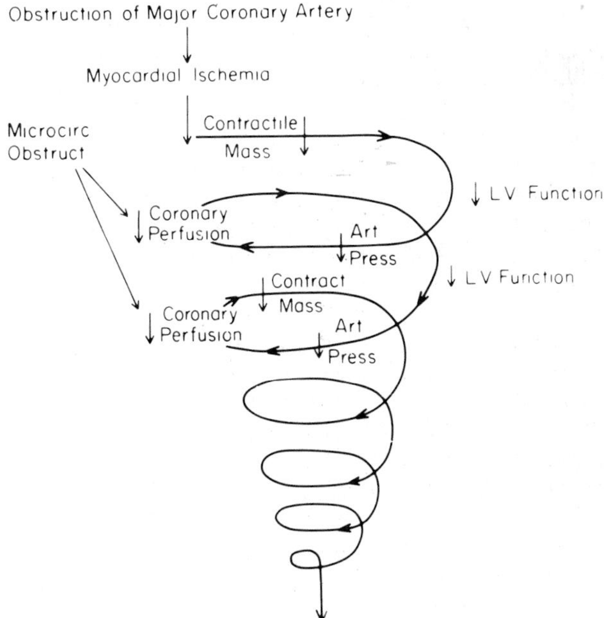

Figure 28-30 Diagram depicting the sequence of events in the vicious cycle in which coronary artery occlusion leads to cardiogenic shock and progressive circulatory deterioration. *[From K. Isselbacher et al. (eds.), Harrison's Principles of Internal Medicine, McGraw-Hill Book Company, New York, 1980, p. 1132.]*

Since some clients with acute MI experience shock but not cardiogenic shock, the following criteria have been defined as necessary for pump failure to exist.[29]

1. An arterial pressure line indicates that the systolic pressure is less than 90 mmHg and has dropped by at least 30 mmHg.
2. Cold, moist skin and cyanosis indicate insufficient peripheral circulation.
3. The sensorium is dulled.
4. The urinary output is less than 20 mL/hour for a 2-hour period.
5. Pain relief and O_2 administration do *not* relieve symptoms.

Management (Table 28-21)

Diagnostic

The client in cardiogenic shock is usually already in the CCU, although some clients are admitted in shock. Diagnostic management involves the use of various hemodynamic monitoring devices to determine the extent of pump failure and the response to treatment. These monitoring devices include arterial pressure lines, a Swan-Ganz catheter, and ECG monitoring.

Therapeutic

The goal of therapy is to interrupt the vicious cycle of pump failure, i.e., to increase coronary circulation, decrease the coronary work load, and increase systemic blood pressure. Since cardiogenic shock results from massive myocardial damage, the prognosis is poor even with aggressive therapy.

The major drugs currently being used are dopamine and dobutamine (see Table 28-15). They have been chosen because of their ability to increase the force of myocardial contraction without increasing the heart rate and the arterial blood pressure. Nitroprusside is also combined with either dopamine or dobutamine for its vasodilating effect and the reduction in afterload to help improve cardiac output.

In recent years, the IABP has been used to improve the hemodynamic status of clients with cardiogenic shock. The nursing management and effects of the IABP were described earlier. Essentially, it is a mechanical device used to assist the left ventricle. If the IABP is instituted early in the occurrence of cardiogenic shock, the prognosis is somewhat improved. However, the overall 1- to 2-year survival rates are poor due to the severity of myocardial disease. Some clients do respond well and live long enough to have revascularization surgery.[30] (Cardiac surgery is discussed in the next section.)

The nursing management of cardiogenic shock begins with the recognition of its onset through observation of vital signs, urinary output, skin condition, level of consciousness, and lung and heart sounds. The circulation is supported as much as possible with medications. These clients are monitored closely and often have arterial and Swan-Ganz monitoring devices. The client will often be in respiratory distress and may need to be intubated and placed on a mechanical ventilator. (The nursing care of clients on ventilators is discussed in Chap. 22.) The care of the client in shock is supportive, including assessment and monitoring of the cardiovascular, respiratory, urinary, neurological, and integumentary systems. Drugs are regulated carefully and titrated to obtain the desired effect.

Table 28-21
Medical Management: Cardiogenic Shock

Diagnostic
1. Place an arterial pressure line in a peripheral artery and take frequent readings (at least every 15 min)
2. Place a Swan-Ganz catheter in a pulmonary artery and take hourly readings of the PCWP or PAW
3. Place client on continuous ECG monitoring
4. Determine cardiac output using thermodilution
5. Measure urine output every 1 h

Therapeutic
1. Administer high concentrations of O_2
2. If client is hypovolemic, administer IV fluids to raise left ventricular filling pressure to 18–20 mmHg
3. Administer dopamine or dobutamine IV (titrating to systolic BP of 90 mmHg)
4. Place on IABP

EARLY MANAGEMENT OF THE CLIENT REQUIRING CARDIAC SURGERY

CCUs are often used as the immediate recovery or post-recovery room site for clients undergoing cardiac surgery. Close monitoring and management of these clients require the specialized skills and knowledge of the CCU nurse. Because clients requiring cardiac surgery need similar types of preoperative and postoperative care, their general management will be described.

Common Cardiac Surgeries in the Adult

Myocardial revascularization

Myocardial revascularization or *coronary artery bypass grafting* is the main surgical treatment for coronary artery disease (Fig. 28-31). It involves a saphenous vein aortocoronary bypass. The saphe-

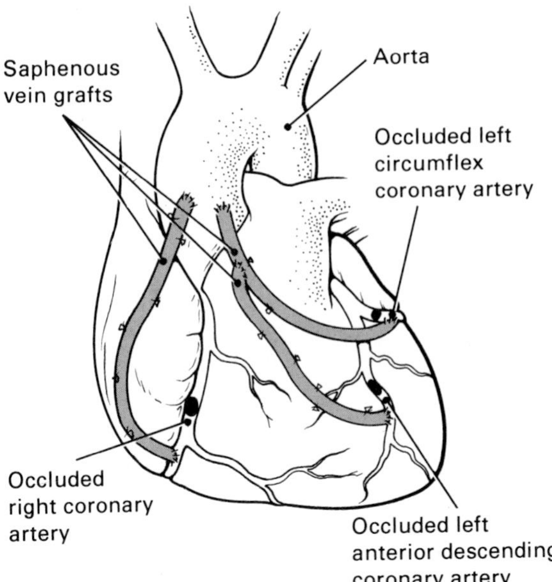

Figure 28-31 Saphenous aortocoronary artery bypass or revascularization involves taking a piece of saphenous vein from the leg and creating a conduit for blood from the aorta to the area below the blockage in the coronary artery. A triple bypass is illustrated. (*Mayo Clinic.*)

nous vein from one of the client's legs is removed and reversed (so that the valves will not obstruct the blood flow). Segments are then sutured in place so that blood may flow from the aorta distal to the obstructed coronary artery. The coronary artery is considered obstructed if its diameter is narrowed by more than 75 to 80 percent. Revascularization surgery has a mortality rate of about 1 to 2 percent, with a 90 percent rate of functional improvement (60 percent of clients have their anginal pain completely eliminated). Some studies have shown improvement in the 5- and 10-year survival rates of clients who have had revascularization surgery as compared with those who were medically treated.[31] Revascularization may be done in conjunction with other cardiac surgeries, such as valve replacement.

Nursing care for these clients involves caring for two surgical sites: the chest and the leg. The care of the leg wound is similar to the postoperative care following the stripping of varicose veins (Chap. 30). The management of the chest wound, which involves a thoracotomy, is similar to that of other chest surgeries. (The nursing management of the client with a thoracotomy is presented in Table 20-19.)

Valvular surgeries

Almost all cardiac valvular surgeries require cardiopulmonary bypass. A closed mitral commissurotomy is the only possible exception. It involves incising the fused leaflets of the mitral valves if there is no significant calcification of the valve (Fig. 28-8). Chap. 29 describes the causes and the medical and surgical management of various valvular diseases.

Both mitral valve disease and aortic valve disease may require valvular replacement when medical management is no longer effective in the presence of increasing heart failure. Many valvular replacements now are heterografts (from a species other than man) from either a pig or a cow. Caged-ball prostheses, used more frequently in the past, are less satisfactory than heterografts because of (1) the high incidence of clotting and thrombosis associated with them and (2) the clicking noise made by the valve as it opens and closes with the changes in pressure and blood flow. (Figure 28-32 shows the replacement of the mitral valve with a ball-in-cage prosthesis.) Disk prostheses are also used as heart valves (Fig. 29-9).

Valvular surgery has a mortality rate of 5 to 10 percent depending on the condition of the client prior to surgery. Four years after surgery, about 55 percent of clients are still in better condition than they were prior to surgery.[32]

Ventricular septal defects

Ventricular septal rupture occasionally occurs as a complication of MI. To repair the damage, the left ventricle is opened in the area of the scar from the MI. If the defect is small, it is closed with heavy sutures. Larger holes are patched with synthetic cloth.

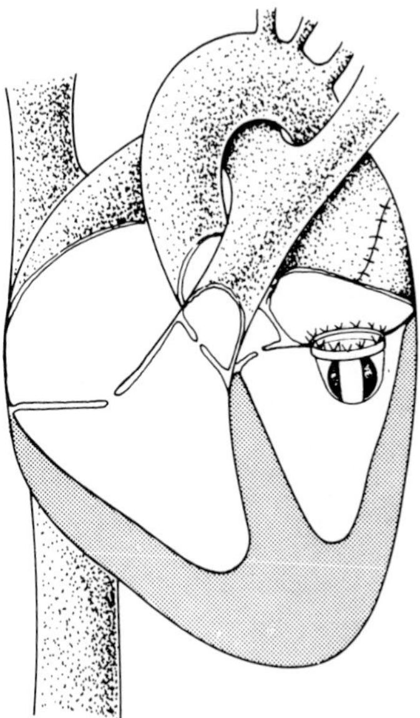

Figure 28-32 Complete replacement of the mitral valve with a ball-in-cage prosthesis. *(From H. Moidell et al., Nursing Care of the Patient with Medical-Surgical Disorders, 2d ed., McGraw-Hill Book Company, New York, 1976, p. 561.)*

Ventricular aneurysmectomy

Ventricular aneurysms located on the anterolateral or apical part of the left ventricle may also be excised. These are large, noncontracting areas which interfere significantly with adequate cardiac contraction. The ventricle is opened and allowed to collapse so that the thinned scar tissue is cut away and any thrombotic material removed before the ventricle is closed (Fig. 27-10).

Cardiac transplantation

The replacement of the heart in the clinical setting of far-advanced cardiac disease is still in the research stage following the first heart transplant in 1967.[33] Efforts have been made to develop mechanical hearts, as well as to refine the transplantation procedure. However, the procedure is considered a last resort because of its complications, the high risk, and the complexity of care.

There are two surgical approaches to cardiac transplantation. The *orthotopic procedure* involves removing the recipient's heart, except for the posterior right and left atrial walls and their venous connections. The recipient's heart is then replaced with the donor's heart, which has been trimmed to match. The *parallel procedure* (also called "piggyback") involves suturing the donor's heart and major blood vessels to the recipient's heart and major blood vessels (Fig. 28-33). The parallel procedure has some advantage over the orthotopic procedure in the presence of pulmonary hypertension and rejection of the donor heart.[34] There are reports of the recipient's own heart recovering after a parallel heart has allowed it to rest.[35]

Nursing care involves a great deal of emotional support and teaching of both the client and his family because transplantation is a last resort. The postoperative care is similar to that of other open heart surgeries. In addition, the amplitude and electrical activity of the ECG are monitored very closely to evaluate the function of the donor heart. The client is also started on immunosuppressive therapy. The nursing management of an immunosuppressed client is the same as that of the client who receives a kidney transplant (Chap. 38). Rejection may be noted by a decrease in myocardial electrical activity and by WBC changes in studies.

Preoperative Management

The preoperative period may vary from a few hours to a month or more depending on the client's physical condition. Some conditions, such as a stab wound to the heart, require immediate surgical intervention. With other conditions, such as heart failure associated with mitral stenosis or regurgitation, the client must be stabilized and prepared for surgery. It is desirable that the client's cardiac and physical condition be stabilized prior to surgery. For example, arrhythmias should be controlled, CHF treated, and anginal pain relieved. In addition, surgery should be postponed for 6 weeks after an acute MI. Table 28-22 lists the most common forms of heart disease that may require cardiac surgery.

Medical management

Extensive diagnostic studies are done before the vast majority of clients undergo cardiac surgery. Most clients will have a cardiac catheterization to measure changes in pressure and blood gases in cardiac chambers and across valves. This is done to look for structural abnormalities or to confirm the diagnosis and to assess the left ventricular function. Coronary arteriography is also done to observe the coronary perfusion of the myocardium. Other diagnostic studies include echocardiograms, phonocardiograms, and stress testing.

In addition, baseline data will be obtained just prior to surgery. These include a chest x-ray, ECG, bleeding studies (clotting time, prothrombin time, fibrinogen, and platelets), complete blood count, urinalysis, serum electrolytes, blood urea nitrogen, creatinine level, and cardiac enzymes. Pulmonary function studies may be done on clients with pulmonary disease or a history of smoking. The client will also have his blood typed and cross-matched.

Other baseline data obtained shortly before surgery include an accurate body weight to aid in fluid management and vital signs, including temperature, because an elevated temperature is an indication for postponement of surgery.

To improve their respiratory status, clients who smoke must stop smoking at least 1 week, and preferably a month or more, prior to surgery. This will help decrease the amount of bronchial secretions and thus reduce the postoperative risk of atelectasis and pneumonia. However, it may be difficult for many clients to stop smoking because of their anxiety over the surgery.

It may be necessary to modify the client's medications to prevent adverse reactions. Digoxin will be discontinued 24 to 36 hours prior to surgery. Digitoxin will be discontinued 3 to 7 days prior to surgery. This is usually done because digitalis toxicity is common in the early postoperative period. (The main exception is atrial fibrillation with a rapid ventricular response.)

If the client can tolerate it (i.e., have no anginal pain), propranolol (Inderal) may be tapered 24 hours to 2 weeks prior to surgery because of its negative

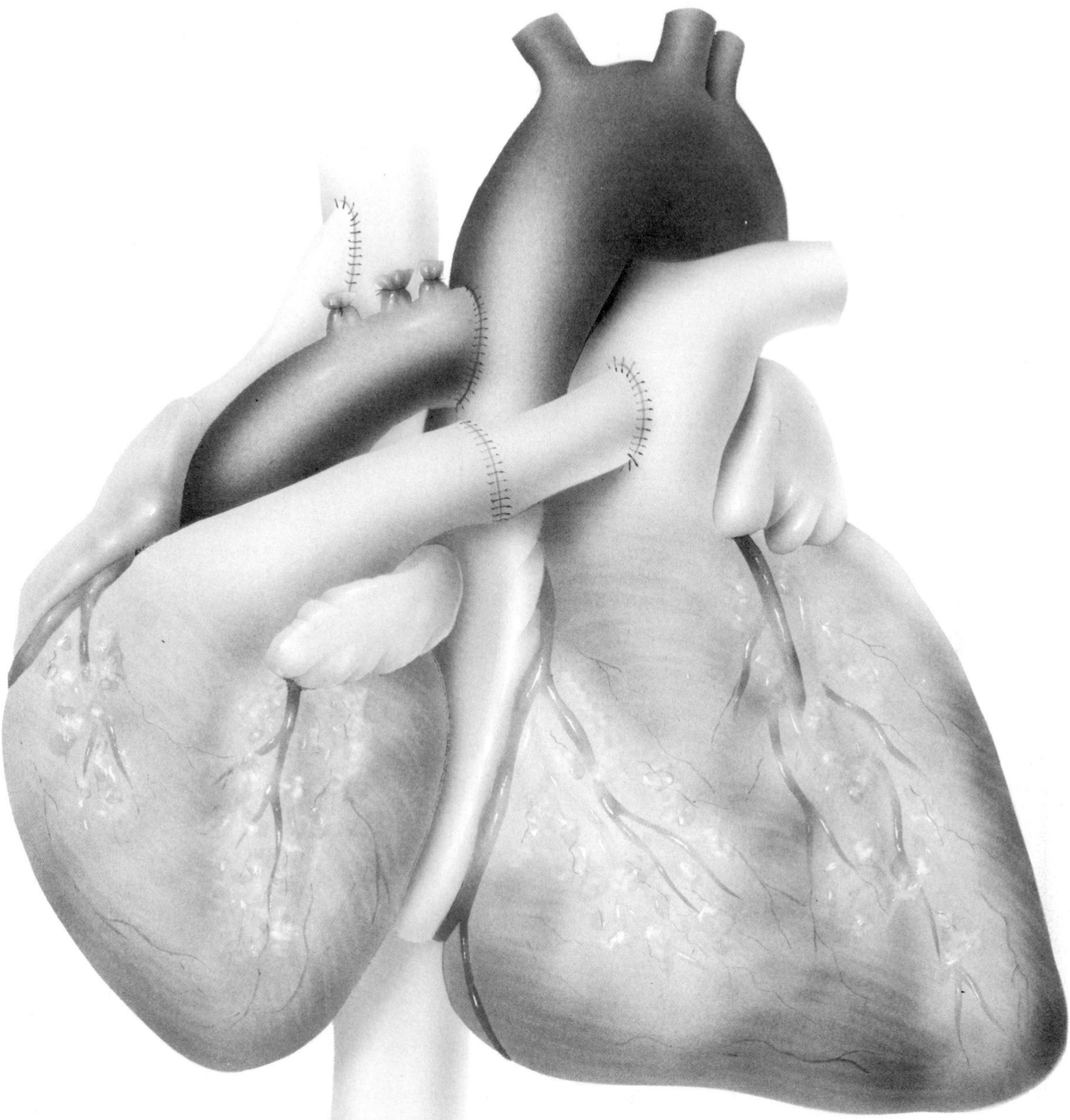

Figure 28-33 Cardiac transplant using the parallel procedure. *[From J. Lamb, "Cardiac Transplantation," Am J Nurs,* ***80:****1787 (1980).]*

chronotropic and inotropic effects. However, clients who require propranolol may be given dopamine, epinephrine, isoproterenol, or glucagon in the early postoperative period to counteract the effects of propranolol.

If the client's heart failure is compensated for, diuretics may be discontinued 24 to 48 hours prior to surgery. This will help reduce potassium loss and hypovolemia. Clients on long-acting insulins will be switched to regular insulin on a sliding-scale basis the day prior to surgery. They will remain on the sliding scale into the postoperative period. Other drugs that may need modification include corticosteroids, anticoagulants, antihypertensives, and phenothiazines. The

Table 28-22
Possible Indications for Cardiac Surgery

Aneurysm of sinus of Valsalva
Aortic stenosis and regurgitation
Atherosclerotic coronary artery disease
Constrictive pericarditis
Dissecting aortic aneurysm
Heart block
Mitral stenosis and regurgitation
Myocardial trauma or rupture
Tricuspid insufficiency or stenosis
Ventricular aneurysm
Ventricular septal defect

Adapted from "Report of the Inter-Society Commission for Heart Disease Sources: Optimal Resources for Cardiac Surgery, Guidelines for Program Planning and Evaluation," *Circulation,* **52**:A-23–A-37 (1975).

nurse should check with the physician about changes in any drug about which there is a question.

To prevent incisional infections, the client will be instructed to shower several times with a basteriostatic soap, such as betadine or hexachlorophene. In addition, the client is usually started on parenteral antibiotics within 12 hours of surgery. The physician also discusses at length with the client and significant others the nature of the surgery, including the procedures, expected outcomes, possible complications, and postsurgical care.

Nursing management

Nursing management complements the various aspects of medical management just described. Extensive preoperative teaching is a major responsibility of the nurse. It deals with general postoperative concerns (see Chaps. 6 and 8) in addition to the specialized concerns related to cardiovascular surgery. A high level of anxiety is common because of the client's perception of the central role of the heart in maintaining life. The purpose of the teaching is to help reduce anxiety. The teaching may be more helpful to the client if the sensations he may experience are described in addition to the procedures he will undergo. Table 28-23 outlines the topics that should be included. The client should be encouraged to ask questions and discuss his concerns. It is essential that the nurse report significant concerns to the physician so that a coordinated approach can be developed to deal with the client's anxiety.

The family should also be involved in the preoperative teaching. This will help to alleviate their anxiety so that they can support the client more effectively during this period. It is important that the family know about the various tubes, lines, monitoring devices,

Table 28-23
Preoperative Teaching List for Cardiovascular Surgery

Operating room	Trip to operating room to see area and meet staff Have family see waiting room Tell client that he may remember conversations and events from the operating room experience
Tour of CCU	If desired, to see area and meet staff
Early postoperative period in CCU	Client may lose track of time and place Client may have hallucinations (visual, auditory, taste) Tubes—discuss location, purpose, and when removed Endotracheal: client cannot talk; devise method of calling a nurse Nasogastric: ice chips provided; client may eat when tube is removed Arterial lines: used for pressure measurements Venous lines: used for fluid or medication administration Chest tubes: red drainage, pulling sensation removed Retention catheter: for input and output, easy voiding Client may feel thirsty
Postoperative routine	Mechanical ventilation Suctioning Coughing and turning Frequent monitoring of vital signs Continuous cardiac monitoring
Pain medications	Client will ask for pain medication to be comfortable for coughing and moving Client will be achy and sore all over for first week postoperatively
IPPB (if used)	Demonstration and return demonstration
Post-CCU routines	Overview of discharge regimens
Emotional reaction	Depression is common

and postoperative routines in order to be aware that these are normal procedures and not an indication of trouble. The family may also be able to help provide comfort and to identify idiosyncracies of the client, such as routines, habits, and foods.

Intraoperative Management

Many cardiovascular surgeries are being performed with the client on a heart-lung machine or a cardiopulmonary bypass. This allows the surgeon to work on the heart, which has been put into asystole or a slowly contracting state. The heart-lung machine serves as a pump to circulate and oxygenate blood. The machine receives blood from catheters in the vena cavae or right atrium, oxygenates it, and returns the blood to the client through a catheter in the aorta. This is usually done in conjunction with hypothermia (about 25° to 28°C for bypass and valvular surgeries).[36] The time on the heart-lung machine is closely monitored and kept to a minimum because the longer the client is on it, the more complications he is likely to have. In addition, careful anesthesia and precise monitoring of the heart rhythm, vital signs, blood gases, electrolytes, and coagulation status are components of the procedure. Often, clients are placed on the IABP, and an LAP line and a left ventricular pacing wire are inserted during the surgery.

Postoperative Management

Complications which may occur as a result of cardiac surgery are outlined in Table 28-24. Much of the postoperative management is directed toward the prevention or early detection of these complications. Postoperative assessment is outlined in Table 28-25. The physician and nurses work very closely during this time, with much overlapping of functions, depending on the policies of the institution.

Table 28-24
Possible Complications of Cardiac Surgery

Early postoperative period
- Low cardiac output syndrome due to hypovolemia, acidosis, acute MI, CHF, drugs such as propranolol, mediastinal tamponade, pulmonary embolism, or incomplete or faulty surgical repair
- Acute MI, especially with aortocoronary bypass surgery
- Cardiac arrhythmias
- Hemorrhage
- Pulmonary embolism, especially with saphenous vein aortocoronary bypass
- Low-grade fever
- Depression
- Less common complications
  - Wound infection
  - Electrolyte disturbances
  - Systemic arterial hypertension
  - Cerebral infarcts due to air or thrombus emboli
  - Confusion, agitation, and disorientation
  - Disseminated intravascular coagulation
  - Adult respiratory distress syndrome
  - Renal failure

Late postoperative period
- Hepatitis
- Postpericardiotomy syndrome
- With valvular surgeries
  - Systemic arterial emboli
  - Infective endocarditis

Table 28-25
Postoperative Assessment

- Nervous system
  - Pupil size and reaction
  - Orientation/level of consciousness
  - Motor functioning
- Respiratory system
  - Placement of endotracheal tube
  - Settings on mechanical ventilator
  - Character of respirations
  - Breath sounds and secretions
  - Arterial blood gases
- Cardiovascular and hematological systems
  - Cardiac rhythm
  - Peripheral pulses
  - Blood pressure
  - Venous or pulmonary artery pressures
  - Temperature
  - Fluid status
  - Chest tubes
  - Coagulation status
  - Cardiac output
- Renal system
  - Urinary output
  - Urine character, color, specific gravity
  - Electrolytes
- Gastrointestinal system
  - Nasogastric secretions
  - Bowel sounds
- Integumentary system
  - Skin breakdown
  - Incisional healing and drainage
- Pain
  - Quality or intensity
  - Location

Upon completion of cardiac surgery, the client is transferred immediately to the CCU. (Some hospitals have separate heart recovery rooms because the CCU and the operating room are not close together.) The CCU staff should have been notified of the client's estimated time of arrival and his status so that all the equipment is ready to provide care.

When the client arrives, he should already be lying on his postoperative bed. He should be transferred directly from the surgical table to the postoperative bed to save time and energy. Usually, a team of two nurses admits the client on arrival to the CCU. This is a crucial time for the client since complications may occur early and during transport. When he arrives, the nurse team will connect the monitoring devices (e.g., ECG, arterial lines) and suction equipment (e.g., chest tubes, nasogastric tubes) so that his hemodynamic parameters can be assessed immediately. The endotracheal tube is checked and the client is attached immediately to a mechanical ventilation preset for the client. As soon as the equipment is properly connected and calibrated, the CCU nurse should immediately assess the client's neurological, respiratory, and cardiac status to determine the level of anesthesia, the ventilation, and the perfusion status. Reports from the anesthesiologist and surgeon are often given during this initial assessment period. Baseline laboratory data are collected, including arterial blood gases, serum electrolytes, complete blood count, and cardiac enzymes.[37]

The CCU nurse also collects baseline data on the cardiovascular status by checking the arterial blood pressure, PAP, PCWP, LAP, (if a line was inserted during surgery), heart sounds, cardiac rhythm, and peripheral pulses. The client's monitoring devices (e.g., Swan-Ganz catheter, left atrial line) are dependent upon the client's preoperative condition, the intraoperative procedures and findings, the surgeon's preference, and the unit's protocol. Many clients return from surgery intubated with only a CVP line, while others may require a Swan-Ganz catheter, an LAP line, and a pacing wire and may be on the IAPB. These variations are of primary importance in preparing for the client and in planning for his care.

Once the initial assessment is made, the client is placed on frequent vital signs (e.g., blood pressure and heart rate initially every 15 minutes for the first 4 hours, then every 30 minutes for 4 hours, and later every hour). Other indicators may be measured at least every hour, such as urinary output, PCWP or PAP, temperature, breath sounds, and respiratory parameters. In addition, the wave patterns for the arterial pressure, Swan-Ganz catheter, LAP, and ECG will be constantly monitored for significant changes. Peripheral pulses also need to be checked every 1 to 2 hours.

Care of the client's chest tubes is indicated by the surgeon's preference and the unit's protocol. Chest tubes must be kept patent so that blood from the mediastinum and pericardium may drain adequately. Plugging or clotting in the chest tube may obstruct the drainage and severely compromise the client. Chest tube drainage (amount and character) is also assessed and recorded frequently (every 15 minutes for the first few hours postoperatively).

The client will also need care to prevent problems associated with immobility. This includes turning from side to side. The head of the bed may be elevated 30° when his vital signs are stable. He may have antiembolic stockings in place. While on the ventilator, the client will need to be suctioned (Chap. 22). When the endotracheal tube is removed, he will need to cough and deep-breathe. Clients can also sit in a chair, usually by the end of the first day postoperatively. Progressive ambulation is then encouraged.

Most tubes and lines are removed within 3 days of surgery. Because rest periods are important, care must be planned to allow for uninterrupted sleep, especially during the early period of intensive care.[38] Pain medications are very important because they allow the client to be active and to participate in coughing and deep-breathing exercises. The client and his family need many explanations and much support. They should be allowed to spend as much time together as the client's condition allows.

After a short period in the CCU, the client is moved to a step-down area if further ECG monitoring or care is necessary, or sometimes to a general surgical unit if his condition is stable. After transfer, the client gradually increases his activity levels and restabilizes his nutritional pattern. Medication regimens are adjusted. He is prepared for discharge, and referrals are made to appropriate community resources. Home regimens and medications are discussed, and the client should be given written instructions. Wound care, diet, and activity levels should be discussed in specific terms with the client and his family. Evaluation should be made of their level of knowledge and of the need for further teaching before discharge.

Postoperative Complications

The possible complications resulting from cardiac surgery are discussed below and are summarized in Table 28-24.

Hypovolemia The most common complication in the early postoperative period is low cardiac output syndrome, usually due to hypovolemia. It is evidenced by hypotension, oliguria, and cutaneous vasoconstriction. If it is due to hypovolemia, the CVP, LAP, and PCWP will be low.

The treatment for hypovolemia is blood replacement in the form of packed red blood cells (see Chap. 26). Blood is often transfused according to the measured loss in the chest tube drainage to prevent hypovolemia. If the client cannot be stabilized with transfusions, he may need to be returned to surgery for hemostasis. Careful recording of all intake and output (IVs, IV flush fluids, chest drainage, gastrointestinal drainage, blood, urine, medications) is essential to monitor fluid balance.

Cardiac Tamponade Mediastinal or cardiac tamponade may be a cause of low output syndrome. Cardiac tamponade is pressure on the heart caused by the accumulation of fluid, such as blood, in the pericardium. Clinical manifestations include a decrease in chest tube drainage, decrease in the precordial pulsation, quiet heart sounds, and increased size of the heart on percussion. A chest x-ray shows an enlarged heart and a widened mediastinum. The ECG may show a decrease in the amplitude of the waves. The PCWP, LAP, and CVP are increased. *Pulsus paradoxus*—the abnormal (more than 8 mmHg) fall in systolic blood pressure on inspiration—may be present. It may be determined by taking blood pressure with a cuff. As the cuff is deflated, it is stopped at the first Korotkoff sound while the client is breathing normally. If the Korotkoff sound is heard during both inspiration and expiration, then no pulsus paradoxus exists. However, if the sound is heard only on expiration, then the cuff is deflated slowly until the first Korotkoff sound is heard on both inspiration and expiration. If the difference in pressure between inspiration and expiration is greater than 8 mmHg, then the client has pulsus paradoxus.

Since the post-heart surgery client already has a mediastinal tube in place, the treatment for cardiac tamponade is one of the following:

1. Disconnect other chest tubes and clean out the mediastinal tube and the fogarty catheter.
2. Remove the tube and break up the clot by inserting a gloved finger into the stoma.
3. Return the client to the operating room, where bleeding can be further assessed or treated.

The other treatment for cardiac tamponade in clients who do not have mediastinal tubes in place is *pericardiocentesis*. This procedure involves the insertion of a needle into the pericardium to remove fluid (Fig. 29-3).

Arrhythmias Arrhythmias are common postoperatively. Frequent PVCs and V tach are managed as described in the section on Common Life-Threatening Arrhythmias. Atrial arrhythmias are common with mitral and aortic valve replacements. Atrial flutter or fibrillation may occur about 36 hours after aortocoronary bypass or about 6 or 7 days postoperatively with pulmonary embolism. These are treated as described in the section on Common Non-Life-Threatening Arrhythmias.

Emboli Pulmonary embolism occurs most often after the third postoperative day. It is common in clients with saphenous aortocoronary bypass surgery. Because the clinical manifestations of pulmonary emboli are not always overt, the nurse should report to the physician any client who has transient weakness,. dyspnea, or faintness. Lung scans are often diagnostic. Anticoagulation is the usual method of treatment. The prevention and treatment of pulmonary emboli are discussed in Chap. 30.

Arterial embolism may occur following aortic or mitral valve surgery. These clients are frequently placed on long-term anticoagulant therapy. The client needs to be observed for evidence of a cerebral embolism, such as a sudden change in the level of consciousness, slurring of speech, or one-sided weakness.

Fever Fever is a very common complication of cardiac surgery and may be the result of pericarditis, which commonly occurs. An elevated temperature increases the work load of the heart because it increases metabolism. The nurse will be involved in preventing potential problems that cause fever as well as assisting in collecting information to assess the cause. The client's body temperature is taken at least every four hours. Causes of a fever may be atelectasis, urinary tract infection, pneumonia, thrombophlebitis, drug reaction, transfusion reaction, and wound infection. Treatment is directed toward curing the infection and reducing the fever.

Another possible cause of fever is endocarditis. However, it rarely occurs in the first weeks postoperatively, probably because of the widespread use of prophylactic antibiotics. However, it can occur with valvular replacements. (Endocarditis is discussed in Chap. 29.)

Intraoperative MI

Of primary importance in all cardiovascular surgery, especially in bypass grafts, is the preservation of myocardial tissue. The incidence of intraoperative and perioperative MI may be as high as 25 percent. Several methods of preserving myocardial tissue during surgery have been developed, primarily cold cardioplegia. Immediately after the aorta is cross-clamped, a cold solution high in potassium is infused around the heart and into the aortic root. This process is repeated whenever the myocardial temperature rises to approximately 19°C. This technique lowers the myocardial oxygen consumption and the metabolic rate to prevent ischemia.

During the immediate postoperative period, serial ECGs are taken and cardiac enzymes are assessed to detect intraoperative infarction. If an infarct has occurred, the prognosis is worsened.

CARE OF THE CLIENT WITH A PACEMAKER

A pacemaker consists of a power source and a catheter electrode inserted into the right ventricle. It is

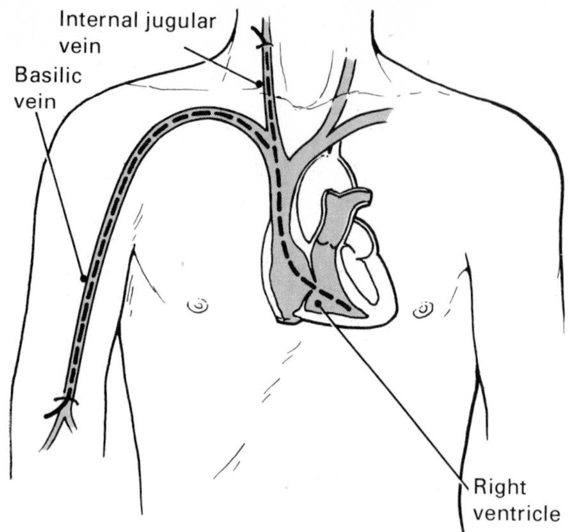

Figure 28-34 Temporary pacemaker catheter insertion.

designed to provide electrical stimulation to the heart when its intrinsic conduction system fails to stimulate a contraction within a specific time period. External temporary pacemakers are inserted in CCUs in emergency situations. A pacing wire is threaded through a convenient vein and attached to the external power source (Fig. 28-34). This may need to be done when a symptomatic heart block or bradycardia develops after an acute MI.

Internal pacemakers with tiny power sources are placed subcutaneously in the chest or abdomen and are attached to pacing catheters placed with the aid of fluoroscopy. They are inserted for a variety of reasons (Table 28-26). Most pacemakers used today are called *demand* pacemakers because they sense the need to stimulate a contraction according to the preset desired rate (Fig. 28-36). Thus, there is less chance of a cardiac stimulus falling on the T wave and stimulating ventricular fibrillation.

Determining the need for a pacemaker, inserting it, and monitoring the pacemaker's performance are the physician's responsibility. Sometimes drug trials and sophisticated electrophysiological studies are performed before permanent pacemakers are inserted. After placement, pacemaking systems may fail to *sense* (the pacemaker does not recognize the client's own heartbeats and continues to send out electrical

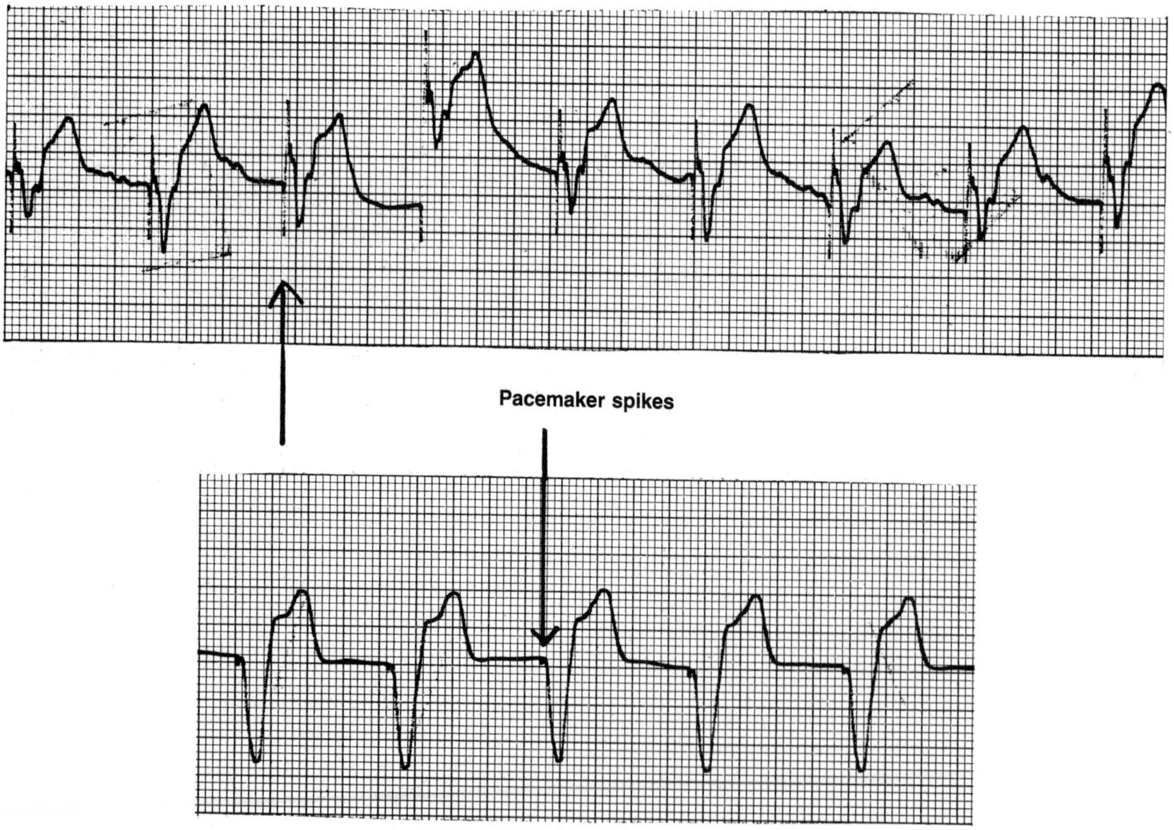

Pacemaker spikes

Figure 28-35 Paced rhythms. Note the pacemaker spike just prior to the ventricular contraction. The QRS complex is also wider than normal because the contraction is initiated in the ventricle.

Table 28-26
Indications for Pacemakers

Temporary (for transient-reversible situations)
- Prophylactic
  - Before general anesthesia
  - After open heart surgery
- Anterior MI with heart block
- Bradycardia with low cardiac output
- Electrophysiological studies
- Control of drug-resistant tachyarrhythmias
- Conversion of arrhythmias

Permanent
- Heart block with low cardiac output, heart failure, or syncope
- Symptomatic sinus bradycardia
- Tachyarrhythmias
- Adverse effects of drugs that the client requires

impulses) or to *capture* (the electrical impulse from the battery does not cause a contraction), and the physician may have to reposition the catheter or replace parts of the pacemaking system.

The client with a permanent pacemaker is followed closely at first. He is usually seen in the office every few weeks to months, and then less often until the predicted life of his battery is near its end. Transtelephone transmitters are often given to clients so that they can periodically send rhythm strips to check pacer function. The ECG in Fig. 28-35 shows a typical pacemaker spike.

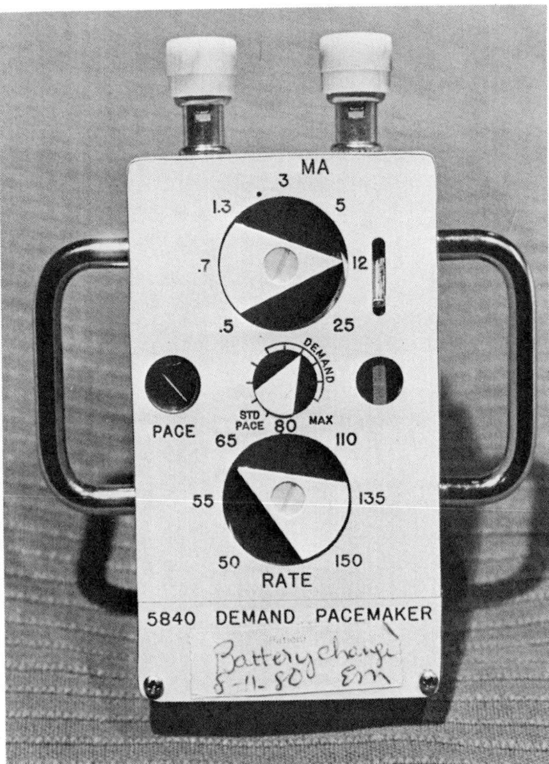

Figure 28-36 Temporary external demand pacemaker.

Complications of pacemaker insertion include infection, failure to capture or sense, perforation of the ventricle, and depletion of the power source before the end of the predicted life span (in permanent pacemakers). Infection may be seen at the site of entrance of the temporary catheter or around the pouch created in the subcutaneous tissue for the permanent battery. Redness, heat, swelling, and a fluid collection will be seen. The infection is treated by using appropriate antibiotics and moving the site. Failure to capture or sense may be helped by (1) adjustment of the client's position to reestablish contact between the catheter and the ventricular muscle or (2) increasing the voltage and sensitivity of the temporary pacemaker. Perforation will be evidenced by a change in the paced QRS shape and possibly by loss of capture.

As batteries of permanent pacers become depleted, the rates usually drop slowly and predictably. If the pacemaker is of the demand mode, a magnet placed over the battery will convert the pacemaker to a fixed-rate mode so that the battery's integrity may be checked. Signs of decreased cardiac output will be seen if the batteries fail abruptly or the catheter breaks.

Besides observing for complications of pacemaker therapy in acute and chronic settings, the nurse must provide client education. Clients and their families need to know why a pacemaker is required, where it is located, how it works, and how they can help to manage the pacemaker. Teaching for clients with permanent pacemakers is outlined in Table 28-27.

Table 28-27
Teaching List for Clients with Permanent Pacemakers

1. Importance of follow-up care.
2. Medications: mechanism of action and side effects.
3. Clinical manifestations of infection.
4. Avoid direct blows to site. Otherwise, activity as tolerated.
5. Good nutrition and special diet if prescribed.
6. Send rhythm strips if appropriate.
7. Avoid high-output electrical generators.
8. Other considerations
   a. Microwave ovens: most pacemakers are well shielded, and microwave will *not* harm them.
   b. Taking pulse: With close follow-up, this is usually not necessary.

REVIEW QUESTIONS

The number of the question corresponds to the same numbered objective at the beginning of the chapter.

1. The most important element for a CCU is
   a. a well-educated, highly motivated nursing staff around the clock
   b. computerized wall banks for collection of vital signs
   c. equipment such as the IABP and Swan-Ganz catheters
   d. rooms with windows, television sets, and bedside commodes

2. Indications for immediate treatment and reporting of PVCs include all the following *except*
   a. a PVC with the R on T phenomenon in 1 minute
   b. multifocal PVCs in 1 minute
   c. two or three nonconsecutive PVCs in 1 minute
   d. paired PVCs in 1 minute

3. Which of the following drugs may cause atrial flutter (due to toxicity) but may also be used to treat atrial flutter?
   a. lidocaine
   b. dopamine
   c. propranolol
   d. digitalis

4. When doing BCLS, which of the following steps must be done *first*?
   a. Ventilate with four quick breaths.
   b. Apply downward pressure on the sternum.
   c. Establish a patent airway.
   d. Check for pupil dilatation.

5. Major risks associated with hemodynamic monitoring include all of the following *except*
   a. hemorrhage
   b. thrombosis with emboli
   c. infection
   d. hepatitis

6. The purpose of an IABP is to mechanically assist left ventricular function by
   a. reducing afterload and increasing diastolic pressure
   b. increasing afterload and augmenting systolic pressure
   c. increasing preload and decreasing diastolic pressure
   d. reducing preload and decreasing systolic pressure

7. Which of the following diagnostic studies are used to diagnose an acute MI?
   a. white blood count, body temperature
   b. cardiac enzymes, myocardial scan
   c. computed tomography scan, cardiac enzymes
   d. ECG, computed tomography scan

8. When managing a client with acute pulmonary edema, which medication will serve to reduce anxiety as well as to improve oxygenation?
   a. morphine sulfate
   b. aminophylline
   c. nitroprusside
   d. furosemide

9. Cardiogenic shock may be managed by all of the following measures *except*
   a. dopamine or dobutamine
   b. mechanical ventilation
   c. IABP
   d. rotating tourniquets

10. Preoperative teaching for the prospective cardiac surgical client should include all of the following *except*
   a. routines in the CCU in which he will be placed
   b. steps of myocardial cellular metabolism
   c. probability of experiencing hallucinations and of depression postoperatively
   d. sensations he may experience postoperatively

11. An emergency indication for a pacemaker is
   a. sinus bradycardia with hypertension
   b. paroxysmal atrial bradycardia with normotension
   c. bradycardia with profound hypotension
   d. complete heart block at 70 bpm with normotension

REFERENCES

1. J. Secor, *Coronary Care,* Appleton Century Crofts, New York, 1981, p. 44.
2. American Heart Association, *Heart Facts,* Dallas, Texas 1981, p. 24.
3. P. M. Zoll and A. J. Linenthal, "Termination of Refractory Tachycardia by External Countershock," *Circulation,* **25:**596 (1962).
4. I. M. Meth, "Electrical Safety in the Hospital," *Am J Nurs,* **80:**1344–1345 (1980).
5. M. E. Hazzard, *Critical Care Nursing,* Medical Examination Publishing Co., Inc., Garden City, N.Y., 1978, pp. 53–54.
6. American Heart Association Council on Cardiovascular Nursing and American Nurses' Association Division of Medical-Surgical Nursing Practice, *Standards of Cardiovascular Nursing Practice,* 1975.
7. J. Thierer et al. (eds.), *AACN Standards for Nursing Care of the Critically Ill,* Reston Publishing Company, Reston, Va., 1981.
8. K. Claus and J. Bailey, *Living with Stress and Promoting Well-Being,* The C. V. Mosby Company, St. Louis, 1980.
9. D. Adler and N. Shoemaker, *AACN Organization and Management of Critical Care Facilities,* The C. V. Mosby Company, St. Louis, 1979, p. xii.
10. Hazzard, op. cit., pp. 88–89.
11. D. Gentry and R. Williams, *Psychological Aspects of Myocardial Infarction and Coronary Care,* The C. V. Mosby Company, St. Louis, 1979.
12. M. R. Kinney et al., *AACN's Clinical Reference for Critical Care Nursing,* McGraw-Hill Book Company, New York, 1981, p. 1086.
13. B. Kozier and G. L. Erb, *Fundamentals of Nursing,* Addison-Wesley Publishing Company, Menlo Park, Calif., 1979, p. 803.
14. Kinney et al., op. cit., p. 1045.
15. P. F. Walter, "Clinical Recognition of Arrhythmias, Shock, Syncope, and Sudden Death (Including a Section on Cardiopulmonary Resuscitation)," in N. K. Wenger, J. W. Hurst, and M. C. McIntyre (eds.), *Cardiology for Nurses,* McGraw-Hill Book Company, New York, 1980, p. 237.

16. Walter, op. cit., pp. 240–241.
17. "Standards for CPR and ECG," *JAMA,* **244**(suppl. 5):467 (1980).
18. Ibid., p. 491.
19. J. F. Pantridge et al., "Electrical Requirements for Ventricular Defibrillators," *Br Med J,* **2:**313 (1975).
20. N. P. Campbell et al., "Transthoracic Ventricular Defibrillation in Adults," *Br Med J,* **2:**1379 (1977).
21. Kinney et al., op. cit., p. 1012.
22. Ibid., p. 934.
23. J. F. Spann and J. W. Hurst, "Treatment of Heart Failure," in J. W. Hurst (ed.), *The Heart,* 4th ed., McGraw-Hill Book Company, New York, 1978, p. 601.
24. K. J. Andreoli et. al., *Comprehensive Cardiac Care*, The C. V. Mosby Company, St. Louis, 1979, pp. 63–64.
25. K. L. MacCannell and D. G. Wyse, "Pharmacologic Management: Cardiovascular Drugs," in Wenger, Hurst, and McIntyre, op. cit., p. 614.
26. Spann and Hurst, op. cit., p. 602.
27. E. Braunwald, T. S. Alpert, and R. S. Ross, "Acute Myocardial Infarction," in K. J. Isselbacher et al. (eds.), *Harrison's Principles of Internal Medicine,* 9th ed., McGraw-Hill Book Company, New York, 1980 p. 1132.
28. R. C. Schlant, "Altered Cardiovascular Physiology of Coronary Arteriosclerotic Disease," in Hurst et al., op. cit., p. 1141.
29. Braunwald, Alpert, and Ross, op. cit., p. 1132.
30. Andreoli, op. cit., p. 85.
31. J. D. Clements, "Coronary Atherosclerotic Heart Disease," in Wenger, Hurst, and McIntyre, op. cit., pp. 312–314.
32. G. I. Litman, "Rheumatic Heart Disease," in Wenger, Hurst, and McIntyre, op. cit., p. 373.
33. J. Lamb, "Cardiac Transplantation," *Am J Nurs,* **80:**1786 (1980).
34. Ibid., p. 1786.
35. C. N. Barnard and J. G. Losman, "Left Ventricular Bypass," *South Afr Med J,* **29:**303–312 (1975).
36. R. B. Logue, P. H. Robinson, C. R. Hatcher, Jr., and J. A. Kaplan, "Medical Management in Cardiac Surgery," in Hurst et al., op. cit., p. 1783.
37. Logue, Robinson, Hatcher, and Kaplan, op. cit., p. 1790.
38. B. Walker, "The Post Surgery Heart Patient: Amount of Uninterrupted Time for Sleep," *Nurs Res,* **21:**164 (1972).

Chapter 29

NURSING ROLE IN MANAGEMENT

Inflammatory and Valvular Heart Diseases

Susan C. Littell
Sharon Mantik Lewis

Learning Objectives

1. Describe the etiology, pathogenesis, clinical manifestations, and medical, pharmacological, and nursing management of infective endocarditis and pericarditis.
2. Identify the indications for prophylactic antibiotic therapy in infective endocarditis.
3. Explain the etiology, clinical manifestations, and management of myocarditis and cardiomyopathies.
4. Describe the etiology, pathogenesis, clinical manifestations, and medical and nursing management of clients with rheumatic fever and heart disease.
5. Identify the etiologies of congenital and acquired valvular heart diseases.
6. Differentiate between the pathophysiology and clinical manifestations of the various types of valvular heart disease.
7. Describe the medical and nursing management of valvular heart disease.

INFLAMMATORY DISORDERS OF THE HEART

Infective Endocarditis

Endocarditis is inflammation of the endocardium, the inner lining of the heart. This lining is contiguous with the heart's valves (Fig. 29-1). The inflammation is usually limited to the membrane lining the valves.

Endocarditis most often occurs when valves have been previously damaged (e.g., in rheumatic heart disease) or are congenitally malformed. However, endocarditis also occurs in individuals with no preexisting valvular disorders. Individuals with other congenital heart abnormalities, such as ventricular septal defects, may also be susceptible to endocarditis.

Before the introduction of antibiotics, endocarditis was almost always fatal. In recent years, both the mortality and the actual incidence of endocarditis have been decreasing. This is due to the widespread use of prophylactic antibiotic treatment in susceptible people and antibiotic treatment of extracardiac infections.[1] However, bacterial endocarditis remains one of the most serious complications of cardiac disease.

Etiology and pathogenesis

The infectious agent may be viral, fungal, or, more commonly, bacterial. The most common infecting agent is Streptococcus viridans. Other bacterial causes are other types of streptococci, pneumococci, and staphylococci.[2] These bacteria enter the bloodstream following dental treatment (most commonly S. *viridans*, a group of alpha-hemolytic streptococci) or procedures involving the upper respiratory, genitourinary, or lower gastrointestinal tract. They may also be introduced via surgical instrumentation. Staphylococcus infections have been related to contaminated intravenous (IV) injections and cardiac surgery. The bacteria lodge on damaged or abnormal valves or on the endocardium in congenital heart defects. It seems that the abnormal structures are predisposed to bacterial implantation. This bacterial invasion initiates an inflammatory response.

*This chapter was reviewed by Marilyn Merz Lowe, R.N., M.S.N., Major U.S. Army Nurse Corps, Chief, Medical Nursing, USA MEDDAC, Ft. Bragg, North Carolina, Consultant to Army Surgeon General in Cardiovascular-Pulmonary Nursing; and Julie M. Dax, R.N., B.S.N., CCRN, Trauma Coordinator, former Assistant Head Nurse—Surgical Intensive and Coronary Care Units, University of New Mexico Hospital, Albuquerque, New Mexico.

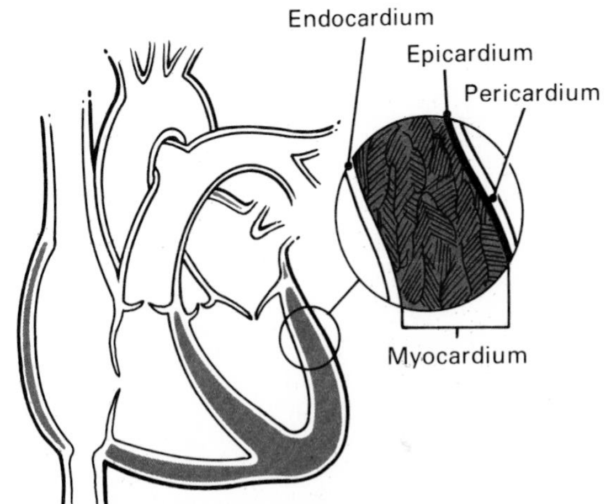

Figure 29-1 Layers of the heart.

The characteristic lesions produced in bacterial endocarditis are friable, irregular, nodular vegetations called *verrucae.* These vegetations adhere to the valve surface or endocardium. Verrucae are composed of bacteria, fibrin, blood cells, collagen, and necrotic material. This mass of material makes it difficult to achieve adequate penetration of antibiotic therapy. The ongoing infective process is capable of causing further damage to the underlying structure (Fig. 29-2).

Emboli may develop from the vegetative structures and travel to almost any body organ. Common sites at which emboli cause infarction are the spleen and kidneys. Other sites for infarction are the peripheral blood vessels, brain, and lungs. Bacterial embolization in the walls of small arteries may result in mycotic aneurysms. These lesions can destroy an organ such as the brain by causing hemorrhage.

Classification of endocarditis

Traditionally, bacterial endocarditis was divided into *acute* and *subacute* forms. The term *acute endocarditis* was used to describe a fulminating, toxic infection with rapid destruction of tissue and almost inevitable death of the person. The term *subacute endocarditis* was used to describe a more prolonged disease process, with the person surviving for a longer period of time. Today this classification system has become artificial because of the introduction of adequate chemotherapy treatment. The term *infective endocarditis* or *bacterial endocarditis* is preferred in describing the disease process.

Clinical manifestations

The early clinical manifestations of bacterial endocarditis may be very nonspecific and resemble those of other diseases. Fever is the most common early manifestation. The degree and pattern of the fever vary from low-grade to high-grade and from continuous to intermittent. The type of fever depends on the infecting organism. Unexplained fever in a person with a cardiac defect should always be investigated for the possibility of endocarditis.

Nonspecific manifestations such as malaise, fatigue, myalgia, and joint pain may be present. Manifestations related to congestive heart failure such as dyspnea (especially on exertion), edema, and cough may occur if the valvular damage has been rapid and extensive.

Usually, a new heart murmur develops or a previous murmur may become more pronounced. The finding of a significant murmur in a person with fever who had a previously normal cardiac examination should create a strong suspicion of endocarditis.

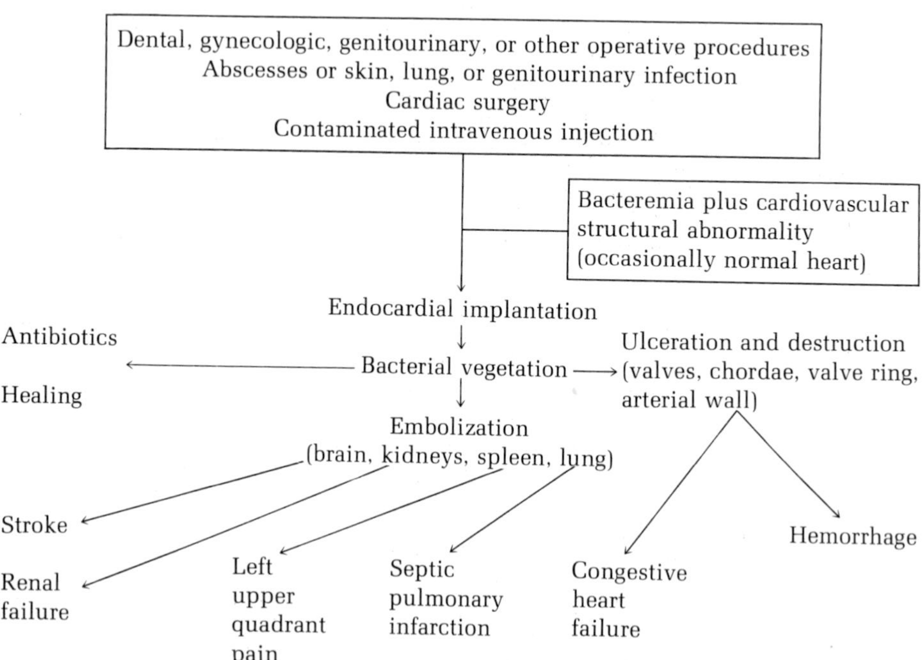

Figure 29-2 A diagram of the sequence of events in infective endocarditis. [*From N. Wenger et al., Cardiology for Nurses, McGraw-Hill Book Company, New York, 1980, p. 440.*]

Manifestations secondary to embolization in various body organs may also be present. Embolic infarction in the spleen may result in sharp left upper quadrant pain and splenomegaly. There may also be local tenderness and abdominal rigidity. Infarction of the kidneys may cause flank pain and hematuria. Emboli may lodge in small peripheral blood vessels and cause gangrene. Embolic infarctions may cause neurological problems such as hemiplegia, loss of vision, and coma. Manifestations resembling those of meningitis may also be present.

Hematological manifestations include anemia, petechiae, and an increased number of monocytes in circulating blood. Petechiae are the most common skin manifestation. There may also be evidence of generalized or localized purpura.

In summary, there are no clear-cut manifestations suggestive of infective endocarditis. The combination of fever, heart murmur, anemia, splenomegaly, and petechiae is suggestive of endocarditis.

Table 29-1
Medical Management: Infective Endocarditis

Diagnostic
1. History and physical examination
2. Blood culture and sensitivity
3. Chest x-ray
4. Echocardiography

Therapeutic
1. Appropriate antibiotic therapy
2. Antipyretics
3. Rest
4. Repeat blood cultures and sensitivity tests
5. Surgical valve replacement (for severe valvular damage)

Medical management (Table 29-1)

Diagnostic Questioning the client about his recent medical history is important in trying to identify the site of bacterial entry. Questions should be asked about any recent dental, urological, or gynecological procedures, as well as any recent skin, respiratory, or urinary tract infections. Other important information includes a previous history of heart disease.

The most important laboratory procedure is a blood culture. Both aerobic and anaerobic cultures are usually obtained. It is possible to have a negative blood culture with a positive clinical picture, especially if the person has recently taken antibiotics.

Anemia may be present, and increased numbers of phagocytic monocytes may be identified in the peripheral blood. There may also be an increased erythrocyte sedimentation rate and a decreased serum complement level. These two findings are also present in many other diseases and are of little diagnostic value.

A chest x-ray is done, and if congestive heart failure is present, it may be detected. An echocardiogram may be ordered, and significant findings may show underlying valvular disease and vegetations.

Therapeutic (Table 29-1) Accurate identification of the infecting organism is the key to successful treatment. The appropriate antibiotic is chosen based on sensitivity studies. Fever may persist for several days after treatment has been started. It is treated with aspirin, fluids, and rest. Complete bed rest is usually not recommended unless the temperature remains elevated or there are signs of heart damage. Subsequent blood cultures may be done to evaluate the effectiveness of antibiotic therapy.

Surgical intervention may be necessary for the client with severe valvular damage secondary to infective endocarditis. Prosthetic valve replacement is not usually performed until a full 6 weeks of antibiotic therapy is completed. Surgery is done earlier if severe heart failure or uncontrollable sepsis develops. (Valve replacement surgery is discussed in Chap. 28.)

Pharmacological intervention

Prophylactic Treatment Prophylactic antibiotic treatment is recommended for high-risk individuals in situations likely to be associated with bacteremia. High-risk individuals include those with a history of rheumatic or other acquired valvular heart disease, congenital heart disease, idiopathic hypertrophic subaortic stenosis, previous cardiovascular surgery, and implanted prosthetic heart valves.

Antibiotic prophylaxis is recommended for all dental procedures (including routine cleaning), upper respiratory tract surgical procedures, genitourinary and gastrointestinal tract surgery or instrumentation, and cardiac surgery.[3] Current recommendations for infective endocarditis prophylaxis in dental or surgical procedures and instrumentation of the upper respiratory tract are presented in Table 29-2.

The recommendations are classified as regimen A and regimen B. Regimen A uses penicillin, and regimen B uses penicillin and streptomycin. For persons allergic to penicillin, vancomycin and enythromycin are used. Regimen B is recommended for individuals with prosthetic valves because of their increased risk for endocarditis. Regimens A or B can be used for most other individuals at risk.

Enterococci (e.g., *Streptococcus fecalis*) are frequently responsible for endocarditis following gastro-

Table 29-2

Endocarditis Prophylaxis for Dental Procedures and Surgical Procedures

Regimen A—Penicillin

For persons not allergic to penicillin
Parenteral-oral combined: aqueous penicillin G (1 million units IM) mixed with procaine penicillin G (600,000 units IM) 30–60 min before procedure. Then 500 mg penicillin V every 6 h times eight doses
Or
Oral: penicillin V 2 g orally 30–60 min before procedure. Then 500 mg penicillin V orally every 6 h times eight doses.

For persons allergic to penicillin
Vancomycin 1 g IV. Then 500 mg erythromycin orally every 6 h times eight doses
Or
Erythromycin 1 g orally 1.5–2 h prior to procedure. Then 500 mg orally every 6 h times eight doses

Regimen B—Penicillin plus Streptomycin

For persons not allergic to penicillin
Aqueous penicillin G (1 million units IM) mixed with procaine penicillin G (600,000 units IM)
Plus
Streptomycin (1 gm IM) 30–60 min prior to procedure. Then penicillin V 500 mg orally every 6 h times eight doses

For persons allergic to penicillin
Vancomycin 1 g IV 30–60 min prior to procedure. Then 500 mg erythromycin orally every 6 h times eight doses

American Heart Association, "Prevention of Bacterial Endocarditis," *Circulation,* **56:**139A (1977).

intestinal tract or genitourinary tract surgery or use of instrumentation. The chemoprophylactic regimens for these procedures include penicillin or ampicillin plus gentamicin or streptomycin. For persons allergic to penicillin, vancomycin plus streptomycin is used.

Antibiotic doses used to prevent recurrences of acute rheumatic fever are not adequate for the prevention of bacterial endocarditis. Acute rheumatic fever is caused by group A beta-hemolytic streptococci. (Prophylactic antibiotic treatment for rheumatic fever is presented in Table 29-11 and is discussed later in this chapter.)

Antibiotic Therapy Penicillin is the primary antibiotic used in the treatment of bacterial endocarditis. For streptococcal endocarditis, treatment is a continuous IV infusion of 10 million units of penicillin G and an intramuscular (IM) infusion of 1 g of streptomycin daily for 3 to 4 weeks. If the person has an allergy to penicillin, clindamycin or vancomycin may be used.

Staphylococcal endocarditis is treated with IV penicillin and streptomycin if the organism does not produce penicillinase. Methicillin or oxacillin IV for 4 weeks is used to treat penicillinase-producing staphylococci.

Gram-negative endocarditis is difficult to treat, and aminoglycosides (e.g., gentamicin, tobramycin) are usually used. Fungal endocarditis is also very difficult to treat. Amphotericin B and 5-fluorocytosine are used, but the results have been unsatisfactory.

Nursing management

Health Promotion and Maintenance One of the most important goals for nurses is to help decrease the incidence of infective endocarditis. This can be done by identifying individuals with a history of heart disease who are at risk (discussed in the section on Pharmacological Intervention). The nurse should evaluate the client's understanding of the disease process. The client needs to understand the need for prophylactic antibiotic therapy when undergoing dental procedures as well as other surgical or instrumentation procedures (as previously discussed). The client should notify his physician prior to any dental procedure in order to be evaluated for prophylactic antibiotic therapy.

Good oral and dental hygiene is essential to prevent unnecessary tooth decay and the need for frequent dental care. (This is further discussed in Chap. 32.) Education of the client is critical to increase his understanding of and adherence to the planned medical regimen.

Acute and Chronic Management Adequate treatment of endocarditis usually requires prolonged hospitalization (2 to 6 weeks). The main reasons are to administer parenteral antibiotics and to monitor the client's response to treatment. Frequent assessment of body temperature is important, as persistent temperature elevations may mean that the drug therapy is ineffective. The nurse needs to provide support and diversion during the long hospitalization period.

Adequate periods of rest are very important. Strict bed rest is usually not necessary. The client needs to be encouraged to eat nutritious meals to facilitate the healing process.

The nurse should observe for complications of endocarditis such as embolization and heart failure. Heart failure may occur either acutely or insidiously secondary to valve damage.

An important responsibility of nursing is client education regarding the nature of the disease. The client needs to be instructed about symptoms that may indicate a relapse, such as fever, fatigue, and malaise.

Pericarditis

Pericarditis is inflammation of the pericardium, the sac that contains the heart. The pericardium consists of an inner serous membrane (visceral pericardium or epicardium) which is adherent to the cardiac muscle and a fibrous sac (parietal pericardium) (Fig. 29-1). Between the two layers is a space called the *pericardial space* or *cavity* which normally contains 15 to 50 mL of clear fluid. The fluid serves as a lubricant to decrease friction between the heart and adjacent structures.[4] The pericardium also limits the sudden dilatation of the ventricles during exercise. The pericardium is not essential to life and can be removed surgically without altering cardiac function. Pericarditis is frequently classified as *acute pericarditis* and *chronic constrictive pericarditis*. Each type will be considered separately.

Acute pericarditis

The causes of acute pericarditis are listed in Table 29-3. The basic mechanism is injury to the pericardial cells and subsequent development of the inflammatory response. Excess fluid accumulates in the pericardial space and fibrin is formed during the healing process.

Table 29-3
Etiologies of Acute Pericarditis

Infection
- Bacterial
- Viral
- Fungal
- Rickettsial

Vasculitis-connective tissue disease
- Lupus erythematosus
- Rheumatoid arthritis
- Ankylosing spondylitis
- Scleroderma

Myocardial Infarction
Uremia
Neoplasms
Trauma
Radiation-induced
Reiter's syndrome
Iatrogenic
- After cardiac surgery
- Pacemaker (temporary or permanent) implant
- Drug reactions
- Cardiac resuscitation

Idiopathic

S. J. Moore, "Pericarditis after Acute Myocardial infarction: Manifestations and Nursing implications," *Heart Lung,* **8:**551–558 (1979)

Clinical Manifestations The most characteristic manifestation of acute pericarditis is *chest pain* (Table 29-4). It typically begins suddenly, is severe and sharp, and is aggravated by inspiration and deep breathing. (This may be due to inflammation of the adjoining diaphragmatic pleura.) The pain is characteristically located in the anterior precordium and

Table 29-4
Common Signs and Symptoms of Acute Pericarditis

Chest pain (increasing with inspiration and movement)
Friction rub
Elevated temperature (usually $< 39°C$, 102.2°F)
Dyspnea, tachypnea, shallow breathing
Dysphagia
Restlessness
Irritability
Weakness, malaise
Anxiety

S. J. Moore, "Pericarditis after Myocardial infarction: Manifestations and Nursing Implications," *Heart Lung,* **8:**551–558 (1979).

radiates to the left shoulder. It is often relieved by sitting up and leaning forward.

A *pericardial friction rub* is often the diagnostic key to acute pericarditis (Table 29-4). Rubs are short, scratchy, or grating sounds heard best with the diaphragm of the stethoscope placed at the left middle to lower sternal border. The sound is caused by the movement of the heart against the inflamed, roughened pericardium. The exudate formed as a result of the inflammatory process roughens the two layers of the pericardium. The rub is often transient, and its quality and intensity may vary. It may even disappear for a few hours. Other common clinical manifestations are also presented in Table 29-4.

Complications Two major complications that may result from acute pericarditis are *pericardial effusion* and *cardiac tamponade*. Pericardial effusion is an accumulation (usually rapid) of excess pericardial fluid. Detection of pericardial effusion is best achieved by echocardiography. Cardiac tamponade develops when the excess pericardial fluid alters the compliance of the heart and impairs diastolic filling and, subsequently, cardiac output.

Cardiac tamponade is caused most frequently by bleeding into the pericardial space (e.g., in postoperative cardiac surgery or trauma), but it can occur with any type of acute pericarditis, especially if anticoagulants are used as part of the client's treatment.

The clinical manifestations of cardiac tamponade are presented in Table 29-5. They are due to decreasing cardiac output and increasing systemic venous congestion, and may develop suddenly or slowly. *Pulsus paradoxus* is an important diagnostic clue to the presence of cardiac tamponade. It is defined as systemic arterial pressure during expiration exceeding the pressure during inspiration by more than 10 mmHg. (Normally, the difference is 10 mmHg or less.) The technique for determining the pulsus paradoxus is outlined in Table 29-6.

Table 29-5
Signs and Symptoms of Cardiac Tamponade

Decreased systolic blood pressure
Narrowing pulse pressure
Pulsus paradoxus (> 10 mmHg)
Increased venous pressure, distended neck veins
Tachycardia
Tachypnea
Possible friction rub
Muffled heart sounds
Low-voltage ECG
Electrical alternation
Rapid enlargement of cardiac silhouette on x-ray
Peripheral cyanosis
Anxiety
Chest pain

S. J. Moore, "Pericarditis after Acute Myocardial Infarction: Manifestations and Nursing Implications," *Heart Lung,* **8:**551–558 (1979).

Diagnostic Study Abnormalities In the early phases, an electrocardiogram (ECG) shows an ST-segment elevation representing injury caused by the inflammatory reaction in the subepicardium. Several days later, ST segments return to normal and T-wave inversion becomes noticeable. Pathological Q waves do not develop, which is an important sign differentiating acute pericarditis from acute myocardial infarction (MI).[5]

Serum enzyme values are usually normal in pericarditis but elevated in acute MI. A chest x-ray is usually normal in acute pericarditis or may show an increased cardiac silhouette if a large pericardial effusion is present. Echocardiography findings may indicate the presence of a pericardial effusion.

Other diagnostic studies may be done to help determine the underlying disease process. For example, a serum creatinine test may be ordered to detect the presence of renal disease.

Medical Management Medical management of acute pericarditis (Table 29-7) includes:[6]

1. Treatment of the underlying disease
2. Rest
3. Symptomatic treatment for pain relief
4. Observation for pericardial effusion with tamponade

Treatment of the underlying disease may involve adequate hemodialysis for the uremic client with pericarditis.[7] If the underlying disease is a malignancy, chemotherapy may help to alleviate the pericarditis. Pericarditis secondary to a bacterial infection usually improves after antibiotics are given. Pericarditis secondary to rheumatic fever and post-MI Dressler's syndrome usually improves following administration of corticosteroids.

The main purpose of drug therapy is to relieve pain. Drug therapy is outlined in the section on Pharmacological Intervention. Bed rest is recommended until the pain and fever have subsided.

If pericardial effusion with tamponade develops, temporary management is directed toward maintain-

Table 29-6
Measurement of Pulsus Paradoxus

1. Determination made during quiet breathing with a stable rhythm.
2. Establish systolic pressure.
3. Inflate BP cuff until no sounds are heard with stethoscope.
4. Deflate cuff slowly until sounds are heard on expiration and note the pressure.
5. Deflate cuff until sounds are heard throughout the respiratory cycle and note the pressure.
6. Determine the difference, which will equal the amount of paradox:

Sounds heard in expiration at	110 mmHg
Sounds heard throughout cycle	82 mmHg
Amount of paradox	28 mmHg

7. The difference is usually less than 10 mmHg. If the difference is greater than 10 mmHg, this may be an indication of cardiac tamponade.

ing adequate blood pressure. This is accomplished by the use of volume expanders (e.g., dextran) and inotropic agents (e.g., dopamine, isoproterenol). More definitive treatment requires a *pericardiocentesis* (Fig. 29-3), which should be done as soon as possible. This is accomplished by inserting a needle into the pericardial space (sac) to aspirate fluid and relieve pressure on the heart. During the procedure, the ECG, blood pressure, and pulse should be monitored, and emergency equipment must be available for resuscitation. Possible complications of needle aspiration include laceration of a coronary artery or myocardium and ventricular fibrillation.

The aspirated fluid is observed for color, turbidity, and the presence of blood. Laboratory examinations of the fluid include culture for the presence of microorganisms, cytology, white blood cell count, and determination of hemoglobin, cholesterol, glucose, and protein.

Table 29-7
Medical Management: Pericarditis

Diagnostic
1. History and physical examination
2. Auscultation of chest
3. ECG
4. Chest x-ray
5. Echocardiography

Therapeutic (for acute pericarditis)
1. Treatment of the underlying disease
2. Bed rest
3. Aspirin
4. Indomethacin (Indocin)
5. Corticosteroids
6. Pericardiocentesis (for large pericardial effusion and/or tamponade)

Therapeutic (for chronic pericarditis)
1. Digitalis
2. Diuretics
3. Pericardiectomy

Pharmacological Intervention Since the pain of acute pericarditis is related to inflammation, anti-inflammatory agents such as aspirin and indomethacin (Indocin) are used to decrease the source of pain. Corticosteroids are used if aspirin or indomethacin is ineffective. Corticosteroids produce dramatic relief from pain, although their use is controversial because of the numerous side effects, such as fluid retention and hypertension.

Chronic constrictive pericarditis

Chronic constrictive pericarditis is characterized by fibrous thickening of the visceral and parietal pericardium. Sometimes there is calcification of the pericardium. Chronic pericarditis may result from acute pericarditis or pericardial effusion. Frequently, the condition presents with no previous history of cardiac disease. The basic pathological problem is inability of the ventricles to fill adequately during diastole because of the limitations imposed by the rigid, thickened pericardium.[8]

Clinical Manifestations The most common clinical manifestations are those of gradually occurring congestive heart failure. These include exertional dyspnea, peripheral edema, hepatomegaly, and ascites. Because of increasing portal pressure and impaired lymphatic drainage from the small intestine, protein may leak into the lumen of the small intestine. This can cause protein malabsorption with diarrhea.

In contrast to acute pericarditis, pain is not a

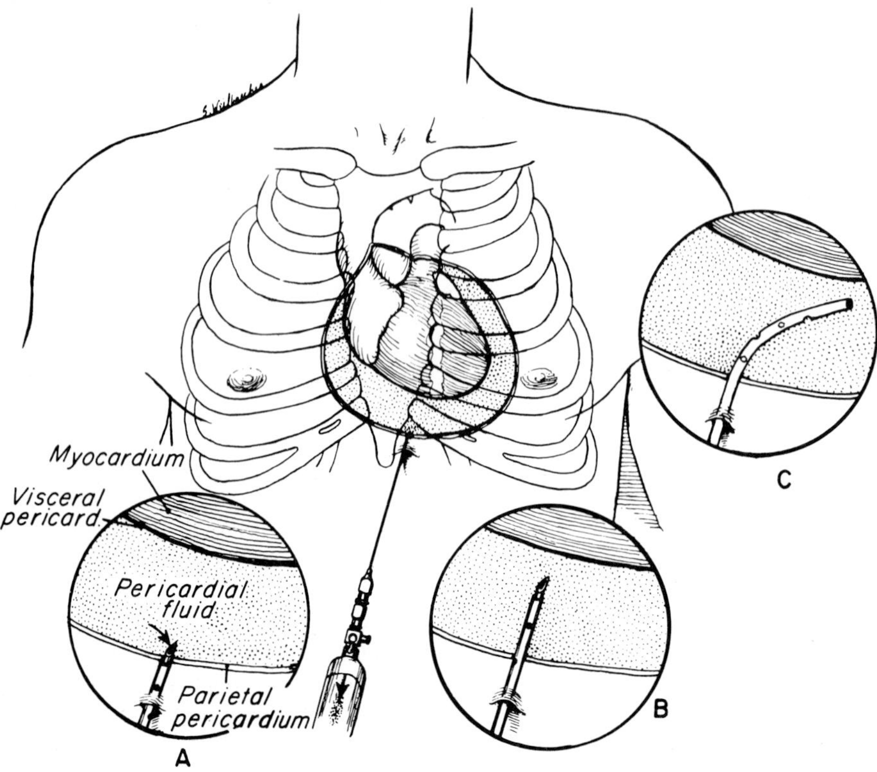

Figure 29-3 The technique for pericardiocentesis. The client's trunk is elevated approximately 45°, and under local anesthesia with lidocaine, a large-bore (17-or 18-gauge thin-wall) needle is inserted between the xyphoid and the left lower costal margin and advanced toward the middle of the left clavice, with the needle making a 20° to 30° angle with the abdominal wall. When the parietal percardium is punctured, a gentle "pop" is usually felt, and fluid is obtained. The aspirated fluid is placed into containers for laboratory analysis. The inserts show the placement of a small catheter in the pericardial space, a technique that is occasionally useful in individuals who have recurring large effusions. [*From N. Wenger et al. (eds.), Cardiology for Nurses, McGraw-Hill Book Company, New York, 1980, p. 481.*]

common manifestation of chronic pericarditis. Pulsus paradoxus occurs less frequently than in cardiac tamponade. A *pericardial knock,* which is a loud, sharp third heart sound, may be heard. Murmurs are usually not present. Systemic manifestations include weakness, fatigue, and weight loss.

Diagnostic Study Abnormalities Common abnormal findings on an ECG in chronic pericarditis are atrial fibrillation, T-wave inversion, and diminished voltage of the QRS complex and T wave. A chest x-ray may show prominent pulmonary blood vessels, absent to minimal cardiac enlargement, and calcium deposits in the pericardium.

Medical Management The only definitive treatment for chronic pericarditis is a *pericardiectomy,* surgical removal of the visceral and parietal pericardium. This surgery is recommended if the client is becoming progressively disabled. (Cardiac surgery is described in Chap. 28.)

Drug therapy consisting of diuretics and digitalis may be a useful supportive measure preoperatively. Digitalis preparations are also used postoperatively to aid the heart in dealing with increased inflow into the ventricles. The postoperative prognosis is good, and improvement is usually quite dramatic.

Nursing management of pericarditis

Nursing management of the client with acute pericarditis is aimed at pain relief. Assessment of pain and appropriate intervention is necessary before the pain becomes too severe. The nurse needs to be aware of the side effects of drugs used to treat pericarditis, such as tinnitus with aspirin administration. Other measures to relieve pain include elevating the head of the bed and placing a table across the bed for the client to lean on.

Another important nursing responsibility is allaying anxiety. The client who has acute pericarditis has often recently experienced an MI. Both processes cause chest pain, but they can be distinguished by the presence of a pericardial friction rub in pericarditis and by the characteristics of the pain. The client may be frightened by the pain, thinking that it is another MI. He may be relieved to know that the pain is due to pericarditis and will probably disappear in a few days.

The nurse needs to observe for manifestations of cardiac tamponade, such as dyspnea, orthopnea, tachycardia, and pulsus paradoxus. A narrowing pulse pressure can also be a sign of cardiac tamponade. Early diagnosis of cardiac tamponade can be essential in saving the client's life.

The conservative nursing management of chronic pericarditis is similar to that of congestive heart failure (Chap. 27). If a pericardiectomy is indicated for chronic pericarditis, postoperative nursing care will be similar to that of other cardiac surgical procedures (Chap. 28).

Myocarditis

Myocarditis, inflammation of heart muscle, is a nonspecific condition which may occur alone or in association with inflammation of tissues throughout the body. Myocarditis occurs during the course of many systemic illnesses, particularly infectious diseases.[9] Disorders commonly associated with myocarditis are acute rheumatic fever, acute pericarditis, sarcoidosis (see Chap. 20), and collagen diseases (e.g., systemic lupus erythematosus). The most frequent etiology of acute myocarditis is viral, particularly Coxsackie B virus and echovirus.

Clinical manifestations

Manifestations of myocarditis may be related to the primary disease or may be nonspecific, such as fatigue, fever, and dyspnea accompanying an infectious process. The clinical manifestations related to congestive heart failure are commonly found in myocarditis. These include dyspnea on exertion, edema, a ventricular gallop (third heart) sound, tachycardia, and hepatomegaly. (Congestive heart failure is discussed in Chap. 27).

Other common manifestations of myocarditis are cardiac arrhythmias and conduction disturbances. In clients with associated pericarditis, chest pain and pericardial friction may be present. Chest x-ray findings will show cardiomegaly and some evidence of pulmonary vein distension. There may be transient ST-T wave changes on the ECG.

Management

The primary goal in the management of myocarditis is to identify and treat the underlying disease. Management is similar to that of congestive heart failure, including the use of digitalis and diuretics, a sodium-restricted diet, and rest. Digitalis should be used cautiously, as the myocardium may be sensitive to its effects. Antiarrhythmic drugs are used in the treatment of cardiac arrhythmias but may not be effective. At times, temporary pacemakers or electrical cardioversion may be needed to treat arrhythmias. Anticoagulant therapy is used because clients with myocarditis are predisposed to systemic and pulmonary emboli. Viral myocarditis is usually self-limiting. The majority of individuals with myocarditis recover spontaneously.

Cardiomyopathy

Cardiomyopathy refers to noninflammatory dysfunctions of the myocardium. Cardiomyopathies are classified according to differences in their pathophysiology and clinical manifestations, as *congestive, restrictive,* or *hypertrophic.*

Congestive cardiomyopathy

Congestive (dilated) cardiomyopathy is characterized by cardiomegaly, congestive heart failure, arrhythmias, emboli, and murmurs. Usually, no specific etiology can be identified. In a few cases, identified etiologies have included beriberi, thyrotoxicosis, daunorubicin (antibiotic used for cancer treatment), muscular dystrophy, diabetes mellitus, and excessive alcohol ingestion. Congestive cardiomyopathy occurs most frequently in men 40 to 60 years of age, especially in blacks.[10]

Treatment is directed toward the underlying disease (if it can be determined). It is also important to treat the clinical manifestations of congestive heart failure with digitalis, diuretics, sodium restriction, and rest. Antiarrhythmic drugs and anticoagulant therapy are usually indicated. In general, the prognosis for clients with congestive cardiomyopathy is poor.

Restrictive cardiomyopathy

Restrictive cardiomyopathy refers to dysfunctions of the heart muscle characterized by restrictions in ventricular filling. Clinically, the manifestations are similar to those of chronic constrictive pericarditis (previously described).

The etiology of restrictive cardiomyopathy is usually unknown. In a few cases, specific etiologies that have been identified include amyloidosis (see Chap. 57), hemochromatosis (increased iron deposits in organs), and sarcoidosis.

Management is initially directed toward differentiating restrictive myocarditis from chronic constrictive pericarditis. Once the diagnosis of restrictive myocarditis is made, treatment is the same as for congestive cardiomyopathy.

Hypertrophic cardiomyopathy

Hypertrophic cardiomyopathy (also called *idiopathic hypertrophic subaortic stenosis*) is characterized by myocardial hypertrophy without ventricular dilatation. The disease process primarily affects the septum but may also extend to involve the free ventricular wall. Obstruction to left ventricular outflow may or may not be present. This disorder has a genetic basis.

Hypertrophic cardiomyopathy without obstruction is often asymptomatic. Arrhythmias, chest pain, exertional dyspnea, and congestive heart failure may develop. Treatment is primarily symptomatic.

Hypertrophic cardiomyopathy with obstruction to left ventricular outflow may cause mitral regurgitation. Clinical manifestations include exertional dyspnea, angina pectoris, syncope, paroxysmal nocturnal dyspnea, and edema. Some individuals are asymptomatic. Treatment may consist of propranolol (Inderal) if angina is present. Propranolol decreases the left ventricular contractile force to the point where outflow obstruction is controlled. Digitalis and nitroglycerin are not usually helpful unless congestive heart failure has developed. In some cases, surgical excision or incision of the hypertrophied portion of the outflow tract may be indicated.[11]

Rheumatic Fever and Heart Disease

Rheumatic fever is an inflammatory disease of the heart potentially involving all layers (endocardium, myocardium, and pericardium). The resulting damage to the heart from rheumatic fever is called *rheumatic heart disease,* a chronic condition characterized by scarring and deformity of the heart valves.

Significance of the problem

The actual incidence of rheumatic fever is not known. Acute rheumatic fever is primarily a disease of childhood, most commonly occurring between the ages of 5 and 15. The attack rate of rheumatic fever following streptococcal pharyngitis in epidemics is about 3 percent. Attacks do occur in adulthood, and recent studies indicate that they are probably more common than previously believed. Recurrent attacks of rheumatic fever are twice as common between the ages of 11 and 22 years as after age 22.[12] The sequela of rheumatic heart disease is primarily seen in young adults.

The attack rate of rheumatic fever following streptococcal infection in individuals with a history of rheumatic fever is increased from 5 to 50 percent. The incidence is especially high in people with rheumatic heart disease. In general, the incidence of rheumatic fever has been decreasing in the past few decades. This finding is due to improved living conditions and to the use of antibiotics in the initial treatment of streptococcal infections.

Etiology

Rheumatic fever occurs as a delayed sequela (usually 2 to 3 weeks) to a group A beta-hemolytic streptococcal infection of the pharynx. Skin infections with these organisms do not cause rheumatic fever. Some strains of group A beta-hemolytic streptococci do not cause rheumatic fever.

In addition to the infecting organism, other factors play a predisposing role in the development of rheumatic fever. These include socioeconomic factors, familial factors, and the presence of an altered immune response. The incidence of rheumatic fever is higher in lower socioeconomic groups. Crowded living conditions may be the major factor contributing to this finding. Neglect or inadequate treatment of streptococcal sore throats may be another factor. Poor nutrition and a lowered state of general health may be other reasons why lower socioeconomic groups are more commonly affected.

There seems to be a familial tendency toward rheumatic fever. This may be genetically related, possibly due to an altered immune response (see the next section).

Pathogenesis

The pathogenesis of rheumatic fever remains unknown. Considerable evidence focuses on the immune response to the streptococcal organism. Antibodies are produced to the streptococci (which are antigenic). These antibodies later may also cross-react with cardiac tissue, joints, and other body tissues. The organism itself is not present in the tissue lesions and has usually been eliminated from the person's body.

Cardiac Involvement In rheumatic fever, all layers of the heart can be involved (*pancarditis*). Endocardial involvement is primarily found in the valves, with swelling and erosion of the valve leaflets. Vegetations, or verrucae, form in areas of erosion from deposits of fibrin and blood cells. (Verrucae were discussed in the section on Etiology and Pathogenesis of infective endocarditis.) These lesions may heal with fibrous thickening of the valve commissures and chordae tendinae. The valves may become stenotic and insufficient. The mitral and aortic valves are most commonly affected; less commonly the tricuspid valve, and rarely the pulmonic valve, are also involved. (Valvular heart disease is discussed below.) There is also resultant thickening of the chordae tendinae and fibrosis of the papillary muscles.

Myocardial involvement is characterized by *Aschoff's bodies,* nodules formed by a reaction to inflammation. There is also accompanying swelling and fragmentation of collagen fibers. As Aschoff bodies age, they become more fibrous, and scar tissue is formed in the myocardium.

Pericarditis may result from rheumatic heart disease, as described in the section on Pericarditis. A serofibrinous effusion may be produced. Pericardial adhesions and calcification may develop, but chronic pericarditis is not common.

The pathological changes in the heart may occur as a result of an initial attack of rheumatic fever. However, recurrent infections may cause further structural damage.

Extracardiac Involvement The lesions of rheumatic fever are systemic, involving especially connective tissue. The joints (polyarthritis), skin (subcutaneous nodules), central nervous system (chorea), and lungs (fibrinous pleurisy and rheumatic pneumonitis) become involved in rheumatic fever.

Clinical manifestations

The clinical manifestations of rheumatic fever vary greatly, and no single sign or symptom is diagnostic. In 1944, Dr. T. D. Jones developed criteria for the diagnosis of rheumatic fever. In 1965, they were modified by the American Heart Association (Table 29-8). If two major and one minor criteria or one major and two minor criteria are present, the diagnosis of rheumatic fever is usually made. With either combination, there must be evidence of an existing streptococcal infection (e.g., positive throat culture for group A streptococci or an increased antistreptolysin O [ASO] titer).

Table 29-8
Modified Jones Criteria for Acute Rheumatic Fever

Major Criteria	Minor Criteria
Carditis	Fever
Polyarthritis	Previous occurrence of rheumatic fever
Chorea	Arthralgia
Erythema marginatum	Abdominal pain
Subcutaneous nodules	Epistaxis
	Prolonged PR interval
	Laboratory findings (see Table 29-9)

Council on Rheumatic Fever and Congenital Heart Disease, "Jones Criteria (Revised) for Guidance in Diagnosis of Rheumatic Fever," *Circulation,* 32:**664** (1965).

Major Criteria *Carditis* is an important manifestation. It presents with four signs:

1. Heart murmurs not previously present, usually of mitral or aortic regurgitation
2. Cardiac enlargement and congestive heart failure
3. Pericarditis manifested as a pericardial friction rub
4. Arrhythmias

Polyarthritis is migratory, usually affecting the larger joints. The joints are red, swollen, warm, and tender. Usually, pain prevents the person from walking.

Chorea is a disorder of the central nervous system characterized by weakness, ataxia, incoordination, and sudden, involuntary movements. It primarily affects children under 18 years of age, especially girls.

Erythema marginatum is a pinkish-red recurring rash originating on the trunk which may spread to other body parts. The erythema fades, leaving clear centers and round margins. The rash is usually transitory (lasting for a few hours) and is exacerbated by heat (e.g., a warm bath).

Subcutaneous nodules are small, hard, painless swellings found most commonly over bony prominences (e.g., knees, elbows, spine, scapula). They frequently are not noticed by the person.

In adults, chorea, erythema marginatum, and subcutaneous nodules are not common presenting manifestations. Polyarthritis and arthralgias are common manifestations.

Minor Criteria The minor clinical manifestations presented in Table 29-8 occur in rheumatic fever but are frequently found in many other diseases as well. They are used as supplemental data to confirm the presence of rheumatic fever.

Complications

The course of rheumatic fever varies greatly. About 90 percent of acute rheumatic attacks subside within 12 weeks, and less than 5 percent persist for more than 6 months. Once acute rheumatic fever has subsided, rheumatic fever does not recur unless a new streptococcal infection occurs.[13] Recurrences are most common within the first 5 years.

A complication that can result from acute rheumatic fever is chronic rheumatic heart disease. It results from changes in valvular structure which may occur months to years after an attack of acute rheumatic fever. As previously mentioned, rheumatic endocarditis can result in fibrous tissue growth to the valve leaflets and chordae tendinae, with scarring and contractures. The mitral valve is most frequently involved (Fig. 25-3). Other valves that can become affected are the aortic and tricuspid valves. (Valvular heart disease is discussed later in this chapter.)

Diagnostic study abnormalities

No single diagnostic study is indicative of rheumatic fever, but the results of combinations of laboratory studies are suggestive (Table 29-9). The ASO titer is most commonly used to demonstrate previous streptococcal infections. The erythrocyte sedimentation rate and C-reactive protein tests are nonspecific tests indicative of an inflammatory process.

An echocardiogram may show valvular and myocardial dysfunction. A chest x-ray may show an enlarged heart if congestive heart failure is present.

Medical and pharmacological management

There is no specific treatment for rheumatic fever. Supportive measures consist of limited bed rest and drug therapy (Table 29-10). The duration of rest and limited activity is governed by the results of laboratory tests and the client's clinical manifestations. Acetylsalicylic acid (ASA) is used to treat the clinical manifestations of inflammation. Corticosteroids are also used as nonspecific anti-inflammatory agents if aspirin is not effective.

Penicillin is used to treat any residual beta-hemolytic streptococcal infection. It is used even if throat cultures are negative. If congestive heart failure develops, it is treated appropriately (Chap. 27).

Table 29-9
Laboratory Test Abnormalities in Acute Rheumatic Fever

ASO titer	> 250 IU/mL
Erythrocyte sedimentation rate	> 15 mm/h—males > 20 mm/h—females
C-reactive protein	Positive
Throat culture	May be positive for streptococci (most commonly is negative)
White blood cell count	Elevated

Table 29-10
Medical Management: Rheumatic Fever

Diagnostic
1. History and physical examination
2. ASO titer
3. Throat culture
4. Erythrocyte sedimentation rate
5. C-reactive protein
6. White blood cell count
7. Chest x-ray
8. Echocardiography

Therapeutic
1. Bed rest (modified)
2. Benzathine penicillin 1.2 million units IM or procaine penicillin 600,000 units IM daily for 10 days
3. ASA
4. Corticosteroids

Nursing Management

Health Promotion and Maintenance Rheumatic fever is one of the few cardiovascular diseases that is preventable. Prevention of rheumatic fever is frequently classified as *primary* and *secondary*. Primary prevention involves early detection and immediate treatment of group A beta-hemolytic streptococcal pharyngitis. Adequate treatment of streptococcal pharyngitis will prevent initial attacks of rheumatic fever. Treatment consists of a single IM injection of 0.6 to 1.2 million units of benzathine penicillin G or 10 days of oral penicillin G. Erythromycin is substituted for individuals allergic to penicillin. Oral therapy requires faithful adherence to the full 10-day course of treatment. The nurse has an important role in educating the community regarding the need to seek medical attention for symptoms of streptococcal pharyngitis. In addition, she can help emphasize the need for adequate treatment of a streptococcal sore throat.

Secondary prevention focuses on the use of prophylactic antibiotics to prevent recurrent rheumatic fever. This is especially important because once a person has had rheumatic fever, he is more susceptible to a second attack following a streptococcal infection. The best prophylactic treatment is monthly injections of benzathine penicillin G. Alternative treatments are presented in Table 29-11.

Prophylactic treatment should continue for life in individuals who developed rheumatic carditis as children. Those who develop rheumatic fever without carditis after the age of 18 may need only 5 years of prophylactic antibiotic therapy.

Table 29-11
Prophylactic Antibiotics Used for Rheumatic Fever

Benzathine penicillin IM 1.2 million units every month
Penicillin G po 250,000 units twice a day
Sulfadiazine po 1 g daily
Erythromycin po 250 mg twice a day

J. W. Hurst et al. (eds.), *The Heart*, McGraw-Hill Book Company, New York, 1978, p. 989.

Individuals with a previous history of rheumatic fever need to be educated to understand the need for continuous prophylactic treatment. They must be made aware of the high risk of recurrence if they develop a streptococcal infection. Rheumatic fever is five times more likely to occur in a person with prior rheumatic fever than in the general population. Nurses need to be made more aware of their role in identifying individuals with a previous history of rheumatic fever and then teaching them the need for and purpose of lifelong prophylactic antibiotic therapy.

The dosage of antibiotics used in prophylaxis of rheumatic fever is not adequate to prevent bacterial endocarditis. If a person with known rheumatic heart disease is having any dental procedures or surgical procedures of the upper respiratory, gastrointestinal, or genitourinary tract, prophylaxis as outlined in the section on Prophylactic Treatment of endocarditis is necessary. It is essential to explain to the client the difference between these two prophylactic programs.

Acute Intervention One of the primary nursing goals for the client with acute rheumatic fever is to provide and encourage optimal rest. Nonstrenuous activities should be encouraged after recovery has begun. Activity restriction is especially difficult for children and young adults.

Relief of joint pain is another important nursing goal. Painful joints should be positioned for comfort and good alignment. It may be necessary to remove the weight of covers from painful joints by using a bed cradle. Heat may be applied to the joints for pain relief.

Psychological and emotional care can be more important than physical care, especially since children and young adults are the primary clients. The heart is often viewed as the center of life, and an alteration in cardiac function may be perceived as a threat to the person's body image.

Chronic Management Secondary prevention, as discussed previously, is concerned with preventing the recurrence of rheumatic fever. The client needs to be taught about the disease process, the possible sequela of rheumatic fever, and the continual need for prophylactic antibiotics. Ongoing client education and reinforcement are essential to encourage good health practices and the continuation of prophylactic antibiotic therapy.

The client needs to be aware of the possibility of developing valvular heart disease. He should be taught to seek medical attention if symptoms such as excessive fatigue, dizziness, palpitations, or dyspnea on exertion develop.

VALVULAR HEART DISEASE

Cardiac valves are located in four strategic places in the heart (Fig. 29-4). They are essentially one-way swinging doors designed to keep blood flowing in the proper direction through the heart's four chambers. The valves are subject to much wear and tear. In addition to normal wearing, they are often damaged by inflammation, infection, and trauma. Valves may also be congenitally abnormal, absent, or malpositioned.

Etiology of Valvular Heart Disease

Congenital heart disease (CHD)

CHD results from disruption during fetal development and has both genetic and environmental causes (e.g., rubella, drugs).[14] CHD occurs in 4 to 10 percent of live births.[15] Mortality related to CHD may occur in the uterus, soon after birth, in infancy, or during or after attempted surgical correction. Sometimes congenital lesions are not detected until later in life. For

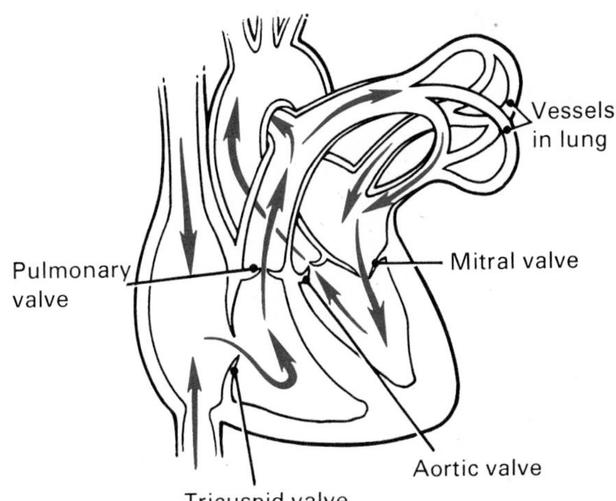

Figure 29-4 Valves of the heart as seen in cross section.

example, a bicuspid aortic valve may function well until calcification develops as a natural occurrence of the aging process. Common congenital lesions are presented in Table 29-12.

Another less serious form of CHD involves a leaflet or cusp of the mitral valve which is weak. This can lead to some degree of mitral valve incompetence. Common terms for this condition are *floppy mitral valve, Barlow's syndrome, click-murmur syndrome,* and *mitral valve prolapse.* Approximately 10 percent of the population has mitral valve prolapse, and it is more common in women than in men.[16] The condition is relatively benign, with symptoms of chest pain and palpitations, although rare fatal arrhythmias have been reported.[17]

Acquired valvular heart disease

Acquired valvular heart disease encompasses all valvular distortions which are not present at birth. The overall incidence of acquired valvular problems is difficult to estimate, as the etiologies are not reportable. Although it is known that valvular damage from rheumatic heart disease is declining due to prevention and improved living conditions, it is still the leading cause of valvular heart disease.

Chronic Rheumatic Heart Disease As described earlier, chronic rheumatic heart disease is a complication of rheumatic fever. Valvular damage occurs when acute inflammation and healing lead to erosion of valve leaflet edges and formation of verrucae along the edges. Valves become *stenosed,* with a reduction in size of the valve opening or orifice, or *insufficient,* with incomplete closure and regurgitation through the valve.

As previously mentioned, the valve most commonly affected is the mitral valve. It is followed by the aortic valve and then by the tricuspid valve. The pulmonic valve is rarely damaged by the rheumatic process.

Infective Endocarditis As described earlier, infective endocarditis can cause structural damage to the valves. When recurrent endocarditis develops, it usually involves the same valve.

Ischemia An insufficient blood supply to portions of the heart caused by atherosclerotic coronary arteries may affect the valves. The valve usually involved is the mitral valve. The papillary muscles which anchor and maneuver the chordae tendinae are often affected. When the papillary muscles are not contracting well, the chordae are not well anchored and valve leaflets become incompetent. These alterations result in insufficiency.

A client may have permanent damage to papillary

Table 29-12
Common Congenital Heart Lesions

Lesion	Description	Incidence (%)*
Ventricular Septal Defect	Hole in septum between two ventricles.	30.5
Atrial Septal Defect	Hole in septum between two atria.	9.8
Patent Ductus Arteriosus	Persistence of opening between aorta and pulmonary artery. Normally closes shortly before birth.	9.7
Pulmonic Stenosis	Narrowing of pulmonic valve.	6.9
Coarctation of Aorta	Stricture and narrowing of aorta caused by infolding of wall of aorta.	6.8
Aortic Stenosis	Narrowing of aortic valve.	6.1
Tetralogy of Fallot	Ventricular septal defect, pulmonic stenosis, aorta overriding two ventricles, and right ventricular hypertrophy.	5.8
Transposition of the Great Vessels	Aorta and pulmonary artery have reversed position. Aorta arises from the right ventricle, and pulmonary artery arises from the left ventricle.	4.2
Tricuspid Atresia	Absence of communication between right atrium and right ventricle.	1.3

*Incidence taken from K. Isselbecher et al. (eds.), *Harrison's Principles of Internal Medicine,* 9th ed., McGraw-Hill Book Company, New York, 1980, p. 1075.

muscles from the infarction process and may be left with chronic mitral insufficiency. At times, usually during or after an MI, the papillary muscles may rupture or a chorda may break, resulting in "flail leaflet." This leads to overwhelming heart failure, a serious and often fatal complication.

Traumatic Damage Valves are infrequently damaged due to trauma. The most common trauma, blunt chest, often leads to contusion of the myocardium. Stab wounds, bullet pathways, and other traumas can distort or destroy valves.

Syphilitic Disease The organism *Treponema pallidum* causes a progressive disruption of the vascular system unless treated. Tertiary syphilis causes aortitis, producing aortic aneurysms and insufficiency of the aortic valve. This cause of aortic valvular disease had decreased in incidence even before the advent of penicillin therapy.[18]

Types of Valvular Heart Disease

Diseased heart valves produce two types of functional alterations, *stenosis* and *regurgitation.* In stenosis the valve orifice is restricted and forward flow of blood is impeded (Fig. 29-5). In regurgitation the valve leaflets fail to close. This allows backflow of blood (Fig. 29-5). *Valvular incompetence* and *valvular insufficiency* are terms used synonymously with *valvular regurgitation.* Regurgitation and stenosis can occur singly or together in the same valve. In addition, multiple valves can be affected, as in rheumatic heart disease.

Cardiac function is significantly altered by valve dysfunction. Valvular regurgitation increases the volume of blood the heart needs to pump. Valvular stenosis necessitates the generation of increased pressure to overcome resistance to flow. Increased volume work leads to chamber dilatation, and increased pressure work leads to muscular hypertrophy. Myocardial dilatation and hypertrophy are compensatory mechanisms intended to increase the pumping capability of the heart.[19]

Mitral stenosis

The mitral valve is the most frequently affected valve in rheumatic heart disease. In most cases, progressive narrowing occurs over 20 to 30 years following the initial attack of rheumatic fever. Frequently, there is a history of more than one attack of rheumatic fever. Symptoms do not usually result until the valve's orifice has narrowed to one-half of its original size. The valve leaflets are thickened with fibrous tissue, and calcium deposits may form. *Mitral stenosis* impedes the flow of blood into the left ventricle. Therefore, the left atrium hypertrophies to generate enough pressure to increase its pumping action. Atrial dilatation also occurs as a result of the increased volume of blood in the left atrium.

The increase in left atrial pressure is reflected backward into the pulmonary veins, resulting in pulmonary congestion. The increased pressure in the lungs is reflected backward into the pulmonary artery and the right side of the heart. Right-sided heart failure is eventually reflected backward into the systemic circulation.

Early in the disease process, a diastolic heart murmur can be detected. In addition, there is increased intensity of the first heart sound (atrioventricular valve closure). Pulmonary involvement, such as dyspnea on exertion, is the usual initial manifestation. Other clinical manifestations are presented in Table 29-13. The most common complications are congestive heart failure, systemic and pulmonary emboli, atrial arrhythmias, and infective endocarditis.

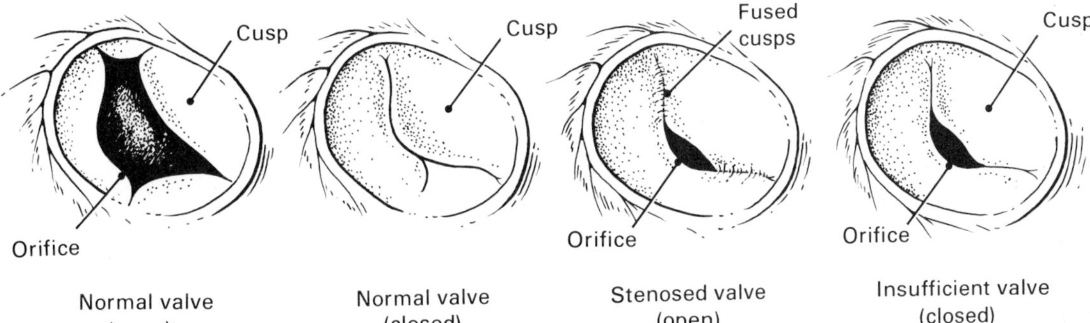

Figure 29-5 A stenosed valve leads to decreased blood flow through the valve and gradual hypertrophy of the preceding chamber (e.g., a stenosed mitral valve leads to a hypertrophied left atrium). An insufficient valve leads to backward flow through the valve and dilation of the preceding chamber (e.g., aortic insufficiency leads to a dilated left ventricle).

Table 29-13
Types of Valvular Heart Disease

Type	Clinical Manifestations	Diagnostic Study Findings
Mitral stenosis	Diastolic heart murmur Dyspnea on exertion Weakness Fatigue Predisposition to respiratory infections Orthopnea Paroxysmal nocturnal dyspnea Palpitations (from atrial fibrillation) Hemoptysis	ECG Left atrial enlargement Prolonged, notched P waves (P mitrale) Right ventricular hypertrophy Chest x-ray Left atrial enlargement Pulmonary venous congestion Interstitial pulmonary edema Right ventricular enlargement Cardiac catheterization ↑ pressure across mitral valve ↑ left atrial pressure ↑ pulmonary capillary wedge pressure Low cardiac output Echocardiogram Decreased excursion of leaflets Diminished E–F slope
Mitral regurgitation	Murmur throughout systole Weakness Fatigue Dyspnea on exertion Palpitations	ECG Left atrial enlargement (P mitrale) Left ventricular hypertrophy Atrial fibrillation Chest x-ray Left atrial enlargement Left ventricular enlargement Pulmonary vascular congestion Cardiac catheterization Angiography and contrast medium used to identify and quantify regurgitation Echocardiogram Left atrial enlargement Hyperdynamic left ventricle
Aortic stenosis	Systolic murmur Syncope (especially on exertion) Angina pectoris Left ventricular failure Fatigue Dyspnea	ECG Left ventricular hypertrophy Chest x-ray Poststenotic aortic dilatation Aortic valve calcification Cardiac catheterization Pressure gradient in systole between left ventricle and aorta (across aortic valve) ↑ diastolic ventricular pressure Normal left atrial and pulmonary pressures Echocardiogram Restricted movement of aortic valve Increased echoes Thickening of left ventricular wall
Aortic regurgitation	Diastolic and systolic murmurs Water-hammer pulse Palpitations Syncope Dyspnea on exertion Chest pain Congestive heart failure	ECG Left ventricular hypertrophy Chest x-ray Aortic valve calcification Left ventricular enlargement Dilatation of ascending aorta Cardiac catheterization Increased pulse pressure Increased diastolic pulse slope

Table 29-13 (Continued)

Type	Clinical Manifestations	Diagnostic Study Findings
		Angiography demonstrates reflux through aortic valve Echocardiogram Left ventricular dilatation Diastolic fluttering of anterior leaflet
Tricuspid valve disease	Murmur throughout systole (tricuspid regurgitation) Diastolic murmur (tricuspid stenosis) Right-sided heart failure Peripheral edema Ascites Hepatomegaly	ECG Tall, peaked P waves Chest x-ray Right atrial enlargement Right ventricular enlargement Cardiac catheterization Pressure gradient across tricuspid valve (stenosis) ↑ right atrial pressure (stenosis) Reflux of contrast medium into right atrium (regurgitation)

Mitral regurgitation

Mitral regurgitation, or insufficiency, allows backward flow of blood from the left ventricle to the left atrium during ventricular systole. During systole, ventricular contraction pushes blood forward into the aorta as well as backward into the left atrium. The left atrium dilates to compensate for the increased volume of blood. The left atrium does not hypertrophy to the extent that it does with mitral stenosis.

The volume of blood increases in the left ventricle at the end of diastole. This increase initially allows a normal cardiac output to be maintained at rest. Eventually, the left ventricle dilates, resulting in left ventricular hypertrophy as well.

As the disease advances, forward flow of blood into the aorta is impaired due to left ventricular failure. In addition, there is backward flow from the left atrium into the pulmonary vasculature. Right-sided heart failure is not as frequent a consequence as it is in mitral stenosis. When it does appear, it frequently occurs late in the disease process.

The clinical manifestations of mitral regurgitation are presented in Table 29-13. Other complications are similar to those of mitral stenosis, including congestive heart failure, atrial arrhythmias, and infective endocarditis. Chronic mitral regurgitation has a more prolonged course than mitral stenosis.

Aortic stenosis

When the aortic orifice becomes narrowed, the left ventricle needs to generate increased pressure to propel blood into the aorta. As a result, left ventricular hypertrophy results. In severe cases of aortic stenosis, left ventricular pressure can increase to 300 mmHg. Eventually, the compensatory ability of the heart is overwhelmed (Figs. 29-6, 29-7).

Myocardial work, as well as myocardial oxygen demand, is increased. When the demand for O_2 exceeds its availability, myocardial ischemia and angina pectoris can result.

Eventually, the left atrium hypertrophies in an attempt to increase ventricular filling at the end of diastole. Left atrial pressure can be reflected backward into the pulmonary vasculature.

The course of aortic stenosis is quite severe once symptoms develop. Congestive heart failure, syncope, angina, and arrhythmias are serious complications. From 10 to 15 percent of clients with symptoms die suddenly. The survival time for clients who develop symptoms of congestive heart failure is often less than 5 years.[20]

Aortic regurgitation

Aortic regurgitation produces a backflow of blood from the aorta into the left ventricle during diastole. Initially, the left ventricle dilates to compensate for the increase in blood volume. Ultimately, the left ventricle hypertrophies as well, resulting in a need for increased myocardial oxygen.

Symptoms of aortic regurgitation do not develop until late in the disease process, when there is marked left ventricular decompensation. The clinical manifestations are presented in Table 29-13. A characteristic finding is a *water-hammer pulse,* which is a rapid rise in arterial pressure during the systolic phase and a rapid fall during the diastolic phase. The pulse pressure becomes widened.

Individuals with aortic stenosis do quite well for a

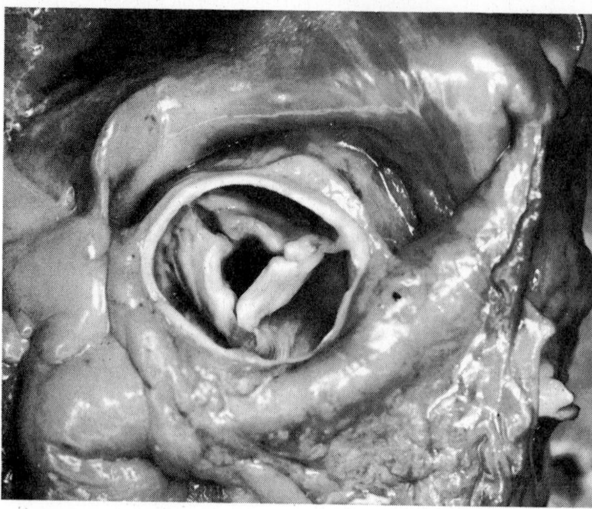

Figure 29-6 Stenotic aortic valve with thickened but noncalcified cusps. The commissures, now fused, are easily identified. This pathological condition suggests that rheumatic fever has caused the lesion. [*From J. W. Hurst et al.* (*eds.*), *The Heart, 4th ed., McGraw-Hill Book Company, New York, 1978, p. 1086.*]

while until heart failure develops. Complications that can occur are congestive heart failure, arrhythmias, and infective endocarditis.

Tricuspid valve disease

Tricuspid stenosis is usually caused by rheumatic fever. *Tricuspid regurgitation* is usually a functional problem resulting from right ventricular failure secondary to left ventricular failure or pulmonary hypertension. As the right ventricle dilates and enlarges, functional tricuspid regurgitation will result.

Both tricuspid stenosis and tricuspid regurgitation cause increased blood volume and increased blood pressure in the right atrium. This is reflected backward into the systemic circulation and typical manifestations of right-sided heart failure, such as ascites, peripheral edema, and hepatomegaly, are seen.

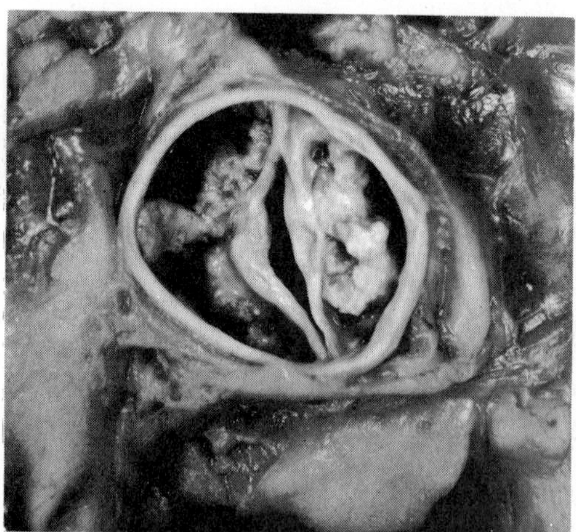

Figure 29-7 Stenotic, calcified aortic valve in an adult male. This probably was a congenitally bicuspid valve which gradually became calcified, rigid, and stenotic. [*From J. W. Hurst et al. (eds.), The Heart, 4th ed., McGraw-Hill Book Company, New York, 1978, p. 1086.*]

Pulmonic valve disease

Pulmonic valve disease is not common and most frequently is due to congenital lesions.

Diagnostic study abnormalities

The most common finding on physical examination in a person with valvular heart disease is a murmur. A murmur occurs when blood flows past an obstruction, dilatation, or unusual opening, and turbulence occurs.

Diagnostic studies that are frequently used in valvular heart disease are an ECG, a chest x-ray, echocardiography, and cardiac catheterization. An ECG shows variation in the heart rate and rhythm, as well as providing information about possible ischemia or chamber enlargement. A chest x-ray shows the heart size and alterations in pulmonary circulation. An echocardiogram provides information on the structure and function of the valves and on enlargement of the chambers. Cardiac catheterization demonstrates pressure changes in the chambers as well as the findings after contrast dye injection. Typical findings for these studies are presented in Table 29-13.

Medical management of valvular disorders (Table 29-14)

Conservative Management An important aspect of conservative treatment of valvular heart disease is prevention of recurrent rheumatic fever and infective endocarditis. These preventive measures have been

Table 29-14
Medical Management: Valvular Heart Disease

Diagnostic
1. History and physical examination
2. Chest x-ray
3. ECG
4. Echocardiography
5. Cardiac catheterization

Therapeutic (Conservative)
1. Digitalis (see Table 27-21)
2. Diuretics (see Table 27-23)
3. Anticoagulants
4. Antiarrhythmic drugs
5. Propranolol (Inderal)
6. Prophylactic antibiotic therapy
   a. Rheumatic fever (see Table 29-11)
   b. Infective endocarditis (see Table 29-2)

discussed in the sections on Nursing Management of rheumatic fever and endocarditis. Specific treatment of valvular heart disease depends on the client's clinical manifestations. If manifestations of congestive heart disease develop, digitalis, diuretics, and a low-sodium diet are recommended. Anticoagulant therapy is used to prevent and treat systemic or pulmonary embolization. It is also used as a prophylactic measure in individuals with atrial fibrillation. Arrhythmias, especially atrial arrhythmias, are common with valvular heart disease. They are treated with digitalis, antiarrhythmic drugs such as quinidine, and electrical cardioversion. Propranolol (Inderal) may be used to slow the ventricular rate in individuals with atrial fibrillation.

Iron preparations and folic acid therapy may be indicated for the treatment of anemia. Hemolytic anemia may result from the breakdown of red blood cells secondary to the trauma of blood turbulence in the area of the diseased valve. If infective endocarditis develops, it needs to be treated promptly. Treatment is based on identification of the organism and appropriate antibiotic therapy.

Surgical Management The types of heart surgery are discussed in Chap. 28. This section will briefly describe specific surgical interventions for valve disease. Surgery is indicated when conservative therapy no longer relieves the client's symptoms or when there is increasing evidence of progressive heart failure (e.g., increasing enlargement of the heart). The type of surgery performed depends on the severity of the disease and on the valves involved.

A *mitral commissurotomy* (valvulotomy) involves surgical splitting of the fused valve leaflets (commissures). It may be performed as a *closed* or *open* operation. The closed commissurotomy may be performed as a transatrial finger fracture (breaking apart); more commonly, however, it is done by the transventricular method (Fig. 29-8). A dilator is inserted through the apex of the left ventricle; guidance is provided by a finger inserted into the mitral orifice. The fused valves are separated, and the mitral orifice is dilated.

An open commissurotomy involves using the heart-lung bypass and provides the surgeon with a better view of the valve. In this approach, a knife is used to split or incise the commissures.

Commissurotomy surgery is a palliative procedure. It is indicated only for pure mitral stenosis with no calcification or history of emboli formation. Over a period of time the disease progresses, and valve replacement is usually necessary.

If the mitral valve shows evidence of calcification or mitral insufficiency, open heart surgery is needed to replace the diseased valve with a *prosthetic valve.* Advanced aortic valve disease is also treated with prosthetic valve replacement.

Prosthetic valves have improved since the first caged-ball valve was introduced in 1952. Early valves disintegrated, stuck, became incompetent, changed the structure of chambers, caused emboli, and traumatized blood cells.[21] Newer valves and improved surgical techniques have made valve replacement safer and long-term valvular functioning more effective.[22] Commonly used prosthetic valves today are pyrolite tilting-disk valves, porcine heterografts, beef pericardial valves, and ball-in-cage valves (Fig. 29-9).

Valvuloplasty (repair of the valve) is another surgical procedure that may be done. It is primarily performed to treat mitral regurgitation. The main advantage of a reparative procedure is that it avoids the risks associated with valve replacement. The disadvantage is that it may not be possible to establish total valve competence.

Nursing management

Health Promotion and Maintenance Prevention of acquired rheumatic valvular disease is achieved by (1) diagnosing and treating the streptococcal infection (see the sections on Diagnostic Study Abnormalities and Medical and Pharmacological Management of rheumatic fever) and (2) providing prophylactic antibiotics for individuals with a history of rheumatic fever (see the section on Health Promotion and Maintenance in rheumatic fever). Individuals at risk for endocarditis must also be treated with prophylactic antibiotics (see the section on Pharmacological Intervention in infective endocarditis).

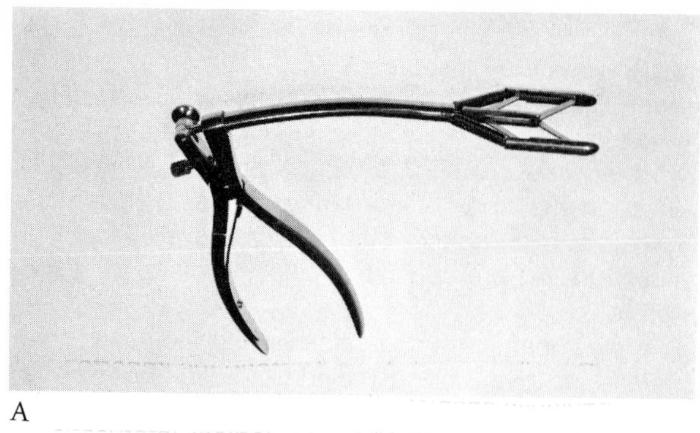

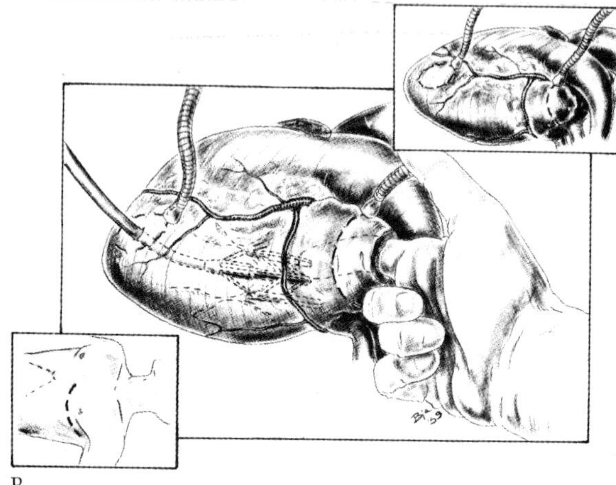

Figure 29-8 Mitral commissurotomy. *(a)* Tubb's mitral valve dilator, used for closed mitral commissurotomy. *(b)* Transventricular mitral valvulotomy. It is important to advance the dilator into the mitral valve under the control of the right index finger. [*From J. W. Hurst et al.* (*eds.*), *The Heart, 3d ed., McGraw-Hill Book Company, New York, 1974, p. 973.*]

Ongoing nursing involvement in client and family education is important to facilitate the client's adherence to these recommended therapies. Individuals with a history of rheumatic fever, endocarditis, and CHD need to know the symptoms suggestive of valvular disease so that they can obtain early medical treatment.

Acute and Chronic Management A client with progressive valvular heart disease may require hospi-

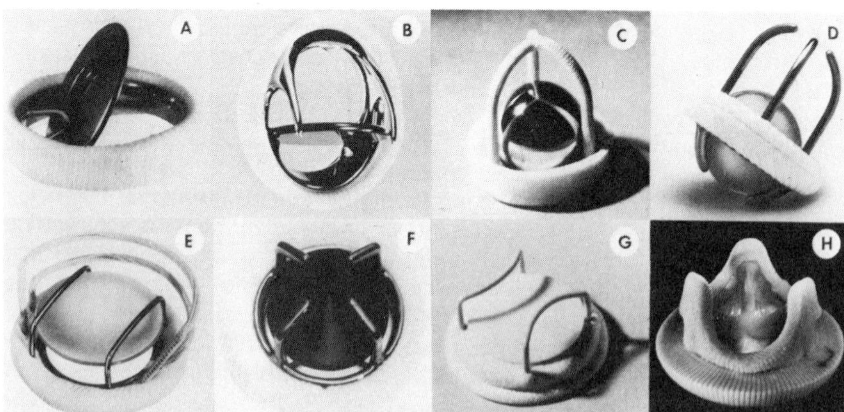

Figure 29-9 Commonly used prosthetic valves. *(a)* Bjork-Shiley aortic. *(b)* Lilehiei-Kaster aortic. *(c)* Starr-Edwards 2320 aortic. *(d)* Smeloff-Cutter. *(e)* Kay-Shiley mital. *(f)* Cooley-Cutter. *(g)* Beall. *(h)* Hancock porcire mitral. [*From J. W. Hurst et al.* (*eds.*), *The Heart, 4th ed., McGraw-Hill Book Company, New York, 1978, p. 1061.*]

talization or ongoing outpatient care for congestive heart failure, endocarditis, embolic disease, or dysrhythmias. Congestive heart failure is the most common reason for ongoing medical care. (See Chap. 27 for Medical and Nursing Management in congestive heart failure.)

Nurses need to help clients achieve and maintain their optimal level of health despite the valvular disorder. Their body weight should be kept within normal limits. The diet should be well balanced nutritionally, with sodium restricted to prevent fluid retention. Daily weights should be taken to detect fluid retention.

Smoking should be discouraged. Exercise should be designed to take account of the client's limitations. An appropriate exercise plan can increase cardiac tolerance. Strenuous physical exercise should be avoided, as damaged valves may not be able to handle the required increase in cardiac output. Vocational counseling may be necessary if the person has a physically or emotionally demanding job. The client should be helped to plan his activities of daily living with an emphasis on conserving energy, setting priorities, and taking planned rest periods.

The nurse has an important role in evaluating the effectiveness of medical therapy. The heart rate and rhythm should be monitored to evaluate the effectiveness of digitalis, propranolol, and antiarrhythmic drugs. Urinary output and daily weight should be monitored when diuretics are used. When anticoagulants are used, the client should be instructed about possible side effects, such as bleeding.

The client needs to understand the importance of prophylactic antibiotic therapy to prevent endocarditis (see the section on Pharmacological Intervention in infective endocarditis). If the valve disease was caused by rheumatic fever, prophylaxis to prevent a recurrence will be necessary.

When valvular heart disease can no longer be managed conservatively, surgical intervention will be necessary. (The surgical treatment of valve disease is discussed in Chap. 28.)

Case Study / Valvular Heart Disease

Mrs. S. is a 54-year-old married woman who has received medical care for 10 years. She was told that she had had strep throat as a child. Her rheumatic valve disease was diagnosed 10 years ago when she complained of a persistent cold, palpitations, and ankle edema. A chest x-ray and ECG revealed an enlarged left atrium. Auscultation revealed murmurs of mitral stenosis, mitral insufficiency, and aortic insufficiency.

Now she presents to the physician's office with an irregular pulse, increasing shortness of breath, and edema. She cannot even make the bed without becoming dyspneic. Her physical examination is unchanged, although she has a few rales in the lung bases. She takes Digoxin 0.25 mg twice a day.

Discussion Questions

1. Explain the etiology of her valvular heart disease. What valves are most likely to become involved with rheumatic heart disease?
2. Differentiate between the pathological characteristics and the clinical manifestations of mitral stenosis and mitral regurgitation.
3. Which other diagnostic procedures would be recommended, and what might they indicate?
4. In addition to Digoxin, what other conservative treatment measures are usually indicated for valvular heart disease?
5. What are the various types of valve surgery? Which ones would be indicated for Mrs. S.?

REVIEW QUESTIONS

The number of the question corresponds to the same numbered objective at the beginning of the chapter.

1. The usual treatment for pericarditis includes
   a. pain relief and anti-inflammatory drugs
   b. antibiotics and aspirin
   c. antipyretics and antifungal agents
   d. nitroglycerin and aspirin

2. Prophylactic antibiotic therapy is indicated to prevent endocarditis for high-risk individuals who
   a. are undergoing any dental procedure
   b. have acquired a viral upper respiratory tract infection
   c. are in the last 3 months of pregnancy
   d. are traveling to a foreign country

3. Myocarditis most commonly is caused by
   a. acute MI
   b. systemic viral infection
   c. congestive heart failure
   d. cardiac tamponade

4. Rheumatic heart disease is caused by
   a. group B beta-hemolytic streptococcal infection
   b. echoviral infection
   c. group A beta-hemolytic streptococcal infection
   d. staphylococcal infection

5. Causes of valvular heart disease may include all the following *except*
a. rheumatic fever
b. infective endocarditis
c. myocarditis
d. idiopathic aortic stenosis

6. Valvular regurgitation of the mitral valve would eventually lead to
a. muscular hypertrophy of the right atrium
b. muscular hypertrophy of the right ventricle
c. dilatation of the left ventricle
d. dilatation of the left atrium

7. Surgical splitting of the valve leaflets is called a
a. curettage
b. leaflet dilatation
c. valvuloplasty
d. commissurotomy

REFERENCES

1. N. K. Wenger et al. (eds.), *Cardiology for Nurses,* McGraw-Hill Book Company, New York, 1980, p. 435.
2. Ibid., p. 438.
3. "Prevention of Bacterial Endocarditis," *Circulation,* **56:**:139A (1977). Reprinted by the American Heart Association.
4. S. J. Moore, "Pericarditis after Acute Myocardial Infarction: Manifestations and Nursing Implications," *Heart and Lung,* **8:**551–558 (1979).
5. E. Braunwald, "Pericardial Disease," in K. Isselbacher et al. (eds.), *Harrison's Principles of Internal Medicine,* 9th ed., McGraw-Hill Book Company, New York, 1980, pp. 1149–1156.
6. Wenger et al., op. cit., p. 475.
7. G. W. Zeluff et al., "Pericarditis in Renal Failure," *Heart and Lung,* **8:**1139–1145 (1979).
8. Braunwald, op. cit., p. 1154.
9. K. Duffy, "A Severe Case of Viral Myocarditis," *AJN,* **81:**1148–1151 (1981).
10. Wenger et al., op. cit., pp. 452–454.
11. G. Glick and E. Braunwald, "The Cardiomyopathies and Myocartides," in Isselbacher et al., op. cit., pp. 1141–1147.
12. Wenger et al., op. cit., p. 352.
13. G. H. Stollerman, "Rheumatic Fever," in Isselbacher et al., op. cit., pp. 1090–1095.
14. A. Moss et al., *Heart Disease in Infants, Children and Adolescents,* The Williams & Wilkins Company, Baltimore, 1977, p. 8.
15. G. B. Avery (ed.), *Neonatology,* J. B. Lippincott Company, Philadelphia, 1975, p. 687.
16. A. C. de Leon, "Mitral Valve Prolapse," *Postgrad Med,* **1:**66 (1980).
17. R. M. Jeresaty, "Sudden Death in the Mitral Valve Prolapse—Click Syndrome," *Am J Cardiol,* **37:**317 (1976).
18. J. W. Hurst et al. (eds.), *The Heart,* 4th ed., McGraw-Hill Book Company, New York, 1978, p. 1660.
19. S. Price and L. Wilson, *Pathophysiology: Clinical Concepts of Disease Processes,* McGraw-Hill Book Company, New York, 1978, p. 358.
20. Wenger et al., op. cit., p. 365.
21. Hurst et al., op. cit., p. 1061.
22. E. Murphy and F. Kloster, "Late Results of Valve Replacement Surgery," *Mod Concepts Cardiovasc Dis,* **48:**53 (1979).

Chapter 30

NURSING ROLE IN MANAGEMENT

Vascular Disorders

Sally J. Ness

Learning Objectives

1. Describe the pathophysiology, clinical manifestations, and surgical management of aortic aneurysms.
2. Describe the preoperative and postoperative care of the client undergoing aortic aneurysmectomy.
3. Describe the pathophysiology, clinical manifestations, and management of aortic dissection and acute and chronic aortic bifurcation occlusion.
4. Describe the pathophysiology, clinical manifestations, and medical and surgical management of peripheral arterial disorders.
5. Explain the nursing management of the client with chronic arterial insufficiency.
6. Describe the pathophysiology, clinical manifestations, and management of acute arterial occlusive disorder, thromboangiitis obliterans, and Raynaud's phenomenon.
7. Describe the risk factors, pathogenesis, clinical manifestations, and medical and surgical management of thrombophlebitis.
8. Explain the purpose and actions of commonly used anticoagulants and the nursing role for clients receiving them.
9. Describe the pathophysiology, clinical manifestations, and medical and nursing management of varicose veins and stasis ulcers.
10. Describe the pathophysiology, clinical manifestations, and medical and nursing management of pulmonary emboli.

Problems of the vascular system include disorders of the aorta, arteries, and veins. *Peripheral vascular disease* is a term used to describe a wide variety of conditions affecting the arteries, veins, and lymphatic vessels of the extremities.

DISORDERS OF THE AORTA*

Aneurysms

Aneurysms are outpouchings or dilatations of the arterial wall and are a common problem involving the aorta. Aneurysms of peripheral arteries can also occur but are far less common. The dilatation may involve one or all layers of the arterial wall (Fig. 25-7 shows the layers of the artery). Aneurysms occur in males more often than in females, and their incidence increases with age.[1] They are seen most often in clients who are 70 to 80 years old, and are considered uncommon before the age of 50. It is significant that one-half of all aneurysms greater than 6 cm ($2\frac{3}{8}$ inches) in diameter rupture within 1 year.[2,3]

Pathophysiology

Although aneurysms have a variety of causes, the two most common are atherosclerosis and syphilis. Atherosclerosis can affect the entire length of the aorta. However, most aneurysms related to atherosclerosis are found in the abdominal aorta below the level of the renal arteries. Plaques composed of lipids adhere to the subintimal layer of the aorta. Plaque formation causes degenerative changes in the medial arterial wall leading to a loss of elasticity, weakening, and eventual dilation of the aorta.[4] (See Chap. 27 for a discussion of the pathogenesis of atherosclerosis.)

At one time, syphilis was considered the major cause of all aneurysm formation. However, today, with early detection and improved health practices, syphilitic aneurysms are uncommon. When they do appear, they primarily involve the thoracic aorta. Atherosclerosis is now a more common cause of thoracic aneurysms than syphilis.[5]

Other causes of aneurysm formation include infections such as tuberculosis and bacterial endocarditis, congenital disorders such as coarctation of the aorta, and trauma.[6] A motor vehicle accident can produce blunt trauma damaging the intima of the aorta. Sharp trauma from needles and gunshot wounds can puncture all three layers of the vessel wall.

Factors common to aneurysms are degeneration of the medial layer of the artery and loss of elasticity. As these conditions occur, the pulsation of the blood places added stress on the already weakened vessel and causes it to increase in size. Aneurysms can grow at a very constant rate. Eventual rupture of the aneurysm is inevitable, but the rate of progression is highly variable.

*This section was written by Barbara G. Whitten, R.N., B.S., CVNS, formerly Cardiovascular Nurse Specialist, Fondren Cardiovascular Intensive Care Unit, The Methodist Hospital, Houston, Texas.

Classification of aneurysms

Aneurysms are generally divided into two basic classifications, *true* and *false*. A true aneurysm is one in which the wall of the artery forms the aneurysm, with at least one vessel layer still intact. Most commonly caused by atherosclerosis, three-fourths of true aneurysms occur in the abdomen and one-fourth in the thoracic aorta (Figs. 30-1 and 30-2). In a false aneurysm (pseudoaneurysm), all the layers of the vessel are involved and the blood escapes into the surrounding area. A clot forms which may or may not pulsate. False aneurysms are usually caused by trauma.

Three basic types of true aneurysms are *fusiform, saccular,* and *dissecting* (Fig. 30-3). The fusiform aneurysm involves the entire circumference of the artery and maintains a uniform shape. The saccular aneurysm is pouchlike and has a narrow neck connecting the bulge to one side of the artery wall. Dissecting aneurysms produce separation of the intima from the medial layer of the artery, and a false lumen is formed as blood is forced between the layers through a small tear in the intima.

Aortic aneurysms are also classified according to their anatomical location. Hence, they are referred to as *thoracic*, *abdominal*, and *thoracoabdominal* aneurysms. The very unusual thoracoabdominal aneurysm is most likely caused by syphilis. The most common location for aneurysm formation is the abdominal aorta below the level of the renal arteries.

Clinical manifestations

When manifestations of aneurysms occur, they are related to the anatomical site of the aneurysms. As the aneurysm increases in size, it causes pressure on surrounding structures resulting in a variety of manifestations.

Abdominal aneurysms are usually asymptomatic. When they are symptomatic, the client may complain of back or abdominal pain. Occasionally, the client may complain of epigastric discomfort or may show symptoms of intestinal obstruction. Males may have problems with sexual function. On physical examination, a mass in the periumbilical area or slightly to the left of the midline is frequently detected. Bruits (pulsatile sounds heard upon auscultation) are usually found over the mass. A pulsation may be felt with gentle palpation of the abdomen. Femoral pulses are diminished in some clients.

Thoracic aneurysms are usually asymptomatic. When manifestations are present, they are quite varied. The most common manifestation is deep, diffuse chest pain. Aneurysms located in the ascending aorta and the arch can produce hoarseness in the client due to pressure on the recurrent laryngeal nerve. Pressure on the esophagus can cause dysphagia. If the aneurysm presses on the superior vena cava, it can cause distended neck veins and edema of the head and arms. Pressure of the aneurysm on pulmonary structures can lead to coughing, dyspnea, and airway obstruction.[7]

Complications

Complications related to aneurysms are catastrophic, the most common being rupture. Constant midabdominal, lumbar, or pelvic pain of recent onset may be a warning sign of impending rupture. Once rupture has occurred, the client will present with pain and manifestations of shock such as tachycardia, hypotension, pale clammy skin, decreased urine output, and altered sensorium.

Paraplegia is also a devastating problem. If the blood supply to the spinal cord is severely compromised secondary to rupture, prolonged hypotension, or prolonged clamp time during surgery, the client may develop permanent paralysis. Paraplegia is generally uncommon in abdominal aortic aneurysms.

Diagnostic study abnormalities

Most aneurysms are found on routine physical or x-ray examination. Chest x-rays are useful in demonstrating the mediastinal silhouette and any abnormal widening. A plain film of the abdomen may show calcification within the wall of the aneurysm.

When an electrocardiogram is performed, it is used to rule out evidence of myocardial infarction since some individuals may present with symptoms related to angina. Echocardiography assists in the diagnosis of aortic insufficiency related to ascending aortic dilatation. Ultrasonography may be used to confirm the presence of an abdominal aneurysm.

Aortography is performed to confirm the diagnosis and to locate the exact position of the aneurysm. Any structures receiving their arterial blood supply from the affected part of the aorta are carefully studied with aortography.

Aortography is done using local anesthesia. A large needle with a stylet is inserted into the femoral artery, although the subclavian, axillary, or brachial arteries may also be used. A catheter is inserted and threaded up the artery through the needle. Contrast medium is then injected, and views are taken under fluoroscopy. When all the films have been taken, the catheter is removed. Pressure is applied over the puncture site for 20 minutes or until the bleeding has stopped.

After the procedure, the client should be kept on

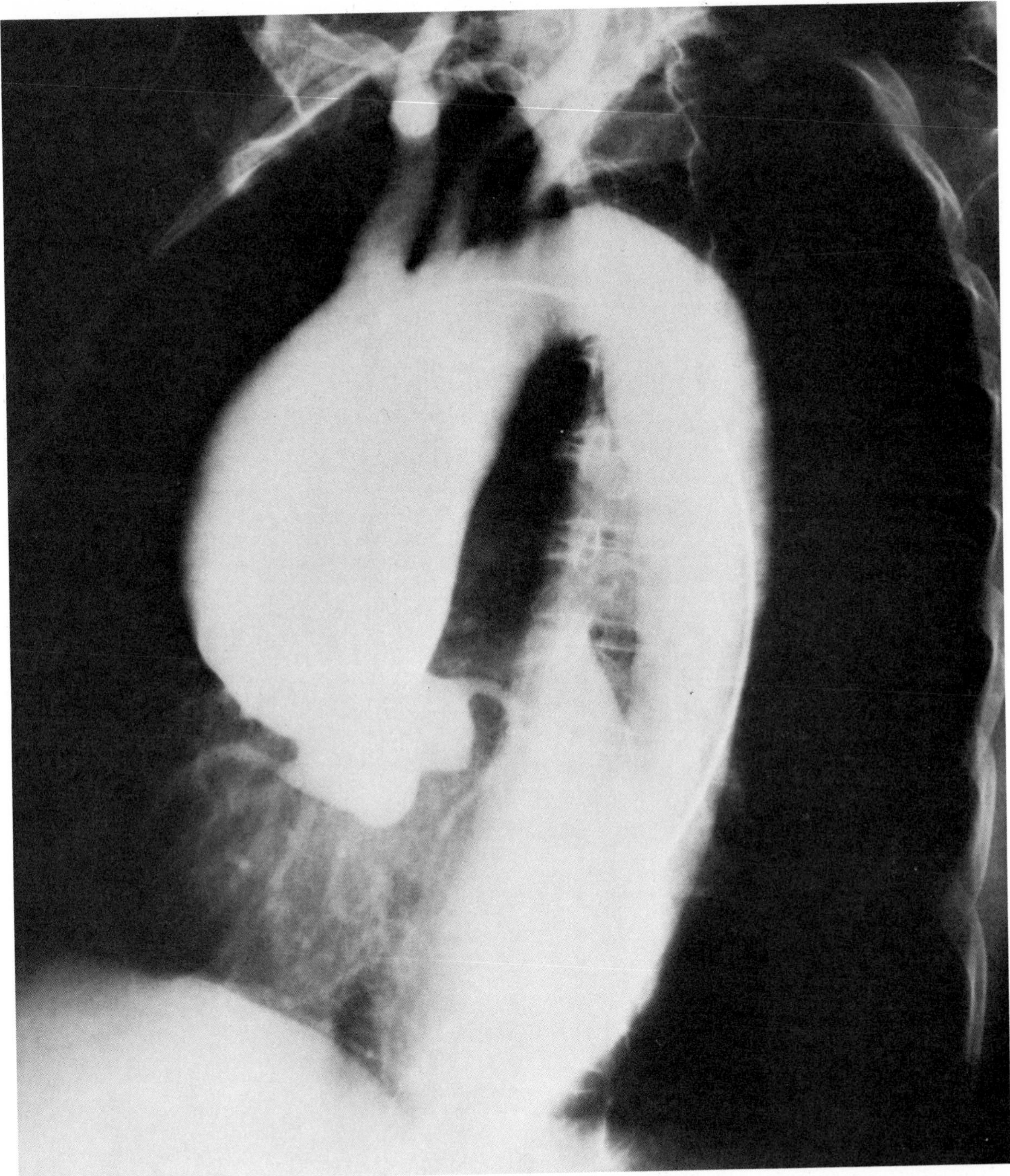

Figure 30-1 Fusiform aneurysm of the ascending aorta. *(Courtesy of Dr. John Roehns, The Methodist Hospital, Houston, Texas.)*

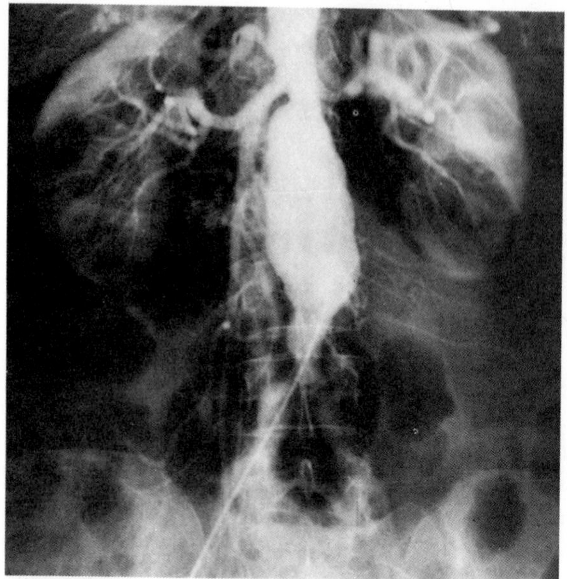

Figure 30-2 Fusiform aneurysm of the abdominal aorta. (*Courtesy of Dr. John Roehm, The Methodist Hospital, Houston, Texas.*)

bed rest and flat if the femoral site is used for injection. Frequent observation of the arterial puncture site is essential in order to detect any bleeding. The peripheral pulses should be checked at the same time since embolism or vasospasm may occur, blocking arterial flow to the involved arm or leg.

Medical and surgical management

The goal of medical management is to prevent rupture of the aneurysm. Therefore, early detection and prompt treatment of the client are imperative (Table 30-1). Once an aneurysm is suspected, studies are performed to determine its exact size and location. A careful review of all body systems is necessary to identify any coexisting disorders. The carotid and coronary arteries should be assessed for indications of atherosclerotic disease. If obstructions in these vessels are present, they may need to be corrected prior to aneurysmectomy.[8] Generally, if no other problems, such as severe debilitation, exist, surgery is the treatment of choice. The type of surgery depends on the location of the aneurysm (Table 30-2).

The only effective treatment of an aortic aneurysm

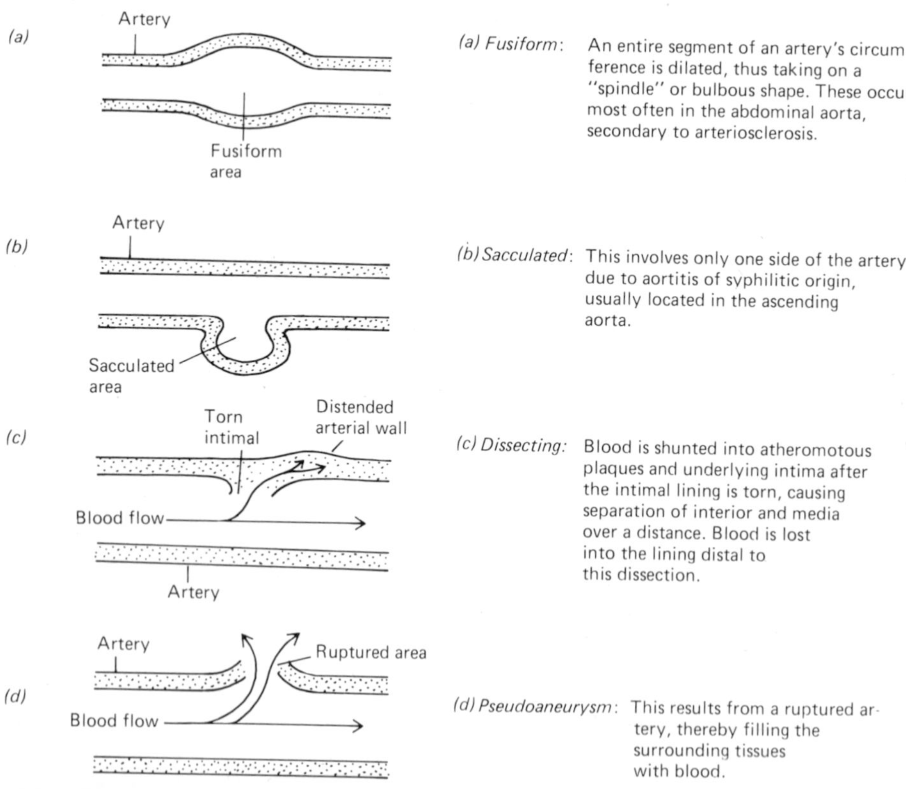

(a)
Artery
Fusiform area
(a) Fusiform: An entire segment of an artery's circumference is dilated, thus taking on a "spindle" or bulbous shape. These occur most often in the abdominal aorta, secondary to arteriosclerosis.
(b)
Artery
Sacculated area
(b) Sacculated: This involves only one side of the artery due to aortitis of syphilitic origin, usually located in the ascending aorta.
(c)
Torn intimal
Distended arterial wall
Blood flow
Artery
(c) Dissecting: Blood is shunted into atheromotous plaques and underlying intima after the intimal lining is torn, causing separation of interior and media over a distance. Blood is lost into the lining distal to this dissection.
(d)
Artery
Ruptured area
Blood flow
(d) Pseudoaneurysm: This results from a ruptured artery, thereby filling the surrounding tissues with blood.

Figure 30-3 Four basic types of aneurysms. *[From J. Barry, Emergency Nursing, McGraw-Hill Book Company, New York, 1978, p. 211.]*

Table 30-1
Medical Management: Aortic Aneurysm

Diagnostic
1. History and physical examination
2. Chest x-ray
3. Plain film of the abdomen
4. Ultrasonography
5. Aortography
6. Echocardiography

Therapeutic
1. Aortic aneurysm resection (see Table 30-2)
2. Control of the atherosclerotic disease process (see Chap. 27 and Table 27-4)

is surgery. In saccular aneurysms, it may be possible to apply an occluding clamp across the narrow neck of the aneurysm and then perform an excision of the lesion. Repair of the aorta is done by using a patch graft if necessary.[9] In a fusiform aneurysm, the entire involved segment of the aorta is removed and replaced by a graft (Fig. 30-4).

Prior to surgery, every effort is made to bring the client to the best possible state of hydration and electrolyte balance. Any abnormalities in coagulation and blood count are corrected. Clients receive antibiotics, enemas, and baths with antiseptics prior to surgery. However, if the aneurysm has ruptured, the treatment of choice is immediate surgical intervention. Even with prompt care, the mortality rate is very high following rupture.

During aneurysmectomy, woven Dacron grafts are used for segmental replacement of the aorta. These grafts come in various sizes and shapes, such as the tube or Y form. All resections require cross-clamping of the aorta proximal and distal to the lesion. Great care is necessary to prevent ischemia to vital organs and to the spinal cord.

If the aorta is cross-clamped above the renal arteries during surgery, these arteries must be evaluated quickly for patency prior to the closure of the operative site. Patency of the renal arteries can be assessed by injection of intravenous indigo-carmine or methylene blue dye following removal of the aortic vascular clamp. If the urinary output is shaded in the dye's color, then adequate perfusion to the kidneys is ensured.

All clients undergoing aneurysmectomy should be placed in an intensive care unit with appropriate support services and equipment. Upon arrival in the intensive care unit, an endotracheal tube, an arterial line, a central venous pressure line, peripheral intravenous lines, a Foley catheter, and a nasogastric tube will be in place. If the thorax was entered during

Table 30-2
Types of Aortic Aneurysm Resection

Location of Aneurysm	Incision Site	Use of Bypass or Hypothermia	Special Considerations
Ascending aorta with aortic valve Insufficiency	Median sternotomy	Cardiopulmonary bypass and hypothermia.	If aortic valvular insufficiency is severe, prosthetic valve replacement is performed.
Aortic arch	Median sternotomy	Cardiopulmonary bypass and hypothermia. If transverse aorta containing brachiocephalic vessels is involved, extracorporeal perfusion of the brain is necessary.	Cold predisposes client to arrhythmias. Watch neurological signs.
Descending thoracic aorta	Posterolateral at 4th intercostal space	Hypothermia. Cardiopulmonary bypass may be used.	Carlen's tube (double-cuffed endotracheal tube) deflates either lung and causes pulmonary stress and atelectasis. Good pulmonary care is important. Ischemia to the spinal cord is common.
Abdominal aortic aneurysm	Xiphoid process to pubis	None. Arterial blood flow to lower extremities can be interrupted for the time needed for the surgical procedure.	Graft is placed within cleaned artery walls. This technique prevents graft from eroding into bowel and causes an aortoduodenal fistula.

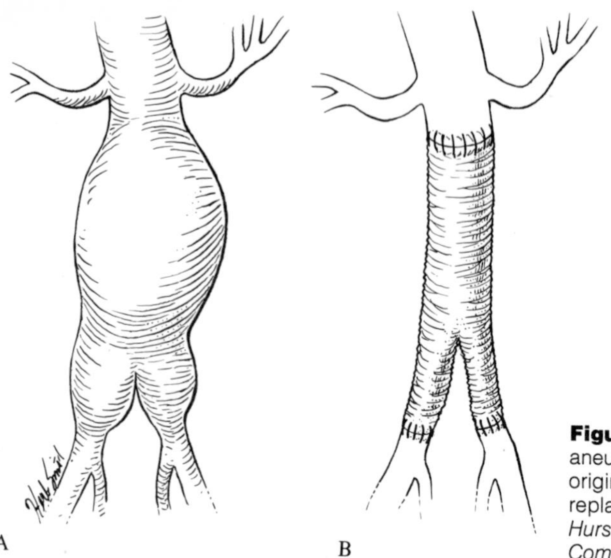

Figure 30-4 (*a*) Characteristic type of arteriosclerotic aneurysm of the abdominal aorta arising just below the origin of the renal arteries. (*b*) Treated by resection and replacement with a bifurcation Dacron graft. [*From J. W. Hurst et al. (eds.), The Heart, 4th ed., McGraw-Hill Book Company, New York, 1978, p. 1919.*]

surgery, chest tubes will be in place. Often, a pulmonary arterial catheter will be inserted.

Nursing management

Health Promotion and Maintenance The client with an aneurysm may present with a variety of manifestations or may be totally asymptomatic. Therefore, the nurse must utilize assessment skills to focus on early detection and treatment. Clients should be urged to receive regular routine physical examinations and should be reminded that any symptom, no matter how minor, must be investigated if it persists.

The incidence of syphilitic aneurysms has declined primarily because people are generally more aware of the manifestations of venereal disease and seek treatment earlier. Nurses need to encourage such individuals and their contacts to obtain appropriate therapeutic intervention in the course of the disease process. (Sexually transmitted diseases are discussed in Chap. 45.)

Nurses must be aware of cardiovascular disease risk factors and alert for opportunities to teach health measures to clients in the hospital and the community. (Risk factors and the prevention of cardiovascular diseases are discussed in Chap. 27.) Trauma victims should be urged to seek medical attention even in the absence of symptoms.

Preoperative Care The nursing role during the preoperative period should include teaching, providing support for the client and his family, and careful assessment of all body systems. It is imperative that problems be identified early and proper intervention instituted. (General preoperative care of the client is discussed in Chap. 6.)

A thorough nursing history and assessment should be performed. Since most aneurysms are atherosclerotic, it is likely that the disease process has spread throughout the body. Therefore, it is important for the nurse to watch for signs of cardiac, pulmonary, cerebral, and peripheral vascular problems. Clients should be monitored for signs of rupture of the aneurysm.

Establishing a data baseline is important for later postoperative assessment and intervention. In addition to gathering data, the nurse should observe the client closely for subtle abnormalities. Special attention should be paid to the character and quality of the peripheral pulses, the voice, and the neurological status. Arterial pulse sites in the lower extremities should be marked prior to surgery.

Postoperative Care General postoperative care is discussed in Chap. 8. In addition to maintaining adequate respiratory function, fluid and electrolyte balance, and pain control, the nurse needs to promote graft patency, adequate renal perfusion, and optimal circulation. The nurse can also assist in preventing ventricular arrhythmias, infections, and neurological complications (Table 30-3).

Maintenance of graft patency

It is important to maintain the patency of the graft. It should not be allowed to leak or to develop clots. An

Table 30-3
Nursing Care Plan for the Client after Aneurysmectomy

Client Problem	Expected Outcome	Nursing Intervention
Decreased blood flow through graft	Patent graft with good arterial blood flow.	Assess BP and all peripherial pulses every hour initially and then with decreasing frequency (e.g., every 2 h, every 4 h). Compare extremities for warmth and color. Administer IV fluids at prescribed rates. Check CVP readings hourly.
Ventricular arrhythmias	Client's normal preoperative rhythm.	Apply hyperthermia blanket to maintain temperature at about 37°C. Administer O_2 as ordered via ventilator or O_2 mask. Monitor the results of ABGs and serum electrolytes. Keep lidocaine 100 mg IV bolus at bedside for PVCs and administer as needed.
Potential hemorrhage	Hct, BP, and pulse rate within normal range.	Keep 4 units of packed RBCs available at all times. Observe drainage of chest tube (if inserted) for excessive bleeding. Monitor CVP, BP, and HR every hour and then with decreasing frequency. Check Hgb and Hct every 4–6 h and prn. Observe abdomen and record girth if distension appears to be developing.
Potential infection	Normal body temperature. No signs of infection.	Administer broad-spectrum antibiotics as ordered. Monitor temperature at least every 4 h. Monitor the results of the WBC count. Use aseptic technique in caring for any indwelling IV line, tubing, or catheter.
Paralytic ileus	Normal bowel sounds.	Attach NG tube to low suction. Irrigate with normal saline as needed and record drainage. Give frequent oral care while client is NPO. Auscultate for bowel sounds every 4–8 h. Palpate abdomen for distension. Encourage early ambulation when possible.
Decreasing level of consciousness	Return to normal neurological status.	Check chart for preoperative neurological status. Assess neurological status, including level of consciousness, pupil size and response to light, movement of extremities, and hand grasp.
Decreasing urinary output	Urine output of ≥ 30 mL/h.	Administer IV fluids as ordered. Check and record hourly urinary outputs and CVP reading. Monitor daily BUN and serum creatinine studies.
Atelectasis	Lungs clear to auscultation.	Initially auscultate lungs every 4 h for breath sounds, then every shift thereafter. Encourage turning, coughing and deep breathing every 2 h. Teach client to cough effectively (Table 21-9). Administer pain medication prior to coughing and deep-breathing exercises. Use IPPB or incentive spirometer as ordered.

adequate systemic blood pressure must be maintained at all times in order to fill the graft and to keep the vessel taut.

Frequent nursing observation of the blood pressure can be accomplished by observation of the oscilloscope since the client should arrive from the operating room with an arterial line in place. The accuracy of monitor readings should be checked at least once each shift by cuff pressure readings. Patency of the arterial line is maintained by irrigation with a heparinized solution.

Intravenous fluids and blood components must be infused at the prescribed rate in order to prevent hypovolemia. Central venous pressure readings should be determined hourly to help assess the client's state of hydration.

Prevention of ventricular arrhythmias

Ventricular arrhythmias are usually caused by hypoxia, hypothermia, or unrecognized electrolyte imbalances. Clients with generalized vascular disease such as atherosclerosis are very prone to arrhythmias. Nursing interventions include cardiac monitoring and monitoring the results of electrolyte studies and arterial blood gas determinations. Individuals who return from surgery with decreased body temperatures should be placed on hyperthermia blankets. Urinary output also needs to be monitored carefully.

Prevention of infection

Clients with prosthetic vascular grafts are very susceptible to infections. Nursing intervention to prevent infection should include ensuring that the client receives a broad-spectrum antibiotic as prescribed to maintain adequate blood levels of the drug. It is important to regularly assess body temperatures and to report any elevations. Laboratory data should be monitored since a rising white blood cell count may be the first indication of an infection.

All intravenous and arterial line sites should be maintained carefully using sterile technique. Incisions should be kept clean and dry.

Maintenance of gastrointestinal status

During abdominal aneurysmectomy, the arterial supply to the bowel may be disrupted, resulting in ischemia or death of intestinal tissue. This is evidenced by lack of bowel sounds, fever, abdominal distension, and diarrheal stool. More commonly, paralytic ileus develops due to the need for displacement of the intestines for long periods of time during surgery. The intestines may become swollen and bruised, and peristalsis may cease for variable intervals.

A nasogastric tube is inserted and connected to low, intermittent suction. This decompresses the stomach and duodenum, prevents aspiration of stomach contents, and decreases pressure on suture lines. The nasogastric tube should be irrigated with normal saline as needed and the amount and character of the drainage recorded. The nurse should auscultate for the return of bowel sounds. The passing of flatus can also be a sign of returning bowel function and should be reported. While the client is NPO, good mouth care should be given every few hours.

Maintenance of neurological status

Neurological complications can occur following surgical procedures on the aorta, especially when the ascending and aortic arches are involved. Nursing intervention should include assessment of neurological signs (hourly initially after surgery and frequently thereafter), including level of consciousness, pupil size and response to light, ability to move all extremities, and quality of hand grasps (see Chap. 48). These should be recorded in detail, with a careful description of the client's response. Any function decreased from the baseline assessment should be reported to the physician immediately.

Clients who develop paraplegia need a great deal of reassurance and the opportunity to express their feelings. Long-term physical therapy and psychological support must be included in the nursing care of these individuals.

Maintenance of optimal circulation

The anatomical location of the aneurysm will indicate the areas of major concern related to circulatory status. All peripheral pulses should be checked and their presence and quality recorded. This should be done every hour for the first 24 hours and routinely thereafter at frequent intervals. Pulses to be assessed include the dorsalis pedis, posterior tibial, popliteal, and femoral as well as the brachial, radial, carotid, and temporal pulses (Fig. 25-8).

When checking the pulses, the nurse should mark their location lightly with a ballpoint or felt-tip pen so that others can find them easily. It is also important to note the temperature, color, and movement of the extremities.

It is common for pulses in the lower extremities to be absent for a brief period following surgery. This is usually due to vasospasm and hypothermia. A decreased or absent pulse in conjunction with a cool, pale, or mottled extremity may indicate embolization or occlusion of the graft.

Maintenance of adequate renal perfusion

One cause of decreased renal perfusion is the possible dislodgment of a fragment from the aortic and subsequent lodging of the bifurcation of the renal arteries. This can cause obstruction and ischemia of one or both kidneys. Hypotension and poor hydration can also lead to decreased renal perfusion.

An accurate record of urinary output should be kept. If it falls below 30 mL/hour for 2 consecutive hours, the physician should be notified. Central venous pressure readings also give important information regarding hydration. Daily blood urea nitrogen (BUN) and serum creatinine studies are performed to evaluate renal function.

Chronic Management The client may be apprehensive about returning home after major surgery involving the aorta. He should be encouraged to express his concerns and should be reassured that he can return to activities of normal living. The client should be taught to observe for changes in color or warmth of the extremities. He can also be taught to take his peripheral pulses and to assess changes in their quality.

If the graft extends into the knee area, prolonged sitting or deep knee bends should be avoided. If the client also has peripheral arterial occlusive disease, he should be taught measures to increase the circulation and to prevent skin breakdown. (See the section on Chronic Arterial Occlusive Disease.)

Aortic Dissection (Dissecting Aneurysm)

Dissecting aneurysm of the aorta is a longitudinal splitting of the medial layer by a column of blood. An aneurysm is often not present prior to the dissection. Aortic dissection affects men more often than women and occurs most frequently between the fourth and seventh decades of life. Among untreated individuals, 50 percent will die within 48 hours of dissection.[10]

Pathophysiology

Dissection of an artery begins when a small tear develops in the intimal layer of the arterial wall. Blood begins to penetrate between the vessel layers, causing the intima and media to be separated. As the heart contracts, each systolic pulsation will cause increased pressure on the damaged area, which further increases the dissection. This splitting of the layers causes a false lumen to be formed. Occasionally, a small tear will develop distally, and the blood flow will reenter the true vessel lumen. Those areas which receive their arterial blood supply from the involved segment of the aortia will develop signs of circulatory insufficiency.

Arterial dissection differs from an aneurysm in that a false lumen is formed by separation of the intima from the media in dissection. In contrast, a true aneurysm is characterized by an outpouching from a weakened medial layer.

The exact etiology of dissection is uncertain. Many authorities believe *cystic medial necrosis* (destruction of the medial layer elastic fibers) to be the leading cause of the problem. Unfortunately, it is asymptomatic and the cause is unknown. Most people with dissection problems have hypertension. Individuals with Marfan's syndrome (a disease of the connective tissue) have a high incidence of dissection. Pregnancy also promotes vascular stress due to increased blood volume. Atherosclerotic ulcerations can produce weakening of the intimal layer and predispose the client to dissection. Areas which seem to suffer from the greatest amount of stress are located above the aortic valve and in the descending aorta near the junction with the left subclavian artery.[11,12]

Classification of dissecting aneurysms

Dissecting aneurysms are usually identified by the DeBakey classification. Type I refers to dissections involving the ascending aorta and the aortic arch and extending into the abdominal aorta. Type II refers to dissections involving only the ascending aorta. Type III aneurysms are located in the portion of the aorta distal to the left subclavian artery and extending distally into the thoracic or abdominal aorta.[13,14]

Clinical manifestations

The client with aortic dissection usually presents with the complaint of severe pain in the back, chest, or abdomen. The pain is described as "tearing" or "ripping." The severe nature of the pain may suggest myocardial infarction. As the dissection progresses, pain may be located both above and below the diaphragm.

If the arch of the aorta is involved, the client may exhibit neurological deficiencies, including an altered level of consciousness, dizziness, and weakened or absent carotid and temporal pulses. An ascending aortic dissection will usually produce some degree of aortic valvular insufficiency, and a murmur will be audible upon auscultation. Severe insufficiency may produce left ventricular failure with the development of dyspnea and orthopnea. When either subclavian artery is involved, pulse quality and blood pressure readings may vary between the left and right arms. As the dissection progresses down the aorta, the lower extremities may begin to demonstrate alterations in circulatory status.

Complications

A severe complication of dissection of the ascending aortic arch is *cardiac tamponade*, which occurs when blood escapes from the dissection into the pericardial sac. Clinical manifestations include narrowed pulse pressure, distended neck veins, muffled heart sounds, and pulsus paradoxus. (Cardiac tamponade is discussed in Chap. 29.)

Because the aorta is weakened by the medial dissection, it may rupture. Hemorrhage may occur into the mediastinal, pleural, or abdominal cavities.

Dissection can lead to occlusion of the arterial supply to many vital organs. The spinal cord, kidneys, and abdominal structures are the organs most commonly affected. Ischemia of the spinal cord produces symptoms of weakness, lack of movement in the lower extremities, and decreased pain sensation. Renal ischemia is usually manifested by low urinary output. The abdomen will show signs of ischemia by decreased bowel sounds and altered bowel habits.

Medical management

Diagnostic The diagnostic studies used to assess dissection of the aorta are similar to those performed for aneurysms (Table 30-4). An electrocardiogram is done to rule out the possibility of a myocardial infarction. Left ventricular hypertrophy is a com-

Table 30-4
Medical Management: Aortic Dissection

Diagnostic

1. History and physical examination
2. Electrocardiography (ECG)
3. Chest x-ray
4. Echocardiography
5. Aortography

Therapeutic

1. Bed rest
2. Pain relief with narcotics
3. Control of BP
   a. Trimethaphan (Arfonad)
   b. Sodium nitroprusside (Nipride)
   c. Methyldopa (Aldomet)
   d. Guanethidine (Ismelin)
4. Propranolol (Inderal)

mon finding and is possibly related to changes caused by systemic hypertension. A chest x-ray may show a widening of the mediastinal silhouette, and left pleural effusion is not uncommon. After the client's condition has stabilized, aortography is necessary to assess the extent of the dissection.

Therapeutic The goal of medical therapy for aortic dissection without complications is to lower the blood pressure and diminish the pulsatile forces within the aorta (Table 30-4). The use of trimethaphan (Arfonad) and nitroprusside (Nipride) intravenously rapidly reduces the blood pressure. Guanethidine (Ismelin) or methyldopa (Aldomet) is administered to provide long-term control. Propranolol (Inderal) is also used to decrease the force of myocardial contractility.

Individuals suffering from dissection without complications can safely be handled medically for a long period of time. Supportive treatment is directed toward pain relief, blood transfusion (if required), and management of heart failure (if indicated). If the dissection is limited to the descending aorta, conservative medical management is usually adequate to treat the problem. If the dissection involves the ascending aorta, surgery is usually indicated.

Surgery is also indicated when drug therapy is ineffective or when complications of aortic dissection (e.g., heart failure, leaking dissection, occlusion of an artery) are present. The aorta is very friable during the acute phase. Therefore, surgery is delayed for as long as possible to allow time for edema in the area of dissection to clear, to permit clotting of the blood in the false lumen, and to allow the healing process to begin.

Surgery for aortic dissection involves resection of the aortic segment containing the intimal tear. The lumen is oversewn at each transected end and conti-channel connecting the true lumen with the false necessary.

Nursing management

Nursing management related to a dissecting aneurysm includes placing the client on bed rest in a semi-Fowler's position and maintaining a quiet environment. These measures assist in keeping the systolic blood pressure at the lowest possible level. Narcotics and tranquilizers should be administered as ordered. Anxiety and pain must be alleviated because they increase the blood pressure.

Continuous intravenous administration of antihypertensive agents require close nursing supervision. The client should be placed on a cardiac monitoring device, and an intraarterial pressure line is usually inserted. (These are discussed in Chap. 28.) The nurse should observe for changes in the quality of peripheral pulses and for signs of increasing pain, restlessness, and anxiety. Vital signs are taken frequently, sometimes as often as every 2 to 3 minutes. A widening pulse pressure may indicate increasing aortic valvular insufficiency. If the blood vessels branching off the aortic arch are involved, decreased cerebral blood flow may alter the sensorium and level of consciousness.

Postoperative care following surgery to correct the dissecting aneurysm is similar to that following any aneurysmectomy procedure (see the section on Postoperative Care of aortic aneurysms). The exception is that most clients require continuation of their intravenous antihypertensive drug therapy.

In preparation for discharge, the nurse needs to focus on client and family teaching. The medical regimen includes antihypertensive drugs, which are usually taken orally. The client needs to understand that he must remain on these drugs to control his blood pressure. Propranolol can be taken orally to continue to decrease myocardial contractility. It is vitally important that the client understand the drug regimen. The nurse should instruct the client that if the pain returns or other symptoms progress, he must immediately return to the health care facility.

Aortitis (Aortic Arch Syndrome, Takayasu's Disease, Pulseless Disease)

These terms describe an inflammatory disorder with occlusion of the aorta and one or more of the large arteries which branch off from the thoracic aorta. The occlusion is commonly a result of atherosclerotic disease. The terms *aortic arch syndrome* and *pulse-*

less disease are used to describe this clinical problem. It occurs with greatest frequency in middle-aged and older people, particularly men.

Occlusion of the carotid and subclavian arteries secondary to aortitis most commonly affects Orientals, particularly young women below the age of 40. This disease syndrome is frequently called *Takayasu's disease*. Aortitis of the lower thoracic and abdominal aorta occurring in young women and children in the tropics is similar to Takayasu's disease.

Aortitis is not common in the United States. The most common infectious form is due to syphilis. Noninfectious aortitis has been associated with Hodgkin's disease, scleroderma, rheumatoid arthritis, and ankylosing spondylitis.

Clinical manifestations

Clinical manifestations vary with the extent and location of the occlusion, the degree of collateral circulation, and the number of vessels involved. Initial manifestations of an acute disorder are fever, joint pain, weight loss, malaise, and headache.

After about 8 years, symptoms of peripheral vascular insufficiency appear in the form of a nonspecific inflammatory process. The vessel intima is markedly proliferated, scarred, and fibrotic, and the media is thickened. Pulse deficits can be detected. Vascular bruits and hypertension are also present. Retinal changes and left ventricular failure may result from the hypertension. The mortality rate is about 18 percent, with the leading causes of death being congestive heart failure and cerebrovascular accidents.

Management

Management is symptomatic for hypertension and congestive heart failure. In general, treatment has not been satisfactory. The role of steroids is not proven. Antibiotics and immunosuppression have not been effective. Surgery may be performed to alleviate the symptoms of local vascular insufficiency.

Chronic Aortic Bifurcation Occlusion (Leriche Syndrome)

This syndrome is produced by slowly progressive atherosclerotic occlusion of the terminal aorta and iliac vessels. It affects mostly men between the ages of 50 and 80. Symptoms depend on location and extent of plaque formation and disease progression.

A characteristic clinical manifestation is pain in the low back, buttocks, or thighs caused by exercise and relieved by rest. *Intermittent claudication* (development of pain in working muscles while walking but subsiding with rest) in the calf or foot may also be present. If atherosclerosis has been continuous over a long period of time, collateral circulation may prevent gangrene of the extremity. Impotence is a common problem. Peripheral pulses in the lower extremities are diminished or absent.

The treatment of choice is surgery, consisting of a bifurcation graft, endarterectomy, or a combination of both. These procedures are discussed in the section on Surgical Treatment of chronic arterial occlusive disease.

Acute Aortic Bifurcation Occlusion

Acute occlusion of the aortic bifurcation is an uncommon but catastrophic event. It may occur as a result of a large embolus (saddle embolus), aortic dissection, or acute thrombosis. A saddle embolus can occur from a myocardial infarction or mitral valve disease with atrial fibrillation. Acute thrombosis may result from abdominal trauma or chronic atherosclerotic disease.[15]

Clinical manifestations include moderate to severe leg pain. The legs are cold, pale, and pulseless. Total paralysis of both legs may occur.

Treatment is immediate surgical intervention. Saddle embolectomy may be performed through a femoral arteriotomy. An *aortofemoral bypass* is usually necessary for aortic thrombosis. Postoperative care is similar to that for abdominal aortic surgery.

DISORDERS OF THE ARTERIES*

Chronic Arterial Occlusive Disease

Peripheral chronic arterial occlusive disease involves narrowing and obstruction of the arteries to the extremities. It may affect the aorto-iliac, femoral, popliteal, tibial, or peroneal vessels or any combination of these areas. Chronic arterial occlusion is a slowly progressive, insidious disease attributed primarily to the atherosclerotic process; hence, the term *arteriosclerosis obliterans* is used. It usually occurs in the fifth and sixth decades of life, primarily affects men, and has a familial tendency. (Arteriosclerosis obliterans of the carotid artery is discussed in Chap. 52.)

Etiology and pathogenesis

The leading cause of chronic arterial occlusion is atherosclerosis, which leads to narrowing of the vessels (Fig. 30-5). Atherosclerosis primarily affects larg-

*This section was written by Thomas P. Ermis, R.N., ADN, CVNS, Cardiovascular Nurse Specialist, Surgical Nursing Service, The Methodist Hospital, Houston, Texas.

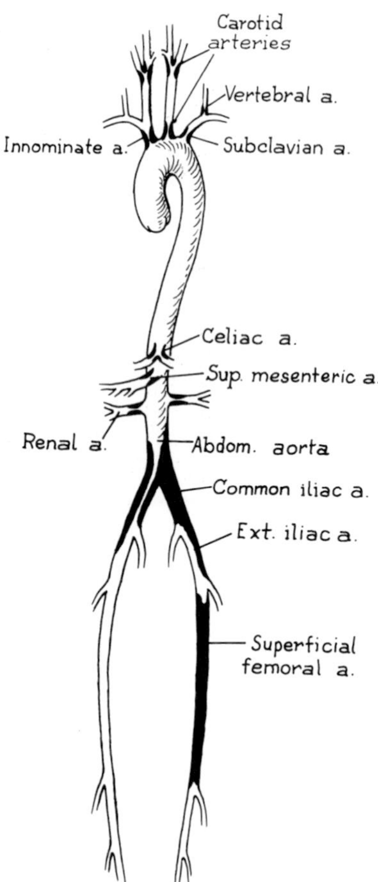

Figure 30-5 Typical patterns of the location and extent of occlusive disease of the aorta and its major branches. [*From J. W. Hurst et al. (eds.), The Heart, 4th ed., McGraw-Hill Book Company, New York, 1978, p. 1925.*]

er arteries. The involvement is generally segmental, with normal segments interspersed between involved ones. By the time symptoms occur, the vessel is 85 to 95 percent occluded.[16] The femoral-popliteal area is the site most commonly affected.

The three most significant risk factors for peripheral arterial disease are smoking, hyperlipidemia, and hypertension. Others are diabetes mellitus, a positive family history, obesity, and a sedentary lifestyle. (The pathogenesis of atherosclerosis is discussed in Chap. 27.)

Chronic arterial obstruction leads to progressively inadequate oxygenation of the tissues supplied by the obstructed arteries. The pain attributable to ischemia is produced by end products of anaerobic cellular metabolism, such as lactic acid. This usually occurs in the larger muscle groups of the legs during exercise. Once the client stops exercising, the metabolites are cleared and the pain subsides. As the disease process becomes advanced, pain develops at rest. This finding indicates insufficient blood flow to the skin and subcutaneous tissues. The client may notice resting foot pain more often at night and achieve partial relief by lowering the limb below heart level.

Clinical manifestations

The severity of the clinical manifestations depends on the site and extent of the occlusion as well as the adequacy of collateral circulation (Table 30-5). The classic symptom of peripheral arterial disease is *intermittent claudication*. Disease involving the femoral or popliteal arteries may cause claudication in the calf or foot. Disease involving the aorto-iliac arteries may produce claudication in the buttocks and upper thigh areas.

Ischemic pain at rest occurs as the disease becomes more severe. Another common manifestation resulting from aorto-iliac arterial disease is impotence. The incidence of sexual dysfunction occurs in 30 percent of cases.[17] *Paresthesia* is manifested as numbness or tingling occurring in the toes at rest.

Peripheral neuropathy occurs more commonly in diabetic clients and in those with extensive, long-standing obstruction. It produces excruciating shooting or burning pain in the extremity. It does not follow any particular nerve roots but may be present near ulcerated areas. Gradually diminishing perfusion to nerve tissue cells produces loss of both sensation and deep pain. Therefore, injuries to the extremity go unnoticed.

The physical appearance of the limb due to postural changes provides important information about the adequacy of blood flow. *Pallor* or blanching and whiteness on elevation indicate occlusion which can cause severe impairment of blood flow. *Hyperemia* or redness and a bluish or dusky appearance are observed when the limb is allowed to hang down in a dependent position. The skin becomes shiny and taut, and there is a loss of hair on the lower legs. Diminished or absent pedal, popliteal, or femoral pulses may be found.

Complications

Chronic peripheral arterial disease progresses slowly. Prolonged ischemia leads to atrophy and fibrosis of the skin and underlying structures. Due to the decreased ability to heal, infection and necrosis may result from trauma to the foot. Ischemic ulcers due to arterial insufficiency most commonly occur on the toes and feet. (This contrasts to ulcers of venous insufficiency, which occur around the malleoli and lower parts of the leg.) If severe ischemia persists, gangrene can develop. Ischemic ulcers and gangrene are the most serious complications of chronic arterial disease.

Medical management

Diagnostic Various tests have been developed to assess blood flow and to outline the vascular system (Table 25-5). A noninvasive test used to determine pulse volume is *oscillometry*. A pneumatic cuff inflated over the artery measures the amplitude of the pulsations.

Doppler ultrasound consists of a transducer containing a crystal which emits sound waves through a probe. It measures the amount of blood flow through a vessel. Directional flow can be measured antegrade or retrograde. The Doppler is extremely sensitive to movement of blood. When arterial palpation is difficult, it can sense a very weak pulsation even when there is severe obstruction. Angiography (aortography and femoral arteriography) is used to delineate the location and extent of the disease process (Fig. 30-6*a*).

Ultrasonic arteriography uses a Doppler system which is capable of systematically mapping the entire region of an artery in which blood is flowing. It provides a picture similar to that of a conventional arteriogram (Table 30-6).

Conservative Treatment Medical management objectives include (1) protecting the extremity from trauma, (2) slowing the progression of atherosclerosis, (3) decreasing vasospasm, (4) preventing and controlling infection, and (5) improving collateral circulation (Table 30-6). The client's risk factors should be assessed and proper intervention begun regarding cessation of smoking, weight reduction (if indicated), and control of lipid disorders[18] (Chap. 27). Hypertension also needs to be properly managed (Chap. 26).

Slow, progressive physical activity should be encouraged to help develop collateral circulation. For example, the client should:

1. Be out of bed at least 4 times per day.
2. Walk for 30 minutes twice a day as tolerated and stop if pain occurs. After a rest break, he should continue walking.
3. Keep the foot of the bed in the reverse Trendelenburg position at 10°.

If ulceration and/or gangrene is present in the foot, special treatment measures are used. To treat or prevent infection, the affected part may be soaked with 3% boric acid or a mild soap (e.g., Ivory Snow) 2 to 3 times daily. Hexachlorophene should not be used on open ulcers. After the lesion is cleansed, lukewarm water should be used to rinse the area. The area is then dried, antibiotic ointment applied, and a dressing used. Antibiotic therapy, local or systemic, is based on the results of cultures of the lesion.

Table 30-5
Comparison of Chronic Venous and Arterial Insufficiency of the Lower Extremities

Venous	Arterial
Edema around ankles. May involve feet.	No edema.
Cyanosis, dermatitis, characterized by brown pigmentation. Scaling eczema.	Loss of hair on legs, feet, toes. Thickening of nail beds. Thinning of skin; overall coolness.
Ulcer around ankle, above or below inner or outer malleoli.	Ulcer around toes or feet.
Dull ache or heaviness.	Claudication (pain with exercise).
Peripheral pulses present.	Peripheral pulses may be present, decreased, or absent.

Surgical Treatment Surgical management is indicated (1) when the symptoms of intermittent claudication become incapacitating or (2) when ulceration or gangrene warrants a limb-salvaging procedure.

Four basic types of surgical therapy for occlusive arterial disease include:

1. Endarterectomy (removal of the obstructing plaque material)
2. Bypass graft using a Dacron prosthetic implant or autogenous veins (Fig. 30-6*b*)
3. Excision of the diseased artery with graft replacement
4. Patch graft angioplasty

These procedures can be used singly or in combination. For example, localized lesions involving the superficial femoral and popliteal arteries can be treated with endarterectomy and patch graft angioplasty. More extensive lesions are usually treated with the end-to-side bypass graft technique (Fig. 30-7).

For individuals who are not suitable candidates for more extensive surgery, blood flow to the periphery may be increased through surgical interruption of sympathetic nerves to the affected part. The purpose of this procedure is to decrease the vasoconstrictor effects when the sympathetic nervous system is stimulated. In the lower extremities a *lumbar sympathectomy* may be performed, and the first, second, and/or third lumbar ganglions are removed. De-

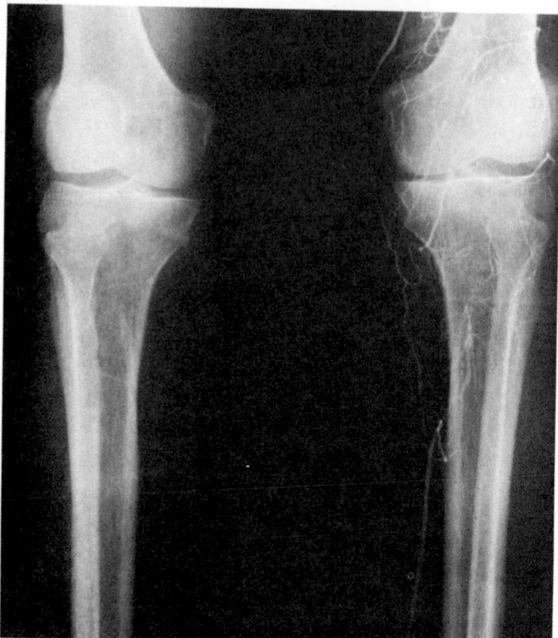

A

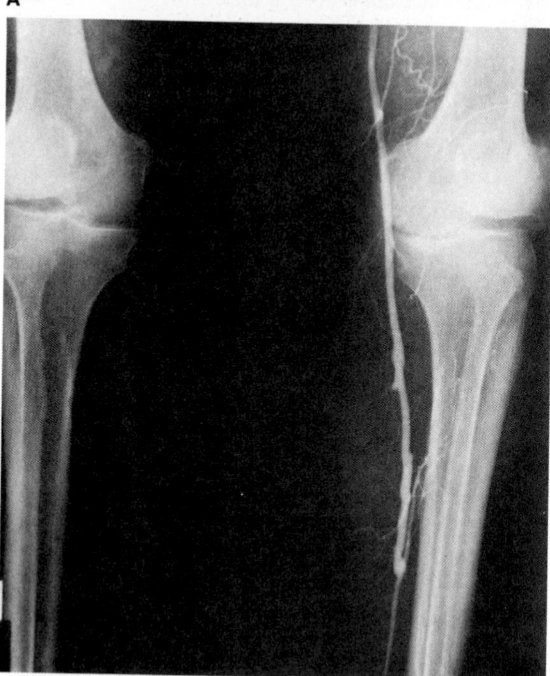

B

Figure 30-6 (*a*) Arteriogram demonstrating occlusion of the femoral and popliteal arteries. (*b*) Postoperative arteriogram showing a bypass by an autogenous vein graft from the femoral to the tibial artery. (*Courtesy of Dr. John Roehm, The Methodist Hospital, Houston, Texas.*)

Table 30-6
Medical Management: Chronic Arterial Occlusive Disease

Diagnostic
1. History and physical examination
2. Palpation of peripheral pulses
3. Doppler ultrasound studies
4. Angiography
5. Fasting blood sugar and 2-h postprandial blood sugar
6. Electrocardiogram
7. Chest x-ray

Therapeutic (conservative)
1. Vasodilator therapy
2. Mild analgesic (e.g., codeine)
3. Reverse Trendelenburg position 10° while in bed
4. Walking exercises 30 min b.i.d. as tolerated
5. Foot care (Table 41-18)
6. Avoidance of extreme temperatures

Therapeutic (surgical)
1. Endarterectomy
2. Bypass graft
3. Excision of diseased artery with graft replacement
4. Patch graft angioplasty

creased sympathetic stimulation increases blood flow and results in enhanced tissue perfusion.

A technique known as *percutaneous transluminal angioplasty (PCTA)* utilizes a special catheter with a cylindrical balloon. When inflated, the balloon dilates the vessel (Fig. 30-8). This procedure is presently being used in selected individuals who have single accessible lesions and whose disease is not diffuse.

Amputation is a last resort when damage to the limb is severe or life-threatening. Amputation is most frequently needed for diabetics with peripheral vascular disease. (The management of clients with amputations is discussed in Chap. 56.)

Pharmacological intervention

Although various agents are employed in the treatment of peripheral vascular occlusive disease, there is no specific drug known to be very effective. Vasodilators are of limited use in relieving the symptoms of claudication. Ethyl alcohol (30 to 60 mL whiskey 3 to 4 times daily) has been administered orally for pain relief, sedation, and its mild peripheral vasodilating effects. Anticoagulants have not proved to be beneficial. Acetylsalicylic acid given in small doses alters platelet aggregation and may be useful in preventing intravascular thrombosis.

Nutritional considerations

If the client has evidence of atherosclerosis, diet changes that should be encouraged are:

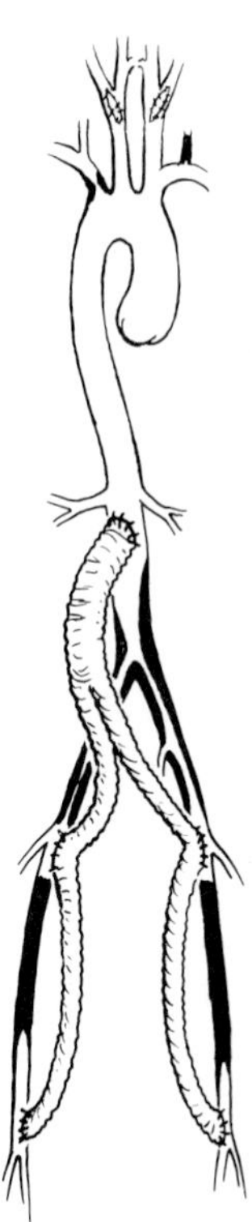

Figure 30-7 Bypass graft used in a client with multiple segmental occlusive lesions of atherosclerotic origin. *[From J. W. Hurst et al. (eds.), The Heart, 4th ed., McGraw-Hill Book Company, New York, 1978, p. 1931.]*

1. Calorie adjustment so that optimum weight can be achieved
2. Decrease in dietary cholesterol to less than 300 mg/day
3. Substantial reduction in saturated dietary fat (see Appendix B, Table 3)

If edema is present, sodium should be restricted to 2 g/day (see Appendix B, Table 2).

Nursing management

Health Promotion and Maintenance The client should be assessed for risk factors and should be taught how to control them (Table 27-4). The nursing role in client education in the inpatient care facility is important in identifying high-risk clients. The nurse should also be involved at the community level, such as in screening clinics for hypertension. Young people and adults need to be educated about the hazards of cigarette smoking. The nurse should also assist in teaching diet modification to reduce the intake of animal fat and refined sugars, proper care of the feet, and the avoidance of injury to the extremities. Individuals with positive family histories of cardiac, diabetic, or vascular disease need to be encouraged to obtain regular follow-up care.

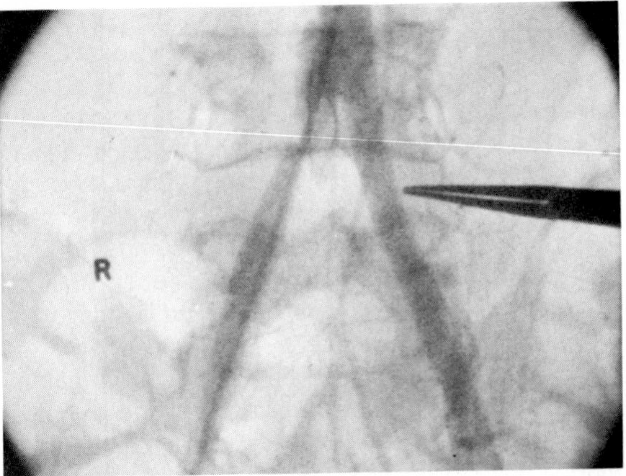

A

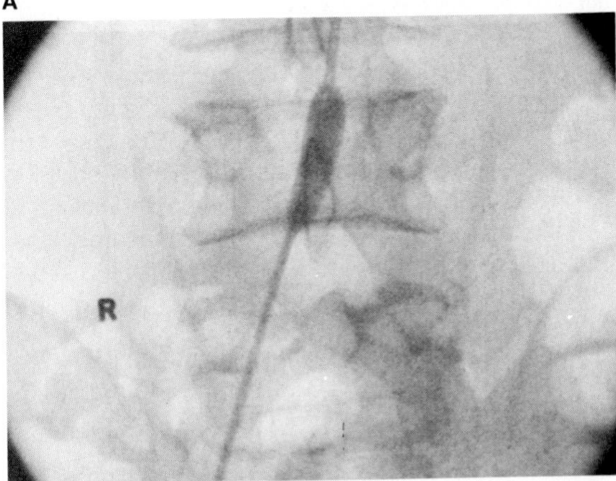

B

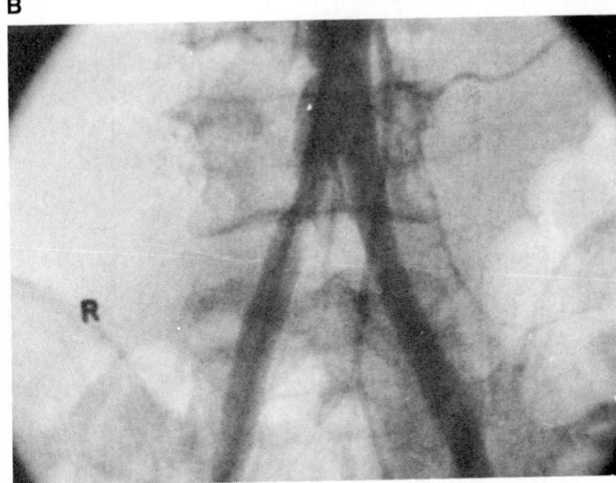

C

Figure 30-8 (*a*) Arteriogram showing partial occlusion of the right ilial artery near its branching off the aorta. (*b*) Dilatation of the right iliac artery by an inflating balloon catheter that compresses the atheromatous material against the arterial wall. (*c*) Following angioplasty, an arteriogram of the iliac artery shows increased patency of the vessel. (*Courtesy of Dr. John Roehm, The Methodist Hospital, Houston, Texas.*)

Acute Intervention Following surgical intervention, the client will be placed in an intensive care unit or recovery area for close observation. (General postoperative care is discussed in Chap. 8.) The extremity should be checked every 15 minutes initially and then hourly for color, temperature, capillary refill, and the presence of peripheral pulses distal to the operative site. These findings should then be compared with findings in the opposite limb. After recovery from anesthesia, the client should be asked to move his toes.

Later, the client should be out of bed at least 4 times a day. Sensation in the affected limb should be assessed during every shift, especially for the presence of numbness and tingling and for recurrence of pain. These symptoms may be indicative of impending graft occlusion or reembolization.

After transfer from the intensive care unit or recovery area, the client is placed on a program of progressive walking for 15 to 20 minutes at a time, 4 to 6 times a day as tolerated. The client should not sit for prolonged periods and should be instructed to use a reclining chair or footstool to minimize pressure on the graft site. The nurse should also tell the client to avoid crossing the legs, as this impedes both arterial flow and venous return.

Chronic Management The overall approach to the control of atherosclerotic chronic occlusive disease involves management of risk factors. Tobacco in any form is totally contraindicated because nicotine causes vasoconstriction and decreases blood flow to the extremities. There is evidence that bypass surgery to the extremity is not a substitute for the cessation of smoking since the long-term graft patency rate in smokers is not as good as it is in nonsmokers. The health care team must consistently agree to inform clients that they must abstain from smoking. The nurse needs to tell clients about various community agencies and support groups, such as behavior modification and antismoking clinics, if they are unable to stop smoking on their own. (The control and management of other risk factors for atherosclerosis, such as obesity, hypertension, and hyperlipidemia, are discussed in Chap. 27 and Table 27-4.)

Once the individual's degree of limitation is assessed by the health care team, a progressive exercise program can be implemented to improve collateral circulation and promote venous return. The most effective physical exercise is walking. The client should be instructed to walk only to the point of distress, to rest, and to allow the discomfort to disappear. Then walking can be resumed until distress recurs. This exercise should be done for the prescribed period of time, usually 30 to 40 minutes.

The client should learn to inspect the extremities daily for skin color, mottling, scabs, alterations in the texture of the skin and subcutaneous fat, and reduction or absence of hair growth. Any ulceration or inflammation needs to be reported to the health care provider. Skin temperature should be noted, and capillary refill of the fingers and toes should be tested.

It has been demonstrated that 20 percent of individuals with peripheral vascular disease have diabetes mellitus.[19] These clients should be instructed in the care of the extremities since their feet are very susceptible to injury due to diminished sensation. (Foot care for the diabetic client is presented in Table 41-18.) These measures also apply to individuals with vascular disease who do not have diabetes.

The client with chronic arterial disease should avoid long periods of standing or sitting. If prolonged sitting or standing is necessary, he should plan periodically to walk a few feet, flex his knees, and rotate his ankles. The legs should not be crossed at the knees because this position occludes the popliteal vessels. Other measures to avoid compromised circulation include avoiding tight nylon hose and garters, tight bands on socks, and tight waistbands. Shoes should not be laced tightly, and new shoes should be broken in gradually.

Acute Arterial Occlusive Disorder

Pathophysiology

Acute arterial occlusion occurs suddenly without warning signs. It can be caused by *embolism*, *thrombosis in situ*, or *trauma*. Embolization of a thrombus from the heart is the most frequent cause of acute arterial occlusion. Heart conditions in which thrombi are prone to develop include infective endocarditis, myocardial infarction, mitral valve disease, atrial fibrillation, cardiomyopathies (see Chap. 29), and prosthetic heart valves. The thrombi become dislodged and may travel to the lungs if they originate in the right side of the heart and to anywhere in the systemic circulation if they originate in the left side of the heart.

Sudden local thrombosis in situ may occur at the location of an atherosclerotic plaque. Traumatic injury to the extremity itself may produce partial or total occlusion of a vessel from compression, shearing, or laceration. Exposure to cold may produce vasoconstriction and, in severe cases, may lead to gangrene. Acute arterial occlusion may also develop as a result of aortic dissection. (See the section on Complications of aortic dissection.)

The emboli tend to lodge at bifurcation sites or in areas of atherosclerotic narrowing. Following an acute arterial occlusion, the blood supply to the extremity decreases. The degree and extent of manifestations produced will depend upon the size and location of the obstruction, the occurrence of clot fragmentation with embolism to smaller vessels, and the degree of peripheral vascular disease already present. Clients with widespread involvement tolerate acute insults poorly.

Clinical manifestations

Symptoms usually have an abrupt onset. If the acute occlusion is superimposed on a chronic occlusive process, symptoms are more insidious or may occur only during exercise. The reason is that collateral circulation provides an accessory pathway for blood if the major vessel is partially or totally occluded. This helps in maintaining sufficient blood flow to prevent symptoms of arterial insufficiency from occurring at rest.

Clinical manifestations include pain and numbness in the affected limb. Varying degrees of paralysis may be present. The limb will be pale and cool, and peripheral pulses distal to the occlusion will be absent. Ischemia may progress to necrosis and gangrene. Ischemic neuropathy is a frequent sequela of sudden arterial occlusion.

Management

Immediate treatment is necessary to save the affected limb. The embolus or thrombus should be removed as soon as possible. Balloon catheters can sometimes be used and are passed distal and proximal to the site in order to remove extensions of the clot material. This procedure can be done under local anesthesia. Direct arteriotomy to perform an embolectomy or thromboendarterectomy may be necessary. The client is usually put on anticoagulant heparin therapy prior to either of these procedures.

Thromboangiitis Obliterans (Buerger's Disease)

Thromboangiitis obliterans (Buerger's disease) is a focal, inflammatory, thrombotic disorder of the medium-sized arteries of the lower extremities. It differs from atherosclerosis in that it tends to involve more distal arteries; veins can also be affected. Occlusion of the vessel occurs, with development of collateral circulation around areas of obstruction. The basic cause is not known. There is a direct relationship to cigarette smoking, as the disease occurs only in smokers. There is usually no lipid accumulation in the vessel media. The disorder, generally asymmetrical, occurs predominantly in men between 25 and 40 years of age who smoke. A familial tendency has also been observed.

The client will complain of the pain of intermittent claudication. The so-called *rest pain* is a premonitory sign of gangrene and develops in advanced stages of the disease process. Other signs and symptoms may include color (rubor, cyanosis) and temperature changes in the affected limb, paresthesia, thrombophlebitis, and sensitivity to cold.

Complications include bone degeneration or osteoporosis. The digits are dissolved or "whittled" away. The client guards the foot, making no attempt to bear weight, since this aggravates the excruciating "electric shocklike" pain.

Treatment includes avoidance of trauma to the extremity and complete cessation of smoking. The client is often told that he has a choice between his cigarettes and his legs; he cannot have both. The disorder is difficult to treat. Anticoagulants and vasodilator therapy have met with little success. Placing the leg in the dependent position and alternating with elevation (Buerger's exercises) was one method to relieve pain through enhancement of arterial flow. Today these exercises are not believed to be effective. Amputation, generally below the knee, is considered as a last resort in some advanced cases.

Arteriospastic Disease (Raynaud's Phenomenon)

Raynaud's phenomenon is an episodic vasospastic disorder of small cutaneous arteries, most frequently involving the fingers. The exact etiology is not known. The disease occurs primarily in young women. It is seen frequently in association with collagen diseases such as rheumatoid arthritis, scleroderma, and lupus erythematosus. Other contributing factors include occupationally related trauma and pressure to the fingertips as noted in typists, pianists, and those who use hand-held vibrating equipment. Exposure to heavy metals may also be a contributing etiological factor.

The symptoms are usually precipitated by exposure to cold, emotional upsets, and tobacco use. The disorder is characterized by three color changes. Initially, the vasoconstrictive effect produces pallor, which is followed by cyanosis. These changes are subsequently followed by rubor or hyperemia. Since Raynaud's phenomenon is a vasospastic disorder, the pulses are never lost. The client usually does not experience pain. The episode typically lasts for about 15 minutes.

If the symptoms persist for several years in the absence of an associated underlying disorder, the diagnosis of *Raynaud's disease* may be made. *Complications* may include punctate (small hole) lesions of the fingertips and superficial gangrenous ulcerations occurring in advanced stages. It is of diagnostic importance to search for an underlying disease. *Treatment* is generally not required since the symptoms are self-limiting. However, treatment with certain catecholamine-depleting antihypertensive drugs has been encouraging. Oral vasodilators have been used with variable success. Sympathectomy is considered only in advanced cases.

Client education should be directed toward reassuring the client that no serious underlying disorder is present and that prevention of recurrent episodes is possible. Warm clothing should be worn as protection from the cold, including gloves when using the refrigerator-freezer or when handling cold objects. Moving to a warmer climate will not necessarily be beneficial since symptoms may still occur during cooler weather. The client should stop smoking and avoid or learn to cope with anxiety-producing stressful situations.

DISORDERS OF THE VEINS*

Thrombophlebitis

The most common disorder of the veins is *thrombophlebitis*, the formation of a *thrombus* (clot) in association with inflammation of the vein. The terms *phlebothrombosis* and *phlebitis* have been used to indicate whether the predominant process is thrombus formation or inflammation. In general, the preferred term is *thrombophlebitis*, as both clots and inflammation are usually present. The initiating event is usually thrombus formation.

It is estimated that at least 5 percent of all surgical clients and about 65 percent of all clients receiving intravenous therapy develop thrombophlebitis. Of greater significance is the fact that embolization of the thrombus to the lungs, heart, and/or brain may be fatal and, at the very least, results in prolonged hospitalization.

Etiology

Three important factors in the etiology of thrombophlebitis are (1) stasis of venous flow, (2) damage to the endothelium, or inner lining of the vein, and (3) hypercoagulability of the blood. Clients who are at high risk for the development of thrombophlebitis are those who have conditions predisposing them to any of these three disorders (Table 30-7). The majority of cases of thrombophlebitis occur in individuals with an underlying medical disease such as myocardial infarction, congestive heart failure, and malignancies.

Venous Stasis Venous stasis occurs in individuals who are obese, have congestive heart failure, have been on long trips without regular exercise, or are immobile over long periods of time (e.g., with spinal cord injuries or fractured hips). Also at risk are pregnant women or women in the postpartum period.

Clients with atrial fibrillation are also at high risk due to stagnation of blood and to the eddying in blood flow caused by the irregular ventricular contractions in response to the fibrillation. Steroid and quinine therapy also predisposes clients to stasis and clot formation.

Endothelial Damage Damage to the endothelium of the vein is caused by trauma or external pressure and occurs any time a venipuncture is performed. Increased endothelial damage is sustained when clients on intravenous therapy are receiving high-dose antibiotics, potassium, chemotherapeutic agents, or hypertonic solutions.

Other factors predisposing to endothelial inflammation and damage include the presence of an intravenous catheter in the same site for longer than 48 hours, the use of contaminated intravenous equipment, a fracture that causes damage to the blood vessels, diabetes, blood pooling, or any unusual physical exertion which results in muscular strain.

Hypercoagulability of Blood Hypercoagulability of blood occurs in many hematological disorders, particularly polycythemia and severe anemias. Clients with systemic infections in which there is a release of endotoxins also have hypercoagulability. Hypercoagulability also seems to be the contributing factor in idiopathic thrombophlebitis.

Clients who take oral contraceptives (especially those containing estrogen) are at increased risk for thromboembolic disease. Recent studies show that women who take contraceptives and smoke double their risk due to the constricting effect of nicotine on the blood vessel wall.[20] Smoking may also cause hypercoagulability. Studies indicate that people taking excessive doses of vitamin E are at high risk for thrombus formation.[21] Hypercoagulability also seems to be the common factor in various malignancies and

*This section was written by Suzanne L. Pixley, R.N., M.S., Head Nurse, General Surgery, Hermann Hospital, Houston, Texas.

the associated higher incidence of thromboembolic disease.

Pathogenesis

Red and white blood cells, platelets, and fibrin adhere to form a thrombus. A frequent site of thrombus formation is the valve cusps of veins, where venous stasis allows accumulation of blood products. As the thrombus enlarges, increased amounts of blood cells and fibrin collect behind it, producing a larger clot with a "tail" which eventually occludes the lumen of the vein. Complications develop as a result of the increasing clot size and the inflammatory process. The gradually dilating vein places pressure upon other blood and lymph vessels.

The inflammatory reaction contributes to the thrombus adhering to the inner surface of the vein, lessening the chance for embolization. Deep vein thrombi usually cause less inflammation and therefore are more likely to result in pulmonary emboli. If the thrombus does not become detached, it will undergo lysis or become firmly organized and adherent within 24 to 48 hours. It is possible that the organized thrombi may detach and give rise to emboli. The turbulence of blood flow past the thrombus is a major factor contributing to its detachment from the vein wall. These emboli generally flow through the venous circulation, back to the heart, and into the pulmonary circulation, where they can cause pulmonary embolism.

Thrombophlebitis can result in local damage to surrounding tissues due to the amount of compression from the distended veins. Ischemia and necrosis can occur in extreme cases unless the clot is dissolved or collateral circulation is developed. The thrombus mass may become fibrotic. If calcification develops, it is then termed a *phlebolith*.

Clinical manifestations

Clinical manifestations of thrombophlebitis vary according to the site and extent of involvement. Thrombophlebitis is usually classified as *superficial* or *deep* (Table 30-8). Clients with superficial thrombophlebitis will usually present with palpable veins. The area surrounding the vein will be tender to the touch, reddened, and warm. There may be a mild temperature elevation and leukocytosis. Edema of the extremity does not usually occur. The most common cause of superficial thrombophlebitis in the arms is an intravenous substance. The most common cause of superficial thrombophlebitis in the legs is related to varicose veins.

Clients with deep thrombophlebitis will have extremely swollen extremities, pain, warm cyanotic skin, and a temperature above 38°C (100.4°F). If the calf is involved, tenderness may be present on palpation. *Homan's sign*, pain on dorsiflexion of the foot, is a classic but not a reliable sign. If the inferior vena cava is involved, both lower extremities may be swollen and cyanotic. If the superior vena cava is involved, both upper extremities as well as the neck and back will become swollen and cyanotic.

Table 30-7
Risk Factors in Thrombophlebitis and Thromboembolism

Prior history of thrombophlebitis
Abdominal and pelvic surgery
Suprapubic prostatectomy
Obesity
Neoplasms, especially hepatic and pancreatic
Congestive heart failure
Advanced age
Atrial fibrillation
Prolonged immobility
- Bed rest
- Long trip without adequate exercise
- Spinal cord injury
- Fractured hip

Myocardial infarction
Pregnancy
Postpartum period
Oral contraceptive agents
IV therapy
Trauma
Sepsis
Venous cannulation/catheterization
Drug abuse
Cigarette smoking
Excessive vitamin E intake
Hypercoagulable states
- Polycythemia vera
- Severe anemias
- Dehydration/malnutrition

Complications

The most serious complications of thrombophlebitis are *pulmonary embolism*, *chronic venous insufficiency*, *phlegmasia cerulea dolens*, and *postphlebitic neurosis*. Pulmonary embolism is discussed later in this chapter. It is the most feared complication of thrombophlebitis because of its lethal potential.

Another common complication is *chronic venous insufficiency* resulting from chronic, persistent thrombophlebitis and recurrent edema which retard blood flow in surrounding veins. Individuals sustaining this complication develop persistent edema, increased pigmentation, secondary varicosities, ulceration, and cyanosis of the limb when it is placed in a dependent position.[22]

Clients with severe thrombophlebitis of the lower

Table 30-8

Summary of Clinical Characteristics of Thrombophlebitis

Clinical Classification	Usual Causes	Usual Location	Clinical Findings	Edema of Extremities	Embolization	Chronic Venous Insufficiency
Superficial	Varicose veins Direct trauma IV injections Thromboangiitis obliterans Malignant disease Blood dyscrasias Idiopathic	Saphenous veins and their tributaries Forearm	Tender, red, inflamed induration along course of subcutaneous vein (visible and palpable)	Almost never	Almost never	Almost never
Deep Small veins and	Postoperative Pre- and postpartum Direct or distant trauma Congestive heart failure Prolonged bed rest Acute febrile disease Sepsis Debilitating disease Malignant disease Blood dyscrasias	Soleal Posterior tibial, other deep calf veins Popliteal Pelvic	Tenderness to deep pressure Induration of overlying muscle Minimal or no venous distension	Occasional	Always a threat	Usually not
Major venous trunks	Systemic lupus erythematosus Pressure of tumors on veins Oral contraceptive drugs(?) Idiopathic	Femoral Iliac Inferior or superior vena cava Axillary Subclavian	Swelling Cyanosis Venous distension of limb with mild to moderate pain Tenderness over involved vein (groin or axilla)	Usual	Always a threat	Frequently

J. W. Hurst et al. (eds.), *The Heart*, 4th ed., McGraw-Hill Book Company, New York, p. 1879.

extremities may develop the complication of *phlegmasia cerulea dolens*. It involves an unusual extension of the thrombosis of the iliofemoral vein. It presents with sudden, massive swelling and intense cyanosis of the extremity. Gangrene may occur due to blocking of blood flow by the massive thrombus.

Postphlebitic neurosis is an inappropriate fear by a client (usually an apprehensive woman) that the veins store clots that may break off and travel to the lungs or brain. These clients have usually developed misconceptions of their problem. They need to understand that once the condition has been adequately treated, a severe problem no longer exists.

Diagnostic study abnormalities

Several diagnostic studies are performed to determine the site and extent of the thrombus and the resulting inflammation (Table 30-9).

Medical management (Table 30-10)

Conservative Therapy The client is usually kept on bed rest, with elevation of the affected extremity until the tenderness has subsided, usually for 7 to 10 days. Warm, moist heat is used to relieve the pain and treat the inflammation. Mild oral analgesics such as aspirin and codeine are used to relieve pain. For more severe pain, phenylbutazone (Butazolidin) has been used to treat the inflammatory process and accompanying pain.

Anticoagulant therapy is usually not indicated for superficial thrombophlebitis but is used for deep vein thrombophlebitis. Intravenous or subcutaneous heparin is usually given for 7 to 10 days, followed by oral anticoagulants for several weeks to 3 to 4 months.

If edema is present when the client becomes ambulatory, elastic stockings are recommended. If edema persists, the use of elastic stockings should be continued after discharge to prevent chronic vein insufficiency.

Surgical Therapy Most clients are managed medically, but a small percentage require surgical intervention (Table 30-10). The primary indication for surgery is to prevent pulmonary emboli. Surgical procedures include *venous thrombectomy*, *femoral vein interruption*, *inferior vena cava interruption*, and *umbrella device insertion*.

Venous thrombectomy involves the removal of a clot in the iliofemoral region. The clot is removed through an incision in the common femoral vein. This

Table 30-9
Diagnostic Study Abnormalities in Thrombophlebitis

Study	Finding
CBC	Elevated RBC count, Hgb, and Hct if polycythemia or dehydration is predisposing factor. Elevated WBC count (due to infectious or inflammatory process).
ESR	Elevated due to inflammatory process.
Coagulation studies	
Platelet count, bleeding time, PT, PTT	Elevated if the client has underlying blood dyscrasia. May be decreased if the client is polycythemic. May be altered due to previous medications.
Phlebogram (venogram)	Radiographic definition of location and size of clot, distension of vein, and development of collateral circulation.
^{125}I fibrinogen scan	Radionuclide tag of fibrinogen which defines location of clot (thrombus) and any emboli that may have moved from thrombus site.
Lung scan (ventilation and perfusion)	Determines presence of pulmonary embolism and extent of resulting lung damage.
Venous pressure measurements	Venous pressure will be high in affected limb until collateral venous circulation is developed or when venous pressure returns to normal.
Ultrasonic Doppler flow detector	Will show impairment of blood flow ahead of thrombus. Most useful as screening procedure in recent thromboses involving the femoral vein.

Table 30-10
Medical Management: Thrombophlebitis

Diagnostic
1. History and physical examination
2. Chest x-ray
3. CBC with differential
4. PT, PTT, platelet count, bleeding time
5. Electrocardiogram
6. Phlebogram of affected limb
7. Lung scan (ventilation and perfusion studies)

Therapeutic (conservative)
1. Heparin IV
2. Bed rest with BRP for BM only
3. Continuous warm, moist soaks to leg (groin to toe) with K-pad
4. Full-length elastic hose
5. Measure and chart the size of both thighs and calves every morning
6. Guaiac test on all stools

Therapeutic (surgical)
1. Inferior vena cava interruption (Fig. 30-9)
   a. Ligation
   b. Clipping
   c. Plication
   d. Filtering
2. Intracaval umbrella insertion

procedure is done to decrease the risk of chronic venous insufficiency subsequent to iliofemoral thrombophlebitis.

Femoral vein interruption is done by ligating the superficial femoral vein. Although this procedure has been used extensively, most surgeons believe that ligation at this level is inadequate because thrombus formation has often extended beyond the femoral level.

Interruption of the inferior vena cava to prevent pulmonary emboli involves various techniques that do not completely occlude blood flow (Fig. 30-9).

If clients are too ill for surgical intervention, an *umbrella device* can be threaded using fluoroscopy into the right internal jugular vein and into the inferior vena cava below the level of the renal veins. The umbrella device is opened, and the spokes penetrate the vessel walls. This device may produce complete occlusion or "sieve type" occlusion, permitting filtration of clots without interruption of blood flow.

Complications after the insertion of the umbrella device are rare. They include air embolism, improper placement, and migration of the filter into the venous system. Venous congestion is common and is caused by accumulation of trapped clots at the filter site. At some point, these clots may clog the umbrella and completely occlude the vena cava. This process is usually so gradual that collateral vessels have a chance to develop and drainage continues from the lower extremities.

Pharmacological intervention

The goals of anticoagulation therapy in the treatment of thrombophlebitis are to prevent (1) propagation of the clot, (2) development of a new thrombus, and (3) embolization. Anticoagulant therapy does not dissolve the clot. Lysis of the clot will begin spontaneously via the fibrinolytic system (see Chap. 23).

The most commonly used anticoagulants are *heparin* and *coumarin compounds* (Table 30-11). Heparin acts directly on both the intrinsic and common pathways of blood coagulation. (The normal coagulation mechanism is outlined in Fig. 23-3.) Heparin inhibits thrombin-mediated conversion of fibrinogen to fibrin. It also potentiates the actions of antithrombin III, inhibits the activation of factor IX, and neutralizes activated factor X by activating factor X inhibitor.[23]

Coumarin compounds, of which warfarin (Coumadin) is the most commonly used, exert their action indirectly on the coagulation pathway. Warfarin inhibits the hepatic synthesis of the vitamin K–dependent clotting factors, II, VII, IX, and X, by competitively interfering with vitamin K. Vitamin K is normally required for the synthesis of these factors.[24]

Oral anticoagulants are begun while heparin is still being administered. An overlap of 3 to 5 days is usually required to maintain therapeutic control of clotting. The clotting status is usually monitored using the partial thromboplastin time (PTT) for heparin therapy and the prothrombin time (PT) for coumarin derivatives. However, other tests can be used (Table 30-12).

Intramuscular injection of any drug is contraindicated for the client on anticoagulant therapy due to the risk of hematoma formation. Another important precaution involves the use of other drugs with anticoagulants. Heparin should not be administered intravenously with most antibiotics, hydrocortisone, or levarterenol (Levophed). Drug interactions can occur with oral anticoagulants (Table 30-13). A careful drug history should be taken from the client prior to anticoagulant therapy administration. In addition, the client on anticoagulant therapy should be told to seek medical advice before starting to take any other medications.

Drugs altering platelet function have also been used in preventing thrombus formation. These drugs have shown potential for use in preventing thromboembolic disease. They include acetylsalicylic acid (aspirin), indomethacin (Indocin), phenylbutazone (Butazolidin), and dipyridamole (Persantine). Their clinical use is still undergoing investigation.

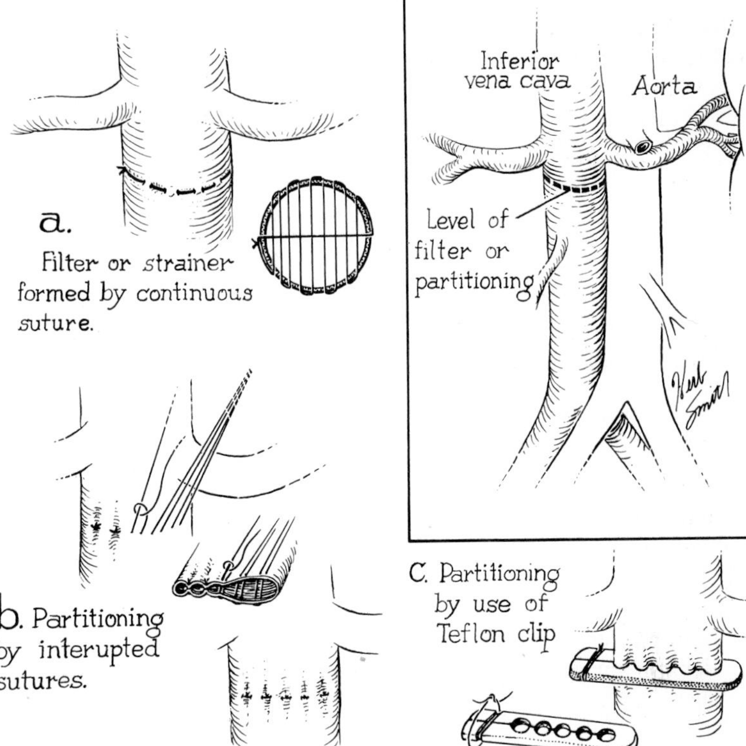

Figure 30-9 Operative procedures designed to prevent passage of pulmonary emboli through the inferior vena cava without complete interruption of blood flow. *[From J. W. Hurst et al. (eds.), The Heart, 4th ed., McGraw-Hill Book Company, New York, 1978, p. 1937.]*

Table 30-11
Anticoagulant Therapy

Drug	Route of Administration	Comments
	Heparin	
Panheprin	Continuous IV infusion via infusion pump	Initial bolus dose of heparin is required. Protamine sulfate should be available as an antidote. Clotting status monitored using whole blood clotting time (Lee-White clotting time), PTT, activated clotting time (ACT), and activated partial thromboplastin time (APTT) (see Table 30-12). Aspirin should not be administered to a client taking heparin. Low-dose prophylactic drugs will not alter clotting studies.
Lipo-Hepin	Intermittent IV infusion every 4 h	
Liquaemin Sodium	Intermittent SC infusion every 6 h	
	Coumarin Derivatives	
Warfarin (Coumadin, Panwarfin) **Dicumarol** **Acenocoumarol** (Sintrom)	Oral	Vitamin K should be available as an antidote. Plasma levels may be maintained for up to 5 days. Clotting status monitored using PT.

Table 30-12
Tests of Blood Coagulation

Test	Drug Monitored	Normal Value	Therapeutic Value
Lee-White whole blood clotting time (WBCT or LWCT)	Heparin	9–14 min	20–30 min
PT	Warfarin	11–12 s	20–25 s
PTT	Heparin	60–90 s	90–180 s
APTT	Heparin	24–36 s	48–60 s
ACT	Heparin	80–135 s	3 min

M. Wiener et al., *Clinical Pharmacology and Therapeutics in Nursing,* McGraw-Hill Book Company, New York, 1979, p. 349.

Low molecular weight dextran can be used as a prophylactic agent in preventing thrombus formation. It reduces platelet adhesiveness and blood viscosity. It is often given as a 500-mL 10% solution every day or every other day until the period of high risk (e.g., dehydration, immobility) is terminated.

Nursing management

Health Promotion and Maintenance Thrombus formation can be prevented in many situations. Prophylactic measures for the surgical client are discussed in Chaps. 6 and 8. They include early ambulation and leg exercises postoperatively, use of elastic stockings (hose), avoidance of dehydration, and low-dose anticoagulant therapy. Heparin (5000 units subcutaneously every 8 to 12 hours) or oral anticoagulants are recommended for high-risk clients who are predisposed to thrombus formation (Table 30-7).

Another important preventive measure is to avoid prolonged standing or sitting in a motionless, dependent position. Frequent knee flexion, ankle rotation, and active walking should be done during periods of sitting or standing.

Table 30-13
Drugs that Interact with Oral Anticoagulants

Drugs Potentiating a Response	Drugs Diminishing a Response
Anabolic steroids (e.g., Dianabol)	Barbiturates (e.g., secobarbital, phenobarbital)
Clofibrate (Atromid-S)	Cholestyramine (Cuemid, Questran)
Dextrothyroxine (Choloxin)	Ethchlorvynol (Placidyl)
Disulfiram (Antabuse)	Glutethimide (Doriden)
Metronidazole (Flagyl)	Griseofulvin (Grifulvin)
Neomycin	Rifampin (Rifadin, Rimactane)
Oxyphenbutazone (Tandearil)	
Phenylbutazone (Butazolidin)	
Phenyramidol (Analexin)	
Salicylates	
Sulfonamides (Gantrisin)	

M. Wiener et al., *Clinical Pharmacology and Therapeutics in Nursing,* McGraw-Hill Book Company, New York, 1979, p. 350.

Acute Intervention Nursing care for thrombophlebitis is directed toward the reduction of inflammation and the prevention of emboli formation (Table 30-14). Intervention includes placing the client on bed rest with elevation of the involved extremity to reduce edema and increase venous return. Mild analgesics such as codeine may be used to reduce pain. Continuous warm, moist soaks are generally accepted as a means of dilating arteries and veins and decreasing lymphatic congestion. In some situations, the acute thrombus formation is treated initially with ice packs and followed later by warm, moist soaks.

While the client is on anticoagulation therapy, the nurse should observe him closely for any indication of bleeding, including epistaxis and bleeding gums. Urine needs to be assessed for gross or microscopic hematuria. A smoky appearance to the urine will sometimes be noted, and a specimen should be checked daily with a laboratory dipstick. Particular attention should be paid to the protection of skin areas which may be traumatized. Surgical incisions should be closely observed for evidence of bleeding. Stools should be tested to determine the presence of occult blood from the gastrointestinal tract.

The nurse should monitor the hemoglobin and hematocrit levels when a client is receiving anticoagulant drugs. (The studies used to monitor the clotting status were discussed in the section on Pharmacological Intervention.) Medication doses are titrated according to the results of clotting studies. The nurse should be cautious about administering either heparin

Table 30-14
Nursing Care Plan for the Client with Thrombophlebitis

Client Problem	Expected Outcome	Nursing Intervention
Painful, swollen leg	Relief of pain and reduction of edema.	Administer analgesics as ordered. Apply continuous warm, moist heat (e.g., K-pad at low heat). Maintain elevated leg. Do not raise knee gatch. Instruct client not to cross legs at knees. Measure thighs and calves every morning.
Possible embolus	No chest pain, dyspnea, or tachypnea.	Take vital signs every 4 h. Report incidence of chest pain or shortness of breath. Use laxative to reduce straining. Maintain adequate hydration. Maintain bed rest to reduce tension on thrombosed vein. Administer anticoagulants as ordered. Use elastic stockings when ambulation is started.
Anxiety over emboli formation	Understanding of disease process and decreased anxiety.	Allow client to verbalize fears and anxieties. Correct any misconceptions of the disease process. Explain normal disease process. Explain all procedures and medications.
Hemorrhage from anticoagulation therapy	Therapy without signs of bleeding.	Administer anticoagulant medications as ordered. Do not give any medication IM. Check PT before giving Coumadin and PTT before giving heparin. Give anticoagulant therapy only if clotting studies are within prescribed limits. Observe client closely for signs of bleeding such as epistaxis, bleeding gums, petechiae, ecchymoses, painful joints, incisional bleeding, or melena. Monitor Hb and/or Hct levels.
Possible development of venous stasis ulcer	No evidence of ulcer formation in the legs.	Teach client to wear elastic stockings when ambulatory. (They should not be worn while client is asleep.) Have client elevate legs when sitting or standing. Teach client to change positions when sitting or standing for prolonged periods.
Lack of knowledge about disease process	Understanding of disease process and treatment, including: a. Anticoagulation management b. Diet and activity b. Clothing to be avoided	Instruct client on the need for routine monitoring of clotting studies. Encourage client to take anticoagulants according to prescribed schedule. Assist client with obtaining Medic-Alert identification to alert others to anticoagulant ingestion. Teach client not to wear garters, girdles, or any constrictive clothing. Encourage dieting to lose weight if indicated.

or coumarin without first checking the results of the clotting studies. The antidote for heparin is protamine sulfate, and for coumarin it is vitamin K. These drugs must be immediately available should hemorrhage occur.

Chronic Management Elastic stockings, properly measured and fitted and evenly applied, should be worn when the client becomes ambulatory. These stockings compress superficial veins and prevent venous stasis. Care should be taken to prevent any pressure under the knee, such as the use of pillows or bed gatches. Clients also need to be taught to avoid crossing their legs at the knees. These measures place pressure on the popliteal space and decrease venous return to the heart.

During all phases of care, the nurse should evaluate the client's psychological response. Many clients are apprehensive that their clots will move to the heart and cause sudden death. All clients should be allowed to verbalize their concerns, and an attempt should be made to clarify misconceptions. Clients hospitalized for long periods of time should be provided with diversion.

Discharge teaching should stress the avoidance of contraceptives for clients with recurrent thrombophlebitis, the hazards of smoking, and the need to avoid constrictive girdles or garters. Exercise programs should be developed with an emphasis on swimming and wading, which are particularly beneficial due to the gentle, even pressure of the water. A balanced program of rest and exercise, along with proper posture, improves both arterial filling and venous return.

Dietary management for the overweight client should be aimed at limiting calorie intake so that the desired weight can be attained. Fat intake may be reduced if lipid or triglyceride levels are above normal for the client's age. Occasionally, sodium limitation is necessary if edema is present. Proper fluid balance is required to prevent additional hypercoagulability of the blood, which may occur in the presence of deficient fluid intake. A well-balanced diet is important, as calcium, vitamin E, and vitamin K all play active roles in the clotting mechanism.

If the client is to be discharged on anticoagulant medication, both he and his family need careful explanations of its dosage, actions, and side effects (Table 30-15).

Varicose Veins

Varicose veins, or varicosities, are dilated, tortuous subcutaneous veins most frequently found in the saphenous system. They may be very small and innocuous or large and bulging. *Primary* varicosities are those in which the superficial veins are dilated and the valves may or may not be rendered incompetent. The condition tends to be familial, is characteristically found bilaterally, and is probably due to congenital weakness of the veins. *Secondary* varicosities result from previous thrombophlebitis of the deep femoral veins and subsequent or antecedent valve damage. Secondary varicose veins may also occur in the esophagus as varices, in the anorectal area as hemorrhoids, and as abnormal arteriovenous shunts (also known as *fistulas* and *malformations*).

Table 30-15
Client Education Related to Anticoagulant Therapy

1. Reasons for and basic mechanism of action of anticoagulant therapy and how long anticipated therapy will last.
2. Need to take medication at the same time each day (preferably in the afternoon or evening).
3. Required close follow-up with blood tests to assess blood clotting and whether a change in drug dosages will be required.
4. Side effects and adverse effects of drug therapy. Client should seek medical attention for the following:
   a. Any bleeding that does not stop after a reasonable amount of time.
   b. Blood in urine or stool.
   c. Unusual bleeding from gums, throat, skin, or nose.
   d. Severe headaches or stomach pains.
5. Avoidance of any trauma or injury that might cause bleeding (e.g., vigorous brushing of teeth, contact sports, improperly fitted shoes).
6. Avoidance of alcohol and aspirin-containing drugs, both of which can prolong coagulation.
7. Wearing of a Medic-Alert bracelet or necklace indicating what anticoagulant is being taken.
8. Use of an electric razor when shaving.
9. Avoidance of marked changes in eating habits such as food fads and crash diets.
10. Need to consult with physician prior to beginning or discontinuing any medication.

Pathophysiology

The basic cause of varicosities is unknown. Superficial veins in the lower extremities become dilated and tortuous with increased venous pressure. The increased venous pressure may be due to congenital weakness of the vein structure, obesity, pregnancy, venous obstruction due to thrombosis or extrinsic pressure by tumors, or occupations that require prolonged standing. As the veins enlarge, the valves are stretched and become incompetent, allowing blood flow to be reversed. As back pressure increases, the *venous pump* (muscle movement that squeezes venous blood back toward the heart) fails, causing further vessel destruction. The increased venous pressure is transmitted to the capillary bed, and edema develops.

Clinical manifestations

Varicose veins produce only mild discomfort unless they are complicated by superficial thrombophlebitis or chronic venous insufficiency. The main problem may be merely an objectionable cosmetic disfigurement. The most common symptom of varicose veins is an ache or pain after prolonged standing which is relieved by walking or by elevating the limb. Some clients feel pressure or a cramplike sensation. Swelling may accompany the discomfort. Nocturnal leg cramps, especially in the calf area, may be noted. The client may not have noticeable pain or swelling but may seek help for the disfigurement caused by the varicose veins (Fig. 30-10).

Complications

Thrombophlebitis is a serious consequence of varicose veins and may occur either spontaneously or following trauma, surgical procedures, or pregnancy. Rupture of varicose veins occurs due to weakening of the vessel wall. Ulceration subsequent to skin infections may also develop.

Areas of *chronic venous stasis ulceration* (damaged dermis due to decreased tissue perfusion) are usually located near the inner aspect of the ankle, above and behind the internal malleolus. This problem is discussed later in the chapter.

Medical and surgical management

Diagnostic Venography (discussed earlier) and the *Trendelenburg test* are two common diagnostic procedures performed for the client with varicose veins. The Trendelenburg test is used to assess valvular competence. The client's leg is elevated to 90°, and

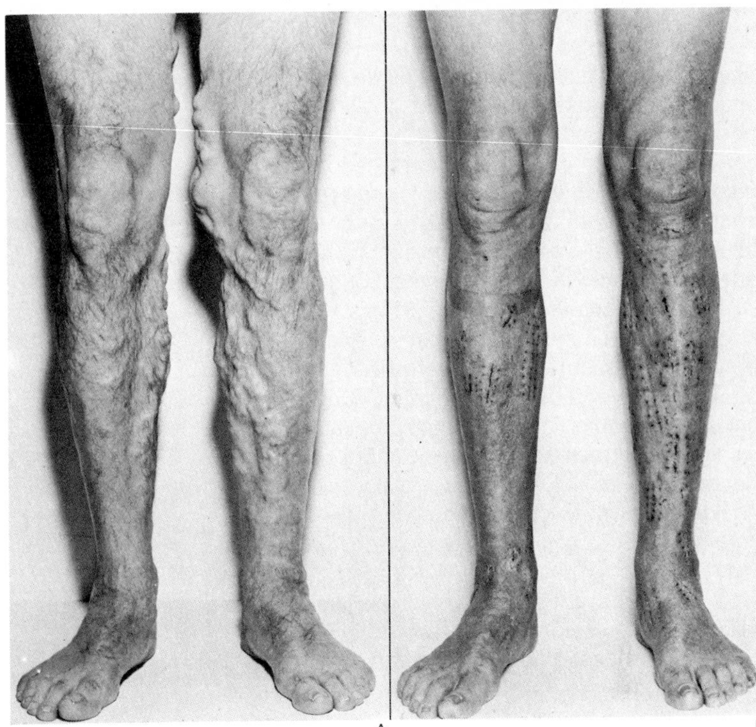

Figure 30-10 Extensive varicosities (incompetency of the greater saphenous systems). (*a*) Appearance preoperatively. (*b*) Appearance 2 weeks postoperatively. *[From K. A. Lofgren, "Varicose Veins," in H. Haimovici (ed.), Vascular Surgery: Principles and Techniques, McGraw-Hill Book Company, New York, 1976, p. 808.]*

a tourniquet is placed around the thigh with sufficient pressure to occlude the great saphenous vein. The client is then asked to stand, and the pattern of filling is observed. No more than 35 seconds should be required for the great saphenous vein to fill with blood from below. If there is no great rush of venous blood at 60 seconds when the tourniquet is removed, the venous valves are competent and the test is considered normal.[25]

Therapeutic Medical treatment is usually not indicated if varicose veins are only a cosmetic problem. If incompetency of the venous system develops, medical management involves rest with the feet elevated, elastic support hose, and walking exercise. These measures will help to prevent chronic venous insufficiency in most situations.

Although no longer a common practice, the injection of sclerosing solutions into varicose veins is still used. The purpose of this measure is to induce aseptic thrombosis and seal off the vein. Two drugs used are sodium tetradecyl sulfate (Sotradecol) and a solution of monoethanolamine oleate (Monolate). Clients are pretested for allergic sensitivity. Unfortunately, the effects of injection therapy are often short-lived, and damage to the surrounding area can lead to local pain from inflammation.[26] This procedure is still used on a limited basis, primarily in small segments of tributary veins. Large varicosities cannot be treated with sclerosing solutions because the thrombosis eventually induces recanalization of the vein.

Surgical management involves ligation of the entire vein (usually saphenous) as well as dissection and removal of its incompetent tributaries. Surgical intervention is indicated when chronic venous insufficiency cannot be prevented or controlled with medical therapy. Recurrent thrombophlebitis in varicose veins is another indication for surgery.

Nursing management

Prevention is a key factor related to varicose veins. The nurse should instruct clients to avoid sitting or standing for long periods of time, to maintain ideal body weight, to take precautions against injury to the extremities, and to avoid wearing constrictive clothing.

Following vein ligation surgery, the nurse should encourage deep breathing, which helps to promote venous return to the right side of the heart. The extremities should initially be checked hourly for color, movement, sensation, temperature, the presence of edema, and pedal pulses. In-bed and other exercises need to be practiced as ordered.

Postoperatively, constant elevation of the extremities at a 15° angle is required (except for limited periods of ambulation) to prevent the development of venous stasis and edema. Elastic stockings or bandages are also used, and should be removed once every 8 hours for short periods and reapplied. The nurse needs to be aware of the signs and symptoms of complications such as pulmonary embolism. She should remember that surgical intervention does not necessarily preclude the development of emboli.

Long-term management of varicose veins is directed toward improving circulation and avoiding complications such as thrombophlebitis and ulceration. Varicose veins can recur in other veins after the surgical procedure. The client should be taught proper care of the lower extremities, including cleanliness and the use of individually measured elastic hose. She should be taught to put on the hose while still lying down just prior to arising in the morning. The importance of periodic positioning of the legs above the heart should be stressed. Overweight clients need assistance with weight reduction (Chap. 60). Those individuals whose employment requires prolonged periods of standing or sitting should be encouraged to change their posture as frequently as possible. Pregnant clients with varicosities need appropriate teaching as prescribed by their obstetricians.

Venous Stasis Ulcers

Chronic venous insufficiency can lead to venous stasis ulceration. This condition usually arises as a complication of thrombophlebitis and varicose veins. The basic dysfunction is incompetent valves of the veins. The ulcers usually develop around the ankles, especially in the area of the medial malleoli (Fig. 30-11). Loss of epidermis occurs and portions of the dermal layer may also be involved, depending upon the degree of venous stasis. A characteristic brownish coloration of the skin develops due to deposition of melanin and hemosiderin. When capillaries rupture, red blood cells are released and disintegrate, with subsequent release of hemosiderin.

Clinical manifestations and complications

The skin texture of the lower leg is leathery, with a characteristic red-brown "brawny" appearance (Fig. 30-11). Edema has usually been present for a long period of time. The ulcer is a concave lesion below the margin of the skin surface and may become extensive. Pain may occur when the limb is in a dependent position or during ambulation. Pain is usually relieved by elevation of the foot.

If the ulcer goes untreated, the lesion will become more extensive, eroding wider and deeper and retarding the healing process. The likelihood of infection is increased. Scar tissue formation around the rim of the ulcer is found. Poor hygiene, debilitation, and inadequate nutritional status contribute to the severity of the ulcerative lesion.

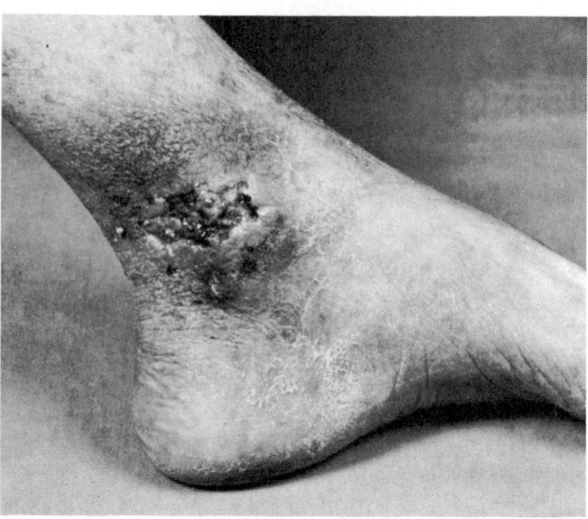

Figure 30-11 Chronic venous insufficiency with typical pigmentation and stasis ulceration overlying the internal malleolus. *[From J. W. Hurst et al. (eds.), The Heart, 4th ed., McGraw-Hill Book Company, New York, 1978, p. 1884.]*

Medical management

The client is placed on bed rest with elevation of the extremity. The wound is cleansed with a bacteriostatic solution several times per day, followed by the application of wet saline dressings. Routine prophylactic antibiotic therapy is not indicated. If there is evidence of infection as manifested by temperature elevation, leukocytosis, or drainage from the site, cultures of the lesion are indicated and appropriate antibiotic therapy is then instituted.

If the ulcer fails to respond to several weeks of conservative therapy, skin grafting may be indicated. The ulcer is debrided, and tissue from a thigh donor site is used. Any varicosities in the area of the lesion are removed. (Skin grafting is discussed in Chap. 13.)

Nursing management

The client with venous stasis ulcers is maintained on bed rest with elevation of the extremity. The nurse should change the dressings as ordered and perform prescribed wound care measures, including observation for signs of infection. A balanced diet is encouraged, with protein and vitamin supplementation to promote wound healing. Once granulation of the wound has begun, the client may sit in a bedside chair with the extremity elevated. Short periods of ambulation in the room are permitted.

Chronic management of venous stasis ulcers should focus on educating the client in self-care measures since the incidence of recurrence of the lesion is greater among these individuals than among those with no prior history of peripheral venous disorders. Discharge planning should include avoidance of trauma to the limbs, proper skin care measures, and application of prescribed elastic support stockings (after complete healing has occurred). Periodic rest periods with elevation of the extremities should also be encouraged. A balanced nutritional program incorporating protein-vitamin supplementation needs to be instituted. Calorie limitation for weight reduction and diabetic diet management are taught when indicated. Once scar formation has occurred, the client may return to his former activity level.

PULMONARY EMBOLISM*

Pathophysiology

Pulmonary embolism is the most common pulmonary complication in hospitalized clients. The exact incidence is difficult to determine. It is known that the incidence of pulmonary emboli has increased in the past 30 years. One major reason for this finding is that more older people are being treated surgically.[27]

Most pulmonary emboli arise from thrombi in the deep veins of the legs. Other sites of origin include the right side of the heart (especially with atrial fibrillation) and the pelvic veins (especially after surgery or delivery). (The etiology and pathogenesis of deep vein thrombophlebitis were discussed in the section on Thrombophlebitis.) Emboli are mobile and generally do not stop moving until they lodge at a narrowed part of the circulatory system. The lung is an ideal location for emboli to lodge due to its extensive arterial and capillary network. The lower lobes are most frequently affected because they have a higher blood flow than the other lobes. Often, the presence of deep vein thrombosis is unsuspected until pulmonary embolism occurs.

The thrombus in the deep veins can dislodge spontaneously. However, a more common mechanism is jarring of the thrombus by mechanical forces, such as sudden standing, and changes in the rate of blood flow, such as those that occur when the Valsalva maneuver is used.

*This section was written by Kemba D. Lowen, R.N., B.A., CVNS, Cardiovascular Nurse Specialist, Surgical Nursing Service, The Methodist Hospital, Houston, Texas.

In addition to dislodged thrombi, pulmonary occlusion can be caused by fat emboli (from fractured long bones), air emboli (from improperly administered intravenous therapy), amniotic fluid, and tumors. Tumor emboli may originate from primary or metastatic sites.

Clinical Manifestations

The severity of clinical manifestations depends on the size of the emboli and the size and number of blood vessels occluded. The most common manifestation of pulmonary embolism is sudden onset of unexplained dyspnea. Other manifestations are cough, chest pain, hemoptysis, tachypnea, rales, tachycardia, fever, and accentuation of the pulmonic heart sound.

Massive emboli may produce sudden collapse of the client with shock, pallor, severe dyspnea, and crushing chest pain. (Some individuals with massive emboli do not experience pain.) The pulse is rapid and weak, the blood pressure is low, and an electrocardiogram indicates right ventricular strain. When there is rapid obstruction of 50 percent or more of the pulmonary vascular bed, *acute cor pulmonale* may result because the right ventricle can no longer pump blood into the lungs. Death occurs in more than 60 percent of individuals with massive emboli.

Medium-sized emboli often cause pleuritic chest pain accompanied by dyspnea, slight fever, and a productive cough with blood-streaked sputum. A physical examination may indicate tachycardia and a pleural friction rub.

Small emboli frequently are undetected or produce vague, transient symptoms. However, repeated small emboli gradually cause a reduction in the capillary bed and eventual pulmonary hypertension. An electrocardiogram and chest x-ray may indicate the presence of right ventricular hypertrophy secondary to pulmonary hypertension.

Complications

Pulmonary infarction

Pulmonary infarction (death of lung tissue) occurs in less than 10 percent of clients with emboli. Infarction is more likely when there is (1) occlusion of a large or medium-sized pulmonary vessel (greater than 2 mm in diameter), (2) insufficient collateral blood flow from the bronchial circulation, and (3) preexisting lung disease. Infarction results in alveolar necrosis and hemorrhage. Occasionally, the infarct becomes infected and an abscess may develop. Concomitant pleural effusion is frequently found.

Pulmonary hypertension

Pulmonary hypertension occurs when more than 50 percent of the cross-sectional area of the normal pulmonary bed is compromised. Pulmonary hypertension also results from hypoxemia. As a single event, an embolus does not cause pulmonary hypertension unless it is massive. However, recurrent small to medium-sized emboli may result in chronic pulmonary hypertension. Pulmonary hypertension eventually results in dilatation and hypertrophy of the right ventricle. Depending on the degree of pulmonary hypertension and its rate of development, death may result rapidly or only mild or transient alterations may be produced. (Pulmonary hypertension is discussed in Chap. 20.)

Diagnostic Study Abnormalities

An *electrocardiogram* is not a very sensitive or specific diagnostic measure to detect pulmonary embolism. With small to medium-sized pulmonary emboli, it may remain normal or show any combination of changes transiently. As an isolated event, pulmonary infarction usually causes no electrocardiographic changes. Arrhythmias are the most common finding related to pulmonary emboli. Recurrent small pulmonary emboli may eventually produce chronic pulmonary hypertension and electrocardiographic changes of right axis deviation with enlargement of the right atrium and right ventricle.

A *chest x-ray* is usually not diagnostic unless an infarction has occurred. Even with pulmonary infarction, the chest x-ray is nondiagnostic in about 50 percent of clients. Positive findings are best visualized 12 to 24 hours after embolism, as variably shaped (round, linear, or occasionally wedge) areas of consolidation are sometimes found in the periphery or lower lobes. Pleural effusions are often noted. The chest x-ray can be valuable in assessing any pulmonary pathology, such as chronic obstructive pulmonary disease or tuberculosis.

A *lung scan* is of value in confirming the diagnosis of initial (or recurrent) pulmonary embolism, assessing the natural history of the lesion, and evaluating the effectiveness of medical or surgical therapy. Lung scanning is therefore indicated in all clients in whom pulmonary embolism is suspected. The lung scan has two components:

1. *Perfusion scanning* involves intravenous injection of a radioisotope. A scanning device reflects the adequacy of the pulmonary circulation.
2. *Ventilation scanning* involves inhalation of a radioactive gas such as xenon. Scanning reflects the distribution of gas through the lung.

A simple, reliable, noninvasive test for detecting deep vein thrombosis in the upper extremities can be performed by using a *bidirectional Doppler blood flow instrument* (discussed in the section on Medical Management of chronic arterial occlusive disorders.) Testing of the legs is best accomplished through the use of *impedance plethysmography (IPG)* and a modified Doppler technique. IPG assesses the capacitance and outflow in the deep venous system by using lower-leg electrodes to measure local blood volume while a thigh blood pressure cuff is inflated and then released. A thrombosed vein will have less distension upon cuff inflation, so the outflow volume will be diminished when the cuff is deflated.

Venography is one method used to delineate the extent of thrombosis. Contrast medium is injected through an 18-gauge needle in a superficial vein of the ankle or dorsum of the foot. A tourniquet above the ankle will retard filling of the superficial veins and direct the flow of contrast medium into the deep veins. Gravity ensures good filling of the veins, and if the client is placed on a tilted surface with the feet down, the return of the dye will be even slower.

Pulmonary angiography is an invasive procedure that involves the insertion of a catheter through the antecubital or femoral vein and advancement to the pulmonary artery. Contrast medium is injected to visualize the pulmonary vascular system. This procedure is usually not necessary to establish a diagnosis of pulmonary embolism. However, it must be used when surgical intervention is planned.

Arterial blood gas analysis is important. The P_aO_2 is always below normal due to inadequate oxygenation secondary to an occluded pulmonary vasculature. The P_aCO_2 is usually below normal due to tachypnea and hyperventilation that occurs with pulmonary emboili. The pH remains normal unless respiratory alkalosis develops due to prolonged hyperventilation or to compensate for lactic acidosis causes by shock.

Medical Management

When the diagnosis of thromboembolic disease has been made, treatment should be instituted immediately (Table 30-16). The objectives of medical treatment are to:

1. Prevent further growth or multiplication of thrombi in the lower extremities

2. Prevent embolization from the lower extremities to the pulmonary arteries
3. Provide cardiopulmonary support if indicated

Conservative therapy

Heparin is the drug of choice for anticoagulant therapy. An initial intravenous bolus is given, followed by intermittent or continuous intravenous heparin administration. Continuous administration provides more uniform blood levels of heparin. Heparin therapy is continued for about 7 to 10 days. (Anticoagulant therapy is discussed in the section on Pharmacological Intervention in thrombophlebitis.)

Supportive therapy for the client's cardiopulmonary status varies according to the severity of the pulmonary embolism. The administration of oxygen by mask or cannula may be adequate for some clients. Oxygen is given in a concentration determined by arterial blood gas analysis. In some situations, endotracheal intubation and/or mechanical ventilation may be needed to maintain adequate oxygenation. Respiratory measures such as turning, coughing, and deep breathing are necessary to prevent or treat atelectasis. If shock is present, vasopressor agents may be necessary to support systemic circulation. If heart failure is present, digitalis and diuretics are used. Pain due to pleural irritation or reduced coronary blood flow is treated with narcotics, usually morphine.

Surgical therapy

If the degree of pulmonary arterial obstruction is severe (usually greater than 50 percent) and the client does not respond to conservative therapy, an immediate embolectomy may be indicated. Pulmonary embolectomy is possible using temporary cardiopulmonary bypass. Preoperative pulmonary angiography is necessary to identify and locate the site of the embolus.

To prevent further pulmonary embolization, the surgical procedures discussed in the section on Surgical Therapy for thrombophlebitis may be used. These include insertion of an intracaval umbrella device and vena cava interruption (Fig. 30-9).

Pharmacological Intervention

Anticoagulant therapy

Properly managed anticoagulant therapy is successful in the management of many clients with pulmonary emboli. Heparin and warfarin (Coumadin) are the anticoagulant drugs of choice. Heparin should be started immediately, and the dosage is reduced as oral anticoagulants are initiated. The dosage of heparin is adjusted according to its effect on the PTT, and that of warfarin is regulated by the PT. Difficulties may be encountered in occasional clients who may bleed or develop thrombosis in spite of an apparently correct dosage. (A detailed discussion of anticoagulant therapy is presented in the section on Pharmacological Intervention in thrombophlebitis.)

Anticoagulant therapy for thromboembolic conditions may not be indicated in the presence of blood dyscrasias, hepatic dysfunction altering the clotting mechanism, injury to the viscera, overt bleeding, a history of cerebrovascular accident, and neurological conditions.

Table 30-16
Medical Management: Acute Pulmonary Embolism

Diagnostic
1. History and physical examination
2. Lung scan (perfusion and ventilation)
3. Chest x-ray
4. Continuous electrocardiographic monitoring
5. Arterial blood gases
6. CBC with differential
7. Pulmonary angiography

Therapeutic
1. Oxygen by mask or cannula
2. Establishment of IV route for drugs and fluids
3. Heparin IV
4. Bed rest
5. Narcotics for pain relief
6. Thrombolytic agents
7. Pulmonary embolectomy

Thrombolytic agents

Thrombolytic agents such as urokinase and streptokinase have been shown to lyse pulmonary emboli within 24 to 48 hours. Streptokinase, obtained from hemolytic streptococci, is thought to activate plasminogen, which is a fibrinolytic enzyme precursor. Urokinase, found in urine, also activates plasminogen. Both of these agents have been suggested for use in clients with massive emboli or in whom surgery is contraindicated. These agents currently are not widely used and are undergoing further investigation.

Nursing Management

Health promotion and maintenance

Nursing measures should be taken to prevent thromboembolic conditions and pulmonary embolism from occurring. Preventive measures are directed toward the major causes of thrombophlebitis, which are *venous stasis*, *hypercoagulability*, and *venous endothelial damage*. Venous stasis can be prevented by proper care of immobilized postoperative clients. Active and passive range-of-motion exercises, frequent turning, and coughing and deep-breathing exercises are important measures that the nurse needs to institute for these clients. The ambulatory client should walk frequently, and antiembolism stockings should be put on before getting out of bed. All hospitalized clients may safely wear elastic stockings except those with severe local disease in the legs such as ischemia, inflammation, or trauma.

Hypercoagulability may be reduced by maintaining a proper fluid balance and by keeping the client adequately hydrated. Alterations in the endothelial lining may be minimized by proper intravenous insertion techniques. Application of heat to a limb diagnosed as thrombophlebitic can help to resolve the inflammatory process. (Other measures to decrease the incidence of thrombophlebitis and pulmonary emboli are discussed in the Nursing Management of thrombophlebitis.)

Acute intervention

The prognosis of a client with pulmonary emboli is very good if therapy is promptly instituted. The client should be placed on bed rest in a semi-Fowler's position to facilitate breathing. A patent intravenous line should be maintained for medications and fluid therapy. The nurse should know the side effects of medications and observe for them. Oxygen therapy should be administered as ordered. (Nursing care for the client receiving oxygen is discussed in Table 20-13.) Careful monitoring of vital signs, electrocardiogram, blood gases, and lung sounds is critical to assess the client's status.

The client is usually very anxious because he is in pain, cannot breathe, and fears death. The nurse should carefully explain the situation and provide emotional support and reassurance to help relieve the client's anxiety. During the acute phase, someone should be with the client as much as possible.

Many clients who develop pulmonary emboli have been hospitalized for a primary problem such as sepsis, acute respiratory failure, or surgical intervention. The nurse needs to focus on management of the problems caused by the primary disorder as well as those related to pulmonary emboli.

Chronic management

Clients affected by thromboembolic processes require much psychological and emotional support. In addition to the thromboembolic problems, they may have an underlying chronic illness requiring long-term treatment. To provide supportive therapy, the nurse must understand and differentiate between the various problems caused by the underlying disease and those related to thromboembolic disease.

Chronic management is similar to that for the client with thrombophlebitis (discussed earlier; see Tables 30-14 and 30-15). Discharge planning is aimed at limiting progression of the condition and preventing complications. Warmth is advised for most clients because it causes vasodilatation and therefore improves circulation to the affected part. Warm compresses may be used at home for thrombophlebitis to reduce inflammation in the involved vessel. With decreased circulation, healing is slowed and the possibility of infection increases. Clients and their families need to be taught that cleanliness and care of the legs and feet is imperative. The nurse must reinforce the need for the client to return to the health care facility for follow-up therapy.

Case Study / Thrombophlebitis

Shirley J., a 34-year-old mother of four, was admitted to the hospital with the diagnosis of thrombophlebitis of the left leg. She is on a regular diet at home, smokes two packs of cigarettes per day, and is obese at 185 lb for her 5-foot 3-inch frame. She knows that she has a bad mitral valve and has previously been treated for "fluttering of the upper portion" of her heart. The only medication she takes is contraceptive pills. She presents with a gradual increase in pain and swelling of her left leg. It appears glossy and warm to the touch. She states that it is very tender from midthigh to toe. She has an elevated white blood cell count and an elevated erythrocyte sedimentation rate. Her temperature is 38°C, and her pulse is irregular at 106 beats per minute.

Discussion Questions

1. Explain the pathogenesis of thrombophlebitis. What risk factors does Shirley have?
2. Compare superficial thrombophlebitis with deep vein thrombophlebitis in terms of the affected veins and clinical manifestations. Which disorder does Shirley have?
3. What complications may result from thrombophlebitis?

4. What are the main features differentiating arterial vascular and venous vascular problems?
5. What diagnostic tests can be utilized for thrombophlebitis?
6. Explain the physiological bases for each of the following treatment measures: leg elevation, hot packs, intravenous heparin, deep-breathing and coughing exercises, elastic hose.
7. What important things should Shirley be taught to prevent recurrent attacks of thrombophlebitis?

REVIEW QUESTIONS

The number of the question corresponds to the same numbered objective at the beginning of the chapter.

1. Which of the following statements accurately characterizes aortic aneurysms?
   a. They are most frequently caused by arteriosclerosis.
   b. They occur exclusively in the descending and abdominal aortae.
   c. They are most frequently caused by syphilis.
   d. They most commonly occur in young women following pregnancy.

2. An important nursing measure following an aneurysm repair is to
   a. administer anticoagulant therapy
   b. position the legs in the Trendelenburg position
   c. apply elastic stockings to both feet
   d. palpate the peripheral pulses frequently

3. Acute aortic occlusion may result from all the following *except*
   a. saddle embolus
   b. acute thrombosis
   c. thromboangiitis obliterans
   d. aortic dissection

4. Intermittent claudication is a manifestation which occurs as a result of
   a. inadequate blood flow to the muscles after exercise
   b. inadequate blood flow to the skin after application of heat
   c. the beginning of gangrene in the toes
   d. dorsiflexion of the foot when thrombophlebitis is present

5. Which of the following instructions would be inappropriate for a client with chronic arterial insufficiency?
   a. Avoid traumatizing or chilling the lower extremity.
   b. Wear an elastic bandage or stocking.
   c. Walk for about 30 to 60 minutes/day or until pain develops.
   d. Check the peripheral pulses daily in both feet.

6. Thromboangiitis obliterans (Buerger's disease) is a condition characterized by
   a. occlusion of arteries and veins secondary to recurring inflammation
   b. inflammation of the large arteries resulting in vasospastic disturbances.
   c. inflammation of the vein secondary to a decrease in muscle tone
   d. atherosclerotic plaque in the medial layer of large arteries

7. Deep vein thrombophlebitis is characterized by
   a. redness, heat, and tenderness of the affected area
   b. generalized edema of the involved extremity
   c. pallor and cyanosis of the involved extremity
   d. paresthesia and coolness of the leg

8. Which of the following describes the rationale for anticoagulant therapy?
   a. dissolves thromboemboli
   b. prevents platelet aggregation
   c. inhibits the clotting mechanism
   d. activates the clotting mechanism

9. Which of the following best describes the manifestations of chronic venous insufficiency?
   a. loss of hair, pallor, and paresthesia
   b. foot pain at rest and ulceration of toes
   c. brownish pigmentation and ulceration around the ankle
   d. thickening of nail beds and coolness of the extremity

10. The most common site of origin of pulmonary emboli is the
    a. right side of the heart
    b. peripheral arterial system
    c. pelvic veins
    d. deep veins of the legs

REFERENCES

1. J. Lindsay and J. W. Hurst, *The Aorta*, Grune & Stratton, Inc., New York, 1979, p. 135.
2. E. Braunwald, *Heart Disease: A Textbook of Cardiovascular Medicine*, W. B. Saunders Company, Philadelphia, 1980, pp. 1600–1603.
3. J. W. Hurst et al. (eds.), *The Heart*, 4th ed., McGraw-Hill Book Company, New York, 1978, p. 1844.
4. Lindsay and Hurst, pp. 56–57.
5. W. E. Stehbens, *Hemodynamics and the Blood Vessel Wall*, Charles C Thomas, Publisher, Springfield, Ill., 1979, p. 472.
6. Ibid., pp. 465, 466.
7. J. Kernicki et al., *Cardiovascular Nursing*, G. P. Putnam's Sons, New York, 1970, pp. 87–88.
8. D. A. Cooley and D. C. Wukasch, *Techniques in Vascular Surgery*, W. B. Saunders Company, Philadelphia, 1979, p. 54.
9. Hurst et al., op. cit., p. 1918.
10. Stehbens, op. cit., p. 501.

11. J. L. Dalen and J. P. Howe III, "Dissection of the Aorta: Current Diagnostic and Therapeutic Approaches," *JAMA*, **242**(14):1530 (1979).
12. W. R. Webb and R. A. Brunswick, "Management of Acute Dissection of the Aorta," *Heart Lung*, **9**(2):84 (1980).
13. M. E. DeBakey and A. Gotto, *The Living Heart*, Grosset & Dunlap, Inc., New York, 1977, p. 175.
14. S. E. Mills et al., "Aortic Dissection: Surgical and Non-surgical Treatments Compared," *Am J Surg*, 137:240 (1979).
15. N. Wenger et al. (eds.), *Cardiology for Nurses*, McGraw-Hill Book Company, New York, 1980, p. 551.
16. R. Zelis, *The Peripheral Circulation*, Grune & Stratton, Inc., New York, 1975, p. 238.
17. Y. Bergman, *Surgery of the Aorta and Its Body Branches*, Grune & Stratton, Inc., New York, 1979, p. 263.
18. J. Juergens et al. (eds.), *Peripheral Vascular Disease*, 5th ed., W. B. Saunders Company, Philadelphia, 1980, p. 857.
19. A. Friedman, "Peripheral Vascular Disease," *Hosp Med*, **15:** 89 (1979).
20. D. B. Pelili et al., "Contraceptive Drug Study, Kaiser Permanente Medical Center, Walnut Creek, Calif.," *Am J Epidemiol*, **1084:**480–483 (1978).
21. "Warning—Megadoses of Vitamin E May Cause Thrombophlebitis," *Nurses Drug Alert*, **3:**123–124 (1979).
22. Kernicki et al., op. cit., pp. 121–124.
23. M. Wiener et al., *Clinical Pharmacology and Therapeutics in Nursing*, McGraw-Hill Book Company, New York, 1979, p. 348.
24. Ibid.
25. B. Bates, *A Guide to Physical Examination*, 2d ed., J. B. Lippincott Company, Philadelphia, 1979, p. 267.
26. Juergens et al., op. cit., pp. 801–802.
27. J. Fitzmaurice and A. Sasahara, "Current Concepts of Pulmonary Embolism: Implications for Nursing Practice," *Heart Lung*, **3:**209–218 (1974).

BIBLIOGRAPHY FOR SECTION 6

Respiratory

Books

Burrows, B., R. Knudson, and L. Kettel: *Respiratory Insufficiency Yearbook*, Year Book, Medical Publishers, Inc., Chicago, 1975.

Burton, George G., Glenn N. Gee, and John E. Hodgkin: *Respiratory Care: A Guide to Clinical Practice*, J. B. Lippincott Company, Philadelphia, 1977.

Criep, L. H.: *Allergy and Clinical Immunity*, Grune & Stratton, Inc., New York, 1976.

DeWeese,' D. D., and W. H. Saunders: *Textbook of Otolaryngology*, The C. V. Mosby Company, St. Louis, 1977.

English, G. M.: *Otolaryngology*, Harper & Row, Publishers, Incorporated, Hagerstown, Md., 1976.

Fishman, A. P. (ed.): *Pulmonary Diseases and Disorders*, McGraw-Hill Book Company, New York, 1980.

Harper, Rosalind: *A Guide to Respiratory Care*, J. B. Lippincott Company, Philadelphia, 1981.

Kinney, M. R. (ed.): *AACN's Clinical Reference for Critical Care Nursing*, McGraw-Hill Book Company, New York, 1981.

Morrison, Martha L. (ed.): *Respiratory Intensive Care Nursing*, 2d ed., Little, Brown and Company, Boston, 1979.

Nursing Inservice Education Programs on Cancer of the Head and Neck: American Cancer Society, New York, 1979.

Petty, T. L. (ed.): *Chronic Obstructive Pulmonary Disease*, Marcel Dekker, Inc., New York, 1978.

Rubin, P. (ed.): *Current Concepts in Cancer: Multidisciplinary Views Cancer of the Head and Neck*, American Cancer Society, New York, 1972.

Sexton, D. L.: *Chronic Obstructive Pulmonary Disease*, The C. V. Mosby Company, St. Louis, 1981.

West, John: *Pulmonary Pathophysiology*, The Williams & Wilkins Company, Baltimore, 1977.

———: *Respiratory Physiology*, 2d ed., The Williams & Wilkins Company, Baltimore, 1979.

Periodicals

Addington, Whitney: "Patient Compliance: The Most Serious Remaining Problem in the Control of Tuberculosis in the United States," *Chest*, **76**(6)(suppl.):741–743 (1979).

Amborn, S.: "Clinical Signs Associated with the Amount of Tracheobronchial Secretions," *Nurs Res*, **25:**121 (1976).

Bates, Joseph H.: "Diagnosis of Tuberculosis," *Chest*, **76** (6)(suppl.):757–763 (1979).

Beahrs, O.: "Complications of Surgery of the Head and Neck," *Surg Clin North Am*, **57:**823 (1977).

Black, L.: "Rhinoplasties under Local Anesthesia," *Nurs Times*, **26:**1304 (1976).

Blues, K.: "A Framework for Nurses Providing Care to Laryngectomy Patients," *Cancer Nurs*, **1:**441 (1978).

Boyer, M. W.: "Treating Invasive Lung Cancer," *AJN*, **77:** 1916–1923 (1977).

Civetta, J.: "Intermittent Mandatory Ventilation and Positive End-Expiratory Pressure in Acute Ventilatory Insufficiency," *Int Anesthesiol Clin*, **18:**123 (1980).

"Continuous or Nocturnal Oxygen Therapy in Hypoxemic Chronic Obstructive Lung Disease," *Ann Intern Med*, **93:**391–398 (1980).

D'Acuti, D. L.: "Eyes, Ears, Nose and Throat Emergencies," *J Emerg Nurs*, **1:**24 (1975).

DeSanto, L., and J. C. Lillie: "Cancers of the Larynx: Supraglottic Cancer," *Surg Clin North Am*, **1:**505 (1977).

Doey, W. D.: "Nasal Obstruction—1," *Nurs Times*, **5:**117 (1976).

———: "Nasal Obstruction—2," *Nurs Times*, **12:**222 (1976).

Dropkin, M. J.: "Compliance in Post-operative Head and Neck Patients," *Cancer Nurs*, **2:**379 (1979).

Dudley, Donald L.: "Why Patients Don't Take Pills," *Chest*, **76**(6)(suppl.):744–749 (1979).

———: "Psychosocial Concomitants to Rehabilitation in Chronic Obstructive Pulmonary Disease Part 2. Psychosocial Treatment," *Chest*, **77:**544–551 (1980).

———: "Psychosocial Concomitants to Rehabilitation in Chronic Obstructive Pulmonary Disease: Part 3. Dealing with Psychiatric Disease (as Distinguished from Psychosocial or Psychophysiologic Problems," *Chest*, **77:**677–684 (1980).

——— et al.: "Psychosocial Concomitants to Rehabilitation in Chronic Obstructive Pulmonary Disease Part 1. Psychosocial and Psychological Considerations," *Chest*, **77:**413–420 (1980).

Epidemiology Standardization Project: *Am Rev Respir Dis*, **188**(6):1–119 (1978).

Ferrer, M. Irene: "Management of Patients with Cor Pulmonale," *Med Clin North Am*, **63:**251–265 (1979).
Fitsgerald, L. M., and G. L. Huber: "Weaning the Patient from Mechanical Ventilation," *Heart Lung*, **5:**228 (1976).
Fox, Wallace: "The Chemotherapy of Pulmonary Tuberculosis: A Review," *Chest*, **76**(6)(suppl.):785–796 (1979).
Gallagher, T., J. Civelta, and R. Kirby: "Terminology Update: Optimal Peep," *Crit Care Med*, **6:**5 (1978).
Gherini, S., R. Peters, and R. Virgild: "Mechanical Work on the Lungs and Work of Breathing with Positive End Expiratory Pressure and Continuous Positive Airway Pressure," *Chest*, **76:**3 (1979).
Greenbaum, D.: "Decannulation of the Tracheotomized Patient," *Heart Lung*, **5:**119 (1976).
"Guidelines for Short-Course Tuberculosis Chemotherapy," *Am Rev Respir Dis*, (1980).
Harris, S. K., et al.: "Gastrointestinal Hemorrhage in Patients in a Respiratory Intensive Care Unit," *Chest*, **72:**301 (1977).
Horoshak, J.: "As Flu Season Approaches: A Call to Battle," *RN*, **38:**17 (1975).
Hutchinson, R.: "The Common Cold Primer," *Nurs 79*, **9:**57 (1979).
"Influenza Vaccine: Recommendations of the Public Health Service Advisory Committee on Immunization Practices," *Ann Intern Med*, **89:**657 (1978).
Johnson, J., et al.: "Toward the Total Rehabilitation of the Alaryngeal Patient," *Laryngoscope*, **89:**1813 (1979).
Keith, R., et al.: "Presurgical Counseling Needs of Laryngectomees: A Survey of 78 Patients," *Laryngoscope*, **88:** 1660 (1978).
Kirilloff, L., and R. Maszkiewicz: "Guide to Respiratory Care in Critically Ill Adults," *Am J Nurs*, **79:**2005 (1979).
Kuzenski, B.: "Effect of Negative Pressure on Tracheobronchial Trauma," *Nurs Res*, **27:**4 (1978).
Levy, M. M., and J. A. Stubbs: "Nursing Implications in the Care of Patients Treated with Assisted Mechanical Ventilation," *Heart Lung*, **7:**299 (1978).
Lyons, H. A.: "Guide to Acute Upper Airway Infections," *Hosp Med*, 0:94, (1976).
Mann, P.: "Marijuana Alert II: More of the Grim Story," *Reader's Digest*, 65–71 (November 1980).
McConnell, E. A.: "How to Truly Help the Patient with a Radical Neck Dissection," *Nurs 76*, **6:**59 (1976).
Minear, D., and F. Lucente: "Current Attitudes of Laryngectomy Patients," *Laryngoscope*, **89:**1061 (1979).
Murray, J.: "Mechanisms of Acute Respiratory Failure," *Am Rev Respir Dis*, **115:**1071 (1977).
Neilsen, L.: "Mechanical Ventilation Patient Assessment and Nursing Care (Home Study Feature)," *AJN*, **80:**2191 (1980).
Pagana, D. K.: "Teaching Your Tracheostomy Patient to Cope at Home," *RN*, 41–64 (1978).
Passey, V., et al.: "Foreign Bodies in the Throat, Nose and Ear," *Hosp Med*, **13:**8 (1977).
Patterson, R.: "Rhinitis," *Med Clin North Am*, **58:**13 (1974).
Pehy, T. L.: "Complications Occurring during Mechanical Ventilation," *Heart Lung*, **5:**112 (1976).
Petty, Thomas L.: "Management of Chronic Airflow Obstruction," *Semin Respir Med*, **1:**30–46 (1979).
Pinney, M.: "Pneumonia," *AJN*, **81:**517–518 (1981).
Powaser and Associates: "The Effectiveness of Hourly Cuff Deflation in Minimizing Tracheal Damage," *Heart Lung*, **5:**740 (1976).
"Proceedings of the Conference on the Scientific Basis of in-Hospital Respiratory Therapy": *Am Rev Respir Dis*, **122:**1–161 (1980).
Promisloff, R. A.: "Administering Oxygen Safely: When, Why, How," *Nurs '80*, **8:**54–56 (1980).
Reichman, Lee B.: "Tuberculin Skin Testing: The State of the Art," *Chest*, **76**(6)(suppl.):764–770 (1979).
——— and R. J. McDonald: "Practical Management and Control of Tuberculosis," *Med Clin North Am*, **61:**1185–1203 (1977).
Sagel, S., et al.: "High Resolution Computed Tomography in the Staging of Carcinoma of the Larynx," *Laryngoscope*, **91:**292 (1981).
Samonds, Rebecca: "Guillain-Barré Syndrome: Helping the Patient in the Acute-Stage," *Nurs 80*, **10:**35-41 (1980).
Sbarbaro, John A.: "Compliance: Inducements and Enforcements," *Chest*, **76**(6)(suppl.):750–756 (1979).
Selecky, P. A.: "Tracheostomy: A Review of Present Day Indications," *Heart Lung*, **3:**272 (1974).
———: "Tracheal Damage and Prolonged Intubation with a Cuffed Endotracheal or Tracheostomy Tube," *Heart Lung*, **5:**733 (1976).
Sobol, S., et al: "Enteral and Parenteral Nutrition in Paitents with Head and Neck Cancer," *Ann Otol*, **88:**495 (1979).
"The Health Consequences of Smoking—the Changing Cigarette—A Report of the Surgeon General": U.S. Department of Health and Human Services, Public Health Service, January 12, 1981.
Thomas, K.: "Carcinoma of the Larynx," *Nurs Times*, **6:**371 (1975).
"Toward Eradication—A Contemporary Tuberculosis Control Strategy," *Am Rev Respir Dis*, **118:**1–4 (1978).
Tuazon, C. U.: "Gram-Positive Pneumonias," *Med Clin North Am*, **64:**343–359 (1980).
Vaugh, C. W., et al.: "Laryngeal Carcinoma: Transoral Treatment Utilizing the Transoral Laser," *Am J Surg*, **136:**490 (1978).
Wang, R.: "Streptococcal Sore Throat," *Am J Nurs*, **77:**1797 (1977).
Westerman, S. T.: "Clinical Experiences with Cryosurgical Tonsillectomy," *Eye Ear Nose Throat J*, **59:**47 (1980).
Wilson, James E.: "Pulmonary Embolism: Diagnosis and Treatment," *Clin Notes Resp Dis*, **19**(4):3–12 (1981).
Wilson, R., and W. Wibbald: "Acute Respiratory Failure," *Crit Care Med*, **4:**78–79 (1976).
Yousuf, M., et al.: "Cryosurgery: Scientific Basis and Clinical Application in Otolaryngology," *Eye Ear Nose Throat J*, **55:**38 (1976).

Organizations

Allergy Foundation of America, 801 Second Avenue, New York, NY 10017
American Academy of Facial Plastic, and Reconstructive Surgery, Inc., 9735 Wilshire Blvd., Beverly Hills, CA 90219
American Lung Association, 1740 Broadway, New York, NY 10019
American Speech and Hearing Association, 9030 Old Georgetown Road, Washington, D.C. 20014
International Association of Laryngectomees, 777 Third Avenue, New York, NY 10017
National Cystic Fibrosis Research Foundation, 202 East 44 Street, New York, NY 10017

Hematology

Books

Linman, J. W.: *Hematology: Physiologic, Pathophysiologic, and Clinical Principles*, The Macmillan Company, New York, 1975.

Williams, W. (ed.): *Hematology*, 2d ed., McGraw-Hill Book Company, New York, 1976.

Wintrobe, M. M., G. R. Lee, D. R. Boggs, T. C. Bitheu, J. W. Athens, and J. Foerester: *Clinical Hematology*, Lea & Febiger, Philadelphia, 1974.

Periodicals

Aisner, J.: "Platelet Transfusion Therapy," *Med Clin North Am*, **61:**1133–1145 (1977).

Alavi, J. B., et al.: "A Randomized Clinical Trial of Granulocyte Transfusions for Infection in Acute Leukemia," *N Engl J Med*, **296:**706–711 (1977).

Barlock, A. L., D. M. Howser, and S. M. Hubbard: "Nursing Management of Adriamycin Extravasation," *Am J Nurs*, **79:**94–96 (1979).

Bingham, C. A.: "The Cell Cycle and Cancer Chemotherapy," *Am J Nurs*, **78:**1201–1205 (1978).

Buickus, B. A.: "Administering Blood Components," *Am J Nurs*, **79:**937–941 (1979).

Crane, L. R., et al.: "Prevention of Infection on the Oncology Unit," *Nurs Clin North Am*, **15:**843–856 (1980).

Cullins, L. C.: "Blood Therapy: Preventing and Treating Transfusion Reactions," *Am J Nurs*, **79:**935–936 (1979).

Dabich, L.: "Adult Acute Nonlymphocytic Leukemias," *Med Clin North Am*, **64:**683–704 (1980).

Daeffler, R.: "Oral Hygiene Measures for Patients with Cancer, I," *Cancer Nurs*, **3:**347–356 (1980).

———: "Oral Hygiene Measures for Patients with Cancer, II," *Cancer Nurs*, **3:**427–432 (1980).

———: "Oral Hygiene Measures for Patients with Cancer, III," *Cancer Nurs*, **4:**29–35 (1981).

DeMoss, C. J.: "Giving Intravenous Chemotherapy at Home," *Am J Nurs*, **80:**2188–2189 (1980).

Desotell, S.: "A Brighter Future for Leukemia Patients," *Nursing*, **7:**19–24 (1977).

Dilworth, J. A., and G. L. Mandell: "Infections in Patients with Cancer," *Semin Oncol*, **2:**349–359 (1975).

Donley, D. L.: "Nursing the Patient Who Is Immunosupressed," *AJN*, **76:**1619–1625 (1976).

Doswell, W. M.: "Sickle Cell Anemia: You Can Do Something to Help," *Nursing*, **8:**65–70 (1978).

Elliott, C.: "Radiation Therapy: How You Can Help," *Nursing*, **6:**34–41 (1976).

Graham, V., and B. J. Rubal: "Recipient and Donor Response to Granulocyte Transfusions and Leukapheresis," *Cancer Nurs*, **3:**97–11 (1980).

Greenberger, J. S., S. E. Come, and R. R. Weichselbaum: "Issues of Controversy in Radiation Therapy and Combined Modality Approaches to Hodgkin's Disease," *Clin Hematol*, **8:**611–624 (1979).

Herzig, R. H., et al.: "Successful Granulocyte Transfusion Therapy for Gram-Negative Septicemia," *N Engl J Med*, **296:**701–705 (1977).

Houlihan, N. G.: "Leukemia: A Hematology Review," *Cancer Nurs*, **4:**61–71 (1981).

Jagathambal, K., H. W. Grunwald, and F. Rosner: "Evaluation and Management of the Bleeding Patient," *Med Clinl North Am*, **65:**133–146 (1981).

Jennings, B. M.: "Improving Your Management of DIC," *Nursing*, **9:**60–67 (1979).

Keaveny, M. E.: "Hodgkin's Disease: The Curable Cancer," *Nursing*, **5:**48–54 (1975).

LeBlanc, D. H.: "People with Hodgkin's Disease: The Nursing Challenge," *Nurs Clin North Am*, **13:**281–300 (1978).

Lerner, R. G.: "The Defibrination Syndrome," *Med Clin North Am*, **60:**871–880 (1976).

Levine, A. S.: "Protected Environment—Prophylactic Antibiotic Programmes; Clinical Studies," *Clin Hematol*, **5:** 409–424 (1976).

Liepman, M. K.: "The Chronic Leukemias," *Med Clin North Am*, **64:**705–727 (1980).

Lister, T. A., and R. A. Yankee: "Blood Component Therapy," *Clin Hematol*, **7**(2):407–423 (1978).

Lovejoy, N. C.: "Preventing Hair Loss during Adriamycin Therapy," *Cancer Nurs*, **2:**117–122 (1979).

Maxwell, M. B.: "Scalp Tourniquets for Chemotherapy—Induced Alopecia," *Am J Nurs*, **80:**900–902 (1980).

Megliola, B.: "Multiple Myeloma," *Cancer Nurs*, **3:**209–218 (1980).

O'Brian, B. S., and S. Woods: "The Paradox of DIC," *Am J Nurs*, **78:**1878–1880 (1978).

Paredes, J. M., and B. S. Mitchell: "Multiple Myeloma," *Med Clin North Am*, **64:**729–742 (1980).

Patterson, P.: "Granulocyte Transfusion: Nursing Considerations," *Cancer Nurs*, **3:**101–104 (1980).

Priesler, H. D., and S. Bjornson: "Protected Environment Units in the Treatment of Acute Leukemia," *Semin Oncol*, **2:**369–377 (1975).

Rodgers, J. M.: "Hodgkin's Disease: Hope Is the Key to Nursing Care," *Nursing*, **5:**55–58 (1975).

Satterwhite, B. E.: "What to Do When Adriamycin Infiltrates," *Nursing*, **3:**37 (1980).

Schiffer, C. A.: "Principles of Granulocyte Transfusion Therapy," *Med Clin North Am*, **61:**1119–1131 (1977).

Schimpff, S. C.: "Therapy of Infections in Patients with Granulocytopenia," *Med Clin North Am*, **61:**1101–1118 (1977).

Schumann, D., and P. Patterson: "Multiple Myeloma," *Am J Nurs*, **75:**78–81 (1975).

Smith, D. S., and T. P. Chamorro: "Nursing Care of Patients Undergoing Combination Chemotherapy and Radiotherapy," *Cancer Nurs*, **1:**129–134 (1978).

Thomas, S. F.: "Transfusing Granulocytes," *Am J Nurs*, **79:**942–944 (1979).

Wagner, L., and M. G. Bye: "Body Image and Patients Experiencing Alopecia as a Result of Cancer Chemotherapy," *Cancer Nurs*, **2:**365–369 (1979).

Welch, D.: "Thrombocytopenia in the Adult Patient with Acute Leukemia," *Cancer Nurs*, **1:**129–134 (1978).

———and K. Lewis: "Alopecia and Chemotherapy," *Am J Nurs*, **80:**903–905 (1980).

Young, R. C., and V. T. DeVita: "Chemotherapy of Hodgkin's Disease," *Clin Hematol*, **8:**625–644 (1979).

Zeluff, G. W., E. A. Natelson, and D. Jackson: "Thrombocytopenic Purpura—Idiopathic and Thrombotic," *Heart Lung*, **7:**327–333 (1978).

Organizations

Foundation for Research and Education in Sickle-Cell Disease, 421–431 West 120 Street, New York, NY 10027

Leukemia Society of America, Inc., 211 East 43 Street, New York, NY 10017

National Hemophilia Foundation, 25 West 39 Street, New York, NY 10018

Cardiovascular

Books

Abramson, D.: *Circulatory Disorders of the Limbs*, Grune & Stratton, Inc., New York, 1978.

Alpert, J. S., and J. M. Rippe: *Manual of Cardiovascular Diagnosis and Therapy*, Little, Brown and Company, Boston, 1980.

Andreoli, K., et al.: *Comprehensive Cardiac Care*, The C. V. Mosby Company, St. Louis, 1979.

Aspinall, M. J.: *Nursing the Open-Heart Patient*, McGraw-Hill Book Company, New York, 1973.

Boarman, C., et al. (eds.): *Current Practice in Critical Care*, The C. V. Mosby Company, St. Louis, 1979.

Conover, Mary H.: *Cardiac Arrhythmias*, 2d ed., The C. V. Mosby Company, St. Louis, 1978.

Constant, Jules: *Bedside Cardiology*, 2d ed., Little, Brown and Company, Boston, 1976.

Cromwell, R. L., et al.: *Acute Myocardial Infarction: Reaction and Recovery*, The C. V. Mosby Company, St. Louis, 1977.

DeLeon, Antonio C., Jr.: *Heart Sounds: What They Teach Us*, Humetrics Corporation, 1975.

Heart Attack! What Now? Georgia Heart Association, Atlanta, 1977.

Hudak, C., et al.: *Critical Care Nursing*, J. B. Lippincott Company, Philadelphia, 1977.

Hurst, J. W., et al. (eds.): *The Heart*, 4th ed., McGraw-Hill Book Company, New York, 1978.

Juergens, J., et al.: *Peripheral Vascular Disease*, W. B. Saunders Company, Philadelphia, 1980.

Kochar, M., and L. Daniels: *Hypertension Control: For Nurses and Other Health Professionals*, The C. V. Mosby Company, St. Louis, 1978.

Lear, M. W.: *Heart Sounds*, Simon and Schuster, New York, 1980.

Madden, J. L., et al.: *Venous Thromboembolism, Prevention and Treatment*, Appleton-Century-Crofts, Inc., New York, 1976.

Rutherford, R. B.: *Vascular Surgery*, W. B. Saunders Company, Philadelphia, 1977.

Storlie, Francis: *Patient Teaching in Critical Care*, Appleton-Century-Crofts, Inc., New York, 1975.

The Hypertensive Handbook: Merck, Sharpe and Dohme in cooperation with the National High Blood Pressure Education Program, 1974.

Tilkian, Ara, and Mary Conover: *Understanding Heart Sounds and Murmurs*, W. B. Saunders Company, Philadelphia, 1979.

Tripp, A.: *Basic Pathophysiologic Mechanisms of Shock*, McGraw-Hill Book Company, New York, 1979.

Wenger, N. K.: *Cardiology for Nurses*, McGraw-Hill Book Company, New York, 1980.

Periodicals

Begley, L. A.: "External Counterpulsation for Shock," *Am J Nurs*, **75:**967 (1975).

Birnbaum, M. L.: "Multisystem Failure: How Almost Everything Can Go Wrong Quickly," *Nurs 78*, **8:**30 (1978).

Bookman, L. B.: "The Early Assessment of Hypovolemia: Postural Vital Signs," *J Emerg Nurs*, **3:**43 (1977).

Bricker, P. L.: "The Intense Nursing Demands of the Intra-aortic Balloon Pump," *RN*, **43:**23–29 (1980).

Buell, J. C., and R. S. Eliot: "The Role of Emotional Stress in the Development of Heart Disease," *JAMA*, **242:**365–368 (1979).

Byrne, D. G., H. M. Whyte, and G. N. Lance: "A Typology of Responses to Illness in Survivors of Myocardial Infarction," *Int J Psychiatry Med*, **9:**135–145 (1978–1979).

Cole, C. M., et al.: "Brief Sexual Counseling during Cardiac Rehabilitation," *Heart Lung*, **8:**124–128 (1979).

Committee on Trauma, American College of Surgeons: "A Guide to the Initial Therapy of Shock," *Consultant*, **8:**94 (1978).

Connors, J. P.: "An Update on Cardiac Surgery," *Heart Lung*, **10:**323–328 (1981).

Cook, R. L.: "Psychosocial Responses to Myocardial Infarction," *Heart Lung*, **8:**130–134 (1979).

Coussons, R. T.: "How to Select the Best Antiobiotic for the Critically Ill Patient," *Res Staff Physician*, **26:**59 (1980).

Cromwell, V., et al.: "Understanding the Needs of Your Coronary Bypass Patient," *Nurs 80*, **10:**34–41 (1980).

Crumlish, C. M.: "Cardiogenic Shock: Catch It Early," *Nurs 81*, **11:**34–41 (1981).

Cukowica, L., and S. Sherry: "Current Status of Thrombolytic Therapy," *Heart Lung*, **7:**97–104 (1978).

DeBusk, R. F., et al.: "Exercise Training Soon after Myocardial Infarction," *Am J Cardiol*, **44:**1223–1229 (1979).

Dehn, M. M.: "Rehabilitation of the Cardiac Patient: The Effects of Exercise," *AJM*, **80:**435–450 (1980).

Dembroski, T. M., J. M. MacDougal, and R. Lushene: "Interpersonal Interaction and Cardiovascular Response in Type A Subjects and Coronary Patients," *J Human Stress*, **5:**28–36 (1979).

Dollery, C. T., et al.: "Drug-Induced Hypertension," *J Applied Med*, **5:**205 (1979).

Elenbaas, R. M.: "Anaphylactic Shock," *Crit Care Q*, **2:**77 (1980).

Eskridge, R. A.: "Septic Shock," *Crit Care Q*, **2:**55 (1980).

Gardner, D., et al.: "The Nurses' Dilemma: Mediating Stress in the Critical Care Unit," *Heart Lung*, **9:**103–106 (1980).

——— and N. Stewart: "Staff Involvement with Families of Patients in Critical-Care Units," *Heart Lung*, **7:**105–110 (1978).

Guglielmo, B. J.: "Evaluation of the Use of Corticosteroids," *Crit Care Q*, **2:**37 (1980).

Hancock, E. W.: "Management of Pericardial Disease," *Mod Concepts Cardiovasc Dis*, **48:**1 (1979).

Hathaway, R.: "Hemodynamic Monitoring in Shock," *J Emerg Nurs*, **3:**37 (1977).

Hill, M.: "Helping the Hypertensive Patient Control Sodium Intake," *Am J Nurs*, **79:**906 (1979).

Hirsh, J.: "Venous Thromboembolism: Diagnosis, Treatment, Prevention," *Hosp Pract*, 53–62 (1975).

Hoffman, M., S. Donckers, and M. Hauser: "The Effect of Nursing Intervention on Stress Factors Perceived by Patients in a Coronary Care Unit," *Heart Lung*, **7:**804–809 (1978).

Hull, R., et al.: "Impedance Plethysmography Using the Occlusive Cuff Technique in the Diagnosis of Venous Thrombosis," *Circulation*, **53:**696 (1976).

Jahre, J. A., et al.: "Medical Approach to the Hypotensive Patient and the Patient in Shock," *Heart Lung*, **4:**577 (1975).

Jarvik, R. K.: "The Total Artificial Heart," *Scientific American*, **244:**74–80+ (1981).

Jelliffe, R. W.: "Electrolytes and Cardiac Arrhythmias," *Crit Care Update*, **7:**5–11 (1980).

Jenkins, D. C.: "Psychosocial Modifiers of Response to Stress," *J Human Stress*, **5:**3–15 (1979).

———, S. J. Zyzanski, and R. H. Rosenman: "Coronary-Prone Behavior: One Pattern or Several?" *Psychosom Med*, **40:**25–43 (1978).

Katsaros, C., and J. Bobb: "Shock—The Critical Hour," *J Emerg Nurs*, **4:**45 (1978).

Kannel, W. B., et al.: "Epidemiological Assessment of the Rise of Blood Pressure in Stroke: The Framingham Study," *JAMA*, **214:**301 (1970).

Klatsky, A. K., et al.: "Alcohol Consumption and Blood Pressure: Kaiser-Permanente Multiphasic Health Examination Data," *N Engl J Med*, **296:**1194 (1977).

Kroncke, G. M., et al.: "What to Do When Your Patient's Pacemaker Stops Working," *Nursing 81*, **11:**74–78 (1981).

Long, G.: "Managing the Patient with Abdominal Aortic Aneurysm," *Nurs 78*, **8:**21–17 (1978).

Maloney, R.: "Helping Your Hypertensive Patients Live Longer," *Nurs 78*, **8:**26 (1978).

Marcinek, M.: "What Hypertension Does to the Body," *Am J Nurs*, **80:**928 (1980).

Matheny, L. G.: "Defibrillation: When and How to Use It," *Nurs 81*, **11:**69–72 (1981).

Mayou, R.: "The Course and Determinants of Reactions to Myocardial Infarction," *British J Psychiatry*, **134:**588–594 (1979).

McCaffree, D. R.: "Shock—How to Recognize Its Early Stages and What to Do about It," *Res Staff Physician*, **26:**27 (1980).

McLane, M., H. Krop, and J. Metha: "Psychosexual Adjustment and Counseling after Myocardial Infarction," *Ann Intern Med*, **92**(4):514–519 (1980).

Mitchell, E. S.: "Protocol for Teaching Hypertensive Patients," *Am J Nurs*, **77:**808 (1977).

Mohr, J. A., and R. T. Coussons: "Septic Shock," *Res Staff Physician*, **26:**49 (1980).

Molyneux-Luick, M., and J. W. Knecht: "The Emergency that Supersedes All Other Duties: Hypovolemic Shock," *Nurs 77*, **7:**32 (1977).

Mondejar, E. S.: "'Last Ditch' Heart Assist Is Producing Survivors . . . Use of the Left Heart Assist Device (LHAD)," *RN*, **43:**54–57+ (1980).

Moser, M.: "How Hypertension Therapy Works," *Am J Nurs*, **89:**937 (1980).

Moyer, J. H., and L. C. Mills: "Vasopressor Agents in Shock," *Am J Nurs*, **75:**620 (1975).

O'Donnell, T. F., and S. C. Belkin: "The Pathophysiology, Monitoring, and Treatment of Shock," *Orthop Clin North Am*, **9:**589 (1978).

Ogden, L. D.: "Activity Guidelines for Early Subacute and High-Risk Cardiac Patients," *Am J Occup Ther*, **33:**291–298 (1979).

Owens, J. F., C. S. McCann, and C. M. Hutelmyer: "Cardiac Rehabilitation: A Patient Education Program," *Nurs Res*, **27:**148–150 (1978).

Pankey, George: "Prevention and Treatment of Bacterial Endocarditis," *Am Heart J*, **98:**102 (1979).

Papadopoulos, C., et al.: "Sexual Concerns and Needs of the Post-Coronary Patient's Wife," *Arch Intern Med*, **140:** 38–41 (1980).

Papper, S.: "The Oliguric Patient," *Res Staff Physician*, **26:**87 (1980).

Park, G. D.: "Cardiogenic Shock," *Crit Care Q*, **2:**43 (1980).

Pearson, R. M., et al.: "Treatment of Severe and Resistant Hypertension," *J Applied Med*, **5:**345 (1979).

Pinneo, R., et al.: "Coronary Care Nursing—The Best Is Yet to Be," *Heart Lung*, **8:**876–81 (1979).

Purcell, J. A., and P. Giffin: "Percutaneous Transluminal Coronary Angioplasty," *Am J Nurs*, **81:**1620–1626 (1981).

Rackley, C. E., et al.: "Cardiogenic Shock," *Res Staff Physician*, **26:**35 (1980).

Richter, J. M., and R. Sloan: "The Relaxation Technique," *Am J Nurs*, **79:**1960 (1979).

Roach, L. B.: "Color Changes in Dark Skin," *Nurs 77*, **7:**48 (1977).

Robinson, W. A.: "Fluid Therapy in Hemorrhagic Shock," *Crit Care Q*, **2:**1 (1980).

Rodman, M. J.: "Drugs for Treating Shock," *RN*, **39:**77 (1976).

———: "Latest Strategies for Post-MI Dysrhythmias," *RN*, **44:**63–64+ (1981).

Rothstein, R. J.: "Hemorrhagic Shock in Multiple Trauma," *Topics in Emerg Med*, **1:**29 (1979).

Scalzi, C. C., L. E. Burke, and S. Greenland: "Evaluation of an Inpatient Educational Program for Coronary Patients and Families," *Heart Lung*, **9:**846–853 (1980).

———and K. Dracup: "Sexual Counseling of Coronary Patients," *Heart Lung*, **7:**840–845 (1978).

Sparks, Colleen: "Peripheral Pulses," *Am J Nurs*, **75:**1132–1133 (1975).

"Standards for Cardiopulmonary Resuscitation and Emergency Cardiac Care," *JAMA*, **227**(suppl):833 (1980).

Stern, M. J., and L. Pascale: "Psychosocial Adaptation Post-Myocardial Infarction: The Spouse's Dilemma," *J Psychosom Res*, **23:**83–87 (1979).

Sweetwood, H.: "Cardiac Tamponade: When Dyspnea Spells Sudden Death," *RN*, **43:**34–41 (1980).

Taylor, C. M.: "When to Anticipate Septic Shock," *Nurs 75*, **5:**34 (1975).

Tharpe, G. D.: "Shock: The Overall Mechanisms," *Am J Nurs*, **74:**2208 (1974).

Thorpe, C. J.: "A Nursing Care Plan—The Adult Cardiac Surgical Patient," *Heart Lung*, **8:**690–698 (1979).

Vij, D.: "A Simplified Concept of Complete Physiologic Monitoring of the Critically Ill Patient," *Heart Lung*, **10:**75–82 (1981).

Visalli, F.: "The Swan-Ganz Catheter: A Program for Teaching Safe, Effective Use," *Nurs 81*, **11:**42–47 (1981).

Waeckerle, J. F.: "Antishock Garments," *Crit Care Q*, **2:**15 (1980).

Ward, G. W., et al.: "Treating and Counseling the Hypertensive Patient," *Am J Nurs*, **78:**824 (1978).

Watson, N.: "Anticoagulant Therapy in the Prevention of Venous Thrombosis and Pulmonary Embolism in Spinal Cord Injury," *Paraplegia*, **16:**265–269 (1979).

Wenger, N. K.: "Research Related to Rehabilitation," *Circulation*, **60**(7):1636–1639 (1979).

Whitsett, T. L.: "Medical Management of Shock—Drugs of Choice and Their Action," *Res Staff Physician*, **26:**73 (1980).

Wilson, R. F.: "The Diagnosis and Management of Severe Sepsis and Septic Shock," *Heart Lung*, **5:**422 (1976).

———: "Diagnosis and Treatment of Shock," *Consultant*, **18:**109 (1978).

———and J. A. Wilson: "Pathophysiology, Diagnosis and Treatment of Shock," *J Emerg Nurs*, **3:**11 (1977).

Young, L. E.: "Nursing Interventions with Obese Cardiac Patients," *Nurs Clin North Am*, **13:**449–456 (1978).

Films

"Sex and the Heart Patient," Synthesis Communications, Inc., 119 West 57 Street, New York, NY 10019. Distributed through Burroughs-Wellcome Company, Research Triangle Park, Durham, NC 27709.

Organizations

American Association of Critical Care Nurses, P.O. Box 5445, Orange, CA 92667

American Heart Association, 44 East 23 St., New York, NY 10010

National Heart and Lung Institute, National Institutes of Health, Bethesda, MD 20014

Section 7

Problems with Ingestion, Digestion, Absorption, and Elimination

Chapter 31

NURSING ASSESSMENT
Gastrointestinal System

Rachel Elrod

Learning Objectives

1. Describe the structures and functions of the organs of the gastrointestinal tract.
2. Describe the structures and functions of the liver, biliary tract, and pancreas.
3. Explain the processes of ingestion, digestion, absorption, and elimination.
4. Explain the process of bile production and excretion.
5. Identify the significant subjective and objective data related to the gastrointestinal system that should be obtained from a client.
6. Describe the appropriate techniques used in the physical assessment of the gastrointestinal system.
7. Differentiate normal from common abnormal findings of a physical assessment of the gastrointestinal system.
8. Describe the purpose, significance of results, and nursing responsibilities related to diagnostic studies of the gastrointestinal system.

The main function of the gastrointestinal (GI) system is to supply nutrients to body cells. This is accomplished through the processes of *ingestion* (taking in food), *digestion* (breakdown of food), and *absorption* (transfer of food products into circulation). *Elimination* is the process of excreting waste products of digestion.

The gastrointestinal system (also called the digestive system) consists of the gastrointestinal tract and its associated organs. Included in the gastrointestinal tract are the mouth, esophagus, stomach, small intestine, and large intestine. The associated organs are the liver, pancreas, and gallbladder with their duct system (Fig. 31-1).

Psychological or emotional factors such as stress and anxiety influence gastrointestinal functioning in many individuals. Stress may be manifested as anorexia, epigastric pain, or diarrhea. However, gastrointestinal problems should not be solely attributed to psychological factors. Organic and psychological-based problems can exist independently or concurrently. Stress can be a predisposing factor for organic diseases of the GI system such as peptic ulcer disease and ulcerative colitis. A complete assessment is essential to determine the psychological factors associated with GI problems.

GASTROINTESTINAL SYSTEM: STRUCTURES AND FUNCTIONS

The gastrointestinal tract is a tube about 9 m (30 ft) long extending from the mouth to the anus. The entire tract is composed of four common layers. Going from the inside to the outside, these layers are: (1) mucous membrane, (2) submucosa, (3) muscle, and (4) serosa. In the esophagus the outer coat is fibrous tissue rather than serosa. The muscular coat consists of two layers: the circular (inner) and the longitudinal (outer).

The GI tract is innervated by the parasympathetic and the sympathetic branches of the autonomic nervous system. The parasympathetic system is mainly excitatory and the sympathetic system is mainly inhibitory. For example, peristalsis is increased by parasympathetic stimulation and decreased by sympathetic stimulation.

The two types of movement of the GI tract are mixing and propulsion. These movements are accomplished by peristalsis and rhythmical movements. The secretions of the GI system consist mainly of enzymes for digestion and mucus for protection and lubrication.

The primary functions of the GI system are: (1) movement of food; (2) digestion; (3) absorption; (4) providing the body with a continual supply of nutrients, electrolytes, and water; and (5) elimination.[1] Each part of the GI system performs different activities in order to accomplish these functions.

Ingestion

Ingestion is the intake of food. *Deglutition* (swallowing) completes the process of ingestion. An individual's appetite or desire to ingest food is a significant factor in how much food is eaten. An appetite center is located in the hypothalamus. It is directly or indirectly stimulated by an empty stomach, decrease in body temperature, hypoglycemia, habit, and the sight, smell, and taste of food. Appetite may be

This chapter was reviewed by Rosemary Lape, R.N., School of Nursing, Syracuse University, Syracuse, New York.

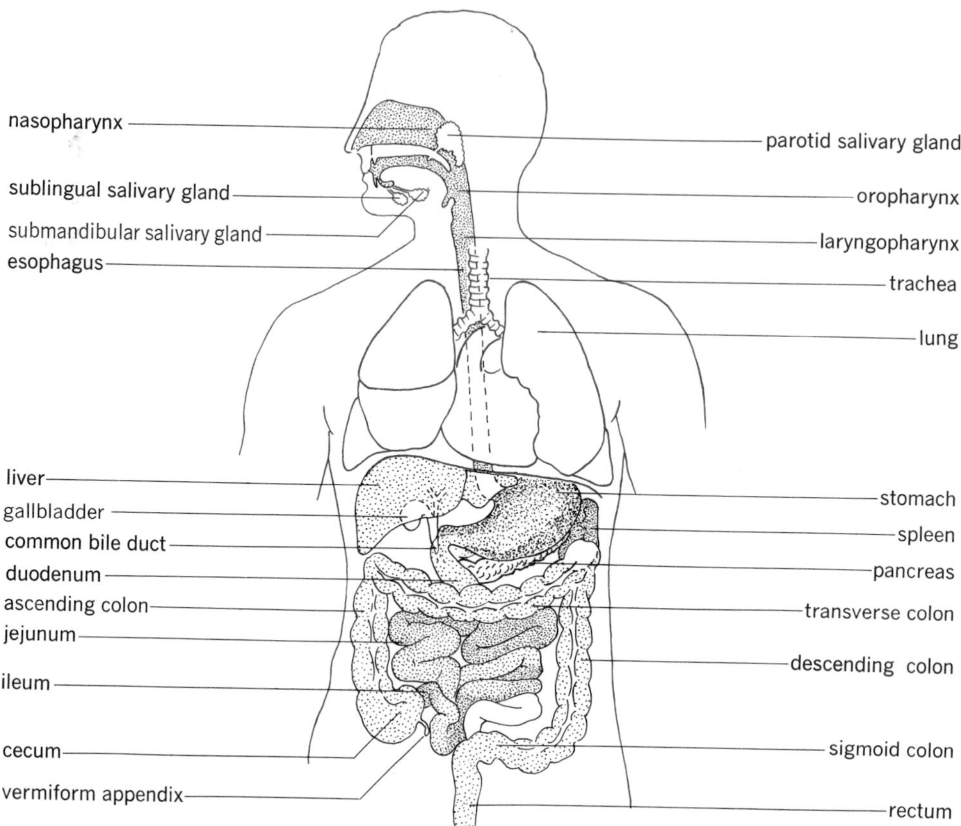

Figure 31-1 Organs of the gastrointestinal system. *(From R. M. DeCoursey and J. L. Renfro, The Human Organism, 5th ed., McGraw-Hill Book Company, New York, 1980, p. 617.)*

inhibited by stomach distension, illness (especially accompanied by fever), hyperglycemia, nausea and vomiting, and certain drugs (e.g., amphetamines). The economic inability to purchase food supplies may be another factor affecting adequate ingestion, especially in the elderly.

Mouth

The mouth consists of the lips and oral cavity. The lips surround the orifice of the mouth and function in speech. The roof of the oral cavity is formed by the hard and soft palate. The oral cavity contains the teeth, used in mastication, and the tongue. The tongue assists in mastication and deglutition by moving the food backward and keeping it between the teeth. Mucus is secreted by glands on the tongue and helps lubricate the food. The tongue is also important in speech and taste sensation.

Within the oral cavity are three pairs of salivary glands: the *parotid*, *submaxillary*, and *sublingual*. These glands, along with the mucous glands in the mouth, produce saliva. Saliva consists of water, protein, mucin, inorganic salts, and salivary amylase.

Pharynx

The *pharynx* is a musculomembranous tube which may be divided into the *nasopharynx*, the *oropharynx*, and the *laryngeal pharynx*. The mucous membrane of the pharynx is continuous with the nasal cavity, mouth, auditory tubes, and larynx. The pharynx functions in the act of swallowing and secretes mucus. The *epiglottis* is a lid of fibrocartilage which closes over the larynx during swallowing. The function of the pharynx in ingestion is to provide a route for the food from the mouth to the esophagus.

Esophagus

The esophagus is a muscular tube that receives food from the pharynx and moves it to the stomach by peristaltic contractions. It is 23 to 25 cm (9 to 10 inches) long and 2 cm in diameter. The esophagus starts behind the trachea at the lower end of the pharynx and extends to the stomach. The muscular layers contract and propel the food to the stomach. The gastroesophageal sphincter at the lower end of the esophagus remains constricted except during swallowing, belching, or vomiting. This sphincter prevents gastric reflux.

Digestion and Absorption

Stomach

The functions of the stomach are to store food, mix the food with gastric juice and mucin, produce chemical changes, and mechanically change the bolus of food. The stomach also absorbs small amounts of water, glucose, alcohol, and electrolytes.

The stomach lies obliquely in the epigastric, umbilical, and left hypochondriac regions of the abdomen (see Fig. 31-7 later in the chapter). The shape and position of the stomach change based on its contents, digestion, and the muscular walls. It always contains gastric fluid and mucus. The three main parts of the stomach are the *fundus*, *body*, and *pylorus* (antrum) (Fig. 31-2). Sphincter muscles guard the entrance to and exit from the stomach. The *cardiac sphincter* is the opening between the esophagus and stomach; the *pyloric sphincter* is between the stomach and the duodenum.

The *serous* (outer) layer of the stomach is formed by the peritoneum. The *muscular* layer which is smooth muscle consists of the longitudinal (outer) layer, circular (middle) layer, and the oblique (inner) layer. The mucous layer forms folds called *rugae* which contain many small glands. In the fundus are the *chief cells* which secrete pepsinogen and the *parietal cells* which secrete hydrochloric acid (HCl), water and the intrinsic factor. The intrinsic factor promotes the absorption of vitamin B_{12} (extrinsic factor). Mucus is secreted by glands in the cardiac and pyloric areas. The stomach also secretes an alkaline substance which is protective and prevents autodigestion.

Branches of the vagus nerve of the parasympathetic nervous system innervate the stomach. Parasympathetic stimulation of the stomach increases both peristalsis and secretions. The stomach is also innervated by the sympathetic nervous system. Sympathetic stimulation inhibits both gastric secretion and motility.

Small intestine

The two primary functions of the small intestine are digestion and absorption of the end products of digestion. The small intestine is a coiled tube about 7 m (23 ft) in length, and from 2.5 cm to 2.8 cm in diameter, diminishing in diameter at the lower end. It extends from the pylorus to the ileocecal valve (Fig.

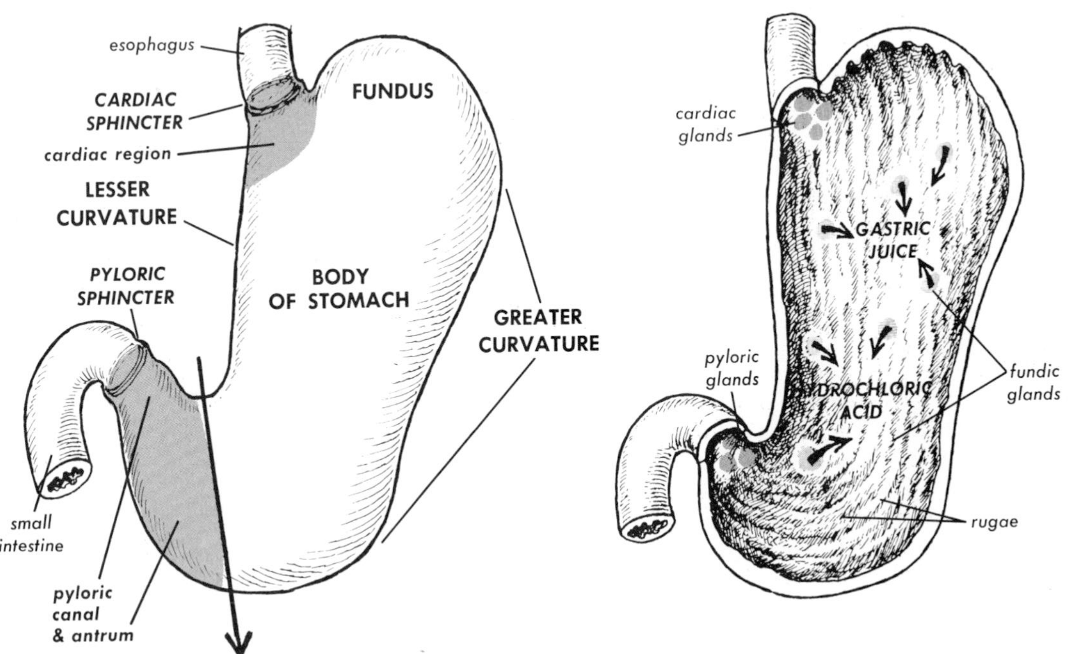

Figure 31-2 Parts of the stomach *(From E. J. Reith et al., Textbook of Anatomy and Physiology, 2d ed., McGraw-Hill Book Company, New York, 1978, p. 308.)*

31-1). The small intestine is composed of the *duodenum*, the *jejunum*, and the *ileum*. The ileocecal valve controls the exit into the large intestine and prevents reflux into the small intestine.

The serous coat of the small intestine is formed by the peritoneum. The mucosa is thick, vascular, and glandular. The circular folds in the mucous and submucous layers provide a greater surface area for secretion of digestive juices and absorption.

The functional units of the small intestine are *villi*. They are present in the entire small intestine. Villi are minute, finger like projections in the mucous membrane. They contain goblet cells that secrete mucus and absorptive cells that absorb digested foodstuffs. The villi greatly increase the surface area for absorption. There are many enzymes on the brush border of the villi which digest food substances as they are being absorbed. The *crypts of Lieberkühn* or *intestinal glands* produce secretions which contain digestive enzymes. *Brunner's glands* in the submucosa of the duodenum secrete mucus.

Both branches of the autonomic nervous system innervate the small intestine. The vagus nerve stimulates motility and secretions and the sympathetic branch inhibits motility. Pain is relayed through sensory fibers of the sympathetic system. The small intestine receives its blood supply from branches of the hepatic and superior mesenteric artery.

Peritoneum

The abdominal viscera are almost completely covered by the peritoneum. The two layers of the peritoneum are the *parietal*, which lines the abdominal cavity wall, and the *visceral*, which covers the abdominal organs. The peritoneal cavity is the potential space between the parietal and visceral layers. The two folds of the peritoneum are the *mesentery* and *omentum*. The *mesentery* attaches the small intestine and part of the large intestine to the posterior abdominal wall and contains blood and lymph vessels. The *lesser omentum* goes from the lesser curvature of the stomach and upper duodenum to the liver, and the *greater omentum* hangs from the stomach over the intestines like an apron. The omentum contains fat and lymph nodes.

Physiology of digestion and absorption

Digestion is the physical and chemical breakdown of food into absorbable substances. The GI system functions in digestion by moving food through the GI tract and by secreting substances to break food into smaller particles (Table 31-1).

The process of digestion begins in the mouth where the food is chewed, mechanically broken down, and mixed with saliva. The saliva lubricates and starts starch digestion. Salivation is stimulated by chewing movements and the sight, smell, thought, and taste of

Table 31-1
Gastrointestinal Secretions

Location	Secretion	Action
Salivary glands	Salivary amylase (ptyalin)	Begin starch digestion
Stomach	Pepsinogen	Protein digestion
	HCl	Protein digestion
	Lipase	Fat digestion
	Intrinsic factor	Essential for vitamin B_{12} absorption in the ileum
Small intestine	Enterokinase	Activates trypsinogen to trypsin
	Amylase	Carbohydrate digestion
	Peptidases	Protein digestion
	Maltase	Maltose to glucose
	Sucrase	Sucrose to glucose and fructose
	Lactase	Lactose to glucose and galactose
	Lipase	Fat digestion
Pancreas	Trypsinogen	Protein digestion
	Chymotrypsin	Protein digestion
	Amylase	Starch to disaccharides
	Lipase	Fat digestion
Liver and gallbladder	Bile	Emulsify fats, aid in absorption of fatty acids and fat-soluble vitamins (A, D, E, K)

food. The food is swallowed and passes into the esophagus where peristaltic waves propel it to the stomach.

In the stomach the digestion of proteins begins with minimal digestion of starches and fats. The food is mixed with gastric secretions which are under nervous and hormonal control (Table 31-2). The stomach also serves as a reservoir for food, slowly passing it into the small intestine. The time food remains in the stomach depends on the nature of the food but average meals remain from 3 to 4 hours. There is some individual variation in stomach emptying time.

Digestion is completed in the small intestine where carbohydrates are hydrolyzed to monosaccharides, fats to glycerol and fatty acids, and proteins to amino acids. The surface area of the small intestine is greatly increased by its circular folds, villi, and microvilli. *Chyme* (food mixed with gastric secretions) in the small intestine causes mechanical or chemical stimulation and mixing and peristalsis occur. Secretions responsible for digestion are *succus entericus* (intestinal juice) from glands in the small intestine, enzymes from the pancreas, and bile from the liver (Table 31-1). Secretions are mainly under nervous and hormonal control.

When food enters the small intestine, hormones are released into the bloodstream. The hormone *secretin* stimulates the pancreas to secrete fluid with a high concentration of bicarbonate which neutralizes acid in the chyme. The duodenum also secretes mucus to neutralize HCl. The hormone *CCK-PZ* (cholecystokinin and pancreozymin), produced by the duodenal mucosa, enters the bloodstream and stimulates contraction of the gallbladder and relaxation of the sphincter of Oddi. These actions permit bile to flow from the common bile duct into the duodenum. CCK-PZ also stimulates the pancreas to release pancreatic juices which contain enzymes for hydrolysis of carbohydrates, fats, and proteins.

Absorption is the transfer of the end products of digestion across the intestinal wall to circulation for use by cells. Most absorption takes place in the small intestine. The movement of the villi keeps the end products of digestion in contact with the absorbing membrane. Simple sugars (from carbohydrates), fatty acids (from fats), amino acids (from proteins), water, electrolytes, and vitamins are absorbed.

Elimination

Large intestine (colon, rectum, anus)

The large intestine is a hollow muscular tube about 1.5 to 2 m (5 to 6 ft) long and 5 cm (2 inches) in diameter. The four parts of the large intestine are: (1) *cecum* with *appendix*, which is a narrow tube at the end of the cecum; (2) *colon*, ascending colon on the right side, transverse colon across the abdomen, descending colon on the left side, and the sigmoid colon; (3) the *rectum*; and (4) the *anus*, which is the terminal portion of the large intestine (Fig. 31-3).

The large intestine is innervated by the parasympathetic nervous system which stimulates secretions and contraction. The sympathetic nervous system inhibits secretions and motility. The large intestine receives its blood supply mainly from the superior and inferior mesenteric artery.

The most important function of the large intestine is the absorption of water and electrolytes. It also forms feces. It serves as a reservoir for the fecal mass until defecation occurs. Feces are composed of water

Table 31-2
The Phases of Gastric Secretion

Phase	Stimulus to Secretion	Secretion
Cephalic (nerve)	Sight, smell, taste of food—before food enters stomach. Occurs from vagal nerve innervation.	HCl Pepsinogen Mucus
Gastric (hormonal and nerve)	Food in antrum of stomach. Vagal stimulation.	Gastrin hormone from antrum released into circulation stimulates increased gastric secretions and motility.
Intestinal (hormonal)	Bulk in duodenum and fats in small intestine.	Intestinal gastrin released into circulation stimulates gastric secretion of pepsin and mucus. Enterogastrone released by intestinal mucosa causes decreased gastric secretion and motility.

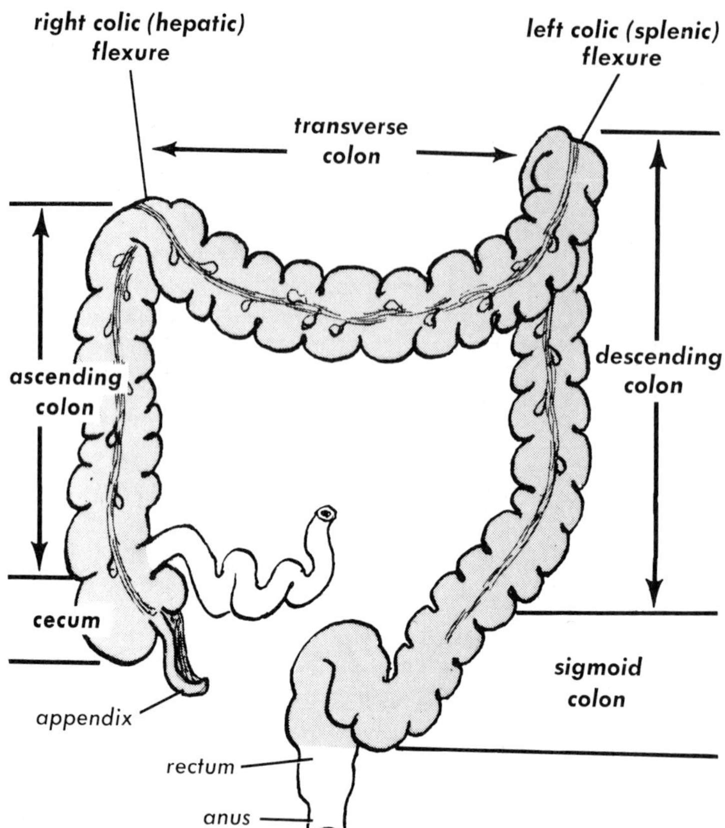

Figure 31-3 Anatonic locations of the large intestine. (*From E. J. Reith et al., Textbook of Anatomy and Physiology, 2d ed., McGraw-Hill Book Company, New York, 1978, p. 312.*)

(75 percent), bacteria, unabsorbed minerals, undigested foodstuffs, bile pigments, and desquamated epithelial cells. The large intestine secretes mucus which acts as a lubricant and protects the mucosa.

Microorganisms in the colon are responsible for the putrefaction of proteins not digested or absorbed in the small intestine. These amino acids are deaminated by the bacteria, leaving ammonia which is carried to the liver and converted to urea. Bacteria in the colon also synthesize vitamin K and some of the vitamin B group. Bacteria also play a part in the production of flatus.

The movements of the large intestine are usually slow. When the circular muscles contract they produce an empty, kneading action called *haustral churning*. Propulsive (mass movements) peristalsis also occurs. When food enters the stomach and duodenum, the gastrocolic and duodenocolic reflexes are initiated, which result in peristalsis in the colon. These reflexes are more active after the first daily meal and initiate defecation reflexes.

Defecation is a reflex action involving both voluntary and involuntary control. Feces in the rectum stimulate sensory nerve endings which produce the desire to defecate. The reflex center for defecation is in the sacral portion of the spinal cord (parasympathetic nerve fibers). These fibers produce contraction of the rectum and relaxation of the internal anal sphincter. When the desire to defecate is felt, the external anal sphincter relaxes voluntarily. Defecation is controlled voluntarily by keeping the external anal sphincter closed.

Defecation can be facilitated by the *Valsalva maneuver*. This maneuver involves contraction of the chest muscles on a closed glottis with simultaneous contraction of the abdominal muscles. These actions result in an increased intraabdominal pressure. The Valsalva maneuver is contraindicated in individuals with head injuries, eye surgery, and cardiac problems (see section on constipation in Chap. 34).

Liver, Biliary Tract, and Pancreas

Liver

The liver is the largest internal organ in the body.

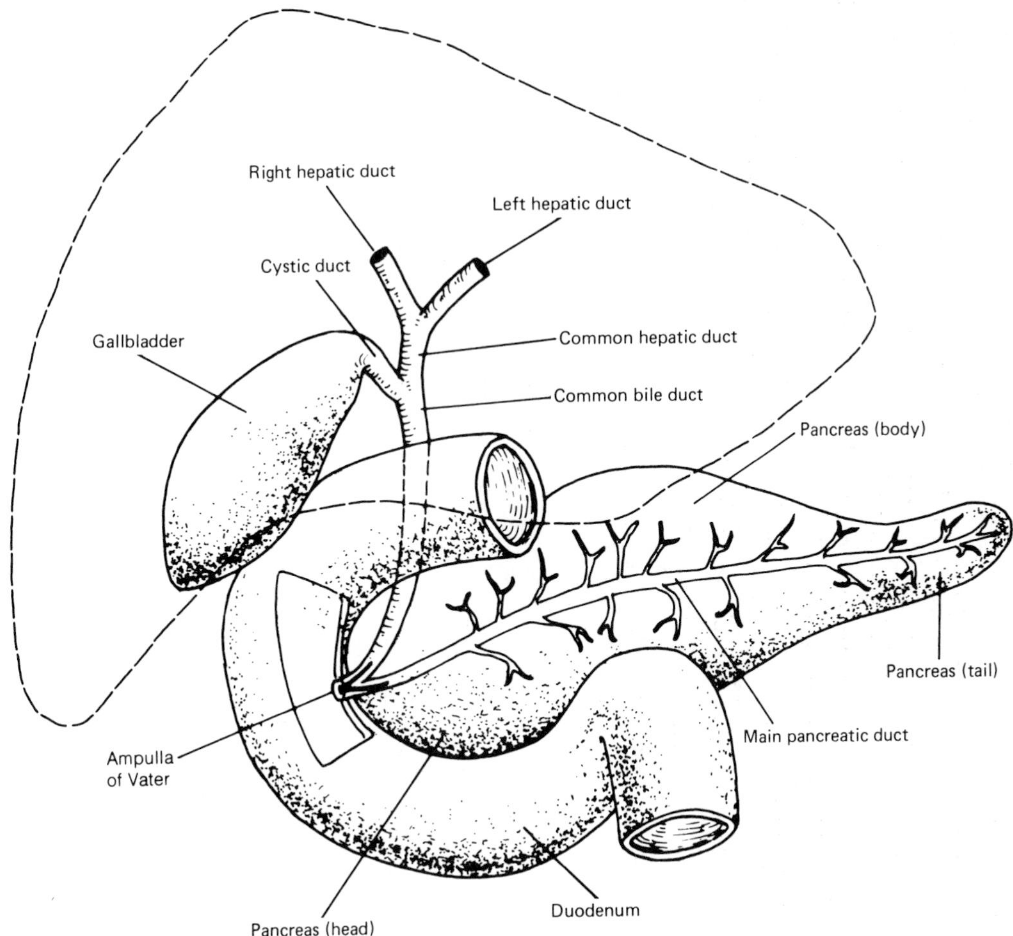

Figure 31-4 Gross structure of the liver, gallbladder, pancreas and their duct system. (*From M. Kinney et al., AACN's Reference for Critical Care Nursing, McGraw-Hill Book Company, New York, 1981, p. 195.*)

It lies in the right hypochondriac and epigastric regions. Most of the liver is enclosed in peritoneum. It has a fibrous capsule which divides it into the right and left lobes (Fig. 31-4).

The functional units of the liver are *lobules* (Fig. 31-5). The lobule consists of rows of hepatic cells arranged around a central vein. The capillaries (*sinusoids*) are located between the rows of hepatic cells and are lined with *Kupffer* cells which carry out phagocytic activity. Interlobular bile ducts form from bile capillaries (*canaliculi*). The hepatic cells secrete bile into the canaliculi.

The nerve supply to the liver is from the left vagus and sympathetic celiac plexus. About one-third of the blood supply comes from the hepatic artery (branch of the celiac artery) and two-thirds comes from the portal vein.

The portal circulatory system brings blood to the liver from the stomach, intestines, spleen, and pancreas. This blood enters the liver via the portal vein. In the liver the portal vein branches and comes in contact with each lobule. The blood in the sinusoids is a mixture of arterial and venous blood.

The liver is essential for life. It is a complex organ with a great number and variety of functions (Table 31-3).

Biliary tract

The biliary tract consists of the gallbladder and the duct system. The gallbladder is a pear-shaped sac on the undersurface of the liver. The function of the gallbladder is to concentrate and store bile. It can hold about 45 mL of bile.

Bile is produced by the hepatic cells and secreted into the biliary canaliculi of the lobules. Bile then drains into the interlobular bile ducts which unite into

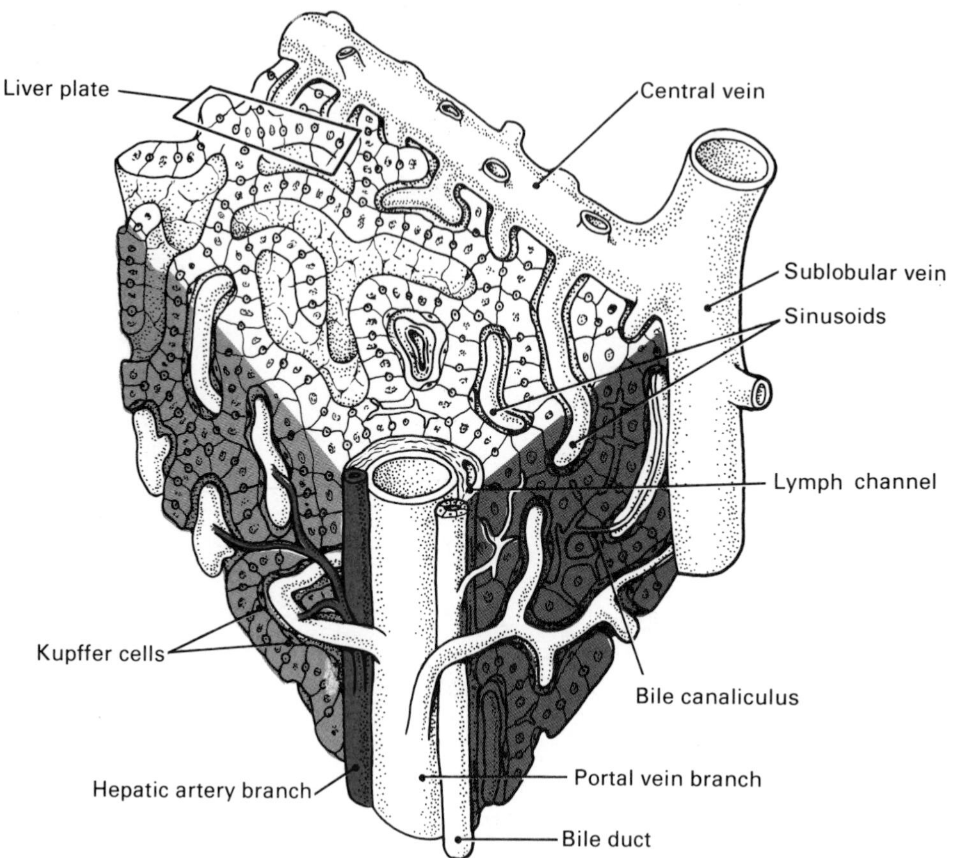

Figure 31-5 Microscopic structure of liver lobule.

the two main left and right hepatic ducts. The hepatic ducts merge with the cystic duct from the gallbladder to form the common bile duct (Fig. 31-4). This duct enters the duodenum at the ampulla of Vater. The sphincter of Oddi keeps the ampulla closed except during digestion.

Bilirubin metabolism

Bilirubin, a pigment derived from the breakdown of hemoglobin, is constantly being formed (Fig. 31-6). It is carried to the liver in an insoluble form as unconjugated bilirubin. The liver conjugates bilirubin with glucuronic acid. Conjugated bilirubin is soluble and is excreted in bile. Bile also consists of water, cholesterol, bile salts, electrolytes, and phospholipids. Bile salts are needed for fat emulsification.

Bile initially enters the duct system in the canaliculi and flows through the interlobular ducts to the hepatic ducts. From the hepatic duct it can move to the cystic duct or down the common bile duct. Most bile is stored and concentrated in the gallbladder. It is then released into the cystic duct and moves down the common bile duct to enter the duodenum at the ampulla of Vater. In the intestines most of the bilirubin is reduced to urobilinogen by bacterial action. This substance accounts for the brown color of stool. A small amount of conjugated bilirubin is reabsorbed by the blood. Some urobilinogen is reabsorbed by the blood and returned to the liver via the portal circulation and excreted in the bile. An insignificant amount of urobilinogen is excreted in the urine.

Pancreas

The *pancreas* is a long, slender gland lying behind the stomach and in front of the first and second lumbar vertebrae. It consists of the head, body, and tail. The anterior surface is covered by peritoneum. The pancreas contains lobes and lobules. The pancreatic duct extends along the gland and enters the duodenum via the common bile duct (Fig. 31-4). The pancreas has both *exocrine* and *endocrine* functions. Its functions as the part of the GI system is the exocrine function. There are exocrine cells in the pancreas which secrete pancreatic enzymes (Table

Table 31-3
Major Functions of the Liver

Function	Description
Metabolic Functions	
1. Carbohydrate metabolism	1. Glycogenesis—conversion of glucose to glycogen Glycogenolysis—process of breaking down glycogen to glucose Gluconeogenesis—formation of glucose from amino acids and fatty acids
2. Protein metabolism	2. Synthesis of nonessential amino acids Synthesis of plasma proteins (except gamma globulin) Synthesis of clotting factors Urea formation from NH_3 (NH_3 is formed from deamination of amino acids and by the action of bacteria on proteins in the colon)
3. Fat metabolism	3. Synthesis of lipoproteins Breakdown of triglycerides into fatty acids and glycerol Formation of ketone bodies Synthesis of fatty acids from amino acids and glucose Cholesterol synthesis and breakdown
4. Detoxification	4. Inactivation of drugs and harmful substances and excretion of their breakdown products
5. Steroid metabolism	5. Conjugation and excretion of gonadal and adrenal steroids
Bile Production and Excretion	
1. Bile production	1. Formation of bile containing bile salts, bile pigments (mainly bilirubin), and cholesterol.
2. Bile excretion	2. Liver excretes about 1 L bile/day
Storage	Glucose in the form of glycogen Vitamins Fat-soluble (A, D, E, K) Water-soluble (B_1, B_2, B_{12}, and folic acid) Fatty acids Minerals (iron and copper) Amino acids in the form of albumin and beta globulins
Reticuloendothelial System (Kupffer cells)	Ingestion of old RBC, bacteria, and other particles Breakdown of hemoglobin from old RBC to bilirubin and biliverdin

31-1). The endocrine function is related to the islets of Langerhans whose beta cells secrete insulin and alpha cells secrete glucagon (Chap. 41).

ASSESSMENT OF THE GASTROINTESTINAL SYSTEM*

Terminology related to the gastrointestinal system is presented in Table 31-4.

Subjective Data: The History

Past medical history

Question the client about the history or existence of the following diseases or problems related to GI functioning:

Hepatitis
Peptic ulcer
Jaundice
Anemia
Gastritis
Diarrhea-constipation
Colitis

The client should be questioned about previous hospitalizations related to the above diseases or problems of the GI system. Gather data related to any abdominal or rectal surgery including year, cause, postoperative course, and possible blood transfusions.

The past medical history should include an assessment of the client's past and current use of medications. This is a very important part of the assessment, particularly in relation to liver problems. It should include over-the-counter and prescription drugs. Many chemicals and drugs are potentially hepatotoxic (Table 31-5). Ask the client if antacids are taken, including the kind and frequency. Many people take baking soda ($NaHCO_3$) for an upset stomach. This can be dangerous because it is a systemic antacid which is readily absorbed and can cause metabolic alkalosis. Assess the client for allergies to any foods and determine what GI symptoms such allergic responses cause.

Family history

It is helpful to determine if there is a family history of certain GI diseases and problems. The presence of

*Refer to Chap. 3 for specific information related to the health history and physical examination.

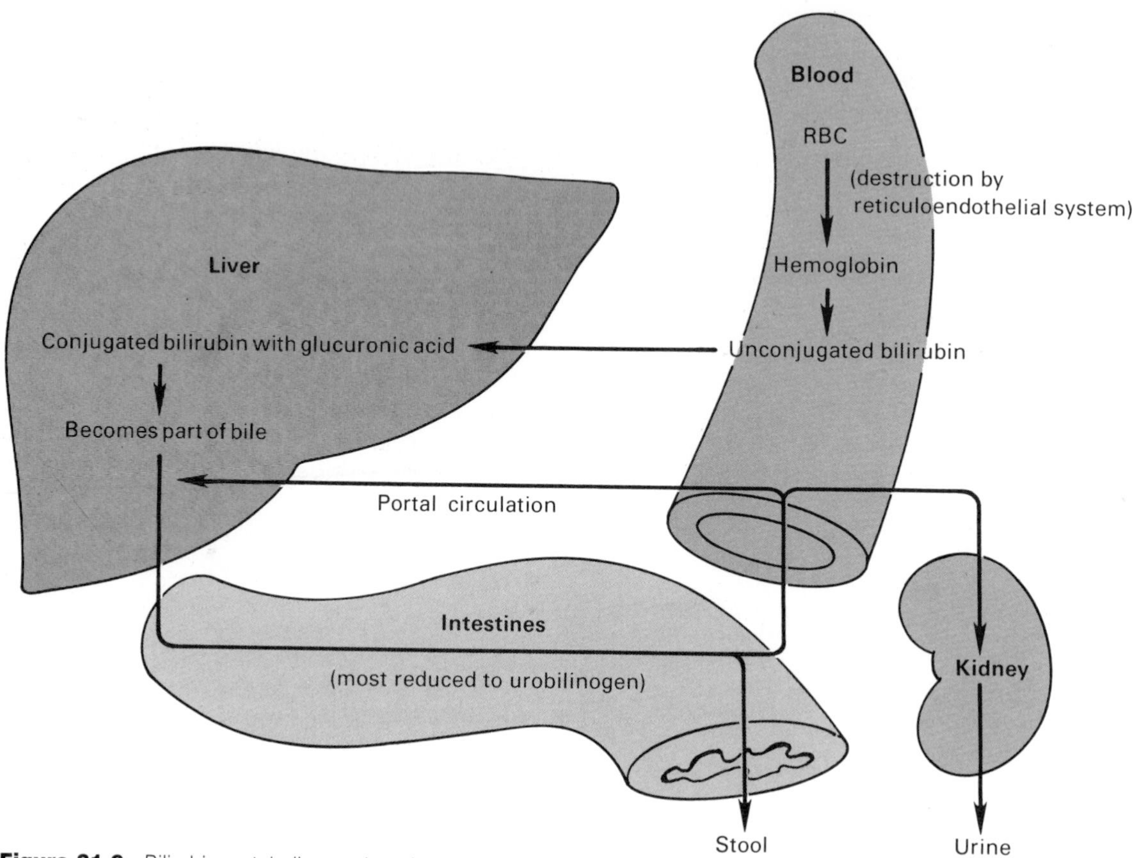

Figure 31-6 Bilirubin metabolism and conjugation.

certain problems may increase the likelihood of similar problems in other family members. Ask the client about the occurrence of such problems as:

- Alcoholism
- Jaundice
- Cancer of GI tract (especially colon)
- Hepatitis
- Peptic ulcers
- Gallbladder disease
- Obesity
- Diabetes

Social and personal history

Background Information The client should be asked about previous occupations in which he could have been exposed to hepatotoxic chemicals such as carbon tetrachloride, arsenic, phosphorus, and mercury. Also ask about foreign travel with possible exposure to hepatitis or parasitic infestation.

Lifestyle

Habits

The client should be assessed in relation to certain habits which have a direct effect on GI functioning. The consumption of alcohol in large quantities has detrimental effects on the mucosa of the stomach and also increases the secretion of acid-pepsin. Alcohol causes fatty infiltration of the liver. Nicotine is very irritating to the entire GI tract mucosa. As previously mentioned, the intake of both prescription and nonprescription drugs by the client is an essential part of the assessment.

Stress and coping

Try to determine what is a stressor for the client and what coping mechanisms the client uses in order to function with these stressors. Many individuals develop GI symptoms such as epigastric pain, nausea, and diarrhea in response to stressful or emotional situations. Some organic GI problems such as peptic ulcers are related to stress.

Table 31-4
Terminology Related to the Gastrointestinal System

Term	Definition
Antrectomy	Removal of the antrum portion of the stomach
Cecostomy	An opening into the cecum
Cholecystectomy	Removal of the gallbladder
Cholecystostomy	An opening into the gallbladder
Choledochojejunostomy	An opening between the common bile duct and the jejunum
Choledocholithotomy	An opening into the common bile duct for the removal of stones
Colostomy	An opening into the colon
Esophagoenterostomy	Removal of a portion of the esophagus with a segment of colon attached to remaining portion
Esophagogastrostomy	Removal of the esophagus and anastomosis of the remaining portion to the stomach
Gastrectomy	Removal of the stomach
Gastrostomy	An opening into the stomach
Glossectomy	Removal of the tongue
Hemiglossectomy	Removal of one-half of the tongue
Ileostomy	An opening into the ileum
Mandibulectomy	Removal of the mandible
Pyloroplasty	Enlargement and repair of the pyloric sphincter area
Vagotomy	Resection of a branch of the vagus nerve

Bowel function habits

Ask the client about his elimination patterns; what is his regular bowel evacuation habit—frequency, time of day, and normal consistency of stool. What activities or emotions change his regular pattern? The development of the "laxative habit" should be determined. How often does the client take a laxative? What kind is it? A similar inquiry should be made related to enemas.

Dietary habits

A thorough nutritional assessment is essential. A diet history of foods eaten should be taken and compared to the basic four food groups. Ask open-ended questions that will allow the client to express his beliefs and feelings about his diet. The nurse may need to ask the client to do a 24-hour dietary recall in order to analyze the adequacy of his diet. Assist the client to recall the preceding day's food intake, being sure to include early morning and night-time intake.

Table 31-5
Hepatotoxic Chemicals and Drugs

Alcohol	Anabolic steroids
Arsenic	Halothane
Carbon tetrachloride	Isoniazid (INH)
Chloroform	Propylthiouracil
Gold compounds	Sulfonamides
Mercury	Thiazide diuretics
Phosphorus	6-Mercaptopurine (6-MP)

The nurse should find out about the intake of snacks, liquids, and vitamin supplements. The nurse must then evaluate the diet in terms of the basic four. Try to determine if the 24-hour recall is typical of the client's usual eating habits. If weekend eating habits vary greatly, obtain a separate weekend diet history. Assess the client's intake for both quality and quantity of food.

Ask the client about the use of salt and sugar substitutes. Also ask how much sodium is used. Determine fluid intake.

Food has many social and emotional values as well as physical ones. What is the emotional atmosphere during meal time? Does the client eat alone? Assess the client's spiritual and cultural beliefs regarding food. Try to determine the economic situation of the client in relation to diet. What percentage of the income is spent on food and how much of this amount is related to culture and how much to economic ability. Remember that food has very different values for each individual but it is essential that all nutrients be included.

Review of systems

This section includes questions related to problems of the GI system which should be explored. (A positive response should be investigated according to the criteria in Chap. 3.) Ask the client questions in the following areas:

1. Mouth
   a. Dental hygiene—caries, condition of teeth and gums, dentures
   b. Bleeding or swelling of gums
   c. Dryness or excessive salivation
   d. Lesions
   e. Odors
   f. Sore tongue
   g. Difficulty chewing
2. Ingestion of food and fluids
   a. Painful swallowing (dysphagia)

b. Appetite (increase or anorexia)
c. Weight change
d. Tolerance to certain foods
e. Nausea and vomiting
f. Indigestion, belching (eructation)
g. Hematemesis
h. Location and type of pain

3. Digestion and absorption
   a. Relationship of pain to eating or specific food
   b. Heartburn (pyrosis)
   c. Burning, indigestion (dyspepsia)
4. Elimination
   a. Constipation, diarrhea
   b. Changes in bowel habits
   c. Gas (flatulence)
   d. Melena
   e. Anal pruritus, burning, pain
   f. Tenesmus
   g. Frothy stool (steatorrhea)
   h. Distension
   i. Hemorrhoids
5. Hepatic and biliary
   a. Yellow skin (jaundice)
   b. Pruritus
   c. Edema (ascites)
   d. Dark urine
   e. Clay-colored stools
   f. Hemorrhagic problems (bruise easily, purpura, bleeding)
   g. Spider angioma
   h. Palmar erythema

Objective Data: Physical Examination

Mouth

Inspection Inspect the lips for symmetry, color, and size. Observe them for abnormalities such as pallor or cyanosis, cracking, ulcers, or fissures. Inspect the tongue. The dorsum (top) should have a thin white coating while the undersurface is smooth. Observe for any lesions. Using a tongue blade inspect the buccal mucosa, noting the color, any areas of pigmentation, and any lesions. Dark-skinned individu-

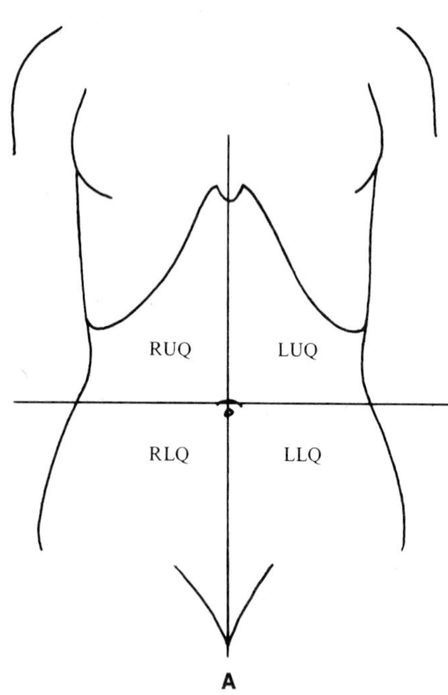

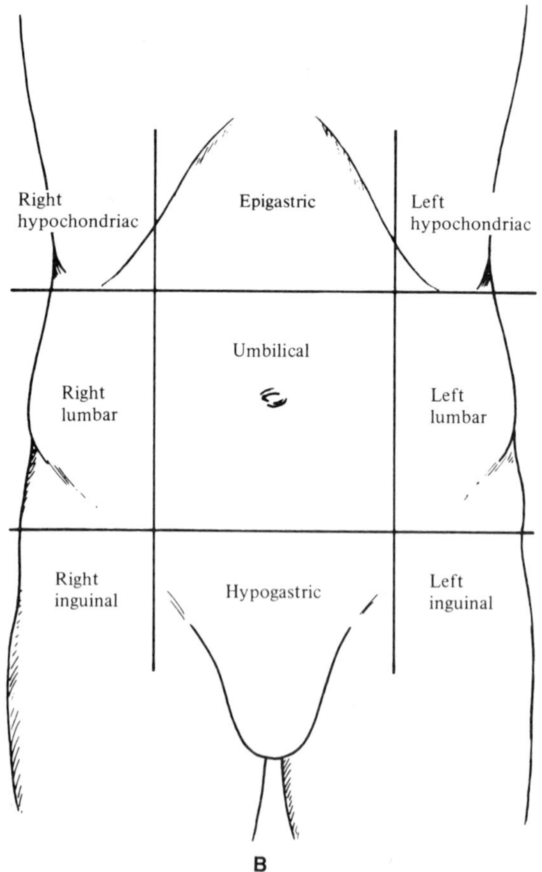

Figure 31-7 (*a.*) Abdominal quadrants. (*b.*) Abdominal regions. (*From L. M. Shortridge and E. J. Lee, Introductory Skills for Nursing Practice, McGraw-Hill Book Company, New York, 1980, pp. 147–149. Used with permission of McGraw-Hill Book Company.*)

als normally have patchy areas of pigmentation. Assess the teeth and gums. Look for caries, loose teeth, abnormal shape and position of teeth, and swelling, bleeding, discoloration, or inflammation of the gums.

Palpation The nurse should palpate any suspicious areas anywhere in the mouth. Palpate any ulcers, nodules, indurations, or areas of tenderness.

Abdomen

Two systems are used to anatomically describe the surface of the abdomen. One system divides the abdomen into four quadrants by a perpendicular line from the sternum to the pubic bone and a horizontal line across the abdomen at the umbilicus (Fig. 31-7 and Table 31-6). The other system divides the abdomen into nine regions (Fig. 31-7), only three of which are commonly referred to: (1) epigastrium, (2) umbilical, and (3) suprapubic.[2]

Inspection The nurse should assess for changes in:

Skin—color, texture, scars, striae, dilated veins, rashes, and lesions
Umbilicus—location and contour
Symmetry
Contour—flat, rounded, concave, protuberant, distension
Observable masses
Movement—pulsations and peristalsis

A normal aortic pulsation may be seen in the epigastric area. Look across the abdomen tangentially for peristalsis. Peristalsis is not normally visible on adults but may be visible in very thin individuals.

Auscultation When examining the abdomen, auscultation is done before percussion and palpation because these latter procedures may alter the bowel sounds. Auscultation of the abdomen includes listening for increased or decreased bowel sounds, and vascular sounds. The diaphragm of the stethoscope is used to auscultate bowel sounds because they are relatively high-pitched. The bell of the stethoscope is used to detect lower-pitched sounds. When listening for bowel sounds, listen for 2 to 5 minutes. Bowel sounds cannot be said to be absent until no sound is heard for 5 minutes. Listen in the epigastrium and in all four quadrants. The frequency and intensity of bowel sounds will vary, depending on the phase of digestion. There may be clicks and gurgles. Very loud gurgles indicate hyperperistalsis and are called *borborygmi*. The bowel sounds will be high-pitched (rushes and tinkling) when the intestines are under tension such as in intestinal obstruction. Listen for decreased or absent bowel sounds. Normally no aortic *bruits* should be heard. This sound resembles a systolic heart murmur.

Percussion The purpose of percussion of the abdomen is to determine the presence of fluid, distension, and masses. Sound waves vary according to the

Table 31-6
Abdominal Structures in Four Regions of the Abdomen

Right Upper Quadrant	Left Upper Quadrant	Right Lower Quadrant	Left Lower Quadrant
Liver and gallbladder	Left lobe of liver	Lower pole of right kidney	Lower pole of left kidney
Pylorus	Spleen	Cecum and appendix	Sigmoid flexure
Duodenum	Stomach	Portion of ascending colon	Portion of descending colon
Head of pancreas	Body of pancreas	Bladder (if distended)	Bladder (if distended)
Right adrenal gland	Left adrenal gland	Ovary and salpinx	Ovary and salpinx
Portion of right kidney	Portion of left kidney	Uterus (if enlarged)	Uterus (if enlarged)
Hepatic flexure of colon	Splenic flexure of colon	Right spermatic cord	Left spermatic cord
Portion of ascending and transverse colon	Portion of transverse and descending colon	Right ureter	Left ureter

From L. M. Shortridge and E. J. Lee, *Introductory Skills for Nursing Practice*, McGraw-Hill Book Company, New York, 1980, p. 148.

density of underlying tissues; the presence of air produces a higher-pitched, hollow sound called *tympany*, while the presence of fluid or masses produces a high-pitched sound called *dullness*. The nurse should lightly percuss all four quadrants of the abdomen, assessing the distribution of tympany and dullness. There is usually more tympany.

To percuss the liver, start below the umbilicus in the right midclavicular line and percuss lightly upward. Determine the lower border of liver dullness. After the lower border of the liver has been determined, start at the nipple line in the right midclavicular line and percuss downward to the area of dullness indicating the upper border of the liver. Measure the height or vertical space between the two areas to determine the size of the liver. The normal range of liver height in the right midclavicular line is 6 to 12 cm.

Palpation *Light Palpation* is used to detect tenderness or cutaneous hypersensitivity, muscular resistance, masses, and swelling. It also helps in relaxation for deeper palpation. Keep fingers together and with the pads of the fingertips press gently, depressing the abdominal wall about 1 cm. Make smooth movements and palpate all quadrants (Fig. 31-8).

Deep palpation is used to delineate abdominal organs and masses. The palmar surfaces of the

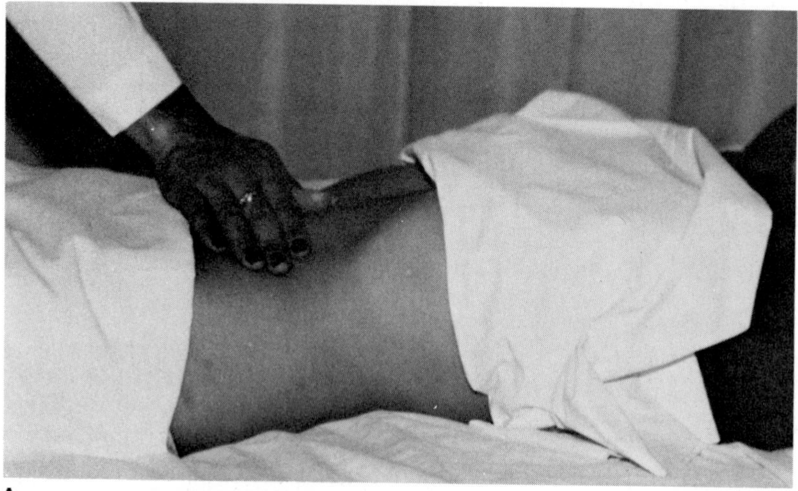

A

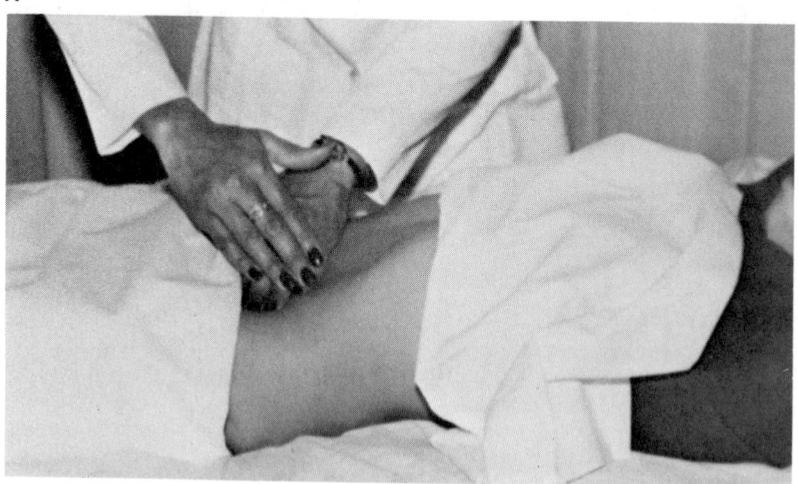

B

Figure 31-8 (*a*) Light palpation of the abdomen. (*Courtesy of Ernest Lee.*) (*b*) Deep palpation of the abdomen (two-hand method). (*Courtesy of Ernest Lee.*)

fingers should be used to press more deeply. Again, palpate all quadrants. When palpating masses, note the location, size, shape, and if tenderness is present.

An alternate method for light and deep abdominal palpation is the *two-hand method* (Fig. 31-8). One hand is placed on top of the other. The fingers of the top hand apply pressure to the bottom hand. The fingers of the bottom hand feel for organs and masses. The examiner should practice both methods of palpation to determine which one is most effective for her.

A problem area on the abdomen can be checked for *rebound tenderness* by pressing in slowly and firmly over the painful site. The palpating fingers are withdrawn quickly. Pain upon withdrawal of the fingers indicates peritoneal inflammation.

To palpate the liver, the examiner's left hand is placed behind the client, supporting the right 11th and 12th ribs (Fig. 31-9). The client may relax on the examiner's hand. Press the left hand forward and place the right hand on the client's right abdomen lateral to the rectus muscle. The fingertips should be below the lower border of liver dullness and pointed toward the right costal margin. Gently press in and up. Ask the client to take a deep breath with the abdomen so the liver will drop and be in a better position to palpate. The examiner should try to feel the liver edge as it comes down to the fingertips. The liver edge should feel firm, sharp, and smooth. Describe the surface and contour and any tenderness.[3]

To palpate the spleen, the examiner's left hand reaches over and under the client and supports and presses the client's left lower rib cage forward. Place the right hand below the left costal margin and press it in toward the spleen. Ask the client to breathe deeply. The tip or edge of an enlarged spleen would be felt by the fingertips. The spleen is usually only palpable if enlarged to three times normal.[4] If palpable, do not pursue as the enlarged spleen may rupture.

Examination of the rectum

The perianal and anal area should be inspected for color, texture, lumps, rashes, scars, excoriations, fissures, and external hemorrhoids. Any lumps or unusual areas should be palpated with a gloved hand.

For the digital examination of the rectum the gloved, lubricated index finger is placed against the anus while the client strains (Valsalva maneuver). Then, as the sphincter relaxes, the finger is inserted. Point the finger toward the umbilicus. Try to get the client to relax. Insert the finger into the rectum as far as possible and palpate all surfaces. Assess for nodules, tenderness, or any irregularities.

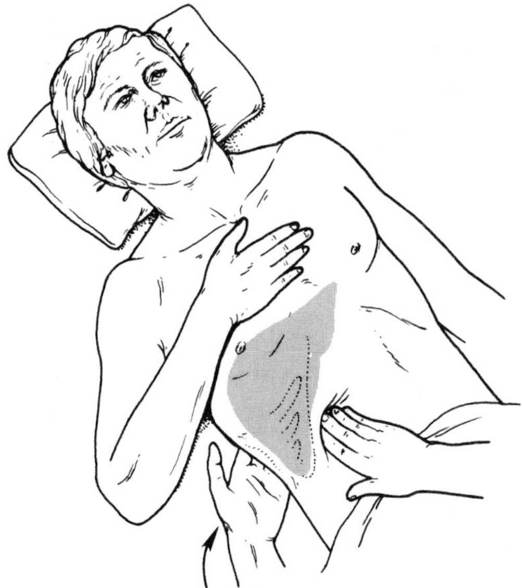

Figure 31-9 Bimanual technique for palpation of the liver.

Recording of the normal physical assessment of the gastrointestinal system is found in Table 31-7. Common abnormal assessment findings are presented in Table 31-8.

DIAGNOSTIC STUDIES OF THE GASTROINTESTINAL SYSTEM

Many of the diagnostic procedures of the gastrointestinal system require measures to cleanse the GI tract as well as ingestion or injection of a contrast medium or a radiopaque dye (Table 31-9). Often the

Table 31-7
Recording the Normal Physical Assessment of the Gastrointestinal System

Mouth

Lips moist and pink. Buccal mucosa and gingiva pink and moist without plaques or lesions. Teeth in good repair. Tongue protrudes in midline without deviation or fasciculations.

Abdomen

Abdomen flat without masses or scars. Bowel sounds present in all four quadrants. Liver and spleen not palpable. Liver 10 cm in right midclavicular line. Generalized tympany.

Anus

No lesions, fissures, or hemorrhoids.

Table 31-8
Common Assessment Abnormalities of the Gastrointestinal System

Finding	Description/Definition	Possible Etiology
	Mouth	
Ulcer, plaque on lips or in mouth	Sore or lesion	Carcinoma
Cheilosis	Softening, fissuring, and cracking at angles of mouth	Riboflavin deficiency
Cheilitis	Inflammation of lips (usually lower) with fissuring, scaling, crusting	Not always known
Geographic tongue	Scattered red, smooth (loss of papillae) areas on dorsum of tongue	Unknown
Smooth tongue	A red, slick appearance	Vitamin B_{12} deficiency
Leukoplakia	Thickened white patches	Premalignant lesion
Pyorrhea	Gums recessed, purulent pockets develop	Periodontitis
	Esophagus and Stomach	
Dysphagia	Difficulty swallowing, sensation of food sticking in esophagus	Esophageal problems
Hematemesis	Vomiting blood	Esophageal varices, bleeding peptic ulcer
Pyrosis	Heartburn, burning in epigastric or substernal area	Hiatal hernia, esophagitis
Dyspepsia	Burning or indigestion	Peptic ulcer, gallbladder disease
	Abdomen	
Distension	Excessive gas accumulation, enlarged abdomen. Generalized tympany	Obstruction, paralytic ileus
Ascites	Accumulated fluid within the abdominal cavity, umbilicus usually everted	Peritoneal inflammation, congestive heart failure, metastatic carcinoma, cirrhosis
Bruit	Sounds like a systolic murmur	Partial arterial obstruction or turbulent flow (aneurysm)
Hyperresonance	Loud, tinkling rushes	Intestinal obstruction
Borborygmi	Waves of loud, gurgling sounds	Hyperactive bowel secondary to eating
Absent bowel sounds	Bowel sounds not auscultated	Peritonitis, paralytic ileus, obstruction
Absence of liver dullness	On percussion becomes very tympanitic	Air from viscus (e.g., perforated ulcer)
Masses	Lump felt on palpation	Tumors, cysts
Rebound tenderness	Sudden pain when fingers are withdrawn quickly	Peritoneal inflammation, appendicitis

Table 31-8 (Continued)

Finding	Description/Definition	Possible Etiology
Nodular liver	Enlarged, hard liver with irregular edge or surface	Cirrhosis, carcinoma
Hepatomegaly	Enlargement of the liver, liver edge more than 1–2 cm below costal margin	Metastatic carcinoma, hepatitis, venous congestion
Splenomegaly	Enlargement of the spleen	Chronic leukemia, hemolytic states, portal hypertension, and some infections
Hernia	A bulge or nodule in the abdomen. Bulge usually appears on straining	Depends on type: 1. Inguinal—in inguinal canal 2. Femoral—in femoral canal 3. Umbilical—herniation of umbilicus 4. Incisional—defect in muscles following surgery
	Rectum	
Hemorrhoids	Thrombosed veins in rectum and anus (may be internal or external)	Portal hypertension, chronic constipation, prolonged sitting or standing, pregnancy
Mass	Firm nodular edge	Tumor, carcinoma
Pilonidal cyst	Opening of a sinus tract. Cyst in midline just above coccyx	Probably congenital
Fissure	Ulceration in anal canal	Straining, irritation
Melena	Blood in stools	Hemorrhoids, cancer, bleeding anywhere in GI tract

client has a series of GI diagnostic tests done. A certain sequence is usually followed; for example, a proctoscopy, then a barium enema, and then an upper GI. The nurse must observe the client closely to assure adequate hydration and nutrition during these series of tests.

Radiologic Studies

Upper gastrointestinal series (upper GI, barium swallow)

The purpose of an upper GI is to observe the movement of a contrast medium (barium sulfate) through the esophagus and into the stomach by means of fluoroscopy and x-ray examination. It is used to identify esophageal and stomach pathology such as esophageal strictures, varices, polyps, tumors, hiatus hernia, and peptic ulcers in the stomach or duodenum (Fig. 31-10).

The procedure consists of the client swallowing barium, after which various positions on the x-ray table must be assumed. The movement of the barium is observed with fluoroscopy and several x-rays are taken (Table 31-9).

Lower gastrointestinal (lower GI, barium enema)

The purpose of a lower GI x-ray is to observe by means of fluoroscopy the filling of the colon with barium sulfate and to take x-rays of the filled colon. This procedure identifies polyps, tumors, and other lesions in the colon. It consists of administering a barium enema and observing the filling of the colon with the barium by fluoroscopy after which x-rays are taken (Fig. 31-10).

Oral cholecystogram (gallbladder series)

The purpose of an oral cholecystogram is to visualize the gallbladder. It is used to determine the gallbladder's ability to concentrate and store dye and to observe the patency of the biliary duct system. It is a common gallbladder test and may be used to detect

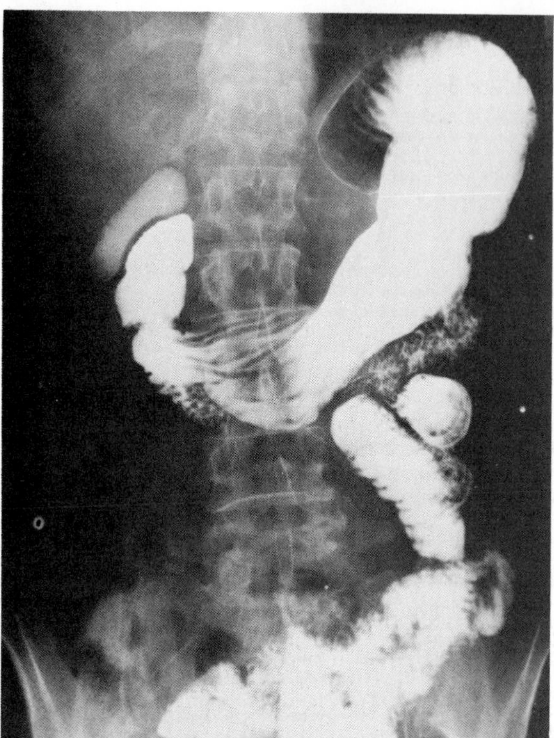

Figure 31-10 Upper gastrointestinal tract x-ray. (*Courtesy of Radiology Department, Lutheran Medical Center, Denver, Colorado.*)

gallstones, obstructions of the biliary tract, and other gallbladder disorders.

The procedure consists of an x-ray examination after a radiopaque dye has been ingested orally. The radiopaque dye used is an organic insoluble iodide such as iopanoic acid (Telepaque, Priodax, or Oragrafin) (Table 31-9).

Cholangiography

The purpose of *cholangiography* is to visualize the biliary duct system. X-rays are taken at intervals following injection of a radiopaque dye. There are several methods for performing cholangiography. First, an intravenous cholangiogram (IVC) is performed by injecting the dye intravenously. Second, a cholangiogram may also be performed during surgery on biliary structures, such as the gallbladder, in which case the contrast medium is injected into the common bile duct. A third method is used postoperatively when the contrast medium is injected into a T-tube (Chap. 35). A percutaneous transhepatic cholangiogram may also be done (Table 31-9).

Endoscopy

Endoscopy refers to the direct visualization of a body structure through a lighted instrument (scope). Most of the GI tract can be visualized by endoscopy, especially with the use of the flexible fiberoptic scopes. The GI structures that can be examined by fiberoptic endoscopy include the esophagus, stomach, duodenum, colon, and even the pancreas and biliary tree, although the last two are not frequently performed. The fiberscopes are equipped with biopsy and cytologic capabilities as well as forceps, electrocauteries, and snare devices which may be utilized through the scopes. Endoscopy of the GI tract is frequently combined with biopsy and cytology. The major complication of GI endoscopy is perforation through the structure being scoped. This complication is decreased with the use of the flexible fiberoptic scopes. The specific endoscopy procedures are discussed in Table 31-9.

Liver Biopsy

The purpose of a liver biopsy is to obtain hepatic tissue to be used in establishing a diagnosis such as cirrhosis, hepatitis, and neoplasms. It may also be useful for following the progress of a disease.

The two types of liver biopsy are *open* and *closed*. The *open* method involves making an incision and removing a wedge of tissue. It is done in the operating room under general anesthesia, often concurrently with another surgical procedure. The *closed* or *needle* biopsy is an invasive procedure in which the site is infiltrated with a local anesthetic and a needle inserted through a small incision between the 6th and 7th or 8th and 9th intercostal spaces on the right side. The client lies supine with a pillow under the left side and the right arm over his head. The client should be instructed to hold his breath while the needle is inserted. Nursing assessment prior to and following a liver biopsy is very important (Table 31-9).

Liver Function Studies

Liver function tests are usually described separately from other GI diagnostic studies. Liver function tests are basically biochemical determinations which reflect hepatic disease.[5] Table 31-10 describes some common liver function tests.

Table 31-9
Diagnostic Studies of the Gastrointestinal System

Study	Description and Purpose	Nursing Responsibility
	Radiology	
Upper gastrointestinal (UGI) or barium swallow	X-ray examination with fluoroscopy of the stomach utilizing contrast medium of barium sulfate. Used to diagnose structural abnormalities of the esophagus and stomach.	Explain procedure to client. Will need to drink barium and assume various positions on the x-ray table. NPO for 8–12 h prior to procedure. After the x-ray, measures need to be taken to prevent barium impaction (fluids, cathartics). Stool may be white up to 72 h after test.
Small bowel series	Barium ingested and flat plate film taken every 20 min until barium reaches the terminal ileum.	Same as for UGI.
Lower gastrointestinal (GI) or barium enema	Fluoroscopic x-ray examination of the colon, using contrast medium (barium sulfate) which is administered rectally (enema). Air contrast studies may also be done in which air is inserted following evacuation of the barium (Fig. 31-11).	*Before procedure:* Colon must be free of stool (laxatives and enemas the evening prior). Enemas until clear morning of procedure. Client NPO for 8 h prior to test or clear liquid breakfast. Instruct client about being given the barium via enema. May experience cramping and the urge to defecate during procedure. May be placed in various positions on tilt table. *After procedure:* Fluids and laxatives given to assist in expelling barium. Observe stool for passage of barium.
Oral cholecystogram (GB series)	X-ray examination to visualize the gallbladder after a radiopaque dye iopanoic acid (Telapaque) has been ingested orally. Determine gallbladder's ability to concentrate and store the dye and the patency of the biliary duct system.	Assess client for sensitivity to iodine. Administer radiopaque dye evening prior to the test. Six tablets (3 g) given one every 5 min. NPO after ingestion of the dye. Observe for side effects of dye such as nausea, vomiting, diarrhea. May be given fatty test meal after the x-ray to check for gallbladder emptying.
Cholangiography 1. Intravenous cholangiogram (IVC)	X-rays to visualize the biliary duct system following intravenous injection of radiopaque dye.	Keep client NPO for 8 h. Assess sensitivity to iodine dye. During injection of dye assess for urticaria, extreme flushing, respiratory distress.
2. Percutaneous transhepatic cholangiogram	Following local anesthesia the liver is entered with a long needle (under fluoroscopy), a bile duct is entered, bile withdrawn, and a radiopaque dye injected. Fluoroscopy used to determine filling of hepatic and biliary ducts.	Observe client for signs of hemorrhage or bile leakage.
	Endoscopy	
Upper GI endoscopy 1. Esophagoscopy 2. Gastroscopy 3. Gastroduodenoscopy	Direct visualization of the esophagus, stomach, duodenum with a lighted scope, usually using a flexible fiberscope. Can observe the mucosa of these structures. May use motion pictures to visualize stomach motility. Inflammations, ulcerations, tumors, varices may be detected.	*Before procedure:* Keep client NPO for 8 h. Obtain signed consent. Give preoperative medication (diazepam or meperidine). Explain to client that local anesthetic may be sprayed on throat prior to insertion of scope. *After procedure:* Keep client NPO until gag reflex returns. Use warm saline gargles for relief of sore throat.
Proctosigmoidoscopy and colonoscopy	Direct visualization of the anus, rectum, sigmoid, and portion of colon with a flexible fiberscope. May include biopsy and cytology.	Enemas the evening before and morning of procedure. Explain to client knee-chest position, need to take deep breaths during insertion of scope, and possible urge to defecate as scope is passed. Observe for rectal bleeding and signs of perforation (malaise, abdominal distension, tenesmus) following test. May experience abdominal cramps due to stimulation of peristalsis.
Peritoneoscopy (Laparoscopy)	Visualization of the peritoneal cavity and contents with a peritoneoscope. May also take biopsy.	Obtain signed permit. Client NPO 8 h before study. Preoperative sedative medication. Bladder and bowel need to be emptied. Instruct client that local anesthesia is used prior to scope insertion.

Table 31-9 (Continued)

Study	Description and Purpose	Nursing Responsibility
	Ultrasound (Sonography)	
Ultrasound	A noninvasive procedure utilizing high-frequency sound waves (ultrasound waves) which are passed into body structures and recorded as they are reflected back.	No special preparation. Explain procedure to client, including use of conductive gel.
Abdominal ultrasound	To detect abdominal masses (tumors and cysts). To assess ascites.	Same as above.
Hepatobiliary ultrasound	To detect subphrenic abscesses, cysts, tumors, cirrhosis. For visualization of biliary ducts.	Same as above.
	Scans (Liver, Pancreas)	
Scans	Purpose is to show size, shape, and position of organ. Functional disorders and structural defects may be identified. A radionuclide (radioactive isotope) is injected intravenously and a counter (scanning) device picks up the radioactive emission, which is recorded on paper. Only tracer doses of radioactive isotopes are used.	For liver scan no special preparation. Explain to client the need to lie flat while scanning is being done. For pancreas scan, client is fasting for 8 h, then has a fat-free breakfast.
	Computerized Axial Tomography (CAT or CT Scan)	
	Noninvasive radiologic examination combining the special x-ray machine used for tomography (exposures at different depths) with a computer.	No special preparation or precautions.
	Liver Biopsy (Closed-Needle)	
	An invasive procedure in which a needle is inserted through a small incision between the 6th and 7th or 8th and 9th intercostal spaces on the right side and a specimen of hepatic tissue is obtained.	*Before procedure:* Check client's coagulation status (prothrombin time, clotting or bleeding time). Client may receive vitamin K and a unit of blood should be ready. Take vital signs as baseline data. Explain holding of breath when needle is inserted. Signed permit required. *After procedure:* Check client frequently for bleeding and make certain pressure dressing on site. Check vital signs every 30 min–1 h. Client kept on bed rest in flat position for 24 h. May lie on right side to splint puncture site. Assess client for complications such as bile peritonitis, shock, pneumothorax.
	Blood Chemistries	
Serum amylase	Measures the secretion of amylase by the pancreas. Very important in diagnosing acute pancreatitis. Peaks in 24 h and then drops to normal in 48–72 h. *Normal:* 60–160 Somogyi units/dL	No special preparation or precautions. Should obtain blood sample in the acute attack of pancreatitis.
Serum lipase	Measures the secretion of lipase by the pancreas. Stays elevated longer than the serum amylase. *Normal:* 0.2–1.5 U/mL	No special preparation or precautions.

Table 31-9 (Continued)

Study	Description and Purpose	Nursing Responsibility
	Miscellaneous	
Gastric analysis	Purpose is to analyze gastric contents for acidity and volume. A nasogastric tube is inserted and gastric contents are aspirated. Contents are analyzed mainly for hydrochloric acid but pH, pepsin, and electrolytes may be determined. Histalog and pentagastrin may be used to stimulate HCl secretion. Exfoliative cytology may be done to determine if malignant cells are present. *Normal:* *Acidity* *Volume* Fasting: 2.5 mEq/L 62 mL/h 30 min after Histalog: 10.5 mEq/L 110 mL/h	Client kept NPO for 8–12 h. Explain insertion of nasogastric tube. Withhold drugs affecting gastric secretions 24–48 h prior to test. No smoking morning of test (nicotine increases gastric secretion). May be responsible for obtaining specimens at 30 min after nasogastric insertion and then at 15-min intervals for an hour.
Fecal analysis (stool exam)	Form, consistency, color noted. Examined for mucus, blood, pus, parasites, and fat content. Tests for occult blood (guaiac test, Hemoccult, Hematest).	Observe client's stools. Responsible for collection of stool specimens. Check stools for occult blood via Hemoccult or Hematest. Diet free of red meat for 24–48 h prior to guaiac test.
D-Xylose tolerance test	An absorption test. Xylose, which is a monosaccharide, is given orally in water. All urine is collected for 5 h and the amount of D-xylose excreted is measured. *Normal*: 20% of xylose excreted in 5 h	Client kept NPO for 10–12 h prior to test. Client to empty bladder before xylose given orally.
Duodenal drainage	Duodenal contents are aspirated via a double lumen nasogastric tube—one lumen in stomach, other one in duodenum. Stimulant drug given IV (usually CCK-PZ). Duodenal contents are analyzed for enzymes, blood, bile, malignant cells, and volume.	Explain procedure to client. Insertion of nasogastric tube.

Table 31-10

Liver Function Tests

Test	Description and Purpose
Bile formation and excretion	
1. Serum bilirubin	These tests measure the ability of the liver to conjugate and excrete bilirubin. Used to differentiate between unconjugated (indirect) and conjugated (direct) bilirubin in plasma.
a. Total	Total bilirubin measures both direct and indirect. (*Normal:* 0.3–1.3 mg/dL)
b. Direct	Measures conjugated bilirubin. Elevated in obstructive jaundice. (*Normal:* 0.1–.3 mg/dL)
c. Indirect	Measures unconjugated bilirubin. Elevated in hepatocellular and hemolytic conditions. (*Normal:* 0.1–1.0 mg/dL)
2. Urinary bilirubin	Measures urinary excretion of conjugated bilirubin. (*Normal:* 0)

Table 31-10 (Continued)

Test	Description and Purpose
3. Urinary urobilinogen	Measures urinary excretion of urobilinogen. Maximum excretion occurs midafternoon to early evening. Total urinary output for 2-h period in afternoon—send to lab immediately as exposure to air oxidizes urobilinogen to urobilin. (*Normal:* 0–4 mg/24 h)
4. Fecal urobilinogen	Measures fecal urobilinogen in a stool specimen. (*Normal:* 30–220 mg/100 g stool)
Dye excretion tests (detoxification)	
1. BSP (Bromsulphalein)	Purpose is to determine liver's ability to excrete a dye given IV. Blood is withdrawn in 30 min and in 1 h. Client is NPO. (*Normal*: less than 5% retention after 1 h)
2. ICG (Indocyanine green)	Sometimes use this rather than BSP to test liver excretion. (*Normal*: 500–800 mL/square meter of body surface/min)
Protein metabolism	Measurement of serum proteins which are manufactured by the liver, such as albumin and globulin:
1. Serum protein levels	Albumin—(*normal:* 3.5–5.5 g/dL) Globulin—(*normal*: 2–3.5 g/dL) Total—(*normal*: 6–8 g/dL) A/G ratio—(*normal*: 1.5:1–2.5:1)
2. Alpha-fetoprotein	Indicative of hepatic cancer. (*Normal*: <25 ng/mL)
3. Blood ammonia levels	The liver normally converts ammonia to urea. Elevated in hepatic encephalopathy secondary to liver cirrhosis. (*Normal*: 30–70 μg/dL)
Hemostatic functions	
1. Prothrombin	Determines prothrombin activity. (*Normal*: 12–15 s)
2. Vitamin K production	Determine the response of the liver to vitamin K. The prothrombin time is checked 24 h after injection of vitamin K.
Serum enzyme tests	These tests measure various enzymes in the blood which are released when there is tissue damage in the liver and/or biliary tree obstruction.
1. Alkaline phosphatase	Liver has high concentrations of this enzyme. It is excreted in bile and is elevated in obstructive jaundice. [*Normal*: 5–13 units (King-Armstrong)]
2. SGOT (serum glutamic-oxaloacetic transaminase) or AST (aspartate aminotransferase)	Elevated in liver damage. (*Normal*: 15–45 U/L)
3. SGPT (serum glutamic-pyruvic transaminase) or ALT (alanine aminotransferase)	There are higher amounts of this enzyme in the liver than SGOT. (*Normal*: 5–36 U/L)
4. LDH (lactic dehydrogenase)	Not as frequently used in assessing liver disease. (*Normal*: 95–200 U/L)
5. Gamma glutamyl transpeptidase	Found in biliary tract (not in skeletal muscle or cardiac). Increased in hepatitis.
6. Other enzymes which may be assessed are:	5'-Nucleotidase, aminopeptidase, and cholinesterase.
Lipid metabolism	
1. Serum cholesterol	Cholesterol is synthesized and excreted by the liver. It is mixed with fatty acids in the liver (esterified). Is increased in biliary obstruction. Is decreased in hepatitis. (*Normal*: 150–270 mg/dL)
Serology for viral hepatitis	
1. Hepatitis B surface antigen (HB_sAg)	May be found in blood in the early stages of hepatitis B. (*Normal:* Negative) Other serology studies for hepatitis are presented in Tables 35–2 and 35–5

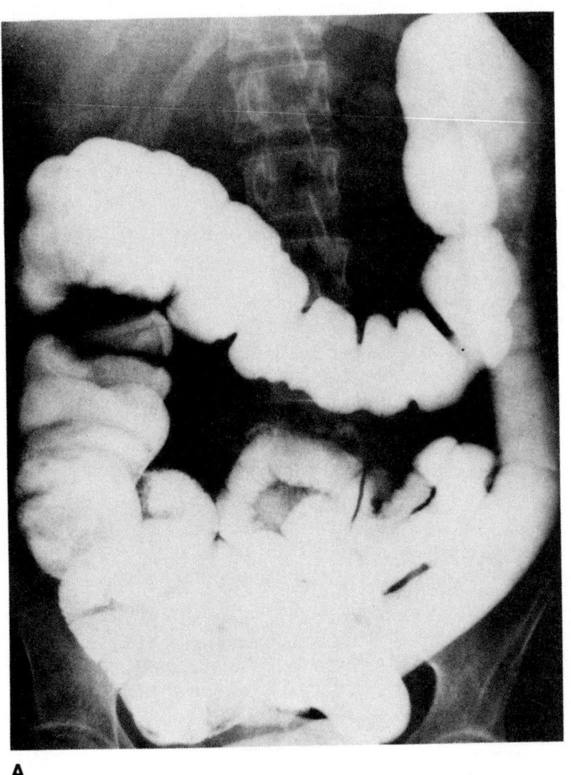

A

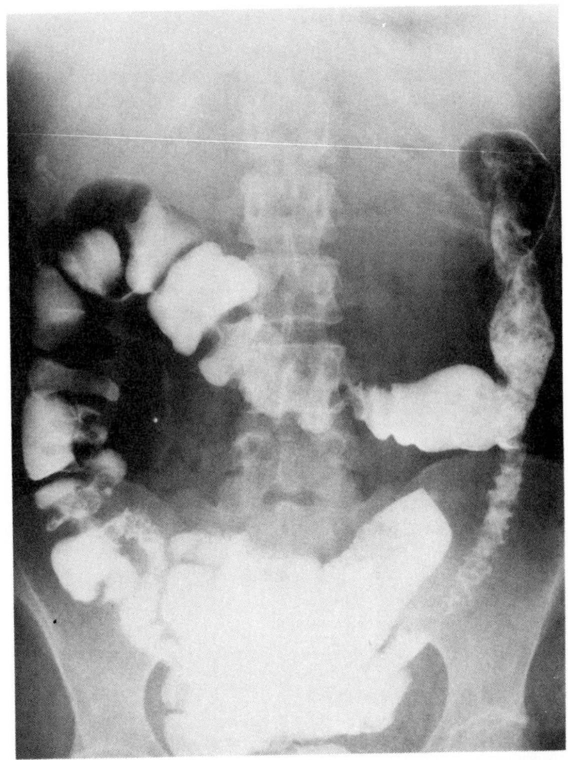

B

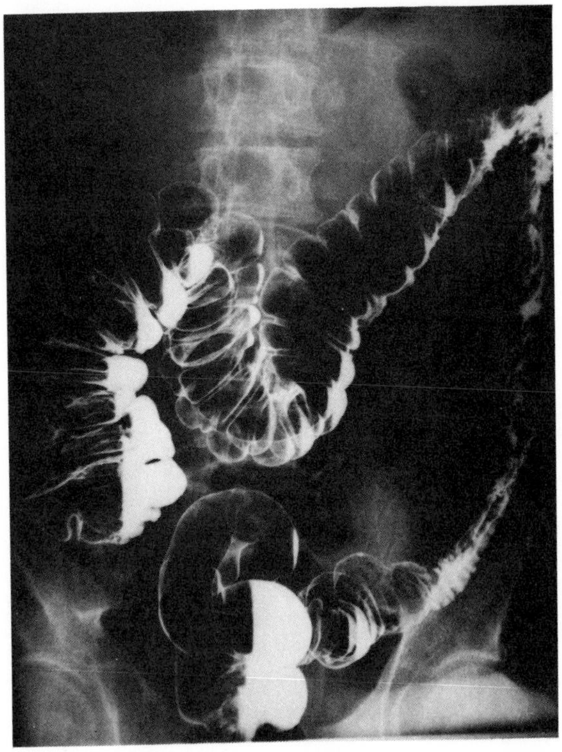

C

Figure 31-11 Barium enema x-ray. (*a*) Colon filled with barium. (*b*) Colon after evacuation of barium. (*c*) Air-contrast study of colon. (*Courtesy of Radiology Department, Lutheran Medical Center, Denver, Colorado.*)

REVIEW QUESTIONS

The number of the question corresponds to the same numbered objective at the beginning of the chapter.

1. The purpose of the villi in the small intestine is to
a. increase the time of digestion
b. slow peristaltic activity
c. phagocytize microorganisms
d. increase absorption area

2. The system which brings blood to the liver from the stomach, intestines, spleen, and pancreas is the
a. portal circulation
b. Kupffer system
c. systemic circulation
d. sinusoid system

3. The Valsalva maneuver facilitates defecation by
a. increasing the intraabdominal pressure
b. decreasing the intraabdominal pressure
c. contracting the anal canal
d. increasing muscle tone of the anal sphincter

4. The basic function of bile is to
a. convert fats to fatty acids
b. dissolve fatty acids
c. emulsify fats
d. absorb fatty acids

5. In the review of systems the client should be questioned about ingestion of food and fluids. A very significant area to include is
a. melena
b. the relationship of pain to eating or to a specific food
c. dark urine and clay-colored stools
d. steatorrhea

6. When percussing the abdomen a high, loud sound called tympany indicates
a. presence of a mass
b. ascites
c. a bruit
d. presence of air

7. Which of the following findings of an abdominal examination is *abnormal*?
a. loud, tinkling rushes on auscultation
b. liver dullness
c. unable to palpate spleen
d. no tenderness on palpation

8. The client who has had a liver biopsy should lie on his right side because this position will
a. apply pressure at puncture site
b. prevent shift of ascitic fluid
c. facilitate blood flow to the liver
d. decrease blood flow to the liver

REFERENCES

1. Arthur C. Guyton, *Textbook of Medical Physiology*, 5th ed., W. B. Saunders Company, Philadelphia, 1976, p. 850.
2. Barbara Bates, *A Guide to Physical Examination*, 2d ed., J. B. Lippincott Company, Philadelphia, 1979, p. 201.
3. Ibid., pp. 207–208.
4. Ibid., p. 210.
5. John Bernard Henry and S. Todd, *Davidsohn Clinical Diagnosis and Management by Laboratory Methods*, 16th ed., W. B. Saunders Company, Philadelphia, 1979, p. 305.

Chapter 32

NURSING ROLE IN MANAGEMENT

Problems of Ingestion

Rachel E. Elrod

Learning Objectives

1. Describe the etiology, prevention, and treatment of common dental problems.
2. Describe the etiology, clinical manifestations, and treatment of common oral inflammations and infections.
3. Explain the etiology, clinical manifestations, complications, and medical and surgical management of carcinoma of the oral cavity.
4. Describe the nursing care of the client having a radical neck dissection.
5. Describe the nursing management following surgical stabilization of a mandibular fracture.
6. Explain the types, pathophysiology, clinical manifestations, complications, and medical and surgical management of hiatal hernia.
7. Describe the nursing management of the client with a hiatal hernia.
8. Explain the pathophysiology, clinical manifestations, complications, and medical and surgical management of cancer of the esophagus.
9. Describe the nursing intervention of the client following surgery for cancer of the esophagus.
10. Describe esophageal diverticula, achalasia, esophageal strictures, and esophagitis.
11. Identify the common types of food poisoning and nursing responsibilities related to food poisoning.

Ingestion is the process of taking food and fluids into the body via the gastrointestinal tract. It begins in the mouth with mastication of food by the teeth. Food then passes down the esophagus and into the stomach. It is important that sufficient nutrients be ingested to meet bodily needs. This chapter discusses problems of ingestion that involve the mouth and esophagus. Oral problems such as poor dental health, infections and inflammations, and cancer interfere with ingestion. Esophageal problems may also interfere with swallowing food and fluids and with passage of the food to the stomach.

DENTAL PROBLEMS

Dental Caries

Dental caries (decay of teeth) is a general term applied to the decalcification of the mineral components and dissolution of the organic matrix of the teeth. Cavity formation is the clinical evidence of the progression of this process.

Development of dental caries

Caries development starts when *plaque* builds up and adheres to the teeth. *Plaque* is a gelatinous like substance consisting of bacteria, saliva, and epithelial cells. The tight adherence of plaque to the teeth provides protection for the bacteria (usually lactobacilli and streptococci). Within 30 minutes after eating, these bacteria produce acids from the breakdown of sugars contained in food deposits on the teeth. The acids destroy the outer enamel and later the underlying dentin of the tooth (Fig. 32-1). The decay proceeds and can progress to the pulp of the tooth.

If the decay is not treated, a *pulpitis* develops and extends to the alveolar bone, forming an abscess. This results in pain, edema of facial structures, and sometimes malaise and fever. During the early stages of pulpitis, pain may result from thermal changes, especially cold drinks. In the later stages of pulpitis, heat or reclining may stimulate the onset of more severe pain. At this stage, damage to the pulp is irreversible. Treatment consists of tooth removal or root canal therapy (removal of pulp and filling pulp canal with inert material).

Periodontal Disease

The *periodontium* is the tissue surrounding and supporting the teeth. It is composed of the gingivae (gums), cementum, alveolar bone, and periodontal ligament which helps to fix the tooth firmly in its bony socket. Periodontal disease begins with gingivitis and eventually involves the periodontal ligament and alveolar bone.

This chapter was reviewed by Gladys Deters, R.N., M.S., Assistant Professor, School of Nursing, University of Virginia , Charlottesville, Virginia.

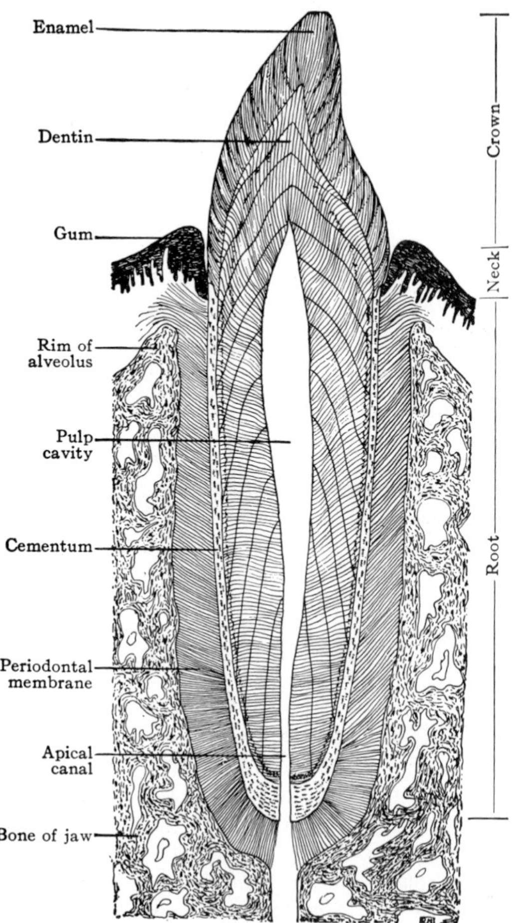

Figure 32-1 Normal tooth structure. (*From L. Weiss and R. Greep, Histology, 4th ed., McGraw-Hill Book Company, New York, 1977, p. 616.*)

Dental plaque is the most important etiologic factor in periodontal disease. When plaque calcifies, it forms *calculus*, which is a hard, tenacious mass on the crowns of teeth. *Malocclusion* (faulty relationships between the teeth when the jaws are closed), margins of overextended fillings, and impacted food are other etiologic factors that can cause local irritation to the gums. Systemic conditions such as diabetes mellitus, thyroid diseases, pregnancy, and nutritional deficiencies may modify the individual's response to the local etiologic factors and make them more susceptible to periodontal disease. The exact role of systemic conditions is not known.[1]

When the gingivae are irritated from any of the above-named local etiologic factors, they become inflamed (Fig. 32-2). The inflammation of the gingiva causes it to separate from the surface of the tooth. Pockets created between the teeth and the gingivae can collect pus and bacteria (periodontitis). At this stage bleeding occurs readily and pus may ooze from the gingiva. Gradually, the bone supporting the teeth is destroyed and the teeth become very loose. As the periodontal pockets deepen and seal themselves off, periodontal abscesses may occur. At this stage, the usual treatment is extraction of the involved tooth or teeth.

Management of Dental Problems

Health promotion and maintenance

Oral Hygiene Proper oral hygiene is essential to prevent caries and periodontal disease. This involves frequent complete cleaning of the teeth and gums with toothbrushing and flossing. The teeth should be brushed after each meal using a soft, rounded-bristle toothbrush. Brushing the teeth should remove food debris and plaque and stimulate the gums. The teeth should be brushed by placing the bristles next to the gum line and then brushed with a motion away from the gum lines.

Flossing should be done at least once a day. It is a useful and important measure for cleaning plaque between teeth, an area that is not easily accessible to brushing. Flossing is done by gently forcing the floss between the teeth and moving the floss up and down the tooth surface a few times, until it reaches the gum line.

During illness the client may not salivate as usual, which reduces the natural cleaning process of the teeth and mouth. The nurse may need to assume responsibility for dental care and oral hygiene. Swabbing the client's mouth or rinsing it with mouthwash are inadequate measures. Mechanical cleansing is essential in order to remove the plaque. Either a regular or electric toothbrush should be used on all surfaces to remove plaque and mechanically stimulate the gingivae to increase blood supply. The client's mouth should be assessed each time oral care is given.

Dental Examinations Regular, periodic dental examinations are important in order to maintain a healthy mouth and teeth. At the time of a dental examination a thorough cleaning with removal of plaque and calculus is done. Caries and early signs of periodontal disease can be detected and treated. For most adults, an examination every 6 to 12 months is adequate. Some individuals may require more frequent visits.

Nutrition Caries develop with increasing frequency in individuals who ingest diets high in refined carbohydrates. Because of this finding, a prevention

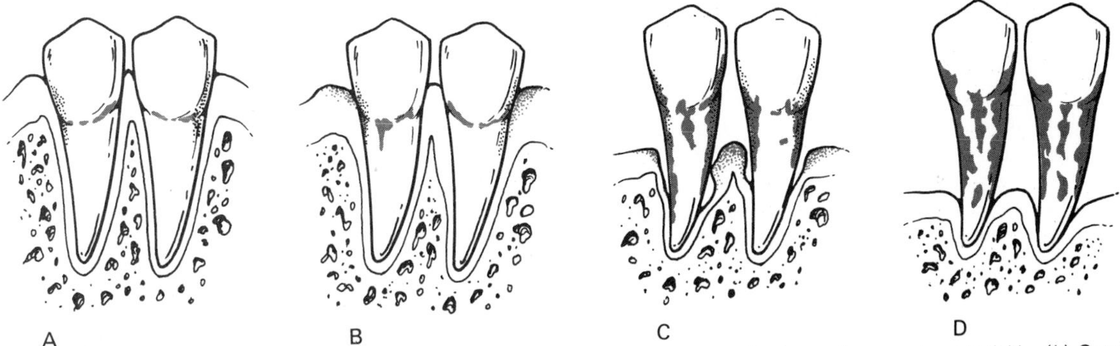

Figure 32-2 Progression of periodontal disease. (*a*) Calculus deposits on teeth at gumline causing gingivitis. (*b*) Gums become swollen and tender with spread of inflammation. (*c*) Inflammation spreads and pockets develop between teeth and gums, which are receding. (*d*) The alveolar bone is destroyed and teeth become loose.

program includes reduction in sugar intake. Another aspect of diet therapy that seems to reduce plaque formation is increased vitamin C intake. If sugars are eaten, the teeth should be brushed within 30 minutes of eating.

Fluoride Fluoridation makes teeth enamel more resistant to the acids produced from the action of bacteria on sugars in the mouth. In drinking water one part of fluoride per million results in a significant decrease in the decay rate.[2] Many communities consider the fluoridation of drinking water a municipal responsibility and have enacted the necessary legislation to do so. A fluoride solution can be applied topically on the teeth during a dental visit. In addition, many toothpastes have fluoride added to them and they are recommended by the American Dental Association.

New Techniques Some chemical methods to inhibit plaque formation and accumulation offer promise. Antimicrobial agents added to mouthwashes, toothpaste, foams, and gels have been tested. They decrease or eliminate bacterial action for a few hours after use. Bonding the teeth with application of a coating substance may protect them from decay.

Acute intervention

The nurse may need to refer the client for acute dental intervention and care. Local manifestations of dental problems include pain (either sensitive to heat or cold stimulation, or dull and continuous), facial swelling, and bleeding or pus drainage from the mouth. Systemic manifestations include fever, nausea, vomiting, and malaise.

If pulpitis and abscess develop, immediate dental care is needed to prevent further spread of infection to the bone. An opening may be drilled into the pulp chamber or the gingivae may need to be incised to provide drainage for the abscess. Sometimes a root canal or extraction is necessary. Following treatment for an abscess, the client can use warm saline rinses. Analgesics may also be required to alleviate the pain.

Extractions may be required for a damaged or defective tooth or one that has a severe abscess. After the extraction, the client should apply cold applications (ice bags, cold washcloth) to the side of the face to reduce swelling and relieve discomfort. Some oozing of blood is expected the first 1 to 2 days. If large amounts of bright red bleeding occur, direct pressure should be applied to the bleeding site and the dentist should be notified.

Sometimes the client is hospitalized for the extraction of several teeth such as impacted molars or when artificial dentures are required. Postoperatively the client will experience pain and soreness. Ice packs and analgesics are used to relieve the discomfort. Nutrients will be liquid to semisoft for a few days. The dentist may order mouthwashes for cleansing and relief of soreness.

Chronic management

Artificial Dentures The decision to obtain artificial dentures is not an easy decision for most people. They are concerned about changes in cosmetic appearance and the ability to chew food. They need to be encouraged that dentures will usually decrease the spread of infection, improve nutritional intake, and improve appearance, especially if they have had excessive dental problems preceding the decision to obtain dentures.

Patience must be stressed in the adjustment phase to dentures. It does take time to get used to a different feel and way of chewing. The gums should be checked for proper fit and any signs of gum irritation. Dentures should be cleaned at least twice a day with salt and sodium bicarbonate or a dentrifice. When the dentures are removed, the client should massage his gums for a few minutes. Some clients prefer to wear their dentures at all times and there is generally no contraindications to this practice. In fact, facial contour is better maintained by this practice. If clients remove their dentures at night, they should be covered with water (especially if the dentures are made with vulcanite) and stored in a safe place.

Clients who wear dentures should be encouraged to obtain regular dental care. Dentures may need to be modified as tissue changes occur from aging, weight changes, or disease processes.

Periodontal Disease Early treatment of periodontal disease consists of curettage under the gum margins. Plaque and calculus should be professionally removed at least twice a year. A *gingivectomy* and *gingivoplasty* may be necessary. In a gingivectomy, gum tissue and deep pockets are removed. A gingivoplasty involves reshaping of gum tissue.

In the later stages of periodontal disease, the bone supporting the teeth is often destroyed. At this stage, treatment is extraction of the teeth and the wearing of artificial dentures.

ORAL INFLAMMATIONS AND INFECTIONS

Oral infections and inflammations which are specific mouth diseases may occur. They may also occur in the presence of some systemic diseases such as leukemia or vitamin deficiency. When oral inflammations and infections occur, they can severely impair the ingestion of food and fluids. Common inflammations and infections of the oral cavity are presented in Table 32-1.

CARCINOMA OF THE ORAL CAVITY

Carcinoma of the oral cavity may occur on the lips or anywhere within the mouth (tongue, floor of the mouth, buccal mucosa, hard palate, soft palate, pharyngeal walls, and tonsils).

Oral carcinoma accounts for about 3 percent of all cancer deaths in the United States and more than 5 percent of all cancers. It is more common in males. Squamous cell carcinoma is the most common oral malignant tumor (90 to 95 percent).[3]

Most of the malignant lesions occur on the lower lip. Carcinoma of the lip has the most favorable prognosis of any of the oral tumors. This is probably due to the fact that lip lesions are more apparent to the client than other types of oral lesions.

Etiology

While the etiology of carcinoma of the oral cavity is not definitive, there are a number of predisposing factors (Table 32-2). Constant overexposure to the sun and wind is definitely a factor in the development of cancer of the lip. Irritation from the pipe stem resting on the lip is a factor in pipe smokers. Factors influencing intraoral cancer include tobacco (cigar, cigarette, pipe, snuff), excessive alcoholic intake, and chronic irritation such as might occur from a jagged tooth and poor dental care. Excessive use of alcohol and tobacco probably causes a decrease in the body's local defense mechanisms.

Clinical Manifestations

Leukoplakia, called "white patch" or "smoker's patch" is usually considered a precancerous lesion. It is described as a whitish patch on the mucosa of the mouth or tongue. The patch becomes keratinized (hard and leathery). Leukoplakia is due to chronic irritation, especially smoking. Currently, a red lesion (*erythroplakia*) in the mouth is considered more likely to be carcinoma than a white lesion.[4]

Cancer of the lip usually presents as an indurated, painless ulcer on the lip (Fig. 32-3). The first sign of carcinoma of the tongue is an ulcer or area of thickening. Soreness or pain of the tongue may occur, especially when eating hot or highly seasoned foods. Some clients experience limitation of movement of the tongue. Later symptoms of cancer of the tongue include increased salivation, slurred speech, dysphagia, toothache, and earache.

Common manifestations of carcinoma of the oral cavity are leukoplakia, erythroplakia, ulcerations, sore spot, and a rough area (felt with the tongue). Later symptoms are pain, dysphagia, and difficulty chewing and speaking.

Diagnostic Study Abnormalities

Biopsy of the suspected lesion with cytologic examination is the best definitive diagnostic measure. Oral exfoliative cytology involves scraping of a suspicious lesion and spreading this scraping on a slide. This procedure can help confirm the presence of a malignancy. Unlike biopsy, a negative cytology cannot be relied on to rule out the possibility of a malignancy.[5]

Two staining techniques have been used as

Table 32-1
Infections and Inflammations of the Mouth

Condition	Etiology	Clinical Manifestations	Treatment
Gingivitis	Neglected oral hygiene. Malocclusion. Missing or irregular teeth. Faulty dentistry. Eating soft rather than fibrous foods.	Inflamed gingivae and interdental papillae. Bleeding during tooth brushing. Development of pus, abscess formation with loosening of teeth (periodontitis).	Focus is on *prevention*. Health teaching. Dental care. Gum massage. Professional cleaning of teeth. Fibrous foods. Conscientious brushing habits.
Vincent's infection (acute necrotizing ulcerative gingivitis, trench mouth)	Fusiform bacteria. Vincenti spirochetes. Predisposing factors: worry, excessive fatigue, poor oral hygiene, nutritional deficiencies (vitamins B and C).	Sore mouth. Eroding necrotic lesions of interdental papillae. Ulcerations which bleed. Increased saliva with metallic taste. Fetid mouth odor. Anorexia, fever, and general malaise.	Rest (physical and mental). Avoidance of smoking and alcoholic beverages. Soft, nutritious diet. Correct oral hygiene habits. Topical applications of antibiotics. Mouth irrigations.
Oral candidiasis (moniliasis or thrush)	*Candida albicans* (a yeastlike fungus). Occurs in debilitated persons. Occurs in persons on prolonged high-dosage antibiotic or corticosteroid therapy.	Pearly, bluish-white "milk-curd" membranous lesions on mucosa of mouth and larynx. Sore mouth. Yeasty halitosis.	Nystatin or amphotericin B as oral suspension or buccal tablets. Good oral hygiene.
Viral infections 1. Herpesvirus (coldsore, fever blister)	Herpesvirus. Predisposing factors: Upper respiratory infections, excessive exposure to sunlight, food allergies, emotional tension, onset of menstruation.	Lip lesions. Mouth lesions. Vesicle formation (single or clustered) Shallow, painful ulcers.	Spirits of camphor. Corticosteroid cream. Mild antiseptic mouthwash. Viscous lidocaine. Removal or control of predisposing factors. Antiviral agents.
2. Aphthous stomatitis (canker sore)	Recurrent and chronic form of infection secondary to herpesvirus, systemic disease; or unknown causes.	Ulcers of mouth and lips.	Steroids (topical or systemic).
Parotitis (inflammation of parotid gland, surgical mumps)	Usually *Staphylococcus*. Streptococcus found occasionally. Debilitated and dehydrated patients with poor oral hygiene. NPO for an extended period of time	Pain in area of gland and ear. Absence of salivation. Purulent exudate from duct of gland.	Antibiotics. Mouthwashes. Warm compresses. Preventive measures such as chewing gum, sucking hard candy (lemon balls), adequate fluid intake.
Stomatitis (inflammation of the mouth)	Trauma. Secondary to pathogens. Irritant (tobacco, alcohol). Renal, liver, and hematologic diseases. Side effect of many cancer chemotherapy drugs.	Excessive salivation. Halitosis. Sore mouth.	Remove or treat cause. Oral hygiene with soothing solutions. Topical medications. Soft, bland diet.

Adapted with permission from H. C. Moidel et al., *Nursing Care of the Patient with Medical-Surgical Disorders*, 2d ed., McGraw-Hill Book Company, New York, 1976, p. 728.

Table 32-2
Comparison of Oral Tumors

Location	Predisposing Factors	Clinical Manifestations	Treatment
Lip	Constant overexposure to sun and wind Fair complexion Irritation from pipe stem	Indurated painless ulcer	Surgical excision Irradiation
Tongue	Tobacco Irritation Syphilis	Ulcer or area of thickening Soreness or pain Later: increased salivation, slurred speech, dysphagia, toothache, earache	Surgery (hemiglosseotomy or glossectomy) Irradiation
Oral cavity	Poor oral hygiene Tobacco (especially pipe and cigar smokers) Chronic alcoholic intake Chronic irritation (jagged tooth)	Leukoplakia Erythroplakia Ulcerations Sore spot Rough area Later: pain, dysphagia, difficulty chewing and speaking	Surgery (mandibulectomy, radical neck dissection, resections of buccal mucosa) Irradiation Chemotherapy

screening tests for oral cancer. One is the mouthwash technique which utilizes a balanced salt solution to irrigate the mouth and obtain a specimen of oral cells which are then stained and studied for malignant cells. The other technique is the toluidine blue test. The toluidine blue is applied topically and will stain an area of carcinoma.[6]

Medical Management

Management of oral carcinoma usually consists of surgery, radiation, chemotherapy, or combinations of these (Table 32-3).

Surgery

Surgery remains the most effective treatment, especially for removing the central core of the tumor. Many of the surgeries are radical procedures involving extensive resections. Various surgical procedures may be performed depending on the location and extent of the tumor. Some examples are partial *mandibulectomy* (removal of the mandible), *hemiglossectomy* (removal of half of the tongue), total *glossectomy* (removal of the tongue), resections of the buccal mucosa and floor of the mouth, and *radical neck dissection*.

Since cancers of the oral cavity metastasize early to the cervical lymph nodes in the neck, a *radical neck dissection* is commonly performed. It includes wide excision of the involved primary lesion with removal of the regional lymph nodes and deep cervical lymph nodes and their lymphatic channels. In addition, the following structures may also be removed or transect-

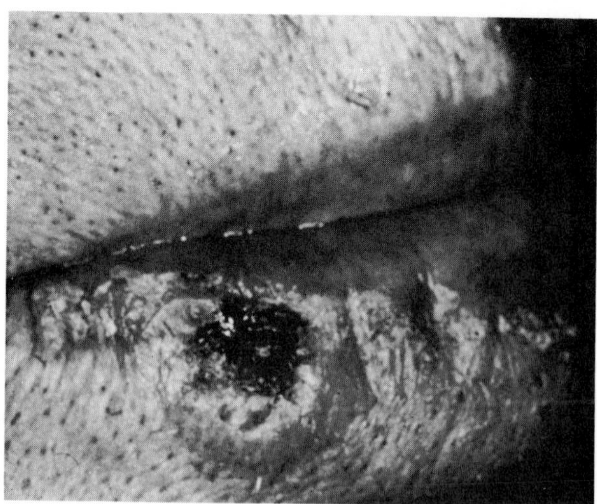

Figure 32-3 Squamous carcinoma of the lip. *(From S. Schwartz et al., Principles of Surgery, 3d ed., McGraw-Hill Book Company, New York, 1979, p. 601.)*

Table 32-3
Medical Management: Oral Carcinoma

Diagnostic
1. Oral exfoliative cytology
2. Biopsy

Therapeutic*
1. Surgical excision of the tumor
2. Radical neck dissection
3. Radiation (internal or external)
4. Combined surgical excision with radiation
5. Chemotherapy

*Any of the following approaches may be used, depending on the primary lesion and the extent of metastasis.

ed (depending on the primary lesion and its extensiveness): sternocleidomastoid muscle and other closely associated muscles, internal jugular vein, mandible, submaxillary gland, part of thyroid and parathyroid glands, and spinal accessory nerve. A tracheostomy is commonly done along with the radical neck dissection. Drainage tubes are inserted into the surgical area and connected to suction to remove fluid and blood (Fig. 32-4). The radical neck dissection usually involves one side of the neck. If the lesion is in the midline of the oral cavity, simultaneous bilateral neck dissection is done.

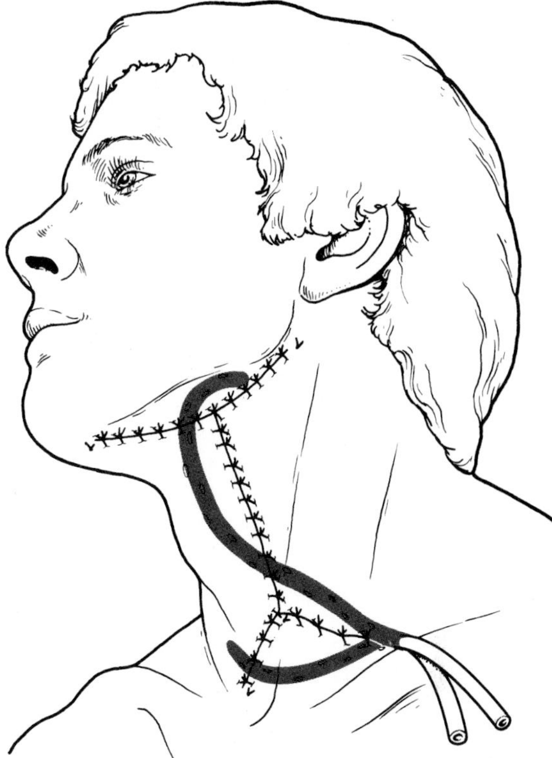

Figure 32-4 Radical neck incision with suction tubing in place.

Complications of Radical Neck Surgery The mortality rate following radical neck surgery is less than 1 percent.[7] However, life-threatening complications may occur, such as *airway obstruction, hemorrhage*, and *tracheal aspiration*. *Airway obstruction* must be prevented. Depending on the degree of surgery, a prophylactic tracheostomy is often done. *Hemorrhage* can occur because of the vascularity of the head and neck area. Another complication is *tracheal aspiration*, which may occur up to a week after surgery. It occurs because the client is unable to swallow saliva or fluids, and aspirates fluid. Other complications include infection, pneumothorax, subcutaneous emphysema or air leak under the skin flaps, and necrosis of the skin flaps. Neural complications can occur due to nerve severing during the surgical procedure. The nerves most commonly severed are the spinal accessory and cervical plexus. The facial nerve (cranial nerve VII) which passes through the parotid gland may be affected if this gland is removed.

Radiation and chemotherapy

Radiation is sometimes used prior to surgery to decrease the size of the tumor. Radiation may also be used postoperatively or palliatively. The type of radiation used may be internal or external. Common forms of internal radiation are the implantation of seeds such as radon seeds in gold tubes or molds. External radiation using x-rays or other radioactive substances may be used.

Chemotherapy and radiation are used together when the lesions are more advanced or involve several structures of the oral cavity. Chemotherapy may be also used when surgery and radiation fail or as the initial therapy for smaller tumors. Methotrexate (MTX) is the most effective chemotherapeutic agent. 5-fluorouracil (5-FU) may be used for small skin lesions. Other chemotherapeutic agents used are cyclophosphamide, bleomycin, vinblastine, and hydroxyurea.

Palliative treatment may be the best management when the prognosis is poor, the cancer is inoperable, or the client decides against multilating surgery. Palliation aims to treat the symptoms and make the client more comfortable. If it becomes difficult to swallow, a gastrostomy may be done to allow for adequate nutritional intake. Analgesic medication should be given freely to these clients. Frequent suctioning of the oral cavity becomes necessary when swallowing becomes difficult. Other nursing measures for the terminally ill client are discussed in Chap. 11.

Dietary Measures

Following radical neck surgery, the client may be unable to take in nutrients through the normal route of ingestion because of swelling, the location of sutures, or difficulty with swallowing. Parenteral fluids will be given for the first 24 to 48 hours. After this time, tube feedings are usually given via a nasogastric tube which was placed during surgery. Sometimes a temporary feeding gastrostomy may be utilized. The nurse must observe for tolerance of the feedings and adjust the amount, time, and formula if nausea, vomiting, diarrhea, or distension occur. The client is usually taught to do the tube feedings himself. When the client can swallow, small amounts of water are given. Close observation for choking is essential. Suctioning may be necessary to prevent aspiration.

Nursing Management

Health promotion and maintenance

The nurse has a significant role in early detection and treatment of carcinoma of the oral cavity. The nurse needs to provide clients with information regarding the predisposing factors such as constant overexposure to the sun and tobacco and other irritants. The nurse should also teach correct oral hygiene and dental care and encourage individuals to seek preventive dental care. Because early detection of oral carcinoma is very important, individuals should be taught to examine their mouths and recognize danger signals of oral cancer. If any of them are present, the client should be instructed to visit his doctor. Danger signals are:

1. Unexplained pain or soreness in mouth
2. Unusual bleeding from oral cavity
3. Dysphagia
4. Swelling or lump in the neck
5. Any ulcerative lesion which does not heal within 1 to 2 weeks.

The last one is very significant and should probably be biopsied. The nurse should assess the client's oral cavity in order to detect suspicious lesions.

Acute intervention

Preoperative care for the client having a radical neck dissection involves consideration of physical and psychosocial needs (Table 32-4). Physical preparation is the same as for any major surgery with special emphasis on oral hygiene. Explanations and emotional support are of special significance and should include postoperative measures relating to communication and feeding. The client should have the surgical procedure explained, and the nurse needs to make sure the information supplied to the client is understood.

Airway Postoperatively, a patent airway is the priority nursing measure. The inflammation in the surgical area may press on and compress the trachea. This is a reason why a tracheostomy is commonly done in conjunction with radical neck surgery. In addition, the client has difficulty swallowing his own saliva and is at risk for aspiration. If the client has a tracheostomy, frequent suctioning is essential. (See Chap. 19 for care of the client with a tracheostomy.) For the client without a tracheostomy, oral or nasopharyngeal suctioning should be done when audible signs of fluid occur or the client indicates a need for suctioning.

Positioning To facilitate drainage from the mouth and prevent aspiration, positioning is essential. In the immediate and early postoperative period, the client should be lying on his side or abdomen, with head turned to one side to prevent aspiration. As soon as the client is awake, the head of the bed is usually elevated to promote venous and lymphatic drainage. The nurse should provide a basin and mouth wipes to assist the client to handle the secretions. The basin should be emptied frequently because of the odor of the secretions.

Oral Hygiene Measures must be taken to prevent infection of the oral cavity. Accumulation of mucus and old blood provides an excellent medium for microorganisms. Oral hygiene will decrease the possibility of infection and also decrease the mouth odor and unpleasant taste for the client. The oral care must be done carefully to prevent trauma. The mouth may be gently irrigated with sterile water, normal saline, or diluted hydrogen peroxide. An applicator soaked with peroxide and saline may be used to cleanse the difficult to reach areas.

Communication One of the client's real fears postoperatively is not being able to talk and easily tell the nurse about pain and request help. Talking is impossible for a person with a tracheostomy. Speech difficulties also arise if part of the tongue or palate has been resected. Alternate means of communication should have been decided on preoperatively. Suggestions include pad and pencil, small chalkboard, and "magic slate." Having the call button within reach

Table 32-4
Nursing Care Plan for the Client Following a Radical Neck Dissection

Client Problem	Expected Outcome	Nursing Intervention
Airway obstruction	Patent airway, no aspiration of saliva.	Position on side or abdomen, with head turned to one side, immediately after surgery. Position in a sitting position as soon as client can tolerate it. Suction client frequently and carefully. Assess client for early signs of respiratory distress. Provide a basin and wipes for saliva and secretions. (For care of tracheostomy see Chap. 19.)
Lung congestion	Lungs clear to auscultation.	Assist client to cough effectively. Support client's neck and head when deep breathing and coughing. Auscultate lungs every 2 h.
Pain	Relief of pain.	Administer mild analgesics. Do not use narcotic analgesics which depress respirations. Provide for comfortable positioning, oral care, and emotional support.
Inability to ingest nutrients	Adequate intake of nutrients.	Administer tube feedings as ordered. Observe for tolerance of feedings. Provide privacy when eating. When client starts taking fluids, observe for choking and have suction available. Offer small, frequent, attractively served meals with adequate fluid intake.
Oral infection	A clean oral cavity with no infection.	Frequent, gentle oral hygiene. Use mouth irrigations with sterile water, normal saline, or diluted peroxide. Suction and provide tissues for drooling of saliva. Use Water Pik or power spray to clean hard-to-reach areas. Apply lubricant to dry lips.
Difficulty communicating	Alternate means of communication.	Plan for and provide alternate means of communication (pad and pencil, small chalkboard, "magic slate"). Place call button within reach. Visit frequently and assure client that help is available to meet his requests.
Altered body image	Acceptance of altered body image.	Assess client's body image concept. Provide privacy. If client drools, instruct to tilt head to side. Encourage attention to personal hygiene and socialization with family and friends. Answer questions honestly about changes in body image. Involve client in self-care.
Feelings of sexual inadequacy and undesirability	Freedom to discuss and analyze these feelings.	Allow discussion regarding sexuality. Encourage client to discuss this problem with sexual partner. Help client realize sexuality involves more than appearance. Refer to counseling services if needed.
Functional and cosmetic deformities	Knowledge about the possibilities of reconstructive surgery.	Provide information about prosthetic devices, speech therapy, and reconstructive surgery. Cooperate with other members of the health care team.

is essential. Added assurance and relief of anxiety is accomplished through frequent visits from the nurse.

Self-Image The nurse should be aware of how the client feels about his altered body. Privacy is important to most clients, especially when eating. The client may have aeroplast protecting the wound with no dressing and therefore be reluctant to go outside his room. If the client drools, instruct him to tilt the head to the side to prevent this. Attention to personal hygiene, socialization with family and friends, and regaining an acceptable self-concept are significant for this client.

Depression Depression is common in clients following radical neck dissections. They cannot speak because of the tracheostomy and cannot control their own saliva. Their neck and shoulders are numb because of the transected nerves. Their facial appearance is grotesque with swelling, edema, and deformities. They need to understand that many of the physical changes are reversible as the edema sub-

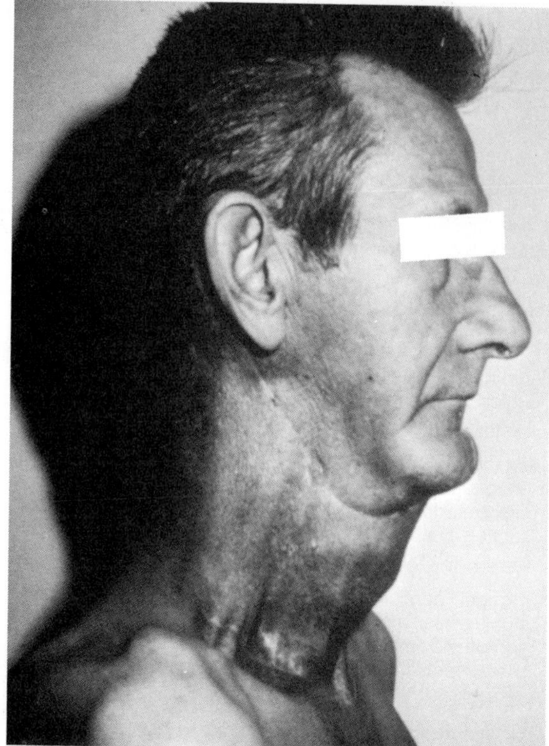

Figure 32-5 Appearance of the neck following healing after a radical neck dissection. This man also had postoperative external radiation therapy. (*Courtesy of R. Doberneck, M.D.*)

sides and the tracheostomy tube is removed (Fig. 32-5). Sometimes it is appropriate to obtain a psychiatric referral for clients who are experiencing prolonged or severe depression.

Rehabilitative management

Facial disfigurement and other mutilating aspects of radical head and neck surgery may have a major long-term impact on the body image. Many of these surgeries leave a deformity, both functionally and cosmetically. It may be difficult for the client to eat and speak, and the altered physical appearance may be embarrassing and depressing. The client may need information about prosthetic devices, speech therapy, and further reconstructive surgery.

Reconstructive surgery should be done soon after the tumor is removed. Various types of skin grafting are used. It may be necessary to rebuild the nose or mandible, or close oral cutaneous openings. Prosthetic materials such as silastic and plastigel (which is very soft) is often used to reconstruct various deformities.[8]

The client may feel less desirable sexually. The nurse can assist the client by allowing discussions regarding sexuality and encouraging the client to discuss this problem with the sexual partner. Helping the client to see that sexuality involves much more than appearance may relieve some anxiety.

MANDIBULAR FRACTURE

Fracture of the mandible may result from trauma to the face or jaws. Maxillary fractures may also occur but are less common than mandibular fractures. The fracture may be simple with no bone displacement or it may involve loss of tissue and bone. The fracture may require immediate and sometimes long-term treatment to both ensure survival and restore satisfactory appearance and function.

Surgical Management

Surgery consists of immobilization, usually by wiring the jaws. Internal fixation may be accomplished with screws and plates. In a simple fracture with no loss of teeth, the lower jaw is wired to the upper jaw. First, wires are placed around the teeth, then cross-wires or rubber bands are used to hold the lower jaw tight against the upper jaw (Fig. 32-6). Arch bars may be used and placed on the maxillary and mandibular arches of teeth. Vertical wires are placed between the arch bars holding the jaws together. When teeth are missing or if there is bone displacement, other forms of fixation such as metal arch bars in the mouth or pin insertion in the bone may be used. Usually the immobilization is only necessary for 4 to 5 weeks since the fractures heal rapidly.

Dietary Management

Ingestion of sufficient nutrients poses a real problem since the diet must be liquid. The client easily tires of sucking through a straw or laboriously using a spoon. The diet must be planned to include an adequate amount of calories and protein. Adequate fluid intake must be included. The nurse needs to work with the dietician and the client to assure adequate nutrition. The low-bulk, high carbohydrate diet and intake of air through the straw creates a problem with flatus and constipation. Ambulation, prune juice, and bulk-forming laxatives may help relieve these problems.

Nursing Management

Preoperative care

The client should be told preoperatively about the surgical procedure; what it involves, how it will look,

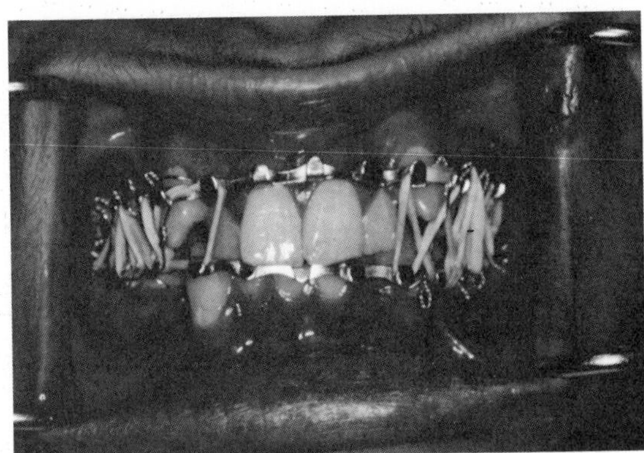

Figure 32-6 Intermaxillary fixation. (*Courtesy of R. A. Weinstein, D.D.S., M.S., Denver, Colorado.*)

and alterations it will cause. He needs to be reassured that he will be able to breathe normally, talk, and swallow liquids. Usually he will only need to be in the hospital for a few days unless there are other bodily injuries or problems.

Postoperative care

Postoperative care should focus on a patent airway, oral hygiene, communication, and adequate nutrition. Because the client cannot open his jaws, measures to assure an airway are essential. The nurse must observe for signs of respiratory distress. The client should be placed on his side with the head slightly elevated immediately after surgery. A wire cutter or scissors (for rubber bands) must be taped to the head of the bed. These are used to cut the wires or elastic bands if the client begins to vomit or choke. Suctioning may be necessary and may be done by the nasopharyngeal or oral route, depending on the extent of injury and type of repair. A nasogastric tube may be used for decompression to remove fluids and gas from the stomach to help prevent aspiration. It will also help prevent vomiting. Antiemetics may also be used. The nasogastric tube can later be used as a feeding tube.

Oral hygiene is a very important part of the nursing care. The mouth should be rinsed frequently, particularly following meals and snacks, to remove food debris. Warm normal saline, water, or alkaline mouthwashes may be used. A soft rubber catheter or a Water Pik is effective for attaining a thorough oral cleansing. The nurse should inspect the mouth several times a day to see if it is clean. A flashlight is necessary and a tongue depressor is used to retract the cheeks.

Communication may be a problem, particularly in the early postoperative period. An effective way of communication must be planned for preoperatively. Some suggestions include a "magic slate," pad and pencil, or a small chalkboard. Usually the client can speak well enough to be understood, especially after the first few postoperative days.

The client is usually discharged with the wires in place. Oral care and feeding must be taught to the client. He must also be instructed on the purpose and use of wire cutters or scissors. The nurse needs to allow the client to verbalize feelings about his appearance.

HIATAL HERNIA

Hiatal hernia is a herniation of a portion of the stomach into the esophagus. It is also referred to as a *diaphragmatic hernia*. Hiatal hernias are classified into two types:

1. *Sliding* in which the junction of the stomach and esophagus is above the hiatus of the diaphragm and a part of the stomach slides through the hiatal opening in the diaphragm. This is the most common type.
2. *Paraesophageal or rolling* in which the esophagogastric junction remains in normal position but the fundus and greater curvature of the stomach roll up through the diaphragm, forming a pocket alongside the esophagus (Fig. 32-7).

Significance of the Problem

The incidence of hiatal hernia is difficult to determine. Although it is said to be the most common abnormality found on x-ray of the upper GI tract, the hernia is often asymptomatic. Hiatal hernias are found most commonly in ages 40 to 70. It occurs more frequently in women (4 to 1) than men.[9]

Pathophysiology

There are many factors that contribute to the development of hiatal hernia. Structural changes such as weakening of the muscles in the diaphragm around the esophagogastric opening are usually a contributing factor. Factors which increase intraabdominal pressure, including obesity, pregnancy, ascites, tumors, tight corsets, and heavy lifting on a continual basis may also predispose to hiatal hernia development. Other predisposing factors are increased age, trauma, poor nutrition, and a forced recumbent position such as a prolonged illness which confines the individual to bed. In some individuals, congenital weakness is a contributing factor.

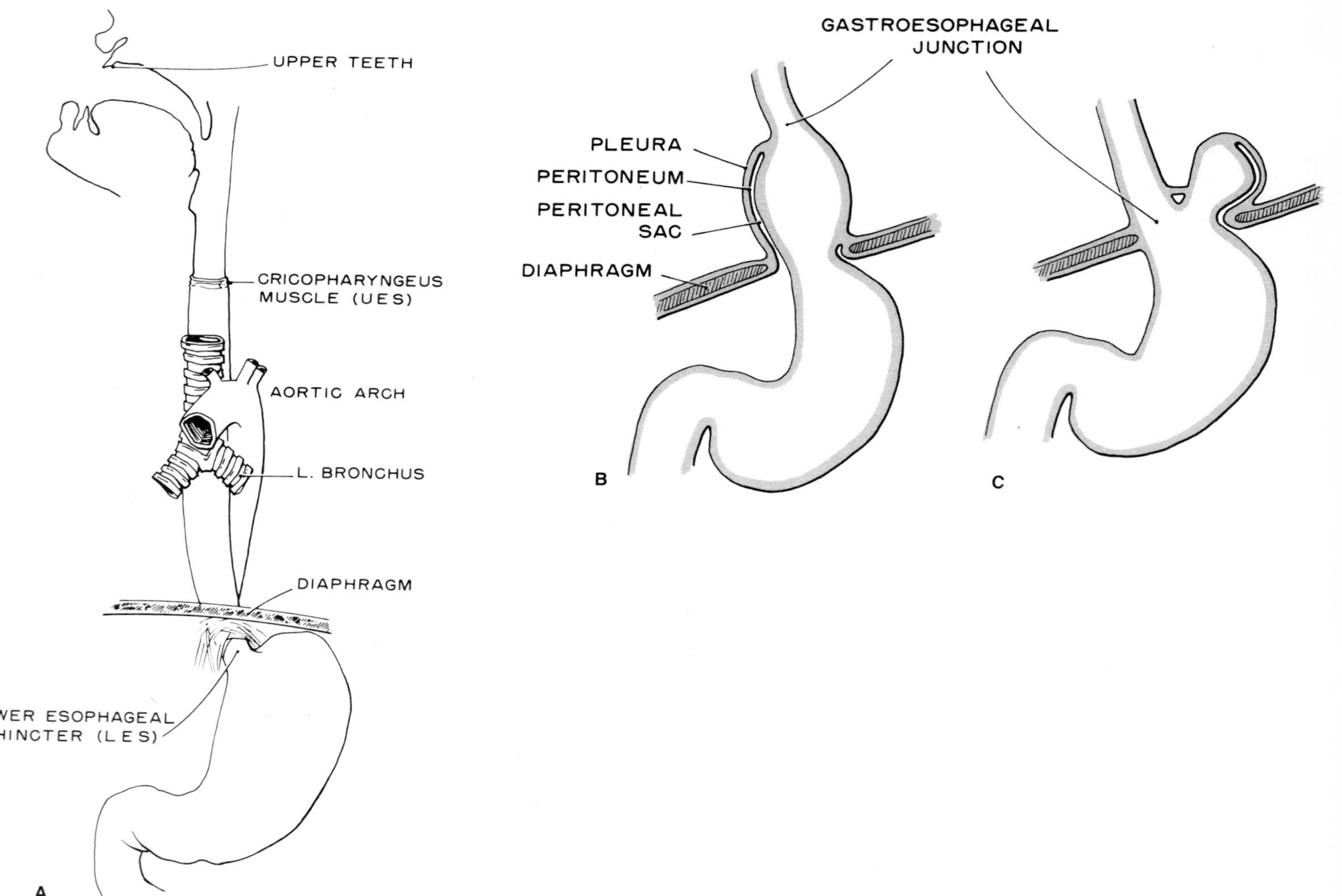

Figure 32-7 (*a*) Normal esophagus. (*b*) Sliding hiatal hernia. (*c*) Rolling or paraesophageal hernia. (*Adapted from S. Price and L. Wilson, Pathophysiology: Clinical Concepts of Disease Process, 2d ed., McGraw-Hill Book Company, New York, 1982.*)

With the accompanying changes of hiatal hernia development, there is frequently reflux of gastric juice into the esophagus. The esophageal mucosa is very sensitive to the acidic gastric secretions. This may cause a *reflux esophagitis*.

Clinical Manifestations

Heartburn (pyrosis, dyspepsia) from reflux esophagitis is the most common clinical manifestation of hiatal hernia. It is due to the irritation of the esophagus by the gastric acids. Heartburn is described as a burning, tight sensation that appears intermittently beneath the lower sternum and spreads upward to the throat or jaw. Heartburn may be aggravated by food or liquid, especially spices and raw foods. It is also associated with position, occurring shortly after or several hours after lying down. Bending over may cause a severe burning pain, but it will be relieved with sitting or standing.

Common precipitating factors of pain include large meals, alcohol, stress, and tension. Nocturnal attacks are common, especially if the individual has eaten before going to sleep. Heartburn is relieved with milk, alkali substances, or water.

Regurgitation (effortless return of material from stomach into esophagus or mouth) is fairly common manifestation of hiatal hernia. It is often described as hot, bitter, or sour liquid coming into the throat or mouth. Other symptoms of hiatal hernia include feelings of a lump in the throat or of food stopping, *dysphagia* (difficulty swallowing), painful swallowing, and bleeding. Frequently the symptoms of hiatal hernia mimic gallbladder disease, peptic ulcer, and angina. Some clients with hiatal hernia are asymptomatic.

Complications

Several complications that may occur with hiatal hernia include problems such as hemorrhage from erosion, stenosis, ulcerations of the herniated portion of the stomach, and regurgitation with tracheal aspiration. Severe chronic esophagitis may follow reflux problems.

Medical Management (Table 32-5)

Diagnostic

A barium swallow is an important diagnostic measure that may show the protrusion of gastric mucosa through the esophageal hiatus. Esophagoscopy is useful in determining the incompetence of the cardiac sphincter and whether gastric reflux is present. Biopsy and cytologic specimens can be taken to differentiate hiatal hernia from carcinoma of the stomach or esophagus. Sometimes esophageal motility studies are done to determine pressure gradients.

Table 32-5
Medical Management: Hiatal Hernia

Diagnostic
1. Barium swallow
2. Esophagoscopy

Conservative therapy
1. Elevate head of bed on 4 to 6-inch blocks
2. Bland diet with six small feedings
3. Antacids
4. Cholinergic drugs

Surgical therapy: Postoperative
1. Nasogastric tube to suction
2. IV fluids with electrolyte replacement
3. I and O
4. Vital signs every 2-4 h
5. Pulmonary physiotherapy (turning, coughing, deep breathing, spirometry)
6. Antiemetic prn
7. Analgesic prn

Conservative management

Medical management consists mainly of various measures to prevent reflux and medications which relieve symptoms. Such methods as administration of antacids, elimination of constricting garments, avoidance of lifting and straining, and elevation of the head of the bed are used to meet these goals. If the client is obese, he is encouraged to lose weight. (Pharmacologic and dietary measures are discussed in the next sections.)

Pharmacologic Intervention

Antacids are used to relieve heartburn by their neutralizing effect on HCl. Cholinergic drugs such as bethanechol (Urecholine) may be used to increase the gastroesophageal sphincter pressure. Sometimes alginic acid and an antacid are given together. The alginic acid reacts with sodium bicarbonate and forms a viscous solution which floats to the surface of gastric contents and will make contact with the esophageal mucosa instead of the gastric secretions if reflux occurs.[10] The effect of histamine antagonists (cimetidine) is not yet known.

The nurse should observe for and instruct the client about side effects of the medications being taken. Antacids have minimal side effects. Antacids containing aluminum tend to cause constipation and those with magnesium tend to cause diarrhea. Several of the antacids are combinations of aluminum and magnesium designed to minimize these side effects. If the client is on bethanechol, side effects to observe for include urinary urgency, increased salivation, abdominal cramping with diarrhea, nausea, vomiting, and hypotension.

Dietary Measures

Since highly seasoned foods usually increase heartburn, a bland diet is recommended. Small, frequent meals are advised to prevent overdistension of the stomach. Clients should be taught to eliminate foods which seem to irritate the hernia and result in heartburn. Most clients find they need to avoid highly seasoned foods, caffeine, and carbonated beverages. Some may need to eliminate fruit juices, fats, and chocolate.

Nursing Management Related to Conservative Therapy

Clients with a hiatal hernia who are being managed conservatively need to avoid factors which bring on symptoms. These factors are tight clothing, bending, and excessive intake of food and alcohol. The client who is overweight should reduce. If the client is a smoker, he should try to stop smoking. Caffeine, nicotine, fats, and chocolate decrease the gastroesophageal sphincter tone and should be avoided.[11] Since stress is a common precipitating factor for the occurrence of symptoms, measures to control stress are helpful to discuss with the client.

Nursing care for the client who is having acute symptoms consists mainly of teaching and encouraging the client to follow the necessary regimen. The nurse should make sure the head of the bed is elevated correctly (usually on 4-to-6-inch blocks) and that the client does not lie down in the first 2 to 3 hours after eating. This position assists gravity in maintaining the stomach in the abdominal cavity and also helps prevent reflux and tracheal aspiration. Teaching the client to avoid food and activities that cause reflux is important (e.g., late night eating should be avoided). The client may be on medications to relieve heartburn (see Pharmacologic Intervention) so the nurse will need to observe for side effects and determine if the medications are relieving symptoms. The client should also be taught possible side effects of medication.

Surgical Management

Surgical intervention for hiatal hernia is indicated when medical therapy fails or for complications such as stenosis, chronic esophagitis, or bleeding. Very large hiatal hernias are frequently repaired surgically.

The objective of surgery is to restore gastroesophageal integrity and prevent gastric reflux. A reinforcement of the sphincter must be done. A *fundoplication* procedure is the type of surgical procedure most commonly done. This procedure involves "wrapping" the upper part of the stomach around the sphincter segment. Fundoplication will prevent reflux. The operations associated with the names of Nissen, Belsey, and Hill are typical of this type of procedure. In a Nissen fundoplication, the fundus of the stomach is wrapped around the distal esophagus (Fig. 32-8). A thoracic or abdominal approach may be used for any of these procedures. The choice depends on the client's condition and the surgeon. An abdominal approach is more commonly performed. Postoperative orders are summarized in Table 32-5.

Nursing Management Related to Surgical Intervention

Postoperative care focuses on concerns related to prevention of respiratory complications, maintenance of fluid and electrolyte balance, and prevention of infection. If the client has a thoracic approach, a chest tube is inserted. Assessment relative to closed chest drainage is important. (Care of chest tubes and thoracotomy clients is discussed in Chap. 20.)

Respiratory complications can occur in clients with an abdominal approach because of the high abdominal incision. Respiratory assessment should include respiratory rate and rhythm, chest reexpansion, pulse rate and rhythm, and signs of pneumothorax (dyspnea, chest pain, cyanosis). Coughing and deep breathing are essential to fully expand the lungs. Pulmonary physiotherapy is necessary. The client

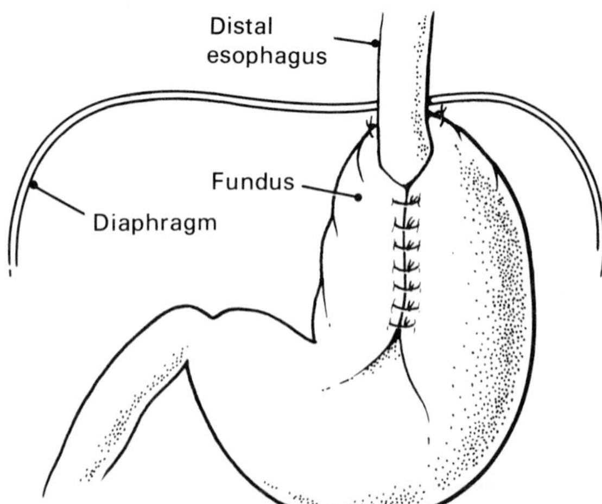

Figure 32-8 Nissen fundoplication for repair of hiatal hernia. Fundus of stomach is wrapped around distal esophagus and sutured to itself.

should not be oversedated with drugs which depress respirations, such as morphine.

The client will receive only intravenous fluids and electrolytes until the return of peristalsis. When peristalsis returns, only fluids will be given for 2 to 3 days. Food will be added gradually so as not to overload the stomach. The nurse must maintain an accurate recording of intake and output and observe for fluid and electrolyte imbalances (see Chap. 12).

Following surgical intervention, the client should not have symptoms of gastric reflux. The client should be instructed to report such symptoms as heartburn and regurgitation. The client should also report dysphagia, epigastric fullness, and bloating. Immediately following the surgical procedure the client cannot voluntarily vomit or belch.

MALIGNANT NEOPLASMS OF THE ESOPHAGUS

About 95 percent of malignant tumors of the esophagus are carcinomas. Carcinoma of the esophagus occurs with more frequency now than in previous years. Part of this increase is probably due to better diagnosis. It accounts for 2 percent of all cancer deaths in the United States. It is predominantly a disease of males (4:1) between the ages of 50 and 70 years. The prognosis of individuals with cancer of the esophagus is very poor.[12]

Pathophysiology

The basic cause of cancer of the esophagus is unknown. Possible predisposing factors are cigarette smoking, excessive alcohol intake, chronic trauma, poor oral hygiene, and spicy foods. Certain conditions of the esophagus such as achalasia, diverticula, and lye burns are considered premalignant lesions.[13]

The malignancy usually appears as an ulcerated lesion. It may have advanced to this stage before symptoms are present. The majority of tumors are located in the middle and lower portion of the esophagus. The tumor may penetrate the muscular layer and even extend outside the wall of the esophagus. Obstruction of the esophagus occurs in the later stages.

Clinical Manifestations

The onset of symptoms is usually late in relation to the extent of the tumor. Progressive *dysphagia* is the most common symptom and may be expressed as a substernal feeling as if food is not passing. Initially the dysphagia occurs only with meat, then with soft foods, and eventually with liquids.

Pain presents later and is described as occurring in the substernal, epigastric, or back areas and usually increases with swallowing. The pain may radiate to the neck, jaw, ears, and shoulders. If the tumor is in the upper one-third of the esophagus, symptoms such as a sore throat, choking, and hoarseness may occur. Weight loss is fairly common. When esophageal stenosis is severe, regurgitation of blood-flecked esophageal contents is common.

Complications

Hemorrhage may occur if the cancer erodes into the aorta. Esophageal perforation with fistula formation into the lung or trachea sometimes develops. The tumor may enlarge enough to cause esophageal obstruction. Esophageal carcinoma has a very poor prognosis due to early lymphatic spread and late development of symptoms. The liver and lung are common metastatic sites.

Diagnostic Study Abnormalities

Barium swallow with fluoroscopy may demonstrate a narrowing of the esophagus at the site of the tumor. Sometimes a crater is visible. Esophagoscopy with biopsy and cytology studies is necessary to make a definitive diagnosis of carcinoma by identification of malignant cells. A bronchoscopy may be done to detect malignant involvement of the trachea.

Medical Management

The treatment for carcinoma of the esophagus depends on the location of the tumor and whether invasion or metastasis has occurred. Surgical removal and radiation are the two methods used. Relatively few individuals are cured. The best results have been obtained by combining surgery and radiation (Table 32-6).

Table 32-6
Medical Management: Carcinoma of the Esophagus

Diagnostic
1. Barium swallow
2. Esophagoscopy with biopsy
3. Bronchoscopy

Therapeutic
1. Surgical resection
   a. Esophagectomy
   b. Esophagogastrostomy
   c. Esophagoenterostomy
2. Radiation
3. Gastrostomy

If the tumor is in the cervical (upper one-third) eosphagus, radiation will probably be used. A tumor in the lower one-third of the esophagus is usually surgically resected. In addition, radiation may be used either before or after surgery.

Several types of surgical procedures that can be performed are: (1) removal of part or all of the esophagus (*esophagectomy*), using a Dacron graft to replace the resected part; (2) resection of a portion of the esophagus and anastomosis of the remaining portion to the stomach (*esophàgogastrostomy*); and (3) resection of a portion of the esophagus and anastomosis of a segment of colon to the remaining portion (*esophagoenterostomy*) (Fig. 32-9). The surgical approaches may be done through the thorax or using both an abdominal and thoracic approach.

A *gastrostomy* may be performed for the purpose of feeding the client. It is the insertion of a retention or mushroom catheter into the stomach. The catheter is sutured to the abdominal wall (Fig. 32-10). (Gastrostomy feedings are discussed in the section on Dietary Measures.)

Surgery may not be done when the client is elderly or has poor physical health. Palliative therapy consists of restoring swallowing and maintaining nutrition and hydration. Various procedures used to accomplish these goals include gastrostomy or esophagostomy, esophageal dilatation, resection, chemotherapy, and radiation.

Nursing Management

Health promotion and maintenance

Since the etiology of esophageal cancer is not definitive, it is difficult to identify preventive measures. Health counseling needs to focus on elimination of smoking and excessive alcohol intake. Maintaining good oral hygiene and dietary habits may also be helpful.

Having the client obtain treatment of esophageal problems such as achalasia and diverticula may be helpful as these are considered premalignant problems. Early diagnosis of esophageal tumors is important but difficult, since the onset of symptoms is usually late. Clients should be encouraged to have regular physical examinations and seek medical attention for any esophageal problems, especially dysphagia.

Acute intervention

Preoperative Care In addition to general preoperative teaching and preparation, particular attention to the client's nutritional needs and oral care is important. Many clients are poorly nourished because of the loss of weight from the inability to ingest adequate amounts of food and fluids prior to surgery. A high calorie, high protein diet should be provided. It may need to be in liquid form. Some clients may need intravenous fluid replacement or hyperalimentation.

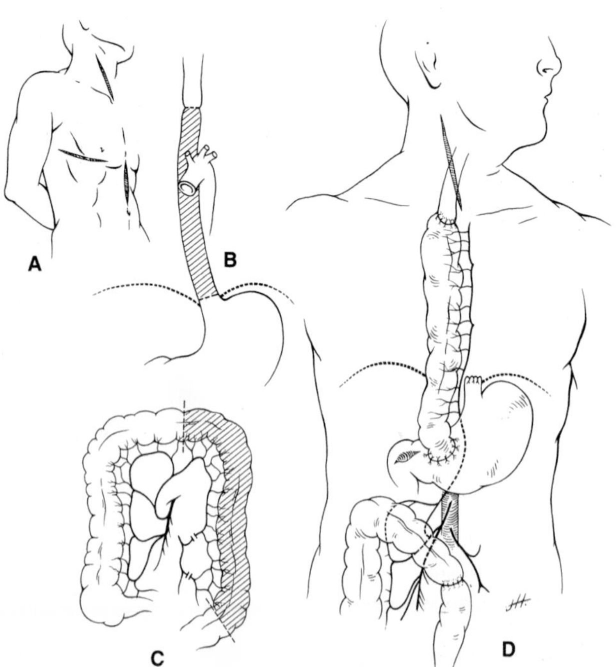

Figure 32-9 Esophagectomy with interposition of the left colon (esophagoenterostomy). (*From S. Schwartz et al., Principles of Surgery, 3d ed., McGraw-Hill Book Company, New York, 1979, p. 1036.*)

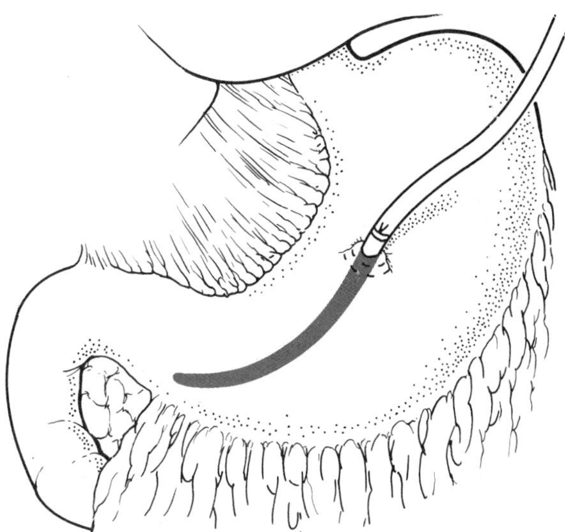

Figure 32-10 Placement of a gastrostomy tube.

The nurse must keep an accurate intake and output record and assess the client for signs of fluid and electrolyte imbalance.

Meticulous oral care is essential. A thorough cleaning of the mouth, including tongue, gums, and teeth or dentures is necessary. It may be necessary to use swabs or a gauze pad and really scrub the mouth, including the tongue. Milk of magnesia with mineral oil may be used to remove crust formation. A mixture of mouthwash, ice, and water makes a very refreshing rinse.

Teaching should include information about chest tubes (if a thoracic approach is used), IVs, nasogastric tube, gastrostomy feeding, turning, coughing, and deep breathing. (See Chap. 6 for preoperative care.)

Postoperative Care The client usually has a nasogastric tube in place which may have bloody drainage for 8 to 12 hours. The drainage will gradually change to greenish-yellow. Assessment of the drainage, maintenance of the tube, and oral and nasal care are nursing responsibilities.

Due to the location of the incision and general condition of the client, special emphasis must be given to prevention of respiratory complications. Turning, coughing, and deep breathing should be done every 2 hours. Intermittent positive-pressure breathing may also be of value.

The client should be positioned in a semi-Fowler's or Fowler's position to prevent reflux of gastric secretions. When the client can drink fluids or eat, the upright position should be maintained for at least 2 hours after eating to assist the movement of food through the GI tract.

Radiation therapy may be done as an adjunct measure to surgery or as a primary therapy. The types of radiation and related nursing care are discussed in Chap. 11.

Chronic management

Many clients require long-term follow-up care following surgery or radiation for esophageal cancer. The client needs encouragement and assistance in maintaining adequate nutrition. The client may need a permanent feeding gastrostomy (see section on Dietary Measures). The client usually has fears and anxieties about a diagnosis of cancer. The nurse should know what the doctor has told the client regarding the prognosis and then provide appropriate counseling. Some communities have resource groups composed of individuals with cancer who can serve as support systems. These groups can usually be contacted through the local American Cancer Society.

A community health nurse referral may be needed for continued care of the client (e.g., gastrostomy teaching and follow-up wound care). Management of the terminally ill client is discussed in Chap. 11.

Dietary Measures

Following esophageal surgery, parenteral fluids will be given for several days. When fluids are allowed after bowel sounds have returned, 30 to 60 mL of water is given hourly, with gradual progression to small, frequent bland meals. The client should be in an upright position to prevent regurgitation of the fluid. The client is observed for signs of intolerance to or leakage of the feeding into the mediastinum. Symptoms to report which indicate leakage are pain, increased temperature, and dyspnea. Symptoms of food intolerance include vomiting and abdominal distension.

Gastrostomy

A gastrostomy bypasses the esophagus and allows for feedings to maintain or restore the client's nutrition. The first gastrostomy feeding is usually only water. Then there is gradual progression to food. The feeding may be blended foods or a special formula. Some tube feeding formulas have created a problem with diarrhea but current lactose-free formulas have decreased this problem to some extent. The feeding should be given at room or body temperature. Privacy should be provided. The head should be elevated in a normal eating position and should remain elevated for 30 minutes to 1 hour after the feeding.

A syringe or funnel is used to introduce the liquid into the tube. A small amount of water is first inserted to make sure the tube is patent. To prevent air from entering the tube, the catheter should be clamped at all times that feedings are not being given. It should not be unclamped until the feeding is placed in the syringe or funnel. The feeding is usually 200 to 500 mL and should be allowed to flow in by gravity over 20 to 25 minutes. After the feeding is finished, the tube should be cleared with water. The client should have an adequate intake of water of up to 2500 mL/24 hours.

Sometimes the catheter is removed after about 2 weeks and reinserted for each feeding. It should be inserted about 4 to 6 inches.

The pleasurable aspects of eating such as smelling, seeing, tasting, and chewing the food are denied the client with a gastrostomy. He may become depressed and needs frequent encouragement. The nurse should allow him to express his feelings about being fed through a tube. The client may experience greater satisfaction with self-feedings and should be taught to do them himself, if possible.

Skin care around the gastrostomy is very important as the action of the gastric juice is irritating to the skin. The nurse must inspect the skin and keep it clean with mild soap and water. A protective ointment such as zinc oxide may be used. A small dressing is sometimes placed around the tube. The nurse should teach the client and family about gastrostomy care.

OTHER ESOPHAGEAL DISORDERS

Esophagitis

Esophagitis (inflammation of the esophagus) may occur as a result of chemical irritation from lye or dust and physical irritants such as smoking, very cold or hot liquids, and excessive alcoholic intake. Trauma to the esophagus may also produce inflammation. Achalasia and carcinoma may lead to esophagitis.

Reflux esophagitis is very common. It is due to the reflux of gastric contents into the esophagus. A sliding hiatal hernia is the most common cause of reflux esophagitis.

Treatment of esophagitis depends on the cause. If strong alkalis or acids cause acute esophagitis, prompt, vigorous treatment is necessary (Chap. 58). The treatment of chronic esophagitis includes oral antacids, bland diet, and sleeping with the head of the bed elevated. The goal of treatment is to prevent gastric juices from damaging the esophageal mucosa.

Diverticula

Diverticula are sac like outpouchings of one or more layers of the esophagus. The main symptoms are dysphagia and regurgitation. Dysphagia occurs because food passes into the diverticulum and compresses the trachea. The client frequently complains of tasting sour food and smelling a foul odor due to the stagnant food. Complications include malnutrition, aspiration, and perforation.

There is no specific treatment for diverticula. Some clients find they can empty the pocket of food that collects by applying pressure at a point on the neck. The diet may have to be limited to foods that pass more readily (e.g., blenderized foods). Surgical removal of the diverticulum may be necessary if nutrition becomes disrupted.

Strictures

The most common cause of esophageal strictures is due to strong acids or alkalis which have been ingested. Traumas such as throat lacerations and gunshot wounds may also cause strictures due to scar formation from healing. The strictures usually develop over a long period of time. Strictures can be dilated using *bougies* (dilatating instruments). Surgical excision with anastomosis is sometimes necessary. The client may have a temporary or permanent gastrostomy.

Achalasia (Cardiospasm)

In achalasia there is decreased motility of the lower two-thirds of the esophagus with absence of effective coordinated peristalsis, resulting in dilatation of the lower esophagus (Fig. 32-11). The lower esophageal sphincter does not relax normally with swallowing and obstruction of the esophagus at or near the diaphragm occurs. Food and fluid accumulate in the lower esophagus. The altered peristalsis is due to impairment of the autonomic nervous system innervating the esophagus. Achalasia affects all ages and both sexes. The course of the disease is chronic.

Dysphagia is the most common symptom and occurs more frequently with liquids. Substernal chest pain (similar to angina pain) occurs during or immediately after a meal. Halitosis and the inability to eructate are other symptoms. Another common symptom is regurgitation of sour-tasting food and liquids, especially when in a horizontal position.

The aim of medical management is to relieve symptoms. Symptomatic treatment consists of sedatives, a semisoft bland diet, eating slowly and drinking fluid with meals, sleeping with the head elevated, and

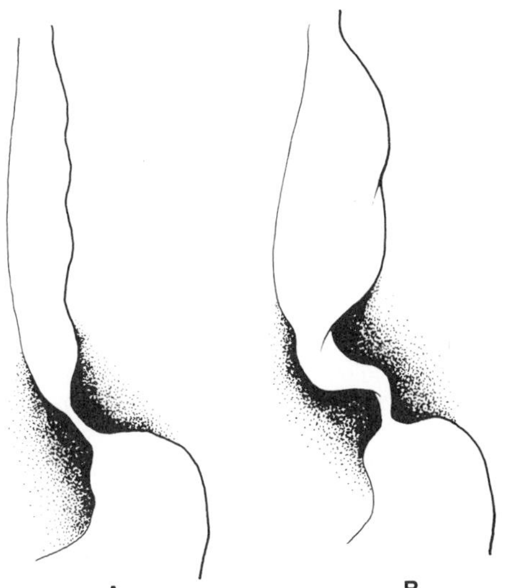

Figure 32-11 Esophageal achalasia. (*a*) Early stage showing tapering of lower esophagus. (*b*) Advanced stage showing dilated, tortuous esophagus. (*From S. Price and L. Wilson, Pathophysiology: Clinical Concepts of Disease Processes, 2d ed., McGraw-Hill Book Company, New York, 1982, p. 208.*)

anticholinergic drugs. The best treatment is forceful dilatation of the entrance into the stomach. Mercury-tipped bougies (dilatating instruments) can be used and will provide temporary relief. A better method is to use bags that can be inflated under pressure (Mosher pneumatic bag). The forceful dilatation does not restore normal esophageal motility but does provide for emptying of the esophagus into the stomach.

Surgical intervention may become necessary. An *esophagomyotomy* may be done in which the muscle fibers that enclose the narrowed area of the esophagus are divided. This allows the mucosa to pouch out through the division in the muscle layer to allow food to be swallowed without obstruction. In combination with the myotomy, a *pyloroplasty* (enlargement of gastric outlet) may be done to help prevent reflux into the esophagus.

FOOD POISONING

Food poisoning is a nonspecific term which describes acute gastrointestinal symptoms such as nausea, vomiting, diarrhea, and abdominal colicky pain due to the intake of contaminated food. Food most commonly causes illness if it is contaminated with microorganisms or their products. The GI tract is frequently the portal of entry for the microorganisms. The two main types of food poisonings are (1) acute gastroenteritis from bacteria, and (2) neurologic symptoms from botulism. The most common bacterial food poisonings are presented in Table 32-7.

Foods may also be contaminated by poisonous chemicals such as mercury, arsenic, zinc, or potassium chlorate. Poisoning can also occur from ingestion of poisonous plants (e.g., certain species of mushroom).

The nursing role in relation to food poisoning is mainly health teaching to prevent its occurrence. Teaching should include correct food preparation and cleanliness, adequate cooking, and refrigeration. If the client is hospitalized, nursing care will focus on correcting fluid and electrolyte imbalance from diarrhea and vomiting. With botulism, additional assessment and care relative to neurologic symptoms are indicated (see Chap. 53).

Table 32-7
Bacterial Food Poisoning

Type	Causative Agent	Sources	Onset of Symptoms	Symptoms	Treatment	Prevention
Staphylococcal	Toxin from *Staphylococcus aureus*	Meat, bakery products, milk Skin and respiratory tract of food handlers	1–6 h	Vomiting Abdominal cramping Diarrhea	Symptomatic Fluid and electrolyte replacement Antiemetics	Immediate refrigeration of foods Control of food handlers
Clostridial	*Clostridium perfringens*	Meat or poultry dishes cooked at lower temperature (stew or pot pie) Rewarmed meat dishes Improperly canned vegetables	6–12 h	Diarrhea Abdominal cramps Vomiting is rare	Symptomatic Antidiarrheal medications	Correct preparation of meat dishes Serve food immediately after cooking or cool rapidly

Table 32-7 (Continued)

Type	Causative Agent	Sources	Onset of Symptoms	Symptoms	Treatment	Prevention
Salmonellae	*Salmonella typhimurium*, grows in gut	Improperly cooked poultry, pork, beef, lamb, and eggs	8–48 h	Nausea, vomiting Diarrhea Abdominal cramps Fever and chills	Symptomatic Fluid and electrolyte replacement	Correct preparation of food
Botulism	Toxin from *Clostridium botulinum*. Ingested toxin absorbed from gut blocks acetylcholine at neuromuscular junction	Improperly canned or preserved food Home-preserved vegetables most common Preserved fruits and fish Canned commercial products	12–36 h	*Gastrointestinal:* Nausea Vomiting Abdominal pain Constipation Distension *Central nervous system:* Headache Dizziness Muscular incoordination Weakness Inability to talk or swallow Diplopia Respiratory embarrassment Paralysis Delirium Coma	Maintain ventilation Polyvalent antitoxin Quanidine HCl (enhances acetylcholine release)	Correct processsing of canned foods Boiling suspected canned foods for 15 min before serving

Case Study / Hiatal Hernia

Mary, 63 years old, has had a sliding hiatal hernia for 10 years. She is 5′2″ and weighs 195 pounds. She used to wear tight corsets but stopped wearing them 2 years ago. In the last year she has had increasing heartburn, especially at night. Mary has currently been on a bland diet and antacids. She does not like the bland diet.

Mary is admitted to the hospital for a hiatal hernia repair. She is not in acute distress but does complain of the substernal pain and heartburn. She has had some regurgitation. Her vital signs are within normal limits. A barium swallow and esophagoscopy revealed a large sliding hiatal hernia. It was determined from the esophagoscopy that she has gastric reflux.

Mary had a Nissen fundoplication through an abdominal approach. Following surgery, she had a nasogastric tube for suction and intravenous fluids. She is reluctant to move or cough.

Discussion Questions

1. Explain the pathophysiology of a hiatal hernia. What is the difference between a sliding and a paraesophageal hiatal hernia?
2. What are the characteristic symptoms of a hiatal hernia? Which of these did Mary have?
3. Describe a Nissen fundoplication procedure. What is the objective of this surgical procedure?
4. What are potential postoperative complications and what are nursing measures to prevent them?
5. What should be included in a teaching plan for Mary?

REVIEW QUESTIONS

The number of the question corresponds to the same numbered objective at the beginning of the chapter.

1. The most effective current method for removing plaque is
   a. physical removal by brushing and flossing
   b. application of a fluoride solution
   c. antimicrobial agents added to toothpaste
   d. large doses of vitamin C

2. Treatment of Vincent's infection includes
   a. topical application of antibiotics
   b. smallpox vaccinations

c. viscous lidocaine rinses
d. amphotericin B suspension

3. Which of the following is *not* considered a predisposing factor for carcinoma of the oral cavity?
a. pipe smoking
b. overexposure to the sun
c. poor dental care
d. herpesvirus

4. Following a radical neck dissection the immediate postoperative goal is
a. communication
b. patent airway
c. prevention of infection
d. nutritional intake

5. If the client begins to vomit or choke following fixation of mandibular fracture, the nurse should first
a. cut the wires or elastic bands
b. suction the client
c. provide oral hygiene
d. give an antiemetic

6. The most characteristic symptom of a hiatal hernia is
a. dysphagia
b. regurgitation
c. heartburn
d. coughing

7. Identify the *false* statement regarding the management of a client with a hiatal hernia.
a. The client should be taught to avoid tight clothing and bending.
b. The overweight client should reduce.
c. The head of the bed may be elevated on blocks.
d. The drug of choice for treatment is an anticholinergic.

8. The most common symptom of esophageal carcinoma is
a. sore thorat
b. dysphagia
c. weight loss
d. hemorrhage

9. Identify the *false* statement about gastrostomy feedings.
a. The feeding may be blended foods or a special formula.
b. The feeding should be warmed to 38°C.
c. The feeding should flow in by gravity.
d. Water should be given preceding and following the feeding.

10. Which of the following is most likely to cause reflux esophagitis?
a. outpouching of the muscular layer
b. impairment of the autonomic nerve plexus
c. incompetent gastroesophageal sphincter
d. stricture of the esophagus

11. The food poisoning in which vomiting is the prominent symptom and food sources are meat, bakery products, and milk is
a. staphylococcal
b. salmonellae
c. botulism
d. clostridial

REFERENCES

1. Kurt J. Isselbacher et al. (eds.), *Harrison's Principles of Internal Medicine*, 9th ed., McGraw-Hill Book Company, New York, 1980, p. 187.
2. Ibid., p. 191.
3. National Institute of Health, "Research Findings of Potential Value to the Practitioner: Oral Cancer," *JAMA*, **237:**19 (1977).
4. S. Schwartz et al., *Principles of Surgery*, 3d ed., McGraw-Hill Book Company, New York, 1979, p. 599.
5. H. W. Baker et al., *Oral Cancer*, American Cancer Society, 1973.
6. Schwartz, op. cit., p. 625.
7. James K. Masson, "Reconstructive Procedures in Head & Neck Surgery," *Surg Clin*, August 1977, pp. 748–749.
8. R. W. Postlethwait, *Surgery of the Esophagus*, Appleton Century Crofts, New York, 1979, p. 195–197.
9. Ibid., p. 218.
10. Ibid., pp. 217–218.
11. Ibid., p. 341.
12. B. Given and S. Simmons, *Gastroenterology in Clinical Nursing*, 3d ed., The C. V. Mosby Company, St. Louis, 1980, pp. 128–129.

Chapter 33

NURSING ROLE IN MANAGEMENT

Problems of Nutrition and Digestion

Gladys Deters

Learning Objectives

1. Describe the essential components for a nutritionally sound diet and why they are necessary to good health.
2. Describe the common etiologies, clinical manifestations, and management of vitamin imbalances and malnutrition.
3. Differentiate between central and peripheral total parenteral nutrition administration, including the indications for use, complications, and medical and nursing management.
4. Explain the pathogenesis, complications, and medical and surgical management of obesity.
5. Describe the nursing care related to conservative and surgical therapy of obesity.
6. Describe the pathogenesis, complications, and medical and nursing management for a client with nausea and vomiting.
7. Differentiate between acute and chronic gastritis, including the causes, pathophysiology, and medical and nursing management.
8. Explain the common etiologies, clinical manifestations, and medical and nursing management of a client with upper gastrointestinal bleeding.
9. Compare and contrast gastric and duodenal ulcers, including pathogenesis, clinical manifestations, complications, and medical and nursing management.
10. Explain the anatomic and physiologic changes and the common complications which result from Billroth I and II surgical procedures.
11. Describe the clinical manifestations and the medical, surgical, and nursing management of a client with cancer of the stomach.

The focus of this chapter is problems with nutrition and digestion. The primary nutritional problems discussed are malnutrition and obesity. The digestive problems discussed are nausea and vomiting, gastritis, peptic ulcers, and gastric cancer.

NUTRITIONAL PROBLEMS

The nurse must be aware that nutritional problems can be found in all age groups, cultures, ethnic groups, socioeconomic classes, and in all parts of the world. Intelligence and wealth do not necessarily preclude the development of poor nutritional habits. The nurse in the roles of care giver, teacher, and resource person can have a profound influence on the health practices of the clients and families with whom she comes in contact. A strong foundation in the principles of sound nutrition is essential. Together with the physician and dietition, the nurse is in a strategic position to assess the dietary practices of her clients and provide important information.

The nutritional state of an individual or family may be influenced by many factors. Attitudes toward the importance of food and eating habits are established early in infancy and childhood as a result of parental behavior. Cultural or religious preferences and requirements frequently are reflected in dietary intake. The financial state of a family or individual will often determine the type and amount of nutritionally sound food that can be purchased. The lower the socioeconomic status, generally the poorer the nutritional state. The availability of food sources also contributes to the nutritional state of individuals. This is usually not a problem in developed countries where agriculture is well established and productive, but it may be a problem in underdeveloped countries.

Normal Nutrition

Nutrition is the process by which the body utilizes food for energy, growth, and maintenance and repair of body tissues. Good nutrition in the absence of any other underlying disease process will result from the ingestion of a balanced diet containing foods from the basic four food groups. The United States Department of Agriculture (USDA) has prescribed the basic four foods to be comprised of milk, meat, fruits and vegetables, and grain. Table 33-1 lists the basic four food groups with daily requirements and examples of common sources.

The essential components of the basic four food groups are carbohydrates, fats, proteins, vitamins, and minerals. *Carbohydrates*, the body's primary source of energy, yield 4 calories per gram. Carbohy-

Table 33-1

Basic Four Food Groups, Recommended Number of Servings

Food Group	Child	Teenager	Adult	Pregnant Woman	Lactating Woman
Milk group 1 cup milk, yogurt; OR calcium equivalent: $1\frac{1}{2}$ slices ($1\frac{1}{2}$ oz) cheddar cheese 1 cup pudding $1\frac{3}{4}$ cups ice cream 2 cups cottage cheese	3	4	2	4	4
Meat 2 oz cooked lean meat, fish, poultry; OR protein equivalent: 2 eggs 2 slices (2 oz) cheddar cheese 1 cup dried beans, peas 4 tbsp peanut butter	2	2	2	3	2
Fruit-vegetable $\frac{1}{2}$ cup cooked or juice 1 cup raw Portion commonly served such as a medium-size apple or banana	4	4	4	4	4
Grain (whole grain, fortified, enriched) 1 slice bread 1 cup ready-to-eat-cereal $\frac{1}{2}$ cup cooked cereal, pasta grits	4	4	4	4	4

Courtesy of National Dairy Council, Rosemont, IL, 60018.

drates are obtained from the ingestion of starches and sugars. They are the chief protein-sparing ingredients in a nutritionally sound diet and comprise about 45 percent of the daily caloric needs of the body. In more affluent countries the amount consumed has reached 60 percent of total calories.

Fats make up about 40 percent of daily caloric needs. One gram of fat yields 9 calories. Fats, when stored, are found as adipose tissue (primarily triglycerides) in the subcutaneous tissues and in the abdominal cavity. Besides being a major source of body energy, fats act as insulation which reduces loss of body heat in cold weather and provides padding and protection for vital organs.

Proteins, the third essential component of a well-balanced diet, are obtained from meat, fish, eggs, dairy products, and other vegetarian-type substances. They provide 15 to 20 percent of daily caloric needs of the body and 1 g of protein yields 4 calories. Proteins are very complex nitrogenous organic compounds, of which amino acids are the fundamental units of structure. An adequate intake of protein is necessary because of the vital role played by the amino acids in biochemical processes in the body. While the body can convert carbohydrates and protein to fat and fat to carbohydrate, the body is incapable of synthesizing protein from either carbohydrates or fat. Protein is totally dependent on a dietary source if it is to be available for tissue repair and maintenance.

Vitamins are organic compounds required in small amounts by the body for normal metabolism. Vitamins primarily function in enzyme reactions that facilitate the metabolism of amino acids, fats, and carbohydrates. The body is capable of synthesizing some vitamins in adequate amounts, but must rely on a dietary source to meet requirements for others such as vitamin B_{12}. Vitamins are divided into two categories: *water-soluble* vitamins (C and B complex) and *fat-soluble* vitamins (A, D, E, K).

Minerals are inorganic ions (e.g., magnesium, iron) that make up about 4 percent of the total body weight. When minerals are present in minute amounts, they are referred to as trace elements or micronutrients. Minerals have a variety of functions in the body, including taking part in enzyme reactions, constituting skeletal structures (calcium, phosphorus, magnesium), and being components of compounds like hemoglobin (iron), thyroxine (iodine), and vitamin B_{12} (cobalt). Some minerals are stored like the fat-soluble vitamins and can be toxic if taken in excess amounts. The amount needed in the daily diet varies a great deal from a few micrograms of trace minerals to a gram or more of the major minerals such as calcium, phosphorus, and sodium.

The *daily caloric requirements* of an individual are influenced by body build, age, sex, and physical activity. Adjustments are necessary dependent upon changes in the health status of the person and his daily activity level. Table 33-2 summarizes recommended daily calorie intake. Table 33-3 gives an example of calorie and protein needs depending on level of activity.

Nutritional Needs of Various Groups

Children and adolescents

Parents are responsible for setting an example of good nutrition for their children. It has been well documented that obese parents will often have obese children. Parental attitudes toward food and eating habits are readily passed on to their children. Parents who have little understanding of what constitutes a well-balanced diet or who cannot or will not learn good nutrition will inevitably influence their children to follow the same poor dietary practices. The nurse must help parents to understand the unique food requirements of their children from infancy through adolescence. Children and adolescents have high caloric requirements because:[1]

1. Their basal metabolic rate is at a high rate.
2. When awake, their activities involve more calories than similar activities in adults.
3. Energy-yielding materials must be stored for growth.

Adolescents are easy prey for food faddism or nutritional quackery. Teenage girls preoccupied with losing weight may adopt one of the many yet unproven

Table 33-2

Recommended Daily Calorie Intake

Category	Age (years)	Weight (kg)	Weight (lb)	Height (cm)	Height (in)	Energy Needs (with Range) (kcal)	
Infants	0.0–0.5	6	13	60	24	kg × 115	(95–145)
	0.5–1.0	9	20	71	28	kg × 105	(80–135)
Children	1–3	13	29	90	35	1300	(900–1800)
	4–6	20	44	112	44	1700	(1300–2300)
	7–10	28	62	132	52	2400	(1650–3300)
Males	11–14	45	99	157	62	2700	(2000–3700)
	15–18	66	145	176	69	2800	(2100–3900)
	19–22	70	154	177	70	2900	(2500–3300)
	23–50	70	154	178	70	2700	(2300–3100)
	51–75	70	154	178	70	2400	(2000–2800)
	76+	70	154	178	70	2050	(1650–2450)
Females	11–14	46	101	157	62	2200	(1500–3000)
	15–18	55	120	163	64	2100	(1200–3000)
	19–22	55	120	163	64	2100	(1700–2500)
	23–50	55	120	163	64	2000	(1600–2400)
	51–75	55	120	163	64	1800	(1400–2200)
	76+	55	120	163	64	1600	(1200–2000)
Pregnancy						+300	
Lactation						+500	

National Research Council, Food and Nutrition Board, *Recommended Dietary Allowances*, National Academy of Sciences, 1980.

Table 33-3
An Example of the Calorie and Protein Needs of a 150-lb (68-kg) Adult Male

Activity	Calories	Protein, Grams
Basal	1400	49
Moderate activity (activities of daily living)	2500	70
Postoperative (no complications)	3150	105
Stress response (e.g., to chemotherapy, radiation therapy)	3500	140
Infection	4500	175+

fad diets that guarantee immediate weight loss if certain foods are either eliminated from the diet or eaten exclusively. Unfortunately, most fad diets do not follow the basic four food groups and are nutritionally unsound. Teenagers are also prone to eating meals on the run or consuming hurried snacks consisting of junk foods. The result may be the ingestion of too much fat, sugar, and cholesterol. Unless parents have a good knowledge of nutrition, practice it in the home, and exert influence over their teenage children, poor nutritional habits may become fixed and lead to a state of chronic inadequate nutrition.

Lower socioeconomic class

Individuals and families from the lower socioeconomic class must spend a greater percentage of their limited income on food. As the cost of food increases, the tendency is to seek out cheaper foods that may not provide adequate nutrition. Conversely, they may prefer to select foods that are more expensive yet marginally nutritious because of their prestige value. The nurse and dietitian can assist the poor in making food choices that will meet nutritional requirements yet stay within their limited resources. See Appendix B, Table 14 for low-cost protein supplements.

Elderly

The nutritional requirements of the elderly are often overlooked. It is more common to find an undernourished older person than an obese one. As one grows older there is a concomitant decrease in the basal metabolic rate and in physical activity which lowers the caloric needs for energy. The older person will frequently reduce his consumption of needed protein, vitamins, and minerals and ingest "empty calories." The reasons given for this alteration in established eating habits can be attributed to living alone, boredom, death of a spouse, disability, and the need to rely on relatives or neighbors for food purchases. When these factors are added to already existing medical problems, it is easy to see why poor dietary patterns develop. Medical conditions involving the gastrointestinal tract such as ulcers, poor dentition, and ill-fitting dentures contribute to the type and amount of foods that can be eaten. The nurse must be aware of these common medical and psychosocial factors of the elderly and suggest interventions for overcoming these problems in her teaching or plan of care.

Clients with physical illnesses

Regardless of the etiology of the illness, the sick person has increased nutritional needs. Pathologic conditions are frequently aggravated by undernutrition while an existing deficiency state is likely to become more severe during illness. Malnutrition is not an unusual complication of illness, surgery, or injury. Diseases of the gastrointestinal tract are accompanied by anorexia, nausea, vomiting, diarrhea, distension, and abdominal cramping. Any combination of these symptoms will interfere with normal food consumption. Many clients restrict their dietary intake to a few foods or fluids that are not nutritionally sound due to fear of aggravating the already disturbed GI function.

The malabsorption syndrome, which reduces the amount of necessary enzymes and bowel surface capable of absorption, can quickly lead to a deficiency state. Extensive administration of antibiotics which change the normal flora of the intestines can result in a decreased ability to synthesize some of the B complex vitamins, especially vitamin B_{12}.

The fever that accompanies many illnesses, injuries, and infections increases the basal metabolic rate by 7 percent for each degree rise in body temperature.[2] Unless there is an increased amount of carbohydrates and fats ingested in the diet, protein will be used to supply calories and protein depletion can become a problem.

Hospitalized clients, especially the elderly, are at risk of becoming malnourished. Prolonged illness, major surgery, sepsis, draining wounds, burns, hemorrhage, fractures, and immobilization can all contribute to malnutrition. The nurse must assume responsibility along with the physician and dietitian for meeting the client's nutritional needs. She must also be mindful of the requirements of clients who are not so overtly ill, but are undergoing diagnostic studies. These clients enter the hospital usually nutritionally fit, yet are deprived of regular nutrition because of restrictions imposed upon them for completion of tests.

Vitamin Imbalances

Vitamin deficiencies are rare in most of the developed countries of the world. When vitamin deficiencies are found, usually several vitamins will be involved rather than a single vitamin deficiency. In the United States the recommended dietary allowances (RDA) for essential vitamins and minerals can be obtained by eating a diet consisting of foods from the basic four food groups. When vitamin imbalances do occur they are found among individuals such as alcoholics, drug addicts, and the very poor who follow poor dietary practices. Followers of fad diets or poorly planned vegetarian diets are also subject to a potential deficiency state. Clinical manifestations of vitamin imbalances are most commonly exhibited as neurologic manifestations. The central nervous system of the growing child is primarily involved while the peripheral nervous system is most affected in the adult.

Vegetarian diets

Vegetarian diets can result in a potential vitamin deficiency state. The two large classes of vegetarians are *vegans*, who are pure or total vegetarians and use only plant food, and *lacto-ova-vegetarians*, who use plant foods and sometimes dairy products and eggs. There are several other types including the *fruitarians* but they comprise only a small percentage of the total group. The commonality among all vegetarians is the exclusion of red meat from the diet.

Vegetarianism cannot be considered a nutritional fad since it is found in all age groups, occupations, and lifestyles. A variety of reasons have been given for following this type of dietary practice including religious or cultural beliefs, a better way of attaining total health, respect for all living beings, ethical-ecological ideals, and economics.

In well planned vegetarian diets the essential vitamins and minerals are easily obtained. Plant protein, although of a lesser quality than that of animal origin, fulfills most of the protein requirements. Table 13 in Appendix B provides an example of vegetable sources of proteins. Lacto-ova-vegetarians do obtain additional protein sources from dairy products and eggs. Milk made from soybeans is an excellent protein source, especially for the true vegan. The one primary deficiency of a strict vegan is lack of vitamin B_{12}. This vitamin can only be obtained from animal protein, special supplements, or foods that have been fortified with the vitamin. Vegans not using vitamin B_{12} supplements are susceptible to the development of megaloblastic anemia and the neurologic signs of vitamin B_{12} deficiency (Table 33-4).

Megavitamin therapy

Megavitamin therapy refers to the administration of high doses of one or more vitamins, usually 10 to 20 times the recommended daily allowances. Unless there are serious vitamin deficiencies, megavitamin therapy has no place in maintaining nutrition. The beneficial effects derived by the ingestion of commercially prepared daily vitamins is negligible if a balanced diet is eaten.

The *water-soluble vitamins* (C and B complex) are absorbed only as needed by the body and the excess is excreted rapidly in the urine. Toxicity from overdoses is rare. The *fat-soluble vitamins* (A, D, E, K) are readily stored and can accumulate to toxic levels. Since most vitamins can be purchased without a prescription, high doses of vitamin A and D can result in serious health hazards since the excess is not eliminated. Toxic levels of the fat-soluble vitamins can be reached within a matter of weeks, especially in infants and children.

Megadoses of vitamin C have received much acclaim in the treatment and prevention of the common cold. While there have been benefits in the prevention and treatment of the common cold, it appears to be of a minor nature.[3] In addition, when vitamin C is taken in doses exceeding 10 g per day, the excess is converted to oxalate and could possibly lead to the formation of renal stones (see Chap. 37).

Malnutrition

Malnutrition may be defined as an excess, deficit, or imbalance in the essential components of a balanced diet. Terms such as *undernutrition* or *overnutrition* are also used to describe malnutrition. *Undernutrition* describes a state of poor nourishment as a result of inadequate diet or diseases that interfere with normal appetite and assimilation of ingested food. *Overnutrition* refers to the ingestion of more food than is required for body needs as in obesity. Undernutrition will be the focus of the section on malnutrition. Obesity is discussed in a separate section.

Malnutrition is most prevalent in the developing countries where abundant food sources do not exist, the inhabitants are not well educated to their nutritional needs, and economic and ethnic conditions often preclude the purchase of a balanced diet. As a result of federal nutritional studies, it is now known that

Table 33-4

Normal Vitamin Requirements and Signs of Imbalance

Vitamin	Biochemical Action	Normal Daily Requirement	Signs of Deficiency or Toxicity	Predisposing Factors
A (retinol)	Maintains epithelial integrity and retinal pigments	5000 IU	1. Night blindness, xerosis 2. Toxicity usually associated with food faddism. Toxicity manifested by malaise, dermatitis, peripheral edema, and yellow tint to skin	Protein deficiency, fat malabsorption
D	Metabolism of calcium and phosphorus	400 IU	1. Rickets 2. Hypocalcemia 3. Toxicity manifested by elevation of serum calcium and phosphorus, soft tissue calcification, and renal calculi	Malnutrition, fat malabsorption
E (tocopherol)	Antioxidant preventing oxidation of polyunsaturated fatty acids	15 IU	1. Hemolytic anemia in children 2. Impaired red cell survival in adults	Fat malabsorption
K	Catalyzes prothrombin synthesis in liver	0.4 mg	1. Decreased prothrombin time	Prolonged antibiotic therapy, bile fistula, obstructive jaundice
C (ascorbic acid)	Maintains intracellular matrixes of cartilage and bone. Important in collagen synthesis	45 mg	1. Poor wound healing 2. Hemorrhage 3. Infection	Malnutrition
Thiamine (B_1)	Decarboxylation of alpha keto acids—requirements proportional to carbohydrate in diet	1.5 mg	1. Beriberi 2. Decreased appetite 3. Cardiomyopathy 4. Neurologic symptoms	Alcoholism Sepsis Trauma
Riboflavin (B_2)	Contributes flavoproteins involved in oxidative process	1.8 mg	1. Cheilosis 2. Bleeding gums 3. Seborrheic dermatitis 4. Magenta-colored tongue	Severe malnutrition
Niacin	Coenzyme in carbohydrate metabolism	20 mg	1. Pellagra 2. Dermatitis 3. Dementia, toxicity manifested by flushing and burning sensations	High-corn diets Diets low or lacking in tryptophan
Pyridoxine (B_6)	Participates in a variety of enzyme systems associated with amino acid metabolism	2 mg	1. Mental depression 2. Dermatitis 3. Increased excretion of tryptophan metabolites	Malnutrition Isoniazid used in treatment of TB
Pantothenic acid	Converted to coenzyme A, which participates in biological acetylation reactions	5–10 mg	1. Decreased antibody production in humans 2. Fatigue 3. Nausea	Severe malnutrition
Folic acid	DNA synthesis, transfer of one-carbon units	0.4 mg	1. Megaloblastic anemia	Malnutrition Malabsorption Folic acid antagonist
Vitamin B_{12}	Maintains normal folic acid metabolism, myelin synthesis, reducing agent, participates in metabolism of fat, carbohydrate, and protein	3 μg	1. Pernicious anemia 2. Neurologic symptoms	Malnutrition Malabsorption Ileal resection HCl and intrinsic factor also necessary for absorption

Adapted from Douglas Wilmore, *The Metabolic Management of the Critically Ill,* Plenum Book Company, New York, 1977, pp. 211–213.

undernutrition does exist in scattered parts of the United States. It is usually found in individuals or groups from the lower socioeconomic class.

Types of malnutrition

Primary malnutrition exists when nutritional needs are not met as a result of poor eating habits. *Secondary* malnutrition is the result of an alteration or defect in ingestion, digestion, absorption, or metabolism. In this type of malnutrition, tissue needs are not met even though the dietary intake would be satisfactory under normal conditions. Secondary malnutrition may occur as a result of gastrointestinal obstruction, surgical treatment (e.g., after peptic ulcer surgery), cancer, malabsorption syndromes, medications, and infectious diseases.

Protein calorie malnutrition (PCM) will be the focus of this discussion on malnutrition. It is the most common form of undernourishment and can result from either primary or secondary factors. PCM is due to the ingestion of foods containing deficient amounts of protein. (The recommended daily calorie intake for adults is summarized in Table 33-4.) In addition to decreased amounts of protein, the diet is generally low in necessary vitamins and minerals. PCM is a serious nutritional problem common throughout the world, affecting any socioeconomic population and any age group. In the United States where protein intake is high and of good quality severe malnutrition is less of a problem, but it can occur in individuals in high-risk groups.

Etiology of malnutrition

Factors that will increase the potential for the development of malnutrition are:

1. Weight loss of one-third to one-half of the initial body weight from any cause
2. Major surgery, radiation therapy, or chemotherapy
3. Severe burns with exudate high in protein
4. Draining wounds
5. Chronic renal and liver diseases
6. Hemorrhage
7. Bone fractures with prolonged immobilization
8. Malabsorption syndrome

It is estimated that nitrogen loss following severe injury or major surgery may be as much as 20 g/day, excreted as urea, creatinine, and creatine. Energy expenditure by the body after major injury or during sepsis may be increased by 50 to 60 percent.[4]

Anorexia Nervosa Anorexia nervosa is a psychiatric condition that results in a severely malnourished state from refusal to eat. This condition is found predominantly in adolescent girls (although it also occurs in males) who are of above-average intelligence and who come from middle-class families. This disturbance is generally considered the result of family conflict with one or both parents, but usually the mother. Sometimes there is a history of obesity in early adolescence which may be followed by a morbid fear of becoming fat.

In anorexia nervosa the eating behavior is severely disrupted, but the appetite is not suppressed. Frequently there is a history of eating binges followed by self-induced vomiting, use of cathartics, or enemas. In addition to refusal of food, the adolescent often engages in intense exercise activities such as calisthenics, jogging, or swimming. Once anorexia nervosa has developed, there is a characteristic power struggle as the parents attempt to force the child to eat, followed by angry responses and devious manipulations by the child to get rid of all forced food.[5]

If the eating pattern is permitted to continue over a prolonged period of time, body wasting and signs of severe malnutrition are evident. Treatment must be a combination of improved nutrition and psychiatric care. Nutritional supervision must be sustained until weight has been regained. The use of tube or parenteral feedings may be necessary. Improved nutrition, however, is not a cure for anorexia nervosa. Resolution of the underlying psychological problem must be accomplished by identification of the disturbed patterns of family interactions followed by individual and family counseling.

Pathophysiology of malnutrition

As the protein depletion continues over a period of time, the individual enters a state of negative nitrogen balance. Liver function is impaired and synthesis of new plasma proteins is diminished. The plasma oncotic pressure is decreased due to decreased protein synthesis. The main function of plasma proteins, primarily albumin, is the maintenance of the osmotic pressure of the blood. Due to this decreased pressure, a shift in body fluids occurs from the vascular space into the interstitial compartment. As protein ingestion decreases and body stores are depleted, albumin eventually leaks into the interstitial space along with the fluid. Edema becomes clinically observable. Often the edema present in the face and legs of the individual will mask the muscle wasting that has occurred.

As the total blood volume is reduced, the skin

appears dry and wrinkled. Along with the shift of fluids to the interstitial space, ions will also move. Sodium (normally an extracellular ion) is found in increased amounts in the cell and potassium (normally an intracellular ion) and magnesium are shifted to the extracellular space. Due to the lack of essential amino acids necessary in all chemical reactions in the body, adenosine triphosphate (ATP) is reduced. ATP is the energy source for the sodium pump. Without ATP the pump fails to function properly, sodium remains within the cell along with water, and the cell expands.[6]

The liver gradually becomes infiltrated with fat, leading to dysfunction in the mobilization of fats. This is believed to be the result of decreased synthesis of lipoproteins which serve as lipid carriers.[7] Lipids accumulate and absorption of fat-soluble vitamins is impaired.

Anorexia and diarrhea are common with PCM. Hair lacks its normal luster, falls out easily, and the color ranges from dull red-brown to gray as a result of pigment changes. Most individuals are anemic and prone to infection. Anemia resulting from PCM may be due to several factors. As cardiac output and blood volume decrease, the perfusion of the kidneys may fall below normal. Without adequate perfusion, the renal erythropoietin system becomes deficient. The red blood cell life span is reduced and very few red blood cells are formed in the bone marrow.

Infection generally occurs due to decreased leukocytes in the peripheral blood. Phagocytosis is altered due to the lack of ATP energy necessary to drive the process. The individual is more susceptible to all types of infectious processes. Both humoral and cell-mediated immunity are deficient in PCM.

Immediate restoration of protein and other necessary constituents to the diet must be instituted or death will rapidly ensue. The most serious problem associated with PCM in the very young is the probability of mental retardation. In severe malnutrition the development of brain cells is greatly reduced. Brain cells increase most rapidly during fetal life and in the first 5 to 6 months after birth. Once this critical time period has passed for brain development, improvement in the nutritional state of the infant will not correct any mental deficiency already incurred.

Clinical manifestations

The adult who is deprived of a diet sufficient in protein and calories will develop many of the clinical manifestations presented in Table 33-5. The most obvious clinical signs on physical examination are apparent in the skin, eyes, mouth, muscles, and nervous system. The speed at which the protein deficiency develops is dependent upon the quantity and quality of the protein intake, caloric value, and the age of the individual.

The clinical manifestations are the result of numerous interactions that take place at the cellular level. A change in one area will almost automatically effect a change in another. As protein intake is severely reduced, the muscles which make up the largest reservoir of protein in the body become wasted and flabby.

Severe PCM has long been recognized in infants and young children throughout the world and identified by such terms as *marasmus* and *kwashiorkor*. In kwashiorkor the principal dietary defect is a lack of protein available in foods ingested after the child is weaned. Marasmus is caused by a deficiency of protein and calories. It is seen most often during the first year of life while kwashiorkor occurs between the ages of 1 to 3 years.

Medical management

Diagnostic The diagnosis of PCM can be determined by a variety of laboratory studies used in conjunction with physical examination. *Total serum protein* is useful in the diagnosis of malnutrition. The degree of protein depletion can be identified by use of the scale in Table 33-6. *Serum electrolyte* levels will demonstrate changes taking place between the intracellular and extracellular space. The serum potassium level will often be elevated and the serum sodium level is decreased. The *red blood cell count* and *hemoglobin* will indicate the presence and degree of anemia. The *total lymphocyte count* will show a decreased level of lymphocytes. The total lymphocyte count is obtained from the differential blood cell count.

Liver enzyme studies will reflect hepatic dysfunction and damage. The *serum bilirubin* level is usually elevated and is related to the fatty liver infiltrate. *Serum vitamin* levels are usually diminished in malnutrition. The lowered levels of the fat-soluble vitamins correlate with the elevated serum bilirubin and the clinical signs of steatorrhea. Water-soluble vitamin levels may also be low.

Therapeutic The management of PCM lies in the immediate restoration of the individual with a diet high in calories and protein. Table 1 in Appendix B gives an example of a high calorie, high protein diet. In severe PCM the individual may be hospitalized for correction of fluid and electrolyte imbalances and treatment of infections. Enteral feeding, both oral and tube feedings, can be used to supplement the diet. In cases of severe PCM, total parenteral nutrition may be

Table 33-5
Signs of Protein Calorie Malnutrition

Body System	Subclinical Signs	Clinical Signs
Integument	Tissue turnover rate slowed Surface temperature 1–2 degrees cooler Febrile response to infection diminished Delayed immune response	Brittle nails Decreased tone and elasticity of skin Xeroderma (dry skin) Pigment changes (brown-gray) Erythematous seborrheic dermatitis Scrotal dermatitis
Hair		Easy loss of hair Color changes Lacks luster
Eye	Night blindness	Blood vessel growth in cornea Bitot's spots (gray keratinized epithelium on conjunctiva) Dryness of conjunctiva and cornea Pale to red conjunctiva
Gastrointestinal		
1. Mouth and lips	Reduced saliva produced	Cheilosis (redness and swelling) Crusting and ulceration at angle of the mouth
2. Tongue	Mucosa more permeable to bacteria	Raw and red—beefy red Edematous and smooth Atrophy
3. Teeth	Improper development Delayed eruption	Caries present Teeth loose Enamel discolored
4. Gums		Periodontal disease Bleed easily Receding, pale, and soft
5. Stomach	Decreased gastric acidity Delayed gastric emptying	Constant hunger Increased incidence of ulcers
6. Intestines	Decreased motility and absorption Normal flora cause of infection from increased permeability of mucosa	Diarrhea and flatulence Protruding abdomen Increased incidence of parasitic diseases
7. Liver–biliary	Fatty liver Decreased absorption of fat-soluble vitamins	Hepatomegaly
Cardiovascular	Decreased cardiac output Decreased circulation time Decreased hemoglobin Shift in heart position Increased risk of thrombophlebitis	Decreased blood pressure and pulse Slight cyanosis Anemia Body edema
Endocrine	Decreased insulin production	Parotid and thyroid enlargement Polydipsia Polyuria Increased sensitivity to cold
Immune	Decreased lymphocyte proliferation Decreased albumin levels Decreased antibody production Decreased total protein	Increased infections Decreased response to skin tests

Table 33-5 (Continued)

Body System	Subclinical Signs	Clinical Signs
Musculoskeletal	Decreased growth rate Decreased body stature with chronic PCM Decreased muscle mass	Prominence of bony structures—face, clavicle, scapula, ribs, iliac crests, spinal vertebrae Arms and legs weak and spindly Buttocks flat Muscles weak and flabby Breasts atrophied Decreased physical activity and work ability Severe weight loss
Neurologic	Loss of ambition Feeling of being old	Depression, confusion Decreased reflexes in legs and ankles Decreased position sense Decreased vibratory sense Paresthesias of hands and feet Syncope
Renal	Negative nitrogen balance Decreased BUN and urine creatinine levels	Nocturia Decreased urinary output
Reproductive	Decreased gonadotrophin levels	Amenorrhea Impotence
Respiratory	Pulmonary edema Decreased strength of respiratory muscles	Prone to respiratory infection Decreased respiratory rate Decreased vital capacity

initiated. These supplemental nutritional measures are discussed in the sections on type of supplemental nutrition.

Nursing management

Acute Intervention Nurses in acute-care settings must be aware of reasons why clients can become undernourished. The most common contributing factors of undernourishment in hospitalized clients are summarized in Table 33-7. Clients at risk to develop malnutrition should be identified and measures instituted to prevent it from happening.

The nurse must have a thorough understanding of nutritional support and the rationale behind orders for such common tasks as daily weights and accurate intake and output records. All too often the busy nurse or the client and family question the need to weigh a person who is in considerable pain and discomfort. Providing the client and family with reasonable explanations can be helpful in gaining their cooperation. Daily weights give an accurate record of body weight gain or loss. These data in conjunction with accurate recording of foods and fluid intake will produce a clearer picture of the client's nutritional state. Obtaining an accurate weight should follow a few simple rules, including weighing the client at the same time each day, on the same scale, with the same type or amount of clothing, and preferably with the bladder recently emptied.

The protein and caloric intake required in the malnourished individual is dependent upon the cause of the malnutrition, what treatment is being employed, and other stressors affecting the client. Table 33-3 gives the requirements of an average 150-pound adult male in various common hospital situations.

If the client is able to take food by mouth, a daily caloric count and/or diet diary should be maintained to give an accurate record of intake. The nurse and dietitian working with the client and family can assist in the selection of high caloric and high protein foods from a selection list. A knowledge of favorite foods preferred by the client will enhance the daily intake

Table 33-6

Degree of Serum Albumin Depletion

Normal value	3.8–4.5 g/dL
Mild depletion	3.0–3.7 g/dL
Moderate depletion	2.5–2.9 g/dL
Severe depletion	< 2.5 g/dL

and permit him to be more involved in his own recovery. Discussion with the client and family about foods that should be eaten to provide high protein, high caloric content is important.

Large amounts of coffee or tea to the exclusion of meats and vegetables will not help the client meet his necessary daily requirements. Visitors should be cautioned not to bring the client carbonated beverages or coffee between meals since they may suppress the appetite for more nutritious foods.

The undernourished client will usually receive between-meal nourishments. They may consist of items prepared in the dietary department or commercially prepared products. Eating these items between meals will increase the total daily intake and will provide extra calories, proteins, fluids, and nutrients. In addition, multiple small feedings improve the tolerance for food intake by distributing the amount throughout the day.

Commercially prepared products that are high in calories and protein content are listed in Table 33-8. A list of some commercial elemental diets are found in Table 33-9. Elemental diets are chemically defined, nutritionally sound diets that contain glucose, glucose derivatives, dextrins, amino acids, essential fatty acids, vitamins, and minerals. They are lactose-free and leave little residue in the lower bowel.

Chronic Management Discharge preparation for both the client and family is important. They must be carefully instructed on the cause of the undernourished state of health and ways to avoid the problem in the future. The client must be made aware that undernourishment, whatever the cause, can recur and that adhering to a diet high in protein and calories for a few short weeks cannot restore him to a normal nutritional state. Many months will be needed to reach this goal. Diet instruction will usually be carried out by the dietitian, but it is important for the nurse to assess understanding and reinforce the information whenever possible. The client's ability to comply with the dietary instructions must be examined in light of his past eating habits, religious and ethnic preferences, age, income, and state of health.

Unless he can be convinced of the necessity for change and has the resources to effect change, it is likely that no long-term benefits will be achieved. Ways should be found in which the client can become involved in his own recovery. Keeping a diet diary or calorie count for a week at a time is one way in which he can analyze his eating patterns. These records will also be helpful to the health care team in the follow-up care. Another means for involving the client in assessing his progress is to have him weigh himself 1 to 2 times a week. The need for continuous follow-up care must be strongly emphasized if rehabilitation is to be accomplished and maintained.

Table 33-7

Factors Contributing to Undernourishment in Hospitalized Clients

1. No height and weight recorded on admission or during hospitalization.
2. Rotation of physicians and nursing staff resulting in no one assuming responsibility for client's nutritional care.
3. Holding meals for tests.
4. Inability to assess the nutritional deficiencies on admission and determine the nutritional requirements of particular disease processes.
5. Delay of nutritional support until the client is in an advanced state of nutritional depletion.
6. Lack of appreciation of the role of adequate nutrition in the prevention, treatment, and resolution of many diseases.

Douglas Wilmore, *The Metabolic Management of the Critically Ill*, Plenum Publishing Company, New York, 1977, pp. 173–174.

Table 33-8

Commercially Prepared Products High in Protein and Calories

Product (Company)	Calories per Liter (1.1 qt)	Protein, Grams per Liter (1.1 qt)
Citrotein (Doyle)	660	39.9
Ensure (Ross)	1000	37
Ensure Plus (Ross)	1420	55
Instant Breakfast (Carnation or Lucerne)	1055 with whole milk	57
Meritene (Doyle)	1000	60 (liquid) 69 (powder with whole milk)
Nutri-1000 (Syntex)	1000	32.5
Sustacal (Mead Johnson)	1000	60
Sustagen (Mead Johnson)	1700	105

Ernest and Isadora Rosenbaum, *A Comprehensive Guide for Cancer Patients and Their Families*, Bull Publishing Company, Palo Alto, Calif., 1980, p. 53.

Table 33-9
Elemental Diets

Product (Company)	Calories per Liter (1.1 qt)	Protein, Grams per Liter (1.1 qt)
Flexical (Mead Johnson)	1000	27
Precision Low-Residue (Doyle)	1100	26
Precision High-Nitrogen (Doyle)	1000	44
Vivonex High-Nitrogen (Eaton)	1000	20
Vivonex High-Nitrogen (Eaton)	1000	41.6

Ernest and Isadora Rosenbaum, *A Comprehensive Guide for Cancer Patients and Their Families*, Bull Publishing Company, Palo Alto, Calif., 1980, p. 54.

TYPES OF SUPPLEMENTAL NUTRITION

Tube Feeding

Tube feedings may be ordered for the client who is unable to take oral nourishment. A nasogastric tube is the most common route utilized for short-term feeding problems. If the feedings are necessary over an extended period of time, other means of feeding may be used, such as a gastrostomy tube inserted directly into the stomach or a jejunostomy giving direct access into the jejunum. (Gastrostomy is discussed in Chap. 32.) These methods are used only when the esophagus or stomach must be bypassed. Both procedures require a surgical incision and may not be appropriate for a nutritionally depleted individual.

The procedure for the administration of tube feeding via a nasogastric tube is standard. The following principles apply:

1. *Position.* Sitting or with the head of bed elevated 30 to 45° to prevent aspiration.
2. *Patency of tube.* If feedings are intermittent, the tube should be irrigated with water after each feeding to prevent blockage of the tube.
3. *Tube position.* Proper placement of the tube in the stomach should be checked prior to each feeding. Methods used may be aspiration of stomach contents or injection of 10 mL of air and auscultating over the gastric area for the sound of air entering the stomach.
4. *Administration of feeding.* The principle of gravity is used with the drip method or use of a funnel with a glass tube adaptor. Applying pressure to force the feeding can damage the gastric mucosa. Pumps may be utilized in some cases. The feeding should be warmed to room temperature before administration.

Problems encountered in clients receiving tube feedings and corrective measures are found in Table 33-10. The use of blenderized foods from a normal diet may be used as tube feedings. The client may psychologically accept these feedings better than commercial products. Normal bowel function is promoted as a result of the fiber and residue content which is similar to that of a normal diet.

When commercial products are used it is necessary for the nurse to be aware that concentration, taste, lactose content, osmolarity, amount of protein, sodium, and fat will vary according to manufacturer. The standard concentration is generally 1 kcal/mL. There are a limited number of flavors available and the overutilization of one or two flavors, even when used as tube feedings, can lead to dislike over time and less tolerance.

Osmolarity higher than normal (normal is 280 mOsm/L) may be poorly tolerated and result in symptoms of the dumping syndrome (cold sweat, dizziness, distension, weakness, tachycardia, nausea, and diarrhea). The dumping syndrome is discussed later in the chapter as a complication of gastric surgery. Protein content greater than 16 percent can lead to dehydration unless the client is sufficiently alert to request additional fluids or is given supplemental fluid intake. The nurse must be aware of this potential problem and provide extra fluids through the feeding tube or by mouth. Tube feedings with high sodium content are contraindicated in clients with cardiovascular problems such as congestive heart failure. High fat content is not advocated for clients suffering from gastrointestinal dysfunction. Some elemental diets use predigested (hydrolyzed) protein and have the advantage of requiring little digestion time and are rapidly absorbed. A disadvantage of predigested protein is the chemical taste and added expense.

Total Parenteral Nutrition

When the gastrointestinal tract cannot be utilized for the ingestion, digestion, and/or absorption of essential nutrients, total parenteral nutrition (TPN) may be substituted. During the past several years parenteral nutrition (also called hyperalimentation) has become a relatively safe and practical method of delivering total nutritional needs by an intravenous route.

Table 33-10
Common Problems of Clients Receiving Tube Feedings

Problem	Possible Causes	Intervention
Vomiting	Tube improperly placed	Replace tube in proper position. Check tube position before beginning feeding.
	Feeding too soon after placement	Give client time to get adjusted to tube before feeding.
	Feeding too fast	Give feeding by slow drip or through funnel slowly. Avoid use of force.
	Client in wrong position	Keep head of bed elevated to 30–45° angle. Have client lie on right side for a half-hour after feeding. Sit up on side of bed or in chair. Encourage ambulation unless contraindicated.
	Feeding too much	Check order for amount and number of feedings.
	Contaminated formula	Refrigerate unused formula and record date opened. Discard outdated formula. Discard formula left standing for long periods of time.
	Air in stomach	Clear tubing of air before feeding. Keep tube feeding container full.
Diarrhea	Feeding too fast	Decrease the rate.
	High concentration of formula	Introduce formula gradually from a quarter to a half of full strength as tolerated.
	Lactose intolerance	Notify physician for change in formula.
Constipation	No fiber in diet	Notify physician to obtain laxative order. Change formula.
	Poor fluid intake	Increase fluid intake.
Dehydration	Excessive diarrhea, vomiting	Slow rate or change formula.
	Poor fluid intake	Increase intake and check amount and number of feedings. May need to increase amount.
	High protein and electrolyte content	Change formula.
	Hyperglycemia due to rapid infusion leading to osmotic diuresis and dehydration	Notify physician. Insulin may be required.
Sore nose and throat	Irritation of tube	Mouth care every 4 h. Cleanse nostrils of crusting. Gargle with saline or xylocaine solution if ordered.

The goal of using TPN is to keep the client in *positive nitrogen balance* and allow for growth of new body tissue, which can be drastically depleted by prolonged inability to eat normally. Regular intravenous solutions of 5% dextrose in water (D5W) or 5% dextrose in lactated Ringer's solution (D5LR) contain no protein and have approximately 200 calories per liter. (5% dextrose/L = 50 g dextrose = 200 cal.) The normal adult requires a minimum of between 1200 to 1500 calories per day to carry out normal physiologic function. Clients immediately after severe injury, surgery, burns, or who are malnourished as a result of medical treatment or disease process have greatly increased nutritional needs. The administration of dextrose solutions sufficient to meet these high caloric requirements would have extreme detrimental effects on the circulatory system, which could result in congestive heart failure or pulmonary edema.

Table 33-11

Possible Indications for Total Parenteral Nutrition

Acute and chronic renal failure*
Alimentary tract anomalies and fistula
Burns
Chronic diarrhea and vomiting
Complicated surgery or trauma
Diverticulitis
Failure to thrive
GI obstruction
Granulomatous enterocolitis
Hepatic failure (reversible)*
Hypermetabolic states (sepsis, fractures)
Inflammatory bowel disease (Crohn's and ulcerative colitis)
Malabsorption
Malnutrition
Pancreatitis
Severe peptic ulcer disease
Severe anorexia nervosa
Short bowel syndrome

*TPN should be used with extreme caution.

Table 33-11 lists the possible indications for the use of TPN.

Composition of total parenteral nutrition

TPN consists of a hypertonic solution of glucose, water, and a nitrogen source. Necessary electrolytes (sodium, potassium, chloride, calcium, magnesium, and phosphate) and trace elements (zinc, copper, chromium, and manganese) are added to meet the client's individual daily needs.

Calories Calories in TPN are supplied primarily by carbohydrates in the form of dextrose (20 to 50 percent). The administration of between 100 to 150 g of dextrose (1g = 4 cal) daily will have a protein-sparing effect. Since most clients receiving TPN are nutritionally depleted, their daily caloric needs are well above the average. These individuals must receive at least 2000 calories or more each day. The administration of 1000 mL of a 50% dextrose solution (50% dextrose/L = 500 g = 2000 calories) or 2000 mL of 25% dextrose will provide about 2000 calories.

Nitrogen The normal healthy adult male needs about 56 g of protein daily. In a nutritionally depleted client under stress of illness or surgery, requirements can exceed 150 g per day in order to ensure a positive nitrogen balance. Providing 150 g of protein (1 g = 4 cal) per day will add an additional 600 calories to the TPN solution.

Electrolytes Individual requirements should be assessed daily at the beginning of therapy and then several times a week as the treatment progresses. The following are normal daily electrolyte requirements:

Sodium, 60 to 200 mEq
Potassium, 50 to 160 mEq
Chloride, 100 to 200 mEq
Magnesium, 20 to 30 mEq
Phosphate, 30 to 100 mEq

The base solutions used by many hospitals already contain electrolytes. If the client requires more or less than this amount, they must be ordered daily by the physician.

Trace elements Zinc, copper, manganese, cobalt, and iodine must be ordered according to the client's condition and needs. Usually they are not added unless intravenous therapy exceeds 1 month.

Vitamins The daily addition of a multivitamin preparation (MVI) to 1 L of TPN will generally meet the vitamin requirements. It is necessary for the physician to order vitamins B_{12}, K, and folic acid separately. With prolonged TPN, B_{12} injections of 100 to 1000 μg IM may be ordered once or twice a month. Folic acid 500 μg is given daily. Vitamin K may be ordered IM depending on the results of the prothrombin time.

Methods of TPN administration

Total parenteral nutrition may be administered by two routes, *central* and *peripheral*. *Central parenteral nutrition* is given through a catheter inserted into the subclavian vein and subsequently threaded into the superior vena cava. Central hyperalimentation is indicated when long-term nutritional support is necessary, when the client has high requirements of protein and calories, and when suitable peripheral veins are not available. *Peripheral hyperalimentation* is administered through a large peripheral vein when nutritional support is needed only for a short time, protein and caloric requirements are not excessively high, the risk of a central catheter is too great, or when nutritional support is used to supplement inadequate oral intake.

Central and peripheral parenteral nutrition differ in their tonicity, which is measured in milliosmoles (mOsm, the concentration of particles in a fluid). Blood which is isotonic measures about 280 mOsm/L. The standard intravenous solutions of D5W and normal saline are isotonic. Central hyperalimentation solutions measure 1600 mOsm/L and are very hypertonic due to the high glucose content, ranging from 20 to 50 percent. It is for this reason that central hyperalimentation must be infused in a large central vein so that rapid dilution can occur. The use of a peripheral vein would cause irritation and thrombophlebitis. Peripheral hyperalimentation is less hypertonic, using 20% glucose, and can be safely administered through a large peripheral vein, although phlebitis can occur. Standard base solutions are now manufactured for parenteral use.

All TPN solutions should be prepared by a pharmacist or trained technician using strict aseptic techniques under a hooded laminar flow unit. Nothing should be added to hyperalimentation solutions after they are prepared in the pharmacy. The danger of drug incompatibilities and contamination is very high. The fewer personnel involved in the preparation and administration of TPN, the less danger of infection for the client. In most hospitals, the physician must order the TPN solution daily. In this way the solution and additives can be adjusted to the client's current needs. Each bottle of solution will indicate the glucose and protein content, all additives, time mixed, and the date and time of expiration. In general, solutions are good for 24 to 36 hours and must be refrigerated until a half-hour before being used.

Complications of TPN

Complications of TPN can be divided into three special categories including sepsis, metabolic problems, and problems with the central catheter line. The major complications of each category are presented in Table 33-12.

Table 33-12
Complications Associated with Total Parenteral Nutrition

Sepsis: Organisms Most Frequently Involved
1. Fungus
Candida accounts for 50–70% of infections
2. Gram-positive bacteria
Staphylococcus aureus
Staphylococcus epidermidis
Streptococcal, alpha or nonhemolytic
Enterococcus
3. Gram-negative bacteria
Klebsiella
Pseudomonas
Escherichia coli
Enterobacter
Proteus
Metabolic Problems
1. Glucose metabolism
Hyper- and hypoglycemia
Glycosuria
Hyperosmolar nonketotic coma
Osmotic diuresis
Ketoacidosis
2. Amino acid metabolism
Serum amino acid imbalances
Elevated serum ammonia
Prerenal azotemia
3. Calcium and phosphorus metabolism
Hypophosphatemia
Hyper- and hypocalcemia
Hyper- and hypovitaminosis (vitamin D)
4. Essential fatty acid deficiency
Central Catheter
1. Insertion
Air embolus
Pneumothorax
Hydrothorax
Hemorrhage
2. Dislodgement
3. Thrombosis of great vein

Nursing management (Table 33-13)

Peripheral hyperalimentation is a source of intravenous nutrition given concurrently with oral nourishment. A large peripheral vein can be used because the solution is less hypertonic and therefore less irritating. The peripheral injection site should be observed for signs of phlebitis. The site is changed at least every 48 hours, depending on established hospital policy. The preparation and administration of peripheral nutrition follows the same criteria as outlined for central hyperalimentation.

Catheter Placement for Central TPN The placement of the catheter into a large central vein will be performed by the physician. The vein most commonly used is the subclavian, although the innominate or jugular veins may be used. The procedure is the same as for the insertion of a central venous pressure line and should be done under strict aseptic conditions (see Chap. 25). The use of sterile gowns, gloves, drapes, and masks is mandatory. The nurse must be ready to clarify or reinforce information already given the client regarding the need for initiating TPN by vein.

During the catheter insertion, the client is placed on his back in Trendelenburg's position with a rolled towel between the scapulae. This position affords the best access route for catheter insertion. Chest and neck hair may be shaved to prevent a source of contamination. The skin is prepped by cleansing with an iodine antiseptic solution over the shoulder, neck, and chest area on the side where the catheter is to be inserted. The iodine must be removed by scrubbing the skin with 70 % alcohol, which will prevent an iodine

Table 33-13
Nursing Care Plan for Clients Receiving Total Parenteral Nutrition

Client Problem*	Expected Outcome	Nursing Intervention
Sepsis	No manifestations of infection. Normal body temperature. Negative blood cultures.	Check the composition of the TPN with orders before administration. Refrigerate solution until a half-hour before using. Use aseptic technique when connecting IV tubing and filter to central catheter. Label tubing and filter with time and date. Change filter every 24 h and tubing with each bottle. Check expiration date. *Do not add anything to TPN solutions* after receiving from pharmacy. *Do not administer blood, blood products, or antibiotics through* the central line. *Do not monitor CVP or draw blood samples* through central catheter. Change occlusive dressing over catheter site three times per week using aseptic technique (sterile gloves, mask). Observe for signs of inflammation and infection. Monitor vital signs every 4 h.
Altered blood sugar levels	Blood sugar within normal range.	Monitor blood glucose level daily. Check urine sugar and acetone every 4 h. Notify physician if 3+ or 4+ readings. Administer regular insulin if ordered. Initial TPN therapy must be gradually increased over 24 to 48 hours. Maintain accurate infusion rate; check every half-hour or use an infusion pump (e.g., IVAC). Watch for kinks and obstruction or disconnected tubing. Never increase flow rate or decrease rate by more than 10%. Observe for signs of *hyperglycemia* (e.g., thirst, polyuria, confusion). Observe for *hypoglycemia* (e.g., sweating, hunger, weakness, tremors). Never stop TPN abruptly unless replaced by another glucose source. Taper TPN gradually.
Electrolyte imbalances	Serum electrolyte levels within normal ranges.	Monitor serum electrolyte levels daily. Check for symptoms of *hyperkalemia* (muscle weakness, flaccid paralysis, cardiac arrhythmias, abdominal cramps, diarrhea) and *hypokalemia* (general weakness, decreased muscle tone, weak or irregular pulse, low BP, shallow respirations, abdominal distension, and ileus). Other manifestations of electrolyte imbalances are discussed in Chap. 12.
Air embolus	No signs of impaired breathing.	On catheter insertion, place client in Trendelenburg's position with rolled towel between scapulae. Instruct client to take a deep breath and hold while needle is inserted into subclavian vein (Valsalva maneuver). Use same position and Valsalva maneuver when changing tubing to prevent air from being sucked into vein. Reconnect catheter to IV tubing immediately. If air embolism is suspected, observe for sudden onset of dyspnea, decreased BP, chest pain, and hemoptysis. Place in Trendelenburg's position with left side down to "trap" air in right atria. Continue to observe for shock, cough, and SOB. Notify physician immediately.
Brachial plexis injury	Normal movement of arms and shoulders.	Observe client for pain in shoulder, chest, and arm due to injury to ventral branch of cervical or thoracic nerve from improper catheter placement. Check vital signs every 1 h. Assess for paresis of upper chest, neck, and arm on side of injury. Notify physician for catheter removal.
Fear and anxiety	Client will accept TPN and understand its benefits to his recovery.	Instruct client on rationale and benefits of TPN. Give approximate length of time he will receive TPN. Illustrate catheter position by drawings and pictures. Reassure client the catheter will not move into the heart. Describe the advantages of physical activity. Provide range-of-motion exercises that client can perform while in bed. Encourage ambulation. Provide oral stimulation and diversional activities during meal times. Suggest family visit at meal times. Provide for frequent mouth care. If allowed some intake, suggest chewing gum or sucking on hard candy. If no oral intake permitted, have client rinse mouth prn with water or mouthwash.

*These problems are all listed as potential problems.

skin burn, reduce any allergic reactions, and help destroy the cell walls of bacteria found on the skin surface.

In some institutions the skin is first scrubbed with soap and water and then followed by defatting the skin with acetone or ether. The use of a defatting agent is of questionable value at the present time because surface lipids possess an antimicrobial property and are known to significantly reduce the number of organisms such as *Staphylococcus aureus* and *Candida albicans*. Use of acetone in the skin preparation is known to remove these antimicrobial substances.

After draping the area and applying a local anesthetic, a silastic catheter is inserted through a large-bore needle into the right or left subclavian vein. The client is instructed to take a deep breath and stop breathing (Valsalva maneuver) when the needle is inserted. This will temporarily stop the positive pressure associated with normal ventilation and prevent air from being sucked into the subclavian vein, which could cause an air embolus or pneumothorax. The catheter is then threaded into the superior vena cava. A skin suture may be employed to stabilize the catheter, although there is not total agreement on its necessity as it is often a source of infection.

A standard isotonic intravenous solution is infused through the central line until x-ray confirms proper placement of the catheter tip in the superior vena cava and not the jugular vein or heart. The catheter insertion site is then covered with an iodine ointment and covered with an occlusive dressing. The date is marked on the dressing. The dressing should be changed three times a week.

Complications frequently associated with catheter placement are hemorrhage and hydrothorax. Proper placement of a catheter for central hyperalimentation is illustrated in Fig. 33-1. Once established, the central catheter should not be used for the administration of blood or antibiotics, drawing blood samples, or for central venous pressure monitoring.

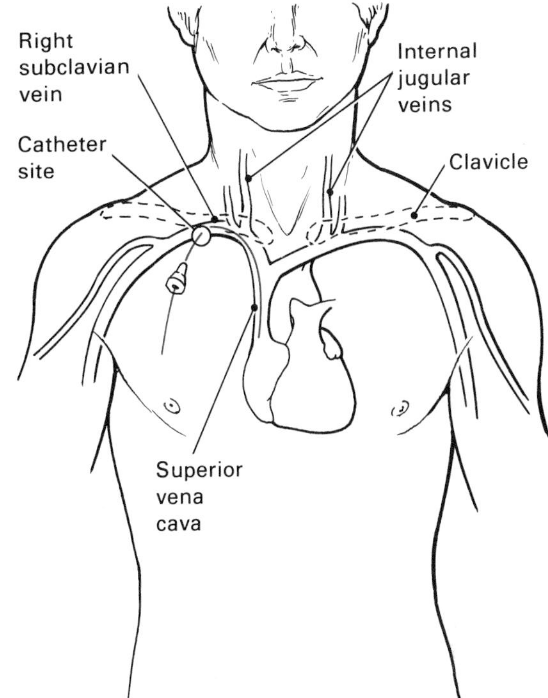

Figure 33-1 Placement of a catheter for total parenteral nutrition.

Administration of TPN Solution Sepsis is one of the major concerns when hypertonic solutions are used for nutrition. It is essential that proper aseptic techniques be followed when inserting the tubing and connecting the millipore filter prior to starting therapy. The filter and tubing are labeled with the date and time. The millipore filter, used to trap bacteria and precipitate from the solution, is placed proximal to the catheter hub. Filters are changed every 24 hours and the tubing is changed with each new bottle of solution hung. When attaching a new tubing or filter to the central catheter, the client should be asked to perform the Valsalva maneuver so that the chance of an air embolus is reduced while the catheter is open and unconnected to an infusion source. All tubing connections should be taped to prevent an accidental break in the continuity of the line.

At the beginning of TPN therapy, the solution will be infused at a gradually increasing rate over a 24- to 48-hour period. In this way the pancreas can adapt to the increased amount of glucose in the circulation by producing more insulin. The urine should be tested for sugar and acetone every 4 to 6 hours while the client is receiving hyperalimentation. Glycosuria of 1+ or 2+ is expected during the first few days of therapy. However, readings of 3+ or 4+ require either the addition of regular insulin to the solution or the administration of insulin on a sliding scale schedule (sliding scale is explained in Chap. 41).

Nurses must be aware that speeding or slowing the infusion rate is contraindicated. Speeding up the rate will result in a large amount of glucose entering the circulation. Endogenous insulin levels will not be adequate to handle this increase in glucose and a hyperosmolar state results. The renal tubules are unable to reabsorb the glucose and it spills into the urine. Conversely, slowing the rate results in a hypoglycemic state, since it takes time for the pancreatic islet cells to adjust to a reduced glucose level. Checking the amount infused and the rate every half-hour is recommended. The use of an infusion pump such as the IVAC regulates the rate accurately and sounds an alarm if the tubing is obstructed or disconnected.

Vital signs should be monitored every 4 hours. Daily weights will give an indication of the client's nutritional status as therapy progresses. Body weight is considered the sum of the changes in protein, fat, and water. Body water fluctuates more from day to day than protein or fat. Analysis must be made as to whether gains or losses in weight are due to fluid gained from edema, fluid lost through diuresis, or actual increase or decrease in true body weight. Blood levels of glucose, electrolytes, protein, a complete blood count, and enzymes studies will be followed on a daily or triweekly basis. Correlation of these important values will assist the nurse in assessing the client's progress toward a more nutritious state.

Dressings covering the catheter site are changed three times a week, usually by specially trained nurses from the IV team or the nutritional support team. Some institutions will allow the staff nurses to carry out dressing changes after special instruction. The procedure for changing the dressing is similar to that followed during the catheter insertion. The site is carefully observed for signs of inflammation and infection. Phlebitis can readily occur in the vein as a result of the hypertonic infusion and can become infected. Most clients receiving central TPN are immunosuppressed and are more susceptible to opportunistic infections. Many are on chemotherapy or corticosteroids and antibiotics which will mask signs of infection.

If sutures are used to anchor the catheter, they frequently become infected. If an infection is suspected during dressing change, a culture of the site and any drainage should be sent for analysis and the physician notified immediately. The use of an occlusive dressing, while protecting the wound from contamination, may also allow the growth of fungi such as *Candida* which account for a large percentage (50 percent) of infections.

If the client exhibits signs and symptoms of a systemic infection, the catheter tip is usually suspect unless another cause can be found. Cultures of blood, sputum, urine, draining wound, and the catheter tip if it has been removed are done at once. A chest x-ray is done to detect any pulmonary infection. The current bottle of TPN solution with tubing and filter should also be cultured and replaced with an entire new setup. When the catheter tip is the infection source, antibiotic therapy is generally not necessary since the removal of the catheter will eliminate the problem. A new central line may be immediately reestablished or replaced by a peripheral route. It is important that a glucose source be given to prevent rebound hypoglycemia.

Weaning from TPN The same precautions should be followed in weaning from TPN as when beginning therapy, except in inverse order. The flow rate must be gradually decreased and oral intake increased. If an emergency situation precludes a slow weaning process, other dextrose-containing fluids should be hung immediately. Clients going to surgery should have their TPN discontinued ahead of the scheduled operation time. At the time the catheter is removed by the physician, the site is immediately covered with iodine ointment and an occlusive dressing is applied. The dressing should be changed daily until the wound heals. Oral nourishments should be encouraged and a careful record of intake be maintained. Daily weights and laboratory analysis of serum levels will continue.

Intravenous Fat Emulsion

The first infusion of fat emulsions was during the 1920s in Japan. Further research was delayed until after World War II. In 1975 the FDA approved the use of Intralipid 10%, a commercially prepared fat emulsion. At the present time Intralipid is the only fat emulsion that can be used in the United States. The contents of Intralipid fat emulsion are listed in Table 33-14. Indications for the use of intravenous fat are:

1. Clients receiving peripheral hyperalimentation who require an additional calorie source
2. Clients receiving long-term (over 5 days) hyperalimentation who require a source of essential fatty acids
3. Clients receiving central hyperalimentation who have excessive caloric needs

The administration of fat emulsion is contraindicated in individuals with a disturbance in fat metabolism and should be used with caution in clients who are in danger of fat embolism, those with pancreatitis, liver damage, pulmonary disease, anemia, and blood coagulation disorders.

Intralipid solution is isotonic and may be infused into a peripheral vein. It can be given in conjunction with peripheral hyperalimentation. When it is used with TPN, the fat emulsion is given as a supplemental source of calories, since essential fatty acids are not included in the standard preparations of TPN. Prolonged use of TPN can lead to a fatty acid deficiency state which is manifested as dermatitis and loss of hair.

Intralipid should be refrigerated until 1 hour before administration. Special tubing is provided by the manufacturer and new tubing is used with each bottle. Nothing is to be added to the solution prior to administration. Intralipid should not be filtered. When running peripheral hyperalimentation at the same time, the fat emulsion should be connected below the filter through a "Y" injection site. As with TPN solutions, fat emulsion should begin at a slow rate, usually 1 mL/min for the first 15 minutes. If no reaction is observed, the rate may be increased to 125 mL/hour. Adverse reactions that can occur are allergic reactions, dyspnea, cyanosis, fever, flushing, and phlebitis. Intravenous fat may be ordered 2 to 3 times per week, depending upon the caloric needs or fatty acid requirements. A major benefit derived from IV fat administration is that a large number of calories can be provided in a relatively small amount of fluid. This is especially good when the client is at risk for fluid overload.

Table 33-14
Standard Contents of Intralipid Fat Emulsion (500 mL)

Soybean triglycerides	10%
Egg yolk phospholipids	1.2%
Glycerin	2.25%
Water	500 mL
mOsm per liter	280 mOsm/L
Electrolytes	None
Total calories	550

OBESITY

Significance of Problem

Obesity is one of the major health problems found in our society. It has been estimated that obesity contributes to more ill health than all the vitamin deficiencies put together.[8] In the United States, obesity affects between 40 to 80 million individuals at the present time. Obesity may be defined as a state in which the intake of food is in excess of the physiologic needs of the body. The term *overweight* has often been used to define obesity, yet the terms are not identical. *Overweight* refers to excess in body weight in relation to a standard for height. *Obesity* refers to excess body fat.

Contrary to common belief, obesity is rarely attributable to hypothalamic damage or organic etiology. Another frequent misconception is that only prosperous middle-aged men and women become obese. Obesity can occur to anyone during the life cycle. A survey conducted in Manhattan confirmed that obesity is found to a greater extent in the lower socioeconomic class.[9]

The Task Force on Risks, Hazards, and Disadvantages of Obesity has provided the following possible implications of obesity from a medical and social standpoint:[10]

1. Increased risk of cardiovascular disease, especially sudden death.
2. Hypertension may be increased by 3 to 5 times in persons who are 50 percent or more above desirable weight.
3. Increased risk of developing gallbladder disease.
4. Increased risk of developing noninsulin-dependent diabetes mellitus.
5. Increased risk of developing endometrial cancer.
6. Aggravation of degenerative joint disease.
7. Economic and social handicap.

Formation of Adipose Tissue

The formation of adipose tissue, unless determined to be secondary to organic etiology, can only occur when an individual consumes more food than is required to carry out normal physiologic function and growth. The excess is stored as adipose tissue in layers beneath the skin surface, the omentum, the mesentery, and in fat pads that normally surround the kidneys and heart. The process of reaching an obese state is usually insidious. The individual may be completely unaware of changes in his eating habits or body size until visualizing himself in a mirror or discovering the need for a larger clothing size.

Adipose tissue present in obesity is of the same composition as fat tissue found normally but in smaller amounts in the same areas. It consists of clumps of fat cells together with supporting tissue such as blood vessels, lymphatic vessels, and fibrous tissue. Although adipose tissue is very high in neutral fat, it also contains water, protein, and a small amount of glycogen.

The size of the adipose tissue mass is the sum of the number of adipose cells and the adipose cell size which is determined by the amount of triglyceride found within the cell. Adipose tissue normally grows by an increase in adipose cell size during the first year of life. After the first year, much of the enlargement of adipose tissue occurs as a result of an increase in cell number.[11]

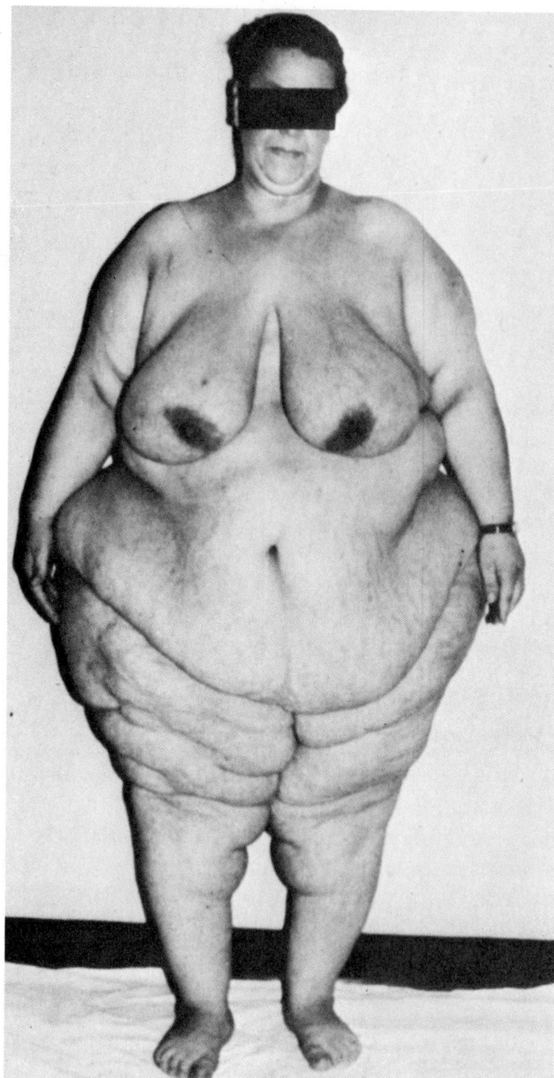

Figure 33-2 Extreme juvenile onset obesity. (*R. Mancini, et al., Medical Complications of Obesity, Academic Press Inc., Ltd., London, 1979.*)

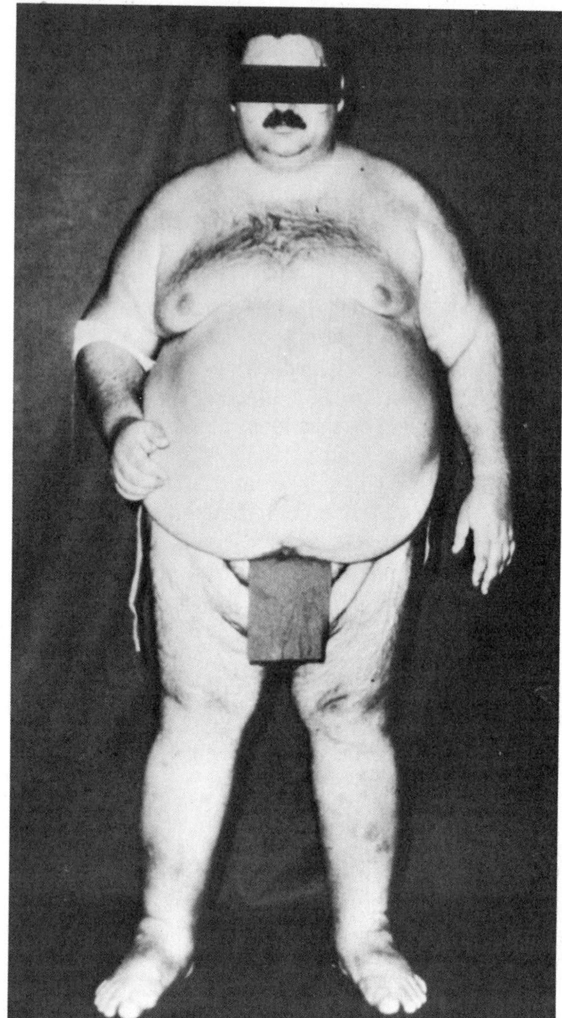

Figure 33-3 Extreme adult onset obesity. (*R. Mancini et al. Medical Complications of Obesity. Academic Press Inc., Ltd., London, 1979.*)

Obesity research has demonstrated that expansion of the tissue mass occurs as a result of an increase in cell size (*hypertrophic obesity*) or by in increase in cell size and cell number (*hypertrophic-hyperplastic obesity*). Adipose hypercellularity is known to occur at two periods of early life, within the first year and at or around the time of puberty.[12] Individuals who become obese in childhood generally have a higher number of fat cells than an individual who becomes obese as an adult. There is considerable evidence that massively obese children continue to increase fat cell number between the ages of 2 to 11 years, whereas fat cell number is usually stable in nonobese children.

Hypercellular obesity tends to occur before age 20, while hypertrophic obesity is generally considered to be adult onset. The adipose tissue mass in early onset obesity is distributed universally over the entire body, while the adipose tissue mass in adult onset obesity is centrally distributed. Figure 33-2 shows a client with extreme juvenile onset obesity. Figure 33-3 shows a client with extreme maturity onset obesity. The understanding and significance of how adipose tissue is formed has considerable implications on weight loss and the reduction of the adipose tissue mass in the adult. Severe dietary restrictions will not decrease the number of fat cells present, but will result in a decrease in the size of the cell. The saying "once a fat cell, always a fat cell" is unfortunately true and is based on scientific fact.

Pathogenesis of Obesity

Many factors have been investigated in order to identify their relationship and influence on the occurrence of obesity. Questions to consider in assessing the client with obesity are:

1. What is the psychological importance of food?
2. Is intake influenced by hunger?
3. Does the taste and appearance and physical factors in the environment make some individuals more sensitive and propel them to excess eating habits?
4. Is there an *emotional* problem that creates a need for oral gratification?
5. Are there *physical stressors* precipitating the individual to overeat?

Although obesity is often familial, research has not as yet discovered any genetic basis for obesity. Until such a link is identified the role of environment and dietary patterns of these families must be considered the basis for the identified familial obesity trend.

There are some *cultures* where obesity is highly prized. It is not uncommon for men of the West Indies or parts of Africa to desire an obese wife. The Sumo wrestlers of Japan receive much notoriety and fanfare for their very large body size in the wrestling arena. In order to achieve this admired status, dietary excess must be a lifelong requirement.

While *endocrine* conditions such as hypothyroidism, hypopituitarism, hypogonadism, and Cushing's syndrome are frequently diagnosed in the obese individual, these conditions may also be found in persons of normal weight. Women at the time of puberty, after childbirth, and at menopause are more prone to obesity. It has been speculated that this tendency might be due to an endocrine influence. However, diagnostic investigations have seldom provided evidence to support this relationship.

The connection between *physical activity* and obesity is well established. Most obese individuals live a sedentary lifestyle, usually having a nonstrenuous indoor occupation, and engage in little or no spirited recreational activities. Their energy needs are considerably less than are the requirements for a construction worker who also plays tennis several times a week. The obese, sedentary person's energy intake usually exceeds his needs and consequently results in a buildup of the adipose tissue mass.

Complications of Obesity

The medical and social problems associated with obesity are numerous. The medical problem may be a direct result of too much fat, or a medical problem may have an adverse effect on obesity. *Cardiovascular* and *respiratory problems* are very common in the obese person. Many clients will develop dyspnea on exertion, orthopnea, paroxysmal nocturnal dyspnea, drowsiness, and somnolence. Heart size increases as body weight increases, since the heart must work harder to maintain adequate circulation. Hypertension is frequently found in obese individuals. A concomitant feature that adds considerable strain on the already overworked heart is an increase in circulating blood volume by an increase in the red cell count and the plasma volume.[13] Therefore, obesity can precipitate chronic volume overload and hypertrophy of the heart, especially of the left ventricle.

The *Pickwickian syndrome*, which is known as obesity-hypoventilation, has been long recognized as a result of extreme obesity. The bellows action of the chest wall is compromised and there is dysfunction of the central respiratory control center. The movement of the muscles of the chest wall and the diaphragm is reduced due to the weight of the fatty tissue mass. Hypoventilation results in hypercapnia. The increased CO_2 level then results in a blunting effect on the respiratory control center and there is a defective response to the high CO_2.[14] The manifestations are cyanosis, dyspnea, edema, and somnolence. In addition, most clients have a reduced vital capacity and polycythemia. Blood gas exchange is also directly affected.

The incidence of *diabetes mellitus* is quite high in obese persons. They are known to secrete large quantities of insulin for an as yet unexplained reason. It is known that obesity is associated with insulin resistance in the adipose cells themselves and in muscle cells, thus creating a noninsulin-dependent diabetic state.

Gallstone formation in the obese client is quite common. The incidence of gallstones rises as the body weight increases. There is a concomitant rise in the serum cholesterol and triglyceride levels as well as an increase in body weight. These levels tend to fall as obesity is corrected. The high levels of cholesterol and triglyceride can also contribute to the formation of coronary heart disease.

Excessive weight on the weight-bearing joints of the hips, knees, and lower spine can cause much pain and discomfort. While obesity has not been implicated as a cause of degenerative joint disease, it is known to be a predisposing factor. It has been postulated that obesity may contribute to the pathogenesis of osteoarthritis in multiple joints that already have the disease process started.

Other medical complications associated with obesity are menstrual irregularities, infertility, endometrial cancer, and fatty liver infiltration. Understandably, the life expectancy of an obese individual can be shortened as a result of the medical problems encountered.

In addition to the many physical complications associated with obesity, the client may suffer from long-standing emotional and social problems. Society puts great emphasis on attaining and maintaining the healthy and vigorous look. Those who deviate from this prescribed standard often meet with discrimination and disdain. The very fat person may find it difficult to obtain a desired job, social acceptance at school, or membership in organizations. Clothing is often limited in style, color, size, and quantity. These socioemotional problems may be manifested in poor self-esteem and body image.

Medical Management

The medical management of obesity must be well planned and have the total commitment of both the physician and the client. While less than 5 percent of all cases of obesity are of organic origin, diagnostic evaluation for such conditions must be a first step in the treatment process. A thorough history and physical examination is necessary and will reveal the extent and duration of the obese state.

Diagnostic

There is no definite agreement on a technique for determining who is obese. Several methods are currently in use. One widely used method is to compare the client's weight to a standardized weight for height chart and then designate the client to be a percentage overweight. Table 33-15 provides a standardized weight for height chart. Normal weight depends largely on body build. A limitation of this method of assessing obesity can be seen from the following example. An individual who inherits a medium frame and bulky muscle mass may be considered 20 percent overweight according to the standardized chart and yet not be obese.

A more scientific method of determining the amount of body fat is by measuring skinfold thickness using special calipers at one of four body sites: biceps, triceps, subscapular, or suprailiac. Accurate estimates of body fat are then derived as a result of correlations established with body density from anthropometric charts. Although considered a more exact technique, this method also has limitations. As a person ages, total body fat increases, as does the skinfold thickness for the fatty tissue at each site. The disadvantage of this method of calculating the degree of obesity lies in the fact that the standards for the skinfold thickness are generally obtained from healthy young men and women aged 20 to 30 years and does not consider age-related changes.

The least reliable technique, yet perhaps the most frequently utilized, is direct observation of the client. A subjective assessment of total body fat is made. The ideal body is one which has only a thin layer of adipose tissue covering the skeletal frame. When a roll of excess subcutaneous adipose tissue is seen, the client is considered obese.

Diagnostic studies may include a chest film and barium contrast studies of both the upper and lower gastrointestinal tract. An oral cholecystogram may be performed, since the incidence of gallstones is high in the obese client.

Laboratory studies must be included in any diagnostic workup. A glucose tolerance test will be needed to determine the presence of or the tendency toward development of diabetes mellitus. Serum cholesterol, triglycerides, red blood cell count, total blood volume, liver and cardiac enzymes, and renal function tests should be included. Alterations in these tests may signify organ dysfunction, but they are also known to be altered in obesity. Arterial blood gases and pulmonary function tests should be carried out when the respiratory status appears to be compromised.

Conservative therapy

When no organic cause can be found for obesity, a supervised plan of care should be devised that will lead to successful weight reduction. The plan should focus primarily on dietary reduction and a sensible exercise program.

A good *reducing diet* should contain foods from the basic four food groups and be as similar to the client's usual eating pattern as is permissible. A diet that includes adequate amounts of fruits and vegetables will provide enough bulk to prevent constipation and meet vitamin A and C daily requirements. Lean meat, fish, and eggs will provide sufficient protein and the B complex vitamins. The amount of caloric intake may need to be restricted to 800 to 1500 calories per day, depending upon the client's age, weight, nutritional status, and length of time estimated for ideal weight to be achieved. Table 4 in Appendix B contains a sample 1200-calorie reducing diet.

Because most obese individuals are sedentary, a *planned exercise program* should be implemented in conjunction with caloric reduction. There is no evidence that exercise promotes an increase in appetite or leads to dietary excess. Walking is considered the best type of exercise for the obese individual, since it is the easiest form of physical activity that can be performed safely. It has been shown that walking for 1 hour a day at 3 mph will expend 4 to 5 kcal/min.[15]

Medications have been used in the treatment of obesity but only as adjuvants to a good dietary and exercise program. These drugs are used to suppress appetite. While a variety of drugs have been used, diuretics, laxatives, antispasmodics, thyroid hormone, amphetamines, and amphetamine-like adrenergic drugs are the most commonly prescribed. Amphetamines do suppress the appetite and facilitate weight loss. However, when the pharmacologic effects of the drug wear off or the drug is discontinued, the appetite generally returns and weight gain will be resumed unless food reduction and the exercise program are maintained. Amphetamines should never be prescribed for extended periods of time or under conditions where supervised control may not be possible. There is always a potential for drug abuse and dependence. These drugs should be used with caution in clients with hypertension, cardiovascular disease, or hyperthyroidism due to the drug's sympathomimetic effects which can aggravate these conditions. Some states have banned the use of amphetamines in the treatment of obesity.

Surgical therapy

Surgical interventions are never the primary method of weight reduction and should be utilized only after the more conventional treatments fail.

In order for a client to be selected for any of the operations for morbid obesity, he must meet the following criteria:

1. Massive obesity of 5 years' duration
2. Failure to reduce weight using other forms of therapy
3. Body weight of 100 pounds above the ideal for age, sex, and height
4. No serious endocrine problem causing the obesity
5. Absence of other medical conditions (liver disease, alcoholism, cardiovascular or pulmonary disease, inflammatory bowel disease)
6. Psychiatric and social stability
7. Availability of a team of physicians to provide immediate and long-term care

Some physicians feel that low intelligence, possible pregnancy, and age are limiting factors to surgical intervention. Clients below the age of 20 or over age 50 are frequently discouraged from seeking surgical treatment. Weight reduction is more difficult to achieve with increasing age and the complications that accompany these procedures are more devastating with age.

Table 33-15
Desirable Weights for Men and Women (According to Height and Frame, Ages 25 and Over)

	Weight in Pounds (in Indoor Clothing)		
Height (in Shoes)*	**Small Frame**	**Medium Frame**	**Large Frame**
Men			
5′ 2″	112–120	118–129	126–141
3″	115–123	121–133	129–144
4″	118–126	124–136	132–148
5″	121–129	127–139	135–152
6″	124–133	130–143	138–156
7″	128–137	134–147	142–161
8″	132–141	138–152	147–166
9″	136–145	142–156	151–170
10″	140–150	146–160	155–174
11″	144–154	150–165	159–179
6′ 0″	148–158	154–170	164–184
1″	152–162	158–175	168–189
2″	156–167	162–180	173–194
3″	160–171	167–185	178–199
4″	164–175	172–190	182–204
Women			
4′10″	92–98	96–107	104–119
11″	94–101	98–110	106–122
5′ 0″	96–104	101–113	109–125
1″	99–107	104–116	112–128
2″	102–110	107–119	115–131
3″	105–113	110–122	118–134
4″	108–116	113–126	121–138
5″	111–119	116–130	125–142
6″	114–123	120–135	129–146
7″	118–127	124–139	133–150
8″	122–131	128–143	137–154
9″	126–135	132–147	141–158
10″	130–140	136–151	145–163
11″	134–144	140–155	149–168
6′ 0″	138–148	144–159	153–173

*1-inch heels for men and 2-inch heels for women

Note: Prepared by the Metropolitan Life Insurance Company. Derived primarily from data of the Build and Blood Pressure Study, 1959, Society of Actuaries.

Adapted with permission of the Metropolitan Life Insurance Company.

The various surgical procedures employed in the treatment of obesity are listed in Table 33-16. Several specific surgeries are discussed in this section.

Lipectomy (Adipectomy) This type of surgery is performed to remove unsightly flabby folds of adipose

Table 33-16
Surgical Procedures Used in the Treatment of Obesity

Purpose	Procedure
Reduction of adipose tissue	Lipectomy
Reduction in food intake	Jaw wiring Gastroplasty
Reduction in food absorption	Gastric bypass Intestinal bypass
Reduction in appetite	Neurosurgery (electrocoagulation of the hunger center in lateral hypothalamus) Truncal vagotomy

tissue. Clients who choose adipectomies do so for cosmetic reasons. In some clients up to 15 percent of the total fat cells have been removed from the breasts, abdomen, lumbar, and femoral areas. There has been no evidence that there is a regeneration of adipose tissue at the surgical sites. However, it must be emphasized to the client that surgical removal does not prevent obesity from recurring since lifetime eating habits remain the same. While body image and self-esteem may be enhanced by such procedures, they are not without complications. The dangerous effects of general anesthesia and the potential for poor wound healing in the obese client cannot be overly stressed. It is more useful for the majority of clients contemplating adipectomies to be instructed on preventive health measures such as slow weight reduction to maintain and preserve tissue integrity, the value of exercise, and behavior modification techniques.

Jaw Wiring During the past few years many obese clients have had their jaws wired in an attempt to achieve weight reduction. The client is able to speak after the procedure but is only able to ingest fluids. This type of obesity treatment does achieve weight loss, but does not change the basic eating patterns of the individual when the wires are removed. Weight is usually regained. While the jaw is wired, the client must carry wire cutters at all times. Both the client and family need to be instructed in the use of wire cutters in times of emergency such as vomiting, choking, and cardiovascular arrest. The nursing care of clients with wired jaws is discussed in Chap. 32.

Surgical Bypass Procedures and Gastroplasty When all other conventional approaches to weight reduction have been exhausted, the client may be considered a candidate for an intestinal bypass (jejunoileal), a gastric bypass, or gastroplasty (gastric partitioning). Generally these surgical procedures are indicated only for clients who are morbidly obese, which is defined as having a body weight two times or more above normal.

The *jejunoileal bypass* procedure results in weight loss by producing malabsorption. In this procedure, the distal end of the jejunum is closed and attached to the omentum. As a result, almost 90 percent of the small intestine is bypassed and malabsorption is achieved. In contrast, the *gastric bypass* operation induces weight loss by reducing food intake and producing only minimal malabsorption. The stomach reservoir is decreased in size to approximately 3 ounces. Weight is lost as a result of both procedures, but at a slower rate following gastric bypass. Table 33-17 compares these bypass surgical procedures.

Gastroplasty (gastric partitioning) is a third type of surgical procedure that is now used to induce weight loss in the morbidly obese person. Two types of gastroplasty are used. The stomach is partitioned into a small upper portion and a large distal portion by dividing the stomach, either by surgical transection or by the placement of two rows of staples at approximately $1\frac{1}{2}$ cm below the gastroesophageal junction.[16] A small channel is left open in both operations so that ingested food and fluid may slowly pass through from the small upper portion into the larger distal end. The new upper gastric pouch holds approximately 2 to 3 ounces of food or fluid at any one time. Figure 33-4 illustrates the three surgical procedures and the anatomic changes that result. Figure 33-5 illustrates gastric partitioning.

Gastric partitioning has several advantages over the gastric bypass operation. It is technically easier to perform, especially when stapling is used. If reversal of the procedure is required, removing the staples is easier than the very difficult procedure of converting the gastric bypass. In addition, symptoms of the dumping syndrome and malabsorption are eliminated.

Nursing Management

The nurse is in a good position to work with the physician, dietitian, and other health care workers. She is involved in providing dietary instruction and clarification, suggesting and supervising exercise programs, encouraging the client during periods of depression and frustration, and carrying out health teaching necessary to help motivation and modify behavior.

Diet teaching

The only effective method of treating obesity is to restrict dietary intake so that it is below energy re-

Table 33-17
Comparison of Bypass Surgical Procedures for Morbid Obesity

Procedure	Mechanism of Weight Loss	Early Complications	Late Complications	Advantages	Disadvantages
Jejunoileal bypass End to end Side to side	Induced malabsorption Reduced food intake	Pulmonary infection Deep vein thrombosis Wound infection and dehiscence Incisional hernia Severe diarrhea Electrolyte imbalance	Anemia Calculi (biliary and renal) Diarrhea, 15–20/day Electrolyte imbalance–K, Na, Ca, Mg Hepatic failure Malnutrition Psychiatric problems Polyarthritis and polymyalgia Steatorrhea Thinning of hair Vitamin deficiency (A, C, D, B_{12})	Weight loss Lowered BP Lowered total lipids, cholesterol Decreased insulin requirements Improved work performance Better body image Decreased mortality Procedure can be reversed	Numerous and severe complications Need of long-term follow-up care Operation still experimental Some clients regain weight
Gastric bypass	Reduced food intake Stomach reservoir decreased 90%	Pulmonary infection Deep vein thrombosis Wound infection and dehiscence Incisional hernia Uncontrolled vomiting Dumping syndrome Leaks at anastomosis Peritonitis	Not sufficient information as yet available	Same as above except for difficulty in reversing In addition: safer for children and adolescents Fewer complications	Same as above In addition: very difficult to reverse surgically

quirements. It is rare to find an overweight individual who has not at some time in his life attempted to lose weight. Some have met with limited and temporary success while others have met only with failure. It is likely that the great majority of these individuals attempted weight loss by trying out one of the many fad diets which offer the enticement to eat and get slim. Fad diets in general claim weight loss quickly and inexpensively. While it is true that body weight is lost initially, it is not fat that is lost but body water. The normal fat cell is composed of neutral fat, protein, glycogen, and water. Glycogen is known to bind with water. Since most slimming diets severely restrict carbohydrate, the body's glycogen stores become depleted within a few days. Included in the body's glycogen loss is the loss from within the fat cell along with water. The amount of fat within the adipose cell is not affected until much later as caloric intake is drastically reduced and sustained. Obese clients must be made to understand that following a well-balanced, low caloric diet is the most sensible approach to weight loss and will have a more satisfying and long-lasting result than fad diets.

The degree of success of any reducing diet depends on the amount of weight to be lost. A moderately obese individual will obviously attain his goal more easily than will a massively obese individual. Adult onset obesity is much more amenable to successful treatment than the obesity of juvenile onset. In juvenile onset obesity, the eating patterns have been present for many years and the number of fat cells is usually much higher. Consequently, more

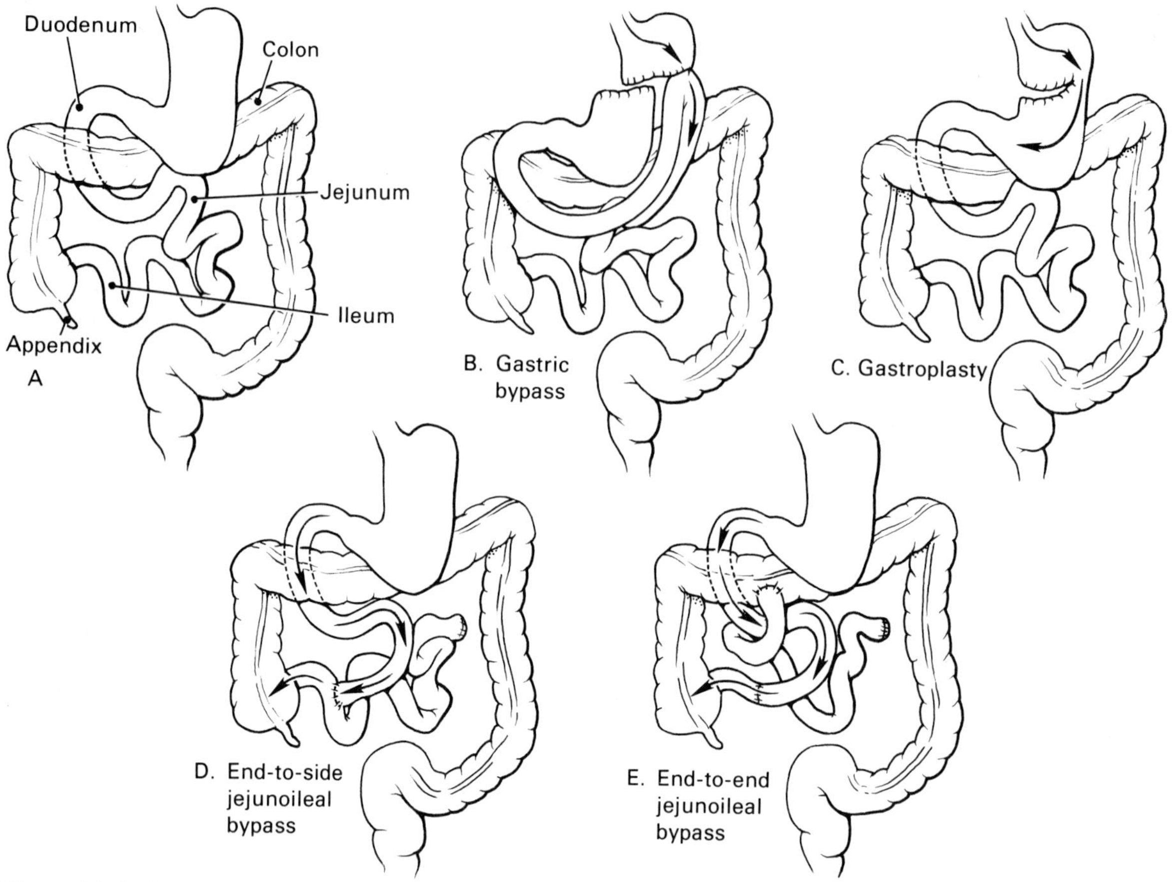

Duodenum
Colon
Jejunum
Ileum
Appendix
A

B. Gastric bypass

C. Gastroplasty

D. End-to-side jejunoileal bypass

E. End-to-end jejunoileal bypass

Figure 33-4 Surgical procedures for morbid obesity and the anatomic changes. (*From R. Hodges, Nutrition: Metabolic & Clinical Applications, Plenum Publishing Co., New York, 1979, p. 384.*)

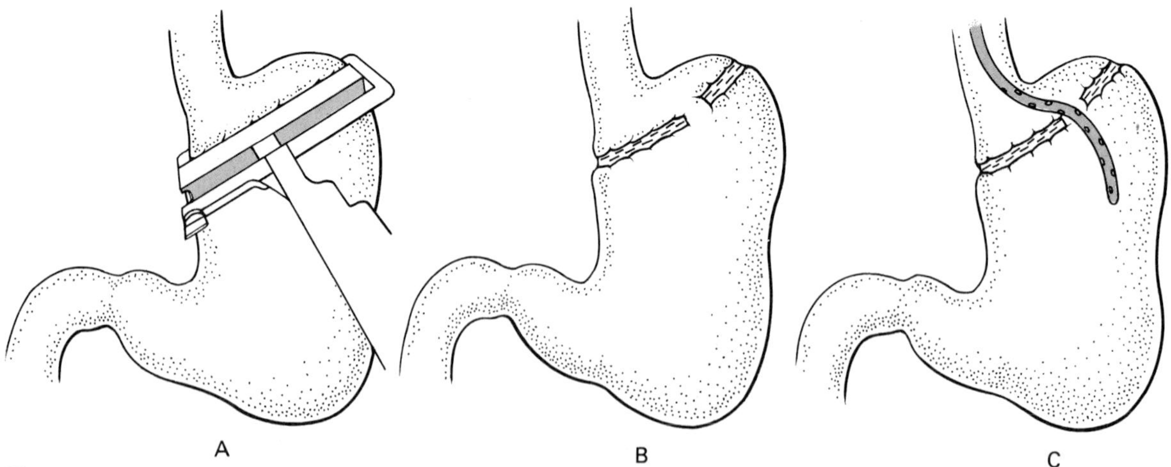

Figure 33-5 Gastric partitioning with staples. (*From C. M. Mojzisik and E. W. Martin, "Gastric Partitioning: The Latest Surgical Means to Control Morbid Obesity," Am J Nurs,* ***81****:571, 1981.)*

drastic dieting efforts and perseverance are necessary to achieve weight reduction.

Motivation is the essential ingredient on the part of the obese client to achieve success. He must see the need for weight loss and the advantages that will accrue. The nurse can assist the client by helping him to look at his eating patterns through a diet diary. How often does he eat? What precipitates his desire to eat? Is it due to boredom, frustration cued from television commercials, or environmental factors? Does the time of day influence this desire for food? Does he snack during the evening hours after eating a large dinner? Does he raid the refrigerator at 2 A.M.? A frank discussion of his eating habits will help the client to realize that he often does not eat because he is hungry, but because of bad habits picked up over time. It is the bad habits that must be changed or weight loss will only be temporary.

Setting a realistic goal such as losing between 1 to 2 pounds per week must be agreed upon at the outset. Trying to lose too much too fast usually results in a sense of frustration and failure for the client. The nurse can help the client understand that losing large amounts of weight in a short period of time causes the adipose tissue to lose elasticity and tone and become unsightly folds of flabby tissue. Slower weight loss will offer better cosmetic results. Frequent checks of body weight is a good method of monitoring progress. Weighing daily is not recommended because of the frequent fluctuations resulting from retained urine and feces. The client should be instructed to weight himself at the same time of day wearing the same type of clothing.

There is no firm agreement on the number of meals to be eaten when on a diet. Some nutritionists advocate eating several small meals a day because the body's metabolic rate is temporarily increased immediately after eating. By ingesting several small meals a day more calories will be burned. There seems to be general agreement that consuming the majority of the daily caloric intake at a large evening meal results in less weight loss than if the calories were evenly distributed throughout the day.

When first starting on a dietary program, food portions should be weighed in order to stay within the dietary guidelines. After a time, weighing will not be necessary as the client can then make accurate judgments of size and weight. A list of permitted foods given to the client serves as a good reference and permits an occasional meal to be eaten at a restaurant. When the client carefully follows the prescribed diet, he will not need to take vitamin supplements. Appropriate fluid intake should be encouraged. Alcoholic beverages are usually not permitted on a reducing diet as they increase the caloric intake and are low in nutritional value.

Exercise teaching

Once an exercise program has been outlined for the client, the nurse can reinforce instruction and assist the client to individualize it to himself, his time schedule, and physical limitations. She should point out that engaging in weekend exercise only or spurts of strenuous activity is not advantageous and could actually be dangerous. Joining a health spa can be one mechanism of getting exercise. However, sitting in a sauna or trying to spot-reduce a specific part of the body do not lend themselves to an appropriate daily program. Walking, swimming, or cycling are more sensible forms of exercise and have more long-range benefits. The combination of a good reducing diet and exercise program can have profound effects on the client achieving his weight loss. A major benefit derived from exercise involving the long muscles is cardiovascular conditioning.

There are many psychological benefits that can be derived from an exercise program. Some of them include reduction in tension and stress, adequate sleep and rest, decreased desire to eat excessively, increased stamina and energy, improved self-concept and self-confidence, better attitudes toward work and play, and increased optimism about the future.

Drug therapy teaching

The role of the nurse in relation to drug therapy should center around teaching about proper administration and side effects. Emphasis should be on the dangers of drug dependence and tolerance. The modification of dosage without consultation with the physician or nurse can lead to detrimental effects. The nurse should reemphasize that the diet and exercise regimens are the cornerstone for permanent weight loss. Medications are only a psychological aid that do not help the client change his eating behavior. The purchase of over-the-counter diet aids should be discouraged.

Behavior modification training

The individual who is on any type of restrictive dietary program is often encouraged to join a group of other obese persons who are receiving professional counseling to help them modify their eating habits. The assumption behind behavior modification is that obesity is a learned disorder due to overeating, and the critical difference between an obese person and a nonobese person is in the way they eat. Therefore, most behavior modification programs deemphasize the diet per se and focus on how the person eats. Participants are taught to restrict their eating to designated meals and to increase the amount of physical activity in their lives. Individuals who have undergone behavior therapy are more successful in maintaining their losses over an extended period of time than persons who followed a diet alone.

Many self-help groups are available to the individual who wants to learn more about successful dieting and who likes the support of others having the same problems and experiences. *TOPS* (*Take Off Pounds Sensibly*) is the oldest nonprofit organization of this type and is patterned after Alcoholics Anonymous. Behavioral modification is an integral part of the program as well as nutrition education. *Weight Watchers International Inc.* is probably the most successful commercial weight reduction enterprise. *Weight Watchers* offers a food plan that is nutritionally balanced and practical to follow. A program of behavior modification, which is reported to have increased average weekly weight loss, was introduced in 1974. Other self-help groups or organizations are *Overeaters Anonymous*, *Weight Losers*, *Trim Clubs, Inc.*, and the *Diet Workshop, Inc.* All these groups offer diet education, exercise plans, and behavior modification.

A new concept of influencing health behavior and better employee health has come about in recent years. Various programs on health teaching and maintenance have been started at the place of employment. The rationale for such programs is that better health repays the cost of the programs through improved work performance, decreased absenteeism, and, eventually, less hospitalization. Weight reduction and hypertension programs have been instituted and are very popular with employees.

Nursing intervention related to surgical therapy

Preoperative Care Special considerations are necessary in the care of clients who are admitted to the hospital for surgical treatment of obesity. Most nursing units are not prepared to meet the needs of a client who is often too large for a typical hospital or recovery room bed or who has arms or legs that even a large-size blood pressure cuff will not fit. Plans for these special needs must be made prior to the client's admission in order to eliminate embarrassment for the client and frustration for the staff. Oversized blood pressure cuffs should be ready for use when the client arrives. A private room may be necessary both for privacy of the client and to accommodate the bed and sitting arrangements. A trapeze bar should be placed over the bed to facilitate movement and positioning. In some cases a specially constructed chair may need to be built and beds joined together to allow the client to sit and sleep in comfort.

Wound infection has been identified as one of the most common complications after surgery. Because of the many layers of flabby skin folds, especially in the abdominal area, the preoperative skin preparation is very important. Frequently, the client is instructed to take several showers a day for a few days prior to hospital admission. Careful cleansing with soap and warm water of the abdominal area from the breasts to below the waist is emphasized.

In order to prevent pulmonary complications after surgery, the client must be instructed on the proper coughing technique, deep breathing, and methods of turning and positioning. The use of a spirometer may be introduced prior to surgery. Since most obese clients breathe shallowly, use of the spirometer will help prevent and alleviate postoperative lung congestion.

All clients will have a nasogastric tube inserted during surgery and attached to suction after surgery. Allowing the client to see a typical tube and telling him why it will be necessary is a good method of involving him in his plan of care and gaining his cooperation. The client should know he will be unable to take oral nourishment for a few days after the surgery and that intravenous fluids will be his main source of intake.

Early ambulation is mandatory for these clients. It is essential the client know that he will usually be expected to get out of bed the night of surgery and with increasing frequency thereafter. The dangers of thrombophlebitis and measures to counteract its development are a routine part of preoperative teaching. He should know that elastic stockings or elastic wraps will be applied to his legs and that active and passive range-of-motion exercises will be a frequent part of his daily care. General preoperative nursing care is discussed in Chap. 6.

Postoperative Care The client will experience considerable abdominal pain. Administration of pain medications should be given as frequently as is necessary during the immediate postoperative period. Since prevention of pulmonary complications is a major nursing goal, it must be anticipated that the client will not fully cooperate if he is having a great deal of discomfort. In addition, the large amount of truncal adipose tissue, especially on the abdomen and chest, will compromise his respiratory ability. Keeping the head of the bed elevated at a 30° angle at all times will facilitate ventilatory efforts. Encouraging and assisting the client to turn, cough, and deep breathe at least every 1 to 2 hours will prevent atelectasis and pneumonia. Frequent mouth and nose care will also help breathing efforts since the nasogastric tube will have been inserted through one nostril.

Position changes and range-of-motion exercises are instituted immediately after surgery and carried out every 1 to 2 hours. Ambulatory efforts are begun the evening of surgery. The nurse should enlist the assistance of other staff during these initial efforts while encouraging the client to help.

The abdominal wound requires frequent observation for amount and type of drainage, condition of the sutures, and signs of infection. The incision must be protected against undue straining that accompanies turning and coughing. Wound dehiscence and wound healing are potential problems with all obese clients. Monitoring the vital signs will assist in identifying problems such as infection.

It is important that the nasogastric tube be kept patent and in the correct position. Vomiting is a common occurrence following gastric bypass and gastric partitioning procedures. If patency is blocked or the tube requires repositioning, the physician should be notified at once. The upper gastric pouch is very small and irrigating the tube with too much solution or manipulating tube position could lead to disruption of the anastomosis or staple line. In most cases, the nasogastric tube can be removed in about 48 hours or when bowel sounds have resumed.

Skin care should be carried out several times each shift. Perspiration may be excessive at times. The many layers of flabby skin should be kept clean and dry so that this source of irritation is eliminated. Clients having jejunoileal bypass encounter severe diarrhea early in their postoperative period. This is due to malabsorption created by surgically shortening the length of the small intestine. Meticulous care of the skin around the anal area and administration of antidarrheal medications must be initiated immediately. Perineal care is important in the client who has an indwelling catheter so that a urinary tract infection is avoided.

Clear liquids will be given orally when tolerance is established. The amount offered at first will necessarily be limited to about an ounce, which is to be sipped slowly. More solid types of food will be given the client having bypass surgery as he progresses through the postoperative recovery period. Clients who have had gastric stapling are kept on a fluid diet in some cases for up to 8 weeks after surgery. The fluid must be of a consistency that can be sipped through a straw. The need for a liquid diet only is based on the rationale that the staple line must be protected from disruption by controlling not only the volume but the consistency of food ingested.[17]

Discharge Teaching Clients who have undergone surgical treatment for their obesity have not been successful in following a prescribed diet. Now they are forced to reduce their oral intake as a result of the anatomic changes brought about by the operative procedure. This is especially so with clients who have had bypasses. These clients find they must adhere to a reduced diet because of their concern for abdominal distension, cramping abdominal pain, increased and foul-smelling flatus, and the need to be near a toilet if food is eaten.[18]

Weight loss will be considerable during the first 6 to 12 months. Most weight is lost by those having intestinal bypass surgery. It is during this period of time that the client must learn to adjust his intake sufficiently to maintain a stable weight. Although behavior modification was not an intended outcome when these surgical procedures were devised, it has become an unexpected secondary gain. The diet generally prescribed should be high in protein, low in carbohydrates, fat, and roughage, and consist of six small feedings daily. Fluids with the meal should be eliminated and in some cases restricted to less than 1000 mL/day. Fluids and foods high in carbohydrate tend to promote diarrhea and symptoms of the dumping syndrome. (The care of the client with dumping syndrome is discussed in the section on postoperative management following gastric surgery for peptic ulcer.)

Vitamin deficiencies are a long-term concern after bypass surgery due to the induced malabsorption and the body's inability to absorb important vitamins such as A, C, D, and B_{12}. Vitamin B_{12} supplements are usually prescribed on a permanent basis because absorption of this vitamin takes place in the ileum. The availability of ileal absorption capacity has been drastically reduced by the surgery for intestinal bypass. The client should be aware of the signs and symptoms of vitamin deficiencies as well as electrolyte imbalances (Table 33-4). It is often necessary to replace iron, calcium, and potassium in order to maintain required physiologic levels.

Diarrhea following intestinal bypass may continue for several years. Some clients still have as many as 6 to 8 stools a day at the end of a year. Proper diet and use of antidiarrheal medications must be clearly understood by the client. Other troublesome problems frequently encountered following intestinal bypass are urinary and biliary stones, polyarthritis, and polymyalgia. Long-term follow-up care must be stressed because of the many complications found late in the recovery period. The client must be encouraged to strictly adhere to the prescribed diet and keep the physician informed of any changes in his physical or emotional condition. Some clients have been known to overeat when they return home and gain rather than lose weight.

Reversal of the surgical procedures may be required for some individuals. Reversal of the gastric bypass is extremely difficult due to the technical nature of the procedure. The jejunoileal bypass can be reversed more easily and has been done for reasons such as hepatic failure, weight loss below ideal weight, debilitating weakness, severe psychiatric problems, intractable electrolyte deficiencies, and pulmonary tuberculosis.[19]

NAUSEA AND VOMITING

Nausea and vomiting are the most common manifestations of gastrointestinal diseases. While each manifestation can occur independently, they are usually closely related and treated as one problem. They are also found in a wide variety of conditions unrelated to gastrointestinal disease. Nausea and vomiting are frequent accompaniments of infectious diseases, central nervous system disorders (e.g., meningitis, central nervous system lesions), circulatory problems (e.g., congestive heart failure), side effects of drugs (e.g., digitalis, antibiotics), metabolic disorders (e.g., uremia), and psychological stimulation (e.g., stress, fear).

Nausea is a feeling of discomfort in the epigastrium with a conscious desire to vomit. Anorexia usually accompanies nausea and is brought on by unpleasant stimulation involving any of the five senses. Generally, nausea occurs prior to vomiting and is characterized by contraction of the duodenum and by slowing of gastric tone and motility.

Vomiting is the forceful ejection of partially digested food from the upper gastrointestinal tract. It occurs when the gut becomes overly irritated, excited, or distended. Immediately before the *act* of vomiting, the person becomes aware of the *need* to vomit. The greatest amount of physiologic changes occur in the stomach and duodenum. In addition, the autonomic nervous system is activated. Sympathetic nervous activation causes tachycardia, tachypnea, and sweating. Parasympathetic activation elicits relaxation of the upper and lower esophageal sphincters, increased gastric motility, and an increase in salivation.[20] These manifestations are experienced immediately preceding the vomiting act.

Vomiting is a complex phenomenon requiring the coordinated activities of several structures including closure of the glottis, deep inspiration with contraction of the diaphragm in the inspiratory position, closure of the pylorus, relaxation of the stomach and cardiac sphincter, and contraction of the abdominal muscles with increasing intraabdominal pressure. These simultaneous activities force the stomach contents up through the esophagus, into the pharynx, and out the mouth. The stomach has a passive role in these activities.

Pathogenesis

Emetic impulses are transmitted to the vomiting center located in the medulla by afferent stimulation of the vagus and sympathetic nervous system. Visceral receptors are located in the gastrointestinal tract, kidneys, heart, and uterus. When irritated, these receptors can stimulate the vomiting center and the vomiting reflex (Fig. 33-6).

In addition, the chemoreceptor trigger zone (CTZ) located on the floor of the fourth ventricle in the brain responds to vestibular impulses associated with motion sickness and chemical stimuli of drugs and toxins. The CTZ then transmits these impulses directly to the vomiting center. Emotions, stress, unpleasant sights and odors, and pain are all capable of triggering vomiting.

Complications of Nausea and Vomiting

When nausea and vomiting are of a prolonged and severe nature, dehydration can rapidly occur. In addition to water loss, essential electrolytes dissolved in body fluids are also lost. As vomiting persists, there may be severe electrolyte imbalances, loss of extracellular fluid volume, decreased plasma volume, and eventually circulatory failure.

Severe nausea and vomiting may precipitate a *metabolic problem* or be the direct result of a metabolic crisis. It is not uncommon to find nausea and vomiting associated with conditions such as uremia, hyperthyroidism, hyper- and hypoparathyroidism, diabetic acidosis, Addison's disease, and hypertensive crisis. When vomiting is severe, metabolic alkalosis results from loss of hydrochloric acid and acids from the extracellular fluids. Metabolic acidosis as a result of severe vomiting is less common than metabolic alkalosis. Acidosis can occur when vomiting contents from the small intestines because of the loss of bicarbonate. Weight loss will be evident within a short time when vomiting is severe.

The threat of *aspiration* is a constant concern when vomiting is severe. This is especially dangerous in the elderly and in the client who is weak and debilitated. In order to avoid this problem, the nurse needs to closely observe and correctly position the client. The client who cannot adequately care for

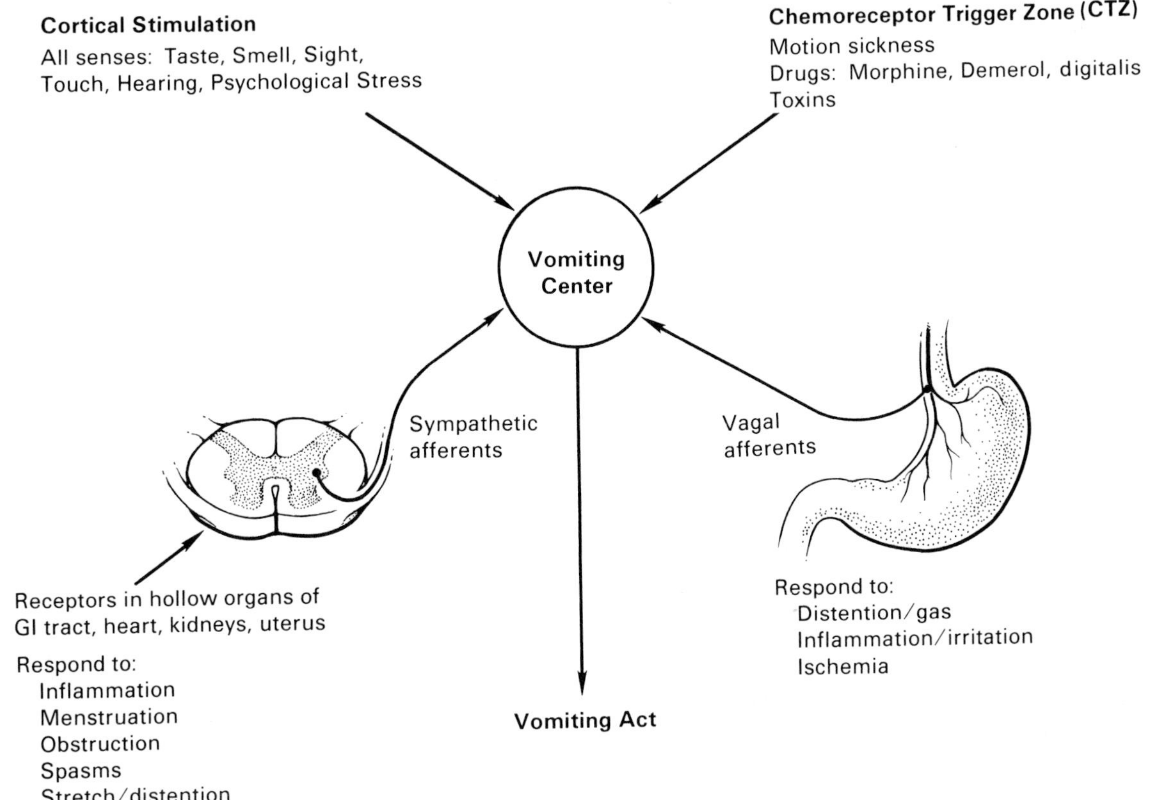

Figure 33-6 Schematic illustration of various stimuli involved in the act of vomiting.

himself should be put in a semi-Fowler's position or side-lying position.

Medical Management

The goals of medical management are to (1) determine and treat the underlying cause of the nausea and vomiting, and (2) provide symptomatic relief for nausea and vomiting. Determining the cause is often difficult because many conditions of the GI tract and disorders of other body systems have nausea and vomiting as presenting manifestations.

A careful history will elicit important information regarding times when the vomiting occurs, what precipitates it, and a description of the contents of the vomitus. A differentiation must be made between vomiting, regurgitation, and projectile vomiting. *Regurgitation* is a process in which partially digested food is slowly brought up from the stomach. *Projectile vomiting* is a very forceful projection of stomach contents without nausea that is characteristic of central nervous system lesions.

The presence of a fecal odor and bile after prolonged vomiting is indicative of intestinal obstruction beyond the pylorus. A functioning ileocecal valve ordinarily prevents the backflow of fecal contents from the colon into the small intestines.

The color of the emesis has value in determining the presence of blood and the location of the blood source. "Coffee ground"-colored vomitus is associated with blood that has remained in the stomach and changed to a dark brown color as a result of its interaction with gastric acid. Bright red blood indicates active bleeding suggestive of a tear in the mucosal lining of the lower esophagus or cardia of the stomach.

Pharmacologic Intervention

The indications for using drugs in the treatment of nausea and vomiting depend on the cause of the problem (Table 33-18). Since the etiology cannot always be readily determined, medications must be used with caution. The use of antiemetics before the cause of the vomiting is established can lead to masking of the underlying disease process and delaying diagnosis and treatment. Drugs inhibiting nausea and vomiting act on the vomiting center, the CTZ, and

Table 33-18
Medications Commonly Prescribed for Relief of Nausea and Vomiting

Classification	Generic Name	Trade Name
Antihistamines	Benzquinamide HCl	Emete-Con
	Cyclizine HCl	Marezine
	Dimenhydrinate	Dramamine
	Diphenhydramine	Benadryl
	Hydroxyzine	Atarax
	Hydroxyzine pamoate	Vistaril
	Meclezine HCl	Antevert
	Promethazine HCl	Phenergan
Phenothiazines	Chlorpromazine	Thorazine
	Perphenozine	Trilafon
	Prochlorperazine	Compazine
	Trifluoperazine	Stelazine
Others	Diphenidol HCl	Vontrol
	Thiethylperazine HCl	Torecan
	Trimethobenzamine HCl	Tigan

peripheral nerves. Antihistamines, phenothiazines, and anticholinergics all have antiemetic properties. These medications are contraindicated for clients with glaucoma, prostatic hypertrophy, pyloric or bladder neck obstruction, and biliary obstruction. They share many common side effects which include dry mouth, hypotension, sedative effects, rashes, and GI disturbances such as constipation.

Nutritional Intervention

Clients with severe vomiting will require intravenous fluid therapy with electrolyte replacement until they are able to tolerate oral intake. In some cases a nasogastric tube and suction may need to be used to decompress the stomach. Once the symptoms have subsided, oral nourishment beginning with clear liquids may be started. Extremely hot or cold liquids are not usually well tolerated. Carbonated beverages at room temperature and with the carbonation gone or warm tea are more easily tolerated. Broth is usually an excellent liquid choice because of its electrolyte content. The addition of dry toast or crackers seems to alleviate the feeling of nausea and helps prevent vomiting.

As the client's condition improves, a diet high in carbohydrate and low in fat foods should be provided. Such items as a baked potato, plain gelatin, cereal with milk and sugar, and hard candy may be added. Foods that are known to be poorly tolerated include coffee, spicy foods, and highly acidic foods. Food should be eaten slowly and in small amounts so that overdistension of the stomach is avoided. Fluids should be taken between meals rather than with meals when solid foods have been reintroduced. It is advised that the client remain quietly relaxed for approximately 1 hour after meals.

Nursing Management (Table 33-19)

An important nursing responsibility relates to client education for those who are at high risk for developing nausea and vomiting. The nurse needs an understanding of the pathophysiology of nausea and vomiting and an awareness of diseases and treatments causing these problems.

Simple explanations of methods for dealing with nausea and vomiting at home can prevent complications and unnecessary discomfort for the client. If the symptoms occur at home, all foods and medications should be stopped until the acute phase is past. If a medication is suspected as the cause, the physician should be notified immediately so that either the dosage can be altered or a new medication can be prescribed. Reminding the client that stopping the drug without consulting the physician may eliminate his immediate nausea and vomiting, but the omission of the prescribed medication may have detrimental effects on his health or disease state over a period of time.

When food is identified as the precipitating cause of nausea and vomiting, the nurse should help the client solve the problem. What food was it? When was it eaten? Has this food caused problems in the past? Is anyone else in the family sick?

If the client believes he can tolerate some foods and fluids, suggestions most helpful would be for him to begin with clear liquids such as warm cola beverages, tea or broth, dry crackers or toast, and then plain Jell-O. Bland foods are generally well tolerated in small amounts. Rest and a relaxed environment free of noxious odors will add to the client's general comfort. An antiemetic drug may be taken only if recommended by the physician. Taking over-the-counter drugs for relief of symptoms may make the condition worse. If nausea and vomiting persist, hospitalization may become necessary to diagnose the underlying etiology.

Hospitalized clients, because of the acute nature of their health problems, are likely to experience episodes of nausea and vomiting. The postoperative client is at high risk due to the surgical procedure, effects of anesthesia, pain, and adverse reactions to medications and treatment. The cancer client may suffer nausea and vomiting as side effects of chemotherapy drugs or radiation treatments. A comprehensive review of nursing care necessary for the client

Table 33-19
Nursing Care Plan for the Client with Nausea and Vomiting

Client Problem	Expected Outcome	Nursing Intervention
Prolonged and persistent vomiting	No nausea and vomiting experienced.	Keep client NPO until able to tolerate foods and fluids by mouth. Monitor amount and type of intravenous fluids. Administer no antiemetic or pain medications unless ordered by physician. Maintain nasogastric tube to low suction if ordered. Maintain accurate I and O records.
Undetermined etiology of nausea and vomiting	Early diagnosis of underlying disease process.	Explain rationale for plan of care and diagnostic tests ordered. Assess relationships between nausea and vomiting with foods, medications, treatment regimen, and psychosocial factors. Routinely test vomitus for bile, blood, and pH. Record amount and frequency of vomitus. Observe for odor and consistency. Notify physician of results and/or changes in vomiting pattern.
Physiologic and emotional distress	Relaxed between episodes of nausea and vomiting.	Offer sympathetic and supportive care. Keep head of bed elevated and avoid sudden changes in position. Remove visual stimuli and source of odors immediately. Provide for mouth care. Change soiled gown and linens. Keep clean emesis basin and tissues within easy reach. Maintain quiet environment, restrict visitors, and avoid unnecessary procedures. Offer reassurance and explanations. Administer antiemetics and pain medications as ordered.
Complications of wound dehiscence, fluid and electrolyte imbalance, dehydration, and aspiration	No complications resulting from nausea or vomiting.	Support abdominal incisions during prolonged and forceful vomiting. Instruct client to take several deep breaths and swallow in order to prevent vomiting. Maintain accurate I and O records. Assess skin tone and turgor for degree of dehydration. Administer IV fluids. Monitor laboratory results of Na, K, Cl. Position conscious client with head of bed elevated. Position unconscious client on side with head dependent. If nasogastric tube in place, check for patency, amount of drainage. Test nasogastric drainage for blood, bile, pH. Provide for frequent mouth care. Remove encrustations around nares. Change tape prn.
Fear of stimulating recurrence of nausea and vomiting	No recurrence of nausea and vomiting.	Encourage client to gradually increase the intake of foods and fluids. Avoid foods implicated as cause of nausea and vomiting. Instruct on a bland diet. Outline instructions or steps to take if nausea and vomiting recurs after going home.

receiving chemotherapy and radiation therapy is found in Chap. 11.

A knowledgeable and understanding nurse can provide the client with emotional and physical support during the critical phase of nausea and vomiting. She can make astute observations and elicit data which will be helpful in determining a diagnosis or a plan of treatment. The nurse should obtain answers to questions such as:

Is there pain or nausea associated with the vomiting?

Does a food or medication precipitate the vomiting?

Is there a particular time of day when the symptoms occur more frequently?

Are there emotional or family problems that bring on the symptoms?

Care of the client is supportive. Nothing by mouth is indicated, including antiemetic drugs, until a thorough evaluation is carried out. Intravenous fluids are administered in order to maintain hydration and fluid and electrolyte balance. A nasogastric tube may be necessary if vomiting is persistent and prolonged. Abdominal surgical incisions must be observed for signs of dehiscence and supported during prolonged and forceful vomiting. Other nursing measures are summarized in Table 33-19.

GASTRITIS

Gastritis is inflammation of the gastric mucosa. It is one of the most common problems affecting the stomach. It has been estimated that approximately 50 percent of adults have mild gastritis during their lifetime.

Types of Gastritis

Gastritis may be acute or chronic and may be diffuse or localized. Table 33-20 lists the types of gastritis.

Acute gastritis is an inflammatory condition that may be the result of ingestion of drugs (e.g., aspirin, digitalis, butazolidin), large amounts of alcohol, contaminated foods (*Staphylococcus* or *Salmonella* organisms), food allergies, and central nervous system lesions. Excesses of spicy, irritating foods and metabolic conditions such as uremia have also been implicated as causing acute gastritis. The symptoms of acute gastritis include anorexia, nausea and vomiting, epigastric tenderness, and a feeling of fullness. Hemorrhage is commonly associated with alcohol abuse and at times may be the only presenting symptom. Acute gastritis is self-limiting, lasting from a few hours to a few days with complete healing of the mucosa expected.

Chronic gastritis has an increasing incidence with age, with most cases occurring after age 50. Chronic irritation and inflammation to the mucosa from repeated alcohol abuse, drugs, stress, and caustic substances can eventually lead to atrophic gastritis and gastric atrophy. Pernicious anemia is known to develop with progressive atrophic gastritis. Symptoms of chronic atrophic gastritis range from an absence of all symptoms to distension, pain, and nausea and vomiting after eating. Misdiagnosis is common since the symptoms are similar to mild indigestion and often go untreated.

Table 33-20

Types of Gastritis

Nonprogressive, usually reversible gastritis

Acute superficial gastritis
Acute erosive gastritis
Gastric erosion
Stress ulcers
Acute hemorrhagic gastritis
Chronic superficial gastritis

Progressive, usually irreversible gastritis

Chronic atrophic gastritis
Gastric atrophy

Miscellaneous gastritis

Corrosive gastritis
Hypertrophic gastropathies
Peptic ulcer

Adapted with permission from R. Hill and F. Kern, *Structure and Function in Disease: The Gastrointestinal Tract*, The Williams & Wilkins Company, Baltimore, 1977, p. 80.

Pathogenesis

There is considerable evidence that gastritis is the result of a breakdown in the normal gastric barrier. Consequently, there is back diffusion of hydrogen and sodium ions from the gastric lumen. The mucosal barrier normally protects the stomach tissue from autodigestion by acid. When the barrier is broken, acid is able to diffuse back into the mucosa, allowing hydrochloric acid to enter and cause injury to small vessels, hemorrhage, and erosion.

Factors that are known to alter the diffusion barrier are chronic alcohol abuse, excess ingestion of aspirin, reflux of duodenal contents after gastric surgery, ischemia, and uremia. The ingestion of two 5-grain tablets of aspirin a day leads to the loss of several milliliters of blood into the gastrointestinal tract in a significant number of susceptible persons.[21] After a severe drinking bout, 75 percent of people will have erosions, petechiae, or hemorrhages in the gastric mucosa. Following some types of gastric surgery, duodenal contents containing bile acids reflux into the stomach and cause gastritis around the gastrojejunal or gastroduodenal stoma.[22]

Progressive gastric atrophy from chronic breakage in the protective mucosal barrier causes the chief and parietal cells to eventually malfunction and disappear. The mucosa then becomes pale, thin, and blue in color as the tiny blood vessels can easily be seen. Not all parts of the stomach are involved to the same degree at the same time.

When the acid-secreting cells do not function, the source of intrinsic factor is lost. Intrinsic factor, which normally combines with vitamin B_{12}, is unavailable and thus B_{12} is not absorbed in the ileum. It is intrinsic factor that protects vitamin B_{12} from digestion by the gastrointestinal enzymes. The body stores of B_{12} in the liver are eventually depleted and a deficiency state exists. Lack of this important vitamin, which is required for growth and maturation of red blood cells, results in the development of pernicious anemia.

The presence of antibodies bound to the parietal cells or freely circulating in the blood has led some researchers to investigate chronic atrophic gastritis as an autoimmune disease. In some instances, there is also cell-mediated immunity against parietal cells.[23] Further research has shown that in relatives of clients with pernicious anemia, the titer of parietal cell antibodies increases with an increasing degree of atrophic gastritis. Cancer of the stomach is closely associated with atrophic gastritis. About 10 percent of clients with achlorhydria develop gastric malignancies.[24]

Medical Management

Diagnostic

Proper diagnosis of gastritis is frequently delayed or completely missed because the symptoms are nonspecific. Endoscopic examination with biopsy must be performed to obtain a definitive diagnosis. Radiographic studies are not helpful since the superficial mucosa is generally involved and changes will not show clearly on x-ray. A complete blood count may demonstrate the presence of anemia from blood loss. Stools are tested for the presence of occult blood. A gastric analysis will demonstrate the amount of hydrochloric acid present, with achlorhydria being a common sign of severe atrophic gastritis. Cytologic examination is done to rule out gastric carcinoma.

Therapeutic

To treat *acute gastritis,* elimination of the cause and its avoidance in the future is generally all that is needed. The plan of care is supportive and similar to that described for nausea and vomiting. Bed rest, nothing by mouth, and intravenous fluids are prescribed. Fluids and electrolytes are replaced according to losses through vomiting and occasionally diarrhea. In severe cases a nasogastric tube and suction may be used. Antiemetics are given for nausea and vomiting. Antacids have proven beneficial in the relief of abdominal discomfort. Clear liquids are resumed when the acute symptoms have subsided with gradual reintroduction of solid, bland foods. Acute gastritis with hemorrhage is treated with transfusion and fluid replacement. Surgical intervention with partial gastrectomy, vagotomy, or pyloroplasty may be necessary if medical treatment fails.

The treatment of *chronic gastritis* focuses on evaluating and eliminating the specific cause (e.g., stop alcoholic intake, abstain from drugs). Pernicious anemia must be treated by regular injections of vitamin B_{12}. (Pernicious anemia is discussed in Chap. 24.) The use of cigarets is contraindicated in all forms of gastritis. An individualized bland diet and use of antacids is recommended.

Nursing Management

Nursing interventions during *acute gastritis* are similar to those described in Table 33-19 for the client with nausea and vomiting. Dehydration can occur rapidly in severe gastritis accompanied by vomiting. Keeping the client NPO, quiet, and monitoring his intravenous fluids is essential. If hemorrhage is considered likely, taking frequent vital signs and testing the emesis for blood is indicated. Elimination of the cause of the gastritis results in rapid improvement in the client's condition. Identification of the causative agent is important to prevent future gastric irritation. A bland diet consisting of six small feedings per day and the use of an antacid after meals will help the client maintain normal gastric function.

The care for the client with *chronic atrophic gastritis* and *gastric atrophy* is also supportive. There is no known cure, although corticosteroids have been somewhat successful in regeneration of parietal cells. With advanced gastric atrophy, vitamin B_{12} injections will be necessary for the lifetime of the individual. Discussion of the continued need for this essential vitamin must be included in the plan of care. The client should also be encouraged to avoid causative factors and follow the prescribed diet and medication regimen. Since the incidence of gastric cancer is higher in clients who have a history of chronic gastritis, especially atrophic gastritis, close medical follow-up should be stressed.

UPPER GASTROINTESTINAL BLEEDING

Etiology and Pathogenesis

While the most serious loss of blood from the upper gastrointestinal (UGI) tract is characterized by a sudden onset, insidious occult bleeding can also be a major problem. The severity of bleeding depends on whether the origin is venous, capillary, or arterial. Suspicion of bleeding from an arterial source may be aroused when the bleeding is profuse and bright red in color. The bright red color indicates the blood has not been in contact with the stomach's acid secretions. In contrast, coffee ground vomitus reveals that the blood and other contents have been in the stomach for some time and have been changed by contact with gastric secretions. This type of bleeding may have come from the slower flow of a venous or capillary origin. Melena (tarry stools) indicates a slow bleed from an upper gastrointestinal source. The darker the color of the stool, the longer the passage of blood through the intestines resulting in further degradation of hemoglobin. Gross melena may occur for 48 to 72 hours after bleeding stops, while occult bleeding may occur up to 8 days after a single bleeding episode.[25]

Discovering the etiology of the bleeding is not always an easy task. There may be a variety of areas in the GI tract involved, as well as many different causes for the blood loss. Table 33-21 lists the common causes of upper gastrointestinal bleeding.

Medication

The overutilization of some medications, either prescribed by the physician or self-administered, have been definitely linked as a cause of UGI bleeding. Clients who take aspirin on a regular basis may be at risk for bleeding episodes.[26] Aspirin and other anti-inflammatory drugs such as phenylbutazone, indomethacin, and corticosteroids can cause irritation and erosion of the gastric mucosa. Erosion into the blood vessels is always a potential danger and a frequent cause of bleeding.

Esophageal origin

Bleeding from an *esophageal source* is most likely the result of chronic esophagitis, esophageal varices, or bleeding from a tear in the mucosa near the esophageal-gastric junction. Chronic esophagitis can be caused by the ingestion of chemicals irritating to the mucosa (e.g., lye) or hot, spicy, irritating foods. Chronic alcohol and cigarette abuse are known irritants to the esophageal mucosa. An incompetent cardiac sphincter which permits reflux of the acidic stomach contents back into the esophagus can lead to chronic irritation and erosion. Severe retching and vomiting have been known to cause a tear in the esophageal mucosa and cause severe bleeding (Mallory-Weiss syndrome). Esophageal varices usually occur secondary to cirrhosis of the liver.

Table 33-21
Common Causes of Upper Gastrointestinal Bleeding

Drug-induced	Salicylates Corticosteroids Phenylbutazone Indomethacin
Esophagus	Esophageal varices Esophagitis Mallory-Weiss Syndrome
Stomach-duodenum	Peptic ulcer disease Stress ulcer Hemorrhagic gastritis Carcinoma Polyps
Systemic diseases	Blood dyscrasias Leukemia Uremia

Branches of the vena cava and azygos veins from the systemic circulation converge with the smaller vessels of the lower esophagus. These vessels are inelastic and become engorged and tortuous due to increased pressure exerted upon them secondary to portal hypertension. Anything that may increase the pressure (e.g., coughing, sneezing, trauma) or result in mechanical irritation (e.g., vomiting) may precipitate a sudden and massive hemorrhage.[27] Esophageal varices are discussed in Chap. 35.

Stomach and duodenal origin

Erosion of a blood vessel by a peptic ulcer located in the *stomach* or *duodenum* must always be considered as a cause of UGI bleeding. Ulcers frequently penetrate through blood vessels. The left gastric artery may be penetrated by a gastric ulcer and the superior pancreaticoduodenal artery by a duodenal ulcer.

Stress ulcers that occur following severe burns, trauma, or major surgery erode more superficial blood vessels than a peptic ulcer but they may also cause bleeding from an eroded blood vessel. Gastritis produced from ingestion of drugs, alcohol, or the reflux of bile contents commonly results in bleeding. Gastric carcinoma can be the cause of a steady blood loss as it grows and ulcerates through the mucosa and blood vessels located within its path. Hematemesis and melena are commonly associated with cancer of the stomach.

Systemic diseases

Systemic diseases (e.g., leukemia, blood dyscrasias) which interfere with normal blood clotting may be a factor that must be considered whenever UGI bleeding occurs.

Medical Management

Even though approximately 75 percent of clients who have massive hemorrhage will stop bleeding spontaneously, the cause must be identified and treatment initiated immediately.

Emergency care and assessment

While a complete history of events leading to the bleeding event is very important in discovering the cause of the blood loss, it should be deferred until emergency care has been initiated. The immediate physical examination must include a systemic evaluation of client condition with emphasis on blood pressure, rate and character of pulse, peripheral perfusion with capillary refill, and the observation for the presence or absence of neck vein distension. Vital signs should be monitored every 15 to 30 minutes. Signs and symptoms of shock must be evaluated and treatment started as soon as possible. (Shock is discussed in Chap. 26.) The client's respiratory status is carefully assessed along with a thorough abdominal examination. The presence or absence of bowel sounds is an important clue in diagnosing the client's condition. A tense, rigid, boardlike abdomen may indicate a perforation and peritonitis.

Laboratory studies will be ordered and will include a complete blood count, blood urea nitrogen, serum electrolytes, blood glucose, prothrombin time, liver enzymes, blood gases, and a type and cross match for possible blood transfusions. All vomitus and stools should be tested for the presence of gross and occult blood. A urinalysis will provide information on the presence of blood in the urine and the specific gravity will give some immediate determination of the client's hydration status.

Therapeutic management

An open intravenous line should be established for fluid and blood replacement. The type and amount of fluids infused is dictated by physical and laboratory findings. It is generally best to begin with an isotonic crystalloid solution (e.g., Ringer's lactate). (The use of volume expanders and blood transfusions is discussed in Chap. 26.) The hemoglobin and hematocrit will not be of immediate assistance in estimating the degree of blood loss, but will provide a baseline for guiding further treatment. The initial hematocrit may be normal and will not reflect the loss until about 4 to 6 hours after fluid replacement has taken place because initially the loss of plasma and red blood cells is equal.

Most clients who are bleeding profusely will have a Foley catheter inserted so urine volume can be accurately assessed on an hourly basis. A central venous pressure (CVP) line may be inserted so that the client's hydration can be monitored more easily. When the client is vomiting blood, a nasogastric tube is indicated. Aspiration of stomach contents through the tube will facilitate the removal of clots from the stomach and alleviate the client's need to vomit.

The use of iced saline lavages into the stomach helps decrease bleeding by causing local vasoconstriction. The amount of iced solution instilled should be no more than 2000 mL/hour. The usual procedure is to instill 100 to 200 mL each time, leave it in place for several minutes, and then aspirate it.[28] The majority of clients bleeding from the stomach will show diminished blood flow in about 30 to 45 minutes using this method.

Diagnostic studies

As soon as the bleeding is under control and the client's condition is more stable (usually within 12 to 24 hours), the exact cause and location of the bleeding should be determined. The most useful diagnostic tools are fiberoptic panendoscopy, angiography, and barium contrast studies.

Fiberoptic Panendoscopy Fiberoptic panendoscopy should be used before either angiography or barium studies. This diagnostic tool is very accurate in identifying the specific source of the bleeding. When performed by a skilled practitioner, bleeding from severe gastritis can be easily distinguished from that of a gastric or duodenal ulcer. The use of the endoscopic examination has been expanded recently by the ability to perform transendoscopic electrocoagulation. In this way bleeding sites can be cauterized locally which prevents the necessity of a surgical procedure. This procedure has proved useful in stopping the bleeding of gastritis, Mallory-Weiss syndrome, bleeding polyps, and gastric ulcer. The use of laser coagulation via endoscopy has also been attempted and holds promise for the future. Only when the endoscopy is unavailable or no skilled operator is at hand should the other diagnostic procedures be utilized.

Angiography Angiography is the next most accurate tool for diagnosing UGI bleeding. It is the most effective procedure when the bleeding is profuse (more than 1 mL/min) and obscures the bleeding site from the endoscope. The procedure is performed by placing a catheter into the left gastric or superior mesenteric arteries and advancing it until the site of bleeding is discovered.

Barium Contrast Studies These studies have less immediate value in the identification of major bleeding sites during the acute phase of treatment. They are of little value if the bleeding is the result of gastritis or a shallow superficial ulcer.

Surgery

Surgical intervention is indicated when bleeding continues regardless of the medical therapy provided. A high percentage of clients are known to have another massive hemorrhage within a 5-year period of time of the first bleeding episode. Some physicans regard surgical therapy as necessary when the client continues to bleed after rapid transfusion of up to 2000 mL of whole blood or the client remains in shock after 24 hours. The choice of operation will be determined by the site of the hemorrhage. In addition, the surgeon must consider the age of the client since mortality rates increase considerably over age 60. It is essential that the operation be performed as soon as possible once the need has been established.

Pharmacologic Intervention

Drug therapy can be started after the bleeding site has been identified and bleeding has slowed or ceased. The drugs most commonly used in the management of UGI bleeding are antacids, histamine H_2 receptor antagonists, and vasopressin. Table 33-22 reviews their mechanism of action in relation to UGI bleeding.

Antacids have long been known to neutralize hydrochloric acid secreted by the stomach parietal cells and therefore are the drugs of choice in the treatment of peptic ulcer. It has only recently been confirmed that antacids help in the healing process as well. Antacids have the ability to neutralize hydrochloric acid, increase the pH of gastric contents to above 5, and therefore inhibit the activation of pepsinogen to pepsin. The most frequently used antacid preparations are magnesium hydroxide, magnesium trisilicate, aluminium hydroxide, calcium carbonate, and sodium bicarbonate (see Table 33-25 later in the chapter). Aluminum hydroxide and magnesium trisilicates are the most useful because they are nonabsorbable. Calcium carbonate and sodium bicarbonate are absorbable and prolonged use can lead to systemic alkalosis.

The neutralizing effects of antacids taken on an empty stomach last only 20 to 30 minutes. When taken after meals the effects may last as long as 3 to 4 hours. After the acute phase of bleeding has diminished from whatever the cause, antacids are generally administered hourly, either orally or through the nasogastric tube. If the tube is in place, the stomach contents should be aspirated and tested for pH periodically. If pH is less than 5, intermittent suction may be employed or the frequency or dosage of the antacid may be increased. Table 33-26 later in the chapter summarizes the adverse reactions seen with antacid therapy. Antacid therapy in relation to ulcer disease is discussed in the section on peptic ulcer disease.

Cimetidine (Tagamet), a histamine H_2 receptor antagonist, is now known to be effective in the control of UGI bleeding from peptic ulcer, esophagitis, or erosive gastritis. This drug inhibits the action of histamine at the H_2 receptors of parietal cells and thereby decreases acid secretion. The neutralizing effects of cimetidine are much longer than regular antacid therapy (lasting up to about 5 hours). Cimetidine is becoming a standard drug in the treatment of peptic ulcers. It has few adverse reactions and has the advantage of being administered orally, intramuscularly, or intravenously.

Vasopressin (Pitressin), which is posterior pituitary extract, can produce vasoconstriction and is used to treat UGI bleeding. When administered intraarterially through the gastric artery, it is effective in controlling bleeding of esophageal varices and erosive gastritis. Since this drug is given through an artery, it is a complex procedure and is not without risk. It should be given with caution to clients with a known history of vascular diseases or hypersensitivity to vasopressin.

Sedatives which are administered for agitation and restlessness should be administered cautiously. They will make accurate assessment of the client's condition more difficult. Anticholinergic drugs are contraindicated in acute UGI bleeding episodes.

Nursing Management

Health promotion and maintenance

While not all cases of UGI bleeding can be anticipated and prevented, the nurse shares responsibility with the physician in trying to identify clients who are at high risk and in carrying out anticipatory guidance. Clients with a history of chronic gastritis or peptic ulcer disease should always be considered in the high-risk category because of the increasing incidence of bleeding associated with chronic irritation or chronic ulcers. Clients who have had one major bleeding episode are very likely to have another within a few years' time. These clients must be instructed to avoid irritating foods, prevent or decrease stress-inducing situations at home or at work, and take only prescribed medications. Over-the-counter medications can be harmful since their contents may include drugs that are contraindicated because of their potential irritating effects on the mucosa. These clients should be instructed on the methods of testing their emesis or stools for the presence of occult blood. Positive results should be promptly reported to the physician or the nurse. Close and frequent follow-up care is very important for all clients diagnosed with ulcers since recurrence rates are high.

The client who requires regular administration of ulcerogenic drugs such as aspirin, corticosteroids, or nonsteroidal anti-inflammatory drugs (e.g., indomethacin) should receive instruction regarding the potential adverse effects they may have on the gastrointestinal mucosa. Enteric coated aspirin tablets can be substituted for regular tablets. Taking the medications at meal times or with snacks will lessen the potential irritating effects. The use of an antacid along with the prescribed anti-inflammatory medication is usually

Table 33-22
Drug Therapy for Gastrointestinal Bleeding

Drug	Source of GI Bleeding	Mechanism of Action
Antacids (see Table 33-25)	Gastric ulcer Duodenal ulcer Hemorrhagic gastritis Esophagitis	Neutralizes acid and maintains gastric pH above 5.5. Elevated pH inhibits the activation of pepsinogen.
Histamine H_2 receptor antagonists (Cimetidine)	Gastric ulcer Duodenal ulcer Esophagitis Hemorrhagic gastritis GI bleeding in cirrhosis	Inhibits the action of histamine at the H_2 receptors of parietal cells and, therefore, decreases acid secretion.
Vasopressin (Pitressin)	Gastroesophageal varices Diverticular disease of the colon Vascular malformation Hemorrhagic gastritis	Vasoconstriction or alteration in splanchnic blood flow decreasing vascular congestion, rupture, and hemorrhage.

Adapted from Norton Greenberger et al., *Drug Treatment of Gastrointestinal Disorders*, Churchill Livingstone, New York, 1978, p. 119.

beneficial. These clients may also be instructed on occult blood tests of emesis and stool and what follow-up measures are necessary if positive results are obtained.

When the nurse is working with the client who has a history of cirrhosis of the liver with esophageal varices, the instructions must be specific regarding the importance of avoiding known irritants such as alcohol and hot, spicy, irritating foods. Even the prompt treatment of an upper respiratory tract infection should be stressed. Severe coughing bouts or sneezing can create increased pressure on the already fragile varices and may result in massive hemorrhage.

Clients who are known to have blood dyscrasias, liver dysfunction, or who are taking cancer chemotherapy drugs have a potential bleeding problem because of the alteration in their normal clotting mechanism. When these clients also have a history of ulcer disease, gastritis, varices, or drug and alcohol abuse, they should be carefully instructed on their disease process and medications and closely observed for potential bleeding.

Acute intervention

The care of the client who is bleeding from an unknown UGI source requires continuous and diligent nursing care and assessment. The client will not be able to provide specific information about the cause of his bleeding until his immediate physical needs are met. An immediate nursing assessment should be performed while getting the client ready for initial treatment. The assessment should include the client's level of consciousness, vital signs, appearance of distended neck veins, skin color, and capillary refill. The abdomen should be checked for distension, guarding, and peristalsis. Immediate determination of vital signs will indicate if the client is in shock from blood loss and will also provide a baseline blood pressure and pulse by which to monitor the progress of treatment. Signs and symptoms of shock include low blood pressure; rapid, weak pulse; increased thirst; cold, clammy skin; and restlessness. Vital signs should be monitored every 15 to 30 minutes and the physician informed of any significant changes.

The client should be approached in a calm and assured manner to help decrease his level of anxiety. Caution should be used before administering sedatives for restlessness as this is one of the warning signs of shock and may be masked by the medication.

Once an infusion has been started, the IV line must be maintained as a vehicle for fluid or blood replacement. An accurate intake and output record is essential so that the client's hydration status can be assessed. Urine output should be measured hourly. A rate of at least 30 mL/hour will provide evidence of adequate renal perfusion. Lesser amounts may indicate renal ischemia secondary to loss of blood volume. Urine specific gravity should be measured as it will give additional information regarding the client's hydration status. Consistent readings greater than 1.025 (normal = 1.005 to 1.025) indicate the urine is very concentrated and that there is probably a low blood volume. The physician needs to be kept informed of these important parameters so that the intravenous solutions can be increased or decreased accordingly. If the client has a central venous pressure line in place, readings must be recorded every 1 to 2 hours. These readings will indicate more accurately the circulating blood volume as it returns to the right heart. Readings below 6 cmH_2O may indicate hypovolemia. Readings of about 15 cmH_2O may indicate that fluid replacement has been administered too quickly or in excess amounts. Elderly clients and those with a history of cardiovascular problems need to be observed closely for signs of fluid overload.

All vomitus and stools must be tested for the presence of blood. It is well to keep in mind that foods such as beets or even swallowed mouthwash can give vomitus a bloody appearance. Unless the contents of the vomitus are checked for occult blood, false information may be recorded. Swallowed blood from a nosebleed must also be accurately noted to avoid misdiagnosis of an UGI bleeding episode. When a nasogastric tube is inserted the nurse must pay special attention to keeping it in proper position and observing the aspirate for blood.

If iced lavages are ordered, the nurse must understand the rationale for this therapy and what results are anticipated. Instillation of approximately 100 to 200 mL at a time into the stomach will generally result in decreased bleeding if the blood is gastric in origin. Instilling too much can increase the client's discomfort, especially if he is already distended. Instilling too small an amount and aspirating too soon will not allow enough time for the cold fluid to cause vasoconstriction in the bleeding area. Charting results of the lavages must be prompt and accurate.

The nurse caring for a client with UGI bleeding should be well informed on what constitutes blood in the stools. Black, tarry stools are not usually associated with a brisk hemorrhage, but do indicate the presence of bleeding of prolonged duration. Bright red blood in the stool is usually from a source in the lower bowel. Menses should be ruled out as a possible source of blood in the stools.

Monitoring the client's laboratory studies will enable the nurse to estimate the effectiveness of therapy. The hemoglobin and hematocrit are usually evaluated every 6 to 8 hours and are accurate in estimating volume lost after rehydration has taken place. Assessing the client's blood urea nitrogen (BUN) level also will provide data on the degree of blood lost, but not for about 24 to 48 hours. The BUN shows the breakdown of blood proteins to urea after they have been absorbed from the gastrointestinal tract.[29] Many clients receive oxygen by mask or nasal prongs so that the circulating blood is assured of an adequate oxygen content. Clients with emphysema should be observed very closely for signs of carbon dioxide narcosis when receiving oxygen. (A further discussion of this problem is found in Chap. 20.)

When oral nourishment is begun, the client is observed for symptoms of nausea and vomiting and a recurrence of bleeding. Feedings are initially either clear fluids or milk and are given hourly until tolerance is determined. These feedings will help to neutralize the gastric secretions and assist in the mucosal repair. Gradual introduction of bland foods will follow if the client exhibits no signs of discomfort.

Antacids are one of the primary medications administered after UGI bleeding. Anticipating the effects of the prescribed preparations can be helpful in providing better care. The nurse should know that preparations containing calcium or aluminum can result in constipation, while those with magnesium cause diarrhea. Although these preparations are nonabsorbable and result in fewer systemic problems, magnesium products must be used with care in clients with renal insufficiency. Administering the antacid preparation accurately and on schedule is important if the stomach pH is to be maintained at a level no lower than 5.

Clients whose hemorrhage was the result of chronic alcohol abuse require close observation for the beginning of delirium tremens as withdrawal from alcohol takes place. Symptoms indicating the beginning of delirium tremens are agitation, uncontrolled shaking, sweating, and vivid hallucinations. (Cirrhosis of the liver is discussed in Chap. 35.)

The client and family need to be taught how to avoid future bleeding episodes. Ulcer disease, drug or alcohol abuse, and liver and respiratory diseases can all result in UGI bleeding. The client and family must be made aware of the consequences of noncompliance with diet and drug therapy. It must be emphasized that no medications (especially aspirin) other than those prescribed by the physician should be taken. Smoking and alcohol should be eliminated as they are a source of irritation and interfere with tissue repair. The client and family should be instructed on what to do if an acute hemorrhage occurs in the future.

PEPTIC ULCER

Peptic ulcer is an erosion of the gastrointestinal mucosa resulting from the digestive action of hydrochloric acid and pepsin. Any portion of the gastrointestinal tract that comes into contact with gastric secretions is susceptible to ulcer development, including the lower esophagus, stomach, duodenum, and the margin of gastrojejunal anastomoses following surgical procedures.

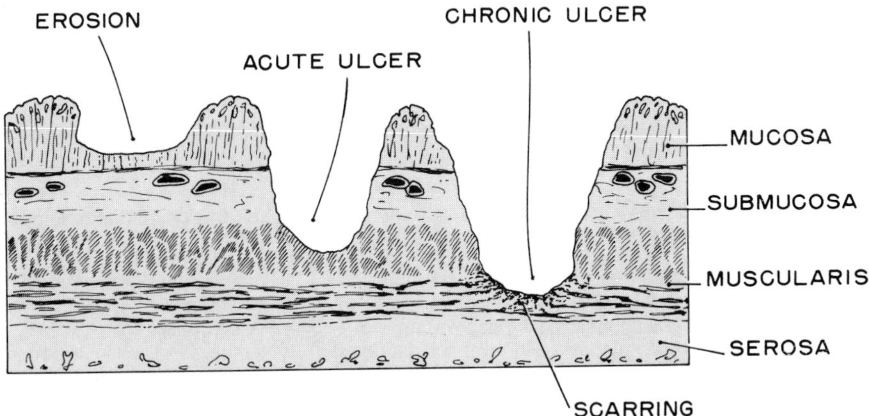

Figure 33-7 Peptic ulcers illustrating an erosion, acute ulcer, and chronic ulcer. Both the acute and chronic ulcer may penetrate the entire wall of the stomach. *(From S. Price and L. Wilson, Pathophysiology Clinical Concepts of Disease Processes, 2d ed., McGraw-Hill Book Company, New York, 1982, p. 220.)*

Types of Ulcers

Peptic ulcers can be classified as *acute* or *chronic*, depending on the degree of mucosal involvement (Fig. 33-7), and *gastric* or *duodenal*, according to location. *Acute* ulcers are associated with superficial erosion and minimal inflammation. They are of short duration and resolve quickly when the cause is identified and removed. A *chronic* ulcer is one of long duration eroding through the muscular wall with the formation of fibrous tissue. They are continuously present for many months, or intermittently present throughout the lifetime of the individual. Gastric and duodenal ulcers, although defined as peptic ulcers, are distinctly different in their etiology, incidence, and treatment (Table 33-23). For these reasons they will be discussed separately.

Gastric ulcers

Although gastric ulcers can occur in any portion of the stomach, they are most commonly found in the antrum. Prior to the beginning of the twentieth century, the incidence of gastric ulcers was more common than duodenal ulcers. They were found predominantly in young women. Since the turn of the century, the incidence of gastric ulcer has decreased and they are now surpassed in incidence by duodenal ulcers by a ratio of 1:10. Gastric ulcers are now found most frequently in men and in the elderly. Although the incidence of gastric ulcer in women is less today than that of men, women continue to have more gastric than duodenal ulcers.

The mortality rate from gastric ulcers is greater than that of duodenal ulcers and is attributed to the fact that the peak incidence occurs between 45 to 54 years of age while the peak incidence of duodenal ulcer occurs a decade earlier. Contrary to common belief, gastric ulcers are not more prevalent among those in executive or managerial positions. Instead, individuals from the lower socioeconomic class and manual or unskilled workers are more prone to gastric ulcers.

Gastric ulcers have been attributed to various factors which lead to acute episodes or to chronic involvement. *Acute gastric lesions* can be precipitated by stressful situations and drugs. The development of *stress ulcers* has been known since the late eighteenth century when they were first described in association with severe body trauma. Later, Curling established the relationship between gastroduodenal ulcers and severe burns. Diffuse superficial lesions including mucosal erosion can be seen in the gastric mucosa within 24 hours after acute burns.[30] Cushing defined ulcers related to central nervous system lesions or trauma. It is now well known that many different major stressors including shock, sepsis, and major traumatic surgery can result in the development of multiple, superficial, acute gastric ulcers.

Drugs that are unwisely prescribed or taken indiscriminately can cause acute gastric ulcers and in some cases can lead to chronic ulcer development. Drugs most often implicated include aspirin, corticosteroids, indomethacin, phenylbutazone, and reserpine. Other known causative factors of gastric ulcer formation are chronic alcohol abuse, smoking, gastritis, and an incompetent pyloric sphincter that allows reflux of duodenal contents back into the stomach.

Table 33-23
Comparison of Gastric and Duodenal Ulcers

	Gastric Ulcer	Duodenal Ulcer
Lesion	Superficial, smooth margins, round, oval, or cone-shaped	Penetrating—associated with a deformity of duodenal bulb from recurrent healing of ulcers
Location of lesion	Antrum predominantly. Also found in body and fundus	First 1–2 cm of duodenum
Incidence	Men and elderly Peak age, 45–54 Number of cases decreasing More common in lower socioeconomic class and in unskilled laborers Increased with smoking, drug, and alcohol abuse, incompetent pyloric sphincter Increased in blood group A Increased in stress ulcers, after severe burns, and head trauma	Younger men. Women equal men after menopause Peak age, 35–45 Number of cases increasing All occupations Increased association with psychosocial pressures. Increased with smoking and alcohol ingestion. Increased in blood group O Increased association with COPD, cirrhosis, pancreatic disease, hyperparathyroidism, Zollinger-Ellison syndrome
Clinical manifestations	Burning or gaseous pressure in high left epigastrium and back Occasional nausea and vomiting Weight loss Pain 1–2 h after meals Pain relieved by food or liquids (if penetrating ulcer, food may aggravate discomfort)	Burning, cramping pressure like pain across midepigastrim Posterior ulcers may cause back pain Pain occurs 2–4 h after meals; midmorning, midafternoon, middle of night Periodic and episodic in nature Pain relief with food Associated with weight gain Occasional nausea and vomiting
Recurrence rate	High	High
Complications	Hemorrhage, perforation, and obstruction	Hemorrhage, perforation, and obstruction

The ingestion of hot, rough, or spicy foods has been suggested as a causative factor but there is no concrete evidence to substantiate this claim.

Research into a genetic cause for ulcers has shown that some members of the same family are more prone to develop gastric or duodenal ulcers. However, evidence is not complete and the ulcer development could just as well be due to the sharing of the same environment. A gastric ulcer personality has not been demonstrated. There is some evidence that individuals having blood group A develope more gastric ulcers than is found in the general population.

The pain associated with gastric ulcer is located high in the epigastrium and occurs spontaneously about 1 to 2 hours after meals. The pain is described as "burning" or "gaseous." The pain can occur either when the stomach is empty or when food has been ingested. If the ulcer has eroded through the gastric mucosa, food will tend to aggravate rather than alleviate the pain. Some persons do not experience any pain until the presence of the ulcer is demonstrated through a serious complication like hemorrhage or perforation.

Duodenal ulcers

Duodenal ulcers account for about 80 percent of all peptic ulcers. While persons susceptible to psychological pressures and anxieties often develop duodenal ulcers, this theory of causation requires more study. It is known that any individual can develop duodenal ulcer regardless of occupation or socioeconomic group. Duodenal ulcers are found more in younger men than women. However, there is evidence that women past the menopause develop ulcers at the same rate as men. This has resulted in a hypothesis that an as yet unidentified endocrine factor offers women protection until menopause.

As with gastric ulcers, some individuals within certain families are more prone to duodenal ulcer formation. Supporting a genetic basis for etiology is the fact that persons with blood group O have an increased incidence of duodenal ulcers.

The development of duodenal ulcers is associated with a high acid secretion by gastric parietal cells. Several diseases have been identified with a high risk of duodenal ulcer development, including chronic obstructive pulmonary disease, cirrhosis of the liver, chronic pancreatitis, hyperparathyroidism, and the Zollinger-Ellison syndrome. A high gastric acid concentration is believed to be the factor common to all these conditions. Alcohol ingestion and heavy smoking habits are also associated with duodenal ulcer formation.

The pain of duodenal ulcer is described as "burning" or "cramplike." It is most often located in the midepigastrium region beneath the xyphoid process. Ulcers located on the posterior aspect of the duodenum can be manifested by back pain. The pain usually occurs 2 to 4 hours after meals and is relieved by food, milk, or antacids which neutralize and dilute the gastric acid. A characteristic of duodenal ulcer is its tendency to occur continuously for a few weeks or months and then disappear for a period of time only to recur some months later. This course of events usually last the entire life span of the ulcer.

Pathogenesis of Peptic Ulcers

Protein digestion can only take place in an acid environment. Hydrochloric acid is secreted by the parietal cells at a pH of 0.8. After mixing with the stomach contents the pH reaches 2 to 3, a highly favorable range of acidity for pepsin activity. Pepsinogen, the precursor of pepsin, is activated to pepsin in the presence of hydrochloric acid and a pH of 2 to 3. The pain associated with both gastric and duodenal ulcers is attributed to (1) spasm of the smooth muscle in the damaged area, and (2) the bathing of the eroded area by hydrochloric acid. When the stomach acid level is neutralized by the presence of food or antacids, the pH of hydrochloric acid is increased to 3.5 or greater. At a pH of 3.5 or more, pepsin has little or no proteolytic activity and soon becomes inactive.

Peptic ulcers develop only in the presence of an acid environment. Hydrochloric acid and pepsin must be present for normal digestion to take place in the stomach. The typical individual with a gastric ulcer has normal to less than normal gastric acidity compared to the person with a duodenal ulcer. However, intraluminal acid does seem to be essential for a gastric ulcer to occur since it has been well established that clients with pernicious anemia and achlorhydria rarely get gastric ulcers. In addition, inhibition of gastric acid secretion by histamine H_2 receptor antagonists accelerates the healing of benign gastric ulcers.[31]

The stomach is normally protected from autodigestion by the gastric mucosal barrier. The gastrointestinal tract has a very high cell turnover rate and the surface mucosa of the stomach is renewed about every 3 days. As a result of this high turnover rate, the mucosa can continually repair itself except in extreme instances when the cell breakdown surpasses the cell renewal rate. Normally, water, electrolytes, and water-soluble substances (e.g., glucose) can pass easily through the barrier. However, the mucosal barrier prevents the back diffusion of acid from the gastric lumen through the mucosal layers to the underlying tissue.

Under specific circumstances the mucosal barrier can be impaired and back diffusion of acid can occur. When the barrier is broken, hydrochloric acid enters the mucosa and causes injury to the tissues.[32] This results in cellular destruction and inflammation. Histamine release in the damaged mucosa causes vasodilatation and increased capillary permeability. The histamine further stimulates acid secretion which will in turn stimulate pepsin secretion.[33]

A variety of agents are known to destroy the mucosal barrier. It is estimated that 5 to 10 percent of all gastric ulcers are drug-induced. Ulcerogenic drugs such as aspirin can inhibit mucous synthesis and cause abnormal permeability. Corticosteroids have the ability to decrease the rate of mucus cell renewal and thereby decrease its protective effects. Cytotoxic drugs which are lipid-soluble can pass through the barrier and destroy it. Other drugs with aspirinlike actions are nonsteroidal anti-inflammatory drugs such as phenylbutazone and indomethacin.

When the mucosal barrier is disrupted, there is a compensatory increase in blood flow. When the increase is sufficient to dilute, buffer, and remove the excess, tissue damage may be minimal or result in no injury at all.[34] Figure 33-8 is a diagrammatic representation of the interrelationship between the mucosal blood flow and disruption of the gastric mucosal barrier.

While gastric ulcers are characterized by a normal to low secretion of gastric acid, the back diffusion of acid is greater with chronic gastric ulcers than that found with duodenal ulcers or in the normal person. Therefore the critical pathophysiologic process in gastric ulcer formation may not be the amount of acid

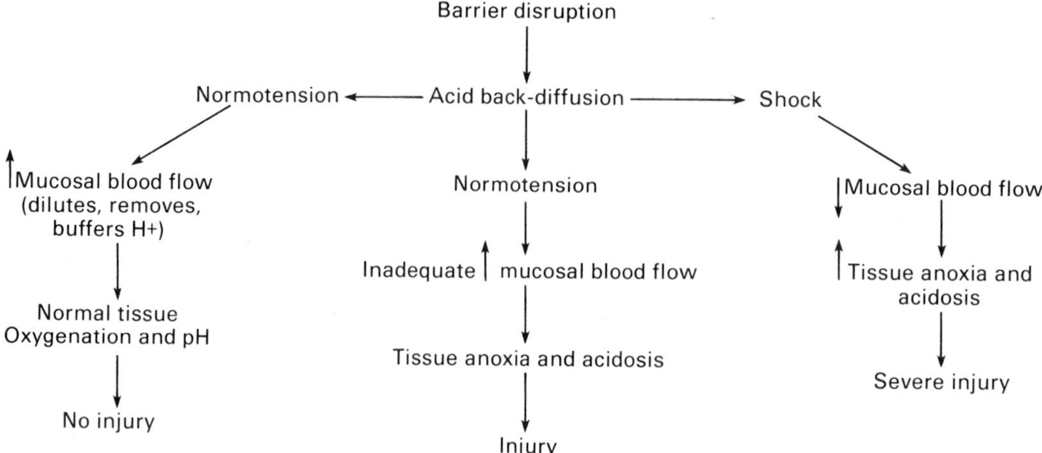

Figure 33-8 Diagrammatic representation of the interrelationship between mucosal blood flow and disruption of the gastric mucosal barrier. (*Adapted from P. H. Guth, "Gastric Mucosal Blood Flow and Resistance to Injury," Advances in Ulcer Disease, Excerpta Medica, 1980, Amsterdam-Oxford-Princeton, p. 107.*)

that is secreted, but the amount that is able to penetrate the mucosal barrier.

Increased vagal nerve stimulation from a variety of causes including emotions causes hypersecretion of hydrochloric acid and pepsin. Increased concentrations of acid can alter the mucosal barrier. Duodenal ulcers are associated with high acid content. Since individuals with duodenal ulcers are prone to the effects of emotional stressors, this may be one reason why acid levels are above normal. It has been suggested that the continual response of the parietal cells to maximal stimulation results in hyperplasia of the cell mass. There is also an increase in gastrin levels in most persons with duodenal ulcer.

Complications of Peptic Ulcer

The three major complications of chronic peptic ulcer disease are hemorrhage, perforation, and gastric outlet obstruction. All of these are considered emergency situations and are initially treated by conservative medical management. However, surgery may be necessary at any time during the course of the therapy.

Hemorrhage

Hemorrhage is the most common complication of peptic ulcer disease. It develops from either erosion of the granulation tissue found at the base of the ulcer during healing or from erosion of the ulcer through a major blood vessel. Duodenal ulcers account for a greater percentage of UGI bleeding than gastric ulcers. For the care of the client with bleeding peptic ulcer refer to the section on UGI bleeding.

Perforation

Perforation is considered the most lethal complication of peptic ulcer. Perforation is commonly seen in large penetrating duodenal ulcers that have not healed and are located on the posterior mucosal wall (Fig. 33-9). Even though duodenal ulcers are more prevalent and perforate more frequently, mortality rates are higher following perforation of gastric ulcers. The older age of the client with gastric ulcers who often has other concurrent medical problems is thought to be the crucial factor. Another possible explanation for this higher mortality rate is that there is a larger population of gastric bacteria found in the hypochlorhydric stomach of gastric ulcer clients. When the stomach perforates, these bacteria may cause intraperitoneal septic complications.

Perforation of a peptic ulcer occurs when the ulcer penetrates through the serosal surface with spillage of either gastric or duodenal contents into the peritoneal cavity. The size of the perforation is directly proportional to the length of time the client has had the ulcer. The larger the perforation, the longer the history of the ulcer. Small perforations will seal themselves and result in a cessation of symptoms while larger perforations require immediate surgical closure. Spontaneous sealing occurs as a result of large amounts of fibrin being produced in response to the perforation. This leads to fibrinous fusion of the duodenum or gastric curvature to adjacent tissue, mainly the liver.

The clinical manifestations of perforation are characterized by their sudden and dramatic onset. The client suffers sudden, severe upper abdominal pain that quickly spreads throughout the abdomen. Shoulder pain may be experienced if the spillage causes irritation to the phrenic nerve. The abdominal muscles are contracted so that they appear rigid and boardlike in an attempt to protect the abdomen from further injury. The client's respirations become shallow and rapid. Bowel sounds are usually absent. Nausea and vomiting may occur but are generally absent. Most clients present with a history of ulcer disease or recent symptoms of indigestion.

The contents entering the peritoneal cavity from the stomach or duodenum contain a variety of ingredients including air, saliva, food particles, hydrochloric acid, pepsin, bacteria, bile, and pancreatic juices. A bacterial peritonitis will occur within 5 to 6 hours followed by paralytic ileus. The intensity of the peritonitis is proportional to the amount and duration of the spillage through the perforation. It is difficult to determine from the sudden onset of symptoms whether gastric or duodenal ulcer is the cause, since the clinical characteristics of perforation are the same. For the care of the client with acute abdomen and peritonitis refer to Chap. 34.

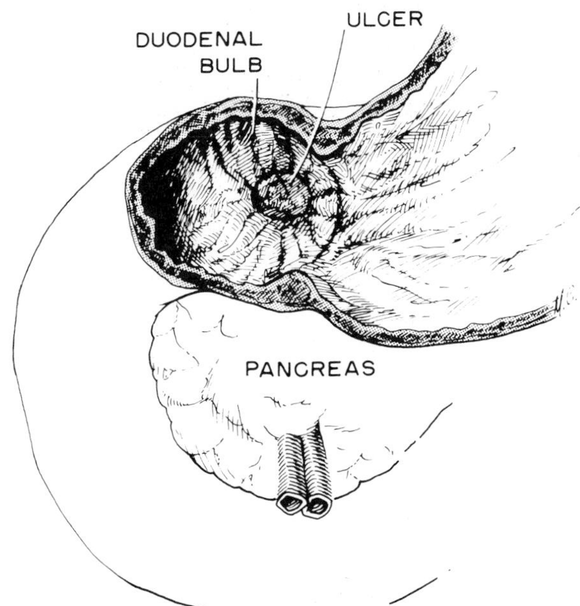

Figure 33-9 Duodenal ulcer of the posterior wall penetrating into the head of the pancreas, resulting in a walled-off perforation. (*From S. Price and L. Wilson, Pathophysiology: Clinical Concepts of Disease Processes, 2d ed., McGraw-Hill Book Company, New York, 1982, p. 224.*)

Gastric outlet obstruction

The most common cause of gastric outlet obstruction is due to duodenal ulceration. At times ulcers located in the antrum, pre-pyloric, and pyloric region may also cause obstruction. In the early phase of obstruction (often referred to as the *compensated phase*), gastric emptying is normal to near normal. This phase may be associated with large peristaltic waves. Over a period of time the excessive peristalsis will create hypertrophy of the stomach wall. After long-standing obstruction, the stomach enters the *decompensated phase*, which results in dilatation and atony. It must be understood that the obstruction is not totally due to fibrous scar tissue because active ulcer formation is associated with edema, inflammation, and pylorospasm, which all contribute to the narrowing of the pylorus.

The client with gastric outlet obstruction generally presents with a long history of ulcer pain. Ulcerlike pain of short duration or complete absence of pain is more indicative of a malignant obstruction. The pain progresses to a more generalized upper abdominal discomfort that becomes more uncomfortable toward the end of the day as the stomach fills and dilates. Relief may be obtained by belching or by self-induced vomiting. Vomiting is very common and often projectile. The vomitus contains food particles that were ingested many hours or even a day or two prior to the vomiting episode. There is often an offensive odor if the contents have been dormant in the stomach for a period of time. If the individual vomits frequently, he will be anorexic with evident weight loss, thirsty, and have an unpleasant taste in his mouth. Constipation is a common complaint that usually results from dehydration and lack of roughage in the diet.

The client with gastric outlet obstruction may show a swelling in the upper abdomen, indicating dilatation of the stomach. Loud peristalsis can be heard and visible peristaltic waves are often observed passing across the abdomen from left to right. If the stomach is grossly dilated, it is possible to palpate it as well.

An upper GI using barium as contrast media is helpful in determining a diagnosis and will demonstrate the presence of an active ulcer crater or scarring from previously healed ulcers. Barium normally should pass from the stomach within 2 hours, but with gastric outlet obstruction 50 percent of the barium will remain on follow-up films up to 6 hours later.

Abnormal Diagnostic Findings

The diagnostic measures utilized to determine the presence and location of peptic ulcer are similar to those discussed with acute UGI bleeding. *Fiberoptic gastroscopy* and *duodenoscopy* are the procedures most often utilized. They are more reliable than barium contrast studies because of the maneuverability of fiberoptic scopes in viewing the entire gastric and duodenal mucosa. These procedures can also be used to determine the degree of ulcer healing after treatment. When gastric malignancy is a possibility, the endoscope can be used in obtaining tissue specimens for biopsy.

Barium contrast studies, although widely used, are not accurate in identifying shallow, superficial ulcers due to failure of the barium to properly fill the ulcer crater. X-ray studies are also ineffective in differentiating a peptic ulcer from a malignant ulcer. Malignant ulcers seldom heal or do so to a degree that will satisfy x-ray study. In addition, x-rays will not readily demonstrate the degree of healing that can be visually determined with the endoscope. Barium studies are of benefit in diagnosing pyloric obstruction due to recurrent ulcers.

Exfoliative cytology is a valuable test when there is need to distinguish between a benign and malignant ulcer. The test consists of examining exfoliated cells that are found in various body secretions or scraped from mucous membranes. A sample of these cells can be obtained during gastroscopic exam. While the accuracy of this examination for determining the presence of a gastric tumor has proven value, it should not stand alone as a diagnostic tool because of the danger of false results.

Gastric analysis has questionable value in the diagnosis of clients suspected of peptic ulcer disease because many clients have normal rates of gastric secretions. However, it can provide important data in (1) identifying clients with a possible gastrinoma (Zollinger-Ellison syndrome), (2) determining the amount of gastric hyperacidity, and (3) evaluating the results of therapy such as vagotomy. Several methods may be used to determine the amount of gastric secretions. A nasogastric tube may be placed into the antrum using fluoroscopy and the secretions collected overnight for a 12-hour period of time. The hydrochloric acid concentration is calculated and compared to equivalents already established for individuals who are ulcerfree, those with gastric and duodenal ulcers, and those with Zollinger-Ellison syndrome. The accuracy of this method is not good since the nasogastric tube may become plugged or aspiration methods may be inconsistent. Augmented histamine or pentagastrin stimulation may be more accurate in estimating the degree of acid secretion. In these tests the stomach's ability to secrete gastric juice is studied after being stimulated by either histalog or pentagastrin.

Laboratory analysis including a complete blood count, urinalysis, liver enzyme studies, and stool examination should be performed. The CBC may indicate the presence of anemia secondary to bleeding from the ulcer. The liver enzyme studies will help to determine any liver problems such as cirrhosis which may complicate the treatment of the ulcer. The urine and stool are routinely tested for the presence of blood.

Medical Management (Table 33-24)

Conservative management

When the client's clinical manifestations and medical history suggest the diagnosis of a peptic ulcer and diagnostic studies confirm its presence, a medical regimen is instituted. The regimen consists of adequate rest, dietary interventions, medications, the elimination of smoking, and long-term follow-up care. The aim of the treatment program is to decrease the amount of gastric acidity and minimize its harmful effects on the mucosa. Hospitalization of the client is not always necessary during the initial treatment phase.

Adequate rest, both physical and emotional, is very important in the treatment process. A quiet, restful environment at home or on the job is not easy to achieve and may require some modification in the client's daily routine. The benefits derived from the elimination of stressors will help to decrease the stimulus for overproduction of gastric secretions. Moderation in daily activity is essential. Excessive physical activity can result in increased gastric secretions through increased motor activity.

Dietary changes will be necessary so that foods and beverages irritating to the client can be avoided or eliminated. An individualized bland diet consisting of six small meals a day is usually prescribed in the regimen. (Diet therapy is discussed under dietary interventions.)

Medications are a vital part of therapy. The client must be well informed on each drug prescribed, why it is ordered, and the expected benefits. Strict adherence to the prescribed regimen of drugs is mandatory. Drug therapy which includes the use of antacids, histamine H_2 receptor antagonists, and anticholinergics will be presented in the section on pharmacologic intervention.

Smoking, while not directly implicated as a cause of peptic ulcer, has an irritating effect on the mucosa, increases gastric motility, and delays mucosal healing. It should be eliminated completely or severely reduced. The combination of adequate rest and the abstinence from smoking has been shown to accelerate ulcer healing.

The healing of a peptic ulcer requires many weeks of therapy. During the healing process, pain disappears after 3 to 6 days but ulcer healing is much slower. About 50 percent of ulcers are healed in 3 weeks, 75 percent in 6 weeks, and 90 percent in 9 weeks.[35] Healing of the ulcer should be assessed using x-ray studies or endoscopic examination. Barium contrast films can be used to measure adequately the healing of a gastric ulcer. However, the endoscope is the only accurate measure of healing of a duodenal ulcer.

Since recurrence of peptic ulcer is frequent, interruption of therapy or discontinuance of therapy could have detrimental results. The client must be encouraged to comply with therapy and continue with follow-up care for at least 1 year. If changes in lifestyle were part of the prescribed therapy, they should be maintained. Antacid and cimetidine are usually stopped after the ulcer has healed. No other medications, unless prescribed by the physician, should be taken since they may have an ulcerogenic effect. Finally, the client and family should be told what to do in the event pain and discomfort recur or if blood is noted in the vomitus or stools.

Acute exacerbation

The recurrence rates for both gastric and duodenal ulcers is high following medical treatment. The client with an acute exacerbation of peptic ulcer can usually be treated with the regimen already outlined under conservative management. However, care of the client is considered a more serious situation due to the chronicity of the ulcer and the possible complications of perforation, hemorrhage, or obstruction.

An acute exacerbation is frequently accompanied by bleeding, increased pain and discomfort, and nausea and vomiting. Symptom relief is achieved by the placement of a nasogastric tube into the stomach with intermittent suction for about 24 to 48 hours. The rationale is to keep the stomach empty and remove any stimulus for hydrochloric acid and pepsin secretion.

If there is a history of an incompetent pyloric sphincter allowing reflux of duodenal contents back into the stomach, maintaining an empty stomach will decrease the stimulus for pancreatic enzyme secretion as well. This period of stomach rest eliminates any causative factors that may have precipitated the acute exacerbation and permits the resolution of edema and inflammation of the mucosa. Fluids and electrolytes are replaced by intravenous infusion until the client is able to tolerate oral feedings without distress.

Blood or blood products may be administered if bleeding has occurred. Careful monitoring of the vital signs, intake and output, laboratory studies, and signs of impending shock are important during this acute episode.

Endoscopic examination is performed as soon as possible to determine the condition of the mucosa. Visual inspection will reveal the degree of inflammation or bleeding as well as the ulcer location. It is important to ascertain the presence of a pre-pyloric or pyloric ulcer that might cause gastric outlet obstruction.

When endoscopic examination reveals no major problems and the client's physical condition stabilizes, the plan of care for the client should follow the

Table 33-24
Medical Management: Peptic Ulcer

Diagnostic

1. Complete blood count
2. Urinalysis
3. Liver enzymes
4. Serum electrolytes
5. Fiberoptic gastroscopy and duodenoscopy
6. Upper GI barium contrast study
7. Gastric analysis
8. Exfoliative cytology

Therapeutic

A. Conservative management
   1. Adequate rest
   2. Bland diet (six small meals a day)
   3. No smoking
   4. Medications
      a. Antacids
      b. Cimetidine
      c. Anticholinergics
   5. Stress reduction

B. Acute exacerbation without complications
   1. NPO
   2. Nasogastric suction
   3. Bed rest to moderate light activity
   4. No smoking
   5. Intravenous fluid replacement
   6. Medications
      a. Antacids
      b. Cimetidine
      c. Anticholinergics
      d. Sedatives

C. Acute exacerbation with complications (hemorrhage, perforation, obstruction)
   1. NPO
   2. Nasogastric suction
   3. Bed rest
   4. Intravenous fluid replacement (whole blood, packed red blood cells, Ringer's lactate)
   5. Iced saline lavages for hemorrhage

D. Surgical intervention
   1. Perforation—simple closure with omentum graft
   2. Gastric outlet obstruction—pyloroplasty and vagotomy
   3. Ulcer cure
      a. Billroth I and II
      b. Vagotomy and pyloroplasty

same regimen of diet, rest, and medications as described with conservative management. A 5-year follow-up program is recommended following acute exacerbation. An increase in the healing rate will be achieved following conservative treatment, but the treatment plan cannot prevent scar formation which can result in gastric outlet obstruction. Approximately 42 to 88 percent of ulcers recur. Duodenal ulcers recur at a rate of 80 to 83 percent.[36]

Perforation

The immediate focus of medical management of a client with a perforation is to stop the spillage of gastric contents into the peritoneal cavity and restore blood volume. In order to halt spillage through the perforation, a nasogastric tube is inserted into the stomach. This will provide continuous aspiration and gastric decompression. Although duodenal aspiration is not achieved as promptly, the placement of the tube as near to the perforation site as possible will facilitate decompression.

Circulating blood volume must be replaced using lactated Ringer's and albumin solutions. These solutions will substitute for the fluids lost from the vascular and interstitial space as the peritonitis develops. Blood replacement in the form of packed red blood cells may be necessary. Unless contraindicated, a CVP line and Foley catheter should be inserted and monitored hourly. Clients with a history of cardiac disease require electrocardiogram monitoring. Broad-spectrum antibiotic therapy should be started immediately to treat the bacterial peritonitis. Administration of pain medications will provide for client comfort.

The medical regimen may be all that is required for some clients whose perforation seals spontaneously. When the perforation cannot be corrected by conservative medical management, surgical closure must be carried out as soon as blood volume is restored. It is generally believed that clients with uncorrected hypovolemia should not be subjected to any surgical procedure for approximately 12 hours. This length of time is viewed as sufficient to adequately initiate decompression measures, restore lost blood volume, and stabilize the client's condition.

The operative procedure involving the least risk to the client is simple oversewing of the perforation and reinforcement of the area with a graft of omentum. The peritoneal cavity is suctioned of the excess gastric contents during the surgical procedure. Prior to surgical closure some surgeons will instill an antibiotic solution into the abdominal cavity to help counteract the peritonitis.

There is controversy regarding the need for more definitive surgical treatment of a perforated ulcer than can be achieved by simple closure. Other types of surgical procedures used depend on the location of the peptic ulcer and the surgeon's preference. If cure of the ulcer is the ultimate goal, the surgical procedures may include gastric resection or vagotomy and pyloroplasty.

Gastric outlet obstruction

The aim of therapy for gastric outlet obstruction is to decompress the stomach, correct any existing fluid and electrolyte imbalances, and improve the client's general state of health. A nasogastric tube is inserted into the stomach and attached to continuous suction in order to remove excess fluids and undigested food particles. By continuous decompression for several days the stomach has the opportunity to regain its normal muscle tone, the ulcer can begin healing, and the inflammation and edema will subside.

The tube will be clamped after several days of suction and gastric residue is measured periodically. The frequency and amount of time the tube remains clamped is proportional to the amount of aspirate obtained and the comfort level of the client. A method commonly followed is to clamp the tube overnight for approximately 8 to 12 hours and measure the gastric residue in the morning. When the aspirate falls below 200 mL, it is considered to be within a normal range and safe to allow the client to begin oral intake with clear liquids. Initially, oral fluids are begun with 30 mL/hour and then gradually increased in amount. The client must be watched carefully for signs of distress or vomiting. As the amount of gastric residue decreases, solid foods may be added and the tube is removed.

Intravenous fluids and electrolytes are administered according to the degree of dehydration, vomiting, and electrolyte imbalance indicated from laboratory studies. Pain relief will result from the decompression measures and analgesics are usually not necessary. Drugs such as anticholinergics are not recommended with gastric outlet obstruction because they reduce gastric motility and gastric emptying. Antacid and cimetidine therapy are an integral part of treatment if the obstruction has been determined to be the result of an active ulcer on endoscopic examination. Surgical intervention may be necessary to remove scar tissue. (Surgical procedures are discussed later in this chapter.)

Pharmacologic Intervention

Antacids

Antacids are the initial drug of choice in the treatment of peptic ulcers. They decrease gastric

Table 33-25
Composition of Antacid Preparations

Ingredient	Trade Name
Single Substance	
Aluminum carbonate	Basaljel
Aluminum hydroxide gel and tablets	Amphojel
Aluminum phosphate	Phosphaljel
Calcium carbonate	Titralac
Dihydroxyaluminum aminoacetate	Robalate
Dihydroxyaluminum sodium carbonate	Rolaids
Magaldrate	Riopan
Magnesium carbonate	Magnesium Carbonate
Magnesium hydroxide	Magnesium Hydroxide
Mixtures of Aluminum Hydroxide and Magnesium Salts	
	Aludrox
	A-M-T
	Bidrox
	Cremalin
	Delcid
	Gaviscon
	Gelusil and Gelusil M
	Maalox
	Mylanta
	Trisogel
	WinGel
Mixtures of Calcium Carbonate, Aluminum and Magnesium Hydroxide	
	Camalox
	Ducon
Mixtures of Calcium Carbonate, Magnesium Carbonate, and Magnesium Trisilicate	
	Tums

acidity and the acid content reaching the duodenum. By raising the pH level to above 3.5, antacids effectively inactivate pepsin's proteolytic activity.

Antacids consist of both systemic and nonsystemic types. Systemic antacids such as sodium bicarbonate are very soluble and are absorbed into circulation. Their long-term use can lead to systemic alkalosis and, therefore, they are rarely used in ulcer treatment. The nonsystemic antacids are insoluble and poorly absorbed. The common commercial nonsystemic antacids consist of calcium carbonate, magnesium hydroxide, or aluminum hydroxide as single preparations or in various combinations (Table 33-25).

The type of preparation may be liquid or tablet. The tablet form requires a large number of tablets to equal the same dose of a liquid preparation. Since the tablets are chewable much of the medication is left coating the teeth and gums instead of the stomach.

It has long been recognized that antacids ingested on an empty stomach are quickly evacuated and only partially utilized. Since their duration of action is only about 30 minutes, best results are obtained when they are prescribed 1 and 3 hours after meals and at bedtime. More frequent administration has resulted in poor tolerance and reduced long-term compliance.

The physician must consider the type and dosage of antacid prescribed because of the adverse effects some of them have on the client's health status or on other medications he might be taking (Table 33-26). Preparations high in sodium such as Titralac, Di-gel, and Amphojel should be used with caution in the elderly and clients with cirrhosis of the liver, hypertension, congestive heart failure, and renal disease. Magnesium preparations should not be prescribed for clients in renal failure because of the risk of magnesium toxicity. The most frequent side effect experienced with magnesium antacids is diarrhea. Aluminum hydroxide causes constipation. The combination of aluminum and magnesium salts seems to lessen the side effects of both.

Antacids have the capacity to interact unfavorably with some medications. They can enhance the absorption of drugs such as dicumarol and amphetamines. The action of digitalis preparations can be potentiated when taken in combination with calcium or magnesium antacids. In some instances antacids may decrease the absorption rates of prescribed drugs.[37] Therefore, it is important to inform the physician of any drugs that are being taken before antacid therapy is begun.

Table 33-26
Adverse Side Effects of Antacid Therapy

Antacid	Reactions
Aluminum hydroxide gels	1. Constipation 2. Phosphorus depletion with chronic use
Calcium carbonate	1. Constipation or diarrhea 2. Hypercalcemia 3. Milk-alkali syndrome 4. Renal calculi
Magnesium preparations	1. Diarrhea 2. Hypermagnesemia 3. Phosphorus depletion syndrome
Sodium preparations	1. Milk alkali syndrome if used with large amounts of calcium 2. Sodium toxicity if on sodium restrictions

The dosage of antacid must often be adjusted by the physician so that the amount prescribed has the capacity of neutralizing the acid present.[38] Alterations such as these must be carefully communicated to the client and family. The adjustment of antacids by the client must be avoided. Taking too much or too little of an antacid can compromise its effectiveness and may lead to unpleasant side effects or an increase in ulcer discomfort.

Compliance with long-term antacid therapy seems to diminish with time. The client fails to take the correct dose or stops taking the drug altogether. Many people stop therapy because they find it inconvenient to keep the necessary daily supply at work, when traveling, or even at home. For some clients it is embarrassing to be seen taking medications generally known to be prescribed for people with ulcers.

Histamine H_2 receptor antagonist

The development of a histamine H_2 receptor antagonist, cimetidine (Tagamet), is looked upon as one of the major advances in the treatment of peptic ulcer. Histamine is believed to be the final intracellular activator of hydrochloric acid secretion. Commonly used antihistamine drugs have no effect on gastric acid secretion. Cimetidine blocks the action of histamine on the H_2 receptors and thus reduces hydrochloric acid secretion. It also accelerates ulcer healing.

Several advantages of cimetidine are that it (1) has few unpleasant side effects; (2) may be administered orally, IV, or IM; and (3) has therapeutic effects for up to 5 hours' duration. The most common side effects are diarrhea, fatigue, dizziness, drowsiness, rash, and gynecomastia.

Anticholinergic drugs

Anticholinergic drugs are often ordered in the treatment of peptic ulcer disease. These drugs decrease cholinergic stimulation of gastric secretions. There is divided opinion on their efficacy in preventing recurrences and their therapeutic effects on alleviating symptoms and preventing complications. Because of their tendency to decrease gastric motility, they should be avoided in gastric ulcer where stasis of secretions will increase the client's pain and discomfort. Their use is associated with a high incidence of side effects such as dry mouth and skin, flushing, thirst, tachycardia, dilated pupils, blurred vision, and urine retention. Anticholinergics must be prescribed with caution in clients with narrow-angle glaucoma, prostatic hypertrophy, and gastric outlet obstruction. It has been predicted that the use of anticholinergics may decline as a result of the histamine H_2 receptor antagonists. Commonly prescribed anticholinergic medications are listed in Table 33-27.

Table 33-27
Anticholinergic Drugs Used in the Treatment of Peptic Ulcer

Trade Name	Generic Name
	Atropine sulfate
Banthine	Methantheline bromide
Bentyl	Dicyclomine HCl
Cantil	Mepenzolate bromide
Daricon	Oxyphencyclimine
Donnatol	Belladonna and phenobarbital
Probanthine	Propantheline bromide
Robinul	Glycopyrolate

Dietary Intervention

There are no specific diets or foods that are totally useful in treating peptic ulcer disease. The client is encouraged to eat as normally as possible. If he is aware that certain foods result in pain or discomfort, they should be avoided. The critical aspect is individualization of the dietary plan.

Food acts as a buffer for gastric secretions. The buffering action of food lasts about 60 minutes and is then followed by an increase in the concentration of acid in the secretions. Dietary orders vary according to the preference of the physician, but there is general agreement that foods eaten should be those well tolerated by the client and eaten on a regular schedule of six meals a day. The rationale for ingesting many meals a day instead of three large ones is so that the stomach is never totally empty. In this way gastric motility is decreased, gastric acid is neutralized, and the digestive action on the mucosa is minimal. Gastric contractions increase in intensity when the stomach is empty or distended with large amounts of food.

Dietary instructions should include a sample diet and a list of foods that usually cause distress and may need to be eliminated from the diet. Foods known to irritate the gastric mucosa include hot, spicy foods and pepper, alcohol, carbonated beverages, tea, coffee, and broth (meat extract) and should not be ingested because they have no known buffering capacity yet are able to stimulate gastric acid secretion. Foods high in roughage such as raw fruit, salads, and vegetables may irritate an inflamed mucosa. If these foods are well chewed, this seems to be less of a problem.

Protein is considered the best neutralizing food, but it also stimulates gastric secretions. Carbohydrates and fats are the least stimulating to acid secretion but do not neutralize well. The client must determine a suitable combination of these essential nutrients without causing undue distress to his ulcer disease.

Milk historically has been an essential part of ulcer therapy. While milk does relieve duodenal ulcer pain, its neutralizing effect is slight compared to meats. The buffering action of milk is outweighed by its ability to stimulate acid production. There are still physicians who prescribe milk therapy along with antacids during the active stage of ulcers.

Nursing Care Related to Conservative Management

Health promotion and maintenance

Clients who have been diagnosed with peptic ulcer disease have specific teaching needs that must be met to prevent and avoid recurrence or complications. General instructions should cover aspects of the disease process itself, dietary therapy, medication administration, possible changes in lifestyle, and regular follow-up care (Table 33-28).

Knowing the cause of his ulcer and understanding the disease process may be a mechanism to get the client more involved in his own care and increase compliance with therapy. The client needs to understand the diet plan and why it is essential for recovery and health maintenance. The nurse and dietitian need to elicit a dietary history from the client and plan for ways in which the ulcer diet can be easily incorporated into the client's home and work setting. When the client is following a diet prescribed for another illness state he will need to know how to balance the two so that both conditions are not harmed by dietary interventions.

The client does not always provide the physician with accurate information regarding his habitual use of alcohol or cigarettes. The nurse may be looked upon as less threatening and more understanding of his habits than the physician. The nurse should use these interactions as opportunities to provide useful information about the detrimental effects of alcohol and cigarettes to ulcer disease.

The nurse needs to instruct the client about prescribed medications including their actions, side effects, and inherent dangers if the drugs are omitted for any reason. The client should know why the ingestion of over-the-counter medications (e.g., aspirin) should not be taken unless approved by the physician. Since antacids are a large part of therapy and may be bought without prescription, clients must be informed that interchanging brands without checking with the physician or nurse can lead to harmful side effects.

Efforts should be made to obtain more information on the client's psychosocial status. Knowledge of his lifestyle, occupation, and coping behaviors can be helpful to the plan of care. The client may be reluctant to talk about himself and the stress he is experiencing at home or on the job. He may not wish to reveal his ordinary method of coping or his dependence on drugs or alcohol. Unfortunately, the client does not often see the relationship between his lifestyle or occupation and his ulcer disease. It is important to listen for subtle clues from his statements or behavior that will help broaden this data base.

When the occupation, related work habits, home, or environment have been implicated as factors in peptic ulcer development, the client must be made aware of these stressors, how to avoid them in the future, or how to successfully cope with them if they cannot be altered. Vocational or psychological counseling may be necessary so that fatigue and repeated emotional upsets can be avoided.

The need for long-term follow-up care must be stressed. Because medical management is frequently followed by a recurrence of the ulcer disease, the client should be encouraged to seek immediate medical intervention if symptoms of the disease recur.

Acute intervention

During the acute exacerbation of an ulcer, the client generally complains of increased pain, and nausea and vomiting, and some may have evidence of bleeding. Initially, many people attempt to cope with the symptoms at home prior to receiving medical assistance.

Very often during this acute phase all that is necessary for the client's immediate recovery is to be kept NPO for a few days with a nasogastric tube to intermittent suction and intravenous fluid replacement. The rationale for this therapy must be conveyed to the anxious client and family. They must be made to understand that the advantages far outweigh any temporary discomfort imposed by the presence of the tube. Regular mouth care will alleviate the dry mouth. Cleansing and lubricating the nares will facilitate breathing and decrease soreness. Gastric contents should be analyzed for acid level, blood, bile, or other irritating substances. When the stomach is kept empty of gastric secretions, the ulcer pain will diminish and ulcer healing will begin. Usually this form of intervention is effective and the client reacts with gratitude and cooperation.

Because the client is NPO, intravenous fluids will

Table 33-28
Nursing Care Plan for the Client with Peptic Ulcer

Client Problem	Expected Outcome	Nursing Intervention
	Conservative Management	
Ulcer pain and discomfort	Expresses no complaints of pain or discomfort	Explain ulcer disease process on client's level of understanding. Help client identify stressors and initiate modifications in his daily routine. Discuss diet plan and assist with implementation at home and in work setting. Provide rationale for the elimination of alcohol, spicy foods, coffee, tea, and carbonated beverages from diet. Encourage and explain the harmful effects of smoking. Provide information on medication actions and side effects. Caution against strenuous exercise and activity.
Noncompliance with medical regimen	Adhere to plan of care	Emphasize that disease process requires commitment to therapeutic regimen and long-term follow-up care. Discuss dangers of dietary indiscretions, alcohol ingestion, and smoking. Discuss why over-the-counter drugs must not be taken without physician's approval. Offer encouragement and helpful ways client can incorporate plan of care into his pattern of living. Inform client what to do if symptoms of ulcers occur.
	Acute Exacerbation	
Increased pain, nausea, and vomiting	No nausea and vomiting	Encourage bed rest or light activity. Provide quiet, relaxed environment and limit visitors. Maintain nasogastric tube to suction and explain rationale. Check patency frequently. Provide nose and mouth care every 4 h. Monitor vital signs every 1 to 2 h. Record I and O. Maintain IV fluids. Observe for possible complications of bleeding, perforation, or obstruction. Monitor laboratory studies. Check vomitus, aspirate, and stools for occult blood.
Depression and frustration	Client will express acceptance of present condition	Assist client and family to understand why the ulcer may have recurred. Reeducate client on diet and drugs. Offer reassurance and faith in plan. Suggest vocational or psychological counseling. Stress need for medical follow-up care for many years.
Potential hemorrhage	No evidence of bleeding. Hemoglobin and hematocrit within normal ranges	Maintain nasogastric tube to suction and ensure its patency. Observe aspirate for amount and color, suggesting brisk or slow bleed. Take vital signs every 15–30 min. Maintain IV infusion line. If blood is replaced, observe for transfusion reaction. Record I and O. Watch for signs of impending shock. Reassure client and family. Remain calm and confident in plan of care. Monitor laboratory studies of hematocrit and hemoglobin. Administer medications as ordered.
Potential perforation	Site of perforation will be located Will be free of pain	Watch for manifestations of perforation such as sudden severe abdominal pain, rigid boardlike abdomen, pain to shoulders, increasing distension, decreasing bowel sounds. Monitor vital signs every 15–30 min. Maintain nasogastric tube to suction. Administer pain medication. Monitor IV fluids. Observe for signs of hypovolemic shock. Prepare client for emergency diagnostic tests and possible surgical intervention. Assess for allergies to antibiotics.
Potential gastric outlet obstruction	Will experience no nausea and vomiting	Maintain nasogastric tube to suction. Check for stomach distension and increasing nausea and vomiting. Monitor IV fluids and maintain client hydration level. When nausea and vomiting subside, check for amount of gastric residue when tube is clamped.

be ordered. The type and amount administered will be directly related to the fluid lost, the manifestations exhibited by the client, and the laboratory results of the hemoglobin, hematocrit, and electrolytes. The nurse should be aware of any other current health problem that could be adversely affected by the type of fluid used or the rate of the infusion. Constant monitoring of all these parameters will provide information on the hydration status and the effectiveness of treatment. Vital signs are initially taken at least hourly so that shock can be detected and treated. This is especially important if the client had a bleeding episode or if blood is present in the gastric aspirate or stool.

Physical and emotional rest are conducive to ulcer healing. The client's immediate environment should be quiet and restful and visitors restricted. The use of a mild sedative or tranquilizer has beneficial effects when the client is anxious and apprehensive. The nurse must use good judgment before sedating a person who is becoming increasingly restless. There is the danger that the medication will mask the signs of shock secondary to upper GI bleeding.

If the client's condition improves without progression of symptoms (e.g., increased pain, vomiting, hemorrhage) the medical regimen outlined for conservative medical management is followed. The nursing care is similar to that described in the previous section. All too frequently an acute exacerbation is accompanied by one or more complications, especially hemorrhage and perforation and to a lesser extent, obstruction.

Hemorrhage It is the early recognition of changes in the vital signs and an increase in the amount and redness of the aspirate that often signals massive UGI bleeding. It is important to maintain the patency of the nasogastric tube so that blood clots do not obstruct the tube. If the tube becomes blocked, the client can develop abdominal distension. When there is an increased amount of blood mixed in the gastric contents, the client's pain is often decreased because the blood helps to neutralize the acidic gastric contents. This is an important point to recognize whenever the pain prior to this time has been constant or unrelieved by suction or drugs.

The nurse needs to monitor the results of the hemoglobin and hematocrit. Her awareness of the significance of the report and her ability to correlate the data to the client's signs and symptoms can be lifesaving. The nursing intervention for upper GI bleeding is discussed in more detail in the section on upper GI bleeding.

Perforation When the client experiences sudden, severe, abdominal pain unrelated in intensity and location to the pain that brought him to the hospital, the nurse must recognize the possibility of ulcer perforation. Any person with an ulcer, particularly one with a chronic duodenal ulcer, who demonstrates these manifestations should be suspected of perforation and the physician notified immediately.

Perforation is indicated by the presence of a rigid, boardlike abdomen with severe generalized abdominal and shoulder pain, drawing up of the knees, and shallow, grunting respirations. The bowel sounds that may have been normal or hyperactive previously may diminish and become absent.

Vital signs are important parameters and should be promptly recorded and taken every 15 to 30 minutes. The nurse should temporarily stop all oral or nasogastric medications and feedings ordered until the physician can be reached and a definite diagnosis made. If perforation does exist, anything taken internally can add to the spillage into the peritoneal cavity and increase discomfort. If intravenous fluids are being administered at the time of the perforation, the rate should be maintained or increased as the plasma volume becomes depleted.

The symptoms experienced by the client are very frightening. The reaction of the nursing staff must be one of calm reassurance in spite of the seriousness of the situation. Simple explanations of the need for chest and abdominal x-rays will help diminish the client's anxiety and give him some insight into the diagnostic plan. Indicating why frequent samples of blood are necessary lessens confusion and resistance.

When perforation is confirmed, the nurse should be sure that any known client allergies have been recorded on the chart. This is important because antibiotic therapy will usually be started and careful observation for allergic reactions must be made. When the perforation fails to seal spontaneously, surgical closure is necessary and is performed as soon as possible. While there is often little time to prepare the client and family thoroughly for the surgical intervention, some instructions can be carried out while the immediate therapy is begun. If major reconstructive surgery is anticipated, the client and his family may question the need if the problem is only a small hole. In order to answer this type of question, the nurse must first have an understanding of the usual operative procedures being utilized. In addition, she must know that unless the surgery can cure the ulcer that caused the perforation, the client may need more surgery in the future. (Nursing management of peritonitis is discussed in Chap. 34.)

Gastric Outlet Obstruction Gastric outlet obstruction is a complication of peptic ulcer disease that can occur at any time. Since the onset of symptoms is usually gradual for most people, the condition is not generally as serious an emergency as hemorrhage or perforation. Obstruction is a possible complication when the client has a history of an ulcer that is located close to the pylorus. Relief of symptoms is easily achieved by constant nasogastric aspiration of stomach contents. This allows edema and inflammation to subside and then permits normal flow of gastric contents through the pylorus.

Obstruction can also occur during the treatment of an acute episode of peptic ulcer exacerbation. If these symptoms are experienced while the client is still NPO, the patency of the nasogastric tube should be suspected. Regular irrigation of the tube with a saline solution will facilitate proper functioning. Repositioning the client from side to side may be helpful so that the tube tip is not constantly lying against the mucosal surface.

When oral feedings have been resumed and symptoms of obstruction are observed, the physician should be promptly informed. Generally, all that is necessary is to resume gastric aspiration so that the edema and inflammation resulting from the acute episode has more time to resolve. Intravenous fluids with electrolyte replacement will keep the client hydrated during this period. Clamping the nasogastric tube and checking for gastric retention will need to be done as described in the medical therapy section. It is important to maintain accurate intake and output records, especially of the gastric aspirate. The client should be kept aware of why he is experiencing these symptoms and that his condition will improve shortly. In some instances where medical treatment is not successful, surgery may be performed after the acute phase has passed.

Chronic management

The client who has recurrence of his ulcer disease following initial healing must learn to live with a disease that is chronic. The client may be angry and frustrated, especially if he feels he faithfully followed the prescribed mode of therapy and it failed to halt the extension of the disease process.

Unfortunately, many clients do not comply with the plan of care originally designed and they experience repeated exacerbations. Clients quickly learn that they experience no discomfort by omitting prescribed medications or having occasional dietary indiscretions. Often they make no or little alterations in their lifestyle. After an acute exacerbation, the client is often more amenable to following the plan of care and open to suggestions for changing his lifestyle. Changes are difficult for most people and may be met with resistance. This reaction, in itself, can result in hypersecretion and hypermotility and cause a delay in ulcer healing.

If the client has been asked to stop smoking or avoid the use of alcohol, the benefits of such a request must be measured against the detrimental physical and emotional outcomes. The client may fare better from a reduction in their use rather than total elimination. While alcohol and smoking are known to interfere with ulcer healing, they frequently serve as coping mechanisms. From the client's point of view, more anguish may be felt than benefits gained. A client with chronic ulcers need to be aware of the complications that may result from the disease, clinical manifestations indicating their presence, and what to do until he can be seen by the physician.

Surgical Management of Peptic Ulcers

The indications for surgical treatment of ulcers are decided on an individual basis. About 20 percent of clients with ulcers will need surgical intervention. Since there is a high recurrence rate for both duodenal and gastric ulcers and complications increase with the duration of the ulcer, many physicians feel surgery is necessary after medical therapy has been tried and been unsuccessful. The following criteria are used as general indications for surgical intervention:

1. Intractibility—failure of the ulcer to heal and/or recurrence of the ulcer following medical therapy
2. Previous history of hemorrhage or increased risk of bleeding during medical treatment
3. Pre-pyloric or pyloric ulcers (both have high recurrence rates)
4. Concurrent illness such as severe burns, trauma, or sepsis
5. Multiple ulcer sites
6. Drug-induced ulcers, especially when withdrawal from the drug may cause a risk for the individual (e.g., aspirin use in an arthritic client)
7. Possible existence of a malignant ulcer

A variety of surgical procedures are used to treat ulcer disease. They usually involve a partial gastrectomy, vagotomy, and/or pyloroplasty. *Partial gastrectomy* with removal of the distal two-thirds of the stomach with anastomosis of the gastric stump to the duodenum is called a *gastroduodenostomy* or *Billroth I*. *Partial gastrectomy* with removal of the distal two-thirds of the stomach with anastomosis of the gastric stump to the jejenum is called a *gastrojejunostomy* or *Billroth II*. In both procedures the antrum and pylorus are removed. Figure 33-10 is a schematic drawing of Billroth I and II procedures.

Vagotomy is the severing of the vagus nerve, either totally (truncal) or selectively at some point in its innervation to the stomach. In a truncal vagotomy the nerve is severed bilaterally in both the anterior and posterior trunk. *Selective vagotomy* consists of

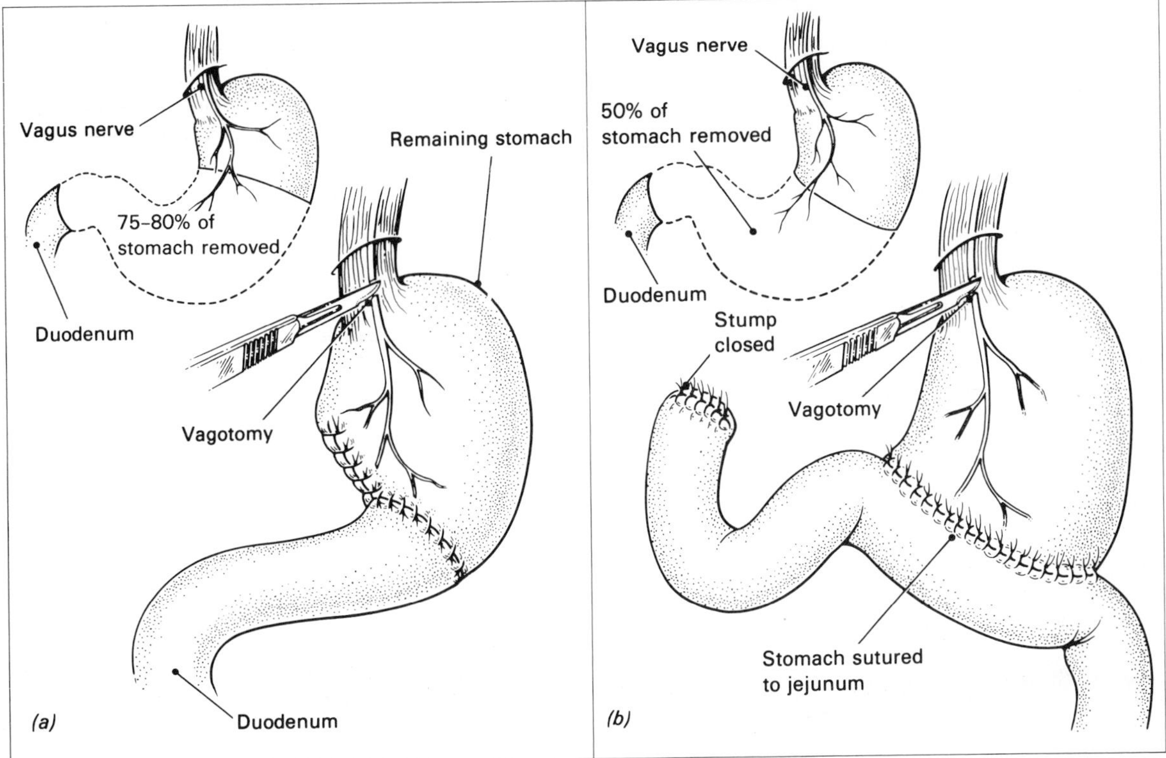

Figure 33-10 *(a)* Billroth I. *(b)* Billroth II. *(From P. Armstrong et al., McGraw-Hill Handbook of Clinical Nursing, McGraw-Hill Book Company, New York, 1978, p. 963.)*

cutting the nerve at a particular branch of the vagus nerve, resulting in denervation of only a portion of the stomach such as the antrum or the parietal cell mass.

Pyloroplasty consists of surgical enlargement of the pyloric sphincter in order to facilitate the easy passage of contents from the stomach. It is most commonly done following vagotomy or to enlarge an opening that has been constricted from scar tissue. A vagotomy causes decreased gastric motility. A pyloroplasty accompanying vagotomy will increase gastric emptying.

The combination of a Billroth I or II with vagotomy has the advantage of eliminating the ulcer and the stimulus for ulcer development. Surgical intervention results in removal of the majority of the parietal cell mass of the stomach and thus decreases the secretion of hydrochloric acid and pepsin. Surgical removal of the antrum results in removal of the source of gastrin secretion. (Gastrin normally stimulates parietal and chief cells.) Vagotomy eliminates the stimulus of hydrochloric acid and gastrin hormone secretion due to vagal stimulation.

Postoperative complications

The most common postoperative complications from peptic ulcer surgery are (1) dumping syndrome, (2) postprandial hypoglycemia, and (3) alkaline reflux gastritis.

Dumping Syndrome The dumping syndrome is the direct result of surgical removal of a large portion of the stomach and the pyloric sphincter. These changes drastically reduce the reservoir capacity of the stomach. Although the dumping syndrome is more commonly experienced after a Billroth II gastrectomy, it can occur after any gastric reconstruction and vagotomy.

The dumping syndrome is associated with meals containing hyperosmolar chyme. Normally, gastric chyme enters the small intestine in small amounts and shifts in fluid from the extracellular space are minimal. However, after surgery the stomach no longer has control over the amount of gastric chyme entering the small intestine. Consequently a large bolus of hypertonic fluid enters the intestine and results in fluid being drawn into the bowel. This creates a decrease in plasma volume. A secondary consequence of this fluid shift is distension of the bowel lumen, which stimulates increased intestinal motility and the urge to defecate.

The dumping syndrome is experienced in approximately one-third to one-half of individuals following peptic ulcer surgery. The onset of symptoms occurs at the end of a meal or within 15 to 30 minutes after eating. The client usually describes feelings of generalized weakness, sweating, palpitations, and dizziness. These symptoms are attributed to the sudden decrease in plasma volume. The client will complain of abdominal cramps, borborygmi, and the urge to defecate. These manifestations occur as a result of the bolus of hypertonic fluid causing extracellular fluid shift into the small intestine. These manifestations usually last for no longer than an hour after meals.

Treatment consists of several simple measures. In most cases the symptoms are self-limiting and disappear completely within several months to a year after surgery. Interventions prescribed for the client are diet instruction, rest, and reassurance. The diet should consist of six small dry feedings daily that are reduced in carbohydrate, restricted in refined sugars, and that contain moderate amounts of protein and fat. Fluids may be taken between meals but not with the meal. The client should plan short rest periods of at least 30 minutes after each meal. The recumbent position is the most beneficial if the client can arrange for it. Reassuring the client that the unpleasant symptoms are usually of short duration is helpful in gaining his cooperation. A small percentage of individuals will experience long-term problems and may require further reconstructive surgery.

Postprandial Hypoglycemia This condition is considered a variant of the dumping syndrome since it is the result of uncontrolled gastric emptying of a bolus of fluid high in carbohydrate into the small intestine. The bolus of concentrated carbohydrate results in hyperglycemia and excessive amounts of insulin released into the circulation. A secondary hypoglycemia then occurs with symptoms appearing about 2 hours after meals. The symptoms experienced are the same observed in any hypoglycemic reaction including sweating, weakness, mental confusion, palpitations, tachycardia, and anxiety.

The immediate ingestion of sugared fluids or candy will relieve the hypoglycemic symptoms. The treatment of this type of hypoglycemia is similar to that of the dumping syndrome. To avoid similar occurrences, the client should be instructed to limit the amount of sugar he consumes with each meal and to eat small, frequent meals with moderate amounts of protein and fat.

Alkaline Reflux Gastritis Gastric surgery that involves the pylorus, either reconstruction or removal, can result in *reflux alkaline gastritis*. It is recognized that prolonged contact of bile, especially bile salts, causes damage to the gastric mucosa. Chronic gastritis of this form may result in the back diffusion of hydrogen ions through the gastric mucosa. Paradoxically, peptic ulcer recurrence may result following surgical treatment that was intended as a cure.

The symptoms associated with reflux alkaline gastritis are continuous epigastric distress that increases after meals. Vomiting relieves the distress but only temporarily. Successful medical treatment has been attained by the administration of cholestyramine resin (Questran) either before or with meals.[39] Cholestyramine binds with the bile salts which are the source of irritation in this condition.

Nursing Care Related to Surgical Management

Preoperative care

Surgical intervention is the treatment of choice for peptic ulcer when conservative medical management has been unsuccessful. Surgery also may be done following an acute remission, when the ulcer is complicated by sudden perforation or increased bleeding, or to relieve gastric outlet obstruction. The wishes of the client for surgical intervention must also be considered, especially when repeated hospitalizations have been required. He may openly request surgery as his only hope for a cure.

When surgery is planned with the goal to cure the ulcer disease, the surgeon should provide necessary information about the procedure and expected outcome so that the client can make an informed decision. The nurse can be helpful to the client and family by clarifying and interpreting their questions. A discussion of the surgical procedure accompanied by a diagram or picture showing the anatomic changes that will result should be incorporated into the preoperative care. Instructions should be clear on what to expect after surgery, including comfort measures, pain relief, coughing and breathing exercises, use of the nasogastric tube, and intravenous fluid administration. General preoperative care of the client is discussed in Chap. 6.

Postoperative care

Care of the client following major abdominal surgery is similar to the postoperative care after abdominal laparotomy (Table 34-6). A nasogastric tube is used to decompress the remaining portion of the stomach so the suture line can be rested and there is time for the resolution of edema and inflammation resulting from surgical trauma.

The gastric aspirate must be carefully observed for color, amount, and odor during the immediate postoperative period. The color of the aspirate is expected to be bright red at first, with a gradual darkening within the first 24 hours after surgery. Normally the color changes to yellow-green within 36 to 48 hours. If the tube should become clogged during this period, the physician may order periodic gentle irrigations with normal saline. If the tube needs to be replaced or repositioned, the physician must be called to perform this task because of the danger of perforating the gastric mucosa or disrupting the suture line.

It is essential that the nasogastric suction is working and the tube remains patent so that increased gastric secretions do not put a strain on the anastomosis. This could lead to distension of the remaining portion of the stomach and could result in (1) rupture of the sutures, (2) leakage of gastric contents into the peritoneal cavity, (3) hemorrhage, and (4) possible abscess formation. A fecal odor from the aspirate is abnormal and may indicate reflux of large intestinal contents into the operative area. The nurse should observe the client for signs of decreased peristalsis and lower abdominal discomfort that may indicate impending intestinal obstruction. Accurate intake and output records must be kept. Vital signs are monitored and recorded every 4 hours.

The client should be kept comfortable and free of pain by the administration of the prescribed medications and by frequent changes in position. The incision is relatively high in the epigastrium and may interfere with deep breathing and coughing measures. Splinting the area with a pillow while gently and persistently encouraging the client to put forth his best efforts will help prevent pulmonary complications. Splinting will also protect the abdominal suture line from rupture during coughing. The dressing must be observed for signs of bleeding or odor and drainage indicative of an infection. Ambulation is encouraged and is increased daily after the first postoperative day.

While the nasogastric tube is connected to suction, intravenous therapy will be maintained. Potassium and vitamin supplements will be added to the infusion until oral feedings are resumed. Sometimes before the nasogastric tube is removed, the client is started on oral feedings of clear liquids to determine tolerance level. The stomach is aspirated within an hour or two to assess the amount remaining and its color and consistency. When fluids are well tolerated, the tube is removed and fluids are increased in frequency with a slow progression to regular foods. The regimen of six small meals a day is begun.

Discharge planning and instruction should be started as soon as the immediate postoperative period is successfully passed. Dietary instructions may be given by the dietitian and reinforced by the nursing staff. Because the stomach's reservoir has been greatly diminished following gastric resection, the meal size must be reduced accordingly. The client must be advised to eliminate drinking fluids with his meals as he has done in the past. Eating dry foods with a low carbohydrate content and moderate protein and fat content is better tolerated until the client has had time to adjust. These dietary changes, with the incorporation of a short rest period after each meal, will facilitate digestion and eliminate most of the problems of the dumping syndrome. The client should be informed that feelings of weakness, palpitations, and dizziness may occur if he does not adhere to the diet instructions. Reassurance that by following these simple dietary measures he will be free of symptoms within a few months is essential to his long-term compliance.

Postprandial hypoglycemic reaction can be avoided if the above dietary instructions are followed with special emphasis on eating foods low in sugar content. While only a very small percentage of clients develop alkaline reflux gastritis, the client must be cautioned to notify his physician if he experiences continuous epigastric distress following meals that is similar to that felt prior to surgery.

Pernicious anemia is a long-term complication that may occur after partial gastrectomy. However, it is seen more often when the entire stomach is surgically removed. The cause of pernicious anemia is the loss of intrinsic factor which is produced by the parietal cells. Depending upon the amount of parietal cell mass removed in surgery, the individual may eventually require regular injections of vitamin B_{12} for the rest of his life. Vitamin B_{12} is normally stored in the liver. Total depletion of vitamin B_{12} stores will usually take several years.

Because the client is generally returning to the same home and work environment and because his basic personality has not changed, there is always the danger of ulcer redevelopment, especially at the site of the anastomosis. Adequate rest, nutrition, and avoidance of known stressors are keys to complete recovery. Avoiding the use of medications not prescribed by the physician should be reemphasized, along with restrictions on smoking and alcohol use. If the client is willing to make these kinds of adjustments in his lifestyle, a successful rehabilitation is more likely.

CANCER OF THE STOMACH

Although the rate of stomach cancer has been steadily declining in the United States since the 1930s, an estimated 23,000 new cases were identified in 1981. Of the gastrointestinal cancers, gastric cancer ranks third behind colorectal and pancreatic cancer in incidence. Japan, Chile, and Costa Rica have the highest incidence rates in the world.[40] Cancer of the stomach is more prevalent in males of the lower socioeconomic class, primarily those living in urban areas. Cancer of the stomach is rarely found in individuals less than 30 years of age. It is most common during the sixth and seventh decades of life.

Etiology

While many factors have been implicated in the development of gastric cancer, no single causative agent has been identified. It is believed that a diet of smoked foods or highly salted or spiced foods may have a carcinogenic effect on gastric cancer development. A genetic etiology has been postulated because of the greater than normal occurrence of stomach cancer in close family members. In addition, there is a greater incidence of stomach cancer in persons with blood group A.[41]

Some other predisposing factors associated with a high incidence of gastric cancer are atrophic gastritis, pernicious anemia, benign gastric polyps, and achlorhydria. The relationship between chronic peptic ulcers of the stomach and the development of gastric cancer is still a controversial topic. Malignant transformation of a benign chronic ulcer does occur, but accounts for less than 5 percent of all gastric cancers. The problem is compounded because of the tendency of gastric cancers to ulcerate and evacuate after necrosis of the center of the tumor, thus giving rise to an ulcer in a cancer. It then becomes difficult to determine which came first, the ulcer or the cancer.[42] It is known that persons with achlorhydria or pernicious anemia are more likely to develop gastric cancer than individuals with normal gastric acid production.

Pathogenesis of Gastric Cancer

Malignant tumors of the stomach may be present for a long time and may have spread to adjacent organs before any distressing symptoms occur. The tumor may grow to large dimensions without obstructing the lumen of the stomach simply because the lumen itself is so large. Gastric cancer can occur in any portion of the stomach. Approximately 60 percent are located in the pyloric area along the lesser curvature and 10 percent at the cardia. The tumors are rarely found along the greater curvature. Adenocarcinoma comprises over 90 percent of the cancers, and sarcomas, comprised of lymphomas and leiomyomas, make up the rest of gastric malignancies.

The malignant lesions may be polypoid, ulcerating, infiltrative, or diffuse. The polypoid lesions grow primarily into the gastric lumen and seldom involve the musculature. Chronic peptic ulcer, on the other hand, commonly involves the muscularis. *Ulcerating lesions* are generally small in size (1 to 2 cm in diameter) and are quite similar in appearance to benign gastric ulcers. *Infiltrative lesions* involve wide areas of the stomach mucosa beyond the ulcer margin. *Diffuse lesions* infiltrate through all mucosal layers of the stomach and in all directions beyond the visible or palpable growth.

The tumor growth is insidious and follows a pattern of continuous infiltration. Cancer of the stomach may spread by direct extension along the mucosal surface and infiltrate through the gastric wall. Once the stomach wall has been penetrated by tumor growth, adjacent organs and structures that may become involved are the esophagus, duodenum, omentum, liver, and pancreas. Distant metastasis is facilitated by the rich lymphatic plexuses in the stomach wall. A typical finding of advanced stomach cancer is involvement of the left supraclavicular lymph node, indicating spread through the thoracic duct.[43] Seeding of tumor cells into the peritoneal cavity may occur late in the course of the disease. Evidence of spread to the peritoneal cavity is manifested by ascites and spread to the ovaries.

Clinical Manifestations

The clinical manifestations exhibited by individuals with gastric cancer can be categorized into three types: those resulting from anemia, those suggesting peptic ulcer, and those resulting from indigestion.[44] Anemia is a common occurrence of stomach cancer due to chronic blood loss as the lesion erodes through the mucosa or as a direct result of pernicious anemia which develops when intrinsic factor is lost. The individual appears pale and weak and complains of fatigue, weakness, dizziness, and in extreme cases, shortness of breath. The stool is positive for occult blood.

The symptoms of gastric malignancy are sometimes identical to those of peptic ulcer. The pain and discomfort can actually be alleviated by belching and the use of antacids and diet restrictions.

Manifestations related to indigestion include vague epigastric fullness with feelings of early satiety after meals. Weight loss, dysphagia, and constipation frequently accompany epigastric distress. When nausea, vomiting, and hematemesis occur, they may indicate obstruction at the gastric outlet or may be a warning of impending hemorrhage.

The early detection of gastric cancer is difficult because of the wide diversity of symptoms. On physical examination the client may be pale and lethargic if anemia is present. When the appetite has been poor and weight loss has been considerable, the client may appear cachectic. A mass can often be detected beneath the abdominal wall and is seen to move with each inspiration. Upon palpation, the mass may be felt in the epigastrium. Masses predominantly in the antrum of the stomach are generally found to the left of the midline. Masses located to the right of midline usually tend to be metastases to the liver or indicate involvement of the perigastric lymph nodes. Supraclavicular lymph nodes that are hard and enlarged and located on the left side are suggestive of metastasis via the thoracic duct from the stomach lesion. The presence of ascites is an obviously unfavorable sign.

Diagnostic Study Abnormalities

The diagnostic studies for gastric malignancy include laboratory analysis of blood, stool, and gastric secretions. Blood chemistries will assist in the determination of anemia and its severity. Liver enzymes and serum amylase may indicate liver and pancreatic involvement or other abnormalities related to their dysfunction. Stool examination will provide evidence of occult or gross bleeding. A gastric analysis indicates the level of hydrochloric acid present in the fasting stomach. Washings obtained during the gastric analysis can be used for the exfoliative cytologic examination. The test will demonstrate the histologic changes indicative of malignancy. However, this test should never be used alone because false readings are sometimes obtained.

The carcinoembryonic antigen (CEA) radioimmunoassay test is used as an adjunctive diagnostic tool for cancer of the gastrointestinal tract. CEA is a glycoprotein that is found in significant amounts in embryonic life, especially in the large intestines. It is also found in some adult clients with GI carcinomas. While elevated levels of CEA may indicate malignancy, CEA is also found to be elevated in persons who smoke and those with benign lesions.[45] Therefore, while the use of the CEA test may be of some use in the preoperative workup of a client with suspected cancer of the stomach, it should never be used as the only diagnostic tool. (CEA is also discussed in Chaps. 11 and 34.)

Barium x-rays may demonstrate defects in peristalsis, tone, secretion, motility, and spasm of the stomach. On x-ray examination the malignant ulcer crater is more irregular around the edges and more elevated than the craters found with benign peptic ulcers. Barium studies do not always detect small lesions of the cardia and fundus.

A gastroscopy should be performed along with barium x-ray studies. Lesions that go undetected on x-ray can be more easily viewed and biopsied when the fiberoptic scope is used. The stomach can be distended with air during the gastroscopy so that the mucosal folds can be stretched. Fixation of the mucosa is indicative of malignancy.

Medical Management

When the diagnosis of gastric malignancy has been confirmed, the treatment of choice is surgical removal of the tumor. The preoperative management of clients with gastric cancer focuses on the correction of nutritional deficits, transfusions for the treatment of anemia, and replacement of blood volume (Table 33-29).

Transfusions of whole blood or packed red blood cells will correct the anemia and increase the blood volume. If a gastric lesion has been located at or near the pylorus and is causing gastric outlet obstruction,

Table 33-29
Medical Management: Gastric Cancer

Diagnostic

1. History and physical examination
2. Complete blood count
3. Urinalysis
4. Stool examination
5. Liver enzymes
6. Serum amylase
7. Upper GI barium study
8. Carcinoembryonic antigen test (CEA)
9. Exfoliative cytology
10. Fiberoptic gastroscopy and esophagoscopy
11. Gastric analysis

Therapeutic

1. Surgery
   a. Subtotal gastrectomy—Billroth I or II
   b. Total gastrectomy with esophagojejunostomy
2. Adjuvant therapy
   a. Radiation therapy
   b. Chemotherapy
   c. Combination radiation therapy and chemotherapy

gastric decompression may be necessary prior to surgery. When the tumor has extended into the transverse colon and partial colon resection is also required, special preparation of the bowel will be necessary. This preparation may include a low residue diet, enemas to cleanse the bowel, and the use of antibiotics to reduce the intestinal bacteria. Clients with achlorhydria who do not have gastric acid available to destroy the bacteria may also need antibiotic bowel preparation.

Surgical therapy

The surgical intervention utilized in the treatment of stomach cancer may consist of any procedure discussed in the section on surgery for peptic ulcer disease. The specific surgery employed is dependent upon the location and extent of the lesion, the client's physical condition, and physician preference. When metastasis is widespread at the time of diagnosis, surgical intervention may only be palliative.

The surgical aim is to remove as much of the stomach as necessary in order to remove the tumor and a margin of normal tissue. When the lesion is located in the cardia or high in the fundus, a total gastrectomy with esophagojejunostomy is done. This procedure involves the anastomosis of the lower end of the esophagus to the jejunum (Fig. 32-11). Lesions located in the antrum or pyloric region are generally treated by either a Billroth I or II procedure. When metastasis has occurred to adjacent organs such as the spleen, ovaries, or bowel, the surgical procedures must be modified and extended as necessary.

The chance of a complete cure by surgical means is decreased considerably when the lymph nodes are involved. Without lymph node involvement it is estimated one-third of clients will have a 5-year cure.[46] Survival rates are considerably shortened when organs adjacent to the stomach show evidence of invasion at the time of surgical intervention.

Adjuvant therapy

Surgery is the only definite means of achieving a cure. However, when the client cannot physically withstand a surgical procedure or when cure is not feasible by surgical means, the use of irradiation or chemotherapy alone or in combination may be used. Neither radiation therapy nor chemotherapeutic agents have been very successful when used as the primary mode of treatment. Radiation therapy has proved to be of little value except in certain instances of obstruction of the cardia. The radiosensitivity of gastric cancers is quite low and it has been estimated that only 10 percent will respond to radiotherapy. Adenocarcinoma occasionally is radiosensitive, while lymphomas frequently respond to treatment.[47]

Preoperative irradiation is usually not done due to the risk of poor wound healing of the anastomosis of the gastric stump to the bowel. When irradiation is used as a palliative measure, the tumor mass can be decreased and thereby temporarily relieve cardia or pyloric obstruction. The use of postoperative radiation has not been widely used nor has it increased survival rates. The combination of chemotherapy and irradiation is now being used for clients who are not candidates for surgical excision. The success rate using 5-fluorouracil (5-FU) and radiation has met with only temporary relief of symptoms and long-term survival rates have not shown significant improvement.

Until recently, single-agent chemotherapy for gastric cancer has proved of little value. Agents which

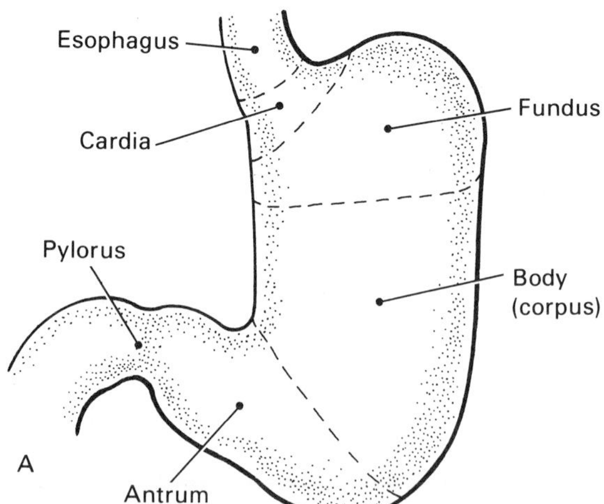

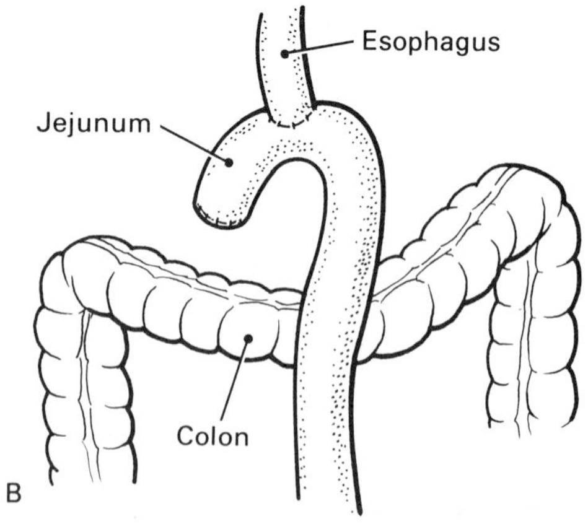

Figure 33-11 Schematic drawing of a total gastrectomy for gastric cancer (total gastrectomy with esophagojejunostomy).

have been identified as having some affect on gastric cancer are 5-FU, Mitomycin C, methyl CCNU, and doxorubicin (Adriamycin). A better response rate in clients with advanced gastric cancer is now found when chemotherapeutic agents are used in combination. The hope for the ultimate cure of clients with gastric cancer now seems to lie in the combined efforts of surgery, irradiation, and chemotherapy. The role of immunotherapy will require more extensive investigation before it can be used with success in gastric carcinoma. These therapies are discussed in Chap. 11.

Nursing Management

Health promotion and maintenance

The nursing role in the early detection of cancer of the stomach is primarily focused on identification of clients who are at high risk. The nurse should be aware of symptoms associated with gastric cancer, method of spread, and the significant findings on physical examination. The nurse should know the cure rate is often quite dismal since symptoms arise late in the course of the disease process, are vague, and often mimic other conditions like peptic ulcer.

The nurse must be alert to problems suggesting gastric cancer such as poor appetite, weight loss, fatigue, and persistent gastric distress. If any of these manifestations are present, medical attention should be obtained and the necessary diagnostic tests performed.

In addition, any client with a positive family history of gastric cancer should be encouraged to undergo diagnostic evaluation if he develops manifestations of anemia, peptic ulcer, or vague epigastric distress. It is imperative that the nurse recognize the possible existence of stomach cancer in a client who is treated for peptic ulcer and who fails to gain relief by diet and prescribed medications after 3 weeks. The ulcer, if it is benign, should show signs of healing on x-ray study.

Acute intervention

Preoperative Care When the diagnostic tests confirm the presence of a malignancy, the client and family generally react with shock, disbelief, and depression regardless of how thoroughly they may have been prepared for this possible outcome. The psychological impact of the diagnosis added to the physical distress already being experienced can be quite devastating. Throughout this period of time the nurse must give emotional and physical support, provide information, clarify test results, and maintain a positive attitude for the client's immediate recovery and long-term survival.

On admission to the hospital, the client may be in poor physical condition. Surgery may need to be delayed while the client is made more physically sound to withstand the strain of major surgery. A positive nutritional state enhances wound healing as well as the ability to withstand infection or other possible postoperative complications. The nursing staff must recognize the necessity for the delay and the advantages to be gained for the client. Many clients have been anorexic for a long time and have lost considerable body weight. The nutritional state will be improved by a well balanced diet along with the administration of supplemental vitamins. It is a challenging situation for the client to eat as much as possible when his appetite and psychological state of mind find eating difficult and unrewarding. Getting the client's family to assist with meals and encourage intake may be beneficial. If the client is unable to ingest oral feedings, it may be necessary to provide for nutritional needs with tube feedings or parenteral hyperalimentation.

If needed, blood replacement and fluid volume restoration may be carried out in the preoperative period. Since anemia is usually present, whole blood may be administered. If the client has cardiovascular problems, the use of packed red blood cells may be substituted so that circulatory overload does not complicate the course of treatment. Close observation for reactions to the transfusions is important. Monitoring the hemoglobin and hematocrit provide information on the progress of therapy.

The preoperative teaching plan prior to gastric surgery for cancer is much the same as that for peptic ulcer surgery. When the anticipated surgery will involve the resectioning of a portion of the colon, the nurse should explain the need for enemas and antibiotic therapy as a bowel prep.

Postoperative Care Postoperative care of the client for gastric carcinoma is similar to that following a Billroth I or II procedure. When the surgical intervention has necessitated a total gastrectomy, the plan of care is somewhat different. The operation performed usually requires some resectioning of the lower esophagus along with the removal of the entire stomach and anastomosis of the esophagus to the jejunum. The chest cavity must be entered and drainage is accomplished by the insertion of chest tubes. (Chest surgery and drainage tubes are discussed in Chap. 20.)

Postoperatively, the nasogastric tube will not drain a lot of secretions because the removal of the stomach eliminates the reservoir capacity. The nasogastric tube is removed in several days when peristalsis has resumed. Small amounts of clear fluids may then be started. The client will need close observation for signs of leakage of the fluids at the anastomosis evidenced by an elevation in the temperature and increasing dyspnea. When fluids are well tolerated without distress, the amount may be increased along with the addition of some solid foods. Meals will consist of six to eight small feedings a day and this pattern will be necessary for the lifetime of the individual.

As a consequence of a total gastrectomy, clients will experience the symptoms of the dumping syndrome. Unfortunately, weight loss is very common and these individuals never do well nutritionally the rest of their lives. Wound healing may be impaired following surgery due to avitaminosis. This will necessitate the intravenous or oral replacement of vitamins B_{12}, C, D, and K, and the B complex vitamins. Because these vitamins are absorbed primarily in the upper small intestine, they must be replaced since the duodenum has been bypassed in the surgical procedure.

Clients who have a Billroth I or II operative procedure should receive the same care postoperatively as that discussed following peptic ulcer surgery. These clients are also subject to the same type of postoperative complications as the dumping syndrome and postprandial hypoglycemia.

Clients who have advanced malignant disease may only be offered palliative treatment. The chemotherapy found most useful for controlling symptoms of gastric cancer is 5-FU. When this medication or any of the combination drugs are prescribed, the nurse must have current information regarding the action and side effects of the drugs. The client should be made aware of the potential benefits and hazards that can result from the chemotherapy prior to its use. (The care of the client receiving chemotherapy is discussed in detail in Chap. 11.)

Radiation therapy can be used as an adjuvant to surgery or for palliation. Clients are generally quite fearful of radiation and may develop many misconceptions regarding its value and dangers. In order to reassure the client and assure his completion of the designated number of treatments, detailed instruction must be provided. Since most therapy is completed on an outpatient basis, the nurse should assess the client's knowledge of irradiation, care of the skin, the need for good nutrition and fluid intake during therapy, and the appropriate use of antiemetic drugs. (Specific care of the individual receiving radiation therapy is discussed in Chap. 11.)

Chronic management

Prior to discharge, the need for teaching should be reviewed. Most dietary measures useful after peptic ulcer surgery are applicable after surgery for gastric carcinoma. Plans should be made for the relief of pain including comfort measures and the judicious use of analgesics. Wound care, if needed, must be taught to the primary care giver in the home situation. The need for dressings, special equipment, or special services may be required for the client's continued care at home. A list of community agencies that are available for assistance can be provided before going home. The services of the American Cancer Society will be especially helpful.

When treatment in the form of chemotherapy or radiation therapy is to be continued after discharge, a referral to the public health nurse may be beneficial. She can provide care to assist with full recovery, determine the degree of client compliance, and be a sympathetic health care provider in whom the client can consult.

Long-term follow-up must be stressed. The client must be encouraged to comply with the prescribed dietary and medication regimens, keep appointments for chemotherapy administration or radiation treatments, and keep the physician informed of changes he is experiencing in his physical condition. (Dealing with the long-term management of the cancer client is discussed in Chap. 11.)

Case Study / Peptic Ulcers

Phyllis, 55, was admitted for a diagnostic workup for recurring epigastric pain. She is 5′2″ and weights 95 pounds. She is a housewife and smokes $1\frac{1}{2}$ packs of cigarettes per day. She has recently undergone many emotional stresses, including a divorce. She is currently taking 15 mg of prednisone every day for rheumatoid arthritis.

Three days after admission she had massive upper gastrointestinal bleeding with hematemesis of bright red blood and melena. She was treated with iced saline nasogastric irrigations and blood transfusions. The bleeding stopped. The next morning she had recurrence of bleeding through her nasogastric tube and bright bleeding from the rectum. A gastroscopy showed a pyloric ulcer. Her hemoglobin was 7.8 g/dL and hematocrit 21%. During the evening, after more emesis of blood clots, she was taken to surgery where a Billroth II (hemigastrectomy and gastrojejunostomy with vagotomy) was performed.

One week after surgery she was started on a bland diet and began to have profuse green diarrhea. She was given frequent small feedings low in carbohydrates and high in protein, moderate in fat.

Discussion Questions

1. What were contributing factors to the development of Phyllis's peptic ulcer?
2. What caused the massive gastrointestinal bleeding? What is the usual treatment for GI bleeding?
3. What was the purpose of her surgery? What phases of gastric secretions were eliminated?
4. Why did Phyllis develop diarrhea and the dumping syndrome? How is it usually treated?
5. What types of anemia could she develop?
6. What types of teaching and/or counseling would be appropriate for Phyllis prior to discharge from the hospital?

REVIEW QUESTIONS

The number of the question corresponds with the same numbered objective at the beginning of the chapter.

1. Which of the following is not essential to the achievement of a good nutritional state of health?
   a. ingestion of foods containing the basic four food groups
   b. megavitamin therapy
   c. energy-producing foods containing fats and carbohydrates
   d. protein foods for tissue repair and maintenance

2. The clinical manifestations commonly exhibited by the person with protein calorie malnutrition include all the following *except*
   a. weak, flabby muscles
   b. severe weight loss
   c. hepatomegaly
   d. normal blood pressure and pulse

3. The nurse working with a client receiving total parenteral nutrition should know that
   a. central hyperalimentation may be administered through the femoral vein
   b. *Pseudomonas* is a frequent cause of sepsis
   c. the rate of administration must never be increased or decreased abruptly
   d. the central catheter can be used for monitoring central venous pressure

4. Which of the following is not appropriate to teach an obese client?
   a. Severe dietary restrictions will help decrease the number and size of the fat cells present.
   b. A well-planned reducing diet and exercise program offers the best long-range results for weight reduction.
   c. Obesity can increase the risk of cardiovascular disease, diabetes, and respiratory problems.
   d. Behavior modification is an essential component of a good weight reduction program.

5. Which of the following statements is not an accurate description of surgical procedures for morbid obesity?
   a. Intestinal and gastric bypasses are still considered experimental procedures.
   b. The intestinal bypass results in many complications, including severe malabsorption.
   c. Jaw wiring is the only surgical procedure that can be reversed at this time.
   d. Gastric partitioning using staples appears to be a safer procedure than the gastric bypass.

6. The least useful measure in the treatment of a client with severe nausea and vomiting is
   a. maintenance of a clean and odor free environment
   b. high carbohydrate and low fat diet
   c. high protein diet and antispasmodics
   d. elevation of head of bed to prevent aspiration

7. Which of the following is not a cause of acute gastritis?
   a. absence of vitamin B_{12} in food intake
   b. ingestion of drugs such as aspirin
   c. contaminated foods with *Staphylococcus* or *Salmonella*
   d. ingestion of large amounts of alcohol

8. When caring for the client who has a sudden, severe upper gastrointestinal bleeding episode, the nursing management would include all the following *except*
   a. administration of anticholinergics and stool softeners
   b. iced saline lavages
   c. central venous pressure monitoring
   d. fluid replacement with volume expanders or blood transfusions

9. Which of the following statements describes the differences between a gastric and duodenal ulcer?
   a. Gastric ulcers are found most often in the fundus of the stomach.
   b. Duodenal ulcers have decreased in incidence over the past 20 years.
   c. Gastric ulcer pain is periodic and episodic.
   d. Duodenal ulcers have a malignant potential.

10. Which of the following statements does not accurately describe the dumping syndrome?
    a. Symptoms arise from a bolus of hyperosmolar fluid entering the intestines.
    b. Symptoms are experienced 2 to 3 hours after meals.
    c. Complaints of weakness, sweating, dizziness, and abdominal cramps are common.
    d. Symptoms are self-limiting and disappear in about 6 to 12 months.

11. Which of the following diagnostic tests is least helpful in accurately diagnosing stomach cancer?
    a. gastroscopy
    b. gastric analysis
    c. carcinoembryonic antigen test
    d. exfoliative cytology

REFERENCES

1. Juanita A. Eagles and Mildred N. Randall, *Handbook of Normal and Therapeutic Nutrition*, Raven Press, New York, 1979, pp. 40–42.
2. Selwyn Taylor (ed.), *Recent Advances in Surgery*, Churchill Livingstone, London, 1977, p. 102.
3. Carol Suitor and Merrily Hunter, *Nutrition: Principles and Application in Health Promotion*, J. B. Lippincott Company, Philadelphia, 1980, p. 199.
4. Selwyn Taylor, op. cit., p. 134.
5. Hilde Bruch, *The Golden Cage: The Enigma of Anorexia Nervosa*, Harvard University Press, Cambridge, Mass., 1978, p. 34.
6. Robert E. Olson (ed.), *Protein-Calorie Malnutrition*, Academic Press, New York, 1975, p. 210.
7. Ibid., p. 124.
8. S. Davidson et al., *Human Nutrition and Dietetics*, 7th ed., Churchill Livingstone, New York, 1979, p. 244.
9. Ibid., p. 245.
10. George A. Bray (ed.), *Obesity in America*, U.S. Dept. of Health, Education, and Welfare, Public Health Service, National Institutes of Health, November 1979, p. 8.
11. Ibid., p. 78.
12. Ibid., p. 79.
13. J. K. Alexander, C. B. Woodard, M. A. Quinones, and W. H. Goosch, "Heart Failure from Obesity," in *Medical Complications of Obesity*, Academic Press, New York, 1979, p. 177.
14. D. F. Rochester and N. S. Arora, "Respiratory Failure in Obesity," in *Medical Complications of Obesity*, Academic Press, New York, 1979, p. 183.
15. Richard B. Stewart, "Exercise Prescription in Weight Management: Advantages, Techniques, and Obstacles," *Obesity and Bariatric Medicine*, Englewood, Colorado, January–February 1975, p. 17.
16. Cathy M. Mojzesik and Edward W. Martin, "Gastric Partitioning: The Latest Surgical Means to Control Morbid Obesity," *Am J Nurs*, **81:**569 (March 1981).
17. Ibid., p. 570.
18. Edward E. Mason, *Surgical Treatment of Obesity*, W. B. Saunders Company, Philadelphia 1981, p. 85.
19. Myron Wenick (ed.), *Nutrition: Metabolic and Clinical Applications*, John Wiley & Sons, Inc., New York, 1980, pp. 181–182.
20. Thomas Sernka, Eugene Jacobson, and Tushar Chowdhury, *Gastro-intestinal Physiology—the Essentials*, The Williams & Wilkins Company, Baltimore, 1979, p. 72.
21. Rolla Hill and Fred Kern, *The Gastrointestinal Tract*, The Williams & Wilkins Company, Baltimore, 1977, p. 79.
22. Norton Greenberger, Constantine Arvanitakis, and Aryeh Hurvitz, *Drug Treatment of Gastrointestinal Disorders*, Churchill Livingstone, New York, 1978, p. 124.
23. Hill and Kern, op. cit., p. 85.
24. Leo Van der Reis (ed.), *The Stomach*, vol. 6, S. Karger, Basel and New York, 1980, p. 159.
25. Cheryl Lamb, Sue Apple, and Zaz Hongo, "The G.I. Bleeder," Nursing Grand Rounds in *Nursing 75*, September 1975, p. 53.
26. Van der Reis, op. cit., p. 65.
27. Barbara Given and Sandra Simmons, *Gastroenterology in Clinical Nursing*, 3d ed., The C. V. Mosby Company, St. Louis, 1979, p. 346.
28. Gail Long, "GI Bleeding: What to Do and When," *Nursing 78*, March, p. 50.
29. Lamb et al., op. cit., p. 53.
30. Rene Menguy, *Surgery of Peptic Ulcer*, W. B. Saunders Company, Philadelphia, 1976, p. 270.
31. Richard Hunt and G. J. Milton-Thompson, "The Epidemiology and Pathogenesis of Gastric Ulcer," in Leo Van der Reis (ed.), *The Stomach*, S. Karger, Basel and New York, 1980, p. 64.
32. Hill and Kern, op. cit., p. 78.
33. Lloyd Nyhus and Christopher Wastell, (eds.), *Surgery of the Stomach and Duodenum*, 3d ed., Little, Brown and Company, Boston, 1977, p. 195.
34. P. H. Guth, "Gastric Mucosal Blood Flow and Resistance to Injury," in *Advances in Ulcer Disease*, Excerpta Medica, Amsterdam-Oxford-Princeton, 1980, p. 107.
35. D. W. Piper, "The Treatment of Chronic Peptic Ulcer," in Leo Van der Reis (ed.), *The Stomach*, S. Karger, Basel and New York, 1980, p. 114.
36. J. R. Malagelada et al., "Pharmacological Basis and Clinical Use of Antacids," in *Advances in Ulcer Disease*, Excerpta Medica, Amsterdam-Oxford-Princeton, 1980, p. 380.
37. Denis McCarthy, "Peptic Ulcer: Antacids or Cimetidine," *Hospital Practice*, December 1979, p. 55.
38. Dexter Mar, "Antacid Therapy," *Am J Nurs*, **81:**788–789 (April 1981).
39. Menguy, op. cit., p. 167.
40. *American Cancer Society: Cancer Facts and figures*, American Cancer Society, Inc., New York, 1981, p. 8.
41. Keiichi Kawai, Minoru Kizu, and Takayuki Miyaoka, "Epidemiology and Pathogenesis of Gastric Cancer," in Leo Van der Reis (ed.), *The Stomach*, S. Karger, Basel and New York, 1980, p. 77.
42. Hill and Kern, op. cit., p. 215.
43. Theodor Grage, Ronald Ferguson, and Richard Simmons, "Gastrointestinal Tract Cancer," in G. J. Hill and J. Horton (eds.), *Clinical Oncology*, W. B. Saunders Company, Philadelphia, 1977, p. 247.
44. Thomas F. Nealon (ed.), *Management of the Patient With Cancer*, 2d ed., W. B. Saunders Company, Philadelphia, 1976, p. 423.
45. Consensus Development Conference Summary, "CEA as a Cancer Marker," vol. 3, no. 7, National Institutes of Health, Bethesda, Md., 1980, p. 2.
46. Grage et al., op cit., p. 250.
47. Carlo Grossi, "Radiotherapy and Chemotherapy of Gastric Tumors," in T. F. Nealon (ed.), *Management of the Patient with Cancer*, 2d ed., W. B. Saunders Company, Philadelphia, 1977, p. 451.

Chapter 34

NURSING ROLE IN MANAGEMENT

Problems of Absorption and Elimination

Earnestine Huffman White

Learning Objectives

1. Explain the common etiologies and medical and nursing management of diarrhea and constipation.
2. Describe common causes of an acute abdomen and nursing care of the client following an exploratory laparotomy.
3. Describe the nursing management for a client with acute appendicitis.
4. Identify the medical and nursing management of peritonitis.
5. Describe the common etiologies, clinical manifestations, and management of gastroenteritis.
6. Compare and contrast ulcerative colitis and Crohn's disease, including pathophysiology, clinical manifestations, complications, and medical and nursing management.
7. Differentiate among mechanical, neurogenic, and vascular bowel obstructions including causes and medical and nursing management.
8. Describe the clinical manifestations and surgical and nursing management of cancer of the colon and rectum.
9. Explain the anatomic and physiologic changes which result from a sigmoid colostomy, a transverse colostomy, and an ileostomy.
10. Describe the preoperative and postoperative medical and nursing management for a client having bowel surgery.
11. Compare and contrast a colostomy and an ileostomy in relation to nursing care and client teaching.
12. Differentiate between diverticulosis and diverticulitis, including clinical manifestations and medical and nursing management.
13. Compare and contrast the types of hernia, including etiology and surgical and nursing management.
14. Describe the types of malabsorption syndrome and appropriate management of sprue syndrome and lactase deficiency.
15. Describe the types, clinical manifestations, and medical and nursing management of anorectal conditions.

DIARRHEA AND CONSTIPATION

Diarrhea

Etiology

Diarrhea is an increase in peristaltic motility resulting in frequent watery or loosely formed stools. Diarrhea is not a disease, but a symptom of a pathologic process. It may result from multiple causes, including coarse and highly seasoned food, antibiotics, diverticulitis, infection, laxatives, malabsorption, neoplasms, diabetic neuropathy, hyperthyroidism, and uremia.

Diarrhea may also result from stress. In acute stress, sympathetic stimulation leads to decreased peristalsis. In chronic stress, parasympathetic stimulation increases peristalsis, causing diarrhea.

Clinical manifestations and complications

In acute cases of diarrhea, the stools are light brown, contain undigested food particles, and are foul-smelling. The client may complain of abdominal cramps, distension, borborygmi (intestinal rumblings), anorexia, and thirst. *Tenesmus* (painful spasms) of the anus may occur with each stool.

Severe diarrhea is debilitating. In diarrhea large amounts of fluids containing sodium, potassium, and other electrolytes are lost. This can eventually lead to hypovolemia, hypokalemia, and shock. If malabsorption is present, nutrients are also lost into the stool. The skin around the anus may become excoriated from frequent stools.

Medical management

Diagnosis of acute diarrhea is determined by client history and examination of the stool for bacteria, pus, or blood. Watery stools are indicative of small bowel disease, whereas loose, semisolid stools indicate a disease of the colon.

The treatment of diarrhea is based on the cause. Symptomatic treatment includes resting the gastrointestinal tract by giving only liquids or foods low in bulk, or giving the client nothing by mouth. If the client is given nothing by mouth, intravenous fluids are administered. Oral fluids are reintroduced gradually. If oral fluids are well tolerated, a bland diet with gradual introduction of other foods is permitted.

This chapter was reviewed by Gladys Deters, R.N., M.S., Assistant Professor, School of Nursing, University of Virginia, Charlottesville, Virginia.

Acute diarrhea is often self-limiting in the adult. The mucous membrane lining is usually not destroyed from the inflammatory process. Hyperperistalsis continues until the irritant or causative agent is excreted.

Chronic or excessive diarrhea can result in serious problems. Excessive loss of fluids containing sodium and potassium occurs. Parenteral hyperalimentation with vitamin supplements may be required.

Most cases of diarrhea are usually not treated with antibiotics since this treatment may alter the bowel flora and increase diarrhea. Antidiarrheal agents are given to delay the passage of food through the intestines and coat the intestinal mucosa (Table 34-1).

Nursing management

Handwashing is the single most important measure to prevent the transfer of microorganisms. Hands should be washed before and after contact with each client and when handling excretions of any kind.

Proper handling as well as cooking and storage of food is important in the prevention of disease. Food handlers should receive instructions on the principles of hygiene, medical asepsis, and the potential dangers of an illness that is infectious to self and others. Precautions should be taken by all personnel to prevent the spread of disease through contamination of hands, linen, feces, vomitus, etc.

Nursing care of the client with acute diarrhea is discussed in Table 34-2. Nursing assessment includes obtaining information on (1) prior bowel habits; (2) number, color, volume, time, and consistency of stools; (3) presence of mucus or blood in the stools; (4) history of loose stools after certain medications or foods; and (5) recent travels in and out of the country. If stress is a factor in causing diarrhea, stress reduction practices such as exercise, biofeedback, diversion, and meditation may be used (Chap. 39).

Strict medical asepsis is important since acute diarrhea is potentially infectious. Enteric isolation precautions are usually instituted if an infection is suspected. All cases of acute diarrhea should be considered infectious until the etiology is determined. Assessment of the client should be done to determine if members of the family or significant others have had diarrhea. If large numbers of persons are affected, the nurse can help in identifying a possible epidemic and report the outbreak to the proper authorities.

Constipation

Etiology

Some people defecate once every 24 hours and some once every 2 to 3 days. Infrequency alone does not necessarily mean a person is constipated. Constipation exists when the interval between bowel movements is longer than that which is normal for the individual, when the volume is small and feces remain in the rectum, and when the consistency of the fecal material is dry and hard.[1]

Occasional constipation may result from inadequate bulk in the diet, a decrease in sufficient fluids, and lack of physical activity. An enema or laxative will usually correct the immediate problem. If proper preventive measures are subsequently taken, this type of constipation should not recur.

Constipation may also be due to diseases within the colon or rectum, side effects of drugs, injury or degeneration of the spinal cord, megacolon, weakness, fatigue, immobility, habitual use of laxatives,

Table 34-1
Antidiarrheal Drugs

Category	Mechanism of Action	Example
Demulcent	Soothing effect. Coats membrane and protects irritated, inflamed walls.	1. Bismuth subcarbonate 2. Kaolin 3. Kaopectate (kaolin with pectin) 4. Activated charcoal
Antispasmodic	Inhibits gastric mobility.	1. Donnagel 2. Donnagel PG (opium added) 3. Diphenoxylate HCl (Lomotil)
Sedatives	Quiets central nervous system.	1. Paregoric (camphorated opium mixture) 2. Opium tincture

Table 34-2
Nursing Care Plan for the Client with Acute Infectious Diarrhea

Client Problem	Expected Outcome	Nursing Intervention
Dehydration due to hypovolemia	Normal skin turgor. Urine output of 1200–1500 mL/day.	Assess for skin turgor changes, sunken eyes, rapid pulse, and anorexia. Monitor intake and output. Record the number and character of stools. Monitor BP and pulse every 4 h. Weigh daily. NPO as ordered. Administer IV fluids as ordered. Increase intake of fluids as tolerated to at least 3000 mL/day. Avoid milk and milk products. When tolerated, diet should be low residue (see Table 7 in Appendix B).
Weakness due to hyponatremia and hypokalemia	Regain stength. Normal serum electrolyte values.	Check lab reports daily for electrolyte values. Identify signs and symptoms of electrolyte imbalances (see Chap. 12). Administer IV with electrolyte replacements as ordered. Resume oral intake as soon as possible. Include foods high in potassium (citrus fruits, bananas, baked potatoes (see Table 11 in Appendix B).
Anal excoriation	Normal skin integrity around rectal area.	Initiate care measures for the skin and mucous membranes of the rectal area. Cleanse the rectal area after each bowel movement with warm water and a mild soap, rinsing well and patting dry with a soft towel. Apply A and D ointment or Desitin to promote healing. Utilize a local anesthetic in ointment or spray form.
Abdominal cramping and loose, frequent watery stools	No abdominal cramping. Normal elimination pattern.	Administer antidiarrheal agents on a scheduled basis (every 4 to 6 h around the clock) or after each bowel movement to effectively relieve diarrhea. Continue to assess the pattern of the bowel movement to determine when a change in dosage or pattern of administration is necessary.
Infectious process	Be free from infectious organisms.	Follow hospital procedure for enteric precautions. Use strict medical asepsis when handling bedpan, linen, or client. Monitor temperature, pulse, and respirations every 4 h. Administer anti-infective medications as ordered. Assess each stool for color, amount, and consistency.
Potential recurrence of diarrhea	No recurrence of diarrhea.	Explain importance of reporting changes in stools. Assist client in identifying factors that precipitated diarrhea. Stress importance of good handwashing techniques. Explain danger signs of diarrhea and when to seek medical care.

limited exercise, changes in diet and environment, and ignoring the urge to defecate. The individual may have developed the habit of delaying the bowel movement so that defecation may occur every 5 to 6 days or significantly less frequently than the normal pattern.

Ignoring the urge to defecate causes the muscles and membranes in the rectal area to become insensitive to the presence of feces. The prolonged retention of feces in the rectum results in drying of stool due to the reabsorption of water from the feces. The harder and drier the feces, the worse the constipation. In response to the presence of the dry feces, the colon produces increased amounts of mucus.

Clinical manifestations

The client may complain of abdominal fullness or distension, sensation of pressure in the rectum, nausea, and increased flatus. Bowel movements are difficult and the stool is expelled as dried fecal masses. Systemic manifestations of prolonged constipation are headache, dizziness, tachycardia, malaise, and lethargy.

Sometimes constipation leads to a fecal impaction, especially in bedridden clients. The client may complain of a feeling of rectal distension, urgency of defecation, and tenesmus. Occasionally the fecal impaction leads to an obstructive process with increased fluid content proximal to the impaction. Diarrhea may result as fluid moves past the obstructing fecal mass. The fecal bulk is not expelled and must be removed manually or with enemas.

Complications

Because constipation causes straining (Valsalva's maneuver), it can be a serious problem for clients with congestive heart failure, cerebral edema, hypertension, and myocardial infarction. Straining by contracting the diaphragm, thoracic, and abdominal muscles can be hazardous to the health of the client. After a deep inspiration, the breath is held, and the glottis closes and traps the air. The abdominal muscles contract and try to push against the colon. In addition to an increase in intraabdominal pressure, there is also an increase in the intrathoracic pressure. This increase in intrathoracic pressure prevents blood from entering the thoracic cavity. Less blood is pumped into the atria and ventricles. The heart slows temporarily (bradycardia) and the cardiac output is decreased with a transient drop in arterial pressure.

When the client relaxes, there is decreased thoracic pressure and a sudden flow of blood into the heart which causes tachycardia. Immediately the arterial pressure rises momentarily. These changes may be fatal for the client who cannot compensate for sudden overload of blood flow to the heart following straining.

Medical management

The underlying cause of constipation is identified and treatment started. Management of constipation includes diet modification (see next section), stool softeners, and laxatives (Table 34-3). If the defecation reflex does not return, a bulk laxative such as psyllium seed (Metamucil) may be given. Enemas should not be used until other measures have been tried. Oil retention enemas may be used to soften fecal impactions.

Dietary intervention

An important role of the nurse is teaching the client the importance of dietary measures to prevent constipation. The diet should include fluid intake of at least 3000 mL/day and high-fiber foods (see Appendix B and Table 34-6). These foods include such products as raw fruits and vegetables, fruits with skins, and whole grain cereals and breads. In addition, natural laxative foods such as prune juice, raisins, and fruit juices may stimulate gastrocolic reflex activity. The client's understanding of the diet is important to ensure compliance.

Nursing management (Table 34-4)

The process of defecation should be explained to the client. Instruction should be given not to suppress the urge to defecate. Emphasis should be placed on establishing and maintaining a regular time to defe-

Table 34-3
Cathartic (Laxative) Drugs

Category	Mechanism of Action	Example
Lubricant (emollient) cathartics	Lubricate intestinal tract and soften feces without increasing bulk.	Mineral oil
Saline cathartics	Increase bulk of stool by osmotic action to retain fluids in the colon.	Magnesium hydroxide mixture (milk of magnesia) Magnesium sulfate sol (epsom salts) Magnesium citrate Fleet enema Phosphate soda
Stimulant (irritant cathartics)	Increase peristalsis by stimulating (irritating) sensory nerve endings in mucosa of the colon.	Castor oil (Neoloid) Cascara sagrada Bisacodyl (Dulcolax) Glycerine suppositories Phenolphthalein (Ex-Lax) Senna (Senokot)
Bulk cathartics	Exert effects by swelling in the presence of water and mechanically stimulating peristalsis.	Methylcellulose (Cologel) Psyllium hydrophilic mucilloid (Metamucil) Agar
Fecal softeners	Soften feces through action of contained wetting agent.	Dioctyl calcium sulfosuccinate (Surfak) Dioctyl sodium sulfosuccinate (Colace, Peri-Colace, Doxinate)

Table 34-4
Nursing Care Plan for the Client with Constipation

Client Problem	Expected Outcome	Nursing Intervention
Accumulation of stool in the rectum	Empty the rectum of stool.	Administer enemas, stool softeners, and mild laxatives as ordered. Encourage high fiber foods (prune juice, fresh fruits, and vegetables—see Table 6 in Appendix B). Encourage fluid intake to at least 3000 mL/day. Gentle massage of the abdomen along the path of the transverse and descending colon.
Possible fecal impaction	No fecal impaction.	Observe for watery diarrhea. Administer oil retention enema as ordered. Digitally break the fecal impaction.
Fatigue and discomfort	Feel rested and comfortable.	Position for comfort when sitting on toilet. Align body correctly when placed on bedpan. Plan long rest periods after rectum is empty.
Recurrence of constipation	No recurrence of constipation.	Teach proper diet therapy (high fiber foods, prune juice, fresh fruit, fresh vegetables, and fluids). Increase fluid intake to 3000 mL/day. Take bulk-forming laxatives as ordered. Establish regular schedule to attempt defecation. Explain factors that may contribute to constipation such as (1) suppression of urge to defecate, (2) overuse of laxatives, and (3) inactivity.

cate. In many individuals the call to defecate occurs after breakfast due to the stimulation of the gastrocolic reflex. The client should be discouraged from using laxatives and enemas to achieve fecal elimination.

Proper position is important when defecating. For a client in bed, the bedpan should be placed and then the head of the bed elevated as high as the client can tolerate. For the person who can sit on a toilet, a footstool may be placed in front of the toilet. Placing the feet on the stool promotes flexion of the thighs which assists in defecation.

The client with poor muscle tone should be encouraged to exercise the abdominal muscles. He can be taught to contract the abdominal muscles several times a day. Sit-ups and straight leg raises can also be used to improve abdominal muscle tone.

INFLAMMATORY DISEASE

Acute Abdomen (Surgical Abdomen)

Etiology

The acute abdomen is any complex of signs and symptoms suggesting an abdominal condition which requires immediate surgery.[2] Causes of an acute abdomen are varied (Table 34-5). Therefore, many disorders must be ruled out until a diagnosis is made.

Clinical manifestations

Symptoms are often varied and nonspecific. Pain is usually the chief complaint. The client may also complain of abdominal tenderness, vomiting, diarrhea, constipation, flatulence, fatigue, bleeding, and an increase in abdominal girth.

Medical management

Diagnostic A complete blood cell count, urinalysis, chest and abdominal x-rays, and an ECG are done initially. The findings of these studies may provide some information as to the cause of the acute abdomen. A sigmoidoscopy may be done if there is rectal bleeding or diarrhea.

Table 34-5
Possible Causes of An Acute Abdomen

Acute urinary retention
Appendicitis
Bowel obstruction
Cholecystitis
Diverticulitis
Enteritis
Fecal impaction
Gastritis
Gastroenteritis
Mesenteric adenitis
Pancreatitis
Pelvic inflammatory disease
Peptic ulcer
Renal calculus
Ruptured ectopic pregnancy
Ruptured ovarian cyst
Sickle-cell crisis
Spinal and nerve root diseases
Ulcerative colitis

The goal of management of the acute abdomen is to identify and treat the cause. If possible, a complete history and thorough physical examination are done, including a pelvic and rectal examination. Each sign and symptom are carefully assessed. The onset, intensity, duration, radiation, acuity, and chronicity of pain are evaluated. The consistency and amount of vomitus and stool are assessed.

The physician attempts to make a differential diagnosis when an acute abdomen occurs, since there are many causes of abdominal pain that do not require surgery. Immediate surgery is more likely if there is acute pain and prolonged vomiting.

Therapeutic In addition to a therapeutic measure, surgery may also be a diagnostic measure. An operative exploration is usually done after a careful examination of the client and is justified when "look and see" is better than "wait and see." The surgical procedure is an *exploratory laparotomy,* an opening made through the abdominal wall into the peritoneal cavity to determine the cause of an acute abdomen.

Nursing management

Preoperative Care of the client for surgery is discussed in Chap. 6. Emergency preparation of the client with an acute abdomen is usually limited to a complete blood count and type and cross match for blood. Catheterization, the abdominal skin prep, and the passage of a nasogastric tube may be done in the emergency room or operating room.

Postoperative Care (Table 34-6) Immediate postoperative care is similar to that discussed in Chap. 8. The nurse prepares the room with equipment for gastric suctioning. When the client returns, the nasogastric tube is connected to suction as ordered and the intravenous infusion checked for patency and drip rate.

The purpose of the nasogastric tube is to empty the stomach of secretions and gas to prevent gastric dilatation. (Gastrointestinal peristaltic activity is impaired due to the manipulative procedures of the surgery.) Low suctioning is ordered to prevent trauma to the gastric mucosa.

Table 34-6
Nursing Care Plan for Client Following Laparotomy

Client Problem	Expected Outcome	Nursing Intervention
Hypoventilation and possible hypostatic pneumonia	Normal respiratory pattern. Lungs clear to auscultation.	Cough and deep breathe 10 times every 2 h for 72-h period. Splint operative site with pillows while coughing and deep breathing. Turn every 2 h. Auscultate lungs every 4 h. Assess breathing pattern and rate. Ambulate at least three times a day beginning the first postoperative day. Have client assume semi-Fowler's position while in bed.
Paralytic ileus and gas pains	Normal bowel sounds. Normal bowel elimination pattern.	Assess for abdominal distension, nausea, and vomiting. Auscultate for bowel sounds every 4 h. Attach nasogastric tube to low suction. Observe for patency of tube and drainage. Irrigate nasogastric tube with 30 mL normal saline solution prn. Provide mouth care using toothbrush, frequent mouth rinses, and lemon swabs. Apply water-soluble lubricant to nasal mucosa.
Potential nausea and vomiting	No nausea and vomiting.	NPO until bowel sounds return. IV fluids with electrolyte replacements ordered at specified rate. Give antiemetic medication as ordered. When bowel sounds return, give sips of water with gradually increasing amounts of fluids.
Potential thrombophlebitis	No tenderness or pain in legs.	Leg exercises in bed 10 times every 2 h. Ambulate three times a day. Apply antiembolic stockings or Ace bandages. Do not raise knee gatch of bed. Teach client not to cross legs or sit with legs in dependent position.
Incisional pain	Relief of pain.	Assess frequently for pain. Give pain medication every 3–4 h prn the first 24–72 h. Splint incision with pillows when coughing and deep breathing. Position in semi-Fowler's.
Potential infection of incision	Clean incision site. Temperature below 37.6°C (99.7°F).	Use aseptic technique when changing dressings. Inspect incision site at this time for signs of inflammation. Keep area around any drains dry. Note and record character of any drainage on dressing and condition of the skin.

Drainage from the tube may be dark brown to dark red for the first 12 hours. Later it should be light yellowish-brown or it may have a greenish tinge due to the presence of bile. If a dark red color continues or bright red blood is observed, the physician should be notified at once of the possibility of hemorrhage. Coffee-ground-like granules in the drainage are due to the presence of small amounts of blood that have been chemically acted on by gastric secretions.

The nasogastric tube is checked frequently for patency. The tube may become obstructed with mucus, sediment, or old blood. An order is usually written to irrigate the tube with 30 mL of normal saline solution if needed. Repositioning the tube may facilitate drainage.

An accurate intake and output including emesis and gastric drainage is essential. The nurse should assess serum electrolyte determinations since prolonged gastric suctioning will result in deficiencies of sodium, chloride, potassium, and bicarbonate.

The nasogastric tube is removed when peristalsis returns, usually 24 to 72 hours after surgery. Peristaltic activity is assessed by auscultation for bowel sounds. The nasogastric tube may need to be reinserted if persistent nausea or vomiting occurs.

Mouth care and nasal care are essential when the nasogastric tube is in place. The client has a tendency to be a mouth breather while the nasogastric tube is in place. In addition, increased nasal secretions and crusting result from the mechanical stimulation of the nasogastric tube.

Parenteral fluids are administered to provide the client with fluids and electrolytes until bowel sounds return. Occasionally, ice chips may be ordered as they aid in the flow of saliva and prevent drying. When bowel sounds return, fluids and food are increased gradually. The diet may be supplemented with vitamin B complex, vitamin C, and iron.

Nausea and vomiting are not uncommon after abdominal surgery. These problems are often self-limiting. Observation is important in determining the cause. Antiemetics such as promethazine HCl (Phenergan), hydroxyzine (Vistaril), or trimethobenzamide (Tigan) may be ordered.

Abdominal distension and gas pains are common after surgery due to swallowed air and impaired peristalsis from immobility, manipulation of abdominal contents during surgery, and side effects of anesthesia. The pain may be so uncomfortable that medications to stimulate peristalsis such as bethanechol (Urecholine) or neostigmine methylsulfate (Prostigmin) may be given. A rectal tube or moist heat on the abdomen may be effective in relieving distension. The physician should be informed of abdominal distension and rigidity. Gradually, as intestinal activity increases, distension and gas pains decrease.

Emotional support from the nursing staff is usually needed. Honest, clear, concise explanations of all procedures in language the client and family can understand will help to allay anxiety.

General postoperative measures for the client with abdominal surgery are presented in Table 34-6. Nursing interventions for specific surgical interventions are discussed elsewhere in this text.

Rehabilitative Management Preparation for discharge begins when the client returns from the operating room. Instructions should include teaching the client and the family any modifications in activity, care of the incision, diet, and drug therapy. Small, frequent meals high in calories should be taken initially with a gradual increase in intake of food as tolerated.

Normal activities should be resumed gradually with planned rest periods. The client should be aware of possible complications following surgery and notify the physician immediately of vomiting, pain, weight loss, incisional drainage, and changes in bowel functions.

Appendicitis

Appendicitis is an inflammation of the appendix, a narrow blind tube that extends from the inferior part of the cecum. It has no known function. An inflammation of the appendix is seen in all ages but is more common between 10 and 30 years of age.[3]

Etiology

The most common cause of appendicitis is obstruction of the lumen by a fecolith (accumulated feces) (Fig. 34-1). As appendicitis progresses, the mucosa ulcerates and the blood supply is impaired by bacterial infection in the wall. The lumen becomes distended with pus, and gangrene and perforation are likely to occur.

Clinical manifestations

Appendicitis typically begins with vague abdominal pain followed by nausea, anorexia, and indigestion. The client may have a slight or moderate temperature elevation, mild changes in bowel function, and vomiting. The pain is persistent and continuous, beginning in the middle of the abdomen and radiating to the right lower quadrant and localizing at McBurney's point (located halfway between the umbilicus and the right iliac crest). Effective assessment of the client will reveal localized tenderness and pain upon palpation or when asked to cough. Rebound tenderness may be

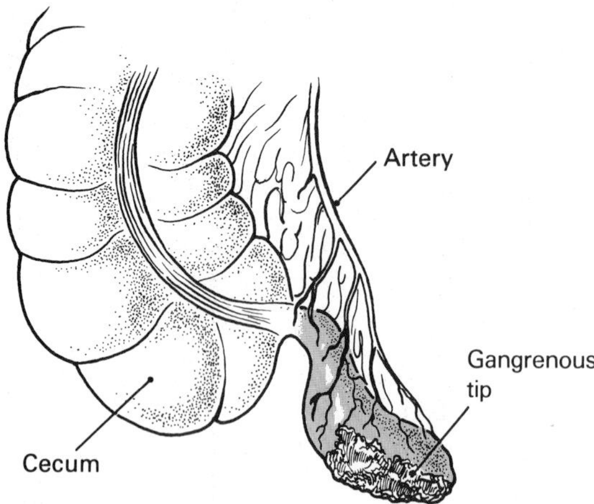

Figure 34-1 In appendicitis the blood supply of the appendix is impaired by bacterial infection in the wall of the appendix. This may result in gangrene.

present and there will be slight muscular rigidity. Rovsing's sign may be elicited by palpating the left lower quadrant, causing pain to be felt in the right lower quadrant. Because of the pain, the client may assume a posture of right flexion. Extension of the right leg is usually very painful.

Complications of acute appendicitis are perforation, peritonitis, and abscesses. Early diagnosis and treatment is important to prevent these serious complications.

Medical management

Examination of the client includes a complete history and physical examination (particularly palpation of the abdomen), and a differential leukocyte count. A urinalysis may be done to rule out genitourinary conditions that mimic the manifestations of appendicitis.

The treatment of appendicitis is immediate surgical removal if the inflammation is localized. If the appendix has ruptured and there is evidence of peritonitis or an abscess, conservative treatment of antibiotic therapy and parenteral fluids may be used to prevent sepsis and dehydration for 6 to 8 hours before doing an appendectomy.

Nursing management

The person with abdominal pain is encouraged to see a physician and to avoid self-treatment, particularly laxatives and enemas. The increased peristalsis from these procedures may cause perforation of the appendix. Until the client is seen by a physician, nothing should be taken by mouth to allow the stomach to be empty in the event surgery is needed. An ice bag may be applied to the right lower quadrant to decrease the flow of blood to the area and impede the inflammatory process. Heat is never used since it may cause the appendix to rupture. Surgery is usually performed as soon as a diagnosis is made. Postoperative recovery is usually short and rapid (4 to 7 days).

Postoperative nursing management is similar to postoperative care of the client after laparatomy (Table 34-6). The client should also be observed for evidence of peritonitis. Ambulation begins the day of surgery or the first postoperative day. The diet is advanced to general as tolerated. The client is usually discharged the fourth or fifth postoperative day and normal activities resumed in 2 to 3 weeks after surgery.

Peritonitis

Peritonitis is a localized or generalized inflammatory process of the peritoneum that may appear in both acute and chronic forms. It may be caused by trauma or rupture of an organ containing chemical irritants or bacteria. The chemicals and bacteria are released into the peritoneal cavity. Examples of a chemical peritonitis include gastric ulcer perforation and ruptured ectopic pregnancy. A chemical peritonitis is commonly followed by bacterial invasion. A bacterial peritonitis is usually caused by a traumatic injury (e.g., gunshot wound, ruptured appendix).

Pathogenesis

The response of the peritoneum to the leakage of contents is localization of the offending agent by attempting to wall it off. If the attempt fails, peritonitis will become worse. The tissue begins to swell and fibrinous exudate develops and adheres. The adhesions may shrink and disappear with the infection. If they do not disappear, they may later cause intestinal obstruction.

Intestinal motility diminishes, gradually progressing to paralytic ileus. The intestinal lumen becomes distended with air and fluid. Fluid accumulates as a result of the inability of the intestines to reabsorb gastrointestinal secretions. Leakage of fluid into the peritoneal cavity causes fluid, electrolyte, and protein losses. These combined losses can lead to rapid depletion of plasma volume, resulting in hypovolemic shock.

Clinical manifestations

Pain is the most constant symptom of peritonitis. A universal sign is tenderness over the involved area. Rebound tenderness is often found. The client has muscular rigidity, abdominal distension, elevated temperature, leukocytosis, increased pulse, nausea, vomiting, anorexia, and hypotension. The respirations may be shallow and rapid, due to the abdominal distension and discomfort. Bowel sounds are absent, because of decreased peristalsis. Hiccups may result from irritation of the diaphragm.

Medical management (Table 34-7)

Diagnostic A complete blood count is done to determine leukocytosis and hemoconcentration. An abdominal paracentesis may be done to determine blood, bile, pus, bacteria, and amylase content. An x-ray of the abdomen shows dilatation of the large and small bowel with edema of the small bowel wall. Air may be seen under the diaphragm.

Therapeutic The goals of medical management of peritonitis are to (1) identify and eliminate the cause, (2) combat the infection, (3) replace fluids and electrolytes, and (4) relieve abdominal distension and paralytic ileus. If the source of peritonitis is a leaking fistula, perforated organ, draining abscess, or ruptured suture anastomosis, surgery is indicated.

Table 34-7
Medical Management: Peritonitis

Diagnostic
1. Complete blood count
2. Serum electrolytes
3. Abdominal x-ray
4. Abdominal paracentesis and culture of fluid

Therapeutic
A. Preoperative or nonoperative
   1. NPO
   2. Fluid replacement
   3. Antibiotic therapy
   4. Preparation for surgery to remove source of infection, drain abscess, close perforation, or remove necrotic tissue
B. Postoperative
   1. NPO
   2. Nasogastric tube to low suction
   3. Semi-Fowler's position
   4. Intravenous fluids with electrolyte replacement
   5. Antibiotic therapy
   6. Blood transfusions as needed
   7. Sedatives and narcotics

Nursing management

Health Promotion and Maintenance Early treatment of clients with a known history of abdominal illnesses such as ulcers, ulcerative colitis, or Crohn's disease may prevent the development of peritonitis. The client with any of these diseases should be instructed to identify signs and symptoms of any complications and seek medical care immediately.

Acute Intervention The client with peritonitis is very ill and needs supportive care. Accurate recording of intake and output is necessary to determine replacement therapy. Nasogastric suction and intravenous fluid replacement (usually sodium chloride or lactated Ringer's solution) are started immediately. Potassium is usually not given initially because of poor renal function from shock and hypovolemia.

The assessment of pain is very important. Identifying the location of pain may assist the physician in determining the cause of peritonitis. Analgesics are given for pain and sedatives are given to allay anxiety. Oxygen may be given to help decrease intestinal anoxia and facilitate diffusion of nitrogen from the intestine to the blood. (Nitrogen tends to accumulate in the lumen of the colon and is not readily absorbed by the blood.)

The nurse should provide rest and a quiet environment, maintain nothing by mouth, monitor vital signs frequently, and assess renal function. An assessment of bowel sounds and increasing distension should be noted. If the client has surgery, drains are inserted to remove purulent drainage and excessive fluid. Care of the client postoperatively is similar to the care of the client with an exploratory laparotomy (Table 34-6).

Gastroenteritis

Gastroenteritis is an inflammation of the mucosa of the stomach and intestines. Clinical manifestations are abdominal cramps, vomiting, diarrhea, fever, and leukocytosis. The causative agents are varied (Table 34-8). Until vomiting has ceased, the client should have nothing by mouth and should remain in bed. If severe dehydration has occurred, intravenous replacement of fluids may be necessary. To replace losses, fluids such as ginger ale, lemonade, 7-Up, liquid Jell-O, and broth are given as soon as possible. If the causative agent is identified, appropriate antibiotic, antimicrobial, or anti-infective medication is given (see Table 34-8).

Nursing management

An accurate intake and output is important to replace fluid lost. Strict medical asepsis and enteric precaution should be instituted when indicated. The client should be instructed in the importance of proper handling and preparation of food to prevent infections such as salmonellosis and trichinosis. The importance of rest and increasing fluid intake should be stressed

Table 34-8
Causes of Gastroenteritis

Types of Infection	Entry Site	Clinical Manifestations	Treatment
		Viral	
Parvoviruses Norwalk agent and Hawaii agent **Rotaviruses**	Mouth	1. Nausea 2. Vomiting 3. Watery diarrhea 4. Low-grade fever 5. Little to no abdominal pain 6. Headache 7. Malaise	1. Usually self-limiting 2. IV fluid replacement if severe dehydration 3. Oral intake to 3000 mL/day
		Protozoan	
Amebic dysentery *(Entamoeba histolytica)*	Mouth From contaminated food and water	1. Fever 2. Weight loss 3. Frequent, small stools with blood and mucus 4. Chills 5. Leukocytosis	1. Diloxamide furoate (Furamide) 2. Metromidazole (Flagyl) 3. IV fluids 4. Low residue bland diet 5. Emetine HCl 6. Dehydroemetine
		Bacterial	
Salmonellosis (Gram-negative *Salmonella* bacillus)	Mouth	1. Gastroenteritis 2. Diarrhea 3. Fluid and electrolyte imbalance 4. Low-grade fever 5. Headaches	1. NPO until abdominal pain subsides 2. Liquids as tolerated 3. Anticholinergics 4. Enteric precautions
Botulism *(Clostridium botulinum)*	(See Table 32-7)	1. Descending paralysis 2. Weakness 3. Vertigo 4. Malaise 5. Fainting 6. Blurring vision 7. Cranial nerve signs 8. Dilated nonreactive pupils	1. Equine antitoxin serums—bivalent A and B and monovalent E 2. Supportive care (see Chap. 53)

as symptomatic treatment measures for gastroenteritis.

Symptomatic nursing care is given for nausea, vomiting, and diarrhea (see Table 33-19 and Table 34-2). The nurse should assess complaints of pain, vomiting, and diarrhea since gastroenteritis is often confused with appendicitis. To allay apprehension, the nurse should explain that gastroenteritis usually runs an acute course with no sequelae. The chronically malnourished, the elderly, and the debilitated are more at risk for complications and should be hospitalized until the gastroenteritis is treated.

Irritable Colon (Irritable Bowel Syndrome, Spastic Colon)

Irritable colon is a chronic, noninfectious irritation believed to be caused by spasticity of the colon associated with tension and psychological stress. The disorder occurs most commonly in clients between 20 to 40 years of age and has a higher incidence in females. Those affected often have tense and anxious personalities.

Clinical manifestations of irritable colon are episodic, colicky abdominal pain, and frequent alternating episodes of diarrhea and constipation. The pain usually is relieved after a bowel movement. The abdomen is frequently distended and borborygmi are heard.

The clinical manifestations are dangerous in that they mimic other conditions and the client may undergo unnecessary diagnostic studies and treatment. The client should be encouraged to verbalize concerns and anxiety. A mild sedative or tranquilizer such as diazepam (Valium) may be ordered for a prescribed period of time. A well-balanced diet with

Table 34-8 (Continued)

Types of Infection	Entry Site	Clinical Manifestations	Treatment
		Parasitic	
Trichinosis (*Trichinella spiralis*)	Mouth Source usually infected pork	1. Symptoms from muscle invasion (edema of eyelids, sclera hemorrhage, generalized pain and sore muscles) 2. Fever 3. Dyspnea 4. Difficulty chewing and swallowing	1. Thiabendazol (Mintezol) 2. Bed rest 3. Analgesics 4. Corticosteroids
Hookworm (*Necator americanus*)	Skin, especially through bare feet	1. Iron deficiency anemia 2. Diarrhea 3. GI symptoms 4. Dry cough 5. Malnutrition 6. Melena	1. Mebendazole (Vermox) 2. Pyrantel (Antiminth) 3. Well-balanced diet 4. Protein and iron supplement
Roundworm (*Ascaris lumbricoides*)	Mouth From feces-contaminated food or raw vegetables	1. GI discomfort 2. Fever 3. Chills 4. Dyspnea 5. Cough 6. Weight loss 7. Pneumonia from migration to lungs	1. Mebendazole 2. Pyrantel 3. Piperazine (Antepar)
Pinworm (*Enterobiasis vermicularis, Enterobiasis oxyuriasis*)	Mouth	1. Intense nocturnal itching around anus 2. Restlessness and nervousness	1. Pyrantel 2. Mebendazole 3. Pyrvinium 4. Pamoate (Povan)
Tapeworm (Beef—*Taenia saginata*, Pork—*Taenia solium*, Fish—*Diphyllobothrium latum*)	Mouth From eating infected beef, pork, and fish	1. Abdominal discomfort 2. Malnutrition symptoms	1. Niclosamide (Yomesan) 2. Quinacrine HCl (Atabrine)

roughage is encouraged. A bulk-producing laxative such as psyllium seed (Metamucil) may be ordered for constipation and an anticholinergic such as propantheline bromide (Pro-Banthine) may be given to decrease spasms of the colon.

Ulcerative Colitis

Significance of problem

Ulcerative colitis is a condition characterized by inflammation and ulceration of the colon and rectum. It may occur at any age but peaks between the ages of 15 and 40. Ulcerative colitis affects both sexes but has a higher incidence in females. Statistics show a low incidence in blacks and a high incidence in Jews. There is a familial tendency believed to be hereditary.[4] It is frequently associated with clients who are identified as immature, dependent, hostile, hypersensitive to criticism, and depressed.

Pathophysiology

The cause of ulcerative colitis is not known. Suggestions for a possible cause include an autoimmune reaction, viral infection, allergies, excessive enzymes, insecurity, and emotional stress. Some individuals with ulcerative colitis are known to have hostile feelings toward self. There has been much controversy concerning the role of psychological factors in the onset as well as for exacerbations of the disease.

The inflammation of ulcerative colitis is diffuse and involves the mucosa and submucosa with alternate periods of exacerbations and remissions (Table 34-9). The disease usually begins in the rectum and

Table 34-9
Comparison of Ulcerative Colitis and Crohn's Diseases

Characteristic	Ulcerative Colitis	Crohn's Disease
Incidence	Five times more common than Crohn's disease Familial tendency	Familial tendency
Location and extent	Starts distally and spreads in a continuous pattern up the colon	Anywhere along GI tract in characteristic skip lesion
Depth of involvement	Mucosa and submucosa	Entire thickness of bowel wall (Transmural)
Rectal involvement	95%	50%
Small bowel involvement	Minimal	80%
Diarrhea	Common	Common
Rectal bleeding	Common	Rare
Malabsorption	Rare	Usual
Predisposition to malignancy	Increased incidence	Minimal incidence

sigmoid and spreads up the colon in a continuous pattern.

The mucosa of the colon is hyperemic and edematous in the affected area. Multiple abscesses develop in the crypts of Lieberkühn (intestinal glands). The edema may cause the mucosa to become so friable that it bleeds with minimal trauma. As the disease advances, the abscesses break through the crypt into the submucosa, leaving denuded areas of colon. The denuded areas are predisposed to the development of a secondary infection. Losses of fluid, protein, and electrolytes occur due to decreased mucosal surface area for absorption. Some of the ulcerative areas heal normally and others form scar tissue.

Clinical manifestations

The three common types of ulcerative colitis are relapsing or recurrent, chronic intermittent, and acute fulminating.

Relapsing or Recurrent Ulcerative Colitis This type of colitis is the mildest type. It is characterized by a gradual onset, malaise, and vague abdominal crampy pain with diarrhea that is not disabling. The client may experience painful straining with defecation resulting in scanty, hard stools. The attack lasts 4 to 12 weeks. Remission occurs and may last weeks to months. Exacerbations usually occur with a gradual decline in health.

Chronic intermittent Ulcerative Colitis This type is manifested by persistent signs of inflammation and edema of the colon. The onset is abrupt and characterized by bloody diarrhea, anorexia, fever, weight loss, abdominal tenderness, and rectal and anal spasticity. This type is usually suspected if the disease is present for 6 consecutive months.

Acute Fulminating Ulcerative Colitis This form of colitis is characterized by an abrupt onset with a rapid course. There is severe bloody diarrhea with mucus (15 to 20 stools per day), nausea, vomiting, and rapid depletion of fluid and electrolytes. It is uncommon, but is the most dangerous type. The client may need surgery because of perforation or hemorrhage. If successful treatment is not achieved, death will ensue.

Complications

Complications of ulcerative colitis may be local or systemic. *Local tissue involvement* causes hemorrhage, obstruction from fibrosis, perforation, perianal and perirectal abscesses, fistulas, and strictures. Cancer of the colon is considered a complication of long-term ulcerative colitis. Megacolon (extreme dilatation of a segment of diseased colon) may result in complete obstruction. The most serious complications of ulcerative colitis are obstruction and perforation.

Systemic complications include uveitis, iritis, erythema nodosum, arthritis, nephrolithiasis, liver disease, pyoderma gangrenosum, and ankylosing spondylitis.[5] Anemia and malnutrition result from malabsorption and iron and vitamin K deficiencies.

Diagnostic study abnormalities

A health history is important because initial attacks may be mistaken for acute gastroenteritis. Physical examination usually reveals abdominal tenderness over the colon and possibly enlargement of the liver. Blood studies usually indicate iron deficiency anemia due to blood loss, low serum albumin due to protein loss, and electrolyte imbalances due to fluid and electrolyte losses. The stools are cultured for bacteria and parasitic infections. The stool is also examined for blood, pus, and mucus.

A sigmoidoscopic examination during an active stage of ulcerative colitis reveals a friable mucosa that bleeds easily and ulcers with purulent exudate. A barium enema may be used to confirm the diagnosis and determine the extent of the disease. The sigmoidoscopic and barium enema are also valuable in distinguishing ulcerative colitis from other inflammatory conditions of the colon.

Medical management

The goals of medical treatment are to (1) rest the bowel, (2) control the inflammation, (3) combat infection, (4) correct malnutrition, (5) alleviate stress, and (6) provide symptomatic relief. Approximately 80 percent of ulcerative colitis clients can be managed with medical treatment.[6] There is no specific medical treatment for ulcerative colitis but certain regimens are used to achieve remission (Table 34-10).

If ulcerative colitis fails to respond to medical treatment or if exacerbations are frequent and debilitating, a total colectomy and ileostomy is performed. For nursing care of the client with an ileostomy refer to the section on ostomy surgery.

Table 34-10
Medical Management: Ulcerative Colitis

Diagnostic
1. Fiberoptic colonoscopy
2. Sigmoidoscopy
3. Barium enema
4. Complete blood count, sedimentation rate
5. Stool for blood, culture and sensitivity, and indirect hemagglutination
6. Complement-fixation test

Therapeutic
A. Mild and moderate disease
   1. Low roughage diet and no milk or milk products
   2. Antimicrobial therapy
   3. Corticosteroids
   4. Anticholinergic therapy
   5. Antidiarrheal agents
B. Severe (fulminant) disease
   1. IV fluids with electrolytes
   2. Blood transfusions
   3. NPO
   4. Nasogastric tube to low suction
   5. Antimicrobial therapy
   6. Corticosteroids
   7. Surgery if no improvement (colon resection with ileostomy)

Pharmacologic intervention

Several drugs are used to treat ulcerative colitis (Table 34-11). Sedatives are ordered to promote rest. Anticholinergics reduce peristalsis, slow motility, and decrease gastrointestinal secretions. Antidiarrheal drugs are given to lessen the frequency of stools (Table 34-1).

Antimicrobial agents may be ordered to prevent or to treat secondary infections. Salicylazosulfapyridine (Asulfidine, Salazopyrin) is the principal drug used. The client must be observed for and taught the side effects of the drug such as skin rash, anemia, nausea and vomiting, leukopenia, anorexia, and headaches. The client should be provided at least 2000 mL of fluid daily to prevent crystalluria. The client should know that the drug will turn the urine orange.

Steroids may be prescribed early in the treatment. They can be given rectally or orally. The relative freedom from side effects, together with the rapid response and the convenience of administration, makes steroid therapy by rectum extremely useful.[7]

Immunosuppressive drugs may be given in addition to steroids. The rationale for using immunosuppressive drugs relates to the possibility that ulcerative colitis is an autoimmune disease. These drugs may be prescribed for clients who do not respond to Azulfidine and corticosteroids. The client taking immunosuppressive drugs must be watched carefully for signs of infection.

Hematinic agents are prescribed to correct the anemia. Oral iron is contraindicated because of decreased absorption in the bowel.

Dietary measures

In the acute phase, the client may receive nothing by mouth. When food is permitted, a well-balanced high caloric, high protein, nonirritating, low residue

Table 34-11
Drugs Used to Treat Ulcerative Colitis

Category	Action	Examples
Anticholinergic	Decrease GI motility and secretions and relieve smooth muscle spasms	Methantheline bromide (Banthine) Propantheline (Pro-Banthine) Oxyphencyclimine HCl (Daricon)
Sedatives	Quiet central nervous system without inducing sleep or analgesia	Diazepam (Valium) Flurazepam (Dalmane)
Antidiarrheal	Decrease GI motility	Diphenoxylate HCl (Lomotil)
Antimicrobial	Prevent or treat secondary infection	Salicylazosulfapyridine (Azulfidine, Salazopyrin)
Steroids	Anti-inflammatory	Corticosteroids (cortisone, prednisone)
Immunosuppressives	Suppress immune response	Azathioprine (Imuran)
Hematinics	Correct iron deficiency anemia	Iron dextran injection (Imferon) Iron sorbetex (Jectofer)

diet with vitamin and iron supplements is frequently prescribed. Some physicians will allow the client to eat anything that does not cause diarrhea. Cold foods, high residue foods (whole wheat bread, cereal with bran, fried foods, nuts, raw fruit), and smoking increase intestinal motility and should be avoided.

Since the client may have serious nutritional problems, the nurse should encourage the client to eat. Mouth care, frequent small feedings, and a conducive environment for eating are helpful. A daily record of weight and intake and output will aid in assessing fluid gains and losses. Supplemental feedings may be given or the client may receive parenteral hyperalimentation.

Nursing management

Nursing care for the client with ulcerative colitis is directed toward an intensive therapeutic and supportive program (Table 34-12). Emotional support is important since clients with ulcerative colitis have a tendency to be insecure, dependent, and sensitive. It is important that the nurse establish a good working relationship and encourage the client to talk about self and daily activities. Honesty, patience, and understanding are crucial in the relationship with the client. An explanation of all procedures and treatment is necessary and may allay some apprehension. Appropriate diversional activity should be used to move the client's attention away from the intestinal tract. Psychotherapy may be indicated if the client is experiencing emotional problems.

Bed rest may be ordered if the client is emaciated. An alternating pressure mattress, foam pads, or sheepskin may be used to prevent skin breakdown around bony prominences. To ensure rest, a sedative or tranquilizer may be prescribed. The client should be kept warm.

The client should be placed in a private room to prevent embarrassment from frequent use of the bedpan or bathroom. The number, amount, character, and color of each stool must be recorded. An accurate intake and output is necessary to monitor for fluid balance. The bedpan should be emptied after each bowel movement and placed near the client in case of urgency. A deodorizer may be placed in the room to remove odors.

Crohn's Disease (Regional Enteritis, Granulomatous Colitis)

Crohn's disease is a chronic, nonspecific inflammatory disease which can affect any part of the gastrointestinal tract. The terminal portion of the ileum is most often involved. Crohn's disease is seen most often in the Jewish population. It may occur at any age but occurs most often between 20 to 40. Both sexes are affected and there is evidence of a familial incidence.

Pathophysiology

The cause of Crohn's disease is unknown. It has been postulated that food allergies, autoimmune factors, lymphatic obstruction, and psychological factors are contributing causes. The emotional aspect is not considered as important as it is in ulcerative colitis (Table 34-9).

Table 34-12
Nursing Care Plan for the Client with Ulcerative Colitis

Client Problem	Expected Outcome	Nursing Intervention
Diarrhea	Absence of loose, watery stools	See Table 34-2
Dehydration	No evidence of dehydration	See Table 34-2
Hyperactivity and inflammation of the bowel	Normal bowel sounds Normal bowel elimination pattern	Administer steroids, sedatives, tranquilizers, and antispasmodics as ordered. Listen to bowel sounds every 4 h. Assess for abdominal distension. Reduce physical activity as much as possible. Provide undisturbed periods of rest. Assist client in turning, getting in and out of bed, and on and off bedpan.
Anorexia	Adequate nutritional intake Maintenance of normal body weight	Administer intravenous fluids with electrolyte replacement. Oral hygiene every 1–2 h and prn. Weigh daily. Obtain accurate intake and output. Give well-balanced bland, low residue diet of small, frequent feedings. Assess for food likes and dislikes. Determine what foods are tolerated by client. Remove tray when peristalsis is stimulated.
Skin breakdown	Maintenance of skin integrity	Change positions frequently. Special care (backrubs, positioning) to bony prominences. Pad rim of bedpan. Wash anal region after bowel movement. Passive range of motion.
Inadequate coping mechanisms	Have healthy coping attitude toward circumstances	Offer psychological support (listen and allow client and family to verbalize). Teach client to avoid emotional stress as much as possible. Help client work through problems and provide realistic encouragement. Accept feelings and reactions of client. Use diversional activity. Include family in assisting client to cope. Offer explanations and reassurance during the acute phase. Know limitations of nursing knowledge and refer to psychiatric counseling when appropriate. Assist client in identifying factor which may cause diarrhea.

Crohn's disease is characterized by inflammation of segments of the gastrointestinal tract. The terminal ileum is the most common location of involvement. The areas of involvement are separated by patches of normal tissue. This pattern of involvement is referred to as *skip* lesions. The intestinal wall in the affected area is edematous and thick, the lumen narrow, and the mucosa has a cobblestone appearance. Ulcerations can develop through the entire wall (transmural) of the intestine.

Clinical manifestations

The onset of Crohn's disease is usually insidious, with presenting manifestations of abdominal pain and tenderness, diarrhea, flatulence, low grade fever, nausea, vomiting, abdominal distension, and melena. As the disease progresses, there is weight loss, malnutrition, dehydration, electrolyte imbalances, anemia, increased peristalsis, and pain around the umbilicus and right lower quadrant. There may be remissions and exacerbations, or the condition may persist. The course is unpredictable.

Complications

Complications are common in Crohn's disease. Scar tissue from the inflammation narrows the lumen of the intestine and may cause obstruction. Perirectal and intraabdominal abscesses as well as perirectal and internal fistulas are common. Inflammation of the intestines may involve all layers, predisposing the client to perforation and generalized peritonitis. Carcinoma may result but is not as frequent as in ulcerative colitis. A higher incidence of cancer is seen in clients who have had Crohn's disease more than 10 years.

Impaired absorption may occur from damaged areas of the intestinal mucosa, causing various nutritional abnormalities. Fat malabsorption causes a deficiency in the fat-soluble vitamins (A, D, E, and K). The client usually has an intolerance to gluten (a protein found in barley, rye, and wheat.)

Medical management

Diagnostic A barium enema reveals a narrowing called "string sign" with areas of strictures separated by segments of normal bowel. Fissures in the lumen may also be identified. A sigmoidoscopy will reveal areas of inflammation and a colonoscopy will aid in identifying the segment of the colon involved. Blood studies are done to determine protein and electrolyte loss.

Therapeutic Medical treatment is generally supportive and symptomatic (Table 34-13). The goals of treatment are to (1) relieve pain, (2) control diarrhea, (3) correct fluid and electrolyte problems (4) treat and control secondary infections, and (5) reduce the client's emotional distress.

The diet is low in residue, roughage, and fat but high in calories and protein. The client usually responds favorably when milk and milk products are excluded from the diet. Lactose, a disaccharide produced from milk digestion, may not be adequately absorbed due to decreased levels of lactose enzyme. The damaged mucosa of the intestine may be unable to produce adequate amounts of lactose. The osmotic action of lactose pulls water into the intestine and perpetuates the problem of loose, watery stools. High fat diets are poorly tolerated due to the malabsorptive deficit caused by loss of absorbing mucosa and altered bile salt metabolism.

Fluids and electrolytes are replaced parenterally if the client has vomiting and diarrhea. Prednisone is given during an exacerbation to suppress the inflammatory response. Salicylazonsulfapyridine (Azulfidine) is given to prevent or treat infections. Iron may be necessary to treat anemia.

Surgery is indicated only for fistulas, perforations, bleeding, and intestinal obstruction. Resection of the involved part is usually done to treat these problems. As much intestine as possible is preserved. The recurrence of the disease after surgery is high.

Table 34-13

Medical Management: Crohn's Disease

Diagnostic

1. Complete blood count
2. Stool for occult blood
3. X-ray of the small bowel
4. Barium enema
5. Protosigmoidoscopic examination
6. Stool for culture and sensitivity

Therapeutic

1. High calorie, high vitamin, high protein, low residue, milk-free diet
2. Antimicrobial agents
3. Corticosteroid drugs
4. Supplementary parenteral nutrition
5. Physical rest

Nursing management

Acute Intervention Nursing care of the client with Crohn's disease is generally supportive and symptomatic. The assistance needed by the client is dependent on the severity of the disease. The physical and mental condition of the client is important in preventing recurrence.

Acute care of the client is very similar to the client with ulcerative colitis (Table 34-12). Special skin care to bony prominences and the perianal region should be given. As the client's condition improves, the nurse should allow for more self-care, provide frequent rest periods, and advise the client of the importance of rest and avoidance or control of emotional stress. This may be difficult initially for the client when he is told the nature of the disease and the limitations of the treatment.

Chronic Management The client should know the nature of the disease and that a relatively normal life is possible. The client and significant others may need help in setting realistic short- and long-term goals. Teaching is important and should include (1) the importance of rest and diet management, (2) perianal care, (3) action and side effects of medications, (4) symptoms of recurrence of disease, (5) when to seek medical care, and (6) use of diversional activities to reduce stress.

INTESTINAL OBSTRUCTION

Intestinal obstruction occurs when intestinal contents cannot pass through the lumen of the bowel. The obstruction may be partial or complete. Intestinal obstruction requires prompt treatment.

Types of Obstruction

The causes of intestinal obstruction are classified as mechanical, neurogenic, and vascular.

Mechanical obstruction (Fig. 34-2)

Mechanical obstruction is most often caused by strangulated hernias and adhesions. Other mechanical causes are *intussusception* (telescoping of a segment of the bowel within itself), which is most commonly found in infants and small children; *volvulus* (twisting of the bowel); inflammatory processes (ileitis, diverticulitis); edema; adhesions; tumors; foreign bodies; and fecal impaction. Cancer of the large bowel is the most frequent cause of obstruction in the older person.

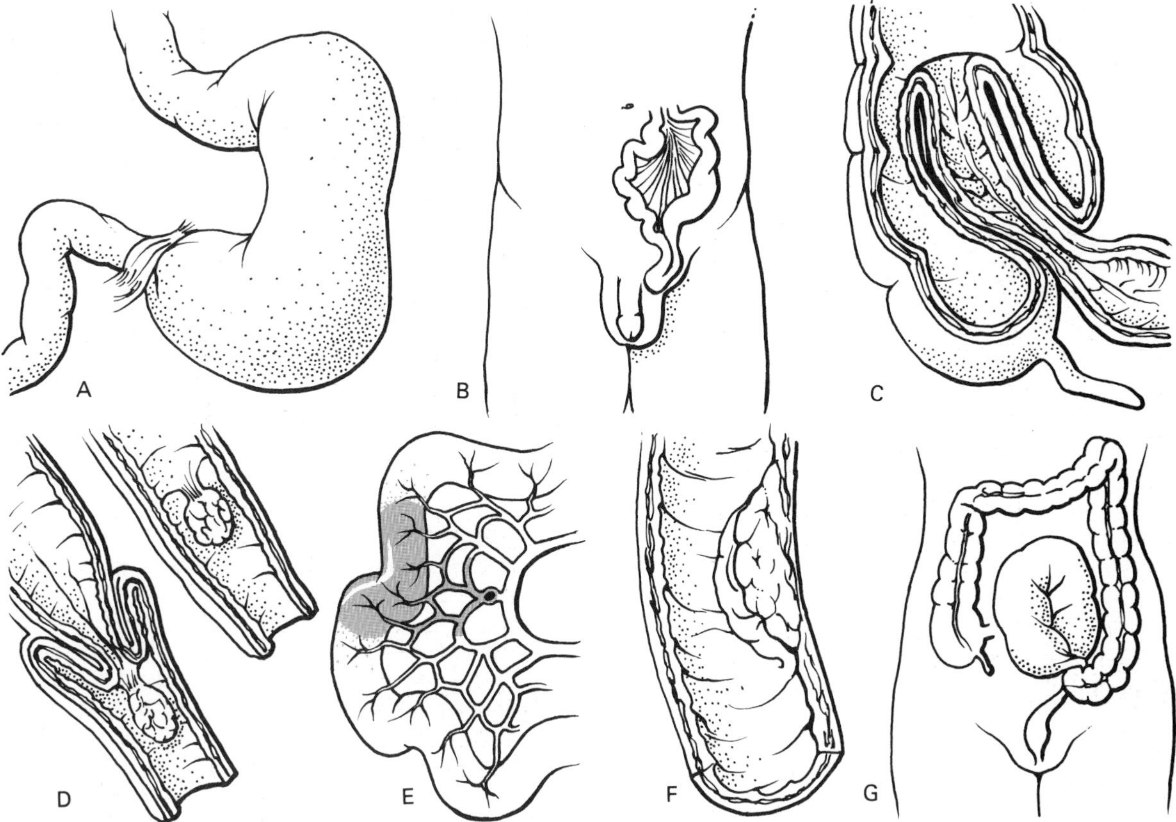

Figure 34-2 Bowel obstructions. *(a)* Adhesions. *(b)* Strangulated inguinal hernia. *(c)* Ileocecal intussusception. *(d)* Intussusception due to polyps. *(e)* Mesenteric occlusion. *(f)* Neoplasm. *(g)* Volvulus of the sigmoid colon.

Neurogenic obstruction

Neurogenic obstruction is caused by decreased or absent peristalsis from an interference in the nerve supply to the intestine *(paralytic ileus* or *adynamic ileus).* Paralytic ileus may result from abdominal surgery, peritonitis, pancreatitis, toxic conditions such as pneumonia or uremia, severe pain, shock, spinal cord lesion, electrolyte imbalance (especially hypokalemia), or trauma to the nerve endings.

Vascular obstructions

Vascular obstructions are rare but are due to an interference with the blood supply to a portion of the intestines. The most common causes are emboli and atherosclerosis. The celiac, inferior, and superior mesenteric arteries supply the blood to the bowel. The superior mesenteric artery is the most commonly affected by an embolus or atherosclerosis. When the blood supply is cut off, the affected areas of the bowel cease to function, peristalsis ceases, the bowel becomes distended, and gangrene rapidly occurs.

Pathophysiology

Fluid, gas, and intestinal contents accumulate proximal to the intestinal obstruction. This causes distension, while the distal bowel may collapse. The distension reduces the absorption of fluids and stimulates intestinal secretions. As the fluid increases, so does the pressure in the lumen of the bowel. The increased pressure leads to an increase in capillary permeability and extravasation of fluids and electrolytes into the peritoneal cavity. Edema, congestion, necrosis from impaired blood supply, and possible rupture of the bowel may occur. The retention of fluid in the intestine and peritoneal cavity can lead to a severe reduction in circulating blood volume and resulting hypotension and shock.

The electrolyte-rich fluids, which are normally reabsorbed in the bowel, are retained in the bowel and subsequently lost into the peritoneal cavity. The location of the obstruction will determine the extent of fluid, electrolyte, and acid-base imbalances. If the obstruction is high, as in the pylorus, metabolic alkalosis may result from the loss of hydrochloric acid from the stomach through vomiting or nasogastric intubation.

If the obstruction is located high in the bowel, dehydration occurs rapidly. Dehydration and electrolyte imbalance do not occur early in large bowel obstruction. If the obstruction is below the proximal colon, most of the gastrointestinal fluids will have been absorbed before reaching the point of the obstruction. Solid fecal material accumulates until symptoms of discomfort appear. Reverse peristalsis may cause vomiting of a fecal nature very late in the bowel obstruction.[8]

Clinical Manifestations

The clinical manifestations vary depending on the location of the obstruction (small or large intestine) and if it is partial or complete (Table 34-14). Vomiting is common in obstructions in the small intestine and occurs earlier and more profusely the higher the obstruction. If the obstruction is in the large intestine, vomiting usually does not occur since the ileocecal valve prevents backflow from the colon into the ileum. Vomiting of fecal material indicates a severe obstruction.

Abdominal distension is a common manifestation of all intestinal obstructions. It is minimally present in high obstructions in the small intestine and markedly increased in colonic obstructions. Abdominal tenderness and rigidity are usually minimal unless strangulation (interruption of blood supply) of the intestine or peritonitis has occurred.

Auscultation of bowel sounds will reveal high-pitched sounds above the area of obstruction. Audible borborygmi are often noted by the client. In adynamic ileus (neurogenic obstruction), colicky pain is usually absent and only discomfort from distension is present. The temperature is rarely above 37.8°C (100°F) unless strangulation or peritonitis has occurred.

Table 34-14
Comparison of Clinical Manifestations of Small and Large Intestinal Obstructions

Clinical Manifestation	Small Intestine	Large Intestine
Onset	Rapid	Gradual
Vomiting	Frequent and copious	Rarely
Pain	Colicky, cramplike, intermittent	Low-grade crampy, abdominal pain
Bowel movement	Feces passed for a short time	Absolute constipation
Abdominal distension	Minimally increased	Greatly increased

Medical Management

Diagnostic

A flat plate x-ray of the abdomen will reveal the presence of gas and fluid. The diaphragm may be elevated due to abdominal distension. A complete blood count is done to assess for leukocytosis and decreased hematocrit from hemoconcentration. A barium enema is usually done to assist in diagnosis. Serum electrolytes and a blood urea nitrogen (BUN) test are also done. Serum sodium, potassium, and chloride values decrease in a small bowel obstruction.

Therapeutic

Mechanical intestinal obstructions are treated surgically. Surgical intervention consists of resecting the occluded bowel and anastomosing the remaining healthy segments. If the client's condition is poor, a temporary cecostomy or colostomy is done to provide immediate treatment. When the physical condition of the client improves, more definitive surgical treatment is planned.

Treatment of neurogenic obstruction consists of intestinal intubation and decompression to remove gas and fluids. This procedure will relieve vomiting and distension. The purpose of intestinal tubes is to decompress the bowel proximal to the obstruction and to prevent distension of the bowel. Different types of intestinal tubes are used, depending upon their purpose and the physician's preference (Fig. 34-3).

The *Cantor tube* is 300 cm (10 feet) long and has a single lumen. At the distal end there is a rubber bag which contains 5 to 10 mL of mercury. Mercury is instilled in the bag before insertion. The weight of the mercury assists in passage of the tube into the intestine. Aspiration of gas and fluid occurs through openings into the tube above the level of the mercury bag.

The *Harris tube* is 180 cm (6 feet) long. It resembles the Cantor tube in that it has a single lumen and a bag with mercury, and the mercury is instilled prior to insertion.

The *Miller-Abbott tube* is 300 cm (10 feet) long and has a double lumen. One lumen is used for aspiration and the other opens into a small rubber bag that is filled with mercury after the tube has been inserted into the stomach. (Nursing management section describes the care of intestinal tubes.)

Parenteral hyperalimentation may be used to replace fluid and electrolyte losses and to supply nutri-

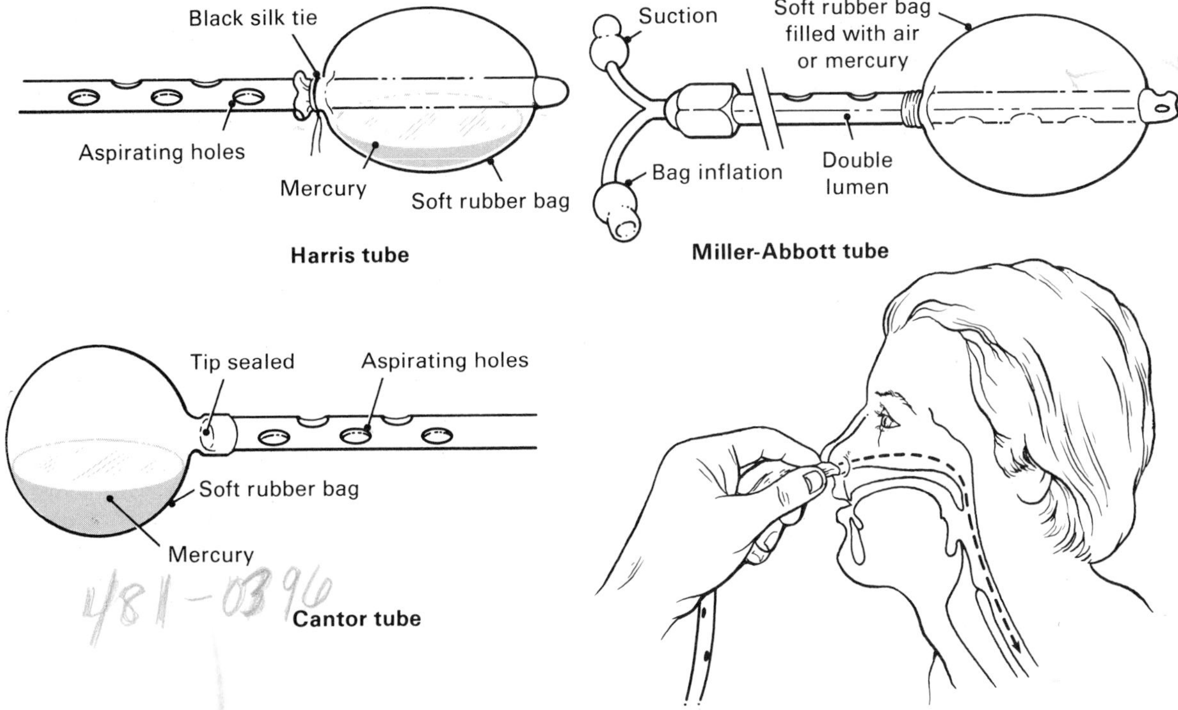

Figure 34-3 Intestinal tubes used for decompression.

ents to improve the client's physical condition for surgery. Special attention is given to the potassium level because hypokalemia can cause adynamic ileus. A retention catheter is inserted to assess hourly output and intravenous fluids are given to maintain an hourly output of at least 60 mL. Antibiotics are given to treat or prevent infection and analgesics are used for pain.

Nursing Management

The role of the nurse during the acute phase is assisting with preparation of the client for diagnostic procedures and maintenance of bed rest in a quiet environment. Nursing care of the client after surgery for an intestinal obstruction is similar to care of the client after a laparotomy (Table 34-6).

Nursing care of intestinal tubes

Although the physician usually inserts intestinal tubes, the nurse assists with the procedure. Insertion is easier if the client relaxes, takes deep breaths, and swallows when instructed.

If rubber tubes are used, they should be placed in ice so that they become stiff and easier to insert. The tube is lubricated with a water-soluble jelly. The tube is inserted similarly to a nasogastric tube. It is threaded through the nose into the stomach. The weight of the mercury facilitates movement of the tube through the pylorus into the intestines. When the intestinal tube reaches the stomach, the client will be asked to lie on the right side until the tube is past the pylorus. After the tube is inserted, it is attached to suction. The tube is not pinned or taped to allow advancement of the tube. The two different inlets of the Miller-Abbott tube at the proximal end must be clearly marked to indicate the lumen for drainage and the lumen for the balloon.

Movement of the tube (which is radiopaque) may be followed by fluoroscopy. The tube is marked in centimeters so that movement of the tube can be determined. The tube can manually be advanced 5 to 10 cm (2 to 4 inches) at regular intervals as determined by the physician. When the tube has reached the desired position, the tube is then secured to the client's face. The tubing should be long enough to prevent tension on the tube when the client moves.

The abdomen is measured for increase in size due to distension and bowel sounds are checked frequently. Fluid trapped in the intestines can only be estimated. Therefore, the client is weighed daily and accurate intake and output measurements are done to aid in fluid balance assessment.

Mouth care of a client with intestinal tubes is very important to provide comfort and to prevent parotitis. The mouth becomes very dry because the client tends to become a mouth breather. The client should be encouraged to brush his teeth and rinse his mouth three to four times per day. Sucking on hard candy or throat lozenges stimulates saliva and promotes comfort. Water-soluble lubricants should be applied to the nostrils and lips.

The intestinal tube may be left in place for several days. When the physician determines that the obstructive process has been relieved, the tube is removed. It can be removed by pulling it back through the nose or it can be allowed to pass through the intestinal tract and come out the rectum.

POLYPS OF THE LARGE INTESTINE

Polyps are structures arising from the mucosal surface of the colon and projecting into the lumen. They are most commonly found in the sigmoid and rectum. They may be single or multiple polyps. They are usually asymptomatic, but there may be painless bleeding.

Types of Polyps

The most common polyp is the *adenomatous polyp,* which may be sessile (flat) or pedunculated (on a stalk). The clinical significance of adenomatous polyps is that they represent premalignant lesions.

Villous adenoma polyps are larger than adenomatous polyps, with a definite malignant potential. They are soft masses and bleed easily.

Familial polyposis is a rare genetic disorder characterized by the appearance of multiple (often greater than 1000) adenomatous polyps in the colon. The probability of cancer of the colon occurring in these individuals is 100 percent by age 40.[9] Therefore, total colectomy with an ileostomy is the treatment of choice.

Medical and Nursing Management

Diagnosis of polyps is made by a sigmoidoscopy, barium enema, and colonoscopy. The polyps are removed (*polypectomy*) through a sigmoidoscope or colonoscope unless there is some contraindication to this procedure. Extensive surgery is not done unless the polyps continue to return and grow or bleeding occurs. After a polypectomy the client is observed for rectal bleeding.

CANCER OF THE COLON AND RECTUM

Significance of Problem

Cancer of the colon and rectum is the most prevalent internal cancer in the United States. Cancer of the colon accounts for about 20 percent of all deaths due to cancer in the United States. The colon is the second most common site for carcinoma in both males and females.[10] Cancer of the colon and rectum may occur at any age, but is most prevalent between 50 to 60 years of age.

The incidence of cancer at specific sites in the colon varies (Fig. 34-4). The distribution of carcinomas in the colon and rectum is characteristic in that about two-thirds of them occur in the rectosigmoid and rectum, with 40 percent of all adenocarcinomas occurring in the rectum alone. The next most common site is the cecum. Over 30 percent of colorectal cancers are within reach of the examining finger, and 60 percent are within reach of the sigmoidoscope.[11]

Pathophysiology

The exact cause of colon cancer is unknown. It occurs with increasing frequency in people over age 40. Familial polyposis and chronic ulcerative colitis are associated with an increased incidence of colon cancer.

Adenocarcinoma is the commonest type of colon

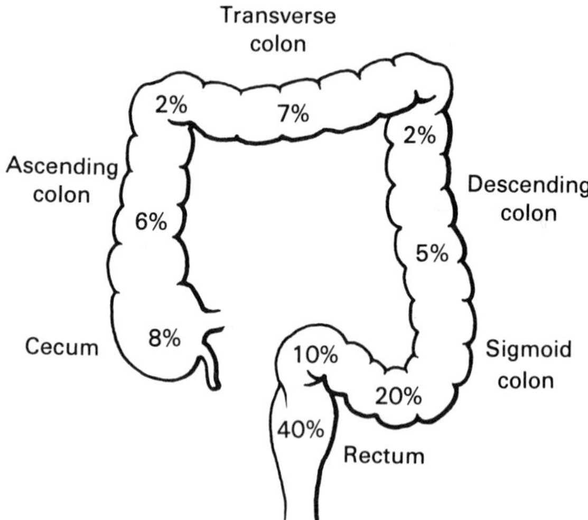

Figure 34-4 Incidence of cancer. Two-thirds of all colon cancers occur in the rectosigmoid and rectum. More than 30 percent of all colon cancers are within reach of the examining finger and 60 percent within reach of a sigmoidoscope. *(Used with permission, from J. Horton and G. Hill, Clinical Oncology, W. B. Saunders Company, Philadelphia, 1977, p. 292.)*

cancer. All tumors tend to spread through the walls of the intestine as well as through the lymphatics and portal vein to the liver.

Clinical Manifestations

Clinical manifestations of colon cancer are usually vague and nonspecific in the early stages. Cancer on the right side of the colon gives rise to different clinical manifestations than those on the left side of the colon (Table 34-15).

Changes in bowel habits are most frequent when the cancer affects the left side. There may be alternating constipation and diarrhea. Cancer of the sigmoid and rectum causes earlier symptoms of partial obstruction than right-sided cancers. The stool will gradually become small "pencil-" or "ribbon-shaped." In rectal cancer, mucous discharge is present and the individual may complain of a sensation of a rectal mass.

Cancers of the right side of the colon are usually asymptomatic because they do not cause visible bleeding or obstruction. Weakness and fatigue from anemia may be the first symptoms of right-sided malignancies. Pain is a late symptom of cancer of the colon and rectum.

Medical Management

Diagnostic

Blood studies, x-rays, and a thorough history and physical examination are essential to the diagnosis (Table 34-16). A carcinoembryonic antigen test (CEA) is not specific for colon cancer and a normal level does not exclude the possibility of a malignancy. This test is used most effectively in following the progress of a client after surgery. Return to normal of a previously elevated CEA indicates successful removal of tumor. In contrast, persistent elevated or increasing CEA levels postoperatively suggest residual tumor or tumor spread.[12] Liver function studies and an intravenous pyelogram are done to assess for possible metastasis.

Table 34-15
Comparison of Right- and Left-Sided Colon Cancers

Right Colon Cancer	Left Colon Cancer
Tumors grow larger before symptoms appear	Tumors tend to be cirrhous and encircling
Late obstructive symptoms due to larger size lumen and liquid consistency of stool	Early obstructive symptoms due to smaller size lumen and formed consistency of stool
Occult bleeding	Rectal bleeding
Diarrhea	Changes in bowel habits
Complaints of vague abdominal discomforts or crampy, colicky pain	Weight loss
Anemia	Narrow, ribbonlike stools
Palpable mass	
Weight loss	

Table 34-16
Medical Management: Cancer of the Colon

Diagnostic
1. Sigmoidoscopy
2. Barium enema
3. Colonoscopy
4. Rectum examination
5. Complete blood count
6. Testing stools for occult blood
7. Carcinoembryonic antigen (CEA test)
8. Liver function studies
9. Intravenous pyelography

Therapeutic
1. Surgery
2. Radiation therapy
3. Chemotherapy

Surgical management

Surgery is the primary form of treatment. The type of surgery performed will depend on the position and extent of cancer. For cancer of the ascending colon, a right colectomy with ileotransverse anastomosis is done. For cancer of the descending colon, a left colectomy with anastomosis of the transverse colon to the descending colon is done. For cancer of the distal sigmoid and rectum, an *abdominal-perineal resection* is done. In the abdominal-perineal resection, an abdominal incision is made and the proximal sigmoid is brought through the abdominal wall in a permanent colostomy. The distal sigmoid, rectum, and anus are removed through a perineal incision. The perineal wound may be closed around a drain or left open with packing to allow healing by granulation.

Radiation therapy and chemotherapy

Radiation may be used preoperatively or as a palliative measure for clients with advanced lesions. As a palliative measure its primary objective is to shrink the tumor size and provide symptomatic relief. (For discussion on radiation therapy see Chap. 11.) Chemotherapy is used as a palliative treatment. No drug has been discovered that can cure malignant tumors. The most commonly used drug is 5-

fluorouracil. Nitrosoureas, BCNU, and MeCCNU are sometimes used in combination with 5-fluorouracil.

Nursing Management

Health promotion and maintenance

Since symptoms of cancer of the colon and rectum are vague, individuals over 40 years of age should have an annual physical examination including a rectal examination and proctoscopy. Special attention should be given to individuals with predisposing conditions to malignancy, such as familial polyposis and ulcerative colitis.

Individuals who experience change in bowel habits or rectal bleeding should seek medical attention. Rectal bleeding is often attributed to hemorrhoids. In the person over age 40 any rectal bleeding should be investigated.

Acute intervention

The acute nursing care for clients with colon resections is like the care of the client having a laparotomy (Table 34-6). Preoperative and postoperative care of the ostomy client is discussed in the next section. This section will focus on the nursing care of the client with an abdominal-perineal resection.

After an abdominal-perineal resection there are three wounds: (1) an abdominal incision through which the colon is severed, (2) a left abdominal incision or stab wound to form the colostomy, and (3) an incision in the perineum. An inflated Foley catheter may be placed in the perineal wound to prevent formation of a hematoma and gradually deflated daily. The perineal wound may be closed with a Penrose drain or left open and packed with gauze. If the wound is packed, the gauze is gradually removed.

The perineal wound is usually irrigated with normal saline solution or hydrogen peroxide to facilitate healing and remove tissue debris. Warm sitz baths are usually given three to four times daily to assist in tissue debridement, provide client comfort, and to increase circulation to the area.

The perineal dressing is reinforced and changed frequently since the drainage is profuse for several hours after surgery. All drainage is carefully assessed for amount, color, and consistency. The drainage is usually serosanguineous. The rectal area is kept as clean as possible to prevent odor and skin irritation. The client's position should be changed frequently from side to side. There is usually considerable pain from the perineal area. Since the dressing is changed often, a T-binder or Fuller shield is used to hold the dressing in place without causing excoriation of the skin and discomfort to the client from using tape.

The perineal wound may not be completely healed before discharge. The client and significant others are taught management of the wound and how to take a sitz bath at home. The client and family should be aware of all community services available for assistance.

Psychological support for the client as well as the family is important. The recovery period is long, and the possibility of recurrence of cancer is present. The overall 5-year survival rate for all individuals undergoing resection for colonic malignancy is 50 percent.[13] Chemotherapy may be used as an adjunct measure for the client with evidence of local or distant metastasis. The special needs of the cancer client are discussed in Chap. 11.

OSTOMY SURGERY

Types of Ostomies (Table 34-17)

An *ostomy* is created when the proximal end of the intestine is brought through the abdominal wall and sutured to the skin. It may be permanent or temporary. The opening is called a *stoma*. Fecal matter is diverted through the stoma to the outside of the abdominal wall.

An *ileostomy* is an opening from the ileum through the abdominal wall. It is most commonly done as the surgical treatment of ulcerative colitis. It may also be done following a colectomy to treat familial polyposis.

A *cecostomy* is an opening between the cecum and the abdominal wall. It is used temporarily to divert feces after some types of bowel surgery to rest the distal portion of the colon.

Colostomies

A *colostomy* is an opening between the colon and abdominal wall. The proximal end of the colon is sutured to the skin (Fig. 34-5). A *temporary colostomy* is usually done to rest the bowel (e.g., diverticulitis) and is usually located in the ascending or transverse colon. A *double-barrel transverse colostomy* is done when an obstruction or tumor is in the descending or transverse colon. The colon is resected and both ends of the colon are brought through the abdominal wall, creating two stomas, a proximal stoma and a distal stoma. The proximal stoma is the functioning colon. The distal portion may be irrigated to remove mucus.

A *loop colostomy* is made when a loop of the colon is brought out above the skin surface and held

Table 34-17
Comparison of Colostomy and Ileostomy

	Colostomy			Ileostomy
	Ascending	**Transverse**	**Sigmoid**	
Stool consistency	Semiliquid	Semiformed	Formed	Liquid to semiliquid
Fluid requirement	Increased	Possibly increased	No change	Increased
Control	Not usually	Maybe	Yes	No
Appliance	Yes	Yes	Depends on control	Yes
Irrigation	Usually	Maybe	Maybe every 72 h	No
Indications for surgery	1. Perforating diverticulitis in lower colon 2. Trauma 3. Inoperable tumors of colon, rectum, or pelvis 4. Rectovaginal fistula	Same as for ascending	Cancer of the rectum or rectosigmoidal area	1. Ulcerative colitis 2. Diseased or injured colon 3. Birth defect 4. Familial polyposis 5. Trauma 6. Cancer

in place by a glass rod (Fig. 34-6). Rubber tubing is connected to the rod to prevent the colon from slipping back into the abdominal cavity. The bowel is not opened until 3 to 5 days after surgery to allow the skin to heal. The bowel is opened by an electric cautery. The client does not experience pain because the bowel has no sensory nerve endings.

The loop colostomy and double-barrel colostomy are usually temporary but they may be permanent. More commonly a *permanent colostomy* consists of a single stoma made when the distal portion of the bowel is removed. Most commonly a permanent colostomy is located in the sigmoid or descending colon and less commonly in the ascending and transverse colon. Permanent colostomies are performed when an abdominal-perineal resection is done. They may also be created following traumatic abdominal injuries and surgical resection of perforated bowel from diverticulitis (Table 34-17).

Nursing Management

Preoperative care

The physician should explain in detail the procedure to be done. Psychological preparation is very important. The family and the client usually have many questions concerning the procedure. If available, an enterostomal therapist can be most helpful. The client and family should understand the extent of surgery as well as the type and care of the ostomy.

If permission is granted by the physician, a visit from a trained ostomee from the Ostomy Association can provide the best psychological support. The client has the opportunity to see a person who has adjusted well and who has experienced some of the same feelings and concerns. The family will also benefit from the visit.

Bowel Preparation The objective of bowel preparation is to decrease the chance of a postoperative infection by cleansing the bowel of feces and bacteria. The client may be admitted several days before the surgery to begin preparation. A high caloric, low residue diet is given if it can be tolerated. Clear liquids are given 24 to 36 hours before the surgery. Stool is removed from the colon by oral cathartics and cleansing enemas.

Antibiotics may be given 3 to 5 days preoperatively to reduce intestinal organisms. Oral antibiotics used to sterilize the bowel are phthalylsulfathiazole (Sulfathalidine), succinylsulfathiazole (Sulfasuxidine), kanamycin sulfate (Kantrex), neomycin, or erythromycin. These drugs are poorly absorbed from the gastrointestinal tract, and remain in the bowel to decrease

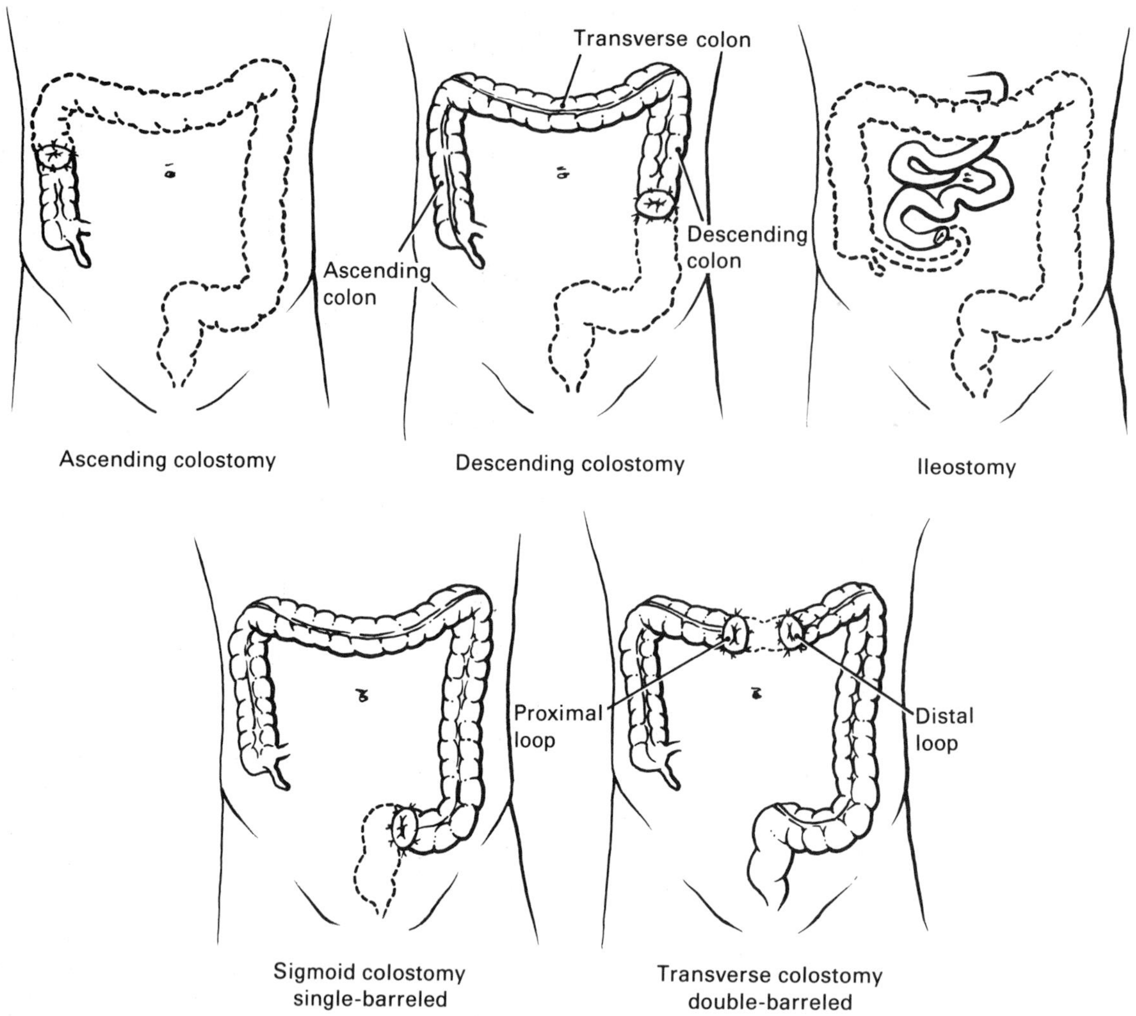

Transverse colon
Ascending colon
Descending colon

Ascending colostomy

Descending colostomy

Ileostomy

Proximal loop
Distal loop

Sigmoid colostomy single-barreled

Transverse colostomy double-barreled

Figure 34-5 Types of colostomies.

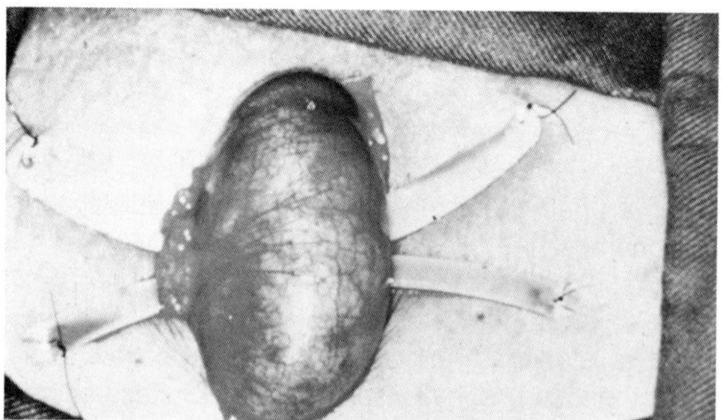

Figure 34-6 Loop colostomy. *(Photo from "Managing the Ostomy Patient," ©Copyright 1980, Hollister Incorporated. All Rights Reserved.)*

the intestinal bacteria. Intravenous antibiotics may be given 1 to 3 hours prior to the surgery to ensure a concentration level in the blood to prevent an infection from possible spillage of the intestinal contents during surgery.

Colostomy care (Table 34-18)

The stoma is dark pink to red (Fig. 34-7*a*). If interference occurs in circulation, the color will become dark red. The first few days the stoma will be edematous and there will be a small amount of drainage.

The skin should be washed with warm water and thoroughly dried. The skin must be kept as free of intestinal juices as possible. A skin barrier such as

Table 34-18
Nursing Care Plan for the Client with a Colostomy

Client Problem	Expected Outcome	Nursing Intervention
Perineal wound (in clients with an abdominal perineal resection)	Wound healing by granulation. No wound infection	Observe carefully for signs of hemorrhage. Irrigate wound as ordered. Observe condition of wound and color, odor, and amount of drainage. Change dressing prn. Sitz baths as ordered. Change position every 2–4 h. Provide pillow or rubber ring for client to sit on.
Potential skin breakdown around stoma	Normal skin integrity around stoma	Cleanse skin around stoma with mild soap and water. Rinse well and dry skin. Assess skin for irritation. Do not apply adhesives on irritated skin. Check the stoma for viability. Instruct client in care of stoma.
Alteration in fecal elimination	Regulation of colostomy	Use plastic stoma bag initially. Teach irrigation procedure (Table 34-20). Teach regulation by irrigation. Allow time for feedback and return demonstration. If client chooses not to irrigate, obtain a permanent appliance to wear.
Malodor	Control of odor	Use deodorizers in bag. Empty or clean bag frequently. Air room after emptying bag. Give oral preparations for control of odor if ordered.
Inadequate nutrition	Reestablishment of normal dietary pattern	Assess return of peristalsis. Observe signs of abdominal distension and pain. Advance diet as tolerated (liquids, soft, and regular). Avoid foods that cause constipation and are gas-forming (Table 34-19). Introduce new foods one at a time. Assess for diarrhea.
Anxiety	Adjustment to loss and altered body image	Encourage verbalization of feelings. Reassure client when progress is made. Be sensitive to clues of grief and denial. Involve client in self-care but do not abandon. Encourage family members to participate in care. Provide thorough instructions (with feedback) regarding skin care, appliance application, complications, Ostomy Association, and where to buy equipment. Assure client that change in lifestyle is not necessary.

topical sprays, ostomy cream, stomahesive, karaya ring, or other products (Fig. 34-7*b*) provide good protection. An open-ended, transparent, disposable plastic bag (Fig. 34-7*c*) makes it easy to protect the skin and observe and collect the drainage. The bag must fit snugly to prevent leakage around the stoma. The size of the stoma is determined by a stoma measuring card (Fig. 34-7*d*). Although the bag is usually applied after surgery, the colostomy does not function until 2 to 4 days postoperatively when peristalsis has been adequately restored.

The volume, color, and consistency of the drainage is recorded. Each time the appliance is changed, the condition of the skin is observed for irritation or excoriation (Fig. 34-7*e*). *An appliance should never be placed directly on irritated skin.*

The *diet* for the client with a colostomy is individualized. The client should be taught to avoid foods that cause gas, diarrhea, constipation, or that are odor-forming or irritating to the skin (Table 34-19). If the client introduces one food at a time, foods that cause problems can be easily identified. Problems with diarrhea may be controlled with medication (Table 34-1). Prune juice or a mild laxative may be used when constipation is a problem.

A colostomy in the ascending and transverse colon has semiliquid stools and is more difficult to control than a colostomy on the left side of the colon. A pouch is worn to collect the drainage. A colostomy in the sigmoid or descending colon has semiformed or formed stools and is easier to regulate. The client may or may not wear a drainage pouch. A cap may be worn over the stoma to help control the odor (Fig. 34-7*f*). Doedorizers such as Nilodar, charcoal, chlorophyl tablets, or oral bismuth subcarbonate (Derifil) will help control odors.

Colostomy irrigations

Colostomy irrigations are similar to an enema with the difference being that the catheter is inserted into

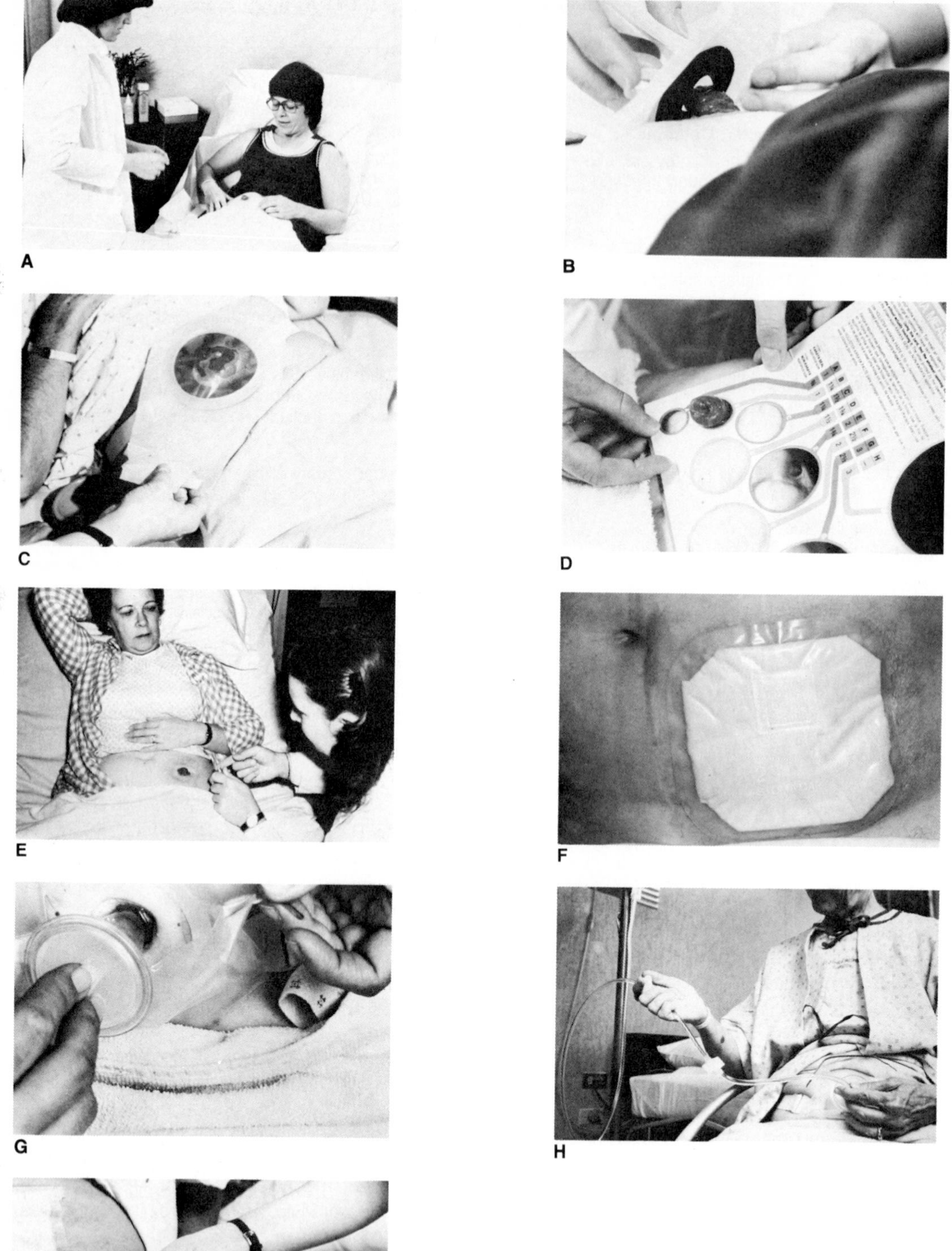

Figure 34-7 *(a)* A stoma. *(b)* Karaya ring. *(c)* Open-ended disposable colostomy bag. *(d)* Stoma measuring card. *(e)* Irritated skin around stoma. *(f)* Stoma cap. *(g)* Cone tip irrigator. *(h)* Client doing irrigation. *(i)* Nurse teaching the client. *(Photos from "Managing the Ostomy Patient," ©Copyright 1980, Hollister Incorporated. All Rights Reserved.)*

Table 34-19
Guide to Food Selection for the Ostomate

Ileostomy	
Foods included	**Foods excluded**
Initially: Clear soups, cottage cheese, tea, coffee, dry cheese, rice, liver, lean meat. Later: The client may experiment with foods to develop a dietary plan satisfactory to his needs.	Initially: Foods high in fiber. Foods high in cellulose. (Beets, leeks, asparagus, artichokes, celery, fruits with seeds.)

Colostomy
The colostomate may start earlier than the ileostomate to experiment with different foods. Initially a bland diet is given. Dietary plan must be individualized.
Constipating foods Dry cheese, nuts, chocolate, coconut, celery, corn, raisins.
Gas-forming foods Legumes, cabbage, onions, beer, carbonated beverages, apples, avocados, watermelon, sourdough bread.
Odor-producing foods Eggs, fish, garlic, mushrooms, asparagus.
Irritating to the stoma Hot spices, citrus fruit juices.

an abdominal stoma instead of into the anus. Colostomy irrigations are a way of trying to regulate a colostomy. If control is achieved, there should be little to no spillage between irrigations. The client who establishes regularity may only need to wear a pad or cover over the stoma. The client who cannot or chooses not to establish regularity by irrigations must wear an appliance at all times.

All equipment should be assembled prior to the irrigation. A commercially obtained irrigation set usually has all the equipment needed. Encourage the client to watch the procedure and explain each step (Table 34-20). The cone tip on the tubing controls the depth of insertion as well as serving as a gentle dilating stoma (Fig. 34-7*g*). If resistance is met, force should not be used because perforation of the intestine can result.

After the irrigation fluid has been inserted, the client may shave, apply cosmetics, read, or do a variety of other things. The irrigation sheath can even be closed off at the bottom to allow ambulation. The procedure should not be rushed and time should be given so that the client will feel relaxed.

Discharge to home should not occur until the client and/or a family member is comfortable with and knows the procedure and has returned the demonstration (Fig. 34-7*h*). The client should be able to identify all necessary equipment and supplies, do skin care, control odor, care for the stoma, identify signs and symptoms of complications, know the importance of fluids and food in the diet, have names and addresses of the Ostomy Association, and know when to seek medical care.

Ileostomy care

An ileostomy stoma protrusion of at least 1 to 1.5 cm makes care easier (Fig. 34-8 and Table 34-21). When the stoma is flat, seepage occurs and the skin becomes excoriated. Regularity cannot be established with an ileostomy because the content of the ileal drainage is liquid and constantly discharged. An appliance needs to be worn at all times. An open-ended drainable pouch is worn by the client so that the drainage can be emptied as needed. The drainable pouch is usually worn for several days before being changed as long as leakage does not occur around the stoma.

Immediately after surgery the intake and output must be accurately monitored. The client should be observed for signs and symptoms of fluid and electrolyte imbalance, particularly potassium deficit. Sodium and fluid deficits may also be present. The ileostomy

Table 34-20
Equipment and Procedure for Colostomy Irrigation

Equipment

1. Lubricant
2. Irrigation set (1000–2000 mL container, tubing with irrigating tip, clamp)
   or
   Bulb syringe (8 oz)
3. Irrigating sheath or sleeve with belt
4. Toilet tissue to clean around the colostomy
5. Bag for soiled dressing

Procedure

1. Place 500–1000 mL of warm water (not to exceed 40.5°C, 105°F) in container. (At first only 500 mL is given.) Amount is gradually increased to 1000 mL.
2. Assure a comfortable position. Client may sit in a chair in front of the toilet.
3. Clear the tubing of all air by flushing it with fluid.
4. Attach tubing to irrigating cone
   or
   Fill the bulb syringe with solution.
5. Hang the container on a hook or IV pole 40–53 cm (18–24 in) above the stoma (about shoulder height).
6. Apply irrigating sheath and place the bottom end in the bedpan or toilet bowl.
7. Lubricate the catheter or bulb syringe.
8. Insert the catheter 7–10 cm (3–4 in). If resistance is met, a digital examination is done to remove feces or check for muscle spasms. *Never use force—the bowel may perforate.*
9. Release clamp or squeeze the bulb to begin the flow. Only 500 mL are given at first. Each day the amount is gradually increased to a 1000 mL maximum.
10. Allow the solution to flow slowly over 7–10 min. The bulb syringe will need to be refilled several times.
11. If cramping occurs, stop the flow of solution for a few seconds. The level of the container can be lowered to lessen the force of flow of the solution.
12. Clamp the tubing and remove irrigating tip when the desired amount has entered.
13. Allow 20–30 min for the solution and feces to be expelled. The irrigating sheath may be closed off at the bottom to allow ambulation.
14. Cleanse, rinse, and dry peristomal skin well.
15. Replace the colostomy drainage pouch.
16. Wash and rinse all equipment and hang to dry.

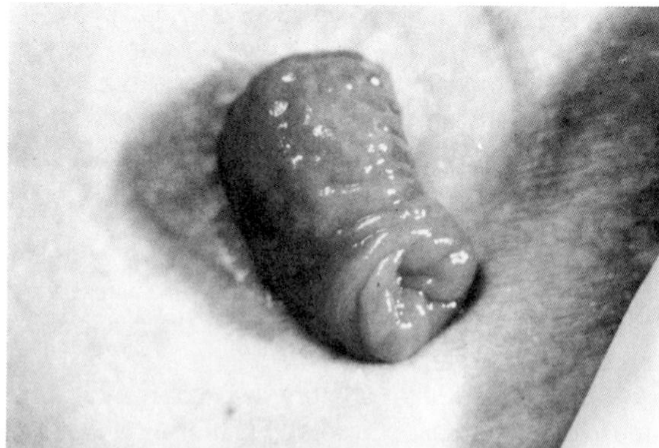

Figure 34-8 Ileostomy stoma. *(Photo from "Managing the Ostomy Patient," ©Copyright 1980, Hollister Incorporated. All Rights Reserved.)*

output may be as high as 4000 mL in 24 hours. The ileal stoma often bleeds easily when it is touched since it is a mucous membrane. The client should be told that minimal oozing of blood is normal.

The importance of fluid and electrolyte balance must be understood by the client. The physician may instruct the client to take an electrolyte solution at home (1 teaspoon of salt and 1 teaspoon of baking soda in 1 quart of water) because diarrhea from the ileostomy produces acidosis from loss of bicarbonate. During the summer, additional fluids are lost through perspiration and supplemental fluid intake is required. A commercial drink, such as Gatorade, is helpful in maintaining electrolyte balance. Usually a low roughage diet is ordered initially, but later there are no restrictions except on foods that are high in fiber (see Table 6 in Appendix B).

Table 34-21
Nursing Care Plan for a Client with an Ileostomy

Client Problem	Expected Outcome	Nursing Intervention
Continual drainage of fecal material	Adequate drainage without leakage	Properly apply ileostomy appliance. Assess appliance for looseness and leakage. Check stoma for retraction, protrusion, and prolapse. Change pouch as needed. Observe color, consistency, and amount of ileostomy drainage. Teach proper techniques of changing ileostomy appliance.
Possible skin breakdown around stoma	Normal skin integrity	Assess skin for irritation. Avoid cement/adhesives directly on irritated skin. Maintain good hygiene by cleansing skin around stoma with mild soap and water, rinsing, and drying.
Potential fluid and electrolyte imbalances	Serum electrolyte values within normal ranges	Record intake and output including fecal drainage. Report signs of watery feces. Ensure fluid intake of at least 3000 mL/day in the initial postoperative period. Teach client to increase fluid intake in very dry, hot climate or when perspiring excessively. Teach client symptoms of sodium, potassium, and fluid deficits (see Chap. 12).
Weight loss	Normal body weight	Reassure client that a normal diet can be tolerated. Gradually introduce food (liquids, soft, bland, low residue). Introduce one food at a time to test tolerance. Teach client to chew food slowly and thoroughly. Give list of foods that are high in fiber, gas-forming, and low residue (Table 34-19). Encourage visits by dietitian for diet instruction. Stress adequate nutritional intake.
Anxiety	Adjustment to loss and altered body image	(For Interventions, see Table 34-18.)

Continent ileostomy

An interesting variation from the traditional ileostomy is the *continent ileostomy* or *Kock pouch*. This method eliminates the need for the client to wear an external pouch or bag over the stoma. The pouch is not used for clients with Crohn's disease because the pouch itself may become diseased. An internal pouch in the distal segment of the ileum is made surgically (Fig. 34-9*a*). The intestine is split, a fold made, and a nipple created and sutured in place on the abdomen (Fig. 34-9*b*, *c*, and *d*). The pouch acts as a reservoir and is drained at regular intervals by inserting a catheter. The capacity of the reservoir increases gradually to approximately 1000 mL in several months. As the capacity increases, there is a decrease in the frequency of drainage.

A continuous leakage of fluid is prevented by a valve created at the internal end of the ileum from the stoma to the ileal pouch. Pressure created by the pouch filling with feces forces the valve to close. When a catheter is inserted, *effluent* (fecal discharge) is released.

During surgery, a catheter is inserted and attached to suction to prevent the pouch from filling before the suture lines heal. Usually 10 to 14 days after surgery, the catheter is removed and client instruction started as soon as possible. Catheter insertions to remove fecal discharge are done every 3 to 4 hours at first and gradually decreased until they are done three times a day. The client will eventually determine the frequency by the changes in sensation of pressure in the pouch. The stoma may be covered with a cap or dressing.

Adaptation to an ostomy

Acceptance of the ostomy is the first step toward total recovery. The client experiences a grief reaction to loss of a body part as well as an alteration in body image. Each individual is different and uses different coping mechanisms. The adjustment period for the ostomy client is dependent upon the individual lifestyle.

Psychological support during the grieving process may be needed. There are usually concerns about body image, sexual activity, family responsibilities, and changes in lifestyle. The client may become resentful and have fears of odor or soiling. Support from the nursing staff, allowing the client to verbalize freely, and talking to another ostomate may help the ostomate work through personal feelings.

The client should not be forced to learn to care for the ostomy. The nurse should watch for clues that the

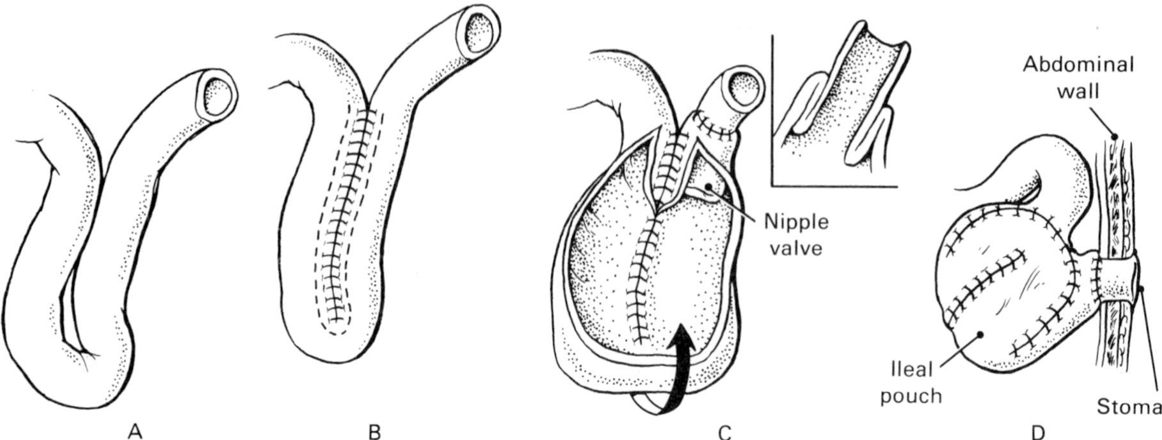

Figure 34-9 Surgical formation of continent ileostomy (Kock pouch). *(a)* Loop of terminal ileum. *(b)* Both limbs sutured together and incised in a U-shaped manner. *(c)* Pouch created with nipple valve. *(d)* Pouch sutured to abdominal wall.

client is ready. Teaching at the appropriate time is a very important part of the care and can contribute to a smooth adjustment process.

Activities of daily living are resumed within 6 to 8 weeks. Very heavy lifting should be avoided. The ostomate's physical condition will determine when sports may be resumed. Bathing and swimming are not prohibited. Water does not harm the stoma and a Band-Aid over the stoma is all that is needed.

Ostomy clients are often confronted with sexual concerns. They fear sexual failure and offending their sexual partner. The capacity to enjoy sexual intercourse is not decreased. Body cleanliness and perfumes may be useful. Impotency is not a common problem except when an extensive abdominal-perineal resection has been done (especially in men). Pregnancy is possible. The pregnant ostomate should have regular medical care.

Sexual concerns should be discussed with the client and partner. If the nurse feels uncomfortable doing this, appropriate counseling help should be obtained.

MECKEL'S DIVERTICULUM

Meckel's diverticulum is a blind tube which usually opens into the distal ileum near the ileocecal valve. It contains all the layers of the intestinal tract. It is a congenital abnormality primarily found as a problem in children and only occasionally in adults.

Clinical manifestations are abdominal pain and dark blood in the stools. Complications include hemorrhage, intestinal obstruction, diverticulitis, and perforation with peritonitis. Bleeding is the most common complication resulting from ulceration of the ileal mucosa. The treatment is usually surgical removal even when found incidentally at the time of another abdominal surgery.

DIVERTICULOSIS AND DIVERTICULITIS

A *diverticulum* is a saccular dilatation or outpouching through a weakened area in the intestinal wall. Diverticula may occur at any point within the gastrointestinal tract but are most commonly found in the sigmoid colon. *Diverticulosis* is a condition in which the individual has multiple diverticula. *Diverticulitis* is an inflammation of the diverticula (Fig. 34-10).

Pathophysiology

Diverticula are usually found in individuals over 40 years of age. It is seen more often in men than women and has a greater incidence in people who are obese. The exact cause is unknown but is believed to be due to congenital weakening. The role of dietary deficiency of fiber and roughage as an etiologic factor in diverticular disease is under investigation.

The cause of diverticulitis is related to the retention in the diverticula of undigested food particles and bacteria, which form a hardened mass called a *fecalith.* This process compromises the circulatory supply to the diverticula and makes them susceptible

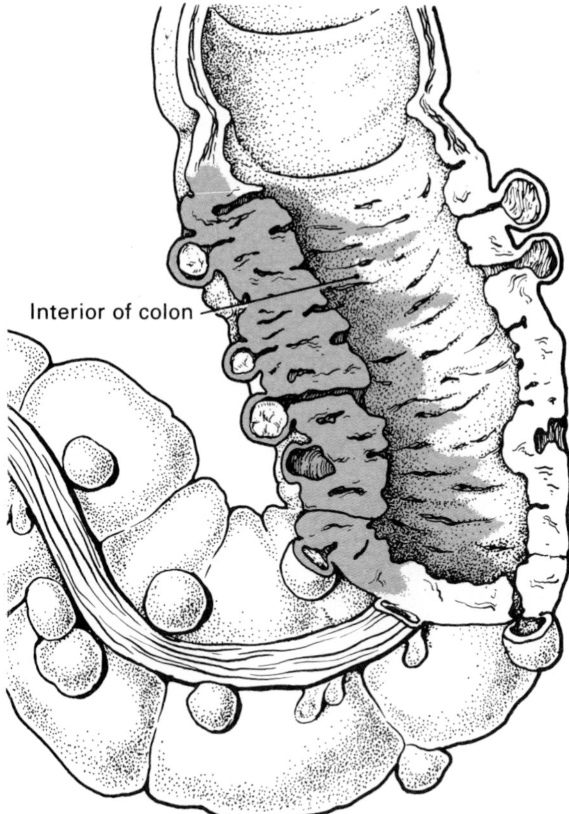

Figure 34-10 Diverticula are outpouchings of the colon. When they become inflamed, the condition is known as diverticulitis. The inflammatory process can spread to the surrounding area in the intestine.

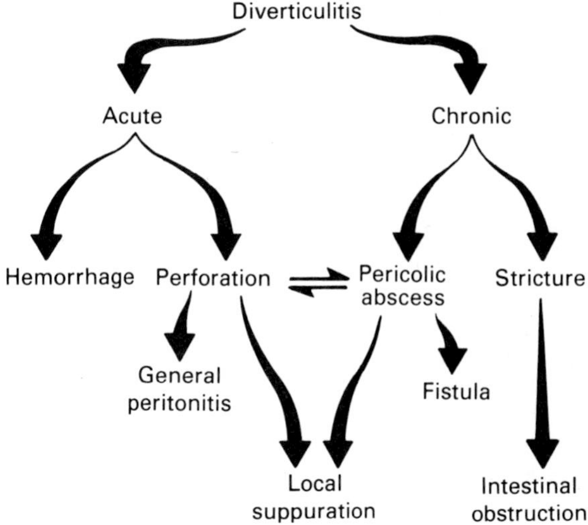

Figure 34-11 Complications of diverticulitis. *(Adapted from S. Price and L. Wilson, Pathophysiology: Clinical Concepts of Disease Processes, McGraw-Hill Book Company, New York, 1978, p. 247.)*

to bacterial invasion and a subsequent inflammatory reaction. Inflammation of the diverticulum spreads to the surrounding area in the intestines (Fig. 34-11). The edema that accompanies the inflammation can occlude the sac, resulting in more swelling and exudate. The bowel becomes irritable, spastic, and highly susceptible to infection.

Clinical Manifestations

Most diverticula are asymtomatic. When present, the symptoms vary with the extent of the inflammatory process. There is intermittent left lower quadrant tenderness, crampy pain, constipation, or alternating constipation and diarrhea. Leukocytosis and fever are commonly present. Occult bleeding may occur, producing iron deficiency anemia. Inflammatory changes in diverticulitis may cause perforation or abscess formation.

Medical Management (Table 34-22)

Diagnostic

The presenting clinical manifestations are similar to those occurring in appendicitis. Differential diagnosis is made on the basis of a thorough history and

Table 34-22

Medical Management: Diverticulosis/Diverticulitis

Diagnostic

1. Stool for occult blood
2. Barium enema
3. Sigmoidoscopy
4. Colonoscopy
5. Complete blood count
6. Urinalysis

Therapeutic

A. Uncomplicated diverticula disease
   1. High residue diet
   2. Bulk laxatives
   3. Stool softeners
   4. Anticholinergics
   5. Mineral oil
B. Acute diverticulitis
   1. Antibiotics
   2. NPO
   3. IV fluids
   4. Possible colon resection for obstruction or hemorrhage

physical examination with a rectal examination and a sigmoidoscopy. A barium enema may be done after signs of inflammation have subsided. This delay is necessary to prevent a possible perforation of the diverticula during the acute inflammatory process.

Therapeutic

Uncomplicated diverticular disease is treated with a high fiber, low roughage diet, bulk additives such as psyllium hydrophilic mucilloid (Metamucil), stool softeners such as dioctyl sodium sulfosuccinate (Colace), and mineral oil. Anticholinergic drugs such as propantheline (Pro-Banthine) and oxyphencyclimine HCl (Daricon) may be used to reduce colonic contractions.

In acute diverticulitis, antibiotic therapy is required. The client is also maintained on bed rest to decrease intestinal motility, is kept NPO, and the white blood count is monitored. A nasogastric tube may be necessary.

Surgical intervention is necessary to drain abscesses or to resect an obstructing inflammatory mass. The usual surgical procedures involve resection of the involved colon with a temporary diverting colostomy. The colostomy is reanastomosed after the colon is healed.

Nursing Management

Clients should be provided a full explanation of their condition. The better they understand the disease process and adhere to the prescribed regimen, the less likely the exacerbation of the disease and the onset of complications.

Uncomplicated diverticular disease is primarily treated by a high fiber diet with avoidance of undigestible roughage (Table 6 in Appendix B) and avoidance of constipation (Table 34-4). Foods such as apples, bananas, bran, prunes, and lettuce are bulk-forming and should be included in the diet. Foods such as nuts, popcorn, and raw celery are high roughage foods and should be avoided. Fluids should be increased because fibers retain water, thus decreasing the amount absorbed by the body. Large meals and the use of alcohol should be avoided. If the client is obese, a reduction in weight is needed.

Increased intraabdominal pressure should be avoided because it may precipitate an attack. Factors that increase intraabdominal pressure are straining at stool, vomiting, bending, lifting, and tight, restrictive clothing.

In acute diverticulitis, the goal of treatment is to allow the colon to rest and the inflammation to subside. The client is kept NPO, put on bed rest, and given parenteral fluids. This client needs good oral hygiene and nursing care to prevent complications from immobility. These measures include turning, coughing, and deep breathing, leg exercises, and skin care. The client needs to be observed for signs of possible peritonitis.

When the acute attack subsides (usually in 5 to 7 days), oral fluids progressing to a semisolid diet are allowed. Ambulation is also permitted. At this stage the client needs to be observed for recurrence of an attack. If the client has surgery for a bowel resection or colostomy, the nursing care is similar to that discussed previously in this chapter.

HERNIAS

A *hernia* is a protrusion of a viscus through an abnormal opening or weakened area in the wall of the cavity in which it is normally contained. A hernia may occur in any part of the body, but usually occurs within the abdominal cavity. If the hernia can be placed back into the abdominal cavity, it is known as *reducible.* The hernia can be reduced by manipulation or it can occur without manipulation when the individual lies down. If the hernia cannot be placed back into the abdominal cavity, it is known as *irreducible* or *incarcerated.* In this situation, the intestinal flow may be obstructed. When the hernia is irreducible and the intestinal flow and blood supply are obstructed, the hernia is *strangulated.* The result is an acute intestinal obstruction.

Types of Hernias

The *inguinal hernia* is the most common type of hernia and occurs where there is a weakness in the abdominal wall where the spermatic cord in men and the round ligament in women emerge (Fig. 34-12). When the protrusion escapes through the inguinal ring and follows the spermatic cord or round ligament, it is termed an *indirect* hernia. When it escapes through the posterior inguinal wall it is a *direct* hernia. An inguinal hernia is more frequent in men.

A *femoral hernia* occurs when there is a protrusion through the femoral ring into the femoral canal. It occurs below the inguinal (Poupart's) ligament as a bulge. It becomes strangulated easily and occurs more frequently in women. The *umbilical hernia* occurs when the rectus muscle is weak or the umbilical opening fails to close after birth. This type of hernia is found most commonly in children.

Ventral or *incisional* hernias are due to weakness of the abdominal wall at the site of a previous incision.

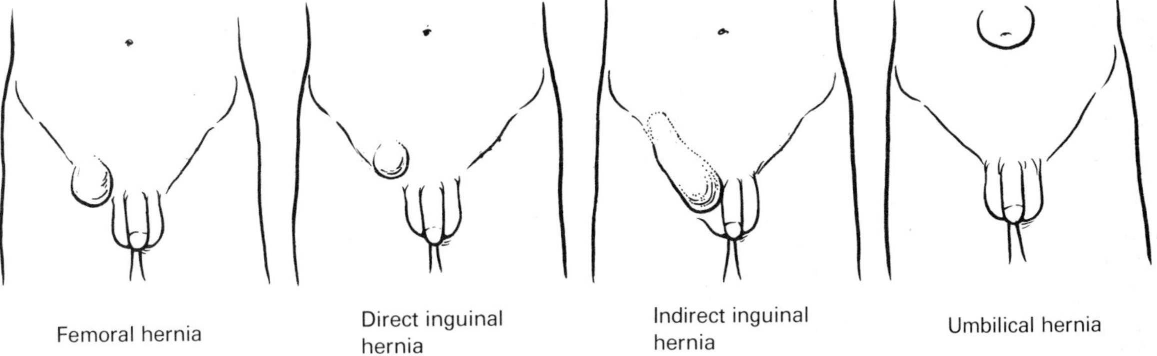

Figure 34-12 Types of hernias.

It is found most commonly in clients who are obese, who have had multiple surgeries in the same area, and who have had inadequate wound healing due to poor nutrition or infection.

Clinical Manifestations

A hernia commonly presents over the involved area when the client stands or strains. There may be some discomfort due to tension. Severe pain is caused if the hernia becomes strangulated. In this situation the clinical manifestations of a bowel obstruction are found such as vomiting, crampy abdominal pain, and distension.

Medical Management

Diagnosis is made by a history and physical examination. Surgery is the treatment of choice for hernias to prevent the possible complication of strangulation. Umbilical hernia is not usually surgically repaired because it may reduce itself if left alone until the child gets older. The surgical repair of a hernia is known as a *herniorrhaphy*. The reinforcement of the weakened area with wire, fascia, or mesh is known as a *hernioplasty*. When there is strangulation, necrosis and gangrene may develop if immediate care is not given. A bowel resection of the involved area or a temporary colostomy may be needed to treat a strangulated hernia.

Nursing Management

Some clients with hernias may wear a *truss* which is a pad placed over the hernia and held in place with a belt. The truss is worn to keep the hernia from protruding. If a client wears a truss, the nurse should check for skin irritation due to the continual rubbing of the truss.

Postoperative nursing care

After a hernia repair, the client may have difficulty voiding. Therefore, the nurse should observe for a distended bladder. An accurate intake and output is important. Scrotal edema is a painful complication after an inguinal hernia repair. A scrotal support with application of an ice bag may assist in relieving pain and edema. Coughing is not encouraged but deep breathing and turning should be done. If the client needs to cough or sneeze, he should splint his incision when coughing and sneeze with his mouth open.

After discharge the client may be restricted from heavy lifting for 6 to 8 weeks. Some surgeons do not put any limitations on physical activities.

MALABSORPTION SYNDROME

The *malabsorption syndrome* is a group of disorders that results from impaired absorption of fats, carbohydrates, proteins, minerals, and water and fat-soluble vitamins. Nutrients are ordinarily broken down in the intestine to smaller molecules to prepare the food for absorption or transport across the intestinal mucosa into the blood. If at any point there is an interruption in the absorption process, malabsorption may occur. A wide variety of problems can cause malabsorption syndrome (Table 34-23).

The most common clinical manifestation of malabsorption syndrome is *steatorrhea* (fatty stools). Other frequently occurring manifestations are diarrhea, weight loss, and flatulence. Two causes of malabsorption, sprue syndrome and lactase deficiency, will be briefly discussed.

Sprue Syndrome

Two closely related malabsorption conditions known as *sprue syndrome* are nontropical sprue and

Table 34-23

Causes of Malabsorption Syndrome

1. Gastric resections
   A. Total gastric resection
   B. Billroth II gastrectomy
2. Pancreatic insufficiency
   A. Chronic pancreatitis
   B. Cancer of the pancreas
   C. Zollinger-Ellison syndrome
3. Sprue syndrome
   A. Celiac disease (nontropical sprue)
   B. Tropical sprue
4. Lactase deficiency
5. Liver disease
   A. Parenchymal liver disease
   B. Biliary tract obstruction
6. Regional enteritis
7. Scleroderma
8. Congestive heart failure

tropical sprue. Tropical and nontropical sprue are found in adults. Celiac disease, which is probably the same pathogenetic disorder as nontropical spruce, is found only in children.

Etiology

In celiac disease (nontropical sprue) there is marked atrophy and flattening of the villi. As a result, absorption within the small intestine is reduced. The proposed reason for the injury to the villi is due to a hypersensitivity response initiated by gluten and gliadin (a breakdown product of gluten). Gluten is a protein found in wheat, rye, barley, and oats. The hypersensitivity leads to an inflammatory response of the mucosa.

Tropical sprue primarily occurs in tropical regions. The exact cause is unknown, but has been linked to an infectious agent. Clinically, it resembles nontropical sprue.

Clinical manifestations

Generalized symptoms include steatorrhea (bulky, foul-smelling, yellow-gray, greasy stools), diarrhea, weight loss, signs of multiple vitamin deficiencies, abdominal distension, and excessive flatulence.

Medical management

Treatment of sprue syndrome is based on the underlying cause. In nontropical sprue, a gluten-free diet will usually lead to clinical recovery. Wheat, barley, oats, and rye products need to be avoided. Soy flours may be used. Corticosteroids are also used to treat nontropical sprue. The basis for this treatment is that the inflammatory response is mediated by an immunologic response.

Tropical sprue is treated with broad-spectrum antibiotics in conjunction with folic acid therapy. After the client responds to this therapy and achieves a remission, he is usually maintained on folic acid.

Lactase Deficiency

Lactase deficiency is a condition in which the lactase enzyme is deficient or absent. This enzyme is needed for the digestion of lactose (the primary carbohydrate of milk) to galactose and glucose. Although primary lactase deficiency seems to be hereditary, milk intolerance may not become clinically evident until late adolescence or early adulthood. This is probably related to a normally found reduction in lactase as the person ages.[14]

About 5 percent of the adult population has primary lactase deficiency. In the United States, those most likely to have lactase deficiency are Afro-Americans, American Indians, Mexican-Americans, Orientals, and some Jews and Arabs.[15, 16]

Acquired lactase deficiency is often seen in other gastrointestinal diseases where the mucosa has been damaged. Some of these conditions include ulcerative colitis, Crohn's disease, gastroenteritis, and sprue syndrome.

Clinical manifestations

The symptoms of lactose intolerance include bloating, flatulence, crampy abdominal pain, and diarrhea. They may occur within one-half to several hours after drinking a glass of milk. The diarrhea of lactose intolerance results from fluid secretion into the small intestines, responding to the osmotic action of undigested lactose.

Medical and nursing management

Many lactose-intolerant individuals are aware they are milk-intolerant and avoid milk. A lactose intolerance test can be done to rule out milk allergies. The client is given 50 to 100 mg of lactose orally. Blood samples are drawn prior to the consumption of lactose and at 15-, 30-, 60- and 90- minute intervals. Failure of the blood sugar to increase more than 20 mg% is suggestive of lactase deficiency.

Treatment consists of eliminating lactose from the diet by avoiding milk and milk products. A lactose-free diet is given initially and gradually advanced to a low lactose diet as tolerated by the client.

The objective of care is to teach the importance of adherence to the diet. Many lactose-intolerant individuals may not exhibit symptoms if lactose is taken in small amounts. In some individuals lactose may be tolerated better if taken with meals.

The client needs to be aware that milk, ice cream, cottage cheese, and cheese have a high lactose content. If the milk has been fermented (e.g., cultured buttermilk, yogurt, sour cream), the client with low lactase levels may tolerate them better.

Lactase enzyme (Lact-Aid) is available commercially as an over-the-counter product. It is mixed with milk and breaks down the lactose before the milk is ingested.

ANORECTAL PROBLEMS

Hemorrhoids

Hemorrhoids are dilated varicose veins of the anus and rectum. They may be internal (occurring above the internal sphincter) or external (occurring outside the external sphincter) (Fig. 34-13). Hemorrhoids occur most frequently between the ages of 20 to 50. In individuals who have them, they appear periodically, depending on the amount of anorectal pressure.

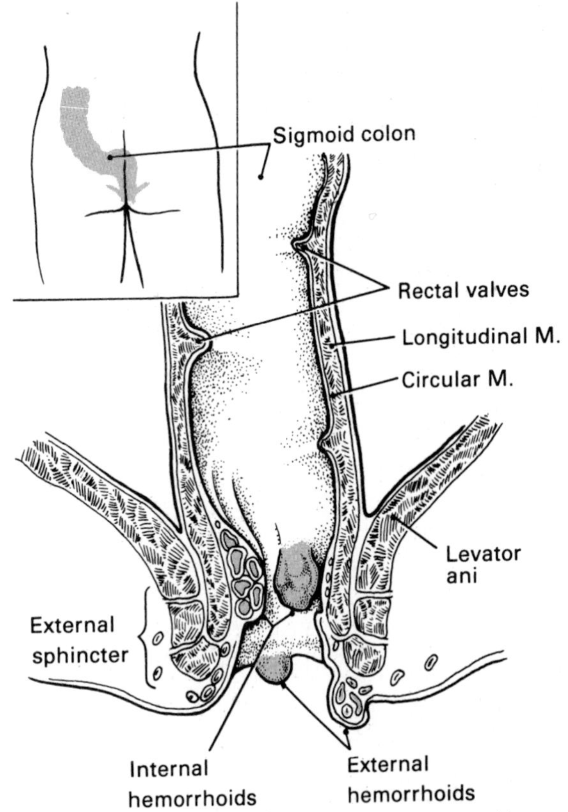

Figure 34-13 Anatomy of the rectum and anus with external and internal hemorrhoids. (*Adapted from S. Price and L. Wilson, Pathophysiology: Clinical Concepts of Disease Processes, McGraw-Hill Book Company, 1978, p. 243.*)

Pathophysiology

Hemorrhoids develop when the flow of blood through the veins of the hemorrhoidal plexus is impaired. Internal hemorrhoids may become constricted and painful and may bleed upon defecation. The amount of blood lost at one time may be small but over a period of time may lead to iron deficiency anemia. External hemorrhoids are reddish-blue in appearance, and seldom bleed or cause pain unless a vein ruptures. If the blood clots in external hemorrhoids they become inflamed, painful, and are said to be *thrombosed*.

Hemorrhoids may be caused by many factors including pregnancy, prolonged constipation, straining in an effort to defecate, heavy lifting, prolonged standing and sitting, and portal hypertension as found in cirrhosis.

Medical management

Hemorrhoids are diagnosed by inspection, digital examination, and proctoscopy. Medical treatment may be symptomatic in mild cases. The objective is to relieve discomfort with good hygiene and avoid excessive straining. Ointments, such as dibucaine (Nupercaine), creams, suppositories, and witch hazel compresses are used to shrink the mucous membrane. Stool softeners or a mild laxative are ordered to keep the stool soft, and a sitz bath is ordered to relieve pain.

Ice packs for a few hours followed by warm packs may be used for thrombosed hemorrhoids. Another conservative treatment is to use a sclerosing solution such as 5% phenol in oil, or a combined solution of quinine and urea may be injected into the submucous tissue surrounding the hemorrhoids, causing a fibrosing and shrinking of the supporting tissues.

Internal hemorrhoids may be ligated with a rubber band. The constrictive effect impairs circulation, and the tissue becomes necrotic, separates, and sloughs off. There is some local discomfort with this procedure, but no anesthesia is required. Aspirin or propoxyphene (Darvon) is usually given for discomfort.

A *hemorrhoidectomy* is the surgical excision of hemorrhoids. Surgery is indicated when there is prolapse, excessive pain or bleeding, or large hemorrhoids. In general, hemorroidectomy is reserved for clients having severe symptoms related to multiple thrombosed hemorrhoids or marked protrusion. Surgical removal may be by cautery, clamp, or excision. One surgical approach is to leave the area open so that healing takes place by secondary intention. In another approach the hemorrhoids are removed, the tissue is sutured, and healing takes place by primary intention wound healing.

Nursing management

Conservative nursing management for the client with hemorrhoids includes teaching measures (1) to prevent constipation (Table 34-4), (2) to avoid prolonged standing or sitting, (3) to properly use over-the-counter medications available for hemorrhoidal symptoms, and (4) to seek medical care for severe symptoms of hemorrhoids (excessive pain and bleeding, prolapsed hemorrhoids) when necessary.

Following a hemorrhoidectomy a common client problem is pain. The nurse must be aware that although the procedure is minor, the pain is severe and narcotics are usually given initially.

Sitz baths are started 1 to 2 days after surgery. A warm sitz bath provides comfort and keeps the anal area clean. A sponge ring in the sitz bath will help relieve pressure on the area. Initially the client should not be left alone in case he becomes weak or faints.

Packing may be inserted into the rectum to absorb drainage. A T-binder may hold the dressing in place. If packing is inserted it usually is removed the first or second postoperative day. The nurse should assess for rectal bleeding. The client may be embarrassed when the dressing is changed and privacy should be provided. The client usually dreads the first bowel movement and often resists the urge to defecate. Pain medication may be given before the bowel movement to reduce discomfort.

A stool softener, such as dioctyl sodium sulfosucinate (Colace) is usually ordered the first few postoperative days. If the client does not have a bowel movement within 2 to 3 days, an oil retention enema is given.

Discharge teaching includes the importance of the diet, care of the anal area, symptoms of complications (especially bleeding), and avoidance of constipation and straining. Sitz baths are recommended for 1 to 2 weeks. The physician may order a stool softener to be taken for a period of time. Hemorrhoids may recur. Occasionally anal strictures develop and dilatation is necessary. Regular medical checkups are important in the prevention of any further problems.

Anal Fissure (Fissure in Ano)

An *anal fissure* is a skin ulcer or a crack in the lining of the anal wall. It is caused by trauma or local infection. It is frequently associated with constipation and subsequent stretching of the anus from hard feces. The most common clinical manifestations are painful spasms of the anal sphincter and severe, burning pain during defecation. Some bleeding may occur and constipation results because of fear of pain associated with bowel movements.

Conservative treatment consists of bowel regulation with mineral oil and stool softeners. Sitz baths and anal anesthetic suppositories (Anusol) are also ordered. Surgical treatment usually consists of excision of the fissure. Postoperative nursing care is the same

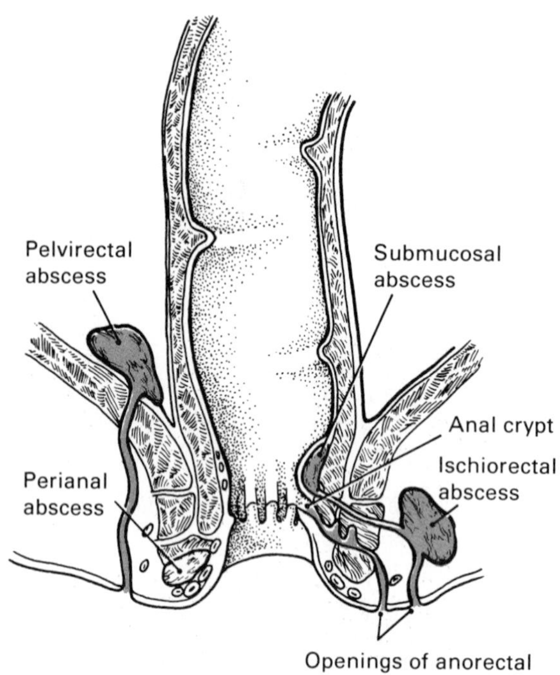

Figure 34-14 Common sites of anorectal abscesses and fistula. *(Adapted from S. Price and L. Wilson, Pathophysiology: Clinical Concepts of Disease Processes, McGraw-Hill Book Company, New York, 1978, p. 252.)*

as the care for the client who has had a hemorrhoidectomy.

Anorectal Abscess

An *anorectal abscess* is a localized infection with pus in the fatty tissue in the anorectal area (Fig. 34-14). It is usually caused by an infection. The most common causative organisms are *Escherichia coli,* staphylococci, and streptococci. Clinical manifestations include pain, foul-smelling pus, tenderness and swelling near the anus, and elevated temperature.

Surgical treatment consists of making an opening into the abscess to drain the pus. If packing is used, it is impregnated with petrolatum jelly and the area allowed to heal by granulation. The packing is changed every day and moist, hot compresses are applied to the area. Care must be taken to avoid soiling the dressing when urinating or defecating. A low residue diet is given. The client may leave the hospital with the area open. Discharge teaching should include wound care, importance of sitz baths, thorough cleaning after bowel movements, and follow-up visits to the physician.

Anorectal Fistula

An *anal fistula* is an abnormal tunnel leading out from the anus or rectum. It may extend to the outside of the skin, the vagina, or the buttocks. Anorectal fistulas are a complication of Crohn's disease. This condition often precedes an anorectal abscess.

Feces may enter the fistula and cause an infection. There is a persistent bloodstained, purulent discharge or stool leak from the fistula. The client may have to wear a pad to prevent staining the clothes.

Surgical treatment is a *fistulotomy* or *fistulectomy.* In a fistulotomy an opening of the fistula is made and healthy tissue allowed to granulate in. A fistulectomy is an excision of the entire fistulous tract. Gauze packing is inserted and the wound allowed to heal by granulation. Care is the same as for the client after a hemorrhoidectomy.

Pilonidal Sinus

A *pilonidal sinus* is a small tract under the skin between the buttocks in the sacrococcygeal area. It is thought to be of congenital origin. It may have several openings and is lined with epithelium and hair, thus the name, *pilonidal* (a nest of hair).

The skin is moist and movement of the buttocks causes the short, wiry hair to penetrate the skin. The irritated skin becomes infected and forms a *pilonidal cyst* or abscess. There are no symptoms unless there is an infection. If it becomes infected, the client complains of pain and swelling at the base of the spine.

The formed abscess requires incision and drainage. The wound may be closed or left open to heal by secondary intention. The wound is packed and sitz baths ordered.

Nursing care includes hot, moist heat applications when an abscess is present. The client is usually comfortable lying on the abdomen or side. Care is taken not to contaminate the dressing when urinating or defecating. Straining should be avoided whenever possible.

Case Study / Ulcerative Colitis

Marie, 37 years old, is admitted for the fifth time in an 11-month period with acute ulcerative colitis. She complains of severe diarrhea (10 to 15 stools a day with blood and mucus), intestinal cramping, anorexia, nausea, and vomiting. She is dehydrated, has a temperature of 38°C (100.4°F), and is crying.

Marie stated she takes Azulfidine and prednisone. During the past 72 hours she has not taken any medication because of the nausea and vomiting.

On physical examination, palpation over the colon revealed abdominal tenderness and an enlarged liver. Blood studies were done upon admission and revealed iron deficiency anemia and a low serum albumin.

Discussion Questions

1. Explain the pathophysiologic changes that occur in ulcerative colitis.
2. How does ulcerative colitis differ from Crohn's disease?
3. Explain the reason for Marie's anemia and low serum albumin.
4. What would a proctosigmoidoscopic examination reveal during the acute phase?
5. List three nursing goals for Marie and your plan for implementation of care to meet these goals.
6. What are the complications of ulcerative colitis and the role of the nurse in preventing their occurrence?

REVIEW QUESTIONS

The number of the question corresponds with the same numbered objective at the beginning of the chapter.

1. Common treatment measures for the client with constipation are
   a. low residue diet and anticholinergic drugs
   b. stool softeners and high residue diet
   c. antiemetics and low fiber diet
   d. enemas and high fluid intake

2. Nursing care of a client following an exploratory laparotomy includes
   a. antacids through nasogastric tube every 2 hours
   b. irrigation of nasogastric tube with sterile water every 2 to 3 hours
   c. assessment of bowel sounds in all four quadrants
   d. assessment of the number and character of stools the first two postoperative days

3. Which of the following is not a common clinical manifestation of acute appendicitis?
   a. prolonged diarrhea
   b. WBC 18,000/mm^3
   c. nausea and vomiting
   d. constipation

4. The physician asks to be notified if any signs of rupture of the appendix occur. He should be notified of which of the following clinical findings?
   a. nausea and vomiting
   b. tenderness in the right lower quadrant
   c. sudden, sharp pain in the right lower quadrant
   d. elevated temperature of 37.8°C (100°F)

5. Common clinical manifestations of gastroenteritis are
   a. abdominal cramps, nausea, and vomiting
   b. fever, diarrhea, and leukopenia
   c. anorexia, pain, and constipation
   d. vomiting, fever, and constipation

6. Which of the following statements regarding the difference between ulcerative colitis and Crohn's disease is accurate?
   a. Crohn's disease is more likely to be treated with a colectomy.
   b. Ulcerative colitis is characterized by skip lesions.
   c. Crohn's disease is more likely than ulcerative colitis to result in cancer.
   d. Both diseases are characterized by remissions and exacerbations.

7. Intestinal obstruction can occur due to
   a. adhesions and paralytic ileus
   b. intussusception and dehydration
   c. volvulus and varices
   d. atresias and telangiectasia

8. In carcinoma of the large intestine there is a higher incidence of bowel obstruction in the
   a. ascending colon because of its narrow lumen
   b. transverse colon because of its semisolid content
   c. ileocecal valve because of the semiliquid content
   d. sigmoid region because of the narrow lumen and fecal consistency

9. Physiologic changes occurring after an ileostomy necessitate
   a. stoma irrigations
   b. skin care around the stoma
   c. avoidance of low residue diets
   d. the need to wear a belted appliance

10. Bowel preparation for a colostomy with nonabsorbable antibiotics is done primarily to
    a. reduce the bacterial flora in the colon
    b. prevent diarrhea
    c. prevent constipation
    d. prevent additional formation of ammonia

11. During a colostomy irrigation the client may experience cramping. If this occurs, the nurse should
    a. reduce the amount of flow by lowering the container
    b. discontinue the irrigation at once
    c. reduce the temperature of the irrigation solution
    d. insert the catheter about 1 inch further

12. In contrast to diverticulitis, the client with diverticulosis
    a. often is asymtomatic
    b. has rectal bleeding
    c. has localized crampy pain
    d. develops abscesses

13. Hernias are commonly found in any of the following sites *except*
    a. epigastrium
    b. inguinal ring
    c. umbilicus
    d. femoral ring

14. In nontropical sprue (celiac disease), the client's diet must be
    a. gluten-free, high protein, high calorie
    b. gluten-free, low fat, low protein
    c. milk-free, high protein, high calorie
    d. low calorie, low protein, high fat

15. Hemorrhoids are characterized by all the following *except*
    a. tendency toward constipation
    b. may be internal or external
    c. bleeding after bowel movement
    d. dilatation of the rectal arteries

REFERENCES

1. B. A. Given and S. J. Simmons, *Gastroenterology in Clinical Nursing,* 3d ed., The C. V. Mosby Company, St. Louis, 1980, p. 38.
2. W. A. Wichen, Jr., "The Surgical Abdomen," *Postgrad Med,* **62:**1–5 (1977).
3. D. Law et al., "The Continuing Challenge of Acute and Perforated Appendix," *Am J Surg,* **131:**533 (1976).
4. H. M. Spiro, *Clinical Gastroenterology,* 2d ed., Macmillan Publishing Company, Inc., New York, 1977, pp. 717–718, 757.

5. S. Price and L. Wilson, *Pathophysiology: Clinical Concepts of Disease Process,* McGraw-Hill Book Company, New York, 1978, p. 14.
6. F. Wheelock, Jr., "Surgical Management of Regional Ileitis, Ulcerative Colitis and Granulomatous Colitis," *Surg Clin North Am,* **54:**680 (1974).
7. M. Patterson et al., "Topical Steroid Therapy of Ulcerative Colitis," *Gastroenterology,* **103:**141–151 (1965).
8. N. Metheney and W. D. Snively, *Nurses' Handbook of Fluid Balance,* 3d ed., J. B. Lippincott Company, Philadelphia, 1979, p. 266.
9. K. Isselbacher et al., *Principles of Internal Medicine,* 9th ed. McGraw-Hill Book Company, New York, 1980, p. 1433.
10. American Cancer Society, Inc., *1979 Cancer Facts and Figures,* New York.
11. J. Horton and G. Helen, *Clinical Oncology,* W. B. Saunders Company, Philadelphia, 1977, p. 292.
12. Isselbacher et al., op. cit., p. 1434.
13. Ibid., p. 1436.
14. T. M. Bayless et al., "Lactose and Milk Intolerance: Clinical Implications," *N Engl J Med,* **292:**1156 (1975).
15. A. D. Neurcomer et al., "Tolerance to Lactose Deficiency in American Indians," *Gastroenterology,* **74:**44 (1978).
16. F. J. Simons, "New Light on Ethnic Differences in Adult Lactose Intolerances," *Am J Digestive Dis,* **18:**595 (1973).

Chapter 35

NURSING ROLE IN MANAGEMENT

Problems of the Liver, Biliary Tract, and Pancreas

Rachel Elrod

Learning Objectives

1. Differentiate between the three types of jaundice, including common causes and diagnostic findings.
2. Differentiate between the types of viral hepatitis, including etiology, pathophysiology, clinical manifestations, complications, and medical management.
3. Describe the nursing management of the client with viral hepatitis.
4. Explain the etiology, pathogenesis, clinical manifestations, complications, and medical and surgical management of cirrhosis of the liver.
5. Describe the nursing management of the client with cirrhosis.
6. Describe the types, clinical manifestations, and management of carcinoma of the liver.
7. Describe the pathophysiology, clinical manifestations, complications, and medical and surgical management of acute and chronic pancreatitis.
8. Describe the nursing management of the client with pancreatitis.
9. Explain the clinical manifestations and management of carcinoma of the pancreas.
10. Explain the pathophysiology, clinical manifestations, complications, and medical and surgical management of gallbladder disorders.
11. Describe the nursing management of the client undergoing medical or surgical treatment of cholecystitis and cholelithiasis.

JAUNDICE

Jaundice (yellowish discoloration of body tissues) results from an alteration in normal bilirubin metabolism or flow of bile into the hepatic or biliary duct systems. It is a symptom rather than a disease. Jaundice results when the concentration of bilirubin in the blood becomes abnormally increased. The bilirubin level has to be about three times the normal for jaundice to occur. Jaundice can usually first be detected in the sclera and skin.

Most of the body's bilirubin is formed from the breakdown of hemoglobin (from erythrocytes) by the reticuloendothelial system. This unconjugated (indirect) bilirubin is released into circulation and is not water-soluble. In the liver the unconjugated bilirubin is conjugated with glucuronic acid to form conjugated (direct) bilirubin which is water-soluble (Fig. 31-6). Conjugated bilirubin is secreted into bile which flows through the hepatic and biliary duct system into the small intestine. In the large intestine bilirubin is converted to urobilinogen, which gives the characteristic color to stool. Some urobilinogen is reabsorbed into the portal circulation and returned to the liver. Normally a very small amount of urobilinogen is excreted in urine.

*This chapter was reviewed by Leslie Ann Rogers, R.N., M.S.N., and Joan Marie Paul, R.N., M.S.N., Assistant Professors, San Antonio College, University of Texas Health Sciences at San Antonio, San Antonio, Texas.

The three types of jaundice are classified as *hemolytic*, *hepatocellular*, and *obstructive*.

Hemolytic Jaundice

Hemolytic jaundice is due to an increased breakdown of red blood cells, which produces an increased amount of unconjugated bilirubin in the blood. The liver is unable to handle this increased load. Consequently, the level of unconjugated bilirubin in the blood rises (Table 35-1). Because unconjugated bilirubin is not water-soluble, it is not excreted in the urine. However, increased urobilinogen is produced due to the liver's increased conjugation and excretion of bilirubin. This may result in darker urine and stool. Causes of hemolytic jaundice include blood transfusion reactions, sickle-cell crisis, and hemolytic anemia.

Hepatocellular Jaundice

Hepatocellular jaundice results from the liver's altered ability to take up bilirubin from the blood, or to conjugate or excrete it. Both unconjugated and conjugated bilirubin serum levels increase (Table 35-1). Because conjugated bilirubin is water-soluble, it is excreted in the urine. The urinary urobilinogen may be normal or increased, depending on the diseased liver's ability to take up urobilinogen from the portal circulation. Fecal urobilinogen will be normal or decreased depending on the degree of intrahepatic

Table 35-1
Diagnostic Findings in Different Types of Jaundice

	Hemolytic	Hepatocellular	Obstructive
Serum bilirubin			
Unconjugated (indirect)	↑	↑	Somewhat ↑
Conjugated (direct)	Normal	↑	Moderately ↑
Urine bilirubin	Negative	↑	↑
Urobilinogen			
Stool	↑	Normal to ↓	Negative
Urine	↑	Normal to ↑	Negative

blockage from fibrosis or inflammation. The most common causes of hepatocellular jaundice are hepatitis, cirrhosis, and hepatic carcinoma.

Obstructive Jaundice

Obstructive jaundice is due to impeded or obstructed flow of bile through the liver or biliary duct system. The obstruction may be *intrahepatic* or *extrahepatic*. Intrahepatic causes of obstruction are due to swelling or fibrosis of the liver's canaliculi and bile ducts. This could be caused by damage from liver tumors, hepatitis, or cirrhosis. Extrahepatic causes of obstruction include common bile duct obstruction from a stone or carcinoma of the head of the pancreas.

Laboratory findings show an elevation of both unconjugated and conjugated bilirubin and urine bilirubin (Table 35-1). Since bilirubin does not enter the intestines, there is decreased to no fecal or urinary urobilinogen.

VIRAL HEPATITIS

Hepatitis is an inflammation of the liver. Acute viral hepatitis is the most common type. The types of viral hepatitis are A, B, and non-A, non-B. Hepatitis may also be caused by drugs and other chemicals (Table 31-5). Occasionally hepatitis is caused by bacteria such as streptococci, *Salmonella*, and *Escherichia coli*. This discussion will focus on viral hepatitis.

Significance of the Problem

Each year there are 40,000 to 70,000 cases of viral hepatitis in the United States. It is more common in children and young adults, with the highest incidence in adolescent girls.[1]

In recent years there has been a decreasing incidence of type A hepatitis. Hepatitis A is most common in children and young adults. About 25 percent of clinical cases of hepatitis in young adults is due to type A. With the increase of drug abuse there has been a rising incidence of hepatitis B, especially in males aged 15 to 34.[2]

Etiology

Increasing knowledge in the past decade regarding viruses causing hepatitis has been due to the discovery of immunologic markers for the various viral antigens and antibodies. Hepatitis viruses A and B have been identified and there is evidence that other viruses (non-A, non-B) exist. The cytomegalovirus and herpesvirus may also cause hepatitis.[3] Current terminology regarding viral hepatitis is presented in Table 35-2.

Hepatitis A virus (HAV)

The hepatitis A virus has been identified as an RNA virus. The virus is found in the serum and stool of clients with hepatitis A. It is found early in the course of the disease, usually before there is an elevated serum glutamic-oxaloacetic transaminase (SGOT) level and prior to jaundice. Anti-HAV (antibody to hepatitis A virus) appears in the serum early in the illness, and stays there indefinitely. The finding of anti-HAV in the serum indicates the client has had a prior sensitization to hepatitis A virus.

Hepatitis B virus (HBV)

Hepatitis B virus, which is a DNA virus, is a complex structure with three distinct antigenic particles:

1. Hepatitis B surface antigen (HB_sAg) is a group of proteins that form the outer coat of the hepatitis B virus. It is produced in large amounts by the host liver cell in response to the virus. It is easily

Table 35-2
Terminology Related to Viral Hepatitis

Term	Description
Hepatitis A virus (HAV)	Agent formerly called infectious hepatitis (IH) virus. Present in stool and serum early in course of hepatitis A. RNA virus.
Type A hepatitis (hepatitis A)	Type of viral hepatitis previously called infectious hepatitis (IH).
Anti-HAV	Antibody to hepatitis A virus (HAV). Detected during acute illness and present indefinitely.
Hepatitis B virus (HBV)	Agent formerly called serum hepatitis (SH) virus. Present in serum. DNA virus.
Type B hepatitis (hepatitis B)	Type of viral hepatitis previously called serum hepatitis (SH).
Hepatitis B surface antigen (HB_sAg)	Group of proteins that form the outer coat of the hepatitis B virus. Former designations were Australian antigen (AuAg) and hepatitis-associated antigen (HAA). Found in serum, body fluids, and hepatocytes in > 80% of clients with hepatitis B.
Anti-HB_s	Antibody to hepatitis B surface antigen (HB_sAg). Usually first detectable in convalescence. Probably protective antibody. Indicates past infection and immunity to HBV.
Hepatitis B core antigen (HB_cAg)	Antigenic determinant of the core of the hepatitis B virus.
Anti-HB_c	Antibody to hepatitis B core antigen (HB_cAg). Detectable during and after acute phase of illness.
Hepatitis B e-antigen (HB_eAg)	Circulating in serum only. Correlates with infectivity of virus.
Anti-HB_e	Antibody to hepatitis B e-antigen (HB_eAg). May not be detectable until late in convalescence. Presence in serum of HB_sAg carrier suggests lower titer of HBV.
Non-A, non-B hepatitis	Forms of viral hepatitis caused by agents other than hepatitis A virus and hepatitis B virus. No immunologic marker or virus particle has yet been satisfactorily demonstrated.

detectable in the serum and persists throughout the clinical course of the disease.

2. Hepatitis B core antigen (HB_cAg) is the antigenic material in the core of the virus. It is probably infectious but is difficult to measure.
3. Hepatitis B e-antigen (HB_eAg) is found in circulating blood. It is only present in Hb_sAg-positive individuals. It seems to be associated with the development of chronic liver disease after having acute hepatitis B. The e antigen is also present in clients with chronic liver disease who are HB_sAg carriers.[4]

Each antigen has a corresponding antibody that is elicited during an attack of acute viral hepatitis (Table 35-2). These antibodies can be detected in the serum of individuals with prior exposure to the antigenic virus.

Non-A, non-B hepatitis

Non-A, non-B hepatitis is caused by a virus or viruses other than hepatitis A virus and hepatitis B virus. Both epidemiologically and clinically it is similar to hepatitis B. It appears to be the cause of 80 to 90 percent of cases of transfusion-associated hepatitis. It also occurs in drug abusers, clients in chronic care institutions, health care workers, and infrequently in hemodialysis clients and renal transplant recipients.[5]

The only way to distinguish the various forms of viral hepatitis is by the presence of the antigens and antigenic subtypes and the subsequent development of antibodies to them. Epidemics of hepatitis are consistently due to HAV while 20 to 60 percent of episodic or sporadic hepatitis is caused by HBV or non-A, non-B virus. Infection with each virus provides immunity to that virus (homologous immunity). The client can still develop another type of viral hepatitis. Characteristics of the hepatitis viruses A, B, and non-A, and non-B are summarized in Table 35-3.

Pathophysiology of Hepatitis

Liver

The pathophysiologic changes in the various types of viral hepatitis are similar. Hepatitis involves widespread inflammation of liver tissue. Liver cell damage consists of hepatic cell degeneration and necrosis. There is proliferation and enlargement of the Kupffer cells. Inflammation of the periportal areas may

Table 35-3
Comparison of Hepatitis A, B and Non-A, Non-B

Characteristic	Hepatitis A	Hepatitis B	Hepatitis Non-A, Non-B
Incubation period	15–45 days (2–6 weeks)	60–180 days (2–6 months)	50 days (average) A wide range
Mode of transmission	Fecal-oral	Parenteral (percutaneous) Nonpercutaneous (saliva, semen, vaginal secretions)	Parenteral (percutaneous)
Sources of infection and spread of disease	Crowded conditions, poor personal hygiene, contaminated food, milk, water, and shellfish Individuals with subclinical infections	Contaminated needles, syringes, instruments and blood products Intimate contact (kissing, sexual intercourse) Asymptomatic carrier	Blood and blood products, needles, syringes, crowded institutions
Virus in feces	Two weeks prior to jaundice	Possible (suspected)	Not identified
Virus in serum	During acute phase During incubation period	HB_sAg is in serum throughout clinical course	Not identified
Gamma globulin (prophylaxis)	Immune serum globulin (ISG)	Hepatitis B immune globulin (HBIG) or ISG	—
Serologic test (specific antigen)	HA Ag	HB_sAg, HB_eAg	Not identified
Vaccine	No	Made from serum containing HB_sAg	No
Antibody	Anti-HAV	Anti-HB_s, anti-HB_c, anti-HB_e	

interrupt bile flow. Cholestasis may occur. The liver cells regenerate in an orderly manner and if no complications occur, they should resume their normal appearance and function during convalescence.

Systemic effects

The antigen-antibody complexes between the virus and its corresponding antibody form a circulating immune complex in the early phases of hepatitis. The presence of circulating immune complexes activates the complement system (Chap. 10). The clinical manifestations of this activation are rash, angioedema, arthritis, fever, and malaise.

Clinical Manifestations

The clinical manifestations of viral hepatitis may be classified into three phases: (1) the *preicteric* or *prodromal phase*, (2) *icteric phase*, and (3) the *posticteric* or *convalescent phase* (Table 35-4).

Preicteric phase

The preicteric phase precedes jaundice and extends from 1 to 21 days. This is the period of maximal infectivity. Gastrointestinal symptoms that are present may include anorexia, nausea, abdominal (right upper quadrant) discomfort and sometimes vomiting, constipation, or diarrhea. The anorexia is frequently severe and is thought to be due to a toxin produced by the diseased liver. The client may find food repugnant and, if a smoker, have a distaste for cigarettes. There is also a decreased sense of smell. Weight loss occurs during the preicteric phase. Other symptoms during the preicteric phase are malaise, headache, fever (low-grade), arthralgias, and skin rashes. Physical examination reveals hepatomegaly, lymphadenopathy, and sometimes splenomegaly.

Icteric phase

The icteric phase lasts 4 to 6 weeks and is characterized by jaundice. Jaundice results from bilirubin diffusing into the tissues. The urine may darken due to excess bilirubin being excreted by the kidneys. If conjugated bilirubin cannot flow out of the liver due to obstruction or inflammation of the bile ducts, the stools will be light or clay-colored. Pruritus sometimes accompanies the jaundice, especially if cholestasis is present. The pruritus occurs due to the accumulation of bile salts underneath the skin.

When jaundice occurs, the fever usually subsides. The gastrointestinal symptoms usually remain and some fatigue may continue. The liver is usually

Table 35-4
Clinical Manifestations of the Three Phases of Hepatitis

Preicteric	Icteric	Posticteric
Anorexia	Jaundice	Malaise
Nausea, vomiting	Pruritus	Easily fatigued
Right upper quadrant discomfort	Dark urine	Hepatomegaly
Constipation or diarrhea	Bilirubinuria	
Decreased sense of taste and smell	Light stools	
Malaise	Fatigue	
Headache	Continued hepatomegaly with tenderness	
Low-grade fever	Continued lymphadenopathy	
Arthralgias	Feeling of well-being	
Urticaria	Weight loss	
Hepatomegaly		
Splenomegaly		
Lymphadenopathy		
Weight loss		

enlarged and tender and there is lymphadenopathy. Toward the end of this phase when the jaundice is receding, the client may experience a feeling of well-being.

Posticteric phase

The convalescent stage of the posticteric phase begins as jaundice is disappearing and lasts weeks to months with an average of 2 to 4 months. During this period the client's major complaint is malaise and easy fatigability. Hepatomegaly remains for several weeks. Splenomegaly subsides during this period. Relapses may occur and the disappearance of jaundice does not mean the client has totally recovered.

Not all clients with viral hepatitis develop jaundice. This is referred to as *anicteric hepatitis* and occurs more frequently in children. A high percentage of individuals with hepatitis A are anicteric.[6]

There is some slight variation in the manifestations between the types of hepatitis. In hepatitis A the onset is more acute and the symptoms are usually mild. In hepatitis B the onset is more insidious and the symptoms are usually more severe. There may be fewer gastrointestinal symptoms. Extrahepatic manifestations of hepatitis B include glomerulonephritis and polyarteritis nodosa. These manifestations are thought to be due to the deposition of circulating HB_sAg and its antibody in tissue and subsequent complement activation.

Complications

Most clients with viral hepatitis recover completely with no complications. The mortality rate is very low (<0.1 percent).[7] The mortality rate is higher in older individuals and those with underlying debilitating diseases. Complications that can occur include chronic persistent hepatitis, chronic active hepatitis, fulminant viral hepatitis, and cirrhosis of the liver.

Chronic persistent hepatitis

The most common complication of viral hepatitis is *chronic persistent hepatitis* in which there is a delayed convalescent period. It is usually benign and is characterized by fatigue and hepatomegaly. Liver function tests may remain abnormal for several years.

Chronic active hepatitis

Chronic active hepatitis is characterized by the persistence of signs and symptoms of hepatitis and abnormal liver function tests for more than 3 months. It is distinguished from chronic persistent hepatitis by liver biopsy. The ongoing process of liver necrosis is likely to progress to cirrhosis. Steroid therapy is usually used to treat chronic active hepatitis.

Recent studies have shown that HB_sAg-positive clients whose serum remains positive for HB_eAg are more likely to develop chronic active hepatitis. In addition, alteration in the client's cellular immune response may be important in the development of the chronic HB_sAg carrier state and consequent progression from acute hepatitis B to chronic active hepatitis.[8] This finding may explain why chronic renal failure clients on hemodialysis who develop hepatitis B are more at risk for developing chronic active hepatitis. (Individuals with chronic renal failure are known to have a depressed cellular immune response.)

Fulminant hepatitis

Fulminant viral hepatitis is an acute hepatitis with an extremely poor prognosis. A very small percentage of clients develop fulminant viral hepatitis (0.5 percent of hepatitis A; 2 to 5 percent of hepatitis B).[9] There is extensive necrosis and inflammation with loss of functioning liver cells. Hepatocellular failure with death usually occurs.

Diagnostic Study Abnormalities

In viral hepatitis many of the liver function tests show significant abnormalities. These findings assist in determining decreased liver function. The common abnormalities are identified in Table 35-5.

Physical assessment will reveal hepatic tenderness, hepatomegaly, and splenomegaly. The liver is palpable. A liver biopsy is not indicated unless the diagnosis is in doubt or if a more severe form of hepatitis is suspected.

The tests for HAV in feces or serum are not routinely available in many clinical laboratories. In these situations, the diagnosis of hepatitis A is based on the finding of negative serologic tests for hepatitis B.

Hepatitis B is confirmed by finding HB_sAg in the serum. The presence of HB_sAg and anti-HB_s aids in the establishment of a definitive diagnosis. In the early stages, hepatitis B can be diagnosed due to the presence of HB_sAg and during the convalescent stage due to the presence of the anti-HB_s.

Medical Management

There is no specific treatment or therapy for viral hepatitis. Emphasis is on measures to rest the body and assist the liver in regenerating (Table 35-6). Adequate nutrients and rest seem to be the most beneficial for healing and liver cell regeneration. The dietary emphasis is on a well-balanced diet which the client can tolerate (see section on dietary measures).

Rest reduces the metabolic demands on the liver, increases the blood supply to the liver, and thus promotes cell regeneration. Strict bed rest may be considered during the icteric phase. Many physicians believe that strict bed rest is not essential but alternating periods of activity and rest are adequate. The type of rest ordered may depend on the severity of symptoms, the client's degree of fatigue, and the degree of

Table 35-5
Diagnostic Findings in Hepatitis

Name of Test	Abnormal Finding	Etiology
Transaminase		
(Aminotransferase)		
SGOT (AST)	Elevated	Liver cell injury
SGPT (ALT)	Elevated in preicteric phase. Decreases as jaundice disappears	Liver cell injury
Alkaline phosphatase	Somewhat elevated	Impaired excretory function of the liver
Serum proteins		
Gamma globulin	Normal or increased	Liver damage
Albumin	Normal or decreased	Liver damage
Serum bilirubin (total)	Elevated to about 8–15 mg/dL	Hepatocellular damage
Urinary bilirubin	Elevated	Conjugated hyperbilirubinemia
Urinary urobilinogen	Elevated 2–5 days prior to jaundice	Diminished reabsorption of urobilinogen
Prothrombin time	Prolonged	Decreased absorption of vitamin K in the intestine with decreased production of prothrombin by the liver
HAV—fecal	Present in hepatitis A until jaundice disappears	Antigen in feces
HB_sAg—serum	Positive in hepatitis B	Surface antigen in serum
Bromsulphalein (BSP) or indocyanine green (ICG) dye clearance	Rate of excretion of dye is decreased	May indicate severity of liver disease or help determine recovery

Table 35-6

Medical Management: Viral Hepatitis

Diagnostic

1. Liver function studies
2. Radioimmunoassay for presence of
   a. HB_sAg
   b. HB_eAg
   c. Anti-HAV

Therapeutic

1. High calorie, high protein, high carbohydrate, moderate fat diet
2. Vitamin supplements
3. Bed rest with BRP

changes in the liver function tests, particularly the enzymes.

Pharmacologic Intervention

There are no specific drug therapies for the treatment of viral hepatitis. Steroid therapy is usually reserved for the client who is extremely ill, has chronic active hepatitis, or seems in danger of developing fulminating hepatitis. Dosage may be as high as 80 mg/day in acute illness. Corticosteroids increase the appetite and improve the sense of well-being. They also improve the metabolism of cholesterol and in this way decrease bilirubin levels and cholestasis. Therefore, jaundice and pruritus are decreased.

Supportive drug therapy may include antiemetics such as dimenhydrinate (Dramamine) or trimethobenzamide (Tigan). Phenothiazines should not be used due to their possible cholestatic and hepatotoxic effects. If the client requires a sedative or hypnotic drug, diphenhydramine (Benadryl) or chloral hydrate may be used.

Immune globulin is used in the prevention and modification of viral hepatitis. Immune serum globulin (ISG) is effective for hepatitis A and offers some protection against hepatitis B since it contains varying amounts of the hepatitis B antibody. ISG is adequate except in a definite contact exposure.

Hepatitis B immune globulin (HBIG) is prepared from plasma of donors with a high titer of anti-HB_s. HBIG is very expensive.

The U.S. Public Health Service Advisory Committee on Immunization Practices recommends the following in relation to ISG and HBIG:[10]

> ISG—Prophylactic passive immunization for clients or health personnel continually exposed to hepatitis B.
>
> HBIG—Immunization for one-time exposure to hepatitis B virus such as accidental needle-stick or contact with mucous membranes.
>
> Dose—0.05 to 0.07 mL/kg—IM within 7 days after exposure. Second dose in 25 to 30 days.

Dietary Measures

No special diet is required in the treatment of viral hepatitis. However, a diet high in carbohydrates with moderate protein and fat content is usually recommended. Adequate calories are important since the client frequently loses weight. Sometimes a diet high in protein is ordered. If fat content is poorly tolerated due to lack of bile in the intestines, it should be reduced. Basically the specific foods on the diet are dictated by the client. Vitamin supplements are frequently used.

If anorexia, nausea, and vomiting are severe, intravenous solutions of glucose or supplemental tube feedings may be used. Fluid and electrolyte balance must be maintained.

Nursing Management

Health promotion and maintenance

Viral hepatitis is a community health problem. The nurse must assume a significant role in the control and prevention of this disease. In order to understand its control and prevention, it is helpful to first discuss the epidemiology of the different types of viral hepatitis before considering appropriate control measures.

Hepatitis A (HAV) Epidemics of viral hepatitis are almost always due to the A virus. The mode of transmission or route of infection of HAV is predominantly fecal-oral and rarely parenteral. Poor hygiene, crowded situations, and poor sanitary conditions are all factors related to hepatitis A. Infected food handlers may be a source of infection. Certain foods such as contaminated milk, water, or shellfish are other sources of infection.

There does not seem to be a chronic carrier state for hepatitis A virus. The virus is present in feces and serum during the incubation period so it can be carried by individuals who have undetectable, subclinical infections. It can also be transmitted by clients with anicteric hepatitis A.

Preventive measures include personal and environmental hygiene and health education to promote good sanitation. The nurse must follow the correct isolation precautions to prevent the spread of the virus. Handwashing is essential and is probably the most important precaution. Disposable dishes and equipment should be used. Any articles contaminated with feces should be sterilized or disposed of properly. Family and significant others should be given clear, concise instructions and explanations regarding the isolation procedures.

Recent studies indicate that the peak excretion of the hepatitis A virus is at about the onset of symptoms and is not detectable by the time the enzymes (such as the SGOT) reach their peak. Therefore, there is no reason to enforce enteric precautions after the client is icteric.[11] Carriers are most infectious just prior to the onset of symptoms. If family members have been exposed, the best prevention for them is immune serum globulin (ISG), given as soon as the diagnosis of hepatitis A is made. ISG may not prevent infection, but it will modify the illness. Immune serum globulin should be given within 2 weeks of exposure. This provides passive protection. ISG may also be used as a prophylactic measure for travelers to foreign countries which have a high incidence of hepatitis.

Hepatitis B (HBV) It was previously thought that HBV was transmitted only by percutaneous inoculation with contaminated needles, instruments, blood, and blood products. Now it is known there are other modes of transmission. HB_sAg has been detected in (1) vaginal secretions, (2) menstrual fluids, (3) semen, (4) saliva, and (5) respiratory secretions. When the HB_sAg was found in these secretions, it was found in even higher concentrations in the blood.

Nonpercutaneous transmission is not as common as percutaneous transmission but it does occur, particularly among sexual partners of both asymptomatic and symptomatic HB_sAg carriers. HBV is definitely transmitted via sexual intercourse. In some areas the incidence among male homosexuals has surpassed intravenous drug abuse as a source of infection. Kissing and sharing of food items may spread the virus via saliva. There is very little if any likelihood of enteric transmission since the HBV is degraded by intestinal mucosal enzymes and enzymes from the bacterial flora.

In summary, the predominant mode of transmission of the HBV is parenteral or percutaneous. The venereal route is probably the most predominant means of nonpercutaneous spread.

There are asymptomatic carriers of the B virus. Three to 4 percent of the population carry the HB_sAg and can transmit it.[12] There is an even higher incidence of carriers in medical and other health care workers. The carriers of hepatitis B may have low-grade disease, a normal liver, or a severe chronic liver disease. A positive test for anti-HB_s in adults indicates they have had hepatitis B.

Control and prevention of hepatitis B focuses on identification of possible exposure via percutaneous and sexual transmission. Other measures include the use of washed red blood cells and the screening of blood donors for HB_sAg. Clients who have anti-HB_s in their blood who receive transfusions seem to be protected from hepatitis B. An added control measure then is to administer blood containing anti-HB_s.

The nurse must be aware of the high-risk groups for developing hepatitis B. These include hemodialysis clients, other clients receiving frequent transfusions, and workers in hemodialysis units and blood chemistry labs.

Disposable needles and syringes should be used and disposed of properly. Good hygienic practices including handwashing and precautions for transmitting contaminated saliva are important. The nurse should instruct clients regarding the transmission of the virus via sexual intercourse to avoid transmission to sexual partners.

Antiviral chemotherapy is being attempted to try to eliminate the chronic HBV carrier state. Passive immunization may be provided with either ISG or hepatitis B immune globulin (HBIG) (see section on pharmacologic interventions). The ISG seems to offer some protection against hepatitis B. There is a formalin-treated hepatitis B vaccine made from purified HB_sAg-containing particles. The vaccine is made from the plasma of chronic HB_sAg carriers.[13] Preventive and control measures for hepatitis A and B are summarized in Table 35-7.

Hepatitis Non-A, Non-B As discussed earlier, this virus or possibly viruses causes the majority of cases of transfusion-associated hepatitis. It also occurs in drug abusers, clients in chronic care institutions, and health care workers. At this time little is known about hepatitis non-A, non-B. Since it resembles HBV epidemiologically, control measures for HBV may apply here.

Acute intervention

Jaundice The nurse should assess for the degree of jaundice. In Caucasians, the jaundice is usually first observed in the sclera of the eyes and later in the skin. In dark-skinned individuals, jaundice is observed in the hard palate of the mouth and inner canthus of the eyes. Ictotest reagent tablets may be used to detect urinary bilirubin. Comfort measures to relieve pruritus (if present), headache, and arthralgias are helpful.

Isolation When the client with suspected viral hepatitis is admitted to the hospital, both enteric and needle precautions should be instituted until the type

Table 35-7
Preventive Measures for Viral Hepatitis

Hepatitis A	Hepatitis B
Handwashing Good personal hygiene Environmental sanitation Control and screening of food handlers (especially while carrying virus) Enteric precautions (prior to jaundice) Immune serum globulin (ISG) a. Given early to exposed individuals (during incubation period) b. Used as prophylaxis for travelers to tropical and developing countries	*Percutaneous* Screen blood donors for HB_sAg Administer washed red blood cells Administer blood containing anti-HB_s when possible Use disposable needles and syringes *Sexual and intimate contact* Avoid kissing individuals who have the disease Avoid having sexual intercourse with individuals who have the disease *General* Registration of carriers Passive immunization a. ISG—for exposure b. HBIG—one-time exposure (needle stick, contact with material from mucous membrane) Active immunization a. Vaccine—limited use currently

of hepatitis can be determined. (Isolation precautions were discussed in the section on health promotion and maintenance.)

Nutrition An important measure in assisting liver cells to regenerate is adequate nutrition (see section on dietary measures). Assuring that the client receives adequate nutrients is not always easy. The anorexia and extreme distaste for food cause nutritional problems. Dietary assessment must be considered. The nurse should try to determine if there is something that appeals to the client in spite of the anorexia. Small, frequent meals may be preferable to three large ones and may also help to prevent nausea. Frequently, clients with hepatitis find that anorexia is not as severe in the morning so that it is easier to eat a good breakfast than a large dinner meal. Measures to stimulate the appetite such as mouth care, antiemetics, and attractively served meals in pleasant surroundings should be included in the nursing care plan. Other measures which may be tried to counteract the anorexia are carbonated beverages and avoidance of very hot or very cold foods.

Rest Rest is essential and is another factor in promoting liver cell regeneration. The nurse must assess the client's response to the rest and activity plan and modify it based on the assessment. The care plan should include appropriate time schedules for rest and activity, with scheduled rest periods uninterrupted by visitors or nursing staff. If the client is on strict bed rest, measures to prevent respiratory and circulatory complications should be initiated. Assessment of the liver function tests and other symptoms should continue as a guide to activity.

Psychological and emotional rest are as essential as physical rest. Strict bed rest may produce anxiety and extreme restlessness in some clients and may be more damaging than reasonable ambulation.

The client should be assisted to understand the temporary nature of symptoms, especially sexual abstinence during the period of communicability. Diversional activities such as reading, and hobbies (knitting, stamp collecting) may help the client.

Chronic management

In order to assist the client to complete recovery, the nurse must assess the client's knowledge of nutrition and provide the necessary dietary teaching. Rest and adequate nutrition are especially important until liver function studies return to normal. The client must be cautioned about overexertion and needs to follow the physician's advice about when it is safe to return to work.

The client should be assessed for any manifestations indicating complications. Bleeding tendencies with increasing prothrombin time, symptoms of encephalopathy, or markedly abnormal liver function tests indicate problems and should be assessed and treated promptly.

The client should be instructed to have regular medical follow-up for at least 1 year following the diagnosis of hepatitis. Since relapses are fairly common, the client should be instructed about symptoms of recurrence. Alcohol should be avoided for 1 year because it is detoxified in the liver and may interfere with recovery.

Clients who remain positive for HB_sAg are carriers and should never be blood donors. The client with hepatitis B should also be instructed to avoid intimate contact such as kissing and sexual intercourse until the enzyme levels are near normal or the HB_sAg is negative.

TOXIC AND DRUG-INDUCED HEPATITIS

Etiology

Liver injury may occur following the inhalation, parenteral injection, or ingestion of certain chemical substances (Table 31-5). The two major types of chemical hepatotoxicity are toxic and drug-induced. Agents producing *toxic hepatitis* (carbon tetrachloride, gold compounds, acetaminophen) are generally systemic poisons or are converted in the liver to toxic metabolites. Liver necrosis generally occurs within 2 to 3 days of acute exposure to a toxic substance.

Idiosyncratic drug reactions produce *drug-induced hepatitis*. Agents such as halothane, isoniazid, chlorothiazides, and alpha methyldopa may produce *idiosyncratic reactions* due to (1) client susceptibility (metabolic reactivity) to these agents or (2) immunologically mediated hypersensitivity responses. Liver injury may occur at any time during or shortly after exposure to the drug. Some responses have been noted to occur 2 to 5 weeks after exposure.

Clinical Manifestations and Treatment

Toxic and drug-induced hepatitis is very similar to viral hepatitis in the pathophysiologic changes in the liver and the clinical manifestations. The usual presenting clinical findings are anorexia, nausea, vomiting, hepatomegaly, splenomegaly, and abnormal liver function studies. Treatment is largely supportive as in acute viral hepatitis. Recovery may be rapid if the hepatotoxin is identified and removed.

CIRRHOSIS OF THE LIVER

Cirrhosis is a chronic progressive disease of the liver characterized by extensive degeneration and destruction of the liver parenchymal cells. The liver cells attempt to regenerate but the regenerative process is disorganized, resulting in abnormal blood vessel and bile duct relationships from the fibrosis. The overgrowth of new and fibrous connective tissue distorts the liver's normal lobular structure, resulting in lobules of irregular size and shape with impeded vascular flow. Cirrhosis may have a very insidious, prolonged course.

Cirrhosis is ranked as the third or fourth cause of death in middle-aged women and men. The highest incidence occurs between the ages of 40 to 60 years and it is twice as common in men as women.[14] Excessive alcohol ingestion is the single most common cause of cirrhosis.

Etiology

The four types of cirrhosis in order of incidence are:

1. *Laennec's cirrhosis* (also called portal, nutritional, or alcoholic cirrhosis) is usually associated with alcohol abuse. The first change in the liver from excessive alcohol intake is an accumulation of fat in the liver cells. Uncomplicated fatty changes in the liver are potentially reversible if the person stops drinking alcohol. If the alcohol abuse continues, widespread scar formation occurs throughout the liver.
2. *Postnecrotic cirrhosis* is a complication of toxic or viral hepatitis. Broad bonds of scar tissue form within the liver.
3. *Biliary cirrhosis* is associated with chronic biliary obstruction and infection. There is diffuse fibrosis of the liver with jaundice as the main feature.
4. *Cardiac cirrhosis* results from long-standing severe right-sided heart failure in clients with cor pulmonale, constrictive pericarditis, and tricuspid insufficiency.

Pathogenesis

In cirrhosis there is cell necrosis and the destroyed liver cells are replaced by scar tissue. The normal lobular architecture becomes nodular. Eventually irregular, disorganized regeneration, poor cellular nutrition, and hypoxia due to an inadequate blood flow and scar tissue result in less and less functioning liver tissue.

The specific etiology of cirrhosis remains a mystery and cannot be determined in many clients. It is known that cirrhosis occurs with greatest frequency among alcoholics. There continues to be some controversy as to whether the cause is the alcohol or the malnutrition that frequently coexists with chronic ingestion of alcohol. There have been cases of nutritional cirrhosis resulting from extreme dieting or malnutrition. It is believed the combined impact of malnutrition and alcohol is especially damaging to liver cells. Alcohol is known to produce necrosis of cells and fatty infiltration with formation of fibrous septae. There is evidence that alcohol alone can cause liver damage.[15] Some individuals seem to have a predisposition to cirrhosis, regardless of their dietary or alcoholic intake.

Clinical Manifestations

Early manifestations

The onset of cirrhosis is usually insidious but may be sudden. Gastrointestinal disturbances are common early symptoms and include anorexia, dyspepsia, flatulence, nausea and vomiting, and change in bowel habits (diarrhea or constipation). These symptoms occur due to the liver's altered metabolism of carbohydrates, fats, and proteins. The client may complain of abdominal pain described as a dull, heavy feeling in the right upper quadrant or epigastrium. The pain is due to swelling and stretching of the liver capsule, spasm of the biliary ducts, and intermittent vascular spasm. Other early manifestations are fever, lassitude, slight weight loss, and enlargement of the liver and spleen. The liver is palpable in many individuals.

Later manifestations

Later symptoms may be severe and result from liver failure and portal hypertension. Jaundice, peripheral edema, and ascites develop gradually. Other late symptoms include skin lesions, hematologic disorders, endocrine disturbances, and peripheral neuropathies (Fig. 35-1). In the advanced stages the liver becomes small and nodular.

Jaundice Jaundice results from the functional derangement of liver cells and compression of bile ducts by connective tissue overgrowth. Jaundice occurs as a result of the decreased ability to conjugate

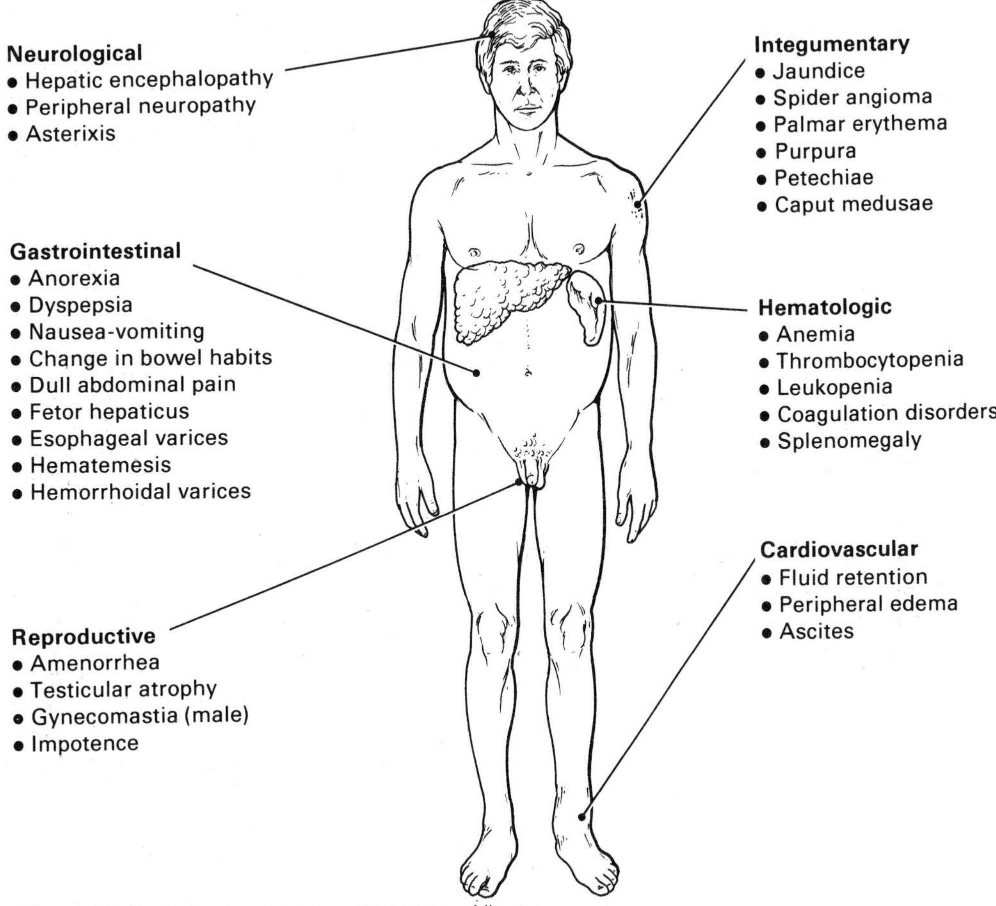

Figure 35-1 Systemic clinical manifestations of liver cirrhosis.

and excrete the bilirubin. The jaundice may be minimal or severe, depending on the degree of liver damage. It is usually *hepatocellular jaundice*. If obstruction of the biliary tract occurs, *obstructive jaundice* also results and will probably be accompanied by pruritus. The pruritus is due to an accumulation of bile salts underneath the skin.

Skin Lesions Various skin manifestations are commonly seen in cirrhosis. *Spider angiomas* (telangiectasia or spider nevi) are small, dilated blood vessels with a bright red center point with spider like branches. They occur on the nose, cheeks, upper trunk, neck, and shoulders. *Palmar erythema* (red areas which blanche with pressure) is located on the palms of the hands. Both of these lesions are attributed to an increase in circulating estrogen as a result of the liver's inability to inactivate it.

Hematologic Problems These include thrombocytopenia, leukopenia, anemia, and coagulation disorders. Thrombocytopenia, leukopenia, and anemia are probably due to the splenomegaly. Splenomegaly results from backup of blood from the portal vein into the spleen. Overactivity of the enlarged spleen results in increased removal of blood cells from circulation. The anemia is also due to inadequate red blood cell production and survival. Other factors involved in the anemia relate to a poor diet, poor absorption of folic acid, and bleeding from varices.

The coagulation problems result from the liver's inability to produce prothrombin and other factors essential for blood clotting. Coagulation problems are manifested by hemorrhagic phenomena or bleeding tendencies such as epistaxis, purpura, petechiae, easy bruising, gingival bleeding, and heavy menstrual bleeding.

Endocrine Disturbances Several symptoms relating to the metabolism and inactivation of adrenocortical hormones, estrogen, and testosterone occur in cirrhosis. Normally the liver inactivates these hormones. When the damaged liver is unable to do this, various manifestations occur. In the male, gynecomastia, loss of axillary and pubic hair, testicular atrophy, and impotency with loss of libido may occur due to estrogen accumulation. In younger females amenorrhea may occur and in older females vaginal bleeding may occur. The liver fails to adequately metabolize aldosterone which results in hyperaldosteronism with sodium and fluid retention.

Peripheral Neuropathy Peripheral neuropathy is a common finding in alcohol-associated cirrhosis. It is probably due to a dietary deficiency of thiamine, folic acid, and vitamin B_{12}. The neuropathy usually results in mixed nervous system symptoms but sensory symptoms may predominate.

Clinical manifestations of cirrhosis of the liver are numerous and may eventually involve the total body (Fig. 35-2).

Complications

Major complications of cirrhosis are portal hypertension with resultant esophageal varices, peripheral edema and ascites, hepatic encephalopathy (coma), and hepatorenal syndrome.

Portal hypertension and esophageal varices

Due to the structural changes in the liver from the cirrhotic process there is compression and destruction of the portal and hepatic veins and sinusoids. These changes result in obstruction to the normal flow of blood through the portal system, resulting in portal hypertension. There are many pathophysiologic changes that result from portal hypertension. Collateral circulation develops in an attempt to reduce this high portal pressure and also to reduce the increased plasma volume and lymphatic flow. The common areas where the collateral channels form are in the lower esophagus (the anastomosis of the left gastric vein and the azygos veins), the anterior abdominal wall, the parietal peritoneum, and the rectum. Varicosities may develop in areas where the collateral and systemic circulation communicate, resulting in *esophageal varices*, *caput medusae* (ring of varices around umbilicus), and *hemorrhoids*.

Esophageal varices are a very common complication, occurring in 60 percent of clients with cirrhosis.[16] These collateral vessels contain little elastic tissue and are quite fragile. They tolerate the high pressure poorly, resulting in distended, tortuous veins which bleed easily.

Clients with bleeding esophageal varices have a high mortality rate. They are the most life-threatening complication of cirrhosis. The mortality rate for adults is 67 percent. Close to 55 percent of the clients who develop bleeding esophageal varices will die within a year. Even with medical intervention only 30 to 33 percent have a survival rate of 5 years.[17]

The varices rupture and bleed due to ulceration and irritation. Factors producing the ulceration and irritation include alcohol ingestion, swallowing poorly masticated food, acid regurgitation from the stomach, and increased intraabdominal pressure due to nausea, vomiting, straining at stool, coughing, sneezing, or lifting heavy objects. The client may present with melena or hematemesis. There may be slow oozing or massive hemorrhage. Massive hemorrhage is a medical emergency.

Peripheral edema and ascites

Peripheral edema sometimes precedes ascites but in some clients its development coincides with or occurs after ascites. Edema results from (1) decreased colloidal osmotic pressure from impaired liver synthesis of albumin, and (2) increased portocaval pressure from portal hypertension. Peripheral edema presents as ankle and presacral edema.

Ascites is the accumulation of serous fluid in the peritoneal or abdominal cavity. It is a very common manifestation of cirrhosis, occurring in approximately 65 percent of clients with Laennec's cirrhosis.[18] When the blood pressure is elevated in the liver as occurs in portal cirrhosis, proteins can be transported from the blood vessels via the larger pores of the sinusoids (capillaries) into the lymph space. When the lymphatic system is unable to carry off the excess proteins and water, they will leak through the liver capsule into the peritoneal cavity. The osmotic pressure of the proteins pulls additional fluid into the peritoneal cavity (Table 35-8).

A second mechanism of ascites is *hypoalbuminemia* due to the liver's inability to synthesize albumin. The hypoalbuminemia results in decreased colloidal osmotic pressure. A third mechanism of ascites, *hyperaldosteronism*, results due to aldosterone not being metabolized by damaged liver cells. The increased level of aldosterone causes increased amounts of sodium to be reabsorbed by the renal tubules. This retention of sodium by cirrhotic clients plus an increase in the antidiuretic hormone (ADH) causes additional water retention in these clients. The fact that the diseased liver does not metabolize estrogen as effectively may also contribute to the edema and ascites.

Hypokalemia is common and is due to an excessive loss of K^+ ions due to the effects of aldosterone. Low potassium levels can also result from diuretic therapy used to treat the ascites.

Ascites is manifested by abdominal distension with weight gain. If the ascites is severe, the umbilicus may be everted. Abdominal striae with distended abdominal wall veins may be present. The client has a dehydrated appearance—dry tongue and skin, sunken eyeballs, and muscle weakness. There is also a decrease in urinary output.

Hepatic encephalopathy (coma)

Hepatic encephalopathy or coma is a frequent terminal complication in liver disease. Encephalopathy is a more descriptive term than coma. Hepatic encephalopathy can occur in any condition in which liver damage causes blood to enter the systemic circulation without liver detoxification. There is a high mortality rate associated with hepatic encephalopathy.

There are a number of etiologic factors involved in hepatic encephalopathy. The main pathogenic agent is nitrogenous ammonia, which is a cerebral toxin. A major source of ammonia (NH_3) is from the bacterial and enzymatic deamination of amino acids in the intestines. The ammonia that results from this deamination process normally goes to the liver via the portal circulation and is converted to urea which is excreted by the kidneys. When the blood is shunted past the liver via the collateral anastomoses or the liver is unable to convert NH_3 to urea, large quantities of ammonia remain in systemic circulation. The ammonia crosses the blood-brain barrier and produces neurologic toxic manifestations.

Other "toxic" substances that may contribute to hepatic encephalopathy are false neurotransmitter substances, methionine, and short-chain fatty acids. It is currently believed that the liver may produce substances necessary to normal brain functioning. When the diseased liver can no longer produce these substances, encephalopathy may result. There are a number of factors that may precipitate hepatic encephalopathy, mostly because they increase the amount of circulating ammonia (Table 35-9).

Clinical manifestations of encephalopathy are

Table 35-8
Factors Involved in the Development of Ascites Associated with Cirrhosis

Factor	Mechanism
Portal hypertension	Increased resistance of blood flow through liver
Increased flow of hepatic lymph	Weeping of protein-rich lymph from surface of cirrhotic liver Results from intrahepatic blockage of lymph channels
Decreased serum colloidal oncotic pressure	Impaired liver synthesis of albumin Loss of albumin into peritoneal cavity
Hyperaldosteronism	Increased aldosterone secretion stimulated by decreased renal blood flow Impaired liver metabolism of aldosterone
Impaired water excretion	Due to reduced renal vascular flow and to excessive serum levels of ADH

Table 35-9

Factors that Precipitate Hepatic Encephalopathy

Factor	Mechanism
GI hemorrhage	Increases ammonia in GI tract
Constipation	Increases ammonia from bacterial action on feces
Hypokalemia	Increases renal production of NH_3, which enters systemic circulation. The brain needs K^+ to metabolize ammonia
Hypovolemia	Increases blood NH_3 by causing hepatic hypoxia. Impaired cerebral, hepatic, and renal function due to decreased blood flow
Infection	Increased catabolism. Increases cerebral sensitivity to toxins
Cerebral depressants (e.g., narcotics)	Cannot be detoxified by the liver. Therefore, higher serum levels of drugs cause increased cerebral depression
Metabolic alkalosis	Facilitates transport of NH_3 across blood-brain barrier. Increases renal production of NH_3
Paracentesis	Loss of Na and K and decrease in blood volume
Dehydration	Potentiates NH_3 toxicity
Increased metabolism	Increases work load of liver
Diuretics	Increases renal formation of NH_3. May eventually lead to azotemia which increases the endogenous NH_3 production. May also cause hypokalemia
Uremia (renal failure)	Retention of nitrogenous metabolites

changes in neurologic and mental responsiveness ranging from lethargy to deep coma. In the early stages, manifestations include euphoria; depression; apathy; irritability; memory loss; confusion; yawning; drowsiness; insomnia; agitation; slow, slurred speech; emotional lability; impaired judgment; hiccups; slow, deep respirations; hyperactive reflexes; and a positive Babinski reflex.

Clinical manifestations of impending coma include disorientation to time, place, or person. A characteristic symptom is *asterixis* or *flapping tremors*. This may take several forms, the most common involving the arms and hands. When the client is asked to hold his arms and hands stretched out, he is unable to hold this position and there will be a series of rapid flexion and extension movements of the hands. Other signs of asterixis are rhythmic movements of the legs with dorsiflexion of the foot and rhythmic movements in the face with strong closure of the eyelids.

Fetor hepaticus occurs in some clients with encephalopathy. It is a musty, sweet odor of the client's breath. This odor is from the accumulation of methionine (an amino acid containing sulfur) due to the liver's inability to metabolize it. Impairments in writing involve difficulty in moving the pen or pencil from left to right and *apraxia* (the inability to construct simple figures). Other signs include hyperventiliation, hypothermia, and grimacing and grasping reflexes.

Hepatorenal Syndrome

Hepatorenal syndrome is a serious complication of cirrhosis. It is characterized by functional renal failure with advancing azotemia, oliguria, and intractable ascites. There is no renal structural abnormality. The exact cause of the renal failure is unknown, but it is thought to be due to altered renal hemodynamics, and possible cortical vessel constriction, which is caused either by a prostaglandin deficiency or increased serum angiotensin. The syndrome frequently follows diuretic therapy, gastrointestinal hemorrhage, or paracentesis. Hepatic encephalopathy is also associated with the renal function deterioration. Treatment measures include salt-poor albumin, salt and water restrictions, and diuretic therapy. Treatment is usually unsuccessful.

Diagnostic Study Abnormalities

A liver profile in cirrhosis will demonstrate abnormalities in most of the liver function studies (Table 31-10). Enzyme levels (alkaline phosphatase, SGOT, SGPT, and lactic acid dehydrogenase) are elevated because of the release of these enzymes from damaged liver cells. Protein metabolism tests will show decreased total protein, decreased albumin, and increased globulin levels. The liver does not synthesize gamma globulins but does synthesize albumin. The globulin level often increases in cirrhosis and indicates increased synthesis or decreased removal. Gamma globulins (antibodies) are produced in the lymphatics, spleen, and bone marrow. Fat metabolism abnormalities are reflected by decreased cholesterol levels. Excretory tests such as the BSP or ICG show retention of the dye. The prothrombin time is pro-

Table 35-10

Bilirubin Metabolism Abnormalities in Cirrhosis*

Serum Bilirubin	Urine Bilirubin	Urobilinogen
Unconjugated: elevated Conjugated: elevated	Increased	Stool: normal to decreased Urine: normal to increased

*These are the bilirubin metabolism abnormalities that occur with *hepatocellular jaundice*, which is the most frequent type of jaundice with cirrhosis of the liver.

longed and bilirubin metabolism is altered (Table 35-10).

Medical Management (Table 35-11)

Rest

Although there is no specific therapy for cirrhosis, there are certain measures which can be taken to promote liver cell regeneration and prevent or treat complications. Rest is very significant in reducing metabolic demands of the liver, reducing the hepatic blood flow, and allowing for recovery of liver cells. At various times during the progress of cirrhosis the rest may need to take the form of complete bed rest.

Ascites

The focus of management of the client with ascites is sodium restriction and diuretics. Rest is very important since bed rest decreases sodium retention. There should also be accurate assessment and control of fluid and electrolyte balance. Salt-poor albumin may be used to help maintain intravascular volume and adequate urinary output. A low sodium diet is prescribed. The client is usually not on restricted fluids unless severe ascites develops. Two diuretics frequently combined are a potassium-sparing agent such as spironolactone (Aldactone) and a thiazide such as chlorothiazide (Diuril). A high potency diuretic such as furosemide (Lasix) may also be used.

If the client does not respond to this treatment regimen, other methods may have to be used. *Paracentesis* (needle puncture of the abdominal cavity to remove fluid) can be dangerous and is infrequently used. It is reserved for clients with acute respiratory or abdominal distress secondary to ascites. Removal of large amounts of ascitic fluid via paracentesis produces loss of albumin, sodium, and potassium and also results in hypovolemia. The client may experience syncope or go into shock. Paracentesis can be a precipitating factor of hepatic coma.

Intravenous reinfusion of the ascitic fluid has been utilized to replace albumin lost in the ascitic drainage. The ascitic fluid is removed at a constant rate through an ultrafiltration device. The fluid passes through a filter that removes crystalloids and fluids. It is then reinjected via an intravenous route.[19]

Peritoneal-Venous Shunt A surgical procedure provides for the continuous reinfusion of ascitic fluid into the venous system. It is called the *LeVeen peritoneal-venous shunt*. It consists of a tube and a one-way valve. The tube runs from the abdominal cavity through the peritoneum, under the subcutaneous tissue, and into the jugular vein or superior vena cava (Fig. 35-2). The valve opens when the pressure in the peritoneal cavity is 3 to 5 cmH_2O higher than that in the superior vena cava. This allows the ascitic

Table 35-11
Medical Management: Cirrhosis of the Liver

Diagnostic
1. Liver function studies
2. Liver biopsy
3. Esophagoscopy
4. Serum electrolytes
5. Prothrombin time
6. CBC
7. Stool for occult blood
8. UGI
9. 24-hour urine for NaCl

Therapeutic
1. 3,000-calorie, high carbohydrate, low to moderate protein, low fat diet (depends on stage)
2. B complex vitamins
3. Complete bed rest with BRP
4. No alcohol
5. Diuretics

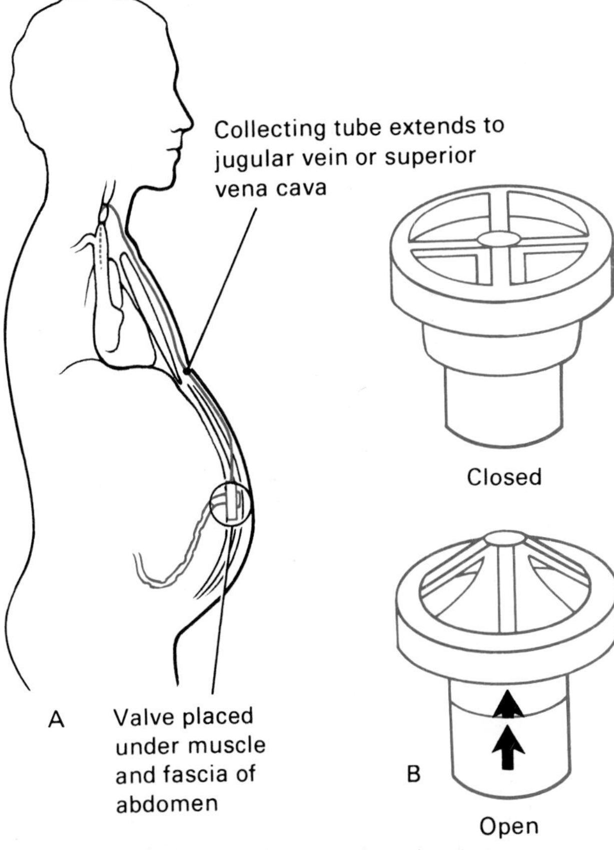

Figure 35-2 LeVeen continuous peritoneal-venous shunt. (*a*) Collecting tube extends subcutaneously from peritoneal cavity to jugular vein or superior vena cava. (*b*) Valve in closed and open position.

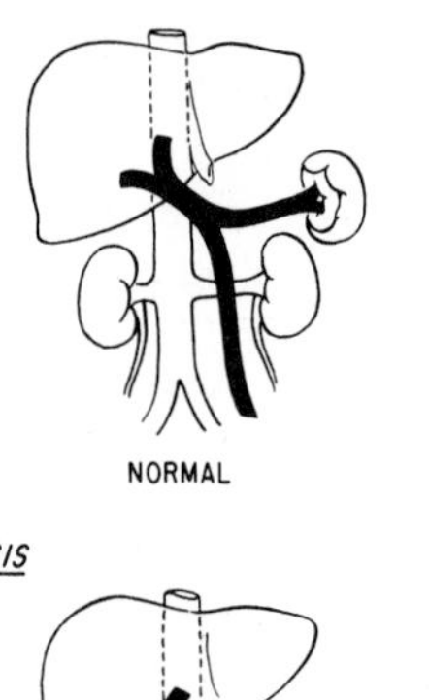

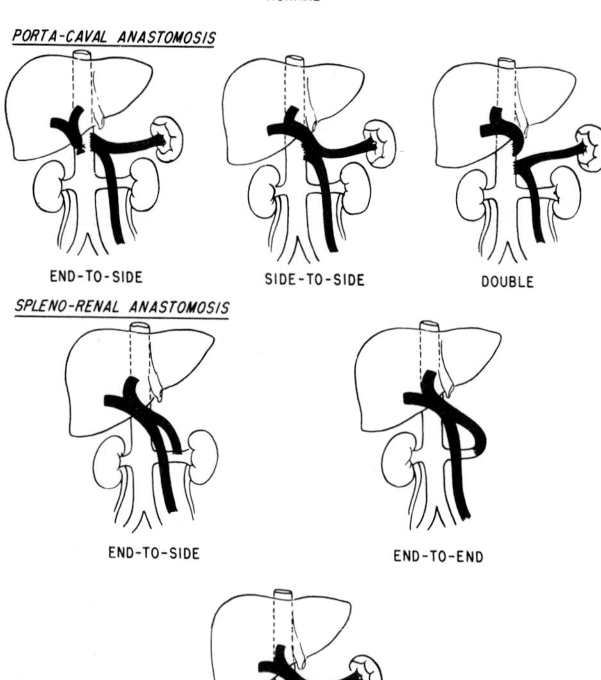

Figure 35-3 Portosystemic shunts. (*From Seymour I. Schwartz, "Surgical Diseases of the Liver," McGraw-Hill Book Company, New York, 1964.*)

fluid to flow into the venous system. The client's inspiration increases the intraperitoneal pressure causing the valve to open. This shunting of the ascitic fluid causes an improvement in hemodynamic factors and increases sodium and fluid excretion. Urine output is also increased.

Esophageal varices

The main medical goal related to esophageal varices is to avoid bleeding and hemorrhage. Individuals who have esophageal varices should avoid ingesting alcohol, aspirin, and irritating foods. Upper respiratory infections should be treated promptly. Coughing should be controlled.

Various surgical shunting procedures (portal to systemic venous shunts) may be used (Fig. 35-3). Their purpose is to decrease portal hypertension by diverting some of the portal blood flow and at the same time allow for adequate liver perfusion. The shunts most distal to the portal vein accomplish this purpose the best. However, thrombosis is a problem with these distal shunts. The shunt procedure is sometimes done as an early treatment measure before a bleeding episode has occurred. It is also performed after the client has stabilized following a bleeding episode. Hepatic encephalopathy is a fairly common problem post shunt because the shunt procedure partially or totally diverts the ammonia past the liver

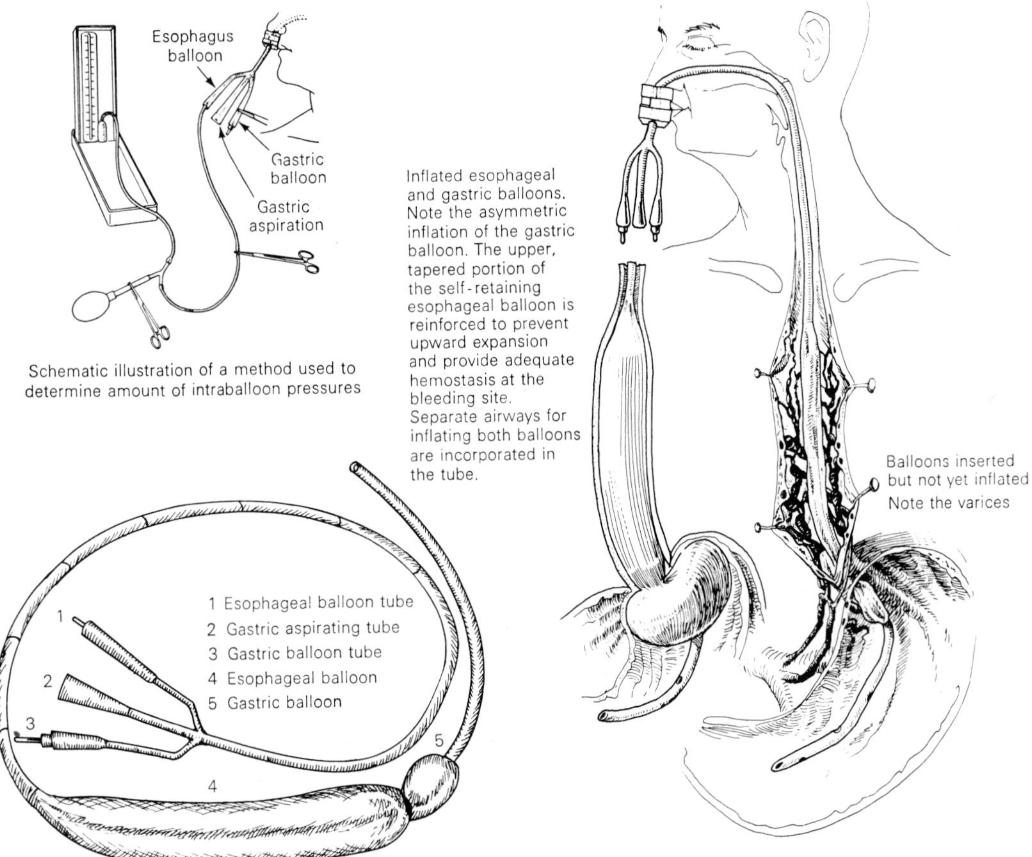
Esophagus balloon
Gastric balloon
Gastric aspiration
Schematic illustration of a method used to determine amount of intraballoon pressures
Inflated esophageal and gastric balloons. Note the asymmetric inflation of the gastric balloon. The upper, tapered portion of the self-retaining esophageal balloon is reinforced to prevent upward expansion and provide adequate hemostasis at the bleeding site. Separate airways for inflating both balloons are incorporated in the tube.
Balloons inserted but not yet inflated
Note the varices
1 Esophageal balloon tube
2 Gastric aspirating tube
3 Gastric balloon tube
4 Esophageal balloon
5 Gastric balloon
1
2
3
4
5

Figure 35-4 Esophageal tamponade accomplished with Sengstaken-Blakemore tube. (*By permission of Davol Rubber Company, Providence, R.I. From H. Moidel et al., Nursing Care of the Patient with Medical-Surgical Disorders 2d ed., McGraw-Hill Book Company, New York, 1976, p. 708.*)

and into the systemic circulation. Other complications of shunts include gastrointestinal bleeding and ascites. Other procedures for treatment of esophageal varices include ligation of the varices or injection of sclerosing drugs via esophagoscopy.

Management of bleeding esophageal varices consists of control of bleeding and restoration of blood volume. Bleeding episodes are a medical emergency. Mechanical compression of the varices is the most effective means of controlling the hemorrhage. This is accomplished with esophageal balloon tamponade using the Sengstaken-Blakemore tube (Fig. 35-4). This tube has two balloons—gastric and esophageal, and three lumina—one for the gastric balloon, one for the esophageal balloon, and one for gastric aspiration. When inflated, the gastric and esophageal balloons put mechanical compression on the varices. The gastric balloon anchors the tube in position and also applies pressure to any bleeding gastric varices.

Blood transfusions may be given to restore blood volume and vitamin K is sometimes administered. Vasopressin (Pitressin) may be used to cause arterial vasoconstriction and lower portal pressure due to constriction of the splanchnic arterial bed. It can be given either intravenously or via intraarterial infusion into the superior mesenteric artery.

Hepatic encephalopathy

The goal of management of hepatic encephalopathy is the reduction of ammonia formation. This consists mainly of protein restriction and reduction of ammonia formation in the intestines. The degree of protein restriction is determined by the client's state of responsiveness. The protein restriction may range from 0 to 40 g/day.

Several measures to reduce ammonia formation in the intestines are used. Sterilization of the intestines using antibiotics such as neomycin sulfate which are poorly absorbed from the GI tract is one method. This reduces the bacterial flora of the colon. Bacterial action on protein in the feces results in ammonia production. Cathartics and enemas are also used to decrease bacterial action.

Lactulose (Cephalac) may also be used to treat hepatic encephalopathy. It is a synthetic keto-analogue of lactose. In the colon it is split into lactic acid and acetic acids, which decrease the pH from 7.0 to 5.0. The acidic environment discourages bacterial growth. The increased availability of H^+ ions encourages conversion of NH_3 to NH_4, which is excreted in the stool.

Levodopa is a recently used drug in the treatment of encephalopathy. It is a precursor of dopamine and norephinephrine. Use of levodopa is based on the theory that there is a deficiency of dopamine and norepinephrine in encephalopathy because they are replaced by false transmitters (amines from breakdown of dietary proteins). Normally these are destroyed by liver enzymes, which the diseased liver can no longer do.

Control of hepatic encephalopathy also involves treating preciptating causes (Table 35-9). This involves controlling gastrointestinal hemorrhage and removing the blood from the gastrointestinal tract in order to decrease the protein in the intestine. Electrolyte and acid-base imbalances and infections should also be treated.

Hemodialysis or peritoneal dialysis may be used to remove the ammonia from the blood by exchanging sodium ions for ammonium ions. Other methods used to correct metabolic and electrolyte disturbances are exchange blood transfusions and cross circulation of blood. In *exchange blood transfusion* the blood volume is replaced with fresh blood. In *cross circulation* the blood is exchanged between the client and a human donor. This allows the client's liver cells to regenerate while the donor's liver detoxifies the client's blood. This procedure raises moral and ethical issues since the donor must be terminally ill or neurologically dead with respirations being mechanically maintained.[20]

In total body perfusion or washout, the substances normally detoxified by the liver are cleared out by perfusion, using a crystalloid plus albumin perfusate with lactated Ringer's solution, albumin solution, sodium bicarbonate, and heparin. The crystalloid perfusion is followed with a blood perfusate of two-thirds whole blood and one-third packed cells.[21]

Pharmacologic Intervention

As previously mentioned, there is no specific drug therapy for cirrhosis. However, there are a number of medications used to treat symptoms and complications of advancing liver disease (Table 35-12).

Dietary Intervention

The diet for the client with cirrhosis without complications will be high in calories (3,000/day), with high carbohydrate content, moderate to high protein, and moderate to low fat. The amount of protein will vary, depending on the degree of liver damage and the danger of encephalopathy. Some physicians will order 1.5 g of protein/kg of body weight in order to maintain plasma osmotic balance and promote liver cell regeneration. In some situations the client may be given a reduced quantity of protein to reduce the risk of encephalopathy. Vitamin supplements are usually given. Foods high in protein include meat, fish, poultry, eggs, and dairy products. High protein nourishments of eggnogs, milkshakes, or protein supplements may be utilized, particularly for the client who is malnourished.

The client with edema formation will be on a low-sodium diet. The degree of sodium restriction will vary, depending on the client's condition. The client needs instruction regarding the degree of restriction. Table salt is the most common source of sodium. Sodium is also present in baking soda and powder and some over-the-counter medications. Foods that are high in sodium content include canned soups and vegetables, salted snacks such as potato chips, nuts, etc., smoked meats and fish, crackers, breads, olives, pickles, catsup, and beer.

The nurse must remember that some medications

Table 35-12
Medications Used in Cirrhosis

Medication	Mechanism of Action
Vasopressin (Pitressin)	Hemostasis and control bleeding in esophageal varices. Constricts splanchnic arterial bed.
Neomycin sulfate	Decreases bacterial flora so formation of NH_3 is decreased.
Lactulose (Cephalac)	In bowel acidifies feces and traps NH_3 so it is eliminated in feces.
Levodopa	Converted to dopamine which has been displaced with amines from protein breakdown.
Diuretics	
a. Spironolactone (Aldactone)	Blocks action of aldosterone. Potassium-sparing.
b. Chlorothiazide (Diuril)	Thiazide that acts on proximal tubule to decrease the reabsorption of Na, K, and H_2O.
c. Furosemide (Lasix)	Rapid-acting on distal tubule and Henle's loop to prevent reabsorption of Na, K, and H_2O.

contain sodium (e.g., antacids). The antacid Riopan is low in sodium. Some carbonated drinks are high in sodium (e.g., colas). Foods high in protein usually have large amounts of sodium. Alternative protein supplements low in sodium may have to be used. The client and family need assistance to make the diet more palatable by the use of seasonings such as garlic, parsley, onion, lemon juice, and spices.

The client with hepatic encephalopathy will be on a very low to no protein diet. Foods allowed include toast, cereal, rice, tea, fruit juices, and hard candies. Sufficient carbohydrate intake must be provided to maintain a caloric intake of 1500 to 2000 calories to prevent hypoglycemia and catabolism. Intravenous or tube feedings may be required.

Nursing Management

Health promotion and maintenance

The client with cirrhosis may be faced with a very prolonged course and the possibility of serious, life-threatening problems and complications. The nurse should be a resource person in helping the client achieve his highest level of wellness. The client and family need to understand the importance of continuous health care and medical supervision. They should be taught symptoms of complications and when to seek medical attention.

Measures to achieve remission and maintain it should be encouraged. These include proper diet, rest, avoidance of potentially hepatotoxic over-the-counter drugs, and abstinence from alcohol. Abstinence from alcohol is very important and results in improvement in most clients. The nurse must realize the difficulty this poses for some clients (Chap. 60). The nurse needs to ascertain her own attitude regarding the client whose cirrhosis is attributed to alcohol abuse. Care should be given without rejection and moralizing. The alcoholic client should be treated with a caring attitude. The nurse also has the responsibility of public education regarding the effects of alcohol and other substances which are toxic to the liver.

Acute intervention

The focus of nursing care for the client with cirrhosis is on conserving the client's strength. Rest assists the liver to restore itself. Complete bed rest may not always be necessary. When the client requires complete bed rest, measures to prevent pneumonia, thromboembolic problems, and decubiti should be taken. The activity and rest schedule may be modified, based on signs of clinical improvement (decreasing jaundice, improvement in liver function studies). Major concerns of the nurse in determining appropriate nursing care measures to meet the need for rest are regulation of the physical, emotional, and social climate (Table 35-13).

Anorexia, nausea and vomiting, pressure from ascites, and poor eating habits all create problems of maintaining an adequate intake of nutrients. Nursing measures relating to nutrition discussed for hepatitis also apply here. Oral hygiene before meals may improve the client's taste sensation. Between-meal nourishments should be available so they can be provided at times when the client can best tolerate them. Food preferences should be provided whenever possible. Explanations to the client and family as to the reason for any dietary restrictions should be provided.

Nursing assessment and care should include the client's physiologic response to cirrhosis. Is jaundice present? Where is it observed—sclera, skin, hard palate (in dark-skinned people)? What is the progression of jaundice? If the jaundice is accompanied by pruritus, measures to relieve itching should be carried out. The color of the urine and stools should be noted (Table 35-10).

Edema and ascites are frequent manifestations of cirrhosis and require nursing assessments and interventions. Accurate calculation and recordings of intake and output, daily weights, and measurements of extremities and abdominal girth help in the ongoing assessment of the location and extent of the edema. If the client can assume a kneeling position when taking abdominal girth measurement, the abdominal fluid will go to the most dependent part of the abdomen. This gives the best measurement of abdominal girth. For many clients girth will need to be measured in the standing or lying position. Where the measurements are taken should be recorded and be a part of the nursing care plan.

Dyspnea is a frequent problem for the client with ascites. A semi-Fowler's or Fowler's position allows for maximal respiratory efficiency. Pillows can be used to support the arms and chest and may increase the client's comfort and ability to breathe.

Meticulous skin care is essential since the edematous tissues are subject to breakdown. An alternating air pressure mattress or other special mattress should be used. A turning schedule (*minimum* of every 2 hours) must be adhered to rigidly. The abdomen may be supported with pillows. If the abdomen is taut, cleansing must be done very gently. This client tends to move very little because of the abdominal discomfort and dyspnea. Therefore, range-of-motion exercises are helpful. The lower extremities may be elevated. If scrotal edema is present, a scrotal support will provide some comfort.

When the client is on diuretics, the serum levels of sodium, potassium, chloride, and bicarbonate should be monitored. The client should be observed for signs

Table 35-13

Nursing Care Plan for Client with Advanced Liver Disease (Cirrhosis)

Client Problem	Expected Outcome	Nursing Intervention
Anorexia, nausea, vomiting	Adequate intake of nutrients. Maintenance of normal body weight.	Provide oral care before meals. Administer antiemetics as ordered. Provide small, frequent meals with nourishments at times the client can best tolerate them. Determine food preferences and allow these whenever possible. Provide attractively served meals in pleasant surroundings.
Jaundice	Normal skin color. Serum bilirubin levels within normal range.	Assess the presence, location, and progression of jaundice. Determine if accompanied by pruritus. Observe color of urine and stools. Assess client's psychological response to the jaundice and intervene appropriately.
Edema and ascites	Control of edema and ascites.	Restrict sodium intake as ordered. Restrict fluids if ordered. Administer prescribed diuretics. Observe for side effects and hypokalemia. Monitor I and O. Assess the location and extent of the edema by weighing the client daily at the same time, taking daily measurements of extremities, and daily measurements of abdominal girth (same location each time). Provide meticulous skin care. Reposition at least every 2 h. Do range-of-motion exercises. Elevate edematous areas. Use special mattress such as alternating air pressure or egg carton.
Dyspnea	Ability to breathe with minimal difficulty.	Place client in semi-Fowler's or Fowler's position. Support the arms and chest with pillows. Auscultate chest for rales.
Peripheral neuropathy	No paresthesia or pain.	Avoid excess stimulation or trauma to extremities. Do not use restrictive bed linens. Avoid tight clothing. Use care with heat and cold applications.
Bleeding tendencies	Minimal bleeding. No hemorrhage.	Provide gentle nursing care. Provide assistance with ambulation. Observe for bleeding from body orifices, urine, and stool. Use smallest gauge needle possible when giving injection and apply gentle but prolonged pressure after injection. Use soft-bristle toothbrush. Teach client to avoid straining at stool, vigorous blowing of nose, and coughing. Observe for signs of thrombocytopenia such as purpura on the forearms, axilla, and skin. Monitor lab results of Hct, Hb, and prothrombin time.
Fatigue	Feeling of being rested.	Conserve client's strength. Provide activity and rest as required by regulating the physical, emotional, and social climate. Monitor hemoglobin and hematocrit readings. Plan scheduled rest periods for the client.
Increased susceptibility to infection	Absence of infections. Normal body temperature.	Monitor client's temperature every 2–4 h. Observe for any local and systemic manifestation of infection. Protect from others with infections. Monitor WBC.
Altered body image	Acceptance of altered body image.	Assess client's response. Present an accepting attitude. Be a supportive listener. Care for the client with concern and warmth. Explain the changes.
Difficulty coping with chronic illness (anxiety and depression)	Ventilates feelings about illness. Progression toward acceptance of chronic disease.	Assess level of anxiety and depression. Provide diversional activities. Provide information regarding community support programs such as AA for help with alcohol abuse. Provide written instructions with explanations to client and family. Listen to concerns of client.

Table 35-13 (Continued)

Client Problem	Expected Outcome	Nursing Intervention
Possibility of progression of disease	Maintain a state of wellness at the highest level possible for client.	Explain to client and family the importance of continuous health care. Teach client and family symptoms of complications and when to seek medical attention. Teach proper diet. Teach to avoid potentially hepatotoxic over-the-counter drugs. Encourage abstinence from alcohol. If client has esophageal varices, avoid ASA and control cough. Avoid spicy and rough foods and activities which increase portal pressure such as straining at stool, coughing, sneezing, and retching and vomiting.
	If Client Develops Bleeding Esophageal Varices	
Possibility of airway obstruction and asphyxiation	Patent airway.	Suction client (oral and pharyngeal) frequently. Position in semi-Fowler's. Have scissors near bed to cut the tube if necessary. (Indications include increased respiratory rate, cyanosis, dyspnea.)
Inability to swallow saliva	Expectorate saliva as necessary.	Encourage client to expectorate. Provide emesis basin and tissues. Provide frequent oral and nasal care to provide comfort from the taste of blood and irritation from mouth breathing.
Possible hypovolemic shock	Blood pressure and pulse within normal limits.	Monitor vital signs every hour. Administer intravenous fluids and blood products as ordered.
	If Client Develops Hepatic Encephalopathy	
Impending coma (alterations in mental functioning)	Prevention of progression to coma.	Assess and record the client's neurologic status at least every 2 h. Include an exact description of the client's behavior. Encourage fluids (if not restricted) and give laxatives and enemas as ordered to decrease the production of ammonia. Provide low or no protein diet as ordered. Limit physical activity. Control factors known to precipitate coma (Table 35-9).

of fluid and electrolyte imbalance, especially hypokalemia. Hypokalemia may be manifested by cardiac arrhythmias, hypotension, tachycardia, and generalized muscle weakness. Hyponatremia is manifested by muscle cramping, weakness, lethargy, and confusion.

Observations and nursing care in relationship to hematologic disorders (bleeding tendencies, anemia, increased susceptibility to infection) are discussed in the nursing care plan for the client with advanced liver disease (Table 35-13).

The nurse must assess the client's response to the altered body image resulting from the jaundice, spider angiomas, palmar erythema, ascites, and gynecomastia. The client may experience a great deal of anxiety regarding these changes. The nurse should explain these phenomena and be a supportive listener. Caring for this client with concern and warmth regardless of physical changes will assist the client to maintain self-esteem.

When the client experiences manifestations of advanced liver disease, other problems such as bleeding esophageal varices and hepatic encephalopathy must be considered.

Bleeding Esophageal Varices If the client has esophageal varices in addition to cirrhosis, the nurse must be observant of any signs of bleeding from the varices, such as hematemesis, and melena. If hematemesis occurs, the nurse should call the physician, take the vital signs, and obtain a Sengstaken-Blakemore tube.

The initial nursing role related to insertion of the Sengstaken-Blakemore tube is to explain the use of the tube and how it will be inserted. The balloons should be checked for patency. Sometimes the stomach is lavaged with iced saline solution prior to insertion of the tube. It is usually the physician's responsibility to insert the tube. The deflated tube is inserted through the nose into the stomach (Fig. 35-5). The gastric balloon is inflated with 150 to 250 mL of air and the tube is retracted until resistance is felt.

Traction may be applied ($\frac{3}{4}$ to $1\frac{1}{4}$ lb) to hold the tube securely in place and prevent downward movement. The tube is secured by placing a piece of sponge or foam rubber at the nostrils. This protects the mucosal surfaces from irritation and injury. The esophageal balloon is then inflated with air. A sphygomomanometer is used to maintain and measure the desired pressure at 20 to 40 mmHg. The position of the balloons is verified by x-ray. Sometimes it is helpful to have the client wear a football helmet with the tube secured to the mouth guard. This stabilizes the tube and applies traction.

Sometimes iced saline lavage is used to assist in controlling the bleeding. The iced saline lavage has a vasoconstrictor effect on the bleeding varices. (Nursing care of upper gastrointestinal bleeding is discussed in Chap. 33). The nurse must assure that the right amount of pressure is maintained for the correct time period. Sometimes the esophageal balloon is deflated every 8 to 12 hours to avoid necrosis. Each lumen must be labeled to avoid confusion.

Nursing care includes monitoring for complications of rupture or erosion of the esophagus, regurgitation and aspiration of gastric contents, and occlusion of the airway by the balloon. If the gastric balloon breaks or is deflated, the esophageal balloon will slip upward, obstructing the airway and causing asphyxiation. If this happens, the nurse must cut the tube or deflate the esophageal balloon. Scissors should be at the bedside. Regurgitation can be minimized by oral and pharyngeal suctioning and a semi-Fowler's position.

The client is unable to swallow saliva due to the inflated esophageal balloon occluding the esophagus. The nurse should encourage the client to expectorate and provide an emesis basin and tissues. Frequent oral and nasal care will provide comfort from the taste of blood and irritation from mouth breathing.

This client is extremely ill at this stage. The crises of the bleeding plus the terrifying ordeal of the Sengstaken-Blakemore tube create a great deal of psychological trauma. The nurse must not get so caught up with the mechanical aspects of nursing care that emotional support and gentle caring are forgotten.

Hepatic Encephalopathy The focus of nursing care of the client with hepatic encephalopathy is sustaining life and assisting with measures to reduce the formation of ammonia. The nurse should assess: (1) the client's level of responsiveness (reflexes, pupillary reactions, orientation), (2) sensory and motor abnormalities (hyperreflexia, asterixis, motor coordination), (3) fluid and electrolyte imbalances, (4) acid-base imbalances, and (5) the effect of treatment measures.

The neurologic status, including an exact description of the client's behavior, should be assessed and recorded at least every 2 hours. Care of the client with neurologic problems should be based on the severity of the encephalopathy.

Nursing measures to prevent constipation should be instituted in order to decrease the production of ammonia. Drugs, laxatives, and enemas should be given as ordered. Encouragement of fluids may also help if not contraindicated. The client should not strain at stool as this may cause bleeding of the hemorrhoidal varices. Any gastrointestinal bleeding may worsen the coma.

Factors which are known to precipitate coma should be controlled as much as possible (Table 35-9). Since exercise produces ammonia as a byproduct of metabolism, the physical activity of the client must be limited. Hypokalemia should be controlled.

The client will be on either a very low or no protein diet, which is not very palatable. Foods and fluids high in carbohydrate should be given since the liver is not synthesizing and storing glucose. The client may require tube feedings or hyperalimentation if an adequate diet cannot be ingested.

Chronic management

The client with cirrhosis has a chronic disease. He is affected not only physically but also psychologically, socially, and economically. Major adjustments may be required to make lifestyle changes, especially if alcohol abuse is the primary etiologic factor. The nurse should provide information regarding community support programs such as Alcoholics Anonymous for help with alcohol abuse.

Adequate explanations along with written instructions related to fluid or dietary restrictions should be given to the client and the family. Other health teaching should include instruction about adequate rest periods, observations to detect early signs of complications, skin care, drug therapy precautions, observation for bleeding, and protection from infection. Counseling information regarding sexual problems may be needed. Community health nurse referral may be helpful to ensure adequate client compliance to prescribed therapy.

CARCINOMA OF THE LIVER

Primary carcinoma (originating in the liver) is quite rare. Metastatic carcinoma of the liver is more common. *Hepatomas*, which are tumors of the parenchymal cells of the liver, are the most common primary tumor (80 to 90 percent). The remaining primary tumors are *cholangiomas*, or bile duct carcinomas. A high percentage of clients (70 to 75 percent) with hepatoma have cirrhosis of the liver.[22] Men have a higher incidence of primary liver cancer.

The liver is a common site for metastatic growth, due to its high rate of blood flow and extensive capillary network. Cancer cells in other parts of the body are commonly carried to the liver via the portal circulation.

The malignant cells cause the liver to be enlarged and misshapen. Hemorrhage and necrosis in the liver are common. Lesions may be singular or numerous, nodular or diffusely spread over the entire liver. Some tumors infiltrate into other organs such as the gallbladder or into the peritoneum or diaphragm. Primary liver tumors commonly metastasize to the lung.

Clinical Manifestations

It is difficult to diagnose carcinoma of the liver. It is particularly difficult to differentiate it from cirrhosis in its early stages as many of the clinical manifestations (hepatomegaly, weight loss, peripheral edema, ascites, and portal hypertension) are similar. Other common manifestations include dull abdominal pain in the epigastric or right upper quadrant region, jaundice, anorexia, nausea and vomiting, and extreme weakness. Clients frequently present with pulmonary emboli. Tests used to assist in the diagnosis are a liver scan, hepatic arteriography, and a liver biopsy. The test for alpha fetoprotein may be positive.

Treatment

Treatment of cancer of the liver is largely palliative. Surgical excision is sometimes utilized if the tumor is localized to one portion of the liver. Usually surgery is not feasible because the cancer is too far advanced when it is detected. The medical management is very similar to that discussed under cirrhosis. Chemotherapy may be used but there is usually a poor response. Hepatic artery perfusion with 5-fluorouracil may be attempted.

Nursing intervention for the client with liver carcinoma focuses on keeping the client as comfortable as possible. Since this client manifests the same problems as any client with advanced liver disease, the nursing interventions discussed for cirrhosis of the liver apply here. (Also refer to Chap. 11 for nursing care of the cancer client.)

The prognosis for cancer of the liver is very poor. The cancer grows rapidly and death may occur within 4 to 7 months, from hepatic encephalopathy or massive blood loss from gastrointestinal bleeding.

LIVER TRANSPLANTATION

Liver transplantation is reserved for chronic end-stage liver disease. Two types of transplant procedures are (1) *orthotopic*, which involves total removal of the person's own liver and replacement with a cadaver liver; and (2) *auxiliary* or *heterotopic*, which involves placing an accessory or second liver in the pelvis or groin. The survival rate is much lower with the heterotopic type and fewer of these have been done.

Changes in technique have led to improved survival in the past few years. In a group of 30 clients the 1-year survival rate was 50 percent.[23] There are a number of liver transplant recipients who have survived for more than 2 years.

Indications for liver transplantation include congenital biliary abnormalities, inborn errors of metabolism, hepatic malignancy, and chronic end-stage liver disease. Cirrhosis of the liver is a major indication in adults. Liver transplants are not recommended for the client with widespread malignant disease.

Problems of liver transplantation include vascular anomalies, coagulation problems such as hemorrhage and thrombosis, rejection, and biliary reconstruction. Rejection is not the major problem. The liver seems to be less liable to severe rejection than the kidney. Tissue typing is frequently not possible but immunosuppressant drugs and antilymphocytic globulin are used.

Changes in technique for biliary tract reconstruction have helped improve survival rates, as this was previously a major problem. An ideal reconstruction procedure is a *choledochocholedochostomy* (direct anastomosis between the common bile ducts of the recipient and donor). This procedure retains the sphincter of Oddi and therefore prevents ascending cholangitis.

The client who has had a liver transplant requires competent and highly skilled nursing care, either in an intensive care unit or other specialized unit. Liver function tests, cholangiograms, and coagulation studies are used to assess functioning of the new liver and to identify complications or problems.

ACUTE PANCREATITIS

Significance of Problem

Acute pancreatitis is an acute inflammatory process of the pancreas. The degree of inflammation varies from mild edema to severe hemorrhagic necrosis.

In the United States the overall prevalence of acute pancreatitis is about 0.5 percent.[24] It is most common in middle-aged men and women. Mortality rate is about 10 percent. The severity of the disease varies based on the extent of pancreatic destruction. Some clients recover completely, others have recurring attacks, and some develop chronic pancreatitis.

Etiology and Pathogenesis

There are many factors that can cause injury to the pancreas. The primary etiologic factors are biliary tract disease and alcoholism. Other less common causes of acute pancreatitis include trauma, viral infections, penetrating duodenal ulcer, cysts, abscesses, certain drugs (corticosteroids, thiazide diuretics, oral contraceptives), and metabolic disorders such as hyperparathyroidism, hyperlipidemia, and renal failure. Pancreatitis may occur following surgical procedures on the pancreas, stomach, duodenum, or biliary tract. In some cases the cause is not known (idiopathic).

The most common pathogenetic mechanism is believed to be autodigestion of the pancreas (Fig. 35-5). The etiologic factors cause injury to pancreatic cells or activation of the pancreatic enzymes in the pancreas rather than in the intestine. It is not clear how the activation of pancreatic enzymes occurs. One possible cause is believed to be the reflux of bile acids into the pancreatic ducts through an open or distended sphincter of Oddi. This reflux may occur due to gallstones impacted at the ampulla of Vater, atony and edema of the sphincter, or obstruction of pancreatic ducts and pancreatic ischemia.

Trypsinogen is an inactive proteolytic enzyme produced by the pancreas. Normally it is released into the small intestine via the pancreatic duct. In the intestine it is activated to trypsin by enterokinase. Normally trypsin inhibitors in the pancreas and plasma bind and inactivate any trypsin inadvertently produced. In pancreatitis activated trypsin is present in the pancreas. This enzyme can digest the pancreas, and also activate other proteolytic enzymes such as elastase and phospholipase.

Elastase and phospholipase A play a major role in autodigestion of the pancreas. The elastase is activated by trypsin and causes hemorrhage by producing dissolution of the elastic fibers of blood vessels. The phospholipase A is probably activated by trypsin and bile acids and causes fat necrosis.

It is not entirely clear how alcohol causes acute pancreatitis. It is known that alcohol stimulates the production of hydrochloric acid and secretin which then stimulate pancreatic secretions. The increased hydrochloric acid also produces spasms in the sphincter of Oddi, resulting in obstruction and edema of the ampulla of Vater. This can lead to increased pancreatic ductal pressure with possible rupture.

The pathologic involvement of acute pancreatitis ranges from *edematous* pancreatitis (which is mild and self-limiting) to *necrotizing* pancreatitis (in which the degree of necrosis correlates with the severity of manifestations).

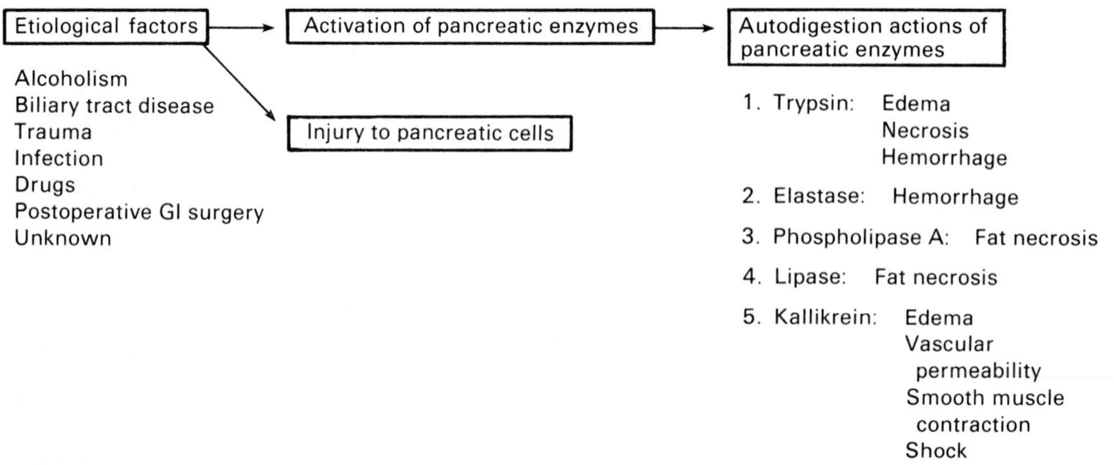

Figure 35-5 Pathogenetic process of acute pancreatitis.

Clinical Manifestations

Abdominal pain is the predominant symptom in acute pancreatitis. The pain is usually located in the left upper quadrant but may be in the mid-epigastrium. It commonly radiates to the back due to the retroperitoneal location of the pancreas. The pain has a sudden onset and is described as severe, deep, and continuous. It is aggravated by eating and frequently has its onset when the client is recumbent. The pain may be accompanied by flushing, cyanosis, and dyspnea. The client may assume various positions involving flexion of the spine in an attempt to relieve the severe pain. The pain is due to distension of the pancreas, peritoneal irritation, and obstruction of the biliary tract.

Other manifestations of acute pancreatitis include nausea and vomiting, low-grade fever, leukocytosis, hypotension, tachycardia, and jaundice. Abdominal tenderness with muscle guarding is common. Bowel sounds may be decreased or absent. Intravascular damage from circulating trypsin may cause areas of cyanosis or greenish to yellow-brown discoloration of the abdominal wall. Other areas of ecchymoses are the flanks (Grey Turner's spots or sign) and the periumbilical area (Cullen's sign). These result from seepage of blood-stained exudate from the pancreas.

Shock may occur due to hemorrhage into the pancreas or toxemia from the activated pancreatic enzymes. The increased formation of kinin peptides (activated by trypsin) such as kallikrein and bradykinin cause vasodilatation, increased capillary permeability, and altered vasomotor tone. Hypovolemia also occurs due to exudation of blood and plasma proteins into the retroperitoneal space.

Complications

Two significant local complications of acute pancreatitis are *pseudocyst* and *abscess*. A *pancreatic pseudocyst* is a cavity continuous with or surrounding the outside of the pancreas. The pseudocyst is filled with necrotic products and liquid secretions such as plasma, pancreatic enzymes, and inflammatory exudates. As pancreatic enzymes escape from the pseudocyst, the serosal surfaces next to the pancreas become inflamed, with subsequent formation of granulation tissue leading to encapsulation of the exudate. Symptoms of pseudocyst are abdominal pain, palpable epigastric mass, nausea, vomiting, and anorexia. The serum amylase level frequently remains elevated. These cysts sometimes resolve spontaneously but may perforate, causing peritonitis, or rupture into the stomach or duodenum. Treatment consists of an internal drainage procedure with a Roux-en-Y anastomosis between the pancreatic duct and the jejunum.

A *pancreatic abscess* is a large fluid-containing cavity within the pancreas. It results from the extensive necrosis in the pancreas. It may become infected or perforate into adjacent organs. Manifestations of an abscess include upper abdominal pain, abdominal mass, high fever, and leukocytosis. Pancreatic abscesses require prompt surgical drainage.

The main *systemic complications* of acute pancreatitis are pulmonary complications (pleural effusion, atelectasis, and pneumonia) and tetany due to hypocalcemia. The pulmonary complications are probably due to the passage of the exudate containing pancreatic enzymes from the peritoneal cavity through transdiaphragmatic lymph channels. Hypocalcemia results from fixation of calcium by fatty acids in areas of fat necrosis and increased levels of circulating glucagon. The glucagon causes an increase in excretion of calcium in the urine.

Diagnostic Study Abnormalities

The primary diagnostic tests for acute pancreatitis are the serum amylase and lipase and the urinary amylase levels. The serum amylase is the most commonly used. It may elevate to levels greater than 200 Somogyi units/dL. The serum amylase is usually elevated early and remains elevated for 24 to 72 hours.

The serum lipase is also elevated in acute pancreatitis and is a helpful complementary test since other disorders (e.g., mumps, cerebral trauma, renal transplantation) may also cause an increase in serum amylase.

There is an increase in urinary amylase which may persist several days beyond the elevation of serum amylase. Urinary amylase may be increased to more than 3600 U/day. Normally a timed collection (e.g., a 2-hour collection) is a more dependable measure than just a randomly collected urinary specimen.

The renal amylase-creatinine clearance test estimates the amount of blood cleared of amylase by the kidney per minute. The finding that the renal clearance of amylase is higher than the creatinine clearance in acute pancreatitis has led to the suggestion that the amylase-creatinine clearance ratio may be a more specific test than urinary amylase. It is a significant finding for assessing acute pancreatitis if the renal clearance of amylase is greater than the clearance of creatinine.

Other laboratory abnormalities include hyperglycemia, hyperlipemia, and hypocalcemia (Table 35-14).

Roentgenographic abnormalities may be found. A flat plate of the abdomen may show a localized paralytic ileus. An upper GI will sometimes show

Table 35-14
Diagnostic Study Abnormalities in Acute Pancreatitis

Laboratory Test	Abnormal Finding	Etiology
	Primary Tests	
Serum amylase	Increased—greater than 200 Somogyi Units/dL	Pancreatic cell injury
Serum lipase	Elevated	Pancreatic cell injury
Urinary amylase	Elevated	Pancreatic cell injury
	Secondary Tests	
Blood glucose	Hyperglycemia	Impaired carbohydrate metabolism due to beta cell damage
Serum calcium	Hypocalcemia	Saponification of calcium by fatty acids in areas of fat necrosis
Serum triglycerides	Hyperlipidemia	Unknown

displacement of the stomach, edematous head of the pancreas, or a pseudocyst. A pancreatic scan may show patchy uptake. A CT scan will show enlargement of the pancreas as well as calcifications and dilatation of bile ducts.

Medical Management

Objectives of medical management of acute pancreatitis include: (1) relief of pain, (2) prevention or alleviation of shock, (3) reduction of pancreatic secretions, (4) control of fluid and electrolyte imbalance, (5) prevention or treatment of infections, and (6) removal of the precipitating cause if possible (Table 35-15).

Table 35-15
Medical Management: Acute Pancreatitis

Diagnostic
1. Serum amylase
2. Serum lipase
3. Two-hour urinary amylase and renal amylase clearance
4. Blood sugar
5. Serum calcium
6. Triglycerides
7. Flat plate of the abdomen
8. Pancreatic scan
9. CT scan of the pancreas

Therapeutic
1. Meperidine IM
2. NPO with nasogastric tube to suction
3. Atropine or cimetidine (IV)
4. Albumin
5. IV calcium gluconate (10%)
6. Lactated Ringer's solution

A primary consideration is the relief and control of pain. Meperidine (Demerol) is preferred because it causes less spasm of the smooth muscles of the ducts than opiate drugs. It may be combined with an antispasmodic such as atropine sulfate. Other medications to relax smooth muscles such as nitroglycerin or papaverine may be used.

If shock is present, blood volume replacements are used. Plasma or plasma volume expanders such as dextran or albumin may be given. Fluid and electrolyte imbalances are corrected with lactated Ringer's solution or other electrolyte solutions. Central venous pressure (CVP) readings may be used to assist in determination of fluid replacement requirements.

It is important to reduce or suppress pancreatic enzymes in order to decrease stimulation of the pancreas and allow it to rest. This is accomplished in several ways. First, the client is kept NPO. Second, nasogastric suction may be used to reduce gastric distension and eliminate gastric digestive juices from entering the duodenum. These measures will suppress pancreatic secretion. Certain drugs may also be used for this purpose (see Pharmacologic Intervention).

The inflamed and necrotic pancreatic tissue is a good source for bacterial growth. Therefore, infections should be prevented. There is some controversy about the prophylactic use of antibiotics. It is important to closely monitor the client so that antibiotic therapy can be instituted early if infection occurs.

Peritoneal lavage or dialysis has been used to remove the kinin and phospholipase A-containing exudate from the peritoneal cavity. This has proved beneficial in some cases of severe acute pancreatitis.[25]

Surgical intervention may be indicated when the diagnosis is uncertain and in clients who do not respond to medical management. Surgery is necessary for an abscess, acute pseudocyst, and severe peritonitis. Surgical treatment of associated biliary tract disease may be necessary.

Pharmacologic Intervention

Several different drugs may be used in the treatment of both acute and chronic pancreatitis (Table 35-16).

Dietary Interventions

Initially the client with acute pancreatitis is NPO in order to reduce pancreatic secretion. When food is allowed, small, frequent feedings are given. The diet is usually high in carbohydrate content because it is the least stimulating food substance to the pancreas. The diet combines the high carbohydrate intake with low fat and high protein. It is bland with no stimulants (caffeine) and no alcohol. Supplemental fat-soluble vitamins may be given. The client may require supplemental commercial liquid preparations. If severe nutritional deficiencies exist, total parenteral nutrition (hyperalimentation) may be used (Chap. 33).

Nursing Management

Health promotion and maintenance

The major factors involved in health promotion are to (1) assess clients for predisposing and etiologic factors of pancreatitis, and (2) encourage early treatment of these factors in order to prevent occurrence of acute pancreatitis. The nurse should encourage the early diagnosis and treatment of biliary tract disease such as cholelithiasis. The client should be encouraged to eliminate alcoholic intake, especially if he has had any previous episodes of pancreatitis. Attacks of pancreatitis become milder or disappear with the discontinuance of alcohol.

Acute intervention (Table 35-17)

Since abdominal pain is a prominent symptom of pancreatitis, a major focus of nursing care is the relief of pain. Giving the prescribed medications before the

TABLE 35-16
Drugs Used in Treatment of Acute and Chronic Pancreatitis

Drug	Indication for Use
	Acute Pancreatitis
Meperidine (Demerol)	Relieve pain
Nitroglycerin or papaverine	Relax smooth muscles and relieve pain
Anticholinergics a. Atropine b. Propantheline (Pro-Banthine)	Decrease vagal stimulation, decrease motility, decrease pancreatic outflow (inhibits volume and concentration of bicarbonate and enzymatic secretion)
Acetazolamide (Diamox) (carbonic anhydrase inhibitor)	Reduce volume level and bicarbonate concentration of pancreatic secretion
Antacids	Neutralize gastric secretions. Decrease hydrochloric acid stimulation of secretin and pancreozymin which stimulates production of pancreatic secretions
Cimetidine (Tagamet)	Decreases hydrochloric acid by inhibiting histamine.
Calcium gluconate	Treat hypocalcemia to prevent or treat tetany
Adrenocortical steroids	Only used for seriously ill clients with hypotension or shock
Aprotinin (Trasylol) (experimental use)	Antitryptic and antikallikreinic. Moderates clinical course
Glucagon (experimental use)	Reduces pancreatic inflammation and decreases serum amylase
	Chronic Pancreatitis
Pancreatin (Viokase)	Replacement therapy for pancreatic enzymes
Insulin	Treat diabetes if it occurs or for hyperglycemia

Table 35-17
Nursing Care Plan for Client with Acute Pancreatitis

Client Problem	Expected Outcome	Nursing Intervention
Abdominal pain	Relief from pain.	Give ordered analgesic and antispasmodic before pain gets too severe. Ascertain how long the medication provides relief. Make assessments regarding the pain, its severity, location, other accompanying symptoms, and precipitating factors. Provide comfort measures such as positioning comfortably with frequent changes in position and diversional activities.
Restlessness	Rests comfortably.	Relieve nausea, vomiting, and pain. Provide comfort measures, both physiologic and psychological. Provide an environment conducive to rest.
Nausea and vomiting	Relief from nausea and vomiting.	Give antiemetics as ordered. Measure and describe emesis. Provide oral hygiene after emesis. Observe for manifestations of metabolic alkalosis in severe vomiting.
Possibility of shock	Blood pressure within normal limits.	Monitor vital signs every 1–2 h. Assess for continuing or increasing signs of shock. Assess hourly output for decreased urinary output.
Electrolyte imbalances	Serum electrolytes within normal ranges.	Observe for manifestations of hypokalemia, hyponatremia and hypochloremia. Monitor serum laboratory results.
Tetany	Absence or control of tetany.	Observe for jerking, irritability, and muscular twitching. Monitor serum calcium laboratory reports. Give calcium gluconate as ordered.
Possibility of respiratory infections	Absence of respiratory infections. Normal breath sounds.	Observe for fever or respiratory symptoms such as dyspnea, tachypnea. Have client turn, cough, and deep-breathe every 1–2 h. Place client in semi-Fowler's position to promote deeper respirations. Auscultate lungs every 2 h.
Discomfort and dry mouth due to nasogastric tube	Moist lips and nares. Absence of parotitis.	Give frequent oral and nasal care every 1–2 h. Moisten nostrils and lips with water-soluble lubricant.
Possibility of future attacks and/or chronic pancreatitis	No recurrent attacks of acute pancreatitis. No progression to chronic pancreatitis.	Teach client to abstain from alcohol. Teach client to restrict fats and utilize more carbohydrates in the diet. Teach client to avoid rich, rough, and stimulating foods. Teach client how to do urinary glucose and acetone levels and to observe for steatorrhea. Make sure client fully understands prescribed regimen.

pain gets too severe makes the medication more effective. The nurse should ascertain how long the pain medication provides relief. Measures such as comfortable positioning, frequent changes in position, and relief of nausea and vomiting assist in reducing the restlessness that usually accompanies the pain. It is important to control the pain and restlessness because they increase body metabolism and subsequent stimulation of pancreatic secretions.

Nursing measures for the client who is NPO or has a nasogastric tube should be employed. Frequent oral and nasal care to relieve the dryness of the mouth and nose is comforting to the client. Oral care is essential to prevent parotitis. If the client is on anticholinergics to decrease gastrointestinal secretions, there will be additional dryness of the mouth due to the side effects of the drug. If the client is on antacids to suppress secretions, they should be sipped slowly or inserted in the nasogastric tube. The nurse must regularly assess the functioning of the suction.

A vital part of the nursing care plan for this client is observation for electrolyte imbalances. Frequent vomiting along with gastric suction may result in decreased chloride, sodium, and potassium. Since hypocalcemia can also occur, the nurse must observe for symptoms of tetany such as jerking, irritability, and muscular twitching. Calcium gluconate as ordered should be given to treat symptomatic hypocalcemia.

The client with acute pancreatitis is susceptible to infections. The nurse should observe for fever and other manifestations of infection. Respiratory infections are common due to the retroperitoneal fluid raising the diaphragm, which causes the client to take shallow, guarded abdominal breaths. Measures to prevent respiratory infections include turning, coughing, deep breathing, and a semi-Fowler's position.

Other important assessments are observation for signs of paralytic ileus, renal failure, and mental changes. Urinary glucose and acetone levels should be determined every 4 hours in order to assess damage to the beta cells of the islets of Langerhans in the pancreas.

Chronic management

Because frequent doses of narcotics may be required for this client during the acute stage, follow-up for assessment of narcotic addiction is indicated. This is a more likely problem with chronic pancreatitis than acute pancreatitis. Counseling regarding alcohol abstinence is very important to prevent future attacks of acute pancreatitis and development of chronic pancreatitis.

Dietary teaching should include restricting fats since they stimulate the secretion of pancreozymin, which then stimulates the pancreas. Carbohydrates are less stimulating to the pancreas so they should be encouraged (see section on Dietary Interventions).

Early detection of mental changes make it possible to correct them by treating the cause before overt psychotic behavior is manifested. Possible causes of mental changes include sepsis, anorexia, toxicity from cellular breakdown products, and withdrawal from alcohol.

The client and family should be given instructions regarding the recognition and reporting of symptoms of diabetes mellitus or steatorrhea (foul-smelling, frothy stools). These changes indicate possible destruction of pancreatic tissue. The nurse should make sure the client fully understands the prescribed regimen. Each aspect must be explained. The importance of taking the required medications and following the recommended diet should be stressed.

CHRONIC PANCREATITIS

Pathophysiology

Chronic pancreatitis is progressive destruction of the pancreas with fibrotic replacement of pancreatic tissue. Strictures and calcifications may also occur in the pancreas. There are actually several types of chronic pancreatitis but they all have a common underlying pathologic disorder. The two major types are *chronic obstructive pancreatitis* and *chronic calcifying pancreatitis*. Chronic pancreatitis may follow acute pancreatitis but may also occur in the absence of any history of an acute condition.

Chronic obstructive pancreatitis is associated with biliary disease. The most common cause is inflammation of the sphincter of Oddi associated with cholelithiasis. Cancer of the ampulla of Vater, duodenum, or pancreas can also cause this type of chronic pancreatitis.

In *chronic calcifying pancreatitis* there is inflammation and sclerosis mainly in the head of the pancreas and around the pancreatic duct. This type of chronic pancreatitis is the most common form. It is also called alcohol-induced pancreatitis. Increases in heavy social drinking have produced a higher incidence in countries in which the disease was previously considered rare. There is an increased incidence in women but it is still predominantly found in men. The mean age for men is 36 to 40 years. It is believed that the prolonged intake of socially acceptable amounts of alcohol is just as likely to produce chronic pancreatitis as is chronic alcoholism.[26]

In chronic calcifying pancreatitis the ducts are obstructed with protein precipitate. This eventually leads to ductal dilatation, acinar cell atrophy, and fibrosis with eventual calcification of the protein plugs.

Clinical Manifestations

As with acute pancreatitis a major manifestation of chronic pancreatitis is abdominal pain. The client may have episodes of acute pain but usually it is chronic (recurrent attacks at intervals of months or years). The attacks may become more and more frequent until they are almost constant or they may diminish as the pancreatic fibrosis develops. The pain is located in the same areas as in acute pancreatitis but is usually described as a heavy, gnawing feeling or sometimes as burning and cramplike. The pain is not relieved with food or antacids.

Other clinical manifestations include symptoms of pancreatic insufficiency, malabsorption with weight loss, constipation, mild jaundice with dark urine, steatorrhea, and diabetes mellitus. The steatorrhea may become quite severe with voluminous, foul, fatty stools. Some abdominal tenderness may be found. Pseudocysts are very common. Cysts and diabetes are sometimes considered complications but due to their frequent occurrence may be considered late manifestations.

Diagnostic Study Abnormalities

Laboratory findings in chronic pancreatitis include increased serum amylase (200 to 600 Somogyi U/dL), increased serum bilirubin, and increased alkaline phosphatase. There is usually mild leukocytosis and an elevated sedimentation rate.

The *secretin stimulation test* is probably the most useful test in diagnosing chronic pancreatitis. Secretin is given intravenously and gastric-duodenal secretions are collected via a double-lumen tube for separate gastric and duodenal aspiration. In chronic pancreatitis there is reduced volume of secretions and reduced bicarbonate concentration (less than 90 mEq per liter). Normally, secretin stimulates the production of pancreatic fluid high in bicarbonate content.

Other abnormal diagnostic findings are hyperglycemia and fatty stools (steatorrhea) found in fecal fat determination. Arteriography and x-rays may demonstrate fibrosis and calcification.

Endoscopic retrograde cholangiopancreatography (ERCP) involves cannulation and visualization of the pancreatic and common bile ducts using a fiberoptic endoscope. It is inserted into the esophagus to the duodenum. The common bile duct and pancreatic duct are then cannulated. Contrast dye can be injected into the ducts for visualization. Changes in the pancreatic ductal system such as gross dilatation and microcysts can be visualized through the use of ERCP.

Medical and Pharmacologic Management

When the client with chronic pancreatitis is experiencing an acute attack, the medical management is identical to that for acute pancreatitis. At other times the focus is on prevention of further attacks, relief of pain, and control of pancreatic exocrine insufficiency. It sometimes requires large, frequent doses of analgesics to relieve the pain, and narcotic addiction may become a problem. Pentazocine (Talwin) may be used instead of a narcotic analgesic in order to avoid potential narcotic addiction.

Diet, pancreatic enzyme replacement, and control of the diabetes are measures utilized to control the pancreatic insufficiency. The diet is bland, low fat, high carbyhydrate, and high protein. The client does not tolerate fatty, rich, and stimulating foods and these should be avoided to decrease pancreatic secretions and demands on the pancreas. Alcohol must be totally eliminated.

Antacids and anticholinergic drugs may be given to decrease hydrochloric acid, which stimulates pancreatic activity. Cimetidine (Tagamet), which inhibits histamine and thus decreases hydrochloric acid secretion, may be used for the same purpose. Pancreatic enzymes such as pancreatin (Viokase) and pancrelipase (Cotazym) contain amylase, lipase, and trypsin and are used to replace the deficient pancreatic enzymes. They are usually enteric-coated to prevent their digestion by gastric acid activity. Bile salts are sometimes given to facilitate the absorption of the fat-soluble vitamins (A, D, E, K) and prevent further fat loss. If the client develops diabetes, it is controlled with insulin or oral hypoglycemic drugs.

Treatment for chronic pancreatitis sometimes requires surgery. When biliary disease is present or if obstruction or pseudocyst develop, surgery may be indicated. Other surgeries performed are various procedures to divert bile flow or relieve ductal obstruction. A *choledochojejunostomy* diverts bile around the ampulla of Vater, which may have spasm or hypertrophy of the sphincter. In this procedure the common bile duct is anastomosed into the jejunum. If the pancreatic sphincter is fibrotic, a *sphincterotomy* enlarges it. Pancreatic drainage procedures relieve ductal obstruction. One type is the Roux-en-Y pancreatojejunostomy in which the pancreatic duct is opened and an anastomosis made with the jejunum.

Nursing Management

Except during an acute episode the focus of nursing management is on chronic care and health promotion. The client should be instructed to take measures to prevent further attacks. Dietary control along with consistency of other treatment measures such as taking pancreatic enzymes is essential. The pancreatic extracts are usually given with meals or can be given with a snack. The nurse should observe the client's stools for steatorrhea to help determine the effectiveness of the enzymes. The client and family need instructions regarding observation of stools.

If the client has developed diabetes, urinary glucose and acetone levels will have to be monitored and the client will need diabetic teaching (Chap. 41). If the client is on antacids to help control gastric acidity, the nurse should instruct him to sip the medication slowly and make certain it is taken as ordered. Both the antacid and pancreatic enzymes may be left at the client's bedside in order to prepare the client for self-management at home.

Alcohol must be avoided and the client may need assistance with this problem. If the client has developed a dependence on alcohol or narcotics, referral to other agencies or resources may be necessary (Chap. 60).

CARCINOMA OF THE PANCREAS

The incidence of carcinoma of the pancreas has tripled in the past 50 years. It is more common in men than women and in the 45 to 65 age group. Cancer of the pancreas is the fourth leading cause of cancer deaths. It accounts for 6 percent of all deaths due to cancer. It is slightly more common in blacks and Jews. There is a high rate of occurrence in Hawaiian natives.[27]

Most of the tumors are adenocarcinomas originating from the epithelium of the ductal system. Over half the tumors occur in the head of the pancreas. As the tumor grows the common bile duct becomes obstructed and jaundice develops. Tumors starting in the body or tail often remain silent until their growth is quite advanced.

It may be difficult to differentiate cancer of the pancreas from chronic pancreatitis. The prognosis of a client with cancer of the pancreas is very poor. Most clients die within 5 to 12 months and the 5-year survival rate is very low.

Etiology

The cause of cancer of the pancreas remains unknown. There seems to be some relationship between pancreatic cancer, diabetes mellitus, and chronic pancreatitis. However, it is not clear whether the cancer follows these diseases or whether these diseases occur as a result of pancreatic cancer. Recently, investigators believe a potential etiologic factor may be a chemical carcinogen. It is known that pancreatic cancer can be induced with chemicals such as nitrosoureas. There is a higher incidence of cancer of the pancreas in urban areas as well as in some metal workers and workers in coke and gas factories.[28] Cigarette smoking (10 to 15 per day) is now firmly established as a significant risk factor in the development of cancer of the pancreas. The carcinogens from the tobacco probably reach the pancreatic ducts by bile reflux or via the bloodstream. Another risk factor is the western diet, particularly the high fat content. Methods of processing foodstuffs may also be involved as a possible risk factor for cancer of the pancreas. The role of coffee as a contributing factor is still being investigated.

Clinical Manifestations

Common clinical manifestations of pancreatic cancer include abdominal pain (dull, aching), anorexia, nausea, rapid and progressive weight loss, and jaundice. Pain is very common and is probably caused by perineural invasion by the tumor. The pain is located in the upper abdomen or left hypochondrium and frequently radiates to the back. It is frequently related to eating and also occurs at night. The weight loss occurs due to poor digestion and absorption caused by lack of digestive juices from the pancreas.

Diagnostic Study Abnormalities

Better diagnostic measures are needed for detecting pancreatic cancer since most of the current methods detect only advanced stages. Cytologic examination of the pancreatic juice may reveal malignant cells. The secretin test will frequently result in decreased volume of pancreatic juice with normal bicarbonate and enzyme production. There are currently no specific blood tests diagnostic of pancreatic cancer. Carcinoembryonic antigen (CEA) is elevated in a high percentage of clients with advanced disease but it is also increased with other types of cancers and even some benign conditions. The CEA plasma level is therefore probably more useful in assessing the client's response to treatment than in diagnosis. The pancreatic oncofetal antigen (POA) has been studied but is still too nonspecific to be of much value.[29]

Ultrasonography will detect abnormalities of the pancreas but will not distinguish cancer from other pancreatic disorders such as pancreatitis. Since it is a noninvasive procedure, it may be used in some situations. CT scans are becoming increasingly useful. Pancreatic arteriography demonstrates occlusion of the celiac axis and the superior mesenteric artery.

With endoscopic retrograde cholangiopancreatography (ERCP) it is possible to get excellent x-ray visualization of the pancreatic ducts. In pancreatic cancer findings include obstruction or narrowing of a major duct and frequently saccular dilatations of smaller peripheral ducts. Material for cytology and biopsy may show malignant cells.

Medical Management

The most effective treatment of cancer of the pancreas is surgery. The classical surgery is a radical pancreaticoduodenectomy or *Whipple's procedure* (Fig. 35-6). This entails the resection of the proximal pancreas (proximal pancreatectomy), the adjoining duodenum (duodenectomy), distal portion of the stomach (partial gastrectomy) and distal segment of the common bile duct. An anastomosis of the pancreatic duct, common bile duct, and stomach to the jejunum is done. Sometimes a simple bypass procedure such as a cholecystojejunostomy to relieve biliary obstruction may be used as a palliative measure. Some surgeons suggest a more radical resection such as a total pancreaticoduodenectomy with splenectomy.

Radiation therapy alters survival very little but is effective for pain relief. External radiation is usually used but implantation of internal radiation seeds into the tumor has been utilized. Chemotherapy has limited success. Combinations of drugs such as 5-FU and BCNU produce a better response than single chemo-

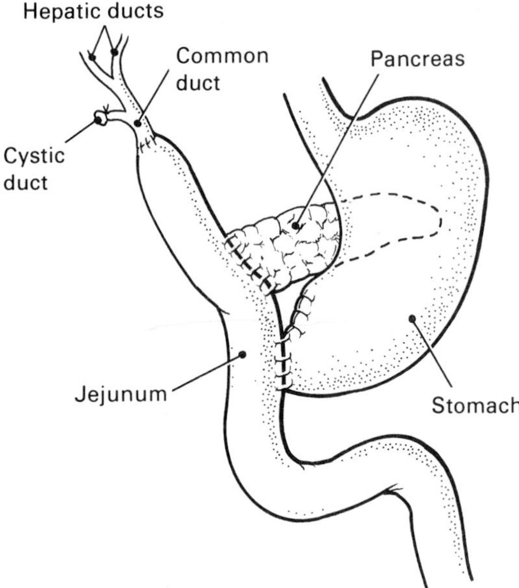

Figure 35-6 Whipple procedure or radical pancreaticoduodenectomy. This surgical procedure involves resection of the proximal pancreas, adjoining duodenum, distal portion of the stomach, and distal portion of the common bile duct. An anastomosis of the pancreatic duct, common bile duct, and stomach to the jejunum is done.

therapeutic agents. Immunotherapy is sometimes attempted (see Chap. 11). Adjuvant therapy which utilizes surgical resection, radiation, and chemotherapy is believed by some to be the most effective way to manage the almost always fatal cancer of the pancreas.

Nursing Management

Since the client with carcinoma of the pancreas has many of the same problems as the client with pancreatitis, nursing care includes the measures previously discussed. The nurse should provide symptomatic and supportive nursing care. Medications and comfort measures to relieve the pain should be provided before the client reaches the peak of pain. Psychological support is essential, especially during times of anxiety or depression which seem to occur frequently in these clients.

Adequate nutrition is an important part of the nursing care plan. Frequent and supplemental feedings may be necessary. Measures to stimulate the appetite as much as possible and to overcome the anorexia, nausea, vomiting should be included in the nursing care. Since bleeding can result from impaired vitamin K production, the nurse should assess for bleeding from body orifices and mucous membranes. If the client is on radiation therapy, the nurse must observe for adverse reactions such as anorexia, nausea, vomiting, and skin irritation.

This client will not live long and this will probably be communicated to him by the physician. A significant component of the nursing care is helping the client and family or significant others through the grieving process.

DISORDERS OF THE BILIARY TRACT

The most common disorder of the biliary system is *cholelithiasis* (stones in the gallbladder) (Fig. 35-7). *Cholecystitis* (inflammation of the gallbladder) is usually associated with cholelithiasis. The stones may be lodged in the neck of the gallbladder or the cystic duct. Cholecystitis may be acute or chronic. Since these conditions usually occur together, they will be discussed together as gallbladder disease with differences identified between the two conditions.

Significance of Problem

Gallbladder disease is a common health problem in the United States. Ten to 20 percent of the adult population have cholelithiasis. The third most common

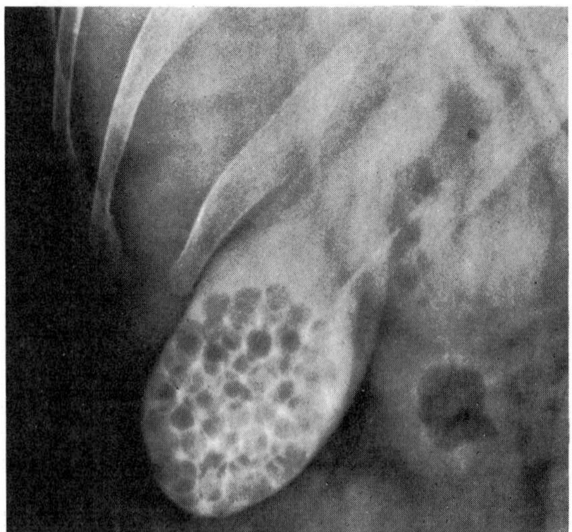

Figure 35-7 X-ray of a gallbladder with gallstones. (*From E. Reith et al., Textbook of Anatomy and Physiology 2d ed., McGraw-Hill Book Company, New York, 1978, p. 326.*)

general surgical procedure performed is a *cholecystectomy* (removal of the gallbladder).[30] The incidence of cholelithiasis is higher in females, multiparous women, and after the age of 40. Postmenopausal women on estrogen therapy are at somewhat greater risk for having gallbladder disease, as are women on birth control pills. Oral contraceptives alter the character of bile, resulting in increased cholesterol saturation. Other factors which seem to increase the occurrence of gallbladder disease are a sedentary lifestyle, a familial tendency, and obesity. Gallbladder disease is more common in the Caucasian racial group than Orientals and blacks. There is an especially high incidence in the Native American Indian ethnic group, particularly in the Navajo and Pima tribes.

Pathophysiology

Cholecystitis

Cholecystitis is most commonly associated with stones. When it occurs in the absence of stones, it is thought to be due to bacteria reaching the gallbladder via the vascular or lymphatic route or chemical irritants in the bile. *Escherichia coli* is the most common bacteria involved. Streptococci and salmonellae are also common causative bacteria. Other etiologic factors include adhesions, neoplasms, extensive fasting, anesthesia, and narcotics.

Inflammation is the major pathology and may be confined to the mucous lining or involve the entire wall of the gallbladder. During an acute attack of cholecystitis, the gallbladder is edematous and hyperemic. It may be distended with bile or pus. The cystic duct is also involved and may become occluded. The wall of the gallbladder becomes scarred after an acute attack. Decreased functioning occurs if large amounts of tissue are fibrosed.

Cholelithiasis

The actual cause of gallstones is unknown. Basically it occurs when the balanace which keeps cholesterol, bile salts, and calcium in solution is altered so that precipitation of these substances occurs. Conditions which upset this balance include infection and disturbances in the metabolism of cholesterol.

It is known that in clients with cholelithiasis, the bile secreted by the liver is supersaturated with cholesterol (lithogenic bile). The bile in the gallbladder also becomes supersaturated with cholesterol. Whenever bile is supersaturated with cholesterol, precipitation of cholesterol will occur.

A high percentage of gallstones are precipitates of cholesterol. Other components of bile which precipitate into stones are bile salts, bilirubin, calcium, and protein. The stones sometimes have a mixed consistency. Mixed cholesterol stones which are predominantly cholesterol are the most common gallstones.

These changes in the composition of bile are probably very significant in the formation of gallstones. Stasis of bile leads to progression of the supersaturation and changes in the chemical composition of the bile. Immobility, pregnancy, and inflammatory or obstructive lesions of the biliary system decrease bile flow. Hormonal factors during pregnancy may cause delayed emptying of the gallbladder.

The stones may remain in the gallbladder or migrate to the cystic duct or to the common bile duct. They cause pain as they pass through the ducts. They may lodge in the ducts and produce an obstruction. Small stones are more likely to move into a duct and cause obstruction. Table 35-18 depicts the changes and manifestations that occur when the stones obstruct the common bile duct. If the blockage occurs in the cystic duct, the bile can continue to flow into the duodenum directly from the liver. However, when the bile in the gallbladder cannot escape, this stasis of bile may lead to cholecystitis.

Clinical Manifestations

Manifestations of cholecystitis vary from indigestion with moderate pain to severe pain, fever, and jaundice. Initial symptoms of acute cholecystitis include indigestion, and pain and tenderness in the right upper quadrant which may be referred to the right shoulder and scapula. Manifestations of inflammation such as leukocytosis and fever occur. Acute cholecystitis may be present with sudden onset of midepigastric or right upper quadrant pain radiating to the back and right shoulder. The pain is accompanied by restlessness, diaphoresis, and nausea and vomiting. Physical findings include right upper quadrant tenderness and abdominal rigidity. Symptoms of chronic cholecystitis include a history of fat intolerance, dyspepsia, heartburn, and flatulence.

Cholelithiasis may produce severe symptoms or none at all. Many clients have "silent cholelithiasis." The severity of symptoms depends on whether the stones are stationary or mobile and whether or not obstruction is present. When a stone is lodged in the ducts or when stones are moving through the ducts, spasms may result. The spasms are the tissue's responses to the stone in an attempt to move it forward. This sometimes produces very severe pain which is termed *biliary colic* even though the pain is rarely colicky. It is more often steady. The pain can be excruciating and accompanied by tachycardia, diaphoresis, and prostration. The severe pain may last up

Table 35-18
Clinical Manifestations Due to Obstructed Bile Flow

Clinical Manifestation	Etiology–Mechanism
Obstructive jaundice	Bile unable to flow into the duodenum.
Dark amber urine which foams when shaken	Soluble bilirubin in urine.
No urobilinogen in urine	No bilirubin reaches small intestine to be converted to urobilinogen.
Clay-colored stools	Same as above.
Pruritus	Deposition of bile salts in skin tissues.
Faulty absorption or lack of absorption of fat-soluble vitamins (A, D, E, K)	Bile not present in small intestine to emulsify fat. Without bile, fatty acids are excreted in stool with a loss of fat-soluble vitamins.
Intolerance for fatty foods (nausea, sensation of fullness, anorexia)	No bile in small intestine for fat digestion.
Bleeding tendencies	Lack of or decreased absorption of vitamin K with decreased production of prothrombin.
Steatorrhea	No bile salts in duodenum so fat emulsion and digestion are prevented.

to an hour and when it subsides there is residual tenderness in the right upper quadrant. The attacks of pain frequently occur 3 to 6 hours after a heavy meal or when the client assumes a recumbent position. When total obstruction occurs symptoms related to bile blockage occur (Table 35-18).

Complications

Complications of cholecystitis include subphrenic abscess, pancreatitis, *cholangitis* (inflammation of biliary ducts), biliary cirrhosis, fistulas, and rupture of the gallbladder, which can produce bile peritonitis.

Many of the same complications can occur from cholelithiasis, including cholangitis, biliary cirrhosis, carcinoma, and peritonitis. *Choledocholithiasis* (stone in common bile duct) may occur, producing symptoms of obstruction.

Diagnostic Study Abnormalities

The main diagnostic tests utilized in diagnosing gallbladder disease are x-ray studies. An oral cholecystogram allows for the visualization of stones when they are radiopaque. An intravenous cholangiogram outlines both the gallbladder and the ducts so that gallstones which have moved into the ductal system can be visualized. Percutaneous transhepatic cholangiography may be used to diagnose obstructive jaundice and to locate stones within the bile ducts.

Laboratory tests may demonstrate abnormalities in some of the liver function tests and an increased white blood cell count due to inflammation. Both the direct and indirect bilirubin are elevated as is the urinary bilirubin if there is an obstructive process present. If the common bile duct is obstructed, no bilirubin will reach the small intestine to be converted to urobilinogen. Serum enzymes such as the alkaline phosphatase, SGOT, and LDH may be elevated. The serum amylase is increased if there is pancreatic involvement.

Medical Management (Table 35-19)

Cholecystitis

During an acute episode of *cholecystitis* the focus of treatment is on (1) control of pain, (2) control of possible infection with antibiotics, and (3) maintaining fluid and electrolyte balance. The treatment is mainly supportive and symptomatic. If nausea and vomiting are severe, gastric decompression may be used to prevent further gallbladder stimulation. Anticholinergics to decrease secretions (which prevent biliary contraction) and counteract smooth muscle spasms may be administered. Analgesics are given to decrease the pain.

Cholelithiasis

Cholelithiasis is most effectively treated surgically. However, the client may be given supportive treatment for a time before surgery. This treatment is similar to the treatment for cholecystitis. If the stones cause an obstruction, additional treatment consists of replacement of the fat-soluble vitamins, administration of bile salts to facilitate digestion and vitamin absorption, and a low fat diet. Chenodeoxycholic acid (CDCA) or bile acid therapy seems effective in the

Table 35-19
Medical Management: Cholelithiasis

Diagnostic
1. Cholecystogram or IV cholangiogram
2. Liver function studies
3. WBC

Conservative treatment
1. IV fluids
2. NPO with nasogastric tube—later, low-fat diet
3. Antiemetics
4. Analgesics (e.g., meperidine)
5. Fat-soluble vitamins (A, D, E, K)
6. Anticholinergics
7. Bile salts
8. Antibiotics

Postsurgical treatment
1. Analgesics
2. Low-Fowler's position
3. Progressive surgical diet
4. Change dressing prn
5. T-tube (if common bile duct exploration performed)

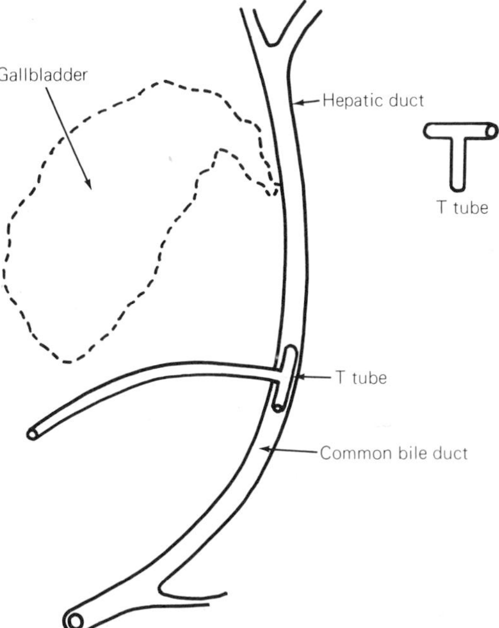

Figure 35-8 Placement of the T-tube. Dotted lines indicate parts removed. (*From H. Moidell, Nursing Care of the Patient with Medical Surgical Disorders, McGraw-Hill Book Company, New York, 1976, p. 719.)*

dissolution of gallstones, particularly cholesterol gallstones. This treatment is still considered somewhat experimental. CDCA reduces the cholesterol secretion in bile, converting bile supersaturated with cholesterol to bile unsaturated with cholesterol.[31]

Surgical intervention

Surgical intervention for cholelithiasis is frequently indicated and may consist of any one of several procedures (Table 35-20). The most common surgical approach is through a right subcostal incision. A T-tube is inserted into the common bile duct during surgery when a common bile duct exploration is part of the surgical procedure (Fig. 35-8). This ensures patency of the duct until the edema produced by the trauma of exploring and probing the duct has subsided. It also allows the excess bile to drain while the small intestine is adjusting to receiving a continuous flow of bile.

Table 35-20
Gallbladder Surgeries

Name	Description
Cholecystectomy	Removal of the gallbladder
Cholecystostomy (usually an emergency)	Incision into the gallbladder (usually for removal of stones)
Choledocholithotomy	Incision into the common bile duct for the removal of stones
Cholecystogastrostomy	Anastomosis between stomach and gallbladder
Cholecystoduodenostomy	Anastomosis between the gallbladder and duodenum to relieve obstruction at distal end of common bile duct

Pharmacologic Intervention

The most common drugs utilized in treatment of gallbladder disease are analgesics, anticholinergics (antispasmodics), fat-soluble vitamins, and bile salts.

To relieve pain, meperidine (Demerol) is used if a narcotic analgesic is required. This causes less spasm in the ducts than opiates such as morphine sulfate. Amyl nitrite and nitroglycerin may be used to relax the biliary tract smooth muscle. If nitroglycerin is given, the nurse should observe for side effects of nausea, vomiting, flushing of the skin, and hypotension.

Anticholinergics such as atropine or other antispasmodics may be used to relax the smooth muscle and decrease ductal tone. Papaverine also has a relaxing effect on smooth muscle. Nursing observations for side effects of drugs and relief of the pain should be made.

If the client has chronic gallbladder disease or any biliary tract obstruction, fat-soluble vitamins (A, D,

E, K) will probably be given. Bile salts may be administered to facilitate digestion and vitamin absorption.

Hydrocholeretic drugs may be administered following gallbladder surgery when a T-tube is in place or with medical management as long as there is no obstruction. These drugs stimulate the production of bile of a low specific gravity. Examples are bile salts such as dehydrocholic acid (Decholin) and florantyrone (Zanchol).

For treatment of pruritus, cholestyramine (Questran) may provide relief. It is a resin which binds bile salts in the intestine, increasing their excretion in the feces. Cholestyramine is administered in powder form and should be mixed with milk or juice. The nurse should observe for side effects of nausea, vomiting, diarrhea or constipation, and skin reactions.

Dietary Measures

The major dietary modification for a client with cholelithiasis and cholecystitis is a low fat diet. If obesity is a problem, a reduced calorie diet is indicated. The low fat diet prevents excess stimulation of the gallbladder. Foods which are avoided include dairy products such as whole milk, cream, butter, whole milk cheese, and ice cream, fried foods, rich pastries, gravies, and nuts. Many clients have fewer problems if they eat smaller, more frequent meals.

Postoperatively, following gallbladder surgery, the client is kept NPO for 24 to 48 hours. The diet is advanced according to the client's tolerance. The amount of fat in the diet postoperatively depends on the client's tolerance to fat. A low fat diet may be helpful if the flow of bile is reduced (usually only in the early postoperative period) or if the client is overweight. Otherwise, there need not be any special dietary instructions other than to eat nutritious meals and avoid excessive fat intake.

Nursing Management

Health promotion and maintenance

The nurse should assume responsibility for recognition of predisposing factors of gallbladder disease in general health screening. Ethnic groups in which the disease is more common, such as Native Americans, should be taught initial manifestations and to seek medical care if they occur. The client with chronic cholecystitis does not have acute symptoms and may not seek medical help until jaundice and biliary obstruction occur. Earlier detection of these clients is beneficial so they can be treated with low fat diet and monitored more closely.

Acute intervention

Nursing objectives for the client undergoing conservative medical management include: (1) relieving pain, (2) relieving nausea and vomiting, (3) providing comfort and emotional support, (4) maintaining fluid and electrolyte balance and nutrition, (5) making accurate assessments for effectiveness of treatment, and (6) observing for complications.

This client is frequently experiencing very severe pain. The medications ordered to relieve the pain should be given as required by the client and before the pain becomes severe. The nurse should assess what medications relieve the pain and how much medication is required. Observations for side effects of the medications must be part of the continued assessment. Nursing comfort measures such as a clean bed, comfortable positioning, and oral care will aid in providing for the client's comfort.

In some clients the nausea and vomiting is more severe than in others. For these individuals it may be necessary to use gastric decompression. The elimination of intake food and fluids also prevents further stimulation of the gallbladder. Oral hygiene, care of nares, accurate I and O measurements, and maintenance of the suction should be a part of the nursing care plan for this client. For clients with less severe nausea and vomiting, antiemetics are usually adequate. When the client is vomiting, comfort measures such as frequent mouth rinses should be provided. Any emesis should be immediately removed from the bedside.

If pruritus occurs with jaundice, measures to relieve itching are necessary. Such measures include baking soda or Alpha Keri baths, lotions such as Calamine, antihistamines, soft old linen, and control of the temperature (not too hot and not too cold). The client's nails should be kept short and clean. Clients should be taught to rub with their knuckles rather than scratch with nails when they cannot control the scratching.

A significant portion of the nursing care plan for this client centers upon accurate assessment for progression of the symptoms and development of complications. The nurse must be knowledgeable of and observe for signs of obstruction of the ducts by stones. These include jaundice, clay-colored stools, dark, foamy urine, and steatorrhea.

When symptoms of obstruction are present, the nurse must be aware of the possibility of bleeding due to decreased prothrombin production. Common sites to observe for bleeding are from the mucous membranes of the mouth and nose, gums, and injection sites. If injections are given, a small-gauge needle should be used and gentle pressure applied after the injection. The nurse should know what the client's prothrombin time is and use this as a guide in the assessment process.

Assessments for an infection include monitoring of vital signs. A temperature elevation with chills and jaundice may indicate choledocholithiasis.

Nursing Care after Surgical Intervention Preoperative care is essentially the same as for any abdominal surgical procedure (see Table 34-6). The nurse should be aware of such variations as whether or not the client will have a nasogastric tube since some surgeons no longer use them for gallbladder surgery.

Postoperative nursing care is discussed in Table 35-21. Adequate ventilation and prevention of respiratory complications are important objectives for this client. The high incision in the right subcostal region is near the diaphragm and the client is reluctant to take deep breaths because of the pain it causes.

If the client has a nasograstric tube, it will probably be in for 24 to 48 hours. When bowel sounds are heard, the client is given clear liquids with progression to surgical soft and to low fat or regular diet. The nurse should observe tolerance to the diet and assist in any required dietary instruction.

The client usually has a Penrose drain inserted into a stab wound near the incision. The Penrose drain allows for drainage and prevents accumulation of fluid and serous drainage in the area from which the gallbladder was removed. Drainage is frequently heavy, with serosanguineous bile-tinged drainage. The dressing may require frequent changing. The wound should be kept dry and clean as the bile is irritating to the skin.

If the client has a T-tube, part of the nursing care plan relates to maintaining bile drainage and observation of the T-tube functioning and drainage. The T-tube is connected to a closed gravity drainage system. Nursing care in relation to the T-tube is summarized in Table 35-22.

Chronic management

When the client is on a conservative medical management program, chronic nursing management depends on symptoms and whether or not surgical

Table 35-21
Nursing Care Plan For Client Following a Cholecystectomy

Client Problem	Expected Outcome	Nursing Intervention
Incisional pain	Relief from pain	Administer ordered analgesic frequently enough to assure that the client will move about. Provide comfort measures. Reposition as needed. Support incision when coughing and deep breathing and getting out of bed.
Possibility of respiratory complications	Normal breath sounds. Respiratory rate 12–16/minute	Assist client to cough and deep-breathe every hour. Auscultate lung sounds every 2–4 h. Plan a schedule with client and assure that analgesic will be given as needed to make it easier to cough, deep-breathe, and move about. Support incision with pillow or hands. Encourage early ambulation. When in bed, place client in low-Fowler's position to reduce pressure on diaphragm.
Paralytic ileus	Normal bowel sounds. Normal nutritional intake	Keep NPO until bowel sounds are present. Maintain IV fluid administration at prescribed rate. Provide oral care every 1–2 h. Auscultate for bowel sounds every 4 h. Encourage ambulation 3–4 times/day if not contraindicated. Start oral fluids gradually after bowel sounds return.
Heavy drainage from surgical area	Maintenance of skin integrity. Wound clean and dry	Change dressing frequently. Use Montgomery straps to reduce skin irritation from frequent removal of tape. Observe and record the type of drainage.
Lack of knowledge about activities and diet upon discharge	Knowledge of activity level and dietary restrictions. Return to normal lifestyle	Instruct client to avoid heavy lifting for at least a month. Discuss sexual activities—client should be able to resume usual sexual activities including intercourse as soon as feels ready (unless physician instructs otherwise). Provide dietary teaching plan if client required to remain on low fat diet or if put on a weight reduction program. Discuss with client when allowed to eat whatever foods tolerated. Encourage client to have the necessary follow-up care.

Table 35-22
Nursing Care of a Client with a T-Tube

Nursing Care	Rationale
1. Observe amount and color of drainage: a. Initially bloody and then greenish-brown after several hours b. Approximately 400 mL/day after first few days. A decrease in amount as the bile begins to follow normal route. If over 1000 mL/day, report to physician	1. To determine excess bleeding and if bile is flowing and not blocking up in liver or leaking into peritoneal cavity Increased bile flow after it has started to decrease may indicate ductal obstruction below tube
2. Observe for drainage around tube	2. Bile very irritating to skin
3. Do not irrigate, aspirate, or clamp the tube without an order	3. Not necessary to irrigate. Want bile to flow freely
4. Low-Fowler's position	4. Promotes bile drainage
5. Keep the drainage bag below the level of gallbladder for first 3–4 days	5. Allow for gravity drainage of bile
6. Raise drainage bag to waist level after 4th postoperative day (when ordered). Later may be raised to shoulder level. Observe for pain, chills, fullness, and nausea	6. To check patency of common bile duct
7. Assist client to turn and ambulate without dislodging or kinking tube	7. Prevent dislodgment and maintain patency
8. If tube is clamped for 1–2 h before and after meals, assess client's response	8. To see if bile is aiding digestion
9. Observe for indications that the bile is flowing through normal channels: a. Brown color to stools b. Decreased amount of drainage from tube	9. Initially most or all bile flows out T-tube. As edema subsides, most of it will flow into duodenum T-tube removed when bile is flowing through normal channels, usually in 7–10 days

intervention is being planned. Dietary teaching is usually necessary. The diet will usually be low fat and sometimes a weight reduction diet is also recommended. The client may need to take fat-soluble vitamin supplements. The nurse should provide instructions regarding observations the client should make indicating obstruction (stool and urine changes, jaundice, and pruritus). Continued health care is important and its significance should be explained and stressed.

Following a cholecystectomy, the client will probably be discharged in 7 to 10 days. If a T-tube has been inserted, hospitalization may be extended to 2 weeks. The client should be instructed to avoid heavy lifting for at least a month. The client should be able to resume usual sexual activities, including intercourse, as soon as he feels ready unless given other instructions by the physician.

Sometimes the client is required to remain on a low fat diet for up to 6 months. If so, a dietary teaching plan is necessary. A weight reduction program may be helpful if the client is overweight. Many clients tolerate a regular diet with no difficulties.

Approximately 5 to 8 percent of clients who have cholecystectomies later have manifestations of biliary tract disease. The problem is called *postcholecystectomy syndrome* and is usually caused by residual calculi, recurring calculi, stricture of the duct, or infection around the common bile duct. Surgical treatment is usually necessary to correct the cause of the problem.[32]

CANCER OF THE GALLBLADDER

Primary cancer of the gallbladder is rare. The majority of gallbladder carcinomas are adenocarcinomas. There seems to be a definite relationship between cancer of the gallbladder and chronic cholecystitis and cholelithiasis. Eighty percent of clients with gallbladder malignancy also have gallstones.

The early symptoms of carcinoma of the gallbladder are insidious and are similar to those of chronic cholecystitis and cholelithiasis, which makes diagnosis difficult. Later symptoms are usually those of biliary obstruction. Cancer of the gallbladder has a very poor prognosis.

Treatment is mainly symptomatic and supportive.

Sometimes the tumor is resected. Chemotherapy and radiotherapy are seldom used because they are neither curative nor palliative.

Nursing management is supportive care with special attention to nutrition, hydration, skin care, and pain relief. Many of the nursing care measures discussed under cholecystitis and cholelithiasis will frequently apply here, as well as nursing care measures for the client with cancer (see Chap. 11).

Case Study / Cirrhosis of the Liver

Ronald is a 42-year-old male admitted with hepatic coma. He has had cirrhosis of the liver for 10 years. He is an admitted alcoholic and has been drinking heavily for 15 years. He says he has been "sober" for the past 2 years. Review of old records reveals progressive weakness, anorexia, weight loss, jaundice, pedal edema, ascites, and mental disorientation.

On admission Ronald is stuporous, has twitching, asterixis, and fetor hepaticus. He appears thin, malnourished, and very ill. Assessment reveals 4+ pitting edema of the lower extremities, ascites, jaundice, spider angiomas, and purpura. The liver and spleen are both palpable.

Previous liver biopsies indicated:

At age 36—fatty liver
At age 40—cirrhosis with some necrosis

Present laboratory values	
Total bilirubin	11 mg/dL
Serum enzymes:	SGOT 180 U/L SGPT 525 U/L LDH 450 U/L
Serum ammonia	220 μg/dL
Hematocrit	24%

Discussion Questions

1. What are possible causes of cirrhosis? What type of cirrhosis does Ronald have?
2. Describe the pathophysiologic changes that occur in the liver as cirrhosis develops. Explain the result of Ronald's two liver biopsies.
3. List Ron's clinical manifestations of liver failure. For each manifestation explain the pathophysiologic bases.
4. Explain the significance of the results of his laboratory values.
5. What is the etiology of hepatic coma? What measures should be instituted to control or decrease the ammonia level?
6. Ronald was being closely observed for the possibility of gastrointestinal bleeding. Why would this be considered as a possible complication?
7. In the early stages of cirrhosis what can be done to control the disease?

REVIEW QUESTIONS

The number of the question corresponds to the same numbered objective at the beginning of the chapter.

1. A major problem in hepatocellular jaundice is with the
   a. production of unconjugated bilirubin
   b. conjugation and excretion of bilirubin
   c. flow of bile through the bile ducts
   d. excessive breakdown of erythrocytes

2. With hepatitis in the prodromal (preicteric) phase you would expect to see
   a. sudden onset of jaundice
   b. weight loss
   c. acute yellow atrophy
   d. flu like symptoms

3. When caring for the client with viral hepatitis the *most* important precaution is probably
   a. gowning and gloving
   b. handwashing
   c. using disposable dishes
   d. getting an injection of immune serum globulin (ISG)

4. A client with cirrhosis of the liver would
   a. have a tendency to bleed and hyperventilate
   b. be prone to infection and metabolic alkalosis
   c. show signs of jaundice and ascites
   d. develop decreased body temperature and pruritus

5. When caring for a client with hepatic encephalopathy the nurse may give enemas, provide a low protein diet, and limit physical acitivity. These measures are done to
   a. eliminate potassium ions

b. decrease the production of ammonia
c. increase the production of ammonia
d. decrease portal pressure

6. Which of the following statements about carcinoma of the liver is *false*?
   a. Surgical excision of the tumor is highly successful.
   b. Nursing intervention focuses on symptomatic and comfort measures.
   c. The prognosis is very poor.
   d. It is difficult to distinguish primary from metastatic tumors.

7. The most common pathogenetic mechanism in acute pancreatitis is
   a. cellular disorganization
   b. lack of secretion of enzymes
   c. autodigestion
   d. overproduction of enzymes

8. Teaching measures for the client with chronic pancreatitis should include all the following *except*
   a. consistency of taking pancreatic enzymes with meals
   b. observation of stools for signs of steatorrhea
   c. monitoring of urinary glucose and acetone levels
   d. high protein, moderate fat, low carbohydrate diet

9. Identify the *false* statement about carcinoma of the pancreas.
   a. Cigarette smoking is a significant risk factor.
   b. Most of the tumors are adenocarcinomas.
   c. The most effective treatment is external radiation.
   d. An important nursing measure is assisting the client with the grieving process.

10. A significant factor in the formation of gallstones seems to be
   a. chemical irritants in the bile
   b. that bile is supersaturated with cholesterol
   c. bacteria reaching the gallbladder via the vascular route
   d. an increase in the bile acid pool size

11. Which of the following measures is appropriate for care of a T-tube following surgery of the common bile duct?
   a. It should drain serosanguineous fluid.
   b. It may be clamped and pinned to his gown when he is up.
   c. It should be irrigated prn.
   d. It should be allowed to drain by gravity.

REFERENCES

1. H. M. Spiro, *Clinical Gastroenterology*, 2d ed., The Macmillan Company, New York, 1977, p. 1139.
2. J. W. Mosley, "Viral Hepatitis—What We Have Learned From Testing," *Current Concepts in Gastroenterology*, **2:**7 (1978).
3. Spiro, op. cit., p. 1139.
4. G. P. Coughlin et al., "Liver Disease and the e Antigen in HB_s Ag Carriers with Chronic Renal Failure," *Gut*, **21:**121 (1980).
5. J. L. Dienstay, "Viral Hepatitis: How Far We Have Come, Where We Are Going," *Drug Therapy*, Biomedical Information Corporation, New York, September, 1978, p. 33.
6. R. D. Aach, "Viral Hepatitis—A to C," *Med Clin North Am*, **62**:59–70 (1978).
7. K. Isselbacher et al. (eds.), *Harrison's Principles of Internal Medicine*, 9th ed., McGraw-Hill Book Company, New York, 1979.
8. Ibid., p. 1462.
9. N. J. Greenberger and D. H. Winship, *GI Disorders: A Pathophysiologic Approach*, Year Book Medical Publishers, Inc., Chicago, 1976, p. 280.
10. The Medical Letter, January 27, 1978, vol. 20, #2, The Medical Letter, Inc., New Rochelle, N.Y.
11. Mosley, op. cit., p. 7.
12. Spiro, op. cit., p. 1143.
13. Hollinger and Graham, op. cit., p. 46.
14. B. A. Given and S. J. Simmons, *Gastroenterology in Clinical Nursing*, 3d ed., The C. V. Mosby Company, St. Louis, 1979, p. 337.
15. E. Rubin and C. S. Lieber, "Fatty Liver, Alcoholic Hepatitis and Cirrhosis Produced by Alcohol in Primates," *N Eng J Med*, **290:**128–135 (1974).
16. Given and Simmons, op. cit., p. 346.
17. Nayereh Shaninpour, "The Adult Patient with Bleeding Esophageal Varices," *Nurs Clin North Am,* **12:**331, 1977.
18. Evelyn Daniel, "Chronic Problems in Rehabilitation of Patients with Laennec's Cirrhosis," *Nurs Clin North Am*, **12:**345–356 (1977).
19. G. Eknoyan et al., "Combined Ascitic-Fluid and Furosemide Infusion in the Management of Ascites," *N Engl J Med*, **282:**713–717, 1970.
20. Kathleen Ann O'Brien, "Cross Circulation for Hepatic Coma," *Am J Nurs*, **77:**1459–1462, 1977.
21. Gerald Klebanoff et al., "Resuscitation of a Patient in Stage IV Hepatic Coma Using Total Body Washout," *J Surg Residency*, **20:**159–165, 1972.
22. Greenberger and Winship, op. cit., p. 333.
23. J. Terblanche et al., "Liver Transplantation," *Med Clin North Am*, **63:**507–521, 1979.
24. Isselbacher et al., op. cit., p. 1503.
25. G. Bolooki and M. L. Gliedman, "Peritoneal Dialysis in Treatment of Acute Pancreatitis," *Surgery*, **64:**466 (1968).
26. I. N. Marks and S. Bank, "Chronic Pancreatitis: Classification, Clinical Aspects, Diagnosis and Management," *Current Concepts in Gastroenterology,* **2:**21–32, 1977.
27. S. D. Leidner, C. J. Lightdale, and P. Sherlock, "Cancer of the Pancreas," *Cur Concepts in Gastroenterology*, **2:**33 (1977).
28. Ibid.
29. F. Gelder, R. Hinter, and C. Reece, "An Oncofetal Antigen Related to Pancreatic Cancer (abstract)." Presented at American Pancreatic Study Group and National Pancreatic Cancer Project Joint Meeting, Chicago, November, 1976.
30. Given and Simmons, op. cit., p. 195.
31. Greenberger and Winship, op. cit., p. 351.
32. C. J. Thorpe and J. A. Caprini, "Gallbladder Disease: Current Trends and Treatments," *Am J Nurs*, **80:**2181–2185, 1980.

BIBLIOGRAPHY FOR SECTION 7

Gastrointestinal Tract

Books

Davidson, Stanley, P. Passmore, J. F. Brock, and A. S. Truswell: *Human Nutrition and Dietetics,* Churchill Livingstone, London, 1979.

Given, Barbara A., and Sandra J. Simmons: *Gastroenterology in Clinical Nursing,* 3d ed., The C. V. Mosby Company, St. Louis, 1979.

Postlethwait, R. W.: *Surgery of the Esophagus,* Appleton-Century-Crofts, New York, 1979.

Rice, H. V.: *Gastrointestinal Nursing,* Medical Examination Publishing Company, Inc., Garden City, N.Y., 1978.

Robinson, Corinne H., and Marilyn R. Lawler: *Normal and Therapeutic Nutrition,* 15th ed., The Macmillan Company, New York, 1977.

Williams, S. R.: *Essentials of Nutrition and Diet Therapy,* 2d ed., The C. V. Mosby Company, St. Louis, 1978.

Wilmore, Douglas, *The Metabolic Management of the Critically Ill,* Plenum Publishing Company, New York, 1977.

Periodicals

Alpers, D.: "Inflammatory Bowel Disease (Ulcerative Colitis)," *Arch Int Med,* **138:**286 (1978).

Baines, A.: "Surgery for Head and Neck Cancer: Keeping Up Good Appearances," *Nurs Mirror,* **149:**38 (1979).

Bass, L.: "More Fiber—Less Constipation," *Am J Nurs,* **77:**254 (1977).

Beck, M. L.: "Two Intestinal Tests: One Oral, One Anal," *Nurs 81,* **11:**20–24 (1981).

Belinsky, I.: "Visualizing the Pancreatic and Biliary Ducts," *Am J Nurs,* **76:**936–937 (1976).

Black, J. M., and P. G. Arnold: "Facial Fractures," *Am J Nurs,* **82:**1086–1088 (1982).

Boyer, C. A., and S. M. Oehlberg: "Interpretation and Clinical Relevance of Liver Function Tests," *Nurs Clin North Am,* **12:**275–290 (1977).

Brindley, G. V., Jr. (ed.): "New Methods of Treatment of Gastrointestinal Disease," *Surg Clin North Am,* **59:**600 (1979).

Broadwell, D., and S. Sorrells: "Loop Transverse Colostomy," *Am J Nurs,* **78:**1029 (1978).

Buchan, D. J.: "Diagnosis and Management of Inflammatory Bowel Disease," *Can Family Physician,* **22:**47 (1976).

Budd, D. C., and W. F. Fouty, Jr.: "Familial Retrocecal Appendicitis," *Am J Surg,* **133:**670 (1977).

Buergel, Nancy: "Monitoring Nutritional Status in the Clinical Setting," *Nurs Clin North Am,* **14:**301–304 (1979).

Buls, J. G., and S. M. Goldberg: "Modern Management of Hemorrhoids," *Surg Clin North Am,* **58:**469 (1978).

Cantrell, R. W.: "Current Concepts: Head and Neck Cancer Surgery," *AORN J,* **22:**253–262 (1975).

Castell, D. O., and B. B. Frank: "Diagnostics: Abdominal Examination, Role of Percussion and Auscultation," *Postgrad Med,* **62:**131 (1977).

Castro, A. F., and P. Tuxen: "Inflammatory Bowel Disease," *Surg Clin North Am,* **58:**573 (1978).

Clark, J. S., et al.: "Preoperative Oral Antibiotics Reduce Septic Complications of Colon Operations," *Ann Surg,* **186:**251 (1977).

Connell, A. M.: "Dietary Fiber and Diverticular Disease," *Hosp Pract,* **11:**119 (1976).

Cotton, C.: "Phillip Was Saved but Not By the Rule Book (Crohn's Disease)," *RN,* **41:**77 (1978).

Craft, M., and B. Folkedahl: "The Story of Melissa's Surgery," *Nurs 80,* **4:**46 (1980).

Curtis, C.: "Colonoscopy: The Nurse's Role," *Am J Nurs,* **75:**430–32 (1975).

Daly, K. M.: "Oral Cancer: Everyday Concerns," *Am J Nurs,* **79:**1415–1417 (1979).

DeLuca, J. D.: "The Ulcerative Colitis Personality," *Nurs Clin North Am,* **5:**23 (1970).

Didich, J. M.: "How to Gauge Abdominal Girth Accurately," *Nurs 81,* **11:**32 (1981).

Dodds, W. J., et al.: "Reflux Esophagitis," *Am J Digestive Diseases,* **21:**49–67 (1976).

Dyer, E. D., et al.: "Dental Health in Adults," *Am J Nurs,* **76:**1156–1159 (1976).

Fay, M. R., and W. R. Snider: "Nonoperative Therapy for Hemorrhoids," *AORN J,* **24:**448 (1976).

Gallagher, D. M., and T. R. Russell: "Surgical Management of Diverticular Disease," *Surg Clin North Am,* **58:**563 (1978).

Gannon, E. P., and E. Kadezabek: "Giving your Patients Meticulous Mouth Care," *Nurs 80,* **10:**70–75 (1980).

Geels, W., et al.: "The Enterocutaneous Fistula: Supplanting Surgery with Meticulous Nursing Care," *Nurs 78,* **8:**52 (1978).

Heindel, M.: "How to Protect Your Ostomy Patients from Post-Op Surgery Skin Problems," *RN,* **41:**43 (1978).

Heyman, E., et al.: "The Pouch Ileostomy," *Nurs 77,* **7:**44 (1977).

"High Fiber Diets and Colonic Disease," *Am J Nurs,* **77:**255 (1977).

Isler, C.: "If the Ileostomy Is Continent, the Benefits Are Obvious," *RN,* **40:**39 (1977).

Kabuto, T., et al.: "Primary Adenoid Cystic Carcinoma of the Esophagus; Report of a Case," *Cancer,* **43:**2452–2456 (1979).

Kim, R. Y., et al.: "Metastatic Carcinoma to the Tongue: A Report of two Cases and a Review of the Literature," *Cancer,* **43:**386–389 (1979).

Kodner, I. J.: "Colostomy and Ileostomy," *Clin Sympos,* **30:**2 (1978).

Kroner, K.: "Are You Prepared for Your Ulcerative Colitis Patient?" *Nurs 80,* **4:**43 (1980).

Lamanske, J.: "Helping the Ileostomy Patient to Help Himself," *Nurs 77,* **7:**34 (1977).

Larsen, G. L.: "Rehabilitation for the Patient with Head and Neck Cancer," *Am J Nurs,***82:**119–120 (1982).

Lee, B. C., E. F. Hansen, and M. R. Poppell: "Facial Fractures Take a Special Kind of Nursing Care," *Nurs 80,* **10:**42–46 (1980).

Literte, J. W.: "Nursing Care of Patients with Intestinal Obstruction," *Am J Nurs,* **77:**1003 (1977).

Mansell, E., et al.: "Patient Assessment: Examination of the Abdomen," programmed instruction, *Am J Nurs,* **74:** 679–1702 (1974).

Masson, J. K.: "Reconstructive Procedures in Head and Neck Surgery," *Surg Clin North Am,* **57:**737–749 (1977).

Matsishe, J. W., and S. F. Phillips: "Chronic Diarrhea," *Med Clin North Am,* **62:**141 (1978).

Mazier, W. P., et al.: "Anal Fissure and Anal Ulcers," *Surg Clin North Am,* **58:**479 (1978).

McNamara, J. P.: "Esophageal Cancer," *Nurs 82,* **12:**64 (1982).
Meissner, J. E.: "A Simple Guide for Assessing Oral Health," *Nurs 80,* **8:**84 (1980).
Mendeloff, A. I.: "Dietary Fiber and Gastrointestinal Diseases," *Med Clin North Am,* **62:**165 (1978).
Miller, Barbara, "Jejunoileal Bypass: A Drastic Weight Control Measure," *Am J Nurs,* **81:**564–568 (1981).
Moss, G.: "Postsurgical Decompression and Immediate Elemental Feeding," *Hosp Pract,* **12:**73 (1977).
Mostyn, M.: "A Quick Look at Botulism: Nursing Care in an Epidemic. Nursing Grand Rounds," *Nurs 78,* **8:**63–69 (1978).
Oser, J.: "Oral Cancer: Coping with the Changes," *Am J Nurs,* **79:**1418–1419 (1979).
Panrucker, R.: "Nursing Care Study. Botulism: A Team Effort to Save the Poison Salmon Victims," *Nurs Mirror,* **147:** 2–35 (1978).
Parker, E. F., and H. B. Gregorie: "Carcinoma of the Esophagus," *JAMA,* **235:**1018–1020 (1976).
Pennel, E.: "Salmonella: What Is—and Isn't," *J Nurs Care,* **11:**20–21 (1978).
Pierch, L.: "Anatomy & Physiology of the Liver," *Nurs Clin North Am,* **12:**259–273 (June 1977).
Raskin, J. B.: "Gastrointestinal Endoscopy," *Postgrad Med,* **57:**85–91 (January 1975).
Rush, A.: "Cancer and the Ostomy Patient," *Nurs Clin North Am,* **11:**405 (1976).
Ryan, A. J.: "Validation of Appendectomy, Can It be Done?" *Postgrad Med,* **65:**19 (January 1979).
Salmond, S. W.: "How to Assess the Nutritional Status of Acutely Ill Patients," *Am J Nurs,* **80:**922–924 (1980).
Schneider, W. R.: "Nutrition in Head and Neck Cancer: Nursing Implications," *Oncology Nurs Forum,* **5:**5–11 (1979).
Schuman, D.: "How to Help Wound Healing in Your Abdominal Surgery Patients," *Nurs 80,* **8:**34 (1980).
Schweiger, J. L., J. W. Schweiger, and J. W. Lang: "Oral Assessment: How to Do It," *Am J Nurs,* **80:**654–657 (1980).
Stahlgren, L., and N. W. Morris: "Intestinal Obstruction," *Am J Nurs,* **77:**999 (1977).
Stevens, L. W.: "Surgical Management of Colonic Diverticulitis and Complicated Diverticulosis," *Postgrad Med,* **85:**122 (1976).
Sweet, K.: Hiatal Hernia—What to Guard Against Most in Postop Patients," *Nurs 77,* **7:**43 (1977).
"Symposium: Esophageal Diseases," *Arch Intern Med,* **37:** 1976. (The entire issue.)
Trowbridge, J., and W. Carl: "Oral Care of the Patient Having Head and Neck Irradiation," *Am J Nurs,* **75:**2146–2149 (1975).
Turnbull, P. C.: "Food Poisoning with Special Reference to Salmonella—Its Epidemiology, Pathogenesis and Control," *Clin Gastroenterology,* **8:**663–714 (1979).
Wah, R. C.: "Colostomy Irrigation: Yes or No?" *Am J Nurs,* **77:**442 (1977).
——— and C. J. Traverso: "Patients with Abdominal Stomas: Critical Care Nursing Considerations," *Crit Care Update,* **4:**5 (1977).
Watson, P. G., et al.: "Comprehensive Care of the Ileostomy Patient," *Nurs Clin North Am,* **11:**427 (1976).
Watt, R. C.: "Ostomies: Why, How and Where, An Overview," *Nurs Clin North Am,* **11:**393 (1976).
Wentworth, A., and B. Cox: "Nursing the Patient with a Continent Ileostomy," *Am J Nurs,* **76:**1424 (1976).
Willacker, J.: "Bowel Sounds," *Am J Nurs,* **73:**2100 (1973).
———: "Cancer in Situ of the Esophagus," *JAMA,* **239:**335–336 (1978).

Liver, Gallbladder, and Pancreas

Books

Bockus, Henry L. (ed.): *Gastroenterology,* vol. 3, 3d ed., W. B. Saunders Company, Philadelphia, 1976.
Chen, T., and P. Chen: *Essential Hepatology,* Butterworth & Co., Boston, 1977.
Gambill, E.: *Pancreatitis,* The C. V. Mosby Company, St. Louis, 1975.
Popper, H., and F. Schaffner (eds.): *Progress in Liver Diseases,* Grune & Stratton, Inc., New York, 1976.
Schiff, L.: *Diseases of the Liver,* 3d ed., J. B. Lippincott Company, Philadelphia, 1972.
Schwartz, S. I. (ed.): *Principles of Surgery,* 3d ed., McGraw-Hill Book Company, New York, 1979.
Sherlock, S.: *Diseases of the Liver and the Biliary System,* 5th ed., F. A. Davis Co., Philadelphia, 1975.
Spiro, Howard M.: *Clinical Gastroenterology,* 2d ed., Macmillan Publishing Co. Inc., New York, 1977.
Vyas, G. N., Cohen, S. N., and R. Schmid (eds.): *Viral Hepatitis,* The Franklin Institute Press, Philadelphia, 1978.

Periodicals

Altshuler, Anne, and Delores Hilden: "The Patient with Portal Hypertension," *Nurs Clin North Am,* **12:**317–329 (1977).
Arvanitakis, C., et al.: "Laboratory Aids in the Diagnosis of Pancreatitis," *Med Clin North Am,* **62:**107–128 (1978).
Bauer, D.: "Preventing the Spread of Hepatitis B in Dialysis Units," *Am J Nurs,* **80:**260–261 (1980).
Bell, J.: "Just Another Patient with Gallstones? Don't You Believe It," *Nurs 79,* **9:**26–33 (1979).
Berk, J. E.: "Acute Pancreatitis: Clinical Features, Diagnosis and Management," *Current Concepts in Gastroenterology,* **2:**14–20 (1977).
Byrne, J.: "Liver Function Studies, Part I: Introduction & Bilirubin," *Nurs 77,* **7:**12–14 (1977).
———: "Liver Function Studies, Part V: Using Enzyme Levels to Assess Liver Function," *Nurs 78,* **8:**50–52 (1978).
Calbreath, D. F.: "The Laboratory. Clinical Enzymology III: Enzymes in Hepatobiliary Disease," *J Nurs Care,* **12:**6 (1979).
Conn, H.: "A Rational Approach to the Hepatorenal Syndrome," *Gastroenterology,* **65:**321–340 (1973).
Corea, A. L.: "A Review of Hepatitis (Cause and Prevention) for Nephrology Nurses," *Nephrology Nurse,* **1:**17–22 (1979).
Czaja, A. J., and W. J. Summerskill: "Chronic Hepatitis: to Treat or Not to Treat?" *Med Clin North Am,* **62:**71–85 (1978).
DiMagno, P., et al., "A Prospective Comparison of Current Diagnostic Tests for Pancreatic Cancer," *N Engl J Med,* **297:**737–742 (1977).
Dolan, P. O., and H. L. Greene II: "Conquering Cirrhosis of the Liver and a Dangerous Complication," *Nurs 76,* **6:**44–53 (1976).

Fortner, J. G.: "Current Management of Tumors of the Liver," *Surg Clin,* **57:**465–472 (1977).

Gocke, D. J.: "New Faces of Viral Hepatitis," *DM,* **1:**32 (1978).

Hepatitis Surveillance Report #41, "Gut Feelings About Hepatitis B," Center for Disease Control (September 1977).

Ihse I., et al.: "Total Pancreatectomy for Cancer," *Ann Surg,* **186:**675 (1977).

Iwatsoki, S., and W. Geis: "Hepatic Complications," *Surg Clin North Am,* **57:**1335–1354 (1977).

Janowitz, H. (guest ed.): "Ultrasonography, Computed Tomography, Endoscopic Retrograde Cholangiography and Angiography in the Diagnosis of Pancreatic Cancer," *Med Clin North Am,* **62:**129–140 (1978).

Johnson, H.: "Liver Transplant," *Nurs Times,* **75:**1358–1361, (1979).

Kosel, K., P. Gibb-Matas, L. Seaborne, and J. Westerberg: "Total Pancreatectomy and Islet Cell Autotransplantation," *Am J Nurs,* **82:**568–571 (1982).

Krugman, S., Friedman, H., and C. Lattimer: "Viral Hepatitis, Type A," *N Engl J Med,* **292:**1141–1143 (1975).

Mazzola, P.: "Nursing Care of the Liver Transplant Patient," *RN,* **39:**34–37 (1976).

McCormack, L. R., et al.: "Pancreatic Carcinoma: Survival Following Detection by Ultrasonic Scanning," *JAMA,* **238:**240 (1977).

McDermott, W. V.: "Portal Hypertension," *Surg Clin North Am,* **57:**375–396 (1977).

McElroy, Diane: "Nursing Care of Patients with Viral Hepatitis, *Nurs Clin North Am,* **12:**305–315 (1977).

Otten, N.: "Drug Evaluation Data: Lactulose," *Drug Intelligence and Clinical Pharmacy,* **11:**604–608 (1977).

Pearlman, B. J., and L. J. Schoenfield: "Gallstones: The Present and Future of Medical Dissolution," *Med Clin North Am,* **62**:87–105 (1978).

Rodman, J.: "Ammonia—Trapping Drug Prevents Hepatic Coma," *RN,* **40:**29–30 (1977).

Segbert, P. L., et al.: "The LeVeen Shunt: New Hope for Ascites Patients," *Nurs 79,* **9:**25–31 (1979).

Sherman, D. W., et al.: "Realistic Nursing Goals in Terminal Cirrhosis," *Nurs 78,* **8:**42–46, (1978).

Stillman, J. J., and R. DeTornyay: "Experiences in Clinical Problem Solving. Nursing Decisions: Nursing Intervention in Acute Pancreatitis," *RN,* **41:**67–73 (1978).

Taylor, P. D.: "Organ Transplantation Series: Liver Transplantation," *Am J Nurs,* **81:**1672–1673 (1981).

———: "Test Yourself—Alcoholic Cirrhosis of the Liver," *Am J Nurs,* **80:**1812 (1980).

Thorpe, C. J., and J. A. Caprini: "Gallbladder Disease: Current Trends & Treatments," *Am J Nurs,* **80:**2181–2185 (1980).

Wapnick, S., et al.: "Le-Veen Continuous Peritoneal–Jugular Shunt," *JAMA,* **237:**131–133 (1977).

Welch, D.: "Nursing the Patient with Advanced Liver Metastasis," *Cancer Nurs,* **2:**297–304 (1979).

Wilson, S. E., and E. Passaro, Jr.: "Guide to the Diagnosis and Management of Acute Pancreatitis," *Hosp Med,* **12:**64 (1976).

Organizations

American Dental Association, 211 East Chicago Avenue, Chicago, IL 60611

American Digestive Society, Inc., 420 Lexington Avenue, New York, NY 10017

Canadian Foundation of Ileitis and Colitis, 294 Spadina Avenue, Toronto, Ontario M5T2E7, Canada

Hollister, Inc., 211 East Chicago Avenue, Chicago, IL 60611

International Association for Enterostomal Therapy, 1701 Lake Avenue, Suite 470, Glenview, IL 60025

National Council on Alcoholism, 2 Park Avenue, New York, NY 10016

National Foundation for Ileitis & Colitis, 295 Madison Avenue, New York, NY 10017

National Institute of Arthritis, Metabolism & Digestive Diseases, National Institute of Health, Bethesda, MD 20205

United Ostomy Association, 1111 Wilshire Blvd., Los Angeles, CA 90017

Section 8

Problems with Urinary Function

Chapter 36

NURSING ASSESSMENT
Urinary System

Sharon Mantik Lewis

Learning Objectives

1. Describe the anatomical location and functions of the kidneys, ureters, bladder, and urethra.
2. Explain the physiological events in the formation and passage of urine from glomerular filtration to voiding.
3. Identify the significant subjective and objective data related to the urinary system that should be obtained from a client.
4. Describe the appropriate techniques used in the physical assessment of the urinary system.
5. Differentiate normal from common abnormal findings of a physical assessment of the urinary system.
6. Describe the purpose, significance of results, and nursing responsibilities related to diagnostic studies of the urinary system.
7. Describe the normal physical and chemical characteristics of urine.

"Bones can break, muscles can atrophy, glands can loaf, even the brain can go to sleep without immediate danger to survival. But should the kidneys fail . . . neither bone, muscle, gland nor brain could carry on."[1] This statement underlines the importance of kidneys to our lives. Adequate functioning of the kidneys is essential to maintaining a healthy body. If the kidneys fail to function and medical care is not given, death is inevitable within 2 to 3 weeks.

The kidney is the principal functional organ of the urinary system. Besides the two kidneys, there are ureters, a urinary bladder, and a urethra in the urinary system (Fig. 36-1). The other organs can be thought of as drainage channels for the urine after it is formed in the kidneys.

The primary function of the kidney is to regulate the volume and composition of extracellular fluid (ECF). Its excretory function is secondary to this regulatory function. The secretory functions of the kidney include renin secretion, erythropoietin production, vitamin D activation, and acid-base balance regulation.

URINARY SYSTEM: STRUCTURES AND FUNCTIONS

Kidneys

Macrostructure

The two kidneys are bean-shaped organs that are retroperitoneal (behind the peritoneum) on either side of the vertebral column. Each kidney weighs 120 to 170 g (4 to 6 ounces) and is usually about 12 cm (5 inches) long. The right kidney, with the liver above it, is lower than the left. The right kidney is at the level of the 12th rib. An adrenal gland lies on top of each kidney.

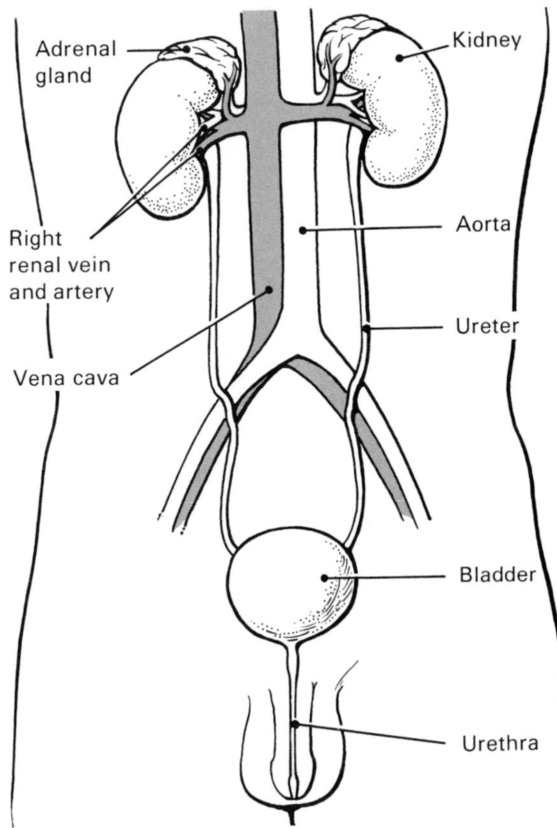

Figure 36-1 Organs of the male urinary system.

*This chapter was reviewed by Linda Stevenson Dillion, R.N., M.S., Renal Clinical Specialist, Methodist Hospitals of Dallas, Dallas, Texas.

Each kidney is surrounded by a considerable amount of fat and connective tissue that serves to support and maintain it in position. The surface of the kidney is covered by a thin, smooth layer of fibrous membrane called the *capsule*. The *hilus* serves as the entry site for the renal artery and nerves and the exit site for the vein and ureter.

On a longitudinal section of the kidney (Fig. 36-2), the internal structure can be visualized. The outer layer is referred to as the *cortex*, and the inner layer is called the *medulla*. The medulla consists of a number of *pyramids*. The apices of these pyramids are called *papillae*. They enter *calyces*. Minor calyces merge to form major calyces. These, in turn, form a funnel-shaped sac called the *renal pelvis*. The lumen of the pelvis decreases to form the *ureter*.

Microstructure

The functional unit of the kidney is the *nephron*. Each kidney has over 1 million nephrons. A nephron is composed of a *glomerulus*, *Bowman's capsule*, and a *tubular system*. The tubular system consists of the *proximal convoluted tubule*, *the loop of Henle*, and the *distal convoluted tubule* (Fig. 36-3). Several nephrons converge into a collecting duct, which eventually merges into a minor calyx.

Blood supply

A blood supply of about 1200 mL/minute, which is 20 to 25 percent of the cardiac output, flows to the two kidneys. It reaches them via the renal artery, which arises from the aorta and enters the kidney through the hilus (Fig. 36-4). The renal artery divides into secondary branches and then into still smaller branches, each of which eventually forms an *afferent arteriole*. The afferent arteriole divides into a capillary network called a *glomerulus*. The capillaries of the glomerulus eventually unite in the *efferent arteriole*. This again splits up to form a capillary network called the *peritubular capillaries*, which, as the name suggests, surround the tubular system.

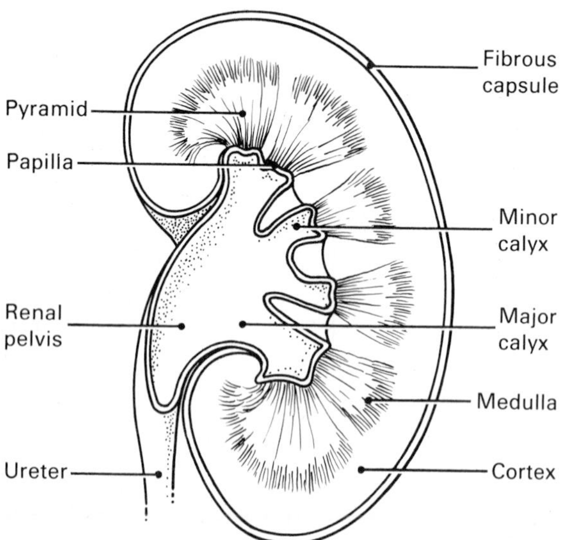

Figure 36-2 Longitudinal section of the kidney.

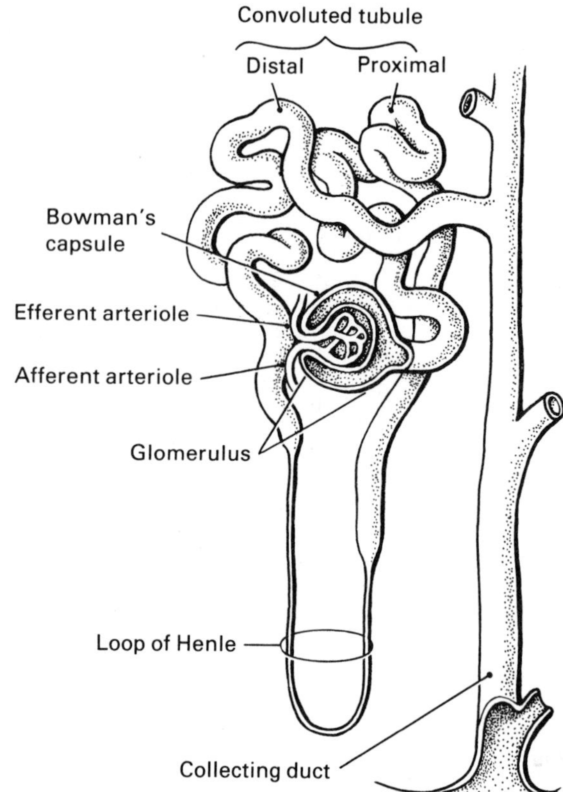

Figure 36-3 Nephron of the kidney.

Physiology of Urine Formation

Glomerulus

Urine formation starts at the glomerulus, where blood is filtered. The blood flow to the glomeruli of both kidneys is about 1200 mL/minute. A semipermeable membrane surrounding the outer surface of the glomerulus allows for filtration. The filtration pressure is supplied by the heart. Filtration in the glomerulus is more rapid than in ordinary tissue capillaries because of the porosity of the glomerular membrane. The ultrafiltrate is similar in composition to blood except

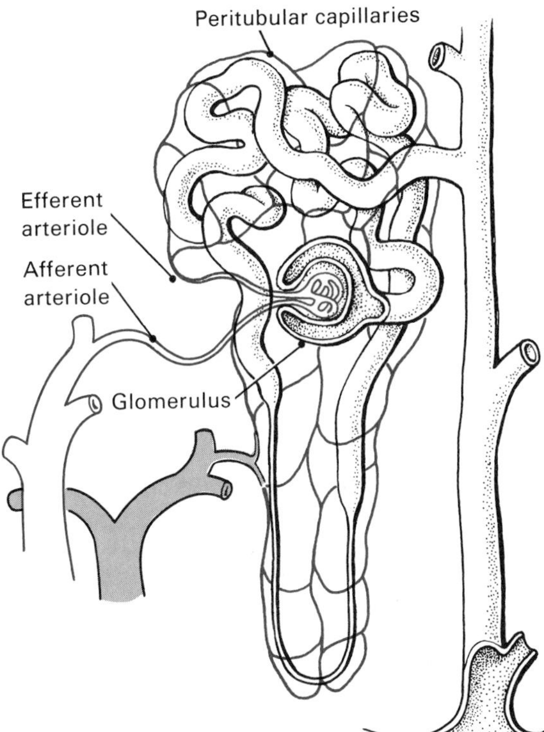

Figure 36-4 Blood supply of the nephron.

that it lacks blood cells, platelets, and large plasma proteins.

The amount of blood filtered by the glomeruli in a given time is referred to as the *glomerular filtration rate (GFR)*. The normal GFR is about 125 mL/minute. However, on the average only 1 mL/minute leaves as urine.

Tubular function

Since the glomerular membrane functions to filter substances chiefly by size, provision is made for the reabsorption of essential materials and the excretion of nonessential ones (Table 36-1). The tubules and collecting ducts carry out these functions by means of *reabsorption* and *secretion* (Fig. 36-5). Reabsorption refers to the passage of a substance from the lumen of the tubules through the tubule cells and into the capillaries. It involves both active and passive transport. Tubular secretion refers to the passage of a substance from the capillaries through the tubular cells into the lumen of the tubule.

In the proximal convoluted tubule, about 80 percent of the electrolytes are reabsorbed. Normally, all the glucose, amino acids, and protein are reabsorbed.

Table 36-1
Functions of the Components of the Nephron

Component	Function
Glomerulus	Filtration
Proximal tubule	Reabsorption of 80% of electrolytes and water Reabsorption of all glucose and amino acids Reabsorption of HCO_3^- Secretion of H^+ and creatinine
Loop of Henle	Na^+ and Cl^- reabsorbed in ascending limb Conservation of water
Distal tubule	Secretion of K^+, H^+, NH_3 Reabsorption of H_2O (regulated by ADH) Reabsorption of HCO_3^- Regulation of Ca^{2+} and HPO_4^- by parathormone Regulation of Na^+ and K^+ by aldosterone
Collecting duct	Reabsorption of H_2O (ADH required)

Hydrogen (H^+) and creatinine are secreted into the filtrate.

In the loop of Henle, reabsorption continues. In the ascending limb, chloride is actively reabsorbed, followed passively by sodium. About 25 percent of the filtered sodium is reabsorbed here. Henle's loop is also very important in conserving water.

Two important functions of the distal convoluted tubule are final regulation of water balance and acid-base balance. In the distal tubule, the role of certain

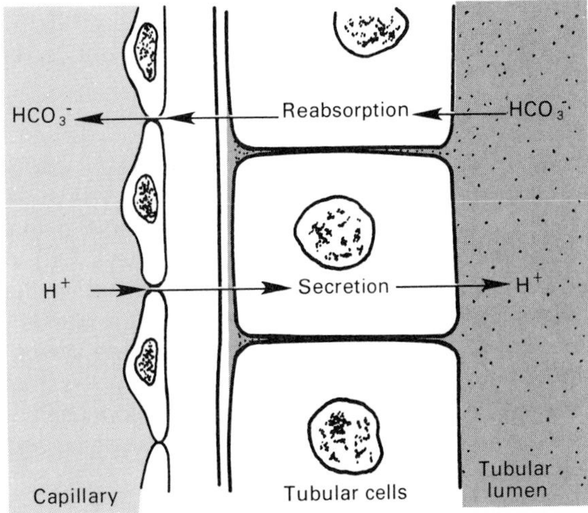

Figure 36-5 Reabsorption and secretion in the tubules.

hormones becomes important. *Antidiuretic hormone (ADH)* released by the posterior pituitary is required for water reabsorption. In the presence of ADH, the tubules become more permeable to water, allowing it to return to circulation. In the absence of ADH, the tubules are practically impermeable to water, and any water in them leaves the body as urine.

In the presence of *aldosterone* (released from the adrenal cortex) at the distal tubule, sodium is reabsorbed, followed by water. In exchange for sodium, potassium is excreted.

Parathormone is released from the parathyroid gland. It is secreted in the presence of low serum calcium levels. It causes increased tubular reabsorption of calcium and decreased tubular reabsorption of phosphate. Therefore, serum calcium levels are increased.

Acid-base regulation involves reabsorbing and conserving most of the bicarbonate (HCO_3^-) and secreting excess hydrogen ions (H^+). The distal tubule functions in different ways to maintain the pH of ECF within a range of 7.35 to 7.45 (see Chap. 12). In the distal tubule, potassium ions are also secreted into the filtrate.

When the filtrate leaves the distal tubule and enters the collecting duct, it is called *urine*. Final concentration of water may occur in the collecting duct.

Summary of nephron function

The basic function of nephrons is to clean or clear blood plasma of unwanted substances. After the glomerulus has filtered the blood, the tubules separate the unwanted from the wanted portions of tubular fluid. The wanted portions are returned to the blood, and the unwanted portions pass into urine.[2] Of every 125 mL filtered, about 1 mL becomes urine; 124 mL is returned to the blood.

Ureters

The ureters are tubes 25 to 35 cm (10 to 12 inches) long and 1 cm (0.4 inch) in diameter that convey urine to the bladder from the kidneys. One to five peristaltic contractions per minute aid in the transportation of urine from the kidneys to the bladder. The ureters receive a nerve supply from the sympathetic vasoconstriction fibers. The afferent fibers from the ureters play an important role in the formation of *renal colic*, which is associated with the lodging and passing of ureteral calculi.

Where the ureters enter the bladder, a fold of mucous membrane serves as a *ureterovesical* valve, which prevents the backflow of urine into the ureters when the bladder contracts. Since the renal pelvis holds only 3 to 5 mL of urine, damage to the kidneys can result from a backflow of urine.

Bladder

The urinary bladder is a collapsible storage bag composed of muscular elastic tissue which is capable of considerable distension. Its primary function is to serve as a reservoir for urine.

On the average, 200 to 250 mL of urine in the bladder will cause moderate distension and the urge to void. When the quantity of urine reaches 400 mL, the person will feel uncomfortable. The bladder's capacity varies with the individual, ranging from 1000 to 1800 mL.

The distension of the bladder stimulates stretch receptors in the bladder wall, causing reflex contraction of the bladder and simultaneous relaxation of the internal sphincter. This is followed by relaxation of the external sphincter and emptying of the bladder.

Voluntary contraction of the external sphincter, which is composed of skeletal muscle, is a learned response. It is dependent on proper neurological function. Injury to the nerves supplying the bladder, urethra, spinal cord, or motor area of the cortex may lead to *incontinence*.

The mucous membrane of the bladder wall has phagocytic ability. The unidirectional flow of urine from the kidney to the bladder also guards against infection.

Normal urine output is approximately 1500 mL/day, which varies with food and fluid intake. The volume of urine produced at night is less than one-half that formed during the day due to hormonal influences. This diurnal pattern of urination is normal. Most people void 5 to 6 times per day and occasionally at night.

Urethra

The urethra is a small tube that leads from the bladder to the exterior of the body. Its primary function is to discharge urine. In the female it is 3 to 5 cm (1 to 2 inches) long and lies behind the symphysis pubis and anterior to the vagina. The male urethra, which is about 20 cm (8 inches) long, originates at the bladder and extends the length of the penis. It serves as the passageway for urine as well as semen.

Normally, the urethra contains some bacteria. The turbulent flow of urine through the urethra flushes it free of debris and bacteria. The mucous membrane lining the urethra secretes mucus that is bacteriostatic.

Renal Functions Not Related to Urine Elimination

The primary function of the kidney is to regulate the volume and composition of ECF. The kidney also functions in erythropoietin production, renin production and secretion, and vitamin D activation.

Erythropoietin is produced and released in response to decreased oxygen tension in the renal blood supply. Erythropoietin stimulates red blood cell production by the bone marrow. A deficiency of erythropoietin leads to anemia in renal failure.

Vitamin D is metabolized by the kidney from a less active form to a more active metabolite. Interference with this function contributes to renal osteodystrophy (see Chap. 38).

Renin is important in the regulation of blood pressure (Fig. 36-6). It is produced and secreted by the *juxtaglomerular apparatus*. This apparatus is located in a portion of the distal tubule, where it comes in contact with the afferent arteriole. In response to renal ischemia, renin is released, which catalyzes the splitting of the plasma protein angiotensinogen into angiotensin I, which is subsequently converted to angiotensin II and angiotensin III. Angiotensin II and III stimulate the release of aldosterone from the adrenal cortex, which causes sodium and water retention. This leads to an increased ECF volume. Angiotensin II and III cause increased peripheral vasoconstriction. The increase in ECF and vasoconstriction cause an elevation in blood pressure, which normally relieves the renal ischemia. Excess renin production may be a contributing factor in the etiology of renal hypertension.

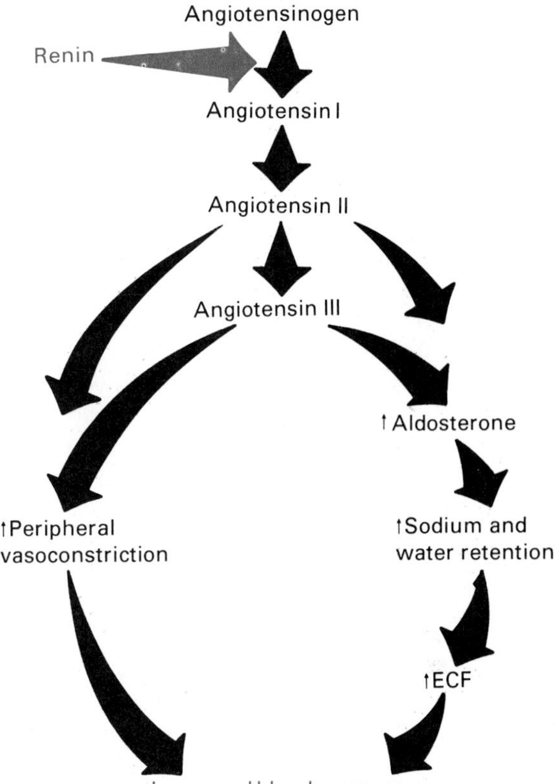

Figure 36-6 Renin-angiotensin mechanism.

Prostaglandins (PGs)

PGs are a structurally related group of 20-carbon fatty acids with a 5-carbon ring. They are synthesized by most body tissues from the precursor, arachidonic acid, in response to appropriate stimuli. PGs, involved in the regulation of cell function and host defenses, exert their influence primarily on cells or tissues located close to the site where they are synthesized.

In the kidney, PG synthesis occurs primarily in the medulla. The kidneys secrete a variety of PGs, most of which are vasodilators. The major purposes of these PGs is to increase renal blood flow and promote sodium excretion. They counteract the vasoconstrictor effect of angiotension and norepinephrine. Renal PGs may have a systemic effect in lowering blood pressure by decreasing peripheral vascular resistance.

The significance of these PGs is related to the role of the kidney in causing hypertension. In renal failure with a loss of functioning parenchymal tissue, these renal vasodepressor factors are also lost. This may be one factor contributing to the common finding of hypertension in renal failure. (Renal failure is discussed in Chap. 38.)

ASSESSMENT OF THE URINARY SYSTEM

This section discusses the data related to assessment of the urinary system that a nurse should elicit from a client in obtaining a health history and performing a physical examination. The nurse should ask not only about the existence of a problem but also about its duration and severity and the client's perception of it.

Subjective Data: The History

Past medical history

The client should be questioned about the existence or history of the following diseases, which are known to be related to renal problems:

Hypertension
Diabetes mellitus
Gout
Systemic lupus erythematosus
Skin or upper respiratory infections (streptococcal origin)
Cystitis
Kidney infections
Renal calculi
Infectious disease

The client should also be questioned about any previous hospitalizations related to the above diseases, as well as any urinary tract problems connected with past pregnancies. If the client has ever been catheterized or has had diagnostic studies involving instrumentation of the urinary tract, this information should be noted.

An assessment of the client's current and past use of medication is very important. This should include over-the-counter drugs as well as prescription drugs. For example, phenacetin contained in APC (aspirin, phenacetin, and caffeine) and marketed as Empirin, taken in quantity over a period of time, is known to cause renal damage. There are many prescription drugs that are known to be nephrotoxic agents (Table 36-2). Certain drugs may alter the quantity and character of urine output. Anticoagulants may cause hematuria, diuretics change the volume of urine output, and drugs such as phanazopyridine (Pyridium) and nitrofurantoin (Macrodantin) change its color.[3]

Family history

The presence of certain renal or urological problems in a family history increases the likelihood of similar problems occurring in a family member. The specific diseases related to renal problems to ask the client about include:

Congenital urinary tract abnormalities
Polycystic renal disease
Urinary tract infection
Urinary calculi
Hypertension
Diabetes mellitus
Gout
Connective tissue disorders (systemic lupus erythematosus, scleroderma, etc.)

Table 36-2
Nephrotoxic Agents

Antibiotics	Other Agents
Amphotericin B	Carbon tetrachloride
Bacitracin	Ethylene glycol
Cephaloridine	Gold
Colistin	Phenacetin
Gentamicin	Quinine
Kanamycin	Rifampin
Neomycin	Salicylates (large quantities)
Polymyxin	
Streptomycin	
Sulfonamides	
Tobramycin	

Social and personal history

Areas of importance to be considered in this category include background information and lifestyle.

Background Information The client should be asked if he has ever been employed in an occupation that involved any exposure to chemicals. Carbon tetrachloride, phenol, and ethylene glycol are examples of nephrotoxic chemicals. The combination of carbon tetrachloride and alcohol is known to cause tubular necrosis.

Lifestyle It has been shown that people living in certain areas of the United States (Great Lakes, southwest, southeast) have a higher than normal incidence of urinary calculi. This may be due to the higher mineral content of the soil and water.

The client's diet may be important in identifying factors contributing to calculi formation. Some people who drink large quantities of milk or ingest other products high in calcium have high concentrations of calcium in their urine. Fluid intake should also be assessed. Dehydration may contribute to calculi formation, urinary infections, and renal failure.

The level of activity should also be assessed. A sedentary person is more likely than an active one to have stasis of urine, which can predispose to infection and calculi formation. Demineralization of the bones may also occur in a person with limited physical activity.

As previously mentioned, a history of past and present drug intake is very important. There are many potentially nephrotoxic drugs that a client may be taking either as a prescription or a nonprescription drug.

Review of systems

A person with a marked decrease in renal function may manifest dysfunctions of multiple body systems. Therefore, it is necessary to discuss the functioning of the total body as well as to ask questions related specifically to the urinary system. The questions related to the general assessment are important because they can reveal common clinical manifestations of renal disease. The occurrence of a combination of these findings increases the likelihood of underlying renal pathology. Clinical manifestations related to general assessment which should be investigated include:

- Fatigue
- Headaches
- Blurred vision
- Elevated blood pressure
- Lack of appetite
- Anorexia
- Nausea
- Itching
- Excess thirst
- Chills

Problems related to the urinary system should then be further explored. These problems can be divided into the following categories:

- Pain
  - Dysuria
  - Flank or costovertebral (CVA)
  - Groin
  - Suprapubic
- Changes in patterns of urination
  - Frequency
  - Nocturia
  - Dysuria
  - Hesitancy of stream
  - Change in stream
  - Urgency
  - Retention
  - Incontinence
  - Stress incontinence
  - Enuresis
- Changes in urine output
  - Polyuria
  - Oliguria
  - Anuria
- Changes in urine consistency
  - Hematuria
  - Pyuria
  - Concentrated
  - Dilute
  - Color (red, brown, yellowish-green)
- Edema
  - Facial (periorbital)
  - Ankle
  - Ascites
  - Anasarca
  - Sacral

Objective Data: The Physical Examination

Inspection

The nurse should assess for changes in the following:

Skin—Pallor, yellowish-gray cast, excoriations, changes in turgor, bruises, urate crystals

Mouth—Stomatitis and urinous breath odor

Face, abdomen and extremities—Generalized edema

Weight gain—secondary to edema

General state of health—Fatigue, lethargy, and diminished alertness

Palpation

The kidneys are posterior organs protected by the abdominal organs, the ribs, and the heavy back muscles. A landmark useful in locating the kidneys is the CVA angle formed by the rib cage and the vertebral column. The normal-sized left kidney is rarely palpable because it is overlaid by the spleen. Occasionally, the lower pole of the right kidney is palpable.

To palpate the right kidney, the examiner's left hand is placed behind and supporting the right side, between the rib cage and the iliac crest. The right flank is elevated with the left hand, and the right hand is used to palpate deeply for the right kidney. The lower pole of the right kidney may be felt as a smooth, rounded mass that descends on inspiration.[4] Kidney enlargement is suggestive of hydronephrosis, neoplasm, or polycystic disease.

The urinary bladder is normally not palpable unless it is distended with urine. If the bladder is full, it may be felt as a smooth, round, firm organ and will then be sensitive to palpation.

Percussion

Tenderness in the flank area may be detected by fist percussion. This is performed by firmly striking the fist (kidney punch) of one hand against the dorsal surface of the other hand, which is placed flat along the posterior CVA margin. Normally, a firm blow in the flank area should not elicit pain. If CVA tenderness and pain are present, a kidney infection may be present.

Normally, a bladder is not percussible until it contains 150 mL of urine. If the bladder is full, dullness

Table 36-3
Common Assessment Abnormalities of the Urinary System

Finding	Definition/Description	Possible Etiology/Significance
Dysuria	Painful or difficult urination	Sign of urinary tract infection and wide variety of pathological conditions
Frequency	Increased incidence of voiding	Acutely inflamed bladder
Enuresis	Involuntary nocturnal voiding	Symptomatic of lower urinary tract disorder
Hesitancy	Delay or difficulty in initiating voiding	Compression of urethra
Hematuria	Blood in the urine	Cancer of GU tract Blood dyscrasias Renal disease Urinary tract infection Stones in kidney or ureter
Burning on urination		Urethral irritation
Pneumaturia	Passage of urine containing gas	Fistula connections between bowel and bladder Gas forming urinary tract infections
Retention	Inability to void even though bladder contains excessive amount of urine	Following pelvic surgery Following childbirth Following catheter removal
Suppression	Kidneys not secreting urine and unable to void	Renal failure
Pain	Over suprapubic area (related to bladder) Urethral pain (irritation of bladder neck) Flank (CVA) pain	Infection Urinary retention Foreign body in canal Urethritis Pyelonephritis Renal colic or stones
Incontinence	Inability to voluntarily control the discharge of urine	Neurogenic disease Bladder infection Injury to external sphincter
Stress incontinence	Involuntary voiding with pressure such as sneezing or coughing	Weakness of sphincter control
Nocturia	Frequency of urination at night	Renal disease with impaired concentrating ability Bladder obstruction Congestive heart failure Diabetes mellitus Renal transplanted client
Polyuria	Large volume of urine voided in a given time	Diabetes mellitus Diabetes insipidus Chronic renal failure Diuretics Excess fluid intake
Urgency	Strong desire to void	Inflammatory lesions in bladder or urethra Acute bacterial infections
Anuria	Technically, no urine voided Considered anuria when 24-h urine output is less than 100 mL	Acute renal disease End-stage renal disease Bilateral ureteral obstruction
Oliguria	Diminished amount of urine voided in a given time Considered oliguria when 24-h urine output is 100–400 mL	Severe dehydration Shock Transfusion reaction Kidney disease

Table 36-4
Recording the Normal Physical Assessment of the Urinary System

No CVA tenderness
Kidney and bladder nonpalpable
No palpable masses

will be heard above the pubic symphysis. A distended bladder may be percussed as high as the umbilicus.[5]

Auscultation

Auscultation is not generally used in the assessment of the urinary system. Table 36-3 presents common assessment abnormalities of the urinary system. Table 36-4 shows here to record the normal physical assessment findings of the urinary system.

DIAGNOSTIC STUDIES OF THE URINARY SYSTEM

Diagnostic studies are important in locating and understanding problems of the urinary system. The accuracy of the findings of these studies is influenced by (1) adherence to the proper procedures related to the study and (2) cooperation of the client in restricting fluids, collecting urine specimens, lying quietly on the x-ray table, etc.

Many of the radiological studies require the use of a bowel preparation the evening before the study. Commonly used bowel preparations include enemas, castor oil, magnesium citrate, bisacodyl (Dulcolax) tablets or suppositories, and sorbitol. Sometimes a further bowel preparation is required the morning of the study. The purpose of bowel preparations is to clear the lower gastrointestinal tract of feces and gas. Since the kidneys lie retroperitoneal, the colon's contents may obstruct visualization of the urinary tract. If a bowel preparation is not properly used, the study may be unsuccessful and will have to be rescheduled.

When a client has repeated diagnostic studies on consecutive days, it is important to prevent dehydration. It is not uncommon to have a client take nothing by mouth after midnight, spend all morning in the x-ray department, return to his room too late for lunch or too tired to eat, sleep all afternoon, and take nothing by mouth after midnight again because of studies the next day. Severe dehydration, especially in a debilitated or elderly client, may lead to acute renal failure. The nurse is responsible for ensuring that a client undergoing diagnostic studies is properly hydrated and given a correct diet between studies.

Another important nursing responsibility related to diagnostic studies is providing the client with an adequate explanation of the procedure. The period during a diagnostic workup is typically a very anxious one for most clients. The fear of not knowing what is wrong is often worse than the diagnosis itself. Additional anxiety is caused by the unknown nature of the procedure. Clients need to know what the procedure involves and its basic purpose, where it will be done, how long it takes, and if it will hurt. These things should be explained at a level appropriate to their understanding. Clients should also be instructed on their responsibility during a particular study (e.g., to lie flat on the table or to keep the legs straight).

Diagnostic studies of the urinary system often cause embarrassment and emotional stress to the client. Examination of the urinary system may be perceived as an intrusion of a very personal body part. The nurse should alleviate anxiety by providing for privacy and protecting the modesty of the client.

Urine Studies

Urinalysis

In evaluating disorders of the urinary tract, one of the first studies done is a urinalysis (Table 36-5). The results of this test may provide a tentative diagnosis, indicate what further studies need to be done, or supply information on the progression of a diagnosed disorder (e.g., diabetes mellitus).

To obtain a routine urinalysis, a specimen may be collected at any time of the day. However, it is best to obtain the first specimen voided in the morning. This concentrated specimen is most likely to contain abnormal constituents if they are present in the urine. The specimen should be examined within 1 hour of voiding. If it is not, bacteria multiply rapidly, red blood cells hemolyze, casts disintegrate, and the urine becomes alkaline due to urea-splitting bacteria. If it is not possible to send the specimen to the laboratory, it should be refrigerated. However, to obtain the best results, the nurse should try to coordinate specimen collection with routine laboratory hours.

The results of a urinalysis usually include a description of the appearance, specific gravity, pH, glucose, ketones, and protein in the urine and a microscopic examination of urine sediment for white blood cells, red blood cells, and casts (see Table 36-6).

Composite urine collections

Composite urine specimens are collected over a period of time that may range from 2 to 24 hours. The purpose of a composite specimen is to examine or measure specific components, such as electrolytes,

Table 36-5
Diagnostic Studies of the Urinary System

Study	Description and Purpose	Nursing Responsibility
	Urine Studies	
Urinalysis	General examination of urine to establish baseline information or to provide data in establishing a tentative diagnosis and determining further studies to be ordered (see Table 36-6).	Try to obtain first voided morning specimen. The specimen should be examined within 1 h of voiding. Perineal area should be washed if soiled with menses, fecal material, etc.
Creatinine clearance	Creatinine is a waste product of protein breakdown (primarily body muscle mass). Clearance of creatinine by the kidney is approximate to the GFR. *Normal*: 85–135 mL/min.	Collect 24-h urine specimen. The person voids, and urine is discarded at the time test is started. Urine from all subsequent voidings for 24 h is saved. At the end of 24 h, the person voids. This specimen is added to collection. Serum creatinine clearance should be determined during the 24-h period. If a urinary specimen is accidentally discarded, the test should be restarted.
Urine culture ("clean catch")	Confirm suspected urinary tract infection and identify causative organisms. Normally, bladder is sterile, but urethra contains bacteria and a few WBCs. If properly collected, stored, and handled: < 10,000 organisms per milliliter indicates no infection. 10,000–100,000 organisms per milliliter is not diagnostic, and test may need to be repeated. > 100,000 organisms per milliliter indicates infection.	Sterile container needed for collection of urine. Only outside of container should be touched. For females: Separate labia with one hand and clean meatus with the other hand, using at least three sponges (saturated with cleansing solution) in a front-to-back motion. For males: Retract foreskin (if present) and cleanse glans with at least three cleansing sponges. After cleansing, instruct client to start urinating, stop, and then continue voiding in sterile container. (The initial voided urine flushes out most contaminants in the urethra and perineal area.) Catheterization may be needed if client is unable to cooperate with this procedure.
Concentration test	Evaluates renal concentration ability. Concentration is measured by specific gravity readings. *Normal:* 1.020–1.035.	Usually, client must fast after a given time in the evening. Three urine specimens are then collected at hourly intervals in the morning.
Residual urine	Determines amount of urine left in bladder after voiding. May be abnormal in problems with bladder innervation, sphincter impairment, or urethral strictures. *Normal*: ≤ 50 mL urine.	If residual urine test is ordered, client should be catheterized immediately after voiding. If a large amount of residual urine is obtained, physician may want catheter left in bladder.
Protein Determination Dipstick (Albustix, Combistix)	Detects protein (primarily albumin) in urine. *Normal*: 0–trace.	End of stick is dipped in urine, and result is read by comparing with color chart on label. Grading is from 0 to 4+. Should be used with caution. A positive result may not indicate significant proteinuria. Some medications may give a false-positive reading.
Quantitative Test	A 12- or 24-h collection gives a more accurate result of the amount of protein in urine. Persistent proteinuria usually indicates renal disease. *Normal*: 0–150 mg/24 h, consisting mainly of albumin.	A 24-h urine collection.

Table 36-5 (Continued)

Study	Description and Purpose	Nursing Responsibility
	Blood Chemistries	
BUN	Most commonly used to diagnose renal problems. Concentration of urea in blood is regulated by rate at which kidney excretes urea. *Normal*: 10–30 mg /dL	In interpretation of BUN, nonrenal factors may cause an increase (e.g., excess protein intake, rapid cell destruction from infections and GI bleeding, trauma, athletic activity with excessive muscle breakdown).
Creatinine	More reliable than BUN as a determinant of renal function. Creatinine is end product of muscle and protein metabolism and is liberated at a constant rate. *Normal*: 0.5–1.5 mg/dL. Results are higher in males.	Explain test and watch for postpuncture bleeding
Sodium	Main extracellular electrolyte determining blood volume. Usually, values stay within normal range until late stages of renal failure. *Normal*: 135–145 mEq/L.	Explain test and watch for postpuncture bleeding
Potassium	Kidneys are responsible for excreting majority of body's potassium. In renal disease, potassium determinations are critical, as potassium is one of the first electrolytes to become abnormal. Elevations of > 6 mEq/L can lead to muscle weakness and cardiac arrhythmias. *Normal:* 3.5–5.5 mEq/L.	Explain test and watch for postpuncture bleeding
Calcium	Main mineral in bone. Aids in muscular contraction, neurotransmission, and clotting. In renal disease, decreased absorption of calcium leads to renal osteodystrophy (see Chap. 38). *Normal:* 9–11 mg/dL (4.5–5.5 mEq/L).	Explain test and watch for postpuncture bleeding
Phosphorus	Phosphorus balance inversely related to calcium balance. In renal disease, phosphorus levels are elevated. Soft tissue calcification may occur if both calcium and phosphorus are elevated. (see Chap. 38). *Normal*: 2.8–4.5 mg/dL.	Explain test and watch for postpuncture bleeding
Bicarbonate	Most clients in renal failure have metabolic acidosis and low serum bicarbonate levels. *Normal*: 20–30 mEq/L.	Explain test and watch for postpuncture bleeding
	Radiological	
Kidneys, ureters, bladder (KUB)	Flat plate x-ray of abdomen and pelvis. (Delineates size, shape, and position of the kidneys).	Bowel preparation may or may not be ordered.
IVP or excretory urogram	X-rays visualize urinary tract after IV injection of radiopaque dye.	The evening before the procedure, cathartic or enema should be given to empty the colon of feces and gas. Client kept NPO 8 h prior to procedure. Prior to procedure, client should be assessed for iodine sensitivity to avoid an anaphylactic reaction. Client instructed that he will lie on table and have serial x-rays taken. After procedure, force fluids (if permitted) to flush out the dye.

Table 36-5 (Continued)

Study	Description and Purpose	Nursing Responsibility
Nephrotomogram	X-ray taken with rotating tubes. Delineates segments of the kidney at different levels. Multiple exposures taken to visualize specific sections of the kidney after IV injection of radiopaque dye.	Explain procedure to client. Preparation similar to that of IVP.
Retrograde pyelogram	X-ray of urinary tract following injection of radiopaque dye into kidneys. A cystoscope is inserted, and ureteral catheters are inserted through it into renal pelvis. Dye is injected through catheters.	Preparation similar to that of IVP. Client may experience pain from distension of pelvis and discomfort from cystoscope. Client may be given general anesthesia for procedure.
Renal arteriogram (angiogram)	Performed by injecting radiopaque dye into renal artery via catheter inserted into femoral artery. Purpose is to visualize renal blood vessels.	Preparation the evening before the procedure requries a cathartic or enema. The morning of the procedure, a preoperative medication to sedate and relax client is given. Prior to injection of dye, client should be tested for iodine sensitivity. After procedure, insertion site should be checked for bleeding and peripheral pulses in leg taken every 30–60 min to detect occluded blood flow.
	Radioisotope	
Renogram	Radioactive isotopes injected IV. Radiation detector probes placed over kidney, and scintillation counter monitors radioactive material in kidney. Purpose is to show blood flow, tubular function, and excretion.	No dietary or activity restriction. Client should feel no pain or discomfort while test is carried out. More commonly done than renal scan.
Renal scan	Radioactive isotope injected IV, and radioactive emissions recorded on paper. Static image of functioning portion of kidney is obtained.	Same as above.
	Endoscopy	
Cystoscopy	Involves use of tubular lighted scope to inspect bladder. Lithotomy position used. May be done with or without anesthesia.	*Before procedure:* Force fluids or give IV fluids if general anesthesia used. Permission slip required. Explain procedure to client. Preoperative medication given 1 h prior to procedure. *After procedure:* Explain to client that burning on urination, pink-tinged urine, and urinary frequency are expected effects after cystoscopy. Do not let client walk alone immediately after procedure, as orthostatic hypotension may occur. Offer warm sitz baths, heat, mild analgesics to relieve discomfort.
Cystogram	Radiopaque dye instilled into bladder via cystoscope or catheter. Purpose is to visualize bladder and evaluate vesicoureteral reflex.	Explain procedure to client. If done via cystoscope, see nursing care related to cystoscopy.
Cystometrogram	Involves inserting catheter and instilling water or saline into bladder. Measurements of pressure exerted against bladder wall are recorded. Purpose is to evaluate bladder tone.	Explain procedure to client. Observe client for manifestations of urinary infection after procedure.

Table 36-5 (Continued)

Study	Description and Purpose	Nursing Responsibility
	Other Tests	
Renal biopsy	Usually done as a skin (percutaneous) biopsy through needle insertion into lower lobe of kidney. Purpose is to obtain renal tissue for examination to determine type of renal disease or to follow progress of renal pathology.	*Before procedure:* Ascertain coagulation status through client history, CBC, hematcrit, prothrombin time, bleeding-clotting time. Type and cross-match client for 2 units of blood. Signed permission slip required. IVP or ultrasound study done prior to biopsy. *After procedure:* Pressure dressing applied to biopsy site and checked frequently for bleeding. Client kept on bed rest for up to 24 h. Vital signs taken frequently. Urine observed for gross bleeding and microscopic bleeding determined by use of dipstick. Client assessed for flank pain.
Ultrasound	Small external ultrasound probe and conductive gel attached to client. Noninvasive procedure involves passing sound waves into body structures and recording images as they are reflected back. Computer interprets tissue density based on sound waves and displays it in picture form.	Requires no preparation other than explanation of procedure to client.

sugar, protein, 17-ketosteroids, catecholamines, or creatinine. These specimens may need to be refrigerated, or preservatives may have to be added to the container used for collecting urine.

To collect a composite urine specimen, the client is instructed to urinate and discard the urine. This time is noted as the start of the test. All urine of subsequent voidings is saved in a container for the designated time period. Finally, at the end of the time period, the client is asked to void, and this urine is added to the container.

Creatinine clearance

One of the most common composite indicators used to analyze urinary system disorders is creatinine clearance. Creatinine is a waste product produced by muscle breakdown. Because almost all creatinine in the blood is normally excreted by the kidneys, creatinine clearance is the most accurate indicator of renal function. The result of a creatinine clearance closely approximates that of the GFR. A blood specimen for serum creatinine should be obtained during the period of urine collection. Creatinine clearance is calculated as follows:

$$\text{Creatinine clearance (mL/min)} = \frac{\text{urine creatinine (mg/mL)} \times \text{urine volume (mL/min)}}{\text{serum creatinine (mg/mL)}}$$

Radiological Studies

Intravenous pyelogram (IVP) or excretory urogram

The purpose of an IVP is to visualize the urinary tract. The presence, position, size, and shape of the kidneys, ureters, and bladder can be evaluated. Cysts, tumors, lesions, and obstructions will cause a distortion in the normal appearance of these structures.

The procedure consists of injecting an intravenous dose of radiopaque dye, which circulates in the blood and is excreted by the kidneys into the urine. During the injection of the dye, the client may experience warmth, a flushed face, and a salty taste. After injection of the dye, films are made every minute for the first 5 minutes, and then at 10 and 15 minutes. A final film, which is taken at 45 minutes, allows for visualization of the bladder. The sequencing of films is

Table 36-6
Normal and Abnormal Findings of a Urinalysis

Test	Normal	Abnormal Finding and Significance
Color	Amber-yellow	Dark-smoky color suggests hematuria. Yellowish-brown to olive green color indicates excessive bilirubin. Orange-red or orange-brown color caused by phenazopyridine (pyridium), urinary antiseptic, or urobilin. Cloudiness of freshly voided urine indicates infection.
Smell	Aromatic	Upon standing, it becomes more ammonialike in smell. In urinary tract infections, the urine smells unpleasant.
Protein	0–150 mg/24 h 0–8 mg/1dL	Persistent proteinuria is characteristic of acute and chronic renal disease, especially involving glomerulus. In absence of disease, may be caused by high protein diet, strenuous exercise, dehydration, or fever. Vaginal secretions may contaminate urine specimen and give a positive reading.
Glucose	None	Glucosuria indicates diabetes mellitus or renal involvement if blood glucose is normal. Small amounts may be found after glucose loading (e.g., glucose tolerance test).
Ketones	None	Altered carbohydrate metabolism, as seen in diabetes mellitus and starvation. Can also be seen in dehydration, vomiting, and diarrhea.
Specific gravity (measures mass and density)	1.003–1.030	A low specific gravity indicates dilute urine and possibly excessive diuresis. A high specific gravity indicates dehydration. If it becomes fixed at about 1.010, indicates renal inability to concentrate urine, suggesting that the kidney is progressing to end-stage renal disease.
Osmolality (measures total solute concentration)	300–1300 mOsm/kg	Deviations from normal indicate tubular dysfunction. Kidney has lost ability to concentrate or dilute urine.
pH	4.0–8.0 (average: 6.0)	If more than 8.0, may be due to standing of urine or urinary tract infections because bacteria decompose urea to form ammonia. If less than 4.5, may indicate respiratory and metabolic acidosis.
RBC	0–4/hpf	Bleeding in urinary tract caused by calculi, cystitis, neoplasm, glomerulonephritis, tuberculosis, kidney biopsy, or trauma.
WBCs	0–5/hpf	Abnormal number of WBCs in urine is called *pyuria*. Indicative of urinary tract infection or inflammation.
Casts	None–occasional	Casts are mucoprotein substances formed by shape of renal tubule. They may contain protein, WBCs, RBCs, and/or bacteria. Casts are indicative of renal dysfunction or urinary tract infections.
Culture for organisms	None	Organisms most commonly found in urinary tract infections are *Escherichia coli, Proteus vulgaris,* staphylococci, and streptococci.

planned so that dye excretion can be followed from the cortex of the kidney to the bladder.

Preparation of the client the evening before the test consists of giving a cathartic or enema to eliminate feces and air from the colon. Fluids are withheld 8 hours prior to testing to produce slight dehydration so that the dye will concentrate. People with significantly decreased renal function should not receive an IVP because the dye will not be properly excreted by the kidneys.

The client should also be assessed for a possible allergic reaction to the dye. The contrast medium is typically an iodine derivative. A person with iodine sensitivity may develop an anaphylactic reaction after dye injection. A person with a known allergy to iodine or seafood should not receive an IVP. During dye injection, the client should be observed for signs of respiratory distress, urticaria, decreasing blood pressure, and other signs of anaphylaxis. Emergency drugs such as epinephrine (Adrenalin) and diphenhydramine (Benadryl) and cardiopulmonary resuscitation equipment should be available in the room.

After the procedure, the nurse should encourage the client to force fluids to assist in flushing out the dye.

Retrograde pyelogram

A retrograde pyelogram evaluates the same structures as an IVP. It is an x-ray visualization of the kidneys, ureters, and bladder following direct injection of a dye into the kidney via a ureteral catheter introduced through a cystoscope. It may be done if an IVP does not visualize the urinary tract, or if the client is allergic to the dye or has decreased renal function.

The dangers associated with a retrograde pyelogram are similar to those related to cystoscopy, including the risk of infection and the use of anesthesia.

Renal arteriogram (angiogram)

The purpose of a renal arteriogram is to visualize the renal blood vessels. Findings of an arteriogram can assist in diagnosing renal artery stenosis, extra or missing renal blood vessels, renovascular hypertension, and in differentiating between a renal cyst and a renal tumor (Fig. 36-7). Renal arteriograms are also done in the workup of a possible renal transplant donor.

The evening before the procedure, the client is given a cathartic to eliminate fecal material from the colon. The morning of the procedure, he receives a preoperative medication to relax and sedate him.

Most arteriograms are done in the x-ray department by a specially trained physician. The client is given a local anesthetic at the site of catheter insertion. A catheter is usually inserted into the femoral artery up the aorta to the level of the renal arteries (Fig. 36-8). A contrast medium (dye) is then inserted to outline the renal blood supply, and x-rays are taken. The client may experience a transient warm feeling along the course of the blood vessel when the dye is injected.

After the catheter is removed, a pressure dressing is placed over the femoral injection site. It is important to observe for bleeding at the site. The client is usually kept on bed rest for 12 to 24 hours. Peripheral pulses in the leg should be taken at least every 30 to 60 minutes to detect occlusion of blood flow due to a thrombus. Complications that may result from a renal arteriogram include thrombus, embolus, local inflammation, and hematoma.

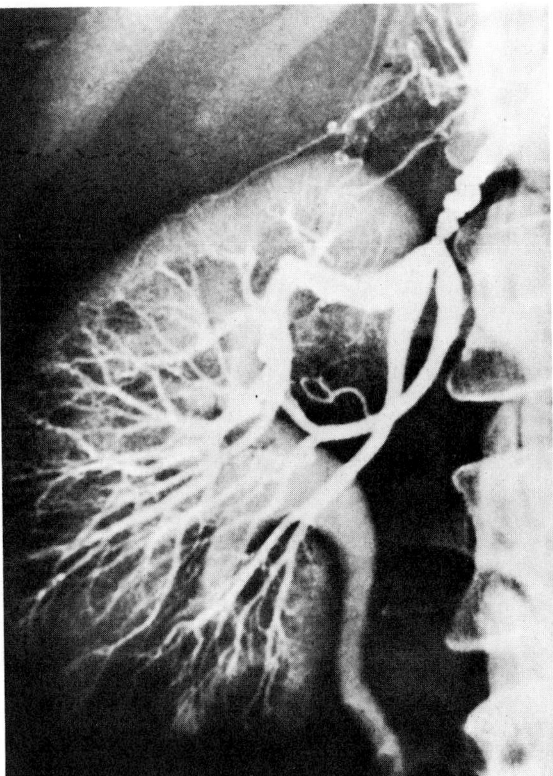

Figure 36-7 Renal arteriogram showing stenosis of the right renal artery. (*From S. A. Price and L. M. Wilson, Pathophysiology: Clinical Concepts of Disease Processes, 2d ed., McGraw-Hill Book Company, New York, 1982, p. 521.*)

Radioisotope Studies

Renogram

The purpose of a renogram is to evaluate renal vascularization, glomerular filtration, and tubular excretion. It is useful in detecting renal vascular disease, acute renal failure, and upper urinary tract obstruction, and in monitoring the function of a transplanted kidney.

The procedure is performed by injecting a radioactive isotope intravenously. Radiation detector probes are placed over the kidney, and a scintillation counter monitors the appearance and disappearance of the radioactive material in the kidney.

The results reveal the difference between the two kidneys with respect to blood flow, tubular function, and excretion. A normal renogram shows symmetrical functioning of both kidneys. Usually, there are no dietary or activity restrictions related to preparation of the client. During the test, the client should feel no pain or discomfort. No special precautions are needed in using radioactive material since only tracer dosages are used.

Renal scan

The purpose of a renal scan is to outline functioning renal tissue showing the location and configuration

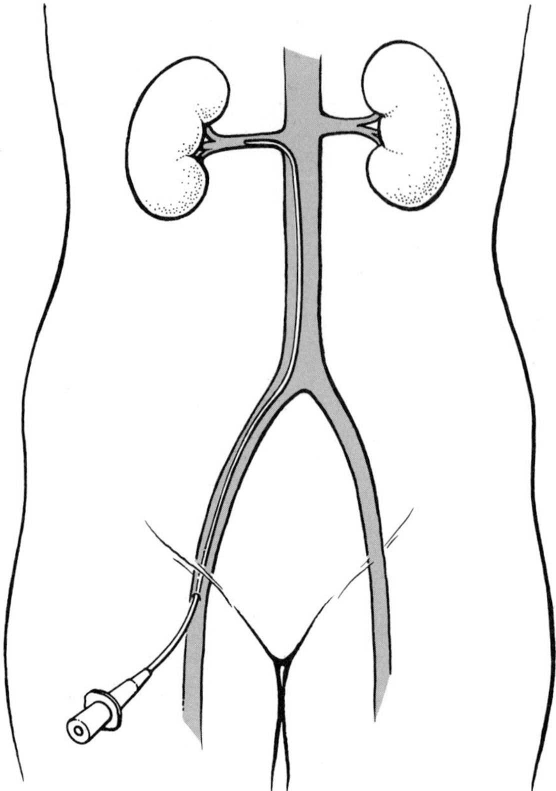

Figure 36-8 Catheter insertion for a renal arteriogram.

of the kidneys. The procedure involves the intravenous injection of a radioactive isotope which is excreted by the kidneys. The area across the back is scanned by probes which detect radioactive emissions and record on paper a static image of the functioning portions of the kidneys.

Normally, the distribution of activity is recorded throughout the kidneys. A lesion (e.g., tumor) is detected by the absence of radioactivity in an involved area and the resultant defect on the scan. In renovascular disease, an area with decreased blood flow can readily be visualized.

Renal Biopsy

The purpose of a renal biopsy is to determine the nature and extent of renal disease. This information can be used in establishing a diagnosis and following the progress of a disease, as well as in determining the treatment. It can be done either through an open biopsy or a closed percutaneous needle biopsy. An open biopsy is rarely done, as it requires a surgical procedure with anesthesia. A percutaneous needle biopsy is more common. It is usually done in the x-ray department, or it may be done in the operating room.

Since one danger of a biopsy is hemorrhage, the client's coagulation status should be assessed prior to the procedure. This includes a health history, complete blood count, hematocrit, prothrombin time, and bleeding or clotting time. The client should also be typed and cross-matched for 2 units of blood.

An IVP or ultrasound examination is done to determine the position and location of the kidneys as a guide to needle insertion. Preparation also includes explaining the procedure to the client and assisting him in discussing his concerns. A signed permission slip is required before a biopsy is performed.

The procedure consists of having the client lie prone, with a pillow or sandbag used to elevate the abdomen and expose the kidneys. Using the IVP or ultrasound findings as a guide, the position of the kidney is marked on the body. Local anesthesia is used, and a biopsy needle is inserted into the kidney just below the 12th rib. The client is instructed to hold his breath while the biopsy is being taken.

After the procedure, a pressure dressing is applied and the client is kept prone for 30 to 60 minutes. Usually, the client should remain on bed rest for 24 hours. Vital signs should be taken every 5 to 10 minutes the first hour and then with decreasing frequency. The biopsy site should be inspected frequently for bleeding. Urine should be assessed for gross and microscopic hematuria. A dipstick can be used to test for bleeding even when hematuria is not obvious. The physician may order all urine sent for laboratory analysis to detect possible hematuria. The client should also be assessed for flank pain.

Complications of a renal biopsy include renal hemorrhage, hematoma, and infection. Even if no complications occur, the client should be instructed to avoid lifting heavy objects for 5 to 7 days.

Endoscopy

Cystoscopy

The main purpose of *cystoscopy* is to inspect the interior of the bladder by use of a tubular lighted scope called a *cystoscope* (Fig. 36-9). Cystoscopies can be used to insert ureteral catheters, to remove calculi, to obtain biopsies of bladder lesions, and to treat bleeding lesions. In most cases, bladder disorders can be determined by cystoscopic examinations.

The client is given a preoperative medication for sedation about 1 hour prior to the procedure. Cystoscopy is usually done in a cystoscope room in the x-ray department or the operating room. A signed permission slip is required. Fluids are usually forced prior to

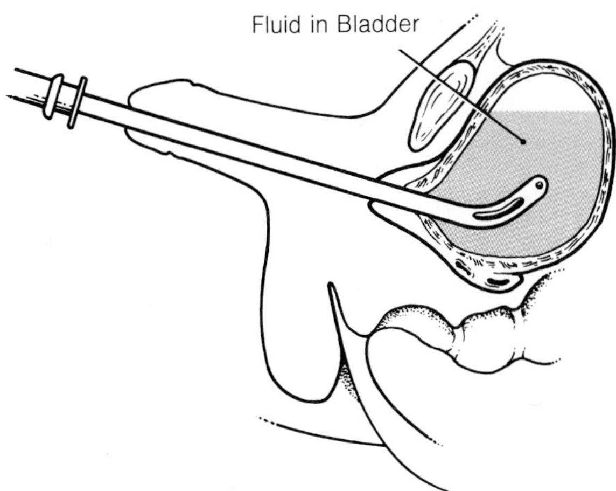

Figure 36-9 Cystoscopic examination of a male bladder.

the procedure to ensure a continuous flow of urine. If general anesthesia is given, intravenous fluids are used to obtain adequate fluid intake.

The cystoscopic examination may be performed with or without anesthesia depending on the needs and condition of the client. The client is put in a lithotomy position. Most of the pain associated with cystoscopy results from spasms and contractions of bladder sphincters. Relaxation and deep breathing by the client alleviate some of the bladder and sphincter spasms. A local anesthetic is instilled into the urethra prior to scope insertion. During the examination, saline is inserted slowly to distend the bladder, which allows for better visualization but will bring about the urge to void.

After the procedure, the client can expect to have burning on urination, blood-tinged urine, and urinary frequency from the irritation of scope insertion and manipulation. The nurse should observe for bright red bleeding since this is not a normal reaction. The client should not be allowed to walk without assistance immediately after the procedure, as postural hypotension may result from blood flow back to the legs after being in a lithotomy position. After the procedure, the nurse is responsible for forcing fluids and administering mild analgesics, sitz baths, and heat to decrease the client's discomfort. Complications that may result from cystoscopy include urinary retention, urinary tract hemorrhage, bladder infection, and perforation of the bladder.

Cystogram

The purpose of a *cystogram* is to outline and visualize the bladder and evaluate the ureterovesical valves for reflux. It can also delineate abnormalities of the bladder such as diverticula or bladder calculi. The procedure involves instilling a radiopaque dye into the bladder, which may be done via a cystoscope or catheter.

A *voiding cystourethrogram (VCU)* is a voiding study of the bladder opening and urethra. The bladder is filled with radiopaque dye. During urination, films are taken to visualize the bladder and urethra. After voiding, another film is taken to assess for residual urine. A VCU can detect abnormalities of the lower urinary tract, urethral stenosis, and bladder neck obstruction.

Cystometrogram

The purpose of a *cystometrogram* is to evaluate bladder tone. It is usually ordered if a client has incontinence or neurogenic dysfunction of the bladder.

The procedure consists of inserting a retention catheter while the client is in a supine position. A liter bottle of saline or water and a cystometer are connected to the catheter. Fluid is instilled at a constant rate, and the pressure exerted against the bladder wall is measured. The client is asked to indicate when he first experiences an urge to void (usually after 100 to 200 mL has been instilled). Fluids are instilled until urgency occurs (350 to 450 mL) or until it is determined that this sensation is absent. After the catheter is withdrawn, the client is asked to empty his bladder, and the amount of residual urine is determined. During the study, a cholinergic drug such as bethanecol (Urecholine) may be given to determine if it will enhance the tone of a flaccid bladder. On the other hand, an anticholinergic drug may be given to promote relaxation of a hyperactive bladder.

REVIEW QUESTIONS

The number of the question corresponds to the same numbered objective at the beginning of the chapter.

1. The main function of the pelvis of the kidney is to
  a. give structural support to the kidney
  b. serve as a collecting chamber for urine
  c. regulate the concentration of the filtrate
  d. serve as the entry and exit site for blood vessels

2. The action of ADH causes
  a. increased sodium reabsorption
  b. decreased sodium reabsorption
  c. increased water reabsorption
  d. decreased water reabsorption

3. A client related a history of the following diseases. Which one is known to be related to renal problems?

a. measles
b. diabetes mellitus
c. gastric ulcer
d. jaundice

4. Which of the following statements regarding the physical assessment of the urinary system is accurate?
a. An empty bladder is palpable as a small nodule.
b. Auscultation is used to listen to urine in the bladder.
c. The client lies prone when the kidneys are palpated.
d. The flank area is percussed with a firm blow.

5. Which of the following findings of a physical assessment of the urinary system is considered normal?
a. easily palpable left kidney
b. CVA tenderness elicited by a kidney punch
c. nonpalpable left kidney
d. bladder palpable to the level of the pubic symphysis

6. An important nursing responsibility following a renal arteriogram is to
a. encourage ambulation 2 to 3 hours after the study
b. apply warm, wet sponges to the insertion site
c. palpate peripheral pulses in the leg
d. give the client nothing by mouth for 4 hours after the study

7. Which of the following is considered a normal constituent of urine?
a. ketones
b. creatinine
c. amino acids
d. bacteria

REFERENCES

1. H. W. Smith, *Fish to Philosopher*, Little, Brown and Company, Boston, 1953, p.4.
2. A. Guyton, *Textbook of Medical Physiology*, 5th ed., W. B. Saunders Company, Philadelphia, 1976, p. 440.
3. D. Brundage, *Nursing Management of Renal Problems*, The C. V. Mosby Company, St. Louis, 1976, pp. 35–36.
4. L. Malasanos et al., *Health Assessment*, The C. V. Mosby Company, St. Louis, 1977, p. 259.
5. S. Schwartz et al. (eds.), *Principles of Surgery*, 3d ed., McGraw-Hill Book Company, New York, 1979, pp. 1671–1672.

Chapter 37

NURSING ROLE IN MANAGEMENT

Renal and Urological Problems

Marie E. Folk-Lighty
Linda Stevenson Dillion

Learning Objectives

1. Describe the pathophysiology, clinical manifestations, and medical and pharmacological management of cystitis, urethritis, and pyelonephritis.
2. Explain the nursing management of urinary tract infections.
3. Describe the immunological mechanisms involved in glomerulonephritis.
4. Explain the clinical manifestations and medical and nursing management of acute poststreptococcal glomerulonephritis, Goodpasture's syndrome, and chronic glomerulonephritis.
5. Describe the common causes, clinical manifestations, and medical and nursing management of nephrotic syndrome.
6. Compare and contrast the etiology, clinical manifestations, and medical and nursing management of various types of urinary calculi.
7. Explain the common causes and management of renal trauma, renal vascular problems, congenital abnormalities, and hereditary renal problems.
8. Describe the mechanisms of renal involvement in metabolic and connective tissue disorders.
9. Describe the clinical manifestations and management of renal and bladder cancer.
10. Describe the common causes and management of bladder dysfunctions.
11. Differentiate among ureteral, suprapubic, nephrostomy, and urethral catheters regarding indications for use and nursing responsibilities.
12. Explain the nursing management of the client undergoing nephrectomy or urinary diversion surgery.

Disorders of the renal and urological systems encompass a broad spectrum of clinical problems. The diverse etiologies of these disorders may involve infectious, immunological, obstructive, metabolic, collagen-vascular, traumatic, congenital, neoplastic, or neurological mechanisms. This chapter will discuss specific disorders of the kidneys, ureters, bladder, and urethra. Acute and chronic renal failure is discussed in Chap. 38.

INFECTIOUS DISORDERS OF THE URINARY SYSTEM

Significance of the Problem

Infections of the urinary tract may present as a variety of disorders. The common factor is a microbial invasion of the tissues of the urinary tract, most often by *Escherichia coli* (Table 37-1). Bacterial counts of 10^5 organisms or more generally indicate urinary tract infection.

The infections may be broadly classified as upper and lower urinary tract infections (Fig. 37-1). Infections may be found in a specific site, such as the kidney (pyelonephritis) or bladder (cystitis), but there is always the possibility that the bacteria may invade the remainder of the urinary tract. Infections that are resistant to treatment are often associated with structural abnormalities of the urinary tract.

It is often difficult to determine the location of the infection based upon the clinical manifestations and diagnostic findings. The client may have both an upper and a lower urinary tract infection. Some clients may be asymptomatic. The frequency of urinary tract infections varies with age and sex and may be acute or chronic.

Etiology of Urinary Tract Infections

Defense mechanisms

The urinary tract above the urethra is normally sterile. There are several physiological and mechani-

Table 37-1
Most Common Bacteria Causing Urinary Tract Infections

Escherichia coli
Klebsiella aerobacter
Proteus mirabilis
Enterobacter
Pseudomonas aeruginosa
Staphylococcus
Streptococcus

*This chapter was reviewed by Jacqueline Zalumas, R.N., M.N., Ph.D. Candidate, Assistant Professor, Nell Hodgson Woodruff School of Nursing, Emory University, Atlanta, Georgia.

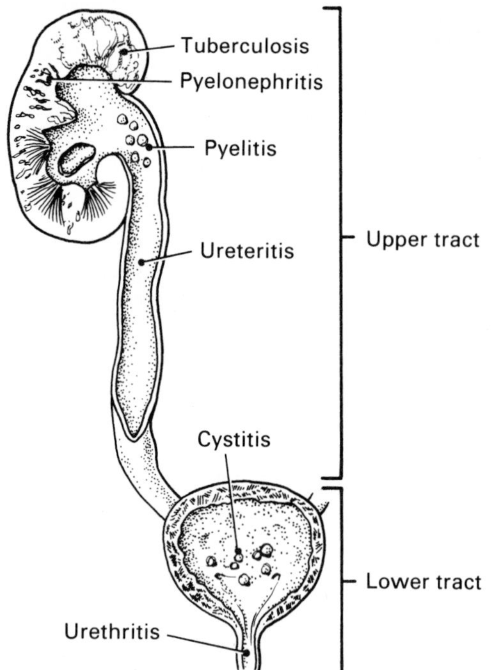

Figure 37-1 Sites of infectious processes in the urinary tract.

cal defense mechanisms that assist in maintaining sterility and preventing urinary tract infections. These defenses include normal voiding with complete emptying of the bladder, normal phagocytic ability of the bladder mucosa, ureterovesical junction competence, and peristaltic activity which propels urine toward the bladder. In the male, the zinc concentration in prostatic fluid provides an antibacterial effect.[1] An alteration in any of these defense mechanisms increases the risk of a urinary tract infection.

The following factors may predispose a client to infection: (1) renal scarring from previous infections, (2) diminished ureteral peristalsis during pregnancy, (3) urinary retention for any reason, (4) the presence of a foreign body such as a stone or urinary catheter, (5) vesicoureteral reflux of urine in a retrograde direction from the bladder toward the kidney, and (6) a humoral or cellular immune deficiency in an otherwise normal urinary tract.

Source of Urinary Tract Infections

The usual source of urinary tract infections is the ascending route from the urethra. Most infections are due to gram-negative aerobic bacilli normally found in the gastrointestinal tract. Two common factors contributing to ascending infection are urological instrumentation (e.g., catheterization and cystoscopic examinations) and urethral trauma. Instrumentation allows bacteria to enter the urethra or bladder. Trauma to the urethra allows bacteria at the opening of the urethra to be introduced into the bladder. This can occur during sexual relations or a pelvic examination.

Rarely do urinary tract infections result from a *hematogenous* route, where blood-borne bacteria secondarily invade the kidneys, ureters, or bladder from elsewhere in the body. For hematogenous spread to cause infection in a kidney, there must be prior injury to the urinary tract such as obstruction of the ureter, damage caused by stones, or renal scars. Lymphatic spread of an infection to the urinary tract is extremely rare.

An important source of urinary tract infections is hospital-acquired, or *nosocomial*, infections. The source of nosocomial infection is often *Staphylococcus* and, less frequently, *Pseudomonas*. Instrumentation of the urinary tract, particularly with the indwelling urinary catheter, is a leading cause of bacteremia and death due to sepsis in hospitals.[2] Over 700,000 cases of urinary tract infection occur among clients in U.S. hospitals each year.[3]

The occurrence of urinary tract infections is often related to the presence of abnormalities of the urinary tract such as strictures and obstructions. In the adult, an untreated urinary tract infection can lead to chronic pyelonephritis and a progressive decrease in renal function. If no abnormality exists, bacteriuria does not usually lead to progressive renal damage and renal failure.

Cystitis

Infections of the *lower urinary tract* include *cystitis* and *urethritis*. It is often difficult to differentiate between infections confined to the bladder (lower urinary tract) and those with renal involvement (upper urinary tract) on the basis of symptoms and diagnostic findings.

Pathogenesis

While the majority of clients with cystitis are adult women, other groups with a high incidence are older men and young children (especially girls). These age and sex variations in the frequency of cystitis are related to anatomical differences and/or pathological changes in the groups at risk. The adult female urethra is short, and its proximity to the rectum and vagina predisposes the client to the risk of easy bladder contamination. Bacterial contamination of the bladder can result from poor personal hygiene practices and sexual intercourse.

In children and older men, urinary tract infections are often associated with other preexisting problems. In children, vesicoureteral reflux is usually the preexisting abnormality. In men, the longer urethra (of which the proximal two-thirds is normally sterile) and the antibacterial property of prostatic secretions provide protection from bacterial infections unless there are predisposing causes. In older men, the infection is usually related to obstruction caused by benign prostatic hypertrophy (see Chap. 46).

Obviously, not all bacterial invasions of the bladder result in urinary tract infection or cause spread to the upper urinary tract (pyelonephritis). Once cystitis has occurred, it may remain localized in the urinary bladder for years without ascension to the kidney. While the bacterial infection may be self-limiting, suspected urinary tract infection should be evaluated even in asymptomatic clients.

Clinical manifestations

The manifestations of cystitis are frequency and urgency of urination, suprapubic pain, dysuria, and foul-smelling urine. In some individuals, hematuria may be present. The presence of fever, nausea and vomiting, and flank tenderness usually indicates pyelonephritis. About one-half of individuals with significant bacteriuria are asymptomatic.

The diagnosis of cystitis is made on examination of a urine Gram stain or by urine culture. The best method for obtaining the urine culture is a *midstream* technique, also called *clean-catch urine* (see Table 36-5 regarding the technique). If a satisfactory specimen cannot be obtained by this method, catheterization may be used. This procedure carries a 1 to 2 percent risk of introducing microorganisms into the bladder and causing a urinary tract infection.

Medical management

Once cystitis has been diagnosed, appropriate antimicrobial therapy is initiated. The medical management of cystitis is summarized in Table 37-2.

Table 37-2
Medical Management: Cystitis

First Infection—Symptomatic
Diagnostic
1. Urinalysis
2. Urine for culture and sensitivity
Therapeutic
1. Antimicrobials for 10–14 days
2. Encourage fluid intake of 3000 mL/day
3. Repeat urine culture
Recurrent Infection
Diagnostic
1. Urinalysis
2. Urine for culture and sensitivity
3. Evaluation of urinary tract (e.g., IVP, voiding cystourethrogram, cystoscopy, pelvic examination)
Therapeutic
1. Antimicrobials for 10–14 days
2. Propylactic drug (e.g., nitrofurantoin)
3. Encourage fluid intake of 3000 mL/day
4. Repeat urine culture

Pharmacological Intervention The pharmacological intervention for cystitis and pyelonephritis is similar. Many drugs are effective against organisms that cause urinary tract infections. Usually a 10- to 14-day course of antimicrobial agents is recommended. If the drugs are taken for less than the recommended period, the client is prone to a relapse.

The most effective and least expensive drugs are the sulfonamides, including sulfisoxazole (Gantrisin) and sulfamethoxazole (Gantanol). Other antiseptic drugs that are used are nalidixic acid (NeGram), nitrofurantoin (Furadantin, Macrodantin), and methenamine mandelate (Mandelamine). Methenamine achieves its desired effect by decomposing to formaldehyde and ammonia. The urinary pH should be less than 6 for methenamine to be effective. The urinary pH should be tested to ensure the activity of the drug.

Systemic antibiotics such as ampicillin, cephalosporins, and aminoglycosides (gentamicin, tobramycin) are sometimes used. Phenazopyridine (Pyridium) may be used in cystitis to provide an analgesic effect on the urinary mucosa. This drug should relieve the burning sensation. The azo dye in the drug stains the urine reddish-orange. It is important to tell clients of the color change so that they do not think something is wrong.

Sulfamethoxazole and trimethoprim (Bactrim, Septra) have proven to be an effective drug combination in the treatment of urinary tract infections, especially recurrent ones. When these drugs are used together, resistance to them seems to develop less rapidly.

Nursing management

Health Promotion and Maintenance Health promotion and maintenance measures include recognizing the groups with a higher than normal incidence of urinary tract infections. Health promotion activities can help decrease the frequency of infections and promote early detection of infection. These activities include teaching preventive measures such as emptying the bladder when the urge to void is first felt, drinking at least eight glasses of water a day, and wiping the perineal area from front to back after urination and defecation. In addition, it is important to teach the client to identify symptoms such as difficulty or pain on voiding, foul-smelling urine, and frequency and urgency of urination.

The nurse can play a major role in the prevention of nosocomial infections. The debilitated, the elderly, the client with severe underlying disease (such as cancer, cirrhosis, or diabetes), and the client being treated with immunosuppressive drugs, long-term corticosteroid therapy, or radiation therapy are at high risk to develop a urinary tract infection. Clients undergoing instrumentation of the urinary tract are also at risk for the development of nosocomial infections.

For clients at risk for nosocomial urinary infections, it is important to provide good perineal hygiene, especially after a bedpan is used. Incontinence should be avoided by answering the call light quickly or offering the bedpan or urinal at frequent intervals to the bedridden client. If a catheter has been inserted, special catheter-care measures need to be employed. These are discussed later in this chapter.

Acute Intervention Acute intervention for the client with cystitis includes forcing fluids if not contraindicated. It is sometimes difficult to get clients to maintain an adequate fluid intake because they think it will increase their feelings of urgency. Warm sitz baths can be used to promote comfort. The treatment of cystitis does not usually require hospitalization.

The client needs to be instructed about the prescribed drug therapy. Common side effects of the drugs should be explained, and the client should be told to notify the physician if they occur.

The urine should be examined for gross or microscopic hematuria, malodor, and sediment. The client should be instructed to observe for any changes in the color or consistency of the urine as a sign of the effectiveness of therapy.

Chronic Management Chronic management of the client with urinary tract infection emphasizes the need for the client's compliance with the medication regimen. It is the nurse's responsibility to educate the client about the need for ongoing care. This includes taking antimicrobial medication as ordered until all the pills are gone and not just until symptoms subside, maintaining adequate fluid intake of 2000 to 3000 mL/day, and emptying the bladder when the urge to void occurs or at least every 2 to 3 hours. In a study of university women, it was found that frequent voiding and adequate hydration could reduce reinfection to less than one-fourth of the expected frequency.[4]

The client must understand the need for follow-up care with urine culture to determine that the infection has been adequately treated. Relapse with bacteria of the same species usually occurs within 1 week after completion of therapy. Frequently, in clients with few or no symptoms, relapse indicates failure to complete an adequate course of medication. If the client has been compliant, relapse suggests possible renal involvement in the infectious process. In clients with uncomplicated cystitis, appropriate treatment with antimicrobials results in resolution of the problem.

Urethritis

The clinical manifestations of inflammation of the urethra (*urethritis*) are the same as those of cystitis. The diagnosis is made by obtaining a sterile urine specimen when the bladder is catheterized, indicating the site of infection in the urethra rather than the bladder. Causes of urethritis include a bacterial or viral infection, *Trichomonas* and monilial infection (especially in women), and gonorrhea (especially in men). (Gonococcal urethritis is discussed in Chap. 45.)

No one specific therapy has been identified to treat urethritis. Treatment is based on identifying the cause and providing symptomatic relief. Hot sitz baths without perfumed bath oil or bath salts may relieve the symptoms. The client should be instructed to avoid the use of vaginal deodorant sprays, to properly cleanse the perineal area after bowel movements and urination, and to avoid intercourse until symptoms subside.

Acute Pyelonephritis

Etiology

Pyelonephritis is an acute or chronic inflammatory process of the renal pelvis and parenchyma of the kidney. Generally, the inflammatory process is caused by bacterial invasion. Most infections are caused by the normal inhabitants of the intestinal tract (e.g., *E. coli*). Pyelonephritis and associated urinary tract infections are responsible for considerable morbidity, especially among young females. Repeated attacks of acute pyelonephritis can result in chronic pyelonephritis, especially if there are abnormalities in the urinary tract.[5]

Pyelonephritis can develop via the ascending route following cystitis. Often, another preexisting factor is present. In children, it is usually associated with vesicoureteral reflux or other urinary tract abnormalities. In adults, common preexisting factors are bladder tumors, prostatic hypertrophy, strictures, and urinary stones.

The infection commonly starts in the renal medulla and then spreads to the adjacent cortex. The infected portion of the kidney may heal by fibrosis and and scarring.

Clinical manifestations

The clinical manifestations of acute pyelonephritis vary from mild lassitude to the sudden onset of chills, fever, vomiting, malaise, flank pain, dysuria, and frequent urination. Symptoms of cystitis may or may not be present.

On the basis of symptoms and clinical findings, it is often difficult to differentiate between clients with infections confined to the bladder and those with renal involvement. Clients with kidney infections may have symptoms related to cystitis or may be asymptomatic. The most promising and practical approach to this problem appears to be the determination of whether antibody-coated bacteria are present in the urine. Their presence correlates well with renal involvement, as confirmed by other methods.[6]

Medical management

The medical management of acute pyelonephritis is summarized in Table 37-3 and the diagnostic findings in Table 37-4. Intravenous pyelograms (IVP) or excretory urograms are usually not obtained early in pyelonephritis to prevent the possible spread of infection.

An essential principle of medical management is to consider factors that may be contributing to the infection, such as an obstruction or urinary tract anomaly. In addition to an IVP, this involves using other diagnostic procedures such as a cystourethrogram and cytoscopy. It is essential to obtain follow-up urine cultures to determine the effectiveness of therapy.

Table 37-3
Medical Management: Acute Pyelonephritis

Diagnostic
1. Urinalysis
2. Urine for culture and sensitivity, Gram stain
3. IVP
4. WBC count, ESR
5. Blood cultures if bacteremia suspected

Therapeutic
- A. Mild symptoms
  1. Outpatient management
  2. Oral antibiotics for 10–14 days (sulfonamide, tetracycline, ampicillin, cephalosporin,)
  3. Fluid intake of 3000 mL/day
  4. Follow-up urine cultures
- B. Severe symptoms
  1. Hospitalization
  2. Parenteral antibiotics (ampicillin, cephalosporin)
  3. Fluid intake of 3000 mL/day
  4. Follow-up urine cultures after discharge

Table 37-4
Diagnostic Findings in Acute Pyelonephritis

Test	Findings
Urinalysis	Cloudy, foul-smelling urine, pyuria Microsopic: large quantities of bacteria, pus, RBCs, and WBCs Antibody-coated bacteria
Blood	Elevated WBC count Possible positive blood cultures
IVP	Enlargement of involved kidney(s) Abscesses in renal tissue

Pharmacological management

The pharmacological management of acute pyelonephritis is the same as that of cystitis.

Nursing management

Health Promotion and Maintenance Health promotion and maintenance measures are similar to those for cystitis. In addition, it is important that the client receive early treatment for cystitis to prevent ascending infections. Because clients with structural abnormalities of the urinary tract are at high risk for infection, the need for regular medical care should be stressed.

Acute and Chronic Intervention Nursing interventions vary depending on the severity of symptoms (Table 37-5). These interventions include teaching the client about the disease process with emphasis on (1) the need to continue medications as prescribed, (2) the need for a follow-up urine culture to ensure proper management, and (3) identification of recurrence of infection. In addition to antibiotic therapy, the client should be encouraged to drink at least eight glasses of fluid every day. Increased fluid intake should be continued even after the infection has been treated.

Chronic Pyelonephritis

Chronic pyelonephritis (also called *chronic interstitial nephritis*) is not the result of an isolated episode of acute pyelonephritis unless there are predisposing factors such as obstruction, neurogenic bladder, or vesicoureteral reflux. Chronic pyelonephritis is usually the end result of long-standing urinary tract infection with recurrences, relapses, and reinfections.

The resultant pathological picture shows a kidney marked by repeated episodes of acute chronic inflammation and scarring. Grossly, both kidneys are irregu-

Table 37-5
Nursing Care Plan for the Client with Acute Pyelonephritis

Client Problem	Expected Outcome	Nursing Intervention
	Acute Management	
Elevated temperature, chills	Normal temperature. No chills.	Monitor vital signs every 2–4 h. Use cooling blanket if indicated and ordered. Administer antipyretics as ordered. Ensure adequate hydration via oral or IV route. Monitor intake and output.
Flank pain	Absence of flank pain.	Palpate abdomen and flank to identify painful area. Position client for comfort. Administer analgesics as ordered.
Frequent urination, dysuria, pyuria	No evidence of infected urine. Normal urination pattern.	Instruct client regarding reason for symptoms. Force fluids—up to 3000 mL/day (e.g., day, 1500 mL; evening, 1000 mL; night, 500 mL). Administer IV fluids as ordered. Obtain urine for culture and sensitivity. Administer antimicrobial medication as ordered. Instruct client about good perineal care and cleansing following each bowel movement. Observe urine for color, odor, amount, and frequency.
Nausea and vomiting	Absence of nausea and vomiting.	Give oral fluids as tolerated. Provide frequent oral hygiene measures. Administer antiemetic medication as ordered. Provide quiet environment.
	Long-Term Management	
Potential for reinfection	Sterile urine. No symptoms of urinary tract infection.	Instruct client about preventive measures, including: Force fluids to 3000 mL/day. Medications—rationale for use, times, and method of administration, effects. Need for follow-up care. Appropriate hygiene—careful cleansing of perineal region, wiping from front to back after voiding; cleansing with soap and water after each bowel movement. Empty bladder before and after intercourse. Void when the urge occurs or at least every 2–3 h. Avoid bath salts, oils, and vaginal sprays, which can irritate the urethral meatus. Observe for symptoms of recurrence to be reported such as changes in voiding habits, character of urine, flank pain, or incontinence.

larly and asymmetrically scarred. The renal pelvis and calyces are deformed, blunted, and dilated.

Clinical features of chronic pyelonephritis include a history of recurrent acute infections and subsequent progressive destruction of functioning nephrons leading to chronic renal insufficiency. In the face of active infection, urine cultures are positive and leukocyte casts are found on urinalysis. End-stage chronic pyelonephritis is not easily distinguished from other causes of chronic renal failure. An IVP and a renal biopsy may be useful in delineating the severity of renal involvement after the infection has been resolved. Since chronic pyelonephritis usually progresses to chronic renal failure, the medical and nursing management is similar to that of the client with chronic renal failure (Chap. 38).

Renal Tuberculosis

Renal tuberculosis is rarely a primary lesion. It is usually secondary to tuberculosis of the lung. In 4 to 8 percent of clients with pulmonary tuberculosis, the tubercle bacilli reach the kidneys via the bloodstream. The onset occurs 5 to 8 years following the primary infection. The most common manifestations include frequent urination, burning on voiding, and epididymitis in the male. Infrequently, renal colic, lumbar and iliac pain, and hematuria may be present. Diagnosis is made after the localization of tubercle bacilli in the urine and by IVP findings.

Long-term complications of renal tuberculosis depend upon the duration of the disease prior to treatment. Scarring of the renal parenchyma and the development of ureteral strictures occur. The earlier treatment is initiated, the less likely is the development of renal failure. (Nursing and medical interventions for the client with tuberculosis are discussed in Chap. 20.)

IMMUNOLOGICAL DISORDERS OF THE KIDNEY

Significance of the Problem

Immunological processes involving the urinary tract predominantly affect the renal glomerulus. Glomerular disease is found in about one-half of all clients with severe renal disease. The disease process results in inflammation of all glomeruli (*glomerulonephritis*). It affects both kidneys equally. While the glomerulus is the primary site of inflammation, tubular, interstitial, and vascular changes also occur.

Glomerulonephritis is divided into a number of classifications which may describe (1) the extent of damage (diffuse or focal), (2) the initial cause of the disorder (lupus erythematosus, scleroderma, streptococcal infection), or (3) the extent of changes (minimal or widespread). Minimal-change glomerulonephritis, which is responsible for 50 percent of all cases of *nephrotic syndrome* in children and about 20 percent of cases in adults, is the only major type of glomerulonephritis which does not involve an immune process. Its etiology is not known.[7]

Etiology and Pathogenesis

Two mechanisms of antibody-induced injury can initiate glomerular damage. In the first type, the antibodies have specificity for antigens within the glomerular basement membrane. These are called *anti-GBM antibodies*. Immunoglobulins and complement are deposited along the basement membrane. The mechanism which causes an individual to develop antibodies against his own glomerular basement membrane is unknown. Production of *autoantibodies* (antibodies to one's own tissue) may be stimulated by a structural alteration in the glomerular basement membrane or by a reaction of the basement membrane with an exogenous agent (e.g., hydrocarbon, viruses).[8]

In the second type of immune process, the antibodies react with circulating nonglomerular antigens and are randomly deposited as immune complexes along the glomerular basement membrane.[9] On electron microscopy of renal tissue sections they appear as "lumpy-bumpy" deposits. In this immune complex process, the antigens do not come from the glomeruli but rather from either endogenous circulating native DNA or exogenous sources (e.g., bacteria, viruses, chemicals, and drugs). Bacterial products appear to be important in poststreptococcal glomerulonephritis as well as in endocarditis. Viral agents have been recognized in certain cases of glomerulonephritis following hepatitis and measles.

All forms of immune complex disease have an accumulation of antigen, antibody, and complement in the glomeruli which can result in tissue injury. The immune complexes activate complement (see Chap. 10). Complement activation results in the release of chemotactic factors which attract polymorphonuclear leukocytes and cause the release of histamine and other vasoactive amines. The intrinsic clotting pathway may also be activated. The end result of these processes is glomerular injury as a result of inflammation and coagulation.

Clinical Features of Glomerulonephritis

There are many clinical manifestations of glomerulonephritis. They may include varying degrees of hematuria (ranging from microscopic to gross) and urinary excretion of various formed elements, including red cells, white cells, and some granular casts. Proteinuria, as well as elevated blood urea nitrogen (BUN) and serum creatinine, are other manifestations. In most cases, recovery from the acute illness is complete. However, when progressive involvement occurs, the result is destruction of renal tissue and marked renal insufficiency.

Glomerulonephritis is most common in children, but all age groups can be affected. The most common cause of glomerulonephritis is a preceding infection of the pharynx and tonsils with group A beta-hemolytic streptococci, certain strains of which are nephrotoxic.

The client's history provides important information related to glomerulonephritis. It is necessary to evaluate his exposure to drugs, immunizations, microbial infections, and viral infections such as hepatitis. It is also important to evaluate the client for more generalized conditions involving immune disorders such as lupus erythematosus and systemic progressive sclerosis (scleroderma).

Acute Poststreptococcal Glomerulonephritis (APSGN)

APSGN develops 5 to 21 days after an infection of the pharynx or skin by certain nephrotigenic strains of group A beta-hemolytic streptococci (e.g., strep throat, tonsillitis, impetigo). The individual produces antibodies to the streptococcal antigen. Although the specific mechanism is not certain, the antigen-antibody complex is deposited in the glomeruli and activates complement. Complement activation causes the inflammatory reaction and injury. The response to injury is a decrease in the filtration of metabolic waste products from the blood and an increase in the permeability of the glomerulus to larger protein molecules. APSGN is twice as frequent in males as in females and occurs most often in children and young adults.

Clinical manifestations and complications

The clinical manifestation of APSGN present as a variety of signs and symptoms including generalized body edema, smoky urine, gross hematuria, proteinuria, and hypertension.

Fluid retention occurs due to decreased glomerular filtration. The edema appears initially in low-pressure tissue, such as around the eyes (*periorbital edema*), but later progresses to involve the total body, as ascites or peripheral edema in the legs. Smoky urine is indicative of bleeding in the upper urinary tract. The degree of proteinuria varies with the severity of the glomerular lesion. Hypertension primarily results from increased extracellular fluid volume.

Clients with APSGN may have abdominal or flank pain. Sometimes the client may be asymptomatic, with the problem being found on routine urinalysis.

Most clients recover spontaneously within days or weeks after only symptomatic therapy. A few develop acute renal failure with severe oliguria and azotemia. They may require temporary dialysis until diuresis begins (see Chap. 38). Ten percent of adults with APSGN develop progressive, irreversible renal failure within 6 months.[10] Children have a more favorable prognosis than adults.

Medical management (Table 37-6)

Diagnostic The diagnosis of APSGN is made by doing a complete history and physical examination to determine the presence or history of a group A beta-hemolytic streptococcus in a throat or skin lesion. An immune response to the streptococcus is often demonstrated by assessing antistreptolysin O (ASO) titers. The finding of decreased complement components (especially C1q, C3, and C4) is indicative of an immune-mediated response. A renal biopsy may be done to confirm the presence of the disease.

Table 37-6

Medical Management: Acute Glomerulonephritis

Diagnostic
1. History and physical examination
2. Urinalysis
3. CBC
4. Serum levels—BUN, creatinine, albumin
5. Complement studies and ASO titer
6. Renal biopsy

Therapeutic
1. Bed rest
2. Sodium and fluid restriction
3. Loop diuretics (furosemide, ethacrynic acid)
4. Antihypertensive therapy
5. Low protein diet

Therapeutic The medical management of glomerulonephritis concentrates on symptomatic relief and/or treatment of acute or chronic renal failure (Table 37-6). Bed rest is recommended until the signs of glomerular inflammation (proteinuria, hematuria) and hypertension subside. Edema is treated by restricting sodium and fluid intake and by giving loop diuretics such as furosemide and ethacrynic acid. Severe hypertension is treated with antihypertensive drugs. Dietary protein intake will be restricted if there is evidence of an increase in nitrogenous wastes (e.g., elevated BUN).

Penicillin or erythromycin should be given only if the streptococcal infection is still present. Steroids and cytotoxic drugs have not been shown to be of value.

Nursing management

Health Promotion and Maintenance One of the most important ways to prevent the development of APSGN is to encourage early diagnosis and treatment of sore throats and skin lesions. If a streptococcus is found in the culture, treatment with appropriate antibiotic therapy (usually penicillin) is essential. The client needs to be encouraged to take the full course of antibiotics to ensure that the bacteria has been eradicated.

Acute Intervention The nursing management of acute glomerulonephritis is specific to the client's symptoms. An important nursing measure is helping the client plan adequate rest to allow the kidneys to heal and regenerate. The client may need assistance in the management of fluid and dietary restrictions. (Low protein, low sodium, fluid-restricted diets are

Table 37-7
Nursing Care Plan for the Client with Acute Glomerulonephritis

Client Problem	Expected Outcome	Nursing Intervention
Acute Management		
Elevated temperature, chills	Absence of fever and chills.	Monitor temperature, pulse, and respiratory rate every 2–4 h. Use cooling blanket as indicated. Keep client warm and dry. Avoid chilling client.
Edema	Absence of edema.	Maintain diet and fluid restrictions as ordered (e.g., low-sodium, low protein diet, limit fluid intake to 1200 mL). Monitor intake and output. Assess skin turgor. Assist client to turn every 2 h. Elevate edematous extremities. Give skin care every 4 h. Give active or passive range-of-motion exercises every 2–4 h. Assess respiratory status every 4 h and observe for pulmonary edema.
Decreased urine output, hematuria	Urine normal in color, amount, and quantity.	Monitor intake and output. Note color and characteristics of urine. If indicated, use dipstick to assess for microscopic hematuria. Limit fluid intake as ordered. Weigh client daily at the same time with the same scale and clothing.
Elevated blood pressure	Blood pressure within normal range.	Monitor blood pressure every 2–4 h. Instruct client to report symptoms related to elevated blood pressure (headaches, blurred vision, loss of balance, nosebleeds). Limit activity as ordered. Administer antihypertensives as ordered. Instruct client about antihypertensives, including rationale for use, method of administration, and side effects.
Apprehension and anxiety	Increased knowledge of disease. Decreased anxiety.	Encourage client to verbalize fears. Instruct client about disease process. Explain treatment prior to implementation. Involve family and client in planning care.
Fatigue	Feeling of being rested.	Monitor vital signs as ordered. Check laboratory values for electrolyte imbalances and anemia. Plan care with client to provide for rest periods. Provide quiet environment. Assist in positioning client for comfort.
Long-Term Management		
Potential for progression of disease	Compliance with medication and health care regimen. Ability to identify symptoms to be reported to physician.	Instruct client during hospital stay to prepare for home self-care, including: Diet and fluid restrictions [e.g., diet of 60 g protein, 2 g Na, 40 mEq K, with fluid restricted to 1200 mL/day (see Appendix B, Table 9)]. Monitoring of client's daily weight. Measurement of urine output and note character of urine. Report any pyuria, dysuria, or hematuria. Rationale, dose, and side effects of medications. Need for rest and relaxation. Need to avoid crowds in cold weather and to avoid people with respiratory infections. Preventive measures for urinary tract infections.

discussed in Chap. 38.) Other nursing measures are described in Table 37-7.

Rapidly Progressive Glomerulonephritis (RPGN)

This form of glomerulonephritis is characterized by renal failure that develops abruptly and progresses rapidly (in weeks to months). It contrasts to chronic glomerulonephritis which develops insidiously and progresses over many years. RPGN involves anti-GBM antibodies. Five percent of all clients with glomerulonephritis may proceed to develop anti-GBM nephritis.[11]

RPGN can occur in a variety of situations: (1) as a

complication of inflammatory or infectious disease (e.g., APSGN), (2) as a complication of a multisystemic disease (e.g., systemic lupus erythematosus, Goodpasture's syndrome), or (3) as an idiopathic disease. Most clients with RPGN progress to end-stage renal disease within 6 to 12 months after the discovery of the illness.

Goodpasture's Syndrome

Goodpasture's syndrome is an antibody-induced anti-GBM glomerulonephritis. It is often accompanied by pulmonary hemorrhage. The pathology of the syndrome results from the binding of anti-GBM antibody to kidney and lung tissue. This binding of antibody causes an inflammatory reaction mediated by complement fixation and activation[12] (see Chap. 10).

Goodpasture's syndrome is a rare disease seen mostly in young men. Clinical manifestations include hemoptysis, gross hematuria, weakness, pallor, rales, rhonchi, and hypertension. Abnormal diagnostic findings include low hematocrit and hemoglobin, elevated BUN and serum creatinine, hematuria, and proteinuria.

Medical and nursing management

Until recently, the prognosis of clients with Goodpasture's syndrome was poor. Medical management consists of high dose steroids, immunosuppressive drugs (e.g., azathioprine), plasmapheresis (see Chap. 10), and dialysis. Renal transplantation can be attempted once the circulating anti-GBM antibody titer decreases. In selected clients with severe pulmonary hemorrhage, bilateral nephrectomy has been helpful. This is based on the theory that the kidneys provide the antigenic source of the anti-GBM antibody.[13]

Nursing management appropriate for a critically ill client who is experiencing symptoms of acute renal failure and respiratory distress is planned. Death is often secondary to respiratory hemorrhage. (Nursing interventions for the client in acute renal failure are discussed in Chap. 38, and nursing interventions for the client with respiratory failure are discussed in Chap. 22.) As this syndrome is rare and primarily affects previously healthy young males, the need for support and understanding of the client and his family is of major importance. The client and family need instruction concerning current therapy, medications, and complications of the disease process.

Chronic Glomerulonephritis

Chronic glomerulonephritis is a syndrome that reflects the end stage of glomerular inflammatory disease. Most types of glomerulonephritis and nephrotic syndrome mentioned in this chapter can eventually lead to chronic glomerulonephritis.

The syndrome is characterized by proteinuria, hematuria, and the slow development of uremic syndrome as a result of decreasing renal function. (Uremic syndrome is described in Chap. 38.) Chronic glomerulonephritis does not usually follow an acute course. It progresses insidiously toward renal failure and uremia over a period of a few to as many as 30 years.

Chronic glomerulonephritis is often found coincidentally when an abnormality on a urinalysis or elevated blood pressure is detected. It is quite common to find that the client has no recollection or history of acute nephritis or any renal problems. A renal biopsy is necessary to determine the exact cause and nature of the glomerulonephritis. (Management of chronic renal failure is discussed in Chap. 38.)

NEPHROTIC SYNDROME

Clinical Manifestations

The term *nephrotic syndrome* describes a clinical picture which results from many causes (Table 37-8). The characteristic manifestations include edema, massive proteinuria, hyperlipidemia, and hypoalbuminemia. The increased glomerular membrane permeability found in nephrotic syndrome is responsible for the massive excretion of protein in the urine. This results in decreased serum protein and subsequent edema formation.

The diminished plasma oncotic pressure from the decreased serum proteins stimulates hepatic lipoprotein synthesis, which results in hyperlipidemia. Initially, cholesterol and low-density lipoproteins are elevated.

Table 37-8
Causes of Nephrotic Syndrome

Membranous, proliferative glomerulonephritis
Diabetic glomerulosclerosis
Systemic lupus erythematosus
Amyloidosis
Congestive heart failure
Renal vein thrombosis
Toxic substances
Syphilis
Malaria
Inherited nephrotic disease
Poststreptococcal glomerulonephritis
Focal glomerulonephritis

Later, the triglyceride level is also increased. Fat bodies (fatty casts) commonly appear in the urine.

Medical Management

Treatment of nephrotic syndrome is symptomatic. The goals are to (1) relieve edema and (2) cure or control the primary disease. Medical management of the edema includes the use of loop diuretics and a low salt, high protein diet. Intravenous albumin has not been beneficial as maintenance therapy because it is rapidly lost in the urine. Albumin is used only in severe *anasarca* (generalized edema).

Corticosteroids and cyclophosphamide (Cytoxan) are used for the treatment of several causes of nephrotic syndrome. Prednisone has been effective to varying degrees in individuals with lipoid nephrosis, membranous glomerulonephritis, proliferative glomerulonephritis, and lupus nephritis. Management of diabetes and treatment of edema are the only measures used for diabetic nephrosis.

Nursing Management

A major nursing intervention of the client with nephrotic syndrome is related to edema. It is important to assess the edema by doing daily weights, accurately recording the intake and output, and measuring abdominal girth or extremity size. The edematous skin needs careful cleaning. Trauma should be avoided. The effectiveness of diuretic therapy needs to be monitored.

The client has the potential to become malnourished from the excessive loss of protein in the urine. Maintaining a high protein diet that is also low in sodium is not always easy. The protein intake should be 1.0 to 1.5 g per kilogram of body weight. The client is usually anorexic. Serving small, frequent meals in a pleasant setting may encourage better dietary intake.

Because the client is susceptible to infection, measures should be taken to avoid exposure to people with obvious infections. Individuals with nephrotic syndrome are often ashamed of their edematous appearance and need support in dealing with their altered body image.

OBSTRUCTIVE UROPATHIES

The outflow of urine from the kidney may be obstructed anywhere along the urinary tract from the ureteropelvic junction to the terminal urethra. As discussed earlier in this chapter, obstruction is a predisposing factor in the development of urinary tract infections and chronic pyelonephritis.

Two general classifications of urinary tract obstructions are *congenital* and *acquired*. Congenital obstructions most commonly involve a stricture, or narrowing, of the ureter. Acquired obstructions include tumors (prostatic or bladder), scar tissue or fibrosis, and foreign bodies such as urinary calculi. Common causes of urinary obstruction are shown in Fig. 37-2. Functional obstruction can occur from neurological lesions which result in a neurogenic bladder. The symptoms and pathological features associated with urinary obstruction depend on the site and on whether the obstruction is partial or complete.

The distension of the renal pelvis and calyces from an obstruction to normal urine flow is termed *hydronephrosis* (Fig. 37-3). *Hydroureter*, dilatation of the ureter, may also result from obstructed urinary flow. In an obstructive process, urine production continues; eventually, sustained or intermittent high pressure may develop, resulting in destruction of renal tissue. If the pressure remains low or moderate, the kidney may continue to dilate, with no noticeable loss of function. There is an increased risk of pyelonephritis because of urinary stasis and reflux. If only one kidney is involved and the other kidney is functioning, the client may be asymptomatic. If both kidneys or only

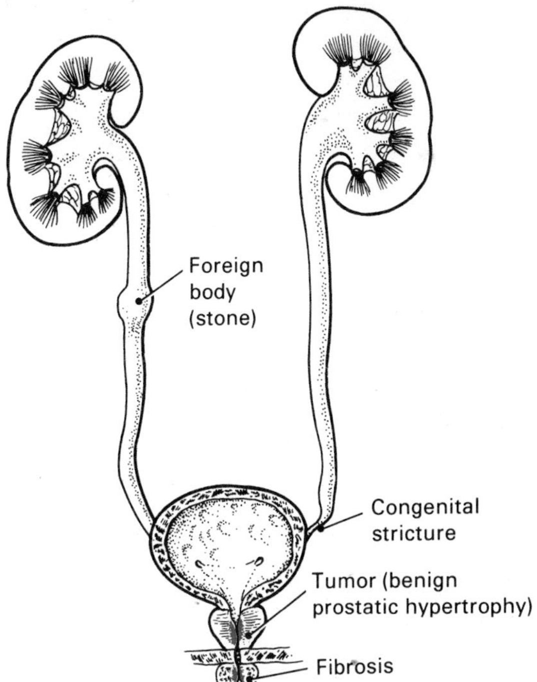

Figure 37-2 Common causes of urinary tract obstruction.

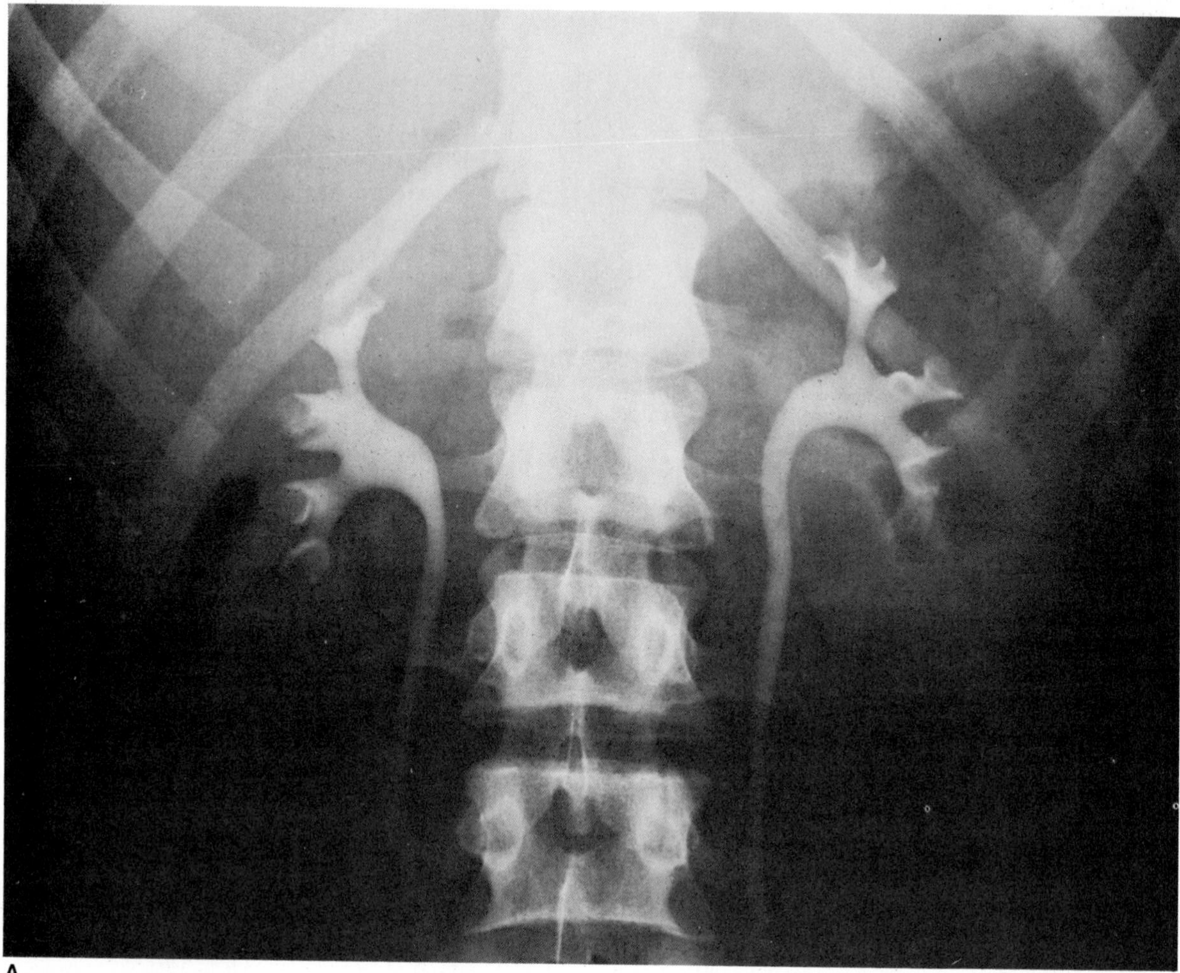

Figure 37-3 (*a*) Normal IVP. (*b*) IVP showing hydronephrosis and mydroureter. (*Courtesy of the Harborview Medical Center, University of Washington.*)

one functioning kidney are involved (e.g., if the client has only one kidney), disturbances in renal function will be found. If the obstruction progresses, the client develops oliguria or anuria. Often there are episodes of oliguria followed by polyuria if the obstruction is a stone that becomes dislodged.

Renal Calculi (Nephrolithiasis)

Significance of the problem

One of the oldest diseases known to humanity is the presence of stones in the urinary tract. There are many factors involved in the incidence and type of stone formation including dietary, genetic, climatic, lifestyle, and occupational influences (Table 37-9).

An annual incidence of 1 or more cases of stones per 1000 population has been identified in the United States. The highest incidence occurs in the southeastern states.[14] Except for *struvite* (an infected stone), which is more common in women, stone disease is more common in men. The majority of clients are between 20 and 55 years of age. Stone formation is more frequent in whites than in blacks. There is a seasonal variation, with stone formation occurring more often in summer months. This raises the question of the role of dehydration in this process. Stone formation also seems to increase as countries become more industrialized.

Etiology

Many theories have been proposed to explain the formation of stones in the urinary tract. No one theory

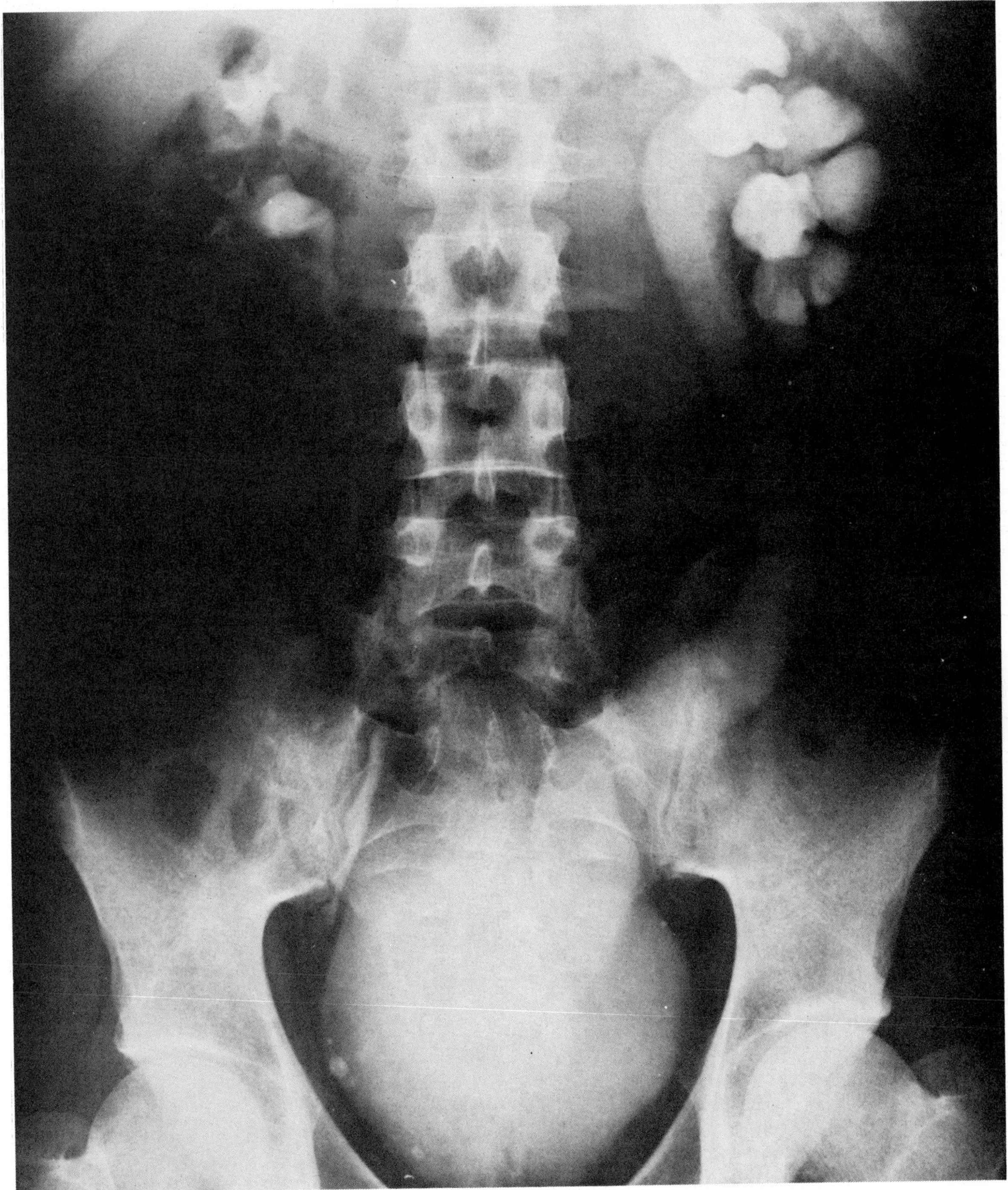

B
Figure 37-3 (Continued)

Table 37-9

Factors in the Development of Urinary Tract Calculi

Climate

High atmospheric temperature resulting in increased fluid loss, low urine volume, and increased solute concentration in the urine.

Diet

Large intake of dietary proteins increasing the uric acid excretion.
Excessive amounts of tea or fruit juices elevating the urinary oxalate level.
Large intake of calcium and oxalate.

Genetic factors

Family history of stone formation, cystinuria, gout, or renal tubular acidosis.

Lifestyle

Sedentary occupation.
Client on bed rest.

can account for stone formation in each case. It is known that in the kidneys of stone formers, a mucoprotein is formed which is the matrix for the stone. Urinary pH, solute load, and inhibitors in the urine affect the formation of stones. The higher the pH, the less soluble are calcium and phosphate. The lower the pH, the less soluble is uric acid. Other important factors in the development of stones include obstruction with urine stasis and urinary infection with urea-splitting bacteria. These bacteria cause the urine to become alkaline and contribute to calcium-phosphate stones. Stones in the lower urinary tract (bladder or urethra) are found primarily in elderly men with prostatic enlargement and urinary tract infection.

Types of calculi

The term *calculus* refers to the stone and *lithiasis* to stone formation. There are five major categories of stones (Table 37-10): (1) calcium phosphate, (2) calcium oxalate, (3) uric acid, (4) cystine stones, and (5) struvite (magnesium ammonium phosphate). Calcium oxalate, calcium phosphate, and magnesium phosphate comprise 95 percent of all upper urinary tract calculi.[15]

Clinical manifestations

Clinical manifestations of calculi include hematuria, abdominal or flank pain, and renal colic. If renal function has been damaged, varying degrees of renal insufficiency may be present.

The type of pain is determined by the location of the stone (Fig. 37-5). If the stone is trapped in a calyx or in the renal pelvis, pain may be absent. If it produces obstruction in a calyx or at the ureteropelvic

Table 37-10

Comparison of the Types of Urinary Calculi

Urinary Stone	Characteristics	Predisposing Factors	Therapeutic Measures
Calcium phosphate	Typically, mixed stones associated with struvite or oxalate stones.	Alkaline urine. Primary hyperparathyroidism.	Usually associated with calcium oxalate and struvite stones. Treat the other stones.
Calcium oxalate	Stones tend to be small and can be trapped in ureter. Occur more frequently in men than in women.	Idiopathic. Secondary calcium disease, hyperoxaluria.	Increase hydration. Reduce dietary oxalate (Table 37-12). Give cholestyramine to bind oxalate. Give calcium lactate to precipitate oxalate in GI tract.
Uric acid	Occurs predominantly in men. Jewish men have high incidence. Accounts for 5–8% of all calculi.	Gout.	Reduce urinary concentration of uric acid. Alkalinize the urine. Administer allopurinol.
Cystine	Accounts for 1–2% of all calculi.	Genetic autosomal recessive defect. Defective absorption of cystine in GI tract and kidney. Excess concentrations cause stone formation.	Increase hydration. Give D-penicillamine to prevent cystine crystallization. Give sodium bicarbonate to maintain alkaline urine.
Struvite	Is 3–4 times as common in women as in men. Tends to be of large staghorn type (Fig. 37-4).	Urinary tract infections.	Use antimicrobial agents. Use surgical intervention to remove stone.

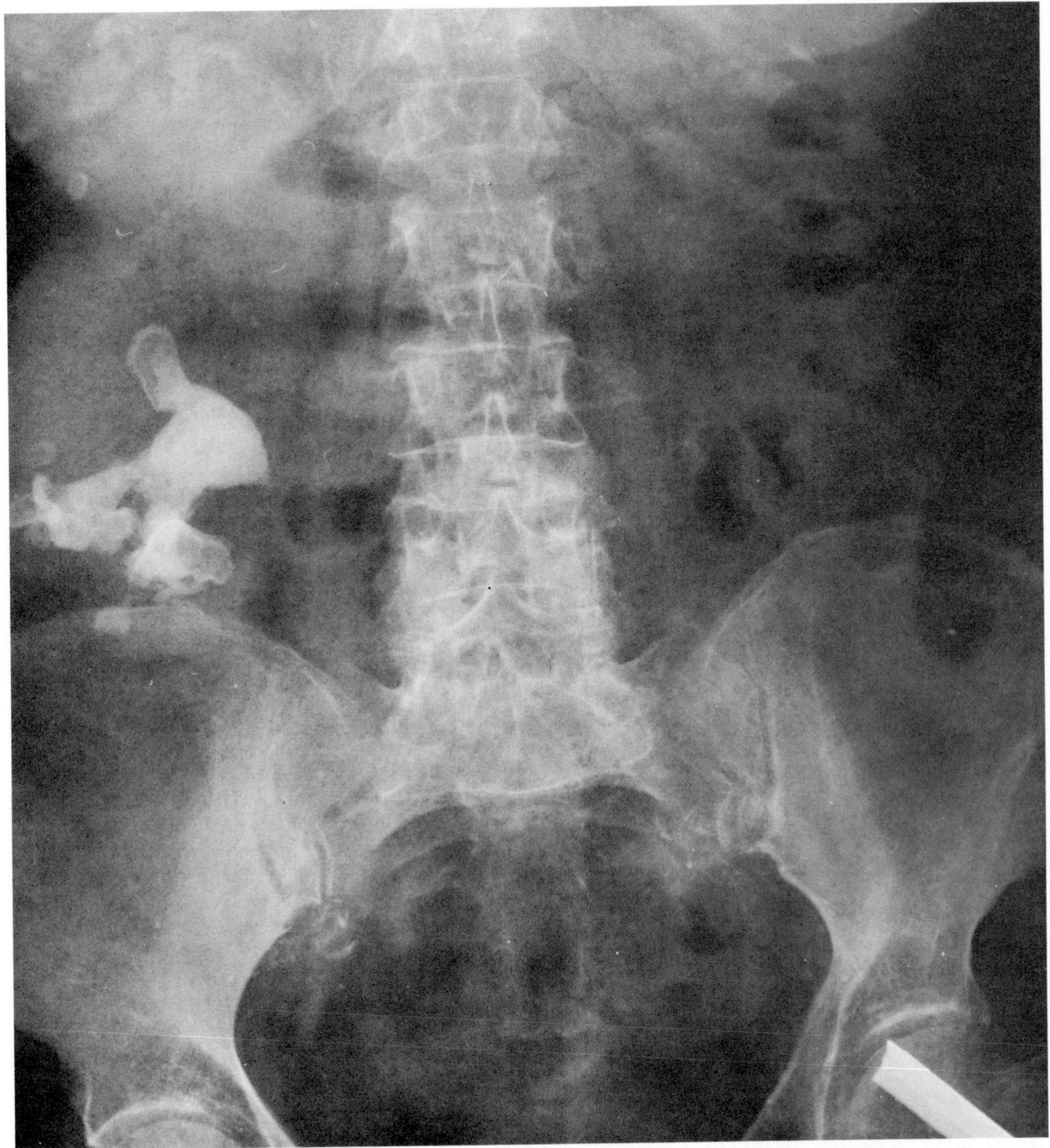

Figure 37-4 X-ray of a staghorn calculus. (*Courtesy of the Harborview Medical Center, University of Washington.*)

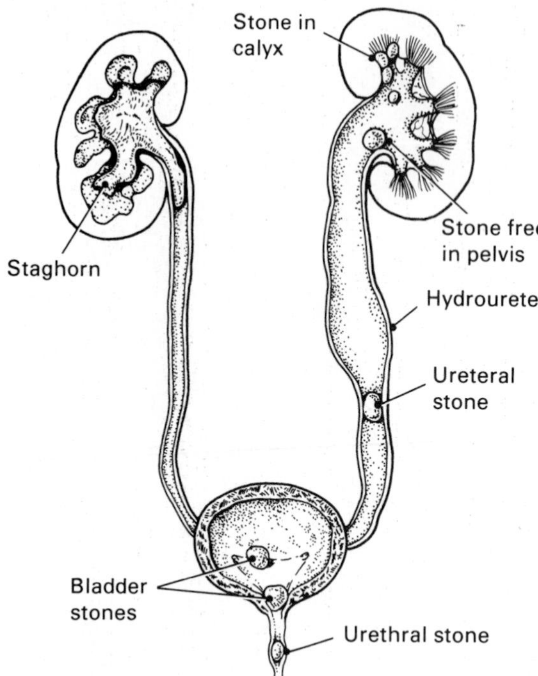

Figure 37-5 Location of calculi in the urinary tract.

junction, the client may experience dull pain or even colic. Pain resulting from the passage of a calculus down the ureter is intense and colicky. The client may be in mild shock with cold, moist skin. Costovertebral tenderness may be present.

Medical management

Diagnostic Studies Diagnostic studies useful in the evaluation and management of renal lithiasis include urinalysis, cystoscopy, IVP, and retrograde pyelogram, stone analysis for metabolic contents, and measurement of the urine and serum levels of various substances involved in stone formation (calcium, oxalate, uric acid). A kidney, ureters, bladder (KUB) x-ray may be done to pinpoint the location, number, and size of radiopaque stones. An IVP or retrograde pyelogram can further localize the degree and site of obstruction and confirm the presence of nonradiopaque stones (uric acid, cystine). Abnormalities in the urinalysis are noted in Table 37-11.

Table 37-11
Abnormalities of Urine Sediment in the Client with Renal Calculi

Abnormality	Significance
Red cells	Suggests injury to urinary tract
White cells	Suggests inflammation or infection
Protein	Suggests glomerular basement membrane injury (e.g., infection or underlying renal dysfunction)
Pus and bacteria	Present in infection (>100,000 organisms per milliliter)
Crystals	Polarized light microscopy can identify type of crystal (urate, cystine, oxalate)

Therapeutic Evaluation and management of the client with renal lithiasis consist of two concurrent approaches. The first approach is directed toward management of the acute attack. This involves treating the symptoms of pain, infection, or obstruction as indicated for the individual client. An adequate fluid intake of 3000 to 4000 mL/day is recommended. About 90 percent of stones pass spontaneously.

The second approach is directed toward evaluation of the etiology of the stone formation. Information to be obtained from the client includes family history, geographic residence, nutritional assessment including the use of vitamins A and D, whether lifestyle is sedentary, history of periods of prolonged illness with immobilization or dehydration, and any history of prior disease or surgery involving the gastrointestinal or genitourinary tract.

Proper therapy for metabolically active stone formers requires a concerted medical and nursing management approach, with primary emphasis on teaching the client and developing a therapeutic regimen with which he can reasonably comply (Table 37-10). Adequate hydration, reduction of dietary oxalate, and reduction in the use of soda and coffee can decrease the incidence of calcium stones. When calcium urolithiasis is associated with hyperuricosuria (even in the absence of hypercalciuria), the use of allopurinol may be helpful. Excessive dietary intake of calcium and vitamins A or D should be evaluated and corrected.

The treatment of *uric acid stones* is aimed at reducing the urinary concentration of uric acid. This can be accomplished by alkalinizing the urine (increasing the intake of bicarbonate), restricting dietary purines, and administering allopurinol. Maintenance of adequate hydration (3 L/day) to reduce the uric acid concentration in urine is helpful. If the urate output is high and results from purine intake, a low purine diet is prescribed (Table 37-12). If the urate output is high as a result of endogenous production, allopurinol is

Table 37-12
Foods High in Purine, Calcium, and Oxalate

Purines

High: sardines, herring, mussels, sweetbreads, liver, kidney, goose, venison, meat soups

Moderate: chicken, salmon, crab, veal, mutton, bacon, pork, beef, ham

Calcium

Milk, cheese, ice cream, yogurt, foods containing flour, all beans (except green beans), lentils, fish with fine bones (sardines, kippers, herring, salmon), dried fruits, nuts, chocolate, cocoa, Ovaltine, sauces containing milk

Oxalate

Spinach, rhubarb, parsley, runner beans, chocolate, cocoa, instant coffee, Ovaltine, tea

given. If the urate output is normal but the urinary pH is low, the treatment is administration of an alkalinizing agent to keep the urinary pH above 5.

Treatment of struvite stones primarily consists of removing all intraurinary foreign bodies, including stones, catheters, and tubes. All infection must then be eradicated. If the stone is large, it may need to be surgically removed.

Surgical Intervention About 10 percent of clients with urinary calculi will need surgery to remove the stone. Either a *transurethral approach* or *open surgery* is used. If the stone is located in the bladder, a transurethral *lithopaxy* may be performed. In this operation, an instrument is inserted into the bladder via the urethra, and the stone is crushed. If the stone is located in the lower third of the ureter, extraction may be attempted transurethrally using instruments which snare the stone. These are referred to as "baskets" and consist of a special catheter with filaments attached so that when the catheter is passed beyond the stone and gradually withdrawn, the stone becomes entangled in the filaments. If this procedure is not successful, one or two ureteral catheters may be left in place to dilate the ureter, and extraction is attempted again in a few days. If extraction is not successful or the stone is above manipulation range in the ureter, open surgery is indicated.

The type of open surgery needed depends on the location of the stone. A *nephrolithotomy* is an incision into the kidney to remove a stone. A *pyelolithotomy* is an incision into the renal pelvis to remove a stone. If the stone is located in the ureter, a *ureterolithotomy* is performed. A *cystotomy* may be indicated for bladder calculi. For open surgery on the kidney or ureter, a flank incision directly below the diaphragm and across the side is usually the preferred surgical approach. (Renal and urological surgery is discussed at the end of this chapter.)

Dietary management

A high fluid intake of 3000 to 4000 mL/day is recommended during or after an attack of urolithiasis. Specific dietary intervention is presented in Table 37-12. Increasing the fluid intake is especially important for clients who are active in sports, living in dry climates, performing physical exercise, or working in occupations that require outdoor work or a great deal of physical activity which could lead to dehydration.

Another preventive measure concerns the client who is on bed rest or is relatively immobile for a prolonged period of time. It is important to maintain a high fluid intake, as well as to prevent urinary stasis by turning the client every 2 hours and helping the client to sit or stand if possible.

Acute Intervention In the acute phase, it is important to determine if the stone has passed. All urine voided by the client should be strained through gauze to detect the stone. Forcing fluids and encouraging ambulation help the stone pass down the urinary tract. The client should not walk if pain is present during an attack of renal colic. Analgesics should be given for renal colic, as the pain is excruciating. Other nursing measures are discussed in Table 37-13.

If the cause of the stone formation is determined, it is important for the nurse to teach the client ways to prevent its recurrence. Dietary restrictions are related to the type of stone. For example, restricting milk and milk products may help those individuals who are at risk for developing calcium phosphate stones. Diets that restrict purines may be helpful to clients at risk for developing uric acid stones.

Stones that do not pass spontaneously will need to be removed by a transurethral approach or surgically through a flank incision and pyelolithotomy or ureterolithotomy. The nursing care of a client with a transurethral approach is discussed in Table 37-14. Nursing care for the client with an open surgical approach is discussed in the section on Renal and Urological Surgery.

Chronic Management Follow-up care includes monitoring the client's compliance with fluid and dietary recommendations. Depending on the situation, periodic urine cultures may be indicated. Testing the pH of the urine is important, especially to assess the

Table 37-13

Nursing Care Plan for the Client with Acute Renal Lithiasis

Client Problem	Expected Outcome	Nursing Intervention
Renal colic or flank pain	Absence of pain.	Encourage fluids to 3000–4000 mL/day unless contraindicated. Assess pain and administer pain medication as ordered. Apply moist heat to flank area prn. Encourage activity as tolerated between attacks of renal colic.
Urinary changes (hematuria, oliguria)	Normal amount and character of urine.	Monitor urine output and fluid intake. Observe for dehydration. Strain all urine. Save stone and send for analysis as ordered. Encourage fluid intake as for renal colic or flank pain.
Inability to pass stone	Stone removal.	Explain surgical procedure (include insertion of ureteral catheters). Allow client to ventilate feelings of anxiety, fear of surgery, etc.
Recurrence of stone formation	Demonstrated adherence to and understanding of health care regimen.	Instruct client during initial hospital stay to prepare for home self-care, including: Force fluids to 3000 mL/day unless contraindicated. Diet restriction and rationale (see Table 37-12). Rationale, dose, frequency, and side effects of medication. If necessary, strain all urine through a piece of gauze. Bring stone to physician for analysis. Symptoms of recurrence to be reported (hematuria, flank pain, etc.).

effectiveness of acidifying or alkalinizing agents. It is important to emphasize the need to avoid inadvertent dehydration from excessive exercise and to increase fluid needs during illness.

Strictures

Strictures may occur in the bladder neck, urethra, or ureters. A stricture is a narrowing of the lumen which is sometimes congenital but usually acquired. Strictures of the neck of the bladder may be congenital or may result from chronic prostatitis in men or cystitis in women. Causes of urethral strictures include trauma from accidents (e.g., fractured pelvis), gonorrheal infections, or urethral instrumentation. Ureteral strictures may be caused by severe or chronic infection, radiation therapy, and retroperitoneal abscess formation from inflammatory bowel disease and perforation.

Strictures may be avoided by proper management of inflammatory processes or traumatic injuries. Treatment of existing strictures includes dilatation, use

Table 37-14

Nursing Care Plan for the Client with Transurethral Extraction of Renal Lithiasis

Client Problem	Expected Outcome	Nursing Intervention
Possible blockage of urethral catheters	Patent catheters.	Monitor urine output every 1 h. Assess patency of catheters hourly. Prevent blockage of catheter. Document amount and character of urine. (Initially, urine may be slightly bloody due to irritation from the stone and the surgical manipulation.)
Possible infection	Absence of infection.	Do not irrigate catheter. Monitor vital signs. Observe for fever. Report any fever or chills to physician. Administer antipyretics if indicated. Force fluids unless contraindicated. Note character and color of urine. Observe for cloudy, foul-smelling urine. Administer antibiotics as ordered.
Bladder spasm and/or flank pain	Absence of and/or relief from pain.	Maintain patency of catheters. Observe for kinks in catheter or lack of urine output. Administer medications for pain as ordered. Explain cause of pain or spasms to client. Assess pain. Persistent pain may be due to perforation of bladder or obstruction of ureteral catheter.

of a catheter for temporary or permanent drainage for ureteral or urethral strictures, and surgery. Nursing interventions include preparing and informing the client about the procedure and assessing the client's need for management, education, and follow-up.

RENAL TRAUMA

The continued increase in the incidence of traumatic renal injuries is related to an increase in the mechanization and speed of transportation and to the growth in violent crimes and injuries. The majority of incidents occur in males less than 30 years of age. Blunt trauma is the most frequent cause. Injury to the kidney should be considered in multiple injuries, traffic accidents, and falls. It is especially likely when the client lands on his abdomen, flank, or back and when fractures of the spine or ribs or penetrating injuries have occurred. The determining factor in the mortality rate is the severity of the associated injuries.

Clinical findings include a history of trauma to the area of the kidneys. Gross or microscopic hematuria may be present. Diagnostic studies include urinalysis, excretory urograms using contrast dye, and tomography. Renal arteriography may also be used. It is important that both the injured and noninvolved kidney be evaluated to provide information for further management. The literature presents varied opinions on when surgical intervention should take place.[16]

Nursing interventions vary with the type and extent of associated injuries. Specific interventions related to renal trauma include monitoring intake and output, observing for hematuria, determining the presence of myoglobinuria, assessing the cardiovascular status, and monitoring potential nephrotoxic antibiotics.

RENAL VASCULAR PROBLEMS

Vascular problems involving the kidney include (1) *nephrosclerosis*, (2) *renal artery stenosis*, and (3) *renal vein occlusion*.

Nephrosclerosis

Nephrosclerosis consists of sclerosis of the small arteries and arterioles of the kidney. There is decreased blood flow which results in patchy necrosis of the renal parenchyma. There is also ischemic necrosis and destruction of glomeruli with subsequent fibrosis.

Benign nephrosclerosis occurs in adults, usually starting after the age of 35.[17] It is due to vascular changes resulting from hypertension as well as from the arteriosclerotic process. The arteriosclerotic vascular changes account for most of the loss of renal function associated with aging. There is a direct relationship between the degree of nephrosclerosis and the severity of hypertension. The client with benign nephrosclerosis may have normal renal function in the early stages. The only detectable abnormality may be hypertension.

Accelerated nephrosclerosis or *malignant nephrosclerosis* is associated with malignant hypertension, a complication of hypertension characterized by a sharp increase in blood pressure with a diastolic pressure greater than 130 mmHg. Clients are usually young adults, with a male predominance of 2:1. Renal insufficiency progresses rapidly, with death occurring secondary to uremia in half the clients.

Treatment of benign nephrosclerosis is the same as that of essential hypertension (Chap. 26). Malignant nephrosclerosis is treated with aggressive antihypertensive therapy (Chap. 26). The availability and use of antihypertensives have improved the prognosis for clients with benign nephrosclerosis. The prognosis for clients with malignant hypertension is poor.

Renal Artery Stenosis

Renal artery stenosis is a partial occlusion of one or both renal arteries and their major branches. It can be due to atherosclerotic narrowing or fibromuscular dysplasia. Renal artery stenosis accounts for 1 to 2 percent of all cases of hypertension.

The primary clinical manifestation of renal artery stenosis is hypertension before 30 or after 50 years of age. This contrasts to the age distribution for essential hypertension, which is 30 to 50 years of age. A renal arteriogram is the best diagnostic study to identify renal artery stenosis.

Surgical revascularization of the kidney is indicated when blood flow is decreased enough to cause renal ischemia or when evidence indicates that renovascular hypertension is present and surgical intervention may cause the client to become normotensive. The surgical procedure usually involves anastomoses between the kidney and another major artery, usually the splenic artery or aorta. In selected cases of unilateral renal involvement with high renin production, unilateral nephrectomy may be indicated.

Renal Vein Thrombosis

Thrombosis of the renal vein may occur unilaterally or bilaterally. Glomerulonephritis, amyloidosis, diabetic glomerulosclerosis, thrombophlebitis of the pelvic and femoral veins, and dehydration resulting from excessive use of diuretics predispose the client to bilateral vein thrombosis. Unilateral thrombosis may result from external trauma, perinephric abscess, retroperitoneal tumors, renal biopsy, renal tumors, surgery near or on the renal hilus, and nephrotic syndrome as a result of membranous glomerulonephritis.

The client presents with symptoms of flank pain, hematuria, or fever, or with nephrotic syndrome. Anticoagulation is the treatment for thrombosis associated with glomerulonephritis. In bilateral involvement, thrombectomy may be indicated.

HEREDITARY RENAL DISEASES

Hereditary renal diseases involve developmental abnormalities of the renal parenchyma. These abnormalities are either isolated or are part of more complex malformation syndromes. The majority of inherited structural abnormalities are cystic. However, cysts may also develop as a result of obstructive uropathies, metabolic derangements, or neurological diseases.

Polycystic Renal Disease

There are two forms of hereditary polycystic renal disease. It may be manifested in *childhood* or *adulthood*. The childhood form of polycystic disease is a rare autosomal recessive disorder that is often rapidly progressive. The infant is either stillborn or dies within a few months of life.[18]

The adult form of polycystic disease is an autosomal dominant disorder. It is latent for many years and is usually manifested at about 40 years of age. It involves both kidneys and occurs in both males and females. The cortex and medulla are filled with thin-walled cysts that are several millimeters to several centimeters in diameter (Fig. 37-6). The cysts enlarge and destroy surrounding tissue by compression. They are filled with fluid and may contain blood or pus.

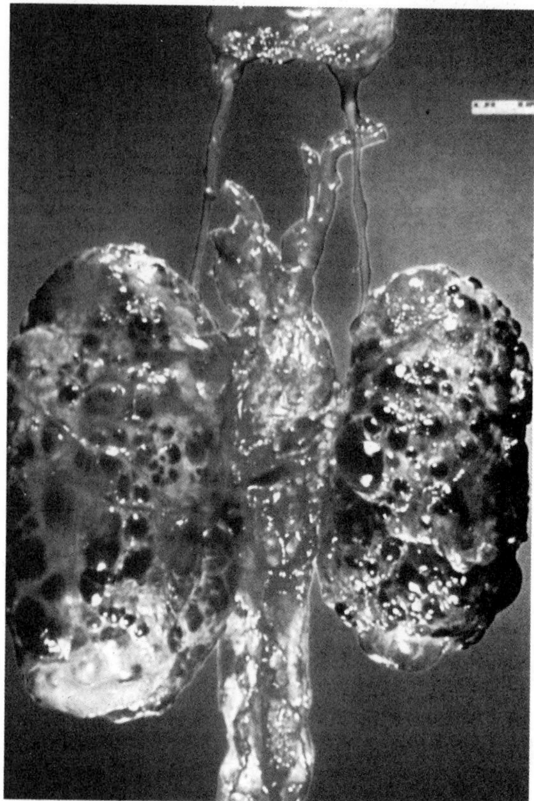

Figure 37-6 Polycystic kidneys. (*From G. Schreiner and R. Heptinstall, Chronic Renal Failure, Famous Teachings in Modern Medicine, MEDCOM, Inc., New York.)*

Clinical manifestations

The client with polycystic disease becomes symptomatic when the cysts begin to enlarge. A common early symptom of adult cystic disease is flank pain which is either steady and dull or abrupt in onset, as well as episodic and colicky. On physical examination, palpable bilateral enlarged kidneys are often found. Other clinical manifestations include hematuria, urinary tract infection, and hypertension. Proteinuria is the most common laboratory abnormality.

Management

There is no specific treatment for polycystic kidney disease. A major aim of treatment is to prevent infections of the urinary tract or, if they occur, to treat them with appropriate antibiotics. Nephrectomy may be necessary if pain, bleeding, or infection becomes a chronic, serious problem.

When the client begins to develop progressive renal failure, the medical and nursing interventions are determined by the remaining renal function. Nursing measures are those discussed in the management of end-stage renal disease (Chap. 38). They include diet modification, fluid restriction, medications, assisting the client to accept the chronic disease process, and assisting the client and his family to deal with the altered body image, financial concerns, and other issues related to the hereditary nature of the disease.

Clients who have adult polycystic disease often have had children by the time they are diagnosed. Each child of the parent with the gene has a 50 percent chance of having the disease. The client will need appropriate counseling regarding plans for having further children. In addition, genetic counseling resources should be available for his children.

Medullary Cystic Disease

Medullary cystic disease is a hereditary disorder that occurs in two forms. The recessive form is associated with renal failure before age 20. The dominant form is associated with renal failure after age 20. Most cysts are located in the medulla. The kidneys are asymmetrical in shape and significantly scarred.

Alport's Syndrome

Alport's syndrome is hereditary nephritis associated with sensoneural deafness. It is inherited as an autosomal dominant or X-linked disorder. Males are more frequently affected than females. The disease is characterized by slow, progressive renal failure leading to end-stage renal disease by 20 to 30 years of age.[18]

The basic defect is altered synthesis of the glomerular basement membrane. Clients most commonly present with hematuria and progressive uremia. Treatment is supportive. Steroids and cytotoxic drugs are not effective. The disease does not recur after transplantation.

CONGENITAL ABNORMALITIES OF THE URINARY SYSTEM

Congenital malformations of the urinary system are of concern for several reasons. An estimated 10 percent of individuals have malformations of the excretory system that are potentially significant.[19] These malformations may be the preexisting causes of infection, hypertension, or the development of calculi. Congenital disorders involve abnormalities in the amount, position, form, and differentiation of renal tissue. Congenital disorders include (1) exstrophy of the bladder, (2) horseshoe kidney, (3) solitary kidney, (4) anomalies of origin and termination of the renal blood vessels, and (5) an abnormal number or structure of the ureters.

Exstrophy of the bladder is a rare condition which can include anomalies of the bladder (located everted on the abdominal wall), pubic bones, and genitourinary system. Initially, the upper urinary tract is not involved. However, if the condition is uncorrected, obstruction with resulting hydronephrosis and hydroureters will develop. Surgical closure should be performed within the first 48 hours of life. Depending on the anomalies involved, some type of urinary diversion surgery may be required.

Horseshoe kidney involves fusion of both kidneys. About half of the individuals with this disorder are symptomatic, and two-thirds require surgical intervention.[20,21] The areas of the kidneys which are fused have poor drainage of urine, which can predispose to stasis of urine, infection, and formation of calculi. Nursing interventions include teaching related to health care follow-up, symptoms to be reported, and proper treatment and prevention of urinary tract infections and the development of calculi.

RENAL INVOLVEMENT IN METABOLIC AND CONNECTIVE TISSUE DISEASES

Various metabolic and connective tissue disease processes may have an effect on renal function. The pathological effects on the renal parenchyma are not always specific to each process. The clinical picture of renal involvement is that of chronic progressive nephropathy which can result in uremia and death. Medical management includes treatment of the primary disorder, along with symptomatic relief of the renal involvement. If renal involvement progresses to chronic renal failure, management will include dialysis and transplantation (Chap. 38). Nursing interventions include teaching the client about the primary disease process, the renal involvement, and the resulting need to comply with dietary and fluid restrictions and medication.

Diabetes mellitus may affect the kidney in several ways. Microangiopathic changes in diabetes consist of diffuse glomerulosclerosis, which involves thickening of the basement membrane, and nodular glomerulosclerosis (Kimmelstiel-Wilson syndrome), which is characterized by nodular lesions. Nodular glomerulosclerosis is reasonably specific for Type I diabetes mellitus. Clients with diabetes are especially susceptible to urinary tract infections. Chronic renal failure is a common cause of death in clients with diabetes.[22] Primary nursing interventions include teaching the client about the increased risk of urinary tract infections, the appropriate preventive measures, and when to seek additional medical care. (Diabetes mellitus is discussed in Chap. 41.)

Gout is a syndrome of acute attacks of arthritis due to hyperuricemia (see Chap. 59). Monosodium urate crystals deposited within joints are responsible for the syndrome. Renal disease may develop as a result of damage caused by deposition of uric acid crystals in the renal interstitium and tubules.

Amyloidosis is a disease manifested by altered structure and function caused by deposition of a *hyaline substance* (amyloid) in a variety of organs. The hyaline largely consists of protein. Kidney involvement is very common in amyloidosis. Proteinura is often the first clinical manifestation.

Systemic lupus erythematosus (SLE) is a connective tissue disorder characterized by the involvement of several tissues and organs, particularly the joints, skin, and kidneys (Chap. 59). Clinical manifestations of lupus nephritis are similar to those of other forms of glomerulonephritis. Most frequently found are microscopic hematuria and significant proteinuria. Renal failure frequently occurs in SLE and has a poor prognosis. Renal biopsy is usually necessary to confirm the diagnosis and to follow the course of the lesions with therapy. The long-term course of SLE is extremely variable.[23]

Scleroderma (progressive systemic sclerosis) is a disease of unknown etiology characterized by widespread alterations of connective tissue and by vascular lesions in many organs (Chap. 59). In the kidney, vascular lesions are associated with fibrosis. An immune complex mechanism has been postulated as a possible etiology. Renal involvement most often occurs within 3 years of diagnosis.[24] A peculiar feature of the renal failure is its rapid onset and progression. Proteinuria is the most common renal manifestation, although hypertension may also occur. The development of azotemia is often associated with a poor prognosis for the client with scleroderma.

NEOPLASTIC DISORDERS OF THE URINARY TRACT

Renal Tumors

Tumors of the kidney are responsible for 1 percent of cancer deaths per year (approximately 6800).[25] They arise from the cortex or pelvis (and calyces). Tumors arising from both areas may be either benign or malignant. Malignant tumors are more frequent. Adenocarcinoma (*hypernephroma*) is the most common type. Epithelial tumors arise from the renal tubules and are called *renal cell tumors*. Adenocarcinoma is twice as frequent in males as in females and is typically discovered when the individual is 50 to 70 years old. There are no characteristic early symptoms. Generalized symptoms of weight loss, weakness, and anemia are the earliest manifestations. The classic manifestations of gross hematuria, flank pain, and a palpable mass are those of advanced disease.

Several studies are used to diagnose adenocarcinoma of the kidney. The excretory urogram and retrograde pyelogram can identify changes in the renal outline (e.g., elongated calyces, invasion of the renal pelvis, calcification). Studies done to differentiate between a tumor and a cyst include nephrotomography, arteriography, ultrasound, percutaneous needle aspiration, and computerized tomography.

The treatment of choice is a radical nephrectomy. Radiation therapy is indicated in inoperable cases, with incomplete tumor removal, or when there are metastases to bone or lungs. Staging of the tumor is presented in Table 37-15. At 5 years, the overall survival is 30 to 50 percent; at 10 years, it is 17 to 28 percent. Studies have found spontaneous regression of lung metastases following nephrectomy.[26] The nursing care following nephrectomy is discussed in the section on Renal and Urological Surgery.

Wilms' Tumor

Wilms' tumor is the most common renal tumor of infants and children, with 75 percent identified before age 5. Forty percent of this type of tumor are hereditary, with an autosomal dominant mode. The most common clinical manifestation is abdominal swelling or distension. This distension is often noticed by the mother or is found on a routine examination. Other symptoms include pain, fever, hematuria, and hypertension. Diagnostic studies for Wilms' tumor include ultrasound and renal arteriography.

Medical treatment includes surgical removal of the involved kidney and radiation therapy. Radiation therapy is used postoperatively as well as for inoperable tumors, bilateral tumors, and metastases. Chemotherapy with actinomycin D is also frequently used. Survival at 2 to 4 years is 78 percent with tumors confined to the kidney, perinephric tissue, and abdominal lymph nodes. Even in stage IV (widespread metastases), a survival rate of 50 percent has been achieved.[26]

Cancer of the Bladder

The most frequent malignant tumor of the urinary tract is carcinoma of the bladder. Most bladder tumors are papillomatous growths within the bladder. Cancer of the bladder is most common in the 50 to 70 age group and is three times more common in males than in females. It accounts for 3 percent of all cancer deaths. The etiology of the tumor can involve cigarette smoking and exposure to dyes used in rubber and cable industries. Chronic bladder infections and calculous disease are involved in the etiology of the squamous cell type.

Table 37-15
Staging of Adenocarcinomas

Stage I—Limited to renal capsule
Stage II—Spread to perirenal fat
Stage III—Regional lymph node involvement
Stage IV—Distant metastases present

Gross hematuria in the most common clinical finding and the first in 75 percent of clients. Bladder irritability with dysuria, frequent urination, and intermittent bleeding may also be noted.[27]

Medical management

Medical management is outlined in Table 37-16. Surgical interventions include four possible procedures. *Cystoscopic resection and fulguration* is used for the diagnosis and treatment of superficial lesions with a slow recurrence rate. This procedure is also used to control bleeding in clients who are poor operative risks or who have advanced tumors. With this technique, the tumor mass is excised using a blade inserted through the cystoscope. The remaining portions of the tumor are cauterized.

A second technique used is *open loop resection* (snaring of polyp-type lesions) or fulguration, which is used for the control of bleeding, large superficial tumors, and multiple lesions. Treatment for large lesions is a *segmental resection* of the bladder.

When the tumor is invasive or involves the trigone (the area where ureters insert into the bladder) and the client has otherwise a good life expectancy and no demonstrated metastases beyond the pelvic area, a *total cystectomy* with urinary diversion is the treatment of choice. (The types of urinary diversion are discussed in the section on Renal and Urological Surgery.)

Radiation therapy is used with cystectomy or as the primary therapy when the cancer is inoperable or surgery is refused. Chemotherapy with local instillation of thiotepa is of some use in the treatment of superficial recurring lesions. Thiotepa is an alkylating agent which is pharmacologically related to nitrogen mustard. It is directly instilled into the client's bladder and retained for about 2 hours. The position of the client is changed every 15 minutes for maximum contact in all areas of the bladder. The usual protocol is once a week for 4 weeks. Cyclophosphamide, adriamycin, and 5-fluorouracil (5-FU) are systemic chemotherapeutic agents used in treating bladder cancer.

Table 37-16
Medical Management: Carcinoma of the Bladder

Diagnostic
1. Urinalysis
2. IVP
3. Cystoscopy with biopsy
4. Cytology studies

Therapeutic
1. Surgical treatment
   a. Cystoscopic resection and fulguration
   b. Open loop resection or fulguration
   c. Segmental cystectomy
   d. Total cystectomy
2. Radiation
3. Chemotherapy

BLADDER DYSFUNCTION

Bladder dysfunction includes the problems of *incontinence* and *retention*. Incontinence is the inability to control the passage of urine. Retention is the inability to urinate in spite of the presence of urine in the bladder. Both problems result from failure of one or more of the three components of bladder function: *storage*, *emptying*, and *control*. Incontinence due to failure of storage may be continuous (gross urethral defect) or intermittent (stress incontinence; see below). When it is due to a failure of emptying and retention of urine occurs, overflow incontinence may occur. This condition may be due to muscle paralysis or obstruction. The most frequent causes of obstruction are vesical neck contracture, prostatic carcinoma, benign prostatic hypertrophy, and urethral stricture. When there is failure of control, involuntary urination is due to a disturbed balance between reflex bladder activity and inhibitory control by higher neurological centers. These include cerebral disorders, nocturnal enuresis (found in 1 to 3 percent of adults), functional urge incontinence, and spinal cord lesions.

Neurogenic bladder is a general term referring to neurological disorders which affect the bladder. Neurogenic bladder can result from disease processes such as tumors, cerebral vascular accidents, multiple sclerosis, diabetes mellitus, and spinal cord injury.

Stress incontinence is involuntary passage of urine as a result of a sudden increase in intraabdominal pressure. It can occur during coughing, heavy lifting, or straining. It is found most commonly in women with relaxed pelvic musculature (frequently from obstetrical complications or multiple pregnancies) and in men following prostate surgery.

The aim of treatment for the client with bladder dysfunction is to preserve renal function by correcting the emptying or storing disorder, thus achieving urinary continence. The incontinent client requires a complete evaluation to determine the etiology. Treatment should correct, if possible, the factors responsible for the retention and/or incontinence. Possible interventions include surgical repair of the urinary sphincter, detrusor muscle, or bladder neck. If surgery is not indicated or is not effective, a bladder-training program can be instituted. This includes such measures as adequate fluid intake with limited intake at bedtime, muscle-strengthening exercises, scheduled voiding times, and protection of skin and clothing while avoiding diapering.

If bladder retraining cannot be achieved, external appliances or intermittent self-catheterization may be indicated. Several external appliances are available for males which prevent soiling, decrease odor, and improve body image. External appliances for females currently are not useful in most situations. Intermittent self-catheterization using a clean technique can be successfully taught to selected clients. (Specific nursing interventions for the incontinent client are described in Chaps. 52 and 53.)

INSTRUMENTATION

A *catheter* is a tubular instrument made of rubber, plastic, metal, or other material which is used to drain or inject gases or fluids through a body passage. The process of inserting the catheter into a body cavity or passage is termed *catheterization*. The nursing responsibility includes understanding the reason for catheterization, the scientific principles involved, and the appropriate care of the client following catheterization.

The reasons for urinary catheterization are listed in Table 37-17. Two reasons which are *not* indications for catheterization are (1) routine acquisition of a sterile specimen for laboratory analysis and (2) convenience of the nursing staff or the client's family. Catheters should be the final means of providing the client with a dry environment for prevention of skin breakdown and protection of dressings or skin lesions.

Urinary catheterization has become common in the management of the hospitalized client. However, it is not without serious risks. The urinary tract is the most common site of nosocomial infections. Urinary catheterization is a major cause of urinary tract infections. In one study, half of the clients with catheterized bladders developed bacteriuria within 14 days.[28] Scrupulous aseptic technique is mandatory when inserting a urinary catheter. Following insertion, maintenance and protection of the closed drainage system is a major nursing responsibility. Irrigation of the catheter should *not* be routinely performed.

Nursing management plans should include assessment of the client's capacity for bladder training or use of external devices and for fluid management. While the client is catheterized, nursing actions should include maintaining patency of the catheter, providing for the comfort and safety of the client, restoring bladder tone in anticipation of catheter removal, and preventing infection. Attention should be given to the psychological implications of urinary drainage. Concerns of the client can include embarrassment related to exposure of the body, an altered body image, and fear concerning the care of the catheter that results in increased dependency of the client.

Catheters vary in construction materials, tip shape (Fig. 37-7), and size of the lumen. Catheters are sized according to the *French scale*. Each French unit equals 0.33 mm of diameter. The diameter measured

Table 37-17
Indications for Urinary Catheterization

1. Relief of urinary retention caused by lower urinary tract obstruction, paralysis, or inability to void
2. Bladder decompression preoperatively and operatively for lower abdominal or pelvic surgery
3. Facilitating surgical repair of the urethra and surrounding structures
4. Splinting of the ureters or urethra to facilitate healing following surgery or other trauma in the area
5. Instillation of medications into the bladder
6. Accurate measurement of urinary output in a critically ill client
7. Following voiding to measure residual urine
8. To study the anatomy of the urinary system

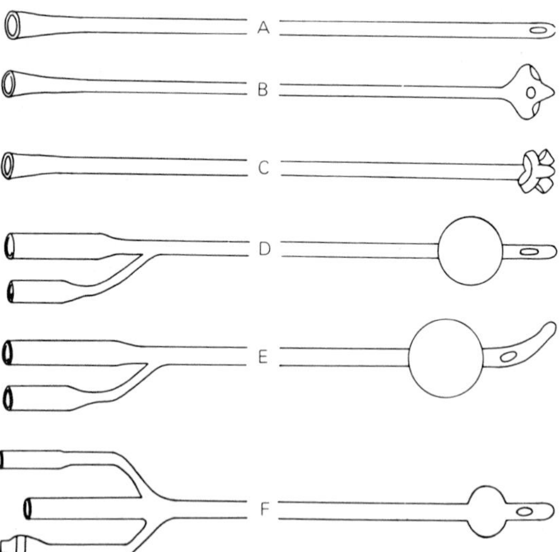

Figure 37-7 Different types of commonly used catheters. (*a*) Simple urethral catheter. (*b*) Mushroom or dePezzar (can be used for suprapubic catheterization). (*c*) Winged-tip or Malecot. (*d*) Foley with inflated bag. (*e*) Foley with Coudé tip. (*f*) Three-way Foley (the third lumen is used for irrigation of the bladder). (*From H. C. Moidel et al., Nursing Care of the Patient with Medical-Surgical Disorders, 2d ed., McGraw-Hill Book Company, New York, 1976, p. 1081.*)

is the internal diameter of the catheter. The size used varies with the size of the individual. In women, urethral catheter sizes 14 to 16 F. are the most common; in men, sizes 16 to 18 F. Problems resulting from too small a catheter include possible obstruction of the urinary flow by blood clots or mucus plugs and difficulty in passing the catheter if resistance is met in the urethra. The primary problem resulting from too large a catheter is tissue erosion secondary to excessive pressure on the meatus or urethra.

Four routes are utilized for urinary tract catheterization. These routes are *urethral*, *ureteral*, *suprapubic,* and via a *nephrostomy tube*.

Urethral Catheterization

The most common route of catheterization is insertion of the catheter through the external meatus into the urethra, past the internal sphincter, and into the bladder. Specific procedures for insertion of the urethral catheter are found in fundamental nursing textbooks. Several principles that should be considered in the management of clients with urethral catheters include the following:

1. Indwelling urinary catheters should be used only when absolutely necessary and *never solely for the convenience of the care givers*. They should be discontinued as early as possible.
2. Catheterized clients, particularly those who are ambulatory, should receive appropriate instruction regarding catheter care.
3. A sterile, closed drainage system should always be used. The distal urinary catheter and proximal drainage tube should not be disconnected except for catheter irrigation (see below). Nonobstructed downhill flow must be maintained. The collecting bag should be emptied regularly and kept below the level of the bladder. Poorly functioning catheters should be replaced. Leg bags should not be used on short-term clients since the risk of bacterial infection is too great.
4. Perineal care (1 to 2 times per day and when necessary) should include cleaning of the meatus-catheter junction with antiseptic soap. Following this, an antimicrobial ointment may be applied. Lotion or powder should not be used near the catheter. The catheter should be properly secured to the leg to prevent movement and urethral traction.
5. Sterile technique must be used whenever the collecting system is opened. Catheter irrigation is performed only when obstruction is suspected. If frequent irrigations are necessary for catheter patency, a triple-lumen catheter, permitting continuous irrigations within a closed system, is preferable. Small volumes of urine for culture can be aspirated from the distal catheter by means of a sterile syringe and a 21-gauge needle. The puncture site must first be prepared with a tincture of iodine and/or alcohol solution. Many drainage systems are now equipped with a sampling port. Silicone or plastic catheters do not self-seal. Urine for chemical analysis (glucose, electrolytes, etc.) can be obtained from the drainage bag.
6. When the client is catheterized for less than 2 weeks, routine catheter change is not necessary. For chronic indwelling catheters, replacement is necessary when concretions can be palpated in the catheter or when malformations of the catheter occur. With long-term use of catheters, leg bags may be used. If the collection bag is reused, it should be washed in soap and water and rinsed thoroughly. When not reused immediately, it should be filled with one-half cup of vinegar. The vinegar, discarded before reuse, is effective against *Pseudomonas* and eliminates odors.

Ureteral Catheters

Ureteral catheters are placed through the ureters into the renal pelvis (Fig. 37-8). The catheters are inserted either by (1) being threaded up the urethra and bladder to the ureters under cystoscopic observation or by (2) surgical insertion through the abdominal wall into the ureters. Ureteral catheters are used after surgery to splint the ureters and prevent them

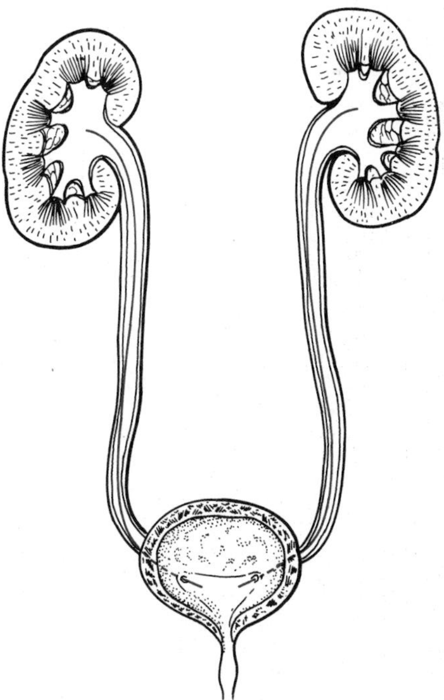

Figure 37-8 Ureteral catheters.

from being obstructed by edema or other trauma. The urine volume from the ureteral catheters should be recorded separately from that of other urinary catheters. Clients are usually kept on bed rest while ureteral catheters are in place until specific orders indicate that ambulation is permissible.

The placement of ureteral catheters should be checked frequently, and tension should be avoided. These catheters drain urine from the renal pelvis, which has a capacity of 3 to 5 mL. If the volume of urine in the renal pelvis increases, tissue damage to the pelvis will result from pressure. Therefore, ureteral catheters should not be clamped or irrigated. If output is decreased, the physician should be immediately notified. Drainage should be checked often (at least every 1 to 2 hours). It is normal for some urine to drain around the ureteral catheter into the bladder. Accurate recording of urine output from both the ureteral and urethral catheters is essential.

Suprapubic Catheters

Suprapubic catheterization is the simplest and oldest method of urinary diversion (Fig. 37-9). The two methods of insertion of a suprapubic catheter into the bladder are (1) through a small incision in the abdominal wall or (2) by the use of a trocar. Suprapubic catheters are placed either under general anesthesia when another surgical procedure is being performed or at the bedside using a local anesthetic. The catheters are usually sutured in place. The nursing responsibility includes taping the catheter to prevent dislodgment. The care of the tube and catheter is similar to that of the urethral catheter. Stomahesive is effective around the insertion site to protect the skin from breakdown.

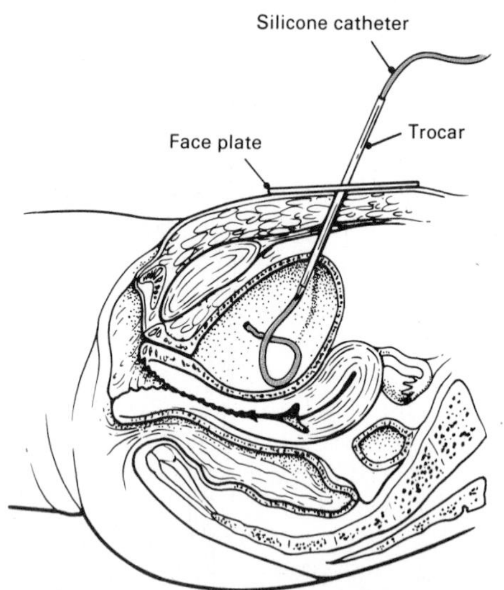

Figure 37-9 Silicone suprapubic catheter in place within the bladder. The catheter is inserted through a small incision or by puncture with a trocar. It is then threaded through the trocar into the bladder. When the catheter is in place, the trocar is removed. The catheter is secured to the abdominal wall with a faceplate, which is sutured to the abdominal wall. The catheter is attached to a drainage system. For permanent use, the catheter should be changed at least every 6 months.

Suprapubic catheters are used in temporary situations such as bladder, vesical neck, prostate, and urethral surgeries. Advantages include a reduced incidence of urinary tract infection and increased comfort and convenience for the client. Suprapubic catheterization may be used instead of urethral catheterization, especially in the young or infant male and when a urethral catheter cannot be inserted.

Suprapubic catheters are prone to poor drainage due to mechanical obstruction of the catheter tip by the bladder wall, sediment, and clots. Nursing interventions to ensure patency of the tube include (1) preventing tube kinking by coiling the excess tubing, (2) having the client turn from side to side, and (3) milking the tube. If none of these measures are effective, the catheter is irrigated using sterile technique after a physician's order has been obtained.

If the client experiences bladder spasms that are difficult to control, urinary leakage may result. Urecholine or belladonna and opium (B+O) suppositories may be prescribed to decrease bladder spasms.

Nephrostomy Tubes

Nephrostomy tubes (catheters) are now inserted on a temporary basis to preserve renal function when there is a complete obstruction of the ureter. They are inserted directly into the pelvis of the kidney and attached to connecting tubing for closed drainage. The principles are the same as those of ureteral catheters. That is, the catheter should never be kinked, laid upon, clamped, or irrigated. If the client complains of excessive pain in the area or if there is excessive drainage around the tube, the catheter should be checked for patency. Infection and secondary stone formation are complications associated with the insertion of nephrostomy tubes.

Intermittent Catheterization

An alternative approach to long-term indwelling catheterization is intermittent catheterization. It is being used with increasing frequency in conditions characterized by neurogenic bladder (e.g., spinal cord injuries, chronic neurological diseases). The main goal of intermittent catheterization is to prevent urinary retention and stasis.

The technique consists of inserting a urethral

catheter into the bladder every 3 to 5 hours. The bladder is emptied and the catheter removed. For females, lubricant is not usually necessary; for males it is. The catheter may be inserted by the individual or the care provider.

In the hospital, sterile technique is used. For home care, clean technique using good handwashing with soap and water is used. There has been no significant increase in infection with the use of appropriate clean technique. The individual is taught to observe for signs of urinary tract infection so that treatment can be instituted early. If indicated, some individuals are placed on prophylactic antibiotics.

RENAL AND UROLOGICAL SURGERY

This section will focus primarily on clients requiring renal and ureteral surgery or urinary diversion surgery.

Renal and Ureteral Surgery

The most common indications for nephrectomy are a renal tumor, polycystic kidneys that are bleeding or severely infected, massive traumatic injury to the kidney, and removal of a kidney from a donor. As mentioned in the section on Surgical Intervention for renal calculi, surgery involving the ureters and kidneys is most commonly done to remove calculi that become obstructed.

The basic needs of the client undergoing renal and ureteral surgery are similar to those of any client who experiences surgery (Chaps. 6 to 8). In addition, it is especially important preoperatively to ensure adequate fluid intake and a normal electrolyte balance. The client needs to be told that he will probably have a flank incision on the affected side and that surgery will be performed with him in a hyperextended, side-lying position. This position frequently causes the client to experience muscle aches after surgery. If a nephrectomy is planned, the client needs to be assured that one working kidney is sufficient to maintain normal renal function.

Specific needs of a client postoperatively are related to urine output, respiratory status, and abdominal distension.

Urine output

In the immediate postoperative period, urine output should be determined at least every 1 to 2 hours. Drainage from various catheters should be recorded separately. (The types of catheters were discussed in the previous section.) Catheters or tubes should not be clamped or irrigated without a specific order. The total urine output should be at least 30 to 50 mL/hour. It is also important to assess for urine drainage on the dressing and to estimate the amount. Daily weighing of the client will assist in monitoring fluid balance.

It is important to observe and monitor the color and consistency of urine. Urine with increased amounts of mucus, blood, or sediment may occlude the drainage tubing or catheter.

Respiratory status

Surgery on the kidneys is usually done through a flank incision just below the diaphragm and frequently involves removal of the 12th rib. Postoperatively, it is important to ensure adequate ventilation. The client is often reluctant to turn, cough, and deep-breathe because of the incisional pain. Adequate pain medication should be given to ensure the client's comfort and his ability to perform coughing and deep-breathing exercises. Frequently, additional respiratory devices such as an incentive spirometer are used every 2 hours while the client is awake. In addition, early and frequent ambulation assists in maintaining adequate respiratory function.

Abdominal distension

Abdominal distension is present to some degree in most clients who have surgery on their kidneys or ureters. It is most commonly due to paralytic ileus from reflex paralysis caused by manipulation and compression of the bowel during surgery. Oral intake is restricted until bowel sounds are present (usually 24 to 48 hours after surgery). Intravenous fluids of at least 3000 mL/day should be given until the client can ingest an equivalent amount of oral fluids. Usually by the fourth postoperative day, clients can eat a regular diet.

Urinary Diversion

Removal of the urinary bladder (cystectomy) with diversion of the urine to an external device may be performed in several conditions including cancer of the bladder, neurogenic bladder, congenital anomalies, strictures, trauma to the bladder, or chronic infections with deterioration of renal function. In the past, several types of surgical procedures were performed (Fig. 37-10 and Table 37-18). The most common type of surgery is the *ileal conduit (ileal loop)*. In this procedure a 6- to 8-inch segment of the ileum is converted into a conduit for urinary drainage. The colon is being used (colon conduit) instead of the ileum with increasing frequency. The ureters are anastomosed into one end of the conduit, and the other end of the bowel is brought out through the abdominal wall to form a stoma (Fig. 37-11). While the segment of bowel remains supported by the mesentery, it is

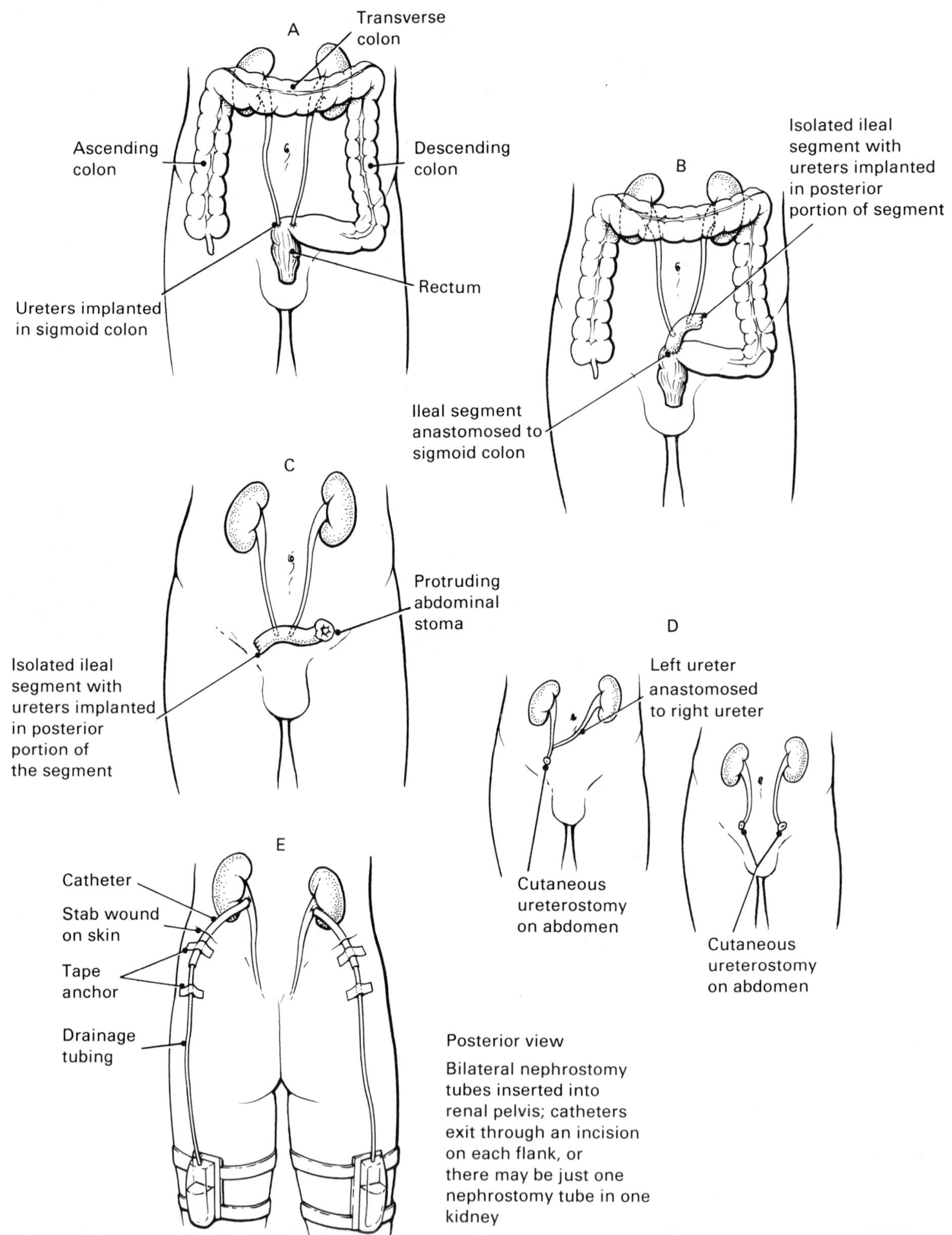

Figure 37-10 Methods of urinary diversion. (*a*) Ureterosigmoidostomy. (*b*) Ureteroileosigmoidostomy. (*c*) Ileal loop (or ileal conduit). (*d*) Ureterostomy (transcutaneous ureterostomy and bilateral cutaneous ureterostomies). (*e*) Nephrostomy. [*From D. Jones et al. (eds.), Medical-Surgical Nursing: A Conceptual Approach, 2d ed., McGraw-Hill Book Company, New York, 1982, p. 235.*]

Table 37-18
Comparison of the Types of Urinary Diversion Surgery

Type	Description	Advantages	Disadvantages	Special Considerations
Ureterosigmoidostomy	Ureters excised from bladder and anastomosed into the sigmoid colon. Urine flows into the colon and empties via the rectum.	No external drainage appliances required. Urinary control via the rectum.	Client needs to urinate via the rectum every 2–3 h. Bowel mucosa absorbs fluid and electrolytes via the bowel mucosa. Hypochloremic acidosis may develop. Possibility of reflux from colon to kidney. High risk of ascending urinary tract infection.	Frequent elimination needed to prevent fluid and electrolyte problems and reflux. Enemas usually are contraindicated. Flatus causes stress incontinence. Flatus needs to be expelled in toilet. A rectal catheter may need to be inserted for drainage while sleeping.
Ileal conduit	Ureters implanted into a part of the ileum or colon that has been resected from the intestinal tract. An abdominal stoma is created.	Relatively good urine flow with few physiological alterations.	External appliance required to continually drain urine.	See text.
Cutaneous ureterostomy	Ureters excised from bladder, brought through abdominal wall, and stoma created. Ureteral stomas may be created from both ureters, or the ureters may be brought together and one stoma created.	Does not require as major surgery as ileal conduit.	Requires external appliance due to continuous urine drainage. Stricture or stenosis of the small stoma may occur.	Periodic catheterizations may be required to maintain patency of the stomas.
Nephrostomy	Insertion of catheter (tube) into pelvis or kidney. May be done to one or both kidneys. May be temporary or permanent. Most frequently done in advanced disease as palliative procedure.	Does not require major surgery.	High risk of renal infection. Catheter predisposes to calculi formation.	Nephrostomy tube may need to be changed every month. Catheter must never be clamped.

completely isolated from the intestinal tract. The bowel is anastomosed and continues to function normally. As there is no valve and no voluntary control over the stoma, drops of urine flow from the stoma every few seconds, requiring the use of a permanent external collecting device.

The disadvantages of this procedure compared to cutaneous ureterostomy or permanent nephrostomy tubes are the extent of the surgical procedure, increased evidence of postoperative complications, reabsorption of urea by the ileum, and attention required to care for the stoma and the collecting device.

Preoperative management

The client awaiting cystectomy and ileal conduit will be given a great deal of information. The nurse must assess his ability and readiness to learn prior to initiating a teaching program. If the client is not ready to learn, the physician should be informed. The client's anxiety and fear may be decreased by the information. However, his anxiety and fear may also interfere with learning. The client's family should be involved in the teaching process. A discussion of the social aspects of living with a stoma (including clothing, changes in body image and sexuality, exercise, and odor) provides the client with facts that may allay some fears. Concerns about the effect on sexual activities should be discussed. A visit from an ostomate may be very helpful at this time. Additional interventions are presented in Table 37-19.

Postoperative management

Nursing interventions during the postoperative period (Table 37-19) should be planned to prevent surgical complications such as postoperative atelectasis and shock (see Chap. 8). Following pelvic surgery, there is an increased incidence of thrombophlebitis. With the removal of part of the bowel, there is an increased incidence of paralytic ileus or small bowel obstruction. A nasogastric tube is necessary for 3 to 5 days.

Specific attention should be given to preventing injury to the stoma and maintaining urine output. Mucus will be present in the urine because it is secreted by the intestines due to the irritating effect of the urine. The client should be told that this is a normal occurrence. A high fluid intake is encouraged to "flush" the ileal conduit.

The skin around the stoma needs meticulous

Table 37-19
Nursing Care Plan for the Client with an Ileal Conduit

Client Problem	Expected Outcome	Nursing Intervention
Lack of information about surgical procedure	Demonstrated knowledge of the surgical preoperative, operative, and postoperative procedures, including both stoma and appliance.	Instruct client in preoperative, operative, and postoperative procedures, including diet, medications, nasogastric tubes, IVs, NPO, enemas, pain management, turning, coughing and deep breathing, and leg exercises. Mark stoma site prior to surgery with consideration of skin folds, old scars, abdominal muscles, clothing lines, and client's predominant use of right or left hand. Demonstrate how to apply appliance and use equipment. Allow client to wear appliance filled with water under clothing to determine how it will feel. Answer questions honestly and provide emotional support. Assess understanding and emotional response of client and significant others. Arrange for visit with person with an ostomy or enterostomal therapist.
Potential for thrombophlebitis	Absence of Homan's sign, swelling, warmth, and pain in legs.	Teach client how to do range-of-motion exercises for legs while in bed and instruct him to keep his legs uncrossed. Turn or assist client to turn every 2 h while in bed. Increase client's activity level gradually and have him ambulate as soon as possible. Provide Ace wraps or support hose for legs as ordered. Administer anticoagulants if ordered.
Potential for paralytic ileus	Normal bowel sounds. Absence of nausea and vomiting.	Maintain patency of nasogastric tube. Encourage early ambulation. Administer IV fluids as ordered. Monitor fluid and electrolyte levels. Assess for presence or absence of bowel sounds, flatus, and bowel movements.
Potential for injury to stoma	Viable pink stoma.	Check appliance position. Observe stoma for any bleeding or eroded areas. Cleanse stoma as ordered. Allow no tight clothing or binders over stoma.
Lack of information about care of stoma and ileal conduit	Demonstrated ability to change stoma bag and cleanse stoma. Demonstrated ability to maintain permanent appliance.	Demonstrate proper method of changing stoma bag and have client give return demonstration. Change temporary bag (Table 37-20). Demonstrate care and procedure to use in changing permanent appliance (Table 37-20). Have client give return demonstration with explanation.
Possible infection or ureteral obstruction	No urinary tract infection. Patent ureters.	Empty appliance every 2–3 h. Use bedside drainage bag at night. Instruct client about symptoms to be reported, including absence of urine, blood in urine, pain in back or abdomen, elevated temperature, malaise, increase in abdominal girth, nausea and vomiting. Encourage high fluid intake—2000–3000 mL/day. No specific diet required. Cranberry juice may help decrease odor. No restrictions on beer and alcohol.

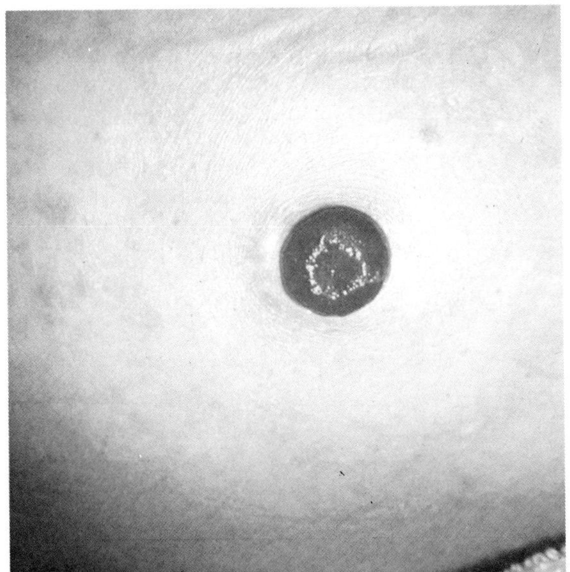

Figure 37-11 Ideal urinary stoma. It is symmetrical, has no skin breakdown, and protrudes about 1.5 cm; the mucosa is a healthy red, and the configuration is flat when the client is upright and supine. (*Courtesy of Lynda Brubacher, R.N., E.T., Virginia Mason Hospital, Seattle.*)

care. Changing of appliances is discussed in Table 37-20. Alkaline encrustations with dermatitis may occur when alkaline urine comes in contact with exposed skin (Fig. 37-12). To prevent skin problems, a properly fitting appliance is essential. The appliance should be about 0.2 cm (0.1 inch) larger than the stoma. It is normal for the stoma to shrink within the first few weeks after surgery. To prevent alkaline encrustations, the urine pH is kept acidic.

Acceptance of the surgery and of alterations in body image is needed to ensure the client's best adjustment. Concerns of the client include fear that the stoma will be offensive to others and will interfere with his sexual, personal, professional, and recreational activities. The client should know that very few, if any, activities will be restricted as a result of the urinary diversion.

Discharge planning includes teaching the client symptoms of obstruction or infection and care of the ostomy. The client will be fitted for a permanent appliance 7 to 10 days after surgery. He may need to be refitted at a later time depending on the degree of stoma shrinkage. Appliances are made of a variety of products, including natural or synthetic rubbers, plastics, and metals. Regardless of the type, all appliances have a faceplate that adheres to the skin, a collecting pouch, and an opening to drain the pouch. The faceplate may be secured to the skin with glues, adhesives, or adhering synthetic wafers. If improperly fitted or applied, the faceplate may cause skin problems (Fig. 37-13). The client needs information on where to purchase supplies, emergency telephone numbers, location of ostomy clubs, and, as indicated, follow-up visits with an enterostomal therapist.

Continent vesicostomy

A relatively new surgical technique called a *continent vesicostomy* is being done as a type of urinary diversion, especially for individuals with neurogenic bladders. The bladder is left intact, the urethral neck is sutured closed, and a vesicostomy with a valve is surgically performed to allow urine drainage. The vesicostomy is created by cutting a flap in the bladder

Table 37-20
Guidelines for Changing Ileal Conduit Appliances

Temporary Appliance

1. Cut a hole in bag to fit over stoma.
2. Remove the old bag.
3. Clean the area gently and remove old adhesive.
4. Wash with soap and water.
5. Place wick (rolled up 4 × 4) over stoma to keep area dry during rest of procedure.
6. Dry skin around stoma.
7. Apply tincture of benzoin or other skin protectant around stoma to area where bag will be placed.
8. Apply bag by first smoothing its edges toward side and lower portion of body.
9. Remove wick and complete application of bag.
10. If client is in bed most of the time, apply bag so that it lies toward side of body.
11. If client is ambulatory, apply bag so that it lies toward center of body.
12. Connect drainage tubing to bag.
13. Keep drainage bag on same side of bed as stoma.

Permanent Appliance Using Skin Cement

1. Appliance may remain in place for 2–14 days.
2. Best time to change appliance is when fluid intake has been restricted for several hours.
3. Have client sit or stand in front of mirror.
4. Moisten edge of faceplate with adhesive solvent and gently remove.
5. Clean skin with adhesive solvent.
6. Wash skin with soap and water. Client may shower.
7. Dry skin and inspect.
8. Place wick (rolled up 4 × 4) over stoma to keep skin free of urine.
9. Apply cement to faceplate and skin.
10. Place appliance over stoma.
11. Wash appliance with soap and lukewarm water. Soak in distilled vinegar; rinse with lukewarm water and air-dry.

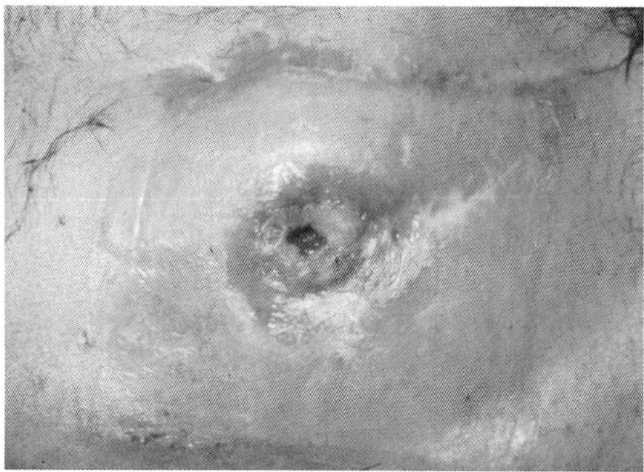

Figure 37-12 Ammonia salt encrustation secondary to alkaline urine. (*Courtesy of Lynda Brubacher, R.N., E.T., Virgina Mason Hospital, Seattle.*)

wall and shaping the flap into a short tube that can be formed into a stoma on the abdominal skin. The valve is formed by taking the other end of the tube and intussuscepting it into the bladder. This fold results in a valve that holds the urine within the bladder.[29]

An external drainage collection pouch is not necessary, as urine is not draining continuously through the stoma. The client needs to learn to perform intermittent self-catheterization in order to drain the urine. Catheterization is usually done every 5 hours. The client is taught a clean technique for inserting and caring for the catheter. Although the continent vesicostomy requires a stoma, it can be reassuring to the client to know that no external appliance is needed.

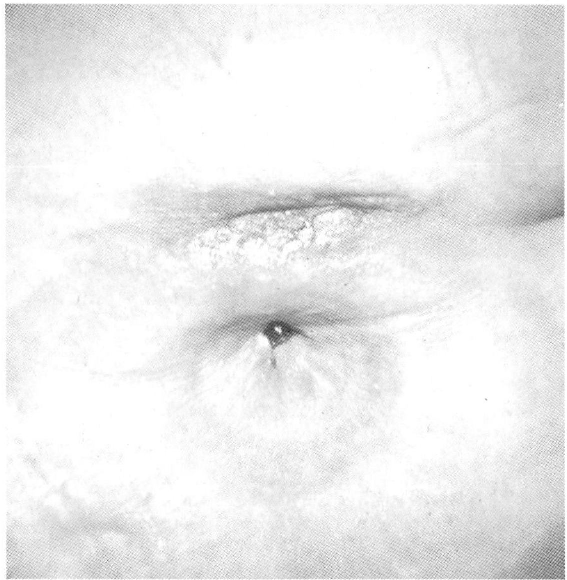

Figure 37-13 Retracted urinary stoma with pressure sore from faceplate above stoma. (*Courtesy of Lynda Brubacher, R.N., E.T., Virginia Mason Hospital, Seattle.*)

Case Study / Urinary Tract Infection

Janet, a 28-year-old woman, has had a history of painful urination for 5 months. Intermittently, she has had fever, chills, and back pain. Recently, she has had frequent urination with the passage of small volumes of urine.

On physical examination, she was in no acute distress. Vital signs revealed a temperature of 38°C (100.4°F), a pulse of 80, and a blood pressure of 100/70. She had bilateral flank pain and upper abdominal tenderness to palpation. A urine specimen for culture and sensitivity was obtained.

Discussion Questions

1. What are the most common organisms that cause urinary tract infections?
2. Identify factors which predispose a client to a urinary tract infection?
3. Identify the clinical manifestations of urinary tract infections. Which symptoms did Janet have?
4. Describe the difference between upper and lower urinary tract infections.
5. What can the nurse do to help Janet prevent further urinary tract infections?

REVIEW QUESTIONS

The number of the question corresponds to the same numbered objective at the beginning of the chapter.

1. The organisms causing pyelonephritis most commonly reach the kidneys by which of the following means?
   a. descending infection
   b. ascending infection
   c. bloodstream
   d. lymphatic system
2. Women who are especially susceptible to urinary tract infections should
   a. take prophylactic sulfonamides for the rest of their lives

b. drink at least 2 to 3 L of fluid per day
c. take tub baths with bubble bath
d. cleanse themselves from the rectum to the urethra after toileting

3. The immunological mechanisms involved in glomerulonephritis include all of the following except
a. activation of complement resulting in release of chemotactic factors
b. deposition of immune complexes along the glomerular basement membrane
c. destruction of glomeruli by proteolytic enzymes contained in the basement membrane
d. release of kinins and vasoactive amines

4. Clinical manifestations of acute pyelonephritis include
a. elevated blood pressure
b. albuminuria and edema
c. bacteria and white blood cells in the urine
d. hematuria and hemoptysis

5. The edema which occurs in nephrotic syndrome is due to
a. increased hydrostatic pressure caused by sodium retention
b. decreased colloidal osmotic pressure caused by loss of serum albumin
c. decreased aldosterone secretion from adrenal insufficiency
d. increased colloidal osmotic pressure caused by increased serum albumin

6. Clinical manifestations of renal calculi include
a. dribbling at the end of urination and pyuria
b. severe flank pain and hematuria
c. frequency of urination and polyuria
d. urgent, uncontrollable urination

7. Which of the following is inherited as an autosomal dominant disorder?
a. adult onset polycystic renal disease
b. horseshoe kidney
c. malignant nephrosclerosis
d. exstrophy of the bladder

8. Renal tissue changes that may occur in diabetes mellitus include
a. glomerulosclerosis and pyelonephritis
b. renal sugar-crystal calculi and cysts
c. lipid deposits in the glomerulus and nephrons
d. uric acid calculi and nephrolithiasis

9. The classic manifestations of advanced renal adenocarcinoma include all the following *except*
a. palpable mass
b. gross hematuria
c. flank pain
d. renal colic

10. Which of the following measures is not appropriate for a bladder-training program for incontinence?
a. limiting fluid intake at bedtime
b. muscle-strengthening exercises
c. scheduled voiding times
d. use of retention catheters during the night

11. A client with a ureterolithotomy returns from surgery with a nephrostomy tube in place. Which of the following should be included in his nursing care?
a. Notify the physician of a nephrostomy tube drainage of more than 30 mL/hour.
b. Irrigate the nephrostomy tube with 10/mL of normal saline as needed.
c. After nausea has subsided, force fluids of at least 2 to 3 L/day.
d. Encourage him to drink fruit juices and milk.

12. A client had a cystectomy and ileal conduit diversion performed. Four days postoperatively, the nurse notices mucus shreds in the drainage bag. She should
a. notify the physician
b. notify the charge nurse
c. chart it as a normal observation
d. irrigate the drainage tube

REFERENCES

1. D. Maude, *Kidney Physiology and Kidney Disease—An Introduction to Nephrology*, J. B. Lippincott Company, Philadelphia, 1977, p. 151.
2. C. Kunin, *Detection, Prevention and Management of Urinary Tract Infections*, 3d ed., Lea & Febiger, Philadelphia, 1979, p. 2.
3. P. Gonick and A. Schwartz, *Nosocomial Urinary Tract Infections*, Projects in Health, Inc., New York, 1976, p. v.
4. K. Adatto et al., "Behavioral Factors and Urinary Tract Infections," *JAMA*, **241:**2525–2526 (1979).
5. Kunin, op. cit., p. 1.
6. K. Isselbacher et al. (eds.), *Harrison's Principles of Internal Medicine*, 9th ed., McGraw-Hill Book Company, New York, 1980, p. 1331.
7. S. Robbins and R. Cotran, *Pathologic Basis of Disease, 2d ed., W. B. Saunders Company, Philadelphia, 1979, p. 1128.*
8. Isselbacher et al., op. cit., pp. 347–351.
9. C. Wilson, "Diagnosis of Immunopathologic Renal Disease," *Kidney Int*, **5:**389–401 (1974).
10. N. Simon and M. Rosenberg, "Medical Treatment of Glomerular Diseases," *Med Clin North Am*, **62:**1157–1181 (1978).
11. G. Berlyne, *A Course in Renal Diseases*, 4th ed., Blackwell Scientific Publications, Ltd., Oxford, 1974, pp. 135–168.
12. K. D. Pagana, "The Intrigue and Challenge of Goodpasture's Syndrome," *Heart Lung*, **9:**700–705 (1980).
13. Ibid.
14. R. Malek, "Calculous Disease of the Genitourinary Tract," in D. Witten et al. (eds.), *Emmett's Clinical Urography*, 4th ed., W. B. Saunders Company, Philadelphia, 1977, pp. 1171–1338.
15. B. Nordin et al., "Urinary Tract Calculi, in J. Hamburger et al. (eds.), *Nephrology*, John Wiley & Sons, Inc., New York, 1979, pp. 1091–1112.

16. N. E. Peterson and L. W. Norton, "Injuries Associated with Renal Trauma," *J Urol*, **109:**766–768 (1973).
17. Berlyne, op. cit., pp. 279–294.
18. R. N. Schimke, "Genetic Aspects of Nephrology," in Hamburger et al., op. cit., pp. 993–995.
19. J. Kissane, "Adult Polycystic Disease," in Hamburger et al., op. cit., pp. 887–891.
20. J. F. Glen, "Analysis of 51 Patients with Horseshoe Kidney," *N Engl J Med*, **261:**684 (1979).
21. J. Seguire et al., "Horseshoe Kidney in Children," *J Urol*, **108:**333 (1972).
22. M. C. Baladimos, "Diabetic Nephropathy," in A. Marble et al. (eds.), *Joslin's Diabetes Mellitus*, 2d ed., Lea & Febiger, Philadelphia, 1971, p. 526.
23. J. Bach, "Systemic Lupus Erythematosus," in Hamburger et al., op. cit., pp. 597–620.
24. P. J. Cannon, "The Kidney in Scleroderma," in Hamburger et al., op. cit., p. 635.
25. *Clinical Oncology: A Multidisciplinary Approach*, 4th ed., American Cancer Society, Rochester, N.Y., 1974, p. 258.
26. H. Abrams, "Tumors and Cysts of the Kidney," in Hamburger et al., op. cit., pp. 1044–1069.
27. *Clinical Oncology*, op. cit., p. 267.
28. Kunin, op. cit., pp. 157–164.
29. N. Barrett, "Continent Vesicostomy: The Dry Urinary Diversion," *AJN*, **79:**462–464 (1979).

Chapter 38

NURSING ROLE IN MANAGEMENT

Acute and Chronic Renal Failure

Sharon Mantik Lewis

Learning Objectives

1. Differentiate between acute and chronic renal failure.
2. Differentiate between the etiological classifications of prerenal, intrarenal, and postrenal acute renal failure.
3. Describe the clinical course of reversible acute renal failure.
4. Explain the medical and nursing management for a client in the oliguric and diuretic phases of acute renal failure.
5. Describe the systemic effects of chronic renal failure.
6. Explain the conservative management of and the related nursing care for clients with chronic renal failure.
7. Differentiate between peritoneal dialysis and hemodialysis in terms of purpose, indications for use, advantages and disadvantages, and nursing responsibilities.
8. Compare common vascular access sites used for hemodialysis.
9. Compare hemodialysis and renal transplantation as methods of treatment of end-stage renal disease.
10. Describe the nursing role for the client in the preoperative, intraoperative, and postoperative stages of kidney transplantation.
11. Explain the long-term problems of the client with a kidney transplant.

Renal failure is severe impairment or total lack of renal function. In renal failure there is an inability to excrete metabolic waste products as well as functional disturbances of all body systems. Renal failure is classified as *acute* or *chronic*. Acute renal failure most commonly has a rapid onset. In contrast, chronic renal failure usually develops insidiously over a period of time.

Although acute renal failure is potentially reversible, the mortality rates remain distressingly high despite advances in treatment. The focus in chronic renal failure has changed from treating a terminally ill client to dealing with a person with a long-term manageable chronic disease. The change in focus is due to the life support system of dialysis and to improved techniques in renal transplantation.

ACUTE RENAL FAILURE

Definition

Acute renal failure is a clinical syndrome characterized by a rapid decline in renal function with progressive *azotemia,* an accumulation of nitrogenous waste products (blood urea nitrogen [BUN], serum creatinine) without decreased urinary output. (*Uremia* is the clinical situation in which azotemia progresses to a symptomatic state.) Acute renal failure is usually associated with a decrease in urinary output to less than 400 mL/day (*oliguria*), although it is possible to have normal or increased urinary output. There is no correlation between the amount of urine produced and the severity of the renal failure.

Acute renal failure may develop insidiously with progressive elevations of BUN, creatinine, and potassium without oliguria. Most commonly, acute renal failure occurs in previously healthy individuals and generally follows an identifiable trauma or contact with a nephrotoxic agent. The most common cause of acute renal failure is related to surgical procedures.[1]

Other terms used synonymously with *acute renal failure* are *renal shutdown, acute tubular necrosis (ATN),* and *acute tubular insufficiency.* Even though *ATN* is often used interchangeably with *acute renal failure,* the former term actually describes a type of acute renal failure.

Etiology and Pathogenesis

The etiologies of acute renal failure are multiple and complex. They are categorized according to similar pathogeneses into prerenal, intrarenal, and postrenal (Table 38-1).

Prerenal causes consist of factors outside the kidneys which impair renal blood flow and lead to decreased glomerular perfusion. Prerenal disease can lead to intrarenal disease because prolonged renal ischemia can lead to tubular necrosis.

Intrarenal causes include conditions of actual damage to the renal tissue leading to malfunctioning of nephrons. Primary renal diseases such as acute glomerulonephritis and acute pyelonephritis may lead to acute renal failure. More commonly, ATN is the predisposing insult. ATN may be caused by hemoglo-

This chapter was reviewed by M. Gail Tyndall, R.N., formerly Coordinator, Kidney Transplant Program, University of New Mexico Hospital, Department of Surgery, Albuquerque, New Mexico.

The section on transplantation was reviewed by Wm. Sterling, M.D., University of New Mexico Hospital, Albuquerque, New Mexico.

Table 38-1
Common Causes of Acute Renal Failure

Prerenal (Inadequate Renal Perfusion)	Intrarenal (Primary Kidney Pathology)	Postrenal (Obstructive Disorders)
Decrease in vascular volume a. Hemorrhage b. Burns c. Prolonged diarrhea or vomiting d. Excessive diuresis Decrease in cardiac output a. Myocardial infarction b. Cardiac arrhythmias c. Congestive heart failure Intravascular pooling of blood a. Septic shock b. Anaphylaxis Renal vascular obstruction a. Thrombosis of renal arteries b. Bilateral renal vein thrombosis	Acute tubular necrosis a. Hemolytic blood transfusion reaction (hemoglobin blocks tubules) b. Severe crushing injury (myoglobin released from muscles blocks tubules) c. Chemicals (ethylene glycol, mercuric chloride, carbon tetrachloride, lead, arsenic) d. Drugs (gentamicin, phenacetin, kanamycin, amphotericin, and radiographic contrast agents) Acute glomerulonephritis Acute pyelonephritis Toxemia of pregnancy Malignant hypertension Systemic lupus erythematosus Acute interstitial nephritis Hepatorenal syndrome	Calculi formation Benign prostatic hypertrophy Neoplasms (bladder and pelvic organs) Renal papillary necrosis Obstruction in collecting ducts (sulfonamides, uric acid crystals) Trauma (to back, pelvis, or perineum) Strictures

bin released from hemolyzed red blood cells (RBCs) or myoglobin from necrotic muscle cells. Hemoglobin and myoglobin block the tubules and cause renal vasoconstriction. Nephrotoxic chemicals and drugs can cause obstruction of intrarenal structures by crystallization or actual damage to the epithelial cells of tubules.

Postrenal causes involve mechanical obstruction of urinary outflow. As the flow of urine is blocked, urine is backed up into the renal pelvis. Usually *anuria,* rather than oliguria, occurs in obstructive disorders. The most common causes are calculi, trauma, and tumors.

The two major mechanisms leading to renal destruction are renal ischemia and nephrotoxic injury (Fig. 38-1). Severe renal ischemia causes a disruption in the basement membrane and patchy destruction of the tubular epithelium. Nephrotoxic agents cause necrosis of tubular epithelial cells, which slough off and plug the tubules. Nephrotoxic injury usually leaves the

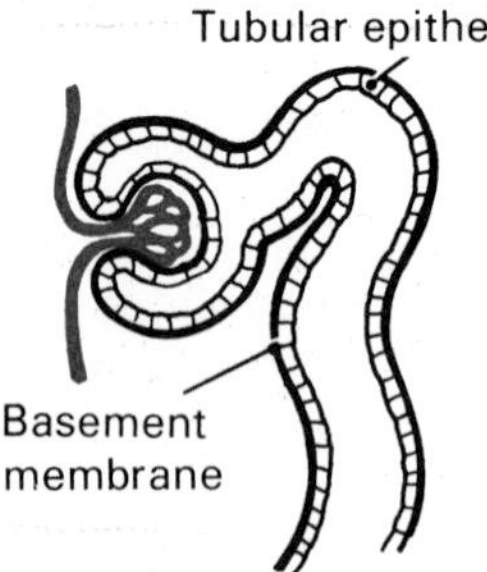

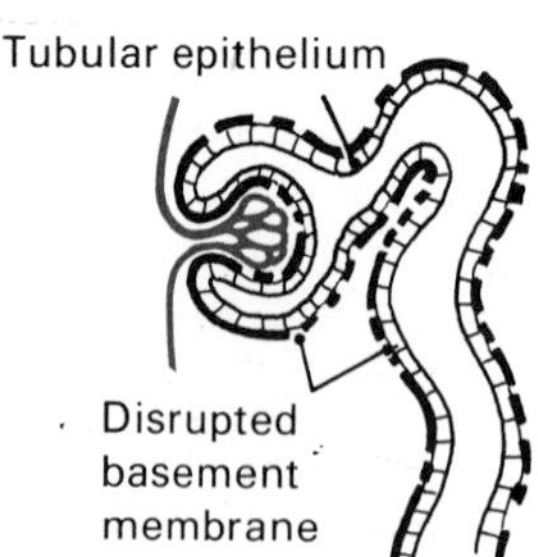

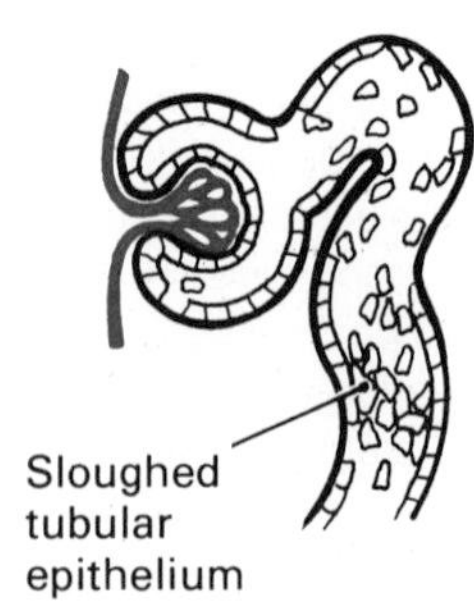

Figure 38-1 Nephron destruction in acute renal failure (*a*) Normal nephron. (*b*) Damage from renal ischemia. (*c*) Damage from nephrotoxic agents.

basement membrane intact. ATN is potentially reversible if the basement membrane is not destroyed and the necrotic tubular epithelium regenerates.

Clinical Course of Acute Renal Failure

Clinically acute renal failure progresses through the phases of oliguria, diuresis, and recovery.

Oliguric phase

The most common initial manifestation of acute renal failure is oliguria caused by a reduction in the glomerular filtration rate (GFR). The oliguria usually occurs within 48 hours of the causative event. Initially, the presence of anuria is rare unless the precipitating cause is a urinary obstructive disorder. (*Acute nonoliguric renal failure* may also occur. In this situation, the onset may be relatively insidious, with hypervolemia or an elevated BUN as the first presenting abnormality.) The duration of the oliguric phase may range from a few days to several weeks. Some cases have lasted for several months. The average duration is about 10 to 14 days. The longer the oliguric phase lasts, the poorer the prognosis.

It is important to distinguish prerenal oliguria from oliguria of acute renal failure. In prerenal oliguria there is no damage to the renal tissue. The oliguria is caused by a decrease in circulating blood volume (e.g., shock, burns, severe dehydration) and is potentially reversible. Prerenal oliguria is characterized by concentrated urine and low urinary sodium. In contrast, oliguria of acute renal failure is characterized by urine with a low specific gravity and a high sodium concentration. Prerenal oliguria can be corrected by fluid, blood, or plasma replacement to increase renal perfusion.

The manifestations of the oliguric phase of acute renal failure are changes in urinary output, fluid and electrolyte abnormalities, and uremia. The nurse needs to be alert for the presenting signs and symptoms related to these changes.

Urinary Changes Urinary output will decrease to less than 20 mL/hour. The urine may be bloody. A urinalysis will show proteinuria, casts, RBCs, WBCs, and a specific gravity fixed at around 1.010. This is the same specific gravity as for plasma. The fixation of the specific gravity at around 1.010 reflects tubular damage with a loss of concentrating ability by the kidney.

Fluid Volume Excess Urinary output decreases and fluid retention occurs. The neck veins enlarge, the pulse becomes more bounding, and edema may develop. Fluid overload can eventually lead to congestive heart failure and pulmonary edema.

Metabolic Acidosis In renal failure, the kidneys cannot excrete acid metabolites or adequately reabsorb bicarbonate. An increased breakdown of fat into ketone bodies also contributes to the acidotic state. The client may develop Kussmaul (rapid, deep) breathing to increase the excretion of carbon dioxide. This is a compensatory mechanism for acidosis.

Sodium Balance Damaged tubules cannot conserve sodium. Consequently, the urinary excretion of sodium increases, resulting in normal or below normal levels of serum sodium. However, excessive intake of sodium can lead to volume expansion, hypertension, and congestive heart failure.

Potassium Excess The serum potassium levels increase since the kidneys' normal ability to excrete 80 to 90 percent of the body's potassium is impaired. If the acute renal failure was caused by massive tissue trauma, the damaged cells release potassium to the extracellular fluid. In addition, acidosis enhances the movement of potassium from intracellular to extracellular fluid.

When potassium levels exceed 6 mEq/L, treatment must be initiated immediately to prevent cardiac arrhythmias. Before clinical signs of hyperkalemia are apparent, the electrocardiogram (ECG) changes will show tall, peaked T waves on a narrow base. This change may be accompanied by ST depression.

Calcium Deficit A low serum calcium level results from decreased gastrointestinal absorption of calcium and elevated serum phosphate levels due to its decreased excretion by the kidneys. Normally, most calcium is found ionized (physiologically active form) or bound to protein. It is unusual for hypocalcemia to be symptomatic because acidosis keeps more calcium in an ionized form. Sometimes a low serum calcium level may cause symptoms of tetany.

Azotemia The BUN and serum creatinine are elevated. If the client is experiencing rapid catabolism (e.g., infections, fever, severe injury, gastrointestinal bleeding), the BUN will be further elevated.

Eventually, all body systems become involved in the acute uremic syndrome (Table 38-2). The extrarenal manifestations are generally similar to those found in clients with chronic uremia (refer to Fig. 38-3).

Table 38-2
Clinical Manifestations of Acute Uremia

Body System	Clinical Manifestations
Urinary	↓ urinary output Proteinuria Casts ↓ specific gravity ↑ urinary sodium
Cardiovascular	Volume overload Congestive heart failure Hypotension (early) Hypertension (after fluid overload develops) Pericarditis Arrhythmias
Respiratory	Pulmonary edema Kussmaul breathing
Gastrointestinal	Nausea and vomiting Anorexia Stomatitis GI bleeding Diarrhea Constipation
Hematological	Anemia (develops within 48 h) Leukocytosis Defect in platelet functioning
Neurological	Lethargy Convulsions Asterixis Memory impairment
Others	↑ susceptibility to infection ↑ BUN ↑ creatinine ↑ K ↓ pH ↓ bicarbonate

Diuretic phase

The diuretic phase begins with a slow, gradual increase in daily urine output, which may reach 3 to 5 L/day. Although urine output is increasing, the kidneys are still not completely healed. The high urine volume is due to osmotic diuresis from the high urea concentration and the inadequate concentrating ability of the tubules.

At this stage, the uremia may still be very severe, as reflected by low creatinine clearances and elevated serum creatinine and BUN. The client needs to be monitored for deficits in sodium, potassium, and water due to excessive losses in the urine. The diuretic phase may last for 2 to 3 weeks.

Recovery phase

Renal function returns to normal when the GFR is adequate to sustain life. Recovery may take 3 to 12 months. Some individuals are left with a permanent reduction in the GFR. Elderly clients recover normal function less frequently than younger clients.

The mortality rate from acute renal failure varies from 25 to 70 percent depending on the cause. The most common cause of death is secondary infection. The incidence of infection is highest in those individuals in whom surgery or traumatic injury contributed to renal failure. The presence of infection may go unrecognized since clients with renal failure have decreased body temperature. This tends to obscure the temperature elevation caused by an infectious process.

Medical Management

The therapy for prerenal oliguria is aimed at restoring blood volume and forcing diuresis. Diuretic therapy consisting of loop-acting diuretics (furosemide and ethacrynic acid) or an osmotic diuretic (mannitol) can be used to increase the renal blood flow and the GFR. These diuretics are used selectively in attempts to prevent acute renal failure. If acute renal failure is already established, forcing fluids and diuresis will not be effective.

There is no direct medical management for acute renal failure. Because the renal lesions are potentially reversible, the primary goal of treatment is to maintain the client in as normal a state as possible while the kidneys are repairing (Table 38-3). The precipitating cause is determined and corrected, if possible. Medical management is concerned with controlling the client's symptoms and preventing complications. Conservative therapy is often all that is necessary until renal function resumes. The general trend now is to initiate early and frequent dialysis to keep the client as symptom-free as possible. Dialysis is more effective in preventing symptoms than in reversing them.

Table 38-3
Medical Management: Acute Renal Failure

Diagnostic
1. History and physical examination
2. Identify precipitating cause
3. Serum creatinine and BUN
4. Serum electrolytes
5. Urinalysis

Therapeutic
1. Treat precipitating cause
2. Fluid restriction (500mL + fluid loss)
3. Dietary management
4. Measures to lower potassium (Table 38-4)
5. Hyperalimentation (if oral intake is limited)
6. Initiate dialysis if necessary

Fluid intake must be closely monitored during the oliguric phase. The common rule for calculating fluid replacement is to consider all losses (urine, diarrhea, vomit, blood, etc.) plus 500 mL for insensible losses in a 24-hour period. For the next 24-hour period, the client's fluid intake would be restricted to the previous day's losses. For example, if a client excreted 300 mL of urine on Tuesday with no other losses, his fluid replacement on Wednesday would be 800 mL.

The various therapies used to decrease potassium are listed in Table 38-4. The current trend in treating acute renal failure is to use dialysis prior to the onset of complications. (The types of dialysis will be discussed later in this chapter.) The most common indications for dialysis include:

1. Volume overload
2. Potassium greater than 6 mEq/L
3. Metabolic acidosis (serum bicarbonate less than 15 mEq/L)
4. BUN greater than 120 mg/dL
5. Any other signs of uremic intoxication (encephalopathy, pericarditis, bleeding)

Nutritional Measures

In the past, the regimen of fluid restriction and dietary therapy was designed so that body weight would decrease by 0.25 to 0.5 kg/day from the loss of body tissue catabolized on the low protein diet. Now, these severe restrictions are usually not necessary except during the interval between the diagnosis of oliguria and the establishment of dialysis and a nutritional regimen. However, a steady weight or weight gain during this interval usually indicates hypervolemia.

If the client does not receive adequate nutrition, catabolism of body protein will occur. This causes increased urea, phosphate, and potassium levels. The major goal of dietary management is to decrease catabolism of the body protein. Carbohydrate intake should be 100 g/day to prevent ketosis from fat breakdown and gluconeogenesis from protein breakdown. Protein intake will be restricted to 20 to 60 g/day. Potassium and sodium will be regulated according to plasma levels. Dietary fat intake is increased so that the client gets at least 2000 calories/day. If a client cannot obtain an adequate oral intake, total parenteral nutrition (TPN) can be used (see Chap. 33). TPN is most commonly used in clients who have had extensive surgical procedures, trauma, burns, or altered gastrointestinal function. The treatment of these clients with essential amino acids and hypertonic glucose has significantly increased their survival.

Table 38-4
Therapies Used to Lower Serum Potassium

Glucose and insulin (IV administration)
Potassium moves into cells with glucose in the presence of insulin.

Sodium bicarbonate (IV administration)
Can correct acidosis and cause shift of potassium into cells.

Calcium gluconate (IV administration)
Generally used in advanced cardiac toxicity. Calcium antagonizes the cardiac effects of potassium.

Dialysis
Hemodialysis can bring K^+ to normal within 1–2 h.
Peritoneal dialysis may take 4–8 h to achieve the same result.

Sodium polystyrene sulfonate (Kayexalate)
Cation-exchange resin (sodium for potassium) administered by mouth or retention enema. Removes 1 mEq K^+/1 g drug. Mixed in H_2O with sorbitol to produce osmotic diarrhea.

Dietary restrictions
Daily K^+ limited to 2 g (50 mEq).

Nursing Management

Health maintenance and promotion

Prevention of acute renal failure is primarily directed toward (1) identifying and monitoring high-risk populations and (2) controlling industrial chemicals and nephrotoxic drugs. In the hospital, the clients at greatest risk for developing acute renal failure are those with massive trauma, major surgical procedures, extensive burns, cardiac failure, sepsis, or obstetric complications. These clients must be monitored carefully for intake and output, fluid and electrolyte balance, and possible blood transfusion reactions.

Streptococcal infections must be identified and treated with antibiotics. Compliance with the antibiotic regimen is critical to eliminate the source of infection. Complications of streptococcal infection include acute poststreptococcal glomerulonephritis and rheumatic heart disease. Recurrent attacks of acute glomerulonephritis are rare. There is little indication for treating the client with prophylactic antibiotics.

Older clients undergoing multiple diagnostic studies need special attention to prevent them from becoming dehydrated. Individuals with urinary tract infections need prompt treatment and careful follow-up care. Other persons considered at risk are those with diabetes, hypertension, connective tissue disorders (e.g., systemic lupus erythematosus) and others taking oncolytic drugs that cause hyperuricemia.

Industrial and agricultural chemicals and products (organic solvents, insecticides, cleaning agents) need continual monitoring regarding their safety for both the employee and the general population. Individuals taking drugs that are potentially nephrotoxic need to have their renal function monitored with serum creatinine and BUN determinations (Table 36-2). Clients should be cautioned about the abuse of over-the-counter analgesics.

Acute intervention

The client with acute renal failure is critically ill. He suffers not only from the effects of a renal disease but often from those of the nonrenal disease (e.g., surgery, obstetric complication) that contributed to the renal failure. The nursing staff may become overly concerned with the client's urinary output and forget to focus on him as a total person with many physical as well as emotional needs. Usually the changes caused by renal failure come on suddenly. Both the client and his family need assistance in understanding that the functioning of the whole body can be disrupted by renal failure. These changes are potentially reversible as the kidneys repair themselves.

The nursing role in managing the fluid and electrolyte balance is important during both the oliguric and diuretic phases. Observing and recording the accurate intake and output of fluids cannot be overemphasized. Daily weights done at the same time each day are essential in evaluating and detecting excessive body fluid gains or losses. The nurse must be knowledgeable about the common signs and symptoms that result from hypervolemia (in the oliguric phase) or hypovolemia (in the diuretic phase), hypernatremia or hyponatremia, hyperkalemia or hypokalemia, and other electrolyte imbalances that may occur in acute renal failure (Chap. 12). Hyperkalemia is the leading biochemical cause of death in acute renal failure. Most typically, hyperkalemia will be manifested with impairment in neuromuscular status and cardiac conduction. Muscle weakness, abdominal cramps, flaccid paralysis, and absence of deep tendon reflexes are signs of neuromuscular impairment. Cardiac conduction abnormalities to watch for include a prolonged PR interval, prolonged QRS interval, peaked T wave, and depressed ST segment.

Because infection is the leading cause of death in acute renal failure, meticulous aseptic technique is critical. The use of an indwelling catheter should be avoided. If acute renal failure is diagnosed in a client, the catheter may be removed. The client should be protected from other individuals with infectious diseases. The nurse should be alert for local manifestations of infection (swelling, redness, pain) as well as systemic manifestations (anorexia, malaise, leukocytosis), since an elevated temperature is not necessarily present. If antibiotics are used to treat an infection, the type and dosage must be considered because the kidney is the route of excretion for many antibiotics.

Respiratory complications, especially pneumonitis, can be prevented. Humidified oxygen, intermittent positive-pressure breathing, turning, coughing, and deep breathing are measures the nurse can use to maintain adequate respiratory ventilation.

Skin care and measures to prevent decubiti should be done since the client usually develops edema as well as muscle loss. Mouth care is important to prevent stomatitis that develops when urea irritates the mucous membranes.

Chronic management

Recovery from acute renal failure is highly variable and depends on the underlying illness, general condition and age of the client, length of the oliguric phase, and management of the client during the oliguric and diuretic phases. Even some individuals who clinically recover have a permanent reduction in their GFR.

The kidneys as well as the rest of the body have suffered a major insult. Good nutrition, rest, and limited activity are necessary to restore the client to a functioning state. The diet should be high in calories and the protein intake regulated according to renal function. Medical follow-up and regular evaluation of renal function are necessary. The client should be taught the signs and symptoms of recurrent renal disease, especially manifestations of fluid and electrolyte imbalances. Measures to prevent the recurrence of acute renal failure need to be emphasized. The long-term convalescence of 3 to 12 months may cause social and financial hardships for the family, and appropriate counseling and referrals should be carried out.

Occasionally, renal function deteriorates after initial improvement, and manifestations of chronic renal failure develop. If the kidneys do not recover, the client progresses to chronic renal failure.

CHRONIC RENAL FAILURE

Definition

Chronic renal failure is progressive, irreversible destruction of both kidneys. The disease process progresses until many nephrons are destroyed and replaced by scar tissue. Chronic renal failure has many etiologies. (The disease processes are discussed in Chap. 37.) Regardless of the cause, there are many similarities in chronic renal failure because the resulting clinical manifestations arise from the loss of functioning nephrons.

The kidneys have a remarkable functional reserve. Up to 90 percent of the GFR may be lost, with few overt changes in the functioning of the body. Humans are born with 2 million nephrons and can survive (with difficulty) with as few as 20,000.[2] In the vast majority of cases, the individual passes through the early stages without recognizing his disease state because the functioning nephrons can compensate. The prognosis and course of chronic renal failure are highly variable. Some individuals live normal, active lives with compensated renal failure, while others may rapidly progress to end-stage renal failure.

Although there are no distinct stages in chronic renal failure, the disease progression may be divided into three stages:

1. *Diminished renal reserve* is characterized by a normal BUN and serum creatinine and an absence of symptoms.
2. *Renal insufficiency* occurs when the GFR is about 25 percent of normal. BUN and serum creatinine are slightly increased. Easy fatigue and weakness are common symptoms. As the renal failure progresses, headaches may occur. Nocturia and polyuria occur due to the kidney's loss of ability to concentrate urine.
3. *End-stage renal failure, or uremia,* occurs when the GFR is less than 10 percent of normal or when creatinine clearances are less than 5 to 10 mL/minute. It is at this stage that most clients become symptomatic.

Significance of the Problem

Each year, about 52,000 people die with various diseases of the kidneys.[3] During the 1970s, there were dramatic changes in the focus of treatment of chronic renal disease. In July 1973, the federal government enacted a law that provided financial assistance for all persons covered by Social Security or their dependents who had end-stage renal disease and required medical treatment.* Prior to 1973, treatment was available only to those who could afford the cost of chronic dialysis or renal transplantation.

Since 1973, many deaths have been prevented through the use of maintenance dialysis and renal transplantation. The majority of clients (>40,000) are treated with dialysis primarily because the shortage of available kidneys has limited the annual rate of renal transplants to less than 5000 (Fig. 38-2). With the expansion of dialysis programs each year, an increasing percentage of older individuals and clients with systemic disease (diabetics and stable cancer clients) are being maintained on dialysis.

*Currently, Medicare pays 80 percent of the cost of dialysis when the client has been on chronic dialysis for 3 months or begins home training.

Clinical Manifestations of Uremia

As renal function progressively deteriorates, every body organ system becomes involved. The clinical manifestations are due to retained uremic toxins including urea, creatinine, phenols, hormones, abnormal electrolyte concentrations, and many other substances.[4] This section will focus on uremic syndrome as a total body disease and will discuss disturbances in the various organ systems (Fig. 38-3). It is important to recognize that the manifestations of uremia vary in different clients.

Urinary system

In the stage of renal insufficiency, the most noticeable sign is polyuria due to the kidneys' inability to concentrate urine. The client notices this most frequently at night, when he must arise several times to urinate (nocturia). Because of the decrease in renal concentrating ability, the specific gravity of urine gradually becomes fixed at around 1.010 (the osmolar concentration of plasma). As renal failure progresses, oliguria and later anuria occur. If the client is still

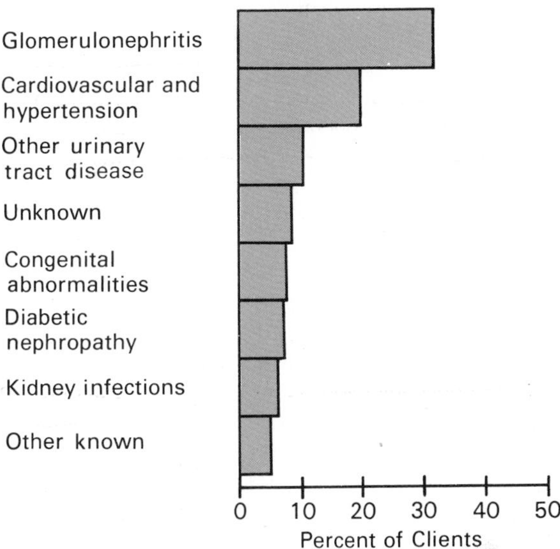

Figure 38-2 Primary disease leading to maintenance dialysis.

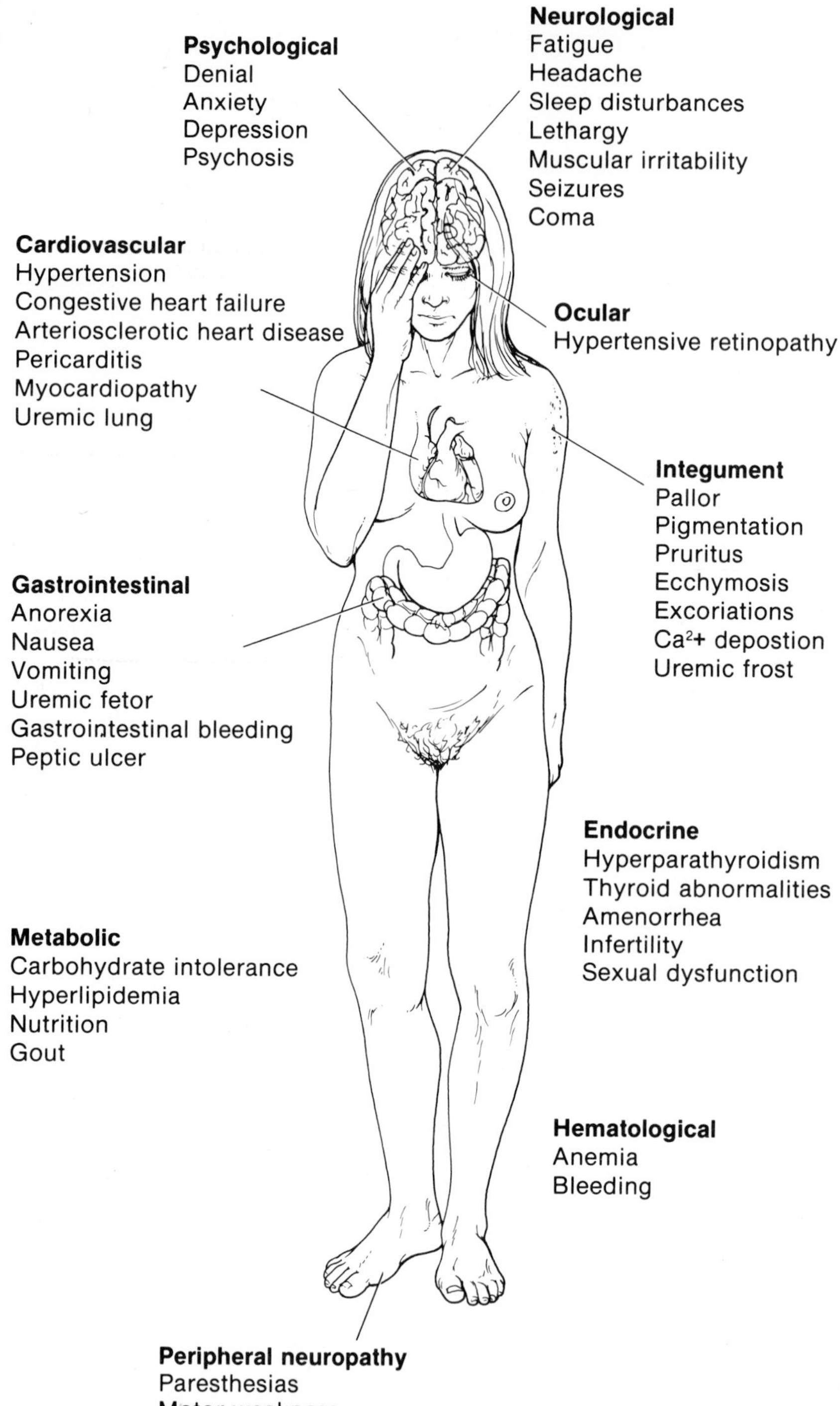

Figure 38-3 Clinical manifestations of chronic uremia. (*Adapted from Nephrology Nursing by Hekelman and Ostendarp. Copyright ® 1979 by McGraw-Hill Inc. Used with permission of McGraw-Hill Book Company.*)

producing urine, common findings are proteinuria with casts, pyuria, and hematuria.

Metabolic disturbances

Azotemia The BUN and serum creatinine levels increase and creatinine clearance decreases. The BUN levels are influenced by protein intake, fever, and catabolic rate. Serum creatinine and creatinine clearance are better indicators of renal function than the BUN. As the BUN increases, nausea, vomiting, diarrhea, and headaches become common complaints. The uric acid level also increases and can lead to precipitation of uric acid crystals causing gouty arthritis. The actual incidence of gout is low.

The initial treatment for azotemia is protein restriction. As the BUN decreases, the nausea, vomiting, and fatigue usually become less noticeable.

Carbohydrate Intolerance Defective carbohydrate metabolism is due to impaired glucose utilization and peripheral antagonists to insulin usage. Moderate hyperglycemia, hyperinsulinemia, and abnormal glucose tolerance tests are found. The insulin dosages of insulin-dependent diabetics need to be individualized and monitored carefully.

Elevated Triglycerides The hyperinsulinemia stimulates hepatic production of triglycerides, while the assimilation of triglycerides by peripheral tissues is diminished. The elevated triglyceride levels cause accelerated atherosclerosis. This dysfunction compounds the problem in diabetics, who already have increased atherosclerotic changes.

Electrolyte imbalances

Potassium Hyperkalemia is the most serious electrolyte problem associated with renal failure. Fatal arrhythmias can result when serum potassium reaches 7 to 8 mEq/L. Hyperkalemia results from the failure of the kidney's excretory ability, the breakdown of cellular protein releasing potassium, and acidosis, which contributes to the shift of potassium from intracellular to extracellular spaces.

Metabolic Acidosis Metabolic acidosis results from the kidneys' impaired ability to excrete the acid load and from defective reabsorption of bicarbonate. Plasma bicarbonate usually stabilizes at a new steady state at around 16 to 20 mEq/L. Kussmaul breathing, less prominent in chronic than acute renal failure, reduces the severity of acidosis by increasing CO_2 excretion.

Magnesium Magnesium is primarily excreted by the kidneys. Hypermagnesemia is generally not a problem unless the client has a sudden intake of magnesium (milk of magnesia, magnesium citrate, antacids containing magnesium).

Sodium Sodium levels can range from low to high. Hypernatremia does not usually develop until the later stages of renal failure. Sodium retention can contribute to edema, hypertension, and congestive heart failure. Sodium intake needs to be individually determined.

Hematological system

Anemia Normocytic, normochromic anemia is typically found. Anemia remains relatively stable at hematocrit levels varying from 15 to 35 percent. The main cause of anemia is decreased production of erythropoietin by the kidney, which results in decreased erythropoiesis by the bone marrow. Other factors contributing to anemia are uremic inhibitors of erythropoiesis, nutritional deficiencies, hypersplenism, increased hemolysis of RBCs, and frequent blood samples. For the client on maintenance dialysis, blood loss in the dialyzer also contributes to the anemic state. Folic acid is dialyzable, and if it is not adequately replaced in the diet or by drugs, megaloblastic anemia may develop in the client on chronic hemodialysis.

Bleeding Tendencies The most common cause of bleeding in uremia is a qualitative defect in platelet function. This dysfunction is due to impaired platelet aggregation and impaired release of platelet factor 3. The altered platelet function, hemorrhagic tendencies, and gastrointestinal bleeding are reversible by hemodialysis or peritoneal dialysis.

Infection Infectious complications are due to changes in leukocyte function and altered immunological response and function. The phagocytic ability of polymorphonuclear cells is impaired. There is also a diminished inflammatory response due to an altered chemotactic response. Both the cellular and humoral immune responses are suppressed. Other factors contributing to the increased risk of infection include protein malnutrition, the uremic effect on mucous membranes, and hyperglycemia.

Cardiovascular system

The most common cardiovascular abnormality is hypertension, which is usually due to hypervolemia. In some individuals, increased renin production contributes to the problem. Hypertension accelerates atherosclerotic vascular disease, produces intrarenal arterial spasm, and eventually leads to left ventricular hypertrophy and congestive heart failure. Hypertension also causes retinopathy and encephalopathy.

Congestive heart failure from left ventricular hypertrophy can lead to pulmonary edema. Peripheral edema is also commonly present. Cardiac arrhythmias may result from hyperkalemia, hypocalcemia, and decreased coronary artery perfusion.

Pericarditis develops due to a fibrinous reaction and occasionally progresses to a hemorrhagic effusion and cardiac tamponade. Pericarditis is manifested by a friction rub, chest pain, and low-grade fever.

The vascular changes from long-standing hypertension and the accelerated atherosclerosis from elevated triglyceride levels result in making cardiovascular complications (myocardial infarction, cerebrovascular accident) the leading cause of death for clients on maintenance hemodialysis.

Respiratory system

Respiratory changes include Kussmaul breathing, dyspnea from congestive heart failure, pulmonary edema, uremic pleuritis (pleurisy), and a predisposition to respiratory infections. The sputum is thick and tenacious. "Uremic lung," or uremic pneumonitis, is typically found in chronic renal failure and shows up as an interstitial edema on a chest x-ray. This condition usually responds to vigorous dialysis treatments.

Gastrointestinal system

Every part of the gastrointestinal system becomes affected due to the inflammation of the mucosa by excessive urea. Mucosal ulcerations, found throughout the gastrointestinal tract, are caused by the increased ammonia produced by bacterial breakdown of urea. Stomatitis with exudations and ulcerations, a metallic taste in the mouth, and a urinous odor of the breath are commonly found. Anorexia, nausea, and vomiting contribute to weight loss. Peptic ulcer disease is found in 25 percent of those with chronic renal failure. Diarrhea may occur due to altered calcium metabolism. Constipation is a frequent complication of aluminum antacids taken to lower phosphate levels.

Neurological system

Neurological changes are expected as the renal failure progresses. The exact cause of these changes is unknown, but they may be partially attributed to increased nitrogenous waste products and electrolyte imbalances.

A *general depression of the central nervous system* results in lethargy, apathy, decreased ability to concentrate, fatigue, and altered mental ability. Convulsions and coma may result from hypertensive encephalopathy and an extremely elevated BUN.

Peripheral neuropathy is initially manifested by a slowing of nerve conduction to the extremities. The client complains of a restless leg syndrome and may describe it as bugs crawling inside the leg. Paresthesia, especially of both legs, may be described by the client as a burning sensation. Eventually, motor involvement may lead to foot drop, various degrees of paralysis, muscular weakness and atrophy, and loss of deep tendon reflexes. Muscle twitching, jerking, asterixis, and nocturnal leg cramps also occur.

There is no treatment for neurological problems except dialysis and transplantation. Sensory impairment is often a signal to start dialysis. Dialysis may reduce the symptoms and halt the progress of neuropathies, but not necessarily. Motor neuropathy may not be reversible. The problem of neuropathy is compounded in the diabetic, who has not only diabetic neuropathy but also the neuropathic changes of renal failure.

Musculoskeletal system

Renal osteodystrophy is a syndrome of skeletal changes found in chronic renal failure. It is due to alterations in calcium-phosphate metabolism. Normally, the calcium-phosphate ratio maintains the electrolytes in an insoluble state. As the GFR decreases, phosphate is not excreted by the kidney (Fig. 38-4). Calcium-phosphate ($CaPO_4$) complexes form and are deposited in various parts of the body (metastatic calcification), leading to a fall in serum calcium levels. The low serum calcium stimulates a rise in parathyroid hormone (PTH), which causes bone resorption of calcium. This eventually leads to demineralization of the bones and an elevated alkaline phosphatase.

Normally, the kidney metabolizes vitamin D (formed in the skin or ingested) to its active form. The active form of vitamin D is needed for adequate calcium absorption from the gastrointestinal tract. In renal failure, the kidney fails to activate vitamin D and calcium absorption is impaired.

The changes resulting from increased phosphate retention, bone resorption of calcium, inadequate calcium absorption, and elevated parathormone lead to the following conditions:

1. *Osteomalacia,* or rickets (in a child), from lack of mineralization of newly formed bone.
2. *Osteitis fibrosa* from calcium resorption from the bone and replacement with fibrous tissue.

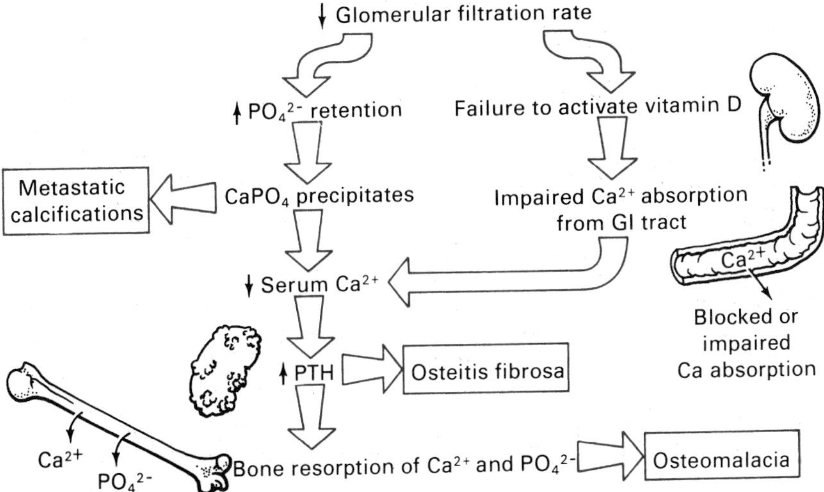

Figure 38-4 Mechanisms of renal osteodystrophy.

3. *Metastatic calcification* (soft tissue calcification) from $CaPO_4$ deposits in soft tissues of the body. Common sites are the blood vessels, joints, lungs, myocardium, and eyes. "Uremic red eye" is due to the irritation of the deposits. Arterial calcification in the fingers and toes may cause gangrene.

Integumentary system

The most noticeable change in the integumentary system is a sallow, yellowish discoloration of the skin. This change is due to the absorption and retention of urinary chromagens that normally give the characteristic color to urine. The skin also appears pale secondary to anemia, and is dry and scaly due to a decrease in oil gland activity. Decreased perspiration results from a decrease in size of the sweat glands.

Pruritus most commonly results from calcium-phosphate precipitations in the skin or from sensory neuropathy. The itching may be so intense that it can lead to bleeding or infection. Pruritus also may be due to *uremic frost*, which results from urea crystallization on the skin. Uremic frost is usually seen only when BUN levels are extremely high.

The hair is dry and brittle and may fall out. The nails are thin, brittle, and ridged. Petechiae and ecchymoses are due to clotting abnormalities.

Reproductive system

Both sexes characteristically experience infertility and a decrease in libido. The female usually develops menstrual changes, with an eventual cessation of menses. Menses and ovulation may return after hemodialysis is started. The male experiences a loss of testicular consistency, decreased testosterone levels, and a low sperm count. Some men become impotent.

Sexual function may improve with maintenance dialysis and is usually restored with successful transplantation. Some dialysis clients and many kidney transplant recipients have parented children.

Endocrine system

All clients with chronic renal failure exhibit some clinical manifestations of hypothyroidism. Tests of thyroid function yield low to low normal levels. The exact reason for these findings is not known.

Psychological changes

Personality and behavior changes, emotional lability, withdrawal, and depression are commonly seen. Fatigue and lethargy contribute to the client's feeling of sickness. The changes in body image caused by edema and integumentary disturbances lead to further anxiety and depression. The decreased ability to concentrate and lessened mental activity make the client appear dull and uninterested in his environment. The client is faced with significant changes in his lifestyle, occupation, family responsibilities, and financial status. His future is dependent on drugs, dietary restrictions, a machine, and possibly another human's kidney.

CONSERVATIVE MANAGEMENT OF CHRONIC RENAL FAILURE

When a client is diagnosed as having chronic renal insufficiency, conservative management is at-

Table 38-5
Conservative Management: Chronic Renal Failure

Diagnostic

1. Identify reversible renal disease
   a. Renal biopsy
   b. Radiographic studies
2. Hematocrit and hemoglobin
3. BUN, serum creatinine, and creatinine clearance
4. Serum electrolytes

Therapeutic

1. Correct extracellular fluid volume overload or deficit
2. Dietary restrictions
3. Multivitamins
4. Hematinics and androgen
5. Phosphate-binding antacids
6. Antihypertensive therapy
7. Measures to lower potassium (Table 38-4)
8. Adjust drug dosages to degree of renal function

tempted before chronic dialysis begins (Table 38-5). Every effort is made to detect and treat potentially reversible causes of renal failure (cardiac failure, dehydration, pyelonephritis, nephrotoxins, lower urinary tract obstruction). Conservative management is directed toward (1) preserving existing renal function, (2) treating the symptoms, (3) preventing complications, and (4) providing for the client's comfort. Conservative management primarily consists of pharmacological and dietary intervention.

Pharmacological Intervention

Hyperkalemia

Acute hyperkalemia is usually treated with intravenous (IV) glucose and insulin or IV 10% calcium gluconate (Table 38-3). Dietary restrictions of protein and foods high in potassium are needed. Sodium polystyrene sulfonate (Kayexalate), a cation-exchange resin, is used to lower potassium levels. The exchange resin, administered orally or rectally, exchanges 1 mEq of sodium for 1 mEq of potassium. The potassium is bound to the resin, which is excreted in the stool. Since Kayexalate is constipating, a bulk laxative (usually sorbitol) is given. The client should be told to expect some diarrhea.

Hypertension

Treatment of hypertension initially consists of sodium and fluid restriction and furosemide (Lasix). Antihypertensive drugs used are methyldopa (Aldomet), hydralazine (Apresoline), guanethidine (Ismelin), propranolol (Inderal), minioxidil (Loniten) and clonidine (Catapres). To effectively monitor the antihypertensive drugs, the blood pressure should be measured in supine, sitting, and standing positions. The blood pressure should be maintained below 150/100 mmHg. However, it should be noted that too vigorous treatment can cause a hypotensive reaction in a client who has compensated for long-standing hypertension.

Renal osteodystrophy

Initially, dietary restriction of protein will also decrease phosphate intake. Aluminum hydroxide antacids (e.g., Amphojel, Basaljel, and Alternagel) are used to bind the phosphate, which is then excreted in the stool. Magnesium-containing antacids should not be given because magnesium is not eliminated by the malfunctioning kidneys and does not bind phosphate. Phosphate binders should be administered with each meal to be effective. Aluminum hydroxide is also available in Alucaps and Amphogel cookies (Phos-Lo cookies). Because aluminum hydroxide does contribute to constipation, stool softeners are usually prescribed.

If hypocalcemia persists in spite of controlled serum phosphate levels, supplemental calcium may be given. The active form of vitamin D is now commercially available in preparations such as calcitriol (Rocaltrol). It is important to lower the phosphate level before administering calcium or vitamin D because these drugs may contribute to soft tissue calcification if both calcium and phosphate levels are elevated. If the renal osteodystrophy remains severe, a subtotal parathyroidectomy may be performed to decrease the synthesis and secretion of parathyroid hormone.

Anemia

There is no cure for the anemia associated with chronic renal failure. Regular maintenance dialysis will marginally increase erythropoiesis. Supplemental folic acid (1 mg or more daily) is usually given. Most clients receive oral iron supplements. Parenteral iron is used if iron deficiencies persist despite oral iron intake. Oral iron should not be taken at the same time as aluminum hydroxide antacids because the aluminum binds the iron.

Androgen therapy (nandrolone decanoate, fluoxymesterone, and testosterone propionate) will stimulate RBC production in some but not all clients. Side effects reported with long-term androgen treatment in males include increased muscular bulk, improved sexual function, and priapism. Side effects in females include hirsutism, voice changes, and acne.

Blood transfusions should be avoided in treating anemia unless the client experiences an acute blood loss or has symptomatic anemia. Undesirable effects of transfusions are suppression of erythropoiesis due to a decrease in the hypoxic stimulus and the transmission of hepatitis. It was once believed that repeated transfusions and sensitization to a variety of transplant antigens would jeopardize the chances of successful kidney transplantation. That theory has been challenged, and it is possible that the precaution is not justified. In fact, transfusions are being used in selected situations in the pretransplant stage to enhance kidney survival in the recipient.[5]

Erythropoietin is being used experimentally. However, it is not yet available commercially. The effectiveness of this product may be limited by the inhibition of erythropoietin and erythropoiesis secondary to uremia.

Drug Therapy in Renal Failure

Most drugs are excreted partially or totally by the kidneys. Drug dosages must be adapted to the degree of renal failure. A complete list of adjusted dosages is available.[6]

Drug toxicity is a serious problem to the client with uremia. Delayed and decreased elimination leads to an accumulation of drugs in the body. Increased sensitivity to the drug may result as the drug becomes concentrated in the urine.

Digitalis preparations are excreted largely by the kidneys. Digitalization and maintenance drug dosages may need to be adjusted. Dialysis does not affect body levels of digoxin, but it does affect potassium levels which can potentiate the action of digitalis.

Aminoglycosides (gentamicin, kanamycin, tobramycin), cephaloridines, penicillin in high dosages, and tetracyclines are potentially nephrotoxic. Aspirin, which inhibits platelet aggregation, can produce clinical bleeding in a uremic client.

Dietary Intervention

Protein restriction

Prior to the use of maintenance dialysis, Giovannetti and Giordano designed a 20-g, high-quality protein diet to prevent the accumulation of nitrogenous waste products.[7] This diet provided the essential amino acids from eggs and milk. No meat was allowed. In addition to eggs and milk, low protein vegetables, noodles, butter balls, and high carbohydrate foods were included. Client acceptance of this dietary regimen was poor, and clients were malnourished as well as vitamin deficient.

Today, the diet is designed to be as normal as possible to maintain good nutrition. For the nondialytic client, one guide is to restrict protein intake to 0.5 g per kilogram of body weight when the creatinine clearance is less than 20 mL/minute. Some treatment centers use a routine 40-g protein diet (Appendix B, Table 9). Because this diet is deficient in vitamins, multivitamins are prescribed. Once the client is started on dialysis, protein intake can be increased to 60 to 80 g of protein per day (and sometimes even as high as 100 g/day). The proteins in eggs, milk, fish, poultry, and meat are considered to have high biological quality because they contain the essential amino acids.

Dietary guidelines for peritoneal dialysis clients differ from those for hemodialysis clients. Because excessive amounts of protein are lost in the dialysate during peritoneal dialysis, the protein intake must be high enough to compensate for the losses to maintain the nitrogen balance.

Sufficient calories from carbohydrates and fat are needed to minimize catabolism of body protein and maintain body weight. Therefore, 100 g of carbohydrates and an appropriate amount of fat are prescribed to maintain an intake of 2000 to 2500 calories/day.

Lowering the protein intake decreases the metabolic end products of urea, potassium, phosphate, and hydrogen. As the BUN decreases, the symptoms of nausea, vomiting, fatigue, and headache become less troublesome.

Commercially prepared products are available that are high in calories and low in protein, sodium, and potassium. Liquid and powder preparations include Cal-Power, HY-Cal, Controlyte, and Polycose. Products containing only the essential amino acids (Amin-Aid) can also be used as dietary supplements.

Water restriction

Water intake is dependent on the daily urine output. Generally, 500 mL (from insensible loss) plus an amount equal to the urine output is allowed. This amount of fluid is in addition to the fluid found in food. Fluid should be counted as anything that is liquid at room temperature. The fluid allotment should be spaced throughout the day so that the client does not become uncomfortable from thirst. With chronic dialysis, fluid intake is adjusted so that ideally the client gains no more than 1.0 to 1.5 kg between dialyses.

Sodium and potassium restriction

The amount of sodium and potassium restriction depends on the kidneys' ability to excrete these electrolytes. Sodium-restricted diets may vary from 500 to 2300 mg (1 mEq = 23 mg Na) depending on the degree of edema and hypertension. (The average daily intake of sodium is 8 to 15 g). Sodium and salt should not be equated since 1 mg NaCl is equivalent to 400 mg Na. The client should be instructed to avoid foods known to be high in sodium such as cured meats, pickled foods, canned soups and stews, frankfurters, cold cuts, soy sauce, and salad dressings. Salt substitutes should not be used because they contain potassium chloride (KCl).

Controlled dietary restrictions of potassium range from 1500 to 2500 mg (1 mEq = 40 mg K). For every 20-g increase in dietary protein, the potassium intake is increased by 500 mg. This makes it virtually impossible to restrict potassium to 40 mEq (1.6 g) in an 80-g protein diet because most protein foods are also high in potassium. Foods with high potassium levels to be avoided are dried fruits, legumes, oranges, bananas, melons, green leafy vegetables, beans, peas, and coffee (unless decaffeinated).

Keto acid supplements

Keto acids of essential amino acids have been used as a dietary supplement in Europe and are now being used on a limited basis in the United States. The rationale for using this treatment is that in the body nonessential amino acids transfer amine groups to the essential keto acids synthesizing essential amino acids. Thus, nitrogen present in nonessential amino acids is utilized, and the total nitrogen intake is kept to an absolute minimum.[8] Keto acid supplements are available in liquid preparations.

Nursing Management

Acute intervention

The specific nursing management related to various problems is included in the nursing care plan for the client with chronic renal failure (Table 38-6). In addition, it is very important to educate the client because he is responsible for his own diet, medications, and follow-up of the progress of his disease. He should take daily weights, learn to take daily blood pressures (if possible), and identify signs and symptoms of edema, hyperkalemia, and other electrolyte imbalances. The client and his family need to understand the importance of strict dietary adherence. The dietician and the nurse need to meet with the client and his family on a continuing basis to assist them in diet planning. A diet history and consideration of cultural variations will make diet planning and adherence more realistic goals.

The client needs a complete understanding of his drugs, the dosages, and the common side effects. It may be helpful to make a list of the medications and the times of administration that can be posted in his home in a convenient location. The client needs to be instructed to avoid certain over-the-counter drugs such as aspirin, laxatives, and antacids containing magnesium.

It is important that the client be motivated to assume a primary role in the management of his disease. The period of conservative management provides a good opportunity to evaluate the client's ability to manage his disease. This is a critical factor in considering him as a candidate for home dialysis or transplantation.

Chronic management

The length of time a client can be maintained on conservative management is highly variable and depends on the progression of the renal failure. When conservative therapy is no longer effective, dialysis and transplantation are the only measures that can be used to prolong life.

While the client is being maintained on conservative management, the decision regarding future therapies, if any, should be made. This must be done before complications such as bleeding, progressive neuropathies, and persistent congestive heart failure occur. Dialysis is more effective in preventing complications than in treating them.

The client and his family need a clear explanation of what is involved in dialysis and transplantation. If alternative treatments are presented early enough in the course of therapy, the client has an opportunity to carefully consider his choices. He needs to be informed that if he decides on dialysis, the option of transplantation still remains. If the transplant does not work, he can return to dialysis. Many people with chronic renal failure have received multiple kidney transplants.

DIALYSIS

Dialysis is begun when the client's uremic state can no longer be adequately managed conservatively. A general guide is to start dialysis when the GFR is less than 5 to 10 mL/minute. However, this varies widely in different clinical situations. Certain uremic complications, such as encephalopathy, neuropathies, uncontrollable hyperkalemia, pericarditis, and accelerated hypertension, indicate a need for immediate dialysis.[9]

Table 38-6
Nursing Care Plan for the Client with Chronic Renal Failure

Client Problem	Expected Outcome	Nursing Intervention
Edema	Absence or control of edema.	Restrict fluid and sodium intake as ordered. Maintain a lo sodium diet. Administer prescribed diuretics. Weigh client dai Monitor intake and output. Observe amount of periorbital, sacr and peripheral edema. Give skin care, with special emphasis o edematous areas. Elevate edematous areas. Reposition clie every 2 h. Auscultate chest for rales. Observe for dyspnea.
Hypertension	Blood pressure maintained below 150/100 mmHg.	Take vital signs every 4 h (lying, sitting, standing). Administe antihypertensive medications as ordered. Observe for orthostatic hypotension and other side effects of medication. Instruct client to change positions slowly.
Nausea, vomiting, anorexia, and weight loss	Maintenance of normal body weight. Maintenance of positive nitrogen balance.	Measure and describe emesis. Administer antiemetics as ordered. Provide frequent mouth care. Provide small, frequent meals. Allow freedom in choosing food and fluid intake within limitations. Provide at least 2000–2500 cal/day with protein restricted. Provide hard candy, gum, and lollipops to improve taste.
Constipation and/or diarrhea	Normal elimination patterns.	Administer stool softeners as prescribed. Record and measure (if diarrhea) the stool. Monitor electrolytes (especially potassium and calcium) with persistent diarrhea. Teach client to avoid over-the-counter laxatives containing magnesium.
Anemia	Feeling of being rested.	Administer hematinics as ordered (at different times than aluminum hydroxide antacids). Administer androgen therapy and observe for side effects. Provide adequate periods of rest. Watch for any bleeding sites. Use soft toothbrush for oral care. Monitor hematocrit readings.
Predisposition to infections (skin, respiratory, etc.)	Absence of infections.	Provide frequent oral and personal hygiene. Avoid people with infections. Client should turn, cough, and deep-breathe every 2 h. Watch for local and systemic manifestations of infection.
Pruritus and dry skin	Freedom from itching and dryness.	Provide skin care every 4–8 h with tepid water, aquaphor, or vinegar baths. Apply ointments or creams as needed. Administer antihistamines and antipruritics as prescribed. Trim client's nails short and keep them clean.
Headaches	Freedom from headache.	Monitor blood pressure every 4 h. Administer analgesics as needed. Provide restful quiet environment.
Peripheral neuropathy	No paresthesia or pain.	Explain reason for neuropathy. Avoid trauma and excess stimulation to extremities. Avoid tight clothing or restricting bed linens. Begin to prepare client for dialysis.
Renal osteodystrophy	Prevention of bone disease. Normal calcium and phosphate balance.	Monitor serum calcium and phosphate levels. Observe for manifestations of bone pain. Provide ROM exercises and encourage ambulation. Administer aluminum hydroxide, calcium supplements, and vitamin D as ordered. (Aluminum hydroxide given with meals.) Observe for and prevent constipation when aluminum hydroxide is used.
Alterations in mental function	Mental alertness and appropriate reaction with environment.	Assess client's level of consciousness and mental status at regular intervals. Discuss significant material for brief rather than long time periods. Allow time to respond. Validate client's understanding of what is discussed. Provide for orientation (calendar, radio, etc.). Teach family how to evaluate mental changes.
Anxiety and depression	Ventilation of feelings about illness and lifestyle changes. Progress toward acceptance of chronic disease.	Listen to concerns of client. Allow time to mourn loss of body function. Include family members in discussions of client's concerns. Provide diversional activities. Discuss alternative therapy approaches (dialysis, transplantation). Offer to introduce client to other renal clients on dialysis or clients who were transplanted.

es

ıovement of fluid and particles ıble membrane from one com- The two methods of dialysis are ɔdialysis. Peritoneal dialysis uses nbrane as the dialyzing surface. , an artificial membrane (cellophane ıs the dialyzing surface which is in client's blood.

used to correct fluid and electrolyte move wastes products and drugs, and function in acute and chronic renal ıs and water move across the membrane ɔd to the dialysate or from the dialysate to accordance with concentration gradients. inciples of *diffusion, osmosis,* and *ultrafil-* involved in dialysis (Fig. 38-5). Diffusion is ment of solutes from an area of greater to an lesser concentration. In renal failure, urea, ne, uric acid, and electrolytes (potassium, nate) move from the blood to the dialysate, with et effect of lowering their concentration in the d. RBCs, WBCs, and large plasma proteins are ıarge to diffuse through the membrane.

Osmosis is the movement of fluid from an area of ɜser to an area of greater concentration. Glucose is dded to the peritoneal dialysate bath, creating a ɉreater concentration gradient in the bath to pull off extra fluid from the blood.

Ultrafiltration is a pressure gradient across the dialyzer membrane created by an increased pressure in the blood component (positive pressure) or a decreased pressure in the dialysate (negative pressure). Extracellular fluid will move to the dialysate because of the pressure gradient. In peritoneal dialysis, excess fluid is removed by increasing the osmolality of the dialysate by adding glucose. In hemodialysis, excess fluid is removed by creating a pressure differential between the blood and the dialysate solution with a combination of positive pressure in the blood compartment (using a blood pump) and/or negative pressure in the dialysate compartment.

The dialysate solution usually contains an electrolyte composition similar to that of normal plasma. Acetate, which is metabolized by the liver to bicarbonate, is used to replace bicarbonate because it is more stable in solution. The concentration of the dialysis solution may be individually determined based on the client's needs.

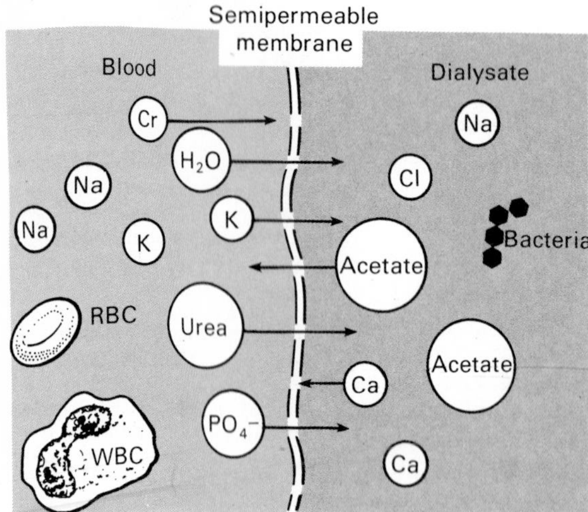

Figure 38-5 Osmosis and diffusion across a semipermeable membrane.

Peritoneal Dialysis

Peritoneal dialysis was first used in 1923 to remove uremic solutes. It has the advantage of simplicity and more widespread availability than hemodialysis. (Table 38-7). The large area of the peritoneum (22,000 cm²) is about equal to the surface area of the skin. Peritoneal access is obtained by inserting a catheter through the anterior abdominal wall with the use of a stylet.

Procedure

Catheter Placement The type of catheter most commonly used was developed by Henry Tenchkhoff (Fig. 38-6). It is made of Silastic tubing and has two Dacron felt cuffs that act to seal out organisms and to prevent their migration down the shaft from the skin. One cuff fits in the subcutaneous tissue above the peritoneum and the other below the skin exit site. The tip of the catheter has many openings and rests in the peritoneal cavity. The catheter is sutured to the skin. Tissue grows into the cuffs in 10 to 14 days, with complete healing in 2 to 4 weeks.

If the client needs only a few dialysis procedures, a stiff plastic catheter may be repeatedly inserted for each procedure. Between procedures, a Deane prosthesis may be inserted when the catheter is removed. The Deane prosthesis is a Teflon rod fused to a retainer disk that is inserted into the sinus tract from the catheter and taped when the catheter is removed. For the next dialysis, a new catheter is inserted after the prosthesis is removed.

Preparation of the client for catheter insertion includes emptying the bladder, weighing the client, and getting a signed consent form. The client should

Table 38-7
Comparison of Peritoneal Dialysis with Hemodialysis

Advantages	Disadvantages
Peritoneal Dialysis	
Instituted immediately in almost any hospital	Slower means of treatment
Technique less complex than that of hemodialysis. Can be used in clients with vascular access problems	Bacterial or chemical peritonitis
Fluid and electrolyte changes more gradual	Protein loss into dialysate
Immediate life-threatening events less likely to occur	Abdominal surgery, ileus, bowel perforation are contraindications to use
Home dialysis possible	Crowding of thoracic organs by large amount of dialysate
Hemodialysis	
Rapid, efficient means of treatment	Specially trained personnel required
Home dialysis possible	Usually available only in larger hospitals
Better biochemical control	Vascular access required
	Transmission of hepatitis
	Heparinization may result in bleeding
	Added blood loss contributes to anemia

have his head raised and should tighten his abdominal muscles immediately prior to catheter insertion. The area 2 to 5 cm (1 to 2 inches) below the umbilicus is anesthetized with a local anesthetic. A trocar (stylet) is inserted into the peritoneal cavity. A catheter is threaded through or over the trocar. When the catheter is in place, the client may feel the urge to defecate. Complications of catheter insertion include perforation of the bladder, bowel, or blood vessel and introduction of bacteria. After the catheter is inserted, the skin is cleaned with an antiseptic solution and a sterile dressing is applied.

Once the catheter incision site is healed, the client may shower. Daily catheter care includes application of an antiseptic solution and sterile dressing, as well as examination of the catheter site for signs of infection. The external end of the catheter is covered by a removable cap. The average life expectancy of the catheter is 9 to 12 months.

Dialysis cycle

Dialysis solutions are available commercially in 2-L bottles or plastic bags (Dianeal, Inpersol, Peridial). Both 1.5% and 4.25% dextrose solutions are used. The electrolyte composition is similar to that of plasma. The concentration of potassium added to the solution depends on the client's needs. A small dose of heparin is added to prevent fibrin from clotting the

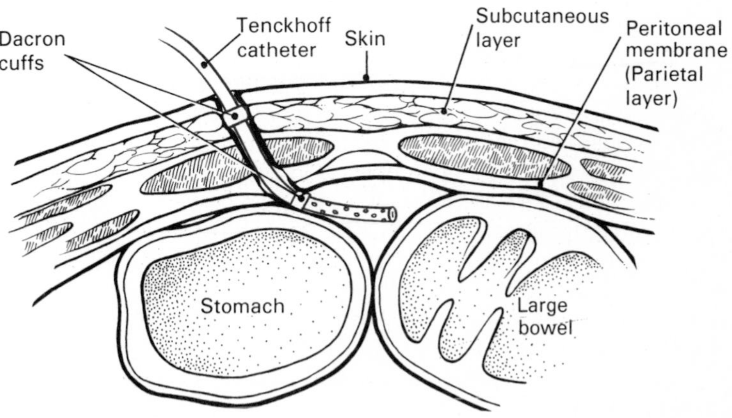

Figure 38-6 Tenckhoff catheter used in peritoneal dialysis.

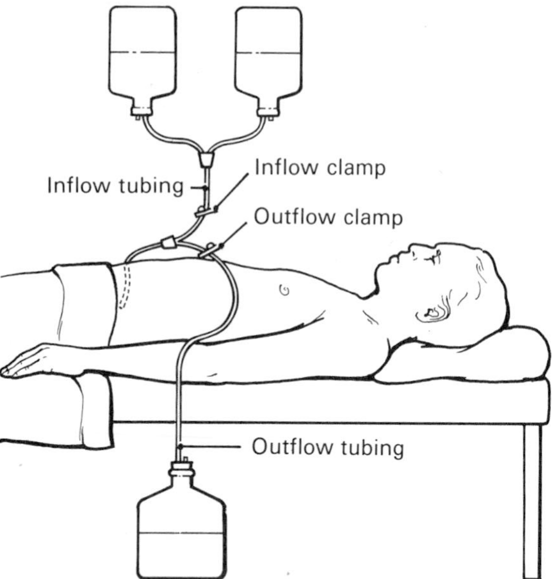

Figure 38-7 Manual peritoneal dialysis setup.

catheter. When adding medications, extreme care must be used to prevent contamination.

The dialysis solution is warmed to body temperature to increase peritoneal clearance, prevent hypothermia, and make the client more comfortable. The peritoneal catheter is connected to the dialysis inflow and outflow tubing by a Y connector after air has been cleared from the tubing (Fig. 38-7). There is an inflow and an outflow clamp on the tubing.

The dialysis cycle is started by closing the outflow clamp and opening the inflow clamp. The three phases of the cycle are *inflow, dwell time* or *equilibration,* and *drain.* During inflow, 2 L of solution is infused in about 10 minutes. The flow rate may be decreased if the client becomes uncomfortable. After the 2 L has been infused, the inflow clamp is closed before air enters the tubing.

The next part of the cycle is dwell time or equilibration, which allows for diffusion and osmosis between the client's blood and the peritoneal cavity. About 20 to 30 minutes are allowed for equilibration, and then the outflow clamp is opened to begin the drain time. Drain time takes 20 to 30 minutes and may be facilitated by gently massaging the abdomen or by changing the client's position. The cycle starts again with the infusion of another 2 L of solution. Acute (short-term) peritoneal dialysis will be performed continually for 24 to 72 hours. A client managed with chronic maintenance peritoneal dialysis will need to dialyze 3 to 5 times per week for 8 to 12 hours.

Nursing intervention

Even though the procedure is not technically difficult, the client often has fears about the tube penetrating into his abdomen. He needs a full explanation of the procedure and the principles involved. The minimal pain associated with the procedure is usually due to the movement and irritation of the catheter. During the dwell time, a feeling of abdominal fullness will be experienced.

There are specific nursing interventions in peritoneal dialysis. Meticulous aseptic technique is needed to prevent peritonitis. The client's weight needs to be checked prior to the procedure. Frequent vital signs should be taken to monitor his progress. A flow sheet (Fig. 38-8) is used to record the fluid exchange. For each exchange, the following should be recorded:

Starting time
Amount of fluid instilled
Concentration of solution
Addition of medications
Finishing time of inflow
Starting time of outflow
Color of outflow
Finishing time of outflow
Amount of negative or positive balance

If the amount of dialysate drained exceeds the amount infused the cumulative balance is negative. If the amount drained is less than the amount infused, the balance is positive. The color of the outflow should be a clear yellow. The first exchange may be pink or slightly bloody. A cloudy color indicates infection and a reddish color indicates bleeding.

The physician will establish guidelines regarding the amount of time needed for the inflow, dwell, and drain phases. Acceptable limits for positive and negative balances will also be determined. If drainage does not occur in the allotted time period, the physician should be notified because the catheter may be blocked or adherent to the peritoneum.

During dialysis the nurse should observe for fluid leaks around the insertion site, and for manifestations of hypovolemia (especially with a 4.25% glucose solution), peritonitis, respiratory distress, and hyperglycemia due to absorption of glucose from the dialysate fluid.

Complications of peritoneal dialysis

Pain Although it is not severe, the most common complication is pain due to the placement of the catheter. Pain results when the tip of the catheter

PERITONEAL DIALYSIS FLOW SHEET

Client ______

Weight Prior ____ Weight on Completion ____

Date	Solution 1.5%	Solution 4.25%	Medication Added to Solution	Other Medication or Remarks	Solution In: Starting Time	Solution In: Finish Time	Solution In: Vol.	Solution Out: Starting Time	Solution Out: Finish Time	Solution Out: Vol.	Difference Plus or Minus	Cumulative Difference
	X				7:00 A.M.	7:10 A.M.	2000	7:40 A.M.	8:00 A.M.	2200	-200	-200
		X	KCl 8 mEq		8:00 A.M.	8:10 A.M.	2000	8:40 A.M.	9:00 A.M.	1900	+100	-100

Figure 38-8 Peritoneal dialysis flow sheet.

touches the bladder, bowel, or peritoneum. A change in the placement of the catheter should correct this problem.

Bleeding Dialysis fluid on the first exchange may be pink or slightly bloody due to the trauma of catheter insertion. Gross bleeding indicates injury to the abdominal wall.

Peritonitis Peritonitis results from contamination of the solution or tubing while preparing the exchange. The clinical manifestations of peritonitis are fever and diffuse abdominal pain. Hyperactive bowel sounds, diarrhea, and vomiting may also be present. Appropriate antibiotic therapy is started both systemically and intraperitoneally. Adhesion formation in the peritoneum can result from repeated infections, which decrease its ability as a dialyzing membrane. Many institutions recommend routine cultures of the outflow fluid at the end of a dialysis period. If the culture shows more than 50 cells per cubic millimeter, antibiotics (cefazolin, gentamicin, or tobramycin) are usually started.

Pulmonary Complications Atelectasis, pneumonia, and bronchitis may occur from repeated upward displacement of the diaphragm, resulting in decreased lung expansion. The longer the dialysis period, the greater the likelihood of pulmonary complications.

Protein Loss Plasma proteins, amino acids, and polypeptides are lost in the dialysate fluid. The amount of loss may be as much as 0.5 to 1.0 g per exchange of dialysate fluid. On chronic peritoneal dialysis, it is possible to lose 30 to 70 g of protein in a week. The client can maintain a positive nitrogen balance with satisfactory protein intake.

Chronic Peritoneal Dialysis

The use and popularity of chronic peritoneal dialysis is increasing. Peritoneal dialysis is indicated especially for those individuals who have vascular access problems and respond poorly to the hemodynamic stresses of hemodialysis. Individuals with cardiovascular complications due to diabetes and those with polyneuropathies seem to do better on peritoneal dialysis than on hemodialysis. Although biochemical control is not as good as in hemodialysis, clients seem to do equally well clinically and sometimes better.

Intermittent peritoneal dialysis

Maintenance peritoneal dialysis has progressed because of automated peritoneal dialysis systems and bacteriologically safer peritoneal catheters. Closed automated dialysate delivery and drainage systems have reduced the amount of time needed and have significantly lowered the incidence of peritonitis compared with manual methods. The automated equipment (Fig. 38-9) can accomplish in 10 to 12 hours the same fluid removal the manual technique took 24 to 36 hours to accomplish.

One type of automated machine sterilizes tap water, mixes the water with the peritoneal dialysate, warms the dialysate, and then pumps it into the

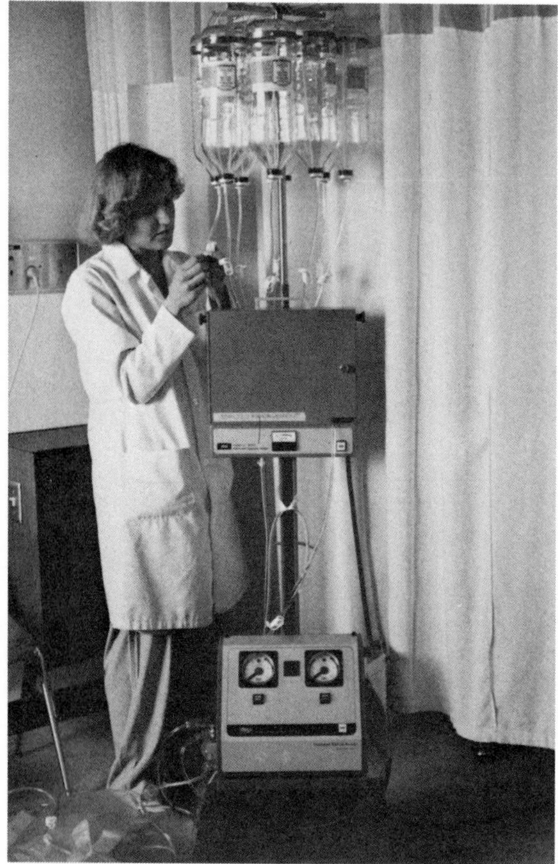

Figure 38-9 Automated peritoneal dialysis machine.

peritoneal cavity at a predetermined rate. Adjustable timers control the duration of each phase, and alarms are activated when preset limits are violated. Some machines weigh the drainage for record keeping.

It is much easier to train clients and their families to use the peritoneal dialysis machines at home compared with hemodialysis equipment. Some clients start the dialysis at bedtime and disconnect in the morning. Dialysis is usually performed for 8 to 12 hours 3 to 5 times per week. A client can manage chronic peritoneal dialysis at home by himself.

Continuous ambulatory peritoneal dialysis

In 1976, a new concept in peritoneal dialysis was developed called *continuous ambulatory peritoneal dialysis*[10] (CAPD) (Fig. 38-10). A permanent peritoneal catheter is inserted and the dialysis exchanges are performed throughout the day. Four exchanges of 2-L dialysate solutions are used each day.[11] Three exchanges remain in the peritoneum for 5 hours at a time, and the fourth exchange remains in overnight. One schedule, for example, starts the three exchanges at 7 A.M., 12 noon, and 5 P.M. and the fourth exchange at 10 P.M. A 2-L plastic bag with tubing is attached to the peritoneal catheter. An inflow time of 6 to 10 minutes is allowed. After inflow the clamps are closed, and the bag and tube are folded into a cloth pouch and concealed under a shirt or blouse. The dwell time lasts for 5 hours or overnight. At the end of dwell time the pouch is removed, the bag and tubing are lowered to the floor, the tubing is unclamped, and the solution drains out in 20 minutes. The bag is discarded and a new 2-L bag is used to start the new cycle. The tubing is changed every 1 to 2 weeks.

The advantages of chronic ambulatory peritoneal dialysis are better urea and biochemical clearance than with intermittent peritoneal dialysis, little or no dietary restrictions (80 to 100 g of protein per day), and greater mobility than with conventional peritoneal dialysis or hemodialysis. The client can dialyze in the car, on an airplane, at work, or while shopping. The major disadvantage is peritonitis, which occurs twice as often as with conventional peritoneal dialysis. As further improvements in the technique are made, the incidence of peritonitis should decrease.

Hemodialysis

In 1943, Willem Kolff in the Netherlands performed the first dialysis on a human using a rotating-drum dialyzer. After coming to the United States during World War II, he established dialysis treatment in the 1950s.

Vascular access sites

Vascular access is one of the major problems with hemodialysis. Prior to 1960, hemodialysis required the insertion of needles into the arterial and venous systems for each dialysis. Long-term dialysis was not possible using this technique. In 1960, Scribner developed a Teflon Silastic cannula that could be inserted into the radial artery and into an adjacent forearm vein (Fig. 38-11). The cannula is implanted subcutaneously and connected by Silastic tubing that exits from the skin. The two ends are connected by a U-shaped shunt. The *external access cannula* is commonly referred to as an *external shunt.* The shunt can be disconnected for dialysis to allow arterial blood to flow through the artificial kidney and return to the venous side. The external shunt is now becoming less common. It is used primarily in treating acute renal failure. (The external shunt is being replaced by femoral and subclavian vein catheterization.)[12]

The main complications with the external shunt

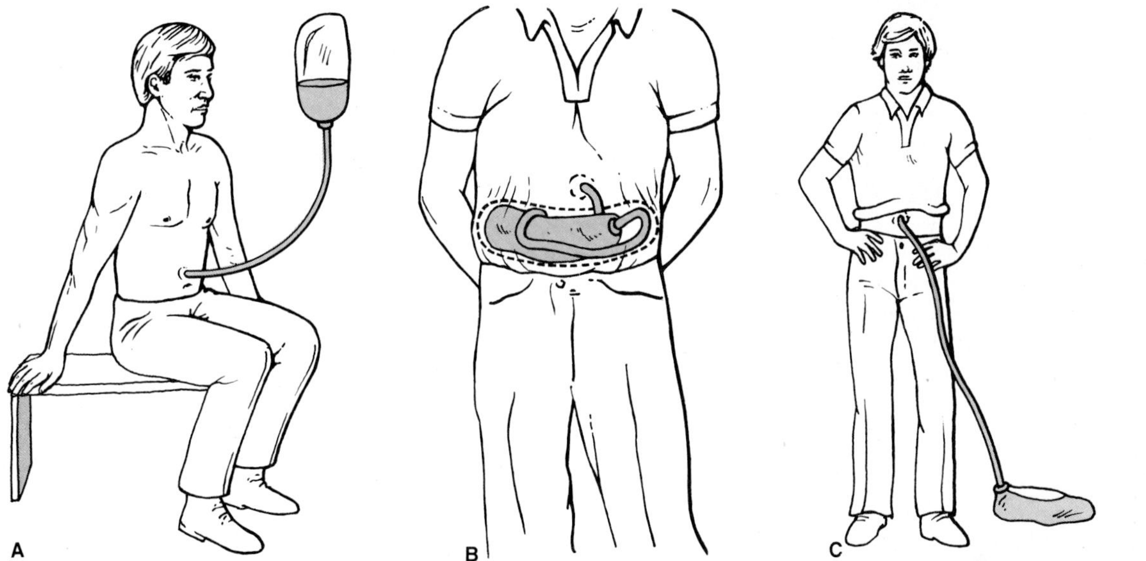

Figure 38-10 Chronic ambulatory peritoneal dialysis. (*a*) Inflow period. (*b*) Bag and tubing placed in cloth pouch during dwell period. (*c*) Drain period.

are clotting, local and systemic infection, erosion of overlying skin, and cosmetic hindrance. The usual life span of a shunt is 6 to 12 months. Daily care for the external cannula consists of cleansing the suture sites with antiseptic solution, observing and palpating blood flow through the shunt, observing for local and systemic signs of infection, and *never* taking a blood pressure or blood sample from the affected extremity. The client has to learn to limit activity with the arm, and avoid swimming and contact sports.

In 1966, the use of the subcutaneous *internal arteriovenous fistula* (Fig. 38-11) was introduced by Cimino and Brescia. An arteriovenous (AV) fistula is created in the forearm or thigh by a side-to-side, end-to-side, or end-to-end anastomosis between an artery (usually radial or ulnar) and a vein. The fistula provides for arterial blood flow through the vein. The increased pressure of the arterial blood flow through the vein makes it accessible for venipuncture. The anastomosis requires about 6 weeks to develop before it can be used. Two 14- to 15-gauge needles are inserted into the engorged vein under local anesthesia. The "venous" needle is placed proximal toward the elbow and the "arterial" needle is placed distal toward the wrist. The venous needle can be placed in any vein for the venous return.

The patency of the internal shunt can be monitored by observing for shunt discoloration. Normally, a thrill can be felt by palpating the area of anastomosis and a bruit can be heard with a stethoscope. Blood pressures and venipuncture should *not* be performed on the affected extremity.

The subcutaneous AV fistula is much less likely to clot and become infected than the external cannula. In fact, good ones seem to get better as the years go by. The main problem is thrombosis due to several years of use. Some people develop distal ischemia (steal syndrome) due to the bypass of arterial blood. Another complication is the development of an aneurysm at the fistula site.

Other vascular access routes that have been developed include autogenous vein grafts, bovine grafts, and the use of synthetic materials. The bovine carotid artery is surgically anastomosed between the brachial artery and any vein (Fig. 38-11). Bovine grafts are also used in femoral vessels. Dacron-Teflon grafts can be similarly inserted and become endothelialized so that they eventually become part of the blood vessel.

In some situations, when temporary vascular access is required, *percutaneous cannulation* of the femoral or subclavian vein is used. A flexible, Shaldon-type catheter is inserted into these large veins and provides easy access to circulation without the need for the client to have surgery or to sacrifice a peripheral artery or vein. The procedure for percutaneous cannulation is similar to the method of insertion of a central venous pressure line (Chap. 25). One catheter which alternates inflow and outflow blood cycles may be used. However, it is preferable to use two catheters

Hemodialysis

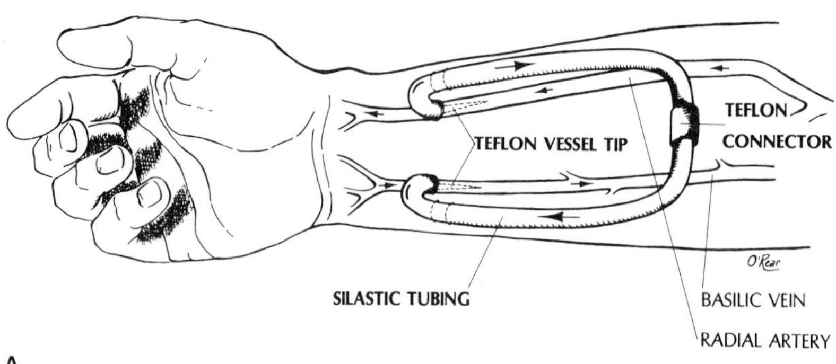

A

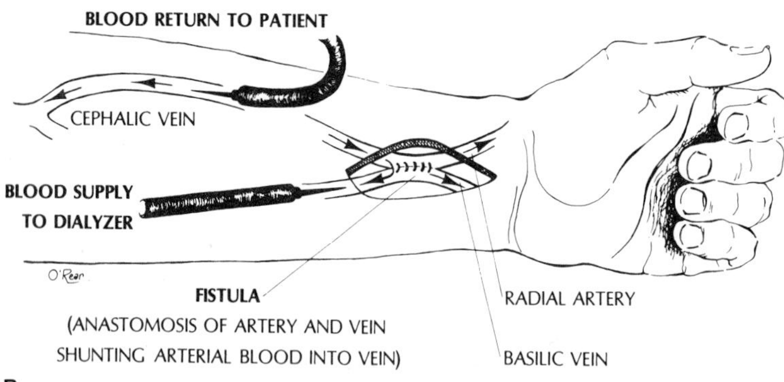

B

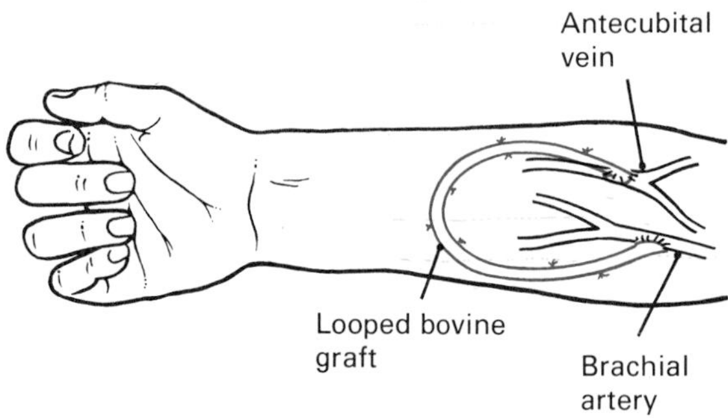

C

Figure 38-11 Methods of vascular access for hemodialysis. (*a*) External cannula or shunt. (*b*) Internal AV fistula. (*c*) Looped bovine graft in forearm. *(a, b from Renal Disease by Kagan. Copyright ® 1979 by McGraw-Hill Inc. Used with permission of McGraw-Hill Book Company.)*

for more efficient dialysis. Access combinations may include two femoral catheters, one femoral and one subclavian catheter, or a femoral or subclavian catheter with a peripheral vein used for blood return. It is preferable to remove the catheters after each use. However, continuous or intermittent heparin administration into the catheter has been successfully used between dialysis periods.

When dialysis is indicated, there are three possible ways to approach treatment. The first procedure consists of simultaneously creating an external shunt and an internal AV fistula. The external shunt can be used until the AV fistula is ready. When the internal shunt is ready, the external one is removed. The second procedure consists of creating a subcutaneous AV fistula and instituting peritoneal dialysis until the AV fistula is ready. The third procedure consists of surgically creating the AV fistula while the client is being maintained on conservative therapy, well in advance of end-stage renal disease.

Dialyzers

In hemodialysis, the semipermeable membrane is a single dialyzer available in various forms (Fig. 38-12). These include a *coil,* in which blood flows through a series of cellophane tubes; a *flat plate (Kiil),* in which blood flows between two sheets of membrane outside of which the dialysate passes; and a *hollow fiber kidney,* which contains thousands of fibers packed in a cylinder. The hollow fiber and coil dialyzers are the types most commonly used. The blood circulates through the fibers and the dialysis fluid between them. Various dialyzers differ in surface area, membrane composition and thickness, clearance of waste products, and removal of fluid.

Procedure

After the venipunctures, the needle closest to the fistula delivers "arterial" blood to the dialyzer. The dialyzer is usually primed with saline. Heparin is added to the blood as it flows into the dialyzer. Once the blood enters the extracorporeal circuit, it is propelled through the dialyzer by a roller pump at a flow rate of 100 to 300 mL/minute, while the dialysate circulates in the opposite direction at a rate of 300 to 900 mL/minute. The dialysate flow rate should be three times the blood flow rate for optimal clearance.

In addition to the dialyzer, the other piece of equipment is a *dialysate delivery and monitoring system* (Fig. 38-13). It pumps the dialysate fluid, as well as the blood, through the dialyzer. Adjustments can be made for ultrafiltration by creating a positive pressure in the venous side or a negative pressure on the dialysate side. The dialysis system has an alarm system to warn of blood or air leaks, alterations in dialysate temperature, concentration, or pressure, and extremes in blood pressure readings.

Dialysis is terminated by turning off the blood flow pump, clamping the arterial inflow line, and flushing the dialyzer with saline to return all blood to the client. The needles are then removed from the client, and firm pressure is applied to the venipuncture sites.

Before dialysis begins, the client is weighed. The difference between the last postdialysis weight and the present predialysis weight will determine the ultrafiltration. Ideally, no more than 1.0 to 1.5 kg should be gained between treatments. While the client is on dialysis, his vital signs should be taken every 30

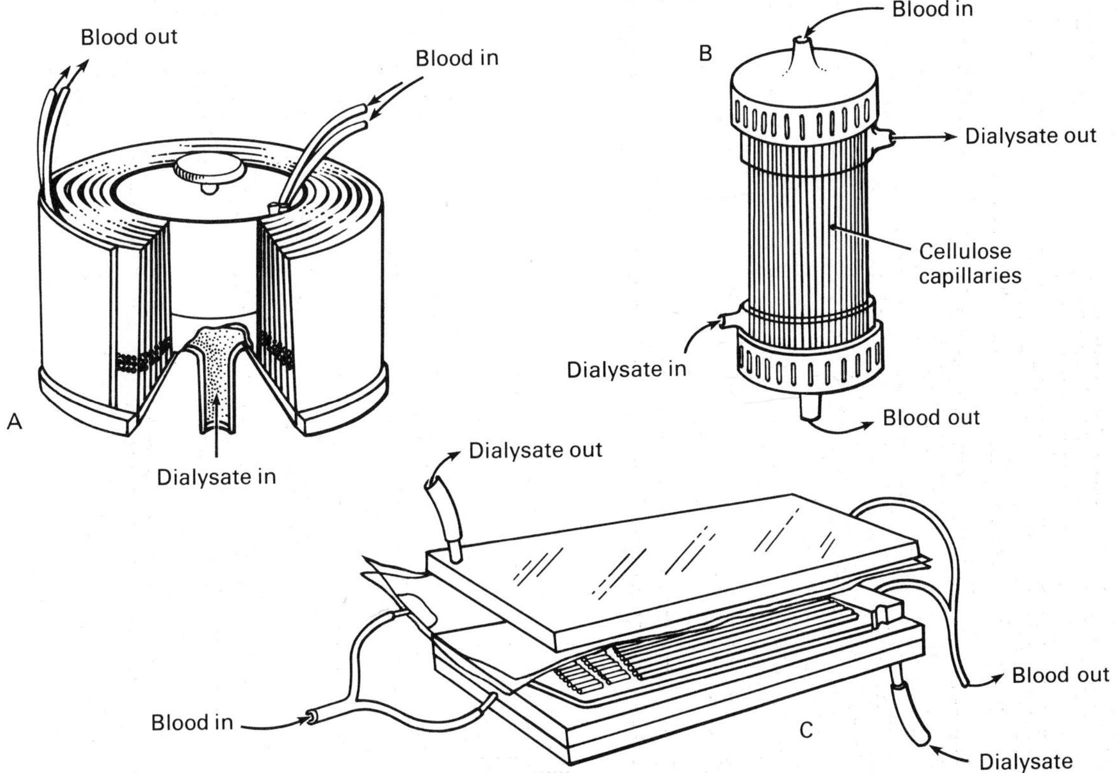

Figure 38-12 Three kinds of dialyzers used for hemodialysis. (*a*) Coil dialyzer. (*b*) Hollow fiber dialyzer. (*c*) Kiil (flat plate) dialyzer.

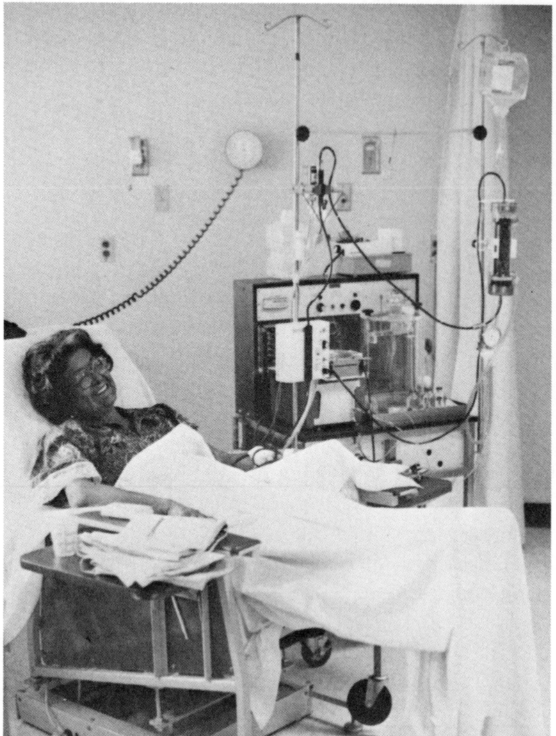

Figure 38-13 Hemodialysis delivery system.

minutes, as rapid changes may occur in the vascular system.

Most dialysis units have reclining chairs, in addition to beds, in an attempt to create a nonhospital environment. Most people sleep, read, talk, or watch television during dialysis. Since one hand is occupied with the procedure, it is difficult to perform other tasks. Hemodialysis usually lasts for 4 to 6 hours and occurs 3 times per week. While the client is attached to the dialysis machine, he can engage in meaningful interaction with the staff. Some units allow meals to be served while the client is on dialysis. This provides an opportunity to allow foods and fluids that would normally be restricted. However, due to the increased risk of hepatitis, many units no longer allow food and fluid to be served.

Settings for dialysis

Dialysis can be done in an inpatient or outpatient setting. Inpatient dialysis is used for treating the seriously ill client. In outpatient dialysis, the client comes to the hospital or a satellite unit for treatment. The client may choose self-care in either of these settings, with backup support from trained personnel if needed.

Another choice of setting is home dialysis. In 1963, home dialysis training was started; today, about 13 percent of clients on hemodialysis use it.[13] One of the main advantages of home dialysis is that it allows greater freedom in choosing dialysis times. People on home dialysis do markedly better and return earlier to normal functioning compared to people on hospital-based dialysis. Hospital dialysis costs about $25,000 per year. Home dialysis costs $21,000 the first year and $11,000 for subsequent years. The main reasons that more people do not use home dialysis are (1) lack of a trained partner, (2) fear of unexpected problems outside of the hospital setting, and (3) medical problems which warrant close supervision while the client is on hemodialysis.

Recent advances in hemodialysis include a portable and wearable artificial kidney. All components of the portable dialyzer are miniaturized and carried in a small case. The device weighs about 3.5 kg. Dialyzing fluid is made by adding electrolytes to tap water. However, this system is not yet a practical means of therapy.

Complications of dialysis

Disequilibrium Syndrome Disequilibrium syndrome occurs when urea is removed more rapidly from the blood than from the brain. The osmotic gradient created by urea in the brain cells allows fluid to pass into cerebral cells, causing cerebral edema. Manifestations include nausea, vomiting, elevated blood pressure, disorientation, leg cramps, and peripheral paresthesias. Treatment consists of slowing the rate of dialysis and infusing mannitol to draw fluid from brain cells back into the circulation.

Muscle Cramps Muscle cramps can result from too rapid removal of sodium and water or from neuromuscular hypersensitivity.

Hepatitis Hepatitis is a major threat on any dialysis unit. Precautions include using gloves to put clients on and off the machine, dialyzing clients with positive hepatitis B surface antigen in a separate area, careful handwashing techniques, and adequate sterilization of equipment.

Hypertension Hypertension can result from fluid overload, disequilibrium syndrome, anxiety, or renin-related causes.

Hypotension Hypotension can result from ultrafiltration or too rapid removal of blood flow from the client to the dialyzer.

Loss of Blood Blood loss may result from accidental separation of cannula tubing or dialysis membrane rupture, or as a side effect of heparinization.

Sepsis Sepsis is usually a consequence of an infected AV fistula. Bacterial endocarditis can occur because of frequent and prolonged access to the vascular system.

Intractable Ascites Intractable ascites is being reported with increasing frequency during the course of chronic dialysis. The etiology is unknown and the prognosis is generally poor.

Effectiveness of dialysis

Dialysis is still an imperfect technique in treating end-stage renal disease. It cannot replace the metabolic and hormonal functions of the kidneys. Dialysis can relieve most of the symptoms of chronic renal failure and, if started early enough, can prevent certain complications. Dialysis does not alter the accelerated atherosclerosis and only partially corrects anemia.

The yearly death rate of people on maintenance dialysis is 5 to 10 percent. The majority of deaths (66 percent) are due to cardiovascular-related disease (cerebrovascular accident or myocardial infarction). Infectious complications account for 13 percent of the deaths.[14] Many of the complications associated with chronic renal failure continue into the transplant period and can affect the success of a kidney transplant.

Adaptation to dialysis

Individual adaptation to maintenance dialysis varies considerably. Initially, many clients feel very positive about the machine because it makes them feel better. People on home dialysis are best adapted to their situation. Some people come to dialysis because they know that if they are not treated, they will get very sick. Dependence on a machine is a reality. Many have dreams of being tied to the machine. The other alternatives are to try a transplant or die. Depression and suicidal tendencies may be manifested as noncompliance with a diet or drug therapy or a large weight gain. A primary nursing goal is to assist the client to regain or maintain positive self-esteem and continue to be productive in society.

TRANSPLANTATION

The first kidney transplant in the United States was performed in 1954 in Boston between identical twins. After 7 years, the recipient died of a myocardial infarction at the age of 29. Advances with immunosuppressives and tissue typing in the 1960s made transplantation available to a broader range of people.

Today, over 30,000 people have received kidney transplants. Although a successful transplant restores all aspects of renal function, its availability depends on having a suitable donor and appropriate tissue matching.

Preoperative Period

Donor selection

Living related donors provide 25 to 30 percent and cadaveric donors 70 to 75 percent of all donated kidneys. Living related donors are usually parents, siblings, or children. Both physiological and psychological assessments of a potential donor are done. Histocompatibility studies (tissue typing) and blood typing are done first. If they match those of the recipient, then the prospective donor receives a complete history and physical examination, intravenous pyelogram, electrolyte studies, BUN, creatinine clearance, and renal arteriogram.

In the psychological assessment done by a psychologist or social worker, the person is asked his motives for wanting to donate a kidney. The risks and complications are discussed. (The one remaining kidney can maintain normal renal function.) Family dynamics are assessed. This is particularly significant because of the importance of knowing the family's strengths and weaknesses. In the event that a rejection occurs, the social worker or psychologist can provide needed support. If the person chooses not to donate a kidney, a plausible excuse is given to the recipient.

Cadaveric donors most commonly are trauma victims. The kidneys are suitable only if they have not suffered ischemia or trauma. Permission from the immediate family is required after proof of brain death. If a living will is in effect or a donor card has been signed prior to death, the family may be able to consent to a donor nephrectomy.

The generally accepted age for donors is 5 to 55 years, although suitable kidneys have been obtained from donors either younger or older. Donors must be free of systemic disease and infection and must have normal kidney function.

A nationwide computerized service for people with end-stage renal disease, containing their blood and tissue types, is available. If a kidney is procured in one area of the country but there is no suitable recipient, the computer service will be used to locate one in another area. Kidneys can be transported within a sterile environment in a compact, watertight package. This method is called *cold preservation.* Using this method, kidneys can be preserved for up to 36 hours.

The development of kidney preservation machines has increased the viability of kidneys. This machine pumps a cold perfusate (plasmanate, albumin, or commercially prepared protein fractions) through the renal artery. The perfusate is cold (10°C; 50°F), which allows for a decreased metabolic rate. Kidneys have been adequately perfused for up to 72 hours, providing additional time for transportation, tissue typing, and preparation of the recipient. The recipient may be dialyzed prior to the surgery, especially if hyperkalemia or hypervolemia is present.

The limited availability of living related donors has turned the focus to cadaveric donors. Although there are over 40,000 people on maintenance dialysis, each year fewer than 4000 transplants are performed due to the lack of available kidneys.

Histocompatibility studies

Histocompatibility testing is performed to determine the degree of similarity between donor and recipient antigens. ABO blood group antigens are important in determining histocompatibility and are matched. In addition, the human leukocyte antigen (HLA) system is the major histocompatibility locus in humans and governs the acceptance or rejection of transplanted tissue. HLA antigens are located on all nucleated cells.

The HLA complex is located on the sixth chromosome in humans. Four major HLA loci (A, B, C, D) have been identified in this region. Each locus may have multiple alleles and more are being discovered (Table 38-8). Each person has two antigens for each locus, one inherited from each parent unless the parents shared an HLA antigen.

The purpose of histocompatibility testing is to identify the antigens at each locus. A *microlymphocytotoxicity test* is used to type for the antigens at HLA-A, -B, and -C loci. The test uses lymphocytes taken from peripheral blood, lymph nodes, or spleen. For kidney transplantation, the antigens at the A and B loci are the only ones considered. Individuals are considered HLA-identical if all four antigens are identical for these two loci. (There is a one-in-four chance that in a given family one child will be identical to another child.) The degree of histocompatibility between donor and recipient is graded according to the criteria outlined in Table 38-8. HLA gradings correlate with graft survivals in living related donors but show little or no correlation with cadaveric transplants.

A *mixed lymphocyte culture (MLC)* assesses the

Table 38-8
Nomenclature for Factors of the HLA System

Recognized Antigens*

A Locus	B Locus	C Locus	D Locus
A1	B5	CW1	DW1
A2	B7	CW2	DW2
A3	B8	CW3	DW3
A9	B12	CW4	DW4
A10	B13	CW5	DW5
A11	B14	CW6	DW6
A25 (10)	B15	CW7	DW7
A26 (10)	B17	CW8	DW8
A28	B18		DW9
A29	B27		DW10
AW19	B37		DW11
AW23 (9)	B40		DW12
AW24 (9)	BW16		
AW30	BW21		**DR Locus†**
AW31	BW22		DR1
AW32	BW35		DR2
AW33	BW38 (16)		DR3
AW34	BW39 (16)		DR4
AW36	BW41		DR5
AW43	BW42		DRW6
	Others (11)		DR7
			DRW8
			DRW9
			DRW10

Match Grades for Living Related Donors

Match Grade	Interpretations	No. of Antigens Mismatched
A	HLA-identical for A, B, C, D antigens. Applies almost exclusively to siblings	0
B	No apparent mismatch (e.g., A, B, C identical) but cross match or mixed lymphocyte culture unrelated	0
C	Incompatibility of one antigen—donor possesses the antigen that recipient lacks	1
D	Donor possesses two antigens that recipient lacks	2
E	Donor possesses three antigens that recipient lacks	3–4
F	Positive cross match	—

For *cadaver transplants,* the match is simply stated as four-antigen match, etc., since compatibility is not comparable to similar match grades in living related donors.

*World Health Organization Committee on Leukocyte Nomenclature, 1980.

†B lymphocyte, D-related antigens.

antigen match at the D locus. In this test, lymphocytes from the recipient are incubated for 4 to 5 days with lymphocytes from the donor. The degree of proliferation of lymphocytes correlates with the degree to which the donor cells are recognized as foreign. A positive MLC may occur in individuals who are identical at the A, B, and C loci. However, this rarely occurs. (Because this test takes about 5 days, it is not used for cadaveric donors.) Grafts from donors who are poor stimulators in the MLC appear to have as good a clinical outcome as do grafts from HLA-A-identical and HLA-B-identical donors.

A *tissue typing crossmatch* uses serum from the recipient mixed with donor cells to test for any preformed cytotoxic antibodies to the donated kidney. The donor may have been exposed to antigens similar to those of the donor by means of prior blood transfusions, pregnancy, a previous kidney transplant, or bacteremia. This procedure takes about 3 to 5 hours and is used in both living related and cadaveric donors. A positive cross match indicates cytotoxic antibodies and is considered an "F" match (Table 38-8). This finding is a contraindication to transplantation. If transplanted, this kidney would immediately undergo hyperacute rejection.

Grading of donors and recipients is commonly done (Table 38-8). The HLA gradings correlate with graft survival in living related donors but show little or no correlation with cadaveric transplants. The value of tissue typing in matching cadaveric donors with recipients is controversial. Even a perfect HLA tissue match does not preclude the possibility of a rejection episode.

Pretransplant blood transfusions

Until recently, in clients with renal failure, an attempt was made to avoid using blood transfusions or using only frozen, washed red cells in which most WBCs and platelets were removed. However, when graft survival was compared in clients who had received transfusions prior to transplantation with those who had not, it was shown that transfusions were associated with increased graft survival. Multiple transfusions are associated in some individuals with an increased incidence of presensitization and the production of cytotoxic antibodies.

However, the beneficial effect of transfusions is demonstrable as long as more than five tranfusions are given and the client does not develop specific antibodies to the donor's antigens. The mechanism by which transfusions act is not well understood. One theory is that enhancing antibodies are made and are directed against D-locus antigens. These antibodies prevent the recipient's immune system from recognizing the donor's D antigens as foreign and thus inhibit an immune response.

Surgical Procedure

For a living related donated kidney transplant, two surgical teams are used. One team carefully removes the donor kidney attached to artery, vein, and ureter. After the kidney is removed, it is core cooled by flushing with an electrolyte solution at approximately 10°C. Frequently, mannitol is added to this solution to increase osmolality. The kidney is then carried to the operating room occupied by the recipient.

The donated kidney is surgically implanted in the iliac fossa on the side contralateral to the side on which the kidney was removed from the donor. For example, a left donated kidney is placed in the right iliac fossa of the recipient (Fig. 38-14). The iliac fossa is used because of the ease of exposing the iliac blood vessels. The renal artery is anastomosed to the internal iliac (hypogastric) artery or external iliac artery. The renal vein is attached to the external iliac vein. The donor's ureter is implanted into the recipient's bladder.

Bilateral nephrectomies of the recipient's kidneys are not performed unless the client has uncontrollable

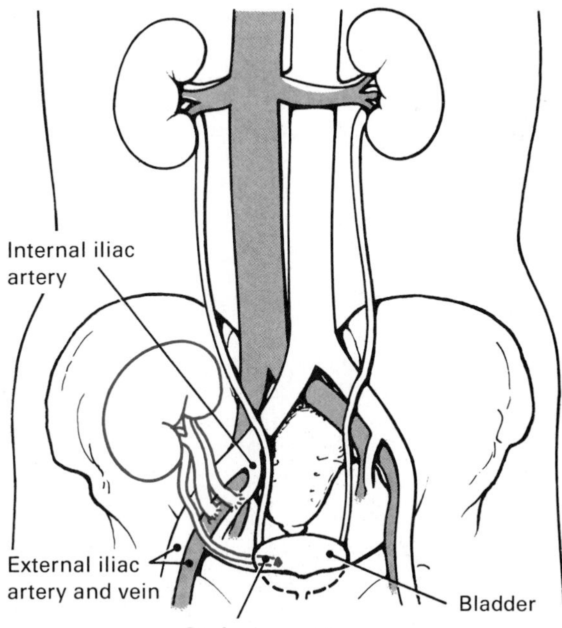

Figure 38-14 Surgical placement of transplanted kidney.

hypertension, infection, bleeding in the kidneys, or ureteral reflux.

Postoperative Care

Recipient

The nursing care is similar to that of any client who has had major surgery. This section will focus on the management of the transplant recipient. The immediate postoperative care consists of careful monitoring of fluid and electrolyte balance and intake and output. A massive diuresis may occur in response to renal ischemia. IV fluids are adjusted hourly according to the urine output and the state of hydration. A common order of magnitude is 30 mL/hour plus urine output. An indwelling catheter is inserted, and urine output is monitored hourly. The catheter is removed as soon as possible, usually the first postoperative day. While the catheter is in place, observing for patency of the tubing and providing catheter care are very important.

The abdominal dressing should be observed for both blood and urine drainage. Urinary leakage may be present if the ureteral anastomosis is not securely implanted into the bladder. It may also result from ureteral obstruction of the newly implanted ureter.

Careful, frequent monitoring of vital signs is critical. A low-grade fever may be a sign of rejection or infection.

Vigorous pulmonary exercises are needed to increase ventilation and drainage of secretions. Coughing and deep breathing can be combined with the use of blow bottles. The client can be turned to the operative side. Usually, frequent and early ambulation is encouraged.

Mouth care is very important because of the ulcerations of the mouth which occur secondary to renal failure as well as steroid therapy. Mycostatin mouthwashes are usually prescribed.

Most clients feel very good as their renal function returns. Occasionally, the new kidney does not release urine immediately. If this occurs, the person must be dialyzed until adequate renal function begins. This is often a time of great discouragement to the hopeful client. The client should be reassured that this is not uncommon, especially in recipients of cadaveric donated kidneys.

Donor

The usual postoperative care is similar to that following a nephrectomy (see Chap. 37). Often, the donor remains the forgotten person as all the attention is focused on "his" kidney in the recipient. The pain of a nephrectomy is greater than that of the iliac fossa incision of the recipient. In contrast to the recipient, who feels better as renal function is restored, the donor feels very sick for 2 to 3 days.

If the kidney does not function immediately or is rejected, the donor may feel disappointed and guilty. The donor is a healthy individual who sacrificed a kidney and took a leave from his occupation and family. He must always face the unanswered question of what happens if his other kidney stops working.

Immunosuppressive Therapy

Immunosuppressive therapy is used to suppress the body's immune response to the foreign kidney (Table 38-9). Azathioprine (Imuran) and corticosteroids are the standard drugs ordered. These drugs are started the day before the transplant. Some transplant centers use total body irradiation and *antilymphocytic globulin (ALG)* in addition to the standard drug therapy. ALG is not uniformly accepted, and its efficacy has been debated. It is prepared in horses, rabbits, and goats immunized with human lymphocytes. The antilymphocytic serum is then purified and given to humans. The antisera destroys human lymphocytes. It suppresses the cell-mediated response more than the humoral response. *Antithymocytic globulin (ATG),* developed more recently, has a more specific and better-established role. Human thymocytes are removed from children at the time of cardiac surgery and utilized to induce antibodies in rabbits. The ATG works better than ALG, but as yet it has not come into widespread use.

The method of administering corticosteroids varies. Most clients are put on prolonged oral prednisone therapy. Some physicians perfer giving corticosteroids only when a rejection crisis is suspected. If a rejection crisis occurs, methylprednisolone (1 to 2 g/day) is given daily or every other day in several doses. Oral prednisone may or may not be increased. Total body radiation can be used in conjunction with the large doses of steroids.

Cyclophosphamide (Cytoxan) has been found to be an adequate substitute for azathioprine. However, it is primarily used to reduce the dose of azathioprine if the client develops liver toxicity.

Cyclosporin A, first used in Europe, is currently under investigation at selected transplant centers. It is classified as a fungicide and is a potent depressant of humoral and cellular immunity. It may be used alone or in conjuction with steroid therapy. Known side effects include an increased incidence of lymphomas, hepatic dysfunction, nephrotoxicity, minor hirsutism, and tremors.

Table 38-9
Immunosuppressive Therapy for Renal Transplant Recipients

Drug	Mechanism of Action	Adverse Side Effects
Azathioprine (Imuran) (IV or PO)	Derivative of 6-mercaptopurine Interferes with purine synthesis and inhibits DNA and RNA synthesis Decreases cell-mediated immune response	Bone marrow suppression (leukopenia, anemia, thrombocytopenia) Drug-induced hepatitis Oral lesions Increased susceptibility to infection
Corticosteroids Prednisone (PO) Methylprednisolone (Solu-Medrol) (IV)	Suppresses inflammatory response Primarily suppresses humoral-mediated immune response	Cushingoid syndrome: Peptic ulcer GI bleeding Aseptic necrosis Sodium and water retention Acne Muscle weakness Fat dystrophy Capillary fragility Delayed healing Hyperglycemia Mood alterations Bacteria, fungal, and viral infections
Cyclophosphamide (Cytoxan) (PO)	Alkylating agent Interferes with DNA, RNA, and protein synthesis	Alopecia Leukopenia Hemorrhagic cystitis
ALG, ALS, ATG (IV, IM)	Exact mechanism unknown Coats lymphocytes Reduces circulating lymphocytes	Serum sickness Fever and chills Anaphylactic shock Rash Hypertension Headache Low back pain

Immunosuppressives affect the entire body, not just the transplanted kidney. This puts the client at great risk for any infection. More specific immunosuppressive therapy aimed only at the foreign kidney and not the total body is needed.

Complications of Transplantation

Rejection

Hyperacute Rejection Hyperacute rejection (humoral-mediated) occurs minutes to hours after transplantation. Renal vessels thrombose and the kidney dies. Preformed humoral antibodies from pregnancy, blood transfusions, or previous transplants react with recipient antigens in the donor kidney. There is no treatment and the transplanted kidney is removed.

Acute Rejection Acute rejection most commonly occurs 4 days to 4 months after transplantation. It is not uncommon to have at least one rejection episode, especially with cadaveric donated kidneys. These episodes are usually reversible with immunsuppressive therapy. However, the prognosis is poor if three or more episodes occur during the first 3 months or if dialysis is needed.

Signs of rejection include decreasing creatinine clearance, increasing serum creatinine, elevated BUN, fever, decreased urine output, increasing blood pressure, and a swollen and painful transplant site.

Chronic Rejection Chronic rejection is a process which occurs over months or years. It is associated with a gradual occlusion of the renal blood vessels. (Signs include proteinuria, hypertension, and increasing serum creatinine.) There is no definitive therapy known to treat this type of rejection. Treatment is mainly supportive therapy (physiological and psychosocial). This type of rejection is difficult to manage and is not associated with the optimistic prognosis of acute rejection.

Infections

Infections are a common and serious complication of immunosuppressive therapy. Respiratory infections are the most frequent cause of death from an infection. The client is at greatest risk during the early months when he is taking maximum dosages of immunosuppressives. The client with a compromised immune system is very susceptible to infection from opportunistic organisms. Bacterial infections (pneumonia, urinary tract, and wound) are usually caused by endogenous organisms. Viral infections (cytomegalovirus) occur frequently after prolonged steroid therapy. Fungal infections can occur anywhere and are difficult to treat.

Malignancies

The incidence of malignancies (5 to 6 percent of clients) due to immunosuppressive therapy is 100 times greater than that of the general population.[15] The malignancies include cancer of the skin, lips, and cervix, and lymphomas.

Recurrence of renal disease

Recurrence of the same type of renal disease that destroyed the original kidney takes place in 15 percent of kidney transplants. It is most common with certain types of glomerulonephritis.

Acceleration of vascular disease

Even if the kidney transplant is successful, the acceleration of atherosclerotic vascular disease continues. The exact reasons this occurs is not known. It may be due to an inability to alter the process that started with the onset of renal failure or to hypertension and hyperlipidemia that is present and is enhanced by steroid therapy. Table 38-10 discusses dietary instruction posttransplantation.

Table 38-10

Dietary Instructions after a Kidney Transplant

Rationale for diet

After you have had a kidney transplant, most of the dietary restrictions you followed before the surgery are no longer needed. However, you will need to follow a salt-restricted, high protein diet with special attention to weight control.

Salt

The low salt diet (2 g sodium) will help to prevent fluid retention and will control blood pressure.

Protein

Your body will need increased dietary protein for two reasons:

1. To repair body tissue damaged during the transplant
2. To replace protein broken down by steroid medications

Calories

Because some of your new medications can cause high blood sugars, increased appetite, and excessive weight gain, you should try to avoid high calorie foods (sweets, sugar, fried foods, soda, potato chips) as much as possible. Snack on low calorie foods (vegetables, fruits, plain yogurt) to help satisfy your appetite.

Contributed by Dietary Department, University of New Mexico Hospitals, Albuquerque, New Mexico.

Adaptation to Transplantation

If a transplant is successful, the client has the potential to return to near-normal functioning. Most clients feel so improved that euphoria predominates for a while. Some of the euphoria is due to the effect of the steroids. The ever-present question of rejection (if and when) is a continual fear. The longer a person goes without rejection, the better the prognosis. Even if a kidney is rejected, the alternatives of dialysis or another transplant are available. The rejection of a first kidney does not greatly appear to jeopardize the success of a second transplant.

Most people who have successful transplants believe that it was worth all the risks to feel so good. It is these people who suffer the greatest depression when the kidney is rejected after many months or years. They need to be reassured that they have done nothing (other than fail to comply with drug therapy) to cause the rejection to occur.

The prolongation of life in chronic renal failure puts the client in an unusual situation. First, he wonders whether he can learn to accept death and then there is hope for life with dialysis. Next, he asks a healthy relative to donate a kidney. Then he lives through months wondering how long this kidney will last.

Effectiveness of Transplantation

During the first year, the mortality rate (5 to 10 percent) for transplanted clients with living related donated kidneys is similar to that of clients on hemodialysis. The mortality rate is higher in cadaveric recipients. The leading causes of death are infection and cardiovascular disease. If the transplant is successful, the quality of life is much better than that offered by maintenance dialysis.

In spite of advances in knowledge and technology, the clinical results of kidney survival have not increased significantly in the past years. The five-year survival is about 75 to 80 percent for living-related kidneys and 50 percent for cadaveric kidneys. But while kidney survival has not improved, client survival has. This is due to the use of less vigorous immunosuppressive therapy and earlier removal of a rejected kidney. Present immunosuppressive therapy is inadequate. More specific and less toxic drugs are needed. The overall goal is client rather than transplant survival.

Case Study / Chronic Renal Failure

Curt had been treated for acute glomerulonephritis at the age of 5. At that time, his urine showed proteinuria and hematuria. At the age of 11, he was diagnosed as having recurring acute glomerulonephritis. He had no follow-up medical care during the next 10 years. At the age of 21, he began noticing weakness on walking, paresthesia, dyspnea on exertion, headaches, diplopia, and swollen hands and feet. His skin was yellowish and sallow. He complained of some itching. A diagnostic workup showed the following:

Serum creatinine	21.6 mg/dL
Creatinine clearance	4.0 mL/minute
BUN	156 mg/dL
Potassium	6.8 mEq/L
Bicarbonate	12.0 mEq/L
Hematocrit	20 percent
Blood pressure	146/100
Chest x-ray	Cardiomegaly and pulmonary edema

He was diagnosed as having chronic glomerulonephritis, and internal (AV fistula) and external cannulas were surgically inserted. He was started on hemodialysis 3 times weekly.

His medical orders consisted of the following:

Alu-caps
Methyldopa (Aldomet)
Multivitamins
Ferrous gluconate
Folic acid
Diet: 60 g protein
2 g sodium
1500 mL fluid

Discussion Questions

1. Explain the basic pathological changes that resulted in the development of chronic glomerulonephritis.
2. Identify the abnormal diagnostic study results and explain why each would occur. What is their significance for nursing observation and care?
3. Explain why Curt developed each of his clinical manifestations. What is the appropriate nursing intervention related to each one?
4. What is the purpose of Curt's medical orders?
5. Explain the principles of hemodialysis and how it works to treat renal failure.
6. Why would both an internal fistula and an external cannula be surgically created at the same time?

REVIEW QUESTIONS

The number of the question corresponds to the same numbered objective at the beginning of the chapter.

1. Which of the following statements best describes acute renal failure?
   - **a.** complete absence of renal blood flow
   - **b.** sudden reduction in renal function
   - **c.** rapid increase in urine output with azotemia
   - **d.** gradual increase in the GFR
2. Common causes of acute tubular necrosis include
   - **a.** septic abortion and acute glomerulonephritis
   - **b.** blood transfusion reaction and carbon tetrachloride inhalation
   - **c.** acute pyelonephritis and ureteral calculi
   - **d.** congestive heart failure and hepatorenal syndrome
3. During the diuretic phase of acute renal failure, which of the following serum electrolyte imbalances are most likely to develop?
   - **a.** increased potassium and decreased sodium
   - **b.** increased potassium and increased sodium

c. decreased potassium and increased sodium
d. decreased potassium and decreased sodium

4. If a client in the oliguric phase of acute renal failure urinated 300 mL during the previous 24 hours, how much fluid should he have during the next 24 hours?
   a. 300 mL
   b. 500 mL
   c. 800 mL
   d. 1000 mL

5. Demineralization of the bones can occur in uremic syndrome because
   a. uremic toxins prevent calcium from combining with bone matrix
   b. secondary hyperparathyroidism causes mobilization of calcium out of the bones
   c. dietary restrictions to combat uremia prevent calcium intake
   d. metabolic acidosis prevents normal bone formation

6. The following measures are used in the management of chronic renal failure. For which one is the correct rationale given?
   a. Kayexalate to reduce peripheral edema
   b. aluminum hydroxide to decrease serum phosphate
   c. calcitriol to decrease serum calcium
   d. methyldopa to increase urine output

7. Nursing intervention for a client receiving peritoneal dialysis would include
   a. keeping warm, moist dressings on the abdominal incision
   b. warming the dialysate solution to 40°C
   c. changing the client's position frequently to facilitate drainage
   d. notifying the physician if dialysate drainage occurs in less than 15 minutes

8. A common complication associated with internal AV fistulas is
   a. infection
   b. palpable thrill
   c. thrombosis
   d. clotting

9. Complications of renal transplantation include
   a. hepatitis and hypertension
   b. malignancies and accelerated vascular disease
   c. steal syndrome and infection
   d. bleeding and osteodystrophy

10. Which of the following factors would have to be compatible in the donor and recipient before a renal transplant would be considered?
    a. sex and HLA
    b. familial relationship and Rh factor
    c. ABO blood groups and tissue cross match
    d. age and ABO blood groups

11. The most common problem associated with immunosuppressive therapy is
    a. anemia
    b. thrombocytopenia
    c. predisposition to infection
    d. hypercoagulation

REFERENCES

1. R. G. Muth, *Renal Medicine,* Charles C Thomas, Publisher, Springfield, Ill., 1978, p. 57.
2. M. Maxwell and C. Kleeman, *Clinical Disorders of Fluid and Electrolyte Metabolism,* McGraw-Hill Book Company, New York, 1980, p. 799.
3. B. T. Burton and G. H. Hirschman, "Demographic Analysis: End-Stage Renal Disease and Its Treatment in the United States," *Clin Nephrol,* **11:**47–51 (1979).
4. G. E. Schreiner and J. F. Winchester, "Uremia—1978 Perspective," *Clin Nephrol,* **11:**52–55 (1979).
5. G. Opelz and P. Terasak, "Improvement of Kidney-Graft Survival with Increased Numbers of Blood Transfusions," *N Eng J Med,* **299:**799–803 (1978).
6. W. Bennett et al., "Drug Therapy in Chronic Renal Failure," *Ann Intern Med,* **86:**754–783 (1977).
7. G. M. Berlyne, "The Place of Dietary Therapy in the Treatment of Chronic Renal Failure," *Clin Nephrol,* **11:** 63–65 (1979).
8. Ibid., p. 64.
9. Muth, op. cit., p. 94.
10. D. G. Oreopoulos et al., "Continuous Ambulatory Peritoneal Dialysis: A New Era in the Treatment of Chronic Renal Failure," *Clin Nephrol,* **11:**125–128 (1979).
11. A. J. Sorrels, "Continuous Ambulatory Peritoneal Dialysis," *Am J Nurs,* **79:**1400–1401 (1979).
12. C. T. Flynn, "Subclavian Vein Catheter and Clockwork Pump," *Dialysis Transplantation,* **9:**556–557 (1980).
13. M. Plonski, "Self-Dialysis and the Government, Legislation, and the Law," *Dialysis Transplantation,* **7:**1040 (1978).
14. Burton and Hirschman, op. cit., p. 49.
15. J. P. Merrill, "Dialysis Versus Transplantation in Treatment of End-Stage Renal Disease," *Ann Rev Med,* **29:**355 (1978).

BIBLIOGRAPHY

Books

Brundage, D.: *Nursing Management of Renal Problems,* 2d ed., The C. V. Mosby Company, St. Louis, 1980.

Earley, L. E., and C. W. Gottschalk: *Strauss and Welt's Diseases of the Kidney,* Little, Brown and Company, Boston, 1979.

Golden, A., and J. Maher: *The Kidney,* 2d ed., The Williams & Wilkins Company, Baltimore, 1977.

J. H. Harrison et al.: *Campbell's Urology,* 4th ed., W. B. Saunders Company, Philadelphia, 1979.

Hekelmann, F. P., and C. A. Ostendarp: *Nephrology Nursing: Perspectives of Care,* McGraw-Hill Book Company, New York, 1979.

Kagan, L. W.: *Renal Disease: A Manual of Patient Care,* McGraw-Hill Book Company, New York, 1979.

Mahoney, J.: *Guide to Ostomy Nursing Care,* Little, Brown and Company, Boston, 1976.

Metheney, N. M., and W. D. Snively: *Nurses' Handbook of Fluid Balance,* 3d ed., J. B. Lippincott Company, Philadelphia, 1979.

Morel, A., and G. Wise: *Urologic Endoscopic Procedures,* 2d ed., The C. V. Mosby Company, St. Louis, 1979.

Witten, D., et al.: *Emmett's Clinical Urography,* 4th ed., W. B. Saunders Company, Philadelphia, 1977.

Periodicals

Butts, P.: "Assessing Urinary Incontinence in Women," *Nurs 79,* **9**:72–74 (1979).

Cass, A., and C. Godec: "Urethral Injury Due to External Trauma," *Urology,* **11**:607 (1978).

DeGroot, J.: "Catheter-Induced Urinary Tract Infections: How Can We Prevent Them?" *Nurs 76,* **7**:34–37 (1976).

———: "Urethral Catheterization," *Nurs 76,* **7**:51–55 (1976).

Denniston, D., and K. Burns: "Home Peritoneal Dialysis," *AJN,* **80**:2022–2026 (1980).

Dericks, V.: "The Psychological Hurdles of New Ostomates: Helping Them Up . . . And Over," *Nurs 74,* **4**:52–55 (1974).

Fisher, J. W.: "Mechanism of the Anemia of Chronic Renal Failure," *Nephron,* **25**:106–111 (1980).

Gault, P.: "Six Patients with Bladder Cancer," *Nurs 77,* **7**:48–55 (1977).

———: "How to Break the Kidney Stone Cycle," *Nurs 78,* **8**:24–31 (1978).

Gruber, P., et al.: "Nursing Panel: Care of the Hospitalized Dialysis Patient," *Dialysis Transplantation,* **9**:443–451 (1980).

Hanley, D. A., and L. M. Sherwood: "Secondary Hyperparathyroidism in Chronic Renal Failure," *Med Clin North Am,* **62**:1319–1335 (1978).

Hartman, M.: "Intermittent Self-Catheterization," *Nurs 78,* **8**:74–75 (1978).

Jensen, V.: "Better Techniques for Bagging Stomas, Part I: Urinary Ostomies," *Nurs 74,* **4**:60–64 (1974).

Juliani, L., and B. Beamer: "Kidney Transplant: Your Role in After Care," *Nurs 77,* **77**:46–53 (1977).

Latos, D. L.: "Chronic Renal Failure: An Overview," *Dialysis Transplantation,* **9**:435–440 (1980).

Lewis, S. (guest ed.): "Symposium on Chronic Renal Failure," *Nurs Clin North Am* **16**:425–526 (1981).

Lim, S. V., et al.: "Endocrine Abnormalities Associated with Chronic Renal Failure," *Med Clin North Am,* **62**:1341–1359 (1978).

Luke, B.: "Nutrition in Renal Disease: The Adult on Dialysis," *Am J Nurs,* **79**:2155–2157 (1979).

Mardis, H., et al.: "Double Pigtail Ureteral Stent," *Urology,* **14**:23–26 (1979).

Mekos, D.: "Evaluation and Management of Anemia in the Dialysis Patient," *Dialysis Transplantation,* **9**:456–457 (1980).

Merrill, J.: "Glomerulonephritis," *N Engl J Med,* **290**:257–266, 313–319, 374–381 (1974).

Moncrief, J. W.: "Continuous Ambulatory Peritoneal Dialysis," *Dialysis Transplantation,* **8**:1077–1080 (1979).

Moore, M.: "Practical Management of Chronic Renal Failure," *Am Fam Physician,* **19**:158–164 (1979).

Morehouse, D., and K. MacKinnon: "Posterior Urethral Injury: Etiology, Diagnosis, Initial Management," *Urol Clin North Am,* **4**:69 (1977).

Riff, L.: "Evaluation and Treatment of Urinary Infection," *Med Clin North Am,* **62**:1183–1199 (1978).

Shapiro, S., et al.: "Catheter Associated Urinary Tract Infections: Incidence and a New Approach to Prevention," *J Urol,* **112**:659 (1974).

Smith, F.: "The Nephrotic Syndrome: Current Concepts," *Ann Intern Med,* **76**:463–477 (1972).

Swanson, J., and S. Balthasar: "Genetic Counseling in Polycystic Kidney Disease," *J Am Assoc Nephrol Nurses Technicians,* **4**:96–99 (1977).

Turner-Warwick, R.: "Complex Traumatic Posterior Urethral Strictures," *J Urol,* **118**:564 (1977).

Vogel, C.: "Keeping Patients Alive in Spite of Postobstructive Diuresis," *Nurs 79,* **9**:50–56 (1979).

Walser, M.: "Keto Acid Therapy in Chronic Renal Failure," *Nephron,* **21**:57–74 (1978).

Walser, N., W. E. Mitch and V. U. Collier: "The Effect of Nutritional Therapy on the Course of Chronic Renal Failure," *Clin Nephrol,* **11**:66–70 (1979).

Whyte, J., and N. Thistle: "Male Incontinence: The Inside Story on External Collection," *Nurs 76,* **6**:66–67 (1976).

Woodrow, M., et al.: "Suprapubic Catheters," *Nurs 76,* **7**:40–42 (1976).

Organizations

American Association of Nephrology Nurses and Technicians (AANNT), Suite 8, 2 Talcott Rd., Park Ridge, IL 60068

National Kidney Foundation, 315 Park Avenue South, New York, NY 10010

Section 9

Problems Related to Regulatory Mechanisms

Chapter 39

GENERAL CONCEPTS

Concepts of Stress

Patricia Palmer Stephens

Learning Objectives

1. Define stress.
2. Describe the three stages of the General Adaptation Syndrome.
3. Describe the role of the nervous system in the mechanism of stress.
4. Describe the role of the endocrine system in the mechanism of stress.
5. Describe behaviors evidenced by a client experiencing stress.
6. List variables that may influence the experience of stress.
7. Describe the nursing management of a client under stress.

DEFINITION

Stress is recognized as a common experience in life. It has been described as specific conditions or events which increase tension in the person. For example, an individual may say, "Stress is becoming a parent, going to school, or falling off a horse." Another view of stress is that it is the *result* of specific conditions or events. For example, an individual may say, "Becoming a parent, going to school, or falling off a horse is a source of stress."

This book utilizes Hans Selye's definition of stress as "the nonspecific response of the body to any demand made upon it."[1] A *stressor* is anything physical or emotional, pleasant or unpleasant, which is perceived to require adaptation by the individual (see Table 39-1). Although stressors are specific events, the physiological response is generalized or nonspecific. This means that the body responds in a generalized manner irrespective of the specific stressor. This response is called by Hans Selye the *General Adaptation Syndrome* (GAS), or Stress Syndrome.

In his recent works, Selye differentiates between *eustress* and *distress*. He describes eustress as normally pleasant experiences and distress as unpleasant experiences. The concept that stressors may be either pleasant or unpleasant events has also been described by Holmes, Rahe, and others involved in research on life changes and illness (see Chap. 1).

GENERAL ADAPTATION SYNDROME (STRESS SYNDROME)

A person cannot live without experiencing stress. Selye comments that the only state without stress is death. The body responds to stress by a local response (Local Adaptation Syndrome, or LAS) which is roughly equivalent to the inflammatory reaction (see Chap. 9). If the local response is inadequate or inappropriate for the stressor, then the body responds by the *General Adaptation Syndrome* (Fig 39-1).

Selye defines three stages of GAS: *alarm reaction, stage of resistance,* and *stage of exhaustion.* The central and autonomic nervous systems and the pituitary, thyroid, and adrenal glands are involved in mediating the GAS.

Alarm Reaction

In the *alarm reaction* the individual perceives a stressor physically or mentally, and the "fight-or-flight" mechanism is initiated. When the stressor is of sufficient intensity as a perceived threat to the steady state of the individual, it calls for a reallocation of energy so that adaptation may occur. This temporarily decreases the individual's resistance to stress and may even result in death. Table 39-2 summarizes the analysis of events associated with 275 sudden deaths by George Engel, an expert in psychosomatic medicine. Although these events do not usually result in or cause sudden death, when sudden death occurs there is some correlation with these emotionally laden situations.

Table 39-1
Examples of Stressors

Physical	Emotional
Noise	Fear of cancer
Amphetamines	Promotion at work
Burns	Watching a loved one die
Running a marathon	Fear of failure
Infectious diseases	Financial loss
Extreme fatigue	Winning a beauty contest
Pain	

This chapter was reviewed by Andrea Mengel, R.N., M.S.N., Associate Professor of Nursing, Community College of Philadelphia, Philadelphia, Pennsylvania.

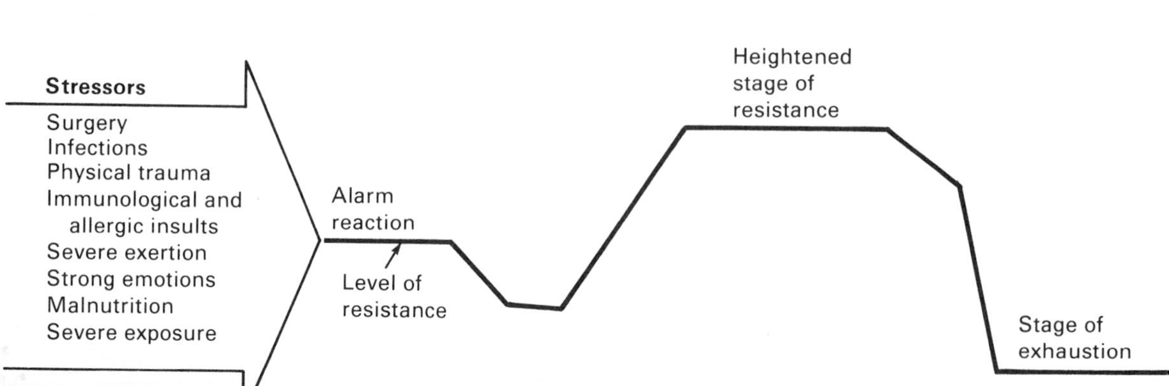

Figure 39-1 Phase of stress. *(From Marjorie L. Byrne and Lida F. Thompson, Key Concepts for the Study and Practice of Nursing, The C. V. Mosby Company, St. Louis, 1978, p. 51.)*

Physical symptoms of the alarm reaction are generally those of sympathetic nervous system stimulation. These symptoms include an increased rate and force of heartbeat, increased blood pressure and respiratory rate, anorexia or nausea, pupil dilatation, and increased perspiration.

Stage of Resistance

Ideally, the individual quickly moves from the alarm reaction to the stage of resistance in which physiological forces are mobilized to increase resistance to stress. This is when adaptation occurs. It may involve modification of the external as well as the internal environment. Resistance is high at this time, as compared to the normal state. The amount of resistance varies among individuals depending on their level of physical functioning, their coping abilities, and the total number of stressors they are experiencing. For example, an individual who has been jogging regularly will have more ability to adapt to the stress of emergency surgery than a person who is very sedentary.

Although there are usually few physical symptoms in this stage, the person is expending energy to adapt. This adaptive energy is limited by the resources of the individual. For example, he may successfully recover from surgery and return to a normal coping state, or he may move to the next stage of the GAS.

Table 39-2
Causes of Sudden Death*

Category	Percentage
Traumatic disruption of a close human relationship or the anniversary of the death of a loved one.	49%
Involvement in a situation of danger, attack, or struggle.	37%
Loss of status or self-esteem due to failure or humiliation and loss of valued possessions.	8%
Sudden moments of triumph, recognition, or reunion, or "happy endings."	6%

*The deaths occurred within minutes to a few hours of the event.
From George Engel, "Emotional Stress and Sudden Death," *Psychology Today*, **11**(6): 114–115, 153–154 (1977).

Stage of Exhaustion

The stage of exhaustion is the final stage of the GAS and results if the stressor is not removed. Exhaustion occurs when all the energy for adaptation has been used. Physical symptoms of the alarm reaction may briefly reappear in a final effort by the body to survive. This is seen in some terminally ill persons who become alert and have stronger vital signs shortly before their death. However, the individual in the stage of exhaustion usually becomes ill and may die if assistance from outside sources is not available. This stage can be reversed by external sources of energy such as medication, blood transfusions, or psychotherapy.

MECHANISM OF STRESS

To simplify a description of the body's perception of stressors and the stress response, the following discussion is divided into the role of the nervous system and the role of the endocrine system. These systems affect and are affected by the other body systems.

Nervous System

As mentioned earlier in this chapter and in Chap. 1, stressors may be physical, psychological, or social. They may be actually or symbolically present for the body to respond with the GAS. The complex process by which an event is perceived as a stressor and the body responds is not fully understood. Fig. 39-2 summarizes what is thought to be the neural control of emotions by the hypothalamus. This is significant because most stressors precipitate an emotional reaction. The major parts of the brain involved in the neural control of emotion are the reticular formation, the hypothalamus, the limbic system, and the cerebral cortex. Their functions are very closely interrelated.

Cerebral cortex

Information that an external event is a stressor is sent to the cerebral cortex via sensory pathways from the peripheral nervous system, the eyes, and the ears. For example, a light touch applied as a restraint could be a stressor. The sensory pathways from the skin to the cerebral cortex are diagrammed in Fig. 39-3. Sensory messages travel through the medulla and thalamus. While the afferent impulse is traveling upward, sensory impulses are sent to the reticular formation in the area of the brainstem. The reticular formation also sends input to the thalamus and cerebral cortex. Activities associated with these afferent impulses are called the *reticular activating system (RAS)*. The RAS functions to maintain wakefulness and alertness.

The cerebral cortex has sensory, motor, and associative functions. Figure 39-4 shows the major cortical areas where these functions are located. The somatic, auditory, and visual associative areas receive data from these senses and do some interpretation. The general interpretive area seems to coordinate information from all the senses and interpret it. The prefrontal area serves to reduce the speed of the

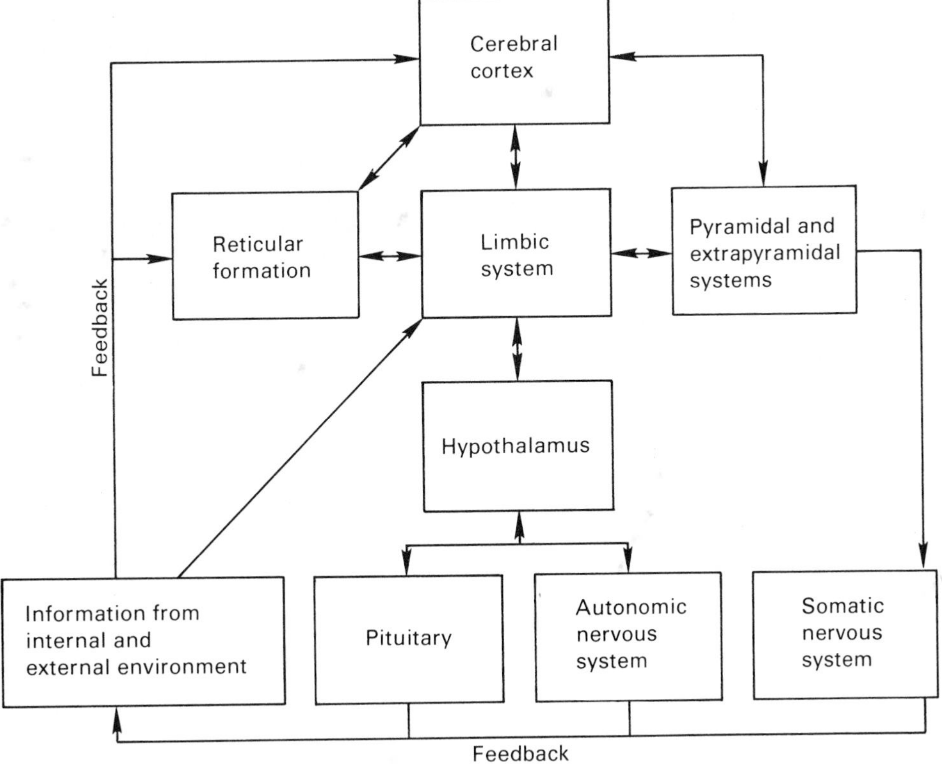

Figure 39-2 Neural control of emotion, *(From T. Cox, Stress, University Park Press, Baltimore, 1978, p. 51.)*

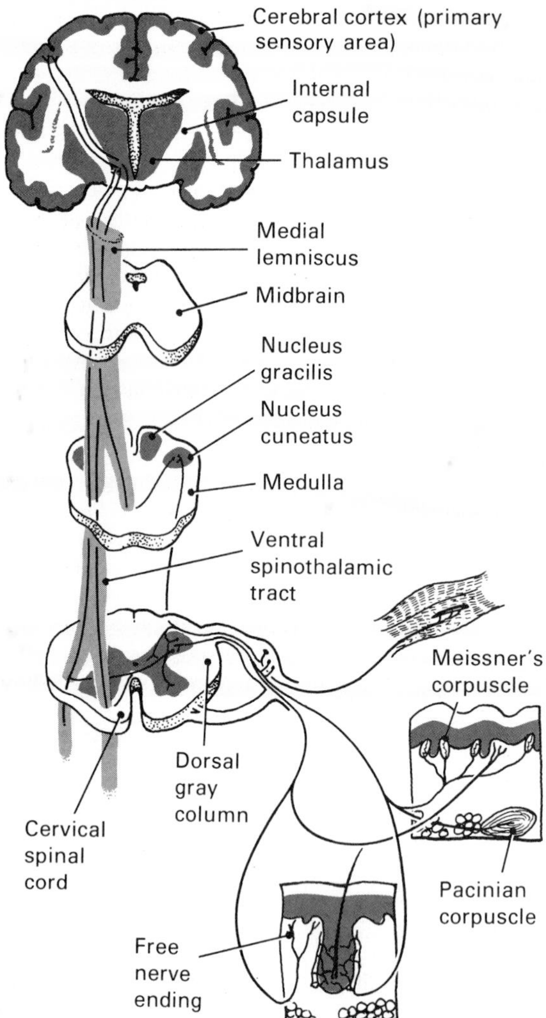

Figure 39-3 Nerve pathway for light pressure illustrating the similarity in pathways for afferent and efferent responses. (*Adapted from L. L. Langley, I. R. Telford, and J. B. Christenson, Dynamic Anatomy and Physiology, 5th ed., McGraw-Hill Book Company, New York, 1980, p. 279.*)

associative functions so that the person has time to evaluate the information in light of past experiences and future consequences and to plan a course of action. All of these functions are involved in the perception of a stressor.[2]

The temporal lobes contain the auditory association areas. These areas have also been found to produce fear when stimulated in the anterior and interior surfaces. Stimulation of the superior and lateral portions of the temporal lobes has resulted in sounds seeming louder or softer, visual displays seeming nearer or farther, and experiences seeming familiar or strange. This effect modifies perception.[3]

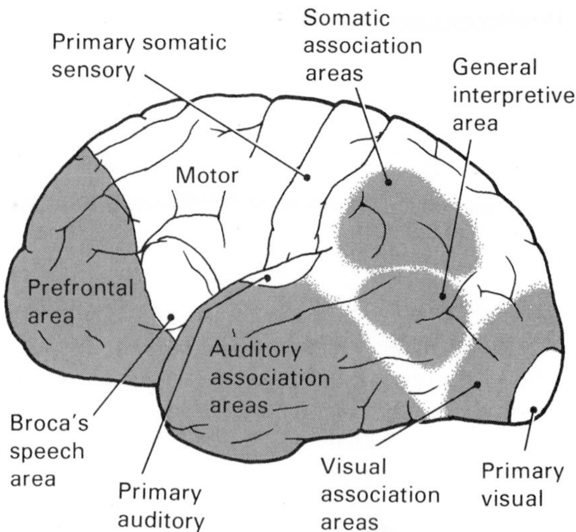

Figure 39-4 The major cortical areas, showing the close relationship between areas where sensory messages are received and areas where messages are interpreted and given meaning. (*From L. L. Langley, I. R. Telford, and J. B. Christenson, Dynamic Anatomy and Physiology, 5th ed., McGraw-Hill Book Company, New York, 1980, p. 279.*)

Limbic system

The limbic system lies in the inner midportion of the brain near the base. It includes the following structures: the septum, the cingulate gyrus, the amygdala, the hippocampus, and the anterior nuclei of the thalamus. The hypothalamus is located in the center of these structures but is not considered a part of the limbic system. The function of the limbic system is thought to be primarily involved with behavior. It has been shown that these structures, when stimulated, lead to emotions, feelings, and behaviors which ensure survival and self-preservation such as feeding, sociability, and sexuality. Tumors in this area have resulted in rage, fear, constant crying, and violent outbursts, as well as passivity. The cerebral cortex and limbic systems interact to serve the experiential and executive functions of emotion.[4] Endorphins (see Chap. 50) are also found in structures of the limbic system. They are known to reduce the perception of painful stimuli.

Reticular formation

The reticular formation is located between the lower end of the brainstem and the thalamus. It contains afferent and efferent connections for the various structures near it. As discussed earlier, it contains the RAS. The RAS sends impulses contributing to alertness to the limbic system as well as the cerebral cortex and thalamus. Impulses from the hypothalamus stimulate the RAS to increase its output of impulses leading to wakefulness. Perceived stress usually increases the degree of wakefulness.

Hypothalamus

The hypothalamus lies just above the pituitary gland. It serves many functions in the body (see Table 39-3). The hypothalamus is a major pathway by which the limbic system sends messages. Since the hypothalamus secretes substances that regulate the release of hormones by the anterior pituitary, it is central to the connection between the nervous and endocrine systems in responding to stress.

In addition, the hypothalamus regulates the function of both the sympathetic and parasympathetic systems of the autonomic nervous system. Thus, when an individual perceives the existence of a stressor, the hypothalamus mediates the response. It does this by activating the sympathetic nervous system (see Chap. 49) and by releasing corticotropin-releasing factor (CRF) to stimulate the pituitary to release adrenocorticotropic hormone (ACTH) (see Chap. 40).

Endocrine System

Once the hypothalamus begins the response to stress, the endocrine system becomes deeply involved. The sympathetic nervous system stimulates the adrenal medullae to release the hormones epinephrine and norepinephrine (catecholamines). These prepare the body for the "fight-or-flight" response, as illustrated by the left side of Fig. 39-5. The level of catecholamines can be measured in the blood or urine. Because of this fact, numerous research studies have used blood and urine tests to determine the impact of various stressors. It has been found that the greater the stressor, the higher the level of catecholamines.

The hypothalamus as mentioned earlier, also secretes CTF which stimulates the pituitary to release ACTH. ACTH, in turn, stimulates the adrenal cortex to release glucocorticoids, aldosterone, and androgens. The glucocorticoids are released in the greatest amounts. Aldosterone acts to increase extracellular fluid (ECF). The pituitary side of Fig. 39-5 diagrams the response to stress by the adrenal cortex. Figure 39-6 relates the *level* of glucocorticoid (corticoid) activity to the stages of the GAS.

It is important to note that stimulating both the adrenal medullae and the adrenal cortex results in an increased blood glucose level. This provides the additional fuel for the increased metabolism needed for fighting or fleeing. In addition, metabolism is facilitated by hormones from the thyroid gland. Thyroid gland secretion is also controlled by the hypothalamus and pituitary.

The physiological stress response prepares the individual to deal with the stressor in a physical manner. The increased cardiac output (due to the increased heart rate, increased ECF, and increased blood pressure), increased blood glucose levels, and increased metabolic rate make the physical response possible. In addition, the dilatation of blood vessels and the resulting increased blood supply to the large muscles and the brain provide for quick movement and increased alertness. The increased blood volume (from increased ECF and the shunting of blood from the gastrointestinal system) and increased clotting time function to help maintain adequate blood volume in case of traumatic blood loss. These are just a few examples of the physiological response to stress that illustrate the complex and interrelated stress phenomenon. A full description is beyond the scope of this chapter.

The physical response to stressors seems better suited to persons living in a primitive society than in the industrialized societies of today. Because of social conventions, much of the physical response to stressors is internalized and produces wear and tear on the body. As a result, many of the diseases experienced by modern people are considered maladaptations to stress (see Chap. 1).

Table 39-3
Hypothalmic Functions

Coordinates impulses for:	Autonomic nervous system Body temperature regulation Food intake Water intake Urine formation Cardiovascular function
Secretes releasing factors	Various hormones of the adenohypophysis Regulates adenohyphophyseal secretions
Affects behavior	Rage Alertness Psychosomatic disorders

Psychological Mechanisms

Psychological mechanisms are mediated in the cerebral cortex. A person responds psychologically to stressors by using *coping* or *defense mechanisms*. These are intrapsychic mechanisms used to deal with

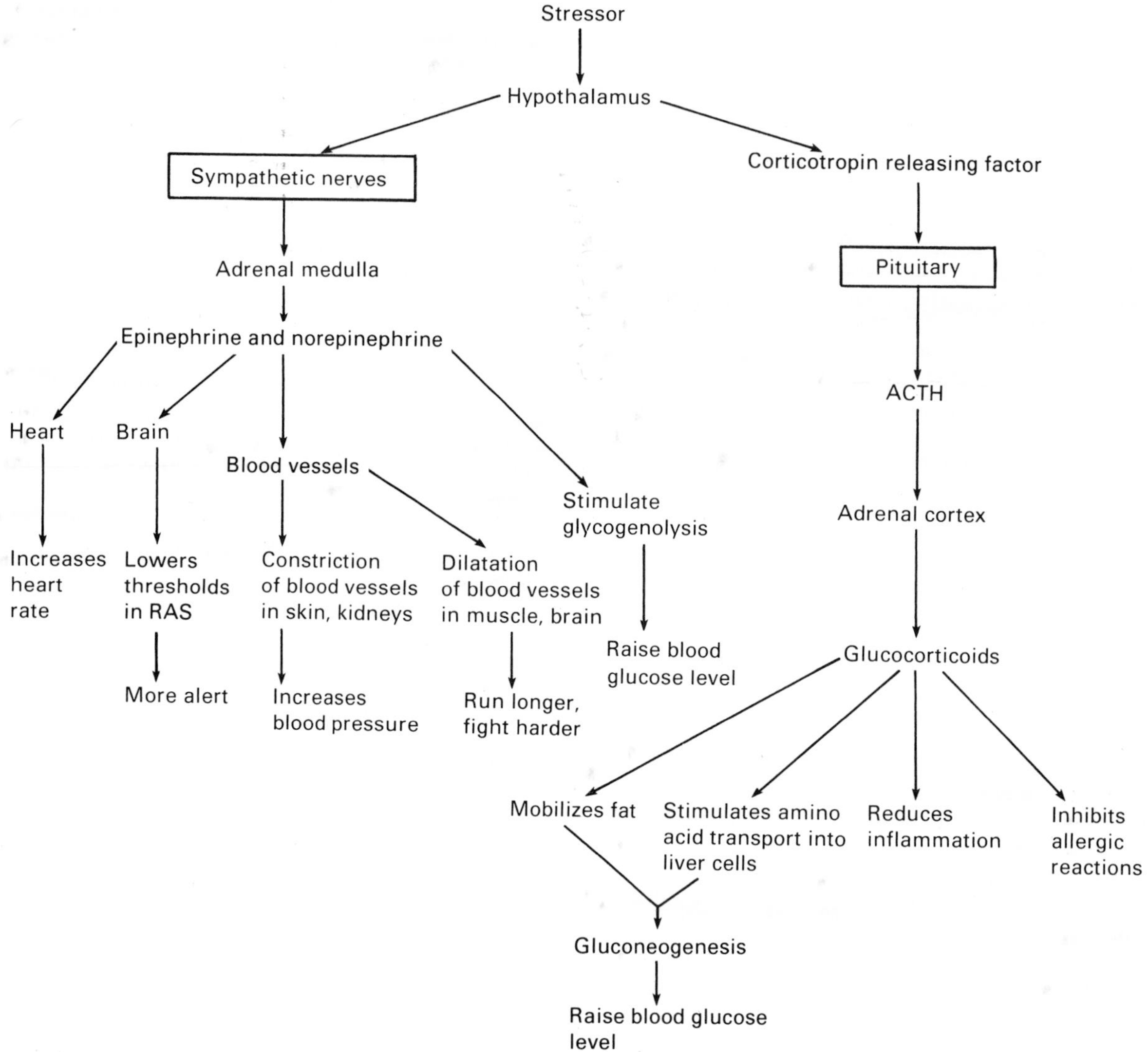

Figure 39-5 Some effects of stress. (*From Eldra Pearl Solomon and William Davis, Understanding Human Anatomy and Physiology, McGraw-Hill Book Company, New York, 1978, p. 535.*)

the demands and goals of life. Coping mechanisms are considered healthy ways to adjust to stressful events or persons. Patterns for coping behaviors are established early in childhood. In positive adaptation, they involve variations of the problem-solving method. As the person solves a problem, he adds to his repertoire of problem-solving skills.

Defense mechanisms, or defensive behaviors, are attempts to deal with stressors by creating long-term alienation from certain circumstances or by avoiding life's demands and goals. They are a form of maladaptation because of their inappropriate use. They may include such behaviors as denial, rationalization, reaction formation, and displacement. The continued use of one or more of these defense mechanisms may result in ineffective coping and neurosis or psychosis.

VARIABLES THAT ALTER THE EXPERIENCE OF STRESS

There are a number of variables that alter the experience of stress.[5] One is the nature of the stressor. The Social Readjustment Rating Scale (SRRS) (see Table 1-4) is an example of a tool that has been

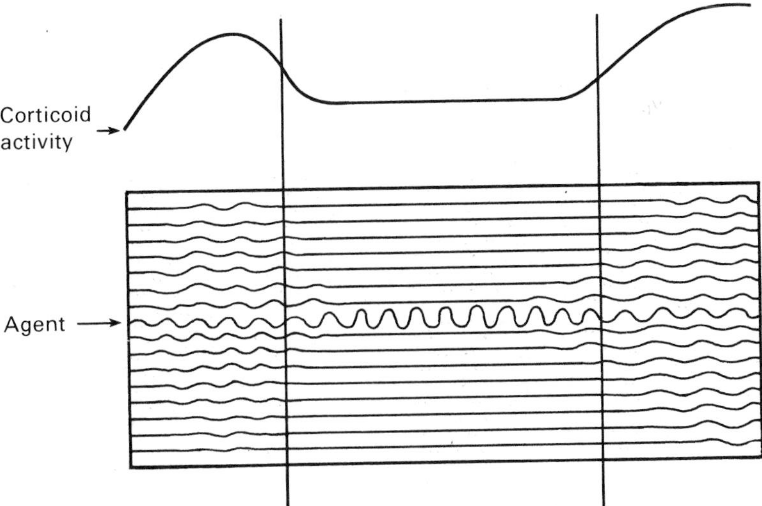

Alarm Reaction

Auxiliary mechanisms are mobilized to maintain life so that the reaction spreads to large territories. No organ system is as yet specially developed to cope with the task at hand.

Stage of Resistance

Adaptation is acquired due to optimum development of most appropriate specific channel of defense. Spatial concentration of the reaction makes corticoid production unnecessary.

Stage of Exhaustion

Reaction spreads again due to wear and tear in the most appropriate channel. Corticoid production rises, but can maintain life only until even auxiliary channels are exhausted.

Figure 39-6 Stress response by the endocrine system. *(From H. Seyle. The Stress of Life, revised edition, McGraw-Hill Book Company, New York, 1976, pp. 36–38.)*

developed to quantify stressors by assigning a number of units to a specific event. The more intense the stressor, the more energy required for adaptation.

A second variable is the total number of stressors with which the individual is coping at one time. This is also reflected in the relationship between the number of life change units and illness, discussed in Chap. 2. The more stressors the individual has to cope with simultaneously, the greater the amount of energy expenditure necessary to adapt. Thus the proverbial "straw that broke the camel's back" may occur when a relatively minor stressor precipitates an emotional or physical crisis.

Third, the longer the duration of the stressor, the less energy the person has available to cope. This variable relates to Selye's stage of resistance. For continued coping, the person's energy level must be maintained by obtaining outside help or by reducing other life stressors.

A fourth variable affecting an individual's response to stress is the previous experience with the stressor. Previous effective adaptation to a stressor usually means that less energy will be necessary to deal with the same or a similar current experience. However, if effective adaptation did not occur, increased stress may be encountered because of the previous experience.

Variables that affect the stress response and resistance are summarized in Table 39-4. Awareness of these variables is important because they aid the nurse in planning interventions for clients who are experiencing stress.

NURSING CARE OF THE CLIENT EXPERIENCING STRESS

Assessment of Stress in a Client

Too much stress in an individual can produce deleterious effects. It is critical that nurses know how to assess the presence of inadequate or inappropriate coping behaviors to stress in a client who is attempting to adapt. Physiological signs of the stress reaction are described in Chap. 40. However, the client may

Table 39-4
Variables that Affect Stress Response and Resistance

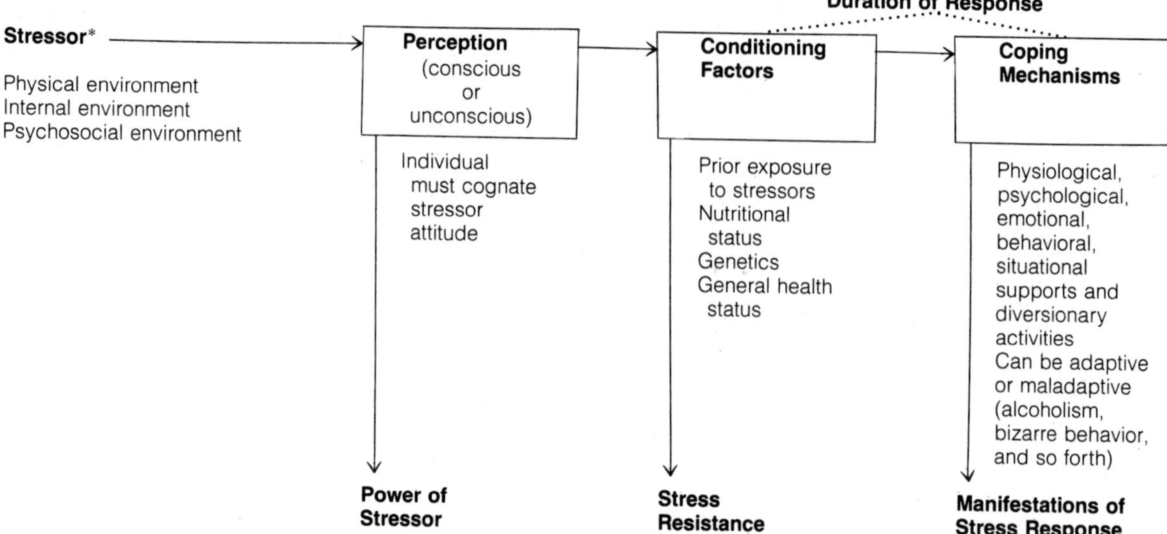

*The impact of a stressor depends on perception of its presence, the state of conditioning factors, and available coping mechanisms. Effects of stress can be reduced by identifying variables and planning nursing actions that will alter the variable in a positive way.
From M. J. T. Smith and H. Selye, "Reducing the Negative Effects of Stress," *Am J Nurs*, **79:**1954 (1979).

also exhibit behavioral clues related to difficulty in coping. When assessing behavioral clues, it is important that nurses validate their impressions with family members so that a habitual activity such as twirling a lock of hair is not misinterpreted. It is also important to recognize that certain crises, such as the death of a spouse, usually result in behavioral changes indicative of stress.

Behavioral clues indicating an increase in stress include:[6]

1. Increased use of one pattern of behavior that is part of the individual's normal behavior. For example, an individual may eat more snacks when stress occurs.
2. A change in the variety of activities in which a person normally participates. This may involve a decrease in activities to provide more energy to cope with stress, as when a normally neat person becomes untidy when a parent becomes seriously ill.
3. A change in behavior that suggests regression to an earlier level of behavior. Purposeless activities such as pacing the floor or nail biting are examples. Another example is the inability of a hospitalized business executive to make a simple decision regarding the next day's menu.
4. Increased sensitivity to factors in the environment, such as noise or light which the client normally does not notice. The response is usually one of irritability directed toward a significant other or others in the setting.
5. Distortion of reality, that is, misperception or misinterpretation of a normal event because the usual level of energy is unavailable for logical thinking. For example, a person who is having diagnostic studies for cancer may interpret a nurse's "I don't know" to mean "you have cancer" when in actuality the nurse may not know.

Physical signs of stress, as compared with behavioral manifestations, are due to activation of the sympathetic nervous system. These include increased heart rate, respiratory rate, blood pressure, and blood glucose, as well as sweating, pupil dilatation, and decreased peristalsis.

Interventions to Promote Adaptation to Stress

Both health professionals and lay persons use many approaches to deal with stress. Table 39-5 lists commonly used measures to reduce stress and indicates whether the measure does or does not require

Table 39-5
Measures Used to Reduce Stress

Used without Professional Help	Require Help of Specialist
Rest and leisure activities (hobbies, sports)	Psychotherapy
Transcendental meditation (related activities resulting in the relaxation response)	Psychoanalysis
Diet, including snacking behavior (e.g., eating junk food, chewing gum)	Hypnosis
Vitamins	Acupuncture
Alcoholic beverages	Chiropractic
Smoking tobacco, marijuana	Psychotropic drugs
Illegal drugs	

From H. Selye, *Stress in Health and Disease*, Butterworth & Co., Publishers, Inc., Boston, 1976, p. 897.

Table 39-6
Aids to Reducing Stress

1. Slow your pace. Do one thing at a time.
2. Develop a more passive attitude toward irritating, frustrating events. Consciously work to remain calm. Deal with problems when you have the emotional strength.
3. Provide for a period of relaxation every day. Try relaxation techniques such as yoga, biofeedback, relaxation response, or meditation.
4. Seek objectivity about problems by talking about feelings to friends, family, or a counselor.
5. Work off the energy of anxiety and relieve tension with physical exercise and recreation. Help others. Develop a fulfilling hobby.
6. Seek to change parts of your life that cause stress or worry.
7. Learn to be satisfied with less when doing your best. Do not hold unrealistic expectations for yourself or others.
8. Analyze what is causing anxiety and try to lessen the impact of the stressor.
9. Accept your own anger response. Accept things which you cannot change.
10. Keep something, such as a religious belief, as the center of your life where you can find a haven of rest.

From R. B. Murray and J. P. Zentner, *Nursing Concepts for Health Promotion*, 2d ed., Prentice-Hall, Inc., Englewood Cliffs, N.J., 1979, pp. 250–251.

the intervention of specially trained health care providers. Even though facts on many of the interventions are available in books on exercise, diet, and relaxation, the nurse needs to be knowledgeable about these topics and familiar with currect literature in order to advise clients on their usefulness.

On the other hand, some measures selected by individuals to reduce stress, such as snacking, smoking, and using drugs, may result in addictive behavior. The stress-reducing technique actually becomes a stressor, and intervention is required to eliminate it both as a stressor and as an addictive behavior.

Table 39-5 also describes approaches to reducing stress which require the intervention of specially trained health care providers. Some of these approaches, such as psychotherapy, are within the traditional medical field, whereas others, such as chiropractic or acupuncture, are within the holistic health field. Research is currently attempting to assess the effectiveness of less traditional approaches to stress reduction.

Nurses should use constructive approaches in dealing with stress in their own lives as well as when planning interventions for clients. Table 39-6 lists some guidelines to aid individuals to reduce stress in their lives. Implementing these principles may require a major change in lifestyle. For this reason, it is better for the nurse to recommend that changes be implemented slowly. Some changes, such as providing for a period of relaxation every day, establishing a regular exercise routine, and developing a hobby involve external action by the client and thus may be easier to implement. Other techniques, such as redefining life goals or developing a more passive attitude, involve internal work by the client. These changes may be facilitated by joining small self-help groups.

One approach the nurse may use to assist clients to cope with stress is seen in the model developed by Smith and Selye (Table 39-7). These researchers define three variables that affect stress response and resistance: perception, conditioning factors, and coping mechanisms (Table 39-4).[7]

Preception of stress

To reduce the client's perception of stress and thus its power, the nurse should assist him to neutralize the intensity of a stressor. This may be done by encouraging him to consciously place less significance on the stressor (e.g., an idea, person, event, or goal) than he has been doing. The client's perspective may be changed if he is made to consider the stressor in terms of time, his personal values and beliefs, and the negative effect that continuation of the stress response has on his life. He may also need to determine if his perception or belief is faulty. For example, an undergraduate college student may feel that he must graduate in 4 years to be a success. However, he has to work his way through school and is experiencing severe personal problems. Thus, in terms of his personal situation, it is unrealistic to expect to

Table 39-7
A Model for Coping with Stress

Variable: Perception 1. The perception of events and agents as stressors. 2. The actual and continued presence of a stressor or a symbolized threat to well-being.	**Approach/action** 1. Neutralizing the intensity of stress by putting events, goals, and ideas in a different perspective through conscious thinking. For instance, saying "I prefer to meet this goal" rather than "I *must* meet this goal." 2. Removing from the environment such stressors as unnecessary visitors, noise, uncomfortable conditions.
Variable: Conditioning factors 1. Self-esteem and control over stressful situations. 2. Sound nutritional habits. 3. Healthy lifestyles. 4. Absence of sudden and profound life changes.	**Approach/action** 1. Education of the client (e.g., teaching biofeedback, meditation, and/or relaxation techniques). 2. Nutritional counseling. General health counseling. 3. Advising and instructing the client as to methods of eliminating such changes.
Variable: Coping mechanisms 1. Situational support: ventilating one's feelings, talking about problems (which dissipates the unchanneled energy of stress reactions or anxiety which, if not relieved, can act as an additional stressor). 2. Diversionary activities (which temporarily distract one's attention from the problem). 3. Physical activity (which utilizes unchanneled energy created by the stress reaction and therefore decreases anxiety).	**Approach/action** 1. Making the client aware of available sources of support (friends, agencies, and so forth) and encouraging him to seek others if necessary. 2. Helping the client to replace maladaptive coping (for instance, alcoholism) with other, more positive behavior. 3. Making suggestions to the client and explaining the benefits of various types of exercise.

From M. J. T. Smith and H. Selye, "Reducing the Negative Effects of Stress," *Am J Nurs*, **79:**1955 (1979).

graduate in 4 years. Counseling by the nurse in Student Health may help him to change his perspective from "I have to graduate in 4 years" to "It's okay for me to take longer than 4 years to graduate."

Another way to reduce the perception of a stressor is to remove the stressor (actual or symbolic threat) from the environment. In the example above, if the source of the severe personal problems is an unsatisfactory living arrangement, then the nurse may help the student explore alternate solutions. In a hospital setting, the nurse has more control over the environment and is often able to directly remove a stressor from the environment. For instance, the nurse could explain the purpose of various pieces of equipment, place the client in a quieter room, administer an analgesic, or assign a different care giver.

Conditioning factors

Conditioning factors are another variable which must be considered by the nurse when assisting a client to cope with stress. An important conditioning factor is the client's feeling of self-esteem and control of a stressful situation. In order to increase the client's sense of control, the nurse should display respect for the client and involve him in the decisions about his care. In addition, the nurse should instruct the client in stress-reducing practices such as biofeedback, meditation, and other ways to elicit the relaxation response (slowed pulse, decreased oxygen use, peripheral warming and flush, lowered voice decibels, decreased muscle tension, and decreased lactic acid leading to an increased galvanic skin response).[8] The type of meditation depends on the client's preference and may include prayer, transcendental meditation, Zen Buddhism, and yoga. In addition, the client may be taught to elicit the relaxation response through the use of relaxation exercises. The client is instructed to sit in a comfortable, well-supported position in a quiet environment and then to progressively tense and relax various muscle groups. It is theorized that there is a close relationship between the muscles and the mind so that muscle contraction is accompanied by psychological tension. Thus, anxiety (psychological tension) "cannot exist when muscles are truly relaxed."[9]

Good nutritional habits also assist the client to resist stress. Thus, if a careful assessment of the client's nutritional status and habits reveals a problem, then nutritional counseling is the appropriate nursing intervention. Generally, clients should eat a well-balanced diet which includes the basic four food groups and avoid foods excessively high in carbohydrates and sodium. They should also be counseled to maintain or achieve their ideal weight (see Chap. 60). A healthy livestyle and avoidance of sudden, major lifestyle changes also help a client resist stress. These topics are discussed in detail in Chap. 1.

Coping mechanisms

A third major variable affecting a client's reaction to stressors is his coping mechanisms. One such coping mechanism may be the support available in a particular situation, which the nurse should encourage the client to use.

The nurse may provide support or may refer the client to others such as family members, friends, a spiritual adviser, or a mental health counselor. The ability to assess a problem and decide on the most appropriate support system for the client is a serious nursing responsibility. Knowledge of community resources is necessary to fulfill this nursing function.

The client may also be assisted to cope with stress by using constructive diversionary activities such as hobbies or involvement in community projects. Specific activities should be based on the client's interest and on economic feasibility. Clients should be channeled away from using maladaptive coping behaviors such as excessive use of alcohol, drugs, or food, smoking, or violent outbursts.

An important coping mechanism for stress, as well as a vital health habit, is participation in regular physical activity. At least part of this activity should consist of aerobic exercise to stimulate cardiovascular and respiratory fitness. The nurse should assist in identifying a physical activity which the client enjoys and can do on a regular basis. If climate, finances, or other factors prevent participation in the activity, the client should select another activity which is better suited to his lifestyle.

If stressors are so great that they are affecting the client's ability to function in society, then he should be referred for professional help. This help may consist of professional counseling or medications such as tranquilizers and sedatives. The use of medications may be crucial in reducing the stress response to a point where other interventions can be initiated. However, medications treat the symptom rather than its cause and, therefore, should be used only on a temporary basis.

In summary, it is important that the nurse have a good data base about her client in attempting to help him manage stress. No one approach will work for everyone. The interventions must be individualized for the client.

REVIEW QUESTIONS

The number of the question corresponds to the same numbered objective at the beginning of the chapter.

1. An example of stress is the
   - **a.** experience of being married at the time of graduation from school
   - **b.** traumatic experience of a car accident upon hearing of the onset of war
   - **c.** incidence of three deaths in one's family due to cancer when one has rectal bleeding
   - **d.** release of catecholamines as a result of stimulation by the sympathetic nervous system

2. All the following statements about the GAS are true *except*
   - **a.** it was first defined by Hans Selye and is different from the local response to a stressor
   - **b.** it involves the central and autonomic nervous systems and the pituitary, thyroid, and adrenal glands
   - **c.** symptoms of the stage of resistance are due to stimulation of the sympathetic nervous system
   - **d.** symptoms of the stage of exhaustion may initially mimic those of the Stage of Alarm

3. The central nervous system is involved in the perception of a stressor by
   - **a.** releasing CRF from the hypothalamus
   - **b.** receiving efferent impulses from the peripheral nervous system
   - **c.** interpreting data received by the somatic, auditory, and visual associative areas
   - **d.** sending data from the cerebral cortex to the thalamus

4. The part of the nervous system which connects it to the endocrine system is the
   - **a.** hypothalamus
   - **b.** cerebral cortex
   - **c.** reticular formation
   - **d.** limbic system

5. The effect of stress on the heart includes
   - **a.** decrease in cardiac output
   - **b.** vasodilatation of peripheral vessels
   - **c.** increase in heart rate
   - **d.** decrease in blood pressure

6. An example of a stressor whose duration may increase a person's stress response is
   - **a.** taking a vacation
   - **b.** unresolved grief following the death of a close friend
   - **c.** receiving a speeding ticket upon leaving a court where he has just been divorced
   - **d.** continued daily care of a severely retarded child

7. When assessing a client, the nurse decides that he is under stress when she determines that
   - **a.** his snacking behavior is the same as it has been for the previous 2 years
   - **b.** since his job promotion, he has increased his sleeping time from 8 to 11 hours per day

c. his wife reports that he is not irritated when his son plays the stereo while the television is on

d. his nail biting has decreased over the last 2 years to the point where he has stopped

REFERENCES

1. H. Selye, *Stress without Distress*, New American Library of World Literature, Inc., New York, 1974, p. 14.
2. L. L. Langley, I. R. Telford, and J. B. Christensen, *Dynamic Anatomy and Physiology*, 5th ed., McGraw-Hill Book Company, New York, 1980, p. 279.
3. T. Cox, *Stress*, University Park Press, Baltimore, 1978, pp. 41–42.
4. Ibid., pp. 47–52.
5. M. L. Byrne and L. F. Thompson, *Key Concepts for the Study and Practice of Nursing*, 2d ed., The C. V. Mosby Company, St. Louis, 1978, pp. 72–77.
6. Ibid., pp. 86–90.
7. M. J. T. Smith and H. Selye, "Reducing the Negative Effects of Stress," *Am J Nurs,* **79** (10):1954–1955 (1979).
8. Dolores Kueger, *The Therapeutic Touch*, Prentice-Hall, Inc., Englewood Cliffs, N.J., 1979, pp. 75–76.
9. D. C. Sutterly, "Stress and Health: A Survey of Self-Regulation Modalities," *Topics Clin Nurs,* **1**:14 (1979).

Chapter 40

NURSING ASSESSMENT

Endocrine System

JoAnn Ganje Congdon

Learning Objectives

1. Explain the common characteristics and functions of hormones.
2. Identify the location of the endocrine glands.
3. Describe the functions of the hormones secreted by the pituitary, thyroid, parathyroid, and adrenal glands and the pancreas.
4. Describe the characteristics and functions of prostaglandins.
5. Identify the significant subjective and objective data related to the endocrine system that should be obtained from a client.
6. Describe the appropriate techniques used in physical assessment of the endocrine system.
7. Differentiate normal from common abnormal findings of a physical assessment of the endocrine system.
8. Describe the purpose, significance of results, and nursing responsibilities of diagnostic studies of the endocrine system.

The endocrine system is a chemical communication system among cells that functions, along with the nervous system, to regulate basic metabolic activities of the body.[1] The endocrine system is composed of the endocrine glands which secrete biologically active chemical substances called hormones. The endocrine glands include the pituitary, thyroid, parathyroids, adrenals, and pancreas, ovaries, testes, and thymus (Figure 40-1). This chapter is concerned with the function of the pituitary, thyroid, parathyroids, adrenals, and pancreas. The normal functions of the testes and ovaries are discussed in Chap. 43. The thymus gland is discussed in Chap. 10.

ENDOCRINE SYSTEM: STRUCTURES AND FUNCTIONS

Types of Glands

Exocrine glands

The two main types of glands are *exocrine* and *endocrine* glands. Exocrine glands pass along their secretions via ducts which empty outside the body or into the lumen of the organ that is lined with the same embryonic epithelium as the gland. For example, the exocrine secretions of the skin glands are discharged directly onto the surface of the skin. Exocrine secretions of the pancreas, the enzymes, are secreted into the pancreatic duct and transported to the intestine.

Endocrine glands

Endocrine glands are ductless glands. Their connecting ducts were lost during embryonic development. Secretions of endocrine glands are called hormones. Endocrine glands secrete their hormones directly into the interstitial fluid surrounding the cells. Then the hormone diffuses into the blood, where it exerts its influence on specific target tissue.

Hormones

Definition and characteristics

A *hormone* is a chemical substance synthesized and secreted by a specific organ or tissue and carried by the blood to other sites in the body where its actions are exerted. Endocrine hormones have certain common characteristics including the following:

1. All hormones circulate in the blood.
2. Hormones are secreted in minute but effective amounts.
3. Most hormones are inactivated or excreted by the liver or kidneys.
4. Hormones act by altering the rate of a physiological response.

Structure of hormones

Structurally, hormones are either steroids or proteins. Steroid hormones are secreted by the adrenal cortices, the ovaries, and the testes. Steroid hormones are lipid soluble, synthesized from cholesterol, and able to penetrate into the cell where specific receptors exist. Protein hormones are unable to penetrate cell membranes because of their large size and lipid insolubility. Instead, they act at receptor sites on the cell membrane which, in turn, activate intracellular processes.

Functions of hormones

Hormones alter the rate of many bodily activities. In general, important hormonal functions are related to

*This chapter was reviewed by Phoebe J. Becktell, R.N., B.S.N., M.A., Assistant Professor, College of Nursing, University of New Mexico, Albuquerque, New Mexico.

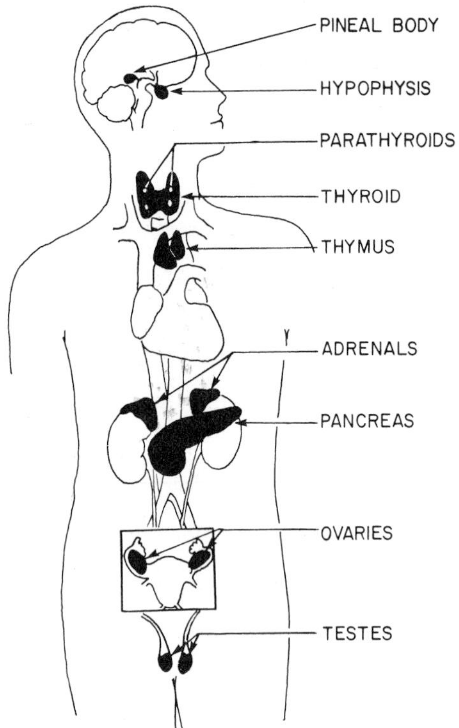

Figure 40-1 Location of the major endocrine glands. Note that the parathyroid glands actually lie on the posterior surface of the thyroid. The thymus atrophies after puberty and is replaced by fatty tissue.

reproduction, responses to stress and injury, ionic metabolism, energy metabolism, and growth and development.[2] Table 40-1 summarizes the major hormones and their corresponding glands and functions. More specific functions will be discussed in terms of the appropriate endocrine gland.

Regulation of Hormonal Secretion

Regulation of endocrine activity is controlled by specific processes which stimulate or inhibit hormone secretion. One such process involves a negative feedback system based on the blood level of a particular hormone. A low circulating level of a hormone causes the stimulating hormone to be produced by the pituitary. This stimulating hormone results in increased hormone production. Conversely, a high circulating level of a hormone will inhibit production of the stimulating hormone. The thyroxine-thyroid-stimulating hormone (TSH) relationship is an example of a negative feedback system (Fig. 40-2).

Another regulator of hormone secretion is a change in the concentration of a plasma substance. The plasma levels of glucose, calcium, and sodium regulate certain hormonal secretions of the pancreas, the parathyroids, and the adrenal cortex, respectively. For instance, insulin is secreted as a direct result of increased glucose in the blood (Fig. 40-3). A decreased level of glucose inhibits insulin secretion. There is no evidence that the pituitary gland controls insulin secretion. The specific mechanisms regulating aldosterone secretion from the adrenal cortex are discussed later in this chapter.

In addition to the chemical regulation mentioned, some endocrine glands are affected directly by autonomic nervous system activity. Nervous stimulation usually results from stress and is mediated by the central nervous system.[3] This interrelationship will be discussed further under the section on the Hypothalamus-Pituitary Complex.

Another regulatory process affecting many hormonal secretions involves the rhythms of secretions. These rhythms originate in brain structures. The menstrual cycle in women is one example. Another type of

Table 40-1
Summary of the Major Hormones

Gland	Hormone	Major function/Control of:
Hypothalamus	Releasing hormones	Secretions of the anterior pituitary
	Oxytocin	(See posterior pituitary)
	Antidiuretic hormone	(See posterior pituitary)
Anterior pituitary	Growth hormone (somatotropin, STH)*	Growth; organic metabolism
	Thyroid-stimulating hormone (TSH)	Thyroid gland
	Adrenocorticotropic hormone (ACTH)	Adrenal cortex
	Prolactin	Breasts (milk formation)
	Gonadotropic hormones:	Gonads
	Follicle-stimulating hormone (FSH)	
	Luteinizing hormone (LH)	

Table 40-1 (Continued)

Gland	Hormone	Major function/Control of:
Posterior pituitary†	Oxytocin	Milk secretion; uterine motility
	Antidiuretic hormone (ADH, Vasopressin)	Water excretion
Adrenal cortex	Cortisol	Organic metabolism; response to stress
	Androgens	Growth and, in women, sexual activity
	Aldosterone	Sodium and potassium excretion
Adrenal medulla	Epinephrine Norepinephrine	Organic metabolism; cardiovascular function; response to stress
Thyroid	Thyroxine (T_4) Triiodothyronine (T_3)	Energy metabolism; growth and development
	Calcitonin	Plasma calcium
Parathyroids	Parathyroid hormone (parathormone, PTH, PH)	Plasma calcium and phosphate
Gonads		
Female: ovaries	Estrogen Progesterone	Reproductive system; growth and development; breasts
Male: testes	Testosterone	Reproductive system; growth and development
Pancreas	Insulin Glucagon	Organic metabolism; plasma glucose
Thymus	Thymus hormone (thymosin)	Lymphocyte development
Pineal	Melatonin	?Sexual maturity

*The names and abbreviations in parentheses are synonyms.

†The posterior pituitary stores and secretes these hormones; they are synthesized in the hypothalamus.

Adapted from D. S. Luciano et al., *Human Function and Structure,* McGraw-Hill Book Company, New York, 1978.

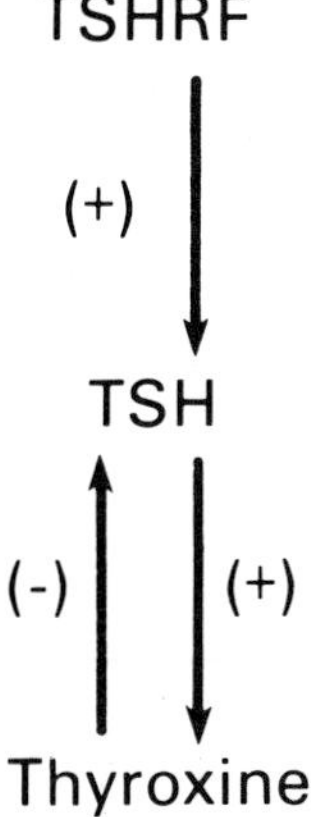

Figure 40-2 Diagrammatic representation of a feedback regulating system. [*From S. Price and L. Wilson (eds.), Pathophysiology: Clinical Concepts of Disease Processes, McGraw-Hill Book Company, New York, 1982.*]

rhythm is referred to as *diurnal* or *circadian*, which means that the level of a hormone fluctuates over a 24-hour period. For example, cortisol rises early in the day, declines later, and rises again during the night to peak by the next morning (Fig. 40-4). These rhythms must be considered when interpreting the result of laboratory data related to hormone levels.

Hypothalamus-Pituitary Complex

Both the nervous and endocrine systems are involved in the communication between organs and tissues of the body. The hypothalamus collects information from these two systems, integrates it, and coordinates the activities of the systems.[4] The hypothalamus regulates the function of the endocrine system by its action on the pituitary gland (Fig. 40-5).

The hypothalamus and the pituitary communicate via blood vessels called the *portal system* (Fig. 40-6).

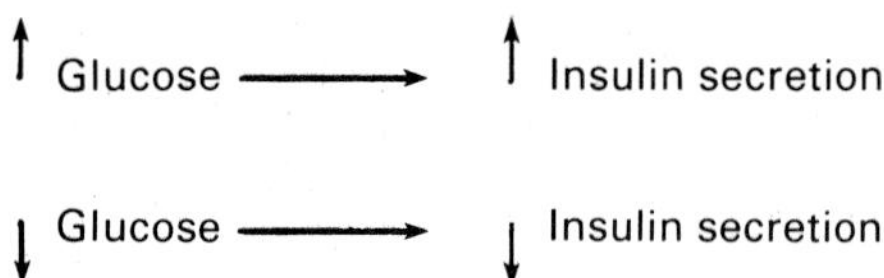

Figure 40-3 Regulation of insulin in response to blood levels of glucose.

The hypothalamus secretes substances which are carried by the portal system to the anterior pituitary. The secretions of the hypothalamus, called *releasing factors,* regulate the release of various hormones of the anterior pituitary. Evidence is now accumulating which shows that some, and perhaps all, of the pituitary hormones are controlled not only by releasing factors but also by inhibiting factors[5] (Table 40-2).

Pituitary Gland (Hypophysis)

The pituitary is a small gland weighing approximately 0.6 g and measuring about 1 cm in diameter. It is located in the sella turcica, situated at the base of the brain above the sphenoid bone. It is connected with the hypothalamus by the infundibular (hypophyseal) stalk. From the standpoint of embryonic development and physiological function, the pituitary consists of two parts: the adenohypophysis (anterior pituitary) and the neurohypophysis (posterior pituitary). There is also a small middle, or intermediate, lobe which does not form a definite autonomic subdivision. Table 40-3 lists the hormones of the three portions of the pituitary.

Anterior pituitary

The anterior lobe comprises about 75 percent of the gland by weight. Blood is supplied via the hypothalamic-hypophyseal portal system. The anterior pituitary is regulated by hypothalamic releasing and inhibiting factors, as well as by a negative feedback system from circulating hormones.

The anterior pituitary secretes six hormones: (1) adrenocorticotropic hormone (ACTH), or corticotropin, which stimulates the secretions of the adrenal cortical hormones, (2) thyrotropin, or thyroid-stimulating hormone (TSH), which stimulates the uptake of iodine and the synthesis and release of thyroid hormones by the thyroid, (3) follicle-stimulating hormone (FSH), which stimulates the growth of the ovarian follicles, (4) lutenizing hormone (LH), which regulates the growth of the gonads and their reproductive activities, (5) growth hormone (GH), or somatotropin, which stimulates growth of all tissues and increases protein synthesis, and (6) luteotropic hormone (LTH), or prolactin, which promotes mammary gland development and stimulates milk secretion plus the corpus luteum of the ovary to secrete progesterone.

Posterior pituitary

The posterior pituitary lies just behind the anterior pituitary in the same body of the sphenoid bone. It is composed of numerous nerve fibers and many small cells termed *pituicytes*. The pituicytes act as supporting structures for the nerve fibers that originate in the hypothalamus. These nerve fibers, or tracts, pass to the posterior pituitary through the hypophyseal stalk. The hormones of the posterior pituitary—antidiuretic hormone (ADH)—and oxytocin are formed in the hypothalamus and move down these nerve fibers to be stored in the posterior lobe. Upon neural stimulation, the stored hormones are released.

ADH has a major physiological role in regulating water metabolism. The usual stimulus to ADH secre-

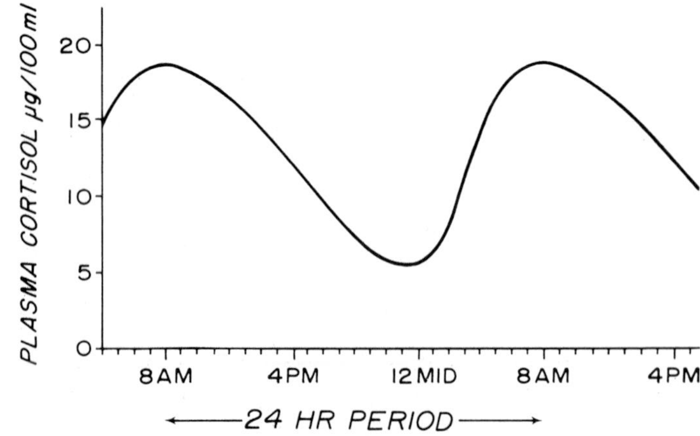

Figure 40-4 Circadian rhythm of cortisol secretion. [*From S. Price and L. Wilson (eds.), Pathophysiology: Clinical Concepts of Disease Processes, 2d ed., McGraw-Hill Book Company, New York, 1982.*]

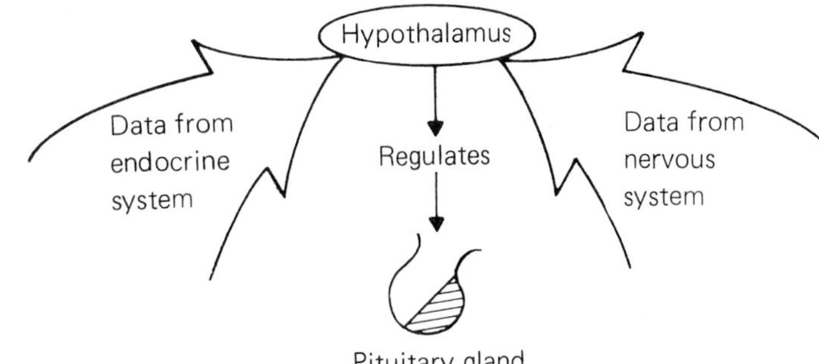

Figure 40-5 The hypothalamus coordinates the activities of the endocrine and nervous systems. *(From A. Tripp, Basic Mechanisms of Endocrine Dysfunction, McGraw-Hill Book Company, New York, 1978.)*

tion is an increase in plasma osmolality. If there is a decrease in extracellular fluid or an increase in sodium concentration, plasma osmolality increases causing the activation of osmoreceptors in the hypothalamus which signal the release of ADH. Therefore, when the body fluids become highly concentrated, ADH is secreted. ADH then acts by increasing the permeability of the cells of the distal tubule and collecting ducts in the kidney to reabsorb water. In the absence of ADH, large amounts of dilute urine are excreted.

Oxytocin has a stimulating effect upon smooth muscles of the pregnant uterus. It is secreted during parturition, causing uterine contractions and active ejection of milk from the alveoli.[6]

Pars intermedia

The pars intermedia is located between the pars distalis and the pars nervosa and secretes melanocyte-stimulating hormone (MSH). Although it is believed to stimulate melanin production, its role in human physiology has not been definitely established.

Thyroid Gland

The thyroid gland is located in the anterior portion of the neck in front of the trachea. It consists of two lateral lobes connected by a narrow isthmus and is a highly vascular organ. It is estimated that about 4 to 5 L of blood per hour circulates through the gland.[7] The function of the thyroid gland is to produce thyroxine

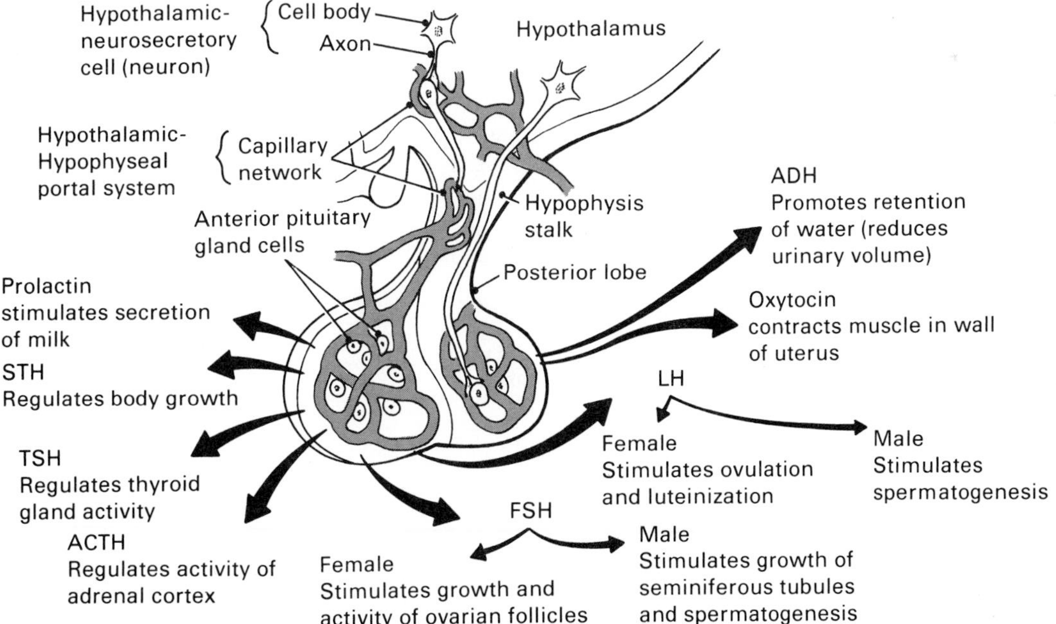

Figure 40-6 The pituitary gland, or hypophysis. (*Adapted from E. Reith et al., Textbook of Anatomy and Physiology, 2d ed., McGraw-Hill Book Company, New York, 1978.*)

Table 40-2
Releasing and Inhibiting Factors of the Hypothalamus

Releasing Factors	Inhibiting Factors
Corticotropin-releasing factor (CRF)	Prolactin-inhibiting factor
Gonadotropin-releasing factor (GRF)	Melanocyte-inhibiting factor
Thyrotropin-releasing factor (TRF)	Growth hormone-inhibiting factor (somatostatin)
Growth hormone-releasing factor (GHRF)	

(T_4) and triiodothyronine (T_3). T_4 is believed to be a precursor of T_3 which is the active hormone. Iodine is necessary for the synthesis of T_3. Thyroxine and triiodothyronine affect metabolic rate, caloric requirement, carbohydrate and lipid metabolism, body growth and development, brain function, and nervous system activity.

Thyroid hormone production is stimulated by TSH. Low serum levels of the thyroid hormones increase the production of thyroid-releasing factor (TRF) by the hypothalamus, which in turn increases the production of TSH by the anterior pituitary. High serum levels of thyroid hormones decrease TRF and TSH secretion in a negative feedback loop.

Calcitonin is also produced by the thyroid gland. Calcitonin inhibits the release of calcium from the bone and renal tubular reabsorption of calcium. Together with parathyroid hormone, calcitonin regulates the concentration of plasma calcium.

Parathyroid Glands

The parathyroid glands are small oval structures located in close proximity to the thyroid gland. Usually, there are four of them, arranged in pairs behind each lobe of the thyroid. Occasionally, they can even be found in the chest. The glands consist of closely packed epithelial cells richly supplied with blood from the branches of the inferior and superior thyroid arteries. The parathyroids secrete parathyroid hormone, or parathormone (PTH). Its major role is to regulate the blood level of calcium and phosphate. PTH acts on three sites: the gastrointestinal tract, the kidney, and the bones. In the intestine, PTH enhances absorption of calcium. The renal effect of PTH is to increase the reabsorption of calcium and promote excretion of phosphate in the renal tubules. In bone, it is believed to stimulate osteoclastic activity to release calcium into the blood.

PTH is free of both pituitary and hypothalamic control. The secretion of this hormone is directly regulated by a negative feedback system. When serum calcium is low, PTH secretion increases; when serum calcium rises, PTH secretion falls.

Adrenal Glands (Suprarenal)

The adrenal glands are small organs located above each kidney. They vary in size, with the average weight for each being 5 to 9 g. Each gland has a medulla and a cortex.

Adrenal medulla

The inner component, the adrenal medulla, constitutes only 10 percent of the total gland. It secretes two hormones, epinephrine and norepinephrine, collectively referred to as *catecholamines*. Their functions are widespread and include almost the same effects produced by direct stimulation of the sympathetic nerves in all parts of the body. A more complete discussion of adrenal medullary hormones can be found in Chap. 49.

Table 40-3
Hormones of the Pituitary Gland

Anterior Pituitary (Adenohypophysis)	Pars Intermedia	Posterior Pituitary (Neurohypophysis)
Growth hormone (GH) (somatotropin)	Melanocyte-stimulating hormone (MSH)	Oxytocin
Luteotropic hormone (LTH)		Antidiuretic hormone (ADH)
Thyroid-stimulating hormone (TSH)		
Adrenocorticotropic hormone (ACTH)		
Follicle-stimulating hormone (FSH)		
Luteinizing hormone (LH)		

Adrenal cortex

The adrenal cortex is the larger outer part of the adrenal gland and secretes about 30 steroid hormones. The most important secretions of the adrenal cortex are the mineralocorticoids, glucocorticoids, and androgens. Aldosterone, the major mineralocorticoid, is essential for the maintenance of sodium and potassium balance. Cortisol and corticosterone are known as glucocorticoids because of their special effect on glucose metabolism. Androgens, or sex steroids, are produced in small but significant quantities in the adrenal cortex. Small amounts of estrogen are also secreted by the adrenal cortex.

Mineralocorticoids Mineralocorticoids mainly affect mineral balance. Aldosterone, the major mineralocorticoid, functions at the renal tubule. It stimulates the reabsorption of sodium, chloride, and water and decreases the reabsorption of potassium. There are several mechanisms which can regulate aldosterone secretion and thus influence the fluid balance. Aldosterone secretion is increased by (1) a decrease in serum sodium concentration, (2) an increase in angiotensin formation, (3) an increase in serum potassium, and (4) ACTH secretion.

Glucocorticoids The major glucocorticoid is cortisol (hydrocortisone). It functions primarily to increase blood glucose levels by increasing the rate of gluconeogenesis and decreasing glucose utilization by the cells. Cortisol facilitates the transport of amino acids into the liver cells. The glucocorticoids reduce protein stores in almost all body cells except those of the liver.

In addition, glucocorticoids support the mobilization of fatty acids and interfere with the utilization of glucose for energy at the peripheral level. Other effects include their anti-inflammatory action and supportive actions in stress situations. Cortisol combats inflammation by stabilizing the membranes of cellular lysosomes and decreasing capillary permeability. This stabilization reduces the destructive effects of proteolytic enzymes on surrounding tissues. A marked increase in the rate of cortisol secretion by the adrenal cortex can aid the body in coping more effectively with stress situations (see Chap. 39). The secretion of cortisol is under the control of ACTH from the anterior pituitary and is maintained by a self-regulating feedback mechanism.

Adrenal Sex Hormones The androgenic hormones (androgen, estrogen, and progesterone) constitute a third functional group of steroids elaborated by the adrenal cortex. It is not definitely known if their function is the same as or different from that of the gonadal secretions. (Secretions of the gonads are discussed in Chap 43.)

Pancreas

The pancreas is a long, tapered, lobular, soft gland weighing between 60 and 90 g. It lies in front of the first and second lumbar vertebrae and behind the stomach. The pancreas has both endocrine and exocrine functions. The exocrine function is concerned with the production of digestive enzymes. The pancreas also contains endocrine gland cells that perform distinct endocrine functions. Within the pancreas are a group of cells called the *islets of Langerhans*, which have two identifiable cell types, alpha and beta cells. The alpha cells secrete glucagon, and the beta cells secrete insulin.

Insulin

Insulin promotes the rate of glucose diffusion across all cell membranes of the body except those of the brain. The brain does not need insulin for glucose diffusion. Insulin is stored in the beta cells in granules and remains there until a stimulus signals its release.

The glucose concentration of the blood is the main stimulus for secretion of insulin. When the glucose level is high, insulin is secreted until a normal glucose level is restored. When the glucose level is low, insulin secretion ceases. In addition to this function, insulin acts on cellular enzymes responsible for the conversion of glucose to glycogen, enhances the transport of glucose into muscle cells, expedites the transfer of amino acids into cells and their incorporation into proteins, augments fatty acid synthesis, and influences many liver enzymes other than those involved in glycogen formation.[8]

Glucagon

Glucagon released from alpha cells causes an increase in blood sugar by increasing both gluconeogenesis and glycogenolysis in the liver. Glucagon is also called the *hyperglycemic factor*. It is secreted in response to low blood sugar levels. The secretion of both insulin and glucagon is influenced by the blood glucose concentration. When the blood sugar falls, glucagon is secreted; when it rises, insulin is secreted. Generally, glucagon and insulin seem to function in a reciprocal relationship to maintain blood sugar in a normal range.

Prostaglandins

The prostaglandins are a group of closely related lipid compounds that were first isolated in semen but more recently have been found to be formed in many other parts of the body such as the lungs, kidneys, uterus, liver, and gastrointestinal tract. Prostaglandins appear to be synthesized in response to appropriate stimuli. Their short half-life makes storage or transport to distant organs ineffective. Although they are not secreted exclusively by endocrine glands, they are hormonelike, exerting a wide range of physiological actions within the body. Prostaglandins exert a more local effect on cells and tissues in which they are synthesized. Several classes of prostaglandins are known, the three main groups being E (PGE), F(PGF), and A(PGA).

The prostaglandins participate in a number of processes, including arteriolar and bronchiolar dilatation, autoregulation of blood flow in a number of organs, blood pressure control, excretion of sodium and water, inhibition of gastric secretion, smooth muscle contraction, nerve function, and fat metabolism. Both treatment with and deprivation of prostaglandins have been shown to have therapeutic effects.[9]

Although the precise role of prostaglandins is complex and not clearly defined, recent work has led to the growing awareness of the importance of these substances. They appear to have potential widespread therapeutic uses in areas ranging from illnesses such as asthma, to electrolyte disturbances, to cardiovascular diseases. At the present time, prostaglandins are being used to initiate labor and induce abortion.[10,11]

ASSESSMENT OF THE ENDOCRINE SYSTEM

The hormones of the endocrine system have diverse systemic effects. Consequently, hypofunction or hyperfunction of an endocrine gland can result in dysfunction of a variety of organs and organ systems. Because many signs and symptoms of endocrine problems have other possible etiologies, the clinician must be alert to subtle manifestations of endocrine disorders. For instance, weight loss may be a sign of diabetes or hyperthyroidism as well as a gastrointestinal or emotional problem. Or, it may be the result of a well-planned, nutritionally sound weight reduction program. A careful health history should yield valuable data related to endocrine problems.

The general survey, as described in Chap. 3 is considered to be the inspection part of an endocrine assessment. It would describe a person who is alert and oriented and whose speech and mannerisms are appropriate for his age, environment and circumstances. The body would be of proper height and weight, with no apparent problems of the skin, nails, or hair. Generally, there would be no gross problems which would alert the clinician to possible endocrine disturbances.

Specific signs and symptoms which reflect excesses or deficiencies of a particular hormone are discussed in the appropriate section. There are, however, nonspecific changes related to endocrine dysfunction which should alert the examiner to possible problems. These include changes in energy level, alertness, personality, appetite, weight, skin, hair, personal appearance, and sexual function.

Subjective Data: The History

Past medical history

The client should be questioned about the existence or history of any of the following problems which are known to be related to endocrine dysfunction:

- Delay or acceleration in growth and development
- Changes in the size of the head, hands, or feet in the adult
- Presence of abnormal secondary sex characteristics (e.g., growth of facial hair in the female)
- Diabetes mellitus or insipidus
- Thyroid disease (exophthalmos, goiter)
- Hypertension
- Kidney stones
- Skin or hair changes
- Appetite or weight changes
- Memory impairment
- Increased sympathetic activity (nervousness, palpitations, sweating, tremors)

The client should be questioned about his general state of health. Has there been any change? Have any of these past problems affected his ability to function at work, at home, or socially? Has he ever been hospitalized, had surgery, or taken medication (specially, hormones or steroids) for any of these problems?

Family history

Hereditary and constitutional factors can play a major role in the cause of endocrine problems. Specific problems related to endocrine dysfunction to ask the client about (which could be familial) include:

Diabetes mellitus or insipidus
Hypertension
Thyroid (cancer, goiter)
Cardiac arrhythmias
Kidney stones
Gout
Obesity
Dermatological disease
Infertility
Growth problems
Mental illness

Further information may be elicited by asking additional questions such as: Are there any other members of your family who have or have had a similar problem? Frequently this will uncover evidence of a familial factor that will not be found in any other way.

Social and personal history

Background Information As discussed in Chap. 39, stressors of all kinds affect the endocrine system. Areas which have the potential for high stress should be investigated. The client should be asked about his place of employment, kind of work, ability to meet the job requirements, and the amount of stress involved. Does the job provide adequate income? What is the client's marital status? What are his usual coping patterns?

Lifestyle If the client presents with a specific problem, then the appropriate history should be taken and the system involved should be assessed. For instance, a chief complaint of tachycardia indicates the need for a cardiovascular assessment as well as information related to stress, diet, exercise, and sleep. The clinician must also remember the possibility of endocrine dysfunction and must assess for hyperthyroidism and stress. The lack of clear-cut endocrine symptoms requires a conscientious and detailed health history.

Review of systems

If an endocrine problem is suspected, the systemic effects of hormones require the nurse to investigate many systems. The client should be specifically questioned about the following:

Skin—Any changes in color, pigmentation, dryness, oiliness, moistness, bruisability, breakdown, rate of healing

Hair—Amount, texture, distribution, and pattern

Nails—Any changes in growth or texture

Head, neck, face, eyes, tongue—Any changes in shape, symmetry, appearance, size, color, position

Cardiovascular—Presence of palpitations; any evidence of light-headedness or syncope related to changes in position (orthostatic hypotension); shortness of breath on mild exertion

Gastrointestinal—Any change in bowel habits or appetite; constipation; presence of abdominal pain

Urinary-reproductive—Any abnormalities in menstruation; changes in sexual desire or activity, or in the size and shape of genitalia; any evidence of kidney stones

Musculoskeletal—Any muscular weakness, or aching when climbing stairs or rising from a chair; any tingling, numbness, cramping, tremors, or fractures

Neurological—Any problem with ability to concentrate; nervousness, irritability, or depression; altered thought and speech patterns; reaction to the interview

Objective Data: The Physical Examination

Mental-emotional status

Throughout the examination, the client's alertness, memory, affect, personality, anxiety, and speech pattern should be objectively assessed.

Inspection

The nurse should look at the client's general appearance, including physical growth and development. Endocrine dysfunction can subtly or markedly affect the size, shape, color, and maturation of the body. Assessment should include the following:

Body size—Height, weight, head, facial features, hands, feet, body alignment, and posture. These should be compared to a table of standard height and weight.

Voice—Husky, hoarse quality, volume, pitch.

Skin—Cold, dry, rough, scaly, velvety soft, warm; enlarged pores; increased sweating or oiliness; bruises, unhealed cuts, patchy erythemas, especially on the face and neck; patchy hyperpigmentation of mucous membranes; generalized hyperpigmentation; pink-purplish striae over the abdomen, thighs, breasts and upper arms; brittle nails or separation of the nails for the nail beds.

Teeth—Condition, repair, mottling.

Body hair—Finer, softer, or straighter than normal; brittle, coarse; less distribution, especially in the axillary and pubic areas in the female; hirsutism.

Edema—Eyelids, hands, feet.

Eyes—Visual acuity, night blindness; shape and color; closeness together; drooping eyelids, nystagmus, lid lag; visual fields, protrusion, signs of exophthalmus. (See Chap. 42 for a description of exophthalmus.)

Neck—Observation of the thyroid gland should be made first in the normal position, next in slight extension, and then while the client swallows. Any unusual bulging of the lobes behind the sternocleidomastoid muscles should be noted. The trachea should be positioned midline.

Muscle strength—Fine tremors can be detected by having the client spread his fingers in the air, palms down, and placing a piece of paper over the fingers. If tremors are present, the paper will move. Muscular weakness and atrophy can be assessed by asking the client, while seated in a chair, to hold one leg out straight in a horizontal position. The thyrotoxic client may be able to do this for 30 seconds or less, whereas the normal person can quadruple this time.

Sexual characteristics—Gynecomastia in men, enlarged clitoris in women.

Palpation

The only endocrine gland examined during a routine physical examination is the thyroid gland. Palpation of the thyroid gland requires care and

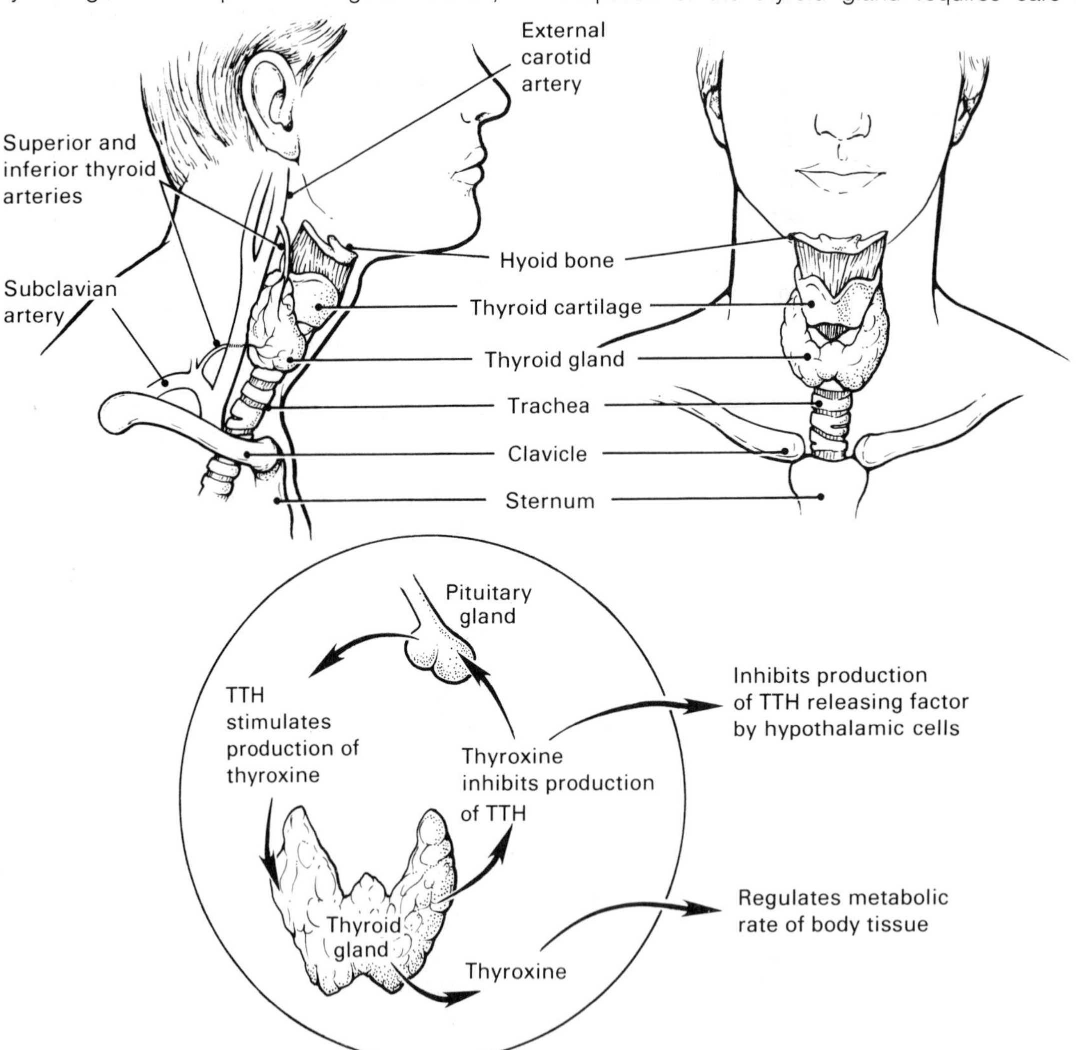

Figure 40-7 Midline structures of the neck. *(Adapted from E. Reith et al., Textbook of Anatomy and Physiology, 2d ed., McGraw-Hill Book Company, New York, 1978.)*

gentleness as well as considerable practice validated by an experienced examiner. In order to palpate the thyroid, other midline neck structures need to be identified. These include the thyroid bone, the thyroid and cricoid cartilages, and the tracheal rings (see Fig. 40-7). There is an anterior and a posterior approach to thyroid palpation.

Anterior Palpation The nurse should stand in front of the client. With the pads of the index and middle fingers, the cricoid cartilage should be palpated for the thyroid isthmus. It is helpful to have the client swallow while feeling for the isthmus rising up under the fingers. Next, the client should flex his head slightly forward and to the right. The right thumb should be placed on the lower portion of the client's thyroid cartilage, gently pressing the client's right side. The tips of the index and middle fingers of the left hand should be hooked behind the sternocleidomastoid muscle while feeling in front of this muscle with the left thumb. As the client swallows, the lateral lobe should be palpated. This procedure is reversed for the other side.

Posterior Palpation The examiner should stand behind the client. With the thumbs of both hands resting on the nape of the client's neck, the index and middle fingers of both hands feel for the thyroid isthmus and for the anterior surfaces of the lateral lobes. In order to facilitate the examination of each lobe and to relax the neck muscles, the client should be asked to flex his neck slightly forward and to the right. The thyroid cartilage is displaced to the right with the left hand and fingers. The nurse should palpate with the right hand after placing the thumb deep and behind the sternocleidomastoid muscle with the index and middle fingers in front of it; the area is palpated with the right hand (Fig. 40-8). While this is done, the client should be asked to swallow. This procedure is then repeated for the left side. The thyroid is palpated for its size, shape, symmetry, and tenderness, and for any nodules. In the average person, the thyroid is generally not palpable. If palpable, it usually feels smooth, with a firm consistency, and is not tender with gentle pressure. Any nodules, enlargement, asymmetry, and hardness are abnormal findings and should be referred for further evaluation.

Vital signs

Assessment should include the following:

Pulse—Heart rate, rhythm, arrhythmias.

Blood pressure—Widening of the pulse pressure, hypotension, or hypertension. Blood pressure should be taken while the client is lying, sitting, and standing, and any orthostatic hypertension should be noted.

Respirations—Rate and quality.

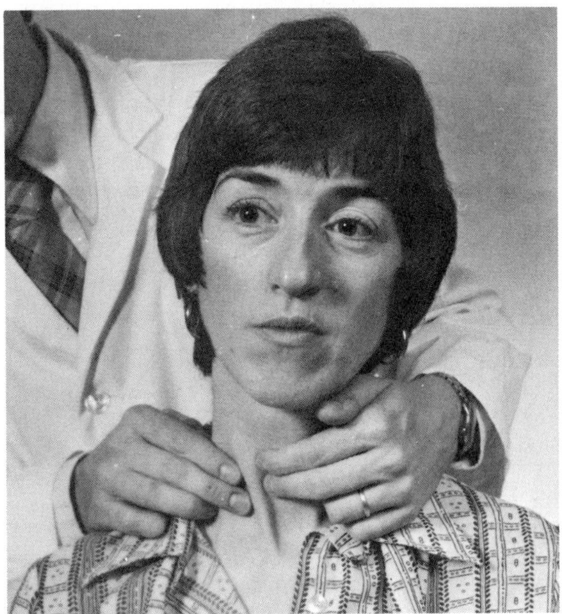

Figure 40-8 Posterior palpation of the thyroid gland.

Percussion and auscultation are not normally part of an endocrine assessment. Additional assessments are appropriate for specific abnormalities and are discussed in Chap. 42.

DIAGNOSTIC STUDIES OF THE ENDOCRINE SYSTEM

Proper diagnosis of endocrine problems can be aided by accurate laboratory tests. The measurement of hormones present in the body is possible because each hormone has unique characteristics. The amount of each hormone present provides an index of the activity of a specific endocrine gland. The value of blood specimen measurement is limited since it does not reflect diurnal variations or temporary changes in the client's status. Blood samples measure hormones only at the time the blood sample is drawn. Collection of a 24-hour urine specimen for analysis of hormones and their metabolites provides more accurate results than a single random specimen and allows for normal fluctuation in hormone secretions.[12]

Three types of tests are available for determining the concentration of the various hormones: bioassay, chemical assay, and displacement assay. The bioassay is relatively insensitive and is used only when more precise tests are not available. The chemical assay is a more direct means of measuring hormone concentration. This test is most commonly used to measure the steroid hormone concentration in urine or blood. The displacement assay is the most common method of hormone measurement, and radioimmunoassay (RIA) is the most extensive and accurate of the displacement methods.

RIA incorporates the use of radionuclides, which makes it possible to detect very small concentrations of hormones. The outstanding features of RIA include sensitivity, specificity, and accuracy.[13]

Specific diagnostic studies related to the endocrine system are summarized in Table 40-4. Because of the interrelatedness of the endocrine system, nursing intervention is focused on reducing the stress and anxiety often associated with diagnostic testing. Unless nursing measures are initiated related to client instruction and expectations, the effect of stress hormones can produce inaccurate and misleading results.

Table 40-4
Diagnostic Studies of the Endocrine System

Study	Description and Purpose	Nursing Responsibility
	Pituitary Studies	
Serum studies		
GH (RIA)	To evaluate GH secretion. After an overnight fast, there should be less than 5 ng/mL in males and less than 8 ng/mL in females.	NPO after midnight.* Bed rest. If samples are drawn from clients who walk to the laboratory or who are stressed from venipuncture, abnormally high levels may result.
Insulin tolerance text	To evaluate clients suspected of having hypopituitarism. Tests GH-secreting capacity. IV injection of regular insulin based on body weight. Blood samples drawn at 0, 30, 45, 60, and 90 min after injection. GH should rise two- to threefold over baseline levels. Response is subnormal or absent in GH deficiency.	Fasting overnight. Bed rest. Have 50 mg of 50% dextrose solution at bedside for use if severe hypoglycemia occurs. Continually assess client's mental status. Seizures and cardiac arrhythmias can result from hypoglycemia. Test is contraindicated in clients with seizure disorders and cardiac disease.
LTH	Levels above 300 ng/mL are indicative of pituitary tumors; levels above 100 ng/mL are associated with pituitary tumors in roughly 50% of clients. *Normal values:* Male: 1–20 ng/mL. Female: 1–25 ng/mL.	Fasting.*
Gonadotropins: FSH, LH	Useful in distinguishing a primary gonadal problem from pituitary insufficiency. Normal levels vary according to age and sex. In females, there are marked differences during the menstrual cycle and in the postmenopausal period. Levels are low in pituitary insufficiency and high in primary gonadal failure.	Nonfasting.* Inform client that three blood samples will be drawn 30 min apart.
Osmolality study		
Urine and serum osmolality	Useful in evaluating ADH control mechanism. Do urine and serum osmolality tests at the same time and compare results. In normal subjects, urine osmolality should be higher than serum osmolality. High levels indicate inappropriate ADH secretion, but urine osmolality should be interpreted in light of what is known about the client's plasma and hydration status. *Normal values:* Serum: 285–295 mOsm/kg. Urine: 300–800 mOsm/kg.	Obtain urine and serum samples. Begin fluid deprivation and continue for 6–12 h as ordered. Weigh client and measure urine volume, specific gravity, and osmolality qh during fluid deprivation. Record values. Send labeled specimens to laboratory at completion of test.
Radiological studies		
Skull x-rays CT scan	Useful in evaluating sella turcica for volume, enlargement, or erosion when disease of the hypothalamic-pituitary axis is suspected. Compare to normal measurement of sella turcica in relation to client's height.	Inform client that tests are painless and noninvasive. Explain procedure to client. No special preparation required.

Table 40-4 (Continued)

Study	Description and Purpose	Nursing Responsibility
	Thyroid Studies	
Serum studies		
T_4 (RIA)	Measures total serum level of T_4. Useful in evaluating thyroid function and monitoring iodine or antithyroid therapy. *Normal values:* 5–12 μg/dL.	Nonfasting.*
T_3 (RIA)	Measures serum levels of triiodothyronine. Helpful in diagnosing hyperthyroidism if T_4 levels are normal. *Normal values:* 110–230 ng/mL.	Nonfasting.*
RT_3U (Resin Triiodothyronine Uptake)	Indirectly measures binding capacity of thyroid-binding protein (TBP). *Normal values:* 0.85–1.15 RT_3U (25–35%).	Nonfasting.*
FT_4I (Free Thyroxine Index)	Combination of T_4 and RT_3U. Provides good index of thyroid hormone status. Normal range calculated by multiplying RT_3U by T_4. *Normal range:* 5.7–13.2% uptake.	Nonfasting.*
Thyroid ^{131}I Uptake (Radioactive Iodine) (RAIU)	Provides indirect measure of thyroid activity. Small tracer dose of ^{131}I given orally or IV. Serum uptake measurements drawn at 6 and 24 h. 24-h urine specimen analyzed. *Normal values for 24-h uptake:* Serum: 8–30%. Urine: 40–80% within first 24 h. Because this test is adversely affected by numerous compounds and iodinized foods, it is unsuitable for diagnosing hypothyroidism.	Instruct client to discontinue thyroid medication. T_3 (Cytomel) 25 mg bid–tid × 4 wk is started. Client to report for further testing in 10–14 days as instructed. Collect 24-h urine specimen. Easily contaminated by drugs, seafoods, certain diagnostic studies.
TSH	Measures level of TSH. From 10 to 14 days after last dose of T_3, TSH measurements and ^{131}I uptake are done. Hypothyroid clients should exhibit an increase in TSH by 20 μU/mL or more. TSH is markedly elevated in hypothyroidism. *Normal values:* 1.9–5.4 μU/mL.	Instruct client regarding dates of follow-up tests.
Calcium	Useful in evaluating possibility of thyroid cancer. Hypercalcemia often associated with malignant tumors of thyroid. *Normal values:* 4.5–5.5 mEq/L or 9.0–11.0 mg/dL.	Nonfasting.*
Radiological test		
Thyroid scan	Useful in determining location, size, and shape of thyroid gland. Tracer dose of ^{131}I given IV. Scanner passes over thyroid and makes graphic recording of radiation emitted. Normal thyroid scan reveals a homogeneous pattern with symmetrical lobes.	Determine if other tests requiring iodine preparation (IVP, SSKI, barium enema) have been done within 30 days. Can invalidate test. Explain procedure to client.
	Parathyroid Studies	
Serum studies		
PTH (RIA)	Measures PTH level in serum. Currently, there is no universal standard for measurement, so normal levels will vary depending on methods used in individual laboratories. Oversecretion causes hypercalcemia and bone demineralization.	Nonfasting.*
Total calcium	Measures total of all three forms of calcium to detect bone and parathyroid disorders. Hypercalcemia can indicate primary hyperparathyroidism. Hypocalcemia can indicate hypoparathyroidism. *Normal values:* 9.0–11.0 mg/dL or 4.5–5.5 mEq/L.	Nonfasting.*
Phosphorus	Measures amount of inorganic phosphorus. Phosphorus excretion dependent on calcium and phosphorus intake. Hyperphosphatemia can indicate hypoparathyroidism or renal failure. Hypophosphatemia can indicate hyperparathyroidism. Inverse relationship between phosphorus and calcium. *Normal values:* 2.8–4.5 mg/dL or 1.8–2.6 mEq/L.	Nonfasting.*

Table 40-4 (Continued)

Study	Description and Purpose	Nursing Responsibility
Urine studies		
Calcium	Used for screening purpose in evaluating parathyroid activity. Estimation of calcium ions in urine. If diet is stable (10–20 mg/kg of calcium per day), normal excretion is <4 mg/kg ideal body weight for males and <3 mg/kg ideal body weight for females.	Collect 24-h urine specimen. Instruct client regarding 24-h urine collection (see Chap. 36).
Phosphorus	Used for screening purposes in evaluating parathyroid activity. Measures phosphorus content in urine. If diet is relatively stable (0.9–1.7 g/day) normal excretion is 1000 mg. Inverse relationship between phosphorus and PTH.	Instruct client regarding 24-h urine collection (see Chap. 36).
Radiological studies		
Skeletal x-rays	To determine bone pathology and osteoporosis. Fractures or deformities can be caused by the demineralization produced by excess parathyroid hormone.	Monitor client's exposure to x-rays. Inform client that tests are painless and noninvasive. No special preparation required.
	Adrenal Studies	
Serum studies		
Plasma cortisol	Measures amount of cortisol in plasma. Evaluates status of adrenocortical function. *Normal values:* 8 A.M. 5–25 μg/dL. 8 P.M. < 10 μg/dL.	Fasting.* Ensure collection of properly timed blood sample. Specimen should be drawn early in the morning, when cortisol levels are highest. Mark time on laboratory slip. Minimize stress to avoid raising level.
ACTH stimulation	Useful in assessing normal or abnormal adrenal function. Two methods are used. After a blood sample is obtained to determine the baseline level: 1. A single dose of ACTH is given IV or IM and blood levels are drawn at 30 and 60 min. 2. There is a continuous infusion of ACTH from 4 to 8 h. Repeated blood samples are taken at 4, 6, and 8 h. In general, there should be at least a twofold increase in plasma cortisol level after 30 min.	Fasting.* Inform client of method to be used. If continuous infusion, monitor site and rate of IV. Ensure collection of specimens at appropriate times.
Dexamethasone suppression test	Assesses adrenal function. Especially helpful if hyperactivity is suspected. Useful in evaluation of Cushing's syndrome. Dexamethasone (Decadron) 2 mg given in evening or at midnight to suppress secretion of CRF. Plasma cortisol sample drawn 8 h later. Low cortisol level indicates normal adrenal response (50% decrease in cortisol production).	Fasting.* Acutely ill clients or those under stress should not be tested. ACTH may override the suppression. Interfering drugs (estrogens, glucocorticoids) may give false-positive results.
Urine studies		
17-Ketosteriods (17-KS)	Measures androgen metabolites in urine. Evaluates adrenal cortical function. *Normal values:* Male: 10–22 mg/day. Female: 6–16 mg/day.	Instruct client regarding 24-h urine collection (see Chap. 36). Must be kept refrigerated or iced during collection. Determine if preservative is required for method used.
17 Hydroxycorticosteroids (17-OHCS)	Measures glucocorticoid metabolites in urine. Evaluates adrenal function. Excessive secretion usually implies adrenal androgen source. Many drugs cause high values. *Normal values:* Male: 3.5–12.0 mg/day. Female: 3–10 mg/day.	Instruct client regarding 24-h urine collection (see Chap. 36). Refrigerate specimen during collection or use appropriate preservative.
Aldosterone	Measures urinary aldosterone level. Not routinely measured to evaluate adrenal function. Useful in determining therapy for hypertension. *Normal values:* 2–26 μg/day.	Client should be on unrestricted diet with normal salt intake and no medication for 3 wk prior to urine collection. Instruct client regarding 24-h

Table 40-4 (Continued)

Study	Description and Purpose	Nursing Responsibility
		urine collection (see Chap. 36).
Metyrapone	Assess pituitary ACTH reserve in clients already shown to have an adrenal response to ACTH. A 24-h urine specimen is collected, and baseline measurements of 17-ketosteroids and creatinine are made. After urine is collected, metyrapone, 750 mg q 4 h × six doses, is given. After last dose of metyrapone, another 24-h urine specimen is collected for 17-ketosteroids and creatinine. A 2 $\frac{1}{2}$- to 3-fold increase in 17-ketosteroids should be observed on day 3 or 4.	Instruct client regarding 24-h urine collection (see Chap. 36). Administer metyrapone as ordered. keep urine refrigerated. Determine if preservative is required for method used.
VMA (vannillylmandelic acid)	Measures urinary excretion of catecholamines. Helpful in diagnosing pheochromocytoma. *Normal value:* <7 mg/day.	A 24-h urine collection to be kept at a pH of 3.0 or less using hydrochloric acid as a preservative. Newer methods of VMA measurement are not affected by dietary intake. Consult with laboratory or physician concerning discontinuance of any drugs 3 days prior to urine collection.
	Pancreatic Studies	
Serum studies		
Fasting blood sugar (FBS)	Measures circulating glucose level. *Normal values:* 70–120 mg/dL.	A 12-h overnight fast.*
Two-hour postprandial glucose tolerance test	Screening test used to evaluate glucose metabolism. Blood glucose levels in healthy people peak at 160–180 mg/dL within $\frac{1}{2}$–1 h after glucose load as described and return to fasting levels or lower in 2–3 h. Normal-plasma glucose of <135 mg/dL. More reliable in detecting diabetes mellitus than FBS.	Diet 3 days prior to test should include 200 g of carbohydrate with an intake of at least 1500 cal/day. After a 12-h overnight fast, the client should (1) eat a high carbohydrate breakfast (100 g) or (2) ingest 100 g of glucose. Ensure collection of a 2-h postprandial blood sample.
Oral glucose tolerance test	Evaluates insulin response to a glucose load. Elevated levels strongly suggest diabetes mellitus. After ingestion of 100 g of glucose, samples for glucose measurement are collected at $\frac{1}{2}$, 1, 2, and 3 h. If indicated, samples can be collected for 4 and 5 h. *General normal ranges:* Fasting 70–120 mg/dL 30 min 30–60 mg/dL above fasting 60 min 20–50 mg/dL above fasting 120 min 5–15 mg/dL above fasting 180 min Fasting level or below	Clients should be active and free of illness. A 12-h fast required. Give oral glucose when indicated. Diuretics, oral contraceptives, nicotinic acid, and phenytoin may impair glucose tolerance. Inform client of time of test and number of blood samples to be drawn.
Urine studies		
Sugar (Clinistix, Labstix, Multistix, Clinitest)	Estimates amount of glucose in urine by using a reducing substance. Amount found parallels blood glucose values.	Use a freshly voided urine specimen collected at the appropriate time. Many different drugs alter glucose readings. Errors are great if directions not followed exactly. Several different types of glucose urine tests available. Follow package directions.
Ketones (Acetest, Ketostix, Labstix, Multistix)	Measures amount of ketone bodies excreted in the urine as a result of incomplete fat metabolism. Positive result can indicate diabetic acidosis. Aids in assessing severity of acidosis and in evaluating effect of treatment.	Use a freshly voided urine specimen. Test often done together with glucose test. Directions must be followed exactly. Certain drugs can produce false-positive and false-negative results.

*Inform client that blood sample will be drawn. Observe venipuncture site for bleeding or hematoma formation.

REVIEW QUESTIONS

The number of the question corresponds to the same numbered objective at the beginning of the chapter.

1. All the following are common characteristics of hormones *except*
   a. hormones are secreted cyclically.
   b. hormones are secreted in large amounts.
   c. hormonal effects are widespread throughout the body.
   d. many hormonal abnormalities give rise to common signs and symptoms.

2. The adrenal glands are located
   a. in the sella turcica
   b. posteriorly in the thyroid gland
   c. above each kidney
   d. behind the stomach

3. Aldosterone secretion is regulated by all the following *except*
   a. serum potassium concentration
   b. renin-angiotensin system
   c. serum sodium concentration
   d. serum hydrogen ions

4. Prostaglandins have all the following characteristics *except*
   a. they are a group of fatty compounds.
   b. they are hormonelike with a wide range of physiological activities.
   c. they suppress inflammation.
   d. they have smooth muscle-stimulating properties.

5. If an endocrine problem is suspected, the client should be specifically questioned about
   a. appetite changes
   b. wheezing
   c. varicosities
   d. hematuria

6. Swallowing will cause the thyroid gland to
   a. rise
   b. fall
   c. stay the same while the trachea rises
   d. stay the same

7. Which of the following endocrine glands can be auscultated if an abnormality is suspected?
   a. pituitary
   b. thyroid
   c. adrenal
   d. parathyroid

8. The dexamethasone suppression test assesses
   a. adrenal function
   b. thyroid function
   c. glucose function
   d. pituitary function

REFERENCES

1. Alice Tripp, *Basic Mechanisms of Endocrine Dysfunction,* McGraw-Hill Book Company, New York, 1978, p. 6.
2. Sylvia Price and Lorraine Wilson, *Pathophysiology: Clinical Concepts of Disease Processes*, 2d ed., McGraw-Hill Book Company, New York, 1982, p. 698.
3. Roberta Spencer, *Patient Care in Endocrine Problems*, W. B. Saunders Company, Philadelphia, 1973, p. 4.
4. Tripp, op. cit. p. 85.
5. Leroy L. Langley et al., *Dynamic Anatomy and Physiology*, 5th ed., McGraw-Hill Book Company, New York, 1980, p. 690.
6. Marjorie Miller, Anna Drakontides, and Lutie Leavell, *Kimber-Gray-Stackpole's Anatomy and Physiology*, 17th ed., The Macmillan Company, New York, 1977, p. 319.
7. Thomas Burns, "Endocrinology," in W. Sodeman and T. Sodeman (eds.), *Sodeman's Pathologic Physiology: Mechanisms of Disease*, 6th ed., W. B. Saunders Company, Philadelphia, 1979, p. 1010.
8. Bernice Muir, *Pathophysiology: An Introduction to the Mechanism of Disease*, John Wiley & Sons Inc., New York, 1980, p. 323.
9. Robert Zurier, "Prostaglandins: Their Potential in Clinical Medicine," *Postgrad Med*, **68**(3):73–81 (1980).
10. Muir, op. cit., p. 323.
11. Robert C. Tarazi and Ray W. Gifford, Jr., "Systemic Arterial Pressure, in Sodeman and Davis, op. cit., p. 207.
12. J. Byrne et al., *Laboratory Tests: Implications for Nurses and Allied Health Professionals*, Addison-Wesley Publishing Company, Menlo Park, Calif., 1981, p. 219.
13. Robert Alsever and Ronald Gotlin, *Handbook of Endocrine Tests in Adults and Children*, 2d ed., Year Book Medical Publishers, Inc., Chicago, 1978, p. 31.

Chapter 41

NURSING ROLE IN MANAGEMENT

Diabetic Client

Sandra Hower Currin
Idolia Cox Collier

Learning Objectives

1. Describe the pathophysiology and clinical manifestations of diabetes mellitus.
2. Describe the differences between insulin-dependent diabetes (type I) and non-insulin-dependent diabetes (type II).
3. Identify the pathogenesis and manifestations of the acute and chronic complications of diabetes mellitus.
4. Describe the medical, pharmacological, and dietary management of diabetes mellitus, ketoacidosis, and hypoglycemia.
5. Describe the purpose and plan of an American Diabetes Association diet.
6. Describe the nursing management of a newly diagnosed diabetic.
7. Describe the nursing management of a diabetic client who has ketoacidosis or hypoglycemia or who is undergoing surgery.
8. Explain the psychological impact of diabetes on the client and his family.
9. Explain the nursing responsibilities in the long-term management of the diabetic client

SIGNIFICANCE OF THE PROBLEM

Diabetes mellitus is a chronic systemic disease characterized by (1) abnormalities of the endocrine secretions of the pancreas resulting in disordered metabolism of carbohydrate, fat, and protein and, in time, (2) structural abnormalities in a variety of tissues.[1] It is a serious health problem throughout the world, with over 10 million diabetics in the United States alone. Diabetes mellitus is one of the leading causes of death in the United States. It is estimated that 1 in 20 people in the United States may have diabetes mellitus. The staggering cost in human suffering and diabetes-related expenses (more than $5 billion annually) warrants a sound knowledge base to provide nursing care for diabetic clients.[2]

PATHOPHYSIOLOGY OF DIABETES MELLITUS

In diabetes mellitus, there is a discrepancy between the amount of insulin available and the amount required by the body. The relative or absolute insulin deficiency may result from abnormal insulin secretion in response to glucose stimulation or from a failure of cell membranes to bind insulin.[3]

This chapter was reviewed by Judith A. Kopper, R.N., M.S.N., Assistant Professor, Nursing Department, Rochester Center, Winona State University, Rochester, Minnesota.

Normal Insulin Metabolism

Insulin is a hormone produced by the beta cells of the islets of Langerhans located in the pancreas. Normally, after food ingestion and absorption, the beta cells are stimulated to release insulin into the bloodstream. The amount of insulin released is dependent upon the blood level of glucose; the higher the blood glucose, the more insulin released.

Insulin's primary function is to promote glucose transport from the bloodstream across the cell membrane to the cytoplasm of the cell. It does this by increasing the cell membrane's permeability to glucose. In the cell, glucose is stored as glycogen, converted into fat, or used for energy.

Insulin is attracted to the cells by receptors on the cell membrane. (Certain organs, such as the brain, skin, heart muscle, and iris, are non-insulin-dependent.) Insulin causes a series of reactions which result in the metabolism of glucose for energy. It also functions in the liver and skeletal muscle to stimulate glycogen formation. In adipose tissue, insulin promotes glucose conversion into fat. Insulin also inhibits glucagon secretion.

There are five other hormones (*glucagon, epinephrine, growth hormone, cortisol,* and *somatostatin*) involved in glucose utilization. Some researchers believe that an abnormal production of any or all of these hormones may be present in diabetes.[4] Glucagon, a hormone produced by the alpha cells of the islets of Langerhans, can inhibit insulin release. One of the most recent hormones to receive attention is somatostatin. It is produced by the delta cells of the islets of Langerhans and has an inhibiting effect on both insulin and glucagon.[5]

Etiology of Diabetes Mellitus

Evidence is mounting that diabetes mellitus is not a single disease but a series of disorders and chronic complications.[6] Diabetes mellitus is a group of syndromes that differ in etiology, clinical characteristics, and progression. Current theories link the cause of diabetes, singly or in combination, to autoimmune, viral, and polygenic (multifactorial) factors, as well as environmental factors such as obesity and stress.[7]

Due to the complexity of factors related to the etiology of diabetes mellitus, it is almost impossible to predict the occurrence of diabetes for the purpose of genetic counseling. It has been demonstrated that the offspring of a diabetic parent is at greater risk for developing diabetes than the population at large. The percentage of risk ranges from slightly greater to four times greater depending on the age of the client and the age of onset of the parent's diabetes.[8]

Types of Diabetes Mellitus

Type I (insulin-dependent)

Insulin-dependent diabetes occurs when there is destruction of the beta cells of the pancreas, resulting in little or no insulin production. Beta cell destruction is attributed to a genetic predisposition to diabetes coupled with one or more viral infections and/or a possible autoimmune reaction. This autoimmune reaction may or may not be triggered by a virus. It is not conclusive that these are the only factors involved. Three viruses that have been implicated are mumps, rubella, and Coxsackie virus B. The clients are usually children or nonobese adults.

Overt insulin-dependent diabetes is accompanied by the signs and symptoms outlined by the American Diabetes Association in Table 41-1. These clinical manifestations all occur in varying degrees depending upon the blood glucose level. Insulin-dependent diabetes is more severe than non-insulin-dependent diabetes in terms of both the difficulty of regulation and the incidence of complications.

Type II (non-insulin-dependent)

Non-insulin-dependent diabetes, the most common form of diabetes, generally occurs in obese people. The main problem seems to be altered insulin receptors on cells. When adults gain weight, their fat and muscle cells become enlarged. As the cell wall enlarges, insulin receptors change and the cells become resistant to insulin. This resistance, coupled with an excessive caloric intake and additional fat tissue requiring glucose, places an extra demand on the pancreas to produce insulin. Often, these clients have elevated insulin levels.

It is believed that if the client has a genetic predisposition to diabetes, the pancreas eventually is unable to meet the extra insulin demand. This is possibly due to beta cell exhaustion. Weight loss can reverse this trend if it occurs before the pancreas is permanently damaged. The maintenance of an ideal body weight is essential for these clients.

The symptoms exhibited by the non-insulin-dependent diabetic are summarized in Table 41-2. Often the presenting complaints are vascular or neu-

Table 41-1

Clinical Manifestations of Insulin-Dependent Diabetes

Insulin-dependent diabetes is characterized by the sudden appearance of:

Constant urination
Abnormal thirst
Unusual hunger
The rapid loss of weight
Irritability
Obvious weakness and fatigue
Nausea and vomiting

Any one of these signals can indicate diabetes. Children usually exhibit dramatic, sudden symptoms and must receive prompt treatment.

From American Diabetes Association.

Table 41-2

Clinical Manifestations of Non-Insulin-Dependent Diabetes

Non-insulin-dependent diabetes may include any of the signs of insulin-dependent diabetes or:

Drowsiness
Itching
A family history of diabetes
Blurred vision
Excessive weight
Tingling, numbness, pain in the extremities
Easy fatigue
Skin infections and slow healing of cuts and scratches, especially of the feet

Many adults may have diabetes with none of these symptoms. The disease is often discovered during a routine physical examination.

From American Diabetes Association, Public Information Pamphlet.

rological. Table 41-3 compares the essential features of the two types of diabetes.

Blood Vessel Changes

The most significant tissue abnormality that occurs in diabetes is related to the structure and function of blood vessels. Although it is still the subject of much controversy, the initial lesion in the blood vessels seems to be a thickened basement membrane.[9] The resulting vascular changes produce the complications of diabetes mellitus which are discussed later.

Although the effect of abnormal glucose levels on blood vessel changes is not known, the management of diabetes is related to this event. If the care provider believes that blood vessel abnormalities are solely the result of wide fluctuations in glucose experienced by diabetics even under good control (Fig. 41-1), then close monitoring and control of blood glucose levels are critical to management. However, if the care provider believes that blood vessel changes are inevitable regardless of overall diabetic control, then strict blood sugar control is much less important.

There are other forms of diabetes that cause glucose intolerance, such as those resulting from pancreatic destruction (e.g., pancreatitis) or endocrine disorders (e.g., acromegaly). This chapter will focus on a discussion of genetic diabetes mellitus.

DEVELOPMENTAL STAGES OF DIABETES MELLITUS

Genetic diabetes has been divided into four stages which describe the progression of the disease. These stages are *prediabetes, subclinical, latent,* and *overt.* Although the disease eventually progresses through each stage, the progression may be rapid or slow, with a possible return to a preceding stage. Specific metabolic and vascular changes are characteristic of the various stages (Fig. 41-2).

Table 41-3
Comparison of the Essential Features of Type I and Type II Diabetes

	Type I	Type II
Other names	Juvenile, growth-onset, ketosis-prone	Adult-onset, maturity-onset, ketosis-resistant
Age of onset	Usually under age 35	Usually over age 35
Type of onset	Abrupt (days to weeks)	Usually gradual (weeks to months)
Nutritional status at onset	Usually undernourished	Usually obese
Manifestations	Polydipsia, polyphagia, and polyuria	Frequently none
Ketosis	Frequent, unless diet, insulin dose, and exercise are properly coordinated	Infrequent except in the presence of infection or stress
Endogenous insulin	Negligible to absent	Present; may be excessive but is relatively ineffective because of obesity
Associated lipid abnormalities	Hypercholesterolemia frequent, particularly when control is suboptimal; all lipid fractions elevated in ketoacidosis	Cholesterol and triglycerides frequently elevated and related to obesity; carbohydrate-induced hypertriglyceridemia common
Insulin	Needed for all clients	Necessary in only 20–30% of clients
Oral agents	Rarely efficacious; should not be used	Efficacious
Diet Regulation	Mandatory, along with insulin for blood glucose control	Diet alone frequently sufficient to control blood glucose

From *Diabetes Mellitus,* 8th ed., Lilly Research Laboratories, Indianapolis, Ind., 1979, p. 2.

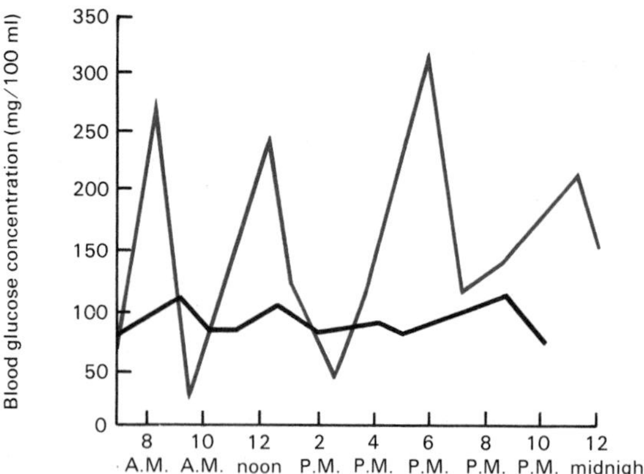

Figure 41-1 Even with insulin therapy, diet, and exercise, the diabetic's blood glucose exhibits wide variations on both sides of the normal range. *[From Alice Chenault Mauer, "The Therapy of Diabetes," Am Scientist,* ***67****:424 (1979).]*

The prediabetes stage begins at conception and lasts until the subclinical stage. During this stage, the client is asymptomatic for diabetes, and all glucose blood tests are normal. However, at this stage there may be some basement membrane thickening in the blood vessels (*microangiopathy*). Commonalities have been identified in clients who develop overt diabetes, including a family history of diabetes, a personal history of obesity, bearing infants over 9 pounds, and having spontaneous abortions. Clients with a history of these situations should be considered at risk for the development of diabetes and followed closely.

Clients in the subclinical stage are also asymptomatic but show some laboratory abnormalities. The oral glucose tolerance test becomes abnormal when the client is under physiological or emotional stress or is pregnant. This is usually a transient situation. The diabetic in the latent stage is usually also asymptomatic. The oral glucose tolerance test is abnormal, but the fasting blood glucose is not elevated.

The final stage is overt diabetes mellitus. The blood glucose is abnormal, and the client is symptomatic for diabetes. Overt diabetes has been traditionally classified as juvenile-onset diabetes or maturity-onset diabetes depending upon the age of onset. Now, juvenile-onset diabetics are referred to as

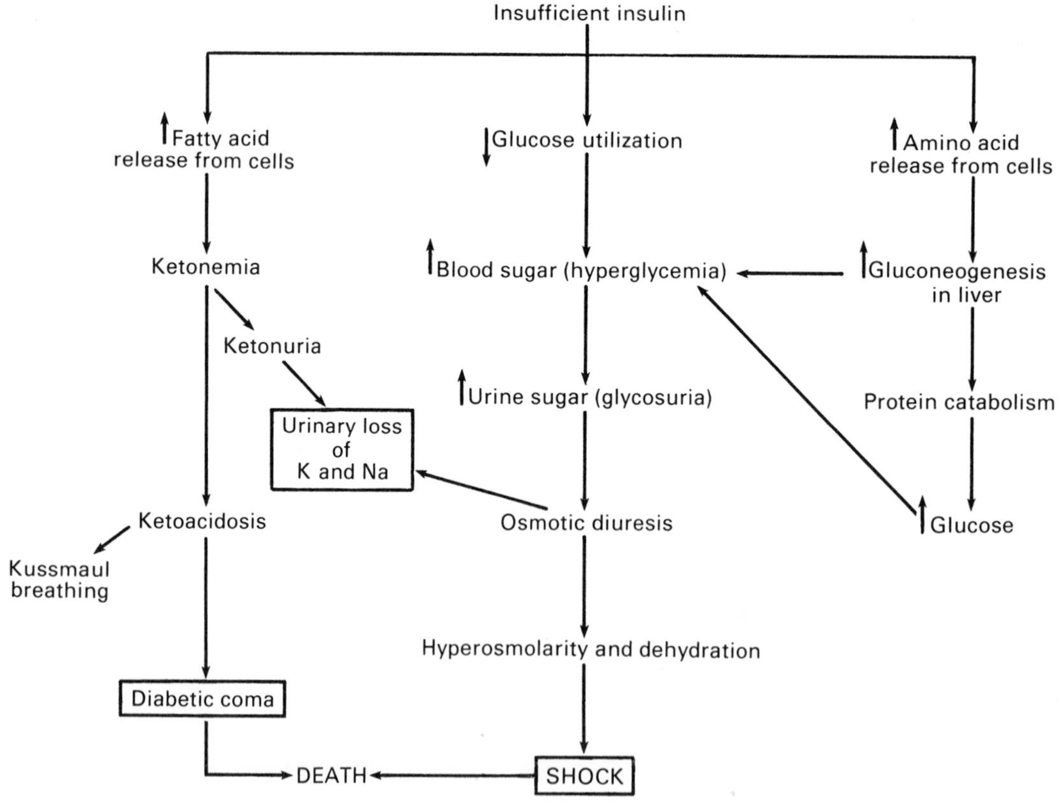

Figure 41-2 Metabolic and vascular changes in various stages of diabetes. *(Adapted from Diabetes Mellitus, 8th ed., Lilly Research Laboratories, Indianapolis, Ind., 1979, p. 9.)*

insulin-dependent diabetics, or *type I.* This group includes all diabetics, regardless of age, who require exogenous insulin to sustain life. Maturity-onset diabetics are referred to as *non-insulin-dependent diabetics,* or *type II,* and are not dependent upon exogenous insulin for life.

CLINICAL MANIFESTATIONS AND COMPLICATIONS OF DIABETES MELLITUS

With the discovery and initial administration of insulin, it was believed that a cure for diabetes had been found. But 60 years of insulin therapy have proven that insulin is not the total answer for the treatment of diabetes. Hyperglycemia-related problems do not cause death as often as they did before insulin was discovered. However, other chronic complications of long-term therapy are responsible for over 75 percent of all diabetic deaths. Prior to 1921, most diabetics did not live long enough to manifest long-term complications.

There is no uniform agreement regarding the complications of diabetes. Some believe that they are unrelated to glucose intolerance. Thus, they are not true complications but concomitants of the diabetic condition. Others believe that the complications of diabetes are a direct result of glucose intolerance and are therefore true complications. A combination of both theories is popular. When the balance between glucose and insulin is disturbed, acute complications of hyperglycemia, ketoacidosis, hyperglycemic hyperosmolar nonketotic coma, or hypoglycemia can develop (Fig. 41-3).

Acute Metabolic Complications

Hyperglycemia

In the early stages of *hyperglycemia,* the blood glucose becomes elevated due to a deficiency in insulin. Thus, glucose does not enter the cell but remains in the bloodstream. When the blood glucose reaches the renal threshold (approximately 180 mg/dL for an adult), it is excreted in the urine (*glycosuria*). Glucose, acting as an osmotic diuretic, carries large quantities of water and electrolytes with it. As a result of the osmotic diuresis, the extracellular fluid volume decreases. Water is drawn from the intracellular fluid to the extracellular fluid, and cellular dehydration and electrolyte imbalance result. The client will manifest an insatiable thirst (*polydipsia*) and will void large quantities of urine (*polyuria*). Sodium and potassium losses cause muscle weakness and fatigue. Abdominal cramping is believed to be due to the loss of electrolytes. Since glucose cannot enter the cell, cellular starvation results. This leads to hunger and an increased appetite (*polyphagia*).

Diabetic stage	Carbohydrate intolerance			Insulin = like activity	Vascular changes
	Fasting blood sugar	Glucose tolerance	Cortisone tolerance		
Prediabetes ↓	Normal	Normal	Normal	May be increased	+
↑ Subclinical ↓	Normal	Normal (abnormal during pregnancy)	Abnormal	Increased	+
↑ Latent ↓	Normal or increased	Abnormal	Test not necessary	Increased	++
↑ Overt	Increased	Test not necessary	Test not necessary	Increased	+++

Figure 41-3 Metabolic relationships in diabetes mellitus.

Often, this set of symptoms (polydipsia, polyuria, polyphagia) will cause the client to seek medical attention. Unless treatment is initiated, ketoacidosis, an advanced stage of hyperglycemia, will develop.

Ketoacidosis

Ketoacidosis, also referred to as *diabetic acidosis* and *diabetic coma,* may develop quickly or over several days or weeks. It can be caused by too little insulin, failure to follow a diet, physical or emotional stress, or undiagnosed diabetes.

In response to cellular starvation, the body releases and breaks down stored fats and protein to provide the needed energy. Free fatty acids from stored triglycerides are released in such large quantities that they are improperly metabolized in the liver and ketones are formed (ketonemia). Protein is broken down into glucose and nitrogen. Due to the insulin deficiency, the cells are still unable to use the ketones and glucose, and the process continues. The additional glucose raises the blood glucose level even higher, adding to the osmotic diuresis and loss of electrolytes. The client's skin becomes dry and loose and the eyeballs soft and sunken. Hypotension with a weak, rapid pulse may develop.

Meanwhile, the excess ketones upset the pH balance and acidosis develops. More water is lost as ketones are excreted (ketonuria) in an attempt to balance the pH. Vomiting caused by the acidosis will also create more fluid and electrolyte losses. The continual bicarbonate loss adds to the acidosis. Finally, Kussmaul respirations (rapid, deep breathing associated with dyspnea) begin to remove carbonic acid through the exhalation of carbon dioxide. Acetone is noted on the breath.

Renal failure may eventually occur to prevent hypovolemic shock from the loss of too much fluid. This failure causes the retention of ketones and glucose, and the acidosis progresses. The client becomes comatose due to the neurological stressors of dehydration, electrolyte imbalance, and acidosis. If the condition is untreated, death is inevitable.

Table 41-4
Pathogenesis of HHNK

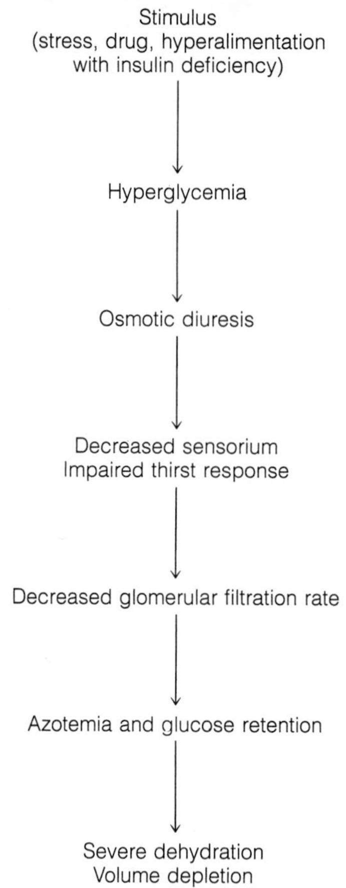

From M. Kinney et al., *AACN's Reference for Critical Care Nursing,* McGraw-Hill Book Company, New York, 1981, p. 647.

Hyperglycemic hyperosmolar nonketotic coma (HHNK)

HHNK occurs in the diabetic client who is able to produce enough insulin to prevent ketoacidosis but not enough to prevent extreme hyperglycemia, osmotic diuresis, and extracellular fluid depletion (Table 41-4). The increasing hyperglycemia causes intracellular dehydration due to a shift of fluid from the intracellular to the extracellular space. This causes neurological abnormalities such as somnolence, coma, seizures, hemiparesis, and aphasia. The client is often elderly and is a non-insulin-dependent or newly diagnosed diabetic. There will usually be a history of inadequate fluid intake, increasing mental depression, and polyuria. HHNK is a medical emergency. This nonketotic coma state has a mortality rate of 40 to 70 percent.[10]

The immediate therapy to reverse this hyperosmolar state is the rapid administration of intravenous (IV) solutions. Hypotonic saline is used unless hypotension is present. From 10 to 20 L of fluid may need to be given over a 24-hour period. The exact amount is titrated. Regular insulin is given IV and/or subcutaneously (SC) to aid in reducing the hyperglycemia. Potassium (K) is supplemented based on serum K^+

levels. The client is usually hypokalemic since potassium enters the cell along with glucose. In addition, potassium is lost in the urine. Once the client is stabilized, attempts to detect and correct the underlying precipitating cause should be initiated. Table 41-5 compares diabetic ketoacidosis and HHNK.

Hypoglycemia (low blood sugar, insulin shock, insulin reaction)

Hypoglycemia, or low blood sugar, occurs when there is proportionately too much insulin in the blood for the available glucose. This causes the blood glucose to drop below 50 to 60 mg/dL. In a nondiabetic, insulin is released according to the glucose level in the blood. In a diabetic, the insulin supply is dependent upon the type of medication and the route of administration. The balance between blood glucose and insulin can be disrupted by the administration of too much insulin, the ingestion of too little food, unusual amounts of exercise, or delayed eating. Although an insulin reaction can occur at any time, most reactions occur when the medication is at its peak of action or when the daily routine is disrupted without adequate adjustments. Hypoglycemia does occur with oral hypoglycemic agents, but less often than with insulin therapy.

The rate of decrease in the glucose level determines which symptoms the hypoglycemic client will exhibit. Rapid-acting insulins and excessive exercise can cause a rapid decrease in glucose. The sympathetic nervous system responds by releasing epinephrine with the resulting manifestations of cold sweats, weakness, trembling, nervousness, irritability, pallor, and increased heart rate. Intermediate- and long-acting insulin cause a slower fall in blood glucose, and the resulting symptoms do not occur until the brain is glucose deficient. The brain is dependent upon a constant supply of glucose because it is unable to store glucose or glycogen. If that supply is inadequate, the client will experience confusion, fatigue, and abnormal behavior which can resemble alcoholic intoxication. Clinical manifestations vary with the individual and do not always appear together.

Hypoglycemia is to be avoided whenever possible by intelligent diabetic management. Although hypoglycemia is reversible, repeated episodes with varying degrees of severity are extremely dangerous. Hypoglycemia can result in hemiplegia, epilepsy, emotional disturbances, intellectual deterioration, and death.[11] Table 41-6 compares hyperglycemia and hypoglycemia.

Chronic Complications

Angiopathy

Angiopathy, or blood vessel disease, is estimated to account for the majority of all deaths among known diabetics. These chronic blood vessel dysfunctions are divided into two categories, macroangiopathy and microangiopathy.

Macroangiopathy Macroangiopathy, or disease

Table 41-5
Comparison of Diabetic Ketoacidosis (DKA) and HHNK

	DKA	HHNK
Age	All ages	Usually over 50 years
Duration of diabetes	Variable	Recent onset
Precipitating events	Infection, stress	Stress, steroids, diuretics
Mortality	5%	50%
Blood sugar	400–800mg/dL	>900mg/dL
Dehydration	Variable (total body weight loss 5–15%)	Severe (total body weight loss 15–25%)
pH	Low	Normal
Breathing	Kussmaul	Normal
Serum acetone	Present	Absent

From M. Kinney et al., *AACN's Reference for Critical Care Nursing.* McGraw-Hill Book Company, New York, 1981, p. 649.

Table 41-6
Comparison of Hyperglycemia and Hypoglycemia

Hyperglycemia	Hypoglycemia
Symptoms*	
Increased thirst Increased urination Increased appetite followed by lack of appetite Weakness, fatigue Blurred vision Headache Elevated urine & glucose Nausea, vomiting Abdominal cramps Progresses to ketoacidosis or HHNK	Sweating Cold, clammy skin Numbness of fingers, toes, mouth Rapid heartbeat Emotional changes Headache Nervousness, tremors Faintness, dizziness Unsteady gait, slurred speech Hunger Vision changes Negative, double-voided urine specimen Seizures, coma
Causes	
Too much food Too little or no diabetic medication Inactivity Emotional, physical stress Poor absorption of insulin	Too little food—delayed, omitted, inadequate intake Too much diabetic medication Too much exercise without compensation Diabetic medication taken at wrong time Loss of weight without change in medication
Treatment	
Requires physician's attention Continue diabetic medication as ordered Check urine specimens frequently and record results Drink fluids hourly	Eat 10 g of simple carbohydrates immediately Repeat in 15 min if no relief obtained Report to physician if no relief obtained Do not take more diabetic medication at that time
Preventive Measures	
Take prescribed dose of medication at proper time Administer insulin accurately Maintain diet Maintain good personal hygiene Follow sick-day rules when ill Check urine specimens as ordered Contact doctor regarding ketonuria Exercise daily	Take prescribed dose of medication at proper time Administer insulin accurately Eat all ordered diet foods at proper time Compensate for exercise Recognize and know symptoms, and treat them immediately Carry simple carbohydrates Educate friends, family, fellow employees about symptoms and treatment Check urine specimens as ordered Wear diabetic identification

*There is a gradual onset of symptoms in hyperglycemia and a rapid onset in hypoglycemia.

of large and medium-size blood vessels, is essentially atherosclerosis, which is common to the general population. However, in the diabetic, atherosclerosis has an early onset. Coronary disease in males or females before age 50 raises the suspicion of diabetes. The degree of vascular damage appears to be related to the duration of the diabetes, not its severity. Although the atherosclerotic plaque formation is believed to have a genetic origin, its development seems to be promoted by the altered lipid metabolism common to diabetes. Tight glucose control may help delay the atherosclerotic process. However, diabetic neuropathy and poor healing, characteristic of diabetes, can further enhance the complications caused by macroangiopathy. Diabetic macroangiopathy, like atherosclerosis, is also responsible for renal failure, cerebral and myocardial infarctions, and peripheral artery disease, which are discussed in other chapters. Although genetic makeup cannot be altered, a diabetic can diminish the risk factors that aggravate macroangiopathy, such as obesity, smoking, hypertension, high fat intake, and low activity levels.

Microangiopathy Microangiopathy, or disease of the small blood vessels, unlike macroangiopathy, is specific to diabetes. Microangiopathy is responsible for the thickening of the basement membranes in the capillaries and arterioles. Although microangiopathy can be found throughout the body, the areas most noticeably affected are the eyes (retinopathy), the kidneys, and the skin. Basement membrane thickening can be present in the prediabetic stage, but the clinical manifestations usually do not appear until 15 to 20 years after the onset of diabetes. It is believed to have a genetic origin.

Retinopathy

Retinopathy, a common problem among diabetics, is classified as *background* or *proliferative.* In background retinopathy, the more common form, partial occlusion of the small blood vessels in the retina causes the development of microaneurysms in the capillary walls. These microaneurysms are so weak that capillary fluid leaks causing retinal edema and eventually hard exudates or intraretinal hemorrhages (Fig. 41-4*a*). The vision may be affected if the macula is involved. Proliferative retinopathy, the more severe form, involves the retina and the vitreous. When retinal capillaries become occluded, new blood vessels (*neovascularization*) are formed to supply the retina with blood (Fig. 41-4*b*). These vessels hemorrhage easily and grow in the retina and vitreous. If the vitreous contracts, these vessels are torn and bleed into the vitreous cavity, preventing light from reaching the retina. The client then sees black or red spots or lines. If these new blood vessels pull the retina while the vitreous contracts, causing a tear, partial or complete retinal detachment occurs. If the macula is involved, vision is lost. The occurrence of retinopathy appears to be correlated with the duration of the diabetes; the longer the disease has been present, the more likely the presence of retinopathy.

Diabetic retinopathy is the leading cause of blindness in the United States in clients up to age 60.[12] The evidence that strict control delays retinal changes is inconclusive. However, some studies show a delay in visual changes secondary to careful diabetic control.[13]

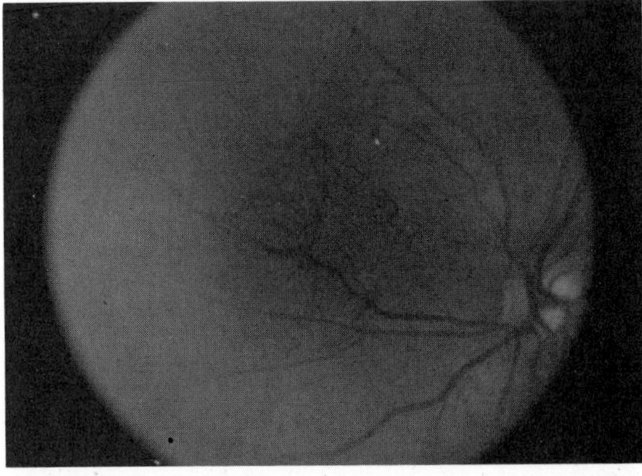

A

B

Figure 41-4 Diabetic retinopathy. *(a)* Hemorrhage and microaneurysms. *(b)* Neovascularizations. *(Courtesy of Dr. Harold Dobson.)*

The two most common forms of treatment of diabetic retinopathy are *photocoagulation* and *vitrectomy.* Photocoagulation converts light energy into heat and coagulates the tissue in the area where the light is directed. It is particularly useful with neovascularization. Vitrectomy is the aspiration of blood, membrane, and fibers from the inside of the eye through a small incision just behind the cornea. This surgery is particularly useful for the treatment of organized vitreous hemorrhage and traction retinal detachments.

Diabetics are also prone to other visual problems. *Glaucoma* occurs due to the occlusion of the outflow channels secondary to neovascularization. This type of glaucoma is difficult to treat and often results in blindness. *Cataracts* occur with increasing frequency in the diabetic. Although the process is similar to that of senile cataracts, it occurs at an earlier age in the diabetic.

Neuropathy

Neuropathy is probably one of the most common complications of diabetes in adults. However, its etiology is unclear. Some believe that it is the result of a decreased blood supply to the nerves due to microangiopathic changes. Others attribute it to metabolic defects in the nerve tissue. Neuropathy can precede, accompany, or follow the diagnosis of diabetes. Individual nerves of the spinal cord or the autonomic nervous system may be involved. Acute-onset neuropathy is usually reversible, while progressive-onset neuropathy is usually irreversible. The two basic types of neuropathy are peripheral (the more common) and visceral.

Peripheral Neuropathy Peripheral neuropathy affects all extremities, but most often the feet and legs. The neuropathy is usually bilateral and symmetrical. Clients complain of *pain* and *paresthesia.* The pain, described as burning, cramping, crushing, or tearing, is usually worse at night and may occur only at that time. It may be relieved by walking.

The paresthesia is associated with tingling, burning, and itching sensations. Complete or partial loss of sensitivity to touch and temperature is common. Clients report that they feel they are walking on pillows or that their feet are numb. At times, their skin becomes so sensitive (hyperesthesia) that even bedding cannot be tolerated. Neuropathy in the hands causes atrophy of the small muscles, limiting fine movement (Fig. 41-5). Peripheral neuropathy also causes foot drop, Charcot's joint (deterioration of the foot or ankle joints), and neuropathic ulcers (Fig. 41-6). These ulcers develop at points of pressure. If the blood supply is adequate, these ulcers will heal once the pressure is removed.

Visceral Neuropathy Visceral neuropathy accounts for changes in the cranial nerves and autonomic nervous system. Involvement of the third, fourth, and sixth cranial nerves affects the extraocular muscles. Headaches, forehead pain, eye pain, and double vision (diplopia) may result.

Neuropathy affecting the autonomic nervous system causes nocturnal diarrhea, postural hypotension, impotence, and neurogenic bladder. Nocturnal diarrhea is not associated with abdominal cramping. It is the result of delayed gastric emptying. It affects few diabetics and does not disturb diabetic control. Antibiotics and antidiarrhea drugs have been used in its control.

Impotence, perhaps the most distressing visceral neuropathy, affects 50 percent of all diabetic men and occurs when the arteries in the penis cannot dilate because of damage to the nerves involved in erection. The onset occurs gradually over 6 months to 2 years and is irreversible. Poorly controlled diabetics can experience temporary impotence until good control is restored. Surgical prosthetic implantations have been developed that make vaginal penetration possible. Decreased libido is a problem with some diabetic women.

A neurogenic bladder develops as sensation in the inner wall decreases, causing urinary retention. Clients with retention complain of infrequent voiding, difficulty in voiding, and a weak stream of urine.

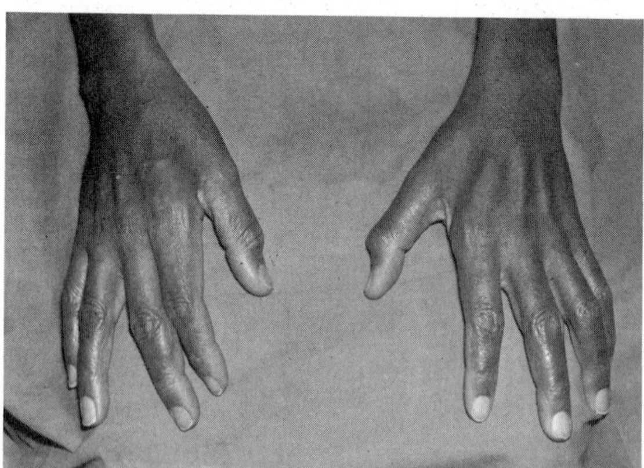

Figure 41-5 Diabetic neuropathy: muscle atrophy. *(Courtesy of Dr. Harold Dobson.)*

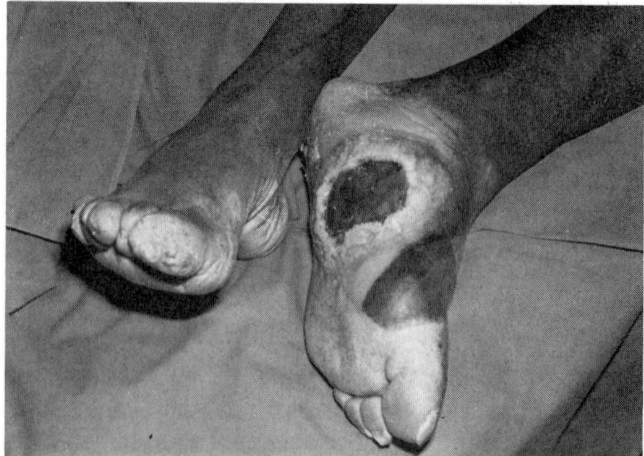

Figure 41-6 Neuropathy: neurotrophic ulcerations. *(Courtesy of Dr. Harold Dobson.)*

Cholinergic drugs may be given to promote the release of urine, and sometimes bladder surgery is indicated.

Treatment of neuropathies involves good diabetic control and supportive care. There is no known cure. Diabetics under relatively good control appear to have a lower incidence of neuropathy than those who are poorly controlled. However, neuropathy can occur during good control.

Nephropathy

Renal Atherosclerosis Nephropathy is the result of vascular changes and infections of the kidney. Renal arteriolosclerosis, diffuse and nodular glomerulosclerosis (microangiopathy), and pyelonephritis occur in diabetes. Atherosclerosis and arteriolosclerosis affect the afferent and efferent arterioles. The most significant tubular lesions can occur within the distal tubules and descending loop of Henle.

Microangiopathy Microangiopathy in the kidneys causes diffuse and nodular glomerulosclerosis. Diffuse glomerulosclerosis affects all the basement membranes of all glomerular capillaries, usually in both kidneys. The basement membranes become thickened and leaky. Total sclerosis of glomerular vascular tufts leads to renal failure. In nodular glomerulosclerosis (Kimmelstiel-Wilson lesions), nodules develop in the glomeruli. In advanced cases, most of the glomeruli are involved.

Pyelonephritis Pyelonephritis, caused by a bacterial infection of the kidneys, spreads from interstitial tissue to the tubules to the glomeruli. Pyelonephritis is a manifestation of the generalized increased susceptibility to infection. Severe renal failure is usually limited to those diabetics who develop the disease at an early age.

If uremia develops, the appetite wanes. Insulin doses must be lowered, and special efforts must be made to find foods palatable to the client. Glycosuria decreases as the renal threshold rises. Treatment is supportive. It is important to protect the kidney as much as possible. Urinary tract and bladder infections must be detected early and treated aggressively.

Indwelling catheters should be avoided when possible. When they are unavoidable, aseptic technique is mandatory. Peritoneal dialysis, hemodialysis, and kidney transplants are often necessary, but their success is complicated by the diabetic state. Renal failure is the second-ranking cause of death among diabetics.

Skin changes

Skin disorders such as *shin spots* and *necrobiosis lipoidica diabeticorum* are caused by microangiopathy (Fig. 41-7). Shin spots are brown spots located on the front surfaces of the lower extremities. They are harmless, painless, and initially measure less than 1 cm in diameter. Shin spots are believed to be the result of trauma and hemorrhaging in the skin.

Necrobiosis lipoidica diabeticorum is also found in the lower extremities. The result of trauma, these lesions are similar to shin spot lesions but are more prone to ulcerations and necrosis. They are reddish yellow in color and atrophic. They sometimes require skin grafts due to slow healing of the skin. Necrobiosis lipoidica diabeticorum is found most often in insulin-dependent females and may precede the onset of overt diabetes.

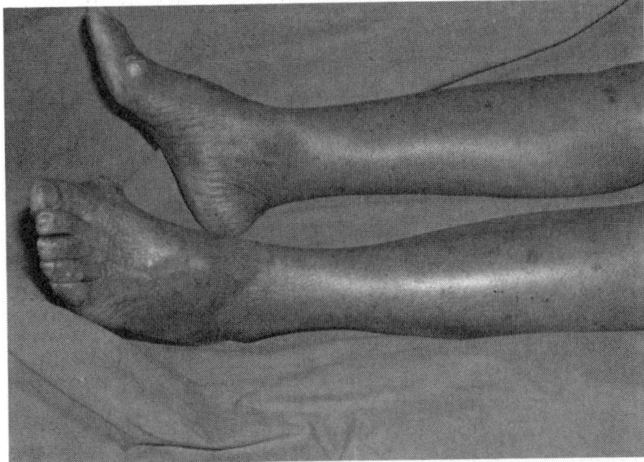

A

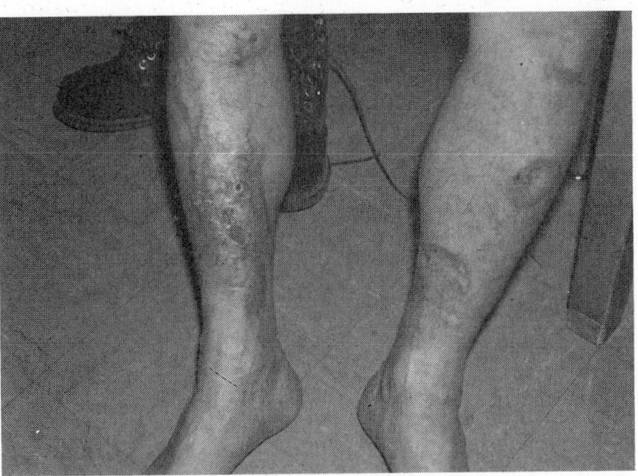

B

Figure 41-7 Microangiopathy. *(a)* Skin spots. *(b)* Necrobiosis lipoidica diabeticorium. *(Courtesy of Dr. Harold Dobson.)*

Infection

Diabetics are more susceptible to infections than nondiabetics. A primary reason for this is a greater than normal accumulation of glucose under the dermis secondary to hyperglycemia. This accumulated glucose is a good medium for bacterial and fungal growth. Recurring or persistent infections such as *Candida albicans,* as well as boils and furuncles, often lead the health care provider to be suspicious of diabetes. Loss of sensation (neuropathy) may delay the detection of an infection.

Excessive amounts of glycosuria encourage bladder infections, especially in a neurogenic bladder. Decreased circulation from angiopathy can prevent or delay the healing process. Protein waste during hyperglycemia and ketoacidosis is also responsible for poor healing. Antibiotic therapy has prevented infection from being a major cause of death in diabetics. The treatment of any infection must be prompt and vigorous.

ABNORMAL DIAGNOSTIC FINDINGS

Since diabetes is a multisystemic, multiproblem disease, all laboratory studies need to be correlated with clinical findings. Table 41-7 summarizes the laboratory findings of common tests when hyperglycemia, ketoacidosis, and hypoglycemia are present.

Glucose determination tests are all abnormal in overt diabetes (Fig. 41-2). Age is important in interpreting blood sugar results. The American Diabetes Association recommends adding 10 mg/dL to the normal value for each decade over 50.

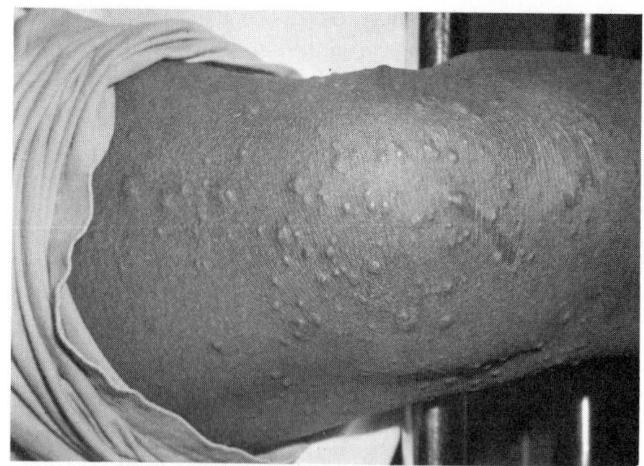

Figure 41-8 Xanthomas of the knee associated with poorly controlled diabetes. *(Courtesy of Dr. Harold Dobson.)*

In the absence of insulin, fat metabolism is altered. This results in elevations of lipids, cholesterol, and triglycerides. These elevations are associated with the vascular disorders of diabetes. Elevated lipids can result in tuberous xanthomas on the buttocks, face, elbows, and knees (Fig. 41-8).

The results of urine tests for sugar and acetone are dependent upon renal function and age. Decreasing renal function and advancing age both raise the renal threshold for glucose and ketone bodies above 180 mg/dL. The higher the threshold, the less likely it is that glycosuria and ketonuria will be apparent. Blood glucose is a better parameter for measuring control than urine testing in the elderly diabetic, as glycosuria may not be evident when hyperglycemia is present.

Table 41-7
Hyperglycemia, Ketoacidosis, and Hypoglycemia

Laboratory Test	Hyperglycemia	Ketoacidosis	Hypoglycemia
Urine glucose	Positive	Positive	Negative to positive depending on time of last voiding
Urine acetone	Negative→positive	Positive	Negative→positive
Plasma glucose	>120 mg/dL	>200 mg/dL	<50 mg/dL
Plasma acetone		Positive	Negative
Plasma bicarbonate		<20 mEq/L	Normal
Blood pH	Normal	<7.35	Normal

Adapted from Stephen Podolsky, *Clinical Diabetes: Modern Management,* Appleton-Century-Crofts, New York, 1980, p. 175.

MEDICAL MANAGEMENT

Appropriate medical management varies depending on the client's clinical manifestations. Specific protocols are outlined in Tables 41-8, 41-9, and 41-10 for the management of a client with suspected diabetes mellitus, ketoacidosis, and hypoglycemia.

The management of diabetes mellitus involves individualized prescriptions for diet, exercise, and medication, if indicated. Specific considerations related to these areas are covered in other sections of this chapter. A more difficult management problem concerns the client in ketoacidosis.

Ketoacidosis

Diabetic ketoacidosis is usually treated in the hospital, as it is a medical emergency. Treatment is aimed at (1) immediate administration of insulin, (2) replacement of fluid to correct hypovolemia, and (3) replacement of electrolytes to correct imbalances.

Insulin

Controversy continues over the two approaches to insulin therapy in ketoacidosis. The conventional method involves an immediate dose of 50 to 150 units of regular insulin, with subsequent doses of 50 to 100 units of regular insulin given IV, SC, or alternated at regular intervals as ordered until the client's condition stabilizes.

Table 41-8
Medical Management: Suspected Diabetes Mellitus

Diagnostic

1. Complete history and physical examination
2. Blood work-fasting blood sugar, 2-h postprandial, oral glucose tolerance test, cholesterol and triglyceride levels, BUN and creatinine, electrolytes
3. Urine for complete urinalysis, culture and sensitivity, glucose and acetone
4. Intake and output
5. Fundoscopic examination
6. Neurological examination
7. Blood pressure
8. Electrocardiogram
9. Monitor weight

Therapeutic

1. Calculated ADA diet
2. Exercise plan
3. Insulin or oral hypoglycemic agent if indicated
4. Dental examination
5. Podiatric examination
6. Specific teaching and follow-up programs

Table 41-9
Medical Management: Diabetic Ketoacidosis

Diagnostic

1. Blood work-stat blood sugar, complete blood count, ketones, pH, electrolytes, BUN, blood gases
2. Urinalysis—specific gravity, pH, sugar, acetone

Therapeutic

1. Regular insulin
2. IV fluids
3. Electrolyte replacement
4. Intake and output
5. Central venous pressure monitoring if indicated
6. Assess diabetic management
7. Cardiac monitoring

The other method is the low-dose infusion method, which is gaining in popularity.[14] In this method, 0.1 unit per kilogram of body weight per hour is administered via an infusion pump. This insulin therapy is continued until a blood glucose level of 250 mg/dL is reached. The risk of hypoglycemia due to stored insulin is reduced by this method.

Fluid and electrolyte replacement

Medical management of ketoacidosis related to fluid and electrolytes is aimed at replacing both extracellular and intracellular water and replacing total body deficits of sodium, chloride, bicarbonate, potassium, phosphate, magnesium, and nitrogen.[15] Assessments of blood pressure, pulse, tissue turgor, and central venous pressure give some indications of the degree of hypovolemia. Plasma expanders such as saline, plasma, albumin, dextran, and whole blood are given initially to correct the hyperosmolarity and hypovolemia of ketoacidosis.

When the blood glucose reaches 250 mg/dL, a 5% to 10% glucose solution is given to prevent

Table 41-10
Medical Management: Hypoglycemia

Diagnostic

1. Stat blood sugar
2. History (if possible)

Therapeutic

1. Stat glucose—20–30 mL 50% glucose IV if comatose
2. Oral carbohydrate snack if conscious
3. IV glucagon
4. Determine cause of hypoglycemia

hypoglycemia. From 1 to 2 L/hour may be given until the clinical picture improves, with a possible total fluid replacement of 6 L in the first 24 hours. Once the client becomes hydrated and the renal output is adequate, potassium and other electrolytes can be added. Early in ketoacidosis, there is a shift of potassium out of the cell as the hydrogen ion moves into the cell. As ketoacidosis progresses, potassium is unable to enter the cell. This is because potassium normally moves into the cell with glucose in the presence of insulin. Osmotic diuresis results in the loss of potassium through the urine. Electrolyte replacement is individualized to the client based on clinical and biochemical assessments. Bicarbonate is usually not given to correct acidosis unless this condition is severe.

Hypoglycemia

The medical management of hypoglycemia is summarized in Table 41-10. Ideally, the client should be able to reverse hypoglycemia before medical assistance is necessary. If this does not occur, aggressive intervention is indicated to raise the blood glucose level. Since the brain needs a constant supply of glucose, hypoglycemia can result in altered cerebral functioning. Repeated episodes of severe hypoglycemia can result in permanent brain damage.

Some clients have difficulty with alternating periods of hypoglycemia and hyperglycemia. This may be a result of the *Somogyi effect.* Initially, hypoglycemia is caused by exogenous insulin. The physiological response is a release of stress hormones (epinephrine, glucagon, cortisol, and growth hormone). As a result, hyperglycemia occurs. If this hyperglycemic state results in an increase in insulin, hypoglycemia recurs. Careful monitoring of urine and blood glucose is necessary. Adjustments in the amount or timing of insulin administration may be necessary to prevent this reaction.

Research Developments

Although in the experimental stage, the artificial endocrine pancreas (AEP) and pancreas transplants are two promising developments in diabetic research. The AEP has two basic designs. One contains a glucose sensor that determines blood glucose, a computer that calculates the needed insulin dose, and a pump that releases insulin or glucose into the bloodstream. The other design contains a preprogrammed insulin pump that provides a steady IV insulin infusion.[16] Both systems provide greater blood glucose control than SC injections.

Pancreas transplants involving either the whole pancreas or islet cells may provide a "cure" for diabetes if immunological rejection of the transplant can be overcome. Successful transplants have restored glucose tolerance and improved vision and kidney function. Islet cell transplantation involves the attachment of islet cells to body tissue, the interior of the liver being the favored site.[17]

PHARMACOLOGICAL INTERVENTION

Insulin

Indication

Exogenous insulin is needed when a client has inadequate insulin to meet specific metabolic needs and the combination of dietary management, exercise, and oral agents cannot maintain a satisfactory blood glucose level. Because insulin is a protein, it is destroyed in the gastrointestinal tract if taken orally. Therefore, insulin must be injected SC or IV.

Exogenous insulin is commonly obtained from the pancreas of pigs and cows. Pork insulin is more similar than beef insulin to human insulin. Most pharmaceutical insulins are a combination of both. Although insulin is still available in U-40 (40 units/mL) and U-80 (80 units/mL), the standard strength is now U-100 (100 units/mL). A unit (U) of insulin, measured by volume, contains a specific quantity, by weight, of pure insulin crystals. Consequently, 1 unit of insulin, regardless of the scale used, contains the same quantity of insulin crystals. Only the quantity of solution differs. U-100 insulin provides for a smaller volume per injection dose. Each concentration has its own color-coded syringes scaled to 1 mL.

Types available

There are several types of insulin. They differ from each other in onset, peak action, and duration (Table 41-11). The specific properties of each type of insulin are correlated with the client's diet and activity. Not all clients respond to insulin as the table indicates. Regular lente and semilente insulin are prescribed when a rapid onset is needed. Only regular insulin can be administered IV and is used in emergencies. Rapid-acting insulins are helpful during surgery, acute illnesses, obstetrical procedures, and the management of poorly controlled diabetes. Regular insulin is used for the sliding-scale or rainbow method. With this method, an insulin dose is administered based on the results of a double-voided urine-glucose test. An order may read, "Give regular insulin accordingly: 1+-5 U, 2+-10 U, 3+-15 U, and 4+-20 U. An additional 5 U if

Table 41-11
Types and Action Times of Insulin

Preparation	Appearance	Onset time (h)*	Peak time (h)*	Duration (H)*
Short-acting				
Regular	Clear	$\frac{1}{2}$–1	2–3	6
Semilente	Cloudy	$\frac{1}{2}$–1	5–7	12–16
Intermediate-acting				
NPH	Cloudy	1–1$\frac{1}{2}$	8–12	24
Lente	Cloudy	1–1$\frac{1}{2}$	8–12	24
Long-acting				
PZI	Cloudy	4–8	14–20	36
Ultralente	Cloudy	4–8	16–18	36

*Times vary with each client.

acetone is present." If the client was 2+ for glucose and positive for acetone, 15 units of regular insulin would be given. The client's fluctuating need for insulin can be met by this individualized method of insulin administration until his condition stabilizes.

The intermediate-acting insulins, NPH and Lente, are the most commonly used insulins for maintenance therapy. They are convenient, as only one injection is usually needed daily. The long-acting insulins, PZI and Ultralente, are rarely used because of their long duration. If one type of insulin does not meet the needs of a client, a combination of rapid-acting and intermediate-acting insulins may be used. Regular insulin can be mixed with any other insulin. The Lentes can be mixed only among themselves. Exogenous insulin is not a cure for diabetes. Even with strict compliance, an insulin-dependent diabetic has wide fluctuations in his blood sugar. A normal blood sugar level cannot be consistently maintained (Fig. 41-1).

Problems associated with insulin therapy

Hypoglycemia, insulin allergies, and insulin antibodies are three problems associated with insulin therapy. Hypoglycemia was discussed earlier. There are two types of cutaneous *allergic reactions* to insulin. The reaction may be a localized wheal at the point of injection or generalized hives. The latter may cause itching and gastrointestinal complaints. These reactions are usually seen in clients new to insulin therapy. If the reactions do not subside, antihistamines or pork insulin are administered. Desensitization is rarely needed.

Clients receiving insulin over several months develop antibodies to the insulin which may interfere with diabetic control.[18] The release of insulin to the tissue is delayed since the serum insulin antibodies bind injected insulin as it is being absorbed into the bloodstream.

Nursing implications

The new diabetic should be taught the proper insulin administration technique (Table 41-12). The diabetic who has been taking insulin should have his technique reviewed at each contact with a health care provider. It should never be assumed that a client knows and practices the correct insulin injection technique. An inaccurate dose is often caused by poor eyesight, a problem clients cannot recognize. Either air bubbles may not be seen or the scale may be read improperly by the visually impaired diabetic.

Superficial injections can cause small wheals resembling mosquito bites which will eventually scar. *Lipodystrophy* (atrophy or hypertrophy at injection sites) can result from a poor rotation technique and the use of cold insulin (Fig. 41-9). Use of lipodystrophic areas for insulin administration can result in erratic insulin absorption. Unaffected areas may absorb insulin more rapidly, causing a hypoglycemic reaction. All clients need a personalized and dated rotation chart drawn according to site preferences and body fat (Fig. 41-10). The chart should include at least 30 dated injection sites 1 inch apart.

Insulin in use does not need refrigeration and should be injected at room temperature. Reserve bottles should be refrigerated. Insulin subjected to freezing or high temperatures should not be used, as it loses its potency. When traveling, clients should always keep insulin and syringes with them in case their luggage is misplaced. Insulin administration gadgets are not needed unless there is visual impairment or a physical handicap which makes this advisable.

Because of the dangerous side effects of insulin-

Table 41-12
Steps to Follow in Preparing for Insulin Injection

1. Wash hands thoroughly.
2. Roll the insulin bottle between the palms of the hands to warm and mix the insulin.
   Note: Always inspect the insulin bottle before using it for the first time. Make sure that it is of the proper type and concentration, that the expiration date has not passed, and that the top of the bottle is in perfect condition.
3. Remove the protective cap from the insulin bottle and clean the rubber stopper top with an alcohol swab.
4. Prepare to fill your syringe.
5. Draw an amount of air into the syringe equal to the insulin dosage.
6. Press the needle through the rubber stopper of the insulin bottle and then push the plunger of the syringe all the way down, expelling the air into the bottle of insulin.
7. Invert the insulin bottle and pull the plunger back to withdraw the proper amount of insulin. Make sure that the needle tip never extends above the level of insulin; this helps to avoid bubbles in the syringe.
8. Check for air bubbles in the syringe and for the proper insulin dosage.
9. If air bubbles are present, tap the barrel with the fingers at the point where bubbles appear. Bubbles should now rise to the top of the syringe barrel. Push the plunger until the bubbles are expelled into the insulin vial. Slowly withdraw the plunger until it is once again lined up with the proper dosage.
10. If no additional air bubbles exist, withdraw the needle from the bottle of insulin.
11. Select a proper injection site (see Fig. 41-10). With the thumb and index finger of one hand, stretch the skin in the area selected for injection and cleanse it with an alcohol swab. Using a circular motion, wipe the injection area from the center out toward the edge.
12. Stretch the skin tight where you are going to make the injection. Keeping the skin stretched, grasp the syringe firmly near its tip with the other hand, taking care not to touch the sterile needle. If the injection is to be made into an area with only a thin layer of fat, pinch a fold of skin between the fingers, rather than stretching the skin. This will keep the needle from penetrating into a muscle.
13. Plunge the needle through the skin quickly up to its hub, and stop stretching or pinching the skin. The needle should enter the skin at an angle of approximately 90°, as straight into the skin as possible.
14. Use the free hand to hold the syringe while the other hand pulls back slightly on the plunger. If blood appears in the bottom of the syringe barrel, pull the unit out of the skin slightly—$\frac{1}{16}$ to $\frac{1}{8}$ inch—to remove the needle tip from the blood vessel. Pull back slightly on the plunger again. If more blood appears, select a new injection site using a sterile syringe and needle.
15. Inject insulin by quickly depressing the plunger. The injection should be completed within 5 s.
16. Place an alcohol swab over the area where the needle entered the skin; remove the needle quickly at the same angle at which it was inserted.
17. Hold the swab in place for a few seconds, but do not rub.
18. Destroy and dispose of the single-use syringe in a safe manner.

From Beckton Dickinson & Co., Rochelle Park, N.J., Patient Information Pamphlet.

induced hypoglycemia, the diabetic teaching program must include the clinical manifestations, causes, prevention, and treatment of this condition.

Oral Hypoglycemic Agents

Indication

Oral hypoglycemic agents are not oral insulin or a substitute for insulin. They act by stimulating the beta cells to release insulin. The client must have some endogenous insulin production for an oral agent to be effective. Clients who benefit most from oral agents are those who are nonobese, older than 40 years of age, require less than 20 units of daily insulin, and have had diabetes for less than 5 years. In the newly diagnosed diabetic, oral agent therapy may be withheld until the client has been given an opportunity to lose weight. Although initially successful, oral agents

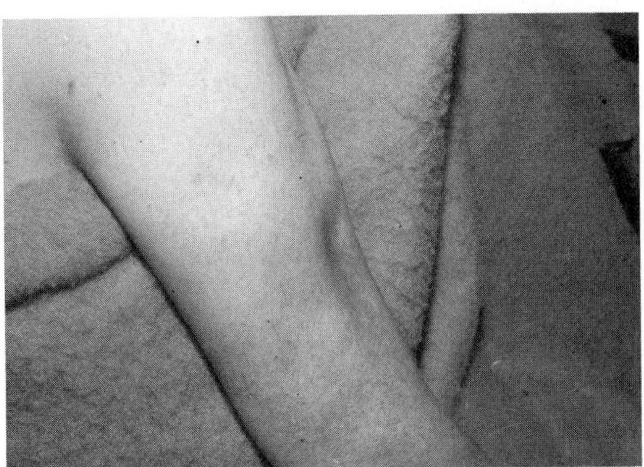

Figure 41-9 Lipodystrophy of the arm. *(Courtesy of Dr. Harold Dobson.)*

may eventually fail to maintain control, and insulin therapy will need to be initiated.

Types available

The sulfonylureas consist of tolbutamide (Orinase), acetohexamide (Dymelor), tolazamide (Tolinase), and chlorpropamide (Diabinese). Like insulin, the sulfonylureas differ in their dosage, absorption time, peak action, and duration (Table 41-13).

Problems associated with therapy

Oral agents became popular because of their convenience. Unfortunately, this convenience has often caused diabetics to underestimate the seriousness of their disease. Diabetics controlled by oral agents are subject to the same complications as insulin-dependent diabetics. Because oral agents stimulate insulin release, hypoglycemia can occur, although less often than with insulin. However, the hypoglycemia may be more severe. This is especially true with the use of chlorpropamide because of its 24- to 36-hour duration. Clients must be warned against taking extra pills for overeating since one pill lasts longer than the digestion of one meal. Oral agents should not be taken at bedtime. The last dose should be taken with supper.

Because chlorpropamide, acetohexamide, and tolazamide are excreted by the kidneys in active form, clients with kidney damage should use tolbutamide to prevent hypoglycemia induced by drug accumulation. Since all sulfonylureas are metabolized in the liver, impaired liver function also causes hypoglycemia by prolonging the drug level. The sulfonylureas can cause side effects such as nausea and vomiting, diarrhea, skin allergies, or hematological disorders. Oral agents are also responsible for prolonging the effects of other medication and can cause an Antabuse effect when mixed with alcohol.

A 1970 study indicated that cardiovascular deaths are more frequent in clients treated with oral agents than those treated with insulin or diet therapy alone.[19] For this reason, many physicians are reluctant to prescribe oral agents and prefer to use other methods of treatment such as diet and exercise.

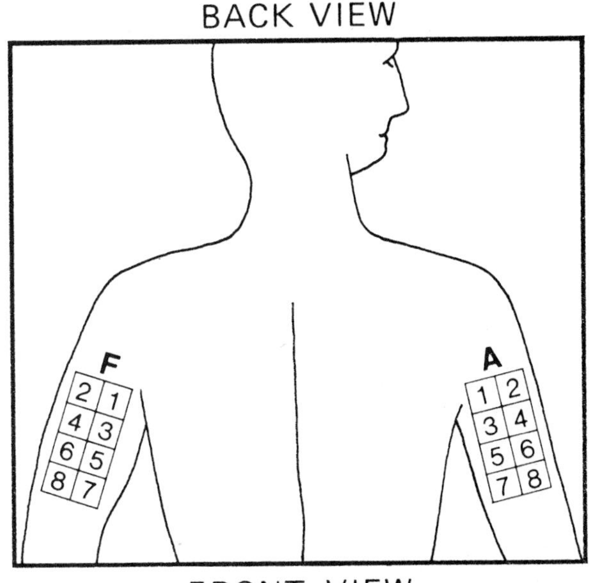

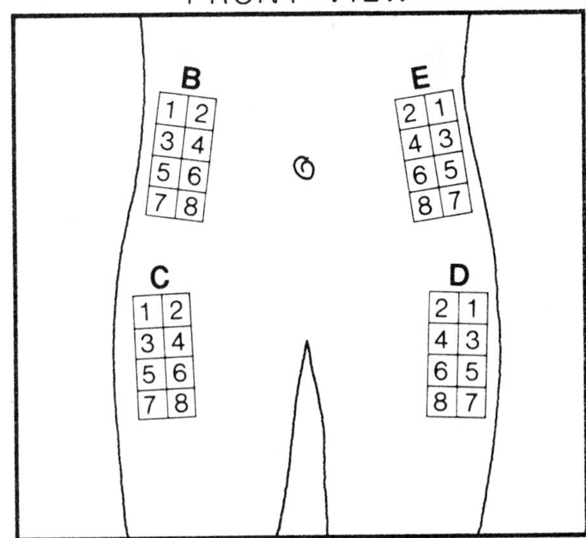

Figure 41-10 Sample rotation chart for insulin injection sites.

Table 41-13
Oral Hypoglycemic Agents

Generic Name	Trade Name	Shape	Color	Size (mg)	Duration (h)	Common Daily Dose (mg)
Tolbutamide	Orinase	Round	White	500	6–12	500–3000
Acetohexamide	Dymelor	Capsule-shaped	White Yellow	250 500	12–24 12–24	250–1500
Tolazamide	Tolinase	Round	White White	100 250	12–24 12–24	100–750
Chlorpropamide	Diabinese	D-shaped	Blue	100 250	12–24 24–36	100–500

Nursing implications

The obese client who loses weight may be able to discontinue the use of an oral hypoglycemic agent. If weight is not lost, however, oral agents may become ineffective. The majority of type II diabetics who lose weight will not need diabetic medication.

Certain clients may refuse insulin therapy or may be unable to learn to administer it. Oral agents may then be the health care provider's only recourse. The nurse must stress the importance of following the total medical prescription, which involves not only medication but also weight and diet control, exercise, and good personal hygiene.

Other Drugs Affecting Blood Glucose Levels

The diabetic concurrently taking other medication must be extremely careful about the hypoglycemic and hyperglycemic effects of certain medications (Table 41-14). Diabetic medications may need to be adjusted if other medications are required.

DIETARY MANAGEMENT

Dietary management is the most important therapy for diabetes. In both type I and type II diabetes, an individually calculated, balanced diet is the primary therapy.

Dietary Compliance

Perhaps the most difficult adjustment for the diabetic client is the need to comply with an individually prescribed diet. Diet and eating patterns have special meanings for each client related to emotions, culture, and religion. Many people are aware that a well-balanced diet is healthy. However, most people can indulge in an occasional indiscretion without serious results. Such is not the case with the diabetic.

The high incidence of obesity among type II diabetes is further evidence that these clients place a high value on food. Reinforcement and encouragement are essential if a successful dietary program is to be followed by the client.

Table 41-14
Medications with Effects on Blood Glucose

Hypoglycemia	Hyperglycemia
Acetaminophen	Acetazolamide
Alcohol	Alcohol
Allopurinol	Amphetamines
Anabolic steroids	Arginine HCl
Clofibrate	Asparaginase
Chloramphenicol	Barbiturates
Chlorpromazine and orphenadrine	Dextrothyroxine
Dicumarol	Diaxoxide
EDTA (and insulin)	Epinephrine
Fenfluramine	Glycerin/glycerol
Guanethidine	Glucagon
Isoniazid	Glucocorticoids
Magnesium (and insulin)	Glucose
MAO inhibitors	Levodopa
Oxyphenbutazone	Marijuana
Oxytetracycline (and insulin)	Nicotinic acid
Pentamidine	Narcotics
Phenylbutazone	Oral contraceptives
Phenyramidol	Phenothiazines
Probenecid	Phenytoin
Propranolol	Potassium depletion
Salicylates	Sympathomimetics
Sulfinpyrazone	Thiazide diuretics
Sulfonamides	
Theophylline	

From Dorothy R. Blevens, *The Diabetic and Nursing Care*, McGraw-Hill Book Company, New York, 1979, p. 203.

Calculating a Diabetic Diet

A diabetic diet is calculated individually according to the client's ideal body weight, occupation, age, and activities. Once caloric needs are determined in relation to the need to lose, maintain, or gain weight, the proportion of carbohydrates, protein, and fat is calculated. The distribution of calories averages 50 percent from carbohydrates, 20 percent from protein, and 30 percent from fat. These percentages are often changed according to individual needs and professional opinion. The spacing of the diet averages $\frac{2}{7}$ at each meal, with $\frac{1}{7}$ of the daily allowance left for a bedtime snack. If the client needs to gain weight, additional daytime snacks may need to be planned in order to reduce the quantity to be eaten at each meal.

Exchange Lists

Individual dietary prescriptions are usually converted into a meal plan based on the exchange list system of the American Diabetes Association. An exchange list divides all foods except concentrated carbohydrates into one of six categories or food groups: milk, meats, vegetables, fats, breads, and fruits. Each food group is calculated to include the specific quantity of food allowed according to standard household measurements. Each food quantity is equal to one food exchange. Calories are not mentioned. The meal plan explains how many food exchanges are allowed from each food group per meal. Any of the foods within the specific food groups are allowed for variety as long as the quantity is observed. Table 41-15 shows a sample 1800-calorie meal plan and an excerpt from the exchange lists. Table 10, Appendix B, shows sample meals for this diet with cultural variations. Complete exchange lists and calculated diets for different caloric requirements are available from the American Diabetes Association.

Areas of Concern

Alcohol

Alcohol is high in calories, has no nutrient value, and promotes hypertriglyceridemia. In addition, it has

Table 41-15
Meal Plan Example and Excerpts from Exchange Lists

Meal Plan Example (1800 cal)

	Breakfast	Lunch	Dinner	HS
Milk, 2%	1	1	1	
Bread	2	2	2	1
Fruit	1	1	1	
Vegetable		1	1	
Meat	2	2	2	1
Fat	2	2	1	1

Excerpts from Exchange Lists

Milk exchange	Amount/serving	Vegetable exchange	Amount/serving
Milk, whole	1 cup	Green beans (plain)	1 cup
Milk, 2%	1 cup	Mushrooms (plain)	1 cup
Yogurt (plain)	1 cup	Tomato Juice	$\frac{1}{2}$ cup
Fruit/juice exchange	**Amount/serving**	**Bread/starch exchange**	**Amount/serving**
Apple juice	$\frac{1}{3}$ cup	Hamburger bun (large)	$\frac{1}{2}$
Banana	$\frac{1}{2}$	Cooked cereal	$\frac{1}{2}$ cup
Cherries	10 large	Corn	$\frac{1}{3}$ cup
Meat/protein exchange	**Amount/serving**	**Fat exchange**	**Amount/serving**
Egg	1	Mayonnaise	1 t
Poultry	1 oz	Bacon	1 strip
Frankfurter	1	Butter	1 t

The exchange lists are based on material in the *Exchange Lists for Meal Planning* prepared by committees of the American Diabetes Association, Inc., and the American Dietetic Association in cooperation with the National Institute of Arthritis, Metabolism and Digestive Diseases and the National Heart and Lung Institute, National Institutes of Health, Public Health Service, U.S. Department of Health, Education and Welfare. Used with permission.

detrimental effects on the liver (see Chap. 35). It is also the leading cause of pancreatitis, which can result in diabetes. Alcohol's inhibitory effect on gluconeogenesis can cause severe hypoglycemia. Alcohol causes an Antabuse effect when ingested with oral hypoglycemic agents.

However, if the client chooses, a drink can be calculated into the diabetic diet. The client can substitute one fat exchange for every 45 calories of alcohol. One drink has approximately 135 calories and would equal three fat exchanges. When possible, diabetic clients should drink on a full stomach, use sugar-free mixes, and drink dry, light wines.

Dietetic foods

The word *dietetic* is confusing because it does not always mean a lack of calories. The caloric value of dietetic foods should be determined by reading the label. If no caloric value is listed, it must be counted in the meal plan as the appropriate exchange. If calories are listed, 15 to 20 free calories per meal of dietetic food are allowed in addition to the food on the meal plan.

Dietetic foods are expensive and, although convenient, are not necessary. The client can be taught to make intelligent decisions regarding the use of nondietetic foods by reading the labels. For instance, foods with sugar, mannitol, or sorbitol listed as the first two ingredients should be avoided. Artificial sweeteners do allow some freedom in the diet. Recipes which use artificial sweeteners are available.

NURSING MANAGEMENT

Health Promotion and Maintenance

Familial tendencies

The most common form of diabetes mellitus is hereditary diabetes. However, the exact method of inheritance is not known. The nurse can inform the client of the strong familial tendency to diabetes mellitus. Families with a strong tendency to diabetes mellitus should have health examinations annually. They need to inform their care provider of the family history of diabetes mellitus so that appropriate testing and surveillance can be done.

Environmental stressors

The high correlation between obesity and type II diabetes indicates a need for client education in the area of weight control. Although weight control after diagnosis is a method of treatment, the loss of weight before diabetes develops is the aim of a weight-control program. Since 80 to 90 percent of diabetics are overweight at the time of diagnosis, this is a major area for nursing intervention.[20]

Environmental stressors of any kind (family, job, friends) can elevate blood glucose levels. Persistent stress can increase the likelihood of developing type II diabetes mellitus. A detailed nursing history can identify stress areas and the need for client education and stress-reduction techniques. Avoidance of aggravating factors such as smoking and a high fat diet should also be taught.

Acute Intervention

Assessment of learning needs

After the initial diagnosis of diabetes has been made, the lifelong process of client education begins. The nurse's understanding of diabetes mellitus is central to a successful teaching program. An assessment of the client's knowledge of diabetes and life-style considerations is a useful beginning in planning the teaching program. Table 41-16 is an example of a diabetes assessment guide which can provide the nurse with valuable information related to the client's learning needs.

Based on an assessment of the client's knowledge of diabetes and his learning needs, an organized teaching plan can be constructed in relation to the major areas listed in the diabetic teaching checklist (Table 41-17). This teaching may take place in an inpatient or outpatient setting, depending on the client's situation. Hospital and community resources should be utilized where appropriate. The goal of diabetic teaching is to allow the client to lead as normal a life as possible.

Diabetic management

Understanding Diabetes Mellitus It is important that the client be taught the actual disease process related to diabetes mellitus. The chronic nature of diabetes must also be understood and reinforced. The diabetic client needs to know that diabetic control is the aim of therapy and is dependent on diet, weight control, exercise, and, for some, medication.

Dietary Management

Diet prescription

The concept of the American Diabetes Association exchange list diet must be understood by the diabetic and his family. Often, the dietician will teach the initial principles of the exchange diet. The nurse

Table 41-16
Diabetic Assessment Guide

Background data

Name ______ Age ______ Date ______
Address ______ Phone ______
Marital status ______ Children ______
Educational level ______
Regular health care provider ______

Past health history

Chronic diseases ______ R_x ______
Current health problems ______
Habits—Smoking ______ Pack years ______
Alcohol ______ Amount ______
Last appointment—Eye ______ PE ______
Dental ______ Podiatric ______

Family history

Do any family members have diabetes mellitus? ______
If yes, what treatment program do they follow? ______

Client profile

Typical day's diet ______
Person responsible for cooking ______
Time of meals ______ Snack pattern ______
Exercise—Type ______
Amount ______
Regularity ______
Stressors—Family ______
Job ______
Social ______
Weekend variations of meals and activities ______
Hygiene practices—Oral ______
Skin ______
Hair ______
Nails ______
Feet ______

Knowledge of diabetes mellitus

Client's explanation of diabetes ______
Family or friends with diabetes ______
Concerns about diagnosis of diabetes ______
Nurse's conclusion about client's perception and understanding of diagnosis of diabetes ______

Table 41-17
Diabetic Teaching Guide

Patient's name ________________
Address ________________ City ________ State ______ Zip ______
Hospital room or clinic number ________________ Phone number ________
Healthcare provider ________________

	Diabetic Teaching Guide							
	Initial instruction	Assessment of understanding	Demonstration (if applicable)	Redemonstration (if applicable)	Reassessment	Reassessment	Reassessment	Reassessment
Definition of diabetes **Diet prescription** 1. ADA exchange lists								
2. Weight control								
3. Alcohol								
Medications 1. Insulin Injection technique								
Type								
Dosage								
Time								
Site rotation								
Storage								
2. Oral hypoglycemics Type								
Dosage								
Time								
Diabetic reactions 1. Hyperglycemia Cause								
Symptoms								
Treatment								
2. Hypoglycemia Cause								
Symptoms								
Treatment								
Urine testing 1. Reason								
2. Timing								
3. Recommended method								
4. Recording results								
5. Interpreting results								
6. Supplies								

Table 41-17 (Continued)

Diabetic Teaching Guide

	Initial instruction	Assessment of understanding	Demonstration (if applicable)	Redemonstration (if applicable)	Reassessment	Reassessment	Reassessment	Reassessment
Exercise 1. Type								
2. Amount								
3. Modifications								
Skin and foot care 1. Reason for special care								
2. Techniques of care								
Stress 1. Identification of stressors								
2. Stress modification								
3. Management modification								
Complications 1. Hypoglycemia—acute								
Emergency R_x								
2. Ketoacidosis								
Cause								
Symptoms								
Treatment								
General health 1. Emotional Acceptance of diabetes								
Understanding of chronicity								
Family concerns								
2. Physical Sick-day guides								
Reasons to contact health care provider								
Miscellaneous 1. American Diabetes Association								
2. Diabetic Alerts card								
Medic-Alert								

should be available and knowledgeable to answer questions which may arise following these teaching sessions. The diabetic should have the opportunity to select meals and design personal meal plans in the hospital to validate his understanding of food selection. The principles of diet control of diabetes were presented under Dietary Management. Principles to teach and reinforce related to the diabetic diet include the following:

1. *Eat according to your individual meal plan.* No two meal plans are alike. A meal plan is individualized to reflect the dietary needs related to ideal body weight, occupation, age, activities, and type of diabetes.
2. *Never skip meals.* Your body needs food at regular intervals throughout the day. Foods cannot be saved up or accumulated for special events or omitted due to time constraints.
3. *Measure your food using the standard measuring utensils specified in the diet plan.* Estimating amounts is not accurate enough and can result in lack of good control.

Weight control

The attainment or maintenance of ideal body weight is a dietary goal of the diabetic. It is most likely that the adult-onset diabetic will be obese. Thus, a reducing diet and a diabetic diet must be calculated and taught. The emotional impact of diabetes on a client who uses food to relieve stress presents a strong challenge to the nurse. Frequently, nurse-client contracts with reinforcement for compliance are helpful. Behavior modification techniques may be successful for long-term weight control. (See Chap. 60 for specific weight-reduction techniques.) Crash or fad diets are to be avoided.

The nurse needs to include the family of the diabetic when teaching the diet plan. Particular attention and teaching efforts should be directed to the person who will be doing the cooking. It is important, however, that the responsibility for maintaining a diabetic diet not fall on the cook, spouse, or other person if that person is not the diabetic. Reliance on another person to make health decisions fosters dependence by the diabetic and should be avoided except in acute situations.

Urine Testing The nurse needs to teach the diabetic that urine testing monitors sugar in the urine. This test gives a rough estimate of the glucose level in the blood and the degree of diabetic control. Specific items which should be included in the diabetic teaching program related to urine testing include the following:

1. *Urine tests cannot be interchanged randomly.* If the usual brand of urine-testing material is changed, the directions should be followed carefully. Directions and results vary from product to product.
2. *Results of urine testing should be charted in percentages.* Table 41-18 compares the reading of various urine-sugar tests with the appropriate conversion to percentages. The higher the percentage, the greater the degree of glucosuria.
3. *Moisture destroys the reliability of testing equipment.* Urine-testing supplies should be kept capped in a dry place.
4. *Medications can affect urine test results.* If a client

Table 41-18
Comparison of Readings with Various Urine-Sugar (Glucose) Tests

	Glucose Concentration							
Product	$\frac{1}{10}$%	$\frac{1}{4}$%	$\frac{1}{2}$%	$\frac{1}{4}$%	1%	2%	3%	5%
Clinitest, 5-drop		Tr	+	++	+++	++++		
Clinitest, 2-drop*			‡		‡	‡	‡	‡
Diastix	Tr	+	++		+++	++++		
Clinistix†	Light (+)	Light (+)	Medium (++)	Medium (++)	Dark (+++)	Dark (+++)		
Tes-Tape	+	++	+++			++++		

*The 2-drop chart provides a "trace" color block without a percent value; a trace result only indicates less than $\frac{1}{2}$%.
†Estimates are relative to the presence of glucose but cannot show the amount in percentages.
‡Measures the percentage at these levels, but equivalent + signs are not available.
Note: Blank spaces indicate that color blocks are absent for these concentrations.
From *Home Urine Testing for the Diabetic,* Ames Company, Division of Miles Laboratory, 1976, p. 7.

is taking medications for other health problems, he needs to know if these medications will influence the results of urine testing. Although there are many such medications, a general listing is not practical since the interaction varies with the urine-testing technique used. Some general drugs which interfere with accurate results include the cephalosporin antibiotics, ascorbic acid, chloral hydrate, isoniazid, L-dopa, probenecid, salicylates, and streptomycin. Most syrup-based medications will have a high sugar content and should be avoided when possible.

5. *Always test your urine before meals and before bedtime.* The technique used will determine if a single- or double-voided specimen is necessary. If a double-voided specimen is necessary, the client should be instructed to empty the bladder 30 minutes prior to the testing time. A full glass of water should be ingested. At the appropriate time, another urine sample is obtained and tested.
6. *Accurate urine records should be kept to review with the health care provider.* The record should provide spaces to record the urine sugar and acetone present. If the results are positive for glucose, the client should be instructed to document possible influencing factors, such as emotional stress, illness, or overeating, to review with the health care provider. The client needs to know that, following an episode of hypoglycemia, urine test results will fluctuate. Such episodes should also be charted.
7. *Medical advice must be sought in certain situations.* When symptoms of hyperglycemia are present in addition to a 1% or greater urine test, the health care provider should be contacted at once. If a 1% or greater urine test is present without symptoms of hyperglycemia, the health care provider should be contacted as soon as possible to discuss adjustments in the diabetic regimen.

Exercise Regular, consistent exercise is considered an essential part of diabetic management. Exercise contributes to weight loss, increased muscle tone, and improved circulation. If the client has not exercised regularly, encouragement will be necessary to promote compliance. Specific facts related to exercise which the diabetic needs to know include the following:

1. *Exercise does not need to be vigorous to be effective.* The blood glucose-reducing effects of exercise can be attained with mild exercise such as brisk walking. The exercises selected should be enjoyable to foster regularity.
2. *Exercise is best done after meals, when the blood sugar is rising.*
3. *Excessive or unplanned exercise can lead to hypoglycemia.* The blood glucose–reducing effects of exercise can result in hypoglycemia if the exercise is more vigorous than usual. The client can be taught to compensate for extensive planned and spontaneous activity by reducing the insulin dose (if taken) or increasing the food intake.
4. *Exercise plans should be individualized for each client and monitored by the health care provider.*

Personal Hygiene The complications of diabetes require that the diabetic be taught to practice good personal hygiene to avoid serious health problems. Specific health care practices which should be taught to the diabetic include the following:

1. *Regular dental care and daily oral hygiene are necessary.* Diabetics are susceptible to periodontal disease and pyorrhea. Consequently, daily flossing and regular dental appointments should be encouraged. The dentist should be informed that the client is a diabetic.
2. *Adjustments in the diabetic routine may be necessary when illness occurs to prevent ketoacidosis.* The diabetic client who has a minor illness such as a cold or the flu should continue drug therapy and food intake (liquid substitution may be necessary). Urine testing should be done frequently to monitor sugar and acetone. Fluid intake should be increased to prevent dehydration. If the client has ketonuria, is unable to eat, is vomiting, or is ill for more than 24 hours, the health care provider should be contacted.
3. *Diabetics are particularly prone to foot problems.* Because of peripheral neuropathy, atherosclerosis, and susceptibility to infections, the diabetic needs to take special care of his feet. Foot-care rules to be taught to the diabetic are listed in Table 41-19. Many of these rules also apply to skin care in general.
4. *Minor scratches, burns, cuts, or injuries should be carefully treated.* Due to the increased susceptibility to infection, the diabetic client should be taught to care for even minor trauma. After the area is carefully washed, an antiseptic ointment can be applied and the area covered with a dry, sterile pad. The pad should be secured with roller gauze rather than adhesive tape. If the injury has not begun to heal within 24 hours, or if signs of infection develop, the health care provider should be notified immediately.

Medication Not all diabetics require medication to keep their condition well controlled. However, for those who do need it, specific information related to

Table 41-19
Rules for Foot Care

1. Wash feet daily with a mild soap and *warm* water. Test water temperature with hands first.
2. Pat feet dry gently, especially between toes.
3. Examine feet daily for cuts, blisters, swelling, and red, tender areas. Do not depend upon feeling the sores. If eyesight is poor, have others inspect feet.
4. Use lanolin on feet to prevent skin from drying and cracking. Do not apply between toes.
5. Use a mild foot powder on sweaty feet. Powder feet only, not shoes.
6. Do not use commercial remedies to remove callouses or corns.
7. Cleanse cuts with warm water and mild soap, covering with a clean dressing. Do not use iodine, rubbing alcohol, or strong adhesives.
8. Report skin infections or nonhealing sores to health care provider immediately.
9. Cut toenails straight across, even at ends of toes. Do not cut down corners. Soak nails before cutting.
10. Separate overlapping toes with cotton.
11. Break in new shoes very slowly. Avoid open-toe, open-heel, and high-heel shoes. Leather shoes are preferred to plastic ones. Wear slippers with soles. Do not go barefooted. Shake out shoes prior to use.
12. Wear clean, absorbent (cotton or wool) socks or stockings that have not been mended. Colored socks must be colorfast.
13. Do not wear clothing that leaves impressions, hindering circulation.
14. Do not use hot water bottles or heating pads to warm feet. Wear socks for warmth.
15. Guard against frostbite.
16. Exercise feet daily either by walking or by flexing and extending feet in a suspended position. Avoid prolonged sitting, standing, and crossing of legs.

the type of medication, amount, and method of administration is necessary.

1. *Oral agents are not insulin.* If the diabetic client takes an oral hypoglycemic agent, he needs to know that it is not insulin. Oral hypoglycemic agents are effective only if the beta cells of the pancreas can be stimulated to produce insulin. The client needs to take the medication at the specified time, and must follow the meal plan and exercise program as outlined.
2. *Insulin can be taken only by injection.* This fact requires a concerted teaching effort by the nurse to ensure that the client is capable of safely administering the correct dose of insulin. Table 41-12 outlines a technique for insulin injection.
3. *Insulin requires special handling.* Insulin that is being used should be at room temperature unless the room temperature is above 23.9°C (75°F) (it should then be refrigerated). Extra insulin should be refrigerated until it is needed. The American Diabetes Association can provide information for special situations such as foreign travel.
4. *Special equipment must be available to inject insulin.* The appropriate syringe to match the unit dose of insulin ordered is necessary. Disposable needles and syringes are convenient and safe. Special instruction is necessary if reusable needles and syringes are to be used. Either cotton balls and rubbing alcohol or prepackaged alcohol pledgets are necessary to clean the injection site. The injection site rotation schedule should be at hand to ensure the use of a different site every day for the insulin injection.

Diabetic Alerts The client should be instructed to carry identification at all times indicating that he is a diabetic. An identification card (Fig. 41-11) can supply valuable information, including the name of the health care provider, dose of insulin, etc. A Medic-Alert bracelet or necklace should be worn by all diabetics. Police, paramedics, and many private citizens are aware of the need to look for this identification when working with sick or unconscious people.

Stressors The newly diagnosed diabetic needs to understand that stressors, both emotional and physical, can increase the blood sugar level and result in hyperglycemia. Adjustments for illness and trauma have already been mentioned. Concepts related to emotional stresses include the following:

1. *Stress-inducing stiuations should be avoided when possible.* A well-kept urine-testing record can help to identify stressful areas for the diabetic—work,

home, family, or certain relationships. If the situation cannot be avoided, then effective coping methods must be tried.

2. *Unavoidable stressful situations require insulin adjustments.* Certain unavoidable life situations, such as deaths in the family, job interviews, and final examinations, may require extra insulin to avoid a hyperglycemic reaction. The diabetic should feel comfortable about contacting his health care provider to discuss necessary adjustments. Eventually, the well-informed diabetic will be able to make most adjustments independently based on past successful experiences.

Complications Another major nursing responsibility in teaching a diabetic is to ensure that the client can recognize signs indicative of problems with control.

Ketoacidosis

The incidence of ketoacidosis is correlated with the client's knowledge of diabetes. The more the client knows about diabetes and diabetic control, the less often ketoacidosis will occur. Ketoacidosis can result from overeating, infection, emotional upsets, or failure to take prescribed medications. Specific signs indicative of ketoacidosis or high blood sugar which the client must know include:

Increased urination
Increasing thirst and dryness of the mouth and skin
Weakness, dizziness, and possible loss of consciousness
Loss of appetite and weight loss
Nausea, vomiting, and abdominal pain
1% or greater glycosuria, or acetone in the urine or on the breath.

Should any of the above signs be present, the client or a reliable other person should call the health care provider. If the client is able, he can drink a cup of broth or tea. If available, a urine specimen should be saved for examination. If the client loses consciousness, he should be transported to the nearest health care facility immediately.

Hypoglycemia

Hypoglycemia results from having too little sugar in the blood. The client needs to know what situations can precipitate hypoglycemia, the signs of this condition, and what to do should it occur.

Certain situations can precipitate hypoglycemia. These include too much insulin or too many pills, too little food, strenuous, unplanned exercise, vomiting or diarrhea, and emotional upsets.

Name Phone
Address
Physician Phone
Address

INSULIN	DOSAGE	TIME	ORAL MEDICATION	DOSAGE	TIME
Regular			Orinase		
PZI			Diabinese		
Globin			Dymelor		
NPH			Tolinase		
Lente			DBI		
Semilente			DBI TD		
Ultralente					

Date

I am a DIABETIC

If unconscious or behaving abnormally, I may be having a reaction associated with diabetes or its treatment.

If I can swallow give me sugar, candy or a sweet drink. If I do not recover promptly, call a physician or send me to the hospital.

If I am unconscious or cannot swallow, do not attempt to give me anything by mouth, but call a physician or send me to the hospital immediately.

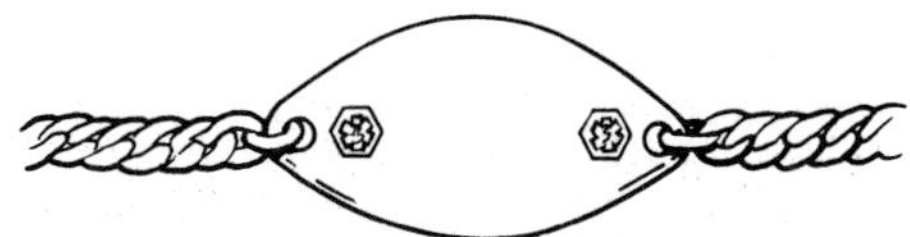

Figure 41-11 Diabetic alerts: Diabetics should carry a card and wear a bracelet or necklace which states that they are diabetics. If the diabetic is unconscious, such measures will ensure prompt and appropriate attention. *(Courtesy of Becton Dickinson Company, Rochelle Park, N.J., and Medic-Alert Foundation International, Turlock, Calif.)*

Diabetics need to recognize the signs of hypoglycemia, which include:

Shaky, nervous, weak feeling
Sweating
Hunger

As the blood glucose level continues to fall, additional signs include:

Irritability, confusion, and sleepiness
Trembling and unsteadiness
Blurred vision and difficulty in speaking
Loss of consciousness

Should these signs be present, the immediate action is to take something high in sugar. The diabetic who takes diabetic medication should always carry some readily available form of sugar, such as Lifesavers or lumps of sugar, which could be taken at this time. One-half glass or more of fruit juice or a sweetened carbonated beverage could be taken. If the client does not feel better within 15 minutes, additional sources of glucose may be used. If the symptoms persist, the health care provider needs to be consulted immediately.

A nursing care plan for the newly diagnosed diabetic is presented in Table 41-20. The role of the nurse in setting the stage for successful adjustment to the diagnosis of diabetes cannot be overemphasized. Demonstrations, redemonstrations, pamphlets, visual aids, tapes, video cassettes, and individual and group teaching sessions are but a few of the strategies the nurse can use to teach the large amount of information required by the diabetic. The new diabetic needs to be encouraged to assume more and more responsibility for self-care. However, even the best-informed clients can lose control and need acute nursing intervention for either ketoacidosis or hypoglycemia.

Table 41-20
Nursing Care Plan for the Newly Diagnosed Diabetic

Client Problem	Expected Outcome	Nursing Intervention
	Acute Management	
Inadequate knowledge of diabetes	State components of diabetic care, including rationale.	Assess client's knowledge of diabetes (Table 41-15). Instruct client and family on self-care related to diabetes (Table 41-16).
Hyperglycemia	Controlled blood glucose.	Administer insulin or oral hypoglycemic agent if ordered. Supervise prescribed diet and exercise regimen. Assess client's return demonstration of insulin injection.
Glycosuria and ketonuria	Mild or no glycosuria or ketonuria.	Test urine and record findings, reporting significant results. Use same methods consistently. Test at designated times. Collect double-voided urine specimens if indicated.
Dehydration	Adequate urine output and good skin turgor.	Monitor intake and output. Encourage fluid intake to 3000 mL daily unless contraindicated. Give good skin hygiene on every shift. Give mouth care after meals and prn. Monitor BP and P qid.
Hypokalemia	Serum potassium within normal range.	Monitor urine output for adequacy of volume. Observe for signs of hypokalemia (Chap. 12).
Grief reaction to diagnosis	Acceptance of and adjustment to diagnosis of diabetes.	Allow client to verbalize feelings in order to work through stages of denial, anger, bargaining, depression, and acceptance.
	Long-Term Management	
Ketoacidosis	Controlled blood sugar and no ketonuria.	Replace fluid and electrolytes. Administer insulin as ordered. Monitor intake and output. Do hourly blood sugar determinations. Perform general nursing care of the unconscious client. Reassess client's learning needs related to diabetes.
Hypoglycemia	Blood glucose <60 mg/dL.	Give glucose replacement (IV dextrose or orally depending on client's level of consciousness). Assess client's neurological status, precipitating factors, and diabetic learning needs.
Infection	No evidence of infection.	Instruct client on hygiene related to foot, dental, and skin care. Teach indications for seeking health care.

Acute care in ketoacidosis

The nurse's role in the acute management of the diabetic in ketoacidosis closely parallels the medical management. The client's condition will be closely monitored by appropriate blood and urine tests. The nurse is responsible for sampling urine for sugar and acetone, as well as using other laboratory test results to direct care.

Areas which need monitoring when ketoacidosis is present are (1) administration of IV fluids to correct dehydration, (2) administration of insulin therapy to reduce blood glucose and serum acetone, (3) administration of electrolytes to correct electrolyte loss, (4) assessment of renal status, particularly the timing of potassium replacement, (5) assessment of the cardiopulmonary status to reflect potassium influences, and (6) monitoring of the level of consciousness.

The IV line must be carefully monitored to regulate both fluid intake and insulin administration. The rate of insulin administration is often readjusted in response to changing levels of blood glucose. The nurse is responsible for marking IV bottles to clearly indicate the dosage of both insulin and potassium which has been added.

The nurse must also monitor the signs of potassium imbalance resulting from osmotic diuresis and a shift of potassium back into the cell when treatment for hyperglycemia is begun. Potassium moves into the cell with glucose in the presence of insulin. Decreased irritability, flabby muscles, distension, loss of deep tendon reflexes, and respiratory depression should alert the nurse to the possibility of hypokalemia. Cardiac monitoring is a useful aid in detecting potassium imbalance. Characteristic changes indicating potassium excess or deficit are observable on electrocardiographic readings.

Vital signs must be assessed frequently to determine the presence of infection, signs of hypovolemic shock, tachycardia, and the rate and depth of respirations. (The nursing management for the client who is unconscious is appropriate and is found in Chap. 52.) Strict sterile technique should be used in all situations which have the potential for initiating infection such as catheterization, injections, and drawing of blood specimens. As insulin replacement becomes effective, the client must be carefully monitored for signs of hypoglycemia.

Acute care in hypoglycemia

Diabetics should be taught self-management of hypoglycemic reactions. However, certain situations, such as sudden severe illness or unavailability of a rapid-acting sugar source, could precipitate a hypoglycemic reaction of such severity that the client loses consciousness. Usually, the client will be brought to the hospital. The Medic-Alert bracelet and diabetic identification card should aid in preventing the unconscious hypoglycemic client from being mistaken for someone who is intoxicated. A blood sample should be obtained to determine the extent of the hypoglycemia and to differentiate the reaction from hyperglycemia, which can also cause unconsciousness.

The treatment of hypoglycemia is the administration of glucose by the most appropriate route. If the client is conscious, concentrated glucose solutions can be given. If the client is unconscious, the IV route must be used. A 50% glucose solution is slowly administered until the client regains consciousness. Glucagon, a hormone that raises the blood glucose level, and epinephrine, which raises the blood sugar level, may also be administered.

With effective treatment, hypoglycemia can be quickly reversed. However, the danger of hypoglycemic reactions must be stressed. The brain can sustain permanent damage due to the lack of necessary glucose. Memory impairment and decreased learning ability can result from hypoglycemia. If treatment is not instituted, death can result.

Once the acute hypoglycemia has been reversed, the nurse needs to explore with the client why the situation developed. Such an assessment may indicate the need for additional education so that the diabetic can avoid future episodes of hypoglycemia.

Both ketoacidosis and hypoglycemia are life-threatening situations and are frightening to the client and his family. The nurse must attempt to keep the family informed of the client's progress during a severe reaction to relieve their anxiety. The nurse's calm, assertive manner in caring for the diabetic provides much assurance to the acutely ill client and his family.

Stress situations

Physical and emotional stress should be avoided by the diabetic whenever possible. Blood glucose and free fatty acid levels increase as part of the sympathetic nervous system's response to stress (see Chap. 39). Such stress-related increases make diabetic management difficult.

Surgery Surgery is a stress situation which requires special management for a diabetic. If the surgery involves a fasting state, the insulin-dependent diabetic will usually be managed by an IV infusion of regular insulin and glucose both preoperatively and intraoperatively. The rate of infusion will depend on blood glucose levels and urine determinations. Postoperatively, the client may be maintained on a sliding scale and regular insulin until the presurgical diabetic regimen can be resumed. The nurse must be particularly alert for signs of hypoglycemia and hyperglycemia until a stable routine is reestablished.

The non-insulin-dependent diabetic may require regular insulin for a short time postoperatively due to the hyperglycemic effects of stress and hormonal changes. This possibility should be explained to the client preoperatively so that the use of insulin is not interpreted as a worsening of his condition.

The nurse should take the opportunity to review previous diabetic instruction with the client during the required hospitalization for surgery. Gaps in knowledge and management errors can be detected and instruction undertaken at this time.

Chronic Management

A critical fact for the diabetic to understand is that diabetes is a chronic disease that can only be controlled, not cured. The initial teaching plan after the diagnosis of diabetes should be aimed at helping the client to understand this fact. The goal of the management program is to allow the client to lead as normal a life as possible while maintaining good control. Over time, however, the complications of diabetes are inevitable. Good control can prevent the occurrence of the more acute complications, such as hypoglycemia and ketoacidosis, and possibly prevent or delay the onset of other complications.

Need for reassessment

The nurse should take advantage of every contact with the client to reassess his understanding of and compliance with the particular diabetic program. The nurse must be alert for changes in the client's life such as pregnancy, infection, additional stress, and major life changes which might necessitate a readjustment in his basic program. Ideally, the client will recognize such situations and seek counsel from the health care provider.

Emotional component

The effect of the diagnosis of diabetes cannot be underestimated by the nurse. Initially, the impact of the diagnosis may not be felt by the client. However, once the basic diabetic education is initiated and the client begins to realize the extent of the problem, the nurse should expect an emotional reaction. (Chap. 1 discusses chronic illness.) The nurse should foster a positive attitude to the discipline imposed on the client by a diabetic regimen. Obviously, the insulin-dependent diabetic will need to make a greater emotional adjustment.

The families of diabetics may also need assistance in adjusting to the chronic nature of diabetes. The nurse can facilitate communication between the family and the client to prevent serious problems from developing.

Self-management

Ideally, the diabetic should be taught and encouraged to manage the disease himself, with only guidance from the health care provider. The more in control the diabetic client can feel, the more likely he is to accept his problem and comply with his management program. The basis of self-management is a sound teaching program related to diabetes. A knowledgeable diabetic should be able to make minor adjustments in his insulin dosage and diet prescription to compensate for special circumstances such as illness or increased exercise.

Not all diabetics are capable of such self-management. If the client is not able to manage the disease, a family member may be able to assume this role. If the client or his family are unable to make decisions related to diabetic management, the nurse must convey a helpful attitude. The client and his family must not be made to feel that they are a bother if they call to ask questions or express concerns about the treatment program.

Outpatient clinics

Diabetics are often managed in outpatient diabetic clinics. Frequently, these clinics are staffed by diabetic nurse specialists. These specialists have preparation beyond the baccalaureate degree in diabetes and work collaboratively with physicians to manage diabetic clients. The diabetic nurse specialist is also available to the nursing staff in the acute-care setting for advice and counsel. The diabetic outpatient clinic can provide specialized instructions, group interaction, and contact with other diabetics. Often, such clinics are run with the team concept. Consequently, an endocrinologist, a diabetic nurse specialist, a dietician, a counselor, and a podiatrist may be available to the client at one visit.

REACTIVE HYPOGLYCEMIA

Many people claim to suffer from reactive hypoglycemia. The symptoms are similar to those of the hypoglycemia of diabetes—sweating, shakiness, trembling, anxiety, tachycardia, hunger, weakness, dizziness, headache, clouding of vision, confusion, abnormal behavior, and loss of consciousness. These symptoms mimic the effects of anxiety and stress, and are often misinterpreted.[21]

Idiopathic hypoglycemia (of no known cause) is particularly difficult to document with postprandial 5-hour oral glucose tolerance examinations. A certain diagnosis can be made only if a plasma glucose concentration of less than 50 dL/100 mL can be demonstrated during a spontaneous attack. The usual treatment is a diet high in protein and low in carbohydrate, with frequent small meals.

If a client claims to have reactive hypoglycemia, the nurse should determine if it was medically or self-diagnosed. Because of the frequent confusion with anxiety reaction, the nurse needs to carefully assess both the symptoms and the treatment. If the symptoms seem to be stress related, the nurse should concentrate on teaching stress-reducing techniques.

Case Study / Diabetic Ketoacidosis

John, a 40-year-old bachelor, was admitted to the emergency room after being found comatose in his apartment by his landlord. He had been diagnosed as diabetic within the last year and was taking 30 units of NPH insulin daily. His landlord stated that John had had stomach flu for the past week and had stopped taking his insulin a few days ago when he was unable to eat.

Upon physical examination, the client was found to be in ketoacidosis. His breathing was deep and rapid, and his breath smelled of acetone. His face was flushed and his skin dry. His serum acetone was 3+ with Acetest tablets and a Dextrostix revealed a glucose level of 1000 mg/100 dL.

Discussion Questions

1. Briefly explain the pathophysiology of ketoacidosis.
2. What are some clinical manifestations of ketoacidosis?
3. What were the precipitating factors in this case? What effect does physical stress have on a diabetic?
4. What distinguished this case history from one of HHNK and hypoglycemia?
5. What educational needs of this client must be met prior to discharge?

REVIEW QUESTIONS

The number of the question corresponds to the same numbered objective at the beginning of the chapter.

1. Which of the following describe diabetes mellitus?
   a. curable
   b. systemic
   c. communicable
   d. idiopathic

2. Insulin-dependent diabetes is the result of
   a. beta cell destruction
   b. high consumption of sugar
   c. insulin resistance at the cell membrane
   d. too much insulin

3. A clinical manifestation indicative of ketoacidosis is
   a. cold sweats
   b. Kussmaul breathing
   c. hyperreflexia
   d. edema

4. The only type of insulin suitable for IV administration is
   a. NPH
   b. regular
   c. Lente
   d. PZI

5. For the diagnosed diabetic, a diabetic diet must be followed
   a. until the blood sugar returns to normal
   b. only for type I diabetics
   c. only during periods of additional stress
   d. as long as the client lives

6. The first topic the diabetic client should be taught is
   a. insulin administration
   b. diet control
   c. disease process
   d. weight loss measures

7. The insulin-dependent diabetic undergoing surgery usually
   a. has the insulin as usual
   b. has the morning dose of insulin omitted
   c. is started on regular IV insulin
   d. receives half the usual dose of insulin

8. The psychological impact of diabetes may require
   a. counseling
   b. adjustments in insulin
   c. use of support systems
   d. all the above

9. The appropriate teaching for the diabetic client related to skin care is
   a. use of heat to increase the blood supply
   b. avoidance of softening lotions and creams
   c. daily inspection of all skin surfaces
   d. use of iodine on cuts and abrasions

REFERENCES

1. Karl E. Sussman and Robert Metz (eds.), *Diabetes Mellitus,* 4th ed., American Diabetes Association, Inc., New York, 1975, p. 1.
2. Stephen Podolsky (ed.), *Clinical Diabetes: Modern Management,* Appleton Century Crofts, New York, 1980, p. XVII.
3. M. I. Drury, *Diabetes Mellitus,* Blackwell Scientific Publications, Ltd., Oxford, 1979, p. 2.
4. Saul Genuth, "Diabetic Ketoacidosis," in Podolsky, op. cit., p. 177.
5. Dorothy R. Blevins, *The Diabetic and Nursing Care,* McGraw-Hill Book Company, New York, 1979, p. 79.
6. Gerald M. Reaven, "Speculations Concerning the Etioloty of Diabetes," in Podolsky, op. cit., p. 33.
7. Gerald M. Reaven, in Podolsky, op. cit., pp. 23–45.
8. *Diabetes Mellitus,* 8th ed., Lilly Research Laboratories, Indianapolis, Ind., 1979, pp. 12–17.
9. Kurt Isselbacher et al. (eds.), *Harrison's Principles of Internal Medicine,* McGraw-Hill Book Company, New York, 1980, p. 566.
10. Stephen Podolsky, "Hyperosmolar Nonketotic Coma: Underdiagnosed and Undertreated," in Podolsky, op. cit., p. 209.
11. Blevins, op. cit., p. 112.
12. *Diabetes Mellitus,* p. 197.
13. C. T. Dollery et al., "Reversal of Retinal Vascular Lesions in Diabetes," *Diabetes,* **14**:121 (1965).
14. *Diabetes Mellitus,* p. 164.
15. Saul Genuth, "Diabetic Ketoacidosis," in Podolsky, op. cit., p. 189.
16. Alice Chenault Maurer, "The Therapy of Diabetes," *Am Scientist,* **67**:426–427 (1979).
17. Ibid., pp. 428–430.
18. Editorial, "Control of Diabetes and Insulin Antibodies," *Br Med J,* **1**:484 (1976).
19. University Group Diabetes Program, "A Study of the Effects of Hypoglycemic Agents on Vascular Complications in Patients with Adult-Onset Diabetes. II. Mortality Results," *Diabetes,* **19**(suppl):789–830 (1970).
20. Blevins, op. cit., p. 274.
21. Isselbacher et al., op. cit., p. 1759.

Chapter 42

NURSING ROLE IN MANAGEMENT
Endocrine Problems

Roberta T. Spencer
JoAnn Ganje Congdon

Learning Objectives

1. Describe the pathophysiology, clinical manifestations, and medical and nursing management of clients with imbalances of hormones produced by the anterior pituitary.
2. Describe the pathophysiology, clinical manifestations, and medical and nursing management related to imbalances of hormones secreted by the posterior pituitary.
3. Describe the pathophysiology, clinical manifestations, and medical and nursing management of clients with enlargement of the thyroid or imbalances of hormones produced by this gland.
4. Describe the pathophysiology, clinical manifestations, and medical and nursing management related to imbalances of the hormone produced by the parathyroids.
5. Describe the pathophysiology, clinical manifestations, and medical and nursing management related to imbalances of glucocorticoids, mineralocorticoids, and androgens produced by the adrenal cortex.
6. Describe the pathophysiology, clinical manifestations, and medical and nursing management related to imbalances of hormones produced by the adrenal medulla.
7. Describe the nursing role in client education related to drug therapy for hormone replacement in endocrine deficiencies.
8. Explain the systemic effects of short- and long-term use of corticosteroid therapy.
9. Explain the nursing role related to monitoring and education for the client receiving steroid therapy.

This chapter focuses on problems related to the hormones produced by the anterior and posterior pituitary, the thyroid gland, the parathyroid glands, and the adrenal glands. Diabetes mellitus is discussed in Chap. 41. Female and male reproductive problems are covered in Chaps. 46 and 47. The concept of stress is discussed in Chaps. 1 and 39.

HEALTH MAINTENANCE AND PROMOTION

The goal of health maintenance activities is to maintain or restore the highest level of health for the individual. For the client with a potential endocrine problem, effort should be directed toward (1) prevention of imbalance, (2) early detection of dysfunction before overt symptoms are produced, and (3) reduction of future risks or complications. The primary nursing interventions related to the accomplishment of these goals are in the areas of health assessment and health education. Specific nursing interventions include the following:

1. Evaluate emotional, physical, and environmental stressors.
2. Evaluate the individual's coping capacities in relation to these present and/or future stressors.
3. Support positive adaptive responses.
4. Teach new methods of response to stressors if needed or if possible.
5. Help the individual modify or eliminate stressors when possible.
6. Reduce potential future stressors.
7. Provide anticipatory guidance in terms of predicting or foreseeing stressful situations, e.g., hospitalization, surgery.
8. Evaluate diet and teach appropriate modification if necessary.
9. Evaluate clients' understanding of medications prescribed to treat an endocrine disorder. (Table 42-1 lists specific information the client must know about medication for an endocrine problem.)

Table 42-1
Information the Client Must Know About Medication for an Endocrine Problem

Does the client know:

1. Correct dosage and time?
2. Correct route and technique of administration?
3. Side effects?
4. Extraneous influences that may interfere with response to medication, e.g., stress?
5. Signs and symptoms that indicate a need to increase, decrease, and/or discontinue the prescribed medication?
6. Signs and symptoms that indicate a need to contact the primary care provider?
7. That lifetime replacement is vital?
8. The plan for regular follow-up care?
9. The necessity of wearing an identification or medical alert device at all times?

*This chapter was reviewed by Phoebe J. Becktell, R.N., B.S.N., M.A., Assistant Professor, College of Nursing, University of New Mexico, Albuquerque, New Mexico.

Persons with early signs of dysfunction should be encouraged to seek medical attention promptly since most endocrine problems become more serious with time and treatment is more effective if begun early. Because hormone imbalances tend to be insidious in onset and often mimic other physiologic and psychological problems, diagnosis is often delayed. The nurse with a sound knowledge base related to endocrine problems and good assessment skills can often detect early endocrine problems. (See Chap. 40, Assessment of the Endocrine System.)

Promotion of endocrine health requires that adequate nutrients be provided for hormone production. The importance of adequate nutrition is most graphically illustrated by the thyroid enlargement and marginal hypothyroidism that develop in individuals with iodine deficiencies. However, iodine is only one of a number of elements required for normal hormone production. Protein hormones and thyroid hormone incorporate amino acids in their molecules. Ascorbic acid is utilized by the adrenal cortex in direct proportion to the production of corticosteroids. To maintain adequate endocrine function, the diet must contain adequate protein of high quality, minerals, and vitamins.

Although steroid hormones utilize cholesterol substrate for their synthesis, the need for a dietary source of cholesterol is uncertain. Cholesterol is produced by the body itself in such organs as the liver. Dietary intake has been associated with degenerative vascular disease (Chap. 27). However, a recent study failed to substantiate the supposed benefits of low cholesterol diets and produced some evidence of harmful effects.[1] A minimal intake of dietary cholesterol may be necessary to support steroid production, especially in individuals whose diets are inadequate in calorie intake. This could include those prone to cachexia due to malabsorption, anorexia nervosa, or debilitating diseases such as cancer.

Disruptions in rhythmic patterns produce an asynchrony between body requirements and hormone production. The distress experienced by both the jet traveler and the shift worker is characteristic of this asynchrony. Changes in routine of living should be minimized in number and degree as much as possible. If sudden marked alterations are unavoidable, the individual should attempt to minimize other stressors as much as possible to keep down the total level of stress.

Stress markedly alters the rate and patterns of hormone production and may disrupt the natural rhythms. It is important that strategies be developed to keep stress within manageable limits. Stress is also an important stimulus to the endocrine system. Many acute endocrine conditions first appear following a major stressor such as the death of a close family member. Unusual stress is also a factor in exacerbations of chronic conditions. (See Chap. 39 for techniques for stress management.)

Most endocrine problems are chronic in nature with symptoms and general reactions that may subside with proper treatment and care. However, without strict adherence to treatment and follow-up care, the problems can become active again. Some individuals will need only periodic medical evaluation and continuing treatment with medication. Others will have episodes of acute illness and require hospitalization. Careful assessment and management can affect the course and outcome of endocrine problems.

PITUITARY GLAND

Disorders of the Anterior Pituitary

Growth hormone excess

An overproduction of growth hormone, usually due to a benign pituitary adenoma, causes rapid overgrowth of the bones. This is associated with either *gigantism* or *acromegaly*. If the onset occurs before the closure of the epiphyses when the long bones are still capable of further longitudinal growth, *gigantism* will result. This is usually associated with early childhood but may not begin until puberty. These giants have disproportionately long limbs and may grow to 8 feet in height and weigh over 300 pounds. These cases are rare, the victims are not healthy, and they usually die in early adult life.

Acromegaly is a more common abnormality due to excessive growth hormone. If the adenoma develops after the epiphyses have closed, longitudinal growth cannot occur. Instead the bones increase in thickness and width. Clinical features include enlargement of the hands, feet, and paranasal and frontal sinuses as well as deformities of the mandible and spine and an overbite (Fig. 42-1). In addition, enlargement of soft tissues (tongue, skin, abdominal organs, etc.) causes symptoms such as difficulty in speaking, coarsening of the features, and abdominal distension. Excessive weight causes increased stress on joints and painful arthritis. Visual disturbances and headaches develop because of increased pressure on surrounding structures by the enlarged pituitary. Because growth hormone mobilizes stored fat for energy, it increases free fatty acid levels in the blood and predisposes to atherosclerosis. The hor-

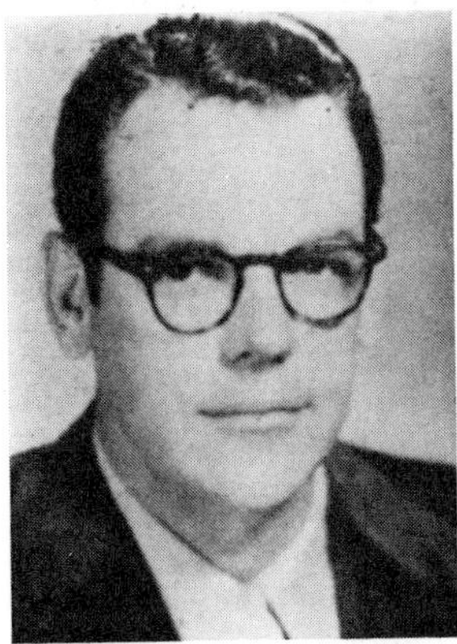
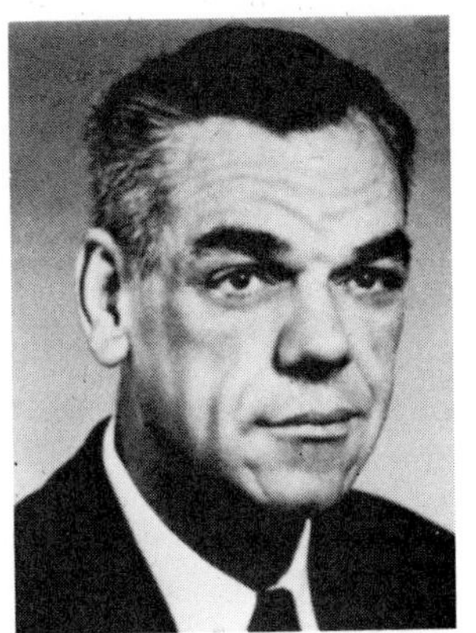
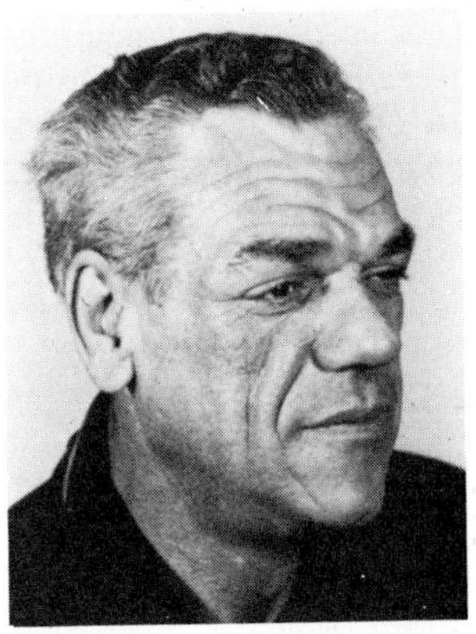

Figure 42-1 Progressive development of acromegalic features. *[From Kurt Isselbacher et al. (eds.), Harrison's Principles of Internal Medicine, 9th ed., McGraw-Hill Book Company, New York, 1980.]*

mone also antagonizes the action of insulin and is diabetogenic.

Medical Management

Diagnostic

Diagnosis requires a thorough history, physical examination, and evaluation of plasma level of growth hormone. Skull x-rays may show a large, distorted sella turcica. Other causes are ruled out by tomograms, pneumoencephalogram, CT scan, and angiography. Peripheral vision and visual fields are checked to determine if there is compression of the optic chiasma.

Therapeutic

Treatment of gigantism and acromegaly is aimed at halting further progression of the disease. Removal or destruction of the pituitary *(hypophysectomy)* by irradiation, surgery, radio-frequency, or freezing is possible. Surgery can be accomplished by a craniotomy or by a transphenoidal approach. In the transphenoidal approach, an incision is made in the inner aspect of the upper lip and gingiva. The sella turcica is entered through the floor of the nose and sphenoid sinuses. Hypophysectomy may also be used as a palliative measure in clients with diabetic retinopathy (stopping secretion of hormones which raise blood sugar) and metastatic cancer of the breast and prostate in whom hormone manipulation has been shown to be effective.

Destruction or removal of the pituitary will result in permanent deficiencies of hormones of the anterior pituitary. Rather than replacing the tropic hormones of this structure, which require parenteral administration, the essential hormones produced by target organs (glucocorticoids, thyroid hormone, and sex hormones) are prescribed. These medications can be administered by mouth. Hormone replacement must be continued throughout life.

Prognosis depends upon the age at onset and the age at which treatment was initiated. Usually bone growth can be arrested and soft tissue hypertrophy reversed. The diabetic and cardiac complications may continue in spite of treatment.

Nursing Management Nurses should be alert for signs and symptoms of abnormal tissue growth in clients of all ages. Assessment of children should include a complete evaluation of growth and development. Markedly accelerated growth, especially if inconsistent with familial patterns, is cause for referral for medical evaluation. Adults should be questioned specifically about increases in hat or glove size. Examination of serial photographs from previous decades may reveal the gradual coarsening of features characteristic of acromegaly.

When first seen, clients usually have experienced undesirable changes in appearance and may have marked alterations in self-image. They also commonly exhibit symptoms of diabetes mellitus. Cardiovascular disease may or may not be present. Clients need unconditional acceptance by health care personnel and considerable emotional support during the period of diagnosis and treatment. They should be carefully monitored for hyperglycemia and cardiovascular symptoms such as angina pectoris, hypertension, and congestive heart failure. Nursing care should be appropriate to the severity of these symptoms.

Individuals treated by hypophysectomy need skilled neurosurgical nursing. Regardless of the surgical approach used, the client must be prepared preoperatively for postoperative care. Discussion of ambulation, pain control, activity, and hormone replacement should be planned. If a craniotomy is performed, nursing care appropriate for the client undergoing a craniotomy is indicated (Chap. 54).

When a hypophysectomy is accomplished by a transphenoidal approach, specific nursing measures are indicated. The client's bed is kept elevated at a 30° angle at all times. This avoids pressure on the sella turcica and decreases the headache which is a frequent postoperative problem. Mild analgesia should be given to control the headache and vigorous coughing, sneezing, and straining at stool is discouraged to prevent cerebral spinal fluid leak in the area where the sella turcica was entered.

Any clear nasal drainage should be tested for glucose. The presence of glucose indicates that the drainage is cerebrospinal fluid. Complaint of persistent and severe generalized or supraorbital headache may indicate cerebrospinal fluid leakage into the sinuses.[2] A cerebrospinal fluid leak usually resolves within 72 hours when treated with head elevation and bed rest. If the leak persists, daily spinal taps may be done to reduce pressure and allow the fossa to heal. Intravenous antibiotics are usually used when there is a cerebrospinal fluid leak to prevent meningitis. The client must avoid bending for any reason for 2 months following a transphenoidal hypophysectomy to avoid disrupting the surgical site. It is important that the client's family be aware of the need for the client to avoid straining and bending so they can assist him whenever necessary. Constipation should be avoided by the use of stool softeners and laxatives.

Following hypophysectomy, hormone replacement is necessary. Immediately postoperatively, the client may exhibit signs of diabetes insipidus due to the loss of ADH which is stored in the posterior lobe of the pituitary. Pitressin IM is given prn based on an output which exceeds 800 to 900 mL/2 hours or if the specific gravity is below 1.004. If the entire pituitary gland was removed, the need to replace pitressin will be permanent.

Since the source of ACTH has been removed, cortisone replacement is also necessary. Careful client education is necessary when cortisone must be taken regularly (see section on glucocorticoid therapy later in this chapter). The tropic hormones of the pituitary are no longer available, so their target glands will develop insufficiency. Lifelong replacement therapy is necessary.

Hypopituitarism is accompanied by infertility. Not only are sex hormones deficient, but the production of gametes (ova and sperm) ceases due to lack of the necessary tropic hormones. If an individual desires to have children, replacement of these hormones by the administration of chorionic gonadotropins may restore fertility. Such treatment involves repeated injections and is not always successful. Women undergoing tropic hormone replacement are at increased risk for multiple and premature births.

Since the decision to destroy the pituitary involves acceptance of altered fertility and permanent hormone deficiencies, clients need assistance in working through the grieving process associated with these losses. It is important that the client be aware of the consequences if surgery is not done, so that an informed decision can be made. The need for continued drug therapy also reduces a client's perception of independence and requires considerable emotional adjustment. The nurse must consider the emotional impact of a hypophysectomy when counseling the client and planning the educational program related to hormone replacement.

Excesses of other tropic hormones

Overproduction of other single anterior pituitary hormones may produce syndromes of single hormone excess. If adrenocorticotropin is involved, Cushing's disease (corticosteroid toxicity) results. If thyrotropin (TSH) levels are excessive, Grave's disease (thyrotoxicity) develops. These conditions are discussed in detail later in this chapter.

In adults hypersecretion of pituitary gonadotropins is characteristic of primary gonadal failure. Lack of sex hormones inactivates the negative feedback control of the pituitary. In this instance the pituitary hypersecretion is not indicative of intracranial pathology. Replacement therapy with sex hormones restores control of pituitary activity but poses risks of side effects from the drugs used (see Chaps. 45 and 46). Excess gonadotropins are believed to be responsible for the vasomotor disturbances and (possibly) emotional fluctuations observed in some menopausal women and middle-aged men.

In other situations, symptoms of excess gonadotropins signify pituitary pathology and are indications for prompt referral for definitive diagnosis. This is true of inappropriate lactation in either sex and precocious puberty in children.

Hypofunction

Hypopituitarism is a relatively rare disorder. As generally seen, it is a decrease in one or more of the anterior pituitary lobe hormones. Primary hypofunction is due to disease, tumor, or destruction of the adenohypophysis. Failure to secrete growth hormone usually occurs first, followed by deficiency in the gonadotropin, then TSH, and finally ACTH.[3] In men and children, the most common cause of hypofunction is a tumor. In women, hypofunction can follow a postpartum hemorrhage. This is called postpartum pituitary necrosis or Sheehan's syndrome.

Sheehan's syndrome develops insidiously over a span of 10 to 15 years. The hypoxic insult resulting from infarction during shock suffered by the pituitary at the time of parturition produces a slow degeneration and necrosis of the gland. The woman usually fails to lactate after childbirth and does not become pregnant again due to failure of prolactin and gonadotropin production. Later, hypothyroidism develops and finally glucocorticoid deficiency. Because of the lethargy and apathy characteristic of the latter two hormone deficiencies, affected women rarely seek medical treatment. They are at high risk for alienation from husbands and other significant others, who may misinterpret the lack of energy and motivation as signs of laziness or mental illness. Inability to fulfill the requirements for gainful employment promotes downward social mobility. Many victims are diagnosed only after an acute Addisonian crisis. Some are never diagnosed or treated because they succumb to this life-threatening condition.

Clinical Manifestations Clinical findings vary with the degree of pituitary dysfunction and are related to the lack of hormones from the target glands. The most common symptoms include weakness, low tolerance to stress, decreased resistance to infection, hypoglycemia, sexual dysfunction, and dry, sallow skin. Orthostatic hypotension may also be present. If the pituitary exerts pressure on the optic chiasm, visual problems also develop.

Hyposecretion of somatotropin during growth results in dwarfism. Growth may be normal in the first year or two and then progressively slows. Intelligence is usually normal. When the hypofunction includes the gonadotropins, sexual development is impaired and the features remain childlike. Replacement therapy with growth hormone is available but because commercial synthesis is not yet possible, the supplies are very limited and difficult to obtain. There are no obvious manifestations of growth hormone deficiency if the hyposecretion occurs in adulthood.

In the adult woman, menstrual irregularities, diminished sexual desire, and decreased secondary sexual characteristics (e.g., pubic hair), are the first signs of adenohypophyseal insufficiency. These are usually due to deficiency of gonadotropin. If the deficiency is due to postpartum necrosis, there may be a failure to lactate and subsequent infertility. Men experience testicular atrophy, diminished spermatogenesis, loss of libido, and impotency as a result of gonadotropin deficiency.

Medical Management Treatment of hypopituitarism consists of surgery or irradiation for removal of a tumor, permanent hormone replacement, and a nutritious diet. Replacement therapy can be carried out with corticosteroids, thyroid hormone, and sex steroids. Gonadotropins can sometimes restore fertility.

If hypopituitarism is not detected and treated, the client eventually develops deficiencies of thyroid hormone and the adrenal corticosteroids. The latter causes a tendency toward shock and may result in an acute episode of Addisonian crisis (refractory shock stemming from sodium and water depletion), which is life threatening.

Nursing Management A primary role of the nurse in relation to adenohypophyseal insufficiency is case finding and referral. This is most clearly illustrated by pituitary dwarfism and Sheehan's syndrome.

Children affected by pituitary dwarfism will exhibit slow but proportional growth. Except for their small size they may appear completely normal. When the age of puberty is reached, sexual maturation may not occur. If it does proceed, the epiphyses will close, ending all possibility of further growth despite hormone replacement. For this reason, and because normal stature and psychosocial development are more likely to be achieved with early initiation of treatment, it is vital that these children be identified and treated early. The reader is referred to a pediatric text for a complete discussion of pituitary dwarfism.

The nurse should be alert for the incidence of postpartum pituitary necrosis (Sheehan's disease) and refer for diagnosis and treatment any woman with the following characteristics:

1. A history of hemorrhage or other hypoxic episode during the birth of the youngest child
2. Failure of lactation after this birth
3. Scanty, irregular, or absent menses
4. A decrease in secondary sex characteristics (or complaint of being "less womanly" than formerly)
5. Signs and symptoms of hypothyroidism
6. Signs and symptoms of Addison's disease without the bronzing of the skin associated with that condition

Although Sheehan's syndrome has been considered a relatively rare condition, there is evidence that it has been seriously underdiagnosed. The disease is devastating on affected women, but is reversible in large part by the administration of oral hormones.

If the disease is not detected and treated early, the woman is likely to need considerable help in rebuilding her life. Marital, vocational, or psychological counseling may be needed. The nature of the physiologic problem should be explained to significant others, and their help in the rehabilitative process enlisted.

Disorders of the Posterior Pituitary

Two hormones secreted by the posterior pituitary are antidiuretic hormone (ADH, vasopressin) and oxytocin. These substances are synthesized by the hypothalamus and secreted into the vascular network connecting this portion of the brain with the neurohypophysis (Fig. 40-6). Because the latter organ does not produce hormones but only controls their release into circulation, pituitary disease rarely causes imbalance of these chemicals, providing the adjacent brain tissue is not injured. Excesses of oxytocin are not recognized as clinical problems. The hormone is administered for pharmacologic effect in the management of labor.

Hyperfunction—Antidiuretic hormone

The syndrome of inappropriate antidiuretic hormone (SIADH) is a disorder in which there is continual release of ADH unrelated to plasma osmolality.[4] Fluids are retained and a dilutional hyponatremia develops. This condition is only considered inappropriate when urine osmolality is above plasma osmolality.

Etiology and Clinical Manifestations Eighty percent of the cases of SIADH are associated with small-cell or oat-cell carcinoma of the lung in which the malignant cells are capable of synthesizing, storing, and releasing ADH into the circulation.[5] Other nonmalignant pulmonary diseases such as tuberculosis can also cause this problem. Many central nervous system disorders such as fracture, encephalitis, and meningitis are also etiologic factors. Several drugs can cause water retention and SIADH (see Table 42-2). Physical and emotional stress, as well as pain often associated with surgery, may precipitate increased secretion of ADH resulting in SIADH.

The clinical picture may include a low urinary output and sudden weight gain without obvious edema. Cerebral edema can cause central nervous system symptoms such as mental confusion, altered levels of consciousness, convulsions, and coma. Muscle cramps due to the sodium imbalance may also be a problem.

Table 42-2
Drugs Which Can Cause SIADH

1. Chlorpropamide
2. Vincristine
3. Cyclophosphamide
4. Carbamazepine
5. Oxytocin
6. General anesthesia
7. Narcotics
8. Barbiturates
9. Thiazide diuretics
10. Tricyclic antidepressants

From Kurt J. Isselbacher et al. (eds.), *Harrison's Principles of Internal Medicine, 9th ed.*, McGraw-Hill Book Company, New York, 1980, p. 1692.

Medical Management The diagnosis of SIADH is made by simultaneous measurement of the urine and serum osmolality. The serum osmolality will be much lower than the urine osmolality, indicating the inappropriate excretion of a concentrated urine in the presence of very dilute serum. There will be low levels of blood urea nitrogen (BUN), serum creatinine, and serum albumin.

Treatment is aimed at restoring normal fluid balance and osmolarity. Fluid intake is limited to 1000 mL daily. If fluid restriction alone does not improve the symptoms, IV administration of 5% saline may be given. If cardiac problems such as congestive heart failure develop, a diuretic such as furosemide might be used to promote diuresis. Because of the increased potassium excretion this hormone causes, potassium supplements may be needed. Syndrome of inappropriate antidiuretic hormone tends to be self-limiting when secondary to head trauma or drugs, but chronic in nature when associated with tumors or metabolic diseases. Treatment of the underlying cause is indicated to improve the clinical picture. No drug is currently available to directly suppress the release of ADH.

Nursing Management When caring for the postoperative client, the nurse should be alert for signs such as low urinary output with a high specific gravity, a sudden gain in weight, or a drop in serum sodium which can indicate excess ADH. Once SIADH has been diagnosed, the nurse can plan other measures, including:

1. Accurate monitoring of intake and output
2. Daily weights
3. Fluid restrictions to 1000 mL daily

4. Frequent neurologic assessments
5. Keeping the head of the bed flat or elevated no more than 10° (This position enhances blood return to the heart and left atrial filling pressure, thus reducing release of ADH.)
6. Administration of prescribed medications and nutritional (electrolyte) supplements

When SIADH is a chronic problem, clients must learn to manage their treatment regimens. Fluid restriction is continued. This may not pose great problems since antidiuretic hormone tends to eliminate the sensation of thirst. If the drinking of liquids is an aspect of socialization, the client should be assisted in planning fluid intake so as to save liquid allowances for social occasions. The diet should be supplemented with sodium and potassium, especially if diuretics are prescribed. Salts of these electrolytes must be well diluted to prevent gastrointestinal irritation or damage. They are best taken at mealtime to allow mixing with and dilution by food. Clients should be taught the symptoms of fluid and electrolyte disturbances, especially those involving sodium and potassium, so they can monitor their response to treatment (see Chap. 12).

Hypofunction—Diabetes insipidus

Diabetes insipidus is an uncommon syndrome of posterior pituitary hormone malfunction characterized by increased thirst and water diuresis. It results from an apparent deficiency of ADH. This can be caused by impaired production of hormone secondary to head trauma, brain surgery, tumors, inflammation within the pituitary and adjacent hypothalamus, or to an inherited sex-linked deficiency of renal ADH receptors in males.

Clinical Manifestations The outstanding characteristic of diabetes insipidus is the excretion of large quantities of urine (up to 5 to 20 L/day) with a very low specific gravity. In a milder form urinary output may be lower (2 to 4 L/day). Some clients are able to compensate for the urine loss by drinking large quantities of fluids so that serum osmolality, which is usually elevated, may be normal or only slightly increased. Severe dehydration will occur if fluids are not replaced to equal output. In addition, if fluid intake is inadequate, marked weight loss, irritability, fatigue, hypothermia, tachycardia, and shock develop. The symptoms are associated with a rising serum osmolality and serum sodium concentration.

Medical Management The first step in diagnosing diabetes insipidus is to determine the cause of the polyuria (usually defined as the production of 100 mL or more of urine per hour). The causes may include a normal renal response to an excessive fluid intake, or it may mean insufficient ADH or impaired renal function.

A complete history and physical is done and the possibility of an emotional disturbance leading to psychogenic polydipsia is ruled out. The latter condition is associated with overhydration and hypervolemia rather than with the dehydration and hypovolemia seen in diabetes insipidus. A dehydration test is generally used to confirm a diagnosis of diabetes insipidus. In this test, fluid is withheld from the client from 2 to 8 hours. At the end of the dehydration period, the osmolality of both the urine and the serum are measured and compared to baseline values. If there is ADH deficiency, the urine will not concentrate. The serum osmolality is high. It must be kept in mind that the water deprivation test may have to be terminated early in some clients with diabetes insipidus because they may develop an intolerable thirst, and/or lose a dangerous amount of body fluid.

A simple and fast test to aid in the diagnosis of diabetes insipidus is to administer ADH by nasal spray. Prompt relief of symptoms strongly suggest the diagnosis of diabetes insipidus.

Diabetes insipidus that is secondary to head trauma or surgery is usually self-limiting and improves with treatment of the underlying problem. The goal of treatment is maintenance of fluid and electrolyte balance. This may be accomplished by the administration of increased amounts of fluid and/or hormone replacement with vasopressin administered by injection or inhalation. Lifelong hormone therapy is required for chronic deficiencies. For long-term treatment, nasal sprays containing vasopressin or pitressin tannate in oil (a slowly absorbed intramuscular preparation) are prescribed.

Nursing Management Nursing care of the client with diabetes insipidus is based on the clinical symptoms. Because of the polyuria, severe dehydration may result. Fluids must be replaced. This can be oral or intravenous replacement, depending on the client's condition or his ability to drink copious amounts of fluids. Accurate recording of intake and output and daily weights is helpful in assessing fluid balance and hydration status. Signs of hypovolemia reflected in changes in blood pressure, pulse, and respiratory rate can be detected early by frequent evaluation. Because of the need to urinate so frequently, sleep and rest are interrupted. This can lead to exhaustion, weakness, and discouragement. Genuine support and a reminder that these symptoms will soon be alleviated should be stressed.

During the dehydration test, the client's blood pressure and weight should be checked hourly because dehydration can be rapid. It is recommended that the test be discontinued if more than 3 to 5 percent of body weight is lost. Protein and salt are usually restricted in the diet in order to reduce the volume of urine through decreasing the amount of solutes in the plasma.

Clients affected by transient diabetes insipidus are usually hospitalized. In this situation, the nurse administers the prescribed antidiuretic hormone. Pitressin tannate in oil should be warmed before use and rolled to thorougly mix the oil and drug. Solutions of protein hormones such as antidiuretic hormone should be protected from excessive heat, freezing, and vigorous agitation to prevent denaturing of the protein molecule. Overmedication can precipitate volume excess and complications stemming from hypervolemia. Intake and output should be monitored for indications of overhydration such as weight gain, headache, listlessness, and angina.

Clients requiring long-term antidiuretic hormone replacement must be taught to manage their own treatment regimen. If pitressin nasal spray is used, clients need to be instructed to use the spray when thirst or polyuria occurs, and to limit its use to two to three times daily. Symptoms to report include nasal irritation, bronchopulmonary allergic reactions, or failure to improve. Clients who use intramuscular solutions need to be instructed in self-injection. In addition, the following features of this form of the drug should be stressed:

1. Pitressin tannate in oil should be warmed before use and rolled to mix the oil and drug thoroughly.
2. It should be stored in a cool, dry place, but protected from freezing.
3. It should be protected from light and high temperatures.
4. It is usually given IM every 1 to 3 days, depending on the response.
5. Report to the physician immediately if angina or any signs of volume excess (weight gain, headache, listlessness) occur.

THYROID GLAND

Dysfunction of the thyroid gland is manifested by hyperfunction, hypofunction, inflammation, or by enlargement (goiter). A goiter interferes with the surrounding structures and can be accompanied by increased, normal, or decreased hormone production.

Hyperthyroidism (Hyperfunction of the Thyroid)

Hyperthyroidism results from excessive circulating levels of thyroxine, triiodothyronine, or both. It is second only to diabetes mellitus among the naturally occurring endocrine diseases. The incidence is six times greater in women than in men, with the highest frequency in the 30-to-50-year-old age group. Iodine deficiency is believed to predispose to this as well as other thyroid disease, with a greater incidence occurring in iodine-poor geographic locations (goiter belt). The two most common forms of hyperthyroidism are Graves' disease and toxic nodular goiter (either single or multiple). Graves' disease is considerably more prevalent than toxic nodular goiter.[6]

Pathophysiology

Graves' Disease Graves' disease is marked by an increased production of thyroid hormone with diffuse hyperplasia and increased vascularity of the gland. Three associated characteristics are excess hormone production, goiter, and exophthalmos. However, Graves' disease can occur in the absence of exophthalmos.

Despite recent extensive research, the exact etiology of Graves' disease is unknown. An immunoglobin LATS (long-acting thyroid stimulator) has been found in the serum of some people with this disease. This immunoglobin has antibody properties against thyroid tissue and stimulates thyroid activity in laboratory animals. Its effects are similar to TSH but it has a slower and a more sustained effect. The exact role of LATS in the etiology of Graves' disease is still a mystery but current thinking is that it represents an antibody produced by the lymphocytes in response to thyroid antigens.[7] What is clear is that this disease is common in young women and may be genetically transmitted. It can go through cycles with remissions and excerabations or can have only a single active period during a person's lifetime. The onset of Graves' disease often follows a period of acute stress, which is considered to be a precipitating factor.

Toxic nodular goiter This condition does not appear to be a disorder of the immune system. It has a tendency to occur more commonly in older individuals with a history of preexisting goiter for years before the onset of demonstrable hyperthyroidism. The manifestations are slower to develop and are usually less severe than those in Graves' disease. More often it is not associated with ophthalmic conditions. Secreting tumors of the thyroid may be benign or malignant.

Clinical manifestations

The clinical manifestations of hyperthyroidism are directly related to the effects that increased thyroid hormones have on body metabolism and on sympathetic activity. The clinical manifestations are summarized in Table 42-3. Only an individual with advanced disease would exhibit all the mentioned symptomatology. Early in the disease the only signs may be increased nervousness and weight loss.

Exophthalmos Exophthalmos, in which the eyeballs protrude from the orbit, is due to increased deposits of fats and fluids in the retroorbital tissues (Fig. 42-2). This condition, characteristic of Graves' disease, may be caused by exophthalmos-producing substance, a fractional part of thyrotropin which has been demonstrated to cause exophthalmos without stimulating thyroid hormone production. In exophthalmos the upper lids are usually retracted and elevated and the eyeballs are forced outward with the sclera above the corners visible. This produces the characteristic stare and protrusion. Exophthalmos is usually bilateral but can be unilateral or asymmetric. When the eyelids do not close completely, the epithelial surfaces become dry and irritated. Serious complications such as corneal ulcers and eventual loss of vision can occur.

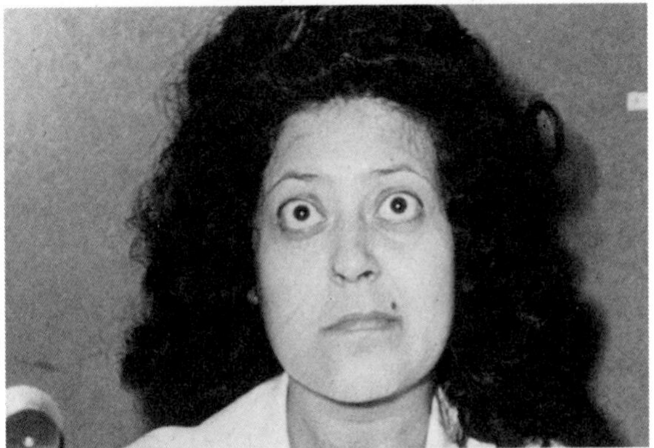

Figure 42-2 Marked exophthalmos in a 38-year old hyperthyroid client. *(From Herbert S. Kupperman and Iven S. Young, Famous Teachings in Modern Medicine, Clinical Endocrinology, Medcom, Inc., New York, 1970.)*

Complications

Thyrotoxic crisis or thyroid storm is an acute exacerbation of all thyrotoxic symptoms. It is a potentially fatal situation but death is relatively rare when antithyroid drugs and radioactive iodine are used. The cause is presumed to be stressors such as infection, trauma, or surgery that produce a massive release of thyroid hormones into the bloodstream. This can happen after a thyroidectomy. Symptoms include severe tachycardia, heart failure, shock, hyperthermia (up to 40.7°C [106°F]), restlessness, agitation, abdominal pain, delirium, and coma. Life-preserving measures must be taken to prevent death.

Diagnostic Study Abnormalities Serum levels of thyroxine (T_4) or triiodothyronine (T_3) can be measured by radioimmunoassay techniques and will be elevated. These tests offer a fairly accurate measure of circulating thyroid hormone.

Special tests are used to determine pituitary involvement in hyperthyroidism. The pituitary normally is inhibited by administration of triiodothyronine. In the T_3 suppression test, thyroid hormone is given daily for 1 week. If thyrotropin (TSH) production drops, radioactive iodine uptake by the thyroid gland drops also. Most clients with active Graves' disease do not respond to this suppression test, indicating that the pituitary is not responsive to the usual negative feedback system. In addition, the ECG may show tachycardia, atrial fibrillation, and P and T wave changes in hyperthyroidism.

Medical management

Treatment is aimed at halting excessive secretion of the thyroid hormones. The methods available today have changed little over the past two decades: (1) subtotal thyroid removal after adequate preparation, (2) thyroid ablation by radioactive iodine, and (3) medical therapy with antithyroid drugs and/or blockers of beta-sympathetic receptors (Table 42-4).

The choice of treatment is influenced by the client's age, severity of the disorder, complicating features (including pregnancy), and the client's preferences. If surgery is to be performed, the client is usually given antithyroid drugs to produce an euthyroid state. Any other associated disorders such as cardiac disease or diabetes mellitus must also be controlled or corrected before surgery.

For thyroidectomy to be effective, approximately 90 percent of thryoid tissue must be removed. If too much tissue is taken, the gland will not regenerate postoperatively and hypothyroidism will develop. During the surgical procedure extreme care has to be taken to avoid injuring the recurrent laryngeal nerves and the parathyroid glands.

Pharmacologic interventions

Antithyroid Drugs The most commonly used an-

Table 42-3
Clinical Manifestations of Thyroid Hormone Dysfunction

System	Hypofunction	Hyperfunction
Cardiovascular	Increased capillary fragility Decreased pulse Varied changes in blood pressure Cardiac hypertrophy, weak contractility Distant heart sounds Anemia Tendency to develop congestive heart failure, angina, and myocardial infarction	Increased blood pressure Increased rate and force of cardiac contractions Bounding pulse Increased cardiac output Cardiac hypertrophy Systolic murmurs Palpitations Arrthymias
Respiratory	Dyspnea	Increased respiratory rate Dyspnea on mild exertion
Gastrointestinal	Decreased appetite Weight gain Constipation Distended abdomen	Increased appetite Weight loss Increased peristalsis Diarrhea Increased bowel sounds
Integumentary	Dry, thick, inelastic, cold skin Thick, brittle nails Dry, sparse, coarse hair Poor turgor of mucosa Generalized interstitial edema	Warm, smooth, moist skin Thin, brittle nails Hair loss Palmar erythema Swelling of legs and feet (dependent edema)
Musculoskeletal	Fatigue Weakness Muscular aches and pains	Fatigue Muscle weakness
Nervous	Apathy Lethargy Forgetfulness Slowed mental process Slow, slurred speech Prolonged relaxation of deep tendon muscles	Difficulty in focusing eyes Nervousness Tremor Insomnia Lability of mood Restlessness Personality changes: irritability, agitation Exhaustion Hyperreflexia of tendon reflexes
Reproductive	Prolonged menstrual periods or amenorrhea Decreased libido Infertility	Menstrual irregularities Amenorrhea Decreased libido Impotence in males
Others	Increased susceptibility to infection Increased sensitivity to narcotics, barbiturates, and anesthesia. Intolerance to cold	Increased sensitivity to warm rooms Increased sensitivity to stimulant drugs Exophthalmos

tithyroid drugs are classified as thioamides. Propylthiouracil (PTU) and methimazole (Tapazole) are the most common drugs used clinically. These antithyroid drugs control the symptoms of hyperthyroidism by depressing the synthesis of thyroid hormone. Although there is considerable variation from person to person, it usually takes about 3 months to achieve an euthyroid state. A more rapid response can be induced by combining antithyroid drugs with iodine therapy.

The two major disadvantages of antithyroid drugs are client noncompliance and a high incidence of recurrence of the disease once the drugs are discontinued. Indications for use include Graves' disease in young clients, thyrotoxicosis during pregnancy, and the need to render a client euthyroid before surgery.

Iodine Iodine used in large doses blocks the release of thyroid hormone. Its maximal effect is usually seen within 1 to 2 weeks. After that time a reduction in therapeutic effect may be seen, and long-term iodine therapy is not effective in controlling hyperthyroidism. A common practice is to administer 5 to 15 drops of a saturated solution of potassium iodide several days prior to surgery. Iodine decreases the size and vascularity of the thyroid gland, making resection safer and easier. Propylthiouracil followed by iodine therapy is a commonly used method of preparing a hyperthyroid person for surgery.

Radioactive Iodine (Radioiodine or RAI) RAI limits the secretion of thyroid hormones by damaging or destroying thyroid tissue. It is administered orally with the dosage determined by estimated thyroid weight. This gives effective treatment, but it may also lead to significant problems related to hypothyroidism. This usually occurs within a decade of therapy. The symptoms of hyperthyroidism should be brought under control with antithyroid drugs prior to RAI administration. RAI has a delayed response and its maximum effects may not be noted for 2 to 3 months. However, it is effective, inexpensive, and can be administered on an outpatient basis. Treatment with *propranolol* is recommended before and during the first month after therapy to help ameliorate the symptoms of hyperthyroidism before the effects of irradiation become apparent. Propranolol, an adrenergic antagonist, relieves the adrenergic effects associated with hyperthyroidism including tachycardia, tremors, and sweating.

Because irradiation is both teratogenic and carcinogenic, radioiodine is used primarily to treat clients beyond the childbearing years. It is contraindicated during pregnancy as radioiodine crosses the placenta and will destroy the thyroid of the fetus.

Table 42-4
Medical Management: Hyperthyroidism

Diagnostic

1. Complete history and physical examination
2. Ophthalmologic examination
3. ECG
4. Laboratory tests
   a. RAIU
   b. Serum T_3 and T_4
   c. Thyroid suppression test (not in elderly)
   d. TRH stimulation test
5. BMR

Therapeutic

A. Graves' disease
   1. Antithyroid drugs
      a. Propylthiouracil
      b. Methimazole
   2. Ablation of thyroid tissue
      a. Partial thyroidectomy
      b. Radioactive iodine
   3. Adrenergic antagonists such as propranolol (Inderal)
   4. High calorie diet

B. Toxic nodular goiter
   1. Antithyroid drugs
      a. Propylthiouracil
      b. Methimazole
   2. Ablation of thyroid tissue by radioactive iodine

Nursing management

Two general objectives in the care of hyperthyroid clients are to (1) assist them in coping with the manifestations of the disorder, and (2) assist them in returning to an euthyroid state. Table 42-5 outlines the general nursing care required by the hyperthyroid client. Specific measures are discussed below.

Environment A restful, calm, quiet room should be provided. Because of the increased body metabolism, there is an increased need for rest. However, this often becomes a challenge if the client exhibits nervousness and irritability. The hyperthyroid client should be placed in a room away from disturbing sights, very ill people, noisy nurses' stations, elevators, and areas of high traffic. The temperature of the room should be adjusted to maintain a cool environment. Only light bed coverings and frequent linen changes should be used if clients are diaphoretic. Sometimes restlessness is marked and exercise is needed to promote the release of nervous tension. Activities should involve use of the large muscles, as tremors can interfere with small muscle coordination. The nurse should try to

Table 42-5
Nursing Care Plan for the Client with Hyperthyroidism

Client Problem	Expected Outcome	Nursing Intervention
Restlessness and insomnia	Decrease in purposeless movements. Restful sleep.	Promote continuation of usual practices related to rest and sleep unless contraindicated. Decrease environmental stimuli. Administer frequent back rubs using effleurage. Approach client with a calm, unhurried demeanor. Work efficiently when with the client. Encourage quiet diversions. Encourage frequent short walks during the day. Encourage maintenance of usual bedtime ritual. Administer antithyroid drugs as ordered. Administer sedatives as needed. Eliminate caffeine (coffee, tea, cola and chocolate) from the diet.
Fatigue and weakness	Decreased perception of weakness and fatigue by client.	Assist client with self-care. Limit ambulation to short walks. Promote rest and relaxation.
Heat intolerance	Decreased perspiration and increased comfort.	Maintain a cool environmental temperature. Provide light, loose clothing. Bathe client frequently. Change linen frequently.
Exophthalmos	No evidence of corneal damage.	Instruct client to wear dark glasses. Restrict salt intake. Raise head of bed at night. Teach client to exercise extraocular muscles daily. Cover eyes with mask or tape shut if eyes will not close.
Increased risk of accidental injury related to fine muscle tremors, fatigue, and incoordination	Prevention of accidental injury.	Assist client as necessary with tasks requiring fine motor skills. Reduce environmental hazards. Assist client when ambulating. Teach client safe practices.
Malnutrition as indicated by weight loss; actual or potential deficiencies of nutrients	Maintenance of weight (or gain in weight); alleviation (or prevention) of signs and symptoms of nutritional deficiency.	Provide a high calorie, high vitamin, high mineral diet which includes between-meal and bedtime snacks. Daily weights. Monitor BUN.
Hypermotility of the bowel	Decreased abdominal discomfort; production of formed or soft rather than liquid stools.	Eliminate from the diet foods with a laxative effect (rhubarb, prunes, bran, large quantities of fruits and vegetables, especially when raw).
Actual or potential hypertension	Reduction in blood pressure toward normal.	Promote rest and relaxation. Teach the client strategies for coping with stress. When ordered, administer antihypertensive medication. Monitor vital signs frequently.
Actual or potential congestive heart failure	Prevention or reduction of congestive failure.	Reduce environmental stressors. Promote rest and relaxation. Assess tolerance to activity. Discourage physical activity which is not well tolerated. Administer cardiotonics as ordered. Monitor vital signs and cardiac status frequently.
Predisposition to anxiety related to increased CNS stimulation	Reduced anxiety.	Explain procedures and medical regimens. Work in a competent manner. Express concern for the client.

Table 42-5 (Continued)

Client Problem	Expected Outcome	Nursing Intervention
Altered self-image, related to changes in appearance and abilities	Improved self-image.	Encourage good grooming and attractive attire. Compliment the client when appropriate. Reassure client that appearance and function will return to normal after reduction of the hormone imbalance.
Potential imbalance of other hormones (diabetes mellitus, glucocorticoid deficiency)	Prompt detection of other endocrine imbalances; early treatment of such conditions.	Monitor urine sugar and acetone. Assess blood chemistries for glucose, sodium, and potassium imbalances. Assess fluid balance. Report promptly any evidence of hyperglycemia, dehydration, or hyperkalemia.

gain the client's confidence and trust as this is helpful in attempting to reduce aggravating events. Whenever possible, the same nurse should care for the client to eliminate a possible source of anxiety.

The nurse should involve the family in efforts to relieve any type of stress. Family members need instruction in the nature of the client's illness so they can better understand the physiologic and emotional symptoms the client has experienced, and can contribute to plans and measures to reduce total stress. Visitors who may be upsetting should be restricted.

Diet and Fluids Because of the increased metabolic rate, there is an increased need for nutrients: 4000 to 5000 calories a day may be required to satisfy hunger and prevent tissue breakdown. Six full meals a day with snacks high in protein, carbohydrates, minerals, and vitamins (especially thiamine and ascorbic acid) are recommended to sustain the high rate of metabolism. The client should be weighed daily to monitor for weight loss or gain. Changes in weight should be toward normal body size for the client. Increased fluids are needed as there is usually increased perspiration, polyuria, and increased metabolic wastes. Highly seasoned or fibrous foods are discouraged because they stimulate the already hypermotile gastrointestinal tract. Stimulants such as coffee, tea, or cola are also omitted since they accentuate the existing overactive autonomic responses.

Eye Care If exophthalmos is present, the cornea must be protected from ulceration, irritation, and infection. Some clients may also suffer from orbital pain. There are a number of nursing measures recommended to help reduce eye discomfort. Methylcellulose drops soothe the membranes and help prevent drying. Elevation of the head improves fluid drainage and reduces congestion. Dark glasses reduce glare and prevent irritation from dust and dirt. If the eyelids cannot be closed, they should be lightly taped shut. To maintain flexibility, the client should be taught to exercise the intraocular muscles by turning the eyes in complete range of motion. Good grooming can be helpful in reducing the loss of self-esteem that occurs due to an altered body image. If the exophthalmos is severe, treatment may involve suturing the eyelids together, administration of corticosteroids, irradiation of retroorbital tissues, orbital decompression, or corrective lid or muscle surgery.

Nursing Care Related to Surgical Intervention

Preoperative care

When a thyroidectomy is the treatment of choice, the client must be adequately prepared to avoid postoperative complications. All exaggerated symptoms should be decreased and cardiac problems controlled. If iodine is used, the client must be observed for signs of iodine toxicity such as swelling of buccal mucosa, excess salivation, coryza, and skin reactions. The drug should be discontinued and the physician notified if these reactions occur.

Preoperative teaching should include comfort and safety measures in which the client can participate. Coughing, deep breathing, and leg exercises should be practiced and their importance explained. The client should be taught how to support the head manually while turning in bed, since this technique will minimize stress on the suture line postoperatively. Range-of-motion exercises of the neck should be practiced. The nurse should explain routine postoperative care such as intravenous infusions. It should be mentioned that talking is likely to be difficult after surgery for a time.

Postoperative care

The client's room needs to be prepared for the client. Oxygen, suction equipment, and a tracheostomy tray should be readily available. A tracheostomy tray is required in the event that airway obstruction occurs. Although this happens rarely, it constitutes an emergency situation. Recurrent laryngeal nerve damage leads to vocal cord paralysis. If there is paralysis of both cords, spastic airway obstruction occurs, which requires an immediate tracheostomy.

Respirations may also become difficult because of excess swelling of the neck tissues, hemorrhage, and hematoma formation, or laryngeal stridor due to tetany. Tetany may occur if the parathyroid glands are accidentally removed during surgery. Calcium gluconate for intravenous administration should be readily available to be used to terminate any episode of tetany.

Additional nursing measures for the postoperative thyroidectomy client include:

1. Assess for any signs of hemorrhage or tracheal compression such as irregular breathing, swelling of the neck, choking, or wetness behind the neck.
2. Place the client in a semi-Fowler's position; support the head with pillows, avoiding flexion of the neck and any tension on the suture lines.
3. Monitor vital signs. Complete the initial assessment by checking for signs of tetany (tingling in toes, fingers, or around the mouth; muscular twitching; apprehension) and assessing difficulty in speaking and hoarseness. (Some hoarseness is to be expected for 3 to 4 days because of edema.)
4. Control postoperative pain. Meperidine or morphine sulfate are commonly prescribed.

If postoperative recovery is uneventful, the client is ambulated the first day, takes fluid as soon as tolerated, and eats a soft diet by the second postoperative day. Discharge is usually in 2 to 6 days after surgery.

Chronic Nursing Management Follow-up medical care is very important for clients who have undergone thyroid surgery. Hyperthyroidism may recur after a period of time, requiring further treatment. Hormone balance should be monitored periodically to assure that normal function has returned. Most clients experience a period of relative hypothyroidism postoperatively, because of the marked reduction in size of the thyroid. The remaining tissue usually hypertrophies, recovering the capacity to produce the hormone needed by the body. The administration of thyroid hormone is avoided since exogenous hormone inhibits pituitary production of thyrotropin and will delay or prevent the restoration of normal gland function.

The client can do much to prevent complications and promote return to normal function during the hypothyroid period following surgery. Calorie intake must be reduced markedly below that which was required preoperatively if weight gain is to be avoided. Some surgeons may suggest avoiding foods containing thyroid-inhibiting substances (Table 42-6). Adequate iodine is necessary to promote thyroid function but excesses will inhibit the thyroid. Seafood once or twice a week or normal use of iodized salt should provide sufficient intake. Regular exercise helps stimulate the thyroid and should be encouraged. Exposure to alternating extremes of temperatures such as hot and cold showers also promotes thyroid hyperplasia, but is not acceptable to many individuals because of cold intolerance. High environmental temperature should be avoided, however, since this will inhibit thyroid regeneration.

To promote comfort and return of full range of motion, the neck incision should be lubricated and range-of-motion exercises carried out three or four

Table 42-6

Exogenous Goitrogens

Foods

- Potent goitrogens
  - Turnips
  - Rutabagas
  - Soybeans (especially when fed to infants in formula)
  - Skins of peanuts
  - Milk from kale-fed cattle
- Less potent goitrogens
  - Seafood
  - Green leafy vegetables
  - Peanuts
  - Peaches
  - Peas
  - Strawberries
  - Carrots
  - Cabbage
  - Mustard seed
  - Radishes

Drugs

- Thyroid inhibitors
  - Propylthiouracil
  - Methimazole
  - Carbimazole
  - Tapazole
  - Iodine in large doses
- Others
  - Sulfonamides
  - Salicylates
  - Para-aminosalicylic acid (PAS)
  - Phenylbutazone

times daily. The client should be taught movements that cause flexion, extension, rotation, and lateral bending of the neck. The appearance of the incision may be quite distressing to the client. The client should be reassured that the scar will fade in color and eventually assume the appearance of a normal neck wrinkle. Scarves, jewelry, or other coverings can effectively camouflage a fresh scar.

Many clients affected by Graves' disease eventually develop hypothyroidism and should be taught to recognize symptoms of hypothyroidism. Regular medical follow-up is to be encouraged twice yearly to monitor for the development of hypothyroidism, hyperthyroidism, or hypoparathyroidism. If a complete thyroidectomy was performed, the client needs instruction on lifelong thyroid replacement. Failure of thyroid function is considered by some authorities to be the normal end stage of this disease. Clients should be taught the signs and symptoms of progressive thyroid failure, and cautioned to seek medical care if these develop. Hypothyroidism is easily controlled by the administration of oral hormone preparations.

Enlargement (Goiter)

Enlargement of the thyroid may be caused by (1) simple goiter, (2) tumors (benign or malignant), and (3) any form of thyroiditis.

Simple goiter

The etiology of goiter includes iodine deficiency or an intrathyroid biochemical defect that can be caused by a variety of factors called *goitrogens*. Goitrogens, which are chemical components of certain foods and drugs, can suppress thyroxine production and inhibit the ability of the thyroid to concentrate iodine (see Table 42-6). Goiters produced by these compounds have the same features as those caused by iodine deficiencies. Treatment is often accomplished by the withdrawal of the particular goitrogen.

In order to determine whether the goiter is associated with hyper- or hypothyroidism, measurements of T_4 and T_3 are necessary. If thyroid hormone levels are normal and glandular enlargement is minimal, no treatment may be attempted. Moderate to marked enlargement may cause pressure on the trachea and esophagus, causing dyspnea and/or dysphagia. In addition, a very large gland causes noticeable disfigurement (Fig. 42-3). When such problems or hormone imbalance are present, treatment is required. This may involve suppression of TSH by the administration of thyroid hormones, the addition of iodine to the diet to promote hormone production, or surgery to remove excess thyroid tissue.

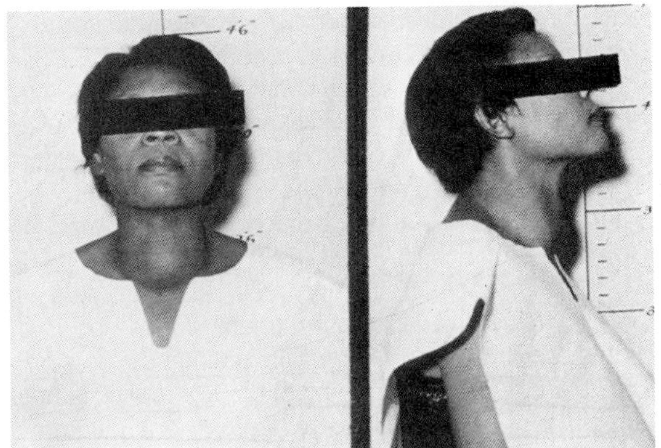

Figure 42-3 Obviously enlarged thyroid secondary to hyperthyroidism. *(From Herbert S. Kupperman and Iven S. Young, Famous Teachings in Modern Medicine, Medcom, Inc., New York, 1970.)*

Tumors

Malignant tumors of the thyroid gland are rare. They account for only 0.5 percent of cancer deaths. The major sign of thyroid cancer is the appearance of a hard, painless nodule in an enlarged thyroid. A thyroid scan will show whether nodules on the thyroid are "hot" or "cold." When a person is given tracer doses of ^{131}I, tumors on the thyroid may take up the radioactive iodine. These are called "hot" nodules and are nearly always benign. Benign nodules are usually not dangerous but they can cause tracheal compression if they become too large. Since few malignancies utilize iodine and many are cystic in nature, they usually show up as "cold" spots in the thyroid scan. Serum thyrocalcitonin is also helpful in diagnosis since increased levels are associated with malignancy.

The treatment of choice for neoplasms is surgical removal. The range of surgical procedures may be from simple removal of the tumor to total thyroidectomy with bilateral neck dissection. Many thyroid cancers are thyrotropin-dependent and thyroid hormone in hyperphysiologic doses is often prescribed to inhibit pituitary secretion of TSH. Nursing care for thyroid tumors is similar to thyroidectomy care and also includes general nursing measures for the client with cancer (Chap. 11).

Thyroiditis

Thyroiditis is an inflammatory disease of the thyroid. It is characterized by painful or nonpainful enlargement. Autoimmune disease is the most common cause, although it can also be due to infection (bacterial or viral) or unknown factors. Hashimoto's thyroiditis, in which thyroid tissue is replaced by lymphocytes and fibrous tissue, has increased in frequency in the past three decades and occurs at present approximately as often as Graves' disease.

T_4 and T_3 are usually elevated in acute and subacute forms of thyroiditis and low or normal in chronic forms. Failure of radioactive iodine indicates a low thyroid reserve and supports the diagnosis. Thyroid biopsy can establish a diagnosis.

Management Recovery may be complete in weeks or months with no treatment. When required, treatment may include specific antibiotics or surgical drainage to eliminate infection, corticosteroids to inhibit the inflammation, nonsteroid anti-inflammatory drugs, analgesics to relieve discomfort or pain, and thyroid hormone to correct deficiencies and reduce TSH stimulation of the gland. Thyroidectomy is rarely required. As many as 10 percent of individuals affected by thyroiditis will eventually develop hypothyroidism and require permanent hormone replacement.

Nursing care of clients with thyroiditis depends in part on the medical regimen. When no treatment is given, clients need support and assistance during the recovery period. Aspirin or acetaminophen may be used to alleviate thyroid discomfort. The client should be urged to remain under close health supervision, and report any change in symptoms so that progress may be monitored.

Clients with thyroiditis of autoimmune etiology are likely to exhibit other allergic tendencies. It is important to avoid exposure to known allergens, as stimulation of immune mechanisms may cause a worsening of thyroid condition. Since stress often triggers allergic reactions, stress management is an important part of client teaching.

Clients receiving thyroid hormone or corticosteroids must be taught the side effects of these drugs and measures to control them. Toxic symptoms should be clearly delineated and the client instructed to report these (Table 42-3). Clients treated surgically need care similar to that outlined for individuals undergoing thyroidectomy.

Hypofunction—Hypothyroidism

Hypothyroidism results from insufficient synthesis of thyroid hormone due to a wide variety of abnormalities. All hypothyroid states have certain features in common, regardless of the cause, and many of these manifestations depend on the age of onset of the deficiency.

Etiology

There are two forms of hypothyroidism—childhood and adult hypothyroidism. *Cretinism* is a disorder in infants and children caused by a deficiency of the thyroid hormone during fetal or early neonatal life. This defect is the result of an inherited recessive trait.

In the adult the most common cause of primary hypothyroidism is atrophy of the thyroid gland, considered to be the end result of both Hashimoto's disease and Graves' disease. These conditions involve autoimmune processes in which the thyroid gland is gradually destroyed by endogenous antibodies. Thyroid deficiency also occurs when pituitary thyrotropin production is inadequate. Iatrogenic causes of hypothyroidism include surgical removal of the thyroid, destruction of the thyroid gland by radiation, or surgical ablation of the pituitary. Occasionally, hypothyroidism develops as a result of ingestion of goitrogens in food or drugs, which inhibit thyroid function.

Although the typical hypothyroid client is a woman over 50, the disease can occur at any age and in either sex. Increased incidence has been correlated with the use of radioactive iodine. As with other thyroid diseases, hypothyroidism is more common in iodine-deficient populations and is associated with high levels of stress.

Clinical manifestations

The major manifestations of *cretinism* are defective physical development and mental retardation. Affected infants exhibit thickened skin and lips, puffy extremities, superclavicular and periorbital edema, enlarged tongue, squinting, and a dull facial expression. Early recognition of symptoms and referral for treatment are essential if physical and mental growth are to be normal.

Failure to treat infants with cretinism causes mental retardation and dwarfism. These complications are irreversible. If begun early (soon after birth), hormone replacement allows for normal growth and near-normal intellectual development.

Hypothyroidism in adults is called *myxedema* and is characterized by a general slowing of body processes, personality changes, and a generalized interstitial nonpitting edema. Characteristic facies are often seen (Fig. 42-4). In addition, constipation, cold intolerance, obesity, and menorrhagia are common. The onset is usually slow, occurring over months to years, unless it occurs quickly following thyroidectomy or during treatment with antithyroid drugs. The symptoms often develop so subtly that medical attention is not sought. The individual's family or friends are often unaware of the changes. The severity of the symptoms depends upon the degree of thyroid hormone deficiency. The manifestations of hypofunction of the thyroid gland are summarized in Table 42-3.

Many of the clinical manifestations associated

with hypothyroidism stem from the long-term physiologic effects of thyroid deficiency. They may involve any body system but tend to affect the cardiovascular, gastrointestinal, reproductive, hematopoietic, and central nervous systems most commonly. In general, the longer and more severe the hypothyroidism, the more severe are the manifestations.

In adults several metabolic changes predispose to accelerated cardiovascular degeneration. Depression of metabolism causes a weakening of cardiac contractility. The resulting decreased cardiac output causes compensatory vasoconstriction, which increases diastolic blood pressure and peripheral resistance. This hypertension coupled with the high serum cholesterol characteristic of hypothyroidism promotes atherosclerotic changes in blood vessels. In myxedema, accumulation of mucopolysaccharides in extracellular fluid causes increased fluid in many body tissues. Pleural, peritoneal, and pericardial effusion commonly develop. These processes culminate in hypertensive arteriosclerotic cardiovascular disease characterized by a dangerously low cardiac reserve and a predisposition to congestive failure.

Gastrointestinal motility and secretion is decreased in hypothyroid individuals. Constipation, which is a common complaint, may progress to obstipation and, rarely, intestinal obstruction. The underlying metabolic disease makes the individual a very high risk surgical candidate.

Hypothyroid women frequently complain of menorrhagia. Some affected individuals have been treated for this condition for long periods of time, and may have undergone hysterectomy, before the underlying endocrine disorder was diagnosed.

Megaloblastic anemia is a feature of hypothyroidism in more than one in ten people with idiopathic thyroid failure. The decrease in red blood cell production by the bone marrow is reflective of the general slowing down of the body processes characteristic of the hypothyroid state.

Inhibition of brain function is manifested by mental sluggishness, lethargy, and changes in affect. Some individuals exhibit an inappropriate lack of concern over the signs and symptoms of the disease. This is not simply apathy, since many exhibit a rather jocular air that may be indicative of inhibition of frontal lobe function. Other individuals appear depressed and express distress and impaired self-image due to the disabilities and altered appearance which develop. Frank psychoses characterized by disorientation, delusions, hallucinations, paranoia, and suicidal tendencies can occur. Administration of replacement hormone usually reduces the psychotic symptoms, indicating that the etiology of this complication is largely organic.

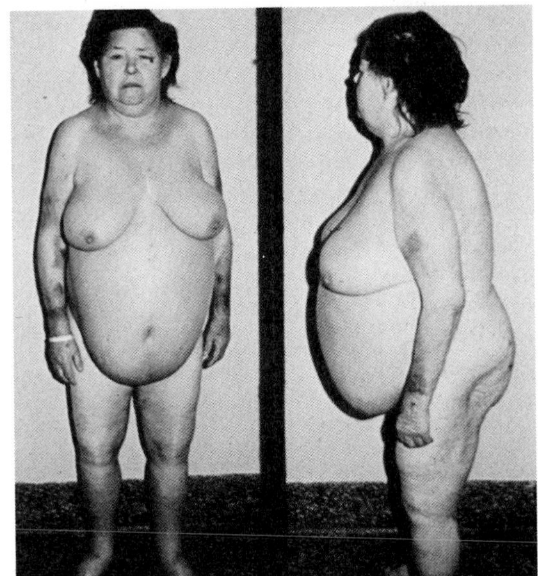

Figure 42-4 Adult myxedema. *(From Herbert S. Kupperman and Iven S. Young, Famous Teachings in Modern Medicine, Medcom, Inc., New York, 1970.)*

Complications—Myxedema coma

The mental sluggishness, drowsiness, and lethargy of hypothyroidism may progress suddenly to marked impairment of consciousness or coma. Myxedema coma can be precipitated by infection, drugs (especially narcotics, tranquilizers, and barbiturates), or exposure to cold or trauma. It is characterized by subnormal temperature, hypotension, and hypoventilation. Vital functions must be supported and intravenous thyroid hormone administered if the individual is to survive.

Diagnostic study abnormalities

The screening laboratory test for hypothyroidism is serum thyroxine concentration. A low value correlated with symptomatology gathered from a thorough history and physical examination may be sufficient to confirm the diagnosis. If other possibilities are suspected, a serum T_3 should be evaluated. This will be low in hypothyroidism.

Serum TSH and TRH stimulation tests can be helpful in distinguishing between primary and secondary hypothyroidism. Serum TSH is high in primary and low in secondary hypothyroidism. A rise in TSH following TRH injection suggests hypothalamic dysfunction. No change is compatible with damage of the anterior pituitary. See Table 42-7 for a summary of diagnostic study abnormalities in hypothyroidism.

Table 42-7
Diagnostic Study Abnormalities in Hypothyroidism

Study	Finding
Serum T_3	Low
Serum T_4	Low
Radioactive iodine uptake	Decreased (below 10% in 24 h)
Serum cholesterol	Increased
ECG	Bradycardia, low voltage
Serum TSH	High in primary thyroidism
TRH stimulation test	Low in secondary disease rise in TSH in hypothalamic pathology, no change in TSH in pituitary hypofunction

Medical management

The primary objective in treating hypothyroidism is the restoration of an euthyroid (normal thyroid gland function) state as safely, rapidly, and inexpensively as possible by replacement therapy. Economic factors are important because severe hypothyroidism is totally disabling. Medical management of adults includes gradual replacement of thyroid hormones and a low calorie diet to promote weight loss and reduction in cholesterol levels. For adults as well as children lifelong therapy is required in most cases.[8]

Pharmacologic management

Levothyroxine is usually the thyroid drug of choice but other commonly used drugs include thyroxine (Levothyroxine, Synthroid), triiodothyronine, desiccated thyroid, purified thyroglobulin and mixtures of T_4 and T_3 in a ratio of 4:1 (Liotrix).

In young clients without evidence of heart disease, the maintenance dose of thyroid replacement can be started at once, but in older clients or those with cardiac complications a small initial dose is recommended. A large dose of thyroid hormone may stimulate metabolic activity to such an extent that the client's circulatory system may be stressed beyond its coping ability and heart failure can result. If there are no contraindications, the dosage may be increased at intervals of 3 to 4 weeks.

Nursing management

Acute Intervention There are several nursing interventions that will contribute to the recovery of the hypothyroid client:

1. Provide a comfortable, warm environment because of the client's intolerance of cold.
2. Take measures to prevent skin breakdown. Use soap sparingly. An alternating pressure mattress may be helpful.
3. Avoid using sedatives. Reduce the dose of any sedative, barbiturate, or anesthetic that must be given. Give half the usual dose and monitor closely.
4. Prevent constipation by gradually increasing exercise, administering stool softeners, increasing bulk in the diet, and promoting regular bowel habits. Enemas are to be avoided because they produce vagal stimulation that could be hazardous in clients with cardiac pathology.
5. Assist the client in adhering to a low calorie diet.
6. Teach the client the nature of the thyroid hormone deficiency, self-care practices necessary to recovery, and signs and symptoms to monitor to assess future health.

To assess the client's progress, vital signs, body weight, fluid intake and output, and visible edema should be monitored. Cardiac assessment is especially important as cardiovascular response to the hormone determines the medication regimen. Note energy level and mental alertness. These should increase within 2 to 14 days and continue to rise steadily to normal levels.

Chronic Management Repeated client education is imperative. Often the hypothyroid client needs more time than usual to comprehend all the information needed. It is important to provide written aids, repeat the information often, and assess comprehension level regularly. The need for lifelong drug therapy must be stressed. The signs of hypo- or hyperthyroidism that indicate hormone imbalance should be included in the treatment plan. Sometimes it is difficult for the client to recognize signs of over- or underdosage. Because of this, a family member or friend should also be instructed on what to look for. Forgetfulness is an early indication of thyroid deficiency.

Because thyroid preparations are cumulative, the client must be taught to contact his physician immediately if any of the following signs or symptoms appear: angina, orthopnea, dyspnea, palpitations, nervousness, or insomnia. Diabetic clients should test their urine for sugar and acetone more frequently as thyroid preparations may require the adjustments of insulin dosages. In addition, thyroid preparations potentiate other common drug groups such as anticoagulants, antidepressants, and digitalis compounds.

With treatment, striking transformations occur in both appearance and mental function. Most adults return to a normal state. Cardiovascular pathology and (occasionally) psychosis may persist despite correction of the hormone imbalance. Relapses will occur if treatment is interrupted, or if thyroid antibodies inactivate the exogenous hormones.

PARATHYROIDS

Hyperfunction—Hyperparathyroidism

Hyperparathyroidism is a condition of excessive secretion of parathyroid hormone. Until recently, this dysfunction had been considered rare. With the advent of routine evaluation of serum calcium levels, true incidence appears to be as high as one case per thousand.[9] Hyperparathyroidism can be classified as either primary or secondary. *Primary disease* may be due to secreting turmors in or hyperplasia of the parathyroid glands. Most cases are attributable to a single adenoma. *Secondary hyperparathyroidism* appears to be a compensatory response to abnormal states which induce or cause hypocalcemia. (Hypocalcemia is the main stimulus to parathyroid activity.) Disease conditions associated with secondary hyperparathyroidism include vitamin D deficiencies, malabsorption, chronic renal failure, and hyperphosphatemia.

Primary hyperparathyroidism occurs most frequently in women between the ages of 35 and 65. It is most common after menopause. Recently, as many as 30 percent of all cases of hyperparathyroidism have been related to head or neck radiation for some benign disease, 20 to 30 years previously.[10]

Clinical manifestations and complications

Hyperparathyroidism has different characteristics and is not always associated with bone disease. Some clients are asymptomatic and show only an increased serum calcium. However, the signs and symptoms that are commonly associated with increased parathyroid hormone are due to hypercalcemia, increased bone reabsorption, decreased serum phosphate, hypophosphaturia, and neuromuscular abnormalities. A summary of common findings is presented in Table 42-8.

The serious complications are those associated with renal and skeletal disturbances such as calcification of kidney parenchyma, collapse of vertebral bodies, and rib fractures. Renal failure and uremia may occur.

Diagnostic study abnormalities

Elevated serum calcium levels with low serum phosphate levels constitute a characteristic combination. Other elevations include parathormone (PTH), urine calcium and phosphate, serum chloride, and serum alkaline phosphatase if bone disease has already begun. If bone changes are present, radiologic studies may reveal subperiosteal reabsorption, bone cysts, demineralization of bones, loss of lamina dura of the teeth, and long bone tumors.

Medical management

The objective of treatment is to relieve symptoms and prevent complications due to excessive secretion of parathyroid hormone. The choice of therapy depends upon the urgency of the clinical situation, the degree of hypercalcemia, the underlying disorder, the status of renal and hepatic function, the clinical presentation of the client, and the particular advantages and disadvantages of the different therapeutic modalities.

Parathyroid tumors should be removed surgically, but this can be somewhat difficult as the parathyroids occasionally lie in ectopic sites such as the mediastinum. This requires a highly skilled surgeon to open the chest and explore the area behind the sternum.

A large fluid intake is necessary to dilute the excess calcium in order to minimize the formation of calcium renal stones. If the disorder is mild, it can be managed by forcing fluids, avoiding immobilization, and by administering certain drugs (discussed in next section). Management of secondary hyperparathyroidism due to chronic renal failure is covered in Chap. 38.

Pharmacologic interventions

The administration of intravenous normal saline solution not only helps to expand the body's fluid volume, but, in addition, the excess sodium promotes excretion of calcium.[11] In severe hypercalcemic states, phosphate may be given to reduce the serum calcium in order to facilitate a positive response to surgery. The phosphate must be given carefully, especially to those clients who are hypotensive. Diuretics such as furosemide or ethacrynic acid can be given to decrease renal tubular reabsorption of calcium. Mithramycin has been shown to effectively lower the serum calcium level within 48 hours. If the client is past menopause, estrogenic hormones may be used.

Nursing management

If surgery is performed, close monitoring of the client's vital signs is required. Other aspects of care are similar to that following a thyroidectomy. The major postoperative complications are tetany and fluid and electrolyte disturbances. Tetany usually is apparent early in the postoperative period but may develop over several days. Mild tetany characterized by unpleasant tingling of the hands and around the mouth may be

Table 42-8
Clinical Manifestations of Parathyroid Dysfunction

System	Hypofunction	Hyperfunction
Cardiovascular	Decreased contractility of the heart muscle Decreased cardiac output ECG changes: prolonged Q-T interval, slurred QRS complex, ST and T changes	Arrthymias Q-T changes on ECG (shortened) Hypertension
Gastro-intestinal	Abdominal cramps	Vague abdominal pain Anorexia Nausea, vomiting Constipation Pancreatitis Peptic ulcer Epigastric distress
Integumentary	Dry, scaly skin Hair loss on scalp and body Brittle nails Changes in teeth: lack of tooth enamel	
Musculo-skeletal	Fatigue Weakness Painful muscle cramps Skeletal x-ray changes: osteosclerosis	Skeletal pain Backache Weakness, fatigue Pain on weight bearing Pathologic fractures
Nervous	Personality changes Psychiatric manifestations: depression, anxiety Irritability Memory impairment Headache Convulsions Positive Chvostek's and/or Trousseau's sign Tremor Paresthesias	Personality disturbances Emotional irritability Psychosis Delirum, confusion Incoordination Hyperactive deep tendon reflexes Abnormalities of gait
Renal	Urinary frequency	Renal colic Renal stones Urinary tract infections Polyuria
Other	Eye changes: lenticular opacities, cataracts, papilledema, photophobia	Eye: Slit-lamp examination of the eye may show corneal calcification

present but should disappear without problems. If tetany becomes more severe, intravenous calcium may be given. Treatment for severe tetany is discussed below in the section on hypoparathyroidism. In order to evaluate fluid and electrolytes, urine output and sodium and potassium levels are assessed frequently. Mobility is encouraged because it promotes recalcification of the bones.

If surgery is not performed, treatment to relieve symptoms and to prevent complications is carried out. Problems requiring attention and appropriate nursing interventions are summarized in Table 42-9.

Hypofunction—Hypoparathyroidism

Hypoparathyroidism is a failure of the parathyroid glands to produce adequate amounts of parathormone (PTH). Affected individuals do not have the

Table 42-9
Nursing Care Plan for the Client with Hyperparathyroidism

Client Problem	Expected Outcome	Nursing Intervention
Fatigue and weakness	Decreased perception of fatigue and weakness by client. Prevention of accidental injury.	Limit ambulation to short walks. Assist client with self-care. Reduce safety hazards in the environment. Maintain bed in low position with siderails up.
Hypercalcemia; predisposition to renal stones	No incidence of renal stones. Prompt detection and early treatment of renal stones.	Provide a low calcium, acid-ash diet. (Omit milk and milk products; include additional cranberries, prunes, and plums.) Consult with the physician concerning possible prescription of ascorbic acid to acidify the urine. Encourage fluid intake to the point of moderate overhydration. Assess client for flank pain and hematuria and report immediately. Strain all urine for stones.
Predisposition to anorexia, nausea, and vomiting	Maintenance of adequate food and fluid intake.	Administer mouth care frequently, using flavored mouthwash or toothpaste. Eliminate noxious odors from the environment. Encourage eating with others, in a sitting or dining room. Serve small amounts of food frequently.
Predisposition to peptic ulcer	No incidence of peptic ulcer. Prompt detection and early treatment of peptic ulcer.	Monitor client for epigastric pain and heartburn. Reduce environmental stressors. Assist client to develop coping strategies for managing stress. Report signs and symptoms of peptic ulcer (epigastric pain, weight loss, vomiting, bleeding) promptly to the physician. Consult with physician regarding diet and medication to treat peptic ulcer. Quaiac stools.
Predisposition to constipation	Regular production, preferably daily, of soft or formed, but not hard, stools. Prompt detection of obstipation or impaction.	Encourage fluid intake to the point of moderate overhydration. Administer prune juice daily. Maintain a diet high in bulk. Request an order for a stool softener from the physician. Encourage frequent short walks. Promote maintenance of a regular habit of defecation.
Potential cardiac arrhythmias	No evidence of cardiac arrhythmias on ECG.	Encourage consumption of potassium-rich foods (orange juice, bananas, meats, and coffee). Avoid digital rectal examinations.
Weakened bone structure	Prevention of deformity. Prevention of accidental injury.	Maintain the client in good body alignment. Assist client when ambulating. Reduce safety hazards in the environment.
Altered self-image and emotional depression	Improved self-image and alleviation of depression.	Encourage client to ventilate feelings about physical and emotional changes. Compliment client when appropriate. Reassure client that fatigability and emotional depression will improve when the hormone imbalance is corrected. Encourage short walks to a sitting room or solarium. Ascertain what activities the client has enjoyed in the past; encourage continued involvement in those activities appropriate to the setting and the client's condition. Reduce gray and blue colors in the environment; increase red, orange, and pure tones of yellow.

hormonal mechanism necessary to maintain a normal level of serum calcium and as a result develop hypocalcemia.

Etiology

Causes of primary hypoparathyroidism vary. In idiopathic hypoparathyroidism, a relatively rare disease, destruction of the glands by autoantibodies is speculated. Other causes include severe magnesium deficiency, which impairs PTH secretion and reduces the response of target cells to PTH, congenital absence of the glands, and sex-linked recessive genetic disorders.

Inadvertent damage or removal of the parathyroid glands during neck exploration, particularly during thyroidectomy, is the commonest cause of hypoparathyroidism. Usually, damage to the vascular supply of the glands, rather than direct physical damage to the parathyroids, is the problem.

Hypoparathyroidism must be distinguished from

other causes of hypocalcemia such as an inadequate intake of calcium due to a poor diet or malabsorption.

Clinical manifestations

The clinical features of hypoparathyroidism are due to a low serum calcium (Table 42-8). Sudden decreases in calcium ion concentration give rise to a syndrome called *tetany*. This state is characterized by paresthesias, stiffness of the hands, feet, and lips; dysphagia; painful tonic spasms of smooth and skeletal musculature; carpopedal spasms; constricting feeling in the throat, and laryngospasms.[12] Respiratory function may be severely compromised as a result of spasm of the accessory muscles and obstruction of the airway due to laryngospasm. The lack of calcium ions also causes weak cardiac contractility and predisposes to serious arrhythmias. Tetany requires immediate treatment by intravenous administration of calcium salts.

Medical management

Abnormal laboratory tests include a decreased serum calcium, an increased serum phosphate, and a decreased PTH level. Two other positive signs may be present: *Chvostek's sign* (a spasm of the facial muscles in response to tapping the muscles or the branches of the facial nerve), and *Trousseau's sign* (carpopedal spasm in response to ischemia of the arm caused by compression of the upper part of the extremity) (see Fig. 12-12).

The main objectives of treatment are (1) to prevent tetany and seizures from hypocalcemia, and (2) to prevent long-term complications by keeping serum calcium levels within normal limits.

The symptoms of acute tetany are relieved by intravenous calcium gluconate. Maintenance therapy can include:

1. Oral calcium salts
2. Vitamin D in large doses
3. Low phosphate diet with increased bulk
4. Aluminum hydroxide, e.g., Amphojel, Basaljel (given in the initial stages of treatment to help lower the serum phosphate level)

Pharmacologic intervention

Emergency treatment of acute tetany requires the administration of intravenous calcium. Generally, 10 to 30 mL of a 10% solution of calcium gluconate are given over a 20-to-60-minute period. This measure increases ionic calcium levels in body fluids and relieves the acute symptoms of hypocalcemia. Calcium chloride is not used because it is irritating to the vein and can cause necrosis and sloughing of tissue if infiltration occurs. For chronic hormone deficiency, calcium supplements are administered orally. Calcium gluconate and calcium lactate are preferred to other salts because of their increased solubility.[13]

Vitamin D must be used in chronic and resistant hypocalcemia due to hypoparathyroidism. Hormone replacement is impractical because parathormone, which must be administered parenterally, is both scarce and expensive. In large doses, vitamin D exerts physiologic effects similar to those of parathormone in respect to absorption of calcium and maintenance of blood calcium levels. Vitamin D or calciferol (Drisdal, Geltabs, Deltalen) is the most useful preparation.[14] Dihydrotachysterol is preferable to vitamin D when a more rapid action is required.

Aluminum hydroxide binds phosphate to the intestines, thus preventing its absorption. It should be given near or with meals. The purpose of this drug is to control the hyperphosphatemia characteristic of hypoparathyroidism.

Nursing management

Acute Intervention Nursing care of the hypoparathyroid client demands close observation and assessment for signs of tetany. These are often first seen when taking the blood pressure, as carpopedal spasm (Trousseau's sign) may occur. Periodic assessment for Chvostek's sign is advisable. Irritability, apprehension, muscle fasciculations, or cramps may precede the advent of acute tetany.

Should tetany or generalized muscle cramps develop, the institution of rebreathing may alleviate symptoms somewhat. If clients can cooperate, they are instructed to breathe in and out of a paper bag. This reduces carbon dioxide excretion from the lungs, increases carbonic acid levels in the blood, and lowers body pH. Since both solubility and degree of ionization of calcium is enhanced in acidic environments, the proportion of total body calcium available in physiologically active form is increased, temporarily relieving the functional hypocalcemia. Clients who are incapacitated by muscle spasms may be rebreathed by the nurse. Rebreathing is accomplished by the nurse placing the open end of a plastic or rubber glove over the victim's mouth and nose at the end of exhalation. The glove inflates with exhaled air which is subsequently rebreathed. To maintain adequate oxygen, the glove should be removed every three or four respirations to allow one inhalation of fresh air.

Intravenous calcium gluconate should be readily available for the treatment of acute tetany. Calcium salts must be infused slowly as high blood levels can cause serious cardiac arrhythmias or cardiac arrest. Clients who have been digitalized are particularly vulnerable. Because ventricular standstill occurs in systole, this type of arrest is less likely than others to respond to resuscitation. ECG monitoring is appropriate.

Until clients are asymptomatic they should be kept in a nonstimulating environment, assisted with hygienic needs, and given psychological support and encouragement.

Chronic Management Clients with chronic hypoparathyroidism need instruction in the management of long-term drug therapy. Calcium supplements are best administered with meals, as food helps moderate the alkalinity of the contents of the small intestine. An alkaline environment normally reduces the solubility of calcium and decreases its absorption. Vitamin D should be taken at the same time to further enhance calcium absorption. The signs and symptoms of hypo- and hypercalcemia should be taught, and the client instructed to report these. The need for lifelong treatment and health supervision should be stressed. Periodic serum calcium levels are required, as changes may necessitate modification of the treatment regimen. Even in the absence of acute symptoms, prolonged hypoparathyroidism predisposes to premature graying of the hair and baldness, degeneration of the teeth, and formation of cataracts in the lens of the eye.

ADRENAL GLANDS

Because the adrenal cortex and the adrenal medulla have different embryonic derivations and entirely different functions, they will be addressed separately.

Hyperfunction of the Adrenal Cortex—Cushing's Syndrome

Cushing's syndrome is caused by an excess of corticosteroids, particularly the glucocorticoids. Several disturbances can produce this condition (Table 42-10). Cushing's syndrome can be seen at any age, but naturally occurring disease is most common in the third to sixth decade of life. Females are affected more often than males. Iatrogenic Cushing's syndrome can result from prolonged use of glucocorticoids or ACTH, which are common treatment modalities administered for their anti-inflammatory effect.

Table 42-10
Causes of Cushing's Syndrome

1. Functional hyperplasia of the adrenals caused by high levels of corticotropin secreted by the pituitary in response to prolonged, excessive stress.
2. A corticotropin-secreting pituitary tumor which is not inhibited by high cortisol levels.
3. A cortisol-secreting neoplasm within the adrenal cortex. This neoplasm can either be a carcinoma or an adenoma.
4. Excess secretion of corticotropin or cortisol by a carcinoma of the lung or other malignant growth outside of either the adenohypophysis or the adrenals.
5. Prolonged administration of high doses of corticosteroids.

Clinical manifestations

The normal function of the adrenal cortex is mobilization of body processes to maintain the increased circulation and energy levels required by the body for adaption to stress. The clinical manifestations of Cushing's disease are exaggerations of the physiologic changes caused by the corticosteroids (Table 42-11). The predominant signs and symptoms are those of glucocorticoid excess, although excesses of androgens and mineralocorticoids are apparent in some individuals.

Glucocorticoid excess produces general debility and marked changes in personality and personal appearance (Figs. 42-5 and 42-6). Diabetes mellitus, peptic ulcers, pathologic fractures, kidney stones, or fulminating infections may be present. Catabolic processes predominate over anabolic ones and healing progresses slowly. A manic type psychosis may develop.

The clinical picture as revealed by the history and physical examination is the first indication that Cushing's syndrome may be present. Of particular importance are: (1) A combination of centripetal obesity and protein wasting (osteoporosis, thin, friable skin), (2) osteoporosis before the age of 50, and (3) unprovoked hypokalemia in the presence of tumors.

In children affected by Cushing's syndrome linear growth ceases. Some degree of androgen excess may accompany cortisol overproduction. This may cause pronounced acne in either sex. In women, menstrual irregularities (oligomenorrhea) and hirsutism develop.

Diagnostic study abnormalities

Abnormal findings in diagnostic tests include a high normal sodium, low potassium, and elevated glucose. Elevated granulocyte, low lymphocyte and eosinophil counts, and a high red cell count will be evident from the complete blood count. Glycosuria will be present, and the chest x-ray will demonstrate osteoporosis of the bone.

In addition, there will be increased plasma cortisol levels, plus the loss of the normal diurnal variations of cortisol levels which remain elevated both morning

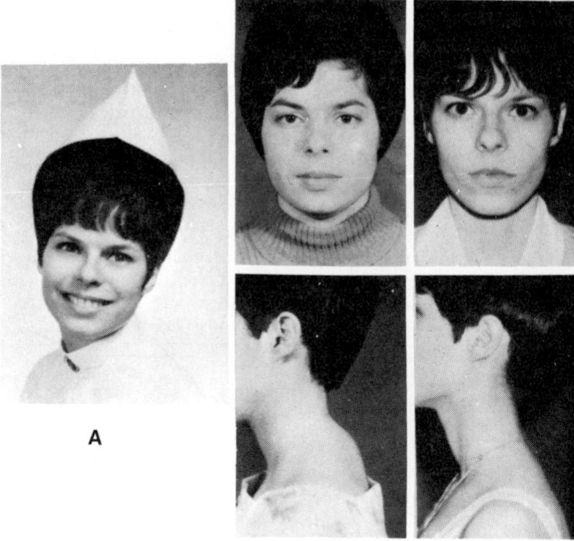

Figure 42-5 A 20-year-old female with Cushing's syndrome due to right adrenal cortical adenoma. *(a)* Two years prior to surgery, age 18. *(b)* One month prior to surgery, age 20. *(c)* One year after surgery. [*From Kurt Isselbacher et al. (eds.), Harrison's Principles of Internal Medicine, 9th ed., McGraw-Hill Book Company, New York, 1980.*]

Table 42-11
Clinical Manifestations of Adrenal Cortex Hormone Dysfunction

System	Hypofunction	Hyperfunction
	Glucocorticoids	
General appearance	Weight loss	Truncal obesity Thin extremities Rounding of the face ("moon face") Fat deposits on back of neck and on shoulders ("buffalo hump")
Skin	If pituitary function is normal: bronzed or smoky hyperpigmentation of the face, neck, hands (especially the creases), buccal membranes, nipples, genitalia, and scars Vitiligo	Thinning of the skin Purplish striae Petechial hemorrhages Bruises Florid cheeks Acne
Cardiovascular	Hypotension Tendency to develop refractory shock	Hypervolemia Hypertension
Gastrointestinal	Anorexia Nausea and vomiting Cramping abdominal pain Diarrhea	Increased secretion of pepsin and hydrochloric acid
Renal		Glycosuria Hypercalcinuria Kidney stones

Table 42-11 (Continued)

System	Hypofunction	Hyperfunction
Musculoskeletal		Muscle wasting Fatigability Osteoporosis Awkward gait
Immune		Inhibition of immune response Suppression of allergy Inhibition of inflammation
Blood	Anemia	Polycythemia Increased coagulability
Fluids and electrolytes	Hyponatremia Dehydration Hyperkalemia	Sodium and water retention Edema Hypokalemia
Metabolic	Hypoglycemia Fatigability	Hyperglycemia Negative nitrogen balance Fatigability
Emotional	Neurasthenia Depression Exhaustion or Irritability Confusion Delusions	Psychic stimulation Euphoria Irritability Mania or Reactive depression Suicidal tendencies
	Mineralocorticoids	
Fluid and electrolytes	Sodium wastage Decreased volume of extracellular fluid Hyperkalemia	Marked sodium and water retention Tendency toward edema Marked hypokalemia
Cardiovascular	Hypovolemia Tendency toward shock Decreased cardiac output Decreased heart size	Hypertension
	Androgens	
Skin	In women, decreased axillary and pubic hair	Hirsutism (male distribution patterns) Acne
Reproductive	No effect in males Decrease libido in females	In women, menstrual irregularities Enlargement of the clitoris
Musculoskeletal	Decrease in size and tone	Increased development

and evening. There is usually no reduction in cortisol levels in response to administration of dexamethasone. Urinary 17-hydroxycorticosteroids are high. 17-Ketosteroids may be low or normal in adrenal adenoma, normal or high in adrenal hyperplasia, and very high in carcinoma. Blood levels of adrenocorticotropic hormone (ACTH) are elevated when a pituitary tumor is present and depressed in adrenal lesions. Abdominal x-rays, intravenous pyelography, and arteriography can help locate adrenal tumors.

Medical management

The management of the syndrome depends upon the etiology. A summary of medical management is given in Table 42-12. The treatment of choice for adrenal adenomas and carcinoma is surgical removal

Table 42-12
Medical Management: Cushing's Syndrome

Diagnostic
1. Complete history and physical examination
2. Plasma cortisol levels for diurnal variations
3. CBC
4. Blood chemistries for sodium, potassium, glucose
5. IVP
6. X-rays of pelvis and spine
7. Dexamethasone suppression test
8. Urinary 17-hydroxycorticosteroids
9. Urinary 17-ketosteroids

Therapeutic
1. Secondary to adrenal adenoma, carcinoma, hyperplasia
   a. Surgical excision of the adrenals
   b. Medical adrenalectomy (metyrapone, *para*—DDD)
2. Secondary to pituitary ACTH hypersecretion
   a. Transphenoidal resection of microadenoma
   b. Radiation
   c Treatment with hypothalamic serotonin antagonist (cyproheptadine)
3. Surgical removal of nonendocrine ACTH-producing tumors
4. Discontinuance or alteration in administration of exogenous corticosteroids

Adapted from Kurt Isselbacher et al. (eds.), *Harrison's Principles of Internal Medicine,* 9th ed., McGraw-Hill Book Company, New York, 1980, p. 1723.

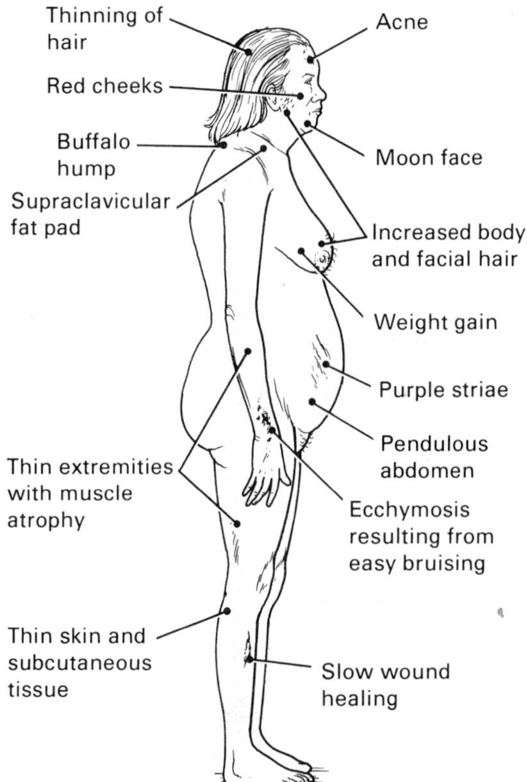

Figure 42-6 Common characteristics of Cushing's syndrome.

of the adrenals. If a pituitary adenoma is demonstrated, a hypophysectomy may be performed.

Clients with nonendocrine tumors that produce excessive amounts of ACTH are usually managed by treating the neoplasm itself. For example, in clients with lung cancer, a pneumonectomy may be done. In inoperable cases, treatment by means of adrenocortical inhibitors have been tried (see the pharmacologic section). The results of these drugs have been variable.

If Cushing's syndrome has developed during the course of prolonged administration of steroids, one or more of the following alternatives may be initiated: (1) discontinuance of the steroid therapy, (2) reduction of the steroid dose, and/or (3) conversion to an alternate-day regimen.

If surgical treatment is not advisable, drug therapy may be used. Mititane (Ortho, Para-DDD) has an unknown mechanism of action but it is thought to inhibit the synthesis of cortisol in the adrenal cortex. Common side effects are gastrointestinal disturbances, lethargy, somnolence, vertigo, skin rashes, and diplopia. It is slow-acting.

Aminoglutethimide (Elipten) was originally used as an anticonvulsant but was found to produce hypocorticoidism. Its action is more rapid than mititane but it has similar side effects.

Nursing management

Acute Intervention The client with Cushing's syndrome is usually seriously ill and debilitated. Nursing care is mainly symptomatic (see Table 42-13). Some helpful interventions include assessment of the client's condition and progress, observing for signs and symptoms of hormone toxicity and complicating conditions such as diabetes mellitus, cardiovascular disease, infection, and pathologic fractures. The nurse should monitor:

1. Signs of severe hypertension and heart failure
2. Daily weight to evaluate edema and obesity
3. Signs and symptoms of infection, especially pain, loss of function and purulent drainage, as other signs and symptoms of inflammation may be minimal or absent
4. Complaints of epigastric pain and hyperacidity
5. Signs of abnormal thromboembolic phenomena
6. Urine glucose and acetone
7. Bone pain or limitation of range of motion, especially in the lower back

Table 42-13
Nursing Care Plan for the Client with Cushing's Syndrome

Client Problem	Expected Outcome	Nursing Intervention
Lowered resistance to infection	Prevention of infection; prompt detection and early treatment of infection. Normal body temperature.	Protect client from exposure to pathogens (maintain meticulous asepsis, prevent contact with contagious individuals). Question the client regarding possible history of tuberculosis or positive tuberculosis test. Consult with the physician regarding the need for a tuberculin test or chest x-ray to screen for latent tuberculosis. If a history indicative of previous contact with the tubercle bacillus is elicited, or tuberculosis test or x-ray is positive, consult with physician regarding antituberculosis medication. Assess client frequently for pain, loss of function, or drainage indicative of infection. Monitor vital signs frequently. Report signs and symptoms of infection promptly to the physician. Administer anti-infective medications when prescribed. Administer applications of heat when ordered. Teach client self-care practices designed to minimize the risk of infection.
Restlessness and insomnia	Decrease in purposeless activity (pacing, repetitive muscle movements). Restful sleep.	Decrease environmental stimuli. Promote continuation of usual rest and sleep practices unless contraindicated. Administer frequent back rubs using effleurage. Encourage maintenance of usual bedtime ritual. Administer sedatives or warm milk as needed (when prescribed). Eliminate caffeine (coffee, tea, cola, and chocolate) from the diet.
Weakness and fatigue	Increased strength and stamina.	Assist client with self-care. Limit ambulation to short walks. Promote rest and relaxation.
Predisposition to accidental injury	No accidental injury.	Assist client as necessary with self-care. Reduce environmental hazards. Assist client when ambulating. Teach client safe practices.
Increased appetite and blunted taste perception	Maintain body weight at, or reduce body weight toward normal.	Control calorie content of the diet. Season food well with herbs or extracts to increase satiety value of the diet. Encourage diversions or activities that the client enjoys to reduce boredom.
Predisposition to hypokalemia	Maintenance of serum potassium levels within normal limits.	Include foods rich in potassium (orange juice, bananas, animal foods) in the diet. Monitor client for signs and symptoms of hypokalemia; if these appear, report promptly to the physician and request an order for potassium supplements.
Predisposition to hypertension and edema	Maintenance of blood pressure within normal limits or reduction of blood pressure toward normal; prevention of edema; prompt detection and early treatment of edema.	Limit sodium content of the diet. Monitor vital signs daily. Assess for edema daily. Weigh daily. Report signs and symptoms of hypertension or edema to the physician promptly. Administer diuretics when prescribed.
Predisposition to hyperglycemia	Maintenance of normal blood sugar.	Provide a diet with controlled levels of calories and carbohydrates. Encourage regular ambulation. Monitor urine glucose and acetone. Administer insulin as ordered.
Predisposition to peptic ulcer	Prevention of peptic ulcer; prompt detection and early treatment of peptic ulcers.	Consult with the physician regarding the need for antacids or prophylactic prescription of cimetidine. Provide a diet high in protein; unless contraindicated feed frequently in small amounts. Monitor client for heartburn and epigastric pain; report these promptly to the physician. Administer antacids or cimetidine as prescribed. Quaiac stools.
Predisposition to pathologic fractures	Prevention of spontaneous fractures; early detection and prompt treatment of fractures.	Provide a diet high in calcium, vitamin D, and protein. Promote weight bearing by encouraging short walks. Monitor client for joint pain, especially low back pain. Report joint pain promptly to the physician. Carry out diagnostic procedures and treatment as ordered.

Table 42-13 (Continued)

Client Problem	Expected Outcome	Nursing Intervention
Alterations in mood (excitation, euphoria, or reactive depression)	Alleviation of excitation or depression.	Select psychological nursing approaches appropriate to the alteration of mood exhibited by the client.
Altered self-image related to the physical, functional, and emotional manifestations of the syndrome	Improved self-image.	Accept and respect the client as a person. Encourage good grooming and attractive attire. Compliment the client when appropriate. Reassure the client that most manifestations of the disease will disappear when the hormone imbalance is corrected.

Clients will need a great deal of emotional support. Changes in appearance can be extremely upsetting. The client may feel unattractive, repulsive, or unwanted. The nurse can help by remaining sensitive to these feelings and offering respect and unconditional acceptance. Clients can be reassured that the physical changes and much of the emotional lability stem from the hormone toxicity and will resolve with a return to normal hormone levels.

Nursing Care Related to Surgical Therapy If treatment involves surgical removal of one or both of the adrenal glands, nursing care will have an additional focus on pre- and postoperative care. Surgery on glandular structures poses risks beyond those of other types of operations. Since glands are highly vascular, there is an increased risk of hemorrhage. Manipulation of glandular tissue during surgery may release large amounts of hormone into the circulation, producing marked fluctuations in the metabolic processes affected by these hormones.

Preoperative management

Before surgery it is essential that the client be brought to optimal medical condition. Nutritional deficiencies of potassium and vitamin C must be corrected. A high protein diet is helpful in correcting the protein depletion caused by excessive glucocorticoid secretion.

Preparation for adrenalectomy involves all the usual measures for clients scheduled for laparotomy. The client should be aware that intravenous infusions and nasogastric suctioning are likely postoperatively. Teaching of exercises, coughing, and deep breathing are particularly important, as these clients are prone to thrombosis and infection. In addition, the abdominal incision will be high in the abdomen, increasing the difficulty in coughing and deep breathing.

Postoperative management

Because of hormone fluctuations, blood pressure, fluid balance, and electrolyte levels tend to be unstable postoperatively. To assure adequate response to the stress of surgery, high doses of cortisone are administered on the day of surgery and several days postoperatively. If large amounts of endogenous hormone have been released into the systemic circulation during surgery, the client is likely to develop hypertension, increasing the risk of hemorrhage. High levels of cortisone also increase the susceptibility to infection and delay healing.

Any rapid or significant changes in blood pressure, respirations, or heart rate should be noted and reported. Fluid intake and output should be monitored carefully and assessed for potential imbalance. The critical period for circulatory instability ranges from 24 to 48 hours postoperatively. Intravenous corticoids are given with the dosage and rate of flow adjusted to the client's clinical manifestations and fluid and electrolyte balance. Oral doses are given as tolerated. The intravenous line may be kept in place after IV corticoids are withdrawn for the purpose of keeping an open line for quick administration of corticoids or vasopressors.

If cortisone dosage is tapered off too rapidly after surgery, corticoid deficiency may develop. Vomiting after the nasogastric tube is removed, increased weakness, dehydration, hypotension, and fever may indicate hypocorticism. These signs and symptoms should be reported so that drug doses may be adjusted. The nurse must constantly be alert for signs of corticoid imbalance in either direction. Following surgery the client is usually maintained on bed rest until the blood pressure stabilizes. The nurse must be alert for subtle signs of infections postoperatively since the usual immune and inflammatory responses are suppressed. Meticulous care must be used when changing the dressing to prevent wound infection.

Chronic nursing management following surgery

The client's discharge instructions are similar to those for clients with Addison's disease. They are to avoid exposure to extremes of temperatures, infections, and emotional disturbances as much as possible. Stress may produce or precipitate acute adrenal insufficiency because the remaining adrenal tissue cannot meet the increased hormonal demands. Many clients can be taught to adjust their corticoid replacement therapy related to their stress level. The nurse should consult with the client's physician to determine the parameters for dosage changes if this plan is feasible. If the client cannot adjust his own medication, or if weakness, fainting, fever, or nausea and vomiting occur, the client should contact his physician for a possible adjustment in corticoid dosage. Lifetime replacement therapy will be required by many clients but it may take several months to adjust the hormonal dose satisfactorily.

Adrenal Cortex—Hypofunction

Hypofunction of the adrenal cortex or adrenocortical insufficiency may be due to (1) bilateral destruction of the adrenal cortex (Addison's disease or primary adrenocortical insufficiency), or (2) lack of ACTH (secondary adrenal cortical insufficiency). In Addison's disease there are reduced levels of all three classes of adrenal steroids: glucocorticoids, mineralocorticoids, and androgens. In secondary hypocortism there is a deficient production of cortisol and of androgens, but rarely of aldosterone, a mineralocorticoid. Deficiency of corticotropin may be due either to pituitary disease or to the suppression of the hypothalamic-pituitary axis by administration of corticosteroids.[15]

Addison's disease—Primary adrenocortical deficiency

Presently the most common cause of Addison's disease is idiopathic atrophy, most likely due to autoimmune disease in which adrenal tissue is destroyed by antibodies formed against the client's own adrenal tissue. Why this happens is unknown, but antibodies to adrenal tissue can be found in most cases of Addison's disease.[16] In the past, tuberculosis was identified as a common cause, but this is now rare. Other less common causes include fungal infections (histoplasmosis), cancer, tumors, and sepsis.[17] Iatrogenic Addison's disease may be caused by anticoagulation therapy causing bilateral adrenal hemorrhage, antineoplastic chemotherapy, or surgical removal of both adrenal glands.

Clinical Manifestations Fatigue, gastrointestinal disturbances (anorexia, nausea, vomiting, weight loss), hypoglycemia, hypotension (with dizziness and fainting), skin pigmentation, and depression are all common characteristics. The most dangerous feature of Addison's disease is the tendency to develop shock, especially when the client is experiencing stress. Circulatory collapse in the hypocorticoid individual is refractory to usual treatment measures (fluid replacement, etc.) and requires the administration of corticoids for stabilization. Skin pigmentation, a striking feature, is due to excessive stimulation of melanocytes by corticotropin and melanocyte-stimulating hormone (MSH). MSH production is stimulated by the same negative feedback loop that stimulates ACTH production. Pigmentation is most prominent in the face, hands (especially in the palmar creases), trunk, buccal membranes, and scar tissue.

Addisonian Crisis Acute adrenal insufficiency or Addisonian crisis is a medical emergency caused by a sudden, marked deprivation or insufficient supply of adrenocortical hormones. It may follow (1) stress (trauma, hemorrhage, surgery, infection, or psychological stress), (2) sudden withdrawal of adrenal cortical hormone replacement, (3) adrenal surgery, or (4) sudden destruction of the pituitary gland.

Severe manifestations of both aldosterone and cortisol deficiencies are exhibited including hypotension, dehydration, cyanosis, confusion, high fever, petechial hemorrhages in the skin and mucosa, hyponatremia, and hyperkalemia. Gastrointestinal signs and symptoms include nausea, vomiting, diarrhea, and abdominal pain.

Diagnostic Study Abnormalities The diagnosis of Addison's disease is made in conjunction with the presence of the clinical features mentioned above, along with low cortisol levels. Other abnormal laboratory findings include hyperkalemia, hypochloremia, hyponatremia, hypoglycemia, and increased BUN. Urinary 17-ketosteroids and 17-hydroxycorticosteroid excretion are low. Failure of cortisol levels to rise in response to corticotropin stimulation indicates primary adrenal disease. A positive response to ACTH points to probable pituitary pathology.

Medical and Pharmacologic Management

Addison's disease (Table 42-14)

The therapy for Addison's disease is steroid replacement. Replacement therapy usually includes a combination of glucocorticoids, mineralocorticoids, and anabolic steroids. Table 42-15 lists some commonly used steroid drugs and their estimated potencies. In mild cases sometimes only cortisone or a combination of cortisone and a mineralocorticoid is

Table 42-14
Medical Management: Addison's Disease

Diagnostic
1. Complete history and physical
2. Plasma cortisol level
3. ACTH stimulation test
4. Serum electrolytes
5. Urinary 17-hydrocorticosteroids
6. ECG

Therapeutic
1. Daily cortisone placement (two-thirds in A.M., one-third in P.M.)*
2. Fluorohydrocortisone daily in P.M.*
3. High-carbohydrate, high-protein, high-sodium diet

*For conditions of normal stress in individuals with usual daytime activity.

adequate. The glucocorticoid dosage is usually divided: two-thirds of the dose is given in the morning and one-third in the afternoon. The mineralocorticoid is given once a day, preferably in the evening. This dosage schedule reflects the normal daily variations in hormone secretion. With the onset of any illness, mild or acute, or the occurrence of any stress (trauma, surgery, etc.), glucocorticoid dosage must be increased to prevent adrenal crisis. If the client takes his medications daily, he can anticipate a normal, active life.

Acute adrenocortical insufficiency

Management of acute adrenocortical insufficiency requires immediate replacement therapy. Treatment must be vigorous and directed toward the management of shock. Intravenous hydrocortisone, sodium, fluids, plasma, vasopressors, and oxygen may be initiated immediately and continued as needed. If infection is present, anti-infectives are also prescribed.

Table 42-15
Estimated Potencies of Corticosteroid Preparations*

Corticosteroid Preparation	Relative to Anti-Inflammatory Activity	Relative to Sodium-Retaining Activity
Short-acting (< 12 hours)		
Hydrocortisone (Hydrocortone)	1	1
Cortisone (Cortone)	0.8	0.8
Intermediate-acting (18–36 hours)		
Prednisone (Deltasone)	4	0.3
Prednisolone (Delta-Cortef)	4	0.3
Triamcinolone (Aristocort/Kenacort)	5	0
Methylprednisolone Medrol	5	0
Long-acting (> 48 hours)		
Betamethasone (Celestone)	25	0
Dexamethasone (Decadron)	30	0
Aldosterone replacement		
Fluorocortisone (Florinef)	10	250

For purpose of comparison, potencies are reported in milligrams and cortisol is used as the standard, with its glucocorticoid and mineralocorticoid properties set as 1 mg.

From Pamela Miller Gotch, "Teaching Patients About Adrenal Corticosteroids," *Am J Nurs*, **81**(1): 80 (January 1981).

Nursing management

Acute Intervention

Management of an adrenal crisis involves those emergency measures appropriate to combat shock as mentioned under the section on medical management. In addition, the following ongoing care should be included in the nursing care plan: regular checking of vital signs, diligent administration of steroids, protection against exposure to infections, assisting with hygiene measures until less fatigued, daily weights, and observation for any signs of electrolyte imbalance. Excessive treatment (intravenous fluids and corticosteroids) may lead to generalized edema, potassium depletion, hypertension, and mental disturbances. Constant observation must be maintained until the client is well out of danger.

When the client is able to take food by mouth, oral cortisone is usually begun. High initial dosages are gradually reduced until maintenance levels are met.

Chronic management

The nurse has an important role in the chronic management of Addison's disease. Because of the serious nature of the disease and the need for lifelong replacement therapy, a well-organized and carefully executed teaching plan is vital to the health of the client. Table 42-16 outlines the major areas which must be included in the teaching plan. The nurse should consult with the client's physician to determine if any special problems or topics need to be included in the plan.

Since the client with Addison's disease is unable to tolerate physical or emotional stress, long-term care revolves around recognizing the need for additional replacement medication and stress management techniques. The client who can control or manage the degree of stress experienced will maintain better hormone balance than one who cannot. The nurse should assist clients to develop good coping skills and techniques for handling stress.

The hormone-deficient client receiving glucocorticoid replacement is less apt to exhibit toxic symptoms from the medication than the client receiving pharmacologic doses of the drugs. Since the aim of replacement therapy is return to normal hormone levels, nursing care is designed to assist the client to maintain hormone balance and manage the medication regimen.

Dosage schedules are designed to mimic the diurnal rhythm of endogenous glucocorticoid production. Two-thirds of the daily dose should be taken upon arising at the beginning of the day. The remaining one-third is taken about 8 hours later. Since glucocorticoids are stimulating to the central nervous system, they cause insomnia if taken late in the day. The need for glucocorticoid hormone is proportional to stress levels. Clients unable to produce endogenous hormone must adjust the dosage of exogenous hormone to stress level. Dosages are usually doubled when minor stress occurs (e.g., a respiratory infection, or a visit to the dentist) and tripled when major stress occurs.

The client must be taught the signs and symptoms of glucocorticoid deficiency and excess. These should be reported to the physician so that dosages may be adjusted to the client's need. It is also important that the client wear an identification band stating that he has Addison's disease, so that appropriate therapy can be initiated should a crisis occur.

Table 42-16

Major Teaching Areas for the Client with Addison's Disease

1. Names and doses of drugs.
2. Effects and actions of drugs.
3. Symptoms of overdosage and underdosage.
4. Conditions requiring increased medication (trauma, infection, surgery, emotional crisis).
5. Course of action to take relative to 3 and 4 above.
   a. Increase dose of glucocorticoid.
   b. Administer large dose of glucocorticoid parenterally.
   c. Consult with physician.
6. Prevention of infection and need for prompt and vigorous treatment of existing infections.
7. Need for lifelong replacement therapy.
8. Need for lifelong medical supervision.
9. Diet high in sodium, carbohydrates, and protein.
10. Need for medical identification device.

Glucocorticoid therapy

Cortisone and related glucocorticoids are used to relieve the signs and symptoms associated with many disease processes (Table 42-17). The chronic administration of glucocorticoids in therapeutic doses often leads to serious complications and side effects from toxicity. For this reason glucocorticoid therapy is not recommended for minor conditions which are chronic in nature. Rather, it should be reserved for diseases in which there is a risk of death or permanent loss of function, and conditions in which short-term therapy is likely to produce remission or recovery. The potential benefits of treatment must always be weighed against the risks.

Effects of Glucocorticoids The therapeutic actions of glucocorticoids are many and include:

Table 42-17
Therapeutic Uses of Glucocorticoids

Replacement therapy
Acute adrenal insufficiency
Chronic adrenal insufficiency
Congenital adrenal hyperplasia
Adrenal insufficiency secondary to anterior pituitary insufficiency

Arthritis
Rheumatoid arthritis
Osteoarthritis

Rheumatic carditis

Renal disease
Nephrotic syndrome

Collagen diseases
Polymyositis
Polyarteritis nodosa
Granulomatous-polyarteritis group
Systemic lupus erythematosus

Allergic diseases
Hay fever
Serum sickness
Urticaria
Contact dermatitis
Drug reactions
Anaphylaxis
Angioneurotic edema

Bronchial asthma
Status asthmaticus
Severe chronic bronchial asthma

Ocular disease
Used to reduce inflammation in the eye

Skin diseases

Diseases of the intestinal tract
Celiac sprue
Chronic ulcerative colitis

Cerebral edema and increased intracranial pressure

Malignancies

Diseases of the liver
Subacute hepatic necrosis
Chronic active hepatitis
Alcoholic hepatitis

Shock

From M. Wiener et al., *Clinical Pharmacology and Therapeutics in Nursing,* McGraw-Hill Book Company, New York, 1979, p. 521.

1. *Anti-inflammatory action* They stabilize lysosomal membranes, thus inhibiting release of proteolytic enzymes during inflammation, and prevent or suppress redness, swelling, tenderness, heat, and local edema.
2. *Immunosuppression* They cause atrophy of lymphoid tissue and decrease production of eosinophils, lymphocytes, and antibodies.
3. *Maintenance of normal blood pressure* They potentiate the vasoconstrictor effect of norepinephrine and act on the renal tubule to increase sodium reabsorption and enhance potassium and hydrogen excretion. Retention of sodium (and subsequently water) increases blood volume and helps maintain blood pressure.
4. *Carbohydrate and protein metabolic effect* They increase blood levels of glucose and facilitate breakdown of protein; increase the activity of enzymes necessary for gluconeogenesis and inhibit glycolytic enzymes; can result in hyperglycemia, glycosuria, and delayed wound healing; and mobilize and redistribute fat in Cushingoid patterns.
5. *Stress effect* They replace normal stress response of release of corticosteroids to support blood pressure and increase blood sugar in the client with decreased adrenal function.

Complications of Glucocorticoid Therapy Both beneficial and toxic effects of the glucocorticoids stem from their physiologic actions. What is beneficial in one situation may be harmful in another. Thus, the hypertensive effect of the hormone is critical in enabling the organism to function in stressful situations but can produce hypertension when the substance is used for drug therapy. Inhibition of cell division is therapeutic and sometimes curative in the treatment of malignancies, but it slows healing following trauma or surgery. Suppression of inflammation and the immune response may help save the life of the victim of anaphylaxis and the transplant recipient, but it causes reactivation of latent tuberculosis and greatly reduces resistance to other infections. Specific side effects related to glucocorticoid therapy are listed in Table 42-18.

In order to minimize the side effects of chronic glucocorticoid therapy the following are recommended:

1. Avoid using glucocorticoid therapy for palliation of non-life-threatening chronic disease (such as arthritis).
2. Use the smallest dose that will obtain the desired therapeutic effect.
3. Administer steroids every other day (alternate-day rotation) to allow some ACTH secretion to avoid adrenal gland atrophy.
4. Gradually reduce steroid dose before its discontinuance.
5. In emergency situations, administer a single parenteral dose, as this is relatively void of side effects.

Table 42-18
Side Effects of Glucocorticoid Therapy

1. Increased susceptibility to infection: Infection develops more rapidly and spreads more widely in the cushingoid individual.
2. Increased blood pressure due to increased blood volume and potentiation of vasoconstrictor effects. Hypertension in turn predisposes to cardiac failure.
3. Diabetes mellitus: Impaired glucose metabolism affects more than 90% of cushingoid individuals.
4. Osteoporosis: Protein depletion decreases bone density and strength and predisposes to pathologic fractures, especially compression fractures of the vertebrae.
5. Peptic ulcer: Decreased mucus production predisposes to stomach and duodenal ulceration.
6. Delayed healing: Clients undergoing surgery are at increased risk for dehiscence and evisceration.
7. Hypokalemia: Potassium supplements may be indicated.
8. Skeletal muscle atrophy: Muscle weakness predisposes to accidental injury.
9. Suppression of pituitary ACTH synthesis: Glucocorticoid deficiency is likely if hormones are withdrawn abruptly.

Nursing Care of the Client Receiving Glucocorticoid Therapy Many clients receive glucocorticoid therapy for problems not related to hormone deficiency. Although drugs in current use have been modified in an attempt to reduce side effects without impairing therapeutic response, the client still needs careful instructions when taking corticosteroids. To reduce complications related to glucocorticoid therapy, the nurse should:

1. Recommend a diet high in protein and potassium but low in concentrated simple carbohydrates.
2. Instruct clients in measures to promote rest and sleep.
3. Monitor vital signs; if blood pressure rises or edema occurs recommend restriction of sodium intake.
4. Monitor urine for glucose and refer to the physician for evaluation of glucose metabolism if glycosuria occurs.
5. Assess for heartburn or epigastric pain. Refer to physician for antacid or cimetidine treatment should signs or symptoms of peptic ulcer occur.
6. Teach the client safety practices to prevent accidental injury.
7. Teach the client to avoid infection and report signs and symptoms of infection promptly.
8. Reassure the client that changes in appearance and mood characteristic of Cushing's syndrome are temporary effects of high hormone levels and will resolve when drug therapy is discontinued.
9. Warn the clients against missing doses or discontinuing drug therapy; acute deficiency of glucocorticoids is likely to follow because of suppressed secretion of corticotropin.

Disorders of Aldosterone Secretion

Primary aldosteronism

Although an excessive production of aldosterone occurs rarely, it can be life-threatening if untreated. It is more common in women and the usual age of onset is between 30 and 50 years of age. Primary aldosteronism is caused by excessive aldosterone secretion by an adrenal adenoma (80 to 85 percent) or by bilateral adrenal hyperplasia (15 to 20 percent). The main effect of aldosterone is to retain sodium and to excrete potassium.

The most striking features are the retention of sodium and excessive loss of potassium through the urine. The sodium retention leads to hypertension, cardiac enlargement, and headaches. The low potassium causes generalized muscle weakness, cardiac arrthymias, polyuria, and metabolic alkalosis. Edema does not usually occur because the elevated blood pressure increases the glomerular filtration rate.

Hypertension with hypokalemia is the hallmark of primary aldosteronism. Once the diagnosis is suspected, it can be confirmed by measuring (1) plasma aldosterone, (2) urinary potassium excretion, and (3) renin concentration. The first two tests will be elevated and the latter suppressed.

Management Treatment consists of surgical removal of the adenoma. Prior to surgery the hypertension and hypokalemia can be treated with spironolactone (Aldactone), potassium supplements, and sodium restriction. Persons with bilateral hyperplasia are usually treated medically unless the hypokalemia is symptomatic. Bilateral adrenalectomy is usually not successful in controlling the associated hypertension.

Nursing care includes monitoring the blood pressure, cardiovascular status, signs of hypokalemia, fluid and electrolyte balance, and preparing the client for surgery.

Clients receiving maintenance drug therapy with spironolactone need instruction regarding the drug's side effects and signs and symptoms of hypo- and hyperaldosteronism. Clients should learn to monitor their own blood pressures, and do so regularly. The need for continued health supervision should be stressed.

Secondary aldosteronism

Secondary aldosteronism is usually found in edematous states such as congestive heart failure, hepatic cirrhosis, and nephrosis. Some persons have peripheral edema, which can be a distinguishing feature between primary and secondary aldosteronism. In addition to treatment of the primary condition, spironalactone or dyrenium is prescribed to alleviate the toxic effects of high aldosterone levels.

Andrenogenital syndrome

In normal subjects the adrenals produce small amounts of androgens. Overproduction of these androgens is called andrenogenital syndrome. This can be caused by both tumors and adrenal hyperplasia which can be secondary to glucocorticoid insufficiency. Symptoms can begin manifesting themselves any time from infancy to early adult life. As a result, males show evidence of precocious sexual development and females show signs of masculinization and menstrual irregularities.

Urinary 17-ketosteroid determination is the most important single test in the diagnosis. Very high levels are assoicated with adrenal tumors. Treatment can involve removal of the tumor, irradiation, or treatment by corticosteroids.

Disorders of the Adrenal Medulla—Pheochromocytoma

Disorders of the adrenal medulla are rare. There are no specific diseases caused by insufficiency of the adrenal medulla. The most common disorder occurs in the form of a neoplasm known as pheochromocytoma, which produces an excessive amount of epinephrine and norepinephrine. Most of these tumors are benign and encapsulated. Pheochromocytoma can occur at any age or sex but it is found most commonly between the ages of 40 to 60.

The most striking clinical features are hypertension, hypermetabolism, and hyperglycemia. The hypertension can be paroxysmal and sustained. Attacks of paroxysmal hypertension are due to sympathetic nervous system stimulation and are usually associated with stress, fear, palpitations, and profuse sweating. The duration of the attacks may vary from a few minutes to several hours. Additional symptoms may be throbbing severe headaches, vasomotor changes (pallor, flushing of the face, pupil dilation), and visual blurring.

Management

Measurement of urinary metanephrines is the simplest and most reliable test. Values are elevated in at least 90 percent of persons with pheochromocytoma. Urinary vanillylmandelic acid (VMA) determination is also helpful. VMA is a major metabolite of epinephrine. In cases of pheochromocytoma it is produced in excess.

Treatment is surgical removal of the tumor. Although rare, this is one of the few conditions in which dangerously high blood pressure can be corrected surgically.

Case finding is an important nursing function. Any client with hypertension accompanied with symptoms of sympathoadrenal discharge should be referred for definitive diagnosis.

Prior to surgery, the client is hospitalized for treatment to correct pathologic symptoms and decrease the risk of surgery. Sympathetic blocking agents are administered to reduce the blood pressure and alleviate the other symptoms of catecholamine excess. Clients need rest, nourishing food, and emotional support during this period. Pre- and postoperative care is similar to that for any clients undergoing adrenalectomy except that blood pressure fluctuations due to catecholamine imbalances tend to be severe.

Case Study / **Graves' Disease**

Jane M., a 45-year-old secretary, saw her physician with complaints of weight loss, hair loss, weakness, and nervousness. Following a complete endocrine workup, Jane was diagnosed as having Graves' disease. She was started on propylthiouracil and a thyroidectomy was planned for 3 months time.

Discussion Questions

What caused the symptoms Jane experienced?

1. What tests were probably done to establish the diagnosis of Graves' disease? What were the probable results?
2. Explain the drug therapy prescribed for Jane.
3. Explain the preoperative and postoperative learning needs of this client.
4. Discuss the chronic management of this client following a thyroidectomy.

REVIEW QUESTIONS

The number of the question corresponds to the same numbered objective at the beginning of the chapter.

1. The client with acromegaly would demonstrate all the following *except*
   a. hypoglycemia
   b. dental abnormalities
   c. abdominal distension
   d. visual changes

2. Clients who have experienced intracranial surgery or head trauma are more likely than clients with other types of surgery or trauma to develop
   a. diabetes mellitus
   b. hyperthyroidism
   c. Cushing's syndrome
   d. SIADH

3. A good position for the postoperative thyroidectomy client to assume is
   a. low or semi-Fowler's position, with head and shoulders supported
   b. on his side, bed flat with one pillow under his head
   c. head of bed raised, small pillow behind neck
   d. on his side, bed flat, no pillow

4. If the parathyroid glands are removed accidentally during neck surgery, the client could develop
   a. kidney stones
   b. difficulty in swallowing
   c. thyroid crisis
   d. tetany

5. An important nursing intervention when caring for a client with Cushing's syndrome is to
   a. administer steroids in equal doses
   b. protect the client from exposure to infection
   c. restrict protein intake
   d. observe for signs of hypotension

6. Following adrenalectomy for pheochromocytoma, the client is most apt to experience
   a. hyperglycemia
   b. marked sodium and water retention
   c. hypokalemia
   d. marked fluctuations in blood pressure

7. The best time to take cortisone for replacement purposes is
   a. every other day, upon awakening
   b. regularly, by the clock, at 6- or 8-hour intervals
   c. on arising and about halfway through the day
   d. once a day, at bedtime

8. The side effects of steroid therapy include all the following *except*
   a. Cushingoid appearance
   b. peptic ulcers
   c. insomnia
   d. hypoglycemia

9. Which of the following symptoms experienced by the client on glucocorticoid therapy should be reported to the health care provider immediately?
   a. low back pain
   b. a reduction in blood pressure
   c. abdominal cramping
   d. "moon face"

REFERENCES

1. J. M. Iacono, et al., "Pilot Epidemiological Studies in Thrombosis," *Advances in Experimental Medicine and Biology,* vol. 10, 1978, pp 309–333.
2. Caroline Camuñas, "Transphenoidal Hypophysectomy," *Am J Nurs,* **80**(10):1822 (October 1980).
3. Bernice Muir, *Pathophysiology: An Introduction to the Mechanism of Disease,* John Wiley & Sons, Inc., New York, 1980, p. 345.
4. Kurt Isselbacher et al. (eds.), *Harrison's Principles of Internal Medicine,* 9th ed., McGraw-Hill Book Company, New York, 1980, p. 1691.
5. Ibid., p. 1692.
6. Monte Greer, "Hyperthyroidism," in Howard F. Conn (ed.), *Current Therapy Nineteen Eighty,* W. B. Saunders Company, Philadelphia, 1980, p. 469.
7. W. Jubiz, *Endocrinology: A Logical Approach for Clinicians,* McGraw-Hill Book Company, New York, 1979, p. 50.
8. Kenneth Sterling, "Hypothyroidism," in Howard F. Conn (ed.), *Current Therapy Nineteen Eighty,* W. B. Saunders Company, Philadelphia, 1980, p. 501.
9. P. Beeson and W. McDermott, *Textbook of Medicine,* 14th ed., W. B. Saunders Company, Philadelphia, 1975, p. 1809.
10. Foster Tah Hsiumg Giraud, "Hyperparathyroidism," in Howard F. Conn and Rex B. Conn (eds.), *Current Diagnosis Six,* W. B. Saunders Company, Philadelphia, 1980, p. 754.
11. T. Doresio, "Hypercalcemic Crisis," *Heart Lung,* **7**:425 (1978).
12. J. Krueger and R. Comptom, *Endocrine Problems in Nursing—A Physiologic Approach,* The C. V. Mosby Company, St. Louis, 1976, p. 125.
13. M. Krupp and M. Chatton, *Current Medical Diagnosis and Treatment,* Lange Medical Publishers, Cal. 1978, p. 701.
14. Giraud, op. cit., p. 754.
15. Patrick Mulrow, "Adrenocortical Insufficiency," in Howard F. Conn (ed.), *Current Therapy Nineteen Eighty, 33 W. B. Saunders Company, Philadelphia, 1980, p. 480.*
16. Jubiz, op. cit., p. 94.
17. M. Tzagournis, "Acute Adrenal Insufficiency," *Heart Lung,* **7**:587 (1978).

Chapter 43

NURSING ASSESSMENT

Reproductive System

Kathy Marquis

Learning Objectives

1. Describe the structures and functions of the male and female reproductive systems.
2. Explain the functions of the major hormones essential to the structural and functional integrity of the male and female reproductive systems.
3. Describe the physiologic and psychological changes of the male and female during the stages of sexual excitement.
4. Identify the significant subjective and objective data related to the male or female reproductive systems and sexual function that should be obtained from a client.
5. Describe the appropriate noninvasive techniques used in physical assessment of the male and female reproductive systems.
6. Differentiate normal from common abnormal findings of a physical assessment of the male and female reproductive systems.
7. Describe the purpose, significance of results, and nursing responsibilities of diagnostic studies of the male and female reproductive systems.

Accurate assessment of the male and female reproductive system is dependent upon a basic understanding of (1) the structure and function of the organs of reproduction, (2) the hypothalamic-pituitary-gonadal axis, (3) the genitourinary system, and (4) the biopsychosocial aspects of sex and sexuality.

MALE AND FEMALE REPRODUCTIVE SYSTEMS: STRUCTURES AND FUNCTIONS

While the physiology of the reproductive system is interrelated with the neuroendocrine system, it must also be discussed from the perspective of being a unique entity itself. First, the reproductive system, like other body systems, is subject to specific physical stresses and illnesses such as choriocarcinoma and hydroceles. Secondly, the reproductive system is responsible for one of the most important functions of all species, the assured continuation of that species through the process of fertilization, pregnancy, and the birth of a new life. Thirdly, the functioning and use of the human reproductive system is intricately interwoven into the complex, highly sensitive, and frequently stress-laden psychosocial mores and values about sex and sexuality. The attention given to human reproduction, sex, and sexuality in our laws, our religions, and our medical and health care texts is sufficient to illustrate the need to study the reproductive system as a distinct though interrelated entity within the person.

This chapter was reviewed by Steve Toussaint, R. N., M. S. N., Instructor, School of Nursing, University of Oregon Health Sciences Center, Portland, Oregon.

Male Reproductive System

Structures

The male reproductive system consists of the external structures—the penis and scrotum—and the internal structures such as the prostate gland, seminal vesicles, and essential linking ducts (Fig. 43-1). The *scrotum* lies within the scrotal sac which is a thin, loose outer layer of skin over a more muscular internal layer. The scrotum is divided by a septum into two halves, each of which contains a *testis*, epididymis, and spermatic cord. The testis is an ovoid, smooth, firm organ measuring 2 to 2.5 cm in depth and 2 to 3 cm in width. Within the testis are the *seminiferous tubules*, where spermatozoa are formed at a rate of 10 to 30 billion per month.[1] The tubules lead into a system of numerous small ducts, which itself conducts them to the *epididymis*. This organ may be considered a large duct. It stores the spermatozoa while they mature and until they are released by ejaculation or until they disintegrate and are reabsorbed by the body (Fig. 43-2).

The epididymis is a soft cordlike structure which measures close to 20 feet in length if stretched out. It lies in the anterior plane and along the posterolateral surface of each testis. The *ductus deferens* extends from the epididymis to a point close to the prostate gland, where it becomes the *ejaculatory duct* and enters the urethra. The duct system emerging from each testis in this way conveys sperm into the urethra.

The spermatic cord contains not only the ductus deferens but also the arteries, veins, and lymph vessels that supply the testis and epididymis. All these are enclosed by the cremaster muscle and by layers of fascia. The cord enters into the inguinal canal

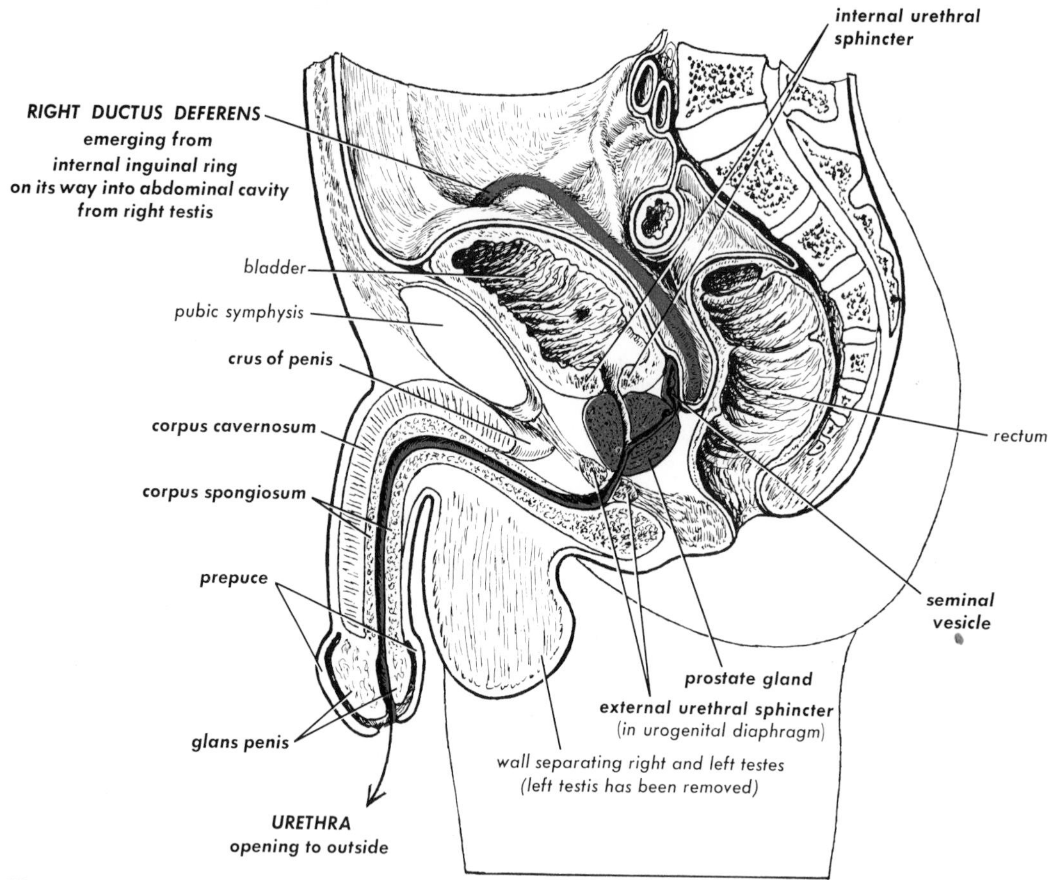

Figure 43-1 Basic structures of the male reproductive system. (*From E. Reith, B. Breidenbach, and M. Lorenc, Textbook of Anatomy, and Physiology, 2d ed., McGraw-Hill Book Company, New York, 1978.*)

through the external inguinal ring. Here the cord ends and its components, primarily the ductus deferens, continue the backward course.

The *prostate, seminal vesicles, and Cowper's (bulbourethral) glands* comprise the accessory glands of the male reproductive system. These glands produce and secrete the seminal fluid, which is a medium and vehicle for sperm. The *prostate gland* is located below the bladder. Its posterior surface approximates the rectal wall. The normal prostate measures 2 × 3 cm and is divided into right and left lateral lobes and an anterior/posterior median lobe. The *seminal vesicles* lie just behind the bladder and between the rectum and bladder. The ducts of the seminal vesicles fuse with the ductus deferens to form the ejaculatory ducts which enter into the prostate gland. *Cowper's glands* lie on each side of the urethra and slightly posterior to it at a point just below the prostate. The ducts of these glands enter directly into the urethra. The secretion from the prostate comprises the largest amount of ejaculate fluid. In comparison, the seminal vesicles and Cowper's glands provide a minimal amount of fluid to the ejaculate. Figure 43-2 follows the route of spermatozoa from production to ejaculation.

The urethra extends from the bladder, through the prostate, and ends in a slitlike opening (meatus) on the ventral side of the *glans*, the terminal portion of the penis. The glans is covered by a fold of skin, the prepuce (or foreskin), which forms at the junction of the glans and shaft of the penis. The broadened segment of the glans at the junction is the *corona*. The prepuce may be absent in the circumcised male. The shaft of the penis consists of (1) the erectile tissue, the corpus cavernosa and corpus spongiosum; (2) the fibrous sheath which encases the erectile tissue; and

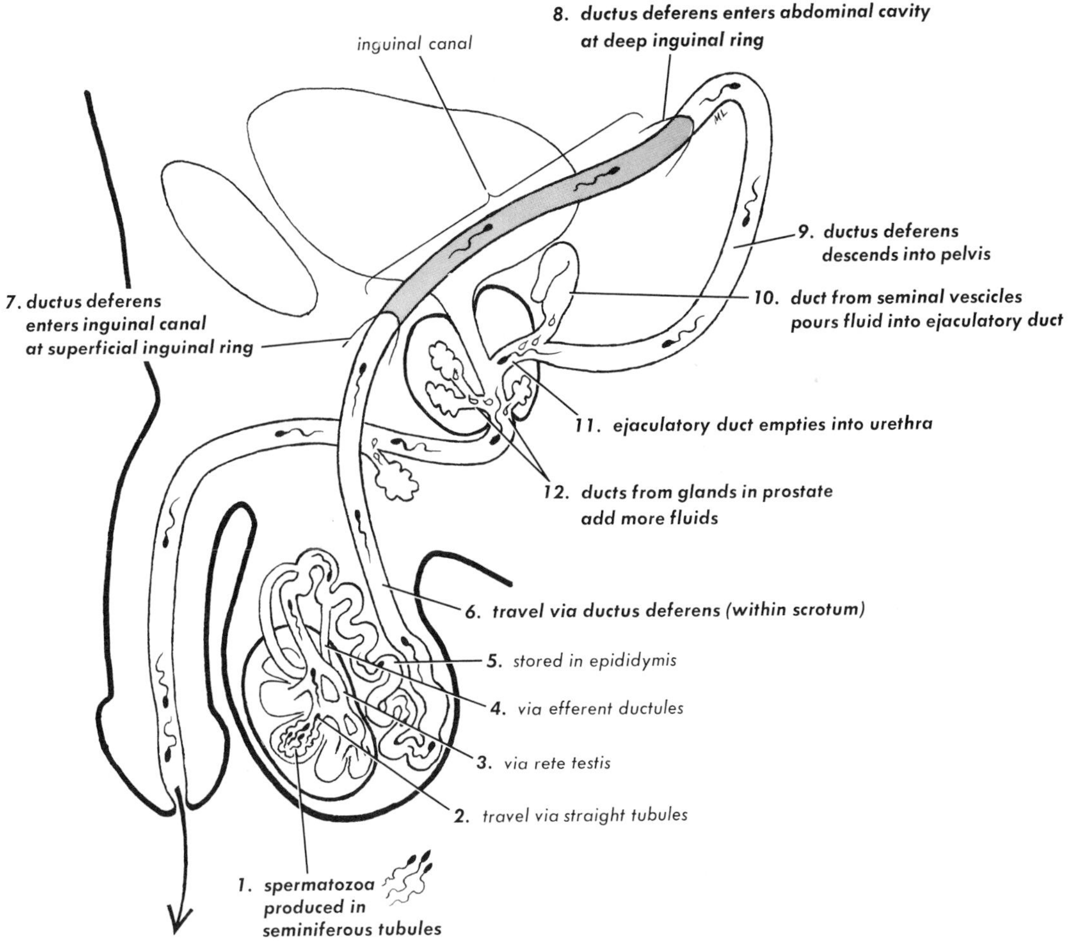
8. ductus deferens enters abdominal cavity at deep inguinal ring
inguinal canal
9. ductus deferens descends into pelvis
7. ductus deferens enters inguinal canal at superficial inguinal ring
10. duct from seminal vescicles pours fluid into ejaculatory duct
11. ejaculatory duct empties into urethra
12. ducts from glands in prostate add more fluids
6. travel via ductus deferens (within scrotum)
5. stored in epididymis
4. via efferent ductules
3. via rete testis
2. travel via straight tubules
1. spermatozoa produced in seminiferous tubules
13. spermatozoa reach exterior via urethra in penis
Route of spermatozoa.

Figure 43-2 Route of spermatozoa. *(From E. Reith, B. Breidenbach, and M. Lorenc, Textbook of Anatomy and Physiology, 2d ed., McGraw-Hill Book Company, New York, 1978.)*

(3) the urethra. The skin covering the penis is thin, loose, and essentially hairless.

Female Reproductive System

The female reproductive system consists of the breasts, uterus, ovaries, fallopian tubes, vagina, and the external genitalia (the vulva). The breasts are generally included in the discussion of the reproductive system because they are a secondary sex characteristic which develop during puberty in response to estrogen. The breasts prepare monthly for lactation following pregnancy should fertilization occur. Also, they are considered a major organ of sexual stimulation and response.

Structure and function of the breasts

The breasts extend from the second to the sixth ribs, with the tail of breast tissue reaching the axilla (Fig. 43-3). The fully mature breast is dome-shaped and contains a pigmented center called the *areola*. The *areolar region* contains *Montgomery's tubercles*, which are sebaceous like glands believed to assist in moistening the nipple. The *nipple* itself contains 15 to 20 minute openings which lead into ducts leading to the *lactiferous sinuses* where milk is stored during periods of lactation. From the lactiferous sinuses, ducts continue extending and branching (secondary tubules) outward, eventually ending in lobules called alveoli or acini of the breasts. The *alveoli* are the

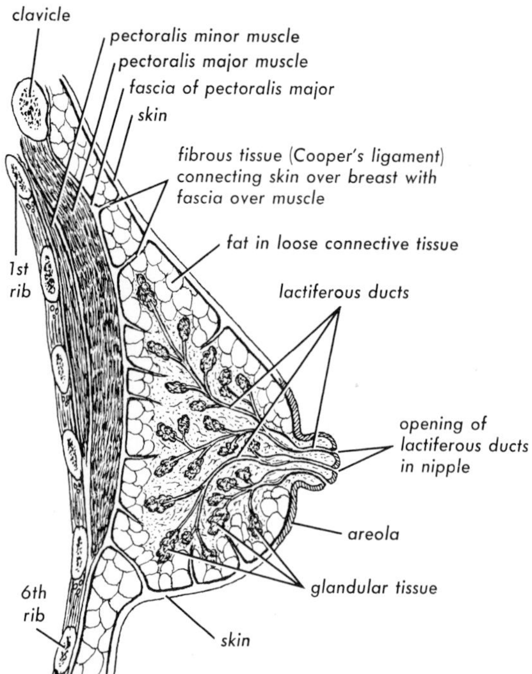

Figure 43-3 The mammary gland. (*From E. Reith, B. Breidenbach, and M. Lorenc, Textbook of Anatomy and Physiology, 2d ed., McGraw-Hill Book Company, New York, 1978.*)

structures which actually secrete milk during the period of lactation.* The breast also has a rich lymphatic network which drains primarily into the axillary, infraclavicular, and supraclavicular channels. It is this rich lymphatic system that is implicated in breast cancer.

The fibrous and fatty tissue which supports and separates the channels of the mammary duct system is primarily responsible for the varying size and shape of the breasts of different individuals. Hence, the importance placed on breast size in western culture is psychosocial rather than functional.

Structure and function of the female pelvic organs

The *ovaries* are usually located on either side of the uterus just behind and below the uterine (fallopian) tubes (Fig. 43-4). They are firm, solid bodies averaging 1.5 × 3 × 2 cm in the mature female. The ovaries carry out the major reproductive functions of the female, i.e., ovulation and hormonal secretions (estrogen and progesterone). The outer zone of the ovary contains approximately 200,000 to 400,000 ovarian follicles in various states of development.[2]

Each follicle contains an immature or primordial ovum which is surrounded by granulosa and theca cells of the follicle. These two layers are responsible for the protection and nourishment of the ovum until follicular maturity is reached and ovulation occurs through the stimulus of the gonadotropic hormones, follicle-stimulating hormone (FSH), and luteinizing hormone (LH).

The *uterine* or *fallopian tubes*, which average about 12 cm in length, extend out from the superior lateral borders of the uterus. It is within the tubes that fertilization usually takes place.

The *uterus* is a pear-shaped, hollow muscular organ consisting of three parts: the fundus, body, and cervix (Fig. 43-4). It is located between the bladder and the rectum. In the mature nulliparous (never pregnant) female the uterus measures approximately 6 cm in length and 4 cm in width. The body forms about 80 percent of the uterus and connects with the cervix at the isthmus. The walls of the uterus are composed of an outer or *serosal* layer; a middle muscular layer, the *myometrium*; and an inner muscosal layer, the *endometrium*.

The *cervix* is the lower portion of the uterus that invaginates into the anterior wall of the vaginal canal. It comprises about 15 to 20 percent of the uterus in the nulliparous female. The columnar epithelium of the cervix, under hormonal influence, provides enough elasticity at labor to stretch sufficiently for the fetus to exit. Otherwise the cervical canal is 2 to 4 cm long and relatively tightly closed. The major function of the cervix is as a passageway (1) to allow sperm entrance into the uterus, and (2) to allow the menses and/or products of conception out.

It should also be noted that sperm entrance into the uterus is facilitated by mucus produced by the cervix under the influence of estrogen. Postovulatory cervical mucus, due to the influence of progesterone, is thick and tenacious and inhibits sperm passage. Knowledge of these physiologic changes are used in natural (noncontraceptive) family planning approaches.

The anterior and posterior peritoneal covering of the uterus is called the *broad ligament*. It separates the uterus from the bladder and rectum. It does not provide any real support for the uterus or adnexa (ovaries and tubes). The *cardinal ligaments* which extend from the isthmus of the uterus to the pelvic wall also offer only minimal support. The *round ligament* which extends anteriorly to the labia majora provides some support but is easily weakened by pregnancy.

*The reader is referred to maternity texts for discussion of breast changes during pregnancy.

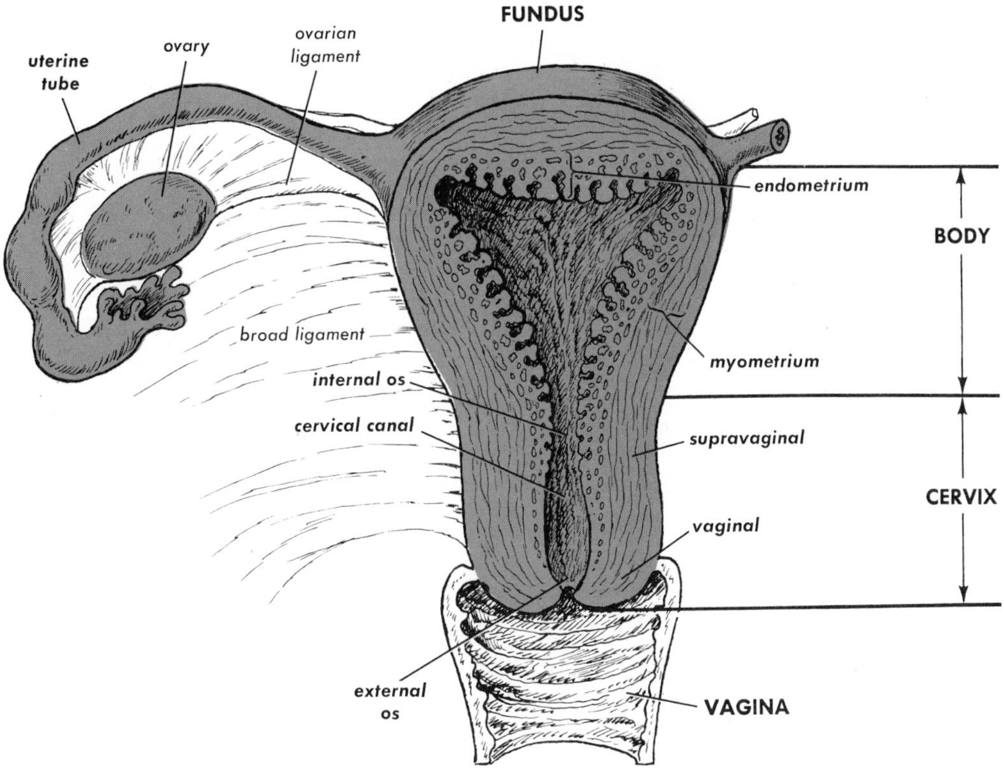

Figure 43-4 The uterine tubes, uterus, and vagina. (*From E. Reith B. Breidenbach, and M. Lorenc, Textbook of Anatomy and Physiology, 2d ed., McGraw-Hill Book Company, New York, 1978.*)

The firmest support for the uterus is provided by the *uterine sacral ligaments*. They pull the uterus back and away from the vaginal orifice.

The *vagina* is a tubular structure 8 to 10 cm in length and lined with squamous epithelium. The secretions of the vagina consist of cervical mucus, desquamated epithelium, and, during sexual stimulation, a direct transudate. These fluids play a protective role against vaginal infection. The major function of the vagina is as a receptacle for the penis and sperm during sexual intercourse, and as the route for exit during childbirth and menstruation. The muscular and erectile tissue of the vaginal walls allows for dilation and contraction sufficient to accommodate the passage of the fetus during labor as well as the penis during intercourse. The anterior vaginal walls lie along the urethra and bladder. The posterior vaginal walls are adjacent to the rectum.

External genitalia

Figure 43-5 depicts the external female genitalia. The external portion of the female reproductive system, commonly called the vulva, consists of the mons pubis, labia majora, labia minora, clitoris, urethral meatus, ducts of Skene's glands, vaginal orifice, and Bartholin's glands.

The *mons pubis* is a fatty layer lying over the pubic bone. It contains coarse hair that lies in an upside-down triangular pattern (the male hair pattern is diamond-shaped). The *labia majora* are folds of adipose tissue which form the outer borders of the vulva. These hair-covered folds contain sweat glands and sebaceous glands. The hairless *labia minora* form the borders of the vaginal orifice and extend anteriorly to enclose the clitoris.

In a virginal female the vaginal orifice usually contains a thin membrane called the *hymen* which varies the size of the vaginal orifice between individuals from pinhole size to an opening large enough to allow two fingers to enter. The hymen is frequently torn during first sexual intercourse and only tags remain. In many societies the bleeding that occurs with this tearing has been used to validate virginity. However, not all hymens are torn by the first intercourse. Some

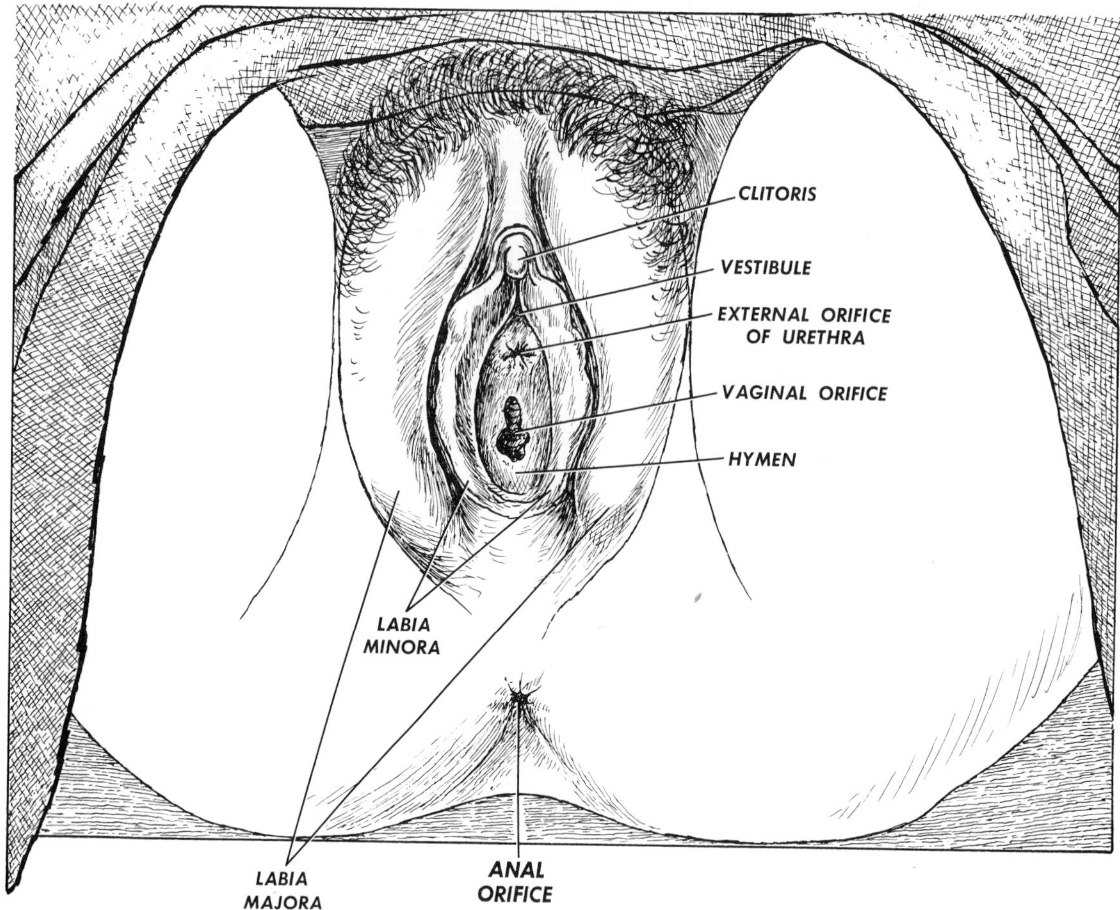

Figure 43-5 External female genitalia. (*From E. Reith, B. Breidenbach, and M. Lorenc, Textbook of Anatomy and Physiology, 2d ed., McGraw-Hill Book Company, New York, 1978.*)

are already well stretched or were minimal to begin with, some were torn through childhood activity or accidents, and some never tear.

The *clitoris* is the female homologue to the male penis, i.e., the erectile tissue which becomes engorged during sexual excitation. It lies anterior to the urethral meatus and vaginal orifice and is usually covered by the prepuce or hood.

Skene's glands and ducts lie alongside the urethral meatus and have no known function. They are a homologue to the male prostate. *Bartholin's glands*, which are located at the posterior and lateral aspects of the vaginal orifice, secrete a thin mucoid material believed to contribute slightly to lubrication during sexual intercourse. These glands are not usually palpable unless sebaceous like cysts form or an infection arises.

Neuroendocrine Regulation of the Female and Male Reproductive Systems

The *hypothalamic-pituitary-gonadal axis* refers to both the anatomic and physiologic relationship of the hypothalamus, the pituitary, and the gonads (organs of reproduction) to reproductive system functioning (Fig. 43-6). Each axis component produces hormones upon which the processes of ovulation, spermatogenesis, fertilization, and secondary sex characteristics of both the male and female are dependent. Chapter 40 discusses the anatomy of the hypothalamus and pituitary.

At the hypothalamic level, gonadotropic-releasing hormones (GRH) are produced and secreted that stimulate the pituitary to secrete the following gonadotropic hormones: follicle-stimulating hormone (FSH),

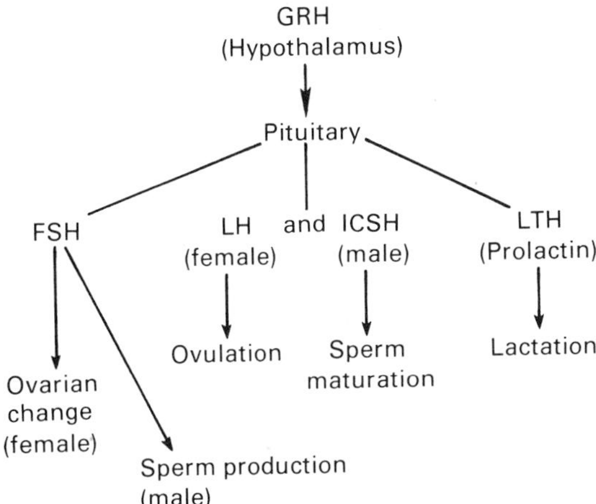

Figure 43-6 The hypothalamic-pituitary-gonadal axis. Only the major pituitary hormone actions are depicted.

luteinizing hormone (LH) in the female and interstitial cell-stimulating hormone (ICSH) in the male, and luteotropic hormone (LTH) in both the female and male, also known as prolactin. Prolactin secretion is controlled by both a hypothalamic-releasing hormone and an inhibiting hormone.[3]

FSH production by the pituitary stimulates ovarian changes in the female which are essential to ovulation and estrogen production. In the male, FSH stimulates the seminiferous tubules of the testes to produce sperm. ICSH is essential for full maturation of sperm as well as production of testosterone by the interstitial cells of the testes. In the female, LH and FSH are responsible for the actual occurrence of ovulation. LH stimulates an estrogen surge which is thought to be the stimulus for ovulation. LH is also essential to the luteinization of the graafian follicle into the mature corpus luteum (see Menstrual Cycle discussion). LTH (prolactin) has no known function in the male but in the female plays a primary role in the process of lactation.

The gonadal hormones of the female are estrogen and progesterone. These two hormones are produced by the ovaries. Estrogen is essential to the development and maintenance of (1) the secondary sex characteristics of the female, (2) the proliferative phase of the ovulatory (menstrual) cycle, and (3) the uterine changes essential to pregnancy. Progesterone also plays a major role in the ovulatory (menstrual) cycle, but most specifically in the secretory phase. Like estrogen, progesterone is involved in the bodily changes associated with pregnancy.

The major gonadal hormone of the male is testosterone, which is produced by the testes. Testosterone is responsible for the development and maintenance of secondary sex characteristics in the male as well as for adequate spermatogenesis. There is some evidence that there may be other male hormones besides testosterone but knowledge on this subject is so sparse as to be of little practical significance at this time. Although estrogen, produced in the adrenal cortex, has been found in the urine of the male, its role and importance are not well understood.

The circulating levels of the above hormones are controlled primarily through a negative feedback process; i.e., receptors within the hypothalamus are sensitive to the circulating blood levels of the hormones produced within the ovary and testes—estrogen, progesterone, and testosterone (Table 43-1). Increased levels of these hormones stimulate a hypothalamic response to *decrease* the high circulating levels. Likewise, low circulating levels of estrogen, progesterone, and testosterone provoke a hypothalamic response which *increase* the low circulating levels. For example, if the circulating level of testosterone is low, the hypothalamus is stimulated to secrete GRH which stimulates the pituitary to secrete greater amounts of FSH and ICSH which in turn causes an increase in the production of testosterone. The high levels of testosterone then stimulate a decrease in the production of GRH and thus of FSH and ICHS.

In the female there is a slight variation. Two centers of control are involved, the tonic center and the cyclic center.[4] The tonic center operates as a negative feedback control mechanism as in the male.

Table 43-1
Gonadal Feedback Mechanisms

Estrogen and progesterone hormones are controlled by both positive and negative feedback mechanisms in the female (a) and (b), depending on the monthly cycle. Testosterone is controlled by a negative feedback mechanism (c).

(a) Tonic Center (negative feedback)

↓ Estrogen estrogen → ↑ GRH (hypothalamus) → ↑ FSH (pituitary) → ↑ estrogen (ovaries)

(b) Cyclic center (positive feedback)

↑ Estrogen → ↑ GRH (hypothalamus) → ↑ LH (pituitary)

(c) Testosterone

↓ Testosterone → ↑ GRH (hypothalamus) →
↑ FSH and ICSH (pituitary) → ↑ testosterone (testes)

When circulating estrogen levels are low, the tonic center of the hypothalamus is stimulated to increase its production of GRH (gonadotropic-releasing hormone). GRH stimulates the pituitary to secrete greater amounts of FSH, which results in higher levels of estrogen production by the ovaries. Reciprocally, *higher* levels of circulating estrogen result in a *decreasing* secretion of GRH and thus a decrease in the secretion of FSH by the pituitary.

In contrast, the cyclic center of the hypothalamus represents a positive feedback control mechanism. Thus, in the presence of high levels of circulating estrogen a greater level of GRH is produced, which results in an increased level of LH from the pituitary. Likewise, lowered levels of estrogen result in a lowered level of LH.

Menstrual Cycle

As previously discussed, the two major functions of the ovaries are the secretion of hormones and ovulation. These functions are accomplished during the normal menstrual cycle. The *menstrual cycle* is a monthly pattern of hormonal activity between the hypothalamus, pituitary, and ovaries which results in menstruation if fertilization does not occur (Fig. 43-7). It is divided into three phases: (1) the *proliferative* (or follicular), (2) *secretory* (or luteal), and (3) *menstrual*. For purposes of discussion a typical cycle of 28 days will be used. The length of the menstrual cycle ranges from 20 to 40 days.

The first day of menstruation is counted as day one of the cycle. Menstruation generally lasts 3 to 5 days. During this time both estrogen and progesterone levels are low but FSH levels are elevated. Under the stimulation of FSH, follicles in the ovary begin to mature until one follicle fully matures. It is not known what mechanism assures that only one follicle reaches maturity. As the follicle matures it secretes estrogen, thus increasing the circulating levels of estrogen and the eventual decrease of FSH secretion.

Although initial follicular maturity is stimulated by FSH, complete maturity and ovulation will occur only with the additional presence of LH. After ovulation, LH promotes the development of the mature corpus luteum.

The fully developed corpus luteum continues to secrete estrogen as well as initiating progesterone secretion. If fertilization does occur, high levels of estrogen and progesterone will continue to be secreted as a result of the continued activity of the corpus luteum from stimulation by human choriotropic hormone (HCG). If fertilization does not occur, menstruation results because of a decrease in estrogen and progesterone production.

During the follicular changes in the ovary, the endometrial lining of the uterus is also undergoing change. As larger amounts of estrogen are produced the endometrial lining proliferates, i.e., there is increased cellular growth, including an increase in the length of blood vessels and glandular tissue. With ovulation and increased levels of progesterone, the luteal or secretory phase begins. In this phase, the blood vessels begin to coil, which increases the surface area of the vascular supply. The glandular tissues mature and secrete a glycogen-rich substance and the glandular ducts dilate. If the corpus luteum regresses (fertilization does not occur) and the estrogen and progesterone levels fall, the endometrial lining can no longer be supported. As a result the blood vessels contract and the tissue begins to slough (fall away). This sloughing is menses.

Menopause

Menopause is the cessation of menses for the remainder of a woman's lifetime. It is usually diagnosed if 1 year of amenorrhea has occurred without signs of other problems. The *climacteric* is the period of time during which symptoms of approaching menopause begin, menopause actually occurs, and equilibrium after menopause is established. In a sense the stage for menopause is set during fetal life. Approximately 6 to 7 million eggs are present in the female during the twentieth week of fetal life. The number actually begins to decline at this time. The average female ovulates only 400 to 500 times during a lifetime. The exact mechanism by which the other germ cells are lost is not well understood.[5] Some 40 to 50 years after birth the full store of germ cells becomes exhausted. As the decline of germ cells reaches lower levels during the climacteric, the amount of estrogen produced also begins to decline.

The reduced level of estrogen leads to a reduced frequency of ovulation. The atrophy of secondary sex characteristics is partially the result of these lowered estrogen levels. Sources of estrogen other than the ovary, such as the adrenal glands, now become very important in maintaining estrogen-dependent tissues. Blood levels of FSH increase as much as ten to twenty fold in response to lower estrogen. These elevated FSH levels may take several years to subside to postmenopausal levels. Though numerous symptoms have been accredited to the climacteric period, Table 43-2 indicates the most common manifestations that occur during the three stages of the climacteric.

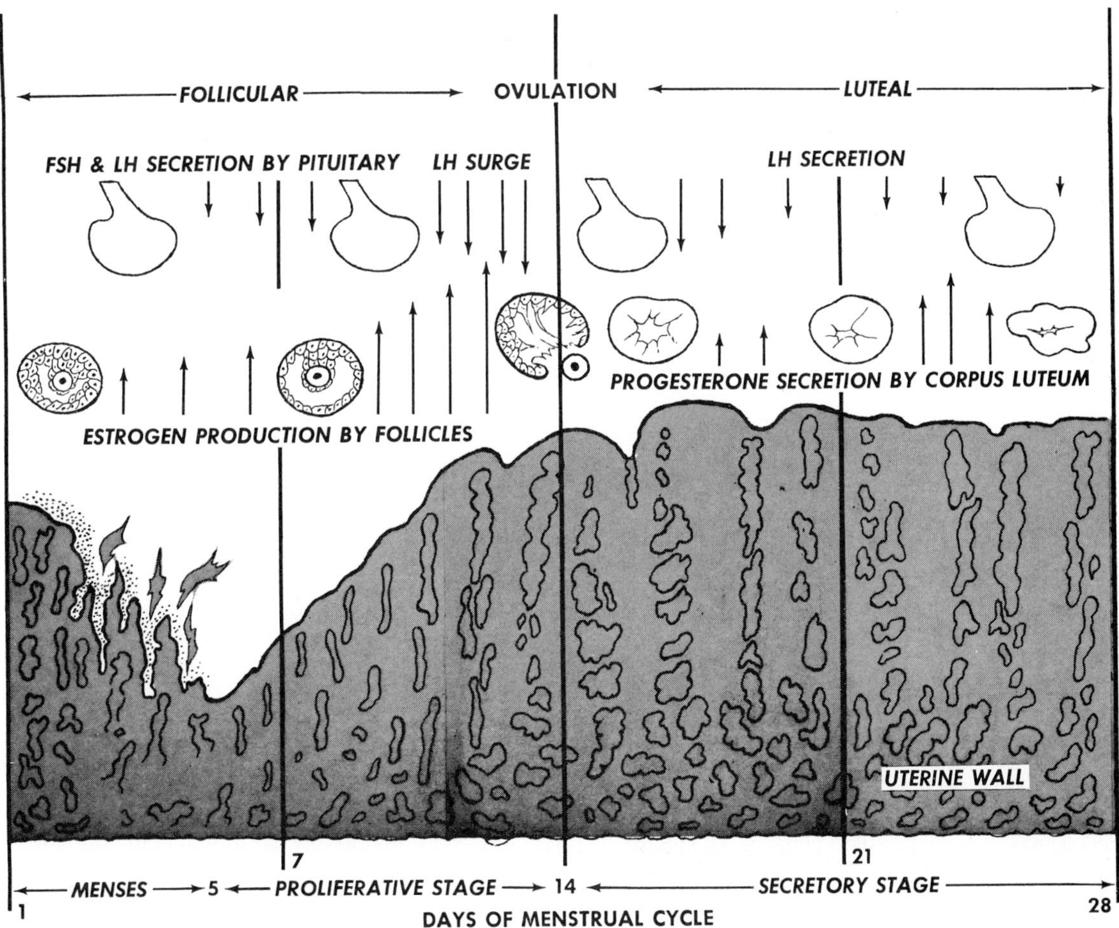

Figure 43-7 The uterine (menstrual) cycle. (*From E. Reith, B. Breidenbach, and M. Lorenc, Textbook of Anatomy and Physiology, 2d ed., McGraw-Hill Book Company, New York, 1978.*)

The reason for "hot flashes" or vasomotor instability is not clearly understood. It is clear, however, that lowered estrogen levels do result in hot flashes and that the more sudden the withdrawal of estrogen, as with oophorectomy, the more likely that the symptoms will be severe (if no replacement is provided). It is also known that these symptoms will subside over time with or without estrogen supplement. Autonomic nervous system instability may also be related to emotional irritability during the climacteric but this "symptom" has been greatly exaggerated both in literature and myth. Atrophy of the vaginal epithelium often causes

Table 43-2
Common Manifestations during the Climacteric

Premenopausal	Menopausal	Postmenopausal
1. Menses are irregular	1. Cessation of menses	1. Atrophic vaginitis
2. Vasomotor instability (hot flashes)	2. Frequent vasomotor symptoms	2. Occasional vasomotor symptoms
3. Nervousness	3. Atrophy of genitourinary tissue (e.g., vaginal epithelium)	3. Atrophy of genitourinary tissue with decreased support
		4. Osteoporosis

vaginal dryness that is responsible for mild to moderate dyspareunia. This could lead to unnecessary and premature cessation of sexual activity. Dryness is a problem easily corrected with hormonal creams. In general, the extent and severity of symptoms of the climacteric vary from individual to individual and are not subject to easy predictability even with a detailed history of family patterns.

Stages of Sexual Excitation

To understand sexual response, it is helpful to look at the structural homologues in the male and female reproductive systems (Table 43-3).

Erection and ejaculation

The penis and urethra are essential to the transport of sperm into the vagina and cervix of the female during intercourse. This transport is facilitated by the erection of the penis. Erection is primarily the result of the filling of the large venous sinuses contained within the erectile tissue of the penis. In the flaccid state, these sinuses hold only a small amount of blood but during the erected state they are literally congested with blood. Since the penis is richly endowed with neurons from the sympathetic, parasympathetic, and pudendal nerve endings, it is readily stimulated to erection. The loose skin of the penis becomes taut as a result of the intense venous congestion. This erectile tautness allows for easy insertion of the penis into the vagina. The subsequent contraction of the penile and urethral musculature during the orgasmic phase of sexual excitation propels the sperm outward through the meatus. This process is *ejaculation*. Thus, the sperm that are produced in the testes and mature in the epididymis are released into the ductus deferens during the contractions of the orgasmic phase. They are advanced through the prostate where they are bathed in fluid from the prostate and seminal vesicles. The sperm continue their path through the urethra, receiving a small amount of fluid from the Cowper's glands, and are finally ejaculated through the urinary meatus.

Table 43-3

Structural Homologues of the Male and Female Reproductive Systems

Male	Female
Penis	Clitoris
Scrotal ridge	Labia minora
Scrotum	Labia majora
Testes	Ovaries
Cowper's glands	Bartholin's glands
Prostate	Skene's ducts
Prostatic utricle (blind pouch of urethra)	Vagina

Female sexual response

The changes which occur in the female during sexual excitation are not dissimilar to those of the male. In response to stimulation the clitoris swells (becomes congested as does the penis) and vaginal lubrication increases (secretion from the cervix, Bartholin's glands, and the sweating of the vaginal walls). This initial response is the excitation phase (erection in the male). As excitation is maintained (plateau phase) the vagina expands and the uterus is elevated (in the male an increase in testicular size). In the orgasmic phase contractions occur in the uterus from the fundus to the lower uterine segment. There is a slight relaxation of the cervical os (conducive to sperm entrance) and rhythmic contractions of the vagina. Both in the male and female, orgasm is marked by the rapid release of the vasocongestion and myotonia which has developed. In other words, in the male the rapid release of muscular tension (through rhythmic contractions) occurs primarily in the penis, prostate, and seminal vesicles; in the female it is the clitoris, vagina, and uterus. This is followed by a resolution phase where the involved organs return to their preexcitation state.

It is important to recognize that not every sexual encounter will terminate in orgasm. Nor is orgasm dependent upon anatomic features such as size of the penis or vaginal canal. Sexual response is a complex interplay of psychological and physiologic phenomena and as such is subject to the effects of everyday stress as well as illness or crisis.

Age-Related Changes

There are gradual changes in both the male and female reproductive systems resulting from advancing age (Table 43-4). These changes occur at different rates and to different degrees among people. The cumulative effects of reproductive system changes plus the negative social attitude toward sexuality in the aging can affect the sexual practices of the elderly.

SUBJECTIVE DATA: THE HISTORY

As in other systems, a thorough review of data for the male and female reproductive system is not confined to the system itself. Because of the potential for problems in areas other than the reproductive system

Table 43-4

Age-Related Changes of the Male and Female Reproductive Systems

Women	Men
1. Estrogen concentration and activity decreases.	1. Slowly decreasing levels of testosterone lead to decreased sexual strength, muscle strength, and viable sperm.
2. The climacteric occurs.	2. Testes become smaller and less firm.
3. Atrophy of uterus and vagina and involution of related genital tissues.	3. Testicular tubules thicken and inhibit production of sperm.
4. Mild regression of secondary sex characteristics.	4. Prostate gland enlarges and becomes weaker.
	5. Reduction in volume and viscosity of seminal fluid results in decreased ejaculatory force.

Adapted from Irene Mortenson Burnside, *Nursing and the Aged,* 2d ed., McGraw-Hill Book Company, New York, 1981, pp. 365–370.

to initiate or enhance stress within the reproductive system, it is important to identify these potential sources of concerns early and accurately.

Past Medical History

Pediatric and adult illnesses

Common pediatric illnesses with specific relevance to male and female reproductive functioning are mumps and rubella, respectively. The occurrence of mumps in the young male has been associated with an increase in sterility. The history should elicit whether the male client has had mumps, has been immunized, or has indications of sterility. Rubella is of primary concern to the female of childbearing age. If rubella occurs in the first 3 months of pregnancy, the possibility of congenital anomalies is greatly increased. For this reason all females of childbearing age who have not been immunized for rubella or have not already had the disease are advised to be immunized if not already pregnant. The female is further advised not to conceive for at least 3 months after immunization.

The presence of chronic disease conditions that have relevance to reproductive system functioning must be assessed. First, the nurse must ascertain if the client has had diabetes. The diabetic male frequently experiences impotency problems in part due to the chemical imbalances of diabetes. In the diabetic female, both pregnancy and the use of oral contraceptives are risks to her health. The morbidity and mortality rates of diabetic females is increased in the presence of pregnancy or with use of oral contraceptives. Likewise, a history of cardiovascular disease in the female, including hypertension, thrombophlebitis, and angina have a higher incidence of morbidity and mortality during pregnancy or when oral contraceptive drugs are used. Anemia is also relevant to the reproductive health of the female. Anemia could be secondary to or aggravated by menstrual flow.

In the male a stroke may cause impotency, either physiologically or psychologically. The male who has suffered a heart attack will frequently experience impotence. Often, this impotence is due to fear of initiating another heart attack. The interviewer must be sensitive to this possible concern of the male. Questions asked relative to the illness may indicate such a fear, and thus indicate a potential need for counseling and support regarding sexual as well as cardiac needs.

In the female of childbearing age who may use oral contraceptives it is extremely important to rule out the presence of neurologic dysfunction such as seizures or migraine headaches. These conditions can be aggravated by oral contraceptives and might be contraindicated depending on the degree of risk from pregnancy. Additionally, cholecystitis and hepatitis are relative contraindications to the use of oral contraceptives. Cholecystitis is often aggravated by oral contraceptives and liver disease generally precludes the use of estrogen products because they are metabolized by the liver. Other relative contraindications to the use of oral contraceptives may be the presence of asthma or other chronic obstructive respiratory problems. This is based on the property of progesterone to thicken secretions.

Questions relating to endocrine disorders, particularly hypo- and hyperthyroidism, also must be raised as they can directly interfere with the menstrual cycle of the female or with sexual performance in the male. Finally, both the male and female should be assessed for kidney and urinary tract disorders, because sexual functioning and reproductive capacity can be impeded in the presence of genitourinary problems.

Hospitalizations and surgeries

Any hospitalizations or surgeries should be noted in the history. However, particular note should be taken of herniorrhaphy, prostatectomy, vasectomy, and testicular torsion in the male. Dilatation and curretage, cryosurgery, tubal ligation, repair of cystocele or rectocele, hysterectomy, oophorectomy, and salpingectomy must be questioned in the female. Pregnancy interruptions, therapeutic or spontaneous, can also be determined at this time.

Medications

A pharmacologic profile of both prescribed and over-the-counter drugs is necessary for all clients. Particularly relevant in reproductive system assessment is the use of diuretics (sometimes prescribed for premenstrual edema), tranquilizers (which may interfere with sexual performance), and antihypertensives (which have been implicated in increased impotency problems). Thus, use of drugs such as methyldopa (Aldomet), clonidine, guanethidine, and hydralazine need to be closely assessed for this problem. Diuretics are least often associated with impotency problems.In the female, use of oral contraceptives and/or other hormones should be noted. Not least important is the need to recognize use of drugs such as marijuana, barbiturates, amphetamines, "angel dust" (PCP), and the like, which can have a serious impact on reproductive system functioning, either behaviorally or physiologically in both the male and female.

Allergies

Three substances are particularly important to evaluate for allergies in assessing reproductive system functioning. These are sulfonamides, penicillin, and rubber. Both sulfonamides and penicillin are frequently used medications in the treatment of genitourinary symptoms, including vaginitis. Rubber is an essential ingredient in diaphragms and some condoms. An allergy to rubber would preclude their use as contraceptive methods.

Family History

A family history of cancer, particularly of the reproductive system organs, is essential to an adequate reproductive history. Determination of a familial tendency to diabetes mellitus, hypothyroidism, hyperthyroidism, hypertension, stroke, angina, myocardial infarction, endocrine disorders, and anemia is also important. In addition, for the female client, it is imperative to obtain data regarding her mother's use of DES (diethylstilbestrol) during the pregnancy with the client. DES was used with some frequency in women with impending abortions during the 1940s and 1950s. Its use declined significantly in the 1960s. However, because of its high correlation with cervical adenosis and cervical and vaginal adenocarcinoma it is extremely important to obtain this data on all females born 1940 and after.

Social History

Lifestyle history is significant to reproductive system assessment, particularly from the viewpoint of sexual behavior and the meaning of reproduction and contraception to a given individual.

Individuals who view sexual performance as an indication of their masculinity or femininity are less likely to consider contraceptive methods such as condoms, foam, or diaphragms. If the number of children one has is important to self-esteem, then family planning will be difficult to advise even if pregnancy threatens the client's health or life. The use of cigarettes, alcohol, caffeine, or other drugs is very important information to obtain in the female of childbearing age. All these substances can be detrimental to the fetus as well as increasing the morbidity statistics in the woman using oral contraceptives. In the male, the primary problem relating to the use of these substances is impotency or decreased libido.

Sexual History

The extent and depth of sexual interviewing will be primarily dependent upon the expertise of the interviewer and the needs and willingness of the client. Prior to taking a sexual history it is important that the interviewer assess his or her own comfort with his or her own sexuality. Discomfort in questioning will be obvious to the client. Sexual interviewing must be done in an environment that provides reassurance, a sense of confidentiality, and a nonjudgmental attitude. It is best to begin questions in the least sensitive areas and move to more sensitive areas. This is why sexual histories are frequently approached at the time of the review of the genitourinary and gynecologic systems. The initial questions can thus relate to such areas as menstruation, onset of puberty, and the presence or absence of genitourinary symptoms. The introduction of the sexual history after these questions has also provided an introductory period for the care provider and client before moving into sensitive areas.

Sexuality questions should alway be asked in a straightforward manner. "*Why*" questions are not conducive to objective interviewing. Questions should be asked in a manner that assumes the individual has done everything. This prevents the individual from feeling guilty or unique. For example, do not ask "Do you masturbate?" Rather, ask "How often do you masturbate?" If the individual does not masturbate, he or she can simply state they do not. If the client does masturbate, he or she is more likely to indicate that fact because the question has been worded without

Table 43-5
Sexual History Format

1. How long have you been sexually active?
2. How frequently do you have vaginal intercourse?
3. How many partners do you have?
4. What is your sexual preference?
5. How frequently do you have oral intercourse?
6. How frequently do you have rectal intercourse?
7. What venereal diseases have you had? (Gonorrhea, syphilis, herpes, other.)
8. What contraceptive method are you using?
9. How often do you use a contraceptive method?
10. Do you consider your sex life satisfactory?
11. How has your sex life changed?
12. How would you like to see your sex life change?
13. How would your partner rate his or her sex life?

implied judgment. Table 43-5 outlines questions related to a sexual history which are appropriate for an initial assessment or annual examination.

Further, the male needs to be questioned about his ability to have and maintain an erection. This may be approached by questioning the frequency with which he finds it difficult to have and/or maintain his erection. Finally, it is important to routinely ask questions related to sexual health because it establishes the fact that the care provider considers sexual health an integral component of overall health. Indications of sexual dysfunction require referral or consultation with a sexual counselor.

In both the male and female a thorough genitourinary history must be collected for the historical assessment of the reproductive system to be complete.

Gynecologic and Obstetric History

Every female who presents to the health care system should have a complete obstetric and gynecologic history (Table 43-6). As is true of most health care needs and problems, the history provides 80 to 90 percent of the data essential to accurate assessment and meaningful nursing care plans and intervention for clients with reproductive system problems.

Breast

The first review questions usually address the breast. First, ask the client if she performs a monthly breast self-examination (Chap. 44). Question the client regarding the presence of breast lumps or masses now or in the past. Cancer of the breast remains the leading cause of death in women between the ages of 30 to 44 years of age.[6] The presence of a breast lump is the single most common presenting sign of cancer. If a lump is present, note its onset, size, and consistency. Ask if there has been either an increase or decrease in size and shape since its onset or discovery. Question as to the presence or absence of breast pain or tenderness. Describe the degree and severity of pain. Breast pain or tenderness is not usually present in the malignant mass, particularly in the early stages.

Nipple discharge in the nonpregnant or nonlactating female is another important symptom to assess. Ask the color, consistency, amount, and odor of discharge. Discharge not related to lactation or pregnancy must be evaluated.

Menstrual history

Menstrual history data are used in the detection of pregnancy, infertility, and numerous other gynecologic concerns. An accurate gynecologic assessment requires obtaining accurate menstrual history. A menstrual history should contain the following data: age at onset of mentruation, average length of cycle, usual duration of menstruation (number of days), and usual amount. The amount is usually best established by ascertaining the number of pads or tampons used per day, noting the extent of saturation (small, medium, large); the presence or absence of dysmenorrhea; and premenstrual symptoms such as headache, tension, and fluid retention.

Changes in the usual menstrual pattern must be explicitly described to determine if the change is transient and unimportant or connected with a more serious gynecologic problem. Intermenstrual spotting or bleeding, excessive menstrual bleeding (menorrhagia), amenorrhea, or postcoital bleeding are potentially significant problems that should be elicited in the history. Any changes in menstrual history created by the use of contraceptive estrogens or intrauterine devices (IUDs) need to be identified. Contraceptive estrogens usually decrease the amount and duration of flow, while IUDs may cause an increase in amount and duration. IUDs also frequently increase the severity of dysmenorrhea.

A general gynecologic history should rule out pelvic pain, venereal disease, vaginal infections, or the presence of symptoms such as vaginal discharge and dyspareunia. Finally, it is important to obtain a clear obstetric history, including therapeutic and spontaneous abortions (pregnancy interruptions). Such data provide the basis for family planning and fertility counseling most relevant to each individual.

Table 43-6
Gynecologic/Obstetric History Format

General gynecologic

External genitalia
___ Pain ___ Rashes ___ Vaginal discharge:
___ During intercourse Amount ______
___ Other Color ______
Consistency ______

___ Bleeding after intercourse
___ Venereal Disease:
___ *Trichomonas* ___ Gonorrhea
___ *Chlamydia* ___ Syphilis
___ *Hemophilus* ___ Herpes
___ Yeast infection *(Monilia)* ___ Other ______
___ Ectopic pregnancy (tubal) ______
Last Pap smear ______ Abnormal Pap ______ (yes or no)
___ Uterine fibroids Treatment of any______
___ Endometriosis ______
___ Ovarian cyst ______

Obstetric

___ # of pregnancies
___ # of deliveries
___ # of live births
___ # of spontaneous abortions (miscarriages)
___ # of therapeutic abortions
Problems during pregnancy (if any): ______

______

______

Breast

___ Breast lumps (describe where) ______

______

______

___ Previous lumps. Identify treatment if any ______

______

___ Previous mammography (when) ______

______

___ Breast pain onset ______
Severity ______
Previous occurrence ______
___ Breast discharge:
Onset ______
Amount ______
Color ______
Odor/consistency______
___ Self-breast exam ______
How often ______

Menstrual

Age of onset ______
LMP ______
Cycle ______ Irregular periods______
How long______
Duration ______
# of pads/tampons on heaviest days ______
Presence of clots ______ Spotting ______
Dysmenorrhea (describe) ______ Rx ______
Change in flow/amt ______
Menopause ______ Hot flashes ______
Other menopausal symptoms ______

______

Birth control method ______
How long ______ Other methods used:

______

OBJECTIVE DATA: THE PHYSICAL EXAMINATION

The examination of the male and female external genitalia utilizes the techniques of inspection and palpation. The reader is again reminded of the extreme importance of observation as an assessment tool.

Both the female and male reproductive examination should begin with the inspection and palpation of the abdomen. This approach provides the opportunity to detect pain or masses which could involve the genitourinary system. The examiner at this point can also evaluate the inguinal regions for rashes, lesions, or lymphadenopathy, which may suggest pelvic organ infection. In the male, examination of the inguinal region may reveal a hernia.

Male Genitalia

The examination of the male may be performed in either a lying or standing position. The standing position is preferred when possible. The examiner should be seated in front of the standing client. The use of a glove is left to the examiner's discretion but if any suspicion of infection exists, gloves should be worn.

Pubes

Observe for the diamond-shaped pattern of male hair distribution. Absence of hair is not normal. Evaluate skin areas as appropriate for any skin area of the body.

Penis

Note the size, skin texture, lesions, scars, swelling. Note location of the urethral meatus; the presence or absence of foreskin; discharge—amount, color, odor. Assess retractability of foreskin; palpate penile shaft for tenderness or mass; observe both ventral and dorsal aspect.

Scrotum, testes, spermatic cord

Perform a complete skin examination. Lift each testis to inspect all sides of the scrotal sac. Palpate the scrotum to note changes in consistency or presence of masses. Teach client self-testicular exam.

Inguinal region

Inspect the inguinal region. Have the client cough or bear down and note any conspicuous bulging in the inguinal canals. Palpate the area as the client again coughs or bears down and feel for any bulging.

Locate the spermatic cord posteriorly in the scrotal sac. Follow the cord on each side. Gently palpate to the inguinal region. Using the forefinger or small finger push up through the loose scrotal skin to the abdominal wall along the inguinal region. The *internal inguinal ring* will meet and impede the finger. At this point, again have the client bear down and cough. Determine if the strain will produce bulging of the intestines through the ring. The presence of hernias requires medical evaluation.

Anus and prostate

The sphincter and perineal regions can be inspected for lesions, masses, and hemorrhoids. Clients with prostate symptomatology and high-risk men require a digital examination.

Female Breasts and External Genitalia*

Breasts

Compare size, shape, and position of both breasts. Note the presence or absence of nipple discharge, amount, color, and consistency. Describe the size, shape, location and consistency of lumps or masses in either of the breasts, axillary, and/or supraclavicular areas. Determine if the lump is movable or stationary.

*See Chap. 44 for technique of breast examination. Remember that the examination should be performed in the same manner in which the care provider will instruct the client to do her own examination.

External genitalia

Inspect the mons pubis, labia majora, labia minora, perineum, and anal region for characteristics of skin, hair distribution, and contour. Note any lesions, swelling, or discharge.

Separate the labia majora and minora to fully inspect the clitoris, urethral meatus, vaginal orifice, hymen, perineum, and anal region. The vagina and cervix can be inspected on speculum examination.

Internal Pelvic Examination

It is during the speculum examination that it is possible to perform the Pap smear and to collect secretions for culture and study under the microscope, i.e., wet smears.

Following the speculum examinations, a bimanual examination is done. This allows for assessment of the size, shape, and consistency of the uterus, ovaries, and tubes. (The tubes are not normally palpable). The reader is referred to a physical examination text for details of the pelvic and bimanual examination. Table 43-7 illustrates the recording format for the physical assessment findings of the male and female reproductive system.

Tables 43-8, 43-9, and 43-10 summarize common assessment abnormalities of the breasts, the female reproductive system, and the male reproductive system.

DIAGNOSTIC STUDIES OF FEMALE AND MALE REPRODUCTIVE SYSTEMS

Many diagnostic tests used to assess problems of other body systems also provide valuable data in the assessment of the male and female reproductive systems. However, only those tests specific to the reproductive system will be discussed in this chapter. Table 43-11 summarizes the most commonly used diagnostic studies in the assessment of male and female reproductive systems and the nurse's responsibility regarding these diagnostic tests. It is to be understood that it is the nurse's responsibility to ensure the client's understanding of the purpose of any test being performed.

Table 43-7

Recording the Normal Physical Assessment of the Male and Female Reproductive System

Male	Female
Penis and scrotum: Normal male hair distribution Skin: No lesions or inflammation Penis circumcised Meatus patent, no discharge Testes smooth, firm, 2 × 3 cm No masses, slight tenderness Epididymis: Nontender, no masses No inguinal hernias	Breast: Symmetrical, nipples everted, no dimpling, no nipple discharge, no masses, lesions, or tenderness Appropriate for age and parity Vulva: Normal female hair distribution No lesions, redness, swelling, or masses. Patent vaginal orifice. No discharge. Skene's ducts and Bartholin's glands nonpalpable, no tenderness. Clitoris and urethral meatus intact

Table 43-8

Common Assessment Abnormalities of the Breast

Findings	Definition and Description	Possible Etiology
Nipple inversion/retraction	Recent onset, reddened, painful, unilateral	Abscess Inflammatory cancer
	Recent onset (usually within past year) unilateral, nontender	Neoplasm
Nipple secretions		
Galactorrhea (female)	Milky secretion which is not related to lactation may be unilateral or bilateral, intermittent or consistent	Drug therapy, particularly phenothiazines, tricyclic tranquilizers, methyldopa Hypo- or hyperfunction of thyroid or adrenals Tumors of the hypothalamos or pituitary axis Excessive estrogen Prolonged suckling or breast foreplay
Galactorrhea (male)	Milky/bilateral	Chorioepithelioma of the testes
Purulent	Gray-green or yellow discharge, usually unilateral in association with pain, erythema, induration, and nipple inversion	Puerperal mastitis or abscess
	Above, but usually without nipple inversion	Infected sebaceous cyst
Serious discharge	Clear, may be unilateral or bilateral, intermittent or consistent	Intraductal papilloma
Dark green or multicolored discharge	Thick, sticky, and almost always bilateral	Mammary duct ectasia
Serosanguineous or bloody drainage	Unilateral	Papillomatosis Intraductal papilloma Carcinoma (both male and female)
Scaling/excoriation of nipple	Unilateral/bilateral, crusting, may be ulceration	Paget's disease Eczema, infection
Nodules, lumps, masses	Multiple bilateral cysts, well-delineated, soft or firm, mobile, painful, premenstrually	Fibrocystic disease
	Rubbery, fluid-filled, painful	Mammary duct ectasia
	Soft, mobile, well-delineated, without pain	Lipoma
	Erythema, tenderness, induration	Infected sebaceous cysts Abscesses

Table 43-9
Common Assessment Abnormalities of the Female Reproductive System

Findings	Definition/Description	Possible Etiology
Vulvar discharge	Cottage cheese consistency, usually accompanied by itching and inflammation, odorless	Candidiasis (*Monilia*/yeast) vaginitis
	Grayish, copious, frothy, with vulvar irritation	*Hemophilus vaginitis* *Trichomonas vaginitis*
	Purulent—grayish green or yellow	*Chlamydia vaginitis* *Gonorrhea vaginitis*
	Bloody	Menstruation, trauma, cancer
Vulvar erythema	Bright or beefy red with itching	*Monilia*
	Reddened base with painful vesicles or ulcerations	Herpes genitalis Chancroid
	Macules or papules with itching	Contact dermatitis Scabies Pediculosis
Vulvar growths	Soft, fleshy growth, nontender	Condyloma acuminatum
	Flat and warty, nontender	Condyloma latum
	May appear as either of above, may be painful	Neoplasm
	Reddened base, vesicles, and small erosions, may be painful	Lymphogranuloma venereum Herpes genitalis Chancroid
	Ulcers nonpainful, indurated, firm	Chancre (syphilis) Granuloma inguinale
Abdominal pain or tenderness	Right or left lower quadrant tenderness, intermittent or consistent	Salpingitis Ectopic pregnancy Ruptured ovarian cyst Pelvic inflammatory disease Tubal or ovarian abscess
	Periumbilical, consistent	Cystitis Endometritis

Table 43-10
Common Assessment Abnormalities of the Male Reproductive System

Findings	Description	Possible Etiology
Penile growths or masses	Indurated, smooth, disklike appearance, nonpainful, singular	Chancre
	Papular to irregularly shaped ulceration with pus, no induration	Chancroid
	Ulceration with induration and nodularity	Cancer
	Flat, wartylike nodule	Condyloma latum
	Elevated, fleshy, moist, elongated projections—single or multiple projections	Condyloma acuminatum
	Localized swelling with retracted, tight foreskin	Paraphimosis Trauma
Vesicles, erosions, ulcers	Painful, erythematous base vesicular or small erosions	Herpes genitalis Balanitis Chancroid
	Painless, singular small erosion with eventual lymphadenopathy	Lymphogranuloma venereum Cancer

Table 43-10 (Continued)

Findings	Description	Possible Etiology
Scrotal masses	Localized swelling of scrotum with tenderness, unilateral or bilateral	Epididymitis Testicular torsion Orchitis (mumps)
	Swelling, tenderness	Incarcerated hernia
	Unilateral or bilateral localized, swelling without pain, translucent cordlike or wormlike, unilateral	Hydrocele Spermatocele Varicocele Hematocele
	Firm, nodular testes or epididymis, most often unilateral	Tuberculosis Cancer
Penile discharge	Clear to purulent, minimal to copious amount	Urethritis or gonorrhea *Chlamydia* Trauma
Penile or scrotal erythema	Macular/papular	Scabies/pediculosis
Inguinal masses	Bulging, unilateral on straining Shotty 1–3 cm nodules	Inguinal hernia Lymphadenopathy

Table 43-11
Diagnostic Studies of the Male and Female Reproductive Systems

Study	Description and Purpose	Nursing Responsibility
	Urine Studies	
Pregnancy testing Pregnosticon Dri Dot (latex inhibition test) Gravindex Pregnosticon Accuspheres (hemagglutination-inhibition)	Detects the presence of human chorionic gonadotropin in urine for the purpose of ascertaining pregnancy. May also be used in the detection of hydatiform mole and of chorioepithelioma (both male and female).	Instruct client to obtain first morning specimen for test. Accuracy of test is greatest 6 weeks after LMP. Obtain thorough menstrual history from client inclusive of birth control methods. Determine presence or absence of presumptive signs of pregnancy, e.g., breast changes, increased whitish vaginal discharge, etc.
Hormone testing Total estrogen levels	Urine estrogens are used to detect ovarian pathology, hyperadrenalism, interstitial cell tumor of the testes, liver disease, and ectopic pregnancy. A 24-h urine collection is required. Normal varies according to menstrual cycle.	Instruct client to save all urine for 24 h. Urine collection bottle must be kept refrigerated for greatest accuracy of results.
Pregnanediol Pregnanetriol	Utilized to assess progesterone levels. Most commonly employed to detect corpus luteum cysts and sometimes threatened abortions. May also be used in ascertaining adrenal cortical function and causes of amenorrhea. Normal varies according to menstrual cycle or length of gestation.	Client should be instructed to collect all urine for 24 h and to keep it refrigerated.
Testosterone	Useful in evaluating tumors of the testes as well as development of anomalies of the testes.	Instruct client to collect 24-h urine specimen. Genitourinary and reproductive system history should be collected.
	Blood Studies	
Prolactin assay	Utilized to detect pituitary dysfunction and causes of amenorrhea.	*Fasting, A.M. specimen.

Table 43-11 (Continued)

Study	Description and Purpose	Nursing Responsibility
Serum androstene-dione **Serum testosterone**	Useful in ascertaining whether elevated androgens are due to adrenal or ovarian dysfunction. Serum testosterones are also drawn as part of the workup to assess the cause of amenorrhea.	It is important to collect a history which eliminates any potential sources of interference with the accuracy of results, i.e., use of steroids, barbiturates, or presence of hypothyroidism or hyperthyroidism.
Serum progesterone-RIA	Most frequently used to detect the presence of a functioning corpus luteum cyst. May also be used in adrenal pathology workup.	*Fasting, A.M. serum. Instruct client that serum needs to be drawn around the 24th or 25th day of cycle for greatest accuracy.
Serum estradiol-RIA	Measures ovarian function. Particularly useful in assessing estrogen-secreting tumors and/or status of precocious female puberty. Normal values are dependent upon laboratory which performs test and should be obtained from the specific laboratory.	*Fasting, A.M. specimen.
	Syphilis Studies	
Nontreponemal serologic tests Wasserman: Complement fixation VDRL: Flocculation RPR: Agglutination	These tests are nonspecific antibody tests used for the detection of syphilis. Positive readings can be made within 1–2 weeks after the appearance of the primary lesion (chancre) or 4–5 weeks after the initial infection.	*Nonfasting. Obtain data ascertaining the presence or absence of problems such as hepatitis and collagen diseases, which may interfere with the accuracy of test results.
Treponemal test FTA-ABS	The fluorescent treponemal antibody absorption test specifically detects syphilis antibodies. Detects early syphilis with great accuracy.	*Nonfasting. Usually performed if results of nontreponemal testing questionable.
	Miscellaneous Studies	
Dark-field microscopy	Direct examination of specimen obtained from potential syphilitic lesion (chancre) for the purpose of observing and detecting treponema.	Avoid direct skin contact with open lesion.
Wet mounts	Direct microscopic examination of specimen of vaginal discharge immediately after collection. Determines presence or absence, as well as number, of trichomonas, bacteria, white cells, monilia buds or hyphae, red cells, and other potential clues or causes of inflammation or infection.	Prepare for collection of specimens, i.e., glass slide, 10–20% KOH solution, NaCl solution, and cotton-tipped applicators. Explain procedure and purpose to client. Instruct client not to douche before examination.
Cultures	Culture of specimens of vaginal, urethral, or cervical discharge. Primarily used to assess the presence of gonorrhea or yeast. Rectal and throat cultures may also be taken dependent upon data obtained from sexual history.	Obtain specific contact and sexual history inclusive of oral and rectal intercourse. Instruct against douching before examination. Obtain urethral specimen from male prior to voiding. Instruct females who are sexually active with multiple partners to have at least a yearly culture. Instruct sexually active males to have any discharge evaluated immediately to rule out gonorrhea strains that do not cause classic symptoms of dysuria.
Gram stain	A presumptive test used for the rapid detection of gonorrhea. The presence of gram-negative intracellular diplococci generally warrants initiation of treatment.	See cultures.

Table 43-11 (Continued)

Study	Description and Purpose	Nursing Responsibility
	Cytologic Studies (Papanicolaou)	
Cervical **Endometrial** **Nipple discharge**	The microscopic study of exfoliated cells via a special staining and fixation technique for the major purpose of detecting a malignancy. Cells most commonly studied are those obtained directly from the endocervix, cervix, vaginal pool, endometrial lining of the uterine cavity, and nipple discharge. A Pap smear most commonly refers to cervical examination while cytologic study is applied when nipple discharge is evaluated.	Instruct all sexually active females or females over the age of 21 to have yearly Pap smears. Arrange for Pap smear at midcycle time. Instruct clients not to douche for at least 24 h before exam. Collect careful menstrual and gynecologic history. Include these data on cytology request. Indicate on the request if any hormonal preparations are being taken by the client. Instruct clients during demonstration of breast self-examination or examination of breasts that nipple discharge should always be evaluated.
	Radiologic Studies	
Soft tissue mammography	X-ray image of breast tissue on photographic film. Used primarily in the assessment of breast masses, recent breast enlargement, and/or nipple discharge to detect the presence of malignancy. Usually an outpatient procedure.	Instruct client on the potential risks and advantages of the examination (radiation).
Contrast mammography	Utilized primarily in the evaluation of abnormal nipple discharge. Particularly effective in detecting intraductal nonpalpable papillomas. The test consists of injection of radiopaque dye into the breast duct.	Determine actual or possible allergy to contrast medium.
Xeroradiography	Similar to mammogram except recordings are made on Xerox paper rather than x-ray film.	Same as mammography.
Ultrasonography (ultrasound)	Measures and records high-frequency sound waves as they pass through tissues of variable density. Very useful in detecting masses greater than 3 cm such as ectopic pregnancies, IUDs, ovarian cysts, and hydatiform moles.	Instruct client that test is performed accurately only with a *full* bladder. Do not empty bladder for at least $1\frac{1}{2}$ –2 h before examination.
	Operative Procedures	
Breast biopsy	Histologic examination of excised breast tissue.	Preoperative preparation includes instruction of operative procedures and sedation. Postoperative care consists of wound care and instruction as needed in breast self-examination.
Hysterosalpingogram	Involves instillation of a radioscopic dye through the cervix into the uterine cavity and subsequently through and out the fallopian tubes. Spot x-rays are taken to detect abnormalities of the uterus and adnexa (ovaries and tubes) as the dye progresses. May be most useful in diagnostic assessment of fertility, i.e., detect adhesions near ovary, an abnormal uterine shape, or blockage of tubal pathways.	Inform client procedure may be fairly uncomfortable. Determine possibility of dye allergy.
Colposcopy	Direct visualization of cervix with the use of binocular microscope allows for study of cellular dysplasia and vascular and tissue abnormalities of cervix. Used as a follow-up study for abnormal Paps and/or in females exposed to DES in utero.	Instruct client in the method of this outpatient procedure and its similarity to the usual pelvic/speculum examination. Inform client that this examination is similar to usual pelvic/speculum exam.

Table 43-11 (Continued)

Study	Description and Purpose	Nursing Responsibility
	A biopsy of cervix may be taken during colposcopic examination. Valuable in decreasing number of false-negative cervical biopsies.	Explain purpose and preparation for procedure.
Conization	Removal of a cone-shaped sample of squamocolumnar tissue of cervix for direct study.	Explain purpose and method of procedure. Requires using surgical facilities and anesthesia. Client should be instructed to rest for at least 3 days following procedure. Also instruct as to necessity for a 3-week follow-up check.
Culdotomy/culdoscopy culdocentesis	Culdotomy consists of an incision made through the posterior fornix of the cul-de-sac. This allows for visualization of the peritoneal cavity (most specifically, the uterus, tubes, and ovaries). A culdoscope visualizing instrument can then be utilized to study these structures closely. This has proved a most valuable technique in fertility evaluations. Withdrawal of fluid (culdocentesis) allows for examination of the type of fluid.	Explanation of purpose and method of procedure. Client is prepared for a vaginal operation with both preoperative instruction and sedation as well as assessment of bleeding and discomfort postoperatively.
Peritoneoscopy (laparoscopy)	Visualizes pelvic structures via special fiberoptic scopes inserted through small abdominal incisions. Instillation of CO_2 into cavity improves general visualization. Useful in the diagnostic assessment of uterus, tubes, and ovaries.	Explanation of purpose and method of procedure. Preoperative preparation includes instruction, abdominal preparation, and sedation. Rest postoperatively for 1–3 days is important.
Dilatation and curretage	Operative procedure which dilates the cervix and allows for curreting the endometrial lining. The curreted material is then studied histologically. Useful in assessing abnormal bleeding patterns as well as for cytologic evaluation of the lining.	Requires preoperative instruction and sedation. Postoperative assessment of degree of bleeding is most important, i.e., frequent pad check first 24 h postoperatively. Overnight hospitalization may be required.
	Fertility Studies	
Semen analysis	Semen is assessed for volume (2–5 mL), viscosity, sperm count (>20 million/mL), sperm motility (60% motile), and/or percent of abnormal sperm (60% have normal morphology). Used in fertility assessments of male.	Instruct client to bring in fresh specimen within 2 h after ejaculation.
Huhner's test	A mucus sample from the woman's cervix is examined within 2 h after intercourse. Total number of sperm is assessed in relation to number of live sperm. Performed to determine if the woman's cervical mucus is "hostile" to passage of sperm from vagina into uterus.	Instruct couples to have intercourse at the estimated time of ovulation and be present for the test *within* 2 h after intercourse.
Endometrial biopsy	Outpatient procedure in which a small curette is utilized to obtain a piece of endometrial lining for the major purpose of assessing endometrial changes common to progesterone secretion after ovulation.	Test must be performed in postovulation portion of cycle. Local anesthesia will be utilized. Procedure should cause only short period of uterine cramping. Instruct client to rest following procedure.

*Inform client that blood sample will be drawn. Observe venipuncture site for bleeding or hematoma formation.

Urine Studies

Pregnancy testing

Detection of pregnancy is generally validated by measuring the output of human chorionic gonadotropin in the urine by means of an immunologic assay test. The three most commonly used methods are latex inhibition, hemagglutination inhibition, and latex agglutination tests. All three utilize the property of agglutination from an antigen-antibody response. The hemagglutination test is the most sensitive but takes 2 hours to perform. The latex methods can be performed in 2 minutes and are considered adequate for screening purposes. The latex methods are most accurate if performed 6 weeks after the last normal menstrual period. Though new tests are being developed for home use which may accurately detect pregnancy within days of conception, their reliability has yet to be validated.

Hormone studies

Although estrogen studies are done, the accuracy of the results is frequently questionable because of the complex metabolic pathways by which estrogen is broken down. Testosterone is a major precursor to estrogen formation and its presence in urine can be measured in both the male and female.

The three-glass urine test may be considered a part of physical assessment by some. Nevertheless, it is frequently a helpful determinant of the presence of infection. The test consists of a collection of three specimens from the male during one uninterrupted voiding: urine I, the first part of the voided specimen, represents the anterior urethra; urine II, the midstream portion of the urine, represents the bladder contents; and urine III, the end of the stream, represents the prostate and seminal vesicles. Theoretically, the site of the infection may be determined by the presence of cells in one of these portions of a single specimen.[7]

In the female, a two-glass urine test can be done to detect the location of infection. Urine I, the first half of the voiding, represents the urethra. Urine II, the second half of the voiding, represents the bladder.[8]

Blood Studies

Prolactin assay is used primarily in the specific protocol for working up the amenorrheic client. High levels of prolactin are normally associated with low levels of estrogen, such as during lactation. However, this same situation can be simulated by the presence of pituitary adenomas.

Serum progesterone and estradiol are commonly tested in ovarian function assessment, particularly the problem of amenorrhea. Finally, hormonal blood studies are essential components of a thorough fertility workup.

Syphilis Studies

There are two types of tests performed to diagnose syphilis, nontreponemal and treponemal tests. Nontreponemal tests such as the Veneral Disease Research Laboratory (VDRL) test and the rapid plasma reagin (RPR) card test are inexpensive and reliable. These tests detect the presence of antibodies which are present in the serum of infected clients.

Treponemal tests such as the fluorescent treponemal antibody absorption test (FTA-ABS) are highly reliable and should be used following a weakly positive VDRL or questionable negative VDRL. This test measures specific antibodies to *Treponema pallidum*. It should be noted that the FTA-ABS is not a test to assess the adequacy of syphilitic treatment. This is because the FTA-ABS will remain reactive even after treatment.

Miscellaneous

The most specific and direct examination to determine the presence of syphilis is dark-field microscopy. Unfortunately, the chancre is frequently gone by the time of client presentation and the test cannot be performed. There are other miscellaneous tests of secretions involving wet mounts, cultures, and stains to detect specific reproductive system problems (Table 43-11).

Cytology

The Papanicolaou smear has been utilized for years as a screening test for cervical cancer. However, little attention has been given to emphasizing the diagnostic implications of specimens obtained from different sites, i.e., cervical as opposed to the vaginal pool.[9] For example, endometrial cancer is more common in the menopausal woman than the premenopausal woman. Therefore, it is more important that the smear contain a sample from the vaginal pool as well as from the cervical and endocervical areas. Timing is another consideration in increasing the accuracy of Pap smears. Smears should be obtained during midcycle or second half of the menstrual cycle. This time is best because it increases the potential of detecting abnormal endometrial cells.[10] Women should be educated to arrange for their annual Pap smear at midcycle time.

A negative Pap test does not rule out endometrial cancer. Specific tests are available to obtain a smear directly from the endometrium. Uterine aspiration or cannulation into the uterine cavity make it possible to obtain endometrial tissue.

Radiology

Mammography has become one of the most frequently used diagnostic tools in reproductive system assessment (See Chap. 44). Unfortunately, its frequent use has been highly criticized because of the concern of the potential risks of radiation. However, increased awareness of the risks from radiographic studies has resulted in valuable improvements in the technique of mammography, particularly in lowering the exposure per examination.[11] General agreement has been reached that mammography should not be routinely administered to women under 35 with little or no risk in their histories and no presenting symptoms. However, women over 50, because of the greatly increased risk of breast cancer, probably should be routinely examined with mammography.[12] At this time the more frequent use of mammography for women under age 50 is generally confined to those women with presenting symptoms such as a mass or discharge, a previous occurrence of cancer, or a strong family history of breast cancer.

REVIEW QUESTIONS

The number of the question corresponds to the same numbered objective at the beginning of the chapter.

1. Which of the following structures comprise the accessory organs of the male reproductive system?
- **a.** scrotum, vas defrens, seminal vesicles, and the urethra.
- **b.** penis, testes, epididymis, and spermatic cord
- **c.** prostate, Cowper's glands, seminal vesicles
- **d.** testes, spermatic cord, prostate, and seminal vesicles
- **e.** penis, prostate, seminal vesicles, and Cowper's glands

2. Which of the following hormones are produced by the male and female gonadal organs?
- **a.** luteotropic hormone, progesterone, testosterone, and follicle-stimulating hormone
- **b.** gonadotropic-releasing hormone, estrogen, and testosterone
- **c.** follicle-stimulating hormone, luteinizing hormone, and interstitial cell-stimulating hormone
- **d.** estrogen, progesterone, and testosterone
- **e.** estrogen, testosterone, and follicle-stimulating hormones

3. Female orgasm is the result of which of the following events?
- **a.** clitoral swelling and increased vaginal lubrication
- **b.** rapid release of vasocongestion and mytonia in both the external and internal reproductive structures
- **c.** clitoral swelling, vaginal lubrication, and uterine elevation
- **d.** vaginal enlargement and secretion with penile insertion
- **e.** fallopian tube and uterine contractions

4. Which of the following data are significant to past history data collection for the assessment of both the male and female reproductive system?
- **a.** the presence or absence of heart disease, diabetes, and hypothyroidism
- **b.** presence or absence of measles, mumps and/or rubella immunizations
- **c.** hypertension, prostate surgery, dilatation and curettage
- **d.** allergies to rubber, breast surgery, and vasectomy
- **e.** anemia, mother's use of DES, and dysmenorrhea

5. Which of the following is not a part of the physical examination of the male?
- **a.** palpation of testes and epididymis
- **b.** palpating for Bartholin's glands and Skene's ducts
- **c.** palpation for inguinal hernia
- **d.** inspection for penile discharge
- **e.** palpation of spermatic cord

6. Vaginal discharge and penile discharge may be indicative of which of the following disease?
- **a.** syphilis
- **b.** gonorrhea
- **c.** balanitis
- **d.** epididymitis
- **e.** endometriosis

7. Because mammography requires the judicious use of radiography, which of the following criteria should be followed for breast mammography?
- **a.** Only women under 35 years of age should have mammography.
- **b.** Women over 35 with a high risk for breast cancer should not have yearly mammographies.
- **c.** Women over 50 with a high risk for breast cancer may have yearly mammographies.
- **d.** Mammography should be performed only when a discernible mass of 3 months' duration is found.
- **e.** A mammography should be performed only in conjunction with breast biopsy.

REFERENCES

1. Diagram Group, *Man's Body: An Owners Manual*, Paddington Ltd., New York, 1976, J-11.
2. S. Phelan, "Reproductive Physiology," Unpublished Module, Center for Continuing Education, Albuquerque, New Mexico, 1980, p. 5.
3. R. C. Benson, *Current Obstetrics and Gynecologic Diagnosis and Treatment*, 2d ed., Lange Medical Publishers, Los Altos, Cal., 1978, p. 56.
4. Phelan, op. cit., p. 2.
5. Benson, op. cit., p. 50.
6. C. J. Anthony, "Risk Factors Associated with Breast Cancer," *Nurse Practitioner* (July–August, 1976), p. 31.
7. *Important Test Groups for the Problem Endocrine Patient,* The Upjohn Company, Kalamazoo, Mich., 1975, p. 12.
8. *Ibid.*
9. V. G. Colon and G. B. Schumann, "Gynecologic Cytology," *Am Fam Physician*, **18**(5):135 (November 1978).
10. *Ibid.*, p. 137.
11. J. R. Guyther, "The Physician's Role in Radiation Protection," *Am Fam Physician*, **18**(6):105 (December 1978).
12. *Ibid.*

Chapter 44

NURSING ROLE IN MANAGEMENT

Breast Disorders

Katherine L. Chipman
Idolia Cox Collier

Learning Objectives

1. Perform breast examination using the proper techniques on both the client and oneself.
2. Teach breast self-examination including rationale, technique, and reasons for referral.
3. Describe the etiology, clinical manifestations, and medical and nursing management of common benign breast disorders.
4. Describe the pathogenesis, clinical manifestations, and medical management of cancer of the breast.
5. Identify the types, indications, and complications of surgical interventions for cancer of the breast.
6. Explain the physical and psychological preoperative and postoperative nursing management for the client undergoing a mastectomy.
7. Describe the indications, types, and management related to mammoplasty.

Breast disorders represent a significant health concern to women. Approximately one in four women will experience some type of breast disorder requiring medical care. In about 7 percent of these situations a malignant growth will be the cause of the breast disorder. Regardless of the cause, intense feelings of shock, fear, and often denial will accompany the initial discovery that a breast problem exists. These feelings are associated as much with the possible loss of a breast from radical surgery with the fear of cancer itself.

Throughout history the female breast has been regarded as a symbol of beauty, sexuality, and motherhood. For many women, identity and femininity are closely related to the breast. The threat of mutilation or loss of a breast is devastating for the woman because of the significant psychological, social, sexual, and body image implications associated with it. This fear has been likened to castration anxiety in the male.[1]

HEALTH PROMOTION AND MAINTENANCE

Breast Self-Examination

Health promotion and maintenance practices apply to all women, regardless of the presence of benign or malignant pathology. The most important practice for a woman related to breast problems is the regular performance of proper breast self-examination (BSE). It is critical that breast lesions be detected early, accurately diagnosed, and promptly treated. Only about 25 percent of breast cancer cases are curable, primarily because they are first seen by the clinician when the disease is already advanced.[2] Vigorous programs to teach breast self-examination to all women could significantly improve this statistic.

Barriers to BSE

A Gallup Poll survey in 1975 revealed that BSE is practiced to a very limited degree because (1) women are ignorant of the importance of the practice, (2) they fear finding a problem, and (3) they lack knowledge of how to perform the examination.[3] Cultural and religious backgrounds are also factors influencing the practice of BSE. Specifically, the fear of cancer and the resultant loss of a breast may prevent a woman from practicing breast self-examination. Nurses, therefore, should stress the fact that most breast lesions are benign. Should the lesion be malignant, the client needs to be informed that early detection and treatment enhance chances of survival. Health professionals, therefore, must direct efforts at teaching women the importance of BSE, how to perform the examination, and what to do if a problem is detected.

Technique

The technique for breast self-examination has been established by the American Cancer Society (Fig. 44-1). BSE should be done monthly at a regular time. In premenopausal women this is best done 7 days after the start of menstruation. At this time the breasts have minimum granularity and are neither enlarged nor excessively tender. Postmenopausal women and women who have had hysterectomies should set a regular date for monthly BSE. The month-

*This chapter was reviewed by Maureen Brady Nash, B.S.N., M.S.N., CPNP, Assistant Professor, College of Nursing, University of New Mexico, Albuquerque, New Mexico. The section on malignant breast problems was also reviewed by John Saiki, M.D., Cancer Research and Treatment Center, Albuquerque New Mexico.

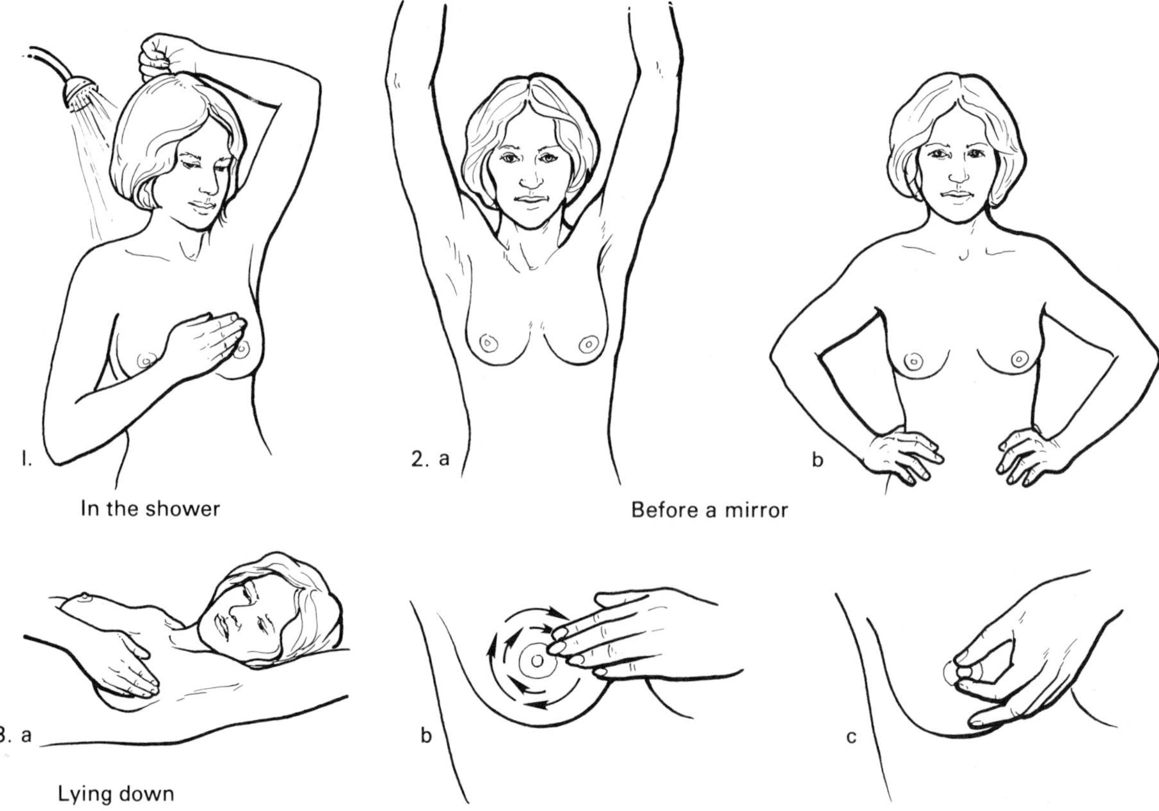

Figure 44-1 Breast self-examination. *(Adapted from "How To Examine Your Breasts," American Cancer Society.)*

ly date of her birthday is a common choice for many women.

The examination should be done in good light and should include both inspection before a mirror and careful, systematic palpation. The entire breast should be examined. The woman should be taught BSE procedure by a nurse or doctor using the woman's own hand on her breast. A gentle stroking motion over wet, soapy skin is particularly useful. The client should be told what to look for such as a lump, nipple discharge, nipple retraction, redness, pain or tenderness, dimpling of the skin, or edema. She should be shown the normal variations in her own breasts so she can detect changes. Finally, she should be reminded that problems discovered are most often benign.

Follow-Up Care

If a problem is suspected, the woman should see her primary care provider immediately. If further diagnostic studies are indicated, they can be initiated immediately. If the problem is not serious, the woman's anxiety can be relieved. Even when the client faithfully practices BSE, she should have an annual breast examination by a nurse or physician. The care evidenced by the clinician in performing BSE will reinforce the practice of BSE by the client. The frequency of these examinations are determined by the client's age and presence of risk factors in her history (Table 44-1). An annual examination by a professional is recommended for all adult females. When birth control pills are begun, a professional BSE should also be done.

BREAST DISORDERS

Statistically, the most frequently encountered breast disorders requiring diagnosis or treatment in women are, in order of frequency:

1. Fibrocystic disease
2. Carcinoma
3. Fibroadenoma

Table 44-1
Factors Influencing Breast Cancer Risk

Lump in breast
Discharge from breast
History of breast surgery
Family history of breast cancer, especially in mother or sister
Early menarche and late menopause
Before age 30, no birth of live child
Endometrial or ovarian cancer

4. Intraductal papilloma
5. Ductal ectasia

In males, gynecomastia is overwhelmingly the most frequently observed disorder.

Assessing a Breast Problem

Multiple factors must be considered when assessing a breast problem. Sex and age are important variables. Only 1 percent of breast carcinoma occurs in males. Benign lesions occur more frequently in premenopausal women. Cancer of the breast is predominantly found in postmenopausal women with the incidence increasing with age.

Risk factors in the client's history must be evaluated. Also, the history of the breast disorder assists in establishing the diagnosis. The presence of nipple discharge, pain, rate of growth, and correlation with the menstrual cycle should all be investigated.

The size and location of the lump or lumps should be carefully documented. Additionally, the physical characteristics of the lesion, such as consistency, mobility, and shape should be assessed. If nipple discharge is present, the color and consistency is noted, as well as whether it occurs from single or multiple ducts.

Diagnostic tests are valuable adjuncts in diagnosing a breast lesion (Chap. 43).

BENIGN BREAST PROBLEMS

Breast Infections

Lactational mastitis

Breast infections occur most frequently in lactating women. *Lactational mastitis* presents as a localized area that is indurated, painful, and tender to palpation. Usually, the infection develops when organisms gain access to the breast through a cracked nipple. Preparation of the breast for nursing by nipple rolling and toughening can decrease the incidence of lactational mastitis. It is not necessary that nursing ceases unless a purulent drainage is noted. The mother may wish to use a nipple shield or hand-express milk from the involved breast until pain subsides. The client should see her physician promptly to begin a course of antibiotic therapy.

Lactational breast abscess

If mastitis persists after several days of antibiotic therapy, a *lactational breast abscess* may have developed. In this condition, the skin may become red and edematous over the involved breast and the client may have an elevated temperature. Antibiotics alone are insufficient treatment for a breast abscess. Surgical incision and drainage is necessary. Following incision and drainage a Penrose drain may be left in place. The drainage is cultured and an appropriate antibiotic is begun. Breast feeding does not have to cease.

Fibrocystic Disease

Fibrocystic disease is a benign breast condition characterized by multiple, bilateral lesions that are determined by aspiration or surgery to be cysts. It is the most frequently occurring breast disorder. Approximately one woman in ten will develop this problem.

Fibrocystic disease occurs most frequently in women between the ages of 35 to 50 years but often begins in women as young as 20 years old. It disappears after menopause. Fibrocystic disease may be unilateral or bilateral, but cysts are usually found widely scattered throughout both breasts. Once the disease begins it may recur periodically through the premenopausal years. The etiology of fibrocystic disease is thought to relate to hormonal influence, because of its relationship to active ovarian function. It is often exacerbated in the premenstrual phase and relieved following menstruation.

Symptomatically, fibrocystic disease presents with one or more palpable lumps that are usually round, well delineated, and movable within the breast. The consistency of the lump is related to the amount of fluid within it. Occasionally there is accompanying pain and/or tenderness. The lump is usually observed to increase in size and perhaps tenderness premenstrually. Cysts may enlarge or reduce in size rapidly. There is rarely a nipple discharge in fibrocystic disease.

Management

Fibrocystic disease is diagnosed and treated by aspiration. With large or frequent cysts, surgical removal of the cysts and even mastectomy may be favored over repeated aspiration. This, however, is not usually recommended. If no fluid is found on aspiration, if the fluid is hemorrhagic, or a residual mass remains, excisional or incisional biopsy should be done.

Although cystic disease and breast cancer may share some common causative factors, cancer does not develop from cysts. Clients with cystic disease should be encouraged to return regularly for follow-up examinations throughout life. They should also be taught BSE so that they may detect any problems. Any new lumps should be evaluated and any changes in symptoms should be pursued. Abstinence from substances containing xanthines such as coffee, tea, and cola beverages is a new treatment approach. This treatment is in the experimental stage.

The role of the nurse in the care of the client with fibrocystic disease is primarily one of teaching. Clients should be told that they may expect recurrence of the cysts in one or both breasts until menopause and that cysts may enlarge or become painful premenstrually. Clients should be reassured that cysts do not "turn into" cancer. They should be instructed to have any new lump examined promptly. The client should be carefully instructed in BSE using the client's own breasts. Teaching breast models can be used if available.

Fibroadenoma

Fibroadenoma is the third most common tumor of the breast in American women. It generally appears any time after puberty and is the most frequent cause of breast tumors in women under 25 years of age.

The lump of a fibroadenoma is usually small, round, well delineated, and very mobile. It may be soft, but is usually solid, firm, and rubbery in consistency. There is no accompanying retraction or nipple discharge. The lump is usually painless. In fibroadenoma the tumor is usually a single, unilateral mass although it can be multiple and occur in both breasts. The tumor grows slowly and often stops growing at 2 to 3 cm. There is no fluctuation in size with menstruation. A relationship with cancer has not been documented.

Management

Diagnosis of a fibroadenoma is made by needle core or excisional biopsy and frozen section. Mammography is of little use diagnostically. Treatment is by excision, which is not urgent in women under 25 years of age. In women over 25 years, all new lesions should be examined by excisional biopsy. Fibroadenomas are not reduced by radiation and are not affected by hormone therapy.

The nurse will frequently have the opportunity to counsel young women with fibroadenomas. During this contact, the benign nature of the lesion should be stressed, follow-up encouraged, and BSE carefully taught.

Nipple Discharge

Nipple discharge may occur spontaneously or as a result of nipple manipulation. A milky secretion is due to inappropriate lactation secondary to such problems as drug therapy, endocrine disorders, or neural problems. It may also be idiopathic.

Secretions can also be serous, grossly bloody, or brown to green, due to either benign or malignant disease. A slide can be made of the secretion to detect specific pathology. Diseases associated with nipple discharge include malignancies, cystic disease, intraductal papilloma, or ductal ectasia. Treatment is dependent on the identification of the cause.

Intraductal papilloma

Intraductal papilloma is a benign disorder manifested by nipple discharge that may be yellow, pink, bloody, or clear. It usually involves a single duct and is found to occur unilaterally. Rarely is a lump present. If one is present, it is mobile, nontender, soft or firm, and located in the periareolar area. Treatment involves excision of the papilloma and involved duct.

Ductal ectasia

Ductal ectasia is a benign breast problem involving the ducts in the subareolar area. It usually involves multiple ducts bilaterally. Nipple discharge is the primary symptom. This discharge is multicolored and sticky. Ductal ectasia usually presents with burning, itching, and pain around the nipple as well as swelling in the areolar area. Inflammatory signs are often found and, in more advanced disease, the nipple may retract and the discharge become bloody. It is not associated with malignancy. Therapy consists of excision of the involved ducts.

Age-Related Breast Changes

Loss of subcutaneous fat and structural support as well as atrophy of mammary glands often result in pendulous breasts in the postmenopausal woman. The nurse should encourage older women to continue to wear a well-fitting bra. Adequate support of sagging breast tissue can prevent backaches and improve physical appearance and mental attitude. It can also prevent *intertrigo* (dermatitis caused by friction between opposing surfaces of skin). Surgical lifting of sagging breasts is possible and may be necessary before breast reconstruction following mastectomy can be attempted. (See section on breast reconstruction.)

The decrease in glandular tissue makes breast masses easier to palpate. Rib margins may be palpable in the elderly woman and cause concern. The nurse needs to encourage the continuation of BSE by the older client, since the incidence of breast cancer increases with age.

Male Breast Problems

Although the vast majority of breast problems occur in women, it is also important that men know how to examine their breasts. A thorough examination of the male breast should be a routine part of a physical examination. *Gynecomastia,* a transient hypertrophy of one or both breasts, is the most common breast problem of men.

Pubertal gynecomastia

Pubertal hypertrophy secondary to increased estrogen production is seen most often in boys between the ages of 13 to 17. It is usually very limited, although occasionally the localized hypertrophy may measure 2 to 3 cm. Pubertal hypertrophy is almost always self-limiting, disappearing in 4 to 6 months from the onset. Parents and the affected boy should be reassured that in almost all cases this is a normal physiologic phenomenon that will disappear spontaneously and will require no treatment. Rarely, unilateral gynecomastia in the young male may be marked and fail to regress. This is the only indication for surgical intervention.

Senescent gynecomastia

Senescent hypertrophy of the breast occurs between the ages of 50 to 70 years. Though initially unilateral, the tender, firm, centrally located enlargement may become bilateral. When gynecomastia is characterized by a discrete, circumscribed mass, it must be diagnosed differentially from the rarer breast cancer in males. Senescent hypertrophy requires no treatment and generally regresses in 6 to 12 months.

Gynecomastia may also be a symptom of other problems. It is seen accompanying developmental abnormalities of the male reproductive organs. It may also accompany organic diseases including testicular tumors, cancer of the adrenal cortex, pituitary adenomas, hyperthyroidism, and liver disease. Gynecomastia may occur as a side effect of drug therapy. Particularly, it may follow administration of estrogens and androgens, digitalis, isoniazid, and spironolactone. Use of heroin and marijuana can also cause gynecomastia.

SUBCUTANEOUS MASTECTOMY

Subtotal mastectomy consists of the removal of breast tissue with preservation of the skin, nipple, and areola. It is considered a prophylactic measure in women with premalignant breast conditions or high-risk situations such as diagnosed cancer of one breast, ductal dysplasia and hyperplasia, papillomas, chronic cystic disease, and suspicious mammogram.

Although this surgical procedure is being done, it is not considered a routine procedure for clients at high risk to develop serious breast problems.[4] Because it is impossible to remove all breast tissue, the risk of cancer still remains.

An implant, usually silastic, can be implanted immediately during surgery or deferred until blood supply to the skin pocket is well established. The survival of the skin over the breast is the major problem associated with this surgery. Although immediate implantation has greater psychological benefits, the added strain on the skin may lead to circulatory problems and eventual necrosis.

MALIGNANT BREAST PROBLEMS

Breast Cancer

Cancer of the breast is a special disease, a special disturbance, not just another cancer. It is a cancer with all the threat of life that cancer means, but it is far more. Treatment has brought such disfigurement that it is a threat to a woman's image of herself.[5]

Incidence

Breast cancer is the most common malignancy of American women. One in 13 women develop this disease. It is the leading cause of death in women between the ages of 39 to 44 years. The mortality rate of 23 per 100,000 women has not changed in 45 years. Each year in the United States approximately 107,000 cases of breast cancer occur and about 35,000 women die of the disease.[6]

Etiology

Although not completely understood, a number of factors are thought to relate to the cause of breast cancer. Heredity or genetically transmitted susceptibility is considered to play a role. Hormonal influences are considered important. A number of external factors seem to be contributory including dietary factors, obesity, viruses, and glucose intolerance. Environmental factors such as cigarette smoke and chemicals may play a part.

Risk factors

Factors placing a client at higher risk for breast cancer have been identified (Table 44-1). Women are at greater risk than men since 99 percent of breast cancer occurs in women. Increasing age also increases the risk of developing breast cancer. Breast cancer is rare in women under 25 years of age and peaks between the ages of 45 to 49.[7] Risk factors are greatest when there is a positive family history, especially if the involved member with breast cancer was premenopausal and had bilateral disease. Identification of risk factors indicates an increased need for careful surveillance of that client as well as careful instruction in BSE.

Clinical manifestations

Breast cancer is usually first detected as a single lump in the breast. It occurs most often in the upper, outer sector of the breast. The rate at which the lesion grows varies considerably. Slow-growing lesions have a lower mortality rate. The lump of breast cancer is characteristically hard, irregular, poorly delineated, and nonmobile. It is painless and nontender in 90 percent of cases. Table 44-2 outlines primary and secondary signs of breast cancer.

Occasionally, breast cancer presents as nipple discharge. The discharge is usually unilateral and bloody. Nipple retraction may occur. Often, there is edema of the skin over the breast, giving it a characteristic appearance like that of an orange peel (peau d'orange). In late stages, infiltration, induration, and dimpling of the overlying skin may occur (Fig. 44-2).

Complications

The main complication of breast cancer is metastatic spread throughout the lymphatic chains, principally those of the axilla (Fig. 44-3). Distant metastasis occurs through the blood stream, either when the end of the lymphatic chain is reached or when the tumor directly invades a vessel. The organs most frequently invaded by metastasis are bone, lung, brain, and

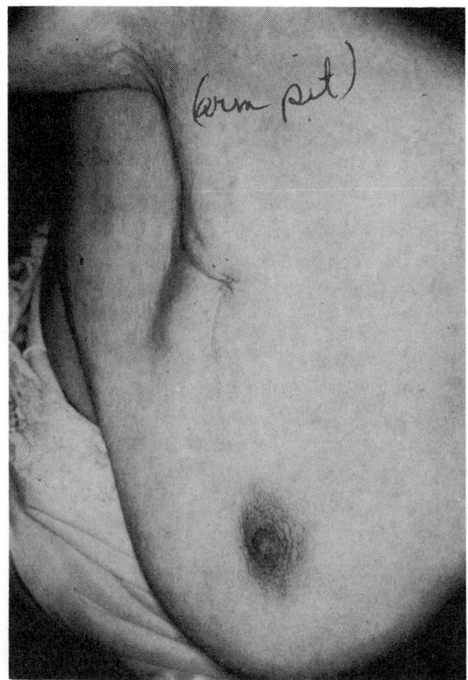

Figure 44-2 Dimpling of skin over primary carcinoma of breast in upper outer quadrant. *(Seymour Schwartz et al., Principles of Surgery, 3d ed., McGraw-Hill Book Company, New York, 1979, p. 571.)*

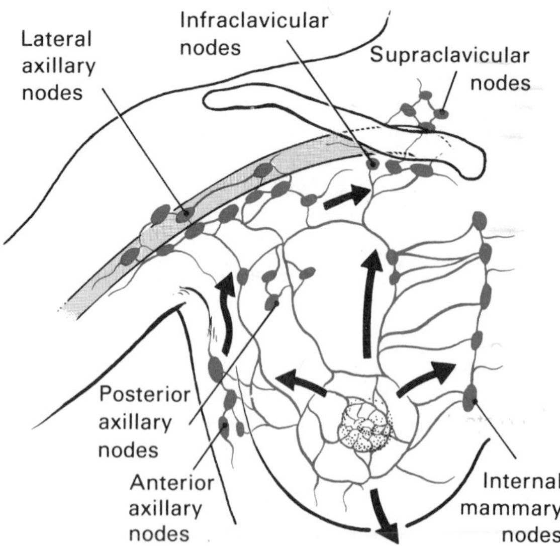

Figure 44-3 Lymphatic drainage of the breast. Arrows indicate direction of drainage.

Table 44-2

Primary and Secondary Signs of Breast Cancer

Primary	Secondary
1. Presence of mass with malignant features	1. Increased vascularity of breast
2. Presence of tumor with microcalcifications	2. Skin edema
3. Segmental ductal prominence in one breast	3. Skin retraction
	4. Nipple retraction
	5. Axillary lymphadenopathy

From Lewis Venet, *A Practical Guide to Diagnosis and Treatment of Breast Cancer*, Spectrum Publications, Inc., New York, 1979, p 17.

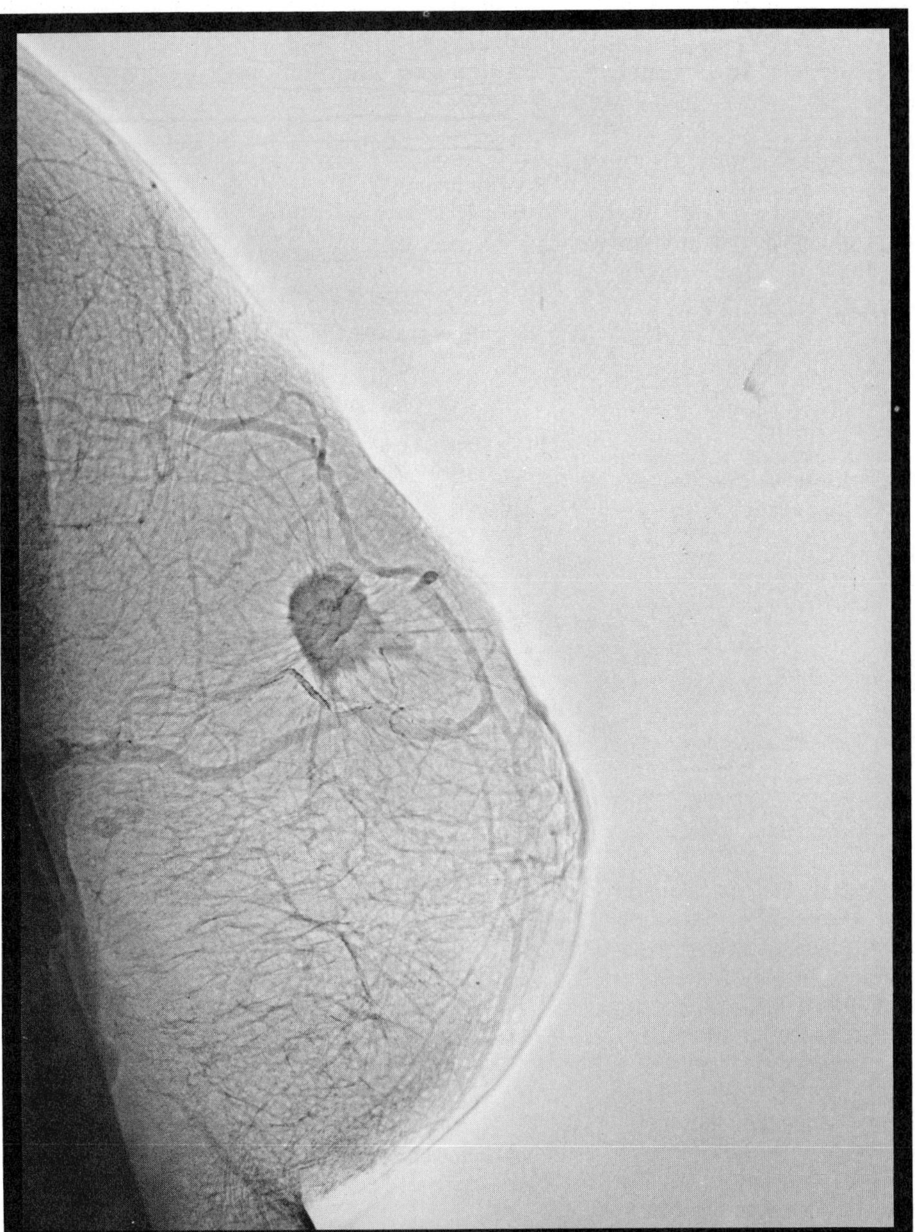

Figure 44-4 Mammogram showing breast cancer and increased vascularity. (*Eldra Pearl Solomon and William Davis, Understanding Human Anatomy and Physiology, McGraw-Hill Book Company, New York, 1978, p. 539.*)

liver.[8] However, metastatic disease can be found in any distant site.

Diagnostic study abnormalities

The discovery of a lump or bloody nipple discharge and the presence of risk factors in the client's history raises the suspicion that cancer exists. Noninvasive techniques such as mammography or xerography may then demonstrate the presence of a tumor mass (Fig. 44-4). Definitive diagnosis of a malignancy is only made by histologic examination of biopsied tissue.

Medical management

There are wide variations in the medical management of cancer of the breast (Table 44-3). The thera-

Table 44-3

Medical Management: Cancer of the Breast

Diagnostic

1. History of risk factors
2. Physical examination of breast and lymphatics
3. Mammography if indicated
4. Biopsy

Staging evaluation of a client with diagnosis of breast cancer

1. CBC, platelet count
2. Calcium, phosphorous, liver function tests
3. Chest x-ray
4. Liver scan
5. Bone scan

Therapeutic

1. Surgery—lumpectomy, simple mastectomy, modified radical mastectomy, radical mastectomy, extended radical mastectomy
2. Radiation therapy
   a. Primary radiotherapy
   b. Adjuvant radiotherapy
   c. Palliative therapy
3. Chemotherapy
   a. Adjuvant chemotherapy
   b. Chemotherapy of recurrent disease
4. Hormonal therapy
   a. Estrogen receptor assay
   b. Hormones—tamoxifen, androgens, estrogens
   c. Surgical hormonal therapy

peutic regimen is often dictated by the clinical stage classification of the cancer (Table 44-4). Although surgical removal of the involved breast has historically been the mainstay of treatment, this is not the case today. (Side effects and appropriate nursing management of specific treatment modalities for cancer are found in Chap. 11.)

Surgery If diagnostic studies indicate that metastatic spread has not occurred beyond the lymphatic system of the breast, surgery is often performed. The recommended surgical procedure is a modified radical mastectomy involving excision of the breast tissue and axillary lymph nodes (Fig. 44-5). An alternative, but not yet proven approach, is the wedge resection and treatment of the breast with primary radiation therapy. Surgical approaches to breast cancer are summarized in Table 44-5.

Recently it has been recommended to perform a biopsy and breast removal in two stages. This allows the pathologist to make a definitive diagnosis. Also, the client does not enter the operating room uncertain of her diagnosis and return to the recovery room with

Table 44-4

Staging and Grouping of Cancer of the Breast

Definitions of T, N, and M

Primary tumor (T)

Clinical-diagnostic classification

TX Tumor cannot be assessed

T0 No evidence of primary tumor

TIS Paget's disease of the nipple with no demonstrable tumor
Note: Paget's disease with a demonstrable tumor is classified according to size of the tumor.

T1* Tumor 2 cm or less in greatest dimension
- **T1a** No fixation to underlying pectoral fascia or muscle
- **T1b** Fixation to underlying pectoral fascia and/or muscle

T2* Tumor more than 2 cm but not more than 5 cm in its greatest dimension
- **T2a** No fixation to underlying pectoral fascia and/or muscle
- **T2b** Fixation to underlying pectoral fascia and/or muscle

T3* Tumor more than 5 cm in its greatest dimension
- **T3a** No fixation to underlying pectoral fascia and/or muscle
- **T3b** Fixation to underlying pectoral facia and/or muscle

T4 Tumor of any size with direct extension to chest wall or skin
Note: Chest wall includes ribs, intercostal muscles, and serratus anterior muscle, but not pectoral muscle.
- **T4a** Fixation to chest wall
- **T4b** Edema (including peau d'orange), ulceration of the skin of the breast, or satellite skin nodules confined to the same breast
- **T4c** Both of above
- **T4d** Inflammatory carcinoma

Nodal involvement (N)

Clinical-diagnostic classification

NX Regional lymph nodes cannot be assessed clinically

N0 No palpable homolateral axillary nodes

N1 Movable homolateral axillary nodes
- **N1a** Nodes not considered to contain growth
- **N1b** Nodes considered to contain growth

N2 Homolateral axillary nodes containing growth and fixed to one another or to other structures

N3 Homolateral supraclavicular or infraclavicular nodes containing growth or edema of the arm†

Distant metastasis (M)

MX Not assessed

Table 44-4 (Continued)

MO	No (known) distant metastasis	
M1	Distant metastasis present Specify ________ Specify sites according to the following notations: Pulmonary —PUL Osseous —OSS Hepatic —HEP Brain —BRA Lymph Nodes —LYM Bone Marrow —MAR Pleura —PLE Skin —SKI Eye —EYE Other —OTH	
	Stage Grouping	
	In situ cancer (in situ lobular, pure intraductal, and Paget's disease of the nipple without palpable mass)	
T1S		
	Invasive cancer	
Stage I		
	T1a or T1b N0 or N1a	**MO**
Stage II		
	T0 N1b	**MO**
	T2a or T1b N1b	**MO**
	T1a or T2b N0 or N1a or N1b	**MO**
Stage III		
	T1a or T1b N2	**MO**
	T2a or T2b N2	**MO**
	T3a or T3b N0 or N1 or N2	**MO**
Stage IV		
	Any T4 Any N	**Any M**
	Any T N3	**Any M**
	Any T Any N	**M1**

*Dimpling of the skin, nipple retraction, or any other skin changes except those in T4b may occur in T1, T2, or T3 without affecting the classification.

†Homolateral internal mammary nodes considered to contain growth are included in N3 for surgical evaluative classification and postsurgical treatment classification.

From *Manual for Staging of Cancer 1978,* American Joint Committee for Cancer Staging and End Results Reporting, Whiting Press, 1978, pp 101–104. Reprinted with permission.

her breast amputated. Such a two-step approach has positive psychological benefits for the client in that she may participate in decision making and benefit from anticipatory support. There have been no adverse effects reported from this two-stage management.[9] One protocol for the use of alternative methods for the treatment of breast cancer is summarized in Table 44-6.

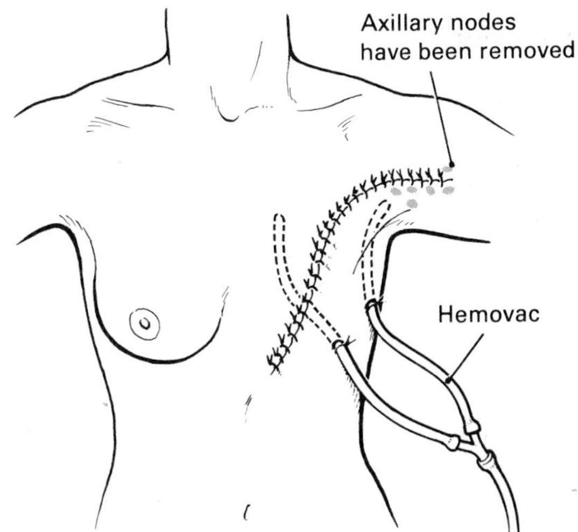

Figure 44-5 Radical mastectomy incision with drains in place.

Lymphedema of the arm on the affected side is a distressing complication following a radical mastectomy. It can occur secondary to the excision or irradiation of lymph nodes. When the axillary nodes cannot return lymph fluid to the central circulation, this fluid accumulates in the arm. This fluid causes pressure on the veins and obstructs venous return. Cellulitis and progressive fibrosis can result from lymphedema.

Following surgery the client must be followed for the remainder of her life at regular intervals. Most clients are seen every 2 to 4 months for 2 years and every 6 months thereafter, in addition to monthly self-breast examination. The client must have yearly mammography of the remaining breast.

Radiation Therapy The three clinical situations in which radiation therapy may be used for cancer of the breast include: (1) the primary treatment, (2) the adjuvant treatment, and (3) the palliative treatment of local recurrences and metastases.

Primary Radiation Therapy

When radiation therapy is the primary treatment, it usually follows local excision of the breast mass. The breast and regional lymph nodes are irradiated over the course of several weeks, using an external beam of radiation. Later, a temporary implant of a radioactive substance such as iridium 192 may be inserted directly into the breast tissue. Hollow needles are inserted into the breast with the client under general anesthesia. The radioactive tube is inserted into the needle when the client returns to her room (Fig. 44-6).

Table 44-5

Surgical Approaches To Breast Cancer

1. Lumpectomy
   Removal of the tumor mass
2. Total mastectomy (simple)
   Removal of the breast, pectoralis major fascia, and axillary tail of the breast
   Noninvasive carcinoma
3. Modified radical mastectomy
   Radical mastectomy with preservation of the pectoralis major muscle
4. Standard radical mastectomy (Halsted procedure)
   Removal of the breast, pectoralis minor and major muscles, and a dissection of the axillary contents
5. Extended radical mastectomy
   Standard radical mastectomy plus resection of the internal mammary chain of lymph nodes with chest wall resection

The radioactive substance remains in place 2 to 3 days. Esophagitis and tracheitis may be temporary side effects of external beam radiation therapy. Chemotherapy is often used systemically to enhance the local effects of irradiation.

Adjuvant Radiation Therapy

Although an uncommon treatment mode, preoperative radiation therapy can reduce the size of a tumor mass to operable proportions by destruction of the cancer cells. Additionally, by partially or completely destroying the malignant cells, the rate of local recurrence will decrease. The disadvantages of potential delayed wound healing and increased lymphedema do not seem to outweigh the advantages.

The decision to use postoperative radiation therapy is made on the probability of the presence of local residual cancer cells. Irradiating the area will not prevent the appearance of metastasis at a later date. The site of radiation therapy (lymph nodes, chest wall, or both) will depend on the degree of spread of the cancer. Although radiation therapy can reduce the local recurrence rate, it has not altered the long-term survival of clients.[10]

Palliative Radiation Therapy

In addition to reducing the primary tumor mass with resultant decrease in pain, radiation therapy is also used to stabilize symptomatic metastatic lesions in such sites as bone, soft tissue organs, the brain, and chest. Radiation therapy affords pain relief and is often successful for long periods of time.

Chemotherapy Improvement in long-term survival rates has been attributed to the use of combination chemotherapy for breast cancer.[11] The five-drug combination (CMFVP) of cyclophosphamide, methotrexate, 5-fluorouracil, vincristine, and prednisone is achieving impressive results in advanced breast can-

Table 44-6

Treatment of Breast Cancer: Alternative Methods Following Surgery

In estrogen receptor-positive patients

Stage I: No apparent metastasis	Observe
Stage II: Axillary metastasis only	Chemotherapy and immunotherapy (more aggressive therapy would add oophorectomy and adrenalectomy or prednisone and antiestrogens). Radiation therapy may be indicated.
Stage III: Distant metastasis (skin, bone, lung parenchyma)	Chemotherapy and immunotherapy plus oophorectomy and adrenalectomy, or aminoglutethimide, cortisol, and antiestrogen if surgical procedures unavailable or unacceptable. Androgens for premenopausal and estrogens for postmenopausal clients are third choice.
Stage IV; Visceral metastasis (brain, liver, pulmonary lymphatics)	Same as stage III, as client's condition allows.

In estrogen receptor-negative patients

Treatment of stages II to IV should be confined to immunotherapy plus prolonged continuous chemotherapy alternating various therapeutic regimens.

Kurt J. Isselbacher et al. (eds.), *Harrison's Principles of Internal Medicine,* 9th ed., McGraw-Hill Book Company, New York, 1980.

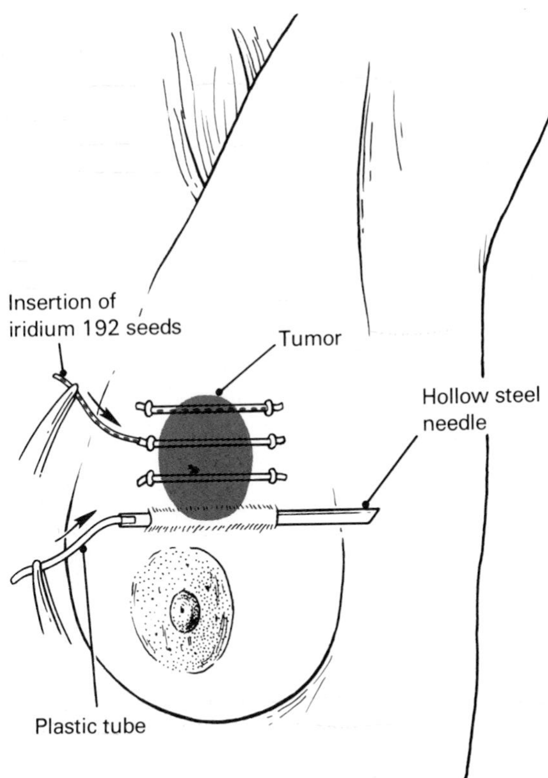

Figure 44-6 Breast radium implant. *(Adapted from Time, The Weekly Newsmagazine. Copyright Time, Inc., 1977. Used by permission.)*

cer. An overall response rate (greater than 50 percent reduction in tumor mass) of 50 percent has been confirmed by several large studies.[12] Currently, the use of cyclophosphamide, methotrexate, and 5-fluorouracil (also called CMF) is recommended in the primary treatment of newly diagnosed breast cancer in premenopausal women who show evidence of lymph node metastasis.

Hormonal Therapy Hormonal therapy can lengthen the time to recurrence, but has no effect on long-term survival. Therefore, it is reserved for the treatment of breast cancer in relapse. The use of the estrogen receptor protein (ERP) assay has refined the use of surgical ablation of estrogen synthesis. It has been found that not all malignant breast tumors are estrogen-dependent. Although normal breast tissue contains receptor sites for estrogen, malignant cell transformation alters these receptor sites in some cells. If the malignant cell retains estrogen receptor sites, it will continue to be regulated by estrogen. Those receptor sites which were altered due to malignant transformation are no longer hormonally controlled. About one-third of breast cancers will be hormone-dependent. If a tumor is found to be ERP-positive, hormone deprivation by bilateral oophorectomy, adrenalectomy, or hypophysectomy can be used successfully as a palliative treatment. If the tumor is estrogen receptor-negative, pointless surgery can be avoided. Antiestrogen drugs (nafoxadine and tamoxifen) which block the estrogen receptor sites of malignant cells, are routinely used in the treatment of recurrent breast cancer.[13] The administration of estrogen and androgens is also effective in reducing tumor mass but has more unpleasant side effects than the administration of antiestrogens. Breast, skin, lymphatic, and bone metastases respond better to endocrine therapy than do organ lesions.

Immunotherapy Although not accepted standard practice, new approaches to immunotherapy with tumor vaccines are being tried experimentally. BCG vaccine is being used to stimulate the immune system (Chap. 11).

Nursing management

Throughout her interactions with the client with breast cancer, the nurse must keep in mind the extensive psychological impact of the disease. All aspects of care must include sensitivity to the client's altered body image. An open environment in which the client may express her fears and feelings is essential. The nurse can help meet the client's psychological needs by

1. Developing within herself a positive, but realistic attitude
2. Realizing that the client is living, and not dying despite the diagnosis of breast cancer
3. Encouraging the client to verbalize her anger and fears of cancer, of disfigurement, and of potential sexual rejection by her partner
4. Encouraging open communication of thoughts and feelings between the client and her family
5. Providing accurate and complete answers to questions

Acute Nursing Management The nursing management of the various cancer treatments is discussed in Chap. 11. The nursing management of the client with a radical mastectomy will be discussed in this section.

Preoperative

The client needs to be provided with sufficient information to ensure informed consent. Some clients need extensive, detailed information. For others, this only increases anxiety. Sensitivity to the individual's needs are essential.

Preoperative diagnostic studies must be completed. The operative site must be prepared and blood ordered for surgery. Teaching in the preoperative phase includes instruction in turning, coughing and deep breathing, a review of postoperative exercises, and explanation of the recovery period from recovery room until discharge. If a radical mastectomy is anticipated, discussing its possibility should not be avoided in the preoperative period.

Postoperative

Physical care. In addition to the usual postoperative nursing measures, the client who has a radical mastectomy needs specific nursing interventions (Table 44-7).

Restoring arm function on the affected side after mastectomy is one of the most important goals of nursing activities. The client should be placed in a semi-Fowler's position with the arm on the affected side elevated. Flexing and extending the fingers should begin in the recovery room with daily increase in activity. Postoperative mastectomy exercises are instituted on the first to seventh postoperative day, depending on the choice of the surgeon (Fig. 44-7). These exercises are designed to prevent contractures and muscle shortening, maintain muscle tone, and improve lymph and blood circulation. The difficulty and pain encountered by the client in performing the

Table 44-7
Nursing Care Plan Following a Radical Mastectomy

Problem	Expected Outcome	Nursing Intervention
		Postoperative
Edema of the arm on the operative side	Usual size and shape of arm	Do not take venipuncture or BP on affected arm. No dependent arm position; arm/hand is elevated on pillows. Avoid abducting arm first week. Start hand and wrist movements and elbow flexion and extension at hourly intervals.
Loss of arm and shoulder function	Return to usual arm and shoulder function	Flex and extend fingers in recovery room and continue throughout postoperative period. Carry out postmastectomy and range-of-motion exercises. Resume ADL gradually. Emphasize bilateral activity of upper extremities.
Tension on incision	Normal incisional healing	Emphasize good posture. Client should use sling when ambulating. Emphasize to client basic motions of abduction and elevation with care to avoid tension. Observe wound and wound drainage.
Disfigurement	Restore external appearance	Explain importance of posture. Introduce client to prosthesis.
Pain	Relief of pain	Distract client with talk and comfort measures. Administer analgesics. Position arm to prevent tension and provide support.
Hematoma	No hematoma formation	Pressure dressing. Client in semi-Fowler's position. Check patency and milk drainage system. Check drainage system insertion site. Measure and assess drainage every 8 h.
Psychological adjustment to altered body image	Acceptance of altered body image	Arrange for *Reach for Recovery* visitor, if available. Include family in discussions. Help client confront deformity. Help client and family anticipate future.
		Long-Term
Persistent lymphedema	Reduce lymphedema	Instruct client on salt-free diet, diuretics, massage, intermittent compression, elastic sleeves.
Inability to adjust to altered sexual and body image	Adjustment to altered body image and satisfying sexual relationships	Refer for counseling. Counsel husband. Refer to *Reach to Recovery* groups.
Potential for metastasis	Early recognition of metastasis	Teach or reevaluate technique of BSE. Instruct client on symptoms to report to physician (e.g., back pain, weakness, constipation, or confusion).

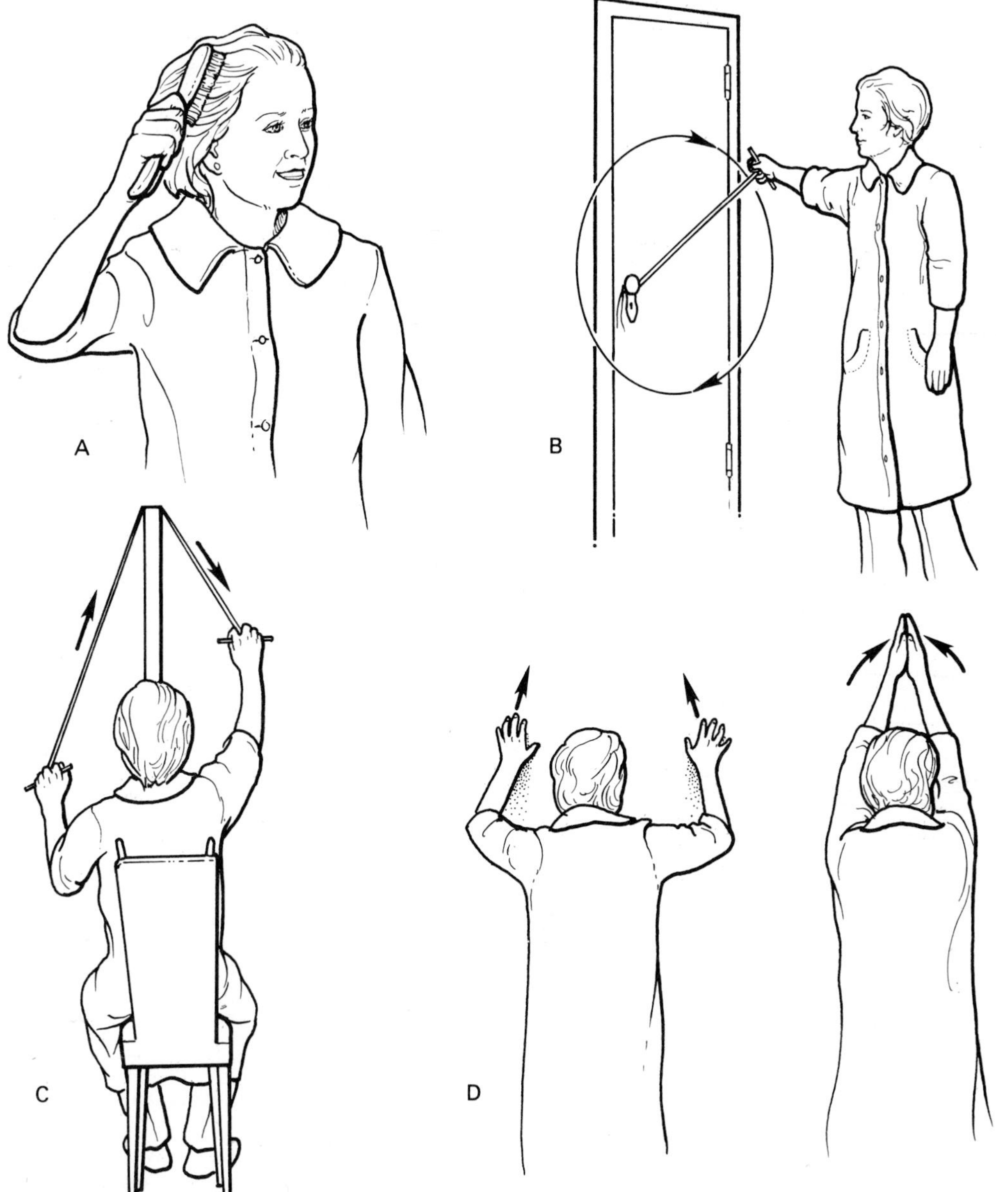

Figure 44-7 Postoperative mastectomy exercises designed to prevent contracture, prevent muscle shortening, maintain muscle tone, and improve lympth and blood circulation. *(a) Hairbrushing:* Until fuller motion is possible, the client can use books to support her arm, gradually reducing the number of books used and increasing range of motion. *(b) Rope Turning:* Attach rope to doorknob on one end and pencil on the other. Hold pencil in palm of hand with rope between middle fingers. Move arm in small circles from shoulder. Circle in both directions, gradually increasing the size of the circle by standing closer to the doorknob. *(c) Pulley:* Tie pencils or tongue depressors to both ends of a rope. Throw rope over a door. Use arm of unaffected side to pull down, raising affected arm as straight and high as possible. *(d) Wall Climbing:* Stand close to wall with feet balanced and forehead touching wall. Hands walk up wall, gradually increasing the height reached until the palms can touch from straight arms.

previously simple tasks included in the exercise program may cause frustration and depression. The nurse will need to encourage the client to perform these exercises regularly in spite of the difficulty encountered. Whenever possible, the same nurse should work with the client with a mastectomy so progress can be commended and problems identified.

Measures to prevent or reduce lymphedema need to be utilized by the nurse and taught to the client. The affected arm must never be dependent, even while the person is sleeping. Blood pressures, venipunctures, and injections should not be done on the affected arm. Elastic bandages should not be used in the early postoperative period because they inhibit collateral lymph drainage. The client needs to be instructed to protect the arm on the operative side from even minor trauma such as a pin prick or sunburn. Should such trauma occur, the incident should be reported to the surgeon immediately. The client needs to know and understand that she can develop lymphedema for the rest of her life following a mastectomy.

When lymphedema is acute, an intermittent pneumatic compression sleeve can be used. This device applies mechanical massage to the arm. Manual massage is also effective in mobilizing subcutaneous accumulations of fluid. Elevation of the arm, diuretics, and isometric exercises may also be used to reduce the fluid volume in the arm. The client may need to wear an elastic pressure-gradient sleeve during waking hours to maintain maximum volume reduction.

Psychological care. The nurse can promote the client's recovery by arranging a visit from a Reach to Recovery volunteer if such a service is available. Medical approval for this visit is necessary. The *Reach to Recovery Program* of the American Cancer Society is a rehabilitation program for women who have had breast surgery. It is designed to help them meet their psychological, physical, and cosmetic needs.[14] The volunteers, all post mastectomy women, can answer questions about what to expect at home, how to tell people about the surgery, and what prosthetic devices are available. If a Reach to Recovery volunteer is not available, it is the nurse's responsibility to be knowledgeable about the needs of the client following a mastectomy. The American Cancer Society can provide excellent material to assist the nurse in meeting the special needs of these clients.

It is critical that the professional staff never underestimate the tremendous psychological impact that the mutilation of a radical mastectomy can have upon the client. Although not all clients will react as dramatically following surgery, anxiety, insomnia, and suicidal thoughts are not uncommon. The nurse's accepting, concerned attitude can do much to relieve the feelings of shame and worthlessness experienced by many clients.

Chronic Nursing Management The nurse should explain the follow-up routine to the client and emphasize the importance of beginning or continuing BSE. Additional symptoms which should be reported to the clinician include back pain, weakness, constipation, or confusion. Brown spots on the involved arm or near the armpit and breast pain that is not associated with menses should also be reported.[15] If adjuvant therapy is to be used, the client should have specific instructions as to appointment times and treatment locations. If lymphedema persists, methods of treating it should be reviewed.

It is important that the nurse impress upon the client the importance of wearing a well-fitting prosthesis. Many fine products are available to meet the specific needs of individual clients. Well-trained saleswomen can assist the client to select a suitable prosthesis. There are both physical and psychological advantages to the use of a prosthesis, especially the return of a normal external appearance.

The implications of a mastectomy on the sexual identity and relationships of the client are variable. A preoperative sexual assessment provides helpful baseline data on which the nurse can plan postoperative interventions. Often, the husband, sexual partner, and/or family may need assistance in dealing with their emotional reaction to the mastectomy surgery. There are no physical reasons for a mastectomy preventing sexual satisfaction. If a problem develops, counseling may be necessary to deal with the emotional component of this problem.

A public health referral may provide the client with follow-up at home to evaluate coping behaviors. The public health nurse also provides an outlet for the patient for whom adjustment is especially problematic. Usually, the initial coping mechanisms begin to lose effectiveness at about 3 months, and a peak period of psychological disorganization occurs for the client. Special nursing interventions are necessary should a recurrence of cancer be found, both in terms of psychological support and teaching.

Paget's Disease of the Breast

Paget's disease is a breast malignancy characterized by a persistent eczematoid lesion of the nipple and areola with or without a palpable mass. Itching and bloody nipple discharge, erosion, and ulceration may be present. Diagnosis of Paget's disease is confirmed by pathologic examination of the surgical specimen. The presence of a palpable mass probably increases the incidence of lymph node metastasis.[16]

The treatment of Paget's disease is a modified radical mastectomy. The nursing care for the client with Paget's disease is the same as if it were a usual breast carcinoma.

MAMMOPLASTY

Mammoplasty is the surgical change in the size and/or shape of the breast. It may be done electively for cosmetic purposes to either enlarge or reduce the size of the breasts. It may also be done to reconstruct the breast following both simple and radical mastectomy.

It is important that the health care providers remain nonjudgmental in their attitude toward the women who desires mammoplasty. The desire to alter the appearance of the breasts has special significance for each client. Their motives should not be questioned. It is important, however, that the client have a realistic idea of what mammoplasty can accomplish as well as the possible complications such as hematoma formation, hemorrhage, and infection. If an implant is involved, there is the possibility of capsular contracture and loss of the implant.

Breast Augmentation

In *augmentation mammoplasty* (the procedure to enlarge small breasts) an implant is placed in a surgically created pocket between the capsule of the breast and the pectoral fascia. Most implants are silastic envelopes filled with a fluid such as dextran, saline, or silicone. Because of their resemblance to the human breast, implants filled with silicone are most widely used. Although physiologically feasible, breast feeding is not generally advised following breast augmentation. Women are often advised to complete their family before undergoing breast augmentation.

Breast Reduction

Contrary to popular opinion, large breasts can be a source of great embarrassment for the client. They can also interfere with normal daily activities such as walking, typing, and driving a car. Overly large breasts can also lead to back and chest problems. They may make stylish dressing more difficult. Reduction in the size of the breasts can have positive effects on both the psychological and physical health of the client. *Reduction mammoplasty* is performed by resecting wedges of tissue from the upper and lower quadrants of the breast. The excess skin is then removed and the areola relocated on the breast.

Breast Reconstruction

Breast reconstruction can be done following mastectomy. Recent strides in techniques have made this surgery a satisfactory alternative for many women. The possibility of breast reconstruction may encourage women to seek professional help if a breast lump is detected.

Indications

The main indication for breast reconstruction is to improve the woman's self-concept and feeling of loss. Present techniques cannot restore lactation, nipple sensation, or erectility.[17] Therefore, the erotic functions of the breast are not present. Although the breast will never return to its premastectomy appearance, the reconstructed appearance is usually an improvement over the mastectomy scar (Fig. 44-8). The contour of the breast is restored without the use of an external prosthesis.

Timing of reconstruction

Controversy exists over the appropriate time lapse from mastectomy to reconstructive surgery. Some surgeons feel reconstruction should not be attempted until there has been a 5-year lapse from surgery.[18] Others feel the timing of reconstruction surgery should be individualized, based on the histologic grading of the tumor, size of the primary tumor, and axillary node metastasis.[19] The timing of reconstruction ranges from 5 days to 5 years postoperatively. It is known that early reconstruction neither retards nor influences further treatment, nor adversely affects predicted survival.

Techniques of reconstruction

The extent of the reconstruction depends on the type of mastectomy done. If extensive chest wall defects are not present, a silastic implant can be used. It is implanted under the subcutaneous tissue to simulate the breast.

If a more extensive mastectomy was performed, dermal fat pads may be used to restore the soft tissue defects. The breast implant is then put in place. Nipple reconstruction may or may not be done.

Nipple reconstruction

If immediate reconstruction is planned following the mastectomy, the nipple of the amputated breast is biopsied for evidence of malignancy. If none is apparent, the nipple can be implanted (banked) in the

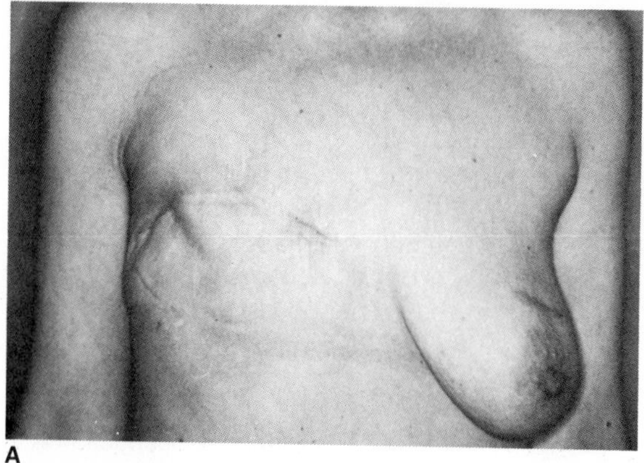

A

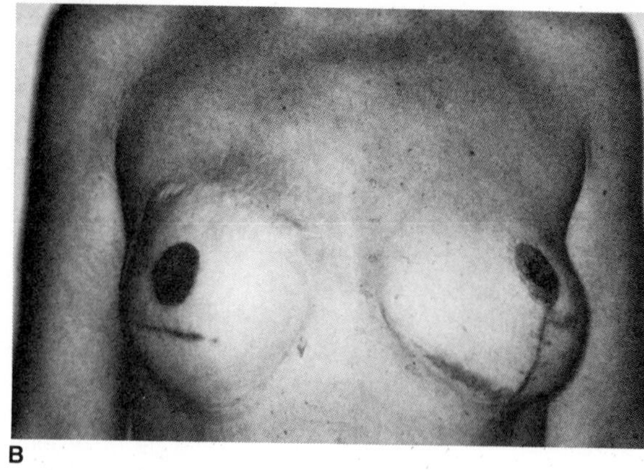

B

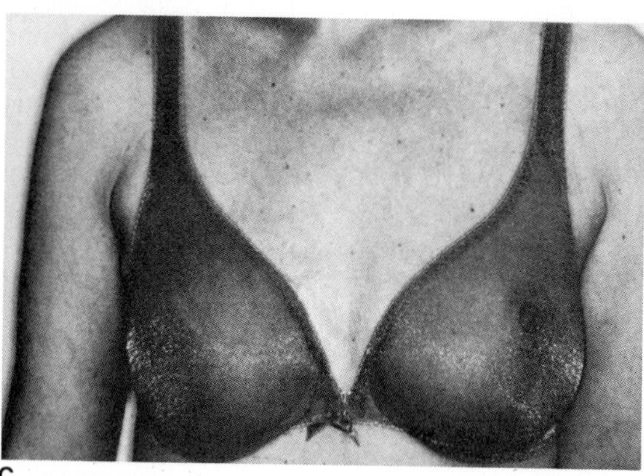

C

Figure 44-8 Breast reconstruction following mastectomy. Three-figure sequence showing pre- and postoperative reconstruction and symmetry in clothing. *(a)* Client with modified radical mastectomy scar and pendulous contralateral breast. *(b)* After right breast and areolar reconstruction and contralateral reduction mammoplasty with nipple-areola repositioning. *(c)* Appearance of the reconstructed client in clothing—an example of what can be achieved. *[Sally Thomas et al., "Breast Reconstruction After Mastectomy," Am. J Nurs,* **77**(9):1440 (1977).*]*

inguinal area at the time of mastectomy. It is transplanted to the newly constructed breast at a later date.

If nipple banking is not feasible, the nipple of the remaining breast can provide material for a nipple on the reconstructed breast. Skin from the labia, skin grafts from other areas, and tattooing are other procedures used. Various techniques are available to build up central nipple projections. In some instances, only the breast will be reconstructed, with no attempt to imitate the nipple.

Nursing Management

Mammoplasty may be done in the outpatient surgical area or it may involve overnight hospitalization. General anesthesia is used. To prevent hematoma formation, drains are generally placed in the surgical site. These are removed 2 to 3 days postoperatively. Drainage must be examined for color and odor to detect postoperative infection. The client's temperature should also be monitored. Dressings should be changed prn using sterile technique *except* when the nipple has been grafted. In these cases, graft dressings should not be disturbed for 7 to 10 days. Postoperatively, the client needs to be assured that the appearance of the breast will improve when sutures are removed and healing is completed. Blackening of the reimplanted nipple immediately postoperatively is to be expected. The client should be instructed to wear a padded bra continuously to support the breasts for 2 to 3 days after mammoplasty. Shoulder and arm movement should be restricted for several weeks, with gradual resumption of normal activities.

Case Study / Breast Cancer

Irene J., a 40-year-old mother of two, discovered a lump in her breast while doing her monthly breast self-examination. She saw her doctor the following day. He confirmed the presence of the lump and ordered a mammogram. The mammogram showed a solid tumor with increased vascularity. Mrs. J. was hospitalized for a biopsy which confirmed the presence of a malignancy. A right radical mastectomy was scheduled in 2 days.

Discussion Questions

1. What risk factors related to cancer of the breast would be asked in taking Mrs. J.'s health history?
2. Describe the characteristics of the malignant growth determined by palpation.
3. Outline the preoperative and postoperative nursing management for Mrs. J.
4. Describe ways to assist Mrs. J. and her family to adjust to the impending change in her body image.
5. Identify the possible complications Mrs. J. might face following a radical mastectomy.
6. Describe the common postoperative exercises which Mrs. J. will need to practice.

REVIEW QUESTIONS

The number of the question corresponds to the same numbered objective at the beginning of the chapter.

1. Included in the BSE procedure recommended by the American Cancer Society is palpation of the breast while lying down using
   a. a top to bottom motion
   b. a left to right motion
   c. a right to left motion
   d. a circular motion

2. In addition to BSE, all adult women should
   a. have their breasts examined by a professional yearly
   b. have their breasts examined and mammography done yearly
   c. have mammography yearly
   d. have no additional examination

3. A round, well-delineated, palpable lump that may increase in size premenstrually each month and disappear entirely when a woman reaches menopause is characteristic of
   a. fibrocystic disease
   b. fibroadenoma
   c. intraductal papilloma
   d. ductal ectasia

4. Breast cancer occurs
   a. with equal frequency in men and women
   b. with equal frequency throughout the life span
   c. more frequently in women who have borne children and lactated
   d. more frequently in postmenopausal women

5. Removal of the breast, pectoralis major fascia, and axillary tail of the breast is called
   a. modified radical mastectomy
   b. lumpectomy
   c. simple mastectomy
   d. standard radical mastectomy (Halsted procedure)

6. Measures to prevent or reduce lymphedema include
   a. keeping the affected arm in a dependent position
   b. protecting the arm on the affected side from trauma
   c. early institution of postmastectomy exercises
   d. early postoperative use of elastic bandages

7. The primary indication for breast reconstruction is to
   a. restore sensation and erectility
   b. restore lactation
   c. improve the client's self-concept
   d. return the breast to its premastectomy appearance

REFERENCES

1. Editorial, "Subcutaneous Mastectomy," *N Engl J Med,* **297**(9):503 (1977).
2. Phillip Strax, "Screening for Breast Cancer," *Clin Obstet Gynecol,* **20**(4):783 (December 1977).
3. A. I. Holleb, "Restoring Confidence in Mammography," *Cancer,* **26**(6):376 (1976).
4. Editorial, "Subcutaneous Mastectomy," *N Engl J Med,* **297**(9):504 (1977).
5. Oliver Cope, *The Breast,* Houghton-Mifflin Co., Boston, 1977, p. 143.
6. American Cancer Society, *Cancer Facts and Figures,* New York, 1979. p. 9.
7. Helmuth Voorhees and Robert Messer, "Breast Cancer: Potentially Predisposing and Protecting Factors," *Am J Obstet Gynecol,* **150**(5):359 (February 1978).
8. *Manual for Staging for Cancer 1978,* American Joint Committee for Cancer Staging and End Results Reporting, Whiting Press, 1978, p. 101.
9. Lewis Venet (ed.), *A Practical Guide to Diagnosis and Treatment of Breast Cancer,* Spectrum Publications, Inc., New York, 1979, p. 108.
10. Venet, op. cit., p. 123.
11. John Saiki, "Adjuvant Chemotherapy of Breast Cancer 1979," unpublished paper, Cancer Research and Treatment Center, Albuquerque, New Mexico, 1979, p. 1.
12. Ibid., p. 2.
13. Ibid., p. 169.
14. Teresa Lasser, *Reach to Recovery,* American Cancer Society, 1969, p. 9.
15. Joanne Tully and Beatrice Wagner, "Breast Cancer," *Nursing 78,* January, p 23.
16. Roy Ashikari et al., "Paget's Disease of the Breast," *Cancer,* **26:**680 (1970).
17. Nicholas Georgiade, *Breast Reconstruction Following Mastectomy,* The C. V. Mosby Company, St. Louis, 1979, p. 148.
18. P. C. Brand (ed.), *Breast Cancer: Psycho-Social Aspects of Early Detection and Treatment,* University Park Press, Baltimore, 1978, p. 69.
19. Georgiade, op. cit., p. 148.

Chapter 45

NURSING ROLE IN MANAGEMENT

Sexually Transmitted Diseases

Linda C. Carnago

Learning Objectives

1. Identify the contributory factors to the high incidence of sexually transmitted diseases.
2. Explain the etiology, clinical manifestations, complications, and diagnostic abnormalities of gonorrhea, syphilis, herpes genitalis, chancroid, lymphogranuloma venereum, and granuloma inguinale.
3. Explain the medical and pharmacologic management of gonorrhea and syphilis.
4. Compare herpesvirus type 1 with herpesvirus type 2.
5. Describe the nursing role in the prevention and control of sexually transmitted diseases.
6. Describe the physiologic and psychological nursing intervention for the client with a sexually transmitted disease.

SEXUALLY TRANSMITTED DISEASES

Sexually transmitted diseases are infectious diseases usually associated with intimate sexual contact. They are often referred to as venereal diseases. Although gonorrhea and syphilis are the most common, there are over 20 diseases which can be sexually transmitted (Table 45-1). Several of the sexually transmitted diseases are more common in tropical and semitropical areas. However, the mobility of present-day society is increasing their occurrence in other areas of the world. Diseases which are associated with sexual transmission can also be contracted by other than sexual means, such as environmental association.

Significance of Problem

In the United States all cases of gonorrhea and syphilis are to be reported to the state or local health officer. In spite of this requirement, there are many unreported and undiagnosed cases (Fig. 45-1). Gonorrhea ranks first and syphilis third among the reported communicable diseases in the United States. The incidence of gonorrhea has steadily increased since 1966 but now may be reaching a plateau. A slight decrease (0.2 percent) was reported in 1977, possibly reflecting the implementation of federally funded programs to control the disease. Teenagers and young adults accounted for 25 to 30 percent of all gonorrhea cases reported. At the present time all but six states have enacted laws allowing for examination and treatment services for minors without parental consent.

The trend of reporting primary and secondary syphilis has changed several times since 1941 (Fig 45-2), presumably due to the availability of penicillin as well as intensive treatment campaigns. While there was a slight decrease in all reported primary and secondary syphilis cases in 1977, there was an increase in the disease involving men. This trend probably reflects the increase in the high-risk population of male homosexuals.[1] In the last 30 to 40 years, treatment of large numbers of clients with syphilis has produced a 98 percent reduction in the complications of syphilis.

A decline in the cases of chancroid, granuloma

Table 45-1

Sexually Transmitted Diseases and Diseases Associated with Sexual Transmission

Syphilis
Gonorrhea
Chancroid
Lymphogranuloma venereum
Granuloma inguinale
Nongonococcal urethritis
Candidiasis
Genital warts (condylomata acuminata)
Trichomoniasis
Genital herpes
Molluscum contagiosum
Cytomegalovirus infection
Viral hepatitis type B
Pubic lice
Scabies
Reiter's syndrome
Corynebacterium vaginale
Nesseria meningitides
Other specific protozoa, helminths, and bacteria

Adapted from T. Fitzpatrick et al. (eds.) *Dematology in General Medicine,* 2d ed., McGraw-Hill Book Company, New York, 1979, pp. 1669–1671.

This chapter was reviewed by Patricia A. Hendrickson, R.N., M.S., CFNP, Instructor, Center for Continuing Education in Women's Health Care, University of New Mexico, Albuquerque, New Mexico.

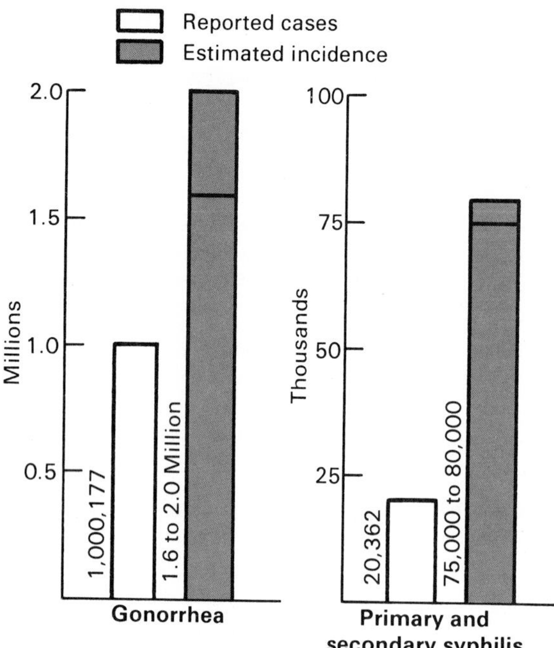

Figure 45-1 Reported and estimated cases of gonorrhea and syphilis. (*Source: CDC 79-8195, HEW-PHS: STD Fact Sheet, 34th ed., Atlanta, 1979, p. 2.*)

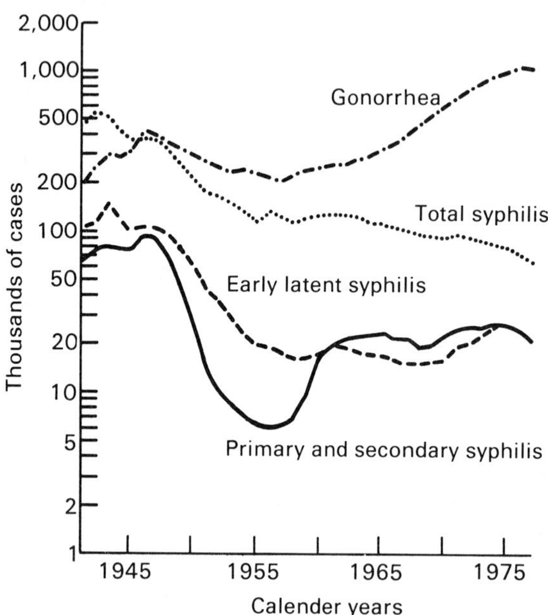

Figure 45-2 Reported cases of syphilis and gonorrhea in the United States: 1941–1977. (*Source: CDC 9, 688, HEW-PHS-CDC-BSS-VD Control Division, Evaluation and Statistical Services Section, Atlanta.*)

inguinale, and lymphogranuloma venereum was reported in 1977 in the United States. The true incidence of herpes genitalis is difficult to determine since it is not a reportable disease. Researchers have estimated that approximately 300,000 new cases of herpes genitalis occur annually.[2] The disease is gaining more attention due to its association with cervical cancer and neonatal infection.

Factors Affecting Incidence

There are contributing factors to the increased incidence of sexually transmitted diseases. Earlier reproductive maturity and expanded longevity have resulted in a longer sexual life span. The increase in the total population has resulted in an increase in the number of susceptible hosts. Greater sexual freedom, decreased social control by religious institutions, and increased emphasis on sexuality by mass media are also factors. In addition, increased leisure time, inexpensive travel, and urbanization have brought people of varying cultural backgrounds and value systems together. Codes of behavior of the new environment are usually adopted and may result in the exploration of new sexual conduct.

Changes in methods of contraception are also reflected in the incidence of venereal disease. The condom is considered to be the only contraceptive device which is prophylactic to venereal disease. Its use has decreased while the use of oral contraceptives has increased. Oral contraceptives cause the secretions of the cervix and vagina to become more alkaline. This change produces a more favorable environment for the growth of venereal disease organisms. It has been demonstrated that women who have gonorrhea and use an intrauterine device have an increased risk of gonococcal salpingitis and pelvic inflammatory disease.[3]

GONORRHEA

Etiology

The causative organism of gonorrhea is *Neisseria gonorrhoeae*, a gram-negative diplococcus. It may invade any mucosal surface of the body but is most likely to invade the moist linings of the urinary and genital organs of both sexes. The disease is spread by direct physical contact with an infected host, usually during sexual activity. Neonates can develop a gonococcal infection after passage through an infected birth canal. The delicate gonococcus is easily killed through drying, heating, or washing with an antiseptic solution. Consequently, indirect transmission by instruments or linens is rare. The incubation period is 3 to 4 days. The disease confers no immunity to subsequent reinfections.

Clinical Manifestations

Men

The initial site of infection in heterosexual men is usually the anterior urethra. Symptoms of urethritis consisting of dysuria and profuse, purulent urethral discharge develop within 3 to 5 days after infection. Males generally seek medical assistance early in the disease because their symptoms are usually obvious and distressing. However, there is increased evidence of asymptomatic disease in males.[4]

Women

Most women who have gonorrhea are either asymptomatic or have minor symptoms which are often overlooked. A small number of women may complain of vaginal discharge, dysuria, or urinary frequency. Changes in menstruation may be a symptom but they are often disregarded by the woman. Following the incubation period, redness and swelling occur at the site of contact, which is usually the cervix or urethra. A purulent exudate often develops with potential for abscess formation. The disease may remain local or can spread by direct tissue extension to the uterus, fallopian tubes, and ovaries. Although the vulva and vagina are uncommon sites for a gonorrheal infection, this may occur when little or no estrogen is present, as is the case in prepubertal girls and postmenopausal women.

General

Anorectal gonorrhea may be present, particularly in homosexual men, and is usually caused by anal intercourse. Gonococcal proctitis in women probably results from rectal coitus as well as from contamination from infected vaginal secretions. Most clients with rectal infections have no significant symptoms. A small percentage of individuals develop gonococcal pharyngitis resulting from orogenital sexual contact. Individuals of either sex in whom the gonococcus can be demonstrated by culture are infectious to their sexual partners.

Complications

Since males often seek treatment early in the course of their disease, they are less likely to develop complications. The complications that do occur in men are prostatitis, urethral strictures, urethritis, and sterility from orchitis or epididymitis. Since asymptomatic females seldom seek treatment, complications are more common and are usually the reason for seeking medical attention. Pelvic inflammatory disease, Bartholin abscess, ectopic pregnancy, and infertility are the main complications of gonorrhea in women. A small percentage of women may develop a disseminated gonococcal infection (DGI). This can result in gonococcal arthritis. The appearance of skin lesions along with arthralgia (due to arthritis) usually leads the client to seek medical help.

Newborn prophylaxis

Almost all states have a health department regulation or law requiring that a prophylactic drug such as 1% silver nitrate or tetraycline be instilled into the eyes of all newborns.[5] Therefore, the incidence of gonorrheal eye infections of newborns (ophthalmia neonatorum) is relatively uncommon today. Untreated infected infants develop permanent blindness.

Abnormal Diagnostic Findings

The most reliable way to confirm gonococcal infection is to demonstrate the organism by smear or culture. The immediate identification of *N. gonorrhoeae* is usually made by means of Gram-stained smears made from the discharge or secretions. It is important that the slides be interpreted by someone with experience in order that a correct diagnosis be made initially, as some clients fail to return for follow-up care. Cultures of the discharge or secretion can provide definitive diagnosis following incubation for 24 to 48 hours. There is no blood test available for diagnosis of gonorrhea.

For males, a presumptive diagnosis of gonorrhea is made if there is a history of sexual contact with an infected individual followed by a urethral discharge within a few days. A typical clinical picture combined with a positive Gram-stained smear of purulent discharge from the penis gives almost certain diagnosis in males. Culture of discharge is indicated for males whose smears are negative in the presence of strong clinical evidence.

Making a diagnosis of gonorrhea in the female on the basis of symptoms is difficult, because most female clients are symptom-free or have complaints that may be confused with a variety of other conditions. Smears of purulent discharge do not establish a diagnosis of gonorrhea in females because their genitourinary tract normally harbors a large number of organisms which resemble *N. gonorrhoeae*. To confirm the diagnosis a culture must be done. Specimens are taken from two or more of the following sites: cervix, urethra, anus, or oropharynx. A specific culture medium (Thayer-Martin) which encourages the growth of the gonococcus is utilized. If laboratory facilities are not readily accessible, special holding media is available.

Medical and Pharmacologic Management

A history of sexual contact with a known case of gonorrhea is considered good evidence for the presence of gonorrhea. Treatment would be instituted without awaiting culture results even in the absence of any sign or symptom.

The treatment of gonorrhea in the early stage is curative. Traditionally, the drug of choice for gonorrheal therapy has been penicillin (Table 45-2). This regimen will also treat coincubating syphilis.[6] In recent years, this practice has been complicated by the emergence of strains of gonococci that have become increasingly penicillin-resistant. Consequently, there is an increase in the required dose of penicillin.

To add to this dilemma, an isolate of *N. gonorrhoeae* was cultured that produced an enzyme (penicillinase) which destroyed penicillin. The worldwide dissemination of *penicillinase-producing N. gonorrhoeae* (PPNG) has profound implications for the control of gonorrhea. At the present time most cases of individuals infected with PPNG in the United States have been cured with spectinomycin 2.0 g intramuscularly in a single injection.[7]

Although the treatment of complications must be individualized, repeated large parenteral doses of aqueous crystalline penicillin G have been shown to be effective. Other drugs such as tetracycline and ampicillin are also utilized. All sexual contacts of clients with gonorrhea must be treated to prevent reinfection upon the resumption of sexual relations. The "ping-pong" effect of reexposure, treatment, and reinfection can cease only when infected partners are simultaneously treated. Additionally, the client should be advised to abstain from sexual intercourse and alcohol for 2 to 4 weeks. Sexual intercourse allows for spread of the infection and can retard complete healing due to vascular congestion. Alcohol has an irritant effect on the healing urethral walls. Men should be cautioned against squeezing the penis looking for further discharge. Follow-up examination and reculture should be done at least once following treatment, usually in 3 to 7 days. Relapse, reinfection, and complications should be treated appropriately.

Table 45-2
Medical Management: Gonorrhea

Diagnostic

1. History and physical examination
2. Smear and culture
3. Serologic testing for syphilis

Therapeutic

1. Initial therapy*
   a. Aqueous procaine penicillin G 4.8 million units divided into 2 doses and injected at different sites
   b. Probenecid (Benemid) 1 g orally, given prior to penicillin injection to delay renal excretion of penicillin
   c. Tetracycline hydrochloride 0.5 g qid for 5 days (used in clients allergic to penicillin or probenecid)
   d. Follow-up cultures 3–7 days after completion of treatment
   e. Test for syphilis
2. Case finding
3. Treatment of contacts
4. Instruct on abstinence from sexual intercourse and alcohol
5. Reexamination and reculture at least once
6. Repeat serologic test for syphilis at 1 month

*Adapted from recommendations of USPHS Center for Disease Control, 1979.

SYPHILIS

Etiology and Pathogenesis

Not all people exposed to syphilis will acquire the disease. Some appear resistant to infection. The causative organism for syphilis is *Treponema pallidum*, a spirochete. It is extremely fragile and is easily destroyed by drying, heating, or washing. The treponema is thought to enter the body through very small breaks in the skin or mucous membrane. Its entrance is facilitated by the minute tissue damage that often occurs during intercourse. In addition to sexual contact, syphilis may be spread by contact with infectious lesions, blood transfusions, sharing of needles among drug addicts, and as congenital syphilis transmitted from an infected mother to the fetus in utero. The incubation period ranges from 10 to 90 days but is usually considered to be 3 weeks. Immunity to reinfection may develop if the disease persists.

Syphilis is a disease of the blood vessels. The host tissues react to the presence of *T. pallidum* multiplying in the lymphatics and perivascular spaces by (1) capillary dilatation and swelling and proliferation of the endothelium, and (2) a perivascular infiltration of lymphocytes, plasma and giant cells, and fibroblasts, with the formation of new blood vessels. Scar tissue formation is the method of healing of syphilis. The severity and extent of the damage vary according to the state of immunity of the host tissue.

Clinical Manifestations

Syphilis presents a variety of signs and symptoms which can mimic a number of less serious diseases. Consequently, it is more difficult to recognize syphilis than it is other venereal diseases. If untreated, there are specific clinical stages characteristic of the disease progression (Table 45-3).

Complications

Complications of the disease occur chiefly in late syphilis. This stage of syphilis is rare today and should never occur since it can be prevented by treatment with antibiotics in the earlier stages. Therapy for complications is symptomatic in nature.

The *gummas* of benign late syphilis may produce irreparable damage to bone, liver, or skin but seldom result in death. In *cardiovascular syphilis* aneurysm formation and scarring of the aortic valve may occur. The resulting aneurysm may press on structures such as intercostal nerves, which results in pain. The possi-

Table 45-3
Stages of Syphilis

Clinical Stage	Characteristic Findings	Communicability	Duration of Stage
Primary	*Chancre*—painless indurated lesion found on penis, vulva, nipples, and lips (Fig. 45-3) as well as in mouth, vagina, or rectum	Highly infectious	2–6 weeks
Secondary	Widespread cutaneous and systemic symptoms appear 6–12 weeks after chancre. Cutaneous eruptions (Fig. 45-4) include bilateral symmetrical rash usually involving palms and soles, mucous patches in mouth, tongue, or cervix, *condyloma lata* (moist papules) in anal and genital areas, *alopecia* (hair loss), and generalized lymphadenopathy. Systemic symptoms include malaise, arthralgia, headache, and occasionally liver and kidney dysfunction	Skin and mucous membrane lesions are highly infectious	2–10 weeks
Latent	Absence of signs or symptoms	Noninfectious after 4 years	Continues throughout life or progresses to late stage
Late	Several forms occur in about 25% of untreated cases, appears 3 to 20 years after initial infection	Noninfectious	Chronic without treatment. May be fatal
1. Benign	*Gummas*—chronic, destructive lesions affecting any organ of the body, especially the skin, bone, liver, and mucous membranes		
2. Cardiovascular	Aortic valve insufficiency or saccular aneurysm of thoracic aorta, aortitis		
3. Neurosyphilis	*General paresis:* Personality changes from minor to psychotic, tremors, physical and mental deterioration *Tabes dorsalis:* Ataxia, areflexia, paresthesias, lightning pains, damaged joints (Charcot's joints)		

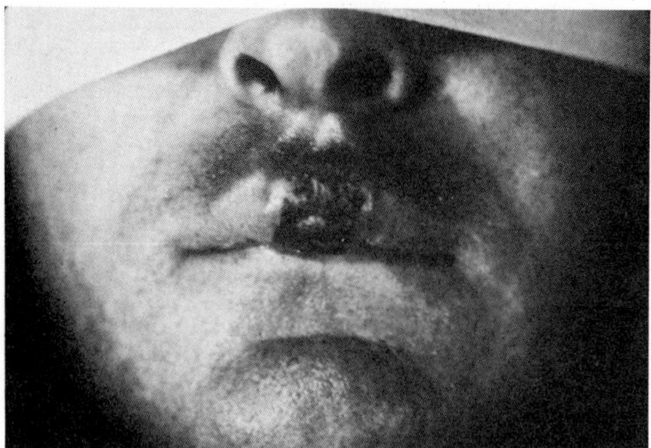

Figure 45-3 Primary syphilis chancre on upper lip. (*Photo by USPHS.*)

bility of rupture exists as the aneurysm increases in size. Scarring of the aortic valve results in aortic valve insufficiency and, eventually, heart failure.

Neurosyphilis (general paresis) is responsible for degeneration of the brain with mental deterioration. Evidence of other neurologic deficits may be present. Problems related to sensory nerve involvement are a result of *tabes dorsalis*. There may be sudden attacks of pain anywhere in the body, which can confuse the diagnosis of conditions such as peptic ulcer. Loss of vision and position sense in the feet and legs can also occur. Walking may become even more difficult as joint stability is lost.

Late syphilis is also discussed in Chap. 51.

Abnormal Diagnostic Studies

The first step in diagnosis is obtaining a detailed history relevant to sexual behavior. A physical examination should be done to identify any suspicious

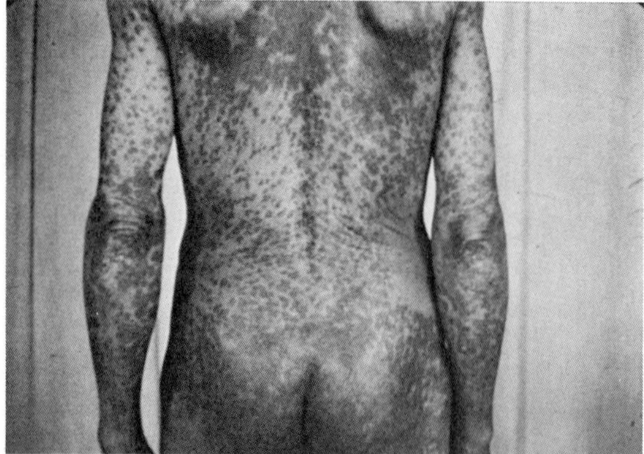

Figure 45-4 Secondary syphilis, generalized posterior cutaneous eruptions. Lesions are bilaterally symmetrical in distribution. (*Photo by USPHS.*)

lesions as well as other significant signs and symptoms.

The presence of spirochetes on *dark-field* microscopy confirms the presence of syphilis. Nontreponemal and treponemal serologic tests are less reliable but are valuable for screening purposes. False negatives and false positives do occur with nontreponemal tests. False negatives may occur during primary syphilis before the body has had time to produce antibody. False positives may occur with other diseases or conditions such as hepatitis, infectious mononucleosis, smallpox vaccination, collagen diseases, narcotic addiction, and aging. Negative nontreponemal test results should be followed by more specific tests to rule out other causes. Specific changes related to cell count, estimation of total protein, cerebrospinal fluid, and one or more tests for antibody are diagnostic of asymptomatic neurosyphilis.

A person may be infected but not show positive serology until antibodies are present in the serum. If a client is treated early in the course of the disease based on history and symptoms, the serologic testing may not indicate the presence of syphilis. Once a person has positive serology for syphilis, indicating the presence of antibodies, it usually remains positive for an indefinite period of time in spite of successful treatment.

Medical and Pharmacologic Management

All syphilitic organisms can be eradicated with adequate treatment (Table 45-4). However, treatment cannot reverse damage already present in the late stage of the disease. Parenteral penicillin remains the treatment of choice for all stages of syphilis. To date, there is no evidence to suggest a decrease in the effectiveness of penicillin against *T. pallidum*.[8] Table

Table 45-4
Medical Management: Primary Syphilis

Diagnostic

1. History and physical examination
2. Dark-field microscopy
3. Nontreponemal or treponemal serologic testing

Therapeutic

1. Appropriate drug therapy (see Table 45-5)
2. Case finding
3. Treatment of contacts
4. Surveillance
   a. Monthly for 6 months
   b. Every 3 months for next 18 months
   c. Examination of cerebrospinal fluid at 1 year

Table 45-5
Drug Therapy for Syphilis

Stage	Benzathine Penicillin (IM)	Aqueous Procaine Penicillin (IM)	Other Antibiotics*
Early syphilis (primary, secondary, and early latent). Includes pregnant women	2.4 megaunits divided in 2 doses at single visit	600,000 U daily for 8 days, totaling 4.8 megaunits	Tetracycline hydrochloride or erythromycin 500 mg orally qid for 15 days†
Syphilis of more than 1 year's duration. Includes pregnant women	Three doses of 2.4 megaunits at 7-day intervals totaling 7.2 megaunits	600,000 U daily for 15 days, totaling 9.0 megaunits	Tetracycline hydrochloride or erythromycin 500 mg orally qid 4 times for 30 days†
Symptomatic neurosyphilis		2–4 million units IV aqueous crystalline penicillin G for 10 days to total of 120–240 million units	

*Given when penicillin is contraindicated.
†Erythromycin estolate and tetracycline are not recommended for syphilitic infection in pregnant women because of potential adverse effects on mother and child.
Adapted from recommendations of USPHS, Center for Disease Control, 1976.

45-5 represents therapy for the various stages of syphilis and is in accordance with the Public Health Service recommendations. All stages of syphilis should be treated.

Appropriate antibiotic treatment of maternal syphilis prior to the eighteenth week of pregnancy prevents infection of the fetus. Appropriate treatment after 18 weeks of pregnancy would cure both mother and fetus since the antibiotics are able to cross the placental barrier.

In the case of neurosyphilis, cerebrospinal fluid examination should be carried out 6 months after treatment, at 1 year, and then annually for several years. Specific medical management is based on the presenting symptoms.

HERPES GENITALIS

There are two types of infection caused by herpesvirus hominis (HVH), type 1 and type 2. In general, type 1 strain (HVH-1) causes infection above the waist, involving infections of the gingiva, dermis, upper respiratory tract, and central nervous system. Type 2 strain (HVH-2) most frequently involves the genital tract and perineum, that is, below the waist. However, either strain can cause disease on either the mouth or the genitals. The primary infection of HVH-2 is usually spread by sexual contact with an infected person. There is a high correlation of infection in sexual partners if one is infected.

The initial infection is usually a type 1 infection occurring in childhood. The primary HVH-2 infection usually occurs when heterosexual activity begins. In contrast to other venereal diseases, the infection can recur completely unrelated to additional venereal contact and produce a syndrome similar to the primary infection. The incubation period is 3 to 7 days.

Clinical Manifestations

Clients with primary genital herpesvirus infections initially complain of burning or tingling at the site of inoculation. Vesicular lesions, which may occur on the penis, scrotum, vulva, perineum, perianal region, vagina, or cervix, contain large quantities of infectious viral particles (Fig. 45-5). The lesions rupture and form shallow, moist ulcerations. Finally, crusting and epithelialization of the erosions occur. Primary infections tend to be associated with local inflammation, pain, inguinal lymphadenopathy, and systemic symptoms including chills, fever, headache, and malaise. Primary lesions are generally present for 2 to 4 weeks. Clients are thought to be noninfectious following the crusting of the ulcers.

Some clients never experience a recurrence whereas others have several. Stress, sexual activity, sunburn, and fever tend to trigger recurrence. Many clients can predict a recurrence by noticing early symptoms of tingling, burning, and itching at the site where lesions eventually arise. The symptoms are less severe and the vesicles heal within 1 to 2 weeks with

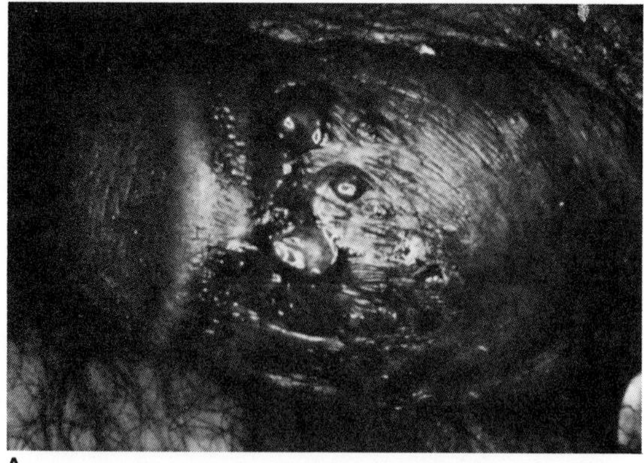

A

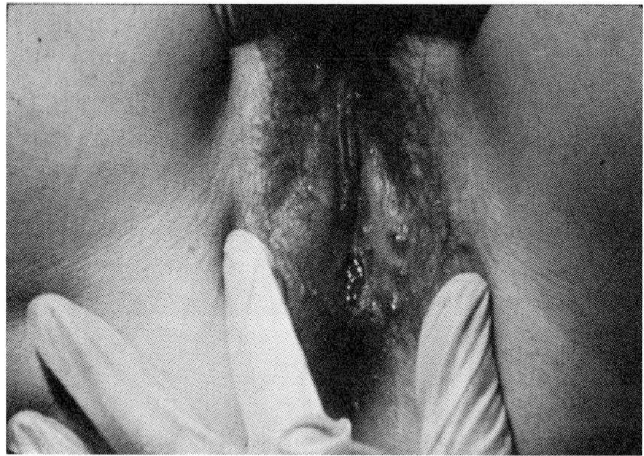

B

Figure 45-5 Herpes genitalis (HVH-2) in male and female. Vesicular lesions on (*a*) penis and (*b*) perineum. (*Photo by USPHS.*)

recurrent episodes. Between recurrences, the virus is thought to be latent in the nerve tissue that innervates the affected sites.

Complications

Pregnancy

Lesions in the pregnant woman persist for a longer time than in the nonpregnant woman. The symptoms seem to be more severe with a higher incidence of secondary monilia infections.[9] The incidence of abortion is higher if a HVH-2 infection is contracted during the first 20 weeks of pregnancy. The development of disseminated neonatal herpesvirus infections carries a high incidence of infant mortality. A positive vaginal viral culture usually indicates the need for a caesarean section.

Cervical cancer

Epidemiologic evidence has linked genital herpesvirus infections in women with carcinoma of the cervix. Both diseases have similar predisposing factors. They occur in young, sexually active women who have early, frequent intercourse and who have multiple partners. The following correlaries seem to support the herpes infection–cervical cancer relationship:

1. More herpesvirus type 2 antibodies have been found in cervical cancer clients than in control groups.
2. Cervical cultures of women with cervical cancer have yielded predominantly herpesvirus type 2.
3. Women who develop cancer of the cervix more often give a history of herpes infections than do control clients.

Although the above data do not say with certainty that herpesvirus initiates a process that results in cervical cancer, the association appears to be a valid one.[10] Therefore, women who have had genital herpesvirus infections should be particularly conscientious about having regular Papanicolaou smears taken.

Abnormal Diagnostic Findings

Diagnosis of herpes genitalis can be confirmed by isolation of the virus in any of several tissue culture systems. Papanicolaou-stained smears from lesions show cellular characteristics of viruses.

Medical Management

The skin lesions of herpesvirus infections will heal spontaneously unless secondary infection supervenes. A condom should be used during intercourse to prevent spread. At this time, treatment is usually symptomatic. Genital hygiene and the wearing of loose-fitting cotton undergarments should be encouraged. There is controversy whether to treat herpetic lesions by wet or dry methods. Some practitioners advocate the use of dry heat, since cool compresses and sitz baths may spread the virus. Others feel Burow's solution or tannic acid (wet teabags) may be therapeutic. Topical anesthetics such as xylocaine ointment and analgesics such as aspirin or codeine can be used for pain relief.

Therapies directed toward viral eradication have met with limited success. These include interferon induction, antimetabolites, photoinactivation, alcohol, ether, smallpox vaccination, bacillus Calmette-Guérin (BCG), and herpesvirus vaccines. Viral chemotherapeutic agents such as acycloguanosine (Acylovir) are now being used to treat recurrence of herpes viral infections. If a secondary infection is present, use of sulfa creams may be helpful.

LYMPHOGRANULOMA VENEREUM (LGV)

Lymphogranuloma venereum is a contagious sexually transmitted disease which is produced by a member of the *Chlamydia* species. It is characterized by a transitory primary lesion followed by suppurative lymphadenitis and much later by serious local complications. The incubation period varies from 1 to 6 weeks but often is about 3 weeks. Relapses after treatment are common. However, proven reinfections have not been observed and immunity probably lasts for life.

Clinical Manifestations and Complications

Primary inoculation may occur at any anatomic site involved in intimate contact. The resulting lesion is usually a small, painless vesicle or superficial nonindurated ulcer which may go unnoticed. Later, regional lymphadenitis develops in the nodes draining the affected site and the disease disseminates further via the lymphatic system. The lymph node involvement in the male is in the inguinal area, while in the female the perianal nodes are most often involved. Lymphatic spread is associated with a variety of constitutional symptoms as fever, chills, anorexia, joint pain, and vague abdominal aches.

Late manifestations of LGV may result in perianal abscesses, multiple fistulous tracts, and rectal strictures. Blockage of the lymphatic drainage of the genital area may lead to chronic edema and ulceration. LGV is usually diagnosed on the basis of clinical signs and symptoms and the presence of elevated serologic complement fixation titer to *Chlamydia* antigen. Aspirates of enlarged nodes may be cultured for the causative organism. The intradermal Frei skin test for LGV is considered to be nonspecific for the infection and is only about 80 percent sensitive.[11] Its usefulness is therefore questionable.

Medical and Pharmacologic Management

Once diagnosed, a client should be questioned about all possible sex contacts. Successful treatment has generally been obtained through the use of tetracycline 500 mg orally four times daily for 2 to 3 weeks.

Suppurating lesions should be aspirated and drainage encouraged from any sinuses or fistulas. Corticosteroids may be used to speed recovery. Abscesses may need to be drained to facilitate healing. The complement-fixation titer is usually negative within 6 to 12 months following effective treatment.

CHANCROID (SOFT CHANCRE)

Chancroid, an infection caused by the *Hemophilus ducreyi* bacillus, is usually sexually transmitted. Postcoital washing with soap and water does not prevent chancroid. The average incubation period is 4 to 5 days. Prior chancroid infections do not result in immunity to reinfection.

The infection begins with a papule of the genitals and/or perianal area. The papule becomes pustular and finally ulcerates. The ulcers have nonindurated borders and are painful. About 50 percent of the clients develop painful inguinal adenitis within 3 weeks after the appearance of skin lesions. In some cases the *bubo* (enlarged lymph node) may soften to form an abscess. Scars due to chancroid infections may narrow the preputial opening, requiring circumcision. Secondary infections may result in destructive ulcerations. Large ulcerating skin lesions may occur if inguinal nodes rupture.

Demonstration of the causative organism through culture and Gram-stained smears of lesions is often difficult and unreliable. Therefore, diagnosis is often made based on clinical suspicion and on attempts to rule out other venereal diseases. There is currently no available serologic test or skin test antigen.

Oral sulfisoxazole (1 g every 6 hours for 10 to 14 days) is the treatment of choice. Resistant cases are treated with kanamycin 500 mg intramuscularly every 12 hours for two weeks. Warm sitz baths will relieve the local discomfort of the lesions and cleanse the infected areas. Attempts to identify sexual contacts should be made.

GRANULOMA INGUINALE (DONOVANOSIS)

Granuloma inguinale is a chronic, sexually transmitted disease caused by *Calymmatobacterium granulomatis*. Little is known about the organism. It is generally accepted that the disease is spread by sexual contact but is considered not to be highly contagious. The incubation period is thought to be 8 to 12 weeks. The possibility of repeated infections is unclear. Individual resistance to this disease varies greatly.

Clinical Manifestations and Complications

The early lesions are subcutaneous nodules found usually on the external genitals and in the perianal region. The nodules soon become painless, well-defined ulcers. The ulcers tend to bleed easily and enlarge slowly. Lymph node involvement is uncommon. The lesions may become secondarily infected.

The complications of the disease are related to the anatomic sites involved. A variety of deformities resulting from scars and adhesions are common. These include stenosis of the urethral, vaginal, and anal orifices. Lymphatic occlusion may lead to elephantoid enlargement of the genitalia.

Diagnotic Findings and Medical Management

Presumptive diagnosis may be made from the clinical picture of the advanced disease. Confirmation requires the demonstration of Donovan bodies, the intracellular stage of the causative organism, in tissue smears or in biopsies, taken from the client. Skin test antigens or serologic tests are not available.

Tetracycline 500 mg orally every 6 hours for 3 weeks or gentamicin 40 mg intramuscularly twice daily for 3 weeks are examples of effective antibiotic regimens. The lesions of Donovanosis should be cleansed at least twice daily with soap and water.

NURSING MANAGEMENT OF SEXUALLY TRANSMITTED DISEASES

Health Promotion and Maintenance

Many approaches to curtailing the spread of venereal disease have been advocated and have met with varying degrees of success. Sexual abstinence is a certain method of avoiding all venereal diseases, but few adults consider this restriction a feasible alternative to sexual expression. Limiting sexual intimacies outside of a well-established monogamous relationship can reduce the risk of contracting venereal disease.[12] There are also specific procedures that, if followed consistently, can aid in preventing a venereal infection. The nurse should counsel clients regarding these measures.

Measures to prevent infection

An inspection of the sexual partner's genitals before coitus is recommended. The presence of a discharge, sores, blisters, or rash should be viewed with concern. The client, aware of specific signs and symptoms of infection, can then intelligently make the decision to continue the sexual interaction with modifications or elect not to have sexual relations. Male clients should know that some protection is afforded them if they void immediately following intercourse and wash their genitalia and the adjacent areas with soap and water. Women may also benefit from postcoital voiding, washing, and douching.

The value of creams, foams, and other preparations in the prophylaxis of venereal disease is currently being assessed. Most attention has been directed toward chemicals placed in the vagina prior to coitus that are bactericidal to the gonococcus and the syphilis spirochete.

Proper use of a condom provides a highly effective mechanical barrier to infection. The condom should be undamaged and correctly in place throughout all phases of sexual activity. The objections to condom usage such as interference with spontaneity and the presence of a barrier will undoubtedly need to be discussed. It should be stressed that most women may not be able to tell the difference when a condom is used. Also, many men find use of condoms objectionable but it need not interfere with sexual satisfaction.

Screening programs

Prevention of certain sexually transmitted diseases is also carried out by a number of screening programs that attempt to find infected clients. For many years there have been various screening programs to find cases of syphilis. Forty-five states have laws requiring premarital blood tests for syphilis and 44 states require serologic testing for syphilis for pregnant women before or during delivery.[13] Other screening programs are carried out by way of preemployment and hospital admissions physicals and when individuals donate blood or are inducted into the military service. This type of screening has successfully detected many cases of sexually transmitted diseases so treatment could be started.

During the past few years new screening programs have been developed and implemented for gonorrhea. The programs involve women since they are more apt to have asymptomatic gonorrhea and thereby serve as sources of infection. Routine gonorrheal cultures for women who are having pelvic exams are being carried out as a major part of the programs. Evidence of the effectiveness of the programs is well documented.

Case finding

Interviewing and case finding are other processes utilized to control venereal disease. These activities are directed toward locating and examining all contacts of each known venereal disease case as soon as possible after sexual exposure so that effective treatment can be initiated. Trained interviewers may often find cases even if they are supplied with limited information. The case workers, who are often nurses, are aware of the social implications of these diseases and the need for discretion. Sexual contacts are often not informed as to the origin of the information naming them as a contact so that greater cooperation and privacy is assured.

Educational and research programs

Nurses can actively encourage their communities to provide better education related to sexually transmitted diseases for its citizens. Teenagers, who are known to have a high incidence of infection, should be a prime audience for such educational programs. Hot-line services, physician extenders, and outreach programs sponsored by the Center for Disease Control have proved effective. Knowledge and understanding of the disease can affect the venereal disease epidemic. Presently, efforts are being made to develop a serologic test for gonorrhea and effective immunizing agents for both syphilis and gonorrhea. The development of venereal disease vaccines is viewed by many as a prerequisite for venereal disease eradication.

Acute Intervention

Psychological

The diagnosis of venereal disease may be met with a variety of emotions such as shame, guilt, anger, or a desire for vengeance. The nurse should try to help clients verbalize their feelings and provide counseling. There is little direct physical nursing care involved when dealing with a client with a sexually transmitted disease. Couples in marital or committed relationships are confronted with an added problem when venereal disease is diagnosed. The realization of sexual activity in one or the other partner outside their relationship must be faced. It is obvious that other concerns relative to their relationship are present and the acute problem may serve as an incentive to do other problem solving. Support and counseling for the couple is needed. A referral to a psychologist where the implications of venereal disease in their relationship can be explored in greater depth may be indicated.

Clients who have contracted herpes genitalis are in a special category. Knowledge that repeated attacks can occur and definitive treatment is unavailable can prove to be frustrating and disruptive to their physical, emotional, and social lives. Helping the client identify and avoid, when possible, any factors that may precipitate the condition is indicated. Specific instructions in preventing secondary infections can provide a degree of support.

Compliance and follow-up

Nurses working in a public health facility, clinic, or other outpatient settings are more apt to care for clients with sexually transmitted diseases. These nurses are in a position to explain and interpret treatment measures such as the effects and possible side effects of prescribed drugs and the need for follow-up care (Tables 45-6 and 45-7).

Single-dose treatment for gonorrhea and syphilis, fortunately, helps prevent noncompliance with drug therapy. Clients requiring multiple-dose therapy should be given special instructions in completing the prescribed regimen and be informed of problems of noncompliance. All clients are to return to the treatment center for a repeat culture from infected site(s) or serologic testing at designated times to determine the effectiveness of the treatment. Informing the client that cures are not always obtained on the first treatment can reinforce the need for a follow-up visit. The client should also be advised to inform their sexual partners, whether they are symptomatic or not, of the need for treatment.

Hygiene measures

The client with venereal disease should have certain hygiene measures emphasized. An important measure is frequent handwashing and bathing, which results in most of the causative organisms of venereal disease being destroyed. Bathing can provide local comfort as well as prevent secondary infection by cleansing the involved areas. Douching may spread the infection and therefore is generally contraindicted. Synthetic materials used in most undergarments frequently increase or exacerbate local irritations because they trap moisture. Cotton undergarments provide better absorption and are cooler and more comfortable for the client with venereal disease.

Sexual activity

Sexual abstinence is indicated during the communicable phase of the disease. If sexual activity occurs before treatment of the client is completed, use of condoms can prevent the spread of infection or reinfection. The client can also choose to relate in a way that avoids either coitus or oral-genital contact.

Chronic Management

The fact that many of the venereal diseases are cured by a single dose or short course of antibiotic

Table 45-6
Nursing Care Plan for the Client with Primary Syphilis

Client Problem	Expected Outcome	Nursing Intervention
	Acute Management	
Painless penile lesion	Absence of lesion	Administer penicillin intramuscularly as ordered and after checking on any allergies. Observe progress of ulcer healing.
Infectious discharge from lesion	Absence of discharge. No spread of infection to others	Instruct in hygienic measures including good handwashing and wearing cotton undergarments. Use precautions regarding linen and handwashing for initial 24 h of treatment. Investigate need for treatment of sexual partner with antibiotics. Instruct regarding abstinence or use of condoms.
Noncompliance with follow-up	Follow appropriate follow-up protocol	Explain the reasons for return visits (of every 3 months for 1 year) to clinic. Inform client that blood samples will be taken at each visit. Assist with case finding.
Emotional reaction to diagnosis of syphilis	Acceptance of diagnosis	Encourage verbalization. Counsel client and sexual partner if indicated.
	Long-Term Management	
Development of further stages	Absence of symptoms of secondary or late syphilis	Describe signs of secondary syphilis as cutaneous eruptions. Reaffirm need for compliance with follow-up care.
Recurrence of symptoms, reinfection	Not become reinfected or symptomatic	Explain precautions necessary to prevent reinfection, such as use of condoms, inspection of partner's genitals, voiding, and washing genitals after intercourse. Inform client that no immunity develops to disease.

Table 45-7
Nursing Care Plan for the Client with Gonorrhea

Client Problem	Expected Outcome	Nursing Intervention
	Acute Management	
Infectious genital discharge	Absence of discharge. No further spread of infection	Administer probenecid and penicillin as ordered after checking on any allergies. Instruct in hygienic measures of handwashing, bathing, and wearing of cotton undergarments.
Dysuria	Absence of burning on urination	Encourage fluids. Monitor intake and output.
Emotional response to diagnosis (e.g., anger, anxiety)	Resolution of conflict	Allow client and sexual partner to verbalize concerns. Investigate need for counseling.
	Long-Term Management	
Prostatitis, urethral strictures, and sterility	Absence of symptoms of complications	Instruct client on symptoms of complications and need to report such problems as difficulty voiding, chills, fever, dysuria, and urethral discharge.
Reinfection	Not become reinfected	Explain precautions to take such as being selective about sexual partners, using condoms, voiding and washing genitals after coitus. Inform client regarding absence of immunity.
Noncompliance with follow-up	Follow appropriate follow-up protocol	Instruct client regarding return to clinic within 3–7 days after completion of treatment for cultures. Assist with case finding.

therapy has caused many individuals to develop a jaded nonchalance about the outcome of these diseases. The consequence of this attitude can result in delays in treatment, noncompliance with instructions, and subsequent development of complications. The complications are most certainly serious and costly. They result in disfigurement and destruction to important tissues and organs.

Surgery and prolonged therapy is indicated for many clients with disease-related deformities. Major surgical procedures such as resection of an aneurysm and aortic valve replacement may be necessary to treat cardiovascular problems. Pelvic surgery could include lysis of adhesions, dilation of strictures, and repair of fistulas. Secondary infections may occur because of the location of the lesions. These infections have been known to be severe, requiring more therapy than the original problem.

Case Study / Syphilis

Mr. Jones, a 48-year-old traveling salesman, is admitted to the hospital following a minor traffic accident. During his physical examination a painless indurated lesion which appeared to be a chancre was discovered on his penis. His sexual history revealed that his only sexual partner other than his wife was a woman he had met 3 weeks ago while on a business trip. A tentative diagnosis of syphilis was made.

Discussion Questions

1. How can the diagnosis of syphilis be established?
2. How could he have prevented the infection?
3. What are the possible complications if he is not treated?
4. What are the implications of this diagnosis for his relationship with his wife?
5. What measures should he have his wife taken?
6. What instructions would you give to him regarding follow-up care?

REVIEW QUESTIONS

The number of the question corresponds to the same numbered objective at the beginning of the chapter.

1. Factors which have led to an increase in sexually transmitted diseases include
   a. longer sexual life span
   b. increased social controls
   c. better reporting of veneral diseases
   d. improved antibiotic therapy

2. If a male goes without treatment for gonorrhea, he may develop
   a. reinfection with the microorganisms
   b. an immunity to the microorganisms
   c. ureteritis, pyelonephritis, nephritis
   d. prostatitis, epididymitis, orchitis

3. Probenecid (Benemid) is used in the treatment of gonorrhea to
   a. reduce the incidence of allergic reactions
   b. decrease the required dose of penicillin
   c. relieve the discomfort of the injection
   d. delay the renal excretion of penicillin

4. Herpesvirus type 1 is characteristically located
   a. on hair-covered surfaces
   b. on mucous membranes
   c. above the waist
   d. below the waist

5. The prime audience for the nurse to reach related to venereal disease control is
   a. primary grade students
   b. teenagers
   c. unmarried adults
   d. homosexuals

6. Emotional support can best be given the client with a venereal disease through
   a. offering many alternatives
   b. concerned listening
   c. isolation from others
   d. emphasizing duration of disease

REFERENCES

1. U.S. Department of Health, Education and Welfare, Public Health Services, STD Fact Sheet, 34th ed., HEW publ. no. (CDC) 79-8195, Atlanta, 1979, p. 2.
2. U.S. Department of Health, Education and Welfare, Public Health Services, "Herpes Genital Infection," publ. no. 00-2939, CDC, 1979, p. 1.
3. W. Faulkner, "Intrauterine Devices and Acute Pelvic Inflammatory Disease," *JAMA,* **235**:1851 (1976).
4. A. M. Harvey, F. J. Johns, A. H. Owens, and R. S. Poss, eds., *Principles and Practice of Medicine*, 19th ed., Appleton Century Crofts, New York, 1976, p. 1283.
5. U. S. Department of Health, Education and Welfare, Public Health Services, "Venereal Disease Control Laws —Summary," CDC, Atlanta, 1972.

6. T. B. Fitzpatrick, et al., *Dermatology in General Medicine*, 2d ed., McGraw-Hill Book Company, New York, 1979, p. 1748.

7. M. S. Siegel et al., "Penicillinase-Producing *Neisseria gonorrhoeae*," *Sexually Transmitted Disease*, **4**:33 (1977).

8. A. H. Rudolph and W. C. Duncan, "Syphilis—Diagnosis and Treatment," *Clin Obstet Gynecol*, **18**:177 (1975).

9. M. S. Amstey, "Genital Herpesvirus Infection," *Clin Obstet Gynecol*, **18**:97 (1975).

10. A. J. Nahmias and B. Roizman, "Infection with Herpes-Simplex Viruses 1 and 2," *N Engl J Med*, **289**:721 (1973).

11. M. F. Rein and T. Chapel, "Trichomoniasis, Candidiasis and the Minor Venereal Diseases," *Clin Obstet Gynecol*, **18**:83 (1975).

12. W. Darrow and P. Wiesner, "Personal Prophylaxis for Veneral Diseases," *JAMA*, **233**:444 (1975).

13. U. S. Department of Health, Education and Welfare, Public Health Services, "Venereal Disease Control Laws—Summary," CDC, Atlanta, 1972.

Chapter 46

NURSING ROLE IN MANAGEMENT

Female Reproductive Problems

Linda C. Carnago

Learning Objectives

1. Describe the etiology, clinical manifestations, and medical and nursing management of common problems of menstruation.
2. Identify the purposes and preoperative and postoperative care for the client having a dilatation and currettage.
3. Explain the physical and psychological alterations and appropriate management during the climacteric and menopause.
4. Compare the advantages and disadvantages of common contraceptive and birth control methods.
5. Differentiate between spontaneous and induced abortion, including medical management and nursing intervention.
6. Describe the effects of rape and appropriate medical, legal, and nursing interventions.
7. Differentiate among the common vaginal, vulvar, and cervical inflammations and infections, including medical and nursing management.
8. Describe the etiology, complications, and medical and nursing management for pelvic inflammatory disease.
9. Describe the clinical manifestations, complications, and medical and nursing management for endometriosis.
10. Explain the manifestations and management for benign tumors of the uterus and ovaries.
11. Identify the clinical manifestations, diagnostic studies, and medical and surgical management for malignant tumors of the uterus, ovaries, and vulva.
12. Describe the preoperative and postoperative nursing intervention for the client requiring major surgery of the female reproductive system.
13. Identify the nursing responsibilities related to internal radiation therapy for uterine cancer.
14. Explain the etiology, clinical manifestations, and medical management of uterine displacements.
15. Identify the clinical manifestations, and medical and nursing management for cystocele, rectocele, and fistulas.

Although problems related to female reproductive organs are discussed and written about more openly today, misconceptions, fears, and embarrassment about gynecologic problems still occur. The nurse plays an important role in (1) disseminating knowledge about health-promoting measures, (2) providing clarification and reassurance where indicated, and (3) assisting in seeking help in order to obtain early recognition and treatment of potentially serious problems.

DISORDERS OF MENSTRUATION

Menstruation is a bloody vaginal discharge which is spontaneous, periodic, and represents endometrial shedding following ovulation.[1] This cycle, which repeats itself approximately every 28 days, can cause many problems for women.

Health Maintenance and Promotion

Before the nurse can begin to do health teaching, the client's knowledge of the characteristics of the menstrual cycle should be assessed. Table 46-1 includes these characteristics and related client education. When this information is discussed and explained, the client will be able to identify that variations do exist for the "normal" menses and that knowledge can help to dispel apprehension and fear. If the client's menstrual cycle pattern does not fall within the range of normal, the nurse should urge her to seek prompt medical attention.

Many old wives' tales are told concerning activities allowed during menstruation. The nurse should be prepared to put an end to them. The client should be assured that bathing and washing hair are safe. A daily warm tub bath can actually relieve some of the associated pelvic discomfort. The woman can swim, exercise, have intercourse, and in short behave like a healthy female.

Frequent changing of tampons or pads will meet comfort and hygiene needs during menstruation. There are many internal as well as external types of protection devices that can be used during menstruation. The selection is a matter of personal preference. Tampons are convenient and make menstrual hygiene easier, whereas pads may provide better protection. The association between the use of tampons and toxic shock syndrome is discussed later in this chapter.

Premenstrual Tension

Premenstrual tension is a syndrome which may appear from 1 to 10 days prior to the onset of menses.

This chapter was reviewed by Steve Toussaint, R.N., M.S.N., Instructor, Health Sciences Center, University of Oregon, Portland, Oregon.

Table 46-1
Characteristics of Average Menstrual Cycle and Related Client Education

	Characteristic	Client Education
Menarche	Occurs between ages of 9–18, the average being 12 or 13.	See physician regarding possible endocrine or developmental abnormality when delayed.
Interval	Usually 27–31 days but regular cycles as short as 17 or as long as 45 days are considered normal if a constant pattern for individual.	Keep written record to identify own pattern of menstrual cycle. Expect some irregularity in premenopausal period. Know that drugs (phenothiazines, narcotics, contraceptives), and stressful events can result in missed periods.
Duration	Menstrual flow generally lasts anywhere from 2–8 days.	Realize that pattern is fairly constant but wide variations do exist.
Amount	Average menstrual flow is 20–30 mL. A very heavy flow is indicated by complete soaking of 2 pads in 1–2 hours. Count pads or tampons used in a day. The average tampon or pad completely saturated absorbs 20-30 mL. A very heavy flow is indicated by complete soaking of 2 pads in 1–2 hours.	Know that flow increases then gradually decreases in premenopausal period. An IUD or drugs such as anticoagulants and thiazides, can produce heavy menses.
Composition	Menstrual discharge is a mixture of endometrium, blood, mucus, and vaginal cells. It is dark red, less viscous than blood, and usually does not clot.	Learn that clots indicate heavy flow or vaginal pooling.

Adapted from L. Martin, *Health Care of Women*, J. B. Lippincott Company, Philadelphia, 1978, p. 103.

It occurs chiefly in women over the age of 35. The symptoms can include a combination of weight gain, painful breasts, abdominal bloating, irritability, depression, nervousness, increased physical and mental activity, craving for sweets, and headache. Some researchers believe that many of the symptoms are a result of sodium retention. As a consequence, water is retained, which, with the sodium, would account for many of the above edema-related symptoms. At present, the problem of premenstrual tension is not well understood and it is thought that other disturbances such as vascular phenomena may be involved.[2]

Symptomatic treatment is directed toward the chief complaints. Salt restriction and diuretics are most useful in relieving the symptoms related to water retention. Potassium may need to be supplemented. Testosterone may be also given to suppress the effects of estrogen excess. Although tranquilizers and other psychotropic drugs can be effective for the symptoms related to emotional instability, their use is not advocated since it is a recurring problem which could lead to drug dependence. Explanation, reassurance, and exploration of any psychological aspects should also be employed.

Dysmenorrhea

Dysmenorrhea is pain or discomfort associated with menstrual flow. The degree of pain and discomfort varies with the individual and may be manifested as lower abdominal cramping pain, backache, and aching of the thighs. These are areas of ovarian and uterine nerve innervation which are referred to other parts of the body. Two types of dysmenorrhea are *primary dysmenorrhea*, where pelvic organs are normal, and *secondary dysmenorrhea*, where a diagnosed pelvic disease or condition is present.

Etiology

Primary Dysmenorrhea Primary dysmenorrhea occurs more frequently than secondary dysmenorrhea. It is the most prevalent symptom requiring women to take off work. Dysmenorrhea is associated with ovulatory cycles and becomes less of a problem with age and pregnancy. Factors such as sedentary occupation, faulty posture, and poor personal hygiene are often concurrently present.

The discomforts of menstruation are now thought to be related to the release of prostaglandins from the endometrium during the luteal phase.[3] Women with dysmenorrhea have been found to have high levels of prostaglandins. Reasons for the overproduction of prostaglandins are still unclear. These hormones stimulate smooth-muscle contractions, which can lead to cramping pain (increased uterine contractility), as well as nausea, vomiting, and diarrhea.

Psychological elements such as dissatisfaction with feminine identity, conflicts, and resentment in familial and marital relations have also been implicated in the etiology of dysmenorrhea. Limited preparation for menarche or a predisposition to overresponding to potentially painful stimuli are known to affect the women's response to menstrual discomforts.

Secondary Dysmenorrhea Secondary dysmenorrhea may occur due to such conditions as large uterine or cervical polyps, submucous fibroids, endometriosis, pelvic infection, a fixed malpositioned uterus, the presence of an intrauterine device, and cervical stenosis following recent gynecologic surgery or procedures.

Clinical manifestations

Primary dysmenorrhea usually occurs within 3 years after menarche and generally lasts only for the first days of the flow. The pain may be sharp and colicky or dull and aching. It has been compared by some to the pain of labor. Nausea, vomiting, and diarrhea are not uncommon.

Secondary dysmenorrhea generally occurs after a pattern of problem-free periods has been present for some time. The pain is generally more constant in nature and continues throughout the period.

Medical management

Diagnostic A careful history can provide data regarding menstrual experiences and emotional factors affecting the client's response to menstrual discomforts. How the client's female relatives dealt with their menses as well as how the women within her family structure carry out their roles can provide valuable information related to the problem. Other information that is important is determining if the discomfort was a sudden or monthly problem, how long it lasts with each period, and if any changes in usual lifestyle or emotional crises have occurred. A thorough physical examination is necessary to rule out the presence of organic disease.

A variety of diagnostic and therapeutic measures are utilized when secondary dysmenorrhea is suspected. These will be discussed later as specific problems are presented.

Therapeutic The extent to which symptomatic, endocrine, or surgical therapy is employed depends upon how much the dysmenorrhea disrupts the client's usual activities. Many cases of dysmenorrhea respond well to symptomatic therapy including rest, reassurance, local heat, and mild drugs which have analgesic, antispasmodic, smooth-muscle relaxing, or sedative effects. The use of narcotics is discouraged since dysmenorrhea is a recurring problem, making drug addiction a possibility. With the discovery of prostaglandins' (PG) relation to menstrual cramps, PG inhibitors such as ibuprofen (Motrin) are now being utilized (see section on Pharmacology).

When the dysmenorrhea is more severe, *endocrine therapy* utilizing oral contraceptives is prescribed. Ovulation, a primary requisite for dysmenorrhea, is suppressed by these drugs. The side effects are an obvious disadvantage of their continued use (see Contraception).

Surgical treatment is limited. Cervical dilatation may provide relief in some clients. Presacral neurectomy (removal of the autonomic nerves to the uterus) may be offered as a last resort to the client whose dysmenorrhea is not relieved by any other means.

Pharmacologic intervention

Prostaglandin inhibitors are useful in the treatment of primary dysmenorrhea. Included in this category of drugs are certain analgesic, antipyretic, and anti-inflammatory agents such as mefenamic acid (Ponstel), ibuprofen (Motrin), indomethacin (Indocin), naproxen (Naprosyn), aspirin, and acetaminophen.

Mefenamic acid and ibuprofen have significantly decreased the frequency and severity of symptoms.[4,5] Both drugs are relatively free of side effects. The nurse should observe for dizziness and gastrointestinal distress. The taking of food with the drug may relieve these problems. A history of asthma or peptic ulcers should be reported to the physician since PG inhibitors are contraindicated in these instances. The nurse should advise the client to take her medication after the menstrual flow begins. If a possibility of pregnancy exists, the use of PG inhibitors is precluded. Since indomethacin is known to have more severe side effects, and aspirin and acetaminophen are weak PG inhibitors, their use is not indicated for dysmenorrhea. Naproxen and similar PG inhibitors such as sulindac are also being studied.

Nursing management

Nurses are often asked what can be done when minor discomforts associated with some cycles occur. The client should be aware that help may be obtained by lying down for short periods, drinking hot beverages, applying heat to the abdomen, and taking a mild analgesic. When medications are prescribed the nurse may be the one who teaches the client regarding their use. Total reliance on drug therapy should be discouraged. The nurse can also suggest noninvasive, pain-relieving practices such as distraction and guided imagery (see Chap. 50). Such practices may increase the client's feeling of control and self-reliance.

Other long-term health care measures which can decrease discomforts of dysmenorrhea are available and should be utilized. These include (1) regular exercise, (2) maintenance of proper nutritional habits, (3) avoidance of constipation, (4) maintenance of good body mechanics, and (5) avoidance of worry, mental strain, and overfatigue, particularly at the time preceding menstrual periods. Staying active and interested in one's activities may also help. The nurse's approach to the problem of dysmenorrhea needs to be thoughtful and sensitive. The counsel and supportive therapy given can provide the foundation for coping with this common female problem.

Menstrual Irregularities

The ovarian cycle is more unstable and vulnerable to disruptive influences in its early phase (adolescence) and late phase (premenopausal). Therefore, abnormal bleeding is more common at the beginning and end of the active menstrual life.

Types

Amenorrhea The absence of menses refers to the failure to menstruate before the age of 18 and cessation of menses for 3 months or more after they have once become established. The common causes of amenorrhea are listed in Table 46-2.

Table 46-2
Causes of Amenorrhea

Physiologic
- Pregnancy
- Breast feeding
- Menopause

Psychogenic
- Emotional shock
- Pseudocyesis (false pregnancy)
- Anorexia nervosa

Systemic
- Chronic diseases (tuberculosis, nephritis)
- Nutritional disorders (malnutrition, obesity)
- Drugs (phenothiazines, narcotics, contraceptives)

Developmental abnormalities
- Genetic conditions (e.g., Turner's syndrome, testicular feminization)
- Congenital conditions (e.g., vaginal atresia, imperforate hymen)

Endocrine disorders
- Pituitary dysfunction (e.g., tumors)
- Thyroid dysfunction (hyper- or hypothyroidism)
- Adrenal dysfunction (e.g., Cushing's disease)
- Ovarian disease (e.g., polycystic disease)
- Premature ovarian failure
- Hyperprolactinemia
- Postpill amenorrhea (pituitary oversuppression)

Menorrhagia Menorrhagia is an increased duration or amount of menstrual bleeding at the time of a normal period. In the early reproductive years it may be associated with an endocrine problem or blood dyscrasia. A single episode of excessive bleeding may indicate a spontaneous abortion or ectopic pregnancy. Uterine tumors including carcinoma are common causes of menorrhagia. Pelvic inflammatory disease, endometriosis, the use of an intrauterine device, and drugs such as anticoagulants and thiazides can also produce heavy menses.

Metrorrhagia Metrorrhagia is bleeding or spotting between menstrual periods. Slight midcycle (mittelschmerz) spotting, associated with the decrease of estrogen levels prior to ovulation, is a common occurrence. Intramenstrual bleeding may be caused by (1) uterine lesions such as fibroids, polyps, hyperplasia, and carcinoma; (2) cervical erosion and carcinoma; and (3) pelvic inflammatory disease. Clients taking contraceptives may have metrorrhagia, which is referred to as breakthrough bleeding.

Reasons for changes in the usual pattern of menstruation will vary as well as the associated degree of concern. One explanation involves a change in lifestyle. Changes in marital status, recent moves, undue excitement, financial stresses, or other emotional crises can cause amenorrhea or unusual bleeding. These effects demonstrate the strong influences that psychological factors have on endocrine function and should be considered when the client presents herself for evaluation. When menorrhagia or metrorrhagia occur, the possibility of pelvic neoplasm must always be considered.

Medical management

Conservative Management Since the cause of menstrual irregularities are multiple and varied, it follows that diagnostic and therapeutic measures will be equally so. Space permits only a broad discussion of them. Initially, a detailed history and careful physical examination, including a pelvic examination, are done. An assessment of the actual loss of blood is attempted. Pregnancy, chronic disease, recent physical or psychic stress, and a possible drug-induced menstrual disturbance are ruled out. A wide range of tests and procedures relative to a tentative diagnosis are then carried out. The client may finally be referred to a gynecologic endocrinologist for further investigation of the problem.

Treatment of menstrual irregularities is directed toward the specific disorder responsible and the age of the client. Conservative treatment consists of hormonal therapy. Progesterone given in a single course for a problem of short duration or for 3 to 4 menstrual cycles has resulted in the return of normal ovarian function and control of excessive bleeding. When estrogen as well as progesterone problems exist, a trial of 3 to 4 months of oral contraceptives are given and often result in normal cycling. The dosage of oral contraceptives is adjusted if breakthrough bleeding occurs.

Treatment for any psychogenic cause of menstrual irregularities involves the giving of ample amounts of reassurance and understanding. Psychotherapy may be indicated for the underlying emotional problem.

Surgical Management Surgical treatment includes a variety of procedures such as dilatation and curettage, polypectomy, cauterization (destruction of tissue by a chemical or by heat), myomectomy (removal of uterine tumor without uterus), and hysterectomy.

Dilatation and curettage (D&C) is the most frequent performed gynecologic procedure. Dilatation is the widening of the cervical canal with a dilator and curettage is the scraping of the lining of the uterus with a curette. A D&C is considered both a diagnostic and a therapeutic measure. A diagnostic D&C is performed to identify a lesion in the endocervix or endometrium. A therapeutic D&C is done for an incomplete abortion and to correct excessive or prolonged bleeding. Dilatation of the cervix may be done to treat dysmenorrhea or sterility due to cervical stenosis. Cramping and mild pelvic and lower back pain occasionally occur. The client is usually discharged on the first postoperative day. In some instances the procedure is done on an outpatient basis.

Nursing management

Acute Intervention The amount of vaginal bleeding that the client experiences should be accurately assessed. The number of pads used as well as the degree of saturation should be reported and recorded. The client's fatigue level along with variations in blood pressure and blood count should be noted, since anemia and hypovolemia may be present.

The client scheduled for a D&C will have her food intake restricted preoperatively, since general anesthesia is required. The perineal area is prepared for surgery according to the policy of the individual institution.

Postoperatively the client returns to the unit with a sterile perineal pad in place. She may also have packing in the cervical and vaginal areas. The client should be observed for excessive bleeding during the first few postoperative hours. The perineal pad is changed as indicated. Since the packing, which generally remains in place for 24 hours, may exert pressure on the urethra, the client is checked for voiding problems. Mild analgesia should relieve any minor discomfort. Persistent pain should be reported to the physician since occasionally the uterus may be perforated during the procedure.

Specific instructions are given the client prior to discharge. They include:

1. Avoid use of tampons and douching and refrain from sexual activity until physician gives consent.
2. Expect a vaginal discharge during the healing process.
3. Avoid strenuous activity for 1 week.
4. Report any signs of infection such as fever, chills, foul-smelling discharge, and heavy bleeding over several hours.

The client should also be told that the subsequent menstrual period is not usually affected.

Chronic Management Treatment for menstrual problems is not always adequate. For instance, a D&C for metrorrhagia may be helpful for a period of time, but then the problem may recur. Continued use of contraceptives may become undesirable because of the client's age or state of health. If the abnormal bleeding persists, the client generally becomes frustrated and worried and wants something done to correct her condition. The client may express her concerns to the nurse and ask questions to help her make the decision for more involved therapy such as a hysterectomy. The woman whose family is complete and who notes little improvement with previous therapy will often accept a hysterectomy as a reasonable solution.

Menopause

The *climacteric* is the transitional period in the life of women during which reproductive function gradually diminishes and then ceases. It occurs generally between the ages of 45 and 55. During this period the monthly menses occur less frequently, are irregular, and the flow decreases in amount (see Table 43-2). The *menopause* is the physiologic cessation of menses associated with decreased ovarian function. It is diagnosed when a year has passed without menstruation.

Clinical manifestations

Physical The most common physical symptoms directly related to menopause are hot flashes and atrophic (senile) vaginitis. The hot flashes are described as a sensation of warmth beginning in the upper part of the chest, spreading to the neck, face, and upper extremities, followed by profuse perspiration and sometimes chilling. Hot flashes, caused by vasomotor instability, have been attributed to both decreased estrogen and increased gonadotropin release from the pituitary. Atrophic vaginitis, secondary to decreased estrogen, is characterized by thinning of the mucosa and disappearance of rugae which increase the possibility of vaginal trauma and infection. Menstrual irregularities are mentioned above.

Many physical changes in menopausal women are frequently associated with the process of aging rather than just decreased ovarian functioning. These changes include a redistribution of fat, a tendency to gain weight more easily, muscle and joint pain, loss of elasticity of skin, and atrophy of the external genitalia and breast tissue.

Psychological During the time of menopause women also begin to reevaluate and redefine their roles. Frustration over lost dreams, guilt feelings about previous failures, boredom with lack of challenge, and discouragement over diminishing horizons can develop into a variety of symptoms. They include emotional lability, anxiety, depression, insomnia, fatigue, palpitations, and headache. Menopause is often more difficult for the woman who perceived her ability to reproduce as her main reason for living and her way to prove her self-worth.

Medical management

The only symptoms of menopause that should be treated with estrogen are hot flashes and atrophic vaginitis, since they are the only symptoms directly attributable to estrogen deprivation. Most women (80 percent) can accept and tolerate the hot flashes without treatment if they are assured that they will eventually stop. If the symptoms are acute, then estrogen in the lowest possible dose that will stop them is prescribed. When atrophic vaginitis is present, intravaginal estrogen creams such as Premarin or vaginal suppositories such as diethylstilbestrol given for 30 nights provide effective and rapid relief.

Controversy exists about the relation between menopause and osteoporosis, arteriosclerosis, and coronary artery disease. There is little substantive evidence at present to warrant the use of estrogen in the prevention of these conditions. Since estrogen predisposes to an increased incidence of breast and endometrial carcinoma, it should only be prescribed for documented need.

A distinction between the menstrual irregularities that are basically physiologic to the menopause and the development of pathology such as polyps and cancer needs to be made. This entails a careful physical as well as pelvic examination, cervical cytology, and curettage of the cervix and endometrium. With pathology ruled out, several months of hormonal therapy (progesterone or oral contraceptives) may be considered.

Symptoms attributed to aging and psychological factors should be treated as such. Tranquilizers and sedatives may be prescribed for symptoms of insomnia and emotional manifestations, *but not at the expense of ignoring the need to resolve the grieving problems that often accompany menopause.* Women need to be listened to in a nonjudgmental fashion. Efforts should be made to help the woman reevaluate her life situation and make realistic plans for the future.

Pharmacologic intervention

While low-dose estrogens provide relief of vasomotor symptoms and atrophic vaginitis in menopausal women, there remains the concern that such therapy also is associated with the development of endometrial carcinoma and possibly breast cancer. The data gathered thus far are suggestive but not conclusive. The following precautions are taken when estrogen is prescribed. The lowest effective dose is used for the shortest possible time. Estrogen is given cyclically with 5 to 7 days per month in which the medication is omitted. The woman is seen by her physician every 6 months, at which time the reproductive organs and breast are examined and a Pap smear and blood pressure (to exclude hormone-induced hypertension) are taken. The therapeutic limits of estrogen replacement therapy and its advantages and disadvantages are also explained to the woman.[6]

Drugs such as Premarin, Amnestrogen, and diethylstilbestrol are administered in the cyclic manner described above. The original dose is tapered and then discontinued after 1 to 2 years of therapy. By this time the acute symptoms have generally subsided. The nurse should be alert to the possible side effects of the drugs and be able to interpret them for the client. The side effects include weight gain, breast and pelvic discomforts due to engorgement, headache, gastrointestinal disturbances, vaginal discharge, and skin pigmentation. These symptoms usually result from an excessive estrogen dosage or are an initial response to therapy. They can be reduced by decreasing the dose or they may resolve spontaneously with continual use. The most potentially significant side effect of estrogen is vaginal bleeding. It often occurs as a withdrawal effect when estrogen is used cyclically. Since postmenopausal bleeding may also be a sign of cancer, any abnormal bleeding should be reported promptly to the physician for investigation.

Nursing management

When menopause occurs women have almost as many years of their adult lives ahead of them as behind them. During this period a woman can choose to foster good health, vitality, and attractiveness, or she can perceive that menopause is the beginning of a prolonged degenerative process. Nurses can help women work through changes that occur by providing health teaching as well as reassurance.

The client's understanding of the physiology of menopause needs to be assessed. She should be made aware that the symptoms she is experiencing are normal and will pass after a reasonable amount of time. Many misconceptions about menopause have been perpetuated and should be clarified by the nurse to reduce unnecessary anxiety. Diet and exercise are important areas of health education. An intake of about 14 calories per pound of body weight while maintaining sound nutrition is recommended for the menopausal woman. A decrease in metabolic rate and careless eating habits, not menopause, result in weight gain and related fatigue. An adequate intake of calcium (1 g/day) and vitamin D (400 to 500 U/day) can maintain healthy bones and thereby counteract the effect of decreased estrogen that tends to make bones grow lighter and more fragile. Supplemental vitamin B complex has been useful in controlling hot flashes. This group of vitamins aids in the detoxification and elimination of the pituitary hormones that may cause the hot flashes.

A regular program of exercise and physical activity can improve circulation, maintain good muscle tone, and delay some aspects of aging for women in menopause. Exercise stimulates osteoblastic activity, thereby delaying osteoporosis. Activities such as brisk walks, swimming, bicycling, and gardening are healthy and enjoyable. Developing new interests can help to ease tension and anxiety.

Sexual function can continue with little change in the vast majority of postmenopausal women. Cessation of menstruation and ability to bear children should not be equated with cessation of sexual intercourse. Femininity and libido do not disappear with menopause. Actually, an older woman is often capable of greater warmth, sensitivity, and humanity in her sexual relationship than she was as a very young woman.[7] Atrophic changes of vaginal epithelium associated with inadequate lubrication may lead to *dyspareunia* (painful coitus). Vaseline or K-Y jelly is often effective in dealing with this problem. The client should be given an opportunity to discuss her concerns candidly.

Some of the symptoms of menopause such as hot flashes are self-limiting, so the concern for them decreases with time. The burden of birth control and fear of pregnancy no longer exist and may be considered as payoffs for this stage of life. A few women may need extended counseling to assist them in resolving their psychological problems. Psychiatric help may also be indicated.

CONTRACEPTION AND BIRTH CONTROL

Problem Identification

The role of women in present-day society is changing. Many of these changes have been brought about and encouraged by the women's liberation movement. Many women wish to pursue careers in addition to family and childbearing roles. Recently, many more avenues have opened up to women and they are eager and willing to explore them. With the advent of effective methods of contraception and abortion, pregnancy is seen as a voluntary experience. Women can now make choices about family size and spacing in keeping with today's newer lifestyles. Poor health or genetic problems of either partner and the mutual desire for fewer children lend themselves to current methods of family planning. Each individual is thereby permitted a personal choice regarding reproduction, based upon his or her own conscience or desire. These practices result in planned pregnancies at desired intervals.

Significance of Problem

The rapid growth of population has been identified as a threat to civilization and to the quality of life for all. Consequently, society as a whole has become increasingly concerned about population control. Although the maternal mortality rate in the United States has declined sharply over the years, it still remains a problem. Those who elect to use birth control measures are being reassured by their relative risk factors.

Illegitimacy, especially during the adolescent period, is on the increase. The increase in population, the risk of death with pregnancy as compared with relatively safe contraception measures, and the illegitimacy rates are all arguments in favor of birth control and contraception. The whole issue of birth control is highly controversial. Many moral and philosophical overtones can be extracted from it.

Contraceptive Methods

An ideal contraceptive is one which is safe, simple to use, inexpensive, reversible, and does not interfere with the act of intercourse. As yet, no single method is available that meets all the preceding criteria. *Temporary* contraceptives provide protection for those individuals who wish to avoid or delay pregnancy. To be effective, they must be used correctly and consistently. *Permanent* methods of birth control or sterilization are becoming increasingly acceptable to men and women. Sterilization is often chosen by individuals who have completed their families or who wish to remain childless. Table 46-3 summarizes the common contraceptive methods used, their use, side effects, and related client education. (Male sterilization is discussed in Chap. 47.)

Nursing Management

Individuals desire to prevent conception for a number of reasons related to personal convenience, economics, social values, and lifestyle. The nurse is in a position to counsel individuals and couples about birth control. The nurse can assist them by presenting concise, factual, unbiased information about methods available, including their benefits and risks. The couple should choose a method which will be most compatible with their personal circumstances. Most certainly this should be the one they will use and feel comfortable in using (Fig. 46-1).

Those women who are considering sterilization as their contraceptive method have common concerns about pain associated with the procedure, effects of sterilization, and possible complications. Counseling

Table 46-3
Methods of Birth Control

Type	Description	Side Effects/Complications	Client Education
		Temporary	
Oral contraceptives	Combination; "the pill"; mixture of estrogen and progesterone taken usually on 5th through 25th day of each cycle; prevents ovulation; changes endometrium; causes alterations in cervical mucus and tubal transport; simple, unobtrusive in use; 97% effective; failure due to irregular or incorrect use	*Minor*—weight gain, nausea and vomiting, spotting and breakthrough bleeding, postpill amenorrhea, breast tenderness, headache, chloasma, irritability, nervousness, depression, and decreased libido *Major*—Thromboembolic disorders *Contraindications*—history of cardiovascular or liver disease, hypertension, breast or pelvic cancer; caution with diabetes mellitus, sickle-cell anemia	Instruct in correct use of pills. Take pill same time each day, when pill is forgotten one day, take two next day. Review side effects, contraindications. Discuss need for periodic (every 6–12 months) checkup—weight, BP, Pap smear, hematocrit; danger signs of drug reviewed. Take drug history—phenytoin, phenobarbital, antibiotic (ampicillin) alter contraceptive action. Inform client usually not recommended for the over-35 age group and use beyond 4 years. Report cramps or swelling of legs, chest pain
Intrauterine device (IUD)	Flexible objects made of nylon, copper, or stainless steel wire inserted into uterus; string usually is attached that protrudes into vagina; contraception probably prevented by inflammatory response in endometrium, preventing implantation; once inserted no further motivation, equipment needed; 95% effective; failure mainly due to undetected expulsion	Increased menstrual flow, intramenstrual bleeding and cramping, especially during early months of use; possible complications of ectopic pregnancy, pelvic infection, and perforation of uterus	Discuss techniques and experience of insertion and removal. Inform client that insertion is difficult and expulsion and complications greater in nulliparous clients. Instruct client to check for string in vagina after each period; report to physician if unable to locate. Discuss need for annual pelvic exam and Pap smear

Table 46-3 (Continued)

Type	Description	Side Effects/Complications	Client Education
Diaphragm	Dome-shaped rubber cup with circular metal spring (vary in size), covers cervix; inner surface is coated with spermicide before insertion; provides mechanical barrier to sperm; prescription method; fitted by professional; recurrent motivation to use needed. 87% effective, failure due to improper fitting or placement of device	Allergy to rubber	Demonstrate how to hold, insert, and remove using model. Allow for insertion and removal practice sessions. Advise insertion may be anytime prior to coitus, but removal should be 6–8 hours after coitus. Give instructions for cleansing and storing, checking for holes or deterioration. Advise client it must be refitted following pregnancy, weight loss, or gain. Advise not suitable with severe degree of pelvic relaxation
Condom ("rubber safe")	Thin rubber sheath which fits over erect penis and provides mechanical barrier to sperm; simple to use; no prescription needed; 85% effective; failure due to tearing or slipping during coitus	Possible allergy to rubber; may decrease sensation and interfere with foreplay	Advise client to roll sheath along entire penis, leaving slack at end to receive semen. Inform client that sharp object, e.g., fingernails, may tear. Advise client to hold sheath in place when penis is withdrawn to prevent emptying of sperm in or near vagina
Spermicide (jellies, creams, foam)	Inserted into vagina by means of applicator or aerosol spray, provides chemical barrier to cervical os, simple method to use; no prescription needed. 80% effective; failure due to uncertain dispersion and retention of agent within vagina	Possible allergies in either partner	Instruct client on proper insertion of spermicide. Advise on application just before *each* act of coitus. Advise client use if chiefly for women with infrequent coitus
Rhythm	Periodic abstinence during fertile portion of menstrual cycle; strong motivation, self-control required; complies with all religious doctrines. 60–65% effective; failure results from difficulty in determining precise day of ovulation; irregularity of menses		Discuss methods to establish baseline menstrual patterns and identify ovulation. Give instructions in use of calendar or basal body temperature method to determine ovulation and fertile period (considered to be day 10 through 17 of 28-day cycle).
		Permanent Sterilization	
Tubal	Variety of abdominal and vaginal surgical procedures (laparotomy, laparoscopy, culdoscopy) which permanently bar sperm and ovum from meeting. Fallopian tubes are crushed, ligated, clipped, or plugged (potentially reversible procedure). 99.96% effective; failure due to recanalization of fallopian tubes, erroneous ligation	Bowel injury, hemorrhage, or infection	Determine if temporary contraceptives were used and reason for their dissatisfaction. Counsel regarding effects of procedure on physiology and sexual performance. Assist in obtaining written informed consent for procedure. Inform client procedure requires short-term hospitalization or can be done on an outpatient basis

Table 46-3 (Continued)

Type	Description	Side Effects/Complications	Client Education
Hysterectomy	Surgical removal of the uterus. 100% effective	Bladder infection, vascular disorders, infection, hemorrhage, pain, psychological adjustment	Assess or counsel client regarding understanding of extent of surgery, altered physiology, complications, and sexual performance. Inform client of increased cost, disability
Vasectomy	Bilateral, surgical ligation and resection of the ductus deferens 100% effective	Hematoma, swelling, psychological adjustment	Inform client this is usually an outpatient procedure taking 15–30 minutes. Need alternate form of contraception until no sperm on examination. Discuss that procedure does not affect maleness

should provide accurate information about these concerns and allow the individuals to explore their feelings about ending reproductive functioning. It is felt that when motives are healthy and the individual is well-adjusted, sterilization will not adversely affect sexual functioning, physiology, or self-concept.

With the increased interest in family planning, nurses should know the available resources for contraceptive referral within their community. *Planned Parenthood* is one such resource that is found in most areas. Literature dealing with contraception should also be provided for those individuals who demonstrate an interest in it.

When the individual(s) has made a decision on the method of contraception, counseling in the proper use of the method needs to be given. The nurse should evaluate the client's real understanding of the method chosen and provide explanations and interpretation if necessary. The client should also be aware of an alternate method of contraception should emergencies such as a missing diaphragm occur at an inopportune time.

Women using contraceptives but wishing to eventually have a family should understand the risks of deferring pregnancy. Infertility increases from 5 percent at age 20 to 30 percent at age 35.[8] Fetal and maternal risks also increase with age. Women with progressive medical conditions such as heart disease should be advised to have their families as early as possible.

INFERTILITY

Infertility is the failure to conceive after a year or more of unrestricted intercourse. Approximately 10 percent of married couples in the United States are infertile. Professional intervention can assist about 40 percent of the couples to achieve a pregnant state.

In determining the cause of infertility and in treating it, both husband and wife must be evaluated. A female factor is found in no more than half of the barren marriages.[9] Proper study and the subsequent therapeutic measures will require time (often a year or more) and patience if results are to be obtained. A trusting relationship between the health professionals and the infertile couple should be established early in the investigative process.

Etiology

A complete list of causes of female infertility would prove to be extensive. The following are found most frequently: anovulation, tubal disease, and abnormalities of the cervical mucus or the uterus. Other possible causes include systemic debility, psychological stress, marital and sexual maladjustment, or lack of knowledge about reproductive functioning. Male infertility is discussed in Chap. 47.

Diagnostic Studies

After a detailed history and general physical examination of the woman are done to rule out any related medical or gynecologic disease, several basic tests are performed to evaluate if the cause is female infertility. These are ovulatory studies, tubal patency studies, and postcoital studies.

Ovulatory studies

A *basal body temperature record* is kept to establish whether or not there is regular ovulation. The

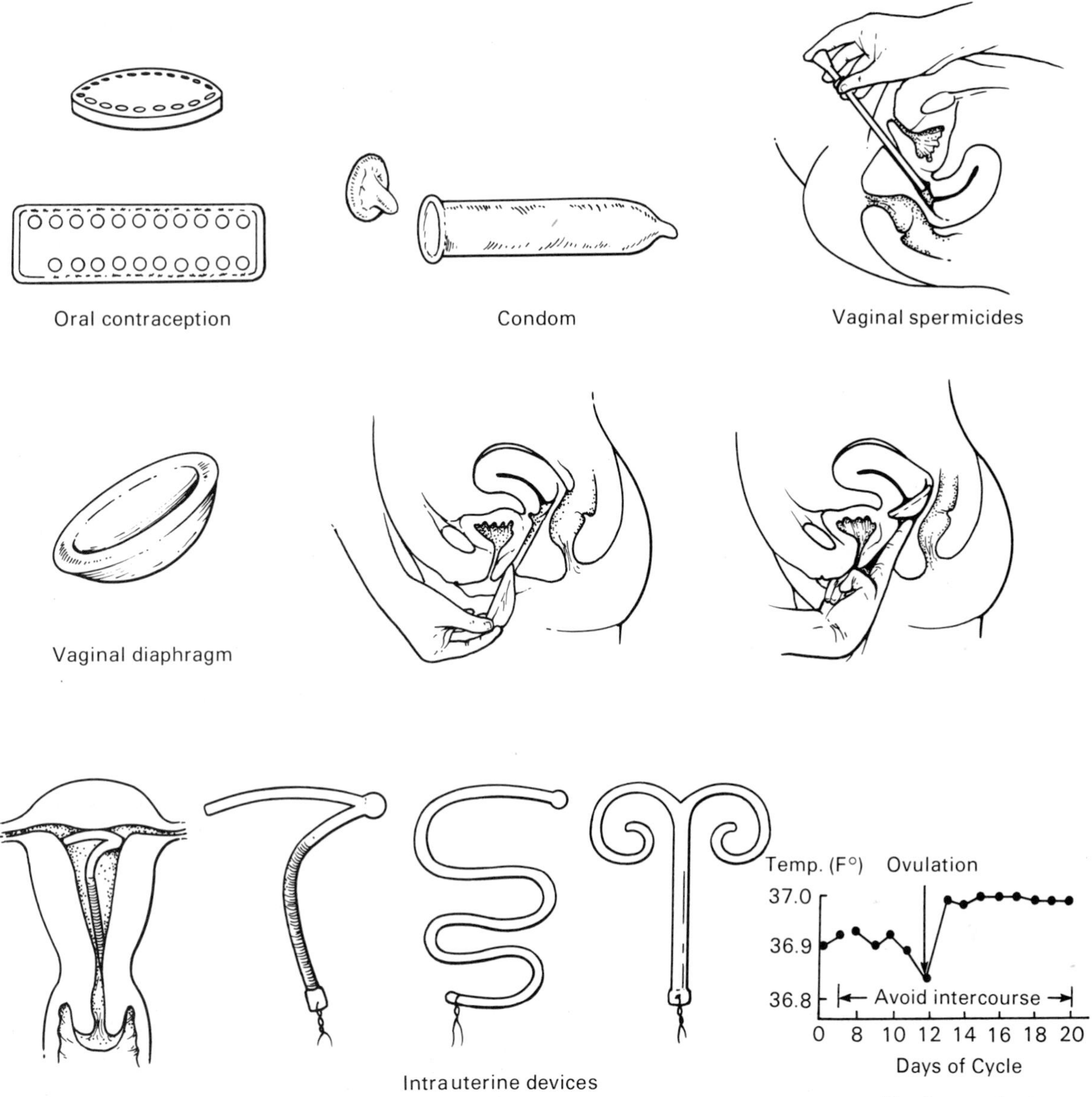

Figure 46-1 Temporary contraceptive methods and devices. (*From M. Garrey, A. D. T. Govan, C. Hodge, and R. Callander, Gynecology Illustrated, 2d ed., Churchill Livingstone Inc., New York, 1979.*)

woman is instructed to take and record her temperature upon awakening and before any activity. The same site, e.g., oral, should be used each time. Any cause for variation such as sleeplessness or illness should be noted. As ovulation approaches, the production of estrogen increases and may cause a drop in temperature. When ovulation occurs, progesterone is produced, causing a 0.3 to 0.4°C (0.5 to 0.7°F) rise in temperature. The temperature graph and the readings (Fig. 46-2) therefore detect ovulation and the timing of intercourse if pregnancy is desired. Other tests for ovulation include cervical and vaginal smears, endometrial biopsy, and plasma progesterone determinations.

Tubal patency studies

Tubal disease (occlusion or lack of peristalsis) can be assessed by two methods, tubal insufflation

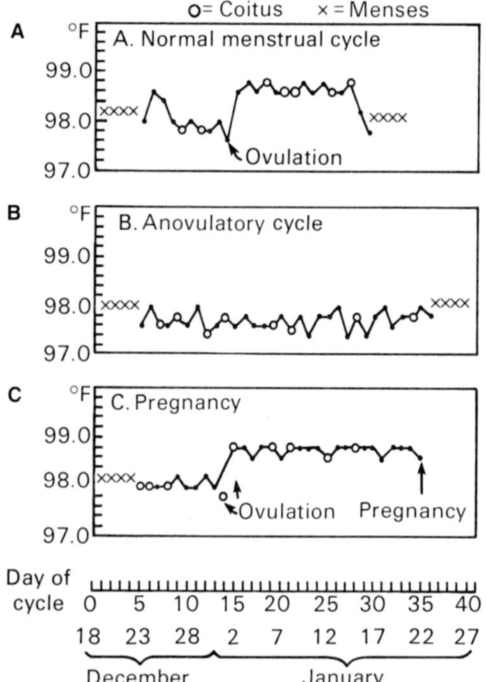

Figure 46-2 Basal body temperature chart. *(a)* Typical biphasic temperature curve indicative of ovulation and normal progesterone effect. *(b)* Irregular monophasic curve characteristic of anovulatory cycles. *(c)* Ovulatory curve with sustained temperature elevation following conception and the first missed period.

and hystosalpingogram. The simplest is *tubal insufflation*, which involves the introduction of carbon dioxide through the cervix via a cannula (Rubin's test). If one or both tubes are patent the gas flows along the uterus and tubes into the peritoneal cavity. This can be heard by auscultation. When the client sits up, the gas rises to the diaphragm, causing referred shoulder pain via the phrenic nerve. This pain should be described to the client prior to the test. A short rest period utilizing the Trendelenburg position, allowing gas to rise in the pelvis, should be provided following the procedure.

Hysterosalpingogram, the second method to evaluate tubal patency, is the radiologic visualization of the uterus and tubes by the injection through the cervix of a radiopaque dye. Tubal patency and any distortions of the endometrial cavity can be determined. A laxative or enema is given the client prior to the test so that distension or gas shadows will be prevented, thereby making the x-ray film easier to read. The client may experience discomforts similar to those following tubal insufflation and should be observed for signs of a possible allergic reaction to the dye. Culdoscopy or laparoscopy in which the tubes may be visualized directly while a dye is injected into the cervix is also being used to detect tubal disease.

Postcoital studies

Examination of the cervical mucus can reveal if it undergoes favorable changes at ovulation enabling penetration, survival, and normal progression of the sperm. A *postcoital examination* can determine if the cervical environment is favorable for the sperm. The woman is asked to have intercourse about the time ovulation is expected and 2 to 4 hours prior to being seen by the physician. Douching or bathing should be avoided before the test. The cervical and vaginal secretions are aspirated and examined for the number and motility of sperm present.

Management

The management of infertility problems depends on the cause. If infertility is secondary to an ovarian disturbance, supplemental hormone therapy to restore and maintain ovulation may be attempted. One drug now being used to induce ovulation is clomiphene citrate (Clomid).

Where actual mechanical tubal block exists, a reparative surgical procedure can be attempted. However, only a small percentage of normal intrauterine term pregnancies have followed tuboplasty.

Poor cervical mucus may be a result of chronic cervicitis or inadequate estrogenic stimulation. Careful cauterization of the cervix may eradicate the chronic cervicitis while the administration of estrogens can improve the quantity and quality of the cervical mucus.

Improving the client's general health may help, especially when a debilitating or chronic illness is present. Removing or reducing psychological stress can improve the emotional climate, making it more conducive to achieving pregnancy. Educating the client (couple) regarding the probable time of ovulation and appropriate coital technique may also be indicated.

In selected cases, *artificial (donor) insemination*, the introduction of semen into the female genital tract, can be an effective treatment. The selection of the donor is carried out with great care, giving attention to his general state of health, genetic background, and blood type. Male sterility is the usual reason for insemination use.

Recently, a new technique in which conception takes place in a test tube rather than the uterus is being investigated. The fertilized ovum is implanted in the natural mother's uterus with subsequent birth of a child. Women who are infertile due to tubal disease may one day opt for this intervention. Both of the preceding methods of conception have social and ethical implications which may preclude their use by some couples.

If it is obvious that an incurable barrier to conception exists or if the program of therapy has failed to achieve pregnancy after a period of a year, the possibility of adoption should be seriously considered.

The nurse has a major responsibility for teaching and providing emotional support throughout the infertility testing period. Feelings of anger and frustration between the partners may heighten as test after test is done. The problem of infertility can generate great tension in a marriage. Shame and guilt may be precipitated when other individuals become involved in this intimate area of a relationship. Recognizing and taking steps to deal with the psychological and emotional factors that surface can assist the couple to better cope with the situation.

Provisions for giving information and emotional support by the nurse continue as therapeutic measures are attempted. Once the cause of fertility is determined, the client with the problem may need help with gender identity related to the inability to conceive. Ample opportunities for the clients to talk over their concerns should also be given.

ABORTION

An abortion is the termination of a pregnancy before the fetus is legally viable. Viability as defined legally varies between 20 and 28 weeks of gestation and between 300 and 1000 g of weight. Abortions are classified as *spontaneous*, occurring naturally with no artificial means; or *induced*, occurring as a result of mechanical or medicinal interruption. *Miscarriage* is the lay term indicating lack of criminal involvement in the termination of the pregnancy.

Spontaneous Abortion

Spontaneous abortion occurs in about 10 to 20 percent of all conceptions. Fetal or maternal abnormalities are the chief causes of these abortions. Spontaneous abortions are subdivided into the categories outlined in Table 46-4 so they can be differentiated clinically.

Table 46-4
Classification of Spontaneous Abortions

Category	Description
Inevitable	History of early pregnancy, then onset of moderate bleeding and cramping. Tissue protrudes from dilated cervix
Complete	All products of conception are expelled
Incomplete	Some products of conception, mainly placenta and membranes, are retained
Missed	Fetal death has occurred but symptoms of abortion cease and products of conception are retained in uterus for more than 4 weeks. Signs and symptoms of pregnancy disappear
Habitual	Occurs when 3 or more consecutive pregnancies end in abortion

Medical management

The presence of uterine cramping serves as an aid to diagnosing the vaginal bleeding as a spontaneous abortion. This symptom is usually absent in vaginal bleeding caused by other conditions such as polyps. Laboratory findings provide little information in establishing a diagnosis. Pregnancy tests may remain positive for about 2 weeks after fetal death.

Treatment for a spontaneous abortion is limited. Bed rest, sedation, and progesterone (although its use is controversial) may be prescribed when a diagnosis of threatened abortion is made. The client is advised to report any bleeding to the physician. It is estimated that 80 percent of the clients will proceed to abortion regardless of management. A D&C is generally done following spontaneous abortions in order to minimize blood loss, reduce chance of secondary infection, and shorten convalescence. The habitual aborter, who is found to have an incompetent cervical os, may have her cervix tightened surgically by placement of a purse-string suture through it. At delivery the suture is removed by the physician and vaginal delivery follows, or the suture is retained and delivery is by caesarean section.

Nursing management

It may be necessary for the client who is threatening to abort to be admitted to the hospital. Vital signs are monitored and an estimation of the blood loss is made. Measures are taken to restrict activity and reduce stress in order to provide the needed physical and mental rest. Any tissue or suspicious clots passed are saved to be examined for traces of fetus and placenta. The possibility of losing the pregnancy may be very distressing to the client. Sympathy, support, reassurance, and someone to talk to are greatly appreciated by these clients.

Induced Abortion

The distinction between the two types of induced abortion, criminal and therapeutic, is a legal one and is not very clear due to the changing law. *Criminal abortions* are generally self-induced or performed by nonprofessionals outside of appropriate medical facilities. Consequently, they are considered illegal. *Therapeutic (legal) abortions* are performed in the hospital or may be done in a clinic on an outpatient basis. Abortion for medical and social reasons is now available to over half the world's population, making it one of the most common medical procedures performed. Since issues surrounding the topic of induced abortion are numerous and complex, only a brief discussion of the law and medical and nursing management is presented here.

In 1973 the United States Supreme Court reached a decision establishing that abortion is a matter between the woman and her physician within certain limits. It was also decided that states could not have laws restricting a woman's access to abortion except during the third trimester of pregnancy and could only regulate second trimester abortion to make the procedure safe. Many states have not revised their laws to allow for the latter so some confusion still remains about the circumstances under which abortions can be legally performed.

Techniques used for abortion

Dilatation and Curettage (D&C) The decision about which technique to employ will depend on the length of the pregnancy. Pregnancies up to 12 weeks gestation are usually terminated by suction curettage (vacuum aspiration) or standard dilatation and curettage (D&C). When suction curettage is utilized, a local or light anesthetic is given. The cervix is dilated and the contents of the uterus aspirated by way of a suction curette. The procedure takes only a few minutes and complications are rare. Many clients experience some cramping after abortion, which is normal and of short duration.

Amnioinfusion The instillation of a substance into the amniotic cavity to induce labor is the method of choice after the sixteenth week of gestation. An 18-gauge spinal needle is introduced into the amniotic cavity and approximately 200 mL of amniotic fluid is removed. A similar amount of 20% sodium chloride (saline abortion) is instilled into the amniotic cavity and the needle is withdrawn. The fetus dies, and the uterus is apparently irritated and begins to contract within 24 to 38 hours. The contractions may need to be assisted with an oxytocic medication given intravenously. When carefully done, the procedure results in few complications, although hypernatremia, water intoxication, amniotic fluid embolism, and retained placental tissues have been known to occur.

Prostaglandins are also being used in amnioinfusion. These compounds stimulate uterine contractions that result in cervical dilatation and expulsion of the fetus and placenta within 24 hours. Side effects of nausea, vomiting, and diarrhea occur when prostaglandins are used but this technique is considered safer than hypertonic saline.[10] Intravaginal, intramuscular, and transcervical instillations of prostaglandins are currently being investigated in terminating pregnancies from 12 to 20 weeks of gestation.[11]

Hysterotomy Hysterotomy is used to terminate late pregnancies of 16 to 20 weeks gestation. In this miniature caesarean section procedure, an incision is made into the uterus and the contents removed. The incidence of morbidity and mortality is greater for hysterotomy than other abortion procedures.

Nursing management

Since physical and psychological complications can arise following abortion procedures, the decision to have an abortion warrants careful consideration. The woman and her significant others will need support and acceptance. Some clients will benefit from counseling beforehand, especially those for whom the abortion involves conflict. The specific procedure planned needs to be explained to each client. At times the overriding need to have the pregnancy terminated does not allow detailed explanations or teaching to be absorbed. Anxiety, loneliness, and fear are emotions often experienced by women before and during the procedure. There may be no friends or family present to support the client. The nurse can be an important factor in the client's experience of the event.

Follow-up care includes instructions on signs and symptoms of possible complications, and avoidance of sex, tampons, or douching until reexamination. The client is instructed to return for reexamination in 2 weeks. Some depression is not uncommon and the client can be prepared for this before discharge. Contraception can be initiated during the client's return visit in accordance with her needs and desires.

ECTOPIC PREGNANCY

An ectopic pregnancy is the implantation of the fertilized ovum anywhere outside the uterine cavity. The most frequent site is in the fallopian tube but it may be ovarian, abdominal, or cervical (Fig. 46-3).

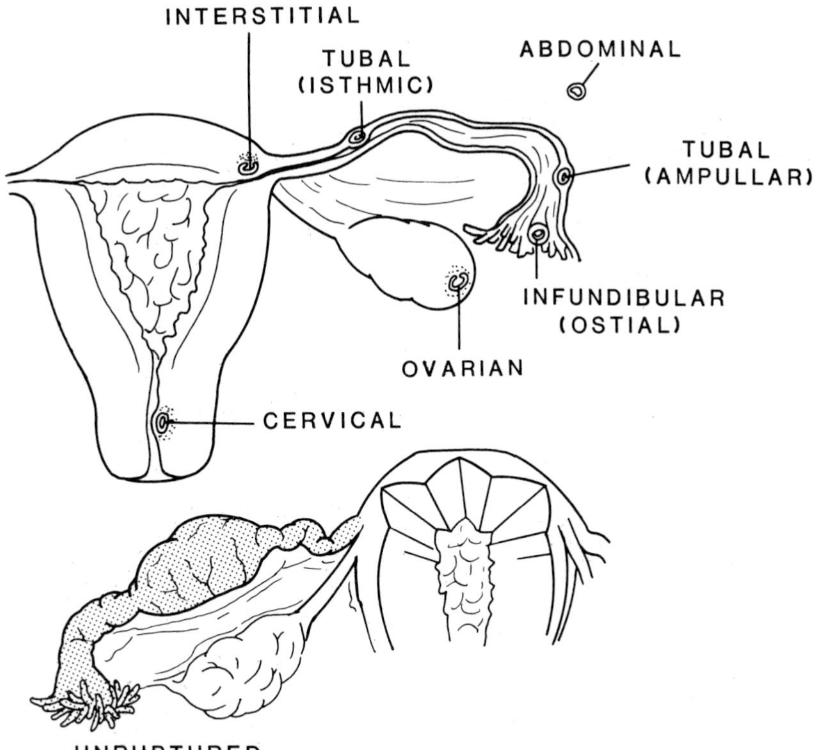

Figure 46-3 Sites of ectopic pregnancy. *[From S. L. Romney et al. (eds.), Gynecology and Obstetrics, The Health Care of Women, 2d ed., McGraw-Hill Book Company, New York, 1981.]*

Any blockage of the tube or reduction of tubal peristalsis will impede or delay the passage of the zygote to the uterine cavity and can result in tubal fertilization. Salpingitis, adhesions, tumors, tubal surgery, and hormonal imbalances as well as the presence of an IUD can predispose to ectopic pregnancy. Ectopic pregnancies occur approximately once in every 200 pregnancies. Even though implantation occurs, the tubal environment is not a favorable one. The thin tubal wall can only expand minimally with growth of the gestational sac before it ruptures, accompanied by tearing into its blood supply and intraabdominal bleeding. The fetus usually dies.

Clinical Manifestations

The majority of women with tubal pregnancy exhibit subacute and atypical symptoms. The chief complaints are menstrual irregularity, vaginal spotting (which occurs after fetal death and estrogen withdrawal), and crampy pain in the lower abdomen (due to tubal distension). Significant pelvic or abdominal tenderness may or may not be present on physical examination. Generally, there is a gradual fall in hemoglobin.

Some women experience vaginal bleeding followed by the sudden development of acute abdominal pain, indicating rupture of the tubal pregnancy. The pain, often accompanied by vomiting and fainting, is associated with referred shoulder pain due to diaphragmatic irritation. The abdomen becomes distended with blood and may be tight and tender to touch. Hypovolemic shock may result as manifested by its classic signs and symptoms. An obvious emergency situation exists.

Management

Ectopic pregnancy generally represents a diagnostic challenge not only because of its vague manifestations but also because of its similarity to a wide variety of other pelvic and abdominal disorders such as salpingitis, abortion, rupture of a cyst, appendicitis, and peritonitis. When the signs and symptoms are more pronounced, a careful history and physical examination can establish the diagnosis of ectopic pregnancy. More often, culdocentesis, a procedure in which the cul-de-sac is tapped for nonclotted blood, or laparoscopy are relied upon to confirm the diagnosis. Ultrasound, a noninvasive procedure, is also currently being utilized as a diagnostic method. A pregnancy test will routinely be done. However, definitive treatment is not based on the results. Often, surgery is necessary before the results of a serum pregnancy test are available.

Once the diagnosis of ectopic pregnancy is made, surgery should proceed immediately. The client may be transfused to relieve shock and restore a satisfactory blood volume for safe anesthesia and surgery. The usual surgical procedure is a salpingectomy.

All the gross abdominal blood and clots are removed to prevent fewer intraperitoneal adhesions. The profuse bleeding that occurs with rupured ectopic pregnancy has made it one of the leading causes of maternal death. Tubal pregnancy has been known to interfere with the future reproductive ability of many females.

Nursing care of the client will depend upon her condition. Before diagnosis has been confirmed the nurse will be alert to signs of increasing pain and vaginal bleeding that may indicate that rupture of the ectopic pregnancy has occurred. Vital signs will be monitored closely, as well as signs of shock. Explanations and preparation for diagnostic procedures will be given where appropriate. Preparation of the client for abdominal surgery may follow rapidly. The client's emotional status will need to be assessed. Reassurance and support for the surgery should be given to both the client and her family.

RAPE

Significance of the Problem

Rape is defined legally as unlawful carnal knowledge of a person by force and without the person's consent. Carnal knowledge can mean completed coitus or even the slightest penetration of the male penis into the female genitalia.

The number of rapes, particularly against women, are increasing at an alarming rate. The Uniform Crime Reports for the United States published by the Federal Bureau of Investigation show that there were 67,131 reported cases of rape in 1978, representing 6 percent of all crimes of violence. The total number of offenses in 1978 increased 21 percent over 1974.[12] At the same time many cases of rape are unreported due to the fear and embarrassment of the victims. Some women feel that they would not be able to withstand the stresses of prosecution or that they would be met with disbelief and humiliation from the police, medical staff, or their peers.

Clinical Manifestations

Physical injuries

Rape, a crime of violence, may result in genital and extragenital injuries, pregnancy, and venereal disease. Genital injuries appear less frequently and are generally of a minor nature, such as bruises and lacerations to the perineum, hymen, vulva, vagina, cervix, and anus. Some women have sustained lacerations of the ligaments supporting the uterus, resulting in uterine displacement, and severe lacerations of the vagina, requiring extensive surgical reconstruction and repair. Dyspareunia and vaginismus (painful spasms of the vagina) have developed as a consequence. Approximately 9 percent of all homicides are related to rape and sex offenses.[13]

In general, the more serious injuries involve the extragenital areas such as the face, neck, and extremities and often occur after the rape. Fractures, subdural hematomas, cerebral concussions, or intraabdominal injuries have resulted in the need for hospitalization. Rape, therefore, is an act of violence with sex as the weapon rather than primarily a sexual act.

Emotional trauma

The emotional trauma of rape victims often affects the victim's future sexual functioning and intimate relationships. The initial reaction of most women to rape is shock, disbelief, and emotional breakdown including crying, agitation, and incoherence. Feelings of anger, fear, embarrassment, and self-blame are commonly expressed. Within several days to weeks after the rape the woman displays controlled behavior and a return to normal life patterns. It is felt that the victim's real feelings at this time may be hidden under her calm, composed affect. The long-term results of the rape include the integration and resolution of the experience.[14,15] Some time is needed for the woman to complete this process; not all are able to achieve full resolution of the rape experience. Many victims develop phobias such as fear of crowds. Others are unable to resume their usual sex style or have frightening dreams which persist for long periods. Counseling may be helpful.

Social effects

The support and acceptance offered rape victims by their significant others is important in reducing the sociological crisis of rape. The men in the victim's life take on a greater significance. How they respond to the situation will affect her future relations with them, and indeed, all men. They, themselves, may have serious problems resolving the incident and need as much help as the victim. Changes in residency and place of employment may result as a consequence of the experience due to fear or inability to maintain previous relationships. Rape trauma dramatically disrupts the homemaking and parenting roles normally performed by the adult woman. Assistance from her husband and other family members is needed. At times, help is given halfheartedly because of reluctance of the individuals to believe in the victim's total innocence.

Medical Management

When the victim of a rape is admitted to the emergency room or clinic, a specific chain of events occurs (Table 46-5). A signed informed consent is obtained from the victim before rape data are collected. All the materials gathered are well documented, labeled, and given to the appropriate person, such as the pathologist or police officer. The materials are handled by as few people as possible and signatures of all responsible for keeping and handling the data are obtained. Much of the data can be used as evidence should the victim choose to file a complaint. Consequently, the integrity of the data must be maintained. The nurse's involvement in the medicolegal process depends on the policies of the individual institution.

A gynecologic and sexual history and history of the assault (who, what, when, where, why), as well as a general physical and pelvic examination add further information about the rape incident. Laboratory tests are done mainly to determine the presence of sperm in the vagina and to rule out the possibility of venereal disease and pregnancy.

During the treatment period, the client's physical injuries are attended to and prophylaxis for venereal disease and pregnancy is administered. The client's immediate and long-term need for emotional support is given special consideration.

The physician is unable to legally (see definition) state that rape occurred but he can swear that his findings show that sexual intercourse took place and injury was inflicted. These findings, along with others such as the police report and examination of the rape scene, can form the foundation for the rapist's conviction.

Nursing Management

All women should be aware of rape prevention tactics (Table 46-6). They should also be encouraged to learn some basic techniques of self-defense. Local high schools or the YWCA usually have self-defense

Table 46-5
Checklist for Evaluation of Alleged Rape

I. Medicolegal
  A. Valid written consent for examination, photographs, lab tests, release of information, and laboratory samples
  B. Two physicians needed for evaluation and slide review
  C. Appropriate "chain of evidence" documentation
  D. Retain typed copies
II. History
  A. Age, marital status, and parity
  B. Menstrual and contraceptive history
  C. Time of last coitus prior to assault
  D. Change of clothes, bath, douche?
  E. Use of drugs or alcohol
  F. Who, what, when, where, why
  G. Penetration, ejaculation, condom, extragenital acts
III. General physical examination
  A. Vital signs and general appearance
  B. Extragenital trauma—mouth, breasts, neck
  C. Cuts, bruises, scratches—photograph
IV. Pelvic examination
  A. Vulvar trauma, erythema, hymen, anal, and rectal status
  B. Matted hairs or free hairs
  C. Vaginal examination—unlubricated speculum; foreign body, discharge, blood, lacerations
  D. Uterine size
  E. Adnexa, especially hematomas
V. Laboratory samples—label carefully
  A. Saline irrigation of vagina—2 mL and swab; acid phosphatase, blood groups
  B. Vaginal smears—Pap and Gram stain
  C. Oral or rectal swabs and smears
  D. Clotted blood, 3 tubes: serology, blood type, alcohol
  E. Cultures—cervix plus other areas, if indicated
  F. Urine—pregnancy test, drugs
  G. Hairs—comb and clip
  H. Fingernail scrapings
  I. Comb pubic hairs
  J. Clip clients' pubic hair
  K. Clip matted hairs
VI. Treatment
  A. Care for injuries and emotional trauma
  B. Consider antibiotic prophylaxis for venereal disease. Probenecid, 1 g orally, preceding procaine penicillin, 4.8 million units IM, or tetracycline phosphate, 3 g PO, if client is penicillin-sensitive
  C. Protect against pregnancy if any risk
    1. Premarin, 50 mg IV
    2. Premarin, 40 mg QD × 3 days
  D. Protect legal rights
  E. Recommend continued follow-up and services of rape crisis center
  F. Repeat gonorrhea culture 7 days later
  G. Repeat gonorrhea culture and serology 6 weeks later
  H. Pregnancy test if appropriate

David Halbert and D. E. Darnell Jones, "Medical Management of Sexually Assaulted Women," *J Reproductive Med*, **20**:272 (May 1978).

Table 46-6

Rape Prevention Tactics

1. See that there are lights at all entrances to your home.
2. Keep your doors locked and do not open them to a stranger. Ask for identification if a service person comes to the door.
3. Do not advertise that you live alone. List only your initials with your last name in the telephone directory or on the mailbox. Never reveal to a caller that you are home alone.
4. Avoid walking alone in deserted areas. Walk to the parking lot with a friend. Be sure you see each other leave.
5. Have your keys ready as you approach your car or home.
6. Keep all doors locked and windows up when driving.
7. Never get on an elevator with a suspicious person. Pretend you have forgotten something and get off.
8. Say what you mean in social situations. Be sure your voice and body language reflect your response.
9. Carry a loud whistle and use it when you think you are in danger.
10. Yell "fire" if you are attacked and run toward a lighted area.

Adapted from Irene Horoshak, "Learn to Fight Rape—Without Hang-Ups," *RN*, **39**:54 (1976).

classes in which formal instruction can be given. Practicing the various techniques with a friend will build up confidence in the ability to fight back. Learning self-defense can make the woman less vulnerable and more self-reliant.

When a rape victim is brought to the clinic or emergency room, she should be given the highest priority for care and treatment. A quiet, private area should be utilized for the initial assessment and examinations that follow. The client should not be left alone. Whenever possible, the same nurse should remain with her throughout her stay and provide needed emotional support. The client's actions and words as she describes the rape incident may be inconsistent, confused, and inappropriate. The nurse should maintain a nonjudgmental attitude, leaving moral and legal judgment to others.

The client usually has many feelings and thoughts about the rape and generally wants to talk about them to an interested listener. Talking may help the client feel better and give understanding to her reactions to the incident. When the nurse listens carefully the client feels she is not alone and is better able to gain control over her situation.

The nurse should assess the client's stress level before preparing her for the various procedures that will follow. The client's coping mechanisms will be supported when she knows what to expect and what is expected of her as well as why the particular procedure must be done. Since the pelvic examination may trigger a flashback of the rape, the nurse should answer all related questions beforehand and urge her to relax as much as she is able.

Following the examinations the client's physical comfort needs should be considered. She may need safety pins, needle and thread for her torn clothing, a cigarette to decrease her anxiety, or a cool drink to relieve her thirst. Most women who have been raped feel dirty and will appreciate a place to wash as well as mouthwash, especially if oral sex was involved.

The nurse can also further emphasize and elaborate on any prescribed medical treatment. The client's understanding of the possible side effects of the medications given should be assessed. The client is urged to see her own physician or return for a follow-up examination and venereal disease testing.

When the client is discharged, the nurse should make certain she has transportation home. If friends or family are not available, the hospital or clinic should attempt to work out an arrangement with an appropriate community resource. The client should not be sent home alone.

Many communities today have rape crisis centers. These public service organizations have trained professional and nonprofessional volunteers who provide an emotional support system for rape victims upon request. Their programs provide advocacy to assure dignified treatment of the victim throughout the medical and police procedures, short-term counseling for the victim and her family, as well as court assistance and public education on rape-related issues. The nurse should be able to give the client the names and local phone numbers of such organizations.

The rape victim generally has many concerns about her sexuality. Long-term counseling may be necessary in order to permit the crisis to stabilize. The nurse can assist the client in obtaining the needed counseling while providing continued reassurance and emotional support.

INFLAMMATION AND INFECTIONS OF THE VAGINA, CERVIX, AND VULVA

Infection and inflammation of the vagina, cervix, and vulva tend to occur when the natural defenses of the acid vaginal secretions and the presence of Döderlein's bacilli are disrupted. Also, the woman's resistance may be decreased due to aging, poor nutrition, and use of drugs which alter the mucosa. The causative organisms gain entrance to the areas through contaminated hands, clothing, douche nozzles, and during intercourse, surgery, and childbirth. Table 46-7 relates the specific etiology, clinical manifestations, and medical management of common inflammations and infections.

Nursing Management

Normally the endocervical glands secrete a clear exudate which may become cloudy and take on a slight odor as it passes through the vagina. The amount of discharge may increase (physiologic leukorrhea) at ovulation, just prior to menstruation, during pregnancy and sexual excitement, and when taking oral contraceptives. When changes in the amount, color, character, or odor of the discharge occur, they usually indicate an infection (pathologic leukorrhea).

Women need to know what situations increase the risk of vaginal, cervical, and vulvar infections. Excessive douching, for instance, can be harmful since it destroys the vagina's natural resistance to disease. Douching more than once every week or two has been known to bring about these results.

Drugs such as oral contraceptives, antibiotics,

Table 46-7
Inflammation and Infection of Vagina, Cervix, and Vulva

Condition	Etiology	Clinical Manifestations	Management
Simple vaginitis	Variety of organisms including *Escherichia coli, Hemophilis vaginalis, Staphlyococcus*	Vulvar irritation; profuse, yellowish mucoid discharge	Appropriate antibiotic, local or systemic. Vinegar douche. Beta lactose vaginal suppository (to restore normal vaginal flora). Sitz baths
Candidiasis	*Candida albicans* (fungus). Associated with pregnancy, poorly controlled diabetes mellitus, oral contraceptives, antibiotics	Inflammation of vaginal mucosa producing internal itching, beefy red irritation White, thick, cheesy discharge adherent to vaginal mucosa Difficult to cure; recurs readily	Nystatin (Mycostatin) vaginal suppositories for 14 days. (Virtually nontoxic and nonsensitizing) Gentian violet (1%) applied locally to vagina. (Low client acceptance due to staining of clothes) Secure medical and drug history
Trichomoniasis	*Trichomonas vaginalis* (protozoan). Can be sexually transmitted. Can survive in wet media several hours, making transmission possible in communal bathing setting[16]	Itching, burning, and excoriation of vulvar tissues. Inflammation of vaginal mucosa. Yellow, thick, foamy, malodorous vaginal discharge	Metronidazole (Flagyl) orally for 10 days. (Produces unpleasant metallic taste, vomiting when taken with alcohol, not used in early pregnancy) or Floraquin vaginal tablets for 30 days preceded by white vinegar douche (few side effects) Evaluate possible role of contraceptive or excessive douching. Hydrocortisone ointment for symptomatic relief of itching
Cervicitis (acute and chronic)	*Gonococcus* *Streptococcus* *Staphylococcus* *Escherichia coli* Repeated episodes of acute cervicitis lead to abnormal healing process	Congestion and edema of cervix. Backache, urinary disturbances. Profuse mucoid vaginal discharge	Appropriate antibiotics. Hot douche. Cervical cauterization or cryosurgery if chronic
Bartholinitis	*Escherichia coli* *Trichomonas vaginalis* *Staphylococcus* *Streptococcus* *Gonococcus*	Erythema around Bartholin's gland Swelling, edema and pain Development of Bartholin's abscess	Appropriate antibiotics Surgical drainage of abscess Excision of gland in clients with chronic Bartholinitis

and steroids may produce changes in the vaginal flora which may trigger an infection. Clients taking these medications need to know of their predisposition to infection. Cleanliness after voiding and defecating is to be stressed. It may be necessary to review the importance of utilizing daily health and hygienic practices with some clients. Instructions to seek medical care when symptoms arise should also be given.

A variety of treatment measures are prescribed for vaginal, cervical, and vulvar infections. Since these measures are usually carried out by the client, her understanding of them and ability to do the treatment correctly must be assessed. Vaginal suppositories, ointments, and creams are often utilized when infection occurs. Instructions in their use are best given when a model of the pelvis is employed. The importance of handwashing before and after their insertion should be stressed. The client should be advised to remain recumbent for 30 minutes after the application to allow for absorption and to prevent loss of the medication from the vagina. There may be some drainage from the vagina. If the client is concerned about this she may want to wear a perineal pad.

Heat in the form of a sitz bath, perineal irrigation, and douche are often prescribed to reduce inflammation, promote healing, and provide comfort. Instructions in their use should be given as indicated. Disposable sitz baths that fit over the toilet bowl are now available although the bathtub serves the same purpose. A fundamentals of nursing text should be consulted for correct douching technique.

Local measures such as avoidance of scratching, excessive moisture (including too frequent bathing), tight clothing (pantyhose) and perineal pads are also advocated. Chafing, increased heat and moisture, and interference with normal ventilation promote favorable conditions for growth of fungal, protozoal, and bacterial agents. The nurse can instruct the client to recognize signs of successful therapy as well as those indicating the need to contact her physician.

When reinfection occurs readily, the possibility of an asymptomatic male carrier or the presence of undiagnosed diabetes mellitus should be investigated. A review of the prescribed treatment measures for possible misunderstandings and a check on compliance with drug therapy may also be indicated.

If the client has cauterization or cryosurgery for chronic cervicitis, specific instructions are necessary. These instructions are similar to those following a D&C. The client should also know that an unpleasant vaginal discharge caused by the sloughing of destroyed cells may persist for 3 weeks. Cryosurgery involves the freezing and removal of abnormal cervical tissue through the use of a probe and liquid nitrogen. The treatment is quick and almost painless. The client will have a watery discharge for 2 weeks. Topical antiseptic creams may be prescribed during the 7 to 8 weeks healing period.

Toxic Shock Syndrome (TSS)

Toxic shock syndrome is a rare disease believed to be due to the toxin of a local infection of *Staphylococcus aureus*. It occurs most commonly in menstruating women. TSS is characterized by the sudden onset of high fever, vomiting, diarrhea, and a diffuse erythematous, macular rash. It may involve multiple organ systems and proceed to hypotension, shock, sepsis, shock lung, disseminated intravascular clotting (DIC), and acidosis. Treatment is symptomatic and supportive.

TSS has been linked to tampon use since it occurs primarily in women during their menstrual period. The exact link has not been identified. The nurse can advise clients to change tampons regularly and use good handwashing techniques prior to tampon insertion to reduce the possibility of this disease. Women who have had TSS should be instructed not to use tampons until *S. aureus* is no longer present in the vaginal flora.

PELVIC INFLAMMATORY DISEASE (PID)

Pelvic inflammatory disease is an infectious condition of the pelvic cavity that may involve the fallopian tubes (salpingitis), ovaries (oophoritis), pelvic peritoneum, or pelvic vascular system.

Etiology

The frequent causative organisms of PID are *Gonococcus, Staphylococcus*, and *Streptococcus*. Any of these organisms generally gain entrance during intercourse or following abortion, pelvic surgery, and childbirth. Intrauterine device users are also at risk for developing the condition. PID is a common complication of gonorrhea. The infection can be acute or chronic.

Clinical Manifestations

The client with acute PID presents a typical picture of a systemic infection with general malaise, fever, leukocytosis, anorexia, nausea, and vomiting. In addition, there is usually bilateral lower abdominal pain which can be quite severe. With gonorrheal or staphylococcal infections the discharge is usually heavy and purulent. Streptococcal infections produce a thinner, more mucoid discharge.

Once introduced, the infection spreads by two

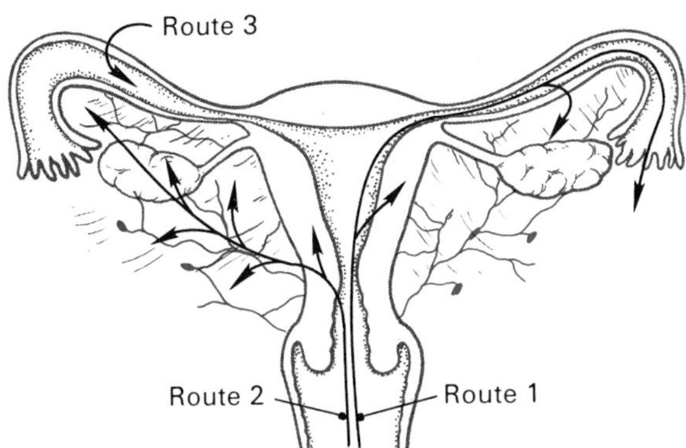

Figure 46-4 Common routes of the spread of pelvic inflammatory disease. Route 1: Commonly *gonococcus* and *staphylococcus*. Route 2: Frequently *streptococcus*. *(From J. Watson, Medical-Surgical Nursing and Related Physiology, W. B. Saunders Company, Philadelphia, 1979.)*

typical routes which are depicted by Fig. 46-4. In route 1 the bacteria spreads along the uterine endometrium to the tubes and into the peritoneum. Salpingitis, pelvic peritonitis, or tubo-ovarian abscess may result. In route 2, the spread is mainly through the uterine or cervical lymphatics across the parametrium to the tubes or ovaries. Pelvic cellulitis and sometimes thrombophlebitis of the pelvic veins can occur.

Chronic PID can result if the acute phase of the condition does not respond to treatment or if treatment was inadequate. Chronic PID is characterized by persistent pelvic pain, secondary dysmenorrhea, dysfunctional uterine bleeding, and periodic bouts of acute symptoms.

Complications

Frequently the client is rendered sterile due to adhesions and strictures that may develop in the fallopian tubes. This may result in closure of the fallopian tubes due to scarring and adhesions. Ectopic pregnancy may result when a tube is partially obstructed since the sperm may pass through the stricture but the fertilized ovum cannot reach the uterus. The pelvic and tubal ovarian abscesses may "leak" or rupture, resulting in pelvic or generalized peritonitis. Embolic episodes may occur following thrombophlebitis of the pelvic veins. Septic shock may result as the general circulation is flooded with bacterial endotoxins from the infected areas.

Medical Management

Diagnostic

The first step in diagnosis of PID is a careful history and physical examination. A history of a recent acute lower genital tract infection is often found. An abdominal examination usually reveals the presence of pain and tenderness in both lower quadrants. Movement of the pelvic organs during vaginal examination increases the pain. Masses that are fixed and poorly defined may be found, indicating enlargement of the fallopian tubes or ovaries or abscess formation.

Cultures and sensitivity studies are done on material taken from the vagina, cervix, or cul-de-sac of Douglas. Culdoscopy is done when abscess formation is suspected in the cul-de-sac. Direct visualization of the reproductive organs through laparoscopy is a helpful diagnostic tool.

Therapeutic

Treatment for PID may be managed on an outpatient basis or may require hospitalization. The client is given appropriate antibiotics and instructions to avoid coitus and douching, to restrict general activities, and to get adequate rest and nutrition. If treatment is not successful or the client is acutely ill or in severe pain, hospitalization is indicated. There, maximal doses of antibiotics can be given. Some physicians feel the addition of cortisone to the antibiotics will serve to reduce the inflammation, allowing for faster recovery and improvement in subsequent fertility. Heat to the lower abdomen or sitz baths may be utilized to improve circulation and decrease pain. Bed rest in the semi-Fowler's position to promote drainage of the pelvic cavity by gravity and analgesics to relieve pain are also prescribed.

Indications for surgery include the presence of residual masses (abscesses) with the potential for rupture and peritonitis, failure of the client to respond to conservative management, or a history of frequent exacerbations. The abscess may be drained without laparotomy or it may be necessary to remove the infected areas along with the uterus, tubes, and ovaries. The extent of the disease, and the age and condition of the client determine the extent of the surgery. Childbearing function in young women is preserved whenever possible.

Nursing Management

Health maintenance and promotion

Prevention, early recognition, and prompt treatment of vulvar, vaginal, and cervical infections can help prevent PID and its serious complications. If the nurse knows the factors that predispose to the development of PID she can identify the clients who are at risk and take appropriate measures.

Gynecologic surgery, childbearing, and abortion tend to lower the resistance of the client and make her more susceptible to infection. Therefore, careful medical and surgical asepsis is imperative in these instances so that the introduction of organisms into the reproductive tract can be prevented. The nurse should counsel the client to seek medical attention for any unusual vaginal discharge or possible infection of the reproductive organs. The client should be encouraged by the fact that some discharges are benign and that early diagnosis and treatment of an infection can prevent complications. Routine cultures for gonorrhea should be taken on every sexually active woman when a pelvic examination is being done. Women should be informed of the methods of preventing infection as well as the signs of infection in their partners.

Acute intervention

See Table 46-8 for the nursing care plan for pelvic inflammatory disease. During the acute phase of the condition, frequent perineal cleansing is indicated to prevent the spread of the infection. The character, amount, color, and odor of the vaginal discharge is recorded. Frequent checks of the vital signs and the degree of abdominal pain can give clues about the effectiveness of therapy. An explanation for the limited activity (bed rest in a semi-Fowler's position) will increase client cooperation.

Efforts need to be made to prevent the spread of the infection to others. Proper handwashing with a germicidal soap and careful handling and disposal of soiled perineal pads are important nursing activities. Disinfection of utensils, bedpans, and all items in direct contact with the client are additional measures that can be utilized to contain the infection. The need for these precautions should be explained to the client and her participation in them encouraged.

Chronic management

The client with chronic PID will experience chronic pelvic discomforts and require repeated treatment.

Table 46-8
Nursing Care Plan for the Client with Pelvic Inflammatory Disease

Client Problem	Expected Outcome	Nursing Intervention
		Acute Management
Heavy purulent vaginal discharge	Decrease in or no vaginal discharge	Observe, report, and record color, amount, character, and odor of discharge. Use strict medical asepsis when in contact with discharge, e.g., proper handwashing, careful handling and disposal of perineal pads. Explain need for precautions related to vaginal discharge and encourage client participation in them. Provide frequent perineal care
Abdominal pain	Decrease in discomfort	Assess degree of pain. Provide comfort measures, e.g., backrub, nonstimulating environment, heat to lower abdomen, administer analgesics as ordered
Anxiety over limited activity	Less concern over restrictions	Maintain bed rest in semi-Fowler's position. Explain need for limited activity. Provide diversional activities. Provide stimulation and orientation, e.g., radio, clock, etc. Allow client to help in planning care. Place in room with clients who are oriented and interested in surroundings
Symptoms of systemic infection such as fever, nausea and vomiting, leukocytosis, and malaise	Body temperature <37°C WBC count WNL. A feeling of wellness	Administer antibiotics as prescribed. Check vital signs every 4 h. Note lab reports for WBC, cultures, and sensitivity studies. Encourage oral fluids. Provide local heat as ordered, e.g., heating pad to abdomen, sitz baths. Provide for rest periods
		Long-Term Management
Guilt feelings about infection and possibility of sterility	Express feelings and make efforts to resolve them	Provide time for client to ventilate feelings. Listen and interact therapeutically. Provide counsel for client and significant others. Clarify about course of disease
Chronic stage of disease	State the importance of maintaining medical supervision. State appropriate action if pain persists and dysmenorrhea and vaginal bleeding occur	Explain factors that may contribute to infection and assist in planning preventive measures. Explain method to evaluate color, amount, character, and odor of vaginal discharge. Review the physician's orders in regard to recurrence of infection

Her emotional response to the disease and the therapy given should be assessed. The client may feel well one day and develop distressing discomforts the next. She may become discouraged and depressed. The nurse will need to be aware of these feelings and provide emotional support as well as clarification about the course of her disease.

The client may have guilt feelings about the problem, especially if it was associated with a venereal disease. She may also be concerned about the possibility of becoming sterile. Discussion with the client and her significant others regarding her feelings and concerns can assist her to cope more effectively with them.

ENDOMETRIOSIS

Endometriosis is a condition characterized by the presence and proliferation of endometrial tissue in sites outside of the endometrial cavity. The most frequent sites are in or near the ovaries, the uterosacral ligaments, and the uterovesical peritoneum, but they can be anywhere, such as the stomach and spleen. The tissue responds to the hormones of the ovarian cycle and undergoes a mini-menstruation just like the uterine endometrium. Active endometriosis is found most commonly in women in their twenties and thirties.

Etiology

Although many theories as to the cause of endometriosis have been advanced, the more commonly held theory concludes that small bits of endometrial tissue are "regurgitated" back up the uterine tube and escape into the abdomen during menstruation. As the ectopic endometrium menstruates, the blood collects in cystlike nodules which have a characteristic bluish-black look. Those in the ovaries are sometimes called "chocolate cysts" because of the thick, chocolate-colored material which they contain.

Clinical Manifestations

The symptoms may be vague and diffuse due to the multiple sites affected. Some clients are asymptomatic and the disease is discovered incidental to abdominal surgery. More commonly, the client complains of pelvic pain which takes the form of secondary dysmenorrhea. The pain is described as dull aching or cramping in the lower abdominal region occurring 1 to 2 days before menses and diminishing after onset of flow. It may be related to hemorrhagic distension of the cyst like nodules or escape of bloody discharge into the peritoneal cavity. Other symptoms include backache, abnormal uterine bleeding, dyspareunia, and painful defecation.

When a cyst ruptures, the pain may be acute and the resulting irritation promotes the formation of adhesions which readily fix the affected area to another pelvic structure. Sometimes the adhesions become severe enough to cause a bowel obstruction or painful micturition. Adhesions involving the uterus, tubes, or ovaries may result in infertility.

Medical Management

Conservative management

Diagnosis is frequently confirmed through a history of the characteristic symptoms of the condition and the presence of firm nodular lumps palpated in the adnexa on bimanual examination. Visualizing the typical bluish nodes by culdoscopy, laparoscopy, or during a laparotomy will establish a definite diagnosis (Fig. 46-5). The treatment of endometriosis is influenced by the client's age, her desire to bear children, and the severity of the symptoms. With menopause, ovarian atrophy begins and hormonal stimulation declines, usually leading to the disappearance of the symptoms.

Observation and mild analgesia are used initially when symptoms are not severe or incapacitating. Regular follow-up examinations at least once yearly to check on further progression of the disease are needed so that necessary changes in the plan of manage-

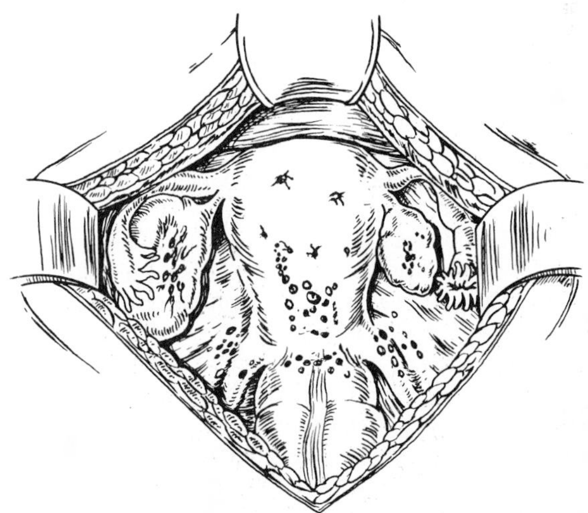

Figure 46-5 Characteristic findings at laparotomy in pelvic endometriosis. (*From Thomas H. Green, Gynecology: Essentials of Clinical Practice, 3d ed., Little, Brown and Company, Boston, 1977.*)

ment can be made. In young women, an ideal treatment is pregnancy since menstruation ceases during this period, resulting in relief of symptoms. Hormonal therapy, which includes the giving of progestogens (e.g., Enovid) or androgens (e.g., methyltestosterone), has resulted in the softening and regression of endometriosis with marked relief of symptoms. Progestogens suppress ovulation, producing a pseudopregnancy. Both drugs produce annoying side effects and the relief obtained is said to be temporary. A new steroid compound, isoxazole ethisterone (Danazol), a substance with an antigonodatropic action, is now available. Danazol has brought about subjective relief of symptoms with minimal side effects but its long-term effects are unknown.

Surgical management

Surgical treatment may be conservative or radical. Conservative surgery is usually utilized in the management of young women. It involves the resecting of as much of the endometriosis as possible while conserving all tissue necessary for reproductive function. Radical surgery is generally carried out in women approaching the menopause. It involves removal of uterus, tubes, ovaries, and as many endometrial implants as possible. Hysterectomy with removal of as many implants as possible but preservation of all or part of ovarian tissue is recommended for the young woman who is not desirous of future childbearing but wishes to have cyclic ovarian function.

Nursing Management

Nurses should encourage women to have regular physical examinations in an effort to identify, if possible, early symptoms of endometriosis. Client education about the disease process can clarify and dispel any false ideas and fears. Dysmenorrhea after years of relatively pain-free menses and infertility after a period of trying to achieve pregnancy may serve as clues to the presence of this disease and should be reported and investigated.

When the symptoms are less severe a "wait and see" approach may be used. Education of the client and reassurance that a health-threatening situation does not exist may permit her to accept the treatment and live with the minor discomforts. The nurse is often the individual who counsels the client in the use of drugs. The action of the prescribed hormones should be explained as well as the possible side effects (see Contraception).

If surgery is the treatment selected, the nursing care is similar to the general pre- and postoperative care of a patient undergoing abdominal surgery (see Surgical Procedures of the Female Reproductive System). The nurse will need to know the extent of the procedure so that appropriate postoperative teaching can be done.

BENIGN TUMORS OF THE FEMALE REPRODUCTIVE SYSTEM

Leiomyomas (Fibroids, Myomas, Fibromyomas)

Etiology

Leiomyomas are the most common benign tumors of the female genital tract. At least 25 percent of women over 35 years of age show some evidence of uterine leiomyomas. The incidence appears higher in black women. The cause of leiomyomas is unknown but they are thought to be dependent upon ovarian hormones, growing slowly during the reproductive years and atrophying with the advent of menopause. These tumors are composed mainly of smooth muscle and fibrous connective tissue.

Clinical manifestations

About half the women with leiomyomas develop symptoms, the most common being menorrhagia. Pain is rarely experienced with leiomyomas but it is associated with infection or twisting of the pedicle from which the tumor is growing. Dysmenorrhea and dyspareunia may occur on occasion. Pressure on surrounding organs may result in rectal, bladder, and lower abdominal discomforts. Large tumors may cause a general enlargement of the lower abdomen. Occasionally, these tumors are associated with abortion and infertility.

Management

Diagnosis is usually made by the characteristic pelvic findings of an enlarged uterus distorted by nodular masses. The presence of a malignancy is ruled out before treatment is begun. Treatment depends on the symptoms, the age of the woman, her desire for more children, and the location and size of the tumor(s). If the symptoms are minor, the physician may elect to follow the client closely for a period of time. In the young woman who wishes children, a myomectomy is done. In cases of large leiomyomas the treatment is hysterectomy (see Surgical Procedures of the Female Reproductive System).

Cervical Polyps

Cervical polyps are benign pedunculated lesions generally arising from the endocervical mucosa and are seen protruding through the external os on speculum examination of the cervix and vagina. Polyps have a characteristic bright cherry-red color, and are soft and fragile in consistency. They are generally small, measuring less than 3 cm in length and may be single or multiple. Their etiology is unknown. No symptoms are usually present but metrorrhagia and bleeding after straining and coitus can occur. Polyps are prone to infection. When the polyp is small, it can be excised as an outpatient procedure. If the point of attachment of the polyp cannot be identified and is not accessible to cautery, a polypectomy is done in an operating room. All tissue removed is sent for pathologic review, since occasionally polyps undergo malignant changes.

Ovarian Tumors

Benign tumors of the ovary are many and varied. The etiology of most is unknown. For purposes of clarity they are divided into non-neoplasms and neoplasms. Non-neoplasms are usually simple cysts surrounded by a thin capsule and are seen mainly during the reproductive years. Neoplasms of the ovaries are fluid-filled cysts which are frequently bilateral and may be benign or malignant. (Malignant tumors of the ovaries are discussed later in this chapter.)

Ovarian tumors are often symptomless until they are large enough to cause pressure in the pelvis. Constipation, urinary frequency, a full feeling in the abdomen, anorexia, and peripheral edema may occur, based on the size and location of the tumor. An increase in abdominal girth may be present. Pelvic pain may be present if the tumor is growing rapidly, and severe pain results when the cyst twists on its pedicle (twisted ovarian cyst).

Pelvic examination will reveal a mass or enlarged ovary that demands further investigation. To confirm the diagnosis, laparoscopy or exploratory laparotomy are often done. During surgical treatment attempts are made to save as much ovarian function as possible. Most often surgery involves removal of the ovary(ies).

MALIGNANT TUMORS OF THE FEMALE REPRODUCTIVE SYSTEM

Health Maintenance and Promotion

Although early diagnosis and treatment of cancer of the genital tract have improved, there still remains a relatively high associated death rate. The chief reason may well be that women do not sufficiently avail themselves of good preventive care. Nurses, in their many contacts with women in a variety of settings, can play a major role in advocating such care. In order to carry out this mission successfully, nurses will need to be well informed about genital tract malignancies, especially their early signs and symptoms, and the various diagnostic studies and treatment measures available.

Cervical Cancer

Carcinoma of the cervix is second only to cancer of the breast as the most frequent malignancy in women. It occurs predominately in women between the ages of 30 and 50. An increased risk of developing cervical cancer is associated with early marriage, early sex life with several partners, multiple pregnancies, a history of untreated chronic cervicitis, herpes genitalis, or venereal disease, and an uncircumcised sex partner. The number of deaths from cervical cancer in the United States has been reduced by roughly 50 percent in the last decade. This is attributed to better early diagnosis with the widespread use of the Pap test.

In the late 1960s several cases of cervical (and vaginal) carcinoma were reported in adolescent females. Subsequent studies revealed that diethylstilbestrol (DES) had been administered to their mothers during pregnancy. Enough evidence has accumulated to recommend that DES not be used during pregnancy. Daughters of women who ingested DES are encouraged to have regular gynecologic examinations.

Women should be taught and motivated to report any abnormal vaginal bleeding, particularly during the menopausal period, to their physicians. A thorough yearly gynecologic examination, including a Pap test, should be urged. The effect of many women having the examination has already decreased the death rate due to uterine cancer.

The fears and anxieties that arise in relation to cancer are many and varied. All women have seen and heard accounts of the disfigurement, the tissue destruction, and the disabilities that seem to follow cancer. Nurses should emphasize the positive fact that early discovery improves the outcome and hinders the occurrence of more serious outcomes. The important goal of disease prevention is again the major concern.

High-risk individuals such as those with family histories of cancer or prolonged local tissue irritation are special cases. These individuals should be sought out and encouraged to have frequent examinations for the appearances of cancer.

Clinical manifestations

Early cervical cancer is generally asymptomatic but eventually leukorrhea and intermenstrual bleeding occur. The discharge is usually thin and watery but

Table 46-9

Classification for Cytologic Findings

Class I	No abnormal or atypical cells present
Class II	Atypical, but no evidence of malignancy
Class III	Suggestive, but not conclusive for malignancy
Class IV	Strongly suggestive of malignancy
Class V	Conclusive for malignancy

becomes dark and foul-smelling as the disease advances, suggesting the presence of an infection. The vaginal bleeding is initially only spotting but as the tumor enlarges it becomes heavier and more frequent. Pain is a late symptom and is followed by weight loss, anemia, and cachexia.

Diagnostic study abnormalities

A Pap test, the Schiller iodine test (see Chap. 43), and a biopsy may be used to diagnose cancer of the cervix. The details of the Pap test are found in Chap. 43. The classification for cytologic findings are given in Table 46-9.

The World Health Organization has developed an international classification of cancer of the cervix with stages from 0 to IV (Table 46-10). Stage 0, the preinvasive stage or carcinoma in situ of the cervix is limited to the epithelial layer. A period of 5 to 10 years may elapse between the preinvasive stage and a stage I lesion, making the prognosis good for early diagnosis. Stage IV involves cancer which has extended outside the reproductive tract.

The finding of an abnormal smear (with the exception of class V) indicates the need for additional procedures such as biopsy and culdoscopy before a definitive diagnosis of cancer can be made.

The type and extent of the biopsy will vary with the abnormality seen. A punch biopsy may be done on an outpatient basis with a special punch biopsy forceps. Since there are few nerve findings in the cervix, little discomfort is experienced by the client. When conization, the excision of a cone-shaped section of the cervix with a scalpel, is utilized surgical facilities are required. The client should be observed for excessive bleeding following a cone biopsy.

Medical management

Treatment for cancer of the cervix is guided by the stage of the tumor, the woman's age, and general state of health (Table 46-10). Conization may be the only type of therapy needed for carcinoma in situ if analysis of the tissue removed demonstrates that a wide area of normal tissue surrounds the excised malignancy. Cautery and cryosurgery may also be utilized. (see Cervicitis.) Fertility is preserved with these three procedures. Invasive cancer of the cervix is treated with surgery, radiation, or a combination of the two in order to remove or destroy the involved areas and lymphatic drainage. Surgical procedures commonly carried out include radical hysterectomy

Table 46-10

World Health Organization International Classification of Carcinoma of the Cervix

Stage	Extent	Treatment	Prognosis for 5-Year Survival
Stage 0 (preinvasive)	Carcinoma in situ (also called preinvasive intraepithelial carcinoma); focal in nature, confined to epithelial layer of cervix	Cervical conization; total hysterectomy with partial vaginectomy	95–100*
Stage I (invasive—stages I to IV)	Confined to endocervix, but has invaded into cervical tissue; small lesion may be present	Wertheim's hysterectomy; irradiation	75–85
Stage IIa	Has extended to vaginal mucosa but not to lower one-third	Irradiation; Wertheim's hysterectomy	65–75
Stage IIb	Has extended to parametrial tissue (tissues around the broad ligament) but not to pelvic wall, or has extended to corpus of uterus	Irradiation	50–65
Stage III	Has reached pelvic wall or lower one-third of vagina	Irradiation	20–30
Stage IV	Has invaded bladder and/or rectum or distant metastasis	Irradiation; surgery, e.g., exenteration	1–10

*Statistics are compiled from a variety of references. Those most generally agreed upon are used.

(Wertheim) and pelvic exenteration (see Surgical Procedures of the Female Reproductive System). Radiation may be external (e.g., cobalt) or internal (e.g., radium). The extent of the radiation depends on the stage of the cancer.

Endometrial Cancer

Cancer of the endometrium (uterus) is second only to cervical cancer as the most common pelvic cancer. During the last 10 to 15 years there has been a sharp rise in the incidence of endometrial cancer in middle-aged women. The prevalence of prolonged use of exogenous estrogen therapy may account for this phenomenon.[17]

Endometrial cancer grows slowly, metastasizes late, and is amenable to therapy if diagnosed early. It is associated with women who are nulliparous, obese, hypertensive, diabetic, or who had a late menopause. The first symptom of endometrial cancer is abnormal uterine bleeding, which is frequently postmenopausal in nature. Pain occurs late in the disease process and other symptoms that may arise are related to metastasis to other organs.

Dilatation and curettage, endometrial biopsy, and smears are utilized to diagnose endometrial cancer. The former requires hospitalization while the latter is an office procedure in which endometrial tissue is "aspirated" from the uterus. The Pap test is not a reliable diagnostic tool for endometrial cancer. Treatment is by total hysterectomy and bilateral salpingo-oophorectomy. Surgery may be preceded by irradiation, either externally with cobalt or internally with intracavitary radium.

Ovarian Cancer

Cancer of the ovary seems to be linked to nulliparity, infertility, and endometriosis. It occurs more frequently in women between the ages of 40 and 65 and has a high familial incidence.

In its early stages, ovarian cancer is asymptomatic. As the malignancy grows, a variety of symptoms such as an increase in abdominal girth, bowel and bladder dysfunction, pain, and ascites accompanied by dyspnea occur. An ovarian malignancy should be considered when abnormal uterine bleeding occurs.

There are no specific tests or procedures to aid in diagnosing ovarian cancer except the pelvic examination. When a suspicious mass in the ovarian area is palpated, an exploratory laparotomy is done to establish the diagnosis. If the mass is malignant, a panhysterectomy (removal of uterus, cervix, fallopian tubes, and ovaries) followed by irradiation is carried out. Unfortunately, many malignancies have metastasized before the discovery of the tumor. Prognosis is poor and surgery may be only palliative. Recurrent ascites will require frequent paracentesis. Chemotherapy has also been used for palliation.

Vulvar Cancer

Cancer of the vulva is relatively rare, occuring mainly among women over 50 years of age. The malignancy is visible, accessible, and relatively slow-growing.

Cancer of the vulva may follow leukoplakia (irregular white patches on vulva mucosa which produce intense pruritus), or other conditions causing chronic irritation of the area. Initially the client may experience pruritus, soreness of the vulva, discharge, or bleeding, but tends to ignore these symptoms. Edema of the vulva and pelvic lymphadenopathy develop as the disease progresses.

Diagnosis of vulvar cancer is by means of pelvic examination and biopsy. Treatment for vulvar cancer is vulvectomy. The extensiveness of the surgery depends upon the size and site of the malignancy. If the lesion is in situ, a simple vulvectomy (surgical excision of the vulva) is done. If the cancer is invasive, a radical vulvectomy with superficial and deep lymph node dissection is indicated. Irradiation is not generally used in this area since the tissues do not tolerate it well.

SURGICAL PROCEDURES OF THE FEMALE REPRODUCTIVE SYSTEM

Types

A variety of surgical procedures are carried out when benign or malignant tumors of the genital tract are found. The definition of terms in Table 46-11 can aid the reader's understanding of them. A hysterectomy may be done either vaginally or abdominally. A vaginal route is used when vaginal repair is to be done in addition to removal of the uterus. The abdominal route is taken when large tumors are present or if the tubes and ovaries are to be removed at the same time. The abdominal route can present more postoperative problems since it involves an incision and the opening of the abdominal cavity.

Nursing Management of Tumors

Acute surgical intervention

All clients experience a degree of anxiety when surgery is contemplated but major gynecologic surgery may heighten their concerns. Some women may fear a loss of femininity and worry about possible changes in their secondary sex characteristics. Oth-

Table 46-11
Surgical Procedures of the Female Reproductive Tract

Type of Surgery	Description
Subtotal hysterectomy	Removal of uterus without the cervix (rarely done today)
Total hysterectomy	Removal of the uterus and the cervix (Fig. 46-6*a*)
Panhysterectomy	Removal of the uterus, the cervix, the fallopian tubes, and the ovaries. It is sometimes abbreviated as TAH-BSO (Fig. 46-6*a*)
Simple vulvectomy	Excision of vulva with wide margin of skin
Radical vulvectomy	Excision of vulva with superficial and deep lymph node dissection
Vaginectomy	Removal of the vagina
Radical hysterectomy (Wertheim)	A panhysterectomy, a partial vaginectomy, and dissection of the lymph nodes in the pelvis
Pelvic exenteration (total)	Radical hysterectomy, total vaginectomy, removal of the bladder with diversion of the urinary system and resection of the bowel with colostomy
Anterior pelvic exenteration	Above operation without the bowel resection
Posterior pelvic exenteration	Above operation without a bladder removal

ers may develop feelings of guilt, anger, or embarrassment. Still others may focus on the effect surgery will have on their reproductive and sexual functions. There are also women who may view the whole process as annoying or who are relieved with the thought of no longer having to worry about becoming pregnant. Each client must be understood in light of her fears and concerns and approached and evaluated individually. The nurse who exhibits an interest and willingness to listen can provide considerable psychological support.

Hysterectomy Preoperatively, the client is prepared physically for surgery utilizing the standard perineal or abdominal preparation and shave. A vaginal douche and enemas may or may not be given according to the preference of the surgeon. The bladder should be emptied before sending the client to the operating room. Often, an indwelling catheter is inserted preoperatively.

Following surgery the client having a hysterectomy will have an abdominal dressing (abdominal hysterectomy) or a sterile perineal pad (vaginal hysterectomy). See Table 46–12 for the nursing care plan for a total abdominal hysterectomy. The dressing should be observed frequently for any sign of bleeding during the first 8 hours following surgery. A moderate amount of serosanguineous drainage is expected on the perineal pad.

The client may develop urinary retention postoperatively because of temporary bladder atony resulting from edema or nerve trauma. This problem is more acute when a radical hysterectomy is done. At times an indwelling catheter is used for 3 to 4 days postoperatively to maintain constant drainage of the bladder and to prevent strain on the suture line. If an indwelling catheter is not used, catheterization may be necessary if the woman has not voided for 8 hours postoperatively. If residual urine is suspected following the removal of an indwelling catheter, catheterization is done to prevent bladder infection due to pooling of urine. A serious urinary complication is the accidental ligation of a ureter. Any complaint of backache or decreased urine output should be reported to the surgeon.

Abdominal distension may develop from the sudden release of pressure on the intestines when a large tumor is removed or from paralytic ileus secondary to anesthesia and pressure on the bowel. Food and fluids may be restricted if the client is nauseated. A rectal tube may be prescribed to relieve abdominal flatus and ambulation is encouraged. Frequently a Fleet enema or suppository is given on the third postoperative day.

Special care needs to be taken to avoid the development of thrombophlebitis of the vessel of the pelvis and upper thigh. Frequent changes of position and the avoidance of high-Fowler's position and pressure under the knees will minimize stasis and pooling of blood. Special attention needs to be given to clients with varicosities. Leg exercises to promote circulation and the application of antiembolic stocklings or elastic bandages can be helpful.

It is not unusual for the woman to feel depressed for several days. This response may be due to hormonal changes. She may experience periodic crying spells, sometimes called "hysterectomy blues," for which she has no explanation. The loss of a body part may bring about grieflike responses that occur when any great loss is sustained. Sympathetic understanding and care is needed during this period. Families, especially husbands, will need to understand and accept these responses.

Before the woman is discharged, the nurse should be certain that the client knows what changes will occur in her body because of the surgery; e.g., she will not menstruate if a total hysterectomy was done. Her discharge planning should include immediate and long-range limitations. Sexual activity should

Table 46-12
Nursing Care Plan for the Client with a Total Abdominal Hysterectomy

Client Problem	Expected Outcome	Nursing Intervention
	Acute Management	
Pain in incisional area and back	Decreased discomfort with periods of rest	Assess pain for type, onset, duration, location. Change position and massage back every 2 h. Maintain correct body alignment. Administer analgesic as ordered. Provide undisturbed rest
Moderate vaginal bleeding	Decrease in vaginal bleeding to spotting. Stable vital signs	Do perineal pad count. Note amount, color, consistency, presence of clots with each pad change. Observe for sudden onset of dizziness, generalized weakness, or unusual symptoms stated by client
Possible urinary retention	Void without difficulty	Measure intake and output. Encourage fluids orally within limitations of diet. Palpate bladder for distension. Catheterize as ordered. Provide privacy during attempts to void. Give perineal care every shift. Report any complaints of backache and decreased output
Abdominal distension	Have soft, flat abdomen and expel flatus	Auscultate, percuss, palpate abdomen for presence of flatus. Encourage ambulation every 4 h. Explain food and fluid restrictions as needed. Insert rectal tube as ordered
Thrombophlebitis of pelvic and upper thigh blood vessels	Have normal circulation with no signs of inflammation of lower extremities	Observe lower extremities for warmth, color, blanching, and sensation every 8 h. Report and record signs and symptoms noted. Change position every 2 h while in bed. Avoid high-Fowler's position and pressure under knees. Do active/passive exercises every 2 h. Reapply antiembolic stockings every shift. Ambulate every 4 h
	Long-Term Management	
Pelvic congestion or vaginal bleeding	Have no complaints of pelvic congestion or vaginal bleeding. State discharge instructions	Explain immediate and long-range limitations including: avoiding heavy lifting for 2 months, avoiding activities such as dancing and horseback riding for several months, avoiding sexual activity for 4–6 weeks; client may wear girdle. Stress need to report any bleeding to physician
Anxiety over change in body image	Will verbalize concerns and take steps to resolve them. Accept altered body image	Be available for client to express possible anxiety. Listen attentively. Encourage client to verbalize concerns with husband. Initiate topic if client needs assistance in doing so. Assess knowledge of effect of surgery on physiology and sexuality. Encourage participation and control over self-care and diversional activities. Explain behavior to significant others and need for their acceptance

be avoided until the wound is healed (about 4 to 6 weeks). However, sexual activity is not contraindicated once healing is complete. Sutures at the top of the vagina can tear and produce considerable bleeding if genital sex is engaged in too early or is too unrestrained. Secondary sex characteristics will not be affected unless the ovaries have been removed. If a vaginal hysterectomy is performed, the woman needs to know that there may be a loss of vaginal sensation and to be reassured that sensation will return in several months.

Physical limitations are short-term. Heavy lifting should be avoided for 2 months. Activities which may increase pelvic congestion such as dancing and walking swiftly should be avoided for several months, whereas other activities such as swimming may be helpful, both physically and mentally. Wearing a girdle is allowed and may provide comfort. Once the client is assured that healing is complete, all previous activity can be resumed.

Salpingectomy and Oophorectomy Postoperative care of the woman who has had a Fallopian tube removed (salpingectomy) and/or an ovary (oophorectomy) removed is similar to that given any client having abdominal surgery. One exception is that if a if a large ovarian cyst is removed there may be abdominal distension due to the sudden release of pressure in the intestines. An abdominal binder may provide relief until the distension subsides.

When both ovaries (bilateral oophorectomy) are removed, postsurgical menopause results. The symptoms are similar to those of regular menopause, but may be more severe because of the sudden withdrawal of hormones. Attempts are made to leave at least a portion of an ovary. Replacement therapy with estrogen is given to most clients to preserve secondary sex characteristics and permit more normal living unless surgery has been done for malignancy (see Menopause for discussion of estrogen).

Vulvectomy Although cancer of the vulva is relatively uncommon, the extent of the required surgery and psychological implications for the client demands the best in nursing management. It is important that the nurse recognize the extent of a vulvectomy and the fact that it is done for a diagnosis of cancer. An honest, open attitude with the client and her husband preoperatively can be most helpful in the postoperative period.

Following a vulvectomy, the client returns to the unit with a wound in the perineal area extending to the groin. The wounds may be covered or left exposed and frequently have drains attached to portable suction (e.g., Hemovac). Often a heavy pressure dressing will be in place for the first 24 to 48 hours. When the perineal wound is covered, a T-binder is utilized. The wounds are cleaned with normal saline or an antiseptic twice daily. A heat lamp is then used to dry the area. Wound care must be meticulous in order to avoid infection, which results in delayed healing.

Special attention to bowel and bladder care is needed. A low-residue diet will prevent straining at stool and wound contamination. An indwelling catheter is used to provide urinary drainage. Great care is taken not to dislodge the catheter because the extensive edema in the area would make its reinsertion very difficult. Often, in order to close the wounds, heavy, taut sutures are used, resulting in severe discomfort for the client. In other instances, the wound may be allowed to heal by granulation. Analgesics may be required frequently to control pain. Careful positioning of the client through the use of strategically placed pillows will provide comfort. Ambulation is usually begun on the second postoperative day but varies with the preference of the surgeon. Anticoagulant therapy to prevent vascular complications is common.

Since the surgery causes mutilation of the perineal area and the healing process is slow, the client is apt to become discouraged. Opportunities for the client to express her feelings and concerns about the operation should be provided. The client will need specific instructions in self-care before her discharge. She should be told to report any unusual odor, fresh bleeding, or perineal pain. Home care nursing can benefit the client during her adjustment period. Sexual function is often retained. Whether or not clitoral sensation is retained may be critical to some women, particularly if it was a primary source of orgasmic satisfaction. A discussion of alternate methods of achieving sexual satisfaction may also be indicated.

Pelvic Exenteration When other forms of therapy prove to be ineffective in checking the spread of cancer and stage IV is identified, pelvic exenteration may be performed. Clients for this procedure are selected on the basis of their likelihood to survive the surgery and their ability to adjust to and accept the imposed limitations.

The postoperative care will involve that of a client who has had a radical hysterectomy, an abdominal perineal resection, and/or an ileal conduit (Fig. 46-6). The physical, emotional, and social adjustments to life on the part of the woman and her family will be great as a result. There will be urinary and/or fecal diversions in the abdominal wall, the sexual function of the vagina will be lost, and menopause may occur (estrogen therapy is frequently contraindicated).

The client's rehabilitative process should keep pace with her acceptance of the situation. Much understanding and support will be needed from the nursing staff. The client should be gently encouraged to regain her independence. She will need to verbalize her feelings about her altered body structure to an interested and concerned listener. The family should be included in the plan of care as the convalescence of the client proceeds.

The client is told to return to her physician or a clinic at specified intervals. Early detection of a recurrence of the cancer can then be identified and treated. At this time her physical and emotional adjustment to the changes in body image produced by the surgery and her ability to carry out any treatment measures can also be assessed. Additional teaching and counseling can then be provided.

RADIATION THERAPY FOR UTERINE CANCER

Internal Radiation

Internal radiation is used in the management of cervical and endometrial cancer because of the ac-

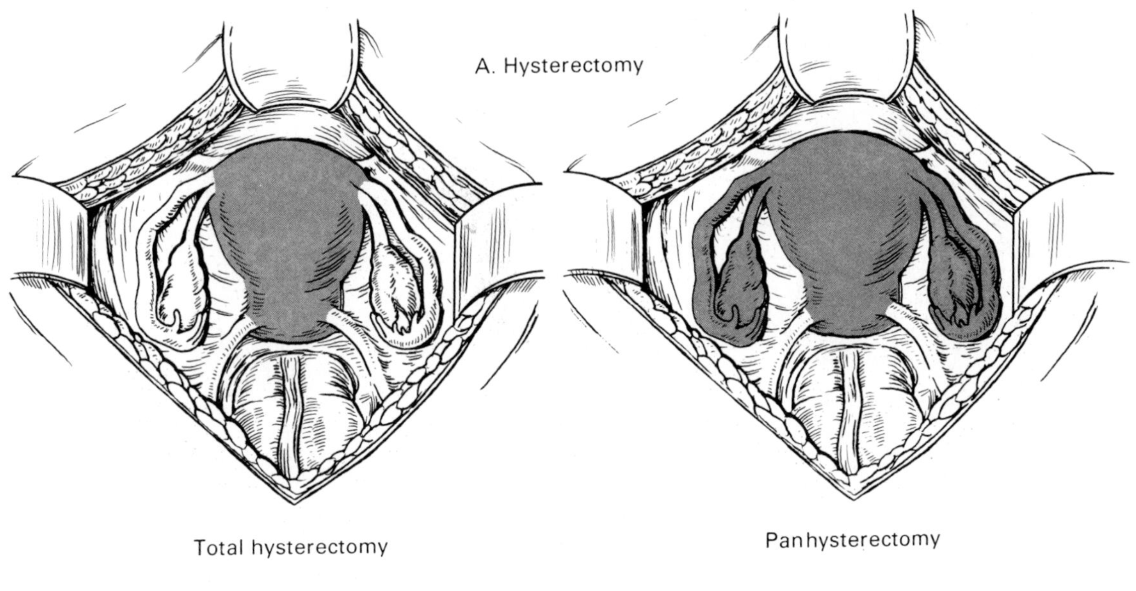

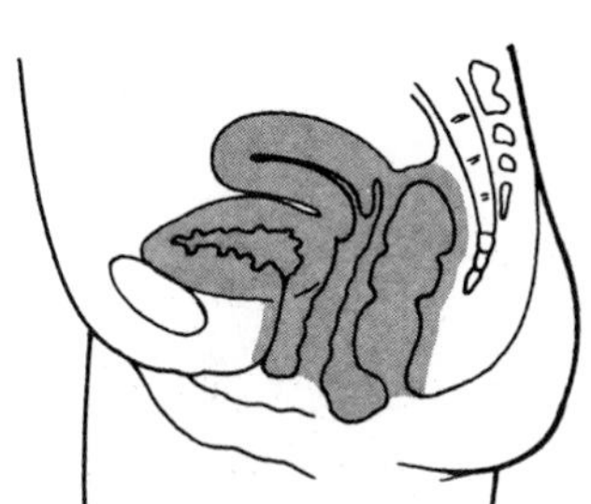

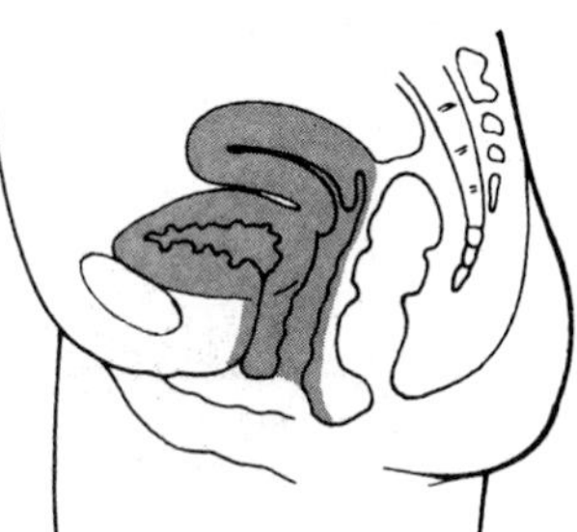

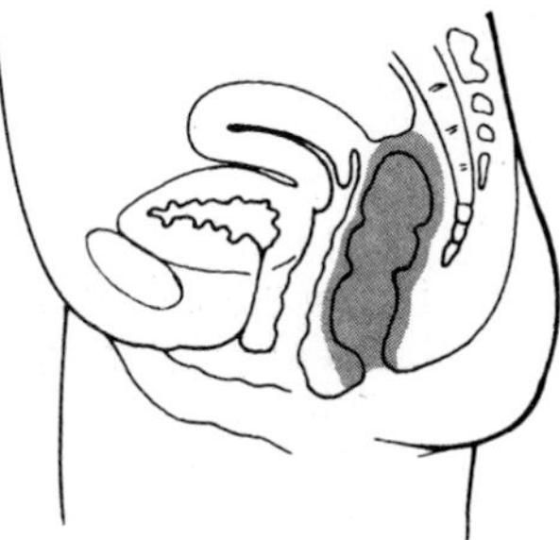

Figure 46-6 Surgical procedures and related organ removal for tumors of female reproductive tract. *(a)* Hysterectomy. *(b)* Pelvic exenteration. (*From M. Garrey A. D. T. Govan. C. Hodge, and R. Callander, Gynecology Illustrated, 2d ed., Churchill Livingstone Inc., New York, 1979.*)

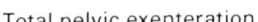

cessibility of these body parts and the favorable results obtained. Radium and cesium are two commonly used isotopes. In preparing the client for the treatment, a cleansing enema is given to prevent displacement of the isotope. An indwelling catheter is inserted to prevent a distended bowel or bladder from coming into contact with the radioactive source.

A variety of applicators have been developed for intracavitary treatment. Some are inserted as multiple small irradiators (e.g., Heyman's capsules, Fig. 46-7*a*) while others consist of a central tube (tandem) with irradiators placed on each side of the cervix (vaginal ovoids).

The applicator may contain the radioactive material when it is inserted into the endometrial cavity and vagina of an anesthetized client in the operating room. This is known as preloading. In the afterloading technique (Fig. 46-7*c*) the applicator is implanted in the operating room but is not loaded with the radioactive material until its correct placement is checked by x-ray and the client has returned to her room. Radiation exposure to the client is precisely controlled and the radiation exposure to the physician and other personnel involved in the implantation is reduced when the afterload technique is utilized. The applicator is secured with vaginal packing and is left in place from 24

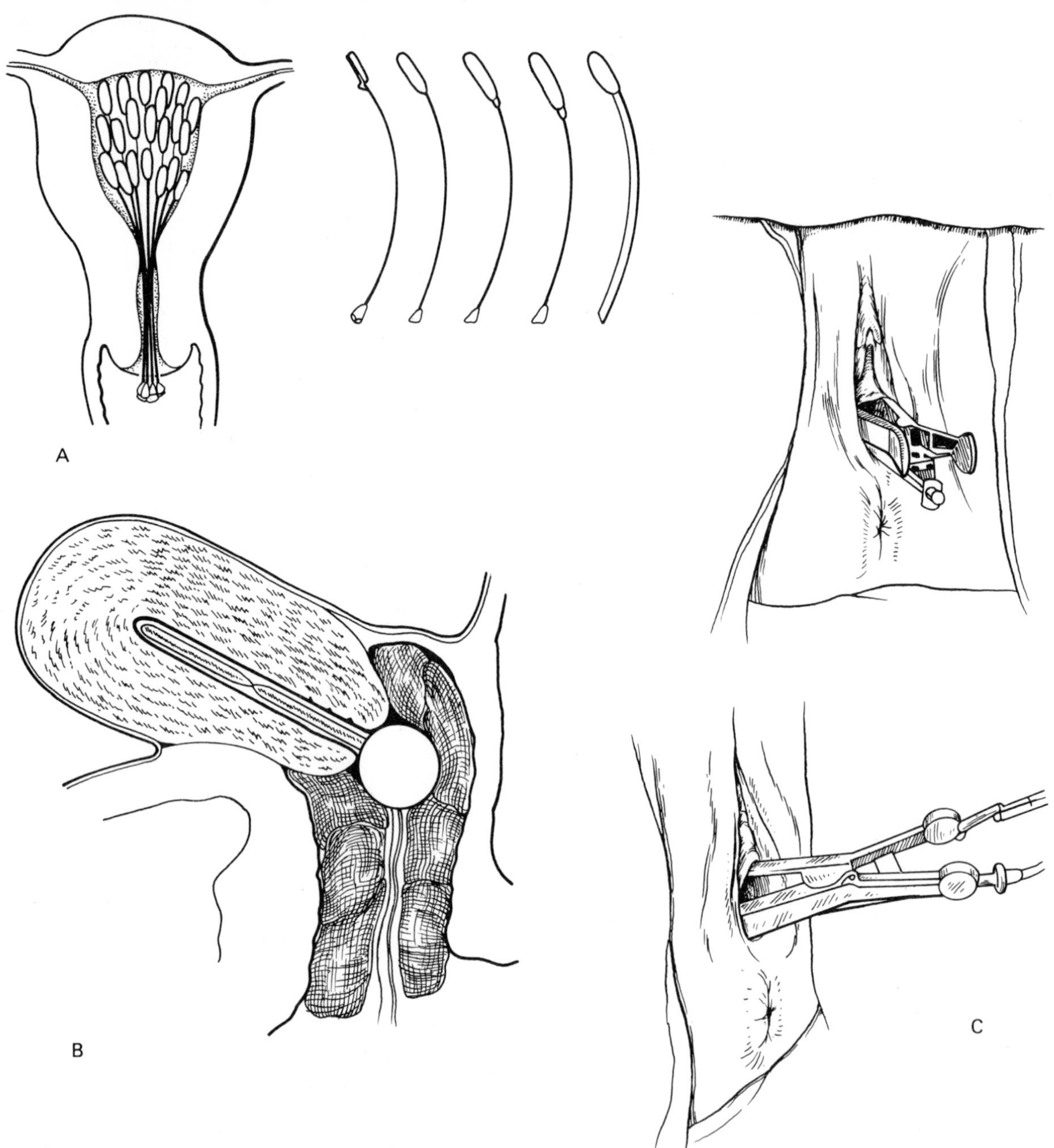

Figure 46-7 Intracavitary radiation for uterine cancer. *(a)* Heyman's capsules: Various sizes and capsules in place. *(From T. Green, Gynecology: Essentials of Clinical Practice, 3d ed., Little, Brown and Company, Boston, 1977.) (b)* Radiation applicator secured in position with gauze packing. *(From M. Garrey, A. D. T. Govan, C. Hodge, and R. Callender, Gynecology Illustrated, 2d ed., Churchill Livingstone Inc., New York, 1979.) (c)* Applicator in position ready to be loaded (after loading). *[From R. Hilkemeyer, "Nursing Care in Radium Therapy," Nurs Clin North Am,* **2***:92 (1967).]*

to 72 hours (Fig. 46-7*b*). The radiologist determines the exact amount of radioactive substance to be used and the hours it will be left in place so that destruction of cancer cells can occur with minimal damage to normal cells.

During the treatment, the client is placed in a private room and is on absolute bed rest. She may be turned from side to side. The presence of an intrauterine applicator produces uterine contractions which may require analgesics. The destruction of cells results in a foul-smelling vaginal discharge; a deodorizer is helpful. Nausea, vomiting, diarrhea, and malaise may develop as a systemic reaction to the radiation.

Nurses should stay in the immediate area no longer than is necessary to give proper care and attention and no nurse should attend the client more than a half hour per day. The nurse may stay at the foot of the bed or at the entrance to the room to minimize radiation exposure. Visitors should stay 6 feet away from the bed and limit the visit to less than 3 hours per day. The reasons for these precautions should be explained to the client and her visitors. (A more detailed discussion of nursing care of the client with an internal implant is in Chap. 11.)

At the end of the prescribed period of radiation, the radioactive material as well as the catheter are removed. A cleansing douche is given. The client is allowed to ambulate and is usually discharged from the hospital within a few days. Complications that may arise following radiation of the uterus include fistulas (vesicovaginal, ureterovaginal), cystitis, phlebitis, hemorrhage, and fibrosis. If fibrosis occurs, the vaginal wall will become smaller in diameter and shorter. Dilation of the vagina through intercourse or the use of an obturator is indicated. The client is urged to report any unusual symptoms or complaints to her physician.

Following internal radiation, the client may be concerned about resumption of sexual activity. Extra lubrication and increased foreplay can aid in vaginal lubrication. Reassurance that intercourse is not contraindicated for either party is important.

External Radiation

Pelvic radiation is delivered by supervoltage equipment like a linear accelerator and cobalt 60. The treatment period usually extends for 4 to 6 weeks. The care of the client receiving external pelvic radiation is the same as it is for treatment elsewhere in the body (see Chap.11). The client should be told to void immediately before the treatment to avoid trauma to the bladder. Radiation side effects, including enteritis and cystitis, may occur. They are natural reactions to radiotherapy and are not due to an overdose. Informing the client in advance of the possible side effects and what measures to employ will lessen their impact when they occur.

UTERINE DISPLACEMENT

Normally the uterus flexes anteriorly about 45 degrees and is movable, and the cervix points downward and posteriorly. The filling of the bladder or bowel may cause a change in uterine position. Displacement of the uterus as well as the bladder and rectum can be either congenital or acquired because of stretching of the muscles of the pelvic floor. The acquired displacement of these structures is frequently due to injuries during childbirth or surgery, repeated close pregnancies, tumors, inflammatory disease, and loss of tissue elasticity due to aging.

Anterior and Posterior Uterine Displacements

The uterus may be displaced anteriorly, posteriorly (Fig. 46-8), and downward. Anterior displacement or *anteflexion* occurs when the body of the uterus is bent forward. Posterior displacements include *retroflexion* (backward bending of the uterus body with the cervix in its normal position) and retroversion (backward rotation of the uterus body and the forward rotation of the cervix). Retroversion occurs most often and has been associated with cul-de-sac disease (e.g., PID, endometriosis) which causes the fundus of the uterus to adhere posteriorly.

Anteflexion is seen in a client with a small, underdeveloped uterus. Usually there are no associated symptoms and it may be treated with appropriate hormones. Symptoms attributed to posterior displacements (retroversion more specifically) include low backache which is generally worse at the beginning of the menstrual period, pelvic pain, fatigue, leukorrhea, dyspareunia, and infertility. Some individuals are asymptomatic.

Treatment is directed toward resolving the underlying cause if it can be found. Other measures include the use of exercise therapy to stretch or strengthen the uterine ligaments. One such exercise has the client assume the knee-chest position (causing the uterus to fall forward) for a few minutes several times a day. A pessary (a rubber or plastic appliance placed in the vagina for uterine support) may be used to treat retroversion (Fig. 46-8*b*). Before inserting the vaginal pessary the uterus is manually replaced in its normal position. Once inserted the pessary holds the cervix in a posterior position, thus allowing the uterus to fall forward. When the pessary is properly positioned, the client is unaware of its presence and experiences no difficulty in voiding or during intercourse. Since a pessary irritates the vaginal mucosa, the client should be instructed to douche regularly to remove excess vaginal debris. Six weeks after the insertion of the pessary the client returns to the physician to report if her symptoms were relieved. The pessary may be changed or removed at this time.

Occasionally surgery is done to correct retroversion. The procedure (uterine suspension) involves the shortening of the round ligaments. These ligaments

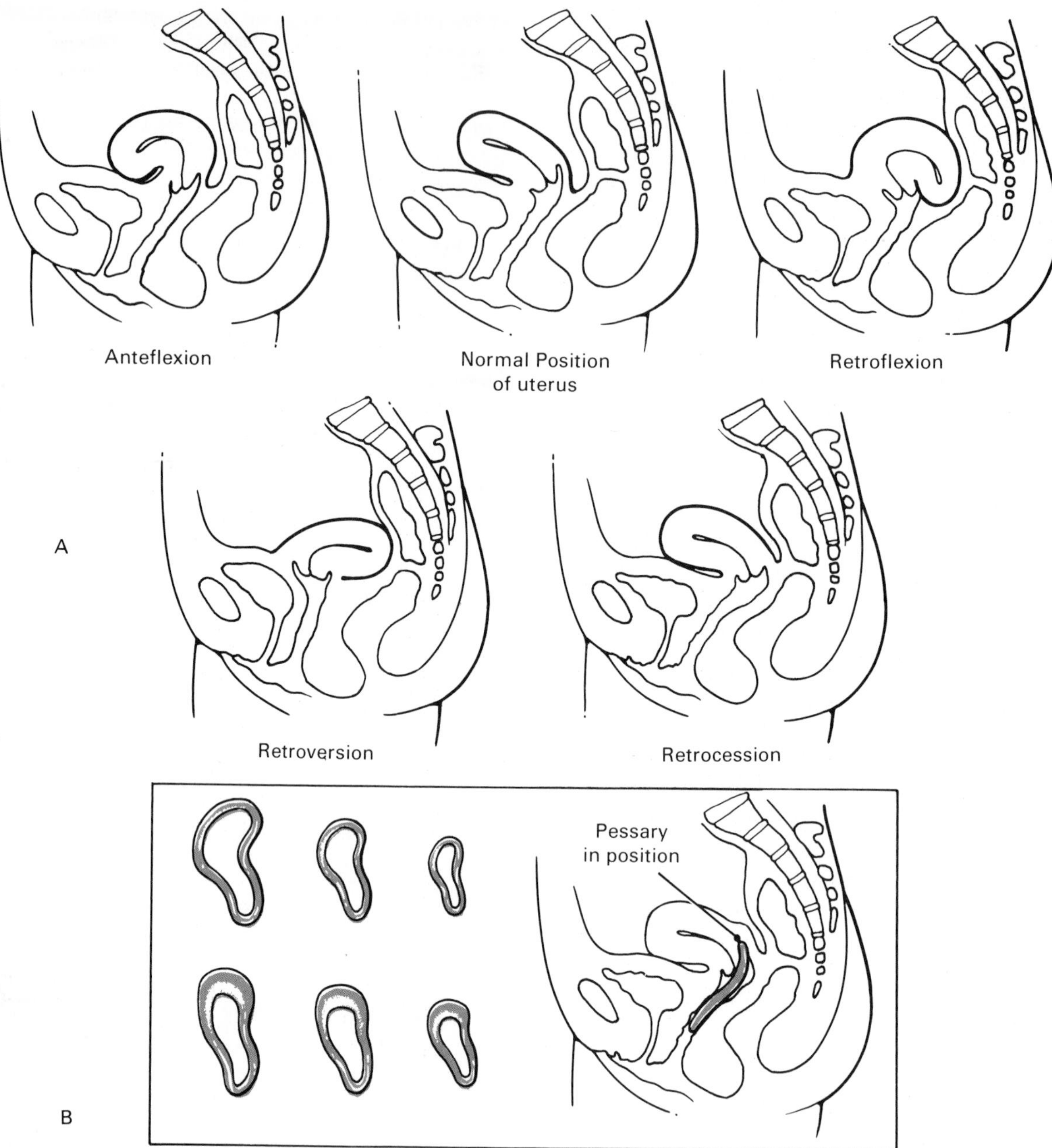

Figure 46-8 *(a)* Types of forward and backward uterine displacements. *(b)* Hard rubber pessaries used in treatment of clients with retroversions. (*From Norman Miller and Hazel Avery, Gynecology and Gynecologic Nursing, 5th ed., W. B. Saunders Company, Philadelphia, 1965.*)

have a considerable capacity for stretching and a permanent correction is not always guaranteed.

Uterine Prolapse

Downward displacement or *prolapse of the uterus* through the pelvic floor and vaginal outlet is traditionally rated as first degree (the cervix comes down to the introitus), second degree (the cervix protrudes through the introitus), or third degree (procidentia, the entire uterus protrudes through the introitus) (Fig. 46-9). The client complains of a feeling of "something coming down." She may have dyspareunia, a drag-

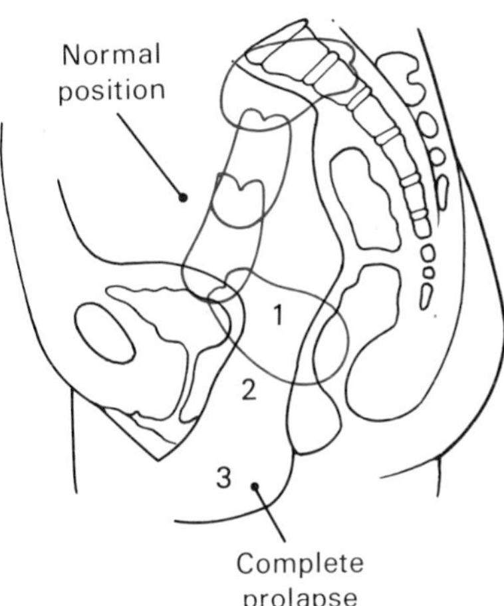

Figure 46-9 Normal position of uterus and course followed as it descends into first-, second-, and third-degree prolapse. (*From Norman Miller and Hazel Avery, Gynecology and Gynecologic Nursing, 5th ed., W. B. Saunders Company, Philadelphia, 1965.*)

ging or heavy feeling in the pelvis, backache, and bowel or bladder problems if cystocele or rectocele are also present. Stress incontinence is a common and troubling problem. When second- or third-degree uterine prolapse occurs, the protruding cervix and vaginal walls are subjected to constant irritation and tissue changes may occur.

In situations in which surgery is contraindicated, pessaries are utilized to correct the prolapse. A variety of pessaries are available for the different degree of prolapse. Every 3 to 4 months the pessary is cleaned and replaced by the client, if possible, or her physician. She is also checked for signs of excessive irritation. Pessaries unattended for long periods of time have been associated with erosion, fistulas, and increased incidence of vaginal carcinoma. Surgery generally involves a vaginal hysterectomy with an anterior and posterior repair of the vagina and underlying fascia.

Cystocele and/or Rectocele

If a prolapse of the uterus occurs, the uterus pulls other structures such as the bladder, rectum, and urethra down or out of position. Such displacements result in disorders such as cystocele, a herniation of the bladder into the vagina, and rectocele, a herniation of the bowel into the vagina (Fig. 46-10).

A cystocele or rectocele may cause a dragging pain in the back and in the pelvis. A cystocele often causes urinary symptoms such as incontinence (especially with activities increasing intra-abdominal pressure such as coughing, lifting), frequency, and urgency. A rectocele may cause bowel symptoms such as constipation and incontinence of gas or liquid feces. Infection, hemorrhoids, and cystitis may result as complications of these conditions.

In the early stages of cystocele or rectocele, perineal exercises may be utilized to strengthen the weakened muscles. A pessary may be used when surgery is contraindicated or refused. Surgery designed to tighten the vaginal wall is generally the method of treatment. A cystocele is corrected with a procedure called an *anterior colporrhapy*, whereas a *posterior colporrhapy* is done for a rectocele. If further surgery is needed to relieve stress incontinence, procedures to support the urethra and restore the proper angle between the urethra and the posterior

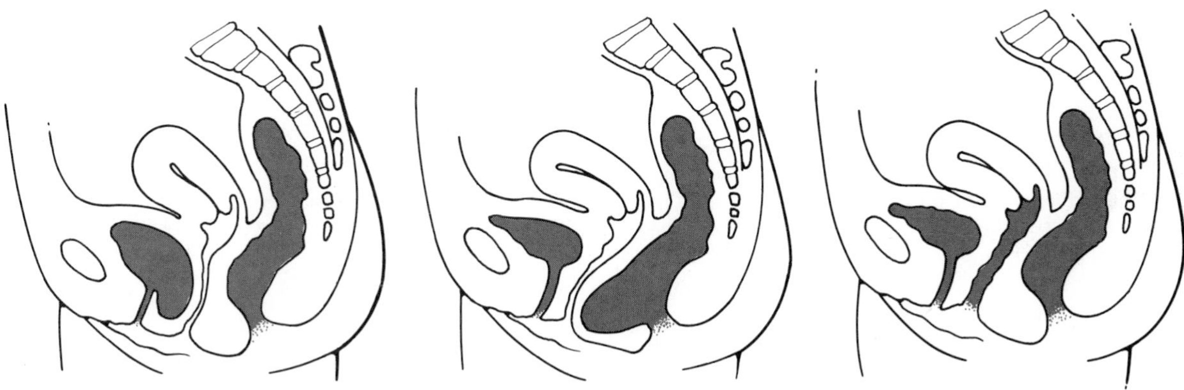

A. Cystocele B. Rectocele C. Normal pelvis

Figure 46-10 Defects of: *(a)* cystocele and *(b)* rectocele compared with normal pelvis. (*From Norman Miller and Hazel Avery, Gynecology and Gynecologic Nursing, 5th ed., W. B. Saunders Company, Philadelphia, 1965.*)

bladder wall are utilized. In a Marshall-Marchetti procedure, the urethra is supported by a series of sutures placed through the anterior vaginal wall on either side of the urethra and then through the periosteum of the pubic bone.

Nursing Management

Nurses can play an active part in preventing the incidence of uterine prolapse. They can encourage pregnant clients to seek qualified obstetrical care early in the pregnancy. Better care during the maternity cycle has helped reduce the occurrence of the problem. Nurses can also teach perineal exercises during the postpartum period. These consist of alternately tightening and relaxing the gluteal and perineal floor muscles. Practicing starting and stopping a stream of urine also helps the client regain good perineal muscle tone. As part of the preoperative preparation for vaginal surgery a cleansing douche may be ordered the morning of surgery. A cathartic and cleansing enema is usually given when a rectocele repair is scheduled. A perineal shave will be done. The nurse can assist the client in understanding any limitations that surgery may impose on sexual and reproductive capacity, since misunderstandings frequently occur.

In the postoperative period, the goals of care are to prevent wound infection and to prevent pressure on the vaginal suture line. This will require perineal care at least twice a day and after each voiding or defecation.

A heat lamp may be used to help dry the area and enhance the healing process. An ice pack applied locally may relieve the initial perineal discomfort and swelling. A disposable glove filled with ice and covered with a cloth works well in these instances. Later, sitz baths are generally employed.

After an anterior colporrhaphy, an indwelling catheter is usually left in the bladder for 4 days to allow for the local edema to subside. The catheter keeps the bladder empty, thereby preventing strain on the sutures. Catheter care utilizing an antiseptic is generally done twice daily. After posterior colporrhaphy, straining at stool is avoided by a low-residue diet and the prevention of constipation. Mineral oil is generally given each night.

Discharge instructions should be reviewed before the client leaves the hospital. They generally include using douches or mild laxatives as needed, restricting heavy lifting and prolonged standing, walking, or sitting, and avoiding intercourse until the physician gives permission. There may be a loss of vaginal sensation that can last for months. The client needs to be reassured that this situation is temporary.

FISTULAS

A fistula is an abnormal opening between internal organs or between an organ and the exterior of the body. Fistulas can occur as a result of injury during delivery, surgery, radiation therapy, and disease processes such as carcinoma. They may develop between the vagina and the bladder, urethra, ureter, or rectum. The following discussion will focus on *vesicovaginal fistulas* (between the bladder and the vagina), and *rectovaginal fistulas* (between the rectum and the vagina), Fig. 46-11. When vesicovaginal fistulas develop, some urine leaks into the vagina, whereas with rectovaginal fistulas flatus and feces escape into the vagina. In both instances excoriation and irritation of the vaginal and vulvar tissues occur and may lead to severe infections. In addition to experiencing wetness, offensive odors may develop, causing embarrassment and severely limiting socialization.

Management

Since small fistulas may heal spontaneously within a matter of months, treatment may be postponed. If the fistula does not heal, surgical excision is required. Inflammation and tissue edema must be eliminated before surgery is attempted. This may involve a wait of up to 6 months for the surgery. The fistulectomy may result in the client having an ileal conduit or temporary colostomy.

Perineal hygiene is of great importance both preoperatively and postoperatively. The perineum should be cleansed every 4 hours. If possible, warm sitz baths should be taken three times daily. Perineal pads should be changed frequently. Deodorizing and comfort measures such as douches or powders and local heat are utilized. Douches should be given with low pressure to avoid further damage to the tissues. A

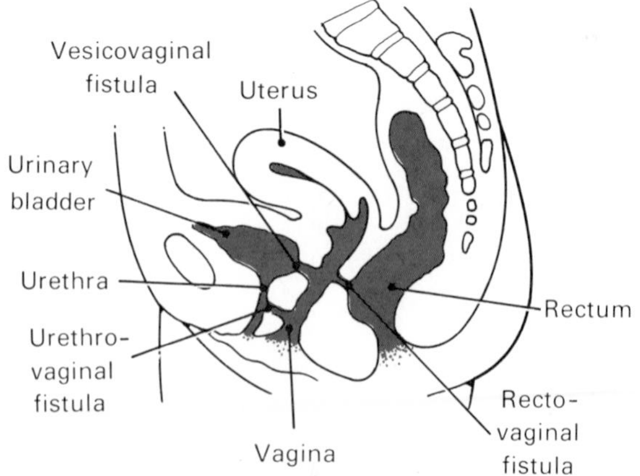

Figure 46-11 Common fistulas involving the vagina.

low-residue diet and high enemas may be given to reduce the constant flow of feces. The client should be encouraged to maintain an adequate fluid intake. Encouragement and reassurance by the staff are needed in helping the client to cope with her problems.

Postoperatively, nursing care emphasis is on avoiding stress on the repaired areas and preventing infection. Care should be taken so that the Foley catheter is draining at all times. Oral fluids should be urged to provide for internal catheter irrigation. Minimal pressure and strict asepsis are utilized if catheter irrigation becomes necessary. The first stool following bowel surgery may be purposely delayed to prevent contamination of the wound. Later, stool softeners or mild laxatives may be given the client. (See Chap. 37 for care of a client with an ileal conduit and Chap. 34 for care of a client with a colostomy.) Surgical repair of fistulas is not always effective even under the best of conditions. Supportive nursing care for the client and her significant others therefore becomes especially important.

Case Study / Total Abdominal Hysterectomy

Mrs. Marion P., a 40-year-old homemaker with two children, has been having menorrhagia and occasionally metrorrhagia for the past 5 months. She consulted her physician who did a complete history and physical examination. On pelvic examination several large, firm masses in the body of the uterus, thought to be leiomyomas, were palpated. Based upon these findings the physician advised Mrs. P. to have a hysterectomy. Initially she was reluctant to undergo such an operation but after deliberating the matter for a week she gave her consent.

Mrs. P. is admitted to the hospital for a total abdominal hysterectomy. She is returned to her room with an indwelling catheter in place and both legs wrapped in full-length antiembolic stockings.

Discussion Questions

1. What are the common causes of menorrhagia and metrorrhagia?
2. What clinical manifestations may result from leiomyomas?
3. State the physical and psychological preoperative preparation that would be given Mrs. P.
4. What observation should be made in Mrs. P.'s immediate postoperative period?
5. What possible complications can arise following abdominal hysterectomy? Include rationale for selection.

REVIEW QUESTIONS

The number of the question corresponds to the same numbered objective at the beginning of the chapter.

1. Primary dysmenorrhea is usually
   - **a.** due to overexertion
   - **b.** rare in the teenager
   - **c.** idiopathic
   - **d.** due to uterine pathology

2. Postoperative care following a D&C includes
   - **a.** observing suture line
   - **b.** checking on bowel activity
   - **c.** doing a pad count
   - **d.** expecting severe cramps

3. The client in climacteric may experience
   - **a.** vasomotor reactions
   - **b.** irregular menstrual periods
   - **c.** dyspareunia
   - **d.** all the above

4. The use of oral contraceptives may result in
   - **a.** perforation of uterus
   - **b.** thromboembolic disorders
   - **c.** infection of the uterus
   - **d.** few side effects

5. An induced abortion
   - **a.** occurs without apparent cause
   - **b.** occurs with mechanical intervention
   - **c.** is always illegal
   - **d.** produces few psychological effects

6. Genital injuries due to rape may include
   - **a.** bruises and lacerations of perineum and cervix
   - **b.** lacerations of the uterine ligaments
   - **c.** a and b
   - **d.** a only

7. A prominent symptom of cervicitis is
   - **a.** leukorrhea
   - **b.** urinary frequency
   - **c.** severe perineal pain
   - **d.** vaginal hemorrhage

8. Symptoms of pelvic inflammatory disease may include
   - **a.** itching, fever, backache
   - **b.** malaise, menorrhagia, polyps
   - **c.** rectal bleeding, nausea, vomiting
   - **d.** vaginal discharge, fever, abdominal pain

9. A complication of endometriosis is
   - **a.** frequent pregnancies
   - **b.** adhesions
   - **c.** dehydration
   - **d.** hemorrhage

10. A common complaint of women with uterine fibroids is
- **a.** constant cramping pain
- **b.** urinary dribbling
- **c.** menorrhagia
- **d.** sterility

11. The diagnosis of endometrial cancer is best made by
- **a.** dilatation and curettage
- **b.** Schiller iodine test
- **c.** Papanicolaou smear
- **d.** culdoscopy

12. Discharge instructions for the patient who has had a hysterectomy include
- **a.** take frequent brisk walks
- **b.** resume normal activities
- **c.** do not wear a girdle
- **d.** avoid sexual activity until wound is healed

13. Nursing responsibilities related to intracavitary radiation for uterine cancer includes
- **a.** allowing the client bathroom privileges only
- **b.** maintaining absolute bed rest of the client
- **c.** remaining at the bedside 1 hour per day for care
- **d.** limiting visitors to 5 hours per day

14. Management of the client with a retroverted uterus includes
- **a.** insertion of pessary
- **b.** immediate uterine suspension
- **c.** vaginal hysterectomy
- **d.** anterior and posterior colporrhaphy

15. A vesicovaginal fistula results in
- **a.** fecal incontinence
- **b.** leakage of urine from the bladder
- **c.** leakage of fecal material into the vagina
- **d.** leakage of urine from the vagina

REFERENCES

1. D. Danforth (ed.), *Obstetrics and Gynecology*, 3d ed., Harper & Row Publishers, Incorporated, New York, 1977 p. 175.
2. S. L. Romney et al., *Gynecology and Obstetrics: The Health Care of Women*, McGraw-Hill Book Company, New York, 1975, p. 166.
3. O. Ylikorkala et al., "New Concept in Dysmenorrhea," *Am J Obstet Gynecol*, **130**:833–839 (1978).
4. P. W. Budoff, "Use of Mefenamic Acid in Treatment of Primary Dysmenorrhea," *JAMA*, **241**:2713–2715 (1979).
5. R. M. Larkin et al., "Dysmenorrhea: Treatment with Antiprostaglandins," *Obstet Gynecol*, **54**:456–458 (1979).
6. N. Kase, "Yes or No on Estrogen Replacement?—A Formulation for Clinicians," *Clin Obstet Gynecol*, **19**:825–832 (1976).
7. L. Rose (ed.), *The Menopause Book*, Hawthorn Books, New York, 1977, p. 113.
8. Romney, op. cit., p. 147.
9. R. M. Wynn, *Obstetrics and Gynecology: The Clinical Core*, 2d ed., Lea & Febiger, Philadelphia, 1979, p. 218.
10. I. Pahl and L. Lundy, "Experience with Midtrimester Abortion," *Obstet Gynecol*, **53**:587–589 (1979).
11. M. Bygdeman et al., "New Prostaglandins E_2 Analogue for Pregnancy Termination," *Lancet*, **8125**:1136 (1979).
12. Uniform Crime Reports, U.S. Federal Bureau of Investigation, 1978, Catalog no. J1.14/7, 1979, p. 14.
13. Ibid., p.15.
14. S. Fox and D. Scherl, "Crisis Intervention with Victims of Rape," *J Soc Work*, **17**:37 (1972).
15. A. Burgess and L. Holmstrom, *Rape Crisis and Recovery* Prentice-Hall, Inc., Englewood Cliffs, N.J., 1979, p.35.
16. M. Rein and T. Chapel, "Trichomoniasis, Candidiasis and the Minor Venereal Diseases," *Clin Obstet Gynecol*, **18**:74 (1975).
17. Z. Rosenwahs et al., "Endometrial Pathology and Estrogens," *Obstet Gynecol*, **53**:403–409 (1979).

Chapter 47

NURSING ROLE IN MANAGEMENT

Male Reproductive Problems

Michael A. Carter

Learning Objectives

1. Describe the pathophysiology, clinical features, and medical management of problems affecting the male reproductive system.
2. Describe the nursing management of problems affecting the male reproductive system.
3. Explain the nursing role in the management of problems related to male sexual functioning.
4. Identify the psychological and emotional implications of problems related to the male reproductive organs.

Problems of the male reproductive tract are a source of anxiety for many men. This anxiety is related to manipulation and exposure of the genitals, discussion of intimate topics, and fear of possible pathology related to the male reproductive organs. Anxiety and fear may cause the client to delay seeking help for a problem or in practicing health-promoting behaviors. Specific nursing measures which can minimize embarrassment for the male client should be used when he seeks health care (Table 47-1). The nursing role in the management of problems of the male reproductive system can involve a wide range of problems of any of the various structures (Fig. 47-1).

PROBLEMS OF THE PROSTATE GLAND

Benign Prostatic Hypertrophy or Hyperplasia (BPH)

Significance of the problem

The most common problem of the adult male reproductive system is benign prostatic hypertrophy or hyperplasia (BPH). This problem occurs in about 50 percent of men over 50 years of age and 75 percent of men over 70.[1] The median and lateral lobes of the prostate are most likely to develop benign prostatic hypertrophy while the posterior lobe is most likely to develop carcinoma (Fig. 47-2).

Pathogenesis

BPH begins with small nodules within the gland. While the cause of the development of these nodules is not completely understood, it is thought that they are an overgrowth of smooth muscle and connective tissue. There is also an increase of glandular tissue. The development of hyperplasia seems to be related to a decrease in the ratio of testosterone to estrogen, which occurs with aging.[2-4]

As the nodules continue to grow in size, there is compression of the normal prostatic tissue to the periphery of the gland. Problems arise when the gland enlarges to the point that the proximal urethra is partially or completely obstructed. This obstruction results in urinary retention. Upon rectal examination, the benign hypertrophic gland will feel firm and enlarged.

Clinical manifestations

The client seeks medical assistance for relief of the symptoms related to urinary obstruction. These symptoms are usually very gradual in onset and may not be noticed by the client until hypertrophy of the prostate gland is rather far advanced. The first symptom experienced by the client is often nocturia (awakening at night to void). This is due to decreasing bladder capacity from an enlarging prostate. A small urinary stream, hesitancy (difficulty in starting the stream), and dribbling at the end of voiding are also symptoms of BPH. A urinary tract infection may be present due to the obstructive process.

Table 47-1
Measures to Minimize Embarrassment for the Male Client

1. Assure privacy for care.
2. Drape carefully so that only the part being examined is exposed.
3. Be sure that client understands terminology being used for his body parts.
4. Use open, nonjudgmental attitude toward client's sexual practices.

*This chapter was reviewed by Steve Toussaint, R.N., M.S.N., Instructor, Health Sciences Center, University of Oregon, Portland, Oregon.

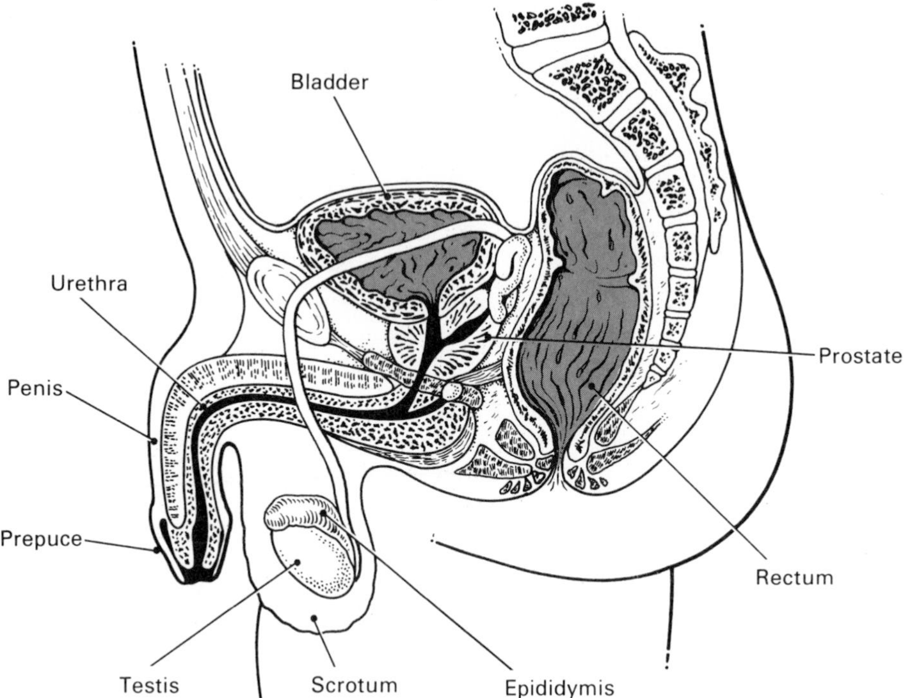

Figure 47-1 Areas of the male reproductive tract likely to develop problems.

Complications

The client with BPH is at increased risk for urinary tract infection because of the failure of the bladder to empty completely. The residual urine provides a favorable environment for bacterial growth. Renal calculi may develop due to the alkalinization of the residual urine. Rupture of overstretched blood vessels of the bladder may produce hematuria.

More serious complications that can result from urinary retention are abnormally distended ureters (hydroureters), destruction of the kidney's parenchyma from the back pressure of the urine (hydronephrosis), and pyelonephritis. These complications can lead to renal failure.

Diagnostic study abnormalities

The most common sign of BPH is enlargement of the prostate upon palpation. Additionally, urinalysis may indicate alkalinity and the presence of infection. In the early stages of BPH, the specific gravity of the urine may be unchanged or elevated as the client may restrict his fluid intake to decrease his need to void. If hydronephrosis has occurred, the specific gravity will be low. If BPH has been a long-standing problem, the blood urea nitrogen (BUN) and creatinine levels may be elevated.

If a cystoscopy is done, the encroachment of the prostate gland into the urethra can be observed. Small hemorrhagic areas may be present in the bladder.

Medical management

The goal of medical management is to restore bladder drainage. This may be temporarily accomplished by catheterization. However, the catheter does not resolve the underlying problem of prostatic enlargement.

The primary medical treatment of BPH is surgery (Table 47-2). There are four surgical approaches to remove the adenomatous tissue. The selection of an approach depends upon the size and position of the prostatic enlargement (Fig. 47-3). Urinary tract infections are usually treated before surgery is attempted.

The type of surgery selected may depend on the degree of debility, reproductive outlook, and degree of obesity of the client. Sometimes, even age is a factor if the health care providers assume the client is too old to care if impotence results. The nurse can assist the client to ask appropriate questions regard-

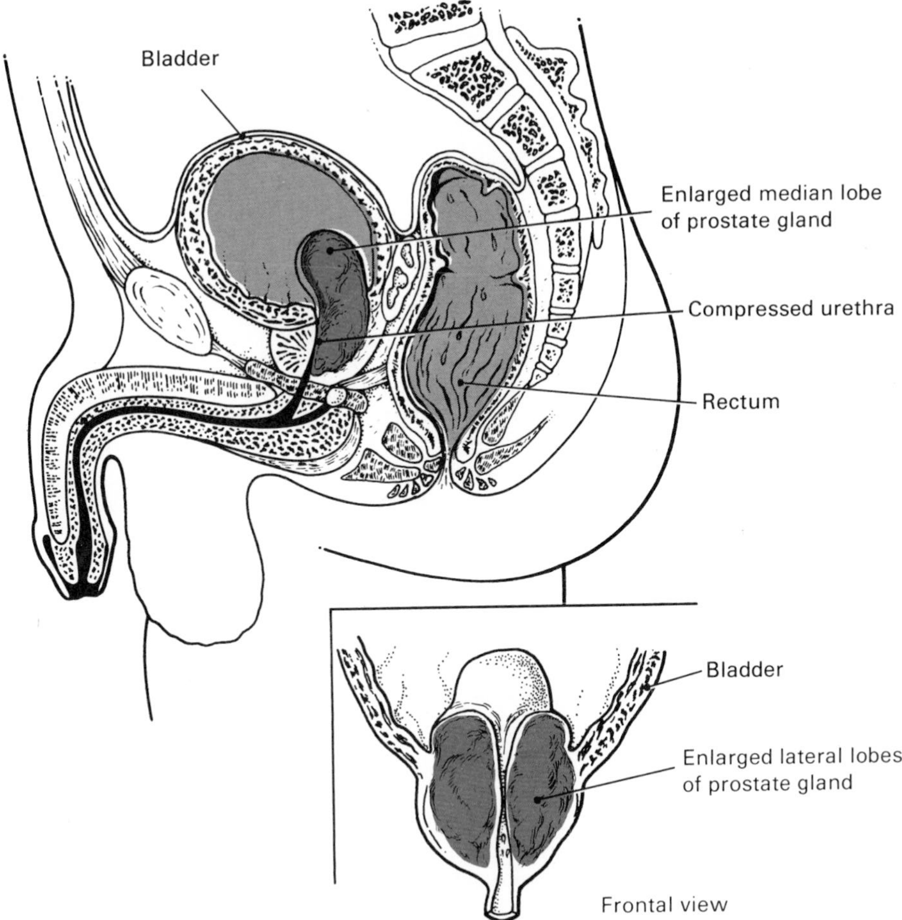

Figure 47-2 Benign prostatic hypertrophy of the median lobe.

ing the impact of a particular type of surgery on sexual functioning.

Transurethral Resection (TUR) The transurethral approach is the most common route for removal of the prostate. This approach is very useful for removal of the medial lobe surrounding the urethra. There is no external surgical incision since a resectoscope is passed through the urethra to excise and cauterize prostatic tissue. A large (no. 18 to 22) three-way Foley catheter with a 30-mL bag is usually inserted into the bladder following the procedure to provide hemostasis and facilitate urinary drainage. Bladder irrigation, continuous or intermittent, is usually done for at least 24 hours to prevent obstruction from mucous threads and blood clots. A TUR is often the surgery of choice for the debilitated client or for the client with moderate prostatic enlargement. The advantage of a TUR is that it does not involve an external incision. A disadvantage is that it does not completely remove all prostatic tissue.

Suprapubic Resection The suprapubic approach is used when an extremely large mass of tissue is obstructing the urethra. The prostate is approached through a low midline abdominal incision through the bladder to the anterior aspect of the prostate. Following surgery a cystotomy catheter is left in place through the abdominal incision to prevent pressure on the suture line. A Foley catheter with a 30-mL bag is placed in the urethra. Although this approach allows better exploration, it carries an increased risk of urinary tract infections and hemorrhage.

Table 47-2
Medical Management: Benign Prostatic Hypertrophy

Diagnostic

1. Rectal examination
2. Cystocopy
3. Urinalysis with culture
4. Renal studies
   a. Blood urea nitrogen
   b. Electrolytes
   c. Intravenous pyelogram

Therapeutic

1. Catheterization
2. Antibiotics
3. Force fluids
4. Surgery
   a. Transurethral resection
   b. Suprapubic resection
   c. Retropubic resection
   d. Perineal resection

Retropubic Resection The retropubic approach is used to remove a large mass located high in the pelvic area. A low midline abdominal incision is made into the prostate gland. Following surgery the client will have a large Foley catheter with a 30-mL bag placed in the urethra. A Penrose drain may be left in the abdominal incision site to aid in the removal of drainage from the area. Both suprapubic and retropubic resections are difficult in the obese client.

The bladder is not incised in this approach and direct visualization of the prostate is possible. The risk of hemorrhage remains high.

Perineal Resection The perineal approach is used to remove a large mass located low in the pelvic area, and is often used with cancer of the prostate. The incision is made between the scrotum and the anus. Since there is a possibility of entering the rectum, the bowel is prepared with enemas, antibiotics, and a low-residue diet. Following surgery a Foley catheter with a 30-mL bag is left in the urethra. There may be a Penrose drain in the incision site to promote drainage of the area. A perineal approach is most likely to result in impotence and urinary incontinence.

A prophylactic vasectomy may be done with an open prostatectomy to decrease the risk of ascending epididymitis. The major postoperative complications of all four types of surgery are hemorrhage, infection, and bladder spasm.

Nursing intervention

Health Maintenance and Promotion Since the cause of BPH is poorly understood, the focus of health promotion is upon early detection and treatment. Men should have a prostate examination at least yearly after 40 years of age.

Some men find that the ingestion of drugs such as alcohol and caffeine tend to increase prostatic symptoms. If this happens, the client should avoid these drugs.

Clients with obstructive symptoms should be advised to void when they first feel the urge in order to minimize urinary stasis and acute urinary retention. Fluid intake should be maintained at a normal level to avoid dehydration or fluid load. The client may believe that if he restricts his fluid intake his symptoms will be less severe, but this will only increase the chance of developing an infection. However, if the client rapidly increases his intake of fluids beyond what the urethra can eliminate, hydronephrosis can develop more readily because of the obstruction to urine elimination.

Acute Management

Preoperative care

The objectives of preoperative care of the client about to undergo prostatectomy are (1) restoration of urinary drainage, (2) treatment of any urinary tract infection, and (3) client education, especially related to sexual functioning.

Urinary drainage needs to be restored before surgery. Prostatic obstruction may have resulted in retention or inability to void. A urethral catheter may be needed to restore drainage. If there is a sizable obstruction of the urethra, a filiform catheter with sufficient rigidity to pass the obstruction may be needed. The insertion of this catheter is usually done by a urologist. Aseptic technique is very important at this time to avoid introducing bacteria into the bladder.

Any infection of the urinary tract must be treated before surgery. Restoring drainage, forcing fluids, and providing a diet high in acid ash producing foods are helpful in clearing the infection. Antibiotics are usually given.

The client is usually concerned about the impending surgery related to his sexual functioning. The data gathered during the health history related to the sexual history will identify possible problem areas. Providing an opportunity for the client to express his concerns is an important nursing role. The client needs to know how the surgery will affect his sexual functioning. The client needs to know if a vasectomy is planned and the

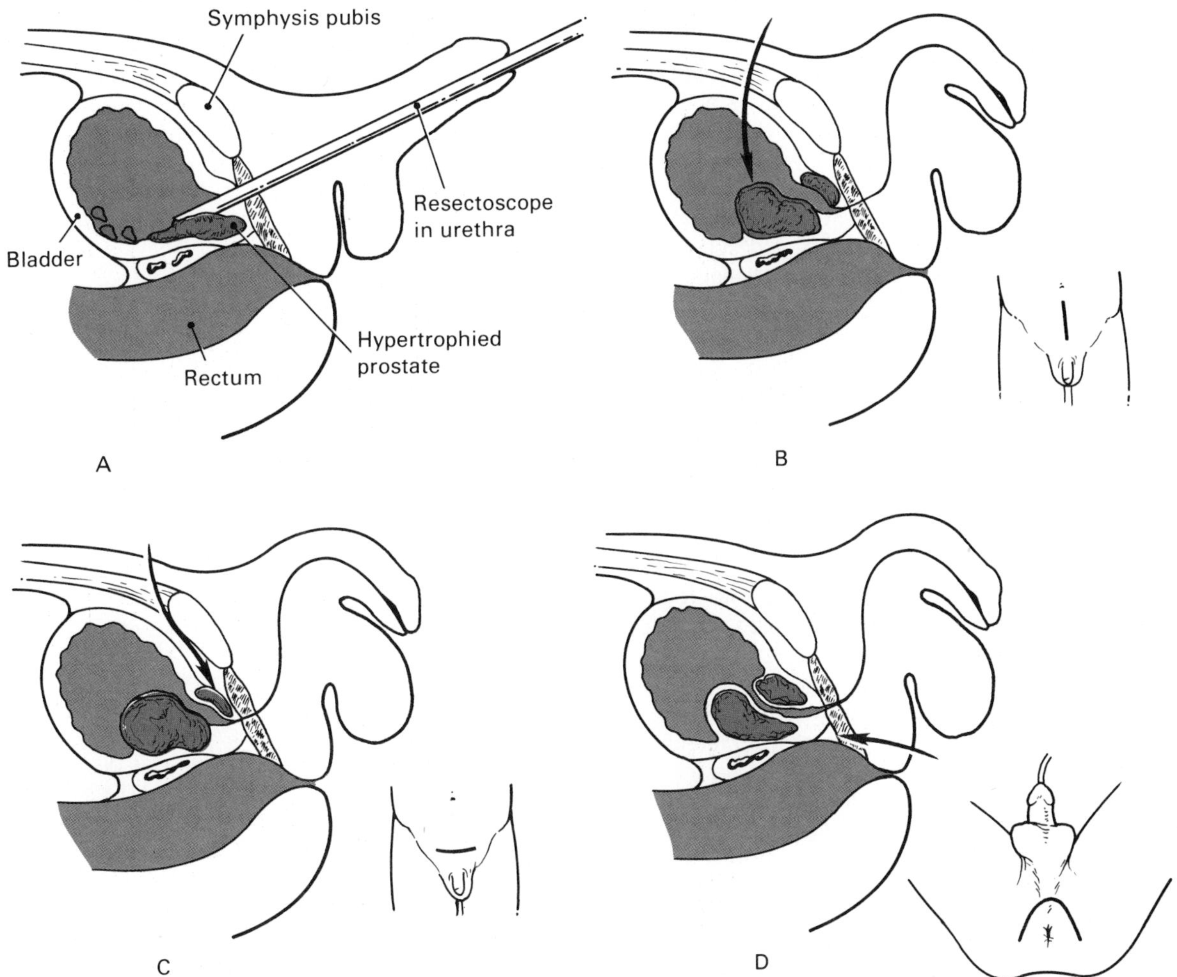

Figure 47-3 Four types of prostatectomy *(a)* Transurethral resection (TUR). *(b)* Suprapubic (transvesical) prostatectomy. *(c)* Retropubic (extravesical) prostatectomy. *(d)* Perineal prostatectomy.

consequences of this related to his ability to father children. The surgical consent form should indicate if a vasectomy is to be performed. Except in the perineal approach, a prostatectomy does not usually result in impotence.

Postoperative care

The nursing responsibilities focus upon assessing and preventing complications and restoring urinary control and sexual expression. The main complications are hemorrhage, bladder spasms, and infection. In designing the plan of care the nurse considers the type of surgery, the reasons for surgery, and the client's response to surgery.

Following prostatectomy the bladder may be continuously irrigated with sterile normal saline or another prescribed solution. This removes clotted blood from the bladder and assures drainage of urine. Some form of irrigation (continuous or intermittent) may be used for 24 hours or until no clots are noted draining from the bladder.

Blood clots are normal following a prostatectomy for the first 24 to 36 hours. However, large amounts of bright red blood in the urine could mean *hemorrhage.* Postoperative hemorrhage may occur from displacement of the catheter or increases in abdominal pressure. Release or displacement of the catheter dislodges the 30-mL bag which provides counter-pressure on the operative site. Slight traction on the catheter will apply counter-pressure on the bleeding site in the prostate, decreasing bleeding. Such traction could result in local necrosis. Consequently, pressure should be relieved on a scheduled basis. Activities that increase abdominal pressure such as sitting for prolonged periods and straining to have a bowel movement should be avoided in the postoperative recovery period.

Bladder spasms are a distressing complication for the client following transurethral and suprapubic prostatectomy. These occur due to irritation of the bladder mucosa from the insertion of the resectoscope, the presence of a catheter, and clots in the catheter. The client should be instructed not to attempt to void around the catheter as this will increase the likelihood of spasm. If the client develops bladder spasms, the catheter should be checked for clots. If present, the clots should be removed so urine can flow freely. Belladonna and opium suppositories are used to relieve the pain and decrease spasm. The catheter is removed from 2 to 6 days following surgery. The client should void within 6 hours after catheter removal. If he cannot void, a catheter needs to be reinserted for a day or two.

Sphincter tone may be poor immediately following surgery, resulting in incontinence or dribbling. This is a very common but distressing situation for the client. Sphincter tone can be strengthened by having the client press the buttocks together, followed by relaxing the muscles, 10 to 20 times per hour. The client may also practicing starting and stopping the stream several times during voiding. Usually it takes several weeks to achieve control. In some instances, control of urine may never be fully regained. Continence can improve for up to 12 months. If continence has not been achieved by that time, the client can be instructed to use a penile clamp, condom catheter, or training pants to avoid embarrassment from dribbling. The nurse should assist the client in developing practices that will allow him to socialize and interact with relatives and friends.

The client should be observed for signs of postoperative infection. If an external wound is present, the area should be observed for redness, heat, swelling, or pus formation. Careful aseptic technique should be used when irrigating the bladder, since bacteria can be introduced into the urinary tract in this manner. The proper care of the catheter is very important. The catheter should be connected to a closed drainage system and should not be disconnected unless it is to be removed, changed, or irrigated. The peri-catheter secretions that accumulate around the meatus should be cleansed at least daily with soap and water. Special care needs to be taken if a perineal incision is present due to the proximity of the anus. Rectal treatments (except belladonna and opium suppositories) such as rectal temperatures and enemas should be avoided as they may initiate bleeding.

Dietary intervention is very important in the postoperative period to prevent the client from straining while moving his bowels. Straining will increase the intraabdominal pressure, which could lead to bleeding of the operative site. A diet high in fiber will produce a soft, easily passed stool (see Appendix B, Table 6).

Rehabilitative Management Following prostatic surgery the client may be concerned about impotence. Physiologic impotence occurs when the perineal nerves are cut during a radical perineal prostatectomy. The other types of prostatic surgery do not usually transect these nerves. The degree of concern is often related to anxiety over loss of sex role, degree of self-esteem, and quality of sexual interaction between the client and his sexual partner. Sexual counseling may be necessary if impotence becomes a chronic problem.

If a vasectomy was performed, the client should have been prepared preoperatively to accept the ensuing sterility. Some men may experience retrograde ejaculation following prostatectomy because of trauma to the internal sphincter. Semen is discharged into the bladder at orgasm and may produce cloudy urine when the client voids following orgasm. In most cases retrograde ejaculation is temporary. The nurse should discuss these problems with the client and his partner and allow them to question her and express their concerns.

The bladder may take up to 2 months to return to its capacity. The client should be instructed to drink at least 1 L of fluid per day to irrigate the urinary tract. Since he may be experiencing incontinence or dribbling, he may believe that decreasing his fluid intake will help his problem.

The client needs to be advised that he should continue to have yearly rectal examinations, particularly if he had a transurethral resection. Hyperplasia can recur in the remaining prostatic tissue and again cause obstruction. Since the entire prostate is not resected during the transurethral resection, he is still at risk for the development of prostatic cancer. Table 47-3 summarizes the nursing care for the client undergoing a TUR.

Prostatic Cancer

Significance of the problem

Although rarely found in men under 60 years of age, cancer of the prostate is a common form of

Table 47-3
Nursing Care of the Client Undergoing Transurethral Resection

Problem	Expected Outcome	Nursing Intervention
	Preoperative	
Urinary retention	Establishment of urinary flow	Insertion of indwelling catheter (usually done by urologist). Monitor intake and output. Percuss every shift for distended bladder.
Urinary infection	Negative urine culture	Monitor temperature. Do urinalysis for culture. Give 8 oz fluid every waking hour. Observe strict aseptic technique for catheter care. Observe color and characteristics of urine.
Anxiety over surgery, diagnosis, and implications for sexual functioning	Reduced anxiety	Standard preoperative teaching. Assess concerns related to sexual functioning. Provide opportunity for private conversation for client to ask personal questions.
	Postoperative	
Acute		
Hemorrhage	No evidence of frank bleeding in first 24 h Clear urine by discharge	Maintain traction on catheter. Observe urinary drainage. Monitor blood pressure, pulse, and respirations. Maintain catheter drainage. No rectal treatments such as enemas or rectal thermometers (except belladonna and opium suppository).
Bladder spasms	No bladder spasms	Irrigate catheter if occluded with clots. Instruct client not to void around catheter. Give belladonna and opium suppository prn.
Infection	No evidence of infection	Take temperature every 4 h. Give 8 oz of water every 8 h. Observe strict aseptic technique for catheter care.
Chronic		
Dribbling	Achieve urinary control	Teach client exercises to control urinary stream. Advise client of devices available to control dribbling.
Potential prostatic cancer	Continue with annual and self-prostatic examination	Explain to client that some prostatic tissue is present which could become malignant. Reinforce need for annual and self-examinations.
Potential hemorrhage	No bleeding	Instruct client to avoid heavy lifting, straining during defecation, prolonged periods of travel.
Potential impotence	Ability to achieve sexual satisfaction	Assure client that a TUR does not usually cause problems in sexual functioning. Assist client and sexual partner to openly discuss concerns.

cancer. There are approximately 25,000 new cases diagnosed each year and about 17,000 deaths each year in the United States from this form of tumor.[5] About one-half of the cases of prostatic cancer can be diagnosed by rectal examination before there are any noticeable symptoms.

There are four stages of prostatic cancer, based upon the tumor's growth:

Stage 1 Entirely intraprostatic, too small to be distinguished by physical examination or laboratory tests

Stage 2 Confined to the prostate but palpable upon rectal examination

Stage 3 Confined to the pelvis but not metastasized to bone or distant points

Stage 4 Has distant metastases

Pathophysiology

Prostatic cancer is a hormone-dependent adenocarcinoma. This means that the growth of the tumor is related to the presence of androgens. The tumor usually develops the ability to continue to grow in the absence of androgens.[6] The exact cause of this form of cancer is not known. There is a higher incidence related to age (60 or older), and in black men and married men.

The tumor usually begins in the posterior or lateral portions of the prostate and spreads by continuity to the seminal vesicles, urethral mucosa, bladder wall, and external sphincter. The cancer spreads later through the perineural lymphatic system to the regional lymph nodes. The veins from the prostate seem to be the mode of spread to the pelvic bones, heads of the femur, the lower lumbar spine, the liver, and the lungs.

Clinical manifestations and complications

The client may have symptoms similar to those of benign prostatic hypertrophy, including urinary obstruction, hesitancy, dribbling, frequency, urgency, hematuria, nocturia, and retention. Upon rectal examination the prostate will feel hard, enlarged, and fixed. The enlargement is usually unilateral.

When coupled with urinary symptoms, pain in the lumbosacral area which radiates down into the hips or legs usually is strongly indicative of metastasis.

The need for early recognition and treatment of this tumor is to control growth and prevent metastasis. As described earlier, the tumor can spread to bone, lungs, and liver. When this occurs, the likelihood of a cure is greatly diminished.

Once the tumor has spread to distant sites, the major problem for the client becomes the management of pain. As the cancer spreads to bone, pain can become very severe, especially in the back and legs (see Chap. 50).

Diagnostic study abnormalities

Blood chemistry and x-rays do not usually show any abnormality through stage 3. In stage 4 serum acid phosphatase is increased due to metastasis. Serum alkaline phosphatase becomes elevated as new bone is formed at the site of bone metastasis. At this stage osteoblastic changes will be seen on x-ray of the bones of the pelvis, spine, ribs, and the skull. Bone scans of metastatic areas will be abnormal.

Medical management

Table 47-4 summarizes the medical management of the four stages of prostatic cancer.

A unique feature of prostatic cancer is that cell growth is initially dependent on the presence of androgens. The usual means of decreasing androgen production in the adult male is orchiectomy (removal of the testis). This procedure has a great many emotional overtones for men, especially if they are sexually active. Estrogens can be substituted for or used in combination with orchiectomy. This treatment can cause regression of the size of the prostate and disappearance of metastatic bone lesions. If estrogens are used, the minimal dose capable of suppressing plasma testosterone to castration levels is used. Estrogens are used to relieve pain or urinary obstruction and not to prolong life. In fact, estrogens in the male may greatly increase the risk of cardiovascular disease. Estrogens are used only for stage 4 prostatic cancer.

Table 47-4
Medical Management: Prostatic Cancer

Diagnostic

1. Rectal examination
2. Biopsy—needle aspiration open biopsy
3. Blood chemistry—serum alkaline phosphatase
4. Radiologic studies

Therapeutic

Stage 1—Total prostatectomy
Stage 2—Radical resection of prostate, seminal vesicles, bladder neck, and lymph nodes
Stage 3—Radical resection of prostate as in stage 2. Radiation to pelvis
Stage 4—TUR
Bilateral orchiectomy
Radiation to pelvis and metastatic bone areas
Estrogen
Cytotoxic agents (cyclophosphamide and methotrexate)

Nursing management

Health Promotion and Maintenance One of the most important roles for nurses related to prostatic cancer is to encourage clients to have an annual prostate examination to increase early detection of this malignancy. Men over 40 years of age should begin the practice of having an annual rectal examination.

Acute Intervention The nursing intervention during the preoperative and postoperative phases of therapy is the same as for benign prostatic hypertrophy. However, an additional consideration is concern for the client's psychological response to a diagnosis of cancer. The nurse needs to provide psychological support for the client and his family, to assist them to cope with the diagnosis of cancer (see Chap. 11).

Rehabilitative Management If the client has stage 4 prostatic cancer, pain management will be the major consideration (see Chap. 50). The use of radiation therapy, orchiectomy, or estrogens will alter sexual functioning and body image. These effects may be more undesirable to the client than the pain that results from no treatment at all. The client and his family should be informed of the benefits and risks of the various treatments and allowed to make the decision as to their use. None of these treatments has been shown to prolong life.

Many of the treatments for prostatic cancer will alter the client's sexual function. Radical prostatectomy, radiation, orchiectomy, and estrogens produce impotence. The client and his partner may need assistance in developing alternative methods of sexual functioning that do not require an erect penis.

Prostatitis

Pathophysiology

A number of inflammatory conditions can affect the prostate gland. The most common form of prostatitis is *abacterial* or *prostatosis.* Acute and chronic prostatitis due to bacterial causes are less common.

Abacterial prostatitis may follow a viral illness or may be secondary to a sudden decrease in sexual activity, particularly in a younger adult. The cause of this problem is presently not known, but it is probably a noninfectious process.

Bacterial prostatitis is commonly associated with urethritis or an infection of the lower urinary tract. Commonly suspected organisms are *Escherichia coli, Enterobacter, Proteus,* and group D streptococci.[7] Organisms are believed to reach the prostate from the bloodstream or the urethra.

Clinical manifestations and complications

Acute bacterial prostatitis most often affects young males. The client may have fever, chills, dysuria, urethral discharge, and a boggy, very tender prostate. Gentle palpation of the prostate results in a copious, purulent urethral discharge.

The symptoms of chronic prostatitis are backache, perineal pain, mild dysuria, and frequency. The prostate will feel irregularly enlarged, firm, and slightly tender when palpated.

The complications of prostatitis are epididymitis and cystitis. Chronic prostatitis can predispose to recurrent urinary tract infections. Sexual functioning may be diminished from the discomfort. A rare complication is a prostatic abscess.

Diagnostic study abnormalities

If the client with prostatitis has a fever, there may be an elevation of the white blood count. The client is instructed to void into two or three separate containers. The first container will show many more white cells and bacteria than subsequent containers.

Medical management

Medical management of acute bacterial prostatitis usually consists of an antibiotic which will concentrate in the prostate. Most antibiotics will not penetrate the prostate because the very low pH of the gland precludes solubility of the drugs. Exceptions are tetracycline and the combination of sulfamethoxazole with trimethoprim.

The medical management of chronic prostatitis is much more controversial (Table 47-5). Long-term antibiotics may be used. Vigorous prostatic massage, sitz baths, and stool softeners are sometimes prescribed. The efficacy of these measures other than for comfort has not been shown.

Nursing management

Early treatment of acute prostatitis can help prevent the development of an abscess. If the client has a sexually transmitted infection, measures should be taken to prevent spreading it to his partner(s).

The client with chronic prostatitis should be instructed regarding the long-term nature of the problem. Since the prostate could serve as a source of urinary tract infection, fluid intake should be kept at a high level. Antibiotics may need to be taken for a number of months. Activities which drain the prostate —intercourse, masturbation, and prostatic massage— will likely be of help in the long-term management of this problem.

Table 47-5
Medical Management: Bacterial Prostatitis

Diagnostic

1. Rectal examination
2. Complete blood count
3. Culture of semen
4. Split specimen urinalysis

Therapeutic

A. Acute bacterial type
   1. Antibiotics:[8] Sulfamethoxazole and trimethoprim—double strength for 30 days (Bactrim DS, Septra DS)
   2. Comfort measures: Analgesics, stool softeners, sitz baths

B. Chronic type
   1. Antibiotics:[8] Sulfamethoxazole and trimethoprim for 12 weeks
   2. Comfort measures: Sitz baths, prostatic massage, intercourse, masturbation

PROBLEMS OF THE PENIS

Health problems of the penis are rare if sexually transmitted infectious diseases are excluded (see Chap. 45). The problems may be divided into congenital problems, problems of the prepuce, problems with the erectile mechanism, and cancer.

Congenital Problems

Hypospadias is present when the urethral meatus is located on the ventral surface of the penis, anywhere from the corona to the perineum. Usually there is no medical treatment for hypospadias unless there is an associated chordee or bending under of the penis during erection which may prevent intercourse.

Epispadias is the opening of the urethra on the dorsal surface of the penis. This condition is a complex birth defect which is usually associated with other genitourinary tract defects. Corrective surgery is usually done in early childhood.

Problems of the Prepuce

Problems of the prepuce rarely occur since circumcision has been so widely practiced in the United States for the past 40 to 60 years. Paraphimosis is edema of the retracted foreskin, preventing normal return over the glans. If this occurs, a circumcision may be required since the blood supply is cut off and necrosis may occur.

Problems of the Erectile Mechanism

Priapism is a long-maintained erection without sexual desire. The erection may be sudden and very painful. The client may be unable to urinate. Causes of priapism include thrombosis of the veins of the corpora cavernosa, leukemia, sickle-cell anemia, diabetes, degenerative lesions of the spine, and neoplasms of the spinal cord. The treatment is aspiration of the corpora cavernosa with a large-bore needle. Following an episode of priapism, the client is often unable to ever have an erection.

Cancer

Cancer of the penis is rare and is seen usually only in men who were not circumcised as infants. The tumor begins as a warty lesion that may be mistaken for a venereal wart. In the early stages, treatment is a partial penectomy. If the cancer has spread, a radical resection may be done.

PROBLEMS OF THE SCROTUM AND ITS CONTENTS

External Problems

The skin of the scrotum is susceptible to a number of common dermatoses. The most common conditions of the scrotal skin are fungal infections (candidiasis), dermatitis (neuro-, contact, and seborrheic), and parasitic infections (scabies and lice). These conditions pose discomfort for the client but have few, if any, severe complications (see Chap. 17).

Internal Problems

Problems that develop inside the scrotum usually are first noticed as a mass or scrotal edema. Some problems produce pain while others do not. Although conditions affecting scrotal contents are rare, those seen most frequently in the adult are epididymitis, hydrocele, spermatocele, varicocele, orchitis, torsion, and testicular cancer.

Epididymitis

Epididymitis is an inflammatory process of the epididymis, usually secondary to an infectious process. Swelling may progress to the point that the epididymis and testis are indistinguishable. The problem is frequently associated with prostatitis and is usually painful. The use of antibiotics is controversial in the absence of a specific infection. Treatment consists of bed rest with elevation of the scrotum and ice packs. Ambulation places the scrotum in a dependent position and increases pain. Most of the tenderness subsides by the end of 1 week, while swelling may last for weeks or months.

Hydrocele

A *hydrocele* results from a problem of lymphatic drainage of the scrotum. There is a swelling of the tunica vaginalis which surrounds the testis. The mass will transilluminate with a bright light. There is no treatment unless the swelling becomes very large and uncomfortable. Treatment is surgical drainage of the mass.

Spermatocele

A *spermatocele* is a firm, sperm-containing cyst of the epididymis. The etiology of this problem is unknown. There is no treatment other than surgical removal. It is important for the client to be able to distinguish this cyst from cancer when performing self-examination. (This procedure is discussed later in this chapter.)

Varicocele

A *varicocele* is a dilation of the veins that drain the testes. The scrotum will feel wormlike when palpated. The etiology of the problem is unknown. The varicocele is almost always located on the left side of the scrotum. Surgery is indicated if the client is infertile and wishes to father children.

Torsion

Although rare, *torsion* involves a twisting of the testes and epididymis and is seen most commonly at puberty. This problem usually follows some form of strenuous exercise. Torsion is a surgical emergency. The client will experience pain, tenderness, nausea, and vomiting. The pain does not subside with rest and elevation of the scrotum.

Tumors of the testes

Significance and Etiology Testicular tumors make up about 0.7 percent of all forms of cancer of the male.[9] They occur in two per 100,000 males per year with the peak age of incidence between 15 and 34 years.[10] Testicular tumors are much more common in clients who have had undescended testicles (cryptorchidism).

Testicular tumors may develop from the cellular components of the testis or from the embryonal precursors (germinal tumors). Nongerminal tumors are very rare, usually benign, and can occur at any age. Germinal tumors are almost always malignant.

Pathophysiology The germinal tumors may have a slow or rapid onset depending upon the type. The client may notice a lump in his scrotum as well as scrotal swelling. The scrotal mass is usually nontender, very firm, and cannot be transilluminated. Back pain or gynecomastia is associated with metastasis. Clients with germinal cell tumors produce increased amounts of chorionic gonadotropin (HCG) which can be measured in the plasma.

The prognosis for clients with advanced stages of testicular cancer is very poor. Only 15 percent are able to obtain complete remission of their disease.[11]

Medical and Nursing Management As with many forms of cancer, survival of the client is closely associated with early recognition of the tumor. The scrotum is easily examined and beginning tumors are usually palpable (Fig. 47-4). The nurse should teach the client how to do a self-examination and should particularly focus upon those clients with a history of an undescended testis or a previous testicular tumor.

The procedure for self-examination is not difficult.

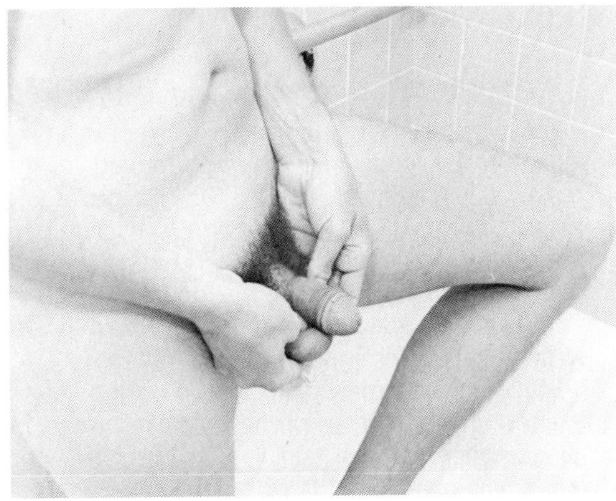

Figure 47-4 Testicular self-examination.

The client may indicate some reluctance to examine his own genitals. With encouragement the client can learn this simple procedure. He should be encouraged to do self-examinations frequently until he is comfortable with the procedure. After that time, the scrotum should be examined once a month.

The guidelines for self-examination of the scrotum are:

1. Do the examination while the scrotum is warm. The testes retract toward the perineum when cold. During a shower or bath is a good time.
2. Use both hands to palpate the scrotal contents. The client should palpate in any manner that is comfortable to him as long as he is systematic and thorough.
3. Identify the structures. Demarcate the testis from the epididymis. The epididymis is not as smooth as the egg-shaped testis. Remember, one testis may be larger than the other. Size is not as important as texture. Also, locate the spermatic cord which is usually firm and smooth.

The nurse should make this procedure as simple and uncomplicated for the client as possible. The client needs to practice to develop familiarity with his body. However he wishes to become familiar is correct for him.

Medical management of testicular cancer involves surgical removal of the affected testis, the cord, and resection of the regional and paraaortic lymph nodes. Radiation of the remaining lymph nodes and single or multiple chemotherapeutic agent regimens are also used following surgery.

SEXUAL FUNCTIONING

Vasectomy

Vasectomy is the bilateral surgical ligation and/or resection of the ductus deferens performed for the purpose of sterilization (Fig. 47-5). The procedure requires only 15 to 30 minutes and is usually performed under local anesthesia on an outpatient basis. Vasectomy is considered a permanent form of sterilization, although some successful reversals (vasovasotomy) have been reported.

Following vasectomy the client will not notice any difference in the quantity of the ejaculate, since its major component is seminal fluid. The client will need to use an alternate form of contraception until semen examination reveals no sperm. This usually requires at least 10 ejaculations or 6 weeks to evacuate sperm distal to the anastomotic site. Sperm cells continue to be produced by the testes but are absorbed by the body rather than passing through the ductus deferens. In rare instances there may be a spontaneous reanastomosis of the vas deferens, resulting in restoration of fertility.

Vasectomy does not usually affect the production of hormones, ejaculation, or the physiologic mechanisms related to sexuality. Occasionally, there is a postoperative hematoma and swelling of the scrotum. The most common complication of vasectomy is a problem with psychological adjustment. It may be very difficult for the client to separate vasectomy from castration at a subconscious level. Some men may develop erectile dysfunction or may feel the need to become much more sexually active than they were in the past to prove their masculinity. Careful discussion of the procedure and its outcome before the surgery can be helpful in detecting those clients who may have problems with psychological adjustment. Surgery should be delayed for these clients.

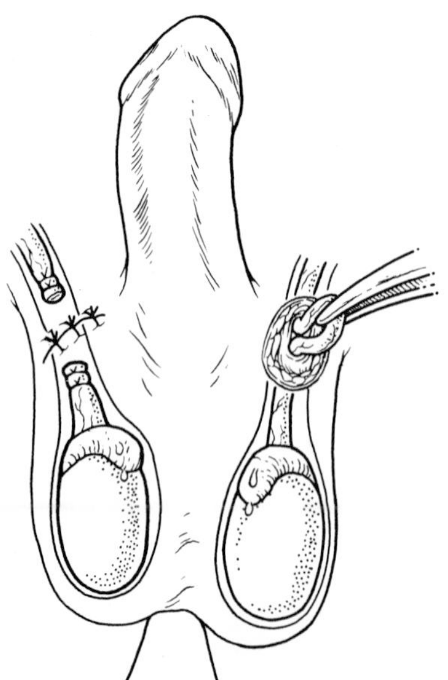

Figure 47-5 Vasectomy procedure.

Erectile Dysfunction

Erectile dysfunction is the inability to attain or maintain an erect penis that allows satisfactory sexual performance. This problem occurs at some time for almost all sexually active males. When the problem occurs during more than 25 percent of sexual encounters, the client is in need of intervention. The problem can occur at any age.

Erection is a vasocongestive engorgement of the corpora cavernosa and corpus spongiosum of the penis. Problems occur when these spaces fail to fill when desired or when they empty prior to orgasm. There are two classifications of erectile dysfunction. *Primary dysfunction* is a form in which the client has never been able to have an adequate erection with any type of sexual experience. *Secondary dysfunction* means the client has lost the ability to perform or is able to have an erection in only a particular way, such as with a full bladder or masturbation, or is able to have an erection with a particular partner and not others.

The causes for the disorder may be physiologic, psychological, or both. The major complication of this problem is that the client's inability to perform sexually can stress his interpersonal relationships and may preclude sex role functioning.

The majority of erectile dysfunctions have psychosocial causes. However, the importance of physical causes should not be overlooked (Table 47-6).

The treatment for erectile dysfunction is based upon the cause. The client with an intact reflex arc and a physiologic cause is treated for the specific problem. The results of these interventions are usually very satisfactory. The client with a neurologic problem may be recommended for a penile prosthesis after careful evaluation of his condition as well as his partner and their relationship. The long-term evaluation of the use of these devices has yet to be reported.

Treatment of psychological causes of erectile dysfunction is usually done by a qualified therapist. The approach may be behavioral or psychological. In most cases the client and his partner will be able to develop a satisfactory sexual relationship following treatment.

Table 47-6
Physiologic Causes of Erectile Dysfunction

Endocrine
1. Testosterone deficiency
2. High levels of prolactin
3. Abnormal hypothalamic-pituitary-gonadal axis
4. Diabetes mellitus
5. Thyroid disorders
6. Adrenal disorders

Cardiovascular
1. Atherosclerosis
2. Leriche's syndrome

Nerve conduction problems
1. Prostatectomy
2. Disk and spinal cord injuries
3. Central nervous system disorders

Drug-induced
1. Antihypertensives
2. Alcohol
3. Narcotics
4. Estrogens

Infertility

The male is the cause of infertility in about one-third of childless marriages. Infertility can be due to disorders of the hypothalamic–pituitary system, disorders of the testes, or abnormalities of the ejaculatory system. A careful history, including sexual practices, and a physical examination are the initial diagnostic measures in an infertility study. The presence of a varicocele, a treatable cause of male infertility, can be detected upon examination.

The first test in an infertility study for the male is a semen analysis. Additional tests helpful in determining the etiology include plasma testosterone and serum luteinizing hormone (LH) and follicle-stimulating hormone (FSH) measurements. A testicular biopsy may be necessary to differentiate between ductal obstruction and maturation arrest. Often the specific cause of infertility is not determined.

Surgery can correct a varicocele or ductal obstruction, and some endocrine problems are treatable. Otherwise, the management of infertility is generally unsuccessful.

The nurse should be concerned and tactful in dealing with the male client undergoing infertility studies. For many men, fertility and masculinity are equated. The nurse must be sensitive to the problem of gender identity with the infertile male. Infertility can seriously strain a marriage, and the couple may require counseling if conception will never be possible. (Female infertility is discussed in Chap. 46.)

Case Study / Benign Prostatic Hypertrophy

Mr. P., 62 years old, has been admitted to the hospital for a suprapubic prostatectomy. Over the past 5 years, he has noticed that he has had increasing difficulty voiding. The problem has been in beginning his urine stream and with dribbling following voiding. He now has to get up at least three times each night to void.

On admission his vital signs revealed a temperature of 38.1°C (100.6°F), pulse 85, respirations 20, and blood pressure 140/86. Palpation of his abdomen showed the bladder to be distended 5 cm above the umbilicus.

Mr. P.'s surgery was uneventful. After 3 hours in the recovery room, he was returned to his room.

Discussion Questions

1. Explain the clinical manifestations of benign prostatic hypertrophy.
2. What are the complications of this problem? Which ones does Mr. P. have?
3. Explain a preoperative teaching plan for this client.
4. Describe Mr. P.'s probable appearance upon return to his room.
5. Describe the possible postoperative complications of this surgery.
6. Prepare a discharge plan for this client.

REVIEW QUESTIONS

The number of the question corresponds to the same numbered objective at the beginning of the chapter.

1. The major risk factor currently identified for the development of benign prostatic hypertrophy is
   a. multiple sexual parnters
   b. smoking
   c. frequent urinary tract infections
   d. age
2. Prevention of bladder spasms immediately following prostatectomy is best done by
   a. forcing fluids
   b. keeping the catheter free of clots

c. elevating the head of the bed
d. ambulation

3. The nurse can inform the client that following vasectomy the client will be
a. immediately sterile
b. unable to ejaculate in a normal manner
c. unable to contract VD
d. able to resume his usual sexual functioning

4. The nurse can decrease the client's discomfort over care involving his reproductive organs by
a. assuring privacy for care
b. assuring that the client understands the terminology being used for his body parts
c. maintaining a nonjudgmental attitude toward his sexual practices
d. all of the above

REFERENCES

1. R. Lytton and F. Epstein, "Tumors of the Urinary Tract," in *Harrison's Principles of Internal Medicine,* 8th ed., G. W. Thorn et al. (eds.), McGraw-Hill Book Company, New York, 1977, p. 1474.
2. B. K. Pradhan and K. Chandra, "Morphogenesis of Nodular Hyperplasia: Prostate," *J Urol,* **113:**210 (February 1975).
3. Lytton and Epstein, op. cit., p. 1474.
4. F. Mostofi and R. V. Thompson, "Benign Hyperplasia of the Prostate Gland," in *Urology,* M. F. Campbell and J. H. Harrison (eds.), W. B. Saunders Company, Philadelphia, 1970, p. 1060.
5. P. K. Bondy, "Medical Treatment of Hormone-Dependent Cancers," in *Cecil Textbook of Medicine,* 15th ed., P. B. Beeson et al. (eds.), W. B. Saunders Company, Philadelphia, 1979, p. 1921.
6. R. J. Shearer et al., "Plasma Testosterone: An Accurate Monitor of Hormone Treatment in Prostatic Cancer," *Br J Urol,* **45:**668 (1973).
7. L. W. Thompson and L. M. Edwards, "Genitourinary Disorders," in *Primary Care,* C. J. Leitch and R. V. Tinker (eds.), F. A. Davis, Philadelphia, 1978, p. 229.
8. *Disease-A-Month,* May 1980.
9. M. B. Lipsett, "The Testis: Tumors of the Testis," in *Cecil Textbook of Medicine,* 15th ed., P. B. Beeson et al. (eds.), W. B. Saunders Company, Philadelphia, 1979, pp. 2174–2175.
10. Thompson and Edwards, op. cit., p. 229.
11. V. T. DeVita, Jr., "Principles of Cancer Therapy," in *Harrison's Principles of Internal Medicine,* 8th ed., G. W. Thorn et al. (eds.), McGraw-Hill Book Company, New York, 1977, p. 1759.

BIBLIOGRAPHY FOR SECTION 9

Endocrine

Books

Alsever, R., and R. Gotlin: *Handbook of Endocrine Test in Adults and Children,* 2d ed., Year Book Medical Publishers Inc, Chicago, 1978.

Antonovsky, A.: *Health, Stress, and Coping,* Jossey-Bass Publishers, San Francisco, 1979.

Benson, H.: *The Relaxation Response,* William Morrow, New York, 1975.

Blevins, D.: *The Diabetic and Nursing Care,* McGraw-Hill Book Company, New York, 1979.

Burns, K., and R. Johnson: *Health Assessment in Clinical Practice,* Prentice-Hall, Inc., Englewood Cliffs, N.J., 1980.

Burns, T.: "Endocrinology," in *Sodeman's Pathologic Physiology Mechanisms of Disease,* W. Sodeman and T. Sodeman (eds.), 6th ed., W. B. Saunders Company, Philadelphia, 1979.

Cohen, E., and D. Etzwiler: *Diabetes Manual,* 4th ed., Health for Living Program Inc., 1975.

Conger, M.: *Endocrine System and Patient Care I,* Concept Media, Irvine, Calif., 1979.

Conn, H.: *Current Therapy,* W. B. Saunders Company, Philadelphia, 1980.

——— and R. Conn: *Current Diagnosis,* W. B. Saunders Company, Philadelphia, 1980.

Cox, T.: *Stress,* University Park Press, Baltimore, 1978.

DeGroot, L., et al.: *Endocrinology,* vol. 2., Grune & Stratton Inc., New York, 1979.

Diabetes Mellitus, 8th ed., Lilly Research Laboratories, Indianapolis, Ind., 1979.

Dolger, H., and B. Seeman: *How to Live with Diabetes,* Pyramid Books, New York, 1968.

Drury, M. I.: *Diabetes Mellitus,* Blackwell Scientific Publications, Oxford, 1979.

Dudley, D. L., and E. Welke: *How to Survive Being Alive,* Doubleday & Company, Inc., New York, 1979.

Ezrin, C., J. Gooden, and P. Walfish: *Clinical Endocrinology, A Survey of Current Practice,* Appleton Century Crofts, New York, 1977.

———, ———, and R. Volpe: *Systematic Endocrinology,* 2d ed., Harper & Row, Publishers, Inc., New York, 1978.

Flynn, P. A. R.: *Holistic Health,* Robert J. Brady Company, Bowie, Md., 1980.

French, R.: *Guide to Diagnostic Procedures,* 5th ed., McGraw-Hill Book Company, New York, 1980.

Galbraigh, R.: *Immunological Aspects of Diabetes Mellitus,* CRC Press Inc., Boca Raton, Florida, 1979.

Grave, G. D. (ed.): *Early Detection of Potential Diabetic: The Problems and the Promise,* Raven Press, New York, 1979.

Groer, M., and M. Shekleton: *Basic Pathophysiology: A Conceptual Approach,* The C. V. Mosby Company, St. Louis, 1979.

Guthrie, D., and R. Guthrie: *Nursing Management of Diabetes Mellitus,* The C. V. Mosby Company, St. Louis, 1977.

Jubiz, W.: *Endocrinology: A Logical Approach for Clinicians,* McGraw-Hill Book Company, New York, 1979.

Krueger, J., and R. Comptom: *Endocrine Problems in Nursing—A Physiologic Approach,* The C. V. Mosby Company, St. Louis, 1976.

Krupp, M., and M. Chatton: *Current Medical Diagnosis and Treatment,* Lange Medical Publishers, Los Altos, Calif., 1978.

Miller, M., A. Drakontides, and L. Leacell: *Kimber-Gray-Stackpole's Anatomy and Physiology,* 17th ed., The Macmillan Company, New York, 1977.

Montgomery, D., and R. Welbourn: *Medical and Surgical Endocrinology,* Edward Arnold (Publishers) Ltd., London, 1975.

Muir, B.: *Pathophysiology: An Introduction to the Mecha-*

nisms of Disease, John Wiley & Sons, Inc., New York, 1980.

Podolsky, S. (ed.): *Clinical Diabetes: Modern Management*, Appleton Century Crofts, New York, 1980.

Selye, H.: *Stress in Health and Disease*, Butterworth Publishers Inc., Boston, 1976.

———: *The Stress of Life*, rev. ed., McGraw-Hill Book Company, New York, 1976.

Skillman, T., and M. Tzagournis: "Diabetes Mellitus," Upjohn Co., Kalamazoo, Mich., 1977.

Sloane, E.: *Biology of Women*, John Wiley & Sons, Inc., New York, 1980.

Spencer, R.: *Patient Care in Endocrine Problems*, W. B. Saunders Company, Philadelphia, 1973.

Stanbury, J., and B. Hetzel: *Endemic Goiter and Endemic Cretinism*, John Wiley & Sons, Inc., New York, 1980.

Sussman, K. E., and R. J. S. Metz: *Diabetes Mellitus*, 4th ed., American Diabetes Association Inc., New York, 1975.

Tindall, G., and W. Collins: *Clinical Management of Pituitary Disorders*, Raven Press, New York, 1979.

Tripp, A.: *Basic Pathophysiological Mechanisms of Endocrine Dysfunction*, McGraw-Hill Book Company, New York, 1979.

Tucker, S., et al.: *Patient Care Standards*, 2d ed., The C. V. Mosby Company, St. Louis, 1980.

Watts, N., and J. Keffer: *Practical Endocrine Diagnosis*, 2d ed., Lea & Febiger, Philadelphia, 1978.

Widmann, F.: *Clinical Interpretation of Laboratory Tests*, 8th ed., F. A. Davis, Philadelphia, 1979.

Periodicals

"ADA Speaks on Combating Diabetes," *Am Dietet Assn J*, **75:**285–286 (S 1979).

Allard, J, and J. George: "Hyponatremia," *Heart Lung*, **7** (4):587–593 (July–August 1978).

Aspinall, M.: "A Simplified Guide to Managing Patients with Hyponatremia," *Nursing 78*, **8**(12):32–35 (December 1978).

Bell, J. M.: "Stressful Life Events and Coping Methods in Mental Illness and Wellness Behaviors," *Nurs Res*, **26**(24):136–141 (March–April 1977).

Benson, H., et al.: "The Relaxation Response: A Bridge Between Psychiatry and Medicine," *Med Clin North Am*, **61:**929 (July 1977).

Benson, W. E., and R. Machemer: "Vitrectomy Update," *Diabetes Forecast* (November–December 1978).

Burchfield, S. R.: "The Stress Response: A New Perspective," *Psychosomatic Med*, **41**(8):661–672 (December 1979).

Cerniglia, J., P. Leapldy, and N. Slater: "Think Thin," *Diabetes Forecast* (September–October 1978).

"Controlling Diabetes Mellitus," *Am J Nurs*, **80**(10):1827–1850 (October 1980).

Cooperman, D., and W. Malarkey,: "Pituitary Apoplexy," *Heart Lung*, **7**(3):425–434 (May–June 1978).

Coughlin, R. W., and A. Patz: "Diabetic Retinopathy," *Diabetes Forecast* (November–December 1978).

Daley, T. J., and E. L. Greenspun: "Stress Management Through Hypnosis," *Topics in Clinical Nursing*, **1**(1):59–65 (April 1979).

DeLaurentis, D.: "The Diabetic and Peripheral Vascular Disease," *Diabetes Forecast* (January–February 1979).

Deluca, H.: "The Vitamin D Hormonal System: Implications for Bone Diseases," *Hosp Pract*, **15**(4):57–63 (April 1980).

Dewitt, C.: "Support Team Helps Patients Cope with Stress," *Hospitals*, **53**(12):93–94 (June 16, 1979).

"Diabetes Due to an Abnormal Insulin," *Am Fam Physician*, **21:**187 (May 1980).

"Diabetic Ketoacidosis," *Am Fam Physician*, **21:**191 (March 1980).

"Diagnosis of Adult-Onset Diabetes Mellitus," *Am Fam Physician*, **19:**92 (February 1979).

Dollery, C. T., et al.: "Reversal of Retinal Vascular Lesions in Diabetes," *Diabetes*, **14:**121 (1965).

Donnelly, G. F.: "Coping: Why You Just Can't Take It Anymore," *RN*, **43**(5):34–37 (May 1980).

Doresio, T.: "Hypercalcemic Crisis," *Heart Lung*, **7:**425 (1978).

Editorial: "Control of Diabetes and Insulin Antibodies," *Br Med J*, **1:**484 (1976).

Ellenberg, M.: "Impotence: What It Is," *Diabetes Forecast* (January–February 1978).

Engel, G.: "Emotional Stress and Sudden Death," *Psychology Today*, **11**(6):114–115 (November 1977).

Ezrin, C., K. Kovacs, and E. Horvath: "A Functional Anatomy of the Endocrine Hypothalamus and Hypophysis," *Med Clin North Am*, **62**(2) (March 1978).

Feek, C., et al.: "Combinations of Potassium Iodide and Propranolol in Preparation of Patients with Graves' Disease for Thyroid Surgery," *N Engl J Med*, **302**(16):883–885 (April 17, 1980).

Fisher, C.: "Impotence: What Can Be Done," *Diabetes Forecast* (January–February 1978).

Frankenhaeuser, M.: "Psychoneuroendocrine Approaches to the Study of Emotion as Related to Stress and Coping," *Nebraska Symposium on Motivation*, **26:**123–161 (1978).

Gavin, L., M. Rosenthal, and R. Cavaliere: "The Diagnostic Dilemma—Isolated Hyperthyroxinemia in Acute Illness," *JAMA*, **242**(3):251–253 (July 20, 1979).

Gottlieb, N., and W. Riskin: "Complications of Local Corticosteroid Injections," *JAMA*, **243**(15):1547–1548 (April 18, 1980).

Greenberg, J. S.: "Stress, Relaxation, and the Health Educator," *J School Health*, **47**(9):522–525 (November 1977).

Guimons, J., and S. G. Wilson: "Postirradiation Thyroid Disorders," *Am J Nurs*, **79**(7):1256–1258 (July 1979).

Guzzetta, C. E.: "Relationship Between Stress and Learning," *Advances in Nursing Science*, **1**(4):35–50 (July 1979).

Hallal, J.: "Thyroid Disorders," *Am J Nurs*, **77**(3):418–432 (March 1977).

Harlin, V. K.: "The Stress Phenomenon," *J School Health*, **48**(8):507 (October 1978).

Hartl, D. E.: "Stress Management and the Nurse," *Advances in Nursing Sciences*, **1**(4):91–100 (July 1979).

Heath, H. III, S. Hoodgson, and M. Kennedy: "Primary Hyperparathyroidism: Incidence, Morbidity, and Potential Economic Impact in a Community," *N Engl J Med*, **302**(4):189–193 (January 24, 1980).

"How Nursing Diagnosis Helps Focus Your Care: Diabetes Out of Control," *RN*, **42:**65–68 (S 1979).

Jeffcoate, W.: "A Guide to the Endocrine System," *Nurs Mirror*, **144**(19):58–60 (May 12, 1977).

Jenkins, E.: "Living with Thyrotoxicosis," *Am J Nurs*, **80** (5):956–958 (May 1980).

Johnson, M. N.: "Anxiety, Stress and the Effects on Disclosure Between Nurses and Patients," *Advances in Nursing Science*, **1**(4):1–22 (July 1979).

Khachadurian, A. K., et al.: "Management of Noninsulin-

Dependent Diabetes Mellitus," *Am Fam Physician,* **21:** 154–160 (February 1980).
Kiser, D.: "Somogyi Effect," *Am J Nurs,* **80**(2):236–238 (February 1980).
Koivisto, V. A., and P. Felig: "Diabetic Athletes Take Note," *Am J Nurs,* **78**(8):1389 (August 1978).
Kolata, G. B.: "Blood Sugar and the Complications of Diabetes," *Science,* **203:**1098–1099 (March 16, 1979).
———: "Controversy Over Study of Diabetes Drugs Continues for Nearly a Decade," *Science,* **203:**986–990 (March 9, 1979); discussion, **204:**362–364 (April 27, 1979).
Krall, L. P.: "To Drink or Not to Drink?" *Diabetes Forecast* (November–December 1977).
Kubo, W., and M. Grant: "The Syndrome of Inappropriate Secretion of Antidiuretic Hormone," *Heart Lung,* **7** (3):469–476 (May–June 1978).
Lidberg, L. A., et al.: "Urinary Catecholamines, Stress and Psychopathy: A Study of Arrested Men Awaiting Trial," *Psychosomatic Med,* **40:**116 (March 1978).
Lipe, H. P.: "The Function of Weeping in the Adult," *Nurs Forum,* **19**(1):26–44 (1980).
"Managing Diabetes Properly," *Nursing 78 Skill Book,* Intermed Communications Inc., Horsham, Pa., 1977.
Marchiondo, K.: "The Very Fine Art of Collecting Culture Specimens," *Nursing 79,* **9**(4):34–43 (April 1979).
Marcinek, M. B.: "Stress in Critically Ill Patients," *Am J Nurs,* **77**(11):1806–1809 (November 1977).
———: "Stress in the Surgical Patient," *Am J Nurs,* **77** (11):1809–1811 (November 1977).
Matthes, M. L.: "Diabetic Day Care," *Am J Nurs,* **79**(1):105–106 (January 1979).
Maurer, A. C.: "The Therapy of Diabetes," *Am Scientist,* **67:**422–431 (July–August 1979).
Miller, E. C.: "Diabetic Emergencies," *Am Fam Physician,* **18:**115–121 (September 1978).
Miller, E. K., and N. E. White: "Diabetes Assessment Guide," *Am J Nurs,* **80**(7):1314–1316 (July 1980).
Morris, C. L.: "Relaxation Therapy in a Clinic," *Am J Nurs,* **79**(10):1958–1959 (November 1979).
Notkins, A. L.: "The Causes of Diabetes," *Scientific American,* **241:**62–73 (November 1979).
Perrin, E. D.: "Laser Therapy for Diabetic Retinopathy," *Am J Nurs,* **80**(4):664–665 (April 1980).
"Principles of Nutrition and Dietary Recommendations for Individuals with Diabetes," *Am Dietet Assn J,* **75:**527–530 (November 1979).
"Researcher Reports New, Easy Method for Diabetes Detection," *Am Fam Physician,* **19:**183–184 (January, 1979).
Richter, J. M., and R. Sloan: "A Relaxation Technique," *Am J Nurs,* **79**(10):1960–1964 (November 1979).
Roberts, A.: "Systems of Life: Hormones and Homeostasis," *Nurs Times,* **75**(5):center page (February 1, 1979).
Sawin, C., D. Chopra, F. Azizi, J. Mannix, and P. Bacharach: "The Aging Thyroid," *JAMA,* **424**(3):247–250 (July 20, 1979).
"Self-Testing of Blood Glucose Helps Diabetics," *Anal Chem,* **51:**1330A (November 1979).
Shaw, K.: "The Nature of the Endocrine System," *Nurs Mirror,* **44**(20):20–22 (May 17, 1977).
———: "The Nature of the Endocrine System: The Pituitary Gland," *Nurs Mirror,* **144**(21):24–26 (May 26, 1977).
———: "The Nature of the Endocrine System: The Thyroid Gland," *Nurs Mirror,* **144**(22):26–28 (June 2, 1977).
——— and A. Bloom: "The Nature of the Endocrine System: The Adrenal Glands," *Nurs Mirror,* **144**(26):32–34 (June 9, 1977).
——— and ———: "The Nature of the Endocrine Glands: The Sex Hormones," *Nurs Mirror,* **144**(26):32–34 (June 30, 1977).
——— and ———: "The Parathyroid and Calcium Balance," *Nurs Mirror,* **144**(25):28–30 (June 16, 1977).
Shubin, S.: "Rx for Stress—Your Stress," *Nursing '79,* **9:**53 (January 1979).
Shultz, D.: "Artificial Pancreas is Closer to Reality," *Science Digest,* **86:**81–82 (December 1979).
Singerland, D., and B. Burrows: "Long Term Antithyroid Treatment in Hyperthyroidism," *JAMA,* **242**(22):2408–2410 (November 30, 1979).
Sirota, D., and R. Segal: "Primary Lymphomas of the Thyroid Gland," *JAMA,* **242**(16):1743–1746 (October 19, 1979).
Smith, M. J. T., and H. Selye: "Reducing the Negative Effects of Stress," *Am J Nurs,* **79**(11):1953–1955 (November 1979).
"Somatostatinoma Syndrome is Clinically Diagnosed," *Am Fam Physician,* **20:**140 (December 1979).
Stephenson, C.: "Stress in Critically Ill Patients," *Am J Nurs,* **77**(11):1806–1809 (November 1977).
Sutterly, D. C.: "Stress and Health: A Survey of Self-Regulation Modalities," *Topics in Clinical Nursing,* **1**(1):1–29 (April 1979).
——— and G. S. Donnelly (eds.): "Stress Management," *Topics in Clinical Nursing,* **1:**1–104 (April 1979).
Tzagournis, M.: "Acute Adrenal Insufficiency," *Heart Lung,* **7**(4):603–609 (July–August 1978).
Urbanci, R., and E. Mazzaferri: "Thyrotoxic Crisis and Myxedema Coma," *Heart Lung,* **7**(3):435–437 (May–June 1978).
"When a Pregnant Woman is Diabetic," *Am J Nurs,* **79** (3):448–460 (March 1979).
Whitehouse, F. W.: "Get Wise—Exercise," *Diabetes Forecast* (March–April 1978).
Wilson-Barnett, J.: "Prevention and Alleviation of Stress in Patients," *Nursing* (Oxford), **10:**432–436 (February 1980).
Wurtman, R.: "The Pineal As a Neuroendocrine Transducer," *Hosp Prac,* **15**(1):82–92 (January 1980).
Zervas, N., and J. Martin: "Current Concepts in Cancer Management of Hormone Secreting Pituitary Adenomas," *N Engl J Med,* **302**(4):210–214 (January 24, 1980).
Zurier, R. B.: "Prostaglandins: Their Potential in Clinical Medicine," *Postgrad Med,* **68**(3):70–81 (September 1980).

Organizations

American Diabetes Association, Inc., 600 Fifth Avenue, New York, NY 10020
American Dietetic Association, Inc., 430 N. Michigan Avenue, Chicago, IL 60611

Male and Female Reproductive Systems

Books

Azzopardi, J. G.: *Problems in Breast Pathology,* W. B. Saunders Company, London, 1979.
Barlow, D.: *Sexually Transmitted Diseases: The Facts,* Oxford University Press, Oxford, 1979.

Benson, R. C.: *Current Obstetric and Gynecologic Diagnosis and Treatment,* 2d ed., Lange Medical Publishers, Los Altos, Calif., 1978.

Berger, K. J., and W. L. Fields: *Pocket Guide to Health Assessment,* Reston Publishing Company, Inc., Reston, Va., 1980.

Bouchard, R., and N. Owens: *Nursing Care of the Cancer Patient,* The C. V. Mosby Company, St. Louis, 1976.

Brand, P. C. (ed.): *Breast Cancer: Psycho-Social Aspects of Early Detection and Treatment,* University Park Press, Baltimore, 1978.

Burgess, A. W., and L. L. Holmstrom: *Rape: Crisis and Recovery,* Prentice-Hall, Inc., Englewood Cliffs, N.J., 1979.

Cope, O.: *The Breast,* Houghton Mifflin Company, Boston, 1977.

Danforth, D. N. (ed.): *Obstetrics and Gynecology,* 3d ed., Harper & Row Publishers, Incorporated, New York, 1977.

Gallager, H. S., et al. (eds.): *The Breast,* The C. V. Mosby Company, St. Louis, 1978.

Garrey, Matthew M., et al.: *Gynecology Illustrated,* 2d ed., Churchill Livingstone Inc., New York, 1978.

Georgiade, N.: *Breast Reconstruction Following Mastectomy,* The C. V. Mosby Company, St. Louis, 1979.

Green, T.: *Gynecology: Essentials of Clinical Practice,* 3d ed., Little, Brown and Company, Boston, 1977.

Keith, L., and J. Brittain: *Sexually Transmitted Diseases,* Creative Infomatics Inc., Aspen, Colo., 1978.

Kemmer, E. J.: *Rape and Rape Related Issues: An Annotated Bibliography,* Garland Publishing Inc., New York, 1977.

King, A., C. Necol, and P. Rodin: *Venereal Diseases,* 4th ed., Bailliere Lindall, London, 1980.

Kunin, C.: *Detection, Prevention, and Management of Urinary Tract Infections,* Lea & Febiger, Philadelphia, 1979.

Malasanos, L., V. Barkauskas, M. Moss, and R. Stoltenbert-Allen: *Health Assessment,* The C. V. Mosby Company, St. Louis, 1977.

Manual for Staging of Cancer 1978, American Joint Committee for Cancer Staging and End Results Reporting, Whiting Press, 1978.

Marchant, D., et al.: *Breast Disease,* Grune & Stratton, Inc., New York, 1979.

Martin, L. L.: *Health Care of Women,* J. B. Lippincott Company, Philadelphia, 1978.

Mayor B., and E. Zingg, *Urologic Surgery,* John Wiley & Sons, Inc., New York, 1976.

Mills, S.: *The Joy of Birth Control,* Emory University Family Planning Program, Atlanta, Ga., 1975.

Morton, B. M.: *VD: A Guide for Nurses and Counselors,* Little, Brown and Company, Boston, 1976.

Noble, R.: *Sexually Transmitted Diseases: A Guide to Diagnosis and Therapy,* Medical Examination Publishing Co., Inc., Garden City, N.Y., 1979.

Ods, S., et al.: *Obstetric Nursing,* Addison-Wesley Publishing Company, Inc., Menlo Park, Cal. 1980.

Phelan, S.: *Reproductive Physiology,* unpublished module, Center for Continuing Education in Women's Health Care, Albuquerque, N. M., 1980.

Reeder, S., L. Mastroianni, and L. Martin: *Maternity Nursing,* 14th ed., J. B. Lippincott Company, Philadelphia, 1980.

Romney, S. L., et al.: *Gynecology and Obstetrics: The Health Care of Women,* 2d ed., McGraw-Hill Book Company, New York, 1981.

Rose, L. (ed.): *The Menopause Book,* Hawthorn Books, New York, 1977.

Schofield, C. B. S.: *Sexually Transmitted Diseases,* 3d ed., Churchill Livingstone, London, 1979.

Schwartz, S. et al.: *Principles of Surgery,* 3d ed., McGraw-Hill Book Company, New York, 1979.

Sherman, J. L., and S. K. Fields: *Guide to Patient Evaluation,* 3d ed., Medical Examination Publishing Co., Inc., Garden City, N.Y., 1978.

Smith, R., et al., *Complications of Urologic Surgery: Prevention and Management,* W. B. Saunders Company, Philadelphia, 1976.

Speroff, L., Glass, R. H., and N. Kase: *Clinical Gynecologic Endocrinology and Infertility,* 2d ed., The Williams & Wilkins Company, Baltimore 1978.

Suave, M. J., and A. Pecherer: *Concepts and Skills in Physical Assessment,* W. B. Saunders Company, Philadelphia, 1977.

Tannenbaum, M.: *Urologic Pathology: The Prostate,* Lea & Febiger, Philadelphia, 1977.

Tilkian, S. M., M. B. Conover, and A. G. Tilkian: *Clinical Implications of Laboratory Tests,* 2d ed., The C. V. Mosby Company, St. Louis, 1979.

Wallach, J.: *Interpretation of Diagnostic Test,* 3d ed., Little, Brown and Company, Boston, 1978.

Winter C., and A. Morel, *Nursing Care of Patients with Urologic Diseases,* The C. V. Mosby Company, St. Louis, 1977.

Woods, N. F.: *Human Sexuality in Health and Illness,* 2d ed., The C. V. Mosby Company, St. Louis, 1979.

Wynn, R. M.: *Obstetrics and Gynecology: The Clinical Core,* 2d ed., Lea & Febiger, Philadelphia, 1979.

Periodicals

"Alternative to Mastectomy," *Time,* March 28, 1977 p. 82.

Anthony, C. J.: "Risk Factors Associated with Breast Cancer," *Nurse Practitioner,* **3**(4):31–32 (July–August 1978).

Bailar, J. C.: "Mammographic Screening: A Reappraisal of Benefits and Risks," *Clin Obstet Gynecol,* **21**(1):1–13 (March 1978).

Birkhoff, J., et al.: "Natural History of Benign Prostatic Hypertrophy and Acute Urinary Retention," *Urology,* **7:**48–52 (January 1976).

Bissada, N. K., and J. F. Redman: "Managing Infections of the Prostate Gland," *Am Fam Physician,* **2**(2):167–173 (February 1975).

Breeding, M. J., and M. Wollin: "Working Safely Around Implanted Radiation Sources," *Nursing '76,* **5:**58 (1976).

Brown, M.: "Syphilis and Gonorrhea: An Update for Nurses in Ambulatory Settings," *Nursing '76,* **6:**71 (1976).

Budoff, P.: "Use of Mefenamic Acid in Treatment of Primary Dysmenorrhea," *JAMA,* **241:**2713 (1979).

Burger, D.: "Breast Self-Examination," *Am J Nurs,* **79:**1088–1089 (June 1979).

Butts, P.: "Meeting the Special Needs of Your Hysterectomy Patient," *Nursing '79,* **9:**40 (1979).

Bygdeman, M., et al.: "New Prostaglandin E_2 Analogue for Pregnancy Termination," *Lancet* **8126:**1136 (1976).

Cohen, S., and R. Gittes: "Patient Assessment: Examination of the Male Genitalia," *Am J Nurs,* **79**(4):689–712 (April 1979).

———, J., Beebe, and M. Duperret: "Patient Assessment: Examination of the Female Pelvis, Part I," *Am J Nurs,* **78**(10):1–26 (October 1978).

———, ———, and ———: "Patient Assessment: Examina-

tion of the Female Pelvis, Part II," *Am J Nurs,* **78**(11):1–28 (November 1978).
Colon, V. F., and G. B. Schumann: "Gynecologic Cytology," *Am Fam Physician,* **18**(5):135–140 (November 1978).
Cowart, M., and D. Neston: "Oral Contraceptives: How Best to Explain Their Effects to Patients," *Nursing '76,* **6**:44 (1976).
Daniels, J.: "Emergency Department Management of Rape," *Ohio State Med J,* **75:**351 (1979).
Dodd, M.: "Theoretical Bases of Immunotherapy," *Am J Nurs,* **78**(2):310–329 (February 1979).
Domenich, N.: "The Methanol Extract Residue (Mer) of Bacillus Calmette-Guérin in Cancer Immunotherapy," *Nurs Clin North Am,* **13**(2):369–380 (June 1978).
Eckert, C.: "How to Evaluate and Manage Breast Lumps," *JAMA,* **234**(8):839–840 (November 24, 1975).
"Estrogen Receptor Guides Treatment of Breast Cancer," *AORN J,* **29**(1):158–159 (January 1979).
Faulkner, W., and H. Ory: "Intrauterine Devices and Acute Pelvic Inflammatory Disease," *JAMA,* **235:**1851 (1976).
Finn, L.: "Augmentation Mammoplasty: The Cosmetic Surgery with a Lift," *Nursing '79,* **9**(2):60 (February 1979).
Foti, A. G., et al.: "Detection of Prostatic Cancer by Solid-Phase Radioimmunoassay of Serum Prostatic Acid Phosphatase," *N Engl J Med,* **297:**1357 (1977).
Freeman, W.: "Not all PID is GC," *Emergency Med,* **10:**47 (1978).
Gorline, L. L.: "Teaching Successful Use of the Diaphragm," *Am J Nurs,* **79:**1732 (1979).
Gorringe, R., M. M. Lee, and A. Voda: "The Mammography Controversy: A Case for Breast Self-Examination, *J Obstet Gyn Nurs,* **7**(4):7–11 (July–August 1978).
Gott, L. J.: "Common Scrotal Pathology; *Am Fam Physician,* **15**(5):165–173 (May 1975).
Greiss, F. C.: "Ovarian Tumors," *Am Fam Physician,* **16:**170 (1977).
Guyther, J. R.: "The Physician's Role in Radiation Protection," *Am Fam Physician,* **18**(6):103–106 (December 1978).
Halbert, D., and D. E. Jones: "Medical Management of the Sexually Assaulted Woman," *J Reprod Med,* **20:**265 (1978).
Hamiliton, M. S., and N. B. Schlapper: "Pelvic Exenteration," *Am J Nurs,* **76:**266 (1976).
Hartgill, J.: "Wertheim's Hysterectomy," *Nursing Times,* **74:** 2061 (December 14, 1978).
Harvey, S.: "New Relief for Menstrual Discomfort," *RN,* **42:**116 (1979).
Haufrect, E., and A. Kaplan: "Answers to Questions on Pelvic Inflammatory Disease," *Hosp Med,* **12:**6 (1976).
Hill, E. C.: "Carcinoma of the Cervix: Diagnostic Guide," *Hosp Med,* **12:**31 (1976).
Holt, J., et al.: "Hormone Receptors and Breast Cancer," *AORN J,* **27**(5):841–848 (April 1978).
Horoshak, I.: "Learn to Fight Rape—Without Hang-ups," *RN,* **39:**52 (1976).
Kagan, J.: "Herpes: It Can Be Treated—But Not Cured," *Ms,* **6:**38 (1978).
Kemp, M., et al.: "Dealing with Depression After Radical Surgery," *Nursing '79,* **9:**47 (1979).
Kennedy, D. (ed.): "Update on Estrogen and Uterine Cancer," *FDA Drug Bulletin,* **9:**2, DHEW, Rockville, Md., 1979.
Kennerly, S.: "What I've Learned About Mastectomy," *Am J Nurs,* **77**(9):1430–1432 (September 1977).
Knapp, R. C., and R. S. Berkowitz: "Gynecologic Cancer: Guide to Diagnostic Approach," *Hosp Med,* **14:**88 (1978).
Koch, S.: "Augmentation Mammoplasty," *Am J Nurs,* **80**(8):1480–1484 (August 1980).
Kremkau, F. W., and L. H. Nelson: "Diagnostic Ultrasound and its Obstetric Applications," *Am Fam Physician,* **17**(5):148–157 (May 1978).
Laatsch, N.: "Nursing the Woman Receiving Adjuvant Chemotherapy for Breast Cancer," *Nurs Clin North Am,* **13**(2):337–349 (June 1978).
Larkin, R. M., et al., "Dysmenorrhea: Treatment with Antiprostaglandins," *Obstet Gynecol,* **54:**456 (1979).
Lasser, T.: "Reach to Recovery," American Cancer Society, 1969.
Leis, H. P.: "Clinical Diagnosis of Breast Cancer," *J Reproductive Med,* **14**(6):231–239 (June 1975).
———, Pilnik, S., and M. M. Black: "Diagnosis of Breast Cancer," *Hosp Med Reprint,* November 1974.
Lester, R. G.: "Risk Versus Benefit in Mammography," *Radiology,* **124:**1–6 (1977).
Letton, A. H., J. P. Wilson, and E. M. Mason: "The Value of Breast Screening in Women Less Than 50 Years of Age," *Cancer,* **40:**1–3 (1977).
Levene, M.: "A New Role for Radiation Therapy," *Am J Nurs,* **77**(9):1443–1444 (September 1977).
Marx, J.: "Dysmenorrhea: Basic Research Leads to a Rational Therapy," *Science,* **205:**175 (1979).
McGowan, L.: "Ovarian Cancer: Improving Survival," *Hosp Med,* **15:**6 (1979).
Mishell, D.: "Current Status of Oral Contraceptive Steroids," *Clin Obstet Gynecol,* **19:**743 (1976).
Mole, R. H.: "The Sensitivity of the Human Breast to Cancer Induction by Ionized Radiation," *Br J Radiol,* **51:**401–405 (1978).
Moran, C.: "Vaginal Hysterectomy," *RN,* **42:**53 (1979).
Moyaihan, B., et al.: "Sexual Assault: A Comprehensive Response to a Complex Problem," *J Emerg Nurs,* **4:**22 (1978).
Pahl, I., and L. Lundy: "Experience with Midtrimester Abortion," *Obstet Gynecol,* **53**:587 (1979).
Pepitone-Rockwell, F.: "Pattern of Rape and Approaches to Care," *J Fam Prac,* **6:**521 (1978).
Prilook, M. E. (ed.): "Roundtable Endometriosis: New Endometriosis Therapies vs. Old, *Patient Care,* **12:**5 (1978).
Puhaty, H.: "Two Rehabilitative Approaches," *Am J Nurs,* **77**(9):1437 (September 1977).
Quirk, B., and L. Huxall: "VD, The Equal Opportunity Disease," *Nurs Digest,* **4:**69 (1976).
Rogers, R.: "Vaginal Discharge: Guide to Diagnosis and Management," *Hosp Med,* **13:**68 (1977).
Rosenwahs, Z., et al.: "Endometrial Pathology and Estrogens," *Obstet Gynecol,* **53:**403 (1979).
Sande, H. A., et al.: "Treating Dysmenorrhea with Anti-inflammatory Agents: A Double Blind Trial with Naproxin Sodium," *Int J Gynecol Obstet,* **16:**250 (1978–1979).
Schwartz, M.: "Hormone Receptor Assay," *Am J Nurs,* **77**(9):1445-1446 (September 1977).
"Semilateral Decubitus Breast Examination," *JAMA,* **243**(17):1713–1714 (May 1980).
Siegel, M., et al.: "Penicillinase-Producing *Neisseria gonorrhoeae," Sexually Transmitted Diseases,* **4:**32 (1977).
Skinner, D. G.: "Non-Seminomatous Testis Tumors: Plan of Management Based on 96 Patients to Improve Survival in all Stages by Combined Therapeutic Modalities," *J Urol,* **115:**65 (1976).

Soteropoulos, G. C., O. S. Cigtay, and M. Kalley: "Localization with Xero-Mammography," *Am Fam Physician,* **20**(3):120–123 (September 1979).

Sredl, D., et al.: "Offering the Rape Victim Real Help," *Nursing '79,* **9:**38 (1979).

Steele, S. J.: "What a Women Fears—Infertility or Disease," *Nurs Mirror,* **147:**46 (October 5, 1978).

Strax, P.: "Screening for Breast Cancer," *Clin Obstet Gynecol,* **20**(4):781–801 (December 1977).

Sutherland, S., and D. Scherl: "Patterns of Response Among Victims of Rape," *Am J Orthopsychiatry,* **40:**503 (1979).

Thomas, S., et al.: "Breast Reconstruction After Mastectomy," *Am J Nurs,* **77**(9):1438–1442 (September 1977).

Timby, B.: Ovulation Method of Birth Control," *Am J Nurs,* **76**:928 (1976).

Tobiason S. J.: "Benign Prostatic Hypertrophy," *Am J Nurs,* **79**(2):286–290 (February 1979).

Todd, A.: Prophylactic Mastectomy," *Am J Nurs,* **77**(9):1447–1449 (September 1977).

Turnbull, E.: "Breast Examination Practices," *Am J Nurs,* **77**(9):1450–1451 (September 1977).

Tyson, M.C.: "Let's Talk About Menopause," *Nursing '78,* **8:**34 (1978).

Uniform Crime Reports, U.S. Federal Bureau of Investigation, 1978. Catalog no. J 1.14/7, 1979.

U. S. Department of Health, Education and Welfare, PHS: "Herpes Genital Infection," publ. no. 00-2939, CDC, 1979.

———: "Recommended Treatment Schedules for Gonorrhea," CDC, 1979.

———: STD Fact Sheet, 34th ed., publ. no. 79-8195, CDC, 1979.

Vorhar, H., and R. Messer: "Breast Cancer: Potentially Predisposing and Protecting Factors," *Am J Obstet Gynecol,* **130**(5):335–356 (February 1978).

WHO: *Neisseria gonorrhoeae* Producing β-Lactamase (Penicillinase)," *Weekly Epidemiological Record,* **52:**357 (1977).

Williams, M. A.: "Earlier Convalescence from Hysterectomy," *Am J Nurs,* **76:**438 (1976).

Winkler, W. A.: "Choosing the Prosthesis and Clothing," *Am J Nurs,* **77**(9):1433–1436 (September 1977).

Woodling, B., et al.: "Sexual Assault: Rape and Molestation," *Clin Obstet Gynecol,* **20:**509 (1977).

Wroblewski, S.: "Toxic Shock Syndrome," *Am J Nurs,* **81**(1):82–85 (January 1981).

Ylikorkala, O., et al.: "New Concepts in Dysmenorrhea," *Am J Obstet Gynecol,* **130:**833 (1979).

Organizations

Planned Parenthood—World Population, 810 Seventh Avenue, New York, NY 10019

Planned Parenthood—World Population, 515 Madison Avenue, New York, NY 10022

Rape Crisis Center, Box 21005, Washington, D.C. 20009

Reach to Recovery Foundation, 19 West 56 Street, New York, NY 10019

Sex Information and Education Council of the United States, 1855 Broadway, New York, NY 10019

The American Cancer Society, 219 East 42 Street, New York, NY 10017

Section 10

Problems Related to Movement and Coordination

Chapter 48

NURSING ASSESSMENT

Nervous System

Judith M. Ozuna

Learning Objectives

1. Describe the function of the two types of cells within the nervous system.
2. Explain the transmission of nerve impulses.
3. Explain the anatomic location and function of the major components of the central nervous system.
4. Describe the arterial blood supply to the brain.
5. Describe the functions of the 12 cranial nerves.
6. Compare the functions of the two divisions of the autonomic nervous system.
7. Identify the significant subjective and objective data related to the nervous system that should be obtained from a client.
8. Describe the techniques used in the physical assessment of the nervous system.
9. Differentiate normal from common abnormal findings of a physical assessment of the nervous system.
10. Describe the purpose, significance of results, and nursing responsibilities related to diagnostic studies of the nervous system.

STRUCTURE AND FUNCTION OF THE NERVOUS SYSTEM

The human nervous system is a highly specialized system responsible for the control and integration of the body's many activities. The nervous system can be divided into a central nervous system (CNS) and a peripheral nervous system. The central nervous system consists of the brain and spinal cord. The peripheral nervous system consists of the cranial and spinal nerves and the autonomic nervous system. Before considering specific organs of the nervous system, the basic structures and functions are discussed.

Cells of the Nervous System

The nervous system is made up of two types of cells, *neurons* and *neuroglia*. While neuroglial cells are more numerous, they are mainly supportive to the neuron, the primary functional unit of the nervous system.

Neuron

Regardless of form, size, or location, all neurons have characteristics common to nerve cells: (1) *irritability*, or the ability to react to stimuli; (2) *conductivity*, or the ability to transmit the reaction to other portions of the cell; and (3) the ability to influence other neurons, muscle cells, and glandular cells. This last characteristic is so vital that the systems are often combined and collectively called the *neuroendocrine system*.

Components of a Neuron A typical neuron consists of a cell body, an axon, and several dendrites (Fig. 48-1). The *cell body*, the largest portion of the neuron, contains the nucleus and cytoplasm. The nerve *axon* projects varying distances from the cell body, ranging from several micrometers to over a meter. Its function is to carry nerve impulses away to other neurons or to end organs. The end organs are smooth and striated muscles and glands. Axons may be myelinated or unmyelinated. Many axons present in the peripheral nervous system are covered by a segmentally interrupted myelin sheath composed of a white, lipid substance which acts as an insulator for the conduction of impulses. Generally, the smaller fibers are unmyelinated. *Dendrites* are multiple tiny processes which extend from the cell body of the neuron. Their function is to receive information from other dendrites.

Neuroglia

Neuroglia or glial cells provide support, nourishment, and protection to neurons and make up about 85 percent of the cells of the central nervous system. Different types of glial cells have specific functions. *Oligodendroglia* produce the myelin sheath of nerve fibers in the CNS (Schwann cells myelinate nerve fibers in the periphery). *Astrocytes* provide nutrition to the neuron and regulate ionic concentrations of interstitial fluid. When neurons are damaged, astrocytes proliferate and form the scar tissue of the nervous system. This is called *gliosis*, or glial scarring. *Ependymal cells* line the brain ventricles and aid in the production of cerebrospinal fluid. *Microglia*, a type of

This work was supported by NIH contract 1-NS-6-2431, National Institute of Neurological and Communicative Disorders and Stroke, PHS/DHEW and grant ID-23-NU-00081-01, Division of Nursing, PHS/DHEW.

This chapter was reviewed by Elizabeth Noroian, R.N., Ph.D., Assistant Professor, School of Nursing, University of Pittsburgh, Pittsburgh, Pennsylvania.

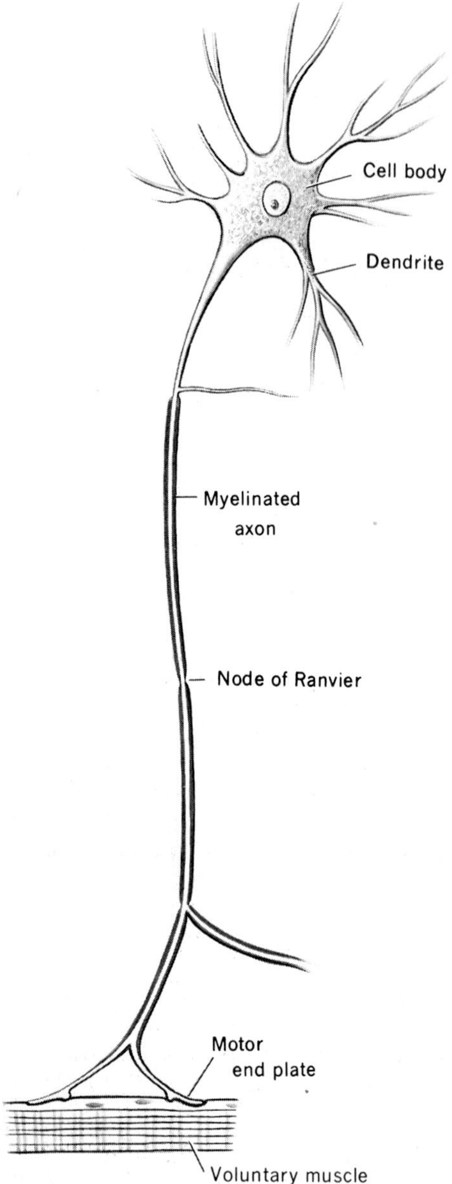

Figure 48-1 A typical neuron. *(From Charles R. Noback and Robert J. Demarest, The Human Nervous System: Basic Principles of Neurobiology, 2d ed., McGraw-Hill Book Company, New York, 1975, p. 47.)*

phagocytic cell, remove and disintegrate the waste products of neurons.

The Nerve Impulse

The nerve impulse transmits information to, from, and within the CNS and is related to transient changes in the physicochemical state of the cell membrane. Action potential and neurotransmitters are basic mechanisms involved in nerve-impulse transmission. An *action potential* is the cycle of electrical changes by which a nerve impulse is transmitted along the nerve axon. When the action potential reaches the end of the axon, the nerve impulse is transmitted to the dendrites of the next neuron at the synapse by the action of chemical substances called *neurotransmitters*.

Action potentials

All cells of the body exhibit a membrane potential oriented so that the inside of the cell is negatively charged relative to the outside. This potential is called the *resting membrane potential*. Consequently, even though a resting neuron is not conducting an impulse, it is considered a charged cell. An action potential occurs when a stimulus is of sufficient magnitude to alter the membrane potential and create a transient physicochemical change.

The cell membrane becomes more permeable to sodium ions, allowing them to move readily into the cell. The inside of the cell temporarily becomes positive relative to the outside. The resulting change in the voltage across the cell membrane is called *depolarization*. *Repolarization* (the inside of the cell becoming negative relative to the outside) is facilitated by a slower increase in potassium permeability, which in turn is caused by the depolarization associated with entry of sodium ions into the cell (Fig. 48-2). The whole process of depolarization and repolarization of the nerve cell membrane takes only 1 to 2 milliseconds. With repeated action potentials the cells would accumulate sodium ions. An active metabolic process within the cell is required to move sodium ions out of and potassium ions back into the cell. This metabolic process is accomplished by the sodium-potassium pump that acquires energy from the breakdown of adenosine triphosphate (ATP).

The action potential has an all-or-none quality. That is, once the cell depolarizes enough to cause an action potential, the size of the action potential is independent of the stimulus magnitude. When an action potential is initiated at one point on a neuron, it is transmitted along the axon without losing its intensity.

The myelination of nerve axons facilitates the conduction of an action potential. Many peripheral nerve axons have gaps, called *nodes of Ranvier*, at regular intervals in the myelin sheath surrounding them. An action potential traveling down one of these axons literally hops from node to node, making the action potential travel much faster than it would other-

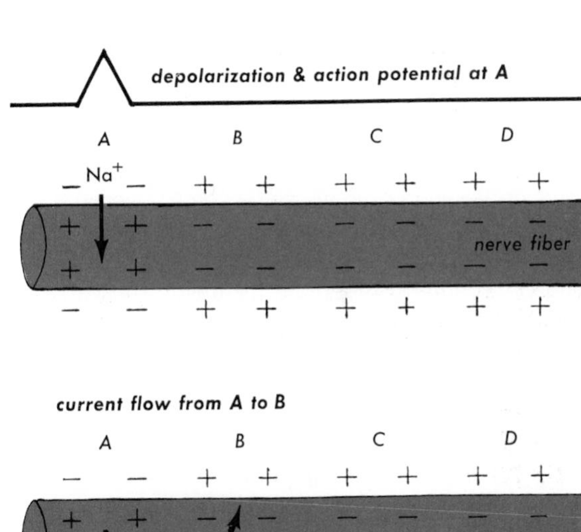

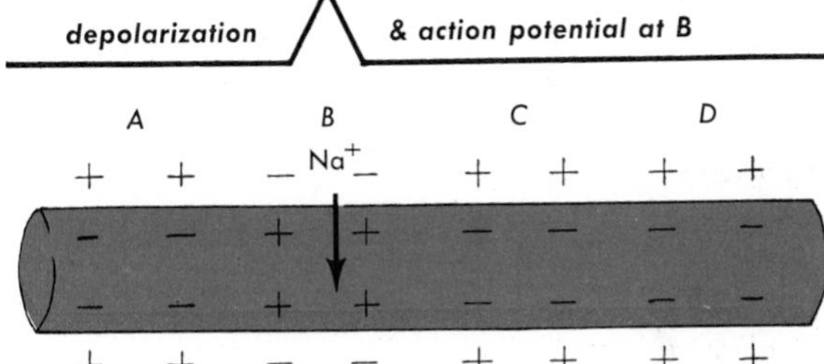

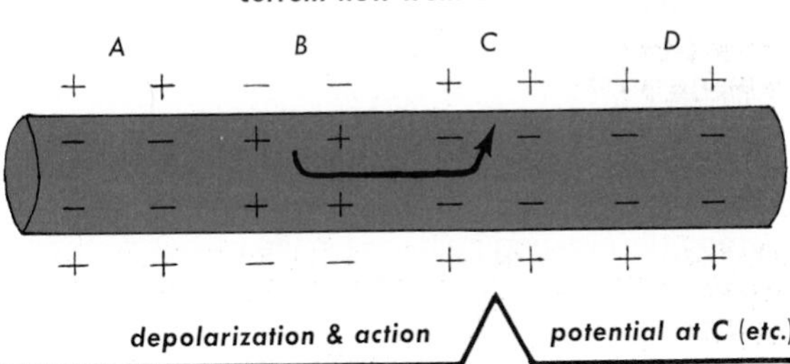

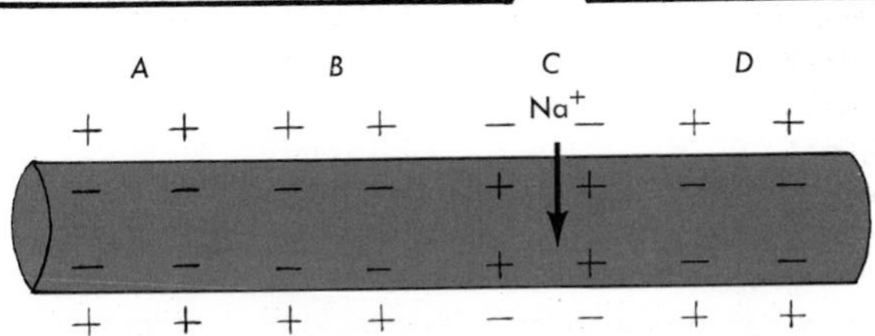

Figure 48-2 Propagation of the nerve impulse along an unmyelinated nerve fiber. *(From E. J. Reith et al., Textbook of Anatomy and Physiology, 2d ed., McGraw-Hill Book Company, New York, 1978.)*

wise. This is called *saltatory* ("hopping") *conduction* (Fig. 48-3).

The synapse

A *synapse* is a region of specialized contact between neurons where an impulse is transmitted. There may be thousands of synaptic junctions on one neuron. In order for this transmission to occur there must be a presynaptic terminal, a synaptic cleft, and a postsynaptic membrane (Fig. 48-4). The *presynaptic terminals* contain synaptic vesicles on the synaptic knob. When an action potential arrives at the synaptic knob, the synaptic vesicles release their contents, neurotransmitters, into the synaptic cleft. Mitochondria in the axon supply the ATP to synthesize new transmitter substances.

The *synaptic cleft* is the microscopic space between the presynaptic terminal and the receptor area of the effector cell. The *postsynaptic membrane* (sometimes referred to as the *subsynaptic membrane*) is the area of the effector membrane that is proximal to the presynaptic terminal.

Neurotransmitters

Neurotransmitters are chemical agents involved in the transmission of an impulse across the synaptic cleft. Some neurotransmitters are excitatory, causing the postsynaptic neuron to depolarize more readily because of increasing permeability to sodium. This type of synaptic input results in an excitatory postsynaptic potential (EPSP). Other neurotransmitters are inhibitory, causing the postsynaptic neuron to become hyperpolarized because of increased permeability to potassium and more resistant to the firing of an action potential. This type of synaptic input results in an inhibitory postsynaptic potential (IPSP). The membrane site determines whether the synapse is excitatory or inhibitory. A given transmitter may be excitatory at one synapse and inhibitory at another.

Every one of the hundreds to thousands of synaptic connections on a single neuron has an influence. Sometimes the net effect of the input is excitatory and sometimes it is inhibitory. The net effect of the synaptic input depends on the number of presynaptic neurons that are releasing neurotransmitters on the postsynaptic cell and their type of influence (excitatory or inhibitory). A presynaptic cell that releases an excitatory neurotransmitter does not always cause the postsynaptic cell to depolarize enough to generate an action potential. But when many presynaptic cells release excitatory neurotransmitters on a single neuron, the sum of their input is enough to generate an action potential. The presynaptic input can be summed by the number of presynaptic cells firing

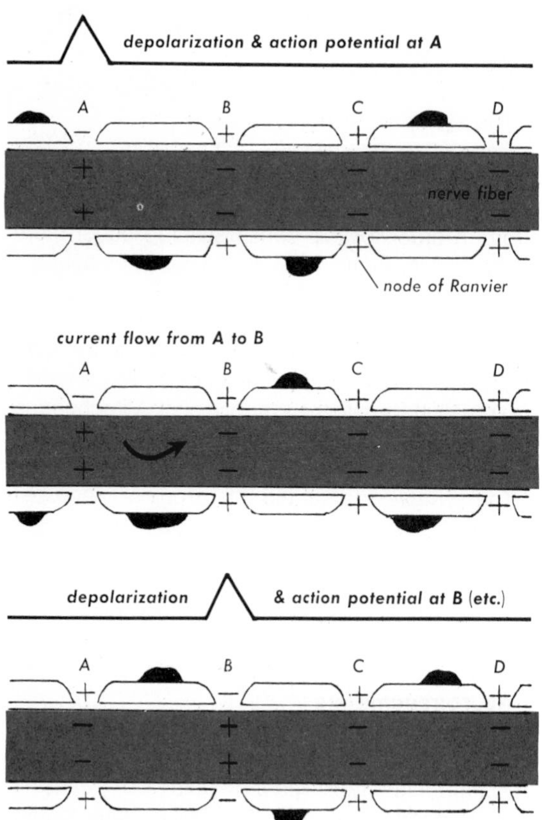

Figure 48-3 Propagation of the nerve impulse along a myelinated nerve fiber. *(From E. J. Reith et al., Textbook of Anatomy and Physiology, 2d ed., McGraw-Hill Book Company, New York, 1978.)*

(*spatial summation*) and/or by the frequency of firing of a single presynaptic cell (*temporal summation*). Summation usually occurs by both events.

Several substances are known to have neurotransmitter properties. The best-known excitatory neurotransmitters in the CNS are acetycholine, norepinephrine, serotonin, dopamine, and histamine. The inhibitory transmitters are gamma-aminobutyric acid (GABA) and glycine. Each neuron can secrete only one type of transmitter substance at its terminals.

Chemical transmitters continue to combine with the membrane sites at the postsynaptic membrane until it is inactivated by another chemical substance, is taken up by the presynaptic endings, or diffuses away from the synaptic region. In addition, the neurotransmitters can be affected by drugs and toxins, which can modify their function or block the membrane site on the postsynaptic membrane and prevent combination.

The most interesting potential neurotransmitter substances, discovered in 1975, are the *enkephalins* and *endorphins*. These are endogenous peptides, all of which are fragments of the hormonal protein β-lipotropin, which have morphinelike properties. After the discovery of opiate receptor sites in the brain and spinal cord during drug abuse research, investigators searched for endogenous opiatelike compounds. They were assumed to exist because there were naturally occurring receptors for them. These compounds were isolated and their chemical makeup identified from brain extracts. They were proved to have morphinelike properties by the fact that their analgesic-anesthetic effects were reversed by the administration of naloxone, a narcotic antagonist. The pituitary gland contains high levels of beta-endorphin. Enkephalins are known to exist in the intestine as well as in the CNS.[1]

Central Nervous System

Spinal cord

Structure Major structural components of the CNS are the cerebral hemispheres, the cerebellum, the brainstem, and the spinal cord. The *spinal cord* is continuous with the brainstem and exits from the cranial cavity through the *foramen magnum*. A cross section of the spinal cord (Fig. 48-5) reveals gray matter which is centrally located in an H shape and is surrounded by white matter. Gray matter contains the cell bodies of voluntary motor neurons and preganglionic autonomic motor neurons, as well as cell bodies of association neurons (*interneurons*). Certain subdivisions within the gray matter have been identified (see Chap. 50). White matter contains the axons of the ascending sensory and descending (suprasegmental) motor fibers. The myelin surrounding these fibers gives them their white appearance. Specific ascending and descending pathways in the white matter can be identified. The spinal pathways or tracts are named for the structures innervated and the direction in which the impulses travel, e.g., spinocerebellar tract (ascending), corticospinal tract (descending). The major spinal pathways are presented in Fig. 48-5.

Ascending Tracts In general the ascending tracts carry specific sensory input to higher levels of the CNS. The *fasciculus gracilis* and the *fasciculus cuneatus* (commonly called the dorsal or posterior columns) carry impulses concerned with touch, deep pressure, vibration, position sense, and kinesthesia (appreciation of movement). The *spinocerebellar tracts* carry subconscious sensations of muscle tension and body position to the cerebellum for coordination of movement in the lower extremities. The *lateral*

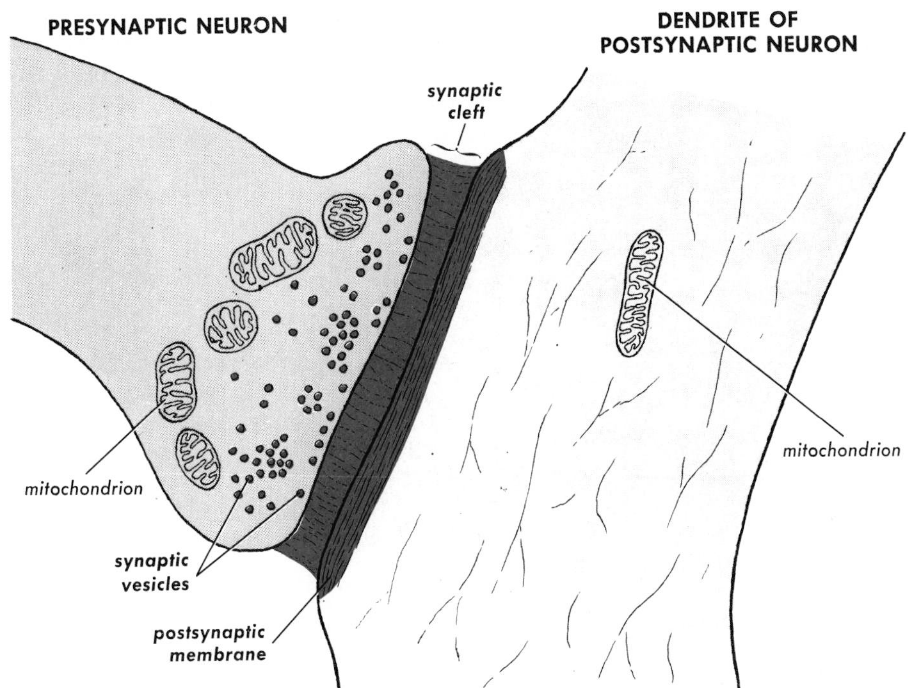

Figure 48-4 A synapse. *(From E. J. Reith et al., Textbook of Anatomy and Physiology, 2d ed., McGraw-Hill Book Company, New York, 1978.)*

spinothalamic, anterior spinothalamic, and spinoreticulothalamic tracts transmit impulses for pain and temperature, while the *anterior spinothalamic* tract is concerned with light touch.

Receptors are located throughout the body to receive incoming stimuli. Receptors are present in the skin for general sensations such as pain and touch. Special sensations such as taste, vision, smell, position, movement, and hearing are received by special receptors. The sensory input received by receptors may be integrated into spinal reflexes, or it may be relayed to the higher centers of the brain via ascending pathways.

While these pathways are generally accepted, there is still some controversy over the possibility that other ascending tracts also carry sensory modalities. The symptoms of various neurological diseases suggests that there are additional pathways for touch, position sense, and vibration besides the ones listed here.

Descending Tracts Descending tracts carry impulses which are responsible for motor movement, the major output of the CNS. Among the most important descending tracts are the *corticobulbar* and *corticospinal* (collectively called the *pyramidal tract*). These tracts carry volitional impulses from the cortex to the cranial and peripheral nerves, respectively. Another group of descending motor tracts carry impulses from the *extrapyramidal system*, which includes all motor systems (except the pyramidal system) concerned with voluntary movement. It includes descending pathways originating in the brainstem, the basal ganglia, and the cerebellum.

Lower and Upper Motor Neurons Both lower and upper motor neurons play a part in motor output. *Lower motor neurons* consist of motor nuclei of cranial nerves, the motor cells in the anterior horns of the spinal cord, and their axons. They are located in both cranial and spinal nerves. The anterior horn motor neuron with its axonal termination in skeletal muscle is the final pathway connecting an impulse from the CNS to skeletal muscle (somatic effectors).[2]

Upper motor neurons are motor cells which originate in the cerebral cortex and project downward. One part (the corticobulbar tract) ends in the brainstem and the other (the corticospinal) crosses in the lower medulla and descends into the spinal cord.[3] Basically, an upper motor neuron is one that connects with the motor neurons of the cranial nerves or the anterior horn cell of the spinal cord.[4] Upper motor

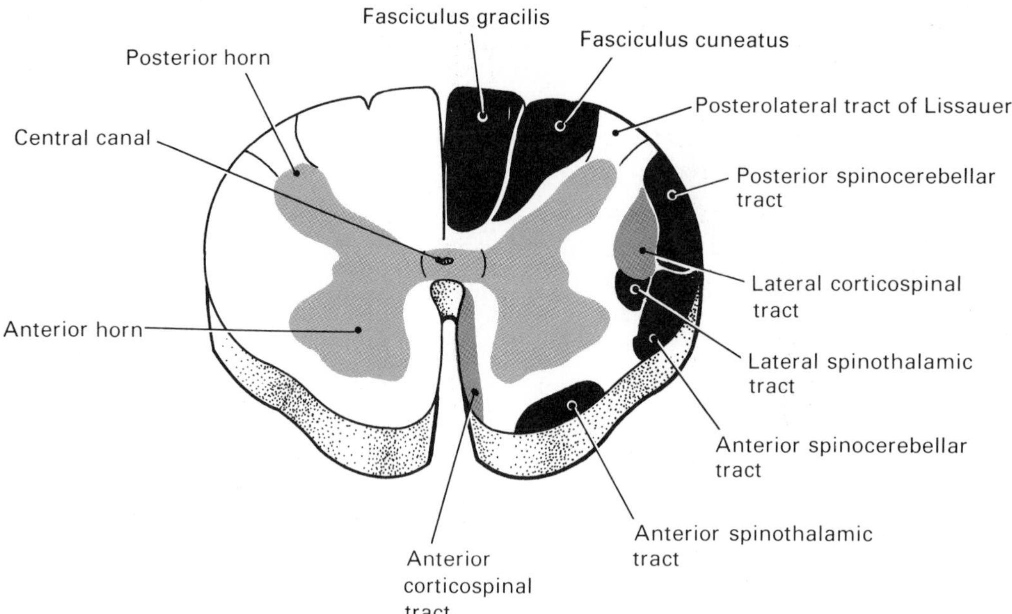

Figure 48-5 Schematic cross section of spinal cord showing arrangement of gray matter and white matter. Major ascending (sensory) tracts of the white matter are indicated in black; major descending (motor) tracts are in color. Zones of the gray matter are discussed in Chap. 50.

neurons are located entirely within the central nervous system. Lesions of the upper motor neurons result in loss of voluntary movement. The different characteristics of muscle response and weakness produced by upper motor neuron and lower motor neuron lesions can help locate the site of disease.

Reflex Arc A motor impulse may reach a skeletal muscle by way of a *simple reflex arc* (Fig. 48-6). These arcs, or loops, are responsible for automatic fixed motor responses to sensory stimuli. The resulting muscle contraction occurs as impulses pass through the lower motor neuron (anterior horn cell) and onto

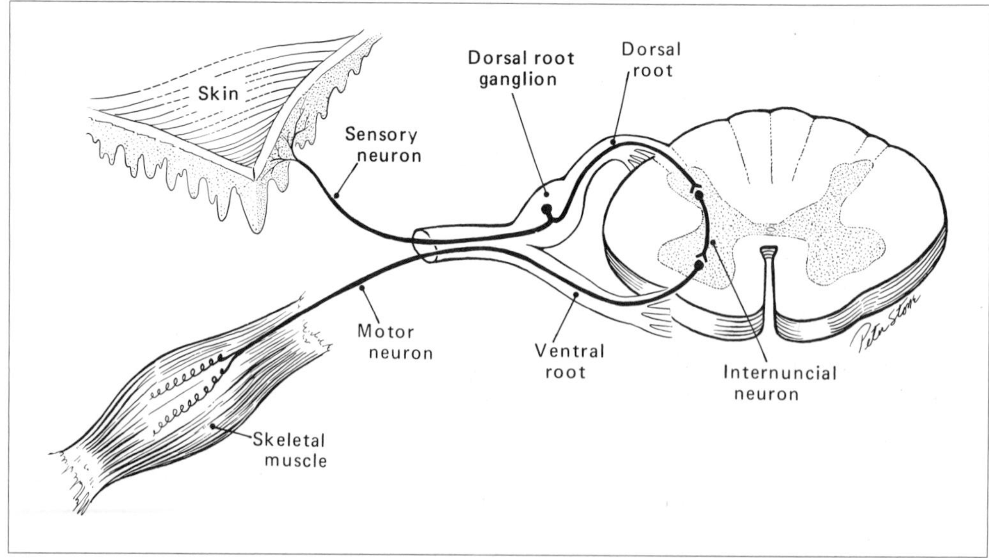

Figure 48-6 Components of a simple reflex: a sensory, an internuncial, and a motor neuron. *(From L. L. Langley et al., Dynamic Anatomy and Physiology, 5th ed., McGraw-Hill Book Company, New York, 1980, p. 287.)*

the effector organ. Although a complex phenomena, a reflex arc basically involves a sensory receptor response to an external stimulus. An afferent root neuron conveys the impulse via peripheral nerves to nuclei within the gray matter of the spinal cord. The afferent root neuron synapses directly with lower motor neurons or with interneurons before synapsing with the lower motor neurons. The lower motor neuron transmits influences to the striated voluntary muscles.[5]

Brain

Cerebrum The brain is divided into the cerebrum, the brainstem, and the cerebellum. Another method of subdividing the brain is shown in Fig. 48-7. The cerebrum and the diencephalon are divided into right and left hemispheres, and each hemisphere is further divided into five lobes: the frontal, parietal, temporal, and occipital lobes and the insula of Reil (Fig. 48-8). Gray matter (cell bodies, nerve fibers, and neuroglia) covers the surface of the brain and is called the *cerebral cortex*. Gray matter is also found deep within the cerebrum. White matter (nerve fibers and neuroglia with myelinated axons) lies between the cortex and basal ganglia.

The functions of the cerebrum are multiple and complex. Specific areas of the cerebral cortex are associated with specific functions. Table 48-1 summarizes the location and function of the parts of the cerebrum.

Brainstem The brainstem includes the midbrain, the pons, and the medulla. Ascending and descending fibers pass through the brainstem going to and from the cerebrum. Discrete areas of white and gray matter are present. The brainstem also contains areas with a mixture of gray and white matter called the *reticular formation*. The reticular formation has specific functions related to excitation and inhibition of motor activity. This area, along with the hypothalamus, is also necessary to initiate and maintain wakefulness. Additionally, the brainstem must be considered when discussing the functions of cranial nerves, since the cranial nerve nuclei are located there.

The vital centers concerned with respiratory, vasomotor, and cardiac function are located in the brainstem. The brainstem also contains the centers for sneezing, coughing, hiccoughing, vomiting, sucking, and swallowing.[6]

Telencephalon (cerebral cortex, basal ganglia) } Cerebrum
Diencephalon* (thalamus and hypothalamus) } Cerebrum

Mesencephalon (midbrain) } Brainstrem
Metencephalon (pons with cerebellum excluded) } Bulb } Brainstrem
Myelencephalon (medulla oblongata) } Bulb } Brainstrem

*Sometimes considered a part of the brainstem

Figure 48-7 Subdivisions of the brain. (*Adapted from Charles R. Noback and Robert J. Demarest, The Nervous System: Introduction and Review, McGraw-Hill Book Company, New York, 1977, p. 7.*)

Cerebellum The cerebellum is located in the posterior cranial fossa under the occipital lobe of the cerebrum. Both white and gray matter are found in the cerebellum. The cerebellum regulates coordination of muscle activity, maintenance of muscle tone, and equilibrium. In order to carry out this function, the cerebellum receives information from the cerebral cortex, muscles, joints, and inner ear.

Ventricles and Cerebral Spinal Fluid There are several nonnervous structures within the CNS which are important for understanding the effects of nervous system dysfunction. The *ventricles* are four fluid-filled cavities within the brain that connect with one another and with the spinal canal. The lower portion of the fourth ventricle becomes the spinal canal in the lower brainstem. The spinal canal extends the full length of the spinal cord and runs down the center of it.

The ventricles and spinal canal are filled with an average of 135 mL of *cerebrospinal fluid* (CSF). This fluid provides cushioning for the brain and spinal cord, allows fluid shifts from the cranial cavity to the spinal cavity, and may serve to carry nutrients. The CSF is formed primarily by dialysis of plasma across the walls of the *choroid plexuses* lining the ventricles; therefore its composition is similar to that of extracellular fluid. Although CSF is continually being formed, many physiological factors influence rate of formation. The CSF circulates throughout the ventricles and seeps into the subarachnoid space surrounding the brain and spinal cord. It is absorbed primarily through the *arachnoid villi*—tiny projections into the subarachnoid space and into the intradural venous sinuses and eventually into the venous system. The analysis of CSF composition provides useful diagnostic information related to certain nervous system diseases.

Peripheral Nervous System

The peripheral nervous system (PNS) includes all the nerve structures that lie outside the CNS. It con-

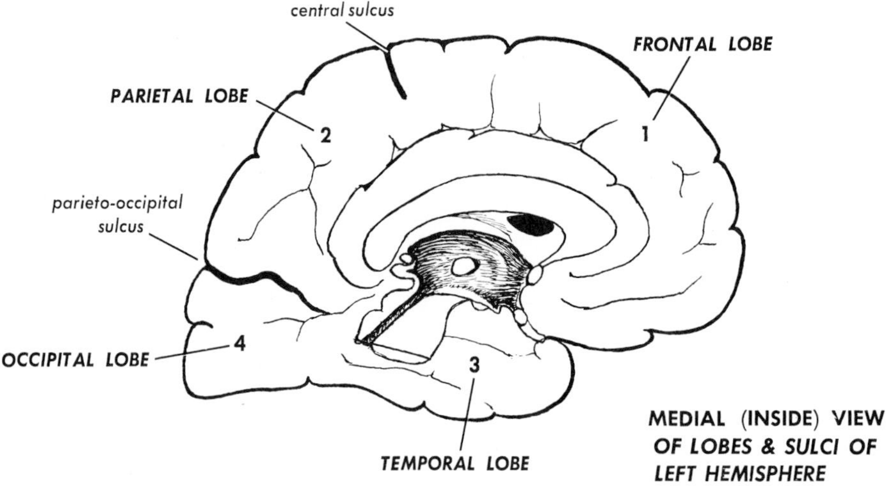

Figure 48-8 Lobes of the cerebrum. *(From E. J. Reith et al., Textbook of Anatomy and Physiology, 2d ed., McGraw-Hill Book Company, New York, 1978.)*

sists of cranial and spinal nerves, their associated ganglia (groupings of cell bodies), and portions of the autonomic nervous system.

Spinal nerves

The spinal cord can be seen as a series of spinal segments, one on top of another. Each segment contains a pair of dorsal (afferent) sensory nerve fibers or roots and ventral (efferent) motor fibers or roots, in addition to their cell bodies, which innervate a specific region of the neck, trunk, or limbs. This combined motor-sensory nerve is called a *spinal nerve* (Fig. 48-9). The cell bodies of the voluntary motor system are located in the anterior horn of the spinal cord gray matter. The cell bodies of the autonomic (involuntary) motor system are located in the anterolateral portion of spinal cord gray matter. The cell bodies of sensory fibers are located in the dorsal root ganglia just outside the spinal cord. Upon exiting the spinal column, each spinal nerve divides into *ventral* and *dorsal rami*, a collection of motor and sensory fibers that eventually go to peripheral structures (skin, muscle, viscera). The sympathetic ganglia are attached to the ventral rami of the spinal nerves by gray and white *rami communicantes*.

A *dermatome* is the area of skin innervated by the sensory fibers of a single dorsal root of a spinal nerve. A *myotome* is a muscle group innervated by the primary motor neurons of a single ventral root. These are simple components in the embryonic stage of human development. However, in the adult the dermatomes and myotomes of a given spinal segment overlap with those of adjacent segments because of the development of ascending and descending collateral branches of nerve fibers. For practical purposes, however, the dermatomes give a general picture of somatic sensory innervation by spinal segments.

Cranial nerves

The cranial nerves are the 12 paired nerves which exit from the cranial cavity. Unlike the spinal nerves, which always have both afferent sensory and efferent motor fibers, some cranial nerves have only afferent and some only efferent fibers. Others have both. Table 48-2 summarizes the motor and sensory components of the cranial nerves. Just as the cell bodies of spinal nerves are located in specific segments of the spinal cord, the cell bodies (nuclei) of the cranial nerves are located in specific regions (segments) of the brainstem. Exceptions are the nuclei of the olfactory nerve and the optic nerve: the primary cell bodies of the olfactory nerve are located in the nasal epithelium, and those of the optic nerve are in the retina. Cranial nerve XI is actually a spinal nerve whose efferent fibers migrate upward before exiting the neuroaxis at the level of the medulla.

Autonomic nervous system

The autonomic nervous system (ANS) governs involuntary functions of cardiac muscle, smooth (involuntary) muscle, and glands. Until recently it was thought that these functions could not be consciously controlled. However, research in biofeedback and studies of Asian cultures indicate that many of these "involuntary" functions can be voluntarily affected.

The ANS is divided into two components,

Table 48-1
The Cerebrum

Part	Location	Function
Cortical areas		
Motor:		
Primary	Anterior central gyrus	Controls activity of skeletal muscle on opposite side of body
Premotor	Anterior to precentral gyri	Involved in movements of a generalized area, e.g., twisting the head
Somesthetic (sensory):	Posterior central gyrus	Registers general sensation such as heat, cold, touch, pressure, pain, and proprioception (muscle sense) from opposite side of body
Visual	Occipital lobe	Receives impressions for vision
Auditory	Superior temporal gyrus	Receives auditory impulses
Smell/taste	Medial surface of temporal lobe; ventral aspect of postcentral gyrus of parietal lobe	Receive impulses for smell and taste
Association areas	Parietal lobe	Integrates sensory information from somesthetic, auditory, visual, and gustatory areas; correlates information about body parts
	Posterior regions of temporal lobe	Integrate sensory data related to vision and hearing
	Anterior portion of temporal lobe	Integrates past experiences
	Anterior part of frontal lobe	Associated with processes of higher order such as judgment, reasoning, and abstraction
Basal ganglia	Masses of gray matter within substance of each cerebral hemisphere	Associated with cerebral cortex and cerebellum to regulate motor activity, provide postural adjustments for specific voluntary acts; involved in habitual voluntary activity
Thalamus	Deep in each cerebral hemisphere	Sensory relay station where impulses synapse on way to cortex; primitive sensory center registering crude sensation
Hypothalamus	Below the thalamus	Produces oxytocin and vasopressin; contains centers which regulate anterior pituitary gland, autonomic nervous system, body temperature, food and water intake; involved in wakefulness and emotion
Limbic system	Alongside the hypothalamus in each hemisphere	Involved in behaviors and associated emotional expressions concerned with self-preservation, e.g., feeding, socializing, sexual activity

Adapted from E. J. Reith et al., *Textbook of Anatomy and Physiology*, 2d ed., McGraw-Hill Book Company, New York, 1978.

sympathetic and *parasympathetic*, which are anatomically as well as functionally different. Together these two systems function to maintain a relatively balanced internal environment. The autonomic nervous system is considered an efferent system and consists of a presynaptic neuron, a synapse, and a postsynaptic neuron.

The preganglionic cell bodies of the sympathetic nervous system (SNS) are located in spinal segments T1 to L2. The sympathetic ganglia, which contain the cell bodies of the postganglionic neurons, lie close to the spinal column, along the vertebral bodies in the rami communicantes. These ganglia and the connecting nerves are called the *paravertebral chain*. The major neurotransmitter released by the postganglionic fibers of the SNS is norepinephrine.

In contrast, the preganglionic cell bodies of the parasympathetic nervous system (PNS) are located in

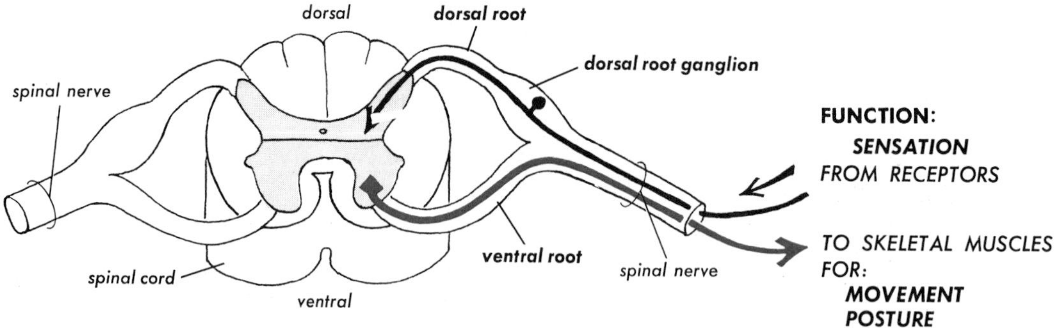

Figure 48-9 A pair of spinal nerves emerging from a spinal cord segment. *(From E. J. Reith et al., Textbook of Anatomy and Physiology, 2d ed., McGraw-Hill Book Company, New York, 1978.)*

the brainstem and the sacral spinal segments (S2 to S4). The parasympathetic ganglia are located in or near the structures which they innervate. Acetylcholine is the neurotransmitter released at both pre- and postganglionic nerve endings.

The ANS provides dual and often reciprocal innervation to many structures. For example, the SNS increases the rate and force of the heartbeat and the PNS decreases the rate and force. The SNS dilates bronchi and bronchioles of the lungs and the PNS constricts them. Some structures are innervated by only one system: e.g., the hair follicles and the sweat glands, which are innervated only by the SNS. Table 48-3 compares the sympathetic and parasympathetic nervous systems.

The result of SNS stimulation is activation of mechanisms required for "fight or flight," a mass response throughout the body. The PNS, on the other hand, is geared to act in localized and discrete regions. It serves to conserve and restore the energy stores of the body.

Cerebral Circulation

The blood supply of the brain comes from the *internal carotid arteries* and the *vertebral arteries*. Knowledge of the distribution of the major arteries of the brain as well as the area supplied is essential for understanding and diagnosing the signs and symptoms of cerebral vascular disease and trauma (Table 48-4).

The internal carotid artery supplies the ipsilateral hemisphere, whereas the *basilar artery*, formed by the junction of the two vertebral arteries, supplies structures within the *posterior fossa* (cerebellum and brainstem). The *circle of Willis* arises from the basilar artery and the two internal carotid arteries. This vascular circle may act as a safety valve when differential pressures are present in these arteries. It also may function as an anastomotic pathway when occlusion of a major artery occurs. In general, the two *anterior communicating arteries* supply the medial portion of the frontal lobes. The two *middle cerebral arteries* supply the outer portions of the frontal, parietal, and superior temporal lobes. The two *posterior communicating arteries* supply the medial portions of the occipital and inferior temporal lobes. Venous blood drains from the brain via the dural sinuses, which form veins that drain into the two jugular veins.

Blood-brain barrier

The *blood-brain barrier* is a physiological barrier between blood capillaries and brain tissue. Brain capillaries are selectively permeable to certain substances, unlike other capillaries in the body. Some substances which normally pass readily into most tissues are prevented from entering brain tissue. This barrier protects the brain from certain potentially harmful agents, while allowing nutrients to enter. The blood-brain barrier affects the penetration of pharmaceutical agents and must be considered when managing problems. Lipid-soluble compounds enter the brain easily, while water-soluble and ionized drugs enter the brain and spinal cord slowly.[7]

Protective Structures

Meninges

The meninges are three layers of protective membranes which surround the brain and spinal cord. The thick *dura* forms the outermost layer, followed by the *arachnoid* and *pia*. The *falx cerebri* which lines the longitudinal fissure and separates the two hemispheres prevents expansion of brain tissue in cases of rapidly growing tumors, acute hemorrhage, and the like. The expanding brain must squeeze under this structure, causing displacement toward the side op-

Table 48-2
Components and Functions of Cranial Nerves

Name	Components	Functions (Major)
I. Olfactory nerve	Special visceral afferent (SVA)	Smell
II. Optic nerve	Special somatic afferent (SSA)	Vision and associated reflexes
III. Oculomotor nerve*	General somatic efferent (GSE)	Movements of eyes
	General visceral efferent (GVE) (parasympathetic)	Pupillary constriction and accommodation
IV. Trochlear nerve*	General somatic efferent (GSE)	Movements of eyes
V. Trigeminal nerve	Special visceral efferent (SVE)	Mastication Swallowing Movements of soft palate and auditory tube Movements of tympanic membrane and car ossicles
	General somatic afferent (GSA)	General sensations from anterior half of head, including face, nose, mouth, and meninges
	General visceral afferent (GVA)	Visceral sensibility
VI. Abducent nerve†	General somatic efferent (GSE)	Movements of eyes
VII. Facial nerve	Special visceral efferent (SVE)	Facial expression Elevation of hyoid bone Movement of stapes
	General visceral efferent (GVE) (parasympathetic)	Lacrimation, salivation, and vasodilatation
	Special visceral afferent (SVA)	Taste
	General visceral afferent (GVA)	Visceral sensibility
VIII. Vestibulocochlear nerve (acoustic)	Special somatic afferent (SSA)	Hearing and equilibrium reception
IX. Glossopharyngeal nerve	Special visceral efferent (SVE)	Swallowing movements Raises pharynx and larynx
	General visceral efferent (GVE) (parasympathetic)	Salivation and vasodilatation
	Special visceral afferent (SVA)	Taste
	General afferent (GSA, GVA)	General senses in region of posterior third of tongue, tonsils, and upper pharynx Receptors of carotid sinus and carotid body
X. Vagus nerve and cranial root of nerve XI	Special visceral efferent (SVE)	Swallowing movements and laryngeal control Movements of soft palate, pharynx, and larynx
	General visceral efferent (GVE) (parasympathetic)	Parasympathetic to thoracic and abdominal viscera
	Special visceral afferent (SVA)	Taste (epiglottis)
	General visceral afferent (GVA)	Sensory from viscera of neck (larynx, trachea, and esophagus), thorax and abdomen
	General visceral afferent (GVA)	Visceral sensibility
XI. Accessory nerve (spinal root)	Special visceral efferent (SVE)	Movements of shoulder and head
XII. Hypoglossal nerve*	General somatic efferent (GSE)	Movements of tongue

*General somatic afferent (GSA)—proprioception from the muscles of the eye and tongue.
†General somatic afferent (GSA)—cutaneous sense from small portion of and just behind external ear and external auditory meatus.
Charles R. Noback and Robert J. Demarest, *The Human Nervous System: Basic Principles of Neurobiology,* 3d ed., McGraw-Hill Book Company, New York, 1981, p. 250.

Table 48-3

Some Comparisons between the Sympathetic and Parasympathetic Nervous Systems

General features	Sympathetic Nervous System	Parasympathetic Nervous System
Outflow from CNS	Thoracolumbar levels	Craniosacral levels
Location of ganglia	Paravertebral and prevertebral ganglia close to CNS	Terminal ganglia near effectors
Ratio of preganglionic to postganglionic neurons	Each preganglionic neuron synapses with many postganglionic neurons	Each preganglionic neuron synapses with a few postganglionic neurons
Distribution in body	Throughout the body	Limited primarily to viscera of head, thorax, abdomen, and pelvis
Metabolism	Energy mobilization during emergency	Conservation and restoration of energy resources
General homeostasis	Central mechanism to obtain mass discharge of system	No central mechanism to obtain mass discharge of system
Specific structures		
Eye:		
Radial muscle of iris	Dilation of pupil (mydriasis)	
Sphincter muscle of iris		Contraction of pupil (miosis)
Ciliary muscle (accommodation)	Relaxation for far vision	Contraction for near vision
Glands of head:		
Lacrimal gland		Stimulates secretion
Salivary glands	Scanty thick, viscous secretion	Profuse, watery secretion
Heart:		
Rate	Increases	Decreases
Force of ventricular contraction	Increases	No direct effect
Blood vessels	Generally constricts*	Slight effect
Lungs:		
Bronchial tubes	Dilates lumen	Stimulates constriction of lumen
Bronchial glands	Inhibits secretion	Stimulates secretion
Gastrointestinal tract:		
Motility and tone	Inhibits	Stimulates
Sphincters	Stimulates	Inhibits (relax)
Secretion	May inhibit	Stimulates
Gallbladder and ducts	Inhibits	Stimulates
Liver	Glycogenolysis increase (blood sugar)	
Spleen (capsule)	Contracts	
Adrenal medulla	Secretion of epinephrine* and norepinephrine	
Sex organs	Vasoconstriction, constriction of vas deferens, seminal vesicle, and prostatic musculature (ejaculation)	Vasodilatation and erection
Skin:		
Sweat glands	Stimulates*	None
Blood vessels	Constricts	Slight effect
Pilomotor	Contracts	
Urinary tract:		
Ureter (motility and tone)	Increases	
Bladder detrusor	Relaxation (usually)	Contraction
Trigone and extension into urethra	Relaxation (see text)	Contraction
Metabolism:		
Liver	Glycogenolysis	
Adipose tissue	Free fatty acid release	
Neurochemical basis		
Neurotransmitter at neuroeffector junction	Usually norepinephrine* Adrenergic	Acetylcholine Cholinergic
Inactivation of transmitter	Slow and re-uptake	Rapid
Reinforcement in body	Secretion of norepinephrine and epinephrine by adrenal medulla	

*Exceptions: Some postganglionic neurons of the sympathetic nervous system are cholinergic neurons. Sympathetic neuroeffector transmission mediated by acetylcholine includes (1) some blood vessels in skeletal muscles and (2) most sweat glands. The sweat glands of the palms are innervated by adrenergic fibers. The adrenal medulla is innervated by preganglionic cholinergic sympathetic neurons.

Charles R. Noback and Robert J. Demarest, *The Human Nervous System: Basic Principles of Neurobiology,* 3d ed., McGraw-Hill Book Company, New York, 1981, p. 224.

Table 48-4
Areas Supplied by Cerebral Circulation

Artery	Area Supplied
Internal carotid	Most of cerebrum (including most of the diencephalon) except those areas supplied by the vertebral arterial system
Vertebral	Medulla, pons, midbrain, caudal portion of the diencephalon, cerebellum, medial and inferior regions of temporal and occipital lobes, and small variable portions of the lateral regions of temporal, parietal, and occipital lobes

Adapted from Charles B. Noback and Robert J. Demarest, *The Human Nervous System: Basic Principles of Neurobiology,* 3d ed., McGraw-Hill Book Company, New York, 1981, pp. 30–31.

posite the lesion. The *tentorium cerebelli* folds under the temporal lobes, separating the cerebral hemispheres from the brainstem and the cerebellum. Expanding mass lesions force the brain to herniate through the only opening in this thick layer, the opening created by the brainstem. This is referred to as *tentorial herniation*.

Although the dura is adherent to the cranial bone, large arteries are present in this area. These vessels pierce the dura and become subdural. A subarachnoid space exists between the dura and arachnoid mater, since these two layers do not follow the fissures as the pia does. The pia continues to be adherent to the spinal cord, resulting in a large subarachnoid space located below the tip of the spinal cord.[8] It is in this area that a spinal tap is performed.

Skull

The bony skull protects the brain from external trauma. It is composed of 8 cranial bones and 14 facial bones.

The skull cavity is significant in the pathogenesis of head injuries (see Chap. 54). Although the top and sides of the inside of the skull are relatively smooth, the bottom surface is very uneven. It has many ridges, prominences, and *foramina* (holes through which blood vessels and nerves enter and exit the brain). The largest hole is the *foramen magnum*, through which the brainstem extends to the spinal cord. This foramen offers the only major space for the expansion of brain contents during increased intracranial pressure.

Vertebral column

The vertebral column protects the spinal cord, supports the head, and provides for flexibility. The vertebral column is made up of 33 individual vertebrae: 7 cervical, 12 thoracic, 5 lumbar, 5 sacral (fused into one), and 4 coccygeal (fused into one). Each vertebra has a central opening through which the spinal cord passes. The vertebrae are held together by a series of ligaments. Intervertebral disks occupy the spaces between vertebrae.

Nerve Regeneration

Once a nerve cell dies, it is not replaced. At the time of birth, the human body contains all the nerve cells it will ever have. The body cannot make new nerve cells. If only the axon of the nerve cell is damaged, however, the cell attempts to repair itself. All nerve cells, when damaged, attempt to grow back to their original destinations by sprouting many branches from the damaged ends of their axons. Unfortunately, excessive scar formation (gliosis) in the central nervous system prevents the new nerve branches from making their former connections to other neurons.

In the peripheral nervous system (outside the brain and spinal cord), injured nerve fibers can successfully regenerate by growing within the protective myelin sheath of the supporting Schwann cells if the cell body is intact. Chances for normal regeneration are greatest when the cut ends of the peripheral nerves are close together. Still, recovery from nerve damage in the periphery is not complete. Motor movements are not as finely tuned as before, and sensory endings are not as sensitive as before.[9]

ASSESSMENT OF THE NEUROLOGICAL SYSTEM

Subjective Data: The History

There are three points to consider in taking the history of clients with neurological problems.[10] One is to avoid suggesting symptoms to the client. Caution must be used not to suggest certain symptoms to the client or ask leading questions like "Is your headache throbbing?" or "Are you weak on the right side?" It is better to ask open-ended questions like "What is your headache like?" or "What is it about your right side that bothers you?" A second point is that the mode of onset and the course of the illness are especially important aspects of the history. Often the nature of a neurological disease process can be described by these facts alone. The third point is that, since many neurological diseases affect a client's mental functioning, mental status must be accurately assessed before assuming that the history is factual. If the client cannot be considered a reliable source, the history should be obtained from a person who has firsthand knowledge of the client's problems and complaints. In many instances a history cannot be obtained and the clinician must proceed with objective data only.

The history helps to guide the approach of the neurological examination—that is, it can direct which parts of the neurological system need to be assessed closely. If the client's primary complaint is dizziness, the examination could be closely focused on visual, vestibular, and cerebellar functions rather than on somatic motor and sensory functions.

Many chief complaints, including behavioral changes, change in level of consciousness, developmental problems, paroxysmal disorders, infectious process, pain, motor or sensory aberrations, and trauma, should alert the clinician to the need for a detailed neurological examination. In addition to being a primary complaint, neurological problems are often secondary to other problems such as herpes zoster and metastatic lesions.

As stated earlier, particular attention should be given to eliciting all pertinent data in the history of the present illness (HPI), especially data related to characteristics and progression of the symptoms.

Past medical history

In eliciting data about past medical history (PMH), the client should be specifically questioned about diabetes, pernicious anemia, cancer, infections, and hypertension, since all these conditions can affect the nervous system. Any hospitalizations, injuries, or surgeries related to the neurological system should be noted. Particular attention should be given to eliciting a careful medication history related especially to the use of sedatives, narcotics, tranquilizers, and mood-elevating drugs, including over-the-counter drugs of these categories.

The perinatal history may reveal exposure to toxic agents such as viruses, alcohol, tobacco, drugs, and x-rays, which are known to adversely influence the development of the nervous system. It may reveal a difficult labor and delivery, which can cause brain damage resulting from such events as hypoxia, forceps delivery, and Rh incompatibility.

Growth and developmental history can be important in ascertaining whether nervous system dysfunction was present at an early age. The nurse should specifically inquire about major developmental tasks such as walking and talking. Success at school or identified problems in an educational setting are other important pieces of developmental data to gather. It is important to remember that often this information is not available when interviewing the older client. If the client cannot provide a detailed developmental history, the nurse should proceed with the history gathering and avoid distressing the client by further probing.

Family history

The purpose of gathering a careful family history is to determine whether the neurological problem might have a hereditary or congenital background. Specifically, the client should be questioned about familial history of such disorders as epilepsy, amyotrophic lateral sclerosis, Parkinson's disease, Huntington's chorea, muscular dystrophy, mental retardation, alcoholism, and emotional problems.

Personal and social history

The standard information gathered in the client profile can provide much information related to actual or potential neurological problems. A major area to assess is the presence of change in any previously established routine of daily living. Changes related to sleep, exercise, recreation, occupation, stressors, and sexual practices can have specific neurological implications and need to be carefully investigated.

Review of Systems

Specific problems to inquire about related to review of systems include the following:

1. General behavior change
2. Mood change
3. Loss of consciousness
4. Anxiety or nervousness
5. Seizures
6. Speech problems
7. Memory deficits
8. Motor problem such as imbalance, paralysis, tic, or tremor
9. Sensory problems such as pain or paresthesea

Following a careful assessment of system information, it is good practice to ask someone who knows the client well if he or she has noted any changes in the client either mentally or physically. Often the client with a neurological problem is not aware of it or is unable to provide enough specific data to aid in the diagnosis.

General survey

The general survey statement can provide much important data related to the neurological status of a client such as grooming, behavioral observations, facies, gait, posture, and communicative patterns. In addition to providing currently useful data, a well-written general survey provides baseline data for future comparison.

Objective Data: The Neurological Examination

There are two approaches to neurological assessment, the medical model and the nursing approach. The primary purposes of the medical neurological examination are to (1) locate the lesion and diagnose the illness; (2) determine the progression, stability, or improvement of neurological dysfunction; and (3) detect life-threatening neurological dysfunction. The choice of particular items of the examination depends on the purpose for which it is done. The approach used to assess an unconscious client who is brought to the emergency room with a head injury is different from that used to assess a conscious ambulatory client who presents with headache.

A different approach to the neurological exam has been proposed for nursing purposes. The primary purposes of the nursing neurological examination are to determine the effects of neurological dysfunction on daily living in light of the client's and his family's ability to cope with the neurological deficits. While the method of gathering data may be the same, the interpretation of the data is different from the medical model. The standard medical model of the neurological exam is presented first, as it can be used for nursing purposes also. This is followed by an explanation of how the assessment data can be interpreted for nursing purposes. It should be noted that nurses share with physicians the responsibility for assessing life-threatening neurological dysfunction. However, it is beyond the scope of this chapter to present that approach.

The standard approach to the neurological examination is primarily by inspection. This examination is usually divided into five parts to assist the examiner to proceed in an orderly manner: mental status, cranial nerves, motor system (including cerebellar functioning and proprioception), sensory examination, and reflexes. It can be adapted for each individual, on the basis of the purpose of the examination.

Mental status (cerebral functioning)

Assessment of mental status gives an indication of how the client is functioning as a whole and how he is adapting to his environment. It involves assessment of complex and high-level cerebral functions which are governed by many areas of the cerebral cortex. Much of the area covered in this part of the examination is assessed during the history and therefore does not need to be further assessed. For instance, language and memory can be assessed when asking the client for details of his illness and significant past events. The client's cultural and educational background should be taken into account when assessing mental status.

Components of the mental status examination are:

1. *General appearance and behavior.* This includes motor activity, body posture, dress and hygiene, facial expression, and speech.
2. *Sensorium.* The client must be conscious before other functions can be determined. Note orientation to time, place, and person. Note memory, fund of information, insight, judgment, problem solving, calculation. Common questions are "Who were the last three presidents?" "What does 'a stitch in time saves nine' mean?" "Subtract 7 from 100, and keep subtracting 7." Ask yourself, "Do the client's plans and goals match his physical and mental capabilities?"
3. *Mood and affect.* Note agitation, anger, depression, or euphoria and appropriateness of these. Questions should be directed to bringing out the feelings of the client.
4. *Thought content.* Note illusions, hallucinations, delusions, paranoia.
5. *Intellectual capacity.* Note retardation, dementia, and intelligence.

Cranial nerves (Table 48-2)

Olfactory Nerve (I) After determination that both nostrils are patent, olfaction is tested by asking the client to close one nostril, close his eyes, and sniff from a bottle containing coffee, spice, soap, or some other readily recognized odor. The same is done for the other nostril. Generally, olfaction is not tested unless the client complains of some disturbance with smell. Chronic rhinitis, sinusitis, and heavy smoking can often decrease the sense of smell.

Optic Nerve (II) Visual fields and visual acuity are assessed to test the function of the optic nerve. Visual fields are assessed by confrontation. The examiner, positioned directly opposite the client, asks the client to close one eye, look directly at the bridge of the examiner's nose, and indicate when he (the client) sees an object (finger, pencil tip, head of pin) presented from the periphery of each of the four visual-field quadrants (Fig. 48-10). The same test is repeated for the other eye. The examiner uses himself as a control because he and the client are sharing the same visual field. Remember that the nasal side of the visual field is narrower because of the nasal bridge. Visual-field defects may be due to lesions of the optic

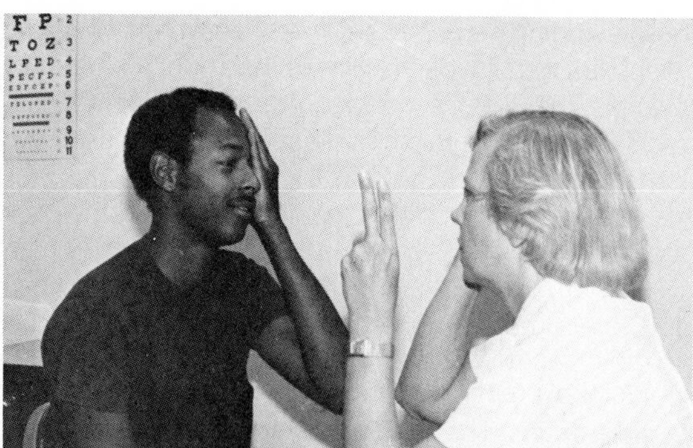

Figure 48-10 Assessing visual fields by gross confrontation.

nerve, optic chiasm, or temporal, parietal, or occipital cortex.

Visual acuity is tested by asking the client to read a Snellen chart from 20 feet away. The number on the lowest line which the client can read with 50 percent accuracy is recorded. The client should wear glasses if he has them, unless they are used only for reading. The eyes should be tested individually and together. If a Snellen chart is not available, the client can be asked to read newsprint for a gross assessment of acuity. The distance required from client to newsprint for accurate reading should be recorded. Acuity may not be testable by these means if the client does not read English, if he is retarded, or if he is aphasic.

Ophthalmoscopy reveals the physical condition of the optic disk (head of the optic nerve) as well as the retina and blood vessels. It is routinely done when the optic nerve is tested. Optic nerve atrophy and papilledema can be detected by this method. Specifics of the ophthalmoscopic exam are beyond the scope of this text.

Oculomotor (III), Trochlear (IV), and Abducens (VI) Nerves Because each of these nerves helps move the eye, they are tested together. The client is asked to follow the examiner's finger as it moves horizontally and vertically (making a cross) and diagonally (making an X). *Nystagmus* (fine jerking movements of the eyes) is noted at this time, even though it is indicative of vestibulocerebellar problems. Other functions of the oculomotor nerve are tested by checking for the pupillary light reflex and for convergence and accommodation. The examiner shines a light into the pupil of one eye and looks for ipsilateral constriction of the same pupil and contralateral (consensual) constriction of the opposite eye. The optic nerve must be intact for this reflex to occur. Convergence (eyes turning inward) and accommodation (pupils constricting with near vision) are tested by asking the client to focus on the examiner's finger as it moves toward the client's nose.

Trigeminal Nerve (V) The sensory component of the trigeminal nerve is tested by having the client identify light touch (cotton) and pinprick in each of the three divisions (ophthalmic, maxillary, and mandibular) of the nerve on both sides of the face. The client's eyes should be closed during this part of the examination. The motor component is tested by asking the client to clench his teeth and palpating the masseter muscles just above the mandibular angle. The corneal reflex test evaluates cranial nerves V and VII simultaneously. It involves having the client look up and applying a cotton wisp strand to the cornea. This reflex is not normally tested in conscious, intact clients because other tests evaluate the same thing. The sensory component of this reflex (corneal sensation) is innervated by the ophthalmic division of cranial nerve V. The motor component (eye blink) is innervated by cranial nerve VII.

Facial Nerve (VII) The facial nerve innervates the muscles of facial expression. Its function is tested by asking the client to raise his eyebrows, close his eyes tightly, draw back the corners of his mouth in an exaggerated smile, and frown. Although taste discrimination of salt and sugar in the anterior two-thirds of the tongue is a function of this nerve, it is not routinely tested unless there is an indication of a peripheral nerve lesion.

Acoustic (Vestibulocochlear) Nerve (VIII) The cochlear portion of this nerve is tested by having the client close his eyes and indicate when he hears a ticking watch or the rustling of the examiner's fingertips as the stimulus is brought closer to the ear. Each ear is tested individually, and the distance from the client's ear to the sound source when first heard is recorded. This test identifies only gross deficits in hearing. For more precise assessment of hearing, an audiometer is used (see Chap. 14). The vestibular portion of this nerve is not routinely tested unless the client complains of dizziness or unsteadiness, or has auditory dysfunction. If this is the case, caloric testing, which is beyond the scope of routine testing, may be done.

Glossopharyngeal (IX) and Vagus (X) Nerves Because both these nerves innervate the pharynx, they are tested together. The glossopharyngeal nerve is primarily sensory. In the gag reflex (bilateral contraction of the palatal muscles initiated by touching either side of the posterior pharynx with a tongue blade), the sensory component is mediated by IX, the major motor component by X. The gag reflex is not routinely tested because of its unpleasantness. Usually the client is asked to phonate by saying "Ah," and bilateral elevation of the soft palate is noted. Swallowing is also assessed.

Spinal Accessory Nerve (XI) The spinal accessory nerve is tested by asking the client to shrug his shoulders against resistance and to turn his head to either side against resistance. There should be smooth contraction of the sternomastoid and trapezius muscles.

Hypoglossal Nerve (XII) This nerve is tested by asking the client to protrude his tongue. It should protrude in the midline. The client should also be able to push his tongue to either side against the resistance of a tongue blade.

Motor system

The motor system examination includes assessment of bulk, tone, and power of the major muscle groups of the body as well as assessment of balance and coordination. The examiner tests strength by asking the client to push or pull against the resistance of the examiner's arm as it opposes flexion and extension of the client's muscle. The client should be asked to offer resistance at the forearm, wrist, knees, and ankles. Tone is tested by passively moving the limbs through their range of motion; there should be a slight resistance to these movements. Abnormal tone is described as *hypotonia* (flaccidity) or *hypertonia* (spasticity). Involuntary movements (tics, tremor, myoclonus, athetosis, chorea, dystonia) should be noted.

Posture, balance, and other acts of coordination are maintained by the proprioceptive system. The neural structures involved are the posterior column of the spinal cord, the cerebellum, and the vestibular apparatus. Posture is assessed by having the client walk to the end of the room and return. Note the posture, balance, and arm and leg movement. On turning, the head should lead the body.

Cerebellar function is tested by assessing balance and coordination. The Romberg test is conducted after observing the client walk. The client should stand with feet together and eyes open. Balance should be easily maintained. Then the client is asked to close the eyes while maintaining the same position. Balance should continue to be maintained with minimum swaying.

Coordination can be easily tested in several ways. Have the client extend the arms and touch the nose with the index finger, keeping the eyes closed. Ask the client to pronate and supinate both hands rapidly. Have the client do a shallow knee bend, first on one leg, then on the other. Test the client's grip by having him firmly grasp your hand. The heel-to-shin test consists in having the client place one heel on the opposite shin below the knee and moving the heel down the shin to the ankle. Repeat for the other leg. These movements should flow smoothly without jerking or hesitation.

Sensory examination

Several modalities are tested in the somatic sensory exam. Each modality is carried by a specific ascending pathway in the spinal cord before it reaches the sensory cortex.

There are some general guidelines for performing the sensory examination. The client should always have his eyes closed, to avoid visual clues. The examiner should avoid giving verbal cues such as "Is this sharp?" The sensory stimulus should be applied in such a way that the client does not expect it; that is, the examiner should avoid rhythmical application of the stimulus. In the routine neurological examination, sensory testing of the four extremities is sufficient.

Light Touch Light touch is usually tested first. The examiner gently strokes a cotton wisp over each of the four extremities and asks the client to indicate when he feels the stimulus by saying "touch." The sensory examination of the face may be delayed until this time, when the materials for testing sensation are brought out.

Pain and Temperature Pain is tested by touching the skin with a sharp end of a pin. This stimulus is irregularly alternated with a simple touch stimulus with the dull end of the pin to determine whether the client can distinguish the two stimuli. Extinction or inhibition is assessed by simultaneously stimulating opposite sides of the body symmetrically with either a pain or a touch stimulus. Normally the simultaneous stimuli are appreciated; appreciation of only one may indicate a parietal lesion.

The sensation of temperature is tested by applying tubes of warm and cold water to the skin and asking the client to identify the stimuli with his eyes closed. If pain sensation is intact, assessment of temperature sensation may be omitted, as both sensations are carried by the same ascending pathways.

Vibration Sense Vibration sense is assessed by applying a vibrating C-128 tuning fork to the fingernails and/or bony prominences of the hands and feet. The examiner asks the client if he feels the vibration, or "buzz." He then asks the client to indicate when the vibration ceases. The examiner stops the vibration with his hand as he desires.

Position Sense Position sense is assessed by placing the thumb and forefinger on either side of the client's forefinger or great toe and gently moving the finger or toe up or down. The client is asked to indicate the direction in which the digit is moved.

Special Sensory Examination Several special tests are done during the sensory exam. *Two-point discrimination* is assessed by placing the two points of a calibrated compass on the tips of the fingers and toes. The minimal recognizable separation is 4 to 5 mm in the fingertips and much more elsewhere. This test is important in diseases of the sensory cortex and in peripheral nerve disease. *Graphesthesia* is tested by having the client identify numbers traced on the palm of his hands. *Stereognosis* is tested by having the client identify the size and shape of easily recognized objects (coins, keys, safety pin) placed in his hands.

Reflexes

Skeletal muscles contract when their tendons are stretched. A simple stretch reflex (deep tendon reflex, or DTR) is initiated by briskly tapping the tendon of a stretched muscle (Fig. 48-11), usually with a reflex hammer. The response (muscle contraction of the corresponding muscle) is measured as follows: 0, absent; 1, weak response; 2, normal response; 3, exaggerated response; 4, hyperreflexia with clonus. Clonus is a continued rhythmic contraction of the muscle after the stimulus has been applied.

In general the biceps, triceps, brachioradialis, and patellar and Achilles tendons are tested. The examiner elicits the *biceps reflex* by striking the biceps firmly with his thumb. The client should have his arms partially flexed at the elbow with the palms down. The normal response is flexion of the arm at the elbow and contraction of the biceps muscle.

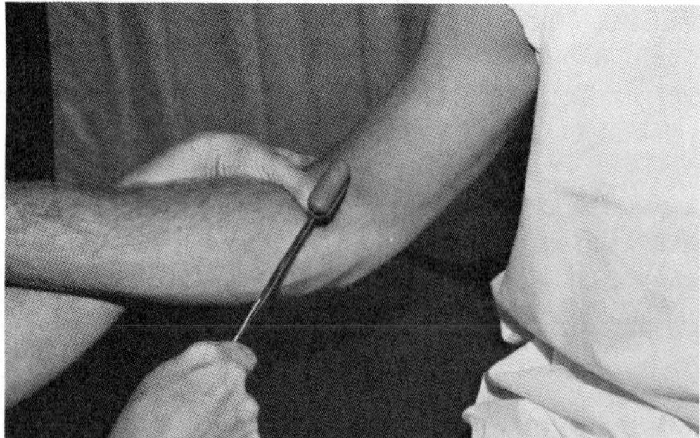

Figure 48-11 The examiner strikes a swift blow over a stretched tendon to elicit a reflex response.

The *triceps reflex* is elicited by striking the triceps tendon above the elbow, with the client's arm flexed. The normal response is extension of the arm.

The *brachioradialis reflex* is elicited by striking the radius 3 to 5 cm above the wrist, with the client's arm relaxed. The normal response is flexion and supination at the elbow.

The *patellar reflex* is elicited by striking the patellar tendon just below the patella. The client can be sitting or lying with the legs hanging freely. The normal response is extension of the leg with contraction of the quadriceps.

The *Achilles tendon reflex* is elicited by striking the Achilles tendon, with the leg flexed at the knee and the foot dorsiflexed at the ankle. The normal response is plantar flexion at the ankle.

Neurological assessment for nursing purposes

A nursing approach to the neurological examination for assessment of the stable, conscious, hospitalized patient has been developed. The premise of the nursing approach is that the primary purpose of nursing is to help clients cope effectively with deficits in self-care and in activities of daily living. Consequently, the neurological examination should be viewed in terms of functional disabilities rather than dysfunction of component parts of the nervous system.

Briefly stated, the nursing approach additionally evaluates the integrated functions of understanding, seeing, eating, speaking, feeling, moving, and eliminating. Consciousness and mentation (higher cortical functions) are assessed by determining whether the client is alert, oriented, aware of his past and present, emotionally stable, able to understand spoken and written words, and able to speak and write. Motor function is assessed by determining whether the client can move his eyes (cranial nerves III, IV, VI), eat (V, IX, X, XII), speak (VII, IX, X, XII), and move his body in a coordinated way (cerebellum, descending motor pathways, basal ganglia). Sensory function is assessed by determining whether the client can smell (I), see (II), hear (VIII), taste (VII, IX) and feel (V, ascending sensory pathways). Bowel and bladder function, which involves both motor and sensory pathways, is assessed by determining whether the client has normal elimination.

Table 48-5 is an example of how to record a normal neurological assessment. Common abnormal

Table 48-5
Recording the Normal Neurological Examination

Mental status	Alert, oriented, orderly thought processes, mood and affect appropriate.
Cranial nerves	Smells soap and coffee, visual fields full to confrontation, visual acuity 20/20 O.U., EOMs (extraocular movements) intact, no nystagmus, PERRLA (pupils equal, round, reactive to light and accommodation), facial sensation intact to touch and pinprick, facial movements full, gag and swallow reflexes intact, soft palate elevates symmetrically, turns head and shrugs shoulders against resistance, tongue protrudes in midline. (May be recorded as: cranial nerves I–XII intact.)
Motor system	Gait and station normal, tandems well, negative Romberg; muscle bulk, tone, and strength normal and bilaterally symmetric; performs finger-nose, heel-shin movements smoothly.
Sensory system	Sensation intact to light touch, position sense, vibration, pinprick, heat and cold, and two-point discrimination; stereognosis and graphesthesia intact.
Reflexes	Biceps, triceps, brachioradialis, patellar and Achilles tendon reflexes 2+ bilaterally, toes downgoing with plantar stimulation (or draw stick figure indicating reflex strength at appropriate site).

Note: If some portion of the neurological examination was not done, indicate this; e.g., "Smell not tested."

assessment findings of the neurological system are presented in Table 48-6.

DIAGNOSTIC STUDIES OF THE NERVOUS SYSTEM (TABLE 48-7)

Laboratory Studies

Cerebrospinal fluid analysis

Cerebrospinal fluid (CSF) analysis provides information about a variety of CNS diseases. Normal CSF fluid is clear, colorless, and free of red blood cells and contains few proteins. Normal CSF values are listed in Table 48-8.

Lumbar puncture

Lumbar puncture (LP) is the most common method of obtaining CSF for analysis. It is contraindicated in the presence of increased intracranial pressure (ICP) or infection at the site of puncture.

Nurses often assist in this procedure because it is usually done in the client's room. Prior to the procedure the nurse should follow the routine preoperative protocol and have the client empty his bladder. The client should lie in the lateral recumbent position, with his back as near as possible to the edge of the bed. The nurse should assist the client to draw up his knees to his abdomen and flex his head to his chest. This helps separate the vertebrae so that the needle can be inserted more easily.

Using strict sterile technique, a needle is inserted between the fourth and fifth lumbar vertebrae. This may cause some local discomfort. There is minimal danger of injuring the spinal cord, because the cord terminates at the second lumbar vertebra. However, the client may experience some pain radiating down the leg if the spinal root is irritated by the needle. The nurse can assure him that this is temporary and that he is not in danger of being paralyzed.

A manometer is attached to the needle and CSF pressure is determined *after* the client is asked to relax and extend legs. If this is not done, the pressure will appear abnormally high. Then CSF is withdrawn in a series of tubes and sent for analysis. Some believe that the client should be kept lying flat for a few hours after the procedure to avoid "spinal headache," which is presumably due to loss of the cushioning effect of CSF secondary to leakage of CSF at the puncture site. The prone position may be effective in preventing CSF leakage. Others do not feel that the lying position is necessary, as some clients seem to develop headache in spite of precautions. Some clients may develop meningeal irritation (nuchal rigidity) or signs and symptoms of local trauma (hematoma, pain).

Radiological Studies

Cerebral angiography

Cerebral angiography is indicated when vascular lesions or tumors are suspected. Two methods are used. In the direct method a radiopaque dye is injected directly into the carotid or vertebral artery. In the indirect method the femoral, brachial, or subclavian artery is used for the catheterization or injection of the carotid or vertebral arteries. By injecting radiopaque contrast medium into the selected artery, the arterial and venous distribution of that vessel can be visualized (Fig. 48-12). This study can help localize and determine the nature of tumors, abscesses, aneurysms, hematomas, arteriovenous malformations, and similar lesions.

Because this is an invasive procedure, untoward

Table 48-6
Common Abnormal Assessment Findings of the Nervous System

Finding	Definition/Description	Possible Etiology/Significance
Altered consciousness	See Table 49-2	Intracranial lesions, metabolic disorder, psychiatric disorders
Anisocoria	Inequality of pupil size	Lesion, injury, or intracranial pressure in area of midbrain
Agnosia	Inability to recognize objects through sensory perceptions	Cerebral cortex lesion
Apraxia	Inability to use an object properly despite knowing its name and function	Cerebral cortex lesion
Aphasia	Loss of language faculty (motor or sensory or both) in any form (hearing, reading, speaking, writing)	Cerebral cortex lesion
Analgesia	Loss of pain sensation	Lesion in spinothalamic tract or thalamus, lack of or damage to sensory nerve endings
Anesthesia (hyperesthesia, hypoesthesia)	Change in sensation	Lesions in spinal cord, thalamus, sensory cortex, or peripheral sensory nerve
Anosognosia	Inability to recognize a bodily defect or disease	Lesions in right parietal cortex, common in right-sided stroke
Astereognosis	Inability to recognize the form of an object by feeling it	Lesions in sensory pathways or parietal cortex
Ataxia	Lack of coordination of muscular movement	Lesions of sensory pathways, cerebellum; anticonvulsant, sedative, hypnotic drug toxicity (including alcohol)
Atrophy (muscle)	Wasting away or diminution in size of muscle	
Disuse atrophy		Suprasegmental lesions
Denervation atrophy		Segmental lesions
Bladder dysfunction		
Atonic	Absence of muscle tone and contractility, enlarged capacity, no sensation of discomfort, overflow with large residual, inability to voluntarily or reflexly empty	Associated with early stage of spinal cord injury
Hypotonic (flaccid)	Varies in degree from atonic bladder	Interruption of afferent pathways from bladder
Hypertonic (spastic)	Increased muscle tone, diminished capacity, reflex emptying, dribbling, incontinence	Lesions in pyramidal tracts (efferent pathways)
Diplopia	Double vision	Lesions affecting nerves of extraocular muscles; cerebellar toxicity
Dysarthria	Lack of coordination in articulating speech	Lesions in cerebellum or pathway of cranial nerves (including brain stem); anticonvulsant, sedative, or hypnotic drug toxicity (including alcohol)
Dyskinesia	Impairment of the power of voluntary movement, resulting in fragmentary or incomplete movements	Disorders of the basal ganglia, idiosyncratic reaction to psychotropic drugs

Table 48-6 (continued)

Finding	Definition/Description	Possible Etiology/Significance
Dysphagia	Difficulty swallowing	Lesions involving motor pathways of IX, X (includes lower brainstem)
Extensor plantar response (Babinski sign)	Upgoing toes with plantar stimulation	Suprasegmental or upper motor neuron lesion
Homonymous hemianopsia	Loss of vision in one side of visual field	Injury or lesions in area of optic tract or its radiations to occipital cortex
Hemiplegia	Loss of motor control in one side of body	Stroke and other lesions involving motor cortex
Nystagmus	Jerking or bobbing of the eyes as they track a moving object	Lesions in cerebellum, brainstem, vestibular system; anticonvulsant, sedative, hypnotic toxicity (including alcohol)
Ophthalmoplegia	Paralysis of the eye muscles	Lesions in brainstem or cranial nerves III, IV, VI
Opisthotonus	Extreme arching of the back with retraction of the head	Meningitis, tonic phase of grand mal seizure
Papilledema	"Choked disk," swelling of optic nerve head	Increased intracranial pressure
Paraplegia	Paralysis of the lower extremities	Spinal cord transection or mass lesion (thoracolumbar region)
Quadriplegia	Paralysis of all four extremities	Spinal cord transection or mass lesion (cervical region)

Table 48-7
Diagnostic Studies of the Nervous System

Study	Description and Purpose	Nursing Responsibility
	Lumbar Puncture	
	Aspiration of CSF via needle insertion in L4–L5 interspace to assess many CNS diseases.	Assist client to assume and maintain lateral recumbent position with knees flexed. Assure maintenance of strict aseptic technique. Assure labeling of CSF specimens in proper sequence. Keep client flat 6 to 24 h depending on physician preference. Encourage fluids. Monitor neurological and vital signs (VS). Administer analgesia prn.
	Radiologic	
Skull films, spine films	Simple x-rays of skull and spinal column to detect fractures, bone erosion, calcifications, abnormal vascularity.	Explain procedure and positions to be assumed. Noninvasive procedure.
Cerebral angiography	Serial x-ray visualization of intracranial and extracranial blood vessels to detect vascular lesions and tumors of brain; radiopaque contrast medium used.	Withhold preceding meal. Explain client will experience hot flush of head and neck when dye injected. Administer premedication. Explain need to be absolutely still during procedure. Monitor neurological and vital signs q 15 to 30 min first 2 h, q h next 6, then q 2 h for 24 h. Maintain pressure dressing and ice to injection site. Maintain bed rest until client alert and VS stable. Report any signs of change in neurological status.

Table 48-7 (continued)

Study	Description and Purpose	Nursing Responsibility
Computerized axial tomography (CAT or CT scan)	Computer-assisted x-ray of several levels or thin cross sections of the brain to detect such problems as hemorrhage, tumor, cyst, edema, infarction, brain atrophy, hydrocephalus.	Noninvasive if no dye used. If dye used, observe for allergic reaction and observe puncture site. Explain appearance of scanner. Instruct client on need to remain absolutely still during procedure.
Myelography	X-ray of spinal cord and vertebral column after injection of dye into subarachnoid space to detect spinal lesions (e.g., ruptured disk, tumor).	Administer preprocedure sedation as ordered. Instruct client to empty bladder. Inform client test is performed with client on tilting table which is moved during test. Specific postprocedural management depends on whether oil- or water-based contrast medium used. Generally, keep client flat first 8–16 h. Encourage fluids. Monitor neurological and vital signs.
Pneumoencephalography	X-ray to demonstrate distribution of air through subarachnoid space and ventricles. Injection of air via lumbar puncture. Detects mass lesions, brain atrophy, or hydrocephalus.	Explain high incidence of postprocedure headache. Withhold preceding meal and premedicate as ordered. Instruct client to remain prone for 12–24 h. Monitor VS; administer analgesia and antiemetics as ordered prn.
Ventriculography	Injection of air directly into ventricles via burr hole or craniotomy flap to visualize ventricles and detect mass lesions, brain atrophy, or hydrocephalus. Preferred over pneumoencephalography in presence of increased intracranial lesions.	Same as for pneumoencephalogram.
Echoencephalography	Use of ultrasound to detect midline shift of intracranial contents due to mass lesions.	Explain that procedure is noninvasive.
Radioisotope brain scan	Specialized scanning of brain after oral, intravenous, or intraarterial administration of radioisotope to detect mass lesions or vascular abnormalities.	Inform client that only tracer dose used so there is no radioactive harm to client. Explain that following administration of radioisotope, scanner will move overhead.
	Electrographic	
Electroencephalography (EEG)	Recording of electrical activity of brain via scalp electrodes to evaluate cerebral disease, CNS effects of systemic diseases, brain death.	Inform client procedure painless and without danger of electrical shock. Withhold stimulants. Inform client that he may be asked to perform various activities such as hyperventilation during test. Determine whether any medications (e.g., tranquilizers, anticonvulsants) should be withheld. Resume medications following test. Assist client to wash electrode paste out of hair.
Electromyography (EMG)	Recording of electrical activity associated with innervation of skeletal muscle via insertion of needle electrodes to detect myopathies and peripheral nerve disease.	Inform client of slight discomfort associated with insertion of needles.

reactions may occur. The client may have an allergic (anaphylactic) reaction to the contrast medium. This reaction usually occurs immediately after injection and may require emergency resuscitation measures in the procedure room. The most common precaution for nurses to take in caring for the client after he returns to his room is observation for bleeding at the catheter puncture site (usually the groin). A pressure dressing and ice are usually placed on the site to aid hemostasis and prevent swelling.

Table 48-8
Normal Cerebrospinal Fluid Values

	Normal value
Specific gravity	1.007
pH	7.35
Appearance	Clear colorless
Red blood cells	None
White blood cells	0–8/μL
Protein	
Lumbar	15–45 mg/dL
Cisternal	15–25 mg/dL
Ventricular	5–15 mg/dL
Glucose	45–75 mg/dL
Microorganisms	None
Opening pressure with lumbar puncture	60–150 mmH_2O

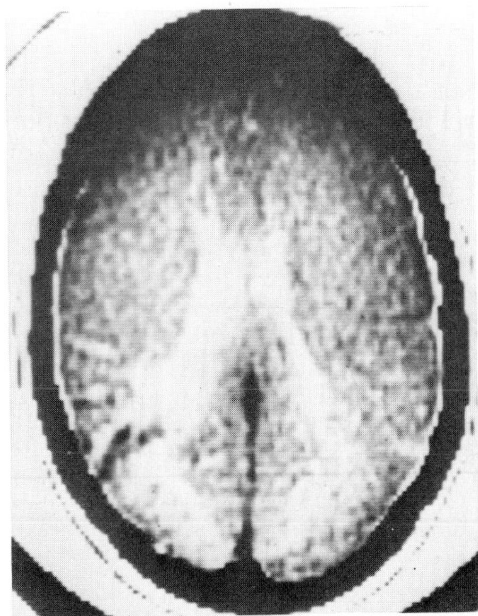

Figure 48-13 CT scan of a client with an arteriovenous malformation (same person as in Fig. 48-12). Note dilated right lateral ventricle and enhancement of arteriovenous malformation just posterior to the right ventricle. (*University of Washington Hospitals.*)

Computerized tomography

Computerized tomography (CT, CAT, EMI scan) has revolutionized neuroradiology. It has greatly reduced the use of other diagnostic studies such as pneumoencephalography, ventriculography, echoencephalography, and radioisotope brain scan. It is noninvasive (although intravenous injection of contrast medium may be used to enhance visualization of the blood vessels and identify disruptions in the blood-brain barrier) and can be done on an outpatient basis. A series of x-rays scanning different levels of the brain are compiled with computer assistance and presented in a series of black and white pictures (Fig. 48-13). These pictures, which literally illustrate "slices" of the brain, can show hemorrhages of all types, tumors, cysts, edema, infarction, brain atrophy, and hydrocephalus. Computerized tomography does not illustrate structures in the posterior fossa and the base of the brain as well as some other tests (e.g., myelography).

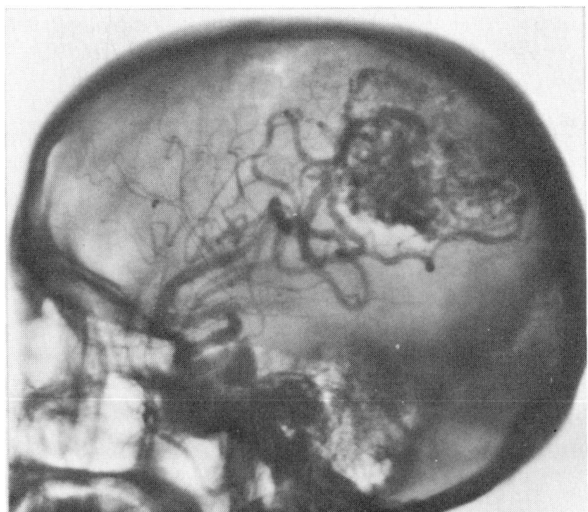

Figure 48-12 Cerebral angiogram illustrating an arteriovenous malformation. (*University of Washington Hospitals.*)

Because CT scanners are so expensive, not all health agencies can afford them. Many times a scanner will be shared by several agencies. This sometimes requires that a nurse accompany a client to another institution for his test. Nursing responsibilities in this case include monitoring of vital signs, communicating with diagnosticians about the nature of the client's problem, and follow-up observation if an untoward reaction to the dye occurs.

Myelography

Myelography is used to visualize the spinal column and the subarachnoid space when a spinal lesion is suspected. The most common lesion for which this test is employed is a herniated or protruding intervertebral disk. Other lesions include spinal tumors, adhesions, syringomyelia, bony deformations, and arteriovenous malformations. The test involves x-ray of the spinal column after injection of the contrast medium iophendylate (Pantopaque) into the subarachnoid space via catheter. Preparation for this procedure is the same as for lumbar puncture. Before the dye is injected, the client must be asked whether he has any

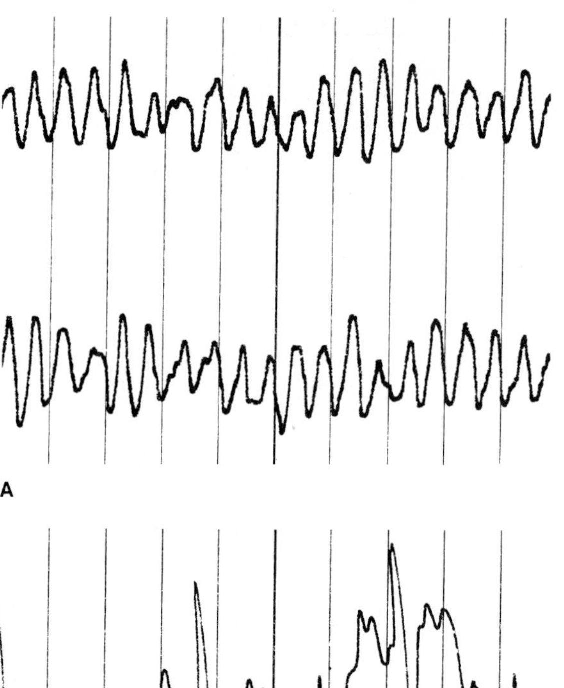

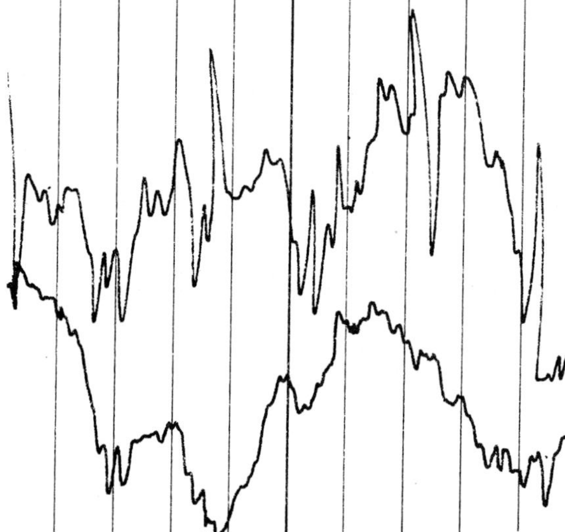

Figure 48-14 (*a*) Normal EEG, posterior head region. (*b*) Abnormal EEG, focal right occipital region. Note epileptiform spikes.

allergies, specifically whether he has had any anaphylactic or hypotensive episodes from other dyes. After the procedure the dye is aspirated so that little is left in the subarachnoid space. If the contrast medium has not been removed, the client's head is kept elevated so that the dye does not gravitate to the brain, causing irritative cerebral meningitis, manifested by severe pain and stiff neck.

Since the CT scan has generally replaced pneumoencephalography, ventriculography, echoencephalography, and radioisotope brain scan, these are only briefly described in Table 48-7.

Electrographic Studies

Electroencephalography

Electroencephalography (EEG) is the recording of the electrical activity of the brain by 8 to 16 electrodes placed on specific areas of the scalp (Fig. 48-14*a*). This test is done not only to evaluate cerebral disease, but also to evaluate the CNS effects of many metabolic and systemic diseases and to determine so-called brain death. Among the cerebral diseases assessed by EEG are epilepsy, mass lesions (tumor, abscess, hematoma), cerebrovascular lesions, and brain injury (Fig. 48-14*b*). The procedure is noninvasive. Clients sometimes have the misconception that the recording electrodes will give them an electric shock. They should be assured that this is not so and that the procedure is similar to electrocardiography (ECG).

Electromyography

Electromyography (EMG) is the recording of electrical activity associated with innervation of skeletal muscle. The recording is displayed on a cathode-ray oscilloscope and may be played on a loudspeaker for simultaneous analysis. Needle electrodes are inserted into the muscle in order to record specific motor units, because recording from the skin is not sufficient. Normal muscle at rest shows no electrical activity. Typical electrical activity occurs when the muscle contracts. This activity may be altered in diseases of muscle itself (myopathies) or in disorders of muscle innervation (segmental or lower motor neuron lesions, peripheral neuropathies). Fibrillations are spontaneous independent contractions of individual muscle fibers which can be detected only by EMG. They appear on EMG 1 to 3 weeks after a muscle has lost its nerve supply.

REVIEW QUESTIONS

The number of the question corresponds to the same-numbered objective at the beginning of the chapter.

1. The primary function of the neuron is to
- **a.** regulate extracellular fluid concentrations
- **b.** supply nutrients to other cells in the CNS
- **c.** transmit information to, from, and within the CNS
- **d.** maintain arousal

2. Nerve impulses are transmitted
- **a.** between neurons by chemical synaptic mechanisms and within a neuron by action potentials
- **b.** within a neuron by action neurotransmitters and between neurons by action potentials
- **c.** between neurons and neuroglia to the periphery
- **d.** between neurons and tiny capillaries

3. Two CNS structures essential for the execution of smooth, coordinated movement are
- **a.** cerebellum and hypothalamus
- **b.** hypothalamus and basal ganglia
- **c.** basal ganglia and occipital cortex
- **d.** basal ganglia and cerebellum

4. The middle cerebral arteries supply
- **a.** the medial portion of the frontal lobes
- **b.** the outer portions of the frontal, parietal, and superior temporal lobes
- **c.** the posterior fossa
- **d.** the occipital lobes

5. Some cranial nerves, unlike spinal nerves
- **a.** have only an efferent motor component
- **b.** have only an afferent sensory component
- **c.** carry "special senses"
- **d.** have all the above

6. The net result of activation of the sympathetic nervous system is
- **a.** hibernation
- **b.** sensory overload
- **c.** seizure activity
- **d.** preparation for fight or flight

7. Data regarding the perinatal and growth and development history are important because they may
- **a.** indicate early damage to the CNS
- **b.** indicate genetic factors
- **c.** reveal aspects of mothering
- **d.** a and b

8. In order to assess for nystagmus, the nurse asks the client to
- **a.** follow the finger as it approaches the nose
- **b.** identify familiar objects placed in the hand with eyes closed
- **c.** follow the nurse's finger laterally and hold
- **d.** bend from the waist with arms hanging freely

9. Disturbances of higher cortical functions include
- **a.** ataxia, agnosia, paraplegia
- **b.** analgesia, ataxia, diplopia
- **c.** apraxia, agnosia, aphasia
- **d.** paraplegia, analgesia, aphasia

10. A common nursing responsibility for studies involving invasive procedures is
- **a.** observation of the puncture site
- **b.** application of pressure bandage to puncture site
- **c.** a and b
- **d.** neither a nor b

REFERENCES

1. Solomon Snyder, "Opioid Peptides in the Brain," in F. Schmitt and F. Worden (eds.), *The Neurosciences*, Fourth Study Program, The M.I.T. Press, Cambridge, Mass., 1979, pp. 1057–1068.
2. Barbara L. Conway, *Carini and Owens' Neurological and Neurosurgical Nursing*, The C. V. Mosby Company, St. Louis, 1978, p. 103.
3. Sylvia A. Price and Lorraine M. Wilson, *Pathophysiology: Clinical Concepts of Disease Processes*, McGraw-Hill Book Company, New York, 1978, p. 589.
4. Joyce W. Taylor and Sally Ballenger, *Neurological Dysfunctions and Nursing Intervention*, McGraw-Hill Book Company, New York, 1980, p. 95.
5. Charles R. Noback and Robert J. Demarest, *The Nervous System: Introduction and Review*, 2d ed., McGraw-Hill Book Company, New York, 1977, p. 46.
6. Edward J. Reith et al., *Textbook of Anatomy and Physiology*, 2d ed., McGraw-Hill Book Company, New York, 1978, p. 165.
7. Betty S. Bergeson, *Pharmacology in Nursing*, 14th ed., The C. V. Mosby Company, St. Louis, 1979, p. 101.
8. Reith, op. cit. p. 169.
9. John Sundsten, "The Neuron, Glia, and Myelin," in Harry D. Patton et al. (eds.), *Introduction to Basic Neurology*, W. B. Saunders Company, Philadelphia, 1976, pp. 31–32.
10. Raymond Adams and Maurice Victor, *Principles of Neurology*, McGraw-Hill Book Company, New York, 1977, p. 4.
11. Pamela Mitchell and Nancy Irvin, "Neurological Examination: Nursing Assessment for Nursing Purposes," *J. Neurosurg Nurs*, **9**(1):23 (1977).

Chapter 49

NURSING ROLE IN MANAGEMENT

Unconscious Client

Idolia Cox Collier

Learning Objectives

1. Explain the mechanism and causes of unconsciousness.
2. Explain how to describe unconsciousness.
3. Describe the nursing management and potential problems of the unconscious client.

The unconscious state implies a void of consciousness and decreased or absent reaction to external stimuli. Unconsciousness is not in itself a disease but rather a manifestation of a wide range of pathological processes. Medical and nursing management is aimed at determining and correcting the cause of the unconsciousness as well as protecting and maintaining the safety and bodily functions of the client.

ETIOLOGY OF UNCONSCIOUSNESS

The basic mechanism of unconsciousness involves interference between the cerebral hemispheres and the reticular activating system (RAS) located in the reticular formation area in the upper brainstem. The RAS is responsible for a state of arousal. The cerebral cortex is responsible for intellectual and emotional functions. These two components account for a state of consciousness.

Many specific causes can result in interference with this state of consciousness. They can be grouped according to pathophysiological mechanisms as metabolic and diffuse cerebral disorders, supratentorial mass lesions, and subtentorial mass or destructive lesions (Table 49-1).[1] Psychiatric disorders can also result in failure to respond to the environment. The only normal form of altered consciousness is sleep.[2]

Metabolic and *diffuse cerebral disorders* of both intracranial and extracranial origin can cause alterations in the conscious state. These disorders can cause disturbances in cerebral metabolism related to nutritional deficiencies, electrolyte imbalances, intoxication, anoxia, or lack of necessary enzymes or cofactors required for essential functions. Specific metabolic problems which can cause unconsciousness include uremia, diabetes, hypoglycemia, alcoholism, barbiturate overdose, and lead poisoning.

Supratentorial mass lesions cause unconsciousness by compressing the brain and causing pressure on the reticular formation in the brainstem. Increasing pressure by the expanding mass can result in herniation of the brain through the tentorial notch. Specific supratentorial mass problems which can cause unconsciousness include trauma resulting in lacerations or contusions, subdural or epidural hematoma, subarachnoid hemorrhage, cerebral hemorrhage or infarction, tumor, or abscess.

This chapter was reviewed by Elizabeth Noroian, R.N., Ph.D., Assistant Professor, School of Nursing, University of Pittsburgh, Pittsburgh, Pennsylvania.

Table 49-1

Causes of Unconsciousness

Supratentorial mass lesions—secondarily encroach upon deep diencephalic structures so as to compress or damage physiological ascending reticular activating system:
- Epidural hematoma
- Subdural hematoma
- Intracerebral hematoma
- Cerebral infarct
- Brain tumor
- Brain abscess

Subtentorial lesions—directly damage the brainstem central core:
- Brainstem infarct
- Brainstem tumor
- Brainstem hemorrhage
- Cerebellar hemorrhage
- Cerebellar abscess

Metabolic and diffuse cerebral disorders—widely depress or interrupt brain function owing to reduction in cerebral metabolism or blood flow:
- Anoxia or ischemia
- Concussion and postictal states
- Infection (meningitis, encephalitis)
- Subarachnoid hemorrhage
- Exogenous toxins
- Endogenous toxins and deficiencies

Gerri Spielman, "Coma: A Clinical Review," *Heart Lung*, **10**(4):702 (July-August 1981).

A *subtentorial mass* causes unconsciousness by direct pressure on or destruction of the reticular activating system anywhere above the midpons. Specific subtentorial causes include pontine or cerebellar hemorrhage, infarction, tumor, or abscess.

Regardless of the cause, two major reactions affecting cerebral metabolism occur: cerebral ischemia-anoxia and cerebral edema. Cerebral ischemia-anoxia, both focal and global, is managed by instituting measures to assure adequate systemic circulation. Cerebral edema and the resulting increased intracranial pressure may be treated by hyperventilation, hyperosmotic drugs, hypovolemia, and steroids. (See Chap. 54 for a more complete discussion of increased intracranial pressure.)

Psychiatric or psychogenic disorders can cause unconsciousness. Although the neurological system is intact, the client does not react to the environment. A psychiatric referral would be appropriate when the possibility of organic disease has been ruled out.

Certain pathological problems such as specific traumas and vascular disturbances can be categorized only after the problem develops, since the site of the problem will determine the specific causative mechanism.

THE UNCONSCIOUS STATE

The client's state of consciousness is defined both by behavior and by the pattern of brain activity recorded by an electroencephalogram. In the most profound state of unconsciousness, the client does not respond to deep pain. Corneal and pupillary

Table 49-2
Levels of Consciousness

Description of Response	Assessment Technique
1. Client aware of self and environment, oriented to time, place, person	Ask client's name in normal voice or touch client
2. Client very sleepy and/or irritable or restless	Ask client's name more loudly, touch with more pressure or shake
3. Client lethargic and sleepy but able to carry out simple commands; following stimulation usually falls back to sleep	Firmly ask client to perform simple task (e.g., shake your hand)
4. Client can be aroused with verbal stimulation but cannot follow simple commands	Firmly ask client to perform simple task (e.g., blink eyes)
5. Arouses to deep pain rather than verbal stimuli; able to carry out simple command	Pinch skin, shake client, prick with pin; firmly ask client to carry out simple command
6. Client aroused with deep pain but cannot follow simple commands; may respond by pushing examiner away, wincing, withdrawing part of body stimulated	Pinch skin, shake client, prick with pin; firmly ask client to carry out simple command
7. Client unresponsive, responds to deep pain only by withdrawal	Apply pressure to underlying tissues of Achilles tendon, supraorbital notch, sternum, or muscles of calves of legs
8. Client responds to deep pain by extension only; may have extensor rigidity of the limbs (decerebration)	Apply pressure to underlying tissues of Achilles tendon, supraorbital notch, sternum, or muscles of calves of legs
9. No response to deep pain; corneal, pupillary, and pharyngeal swallowing and cough reflexes absent; incontinence of urine and feces	Apply pressure to underlying tissues of Achilles tendon, supraorbital notch, sternum, or muscles of calves of legs; test corneal, pupillary, pharyngeal reflexes

In recording the level of consciousness, both a description of the response and the assessment technique used should be recorded.

Adapted from M. C. Slater, "Nursing Assessment and Intervention for the Patient with Central Nervous System Dysfunction," in K. C. Kintzel (ed.), *Advanced Concepts in Clinical Nursing*, 2d ed., J. B. Lippincott Company, Philadelphia, 1977, p. 668.

reflexes are absent. The client is unable to swallow or cough and is incontinent of urine and feces. The EEG pattern is almost flat.

Describing Behavior

The nurse may find it helpful to perceive states of consciousness as a continuum. This continuum of electrical activity in the brain ranges from the hyperexcitable state of seizure to the hypoexcitable state of coma. The normal level of alertness is between these two states. A variety of terms have been used to describe points on the continuum. They tend to be confusing; for example, the term *lethargy* has a variety of meanings. Rather than relying on these terms, the nurse needs to learn appropriate assessment techniques and how to describe the level of consciousness by noting the specific behaviors observed (Table 49-2).

Glasgow Coma Scale

Because of the confusion and ambiguity which surround terms describing altered states of consciousness, the Glasgow Coma Scale (GCS) was developed in 1974. The three areas assessed in this method are eye opening, best verbal response, and best motor response. Specific behaviors in each of these three areas are given a numerical value and can be plotted on a graph (Table 49-3). The graph visually plots the client's place on the consciousness continuum to determine whether he is stable, improving, or deteriorating. Additionally, the score for each area can be added to give a sum. This sum can be interpreted

Table 49-3

Glasgow Coma Scale

Category of Response	Appropriate Stimulus	Response	Score
Eyes open	Approach to the bedside	*Spontaneously*	4
	Verbal command	*To speech.* Eyes open to name or to command	3
	Pain (pressure on the proximal nail bed)*	*To pain.* Does not open eyes to previous stimuli, but does to pain	2
		None. Does not open eyes to any stimulus	1
Best verbal response	Score best response client makes with maximum arousal. Painful stimulus may be needed	*Oriented.* Converses; knows who he is; where he is; year and month	5
		Confused. Converses but disoriented in one or more spheres	4
		Inappropriate words. Without sustained conversation; words disorganized or inappropriate (for example, cursing)	3
		Incomprehensible. Makes sounds (for example, moaning) but no recognizable words	2
		None. No sound even with painful stimuli	1
Best motor response	Verbal command (for example: "raise your arm; hold up two fingers")	*Obeys command*	6
	Pain (pressure on proximal nail bed)	*Localizes pain.* Does not obey, but "finds" offending stimulus and attempts to remove it	5
		Flexion withdrawal.† Flexes arm in response to pain without abnormal flexion posture	4
		Abnormal flexion. Flexes arm at elbow and pronates, making a fist	3
		Abnormal extension. Extends arm at elbow, usually adducts and internally rotates arm at shoulder	2
		None	1

*Produces least inter-rater variability
†Added to the original scale by many centers

Table 49-4

Nursing Care Plan for the Unconscious Client

Client Problem*	Expected Outcome	Nursing Intervention
Airway obstruction	Patent airway	Initially, loosen all tight clothing. Assure patent airway by positioning on side, suctioning, or use of oral airway. Do not hyperextend neck unless spinal cord injuries have been ruled out. Place in lateral or semiprone position. Do not position on back. Avoid acute flexion of neck in positioning. Monitor maintenance of proper position. May use oral airway for up to 48 h if necessary. Have suction machine and O_2 immediately available. Monitor blood gases. Observe for signs of inadequate oxygenation such as cyanosis and restlessness.
Atelectasis or pneumonia	Aeration in all lobes upon auscultation. No adventitious sounds. Temperature 36 to 38°C (96.8 to 100.4°F)	Auscultate breath sounds at least every 4 h. Turn every 2 h. Keep hydrated, unless contraindicated. Suction prn. Take rectal temperature every 4 h.
Malnutrition	Body weight within normal limits	Maintain IV or tube feeding rate as ordered. Record changes in muscle mass. Observe good technique in administering tube feedings. Weigh daily. Monitor BUN. Record intake and output. Assure adequate caloric intake for size, age, and condition.
Oral infection	Moist, clean oral mucous membranes without evidence of infection	Give oral hygiene every 4 h. Insert padded tongue blade to keep teeth apart. Use toothbrush and toothpaste 3 times/day using catheter and suction. Coat lips with water using soluble lubricant.
Urinary incontinence	Dilute, clear urine free of bacteria Clean, dry perineal area free of excoriation	Use diapers or condom catheter if coma is short term. Otherwise insert internal catheter using sterile technique. Maintain closed gravity drainage. Give catheter care according to protocol at least 2 times/day. Force fluids unless contraindicated. Monitor intake and output.
Fecal impaction	Regular, soft, formed bowel movements	Monitor and record bowel movements. Maintain hydration unless contraindicated. Administer stool softeners and laxatives as ordered.
Decubitus ulcers	Intact, warm skin	Bathe daily. If skin is dry, bathe with emollient q 4 to 5 days. Keep nails clean and short. Place on alternating-pressure mattress. Keep sheets dry and free of wrinkles. Turn every 2 h. Massage pressure points. Check ears for signs of pressure.
Joint contractures and muscular atrophy	Full range of motion (ROM) in all joints. No muscular atrophy	Give passive ROM every 2 to 4 h. Position in correct body alignment, avoiding dependent edema.
Corneal ulceration	Clear, moist eyes free of ulceration	Inspect eyes every 4 h for signs of irritation. Apply protective eye shield if eye remains open. Irrigate with sterile normal saline solution and/or apply methycellulose drops 4 times/day.
Irritation of nose or ears	Patent nose and ears, no redness or excoriation of nose or ears, no abnormal drainage	Observe for bleeding or leakage of cerebrospinal fluid. Do not introduce anything into eyes or ears until trauma ruled out. Clean nose with normal saline. May apply lubricant. Clean and dry folds of ears carefully.
Hyperthermia	Temperature ranging from 36 to 37°C (96.8 to 98.6°F)	Take temperature every 4 h. Keep client lightly covered. Sponge with tepid water. Use hypothermic blanket as ordered.
Seizure	No seizures	Keep side rails up at all times. Pad if necessary. Remove extraneous objects from bed. Carefully note and record seizure activity.
Anxiety secondary to overhearing conversations	No anxiety generated by staff	Address client by name. Explain all activities. Do not talk about client within hearing distance. Support by touch.

*The general nursing care plan for the unconscious client is based on maintenance of function and prevention of complications; therefore all problems listed are potential. For a more definitive plan, knowledge of specific causation is necessary.

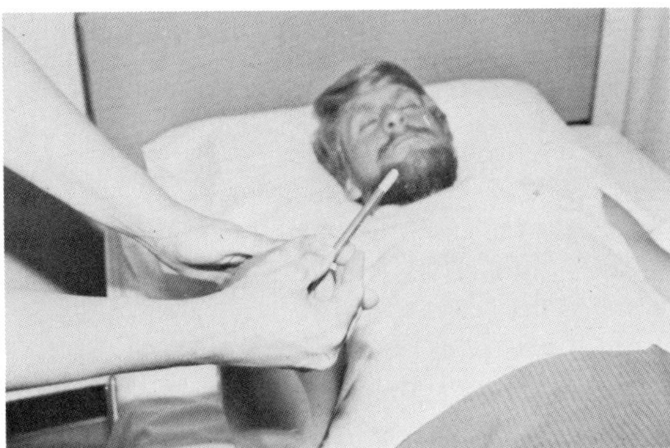

Figure 49-1 The nurse is assessing motor response by assessing reaction to pain. This client shows no response to firm pressure applied to the nail bed and would score 1 on this area of the Glasgow Coma Scale.

by comparing it to the score of 15 for a fully alert person and the lowest possible score of 3. A score of 7 or less is generally considered coma level. While the GCS does not replace a complete neurological assessment, its simplicity and validity make it a valuable assessment tool.[3] (Refer to Fig. 54-6.)

NURSING MANAGEMENT OF THE UNCONSCIOUS CLIENT

Regardless of the cause of unconsciousness or the method of assessment used to determine it, the unconscious state indicates a need for specific nursing management. The goals of this nursing management of the unconscious client are to (1) maintain function, (2) monitor neurological changes, and (3) prevent complications secondary to immobility and the comatose state.

The nursing care of the unconscious client is presented in Table 49-4. The problems presented are potential problems which could develop should excellent nursing care not be provided. Additional nursing interventions might be appropriate on the basis of the cause of the unconscious state. For instance, if unconsciousness is due to a deep head wound, the nurse will also need to observe the dressing for signs of hemorrhage.

REVIEW QUESTIONS

The number of the question corresponds to the same-numbered objective at the beginning of the chapter.

1. The basic mechanism of unconsciousness is interference between the cerebral hemispheres and the
  a. pons
  b. reticular activating system
  c. medulla
  d. autonomic nervous system

2. A score of 6 on the GCS indicates
  a. brain death
  b. alertness
  c. coma
  d. seizure state

3. Appropriate nursing management for the unconscious client with a problem related to airway obstruction includes all the following *except*
  a. suction as needed
  b. keep in side-lying position
  c. use oral airway up to 48 hours
  d. hyperextend the neck

REFERENCES

1. G. Spielman, "Coma: A Clinical Review," *Heart Lung,* **10**(4):72 (July–August 1981).
2. Ibid., p. 701.
3. Cathy Jones, "Glasgow Coma Scale," *Am J Nurs,* **79**(9):1551 (September 1979).

Chapter 50

NURSING ASSESSMENT AND ROLE IN MANAGEMENT

Pain

Barbara J. Boss
Joan W. Goloskov

Learning Objectives

1. Describe the components of pain.
2. Describe the anatomical and physiological basis of pain.
3. Describe the physiological and chemical modulating influences related to pain.
4. Compare the theories of pain.
5. Describe individual factors that affect the pain experience.
6. Differentiate between acute and chronic pain syndromes.
7. Describe subjective and objective data that should be obtained related to pain assessment.
8. Describe therapeutic pain management techniques.
9. Describe the nursing management of the client experiencing pain.

Pain is a complex phenomenon. The understanding of this phenomenon has undergone and is still undergoing dramatic change. Increased knowledge plus the demonstrated need and demand for an integrated, holistic approach to pain management has led to (1) a revolutionary increase in the number and types of therapeutic modalities used to manage pain; (2) an emphasis on approaching the client experiencing pain from a whole-person perspective; and (3) the recognition that pain management is a specialty area of health care practice. The nurse's role in assessing and managing pain has therefore become more complex.

DEFINITION OF PAIN

Pain must be understood as a complex biopsychosocial phenomenon. There is no simple, clear-cut definition. Pain cannot be reduced to a purely physiological definition such as "Pain is a protective mechanism." The behavioral manifestations of pain are socially and culturally determined.

Nor can pain be viewed as having no positive value. Often pain serves as a warning signal that the body is experiencing tissue damage. This prevents a person from continuing a task that would perhaps cause serious injury to body structures and results in ways being sought to reduce the discomfort. Pain may aid in locating and diagnosing the cause of a problem as well as serving as a measure of treatment effectiveness. Fear of pain not only prevents some persons from pursuing potentially harmful experiences but encourages them to take care of themselves.

This chapter was reviewed by Margaret Armstrong, Associate Research Professor, College of Nursing, University of Utah, Salt Lake City, Utah; and Daniel A. Dansak, M.D., Assistant Professor of Psychiatry, School of Medicine, University of New Mexico, Albuquerque, New Mexico.

Since pain is a complex concept and experience, a useful definition to guide nurses in the assessment and management of clients experiencing pain is: *Pain is whatever the person experiencing the pain says it is, existing whenever he says it does.*[1] This definition recognizes pain as a personal, private experience.

COMPONENTS OF PAIN

Sensory-Discriminative

Generally pain is conceptualized as having three components: a sensory-discriminative component, an affective-motivational component, and a cognitive component, which are integrated into a total pain experience. The sensory-discriminative component involves the perception of pain, which is the recognition of the sensation as painful. It ordinarily involves the transmission of a nerve impulse from a receptor through a sensory pathway to the thalamus. At the thalamic level, the sensation of pain is experienced and the temporal, spatial, and intensity dimensions of the sensation are distinguished.

Affective-Motivational

The affective-motivational component of pain comprises the emotional and behavioral dimensions of the pain experience. Structures in the limbic system and the hypothalamus mediate these emotional and behavioral responses to pain.

Cognitive

The cognitive component mediated by the cerebral cortex involves responses to the pain experience that are determined by memories of past experiences, learned behaviors, conditioned responses, and the person's analysis and interpretation of the situation (the meaning the pain experience has for him).

Other Concepts

Pain can also be conceptualized as having a perceptive component and a reactive component. By the *perceptive component* the sensation being experienced is perceived as one of pain, hence it is equivalent to the sensory-discriminative component. The *reactive component* comprises responses elicited by the pain perception and involves physiological, psychological, behavioral, and cognitive responses to pain. The affective-motivational and the cognitive components of pain are part of this reactive component.

ANATOMICAL AND PHYSIOLOGICAL BASIS OF PAIN

Pain Stimuli

An analysis of the pain experience should start at the biological level. At this level pain may be due to actual or potential tissue damage and is caused by a physical stimulus. Noxious (pain) stimuli may result from a mechanical, thermal, electrical, or chemical source. The *mechanical* sources that may serve as stimuli for initiating painful sensations include distension, spasm, obstruction, edema, traction, tearing, inflammation, infection, and pressure. An excessive degree or amount of radiant heat may serve as a noxious *thermal* stimulus. Electrical current, often experienced as an electrical shock, serves as a noxious *electrical* stimulus. *Chemical* mechanisms that produce painful sensations include exogenous substances such as acids, bases, and other caustic chemical agents and endogenous pain-producing substances released from damaged cells. The endogenous pain-producing substances, such as potassium, histamine, serotonin, the plasma kinins (for example, bradykinin), and the prostaglandins are the specific chemical mediators of pain regardless of the nature of the initial source.

Pain Receptors

Receptors act as transducers converting the electrical, mechanical, thermal, or exogenous chemical stimuli into electrical impulses. It is currently believed that free, or undifferentiated, nerve endings are probably the noxious stimulus (pain) receptors.[2–4] This belief is supported by the fact that free nerve endings are the only type of nerve ending present in such potential pain-producing sites as the pulp of the tooth and the cornea of the eye. Some receptors respond to only one type of noxious stimuli, such as noxious mechanical stimuli or noxious thermal stimuli; these are called *unimodal nociceptors*.

Other receptors not only respond to noxious stimuli but also serve as receptors for other innocuous (non-pain-producing) stimuli such as temperature and pressure; these are called *polymodal nociceptors*.[5] Current thinking among pain experts is that any stimulus can probably evoke a pain-impulse transmission via any receptor if the stimulus is strong enough.

Transmission of Pain Impulses

The typical means of nociceptor (pain receptor) excitation apparently involves the release of cellular chemicals such as histamine and bradykinin from the damaged cells. These chemicals stimulate a burst of action potentials at the nerve ending. If the action potentials reach the threshold level, transmission of a nerve impulse begins. The pain threshold (nociceptive threshold) is "the lowest intensity stimulus that will excite the sensation of pain."[6] The nociceptive (pain) threshold does not normally differ among individuals even of different racial or cultural backgrounds.[7] However, the nociceptive threshold can be lowered or raised in an individual under certain circumstances.[8–10] Lowering the nociceptive threshold means that a stimulus of lower than normal intensity can initiate a nerve-impulse transmission. Raising the nociceptive threshold means that a stimulus would have to be of greater than normal intensity to evoke a nerve impulse. Factors that raise or lower the nociceptive threshold are discussed later in the chapter.

Pain Pathways

Pain impulses spread along the nerve fiber ascending toward the spinal cord (or the brainstem in the case of the head region) by way of afferent nerve fibers. A first neuron ascends from the receptor to the spinal cord, where it synapses. This afferent component is either a fine, myelinated A-delta fiber or an unmyelinated C fiber. A-delta fibers mediate sharp, pricking pain. C fibers mediate a burning type of sensation.[11] Both types of fiber pass through the dorsal root of the spinal nerve, enter the posterolateral tract of Lissauer and then synapse in the lamina I, the marginal zone of the dorsal horn, with a second neuron.

Direct spinothalamic tract

Currently it is thought that pain is predominantly conveyed via two spinal cord–brainstem pathways,

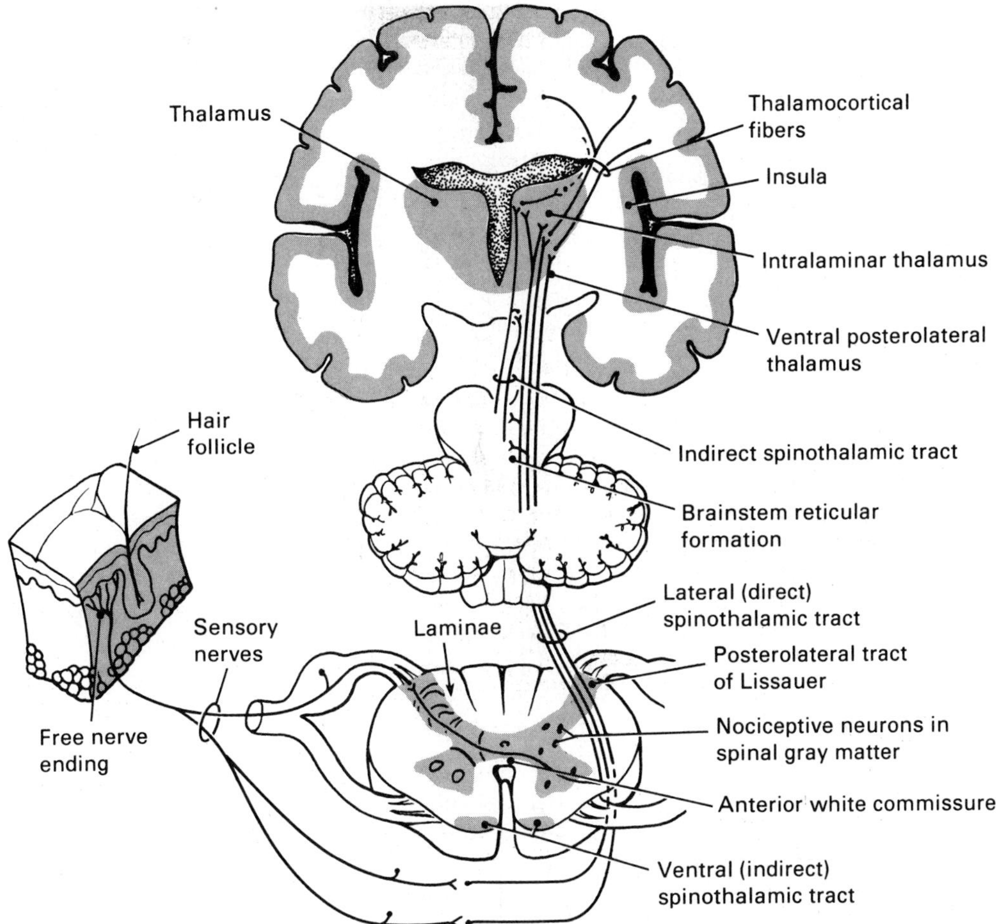

Figure 50-1 The pain pathways. The direct spinothalamic pathway is composed of (1) neurons ascending from the receptors to the spinal cord; (2) neurons from the posterior horn of the spinal cord which decussate and ascend as the lateral spinothalamic tract to the thalamus; and (3) neurons projecting from the thalamus to the cerebral cortex. The indirect spinothalamic pathway is composed of (1) neurons ascending from the receptors to the spinal cord; (2) a sequence of several neurons that project through the brainstem reticular formation to the intralaminar thalamic nuclei; and (3) neurons projecting from the thalamus to the cerebral cortex (the latter is represented in broken line because the course is not precisely known).

the direct (lateral) spinothalamic tract and the indirect (ventral) spinoreticulothalamic tract (Fig. 50-1). The direct (lateral) spinothalamic tract is composed of neurons that originate in the dorsal horn and the intermediate and ventral gray matter of the spinal cord, decussate (cross) at about the same level of the cord by passing through the anterior white commissure, and then ascend as the lateral spinothalamic tract. These neurons synapse primarily in the posterior thalamus. This tract is thought to convey information about the spatial and temporal aspects of pain sensations. Pain sensations conducted by this pathway are experienced as sharp and well localized in nature.

Indirect spinothalamic tract

The indirect (ventral) spinothalamic pathway, called the *spinoreticulothalamic pathway*, is a complex pathway whose neurons are also found in the dorsal horn and the intermediate and ventral gray matter. After decussating, the fibers ascend as the ventral spinothalamic tract through the reticular formation of the brainstem, where many of the fibers terminate in the reticular formation nuclei. The remaining fibers that do not synapse in the reticular formation continue to ascend upward to terminate in the medial thalamus.

Since the reticular formation has numerous connections with the hypothalamus, and the limber system, it is believed that the indirect spinothalamic pathway plays an important role in the affective-motivational component of pain. It is also theorized that the connections to the hypothalamus are responsible, at least in part, for the autonomic nervous system activity that constitutes part of the response to pain. This pathway is concerned with unpleasant sensations of a diffuse and burning nature. Visceral sensations are thought to be conveyed in this system as well.

Pain Perception

Pain perception is the threshold for recognition (awareness) of pain—that is, the point at which a person experiences pain. Pain perception takes place at the thalamic level. As with the pain threshold, pain perception does not vary among persons of different racial or cultural backgrounds. Pain perception within an individual, however, can be raised by decreasing cerebral function, as in cerebral trauma or cerebral hypoxia, or through the use of analgesics or anesthetics.

Cortical Areas Involved in Pain

From the posterior thalamic neurons, pain impulses are probably transmitted to a somatic sensory area of the cortex. The medial thalamic neurons also have fibers that project to the cortex.[12] The significance of these cerebral cortical areas in the pain experience is not yet clear and is a matter of considerable controversy. The cortex is presumed not to be an important part of a specific pain pathway but to provide analysis and interpretation of the pain experience.[13] This interpretation of the type, quality, and meaning of the pain is dependent on such factors as personality, cultural background, past experiences, physical and psychological conditioning, and motivation.[14]

Pain Tolerance

Pain tolerance is the point at which a person feels he can no longer tolerate the pain.[15] It varies both among individuals and within the same individual. This highly individual dimension has a large component of social and cultural conditioning. Pain tolerance is essentially a learned response.

Descending Systems Involved in Pain

Besides the pain-impulse transmission upward to higher brain centers, some impulses synapse with motor neurons in the same and adjacent spinal cord segments to produce reflex responses, including skeletal muscle spasm, vasoconstriction, and decreased gastrointestinal and genitourinary function. Other automatic reflexes elicited higher in the nervous system by the pain impulse alter the rate and depth of breathing. Increased hypothalamic activity results in increased sympathetic tone, tachycardia, increased cardiac output, and hypertension.[16]

In addition, as nociceptive information is transmitted in the afferent system, various central nervous system structures function to select, modulate, and control the ascending information. This is accomplished through a descending (efferent) system that can alter or inhibit the pain (nociceptive)-impulse transmission. The cerebral cortex, the gray matter of the midbrain surrounding the aqueduct of Sylvius (the periaqueductal gray matter), and certain neurons in the pons and medulla exert profound modulating effects on pain-impulse transmission.[17]

The anxiety, apprehension, and suffering experienced by the person is triggered by the release of stress hormones, the activation of the limbic system, and the interpretation the person places on the pain experience. These emotional responses activate the voluntary motor system, and overt behavior is manifested.[18]

PHYSIOLOGICAL MODULATING INFLUENCES ON THE PAIN-IMPULSE TRANSMISSION

Facilitating Mechanisms

Within the nervous system there are both facilitating and inhibiting mechanisms that modulate pain-impulse transmission. Facilitating mechanisms generally can be defined as those factors which lower pain threshold or pain perception. Facilitating mechanisms that influence pain-impulse transmission include the phenomenon of facilitation and the release of large amounts of endogenous pain-producing substances.

Facilitation is the phenomenon whereby a stimulus from a preceding neuron that is normally not strong enough to produce a nerve impulse "primes" the succeeding neuron so that a second similar stimulus can evoke a nerve impulse. The threshold of excitation of the succeeding neuron is lowered by the preceding neuron's activity. Thus the person's experience of pain can be intensified even when the degree of stimulation and the extent of tissue damage remain constant. Facilitation is a major component in many chronic pain syndromes.

Also, massive local mobilization of the endogenous pain-producing substances such as histamine, serotonin, the kinins, and the prostaglandins lowers the nociceptive threshold. These mediator agents can so lower the nociceptive threshold that they will fire at normal touch.[19] Thus pain impulse transmission is enhanced.

Inhibiting Mechanisms

Inhibiting mechanisms generally are those factors which increase nociceptive threshold and pain perception. Inhibitory mechanisms that influence pain-impulse transmission include the phenomenon of adaptation and the release of endogenous opiates.

Adaptation

Adaptation is the phenomenon by which, in response to steady, constant stimulation, a receptor exhibits decreased sensitivity. Initially, when an unchanging, constant stimulus is applied, the receptor will discharge rapidly. Over time, the frequency of the discharge will decrease. Pain receptors, however, are slowly adapting receptors. They maintain a rate of discharge over minutes and often hours. Since the primary purpose of pain is protective in nature, this slowness to adapt is useful in acute tissue injury, as it urges the individual to take measures to stop the tissue damage. But in ongoing acute or chronic pain in which tissue damage is not continuing, this feature of slow adaptation is not to the person's advantage.

Endogenous opiates

In recent years, a group of neuropeptides with morphinelike (opiate) properties have been discovered. Called *endorphins* (from "endogenous" and "morphine"), these natural constituents of the brain play a major role in the body's own chemical defense against pain. These endogenous opiates inhibit the transmission of nociceptive impulses. Many of these substances have similar actions, although they differ in molecular size, site of origin, and site of action. Presently the endogenous opiates are grouped into two categories: the enkephalins (short-chain peptides) and the endorphins (long-chain peptides).

Enkephalins Within the nervous system, the enkephalins have been found in high concentration in several areas of the brain and in the dorsal horns of the spinal cord, where pain transmission is mediated. Highest concentrations of enkephalins are found in the caudate nuclei of the basal ganglia, the anterior hypothalamus, the central gray matter of the brainstem, and the substantia gelatinosa. They are also found in the thalami at sites of termination of the spinothalamic systems.[20]

The enkephalins are released into the synaptic cleft. The released enkephalins are either rapidly inactivated by specific enzymes or they are attracted to and bind with specific cellular attachment sites (opiate receptors). Ordinarily the activity of the cell with the opiate receptors is depressed.[21] For example, in the dorsal horn of the spinal cord, the presence of enkephalin attached to the opiate-receptor site partially depolarizes the neuronal membrane, resulting in a reduction in the amount of transmitter substance released from the neuron's terminal endings. This results in a decrease in the intensity and firing rate of the impulses transmitted to the next ascending neuron (Fig. 50-2).

Endorphins Beta endorphin is contained in all cells composing the intermediate lobe of the pituitary and in scattered cells of the anterior pituitary. Beta endorphin binds firmly to the opiate receptor, but it is not inactivated nearly as rapidly as the enkephalins. Beta endorphin has a wide range of effects. Its actions include analgesia, catatonia, and behavioral disturbances. Beta endorphin appears to be released in combination with adrenocortical hormone (ACTH) in response to stress. This would account for the analgesia seen in some cases of severe trauma.[22]

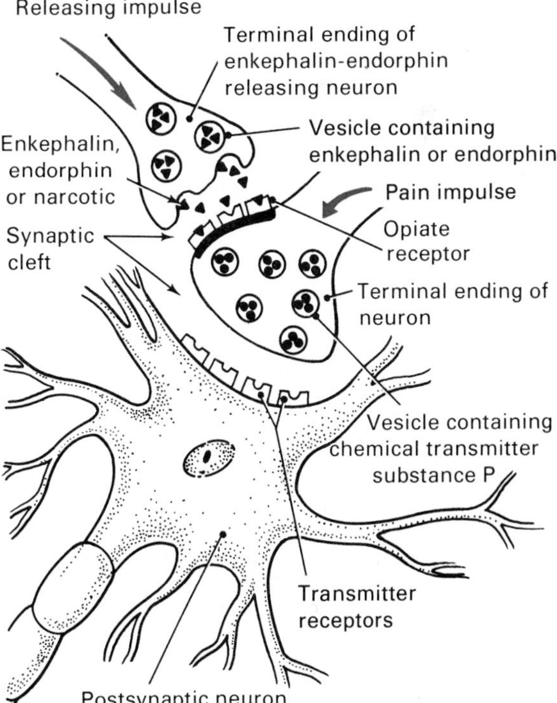

Figure 50-2 The enkephalin-endorphin receptor sites.

Evidence now exists to indicate that the placebo response is due to the release of endogenous opiates. The placebo somehow causes the individual to mobilize his own endogenous opiates.

It is now hypothesized that persons who have a deficiency of endogenous opiates are far more likely to develop chronic pain syndromes. With the development of radioimmunoassay techniques, measurement of the opiate-receptor binding level is now possible, and persons suffering from chronic pain syndromes have been found to have significantly lower endogenous opiate levels.[23]

The opiate receptors have also been identified as the same receptor sites at which morphine and other narcotic molecules act to block the transmission of nociceptive impulses. The activity of the endogenous opiates can be blocked by opiate antagonists such as naloxone (Narcan). Research findings have led some pain experts to suggest that exogenous narcotics may compete with the endogenous opiates as well as delay their mobilization.[24]

PAIN THEORIES

Three theories of pain have predominated—the specificity theory, pattern theories, and the gate-control theory. Recently the thalamic neuron theory and the endogenous pain-control theory have gained recognition.

Specificity Theory

The specificity theory, the earliest of the pain theories, proposed first by Descartes in the seventeenth century, is founded on the postulate that there are distinct pain receptors, which are free nerve endings, in the tissues. The theory implies that these peripheral pain receptors are stimulated only by a specific type of sensory input and function only as pain receptors (Fig. 50-3*a*). No other type of receptor generates nerve impulses that are experienced as pain. In its current state of development, this theory also postulates that pain impulses are transmitted by A-delta fibers and by C fibers through the peripheral nerves entering the spinal cord via the dorsal roots, where the fibers ascend or descend in the tract of Lissauer and synapse with neurons in the dorsal horn. The fibers then cross to the opposite (contralateral) side of the cord through the anterior commissure, ascending to the brain in the spinothalamic pathways. As the tracts travel through the brainstem, a predominantly A-delta-fiber pathway associated with pricking pain and a predominantly C-fiber pathway associated with burning pain separate. The C-fiber tract terminates in the reticular area of the brainstem and in the medial portion of the thalamus. The A-delta tract terminates in the posterior thalamus.

Although some receptors are specialized, it is doubtful that such specific receptors have direct constant channels to the higher brain centers. Each

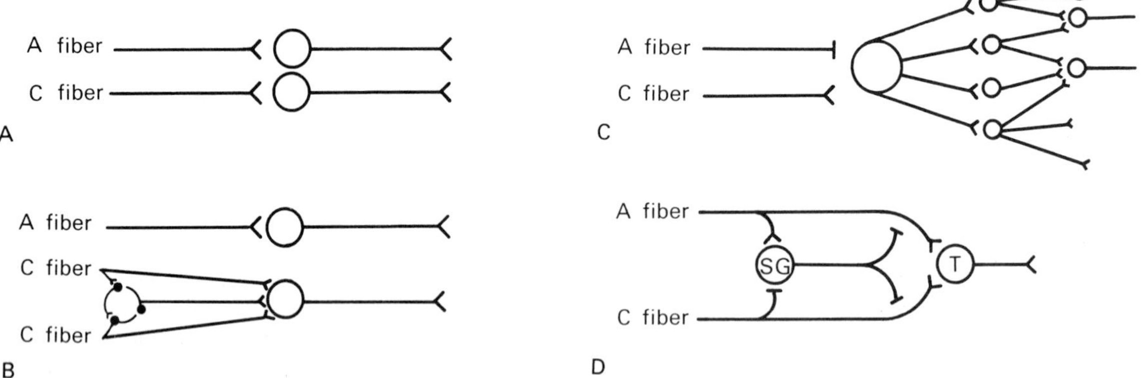

Figure 50-3 Schematic representation of the pain theories. (*a*) Specificity theory: Large A fibers transmit touch and small C fibers transmit pain in separate pathways to the thalamic centers for touch and pain respectively. (*b*) Central summation pattern theory: Large A fibers transmit touch. Small C fibers project both onto a posterior horn cell and to a central group of cells, creating a reverberating circuit. (*c*) Sensory interaction pattern theory: Large A fibers inhibit central transmission neurons. Small C fibers excite central transmission neurons that in turn have multiple synapses with other transmission cells. (*d*) Gate control theory: Both large A fibers and small C fibers project to the substantia gelatinosa (SG) and transmission (T) cells: Large A fibers excite the SG cells that in turn inhibit the T cells. Small C fibers inhibit the SG cells.

impulse is probably not automatically interpreted as pain and only pain. The theory is adequate to explain physiological reception in the peripheral tissues. It does not satisfactorily explain pain tolerance, especially the modulation of the pain experience by variables such as social factors, cultural influences, personality, and previous pain experiences. Nor does the theory account for many of the clinical pain syndromes such as causalgia, phantom-limb pain, or peripheral neuralgia.[25]

An understanding of the specificity theory remains important because it provides the rationale for many neurosurgical interventions such as cordotomy and tractotomy used to treat intractable pain syndromes.

Pattern Theories

The pattern theories of pain were proposed because the specificity theory was inadequate to explain all aspects of the pain experience. These theories do not hold that there are specific receptors for pain. Pain is experienced because various sensory receptors are stimulated in a certain pattern. Pain is the result of intense receptor stimulation producing a certain pattern of nerve impulses that is centrally coded to signify pain. To account for causalgia, phantom-limb pain, and the neuralgias, the *central summation pattern theory* proposes that initial extreme stimuli result in the development of reverberating circuits within the spinal cord that so hypersensitize the pain-transmission neurons that innocuous (low-intensity, weak) stimuli are able to generate transmission of the pain pattern (Fig. 50-3*b*).

As a further development, the *sensory interaction pattern theory* hypothesized that small-diameter fibers carry pain patterns while large-diameter fibers inhibit pain transmission (Figure 50-3*c*). In abnormal syndromes such as neuralgias and postinfectious pain, it is theorized that the large inhibitory fibers are lost.

The pattern theories have contributed to the understanding of pain, but the alteration of pain perception by psychological factors is not explained by any of the pattern theories.

Thalamic Neuron Theory

The thalamic neuron theory places the origin of a chronic pain syndrome in the thalamus. The theory suggests that intermediate neurons normally transmitting sensory impulses become autonomous, and a state of prolonged hypersensitivity develops. Normal sensory impulses are then experienced as pain when transmitted by these hyperexcitable intermediate neurons. The theory proposes that the thalamic neurons are more prone to develop a hyperexcitable state, especially when repeatedly stimulated.

This theory moves pain generation from the periphery or the spinal cord to the thalamus. It suggests that continuous or repeated stimulation—for example, an acute tissue injury—can generate a hyperexcitable state; and implies that it is essential to prevent large numbers of pain impulses from reaching the thalamus after acute injury.

Gate-Control Theory

In 1965 the gate-control theory of pain was proposed. According to this theory, the perception of pain is not dependent on specific pain receptors. Pain results from enhanced sensory input through pathways that normally conduct touch and pressure sensations. Stimuli interpreted as pain are carried to the central nervous system by small C and A-delta fibers. Touch and pressure are carried over larger A fibers. Large fibers entering the spinal cord synapse with both transmission (T) cells and substantia gelatinosa (SG) cells. Excitation of SG cells inhibits further large A-fiber and small C-fiber transmissions. The small C fiber also synapses on both the T and SG cells. The C fibers inhibit the SG cells (Fig. 50-3*d*).

The gate theorists have postulated two other pain-inhibiting mechanisms besides stimulating large-A-fiber inhibitory transmissions—the *central biasing mechanism*, thought to be located in the reticular formation of the brainstem, and the *central control mechanism*, located in the thalamus and cerebral cortex. The central biasing mechanism functions in the presence of maximal amounts of visual, auditory, or other sensory stimuli. It is postulated to be capable of sending efferent impulses down the spinal cord to close the pain gate in the dorsal horn, thus inhibiting pain-impulse transmission.

The central control mechanism is postulated to be activated by stimulation of the dorsal horn transmission (T) cells, thus triggering selective brain processes that regulate or modulate the gate-control system. At this level attention, past experience, emotions, anxiety, anticipation, culture, expectations, suggestion, distraction, and other factors are able to regulate and therefore exert control over the sensory input.

The theory has clinical significance because it provides insight into previously unexplained phenomena regarding pain, such as how the meaning of a pain-producing situation for the individual, a person's unique history of pain, and his present state of mind cannot only influence his reaction to pain but greatly affect his perception of pain.[26] Since its publication in 1965, the gate-control theory has generated fruitful search for additional pain-management techniques. It gave support to such therapies as rubbing, massage, touch, acupuncture, and electrical stimulation prior to the discovery of the endogenous opiates. The theory still gives support to the behavioral therapies such as behavior modification and Lamaze training.

Endogenous Pain-Control Theory

The endogenous pain-control theory proposes the existence of a trilevel pain-inhibiting system. A descending efferent pathway activated by ascending nociceptive impulses functions to inhibit the lower pain-transmission neurons. This system is thought to be mediated in part by endogenous opiates. At the midbrain level, endogenous opiates are released from periaqueductal gray matter. These endogenous opiates are capable of producing analgesia in themselves. They also can serve as transmitter substances that excite descending (efferent) fibers, which in turn activate a system of serotonin-containing cells at the medullary level. This system transmits inhibitory impulses to the pain-transmission cells in the dorsal horn.

TYPES OF PAIN SYNDROME

Acute Pain Syndromes

Acute pain can be described as "an unpleasant sensory, perceptual, and emotional experience produced by tissue damage [that is] caused by disease, accidental injury, surgical operation or certain other therapeutic procedures."[27] Once the cause of the pain is known, acute pain has no useful purpose. Such pain is only a source of anxiety and suffering, and if the pain is not stopped, it elicits autonomic reflex responses that promote physiological dysfunction.[28] The uncontrolled acute pain cycle is diagrammed in Fig. 50-4. Increased sympathetic nervous system activity results in significant increases in cardiac output and blood pressure, thus increasing cardiac work load, metabolism, and oxygen consumption.[29] This cycle must be broken by an effective pain management protocol.

If pain is very severe or continuous over a prolonged time, parasympathetic activity may predominate over the sympathetic nervous system activity. With increased parasympathetic activity there is a decreased heart rate, decreased blood pressure, weakness, fainting, pallor, nausea, and vomiting.

Postoperative pain

A prototype for an acute pain syndrome is postoperative pain. The quality, quantity, and duration of pain is related to the nature of the surgical procedure.[30,31] Any trauma, including surgical trauma, results in tissue damage. Pain-producing substances released in the traumatized tissue lower the pain threshold; thus normally innocuous (nonnoxious) stimuli are experienced as painful. The length of the incision contributes directly to the amount of pain-producing substance released. The duration and extent of the surgery also contribute directly to the amount of trauma.[32] A transverse incision generally produces less postoperative pain than a vertical or diagonal incision, because fewer nerves and muscles and less fascia are severed.[33,34] Incisions involving the thoracic and upper abdominal areas are frequently associated with greater postoperative pain because of movement with each respiration. Clients with anorectal

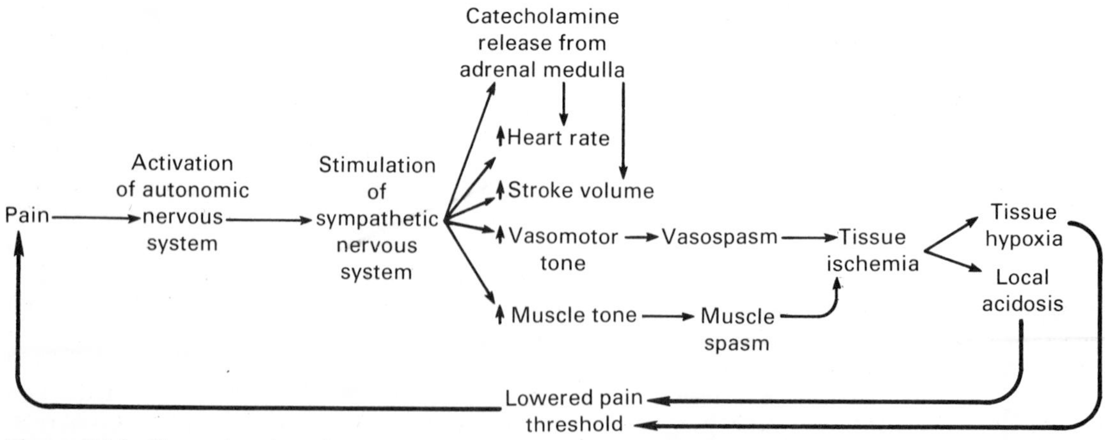

Figure 50-4 The acute pain cycle.

surgery and surgery involving the back region often experience greater postoperative pain because of muscle spasm.[35]

Since skin and soft tissues are well supplied with free nerve endings, incisional pain is experienced as sharp and well localized. Clients describe incisional pain as sharp, cutting, tearing, or stabbing. With prolonged stimulation such as that from tension on the sutures, the pain tends to develop a burning quality. Deeper tissues such as muscles, tendons, ligaments, joints, bones, and arteries have fewer nerve endings; thus the ability to clearly localize the pain is diminished. Pain is experienced as more diffuse and tends to radiate to adjacent areas. Clients tend to describe somatic pain as dull and aching. Pain from various deep structures differs: for example, pain associated with a punctured artery tends to be diffuse and dull, whereas pain from periosteum damage is sharp.[36] Trauma to visceral structures, pleura, or peritoneum can produce sharp but diffuse tenderness, pain, or intense referred pain. The phenomenon of referred pain is discussed in the following section.

Fear and anxiety are both part of the affective-motivational component of postoperative pain. These aspects are discussed in Chap. 8.

Referred pain

Acute pain syndromes may arise from ischemia of a viscus due to pressure or impaired blood supply. Visceral pain is often experienced as a vaguely localized but often severe pain on the surface of the skin, and the affected skin surface area may be distant from the damaged viscus. This phenomenon is known as *referred pain*. Several explanations have been offered to account for the misinterpretation of the source of the pain. Currently the most accepted one states that the afferent pathway from the involved viscus and the somatic afferents from the involved skin areas share common dorsal horn cell synapses. Thus the visceral impulses stimulate a group of neurons within the central nervous system that normally conduct cutaneous pain sensations. Impulses transmitted from this pool lead to misinterpretation of the location of the pain (Fig. 50-5).

Chronic Pain Syndromes

Chronic pain is a continuous or regularly recurring pain that extends over a period of 6 months or more. *Intractable pain* is severe chronic pain that is incapacitating and resistant to the usual therapeutic measures.

Chronic pain is different from acute pain and presents additional problems (Table 50-1). In chronic pain syndromes there may be a disease factor or pathological state that is persistent. In such instances the pain serves as a constant reminder of the threat to functional integrity and possibly to life itself. But chronic pain is also a disease in itself. The client becomes anxious and frustrated. Chronic pain affects his entire life: life begins to revolve around the pain, and the total being is affected. The client's family is also affected by the chronic pain state.

The causes of chronic pain syndromes can be categorized under the headings of posttraumatic, postinfectious, degenerative, vascular, cancer, and idiopathic (cause unknown). Two of the most common causes of chronic pain syndromes are discussed further as prototypes of the chronic pain syndromes.

Posttraumatic pain syndromes

Posttraumatic pain syndromes often occur after accidental injuries and are characterized by persistence of the pain long after the damaged tissues are presumed to have healed. The severity of the posttraumatic pain experience exceeds what would normally be expected following that degree of tissue injury. Posttraumatic pain syndromes include such conditions as chronic low back pain, herniated disk syndromes, posttraumatic head pain, postsurgical pain syndromes, and causalgias. If the pain is not brought under control, trigger zones surrounding the painful areas may extend, involving other body parts.

Pain associated with cancer

The pain associated with cancer may take the form of acute pain at some points and chronic pain at other times. Most persons suffering from cancer do not initially experience pain. Some never suffer physiological pain from the malignant process. However, many experience pain in the later stages of their disease, and this is commonly associated with tumor recurrence or metastasis.[37] Some 60 to 80 percent of hospitalized cancer patients suffer severe pain.[38]

Stages Three stages of cancer pain have been described—early stage, intermediate stage, and late stage.[39] *Early-stage pain* most frequently occurs with diagnostic testing or follows surgery to establish a diagnosis or to treat the primary lesion. This pain resembles an acute pain process, with the pain being short-lived and temporary, resolving rather rapidly over the first few postoperative days and often disappearing entirely.

Intermediate-stage pain may occur for several reasons, such as postoperative scar contracture with or without nerve entrapment, tumor recurrence, development of metastatic lesions, repeated surgical inter-

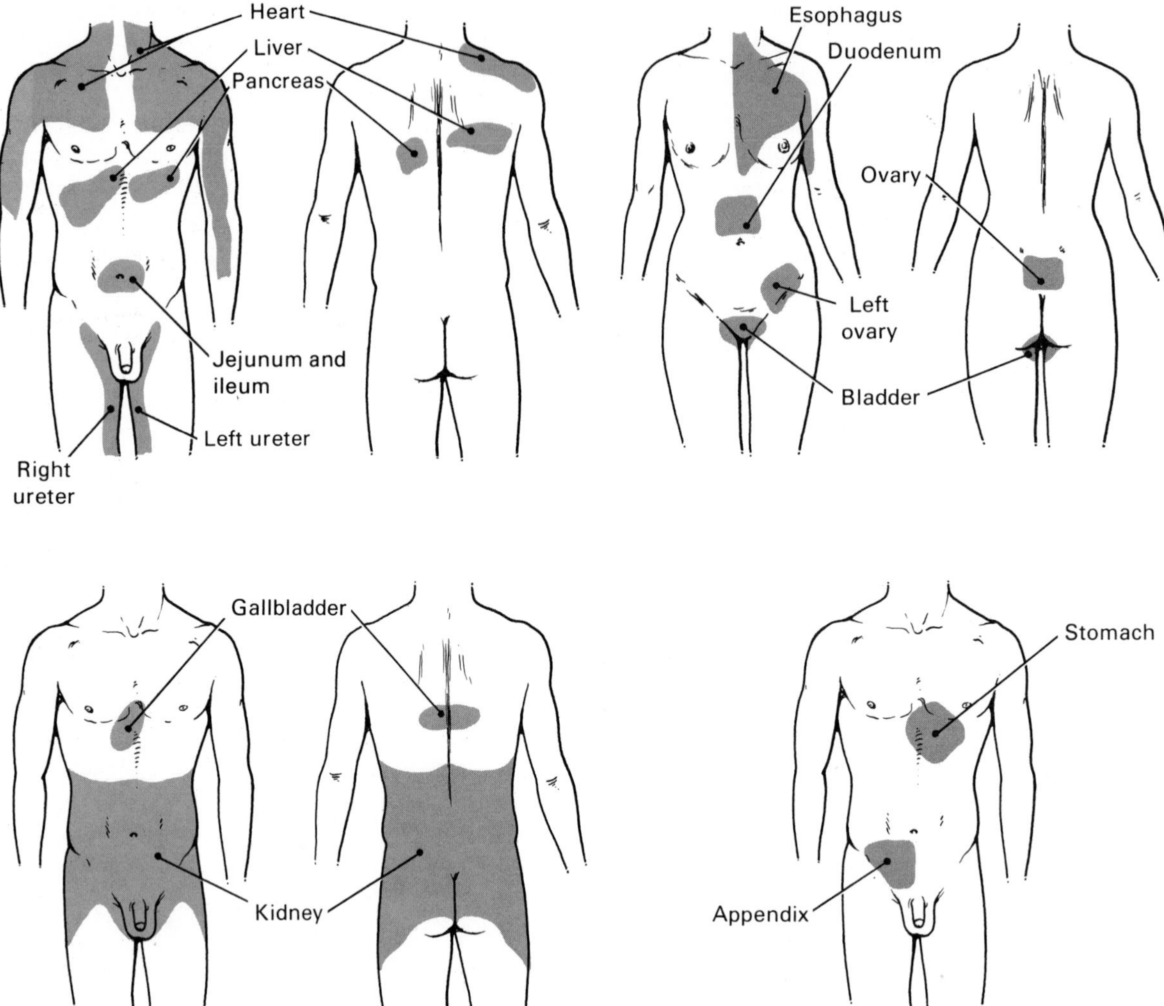

Figure 50-5 Typical surface locations of pain originating from stimuli in visceral organs.

vention, further diagnostic testing, or side effects from chemotherapy or radiotherapy. This pain may or may not subside, and the anxiety the individual experiences almost certainly will increase. Often palliative measures used to control persistent pain themselves produce discomfort and painful side effects.[40]

When the progress of the cancerous process can no longer be controlled by medical treatment, *late-stage pain* may occur. Continuous intractable pain may predominate that has the potential to impinge on all aspects of the person's life.

Causes The pain associated with a progressive cancerous process may involve several physiological mechanisms that induce pain. The compression of neural tissues produces a continuous, stabbing or sharp, well-localized pain that follows the neural distribution of the involved nerve. Paresthesias (abnormal sensations such as pins and needles or burning sensations) are often experienced. Infiltration of the integument, fascia, or other tissues results in localized pain that is initially dull and aching but becomes more severe as the tumor enlarges. Obstruction of a viscus causes a true visceral pain described as full, diffuse, boring, and poorly localized.

Sudden occlusion of a tube such as the ureter may produce a severe, cramping, colicky pain. The pain associated with obstruction of a blood vessel depends on the type of vessel occluded: occlusion of an artery results in ischemic pain, while occlusion in the venous system or the lymphatic system results in dull, diffuse, burning, and aching pain. Tissue damage results in inflammation, and the inflammatory process produces tenderness and sensitivity to touch.

Table 50-1
Classical Peripheral and Central Pain Syndromes

Pain	Description	Precipitating Factors
	Peripheral Nerve Pain	
Causalgia	Spontaneous severe burning pain felt in distal portion of the extremities; initially vasodilatation but later vasoconstriction and trophic skin, subcutaneous tissue, bone and joint changes appear.	Follows acute peripheral nerve injury (often develops more than 6 months after injury. Aggravated by cold, touch, emotions, visual stimuli, auditory stimuli, or startle response).
Nerve-root compression	Intermittent, radicular, stabbing pain along one or more nerve roots.	Any activity that stretches the nerve intensifies the pain.
Neuralgias		Caused by viral infections and conditions such as diabetes mellitus, vitamin deficiency, ischemia, and ingestion of toxins, in which the axons degenerate.
Trigeminal neuralgia (tic douloureux)	Brief, paroxysmal, extreme pain usually along one division of the trigeminal nerve.	Triggered by eating, talking, cold, air currents, or may occur spontaneously.
Postherpetic pain	Sudden explosive pain occurs along the cutaneous distribution of the nerve.	Following herpes zoster, the pathway from the skin surface becomes hyperesthetic as the skin lesions improve. Aggravated by cutaneous stimuli, noise, and stress.
Phantom-limb pain	May be experienced as tingling, pins and needles sensations (parasthesias), feelings of coldness and heaviness, cramping, shooting, burning, or crushing pain.	Trigger zones may develop on the skin surface or in deeper structures; the syndrome is more likely to develop if the person experienced pain in the limb prior to amputation.
	Central Pain	
Spinal cord		
Tabetic pain	Paresthesias (dysesthesias), poorly localized pain sensations.	Involvement of the sensory fibers entering the spinal cord.
Multiple sclerosis	Paresthesias (dysesthesias, poorly localized pain sensations.	Involvement of the ascending sensory pathway.
Trauma	Paresthesias (dysesthesias), poorly localized pain sensations.	Involvement of ascending sensory pathways.
Low back pain	Highly variable pain syndrome.	Trauma, scar tissue formation, traction on tissues, pressure.
Brainstem		
Direct tissue damage	Highly variable pain syndrome.	Sensory pathways stimulated, initiating transmission of impulses interpreted as pain.
Thalamic pain syndrome	Deep, paroxysmal, and excruciating pain, often burning and causalgialike, in the contralateral extremities.	Damage to the ventroposterior lateral nucleus of the thalamus.
Cerebrum		
Pain of cortical origin	Disturbed sensations on the contralateral side of body similar to nerve-root pain.	Inadequately understood at present.
Headache	Highly variable pain syndrome.	Vasodilatation of cerebral vessels, muscle contraction, traction on pain-sensitive structures, meningeal irritation, pressure.

Adapted from Barbara L. Conway, *Carini and Owens' Neurological and Neurosurgical Nursing,* The C. V. Mosby Company, St. Louis, 1978, p. 529.

Often this inflammation is complicated in the person with late-stage cancer by infection and necrosis of the involved tissues.

The pain associated with necrosis is severe and often excruciating and tends to be refractory to most treatment. The bone destruction often resulting from metastasis is another frequent cause of cancer pain. The pain is sharp and lancinating in nature. Although it is often continuous, the pain is more severe on movement.

The physiological and psychological impact of pain associated with cancer is often greater than that of nonmalignant chronic pain syndromes. Physical deterioration is usually more severe, since the person is often anorectic as a result of chemotherapy or radiation therapy.

PAIN-MANAGEMENT TECHNIQUES

Therapeutic techniques to manage pain syndromes are generally directed at altering either the sensory-discriminative or the affective-motivational and cognitive components of pain. Comprehensive, holistic pain-management programs employ a combination of techniques directed at all components of pain.

Techniques to Alter the Sensory-Discriminative Pain Component

Many techniques to alter the sensory-discriminative pain component induce an analgesic or an anesthetic state. Analgesia can be achieved through dermal stimulation using techniques such as massage, pressure, vibration, heat, cold, externally applied preparations, and transcutaneous electrical nerve stimulation (TENS). Deep-structure stimulation via percutaneous electrical nerve stimulation, acupuncture, dorsal cord stimulation, and deep brain stimulation also produce analgesia. Endogenous opiate mobilization has been demonstrated to account for the analgesia produced by TENS, acupuncture, and deep brain stimulation.[41] Narcotic analgesics provide exogenous opiates. An anesthetic state can be produced by nerve block or by ablative neurosurgical or radiological interruption of the pain pathway.

Another means to alter the sensory-discriminative pain component is to block release of endogenous pain-producing substances. Many nonnarcotic analgesics act to inhibit activation or release of these mediator substances.

Dermal stimulation to induce analgesia

Types of Dermal Stimulation Dermal (cutaneous) stimulation to produce analgesia is defined as noninjurious stimulation of the client's skin for the purpose of pain relief.[42] Dermal stimulation may be provided by the client himself or by someone else. The dermal stimulation methods differ as to convenience, cost, need for a physician's prescription, precautions, and contraindications. A major difference from the client's perspective is that the various methods produce different sensations; they feel different to the client.

Pressure is an instinctual response to pain. An injured part is reflexly clutched and pressure applied. Dermal stimulation utilizing a pressure method harnesses this automatic response in deliberate fashion. Pressure may be applied with the fingertips, the ball of the thumb, the heel of the hand, the entire hand, or the knuckles. At times both hands are used. Occasionally a hard but smooth object such as a sandbag may be used to apply pressure.

Acupressure is a specific pressure technique that involves applying pressure, massage, or both to specified points on the skin. These points are the same as the traditional acupuncture points. Pressure is applied using the thumb, tip of the index finger, palm of the hand, or fingernail/thumbnail.

Massage of an injured body part by rubbing is also an instinctual response. Again, this response can be deliberately tapped to manage pain. Many massage techniques exist. Examples include moving the hands or fingers over the skin slowly or briskly with long strokes or in circles or applying firm pressure to the skin to maintain contact while massaging the underlying tissues. Relaxation is also often induced by massage. Specific massage techniques are involved in some forms of acupressure and in trigger-point massage. Cold massage to trigger points is also used.

The application of *cutaneous vibration* to induce pain relief is currently gaining more recognition. The pain relief may be immediate or may require several minutes to occur. The duration of the pain relief is highly variable. Many different vibration devices exist, varying in size and shape to meet individual need. A physician's prescription is not necessary to purchase a vibratory device.

Heat therapy consists in applying either moist or dry heat to the skin. Heat therapy can be either superficial or deep. Superficial dry heat can be applied by using an electrical device such as a heating pad, a heat cradle, or a gooseneck lamp or by nonelectrical means such as hot-water bottles and exposure to the sun. Superficial moist heat can be obtained nonelectrically from hydrocollator (moist heat) packs, soaks, showers, baths, whirlpools and Hubbard tanks and by wrapping the body part in plastic to trap body heat.[43] Electric heating pads designed to provide moist heat are also available. Physical therapy departments provide deep-heat therapy through such techniques as short-wave diathermy, microwave diathermy, and ultrasound therapy (Fig. 50-6).

Heat therapy generally involves intermittent applications of heat for short periods of time, but some therapy methods, such as trapping the body heat, may be continued for prolonged periods or be continuous.

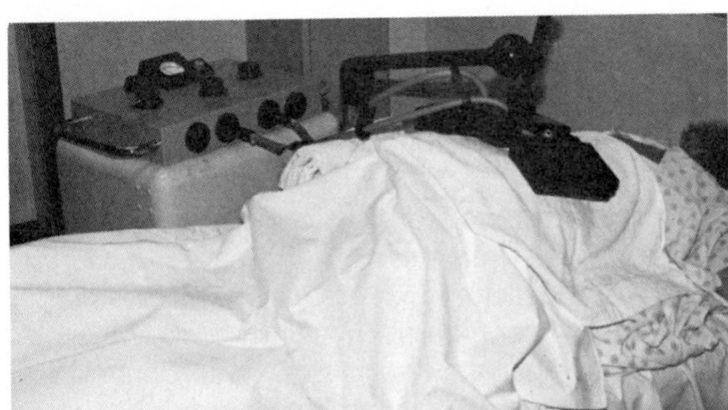

Figure 50-6 Client receiving heat treatment by diathermy.

Cold therapy involves the application of either moist or dry cold to the skin. Dry cold can be applied by using an ice bag, moist cold by using towels soaked in ice water, cold hydrocollator packs, or immersion in a bath or under running cold water. *Icing*, with ice cubes or blocks of ice made to resemble Popsicles, is another technique used for pain relief. *Ice massage* is a technique combining cold therapy and massage; the ice is applied evenly over the area of pain with slow up-and-down strokes for about 10 minutes.[44] Physical therapists sometimes use ethyl chloride or "vasocoolant" sprays as part of a cold-therapy regimen.

Cold therapy is used for a variety of painful conditions including posttraumatic pain and postoperative pain, especially that following orthopedic procedures, with bursitis, osteomyelitis, and muscle spasms. Cold therapy has been found to be more effective in the management of pain syndromes than heat therapy.[45]

Externally applied preparations such as ointments, lotions, gels, liniments, and balms, most of which are over-the-counter products, are sometimes applied to the skin to achieve pain relief. Although these agents contain various substances, two common ingredients are menthol and methyl salicylate (oil of wintergreen). The salicylate component is absorbed from the skin. On application, these agents usually produce a strong hot or cold sensation, generally intensified when the skin pores are open, as after a hot shower. Massage also intensifies the sensation. Skin testing is advisable when the client has not used the particular agent before, since the strengths of the agents vary and they produce various intensities of sensation. Relief of pain is reported for muscle pain, joint pain, headache, and visceral pain associated with gas, distension, and endometriosis.

Transcutaneous electrical nerve stimulation (TENS) involves the delivery of an electrical current through electrodes applied to the skin surface over the painful region or over a peripheral nerve. A TENS system consists of two or more electrodes connected by lead wires to a stimulator (Fig. 50-7). The stimulator is generally about the size of a pack of cigarettes and is battery-operated. Usually the batteries are rechargeable. Most stimulators may be worn and used 24 hours a day. For intermittent use the system can also be disassembled by detaching the stimulator and wires while leaving the electrodes in place. A physician's order is required to initiate this therapy.

Experimentation with different stimulators and different electrode placements is frequently necessary to achieve therapeutic results with TENS. If one stimulator is not effective in providing pain relief, another should be tried. Multiple sites of stimulation may also be tried during successive trials to determine the most effective site for pain modulation.

The person receiving TENS experiences paresthesias (tingling, burning, or vibratory sensations) during the treatments. The voltage and rate of stimulation are altered according to the client's response to the paresthesias.

Research has now clearly demonstrated that the pain relief produced by TENS is due to the mobilization of endogenous opiates.[46] TENS is used most commonly to treat chronic pain in adults. Pain relief has been reported in low back pain, cervical (neck)

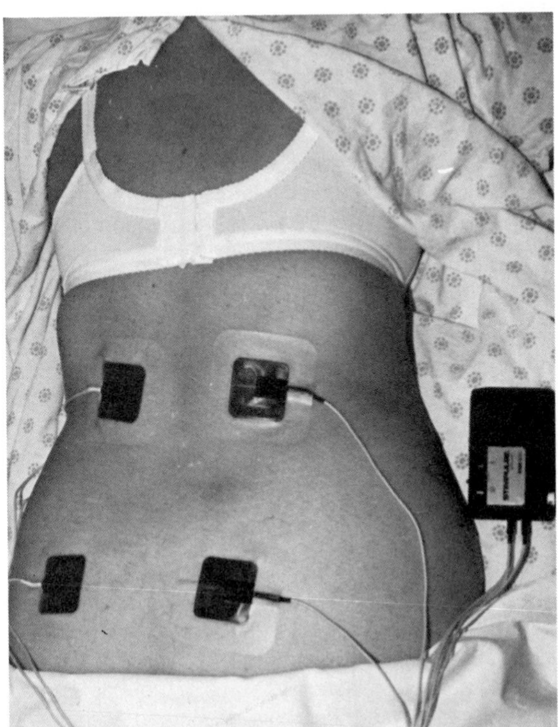

Figure 50-7 Initial TENS treatment being given by physical therapy department to assess value in pain relief.

syndrome, arthritis, sciatica, causalgia, headache, tic douloureux, postherpetic neuralgia, postsurgical neuralgia, peripheral neuropathy, chronic pancreatitis, and various types of cancer pain.[47] Recently TENS has been used in children with a chronic pain syndrome or with acute pain. Recent evidence suggests that during the actual application of TENS, acute postoperative pain is reduced. Postoperative pulmonary and gastrointestinal tract complications can also be minimized with the use of TENS. Pain relief after discontinuance of TENS has been highly variable in the research studies.[48-52]

Contraindications for the use of TENS have not yet been firmly established. Currently TENS is not recommended for clients with cardiac pacemakers or with a history of myocardial ischemia or arrhythmias.[53]

General Guidelines for Dermal Stimulation Any type of dermal stimulation should initially be of moderate intensity, then increased or decreased to achieve optimal pain relief. The most effective intensity for dermal stimulation has been found to be slightly less than that which produces discomfort in persons with normal skin[54,55]—frequently a stimulation of slightly above moderate intensity.[56]

Dermal stimulation may be continuous or intermittent. The duration of most cutaneous stimulation is usually 10 to 30 minutes; however, ice massage rarely last longer than 10 minutes. When firm pressure is applied to trigger points or acupuncture points, steady pressure is usually not maintained more than a few seconds.

The frequency of dermal stimulation is determined ideally by how long pain relief persists following stimulation. When the pain recurs, the dermal stimulation is reapplied. An arbitrary schedule such as tid or qid may be established in an institutional setting. On an outpatient basis, dermal stimulation is scheduled by appointment.

Continuous application of most dermal stimulation methods is impractical. If the client needs continuous stimulation to achieve pain relief, TENS or a menthol product may be the most practical solution.[57]

Generally, dermal stimulation is applied directly over the painful area, around the painful site, or just proximal and distal to the painful area. *Trigger-point stimulation* is an effective alternative in some instances. A trigger point is "a small hypersensitive region in the muscle or connective tissue, often just below the skin, that causes pain when it is stimulated sufficiently."[58] Trigger points may exist in the painful area or at a point distant from the actual pain. It has been demonstrated that there is a strong association between trigger points and acupuncture points for pain.[59] Although pressure on a trigger point may produce a dull, aching discomfort, continued pressure may relieve the pain. Pressure with massage and ice massage are also used for trigger-point stimulation.

Another possible area of stimulation is over peripheral nerves that innervate the painful area. This type of stimulation is most readily accomplished by TENS. Tingling or burning sensations are experienced in the area innervated by the nerve(s). Contralateral stimulation may be necessary when a painful area is too sensitive to be directly stimulated or when the painful area is not accessible because of some covering. Contralateral stimulation is also used with phantom-limb pain. If all the above alternatives are unacceptable, then unrelated areas can be stimulated.

Summary Utilization of cutaneous stimulation techniques must be individualized to the client and his particular type of pain. The client may have strong preferences regarding the type of dermal stimulation used and the area to be stimulated. He will have individual needs related to cost, convenience, intensity of stimulation, and duration of stimulation. Although success rates vary, 50 percent of persons using some type of dermal stimulation achieve 50 to 100 percent reduction of their pain.[60]

Deep-structure stimulation to induce analgesia

Percutaneous Electrical Nerve Stimulation Deeper peripheral tissues can be stimulated through percutaneous electrical nerve stimulation or acupuncture. Percutaneous electrical nerve stimulation is a preliminary step designed to evaluate the potential usefulness of a permanently implanted device. It is accomplished by inserting a needle to which a stimulator is attached near a large peripheral or spinal nerve. The amount of electrical current is regulated to provide the maximum pain relief. If the percutaneous stimulation successfully reduces the client's pain, a permanent peripheral nerve stimulator is surgically implanted. A special electrode is placed around the nerve, and an internal receiver is implanted subcutaneously at waist level on the anterior chest wall. The client activates the receiver by means of a special transmitter and antenna as needed for optimum pain relief.

Acupuncture Acupuncture involves the insertion of needles at specified cutaneous sites. The needles are activated by hand, low-voltage electrical current, or heat through moxibustion (burning of herbs). Onset of analgesia may not be immediate, but once the endogenous opiates have been mobilized, the technique's pain-relieving capacities extend beyond the period of actual stimulation.

Dorsal Cord or Deep Brain Stimulation Central nervous system stimulation can be achieved through dorsal cord stimulation or deep brain stimulation. Dorsal cord stimulation is an alternative pain-management technique to percutaneous electrical nerve stimulation when the pain involves large areas such as both lower extremities or the back. During a laminectomy, electrodes are implanted intradurally in the dorsal aspect of the spinal cord. The level of implantation is determined by the pain location. A receiver is implanted subcutaneously on the anterior chest wall at waist level. The antenna and transmitter system are similar to those used in permanent peripheral nerve stimulation.

Electrical stimulation of certain regions of the brain, including areas of the frontal lobes, thalamus, midbrain, lower brainstem, caudate nucleus of the basal ganglion, and internal capsule, produces long-lasting analgesia, called *stimulus-produced analgesia (SPA)*. This analgesia is specific to pain. Motor function, affect, and other behavior responses are unaffected. The release of enkephalin is hypothesized to activate neurons that exert an inhibitory action on small pain afferents. To explain the long-lasting effects of this deep brain stimulation, the SPA is hypothesized to also activate the release of beta endorphin from the anterior hypothalamic beta-endorphin fibers.[61]

Analgesic therapy

Analgesic agents used in pain management interfere with pain transmission at peripheral, spinal cord, or lower brain center sites by blocking release of endogenous pain-transmitter substances. Some drugs also alter perception and response to pain.

Narcotic Analgesics In view of the previous endogenous opiate discussion, the narcotic/nonnarcotic classification scheme is used to present this section. Narcotics include natural, semisynthetic, and synthetic drugs that bind to opiate-receptor sites in the central nervous system to block pain transmission (Table 50-2). For example, in the dorsal spinal cord such binding blocks the release of pain-transmitter substances such as substance P. Most narcotic drugs are capable of relieving severe pain. However, toler-

Table 50-2
Analgesic Medication

Medication	Drug Action	Comments
	Narcotic Analgesics	
Opium (natural alkaloids)		
Morphine sulfate	Depresses cerebral cortex and probably thalamus; adheres to opiate receptors in the CNS. Interferes with perception of pain and influences affect, or emotional response to pain.	Used to relieve pain, induce sleep (especially when sleep is prevented by pain). Useful with moderate to severe pain.
Codeine phosphate, codeine sulfate	Similar to morphine.	Weaker and less habit-forming than morphine. Used for mild to moderate pain.
Hydromorphine hydrochloride (Dilaudid, Hymorphan)	Similar to morphine.	Used in moderate to severe pain.
Meperidine group (synthetic preparations)		
Meperidine hydrochloride (Demerol, Dolosal)	Descending central nervous system depressant; action similar to morphine.	Used as an analgesic and sedative. Can be given orally but is less effective.
Anileridine (Leritine)	Similar to meperidine.	Used like meperidine. Comes as phosphate salt for oral use, hydrochloride for parenteral use.
Methadone group		
Methadone hydrochloride (Adanon, Dolophine, Miadone, Polamidon)	Similar to morphine.	Used to relieve pain in trauma, myalgia, dysmenorrhea, and cancer; also in opium withdrawal and maintenance programs.

Table 50-2 (Continued)

Medication	Drug Action	Comments
Miscellaneous synthetic analgestics		
Pentazocaine (Talwin)	Similar to morphine.	Has properties of a narcotic although originally labeled nonnarcotic. 30 mg as effective as 10 mg morphine or 75 to 100 mg meperidine. Duration of action may be less than morphine. Should not be mixed in syringe with soluble barbiturates as precipitate will occur.
Propoxyphene (Darvon)	Similar to codeine.	Narcotic used in mild to moderate pain. Not useful in severe pain. Less potent and less habituating than codeine.
	Nonnarcotic Agents	
Analgesics-antipyretics		
Acetaminophen (Anapap, Apamide, Febrolin, Fendon, Nasprin, Nebs, Pyrapap, Sk-Apap, Tempra, Tylenol, Valadol)	Inhibits release of kinins at tissue level. May decrease brain activity.	Relieves various pains, headache, myalgia, arthralgia, nervous irritability; reduces fever. Prepared in flavored liquid for children.
Phenacetin (Acetophenetidin)	Similar to acetaminophen.	Used for acute or chronic pain associated with inflammatory process, headache, neuralgia, dysmenorrhea and to reduce fever. Has been implicated in some blood dyscrasias and may be harmful to the kidneys on long-term use.
Aspirin (acetylsalicylic acid, A.S.A.)	Inhibits release of kinins at tissue level.	Common analgesic and antirheumatic drug used alone and in combination. Clients should be cautioned against too high a dosage as well as indiscriminate use.
Antispasmodics (skeletal muscle relaxants, synthetic)		
Meprobamate (Equanil, Meprospan, Meprotabs, Miltown, Vio-Bamate)	Blocks synaptic passage of impulse and reduces sensitivity of the thalamus.	Used as muscle relaxant or tranquilizer alone and in combination.
Methocarbamol (Robaxin)	Depresses basal ganglion, brainstem, and synaptic connections in spinal cord.	Muscle relaxant and analgesic for back pain, sprains, and traumatic injuries.
Compounds used to potentiate analgesia (synthetic preparations)		
Promethazine hydrochloride (Ganphen, Phenergan)	Antihistamine action: blocks receptor sites.	Used for preoperative sedation and to potentiate action of analgesics.

Adapted from Mary W. Falconer, H. Robert Patterson, and Edward A. Gustafson, *Current Drug Handbook 1976–78*, W. B. Saunders Company, Philadelphia, 1976, pp. 86–133.

ance to the analgesic effects and physical dependence may occur. These drugs also tend to alter perception of the pain experience and behavioral response to the pain. In addition, the common side effects of respiratory suppression, nausea, vomiting, ileus, and urinary retention encourage the use of alternate pain-relief methods.

Nonnarcotic Analgesics Nonnarcotic analgesics tend to act at peripheral sites to reduce pain, often by inhibiting transmitter-substance mobilization. These drugs do not bind to opiate-receptor sites. Nonnarcotic agents relieve mild to moderate pain and do not cause drug tolerance or physical dependence.

Because of the differing actions and sites of action for these two categories of analgesic drugs, narcotic and nonnarcotic agents are often used simultaneously. Thus several sites and two components of pain are attacked at one time. Also there is an additive effect as to the degree of analgesia.

Potentiators Another group of drugs called *potentiators* are used to intensify the action of narcotic agents, thus increasing the degree and duration of analgesia. Drugs commonly used as potentiators include promethazine (Phenergan), hydroxyzine (Atarax, Vistaril), meprobamate (Equanil, Miltown) and diazepam (Valium). In actuality, these drugs have an additive effect or are antianxiety agents rather then true potentiators.

Techniques to induce anesthesia

Nerve blocks and neurosurgical or radiological procedures to reduce pain are destructive in nature. A functional part of the nervous system is deliberately destroyed to interrupt pain transmission.

Nerve Blocks Nerve blocks are accomplished by using local anesthetics or neurolytic agents. Initially, temporary nerve blocks using local anesthetics are employed to isolate the involved pain pathway and to determine the possible effectiveness of a permanent blocking procedure for the particular individual. Typically the local anesthetic effects last for only a few hours. The effects of neurolytic agents such as alcohol, phenol, or saline last for weeks to months; therefore these agents are used for a more long-lasting effect.

Nerve blocks have been a successful pain-management technique for more localized chronic pain states such as peripheral vascular disease, trigeminal neuralgia, causalgia, and some cancer pain. Formerly a nerve block was advantageous in managing localized pain due to malignancy and in debilitated clients who could not withstand a surgical procedure for pain relief.[62] Today, with other available therapeutic modalities, the use of nerve blocks has been reduced.

Neurosurgical Interventions Neurosurgical interventions are accomplished by surgical resection or thermocoagulation, including radiofrequency coagulation (Table 50-3). Interventions that destroy the sensory division of a peripheral or spinal nerve are classified as neurectomies, rhizotomies, and sympathectomies. Neurosurgical procedures that ablate the lateral spinothalamic tract are classified as cordotomies if the tract is interrupted in the spinal cord or tractotomies if the interruption is in the medulla or the midbrain of the brainstem. (Fig. 50-8 identifies the sites of neurosurgical procedures for pain relief.) Surgical resection of the lateral spinothalamic tract is becoming more rare today since a percutaneous approach is available. Both cordotomy and tractotomy can be done under local anesthesia, using a percutaneous technique in which the pain fibers are isolated by fluoroscopy and a radiofrequency lesion is created.

Neurosurgical interventions involving the thalamus or frontal lobe region of the brain are accomplished through a stereotaxic procedure. Long electrodes or other probes are inserted deep into the brain tissue and positioned by the use of external points or landmarks of the skull. The tissue is then destroyed by thermocoagulation or other means. These procedures are used only for severe, intractable pain that does not respond to other therapeutic measures. Ablative procedures are less frequently utilized today, with the availability of good analgesic methods to control pain.

Techniques to Alter the Affective-Motivational and Cognitive Components of Pain

Techniques to alter the affective-motivational and cognitive components of pain include a variety of cognitive strategies, behavioral approaches, and hypnosis. Many of the behavioral approaches such as biofeedback, autogenic training, and relaxation strategies involve biogenic training.

Cognitive strategies

Distraction Cognitive strategies that are designed to affect the affective-motivational and cognitive components of pain include distraction, imagery, and meditation. Distraction involves "focusing attention on stimuli other than the pain."[63] The distraction

Table 50-3
Neurosurgical Procedures for Pain Management

Description	Indications for Use	Remarks
Neurectomy		
Sensory fibers of a peripheral nerve or a cranial nerve are isolated and interrupted.	Phantom-limb pain, neuralgias, pain of deep origin, and occlusive vascular pain.	Isolation of only sensory fibers is often difficult to accomplish. Nerve fibers tend to regenerate over time.
Rhizotomy		
Surgical resection approach: Interruption of the posterior roots as they enter the spinal cord proximally but distal to the posterior horn cell or interruption of the cranial nerve at its entrance into the brainstem.	Traumatic nerve injury, degenerative orthopedic disorder, trigeminal and glossopharyngeal neuralgias, pain associated with head and neck cancers.	Eliminates all sensations. Severing posterior roots requires a laminectomy. Severing a cranial nerve requires a posterior fossa craniotomy. 2 or 3 segments on either side of involved areas must be resected to achieve pain relief.
Percutaneous approach: Specific pain fibers are isolated and destroyed by creating radiofrequency lesions under local anesthesia.	Same as surgical resection.	Laminectomy and general anesthesia not required. Touch and temperature sensations can be preserved.
Surgical ablation of the sympathetic ganglia along the thoracic and lumbar vertebrae.	Intractable pain involving a sympathetic component such as vascular disorders, causalgias, phantom-limb pain, and visceral pain.	Often satisfactory relief is not achieved. Peripheral pathway may regenerate over time.
Cordotomy		
Surgical resection approach: Interruption of the lateral spinothalamic tract in the cervical or thoracic area.	Intractable pain from a large area or deep midline structure.	Because the cervical area pathway is more distinct, it can be resected with fewer side effects. Loss of bladder, bowel, and sexual functions may occur. Respiratory failure may occur with high cervical cordotomies. Pain usually recurs as other pathways take over the function of the lateral spinothalamic tract.
Percutaneous approach: Interruption of the lateral spinothalamic tract in the cervical and thoracic area by creating radiofrequency lesions under local anesthesia.	Same as surgical resection.	Same as for surgical resection.
Thalamotomy		
Surgical resection approach: Interruption of the lateral spinothalamic tract in the medulla or midbrain of the brainstem.	Intractable pain of the head, neck, and arm.	May have visual and auditory side effects. Painful dysesthesias may occur.
Percutaneous approach: Interruption of the lateral spinothalamic tract in the medulla or midbrain of the brainstem by creating radiofrequency lesions under short-term anesthesia.	Same as surgical resection.	Fewer side effects than with surgical resection.
Thalamic nuclei thermocoagulated by implantation of electrodes in them via Burr holes.	Severe, intractable pain unresponsive to other therapeutic measures.	Pain relief tends to diminish with time. A thalamic pain syndrome may develop if destructive lesion not extensive. Temperature sensation is lost also.
Cingulotomy		
Interruption of the cingulum (frontal white matter) through which pain is transmitted to the cortical areas of the frontal lobe by stereotaxic procedures.	Client with a strong psychogenic component with the intractable pain.	Affective response to pain altered. Person loses characteristics that distinguish him as an individual. Produces apathy, lack of consideration for others, appearance of unacceptable behavior.

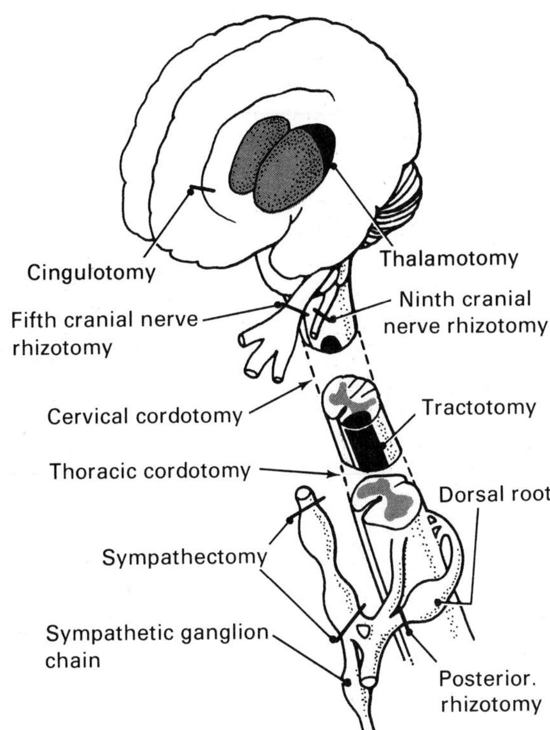

Figure 50-8 Sites of neurosurgical procedures for pain relief.

stimuli may be external events, internal activities, or bodily sensations. Distraction techniques help the client cope with the pain he is experiencing.

Imagery Guided imagery is "the purposeful or therapeutic use of images, that is, use of one's imagination as a therapeutic tool."[64] For pain relief, the individual's own imagination is used to develop sensory images that focus away from the pain sensation and emphasize other sensory experiences and pleasant memories. Specific images have been developed for use in pain relief to bring about removal of the pain. These include the techniques of breathing out the pain, the ball of healing energy, the healthy body image, and the glove anesthesia image.[65]

Another imagery technique is to give conversational images. For example, the client is helped to relax by telling him to "pretend your body is a puppet on a string," "let your body go limp all over," or "try to feel like a limp dishrag." To explain a therapeutic measure, the client may be told that "this will loosen the knots you describe in the back of your neck," "this is stretching out the back muscles to stop the spasms," "the heat is melting away the pain," or "the heat is driving away the pain." Using images such as the client himself has used to describe the pain may be particularly effective.

A similar imagery technique is brief instruction. The client is told to "think of the sensation as unusual, not painful," "concentrate on other things," "think of your hand as dull and insensitive," or "think of your hand as a wax hand or a rubber hand and not really part of your body."[66]

Images that suggest return to health are also helpful. They increase therapeutic physiological functioning. Examples of such images are "the food is supplying nutrients to repair the damaged tissues" or "the heat is bringing increased blood flow to the area to cleanse the tissues and carry away the wastes."

Hypnosis Hypnosis is a state of altered consciousness characterized by extreme responsiveness to suggestion. Through hypnosis the client is separated from the analytical and judgmental component of his thought processes so that acceptance of suggestion is possible.[67] Hypnosis is induced artificially in a subject by means of verbal suggestion from the hypnotist or by the subject's concentration upon some object.[68] Although to utilize hypnotic suggestion requires training, hypnosis can be used successfully by some persons whose pain syndromes involve a tension component or a psychogenic-based set of symptoms. This technique decreases tension by reducing fear and anxiety and by enhancing the person's optimism and sense of well-being. Hypnotic suggestion can also be used to induce analgesia, for sensory-imagery conditioning, and to induce a relaxation state.

Behavioral approaches

Relaxation strategies elicit the relaxation response. The positive effects of relaxation include reducing the effects of stress, decreasing acute anxiety, acting as a distraction from the pain, alleviating skeletal muscle tension or contraction, producing a state of increased susceptibility to suggestions of comfort, combating fatigue, facilitating sleep, and enhancing the effectiveness of other pain-relief measures.[69] To elicit the relaxation response requires a quiet environment, a comfortable position, a mental device, and a passive attitude.[70] Relaxation strategies include deep-breathing regimens, heartbeat breathing, music, slow rhythmic breathing, and progressive relaxation exercises with a trainer.

Relaxation techniques are utilized in biofeedback, autogenic training, meditation, yoga, Zen practices, imagery, and hypnosis. *Autogenic training* is learning to self-regulate bodily functions such as heart rate, breathing rate, and blood flow.

Biofeedback applies operant conditioning principles. Through an attached monitoring device such as an electrocardiograph, electroencephalograph, or electromyelograph, the client is provided with information about a physiological function that he would not normally have available. The physiological signal itself is transformed, amplified, and then displayed on a monitor or via an auditory feedback system. With this increased awareness of his physiological state and special training, the individual can learn to modify his particular physiological state.

Several principles of pain control seem to be involved in biofeedback, including the principle of distraction, induction of a relaxed state, and development of control over the pain. Biofeedback has been used to treat chronic pain syndromes with a stress-related component. The effectiveness of EMG biofeedback in controlling tension headache and low back pain has been demonstrated. Use of this technique for other disorders involving abnormal muscle tension is currently under investigation.

Comprehensive pain management programs

Recently there has been a movement toward a holistic view of pain and emphasis on comprehensive pain management that recognizes the need to rehabilitate the person who has lived with chronic pain. Most comprehensive pain-management programs have come into existence since the early 1970s. This approach involves comprehensive assessment and problem identification. The treatment plan includes elimination of drug addiction, therapeutic measures to reduce the pain, physical rehabilitation, psychological rehabilitation for the client and his family, and the return of control over the pain-management program to the client. A comprehensive multidisciplinary pain assessment and pain profile along with a complete physical and laboratory evaluation are the first steps. Whether the client is withdrawn from the medication he has been using and a new drug regimen initiated or whether his current drug regimen is simply titrated downward depends on the individual pain center.

Generally treatment is aimed at achieving maximum mobilization and relief of pain by the use of physical and psychological treatment techniques. Physical reconditioning is initiated slowly. Gradually, a sound and reasonably vigorous exercise program is established. Physical treatment modalities initiated may include massage, pressure, heat therapy, cold therapy, vibration, TENS, and acupuncture. An equally important component in chronic pain management is what some have called *psychophysiological therapy*.[71] The client is taught mental exercises such as "relaxation, psychophysiological balance of sensation, balancing emotional distress, special goal-oriented phrases and imagery, and spiritual attainment."[72] Often biofeedback training is used. Psychological counseling is a critical component. Persons who have been in pain for a prolonged period of time have markedly altered their interpersonal relationships and communication patterns with family, friends, and health care personnel. The chronic stress of the pain has left their lives in shambles. Some authorities recommend an intensive program of psychological therapy over a short period of time rather than the more traditional prolonged therapy.[73]

In a holistic pain-management program, the client learns to draw upon his own inner resources and to assume responsibility for practicing skills that will help him cope with his pain. He is helped to use family and significant others effectively. He learns to manage his own pain.

ASSESSMENT OF PAIN

The goals in pain assessment are (1) to attempt to truly understand the client's pain experience, (2) to identify the causative factor or factors, and (3) to identify modulating factors that are influencing the pain experience.

Detecting Physical Sources

When a client is experiencing pain, the cause for the pain should be sought so that, if possible, it can be removed. The nurse should observe for signs of physical sources of pain, including trauma, inflammation, ischemia, distension (especially of a viscus), perforation of a viscus and muscle spasm. In many cases there may be a secondary pain source. For example, the postoperative client may have a distended bladder that needs to be decompressed. Searching for the cause of pain is especially important with the onset of an acute pain episode. But it must be remembered that clients with chronic pain syndromes may also have a related or unrelated acute pain experience.

Data Collection

The following data should be collected from the client experiencing pain, whether acute or chronic:

1. Brief but thorough discussion of pain location
2. Mode of onset

3. Precipitating or associated factors
4. Detailed description of how pain evolved
5. Quality and characteristics of pain (dull, aching, shooting, etc.)
6. Duration, intensity, and severity of pain
7. Change in pain since it was first perceived
8. Measures that relieve the pain
9. Associated signs and symptoms such as autonomic nervous system responses
10. Meaning of pain experience to the client.[74]

Clinical observation should be used to expand or clarify the data collected from the client. The nurse should also conduct a general survey of the client that includes

1. Client's appearance
2. Client's motor behavior (e.g., facial expression, posture, gait, motor activity)
3. Client's affective behavior (e.g., affect, crying, withdrawal, irritability)
4. Client's verbal behavior (e.g., expressions of anger, frustration, hopelessness or despair, fear, anxiety)

Responses elicited by a pain stimulus should be noted, including

1. Brainstem-level automatic responses: rise in blood pressure, increased heart rate, increased cardiac output, rapid irregular respirations, dilated pupils
2. Spinal-level reflex responses: decreased gastrointestinal motility resulting in nausea, vomiting, and distension; decreased urinary output; bronchospasm; increased muscle tension

Besides collecting the above assessment data, the nurse may need to

1. Inspect and palpate the painful area
2. Identify trigger points of pain
3. Test the range of motion of involved joints
4. Test the location, degree, and type of decreased sensation or increased hypersensitivity

Trigger points can be identified by pressing carefully and systematically throughout the painful area and at distances from the area of pain.[75]

In chronic pain situations, the following assessment data should also be collected:

1. Brief but thorough review of past history and past experiences with pain
2. Past treatments and results of those treatments[76]
3. Current pain-management protocol
4. Effect of pain on activity level and lifestyle in general
5. Methods client uses to cope with pain of various intensities

NURSING MANAGEMENT FOR PAIN SYNDROMES

The nursing goals for pain management are the same as those of other members of the health team: (1) to alter the sensory-discriminative pain component and (2) to alter the affective-motivational and cognitive components of pain. A critical element in the nursing management of a client with a pain syndrome is the establishment of a trusting relationship and a good rapport with the client. The client needs to know that (1) the nurse considers his pain significant; (2) the nurse's goal is to help him cope with the pain by using techniques to help him relax, by making him more comfortable, by minimizing his sense of aloneness and isolation, and by protecting him from depersonalization; and (3) the nurse will help him maintain or regain control over his environment.

Establishing a Nurse-Client Relationship

Nursing actions that will promote the establishment of an effective relationship with the person who is experiencing pain should include:

1. Clarify responsibilities in pain relief. What is the nurse going to do? What are the client and the family expected to do?
2. Believe the client. This person needs to be able to trust the nurse to believe in his pain. Nursing activities to relieve pain convey concern and trustworthiness. This message can also be conveyed verbally to the client by saying "I know you are in pain."
3. Respect the client's response to pain. Accept the client's right to respond to his pain in the manner that he needs to. The client may also need help to accept his own response to the pain; his behavior may be less than he expects of himself.
4. Collaborate with the client. Encourage the client to use coping techniques that have been effective for him in the past. Assist the client to utilize his own resources more effectively. Also meet the client's expectations of a nurse even if those expectations do not entirely conform to the job description or to one's own role perception. Help the client to actively participate in setting goals for his pain relief.

5. Explore with the client his pain. Find out the meaning of the pain to the individual enduring the pain.
6. Be with the client. Act as a buffer for the client during difficult times as well.[77]

Nursing Measures to Alter the Sensory-Discriminative Pain Component

Physical measures

Nursing measures to alter the sensory-discriminative pain component include those nursing actions which stimulate large-diameter A fibers, such as (1) applying electrical stimulation, vibration, or counterirritation via heat or cold therapy as ordered by the physician and (2) providing cutaneous stimulation through pressure, massage, bathing, and trapping of body heat (Fig. 50-9). This aspect of nursing management cannot be overemphasized.

Anxiety, pain, and immobility increase muscular tension. Nursing management of pain syndromes must include measures to reduce this muscular tension, including frequent position changes, positioning that supports body parts, early ambulation, heat applications, and measures to promote relaxation such as massage and back rubs.

Use of analgesia

The nursing management of pain syndromes also involves establishing and maintaining an effective analgesic regimen. The use of a preventive approach to pain is crucial. The client should be medicated prior to painful procedures and before activities that can be expected to produce pain. If these procedures or activities are planned so that they occur when the client's analgesic has reached its peak effectiveness, his pain will be decreased and his ability to participate will be increased. Moreover, if the client is medicated before the pain begins to increase rather than waiting until it becomes severe, far less medication is required. This may minimize the drug side effects that often aggravate the pain. The client may need to be taught when to ask for his pain medication. Administration may also be time-controlled, with the medication given regardless of the presence or absence of pain.

Nurses need to remember that an injection is not necessarily the only or best route of administration of pain medication. The oral route is an alternate route in almost all pain syndromes, including acute pain experiences. Good pain control can be achieved by this approach, and it avoids the problems inherent in the prolonged use of intramuscular injections. It must be remembered, however, that a larger dose must be ordered to achieve effective pain relief when the oral route is used.

Another route often overlooked but particularly useful when the client cannot take his analgesic by mouth is the rectal route. The rectal suppository that has been shown to be most effective for pain relief is oxymophone (Numorphan), a narcotic agent.[78]

A preventive approach should be employed when utilizing either the oral or the rectal route. Absorption of the drug is slower than with intramuscular injections, and therefore more time is needed for the drug to provide effective pain relief.

Currently there are also available creams and lotions containing 10% triethanolamine salicylate (Aspercreme, Myoflex Cream). These agents have been recommended by the manufacturers for joint and muscle pain. Although no sensation is experienced when they are applied at or near the pain source, the aspirinlike substance is absorbed locally. This route of administration avoids gastric irritation, but the other side effects of high-dose salicylate are not necessarily prevented.[79]

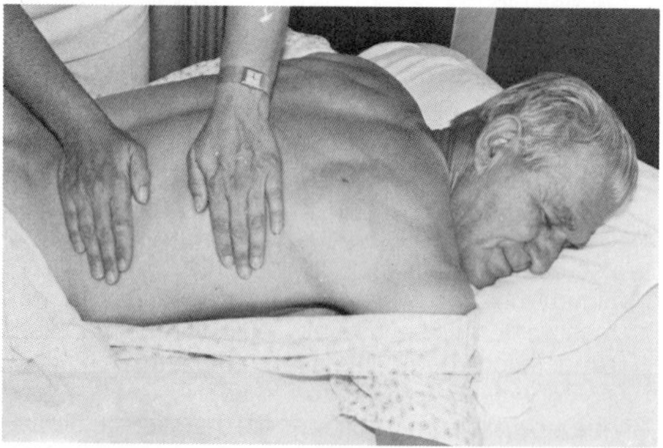

Figure 50-9 A back rub is a time-honored method of providing cutaneous stimulation.

Preventive measures

Institution of preventive measures to minimize joint and muscle stiffness is important to the pain-management regimen. As severe pain subsides, the client will tend to become more aware of the pain associated with joint and muscle tenderness. The nurse should establish a passive range-of-motion program and, if not contraindicated by the client's condition, an active exercise regimen for the client. The exercise program reduces the stiffness and helps to release muscle spasms if present. Both client and family should be taught the exercise regimen. The client should be encouraged to move about as much as possible within the medically prescribed activity order.

The nurse must also prevent painful complications that result from immobility, including decubiti, contractures, and thrombophlebitis. Since pain can be intensified by distension of a viscus, constipation should be prevented by ensuring that the client is well hydrated, mobilized as soon as possible, and given laxatives as necessary. Since urinary retention can cause or increase pain, intake and output should be monitored and the bladder percussed to assess the degree of distension. Foley catheters should be checked frequently to assure patency and free flow of urine.

The client should be helped to identify precipitating factors causing pain. Then measures to prevent the pain should be instituted and taught to the client and family.

Pain management must include methods to promote rest and sleep. Research has clearly established that persons deprived of REM sleep and deep sleep become irritable and fatigued and have increased sensitivity to pain. Not only must the client be allowed to sleep undisturbed for at least 2 hours at a time, but comfort measures, analgesics and hypnotics, and relaxation techniques should be employed to promote sleep.

A well-balanced diet high in the B-complex vitamins and tryptophan is now being recommended by experts in the field of chronic pain management. The B-complex vitamins and tryptophan enhance optimal neurologic functioning and nervous system repair. It is recommended that sugars, caffeine, nicotine, and alcohol be kept to a minimum.[80]

Nursing Measures to Alter the Affective-Motivational and Cognitive Pain Components

Behavorial measures

Nursing actions designed to alter the affective-motivational and cognitive components of pain include anticipatory guidance, effective use of others, and assisting the client to use behavioral approaches involving relaxation and conditioning and cognitive strategies such as distraction and imagery.

Anticipatory Guidance The client should be prepared as much as possible regarding pain experiences. This is referred to as *anticipatory guidance*. By preparing the client for what to expect, the nurse can help to reduce his anxiety and clarify misinformation and misinterpretation. Knowing what to expect helps the client to cope with the unknown. The following are areas of client teaching:[81]

1. Occurrence, onset, and duration of pain
2. Quality, location, and severity of pain
3. Information on how his personal safety is being assured
4. Underlying cause of pain
5. Methods of pain relief

In the anticipatory phase of the pain experience, some anxiety mobilizes the development of coping strategies. This is an important point when dealing with clients who are to have a painful experience. They cannot be reassured that there will be little or no pain but must be helped to identify ways to cope with the pain that will be experienced.[82]

Family teaching and family-nurse relationships are extremely important. Assessment of the family and friends and their interaction with the client is essential in the presence of a pain syndrome. The interpersonal dynamics are often inappropriate and stressful. Nursing intervention to teach the family and friends and to provide information on more effective coping techniques for themselves as well as strategies to help the client are essential.

Relaxation Technique In the area of assisting the client to use behavioral approaches, the client should be encouraged to continue to do what he has found helpful in terms of relaxing. He should be taught to use those relaxation techniques that appeal to him. Teaching the client relaxation techniques is beginning to assume a larger role in the nursing management of pain.

Conditioning Certain pain-relief measures result in relief frequently enough for *classical conditioning* to take place. Nurses can help the client benefit from this phenomenon by deliberately pairing relief methods. For example, teach a relaxation technique to be utilized each time a pain medication is given. One result of this is the additive effect gained from two measures used simultaneously. A second result is the conditioned response gained over time, so that eventually the relaxation technique will have the same effect as receiving the pain medication.[83]

Behavior modification (*operant conditioning*) is based on the principle that the frequency of a behavior may be increased or decreased by the use of reinforcement. Positive reinforcement results in an increase in the frequency of the behavior. Nurses can utilize behavior modification by giving praise and attention to the client when he tries new pain-relief methods or when he engages in behaviors unrelated to pain. He should be praised and noticed when he attempts to progress toward recovery.

Cognitive Strategies In assisting the client to use cognitive strategies, it must first be emphasized that the fact that the client can use distraction effectively to decrease his pain experience does not mean that the pain is not severe. Clients and family members, as well as some health care personnel, need to understand this. Distraction techniques remove pain from the center of attention; this increases pain tolerance and decreases the response to the pain experience.

Part of the nurse's role is to encourage the client to utilize the distraction techniques that he has found helpful in the past. The nurse should also assist the client to utilize distraction techniques. Family members need to be taught how to assist him to effectively use distraction techniques, and both client and family need support to utilize such techniques.

The nurse should utilize imagery in conversation with the client. Another part of the nurse's role is to assist the client with his own imagery. Encourage him to relive past events; ask him for a detailed description of a pleasant event or scene from his life. When he focuses on only one sensory modality—for example, what the mountain looked like—ask him about other sensory modalities such as the sound, smell, or temperature. This technique can also be taught to family members.

Another point should be made about imagery at this time. Clients, especially children, are often more accepting of the use of imagery than health care professionals. Nurses are sometimes resistant to teaching clients these techniques for fear of disapproval from physicians or other nurses or because they seem unscientific.

Many of the above techniques elicit behaviors that are incompatible with pain. For example, relaxation is incompatible with muscle tension. Talking about a scenic view is incompatible with thinking about pain. Rhythmic breathing is incompatible with the breath holding and gasping that are associated with pain. Such eliciting of behaviors that are incompatible with pain is part of the nursing management of the client experiencing pain.

Emotional considerations

Depression and anger are often experienced by the person in pain. These feelings of anger and depression can often be reduced by helping the client to gain control over his pain and to feel less isolated and alone. The nurse should encourage the client to express his feelings. He needs to be assured that these feelings are common, and he may need assistance to maintain a reality orientation about the direction of his anger. The establishment of an activity program such as an exercise, occupational therapy, or recreational therapy regimen can be an effective measure to reduce depression. The client may need antidepressant or mood-elevating drugs as much as or more than he needs pain medication.

Preserving the client's energy for activities he enjoys is also important. The nurse must first identify the activities that are most important or pleasurable for the client. Then together they must find ways for him to carry out these activities by reorganizing priorities and schedules and perhaps changing some rules and regulations. Providing periods of rest and sleep may also be necessary to allow the client to have the energy he needs for those activities important to him.

EVALUATING THE PAIN-MANAGEMENT PROTOCOL

In both the acute and the chronic pain situations, the nurse should evaluate the effectiveness of the pain-relief measures taken by nursing and other health care personnel. The effectiveness of individual pain-relief measures and of the total pain-management protocol must be judged. Such judgments are made by comparing the client's motor, autonomic, affective, and cognitive responses prior to the intervention with his responses following the intervention. Both subjective and objective data enter into the evaluation. But it must be remembered that the client is the final judge.

If the client says that the relief measures are not adequate, reassess the pain and in addition ask the following questions:

1. Are a variety of pain-relief measures being used? (If not, add additional measures.)
2. Are the pain-relief measures being used before the pain becomes severe? (If not, implement an anticipatory analgesia regimen.)
3. Is what the client believes will be effective included in the pain-management protocol? (If not, why not?) Can classical conditioning be used if the client cannot keep receiving what he believes is most effective?
4. Is the client willing and able to be a more active participant in his pain management? (If not, why not?) How can he be helped to become more active?
5. Can the client be encouraged to try the pain-relief measure one or two more times, especially if some additional measures are implemented?[84]

A revised pain-management protocol should then be formulated and implemented.

SUMMARY

The client has several rights with regard to pain. He has the right "(1) to decide the duration and intensity of the pain he is willing to tolerate, (2) to be informed of all the possible methods of pain relief, along with the favorable and unfavorable consequences, as well as the controversial aspects, (3) to choose which method he wishes to try, and (4) to choose to live without pain."[85]

Pain relief is a legitimate therapeutic goal and contributes significantly to the client's total well-being. The client has the right to pain relief, and that relief should have high priority in his care.[86]

Case Study / Acute Head Pain

Mrs. M. is a 26-year-old white woman admitted from the emergency room with incapacitating head pain of 3 days' duration. She complains of generalized pounding pain involving her entire head and neck that has become gradually worse over the last 3 days. She is now curled up in bed on her left side and refuses to move. She states that moving "makes the pain unbearable." She has been unable to eat or drink because of nausea and vomiting for the past 48 hours. Her vital signs are: T = 37.7°C (99.8°F), BP = 90/50, P = 125, R = 24. The muscles of her neck and upper back are tense. She has been crying since admission.

Mrs. M. is married to a first-year general surgery resident. She has a 6-month-old daughter and a 2-year-old son. She and her husband are from the Northeast and moved to this southern university town 9 months ago when her husband started his residency program. Both families live in New York State.

Discussion Questions

1. Explain the components of pain specifically related to Mrs. M.
2. What physiological factors are contributing to the head pain? What can be done to decrease or eliminate these factors?
3. What are the clinical manifestations of an uncontrolled acute pain cycle? Which of these does Mrs. M. manifest?
4. What can the nurse do to help alleviate Mrs. M.'s pain?
5. What other nursing problems besides pain does this client have? Describe the appropriate nursing interventions for each.

REVIEW QUESTIONS

The number of the question corresponds to the same-numbered objective at the beginning of the chapter.

1. Choose the most comprehensive definition of pain.
   - **a.** A harmful stimulus that signals current or impending tissue damage.
   - **b.** A pattern of responses that operate to protect the individual from harm.
   - **c.** An unpleasant sensation or sense of hurt experienced by the individual.
   - **d.** An individualized experience that has a perceptual component and a response component.

2. Pain perception occurs at the level of the
   - **a.** spinal cord
   - **b.** reticular activating system
   - **c.** thalamus
   - **d.** cerebral cortex

3. A modulating factor that increases the pain threshold is
   - **a.** the phenomenon of facilitation
   - **b.** enkephalin-endorphin release
   - **c.** slow adaptation of pain receptors
   - **d.** decrease in cerebral function

4. The gate-control theory of pain provides a theoretical basis for all the following therapeutic modalities *except*
   - **a.** ablative neurosurgical procedures
   - **b.** massage
   - **c.** electrical nerve stimulation
   - **d.** exercise regimens

5. Factors that may cause pain perception to vary within the same individual are
   - **a.** presence of fatigue
   - **b.** degree of motivation
   - **c.** level of anxiety
   - **d.** all of the above

6. Pathophysiological consequences of an untreated acute pain syndrome include
   - **a.** local alkalosis
   - **b.** increased urinary output
   - **c.** decreased peristalsis
   - **d.** decreased muscle tone

7. What assessment data are *not* critical to planning care for the client who is experiencing a chronic pain syndrome?
   - **a.** cause of the pain
   - **b.** the client's past experiences with pain
   - **c.** methods used by the client to cope with the pain
   - **d.** factors precipitating or associated with the pain

8. Mobilization of the endogenous opiates is *not* achieved by which of the following management techniques?
   - **a.** narcotic analgesics
   - **b.** electrical nerve stimulation
   - **c.** acupuncture
   - **d.** deep brain stimulation

9. A method of cutaneous stimulation that is an independent nursing action is
   - **a.** electrical nerve stimulation
   - **b.** acupuncture
   - **c.** pressure, rubbing, and massage
   - **d.** application of external counterirritants

REFERENCES

1. Margo McCaffery, *Nursing Management of the Patient with Pain*, J. B. Lippincott Company, Philadelphia, 1979, p. 11.
2. Arthur C. Guyton, *Textbook of Medical Physiology*, W. B. Saunders Company, Philadelphia, 1976, p. 663.
3. Charles R. Noback and Robert J. Demarest, *The Human Nervous System: Basic Principles of Neurobiology*, 2d ed., McGraw-Hill Book Company, New York, 1975, p. 70.
4. Beverly Bishop, "Pain: Its Physiology and Rationale for Management," *Phys Ther*, **60:**14 (1980).
5. Ibid.
6. Guyton, op. cit., p. 663.
7. Ibid.
8. Ibid., p. 664.
9. William B. McCullough, "A General Surgeon's Perspective," in John J. Bonica (ed.), *Pain Overview 1980*, HP Publishing, New York, 1980.
10. John J. Bonica (ed.), "Introduction," *Pain Overview 1980*, HP Publishing, New York, 1980, p. 4.
11. Bishop, op. cit., p. 14.
12. Ibid., p. 19.
13. Ibid.
14. Bonica, op. cit., p. 3.
15. Margaret E. Armstrong, "Current Concepts in Pain," *AORN J*, **32:**385 (1980).
16. Bonica, op. cit., p. 3.
17. Bishop, op. cit., p. 20.
18. Bonica, op. cit., p. 3.
19. McCullough, op. cit., p. 14.
20. Bishop, op. cit., pp. 21–22.
21. Ibid., p. 22.
22. Ibid., p. 23.
23. Bella Almay, G. I. Johanson et al., "Endorphins in Chronic Pain," in *Pain #5*, Elsiever Press, North Holland, 1978, pp. 153–162.
24. C. Richard Chapman, "The Role of Anxiety in Acute Pain," in John J. Bonica (ed.), *Pain Overview 1980*, HP Publishing, New York, 1980, p. 6.
25. Barbara L. Conway, *Carini and Owens' Neurological and Neurosurgical Nursing*, The C. V. Mosby Company, St. Louis, 1978, p. 523.
26. Dorothy S. Siegele "The Gate Control Theory," *Am J Nurs*. **74:**501 (1974).
27. Bonica, op. cit., p. 3.
28. Ibid.
29. Ibid., pp. 4–5.
30. Kathleen McCauley and Rosemary C. Polomano, "Acute Pain: A Nursing Perspective with Cardiac Surgical Patients," *Topics Clin Nurs*, **2:**46 (1980).
31. Sandra S. Sweeney, "OR Observations: Key to Postop Pain," *AORN J*, **32:**394–396 (1980).
32. Ibid., p. 395.
33. Ibid.
34. Bonica, op. cit., p. 5.
35. Sweeney, op. cit., p. 395.
36. McCauley and Polomano, op. cit., p. 46.
37. M. Oster, N. Vizel, and L. Turgeon, "Pain of Terminal Cancer Patients," *Arch Intern Med*, **138:**1801–1802 (1978).
38. John J. Bonica, "Cancer Pain: A Major National Health Problem," *Cancer Nurs*, **1:**313–316 (1978).
39. G. Mathews, V. Zarro, and J. Osterholm, "Cancer Pain and its Treatment," *Semin Drug Treat*, **3:**45–52 (1973).
40. Margaret Rankin, "The Progressive Pain of Cancer," *Topics Clin Nurs*, **2:**58 (1980).
41. Bishop, op. cit., pp. 24–27.
42. McCaffery, op. cit., 1979, p. 116.
43. Ibid., p. 123.
44. Ibid., p. 125.
45. C. Norman Shealy, "Holistic Management of Chronic Pain," *Topics Clin Nurs*, **2:**6 (1980).
46. Bishop, op. cit., pp. 24–27.
47. McCaffery, op. cit., 1979, p. 128.
48. A. C. Hymes, D. E. Raab, E. G. Yonehiro, G. D. Nelson, and A. L. Printy, "Electrical Surface Stimulation for Control of Acute Postoperative Pain and Prevention of Ileus," *Surg Forum*, **24:**447–448 (1973).
49. A. C. Hymes, D. E. Raab, E. G. Yonehiro, G. D. Nelson, and A. L. Printy, "Acute Pain Control by Electrostimulation: A Preliminary Report," in John J. Bonica (ed.), *Advances in Neurology #4*, Raven Press, New York, 1974, pp. 761–767.
50. A. C. Hymes, E. G. Yonehiro, D. E. Raab, G. D. Nelson, and A. L. Printy, "Electrical Surface Stimulation for Treatment and Prevention of Ileus and Atelectasis," *Surg Forum*, **26:**77–78 (1975).
51. A. M. Cooperman, B. Hall, E. S. Sadar, and R. W. Hardy, "Use of Transcutaneous Electrical Stimulation in Control of Postoperative Pain," *Surg Forum*, **26:**77–78 (1975).
52. G. D. Vanderark and K. A. McGrath, "Transcutaneous Electrical Stimulation in Treatment of Postoperative Pain," *Am J Surg*, **130:**338–348 (September 1975).
53. D. M. Long and M. T. Carolan, "Cutaneous Afferent Stimulation in the Treatment of Chronic Pain," in John J. Bonica (ed.), *Advances in Neurology #4*, Raven Press, New York, 1974, pp. 755–759.
54. G. D. Gammon and I. Starr, "Studies on the Relief of Pain by Counterirritation," *J Clin Invest*, **20:**13–20 (January 1941).
55. R. Melzack, "Prolonged Relief of Pain by Brief, Intense Transcutaneous Somatic Stimulation," *Pain*, **1:**357–273 (1975).
56. McCaffery, op. cit., 1797, p. 132.
57. Ibid., p. 133.
58. Ibid.
59. Ibid.
60. Shealy, op, cit., p. 6.
61. Bishop, op. cit., p. 25.
62. Maureen P. Terzian, "Neurosurgical Interventions for the Management of Chronic Intractable Pain," *Topics Clin Nurs*, **2:**77 (1980).
63. McCaffery, op. cit., 1979, p. 92.
64. Ibid., p. 157.
65. Ibid., p. 31.
66. Ibid., p. 173.
67. Thomas J. Daly and Eric L. Greenspun, "Stress Management Through Hypnosis," *Topics Clin Nurs*, **1:**59 (1979).
68. Margaret E. Armstrong, Jeanne Howe, Ann P. Smith, Marilyn M. Smith, and M. Josephine Snider (eds.), *McGraw-Hill Nursing Dictionary*, McGraw-Hill Book Company, New York, 1979, p. 447.
69. McCaffery, op. cit., 1979, p. 143.
70. H. Benson, *The Relaxation Response*, William Morrow Publishing, New York, 1975.
71. Shealy, op. cit., p. 6.
72. Ibid.
73. Ibid., p. 7.
74. Conway, op. cit., pp. 526–527.

75. McCaffery, op. cit., 1979, p. 133.
76. Conway, op. cit., pp. 526–527.
77. McCaffery, op. cit., 1979, pp. 43–56.
78. Margo McCaffery, "How to Relieve Your Patients' Pain Fast and Effectively with Oral Analgesics," *Nursing*, **10:**63 (November 1980).
79. McCaffery, op. cit., 1979, p. 126.
80. Shealy, op. cit., p. 7.
81. McCaffery, op. cit., 1979, pp. 57–73.
82. Ibid., p. 3.
83. Ibid., pp. 27–29.
84. Ibid., p. 42.
85. Ibid., p. 3.
86. Ibid.

Chapter 51

NURSING ROLE IN MANAGEMENT

Chronic Neurologic Problems

Judith M. Ozuna

Learning Objectives

1. Explain the potential impact of chronic neurologic disease on physical and psychological well-being.
2. Compare and contrast muscle-contraction, migraine, and cluster headaches in terms of pathophysiology, clinical manifestations, and treatment.
3. Describe the etiology, clinical manifestations, diagnostic study abnormality, and management of epilepsy, multiple sclerosis, Parkinson's disease, and myasthenia gravis.
4. Explain the nursing role in the acute and long-term care of a client with a chronic neurological disease.
5. Describe the clinical manifestations and management of amyotrophic lateral sclerosis, Huntington's chorea, muscular dystrophy, and syringomyelia.
6. Identify common physical complications in a person who is immobilized by chronic neurologic disease.
7. Outline the major goals of treatment for the client with a chronic, progressive neurologic disease.

Management of chronic neurologic disease can be challenging for both clients and health care providers. Many neurologic disorders involve progressive deterioration in physical and/or mental capabilities, which can be devastating to both the client and his family. The client may experience psychological upheaval in the form of depression, fear, anxiety, anger, or withdrawal. This is compounded by a change in body image and self-esteem. In addition, the physical disabilities resulting from degenerative disease necessitate varying, and sometimes extreme, alterations in lifestyle which add to the emotional trauma of the client. Families are torn between their sense of obligation to care for the ill person and the need to lead their own lives. They are simultaneously pushed and pulled by feelings of guilt, love, despair, hope, resentment, and empathy.

The challenge of chronic neurologic illness is equally great for health care providers. Many of these diseases have no cure, so health care professionals can only attempt to alleviate physical symptoms, prevent complications, assist clients in maximizing self-care abilities in the face of neurologic deficits, and help them in the difficult task of adjusting to their illness. Nurses, by virtue of their provision of continuous care in health institutions and their widespread presence in so many community health agencies, can and should greatly infuence these aspects of management.

This work was supported by NIH Contract No. 1-NS-6-2431, National Institute of Neurological and Communicative Disorders and Stroke, PHS/DHEW, and grant No. ID-23-NU-00081-01, Division of Nursing, PHS/DHEW.

This chapter was reviewed by Jane Ellen Mead, R.N., M.S.N., Assistant Professor, The Catholic University, Washington, D.C.

HEADACHE

Headache is a common subjective complaint which annually causes over 42 million Americans to seek health care.[1] Of all those with headache, 90 percent have *functional* headaches, which include migraine, cluster, tension, and psychogenic headaches; the remaining 10 percent suffer *organic* headaches due to significant intracranial or extracranial disease. Headaches from organic causes are discussed under the causative diseases.

Not all tissues of the cranium are pain-sensitive. The pain-sensitive structures in the head which can cause headache are the intracranial and extracranial blood vessels, the venous sinuses, portions of the dura (near large blood vessels), muscles of the scalp and neck, and cranial nerves V, VII, IX, and X and cervical nerves 2 and 3. Pain can result from (1) vascular stretching and dilatation, displacement of cerebral contents, inflammation, and direct pressure on cranial and cervical nerves; (2) sustained contraction of skeletal scalp and neck muscles; and (3) noxious stimulation from diseases of the eyes, nose, ears, and sinuses.

Chronic functional headache is the most common and perhaps the least effectively treated physical disorder. The history and neurologic examination are the keys to diagnosis.

Types of Headache

Muscle-contraction headache

Headache due to sustained contraction of the head and neck muscles is the most prevalent type of headache and may occur in up to 50 percent of men and 70 percent of women.[2] Muscle-contraction headache, also called tension, psychogenic, nervous, or rheumatic headache, is also the most difficult headache to treat.

Etiology It is generally accepted that the pain of muscle-tension headache is a result of sustained contraction of skeletal muscles in the neck, scalp, and jaws. Some clients may have actual structural alterations in muscle, joint, or connective tissue which contribute to headache pain. However, most clinicians agree that the headache is usually a part of the individual's "reaction during life stress."[2] Psychoemotional factors associated with tension headache include attempts to control hostile impulses toward family members, unconscious dependency wishes, need for love and attention, depression, and problems with sexuality.[3]

Clinical Manifestations There is no prodrome (early manifestation of impending disease) in tension headache. The pain is usually bilateral, occurring most often in the back of the neck. It usually does not interfere with sleep. The pain is often described as a tight, squeezing, bandlike pressure. It is sustained, chronic, dull, and persistent. It may last weeks, months, or even years. Of note is that many clients can have a combination of migraine and muscle-contraction headaches with features of both headaches occurring simultaneously. People with migraine may experience muscle-contraction headaches between migraine attacks.

Diagnostic Study Abnormalities Careful history taking is probably the single most important diagnostic tool for muscle-contraction headache. Electromyography (EMG) may reveal sustained contraction of neck, scalp, and/or facial muscles, but many clients may not show increased muscle tension with this test, in spite of having the test during the actual headache. Conversely, clients with diagnosed migraine headaches may show increased muscle tension on EMG. If muscle-contraction headache is present during physical examination, one may find increased resistance to passive movement of the head and tenderness of the head and neck.

Migraine

Migraine headache usually starts in adolescence. Females are affected more frequently than males. A family history of migraine can be found in 65 percent of people with migraine. Although migraine has often been associated with people who are high achievers and who suppress expressions of aggression and hostility, no single personality type describes all migraine clients.

Etiology Migraine headache is of vascular origin and involves the intracranial and extracranial arteries of the head. Recent studies have confirmed the classical theory of migraine, which is that the *prodromal* or *aural phase* is associated with decreased blood flow and vasoconstriction and the *headache phase* is associated with increased blood flow and vasodilatation.[4] Recent evidence suggests that a mechanism other than vasoconstriction may be involved in the prodrome of migraine. Increased platelet aggregation found in the circulation during the prodromal phase is thought to be triggered by a stress response and release of epinephrine in some cases.[5] Some believe there is a profound instability of blood vessel regulation mechanisms. Studies suggest that the dilated artery is hyperpermeable and involved in a sterile local inflammatory reaction. Several vasoactive substances have been implicated in this process, including cathecholamines, histamine, serotonin, peptide kinins, and prostaglandins. It is thought that accumulation of these substances around the artery sensitizes it to pain.

Clinical Manifestations There are two major types of migraine, classical and common. *Classical migraine* occurs in only 10 percent of migraine clients. The sharply defined prodrome may last 10 to 30 minutes before the headache begins and may include sensory dysfunction (visual-field defects, tingling or burning sensations or paresthesias), motor dysfunction (weakness, paralysis), dizziness, confusion, or even loss of consciousness. The classical preheadache symptom is perception of flashing lights in one quadrant of the visual field, often referred to as *scintillating scotomata*. This type of migraine usually peaks in 1 hour and may last several hours.

Common migraine is the second and most common type of migraine. The prodrome is not sharply defined and it can involve psychic disturbances, gastrointestinal upset, and changes in fluid balance. The prodrome may precede the headache by several hours or days. The headache itself may last several hours or days.

Clinical manifestations which occur in both classical and common migraine are generalized edema, irritability, pallor, nausea and vomiting, and sweating. During the headache phase, people with migraine tend to "hibernate"; that is, they seek shelter from noise, light, odors, people, and problems. The headache itself is described as a steady, throbbing pain which is synchronous with the pulse. Although the headache is usually unilateral, it may switch to the opposite side in another episode. The diagnosis of migraine is usually made from the history. The neurologic and other diagnostic examinations are often normal.

Cluster headache

Cluster headache is sometimes associated with migraine headache because of its similar vascular origin. It stands in a 1:10 ratio to migraine in frequency of occurrence and is more frequent in males than in females by 5:1. The onset is usually between the ages of 30 and 60.

Etiology Although the vasodilatation in cluster headache is similar to that of migraine headache, the pathogenesis is not quite the same. There is no fall in plasma serotonin as there is in migraine, but there is a rise in plasma histamine during the cluster headache. Neither the etiology nor the pathophysiology of cluster headache is fully known. However, it is clear that paroxysmal recurring discharge of the parasympathetic nervous system is involved.

Clinical Manifestations The headache has an abrupt onset, usually without a prodrome. It peaks in 5 minutes and lasts 30 to 90 minutes. It may recur several times a day over several days and usually affects only one side of the face and head. Signs of parasympathetic discharge accompany the headache: conjunctivitis, increased lacrimation (tearing), and nasal congestion on the side of the headache. The headache is described as deep, steady, and boring but not throbbing, which may imply involvement of larger blood vessels. It involves the upper face, periorbital region, and forehead on one side. Attacks commonly occur upon awakening from a nap or from a night's sleep. They can occur during sleep and often wake the person after a few hours of sleep. Unlike the person with migraine, who seeks isolation and quiet, the person with a cluster headache paces the floor, cries out, does bizarre things, and resents being touched. As with migraine, there are usually no complications. However, an increased incidence of peptic and duodenal ulcer has been reported by some investigators.[5]

Diagnostic Study Abnormalities In addition to the history, thermography is useful in the diagnosis of cluster headache. This procedure involves assessment of blood flow by determining the body temperature and measuring the variation from the normal physiologic state. The thermogram is specific for cluster headache and will reveal areas of coolness in the supraorbital region on the side of the headache.[6] These cool spots are apparently along the distribution of a division of the ophthalmic artery, a terminal branch of the internal carotid artery.

Other headaches

Although migraine, cluster, and tension headaches are by far the most common, other types of headache can occur. They may be the first symptom of a more serious illness. Headache can accompany subarachnoid hemorrhage, brain tumor, other intracranial masses, arteritis, vascular abnormalities, trigeminal neuralgia (tic douloureux), diseases of the eyes, nose, and teeth, and systemic illness (bacteremia, carbon monoxide poisoning, mountain sickness, polycythemia vera). The symptoms and mechanisms of these headaches vary greatly from one illness to another. Because of the variety of causes of headache, the clinical evaluation must be thorough. It should include evaluation of personality, life adjustment, environment, and family situation as well as comprehensive evaluation of physical status.

Medical management of headaches

Table 51-1 outlines the general medical workup for a client presenting with headache in order to rule out any intra- or extracranial disease. Table 51-2 compares muscle-contraction headache, migraine, and cluster headache. If no disease is found, therapy is directed toward the functional type of headache. Table 51-3 summarizes the current therapies for symptomatic and therapeutic relief of common headaches. Because drug therapy has not been totally successful, new *holistic* therapies (affecting both mind and body)

Table 51-1
General Diagnostic Workup for Client with Headache

1. Complete history
2. Clinical examination (often negative)
   a. Inspection: local infections
   b. Palpation: tenderness, hardened arteries, bony swellings
   c. Auscultation: bruits over major arteries
3. Routine laboratory studies to rule out underlying causes of headache
   a. CBC
   b. Electrolytes
   c. Urinalysis
   d. Serology
4. Skull x-ray, lateral and frontal views
5. Special studies (CT scan, angiography, myelography, electroencephalography) if structural disease is suspected

Table 51-2
Comparison of Muscle-Contraction, Migraine, and Cluster Headaches

Pattern	Muscle-Contraction	Migraine	Cluster
Site	Bilateral, bandlike at base of skull, in face, or both	Unilateral (in 60%), may switch sides, commonly anterior	Unilateral, radiating up or down from one eye
Quality	Constant, squeezing tightness	Throbbing, synchronous with pulse	Severe, bone-crushing
Frequency	Dull, persistent, no specific pattern	Periodic	May have months or years between attacks
Duration	Intermittent for months or years	Continuous for hours or days	30 to 90 min
Time and mode of onset	Not related to time	May be preceded by prodrome	Nocturnal, may awaken after nap or few hours of sleep
Associated symptoms	Palpable neck and shoulder muscles, stiff neck, tenderness	Nausea/vomiting, edema, irritability, sweating, photophobia; prodrome of sensory, motor, or psychic phenomena; family history (65%)	Tearing and nasal congestion on ipsilateral side

have been developed and have proved effective in both muscle-contraction and vascular headaches. These therapies include meditation, yoga, biofeedback, and muscle-relaxation training.

Biofeedback involves the use of physiologic monitoring equipment to give the client information regarding his muscle tension and/or peripheral blood flow (skin temperature of the hand). The client is trained to relax his muscles and raise his hand temperature and is given reinforcement (operant conditioning) in accomplishing these physiologic alterations.

Other therapies for muscle-contraction headache include physical therapy (massage, hot packs, cervical collar), injection of local anesthetic into spastic

Table 51-3
Specific Medical Management of Headache

	Tension Headache	Migraine	Cluster Headache
Diagnostic	History; neck and head tenderness, resistance to movement; EMG	History	History, thermography
Therapeutic: Symptomatic	1. Nonnarcotic analgesics (aspirin, acetaminophen) 2. Analgesic-sedative/tranquilizer combinations (Fiorinal) 3. Muscle relaxants	1. Nonnarcotic analgesics (aspirin, acetaminophen); 2. Alpha-adrenergic blockers: ergotamine tartate (Cafergot) 3. Analgesic combinations (Fiorinal) 4. Vasoconstrictors (Midrin)	1. Alpha-adrenergic blockers: ergotamine tartate (Cafergot) 2. Analgesic combinations (Fiorinal) 3. Vasoconstrictors (Midrin) 4. Oxygen
Prophylactic	1. Muscle relaxants: tranquilizers a. Cyproheptadine HCl (Periactin) b. Methysergide maleate (Sansert) c. Chlordiazepoxide HCl (Librium) d. Diazepam (Valium) 2. Antidepressants 3. Biofeedback 4. Muscle-relaxation training 5. Psychotherapy	1. Serotonin antagonists: methysergide maleate (Sansert) 2. Analgesic combinations 3. Antidepressants: imipramine HCl (Tofranil), amitryptyline HCl (Elavil) 4. Anti-inflammatory agents 5. Biofeedback 6. Yoga 7. Meditation 8. Electrical counterstimulation	1. Serotonin antagonists: methysergide maleate (Sansert) 2. Analgesic combinations 3. Antidepressants: imipramine HCl (Tofranil), amitryptyline HCl (Elavil) 4. Anti-inflammatory agents 5. Lithium

muscles, and correction of faulty posture. Acupuncture and hypnosis are successful innovative therapies, although acupuncture provides only temporary relief. Most clients can benefit from psychotherapy aimed at helping them recognize conflicts and deal with them more effectively.

Pharmacologic intervention

Drug treatment for muscle-contraction headache usually involves a nonnarcotic analgesic (aspirin or acetaminophen) used alone or in combination with a sedative, a muscle relaxant, a tranquilizer, or codeine. However, many of these drugs have potentially dangerous side effects. Clients should be cautioned about long-term use of aspirin and aspirin combination drugs, as they can cause gastric bleeding and coagulation abnormalities in susceptible persons. Long-term use of Fiorinal should be avoided because it contains a barbiturate (habit-forming) and phenacetin (may cause kidney damage) in addition to aspirin. Drugs containing acetaminophen (Tylenol, Phenaphen, Midrin) can cause liver damage with chronic use. Narcotics and tricyclic antidepressants (benzodiazepines) can cause addiction and habituation.

Drug treatment of the acute migraine attack is aimed at preventing the painful dilatation of the cranial blood vessels. Ergotamine tartate (Cafergot) is considered the most effective drug for this. Ergotamine inhibits the reuptake of neuronally liberated norepinephrine into storage sites of the postganglionic nerve terminal of the sympathetic nervous system. This allows more norepinephrine to attach to alpha-adrenergic sites on smooth muscle in the artery wall, thereby causing prolonged vasoconstriction of cranial vessels. Relief of headache with ergotamine treatment usually confirms the diagnosis of vascular headache. Ergotamine can be administered orally, sublingually, parenterally, rectally, or by inhalation. The usual dose is 1 to 2 mg (oral, rectal) at the onset of the headache, followed by 2 mg within 1 hour. Not more than 6 mg is given for any single attack. Other drugs which may relieve migraine headache include Fiorinal, Midrin, aspirin, acetaminophen (Tylenol, Datril), meperidine (Demerol), and codeine.

A variety of drugs are employed to prevent further migraine attacks. These drugs are taken during the interval between attacks rather than during the actual headache. Methysergide maleate (Sansert) is often prescribed for clients whose headaches are more frequent than once a week. Methysergide is chemically related to a drug which is a potent antagonist of serotonin. It may act by substituting at serotonin receptor sites whenever small reductions in serotonin occur.[7] Because this drug can cause fibrosis of the kidneys, heart, and lungs, it is recommended that after 6 months' use it be discontinued for a 2-month period before being reinstituted. Yearly intravenous pyelogram, chest X-ray, ECG, and blood chemistry studies are advised. Other drugs sometimes used in prophylaxis of migraine headache are Bellergal which corrects imbalance of autonomic nervous system; cyproheptadine hydrochloride (Periactin; serotonin antagonist), propranolol hydrochloride (Inderal), tricyclic antidepressants (Tofranil, Elavil), and tranquilizers such as chlordiapoxide and diazepam (Librium and Valium).

Nursing management

Since the history provides the key to assessment of headache, it should include specific details of the headache itself: location and type of pain, onset, frequency, duration, relation to events (emotional, psychological, physical), and time of day. Information about previous illnesses, surgery, trauma, allergies, family history, and response to medication should also be obtained. The nurse can suggest that the client keep a diary of headache episodes with details of the above information. Such a record can be of great help in determining the type of headache as well as precipitating events.

Clients with chronic headache present a great challenge to health care providers. Their headache often results from inability to cope with daily stresses. The most effective therapy may be to assist clients to examine their lifestyle and to recognize stressful situations and learn to cope with them more appropriately. Precipitating factors can be identified and ways of avoiding them developed. Daily exercise, relaxation periods, and socializing can be encouraged, as each of these can help reduce recurrence of headache. The nurse can suggest alternative ways of handling the pain of headache through relaxation, meditation, yoga, and self-hypnosis.

Besides the use of analgesics and analgesic combination drugs for symptomatic relief of headache, clients should be encouraged to employ relaxation techniques, as these have proved effective in both muscle-contraction and vascular headaches. Migraine sufferers often need a quiet, dimly lit environment. Massage and moist hot packs to the neck and head can help clients with muscle-contraction headache.

The client should learn about the medications prescribed for prophylaxis and symptomatic treatment of his headache. He should be able to describe the purpose, action, dosage, and side effects of his medication. It is often good practice to have the client write down each time he takes a medication for headache relief, to prevent accidental overdose.

SEIZURE DISORDERS/EPILEPSY

Seizures are frequently a symptom of an underlying illness. They may accompany a variety of disorders or may occur spontaneously without any apparent cause. Seizures resulting from systemic and metabolic disturbances are not considered epilepsy if the seizures cease when the underlying problem is corrected. Metabolic disturbances in the adult which cause seizures include acidosis, electrolyte imbalance, hypoglycemia, hypoxia, alcohol and barbiturate withdrawal, dehydration, and water intoxication. Extracranial disorders that can cause seizures are heart, lung, liver, and kidney disease, systemic lupus erythematosus, diabetes, hypertension, and septicemia.

Epilepsy connotes spontaneously recurring seizures. There are an estimated 1 to 2 million people with epilepsy in the United States, and 80 percent experience their first seizure before the age of 20. After this age the incidence decreases.

Etiology

From birth to 6 months the most common causes of epilepsy are severe birth injury, congenital defects involving the CNS, infections, and inborn errors of metabolism. Between the ages of 2 and 20 the primary factors are birth injury, infection, trauma, and genetic factors. From ages 20 to 30 epilepsy occurs usually as the result of structural lesions such as trauma, brain tumors, or vascular disease. After the age of 50 the primary causes of epilepsy are cerebrovascular lesions and metastatic brain tumors. Although many causes of epilepsy have been identified, three-fourths of all epilepsy cases cannot be attributed to a specific cause and are termed *idiopathic*.

The role heredity plays in the etiology of epilepsy has been difficult to determine because of the problem of separating hereditary from environmental or acquired influences. However, it is known that certain normal and abnormal EEG patterns are genetically transmitted. It has been determined that typical absence seizures (petit mal epilepsy) are inherited as an autosomal dominant trait.[8] Although some have disputed the conclusion, it is generally accepted that typical absence seizures run in certain families, indicating some type of inherited link. Some families carry a predisposition to epilepsy in the form of an inherently low threshold to seizure-producing stimuli such as trauma, disease, or high fever. For instance, an inherently low seizure threshold may explain why some people develop seizures after a head injury or similar insult, while others do not.

Pathophysiology

Seizures are paroxysmal, uncontrolled electrical discharges of neurons in the brain that interrupt normal function. Seizures can be the result of a variety of physical alterations. Because the brain transmits information by electrical and chemical processes, anything that disrupts these processes can cause a seizure. Researchers have found that in recurring seizures (epilepsy) a group of abnormal neurons (*seizure focus*) supposedly undergo spontaneous firing (Fig. 51-1). This firing then spreads by physiologic pathways to involve adjacent or distant areas of the brain. If this activity spreads to involve the whole brain, a generalized seizure occurs. Just what causes this abnormal firing is not clear. Anything that depolarizes the nerve cell dendrites or the cell membrane will induce a tendency to spontaneous firing.

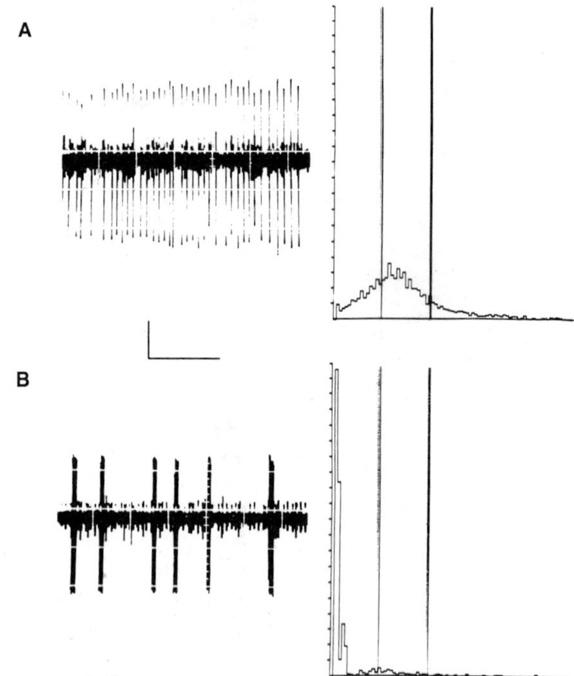

Figure 51-1 *(a)* Firing pattern of a normal neuron in motor cortex. The action potentials (APs) seen as spikes occur at regular intervals (most are 30 to 60 milliseconds apart). *(b)* Spontaneous firing pattern of an epileptic cell. Unlike the single APs seen above, these APs are so close together (less than 10 milliseconds apart) that they cannot be discriminated. Instead one sees several APs in a burst (burst firing). *(Courtesy of Allen Wyler, M.D., University of Washington.)*

Several theories on the etiology of epilepsy have been advanced. One of the most popular explanations for the formation of an epileptic focus is formation of scar tissue in the brain. This scar tissue formation is the physiologic response to such problems as brain tumors, head injuries, infections, and degenerative diseases. Since neurons do not regenerate after injury, astrocytes (a type of glial cell) proliferate. It is postulated that this proliferation of glial tissue alters the extracellular potassium concentration, allowing it to increase beyond its normally low level. An increase in extracellular potassium is known to cause seizures by allowing the neuron to depolarize more readily than usual.

There is evidence that gliosis occurs during the birth process and that this may later lead to epilepsy in some people. It is believed that as the infant's head passes through the pelvic opening the medial sides of the temporal lobes are squeezed against the rigid tentorium, causing hypoxic damage to some neurons and subsequent gliosis.

Another structural change which may be the result of scarring is the loss or alteration of the tiny prominences, called *spines*, on the dendrites of epileptic cells. These are believed to be the primary structures for receiving synaptic input. Investigators have suggested that because of this loss of dendritic spines, the cell, which has thus lost some of its synaptic input, becomes hyperexcitable. It is thought that the naked dendrite is more susceptible to the surrounding interstitial neurotransmitters and that the excitatory ones have a greater influence. The actual mechanism of this structural alteration is still conjecture.

Another theory is that hypoxia resulting from some alteration in the vascular supply within the brain can cause certain cells to die out. The cells most susceptible to this oxygen deprivation are those with an inhibitory influence, some interneurons of the cortex, and the Purkinje cells of the cerebellum. If these cells die out, a decrease in the inhibitory modulation of neuronal action potentials occurs, allowing neurons to fire unchecked.

It appears that repetitive electrical discharges from an epileptic focus in experimental animals can produce long-lasting and possibly permanent changes in neuron excitability, both locally and in distant areas of the brain. This effect is called *kindling*, and it presents an interesting and important implication for epilepsy in humans: seizures can beget more seizures. Clinical experience indicates that the longer one goes without good seizure control, the less likely the seizures are to be controlled. Therefore a vigorous attempt must be made to control recurring seizures.

Clinical Manifestations

The preferred method of classifying seizures is the International Classification System proposed by Gastaut in 1970 [9] (Table 51-4). It is based on the clinical and electroencephalographic manifestations of seizures and is currently undergoing revision. In this system seizures are divided into two major classes, generalized and partial.

Generalized seizures

Generalized seizures are characterized by bilateral synchronous epileptic activity in the brain from the onset of the seizure. Because the entire brain is affected at the onset of the seizures, there is no warning or aura. The person loses consciousness for a few seconds to several minutes.

Grand Mal Seizures The most familiar generalized seizure is the generalized tonic-clonic, or grand

Table 51-4

International Classification of Epileptic Seizures*

I. Partial seizures (seizures beginning locally)
   A. Partial seizures with elementary symptomatology (generally without impairment of consciousness)
      1. With motor symptoms (include Jacksonian seizures)
      2. With special sensory or somatosensory symptoms
      3. With autonomic symptoms
      4. Compound forms
   B. Partial seizures with complex symptomatology, generally with impairment of consciousness (temporal lobe or psychomotor seizures)
      1. With impairment of consciousness only
      2. With cognitive symptomatology
      3. With affective symptomatology
      4. With psychosensory symptomatology
      5. With psychomotor symptomatology (automatisms)
      6. Compound forms
   C. Partial seizures secondarily generalized

II. Generalized seizures (bilaterally symmetrical and without local onset)
   1. Absences (petit mal)
   2. Bilateral massive epileptic myoclonus
   3. Infantile spasms
   4. Clonic seizures
   5. Tonic seizures
   6. Tonic-clonic seizures (grand mal)
   7. Atonic seizures
   8. Akinetic seizures

III. Unilateral seizures (or predominantly unilateral)

IV. Unclassified epileptic seizures (incomplete data)

*Currently undergoing revision by the International League Against Epilepsy.

mal, seizure. This seizure is characterized by loss of consciousness and falling to the ground if upright, followed by stiffening of the body for 10 to 20 seconds and subsequent jerking of the extremities for another 1 to 3 minutes. Cyanosis, excessive salivation, tongue biting, and incontinence may accompany the seizure.

In the postictal phase (following a seizure) the person usually has muscle soreness, is very tired, and may sleep for several hours. Some people may not feel normal for several hours or days after a seizure.

Typical Absence (Petit Mal) Seizures The other familiar generalized seizure is the typical absence (petit mal) seizure. This seizure usually occurs only in children and rarely continues beyond adolescence. It may cease altogether as the child matures, or it may evolve into another type of seizure. The typical clinical manifestation is a brief staring spell lasting only a few seconds, which is why it often occurs unnoticed. These seizures may occur up to a hundred times a day. The EEG demonstrates a three-per-second spike-and-wave pattern which is unique to this type of seizure. Absence seizures can often be precipitated by hyperventilating and by flashing lights.

Atypical Absence Seizures Another type of generalized seizure is the staring spell accompanied by other signs and symptoms, including brief warnings, peculiar behavior during the attack, and/or confusion after the attack. The EEG demonstrates atypical spike-and-wave patterns, usually greater or less than three cycles per second.

Other Types Other generalized seizures are myoclonic and akinetic seizures. A myoclonic seizure is characterized by a sudden, excessive jerk of the body or extremities. The jerk may be forceful enough to hurl the person to the ground. These seizures are very brief and may occur in clusters. The terms *akinetic* (arrest of movement), *atonic* (loss of tone), and *astatic* (loss of balance) have been used interchangeably to describe drop attacks or falling spells. This type of seizure begins quite suddenly with the person falling to the ground. He usually is conscious by the time he hits the ground and is ready to resume normal activity immediately. Persons with this type of seizure are at great risk for head injury and often have to wear protective helmets. A less severe akinetic seizure involves brief loss of muscle tone without falling.

Partial seizures

Partial (focal) seizures are the second major class of the International Classification System. Partial seizures begin in a specific region of the cortex, as indicated by the EEG and usually by the clinical manifestations. For instance, if the discharging focus is located in the medial aspect of the postcentral gyrus, the person may experience paresthesias and tingling or numbness in the leg on the side opposite the focus. If the discharging focus is located in the part of the brain which governs a particular function, sensory, motor, cognitive, and emotional phenomena may occur.

Partial seizures may be confined to one side of the brain and remain partial or focal in nature, or they may spread to involve the entire brain, culminating in generalized tonic-clonic seizure. Any tonic-clonic seizure that is preceded by an aura or warning is a partial seizure which secondarily generalizes. Many tonic-clonic seizures which appear to be generalized from the outset may actually be secondarily generalized seizures, but the preceding partial component may be so brief that it is undetected by the client, the observer, or even the EEG. Unlike the primary generalized tonic-clonic seizure, the secondarily generalized seizure may result in transient residual neurologic deficit postictally. This is referred to as Todd's paralysis (focal paresis); it resolves after varying lengths of time.

Partial seizures are further divided into those with elementary symptomatology (simple motor or sensory phenomena) and those with complex symptomatology (also called *temporal lobe* or *psychomotor seizures*). Partial seizures with elementary symptomatology usually do not involve loss of consciousness and rarely last longer than 1 minute. They may involve motor, sensory, or autonomic phenomena or a combination of these. The terms *focal motor, focal sensory,* and *Jacksonian* have been used to describe seizures of the partial elementary type.

Partial seizures with complex symptomatology, as the name implies, can involve a variety of behavioral, emotional, affective, and cognitive functions. The location of the discharging focus is usually in the temporal lobe, hence the term *temporal lobe seizure.* These seizures usually last longer than 1 minute and are frequently followed by a period of postictal confusion. Partial complex seizures are distinct from partial elementary (focal motor, focal sensory) seizures in that they usually involve some alteration in consciousness. In fact, the sole manifestation may be clouding of consciousness or a confused state without any motor or sensory components. This type of attack is sometimes called *temporal lobe absence.* There is rarely the complete loss of consciousness which is typical of the generalized absence (petit mal) attack, nor does the person snap back to his previous state as does one who has had a generalized absence attack.

The most common partial complex seizure involves lip smacking and *automatisms* (repetitive movements which may not be appropriate). These are often called *psychomotor seizures*. The person may continue an activity which was initiated before the seizures, such as counting out change or picking items from a grocery shelf; but after the seizure, he does not remember the activity performed during the seizure. Other automatisms are less organized, such as picking at clothing, fumbling with objects (real or imaginary), or simply walking away. Many say they can hear others call to them during their seizure but cannot respond verbally or physically to commands. If they do speak, it is gibberish or mumbling. If someone tries to restrain them during a seizure, they may become combative and agitated. They are not malicious, nor are they directing their aggression to any one person. It is as if their brains were driving them to execute a behavior, and if someone tries to prevent them from doing it, they resist to the point of becoming aggressive. People who exhibit this behavior during a seizure are often misunderstood and sometimes erroneously committed to psychiatric or corrective institutions.

Autonomic symptoms usually occur during partial seizures of complex symptomatology, rarely as the sole feature of a partial elementary attack. The symptoms may include gastrointestinal (GI) disturbances, cardiovascular and respiratory alterations, or enuresis. Hypersalivation, masticatory movements with lip smacking and swallowing, or a feeling of epigastric discomfort and nausea may accompany the GI symptoms. Many clients describe the feeling as a "rise" in the stomach, "butterflies in the stomach," or a "rush."

A variety of psychosensory symptoms may occur during a partial complex seizure, including distortions of visual or auditory sensations and vertigo. There may be alterations in memory such as a feeling of having experienced an event before *(déjà vu)* or alterations in thought processes such as forced thinking.

Complications

Physical

Status epilepticus is the most serious complication of epilepsy. This is a state in which seizures recur in rapid succession and the person does not regain consciousness or normal function between seizures. Status epilepticus can involve any type of seizure (see preceding sections). During repeated seizures the brain uses more energy than can be supplied. Neurons become exhausted and cease to function. Permanent brain damage may result. Grand mal status is the most dangerous, because it can cause ventilatory insufficiency, hypoxemia, cardiac arrhythmias, and systemic lactic acidosis which can be fatal.

Another complication of epilepsy is severe injury, and even death, due to trauma suffered during a seizure. Persons who lose consciousness during a seizure are at greatest risk for this. Death can result from head injury incurred in a fall, from drowning in the bathtub, or from severe burns.

Psychosocial

Perhaps the most common complication of epilepsy is the effect it has on a person's lifestyle. Although attitudes have improved in recent years, epilepsy still carries a social stigma.[10] In the past it was associated with supernatural powers, possession by the devil, and insanity. Today the stigma probably exists because the characteristics of seizures are in direct conflict with modern societal values of self-control, conformity, and independence. The person with epilepsy may experience discrimination in employment[11] and educational opportunities. He may find transportation difficult because of the legal sanction against driving. He may develop inadequate methods of coping. Several articles and books relating to these difficulties are available (see Bibliography for Section 10).

Diagnostic Study Abnormalities

The most useful diagnostic tool is an accurate and comprehensive description of the seizure(s) and the past history. The EEG is a useful diagnostic adjunct to the history, but only if it shows abnormalities. Unfortunately, only a small percentage of people with epilepsy have abnormal EEGs the first time the test is done. Many times several EEGs need to be done before abnormalities are detected, if they ever are, because abnormal discharges may not occur during the 30 to 40 minutes of EEG sampling. The EEG is not foolproof. Some people without epilepsy have abnormal EEGs, and many people with epilepsy have normal EEGs. Abnormal findings help to determine the seizure type and to pinpoint the seizure focus.

Medical Management

The diagnostic and therapeutic management of seizure disorders is summarized in Table 51-5. Treatment of epilepsy is primarily by antiepileptic medication. Therapy is aimed at preventing seizures, since cure is not possible. Medications generally act by stabilizing nerve cell membranes and preventing spread of the epileptic discharge. Alternative therapies for epilepsy are surgical removal of the epileptic focus and biofeedback or operant conditioning in selected cases. Potential candidates for cortical resection must have a clearly identifiable epileptic focus located in the nondominant hemisphere and/or in an

Table 51-5

Medical Management: Seizures

Diagnostic

1. Complete history and physical examination
   a. Birth and development history
   b. Significant illnesses and injuries
   c. Family history
   d. Febrile seizures
   e. Comprehensive neurologic assessment
2. Seizure history
   a. Precipitating factors
   b. Antecedent events
   c. Seizure description (include onset, duration, frequency, postictal state)
3. Diagnostic studies
   a. CBC, urinalysis, electrolytes, BUN, fasting blood sugar
   b. Lumbar puncture
   c. CT scan
   d. EEG

Therapeutic

1. Antiepileptic medication (see Table 51-6)
2. Surgery (cortical resection, stereotactic lesions, corpus callosum resection)
3. Biofeedback (operant conditioning)
4. Psychosocial counseling

Table 51-6

Antiepileptic Drugs and Drug Interactions

Drug	Known Drug Interactions
Grand Mal, Focal, and Psychomotor Seizures	
Phenytoin (Dilantin)	Aspirin, benzodiazepines, bishydroxycoumarin, carbamazepine, clonazepam, coumarin, chloramphenicol, dexamethasone, disulfiram; ethosuximide, ethanol, isoniazid, methylphenidate, phenothiazines, phenylbutazone, valproic acid, birth control pills
Carbamazepine (Tegretol)	Phenytoin, birth control pills
Phenobarbital	Bishydroxycoumarin, clonazepam, diazepam, phenothiazines, phenylbutazone, phenytoin, valproic acid, birth control pills
Primidone (Mysoline)	Isoniazid (see also phenobarbital interactions)
Absence, Akinetic, and Myoclonic Seizures	
Ethosuximide (Zarontin)	None known
Valproic acid (Depakene)	Clonazepam, phenytoin, phenobarbital
Clonazepam (Clonopin)	Valproic acid

area which will not leave the client with permanent neurologic deficits after resection. Biofeedback to control seizures is aimed at teaching the client to maintain a certain brain-wave frequency which is refractory to seizure activity. This method is still in the experimental stage.

Pharmacologic Intervention

The primary goal of antiepileptic therapy is to obtain maximum seizure control with a minimum of toxic side effects. The principle of drug management is to begin with a single drug and increase the dose until a therapeutic serum level is reached. The therapeutic range for each drug indicates the serum level above which most clients experience toxic side effects and below which most continue to have seizures. If seizure control is not achieved with a single drug, a second drug is added.

The primary drugs for treatment of generalized tonic-clonic (grand mal) and partial (focal) seizures are phenytoin (Dilantin), carbamazepine (Tegretol), phenobarbital, and primidone (Mysoline). The primary drugs for treatment of absence (petit mal), akinetic, and myoclonic seizures are ethosuximide (Zarontin), valproic acid (Depakene), and clonazepam (Clonopin). Table 51-6 summarizes the known drug interactions of the major antiepileptic drugs. Because many of these drugs have a long half-life (phenytoin, phenobarbital, ethosuximide), they can be given in once- or twice-daily doses. This aids medication-taking compliance by simplifying the drug regimen and avoiding the need to take medication at work or school. These drugs should not be discontinued abruptly, as this can precipitate seizures.

Toxic side effects of antiepileptic drugs involve the central nervous system (CNS) and include diplopia, drowsiness, ataxia, and mental slowing. Neurologic assessment for dose-related toxicity is simple and objective: the eyes are tested for nystagmus. Mild nystagmus confirms that the drug is being taken. If it is associated with diplopia, the dose may need to be decreased. Hand and gait coordination should be assessed as well as cognitive functioning and general alertness.

Idiosyncratic side effects involve organs outside the CNS. These include the skin (rashes), gums (hypertrophy), bone marrow (blood dyscrasias), liver, and kidney. Nurses should be knowledgeable about these side effects so that clients can be informed and proper treatment instituted. A common idiosyncratic side effect of phenytoin is hypertrophy of the gums. This can be limited by good dental hygiene, including regular tooth brushing and flossing. If extensive, the hypertrophied gum tissue may have to be surgically removed (gingivectomy) and phenytoin may have to be replaced by another antiepileptic drug.

Nursing Management

Health promotion and maintenance

Many cases of epilepsy can be prevented by promotion of general safety measures such as wearing helmets in situations involving risk of head injury. Improved prenatal, labor, and delivery care has reduced fetal trauma and hypoxia and thereby reduced brain damage leading to epilepsy. Children with fever should be treated quickly to avoid high temperatures which might cause seizures.

Clients with epilepsy, like everyone else, should practice good general health habits (proper diet, adequate rest, and exercise). They should be helped to identify events or situations which precipitate their seizures and be given suggestions to avoid them or handle them better. Clients should avoid excessive alcohol intake, fatigue, and loss of sleep. They should be helped to handle stress constructively.

Acute intervention

Nurses caring for hospitalized epileptic clients or clients who have had a seizure due to any of a variety of metabolic causes have several responsibilities, including observation and treatment of the seizure, education, and psychosocial intervention. Table 51-7 summarizes the nursing care for the client with seizures.

When a seizure occurs, the nurse should carefully observe and record it, because the diagnosis and subsequent treatment often rest solely on the seizure description. All aspects of the seizure should be noted. What events preceded the seizure? When did the seizure occur and how long did each phase of it (aura, if any; ictus, or seizure; postictal period) last? What occurred during each phase? Both subjective data (usually the only type of data in the aural phase) and objective data are important. Objective data should include the exact onset of the seizure (which body part was affected first and how), the course and nature of the seizure activity (loss of conciousness, tongue biting, automatisms, stiffening, jerking, total lack of muscle tone), what body parts were involved and in what sequence, what autonomic signs were present (dilated pupils, excessive saliva, altered breathing, cyanosis, flushing, diaphoresis, incontinence). Assessment of the postictal period should include level of consciousness (coma, stupor, lethargy), vital signs, memory loss, muscle soreness, speech disorders (aphasia, dysarthria), weakness or paralysis, sleep period, and the duration of each.

A seizure can be a frightening experience for the client and for others who may witness it. The nurse should assess the level of their understanding and inform both about how and why the event occurred. This is an excellent opportunity for the nurse to dispel many common misconceptions about seizures. Misunderstanding is perhaps at the root of many psychosocial problems that clients with epilepsy and their families experience.

Chronic management

Prevention of recurring seizures is the major goal in the treatment of epilepsy. Because epilepsy cannot be cured, medication must be taken regularly and continuously, often for a lifetime. The nurse should make sure the client knows this as well as the specifics of his medication regimen and what to do if he misses a dose (usually he should make up the dose if he remembers it within 24 hours). He should be cautioned not to adjust medications on his own, as this can increase seizure frequency and even cause status epilepticus. He should be encouraged to report any medication side effects and to keep regular appointments with his health care provider.

Nurses should teach family members and significant others the first-aid treatment of tonic-clonic (grand mal) seizures. They should be reminded that it is not necessary to call an ambulance or send a person to the hospital after a single seizure unless it is prolonged, another seizure immediately follows, or extensive injury has occurred.

Perhaps the greatest challenge epilepsy presents to the client is adjusting to the limitations placed on him by his illness. Discrimination in employment was the most serious problem facing the person with epilepsy in a recent national survey.[11] Clients can be informed that the Rehabilitation Act of 1973 was designed to protect handicapped (including epileptic) persons from discrimination in employment. For issues relating to job discrimination, clients can be referred to the State Human Rights Commission or the State Department of Vocational Rehabilitation.

A variety of other resources can be offered to the client with epilepsy who has a specific problem. If the nurse feels that the client can benefit from associating with others who have epilepsy, she can refer him to the local chapter of the Epilepsy Foundation of America (EFA), a voluntary agency that offers a variety of services to clients with epilepsy. If the client is a veteran, she can refer him to the Veterans' Administration Hospital which provides comprehensive care.

The client should be informed that medical alert bracelets, necklaces, and identification cards are

Table 51-7
Nursing Care Plan for the Client with Seizures

Client Problem	Expected Outcome	Nursing Intervention
	Acute Management	
Generalized tonic-clonic seizure	Absence of injury after the seizure	Remove objects from person's surroundings. Loosen tight clothing. If client is in bed, siderails should be padded and in the raised position. If client gives enough warning before teeth become clenched, place soft cloth between teeth; do not force objects between teeth. If client is on floor, place soft padding under his head (pillow, or put head on your legs as you kneel on floor). As client relaxes from seizure, turn his head to the side to allow secretions to drain from mouth, preventing aspiration. Do not restrain client. Remain with client until seizure is over. Offer comfort and assistance. Assess neurologic status and vital signs postictally. Record seizure events (preictal, ictal, and postictal) (see Table 51-5). If client begins to have another seizure before regaining consciousness, call for medical assistance immediately, as this may signal status epilepticus.
Partial complex seizure	Absence of injury and embarrassment	Stay with client until seizure is over. Speak calmly and reassuringly during seizure, as client may be able to hear. Do not restrain unless he may put himself in danger. Record seizure events (see Table 51-5).
Status epilepticus	Cessation of seizures and absence of injury	Implement same first-aid measures as described above for general tonic-clonic seizure. Prepare medication (Valium, Dilantin, phenobarbital). Prepare oxygen delivery equipment; assure availability of emergency respiratory tray. Place oral airway if possible. Insert nasogastric tube to prevent vomiting and aspiration. Establish IV route. Assess neurologic status.
	Chronic Management	
Denial of disorder	Acceptance of disorder as evidenced by using *epilepsy* to describe illness and admitting seizures when they occur	Explore reasons for denial. Implement and individualize teaching plan about causes and mechanisms of seizures, effectiveness of drugs in controlling seizures, inaccuracy of myths about epilepsy, avoidance of precipitating factors, state law regarding driving, pros and cons of medical ID tags, using moderation in drinking and eating, exposure to stress, and avoiding hazardous activities.
Noncompliance	Regular taking of medications	Assess compliance by interview and drug levels. Assess reasons for noncompliance and implement counseling approach accordingly. Tailor regimen to daily activities. Use medication and seizure calendar. Use special pill containers. Use support by family, significant others.
Psychosocial problems (depression, anxiety, anger, withdrawal, employment discrimination, dependency, lack of social skills)	Effective and appropriate coping and social skills	Counseling, referral to appropriate agencies (see Bibliography for Section 10.)

available through the EFA, local pharmacies, or companies specializing in identification devices. However, the use of these medical identification tags is optional. Some clients have found them beneficial, but others have found them to be more a burden than a help; they prefer not to be identified as epileptic.

Social workers and welfare agencies can help with financial problems and living arrangements. The state services for those with developmental disabilities can offer assistance with job placement and training for clients whose seizures are not well controlled. It can offer sheltered housing and provide funding for special needs such as medical evaluation, psychological evaluation, and transportation State agencies specializing in vocational rehabilitation services can offer vocational assessment, counseling, funding for training, and assistance with job placement. They can also offer financial assistance for transportation and medical costs that are necessary for either vocational rehabilitation or job maintenance. If intensive psychological counseling is needed, the nurse can refer the client to a community mental health center.

The client should be encouraged to learn more about epilepsy through self-education materials. The EFA provides several information pamphlets. Many agencies offering services to epileptic persons, as well as local chapters of the organization, have these available as teaching aids.

MULTIPLE SCLEROSIS

Multiple sclerosis (MS) is a degenerative disorder of the CNS which affects approximately 500,000 people in the United States. It is considered a disease of young adults, with the onset usually between 20 and 40 years of age. Females are affected almost twice as often as males.

Etiology

Epidemiological factors

Multiple sclerosis primarily affects whites of northern European descent, which means that the disease is associated with certain environmental and familial factors. Incidence is highest in the temperature zones of the globe (between 45 and 65° latitude), especially northern Europe, Canada, and northern United States, and it is associated with the place of birth: if someone born and raised in one of the regions listed moves to a warmer climate (nearer the equator) after the age of 15, he carries the same risk for MS as others in his country of origin. Of interest is that blacks and Asians have a lesser incidence of MS than whites; some believe that these peoples do not carry certain histocompatibility antigens found in persons of northern European descent.[12] Relatives of persons with MS have a greater chance of getting the disease because of an apparent familial predisposition to defects of the immune system (see below).

Immunological factors

A current theory is that MS is the result of childhood infection by a "slow virus" which later triggers an autoimmune process. This produces antibodies which attack and destroy the myelin sheath of neurons in the CNS. Many investigators have found higher concentrations of measles antibodies in MS clients than in controls. However, measles has not been proved to be a cause of MS.[13] In addition, other virus antibodies have been found to be elevated in MS clients.

Recent research suggests that there is a defect in the T lymphocytes of the immune system in people with MS. Normally a type of T cell assists in the regulation of the immune system by suppressing production of antibodies. It is thought that there is a correlation between the failure of T suppressor cells and the autoimmune process in MS.[14]

Precipitating factors

The concept of precipitating factors is controversial. It is possible that their association with MS is pure chance. Possible precipitating factors include infections, physical injury, emotional stress, excessive fatigue, pregnancy, and lowered state of health.

Pathogenesis

In MS the myelin sheaths of the neurons in the brain and spinal cord are attacked (Fig. 51-2*a, b*). An inflammatory process accompanies the destruction of myelin. Early in the disease the myelin sheath is damaged, but the nerve fiber is not affected and nerve impulses are still transmitted (Fig. 51-2*c*). At this point the client may complain of noticeable impairment of function (e.g., weakness). However, the myelin can regenerate and the symptoms can disappear, resulting in a remission.

As the disease progresses, the myelin becomes totally disrupted and the axon becomes involved (Fig. 51-2*d*). Myelin is replaced by glial scar tissue, which forms hard, sclerotic plaques in multiple regions of the CNS. Without myelin, nerve impulses slow down, and with destruction of nerve axons, impulses are totally blocked, resulting in permanent loss of function.

The disease process has a spotty distribution in the CNS. Therefore the signs and symptoms vary from person to person and within the same person over time. The disease is characterized by remissions and exacerbations. With repeated exacerbations, however, progressive scarring of myelin occurs, and the overall trend is progressive deterioration in neurologic function.

Clinical Manifestations

Because the onset is often insidious and gradual, with vague symptoms occurring intermittently over a period of months or years, the disease may be diagnosed long after the onset of the first symptom. The clinical manifestations vary according to the areas of

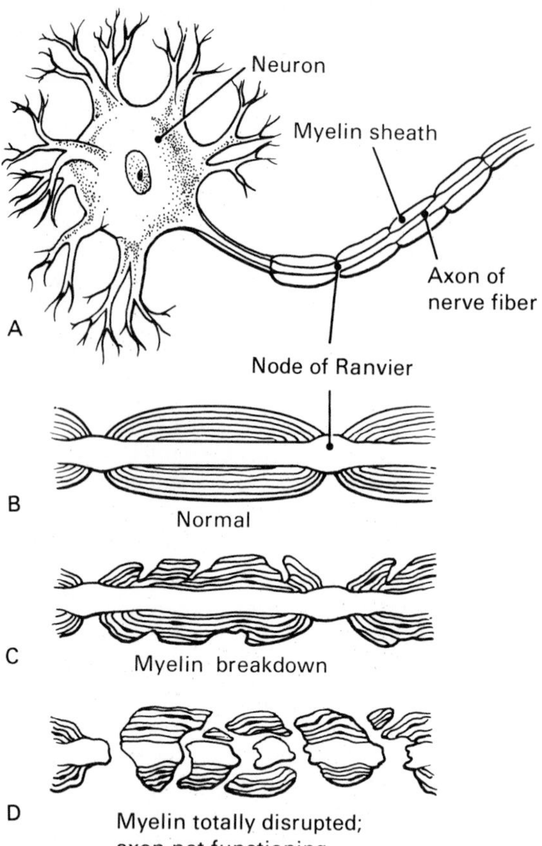

Figure 51-2 *(a)* Normal nerve cell with myelin sheath. *(b)* Normal axon. *(c)* Myelin breakdown. *(d)* Myelin totally disrupted, axon not functioning.

the CNS involved. Some clients have severe, long-lasting symptoms early in the course of the disease, while others may experience only occasional and mild symptoms for several years after onset.

Common signs and symptoms may include motor, sensory, cerebellar, and emotional phenomena. Motor symptoms may include weakness or paralysis of limbs, trunk, or head, diplopia, or spasticity of muscles which are chronically affected. Sensory symptoms include numbness and/or tingling and other paresthesias, patchy blindness (scotomas), blurred vision, vertigo, tinnitus, and decreased hearing. Cerebellar signs include nystagmus, ataxia, dysarthria, and dysphagia. Bowel and bladder function can be affected if the sclerotic plaque is located in areas of the CNS controlling elimination. Problems with defecation usually involve constipation (due to loss of tone in the external sphincters) rather than fecal incontinence.

Urinary problems are variable. A common problem in MS clients is a spastic (uninhibited) bladder. This indicates a lesion above S_2 which cuts off suprasegmental inhibiting influences on bladder contractility. The bladder has a small capacity for urine, and it contracts unchecked. This is accompanied by urinary urgency and frequency and results in dribbling or incontinence. A flaccid (hypotonic) bladder (another type of bladder problem in MS clients) indicates a lesion of sensory input from the bladder to the CNS. The bladder has a large capacity for urine because there is no sensation or desire to void, no pressure, and no pain. Consequently urinary retention occurs, but urgency and frequency may occur with this type of lesion also. Urinary problems cannot be adequately diagnosed and treated unless urodynamic studies are done.

Although intellectual functioning generally remains intact, emotional stability may be affected. People may be easily angered, depressed, or euphoric. Sexual function may also be affected. Physiologic impotence may result from spinal cord involvement in the male. Diminished sensation can prevent normal sexual response in both sexes. The emotional effects of chronic illness and loss of self-esteem also contribute to loss of sexual response. Signs and symptoms of MS are aggravated or triggered by physical and emotional trauma, fatigue, and infection.

The average life expectancy after onset of symptoms is more than 25 years. The leading causes of death are related to respiratory and urinary infections and complications of decubitus ulcers. The life expectancy of MS clients is about 80 percent of that of the general population.

Diagnostic Study Abnormalities

Because there is no definitive diagnostic test for MS, diagnosis is primarily based on the history and clinical manifestations. Certain laboratory tests are currently used as major adjuncts to the clinical examination. In some clients, CSF analysis may show an increase in lymphocytes during the active phase of the disease and an increase in oligoclonal immunoglobulin G (IgG). The visual evoked response (VER), determined by EEG recording of occipital lobe discharges in response to a flash of light in the eye, is often delayed in persons with MS because of decreased nerve conduction from the eye to the brain. Computerized tomography (CT scan) may be helpful, as sclerotic plaques as small as 3 to 4 mm in diameter can be detected. The "hot bath test," which causes aggravation of symptoms in persons with MS, is sometimes used as a diagnostic tool, although positive results occur in other neurologic disorders as well.

Medical Management

Since there is no cure for MS, medical management is aimed at treating the disease process and providing symptomatic relief (Table 51-8). The disease process is treated with certain drugs (see below) and the symptoms with a variety of medications and therapies. Spasticity can be treated with antispasmodic drugs, surgery (neurectomy, rhizotomy, or cordotomy), or dorsal-column electrical stimulation. Intention tremor that becomes unmanageable is sometimes treated by stereotactic surgery on the thalamus. This involves selective destruction of the ventrolateral nucleus in the thalamus. Two methods may be employed: freezing (cryothalamectomy) and radiofrequency current (thalamotomy). Neurologic dysfunction sometimes improves with hypothermia, physical therapy, and speech therapy.

Table 51-8
Medical Management: Multiple Sclerosis

Diagnostic
1. History and physical examination
2. CSF analysis
3. Visual evoked response (VER) test
4. CT scan
5. "Hot bath" test

Therapeutic
1. Drugs
   a. Anti-inflammatory
   b. Immunosuppressive
   c. Anticholinergic
   d. Cholinergic
   e. Antispasmodic
2. Surgery
   a. Thalamotomy (for unmanageable tremor)
   b. Neurectomy, rhizotomy, cordotomy (for unmanageable spasticity)

Pharmacologic Intervention

ACTH and prednisone have been helpful in rapidly improving acute exacerbations by reducing edema and acute inflammation at the site of demyelination. The treatment regimen usually consists of parenteral administration of ACTH 40 U twice a day for 7 days, followed by 20 U twice a day for 4 days, then 20 U/day for 3 days. Immunosuppressive drugs such as azathioprine (Imuran) have been tried, but so far they have not shown clear-cut beneficial effects in controlled studies. Table 51-9 summarizes the drugs commonly used for symptomatic treatment of MS.

Dietary Measures

Various dietary measures that have been advocated in the management of MS include megavitamin therapy (vitamin B_{12}, vitamin C) and diets of high-fat, low-fat, and gluten-free food and raw food or vegetables. These particular dietary measures have not come into widespread use because of lack of proof of their effectiveness.

A nutritious, well-balanced diet is essential. Although there is no standard prescribed diet, a high protein diet with supplementary vitamins is often advocated. A diet high in roughage may help relieve the problem of constipation. Vitamins are merely supplementary and not curative.

Nursing Management

Acute intervention

The most common reasons for hospitalization of the multiple sclerosis client are diagnostic workup and treatment of an acute exacerbation of complications such as bladder dysfunction. During the diagnostic phase the nurse has an important role in reassuring the client that even though he may have been admitted with a tentative diagnosis of MS, certain diagnostic studies must be made to rule out other neurologic disorders. The nurse needs to assist the client in dealing with the anxiety caused by a diagnosis of disabling illness. Recently diagnosed clients may need assistance with the grieving process.

During an acute exacerbation the client is often immobile and confined to bed for 2 to 3 weeks. The focus of nursing intervention at this phase is to prevent major hazards of immobility such as respiratory and urinary infections and decubitus ulcers. Specific measures are discussed in the nursing care plan (Table 51-10).

Rehabilitative management

Rehabilitative management is aimed at (1) helping the client adjust to his illness, (2) client education on avoidance of factors which precipitate exacerbations, (3) maximizing self-care in light of current neurologic deficits, and (4) meeting the needs for activities of daily living. The main goal is to keep the client active and functionally useful.

Physical therapy is an important measure for keeping the client as functionally active as possible. The purpose of therapy is to relieve spasticity, increase coordination, and train the client to substitute nonaffected muscles for impaired ones. An especially beneficial type of physical therapy is water exercise. Water gives buoyancy to the body and allows the client to perform activities that would normally be

Table 51-9
Drugs for Symptomatic Treatment of Multiple Sclerosis

Drug	Symptoms Relieved	Precautions	Side Effects	Education Needs
Corticosteroids ACTH, Prednisone, Dexamethasone, Hydrocortisone	Exacerbations	These have widespread effects on many enzymes and metabolic processes. If used for less than one month at a time, few adverse effects will occur.	Edema, mental changes (euphoria), weight gain, redistribution of body fat (see Chap. 42 for effects of long-term steroid therapy)	Restrict salt intake. Do not abruptly stop therapy. Know drug interactions.
Cholinergic drugs Bethanicol chloride (Urecholine) Neostigmine methylsulfate (Prostigmine methylsulfate)	Urinary retention (flaccid bladder)	History of hypotension, cardiac dysfunction, allergies, hyperthyroidism, stomach and intestinal problems. Avoid use with adrenergic drugs (antiasthmatic drugs), may cause serious asthma attach.	Hypotension, diarrhea, diaphoresis, salivation, muscle weakness	Consult physician before using other drugs.
Anticholinergic drugs: Propantheline bromide (Pro-Banthine) Oxybutynin chloride (Ditropan)	Urinary frequency* and urgency (spastic bladder)	History of glaucoma, prostatic hypertrophy, cardiac dysfunction, intestinal obstruction.	Dry mouth, blurred vision, constipation, hypertension, flushing, urinary retention (if dose too high)	Consult physician before using other drugs, esp. sleeping aids, antihistamines (can be potentiated).
Antispasmodics Diazepam (Valium)	Spasticity	History of narrow-angle glaucoma.	Drowsiness, ataxia, fatigue	Avoid driving and similar activities because of CNS-depressant effects. Addictive, avoid long-term use. Avoid concomitant use of phenothiazines, narcotics, barbiturates, MAO inhibitors, other antidepressants.
Baclofen (Lioresal)	Spasticity	Known hypersensitivity, renal damage. Avoid use in pregnancy. May exacerbate seizures in clients with epilepsy.	Drowsiness	Do not abruptly stop therapy (can get hallucinations). Avoid driving and similar activities (sedative). Avoid use with other CNS depressants.
Dantrolene (Dantrium)	Spasticity	History of respiratory or cardiac dysfunction. May cause abnormal liver function, hepatitis. Avoid use with estrogen therapy since it predespOses to hepatotoxicity.	Drowsiness, dizziness, malaise, fatigue, diarrhea	Avoid driving. Avoid use with tranquilizers. May cause photosensitivity.

*Remember that urodynamic studies must be done before instituting therapy, because multiple sclerosis clients have multiple lesions, and bladder dysfunction cannot be diagnosed from symptoms alone.

Table 51-10
Nursing Care Plan for the Client with Multiple Sclerosis*

Client Problem	Expected Outcome	Nursing Intervention
	Acute Management	
Respiratory infection	Absence of infection. Optimal respiratory function.	Encourage coughing and deep breathing q 4 h while awake. Turn q 2 h. Protect from infectious illnesses of clients, staff, family. Feed in upright position.
Urinary tract infection	Absence of urinary infection. Optimal urinary function.	Sterile technique with catheter care. Regular cleansing of perineal area. Encourage fluids to 2–3 L daily. Teach symptoms of UTI.
Skin breakdown	Skin remains intact and free of redness	Assess skin every shift. Turn q 2 h. Keep bed free of crumbs. Use circular massage of bony prominences with each turning. Provide high protein diet. Cleanse back and buttocks if incontinent.
	Rehabilitative Management	
Muscle spasticity	Decreased duration of muscle spasms	Administer medications as ordered. Perform stretching exercises every shift.
Difficulty walking	Absence of injury	Use assistive device as indicated. Initiate gait training. Arrange PT consult. Encourage ambulation.
Urinary retention	Voiding qs with residual of less than 150 mL	Administer medications as ordered. Follow intermittent catheterization protocol, Credé maneuver, or use reflex stimulation (manual stimulation). Encourage fluid intake to 3000 mL per day.
Urinary incontinence	Urinary continence	Administer medications as ordered. Initiate bladder training program. Ensure client is protected and will not be embarrassed by incontinence.
Constipation	Normal bowel movement q 2–3 days	Maintain fluid intake (3000 mL/day). Use prune juice at same time of day. Encourage high-residue diet. Administer stool softeners, suppositories as ordered. Initiate and maintain a bowel program.
Visual disturbances	Visual function satisfactory for ADL	Patch eyes alternately q 4 h. Assess visual acuity monthly. Encourage use of large-print reading material and talking books.
Impotence	Optimal sexual functioning	Initiate sexuality counseling if indicated. Suggest alternative methods of sexual gratification.
Poor self-esteem, altered body image, depression	Positive emotional attitude	Encourage positive attitude toward effects of treatment in client, family, significant others. Assist in grieving process. Encourage use of support systems: religion, meditation, yoga, referral agencies: a. M. S. societies b. Self-help groups c. Financial agencies d. Vocational agencies Focus on remaining abilities.

*For a comprehensive nursing care plan, see M. McDonnell et al., "Multiple Sclerosis: Problem Oriented Nursing Care Plan," *Am J Nurs,* **80**(2):292–297, (February 1980).

impossible. In water the client experiences more control over his body.

Client education should focus on building general resistance to illness. This includes avoiding fatigue, extremes of heat and cold, and exposure to infection. The latter involves avoiding exposure to ill people and cold climates, as well as vigorous and early treatment of infection when it does occur. It is important to promote a good balance of exercise and rest, nutritious and well-balanced meals, and avoiding the hazards of immobility (contractures and pressure sores). Clients should know their treatment regimens, the side effects of medications and how to watch for them, and drug interactions with over-the-counter medications. The client should consult a health care provider before taking nonprescription medications.

The MS client and family must make many emotional adjustments because of the unpredictability of the disease, the need to change lifestyles, and the challenge of avoiding or decreasing precipitating factors. The National Multiple Sclerosis Society and its local chapters can offer a variety of services to meet the needs of MS clients (see bibliography).

PARKINSON'S DISEASE (PARALYSIS AGITANS)

Parkinson's disease is named after James Parkinson, who in 1817 wrote a classic essay on the "shaking palsy," a disease whose cause is still unknown today. Many other disorders resemble this disease, but their causes are known. These include drug-induced parkinsonism, postencephalitic parkinsonism, and arteriosclerotic parkinsonism. The pathogenesis of all these disorders is the same. There is injury or impairment of the dopamine-producing cells of the substantia nigra in the midbrain. The substantia nigra is part of the extrapyramidal system, which influences the initiation, modulation, and completion of movement and regulates unconscious automatic movements (see Chaps. 48, 49).

About 250,000 to 500,000 (some estimates are as high as 1 million) people in the United States have Parkinson's disease, making up approximately 1 to 2 percent of neurologic disorders.[15] The disease shows no sexual, socioeconomic, or cultural preference, and symptons most commonly occur after age 50. There is no apparent genetic cause, nor is there a known cure. It rarely occurs in the black population.

Etiology and Pathophysiology

There are many causes of parkinsonism. Encephalitis lethargica, or type A encephalitis, has been clearly associated with the onset of parkinsonism. However, the incidence of postencephalitic parkinsonism has dwindled since the 1920s, when there was a large outbreak of this infectious illness. Parkinsonlike symptoms have followed intoxication by a variety of chemicals, including carbon monoxide and manganese (among copper miners). Drug-induced parkinsonism can follow reserpine, methyldopa, haloperidol, and phenothiazine therapy. Although clients with cerebrovascular disease may develop parkinsonlike symptoms, there is little evidence that parkinsonism is caused by arteriosclerosis. Distinguishing arteriosclerosis from true Parkinson's disease is important for prognostic purposes. Clients with the former do not respond as well to treatment and are more likely to experience side effects of drug therapy. Most clients with parkinsonism have the degenerative or idiopathic form, for which the term Parkinson's disease is usually reserved.

The pathogenesis of Parkinson's disease is associated with degeneration of the dopamine-producing neurons in the substantia nigra of the midbrain (Fig. 51-3). It is hypothesized that there is normally a balance between the effects of acetycholine (Ach) and dopamine in the basal ganglia. Any shift in the balance of activity (increase in effects of Ach or decrease in effects of dopamine) supposedly leads to parkinsonlike symptoms. Dopamine is a neurotransmitter essential for normal functioning of the extrapyramidal system. Levels of enzymes and dopamine metabolites are reduced. Postmortem cross sections of the midbrain show loss of the normal melanin pigment in the substantia nigra and loss of nerve cells there and elsewhere in the brain. In addition, deficient amounts of gamma-aminobutyric acid (GABA), serotonin, and norepinephrine have been found in the basal ganglia as well as in the substantia nigra.

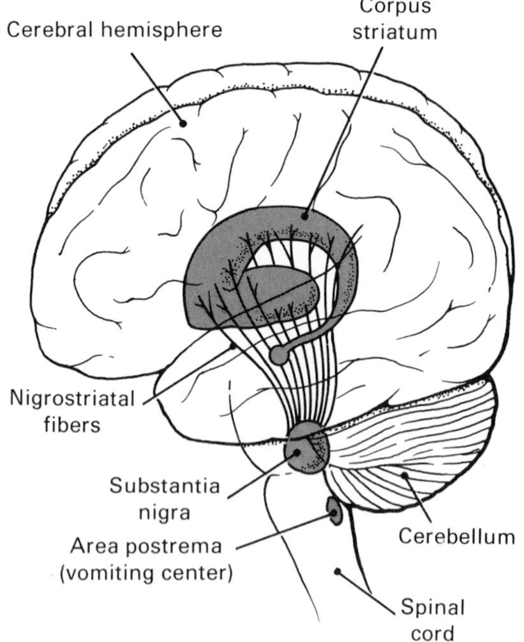

Figure 51-3 Left-side view of the human brain showing schematically the substantia nigra and the corpus striatum (shaded area) lying deep within the cerebral hemisphere. For simplicity, only one side is shown. Nerve fibers extend upward from the substantia nigra and, dividing into many branches, carry dopamine to all regions of the corpus striatum.

Clinical Manifestations

The onset of Parkinson's disease is gradual and insidious. In the beginning stages only a mild tremor, a slight limp, or a decreased arm swing may be evident. In some there may be a slight change in speech patterns. None of these alone is sufficient evidence for a diagnosis of the disease.

Because there is no specific diagnostic test for Parkinson's disease, the diagnosis is based solely on the history and the clinical picture. A firm diagnosis can be made only when at least two of the three characteristic signs, the classical triad are present: tremor, rigidity, and bradykinesia (slow or retarded movement). Unfortunately, many persons with benign essential tremor have mistakenly been diagnosed as having Parkinson's disease. Essential tremor occurs during voluntary movement and is a familial disorder. The ultimate confirmation of Parkinson's disease is a positive response to antiparkinsonian medication.

Tremor

Tremor, often the first sign, may be minimal initially, so that the client is the only one who notices it. This tremor can affect handwriting, causing it to become smaller, particularly toward the end of words *(micrographia).* Parkinsonian tremor is more prominent at rest and is aggravated by emotional stress or increased concentration. The hand tremor is described as "pill rolling," because the thumb and forefinger appear to move in a rotary fashion, as if rolling a pill, coin, or other small object. Tremor can involve the diaphragm, tongue, lips, and jaw but rarely causes shaking of the head.

Rigidity

Rigidity, the second sign of the triad, is increased resistance to passive motion when the limbs are moved through their range of motion. Parkinsonian rigidity is typified by a jerky quality, as if there were intermittent catches in the movement of a cogwheel, when the joint is moved. This is called *cogwheel rigidity.* The rigidity is due to sustained muscle contraction and consequently elicits a complaint of muscle soreness, tired and achy feelings, or pain in the head, upper body, spine, or legs. Another consequence of rigidity is slowness of movement, because it inhibits the smooth alternation of contraction-relaxation in opposing muscle groups (e.g., the biceps and triceps).

Bradykinesia

Bradykinesia is particularly evident in the loss of automatic movements which is secondary to the physical and chemical alteration of the basal ganglia and related structures in the extrapyramidal system of the CNS. In the unaffected client, automatic movements are involuntary and occur subconsciously. They include blinking the eyelids, swinging the arms while walking, swallowing saliva, expressing oneself via facial and hand movements, and minor movements of postural adjustment. The client with Parkinson's disease does not execute these movements, and there is a poverty of spontaneous activity. This accounts for the stooped posture, masked facies ("deadpan" expression), drooling of saliva, and shuffling gait *(festination)* so characteristic of a person with this disease. In addition, there is difficulty initiating movement. Movements such as getting out of a chair cannot be executed unless they are consciously willed.

Complications

Many of the complications of Parkinson's disease are a result of the decomposition and loss of spontaneity of movement. Swallowing may become very difficult (dysphagia), in severe cases leading to malnutrition or aspiration. General debilitation may lead to pneumonia, urinary tract infections, and skin breakdown. Mobility is greatly decreased. The gait is slowed down, and turning is especially difficult. Some may experience "freezing" and cannot initiate a step, even though they may have walked to their present position. The gait is usually composed of rapid, short, shuffling ministeps. The posture is that of the "old man" image, with the head and trunk bent forward and the legs constantly flexed (Fig. 51-4). The lack of mobility may lead to constipation, ankle edema, and, more seriously, contractures. Hypotension may occur in some. Bothersome complications include seborrhea (increased oily secretion of the sebaceous glands of the skin), dandruff, excessive sweating, conjunctivitis, difficulty in reading, insomnia, incontinence, and depression.

Medical management

Because there is no cure for Parkinson's disease, medical management (Table 51-11) is aimed at relieving the symptoms. Antiparkinsonian medication is the most common form of symptomatic treatment. The lack of dopamine is thought to allow acetylcholine (Ach) to circulate unchecked in the brain. Two major types of drugs used are therefore *dopaminergic* (agents to enhance dopamine secretion or supply) and *anticholinergic* compounds (to antagonize effects of Ach).

The only other treatment for Parkinson's disease

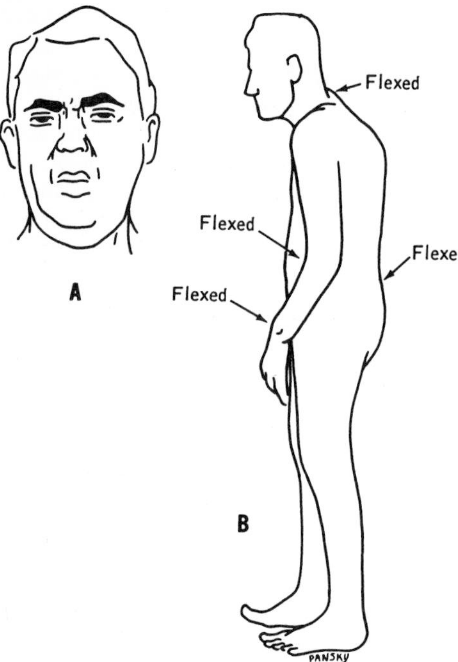

Figure 51-4 Parkinson's disease. Note the flexed posture of the head and trunk and the flexion of the arms. A masked facial expression is common. *(From E. L. House, B. Pansky, and A. Siegel, A Systematic Approach to Neuroscience, 3d ed., McGraw-Hill Book Company, New York, 1979. Used with permission of McGraw-Hill Book Company.)*

is *cryothalamectomy* or *thalamotomy.* Surgical treatment is most effective in younger clients whose major problem is unilateral tremor. A greater risk of complications and residual neurologic deficits preclude the use of this treatment in older clients with more severe disease. Because the long-term benefits of surgery vary widely, the role of surgical intervention is limited.[16]

Pharmacologic aspects

Of the dopaminergic drugs, levodopa (L-dopa) and levodopa with carbidopa (Sinemet) are the only ones proved effective so far. Levodopa is a precursor of dopamine and can cross the blood-brain barrier. Sinemet is the preferred drug in the biochemical sense because it contains carbidopa, an agent which inhibits the enzyme dopa-decarboxylase (which breaks down dopa before it reaches the brain). The net result is that more dopa reaches the brain and therefore less drug is needed. In addition to the two major drug types, antihistamines are sometimes employed to relieve tremor and rigidity. The antiviral agent amantadine hydrochloride (Symmetrel) is also

Table 51-11

Medical Management: Parkinson's Disease

Diagnostic

1. History
2. Physical exam—presence of two or more of the triad of symptoms:
   a. Tremor
   b. Rigidity
   c. Bradykinesia
3. Positive response to antiparkinsonian medication (Table 51-12)
4. Rule out side effects of phenothiazines, reserpine, benzodiazepines, haloperidol

Therapeutic (symptomatic only)

1. Antiparkinsonian medication
2. Surgical destruction of ventrolateral nucleus of the thalamus

an effective antiparkinsonian drug, although its mechanism of action is not known. Table 51-12 summarizes the drugs commonly used in Parkinson's disease, the symptoms they relieve, and their common side effects. The use of one drug is preferred, as there are fewer side effects and the medication is easier to adjust. It should be noted that excessive amounts of dopaminergic drugs can lead to paradoxical intoxication (aggravation rather than relief of symptoms).

Dietary measures

Diet is of major importance to the client with Parkinson's disease because malnutrition and constipation can be serious consequences of inadequate nutrition. Clients who have dysphagia and bradykinesia need appetizing foods that are easily chewed and swallowed. The diet should contain adequate roughage and fruit to avoid constipation. Food can be cut into bite-sized pieces *before* it is served, and it should be served on a warmed plate to preserve its appeal. Eating six small meals a day may be less exhausting than eating three large meals a day. Ample time should be planned for eating to avoid frustration and encourage independence.

Nursing management

Promotion of physical exercise and a well-balanced diet are major concerns for nursing care (Table 51-13). Exercise can limit the consequences of decreased mobility which are muscle atrophy, contractures, and constipation. The American Parkinson's Disease Association publishes a booklet, "Home Exercises of Patients with Parkinson's Disease," which illustrates a variety of exercises and can be used by family members as well as health professionals.

Table 51-12
Drugs for Symptomatic Treatment of Parkinsonism

Drug	Symptoms Relieved	Side Effects/Precautions
Dopaminergic		
Levodopa (L-dopa)	Bradykinesia, tremor, rigidity	Nausea, dyskinesia, hypotension, palpitations, arrhythmias. In older clients: agitation, hallucinations, confusion. Avoid vitamin pills and diet high in vitamin B_6 (reverses levodopa effect)
Levodopa + carbidopa* (Sinemet)	Bradykinesia, tremor, rigidity	Less nausea but greater chance of dyskinesia, confusion, and hallucinations. Periodic check of BUN, SGOT, WBC, Hct for both drugs. Contraindications: melanoma, narrow-angle glaucoma, clients taking MAO inhibitors, reserpine, methyldopa, guanethidine, antipsychotics
Anticholinergic	Tremor	Dry mouth, blurred vision, constipation, delirium, anxiety, agitation, hallucinations
Trihexyphenidyl (Artane)		
Procyclidine (Kemadrin)	Tremor	Avoid drugs with similar actions: over-the-counter drugs containing scopolamine or antihistamines (e.g., Sominex), antispasmodics (e.g., Donnatal, Bellergal), tricyclic antidepressants (Tofranil, Elavil, Norpramin, Vivactil)
Benztropine mesylate (Cogentin)		
Biperiden (Akineton)		
	Tremor, rigidity	Sedation; same precautions as for anticholinergic drugs
Antihistaminic		
Diphenhydramine (Benadryl)		
Orphenadrine (Disipal)		
Chlorphenoxamine (Phenoxene)		
Phenindamine (Thephorin)		
Amantadine HCl (Symmetral)	Rigidity, akinesia	Nervousness, insomnia, confusion, hallucinations, dry mouth, nausea, ankle edema

*Carbidopa is now available as a single drug (*FDA Bulletin*, November 1979).

Adapted from F. McDowell, F. J. Lee, and R. Sweet, "Extrapyramidal Disease," in A. B. Baker and L. H. Baker (eds.), *Clinical Neurology*, vol. 2, Harper & Row, Publishers, Incorporated, New York, 1978, chap. 26, p. 29.

Also, P. Mitchell, personal communication.

Because Parkinson's disease is a chronic degenerative disorder with no acute exacerbations, health teaching and nursing care are directed toward maintaining good health, encouraging independence, and avoiding complications such as contractures.

Problems secondary to bradykinesia can be alleviated by employing relatively simple measures. The following are helpful hints for clients who tend to "freeze" while walking: consciously think about stepping over imaginary or real lines on the floor, drop rice kernels and step over them, rock from side to side, lift the toes when stepping, take one step backward and two steps forward. Getting out of a chair can be facilitated by using an upright chair with arms and placing the back legs on small (2-inch) blocks. Other aspects of the environment can be altered. Rugs and

Table 51-13
Nursing Care Plan for the Client with Parkinson's Disease

Client Problem	Expected Outcome	Nursing Intervention
Muscular rigidity and bradykinesia	Ability to perform daily activities	Administer antiparkinsonian drugs as prescribed. Provide suggestions if client "freezes" while walking. Use upright chair for sitting. Alter clothing to facilitate ease of dressing. Apply heat (hot packs) and massage to lessen rigidity.
Drooling	Minimal or absent drooling	Suggest chewing gum or eating hard candy to remind client to swallow.
Tremor	Minimal interference with or embarrassment from tremor	Suggest method to decrease tremor at rest, such as carry an object in hand, put hand in pocket, change positions. Educate client and others about resting tremor and that it is not due to "nerves."
Contractures, deformities	Full range of motion, absence of contractures	Encourage ambulation as tolerated. Perform active or passive exercises in all extremities, head, and neck q 4 h.*
Constipation	Normal bowel movement q 2–3 days	Maintain fluid intake (3000 mL/day). Include fruit juices. Encourage high-residue diet. Administer stool softeners, suppositories as ordered. Establish regular bowel routine.
Weight loss	Maintenance of weight	Monitor weight. Encourage high calorie, high protein easily chewable diet in frequent small feedings. Provide pleasant atmosphere for meals.
Difficulty communicating	Verbalizes needs and desires. Corresponds in writing	Use patience, encourage verbalization, anticipate needs. Have client use "pacing" board.† Suggest use of typewriter.
Depression secondary to altered body image and loss of self-esteem	Emotional adjustment and acceptance of disease	Explore reasons for depression with client and family. Encourage independence, setting realistic goals. Encourage diversional activities, hobbies.

*See "Home Exercises for Patients with Parkinson's Disease," a booklet prepared by the American Parkinson's Disease Association.
†See N. Helm, "Management of Palilalia with a Pacing Board," *J Speech Hear Disord,* **44:**350–353 (August 1979).

excess furniture can be removed to avoid stumbling. An ottoman can be used to elevate the legs and avoid dependent ankle edema. Clothing can be simplified by using slip-on shoes and Velcro fasteners or zippers on clothing instead of buttons and hooks.

MYASTHENIA GRAVIS

Myasthenia gravis (MG) is a disease of the neuromuscular junction characterized by fluctuating weakness of certain skeletal muscle groups (of the eyes, face, and, to a lesser degree, the limbs). Prevalence varies from 1 in 10,000 to 1 in 50,000 of the population. The peak age of onset is 20 to 30 years. Women are affected slightly more often than men, although a majority of persons with both thymoma and myasthenia (15 to 20 percent of all persons with myasthenia) are male and over the age of 50.

Etiology and Pathophysiology

Investigators have detected a reduced number of acetylcholine (Ach) receptor sites of the neuromuscular junction of myasthenic clients.[17] When examined under electron microscopy, the number of postsynaptic folds is found to be reduced and the synaptic cleft widened. An autoimmune process may be associated with this disease. The most popular explanation, which has been supported by studies of laboratory animals, is that antibodies, probably formed by the thymus gland, combine with end-plate receptors. This prevents Ach molecules from attaching and causing muscle contraction. A single specific cause for all myasthenia, however, has not yet been found.

There are two theories about the role of the thymus gland in MG. One is that the thymus oversecretes thymine, a compound which interferes with neuromuscular function but is present normally in small amounts. The other is that the thymus is responsible for producing antibodies that attack the neuromuscular junction. Neither of these theories has been proved, and, as in other autoimmune diseases, evidence of persistent viral infection is being sought.[17]

Clinical Manifestations

The primary feature of MG is that skeletal muscle becomes easily fatigued. Strength is usually restored after a period of rest. The muscles most often involved are those for moving the eyes and eyelids, chewing, swallowing, speaking, and breathing. The cell bodies (nuclei) of all these are located in the brainstem. The muscles are generally strongest in the morning and become exhausted with continued activity. Consequently, by the end of the day, muscle fatigue is prominent.

The first manifestations of MG are ptosis (drooping eyelid) and diplopia in 90 percent of cases. Facial mobility and expression can be impaired. There may be difficulty in chewing and swallowing food. Speech is affected, and the voice often fades after a long conversation. The muscles of the trunk and limbs are less often affected. Of these, the proximal muscles of the neck, shoulder, and hip are more often affected than the distal muscles. No signs of neural disorder accompany myasthenia gravis; there is no sensory loss, reflexes are normal, and muscle atrophy is rare.

The course of this disease is highly variable. Some persons may have short-term remissions, others may stabilize, and others may have severe progressive involvement. Restricted ocular myasthenia, usually seen only in adult men, has a good prognosis, whereas myasthenia which has a remission period of a year or more tends to be progressive.[17] Myasthenia exacerbations can be precipitated by emotional stress, pregnancy, menses, secondary illness, and surgery. In some cases the onset of myasthenia occurs after one of these events.

Complications

The major complications of MG result from muscle weakness in areas which affect swallowing and breathing. An acute exacerbation of this type is sometimes called *myasthenic crisis*. Aspiration, respiratory insufficiency, and respiratory infection are the major complications.

Diagnostic Study Abnormalities

The simplest diagnostic test for myasthenia is to have the client look at the ceiling for 2 to 3 minutes. There will be an increased droop of the eyelids, so that the person can barely keep the eyes open. After a brief rest the eyes can open again. Other tests may be employed if the diagnosis is still in doubt. Electromyography may show a decrementing response to repeated stimulation of the hand muscles, indicative of muscle fatigability. Use of pharmacologic agents may also aid the diagnosis. The Tensilon test in a myasthenic client reveals improved muscle contractility after intravenous injection of edrophonium chloride (Tensilon chloride). This test also aids in the diagnosis of *cholinergic crisis* (secondary to overdose of neostigmine). In this condition, Tensilon, a cholinergic agent, does not improve muscle weakness but may actually increase it.

Medical Management

Since there is no cure, medical management is palliative and usually lifelong. Two classes of drugs and a surgical procedure constitute the current therapy. Table 51-14 summarizes these therapies. Thymectomy is considered for clients who do not respond to drugs. Although this is a major treatment and results in improvement in many clients, controlled prospective studies have not been done to validate its efficacy.[17]

Plasmapheresis is a relatively new therapy for MG, having first been reported in 1976. This procedure involves separation of plasma from blood by a machine called a cell separator which is connected to the client by a vascular cannula similar to a dialysis cannula. This process supposedly "cleans" the plasma of myasthenia antibodies. It is still in the experimental stage, is not a cure, and does not work for all clients. However, it can produce short-term improvement in clinical status in conjunction with immunosuppressive therapy.[18]

Table 51-14
Medical Management of Myasthenia Gravis

Diagnostic
1. History
2. Physical examination
   a. Fatigability with prolonged upward gaze (2–3 min)
   b. Muscle weakness
3. EMG
4. Tensilon test

Therapeutic
1. Drugs
   a. Anticholinesterase agents
   b. Corticosteroids
2. Surgery (thymectomy)
3. Plasmapheresis

Pharmacologic Aspects

One of the two classes of drug for treatment of MG is the anticholinesterase group. Neostigmine (Prostigmin) and pyridostigmine (Mestinon) are the most successful drugs of this group. The anticholinesterase drugs improve myasthenic weakness by inhibiting the destruction of Ach by acetylcholinesterase, thus facilitating transmission of impulses across the neuromuscular junction. If this treatment is unsuccessful, corticosteroids (specifically prednisone) may be helpful because of their immunosuppressive action.

Many drugs are contraindicated or must be used with caution in myasthenic clients. Classes of drug that should be cautiously evaluated before use include corticosteroids, anesthetics, antiarrhythmics, antibiotics, quinine, antipsychotics, barbiturates and sedative-hypnotics, cathartics, diuretics, narcotics, muscle relaxants, thyroid preparations, and tranquilizers.

Table 51-15
Myasthenic Crisis and Cholinergic Crisis

Myasthenic Crisis	Cholinergic Crisis
Causes	
Exacerbation of myasthenia (following precipitating factors or failure to take medication as prescribed)	Overdose of anticholinesterase drugs, remission (spontaneous or following thymectomy)
Signs and Symptoms	
Increased weakness Ptosis Bulbar signs: Dysphagia Dysarthria Dyspnea	Nicotinic signs: Bulbar signs, ptosis Muscarinic signs: Increased diaphoresis Diarrhea Fasciculations Increased salivation Nausea/vomiting Miosis Cramps

Nursing Management

Clients with myasthenia who are admitted to the hospital usually have a respiratory infection or are in an acute myasthenic crisis. Nursing care is aimed at maintaining adequate ventilation, continuing drug therapy, and watching for side effects of therapy. The nurse should be able to distinguish cholinergic from myasthenic crisis, as the causes and treatment of the two differ greatly (see Table 51-15).

As with other chronic illnesses, rehabilitative care focuses on the neurologic deficits and their impact on daily living. A good diet that can be chewed and swallowed easily should be developed. Diversional activities that require little physical effort and match the interests of the client should be arranged. Education should focus on the importance of following the medical regimen, on potential adverse reactions to specific drugs, on planning activities of daily living to avoid fatigue, on availability of community resources, and on complications of the disease and therapy (crisis conditions) and what to do about them.

OTHER NEUROLOGIC DISORDERS

Amyotrophic Lateral Sclerosis

Loss of motor neurons is the major morphologic change in amyotrophic lateral sclerosis (ALS), a rare progressive neurologic disease which usually leads to death in 2 to 6 years. This disease became known as Lou Gehrig's disease when the famous baseball player developed it in the early 1940s. The onset is between the ages of 40 and 70, and twice as many men as women are affected.

Typically, motor neurons in the cervical spinal cord and the lower cervical nerves are affected. Consequently the primary symptoms are weakness of the upper extremities, dysarthria, and dysphagia. Muscle wasting and fasciculations result from the denervation of muscles. Death usually results from respiratory infection secondary to compromised respiratory function. Unfortunately, there is no cure and no treatment for ALS. This illness is devastating because the client remains cognitively intact while he watches himself literally waste away. The challenge of nursing care is to support the client's cognitive and emotional functions by providing diversional activities such as reading and human companionship.

Huntington's Chorea

Huntington's disease is a genetically transmitted, autosomal dominant disorder which affects both men and women of all races. The offspring of a person with this disease has a 50 percent risk of inheriting it.

Like Parkinson's disease, the pathology of Huntington's disease involves the basal ganglia and the extrapyramidal system. However, instead of a deficiency of dopamine, Huntington's disease involves a deficiency of the neurotransmitters acetylcholine (Ach) and gamma-aminobutyric acid (GABA). The net effect is an excess of dopamine, which leads to symptoms opposite to those of parkinsonism. The clinical manifestions, the onset of which is between the ages of 35 and 45, are characterized by abnormal and excessive involuntary movements *(chorea)*. These are writhing, twisting movements of the face, limbs, and body. The movements get worse as the disease progresses. Facial movements (involving speech, chewing, and swallowing) are affected and may cause aspiration and malnutrition. The gait deteriorates, and ambulation eventually becomes impossible. Perhaps the most devastating deterioration is in mental functions, which include intellectual decline, emotional lability, and psychotic behavior. Death usually occurs 10 to 20 years after the onset of symptoms.

Since there is no cure, medical management is palliative. Antipsychotic, antidepressant, and antichorea medications are prescribed and have some effect. However, the course of the disease is not altered by these therapies. This disease presents a great challenge to health care professionals. The goal of nursing management is to provide the most comfortable environment for the client and family by maintaining physical safety, treating the physical symptoms, and providing emotional and psychological support. Genetic counseling is of paramount importance.

Muscular Dystrophy

The many types of muscular dystrophy (MD) are all progressive, hereditary, degenerative disease of skeletal muscle. There is no involvement of the nerves; rather, the pathology lies within the muscle fibers themselves. For unknown reasons a genetic abnormality induces degeneration of muscle fibers. The common feature of MD is symmetrical muscle weakness and atrophy. There is no treatment for MD, and, as in ALS, the client experiences progressive muscle weakness and wasting. Medical management is purely symptomatic. Quinine, procainamide, and phenytoin can relieve myotonia, although side effects may outweigh the benefits of drug therapy. Surgical procedures such as fasciotomy or tendon lengthening and leg braces may preserve ambulation for several additional years. Complications include fractures, respiratory infections, and cardiac decompensation. Nursing care should be directed toward maintaining normal daily activity as much as possible and avoiding contractures, skeletal deformities, and obesity.

Syringomyelia

Syringomyelia is a rare neurologic disorder involving cavitation of the spinal cord, usually in the cervical region. The cavity, or *syrinx* (Greek word for tube or pipe) is filled with CSF and slowly expands, destroying central gray matter. Syringomyelia may be congenital or acquired. Clinical features involve lower motor (segmental) neurons as well as ascending and descending spinal cord tracts, depending on the location and extent of the lesion. The syrinx may extend longitudinally and involve the lower brainstem, producing respiratory, swallowing, and articulation difficulties ("bulbar crises").

Diagnosis is based on neurologic examination, myelography, and sometimes body CT scan. CSF analysis is usually normal. Surgical intervention is the only treatment, and results are variable. The type of surgery depends on the morphologic abnormality, which varies from person to person. Many feel that the risks of surgery in the cervical region and posterior fossa outweigh the potential benefits. Nursing care is aimed at assisting the client to preserve independence in the activities of daily living, avoid the hazards of immobility, ensure physical safety, and cope with the disability.

Case Study / Epilepsy

W. G. has been diagnosed as having partial elementary and secondarily generalized tonic-clonic seizures. His medical records indicate that he has been seizure-free for several months. He is admitted to the hospital for treatment of lacerations after reportedly having a seizure at his job as a gas station attendant. He denies having a seizure and says he just fell and hurt himself. His serum anticonvulsant level is well below the therapeutic range. His wife states that, in fact, W. G. has had several seizures in his sleep over the past month. She says he denies having them, even though they wake him up and cause him to be incontinent and injure his tongue. He still drives a car.

Discussion Questions

1. Explain the pathophysiology of the type of epilepsy W. G. has.
2. What is the probable reason for W. G. having these recent seizures?
3. What kind of seizure is W. G. having in his sleep?
4. What psychological defense mechanism is W. G. exhibiting?
5. How would you counsel W. G. and his wife?

Case Study / Parkinson's Disease

T. L. noticed that he required a progressively longer time to perform activities of daily living. His family observed that he had problems getting in and out of chairs. They also found it difficult to interpret his facial expressions, as they did not seem to reflect his mood. Customers on the phone frequently had to ask him to repeat words.

T. L. went to his physician, who prescribed anti-parkinsonian medication. However, now he is having problems with nausea and visual hallucinations at night, and he is still having some difficulty dressing himself.

Discussion Questions

1. Explain the pathophysiology of Parkinson's disease.
2. What are the typical symptoms of this disease?
3. How many symptoms have to be present before the diagnosis is made?
4. In relation to the communication problem, how would you counsel T. L. and his family?
5. How would you handle the side effects of antiparkinsonian medication?
6. What suggestions would you make to T. L. and his family about dressing himself?

REVIEW QUESTIONS

The number of the question corresponds to the same numbered objective at the beginning of the chapter.

1. Chronic neurologic disease often involves
   a. long-term use of medication
   b. progressive physical deterioration
   c. a and b
   d. neither a nor b

2. Differentiate migraine from muscle-contraction headache by choosing the correct statement.
   a. Migraine headache involves contraction of the scalp and neck muscles.
   b. Muscle-contraction headache is described as a throbbing, usually unilateral pain.
   c. The prodrome of migraine is associated with vasoconstriction, the actual headache with vasodilatation.
   d. Cluster headache is associated with recurrent discharge of the sympathetic nervous system.

3. The triad of symptoms common in Parkinson's disease is
   a. diplopia, tremor, bradykinesia
   b. tremor, rigidity, bradykinesia
   c. spasticity, diplopia, tremor
   d. ataxia, drowsiness, dysarthria

4. Nursing intervention for the client with multiple sclerosis is aimed at management of
   a. incontinence, depression, spasticity
   b. incontinence, hallucinations, tremor
   c. bradykinesia, rigidity, tremor
   d. rigidity, incontinence, diplopia

5. The most common cause of death in amyotrophic lateral sclerosis is
   a. cerebral infarction
   b. renal failure
   c. pulmonary embolus
   d. respiratory infection

6. Common physical complications of a person who is immobilized by chronic neurologic disease are
   a. constipation, skin breakdown
   b. contractures, pneumonia
   c. urinary tract infections
   d. all the above

7. A major goal of treatment for the client with a chronic, progressive neurologic disease is
   a. prevention of extension of the disease
   b. acceptance of the disease by client and family
   c. treatment of complications
   d. continuation of usual lifestyle

REFERENCES

1. Seymour Diamond, "Headache, Its Diagnosis and Management," *Headache,* **9**(3):113 (April 1979).
2. Arnold Friedman and Merritt Houston, *Headache: Diagnosis and Treatment,* F. A. Davis Company, Philadelphia, 1959, p. 209.
3. Dewey Ziegler, "Tension Headache," *Med Clin North Am,* **62**(3):495–505 (May 1978).
4. Donald Dalessio, "Mechanisms of Headache," *Med Clin North Am,* **62**(3):429 (May 1978).
5. Otto Appenzeller, "Cerebrovascular Aspects of Headache," *Med Clin North Am,* **62**(3):467 (May 1978).
6. Lee Kudrow, "Cluster Headache: Diagnosis and Management," *Headache,* **19**(3):142–150 (April 1979).
7. Arnold Friedman, "Headache," in A. B. Baker and L. H. Baker (eds.), *Clinical Neurology,* Harper & Row, Publishers, Incorporated, New York, 1979, p. 12.
8. K. Metrakos and J. D. Metrakos, "Genetics of Convulsive Disorders: II. Genetic and Centrencephalic Epilepsy," *Neurology,* **11**:474–483 (1961).
9. Henri Gastaut, "Clinical and Electroencephalographical Classification of Epileptic Seizures," *Epilepsia,* **11**:102–113 (1970).
10. W. F. Caveness, H. H. Merritt, and G. H. Gallup, Jr., "A Survey of Attitudes Toward Epilepsy in 1974 with an Indication of Trends over the Past Twenty-five Years," *Epilepsia,* **15**:523–536 (1974).
11. L. Perlman, *The Person with Epilepsy: Life Style, Needs,*

Expectations. A Needs Assessment Survey of the Clients of the National Epilepsy League, S. Pietch (ed.), National Epilepsy League, Chicago, 1977.

12. Howard Weiner, "Multiple Sclerosis," in H. R. Tyler and D. Dawson (eds.), *Current Neurology,* Houghton Mifflin Professional Publishers, Boston, 1978, p. 56.

13. Charles Poser, "Diseases of the Myelin Sheath," in A. B. Baker and L. H. Baker (eds.), *Clinical Neurology,* Harper & Row, Publishers, Incorporated, New York, 1978, p. 20.

14. R. P. Lisak, "Multiple Sclerosis: Evidence for Immunopathogenesis," *Neurology,* **30**:99–105 (1980).

15. F. McDowell, J. Lee, and R. Sweet, "Extrapyramidal Disease," in A. B. Baker and L. H. Baker (eds.), *Clinical Neurology,* Harper & Row, Publishers, Incorporated, New York, 1978, p. 20.

16. Ibid. p. 34.

17. Lewis Rowland and Robert Layzer, "Muscular Dystrophies, Atrophies, and Related Diseases," in A. B. Baker and L. H. Baker (eds.), *Clinical Neurology,* Harper & Row, Publishers, Incorporated, New York, 1977.

18. Alister Finlayson, "Syringomyelia and Related Conditions," in A. B. Baker and L. H. Baker (eds.), *Clinical Neurology,* Harper & Row, Publishers, Incorporated, New York, 1971, pp. 3–4.

Chapter 52

NURSING ROLE IN MANAGEMENT

Stroke Client

Naomi R. Ballard

Learning Objectives

1. Describe the incidence and risk factors of stroke.
2. Explain the mechanisms that affect cerebral blood flow.
3. Describe the atherosclerotic process.
4. Compare and contrast the pathophysiology of strokes caused by thrombosis, embolus, and intracranial hemorrhage.
5. Correlate the clinical manifestations of stroke with the underlying pathology.
6. Describe the diagnostic study abnormalities found in stroke.
7. Describe the medical, pharmacological, and dietary management of the stroke client.
8. Outline a behavior-modification program designed to reduce the risk factors related to stroke.
9. Describe the acute and chronic nursing management of the stroke client.
10. Explain the emotional impact of a stroke upon clients and their families.

A stroke is the most common neurological cause of problems related to mobility and coordination. The clinical manifestations of a stroke are the result of neurological deficits that occur when cerebral blood flow is impaired. This condition is also called *acute brain infarction* (ABI), *cerebrovascular accident* (CVA), or *apoplexy*. These terms are misleading because they imply a cataclysmic event. Although a stroke can be devastating, it rarely strikes without warning. In many cases it can be predicted and prevented.

SIGNIFICANCE OF THE PROBLEM

The challenge of the 1980s, as outlined in the Surgeon General's Report, *Health People,* is to reduce the risk factors of stroke through health promotion and disease prevention.[1] Some progress in this area has been made; the incidence of stroke decreased almost 30 percent in the last decade. This has occurred despite an increase in the number of aged people, in whom strokes are more common. The change has been primarily attributed to improved detection and treatment of hypertension. Yet in 1977, over 180,000 people died from stroke. Two million people suffer residual effects of stroke.[2] These effects range from decreased ability to work to the need for complete custodial care. Both the cost in human suffering and the cost to the economy are almost inestimable. Better control of the risk factors of stroke is critical.

This chapter was reviewed by Elizabeth L. Noroian, R.N., Ph.D., Assistant Professor, School of Nursing, University of Pittsburgh, Pittsburgh, Pennsylvania.

RISK FACTORS

Stroke is closely associated with certain risk factors, many of which are related to the poor health habits of many Americans. The risk factors that are correlated with stroke may be divided into three categories: (1) nonreversible, (2) partially reversible, and (3) reversible (Fig. 52-1). The *nonreversible* risk factors include sex, age, race, and heredity. Men are more prone to strokes than women. Advancing age generally increases the chance of strokes. Blacks are more likely to have a stroke than whites, probably because of their higher incidence of hypertension. There is often a hereditary pattern to the occurrence of strokes. For example, an elderly black male with a family history of cerebrovascular disease is at high risk of a stroke. However, nothing can be done to alter nonreversible risk factors.

The *partially reversible* risk factors are hypertension, diabetes mellitus, cardiac impairments, and blood lipid abnormalities. Any one of these diseases doubles the risk of stroke. When they occur in combination, the risk is compounded. The incidence of stroke may be reduced by improved detection and management of these specific conditions.

The *reversible* risk factors include smoking, obesity, stress, salt intake, inactivity, and the use of oral contraceptives. They are related to lifestyle and are potentially alterable. (See Table 27-4 related to modifi-

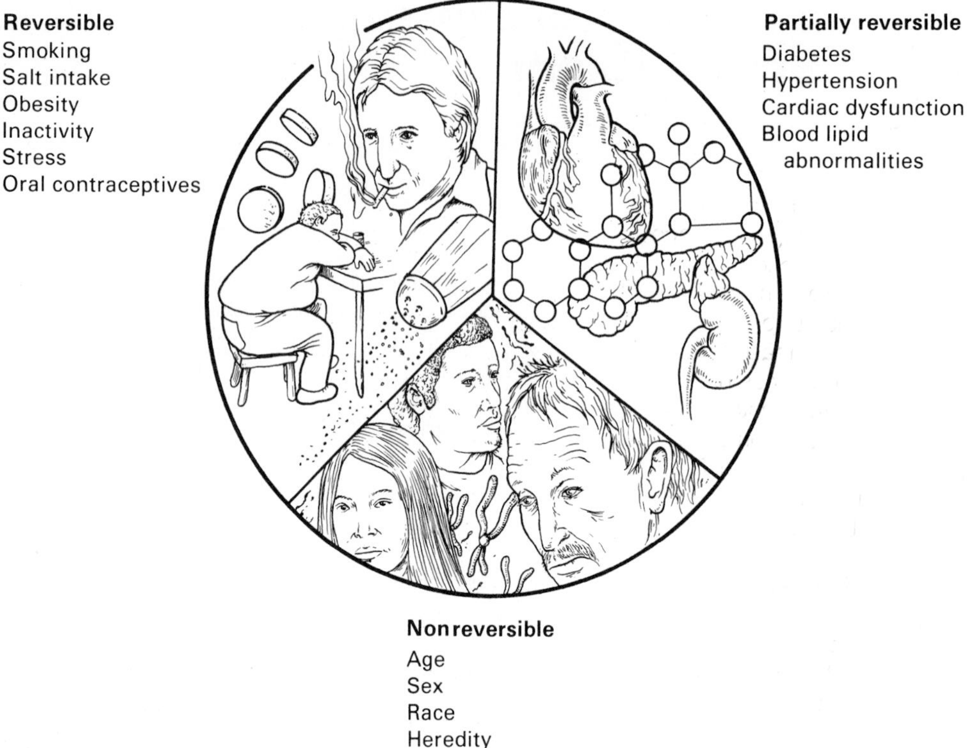

Figure 52-1 Risk factors in stroke.

cations of risk factors related to coronary artery disease.)

PATHOPHYSIOLOGY

Factors Affecting Regulation of Cerebral Blood Flow

Because the neurons of the brain do not have regenerative capabilities, the prevention of cerebral damage is important. For adequate cerebral functioning, blood flow must be maintained at 750 to 1000mL/minute, which is one-fifth of the cardiac output. If this blood flow is interrupted, as in a stroke, neuronal metabolism is altered in 30 seconds, metabolism ceases in 2 minutes, and cellular death occurs in 5 minutes.[3] Once the neuron is dead, its function is lost unless another part of the brain can be trained to take over the lost function.

The cerebrovascular system is very adaptive. It is able to maintain a constant blood flow to the brain despite marked changes in the systemic circulation. The factors that affect cerebral blood flow can be divided into extracranial and intracranial factors.

Extracranial factors

The extracranial factors are primarily related to the circulatory system. They include (1) systemic blood pressure, (2) cardiac output, and (3) viscosity of the blood. During activities of daily living marked variations in local oxygen requirements occur. Alterations in cardiac output, vasomotor tone, and distribution of blood flow are effective in maintaining constant cerebral perfusion. The mean arterial blood pressure has to fall below 70 mmHg or rise above 160 mmHg before the cerebral blood flow is altered,[4] and cardiac output has to be reduced by one-third before cerebral blood flow is reduced. Changes in blood viscosity either increase or decrease cerebral blood flow. Anemia increases flow and polycythemia reduces it.

Intracranial factors

Metabolic Factors Metabolic alterations are important intracranial factors involved in the regulation of cerebral blood flow. Metabolic factors which result in vasodilatation with restoration of blood flow toward normal include high carbon dioxide concentration and low oxygen tension. An increase in hydrogen ion concentration also increases cerebral blood flow. Singly or in combination, these metabolic factors can maintain adequate cerebral blood flow in normal situations.

Blood Vessels The condition of the blood vessels supplying the brain also influences the cerebral blood flow (Chap. 48). Many people have congenital anomalies in the cerebrovascular system. These anomalies include tortuosity, coiling, kinking, and arteriovenous malformations. These congenital anomalies interfere with cerebral blood flow and are common sites for the development of atherosclerotic diseases. Atherosclerosis from any cause increases resistance in the blood vessels and further reduces blood flow.

Collateral circulation is another factor related to cerebral blood flow. Collateral circulation develops in response to a decrease in normal blood flow. The circle of Willis contains many collateral circulatory connections and is responsible for the greater part of collateral circulation.

Collateral vessels should be able to maintain cerebral blood flow in the event of damage to the main blood supply. However, they cannot always do so. Individual differences in the state of the collateral circulation when a stroke occurs are the factors determining whether major loss of function will result or collateral circulation will prove to be adequate.

Intracranial Pressure Intracranial pressure is another factor that influences cerebral blood flow. Increased intracranial pressure compresses the brain and reduces cerebral blood flow. Among the causes of increased intracranial pressure are stroke, neoplasms, trauma, and hydrocephalus. Greatly reduced cerebral blood flow may result in cerebral infarction.

Both extracranial and intracranial factors may be involved in a stroke. The initial insult may be related to one or more of these factors. For example, when an intracranial hemorrhage occurs the continuity of the vascular system is interrupted. The lost blood and the edema secondary to the inflammatory process cause an increase in intracranial pressure. This interferes with cerebral perfusion, and carbon dioxide and hydrogen ion concentration increase. This results in vasodilatation unless the process is complicated by vasospasm, a common occurrence following hemorrhage.

Atherosclerosis

Atherosclerosis, a common pathophysiological process in stroke (also discussed in Chap. 27), is usually involved in the development of a thrombosis and is often implicated in strokes caused by emboli or hemorrhage. The role atherosclerosis plays in the development of thrombosis and emboli is traced in Fig. 27-3. Initially, an abnormal infiltration of lipids occurs in the intima of the arteries. This fatty streak may develop into an atherosclerotic plaque. These plaques often develop where there is increased turbulence in the blood, as at the bifurcation of an artery or a tortuous area (Fig. 52-2). Later, turbulence may damage the atherosclerotic plaque, resulting in a loss of intimal continuity or ulceration. Platelets and fibrin aggregate on the roughened surface. Parts of the plaque may break off and travel to a distal artery. Cerebral infarction occurs at the point where the blood supply is cut off.

Types of Stroke

The three most common types of stroke are thrombosis, embolism, and intracranial hemorrhage (Table 52-1).

Thrombosis

Thrombosis is the formation of a blood clot or coagulum which results in the narrowing of the lumen of a blood vessel with eventual occlusion. It is the most common cause of cerebral infarction and is considered a disease of the elderly. Two-thirds of the strokes due to thrombosis are associated with hypertension or diabetes, which are both conditions that accelerate the atherosclerotic process. In 80 percent

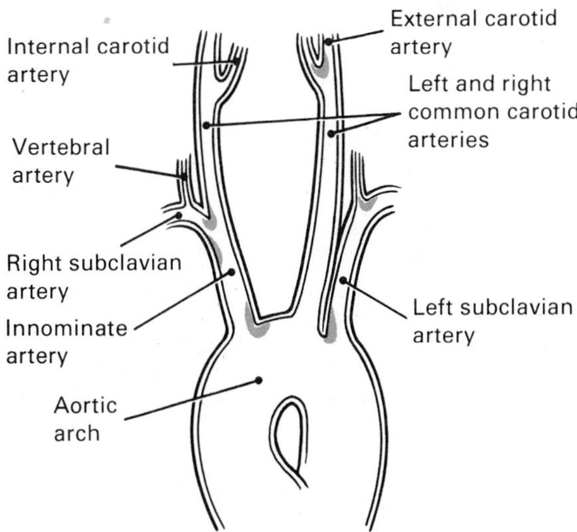

Figure 52-2 Common sites for the development of atherosclerosis in extracranial and intracranial arteries. The main locations are the carotid bifurcation and the takeoff points of the branches from the aorta, innominate, and subclavian arteries.

Table 52-1
Comparison of Types of Strokes

Characteristics	Thrombosis	Embolism	Intracranial Hemorrhage
Related diseases	Diabetes Hypertension Atherosclerosis	Cardiac disease Atherosclerosis Metastatic lesion	Hypertension Aneurysm Trauma
Prodromal warning	TIA	TIA (occasionally)	Headache (occasionally)
Time of onset	Sleep; repose	Unrelated to activity	Activity
Course	Stepwise progression	Single attack	Progressive; peaks in 24 h
Prognosis	Usually some improvement	Usually some improvement	Poor

of the cases, thrombosis is preceded by prodromal warnings such as paresthesias (abnormal sensations), paresis (decreased strength and motility of an extremity), and aphasia (disturbance of language function). These transient periods of neurological deficit called *transient ischemic attacks (TIAs)* can signal a developing lesion.

A stroke caused by thrombosis usually occurs after a period of repose or sleep. It is characterized by intermittency or erratic progression of signs and symptoms. The resultant ischemia leads to edema and congestion of the affected area. The manifestations usually peak within 70 hours and are often secondary to the developing edema. The degree of involvement depends upon the rapidity of onset, the size of the lesion, and the presence of collateral circulation. As edema subsides, some improvement will usually be apparent within 2 weeks. In most cases, maximum improvement is attained in 12 to 24 weeks.

Embolism

Cerebral embolism is the occlusion of a cerebral artery by an embolus, resulting in necrosis and edema of the area supplied by the involved blood vessel. Embolism is the second most common cause of stroke. The majority of emboli originate in the endocardial (inside) layer of the heart, with plaques or tissue breaking off from the endocardium and entering the circulation. The embolus lodges at the point where an artery becomes too narrow for it to pass and causes ischemic infarction. Cardiac diseases or situations that contribute to the development of emboli include chronic atrial fibrillation, myocardial infarction, valve replacements, rheumatic heart disease, and infective bacterial endocarditis. Atherosclerotic plaques in the extracranial arteries are a second source of emboli. The emboli from the heart or extracranial arteries usually travel up through the carotid system and lodge in the middle cerebral artery or its branches.

The clinical picture of an embolic stroke is more varied than that of a thrombotic stroke. It can affect any age group. An embolic stroke secondary to rheumatic heart disease may involve young to middle-aged adults. An embolus arising from an atherosclerotic plaque is more common in the elderly. A prodromal warning is less common than with thrombosis. Emboli are increasingly being implicated in transient ischemic attacks. However, a sudden loss of neurological function usually occurs. The onset of the stroke is unrelated to activity. The client usually maintains consciousness, although a headache may develop on the side where the embolus is lodged. Because the damage may be more extensive than with a thrombotic stroke, the prognosis is poorer.

Intracranial hemorrhage

Intracranial hemorrhage is the third most common type of stroke. It can be caused by rupture of (1) cerebral arteries secondary to hypertension or trauma or (2) an aneurysm. (Head trauma is covered in Chap. 54.) The blood extravasates into the brain or the subarachnoid space. A mass is created that compresses and displaces the brain. In a large hemorrhage, herniation of the brain tissue may occur, usually resulting in coma and death. Approximately half the clients do not survive a stroke caused by an intracranial hemorrhage.

The clinical pictures of hypertensive hemorrhage and of ruptured aneurysm are similar. Both tend to occur in a younger population than thrombotic strokes. Blacks have a higher incidence of hypertensive hemorrhage than whites. Often there is no prodromal warning. In some cases, the client may be able to recall a recent severe headache. Intracranial hemorrhage is usually related to increased activity. Coma is common. The prognosis for recovery is usually poor and is related to the extent of the initial bleeding.

Initially a clot forms at the site of a ruptured aneurysm. As the clot begins to dissolve and vasospasm subsides, the chance of renewed bleeding increases. Reduced activity and the prevention of straining are critical parts of the management of a ruptured aneurysm, to decrease the possibility of clot disruption.

Stroke Syndromes

Strokes are also classified, according to their stage of development, as transient ischemic attack, stroke in evolution, and completed stroke. A knowledge of these syndromes is useful in planning nursing care.

Transient ischemic attack

A transient ischemic attack (TIA) is a syndrome of brief episodes of neurological deficit that pass without apparent residual effects. A TIA is considered a warning signal and is usually a sign of advanced atherosclerotic disease of cerebral arterial supply. If untreated, approximately one-third of the clients will develop a cerebral infarction, one-third will remain the same, and one-third will improve. A widely held hypothesis is that TIAs are caused by microemboli breaking off from atherosclerotic plaques in the extracranial arteries and temporarily interrupting cerebral oxygenation.

A TIA must be differentiated from other causes of cerebral ischemia such as a developing subdural hematoma or an increasing tumor mass. The signs and symptoms vary according to the part of the brain affected. The anatomic location of the neurological deficit can be identified on the basis of clinical manifestations. If the carotid system is involved, the client may report a temporary loss of vision in one eye, a transient hemiparesis, or a sudden inability to speak. The most common symptoms of TIA related to basilar artery insufficiency are tinnitus and vertigo. The deficits usually last less than 30 minutes but may last for up to 24 hours. No sign of permanent neurological deficit is present between attacks. A client with TIAs needs to be encouraged to seek medical care promptly.

Stroke in evolution

A stroke in evolution, or progressive stroke, develops over a period of hours or days. This pattern of progression is most characteristic of an enlarging intraarterial thrombus. A stepwise or intermittent progression of deteriorating neurological findings is common. However, any stroke may have a gradual progression of manifestations for up to 70 hours after the infarct. The progression of manifestations correlates with the degree of edema secondary to the inflammatory process.

Completed stroke

When the neurological deficit remains unchanged over a 2- to 3-day period, the stroke is called a *completed stroke.* An embolic stroke may demonstrate this characteristic from the beginning. With the exception of stroke secondary to a ruptured aneurysm, a completed stroke signals readiness for more aggressive rehabilitative treatment. If a ruptured aneurysm is the suspected cause, activity continues to be restricted for as long as 4 to 6 weeks to reduce the possibility of additional hemorrhage resulting from clot disruption.

CLINICAL MANIFESTATIONS OF STROKES

The concept of stroke evokes a common mental picture. In reality, however, this picture varies markedly from client to client. The manifestations of stroke depend upon (1) the anatomic site of the lesion, (2) the rate of onset, (3) the size of the lesion, and (4) the presence of collateral circulation. Table 52-2 lists symptoms seen when specific cerebral arteries are involved, regardless of whether the cerebrovascular accident is due to thrombosis, embolus, or hemorrhage. Consequently, the nurse must make a complete assessment before planning care. The physical disabilities are usually easy to idenfity. The language and spatial-perceptual problems are more subtle and difficult to recognize; consequently, these problems are often ignored or misunderstood. Figure 52-3 illustrates the manifestations of right-sided and left-sided stroke. General manifestations of stroke are discussed below.

Neuromuscular

Neuromuscular deficits are the most obvious manifestations of stroke. These symptoms are caused by the destruction of motor neurons in the pyramidal pathway. This destruction can result in the loss of skilled voluntary movements (akinesia), impairment of integration of movements, and exaggeration of reflexes (hyperreflexia).

These losses follow characteristic patterns. Be-

Table 52-2
Clinical Manifestations Related to Specific Cerebral Artery Involvement

Manifestations Seen with Middle Cerebral Artery Involvement

A. General (main stem blocked)
   1. Contralateral paralysis
   2. Contralateral anesthesia: loss of proprioception, fine touch, localization
   3. Dominant side: aphasia
   4. Nondominant side: neglect of opposite side, dysmetria
   5. Visual: homonymous hemianopsia, conjugate-gaze paralysis
   6. Alertness: decreased
B. Specific (branches blocked)
   1. Superior branch (rolandic and prerolandic areas)
      a. Alert
      b. Severe contralateral motor and sensory deficits of face, arm, and leg. Leg may improve, enabling patient to walk; arm and face seldom regain function.
      c. Left side: global aphasia initially, later motor aphasia only
   2. Inferior branch (temporoparietal area): homonymous hemianopsia: usually
      a. Left side: Wernicke's aphasia: severe defect in comprehension of spoken and written language with paraphasia and paragraphia
      b. Right side: opposite-side neglect

Manifestations Seen with Anterior Cerebral Artery Involvement

A. General (stem occluded)
   1. Usually no problem if stem occluded near the anterior communicating artery (allows for perfusion from the opposite side)
   2. If both anterior cerebral arteries come from one stem:
      a. Infarction of the medial aspect of both hemispheres
      b. Paraplegia
      c. Urinary incontinence (unknowing)
      d. Severe mental symptoms
B. Occlusion distal to the anterior communicating artery
   1. Contralateral sensory and motor deficits of leg and foot
   2. Contralateral paresis: arm
   3. Possible unknowing urinary incontinence
   4. Contralateral grasp and sucking reflexes
   5. Paratonic rigidity
   6. Abulia
   7. Laconic spoken responses
   8. Tendency to speak in whispers
   9. Distractibility
   10. Amnesia
C. Smaller branches: further limits and decreases the area of deficit

Manifestations Seen with Posterior Cerebral Artery Involvement*

A. Anterior and proximal occlusion
   1. Thalamogeniculate branch occlusion (thalamic syndrome. Déjèrine-Roussy syndrome)
      a. Contralateral sensory loss: deep and cutaneous with varying degrees, i.e., pain and temperature loss may be greater than touch or position sense (or the reverse), or the loss may occur in only a given part of the body
      b. Hemiparesis: temporary
      c. Homonymous hemianopsia
      d. Thalamic pain: later with recovery. Unpleasant, diffuse, contralateral. Can occur spontaneously or after stimulus. Depression and distortion of taste may also be present.
   2. Paramedian branch occlusion: central midbrain and subthalamus
      a. Weber's syndrome: oculomotor palsy with contralateral paralysis
      b. Stupor or coma
      c. Contralateral ataxic tremor: possible
   3. Thalamoperforating branch occlusion: anteromedial-inferior thalamus
      a. Hemiballismus or hemichoreoathetosis
      b. Sensory loss: deep
      c. Hemiataxia or tremor

Table 52-2 (Continued)

B. Cortical occlusion
   1. Branches to the temporal and occipital lobes
   2. Homonymous hemianopsia: may be incomplete, usually in upper fields
   3. Dominant hemisphere
      a. Alexia
      b. Anomia: most severe for colors
      c. Recent memory deficit: moderate
   4. Nondominant hemisphere
      a. Topographic disorientation (surroundings)
      b. Anomia: faces

C. Upper basilar artery occlusion—bilateral
   1. Eye deficits
      a. Homonymous hemianopsia: bilateral
      b. Total blindness (cortical)
      c. Central vision loss } Those with some vision may have
      d. Paracentral vision loss } difficulty seeing to and fro
      e. Visual hallucinations
      f. Apraxia of ocular movement
   2. Memory loss: may be severe
   3. Inability to count or name objects

Manifestations Seen with Vertebral Artery Involvement†

1. Lateral medulla block (may involve one or more arteries) (most frequent in occurrence)
   a. Contralateral decrease in pain, temperature sense
   b. Ipsilateral Horner's syndrome: miosis, ptosis, decreased sweating
   c. Hoarseness
   d. Dysphagia
   e. Ipsilateral paralysis of palate and vocal cord
   f. Decreased gag reflex
   g. Nystagmus, diplopia, oscillopsia, vertigo, nausea, vomiting
   h. Ipsilateral ataxia of limbs: falling or toppling to ipsilateral side
   i. Pain, numbness, decreased sensation of face: ipsilateral
   j. Loss of taste
   k. Ipsilateral arm numbness
   l. Hiccups
2. Posterior medulla block
   a. Ipsilateral cerebellar ataxia
3. Medial medulla block (rare)
   a. Contralateral paralysis of arm and leg
   b. Contralateral loss of position and vibration sense
   c. Ipsilateral paralysis and atrophy of tongue
4. Posterior inferior cerebellar artery occlusion: sudden vertigo, nausea, vomiting, ataxia, nystagmus

Manifestations Seen with Basilar Artery Involvement‡

A. General or stem
   1. Bilateral motor and sensory deficits: all extremities
   2. Diplopia
   3. Nystagmus
   4. Blindness or lesser degree
   5. Ataxia
   6. Coma

B. Branches
   1. Superior cerebellar
      a. Ipsilateral cerebellar ataxia: severe
      b. Nausea and vomiting
      c. Slurred speech
      d. Contralateral loss of pain and temperature including face
      e. Deafness: partial
      f. Static tremor: ipsilateral, upper extremity
      g. Horner's syndrome: ipsilateral

Table 52-2 (Continued)

2. Anterior inferior cerebellar
   a. Ipsilateral deafness
   b. Vertigo, nausea, vomiting
   c. Nystagmus
   d. Tinnitus
   e. Cerebellar ataxia
   f. Horner's syndrome: ipsilateral
   g. Conjugate lateral-gaze paralysis
   h. Contralateral pain and temperature loss
   i. Hemiplegia: depending on location of infarction

**Note:* The site of occlusion, the origin of the basilar arteries, and the arrangement of the circle of Willis are involved in the type of deficit seen. Can occur from thrombus or embolus.

†*Note:* If both vessels are of adequate size and there is contralateral blood flow, there may be no visible deficit.

‡*Note:* If the occlusion is due to a thrombus, it usually involves only a branch. If the occlusion is due to an embolus, it frequently lodges at the upper bifurcation of the basilar artery or in one of the posterior cerebral arteries.

Joyce W. Taylor and Sally Ballenger, *Neurological Dysfunctions and Nursing Intervention,* McGraw-Hill Book Company, New York, 1980, pp. 395–397.

cause the pyramidal pathway decussates at the lower end of the medulla, a stroke in the right hemisphere of the brain will cause paralysis of the left side. Both upper and lower extremities of the involved side are affected. The shoulder tends to rotate internally and the hip rotates externally. The foot is plantar-flexed and inverted. A period of flaccidity (hypotonia) may last for a few days to several weeks. Flaccidity is followed by spasticity (hypertonia). During the spastic stage, the deep tendon reflexes are exaggerated. The Babinski reflex is positive.

Problems with neuromuscular control may affect nutrition and respiration. In addition to experiencing difficulty with self-feeding, the client may be unable to swallow. This is a very difficult problem when the stroke affects both sides of the internal capsule. The client may be unable to swallow his own secretions and consequently is susceptible to aspiration pneumonia.

Problems related to the neuromuscular control of elimination are more complex. Fortunately, they are usually transient. When the stroke is confined to one hemisphere, the prognosis for return to normal bladder function is excellent. The reflex arc remains intact, a partial sensation of bladder filling remains, and the client maintains partial voluntary control over voiding.[5] Initially the client may experience frequency, urgency, and incontinence. Bladder training is facilitated if started immediately. A retention catheter may interfere with this process; it should be used only during the most acute period of the stroke if absolutely necessary. Neuromuscular control of the bowel is usually not a problem. However, the client is prone to constipation. This is attributed to immobility, weakened abdominal muscles, decreased oral intake, inability to communicate the need to defecate, and lack of response to the defecation reflex.[6] (See Chronic Management for bowel and bladder training.)

Communicational

The left hemisphere is dominant for the 93 percent of the population who are right-handed. When the stroke occurs in the dominant hemisphere, the client experiences communication difficulties or aphasia, since the speech center is located in the left hemisphere in right-handed people. Language disorders involve both the expression and the comprehension of written or spoken words. When the lesion involves Wernicke's area of the brain, the client experiences *receptive aphasia:* neither the sounds of speech nor its meaning can be distinguished, and comprehension of both written and spoken language is impaired. The lesion causing *expressive aphasia* affects Broca's area; this client has difficulty in both speaking and writing. In *nonfluent aphasia,* the client speaks very little. In *fluent aphasia,* he speaks meaningless phrases. A massive lesion may affect both areas, resulting in *global aphasia,* in which all language function, both expressive and receptive, is lost. The client cannot understand what he hears or reads nor can he communicate his thoughts in speech or writing.

Affective

Clients with a stroke may demonstrate loss of control of their emotions, probably related to edema

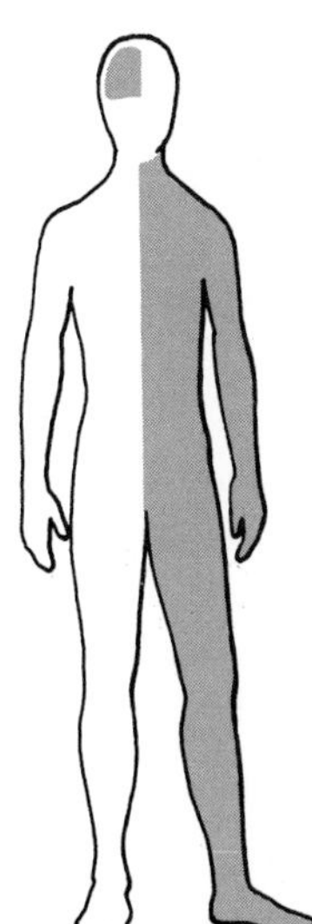

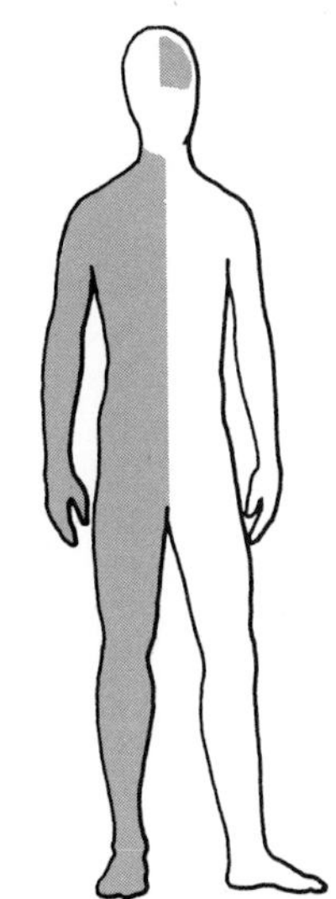

Figure 52-3 Manifestations of right-sided and left-sided stroke. Speech language deficits (aphasia) result only if the right side is dominant.

and pressure on the frontal lobe. Their emotional responses may be exaggerated or unpredictable. This is compounded by the depression experienced with the change in body image and the frustration related to communication problems. It may be difficult to tell if the client is crying because of emotional lability or depression. Distraction is usually effective in coping with emotional lability. Depression requires sensitive, therapeutic communication between the client and the nurse. Frequent reassurance that improvement is possible helps the client maintain a positive attitude.

Intellectual

Both memory and judgment may be impaired in a stroke. These impairments are experienced in both right- and left-sided lesions. A left-sided lesion is more likely to result in memory problems related to language; a right-sided lesion, in problems related to spatial-perceptual content. The client with a left-sided lesion tends to be overly cautious in matters of judgment. In contrast, the client with a right-sided lesion is quick and impulsive. Both may experience difficulty in making generalizations, which interferes with ability to learn.

Spatial-Perceptual

A stroke in the right hemisphere is most likely to cause deficits in spatial-perceptual orientation. These spatial-perceptual deficits may be divided into four categories.[7] The first relates to the client's perception of self and illness. This deficit follows lesions of the parietal lobe. Clients may deny their illnesses or their own body parts. The second category concerns the client's perception of himself in space. He may neglect all input from the affected side. This may be caused, in part, by *homonymous hemianopsia.* In this condition, blindness occurs in the corresponding halves of the visual fields of both eyes. In addition, the client has difficulty with spatial orientation in matters such as judging distances. The third spatial-perceptual deficit is *agnosia,* the inability to recognize an object by sight, touch, or hearing, and the fourth is *apraxia,* the inability to carry out learned movements.

DIAGNOSTIC STUDY ABNORMALITIES

A number of diagnostic-study abnormalities may occur as a result of a stroke. Although the skull x-ray is usually normal, there may be a pineal shift with a massive infarct. A brain scan will show increased uptake of radioactive media in infarction.

A lumbar puncture may show a transient increase in leukocytes in the cerebrospinal fluid (CSF). The presence of blood in the CSF is indicative but not diagnostic of hemorrhage. A lumbar puncture is usually not attempted in the presence of increased intracranial pressure because of the danger of herniation from a sudden decrease in pressure.

An electroencephalogram (EEG) may show low-voltage slow waves in ischemic infarction. If hemorrhage is the cause of the stroke, the EEG may show high-voltage slow waves. The increased density on computed tomography (CT) can indicate the size and location of the lesion. This test can also aid in differentiating ischemic infarction and hemorrhage. Arteriography can demonstrate areas of cervical and cerebrovascular occlusion, atherosclerotic plaques, and malformation of vessels.

MEDICAL MANAGEMENT

Prevention

Once a stroke has occurred, the impact of medical management is limited. The priority of medical therapy is therefore prevention—both the prevention of infarction in clients with TIAs and the prevention of recurrence in clients who have had a stroke. Clients with known risk factors such as diabetes, hypertension, or cardiac dysfunction should be followed closely. Measures designed to prevent the development of a thrombus or embolus are utilized. For males, the administration of aspirin (A.S.A.) or dipyridamole (Persantine) has decreased the incidence of stroke. However, these antiplatelet aggregants have been of questionable benefit in the treatment of females, although the reason for this is not known. Anticoagulants are also used for clients with TIAs, although the possibility of hemorrhage has to be considered should a rupture occur.

The most common surgical procedures used to reduce the frequency of TIAs and the danger of impending stroke are endarterectomy and cerebral artery bypass. Both are designed to maintain cerebral blood flow, and both must be performed before an infarction occurs or the hazards will outweigh the benefits. An endarterectomy is used to remove an atherosclerotic plaque from an extracranial artery. The most common site of atherosclerotic plaque development is the region of the carotid bifurcation and the arch of the aorta. During the procedure the arteries are clamped above and below the plaque. An incision slightly larger than the plaque is made and the plaque is removed. During this period the brain receives blood through the vertebral-basilar system and the other internal carotid (Fig. 52-4). If these blood vessels have a compromised blood flow due to atherosclerosis, the procedure is undertaken at risk.

The cerebral artery bypass is used for intracranial problems. Although there are a number of variations, the procedure usually involves anastomosing a branch of the external carotid artery to an intracranial artery. Branches of the middle cerebral artery are most commonly used. A burr hole is drilled in the skull, and the two arteries are connected through it. In this way an intracranial occlusion is bypassed.

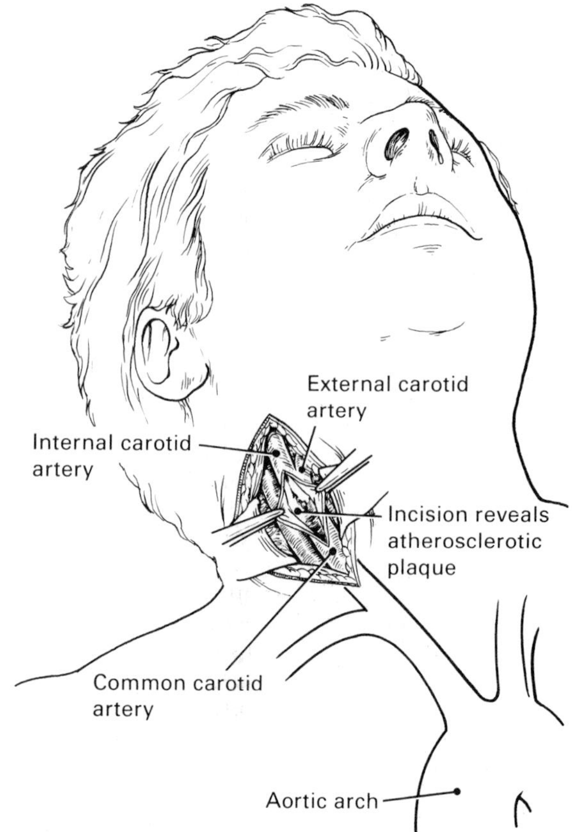

Figure 52-4 Carotid endarterectomy. The atherosclerotic plaque in the internal carotid artery is removed to prevent impending cerebral infarction.

Acute Medical Management

The focus of medical management of the stroke client is (1) the preservation of life, (2) the prevention of additional brain damage, and (3) the lessening of disability. The diagnostic tests used to determine the cause of the stroke are the same for all types of stroke; the medical treatment differs according to whether the stroke is in the acute or chronic phase (Table 52-3).

The first goal of medical management is to maintain a patent airway. The client is monitored closely for signs of increasing neurological deficit. Because of cerebral edema, the fluid and electrolyte balance must be carefully controlled. Initially, the client will retain fluids because of the stress response (increased antidiuretic hormone and aldosterone). Inappropriate secretion of antidiuretic hormone may occur. This may be partially offset by the client's inability to drink or by highly concentrated tube feedings. All these factors must be considered before ordering

Table 52-3
Medical management: Cerebal Vascular Accident

Diagnostic
1. Neurological examination
2. Skull x-ray
3. Electroencephalogram
4. Lumbar puncture
5. Arteriography
6. Brain scan
7. Computed tomography

Therapeutic
A. Acute
 1. Maintain oral airway
 2. Neurological checks q 2 h
 3. Vital signs q 2 h
 4. Suction prn
 5. NPO
 6. Measure intake and output
 7. 1000 mL D5/W q 24 h
 8. Bed rest
 9. Passive ROM exercises
 10. Dexamethasone
B. Chronic
 1. Diet as tolerated
 2. Physical therapy
 3. Occupational therapy
 4. Speech therapy
 5. Aspirin
 6. Dipyridamole
 7. Dioctyl sodium sulfosuccinate
 8. Refer to public health nurse for evaluation of home environment

Surgical Management—of Cerebral Hemorrhage Due to an Aneurysm
1. Clipping
2. Muscle wrap
3. Crutchfield clamp on carotid artery

fluids. The physician usually tries to keep the client slightly dehydrated yet provide enough fluids to prevent capillary sludging. Adequate fluid intake during the acute phase is usually 1000 mL/day. When the period of acute stress is over, the fluid requirements increase as diuresis starts. Fluid requirements may be met with an additional 1000 mL D5/W per day. If the client is unable to eat within a week to 10 days, parenteral hyperalimentation or tube feedings are instituted.

To prevent additional brain damage, three therapeutic approaches have been utilized with varying success. The first and most effective is the use of measures designed to reduce cerebral edema, which interferes with the metabolism of the viable cells. Although a temporary phenomenon, this interference may result in the death of additional cells or even of the person. Dehydrating agents such as mannitol, glycerol, or urea may be employed. These hyperosmotic agents tend to draw fluid from the interstitial spaces into the vascular system. Corticosteroids are also used to reduce cerebral edema. The second approach used to prevent additional brain damage involves measures designed to reduce the metabolic needs of the brain. Hypothermia and barbiturate therapy are among the treatments used for this purpose; neither has proved effective. The third therapeutic approach is designed to promote cerebral blood flow. Vasodilators, hypertensive agents, and hyperventilation therapy have been used but have been of little proven value.

When a cerebral hemorrhage is due to rupture of an aneurysm, surgical intervention may be appropriate. Surgery is usually indicated only when the client's condition has stabilized, when the bleeding has been mild, or when minimal neurological impairment is present

Clips may be placed on either side of the aneurysm. The aneurysm may be wrapped or reinforced with muscle. These internal repair procedures carry great risk for the client.

If the client's condition or the location of the aneurysm indicate that internal repair is inadvisable, external repair may be attempted. This involves clamping of the common carotid, a procedure that requires perfusion of the affected hemisphere by circulation from the opposite side. The adequacy of this circulation is determined by angiogram and isotope blood-flow studies.

Chronic Medical Management

After the stroke has stabilized for 12 to 24 hours, medical management shifts from the preservation of life to the lessening of disability. At this point other members of the health team—physical therapist, occupational therapist, social worker, and public health nurse—join in the effort. An aggressive program is designed to return the client to optimal functioning.

PHARMACOLOGICAL MANAGEMENT

Hyperosmotic Agents

When the cerebral edema accompanying a stroke threatens to cause herniation, intravenous *mannitol* is the drug of choice. This hyperosmotic agent reduces the intracranial pressure due to edema. It must be used with caution in clients with renal dysfunction, as the increased circulatory volume may compromise damaged kidneys. Side effects of mannitol include fever, angina, pulmonary congestion, headache, and blurred vision.

Urea and *glycerol* may also be used as hyperosmotic agents. However, urea has a rebound effect which may eventually increase the intracranial pressure. Glycerol is metabolized into sugar and cannot be used for diabetics. These drugs are not used as often as mannitol. With any of these agents, the nurse must carefully monitor intake and output, body weight, and electrolytes. The client can become dehydrated.

Corticosteroids

Dexamethasone (Decadron) is also used to treat the client with a stroke. When this drug is used, the initial dose is tapered over a period of 7 to 10 days. Dexamethasone acts as an anti-inflammatory agent to break the cycle of increasing intracranial pressure by reducing the inflammatory reaction. Although commonly used, its benefit in the treatment of stroke is questionable. Additional research is needed.

Anticoagulants

Heparin is used as an anticoagulant in the treatment of TIAs, thrombotic strokes, and strokes in evolution. It exerts its effect by the activation of plasma antithrombin and the subsequent inactivation of thrombin. Heparin is used as the first step in anticoagulation. It is most effective when administered by continuous intravenous infusion at a rate of 1000 U/hour or until the partial thromboplastin time (PTT) is 2 to 3 times normal. The duration of treatment is usually 7 to 10 days. Complications include bleeding and easy bruising. Since its effectiveness in the treatment of stroke syndromes is controversial, the risk of bleeding has to be weighed in terms of benefits.

Long-term anticoagulation is accomplished by the oral administration of *warfarin* (Coumadin, Panwarfin), which inhibits prothrombin synthesis and decreases the vitamin K–dependent clotting factors. The usual dosage is 5 to 10 mg/day. A prothrombin time (PT) of 2 to $2\frac{1}{2}$ times normal is desirable. The duration of treatment in stroke syndromes is 3 to 6 months. Excessive bleeding is the primary complication. Table 30-15 lists the nursing implications related to anticoagulant therapy and client education.

A client taking warfarin on a long-term basis needs to know the following:

1. Signs of anticoagulant overdosage
2. Drugs with which warfarin interacts
3. Rationale for avoiding modifications in diet
4. Importance of avoiding trauma
5. Importance of a Medic-Alert bracelet
6. Need for routine blood testing

Antiplatelet Aggregants

Acetylsalicylic acid (aspirin, A.S.A.) is used to prevent platelet aggregation at the site of an atherosclerotic plaque in men. The dosage of 320 mg qid or 640 mg bid is administered orally. The complications of gastrointestinal bleeding may be reduced by administering the aspirin with meals. It is contraindicated in clients with peptic ulcer and must be used with caution when anticoagulants are also being taken. The duration of treatment is indefinite.

Dipyridamole (Persantine) also inhibits platelet aggregation. It is used alone or with aspirin in treating TIAs. It is administered orally in doses of 50 to 75 mg qid (or tid with aspirin). Complications include nausea and vomiting. Duration of treatment is indefinite.

NUTRITIONAL CONSIDERATIONS

A diet containing 1200 to 1500 calories per day is usually adequate for the client with a stroke once the acute phase is over. If the client is unable to take this orally, tube feeding may be initiated, usually by the nasogastric route. Most commercially prepared formulas provide about 1000 calories/100 mL. Sustagen, Isocal, and Ensure are examples of complete nutritional formulas. The latter two are also low in lactose and residue. Since tube feedings tend to be hyperosmotic, they may dehydrate the client. If a quantity is given at one time, it needs to be preceded and followed by water. A continuous feeding of 80 to 150 mL/hour is ideal. Cramping and diarrhea are common side effects of tube feedings. (Tube feedings are discussed in Chap. 33.)

Although the client may experience diarrhea from the tube feedings, more commonly the client with a stroke tends to be constipated. The following dietary measures aid in the prevention of constipation:

1. Fluid intake of 2500 to 3000 mL daily unless contraindicated
2. Prune juice 120 mL or stewed prunes daily
3. Cooked fruit 3 times daily
4. Cooked vegetables 3 times daily
5. Whole-grain cereal or bread 3 to 5 times daily

In combination with a regular schedule, privacy, a footstool to increase abdominal pressure, and exercise, these measures are very effective in preventing constipation.

NURSING MANAGEMENT

Health Promotion and Maintenance

To reduce the incidence of strokes, the nurse needs to focus teaching efforts on the partially reversible and reversible risk factors of stroke. A behavior-modification program designed to reduce reversible risk factors of smoking, obesity, stress, and inactivity is outlined below. For the nurse's role in the management of partially reversible factors, see Chap. 26 (hypertension), Chap. 27 (coronary artery disease), and Chap. 41 (diabetes). Table 27-4 lists ways to reduce risk factors related to coronary artery disease which also apply to stroke. For many clients these modifications represent difficult and drastic changes in lifestyle. A program designed to facilitate risk reduction includes the following:[8]

1. Assessing and identifying the problem
2. Building confidence and commitment to change
3. Increasing awareness of behavioral patterns by self-observation
4. Developing and implementing an action plan
5. Evaluating the plan
6. Maintaining the change

Assessing and identifying the problem

To assist the client in identifying the problem, the nurse can use one of the many assessment tools available related to risk of heart attack and stroke. After the high-risk areas are identified, the client needs to select one risk area which he wants to modify. Then a more thorough assessment of the behavior is necessary, including duration, frequency, type, and emotional reaction to cessation of the particular risk selected. When the client is ready to make a commitment to change, a written contract may be helpful. The nurse or a friend may be included in the contract as helpers in meeting the goals.

Building confidence and commitment to change

To build confidence and commitment to change, the barriers to change must be identified. Since these usually include both attitudes and behaviors, change is likely to take a long time. The client needs to be aware of this time frame and not be overly critical of lapses. The client may find that recording and analyzing his internal monologues related to the specific behavior is helpful. Negative thinking can be identified by this method, for example, "I don't have the will power to stick to a diet." Initiating and succeeding at small changes such as removing the salt shaker from the table helps build confidence.

Building awareness of behavioral patterns

Since behavior patterns are complex, a complete and systematic analysis may identify relationships (for example, always eating on the run). Keeping a log of the activities may be helpful. However, the method needs to be individualized for each client. An accountant might enjoy keeping a systematic written record; an office worker might move a penny from his right to left pocket when he feels stress. The goal is to identify the behaviors, not to keep a record book.

Building an action plan

In building an action plan, both short-term and long-term goals need to be identified. For example, if an objective requires 6 months to meet, break it down into a series of steps. In the early phase, the initial objectives need to be readily obtainable in order to build confidence. Careful consideration needs to be given to selecting a helper in implementing the plan. The purpose of the helper is to provide social support. The person chosen is, therefore, also in a position to undermine the planned behavioral change. A reward system needs to be built in that is consistent with the overall plan. A chocolate sundae may be deemed a just reward for a week of dieting, but it would reinforce the use of food as a reward. A daily reward may be more reinforcing than a long-term one. A daily reward of points or pennies may be used to build toward a long-term goal such as a vacation in Hawaii.

Evaluation of the action plan

Encourage the client to evaluate the plan daily. Flexibility needs to be encouraged. If the goal is unrealistic, the client may need to return to an earlier phase. Avoiding a climate of chastisement is necessary for long-term progress. Both expected and unexpected outcomes need to be considered in the evaluation.

Maintenance

The maintenance stage is often the most difficult, even though the daily expenditure of effort is less. Setting up a regular checkup time to evaluate the long-term effect of the behavior modification is recommended. A gradual change of behavior tends to result in more long-lasting behavioral changes than more drastic, sudden changes.

Acute Intervention

Respiratory problems

During the acute phase of a stroke, the nursing priority is management of respiratory function. Stroke clients are particularly vulnerable to respiratory problems. Advancing age and immobility make them particularly susceptible to atelectasis. With dysphagia or coma, aspiration pneumonia may develop. In coma the tongue tends to fall back and obstruct the airway. This problem requires that the client be positioned in a side-lying position.

An oropharyngeal airway may be used during the first 24 to 48 hours. This airway holds the tongue in place, preventing airway obstruction and providing access for suctioning. If the client is unable to breathe without an airway after 48 hours, a tracheostomy is performed. A suction machine should be available in the room. Coughing and deep breathing are helpful to the client with a stroke. Since these activities increase intracranial pressure, they should be used with caution in a hemorrhaging client or when the possibility of herniation of the uncus is present. However, in most clients with a stroke, an obstructed airway is more harmful than increased intracranial pressure secondary to coughing.

Neurological problems

The client's neurological status needs to be monitored closely to detect stroke in evolution or increased intracranial pressure. The level of consciousness, vital signs, pupillary responses, and muscular strength are checked at regular intervals. The frequency of neurological checks (Chap. 54) depends upon the condition of the client. A decreasing level of consciousness, a sign of increasing ischemia in the brain, should cue the nurse to check the client more frequently. Careful recording of the neurological status provides an accurate record of client progress.

Cardiovascular problems

Nursing goals for the cardiovascular system are designed to maintain homeostasis. Because of advancing age or heart problems, many clients with a stroke have decreased cardiac reserve. Fluids are retained because of increased production of antidiuretic hormone and aldosterone secondary to stress. Fluid retention plus overhydration can result in fluid overload. It can also increase cerebral edema. The nurse therefore should closely monitor intake and output. Intravenous therapy is also carefully regulated. In the initial stages, fluids may be limited to 1000 mL/day or approximately 42 mL/hour. Every effort needs to be made to ensure a constant flow rate and to avoid a sudden rush of intravenous fluid. Manifestations of fluid overload are rales, dyspnea, shortness of breath, and coughing. In addition, the nurse should regularly assess for other cardiovascular problems such as hypertension and cardiac arrhythmias.

Musculoskeletal problems

The nursing goal for the musculoskeletal system is to maintain function. This is accomplished by the prevention of joint contractures and muscular atrophy. In the acute phase, range-of-motion exercises (ROM) and positioning are important nursing interventions. Passive ROM is begun on the first day of hospitalization. If the stroke is due to a cerebral hemorrhage, the movements are limited to the limbs. As soon as possible, the client is taught to actively exercise the affected limbs. (Muscle atrophy secondary to lack of innervation and inactivity can develop in as little as a month.)

The paralyzed side needs special attention when positioning the client. Each joint should be positioned higher than the joint proximal to it. Specific deformities on the affected side of the hemiplegic client which nurses must be aware of are shoulder adduction; flexion contractures of the hand, wrist, and elbow; external rotation of the hip; and plantar flexion of the foot. A shoulder sling may be useful when the client is sitting up. This technique helps to prevent subluxation of the shoulder with resultant pain and loss of function. A cone-shaped, hard-hand device is useful in maintaining the hand in a functional position. A trochanter roll can prevent external rotation of the hip. When the client is in a supine position, a footboard is used to prevent plantar flexion of the feet. However, even therapeutic interventions can be detrimental if the client is allowed to stay in any one position too long.

Integumentary problems

The skin of the client with a stroke is particularly susceptible to breakdown because of loss of sensation and diminished circulation. This results from interference with the nerve supply to the blood vessels of the affected side. The problem is compounded by the age of the client and possible incontinence. Pressure points should be examined and massaged with each turning. Should an area of redness develop, the client should be turned more frequently. The client should not be left in any position longer than 2 hours. In addition, the skin needs to be kept clean and dry. An emollient may be beneficial for the elderly or dehydrated client. An alternating-pressure mattress or special pads are helpful in relieving pressure areas. A protective coating such as tincture of benzoin may be used on reddened areas. Vigilance is critical if pressure sores are to be avoided.

Gastrointestinal problems

In the acute phase of stroke, the nutritional needs of the client are a secondary concern. The client may be maintained for up to 10 days on intravenous fluids. Facial weakness on the affected side and dysphagia (difficulty in swallowing) present special problems. If the client is conscious, oral feeding is encouraged.

The first oral feeding should be approached with caution, as the gag reflex may not be intact. In order to check this before initiating a feeding, the back of the throat may be gently stimulated with a tongue blade (Fig. 52-5). If the gag reflex is present, the client will gag spontaneously. If it is absent, the feeding should be deferred and exercises to stimulate swallowing begun. The speech therapist, occupational therapist, or physical therapist is usually responsible for designing this program. However, the nurse may be called upon to develop this program in certain clinical settings.

If the gag reflex is present, the nurse may proceed with the feeding. The client should be placed in a high-Fowler's position for the feeding as well as for 15 minutes before and after the feeding. For the first feeding, foods should be selected that are easy to swallow, such as pureed food. Liquids often promote coughing. Milk products should be avoided, as they tend to increase the viscosity of mucus and increase salivation. Food should be placed on the unaffected side of the mouth. Stroking the neck or pressing down on the top of the head decreases laryngeal tension and promotes swallowing. The nurse should ensure that the atmosphere is unrushed and nonstressful. Each feeding must be followed by scrupulous oral hygiene, as food tends to collect on the affected side.

The most common bowel problem is constipation. The client should be checked every 2 days for impaction. Since diet, fluids, and exercise are limited during the acute phase of stroke, a laxative such as milk of magnesia or a stool softener may have to be used. It is often the responsibility of the nurse to request these medications. Enemas are a last resort to relieve constipation and impaction.

Genitourinary problems

In the acute stage of stroke, the primary genitourinary problem is poor bladder control resulting in incontinence. An indwelling catheter is helpful initially. However, chronic use of a catheter prolongs bladder retraining and promotes the development of urinary tract infections. Efforts to avoid the use of an indwelling catheter should be initiated. An adequate fluid intake is critical for bladder retraining. A bedpan or urinal should be offered every 2 hours. Disposable

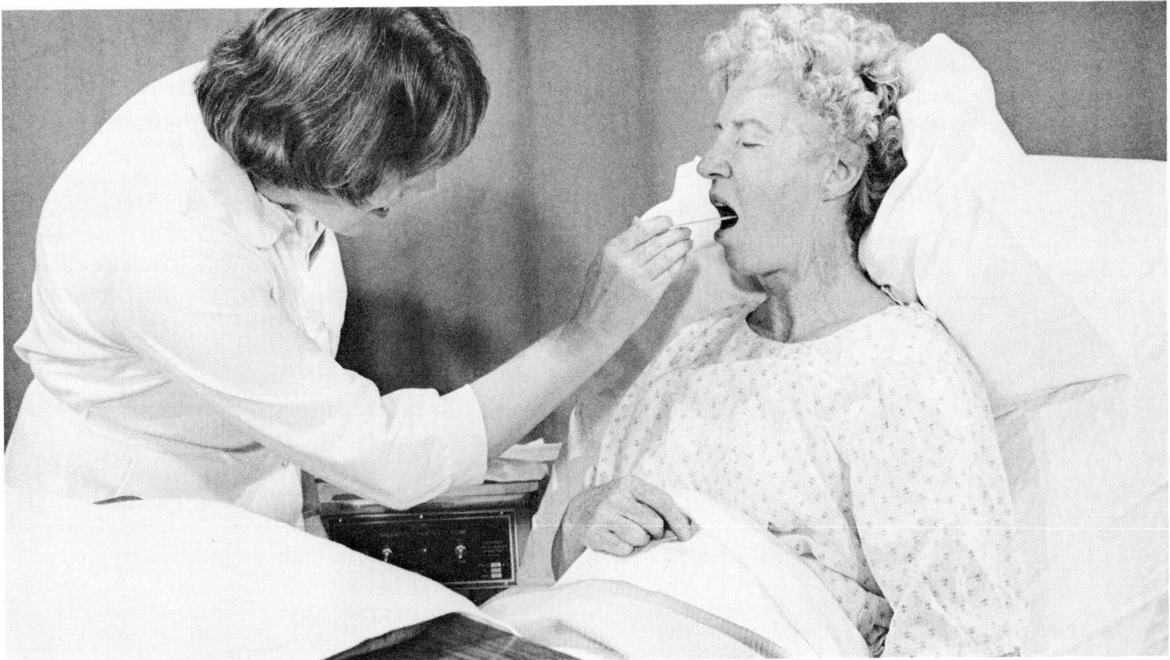

Figure 52-5 Before initiating oral feeding, the nurse should check for the presence of a gag reflex.

diapers for adults are easy to change and keep linens dry. The nurse must explain to the client that the diapers are for short-term use only, to prevent emotional trauma due to the suggestion of infantile behavior. Their short-term use may prevent long-term problems. For male clients, a condom catheter may be used.

Psychological/communication problems

During the acute stage, the nurse's role in meeting the psychological needs of the client is primarily supportive. An alert client is usually very anxious because of lack of understanding of what has happened and inability to communicate. This is not the time for an extensive assessment of language abilities. The client's response to one or two simple questions should give the nurse a guideline for structuring explanations and instructions. If the client cannot understand words, pantomime may be used to support the verbal cues. Tone, demeanor, and touch may also be supportive to the client. Explain to the client, slowly and in simple terms, what has happened. If the prognosis is promising, assure the client that some function will return and that the health team will be available for help during this time of crisis.

Any stroke client may have homonymous hemianopsia (blindness in the same half of each visual field) (Fig. 52-6). Persistent disregard of objects in part of the visual field should alert the nurse to this possibility. The client needs to be trained to compensate for these deficits. After the initial stress of the illness, the nurse may begin placing items necessary for activities of daily living on the affected side. Initially, the nurse compensates for the perceptual problem by arranging the environment within the client's perceptual field. Later, the client is instructed to consciously attend to the neglected side. The position of the affected arm or leg in space must be checked by the client to prevent unfelt trauma. Other visual problems may include diplopia, loss of the corneal reflex, and ptosis.

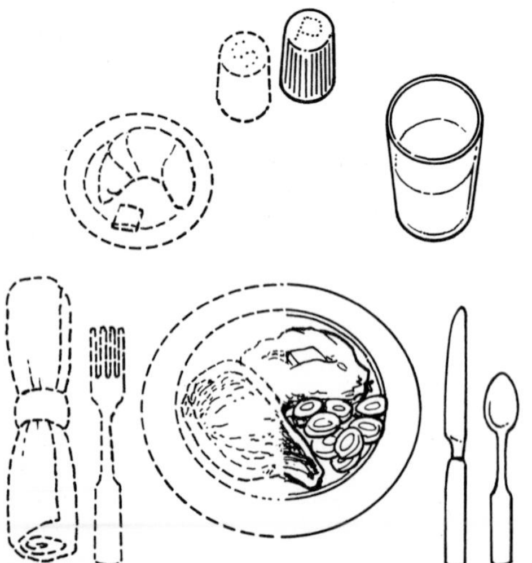

Figure 52-6 Spatial-perceptual deficits in stroke. This illustrates the perception of a client with homonymous hemianopsia. Food on the left side is not seen and is thus ignored.

Family problems

The client's family needs a careful, detailed explanation of what has happened to the client. However, if the family is extremely anxious and upset during the acute phase, explanations may need to be repeated at a later time. Since the family usually has not had time to prepare for the illness, they may need assistance in arranging care for family members or pets, transportation, or finances. A social service referral is often helpful.

Rehabilitative Management

Rehabilitation is the process that enables a disabled or ill client to achieve maximum functioning related to physical, mental, and social well-being. The three goals of rehabilitative management are to prevent deformity, to maintain function, and to restore function. Work toward the first two goals begins at the time the client enters the health care system. For example, upon admission the nurse attempts to prevent deformity in the hemiplegic client by passive exercises, ROM, and proper positioning. In addition, measures to maintain the function of the respiratory and gastrointestinal system are implemented. With the physiological stabilization of the client, the focus shifts to restoration of function. During this stage the client begins to relearn and regain control over bodily actions and functions which are deficient or lost because of the stroke. Such activities might focus on speech, walking, bowel and bladder control, and activities of daily living.

Because no member of the health team possesses all the knowledge and skills necessary for rehabilitation, a team approach is usually used. In this method the health team works together, usually under the direction of the physician, to achieve the rehabilitation goals. This requires a great deal of communication and coordination. The nurse is in a good position to facilitate this process and is often the key person in successful rehabilitation efforts.

The chronic management of the stroke client is focused on rehabilitation. All the problems the stroke client has are caused by or are a response to a neurological deficit. However, for clarity, they will be listed under the system to which the intervention is directed.

Musculoskeletal system

In the rehabilitation of the musculoskeletal system, the nurse initially emphasizes the functions the client needs to feed himself, to toilet, and to walk around the room. This mobility gives the client a psychological boost in preparation for harder tasks later. To achieve these goals, the client needs sitting and standing balance and some function in the affected leg.

Before beginning any intervention, the nurse needs to assess the stage of recovery of muscle function. If the muscles are still flaccid after several weeks, the prognosis for regaining function is poor; the focus of care will be on preventing additional loss. Most clients begin to show signs of spasticity with exaggerated reflexes within 48 hours. This actually denotes progress. As improvement continues, small voluntary movements of the hip or shoulder may be accompanied by involuntary movements in the rest of the extremity (synergy). In the final stage of recovery, the client acquires voluntary control of isolated muscle groups.

Balance training is an initial rehabilitative effort and begins with the client sitting up in bed or on the edge of the bed. The nurse may teach the client to compensate by leaning slightly toward the affected side. The nurse must be alert for dizziness or syncope as a result of vasomotor instability.

Next the client needs to learn to transfer from the bed to an armchair or wheelchair (Fig. 52-7). The chair is placed by the bed on the client's unaffected side. First the client rises to a standing position. When he is stable in the standing position, the unaffected hand is placed on the far arm of the chair. The client turns on the strong foot and sits down. The nurse may provide minimal assistance by standing at the client's weak side supporting the affected arm and blocking the affected knee to keep it from buckling.

Usually some support or assistive device, such as a cane, walker, or leg brace, is needed when the client begins to walk (Fig. 52-8). The physical therapist usually selects the one most appropriate for the client. The nurse needs to incorporate physical therapy activities into the daily routine of the client for additional practice and repetition of the rehabilitative efforts. When walking the stroke client, the nurse generally offers support on the unaffected side.

Gastrointestinal system

Inability to feed oneself and lack of bowel regularity are two common gastrointestinal problems following a stroke. The inability to feed oneself is very frustrating and may result in malnutrition. The easiest solution is to have the client switch hands for eating. The unaffected hand may be clumsy at first, but the end result is usually better than using assistive devices. However, eating with only one hand is still a challenge. Assistive devices such as a rocker knife, a plate guard, and a nonslip mat to keep the plate from sliding are particularly useful eating aids (Fig. 52-9). Removing unnecessary items from the tray or table can reduce spills and resulting embarrassment. Careful attention to aesthetic and environmental detail are important nursing considerations related to improving appetite.

Problems with bowel control may be alleviated by implementing a bowel training program. A high-fiber

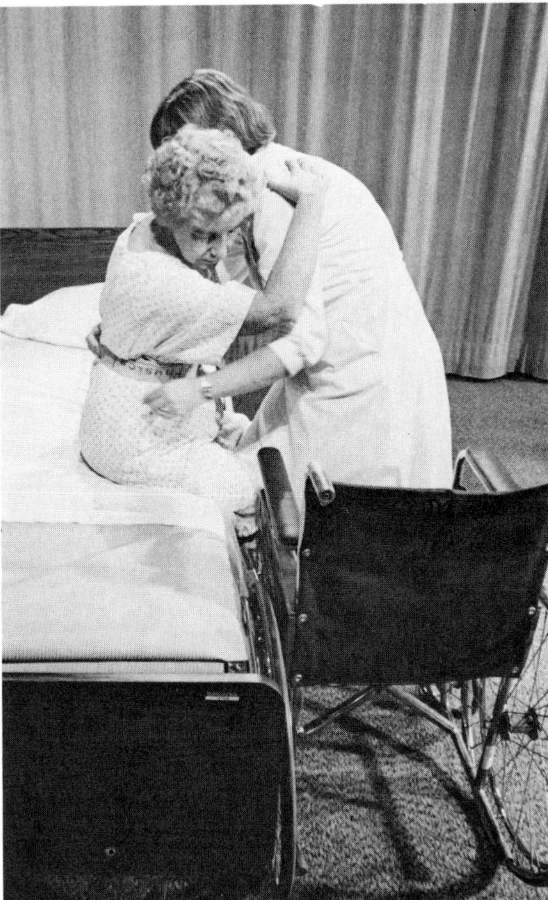

Figure 52-7 Transferring a client with a stroke to a chair. When assistance is needed, the nurse places her right knee against the client's strong knee. The client is grasped around the waist with both arms and pulled forward. Pressure of the nurse's knee forces the client to straighten the strong knee and to bear weight on it. The nurse's right leg and the client's strong leg are used as a pivot. The client is lowered to the chair.

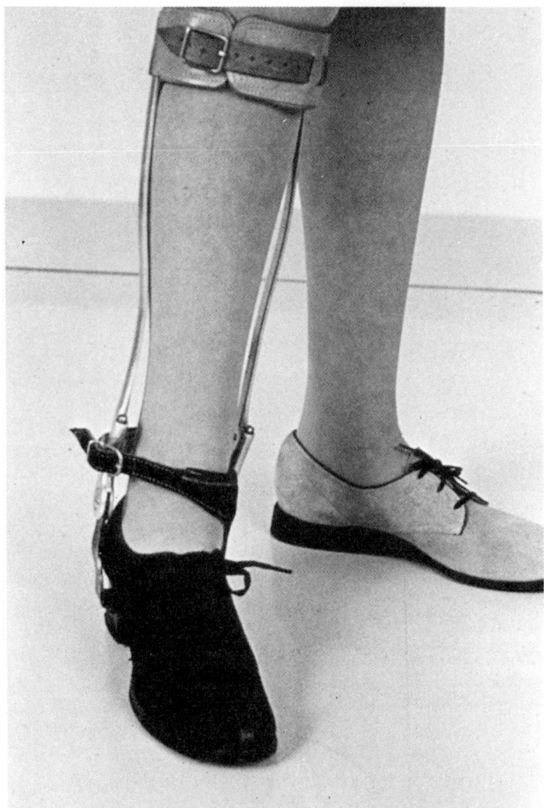

Figure 52-8 This short leg brace is an example of an assistive device which might be needed by the poststroke client. *(J. Sarno and H. Rush, "Rehabilitation of the Stroke Patient," Famous Teachings in Modern Medicine, Medcom, Inc., New York, 1971.)*

diet (see Appendix B, Table 6) and adequate fluid (2000 to 3000 mL/day), as well as the dietary inclusions listed under Nutritional Considerations, should be given unless contraindicated. The client should be put on a bedpan, assisted to a bedside commode, or walked to the bathroom at a regular time daily to assist with reestablishment of bowel regularity. A good time to establish this pattern is within 30 minutes after breakfast each day if the hospital routine and physical therapy schedule do not conflict. If the client's usual bowel habits differ from this pattern, efforts should be made to adhere to his individual timing. Stool expanders and stool softeners are often used in addition to diet and habit retraining.

If these techniques are ineffective in reestablishing bowel regularity, a Dulcolax or glycerine suppository may be inserted 15 to 30 minutes before the usual evacuation time. This stimulates the anorectal reflex and often can be discontinued when a regular pattern is reestablished.

Genitourinary system

If the client is unable to monitor his own urination, the nurse should assist with this activity. An indwelling catheter is not practical for long-term use because of the possibility of urinary tract infection and later problems with reestablishing bladder control. Incontinence often results from the client's inability to make his needs known. Nursing measures aimed at maintaining urinary continence include frequent palpation to assess for bladder distension and offering the urinal every 2 hours around the clock. In addition, the nurse should ensure that the client maintains a high fluid intake during the day. Assuming the usual position for urination (standing for the man and sitting for the woman) and applying pressure over the bladder area often aid in urination.

The use of fluid restriction, diapers, or a urinal in place at all times are only temporary measures to reduce the occurrence or effects of incontinence. Long-term use of these measures discourages continence and can lead to dehydration and skin problems. Intermittent catheterization or external devices may be used for short periods of time until bladder retraining can be attempted.

If the client is unable to regain bladder control, a serious care problem develops. A coordinated retraining program by all members of the nursing staff is a major nursing responsibility. Until bladder and bowel control are attained, further rehabilitation efforts will be hampered.

A client with a stroke may be concerned about loss of sexual function. Many are comfortable in expressing their fears if the nurse provides an atmosphere in which sexuality can be discussed. Sometimes the nurse has to initiate the conversation. Fear that sexual activity will bring on another stroke, alternative positions for intercourse, and the possibility of impotence are common concerns. Impotence, if it occurs, is more likely to be due to psychological factors than to neurological deficits. The client can be referred to *The Source Book for the Disabled* for reassurance in this area.[9]

Psychological considerations

Frequently clients who have had a stroke are viewed as uncooperative by nurses. This labeling often indicates a lack of understanding of the spatial-perceptual deficits with which the clients must cope. Clients with a stroke on the right side of the brain are more likely to have these problems. They have difficulty judging position, distance, and rate of movement.

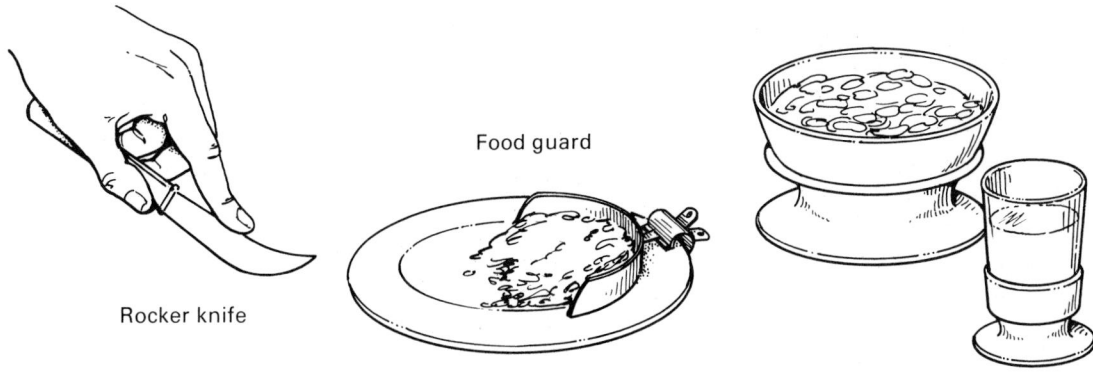

Figure 52-9 Assistive devices for eating.

Furthermore, they tend to *deny* these difficulties and are assertive in tackling unfamiliar tasks. Sometimes these clients have two or three automobile accidents before they realize that they cannot drive a car. They fail to correlate spatial-perceptual problems with their inability to perform certain activities such as getting their wheelchair through a wide doorway. They should be supervised in all activities before being allowed to pursue them independently. Directions should be given verbally, breaking them into small steps. Distracting clutter in the environment should be reduced, and it should be kept well lighted and free of obstacles. A mirror may help the client to orient himself in relation to his environment. One-sided neglect is more common with left hemiplegics. The nurse may need to remind the client to care for the affected side.

Emotional lability may continue into the rehabilitative phase. The client continues to be unable to control his emotions and may burst out in tears or laughter. The behavior is out of context and often unrelated to the underlying emotional state of the client. Inappropriate behavior can be alleviated by distraction. Indeed, the client is usually uncomfortable with this lack of control and will appreciate the intervention.

In addition to the psychological problems secondary to neurological deficit, the client with a stroke may need to be assisted to cope with permanent loss of function secondary to the stroke. Clients often go through all the stages associated with grief and mourning. Many clients are plagued by long-term depression. Inability to resume prestroke role tasks is often a cause of depression. In addition, the time and energy required to perform previously simple tasks can result in anger and frustration.

The family and friends of a client with a stroke also need assistance from the nurse. The poststroke physical, mental, and emotional capabilities of the client may differ markedly from those of the prestroke person. The family needs to understand the true significance of residual stroke damage so that they can make realistic plans regarding both their own and the client's welfare.

It is a nursing responsibility to instruct the care givers on the client's exercise, diet, activity, bowel and bladder activities, skin care, oral hygiene, and occupational therapy. A public health referral will assure continuity of care and provide a support system for the family.

Social

Speech and language deficits constitute one of the most difficult problems for the social system to handle. Speech therapy is only a partial answer. The nurse needs to be a role model for the client's family and avoid making common mistakes when communicating with the aphasic client (Table 52-4). The client needs frequent, meaningful verbal stimulation. A common phenomenon is the client who does not read the cue cards with *dog* and *cat* written on them, but can read a menu. The well-meaning intervention is perceived as a childish game, and the client refuses to play. A better approach for the nurse and the client's family is to talk about the activities of daily living (ADL) which would be familiar to the client. The client should always be allowed sufficient time to answer. A relaxed atmosphere should be maintained, and the client should not be pressured to respond. Reinforcing the use of simple responses such as yes or no may give the client enough confidence to tackle more difficult communication.

In their communication with the client and in the rest of their relationship, families tend to develop patterns of interaction. Sometimes these are detrimental to the long-term health of the client. Families that

Table 52-4

Common Mistakes in Working with the Aphasic Client

1. Finishing his attempts at sentences.
2. Displaying impatience.
3. Anticipating every need so that the client need not talk.
4. Giving care without talking to the client.
5. Talking about the client in his presence as if he does not understand.
6. Talking too loudly or too rapidly.
7. Giving too many directions at one time.
8. Introducing extraneous material while giving instructions.
9. Treating the client as though he were a child.
10. Not giving the client enough time to answer or participate in conversations.
11. Assuming that the client cannot understand any form of communication at all.
12. Assuming that the client's intellect has been impaired.

Adapted from Margot J. Stillman, "Stroke! How to Care for a Recovering Patient," *RN*, November 1979, p. 49.

overreact to the stroke may respond by keeping the client in the dependent, sick role. A common example of a family problem secondary to stroke is rejection of the client's illness; the family expects the client to perform in his normal manner. The preferred solution is a compromise between these two ends of the continuum.

The family has to cope with three aspects of the client's behavior. First, they must recognize those changes that are secondary to neurological deficits and that cannot be changed. Second, they must cope with the client's response to the object loss at the same time that they are dealing with their own response. Third, they must deal with behavior that they have reinforced in the early stages of the illness. For example, the client may be reluctant to resume dressing himself, and the family unconsciously reinforces the behavior by continuing to dress him. This is due both to lack of knowledge and to guilt. Internal dialogues demonstrate the latter: "He wouldn't have had the stroke if I had been a better wife"; "I should have made him see the doctor." Consequently, the family may be hesitant to assert themselves because they are afraid of a recurrence.

Family therapy is a helpful adjunct to a rehabilitation program. The family needs support and reassurance. Open-ended statements like "I imagine this is pretty confusing" may help the family express their feelings. In addition, the family needs accurate and complete information about the disease and treatment. They also need assistance in problem solving in this crisis period.[10]

Discharge planning

Discharge planning should begin as soon as the acute phase of the stroke is over. The family may need assistance in arranging transfer to an intermediate-care facility once hospital care is not required. Such a transfer may be temporary or permanent, depending on the condition of the client and the situation of the primary care provider.

The care provider needs instruction and practice in necessary areas of care while the client is hospitalized. This allows for support and encouragement as well as opportunities for feedback. Adjustments in the home environment such as removing a door to accommodate a wheelchair can be made before discharge.

Specific areas for instruction related to home care of the stroke client include exercise and ambulation techniques; dietary requirements; recognition of signs indicating another stroke, such as headache, vertigo, numbness, and visual disturbances; understanding of emotional lability and the possibility of depression; medication routine; and time, place, and frequency of follow-up activities such as occupational therapy and physical therapy.

Community resources can be an asset to clients and their families. The American Heart Association has information about stroke, hypertension, diet, exercise, and assistive devices. They also sponsor self-help groups in many locales. The Easter Seal Society may provide wheelchairs and other assistive devices. Other local groups are often available to aid with meals and transportation. Referral to a community health nurse will promote continuity of care.

Case Study / Chronic Stroke

Minnie, a 70-year-old white female, is recuperating from a thrombotic stroke of the right hemisphere. She is 5 feet tall and weighs 200 pounds. Eight years ago she was diagnosed as having adult-onset diabetes.

Despite her physical limitations, Minnie had maintained a very active lifestyle. She gardened, kept house for her husband, and painted. In the past 2 years, she had had two one-man shows of her art. Now she is concerned that she will be unable to paint again (she is left-handed). She also verbalized fear about taking care of herself at home. She said, "I don't want to be a burden on my husband."

Discussion Questions

1. What is the relationship between stroke and diabetes?
2. How can a recurrence of Minnie's stroke be prevented?
3. What perceptual deficits might be anticipated with a stroke in the right hemisphere?
4. How can the nurse facilitate Minnie's coping with object loss?
5. What nursing measures may be utilized to promote ADL for Minnie?
6. What changes in the home setting might be useful to Minnie?
7. What community resources are available to help her cope?

REVIEW QUESTIONS

The number of the question corresponds to the same-numbered objective at the beginning of the chapter.

1. Which of the following clients is most likely to have a stroke?
   a. a black 65-year-old male with hypertension
   b. a white 20-year-old female on oral contraceptives
   c. an obese 15-year-old Native American male
   d. an oriental 35-year-old female who smokes

2. Which of the following is the *most* potent regulator of cerebral blood flow?
   a. oxygen
   b. carbon dioxide
   c. bicarbonate
   d. lactic acid

3. In which of the following sites is an atherosclerotic plaque most likely to develop?
   a. left ventricle of the heart
   b. bifurcation of the carotid artery
   c. aortic arch
   d. ophthalmic artery

4. A stroke due to thrombosis
   a. is associated with hypertension
   b. occurs following activity
   c. evolves in a stepwise fashion
   d. is associated with cardiac dysfunction

5. A right-sided hemiplegia may be caused by a lesion in the
   a. lateral spinothalamic tract
   b. motor area of the left frontal lobe
   c. medial superior area of the paracentral lobule
   d. posterolateral nucleus of the thalamus

6. In the diagnosis of stroke, arteriography is used to determine the
   a. site and size of the infarction
   b. patency of the cerebrovascular system
   c. presence of increased intracranial pressure
   d. presence of blood in the CSF

7. For a client with TIAs, the goal of medical therapy is the
   a. prevention of stroke
   b. reduction of disability
   c. reduction of cerebral edema
   d. prevention of complications

8. The first step in developing a plan to prevent stroke is
   a. identifying the risk factors
   b. stating the goals
   c. making a complete assessment
   d. writing a contract

9. For a stroke client with hemiplegia, the nurse positions each joint
   a. higher than the proximal joint
   b. lower than the proximal joint
   c. at the same level as the proximal joint
   d. at the same level as the distal joint

10. The most common response of the stroke client to the change in body image is
    a. denial
    b. depression
    c. disassociation
    d. intellectualization

REFERENCES

1. *Healthy People: The Surgeon General's Report on Health Promotion and Disease Prevention,* U. S. Department of Health, Education and Welfare, Washington, D.C., 1979.
2. *Heart Facts,* 1980, American Heart Association, Dallas, 1979, p. 19.
3. J. F. Toole and A. R. Patel, *Cerebrovascular Disorders,* 2d ed., McGraw-Hill Book Company, New York, 1974, p. 53.
4. Ibid., p. 54.
5. M. T. O'Brien and P. J. Pallett, *Total Care of the Stroke Patient,* Little, Brown and Company, Boston, 1978, p. 263.
6. Ibid., p. 272.
7. Ibid., pp. 135–144.
8. J. W. Farquhar, *The American Way of Life Need Not Be Hazardous to Your Health,* Stanford Alumni Association, Stanford, 1978, p. 39.
9. G. Hale (ed.), *The Source Book for the Disabled,* Imprint Books, New York, 1979.
10. C. M. Cole, "The Role of Brief Family Therapy in Medical Rehabilitation," *J. Rehabil,* **4**:31 (1978).

Chapter 53

NURSING ROLE IN MANAGEMENT

Peripheral Nerve and Spinal Cord Problems

Maureen Brady Nash
Sharon Wahl

Learning Objectives

1. Explain the causes, clinical manifestations, and medical and nursing management of the client with trigeminal neuralgia and Bell's palsy.
2. Describe the pathophysiology, risk population, and significance of spinal cord injury.
3. Describe the clinical manifestations and medical and nursing management of spinal cord shock.
4. Compare the experimental and conventional medical management of spinal cord injury.
5. Correlate the clinical manifestations of spinal cord injury with the level of disruption and rehabilitation potential.
6. Explain the nursing management for the major physical and psychological problems resulting from spinal cord injury.
7. Explain the types, clinical manifestations, and medical and nursing management of spinal cord tumors.
8. Explain the causes, clinical manifestations, and treatment of Guillain-Barré syndrome, botulism, tetanus, and neurosyphilis.

In general, cranial nerve disorders come under the classification of peripheral neuropathies but are distinguished as *mononeuropathies* since they usually involve motor and/or sensory branches of a single nerve. Causes of cranial nerve problems include tumors, trauma, infectious or inflammatory processes, or idiopathic (unknown) causes. Common cranial nerve disorders discussed in this section are trigeminal neuralgia (tic douloureux) and acute peripheral facial paralysis (Bell's palsy).

In contrast, the *polyneuropathies* affect multiple peripheral nerves, with more generalized symptoms, and are more often due to metabolic or chemical toxins than to infectious processes. Examples of these include Guillain-Barré syndrome, botulism, tetanus, and neurosyphilis, which are discussed in this chapter. Problems related to the spinal cord are also covered.

SPECIFIC CRANIAL NERVE DISORDERS

Trigeminal Neuralgia (Tic Douloureux)

Trigeminal neuralgia is a relatively common cranial nerve disorder affecting 2 percent of the population. It usually begins in the fifth or sixth decade of life and occurs with increasing frequency with aging. While the trigeminal nerve (cranial nerve V) has both motor and sensory branches, only the sensory branches (usually the maxillary and mandibular branches) are involved in trigeminal neuralgia (Fig. 53-1). Although no specific cause has been identified, nerve compression by blood vessels, demyelinating plaques, and the herpes-virus have been suggested.[1] The effectiveness of antiepileptic drug therapy in shortening or suppressing the duration of an attack suggests a similar cause as epilepsy.[2]

Clinical manifestations

The classic picture of trigeminal neuralgia is an abrupt onset of paroxysms of excruciating pain described as burning, knifelike, or a lightning like shock in the lips, upper or lower gum, cheek, or side of the nose. During the acute attack, intense pain, twitching, grimacing, and frequent blinking and tearing of the eye is observed (giving rise to the name *tic*). The attacks are usually brief, lasting seconds to 2 to 3 minutes. Recurrences are unpredictable; they may occur several times a day or weeks or months apart. However, after the refractory (pain-free) period, a phenomenon known as clustering can occur. It is characterized by a cycle of pain, refractoriness, and pain which can continue for hours. Remissions decrease as the client ages.

The painful episodes are usually initiated by a triggering mechanism of light cutaneous stimulation at a specific point along the distribution of the nerve branches. Precipitating stimuli include chewing, tooth brushing, a hot or cold blast of air on the face, washing the face, or even talking; touch and tickle seem to predominate as causative factors rather than pain or temperature. As a result, the person may not eat

This chapter was reviewed by Jane Ellen Mead, R.N., B.S.N., M.S.N., Assistant Professor, The Catholic University of America, Washington, D.C.

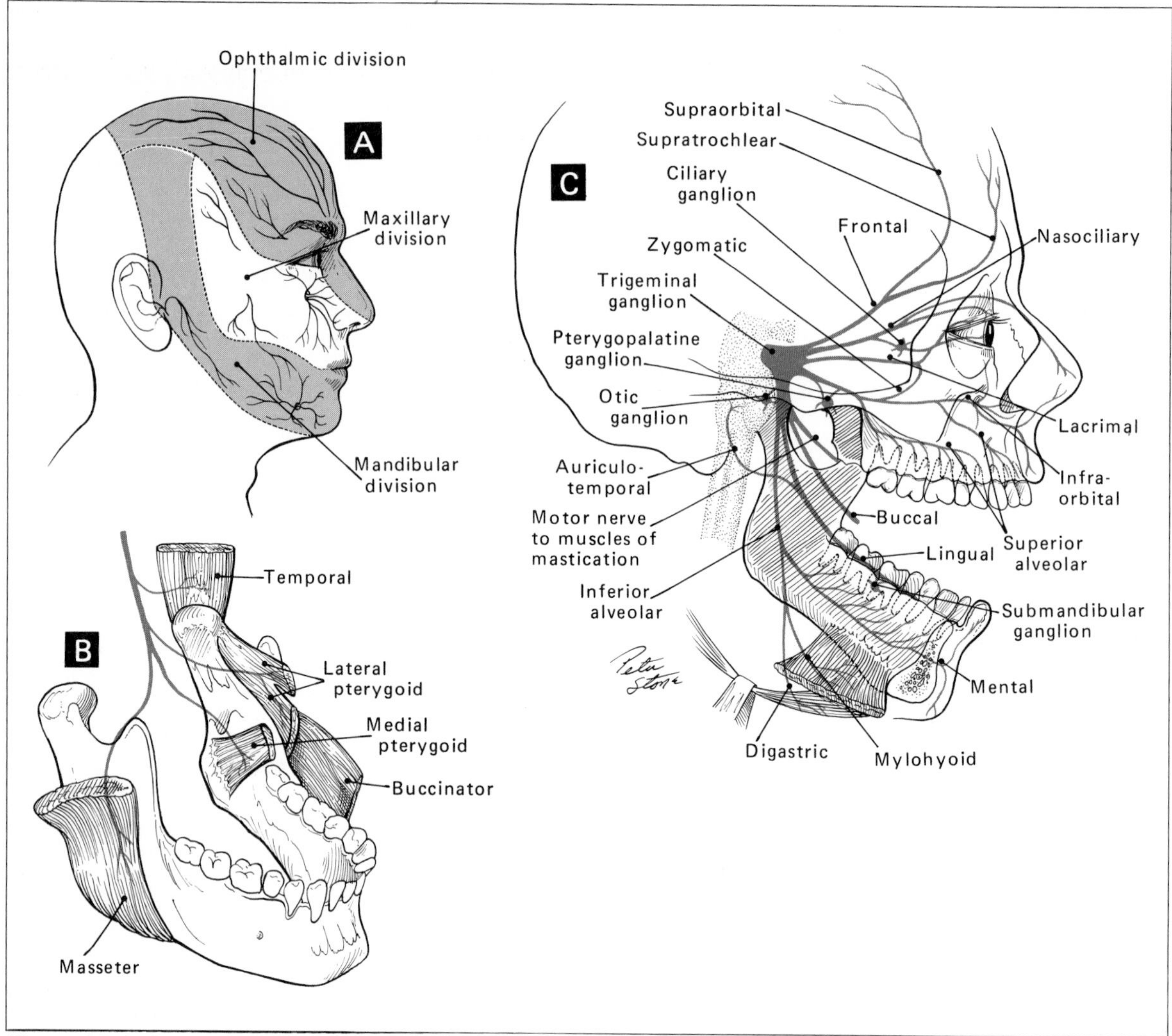

Figure 53-1 Branches of the trigeminal nerve (cranial nerve V) and the areas they serve. (*From L. L. Langley, L. R. Telford, and J. Christensen, Dynamic Anatomy and Physiology, 5th ed., McGraw-Hill Book Company, New York, 1980.*)

properly and may neglect the practice of hygiene, wear a cloth over the face, and withdraw from interaction with other people. Fortunately, the attacks are rarely nocturnal, so sleep is not interrupted. However, the client may use excessive sleep as a means of coping with the pain.

Although this condition is considered benign, the severity of the pain and the disruption of lifestyle can result in almost total physical and psychological dysfunction or even suicide.

Medical management (Table 53-1)

Initially, the physician must rule out other problems with similar manifestations such as other forms of facial and cephalic neuralgias as well as pain arising from the sinuses, teeth, and jaws. A complete neurological workup will usually be done. Once the diagnosis is made, the goal of treatment is relief of pain, either medically or surgically. Between 70 and 80 percent of all clients get adequate relief through anticonvulsant drug therapy.[3] Anticonvulsant drugs such as diphenylhydantoin (Dilantin) and carbamazepine (Tegretol) have been quite effective in many clients with trigeminal neuralgia. They may prevent an acute attack or cause a remission of symptoms. Blood abnormalities such as a decreased WBC associated with these drugs require routine CBC studies. Unfortunately, these drugs may lose their effectiveness and are not a permanent solution. Other clients may seek help repeatedly through otolaryngology or such therapies as acupuncture and use of megavitamins.[4]

If a medical regimen is not effective, surgical re-

Table 53-1
Medical Management: Trigeminal Neuralgia

Diagnostic
1. History and physical examination
2. Brain scan or CT scan
3. Audiological evaluation
4. Electromyography (EMG)
5. Spinal tap
6. Arteriography
7. Pneumoencephalography
8. Posterior myelography

Therapeutic
1. Anticonvulsant therapy (e.g., diphenylhydantoin and carbamazepine)
2. Local nerve blocking
3. Surgical intervention (see Table 53-2)

lief is available (Table 53-2). Percutaneous radio-frequency rhizotomy and microvascular decompression afford the greatest relief of pain. *Percutaneous radio-frequency rhizotomy* consists of placing a needle into the trigeminal rootlets adjacent to the pons and destroying the area by means of a radio-frequency current. This results in paresthesias of the face. Prior to surgery, injection of a lidocaine nerve block is recommended. This trial period allows the client to experience the effectiveness of the treatment and the local anesthesia of the face, which some may find intolerable. Irritation or inadvertent destruction of the ophthalamic branches can result in loss of the corneal reflex. *Microvascular decompression* of the trigeminal nerve is accomplished by displacing and repositioning vessels which appear to be compressing the nerve at the root-entry zone (where it enters the pons). This procedure relieves pain without residual sensory loss but requires great skill on the part of the neurosurgeon. It is potentially dangerous, like any surgery in the posterior fossa (see Chap. 54 regarding care of the client having a craniotomy). It is poorly tolerated in the elderly.

Local nerve blocking is another treatment possibility. The pain relief is only temporary and lasts from 6 to 18 months. Complete anesthesia of the area supplied by the injected branches results. This treatment choice is usually well tolerated by the elderly.

Nursing management

Acute Intervention Assessment of the nature of the attacks, the triggering factors, and pain management techniques help the nurse plan for client care.

Table 53-2
Surgical Intervention for Trigeminal Neuralgia

Procedure	Technique	Benefit
	Peripheral	
Alcohol or phenol injection into one or more branches of trigeminal nerve	Dehydration of nerve	Complete anesthesia of affected area for 6–18 months
Avulsion or resection of peripheral branches of facial nerve	Preganglionic section of sensory portion	Permanent; good for poor surgical risk
	Intracranial	
Retrogasserian rhizotomy	Temporal craniotomy (section of sensory root in middle cranial fossa)	Permanent anesthesia (with sparing of adeptness, corneal reflex and touch)
Suboccipital craniotomy	Sectioning of sensory root in posterior fossa	Permanent anesthesia
Percutaneous radio-frequency rhizotomy	Low-voltage current destroys sensory fibers	Total pain relief; spares touch and corneal reflex; few residual problems
Microvascular decompression (Janetta procedure)	Operating microscope lifts the artery pressing on the nerve root in the posterior fossa with a wedge of sponge, removes pressure at nerve-root entry zone	Permanent pain relief with no loss of sensation

Modified from Sharon C. Sell, "The Treatment of Tic Douloureaux by Vascular Decompression of the Trigeminal Nerve," *J. Neurosurg Nurs*, **9**(1): 20–22 (March 1977).

The nursing assessment should include the client's nutritional status, hygiene (especially oral), and behavior, including withdrawal. The nursing assessment should also include evaluation of the degree of pain and its effects on the client's lifestyle, emotional state, and suicidal tendencies.

Pain relief is primarily obtained by administration of recommended drug therapy. The client's response should be monitored and any side effects noted. While strong narcotics such as morphine may relieve pain, they should be avoided because of the potential for addiction. Propoxyphene (Darvon) or Pentazocine (Talwin) may be used in moderation. Alternative pain relief measures such as bio feedback or pain clinics should be explored for the client who is not a surgical candidate and whose pain is not controlled by other medical measures. Careful assessment of pain history and drug dependency can assist with appropriate interventions.

Environmental management is essential to lessen triggering stimuli. The room should be kept at an even, moderate temperature and free from drafts. A private room is preferred during the acute period. The nurse must use care to avoid touching the client's face or jarring the bed. Many clients prefer to carry out their own care, fearing to be inadvertently hurt by another.

The client needs instruction about the importance of nutrition, hygiene, and oral care. The nurse should convey her understanding of the cause if previous neglect is apparent. Lukewarm water and soft cloths or cotton for cleansing the face should be made available. They may be saturated with solutions not requiring rinsing. Offering a small, very soft (boiled) toothbrush or warm mouthwash will assist in promoting oral care. All these activities are best carried out after medication or analgesics are given.

The client will probably not engage in extensive conversation during the acute period. Alternative communication methods such as paper and pencil should be provided.

Food should be nonchewy, served lukewarm, offered frequently, and be high in protein and calories. The diet should be individualized according to personal, cultural, and religious preferences. In severe cases, insertion of a nasogastric tube on the unaffected side may be necessary.

If surgery is planned, the nurse is responsible for the preoperative teaching and instruction related to diagnostic studies planned to rule out other problems such as acoustic neuroma and neoplasms. The nurse may also need to reinforce the surgeon's instructions related to postoperative expectations. Appropriate teaching of postoperative activities depends upon whether a craniotomy or a local procedure is planned. The client needs to know that he will be awake during a local procedure so that he can cooperate when corneal and ciliary reflexes and facial sensations are checked.

Postoperatively, the client's pain is compared to the preoperative level. The corneal reflex, extraocular muscles, and facial nerve are evaluated at frequent intervals, using the techniques outlined in Chap. 48. The general postoperative nursing care following a craniotomy is appropriate (Chap. 54) if intracranial surgery was performed. Diet and ambulation should be increased according to client progress or specific orders.

If radio-frequency percutaneous electrocoagulation is the procedure used, an ice pack is applied to the operative side on the jaw for 3 to 5 hours. To avoid injuring the mouth, the client should be warned not to chew on the operative side until the paresthesia has diminished.

Chronic Management If treatment is pharmacological, the client will need instruction regarding the dosage and side effects of medications. Regular follow-up care should be planned. Even though relief of pain may be complete, the client should be encouraged to keep environmental stimuli to a moderate level and to use stress reduction methods. Herpes simplex (cold sores) can occur from manipulation of the gasserian ganglion. Treatment usually is topical.

Chronic management following surgical intervention depends on the residual effects of the procedure used. If anesthesia is present or the corneal reflex is altered, the client should be taught to (1) chew on the unaffected side, (2) avoid hot foods or beverages that could burn the mucous membranes, (3) check the oral cavity after meals to remove particles, (4) practice meticulous oral hygiene and continue with semiannual dental visits, (5) protect the face against extremes of temperature, (6) use an electric razor, and (7) provide protective eye care.

Since the client may have developed a whole series of protective devices to prevent pain, he may need counseling or even psychiatric assistance in personality readjustment, especially in reestablishing personal relationships. Some persons will grieve the loss of the pain, especially if it had a special significance such as relieving guilt or anxiety. Occasionally a client may have used his pain to manipulate family and friends and may not adjust following successful pain relief.[5] Careful management in the rehabilitative period can prevent "phantom pain."

Bell's Palsy (Peripheral Facial Paralysis, Acute Benign Cranial Polyneuritis)

Bell's palsy is a disorder characterized by a disruption of the motor branches of the VIIth cranial (facial) nerve on one side of the face in the absence of any other disease such as a stroke. While it can affect any age group, it is more commonly seen in the 20 to 40 age range. The cause is still unknown, but current theories suggest that the herpes simplex virus may cause inflammation and demyelination of the nerve. Mumps and emotional trauma with resultant vasoconstriction have also been suggested as causes.[6]

The onset of Bell's palsy is often accompanied by an outbreak of herpes vesicles in or around the ear. Bell's palsy is considered benign, with full recovery after 3 to 4 months in about 85 percent of cases, especially if treatment is instituted immediately. A small number of clients may have some residual effects. Failure to evidence spontaneous recovery after 6 months indicates that the problem is not Bell's palsy.[7]

Clinical manifestations and complications

The paralysis of the motor branches of the facial nerve typically demonstrates a flaccidity of the affected side of the face with drooping of the mouth accompanied by drooling. A lag or inability to close the eyelid, with an upward movement of the eyeball when closure is attempted, is also evident. A widened palpebral fissure, flattening of the nasolabial fold, and inability to smile, frown, or whistle are also common. Taste sensation is often lost over the anterior two-thirds of the tongue. There may be pain behind the ear on the affected side, especially before the onset of paralysis.

Interventions are primarily supportive until the client has a return of function. Complications can include psychological withdrawal due to change in body image, malnutrition and dehydration, trauma to the mucous membrane, muscle stretching, and facial spasms and contractures.

Medical management

Bell's palsy is diagnosed and the prognosis indicated by (1) observation of the typical pattern of onset and signs, (2) percutaneous nerve excitability testing, and (3) a Schirmer tear test for the presence of decreased tearing on the affected side.[8] The use of the Schirmer tear test is controversial. Corticosteroids, especially prednisone, are started immediately. Results are best if corticosteroids are initiated before paralysis is complete. When the client improves to the point that the corticosteroids are no longer necessary, they should be tapered off over a 2-week period. Usually the steroid treatment decreases the edema and pain, but mild analgesics can be used if necessary. Electromyographic biofeedback may prove to be a new modality for clients with Bell's palsy.[9] It is believed that stimulation maintains muscle tone and prevents atrophy. Vasodilators have been used to stimulate and promote circulation to the affected area. Care is primarily focused on relief of symptoms and prevention of complications.

Nursing management

Health Promotion and Maintenance Early recognition of the possibility of Bell's palsy is important. Since herpes simplex is implicated as a possible etiologic factor, any person who is prone to herpes simplex should be alerted to seek immediate health care if pain occurs in or around the ear. Any evidence of facial weakness should be reported. Persons having active herpes simplex should avoid intimate contact with others. Herpes simplex is discussed in Chap. 17.

Acute Intervention The nurse should regularly assess facial nerve function using the techniques described in Chap. 48. Careful recording of assessment data provides information related to progress.

Pain may be relieved by mild analgesics. Hot wet packs can reduce the discomfort of herpetic lesions as well as aid circulation and relieve pain. The face should be protected from cold and drafts, since trigeminal hyperesthesia may accompany the syndrome. Maintenance of good nutrition is important. The client should be taught to chew on the opposite (functional) side of the mouth to avoid trapping food and to improve taste. Thorough oral hygiene must be carried out after each meal to prevent the development of parotitis and dental caries from accumulated residual food.

Dark glasses may be worn for protective as well as cosmetic reasons. Artificial tears (methylcellulose) should be instilled frequently during the day to prevent drying of the cornea. Ointment and an eye patch should be used at night (see Chap. 15 for special eye care).

A facial sling may be helpful to support affected muscles, improve lip alignment, and facilitate eating. Vigorous massage can break down tissues, but gentle upward massage has psychological benefits even if physical effects other than the maintenance of circulation are questionable. When function begins to return, active facial exercises several times a day are started.

The change in physical appearance as a result of Bell's palsy can be devastating. The client needs to be reassured that he did not have a stroke and that changes for a full recovery are good. While the client's need for privacy should be respected, especially during meals, assistance in adjusting to the change should not be delayed too long. Enlisting support from family and friends is important. If it becomes evident that the altered facial appearance is permanent, more intensive counseling may be indicated.[10]

SPINAL CORD TRAUMA

Problem Identification

Spinal cord problems are generally the direct result of trauma which causes edema, possible cord severance, or cord compression. Prior to World War II, life expectancy for the person with a spinal cord injury was only 10 years from the onset of injury. Presently, even the very young client with spinal cord injury can anticipate a long life. Quadraplegics have a higher incidence of death due to respiratory involvement, but generally prognosis for life is only about 5 years less than for peers without spinal cord injury.

Spinal cord injury can result in complete or partial paralysis (paresis). A complete lesion above T_1 results in loss of function of C_8 and higher and quadriplegia (paralysis involving all four extremities). Lesions below this level can result in paraplegia (paralysis of the lower half of the body involving both legs). However, many consider this designation arbitrary and claim that the distinction lies in the extent of involvement of the brachial plexus and the completeness of the cord lesion.

Health care providers often consider spinal cord disability to be one of the most devastating of physical disabilities. However, survey of the literature reveals that clients with spinal cord injury are remarkably resourceful, with impressive resilience and an ability to work out new patterns of living and coping. Staff members often underestimate the client's potential for independence. Misplaced sympathy and overidentification can compromise the nurse in her attempt to give the involved and complex care required by this person for optimal rehabilitation. Recovery is prolonged, and nurses must learn to gauge progress in inches rather than miles. Skilled, persistent care draws upon every known nursing intervention until the client achieves a maximal level of independence.

Significance

The disruption of individual growth and development, altered family dynamics, economic loss in terms of absence from work, and the high cost of rehabilitation and/or maintenance make spinal cord trauma a devastating problem. With regional variations, initial rehabilitation for a spinal-cord-injured person is approximately $30,000. The United States armed forces estimates that the care for military personnel with spinal cord injuries approaches 1 billion dollars.[11]

Although many spinal-cord-injured clients are able to care for themselves with minimal assistance, a larger number are confined to nursing homes, care centers, and rehabilitation units. Quadriplegics spend an average of 25 days per year in the hospital, while paraplegics spend 15 days.[12] The cost in terms of lost manpower is inestimable.

Etiology and Classification

The risk population for spinal cord injury is primarily young adult males between the ages of 15 and 29 and those who are impulsive or take risks in daily living. A history of numerous injuries prior to the cord injury is common. There is high correlation between alcohol abuse and spinal cord injury. Others at high risk for spinal cord injury include motorcycle racers, sky divers, football players, policemen, divers, and the military. In decreasing order of prevalence, the causes of spinal cord injury include auto accidents, diving, falls (stairs), industry, gunshot wounds, and sports.[13] The resulting spinal cord injury can be due to cord compression by bone displacement, interruption of blood supply, or traction resulting from pulling on the cord. Nontraumatic causes such as tumors, hematomas, and aneurysms can also result in damage to the spinal cord.

Spinal fractures are of four types: flexion, flexion-rotation, compression, or extension (Fig. 53-2). Flexion fractures which include dislocation are the most unstable, since the ligamentous structures stabilizing the spine are severed. These are most often implicated in severe neurological deficits.

Pathophysiology

Initial injury

Research has shown that the cord is physically very tough and is rarely torn or transected by indirect trauma. The complete cord dissolution (previously thought to be transection) in severe trauma is related to auto destruction. Shortly after the injury, petechial hemorrhages are noted in the central gray matter of the cord. This is followed in 1 to 2 hours by extravasation of red blood cells, fluid, and polymorphonuclear leukocytes, which extend throughout the gray matter. Vascular stasis occurs, and the endothelium of vessel walls is damaged. Hemorrhage, edema, and metabolites all act together to produce ischemia, which progresses to necrotic destruction of the cord. The resulting hypoxia reduces the O_2 tension below a level which will meet the metabolic needs of the cord. Lactate metabolites and a gross increase in norepinepherine is noted. In toxic doses, norepinephrine caus-

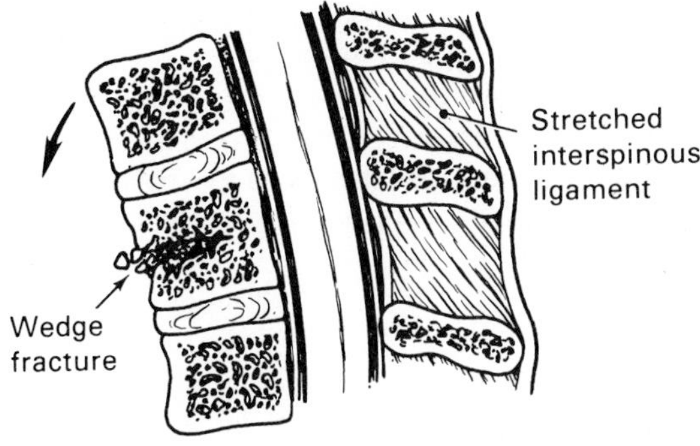

A. Flexion injury

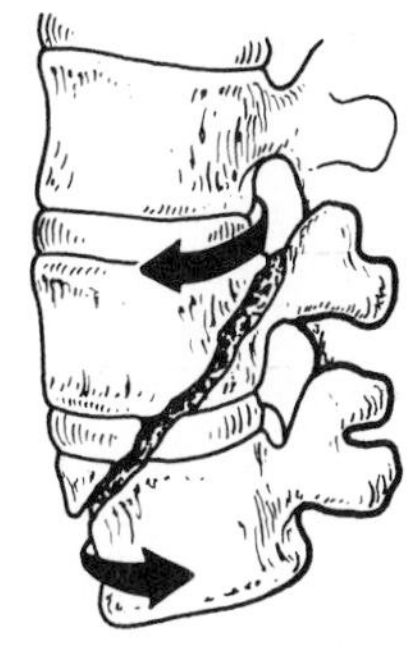

C. Flexion-rotation injury

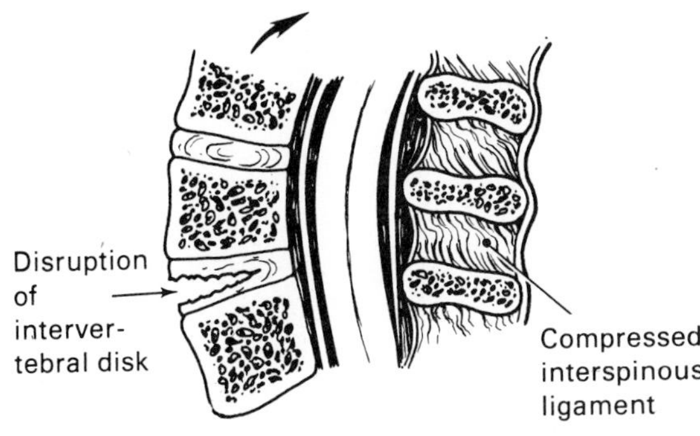

B. Extension injury

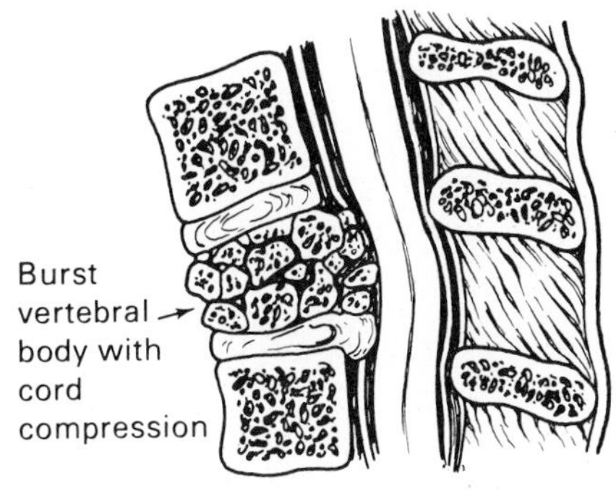

D. Compression injury

Figure 53-2 Types of spinal injury.

es vasospasms, hypoxia, and subsequent necrosis. Unfortunately, the spinal cord has minimal ability to adapt to vasospasm by means of increased flow from anastomotic areas. By 4 hours after injury, this process has progressed to coagulation necrosis of up to 40 percent of the gray matter and subjacent white matter.

By 24 hours after injury, this destructive process has progressed to the point where the spinal cord is composed mainly of necrotic tissue and aggregated red blood cells, with only a small rim of identifiable white matter.[14] Edema secondary to the inflammatory response is particularly deleterious because of lack of space for tissue expansion. The resultant compression of the cord and extension of edema above and below the injury therefore increases the ischemic damage. The end result is no different from mechanical severance of the cord.

Because of the hemorrhagic necrosis, the lesion is complete after 48 hours, and any function of nerves that arise in and pass through this level is destroyed. Additional edema will extend the level of injury beyond the level of destruction for 72 hours to 1 week, so the exact extent of injury cannot be determined before that time.

Spinal cord shock or areflexia

In addition to the discrete damage done at the trauma site, the entire cord below the level of the lesion goes into spasm immediately after injury because of loss of communication with the higher centers. As a result, all functions (motor, sensory, autonomic, and reflex) cease for a period of from 72 hours up to 3 months (the average is 4 weeks). There is a flaccid paralysis, lack of sensation and reflexes, and autonomic disruption specific to the level of injury. In addition to spinal cord shock, systemic shock is present (see Chap. 26). However, since some of the physiological responses of the two types of shocks are antagonistic, the manifestations of spinal cord shock will override the manifestations of systemic shock. For example, vaso constriction will not occur, since sympathetic fibers to vessels are blocked. Symptoms of spinal cord shock (areflexia) include flaccid paralysis, bowel and bladder dysfunction, hypotension with bradycardia, priapism in the male, and absence of reflexes, temperature control, and pain below the level of the injury.

After spinal shock subsides, reflex and autonomic activity returns. Spasticity is evident in the client with an upper motor neuron lesion. No reflex activity is present in lower motor neuron lesions.[15] If the lesion is complete, reflexes are no longer controlled and coordinated by the central nervous system and therefore are often inappropriate and excessive. However, they do form the basis for bowel, bladder, and sexual retraining.

Clinical Manifestations

The manifestations of a spinal cord injury can be predicted on the basis of the site of the injury (Fig. 53-3). There are also cases of incomplete lesions in which mixed symptomatology is present. The higher the injury, the more serious are the sequelae, because of the proximity of the cervical cord to the brainstem and medulla. Table 53-3 describes the movement and rehabilitation potential related to specific locations of the spinal cord injury. In general, sensory function parellels motor function at all levels.

Cervical

Persons with lesions at C1 to C3 are seldom seen in hospitals; they usually die at the scene of the accident from respiratory arrest due to loss of phrenic nerve function or disruption of vital centers in the medulla. At C4 there is flaccid paralysis and sensory loss below the neck. If edema extends above C4, the

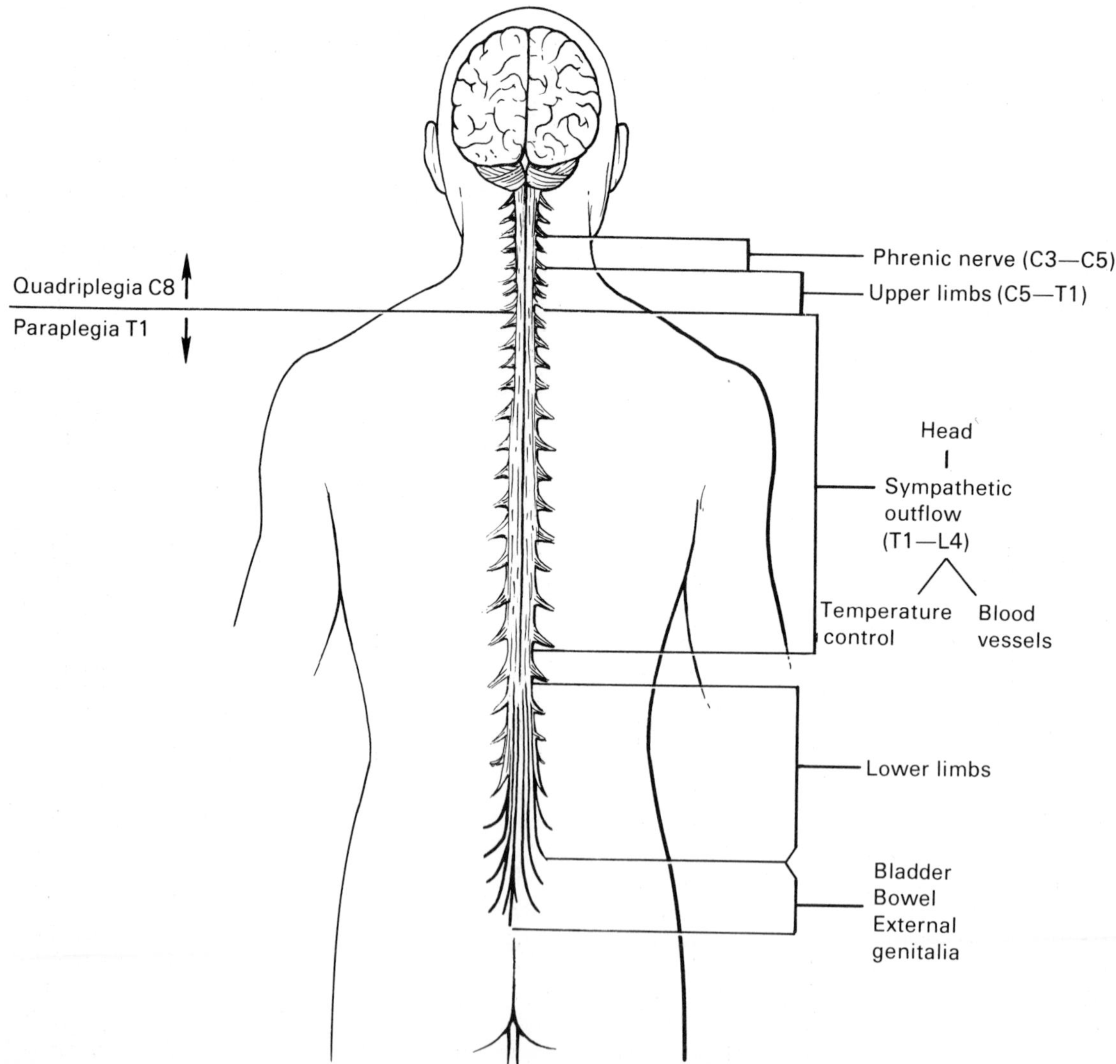

Figure 53-3 Symptoms, degree of paralysis, and potential for rehabilitation depend on the level of the lesion.

Table 53-3

Functional Level of Spinal Cord Disruption with Rehabilitation Potential

Cord Segment	Autonomic	Movement Remaining	Rehabilitation Potential
		Quadriplegia	
C1–C3	Usually fatal. Vagus domination of heart, respiration, blood vessels, all organs below	Neck and above. Innervation to diaphragm lost, no independent respiratory function.	Drive electric wheelchair equipped with portable respirator by using chin control or mouth stick. No bowel or bladder control.
C4	Vagal domination of heart, respirations, and all vessels and organs below.	Sensation and movement above neck.	Drive electric wheelchair by using chin control or mouth stick. No bowel or bladder control.
C5	Vagus domination as C4	Full neck, partial shoulder, back, biceps. Gross elbow-cannot roll over or use hands. Decreased respiratory reserve.	Drive electric wheelchair with mobile hand supports. Some can utilize powered hand splints. No bowel or bladder control.
C6	Vagus domination as C4	Shoulder and upper back—abduction and rotation at shoulder, full biceps-elbow flexion. Wrist extension. Thumb—weak grasp. Decreased respiratory reserve.	Assist with transfer and some self-care. Feed self with hand devices. Push wheelchair on smooth, flat surface. No bowel or bladder control.
C7–C8	Vagus domination as C4	All triceps-elbow extension. Finger extensors and flexors. Good grasp though still decreased strength. Can roll over and sit up in bed. Decreased respiratory reserve.	Transfer self to wheelchair, push self on most surfaces, most self-care. Wheelchair-independent. Some can drive car with powered hand controls. No bowel or bladder control.
		Paraplegia	
T1–T6	Sympathetic innervation to heart, vagus domination of rest	Full innervation of upper extremities and back plus essential intrinsic muscles of hand. Full strength and dexterity of grasp. Decreased trunk stability and decreased respiratory reserve.	Fully independent in self-care and in wheelchair. Most can drive car with hand controls. Full body brace for exercise but not for functional ambulation. No bladder or bowel control.
T6–T12	Vagus domination only of leg vessels, GI-GU organs	Full, stable thoracic muscles and upper back. Intercostals functional so increased respiratory reserve.	Wheelchair-independent. Can stand erect with full body brace; can ambulate on crutches, with swing-through gait difficult. Cannot climb stairs. No bladder or bowel control.
L1–L2	Vagus domination of leg vessels as above	Varying control of legs and pelvis. Low back instability.	Good sitting balance. Full use of wheelchair.
L3–L4	Partial domination of leg vessels and organs as T6	Quadriceps and hip flexors, no hamstrings. Flail ankles.	Completely independent ambulation with short leg braces and canes. Cannot stand for long periods. Bladder and bowel continence.

client is at risk for respiratory arrest due to loss of innervation of the phrenic nerve, which is formed by spinal nerves C1 to C4. At this level, autonomic control is mainly parasympathetic, with vagal domination of the heart, respirations, and all vessels and organs below. This results in bradycardia, mild bronchial constriction, nasal stuffiness, vasodilatation with subsequent postural hypotension, venous pooling and reduced blood volume to vital organs, and absent perspiration or piloerection, leading to decreased ability to control body temperature. Gastrointestinal function is normal once the period of acute systemic stress is over. Urine and feces are retained. The eyes maintain their normal sympathetic intervention, and some fibers are still functional to the nose and heart. All reflexes are initially absent but may later become hyperactive and unresponsive to normal stimuli.

At C5, shoulder, trapezius, and gross elbow and partial bicep flexion movement are present. Respiratory function is the same as at C4, since intercostal control does not occur until about T6 and abdominal control at T12. Vagus domination of the heart, respiration, and blood vessels continues. Perspiration and piloerection parallel motor and sensory levels. An elbow reflex can be elicited.

Injuries at C6 represent a substantial gain, as the biceps, thumb, and high upper back are now functional and the triceps are partially functional. Shoulder strength is increased, allowing for gross arm movements and grasp with the opposite thumb, but fine control is absent. Respiratory reserve is still decreased.

At the C7 to C8 level, triceps, biceps, and fingers are innervated but strength is still diminished. The upper one-third of the chest and back is innervated. There is no change in vital capacity, and vagal dominance persists. Reflexes are now noted in the arms and upper chest.

Thoracic

The manifestations of T1 injury are similar to C7 to C8 injury except that full innervation and strength are present in all upper extremities. Respiratory function is still the same as at C4, and the trunk has decreased stability. Vagus domination still persists in the respiratory system and lower extremity vessels, but the heart is no longer subject to strictly vagal control. Lower thoracic injuries show stability of thoracic muscles and improvement in respiratory function to about three-fourths of normal because of the action of the intercostal muscles. The vagus nerve now dominates the leg vessels and gastrointestinal and genitourinary systems. Bronchial constriction and nasal stuffiness are no longer a problem.

Lumbar

The L1 level demonstrates full abdominal muscle and sensory innervation, so respiratory vital capacity is normal. Some low back instability is present. Paralysis and sensory loss extend downward from the flank area in back and the pubis in front. The vagus nerve dominates leg vessels, small intestine, rectum, bladder, and genitalia. Abdominal reflexes are present.

At L4 to L5, quadriceps muscles and hip flexors are functional, but the hamstrings, gluteus maximus, ankles, and soles of the feet are paralyzed. In general, the anterior leg is functional but the posterior aspect and buttocks are not. Leg vessels, bladder, rectum, and genitalia now have sympathetic control even though sensation is not present. The knee reflexes are present.

Sacral lesions are rare, but when they occur at S3, only the genitalia and rectum are affected. However, vagal control is lost, resulting in sympathetic dominance and incontinence.

The types of accident causing spinal cord trauma can also result in head injury. The client should therefore be assessed for signs of concussion and increased intracranial pressure (see Chap. 54). In addition, he should be carefully assessed for musculoskeletal injuries and trauma to internal organs. Since there are no muscle, bone, or visceral sensations, the only clue to internal trauma with hemorrhage may be a rapidly falling hematocrit.

Medical Management

Medical

The initial medical goals for the client with a spinal cord injury are to sustain life and prevent further cord damage. Systemic and spinal cord shock must be treated. If the injury is at the cervical level, all body systems must be maintained for the client until the full extent of the damage can be evaluated. Treatment of a spinal cord injury may be medical or surgical. Table 53-4 describes the medical management for the client with a cervical injury. The systemic support required by the client is less intense for thoracic and lumbar injuries. Respiratory care is not as intense, and bradycardia is not a problem. Specific problems that arise are treated symptomatically.

Surgical

The decision to perform surgery on a client with a spinal cord injury often depends on the preference of a particular clinician. The aim of surgery is stabilization of the spinal column. In general, the following are accepted criteria for the scheduling of early surgery:[16]

1. Evidence of cord compression
2. Progressive neurological deficit
3. Compound fracture of the vertebra (bony fragments may dislodge and penetrate the cord)
4. Penetrating wounds of the spinal cord or surrounding structures
5. A bone fragment in the spinal canal

The more common surgical procedures include decompression laminectomy by anterior cervical and thoracic approaches with fusion, posterior laminectomy with use of acrylic wire mesh and fusion, and insertion of Harrington rods with correction and stabili-

Table 53-4
Medical Management: Cervical Cord Injury

Diagnostic
1. Complete neurological examination
2. Arterial blood gases
3. Electrolytes, glucose, hemoglobin, and hematrocrit
4. Anteroposterior and lateral spine x-rays
5. Urinalysis

Therapeutic
1. Immobilization of vertebral column b y skeletal traction
2. Maintenance of heart rate (e.g., atropine) and blood pressure (e.g., dopamine)
3. Corticosteroid therapy to reduce edema
4. Insertion of nasogastric tube with regular administration of antacids
5. Intubation if indicated by arterial blood gases
6. Oxygen per high-humidity mask
7. Foley catheter to gravity drainage
8. IV fluids with moderate fluid restriction first 72h

zation of thoracic deformities. Specific surgical and nursing interventions for these techniques are discussed in Chap. 56.

Experimental

The management of spinal cord injury has changed dramatically within recent years. Although many of the methods used are still experimental, the prognosis for the client with indirect trauma appears brighter. Methods presently being tested include:

1. *Myelotomy*—The cord is opened and blood, edema, and metabolites are drained.
2. *Norepinephrine counteractants*—Counteract the effects of norepinephrine when injected within 15 minutes of injury. Effective only at toxic levels. Include alpha methyltyrosine (AMT) (prevents hemorrhagic necrosis), reserpine (depletes catecholamines in peripheral nerves and central nervous system), levodopa (competes with norepinephrine for nerve cell receptor sites), and steroids (maintain vascular integrity and protect cellular membranes during decreased perfusion; reduce edema).
3. *Aminocaproic acid (Amicar)*—Antifibrinolytic that inhibits bleeding by clot stabilization (decreases fibrinolytic activity).
4. *Hypothermia*—Perfusion of cord with 4°C normal saline. Slows neural enzymatic processes; reduces cellular metabolic rates and oxygen requirements.
5. *Hyperbaric oxygen*—While in a hyperbaric chamber, the client breathes pure oxygen under increased atmospheric pressure. This results in increased oxygen to tissues and facilitates penetration of oxygen into hypoxic areas.

Pharmacologic Interventions

A variety of drugs are useful in the treatment of the client with a spinal cord injury, including nonnarcotic analgesics, parasympatholytics, anticholinergics, sympathomimetics, and corticosteroids. Specifics of these drugs are discussed under the appropriate system elsewhere in this text.

Because the pharmacology of drug metabolism is altered in spinal cord injury, an awareness of possible drug interactions is important. For instance, besides its analgesic effect, propoxyphene (Darvon) is believed to enhance vasodilatation and possibly aggravate orthostatic hypotension. These actions could enhance these problems in the neurologically disabled client. Drug-induced sedation could also mask a decreasing level of consciousness.

Pharmacologic agents are used to treat specific autonomic dysfunctions such as gastrointestinal hyperactivity, bleeding, bradycardia, orthostatic hypotension, inadequate bladder emptying, and autonomic dysreflexia. The nurse must be an astute observer of the response to these drugs, provide specific interventions if untoward reactions are noted, and work closely with the pharmacologist in planning for future care.[17]

Nursing Management

Health promotion and maintenance

Nursing interventions related to health promotion and maintenance include identification of the risk population, counseling, and education. Professional risk takers are less likely to have such accidents, but identification of the "accident-prone" person can enable the nurse to counsel him in terms of thinking before he acts, finding alternative means for proving himself, reducing stress, and not undertaking physical activities when using alcoholic beverages. In addition, the nurse can reinforce and participate in community education programs emphasizing the use of seat belts, child car seats, and helmets and not driving when drinking. A coordinated community program for the training of emergency personnel is essential.

Acute intervention for the cervical injury

Interventions are discussed for the high cervical injury due to flexion-rotation which is the most complex spinal cord injury (Table 53-5). This care can be modified for those with less severe problems.

Emergency Room Care After stabilization at the accident scene, the victim is transferred to a medical facility (see Chap. 58). A thorough assessment is

Table 53-5

Nursing Care Plan for the Client with Quadriplegia

Client Problem	Expected Outcome	Nursing Intervention
Respiratory dysfunction	ABG WNL. Lungs clear. No respiratory distress. No respiratory infection	Assess respiratory parameters every 2 h early, later every 4–8 h. Give O_2 per Maximyst-mask or nasal prongs until ABG stable. Suction prn. Use incentive spirometry, "blow bottles," IPPB every 4 h. Assist coughing by pushing up on abdominal muscles. Administer bronchial dilators and nasal decongestants prn. Use tracheostomy and artificial ventilation if necessary. Culture sputum if indicated. Administer antibiotics if indicated.
Cardiovascular instability	Heart rate >50. Blood pressure >80/50. No fainting, arrhythmias, thrombophlebitis, or pulmonary emboli	Monitor vital signs every 2 h early, later every 4–8 h. Monitor ECG until stable rhythm. Administer dopamine or other adrenergic if BP <80, atropine or isoproterenol if <50. Apply antiembolic hose or elastic bandages to legs thigh-high; remove every 4 h for skin care. Use care with postural changes. Perform ROM–heel-cord stretch exercises every 2–4 h. Assess for signs of phlebitis daily. Give heparin 5000 U every 12 h if ordered.
Systemic stress reaction: catabolism, edema, GI shutdown	Weight loss <4.5kg (10 lb). Minimal negative nitrogen balance. No gastric distension with eventual return of GI function. Minimal edema	Keep NPO. Give IV fluids: 2000 mL D5/0.25 NaCl every 24 h for 72 h—if not able to take oral, then TPN 2000–3000 mL with vitamins every 24 h. Test urine for glucose every 4 h if on TPN. Use nasogastric (sump) tube to suction until return of bowel sounds. Administer diuretics and corticosteroids as ordered. Monitor and record intake and output. Weigh daily.
Unstable vertebral fracture	No increase in neurological deficit	Keep skull tongs-halo traction at ordered amount of traction. Do not allow head or neck to be in position of fracture (e.g., no flexion with a flexion fracture). Turn side to side "in one piece" with several nurses. Turn on frame-circular electric bed with safe procedure, using several nurses.
Immobility	No decubiti, renal calculi, or contractures. Good respiratory function	Turn every 2–4 h when stable. Massage skin every 1–2 h; keep bed free of debris. Use alternating-pressure mattress. Keep pressure on feet—use tilt table. Perform passive-active ROM every 2–4 h. Inspect areas of pressure regularly.
Pain: Headache, neck, muscle spasms	Pain relieved. Adequate rest	Assess type, location, and degree of pain. Change position as appropriate. Medicate with mild analgesics prn. Medicate with muscle relaxants prn. Provide diversion, therapeutic touch.
Potential infection: bladder, respiratory, tong sites, decubiti	No signs of systemic or location infection. Ability to identify site(s) of infection	Assess temperature every 4 h. Check secretions and drainage for color, odor, and consistency. Send specimens of any suspicious drainage or secretions to lab for culture and sensitivity tests. Use aseptic catheter care. Give good pulmonary hygiene. Wash tong sites with antiseptic solution; apply antibiotic ointment and dress daily. Prevent decubiti (see Immobility, above); initiate vigorous treatment if it occurs. Encourage fluids, keep urine acid with acid ash juices and/or ascorbic acid. Teach client signs and symptoms of infection. Administer antibiotics as ordered.
Loss of bladder control	Ability to maintain bladder function. No kidney or bladder infection	Use of Foley catheter or intermittent catheterization. Teach client clean catheter technique if able to do. Teach client care of other types of catheters. Force fluids 3–4 L/day. Give acid ash juices such as cranberry or grape. Keep catheter patent. Administer ascorbic acid and urinary antiseptic (Mandelamine) if ordered. Check pH of urine and serum calcium daily.
Loss of bowel control	Ability to establish a regular evacuation pattern. No constipation	Include adequate roughage in diet. Provide adequate fluid intake. Administer stool softeners. Institute digital stimulation or use of suppositories q 2 days at same time each day. Teach client bowel regimen if able to carry out this function.
Loss of temperature control	Temperature >36–38°C (96.8–100.4°F)	Check temperature every 4 h. Keep room at 21.1°C(70°F). Avoid excess covering or excessive exposure, especially at bathing. Use hypothermia blanket if temperature >40°C (104°F).

Table 53-5 (Continued)

Client Problem	Expected Outcome	Nursing Intervention
Potential for stress ulcers	No stress ulcer	Give antacids via nasogastric tube or per os. Give corticosteroids with food. Guaiac stool test and gastric drainage. Check hematocrit regularly. Manage predisposing factors-reduce physical and psychological stress.
Increased need for fluid and nutrition	No kidney-bladder complications. Weight loss <4.5kg (10 lb). Ability to select a variety of high protein, high-CHO, high calorie foods in planning meals	Force fluids to 3–4 L/day. Encourage high protein, high-CHO, high calorie meals with high bulk. Give between-meal snacks. Incorporate client's personal and cultural preferences in meal planning. Teach client to select appropriate foods. Encourage family to bring in favorite foods. Provide pleasant environment, allow plenty of time for eating. Let client feed self as able. Keep calorie count; weigh twice a week. Give vitamin-mineral supplements.
Autonomic dysreflexia (hyperreflexia)	No serious sequelae if autonomic dysreflexia occurs	Teach client about reflex activity. Reduce incidence by keeping client adequately warm and decreasing cutaneous stimulation. Relieve discomfort of muscle spasms by warm baths or whirlpool. Administer muscle relaxants and antispasmodics prn. Assess for autonomic dysreflexia. If it occurs, elevate head of bed and eliminate stimulation. Administer hexamethonium or phentolamine prn.
Grieving: denial, anger, depression	Orderly progression through stages of grieving	Assess level of grieving state. Support client through level. Encourage verbalization of feelings and concerns. Involve in self-care activities—give control over environment. Treat client as an adult. Do not react to anger or manipulation. Negotiate care plan with client but insist care be done. Involve family in care—encourage them to promote independence in client. Be alert to clues regarding suicidal thoughts. Develop rapport through primary nurse relationship. Avoid sympathy and overidentification.
Disruption of developmental tasks	Ability to meet developmental tasks as fully as able with minimal delay	Provide sexual and family counseling. Teach about potential for sexuality and children. Provide books, teachers, other educational resources for expanding mind. Discuss potential abilities with available rehabilitation resources. Discuss vocational rehabilitation. Encourage sense of humor. Put with clients with similar problems.

done to specifically evaluate the degree of deficit and to establish the level and degree of injury. A history is obtained with emphasis on how the accident occurred and the degree of disruption as perceived by the client immediately after the accident. The assessment is carried out in the following order:[18]

1. Ask the client to move his legs. If he cannot, then request him to move his hands.
2. Have him spread his fingers; check the strength.
3. Check the quality of his grasp.
4. Check wrist extension.
5. Evaluate the function of biceps and triceps.
6. Determine whether he can shrug his shoulders and how well.
7. Make a complete sensory examination, including touch, pain, position, two-point discrimination, and vibration, starting with the toes and moving upward. A dermatome chart will help with localization.
8. Check deep tendon reflexes; these will be suppressed below the level of injury.
9. Carefully document all findings, using exact descriptions.

Respiratory, cardiac, and gastrointestinal functions should be monitored. The client will probably have x-rays to document the injury. It is critical that the client be handled carefully during the x-ray procedure to prevent further injury. The client then goes either to surgery or directly to an intensive care unit for monitoring and treatment.

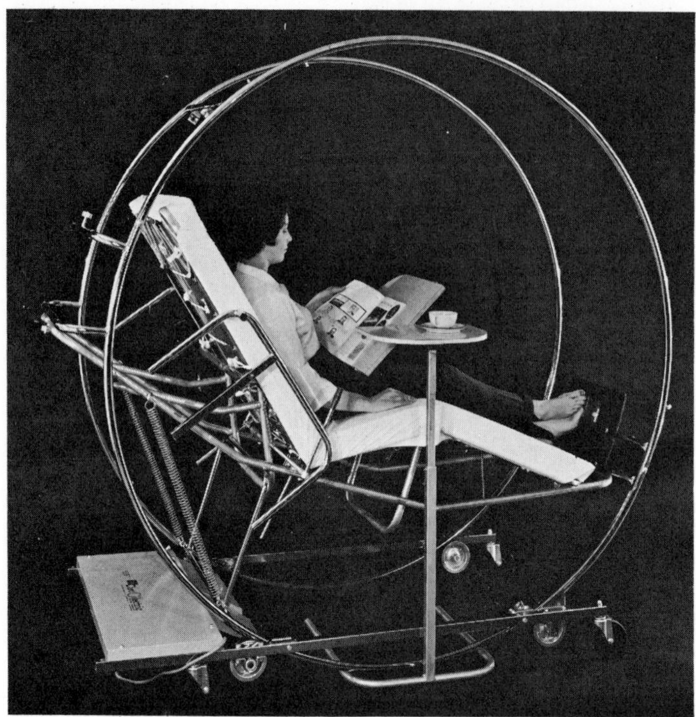

Figure 53-4 Stryker frame (*Orthopedic Frame Co., Kalamazoo, Mich.*)

Often some type of cervical tongs or a halo device will be applied in the emergency room to immobilize the cervical region. The client may be placed on a Stryker or Foster frame (Fig. 53-4) or a circular electric bed (Fig. 53-5) prior to beginning traction. If a regular hospital bed is used, it should have a firm mattress and a bed board. These measures may be delayed until admission to the ICU.

Respiratory Dysfunction During the first 48 hours after injury, edema may increase the level of dysfunction, and respiratory distress may occur. If the client is exhausted from labored breathing or if blood gases deteriorate, indicating inadequate oxygenation, endotracheal intubation or tracheostomy and mechanical ventilation should be initiated. Respiratory arrest is a possibility requiring careful monitoring and prompt action. All nurses who care for spinal-injured clients should be competent at cardiopulmonary resuscitation. Pneumonia and atelectasis are potential problems because of the loss of vital capacity, loss of intercostal and abdominal muscles leaving only diaphragmatic breathing, pooled secretions, and ineffectual coughing. Nasal stuffiness and bronchospasms also present problems.

The nurse should regularly assess (1) breath sounds; (2) arterial blood gases (ABG); (3) skin color; (4) breathing patterns, especially use of sternocleidomastoid (SCM) muscles or rapid shallow respirations; (5) client's subjective comments about ability to breathe; and (6) amount and color of sputum. A P_aO_2 above 60 mmHg and a P_aCO_2 below 45 mmHg are acceptable values in a client with uncomplicated quadraplegia.[19] It is especially important to note the effect of the prone position, since this can reduce vital capacity significantly and result in respiratory arrest. A client who is unable to count to ten without taking a breath needs immediate attention.

In addition to monitoring activities, the nurse can intervene in maintaining ventilation. Oxygen is administered until arterial blood gases stabilize. Chest physiotherapy and "quad coughing," a technique of placing the palm of the hand under the diaphragm and pushing down forcefully during exhalation, facilitate the raising of secretions. Tracheal suctioning should be carried out when indicated by auscultation of rales or rhonchi. Incentive spirometry, "blow bottles," and intermittent positive-pressure breathing (IPPB) are additional techniques to improve the client's respiratory status (see Chap. 21 for details). Other more vigorous methods of pulmonary toilet are not indicated until the client's condition is stable, because of the potential for increasing vagal stimulation, increasing intracranial pressure, or extending injury to vertebrae.

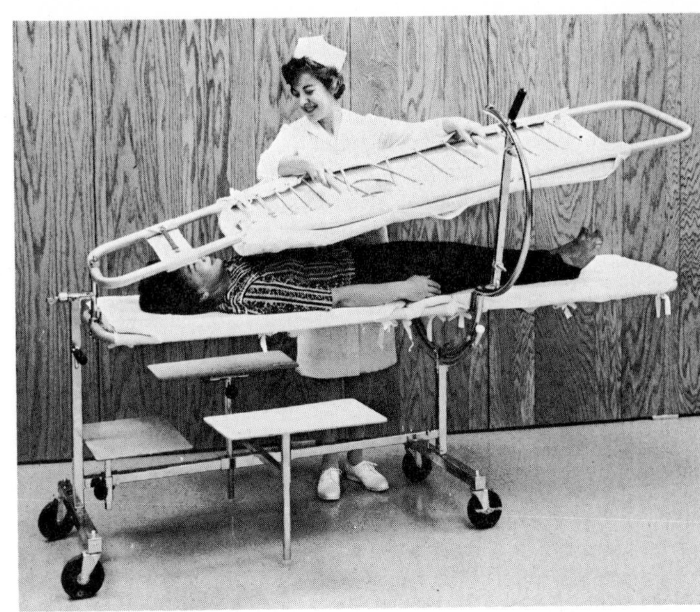

Figure 53-5 Circular electric bed. (*Orthopedic Frame Co., Kalamazoo, Mich.*)

Cardiovascular Instability Because of unopposed vagal response, the heart rate is slowed, often below 60. Any increase in vagal stimulation such as turning or suctioning can result in cardiac arrest. Loss of sympathetic tone in peripheral vessels results in chronic low blood pressure (BP) with potential postural hypotension. Lack of muscle tone to aid venous return can result in sluggish blood flow and predisposition to deep-vein thrombosis.

Vital signs need to be assessed frequently. If bradycardia is symptomatic, a medication such as atropine is administered. A temporary arterial pacemaker may be inserted in some instances. Hypotension is managed with a vasopressor agent such as dopamine.

If the client is on a circular electric bed, care must be exercised the first few times he is turned. Turning should be done slowly and the client observed closely. Vital signs should be monitored every 5 minutes. If the client faints, complete the turn until he is flat. The physician may order gradual elevation. The client will usually be anxious until he adjusts to the new sensations, but the nurse should heed complaints of vertigo, heart palpitations, or shortness of breath. Often Stryker frames which turn side-to-side are preferred, since there is less chance of alteration of vascular dynamics. The legs should be wrapped to the thighs with elastic bandages or antiembolic elastic stockings to prevent thromboemboli and promote venous return. These leg wraps need to be removed every 4 hours for skin care. An abdominal binder may also be beneficial. The nurse should also give range-of-motion exercises and heel-cord stretching regularly. The calves of the legs should be assessed every shift for signs of thrombophlebitis.

If blood loss has occurred from other injuries, the hemoglobin and hematocrit should be monitored and blood administered according to protocol. The nurse will need to monitor the client for indications of hypovolemic shock secondary to hemorrhage.

Fluid and Nutritional Maintenance During the first 48 to 72 hours the gastrointestinal tract may cease to function (paralytic ileus); a nasogastric tube must then be inserted. Because the client cannot have oral intake, fluid and electrolyte needs must be carefully monitored. Specific solutions and additives are ordered by the attending physician. Once bowel sounds are present or flatus is passed, oral food and fluids can gradually be introduced. If the client is unable to resume eating within 3 to 4 days, total parenteral nutrition (TPN) may be started to provide nutritional support (see Chap. 33).

Because of severe catabolism, a high protein, high calorie diet is necessary. Calcium may be limited if serum levels are high. Experts vary on the use of milk to balance the nitrogen depletion. Many fear the potential for renal calculi, and most agree that some restriction of milk is necessary beyond the intermediate stage of recovery.[20]

Increased roughage should be included to promote bowel function. Some clients experience anorexia, which can be due to psychological depression, boredom with institutional food, or discomfort at being fed (often by a hurried nurse). Some clients have a normally small appetite. Occasionally, not eating is used as a means of maintaining control over one's environment, since body control is diminished or absent. If the client is not eating adequately, a thorough assessment of the cause should be undertaken. On the basis of this assessment, a contract may be made with the client regarding diet, utilizing mutual goal setting. This gives the client increased control of the situation and often results in improved nutritional intake. General measures such as providing a pleasant eating environment, allowing adequate time to eat (including any self-feeding the client can achieve), encouraging the family to bring in special foods, and planning social rewards for eating may be useful. A calorie count should be kept and the client's weekly weight recorded as a means for evaluating progress. If feasible, the client should participate in recording caloric intake. In particular, the nurse should avoid allowing the client's nutritional intake to become the basis for a power struggle.

After the risk of edema has subsided, fluid intake should be encouraged up to 3 to 4 L daily. This assists the bowel to function and helps to prevent urinary tract infection and renal calculi.

Immobilization of Fracture Proper immobilization of the neck involves the maintenance of a neutral or extension position, never flexion. The body should always be correctly aligned, and turning should be done "in one piece." For cervical injuries, skeletal traction is usually provided through the use of devices like Crutchfield or skull tongs (Fig. 53-6). These are inserted through parietal burr holes, and the insertion sites are covered with sterile dressings. Traction is provided from a rope extended from the center of the tongs over a pulley with weights attached at the end. Traction must be maintained at all times. Skull tongs present the problems of easy displacement of the skull screws and site infection. If displacement should occur, hold the head in a neutral or extended position and call for help. Sandbags can be applied to stabilize the head and the physician called to reinsert the tongs (see Chap. 56 regarding principles of traction).

Two frames are in common use for the long-term management of the spinal-cord-injured client, the circular electric bed and the Stryker frame. The Stryker frame employs a side-to-side, lateral turn, whereas the circular electric bed turns on an arc of a circle. Some question the therapeutic benefit of the circular electric bed because of increased spinal compression, as from axial loading in the vertical position.[21] (See Table 53-6 for summary of principles in management of these frames.)

A physician should be readily available the first time the client is turned. Continue the turn even if the client faints. Some clients never adjust to the use of a turning frame, and other techniques will need to be planned.

Infection at the tong insertion sites is another potential problem. Preventive care includes (1) dressing the sites daily after cleansing the area with an

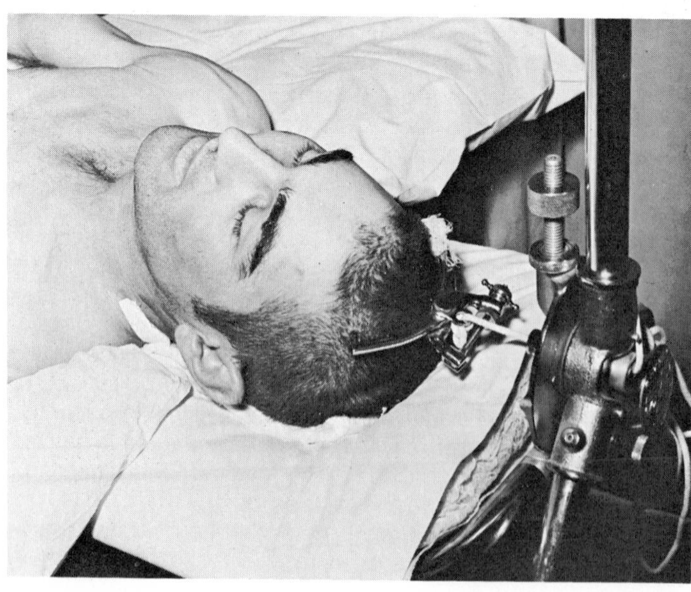

Figure 53-6 Cervical traction is attached to tongs inserted in the skull. (*Orthopedic Frame Co., Kalamazoo, Mich.*)

Table 53-6

General Guidelines for Use of Turning Frames

(For specific guidelines refer to operating manuals or hospital procedure manual.)

1. Explain to client and family the purpose of the turning frame.
2. Properly secure all equipment, IV tubing, catheters, respirator tubing.
3. Periodically check for intactness of mattress, lacing tautness, etc.
4. Maintain alignment with full complement of equipment, rest wings, etc.
5. Place prone for meals, careful to note respiratory problems and provide for expectoration if necessary.
6. Maintain sensory stimulation when prone, provide reading materials, fluids, etc.
7. Place supine for bowel program. Use accessory equipment for increased visual stimuli, prism glasses, mirrors, etc.
8. Maintain traction with special caution during turning.
9. Although this equipment was designed for reduced need for personnel, always have an assistant.

antiseptic solution such as povidone-iodine (Betadine) and (2) applying an antibiotic ointment which will act as a mechanical barrier to the entrance of bacteria.

After 2 to 4 weeks, the tongs and traction are removed and a neck collar or halo traction is applied to allow the client more activity and rehabilitation efforts. Since the head has been shaved, the client may find that a wig or colorful surgical cap will enhance his self-image.

Pain from muscle spasms in the neck or from injury can be quite troublesome during traction. Mild analgesics such as propoxyphene (Darvon) or codeine are helpful.

Immobilization of the neck of the spinal-cord-injured client will prevent further injury but creates a problem in that the effects of immobility for this client are profound. Unlike the nonparalyzed immobilized client, the lack of any movement increases catabolism greatly, and other problems of immobility are accentuated. The paralysis and psychological stress cause a lifelong problem related to nitrogen balance. Meticulous skin care is critical, since decreased sensation and circulation make the client particularly susceptible to skin breakdown. Tilt-table activities should be started as soon as possible to retard problems related to immobility.[22]

Bowel and Bladder Management Urine is retained because of the loss of autonomic and reflex control of the bladder and sphincter. Since there is also no sensation of fullness, overdistension of the bladder can result in reflux into the kidney, with eventual kidney failure or even rupture of the bladder. Consequently an indwelling catheter is usually inserted as soon as possible after injury. Its patency must be ensured by irrigation and frequent inspection. In some institutions a physician's order is required for this procedure. Strict aseptic technique for catheter care is essential to avoid introducing infection. After the client is stabilized, the best means of managing long-term urinary functions will be assessed.

Urinary tract infections are a common problem. To combat these infections a large fluid intake and the liberal use of juices such as cranberry, grape, and apple should be planned. These juices leave an acid ash in the urine which discourages bacterial growth. Citrus juices should be used sparingly. Sometimes ascorbic acid and a urinary antiseptic such as methenamine mandelate (Mandelamine) are given. The pH of the urine should be tested daily to evaluate acidity. If the appearance or odor of the urine is suspicious, a specimen should be sent for culture.

During spinal cord shock there is no voluntary or involuntary evacuation of the bowels. Soapsuds or saline edemas are given every 3 days until reflex control can be attained. Bowel training or controlled evacuation is instituted as soon as the client is started on a full diet regimen.

Loss of Temperature Control Since there is no vasoconstriction, piloerection, or heat loss through perspiration below the level of injury, temperature control is largely external to the client. Therefore the nurse needs to monitor the environment closely to maintain an appropriate temperature. Body temperature should be monitored on a regular basis. Overloading the client with covers or unduly exposing him, as when bathing, should be avoided. If the client develops an infection, more extensive means of temperature control such as a cooling blanket may be necessary.

Stress Ulcers Ulcers are a problem to the cord-inured client because of the physiological response to severe trauma and psychological stress. Peak incidence is between day 6 and day 14 after injury.[23] Shoulder pain may be an indication of referred pain from an ulcer and should be investigated. Stool and gastric content should be tested daily for blood and the hematocrit observed for a slow drop. If steroids are given, they should be accompanied by antacids and/or food. Such drugs as cimetidine (Tagamet) and propantheline bromide (Pro-Banthine) may be given prophylactically to decrease the secretion of HCl.

Sensory Deprivation The nurse must compensate for the client's absent sensation to prevent sensory deprivation. This is done by stimulating the senses that are intact as much as possible. Such measures as touching the client above the level of injury, conversation, music, strong aromas, and interesting flavors should be a part of the nursing care plan. Prism glasses should be provided so the client can read and watch television. Every effort should be made to prevent him from withdrawing from the environment.

Rehabilitation and chronic care

Grief For the person with a spinal cord injury, awareness of the extent of injury is coupled with a sense of overwhelming loss. No longer in control, he is dependent on others not only for all activities of daily living but for his very life. The client may feel useless and a burden on his family. At a stage when independence is often of the greatest importance developmentally, he is totally dependent.

This client's response and recovery differ in some important aspects from those experiencing loss from amputation or terminal illness. First, regression can and does occur at different stages. The usual 2-year limit for healthy adjustment to loss cannot be applied to the spinal-cord-injured client. Working through grief is a difficult, lifelong process with which the client will need support and encouragement. With recent advances in rehabilitation, it is not unusual for the client to be independent physically and discharged from the rehabilitation center prior to accomplishment of his grief work. Another phenomenon involves that of triggering experiences—new experiences such as marriage that recall earlier unresolved difficulties. Depending on the success of previous grief work, the new demand for grief work may be shortened or prolonged.

The goal of recovery is perhaps best described in terms of adjustment rather than acceptance. Adjustment implies the ability to go on with living given certain limitations. Some severely disabled persons find a more meaningful life after their injury than they experienced prior to the injury.

Although the cooperative, accepting client is easier to treat, the nurse should expect a wide fluctuation of emotions from the client with a spinal cord injury. Often it is the nursing staff which has difficulty accepting the client's limitation.[24] Depression itself may not be a component of the recovery process. Societal norms allow depression after severe loss and almost impose it on those confronted with death or radical life style change. However, this client may not experience depression. Staff must learn not to impose their need to feel sorry for the client and expect the client to respond appropriately.[25]

The nurse's role in grief work is to allow mourning to take place as a component of the rehabilitation process. Table 53-7 summarizes the mourning process and appropriate nursing interventions. During shock and denial stages the nurse should be reassur-

Table 53-7
Mourning Process and Nursing Interventions in Spinal Cord Injury

Stage	Client Behaviors	Nursing Action
Shock and denial	Actual struggle for survival; complete dependence; excessive sleep; withdrawal; fantasies; unrealistic expectations	Use meticulous nursing care. Be honest. Use simple diagrams to explain injury. Encourage client to begin the long road to recovery.
Anger	Refusal to discuss paralysis; decreased self-esteem; manipulation; hostile and abusive language	Place in room with another SCI client further along in the rehabilitation process; encourage self-care. Coordinate care with the client. Support the family; prevent alleviation of guilt by supporting dependency. Use humor liberally. Allow outbursts. Do not allow fixation at this stage.
Depression	Sadness; pessimism; anorexia; nightmares; insomnia; agitation; psychomotor retardation; "blues"; suicidal preoccupation; refusal to participate in any self-care activities.	Encourage family involvement and resources. Plan graded steps in rehabilitation to give success with minimal opportunity for frustration. Give cheerful and willing assistance with ADL. Avoid sympathy. Use firm kindness.
Adjustment	Planning for the future; active participation in therapy; may find personal meaning in the experience and continue to grow; return to premorbid personality	Remember SCI clients are not homogeneous in their personalities and must be considered as individuals. Balance support systems to encourage independence. Set goals with client input. Emphasize potentials as achieved by others. Avoid use of clichés.

ing and stress the expertise of the entire health care team. During the stage of anger, the client should be assisted to achieve control over his environment, particularly by being allowed input into his plan of care. The nurse should not respond to anger or manipulation or become involved with a power struggle with the client. As self-care abilities increase, so will independence.

The client's family will also need counseling to avoid promoting dependency in the client through guilt or misplaced sympathy. During the stage of depression, the nurst must keep her own sense of humor and be patient and persistent. Sympathy is not helpful. She should treat the client in an adult manner and involve him in decision making about care but insist that the care be done. A primary nurse relationship is helpful, but the nurse herself will need some relief from the intense stress of continual interaction with this client. Staff planning and rap sessions are helpful in providing consistency of care and in allowing staff to safely vent their feelings and frustrations. To achieve the stage of adjustment the client will need continual support throughout the rehabilitation in the form of acceptance, affection, and caring. The nurse must allow time to be attentive when the client needs to talk and must be sensitive to needs at the various stages of the grief process.

Reflexes Once spinal cord shock is resolved (approximately 4 weeks), the return of reflexes may complicate rehabilitation. Lacking control from the higher brain centers, reflexes are inappropriate and often excessive. Erections can occur from a variety of stimuli, causing embarrassment and discomfort. Spasms ranging from mild twitches to convulsive movements below the level of the lesion may also occur. This reflex activity may be interpreted by the client or family as a return of function. The fact that it is not should be tactfully explained. The client may be informed of the positive use of these reflexes in sexual, bowel, and bladder retraining. Spasms may be relieved with warm baths, whirlpool treatments, antispasmodics, and muscle relaxants. Peak spasticity occurs after 2 years, and if it is severe, destruction of the reflexes (chordotomy) may be necessary. This compromises retraining and should be done as a last resort.

Autonomic Dysreflexia (Hyperreflexia) For 85 percent of all clients injured at T6 and higher, an excessive inhibited response to stimuli may occur following return of reflexes. This is called *autonomic dysreflexia* (AD). A full bladder, excessive skin stimulation, or digital stimulation may trigger a massive autonomic discharge resulting in severe hypertension (up to 300 mmHg systolic) and severe bradycardia (down to 30 to 40 beats/minute). The first sign is a complaint by the client of severe headache, accompanied by flushing, diaphoresis, and piloerection above the level of injury. Nasal stuffiness may also be present. Since the client could have a cerebral infarction, the nurse must take immediate action. She should immediately elevate the head of the bed to 45° and eliminate the cause of the stimulation. For instance, a plugged catheter may result in a full bladder. Irrigating the catheter and ensuring patency should eliminate the stimulation. If the symptoms persist for 1 to 2 minutes following removal of the stimulation, an alpha-adrenergic blocker such as phentolamine (Regitine) or an arteriolar vasodilator such as hydralazine (Apresoline) may be given. Lastly, a low spinal anesthetic to block stimulation may be lifesaving.[26] Careful neurological monitoring must continue until vital signs stabilize.

To prevent future episodes, instillation of tetracaine (Pontocaine Hydrochloride) for bladder excitability may be ordered. Gentle removal of an impaction followed with dibucaine (Nupercaine ointment) may prove beneficial. Clients and their families should be taught to be alert to symptoms of autonomic dysreflexia and to report immediately should they occur. For intractable episodes, severance of the nerves may be a last resort.

Sexuality Since the majority of spinal-cord-injured clients are males between 18 and 35, sexual rehabilitation is a major issue. For the nurse working with these clients, an awareness and acceptance of her own sexuality and knowledge of the human sexual response are essential. When discussing sexual potential the nurse should use scientific terminology rather than street language whenever possible. Knowledge of the level of the lesion is needed in order to understand the client's potential for orgasm, erection, and fertility and the capacity for sexual satisfaction for himself and his partner (Table 53-8). Spinal-cord-injured women lack sensation during intercourse regardless of the type of lesion.

Sexual rehabilitation should begin in an informal way once the acute phase of the injury has passed. Questions such as "Have you had an erection since your accident?" or "Have your menstrual periods continued since the accident?" are generally nonthreatening ways to introduce the topic of sexual functions; or the client may pose a question such as "Can I ever be a man again?"

Frank, open discussion with the client is essential. This important aspect of rehabilitation should be sen-

Table 53-8
Potential for Sexual Activity in the Cord-Injured Male

Type of Lesion	Erections	Ejaculation	Orgasm
Upper motor neuron:			
Complete	Frequent (93%), reflexogenic only	Rare	Absent
Incomplete	Most frequent (99%) Reflexogenic (80%) Reflexogenic and psychogenic (19%	Less frequent (32%) after reflexogenic erection (74%), after psychogenic erection (26%)	Present if ejaculation occurs
Lower motor neuron:			
Complete	Infrequent (26%)	Infrequent (18%)	Present if emission occurs
Incomplete	Psychogenic and reflexogenic	Frequent (70%) after psychogenic and reflexogenic erections	Present if ejaculation occurs

sitively handled by someone specially trained in sexual counseling. Unless the nurse has such training, she should not attempt to direct the plan for sexual counseling.

The properly trained nurse will work with both partners or provide support during new relationships, emphasizing open communication. The nurse's educational role requires respect for each couple's own standards of religious and cultural beliefs. Alternative methods of obtaining sexual satisfaction such as oral-genital sex (cunnilingus and fellatio) may be suggested. Explicit films, e.g., *Touching*, may also be used. This film demonstrates the sexual activities of a paraplegic client and his normal partner.[27] Graphics should be used cautiously, as they may be too limiting or focus too much on the mechanics of sex rather than the relationship.

Sexual activities may require more planning and be less spontaneous than previously. For instance, it may be necessary to have an attendant undress the client and remove equipment.

Care should be taken not to dislodge the Foley catheter during sexual activity. If a Texas catheter is used, it should be removed 1 hour before sexual activity and the client should refrain from fluids. The bowel program should include evacuation the morning of sexual activity. The partner should be informed that having an accident is always a possibility. Illustrations for teaching management of urinary equipment are available.[28] In the female a water-soluble lubricant may be needed to supplement inadequate vaginal secretions and facilitate vaginal penetration.

Menses may temporarily cease for as long as 6 months. If sexual activity is resumed, protection from an unplanned pregnancy is necessary. A normal pregnancy may be complicated by urinary tract infections, anemia, and autonomic dysreflexia. Since uterine contractions will not be felt, precipitate delivery is always a danger. In the male, fertility is reduced because of decreased number and motility of the sperm. For those desiring children, alternative methods include adoption, artificial insemination, and the newer techniques of electrostimulation.[29]

A relaxed, unhurried environment can do much to encourage sexual satisfaction. Wine, music, and perfume can help create such an atmosphere. Ample time for caressing, fondling, and kissing is essential. The partners should be encouraged to explore each other's erogenous areas such as the lips, neck, and ears, which can arouse them to psychogenic erection or orgasm. Demands from each other initially should be few.[30]

Neurogenic Bladder Once spinal cord shock and its resulting bladder atony are no longer a problem, the client is left with a neurogenic bladder. Spinal cord injury is only one cause of neurogenic bladder. A *neurogenic bladder* is any type of bladder dysfunction related to abnormal or absent bladder innervation. It may lead to a residual urine problem, stone disease, or infection and is often associated with progressive renal deterioration. It is frequently associated with urinary incontinence. Depending on the lesion, a neurogenic bladder may have no reflex detrusor contractions (areflexic, flaccid) or may have hyperactive reflex detrusor contractions (hyperreflexic, spastic). The common symptoms of a neurogenic bladder include urgency, frequency, incontinence, inability to void, and obstructive-type symptoms.

Neurogenic bladder can be classified according

to reflex detrusor activity, intravesical filling pressure, and continence function. Types of neurogenic bladder include:

1. *Uninhibited neurogenic bladder*—This lesion is due to a defect in the corticoregulatory tracts. The uninhibited neurogenic bladder behaves as though there were no inhibitions influencing the time and place of voiding. This is the bladder seen in the newborn child. It may occur after cerebrovascular accident and with multiple sclerosis, syphilis, brain trauma, and brain tumor. The usual symptoms are increased frequency, urgency, and incontinence.
2. *Reflex neurogenic bladder*—This behaves as part of the spinal reflex arc, with no connections to the brain. It is a lesion which affects both the sensory and motor tracts to and from the higher nerves above the conus medullaris and is occasionally seen in multiple sclerosis and pernicious anemia. Symptoms are reflex involuntary voiding.
3. *Autonomous neurogenic bladder*—This bladder behaves as if it were completely cut off from the brain and the spinal cord and thus autonomous. It is seen in spina bifida and myelomeningocele, also in cases of trauma or neoplasm involving the conus medullaris, cauda equina, or pelvic nerves. It is occasionally seen after exenterating types of radical pelvis surgery and occasionally with a herniated intervertebral disk. These clients cannot initiate micturition in a normal way, and they may be incontinent.
4. *Motor paralytic bladder*—This bladder acts as if there were paralysis of all motor function. It is seen in poliomyelitis and with herniated intervertebral disks. It is also seen with trauma or neoplasms involving sacral roots 2, 3, and 4 (parasympathetic fibers). Symptoms may be similar to those seen in a patient with outlet obstruction.
5. *Sensory paralytic bladder*—This bladder is seen in diabetes mellitus, tabes dorsalis, pernicious anemia, and multiple sclerosis. It acts as if there were paralysis of all sensory modalities. There are no particular symptoms except for poor bladder sensation, infrequent voiding, and large urine volume when the detrusor muscle ultimately decompensates.

The cord-injured client with a neurogenic bladder requires a comprehensive program to manage bladder function. Such a program should include:

1. *Diagnostic evaluation*—After the client's overall condition is stable and there is evidence of neurologic reflexes, a cystometrogram, an intravenous pyelogram, and a urine culture are taken.
2. *Pharmacologic*—Drugs to increase the strength of bladder contractions (detrusor), acidify the urine, and relax the urethral sphincter are utilized.
3. *Nutrition*—A low-calcium diet (1 g) to reduce the possibility of kidney and bladder stones is advocated.
4. *Fluids*—A fluid intake of 1500 to 2000 mL/day must be maintained to prevent stone formation and to ensure adequate urine flow.
5. *Urine drainage*—The method used for urinary drainage depends on the condition of the client as well as the preference of the physician, the nursing staff, and the policy of the institution. The four possible drainage systems include reflex training, indwelling catheter, intermittent catheterization, and urinary diversion surgery.

With the return of the reflex arc, bladder function may be reflex. However, since there is an interruption in the pathways to the brain, the client has no control over voiding. This results in a bladder with a small capacity, hyperirritable detrusor muscle and sphincter, and loss of inhibition of the reflex by the brain. The client or the nurse can use techniques such as the Credé and Valsalva maneuvers or a rectal stretch to facilitate complete emptying of the bladder. The Credé maneuver involves the exertion by the nurse or client of downward pressure over the bladder with a pumping motion. In the Valsalva maneuver, the client inhales deeply, holds the breath, and bears down. The rectal stretch is the insertion of a gloved finger into the rectum, gently pulling to exert pressure on the sphincter to cause a relaxation of the perineal floor. Combining the Valsalva maneuver with rectal stretch results in more complete emptying of the bladder. The client should be regularly assessed for residual urine following reflex bladder emptying. Residual urine should be maintained below 100 mL. Many drugs affect urinary retention and indicate reassessment for residual. The ultimate goal for this technique is for the client to be catheter-free.

The long-term use of an indwelling catheter should be carefully evaluated because of the associated high incidence of urinary tract infection, fistula formation, and diverticula. Adequate fluid intake and patency of the catheter should be ensured. The frequency of catheter changing ranges from 1 week to 1 month, depending on the type of catheter used and agency policy.[31]

Intermittent catheterization is an increasingly popular method of bladder management (see Chap. 37). Nursing assessment is important in selecting the time interval between catheterizations. Initially, catheterization is done every 4 hours. If less than 200 mL of urine is drained. the time interval may be extended. If 500 mL or more of urine is obtained, the time interval should be shortened. Clients often experience diuresis at a regular time during a 24-hour period, which may require an extra catheterization. The number of intermittent catheterizations per day is usually five or six.

Urinary diversion surgery may be necessary if the client has repeated urinary tract infections with renal involvement or repeated stones. (Table 37-18 compares types of urinary diversion surgery.)

Bowel Evacuation Bowel evacuation needs careful management in the cord-injured client, since voluntary control of this function may be lost. The usual measures for preventing constipation such as a high-fiber diet (Appendix B, Table 6) and adequate fluid intake are appropriate. In addition, suppositories or digital stimulation by the nurse or client may be necessary. Digital stimulation combined with the Valsalva maneuver and a regular schedule facilitate regularity.

Generally, a bowel movement every other day is considered adequate. However, preinjury patterns should be considered. Incontinence can result from too much stool softener or a fecal impaction. Careful recording of bowel movements, including amount, time, and consistency, are important to the overall success of the program.

Rehabilitation The physiological and psychological rehabilitation of the spinal-cord-injured person is very complex and involved. With quality physical and psychological care the spinal-cord-injured person will be able, through intensive and specialized rehabilitation, to function at his highest level of wellness. This phase is often carried out at special rehabilitation centers where clients must demonstrate adequate motivation for self-care in order to be admitted.

Many of the problems identified in the acute period become chronic and continue throughout life. Rehabilitation is concerned with refined retraining of physiological processes. Braces, electronic wheelchairs, and a variety of mechanical apparatuses are utilized to maximize what function the client has. Mobility has greatly increased for the high cervical spinal-cord-injured client with electronic diaphragmatic pacemakers and the Bantam respirator. While rehabilitation and the special equipment needed are very costly, many of these programs are state and federally funded.

If the client can be successfully brought through the acute period, his life can be fuller and richer than previously possible because of exciting advances and technical innovations. Some spinal-cord-injured clients find, like other persons who have been close to death, that their lives are richer and more meaningful than before their injury. For others, unfortunately, the future is not so positive. It cannot be stressed enough how important the pivotal role of the nurse is to the coordinated efforts of the whole health team to effect a positive outcome.

SPINAL CORD TUMORS

Tumors which affect the spinal cord account for only 0.5 to 1 percent of all neoplasms. These tumors are classified as primary (arising from some component of cord, dura, nerves, or vessels); secondary (due, to intraspinal extension of osteosarcomas of vertebrae or invasion of neck or to thoracic or abdominal tumors); and metastatic (from primary growths in the breast, thyroid, lung, kidney, and other sites). They are seen as extradural, intradural-extramedullary, and intradural-intramedullary (Fig. 53-7; Table 53-9). Neurofibromas, meningiomas, gliomas, and hemangiomas are the most frequently occurring neoplasms.

Since many of these tumors are slow-growing, their symptomology is related to mechanical effects of slow compression and irritation of nerve roots, displacement of the cord, and/or gradual obstruction of vascular supply. The slowness of growth does not cause autodestruction as in traumatic lesions; therefore as complete functional restoration is possible when the tumor is removed.

Clinical Manifestations

The most common early symptom of a spinal cord tumor is pain in the back with radiations simulating intercostal neuralgia, angina, or herpes zoster. The location of the pain is dependent on the level of compression and worsens with activity, coughing, straining, and lying down. Later, sensory disruption is manifested by coldness, numbness, and tingling in an extremity or extremities, slowly progressing upward until it reaches the level of the lesion. Impaired sensation of pain, temperature, and light touch precedes a deficit in vibration and position sense, which may go on to complete anesthesia. Motor weakness accompanies the sensory disturbances and consists of slowly increasing clumsiness, weakness, and spasticity. Sphincter disturbances are marked by urgency, with difficulty in starting to void and progressing to retention with overflow incontinence.

Extradural tumors are seen early on routine spinal

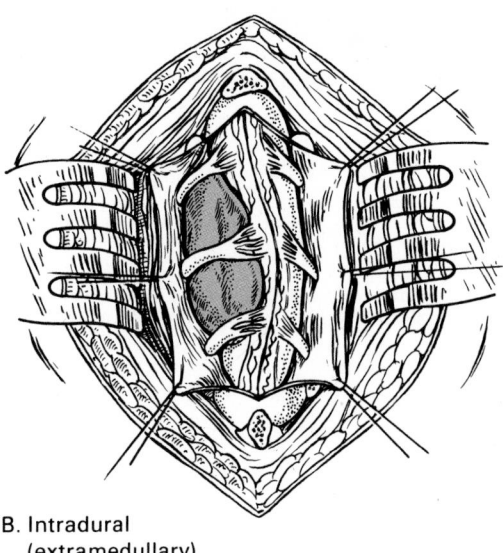

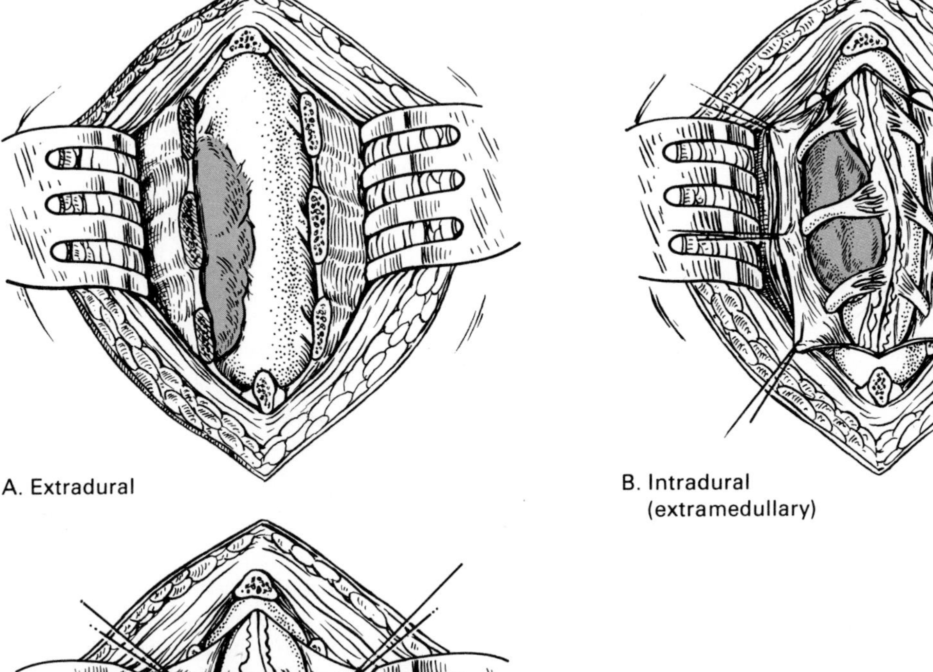

Figure 53-7 Types of spinal cord tumor.

x-rays, while intradural and intramedullary tumors require myelography for detection. Spinal fluid analysis may reveal tumor cells.

The cord is decompressed by removal of the tumor by a laminectomy (see Chap. 56). Over 85 percent of primary neoplasms are benign and can be completely resected, with 90 percent of the clients recovering without residual problems.

Management

Metastatic neoplasms frequently are manifested only by intense, intractable back pain as a symptom for months. The problem progresses to collapse of the vertebrae with immediate cord compression and dissolution. Early radiation and/or chemotherapy is sometimes effective. Laminectomy can effect pain relief. Narcotics such as morphine sulfate or meperidine (Demerol) are used as well as physical measures for pain relief. Psychological care is dependent on the prognosis. If the tumor is benign, adjustment to disability may not be necessary, depending on the degree of damage prior to surgery and the surgery itself. The focus should be on support of fear and anxiety in facing possible cancer, but with a generally optimistic note. The client with metastatic disease will need the special comfort and psychological care discussed in Chap. 2.[32]

Table 53-9
Classification of Spinal Cord Tumors

Type	Incidence	Treatment	Prognosis
Extradural (from bones of spine, in extradural space, or in paraspinal tissue)	20–50% of all intraspinal tumors; mostly malignant metastatic lesions	Relieve cord pressure by surgical laminectomy, radiation, chemotherapy, or a combination approach.	Poor
Intradural (within or under dura):			
Extramedullary (within dura mater, outside cord)	Most frequent—40% of intradural tumors; mostly benign meningiomas and neurofibromas	Complete surgical removal of most is possible; if not, partial removal followed by radiation.	Usually very good if cord not damaged by compression
Intramedullary (within cord)	Least frequent—5–10% of intradural tumors	Most cannot be completely removed surgically. Radiation therapy shows only some temporary improvement.	Very poor

MISCELLANEOUS NEUROLOGICAL DISORDERS (POLYNEUROPATHIES)

Guillain-Barré Syndrome

Problem identification

Guillain-Barré syndrome (Landry-Guillain-Barré-Strohl syndrome, infectious polyneuropathy, ascending polyneuropathic paralysis, radiculoneuropathy) is an inflammatory polyneuritis of unknown cause. It is considered to be an immunologic reaction directed primarily at the peripheral nerves, specifically the myelin sheath. This syndrome is frequently preceded by a mild upper respiratory or gastrointestinal infection or flu. While it may affect any age group, it is more commonly seen in adults (ages 20 to 50) of both sexes.[33] There has also been some recent evidence associating the occurrence of Guillain-Barré syndrome with swine flu immunization. During the mass screening against swine flu in 1976 there was an 8 to 10 times greater occurrence of this syndrome in those immunized. It is not known whether this was attributable to this specific vaccine or would have occurred with other vaccines as well.[34]

The process involves segmental demyelination of ventral and dorsal nerve roots in the spinal cord and medulla. The demyelination leads to inflammation, edema, and nerve root compression, which causes decreased nerve conduction and rapidly ascending paralysis which may be partial or complete. With meticulous supportive care, mortality can be held to 5 percent.

Clinical manifestations and complications

Typical clinical manifestations of Guillain-Barré syndrome include weakness, ataxia, and bilateral paresthesia of the lower extremities progressing to complete paralysis. This paralysis may involve the respiratory musculature. Further progression can produce bulbar signs (lower brainstem) such as difficulty with respiration, talking, and swallowing and cranial nerve involvement. The manifestations may progress rapidly (24 hours) or take up to 2 to 3 weeks to develop. Muscle atrophy is minimal. Recovery is usually spontaneous and may occur at any time, but a range of 6 to 18 months is not uncommon. If respiratory involvement occurs, rapid intervention is needed to prevent death. Some clients may have residual loss of function, but this can often be resolved by intensive physiotherapy.

Medical and nursing management

The diagnosis is made primarily on clinical signs. The cerebral fluid is normal except for elevated protein. Sedimentation rate and leukocyte count are usually normal. Nerve conduction velocity is reduced.

Medical management is aimed at supportive care. Corticosteroids are often used, and experimentation with use of measles vaccine is promising. The arterial blood-gas measurements must be carefully monitored to determine whether a tracheostomy and artificial ventilation are necessary.

There are many similarities between Guillain-Barré syndrome and spinal cord injury (Table 53-5). The main difference involves the assessments the nurse must make related to respiratory and cardiovascular status and cranial nerve function. A tracheostomy set and respirator should be immediately available. Special nursing interventions are needed if the client has a tracheostomy and is on a respirator (see Chap. 22).

It is important to assess the gag reflex before

each feeding to determine the client's ability to swallow. The nurse should stay with the client during eating and have suction equipment available. Thicker fluids are easier to swallow. Soft grains, fruits, and vegetables and pureed meats are often recommended.

Throughout the course of the illness, the nurse should provide support and encouragement to the family and client. Since residual problems are not common, the family can be assured that complete recovery can be anticipated.

Botulism

Botulism is the most serious type of food poisoning. It is caused by gastrointestinal absorption of the neurotoxin produced by *Clostridium botulinum*. This organism can grow in any food contaminated with the spores. Improper home canning of foods is often the cause. It is thought that the neurotoxin destroys or inhibits the neurotransmission of acetylcholine at the myoneural junction. The first symptoms are usually nausea, vomiting, and abdominal cramps, usually within 12 to 36 hours after consumption of the contaminated food. Neurological manifestations develop slowly (4 to 8 days) and include difficulty in convergence of the eyes, photophobia followed by ptosis and paralysis of extraocular muscles resulting in blurred vision, dry mouth, sore throat and difficulty in swallowing, ileus, mild muscle weakness, and respiratory symptoms which can rapidly deteriorate to arrest.

Medical management

The initial treatment of botulism is intravenous administration of botulinum antitoxin as soon as botulism is suspected. Prior to administering the antitoxin, possible sensitivity should be assessed by instilling a drop of antitoxin into one eye. A rapidly occurring conjunctivitis indicates sensitivity, in which case the antitoxin is not given.

The gastrointestinal tract is purged to decrease absorption of the toxin by the use of laxatives, high colonic enemas, and gastric lavage. Botulism is a reportable disease, so local, state, and federal health agencies, particularly the Communicable Disease Center in Atlanta, should be notified. Prophylactic penicillin may be ordered to halt the release of toxin in the gastrointestinal tract.

Nursing management

The nurse should educate the public to be alert to situations that could result in botulism. Particular attention should be given to foods which are of high pH—that is, low in acid, which destroys or prevents spore formation. These include fish, tuna, vichyssoise, and peppers. All varieties of spores are destroyed by boiling for 10 minutes or maintaining at a temperature of 80°C for 30 minutes. Specific suggestions related to the preparation, storage, and use of food include:[35]

1. In home canning, follow the equipment manufacturer's directions; use only fresh fruits and vegetables with questionable spots removed; cleanse all containers and utensils; make certain that the seal is airtight; store canned foods properly in a cool, dry place.
2. Never use a can with a swollen end; this could be caused by gases from *C. botulinum*.
3. When opening a container, if the food is forcefully expelled, discard it without tasting.
4. If, after opening a can, its contents look or smell bad, discard it without tasting.

Suspicious materials should have lye added to them and be stored for 24 hours prior to burying in order to destroy bacteria and toxins and prevent further contamination. Flushing down the toilet or in the garbage disposal are also appropriate if followed by large amounts of water.

Nursing care during the acute illness is similar to that for Guillain-Barré syndrome. Supportive nursing interventions include rest and activities to maintain respiratory function, adequate nutrition, and muscle mass.[36] Since the recovery process is slow, the client may develop problems related to a feeling of helplessness, boredom, and low morale.

Tetanus

Tetanus is an extremely severe polyradiculitis and polyneuritis affecting both peripheral and cranial nerves. It results from the effects of the neurotoxin released by the anaerobic bacillus *Clostridium tetani*. The spores of the bacillus are present in the soil, garden mold, and manure. They gain entry into the body through a traumatic or suppurative wound which provides an appropriate low-oxygen environment for spores to mature and produce toxin. Other causes include dental infection, heroin injections, human and animal bites, abortion, pregnancy, frostbite, compound fractures, and gunshot wounds. The incubation period is 2 days to 3 weeks, with symptoms frequently appearing after the original wound is healed.

Worldwide, 50,000 people die annually from tetanus, with an incidence of 300,000 to 500,000 reported cases.[37] Mortality varies according to age, with infants and those over 60 most seriously afflicted. Overall mortality ranges from 45 to 55 percent.

Clinical manifestations

The clinical manifestations of tetanus include a prickly sensation in the jaw muscles stimulating excessive yawning early in the disease. Within 24 hours the jaw muscles become tender and stiff (lockjaw). There is dysphagia and generalized tonic spasms. As the disease progresses, the neck muscles, back, and extremities become progressively rigid. In severe forms, continuous tonic convulsions may occur, with opisthotonus (extreme arching of the back and retraction of the head). Laryngeal and respiratory spasms cause apnea and anoxia. The slightest noise, jarring motion, or bright light can set off the convulsion. In the severe form, mortality is almost 100 percent. Residual damage such as vertebral fractures, muscular contraction, or brain damage due to hypoxia may remain.

Medical and nursing management

The medical management of tetanus includes administration of tetanus toxoid booster (Td) and tetanus immune globin human [TIG(H)] before the onset of symptoms to neutralize circulating toxin. Once neurological signs have appeared these injections are ineffective, since the neurotoxin is permanently fixed once it is attached to the neuromuscular end plate.

Serum electrolytes, CBC, albumin, clotting factors, glucose, and arterial blood gases are monitored. Cardiac function is monitored by ECG and auscultation. As larger numbers of nerve cells are attacked, their inhibitory control over muscle activity decreases and symptoms develop. Prompt control of spasms is essential and is managed by deep sedation, usually with diazepam, barbiturates, or chlorpromazine.

Usually a tracheostomy is performed early and the client maintained on artificial ventilation. If the above drugs do not control convulsions, skeletal-muscle-paralyzing drugs such as tubocurare are used. Pain is relieved by codeine or meperidine, often with the addition of promethazine. Antibiotics may be given to prevent secondary infections. Nutrition is maintained through intravenous or nasogastric feeding. Even with the best of care mortality is 50 percent, and those recovering have a long convalescence, including extensive physiotherapy.[38,39]

Nursing management

Health teaching should include immediate thorough cleansing of all wounds with soap and water. If an open wound occurs and the client has not been immunized within 10 years, the primary care provider should be contacted to give a tetanus booster. The military services have an outstanding record in that only a few cases of tetanus have occurred in the combined services since World War II. Treatment protocols are summarized in Table 53-10.

If equine tetanus antitoxin is to be used, the client should be tested for sensitivity. Experts do not recommend administration of equine antitoxin if sensitivity occurs; anaphylactic shock is more dangerous than the threat of tetanus, and desensitization is ineffective.[40] The side effects of routine administration are mild, such as a sore arm, swelling at the site, or itching. Serious side effects occur rarely. Routine administration of a booster shot to an adequately immunized client can cause extreme arm swelling, lymphadenopathy, or severe hypersensitivity.

All clients should receive a written record of immunizations and be encouraged to complete their active immunization schedule. To protect the client and care providers it is recommended that the client's immunization history be accurately recorded.

The acute nursing management of the client with tetanus is aimed at supportive care based on manifestations. The client should be placed in a quiet room insulated against noise and kept dark. Nursing care should be administered with the utmost caution to avoid triggering spasms. Nursing care related to

Table 53-10
Tetanus Prevention and Immunization Protocols

Client Was Actively Immunized in Past 10 Years	
Majority of wounds	Td* or 0.5 mL adsorbed tetanus toxoid *unless* client had a booster of completed initial immunization within past 5 years
Wounds that are severe (involve extensive injury), neglected, or old (more than 24 h)	Td* *unless* client had a booster within past year
Client Was Immunized More Than 10 Years Ago	
Majority of wounds	Td*
Wounds that are severe, neglected, or old	Td*; 250 or more units TIG(H)†
Client Was Never Immunized	
Clean, minor wound—possibility of tetanus unlikely	Td*; consider as first in series of basic immunizations
Majority of tetanus-prone wounds	Td*; 250 units TIG(H)†
Wounds that are severe, neglected, or old	Td*; 500 or more units TIG(H)†

*If there is any reason to suspect hypersensitivity to diptheria toxoid, substitute adsorbed tetanus toxoid.

†When administering Td or adsorbed tetanus toxoid and TIG(H) concurrently, use separate needles, syringes, and injection sites.

J. Cutting et al., "Tetanus: Not Too Rare to Be Wary of," Patient Care, April 30, 1979, p. 193.

tracheostomy and mechanical ventilation is appropriate. Problems related to bowel and bladder function and immobility must be planned for.

The client will need support during the acute phase, since fear for survival is real. The family will also need support and explanation.

Neurosyphilis

Neurosyphilis is an infection of any part of the nervous system by the organism *Treponema pallidum*. It is the result of untreated or inadequately treated syphilis (see Chap. 45). The organism can invade the central nervous system within a few months of the original infection. Except for causing some changes in the cerebrospinal fluid, including increased white cells, increased protein, and positive serologic reaction, the organism lies dormant for many years. Although not contagious, untreated neurosyphilis can be fatal. Penicillin therapy is effective for syphilitic meningitis, but the neurological deficits remain.

Late neurosyphilis results from degenerative changes in the spinal cord (tabes dorsalis) and brainstem (general paresis). *Tabes dorsalis* (progressive locomotor ataxia) is characterized by vague, sharp pains in the legs, ataxia, "slapping" gait, loss of proprioception and deep tendon reflexes, and zones of hyperesthesia. Charcot's joints, which are characterized by enlargement, bone destruction, and hypermobility, also occur as a result of effusion and edema.

Dementia paralytica is an ongoing spirochetal meningoencephalitis which causes a general dissolution of mental and physical capabilities. This disorder may mimic any number of major or minor psychoses. Management includes treatment with penicillin, symptomatic care, and protection from physical injury.

Case Study / Spinal Cord Injury

John M. is a 22-year-old male who sustained a fractured neck at C5 when he ran his motorcyle into a guardrail on the interstate highway. This was John's third accident in the past 2 years. He had sustained a fractured femur and was hospitalized for 22 days 6 months ago in a similar accident. His wife of 4 years has just come home from the hospital with their third child. John is an unemployed sheet-metal worker.

John is admitted directly to ICU, where the neurosurgeon is waiting to put in Crutchfield tongs with 20 lb of traction. As he arrives John says to you: "Tell the doctor to hurry, I am going to be late for a motorcycle race." John has no movement or sensation below his neck at this time.

Discussion Questions

1. What do you say to John in response to his comment?
2. What are your first activities when John arrives in the ICU?
3. What physiological problems do you anticipate from his C5 injury?
4. What psychological problems do you anticipate with John?
5. What questions do you need to ask John in order to plan his long-range care?
6. How can you best help his wife at this time?
7. What data do you need to collect regarding her needs?

REVIEW QUESTIONS

The number of the question corresponds to the same-numbered objective at the beginning of the chapter.

1. The client with trigeminal neuralgia will present with
   a. flaccid muscles of the neck
   b. vertigo, nausea, and vomiting
   c. paroxysms of excruciating facial pain
   d. dysphagia and respiratory distress

2. The person most likely to sustain a spinal cord injury is a
   a. 30-year-old pregnant woman
   b. 50-year-old obese diabetic
   c. 42-year-old policeman
   d. 19-year-old unemployed male

3. Which one of the following statements is true about the pathophysiology of indirect spinal cord trauma?
   a. The cord is very delicate and is readily transected (torn) by indirect trauma.
   b. Hemorrhage, edema, and excessive metabolites produce ischemia and progressive necrotic destruction.
   c. Oxygen tension in the cord is usually normal.
   d. The injury process starts in the white matter.

4. The reason new drug treatment for spinal cord injury is still not effective is that
   a. the dosage has not been determined
   b. clients are refusing the treatment
   c. they need to be injected within 15 minutes of injury
   d. the effect of all drugs is unknown

5. A client with a C6 injury would be able to
   a. assist with transfer activities
   b. repair watches for a living
   c. walk with braces
   d. catheterize self

6. The initial nursing intervention for the client exhibiting symptoms of autonomic dysreflexia is to
  a. elevate the head of the bed 45°
  b. increase the rate of intravenous infusion
  c. notify the attending physician
  d. retake the blood pressure in 5 minutes

7. Spinal cord tumors are usually
  a. fast-growing
  b. slow-growing
  c. untreatable
  d. rapidly fatal

8. Which of the following is *not* true of Guillain-Barré syndrome?
  a. Cerebrospinal fluid may show increased protein.
  b. It is only mildly contagious.
  c. The onset of symptoms is gradual.
  d. Respiratory failure is a major cause of death.

REFERENCES

1. R. Apfelbaum, "Microvascular Decompression of the Trigeminal Nerve for the Treatment of Trigeminal Neuralgia," *J Neurosurg Nurs,* **10**(2):77–82 (June 1978).
2. W. E. Crill, "Carbamazepine," *Ann Intern Med,* **79:**844–847 (1973).
3. N. Wachter-Shikora, "Trigeminal Neuralgia: Current Concepts and Nursing Implications," *J Neurosurg Nurs,* **9**(2):78–83 (June 1977).
4. J. Tew, "Trigeminal Neuralgia," in H. Coon (ed.), *Current Therapy,* J. B. Lippincott Company, Philadelphia, 1979, p. 718.
5. Sharon Sell, "The Treatment of Tic Douloureaux by Vascular Decompression to the Trigeminal Nerve," *J Neurosurg Nurs,* **9**(1):20–22 (March 1977).
6. M. J. Goldberg, "Emotional Factors Contributing to Facial Paralysis," *J Geriat Soc,* **20:**324–329 (July 1962).
7. Ugo Fisch, "Current Surgical Treatment of Intratemporal Facial Palsy," *Clin Plast Surg,* **6**(3):377–395 (July 1979).
8. K. K. Adour et al., "The True Nature of Bell's Palsy: Analysis of 1000 Consecutive Patients," *Laryngoscope,* **88**(2):787–801 (May 1978).
9. D. Brown et al., "Electromyographic Biofeedback in the Reeducation of Facial Palsy Patients," *Am J Phys Med,* **57**(4):183–189 (April 1978).
10. H. Cantor et al., "Help for the Patient with Bell's Palsy," *Patient Care,* Oct. 1, 1975, pp. 99–102.
11. Rosemarie King and Susan Dudas, "Rehabilitation of the Patient with a Spinal Cord Injury," *Nurs Clin North Am,* **15**(2):225–243 (June 1980).
12. Samuel Webb et al., "Spinal Cord Injury: Epidemiologic Implications, Costs, and Patterns of Care in 85 Patients," *Arch Phys Med Rehab,* **60:**335 (August 1979).
13. Mary Jane Oliveto, Susanna Wilson and Harold A. Mackinnon, "Sara: Her Rehabilitation and Its Cost," *Am J Nurs,* **77**:1340 (1977).
14. Diana DeJesus-Greenberg, "Acute Spinal Cord Injury and Hyperbaric O_2 Therapy: A New Adjunct in Management," *J Neurosurg Nurs,* **12**(3):155–160 (September 1980).
15. Marilyn Pires, "Spinal Cord Injuries," in *Coping with Neurological Problems Proficiently: Nursing Skillbook,* Intermed Communications, Horsham, Pa., 1979, chap. 6, p. 105.
16. Joanne V. Hickey, *The Clinical Practice of Neurological and Neurosurgical Nursing,* J. B. Lippincott Company, Philadelphia, 1981, p. 271.
17. Laura Halstead et al., "Neurologically Active Drugs in Spinal Cord Injury: A Clinical Coding System," *Arch Phys Med Rehabil,* **59**(8):358–366 (August 1978).
18. S. Ginnity, "Assessment of Cervical Cord Trauma by the Nurse Practitioner," *J Neurosurg Nurs,* **10:**193–197 (December 1978).
19. Pires, op. cit., p. 107.
20. Larrabee, op. cit., p. 1328.
21. King, op. cit., p. 226.
22. P. Kaplan et al., "Calcium Balance in Paraplegic Patients: Influence of Injury Duration and Ambulation," *Arch Phys Med Rehabil,* **59:**448 (October 1978).
23. Pires, op. cit., p. 108.
24. Edith Kowalsky, "Grief: A Lost Life-Style," *Am J Nurs,* **78**(3):418 (March 1978).
25. G. Bartol, "Psychological Needs of the Spinal Cord Injured Person," *J Neurosurg Nurs,* **10**(4):171–175 (December 1979).
26. Linda L. Lazure, "Autonomic Dysreflexia," *Nursing 80,* **10**(9):52–54 (September 1980).
27. W. Johnson, *Sex Education and Counseling of Special Groups,* Charles C Thomas, Publisher, Springfield, Ill., 1975.
28. T. Mooney et al., *Sexual Options for Paraplegics and Quadraplegics,* Little, Brown and Company, Boston, 1975.
29. R. Baxter, "Sex Counseling and the SCI Patient," *Nursing 78,* **8**:46–52 (September 1978).
30. L. Hodges, "Human Sexuality and the Spinal Cord Injured: Role of the Clinical Nurse Specialist," *J Neurosurg Nurs,* **10**(3):125–129 (September 1978).
31. Martha Hartman, "Intermittent Self-Catheterization," *Nursing 78,* **8**(11):72–75 (November 1978).
32. Norma Isaacs, "Intraspinal Tumors," in *Coping with Neurological Problems Proficiently, Nursing 79 Skillbook,* Intermed Communications, Horsham, Pa., 1979, chap. 8, pp. 139–148.
33. R. J. Samonds, "Guillain-Barré Syndrome," *Nursing 80,* **10**(8):35 (August, 1980).
34. Vernon Knight, "Influenza," in Kurt Isselbacher et al. (eds.), *Harrison's Principles of Internal Medicine,* McGraw-Hill Book Company, New York, 1980, chap. 179, p. 786.
35. K. Cramer et al., "Botulism: Nursing Care in an Epidemic," *Nursing,* **8**(11):62–71 (November 1978).
36. S.C. Sell, "Neurologic Infections," in *Coping with Neurologic Problems Proficiently, Nursing Skillbook,* Intermed Communications, Horsham, Pa., 1979, chap. 10, pp. 169–172.
37. R. J. Rothstein and F. J. Baker, "Tetanus: Prevention and Treatment," *JAMA,* **240**(7):675–676 (Aug. 18, 1978).
38. W. Furst and A. Aguirre, "Preventing Tetanus, *Am J Nurs,* **78**:834–837 (1978).
39. D. Nicholson, "Tetanus—Still a Therapeutic Challenge," *Heart Lung,* **5**(2):226–227 (March–April 1976).
40. S. Peters and N. Vogel, "Physiological and Psychological Aspects of Tetanus: Report of a Case," *Heart Lung,* **5**(2):297–300 (March–April 1976).

Chapter 54

NURSING ROLE IN MANAGEMENT

Critical of the Client with Increased Intracranial Pressure

Maureen Brady Nash
Sharon Wahl

Learning Objectives

1. Define intracranial pressure.
2. Identify the regulatory mechanisms in the maintenance of normal intracranial pressure.
3. Identify the common causes, clinical manifestations, and medical management of increased intracranial pressure.
4. Describe the downward progress model related to levels of consciousness.
5. Identify the nursing interventions for the client with increased intracranial pressure.
6. Differentiate between the main causes and types of head injury.
7. Correlate the clinical manifestations with the pathophysiological problems occurring with head injury.
8. Describe the medical and nursing management of head injury.
9. Describe the types, clinical manifestations, and medical management of intracranial tumors.
10. Identify the nursing interventions for the client with an intracranial tumor.
11. Describe the nursing care for the craniotomy client.
12. Compare the causes, medical management, and prognosis of common cerebral inflammatory problems.
13. Explain the nursing interventions for the client with a cerebral inflammatory problem.

Increased intracranial pressure (IICP) occurs when there is an increase in any of the major intracranial components—brain tissue, cerebrospinal fluid, or intravascular blood. Figure 54-1 shows the percentage constituted by each of these components. Because the cranial cavity is nonexpansive, only a very narrow shift in any of these components can occur before symptoms of IICP appear. Without intervention, IICP can progress to loss of consciousness, brain herniation, and death. Normal intracranial pressure is 0 to 15 mmHg (110 to 140 mmH_2O) reclining and 30 mmHg sitting. Coughing, straining, and sneezing cause transient elevations to 100 mmHg in the normal person without apparent distress. While causes of IICP are varied, general categories include trauma, space-occupying lesions, obstruction, and inflammation.

Following a discussion of the common problems associated with IICP, each of the possible causes will be addressed. It is important to remember that IICP is a pathological process of multiple causes and not a disease in itself.

This chapter was reviewed by Jane Ellen Mead, R.N., B.S.N., M.S.N., Assistant Professor, the Catholic University of America, School of Nursing, Washington, D.C.

INCREASED INTRACRANIAL PRESSURE

Intracranial Pressure and Cerebral Blood Flow

The cerebral perfusion pressure (CPP) must be at least 50 mmHg if the brain is to receive adequate blood. (The average range is 80 to 100 mmHg.) The CPP is the difference between the mean arterial blood pressure of blood flow to the brain and the intracranial pressure. Table 54-1 shows how to calculate the CPP. A CPP of 30 mmHg is incompatible with life.

Normal Regulatory Mechanisms of Intracranial Pressure

Autoregulation

The brain has the ability to regulate its own blood flow (called autoregulation). This is critical, since the brain needs a constant supply of oxygen and glucose. The brain uses 20 percent of the body's oxygen and 25 percent of its glucose.[1]

Autoregulation maintains a constant cerebral blood flow and perfusion pressure despite systemic, cardiovascular, or hormonal variations. This is accom-

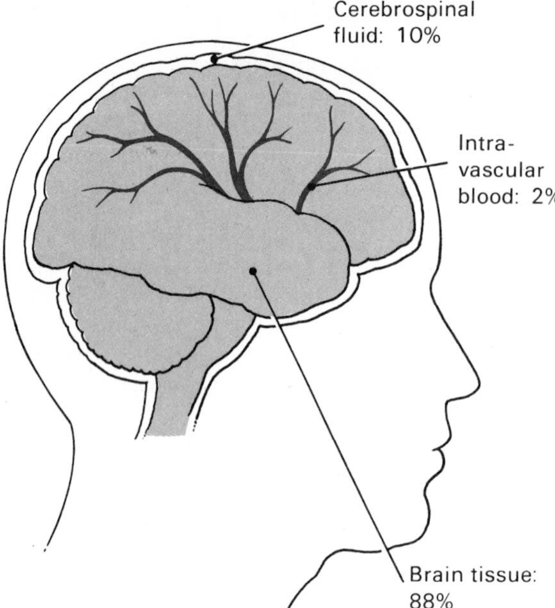

Figure 54-1 Components of the brain.

plished by three main mechanisms: pressure changes, cerebral vasodilatation, and metabolic factors.

Pressure Changes As intracranial pressure increases, systemic arterial pressure also rises to maintain a constant cerebral blood flow. Conversely, if the systemic arterial pressure rises, there is compensatory vasoconstriction in the resistance vessels, causing the pressure within the vessels to increase. Decreased systemic arterial pressure causes vasodilatation.

These pressure changes can compensate only to a critical point. The critical point at which autoregulatory mechanisms are impaired occurs when intracranial pressure reaches a level of approximately 33 mmHg.[2] At this point intracranial pressure would begin to rise.

Table 54-1
Calculating Cerebral Perfusion Pressure

CPP = mean arterial pressure − intracranial pressure

Mean arterial pressure = diastolic pressure + $\frac{1}{3}$ pulse pressure

Example: Systemic blood pressure = 122/84
Mean arterial pressure = 97
Intracranial pressure = 12 mmHg
CPP = 85 mmHg

Cerebral Vasodilatation Cerebral arteries dilate when the cerebral oxygen tension falls below 50 mmHg. This dilatation decreases cerebral vascular resistance. If this is not sufficient to raise oxygen tension, anaerobic metabolism will begin, resulting in lactic acid accumulation and making the blood more acid. This acidity causes vasodilatation, which in turn increases cerebral blood flood.

Metabolic Factors Oxygen tension, carbon dioxide tension, and hydrogen ion concentration affect cerebral vessel tone. High PCO_2, low PO_2, and high hydrogen ion concentration (acidosis) are potent cerebral vasodilators. High P_aO_2 and low P_aCO_2 produce mild vasoconstriction.

Extreme cardiovascular changes such as asystole or pathological states such as diabetic coma can alter or abolish autoregulation. When it is lost, cerebral vessels are directly influenced by any systemic change in blood pressure, by hypoxia, or by effects of catecholamines.

Compensatory mechanisms for changes in intracranial pressure

The cranial contents can shift in volume only within narrow limits without damaging cranial tissue. Three situations require adjustments in the cranial compartment:

1. *Expansion of brain tissue*—When this occurs, there is an increase in absorption of cerebrospinal fluid into the venous sinuses, since this system is pressure-dependent. There is also a compensatory escape of blood into the systemic vascular system.
2. *Increase in cerebrospinal fluid*—When this occurs, blood moves into the systemic circulation and results in an increase in blood volume. This in turn leads to increased absorption of cerebrospinal fluid.
3. *Failure of all compensatory mechanisms*—If the previously mentioned compensatory mechanisms are ineffective in preventing an elevation in intracranial pressure, brain tissue may herniate through openings in the cranium. These sites include the midline, the tentorial notch, and the foramen magnum. This herniation puts pressure on the vital structures of the midbrain, pons, and medulla, interfering with cranial nerves, nerve tracts, and vital life centers. This is a life-threatening situation and is discussed in detail later in this chapter.

Pathophysiology of Increased Intracranial Pressure

Regardless of the cause, almost all insults to the brain such as trauma, tumors, anoxia, and hypertension result in cerebral edema, an increase in the water content of the brain leading to an increase of tissue volume. The edema may be the primary cause of IICP or may be secondary to another cause such as inflammation. Edema is a normal physiological response to trauma. Because of the brain's inability to expand within the cranial cavity, however, cerebral edema assumes grave significance. Cerebral edema affects the permeability of the blood-brain barrier and hence the brain's protection from potentially damaging substances.

The extent of the original insult determines the degree of cerebral edema. Cerebral edema reaches its peak in 2 to 4 days and begins to subside after 2 weeks. The rate of development is accelerated by elevated systemic blood pressure, fever, and lesions interfering with venous drainage. Figure 54-2 illustrates the progression of IICP unless intervention occurs.

Clinical Manifestations

Signs and symptoms

Regardless of the cause, IICP will result in progressive neurological deficiences based on the location of the source of pressure (Table 54-2). The pressure causes compression of the brain tissue and structures, which interferes with blood supply to the involved areas. This results in ischemia and anoxia of the nerve cells, with eventual necrosis and cell death. Dysfunctions of the reticular activating system, the pons, and the medulla account for most of the manifestations of IICP.

There is disagreement over which of the symptoms constitute the triad of IICP, but most authors seem to agree that rising systolic pressure, widening of the pulse pressure, and bradycardia are the classic symptoms.[3] Other common manifestations of increased intracranial pressure are as follows:

1. *Decrease in level of consciousness* (LOC)—This may occur as a subtle change such as flattening of affect or a more dramatic change such as coma. Change in the LOC is due to the sensitivity of the cerebral cortex to a decreased oxygen supply secondary to the IICP.
2. *Change in vital signs*—The initial changes seen in the compensatory phase of IICP include an increase in systemic arterial pressure due to ischemia of the vasomotor center. A decrease in rate of a

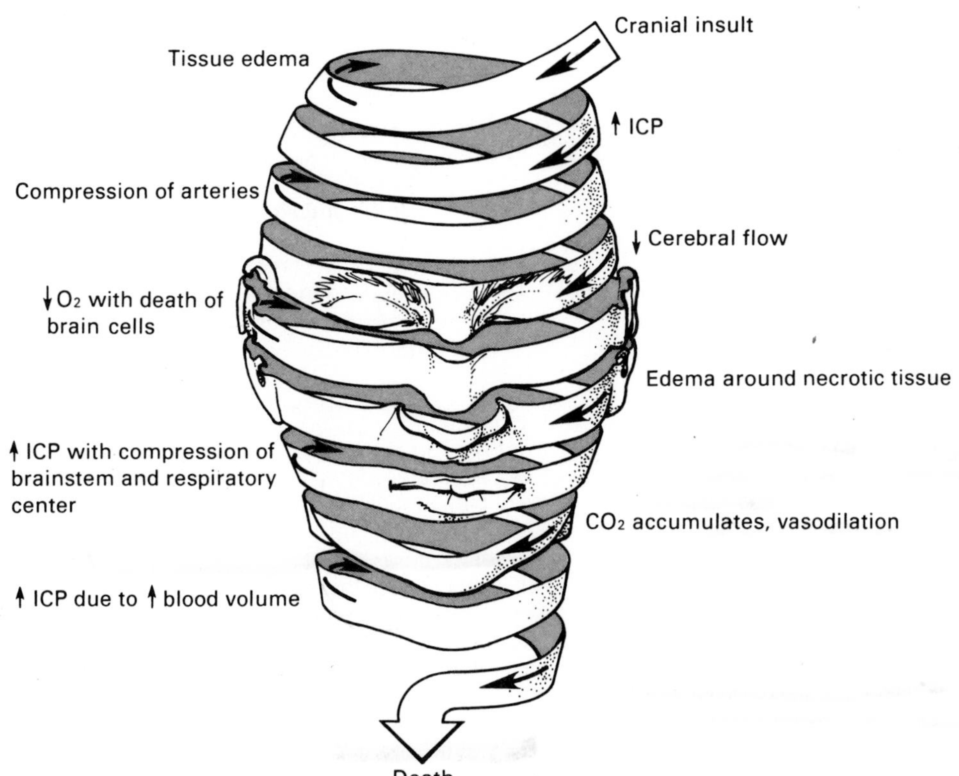

Figure 54-2 Progression of IICP. (*From M. Snyder and M. Jackle, Neurologic Problems: A Critical Care Nursing Focus, Robert J. Brady Co., Bowie, Md., 1981, p. 52.*)

Table 54-2
Symptoms of Supratentorial IICP

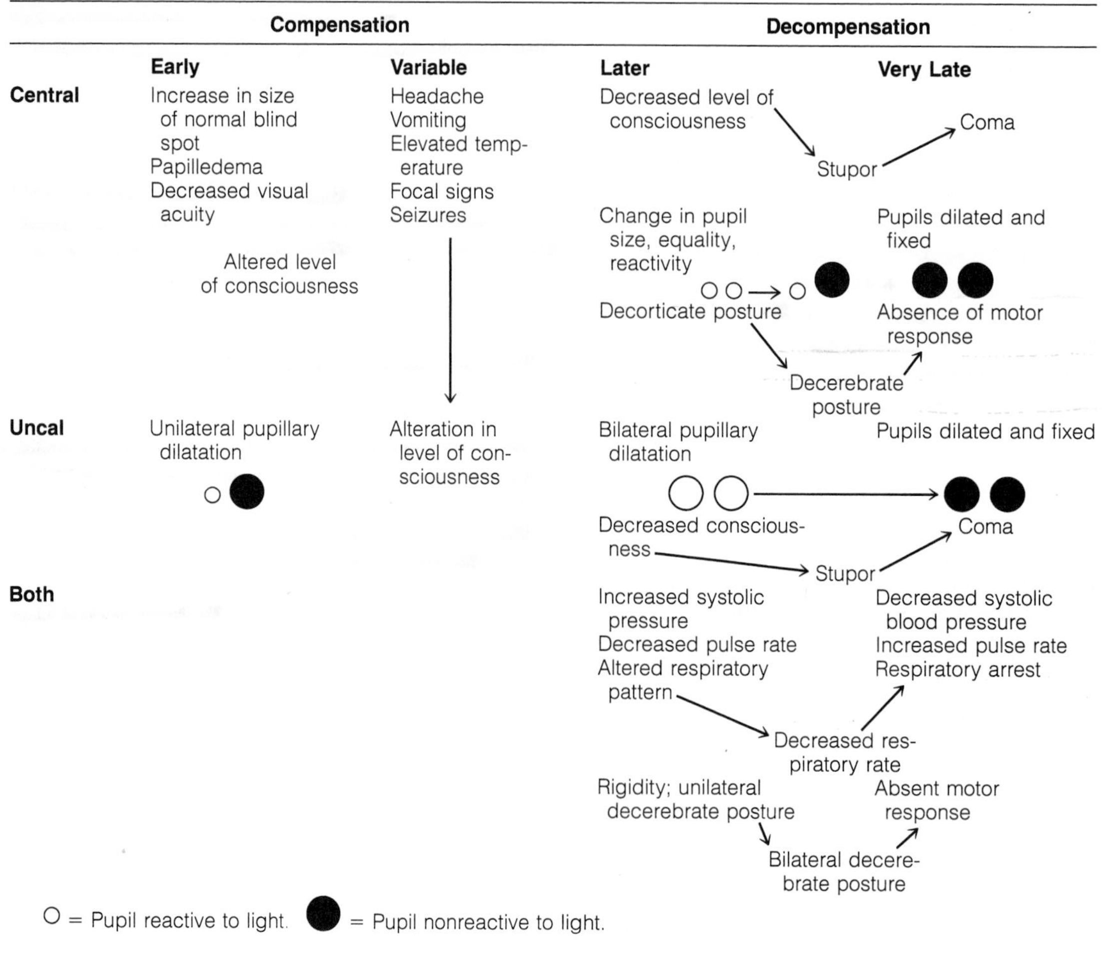

	Compensation		Decompensation	
	Early	**Variable**	**Later**	**Very Late**
Central	Increase in size of normal blind spot Papilledema Decreased visual acuity Altered level of consciousness	Headache Vomiting Elevated temperature Focal signs Seizures ↓	Decreased level of consciousness ↘ Stupor Change in pupil size, equality, reactivity ○○ → ○● Decorticate posture ↘ Decerebrate posture	↗ Coma Pupils dilated and fixed ●● Absence of motor response ↗
Uncal	Unilateral pupillary dilatation ○●	Alteration in level of consciousness	Bilateral pupillary dilatation ○○ → Decreased consciousness → Stupor	Pupils dilated and fixed ●● ↗ Coma
Both			Increased systolic pressure Decreased pulse rate Altered respiratory pattern ↘ Decreased respiratory rate Rigidity; unilateral decerebrate posture ↘ Bilateral decerebrate posture	Decreased systolic blood pressure Increased pulse rate Respiratory arrest ↗ Absent motor response ↗

○ = Pupil reactive to light. ● = Pupil nonreactive to light.

H. C. Moidel et al., *Nursing Care of the Patient with Medical-Surgical Disorders,* McGraw-Hill Book Company, New York, 1976, p.868.

full and bounding pulse and alterations in respiratory pattern related to the level of brain dysfunction are also evident (Fig. 54-3). As the decompensation phase begins, the blood pressure begins to drop. The pulse becomes rapid, irregular, and thready as it tries to pump blood into resistant vessels. The temperature, normal to this point, may reach high levels if the hypothalamus is affected.

3. *Ocular signs*—Compression of cranial nerve III results in various ocular changes ranging from constriction on the ipsilateral side to dilatation. The pupils deteriorate to the point of being bilaterally fixed. Reaction to light ranges from sluggishness to nonresponsiveness. Blurred vision, diplopia, and changes in extraocular movements may also be evident. Papilledema indicates IICP but is not usually present until intracranial pressure is markedly elevated.
4. *Decrease in motor and sensory function*—As the IICP continues, the client manifests deteriorating motor and sensory function related to movement, pain perception, temperature, and proprioception. Decorticate and decerebrate posture (Fig. 54-4) may occur when any noxious stimulus is presented to the client, such as suctioning or repositioning. Decorticate posture consists of extension of the legs and internal rotation and adduction of the arms, with flexion of the elbows, wrists, and fingers;

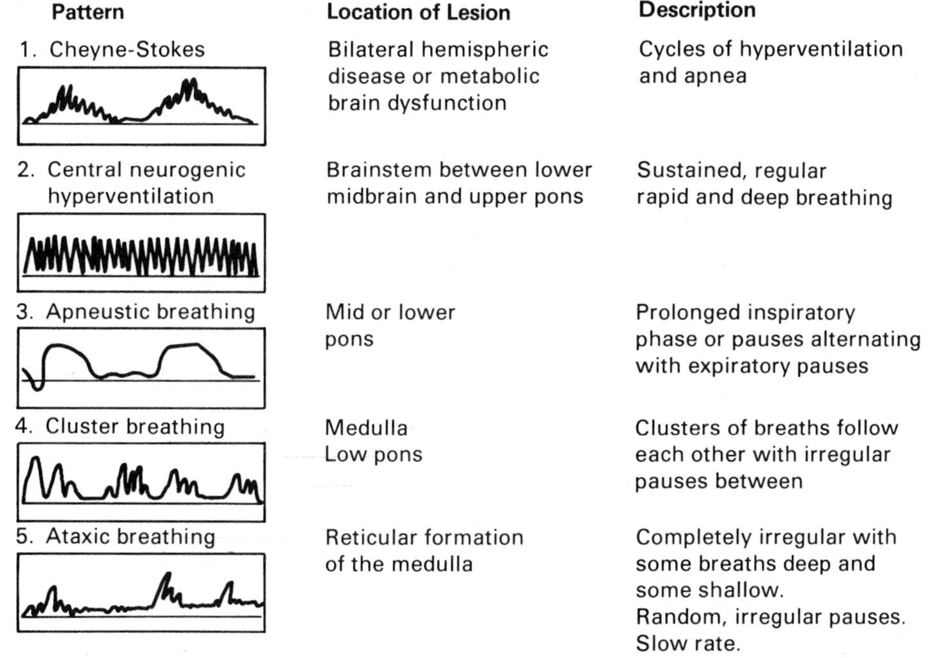

Pattern	Location of Lesion	Description
1. Cheyne-Stokes	Bilateral hemispheric disease or metabolic brain dysfunction	Cycles of hyperventilation and apnea
2. Central neurogenic hyperventilation	Brainstem between lower midbrain and upper pons	Sustained, regular rapid and deep breathing
3. Apneustic breathing	Mid or lower pons	Prolonged inspiratory phase or pauses alternating with expiratory pauses
4. Cluster breathing	Medulla Low pons	Clusters of breaths follow each other with irregular pauses between
5. Ataxic breathing	Reticular formation of the medulla	Completely irregular with some breaths deep and some shallow. Random, irregular pauses. Slow rate.

Figure 54-3 Common abnormal respiratory patterns associated with coma.

it is due to interruption of voluntary motor tracts. Decerebrate posture (Fig. 54-4) indicates more serious brain damage and results from disruption of motor fibers in the midbrain and brainstem. In this position the teeth are clenched and the arms are stiffly extended, adducted, and hyperpronated. There is hyperextension of the leg with plantar flexion of the foot.

5. *Headache*—Although not always present, headache may be a sign of IICP. If present, it is usually worse upon rising in the morning after REM sleep, when intracranial pressure normally rises.
6. *Vomiting*—Projectile vomiting not preceded by nausea may be present with IICP. This results when the afferent limb on the vomiting mechanism is short-circuited by the lesion, producing vomiting without nausea.[4]

Downward progress model

Another way to look at manifestations of IICP is the downward progression model. The model correlates clinical signs and symptoms with the location of the increased pressure. The manifestations are cumulative as the pressure increases. Table 54-3 outlines this model.

Complications

The major complication of uninterrupted IICP is brain herniation (Fig. 54-5). Uncal or tentorial herniation results from increased supratentorial pressure, which causes herniation of the uncus of the temporal lobe through the tentorial notch. This results in ischemia and hemorrhage in the brainstem. It may also cause obstruction of cerebrospinal fluid, resulting in increased cranial volume. Foramen magnum and in-

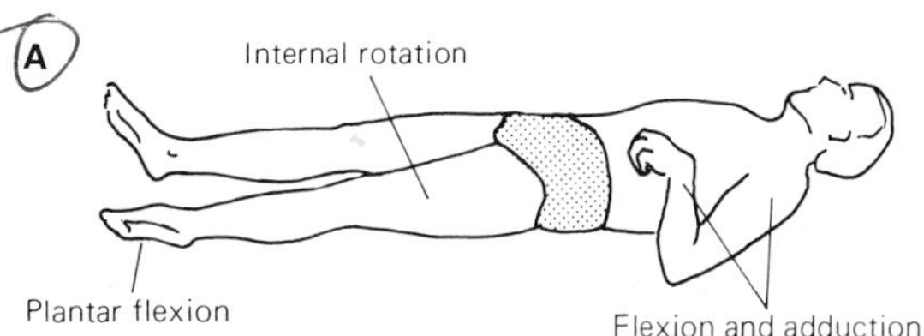

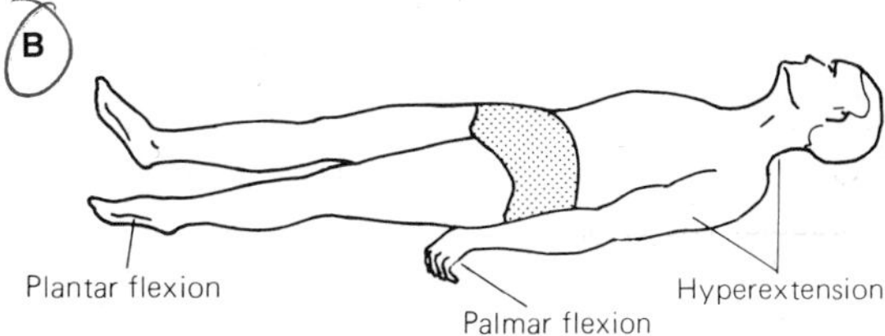

Figure 54-4 *(a)* Decorticate posture. *(b)* Decerebrate posture. [*From H. C. Moidel et al. (eds.), Nursing Care of the Patient with Medical-Surgical Disorders, 2d ed., McGraw Hill Book Company, New York, 1976.*]

Table 54-3
Downward Progression Model of IICP

Site of ICP	Clinical Manifestations
Cortical level	Persistent headache; vomiting; papilledema; decrease in LOC such as mental fogginess, increased restlessness; agitation; vital signs not significantly affected; reflexes normal; seizures may occur.
Diencephalon level	Difficult to arouse; more loss of strength and sensation; difficulty following commands; agitation or apathy; may assume decorticate or decerebrate posture; pupils small and briskly reactive; abnormal respiration with increased blood pressure; widening pulse pressure and bradycardia; positive Babinski, grasp, oculocephalic (doll's eyes), and oculovestibular (caloric) reflexes appear.
Midbrain–upper pontine level	Semicomatose, responds only to noxious stimuli, difficult to elicit abnormal reflexes except Babinski; wide fluctuations in body temperature; diabetes insipidus may occur; central neurogenic hyperventilation present; pupils midsize and sluggish.
Lower pontine–upper medullary level	Coma; flaccid skeletal muscles; respirations slow and regular or fast and shallow; only positive reflex is Babinski; vital signs stable; pupils dilated and less responsive.
Medullary level	Deep coma, reflexes absent, pupils dilated and fixed, temperature subnormal, blood pressure low, pulse slow, respirations cease.

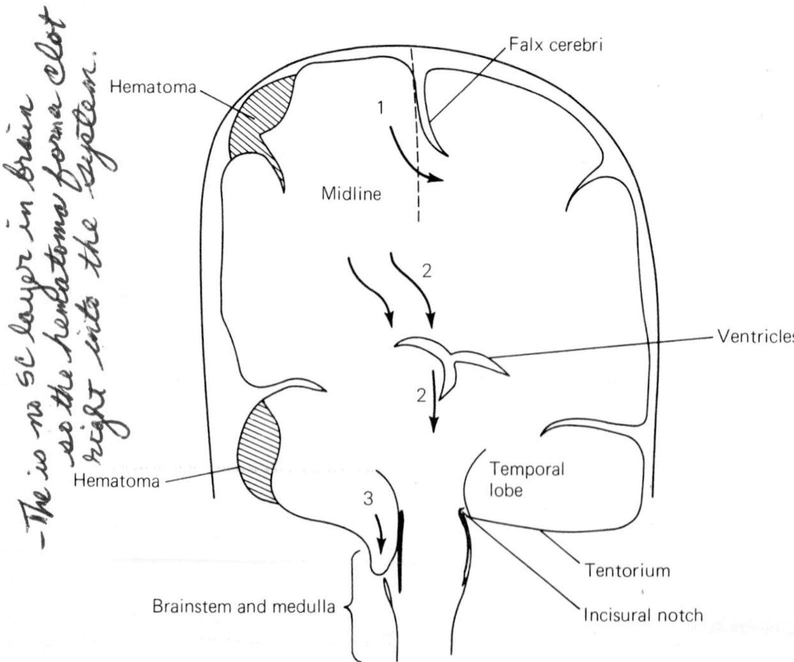

Figure 54-5 Schematic representation of the anatomical boundaries of the brain, with composite representation of the three supratentorial herniation syndromes. Note displacement of the falx cerebri by the hematoma mass—cingulate herniation. (1) Central herniation is shown by the central arrows. (2) Displacement of the ventricles. (3) Uncal herniation (also called temporal lobe herniation) and stretching of cranial nerve III. [*From H. C. Moidel et al. (eds.), Nursing Care of the Patient with Medical-Surgical Disorders, 2d ed., McGraw-Hill Book Company, New York, 1976.*]

fratentorial herniation result from increased infratentorial pressure. Compression of the medulla often results in respiratory arrest. Specific manifestations are associated with different types of herniation but always include a sharp decrease in level of consciousness. Regardless of the site of the herniation, it is a grave occurrence with a poor prognosis.

Diagnostic Studies

Diagnostic studies are aimed at identifying the underlying cause of the IICP and vary according to the suspected cause. Tests which might be ordered include a CT scan, electroencephalogram, and cerebral angiogram. In general, a lumbar puncture is not done when IICP is suspected because of the possibility that the drop in pressure could precipitate brain herniation.

Direct measurement of intracranial pressure is possible. Since it is also used on a continuous basis to monitor intracranial pressure, it is discussed under acute nursing intervention.

Medical Management

The goals of medical management (Table 54-4) are to identify and treat the underlying cause of IICP and to treat the effects of cerebral edema. A careful history is an important diagnostic aid which can direct the search for the underlying cause. Friends and relatives may need to be questioned regarding subtle behavorial cues.

Table 54-4
Medical Management: Increased Intracranial Pressure

Diagnostic

1. Complete history and physical examination
2. Vital signs, neurological checks, and intracranial pressure measurements every hour
3. Chest, spinal column, and skull x-rays
4. EEG, CT scan, ECG, cerebral arteriography
5. CBC, BUN, creatinine, glucose, electrolytes, ABG, ammonia level; general drug and toxin screening, especially for blood alcohol level; CSF protein, glucose, and C&S

Therapeutic

1. Maintenance of a patent airway and adequate ventilation
2. Fluid restriction
   a. Intake and output
   b. Daily weight
3. Temperature control—e.g., hypothermia blanket
4. Drug therapy
   a. Osmotic diuretics—e.g:, mannitol, glucose
   b. Corticosteroids—e.g., dexamethasone
   c. Anticonvulsants—e.g., phenytoin
5. Possible ventricular drainage
6. Possible continuous intracranial monitoring

Even while the underlying cause is being sought, IICP must be aggressively treated if the cycle is to be interrupted. In order to maintain adequate ventilation, an endotracheal tube or tracheostomy may be necessary. Blood gas analysis will guide oxygen therapy. Nonsurgical intervention to reduce edema includes (1) corticosteriods (e.g., dexamethasone), (2) diuretics, (3) limited fluid intake and (4) hyperventilation. Care must be taken to avoid severe dehydration, especially if diabetes insipidus is evident. Fluids are generally limited to 75 to 100 mL/hour or calculated to be replaced at a rate to equal urine output of 500 mL/day. An intravenous solution containing water should never be given to clients with IICP, since water crosses the blood-brain barrier and increases cerebral edema. Lactated Ringer's or sodium solutions are preferred, as the sodium will keep fluid within the vessels.[5] Passive artificial hyperventilation may be used to keep the P_aCO_2 to 25 to 30 mmHg. This causes cerebral vasoconstriction with a resultant decrease in intracranial pressure.

Pharmacological Intervention

Drug therapy plays an important part in the management of IICP. Generally, the three classes of drugs used are osmotic diuretics, corticosteroids, and anticonvulsants.

Osmotic diuretics such as mannitol (Osmitrol), 50% glucose, and urea are used to draw fluid from the cells to the extracellular fluid. Fluid and electrolyte balance should be monitored when these drugs are used. Mannitol and urea are contraindicated if renal disease is present. The effect of these hypertonic solutions is rapid and short-lived, so corticosteroids may also be administered.

Dexamethasone (Decadron) is the usual corticosteroid used to treat IICP. It helps to stabilize the capillary membrane and decrease permeability. This prevents edema from increasing and facilitates diuresis. The benefit of dexamethasone is variable; it is considered more useful in tumors and hematomas and less effective in head injury. However, recent research indicates that megadoses of dexamethasone used in head injury may serve a role in decreasing intracranial pressure.[6] The nurse should monitor fluid intake carefully because of the potential for hyponatremia. She should also observe for infection and monitor for evidence of hyperglycemia. The glucose levels of blood and urine should be monitored regularly because of the hyperglycemic effect of corticosteroids.

Phenytoin (Dilantin) is the usual anticonvulsant used to prevent seizures. Barbiturates in high doses have been demonstrated to decrease intracranial pressure within 1 to 2 minutes of administration; pentobarbital (Nembutal) is the drug most commonly used. New research has shown that ethacrynic acid (Edecrin) also reduces cerebral edema by decreasing astroglial swelling.

Nutritional Considerations

A nasogastric tube attached to suction is usually kept in place until the client's condition stabilizes and bowel sounds are present. When the tube is removed, the client can be started on high calorie, high protein fluids, progressing to a full high protein diet as soon as tolerated. Meals should be divided into six or more small feedings to avoid overdistension of the stomach. Antacids should be continued as long as the client remains on corticosteroids. If the client is unable to take oral feedings after 4 to 5 days, either total parenteral nutrition (TPN) or tube feedings are instituted.

When there is inappropriate secretion of ADH (SIADH) secondary to stimulation of the hypothalamic-neurohypophyseal system, tube feedings should be administered with great care since the free water can increase cerebral edema if IV fluids are not restricted. The nurse should familiarize herself with the type of feeding being administered, since some types are low in sodium and added salt may be necessary. Since malnutrition is known to promote continued cerebral edema, maintaining optimal nutrition is imperative.[7]

Nursing Management

Acute intervention

Since the nursing management of IICP is the same regardless of the cause, the general nursing measures are included here; specific interventions are discussed in later sections. Table 49-3, Nursing Care Plan for the Unconscious Client, contains much of the nursing care appropriate for the client with IICP. If the client is unconscious, the problems in that care plan would be the basis for nursing intervention. Additional problems specific to the nursing management of the client with IICP are discussed here.

Neurological Assessment The neurological assessment is an important nursing responsibility for the client with IICP. Careful recording of the assessment is equally important. Figure 54-6 illustrates a typical neurological clinical flow sheet used to graphically display a client's neurological status over time. The usual components of a neurological check are vital signs, pupil size and eye movement, level of consciousness, and limb movement. The frequency of neurological checks is a matter of nursing judgment.

When recording vital signs, it is important to note trends. Respirations vary according to the degree of pressure in the cranial cavity (see Fig. 54-3). Temperature should not be elevated because of the increased metabolic demands that occur. A hypothermia blanket is an effective way to reduce temperature.

Pupil size and reaction are also assessed during a neurological check. The nurse looks at the size of each pupil and compares the two (Fig. 54-7). Initially, only the pupil on the side of the lesion is affected. If the intracranial pressure continues to increase, both pupils dilate. If the corneal reflex is absent, routine eye care should be initiated (see Chap. 15).

Following examination of the pupil for size, pupillary reaction is assessed. After the room is dimmed, a flashlight is shone into each eye. Both direct reactions and consensual reactions (constriction of pupil when light is shined into the other eye) are assessed. The nurse should also note whether the reaction is brisk (normal) or sluggish (indicating pressure on the nerve).

Level of consciousness is assessed during the neurological check and is an important indicator of changing intracranial pressure. Whether the Glasgow scale (Table 49-3) or a descriptive statement (Table 49-2) are used, the nurse should be as explicit as possible regarding the level of consciousness.

Limb movement is assessed by asking the conscious client to squeeze the nurse's hand and press his feet against her hands. The equality and strength of both upper and lower extremities are noted. If the client is unconscious, the position assumed should be noted.

Maintaining Respiratory Function P_aCO_2 should be kept at normal levels because of its vasodilating effect on cerebral vessels when elevated, which increases intracranial pressure. This is accomplished by maintaining a patent airway. Specific nursing interventions depend on the level of consciousness of the client. If the client can cooperate, turning and deep breathing at regular intervals should be planned.

As the LOC decreases, the client is at increased risk for obstruction by the tongue dropping back and by the accumulation of secretions. Altered breathing patterns may become evident. Airway patency can be aided by keeping the client on his side with frequent position changes, avoiding the supine position. Suctioning should be done as necessary. An airway will facilitate breathing and provide an easy suctioning route in a comatose client. Since suctioning and

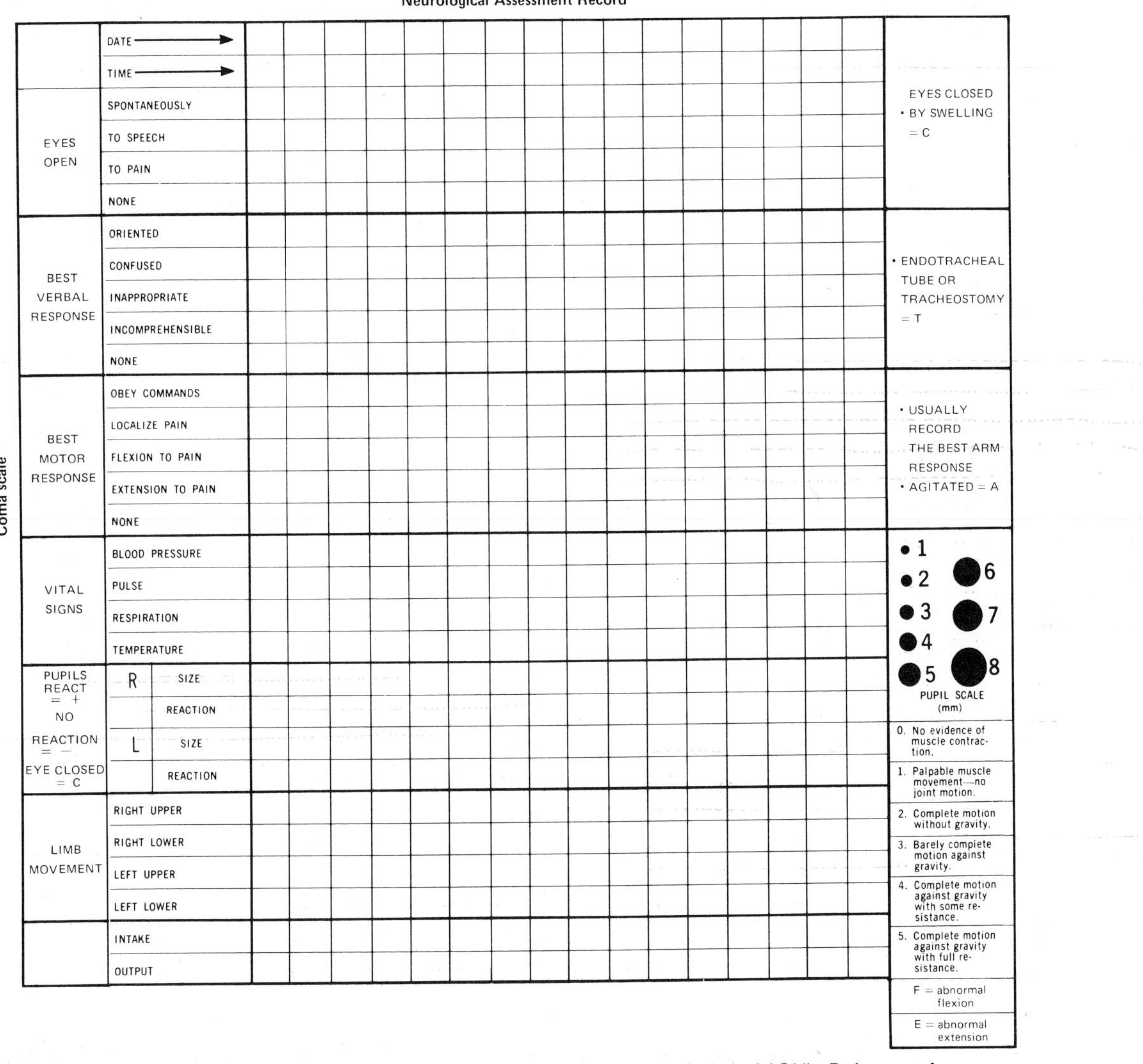

Neurological Assessment Record

Coma scale

	DATE →	
	TIME →	
EYES OPEN	SPONTANEOUSLY	EYES CLOSED • BY SWELLING = C
	TO SPEECH	
	TO PAIN	
	NONE	
BEST VERBAL RESPONSE	ORIENTED	• ENDOTRACHEAL TUBE OR TRACHEOSTOMY = T
	CONFUSED	
	INAPPROPRIATE	
	INCOMPREHENSIBLE	
	NONE	
BEST MOTOR RESPONSE	OBEY COMMANDS	• USUALLY RECORD THE BEST ARM RESPONSE • AGITATED = A
	LOCALIZE PAIN	
	FLEXION TO PAIN	
	EXTENSION TO PAIN	
	NONE	
VITAL SIGNS	BLOOD PRESSURE	1 2 3 4 5 6 7 8 PUPIL SCALE (mm)
	PULSE	
	RESPIRATION	
	TEMPERATURE	
PUPILS REACT = + NO REACTION = − EYE CLOSED = C	R SIZE	
	R REACTION	0. No evidence of muscle contraction.
	L SIZE	1. Palpable muscle movement—no joint motion.
	L REACTION	2. Complete motion without gravity.
LIMB MOVEMENT	RIGHT UPPER	3. Barely complete motion against gravity.
	RIGHT LOWER	4. Complete motion against gravity with some resistance.
	LEFT UPPER	5. Complete motion against gravity with full resistance.
	LEFT LOWER	F = abnormal flexion
	INTAKE	E = abnormal extension
	OUTPUT	

Figure 54-6 Neurological clinical flow sheet. [*From M. R. Kinney et al. (eds.), AACN's Reference for Critical Care Nursing, McGraw-Hill Book Company, New York, 1981.*]

coughing cause transient increases in intracranial pressure as well as decreases in P_aO_2, hyperinflation and hyperoxygenation with an Ambu bag and 100 percent oxygen should precede each suctioning period. However, this procedure can increase intrathoracic pressure if the Ambu bag does not have a controlled pressure valve. Recent studies indicate that limiting the length of suctioning to 15 seconds or less limits the buildup of CO_2 and is more important than hyperinflation. If copious secretions need removal, coughing or suctioning should be of short duration, with rest periods in between. Abdominal distension should be avoided, since the pressure on the diaphragm can cause respiratory difficulty. Insertion of a nasogastric tube can prevent distension, vomiting, and possible aspiration.[8]

The use of sedatives or opiates should be avoided unless sedation is part of the pharmacological management. Restlessness and agitation in the client with IICP may indicate cerebral hypoxia. The use of sedatives may depress respiration further, which only compounds the problem. Small doses of codeine may be used for obvious pain.

Blood gases should be measured and evaluated regularly. Low-flow O_2 is useful in most clients. If the client is not ventilating well or is dusky, the physician

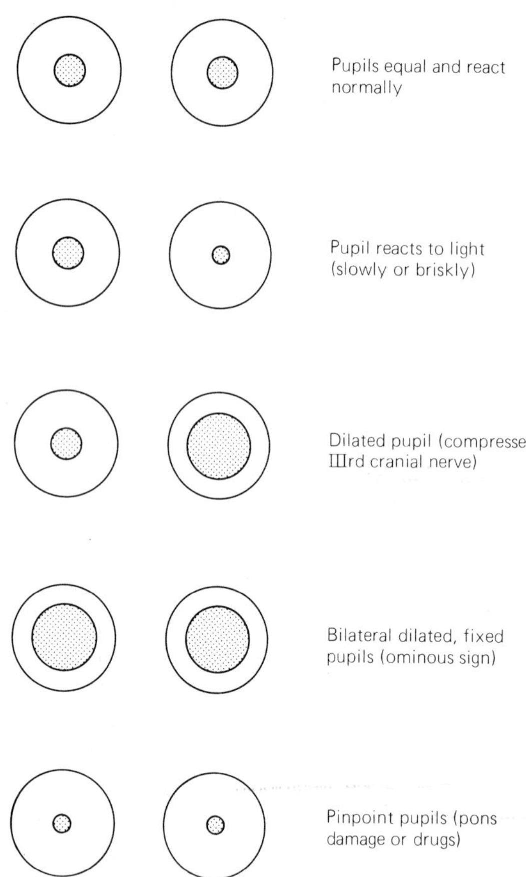

Figure 54-7 Pupillary check for size, movement, and response. [*From H. C. Moidel et al. (eds.), Nursing Care of the Patient with Medical-Surgical Disorders, McGraw-Hill Book Company, New York, 1976, p. 278.*]

should be notified immediately, since intubation and artificial ventilation may be indicated. Neurogenic hyperventilation affects the acid-base balance and is notoriously difficult to manage even with a respirator. Generally, the client is treated supportively. If this pattern continues over a long period, the client is put on a respirator and a skeletal muscle relaxant such as pancuronium bromide is used to normalize blood gases. (See Chap. 22 for nursing management of the client on a mechanical ventilator.)

Fluid and Electrolyte Balance Fluid intake is carefully calculated to equal output plus 500 mL to account for insensible loss. If the client is conscious, oral intake must be considered in the 24-hour total. The fluid intake should be spread evenly over the 24-hour period. IVs should be closely monitored, using a limited-volume device or a volume control apparatus for accuracy. Accurate intake and output measurement and daily weights are important parameters to assess fluid balance. Diarrhea and diaphoresis should be included as output.

Output is monitored to detect problems related to diabetes insipidus (increased urinary output) and inappropriate secretion of ADH (SIADH; decreased urinary output). Diabetes insipidus may result in severe dehydration unless treated. The usual treatment is pitressin (see Chap. 42). SIADH results in dilutional hyponatremia, which adversely affects LOC. Electrolyte determinations should be made daily and any abnormal values discussed with the physician.

Monitoring Intracranial Pressure It is possible to directly measure intracranial pressure by the use of a monitoring device in the subarachnoid, epidural, or subdural spaces and the ventricles of the brain (Fig. 54-8). Several techniques are available, but in general a catheter or screw is placed through a hole drilled in the skull and positioned in the proper place. A stopcock and tubing are attached. A transducer is connected to convert the pressure waves into electrical currents which can be displayed on an oscilloscope or a recording instrument. Complications related to the insertion and placement of the equipment include CSF leak and infection.

Intracranial pressure is a fluctuating measurement with three distinct, identified pressure waves (Fig. 54-9). *A, or plateau, waves* are present when intracranial pressure is greatly elevated and may last for 5 to 20 minutes. *B waves* indicate intracranial pressure in the 20 to 50 mmHg range and are present for $\frac{1}{2}$ to 2 minutes. The significance of *C waves* has not yet been determined.

Inaccurate intracranial pressure readings can be caused by leaks, obstruction of the screw, difference in height of the screw and the transducer, kinks in the tubing, and the Valsalva maneuver.[9] It may be necessary to flush the tubing, using sterile technique, if it is suspected that readings are not accurate. It is important to provide enough tubing to allow for nursing activities and client movement; but lengths over 4.25 m (14 feet) can cause inaccurate readings. Daily cleansing of the site is important to reduce the possibility of infection.

Certain equipment used for intracranial pressure monitoring can also be used to drain CSF for relief of cerebral edema. If this is not possible, a ventriculostomy can be done and a drainage system instituted. It is important that the amount of CSF removed be carefully monitored to avoid brainstem herniation due to a sudden decrease in pressure. As with intracranial monitoring equipment, it is the responsibility of the

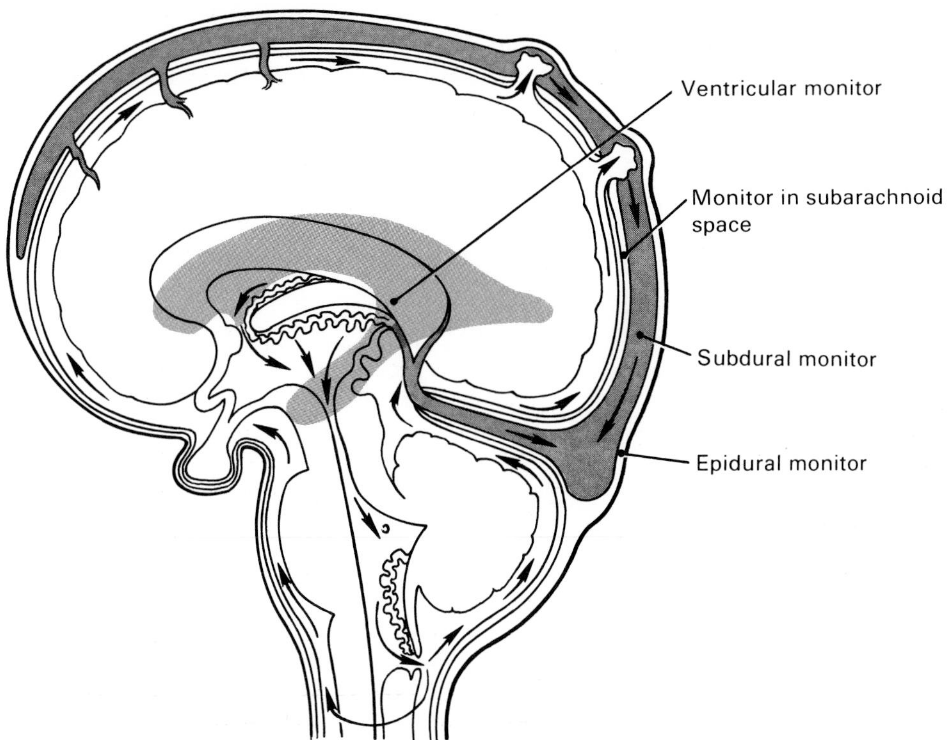

Figure 54-8 Location of CSF and CSF Monitor points. (*From M. Snyder and M. Jackle, Neurologic Problems: A Critical Care Nursing Focus, Robert J. Brady Co., Bowie, Md., 1981, p. 177.*)

nurse to maintain strict sterile technique when handling the equipment to ensure intactness of the system and to carefully record results.

Body Position and Function The cerebral venous system does not have valves, so it is dependent upon gravity for proper drainage. The prone position has been demonstrated to increase intracranial pressure. Elevation of the head of the bed assists cerebral venous drainage and aids in reducing cerebral edema and IICP. Because intracranial pressure is normally increased in a sitting position, the client should not be put in Fowler's position. The head of the bed should usually be elevated about 30° unless ordered otherwise. This elevation is used for both back and side-lying positions.

Since rapid position changes cause an increase in intracranial pressure, the client should be turned and handled with slow, gentle movements. Every care should be used to prevent discomfort in turning and in positioning, since pain or agitation also increases pressure. Hip flexion and neck flexion should be avoided. Every-4-hour turning and skin care offers a good balance between adequate care and reduced stimulation. If pressure-monitoring equipment is in place, care must be used not to dislodge it. With decerebrate or decorticate posture or with the client unable to move, passive range-of-motion (ROM) exercises are carried out to avoid contractures. Slow, gentle, movements will prevent pain in rigid muscles and not unduly increase pressure.

Protection from Injury and Environmental Management The client often needs protection from self-injury due to confusion or seizures. Restraints

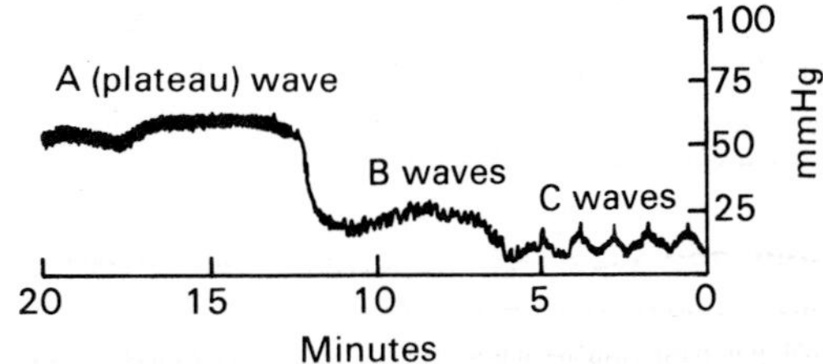

Figure 54-9 Intracranial pressure waves. Composite diagram of A (plateau) waves, B waves, and C waves. (*From N. Holloway, Nursing the Critically Ill, Addison-Wesley Publishing Company, Inc., Menlo Park, Calif., 1978.*)

should be used judiciously but may be necessary to keep the client from removing tubes or falling out of bed. If the client becomes agitated or struggles against the restraints, they should be removed and alternative methods of protecting him instituted. Ideally it is best to have someone with the client, either a nurse or a family member. Seizure procautions should be taken for all persons with IICP, such as administration of anticonvulsants, padded siderails, and close observation.

The client will benefit from a quiet, nonstimulating environment with a decreased light level. The nurse's approach should be calm and reassuring. At the same time sensory deprivation must also be avoided. Touching and talking to the client, even the comatose one, are appropriate. There is need for a balance between deprivation and overstimulation based on the individual client situation.

Psychological Considerations If the client is conscious, he will probably be aware of the concern of the staff related to his neurological status. The neurological checks are a regular reminder of a potential worsening of his condition. The family is also usually extremely anxious and concerned about the client's condition. The nurse's competent and assured manner as she goes about her duties is reassuring. Short, simple explanations to client and family are appropriate.

If the client is in an altered state of consciousness, the nurse must recognize the anxiety and confusion this causes him. It is often at this point that the client with IICP is transferred to a critical care unit—a move that adds to his anxiety and confusion. The family needs to be assured that the transfer is made to provide opportunity for more individualized care than is available on a general unit.

The client who is unconscious from IICP is often admitted directly to a critical care unit. If the neurological problem is related to trauma, other injuries may be present. In spite of the client's apparently unconscious state, the nurse should carefully explain all treatments and contacts to him. The client's family will need support and consideration during this time. The nurse should assess the family and involve them in the client's care on the basis of this assessment and should determine whether spiritual counseling is appropriate.

Factors Contributing to IICP Nurses need to be alert for activities and situations which are known to increase intracranial pressure. Interventions aimed at eliminating these are an important part of the care for the client with IICP. Table 54-5 lists factors which contribute to IICP.

Table 54-5

Contributory Factors in Increased Intracranial Pressure

1. Hypercapnia (P_aCO_2 more than 42 mmHg)
2. Hypoxemia (P_aO_2 less than 50 mmHg)
3. Certain cerebral vasodilating agents such as halothane anesthesia and antihistamines
4. Valsalva's maneuver
5. Certain body positions (prone, flexion of neck, or extreme hip flexion)
6. Isometric muscle contractions
7. Coughing or sneezing
8. REM (rapid eye movement) sleep
9. Emotional upset
10. Arousal from sleep

Joanne Hickey, *The Clinical Practice of Neurological and Neurosurgical Nursing,* J. B. Lippincott Company, Philadelphia, 1981, p. 152.

HEAD TRAUMA

Head injury includes any trauma to the scalp, skull, or brain. For the purpose of this section, the term *head trauma* is used primarily to signify craniocerebral trauma, which includes an alteration in consciousness no matter how brief.

Significance

Statistics regarding the actual occurrence of head injuries are incomplete because many victims die at the scene of the accident or the condition is considered minor and health care is not sought. Mortality related to head injury is approximately 24 per 100,000 population in the United States.[10] Car accidents are the most common cause. Other common causes of head injury include assaults, boxing, football, horseback riding, and alcohol-related accidents.

Etiology and Pathophysiology

Head trauma is classified as indirect or direct. Indirect injury is secondary to compression or rebounding of the contents of the brain. Direct trauma results from penetration or impact immediately causing craniocerebral damage. Direct injuries may be further classified as (1) *closed*—no fractures present; (2) *open*—the skull may have a simple fracture or a depressed (compound) fracture with bone fragments lacerating the vessels, meninges, or brain tissue; or (3) *penetrating*—the cranial cavity is entered by an external object.

A closed injury is potentially more dangerous than an open injury. Trauma to the head transmits shock waves to the brain tissue, causing varying degrees of damage in the form of contusion, hemorrhage, and cerebral edema. In an open injury from a skull fracture, much of the impact is absorbed and not transmitted, so that, while bleeding and local damage to brain tissue may occur, generalized internal damage to the brain and the risk of IICP are reduced.

In closed head injuries two phenomena may occur. First, the *acceleration-deceleration* phenomenon occurs when the head is thrown forward and then backward. An example of this is the sudden stopping of a car and the resulting impact. In this type of injury, contents of the cranial vault are moved about from within, striking bony prominences in the temporal-parietal or frontal areas of the inner skull. The second phenomenon, the *coup-contrecoup*, involves damaged areas both below the site of impact (coup) and on the opposite side away from the injury (contrecoup). The impact causes the brain to rebound off the opposite side of the inner skull, thus causing more generalized damage. Additionally, the upper brain may rotate on its axis (brainstem), causing torsion and stretching of blood vessels and nerve tracts. These shearing stresses may result in rupture, hemorrhage, and nerve disruption.

With penetrating head injuries, the extent of the damage depends on the type of missile entering the skull as well as the depth and location of the injury. Head injuries may result in various pathological problems including concussion, contusions or bruising, laceration, hemorrhage, and fractures. Some degree of cerebral edema accompanies almost all these injuries. The edema results from both a cellular inflammation and increased production of cerebrospinal spinal fluid. Intracranial pressure may be increased, depending on the extent and site of the injury.

Clinical Manifestations

Concussion

Concussion is a head injury accompanied by an immediate, brief period of unconsciousness without normal neurological signs. There may be a brief period of respiratory arrest and bradycardia. Reflexes are absent. Spontaneous recovery is usual.[11]

Headache is a common complaint following concussion, with a brief period of nausea, vomiting, and diplopia. These problems do not persist. If the client is alert and responsive, he will be discharged from the health care setting with instructions to consult a physician if symptoms persist or if behavior changes are noted. However, if the accident was very serious or if behavioral changes are present, the client may be admitted for diagnostic tests and observations.

Behavioral changes are related to the areas of the brain affected as described in the coup-contrecoup phenomenon. While it is not fully understood what actually occurs within the brain, it has been suggested that when the brain hits the bony prominences within the skull there is mild edema and "shock" to the lobes underlying that area. Disruption of the prefrontal lobes results in irrational, bizzare behavior that is often immature and without social restraint. Swearing, combativeness, restlessness, and irritability are common. Temporal lobe disruption produces temporary amnesia, altered perception, and confusion. Thus the client does not remember the accident and may be disoriented to time, place, and occasionally person. Because of the altered perception and memory loss, the client may be confused and frightened by the environment and may misinterpret the actions of those who are trying to help.

While concussion is generally benign and resolves spontaneously within minutes to days, the signs and symptoms may be preliminary to more serious, progressive disease. Poor management may fail to detect evidence of IICP, thus increasing brain damage.

Contusion

A contusion is a bruise serious enough to cause hemorrhage of the vessels on the surface of the brain without penetrating the pial covering. It frequently occurs at the site of fracture or as the result of contrecoup injury. The bleeding is usually minimal and contained at the area of injury and is reabsorbed slowly. This may cause a focal deficit such as a temporary weakness of an extremity or a focal seizure.

Laceration

A laceration involves tearing of the cortical surface of the brain and occurs most commonly with a depressed, compound skull fracture or as a result of a penetrating injury. External bleeding may be quite profuse, but unless brain tissue is severely damaged, signs of neurological disruption are uncommon. If bleeding is deep within the brain parenchyma, focal signs or seizures will be present, as with contusion.

Intracranial hemorrhage

Intracranial hemorrhage may occur into the extradural, subdural, or subarachnoid spaces or into the brain or ventricles. Depending upon the site and rate of bleeding, symptoms may occur immediately or several months after the injury.

Epidural Hematoma When a large vessel (usually an artery) which lies in the dura mater is severed, either by a skull fracture or by a severe direct blow, an epidural or extradural hematoma forms (Fig. 54-10*a*). Hemorrhage occurs into the epidural space which lies

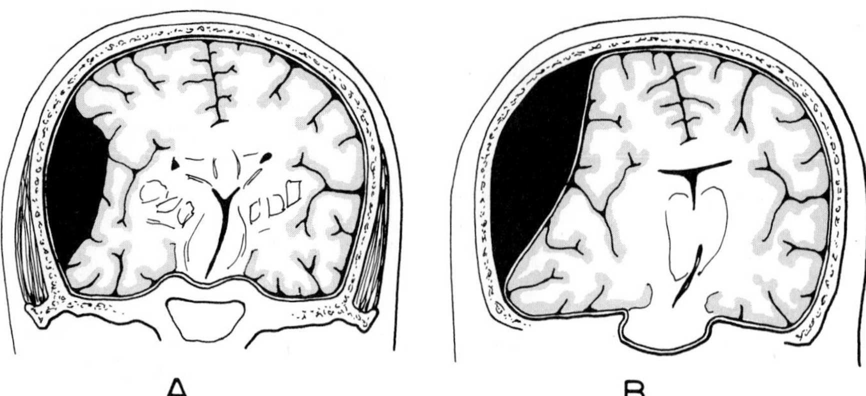

Figure 54-10 *(a)* Subdural hematoma, usually a result of laceration of the subdural veins. *(b)* Epidural hematoma in the temporal fossa, usually a result of laceration of the middle meningeal artery. [*From S. A. Price and L. M. Wilson (eds.), Pathophysiology: Clinical Concepts of Disease Processes, 2d ed., McGraw-Hill Book Company, New York, 1982.*]

between the dura and the surface of the skull. The more common site for epidural hemorrhage is where the middle meningeal artery lies close beneath the thin temporal bone. Since this is an arterial hemorrhage, the hematoma forms rapidly, and ipsilateral (same side) signs of increased pressure occur quickly. Memory loss and confusion are seen, followed by rapid decrease in LOC. Without immediate intervention, mortality approaches 100 percent.[12] Tentorial herniation occurs with contralateral decerebrate activity and pupil dilation and fixing on the affected side. Death follows shortly. The person with a temporal injury will often present with obvious bruising at the site.

Subdural Hematoma A subdural hematoma usually results from injury to the brain substance and its parenchymal vessels. The veins that drain the brain's surface into the sagittal sinus are the source of most subdural hematomas (Fig. 54-10*b*). The sagittal sinus lies in a potential space between the inner aspect of the dura and the arachnoid space where the CSF circulates. Veins may bleed into this space and produce a typical hematoma. Unlike the arterial epidural hematoma, the subdural hematoma is venous in origin and therefore is much slower in developing a mass large enough to produce symptoms. However, a subdural hematoma may be caused by an arterial hemorrhage, in which case it develops more rapidly.

Subdural hematomas may be acute, subacute, or chronic (Table 54-6). An acute subdural hematoma manifests signs within 48 hours of the injury. The signs and symptoms are similar to those associated with IICP and include decreasing LOC and headache. The client appears drowsy and confused. The ipsilateral pupil dilates and becomes fixed. A subacute subdural hematoma usually occurs within 2 to 14 days of the injury. Failure to regain consciousness may point to this possibility.

A chronic subdural hematoma develops over weeks or months following a seemingly minor head injury. The peak incidence of chronic subdural hematoma is in the sixth and seventh decades of life, because brain atrophy with age allows more room for expansion. With atrophy, the brain remains attached to the various supportive structures, but with increased tension it is subject to tearing. The larger size of the subdural space also accounts for the focal symptoms rather than the signs of IICP as the presenting complaint.[13] Chronic alcoholics are also prone to cerebral atrophy and subsequent development of subdural hematoma.

Delay in diagnosis in the older adult can be attributed to the fact that the symptoms mimic other health problems in the elderly, including vascular disease and senile dementia; somnolence, confusion, lethargy, and memory loss are associated with other health problems in addition to subdural hematoma. The client history includes head trauma in only 60 to 70 percent of cases.[14]

Other Hemorrhages Severe head injury may also result in intracerebral hematoma and subarachnoid hemorrhage. An intracerebral hematoma manifests as a space-occupying lesion with unconsciousness, hemiplegia on the contralateral side, and a dilated pupil on the side with the clot. As the hemato-

Table 54-6
Comparison of Acute, Subacute, and Chronic Subdural Hematomas

	Acute	Subacute	Chronic
Occurrence in relation to time of accident	24–48 h	48 h–2 weeks	Weeks, months, years; longer than 20 days
Progression of symptoms	Immediate deterioration	Initially unconscious, gradual improvement, then deterioration over hours; dilated pupils; ptosis	Nonspecific; nonlocalizing; progressive alterations in LOC
Incidence of bilaterality	50 percent	Many	Many
Treatment	Evacuation and decompression	Evacuation and decompression	Evacuation and decompression; membranectomy
Type of trauma	Severe	Severe	Trivial; nonexistent or forgotten; incident known by only 60–71%; most common 6th and 7th decades of life

ma expands, symptoms of IICP become more severe. Prognosis is poor. Subarachnoid hemorrhage produces signs and symptoms of nuchal rigidity, headache, deteriorating LOC, hemiparesis, and ipsilateral dilated pupil. It may produce an intraventricular hemorrhage.

Fracture

There are four types of skull fracture (Table 54-7). A fracture may be closed or open, depending on the presence of a laceration of the scalp or an extension of the fracture into the middle ear or paranasal sinuses. The type and severity of a skull fracture depends upon the velocity, momentum, and direction of the injuring agent and the location of the impact.[15] Specific manifestations of a skull fracture depend on the location of the injury (Table 54-8). The type of fracture and severity of injury must be considered before the total clinical picture is clear.

It is often necessary to determine whether there is drainage of cerebrospinal fluid. Cerebrospinal fluid drainage from the ear or nose can be differentiated from mucoid or purulent drainage by the use of Testape or other agent which tests CSF for the presence of glucose. Cerebrospinal fluid will give a positive reading for sugar.

Medical Management

In addition to measures to prevent or manage IICP and to maintain bodily functions, the principal

Table 54-7
Comparison of Types of Skull Fractures

Type	Description	Cause
Linear	Break in continuity of bone without altering relationship of parts	Low-velocity injuries
Comminuted	Multiple linear fractures with fragmentation of bone into many pieces	Direct, high-momentum impact
Depressed	Displacement of comminuted fragments	Indentation due to powerful blow
Compound	Depressed skull fracture and scalp laceration with communicating pathway to intracranial cavity	Severe head injury

Table 54-8
Clinical Manifestations of Skull Fractures by Location

Location	Symptoms/Sequelae
Frontal fracture	Exposes brain to contaminants through frontal sinus; may be associated with air in the forehead tissue, CSF or cortex rhinorrhea, or pneumocranium
Orbital fracture	Periorbital ecchymosis (Coon's eyes)
Temporal fracture	Boggy temporal muscle due to extravasation of blood, benign oval-shaped bruise behind the ear in mastoid region (Battle's sign), CSF, or cortex otorrhea
Parietal fracture	Deafness, CSF or brain otorrhea, blood or CSF bulging the tympanic membrane, facial paralysis, loss of taste, and Battle's sign
Posterior fossa fracture	Occipital bruising resulting in cortical blindness, visual field defects; rarely ataxia and other cerebellar signs
Basilar skull fracture	CSF or brain otorrhea, blood or CSF bulging the tympanic membrane, Battle's sign, tinnitus or hearing difficulty, facial paralysis, conjugate deviation of gaze, and vertigo

Adapted from Joan E. Davis and Celestine B. Mason, *Neurologic Critical Care,* Van Nostrand Reinhold Company, New York, 1979, pp. 111–112.

treatment of head injuries is quick diagnosis and surgery. For the client with concussion and contusion, observation and management of IICP are all that is usually necessary.

For lacerations, bleeding is arrested and the wound sutured if necessary. If the skull is depressed and loose fragments are present, these are removed and the bone elevated. It may be necessary to perform a cranioplasty, with insertion of a bone or artificial graft. If cerebral edema is present, this treatment may be deferred for several months. Antibiotics may be given to prevent infection.

For epidural and subdural hematomas, the blood may be removed through burr holes (openings into the skull made by a twist drill) in the rostral part of the subdural collection. The dura and outer membrane of the subdura are perforated and the hematoma evacuated. Bone wax, gel foam, and electrocoagulation can be used through the burr holes for prolonged bleeding. A Jackson-Pratt drain (similar in function to a Hemovac) may be left in place for several days.[16]

In some cases of epidural and subdural hematoma a craniotomy may be necessary. A craniotomy is an opening of the skull by surgically creating a bone flap. It is done in order to provide direct visualization of the brain. The bone flap may remain attached to other muscles or be completely removed for greater operative access. A cranioplasty may be done later (6 months to 1 year) to repair the defect. When a craniotomy is necessary, it is usually performed to ligate bleeding blood vessels. Since manipulation of the brain tissue causes an increase in cerebral edema, a flap of bone may be removed to allow the brain to expand outward until the edema subsides. The scalp is loosely attached over this site, but the area remains vulnerable to external pressure.

Basal skull fractures may cause CSF drainage from the nose or ears. It is important to observe for signs of meningitis because of the potential entry for infection. Nose and throat cultures are done to establish flora. Since these leaks usually seal off in 10 to 14 days, no further treatment is necessary. The client is instructed not to plug up the nose or ear with cotton, but a loose "snuffer"-type gauze dressing may be used.

Nursing Management

Health maintenance and promotion

One of the best ways to prevent head injuries is to prevent car and motorcycle accidents. The nurse can be active in campaigns promoting driving safety and can speak to driver's education classes regarding the dangers of unsafe driving and driving after drinking. Wearing seat belts in cars and helmets with motorcycles is the greatest measure for survival during accidents. The speed limit of 55 mph has dramatically reduced fatalities within the United States. Wearing of protective helmets by lumberjacks, construction workers, miners, horseback riders, and sky divers is also recommended. The nurse should be familiar with data on outcomes with and without safety devices in working with groups who oppose safety legislation as an infringement of personal freedom. Young parents should be educated in the proper use of car seats and restraints for their children. The nurse should also teach younger children about safety in bicycle riding, skateboarding, and contact sports.

Acute intervention

The general nursing management of the head-injured client may be only observation for changes in neurological status; or the client's condition may deteriorate rapidly, leading to emergency surgery requiring appropriate pre- and postoperative nursing interventions.

It is important that the nurse explain the need for frequent neurological assessments to both the client and the family. Behavioral manifestations associated with head injury can result in a frightened, disoriented client who is combative and resistive to help. The nurse's approach should be calm and gentle. Restraints should be avoided if possible, since they often produce agitation, which further elevates intracranial pressure. A family member may be available to stay with the client to prevent increasing anxiety and fear.

The nurse should perform neurological checks at intervals based on the client's condition. The Glasgow Coma Scale is a useful tool in assessing level of consciousness (see Fig. 49-1). Indications of a deteriorating neurological state such as decreasing LOC or lessening of motor strength should be reported to the physician and the client's condition closely monitored.

Much of the nursing care for the brain-injured client relates to the unconscious state and IICP (Table 49-3). (Nursing care for these problems is presented elsewhere in this text.) However, specific problems may occur which require nursing intervention.

Eye problems may include loss of the corneal reflex, periorbital ecchymosis and edema, and diplopia. Loss of the corneal reflex may necessitate taping the eye shut to prevent abrasion and using eye drops to lubricate. Periorbital ecchymosis and edema will disappear spontaneously, but warm and cold compresses provide comfort and hasten the process. Diplopia can be relieved by using an eye patch.

Hyperthermia may occur from infection or injury to the hypothalamus. Increased metabolism secondary to hypothermia increases metabolic waste, which in turn produces further cerebral vasodilatation. Specific nursing measures for the febrile client are presented later in this chapter.

Nursing measures specific to the care of the immobilized client such as those related to bladder and bowel function, skin care, and infection, are also indicated.

If clear rhinorrhea occurs, the nurse should elevate the head of the bed 30° and test for sugar. A positive test for sugar indicates leakage of CSF, and the physician should be notified immediately . The client should remain quietly in bed. For comfort and to collect drainage, the nurse should place a wick of gauze in the nostril or tape a rolled dressing at the outlet of the nasal orifice. The client should be cautioned not to blow his nose. To prevent aspiration of brain tissue, the nurse should never perform nasal suction when fracture of the cribriform plate is suspected. Any discharge from the ear should also be tested and a loose dressing secured to collect the drainage.

Nausea and vomiting may be a problem and can be alleviated by antiemetic medication. Headache can usually be controlled with aspirin or small doses of codeine.

If the client's condition deteriorates, intracranial surgery may be necessary. A burr hole or craniotomy may be indicated, depending upon the underlying injury which is causing the symptoms. (Nursing care of the client undergoing intracranial surgery is discussed under Intracranial Tumors.)

Often the client will be unconscious prior to surgery, making it necessary for a family member to sign the consent for surgery. This is a difficult and frightening time for the client's family and requires sensitive nursing management. The suddenness of the situation makes it especially difficult for the family to cope.

The emergency nature of the surgery may prevent the usual careful preoperative preparation. The nurse should consult with the neurosurgeon to determine specific preoperative nursing measures.

Chronic management and sequelae of head injury

Once the client's condition has stabilized, he will usually be transferred to a general neurological unit for rehabilitation. As with any craniocerebral problem, chronic problems may result related to motor and sensory deficits, communication, and memory and intellectual functioning. Many of the principles of nursing management of the client with a stroke (Chap. 52) are appropriate. With time and patience, many of the chronic problems subside or disappear.

Specific manifestations of posttraumatic syndrome include nervous instability, epilepsy, and mental and emotional problems. Nervous instability includes such problems as headache, dizziness, intolerance of noise, emotional excitement in crowds, tenseness, restlessness and apprehension, inability to concentrate, and intolerance of usual amounts of alcohol.[17]

Clients describe the headache as like a tight

Table 54-9
Comparison of Major Intracranial Tumors

Tumor	Tissue of Origin	Percent of All Brain Tumors	Usual Locations	Malignant/Benign
Gliomas				
Astrocytoma	Supportive tissue: glial cells and astrocytes	20	White matter of frontal and temporal lobes in adults, lateral cerebellar lobes in children	Moderately malignant grades I and II
Glioblastoma multiforme	Primitive stem cell (glioblast)	20	Cerebral hemispheres	Highly malignant and invasive, grades III and IV
Oligodendroglioma	Glial cells and dendrites	2	Cerebral hemispheres: most in frontal lobe, some in basal ganglia and cerebellum	Benign—encapsulates and calcifies
Ependymoma	Ependymal epithelium	1	Lateral and fourth ventricles—usually in children and young adults	Varies from benign to highly malignant; most benign and encapsulated
Medulloblastoma	Supportive tissue	1	Posterior fossa, 4th ventricle, brainstem; almost exclusively in children	Highly malignant, invasive, metastatic to spinal cord and remote areas of brain
Meningioma	Endothelial cells, fibrous tissue elements, transitional cells, angioblasts	25	Arachnoid villi, dura; half located over convexity of hemisphere and half at base of hemisphere	Benign, encapsulated; outside of brain substance
Acoustical neuroma (Neurofibroma)	Sheath of vestibular portion of VIIIth cranial nerve	5	Between pons and cerebellum	Benign or low-grade malignancy; encapsulated
Pituitary adenoma	Pituitary glandular tissue	10	Pituitary gland	Usually benign
Vascular tumors Arteriovenous malformation	Overgrowth of arteries and veins which steal blood and enlarge from feeder vessels	3	Parietal cortex near middle cerebral vessels	Benign
Metastatic tumors	Primary sites in lungs, breast, kidney, thyroid, prostrate	8	Cerebral cortex, diencephalon	Malignant

Rate of Growth	Prognosis with Treatment
Moderately slow	Rarely cured—death by 2 years from time of surgery; slightly longer with radiation and chemotherapy
Rapid	Incurable: death 6–9 months after surgery, 1–1½ years with radiation and chemotherapy
Very slow	Cure with surgical removal but usually cannot remove totally because of location—3–5 years survival with partial surgery and radiation
Moderate	Cure with complete removal, extended survival with partial removal and radiation
Rapid	Complete removal impossible; 2–3 years survival with radiation
Very slow	Complete removal possible but because of size may need to be done in two stages. Cure with complete removal—occasionally only partial—only because of location, but still long survival
Slow	Complete surgical removal accompanied by high operative mortality and complete facial paralysis; intracapsular enucleation has less neurodeficit but higher recurrence; mental disruption and deafness may persist
Very slow	When involving only pituitary, good results with radiation; if extended to sella turcica, surgical removal restores vision
Slow	Clipping or cryosurgery of feeder vessels and removal of "tumor" may result in minimal disability
Related to primary tumor	Surgery only palliative, extends life 2–3 months; good response of some tumors to radiation and chemotherapy with 1–2 years life extension

band around the head, similar to a tension headache. The onset of the headache may be as much as 6 months after the injury. Localization is frequently in the occipital or neck regions, and for some the severity of symptoms is incapacitating. Etiological theories for headache include pain in the scalp scars, neuralgia of the occipital or supraorbital nerves, hydrocephalus, precipitation of migraines in susceptible persons, trauma to the soft tissue, or irritation of preexisting spondolysis.[18]

Dizziness, another symptom occurring after minor to severe trauma, is hypothesized to originate from labyrinthine concussion and damage to the hearing mechanism. Seizure disorders occur in approximately 5 percent of those clients with nonpenetrating injuries. In 25 percent of cases, seizure disorders have their onset 4 years or more after the initial injury.[19] Anticonvulsant therapy is usually effective. Most of the manifestations related to nervous instability wane with time.

The mental and emotional sequelae of brain trauma are often the most incapacitating problems. It is estimated that over 60 percent of all head-injured clients who have been comatose for more than 6 hours undergo some personality change. They may suffer loss of concentration, memory loss, and defective memory processing. Personal drive may decrease, while apathy and apparent laziness may increase. Euphoria and lability, along with a seeming lack of awareness of the seriousness of the injury, mark their affect. The client's behavior may indicate a loss of social restraint, judgment, tact, and emotional control.[20]

Progressive recovery may continue for 6 months or more before a plateau is reached and a prognosis for recovery can be made. Specific nursing management in the posttraumatic phase depends on specific residual deficits.

In all cases the family must be given special consideration. They need to understand what is happening to their loved one, be taught appropriate interaction patterns, given guidance and referrals for financial, child care, or other personal needs, and be assisted to involve the client in family activities whenever possible.

INTRACRANIAL TUMORS

Description

Tumors within the cranial cavity cause approximately 2 percent of all deaths.[21] There are 15,000 cases of brain tumor diagnosed each year, accounting for 10 to 15 percent of all malignant disease. Brain tumors rank tenth in men and twelfth in women as a cause of cancer death.

Tumors of the brain may be primary, arising from some tissue within the brain, or secondary, due to metastasis from a malignant neoplasm elsewhere in the body. They may be malignant or benign. Brain tumors arise from any tissue within the brain and may be found in any location. They are generally classified according to the tissue from which they arise. If malignant, the tumor is graded according to general cancer staging procedures (Table 11-9). Brain tumors may be classified as (1) inside the brain substance (e.g., gliomas or vascular tumors) or (2) outside the brain substance (e.g., meningiomas or cranial nerve tumors). Probably more than half the intracranial tumors are malignant, infiltrate the brain parenchyma, and are not amenable to complete surgical removal. Other tumors may be benign histologically but are so located that complete removal is not possible. Brain tumors are more commonly seen in middle age but may occur at any age.

Unless treated, all intracranial tumors would eventually cause death from increasing tumor volume leading to IICP. Brain tumors rarely metastasize outside the central nervous system because of their containment by structural (meninges) and physiological (blood-brain) barriers. Table 54-9 compares the major intracranial tumors.

Clinical Manifestations

The clinical manifestations of intracranial tumors are generally due to the local destructive effects of the tumor and the resulting accumulation of metabolites and to IICP. Table 54-10 summarizes the general manifestations of intracranial tumors. The rate of growth and appearance of manifestations depend upon the location and type of the tumor. Table 48-1 describes the functional areas of the cerebrum. Figure 54-11 illustrates the functional areas of the cerebral cortex and can be used as a guide to correlate manifestations with location to aid in locating the site of a tumor.

Complications

If the tumor mass obstructs the ventricles or occludes the outlet, ventricular engorgement can occur (hydrocephalus). Surgical treatment is needed to relieve the pressure and involves placement of either a ventriculoatrial or ventriculoperitoneal shunt. A catheter is placed in the ventricle to provide drainage and a distal catheter tunneled through the skin to drain into either the right atrium or the peritoneum. Rapid decompression can cause prostration and headache, so the client is gradually introduced to the upright position. The client should be instructed to avoid contact sports to prevent a blow to the valve or severing of the catheter. If signs of IICP such as headache, blurred vision, vomiting without nausea, decreasing LOC, or restlessness occur, the physician should be notified. Signs of an infected shunt such as high fever, persistent headache, or stiff neck warrant investigation.[22]

Table 54-10

Clinical Manifestations of Intracranial Tumors

Headache, vomiting, papilledema
Focal neurological deficits (motor, sensory, cranial nerve dysfunction)
Seizure activity
Endocrine dysfunction secondary to pituitary dysfunction
Cerebrospinal fluid obstruction
Personality changes

Medical Management (Table 54-11)

Treatment goals are aimed at (1) identification of tumor type and location; (2) removal or decreasing of the tumor mass; and (3) preventing or managing IICP.

The type and location of the tumor are determined by a variety of diagnostic measures. A careful history and physical examination may provide data as to location. CT scan and brain isotope scan provide the most reliable diagnostic information. The EEG is useful but of less importance. A lumbar puncture is seldom diagnostic and carries with it the risk of uncal herniation.

Surgery

Surgery is the best form of treatment for brain tumors. However, the outcome depends on the type and location of the tumor. Meningiomas and oligodendromas are usually amenable to complete removal, while the more invasive gliomas and medulloblastomas can be only partially removed. Surgery will reduce tumor mass, which decreases intracranial pressure and provides relief of symptoms, with an extension of survival time. Tumors located in the deep central areas of the dominant hemisphere, posterior corpus collosum, or upper brainstem cause extensive neurological damage and are considered inoperable.

Radiation and chemotherapy

Radiation therapy has been found to lengthen survival in clients with malignant gliomas, expecially when radiation is combined with partial surgical removal. Less malignant tumors have responded to

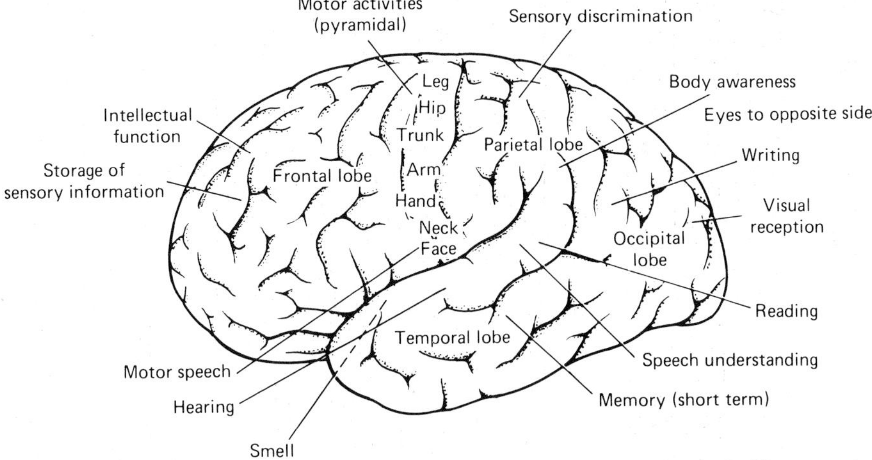

Figure 54-11 Localized functional areas of the cerebral cortex. [*From M. R. Kinney et al. (eds.), AACN's Reference for Critical Care Nursing, McGraw-Hill Book Company, New York, 1981, p. 119.*]

radiation with longer survival time and decreased tumor recurrence. Edema and rapidly increasing intracranial pressure may be a complication of radiation therapy but can be managed with high doses of corticosteroids.

Normally the blood-brain barrier will prohibit the entry of most drugs into the brain. However, it has been shown that the tumor abolished the blood-brain barrier at the specific tumor location, so chemotherapeutic drugs can be used to treat the tumor.[23] Different chemotherapeutic drugs are used to attach tumor growth in different stages. Currently used drugs include amethopterin (methotrexate), vincristine sulfate (Oncovin), and benzamide (Procarbazine). Brain tumors which cannot be totally removed may be treated with a combination of surgery, radiation, chemotherapy, and steroids. While progress in treatment has increased both length and quality of survival of clients with malignant gliomas, death is inevitable, because the tumor grows at a faster rate than it can be destroyed. The medical management of IICP is summarized in Table 54 -4.

Nursing Management

Acute intervention

Assessment The initial assessment of the client with a brain tumor is made to provide baseline data. Specific areas to assess include:

Functional abilities;
Localizing manifestations
Neurological status, including mental, motor, sensory, proprioceptive, reflexes, and cranial nerves
Chronology of symptoms
Pain
Seizure activity
Manifestations of IICP

Table 54-11
Medical Management: Intracranial Tumors

Diagnostic
1. History and physical examination
2. Neurological examination
3. EEG
4. CT scan
5. Skull x-rays
6. Visual field examination
7. Brain scan
8. Biopsy

Therapeutic
1. Dexamethasone IV
2. Anticonvulsant therapy
3. Surgical excision
4. Radiation therapy
5. Chemotherapy

Pain Management Pain, especially headache pain, can be so severe that the person may consider suicide for relief. Care must be taken to find a method of relief that will not severely alter the LOC or dangerously depress respiration. Some clients receive relief from mild analgesics such as aspirin or codeine, while others seem to be unaffected by any drugs. "Brompton's cocktail," a mixture of morphine, cocaine, alcohol, and flavoring syrup, has been found particularly useful. The use of marijuana is still in the initial stages of experimentation, and more time is needed to document its effectiveness.[24] Phenothiazines such as prochlorperazine (Compazine) and chlorpromazine (Thorazine) may be useful adjuncts to analgesics. Other pain-relieving measures are discussed in Chap. 50.

Behavioral Changes Behavioral changes can be quite devastating for both client and family. Frontal lobe tumors cause loss of emotional control, which may result in behavior ranging from catatonic apathy to intermittent rages. The client may demonstrate purposeless, continuous activity, be confused and wander from his familiar environment, cease any self-care activities, and no longer recognize family or friends. In the early stages, when behavior swings are intermittent, the client may recognize that he is "not himself" and may experience shame, depression, and fear of hurting himself or others. Later, the impact of this behavior falls on the family, who may become afraid of the client and avoid him or may carry the burden of protecting him from self-harm and carrying out all the activities of daily living, including toileting. Some families take the behavior personally and become angry or depressed. The end result can be a loss of the love, caring, and support which the client so desperately needs.

It is important for the nurse to help the family understand the reason for the behavior changes and encourage them to support the medical treatment. They need assistance in designing a care program for managing the client's needs and in continuing to give him closeness and love. When the behavior becomes unmanageable to them or adversely affects children, the client needs to be hospitalized.

During hospitalization the nurse must provide optimal safety for the client. Techniques that may be useful include close supervision of activity; labeling the wanderer; siderails and body restraints as needed; padded, locked rooms for the very violent; and attending to physiological and hygiene needs. The nurse needs to manage her own fear and aversion to these behaviors so that she can deal with the client with caring, gentleness, and objectivity. The family and client need an opportunity to discuss feelings and concerns and receive nonjudgmental support from the nurse. Mental health referral may be useful for the more disturbed families. If the client is in a terminal condition working through the stages of grieving is desirable.

Suicide should be considered a potentially significant problem, since these clients are at risk because of pain, depression, and altered perception. Close observation, counseling, and crisis intervention techniques are useful.[25]

Physical Changes Seizures frequently occur with brain tumors and are managed by anticonvulsant drugs and seizure precautions. It should be recognized that some of the behavioral disorders are in fact seizure disorders (see Chap. 51) and show much improvement with medication.

Motor and sensory dysfuntions are problems which interfere with activity and self-care abilities. Problems of immobility need to be managed and the client assisted to do as much for himself as possible within his limitations. The unconscious client needs total care. See Chap. 49 for nursing management of these problems.

Adequate nutrition must be maintained, especially if surgery is anticipated. The client may need encouragement to eat or in some cases may need feeding orally, parenterally, or by nasogastric tube.

Language and perceptual defects may occur and may be manifested by expressive or receptive aphasia, agnosia, apraxia, loss of stereognostic perception, and so on (see Chap. 52 for definition and management). Clients receiving radiation and chemotherapy have special needs which are discussed in Chap. 11.

Surgical Intervention The general pre- and postoperative nursing care for the client undergoing cranial surgery is similar whether the underlying cause is tumor or trauma.

The family and client (if conscious and coherent) will be gravely concerned about the potential physical and emotional problems that could result from the surgery. The uncertainty regarding prognosis and outcome requires compassionate nursing care in the preoperative period.

The nurse should be providing emotional support while completing the usual preoperative preparation (see Chap. 6) and activities specific to cranial surgery. In addition to a complete diagnostic workup and gathering of baseline assessment data, the client's hair is washed according to procedure. It is important that the client understand that the scalp must be shaved to allow better exposure and prevent contamination. The family should be informed of the expected length of the operation and that the client will be taken to the intensive care unit following a short stay in the recovery room.

The care of the client following a craniotomy is summarized in Table 54-12. Positioning and turning of

Table 54-12
Nursing Care Plan for the Client with Craniotomy

Client Problem	Expected Outcome	Nursing Intervention
Increased Intracranial pressure	No permanent decrease in neurological functioning	Establish baseline of neurological function immediately upon return from OR. Neurological checks q h until stable; then q 4 h for at least 72 h postop. Report significant changes. Measure and record intracranial pressure q 1–4 h. Maintain monitoring equipment in functioning condition. Aseptic care of insertion site. Protect equipment from being dislodged. Administer diuretics and corticosteroids as ordered. Position with head-of-bed angle increased to 30°. Avoid neck and hip flexion. Handle gently—turn only q 4 h. Prevent constipation and straining with defecation (see Possible constipation, below). Manage elevated temperature (see Table 54-15). Use measures to decrease agitation and hyperactivity (see Headache and Potential seizures, below).
Respiratory dysfunction: atelectesis, possible respiratory depression, possible alterations in respiratory patterns	Patent airway. No rales or rhonchi. Aeration of all lobes. ABS within normal limits. No respiratory distress or infection	Assess all respiratory parameters q 2 h for 72 h, then q 4–8 h. Draw and evaluate ABG regularly. O_2 per prongs or mechanical ventilator until ABG stable—at least 24–72 h. Gentle coughing and turning—position on side with head slightly hyperextended if LOC decreased. Suction gently and for only brief periods if necessary. Hyperventilate and hyperoxygenate with Ambu bag before and after each coughing or suctioning session. Avoid sedatives or narcotics. Observe for gastric distension—insert nasogastric tube if indicated and maintain patency. Report any consistent alterations in breathing patterns such as apnea, central neurogenic hyperventilation. Tracheostomy or endotracheal tube with artificial ventilation if necessary. Culture any abnormal secretions. Avoid suctioning through nose if sinus fractures are present.
Headache	Decreased complaints of pain. No decrease in LOC. Able to rest	Assess location, type, duration, degree, and severity of pain. Administer mild analgesics as ordered and evaluate effects. Position as comfortably as possible (see IICP, above). Keep environment quiet, darken room, put cool cloth on eyes.
Possible fluid, electrolyte, and nutritional imbalance	No dehydration or overhydration. No cerebral edema. Electrolytes normal. No negative nitrogen balance or excessive weight gain or loss	Assess fluid status regularly: orthostatic BP, skin turgor, urine output, urine sp. gr., eyeball turgor, mucous membranes, edema. Keep accurate fluid balance evaluation. Monitor electrolytes. Weigh daily. Maintain fluid restrictions as ordered. Oral fluids when tolerated—evaluate ability to swallow. Advance to high protein, high calorie, small frequent feedings as tolerated. Feed client if necessary. If unable to eat, administer tube feedings q 3–4 h or TPN prn.
Possible incontinence and constipation	No incontinence. Soft, formed stools. No straining	Insert indwelling catheter in acute period if necessary for fluid management or control ability altered. Use condom catheter (male) or bedpan-urinal training for chronic management. Use stool softeners, suppositories, small enemas as necessary to prevent constipation. Include roughage and cellulose in diet. Instruct client not to strain at stool.
Potential infection; potential brain injury	No wound infection. No pressure injury to exposed brain tissue	Observe dressing for excessive drainage, circle area each shift, report if excessive, describe type. Observe for cerebrospinal fluid: pale yellow halo around serum or blood. Reinforce dressing when wet, and change reinforcements prn. Consult with surgeon before changing primary dressing. When able, observe wound for healing, redness, induration, swelling. If bone flap removed, identify area and do *not* allow client to lie on the site. Keep any drainage tubes free from kinking and protect from dislodging. Assess for pain at incision site and report (usually insensitive).

Table 54-12 (Continued)

Client Problem	Expected Outcome	Nursing Intervention
Potential seizures; altered LOC	No seizure activity. No self-injury. Decreased anxiety or restlessness	Administer anticonvulsive medications as ordered. Use seizure precautions with careful observations and documentation if seizure occurs. Use siderails prn and at night. Avoid restraints if possible; family or nurse should stay with client if very agitated or confused. Use calm, gentle, reassuring approach. Give frequent reorientation and simple explanation of procedures. Plan balance of quiet and sensory stimulation. Reduce noise and activity near client. Touch frequently and talk to client, even if nonresponsive.
Decreased mobility; possible motor-sensory loss	No complications of immobility. Optimal functioning based on residual abilities. No injury from falls	Assess level of motor-sensory abilities. Ambulate as soon as possible postop (within 8 h for uncomplicated surgery) at least q 4 h. Assist with ambulation to protect from falls—have enough help! Up in chair frequently if unable to ambulate, especially for meals. Give frequent skin massage, alternating pressure mattress heel protectors, etc., for bed clients. Teach client safe transfer procedures. Assist client to understand limitations and abilities. Give gentle ROM, especially with decorticate-decerebrate rigidity. Consult with physiotherapist for best rehabilitation program for client—carry out and assist in teaching client.
Possible CSF leak from nose and/or ears	Leak sealed up in 1–2 weeks. No meningitis	Assess for clear or slightly yellow drainage from ears or nose. Clinitest drainage, report to physician if positive. Carry out cultures of nose and throat. *Do not* plug nose or ears with cotton—loose "snuffer"-type gauze dressing can be used for comfort (change frequently). Watch for temperature elevation, irritability, headache, or nuchal rigidity and report state. Administer antibiotics if ordered.
Anxiety over prognosis	Understanding of disease and prognosis. Evidence of decreased anxiety. Acceptance of disabilities. Participation in rehabilitation. Ability to move through stages of grieving if indicated	Assess client's level of understanding of illness—what physician has told him. Collect best information about client's status, prognosis, and predicted functional abilities. Explain to client and family, using multiple teaching techniques; evaluate client's and family's level of comprehension. Share information on rehabilitation programs and community resources. Assist family to use resources and support groups. Encourage participation in self-care. Assist in ventilation of feelings and concerns.
Alteration of body image: hair loss, possible alteration of motor-sensory function or facial appearance	Positive self-image. Acceptance of disabilities	Save hair removed before surgery and give to family or client. Provide attractive surgical caps when dressings removed. Encourage wigs until hair grows out. Inform client of *possible* change in color, texture, etc., of new hair. Promote use of cosmetics to enhance appearance for women, shaving for men. Assist in adjustment to other body changes by patience and nonjudgmental handling of anger, etc. Be honest about appearance but focus on remaining positive qualities and abilities and encourage their development. Assist through grieving process.

the client depend on the site of the operation. If it is infratentorial (incision slightly above the nape of the neck), the client will usually be kept off his back for 48 hours. Flexion is contraindicated to prevent tearing of the suture line. The head of the bed is gradually elevated over a period of days. With supratentorial incision (above the tentorium and directly over the operative area), the head of the bed is elevated 30 to 45°. If the surgeon has removed part of the skull (craniectomy) to allow for swelling, the client should be positioned on the operative side to avoid direct pressure on the brain. Neurological signs should be monitored closely, with frequency determined by client status.

The dressing should be observed for color, odor, and amount of drainage. The physician should be notified immediately of excessive bleeding or clear drainage. A too tightly wrapped dressing can cause increased cerebral edema. Fluids and electrolytes are monitored closely in order to detect inappropriate ADH or the onset of diabetes insipidus. Before the diet is increased, the client should be tested for the presence of swallow and gag reflexes, especially following infratentorial surgery. Medications are given to reduce edema, prevent seizures, reduce straining during elimination, and minimize pain. Respiratory management is discussed at the beginning of the chapter.

Scalp care should include meticulous care of the incision to prevent meningitis. The area should be cleansed with povidone-iodine (Betadine), and followed by application of an antibiotic ointment. Use of an antiseptic soap for washing the scalp may also be beneficial. The psychological impact of baldness may be alleviated by a wig, turban, or surgical cap. The itching that occurs when the hair growth returns may be most uncomfortable for the client. For the client receiving radiation, use of a sunblock and head covering is advocated when sun exposure is planned.[26]

Chronic management

The rehabilitative potential for a client after intracranial surgery is dependent upon the reason for the surgery, the postoperative course, and the client's general state of health. The nursing intervention must be based on a realistic appraisal of these factors. An overall goal for the nurse is to foster independence for as long as possible and to the highest degree possible.

Specific rehabilitation potential cannot be determined until cerebral edema and IICP subside postoperatively. Care must be taken to maintain as much function as possible through such measures as careful positioning, meticulous skin and mouth care, regular range-of-motion exercises, bowel and bladder care, and adequate nutrition.

Referrals may need to be made to other specialists on the health care team. For instance, the speech therapist may be helpful in assisting the client with a speech problem. The needs and problems of each client should be addressed individually, since many variables affect the plan.

Mental and emotional residual deficits are often more difficult for the client and family to accept than motor and sensory losses. The nurse can provide much help and support during the adjustment phase and for long-range planning.

The mental and physical deterioration, including seizures, personality disorganization, apathy, and wasting, is hard for both family and health professionals to endure. Although progress is being made for the client with a brain tumor in chemotherapy, conventional and interstitial radiation, and immunotherapy, the prognosis remains grim.

INFLAMMATORY CONDITIONS OF THE BRAIN

Meningitis, encephalitis, and brain abscesses are the most common inflammatory conditions of the brain and spinal cord. These can be caused by bacteria, viruses, fungi, cancer necrosis, rupture of tumors, and chemical irritation (e.g., contrast media used in diagnostic tests). Bacteria are the most common cause and include organisms such as *Streptococcus pneumoniae*, *Hemophilus influenzae*, *Neisseria meningitidis*, and *Staphylococcus aureus*. Bacterial meningitis is the most common problem and has the highest mortality; it is considered a medical emergency. Central nervous system infections may enter from the bloodstream, by extension from a primary site, by the oral and nasopharyngeal route, through the cerebrospinal fluid, by extension along cranial and spinal nerves, and in utero.[27]

Meningitis

Pathogenesis

Meningitis is an inflammation of the meninges of the brain and spinal cord. The subarachnoid space is secondarily involved. The organisms usually gain entry to the central nervous system through the upper respiratory tract but may also enter by direct extension from penetrating wounds of the skull or through fractured sinuses in basal skull fractures.

Meningitis usually occurs in the fall, winter, or early spring and is often secondary to viral respiratory diseases. Children under 6, the elderly, and the debilitated are more often affected. *Streptococcus pneumoniae* causes about 30 percent of the cases.

The inflammatory response to the infection tends to increase cerebrospinal fluid production, with a moderate increase in pressure. The purulent secretion produced quickly spreads to other areas of the brain via the cerebrospinal fluid. If this process extends into the brain parenchyma or a concurrent encephalitis is present, cerebral edema and IICP become more of a problem. All clients with meningitis must be observed closely for manifestations of IICP. These manifestations are thought to be due to swelling around the dura, increased CSF volume, and endotoxins produced by the bacteria.

Clinical manifestations

Severe headache with photophobia accompanied by fever of 39 to 41°C (102.2 to 105.8°F) are primary clues to meningitis. Signs of meningeal irritation such as nuchal rigidity (stiff neck) and flexion rigidity of the muscles of the legs are seen, as well as general irritability, anorexia, nausea and vomiting, malaise, and photophobia. Brudzinski's signs and Kernig's sign are positive (see Chap. 48). Confusion and seizures are present in some cases. Petechiae on lower extremities and trunk occur in 75 percent of meningococcal infections. The history usually reveals a respiratory infection or "flu" prior to onset. Any client with a basal skull fracture or penetrating injury to the head should be observed for signs of meningitis.

Mumps and measles viruses can cause both meningitis and encephalitis. Early back and leg aching and sore throat are common manifestations of these following mumps and measles immunizations.

Abnormal diagnostic findings

Changes in cerebrospinal fluid due to bacterial meningitis are described in Table 54-13. Serum lactic dehydrogenase (LDH) is greater than 40U/L, a finding that helps to differentiate bacterial from viral infections. Serum white count is elevated to 20,000 to 40,000 uL, with a predominance of neutrophils in bacterial infection and lymphocytes in viral infections. Sedimentation rate and blood glucose are elevated. RBC, hemoglobin, and hematocrit may show anemia if the client is not well dehydrated.

Complications

Disseminated intravascular coagulation (DIC) is a serious complication in 10 to 20 percent of meningitis clients, especially in meningitis caused by gram-negative organisms. It is a cause of death in only about 1 percent. Abnormal coagulation studies demonstrate this problem, as well as evidence of increased bruising or bleeding from an area of the body (urinary tract, GI tract, gums, etc.) For a more complete discussion of DIC, see Chap. 24.

Medical management (Table 54-14)

Rapid diagnosis based on history and physical examination is crucial, since the client is usually in a crisis state when health care is sought. When meningitis is suspected, antibiotic therapy is instituted even before the diagnosis is confirmed. Diagnostic measures include lumbar puncture and analysis of cerebrospinal fluid. Eye grounds should be examined for papilledema prior to the lumbar puncture for identification of possible IICP.

Penicillin and ampicillin are the drugs of choice, with chloramphenicol used for persons allergic to penicillin. Nafcillin can be used for gram-negative organisms. These drugs are effective because of their ability to penetrate the blood-brain barrier.

Nursing management

Health Promotion and Maintenance Prevention of respiratory infections through vaccination programs for pneumococcal pneumonia and influenza should be supported by nurses. In addition, early and vigorous treatment of respiratory and ear infections is important. Persons in close contact with anyone with meningitis should be given prophylactic antibiotics.

Table 54-13
Comparison of Cerebral Inflammatory Conditions

	Meningitis	Encephalitis	Brain Abscess
Causative organisms	Bacteria, yeasts, fungi, viruses, pneumococcus, meningocococcus, streptococcus	Bacteria, fungi, parasites, herpes simplex virus, other viruses	Streptococcus, staphylococcus via the bloodstream
Cerebrospinal fluid			
Pressure (60–150 mmH_2O)	Increased	Normal to slight; increased if severe IICP	Increased
Cells (WBC: 0–8 μL, RBC: none)	500/μL, mainly polymorphonuclear (PMN)	Less than 500; early PMN, later lymphocytes	25–300/μL neutrophils and lymphocytes
Protein (lumbar: 15–45 mg/dL)	High	Slight increase	75–300/μL
Glucose (45–75 mg/dL)	Low or absent	Normal	
Appearance	Turbid	Clear	Clear
Diagnostic studies	Stained smears and cultures	Viral studies with specialized techniques to isolate	CT scan, EEG, skull x-ray
Treatment	Antibiotics with sensitivity tests	Supportive, prevent symptoms of IICP; Vidarabine (Vira-A)	Antibiotics, incision and drainage

Rifampin is effective for this purpose and prevents a carrier state but is very expensive.

Acute Intervention The client with meningitis is usually acutely ill. The fever is high and resistant to aspirin. Head pain is severe. Irritation of the cerebral cortex may result in seizures. Mental status and level of consciousness are dependent on intracranial pressure.

Initial assessment should include vital signs, neurological checks, intake and output, breath sounds, and skin. These should be measured at intervals based on the client's condition and recorded carefully.

Headache pain and neck pain secondary to movement require attention. Codeine provides some pain relief without undue sedation for most clients. The client should be assisted to a position of comfort, often curled up with head slightly extended. The head of the bed should be slightly elevated when permitted after lumbar puncture. Keeping the room darkened and a cool cloth over the eyes relieves the discomfort of photophobia.

For the delirious client, additional low light may be necessary to decrease hallucinations. All clients suffer some degree of mental distortion and hypersensitivity and may be frightened and misinterpret their environment. Every attempt should be made to minimize environmental stimuli and the resulting exaggerated perception. Restraints should be avoided. Padded siderails with sheets tied to the four corners may be used to prevent injury to the client. Arm boards secured with multiple layers of stretch gauze such as Kerlix will protect the IV infusion site. A familiar person at the bedside will have a calming effect. The nurse needs to be efficient with care but also to project an attitude of caring and of unhurried gentleness. The use of touch and a soothing voice to give simple explanations of activities is helpful. If seizures occur, appropriate observations should be made and protective measures taken. Anticonvulsant medications are administered as ordered. Problems associated with IICP are managed as described earlier in this chapter.

Fever must be vigorously managed by the nurse because of its effect of increasing cerebral edema and seizures (Table 54-15). In addition, neurological damage may result from an extremely high temperature over a prolonged time. Aspirin should be administered, since it is useful in reducing fever and its anti-inflammatory effects are therapeutic. However, if the fever is aspirin-resistant, more vigorous means are necessary. The automatic cooling blanket is the most efficient method. Care should be taken not to reduce the temperature too rapidly, since shivering may result, causing a rebound effect and increasing the temperature. The extremities should be protected from "frostbite" by wrapping them in sheepskin, soft towels, or a blanket covered with a sheet. Skin care should be given frequently to prevent breakdown. If a cooling blanket is not available or desirable, tepid sponge baths with a mixture of alcohol and water may be effective in lowering the temperature. The skin needs to be protected from excessive drying or injury.

Table 54-14
Medical Management: Cerebral Inflammatory Problems

Diagnostic

1. History and physical examination
2. Analysis of cerebrospinal fluid
3. CBC, electrolytes, glucose, prothrombin time, platelet count
4. Routine urinalysis
5. Blood cultures × 2
6. Urine specific gravity q 4 h
7. CT scan
8. EEG
9. Skull x-rays
10. Brain scan

Therapeutic

1. Strict bed rest
2. IV fluids
3. Penicillin IV
4. Chloramphenicol IV
5. Codeine for headache
6. Aspirin for temperature of 38°C (100.4°F)
7. Hypothermia
8. Clear liquids as desired/tolerated
9. Phenytoin IM

Since high fever greatly increases the metabolic rate and thus insensible fluid loss, the client should be assessed for dehydration and adequacy of intake. Diaphoresis further increases fluid losses, which should be estimated and included in an intake-and-output recording. Replacement fluids should be calculated as 800 mL for respiratory losses and 100 mL for each degree of temperature above 38°C (100.4°F). It is essential that the designated antibiotic schedule be followed to maintain therapeutic blood levels. Observations should be made for side effects of the drugs used.

With the exception of meningococcal meningitis, meningitis usually no longer requires isolation. However, good aseptic technique is essential to protect both the client and the nurse. It is recommended that a mask be worn for direct client contact and be changed with each contact. Visitors should also be masked, and no young children should be allowed in the room.

Table 54-15
Nursing Care Plan for the Febrile Client

Client Problem	Expected Outcome	Nursing Intervention
Core body temperature >37.8°C (100°F)	Core body temperature 37.8°C (100°F). No damage to skin as a result of antipyretic measures	Take temperature q 2–4 h, more often if hypothermia used. Administer antipyretic drugs orally or rectally q 4 h. Keep environment temperature 21.1°C (70°F). Avoid heavy layers of clothing or bed covers. Give tepid sponge baths (half alcohol-half water). Use skin lotion to prevent drying. Change linen frequently if profusely diaphoretic. Use hypothermia blanket. Reduce temperature gradually. Protect extremities by sheepskin or wrapping in soft towels. Frequent application of lotion to entire body. Sedate if necessary to prevent chilling.
Increased metabolic rate	Normal metabolic rate	Force fluids to 3–4 L/day if tolerated. Monitor vital signs q 2–4 h. Administer IV fluids if necessary. Accurate intake and output, careful estimate of insensible losses. Assess for dehydration. Weigh daily. High calorie, high protein, easily digested food and fluids. Conserve energy. Keep balance between activity and rest.
Delirium/seizures	Minimal or no seizure activity. No evidence of physical injury	Administer anticonvulsant and sedative medication as ordered. Keep room quiet, dim lights. Use calm, reassuring approach. Avoid use of restraints. Keep siderails padded. Assist and support patient during uncomfortable or frightening diagnostic procedures.
Discomfort due to anxiety, headache, muscle-joint aches, malaise	Minimal or no pain. Decreased restlessness and anxiety	Administer mild analgesia prn. Assist to position of comfort in bed. Encourage gentle ROM and leg exercises. Massage muscles prn. Environmental control to encourage rest.

Chronic Rehabilitative Management After the acute period has passed the client will require several weeks of convalescence before normal activities can be resumed. In this period good nutrition should be stressed, with emphasis on a high protein, high calorie diet in small, frequent feedings.

Muscle rigidity may persist in the neck and the back of the legs. Progressive range-of-motion exercises and warm baths are useful. Activity should be gradually increased as tolerated, but adequate bed rest and sleep should be encouraged. A variety of quiet activities, based on an assessment of individual interests, should be encouraged to prevent boredom.

Residual effects are uncommon in meningococcal meningitis, but pneumococcal meningitis results in sequelae such as dementia, epilepsy, deafness, hemiplegia, and hydrocephalus in 30 percent of affected clients.[28] Vision, hearing, cognitive skills, and motor and sensory abilities should be assessed after recovery, with appropriate referrals as indicated. Meningitis in infancy may have "silent" neurological sequelae which manifest as learning and behavior problems when the child reaches school age.[29]

Throughout the acute and convalescent periods, the nurse should be aware of the anxiety and stress experienced by the client's significant others. The public considers spinal meningitis a serious and usually fatal illness. The family need to be supported and involved in care as much as possible.

Encephalitis

Encephalitis is an acute inflammation of the brain usually caused by virus. Many different viruses have been implicated in encephalitis, some of them endemic to certain seasons and geographical areas. Epidemic encephalitis is transmitted by ticks and mosquitoes. Nonepidemic encephalitis may occur as a complication following measles, chicken pox, or mumps.

Encephalitis is a serious, sometimes fatal, disease. Mortality ranges from 5 to 20 percent, with the highest fatality in encephalitis due to herpes simplex and eastern and Venezuelan equine viruses. Manifestations resemble those of meningitis but have a more gradual onset and include headache, high fever, convulsions, and change in LOC. Medical and nursing management is symptomatic and supportive. Cerebral edema is a major problem, with hypertonic solutions and steroids used to control it. The pathology is characterized by diffuse damage to the nerve cells of the brain, perivascular cellular infiltration, proliferation of glia, and increasing cerebral edema.[30] Idoxuridine, cytosine arabinoside (ara-C), and vidarabine suspension (Vira-A) have been approved for treatment of herpes simplex encephalitis. Vidarabine appears to be the most promising, with mortality reduced from 70 to 28 percent. For maximal benefit the medication must be started prior to the onset of coma.

The potential toxicity of vidarabine requires that nurses be knowledgeable about the method of administration and side effects.[31] The sequelae of encephalitis include mental deterioration, amnesia, personality changes, and hemiparesis.

Brain Abscess

Brain abscess is an accumulation of pus within the brain tissue which can result from a local or systemic infection (Fig. 54-12). Direct extension from ear, mastoid, or sinus infection is the primary cause. Other foci include septic venous thrombosis from pulmonary infection, bacterial endocarditis, skull fracture, and unsterile neurological procedures. Streptococcus and staphylococcus are the primary infective organisms.

Manifestations are similar to meningitis and encephalitis and include headache and fever. Signs of IICP may include drowsiness, confusion, and seizures. Focal symptoms may be present and reflect the local area of the abscess. For instance, visual field defects or psychomotor seizures are common in temporal lobe abscess, while occipital abscess may present with visual impairments and hallucinations.

Antimicrobial therapy is the primary treatment for brain abscess. Other manifestations are treated symptomatically. If pharmacological management is not effective, the abscess may need to be drained or removed if encapsulated. In untreated cases mortality approaches 100 percent. Epilepsy occurs in approximately 30 percent of the cases. Nursing measures parallel those for meningitis or for IICP.

Other infections of the brain include subdural empyema, osteomyelitis of the cranial bones, epidural abscess, and venous sinus thrombosis after periorbital cellulitis.

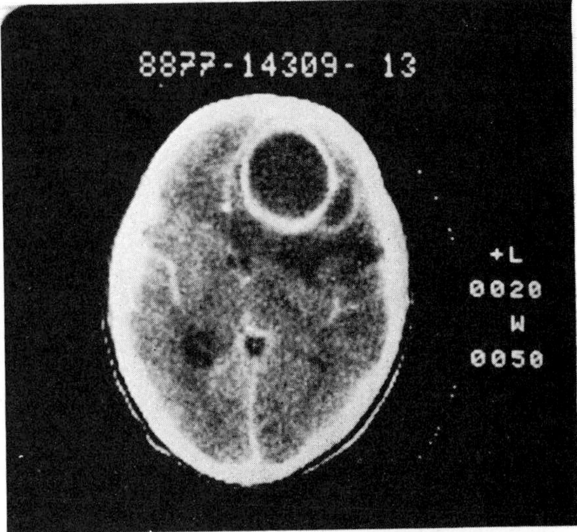

Figure 54-12 Brain scan showing frontal lobe abscess with adjacent daughter abscess and edema of surrounding brain. [*From K. Isselbacher et al. (eds.), Harrison's Principles of Internal Medicine, 9th ed., McGraw-Hill Book Company, New York, 1980, p. 1907.*]

Case Study / Head Injury

Thomas M. is a 44-year-old college professor who was admitted to the intensive care unit with a diagnosis of head injury and possible concussion due to a motor vehicle accident. Information from the ambulance attendant suggests that he may have fallen asleep while driving home, run off the road, and hit a telephone pole. He was unconscious briefly after the accident but alert on admission, though he did not remember what happened to him or why he was at the hospital. During morning report, the staff reported that he became very agitated and verbally and physically abusive, requiring the use of full leather restraints. His wife went home in tears, distressed by his aggressive behavior. He became increasingly noisy, so IV diazepam was ordered. The nurse reported next morning that he was "nice and quiet," with vital signs and laboratory tests within normal limits. Neurological checks had not been done, since staff did not want to wake him up.

When he is assessed at 8 A.M. it is noted that he cannot be roused except by noxious stimuli. Observation shows Cheyne-Strokes respiration, and during the apneic phase he assumes decorticate posture. His pupils are small but reactive. The Babinski sign is positive. Blood pressure is 150/62, pulse 60.

Discussion Questions

1. What was the cause of Mr. M.'s combative behavior?
2. Analyze the management he received in the first 12 hours. What, if anything, would you do differently?
3. What were the causative factors in his change of status by morning?
4. What level of brain function seems to be affected?
5. On the basis of the nursing assessment, what are priority interventions?
6. What could be said to Mrs. M. about her husband's condition? What additional data might be elicited from her?

REVIEW QUESTIONS

The number of the question corresponds to the same-numbered objective at the beginning of the chapter.

1. Clinically significant increased intracranial pressure is defined as
   a. any pressure elevation over 15 mmHg
   b. sustained pressure of 50 mmHg for at least 2 hours
   c. transient pressures over 100 mmHg when sneezing
   d. sustained pressure of 100 mmHg for more than 15 minutes

2. Which of the following compensatory mechanisms is *not* physiologically useful in managing pressure changes within the cranial cavity?
   a. displacement of CSF into the spinal subarachnoid space
   b. herniation of the temporal lobes through the tentorial notch
   c. increased absorption of CSF by the venous system
   d. compression of the venous system

3. Which one of the following admitting medical orders might be written for a client with proven or suspected IICP?
   a. Ambulate every 4 hours.
   b. IV's of D5/W at 150mL/hour
   c. Place on hypothermia blanket and keep temperature at 36°C (96.8°F).
   d. Meperidine hydrochloride 100 mg prn for pain.

4. At the lower pontine-upper medullary level, which of the following abnormal signs would most often be noted?
   a. high blood pressure with wide pulse pressure
   b. decorticate posture
   c. pinpoint, reactive pupils
   d. neurogenic hyperventilation

5. The best position for the client with IICP is
   a. head of bed angle increased to 30°, on back or side-lying without neck or hip flexion
   b. supine with bed flat, head turned to left
   c. high-Fowler's position with knee flexion and legs elevated
   d. head of bed angle increased to 30° side-lying with hips and knees flexed

6. Shock waves are strongly transmitted to the brain through the skull in which of the following types of direct head injury?
   a. depressed fracture (open)
   b. linear fracture (open)
   c. closed
   d. penetrating

7. The most common manifestations of concussion are
   a. paresthesias
   b. field cuts
   c. seizures
   d. behavoral changes

8. The main general focus of medical treatment for the client with head injury is
   a. preventing or managing IICP
   b. preventing future head injuries
   c. preventing infection
   d. surgery

9. The combination treatment of choice for brain tumors which cannot be totally removed surgically includes all the following *except*
   a. radiation
   b. chemotherapy
   c. cryosurgery
   d. steroids

10. Effective management of behavioral manifestations should focus on
    a. teaching the wife or husband assertive behavior
    b. isolating the client for his own safety and that of others
    c. explaining to the client how disturbing his behavior is to others
    d. assisting the family in handling their feelings

11. Postsurgical care after a craniotomy includes which of the following nursing orders?
    a. frequent neurological checks, keeping the client flat in bed for 48 hours, limited IV fluids progressing to oral feedings
    b. intracranial pressure measurements, ambulation as soon as tolerated, suctioning every 2 hours
    c. neurological checks, changing of head dressing every 4 hours, gentle pulmonary toilet
    d. frequent neurological checks, elevation of head of bed to 30° and avoidance of neck and hip flexion

12. The three key signs and symptoms which are primary clues to meningitis are
    a. severe headache, fever 39°C(102°F), nuchal rigidity
    b. general irritability, nausea and vomiting, fever 39°C(102° F)
    c. severe headache, fever 37.2 to 37.8°C (99 to 100°F), anorexia
    d. nuchal rigidity, normal temperature, lassitude

13. The most critical assessments for the nurse to perform for the client with a cerebral inflammatory problem include
    a. pain, neurological checks, GI functions
    b. neurological checks, seizures, breath sounds
    c. pain, seizures, skin
    d. neurological checks, breath sounds, skin

REFERENCES

1. Mariah Snyder and Mary Jackle, *Neurologic Problems: A Critical Care Nursing Focus,* Robert J. Brady Co., Bowie, Md., 1981, p. 42.
2. Joanne Hickey, *The Clinical Practice of Neurological and Neurosurgical Nursing,* J. B. Lippincott Company., Philadelphia, 1981, p. 145.
3. Hickey, op. cit., p. 146.
4. F. Plum and J. Posner, *The Diagnosis of Stupor and*

Coma, 2d ed., F. A. Davis, Philadelphia, 1972, pp.72–92.

5. K. Jamieson, *A First Notebook of Head Injury,* Butterworth Scientific Publications, London, 1971.

6. Jean Kaktis and Lawrence Pitts, "Complications Associated with Use of Megadose Corticosteroids in Head-Injured Adults," *J Neurosurg Nurs,* **12**(3):166–179 (September 1980).

7. Ibid.

8. Pamela Mitchell, "Intracranial Hypertension: Implications of Research for Nursing Care," *Neurosurg Nurs,* **12** (3):152 (September 1980).

9. Snyder and Jackle, op. cit., p. 184.

10. Bryon Jennett, and Graham Teasdale, *Management of Head Injuries,* F. A. Davis Company, Philadelphia, 1981, p. 60.

11. Jamieson, op. cit.

12. Barbara Krajewski, "Head Injury: Preventing Life Threatening Complications, in *Coping with Neurologic Problems proficiently, Nursing Skillbook,* Intermed Communications, Horsham, Pa., 1979, chap. 5, pp. 85–98.

13. Willa Adelstein, "Chronic Subdurals," *Neurosurg Nurs,* **12** (1):36–45 (March 1980).

14. Ibid.

15. Joan Davis and Celestine Mason, *Neurologic Critical Care,* Van Nostrand Reinhold Company, New York, 1979, p. 108.

16. J. Kunkel and J. Wiley, "Acute Head Injury: What to do When . . . and Why," *Nursing,* **9**(3):33 (March 1979).

17. Hickey, op. cit., p. 247.

18. Jennett, op. cit., pp. 256–272.

19. Ibid., pp. 272–278.

20. Ibid., pp. 289–299.

21. A. Lieberman and J. Ransohoff, "Treatment of Primary Brain Tumors," *Med Clin North Am,* **63**(4):835–46 (July 1979).

22. Carol Mayberry, "Intracranial Tumors: Giving Expert Pre and Post Op Care," in *Coping with Neurologic Problems Proficiently, Nursing Skillbook,* Intermed Communications, Horsham, Pa., 1979, Chap. 7, p. 137.

23. Lieberman, op. cit.

24. A. Lipman, "Drug Therapy in Cancer Pain," *Cancer Nurs,* **3**(1):39–46 (February 1980).

25. M. Maxwell "Cancer and Suicide," *Cancer Nurs,* **3**(1):33–36 (February 1980).

26. Mayberry, op. cit, pp. 127–138.

27. Hickey, op. cit., p. 432.

28. Kurt Isselbacher et al. (eds.), *Harrison's Principles of Internal Medicine,* 9th ed., McGraw-Hill Book Company, New York, 1980, p. 1962.

29. J. Picardi, "Bacterial Meningitis," *Continuing Educ,* **10** (4):53–65 (April 1979).

30. Barbara L. Conway, *Carini and Owens' Neurological and Neurosurgical Nursing,* The C. V. Mosby Company, St. Louis, 1978, p. 343.

31. Carol Swisher and Alice Williams, "Herpes Encephalitis: A Nursing Challenge," *J Neurosurg Nurs,* **13**(1):34–37 (1981).

Chapter 55

NURSING ASSESSMENT
Musculoskeletal System

Kenneth J. Webb
Sharon Mantik Lewis
Idolia Cox Collier

Learning Objectives

1. Describe the gross anatomical and microscopic structure of bone.
2. Explain the classification system of joints and movements at synovial joints.
3. Describe the function of cartilage and soft-tissue structures of the musculoskeletal system, including muscle, ligaments, tendons, fascia, and bursae.
4. Identify the significant subjective and objective data related to the musculoskeletal system that should be obtained from a client.
5. Describe the appropriate techniques used in the physical assessment of the musculoskeletal system.
6. Differentiate normal from common abnormal findings of a physical assessment of the musculoskeletal system.
7. Describe the purpose, significance of results, and nursing responsibilities related to diagnostic studies of the musculoskeletal system.

Human beings are capable of performing complex and precise movements. Proper functioning of the musculoskeletal system allows such movements, permitting interaction and adaptation to the environment. The musculoskeletal system consists of bones (skeletal system), muscles (muscle system), joints (articular system), cartilage, ligaments, tendons, fascia, and bursae.

The musculoskeletal system is particularly vulnerable to external environmental forces. These forces can cause alteration in the structure of bone or soft connective tissue, resulting in functional disruption. The consequences may be deformity, alteration of body image, pain, or permanent disability. These problems often produce long-term health problems which interfere with activities of daily living and the quality of life.

MUSCULOSKELETAL SYSTEM: STRUCTURES AND FUNCTIONS

Bone

Function of bone

The three main functions of bone are support, protection, and movement. Bone supports the skeletal framework and the surrounding tissues. Without this support the body would collapse. A second function of bone is protection of the vital organs and soft tissue. For example, the skull protects the brain and the rib cage protects the lungs and heart. A third function, movement, occurs as a result of the functioning of bone as a lever for muscles. Muscles are anchored to bones by tendons. Movement occurs as a result of muscular contraction force applied to the levers. The joint serves as a fulcrum.

Bone tissue also has physiological functions. Bone contains marrow which is involved in hematopoiesis. It also serves as a site for the storage of calcium and phosphate.

Gross structure of bone

Bone is a dynamic tissue which changes form and substance continually. It is composed of both organic (collagen) and inorganic material (calcium, phosphate). Internal and external growth and remodeling are continuous processes.

Bone is classified according to structure as compact (dense) or cancellous (spongy). In compact bone, haversian systems (see Microscopic Structure of Bone) fit closely together, giving a dense consistency to the bone structure. In cancellous bone there are many open spaces between thin processes and networks of bone tissue.

The best example of the anatomical structure of bone is the typical long bone (e.g., femur). Each long bone consists of epiphysis, articular cartilage, diaphysis, periosteum, and medullary (marrow) cavity (Fig. 55-1).

The *epiphysis* is the end of long bones and is composed of cancellous bone. It is the location for

This chapter was reviewed by Phyllis Gappa Jensen, M.S.N., Teacher in Associate Degree Nursing, Madison Area Technical College, Madison, Wisconsin.

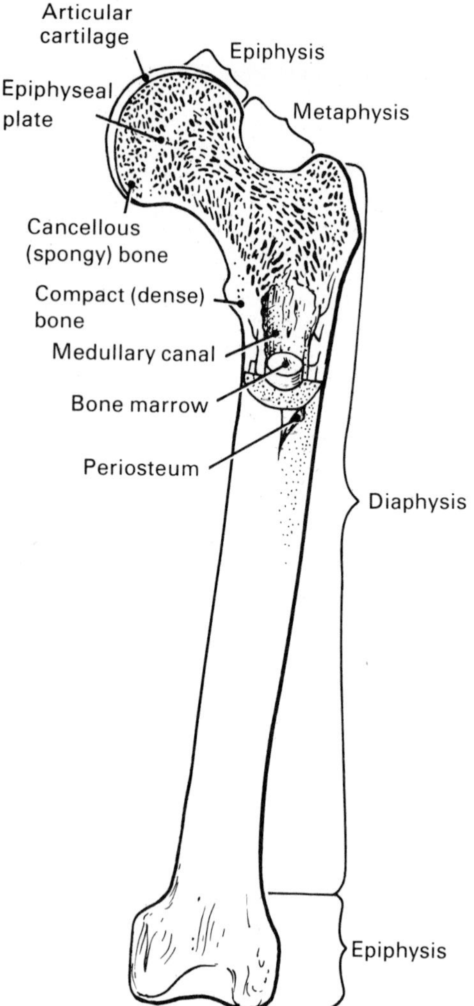

Figure 55-1 Anatomical structure of a typical long bone (femur).

muscle attachment and increases the stability of the joint. *Articular cartilage* covers the ends of bone and provides smooth surfaces for joint movement.

The *diaphysis* is the main shaft of bone and provides structural support. It is composed of compact bone. The *metaphysis* is the flared area between the epiphysis and diaphysis. During bone development it contains the growth zones. In the adult the metaphysis is joined to the epiphysis. The *epiphyseal plate* in children is the cartilaginous area which actively produces bone and results in longitudinal growth. In the adult this plate hardens to mature bone and longitudinal growth ceases.

The *periosteum* is fibrous connective tissue that covers the bone. Musculotendinous fibers attach to the outer layer of the periosteum. The inner layer of the periosteum contains osteoblasts (bone-forming cells) that are essential for transverse bone growth and fracture repair.

The *medullary (marrow) cavity* is in the center of the diaphysis. In the adult the medullary cavity of long bones contains yellow bone marrow. In the growing child, red bone marrow in the medullary cavity is actively involved in hematopoiesis. In the adult, hematopoiesis normally occurs only in the red bone marrow of the cranium, ribs, sternum, vertebrae, and proximal ends of the humerus and femur.

Microscopic structure of bone

Bone is a special kind of connective tissue in which organic matter (collagen) has become mineralized. The structural unit of compact bone is the haversian system (Fig. 55-2). It consists of lamellae (concentric layers) of calcified collagen matrix that enclose a long canal (*haversian canal*). The main function of the haversian canal is to transport blood to bone tissue. Blood vessels from the periosteum go through Volkmann's canals to the blood vessels of the haversian canals.

Osteocytes (bone cells) lie in small spaces called *lacunae* between lamellae. *Caniculi* (tiny canals) extend from lacunae to connect the osteocytes to one another and to the haversian canal.

In compact bone the haversian systems are arranged in a tight and compact manner. In cancellous bone, large spaces filled with either red or yellow marrow are present between thin processes of bone.

The three types of bone cell are osteoblasts, osteocytes, and osteoclasts. The osteoblast synthesizes organic bone matrix (collagen) and is the basic bone-forming cell. The osteocyte is the mature bone cell and resides in a lacuna. The osteoclast is involved in resorption of bone tissue and participates in bone remodeling.

Types of bones

The 206 named bones in the body are classified according to shape as long, short, flat, or irregular. *Long bones* are characterized by a central shaft (diaphysis) and two epiphyseal ends (Fig. 55-1). Examples include the femur, humerus, and radius. *Short bones* are characterized by cancellous (spongy) bone covered by a thin layer of compact (dense) bone. Examples include the carpals and tarsals.

Flat bones are characterized by two layers of compact bone separated by a layer of cancellous bone. Examples include the ribs, skull, scapula, and sternum. The spaces in the cancellous bone contain bone marrow. *Irregular bones* have a variety of shapes and sizes. Examples include the vertebrae, sacrum, and mandible.

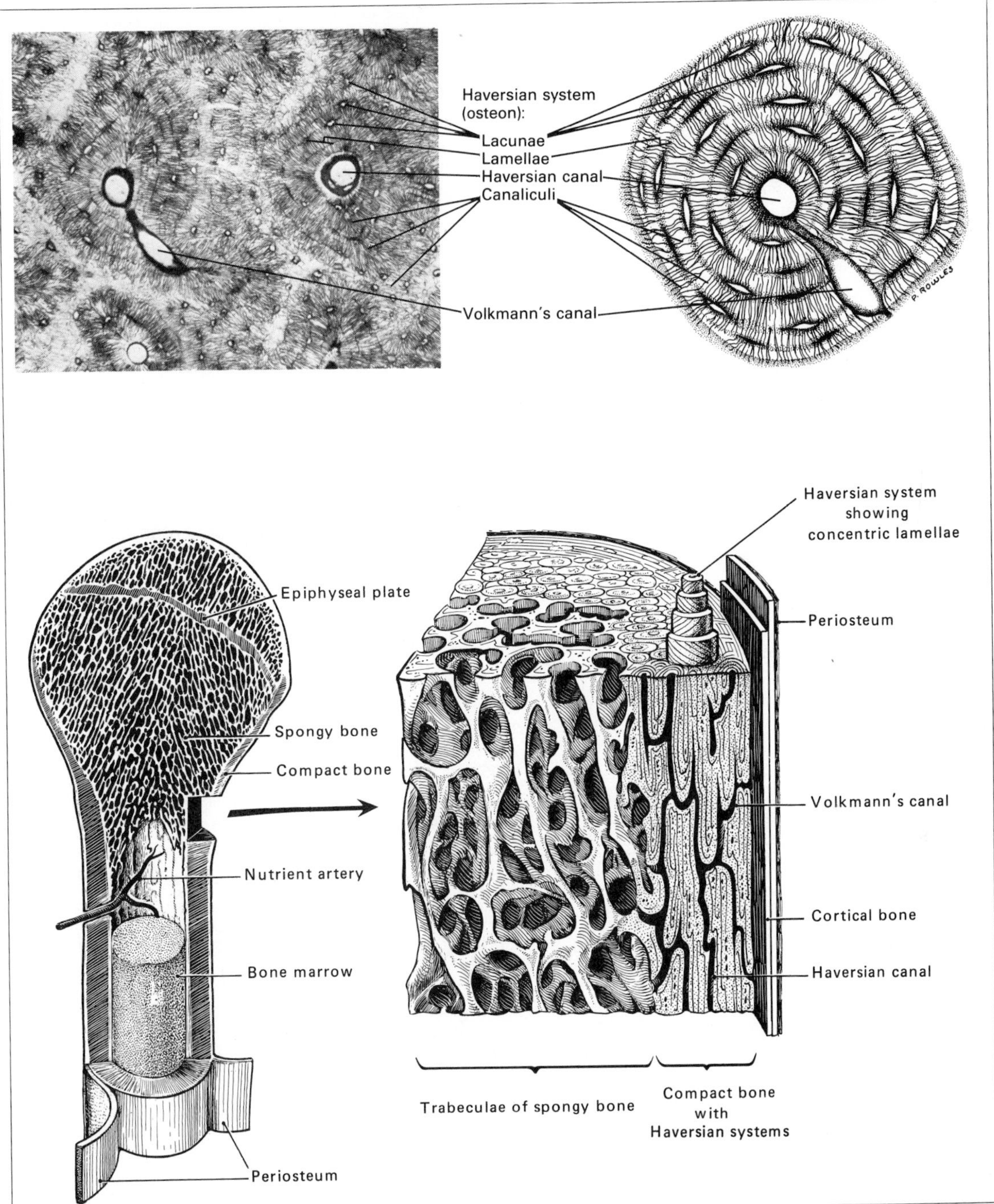

Figure 55-2 Structure of bone showing haversian system. (*From L. Langley, I. Telford, and J. Christensen, Dynamic Anatomy and Physiology, 5th ed., McGraw-Hill Book Company, New York, 1980.*)

Joints

Bones are connected to one another by means of structures called *joints (articulations)*. Rigid bone is capable of changing position and permitting movement by the action of joints. Joints are commonly classified according to their degree of movement (Fig. 55-3).

The diarthrodial (synovial) type, the most common, consists of a joint cavity between the articular surfaces of the bones that make up the joint (Fig.

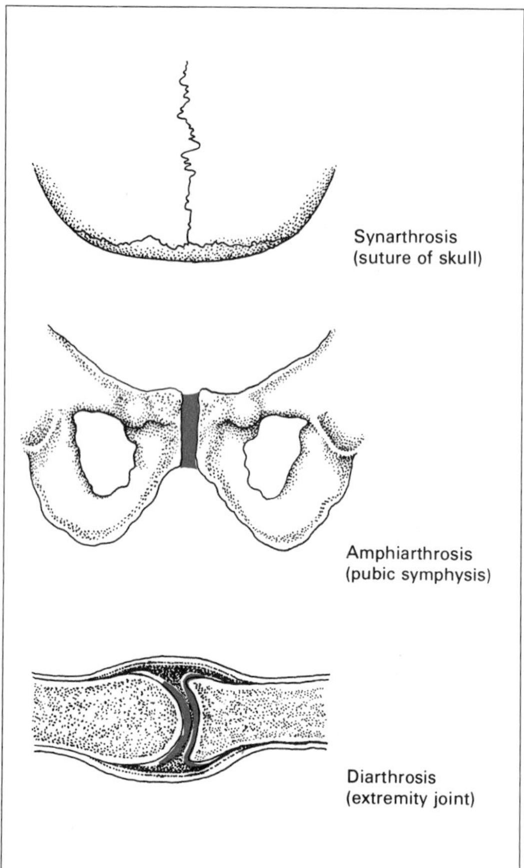

Figure 55-3 Classification of joints. (*From L. Langley, I. Telford, and J. Christensen, Dynamic Anatomy and Physiology, 5th ed., McGraw-Hill Book Company, New York, 1980.*)

55-4). The ends of the bone are covered with articular (hyaline) cartilage. A capsule of connective tissue called the *fibrous capsule* joins the two bones together, forming a cavity. The capsule is lined by a synovium, or synovial membrane, which secretes a thick synovial fluid to lubricate the joint and reduce friction. Types of diarthrodial joints are illustrated in Fig. 55-5.

Cartilage

Cartilage is a type of rigid connective tissue. It functions to support soft tissue, provide the articular surfaces for joint movement, and protect underlying tissues. Cartilage making up the epiphyseal plate is also essential for the growth of long bones prior to maturity.

Cartilage is avascular and nourished by the diffusion of material from capillaries in adjacent connective tissue. The lack of a direct blood supply is related to the fact that cartilage cells are slow to reproduce. Damaged cartilage therefore heals slowly.

The three types of cartilage tissue are hyaline, elastic, and fibrous. Hyaline cartilage, the most common, contains a moderate amount of collagen fibers. It is found in the trachea, bronchi, nose, and articular surfaces of bones. Elastic cartilage, containing collagen and elastic fibers, is more flexible than hyaline cartilage. It is found in the ear, epiglottis, and larynx. Fibrocartilage, consisting mostly of collagen fibers, is a very tough tissue often functioning as a shock absorber. It is found between vertebral disks and in the knee. Fibrocartilage also forms a protective cushion between the bones of the pelvic girdle.

Soft-Tissue Structures

Muscle

Types of Muscle The three types of muscle tissue are cardiac, smooth, and skeletal (striated) muscle. Cardiac muscle is found only in the heart and is controlled by involuntary nerve activity. In fact, cardi-

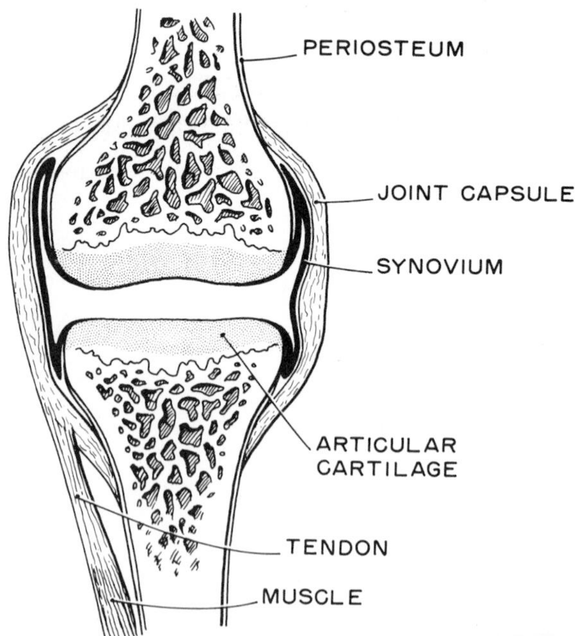

Figure 55-4 Normal diarthrodial (synovial) joint (knee). (*From S. Price and L. Wilson, Pathophysiology: Clinical Concepts of Disease Processes, 2d ed., McGraw-Hill Book Company, New York, 1982.*)

Joint	Movement	Examples	Illustration
Hinge joint	Flexion, extension	Elbow joint (shown), knee joint, interphalangeal joints	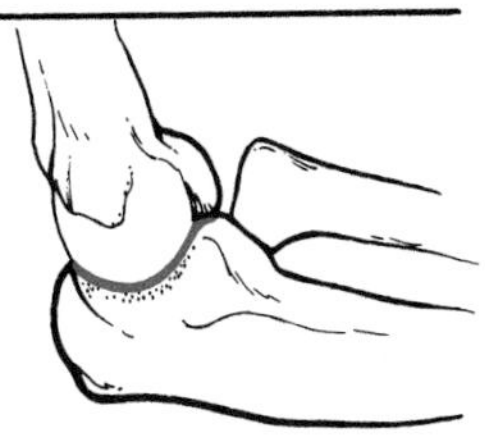
Ball and socket	Flexion, extension; adduction, abduction; circumduction	Shoulder (shown), hip	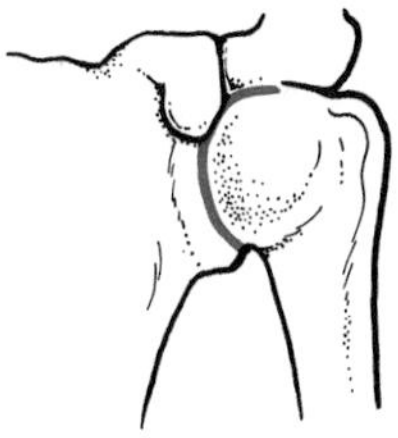
Pivot	Rotation	Atlas-axis, proximal radial and ulnar joint (shown)	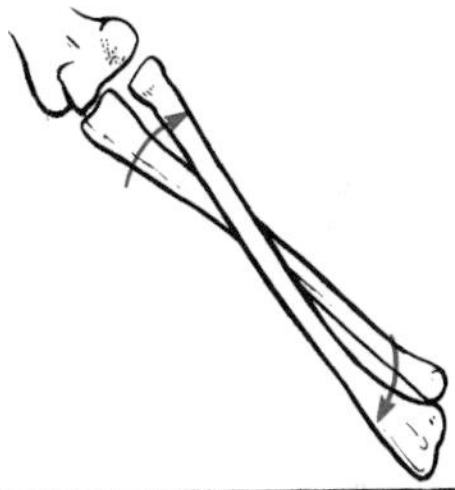
Condyloid	Flexion, extension; abduction, adduction; circumduction	Wrist joint (between radial and carpals) (shown)	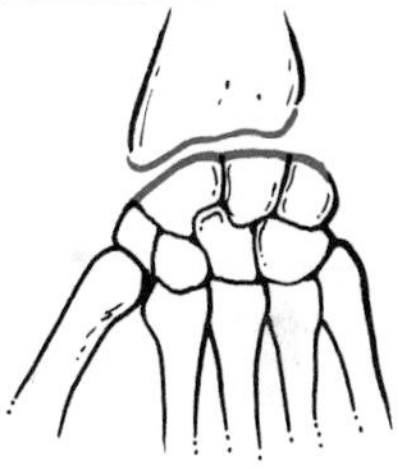
Saddle	Flexion, extension; abduction, adduction; circumduction	Carpal-metacarpal joint of thumb	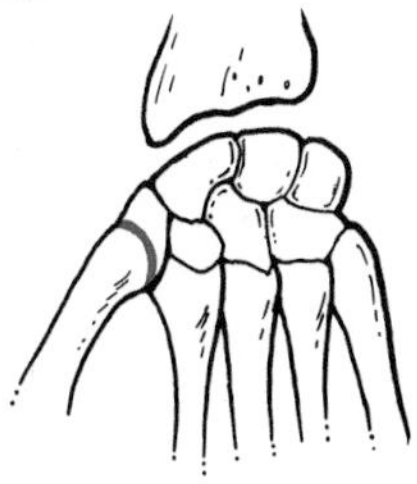
Gliding	One surface moves over another surface	Between carpal bones (shown), between tarsal bones, sacroiliac joint	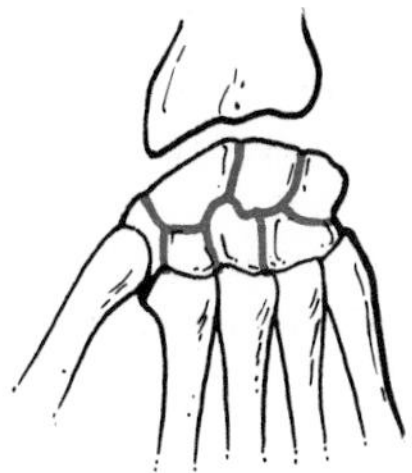

Figure 55-5 Types of diarthrodial joints.

ac muscle can function without being stimulated by nerve impulses (Chap. 25).

Smooth muscle is found in the walls of hollow structures such as the gastrointestinal tract, urinary bladder, uterus, and blood vessels. Smooth-muscle contractions result from involuntary nerve stimulation from the autonomic nervous system. Smooth muscle usually cannot be controlled by conscious efforts.

Most skeletal (striated) muscles are attached to bones. Contraction of skeletal muscle accounts for movement of the skeletal system. It is considered voluntary muscle because it can be controlled by conscious effort.

Structure of Skeletal Muscle The structural unit of muscle tissue is the muscle cell, which is also called a *muscle fiber*. Each skeletal muscle fiber is a cylinder containing many nuclei which may extend up to 30 cm (1 foot) in length.[1] Muscle is composed of numerous muscle fibers bound together by connective tissue. Muscle fibers are composed of myofibrils, which, in turn, are made up of filaments (Fig. 55-6).

Under a microscope, skeletal muscle shows alternating banding which accounts for the striated appearance. This appearance is due to a repeating pattern of filaments seen in the myofibrils. The sarcomere is the contractile unit of the myofibril. Each sarcomere contains myosin (thick) filaments and actin (thin) filaments. The arrangement of the thin and thick filaments accounts for the banding. (For example, the thick filaments located in the central area give rise to a dark band called the *A band*.) The sarcomere is defined as the Z to Z distance within a myofibril.
of a sarcomere slide past each other, pulling the Z lines closer together. As all the sarcomeres become shorter, the muscle fibers and hence the muscle itself is shortened (contracted).

Neuromuscular Junction Skeletal muscles require a nerve supply in order to contract. The nerve cell and the muscle fibers it supplies are called a *motor unit*. The junction between the axon of the nerve cell and the muscle cell it supplies is called the *myoneural* or *neuromuscular junction*.

When acetycholine is released from the motor end plate of the neuron, it diffuses across the neuromuscular junction and travels into the muscle fibers. In response to this stimulation, the sarcoplasmic reticulum releases calcium ions into the cytoplasm. The presence of these ions triggers the contraction in the myofibrils.

Energy Source The energy source used in muscle fiber contractions comes from adenosine triphosphate (ATP). ATP is synthesized by cellular oxidative metabolism in numerous mitochondria located close to the myofibrils. A second energy source is creatine phosphate, which can easily be converted to ATP. Creatine phosphate is synthesized and stored in muscle tissue.

Ligaments and tendons

Ligaments and tendons are both composed of dense, fibrous connective tissue. This type of connective tissue contains large numbers of collagen fibers that are closely packed together. Tendons attach muscles to bones. They are an extension of the muscle sheath that attaches to the periosteum. Ligaments connect bones to bones at joints (e.g., knee joint). They provide stability while permitting movement.

Fibrous connective tissue has a relatively poor blood supply. Although the tissue can repair itself following injury, it may be a slow process. This explains why a sprain (injury to tissue around a joint), a relatively minor injury, may take time to heal.[2]

Fascia

Fascia is the term used for layers of connective tissue. It is classified as superficial or deep. Superficial fascia is the loose connective tissue located immediately under the skin. Deep fascia (dense fibrous connective tissue) is found surrounding muscle, between muscles, and surrounding and binding bundles of nerves and blood vessels together.

Fascia separates one muscle from another in order to permit independent muscle action. Fascia also allows gliding of one muscle upon another. In addition, fascia provides strength to muscle tissues.

Bursae

Bursae are small sacs of connective tissue lined with synovial membrane and synovial fluid. They are commonly located at joints to prevent friction where one body part moves upon another. Bursae function as cushions to relieve pressure between the moving parts. They are found between the patella and the skin (prepatellar bursa), between the olecranon process and the skin (olecranon bursa), and between the head of the humerus and the acromion process (subacromial bursa) (Fig. 55-7). Bursitis (inflammation of the bursa) may be due to mechanical injury to the bursa or excessive use of a joint. "Tennis elbow" is a form of bursitis involving the olecranon process.

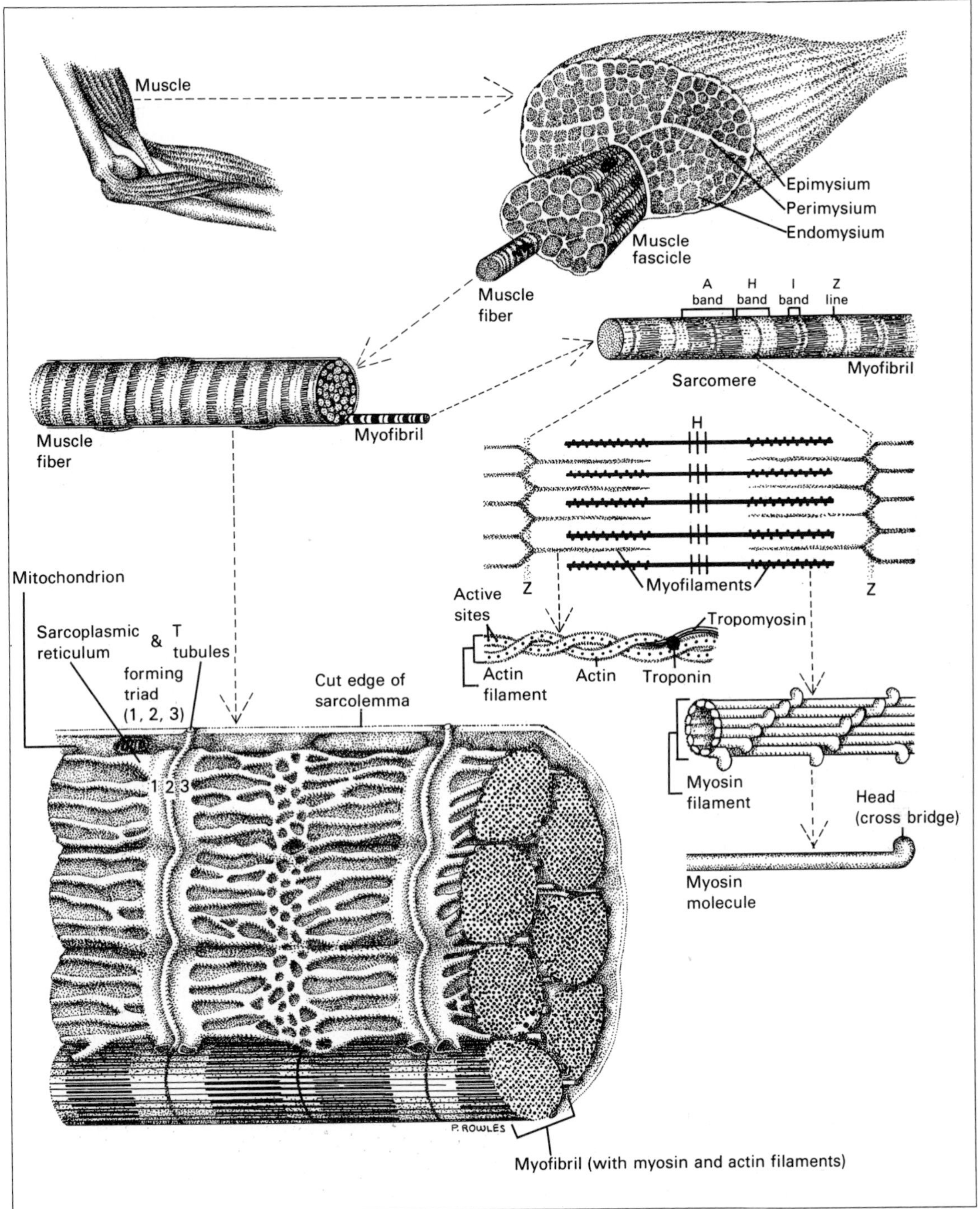

Figure 55-6 Levels of organization within a striated muscle. (*From L. Langley, I. Telford, and J. Christensen, Dynamic Anatomy and Physiology, 5th ed., McGraw-Hill Book Company, New York, 1980.*)

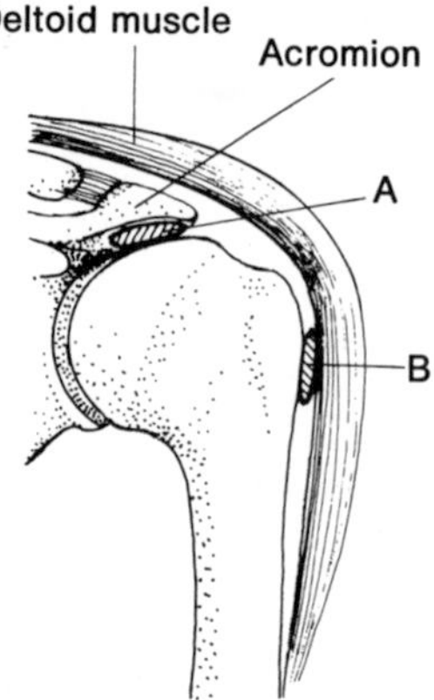

Figure 55-7 A pair of bursae in the shoulder region *(a)* Subacromial. *(b)* Subdeltoid. (*From L. Elson, It's Your Body, McGraw-Hill Book Company, New York, 1975.*)

ASSESSMENT OF THE MUSCULOSKELETAL SYSTEM

Subjective Data: The History

A musculoskeletal assessment can be made on a specific body part, as part of a general physical examination, or as an examination in itself. Judgment must be used in selecting all or part of the components of the musculoskeletal history and physical examination on the basis of the client's presenting problem.

The chief complaints which alert the nurse to obtain subjective and objective data related to the musculoskeletal system include joint pain or swelling, decreasing strength, change in size of an extremity or muscle, deformity, spasms, changes in sensation, and changes in gait. Many accidents result in trauma to the musculoskeletal system and require a thorough assessment. If the injury is serious or life-threatening, a complete health history is deferred and only pertinent information related to the accident is obtained.

Past medical history

Pediatric and Adult Illnesses Certain illnesses are known to affect the musculoskeletal system either directly or indirectly. The client should be questioned specifically about a past history of tuberculosis, coccidioidomycosis, poliomyelitis, diabetes mellitus, gout, inflammatory and degenerative arthritis, rickets, osteomalacia, scurvy, osteomyelitis or soft-tissue infection, fungus infection of the bones or joints, and neuromuscular disabilities. If the client has a history of any of these problems, a detailed account should be obtained (see Chap. 3). In addition, the client should be questioned about possible sources of secondary bacterial infection such as ears, tonsils, sinuses, genitourinary tract, or pelvic inflammatory disease.

Immunizations The client should be specifically questioned about immunizations related to tetanus and polio. The date and reaction to a tuberculin skin test should also be obtained. Failure to be properly immunized or tested can result in serious musculoskeletal problems.

Hospitalization Information should be obtained about hospitalizations necessitated by a musculoskeletal problem. The reason for the hospitalization, the date and duration, and the treatment should be carefully documented, as well as specifics of any surgical procedure and the postoperative course.

Injuries The list of minor and major injuries of the musculoskeletal system can be extensive in the client who is a good historian. The information should be recorded chronologically and should include:

Circumstances related to the injury
Diagnostic evaluations
Method of treatment
Duration of treatment
Current status related to the injury
Need for assistive devices
Interference with activities of daily living

Medication History The client should be questioned carefully regarding both prescription and over-the-counter drugs used to treat a musculoskeletal problem. Information on the reason for taking the medication, its name, the dose and frequency, how long it was taken, its effect, and any side effects should be obtained. Specific inquiry should be made related to skeletal muscle relaxants, antirheumatoid agents, salicylates, nonsteroidal anti-inflammatory agents, and systemic steroids.

In addition to drugs taken for treatment of a musculoskeletal problem, the client should be questioned about drugs which can have detrimental effects on this system. Such drugs would include anticonvulsants (osteomalacia), phenothiazines (gait disturbances), estrogen (osteoporosis), steroids (abnormal fat distribution and muscle weakness), and potassium-depleting diuretics (cramps and muscle weakness). Amphetamines and caffeine can cause a generalized increase in motor activity.

Allergies Food or contact allergies are of little consequence in relation to musculoskeletal problems, but the general malaise often associated with allergic reactions can manifest itself in musculoskeletal stiffness and lethargy. Allergic reactions to drugs used to treat musculoskeletal problems can interfere with therapy, and an alternative treatment method may have to be employed if the allergic reaction is severe.

Family history

A three-generation family history should be obtained related to arthritis and gout, since these two problems have a familial predisposition.

Social and personal history

Although all facets of the client as a unique individual need to be considered, several categories of the client profile are particularly important to explore in depth.

Occupation Extremes of activity related to occupation can affect the musculoskeletal system. A sedentary occupation does not allow for keeping the body flexible and loose. Jobs that require extreme effort and use of the body for heavy lifting and pushing can result in damage to the joints and supporting structures of the body.

Exercise and Recreation A detailed account of the type, duration, and frequency of activities related to exercise and recreation should be obtained and assessed as to adequacy. This information is readily obtained when the client recounts a typical day. Daily, weekend, and seasonal patterns should be compared, as occasional or sporadic exercise can be more problematic than regular exercise.

Safety Practices Specific questions should be asked related to the safety practices of the client as they relate to the job environment, recreation, and exercise, regarding, for example, the kind of shoes worn for jogging. The high incidence of trauma to the musculoskeletal system requires a careful investigation of the area of safety practices. Identification of problems in this area will identify the need for client education.

Diet The client's recounting of a typical day's diet could provide clues to two areas of concern in relation to the musculoskeletal system. Obesity predisposes to ligamentous instability, particularly in the lower back region. It also adds additional stress to weight-bearing joints. The maintenance of normal weight should be a goal for client education.

Abnormal nutritional states can predispose to musculoskeletal problems such as osteoporosis and osteomalacia. Adequate amounts of vitamins C and D, calcium, and protein are essential for a healthy, intact musculoskeletal system.

Review of systems

The review of systems is the final step in acquiring subjective data before beginning the physical examination. The client should be asked if he has ever had any problems related to muscle pains or cramps, joint pain, redness, or stiffness, backache, limited range of motion, or any change in the bones or joints which causes him trouble in his daily activities. Any positive response to the review of systems must be carefully investigated and documented, including the psychological effect of the disability or deformity.

Objective Data: The Physical Examination

The primary methods used in the physical examination of the musculoskeletal system include inspection and palpation. The data gathered from a careful health history will provide the clinician with clues as to where to concentrate the examination.

Inspection

Inspection begins with the nurse's first contact with the client. Any apparent asymmetry, the stance

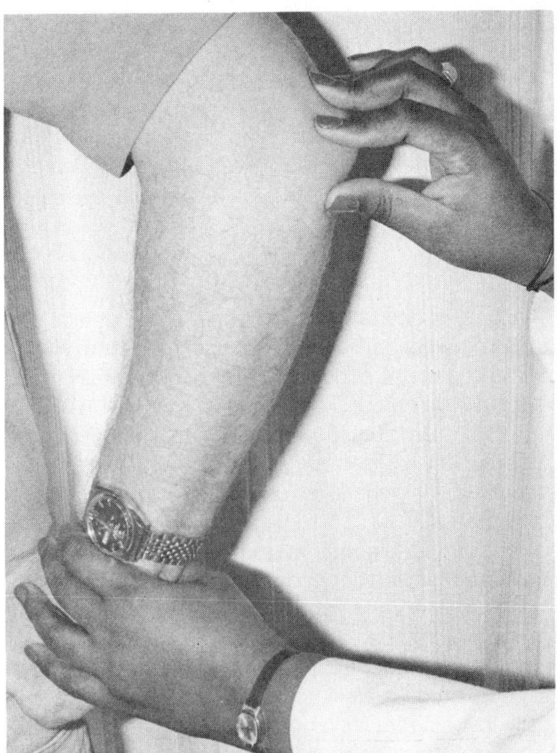

Figure 55-8 Palpation of elbow.

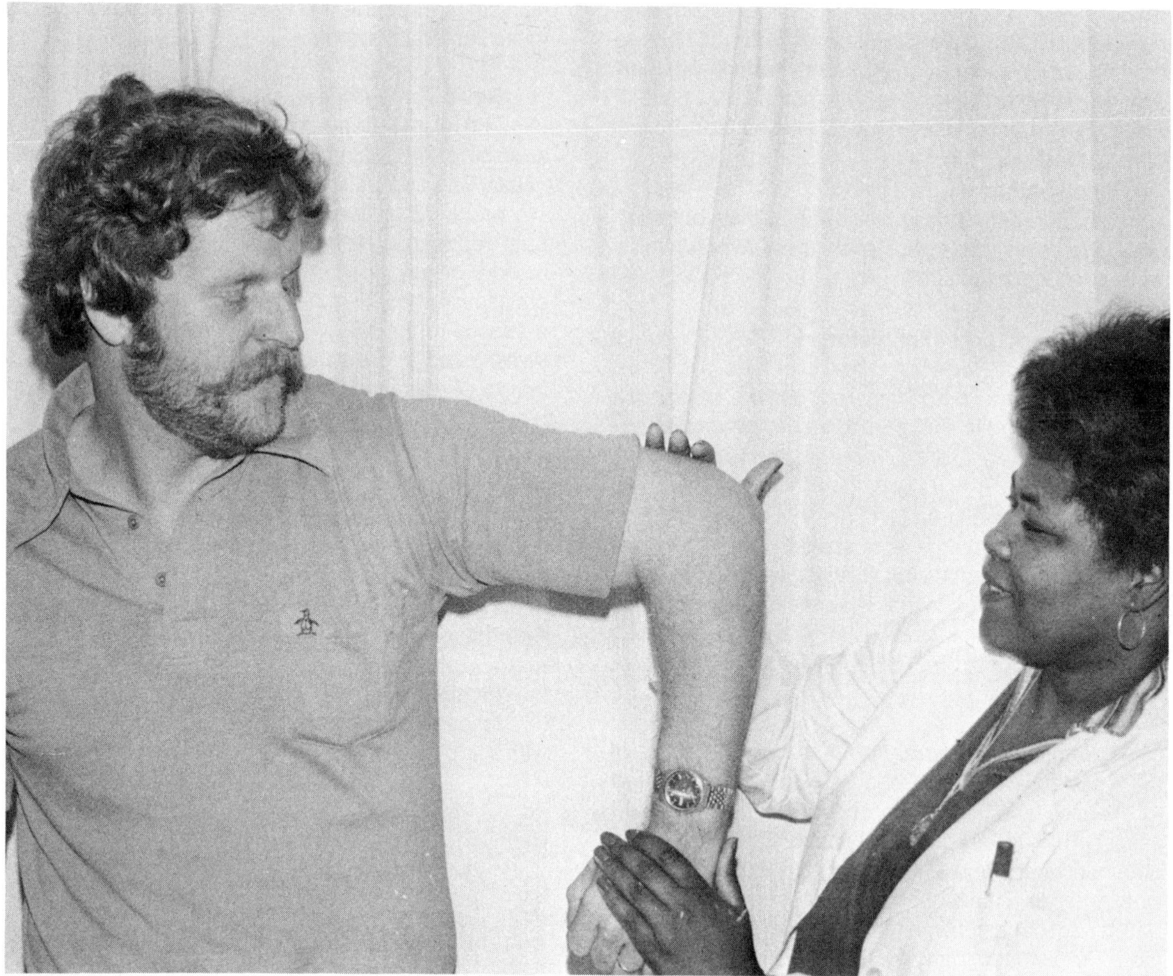

Figure 55-9 Measuring joint range of motion: internal rotation of shoulder.

and gait, ability to perform normal activities such as dressing and undressing and standing and sitting, and the general body build and configuration of the muscles are noted.

The client should be appropriately exposed with due respect for modesty. The condition of the skin is observed for general color, scars, or overt signs of previous injury or operations. A systematic inspection is performed starting at the head and neck and proceeding to the upper extremities, the lower extremities, and finally the back. Although the order is not of great importance, the regular use of a systematic approach is important to avoid missing important aspects of the examination. The nurse should specifically inspect for joint motion and asymmetry of movement, swelling, deformity, masses, and evidence of limb-length or muscle-size discrepancies. The client's own opposite body part is used for comparison when an abnormality is suspected.

Palpation

Any area which has aroused concern because of a subjective complaint or been noted on inspection should be carefully palpated. The examiner's hands should be warm in order to prevent muscle spasm which could interfere with identification of essential landmarks or soft-tissue structures. Palpation of the soft tissues, including muscles and joints, will enable the examiner to evaluate skin temperature and areas of local tenderness, swelling, or crepitation. It is important to establish the relationship of adjacent structures and to evaluate the general contour, abnormal prominences, and local landmarks (Fig. 55-8). The usual sequence is to begin at the neck and proceed cephalopedally (head to feet) to examine the neck, shoulders, elbows, wrists, hands, back, hips, knees, ankles and feet. Although the different types of palpation are discussed separately, they are usually performed concurrently.

Movement When examining joint movement the nurse must carefully evaluate passive and active range of joint motion (Fig. 55-9). Active motion occurs as the result of the client's own movement of the musculature. It is usually examined first. Passive motion occurs as the result of movement of the extremity by the examiner. Normally the active and passive joint motions are similar. Joint motion is most accurately measured by a goniometer (Fig. 55-10). Caution is required when testing passive joint motion because of the possibility of injury to the underlying soft-tissue structures. Manipulations must cease immediately when pain or resistance is encountered. Specific degrees of range of motion for particular body parts can be obtained from a physical assessment manual. Range of motion of all joints is usually not measured unless a musculoskeletal problem has been identified. A less accurate but nevertheless valuable assessment is to compare the range of motion of one extremity with the range of motion on the opposite side. The common movements at synovial joints and the ones most commonly tested for joint motion are listed in Table 55-1 and illustrated in Fig. 55-11.

Measurement Limb length and circumferential measurement of muscle mass are often determined when subjective problems so indicate, especially in disorders related to gait. Limb length is measured between two bony prominences and compared with the similar measurement of the opposite extremity. Muscle mass is measured circumferentially at the maximum area of the mass. Any muscle which appears hypertrophied or atrophied should be measured and compared with the opposite extremity. When recording measurements the nurse should record the exact location at which the measurements were obtained. This informs the next examiner of the exact area to be measured and ensures consistency of measurements in future examinations.

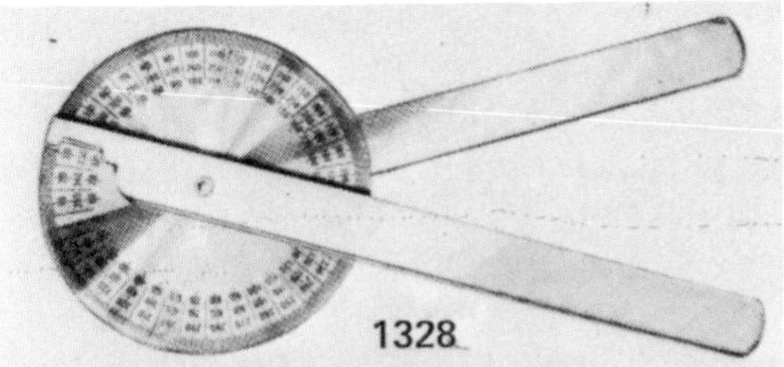

Figure 55-10 Goniometer used in measurement of joint range of motion. (*Graham-Field Surgical Co., Inc.*)

Table 55-1
Movement at Synovial Joints

Movement	Description
Flexion	Bending of a joint that decreases the angle between two bones
Extension	Bending of a joint that increases the angle between two bones
Hyperextension	Extension in which the angle exceeds 180°
Abduction	Movement of a part away from the midline
Adduction	Movement of a part toward the midline
Rotation	Movement about a longitudinal axis
Supination	Turning of the palm upward or the sole inward
Pronation	Turning of the palm downward or the sole outward
Circumduction	Combination of flexion, extension, abduction, and adduction such that the body part moves in a circular motion

Muscle Strength Testing The strength of individual muscles or groups of muscles is graded in performance of movements during contraction against applied resistance. Table 55-2 shows two scales for grading muscle strength. The examiner should instruct the client to apply counterresistance to the force exerted by the examiner. For instance, if the examiner tries to pull the bent arm down, the client will try to raise it up (Fig. 55-12).

Gait The nurse assesses the client's gait by having him walk across the room and back. The normal gait is divided into two separate phases, the stance phase and the swing phase (Fig. 55-13). The two occur simultaneously: while one limb is in stance phase, the other is in swing phase.

Table 55-3 is an example of how to record a normal physical asssessment of the musculoskeletal system.

Common abnormal assessment findings of the musculoskeletal system are presented in Table 55-4.

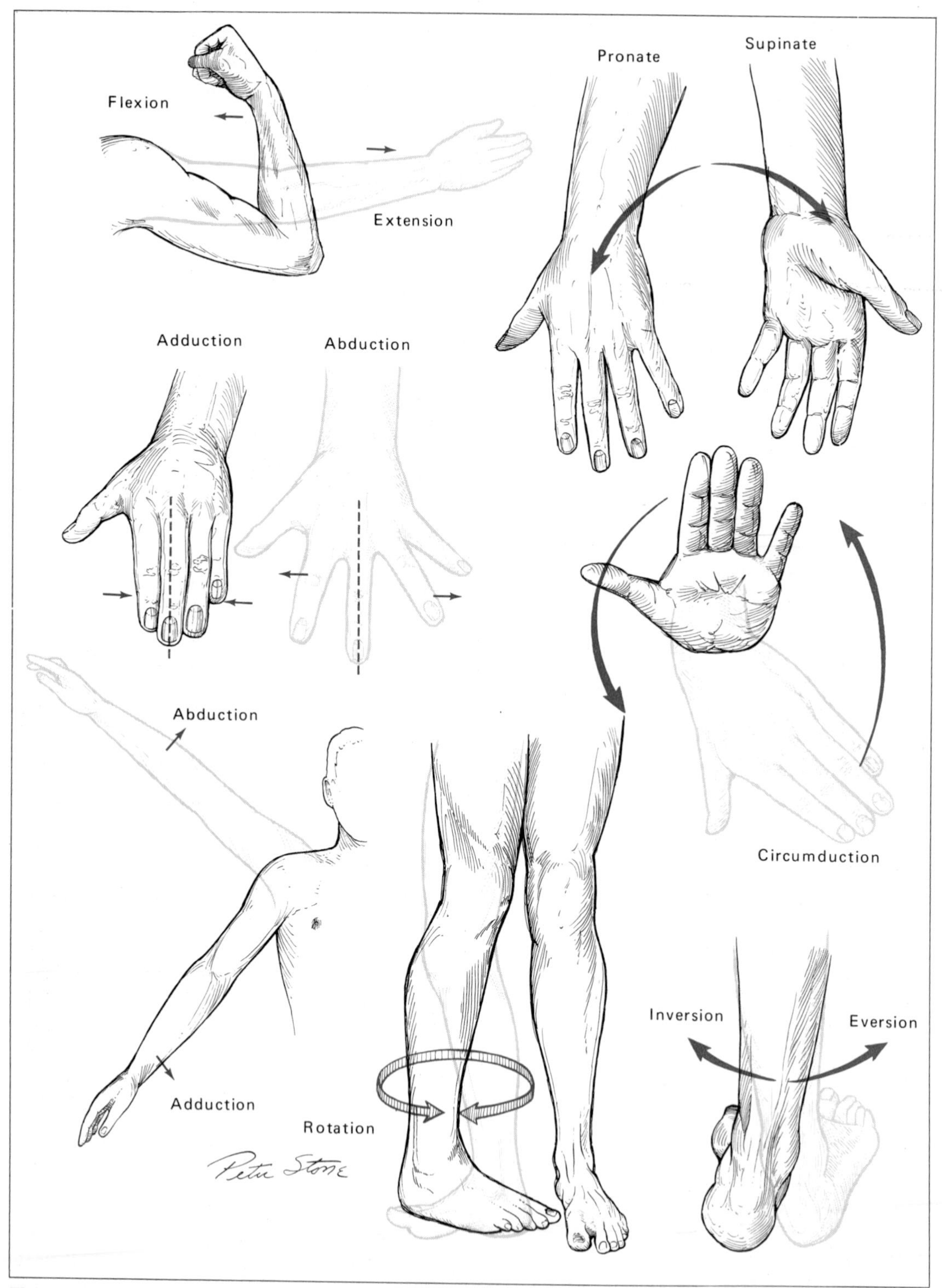

Figure 55-11 Joint movements. (*From L. Langley, I. Telford, and J. Christensen, Dynamic Anatomy and Physiology, 5th ed., McGraw-Hill Book Company, New York, 1980.*)

Table 55-2
Muscle Strength Scale

100%	N (Normal)	Complete range of motion against gravity with full resistance
75%	G (Good)	Complete range of motion against gravity with some resistance
50%	F (Fair)	Complete range of motion against gravity
25%	P (Poor)	Complete range of motion with gravity eliminated
10%	T (Trace)	Evidence of slight contractility but no joint motion
0	O (Zero)	No evidence of contractility

H. Robert Brashear, Jr., and R. Beverly Raney, Sr., *Shands' Handbook of Orthopaedic Surgery*, 9th ed., The C. V. Mosby Company, St. Louis, 1978.

DIAGNOSTIC STUDIES OF THE MUSCULOSKELETAL SYSTEM

Radiological Studies

The most common diagnostic study used to assess musculoskeletal problems is the x-ray. Radiological studies are important to establish the presence of a musculoskeletal problem and to follow its progress and the effectiveness of treatment.

A standard x-ray is a film produced by the action of x-rays emitted from a cathode tube directed through an anatomical structure onto a photosensitive surface. X-rays can be thought of as shadows of

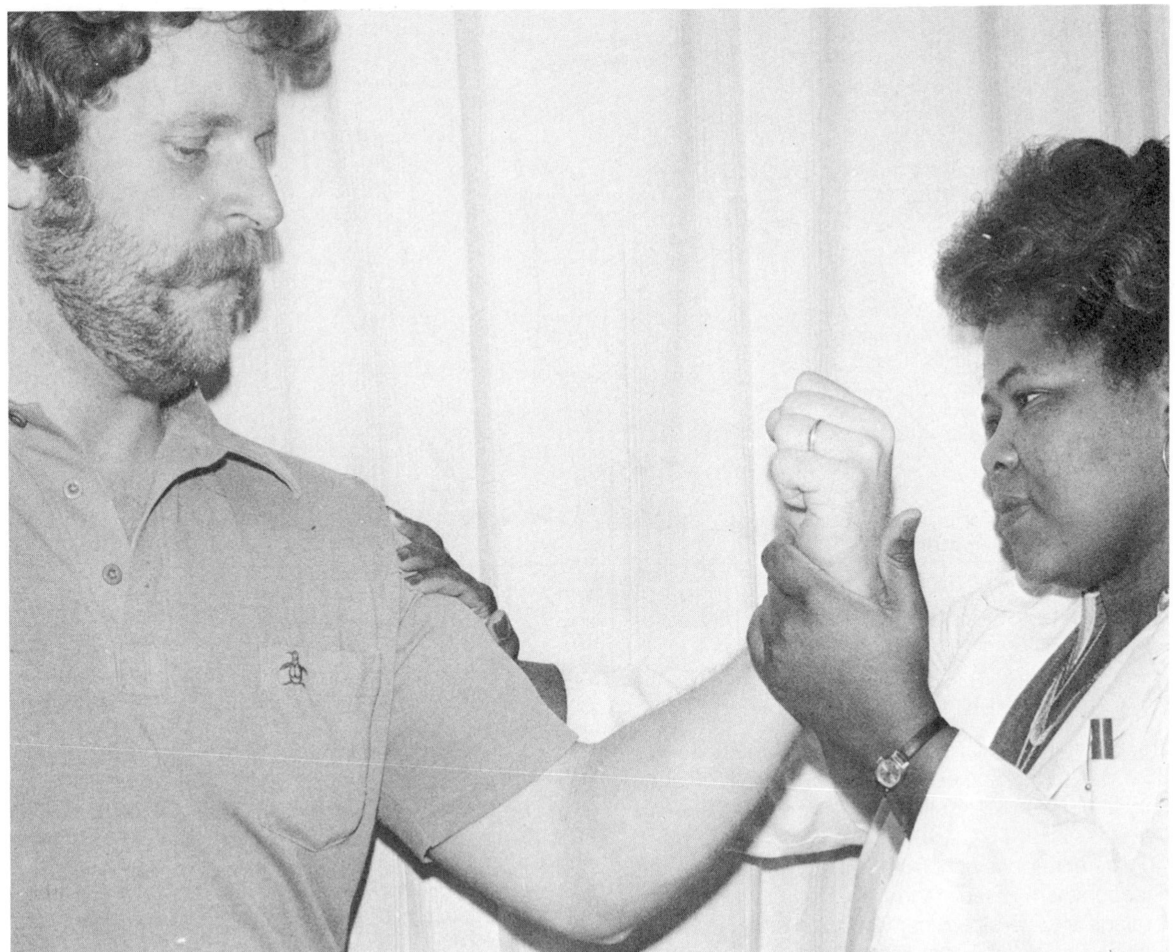

Figure 55-12 Muscle strength testing of biceps.

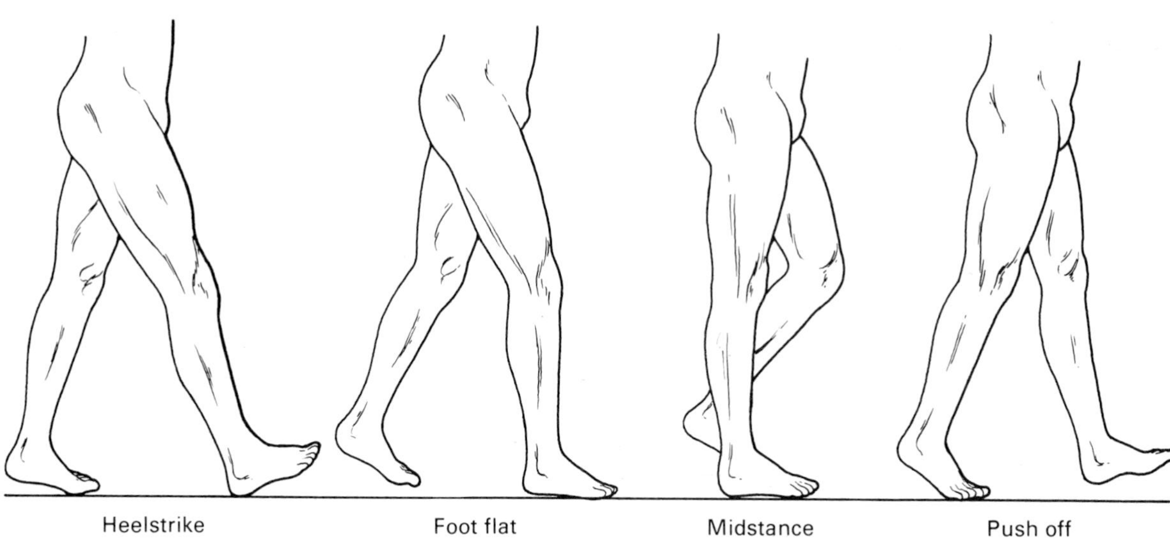

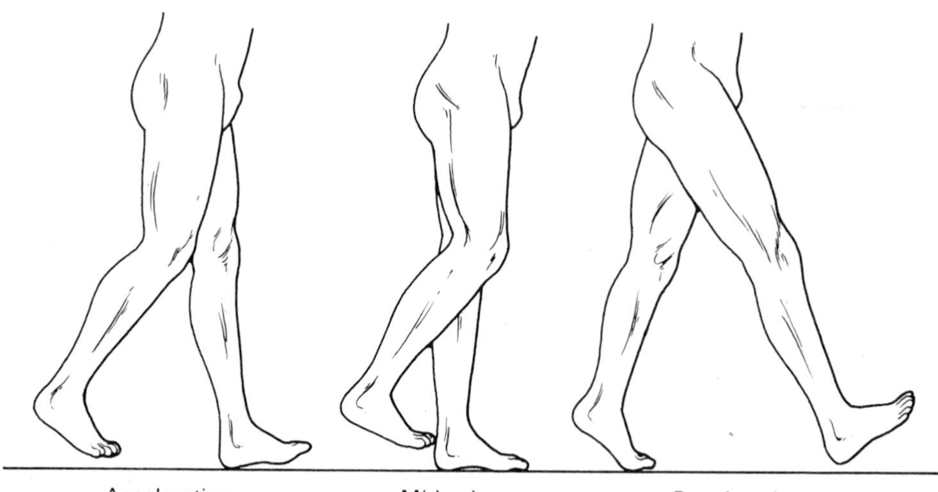

Figure 55-13 Phases of gait. (*From Stanley Hoppenfield, Physical Examination of the Spine and Extremities*, Appleton Century Crofts, New York, 1976.)

structures, particularly bony structures. Bones are more dense than other tissues and do not allow the x-ray to penetrate. The standard x-ray develops dense areas as white.

The anteroposterior (AP) and lateral views are the most commonly used standard x-rays. Since disk and cartilage structures are not visible on standard x-ray, special x-rays (arthrogram, diskogram) involving the use of contrast media are used to visualize them.

Table 55-3

Recording the Normal Physical Assessment of Musculoskeletal System

Full ROM of all joints. No joint swelling, deformity, or crepitation. Normal spinal curvatures. No tenderness on palpation of spine. No muscle atrophy or asymmetry. Muscle strength 100 percent.

Table 55-4
Common Assessment Abnormalities of the Musculoskeletal System

Findings	Definition/Description	Etiology/Significance
Ankylosis	Scarring within a joint leading to stiffness or fixation	Chronic joint inflammation
Atrophy	Wasting of muscle, characterized by decrease in circumference and flabby appearance. Result is decrease in function and muscle tone	Prolonged disuse, contraction, immobilization, muscle denervation
Contracture	Resistance to movement of muscle or joint produced by fibrosis of supporting soft tissues	Shortening of muscle or ligament structure, tightness of soft tissue, immobilization, incorrect positioning
Crepitation	Crackling sound or sensation produced by friction between bones	Fracture, chronic inflammation, dislocation
Effusion	Escape of fluid into a body part; may be accompanied by swelling and pain	Trauma, especially to knee
Felon	Purulent bacterial infection of pulp space (tissue mass) of distal phalanx of a finger	Minor hand injury, puncture wound, laceration
Ganglion	Small, fluid-filled cyst usually observed on dorsal surface of wrist and foot	Degeneration of connective tissue close to tendons and joints leading to formation of small cysts
Hypertrophy	Increase in size of a muscle produced by enlargement of existing cells	Exercise, increased androgens, increased stimulation or use
Kyphosis (round back)	Anteroposterior or forward bending of spine in which convexity of curve is directed posteriorly; commonly occurs in thoracic and sacral levels	Poor posture, tuberculosis, chronic arthritis, growth disturbance of vertebral epiphysis
Lordosis	Deformity of spine resulting in anteroposterior curvature with concavity in posterior direction; commonly occurs in lumbar spine	Secondary to other deformities of spine; other causes: muscular dystrophy, obesity, flexion contraction of the hip, congenital dislocation of the hip
Pes planus	Flatfoot	Congenital, muscle paralysis, mild cerebral palsy, early muscular dystrophy
Scoliosis	Deformity resulting in lateral curvature of spine	Idiopathic, congenital, fracture/dislocation, osteomalacia, functional
Subluxation	Partial dislocation of joint	Instability of joint capsule and supporting ligaments, e.g., trauma, arthritis

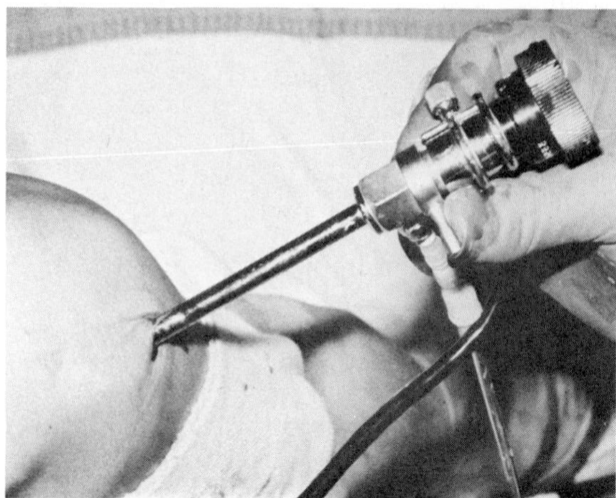

Figure 55-14 Arthroscopy.

Arthroscopy

Endoscopy of the joints involves the use of an arthroscope for direct visualization of the interior of a joint cavity. It is usually performed in the operating room under sterile conditions. Following local or general anesthesia, a large-bore needle is inserted into the joint pouch and the joint distended with saline (see Fig. 55-14). The arthroscope is then inserted and the joint cavity examined. Photographs can be made through the scope, and a biopsy of the synovium or cartilage can be obtained. The procedure is particularly useful in the diagnosis of disorders of the meniscus.

Arthrocentesis and Synovial Fluid Analysis

An arthrocentesis is usually performed to obtain synovial fluid for examination. It may also be used to instill medications and remove fluid to relieve pain. After the skin has been cleaned, a local anesthetic is instilled. An 18-gauge or larger needle is inserted into the joint and all fluid is aspirated.

The fluid is examined grossly for volume, color, clarity, viscosity, and mucin clot formation. Normal synovial fluid is clear, light yellow in color, and scanty (1 to 3 mL). Septic joint fluid may be purulent and thick or gray and thin. In gout the fluid may be whitish yellow. Blood may be aspirated if there is hemarthrosis. The mucin clot test indicates the character of the protein portion of the synovial fluid. Normally a white, ropy mucin clot is formed. In an inflammatory process the clot breaks apart easily and fragments.

The fluid is examined microscopically for cell count and identification of the cells. The normal white blood count (WBC) is less than 200 cells/μL and no bacteria are found. The WBC and protein are increased in an inflammatory process.

Muscle Enzymes

Muscle enzymes are released from injured or dead muscle cells. Determinations of muscle enzyme values are used to distinguish between muscle weakness due to nerve innervation problems and dystrophic disease of the muscle itself. The level of enzymes reflects both the progress of the disorder and the effectiveness of treatment. Serum glutamic-oxaloacetic transaminase (SGOT; also known as aspartate aminotransferase, AST) levels are the least sensitive indicators of muscle disease and creatine phosphokinase (CPK) the most sensitive.

Serology

Rheumatoid factor

About 85 percent of people with rheumatoid arthritis have an autoantibody known as rheumatoid factor in their serum. This factor is an anti-gamma-globulin factor. The test used to determine the presence of this antibody is the *latex fixation test.* Latex particles are coated with denatured immunoglobulin G (IgG). If serum containing rheumatoid factor is mixed with these latex particles, it reacts with the latex particles and causes agglutination.

Other diagnostic studies of the musculoskeletal system are summarized in Table 55-5.

Table 55-5
Diagnostic Studies of the Musculoskeletal System

Study	Description and Purpose	Nursing Responsibility
	Radiological Studies	
Standard roentgenogram	X-ray to determine density and texture of bone. Evaluates structural or functional changes of bones and joints. In anteroposterior (AP) view x-ray beam passes from front to back, allowing one-dimensional view; lateral view provides two-dimensional view.	Avoid excessive exposure of client and nurse. Prior to procedure remove any radiopaque objects which could interfere with results. Explain procedure to client.

Table 55-5 (Continued)

Study	Description and Purpose	Nursing Responsibility
Arthrogram	Involves injection of contrast media and/or air into joint cavity, which permits visualization of joint structures. Joint movement followed with series of x-rays.	Assess client for possible allergy to contrast media. Explain procedure. Area to be injected is prepared aseptically. Contrast dye injected into joint structure using sterile technique.
Diskogram	X-ray of cervical or lumbar intervertebral disk after injection of contrast dye into nucleus pulposus. Permits visualization of intervertebral disk abnormalities.	Same as for arthrogram.
Laminogram (tomogram)	Multiple x-ray views of body region, focused at successively deeper layers of tissue lying in predetermined planes. Focuses on certain tissues, eliminating or blurring surrounding structures. Useful in locating bone destruction, small body cavities, foreign bodies, and lesions overshadowed by opaque structures.	Explain procedure to client. No special preparation.
Sinogram	X-ray made after injection of contrast dye into sinus tract (deep draining wound). Visualizes course of sinus and tissues involved.	Same as for arthrogram.
	Radioisotope Studies	
Bone scan	Involves injection of radioisotope (usually sodium pertechnetate, Tc 99m) that is taken up by bone. Camera scans entire body front and back, and recording is made on paper. Degree of uptake is related to blood flow to bone. Increased uptake seen in osteomyelitis, osteoporosis, primary and metastatic malignant lesions, and certain fractures.	Explain procedure to client. Calculated dose of radioisotope given 2 h before procedure. Bladder should be emptied before scan. Procedure requires 1 h while client lies supine. Causes no pain or harm from isotopes. No follow-up scans required.
	Endoscopy	
Arthroscopy	Involves insertion of arthroscope into joint (usually knee) for visualization of structure and contents. Can be used for exploratory surgery (removal of loose bodies and biopsy) and diagnosing abnormalities of meniscus, articular cartilage, ligaments, or joint capsule.	Explain procedure to client. Performed in OR with strict asepsis. Either local or general anesthesia used. After procedure wound is covered with sterile dressing. Leg is wrapped from midthigh to midcalf with compression dressing for 24 h. Client instructed to limit activity for a few days.
	Arthrocentesis	
	Incision or puncture of joint capsule to obtain samples of synovial fluid from within joint cavity or remove excess fluid. Local anesthesia and aseptic preparation before needle is inserted into joint and fluid aspirated. (See text for analysis of synovial fluid.) Useful in diagnosing joint inflammation.	Explain procedure to client. Usually done at bedside or in examination room. After procedure compression dressing applied and joint rested for 8–24 h. Observe for leakage of blood or fluid on dressing.
	Electromyogram (EMG)	
	Evaluates electrical potential associated with skeletal muscle contraction. Long, small-gauge needles are inserted into certain muscles. Needle probes are attached to leads which feed information to EMG machine. Recordings of electrical activity of muscle are traced on audiotransmitter as well as oscilloscope and recording paper. Useful in providing information related to lower motor neuron dysfunction and primary muscle diseases.	Procedure usually done in EMG lab while client lies supine on special table. Client awake to cooperate with voluntary movement. Procedure involves some discomfort from needle insertion. Stimulants and sedatives should be avoided 24 h before procedure.

Table 55-5 (Continued)

Study	Description and Purpose	Nursing Responsibility
	Muscle Enzymes	
Creatine phosphokinase (CPK)	Highest concentration found in skeletal muscle. Increased values found in progressive muscular dystrophy, polymyositis, and traumatic injuries. *Normal*: Male: 5–55 U/L, female: 5–35 U/L.	Nonfasting.*
Aldolase	Useful in monitoring muscular dystrophy and dermatomyositis. *Normal*: 1.0–7.5 U/L.	Nonfasting.*
SGOT or AST	Found in skeletal muscle but primarily an enzyme of cardiac and hepatic cells. *Normal*: 15–45 U/L.	Nonfasting.*
	Mineral Metabolism	
Alkaline phosphatase	Enzyme produced by osteoblasts of bone; needed for mineralization of organic bone matrix. Elevated levels found in healing fractures, bone cancers, osteoporosis, osteomalacia, and Paget's disease. *Normal*: 5–13 King-Armstrong units, 2–5 Bodansky units, 3–10 Gutman units.	Explain procedure to client. Blood samples obtained by venipuncture.
Calcium	Bone is primary organ for calcium storage. Calcium provides bone with rigid consistency. Decreased level found in osteomalacia, renal disease, and hypoparathyroidism, increased level in hyperparathyroidism, bone tumors, and acute osteoporosis. *Normal*: 9–11 mg/dL, 4.5–5.5 mEq/L.	Nonfasting.*
Phosphorus	Directly related to calcium metabolism. Decreased level found in osteomalacia. Increased level found in chronic renal disease, healing fractures, osteolytic metastatic tumor. *Normal*: 2.8–4.5 mg/dL.	Nonfasting.*
	Serology	
Rheumatoid factor (latex fixation)	Assesses presence of autoantibody (rheumatoid factor) in serum. Not specific for rheumatoid arthritis and seen in other connective tissue diseases as well as small percentage of normal population. *Normal*: Negative or titer <1:20.	Nonfasting.*
Erythrocyte sedimentation rate (ESR)	Nonspecific index of inflammation. Measures rapidity with which RBC settle out of unclotted blood in 1 h. Results influenced by physiological factors as well as diseases. Elevated levels seen with any inflammatory process (especially rheumatoid arthritis, rheumatic fever, and respiratory infections). Normal: <20 mm/h.	Nonfasting.*
Lupus erythematosus cells (LE prep)	LE cells seen in about 80% of cases of lupus erythematosus; normally no LE cells present.	Blood obtained from client and blood smear made on slide.
Antinuclear antibody (ANA)	Assesses presence of antibodies capable of destroying nucleus of body's tissue cells. Positive in 95% of people with lupus erythematosus; may also be positive in scleroderma, rheumatoid arthritis, and small percentage of normal population.	Nonfasting.*

Table 55-5 (Continued)

Study	Description and Purpose	Nursing Responsibility
Anti-DNA	Detects serum antibodies which react with DNA. Most specific test for systemic lupus erythematosus.	Nonfasting.*
Complement fixation	Complement, a normal body protein, is essential to both immune and inflammatory reactions (see Chap. 10). Complement used up in these reactions said to be *fixed*: subsequent test applied to serum yields little or no serum complement. Complement may be fixed in rheumatoid arthritis and systemic lupus erythematosus.	Nonfasting.*
Uric acid	End product of purine metabolism that is normally excreted in urine. Although not specific, usually elevated in gout. *Normal*: Male: 4.5–6.5 mg/dL, female: 2.5–5.5 mg/dL.	Nonfasting.*
	Miscellaneous	
Thermography	Uses infrared detector that measures degree of heat radiating from skin surface. Useful in investigation of cause of inflamed joints and following client's response to anti-inflammatory drug therapy.	Inform client that it is painless and noninvasive.
Plethysmography	Recording of variations in volume and pressure of blood passing through tissues. Nonspecific and quantitative.	Inform client that it is painless and noninvasive.

*Inform client that blood sample will be drawn. Observe venipuncture site for bleeding or hematoma formation.

REVIEW QUESTIONS

The number of the question corresponds to the same-numbered objective at the beginning of the chapter.

1. Which of the following statements best describes the diaphysis?
   a. end of long bone
   b. main shaft of long bone
   c. flared area of long bone
   d. fibrous covering of bone

2. The type of synovial (diarthrodial) joint permitting the greatest degree of movement is the
   a. hinge joint
   b. pivot joint
   c. ball-and-socket joint
   d. gliding joint

3. The main function of ligaments is to
   a. attach muscles to muscles
   b. attach muscles to bones
   c. attach bones to bones
   d. support underlying muscle tissue

4. A musculoskeletal problem which often has a familial predisposition is
   a. osteomalacia
   b. arthritis
   c. osteomyelitis
   d. poliomyelitis

5. Limb length is measured by
   a. measuring circumferentially at the largest muscle mass
   b. having the client bend from the waist
   c. measuring between two bony prominences on a limb
   d. having the shortest distance as the baseline

6. Wasting of a muscle is called
   a. contracture
   b. effusion
   c. atrophy
   d. osteoporosis

7. Serum alkaline phosphatase levels would most probably be elevated in
   a. severe muscle damage
   b. metabolic disorders of the bone
   c. increased osteoblast activity
   d. general body response to trauma

REFERENCES

1. Arthur J. Vander et al., *Human Physiology: The Mechanisms of Body Function*, 3d ed., McGraw-Hill Book Company, New York, 1980, p. 212.
2. John W. Hole, Jr., *Human Anatomy and Physiology*, Wm. C. Brown Company Publishers, Dubuque, Iowa, 1978, p. 93.

Chapter 56

NURSING ROLE IN MANAGEMENT
Musculoskeletal Problems

Kenneth J. Webb
Phyllis Gappa Jensen

Learning Objectives

1. Explain the pathophysiology, clinical manifestations, and management of soft-tissue injuries: strains, sprains, dislocations, subluxation, bursitis, and muscle spasms.
2. Describe the sequential events involved in fracture healing.
3. Describe the management and common complications associated with fracture injury and fracture healing.
4. Differentiate among open reduction, closed reduction, traction, and plaster immobilization as to purpose, complications, and nursing care.
5. Explain the neurovascular assessment of an injured extremity.
6. Describe the medical and nursing management of specific fractures.
7. Explain the etiology and medical and nursing management of osteomyelitis.
8. Describe the indications and medical and nursing management for an amputation.
9. Describe the pathophysiology, clinical manifestations, and treatment of neoplasms of the bone.
10. Describe the causes and characteristics of acute and chronic low back pain.
11. Describe the conservative and surgical treatment of low back pain.
12. Describe the postoperative nursing management of laminectomy.
13. Explain the etiology and management of common foot disorders.
14. Describe the pathophysiology, clinical manifestations, and management of metabolic diseases of bone.

The most common cause of injury to the musculoskeletal system is accidents, which result in fracture, dislocations, and associated soft-tissue injuries. Although most of these injuries are not fatal, the expense in terms of pain, disability, medical expense, and lost wages is enormous. For all ages, accidents as the cause of death are exceeded only by diseases of the heart, malignant neoplasms, and strokes. Between the ages of 5 and 44, accidents are the leading cause of death.

SOFT-TISSUE INJURIES

Soft-tissue injuries include sprains, strains, dislocations, and subluxation. These common injuries are usually caused by trauma.

Sprains and Strains

Sprains and strains are the two most common types of injury affecting the musculoskeletal system. These injuries are usually associated with the abnormal stretching forces which may occur during vigorous activities. A *sprain* can involve all degrees of tearing. It is classified as first degree (minor tears), second degree, or third degree (almost complete) according to the severity of the tear. This injury affects the joint capsule and synovial membrane as well as the ligaments. Since these areas are rich in nerve endings, the injury can be quite painful. A *strain* is a stretching of a muscle.

The clinical manifestations of the two injuries are similar and include pain, edema, decrease in function, and bruising. Pain aggravated by continued use is common. Edema develops in the injured area because of minute hemorrhages within the disrupted tissues and the ensuing inflammatory response. The client will usually recount a history of traumatic injury.

Minor sprains and strains are usually self-limiting, with full function returning within 3 to 6 weeks. A severe sprain, however, may result in an *avulsion fracture*, in which the ligament pulls loose a fragment of bone. Alternatively, the joint structure may become unstable and result in dislocation. The external force causing the sprain or strain may also cause *hemarthrosis* (bleeding into a joint space or cavity), or disruption of the synovial lining. An acute strain may involve rupture of a muscle.

Management

The use of elastic support bandages or adhesive tape wrapping prior to beginning a vigorous activity can significantly reduce the occurrence of sprains. Preconditioning, stretching, and warming up prior to vigorous activity also help prevent strains. Precondi-

This chapter was reviewed by Cindy Gregory, P.T., M.S., Instructor, Division of Physical Therapy, School of Medicine, University of New Mexico, Albuquerque, New Mexico.

tioning exercise protects an inherently weak joint, since slow stretching is tolerated better by biological tissues than quick stretches. Warm-up exercises "prelengthen" potential strained tissue by avoiding the quick stretch often encountered in sports.

Warm-up exercises also increase the temperature of muscle, which increases the speed of cell metabolism as well as the speed of nerve impulse transmission. The increased metabolism contributes to better oxygenation of muscle fiber during work. Stretching is also thought to improve kinesthetic awareness, thus lessening the chance of uncoordinated movement.

If an injury occurs, the immediate care focuses on (1) limiting movement and use, and (2) elevation of the affected extremity. Ice packs can be used to limit swelling by exerting a vasoconstrictor effect. The pressure of the pack can also decrease edema and bleeding. These measures will usually minimize pain and swelling, but mild analgesia may be necessary.

The affected part is usually x-rayed to rule out fracture or widening of the joint structure. Surgical repair may be necessary if the injury is significant enough to produce severe disruption of either ligamentous or muscle structures, fracture, or dislocation. After the acute phase (usually lasting 24 to 48 hours) warm, moist heat can be applied to the affected part to reduce swelling. If the joint is protected from recreating the position of the injury by casting, taping, or splinting, the client is encouraged to use the limb. Movement of the joint surfaces maintains cartilage nutrition, while muscle contraction speeds circulation and phagocytosis of the hematoma.

Dislocation and Subluxation

A *dislocation* is a severe injury of the ligamentous structures that surround a joint. It results in the complete displacement or separation of the articular surfaces of the joint. A *subluxation* is a partial or incomplete separation of the joint surface. The clinical manifestations of a subluxation are similar to a dislocation but less severe. Treatment of subluxation is similar to that of dislocation, but subluxation requires less healing time.

Dislocations characteristically result from overwhelming forces transmitted to the joint, causing a disruption of the soft tissues of the joint. The joints most frequently dislocated in the upper extremity include the thumb, elbow, and shoulder. In the lower extremity the hip is vulnerable to dislocation, which occurs as a result of severe trauma often associated with motor vehicle accidents (Fig. 56-1).

The most obvious clinical manifestation of a dislocation is asymmetry of the musculoskeletal contour. For example, if a hip is dislocated, the limb is shorter on the affected side. Additional manifestations include local pain, tenderness, loss of function of the injured part, and swelling of the soft tissues in the region of the joint. The major complications of a dislocated joint are open joint injuries, intraarticular fractures, fracture dislocation, and damage to adjacent neurovascular tissue.

Management

Radiological studies are performed to determine the extent of shifting of the involved structures. The joint may be aspirated to determine the presence of fat cells. If fat cells from the exposed marrow are found in the synovial fluid, an intraarticular fracture is present.

A dislocation requires prompt medical intervention. The longer the joint remains unreduced, the greater is the possibility of *avascular necrosis* (bone cell death secondary to inadequate blood supply). The first goal of medical management is to realign the dislocated portion of the joint in its original anatomical position. This can usually be accomplished by a closed reduction under general anesthesia. Anesthesia is necessary to produce muscle relaxation so the bones can be manipulated. In some situations, open reduction may be necessary.

After reduction the extremity is usually immobilized by taping or use of a sling to allow the torn ligaments and capsular tissue to heal. Nursing care is directed toward the symptomatic relief of pain and the support and protection of the injured joint. Following immobilization, joint motion is usually restricted. A carefully regulated rehabilitation program can prevent the formation of contractures. It is essential that the client not stretch the joint beyond its limits. The torn capsule and ligament heal in a shortened position and with fibrous scar that is not as strong as the original tissue. Therefore, a carefully regulated exercise program is required to slowly and methodically restore the joint to its original range of motion without redislocation.

Carpal Tunnel Syndrome

Carpal tunnel syndrome is a condition caused by compression of the median nerve beneath the transverse carpal ligament within the narrow confines of the carpal tunnel located at the wrist. This condition is frequently due to pressure from trauma or edema caused by inflammation of a tendon (tenosynovitis), neoplasm, rheumatoid synovial disease, or soft-tissue masses such as ganglia. Carpal tunnel syndrome occurs most frequently in middle-aged or postmenopausal females. The clinical manifestations are weak-

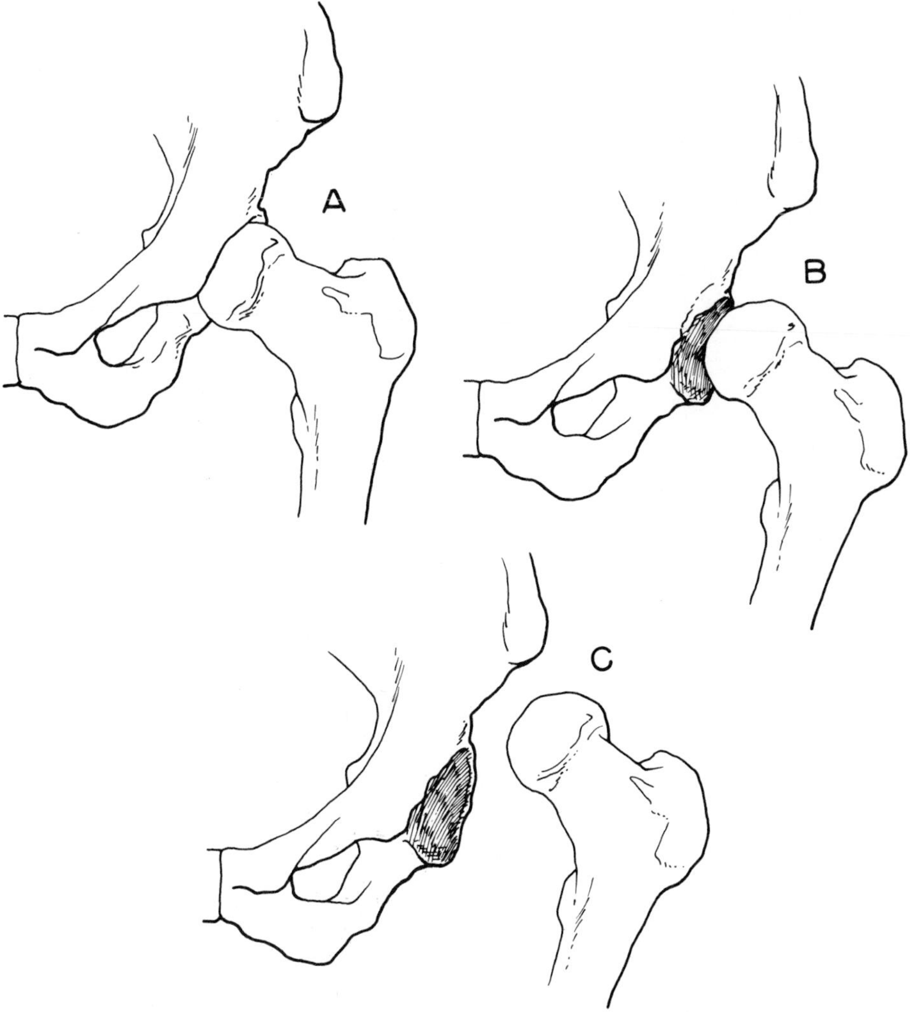

Figure 56-1 Soft-tissue injury of the hip. *(a)* Normal. *(b)* Subluxation. *(c)* Dislocation. (*From S. Price and L. Wilson, Pathophysiology: Clinical Concepts of Disease Processes, 2d ed., McGraw-Hill Book Company, New York, 1982.*)

ness or atrophy of the thenar muscles of the hand, impaired sensation in the distribution of the median nerve, and clumsiness in performing fine hand movements. Carpal tunnel syndrome can result in recurrent pain and eventual dysfunction of the hand.

Management

Medical management is directed toward relieving the underlying cause of the nerve compression. The early symptoms associated with carpal tunnel syndrome can usually be relieved by placing the hand and wrist at rest by immobilization in a plaster hand splint. If the cause is inflammation, injection of hydrocortisone directly into the carpal tunnel may bring relief. If the problem continues, the median nerve may have to be surgically decompressed by longitudinal division of the transverse carpal ligament.

Meniscus Injury

Meniscus injuries are closely associated with ligament sprains commonly occurring in young athletes engaged in sports such as basketball, rugby, football, soccer, and hockey. These activities produce a rotational stress when the knee is in a flexed position and the foot is fixed. A blow to the knee can cause the meniscus to be trapped between the femoral condyles and the plateau of the tibia, resulting in a torn

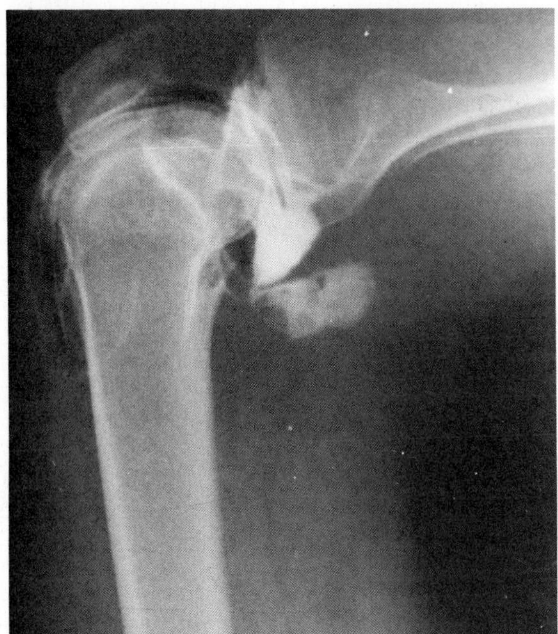

Figure 56-2 Double-contrast arthrogram in the lateral projection. Note the popliteal cyst projecting posteriorly to the knee joint. Iodine contrast medium and air were used.

meniscus (Fig. 56-2). There is a causal relationship between occupations which require working in a squatting or kneeling position and meniscus injuries.

Meniscus injuries alone do not usually cause chronic edema or even pain, since cartilage is avascular and aneural. The usual clinical picture is a feeling by the client that the knee is unstable and may click and lock periodically. Quadriceps atrophy is evident if the injury has been present for some time. Degenerative joint disease can occur if a damaged, roughened meniscus is not surgically removed. Usually the instability and locking causes the person to seek care.

Management

An arthrogram or arthroscopy is always diagnostic. Initial treatment includes exercises aimed at strengthening the stability of the knee, such as straight leg raising. The knee may also be unlocked by manipulation, followed by immobilization by a removable splint or cast. If conservative treatment is not effective in relieving symptoms, surgical excision of the meniscus (*meniscectomy*) may be necessary.

Bursitis

Bursae are closed sacs which are lined with synovial membrane and contain a few drops of synovial fluid. They are located beneath the skin at sites of friction, as between tendons, bones, and overlying joints. A bursa may become inflamed (*bursitis*) because of repeated or excessive trauma or friction, gout, rheumatoid arthritis, or infection. The primary clinical manifestations of bursitis are pain and swelling due to edema in the affected part. Sites at which bursitis commonly occurs are the hand, knee, trochanters, shoulder, and elbow.

Management

Attempts are made to determine and correct the cause of the bursitis. Rest is often the only treatment needed. The affected part is often immobilized in a compression dressing or plaster splint. Aspiration of the bursal fluid and injection of hydrocortisone may be necessary. If the bursa wall has become thickened and continues to interfere with normal joint function, surgical excision may be necessary. For example, subacromial bursal thickening causes pain and loss of range of motion on abduction of the shoulder. Septic bursae usually require surgical drainage.

Muscle Spasm

Local muscle spasms are a common condition often associated with overdoing everyday activities. Injury to a muscle stimulates free pain endings, resulting in muscle excitation and spasm. The spasm produces additional pain, and a cycle is established. The clinical manifestations of muscle spasm of local origin include local pain, palpable muscle mass in spasm, tenderness, diminished range of motion of the affected site, and limitation of daily activities.

Management

A careful history should be taken and physical examination made to rule out central nervous system problems. The muscle spasm can be managed with drug therapy, physical therapy, or a combination of both. A physical therapy program might include heat, rest plus exercise, massage, hydrotherapy, local heat-producing applications, ultrasound (deep heat), manipulation, and bracing. Drugs used for treatment of local muscle spasm include analgesics, tranquilizers, skeletal muscle relaxants, and cyclobenzaprine.[1]

Nursing Management of Acute Soft-Tissue Injuries

The major nursing responsibility related to acute soft-tissue injury involves client education related to care of the injured part. Such teaching often takes place in an outpatient setting, where most soft-tissue injuries are diagnosed and treated. The client should be instructed to reduce swelling by the use of ice which causes vasoconstriction. Initially, ice should be applied intermittently for the first 24 hours. Ice applications should not exceed 20 to 30 minutes per application, allowing a "warm-down" time of 10 to 15 minutes between applications. Most clients can be taught to do this themselves. The effect of leaving ice on the skin too long is reflex vasodilatation. Also, cold application to muscle in spasm for over 1 hour will increase the spasm. The ice applications should be cold enough to produce reddening of the skin (hyperemia) followed by blanching and sensory anesthesia. Both ice and commercial cold packs can be made colder by wrapping them in a wet towel.

After the swelling has stabilized, warm moist heat can be applied several times a day to provide comfort and aid in regaining joint mobility. Heat applications likewise should not exceed 20 to 30 minutes, allowing a cool-down time between applications. The heat can be applied in the form of a wrap or soak, depending upon the area affected. The temperature of the water should not exceed 37.8°C (100°F). Prolonged heat application will slow circulation rather than enhance it. Heat should be avoided during the first 24 to 48 hours, as the resulting vasodilatation increases edema and also increases any active hemorrhaging.

Utilization of an elastic bandage will provide support and limit edema. The client should have careful instruction on the application of an elastic bandage to prevent circulatory impairment. Pain relief can usually be obtained by mild analgesic agents such as aspirin or acetaminophen. Rest and support of the injured part also help.

FRACTURES

Classification and Etiology

A fracture is a disruption or break in the continuity of the structure of bone or cartilage. Traumatic injuries account for the majority of fractures, although some fractures are secondary to a disease process (pathological fractures). Fractures are described and classified according to (1) type (Table 56-1), (2) location of the fracture (Fig. 56-3), and (3) communication or noncommunication with the external environment (Figs. 56-4 and 56-5). Fractures are also described as stable or unstable. A *stable fracture* occurs when

Table 56-1
Types of Fracture

Type	Description	Appearance
Avulsion	Fracture of bone resulting from strong pulling effect of tendons or ligaments at bone attachment	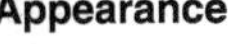 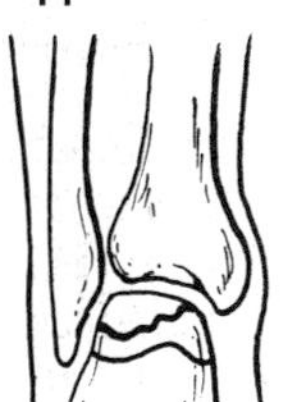
Bayonette (overriding)	Displaced fracture fragment which is overriding other bone	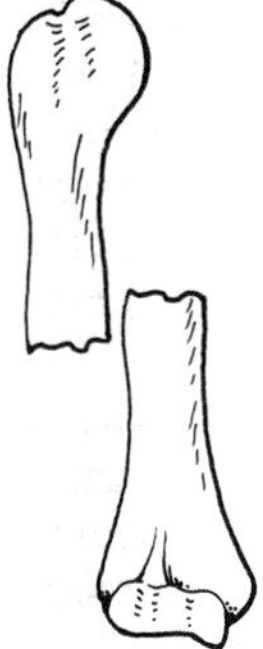

Table 56-1 (Continued)

Type	Description	Appearance
Butterfly	Comminuted fracture in which main fragment is triangular and resembles butterfly with wings	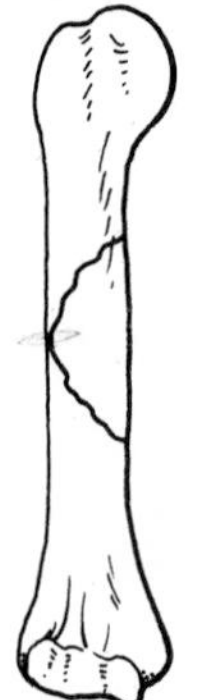
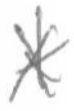 Comminuted	Fracture with many fragments	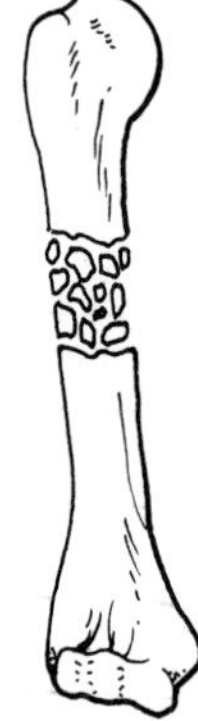
Impacted	Fracture fragments of one bone driven into another	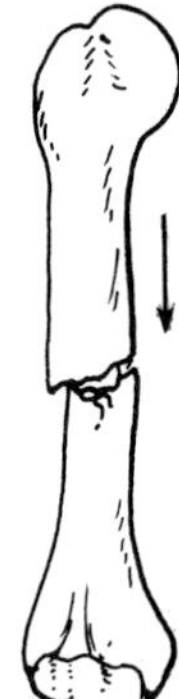
Intraarticular	Fracture extending to articular surface of bone	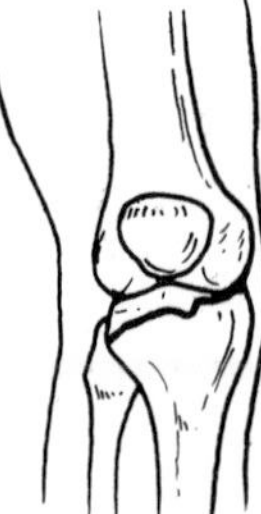

Table 56-1 (Continued)

Type	Description	Appearance
Nondisplaced/ displaced	A fracture is nondisplaced or displaced according to the separation of the fragments	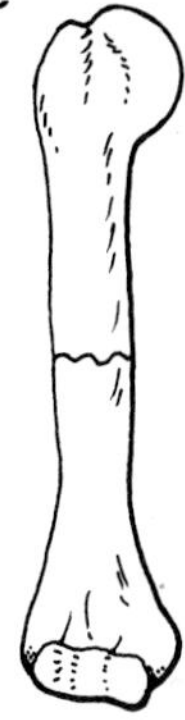
Oblique	Line of fracture extends in oblique direction	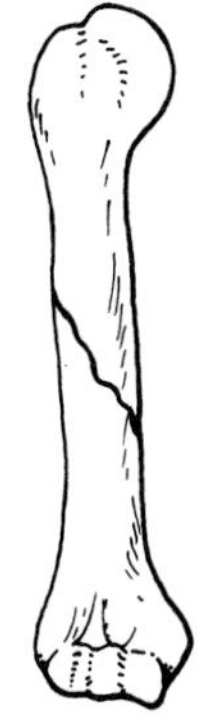
Pathological	Spontaneous fracture usually caused by disease process such as neoplasm	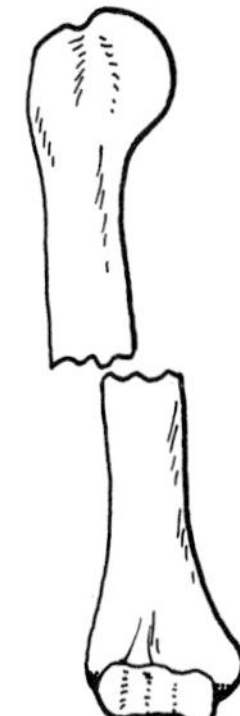
Segmental	Fracture which results in three or more bone fragments	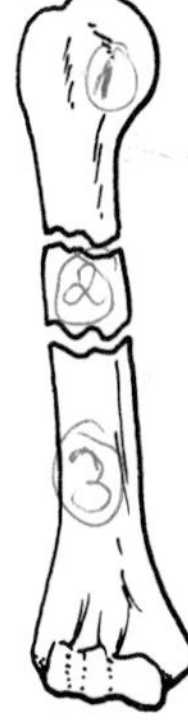

Table 56-1 (Continued)

Type	Description	Appearance
Spiral	Line of fracture extends in spiral direction along shaft of bone	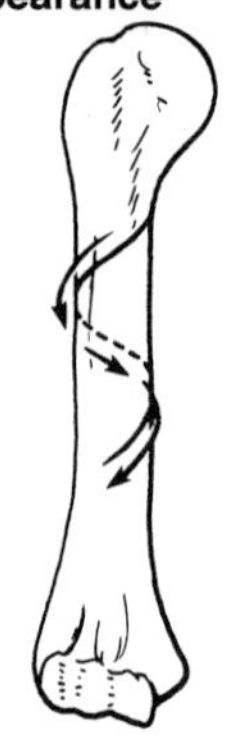
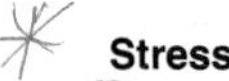 **Stress**	Prolonged or repeated stress which causes fracture	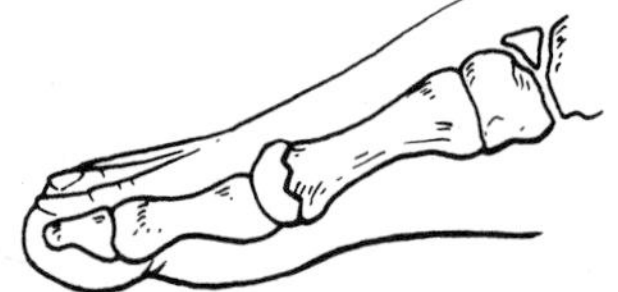
Transverse	Line of fracture extends across bone at a right angle	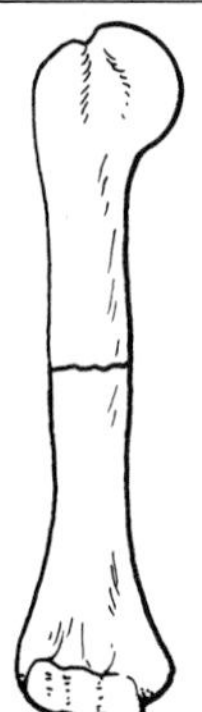

some of the periosteum is intact across the fracture; either external or internal fixation has rendered the fragments stationary. Stable fractures are usually transverse, spiral, or greenstick. An *unstable fracture* is grossly displaced at the time of injury and is a site of poor fixation. Unstable fractures are usually comminuted or oblique.

Clinical Manifestations (Table 56-2)

The client's history will indicate injury associated with immediate localized pain, decreased function, and inability to use the affected part. The client will guard and protect the part against movement. It is possible that the fracture may not be accompanied by obvious bone deformity. If a fracture is suspected, the affected part should be immobilized. Unnecessary movement increases soft-tissue damage and may convert a closed fracture into an open fracture. Careful management is particularly important for fractures through the epiphyseal plate in children. If fixation is not solid, the entire long bone may cease its longitudinal growth at all or part of the plate .

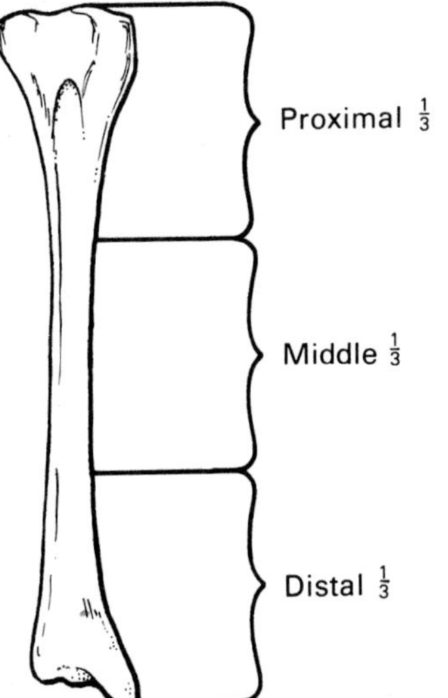

Figure 56-3 Fracture classification according to location.

Complications

The majority of fractures heal without complications. If death occurs after a fracture, it is usually the result of damage to underlying organs and soft tissue or of certain complications of the fracture. Complications of fractures may be either direct or indirect. Complications directly related to fractures include problems with bone union, avascular necrosis, and bone infection. Skeletal complications of fracture healing are summarized in Table 56-3. Indirect complications of fractures are associated with blood vessel and nerve damage—e.g., compartment syndrome, venous thrombosis, fat embolism, and traumatic or hypovolemic shock. Although most musculoskeletal injuries are not life-threatening, an open fracture accompanied by severe blood loss and fractures which damage vital organs are medical emergencies which require immediate attention.

Infection

Open fractures and soft-tissue injuries have a high incidence of infection. An open fracture usually results from the impact of severe external forces. The soft-tissue injury often has more serious consequences than the fracture. Devitalized and contaminated tissue is an ideal medium for many common pathogens, including gas-forming bacilli. Treatment of infections is costly in terms of extended nursing, medical care, treatment, and loss of client income.

Management Open fractures require surgical intervention. The wound is thoroughly cleaned by extensive irrigation, usually with sterile normal saline, and gross contaminants are mechanically removed. Contused, contaminated, and devitalized tissue such as muscle, subcutaneous fat, skin, and fragments of bone are surgically excised (*debridement*). The extent of the soft-tissue damage will determine whether the wound will be closed at the time of surgery, whether closed suction drainage will be used, and whether skin grafting will be necessary. Depending on the location and extent of the fracture, reduction may be

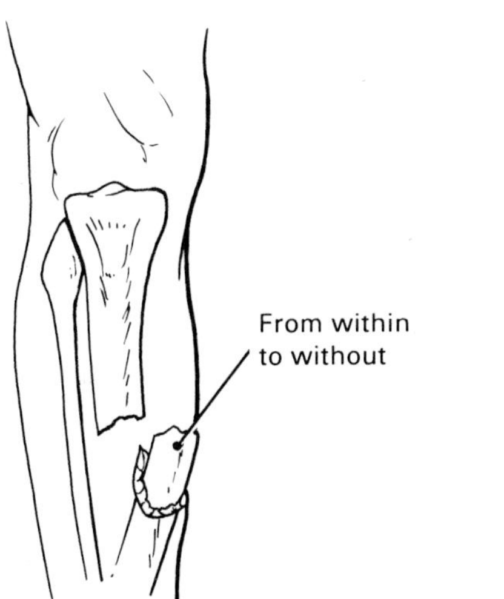

A. Open fracture

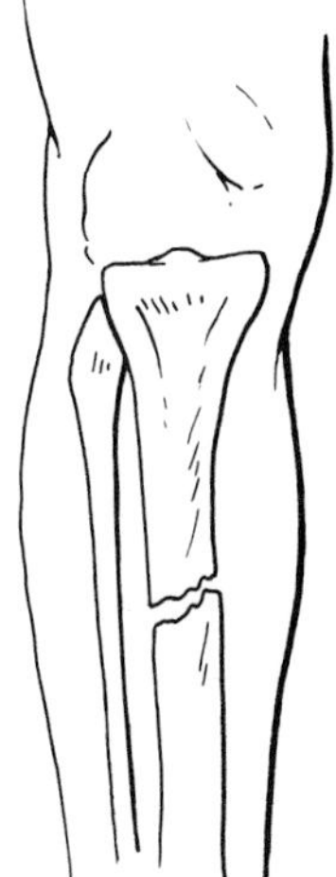

B. Closed fracture

Figure 56-4 Fracture classification according to communication.

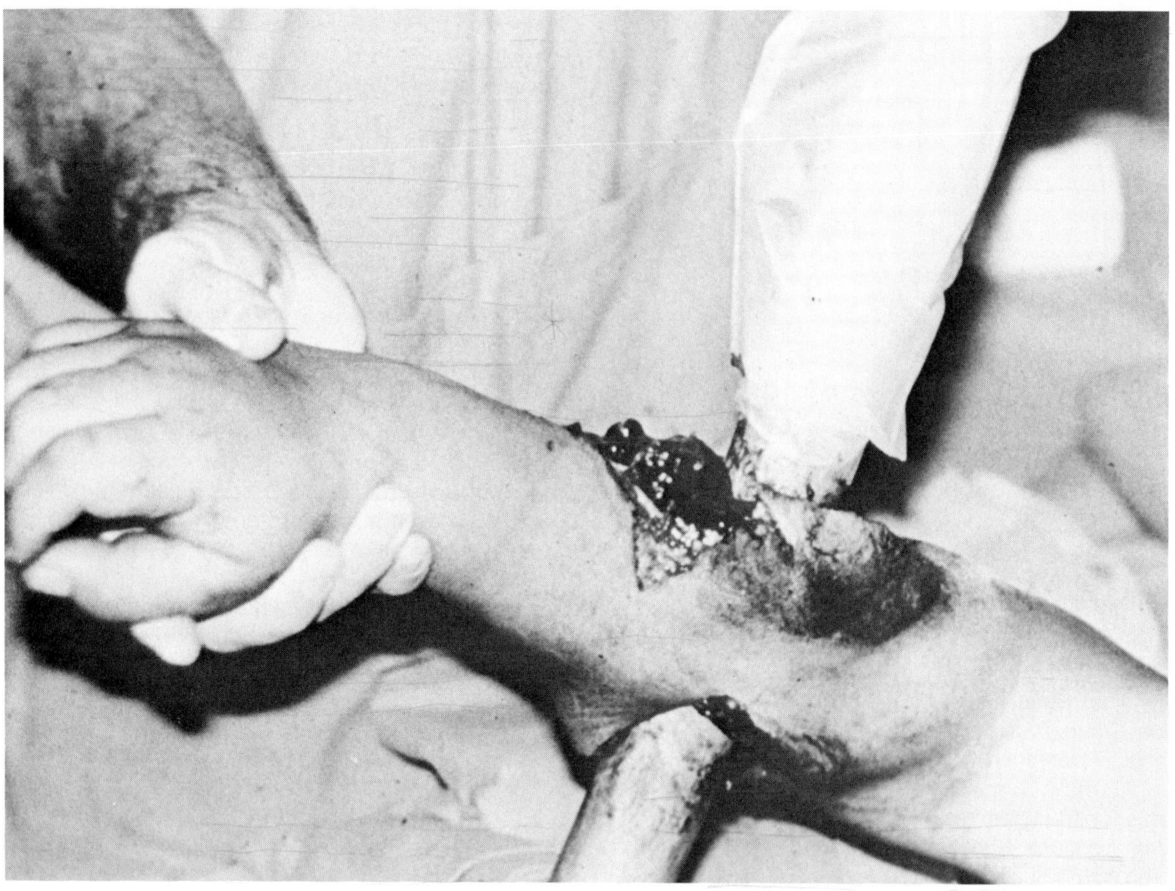

A

Figure 56-5 Open fracture. *(a)* Penetration from the outside environment to within. *(b)* Displacement of fracture fragments from within to the outside environment. Note soft-tissue disruption.

maintained by either a plaster cast or traction. During surgery the open wound may be irrigated with antibiotic solution. During the postoperative phase the client may have antibiotics administered intravenously, intramuscularly, or orally for a 7- to 10-day period. Antibiotics, in conjunction with aggressive surgical management, have greatly reduced the occurrence of infection.

Compartment syndrome

Compartment syndrome is the compression of structures within a defined area formed by fascial walls resulting from secondary edema. Development of a compartment syndrome requires immediate attention. Normally there is some increase in edema secondary to soft-tissue injury in the general region of the injury. If edema continues, there may be an increase of pressure within the closed spaces of the tissue compartments formed by the nonelastic fascia. This can cause sufficient pressure to obstruct venous circulation and cause arterial occlusion, resulting in inadequate circulation to the extremity, or ischemia. It can cause muscle infarction, with a gradual binding down of tendons and nerves with scar tissue, resulting in permanent anesthesia and paralysis of the affected part of the extremity.[2]

Compartment syndrome is associated with fractures or extensive soft-tissue damage in an extremity, most commonly the forearm or lower leg. Fractures of the distal humerus and proximal tibia are identified as the most common fractures associated with compartment syndrome. In the upper extremity this condition is referred to as *Volkmann's contracture* (Fig. 56-6) and in the lower extremity as the *anterior compartment syndrome*, although the underlying pathophysiology is similar.

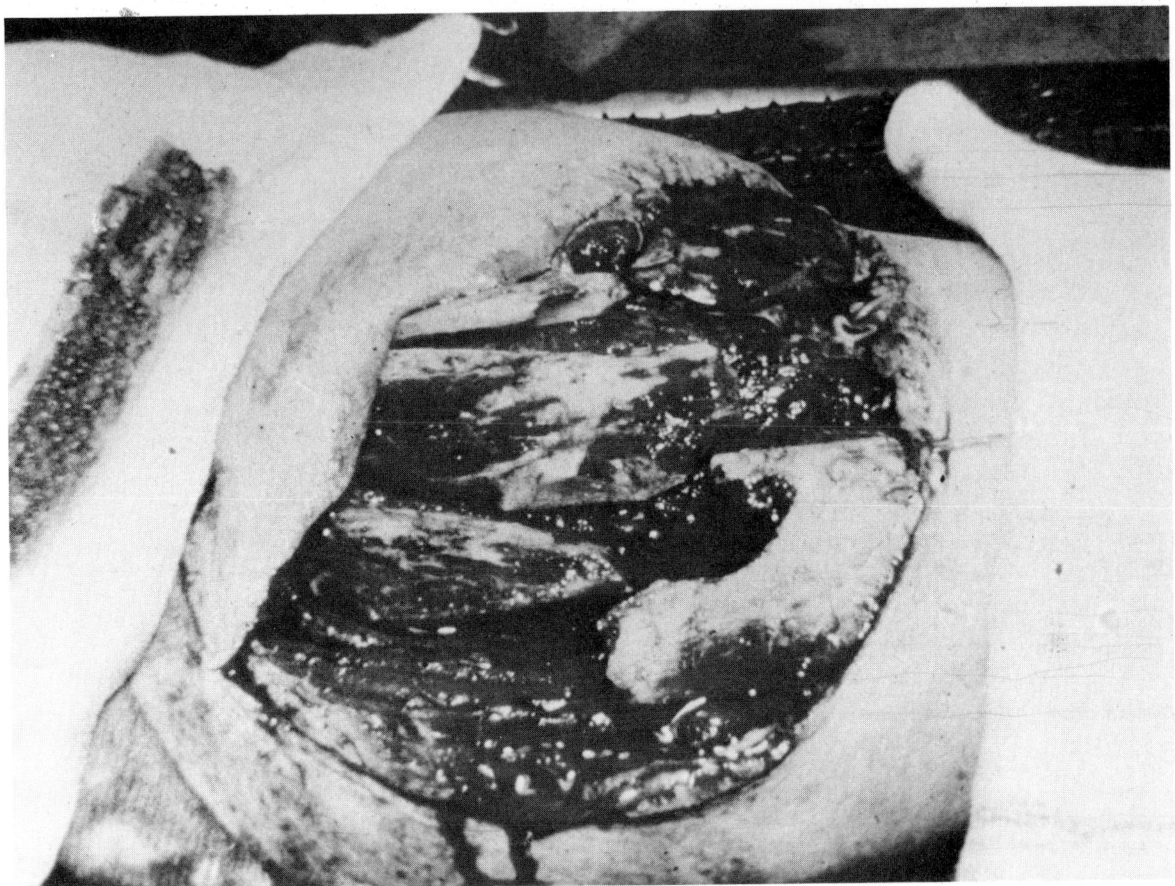

B

Figure 56-5 (Continued)

Clinical Manifestations The earliest sign of a developing compartment syndrome is progressive pain which is not relieved by the usual analgesics. The overlying skin may appear normal, since surface vessels are not occluded. In addition to inability to actively extend the digits, pain results from passive movement of the digits. Other symptoms as the condition progresses include numbness and tingling, loss of sensation and function, pallor and coolness of the extremity, and diminished or absent peripheral pulses. Absence of a peripheral pulse is an ominous sign which indicates severe disturbance of circulation. Regular neurovascular assessments (Fig. 56-7) should be carried out on all clients with injury of the distal humerus or proximal tibia or soft-tissue disruption in these areas.

Because of the possibility of muscle damage, the urine output should be assessed. Myoglobin, released from damaged muscle cells, can get trapped in renal tubules because of its high molecular weight. Common signs of myoglobinuria are (1) dark urine associated with a positive benzidine test in the absence of hematuria and (2) the manifestations associated with acute renal failure (see Chap. 38).

Management Prompt, accurate diagnosis of compartment syndrome is critical. Prevention is a key. The extremity should be elevated and ice applied to enhance venous return and decrease edema. It may be necessary to remove or loosen the bandage or cast or to reduce poundage on traction to prevent edema formation. It may be necessary to relieve compression and restore blood supply by surgically incising the fascia (*fasciotomy*).

Venous thrombosis

The veins of the lower extremities and pelvis are highly susceptible to thrombus formation after fracture

Table 56-2
Clinical Manifestations Suggestive of Fracture

Sign	Cause	Significance
Edema and swelling	Disruption of soft tissues or bleeding into the surrounding tissues	Unchecked swelling in a close space can occlude circulation and damage nerves
Pain and tenderness	Muscle spasm due to involuntary reflex action of muscle; direct tissue trauma; increased pressure on sensory nerve	Encourages splinting of fracture with reduction in motion of injured area; muscle spasm may displace a nondisplaced fracture or prevent it from spontaneously reducing
Deformity	Abnormal position of bone caused by original forces of injury and by action of muscles pulling fragment into abnormal position	Cardinal sign of fracture; uncorrected deformity may result in problems of bony union and restoration of function of injured part
Loss of function	Disruption of bone prevents functional use	Fracture must be managed properly to assure restoration of function
False motion	Motion which occurs at site of fracture	Cardinal sign of fracture; normally there is no movement of bone except at joint
Crepitation	Grating or crunching together of bony fragments producing palpable or audible crunching sensation	May increase soft-tissue damage
Ecchymosis	Discoloration of skin by extravasation of blood in subcutaneous tissues.	Usually appears several days after injury; may appear distal to injury; reassure client process is normal

Table 56-3
Complications of Fracture Healing

Problem	Description
Delayed union	Fracture healing is progressing more slowly than expected. Healing eventually occurs.
Nonunion	Fracture fails to heal properly despite treatment. Results in fibrous union or pseudarthrosis.
Malunion	Fracture heals in expected time but in unsatisfactory position which may result in deformity or dysfunction.
Angulation	Type of malunion in which fracture heals in abnormal position in relation to midline of the structure.
Pseudarthrosis	Type of malunion occurring at the fracture site, with each bone end being covered with fibrous scar.
Posttraumatic osteoporosis	Loss of mineral (bone substance) secondary to immobilization and/or disuse.
Refracture	Occurrence of new fracture through original fracture site.
Myositis ossificans	Response to hemorrhage in muscle caused by trauma. This hematoma ossifies. Has been known to occur in arm, elbow, and thigh.

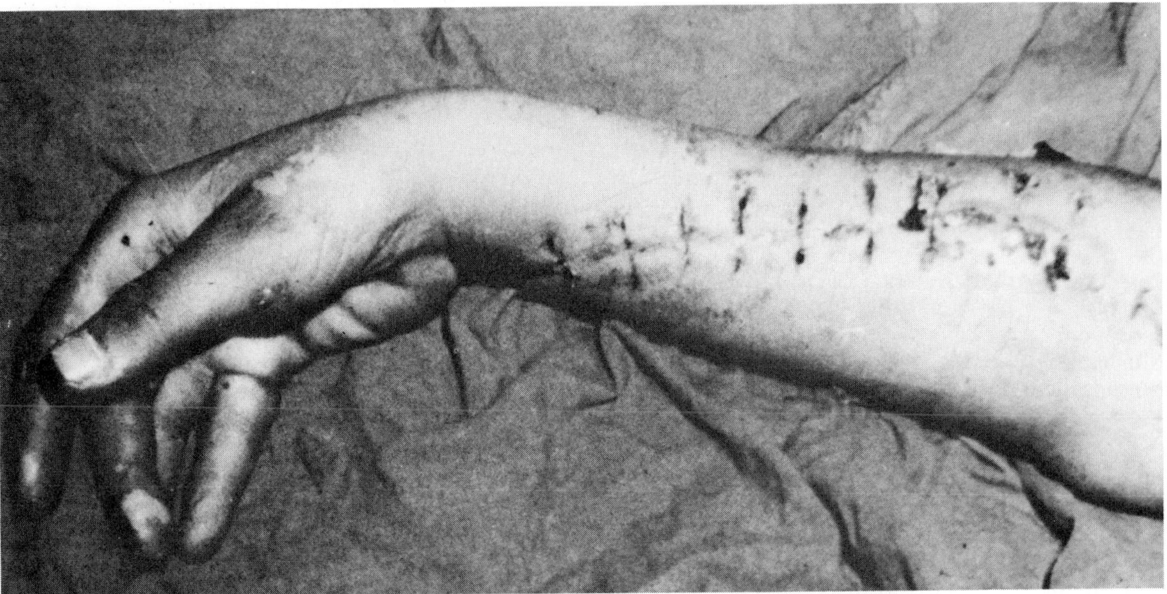

Figure 56-6 Volkmann's ischemic contracture of the forearm secondary to a supracondylar fracture of the humerus. Note the incision line of an unsuccessful fasciotomy.

injury. Precipitating factors are venous stasis caused by incorrectly applied casts or traction, local pressure on a vein, or prolonged bed rest. Venous stasis is aggravated by inactivity of the muscles which normally assist in the pumping action of venous return of blood in the extremities. In addition to wearing antiembolic (compression) stockings, the client should be instructed to move the fingers or toes of the affected extremity against resistance and to perform range-of-motion (ROM) exercises on all unaffected extremities. Assessment and management of venous thrombosis have been previously discussed in Chap. 30.

Fat embolism

Fat emboli, often associated with fractures of long bones, are a contributory factor in many deaths associated with fractures. There are two theories related to the origin of fat emboli.[3] The *mechanical theory* suggests that fat is liberated from the marrow of injured bone. It is driven out by an increase in intramedullary pressures and transmitted via draining veins to pulmonary capillaries, where it lodges. Some fat droplets traverse the capillary bed to enter systemic circulation and embolize to other sites. The *metabolic theory* postulates that the embolus arises in the plasma from conglomeration and fusion of a preexisting suspension of tiny chylomicrons. This is possibly due to some biochemical change initiated by the injury. The tissues of the lungs, brain, heart, kidneys, and skin are most frequently affected.

Clinical Manifestations Initial manifestations usually occur 12 to 72 hours after injury. The fat globules transported to the lungs cause a hemorrhagic interstitial pneumonitis that produces symptoms of adult respiratory distress syndrome, e.g., chest pain, tachypnea, cyanosis, dyspnea, apprehension (tachycardia), and decreased P_aO_2. All these are caused by poor oxygen exchange. The changes in the mental state are very important. Memory loss, restlessness, confusion, elevated temperature, and headache prompt further investigation so that central nervous system involvement is not mistaken for alcohol withdrawal. The continued change in level of consciousness and the petechiae located around the neck, anterior chest wall, axilla, buccal membrane of the mouth, and conjunctiva of the eye help distinguish between the two (Fig. 56-8).

The clinical course of a fat embolism may be brief and acute. Not infrequently the client expresses a feeling of impending disaster, and in a short period of time his color changes from pallor to cyanosis. He may become comatose. There are no specific laboratory examinations to aid in the diagnosis. However, certain diagnostic abnormalities may be present. These include fat cells in the urine or sputum, a decrease of the

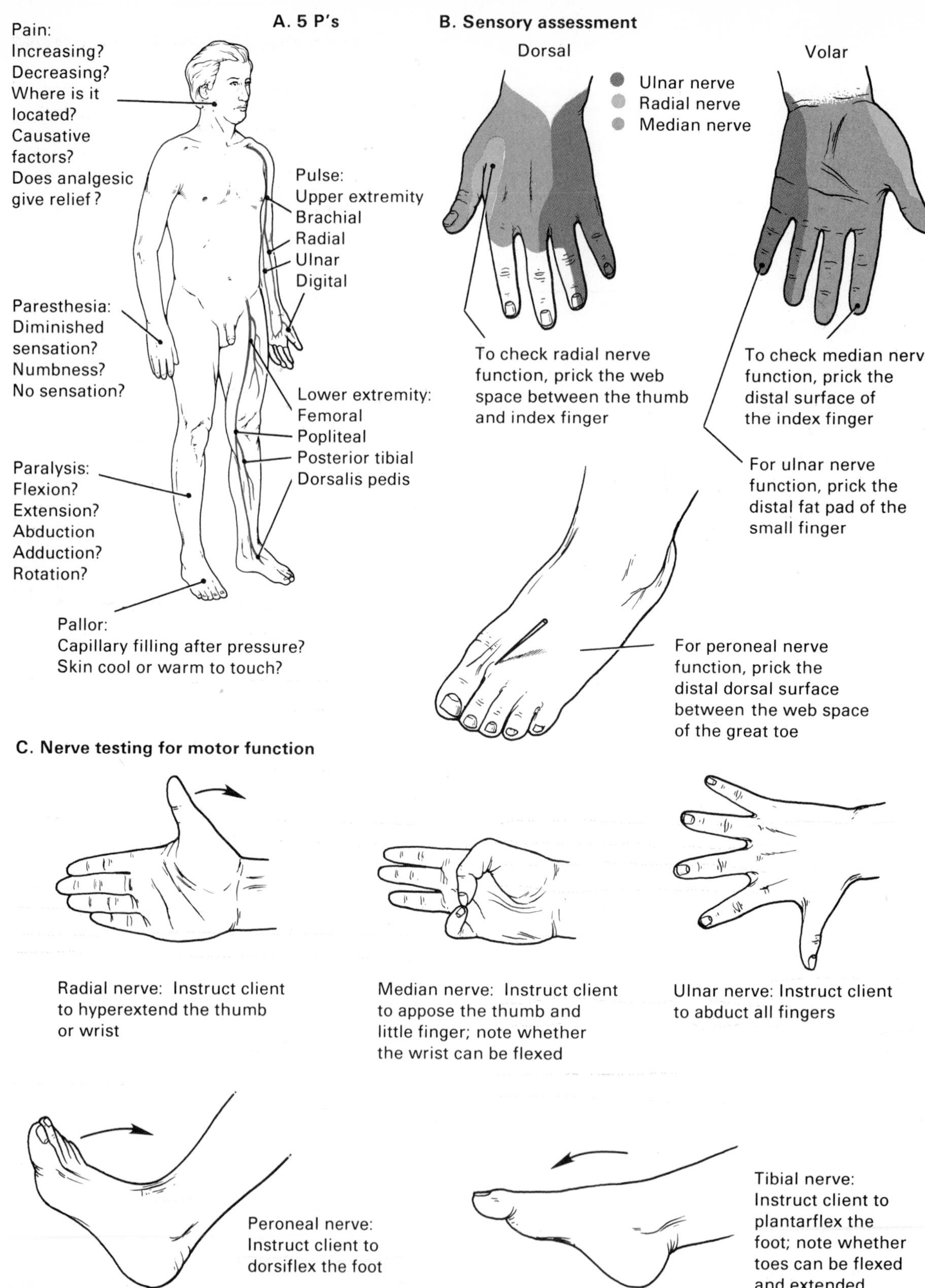
A. 5 P's
Pain:
Increasing?
Decreasing?
Where is it located?
Causative factors?
Does analgesic give relief?
Pulse:
Upper extremity
Brachial
Radial
Ulnar
Digital
Paresthesia:
Diminished sensation?
Numbness?
No sensation?
Lower extremity:
Femoral
Popliteal
Posterior tibial
Dorsalis pedis
Paralysis:
Flexion?
Extension?
Abduction
Adduction?
Rotation?
Pallor:
Capillary filling after pressure?
Skin cool or warm to touch?
B. Sensory assessment
Dorsal
Volar
Ulnar nerve
Radial nerve
Median nerve
To check radial nerve function, prick the web space between the thumb and index finger
To check median nerve function, prick the distal surface of the index finger
For ulnar nerve function, prick the distal fat pad of the small finger
For peroneal nerve function, prick the distal dorsal surface between the web space of the great toe
C. Nerve testing for motor function
Radial nerve: Instruct client to hyperextend the thumb or wrist
Median nerve: Instruct client to appose the thumb and little finger; note whether the wrist can be flexed
Ulnar nerve: Instruct client to abduct all fingers
Peroneal nerve: Instruct client to dorsiflex the foot
Tibial nerve: Instruct client to plantarflex the foot; note whether toes can be flexed and extended

Figure 56-7 Peripheral nerve and vascular assessment *(a)* The five P's. *(b)* Sensory assessment *(c)* Motor assessment *[From Kenneth J. Webb, "Early Assessment of Orthopedic Injuries," Am J Nurs, **74:**1054 (June 1974).]*

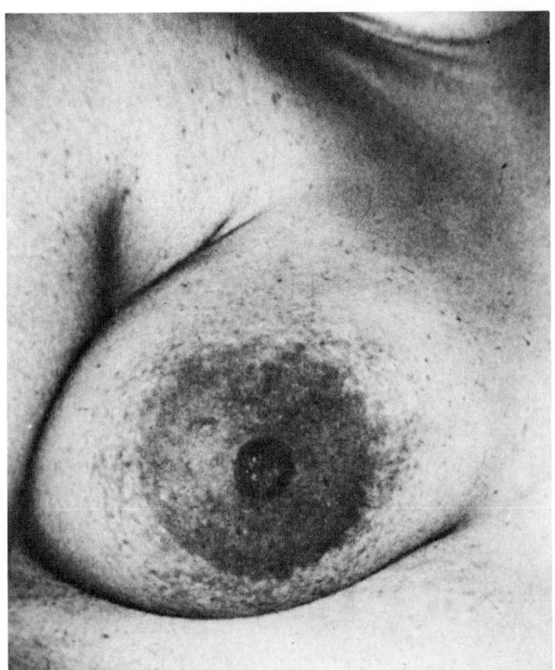

Figure 56-8 Formation of petechiae secondary to a fat embolus in the region of the breast and axilla 24 hours after distal femoral shaft fracture in a 43-year-old female.

P_aO_2 to less than 60 mmHg, and a decrease in the platelet count. A chest x-ray may reveal areas of pulmonary infiltrate or multiple areas of consolidation.

Management Careful immobilization of long-bone fractures is thought to be helpful in reducing the occurrence of fat embolism. Although there is no specific treatment for it, oxygen is administered to treat hypoxia. Steroids, anticoagulants, and low-molecular-weight dextran have proved beneficial in conjunction with the maintenance of alveolar gas exchange.[4] Management is essentially symptomatic and supportive and includes restriction of fluid intake, correction of acidosis, and replacement of any blood loss. Coughing and deep breathing should be encouraged. The client should be repositioned as little as possible during the acute phase because of the danger of dislodging more fat droplets into the general circulation.

Fracture Healing

In order to provide appropriate and therapeutic interventions, it is important to understand the principles of fracture healing (Fig. 56-9). The reparative process of bone healing (called *union*) occurs in the following stages:

1. *Fracture hematoma*. When a fracture occurs, bleeding and edema precede the development of a hematoma, which surrounds the ends of the fragments. The hematoma is extravasated blood which changes from a liquid to a semisolid clot.
2. *Granulation tissue*. During this stage there is active phagocytosis to absorb the products of local necrosis. The hematoma changes into new tissue known as granulation tissue. Granulation tissue, consisting of young blood vessels, fibroblasts, and osteoblasts, produces a new bone substance called osteoid.
3. *Callus formation*. As minerals are deposited in the osteoid, it forms an unorganized network of bone which is woven about the fracture parts. Callus is primarily composed of cartilage, osteoblasts, calcium, and phosphorus and usually begins to appear by the end of the first week after injury. Evidence of callus formation can be verified by x-ray.
4. *Clinical union*. Clinical union is the stage in which a client can come out of the skeletal traction or cast and start being more mobile. This stage is marked by enough ossification of the callus that no movement occurs at the fracture site when the bones are gently stressed. However, the fracture is still evident radiographically.
5. *Consolidation*. As callus continues to develop, the distance between bone fragments diminishes and eventually closes. This stage is called consolidation or ossification. It can be equated with radiographic union.
6. *Remodeling*. Excess cells are absorbed in the final stage of bone healing and union is complete. There is gradual return of the injured bone to its preinjury structural strength and shape. Remodeling of bone is enhanced as it responds to physical stress. At first such stress is provided through exercise. Weight bearing is gradually introduced. New bone is deposited in sites subjected to stress and resorbed at areas where there is little stress. *Radiographic union* occurs when there is radiographic evidence of complete bony union.

Many factors such as age, initial displacement of the fracture, site of the fracture, and blood supply to the area influence the time required for fracture healing to be complete. It may be disrupted or delayed if blood supply is not adequate, if immobilization is poor, if infection develops, or if traction is excessive. Healing time for fractures increases with age; for example, an uncomplicated midshaft fracture of the femur heals in 3 weeks in a newborn and requires 20 weeks in an adult.

Medical Management

The overall goals of fracture treatment are (1) anatomical realignment of bone fragments; (2) immo-

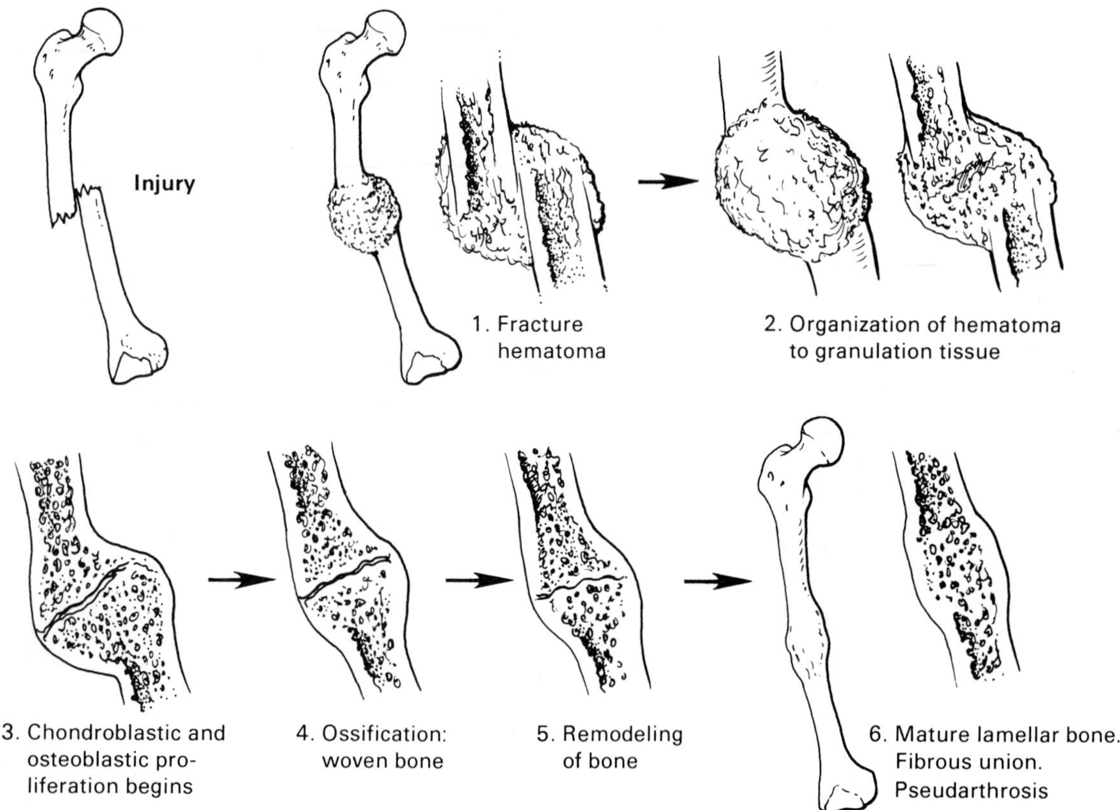

Figure 56-9 Stages in fracture healing. *(From F. Richard Schneider, Handbook for the Orthopaedic Assistant, The C. V. Mosby Company, St. Louis, 1978, vol. 2, p. 47.)*

bilization to maintain realignment; and (3) restoration of function of the part. Table 56-4 summarizes medical management of fractures.

Fracture reduction

Manipulation or Closed Reduction This is a nonsurgical, manual realignment of bones to their previous anatomical position. Local or general anesthesia may be required. Traction and countertraction are manually applied to the bone fragments to restore position, length, and alignment. Closed reduction is usually performed under some type of anesthesia. After reduction, the injured part is immobilized by casting or traction in order to maintain alignment until healing occurs.

Open Reduction Open reduction is the correction of bone alignment through a surgical incision. It may include internal fixation of the fracture utilizing various types of rods, wire, screws, pins, intramedul-

Table 56-4

Medical Management: Fractures

Diagnostic

1. History and physical examination
2. X-ray examination

Therapeutic

1. Fracture reduction
   a. Manipulation (closed reduction)
   b. Open reduction
   c. Traction devices
      (1) Skin traction
      (2) Skeletal traction
2. Fracture immobilization
   a. External fixation: casting
   b. Internal fixation devices
   c. Maintenance traction
3. Open fractures
   a. Surgical debridement
   b. Tetanus immunization
   c. Prophylactic antibiotic therapy
   d. Immobilization

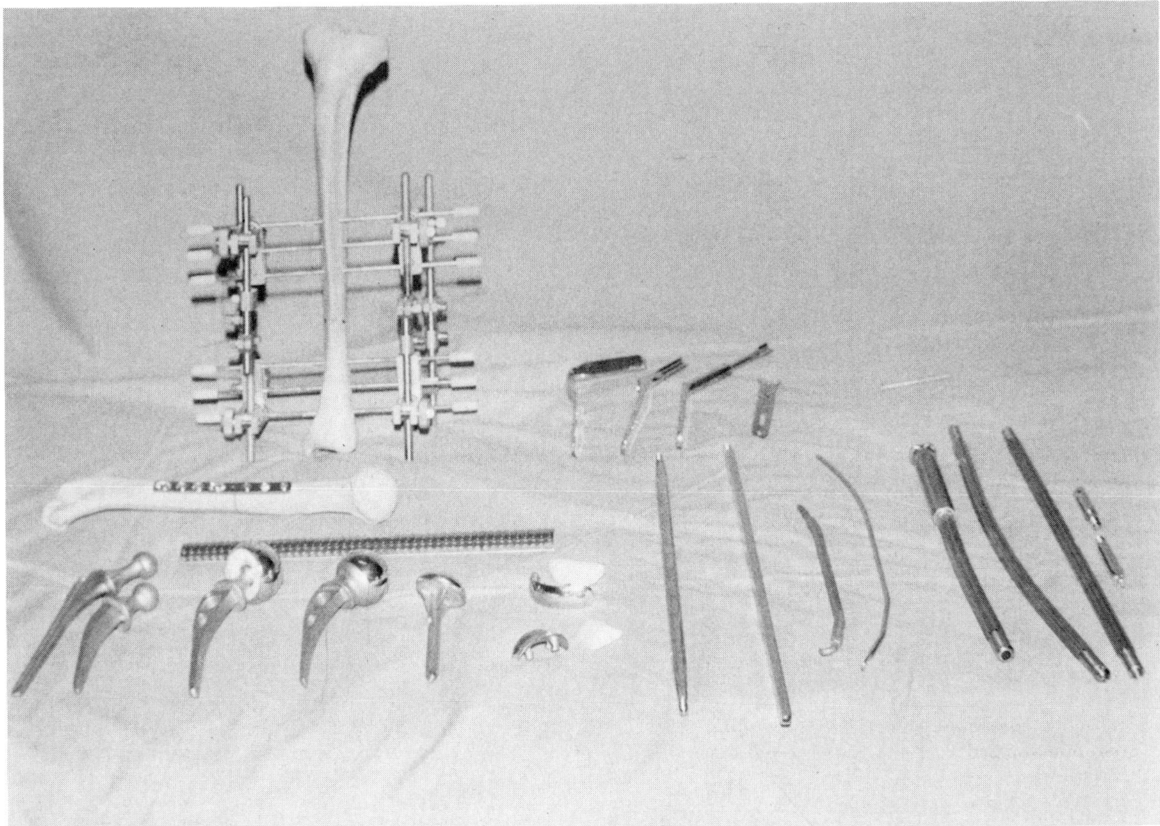

Figure 56-10 Common surgical appliances utilized in orthopedic surgery. From left to right: *Top row:* External fixation appliance, intercondylar blade plate, Jewett hip nail, telescoping compression hip nail, bone plate, cancellous bone screw. *Middle row:* Compression plate, titanium bone plate, *Bottom row:* Straight solid Moore-type Bateman stem, endoprosthesis, Nee shoulder prosthesis patellar emoral resurface, Schneider straight rod, Hanson straight nail, upper-extremity boat nail, Ender flexible pin, Sampson subtrochanteric fluted nail, Sampson curved fluted nail, Sampson straight fluted nail, extrator cap.

lary rods, or nails (Fig. 56-10). The type and location of the fracture, as well as the result of attempted closed reduction or traction, influence the decision to use open reduction. The chief disadvantages of this form of treatment are the possibility of infection and the complications associated with general anesthesia.

Traction Traction devices apply a pulling force on the fractured extremity and result in realignment. The force can be applied through adhesive applied directly to the skin (*skin traction*) or through a metal pin or wire inserted directly into or through a bone (*skeletal traction*). Traction has several therapeutic purposes: (1) to reduce, align, and immobilize fractures until bony union occurs; (2) to lessen, prevent, or correct deformity associated with bone injury and muscle disease; and (3) to reduce muscle spasms in fracture of a long bone or back injury.

When traction is utilized to treat fractures, the traction forces are usually exerted on the distal fragment in order to obtain alignment with the proximal fragment. Several different types of traction are used for this purpose (Table 56-5). Fracture alignment is dependent upon the correct positioning and alignment of the client while the traction forces remain constant. For extremity traction to be effective, there must be forces pulling in the opposite direction (*countertraction*) to prevent the client from sliding to the end of the bed. Countertraction may be obtained by elevating the end of the bed 8 to 12 inches and by the weight of the client's own body. In the case of a light person, the trunk may need fixation with vest immobilizers.

Table 56-5
Common Types of Traction

Type	Indications	Nursing Implications	Appearance
Skin			
Buck's	Used for wide variety of conditions affecting hip, femur, knee, or back. Generally used for temporary immobilization.	Assess for nerve and circulatory disturbances caused by circumferential bandages, especially over bony prominences, also for skin necrosis, allergic reaction to adhesive material, rotation of extremity, and constant traction and countertraction forces. (Applies to Buck's and Russell's types.)	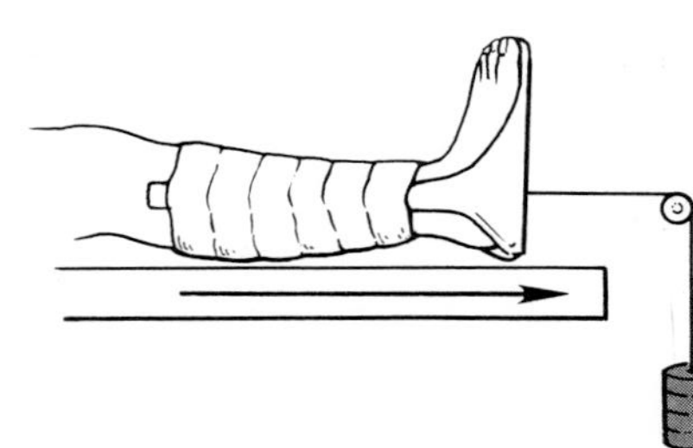 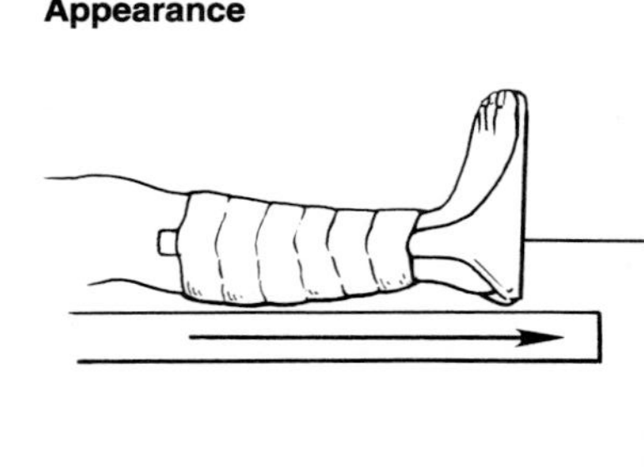
Russell's	Utilized for basically same conditions as Buck's traction. Resultant force is in line with femur.		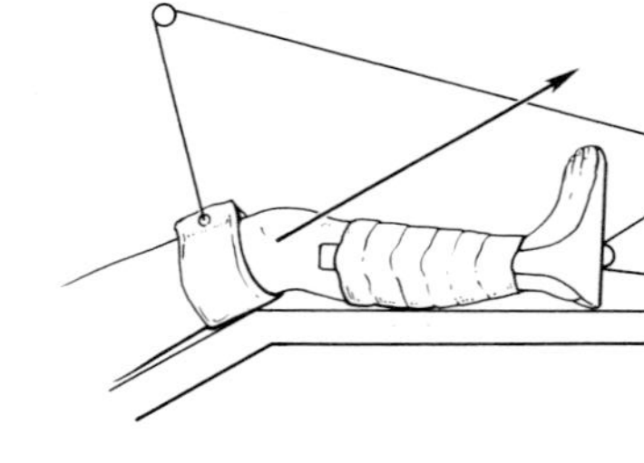
Bardenheuer's (lateral arm traction)	Utilized for fracture in upper extremity, usually supracondylar fracture of distal humerus.	This type of fracture usually manifested by severe swelling. Assess circulatory status carefully to avoid Volkmann's contracture.	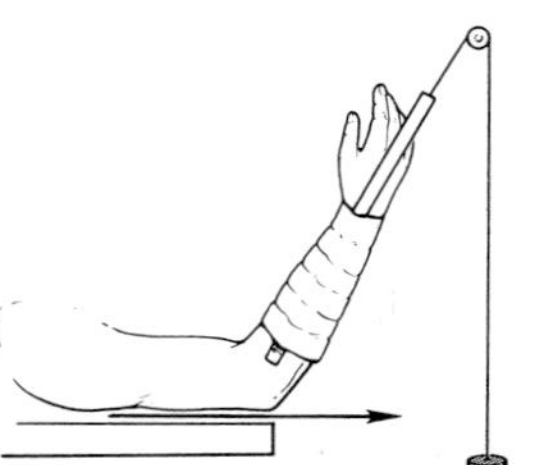
Circumferential			
Head halter	Soft-tissue disorders or degenerative disk disease of cervical spine. Not commonly used for unstable fractures of cervical spine.	Assess for alignment with trunk, for areas of local pressure under chin and occipital area, and for pain or dysfunction in temporomandibular joint.	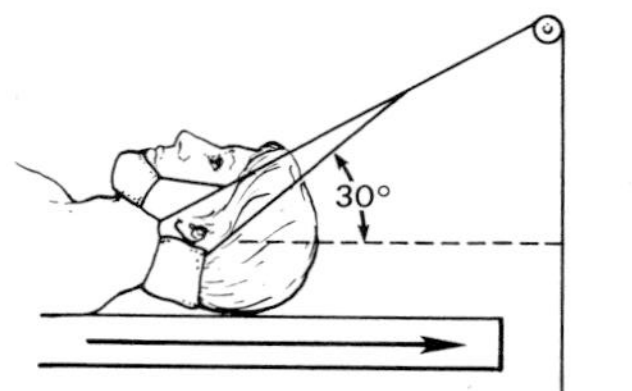

Pelvic traction	Acute or low back pain.	Check securing of pelvic belt around iliac crests: frequent complaint of pressure from being applied too tight. Administer good skin care in region of traction belt.	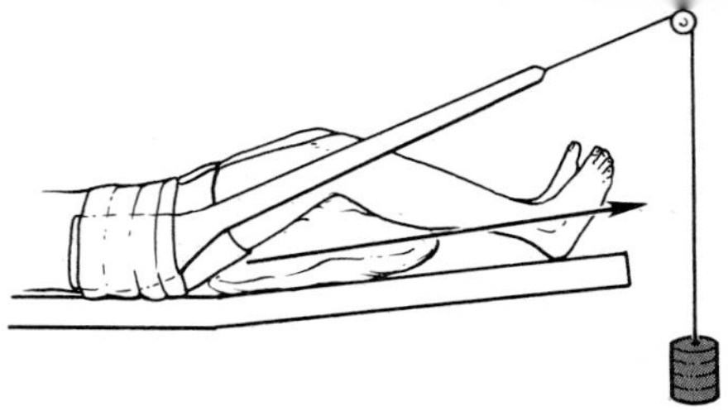
Skeletal Overhead arm	Commonly utilized in treatment of fractures of middle or proximal humerus and dislocations of shoulder.	Encourage motion of hand and fingers of affected part; observe for motion of skeletal pin or signs of loosening; assess peripheral nerve function. Bed in flat position at all times. Decubitus and antiembolic precautions. Encourage active movement of uninvolved extremities, coughing and deep-breathing exercises. (Applies to overhead arm and lateral arm types.)	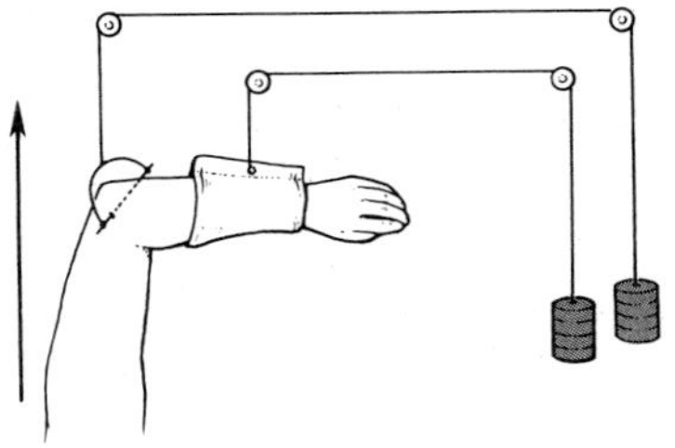
Lateral arm	Commonly utilized in treatment of fractures of distal humerus.		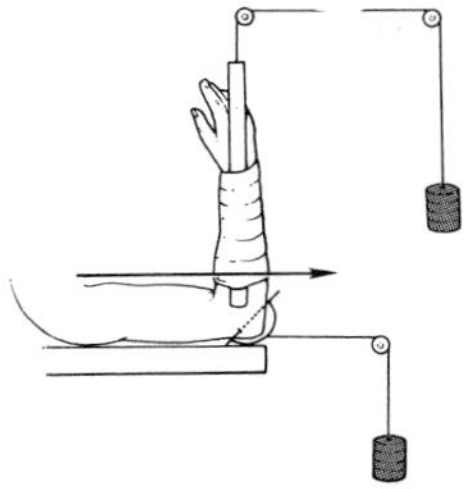
Balanced suspension traction	Injury or fracture of middle or distal third of femur, fracture of acetabulum, or hip dislocation.	Utilizes half-ring Thomas splint (1) and Pearson attachment (2). Suspension of extremity (A) and direct traction (B) applied. Frequent skin care of groin area necessary to prevent irritation. Daily inspection of pin site. Head of bed should not be elevated more than 25° because of interference with countertraction forces. Special nursing measures to prevent foot drop.	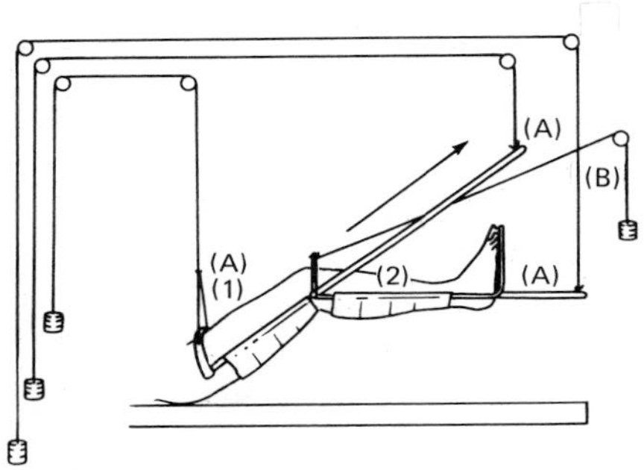

Fracture immobilization

External Fixation or Casting This is a common treatment following closed reduction. Casting allows the client to perform many normal activities of daily living while providing sufficient immobilization to ensure stability. Cast materials include plaster of paris, fiberglass, and thermolabile plastic.

Plaster of paris continues to be the material most widely used for casting. It is anhydrous calcium sulfate embedded in gauze of varying widths and sizes. When water is added the plaster assumes a crystalline state and can be molded or wrapped around the affected part (Fig. 56-11). The strength of the cast is determined by the number of layers of plaster bandage and the technique of application. During the process of crystallization, the cast becomes warm as it dries and hardens. After the cast is completely dry, it is strong, firm, and able to withstand stresses. The plaster is hard within 15 minutes, so the client can move around without problems. It is not strong enough for weight bearing until it is dry, about 24 to 48 hours. There is also a danger of increased edema due to the increased circulation produced by the heat of the drying cast.

Thermolabile plastic (Orthoplast) comes in large squares. After being heated, it is molded to fit the torso or extremity. *Fiberglass* cast material is supplied in rolls of tape which has been impregnated with a photosensitive resin. The fiberglass material is exposed to ultraviolet light to cure it, and the result is a hard, lightweight cast. These two newer cast materials permit great mobility and comfort. They are very strong, do not soften in water, and are radiolucent. Clients can bathe with casts of these types. The major deterrent to their use is higher cost.

Internal Fixation Internal fixation devices are surgically inserted at the time of realignment. They are biologically inert devices which are used to realign as well as maintain bony fragments. Proper alignment is evaluated by x-ray at regular intervals.

Maintenance Traction Maintenance traction is initiation or continuation of traction and countertraction. A continuous pulling force can be applied directly to bone with wires and pins (skeletal traction) or can be applied indirectly by weights that are attached to the skin with adhesive straps or boots. Skin traction is usually applied directly to the extremity by adhesive material which is circumferentially wrapped with a bandage or a special garment with straps which is attached to a rope with a weight. Skin traction is applied for a short period of time and usually consists of not more than 7 to 10 pounds of traction weight because of skin intolerance to pressure.[5] Skeletal traction is usually indicated when the traction forces are expected to exceed 10 lb or the traction will be utilized for a long period of time. The use of too much weight to maintain traction can result in delayed union or nonunion. The major disadvantages of skeletal traction are the possibility of infection in the area of bone where the skeletal pin has been inserted and the complications of prolonged immobility.

Open fracture

An open fracture is treated as previously discussed under complications. In addition, tetanus prevention should be assured by the used of tetanus toxoid or tetanus antitoxin for a client not previously immunized. A broad-spectrum antibiotic is usually used prophylactically. A decision on whether to close the wound or leave it open is based on the degree of contamination and the time elapsed before treatment was initiated.

The overall long-term goal of medical treatment is the correction of the fracture and return of the client to the preinjury level at the earliest possible time. Discharge planning should include referral to the appropriate human service agency for assistance in the transition to the home environment.

Pharmacological Intervention

Persons with fractures often experience varying degrees of pain associated with muscle spasms. These spasms are caused by involuntary reflex secondary to the muscle injury. Muscle relaxants are often prescribed for the relief of pain associated with muscle spasm. Muscle relaxants are categorized according to whether they primarily control muscle relaxation only or are combinations of muscle relaxant and sedative.[6]

Medications primarily used as muscle relaxants include carisoprodol (Rela, Soma), chlorphenesin carbamate (Maolate), chlorzoxazone (Paraflex), dantrolene sodium (Dantrium), metaxalone (Skelaxin), methocarbamol (Robaxin), mephenesin (Atensin), orphenadrine (Disipal), and styramate (Sinaxar). Medications which combine a sedative action with muscle relaxant properties include chlormezanone (Trancopal), diazepam (Valium), meprobamate (Equanil, Miltown), and tybamate (Solacen, Tybatran).

Common side effects associated with muscle relaxants are drowsiness, lassitude, lethargy, headache, weakness, fatigue, blurred vision, ataxia, and gastrointestinal upset. Hypersensitivity reactions may include skin rash or pruritus. Ingestion of large doses may cause hypotension, tachycardia, or respiratory

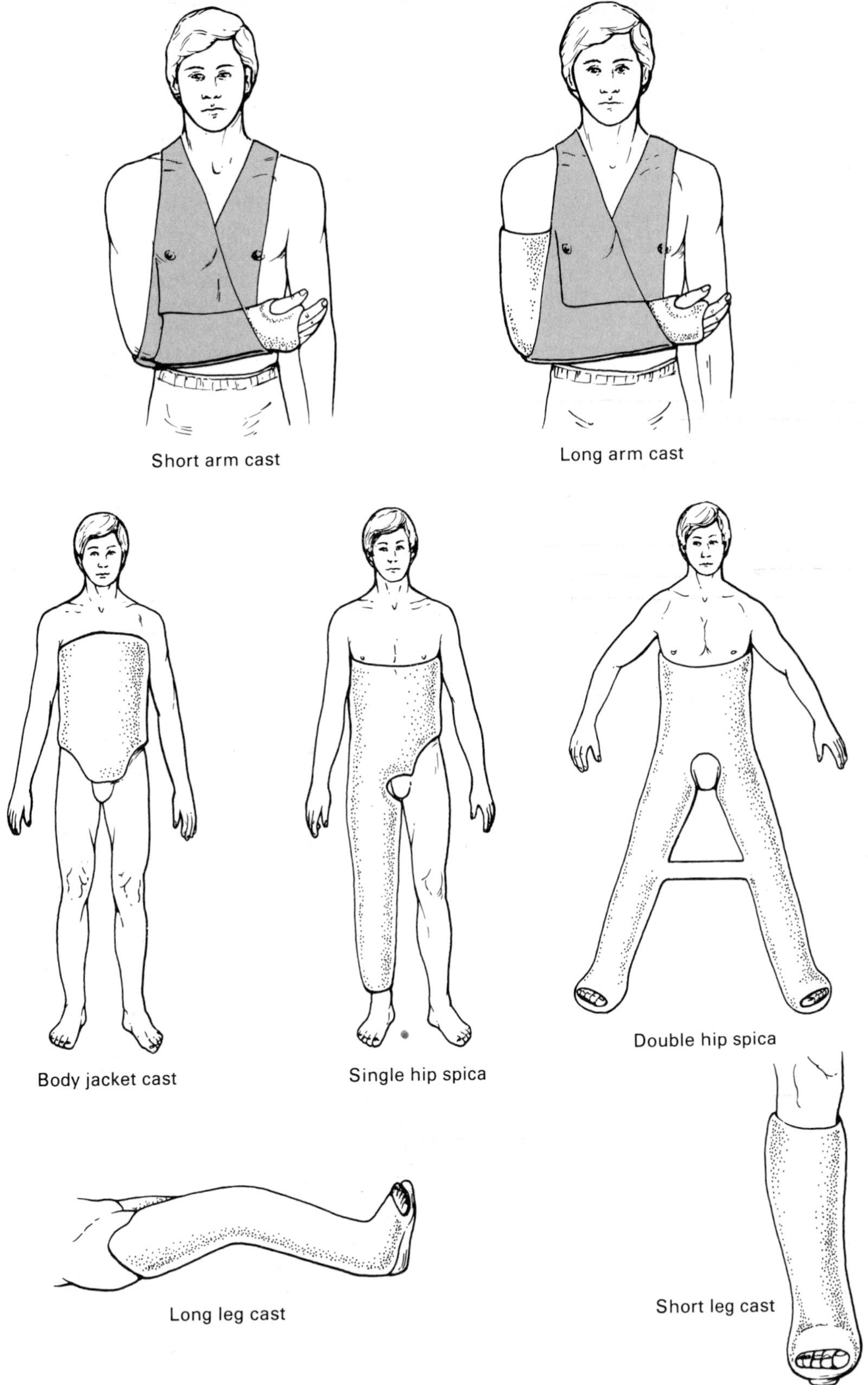

Figure 56-11 Common casts utilized in treatment of disorders of the musculoskeletal system.

depression. The possible habituating effects associated with chronic use or abuse must be carefully considered.

Some physicians do not believe in the use of muscle relaxants for relief of muscle spasms. They feel that the reflex spasm will continue as long as the precipitating pain persists, and that if the pain is controlled by the use of appropriate analgesia, the muscle spasms will cease.

Dietary Measures

Proper nutrition is an essential component of the reparative process in injured tissue. An adequate energy source is needed to meet the requirements for recovery such as (1) promotion of muscle strength and tone, (2) building endurance, and (3) ambulation and gait-training skills. To ensure optimal soft-tissue and bony healing, the client's dietary requirements must include ample protein (e.g., 1 g per kilogram of body weight) and vitamins, especially B and C. Low serum protein levels and vitamin C deficiencies interfere with tissue healing. Three well-balanced meals a day will usually provide the necessary nutrients. The well-balanced diet should be supplemented by an intake of fluid of 2000 to 3000mL/day to promote optimal function of the bladder and the bowel. Adequate fluid and a high fiber diet (see Appendix B, Table 6) will prevent constipation. If immobilized in a body jacket or hip spica cast, the client should be instructed not to overeat to avoid pressure and cramping.

Nursing Management of the Client with a Fracture

Health promotion and maintenance

The nurse has an important role in educating the public in the basic principles of safety and accident prevention. The morbidity associated with accidents could be significantly reduced if people were aware of environmental hazards, utilized existing safety equipment, and applied safety and traffic rules. In the industrial setting, the nurse should stress the use of appropriate safety equipment and avoidance of hazardous working situations.

In the home environment, falls account for many musculoskeletal injuries. Preventive education should be directed toward the importance of wearing shoes with functional soles and heels, avoiding wet or slippery surfaces, careful placement of throw rugs, and removal of obstacles from the pathway of persons with impaired vision or those who use an assistive device for ambulation.

Acute intervention

The client with a fracture may be treated in an emergency room or physician's office and released to home care, or the fracture may require hospitalization for varying amounts of time. Specific nursing measures are dependent upon the type of treatment used and the setting in which the client is placed for healing to take place. Table 56-6 summarizes general nursing measures for the client with a fracture.

Assessment Assessment and intervention at the scene of an accident or acute injury are covered in Chap. 58. This section deals with nursing management of the client with a fracture who is in a setting where definitive treatment will take place.

The nurse is responsible for regular assessment of the client until management is initiated. Assessment of neurological and vascular status should follow the guidelines known as the 5 P's (Fig. 56-7):

Pain—Changes in the intensity of pain should be noted. Increased pain can be caused by an incorrectly applied immobilization device, constrictive dressings, or excessive movement of the extremity.

Pulse—The peripheral pulses distal to the site of injury should be regularly evaluated to determine circulatory adequacy.

Paresthesia—The sensory status of the injured extremity can be assessed by asking the client if he feels a touch or pinprick. Sensation is described as fully present, abnormal (paresthesia), or numbness and tingling.

Paralysis—Inability to move a part distal to the site of injury should be noted.

Pallor—Absence of skin coloration or evidence of cyanosis or temperature change of the extremity should be regularly evaluated.

Special emphasis must be focused on the region distal to the site of injury. The involved extremity should be compared with the uninvolved extremity. Clinical findings must be recorded before fracture treatment is started in order to avoid any doubts as to whether a problem discovered later was caused by the treatment or by the original injury.[7]

Surgical Management: Preoperative If surgical intervention is required to treat the fracture, the client will need preoperative preparation. In addition to the usual preoperative nursing measures (Chap. 6), the nurse should inform the client of the type of immobilization device that will be used and the expected activity limitations. The client must be assured that his

Table 56-6
Nursing Care Plan for the Client with a Fracture

Client Problem	Expected Outcome	Nursing Intervention
Edema	Absence of swelling	Elevate extremity above heart level. Apply ice compresses as ordered. Assess nerve and vascular status of affected extremity q 2 h.
Pain	Decrease or absence of pain	Gently and correctly position fractured extremity. Assess for constriction or pressure caused by immobilization. Give analgesics as indicated.
Infection (open fracture)	No evidence of wound infection	Use sterile technique when providing wound care or dressing change. Observe for wound drainage. Obtain culture and sensitivity test of wound. Administer antibiotics as ordered. Monitor temperature q 2 h. Isolate client to prevent dissemination of pathogen or cross-contamination of wound.
Muscle spasms	Decrease in muscle spasms and resulting pain	Correctly position and align extremity. Change position of client q 2 h. Administer muscle relaxant as ordered (e.g., diazepam).
Weakness	Preinjury strength and endurance	Encourage active range-of-motion exercise of joints not immobilized. Perform resistive exercises of unaffected extremities. Plan rest periods between activities. Encourage client participation in ADL and exercises.
Immobilization of fracture	Maintenance of bony alignment until healing is complete	Give cast care (see Table 56-7). Ensure adequate drying without development of pressure points. Keep cast clean and dry. Protect skin by tape or moleskin to petal edges. Monitor amount and type of drainage. Give appropriate traction care. Examine traction equipment regularly for frays or slippage. Maintain free-hanging weights. Assess skin areas at traction sites for signs of infection or irritation.
Skin breakdown	No evidence of skin breakdown	Use alcohol at cast edges and over bony prominences. Examine and massage casted areas and pressure areas regularly. Petal cast edges. Turn q 2 h. Keep bed free of wrinkles and crumbs.
Ambulation difficulties (with lower extremity fractures)	Resume normal gait cycle	Teach client principles of gait training (non-weight-bearing gait status unless otherwise ordered by physician): sit with feet over edge of bed; stand with no weight on affected extremity; measure and adjust crutches; start gait training on parallel bars; correct gait compatible with weight-bearing status.
Looseness of cast	Notify clinician if cast becomes too loose	Explain that cast will sometimes become loose because of muscle atrophy. Seek medical attention if cast becomes loose and permits rotation or flexion or begins skin abrasion.
Muscle atrophy	Minimal loss of muscle bulk of affected extremity	Cooperate with physical therapist regarding exercise and gait training. Explain importance of activity of affected extremity as tolerated. Reinforce exercise program as prescribed by physician. Explain factors which contribute to disuse atrophy.
Decreased range of motion (ROM)	No decrease in ROM of affected extremity	Plan regular ROM exercises. Perform passive or active exercises depending on status of client, method of immobilization, and type and location of fracture. Instruct client not to exercise beyond point of comfort.
Soiled cast	Cast remaining clean and strong to effectively immobilize fracture	Instruct client in proper cast care (see Table 56-7).

needs will be met by the nursing staff until he can again assume this role. Assurance that pain medication will be available, if needed, is often beneficial.

Proper skin preparation is an important part of preoperative preparation before surgery. The protocol for skin preparation varies among agencies and may or may not be the responsibility of the nursing staff. The aim of skin preparation is to clean the skin and remove hair by shaving. Careful attention to this preoperative treatment can influence the postoperative course by reducing the possibility of infection.

Surgical Management: Postoperative In general, postoperative nursing care and management is directed toward monitoring vital signs and applying the general principles of postoperative nursing care (Chap. 8). Any limitations of movement or activity in relation to turning, positioning, and extremity support should be followed closely. Pain and discomfort can be kept to a minimum by correct alignment and positioning. Dressings or casts should be carefully observed for any overt signs of excessive bleeding or drainage. An acceptable method of detecting increases in bleeding is to draw a circle on the cast around an area of drainage, noting the date and time. Rapid enlargement of the drainage area should be reported. If a wound-drainage system is in place, the patency of the system and the volume of drainage should be assessed at least once each shift. Whenever the contents of a drainage system are measured or emptied, the nurse should utilize sterile technique to avoid contamination of the site. Additional nursing responsibilities depend upon the type of immobilization that is used.

Nursing Care of the Client with a Cast Immediately after the application of a plaster of paris cast, there is a short period of exothermic reaction when heat is released from the plaster. The client should be alerted to this occurrence, since it can increase edema. Evaporation of water and dissipation of heat from the cast can be hastened by encouraging circulation of room air around the cast. A fresh cast should never be covered with a blanket, since air will not circulate and heat will build up in the cast. The client should be turned every 2 hours in order to reduce continuous pressure and promote even drying of the cast. The drying process is usually complete in 24 hours. During the drying period the cast should not be subjected to any abnormal stresses, wetness, or soiling which could cause weakening or a break in it. It should be carefully handled to avoid indentations which will dry and become potential pressure areas.

A cast can interfere with circulation and nerve function either because of being applied too tightly or because of excessive edema development after application. Frequent neurovascular assessments of the immobilized extremity are critical. The client needs to know the signs of cast complications so that he will know what needs to be reported (Fig. 56-7). Elevation of the extremity above the heart level to promote venous return and application of ice are frequently utilized to control or prevent edema during the initial phase of immobilization. The nurse should instruct the client to exercise the joints above and below the cast. Pulling out cast padding and scratching or placing foreign objects under the cast should be forbidden.

If the client will be immobilized for a period of time as a result of the fracture, the nurse must plan care to avoid the occurrence of constipation and renal calculi. Constipation can be avoided by maintaining a high fluid intake and a diet high in bulk and roughage. If these measures are not effective in maintaining the client's normal bowel pattern, stool softener, laxatives, or suppositories may be necessary. Maintaining a regular time for a bowel movement in spite of bed rest is effective in promoting regularity.

Renal calculi can develop as a result of bone demineralization. The resulting hypercalcemia causes a rise in urine pH and stone formation resulting from the precipitation of calcium. Unless contraindicated, a fluid intake of 2100 to 2800 mL per day is recommended.[8] Cranberry juice is often recommended to acidify the urine and discourage the development of stones.

Rapid deconditioning of the circulatory system can occur as a result of bed rest. These effects can be diminished by letting the client sit up in bed with the lower limbs dangling over the side and perform standing transfer, if treatment allows.

Immobilization of an acute fracture or soft-tissue injury of the upper extremity is frequently accomplished by utilization of three common types, or various modifications of plaster casts or splints. Splints are removable, whereas casts are not. These types include (1) the sugar-tong splint, (2) the short arm cast, and (3) the long arm cast. The *sugar-tong splint* is utilized for acute injuries of the wrist. Multiple layers of plaster splints are applied to the padded forearm, beginning at the phalangeal joints of the hand and extending up the dorsal aspect of the forearm around the distal humerus and then extending down the volar aspect of the forearm to the distal palmar crease. The splinting material is wrapped with either elastic bandage or bias stockinet. The major advantage of the sugar-tong cast is avoidance of the circumferential effects of a nonelastic cylinder.

The *short arm cast* is frequently utilized for the

treatment of stable injuries of the wrist or metacarpals. An aluminum finger splint can be fabricated into the short arm cast for treatment of phalangeal injuries. The short arm cast is a circular plaster cast extending from the distal palmar area to the proximal forearm. This cast provides wrist immobilization and permits unrestricted motion of the elbow.

The *long arm cast* is commonly utilized for stable fractures of the forearm or elbow and unstable fractures of the wrist. The long arm cast is similar to the short arm cast but extends to the mid- to proximal humerus. The long arm cast restricts motion in the wrist and elbow. It is important that nursing measures be directed toward supporting the extremity and reducing the effects of edema by maintaining elevation with a triangle sling. When a triangle sling is utilized, the nurse must ensure that the axillary region is well padded to prevent the skin maceration associated with direct skin-to-skin contact. Placement of the sling should not put undue stress on the neck. Movement of the fingers should be encouraged in order to more effectively enhance the pumping action of the veins to lessen edema development. The nurse should also encourage the client to actively move the joints of the affected upper extremity which are not immobilized, to prevent stiffness and atrophy.

The *body jacket cast* is frequently utilized for immobilization and support of stable spine injuries of the thoracic or lumbar spine or postoperative spinal surgery. This type of cast is applied around the chest and abdomen and extends from above the nipple line to the pubis. After application of the cast, the nurse must assess the client for the development of a *cast syndrome*. This condition occurs if the body cast is applied too tightly and the cast compresses the superior mesenteric artery against the duodenum. The client will generally complain of abdominal pain, abdominal pressure, nausea, and vomiting. Treatment includes gastric decompression with a nasogastric tube and suction. The cast may need to be removed. Nursing assessment also includes observation of respiratory status, bowel and bladder function, and areas of pressure over the bony prominences, especially the iliac crest. During the time required for the cast to dry, the nurse should reposition the client every 2 to 3 hours in order to promote even drying of the cast and to relieve pressure and discomfort.

The *hip spica cast* is commonly utilized in the treatment of femoral fractures. The purpose of the hip spica cast is to securely immobilize the affected extremity to the adjoining trunk. It includes two separate casts joined together: (1) the body jacket and (2) the long leg cast. The location of the femoral fracture will determine whether the unaffected extremity will have to be immobilized in order to restrict rotation of the pelvis and possible hip motion. The hip spica cast extends from above the nipple line to the base of the foot (single spica) or may include the opposite extremity to above the knee (spica and a half) or both extremities (double spica). The nurse should assess the client for the same problems associated with the body jacket cast. During the initial drying stage the client should not be placed in the prone position because of the possibility of breaking the cast. Instead, he should be slightly turned from side to side and supported with pillows. When the client is repositioned, the support bar must never be utilized to assist, because the bar can break and cause disruption of the cast. After the cast has dried, the nurse, with assistance, can turn the client to the prone position and provide pillow support under the chest and immobilized extremity. Skin care around the edges of the cast and the areas not encompassed by plaster is very important to prevent any pressure sores. It is important that the nurse instruct the client in the positioning activities required to get on and off the fracture bedpan. After the hip spica cast has dried sufficiently, the client will be instructed by the physical therapist in the techniques of ambulation.

Injuries to the lower extremity are frequently immobilized by either a long leg cast or short leg cast. The usual indications for the application of a long leg cast are an unstable ankle fracture, soft-tissue injuries, fracture of the tibia, or injuries of the knee. The cast will usually extend from the base of the toes to the groin and gluteal crease. The short leg cast can be utilized for a wide variety of conditions but is usually used for stable injuries of the ankle and foot. After application of a lower-extremity cast the extremity should be elevated with pillows above the heart level for the first 24 hours. After the initial phase the cast should not be placed in a dependent position because of the possibility of excessive edema. Initially, no weight can be put on the injured extremity. Later, a walking heel or cast shoe will be added to the cast. The nurse should observe for signs of pressure, especially in the regions of the fibular head and malleoli.

Since many fractures are casted in an outpatient setting, the client often requires only a short hospitalization. Therefore, *client education* is an important nursing responsibility. In addition to specific instructions related to the care of the cast and recognition of complications, the nurse should encourage the client to contact the clinic or care provider should questions arise. Table 56-7 summarizes client instructions for cast management. The nurse should validate the client's understanding of these instructions prior to discharge from the clinic or hospital.

Table 56-7

Client Instructions for Cast Care

Do not

1. Get cast wet
2. Remove any padding
3. Insert any foreign object under cast
4. Bear weight on cast for 48 h
5. Cover cast with plastic for prolonged periods of time

Do

1. Elevate extremity above level of heart for first 48 h
2. Move joints above and below cast regularly
3. Apply ice directly over fracture site for first 24 h (avoid getting cast wet by keeping ice in plastic bag and protecting cast with cloth)
4. Report any of following signs to health care provider:
   a. Increasing pain
   b. Swelling associated with pain and discoloration of toes
   c. Pain on motion
   d. Burning or tingling under cast
5. Keep appointment to have fracture and cast checked

Nursing Care of the Client in Traction The nurse is responsible for client comfort and safety while traction is used, as well as assuring proper functioning of the traction equipment. The equipment should be regularly examined for frayed ropes, loose knots, ropes out of the groove of the pulley, pulley clamps not fastened firmly to the bed frame, and weights not hanging freely.

When slings are used with traction, the nurse should inspect the sling skin area regularly. Pressure over a bony prominence or a wrinkled area can impair blood flow, causing injury to the peripheral neurovascular structures. Skeletal traction pin sites must be observed for signs of infection. Pin-site care varies according to the preference of the physician but usually includes regular cleaning and the use of an antibiotic ointment. External rotation of the hip is a common problem when skin traction is used to treat lower-extremity disorders. The nurse can correct this position by placing a pillow, sandbag, or rolled-up drawsheet along the outer aspect of the femur. Whenever traction is utilized the nurse should ensure that there is always correct body alignment with the traction device.

In order to offset some of the problems associated with prolonged recumbency, the nurse should discuss specific activity with the physician. If exercise is permitted, the nurse should encourage participation by the client in a simple exercise regimen including:[9]

1. Participation in feeding and bathing activities
2. Use of the trapeze bar to get on and off the bedpan and for change of linens
3. Performance of simple range-of-motion exercises of all unaffected joints several times a day
4. Performance of isometric exercises and deep-breathing exercises several times a day
5. Change of position frequently to prevent decubiti

Active exercises that move the joints through their range of motion is the preferred activity, if allowed. Frequent exercise of the trunk and extremities is an excellent stimulus to respiratory activity.

Rehabilitative management

Psychosocial Problems The short-range rehabilitative goals are directed toward the transition from dependence to independence in the performance of simple activities of daily living and preserving or increasing strength and endurance. The long-range goals are prevention of problems associated with musculoskeletal injury (Table 56-8). An important part of nursing care during the rehabilitative phase is assisting the client to adjust to any psychosocial problems caused by the injury, possible separation from family unit, financial impact of medical care, and loss of income from inability to work. The nurse must exhibit gentleness, support, and encouragement as well as actively listening to the client's fears.

Progressive Ambulation The physical therapist often assumes primary responsibility for directing the client during the strengthening phase of care. The nurse must be aware of the overall goals of physical therapy in relation to the client's abilities, needs, and tolerance. Mobility training and instruction in the use of assistive aids constitute one of the major areas of responsibility of the physical therapist. The client with dysfunction of the lower extremity is usually started in mobility training when able to sit up in bed and dangle the feet over the side. This activity should be done two or three times per day for 10 to 15 minutes, with the nurse assisting as necessary. As endurance increases the client will be instructed in the techniques of transferring from bed to chair. Progressive ambulation is usually started with parallel bars and progresses to ambulatory assistive devices. When the client begins to ambulate, the nurse must know the weight-bearing status of the affected extremity and the correct technique if the client is using an assistive device. There are different degrees of weight-bearing status: (1) *non-weight-bearing* (NWB), (2) *partial weight-bearing* (PWB), and (3) *full weight-bearing* (FWB).

Assistive Devices Devices for ambulation range from a cane, which can relieve a maximum of only 40 percent of the weight normally borne by a lower limb, to crutches or walker, which allow complete non-

Table 56-8
Problems Associated with Injury of the Musculoskeletal System

Problem	Description
Muscle atrophy	Decrease of muscle mass which normally occurs as a result of disuse secondary to prolonged immobilization. Isometric muscle-strengthening exercise regimen within the confines of the immobilization device assists in reducing the amount of atrophy. Muscle atrophy interferes with and prolongs the rehabilitation process.
Contracture	Abnormal shortening of a muscle due to improper support and positioning. Occurs as a result of imbalance of muscle or ligament, which adaptively adjusts to a shortened position in the region of a joint. This condition can be prevented by frequent change of position, correct body alignment, and active-passive range-of-motion exercises several times a day. Contracture of a joint immobilized for a long period of time with a plaster cast is common. Intervention requires gradual and progressive stretching of the muscles or ligaments in the region of the joint.
Dropped foot	Plantar-flexed position of the foot which occurs when the foot is allowed to assume an unsupported position and the Achilles tendon shortens. May signify damage to the perineal nerve. Nursing management of the client with long-term injuries must include measures of prevention by supporting the foot. Once foot drop has developed, ambulation and gait training can be significantly hindered.
Pain	Frequently associated with fractures, ensuing edema, and muscle spasm. Pain varies in intensity from mild to severe and is usually described as aching, dull, burning, throbbing, sharp, or deep. Important causal factors of pain include incorrect positioning and alignment of the extremity, incorrect support of the extremity, sudden movement of the extremity, immobilization device applied too tightly or in incorrect position, constrictive dressing, motion occurring at the fracture site, and psychosocial factors. Pain is a valuable assessment guide, and the underlying causes should be ascertained and corrective nursing action taken before analgesics are administered.
Muscle spasms	Caused by involuntary muscle contraction after fracture which may last as long as several weeks. Pain associated with muscle spasm is often intense. The duration varies from several seconds to several minutes. Nursing measures to reduce the intensity of the muscle spasms are similar to the corrective actions for control of pain. (Do not massage the area involved in muscle spasm.)

weight-bearing ambulation. The decision as to which device is appropriate for a client involves weighing the trade-off between providing maximum stability and safety and providing the maneuverability required in small spaces like bathrooms and buses. The decision is made easier by discussing with the client the requirements of his lifestyle and determining the device with which he feels most secure and independent.

Although the technique for the use of devices varies, usually the involved limb is advanced at the same time or immediately following the advance of the device and the uninvolved limb is advanced last. With only a few rare exceptions, canes are held in the hand opposite the involved extremity.

The common gait patterns with assistive devices are:

Two-point gait—Crutch on one side advances simultaneously with the opposite foot; used also with cane ambulation

Four-point gait—A slower version of the two-point

gait, in which each "point" is advanced separately

Swing-to gait—Both crutches are advanced together, followed by the lifting of both lower limbs to the same place; used with walkers

Swing-through gait—Similar to the swing-to gait, but the client swings body past the crutches

Clients in the learning stages may best be guarded by grasping a belt secured around the waist. The clinician should discourage the client's reaching for furniture or relying on companion support. With inadequate upper limb strength or poorly fitting crutches, a client will bear weight at the axilla rather than the hands, endangering the neurovascular bundle that passes across the axilla. If verbal coaching does not correct the problem, the client should be kept from further ambulation until strength is adequate.

The client who must ambulate without weight bearing requires sufficient strength of the upper limbs to lift his weight at each step. As the muscles of the shoulder girdle are not accustomed to this work, they require vigorous and diligent training in preparation for the task. Common exercises advocated for this purpose are wheelchair "push-ups" using pulleys attached to the bed frame and "pull-ups" using an overhead trapeze bar.

Counseling and Referrals During the rehabilitative process the client's family assumes an important role in the provision and follow-through of long-term-care plans. The family must be instructed in the techniques of strength and endurance exercises, assistance with mobility training, and promoting activities which enhance the quality of daily living. Sexual counseling should be included in discharge planning. Stress needs to be placed on the nurse's role in relation to the psychosexual needs of clients.. The nurse is in a key position to listen to and assess the client's sexual needs. Unless the nurse has specific preparation for sexual health counseling, she should keep in mind that wrong answers are usually more harmful than no answers. For referral purposes the nurse must know whether sexual activity is compatible with the degree of injury and whether any restrictions are imposed by an immobilization or support device.

Medical and Nursing Management of Specific Fractures

Colles' fracture

A Colles' fracture is a fracture of the distal radius and is one of the most common fractures of adults. The ulnar styloid process may be involved as well. The injury usually occurs when the client attempts to break a fall with the hand open. This type of fracture often occurs in conjunction with minor injuries through bone weakened by osteoporosis and is more common in females over 50 years of age. The clinical manifestations of a Colles' fracture are pain in the immediate area of injury, pronounced swelling, and dorsal displacement of the distal fragment (dinner-fork deformity; Fig. 56-12). The major complication associated with a Colles' fracture is vascular insufficiency secondary to edema.

Management A Colles' fracture is usually managed by closed manipulation of the fracture and immobilization by either a sugar-tong splint or a long arm cast. The elbow must be immobilized to prevent supination and pronation. Nursing management should include antiedema measures and accurate neurovascular assessment. Support and protection of the extremity should be provided while encouraging

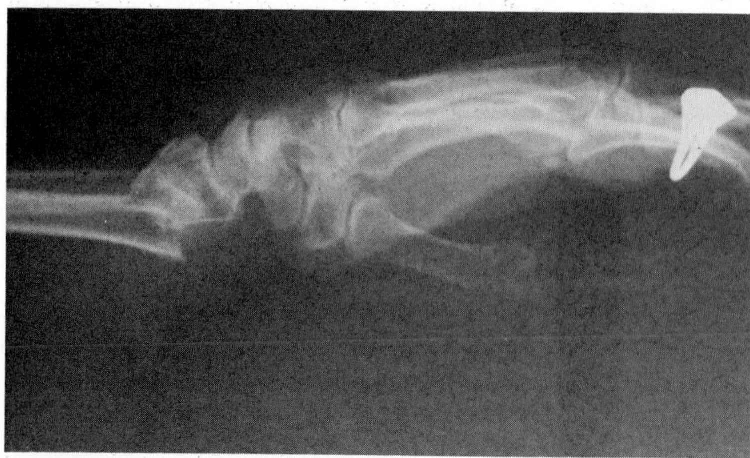

Figure 56-12 Comminuted fracture of the distal radius and ulnar (Colles' fracture). Note the fork deformity of the hand.

active movement of the thumb and fingers. Such movement helps reduce edema and increases venous return. The client should be instructed to perform active movements of the entire upper extremity, especially the shoulder, to prevent stiffness or contracture.

Fracture of the humerus

Fractures involving the shaft of the humerus are a common injury of young and middle-aged adults. The prominent clinical manifestations are an obvious displacement of the humerus shaft, shortened extremity, abnormal mobility, and pain (Fig. 56-13). The major complications associated with fracture of the humerus are radial nerve injury and vascular injury to the brachial artery secondary to laceration, transection, or spasm.

Management The treatment of a fracture of the humerus depends on the location and displacement of the fracture. Treatment may include the hanging

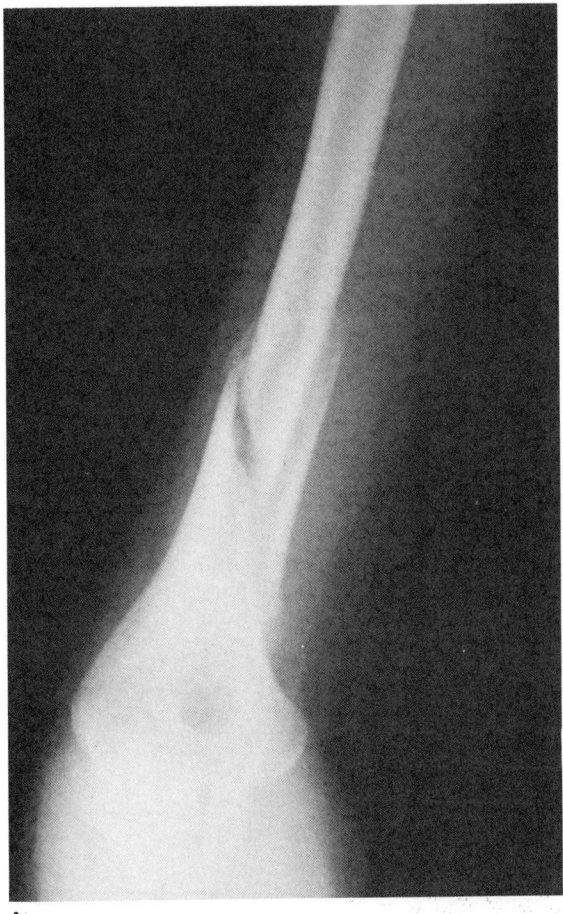

A

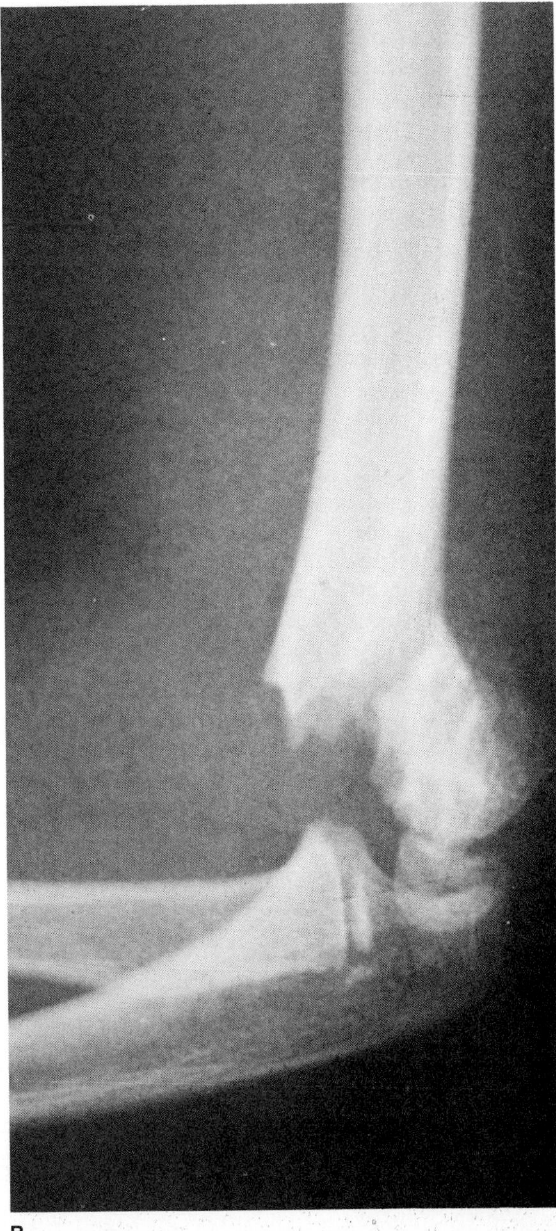

B

Figure 56-13 *(a)* Supracondylar fracture of the humerus. This type of injury would result in the formation of a large hematoma. *(b)* Fracture of distal shaft of humerus.

arm cast and the sling and swathe—a type of immobilization that prevents glenohumeral movement. The swathe encircles the trunk and humerus as an additional binder. It is often used for surgical repairs and dislocation of the shoulder.

When these devices are used, the head of the bed must be elevated to assist gravity in reduction of the fracture. The nursing plan should include measures to protect the axilla and prevent skin maceration. Skin or skeletal traction may also be utilized for purposes of reduction and immobilization.

During the rehabilitative phase, an exercise program to gain strength and motion of the injured extremity is extremely important. This should include assisted motion of the hand and fingers. The shoulder can also be exercised if the fracture is stable.

Fracture of the pelvis

Pelvic fractures are usually caused by vehicular accidents. Elderly clients may sustain this injury as a result of a fall. Although only 3 percent of all fractures are pelvic fractures, this type of injury accounts for 5 to 20 percent of the mortality from fractures.[10] Preoccupation with associated injuries at the time of an accident may result in neglect of pelvic injuries. Pelvic fractures may cause serious intraabdominal injury such as laceration of the colon, paralytic ileus, intrapelvic hemorrhage, and rupture of the urethra or bladder.

Physical examination demonstrates local swelling, tenderness, deformity, and ecchymosis. The neurovascular status of the lower extremities and manifestations of associated injuries should be assessed. Fractures of the pelvis are diagnosed and classified by x-ray. They may range from simple undisplaced fractures to more serious fracture dislocations with potential for serious complications (Fig. 56-14).

Management Treatment of a pelvic fracture depends on the severity of the injury. Bed rest for stable pelvic fractures is maintained from a few days up to 6 weeks. More complex fractures may be treated with pelvic slings, skeletal traction, hip spica casts, open reduction, or a combination of these methods. Extreme care in handling or movement of the client is important to prevent serious injury from a displaced fracture fragment. Since pelvic fracture can damage other organs, appropriate assessments are important nursing activities in the early care of the client.

The client should be turned only with specific orders. Back care is given with the client raised from the bed by use of the overhead trapeze or adequate assistance. Weight bearing on the affected side should be avoided until healing is complete. If the pelvic fracture is undisplaced, the client is usually allowed to ambulate, using a walker or crutches to distribute the weight bearing between the upper and lower extremities. Elimination needs may require the use of an indwelling catheter in female clients if a pelvic sling is used.

Fracture of the hip

Hip fractures are a common trauma in the elderly, particularly in women over 60 years of age. Fractures which occur within the capsule are called *intracapsular* fractures. Intracapsular fractures are

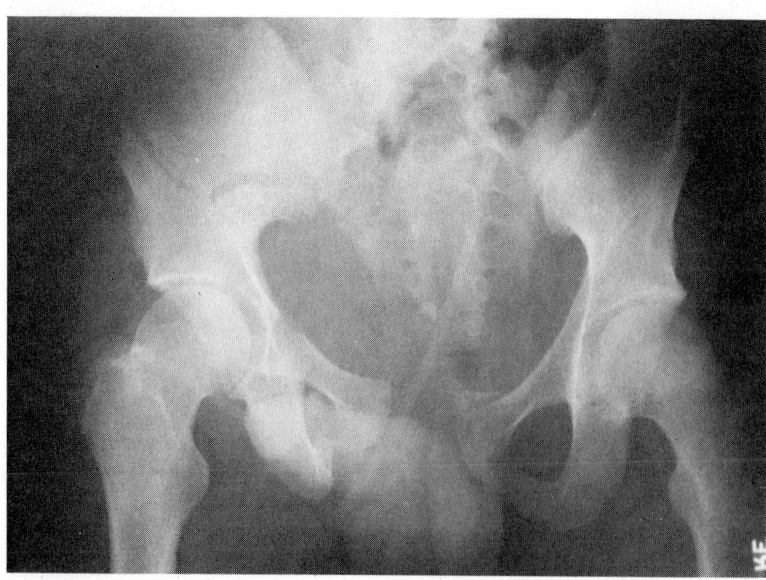

Figure 56-14 Fracture of the pelvis. Note the separation of the pubis and fracture of the left sacroiliac joint.

further identified by a name taken from their specific location: (1) subcapital, (2) transcervical, and (3) basilar neck. These fractures are often associated with osteoporosis and minor trauma. *Extracapsular* fractures occur below the capsule and are termed *intertrochanteric* if they occur in a region between the greater and lesser trochanter and *subtrochanteric* if in the region below the trochanter (Fig. 56-15). Extracapsular fractures are usually caused by severe direct trauma or a fall.

Clinical Manifestation The clinical manifestations of fracture of the hip are external rotation and shortening of the affected extremity and severe pain and tenderness in the region of the fracture site. Displaced femoral neck fractures cause serious disruption of the blood supply to the femoral head which can result in avascular necrosis.

Management Surgical repair is the preferred method of managing intracapsular and extracapsular fractures of the hip. Surgical treatment permits the client to be out of bed sooner and prevents the major complications associated with immobility. By comparison, treatment with traction requires from 12 to 16 weeks of immobilization for healing to occur, even if the blood supply to the region is intact. Initially the affected extremity may be temporarily immobilized by either Buck's or Russell's traction until the client's physical condition is stabilized and surgery can be scheduled. Traction also helps relieve painful muscle spasms.

Repairs are accomplished with the use of a prosthesis or pins. The intracapsular fracture is slow to heal because of interruptions of blood supply. When avascular necrosis appears imminent, the surgeon may elect to resect the femoral head and neck and insert an endoprosthesis such as the Austin Moore or Thompson type. A variety of devices in the form of screws, nails, and pins are available to the surgeon for the purpose of repairing fracture of the hip by pinning. Intracapsular fractures are usually repaired by using a hip prosthesis, while extracapsular fractures are usually pinned (Fig. 56-16). The principles of client care are similar (Table 56-9).

Preoperative Care Since older people are most prone to fractures of the hip, chronic health problems must often be considered when planning treatment. Diabetes, hypertension, cardiac decompensation, and arthritis are chronic problems which may complicate the clinical picture. Surgery may be delayed until the client's general health improves.

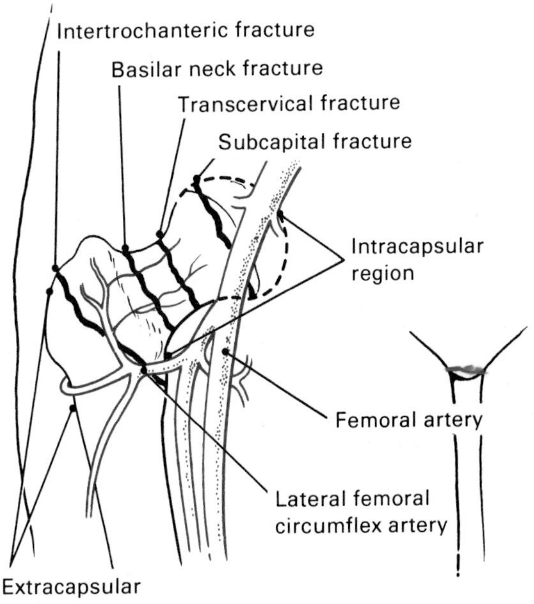

Figure 56-15 Innominate bone, with location of various types of fracture.

Preoperatively, severe muscle spasms can increase pain. These spasms are managed by appropriate medications, positions of comfort unless contraindicated, and properly adjusted traction if it is being used.

Careful preoperative teaching can affect future mobility. The client should know how and how often the unaffected leg and both arms are to be exercised. He will be instructed how to utilize the trapeze bar and opposite siderail to assist in changing position. He can expect to be out of bed by the second postoperative day. Practice in getting out of bed and transferring to a chair should be discussed and demonstrated preoperatively. The family should be informed about the client's weight-bearing status following surgery. Plans for discharge may need to be discussed and arrangements initiated.

Postoperative Care The initial postoperative management of a client following surgical repair of a hip fracture is similar to that of any geriatric surgical client: monitoring vital signs and intake and output, supervising respiratory activities such as deep breathing and coughing, administering pain medication cautiously, and observing the dressing for signs of bleeding and infection.

In the early postoperative period there is a potential for impairment of circulation, movement, and sen-

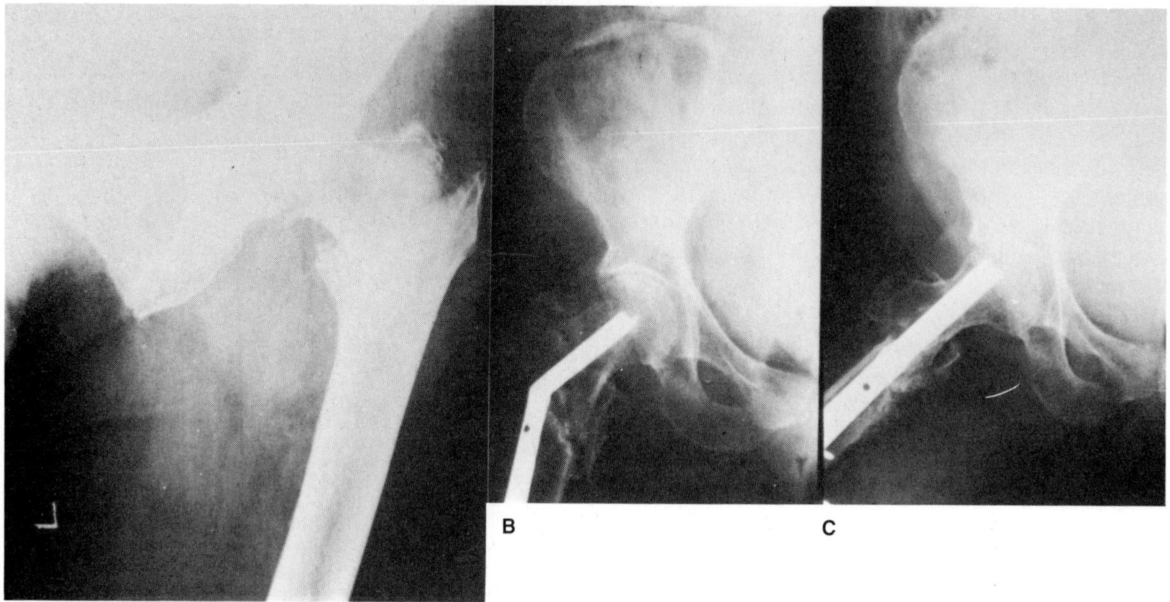

Figure 56-16 (*a*) Intertrochanteric fracture. (*b*) Anteroposterior radiograph demonstrating surgical fixation with Neufeld hip nail. (c) Lateral radiograph. (*Courtesy of Herman Epstein, M.D., University of Southern California School of Medicine.*)

Table 56-9

Nursing Care Plan for the Client with Fracture of the Hip

Client Problem	Expected Outcome	Nursing Intervention
Pain	Pain decreased or absent	Align and position extremity and client correctly. Use gentleness when positioning or turning. Maintain constant traction forces. Administer analgesics as indicated.
Venous stasis	No evidence of thrombosis or embolism	Apply antiembolic stockings to unaffected lower extremity. Teach resistive range of motion of unaffected extremities, especially ankle plantar flexion against footboard. With assistance, change position utilizing trapeze bar or opposite siderail q 1–2 h. Encourage client to feed and wash self.
Skin breakdown	No pressure sores or skin breakdown	Change position q 2 h. Keep skin clean and dry. Massage skin over bony prominences every shift. Keep bed linen free of wrinkles.
Dehydration	Normal skin turgor and adequate urine output	Monitor intake and output. Administer IV fluids as ordered. Soft diet supplemented by 2000–3000 mL fluids per day.
Possible respiratory problems (e.g., pneumonia)	No evidence of pulmonary infection	Perform coughing and deep-breathing exercises q 2 h. Monitor temperature q 2–4 h. Auscultate lungs q 4 h. Obtain sputum specimen for culture and sensitivity testing if cough productive. Administer antibiotics as ordered. Administer respiratory therapy as ordered. Give mouth care q 2 h and prn.
Maintenance of traction	Affected extremity maintained in correct alignment without complications	Keep head of bed flat if possible. Maintain unobstructed pulleys and traction force. Examine traction regularly.
Limited ROM of adjacent joints of affected extremity	No evidence of restriction of adjacent-joint motion	Passive-active exercises of joints q 4 h.

Table 56-9 (Continued)

Client Problem	Expected Outcome	Nursing Intervention
Decreased muscle strength	Sufficient muscle strength to participate in gait-training program	Cooperate with physical therapist in muscle-strengthening program. Teach and assist client in exercise program, including resistive strengthening exercises of uninvolved lower and both upper limbs, including elbow extension, shoulder depressors, and knee and hip extension.
Urinary and bowel elimination difficulty	Position self on fracture bedpan with minimum discomfort	Encourage client participation in positioning self on bedpan by utilizing trapeze bar in conjunction with adequate assistance. *Always use the fracture bedpan.*
Malposition of affected extremity	Correct position and alignment of affected extremity	Know and follow surgeon's protocol for positioning extremity.
Urinary tract infection	No evidence of urinary tract infection. Normal temperature	Ensure liberal fluid intake. Avoid catheterization if possible. Assess urinary output for volume, color, and odor.
Wound infection	No evidence of wound infection. Normal temperature	Use sterile technique when changing dressing or providing wound care. Assess wound site for erythema and drainage. Monitor temperature. Obtain wound culture and sensitivity tests as indicated, then administer antibiotics as ordered.
Contracture of hip, knees, and ankles	No contracture	Teach client about contracture prevention: (1) while in bed, keep legs in extension; (2) passive-active exercises of knee and ankle; (3) do not sit in chair for extended periods of time with hip and knee flexed.
Ambulation dysfunction	Function at optimal level with ambulatory assistive appliance, usually walker	Increase activities as tolerated. Assist with standing at side of bed. Encourage quadriceps exercises, arm-strengthening exercises, and abdominal and gluteal contraction exercises. Instruct client about ambulatory training program. *(A non-weight-bearing status of the involved extremity must be maintained unless changed by an order from the physician.)* Get client out of bed and into chair, usually 24–48 h after surgery. Instruct and assist client with transfer from bed to chair. Instruct and assist with utilization of ambulatory assistive appliance. Explain ambulatory management program. Explain and demonstrate getting up; demonstrate transfer and pivot activities. Teach use of ambulatory assistive aid with non-weight-bearing gait.
Confusion	Remains oriented	Orient as necessary. Keep siderails up if family or staff not present. Keep light on at night. Minimize pain. Give careful explanation of procedures.
Depression	Maintains an optimistic attitude about recovery	Ambulate as prescribed and tolerated. Allow as much independence and decision making as possible. Talk about future activities with a positive attitude. Involve client and family in planning of care.

sation. The nurse should assess the client's toes for (1) ability to move, (2) warmth and pink color, (3) numbness or tingling, and (4) edema. Edema, which may develop after the client is out of bed, will be alleviated by elevating the leg whenever the client is in a chair. The pain resulting from poor alignment of the affected extremity can be prevented by keeping pillows (or an abductor splint) between the knees when turning to either side. Sandbags and pillows are also used to prevent external rotation.

The physical therapist usually supervises active assistive exercises of the affected extremity and ambulation when the surgeon permits it. The nurse needs to be aware of the client's ambulation status and to monitor for proper crutch-walking or use of the walker. The client must be able to demonstrate safe use of

Table 56-10

Client Instructions Following Total Hip Replacement

Do not

1. Force hip into more than 90° flexion*
2. Cross legs
3. Put on own shoes or stockings until 8 weeks after surgery
4. Sit on chairs without arms to aid rising to a standing position*

Do

1. Use toilet elevator on toilet seat*
2. Place chair inside shower or tub and remain seated while washing
3. Use pillow between legs for first 8 weeks after surgery when lying on "good" side*
4. Keep hip in neutral, straight position when sitting, walking, or lying*
5. Lie prone once a day for 15 min
6. Notify surgeon if severe pain, deformity, or loss of function occurs*

*These precautions apply following a hip pinning.

crutches or a walker prior to discharge. Table 56-10 summarizes client-family instructions related to discharge.

If the hip fracture has been treated by use of a femoral-head prosthesis, measures to prevent dislocation must be used at all times. The client and family must be fully aware of positions and activities which encourage dislocation (flexion adduction with internal rotation, known by the acronym FLADIR). Many daily activities may reproduce these positions: putting on shoes and socks, crossing the legs while seated, side-lying incorrectly, standing up or sitting down while the body is flexed relative to the chair, and sitting on low seats. These activities have to be strictly avoided for at least 6 weeks, until the soft tissue surrounding the hip has healed sufficiently to withstand stressing. Sudden severe pain and extreme external rotation indicate prothesis displacement.

In addition to teaching the client and family how to prevent prosthesis dislocation, the nurse should (1) place three pillows between the client's legs when turning; (2) keep leg abductor splints on the client except when bathing; (3) avoid extreme hip flexion, and (4) not turn the client on the affected side.

If the hip fracture is treated by pinning, dislocation precautions are not necessary. Usually the client is encouraged to be out of bed on the first postoperative day. Weight bearing on the involved extremity is not allowed until radiographic examination indicates adequate healing, usually within 3 to 5 months.

Complications of fracture of the femoral neck include nonunion, avascular necrosis, and degenerative arthritis. Following an intertrochanteric fracture, the client may develop shortening of the affected leg.

The nurse must assist both the client and the family to adjust to the restrictions and dependence imposed by the hip fracture. Depression can easily occur, but creative nursing and awareness of the problem can do much to prevent it. The client and family may need to be informed about community referral services which can assist in the posthospital rehabilitation phase. Regular follow-up care should be arranged.

Femoral shaft fracture

Fracture of the femoral shaft is a common injury occurring particularly in young adults. Severe direct force is required to produce this type of injury, because the femur can bend approximately 2 inches prior to actual fracture. The force exerted to cause the fracture frequently causes damage to the adjacent soft-tissue structures which may be more serious than the bone injury. Displacement of the fracture fragments frequently results in open fracture and increases soft-tissue damage. This can result in considerable blood loss.

The clinical manifestations of a fracture of the femoral shaft are usually obvious. They include marked deformity and angulation, shortening of the extremity, inability to move either the hip or knee, and pain. The common complications associated with fracture of the femoral shaft include fat embolism, nerve and vascular injury, problems associated with union, open fracture, and soft-tissue damage.

Management Initial management is directed toward stabilization of the client and immobilization of the fracture. Nonoperative treatment may consist of tibial pinning with balanced skeletal traction. Traction will continue for a period of 8 to 12 weeks. The nurse must encourage the client to perform exercises and range-of-motion activities of the uninvolved extremities and joints. The physician will determine when active exercise can be instituted on the affected extremity. When there is sufficient evidence of clinical union, a hip spica cast is usually applied. Nursing care of a client in a hip spica cast is discussed earlier in this chapter.

Internal fixation is another way to manage a fracture of the femur. It is carried out with an intramedullary rod or compression plate (Fig. 56-17). Internal fixation is frequently the treatment of choice because

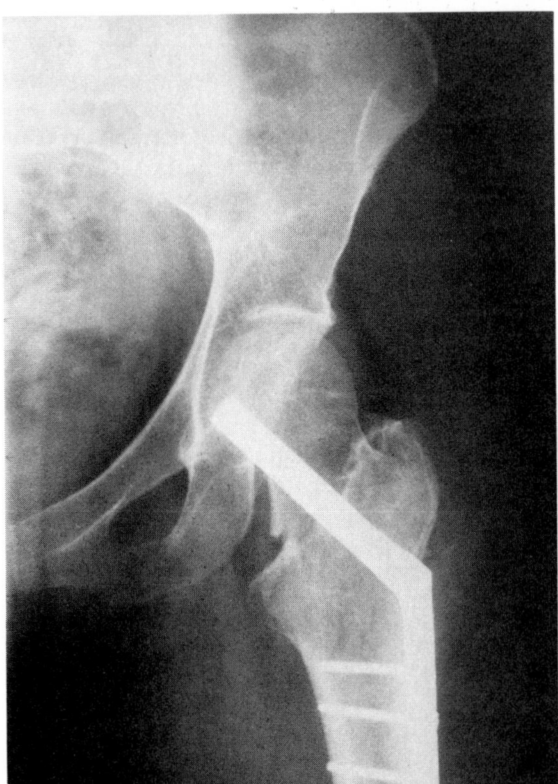

Figure 56-17 Intertrochanteric fixation of the femur with a Jewett nail in place.

of the significant reduction in the length of hospitalization and the complications associated with prolonged bed rest. Other indications for internal fixation are failure to obtain satisfactory reduction by nonoperative methods and multiple associated injuries. During the postoperative phase the surgically repaired femur is usually supported by suspension traction for 3 to 4 days to prevent excessive movement of the extremity and control rotation. Then non-weight-bearing gait training is begun.

Exercises which promote and maintain strength in the affected extremity usually include gluteal and quadriceps exercises. It is important to ensure performance of range-of-motion and strengthening exercises of all uninvolved extremities in preparation for ambulation. The client may be immobilized in a hip spica cast and gradually progress to an articulating cast brace, or he may be allowed to begin non-weight-bearing activities with an ambulatory assistive device. Full weight bearing will usually be restricted until there is radiological evidence of bony union of the fracture fragments.

Fracture of the tibia

The tibia is very vulnerable to injury because of the lack of anterior muscle covering. Strong force is required to produce a fracture of the tibia; as a result, soft-tissue damage, devascularization, and open fracture are frequent. Other complications associated with tibial fractures are compartment syndrome, fat embolism, problems associated with bony union, and the possibility of infection associated with open fracture.

Management The recommended management of closed tibial fractures is closed reduction followed by immobilization in a long leg cast. Open reduction may be achieved with a compression plate. With either method of reduction, emphasis is placed on maintaining the strength of the quadriceps, since delayed union is frequent.

The neurovascular status of the affected extremity must be assessed at least every 2 hours during the first 48 hours. The client will be instructed to perform active range-of-motion exercises of all uninvolved extremities and exercises of the upper extremity to build the strength required for crutch-walking. When the physician has determined that the client is ready for gait training, he is instructed in the principles of crutch-walking. If the fracture is stable, partial weight bearing (PWB) as tolerated is usually permissible. Compression across a stable fracture site will stimulate healing. However, an unstable tibial fracture may permit only partial weight bearing or none at all. A non-weight-bearing gait such as the swing-through gait should be used. When fracture healing has progressed sufficiently (usually around 2 to 4 weeks), a walking heel is applied to the cast and full weight bearing allowed.

Stable vertebral fractures

A stable fracture of the vertebral column is usually caused by motor vehicle accidents, falls, diving, or athletic injuries. A stable fracture is one in which the fracture or the fragment is not likely to move or cause spinal cord damage. This type of injury is frequently confined to the anterior element (vertebral body) of the spinal column in the lumbar region, less frequently the cervical and thoracic regions. The vertebral bodies are usually protected from displacement by the intact spinal ligaments.

Most clients with spinal fractures have stable fractures and experience only brief periods of disability. If the ligamentous structures are significantly disrupted, however, there may be dislocation of the vertebral structures, resulting in instability and injury to the spinal cord (unstable fracture). The most common injury to the vertebral body is the compression type of fracture caused by excessive vertical load, such as a severe fall on the buttocks or injury resulting from sudden flexion which forces the spine beyond its normal range of motion. The most serious complication of vertebral fractures is displacement of the fracture, which can cause damage to the spinal cord. (Fractures involving spinal cord injury are covered in Chap. 53.) Although stable vertebral fractures are not associated with abnormal spinal cord pathology, all injuries of the spine should initially be considered unstable and potentially serious.[11]

The client will usually complain of pain and tenderness in the affected region of the spine. Compression fractures are associated with a gibbus deformity (flexion angulation localized to one vertebral level). This deformity may be noted on physical examination. Bowel and bladder dysfunction may be an indication of a temporary interruption of the sympathetic nervous system or injury to the spinal cord structure.

Management The overall goal in management of stable fractures of a vertebral body is to keep the spine in good alignment until union has been accomplished. Many of the nursing interventions are aimed at assessing for the possibility of spinal cord trauma. Vital signs, color, and bowel and bladder function should be evaluated regularly, as should the motor and sensory status of the peripheral nerves distal to the region of the injury. Any deterioration in the client's neurovascular status should be promptly reported.

Treatment includes support, heat, and traction. The client is usually placed in a standard hospital bed with firm support from the mattress or a bedboard. The aim is to support the spinal cord, relax muscles, and release any compression on nerve roots. Heat and traction may be used to relieve muscle spasms due to the fracture, and traction may be used to reduce and immobilize fracture fragments. A trapeze is not usually allowed because its use disrupts alignment and immobilization. Both an upright position and torsional turning are prohibited. When turning, the client should be taught to keep the spine straight by turning shoulders and pelvis together. Nursing assistance is necessary for the client to turn in this logrolling fashion.

Several days after the initial injury, if there is no evidence of neurological deficit, the physician may apply a specially constructed orthotic device, a jacket-type cast, or a removable corset. This will immobilize the spine in the fracture area but allow client mobility. The client is discharged after (1) regaining ambulation skills, (2) learning care of the cast or orthotic device, and (3) learning how to cope with interferences in safety and security imposed by injury and treatment.

OSTEOMYELITIS

Etiology and Pathogenesis

Osteomyelitis is an infection of bone by either direct or indirect invasion by an organism. Direct entry results from contamination due to an open fracture or surgical intervention. Indirect inoculation results from a blood-borne infection from a distant site such as infected tonsils or furuncles. The most common infecting organism is *Staphylococcus aureus* and less commonly, *Escherichia coli*, *Pseudomonas*, or *Proteus*. The course and virulence of osteomyelitis are influenced by the blood supply to the affected bone. The widespread use of antibiotics in conjunction with surgical treatment has significantly reduced the mortality associated with osteomyelitis. The incidence and morbidity remain relatively unchanged, however, because of new, drug-resistant strains of organisms.

The *indirect entry* variety of osteomyelitis (also called *hematogenous*) most frequently affects growing bone of male children and is associated with local trauma. The most common site of indrect-entry osteomyelitis is the long bones of the leg.

The *direct-entry* type of osteomyelitis can happen at any age when there is an open wound. After gaining entrance to the bone by way of arterial supply, the bacteria lodge in an area of bone where circulation slows, usually the metaphysis. The locus of bacteria grows, resulting in an increase in pressure because of the nonexpanding container of tubular bone. This increasing pressure eventually leads to ischemia and vascular shutoff. Once ischemia occurs, the bone dies. The areas of devitalized bone eventually separate from the surrounding living bone, forming *sequestra*. These sequestra form havens for bacteria, and chronic osteomyelitis develops.

Once formed, a sequestrum will continue to be an infected island of bone, surrounded by pus and unreachable by any arterially carried antibiotics or leukocytes. It will enlarge and serve as a source of bacteria for metastasis to other sites, even the lungs and brain. Two situations are possible. The sequestrum may extrude through a defect in tubular bone. However, this is hindered by the formation of new bone laid down by the elevated periosteum called *involucrum*. Once outside the bone, the sequestrum may revascularize and undergo removal by normal defense processes. The other possibility is surgical removal. Unless resolved naturally or surgically, the necrotic sequestrum may develop a sinus tract, resulting in chronic wound drainage.

Clinical Manifestations

The clinical manifestations of osteomyelitis are both systemic and local. The systemic manifestations include fever and symptoms of acute illness. The local manifestations are local tenderness, swelling, and warmth. Drainage from the wound site may be present. Wound cultures will determine the causative organism. Frequently the client's blood cultures are positive. An elevated leukocyte count and sedimentation rate may also be found. Radiological signs suggestive of osteomyelitis usually do not appear until 10 to 21 days after the appearance of clinical symptoms, by which time the disease will have become chronic.

Chronic osteomyelitis can represent either a continuous, persistent problem or a process of exacerbations and quiescence. Chronic osteomyelitis results from inadequately treated acute osteomyelitis. Pus accumulates, causing ischemia of the bone. Over time, granulation tissue turns to scar tissue. This avascular scar tissue provides an ideal site for bacterial growth and is impenetrable to antibiotics.

Medical Management

Acute

Vigorous antibiotic therapy is the treatment of choice for acute osteomyelitis, provided ischemia has not yet occurred. Wound cultures should be taken before antibiotic therapy is initiated so that the specific antibiotic can be determined by sensitivity studies. If antibiotic therapy is not started early in the course of the illness, surgical decompression is usually necessary to relieve pressure within the bone and prevent ischemia. Some type of immobilization of the affected part is usually indicated. Oral antibiotic therapy is usually continued for 4 to 8 weeks following discharge.

The most serious, and potentially a fatal, complication of osteomyelitis is the development of overwhelming sepsis from metastasis of bacteria to other sites. Pathological fractures may occur through weakened, devitalized bone. Healing of soft tissues and bone occurs slowly in the presence of infection, and the client may develop subsequent deformity of the extremity.

Chronic

Treatment of chronic osteomyelitis includes surgical removal of poorly vascularized tissue and dead bone in conjunction with extended use of antibiotics. Following surgical debridement of devitalized and infected tissue, the wound may be closed, with the insertion of a suction irrigation system for drainage of any devitalized tissues remaining in the wound area. Usually, regional perfusion involving constant irrigation of the affected bone with antibiotics is initiated. Hyperbaric oxygen therapy may be attempted when available.

Saucerization, a type of decompression surgery, removes a window (saucer) of bone to decrease pressure. Skin and bone grafting may be necessary if destruction is extensive. The use of pulverized bone to stimulate growth of healthy bone is another management possibility.[12] The infection and bone destruction may be so extensive that amputation of the extremity is necessary to preserve life.

Nursing Management

The nursing management of the client with osteomyelitis is challenging and demanding. Often a prolonged hospital stay is required to ensure adequate treatment. Nursing care for the client with osteomyelitis is summarized in Table 56-11.

The involved extremity should be handled carefully to avoid excessive manipulation with increased pain and the possibility of pathological fracture. Control of any draining wound is usually managed by the application of various types of sterile dressings. Dressings, besides protecting the wound area, are also utilized as adjuncts in the mechanical debridement of devitalized tissue from the wound area by extracting the exudate from the wound site when they are removed. Types of dressings used include dry sterile dressings, dressings saturated in saline or antibiotic solution, and wet to dry dressings. Soiled dressings should always be disposed of carefully to prevent cross-contamination of the wound or spread of the infection to other clients. When the dressing is changed, sterile technique is essential; it should always include sterile dressing sets, gloves, and surgical cap, gown, and mask to reduce wound contamination from external sources.

Good body alignment and frequent position changes prevent complications and promote comfort. Flexion deformity, especially of the hip or knee, is a common sequela of osteomyelitis because the client will frequently position the affected extremity in a flexed position to promote comfort. This can lead to

Table 56-11

Nursing Care Plan for the Client with Osteomyelitis*

Client Problem	Expected Outcome	Nursing Intervention
Infected bone tissue	Absence of infected bone tissue. Normal WBC and sedimentation rate. No bacteremia after 48 h of antibiotics	Have client use assistive device for ambulation if needed. Give appropriate antibiotic as ordered, diluted in appropriate solution, over recommended span of time. Assure administration of antibiotic therapy. Assess IV site q h. Assess symptoms of antibiotic toxicity such as pruritus, urticaria, and diarrhea.
Pain, redness over affected bone, tenderness	Minimal discomfort after 3 weeks of therapy	Avoid activities which increase circulation, such as heat or exercise. Use gentle handling and support when moving extremity. Maintain in correct alignment and positioning. Keep client in bed. Avoid jarring bed. Use bed cradle if covers cause discomfort. Give analgesics as indicated.
Fever	Normal temperature	Take temperature q 4 h. Provide comfort with cool environment, light clothing and bedding, antipyretic drugs as ordered, and sponge bath or tub bath. Prevent dehydration from insensible fluid loss by offering fluids q h and observing skin turgor and moistness of mucous membranes.
Edema	Decrease or absence of edema in affected extremity	Measure circumference of affected extremity daily. Elevate affected extremity unless contraindicated.
Potential deformity of affected bone	No deformity	Enforce absolute rest of affected part. Maintain proper positioning and good alignment.
Wound drainage	No drainage from wound	Follow hospital procedures for isolation techniques. Use proper technique for dressing changes and disposal of soiled dressings.
Depression	Optimistic attitude toward recovery	Allow client and family to participate in care and decision making. Encourage client to verbalize concerns. Keep client informed of treatment plans and progress.

*Management of chronic osteomyelitis is similar to management of acute osteomyelitis.

the development of contracture, which may progress to a deformity. In the lower extremity dropped foot can develop quickly if the foot is not correctly supported. A splint is frequently applied to the involved extremity in an attempt to maintain immobilization, support, and comfort. The client should be instructed to avoid any activities such as exercise or heat application that would speed circulation and serve as a stimulus to the spread of infection.

The client is frequently frightened and discouraged because of the serious nature of the disease, systemic illness, pain, and the length and cost of treatment. Continued psychological support is an integral part of the nursing management.

If the osteomyelitis becomes chronic, the client will need both physical and psychological support over a prolonged period of time. He may become suspicious of and hostile to the care givers when treatment plans do not effect a cure. A well-informed client will be better able to participate in decisions and ccoperate in treatment plans.

AMPUTATION

During the past two decades major advances have been made in surgical amputation techniques, prosthetic design, and rehabilitation programs. These advances are enabling the amputee to return to a productive and nearly normal social role. There are an estimated 400,000 amputees in the United States, with an annual increase of 20,000.[13] The middle and older age groups have the highest incidence of amputation secondary to the effects of peripheral vascular disease, especially atherosclerosis and diabetes mellitus. Traumatic injury is the usual cause for amputation in the younger adult. Amputation is required more often in persons engaged in hazardous occupations, and since males are more often involved in such occupations, the incidence in males is greater.

Clinical Indications

The clinical features which indicate the need for an amputation depend upon the underlying disease or trauma. Common indications for amputation include circulatory impairment resulting from a peripheral vascular disorder, traumatic and thermal injuries, malignant tumors, uncontrolled or widespread infection of the extremity, and congenital disorders. These conditions may manifest as loss of sensation, inadequate circulation, pallor, swelling, and local or systemic infection. Although pain is often present, it is not usually the primary reason for an amputation. The underlying disease will dictate whether the amputation is performed as elective or emergency surgery.

Medical Management (Table 56-12)

Diagnostic abnormalities will depend upon the underlying disease which makes the amputation necessary. Often the white blood cell count will be elevated, indicating infection. Vascular studies such as arteriography provide information about the circulatory status of the extremity. The potential for revascularization surgery rather than amputation can be assessed on the basis of these vascular studies.

If an elective amputation is to be performed, the client's general health is carefully monitored. Chronic illnesses and infection are treated when possible. The client and family should be helped to understand the need for the amputation and assured that rehabilitation can result in an active, useful life. If the amputation is done on an emergency basis as a result of trauma, the management is both physically and emotionally more complicated.

The goal of amputation surgery is to leave as long and as functional a stump as possible. This improves the possibility of good prosthetic, cosmetic, and functional satisfaction. Levels of amputation of upper and lower extremities are illustrated in Fig. 56-18. The type of amputation depends upon the reason for the surgery. A *closed amputation* is performed to create a stump that can be used with a prosthesis. Skin flaps with dissected soft-tissue padding cover the bone stump. Special care is necessary to prevent the accumulation of drainage, which can produce pressure and infection. *Disarticulation* is an amputation performed through a joint.

An *open amputation* leaves a stump surface that is not covered with skin. This type of surgery is generally indicated for control of actual or potential infection. The wound is usually closed later by a secondary surgical procedure or closed by skin traction surrounding the stump. This type of amputation is often referred to as a *guillotine amputation*.

The surgeon must decide what type of prosthetic fitting will be used postoperatively: an immediate fitting or a delayed fitting. The *immediate prosthetic fitting* is done in the operating room following the amputation. A rigid plaster bandage is applied around the closed stump with (in the case of a leg amputation) attachment of a prosthetic pylon and foot-ankle assembly (Fig. 56-19). While the client is still anesthetized, the prosthetic pylon and ankle-foot assembly are aligned and adjusted for smooth gait and avoidance of excessive pressure on the stump area. A strap is placed on the proximal anterior surface of the rigid plaster bandage and attached to a waistband to prevent slippage. The main advantage of this type of device is reduction of edema and the psychological lift of early ambulation. A disadvantage is the inability to directly visualize the operative site.

The *delayed prosthetic fitting* may be the best choice for certain clients. Individuals with amputations above the knee or above the elbow, the elderly and

Table 56-12

Medical Management: Amputations

Diagnostic

1. Physical examination
   a. Physical appearance of soft tissues
   b. Temperature of skin
   c. Sensory function
   d. Presence of peripheral pulses
2. Arteriography
3. Thermography
4. Plethysmography
5. Transcutaneous ultrasonic Doppler recordings

Therapeutic

1. Medical
   a. Appropriate management of underlying disease process
   b. Stabilization of trauma victim
2. Surgical
   a. Appropriate type of amputation, leaving as long a stump as possible
   b. Stump management
      (1) Immediate prosthetic fitting
      (2) Delayed prosthetic fitting
3. Rehabilitation
   a. Coordinate prosthesis-fitting and gait-training activities
   b. Coordinate muscle strengthening and physical therapy regimen

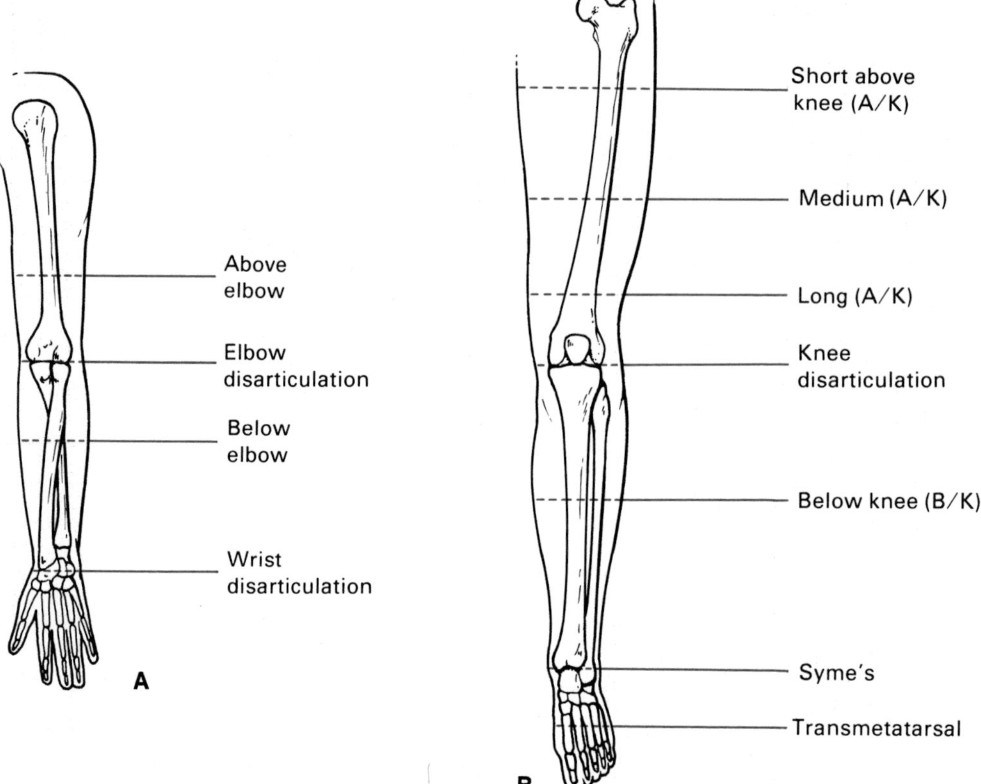

Figure 56-18 Levels of amputation. *(a)* Upper extremity. *(b)* Lower extremity.

debilitated, and those with infection usually have delayed prosthetic fitting. The timetable for use of a prosthesis depends upon satisfactory healing of the stump as well as the general condition of the client. A temporary prosthesis may be used for partial weight bearing once the sutures are removed. Barring any problems, the client can bear full weight on a permanent prosthesis by 3 months after amputation.

Not all clients are candidates for a prosthesis. It is important that the surgeon discuss ambulation possibilities frankly with the client and family. The seriously ill or debilitated client may not have the energy required for use of a prosthesis. Use of a wheelchair for mobility may be the most realistic goal for this type of client.

Medical management also includes the direction and coordination of the rehabilitation program for the amputee. The degree of success is dependent upon the physical and emotional health of the client. Chronic illness and debility will complicate aggressive rehabilitation efforts.

Nursing Management

Health promotion and maintenance

The nurse needs to be aware that most lower-limb amputations result from peripheral vascular disease, while most upper-limb amputations result from severe trauma. This knowledge gives direction for client education related to prevention of amputation. Control of causative illnesses such as peripheral vascular disease, diabetes, chronic osteomyelitis, and ulcers can reduce or delay the need for amputation. Clients with these problems need to be taught to carefully examine their lower extremities daily for signs of impending problems. If the client cannot assume this responsibility, a family member should be instructed on the procedure. The client or family needs to be instructed to report immediately to the health care provider such problems as change in skin color or temperature, decrease or absence of sensation, tingling, pain, or the presence of a lesion.

Instruction in proper safety precautions related to

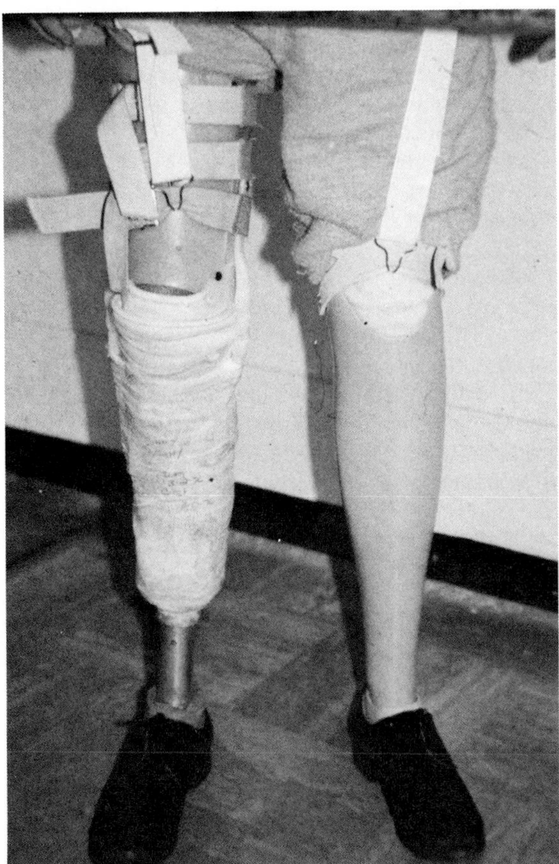

Figure 56-19 Two types of prosthesis. *Left:* Patellar tendon-bearing (PYB)-type, below-the-knee prosthesis with cuff suspension. *Right:* Early-fitting below-the-knee rigid plaster dressing with pylon.

recreation and occupation are a nursing responsibility of major importance. Prevention of amputation of a mutilated limb is only one of the serious consequences of trauma which might be avoided by such instruction.

Acute intervention (lower-limb amputation)

The nurse must recognize the tremendous psychological and social implications of an amputation for the client. The disruption in body image caused by an amputation often causes a client to go through psychological stages similar to the grieving process. Allowing the client to go through a period of depression and recognizing it as a normal consequence of the amputation may do much to aid the client's acceptance of the amputation. The client's family must also be helped to work through the process to arrive at a realistic and positive attitude about the future. The implications of an amputation and the rehabilitation potential are dependent upon age, diagnosis, occupation, personality, resources, and support systems.

Preoperative Care Preoperatively, the nurse should reinforce the information the client and family have received related to the reasons for the amputation, the proposed prosthesis, and the mobility training program. In addition to the usual preoperative instructions, the client undergoing an amputation has special education needs. In order to meet these needs, the nurse must know the level of amputation, the type of postsurgical dressing, and the type of prosthesis planned. The client should receive instruction in the performance of upper-extremity exercises, such as push-ups in bed to promote arm strength, which will be essential for later crutch-walking and gait training. If conditions permit, the nurse should instruct the client in the technique of crutch-walking and the type of gait which will be utilized postoperatively and during gait training with the prosthesis. The general postoperative nursing care should be discussed, including positioning, support, and care of the stump. If a compression type of postoperative bandage is to be used, the client should be instructed as to its purpose and how it will be applied. If an immediate prosthesis is planned, the general ambulation program should be discussed.

The client needs to be warned that he may feel as if his limb is still present following amputation. This *phantom sensation* usually disappears but may cause the client grave concern unless he is forewarned. Phantom-limb pain can also be mentioned. This is a sensation of aching, burning, or cramping in the amputated limb. (See Chap. 50 for discussion of phantom-limb pain.) As recovery progresses, phantom-limb pain usually subsides. Some surgeons believe phantom sensations occur less often if the client is *not* forewarned.

Postoperative Care General postoperative care of the client who has had an amputation depends largely upon the client's general state of health, the reason for the amputation, and the client's age. Nursing care must be individualized on the basis of these factors. For instance, an elderly client would need particularly careful monitoring of respiratory status; a victim of a motorcyle accident might need careful neurological monitoring.

Specific nursing intervention for the client who has undergone an amputation involves prevention of complications, stump care, and muscle strengthening of both stump and uninvolved extremities. Hemorrhage is a serious complication of amputation. Regular assessment of the surgical area is essential. If an immediate prosthesis has been applied, the nurse must monitor vital signs carefully, since the surgical site is heavily covered. A surgical tourniquet must always be available for emergency use. Should hemorrhage occur, the surgeon should be notified immediately while efforts to control the hemorrhage are begun.

Flexion contractures are another complication of amputation which may delay the rehabilitation process. The most common and debilitating contracture is hip flexion. Hip adduction contracture is rare and is usually prevented by the client's normal bed mobility. The client should avoid sitting in a chair with hips flexed for long periods of time to prevent a flexion contracture. Unless specifically contraindicated, the client should turn onto the abdomen several times a day and position the hip in extension while prone.

A hematoma may develop at the surgical site from oozing blood vessels. Aspiration is usually necessary to prevent infection and disruption of the wound edges. Delayed healing of the wound or infection and necrosis of the wound edges may require revision of the stump.

Proper bandaging of the stump fosters shaping and modeling for eventual fitting of the prosthesis (Fig. 56-20). The physician will usually order a compression bandage applied immediately after surgery in order to support the soft tissues, reduce edema, hasten healing, and promote stump shrinkage and maturation.

Initially the compression bandage is worn 24 hours a day except for physical therapy and bathing. The bandage is taken off and reapplied several times a day, taking care that it is applied snugly but not so tight as to interfere with circulation. Shrinker bandages should be washed and changed daily. After the stump has matured, it is bandaged only when the client is not wearing the prosthesis. The client should be instructed to avoid dangling the stump over the side of the bed, to avoid edema formation.

As the client's overall condition improves, the nurse begins instruction in the principles and techniques of transferring from bed to chair and vice versa. Active exercises and conditioning are essential in developing ambulation skills. The exercise regimen is normally started under the supervision of the physician and physical therapist. The nurse must have a clear understanding of the exercise regimen in order to reinforce and ensure that the exercises are performed correctly. Active range-of-motion exercises of all joints within the client's pain tolerance and medical status should be started as soon as possible following surgery. In addition, the client needs to increase triceps strength, shoulder depressors, and support of lower limbs, as well as practice with balance. The loss of the weight of a limb requires a retuning of the client's proprioceptive mechanisms in order to prevent falls and frustration.

Crutch-walking is started as soon as the client is physically able. If he has had an immediate postsurgical fitting, orders related to weight bearing must be carefully followed to avoid disruption of the skin flap and delay in the training process. Initial periods of ambulation should not exceed 5 minutes to prevent edema.

Prior to discharge, the client and family must have careful instruction related to stump care, ambulation, exercise, and follow-up care. Table 56-13 outlines appropriate stump care for the client to follow.

Rehabilitative management

When the stump has healed satisfactorily and is well molded, the client is ready for fitting of the prosthesis. Matching a client with a suitable prosthesis involves many factors including age, general health, intelligence, motivation, occupation, and finances. After the physician makes his recommendation, the client is referred to a prosthetist, who initially makes a mold of the stump and measures landmarks for the fabrication of the prosthesis. The molded stump socket allows the stump to fit snugly into the prosthesis. The stump is covered with a stump sock to ensure better fit and prevent skin breakdown. The nurse should be aware that the stump may continue to shrink, causing a loose fit, in which case a new socket has to be fabricated. Excessive movement of a loose prosthesis can cause severe skin irritation and breakdown. To ensure a normal gait with minimum expenditure of energy, the prosthesis and limb have to be accurately aligned. Alignment of the prosthesis in relation to the stump and the rest of the body is one of the more important factors determining its successful use.

Before the client begins gait training, control of the prosthesis must be mastered. After initial evaluation by the physician and direction of mobility and strength training by the physical therapist, the client is taught the correct sequence of gait cycle and the use of the prosthesis. Learning to use a prosthesis is frustrating, and the client may easily become discouraged. The nurse must continually offer support and encouragement until the client is able to manage by himself.

Artificial limbs become an integral part of the client's body image. Proper care ensures their long life

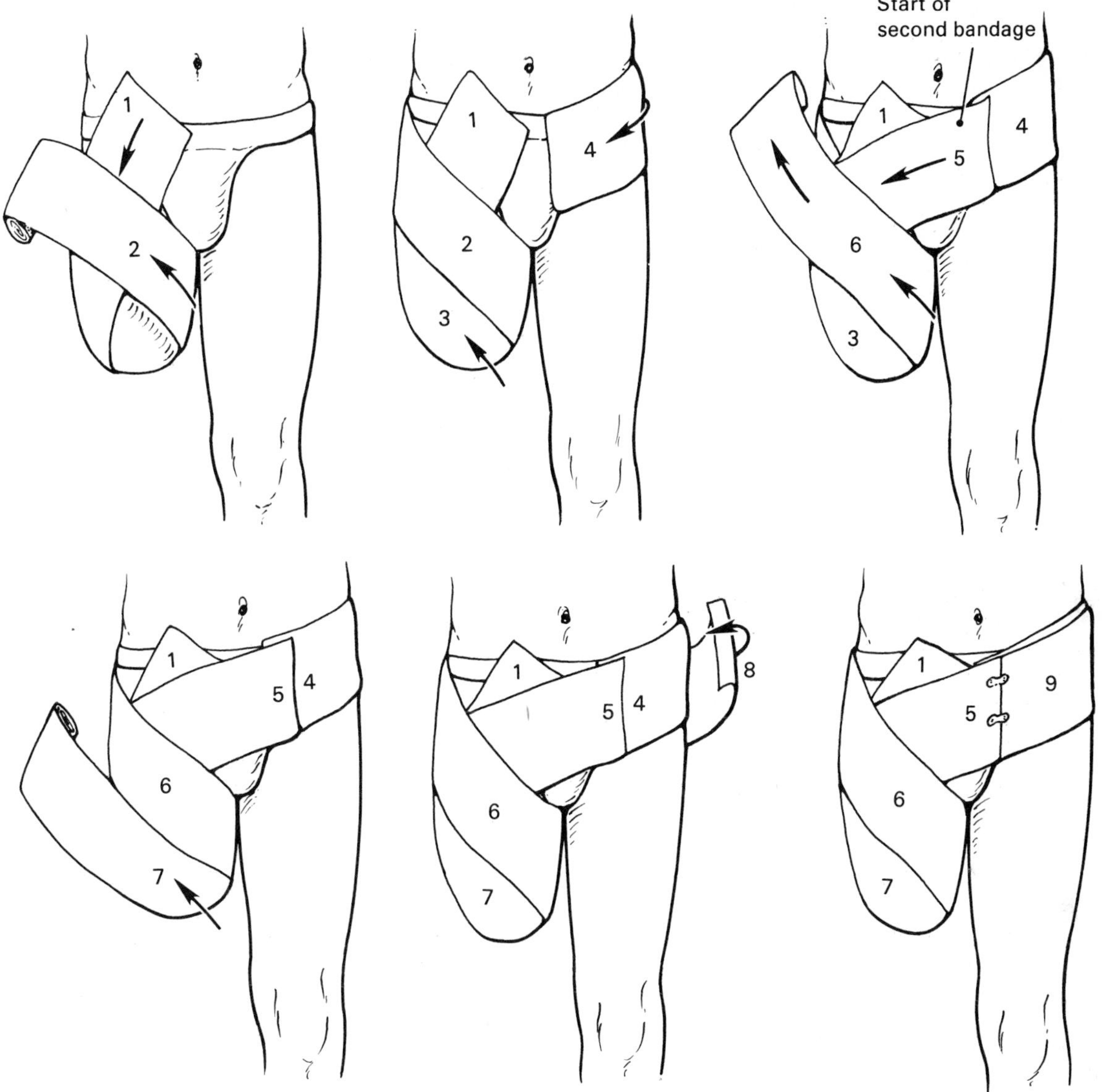

Figure 56-20 Proper stump bandaging for above-the-knee stump: figure-of-eight style that covers progressive areas of stump. Two bandages are required.

and useful functioning. The client should be instructed to clean the socket daily with a mild soap and rinse thoroughly to remove irritants. The leather and metal parts of the prosthesis should not get wet. Regular maintenance by the prosthetist should be encouraged. The client should also consider the condition of the shoe: a badly worn shoe will throw the gait off and may cause damage to the prosthesis.

Some shrinkage of the stump is to be expected, and the client may need to have his prosthesis adjusted to prevent rubbing and friction between the stump and the socket.

The long-term goals of nursing intervention are not usually achieved in the hospital setting. It takes time, determination, and energy to successfully master the use of an artificial limb. The psychological impact may take more time to accept than the limb itself. The community health nurse can do much to foster both physical and emotional adjustment to the amputation.

Table 56-13
Client Instruction for Stump Care

1. Inspect the stump daily for signs of skin irritation, especially redness.
2. Discontinue use of the prosthesis if an irritation develops. Have the area checked before resuming use of the prosthesis.
3. Wash thoroughly each night with warm water and a bacteriostatic soap. Rinse thoroughly and dry gently.
4. Do not use any irritating substance such as lotions, alcohol, or powders.
5. If you wear a stump sock, wear only the one supplied by your prosthetist. Change daily. Launder in a mild soap, squeeze dry, and lay flat to dry.

Special Considerations in Upper-Limb Amputation

The emotional implications of an upper-extremity amputation are often more devastating than those of a lower-limb amputation. The enforced dependency brought about by one-handedness is both frustrating and humiliating to many clients. Also, since most upper-extremity amputations result from trauma, the client has not had the opportunity to adjust psychologically to the possibility of an amputation or to participate in the decision.

Both immediate and delayed prosthetic fittings are possible for the below-the-elbow amputee. Prosthetic fitting is delayed for the above-the-elbow amputee. The usual functional prosthesis is the arm and hook. A cosmetic hand is available but has limited functional value. As with the lower-limb prosthesis, client motivation and endurance are major factors in a satisfactory outcome.

CANCER OF THE BONE

Primary malignant bone neoplasms are rare in adults and account for less than 1 percent of all deaths attributed to cancer. These neoplasms are characterized by their rapid metastasis and destruction of bone. Primary neoplasms occur more frequently in the period of childhood through young adulthood.

Multiple Myeloma

In adults multiple myeloma (plasma cell myeloma) is the most frequently occurring primary tumor arising in bone. It is a malignant neoplasm of plasma cells causing widespread infiltration and destruction of bone marrow and cortex and producing osteolytic lesions throughout the skeletal system. The bones of the axial skeleton, such as the skull, vertebrae, ribs, pelvis, and flat bones, are commonly invaded by plasma cell myeloma. Other sites of involvement may include the spleen, liver, kidney, and lymph nodes. As the bones become affected by proliferating plasma cells, there is painful destruction of bone cortex leading to generalized weakening of bone. This may cause spontaneous fracture or collapse. Continued destruction of normal marrow components causes the development of anemia and thrombocytopenia. During the course of the disease there is a tendency to bleed because of platelet deficiency and dysfunction. Pronounced anemia, increased debility, and increasing pain are also common.

Multiple myeloma occurs more frequently in males over 50.[14] It has an insidious onset, with the lesions often remaining localized for an extended period of time before disseminating. The client's history will usually indicate progressive weakness, malaise, vague bone pains particularly in the lower back, weight loss, and periods of immobility.

The diagnosis of multiple myeloma is confirmed by biopsy or bone marrow aspiration. Radiographic examination of the axial skeleton usually reveals destructive osteolytic defects which appear as punched-out areas. Bence-Jones protein in the urine is indicative of multiple myeloma but is not always found in the urine of all clients with the disease.

The overall prognosis is poor, because by the time diagnosis has been confirmed the disease has usually invaded the axial skeleton. The median life expectancy for the untreated client is approximately 17 months and for the treated client from 26 months to not more than 5 years. Chemotherapeutic treatment of multiple myeloma has limited usefulness; it is primarily directed toward suppressing plasma cell growth by use of melphalen (Alkeran), cyclophosphamide (Cytoxan), doxorubicin (Adriamycin), and methotrexate (A-Methopterin). Steroids are commonly used in conjunction with melphalan and cyclophosphamide. Steroid therapy increases the client's susceptibility to infection. Death usually results from complications attributable to infection and renal failure. (Multiple myeloma is also discussed in Chap. 24.)

Osteogenic Sarcoma

Osteogenic sarcoma (osteosarcoma) is a primary neoplasm of bone which is extremely malignant and is characterized by rapid growth and metastasis (Fig. 56-21). The usual site of occurrence is the metaphyseal region of the long bones of the extremities, particularly in the regions of the distal femur, proximal tibia, and proximal humerus. Osteogenic sarcoma has its highest incidence in the 10- to 25-year-old range and more commonly occurs in males.

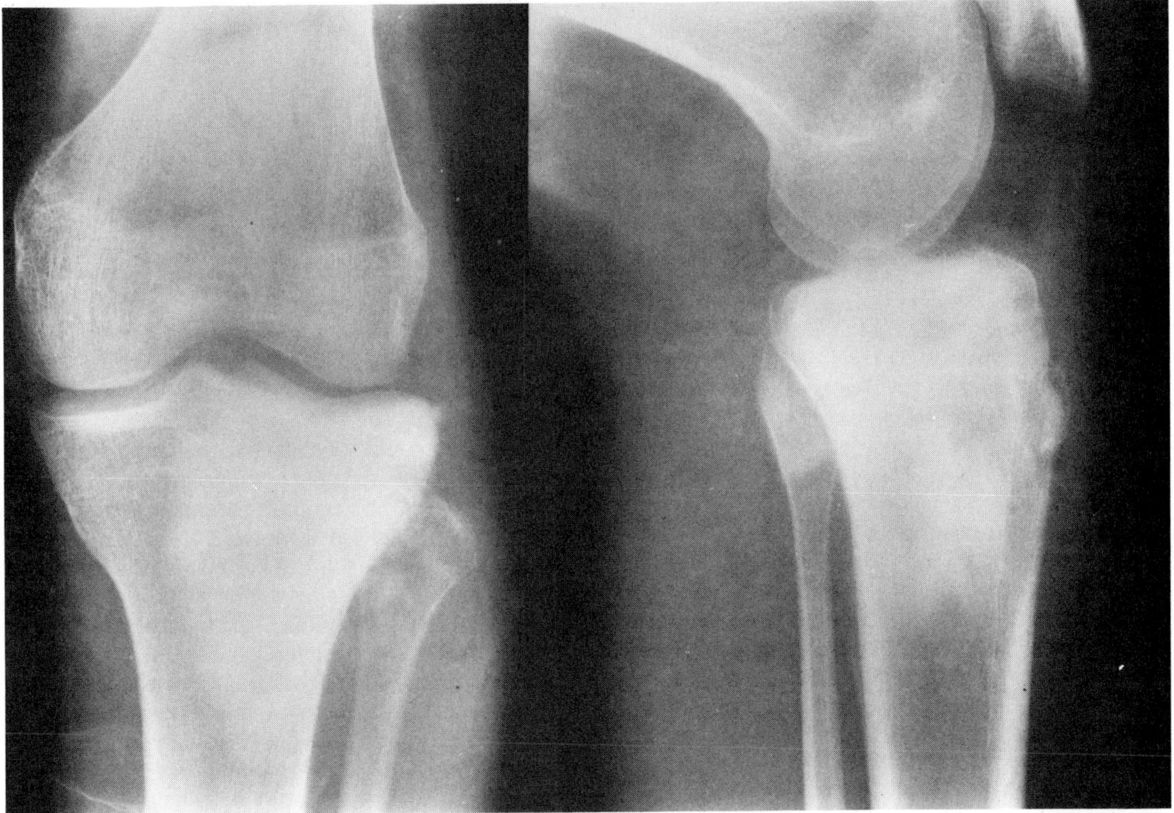

Figure 56-21 Locally advanced sclerotic type of osteogenic sarcoma of the proximal tiba, anteroposterior and lateral views. (*Courtesy of T. M. Moore, M.D., University of Southern California School of Medicine.*)

The clinical manifestations of osteogenic sarcoma are usually associated with a past history of minor injury and gradual onset of pain and swelling. The injury does not cause the neoplasm but rather serves to bring the preexisting condition to medical attention. The neoplasm grows rapidly and produces a noticeable increase in the size of the general region, which can restrict joint motion if the lesion is close to a joint structure. The diagnosis is confirmed from biopsied tissue specimens, elevation of the serum alkaline phosphates and calcium levels, and radiographic findings. Amputation is usually the treatment of choice, in combination with irradiation and chemotherapy. Early metastasis to the lungs is responsible for a poor prognosis and the survival rate of 15 to 20 percent.

Osteoclastoma

True osteoclastoma (giant cell tumor) is a malignant, destructive neoplasm that arises in the cancellous ends of long bones in young adults. Some variant giant cell tumors which have been put in this class of neoplasm are usually benign. Giant cell tumors most commonly occur between the ages of 20 and 35. The common sites are the distal end of the femur, proximal tibia, and distal radius. The giant cell tumor is a locally destructive lesion whose growth extends from a few months to several years. The clinical manifestations are usually swelling, local pain, and some disturbances of joint function. Radiographic evidence of giant cell tumor is variable but usually reveals local areas of bone destruction and eventual expansion of the bone ends. Medical treatment initially includes biopsy to establish the diagnosis, followed by surgical curettage of the lesion with bone grafting. After treatment there is a greater than 50 percent chance of recurrence. Recurrent giant cell tumors may subsequently make amputation necessary. Advances in chemotherapy have recently improved the overall statistics.

Ewing's Sarcoma

Ewing's sarcoma is the third most common primary malignant neoplasm of bone, occuring most frequently in males under 30 years of age. This neoplasm is characterized by rapid growth within the medullary cavity of long bone, especially the femur and tibia, and early metastasis. The most frequent site of metastasis is the lungs. Ewing's sarcoma has a poor prognosis, with survival estimated at only 5 percent. Common manifestations are progressive local pain, swelling, palpable soft-tissue mass, noticeable increase in size of the affected part, fever, and leukocytosis. Initially, radiographic evidence usually indicates periosteal elevation, which progresses to extensive areas of bone destruction. Medical treatment usually involves radiation therapy and surgical resection or amputation. Chemotherapy agents commonly utilized are cyclophosphamide (Cytoxan), dactinomycin, vincristine (Oncovin), methotrexate, and doxorubicin (Adriamycin). New chemotherapeutic techniques hold promise of improvement in survival rates.

Metastatic Lesions of Bone

The most common type of malignant bone tumor occurs secondary to metastasis from a primary tumor. Common sites for the primary tumor include the breast, intestinal tract, lungs, prostate, kidney, ovary, or thyroid. The metastatic lesion is commonly found in the spine, pelvis, or ribs. Pathological fractures at the site of metastasis are common owing to weakening of the involved bone.

Once a primary lesion has been identified, bone scans are often done to detect metastatic lesions before they are visible on x-ray. Treatment is palliative and consists in pain management and irradiation. Prognosis is poor.

Nursing Management

The nurse needs to educate the public to recognize the warning signs of bone cancer, including swelling, pain of unexplained origin, limitation of joint function, and changes of skin temperature. As with all forms of cancer, health promotion should stress the importance of periodic health examinations.

Nursing care of the client with malignant bone neoplasm does not differ significantly from the care given to the client with a malignant disease of any part of the body. However, special attention is required to reduce the complications associated with prolonged bed rest and prevention of pathological fractures. Often the client is reluctant to participate in therapeutic activities because of weakness and fear of pain. Regular rest periods should be provided between therapeutic activities. Careful handling of the affected extremity is important in the prevention of pathological fractures.

The nurse must be able to assist the client in accepting the guarded prognosis associated with bone cancer. Inability to accomplish age-specific developmental tasks can increase the frustrations of this condition. General principles related to cancer nursing are applicable (Chap. 11). Special attention is necessary for the problems of pain and dysfunction, chemotherapy, and specific surgery such as cord decompression and amputation.

LOW BACK PAIN

Etiology and Pathogenesis

Low back pain is a common symptom related to the musculoskeletal system. This problem has probably affected every adult at least once. In industry, low back pain is responsible for more lost working hours than any other medical condition and represents one of the nation's costliest symptoms. Each year about 18 million visits are made to physicians for treatment of this condition.[15] Pain in the lumbar region is a common problem because this area bears most of the weight of the body, is the most flexible region of the spinal column, contains nerve roots which are vulnerable to injury or disease, and has an inherently poor structure.

Low back pain is most often due to a musculoskeletal problem. However, other causes such as metabolic, urologic, or psychosomatic problems must not be overlooked. The causes of low back pain of musculoskeletal origin include (1) acute lumbosacral strain, (2) unstable lumbosacral bony mechanism, (3) osteoarthritis of the lumbosacral spine, and (4) intervertebral disk degeneration. Of these, the most common cause of low back pain is mechanical strain of paravertebral muscles. Degeneration and herniation of the nucleus pulposus is another common cause of low back pain.

Acute Low Back Pain

Clinical manifestations

Acute low back pain is usually associated with some type of activity which causes undue stress on the tissues of the lower back. Often symptoms will not appear at the time of the injury but develop later because of gradual buildup of paravertebral muscle spasms. The client will complain of pain on walking, turning, straining, and coughing. Guarding is seen in any activities which might aggravate the pain. Upon palpation, tenseness and tightening of the paravertebral muscles may be apparent. Few definitive diagnostic abnormalities are present with acute low back pain. The straight leg raise will produce pain in the lumbar area without radiation along the sciatic nerve.

Medical management

If the muscle spasms are not severe, the client may be treated on an ambulatory basis with analgesics, muscle relaxants, and strapping or use of a corset. Strapping and a corset prevent movement of the joint into a position that would stretch damaged tissue. Strapping is less often used because of skin sensitivity to adhesive tape.

If the spasms and pain are severe, however, a period of hospitalization is often required. Since paravertebral muscle spasms are worse when the client is upright, bed rest is the prime treatment for acute low back pain. Bathroom privileges are usually allowed. Bed rest is maintained until the client can turn from side to side with minimal discomfort. At this time, gradually increasing activity is initiated. The period of complete bed rest usually lasts for 5 to 10 days.

Nursing management

Health Promotion and Maintenance The nurse has a place as both role model and teacher with clients with low back problems. As a role model, the nurse should use proper body mechanics at all times. Proper body mechanics should be a prime consideration when teaching both clients and care providers transfer and turning techniques. The nurse should assess the client's use of body mechanics and offer advice when movements which could produce back strain are used.

The position assumed while sleeping is also important in prevention of low back pain. Sleeping on the stomach should be forbidden, because it produces excessive lumbar lordosis. The mattress should be firm, and the sleeping position should be either on the back or in a side-lying position with the knees and hips flexed. Maintenance of optimal body weight is also important in preventing unnecessary pressure on supporting muscles, ligamentous structures, and lumbosacral joints.

Acute Intervention The prime nursing responsibility in acute low back pain is to assist the client to maintain bed rest. Whether the client is at home or hospitalized, measures to ensure bed rest should be enforced. Other nursing interventions related to acute low back pain are summarized in Table 56-14.

Muscle-strengthening exercises are often ordered. Although the actual exercises are often taught by the physical therapist, it is the nurse's responsibility to ensure that the client understands the kind and frequency of exercise prescribed.

Many different types of low back exercise may be prescribed; Fig. 56-22 illustrates some common ones. Typical instructions for a low back exercise program include: start with doing each exercise 5 times twice a day; add one exercise every 2 days until each exercise is done 10 times twice a day; perform the exercises slowly and smoothly; perform the exercises on a hard surface such as the floor or a table.

Chronic Management Management seeks to make an episode of acute low back pain an isolated incident. If the lumbosacral mechanism is unstable, repeated episodes can be anticipated. The lumbosacral spine may be unable to meet the demands placed on it without strain because of obesity, poor muscular support, advancing age, or local trauma. Intervention is then aimed at strengthening the supporting muscles by exercise and use of a corset to limit extremes of movement. In addition, weight control reduces the mechanical demands on the lower back.

Persistent use of poor body mechanics may also result in repeated episodes of low back pain. If the strain is work-related, occupational counseling may be necessary. The frustration, pain, and disability imposed by low back problems requires emotional support and understanding care by the nurse.

Chronic Low Back Pain

Pathogenesis

The multiple causes of chronic low back pain include degenerative disk disease, lack of physical exercise, obesity, structural and postural abnormalities, and systemic disease. The focus of this section is on structural degeneration of the intervertebral disk, resulting in degenerative disk disease manifested by low back pain. This degeneration can also occur in the cervical spine area. The degeneration results in intervertebral narrowing and a lessening of the efficiency of the intervertebral disk in acting as shock absorbers. The resulting poor biomechanics results in chronic low back pain which may or may not be associated with leg pain. As the stresses on the degenerated disk continue and eventually exceed the strength of the disk, a herniated intervertebral disk may result (Fig. 56-23). Nuclear material from the intervertebral disk herniates into the spinal canal, causing compression or tension on a lumbar or sacral spinal nerve root.

Clinical manifestations

The most characteristic feature of a herniated intervertebral disk is back pain associated with buttock and leg pain along the distribution of the sciatic nerve. The straight-leg-raise test will be positive, with pain reproduced by raising the leg. Neurologically, the Achilles reflex may be depressed or absent, depending on the spinal root involved, with numbness or

Table 56-14
Nursing Care Plan for the Client with Low Back Pain

Client Problem	Expected Outcome	Nursing Intervention
	Acute Management	
Pain and muscle spasm	Decrease of pain and muscle spasm	Enforce bed rest. Keep head of bed elevated 20° and knee of bed flexed. Maintain pelvic traction as ordered, correctly aligned. Examine skin for pressure over iliac crest. Apply moist heat to lower back qid. Administer analgesics or muscle relaxants as ordered.
Constipation or painful straining	Regular bowel movement, absence of pain associated with straining	Give high bulk, high fiber diet (Table 6, Appendix B). Administer stool softeners as ordered.
Decreased mobility	Unrestricted gait and ambulation within normal limits	Perform ROM exercises daily. Ambulation program should start slowly and progress with assistance. Avoid having client bend, sit, or lift. Report leg or back pain and change in sensation.
Alteration of body image	Positive self-concept	Provide psychological support, active listening, and encouragement. Assist client to be as independent as possible.
	Long-Term Management	
Chronic pain	Development of effective methods of handling pain	Instruct client and family about home care and alternative methods of pain control, including use of heat, activity, and massage, avoiding strenuous activities. Assist in identifying activities which exacerbate pain and develop plans to prevent.
Stiffness and contractures	Remains active and ambulatory	Assess for development of joint contracture or instability and decreasing muscle strength. Teach low-back exercises. Encourage activity and ambulation within limitations.
Disability-related behavior	No development of chronic sick-role behavior	Explain factors that may contribute to development of maladaptive coping behavior. Explain how to develop therapeutic coping skills and activities which enhance self-concept and social interaction.
Poor body mechanics	Use of proper body mechanics at all times	Assess body mechanics. Instruct client on proper body mechanics and use of firm mattress or bedboard.
Unstable lumbosacral mechanism	No episodes of back strain	Reinforce need for trunk-strengthening exercises. Instruct on weight reduction and use of corset if indicated.

tingling in the toes and feet. Myelograms are helpful in localizing the site of herniation. If the disk ruptures in the cervical area, the clinical manifestations are stiff neck, shoulder pain radiating to the hand, and paresthesias and sensory disturbances of the hand.

Medical management

Degenerative disk disease is managed conservatively with heat, pelvic traction, rest, limitation of extremes of spinal movement (corset), and anti-inflammatory medication. If herniation of the disk occurs, more aggressive treatment is indicated (Table 56-15). Conservative treatment sometimes results in a healing over of the herniated area with a decrease in the pain of the nerve root irritation. Complete bed rest is often encouraged by the use of traction. Once the symptoms subside, back-strengthening exercises are begun to make the client aware of good posture. Extremes of flexion, extension, and torsion are strongly discouraged. If the disk ruptures directly into the spinal canal, surgery is often the treatment required to reduce the sciatic pain.

Many clients with herniated disks will recover after a 2-week period of bed rest. However, if the client continues to have pain even with analgesics and muscle relaxants and there is evidence of decreasing sensory and motor status, surgery is indicated. The usual procedure is a *laminectomy* with or without a *spinal fusion*. A laminectomy is the surgical excision of part of the posterior arch of the vertebra in order to gain access to part or all of the protruding disk. Spinal fusion is often performed at the time of laminectomy,

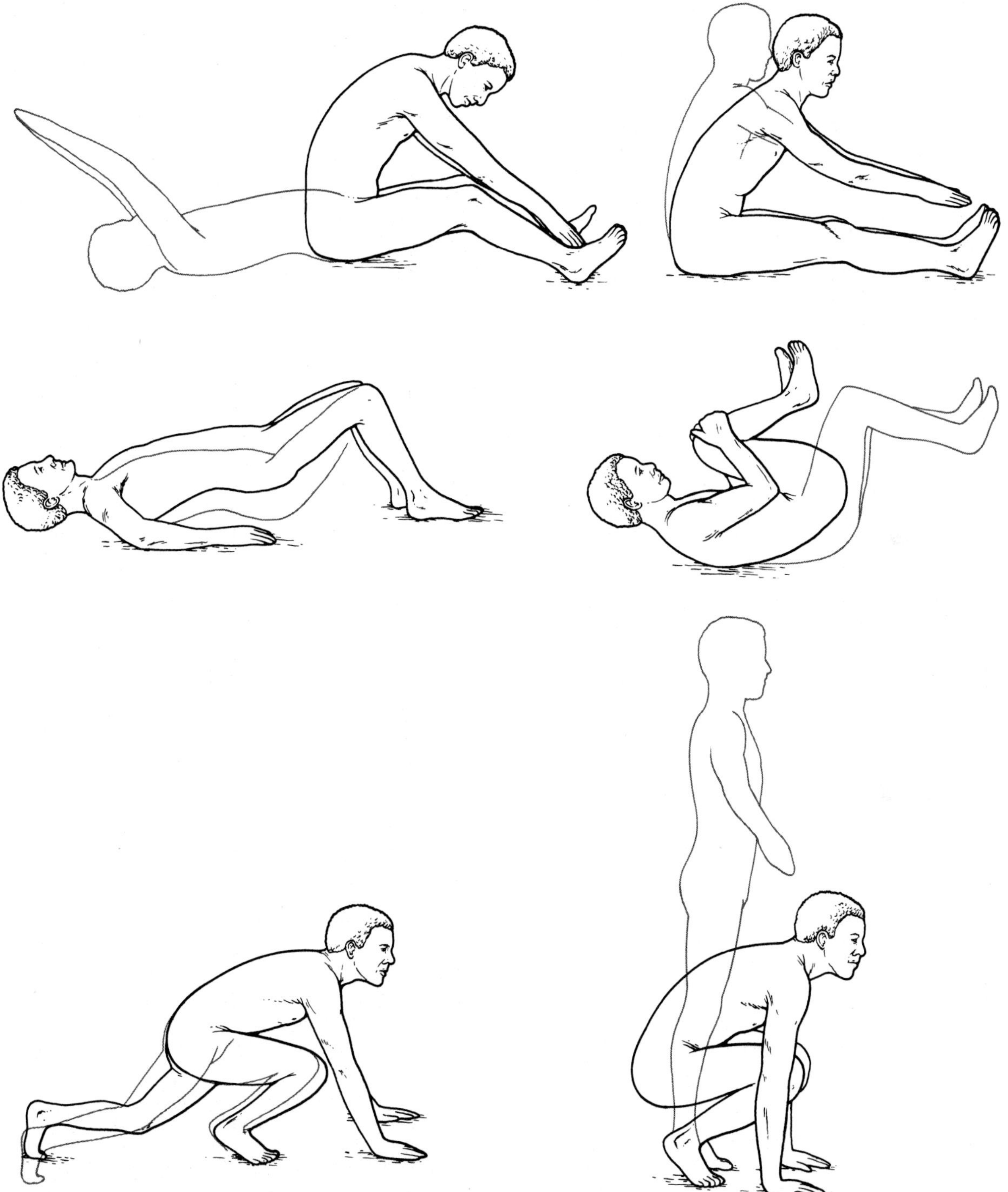

Figure 56-22 Williams flexion exercises for low back pain.

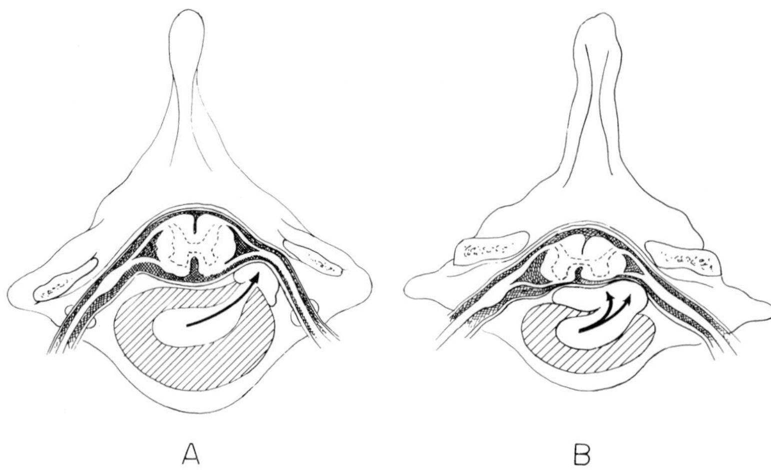

Figure 56-23 Diagram of herniated nucleus pulposus (HNP) as seen from the back, with the spinous processes and laminae removed from the pedicles. Note that the disk protrusion between the fourth and fifth lumbar vertebrae impinges on the fifth lumbar nerve root. *(From R. Adams and M. Victor, Principles of Neurology, 2d ed., McGraw-Hill Book Company, New York, 1980.)*

particularly if the protrusion is at the lumbosacral interspace. In a spinal fusion, the spine is stabilized by creating an ankylosis of contiguous vertebrae using a bone graft from the client's tibia or iliac crest.

Nursing management

Acute Intervention The postoperative management of the client who has undergone spinal surgery requires vigilant routine postoperative care. In addition, nursing intervention is aimed at maintaining proper alignment of the spine at all times until healing has taken place. The bed must always be in a flat position. Logrolling the client when turning him is essential to maintain proper body alignment. Use of pillows to support the full leg when supine and between the legs when side-lying provides for both comfort and safety.

Severe muscle spasms in the surgical area can be controlled with medication and correct turning and positioning. The client is often fearful of turning or any movement which increases pain by straining the surgical area. It is critical that enough staff be available to move the client without undue pain or strain.

Since the spinal canal is entered during surgery, there is a potential for spinal fluid leakage. Severe headache and leakage of fluid are to be reported immediately. Frequent monitoring of neurological changes is a routine postoperative nursing responsibility following a laminectomy. The client is expected to have normal movement of arms and legs as well as normal response to pinprick sensation. Table 56-16 summarizes a lumbar laminectomy check appropriate for the client with back surgery. This check is repeated 4 times a day and findings compared with the original assessment.

Interference with bowel and bladder function may occur for several days and requires careful monitoring to prevent constipation and distension. A potential for paralytic ileus can be evaluated by noting whether the client is passing flatus, is nauseated, has a flat, soft, abdomen, and has bowel sounds.

Activity prescriptions vary with surgeons, but the laminectomy client often ambulates early in the postoperative period. It is a nursing responsibility to know the specific orders related to activity for any given client.

In addition to the nursing care appropriate for a client who has had a laminectomy, there are additional nursing responsibilities if the client has also had a spinal fusion. Because a bone graft is involved, the

Table 56-15
Medical Management: Herniated Intervertebral Disk

Diagnostic
1. History
2. Physical examination with emphasis on neurological deficits, straight leg raising, and sitting root test
3. Electromyography
4. Myelogram

Conservative Therapeutic
1. Absolute bed rest
2. Medication
   a. Analgesics
   b. Anti-inflammatory agents
   c. Muscle relaxants
3. Diathermy and local heat
4. Traction

Surgical
Laminectomy with or without spinal fusion

Table 56-16
Lumbar Laminectomy Check

Indications

1. Low back pain
2. Lumbar laminectomy and lumbar fusion
3. Lumbar fracture
4. Paralysis
5. Suspected spinal injury in trauma patients

Areas of evaluation

1. *Pain*—Locate the pain and the area of radiation of the pain exactly
2. *Neurological status*—Check for normal sensation, numbness, or tingling
3. *Circulatory status*—Check the color and temperature of the lower extremities
4. *Movement*—Check the ability to dorsiflex and plantarflex the ankle and the ability to wiggle the toes
5. *Muscle tone*—Check the quadriceps muscles on the upper anterior thigh

Adapted from Barbara Gilbertson, "Low Back Pain: What to Look For—What to Do," *RN*, October 1978, p. 76.

postoperative healing time is greatly prolonged compared to a laminectomy. Immobilization over an extended period of time is necessary. Often, a rigid orthosis ("chairback brace") is used during the period of immobilization. The client must be taught to take it on and off by logrolling in bed. The extended immobilization required by a spinal fusion carries with it all the potential problems related to this inactive state.

In addition to the primary surgical site, the donor site for the bone graft must be regularly assessed; often the donor site may cause greater postoperative pain than the fused area. The donor site is bandaged with a pressure dressing to prevent hemorrhage. If the donor site is the tibia, neurovascular assessments of the extremity are a routine postoperative nursing responsibility.

If the surgery has involved the cervical spine, the nurse must be alert for symptoms of cord edema such as respiratory problems and a worsening neurological status of the upper extremities.

Chronic Management As the bone graft heals, the client will need to adjust to the permanent immobilization of the surgical area. Instruction in proper body mechanics is essential and should be evaluated during the hospital stay. The client should learn to mentally think through an activity before starting any potentially injurious task such as bending, lifting, or stooping. A firm mattress or bedboard is essential. When sitting, a straight-backed, firm-seated chair with arms is preferable to a low, overstuffed chair. The surgeon's preference as to the use of a corset, brace, or cast should be carefully explained to both client and family. The extended convalescence associated with a spinal fusion require careful assessment of the client's psychological state, with appropriate intervention if depression or anxiety develop. Follow-up care should be planned and understood by the client.

COMMON FOOT PROBLEMS

The foot is the platform which provides support for the weight of the body and absorbs considerable shock in ambulation. It is a complicated structure composed of numerous bony structures, muscles, tendons, and ligaments and can be affected by (1) congenital conditions, (2) structural weakness, (3) traumatic injuries, and (4) systemic conditions such as diabetes and rheumatoid arthritis. Abnormalities of the foot affect over 80 million persons in the United States.[16] Much of the pain, deformity, and disability associated with foot disorders can be directly attributed to or accentuated by improperly fitted shoes, which can cause crowding and angulation of the toes, inhibit the normal movement of the foot muscles, fail to provide foot support, and promote areas of excessive pressure and friction.[17] Table 56-17 summarizes common foot problems and their treatment.

Nursing Management

Well-constructed and properly fitted shoes are essential for healthy, pain-free feet. Fashion styles, especially women's, often influence selection of footwear instead of considerations of comfort and support. Client education should stress the importance of having a shoe that conforms to the foot rather than to current fashion trends. The shoe must be long enough and wide enough to prevent crowding of the toes and forcing the great toe into a position of hallux valgus. At the metatarsal head, the width of the shoe should be sufficient to allow free movement of the foot muscles and permit bending of the toes. The shank of the shoe should be rigid enough to give optimal support. The height of the heel should be realistic in relation to the purpose for which the shoe will be worn. Ideally, the heel of the shoe should not rise more than 1 inch higher than the forefoot support.

Care of the feet should include daily hygenic care, including the wearing of clean stockings. Stockings should be long enough to avoid wrinkling and areas of pressure. Trimming the toenails straight across will help to prevent ingrown toenails and reduce the possibility of infection. Persons with impaired

Table 56-17
Common Foot Problems

Disorder	Definition	Treatment
	Common Disorders of the Foot	
Forefoot		
Hallux valgus (bunion)	Painful deformity of large toe consisting of lateral angulation of large toe toward second toe, bony enlargement of medial side of first metatarsal head, and formation of a bursa or callus over bony enlargement.	Conservative treatment includes wearing shoes with wide forefoot or "bunion pocket" and use of bunion pads to relieve pressure on bursal sac. Surgical treatment is removal of bursal sac and bony enlargement and correction of lateral angulation of large toe.
Hallux rigidus	Painful stiffness of first metatarsophalangeal joint due to osteoarthritis or local trauma.	Conservative treatment includes intraarticular corticosteroids and passive manual stretching of first metatarsophalangeal joint. A shoe with a stiff sole will decrease pain in the joint when walking. Surgical treatment is joint fusion or arthroplasty.
Hammertoe	Deformity of second toe including dorsiflexion of metatarsophalangeal joint, plantar flexion of proximal interphalangeal joint, and callus on dorsum of proximal interphalangeal joint and end of involved toe. Complaints related to hammertoe are burning on bottom of foot and pain and difficulty walking when wearing shoes.	Conservative treatment consists in passive manual stretching of proximal interphalangeal joint and use of metatarsal arch support. Surgical correction consists in resection of base of middle phalanx and head of proximal phalanx and bringing these raw bone ends together. A Kirschner wire maintains straight position.
Morton's neuroma (Morton's toe or plantar neuroma)	Neuroma in web space between third and fourth metatarsal heads causing sharp sudden attacks of pain and burning sensations.	Surgical removal.
Midfoot		
Pes planus (flatfoot)	Breakdown or lowering of metatarsal arch causing pain in foot or leg or referred to other parts of body.	Symptoms relieved by use of resilient longitudinal arch supports. Surgical treatment by triple arthrodesis, fusion of subtalar joint.
Pes cavus	Elevation of longitudinal arch of foot resulting from contracture of plantar fascia or bony deformity of arch.	Before age 6, treated by manipulation and casting. After age 6, surgical correction if interfering with ambulation.
Hindfoot		
Painful heels	Complaint is pain in heel with weight bearing. Commonly caused in adult by plantar bursitis or calcaneal spur.	Local injection of corticosteroids into inflamed bursa and sponge rubber heel cushion; surgical excision of bursa or spur.
	Local Foot Problems	
Corn	Localized thickening of skin caused by continual pressure over bony prominences, especially metatarsal head, which frequently causes localized pain.	Soften with warm water or preparations containing salicylic acid; trim with razor blade or scalpel. Relieve pressure by shoes on bony prominences.
Soft corn	Painful lesion caused by bony prominence of one toe pressing against adjacent toe. Usually located in web space between toes. Softness is produced by secretions that keep web space relatively moist.	Pain relieved by placing cotton between toes to separate them. Surgical treatment is excision of projecting bone spur.
Callus	Formation similar to corn but covering wider area and usually located on weight-bearing surface of foot.	Same as for corn.
Plantar wart	Painful papillomatous growth, caused by virus, that may occur on any part of skin on sole of foot.	Excision with electrocoagulation or surgical removal; ultrasound.

circulation or diabetes require detailed instruction to prevent serious complications associated with blisters, pressure areas, and infections (see Table 41-18).

Acute intervention

Many problems of the feet require surgery. When surgery is performed, the foot is usually immobilized by a bulky dressing or short leg cast or a platform "shoe" that fits over the dressing and has a rigid sole. To help reduce discomfort and prevent edema, the foot should be elevated with the heel off the bed. The neurovascular status should be assessed at frequent intervals during the immediate postoperative period. Depending on the type of surgery, pins or wires may extend through the toes or a protective splint which extends over the end of the foot may be in place. Care must be taken not to jar these devices and produce pain. The devices will interfere with or preclude assessment for movement. The nurse should be aware that sensation may be difficult to evaluate, because postoperative pain can interfere with the client's ability to differentiate pain secondary to the surgical procedure from pain secondary to nerve pressure or circulatory impairment.

The type and extent of surgery will determine the ambulation allowed. Crutches may or may not be necessary. The client may initially experience pain or a throbbing sensation when starting ambulation. The nurse should reinforce instructions given by the physical therapist and be careful that the client does not develop a faulty gait pattern such as walking on the heels in an attempt to avoid excessive pain or pressure. The nurse must reinforce the importance of walking with an erect posture and with proper weight distribution. Dysfunction of gait or continued pain should be reported to the physician. It is important that the nurse instruct the client on the importance of frequent rest periods with the feet elevated.

METABOLIC DISEASE OF BONE

Normal bone metabolism is dependent upon adequate intake, absorption, and utilization of calcium, phosphorus, protein, and vitamins. When there is dysfunction in one of these critical factors, generalized reduction of bone mass may result.

Osteomalacia

Osteomalacia is an uncommon disorder of adult bone associated with vitamin D deficiency, resulting in decalcification and softening of bone. This disease is the same as rickets in children except that the epiphyseal growth plates are closed in the adult. Vitamin D is required for the absorption of calcium from the intestines. Insufficient vitamin D intake can interfere with the normal mineralization of bone, causing failure or insufficient calcification of bone, which results in softening of bone and deformities. Lack of exposure to ultraviolet rays, gastrointestinal malabsorption, chronic diarrhea, pregnancy, or kidney disease are etiological factors in the development of osteomalacia.

The leading clinical feature of osteomalacia is persistent skeletal pain. Other clinical manifestations include progressive muscular weakness, weight loss, and progressive deformities of the spine (kyphosis) or extremities. Pathological fractures are uncommon and demonstrate delayed healing when they occur.

The most common laboratory findings associated with osteomalacia are decreased serum calcium and phosphorus levels and elevated serum alkaline phosphates. Radiographic examination may demonstrate the effects of generalized bone demineralization, especially loss of calcium in bones of the pelvis and the presence of associated bone deformity. Looser's zones (ribbons of decalcification in bone found on x-ray) are diagnostic of osteomalacia.

Medical management of osteomalacia is directed toward correction of the underlying cause. Vitamin D is usually supplemented and the client often shows dramatic response. Calcium and phosphorus intake may also be supplemented.

Osteoporosis

Osteoporosis (porous bone) is a general term for disorders of bone, commonly occurring in older persons, especially females past 60 years of age. It is characterized by a rate of bone resorption (loss of substance) which exceeds bone formation. This, in turn, results in a decrease in the density of bone. Among the many causes of osteoporosis are (1) disturbances of protein metabolism or protein deficiency, (2) disuse of bones or prolonged periods of immobilization, (3) estrogen deficiencies associated with menopause, (4) a diet deficient in vitamins or calcium, and (5) long-term administration of high doses of corticosteroids.

The client with osteoporosis frequently complains of bone pain, most commonly in the back, which may be caused by repeated microscopic fractures. Deformity associated with osteoporosis usually occurs as the result of spontaneous fractures. Radiographic studies demonstrate irregular loss of bone, often most marked in the vertebral bodies. Thin areas of porous bone are also evident. Serum calcium, phosphorus, and alkaline phosphatase levels usually remain normal.

Medical management is directed toward correcting the cause of the problem, because there is no specific treatment for osteoporosis. Estrogen and androgen therapy may be indicated in postmenopausal women to retard the rate of bone loss.

Efforts are made to keep clients with osteoporosis ambulatory in order to prevent further loss of bone substance secondary to immobility. Treatment also involves protecting areas of potential pathological fractures, as by the use of a corset to prevent kyphosis.

Paget's Disease

Paget's disease (osteitis deformans) is a skeletal bone disorder in which there is excessive bone removal and replacement with associated skeletal deformity. It usually occurs after the fourth decade, most commonly in males. It is characterized by deformities of bone caused by unexplained abnormal regeneration and resorption of bone, fibrotic changes, and remodeling with structurally uneven bone (Fig. 56-24). The regions of the skeleton commonly affected are the pelvis, long bones, spine, and cranium.

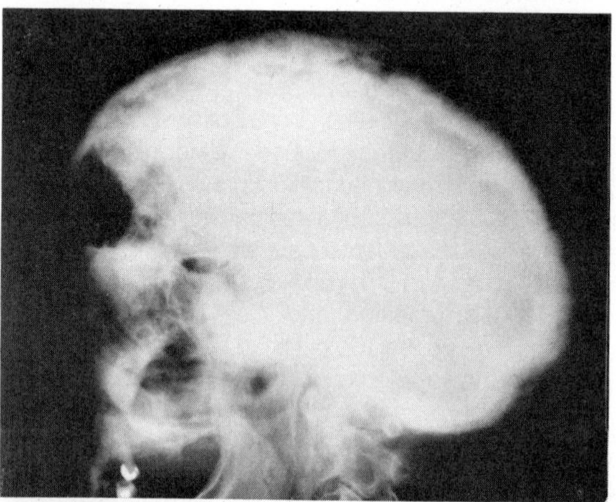

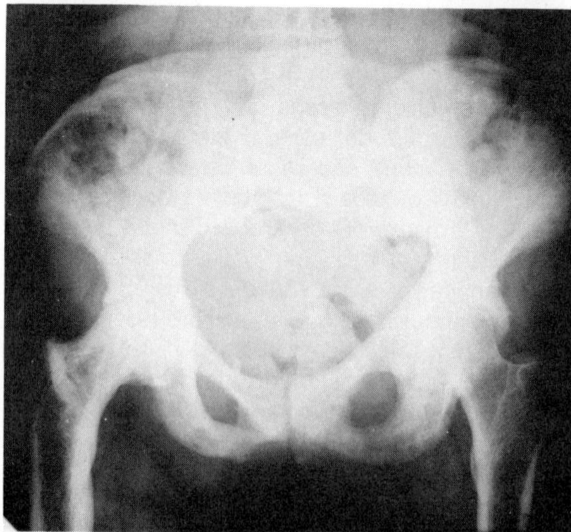

Figure 56-24 Paget's disease (osteitis deformans). Note thickening of the skull and unevenness and widespread changes in the density of bone. *(Courtesy of Herman Epstein, M.D., University of Southern California School of Medicine.)*

In milder forms of Paget's disease, the client may remain asymptomatic and the disease may be discovered incidentally on radiographic examination. The initial clinical manifestations are usually insidious development of skeletal pain, which may progress to severe intractable pain, complaints of fatigue, and progressive development of bowleg. The client may complain that he is becoming shorter or his head is becoming larger. The serum alkaline phosphatase is markedly elevated in advanced forms of the disease. Radiographic examination reveals that the normal contour of the affected bone is curved and the bone cortex thickened, especially the weight-bearing bones and the cranium. Pathological fracture is the most common complication of Paget's disease and may be the first indication of the disease. Other complications include malignant degeneration of Paget's disease to an osteosarcoma, chondrosarcoma, or fibrosarcoma. Medical management of Paget's disease is usually limited to symptomatic and supportive care and correction of secondary deformities by either surgical intervention or braces. Bone resorption, relief of acute symptoms, and lowering of the serum alkaline phosphatase levels may be significantly influenced by the administration of calcitonin. X-ray therapy may be utilized for the control of pain, and local operative procedures such as periosteal stripping will ease pain.

Nursing Management of the Client with Metabolic Bone Disorders

Since metabolic bone disorders increase the possibility of pathological fractures, the nurse must use extreme caution when the client is turned or moved. It is important to keep the client as active as possible in order to retard demineralization of bone resulting from disuse or extended immobilization. A supervised exercise program is an essential part of the treatment program. If the client's condition permits, ambulation must be encouraged without causing fatigue.

A firm mattress should be used both for back support and to relieve pain. The client may be required to wear a support corset or light brace to relieve back pain and provide support when in the upright position. The client should be proficient in the correct application of such devices and know how to regularly examine possible friction areas. Activities such as lifting and twisting should be discouraged. Good body mechanics is essential. Analgesics and muscle relaxants are administered to relieve pain. A properly balanced dietary program is very important in the management of metabolic disorders of bone, especially vitamin D, calcium, and protein, which are necessary to ensure the availability of the components for bone formation.

Case Study / Fracture

Henry A., a 30-year-old male, was seen in the emergency room following an auto accident. The right lower extremity was splinted with a cardboard splint and large bulky dressing. Avulsion of soft tissue on the anterolateral aspect of the tibia was present with obvious deformity, marked swelling, and ecchymosis in the region of the injury. The client complained of severe pain.

Discussion Questions

1. Describe the appropriate nursing neurovascular assessment of the injured extremity.
2. Differentiate an open fracture from a closed fracture.
3. Describe the probable medical and nursing interventions to prevent infection.
4. Describe specific nursing activities which the nurse can carry out to alleviate this client's pain.
5. Explain the stages of healing which will occur as this fracture heals.

REVIEW QUESTIONS

The number of the question corresponds to the same-numbered objective at the beginning of the chapter.

1. Which statement most accurately describes a strain?
   a. musculotendinous injury caused by use of the structure beyond its capacity
   b. overstretching of ligament fibers in the region of a joint
   c. minor injury of muscle tissues caused by blunt trauma
   d. torsional stress applied to the musculotendinous unit which causes hemarthrosis

2. The remodeling phase of bone healing is characterized by
   a. absence of movement at the fracture site
   b. conforming of the callus mass to the contour of the bone
   c. radiographic evidence of bony union
   d. gradual return of the structural strength and shape of the injured bone

3. Pseudarthrosis is a type of nonunion which is characterized by
   a. fracture healing in an abnormal position
   b. failure of the fracture to heal despite surgical intervention
   c. formation of fibrous tissue at the fracture site which permits movement
   d. slow healing

4. Instruction of the client in care of the cast should include
   a. awareness of signs of developing peripheral nerve and vascular complications
   b. hazards of walking on a "green" cast
   c. joint exercise above and below the plaster immobilization device
   d. all the above

5. Changes in pain which could include a neurovascular problem include
   a. increase in pain
   b. decrease in pain
   c. absence of pain
   d. all the above

6. The major complication associated with fracture of the humerus is
   a. radial nerve injury
   b. nonunion
   c. bursitis
   d. carpal tunnel syndrome

7. The most common infecting organism associated with osteomyelitis is
   a. *Streptococcus*
   b. *Escherichia coli*
   c. *Staphylococcus aureus*
   d. *Proteus*

8. During the postoperative period the amputee client should be instructed that the amputated extremity should not be positioned in a flexed position because
   a. this position promotes thrombosis formation
   b. unnecessary movement of the extremity can cause wound separation
   c. the flexed position can promote flexion contracture
   d. this position increases pain and edema

9. Osteogenic sarcoma is characterized by
   a. rapid growth and early metatasis
   b. rapid destruction of plasma cells
   c. destruction of red marrow within the medullary cavity
   d. slow growth which can be controlled by chemotherapy

10. The most common cause of acute low back pain is
   a. osteoarthritis of the lumbosacral spine
   b. acute lumbosacral strain

c. herniated nucleus pulposus
d. degenerative disk disease

11. A major nursing responsibility related to prevention of low back pain is the teaching of
a. proper body mechanics
b. use of a foam rubber mattress
c. sleeping on the stomach
d. traction application

12. Important nursing interventions following a laminectomy include
a. maintenance of proper body alignment
b. prevention of constipation and distension
c. assessing for paralytic ileus
d. all the above

13. Lateral angulation of the great toe in relation to the first metatarsal head is a condition of the foot known as
a. hallux rigidus
b. hallux varus
c. hallux valgus
d. none of the above

14. A common cause of bone pain associated with osteoporosis is
a. increased bone formation
b. repeated microscopic fractures
c. decreased blood supply
d. compression of nerves

REFERENCES

1. Jesse C. Delee and Charles A. Rockwood, "Skeletal Muscle Spasm and a Review of Muscle Relaxants," *Ther Res,* **27**(1):67 (January 1980).
2. J. J. Garland, *Fundamentals of Orthopaedics*, 3d ed., W. B. Saunders Company, Philadelphia, 1979, p. 280.
3. Alan R. Gurd and R. I. Wilson, "The Fat Embolism Syndrome," *J Bone Joint Surg [Br]*, **56-B**(3):412 (August 1974).
4. C. A. Donahoo and J. H. Diamond, *Orthopedic Nursing*, Little, Brown and Company, Boston, 1977, p. 210.
5. R. F. Schneider, *Handbook for the Orthopaedic Assistant*, 2d ed., The C. V. Mosby Company, St. Louis, 1976, p. 135.
6. DeLee, op. cit., p. 67.
7. R. B. Salter, *Textbook of Disorders and Injuries of the Musculoskeletal System*, The Williams & Wilkins Company, Baltimore, 1970, p. 355.
8. Nancy Hilt and Shirley Cogburn, *Manual of Orthopedics*, The C. V. Mosby Company, St. Louis, 1980, p. 134.
9. G. Schmeisser, Jr., *A Clinical Manual of Orthopaedic Traction Techniques*, W. B. Saunders Company, Philadelphia, 1963, p. 2.
10. Gartland, op. cit., p. 373.
11. Salter, op. cit., p. 489.
12. C. A. Rockwood and D. P. Green, *Fractures*, J. B. Lippincott Company, Philadelphia, 1975, p. 210.
13. A. H. Crenshaw (ed.), *Campbell's Operative Orthopaedics*, 5th ed., The C. V. Mosby Company, St. Louis, 1971, p. 838.
14. L. Diehl, P. Nugent, M. Brown-Stanley, and C. Witherell, "Achieving Pain Control in the Patient with Multiple Myeloma: A Team Approach," *Nursing 79*, 36 (November 1979).
15. L. Donovan, "Low Back Pain: Where Care is the Key to Recovery," *RN*, 71 (October 1978).
16. R. D. D'Ambrosia, *Musculoskeletal Disorders: Regional Examination and Differential Diagnosis*, J. B. Lippincott Company, Philadelphia, 1977, p. 497.
17. I. Haslock, V. Wright, and B. Champney, "Disorders of the Foot," *Nurs Mirror*, 49 (April 29, 1976).

Chapter 57

NURSING ROLE IN MANAGEMENT

Joint and Connective Tissue Problems*

Gayle L. Ziegler

Learning Objectives

1. Describe the pathophysiology, clinical manifestations, and medical management of degenerative joint disease, rheumatoid arthritis, gout, systemic lupus erythematosus, and progressive systemic sclerosis.
2. Describe the clinical manifestations and management of juvenile rheumatoid arthritis, associated rheumatic diseases, septic arthritis, polymyositis, and dermatomyositis.
3. Describe the sequence of events leading to joint destruction in degenerative joint disease and rheumatoid arthritis.
4. Compare degenerative joint disease with inflammatory joint disease as to clinical manifestations, treatment, and prognosis.
5. Identify the nursing role in the conservative management of joint and connective tissue problems.
6. Describe the various types of reconstructive surgery associated with joint and connective tissue problems.
7. Identify the preoperative and postoperative teaching and management of the client with reconstructive surgery associated with joint and connective tissue problems.
8. Describe the pharmacological interventions and nursing considerations related to joint and connective tissue problems.

DEGENERATIVE JOINT DISEASE (OSTEOARTHRITIS)

Degenerative joint disease (DJD) is a slowly progressive, noninflammatory disorder of mobile joints, particularly weight-bearing articulations, and is characterized by degeneration of articular cartilage.[1] The damage from osteoarthritis is confined to the joints and surrounding tissues. Osteoarthritis may be primary or secondary. *Primary osteoarthritis* begins without any known or apparent cause. The speed with which it progresses may be influenced by genetic, mechanical, and chemical factors. *Secondary osteoarthritis* is due to wear and tear on or injury to the joint.

Significance

It is estimated that over 40 million Americans have some evidence of osteoarthritis. Nearly 90 percent of persons over age 40 exhibit typical changes on x-ray.[2] Over one-third of these have clinical manifestations including pain, stiffness, and limited range of motion. There is a wide spectrum of severity, ranging from annoying and uncomfortable symptoms to significantly disabling disease. The incidence of degenerative joint disease increases with age, and men and women are affected equally.

Etiology and Pathology

Degenerative changes cause the normally smooth, white, translucent cartilage to become yellow and opaque, with rough surfaces and areas of malacia (softening). As the cartilage breaks down, fissures may appear and fragments of cartilage become loose in the joint space. Secondary inflammation of the synovial membrane may follow. As the articular surface becomes totally denuded of cartilage, subchondral bone increases in density and new bone (osteophytes) is formed at joint margins and at the attachment sites of ligaments and tendons.

There are several theories concerning the cause of cartilage deterioration. The enzyme hyaluronidase, which is normally found in the synovial fluid, may be responsible for digestion of protein polysaccharide through cracks in the surface layer of articular cartilage. Another theory suggests that inadequate nutrition may result in cartilage degradation. Since cartilage is avascular, nutrients are provided by the synovial fluid.

Specific predisposing factors, such as excessive use of or stress on a joint, have been identified as accelerating osteoarthritic changes, as in, for example, the knees of football players and the feet and ankles of ballet dancers. Other factors leading to the development of osteoarthritis include congenital structural defects (e.g., Legg-Calvé-Perthes disease

*Joanne White, R.N., M.S.N., assisted in the preparation of selected sections of this chapter.

This chapter was reviewed by Janice Smith Pigg, R.N., B.S.N., Nurse Consultant Rheumatology, Rheumatic Disease Program, Columbia Hospital, Milwaukee, Wisconsin.

and genu varum), metabolic disturbances (e.g., alkaptonuria and acromegaly), repeated intraarticular hemorrhage (e.g., hemophilia), neuropathic arthropathies, and inflammatory and septic arthritis.

Clinical Manifestations

Systemic

Constitutional symptoms such as fatigue or fever are not present in osteoarthritis. There is an absence of other organ involvement as well.

Joints

Articular manifestations are related to the particular joint involved. The client complains of pain on motion and weight bearing, generally relieved by rest. The pain is caused by irritation and pressure on nerve endings, muscle tension, and muscle fatigue. The joint may ache before inclement weather and feel stiff after immobility. Rising humidity with falling barometric pressure seems to aggravate arthritic symptoms. Loss of mobility is another common manifestation. Overall body coordination and posture may be affected as a result of the pain and loss of mobility. Crepitation on joint motion and malalignment of the extremity may be noted on physical examination.

The joints most frequently involved are the distal interphalangeal (DIP) joints of the fingers, first carpometacarpal (CMC) joint, hips, knees, first metatarsophalangeal (MTP) joint, and lower lumbar and cervical vertebrae (Fig. 57-1). Degenerative changes are rarely seen in metacarpophalangeal (MCP) joints, wrists, elbows, or shoulders.

Nodules

Heberden's nodes are another common manifestation of osteoarthritis, particularly common in women with primary osteoarthritis. These nodes are reactive bony overgrowths located at the distal interphalangeal joints (Fig. 57-2). Heberden's nodes are palpable protruberances which are often associated with flexion and lateral deviation of the distal phalanx, occur more frequently in women, and tend to appear in families. Bouchard's nodes, seen less commonly in osteoarthritis, involve the proximal interphalangeal joints.

Heberden's nodes may present with redness, swelling, tenderness, and aching. They often begin in one finger and spread to others. Although there is usually no significant loss of function secondary to the bony enlargements, clients are often distressed by the resulting disfigurement of their hands. Little can be done to prevent the occurrence of these nodes.

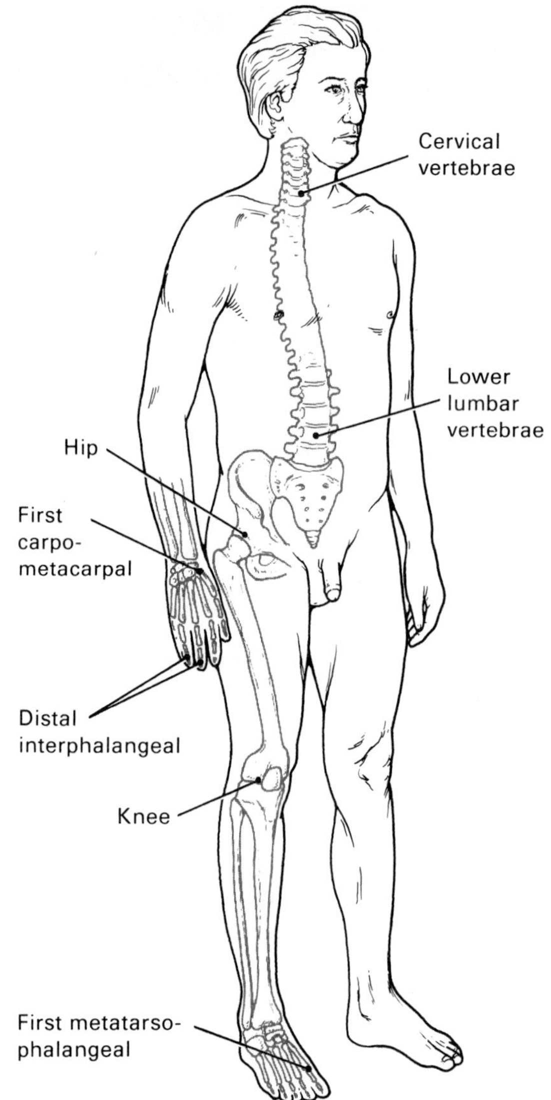

Figure 57-1 Joints most frequently involved in degenerative joint disease.

Complications

Advanced disease is complicated by gross deformity and subluxation due to deterioration of cartilage, collapse of subchondral bone, and extensive bony overgrowth.

Hips

Degenerative joint disease of the hips (Malum coxae senilis) may be extremely disabling. Congenital or structural abnormalities are frequent antecedent causes. This problem occurs more frequently in men

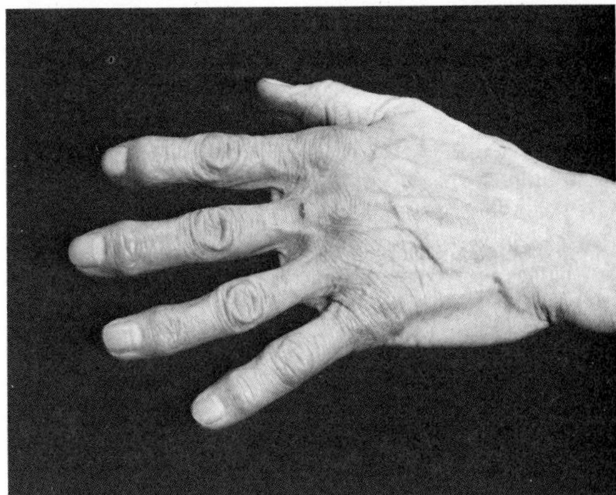

Figure 57-2 Left hand of a 71-year-old woman with osteoarthritis and Heberden's nodes. [*From G. P. Rodnan (ed.), Primer on the Rheumatic Diseases, Arthritis Foundation, Atlanta. Reprinted by permission of the Arthritis Foundation.*]

than in women and may be unilateral or bilateral. Hip pain may be perceived as pain in the groin, buttock, or medial side of the thigh or knee, so that the client may find it difficult to correctly localize the problem. Pain on motion or on weight bearing may become progressively severe, and pain on rest may ensue. Sitting down is difficult, as is rising from a chair. The client learns to sit in a high seat with firm support and arm rests. Eventually there is significant loss of range of motion (ROM) with marked limitation of extension and internal rotation.

Knees

Softening of the posterior surface of the patella (chondromalacia patellae) is seen most commonly in young people. Degeneration of the weight-bearing surfaces of the femoral and tibial condyles is usually seen in older women and is associated with limitation of motion, crepitus, and flexion deformity.

Vertebral column

Osteoarthritis in the spine may produce localized symptoms of stiffness and pain. Degenerative disease of the intervertebral disks results as the nucleus pulposus deteriorates, becoming brittle and inelastic. Herniation of the degenerating nucleus most often occurs posteriorly or laterally, compressing a nerve root and causing muscle spasm or radicular pain. In contrast, the client may develop degenerative disease of the intervertebral (apophyseal) joints, which generally follows disk disease by a number of years. Marginal osteophytes also appear at vertebral attachments of the anulus, periosteum, and longitudinal ligaments. Spurs may fuse and limit range of motion, or they may press against intervertebral foramina, producing symptoms of nerve root compression. Osteophyte formation in the posterior aspect of the cervical spine may rarely produce vascular compression and insufficiency, resulting in intermittent dizziness, visual disturbances, headaches, and ataxia.

Diagnostic Study Abnormalities

No specific laboratory abnormalities are useful in the diagnosis of osteoarthritis. In late disease, x-ray examination shows joint space narrowing, bony sclerosis, spur formation, and, in some cases, subluxation. It is important to note that x-ray changes do not always indicate the degree of pain the client experiences. Often degenerative disease is present and the client is completely asymptomatic. Conversely, some clients complain of severe pain with only moderate x-ray changes. The sedimentation rate is normal except in instances of erosive osteoarthritis, in which moderate elevation may be noted. Synovial fluid aspirated from an involved joint may be increased in volume but is clear yellow and viscous. Analysis of the fluid reveals little or no sign of inflammation.

Medical Management

There are no specific therapies for the management of osteoarthritis. Therapy is aimed at pain control, prevention of progression and disability, and restoration of joint function (Table 57-1). Once the

Table 57-1
Medical Management: Degenerative Joint Disease

Diagnostic
1. Complete history and physical examination
2. X-ray examination of involved joints
3. Sedimentation rate
4. Synovial fluid analysis

Therapeutic
1. Rest and joint protection
2. Heat and exercise
3. Mild analgesia
4. Assistive devices
5. Orthopedic surgery
   a. Debridement
   b. Arthrodesis (joint fusion)
   c. Arthroplasty
   d. Osteotomy
   e. Total joint replacement

diagnosis is confirmed, the client should be assured that osteoarthritis is likely to remain confined to a few joints and does not cause extensive crippling. Specific orthopedic surgical modes of treatment are discussed later in this chapter.

Pharmacological Intervention

Aspirin remains the most commonly used drug for the treatment of osteoarthritis. It is generally prescribed in larger than usual doses and is given on a regular basis. In addition to relieving pain, aspirin reduces inflammation and consequently reduces swelling, stiffness, and joint damage. An overdose of aspirin may cause ringing in the ears and slight deafness. These symptoms disappear if the dosage is reduced. Gastrointestinal problems related to aspirin can be alleviated by giving the drug with meals and by the use of antacids.

Phenylbutazone (Butazolidin) and indomethacin (Indocin) are useful drugs but have more serious side effects. Intraarticular injections of corticosteroids are useful in treating a severely inflamed joint. Systemic use of corticosteroids should be avoided, as it may actually accelerate the disease process.

Dietary Intervention

There is no specific diet for osteoarthritis except that which maintains optimal health. However, if the client is obese, a weight-reduction program becomes an important part of the total treatment plan. Body weight is magnified 5 times through the hips and 3 times through the knees. The additional strain of extra pounds can greatly increase pain and loss of function in osteoarthritis. (See Chaps. 33 and 60 on ways to assist the client in obtaining and maintaining ideal body weight.)

Nursing Management

Health promotion and maintenance

Prevention of primary osteoarthritis is not possible. However, preventive education may include elimination of excessive strain by reduction of occupational and recreational hazards and nutritional counseling for obesity. Congenital conditions such as Legg-Calvé-Perthes disease, known to predispose to development of osteoarthritis, should be treated promptly.

Acute intervention

The client is often hospitalized for treatment if persistent pain or a disabling deformity is present. The goals of therapy are to relieve pain, protect joints from further stress, and restore mechanical function and alignment. The nurse should assess the client's range of motion and degree of discomfort. Proper body alignment must be maintained. Traction should be properly applied, if necessary. Medications are administered for the relief of pain and, to the extent that inflammation is also present, for its control. The nurse should educate the client concerning the nature of the disease and usual modes of therapy. Diagnostic and surgical procedures should be thoroughly explained. The nurse should assist the client with activities of daily living and provide planned rest periods during the day. Nursing intervention includes teaching correct posture and body mechanics and observing the correct and safe use of assistive devices such as walkers and canes. The client should demonstrate his understanding of joint protection and energy-conservation techniques as well as a therapeutic exercise program. Nursing care should include emotional support for the client and family.

Chronic management

The health professional must work closely with the client to develop a home care program specific to individual needs. The nurse's explanation of degenerative joint disease will reassure the client that his disease is localized and that severe deforming arthritis is not the usual course. The client should be instructed to wear well-fitting supportive shoes. Safety measures at home are important, including removal of scatter rugs, provision of rails at stairs or bathtub, and use of night-lights. Assistive devices such as canes, walkers, elevated toilet seats, and grab bars may be helpful as well. The client should demonstrate the proper self-administration of analgesics and anti-inflammatory medications and recognize their side effects. The nurse can suggest alternative ways to minimize weight-bearing activities by reviewing joint protection and energy-conservation techniques (Table 57-2). Vocational rehabilitation may begin by altering work habits which may produce chronic strain on the joints (e.g., sitting on a stool instead of standing). Physical therapy is essential for promotion of muscle strength and maintenance of joint motion. Generally a daily program of moist heat to joints by hot bath and hot packs followed by active exercise relieves pain and stiffness and improves joint function. Rehabilitation by surgical intervention is discussed later in this chapter.

RHEUMATOID ARTHRITIS

Rheumatoid arthritis (RA) is a chronic, systemic disease characterized by recurrent inflammation of

Table 57-2
Principles of Joint Protection

Maintain good posture and proper body mechanics
Maintain normal weight
Use daily heat and exercise
Use assistive devices if indicated
Avoid positions of deviation and stress
Find less stressful ways to perform tasks
Avoid tasks that cause pain
Develop organizing and pacing techniques
Avoid forceful repetitive movements
Schedule frequent rest periods

the diarthrodial joints and related structures. It is frequently accompanied by a variety of extraarticular manifestations.[3] Rheumatoid arthritis is characterized by periods of remission and exacerbation of disease activity. The course of illness varies from person to person, ranging from episodes of illness separated by periods of remission to a more continuous, progressive disease.

Significance

Of the approximately 6 million Americans who have rheumatoid arthritis, 75 percent are women. There are no geographical or racial predispositions. Although rheumatoid arthritis can occur at any age, incidence increases with age, peaking between 35 and 45 years.[4]

In terms of its potential for chronic disability, rheumatoid arthritis is the most serious form of arthritis and is considered a significant national health problem. Arthritis is second only to heart disease as a major cause of chronic limitation, although death from it is rare.

Etiology and Pathogenesis

Etiology

The cause of rheumatoid arthritis remains unknown. In fact, it is unclear whether a single causative factor is responsible or multiple factors are involved. There are several etiologic possibilities:

Infection—Vigorous research continues to probe the possibility of specific infectious pathogens, particularly viruses, which may trigger the process.

Autoimmunity—Altered immune responses result in the formation of antigen-antibody complexes which activate complement components and attract polymorphonuclear leukocytes to the affected joints (see Chap. 10 for an explanation of complement activation.) These leukocytes are responsible for ingesting the immune complexes and releasing destructive enzymes, which then damage articular cartilage.

Genetic factors—Certain familial factors may influence the expression of the disease. One particular HLA type has been identified which correlates with the presence of RA.

Other factors—Metabolic and biochemical abnormalities, nutritional and environmental factors, and occupational and psychosocial influences may play a part in the cause and/or expression of the disease, but their contribution is entirely speculative at present.

Pathogenesis

The pathogenesis of RA is more clearly understood than its etiology. If unarrested, the disease progresses through four stages:

First stage—The unknown etiologic factor initiates joint inflammation, or *synovitis*, with swelling of the synovial lining membrane and production of excess synovial fluid.

Second stage—*Pannus* (granulation inflammatory tissue) is formed at the juncture of synovium and cartilage. This extends over the surface of the articular cartilage and eventually invades the joint capsule and subchondral bone.

Third stage—Tough fibrous connective tissue replaces pannus, occluding the joint space. *Fibrous ankylosis* results in decreased joint motion, malalignment, and deformity.

Fourth stage—As fibrous tissue calcifies, *bony ankylosis* may result in total joint immobilization.

Clinical Manifestations

Joints

Rheumatoid arthritis typically develops insidiously. Nonspecific manifestations such as fatigue, anorexia, weight loss, and generalized stiffness may precede the onset of arthritic complaints. The stiffness becomes more localized over a period of weeks to months. Some clients report a history of precipitating stressful events such as infection, overwork, childbirth, surgery, or emotional upset. However, there are no data correlating these events and the onset of rheumatoid arthritis.

Specific articular involvement is manifested clinically by pain, stiffness, limitation of motion, and signs of inflammation (heat, swelling, and tenderness). Joint symptoms are generally bilaterally symmetrical and frequently affect small joints of the hands—proximal

Table 57-3
Comparison of Rheumatoid Arthritis and Degenerative Joint Disease

	Rheumatoid Arthritis	Degenerative Joint Disease
Age	Young and middle-aged	Usually over age 40
Sex	Female more often than male	Female and male have same incidence
Weight	Weight loss common	Usually overweight
Illness	Systemic manifestations	Local joint manifestation
Joints affected	PIPs, MCPs, MTPs, wrists, knees, subtalar; symmetrical, many joints	DIPs, CMCs, thumbs, MTPs, knees, spine, hips; asymmetrical, one or more joints
Effusions	Common	Uncommon
Nodules	Present	Heberden's nodes
Synovial fluid	Inflammatory	Noninflammatory
X-rays	Osteoporosis, narrowing, erosions	Osteophytes, subchondral cysts, sclerosis
Anemia	Common	Uncommon
Rheumatoid factor	Positive	Negative
Sedimentation rate	Elevated	Normal

interphalangeal (PIP), metacarpophalangeal (MCP)—and feet—metatarsophalangeal (MTP)—as well as larger peripheral joints, including wrists, elbows, shoulders, knees, hips, ankles, and the jaw. Table 57-3 compares the manifestations of rheumatoid arthritis and osteoarthritis.

The client characteristically complains of stiffness upon arising in the morning and after periods of inactivity. This morning stiffness usually lasts for 30 minutes to several hours or more, depending upon disease activity. Proximal interphalangeal joints are typically swollen. The fingers may become spindle-shaped from synovial hypertrophy and thickening of the joint capsule (Fig. 57-3). Joints become tender, painful, and warm to the touch. The pain is more pronounced on motion, varies in intensity, and may not be proportional to the degree of inflammation. Tenosynovitis frequently affects the extensor and flexor tendons around the wrists and may produce symptoms of carpal tunnel syndrome (see Chap. 56).

As disease activity progresses, inflammation and fibrosis of the joint capsule and supporting structures may lead to deformity and disability. Atrophy of muscles and destruction of tendons around the joint cause one articular surface to slip past the other (subluxation). Typical deformities of the hand include "ulnar drift" and "swan-neck" and boutonniere deformities (Fig. 57-4). Metatarsal-head subluxation and hallux valgus (bunion) may cause pain and walking disability.

Extraarticular manifestations

Rheumatoid nodules are present in 25 percent of all clients with rheumatoid arthritis. Small-vessel vasculitis is considered to be the initiating event in the

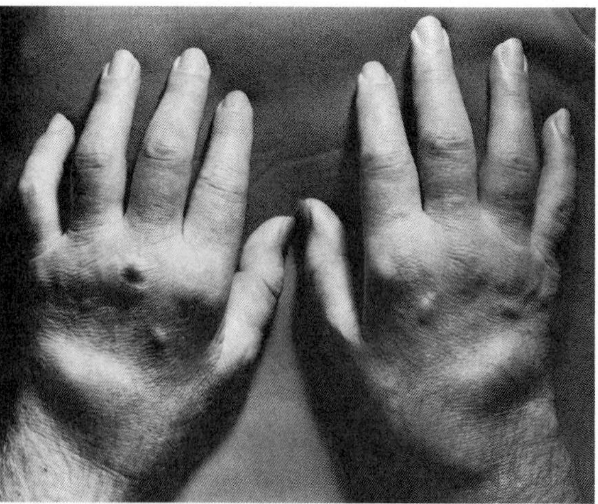

Figure 57-3 Rheumatoid arthritis of 2 years' duration. This 45-year-old man has MCP and PIP swelling, as well as tenosynovitis. [*From G. P. Rodnan (ed.), Primer on the Rheumatic Diseases, Arthritis Foundation, Atlanta. Reprinted by permission of the Arthritis Foundation.*]

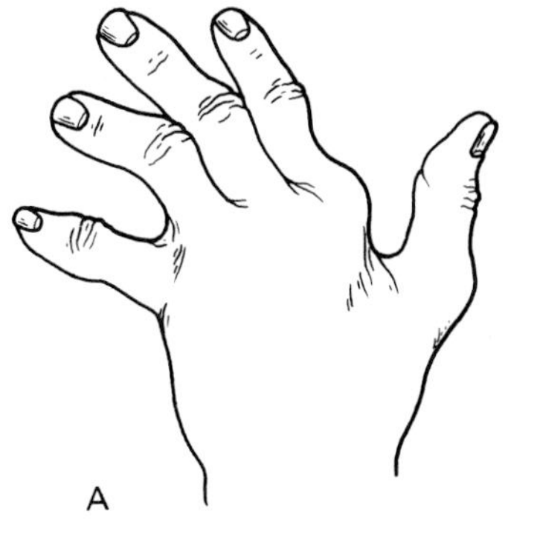

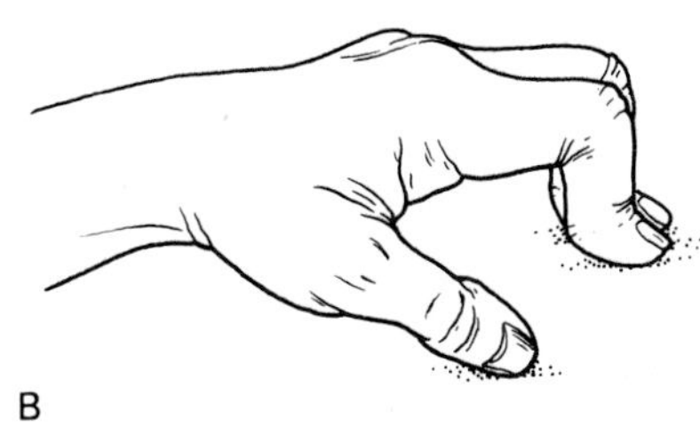

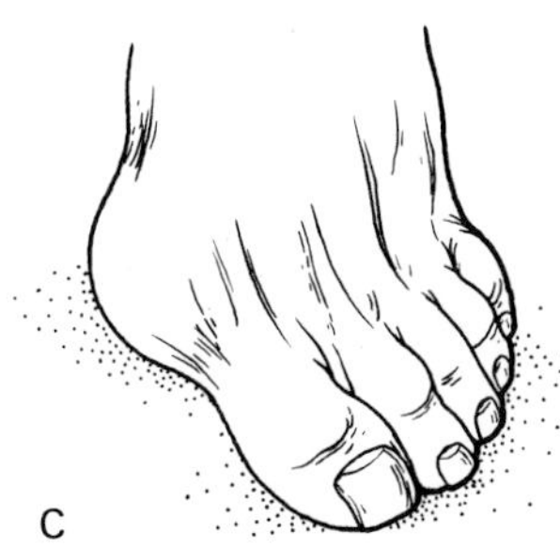

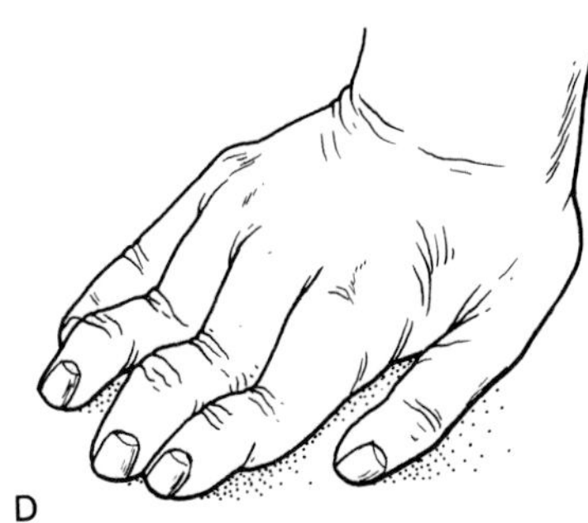

Figure 57-4 Typical deformities of rheumatoid arthritis. *(a)* Ulnar deviation. Chronic synovitis results in volar subluxation of MCPs, stretching extensor tendons which slide laterally toward the ulnar side of the joint. *(b)* Boutonniere deformity. Flexion contracture of PIP joints and rupture of the extensor digitorum tendon causing dorsal migration and hyperextenson of the DIP joints. *(c)* Hallux valgus. Characterized by prominent bunion and displacement away from other toes. Metatarsal arch collapses, causing weight bearing on MTP heads. Overlapping toes (hammertoes) are common. *(d)* Swan-neck deformity. Hyperextension of PIP joint with volar subluxation and flexion of DIP joint (opposite of boutonniere deformity).

formation of these nodules. They appear subcutaneously as firm, nontender masses usually found on olecranon bursae, or along the extensor surface of the forearm. These nodules are usually not removed unless they are creating a problem, because of the high probability of recurrence. Nodules may also appear on the eye or lungs; these indicate active disease and a poor prognosis.

Vasculitis (inflammation of blood vessels) may be responsible for a variety of systemic complications including peripheral neuropathy, myopathy, cardiopulmonary involvement, and ischemic ulcerations of the skin. Figure 57-5 shows the variety of extraarticular manifestations of rheumatoid arthritis.

Complications

Potential complications include infection, osteoporosis, amyloidosis, and Sjögren's syndrome. Spinal cord compression may occur from instability of articulations in the cervical spine.

Diagnostic Study Abnormalities

Although no single laboratory test is conclusive, several findings are helpful in diagnosing rheumatoid arthritis, in conjunction with the history and physical examination. Moderate anemia is common. The sedimentation rate (ESR) is elevated in 85 percent of clients and is useful in monitoring the response to therapy. Serum rheumatoid factor, a circulating antibody of the immunoglobulin-M class, is present in titers greater than 1:160 in nearly 80 percent of cases. ANA and LE cell tests may be positive in a smaller percentage of clients.

Synovial fluid analysis may show increased volume and turbidity but decreased viscosity. The WBC is elevated (often as high as 30,000 per microliter) and

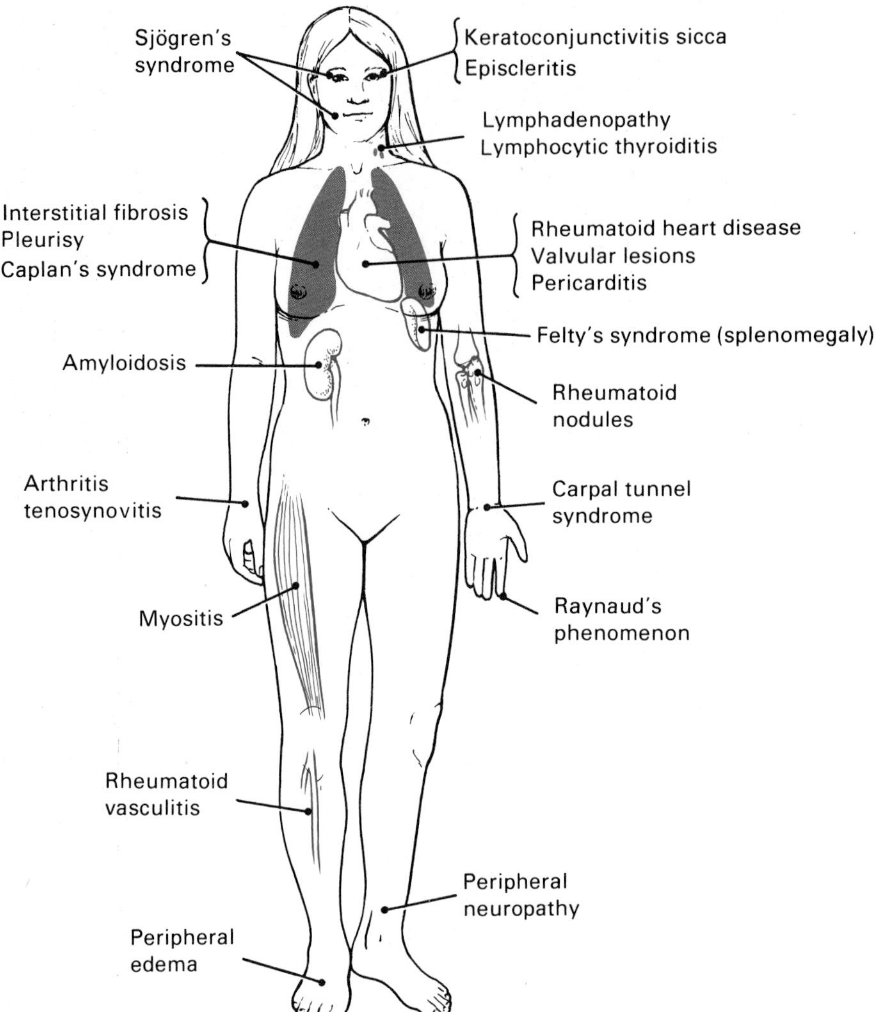

Figure 57-5 Common clinical features of rheumatoid arthritis.

consists predominantly of polymorphonuclear leukocytes. Inflammatory changes in the synovium can be confirmed by tissue biopsy.

X-ray findings (not specifically diagnostic) may reveal only bone demineralization and soft-tissue swelling during the first 6 months of the disease. Later, narrowing of the joint space, destruction of articular cartilage, erosion, subluxation, and deformity are present. Table 57-4 describes RA stages according to bony erosion and joint deformity.

Medical Management

It is important that the client understand the chronic nature of rheumatoid arthritis. Treatment is available to reduce joint inflammation and pain, maintain motion and strength, and prevent and correct deformities (Table 57-5). Personal attention and an individualized treatment program should help prevent the client from seeking relief through quack remedies.

In planning a treatment program, several factors need to be considered: (1) status of joint function; (2) degree of disease activity; (3) age, sex, occupation, and family responsibilities of the client and individual response to treatment; and (4) results of previous treatment.[5]

Pharmacological Intervention

The foundation for the pharmacological treatment of rheumatoid arthritis is aspirin at dosages adequate to maintain an anti-inflammatory effect (Table 57-6).

Table 57-4

Stages of Rheumatoid Arthritis

Stage 1
No destructive changes on x-ray
May have evidence of osteoporosis

Stage 2
X-ray evidence of osteoporosis, may have slight subchondral bone and/or cartilage destruction
May have limitation of motion but no joint deformity

Stage 3
X-ray evidence of cartilage and bone destruction
Joint deformity without ankylosis

Stage 4
X-ray evidence of fibrous or bony ankylosis
Extensive muscle atrophy and soft-tissue lesions such as nodules may be present

Modified from O. Steinbrocker, C. H. Traeger, and R. C. Batterman, "Therapeutic Criteria in Rheumatoid Arthritis," *JAMA,* **140:** 659-662 (1949).

Table 57-5

Medical Management: Rheumatoid Arthritis

Diagnostic

1. Complete history and physical examination
2. Laboratory studies
   a. CBC
   b. ESR
   c. Protein electrophoresis
   d. Latex agglutination test for rheumatoid factor
   e. Antinuclear antibodies
3. Joint x-ray examination

Therapeutic

1. Rest and joint protection
2. Drug therapy
   a. Anti-inflammatory medication
   b. Chloroquine, gold salts, penicillamine
   c. Intraarticular and systemic steroids
3. Well-balanced diet
4. Splints
5. Physical therapy
6. Orthopedic surgery

Table 57-6

Pharmacological Management of Rheumatoid Arthritis

Drug	Mechanism of Action	Common Side Effects	Nursing Considerations
		Salicylates	
Aspirin	Anti-inflammatory, analgesic, antipyretic	GI irritation (ulcer and hemorrhage) Hypersensitivity Salicylism (nausea, tinnitus, dizziness, hyperpnea) Prolonged bleeding time	When drug is taken for anti-inflammatory effect, should not be discontinued if pain decreases Take drug with food, milk, antacids as prescribed, or full glass of water Report signs of bleeding (tarry stool, bruising, petechiae, melena)
		Nonsteroidal Anti-Inflammatory Drugs (NSAID)	
Fenoprofen calcium (Nalfon)	Anti-inflammatory analgesic	Headache Nervousness GI irritation	General considerations for NSAID: Take drug with food, milk, or antacids as prescribed
Ibuprofen (Motrin)	Anti-inflammatory analgesic	GI irritation Dizziness Rash	Report signs of bleeding, edema, skin rashes, persistent headaches, or visual disturbances
Indomethacin (Indocin)	Anti-inflammatory analgesic	GI irritation Headache Visual disturbances	Use cautiously in clients with GI, renal, or cardiac disease and those with bleeding disorders
Naproxen (Naprosyn)	Anti-inflammatory-analgesic	GI irritation Headache Tinnitus Pruritus	Check renal and hepatic function periodically in long-term therapy
Oxyphenbutazone (Tandearil)	Anti-inflammatory analgesic	Gi irritation Blood dyscrasia Fluid retention	
Phenylbutazone (Butazolidin)	Anti-inflammatory-analgesic	GI irritation Blood dyscrasia Fluid retention	

Table 57-6 (Continued)

Drug	Mechanism of Action	Common Side Effects	Nursing Considerations
Sulindac (Clinoril)	Anti-inflammatory analgesic	GI irritation Rash Dizziness Headache	
Tolmetin sodium (Tolectin)	Anti-inflammatory analgesic	GI irritation Dizziness Rash Tinnitus	
		Remission-Producing Agents	
Chrysotherapy:			
Gold sodium thiomalate (Myochrysine) **Aurothioglucose (Solganal)**	Unknown; Inflammatory-suppressive effect	Dermatitis Pruritus Stomatitis Blood dyscrasia Nephrotoxicity	Regular blood and urine testing essential for long-term therapy Check urine for blood and protein before each dose and delay injection until negative Mix drug well and give deep IM injection in buttocks Symptomatic improvement not expected for 3–6 months; therapy may be continued indefinitely
Antimalarials:			
Chloroquine phosphate (Aralen)	Anti-inflammatory	Asymptomatic retinopathy Corneal opacity Headache	Ophthalmologic examination including slit lamp studies required every 3–6 months
Hydroxychloroquine sulfate (Plaquenil Sulfate)	Anti-inflammatory	Dizziness GI irritation Blood dyscrasia Pruritus	Take drug with meals, milk or antacid as prescribed Report all skin eruptions and visual disturbances Avoid excessive sun exposure Contraindicated for clients with psoriasis Monitor CBC and liver function studies periodically
Penicillamine (Cuprimine)	Unknown	Blood dyscrasia Glomerulonephropathy	Give drug on empty stomach before meals (not with) Monitor CBC, urinalysis, and liver function studies Report fever, sore throat, chills, bruising, or bleeding. Contraindicated with gold therapy
		Corticosteroids	
Intraarticular injections:			
Methyl-prednisolone acetate (Depo-Medrol)	Anti-inflammatory, analgesic	Suppression of local infection Local osteoporosis or neuropathic arthropathy from repeated injection	Use strict aseptic technique as joint fluid is removed and steroids are injected Joint may feel worse immediately following injection
Triamcinolone hexacetonide (Aristospan)	Anti-inflammatory, analgesic		Improvement lasts weeks to months after injection Weight bearing should be minimized for 2–6 weeks after injection

Table 57-6 (Continued)

Drug	Mechanism of Action	Common Side Effects	Nursing Considerations
Systemic:			
Hydrocortisone sodium succinate (Solu-Cortef)	Anti-inflammatory	Cushing's syndrome: fluid retention, GI irritation, osteoporosis, hypertension, diabetes, acne, menstrual irregularities, hirsutism, risk of infection, bruising, iridocyclitis in children	Use only when symptoms persist with less potent anti-inflammatory drugs or in life-threatening situations Administer for limited time only, tapering dose slowly Exacerbation of symptoms with abrupt withdrawal Monitor blood pressure, weight, and CBC and potassium Limit salt intake Report signs of infection Report corticosteroid use to surgeon or dentist, as booster dose may be required to avoid postoperative adrenal insufficiency
Methyl prednisolone succinate sodium (Solu-Medrol)	Anti-inflammatory		
Dexamethasone (Decadron)	Anti-inflammatory		
Prednisone (Deltasone)	Anti-inflammatory		
Triamcinolone (Aristocort)	Anti-inflammatory		
		Immunosuppressive	
Azathioprine (Imuran)	Unknown; suppresses autoimmune mechanism	GI irritation and ulceration Alopecia Oral lesions Dermatitis Blood dyscrasia Bone marrow depression	Informed consent required Limited to those clients not responsive to conventional therapy Teratogenic potential cautions against use for children or adults of childbearing age Monitor CBC and urinalysis
		Cytotoxic Therapy	
Cyclophosphamide (Cytoxan)	Unknown; suppresses autoimminue mechanism	GI irritation and ulceration Alopecia Oral lesions Dermatitis Blood dyscrasia Bone marrow depression	Informed consent required Monitor CBC and urinalysis Teratogenic potential cautions against use for children or adults of childbearing age

Other recently available nonsteroidal anti-inflammatory agents may also be used successfully but usually have more serious side effects. Remission-producing agents include antimalarials, penicillamine, and chrysotherapy. Antimalarials may be prescribed for those clients with persistent arthritis but take 4 to 6 weeks for effects to become evident. The possibility of rare irreversible retinal degeneration due to deposition of these drugs in the pigment layer of the retina requires ophthalmologic examination at 4- to 6-month intervals. Intramuscular gold (chrysotherapy) may be recommended for those clients whose disease activity continues despite more conservative therapy. This drug should be considered only when the client is willing to commit himself to a lengthy treatment regimen, including frequent laboratory evaluations. The exact mechanism for the effectiveness of gold and penicillamine in the treatment of rheumatoid arthritis is not known.

Corticosteroids may be required for suppression of severe disease activity or extraarticular manifestations. Since serious side effects are generally dose-related, steroids must be given in low maintenance doses with consideration of the need for long-term therapy. Like gold, penicillamine may induce remission of symptoms, requires several months to take effect, and needs careful laboratory monitoring.

Diet

There is no special diet for rheumatoid arthritis. Balanced nutrition is important. Clients are vulnerable to fad claims for improvement through health foods and vitamins. A sensible weight-loss program should be undertaken by the obese client to relieve stress on affected joints.

Limited salt intake may help minimize weight gain if the client is taking corticosteroids. Steroids also increase the appetite and may result in a higher caloric intake. Clients should be aware of this and should monitor their caloric intake. Excessive weight gain may result as a side effect of steroids despite attempts to control caloric intake.

Nursing Management

Health promotion and maintenance

Prevention of rheumatoid arthritis is not possible at this time. However, community education programs should include information concerning the symptoms of rheumatoid arthritis to promote early diagnosis and treatment. Many fine publications for laymen are available through the Arthritis Foundation, 3400 Peachtree Road, N.E., Atlanta, GA 30326.

The nurse should be a strong advocate of a thorough workup when rheumatoid arthritis is suspected. Once the diagnosis is confirmed, the nurse should support the client in following the individualized treatment program. Quackery and fads should be exposed whenever possible by the nursing community.

Acute intervention

The primary objectives in the management of rheumatoid arthritis are reduction of inflammation and pain, preservation of joint function, and prevention or correction of joint deformity. These may be approached by a comprehensive program of daily anti-inflammatory medication, rest and joint protection, therapeutic heat and exercise, and thorough patient and family education (Table 57-7; Fig. 57-6). The nurse is an integral member of the health team, working closely with the physician, physical and occupational therapists, and social worker to restore function and to help the client make lifestyle adjustments to chronic illness.[6]

The newly diagnosed client may be hospitalized for control of acute inflammation, evaluation of systemic involvement, and comprehensive education by the health team. Hospitalization may also be necessary for those with extraarticular complications or advanced disease requiring reconstructive surgery for disabling deformities (nursing care discussed later).

Nursing intervention begins with a careful assessment of joint pain, swelling, and range of motion. The physical assessment should include presence of extraarticular manifestations such as nodules, vasculitic ulceration, or symptoms of Sjögren's syndrome (discussed later). Psychosocial problems such as poor family understanding and cooperation, financial and vocational limitations, emotional distress, and environmental restrictions (e.g., cannot turn doorknob) should be identified. Following the identification of problems, a carefully planned educational program should be initiated.

Morning care and procedures should be planned around the client's morning stiffness and may need to be delayed. Standing in a warm shower, sitting in a tub with warm towels around the shoulders, or simply soaking the hands in a basin of warm water may help to relieve joint stiffness and allow the client to comfortably perform the activities of daily living. Careful skin care should be offered, particularly if the client is confined to bed.

Lightweight splints are sometimes used to rest an inflamed joint and prevent deformity from muscle spasms and contractures. These splints should be removed, skin care given, range-of-motion exercises performed, and splints reapplied as prescribed. Occupational therapy may help to identify self-help devices which can assist in the activities of daily living.[7]

As the nurse administers each medication, the client should be informed of its name, dose, proper administration, action, side effects, and any laboratory studies required for purposes of monitoring. Often there is poor understanding of the value of aspirin as an important anti-inflammatory drug. The client should understand that aspirin is given for its anti-inflammatory property. Regular administration provides a therapeutic blood salicylate level which can be measured and adjusted.

The professional nurse acts as liaison among the client, family, and other members of the health team, coordinating services and evaluating the client's understanding of the total home management program. (See Table 57-7 for the nursing care plan for rheumatoid arthritis, also points for education included in chronic care section.)

Rehabilitative management

Rest Regularly scheduled rest periods alternated throughout the day help to relieve fatigue and pain and minimize excessive weight bearing. The amount of rest necessary will vary according to the severity of the disease and each client's limitations. Total bed rest is rarely necessary and should be avoided to prevent stiffness and immobility. A client with mild disease usually requires daytime rest in addition to 8 to 10 hours of sleep at night. The nurse should help the client identify ways to modify daily activities, since overexertion can lead to fatigue and a flare-up in

Table 57-7

Nursing Care Plan for the Client with Rheumatoid Arthritis

Client Problem	Expected Outcome	Nursing Intervention
		Acute Management
Inflammation	Decreased pain, swelling, and erythema of joints	Provide decreased activity, increased rest, and supportive resting splints for affected joints. Administer anti-inflammatory medications as ordered (e.g., aspirin, indomethacin). Maintain aseptic technique while assisting with joint aspiration procedures. Monitor ESR for response to therapy.
Limitation of motion	Increased ROM and function. Decreased stiffness	Apply moist heat, e.g., paraffin bath, hot packs, warm shower. Encourage ROM exercises when pain and swelling have subsided. Schedule morning care and procedures later in the day after A.M. stiffness subsides. Assist with daily hygienic care. Teach client to use assistive devices to promote independence.
Fatigue	Increased stamina and decreased fatigue	Plan rest periods throughout the day. Avoid multiple procedures in one day. Monitor BP, heart rate, respirations, and RBC and WBC.
Low-grade fever	Normal body temperature	Monitor temperature q 4 h and assess fever pattern. Encourage fluid intake (2–3 L/day). Monitor blood studies, e.g., WBC.
Weight loss	Stable weight and good appetite	Weigh daily and accurately measure intake and output. Provide clean, cheerful environment for eating. Assist client with tray while food is still hot. Provide nutritious diet.
Anxiety about illness	Decreased anxiety related to diagnosis	Introduce client to staff and hospital environment. Listen to client's fears and assess knowledge of the disease. Plan and initiate program of education based on client readiness. Include client's family in discussion of nature and treatment of RA. Explain importance of laboratory tests and procedures. Evaluate client's understanding through verbalization and demonstration.
		Long-Term Management
Inflammation	Decreased joint pain, swelling, and erythema	Teach self-administration of anti-inflammatory medications as prescribed. Teach client about home care, including names, action, side effects, dose, and administration of prescribed drugs; resting joint until symptoms have subsided; daily rest periods and protective techniques which limit stress to joints; and avoiding undue physical and emotional stress.
Exacerbation of active disease	No guilt related to exacerbations, early recognition of exacerbation	Make clear that despite adherence to home management program, unpredicted exacerbations of disease activity are part of nature of RA. Teach client to recognize and identify signs of exacerbation: increased A.M. stiffness, increased pain and fatigue, signs of inflammation.
Increasing limitation of motion	Improved joint function and muscle strength	Teach use of moist heat prior to ROM exercises. Instruct on ROM exercises and joint protection techniques.
Deformity	Minimal deformity; proper posture and body alignment	Instruct client on correct application of resting splints, selection of properly fitting footwear, maintenance of proper posture and body alignment, and selection and use of assistive devices. Assist client to develop less stressful ways to do tasks.
Depression	Accept body changes and maintain interest in life	Allow client to ventilate feelings about disease. Offer psychological support to client and family. Assist client to recognize need for regular medical management and resist false advertising and forms of quackery.
Lifestyle change	Successful adjustment of client and family to disease	Discuss possible adjustments related to occupation, home, recreation, and sex with client and family. Refer client to appropriate community resources for additional support.
Long-term management and drug therapy	Knowledge of disease process and management	Instruct client on chronic nature of RA. Teach importance of continued medical and laboratory follow-up. Stress that medications must be taken regularly as ordered, and review side effects related to long-term drug therapy.

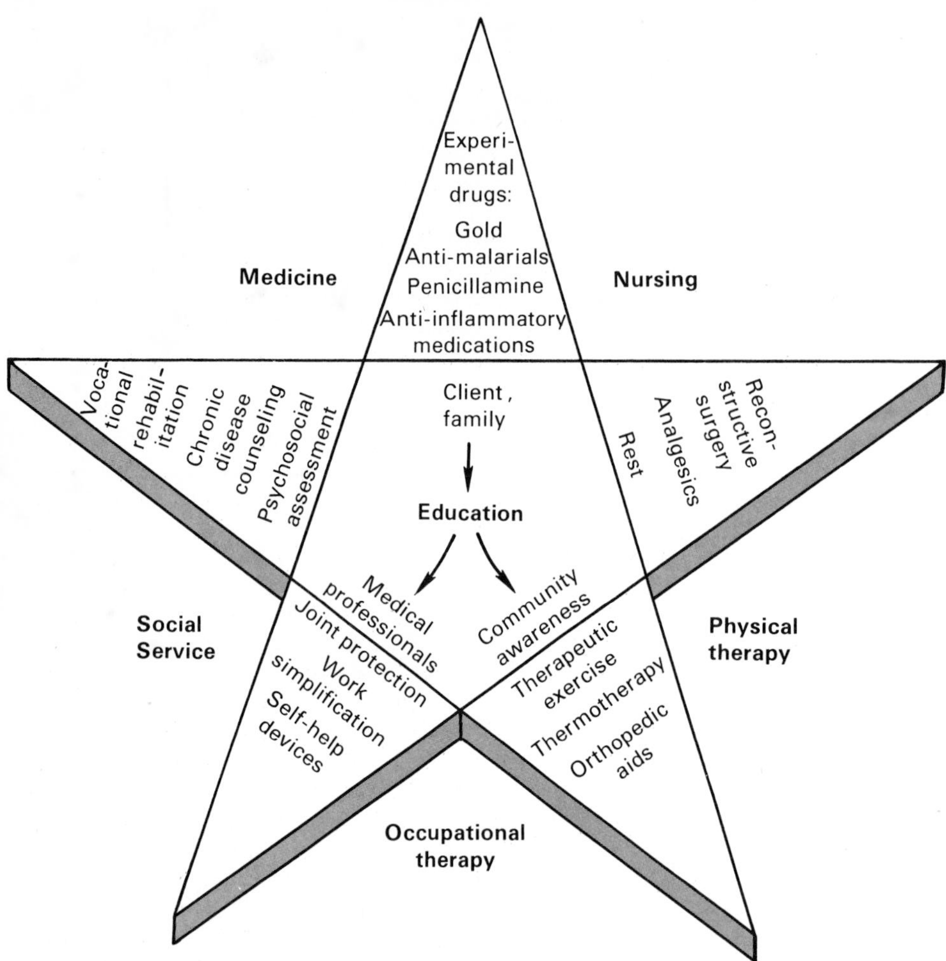

Figure 57-6 Team approach to the management of rheumatoid arthritis. The level closest to the core indicates the most basic treatment. Each level builds on therapy.

disease activity. Clients should rest *before* becoming exhausted. The nurse should assist the client in pacing and setting priorities on activities on the basis of realistic goals.

Good body alignment while resting is important. A firm mattress or bedboard should be used. Positions of extension should be encouraged and positions of flexion avoided. Lying prone for a half hour twice daily is recommended. Pillows should never be placed under the knees. A small, flat pillow may be used under the head. Splints and casts may be helpful in maintaining proper alignment, especially when joint inflammation is present.

Joint Protection Protecting joints from stress is as important as taking medications regularly. Nursing intervention includes helping the client identify ways to modify tasks. Each client needs to learn less stressful ways to accomplish the activities of daily living. The emphasis is on changing the way the task is done and work-simplification techniques.

Energy conservation requires careful planning. Work should be done in short periods with scheduled rest breaks to avoid fatigue. Chores should be spread through the week rather than concentrated (e.g., do not do all the cleaning on the weekend). Activities should be organized to avoid running up and down stairs. Carts should be used to carry things. Materials used often should be stored in a convenient, easy-to-reach area. Time-saving devices should be employed, if possible (e.g., electric can opener). Chores should be delegated to other family members, and sitting instead of standing for long periods should be encouraged.

The nurse should instruct the arthritic client in activities which will protect the small joints from stress. Observing the client perform activities both in the hospital and in the home situation will identify activities which need to be revised. Activities which are joint-saving should be reinforced. Table 57-8 lists sample activities which protect small joints.

Client independence may be reinforced by using assistive devices which help simplify tasks: built-up utensils, buttonhooks, modified drawer handles, lightweight plastic dishes, and raised toilet seats are examples. Wearing clothing with buttons or a zipper down the front instead of the back makes dressing easier. The nurse can refer the client to the Arthritis Foundation self-help book.

Daily Heat and Exercise Heat and cold therapy help to relieve stiffness, pain, and muscle spasm. Application of ice may be beneficial in an acute episode, while moist heat appears to offer better relief of chronic stiffness. Superficial heat sources such as heating pads, moist hot packs, paraffin baths, whirlpool baths and warm baths or showers relieve stiffness prior to therapeutic exercises; the modality should be selected according to disease severity, ease of application, and cost. The nurse should alert the client to the possibility of a burn, especially if a heat-producing liniment is used with another external heat device.

Table 57-8

Activities To Protect Small Joints

1. Avoid positions of deformity:
   a. Press water from a sponge instead of wringing
   b. Do not use pillows under the knees
2. Use strongest joint available for any task:
   a. When rising from chair, push with palms rather than fingers
   b. Carry laundry basket in both arms rather than with fingers
3. Distribute weight over many joints instead of stressing a few:
   a. Slide objects instead of lifting them
   b. Hold packages close to body for support
4. Change positions frequently:
   a. Don't hold book or grip steering wheel for long periods without resting
   b. Avoid grasping pencil or cutting vegetables with knife for extended periods
5. Avoid repetitious movements:
   a. Do not knit for long periods of time
   b. Rest between rooms when vacuuming
6. Modify chores to avoid stress on joints:
   a. Avoid heavy tasks
   b. Sit on stool instead of standing

Individualized exercise is an integral part of the treatment plan and must be carefully balanced. Inadequate joint movement can result in progressive joint immobility and muscle weakness; too much exercise can result in increased pain, inflammation, and joint destruction.

Gentle range-of-motion exercises are usually done daily (Table 57-9) to keep the joints functional. *The nurse needs to emphasize that usual daily activities do not provide adequate exercise to maintain joint motion.* Careful adherence to the prescribed exercise program should be a prime goal of the teaching program. The client should have the opportunity to practice the exercises with supervision.

If the client is experiencing an acute inflammatory episode, the joints are at risk for damage from overaggressive exercise. One or two repetitions of range-of-motion exercises are sufficient until the acute episode subsides.

Psychological Support Self-management and adherence to an individualized home program are contingent upon a thorough understanding of rheumatoid arthritis, the nature and course of the disease, and the objectives of treatment. In addition, the client's perception of the disease and value system must be considered. The client should be able to recognize false advertising and quackery despite claims of cure and relief of chronic pain, as well as obtain medical information from health professionals, the media, and community agencies.

A treatment program tailored to individual problems and lifestyle increases adherence. The nurse can help the client recognize common fears and concerns faced by all clients living with a chronic illness. Evaluation of the family support system is important. The client is constantly threatened by problems of limited function and fatigue, loss of self-esteem, and fear of disability and deformity. Alterations in sexuality should be discussed. Financial planning may be necessary. Community resources such as the Visiting Nurse Association, homemaker services, and vocational rehabilitation may be considered. Self-help groups are beneficial for some clients.

JUVENILE RHEUMATOID ARTHRITIS

Juvenile rheumatoid arthritis (JRA), the major rheumatic disease of youth since rheumatic fever has been controlled, is defined as rheumatoid arthritis beginning before age 16 and may be classified on the basis of the type of onset: systemic, pauciarticular, and polyarticular.[8] The last form most closely resem-

Table 57-9

Home Program for the Arthritis Client: Exercise Regimen

Hip and trunk extension exercises

1. Lie on stomach; squeeze buttocks together.
2. Lie on stomach; lift one leg at a time, keeping knee straight.
3. Lie on stomach; with arms straight at your sides, arch your back, lifting head, shoulders, and both legs at the same time; keep knees straight.

Trunk flexion exercises

1. Lie on back with knees straight; lift head and reach arms towards knees; hold to the count of 5.
2. Same as above but do 20 times.
3. Lie on back with knees straight; come to a sitting position, reaching to the right. Repeat, reaching to the left.
4. Lie on back with knees bent, feet flat; come to a sitting position, reaching to the right. Repeat, reaching to the left.
5. Lie on back with knees bent; with arms folded across chest, come to a sitting position, reaching to the right. Repeat, reaching to the left.

Hip abduction exercises

1. Lie on back with knees straight and feet pointing together; spread legs apart, keeping feet pointing toward each other.
2. Lie on left side and bend left knee up toward chest; keep right leg straight and in line with your body. Lift right leg up toward the ceiling. After doing this 10 times, turn to right side and repeat with left leg.
3. Same as exercise 1, but place elastic strap above both knees.
4. Same as exercise 1, but keep both legs straight and place elastic strap above both knees.
5. Same as exercise 1, but place elastic strap around both ankles.

Knee extension exercises

1. Lie on back; tighten quadriceps muscles 20 times. (Straighten knees as much as possible.)
2. Lie on back; first tighten quadriceps muscles, then lift leg into air, keeping knee straight. Alternate legs.
3. Same as exercise 2, except do in a sitting position, with legs straight.
4. Do this exercise with weights as directed by the physical therapist.

Dorsiflexion and eversion of feet

Sitting with feet on floor or on a stool, keep heels on floor and lift forefoot up and then turn forefoot out to the side. Keep knees from moving. All motion should be at the ankles.

Shoulder and elbow exercises

1. With elastic strap looped *above* both elbows, lift one arm up as you push opposite arm down. Try to keep elbows straight.
2. With elastic strap looped *above* both elbows, lift both arms up in front of you and spread them apart. Try to keep elbows straight.
3. With elastic strap looped *below* both elbows, bend one elbow as you straighten the opposite elbow.

Breathing

Lie on back; hold broomstick with palms of hands facing the ceiling. Lift broomstick overhead, keeping elbows straight. Breathe in deeply as arms go up; force air out as arms go down.

Shoulder external rotation exercises

1. Sit; hold on to broomstick with right hand on one end. Bend right elbow and try to push right hand in back of head, pushing with the left hand. Do same with left hand.
2. Sit; hold on to broomstick with both hands; lift broomstick in back of head.
3. Stand in a corner with hands clasped behind head and elbows out to the sides. Place one elbow on each wall of the corner. Don't allow elbows to move. Lean the body into the corner.

Finger exercises

1. Sit; place hand on flat surface, palm down. Lift each finger, one at a time.
2. Using a can of sand, bury five marbles. Then dig up five marbles.

Physical Therapy Department, University of New Mexico/Bernalillo County Medical Center, Albuquerque, New Mexico.

bles adult RA, while the others may represent other types of arthritis with onset during childhood. Children as young as 6 months of age may be affected, with the peak ages of onset between 1 and 5 years and again between 9 and 12 years. Prognosis is generally favorable, with nearly 70 percent of the children having few or no inflammatory symptoms by adulthood.[9] Residual deformity, however, may be a severe problem for some.

JRA may occur with arthritis confined to one joint (*pauciarticular*) or in several (*polyarticular*). Children most often do not complain of joint pain but may assume a position of flexion to minimize pain, carefully limit movement, or refuse to walk at all. A more constitutional variant, known as *Still's disease* (systemic onset) occurs with high spiking fever, vague arthralgias, generalized rash, hepatosplenomegaly, lymphadenopathy, and pleuritis or pericarditis. Complications of JRS include retarded growth and development and chronic, asymptomatic (and at times vision-threatening) eye inflammation.

The diagnostic measures are similar to those for rheumatoid arthritis. Leukocytosis is common, while rheumatoid factor is present in only 15 percent of those afflicted. Long-range management includes client and parent education and psychosocial assessment. Aspirin suppresses inflammation in the majority of cases, saving chrysotherapy for more unresponsive arthritis.

Nursing intervention requires an individualized, written home program with emphasis on compliance. Growth and development should be documented. Slit-lamp ophthalmologic examinations must be done routinely for those clients at highest risk to develop ocular complications (pauciarticular group). The school nurse should be involved in the child's care. Parents are encouraged to treat the child as normally as possible, avoiding infantilizing or overprotection. (For more specific information on juvenile rheumatoid arthritis, refer to a pediatric text.)

HLA-ASSOCIATED RHEUMATIC DISEASE

Tissue typing is used in the field of human organ transplantation because specific tissue factors called *histocompatibility antigens* are responsible for the eventual acceptance or rejection of a donor organ. These antigens reside on the cell surfaces of all nucleated cells and were first described on leukocytes; hence they were called *human leukocyte antigens* (HLA). It soon become apparent that there was an association between a number of autoimmune diseases and HLA antigens. An unusually high frequency of HLA-B27 is found in ankylosing spondylitis, psoriatic arthritis, and Reiter's syndrome, known as the *seronegative spondyloarthritides*.[10] Detection of this marker is an important aid to early diagnosis of these diseases.

Ankylosing Spondylitis

Ankylosing spondylitis (Marie-Strümpell disease) is a chronic inflammatory disease which primarily affects the sacroiliac joints, apophyseal and costovertebral joints of the spine, and adjacent soft tissues. Approximately 90 percent of white clients with ankylosing spondylitis are HLA-B27-positive.[11] The disease typically appears in adolescence or young adulthood. Males are affected much more frequently than females, and there appears to be a definite familial tendency. The condition is unusual in blacks.

Etiology and pathogenesis

The cause is unknown. Genetic predisposition appears to play an important role in the disease pathogenesis, but the precise mechanisms are unknown.[12] Inflammation in joints and adjacent tissue causes the formation of granulation tissue, eroding vertebral margins and resulting in spondylitis. Calcification tends to follow the inflammation process, leading to bony ankylosis.

Clinical manifestations and complications

The client typically complains of low back pain, stiffness, and limitation of motion which is worse during the night and in the morning but improves with mild activity. General constitutional features such as fever, fatigue, anorexia, and weight loss are rarely present. Other symptoms depend on the stage of the disease and may include peripheral arthritis of the shoulders, hips, and knees and occasional ocular inflammation (iritis).

Involvement of costovertebral joints leads to a decrease in chest expansion. Advancing kyphosis leads to a bent-over posture, and compensating hip-flexion contractures may occur (Fig. 57-7). Atlantoaxial subluxation of the lower cervical spine is a rare but serious complication resulting in spinal cord or brainstem compression. Extraskeletal involvement may include iritis, aortic valvular regurgitation, and apical pulmonary fibrosis.

Diagnostic study abnormalities

Changes on x-ray may not become apparent for months to years after the onset of symptoms. When abnormalities are present, they include sacroiliac joints that show pseudowidening of the joint space

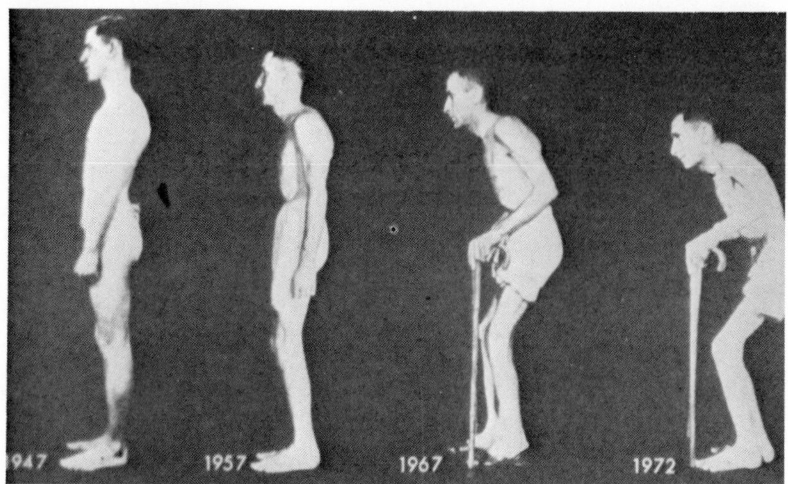

Figure 57-7 Progression of ankylosing spondylitis.

and later obliteration with ankylosis. New bone formation (syndesmophytes) may be spotty or generalized (classical "bamboo spine"). The sedimentation rate is usually elevated. Tissue typing is positive for HLA-B27.

Management

Prevention of ankylosing spondylitis is not possible at this time. However, families with diagnosed HLA-B27-positive rheumatic diseases should be alert to signs of low backache and arthritis symptoms, especially in male offspring.

Medical management is aimed at maintaining a maximum skeletal mobility. Proper posture is important in all activities. Although drugs will not halt the progression of the disease, such drugs as phenylbutazone and indomethacin can provide pain relief which makes proper posture easier. Surgery to correct extreme flexion deformities may be attempted in certain cases. A total hip replacement is performed for clients with crippling hip ankylosis.

Nursing responsibilities for the client with ankylosing spondylitis include education about the nature of the disease and principles of therapy. The degree of limitation of motion should be assessed for baseline data. Pain should be managed by appropriate medication as well as by heat, massage, and gentle exercise. A continuing physiotherapy program must be vigorously followed by the client to prevent deformity and preserve range of motion. Excessive physical exertion during periods of active inflammation should be discouraged. The client must understand the importance of a home management program and should demonstrate proper use of medications, local heat, and exercise. Proper positioning at rest is essential. The mattress should be firm, and pillows must be avoided. The client should sleep on his back, avoiding positions which encourage flexion deformity. Postural training must include emphasis on avoiding forward flexion (leaning over a desk), heavy lifting, and prolonged walking, standing, or sitting. Application of moist heat should be followed by range-of-motion exercises and daily chest expansion and deep-breathing exercises (Fig. 57-8). Sports which facilitate natural stretching, such as swimming and racquet games, should be encouraged. Family counseling and vocational rehabilitation are important.

Psoriatic Arthritis

Psoriatic arthritis can be defined as an association of clinically apparent psoriasis with inflammatory polyarthritis.[13] (Psoriasis is discussed in Chap. 15.) Psoriatic skin changes may antedate or follow articular symptoms. Approximately 10 to 15 percent of persons with psoriasis have such an arthritis, which is generally mild, with intermittent flare-ups affecting only a few peripheral joints. However, a severe erosive form indistinguishable from RA is also seen. Psoriatic clients are subject to spondylitis, associated with an 80 percent frequency of HLA-B27 positivity. Hyperuricemia often accompanies the disease. Forms of treatment include splinting, joint protection, physical therapy, and nonsteroidal anti-inflammatory medications. Antimalarials may aggravate skin disease and should be avoided.

Reiter's Syndrome

Reiter's syndrome is a self-limiting disease associated with arthritis, urethritis, conjunctivitis, and mu-

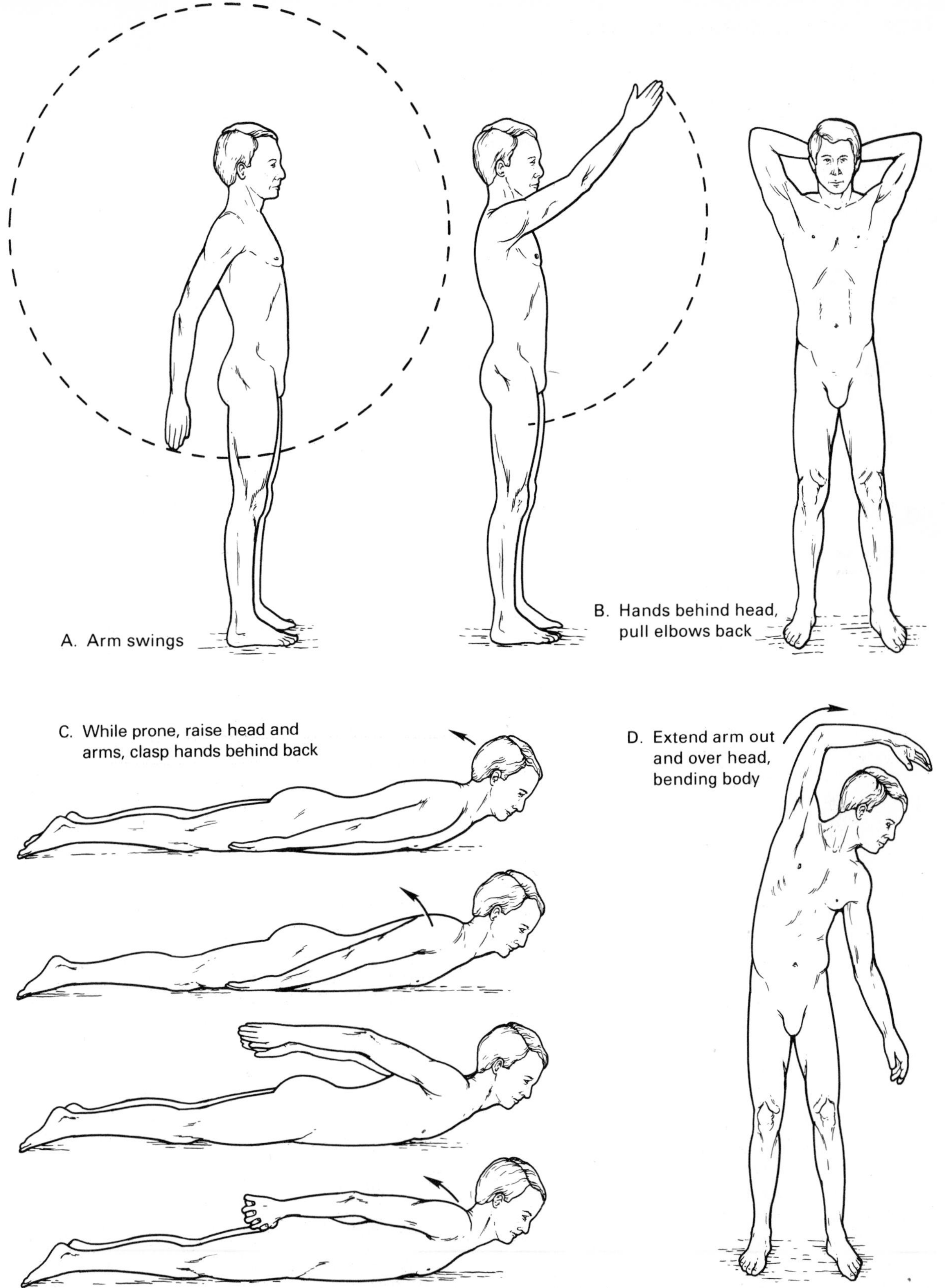
A. Arm swings
B. Hands behind head,
pull elbows back
C. While prone, raise head and
arms, clasp hands behind back
D. Extend arm out
and over head,
bending body

Figure 57-8 Typical chest-case stretching and deep chest breathing exercises.

cocutaneous lesions. While the exact etiology is unknown, Reiter's appears to be a reactive arthritis following certain enteric (e.g., *Shigella*) or venereal infections.[14] The disease usually affects males, and 85 percent of clients with Reiter's are HLA-B27-positive. Arthritis tends to be asymmetrical, frequently involving the weight-bearing joints of the lower extremities and sometimes the lower back. Soft-tissue manifestations commonly include Achilles tendinitis. Prognosis is favorable, with most clients recovering after 2 to 16 weeks. Lesions heal without a trace, and many clients experience complete remission with full joint function. Half the clients, however, have recurring acute attacks, while others follow a chronic course, experiencing continued synovitis and progression of x-ray changes closely resembling those of ankylosing spondylitis.

SEPTIC ARTHRITIS

Manifestations

Septic arthritis (infectious or bacterial arthritis) is caused by invasion of the joint cavity with microorganisms.[15] Various bacteria are commonly responsible, including *Staphylococcus aureus, Streptococcus hemolyticus, Diplococcus pneumoniae,* and *Neisseria gonorrhoeae*. Factors increasing the risk of such infections include previous joint trauma or arthritic disease, decreased-host-resistance diseases such as leukemia, treatment with corticosteroids or immunosuppressives, and serious chronic illness. Infants, young children, and the elderly appear to be more frequently affected by the infectious arthritides, with the exception of gonococcal arthritis, which affects sexually active young adults. A site of active infection is often responsible for bacteremia (microorganisms reaching the bloodstream), leading to hematogenous seeding of joints.

Inflammation of the joint cavity causes severe pain, erythema, and swelling of one or several joints. Fever and/or shaking chills often accompany articular symptoms. Precise diagnosis is made by aspiration of the joint and culture of the synovial fluid.

Management

Septic arthritis is a medical emergency which requires prompt diagnosis and treatment if joint destruction is to be prevented. Treatment is immediate administration of an appropriate antibiotic. Open surgical drainage may be required. Nursing intervention includes careful observation of the progression of joint inflammation. Gentle range-of-motion exercises should be done. Pain and fever should be monitored and treated appropriately. Strict aseptic technique should be used while assisting with joint aspiration procedures. The affected joint(s) should be immobilized with splints or traction. The necessity of antibiotics should be explained and the importance of their continued use should be stressed. Support should be offered to the client requiring repeated arthrocentesis or operative drainage. The extent of joint damage is generally related to the invading microorganism and the time period between infection onset and initiation of treatment.

GOUT

Gout is characterized by recurrent attacks of acute arthritis in association with increased levels of serum uric acid. It may be classified as primary or secondary. In primary gout, a hereditary error of purine metabolism leads to the overproduction or retention of uric acid. Secondary gout may be related to another, acquired disorder or may be the result of medications known to inhibit uric acid excretion (Table 57-10). Secondary gout may also be caused by medications which increase the rate of cell death, such as the chemotherapeutic agents used in leukemia.[16]

Significance of Problem

Primary gout occurs predominantly (90 percent) in middle-aged males, with relative sparing of premenopausal women. There is an increased frequency of hyperuricemia in the families of primary gout clients. Although some races have been identified as having a low incidence of gout, these same peoples living in another country may exhibit higher mean serum uric

Table 57-10

Associated Conditions Leading to Hyperuricemia

Obesity
Diabetes mellitus
Hyperlipidemia
Hypertension
Atherosclerosis
Myeloproliferative disorders
Malignant disease
Sickle cell anemia
Cytotoxic drugs
Intrinsic renal disease
Drug-induced renal impairment
Acidosis or ketosis

acid levels, indicating that both genetic and environmental factors contribute to the pathogenesis.

Etiology and Pathogenesis

Uric acid represents the major end product of the catabolism of purines and is primarily excreted by the kidneys. Thus hyperuricemia may be the result of increased purine synthesis or decreased renal excretion or both. About half the clients with primary gout can be shown to produce excessive amounts of uric acid. Folklore has long associated excesses of food and drink with acute attacks of gouty arthritis. Although high dietary intake of purine alone has relatively little effect on uric acid levels, it is clear that hyperuricemia may result from prolonged fasting or excessive drinking because of increased production of keto acids, which then inhibit normal renal excretion of uric acid.[17]

Clinical Manifestations

In the acute phase, gouty arthritis may occur in one or more joints but usually less than four. Affected joints may appear dusky or cyanotic and are extremely tender. Inflammation of the great toe (*podagra*) is most commonly the initial involvement and occurs in 75 percent of all patients. Other joints affected are the midtarsal, ankle, knee, and wrist joints and the olecranon bursa. Onset of symptoms is usually rapid, with swelling and pain peaking within several hours, often accompanied by low-grade fever. Individual attacks usually subside, treated or untreated, in 2 to 10 days. The affected joint then returns entirely to normal, and patients are often symptom-free between attacks.

Chronic gout is characterized by multiple joint involvement and deposits of sodium urate crystals (*tophi*). These are typically seen in the synovium, subchondral bone, olecranon bursa, vertebrae, along tendons, and in the skin and cartilage (Fig. 57-9). Tophi are rarely present at the time of the initial attack and are generally noted only many years after the disease onset.

The severity of gouty arthritis is variable. The clinical course may consist of infrequent mild attacks or multiple severe episodes associated with a slowly progressive disability. In general, the higher the serum uric acid level the earlier the appearance of tophi and the greater the tendency toward more frequent and severe episodes of acute gout.

Complications

Chronic inflammation may result in joint deformity. Destruction of the cartilage may predispose the joint to secondary osteoarthritis. Tophaceous deposits may be large and unsightly and may perforate overlying skin, producing draining sinuses which often become secondarily infected. Excessive uric acid excretion may lead to kidney stone formation. Pyelonephritis associated with intrarenal sodium urate deposits and obstruction may contribute to renal disease.

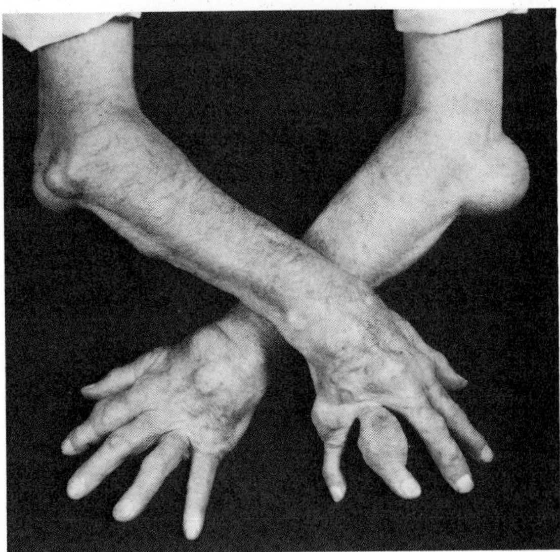

Figure 57-9 Tophaceous gout.

Diagnostic Study Abnormalities

The diagnosis can be established by finding monosodium urate monohydrate crystals in the synovial fluid of an inflamed joint or tophus. Serum uric acid levels are almost always elevated to 8 mg/dL or higher. It is important to note that hyperuricemia is not specifically diagnostic of gout, since increased levels may be related to a variety of drugs or may exist as a totally asymptomatic abnormality in the general population.

Medical Management

Medical management of gout (Table 57-11) has several goals. The first is to terminate an acute attack. This is accomplished by the use of an anti-inflammatory agent such as colchicine. Future attacks are prevented by a maintenance dose of colchicine, weight reduction if necessary, a diet low in purines and alcohol, and the use of drugs to reduce the serum urate concentration.

Treatment is also aimed at preventing the formation of uric acid kidney stones and other associated

Table 57-11
Medical Management: Gout

Diagnostic
1. History and physical examination
2. Family history of gout
3. Presence of monosodium urate monohydrate crystals
4. Elevated serum uric acid levels

Therapeutic
1. Bed rest and joint immobilization
2. Local application of heat or cold
3. Joint aspiration and intraarticular corticosteroids
4. Analgesics
5. Drug therapy—colchicine, probenecid, allopurinol

conditions such as hypertriglyceridemia and hypertension.

Pharmacological Intervention

Although medication does not cure gout, it can control its symptoms. Oral administration of colchicine will generally produce dramatic pain relief within 24 to 48 hours. Phenylbutazone and indomethacin are also effective in the control of joint inflammation. These medications may produce gastrointestinal irritation. Prophylactic doses of colchicine will reduce the frequency of attacks but will not alter the serum uric acid level.

For many years the standard therapy for hyperuricemia was a uricosuric drug (e.g., probenecid), which acted by increasing urinary uric acid excretion. The ability of salicylates to increase the excretion of uric acid is dose-related. Acetylsalicylate (aspirin) inactivates the effect of uricosurics, resulting in urate retention, and should be avoided while taking probenecid and other uricosuric drugs. Adequate urine volume must be maintained in order to prevent precipitation of uric acid in the renal tubules. Now a more potent drug, allopurinol (Zyloprim), which blocks the production of uric acid, may control the serum level and is particularly useful in those clients with uric acid stones or renal impairment, in whom uricosuric drugs may be either ineffective or potentially dangerous. Regardless of which drug or combination of drugs is prescribed, it is essential that the concentration of serum urate be checked regularly to monitor the effectiveness of treatment.

Diet

Dietary restrictions may include limiting the use of alcohol and of foods high in purine (shellfish, liver, brains, sweetbreads). (See Table 37-12 for foods high in purine.) However, medication is generally capable of controlling the situation without requiring these limitations. Obese clients should be instructed in a carefully planned weight-reduction program.

Nursing Management

Acute gouty arthritis may be prevented by maintaining the serum uric acid at normal levels. Nursing intervention is directed at supportive care of the inflamed joints. Bed rest may be appropriate, with affected joints properly immobilized. The limitation of motion and degree of pain should be assessed. Treatment effectiveness should be documented. Special care should be taken to avoid causing pain to an inflamed joint by careless handling.

The client and his family should understand that hyperuricemia and gouty arthritis are chronic problems which can be controlled, but that adherence to a treatment program is necessary to achieve this goal. Thorough explanations should be given concerning the importance of drug therapy. The client should be able to demonstrate his knowledge of precipitating factors which may cause an attack including alcohol, overindulgence, starvation (fasting), medication (aspirin, diuretics), and major medical events (surgery, myocardial infarction). The need for periodic determination of blood uric acid levels should be stressed. All clients should understand the importance of moderation in their intake of calories, purines, and alcohol.

SYSTEMIC LUPUS ERYTHEMATOSUS

Systemic lupus erythematosus (SLE) is a chronic multisystem inflammatory disease of connective tissue which often involves the skin, joints, serous membranes (pleura, pericardium), kidney, and hematologic and central nervous systems.[18] Discoid lupus erythematosus is a cutaneous form of the disease characterized by raised, red, scaly lesions, frequently appearing on the face, and irregular patchy hair loss on the scalp (*alopecia*). Estimates suggest that 1 out of 20 clients with discoid lupus will develop systemic involvement. Generally speaking, systemic features are more likely to develop in a discoid client with abnormal blood findings.

Significance of Problem

In 1948 Hargraves and others described the LE cell, an abnormal-appearing cell on blood smear, and this has led to a broadened concept of lupus and an increased awareness of its frequency.[19] Recent studies suggest an annual incidence as high as 75 per million population at risk.[20]

SLE affects females approximately 7 times more frequently than males, with the ratio increasing to 15:1

during the childbearing years (age 15 to 45). The disease also occurs in children and the elderly, although the average age at diagnosis is 30 years. Lupus affects all races but occurs more frequently in black Americans and Asians than in whites. Family members of some clients may have diagnosed SLE or may demonstrate laboratory abnormalities without clinical evidence of disease activity, suggesting a somewhat greater than chance familial occurrence.[21]

Etiology and Pathogenesis

The cause of systemic lupus erythematosus is unknown, although various triggering mechanisms have been identified. Genetic susceptibility is suggested by an increased frequency in the identical twins of persons having the disease and by the spontaneous occurrence of SLE in certain inbred strains of mice. Environmental factors such as viruses, overexposure to ultraviolet light, stress, pregnancy, or vaccines may be predisposing factors in persons susceptible to lupus. Certain drugs have been associated with the onset or exacerbation of lupus including procainamide, hydralazine, and anticonvulsants. It is not clear whether these agents uncover latent lupus or induce the disease. However, manifestations usually resolve as the medications are withdrawn. Current evidence points to a multifactorial origin of SLE, suggesting that a combination of events may bring about the clinical manifestations.

Immunological abnormalities include a variety of autoantibodies in the serum directed against components of the cell nucleus (antinuclear antibodies, or ANA) and against circulating proteins, blood cells, and solid organs. Histological examination of involved tissue reveals electron-dense deposits of immunoglobulin and complement components.

Clinical Manifestations

General

Lupus erythematosus is extremely variable in its severity, ranging from a relatively mild disorder to a rapidly progressive one affecting many organ systems (Fig. 57-10). SLE is characterized by alternating periods of remission and exacerbation. General constitutional complaints include fever, weight loss, and excessive fatigue and may precede an exacerbation of disease activity.

Dermatological manifestations

The most common cutaneous feature of SLE is an erythematous rash which can occur on the face, neck, or extremities. The classic butterfly rash, distributed across the bridge of the nose and cheeks, occurs in about 40 percent of clients (Fig. 57-11). The rash may appear as discoid (coinlike) lesions (Fig. 57-12) or as a diffuse maculopapular rash; it may occur anywhere on the body, but is most frequently seen on the face and chest.

Exposure to sunlight and other sources of ultraviolet radiation can cause a severe skin reaction and may even precipitate a flare-up of disease activity in those who are photosensitive. Ulcerations of the oral or nasopharyngeal membranes occur in up to one-third of SLE clients. Transient diffuse or patchy hair loss (alopecia) is common, with or without underlying scalp lesions; eventual regrowth is expected.

Musculoskeletal problems

Polyarthralgia with morning stiffness is often the client's first complaint and may precede the onset of multisystem disease by many years. Joint symptoms tend to be transitory and typically produce pain without objective signs of inflammation. True arthritis is occasionally seen but joint destruction is unusual.

Cardiopulmonary involvement

Pericarditis is present in nearly one-quarter of SLE clients, but myocarditis is rare. Pleurisy with or without effusion is encountered in nearly 40 percent of clients at some time during their illness. Raynaud's phenomenon occurs in 20 percent.

Complications

Renal disease

Clinical evidence of renal involvement is present in nearly half the clients with SLE and includes microscopic hematuria, excessive cellular casts in the urine sediment, proteinuria, and elevation of the serum creatinine. Kidney involvement varies in degree but may eventually end in renal failure. Regardless of whether renal manifestations are evident, nearly all clients with SLE show renal histological abnormalities in renal biopsy studies or autopsy results. Renal failure is the leading cause of death.

Clinical parameters, including blood pressure, urinalysis, serum creatinine, serum complement, and anti-DNA antibody levels should be monitored carefully and frequently over prolonged periods of time, since renal involvement in the earliest stages is asymptomatic.

CNS disease

Central nervous system involvement ranks close behind kidney disease and infection as a leading cause of death in lupus. Seizures are the single most common neurological manifestation and occur in as

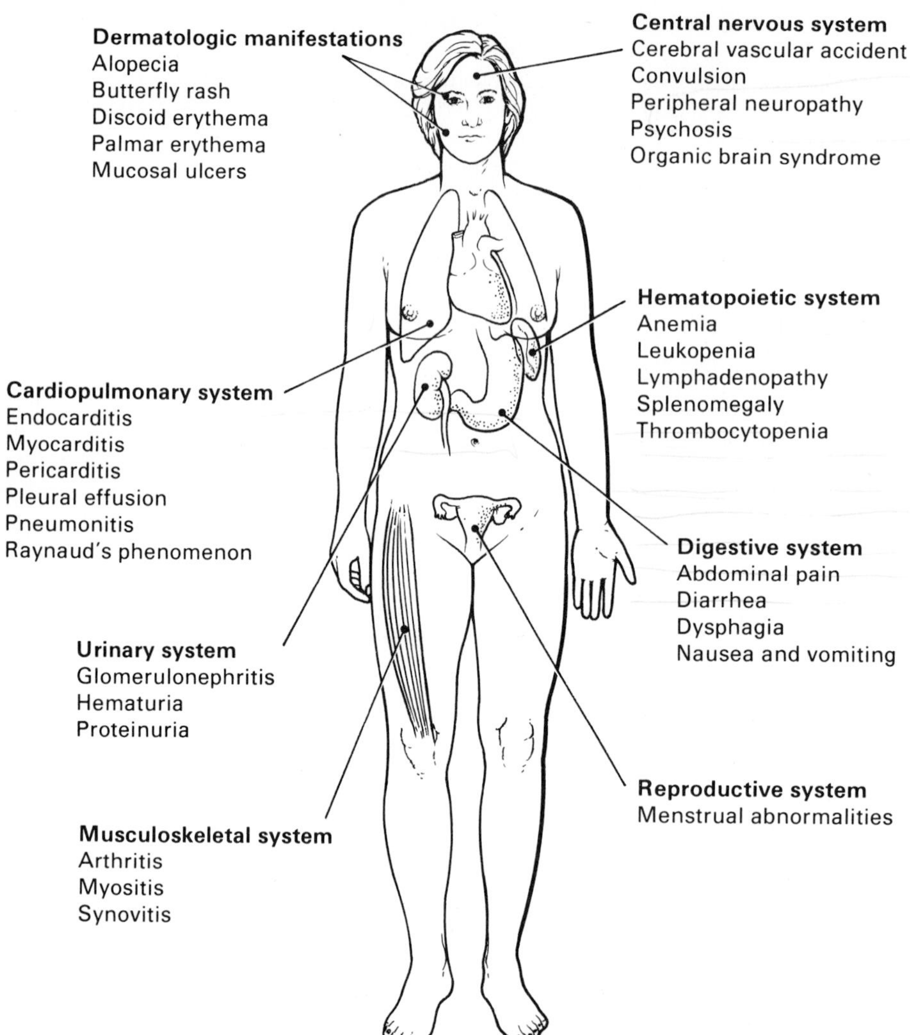

Figure 57-10 Systemic involvement in lupus erythematosus.

many as 15 percent of SLE clients by the time of diagnosis. They may be of the grand mal, petit mal, or psychomotor type and are generally controlled by corticosteroids or anticonvulsant therapy.

Organic brain syndrome, another recognized CNS manifestation of SLE, is characterized by disordered thought process, disorientation, memory deficits, and psychiatric symptoms such as severe depression and psychosis. Recovery from organic brain disease is expected, although some residual impairment may result. Occasionally a cerebrovascular accident (stroke) or aseptic meningitis may be attributable to lupus.

Infection

SLE clients appear to have increased susceptibility to infections, possibly related to defects in their ability to phagocytize invading bacteria, deficiencies in production of antibodies, and the immunosuppressive effect of many anti-inflammatory drugs. Any fever should be considered serious, as it may indicate an underlying infectious process rather than lupus activity alone.

Diagnostic Study Abnormalities

The diagnosis of SLE is based on the history and physical examination and laboratory findings (Table

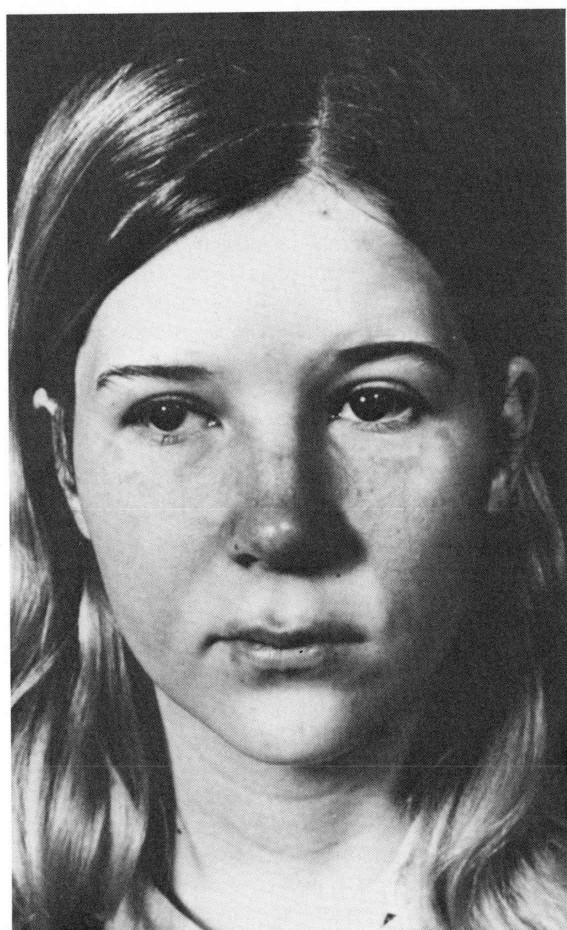

Figure 57-11 Malar erythema across nose and cheeks (butterfly distribution) typical of lupus erythematosus. [*From G. R. Rodnan (ed.), Primer on the Rheumatic Diseases, Arthritis Foundation, Atlanta. Reprinted by permission of the Arthritis Foundation.*]

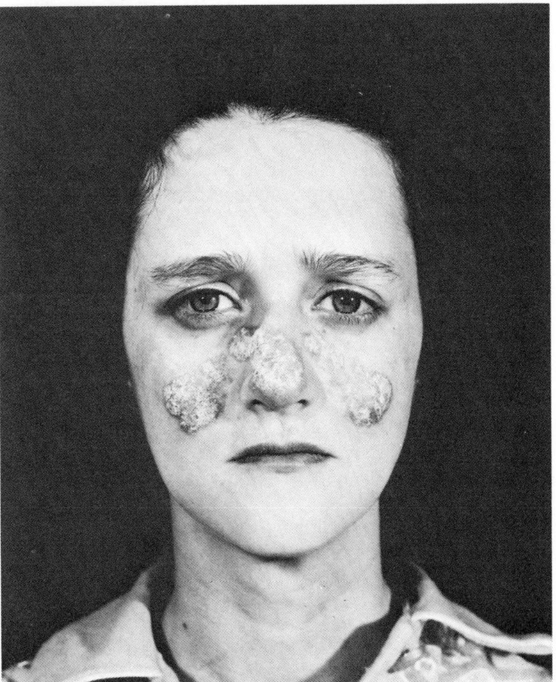

Figure 57-12 Discoid lesions of lupus erythematosus. Plaques seen typically on face, neck, scalp, and sun-exposed areas. Note here the butterfly distribution. (*Courtesy of Dr. Gerald P. Rodnan.*)

57-12). A variety of abnormalities may be present in the blood of clients with SLE, including elevated sedimentation rate, increase in gamma-globulin levels, anemia, decreased WBC and platelet counts, ECG or chest x-ray evidence of pericarditis or pleural effusion, and a biologic false-positive serological test for syphilis. Abnormalities in urine sediment (cellular casts, proteinuria), reduced serum complement activity, and tissue specimens demonstrating changes compatible with SLE are other confirmatory findings.

More specific tests which identify circulating antibodies directed against cell nuclei include:

ANA (antinuclear antibody) test—This test is positive in nearly 95 percent of clients with SLE, thus it is a sensitive screening test. A positive test is not specific, however, since persons with a variety of other autoimmune disorders may also have serum antinuclear antibodies.

LE cell test—This test is positive in over 80 percent of cases at one time or another and demonstrates the presence of the LE factor—an antinuclear antibody of the immunoglobulin-G class. This test is occasionally positive in other conditions but is more specific than the ANA.

Anti-DNA test—This test detects serum antibodies which react with DNA and is found in especially high titer when renal involvement is associated with SLE. It is the most specific test available for the diagnosis of SLE, since it is rarely positive in other disorders. Unfortunately, it is less sensitive, since these antibodies are detectable in the serum of only 60 percent of SLE clients.

Medical Management

There is a high rate of spontaneous remission in SLE. Corticosteroids remain the mainstay for clients with more severe illness. Their use should be reserved for acute generalized exacerbation or serious organ involvement, although a reduced maintenance dose is

Table 57-12

Systemic Lupus Classification

The following 14 manifestations, as proposed by the American Rheumatism Association, are useful in the *classification of patients in population surveys* and other epidemiology studies. A person shall be said to have SLE if any 4 or more of the following 14 manifestations are *observed during any period* of evaluation.

1. Facial erythema (butterfly rash)
2. Discoid lupus
3. Raynaud's phenomenon
4. Alopecia
5. Photosensitivity
6. Oral or nasopharyngeal ulceration
7. Arthritis without deformity
8. LE cells*
9. Chronic false-positive STS
10. Profuse proteinuria
11. Cellular casts
12. Pleuritis and pericarditis (one or both)
13. Psychosis and convulsion (one or both)
14. Hemolytic anemia, leukopenia, and thrombocytopenia (one or more)

*Some believe positive serum antinuclear antibody test can be substituted.

Modified from A. S. Cohen et al., "Preliminary Criteria for the Classification of Systemic Lupus Erythematosus," *Bull Rheum Dis,* **21**:643 (1971).

sometimes used. Immunosuppressive drugs may be used for clients who are resistant to corticosteroid therapy (Table 57-13).

The variability in seriousness of SLE makes education and support of the client very important. The overall survival rate is about 90 percent in 10 years.[22] The survival rate has significantly improved with early diagnosis and better treatment regimens. The prognosis is more favorable for those who do not have renal or CNS involvement or a superimposed bacterial infection.

Table 57-13

Medical Management: Systemic Lupus Erythematosus

Diagnostic

1. History and physical examination
2. Positive ANA or LE cell tests

Therapeutic

1. Nonsteroidal anti-inflammatory drugs
2. Corticosteroids for exacerbations and severe disease
3. Alternate therapies:
   a. Immunosuppressive drugs
   b. Plasmapheresis (plasma exchange)
   c. Steroids

Pharmacological Intervention

Therapeutic programs for SLE are prescribed to control inflammation and depend almost entirely on disease activity. Aspirin or other nonsteroidal anti-inflammatory drugs may reduce mild symptoms such as fever and arthritic complaints. Gastrointestinal upset and tinnitus which are recognized adverse effects of these agents, should be reported. Antimalarial drugs such as hydroxychloroquine sulfate (Plaquenil Sulfate) may be used to improve skin problems, but eye examinations must be scheduled periodically during this therapy, since visual loss is a rare but serious side effect. Topical steroid preparations and intralesional steroid injections are effective treatments for skin lesions.

Corticosteroids are potent anti-inflammatory medications used for acute generalized exacerbations of SLE and for the treatment of serious involvement of vital organs. As clinical and laboratory parameters improve, these drugs are gradually tapered off. Client education must include indications for use and proper administration of steroids and possible side effects. The client should understand that abrupt cessation may precipitate recurrence of disease activity. Immunosuppressive drug therapy such as azathioprine (Imuran) and cyclophosphamide (Cytoxan) remains controversial but is occasionally employed in life-threatening situations for those clients unresponsive to more conservative treatment. (See Chap. 42 for the nursing care of the client on steroid therapy.)

Nursing Management

Acute intervention

Prevention of SLE is not possible at this time. Education of the health professional and the community may promote a clearer understanding of the disease and earlier diagnosis.

During an exacerbation clients may become abruptly and dramatically ill. The nurse must monitor the vital signs closely. Nursing intervention includes accurately recording the severity of symptoms and documenting response to therapy. Fever pattern, joint inflammation, limitation of motion, location and degree of discomfort, and fatigability should be specifically assessed. The client's weight and fluid intake and output should be monitored because of the fluid-retention effect of steroids and the possibility of renal failure. Careful collection of 24-hour urine may be required. Seizure precautions, safety measures, and restraints may be indicated for CNS involvement. The nurse should observe for signs of bleeding secondary to drug therapy such as pallor, skin bruising, petechiae, or tarry stools. Careful assessment of neurological status includes observation for visual disturbances, headaches, personality changes, or forgetfulness. Psychosis may indicate CNS disease or may be the effect of corticosteroid therapy. Irritation of the nerves of the extremities (peripheral neuropathy) may produce numbness, tingling, and weakness of the hands and feet. Less frequently a stroke may result.

The nurse must explain the nature of the disease and modes of therapy and prepare the client for numerous diagnostic procedures. Emotional support for the client and family is essential.

Chronic management

With increased understanding of SLE, better diagnostic techniques, and improving prognosis, nursing intervention must emphasize health teaching and home management. The client should be taught to live *with* the disease, not *for* it.

The client must understand that even perfect adherence to the treatment plan is not insurance against exacerbation, since the course of the disease is unpredictable. However, a variety of factors may encourage exacerbation, such as fatigue, sun exposure, emotional stress, infection, drugs, and surgery. Nursing intervention should be directed at eliminating or minimizing exposure to precipitating factors. Client understanding and cooperation are important to this goal.

Nursing education should include the following points to promote understanding and improved adherence to home management:

1. Client and family education on the disease process
2. Names of medications and actions, side effects, dose, and administration
3. Energy-conservation and pacing techniques
4. Daily heat and exercise program (for arthritis)
5. Avoidance of physical and emotional stress
6. Avoidance of overexposure to ultraviolet light
7. Avoidance of unnecessary exposure to infection
8. Regular medical and laboratory follow-up
9. Marital counseling if necessary
10. Referral to community agencies and other medical resources

Since SLE is diagnosed in the majority of women during the childbearing years, many questions regarding pregnancy will be asked. Menstrual periods are frequently irregular or absent during active disease, returning to normal during a remission. The nurse should explain that pregnancy must be planned with the cooperation of the primary physician and obstetrician at a point when disease activity is minimal. Although the client often enjoys a degree of remission during pregnancy, exacerbation is common during the postpartum period. Fetal risks include increased rates of miscarriage, prematurity, and stillbirth.[23] Babies may have low birth weight but are generally healthy. Regular clinical and laboratory monitoring is essential for the pregnant woman with SLE.

Chronic disease has many effects on the client and family. Pain, fatigue, absence from work, multiple medications, hospital costs, inability to keep up with family routines, and side effects of treatment are all possible problem areas. The nurse must offer psychological support when needed and encourage help from community resources. Vocational rehabilitation may be necessary. The nurse should help the client to recognize nontraditional and unproven methods of treatment and obtain accurate information from the health care team and medically supported self-help organizations such as the Lupus Foundation and the Arthritis Foundation.

PROGRESSIVE SYSTEMIC SCLEROSIS

Progressive systemic sclerosis (PSS, scleroderma) is a disorder of connective tissue characterized by fibrotic, degenerative, and occasionally inflammatory changes in the skin, blood vessels, synovium, skeletal muscle, and internal organs.[24] Skin thickening and tightening is the cardinal feature. The disease may range from a diffuse cutaneous thickening with rapidly progressive and fatal visceral involvement to a more benign variant called CREST (calcinosis, *R*aynaud's phenomenon, *e*sophageal dysfunction, *s*clerodactyly, and *t*elangiectasis) syndrome.

Significance of Problem

PSS affects women 4 times more frequently than men, with the female to male ratio increasing to 15:1 during the childbearing years. Scleroderma has been reported in all races. Although symptoms may begin at any time, the usual age of onset is between 30 and 50 years. The average annual incidence is approximately 10 new cases per million population at risk.[25]

Etiology and Pathogenesis

The exact cause of PSS remains unclear. Abnormal serological and cellular immune reactions suggest that immunological mechanisms play an important role in pathogenesis. Fibrosis of the skin and internal organs is probably the result of the overproduction of collagen, as evidenced by an increase of compact collagen fibers in skin biopsy specimens. Histologically the gastrointestinal tract shows increased deposits of collagen as well as extensive replacement of the muscular layers by fibrous tissue. Kidney disease is marked by fibrinoid necrosis and fibrosis of small vessels, along with subintimal proliferation of mucopolysaccharide-rich material.[26]

Clinical Manifestations

Raynaud's phenomenon

The initial complaint is generally Raynaud's phenomenon (paroxysmal vasospasm of the digits), occurring in nearly 98 percent of all PSS clients. Clients experience diminished blood flow to fingers and toes on exposure to cold (blanching, or white phase) followed by cyanosis as hemoglobin releases oxygen to the tissues (blue phase), then erythema on rewarming (red phase). The color changes are often accompanied by numbness and tingling. Raynaud's phenomenon may precede the onset of systemic disease by months, years, or even decades.

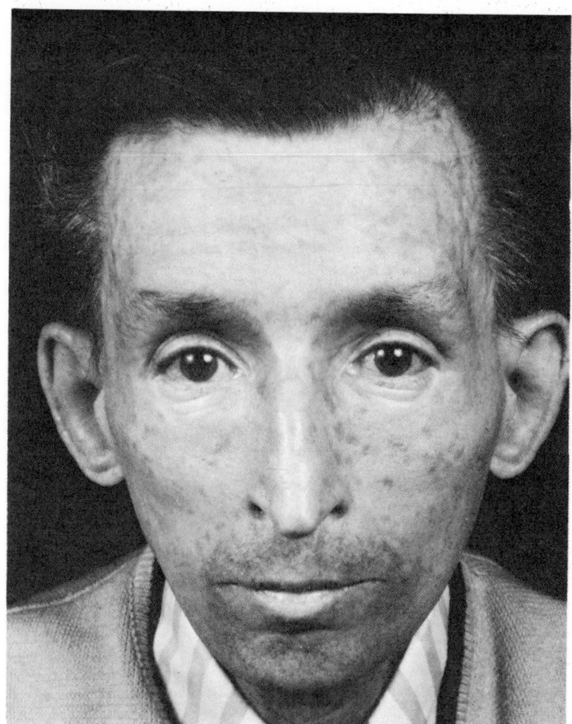

Figure 57-13 Facies of man with PSS. Note tight, shiny skin showing loss of normal skin folds and multiple telangiectases. (*Courtesy of Dr. Gerald P. Rodnan.*)

Skin and joint changes

Symmetrical painless swelling or thickening of the skin of the fingers and hands may progress to diffuse scleroderma of the trunk. The skin loses elasticity and becomes taut and shiny, producing the typical expressionless facies with tightly pursed lips (Fig. 57-13). Digital tuft resorption, flexion contractures, and atrophy of soft tissue may give the hands a clawlike appearance (Fig. 57-14). Polyarthralgias and morning stiffness may be early symptoms. Tendon friction rubs may be present.

Internal organ involvement

Esophageal dysfunction causes frequent reflux of gastric acid, causing heartburn, and substernal dysphagia for solid foods. If swallowing becomes difficult, the client often decreases food intake and loses weight. Gastrointestinal complaints may also include abdominal distension, diarrhea, malodorous floating stools (malabsorption syndrome) due to small bowel disease, and constipation secondary to colonic involvement.

Renal disease is a major cause of death in PSS. Often, malignant arterial hypertension associated with rapidly progressive and irreversible renal insufficiency is present. Recent improvements in hemodialysis, bilateral nephrectomy in those clients with uncontrollable hypertension, and the advent of renal transplantation have offered some hope to those with this serious complication of PSS.

Complications

The overall mortality approaches 50 percent at 10 years after initial diagnosis.[27] In advanced disease, heart and lung involvement may produce heart disease, arrhythmia, dyspnea, and pulmonary fibrosis. The prognosis for "scleroderma kidney," usually accompanied by malignant hypertension and renal failure, is especially grave.

Diagnostic Study Abnormalities

Blood studies may reveal a mildly elevated sedimentation rate and occasionally hypergammaglobulinemia. The ANA is frequently positive in low titer in a speckled pattern. If renal involvement is present, urinalysis may show proteinuria, microscopic hematuria, and casts. X-ray evidence of subcutaneous calcification, digital tuft resorption, distal esophageal hypomotility, and/or bilateral pulmonary fibrosis are diagnostic of PSS. Pulmonary funcation studies reveal

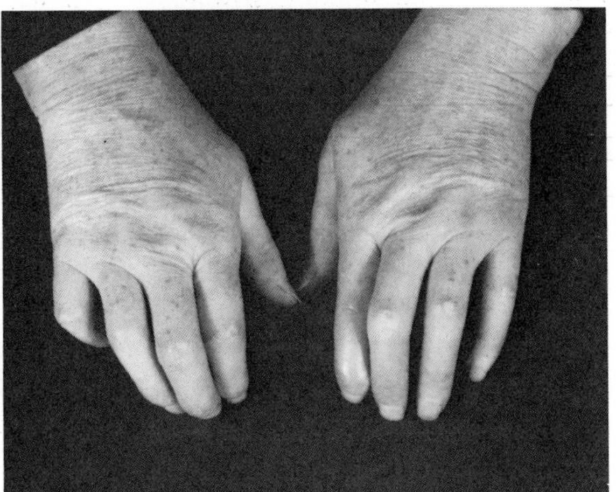

Figure 57-14 Hands of a woman with PSS CREST syndrome. Flexion contractures and soft-tissue atrophy give fingers a clawlike appearance. Notice multiple telangiectases. [*Reprinted by permission of G. P. Rodnan, from "Progressive Systemic Sclerosis: Arthritis and Allied Conditions," in D. J. McCarty, Jr. (ed.), Arthritis and Allied Conditions: A Textbook of Rheumatology, 9th ed., Lea & Febiger, Philadelphia, 1979, p. 765.*]

decreased vital capacity and diffusion capacity for carbon monoxide. Skin biopsy features dermal collagen thickening, condensation, or homogenization.

Medical Management

The medical management of PSS (Table 57-14) offers no specific treatment with long-range effect. Various drugs such as corticosteroids, para-aminobenzoic acid (PABA), D-penicillamine, and colchicine have been used with varying degrees of success.

Contractures cannot be prevented by physical therapy, but therapy can help to preserve muscle strength. The symptoms of Raynaud's phenomenon may be temporarity relieved by a thoracic sympathectomy. Additional measures to prevent vasospasm and increase digital blood flow should be initiated (see Chap. 30).

Pharmacological Intervention

No specific drugs or combination of drugs have been proved effective as treatment for systemic sclerosis. Corticosteroids are generally reserved for clients with myositis or overlap syndromes (e.g., mixed connective tissue disease). Penicillamine (Cuprimine) increases the solubility of dermal collagen and causes thinning of the skin in some clients but has several potentially serious side effects. Colchicine has recently been used to inhibit the accumulation of collagen, but there is still insufficient evidence to prove its therapeutic worth. The use of immunosuppressive agents is under investigation.

Supportive measures include oral vasodilating drugs and intraarterial injections of reserpine. Infected ulcerations of the fingertips may be treated by soaking with hyaluronidase and using bactericidal antibiotic ointment. Joint complaints may be relieved by aspirin and other nonsteroidal anti-inflammatory drugs. Antacids may be useful for heartburn. Tetracycline and other broad-spectrum antibiotics may improve intestinal malabsorption. Various combinations of antihypertensive medications, including hydralazine, guanethidine, propranolol, and methyldopa, have been used in the treatment of hypertension and renal failure.

Table 57-14
Medical Management: Progressive Systemic Sclerosis

Diagnostic
1. History and physical examination
2. Serological testing
3. X-rays of chest, hands, GI tract
4. Skin and/or visceral biopsy

Therapeutic
1. Vasodilator and antihypertensive drugs
2. Anti-inflammatory agents
3. Physical therapy
4. Antacids

Nursing Management

Since prevention is not possible at this time, nursing intervention often begins during a hospitalization for diagnostic purposes. Vital signs, weight, intake and output, respiratory function, and limitation of joint motion should be assessed daily. Emotional stress and air conditioning may aggravate Raynaud's phenomenon. These clients should not have finger-stick blood testing done because of compromised circulation and poor digital healing. Diagnostic studies should be thoroughly explained. The nurse may help the client to eliminate some feelings of helplessness by explaining the illness and treatment with the help of pictures and literature. Whenever possible, the client should be encouraged to participate in planning his own care.

Health teaching is a major nursing concern as the client and his family begin to live with a chronic disease. They should be helped to adjust to a new body image and the limitation of motion. Expressing fears and setting realistic goals is to be encouraged. The client should understand the action and side effects of all medications; he should be instructed in heat therapy, daily range-of-motion exercises, the use of assistive devices, and pacing and organizational activities. Hands and feet should be protected from cold exposure and possible burns or cuts that might heal slowly. Signs of infection should be reported immediately. Smoking should be discouraged. Lotions and oils may help to alleviate skin dryness and cracking but must be rubbed in for an unusually prolonged time because of the thickness of the skin. Dysphagia may be reduced by eating small, frequent meals, chewing carefully and slowly, and drinking fluids. Heartburn may be minimized by using antacids 45 to 60 minutes after each meal and by sitting upright for 30 to 45 minutes after eating. Using additional pillows or raising the head of the bed on blocks may help to reduce nocturnal esophageal reflux.

POLYMYOSITIS AND DERMATOMYOSITIS

Polymyositis and dermatomyositis are diffuse inflammatory myopathies of striated muscle, producing symmetrical weakness primarily in the proximal muscles of the pelvic and shoulder girdle.[28] Table 57-15 lists the classification of polymyositis and dermatomyositis. Dermatomyositis is a myopathy with a characteristic skin rash. Both disorders have been classified according to treatment response and prognostic considerations.

Polymyositis and dermatomyositis occur twice as frequently in women as in men and are seen predominantly during midadult life. The incidence is slightly greater than that of muscular dystrophy in adults. In cases of dermatomyositis, especially among older persons, there appears to be an increased frequency of malignancy.

Table 57-15
Classification of Polymyositis/Dermatomyositis

Adult polymyositis
Adult dermatomyositis
Polymyositis associated with malignant disease
Childhood polymyositis/dermatomyositis
Polymyositis/dermatomyositis associated with another connective tissue disease

Modified from C. M. Pearson, "Polymyositis," *Ann Rev Med.*, **17**:63 (1966).

Etiology and Pathogenesis

The exact cause of polymyositis and dermatomyositis is unknown. Theories include presence of an infectious agent, a hypersensitivity response, and cell-mediated immune system abnormalities. Close association with neoplastic disease suggests an autoimmune reaction. Histopathological study typically reveals the presence of inflammatory infiltrates, degeneration, regeneration, necrosis, and fibrosis of muscle fibers.

Clinical Manifestations and Complications

Muscular

The client usually experiences an insidious onset of proximal muscle weakness, primarily of the shoulder and pelvic girdle, and has difficulty arising from a chair or bathtub, climbing stairs, combing the hair, or reaching into a high cupboard. Neck muscles may become so weak that the client is unable to raise his head from the pillow. Muscle discomfort or tenderness is the exception rather than the rule. Muscle examination reveals inability to move against resistance or even against gravity. Weak pharyngeal muscles may produce proximal dysphagia (regurgitation of fluids through the nose) and dysphonia (nasal or hoarse voice).

Dermal

The typical skin rash appears as a dusky erythema of the face, neck, shoulders, anterior chest, upper back, and arms and occurs in nearly 40 percent of clients with muscular disease. Nearly pathognomic for dermatomyositis is heliotrope rash over the eyelids (lavender hue) and periorbital edema. The rash is prominent on the extensor surfaces of the forearms, elbows, knuckles, periungual areas, knees, and ankles. Scaling is a characteristic feature and may easily be confused with that of psoriasis or seborrheic dermatitis.

Other

Nearly half the clients with polymyositis experience mild or transient arthritis and/or Raynaud's phenomenon. Calcinosis, contractures, and muscle atrophy may occur with advanced disease. Aspiration pneumonia may result from weak pharyngeal muscles. Childhood dermatomyositis appears to have a more progressive, crippling course, and dermatomyositis diagnosed in males over age 40 is more frequently associated with concurrent malignant disease.

Diagnostic Study Abnormalities

Elevations in serum muscle enzymes (CPK, aldolase, and SGOT) are most valuable in determining diagnosis and response to treatment. Antinuclear antibody (ANA) and antibodies to extractable nuclear antigen (ENA) are frequently found, as well as an elevation in sedimentation rate. The EMG shows polyphasic, short-duration potentials, fibrillation, and positive spike waves. Muscle biopsy reveals necrosis, degeneration, regeneration, and interstitial chronic inflammatory cell infiltration (primarily lymphocytes).

Medical Management

Polymyositis and dermatomyositis can be treated with some degree of success by the use of corticosteroids and, occasionally, cytotoxic-immunosuppressive drugs such as cyclophosphamide (Cytoxan). Improvement is generally achieved with prompt institution of corticosteroid therapy. Topical steroids may be applied to the skin rash. Clients who respond poorly to corticosteroids may improve with immunosuppressives (e.g., intermittent intravenous or daily oral cyclophosphamide). Corticosteroid therapy may cause potassium, which is necessary for normal muscle contraction, to be released from damaged muscle cells and lost in the urine. Supplemental dietary potassium (e.g., orange juice, bananas) is encouraged.

Physical therapy can be helpful and should be tailored to the activity of the disease. Massage and passive movement would be appropriate during active disease, with more aggressive exercises reserved for periods when disease activity is minimal, as evidenced by low serum enzyme levels.

A careful search for possible malignant lesions should be undertaken for the client over 40. If malignant disease is found, it should be treated appropriately (see Chap.11). Complete remission of dermatomyositis may occur if the malignant lesion is removed.

Nursing Management

Although prevention is not possible at this time, greater recognition of polymyositis and its insidious onset resembling muscular dystrophy may favorably influence prognosis by more rapid diagnosis and institution of therapy.

Nursing intervention should include assessment of muscular weakness and limitation of motion. The nurse should promote bed rest and assist the client with activities of daily living. Emotional support should be offered to the client and family concerning fears of inability to move against gravity. Special attention should be provided at mealtime to prevent aspiration. The nature of the disease and modes of therapy should be thoroughly reviewed and the diagnostic tests explained. Understanding that the benefits of therapy are often delayed is important (for example, weakness may increase during the first few weeks of corticosteroid therapy).

The client should have a thorough understanding of the chronic nature of this disorder, the usefulness and the side effects of all prescribed medications, and the importance of regular medical appointments and serial laboratory testing. The nurse should provide guidelines for conserving energy by means of organizing activities and pacing techniques. Daily range-of-motion exercises should be encouraged to prevent contractures, and when there is no evidence of active inflammation, muscle-strengthening (repetitive) exercises may be begun.

MISCELLANEOUS ASSOCIATED DISORDERS

Sjögren's Syndrome

Sjögren's syndrome is a chronic inflammatory disease characterized by decreased lacrimal and salivary secretion.[29] More than 90 percent of the clients are women, and half have rheumatoid arthritis or other connective tissue disease. Decreased tearing leads to a "gritty" sensation in the eye, burning, and photosensitivity. Dry mouth produces buccal membrane fissures, dysphagia, and frequent dental caries. Dry nasal and respiratory passages are common and can result in a cough. Often the parotid glands are enlarged. Other exocrine glands may also be affected —for example, vaginal dryness may lead to dyspareunia.

Histological study reveals lymphocyte infiltration of salivary and lacrimal glands, but the disease may become more generalized and involve lymph nodes, bone marrow, and visceral organs (pseudolymphoma). Extraglandular proliferation may become frankly malignant (e.g., lymphoma). Rheumatoid and antinuclear factors are present in the majority of clients. Anemia, leukopenia, hypergammaglobulinemia, and elevated sedimentation rate are also usually found. Ophthalmologic examination (Schirmer test), salivary flow rates, and lower lip biopsy of minor salivary glands confirm the diagnosis. The treatment is symptomatic, including artificial tears and increased fluids with meals. Dental hygiene is important. Increased humidity at home may reduce respiratory infections.

Corticosteroids and immunosuppressive drugs are indicated for treatment of pseudolymphoma.

Mixed Connective Tissue Disease

Clients having a combination of the clinical features of several rheumatic diseases are described as having mixed connective tissue disease.[30] The symptoms include overlapping features of systemic lupus erythematosus, progressive systemic sclerosis, and polymyositis (Fig. 57-15). Serological studies indicate unusually high titers of antinuclear antibody, consisting chiefly of antibodies to ribonucleoprotein (anti-RNP). Mild disease may be controlled by nonsteroidal anti-inflammatory medications, while major organ involvement generally responds to corticosteroid therapy. The prognosis is generally good, although some clients develop renal involvement more typical of SLE or PSS.

Amyloidosis

Amyloidosis is a disorder characterized by an accumulation of amyloid, an extracellular filamentous glycoprotein.[31] Deposits may be limited, with little effect on health, or widespread, affecting major organ systems. Primary amyloidosis is unrelated to any other disease, while secondary amyloidosis may be associated with chronic infections, neoplasms, and inflammatory disorders such as rheumatoid arthritis, ankylosing spondylitis, tuberculosis, osteomyelitis, and multiple myeloma.

Clinical manifestations vary with the organ system involved. Primary amyloidosis commonly affects the peripheral nerves, joints, heart, and integumentary system, while secondary amyloidosis affects the liver, spleen, and kidney. The diagnosis is established by biopsy examination. Treatment of the underlying infection or inflammation may combat secondary amyloidosis, but the primary form remains untreatable. Conservative and supportive measures are the mainstay of both medical and nursing management. Emotional support of both the client and the family is an important consideration.

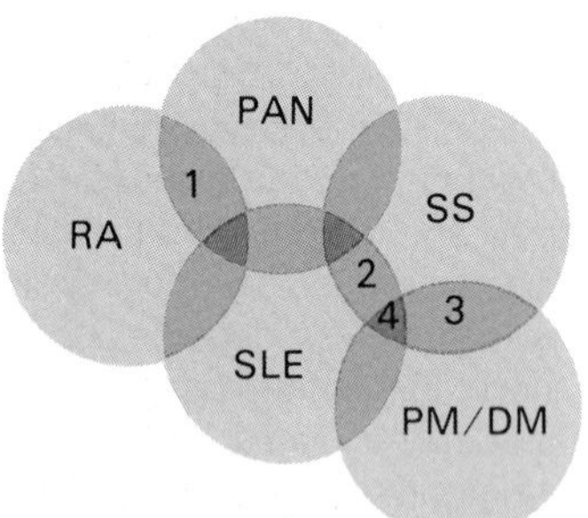

Figure 57-15 Clinical overlaps in connective-tissue diseases: (1) Rheumatoid vasculitis. (2) "Lupoderma." (3) "Scleromyositis." (4) Mixed connective-tissue disease. [*Reprinted by permission of T. A. Medsger, from "Epidemiology of Rheumatoid Diseases in Arthritis and Allied Conditions," in D. J. McCarty, Jr. (ed.), Arthritis and Allied Conditions: A Textbook of Rheumatology, 9th ed., Lea & Febiger, Philadelphia, 1979, p. 27.*]

COMMON JOINT SURGICAL PROCEDURES*

Joint surgery dates back to 1891, when hip, finger, and thumb joints were implanted.[32] In the following years the technology of joint replacement was actively pursued. Rejection of the prosthesis material and loosening of the parts were two persistent problems. The discovery of Vitallium, an alloy, and methylmethacrylate cement to fix the prosthesis in place were significant advances in the field of joint surgery. Since that time, improvements have been made in prosthetic design and materials and in surgical techniques.

Indications for Joint Surgery

Joint surgery may be indicated for conditions related to trauma, arthritic processes, or other painful conditions resulting in functional disability. Surgery is aimed at relieving pain, improving joint motion, correcting deformity and malalignment, reducing vertical loads and shear stresses, and removing intraarticular causes of erosion.

Pain is one of the primary reasons for joint surgery. In addition to the effects of chronic pain on the physical and emotional well-being of the client, any movement of the painful joint is often avoided. If this lack of movement is not corrected, contraction with limitation of motion often occurs. Limitation of motion at any joint can be demonstrated on physical examination and by joint space narrowing on radiological examination.

There may also be a slow loss of cartilage in affected joints which may or may not be related to loss of motion. Synovitis can cause tendon damage, resulting in rupture or subluxation of the joint and subsequent loss of function. Continuing disease activity may cause loss of cartilage and bony surface and result in mechanical barriers to movement requiring surgical intervention.

*This section written by Candelario Garcia, R.N., CFNP.

Types of Surgical Procedures

Synovectomy

Synovectomy (removal of synovial membrane) is used as a prophylactic measure as well as a palliative treatment of rheumatoid arthritis. Removal of synovial membrane, thought to be the location of the basic pathological changes in joint destruction, helps to prevent further damage. A synovectomy is often performed early in the disease process to prevent serious destruction of joint surfaces. Removal of the thickened synovium prevents extension of the inflammatory process into the adjacent cartilage, ligaments, and tendons.

It is impossible to surgically remove all the synovium in a joint. The underlying disease process is still present and will again affect the regenerating synovium. However, the disease appears to be milder following synovectomy; definite improvement in pain, weight bearing, and range of motion can be expected. Common sites for this surgery include the knees, elbow, wrist, and fingers.

Osteotomy

An osteotomy is performed by cutting a bone to change its alignment and thereby correct deformity and relieve pain. It is used in osteoarthritis and chronic rheumatoid arthritis mainly after a joint becomes ankylosed in a nonfunctional position. The postoperative care is similar to the treatment of an internal fixation of a fracture at a comparable site. Usually the osteotomy is fixed by internal measures such as wire, screws and plates, bone grafts, or fixation material. (For management of internal fixation of fractures see Chap. 56.)

Arthroplasty

Arthroplasty is the reconstruction or replacement of a joint. This surgical procedure is performed to relieve pain, to improve or maintain range of motion, and to correct deformity—conditions that could result from osteoarthritis, rheumatoid arthritis, avascular necrosis, congenital deformities or dislocations, and other systemic problems. There are several types of arthroplasty including replacement of part of a joint, surgical reshaping of the bones of the joints, and total joint replacement.[33] Innovative procedures as well as prosthetic devices offer exciting possibilities for future reconstructive joint surgery. Replacement arthroplasty is available for the elbow, shoulder, phalangeal joints of the fingers, hip, knee, and ankle (Fig. 57-16).

Hip Hip reconstruction is frequently used in the treatment of clients with rheumatoid arthritis and osteoarthritis as well as for fractures of the hip. This surgery is usually performed on clients over 60 years of age. It is occasionally done in younger clients, but the long-term effects and durability of the joint have not been established. It is also done on clients who have had previously unsuccessful surgery for fracture repair. A detailed discussion of the client undergoing a total hip replacement can be found in Chap. 56.

Knee Unremitting pain as a result of severe destructive deterioration of the knee joint is the main indication for knee arthroplasty. Either part or all of the knee joint may be replaced with a metal and plastic prosthetic device. There is great emphasis on postoperative exercising, which requires a high degree of motivation on the part of the client because of the pain involved. Within 2 to 5 days after surgery, the client is instructed to perform quadricep-setting exercises and straight leg raising. When the bulky dressing is removed, active flexion exercises are begun. Weight bearing is begun when the client can use a walker or crutches. The usual hospital stay is around 2 weeks, so the client can participate in a supervised muscle-strengthening program.

Finger Joints A silicone rubber arthroplastic device is used to help replace function in the client with rheumatoid arthritis. The metacarpophalangeal and proximal interphalangeal joints are most commonly involved. Ulnar deviation is often present, which limits the client to essentially a nonfunctional use of the hand. Prior to surgery the client is instructed in hand exercises including flexion, extension, abduction, and adduction of the fingers. Postoperatively, the hand is kept elevated with a bulky dressing in place. The operative area and the hand should be checked for sensation, temperature, pulse, and signs of infection. Once the dressing is removed, a guided splinting program is initiated. The client will be discharged with splints to use while sleeping and hand exercises to do for 10 to 12 weeks at least 3 or 4 times a day. The client is also instructed to avoid lifting heavy objects.

Elbows and Shoulders Total replacement of elbow and shoulder joints, although available, is not as common as other forms of arthroplasty. The shoulder replacement is usually considered if the client has adequate surrounding muscle strength. Shoulder and elbow replacements have less satisfactory results than other joint replacements, but further developments are possible for the future.

Arthrodesis

Arthrodesis is the surgical fusion of a joint. This procedure will relieve pain and provide a stable joint

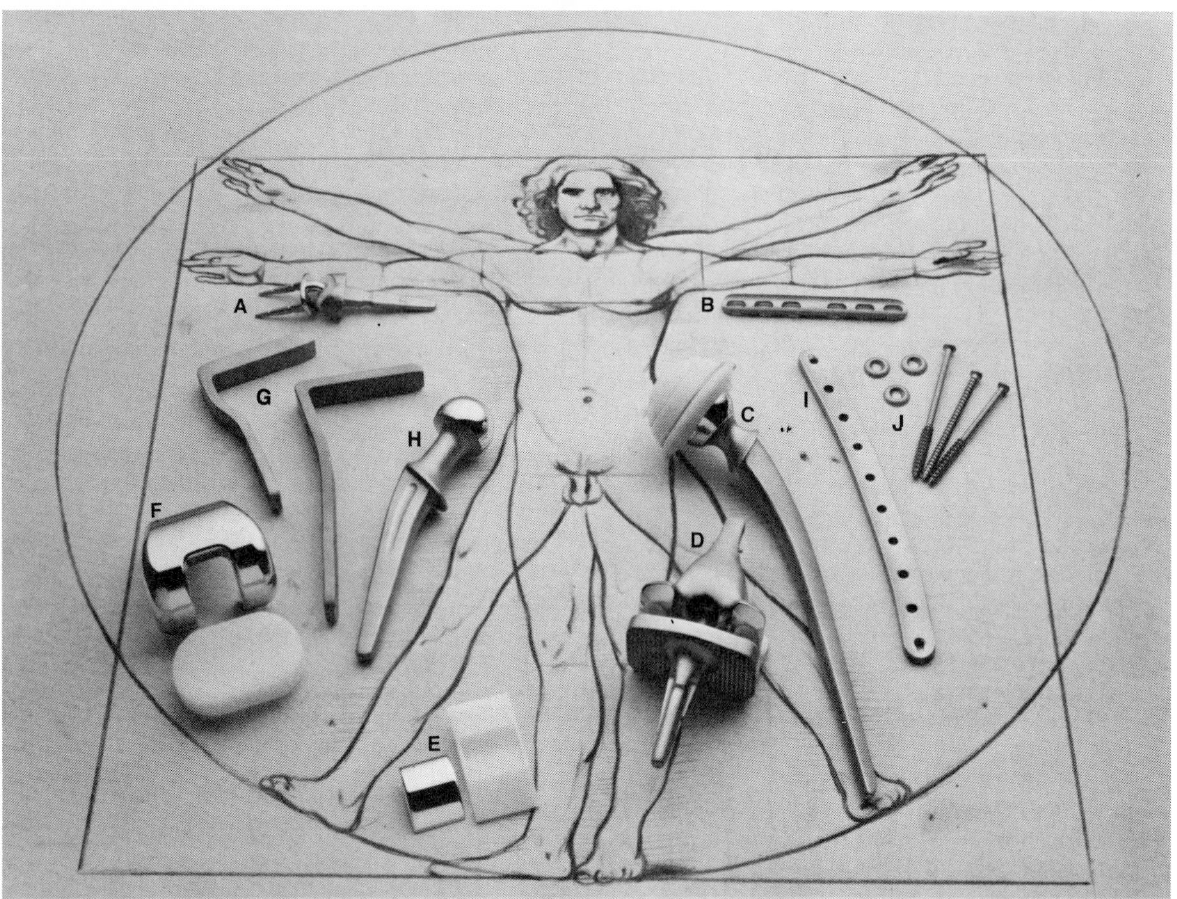

Figure 57-16 Vitallium alloy group. Examples of special processes for special application. *(a)* AMC total wrist. *(b)* Harris osteotomy blade plate. *(c)* CAD Muller hip. *(d)* Freeman-Swanson knee. *(e)* Scholz ankle. *(f)* Spherocentric knee. *(g)* Tetoirrnel hip. *(h)* Vitallium alloy curved compression plate. *(i)* Bagby plate. *(j)* Vitallium alloy bone screws and washers. *(Howmedica, Inc., Rutherford, N.J.)*

by eliminating the range of motion of a particular joint. The fusion is usually accomplished by removal of the articular hyaline cartilage and the addition of bone grafts across the joint surface. The affected joint must be immobilized until bone healing has taken place.

Common areas of fusion are the wrist, ankle, cervical spine, and lumbar spine. It must be stressed to the client that the fused joint will have no motion. Arthrodesis is usually considered after other forms of surgical intervention such as synovectomy, osteotomy, and arthroplasty have proved unsuccessful.

Management of the Surgical Client

The surgeon will complete a careful preoperative assessment before deciding on the most appropriate type of joint surgery. In addition to a careful evaluation of the problem underlying the surgery (e.g., rheumatoid arthritis, osteoarthritis, deformity), a careful cardiovascular and respiratory assessment is essential. Any additional situations which could affect the success of the surgery, such as previous long-term steroid use or the presence of osteoporosis, should be evaluated.

Careful timing and preparation of the client are important if surgery is to be performed on the client with rheumatoid arthritis. The client with rheumatoid arthritis should be strong constitutionally, preferably with a low ESR, and should be watched for postoperative anemia. Transfusions and iron preparations are often given preoperatively. Clients who have been on prolonged steroid therapy must be monitored carefully, as they may be susceptible to shock after surgery because of adrenal insufficiency.

Postoperatively, the surgeon will be concerned with nerve function and circulatory status. Generally the affected joint is exercised as early as possible, and ambulation is encouraged. Specific details regarding exercise and ambulation vary among surgeons, so detailed directions should be requested.

The nursing management of the client undergoing joint surgery includes both preoperative and postoperative activities. Preoperatively the nurse should reinforce the surgeon's explanation of the intended procedure and help the client set realistic expectations. It is important that the client understand and accept the limitations of the proposed surgery and realize that it will not remove the underlying disease process. Client activities such as exercises, turning, coughing, and deep breathing should be explained and opportunities for practice provided. The client should be reassured that pain relief will be available if necessary. A preoperative visit from a physical therapist should be arranged by the nurse. The physical therapist can explain in detail the postoperative exercise program, measure for crutches or other assistive devices, let the client see the tilt table if one is indicated, and introduce the client to some of the more frightening elements of rehabilitation. The nurse can explain her role in the therapy program for the client. The spirit of respect and cooperation displayed between the physical therapist and the nurse can do much to reassure an anxious client.

The nurse should begin discussion of discharge planning with the client and family. The family should be instructed to examine the home for any obstacles which could cause a fall, such as scatter rugs and electric cords. The duration of the hospital stay and the expected postoperative events should be discussed so that the client and family can plan ahead.

The general postoperative care for a surgical client is appropriate (see Chap. 8). The nerve and circulatory status of the operated areas should be assessed every hour for the first 24 hours. Anesthesia, parasthesias, coldness, pallor, excessive pain, and swelling should be reported immediately to the surgeon. Specific directions related to activity and positioning should be followed carefully. Nursing measures for pain control such as massage, positioning, and distraction should be used in addition to pain

Table 57-16
Nursing Care Plan for the Client Undergoing Joint Surgery

Client Problem	Expected Outcome	Nursing Intervention
		Acute Intervention
Limitation of movement	Functional ROM of operated joint	Begin exercise program as directed. Cooperate with physical therapist to increase client compliance. Give pain medication prior to exercise.
Pain	Minimal pain on movement of operated joint	Give pain medication as ordered. Use nursing measures to relieve pain such as massage, positioning, distraction.
Edema	No evidence of nerve damage or circulatory impairment	Assess neurovascular status q h × 24 h, then q 4 h. Instruct client to report any sensory or motor changes in involved extremity.
Potential adrenal insufficiency (secondary to long-term steroid therapy)	No evidence of postoperative adrenal insufficiency (e.g., peripheral circulatory collapse)	Administer additional steroid doses preoperatively and postoperatively as ordered. Monitor vital signs q h first 24 h then q 4 h.
Potential infection	No evidence of infection (fever, increased pain, or drainage)	Monitor vital signs q 4 h. Assess dressing for amount and character of drainage q 4 h. Assess level of pain. Use strict aseptic technique for dressing changes.
		Rehabilitative Management
Modification of ADL	Appropriate modifications made in occupation and recreation	Make clear to client that joint surgery does not alter underlying disease process. Assist him to identify activities which require modification. Refer for vocational counseling if indicated.
Limitation of function and strength	Acceptance and adjustment to limitations of function and strength	Discuss realistic posoperative expectations with client. Identify possible areas requiring adjustments. Initiate visiting nurse referral.

medication. Careful timing of exercise activity to follow pain medication will improve client cooperation in the necessary procedures. The family should be encouraged to accompany the client to the physical therapy department to observe his exercise program and offer support and encouragement. The nurse should consult regularly with the physical therapist on ways to implement the exercise program on the nursing unit.

The nurse should be alert for the possible need for referral prior to discharge. A social worker may be able to assist the client with transportation and financial concerns. A visiting nurse can ease the transition from hospital to home and provide both physical and emotional support to the client and family. Since many surgical procedures require long-term exercise programs, the visiting nurse can monitor this program and assess and refer any problems which arise.

The client should be instructed on specific complications to report, including infection (fever, increased pain and drainage), and dislocation of the prosthesis (pain, loss of function, shortening or malalignment of an extremity). The client should clearly understand the need to continue medical supervision for the underlying disease process as well as the need for postoperative follow-up by the surgeon. Specific nursing intervention related to joint surgery is summarized in Table 57-16.

Case Study / Rheumatoid Arthritis

Mrs. Betty M. is a 36-year-old, obese, white, married homemaker who has rheumatoid arthritis. Mrs. M. has three children aged 4, 7, and 10. Her husband Jack is a truck driver who works steady nights. About a year ago she noticed that her hands and feet were painful and some of the small joints were swollen. Some mornings she found it rather hard to get out of bed because she felt generally tired and stiff. She also thought at times that she was running a slight fever. Only when her symptoms began to interfere with her activities to such an extent that her friends began to notice did she seek help. By this time she was having increased pain and stiffness, and her hands at times were so swollen that she could not open jars or work in the yard without great difficulty.

Mrs. M. was admitted to the hospital for evaluation and a comprehensive treatment program. She stated on admission that she had arthritis but did not know what type. Her medication program consisted of the following: Ascriptin iii qid and indomethacin 75 mg. h.s. Gold injections were being considered. She was wearing a copper bracelet that her neighbor gave her to wear upon hearing of her recent diagnosis of arthritis. She also stated that for the past year she had been taking "arthritis strength" Anacin that she saw advertised on television for "aches and pains of arthritis" because her symptoms sounded similar.

Discussion Questions

1. How might the nurse explain the pathophysiology of RA to Mrs. M.?
2. What manifestations did Mrs. M. experience which suggested the diagnosis of RA?
3. What results may be expected of gold therapy? What are the nursing responsibilities related to gold therapy?
4. What are some suggestions that may be offered concerning home management and joint protection?
5. How can the nurse help Mrs. M. to recognize ineffective, unproven methods of treatment?
6. What other sources of information regarding arthritis might the nurse suggest to Mrs. M.?

REVIEW QUESTIONS

The number of the question corresponds to the same-numbered objective at the beginning of the chapter.

1. A common manifestation of degenerative joint disease is
   a. fever
   b. fatigue
   c. pain
   d. elevated ESR

2. The most common site of muscle weakness in polymyositis is the
   a. chest and thorax
   b. shoulder and pelvic girdle
   c. upper legs and hips
   d. knees and ankles

3. The final stage in the pathogenesis of rheumatoid arthritis is
   a. fibrous ankylosis
   b. pannus formation
   c. bony ankylosis
   d. synovitis

4. Degenerative joint disease is characterized by
   a. systemic joint manifestations
   b. usually overweight client
   c. presence of sepsis
   d. anemia

5. When caring for the client with SLE, the nurse should
   a. observe for CNS involvement
   b. monitor and record fever pattern
   c. assess limitation of movement
   d. all the above

6. The purpose of a synovectomy is to
   a. prevent further joint damage
   b. ankylose a joint

c. correct a deformity
d. replace a joint

7. Prior to surgery, the client with rheumatoid arthritis should have
   a. a cardiovascular and respiratory assessment
   b. a low ESR
   c. an assessment of steroid use
   d. all the above

8. Drugs commonly used in the treatment of rheumatoid arthritis include all the following *except*
   a. penicillamine
   b. antibiotics
   c. aspirin
   d. corticosteroids

REFERENCES

1. D. S. Howell et al., "A View on the Pathogenesis of Osteoarthritis," *Bull Rheum Dis,* **29**:996–1000, (1979).
2. R.W. Moskowitz, "Management of Osteoarthritis," *Hosp Pract,* **14**:75–86, July 1979.
3. N. J. Zvaifler, "Etiology and Pathogenesis of Rheumatoid Arthritis," in D. J. McCarty (ed.), *Arthritis and Allied Conditions: A Textbook of Rheumatology*, 9th ed., Lea & Febiger, Philadelphia, 1979, chap. 28, pp. 417–428.
4. A. T. Masi and T. A. Medsger, Jr., "Epidemiology of the Rheumatic Diseases," in D. J. McCarty (ed.), *Arthritis and Allied Conditions: A Textbook of Rheumatology,* 9th ed., Lea & Febiger, Philadelphia, 1979, chap. 3, pp. 11–35.
5. R. Wallace et al., *Staff Manual for Teaching Patients about Rheumatoid Arthritis*, American Hospital Association, Chicago, 1980.
6. *An Interdisciplinary Educational Program for Patients with Rheumatic Diseases: A Guide for Professional Staff,* Columbia Hospital, Milwaukee,1980.
7. H. Gruen and B. Wingert, *Joint Protection and Energy Conservation for the Early Rheumatoid Arthritis Patient*, Graphics Plus Associates, 1980.
8. J. J. Calabro et al., "Juvenile Rheumatoid Arthritis: A General Review and Report of 100 Patients Observed for 15 Years," *Semin Arthritis Rheum,* **5**:257–298 (1976).
9. J. G. Schaller, "Juvenile Rheumatoid Arthritis," *Arthritis Rheum,* **20** (2, Suppl.): 165–170 (1977).
10. R. Bluestone, *Histocompatibility Antigens and Rheumatic Diseases: Current Concepts*, Upjohn Company, Kalamazoo, Mich., 1978.
11. D. A. Brewerton et al., "Ankylosing Spondylitis and HLA-27," *Lancet,* **1**:904–907 (1973).
12. D. H. Neustadt, "Symposium on Ankylosing Spondylitis," *Postgrad Med,* **61**:124–135 (1977).
13. J. M. H. Moll and V. Wright, "Psoriatic Arthritis," *Semin Arthritis Rheum,* **3**:55–78 (1973).
14. V. Wright, "Arthritis Associated with Venereal Disease: A Comparative Study of Gonococcal Arthritis and Reiter's Syndrome," *Ann Rheum Dis,* **22**:77–90 (1963).
15. D. L. Goldenberg and A. S. Cohen "Acute Infectious Arthritis," *Am J Med,* **60**:369–378 (1976).
16. J. B. Wyngaarden and W. N. Kelley, *Gout and Hyperuricemia,* Grune & Stratton, Inc., New York, 1976.
17. M. J. Maclachlan and G. P. Rodnan, "Effects of Food, Fast and Alcohol on Serum Uric Acid and Acute Attacks of Gout," *Am J Med,* **42**:38–57 (1967).
18. E. L. Dubois, *Lupus Erythematosus*, University of Southern California Press, Los Angeles, 1974.
19. M. M. Hargraves et al., "Presentation of Two Bone Marrow Elements: The "tart cell" and the "LE cell," *Mayo Clin Proc,* **23**:25 (1948).
20. A. T. Masi and T. A. Medsger, Jr., "Epidemiology of Various Arthritis Conditions," in A. S. Cohen (ed.), *Science and Practice of Clinical Medicine*, vol. 4, Grune & Stratton, Inc., New York, 1979, p. 66.
21. A. T. Masi and T. A. Medsger, Jr., "Epidemiology of Rheumatic Diseases," in D. J. McCarty (ed.), *Arthritis and Allied Conditions: A Textbook of Rheumatology*, 9th ed., Lea & Febiger, Philadelphia, 1979, chap. 3, pp. 11–35.
22. E. Ginsberg, H. Diamond, and the Lupus Survival Study Group, "A Multicenter study of Survival in systemic lupus erythematosus (SLE)," *Arthritis Rheum,* **22**:613 (1979).
23. J. Zulman et al., "Problems Associated with the Management of Pregnancies in Patients with Systemic Lupus Erythematosus," *J Rheumatol,* **7**:1 (1980).
24. G. P. Rodnan, "Progressive Systemic Sclerosis (Scleroderma)," in D. J. McCarty (ed.), *Arthritis and Allied Conditions: A Textbook of Rheumatology*, 9th ed., Lea & Febiger, Philadelphia, 1979, chap. 53, pp. 762–809.
25. T. A. Medsger, Jr., and A. T. Masi, "Epidemiology of Systemic Sclerosis (Scleroderma)," *Ann Intern Med,* **74**:714–721 (1971).
26. W. A. D'Angelo et al., "Pathologic Observation in Systemic Sclerosis (Scleroderma): A Study of 58 Autopsy Cases and 58 Controls," *Am J Med,* **46**:428–440 (1969).
27. T. A. Medsger, Jr., "Systemic Sclerosis," in J. F. Fries and G. E. Ehrlich (eds.), *Prognosis: Contemporary Outcomes of Disease,* Charles Press Publishers, Bowie, Md., 1981, chap. 104.
28. C. M. Pearson, "Polymyositis and Dermatomyositis," in D. J. McCarty (ed.), *Arthritis and Allied Conditions: A Textbook of Rheumatology*, 9th ed., Lea & Febiger, Philadelphia, 1979, chap. 52, pp. 742–761.
29. M. A. Shearn, *Sjögren's Syndrome*, W. B. Saunders Company, Philadelphia, 1971.
30. G. C. Sharp et al., "Mixed Connective Tissue Disease," *Am J Med,* **52**:148–159 (1972).
31. A. S. Cohen, "Amyloidosis," *N Engl J Med,* **277**:522– 530 (1967).
32. P. S. Walker, "Human Joints and Their Replacement," Charles C Thomas, Publisher, Springfield, Ill. 1977, p. 253.
33. V. Wright, "Rheumatoid Arthritis—Surgical Treatment," *Nurs Times*, Dec. 15, 1977.

BIBLIOGRAPHY FOR SECTION 10

Neurological

Books

Adams, R., and M. Victor: *Principles of Neurology*, McGraw-Hill Book Company, New York, 1977.

Albanese, J.: *Nurses' Drug Reference*, McGraw-Hill Book Company, New York, 1979.

American Heart Association, *Diagnosis and Management of Stroke*, Dallas, 1979.

———: *Heart Facts: 1980*, Dallas, 1979.

Becker, D. P., et al.: "Head Injury Management," in A. J.

Popp et al. (eds.), *Neural Trauma*, Raven Press, New York, 1979.

Bonica, J. J. (ed.): *Pain Overview 1980*, HP Publishing, New York, 1980.

Boroch, R. M.: *Elements of Rehabilitation Nursing: An Introduction*, The C. V. Mosby Company, St. Louis, 1976.

Chusid, J.: *Correlative Neuroanatomy and Functional Neurology*, Lange Medical Publications, Los Altos, Calif.,1976.

Conway, B. L. (ed.): *Carini and Owens' Neurological and Neurosurgical Nursing*, The C. V. Mosby Company, St. Louis, 1978.

Cooper, I. S.: *Living with Chronic Neurologic Disease*, W. W. Norton & Company, Inc., New York, 1976.

Core Curriculum, American Association of Neurosurgical Nurses, Baltimore, 1977.

DeMyer, W.: *Technique of the Neurologic Examination*, McGraw-Hill Book Company, New York, 1980.

Duvoisin, R.: *Parkinson's Disease: A Guide for Patient and Family*, Raven Press, New York, 1978.

Farquhar, J. W.: *The American Way of Life Need Not be Hazardous to Your Health*, W. W. Norton & Company, Inc., New York, 1978.

Friedman, A.: "Headache," in A. B. Baker and L. H. Baker (eds.), *Clinical Neurology*, Harper & Row, Publishers, Incorporated, New York, 1979.

Goldberg, S.: *Neuroanatomy Made Ridiculously Simple*, Med Master, Inc., Miami, 1979.

Goldenson, R. M. (ed.): *Disability and Rehabilitation Handbook*, McGraw-Hill Book Company, New York, 1978.

Hale, G. (ed.): *The Source Book for the Disabled*, Imprint Books, New York, 1979.

Hickey, J.: *The Clinical Practice of Neurological and Neurosurgical Nursing*, J. B. Lippincott Company, Philadelphia, 1981.

Holloway, N.: *Nursing the Critically Ill Adult*, Addison-Wesley Publishing Company, Inc., Menlo Park, Calif., 1979.

House, E. L., et al.: *A Systematic Approach to Neuroscience*, 3d ed., McGraw-Hill Book Company, New York, 1979.

Hunt, W.: "Spinal Cord Injury and Outcome," in A. J. Popp et al. (eds.), *Neural Trauma*, Raven Press, New York, 1979, pp. 201–204.

Jacox, A. E.: *Pain: A Source Book for Nurses and Other Health Professionals*, Little, Brown & Company, Boston, 1977.

Krause, M. V., and L. K. Mahan: *Food, Nutrition and Diet Therapy*, 6th ed., W. B. Saunders Company, Philadelphia, 1979.

Matthews, W. B.: *Multiple Sclerosis: The Facts*, Oxford University Press, New York, 1978.

McCaffery, M.: *Nursing Management of the Patient with Pain*, J. B. Lippincott Company, Philadelphia, 1979.

Medical Clinics of North America, *Headaches and Related Pain Syndromes*, W. B. Saunders Company, Philadelphia, 1978.

Mooney, T., et al.: *Sexual Options for Paraplegics and Quadriplegics*, Little, Brown and Company, Boston, 1975.

Mossman, P. L.: *A Problem-Oriented Approach to Stroke Rehabilitation*, Charles C Thomas, Publisher, Springfield, Ill., 1976.

O'Brien, M. I., and P. J. Pallett: *Total Care of the Stroke Patient*, Little, Brown and Company, Boston, 1978.

Pierce, D., and V. Nickle: *The Total Care of Spinal Cord Injuries*, Little, Brown and Company, Boston, 1977.

Plum, F., and J. Posner: *Diagnosis of Stupor and Coma*, 2d ed., F. A. Davis Company, Philadelphia, 1978.

——— et al.: "Surgical Intervention in Spinal Cord Injury," in A. J. Popp et al. (eds.), *Neural Trauma*, Raven Press, New York, 1979.

Restak, R. M.: *The Brain: The Last Frontier*, Doubleday & Company, Inc., Garden City, N.Y., 1979.

Rusk, H. A.: *Rehabilitation Medicine*, 4th ed., The C. V. Mosby Company, St. Louis, 1977.

Sahs, A. L., et al.: *Guidelines for Stroke Care*. U.S. Department of Health, Education and Welfare, 1976.

Sands, H., and F. Minters: *The Epilepsy Fact Book*, F. A. Davis Company, Philadelphia, 1979.

Sine, R. D., et al. (eds.): *Basic Rehabilitation Techniques: A Self-Instructional Guide*, Aspen, Germantown, Md., 1977.

Solomon, G., and F. Plum: *Clinical Management of Seizures*, W. B. Saunders Company, Philadelphia, 1976.

Sternback, R.: *The Psychology of Pain*, Raven Press, New York, 1978.

Svoboda, W.: *Learning About Epilepsy*, University Park Press, Baltimore, 1979.

Tator, C.: "Spinal Cord Cooling and Irrigation for Treatment of Acute Cord Injury," in A. J. Popp et al. (eds.), *Neural Trauma*, Raven Press, New York, 1979, p. 363–369.

U.S. Department of Health, Education and Welfare, *Healthy People: The Surgeon General's Report on Health Promotion and Disease*, 1979.

Willman, V. L., and H. B. Barnes: "Carotid Occlusive Disease," in D. C. Sabiston (ed.), *Textbook of Surgery: The Biological Basis of Modern Surgical Practice*, 11th ed., W. B. Saunders Company, Philadelphia, 1977.

Wittrock, M. C., et al.: *The Human Brain*, Prentice-Hall, Inc., Englewood Cliffs, N.J., 1977.

Periodicals

Adolphus, P.: "Sunnybrook Stroke Team: An Innovative Experience," *Can Nurse,* **72:**16 (1976).

Allmond, J.: "Management of Cervical and Thoracic Spine/Cord Injured Patients," *J Neurosurg Nurs,* **13**(2):97–101 (April 1981).

Altshuler, A., and J. Meyer: "Clean Intermittent Self Catheterization," *Crit Care Update,* **6:**8–11 (April 1979).

Anderson, D. C., and R. D. Cranford: "Corticosteroids in Ischemic Stroke," *Stroke,* **13:**19 (1978).

Anderson, T. P., et al.: "Quality of Care for Completed Stroke without Rehabilitation: Evaluation by Assessing Patient Outcomes," *Arch Phys Med Rehabil,* **60:**96 (1979).

Armstrong, M.: "Current Concepts in Pain," *AORN J,* **32:**383 (September 1980).

Arseenault, L.: "Primary Spinal Cord Tumors: A Review and Case Presentation of a Patient with an Intramedullary Spinal Cord Neoplasm," *J Neurosurg Nurs,* **13**(2):53–58 (April 1981).

Bahrenda, E.: "Superficial Temporal Artery Anastomosis to the Middle Cerebral Artery (STA-MCA)," *J Neurosurg Nurs,* **8:**113 (1976).

Bassler, S. F.: "Achieving Continuity of Care for the Spinal Cord Injured Patient through the Problem-Oriented Approach," *J Neurosurg Nurs,* **13**(2):61–71 (April 1981).

Beeken, J.: "Body Image Changes in Plegia," *J Neurosurg Nurs,* **10:**20–23 (March 1978).

Benvenuti, C. S.: "Independence for the Quadriplegic: The Bantam Respirator," *Am J Nurs,* **79:**918–920 (May 1979).

Berkman, A., et al.: "Sexual Adjustment of the Spinal Cord Injured Veterans Living in the Community," *Arch Phys Med Rehabil,* **59:**29–33 (January 1978).

Bishop, B.: "Pain: Its Physiology and Rationale for Management," *Phys Ther,* **60:**14 (January 1980).

Breu, C., and K. Dracup: "Helping the Spouses of Critically Ill Patients," *Am J Nurs,* **78:**50 (1978).

Buckley, J. E., et al.: "Feeding Patients with Dysphagia," *Nurs Forum,* **15:**69 (1976).

Caronna, J. J., and S. Finkelstein: "Neurological Syndrome after Cardiac Arrest," *Stroke,* **13:**9 (1978).

Catanzaro, M.: "Multiple Sclerosis: Exploding Myths That Compromise Patient Care," *RN,* **40**(12):42 (December 1977).

Cole, C. M.: "The Role of Brief Family Therapy in Medical Rehabilitation," *J Rehabil,* **44:**29 (1978).

Cook, D. W.: "Psychological Aspects of Spinal Cord Injury," *Rehabil Counseling Bull,* **19:**535–543 (1976).

Crewe, N., et al.: "Spinal Cord Injury: A Comparison of Preinjury and Post Injury Marriages," *Arch Phys Med Rehabil,* **60:**252–256 (June 1979).

Cummings, D.: "Stopping Chronic Pain before It Starts," *Nursing,* **11:**60 (January 1981).

Cutting, J., et al.: "Tetanus: Not Too Rare To Be Wary of," *Patient Care,* **13**(7):178–193 (Apr. 30, 1979).

Daley, T. J., and E. R. Greenspun: "Stress Management through Hypnosis," *Topics Clin Nurs,* **1:**59 (April 1979).

David, A., et al.: "Survival in Marriage in the Paraplegic Couple: Psychological Study," *Paraplegia,* **15:**198–201 (1977–1978).

DeJesus-Greenberg, D.: "Acute Spinal Cord Injury and Hyperbaric O_2 Therapy: A New Adjunct in Management," *J Neurosurg Nurs,* **12**(3):155–160 (September 1980).

Dyken, M. L.: "Assessment of the Role of Antiplatelet Aggregating Agents in Transient Ischemic Attacks, Stroke, and Death," *Stroke,* **14:**9 (1979).

Edmonds, V.: "The Role of Laboratory Research in the Clinical Treatment of Acute Spinal Cord Injuries," *J Neurosurg Nurs,* **10**(13):18–21 (July 1976).

———: "Electrophysiologic Analysis of the Motor System after Stroke: The Suppressive Effect of Vibration," *Arch Phys Med Rehabil,* **60:**13 (1979).

Feustel, D.: "Autonomic Hyperreflexia," *Am J Nurs,* **76:**228–230 (January 1976).

Fisher, M., et al.: "Electrophysiologic Analysis of the Motor System after Stroke: The Flexor Reflex," *Arch Phys Med Rehabil,* **60:**4 (1979).

Frost, M.: "The Importance of Being Ernest," *Nurs Times,* **75**(31):1329 (Aug. 2, 1979).

Gillingham, F. J., et al.: "Acute Cervical Spinal Cord Injury: Early Management and Long Term Results," *Acta Neurochir (Wien),* **41:**73–85 (1978).

Gilmor, R.: "Computerized Axial Tomography in Head Trauma," *Crit Care Q,* **2**(10):61–66 (June 1979).

Goldstone, J., and W. S. Moore: "A New Look at Emergency Carotid Artery Operations for the Treatment of Cerebrovascular Insufficiency," *Stroke,* **13:**15 (1978).

Goloskov, J., et al.: "The Role of the Nurse in Quantitative Intracranial Pressure Determinations," *J Neurosurg Nurs,* **10**(1):17–19 (March 1978).

———and P. Leroy: "The Role of the Nurse in the Treatment of Chronic Intractable Pain," *J Neurosurg Nurs,* **7:**107 (December 1975).

———and———: "Use of Dorsal Column Stimulator," *Am J Nurs,* **74:**506 (March 1974).

Graham, H., et al.: "Epidemiologic Profile of Long-Term Stroke Disability: The Framingham Study," *Arch Phys Med Rehabil,* **60:**487 (1979).

Granger, V. C., et al.: "Stroke Rehabilitation: Analysis of Repeated Barthel Index Measures," *Arch Phys Med Rehabil,* **60:**14 (1979).

Haerer, A.: "Coma: Some Differential Considerations in the Diagnosis and Management," *Hosp Med,* **2**(4):68 (April 1976).

Haring, M., and L. Meyerson: "Attitudes of College Students toward Sexual Behavior of Disabled Persons," *Arch Phys Med Rehabil,* **60:** 260–262 (June 1979).

Headache, **19**(3) (1979). (Official Publication of the American Association for the Study of Headache.)

Hinterbuchner, L.: "Evaluation of the Unconscious Patient," *Hosp Med,* **13**(2):83 (February 1977).

Holbach, K. H., et al.: "The Use of Hyperbaric Oxygenation in the Treatment of Spinal Cord Lesions," *Eur Neurol,* **16:**213–221 (1976).

Huffman, A. L.: "Biofeedback Treatment of Orofacial Dysfunction: A Preliminary Study," *Am J Occup Ther,* **32:**149 (1978).

Isaacs, N.: "The Treatment of Acute Spinal Cord Injury Using Local Hypothermia," *J Neurosurg Nurs,* **10**(3):95–101 (September 1978).

Jacobs, S., and J. Kaufman: "Complications of Permanent Bladder Catheter Drainage in Spinal Cord Injured Patients," *J Urol,* **119:**740–741 (June 1978).

Jacox, A. E.: "Assessing Pain," *Am J Nurs,* **79:**895 (May 1979).

Johnson, A., et al. "Help for the Patient with Facial Pain," *Patient Care,* **11:**46–58 (May 1, 1977).

———et al.: "Meeting Three Severe Neurologic Challenges," *Patient Care,* **11:**128–129 (June 1, 1977).

Kamelhar, D., et al.: "Plasma Renin and Serum Dopamine-Beta-Hydroxylase during Orthostatic Hypotension in Quadriplegic Man," *Arch Phys Med Rehabil,* **59:**212–216 (May 1978).

Kannel, W. B.: "A General Cardiovascular Risk Profile: The Framingham Study," *Am J Cardiol,* **38:**46 (1976).

Kerber, C.: "Use of Balloon Catheters in the Treatment of Cranial Arterial Abnormalities," *Stroke,* **14:**13 (1979).

Kinash, R.: "Experiences and Nursing Needs of Spinal Cord Injured Patients," *J Neurosurg Nurs,* **10:**29–32 (March 1978).

Kline, D., et al.: "The Battered Brain," *Emerg Med,* **11**(3):15–32 (Mar. 15, 1979).

Kolb, D.: "Understanding Aphasia and the Aphasic," *J Neurosurg Nurs,* **9:**15 (1977).

Kunkel, J., and J. Wiley: "Acute Head Injury: What to do When . . . and Why," *Nursing,* **9**(3):23–33 (March 1979).

Langan, R.: "Parkinson's Disease: Assessment Procedures and Guidelines for Counseling," *Nurse Pract,* **2:**13–16 (November–December 1976).

Laws, E. R.: "An Injured Skull," *Emerg Med,* **7**(1):219–235 (January 1975).

Lawson, N. C.: "Significant Events in the Rehabilitation Process: The Spinal Cord Patient's Point of View," *Arch Phys Med Rehabil,* **59:**573–579 (December 1978).

MacVicar, M. G., and P. Archbold: "A Framework for Family Assessment in Chronic Illness," *Nurs Forum,* **15:**180 (1976).

Maury, M.: "About Pain and Its Treatment in Paraplegia," *Paraplegia,* **15:**349–352 (1977–1978).

McCaffery, M.: "Patients Shouldn't Have To Suffer: How To Relieve Pain," *Nursing,* **10:**34 (October 1980).

———: "Relieve Your Patients' Pain Fast and Effectively with Oral Analgesics," *Nursing,* **10:**58 (November 1980).

———: "Relieving Pain with Noninvasive Techniques," *Nursing,* **10:**55 (December 1980).

———: "Understanding Your Patient's Pain," *Nursing,* **10:**26 (September 1980).

McOuat, F.: "The Insidious Spinal Cord Tumor," *J Neurosurg Nurs,* **13**(1):18–22 (February 1981).

Melnyk, B. A., et al.: "Attitude Changes Following a Sexual Counseling Program for Spinal Cord Injured Persons," *Arch Phys Med Rehabil,* **60:**601–604 (December 1979).

Middaugh, J. P.: "Side Effects of Diptheria-Tetanus Toxoid in Adults," *Am J Public Health,* **69**(3):246–249 (March 1979).

Miller, L. S., and A. T. Mujamoto: "Computed Tomography: Its Potential as a Predictor of Functional Recovery Following Stroke," *Arch Phys Med Rehabil,* **60:**108 (1979).

Mills, N., and P. Hiram: "Guillain-Barré Syndrome: A Framework for Nursing Care," *Nurs Clin North Am,* **15**(2):257–264 (June 1980).

Mitchell, P., and N. Morse: "Intracranial Pressure: Fact and Fancy," *Nursing,* **6**(6):53–57 (June 1976).

"Multiple Sclerosis" (continuing education course), *Am J Nurs,* **8:**273 (February 1980).

Munley, M. J., and M. C. Keane: "Impressions of Pain: A Nursing Diagnosis," *Nurs Clin North Am,* **12:**609 (December 1978).

Pallant, C.: "Acute Nursing Care in the Stroke Unit," *Can Nurse,* **72:**18 (1976).

Pepper, G.: "The Person with a Spinal Cord Injury: Psychological Care," *Am J Nurs,* **77:**1326–1330 (August 1977).

Quest, D. O.: "Dehydrating Agents Commonly Used in Neurosurgery: Advantages and Disadvantages," *J Neurosurg Nurs,* **11:**141 (1979).

Ransohoff, J., and A. Fleischer: "Insult and Injury: Head Injuries," *Emerg Med,* **7**(4):147–151 (April 1975).

Reinmuth, O. M.: "Intracranial Bypass Surgery for Cerebral Artery Diseases and the Responsibility of the Practicing Physician," *Stroke,* **14:**1 (1979).

——— et al.: "Stroke," *Patient Care,* **10:**68–73 (Apr. 1, 1976).

Ricci, M. M.: "Intracranial Hypertension: Barbiturate Therapy and the Role of the Nurse," *J Neurosurg Nurs,* **11:**247 (1979).

Rodman, M.: "How To Coax Maximum Pain Relief from Standard Drugs," *RN,* **43:**83 (September 1980).

Roglitz, C.: "Team Approach in the Acute Phase of Spinal Cord Injury," *J Neurosurg Nurs,* **10**(3):117–120 (September 1978).

Rusinski, P. S.: "Neurological Assessment of the Hemiplegic Patient," *Nurse Pract,* **4:**26 (1979).

Sather, M., et al.: "Pressure Sores and the Spinal Cord Injury Patient," *Drug Intell Clin Pharm,* **78:**155–168 (March 1978).

Schwartzman, S. T.: "Anxiety and Depression in the Stroke Patient: A Nursing Challenge," *J Psychiatr Nurs,* **14:**13 (1976).

Shields, C. B.: "Cerebral Revascularization," *AORN J,* **27:**909 (1978).

Shoenfeld, Y., et al.: "Orthostatic Hypotension in Amputees and Subjects with Spinal Cord Injuries," *Arch Phys Med Rehabil,* **59:**138–141 (March 1978).

Shontz, F.: "Psychological Adjustment to Physical Disability: Trends in Theories," *Arch Phys Med Rehabil,* **59:**251–254 (June 1978).

Silverman, E. M., and I. R. Elfant: "Dysphagia: An Evaluation and Treatment Program for the Adult," *Am J Occup Ther,* **33:**382 (1979).

Simmons, S. A.: "Evaluating Hidden Intracerebral Bleeds," *J Emerg Nurs,* **4:**9 (1978).

Snyder, J., and D. Powner: "Considerations in the Medical Care of Neurologically Impaired Patients," *Heart Lung,* **8**(6):1065–1072 (November–December 1979).

Spielman, G.: "Cerebral Vasospasm Following Subarachnoid Hemorrhage," *Crit Care Q,* **2:**77 (1979).

Standish, V., and W. S. Welborn: "Evaluating the Unconscious Patient," *Patient Care,* **12**(3):158–172 (Feb. 15, 1978).

Sweeney, S. S.: "OR Observation: Key to Postop Pain," *AORN J,* **32:**391 (September 1980).

Teasdale, G., and B. Jennett: "Assessment of Coma and Impaired Consciousness: A Practical Scale," *Lancet,* **2:**81–84 (July 13, 1974).

Turner, M.: "Intracranial Hypertension," *Crit Care Q,* **2:**67 (1979).

Tyson, G., et al.: "Acute Care of the Head-Injured Patient," *Crit Care Q,* **2**(1):23–44 (June 1979).

Wahl, S.: "Only a Concussion," *Nursing,* **6**(8):44–45 (August 1976).

Wahlquist, G. I.: "Regaining Urinary Continence through Intermittent Catheterization," *J Neurosurg Nurs,* **12**(2):73–75 (June 1980).

Webb, S. B., et al.: "Spinal Cord Injury: Epidemiologic Implications, Costs and Patterns of Care in 85 Patients," *Arch Phys Med Rehabil,* **60**(8):335–338 (August 1979).

Weinberg, N., and J. Williams: "How the Physically Disabled Perceive Their Disabilities," *J Rehabil,* **44:**31 (1978).

West, B. A.: "Understanding Endorphins: Our Natural Pain Relief System," *Nursing,* **11:**50 (February 1981).

Wiley, L.: "Pitfalls of Emotional Involvement: Sympathetic Nursing Care of a Patient with Cervical Spine Injury," *Nursing '76,*, **6:**42–47 (1976).

Wolf, S. L., et al.: "EMG Biofeedback in Stroke: Effect of Patient Characteristics," *Arch Phys Med Rehabil,* **60:**96 (1979).

Wolf, Z. R. (ed.): "Pain Management," *Topics Clin Nurs,* **2:**1 (April 1980).

Yashon, D.: "Pathogenesis of Spinal Cord Injury," *Orthop Clin North Am,* **9**(2):247–261 (April 1978).

Unpublished

Yatsu, F. M., et al.: "Prevention and Diagnosis of Stroke: A Circuit Course Program," School of Medicine, University of Oregon Health Science Center, Portland, 1978.

———: "Syllabus: First Annual Update on Current Concepts of Stroke," Comprehensive Stroke Program of Oregon, Portland, 1979.

Pamphlets

Pamphlets available from the American Heart Association for the instruction of clients and their families:

"Aphasia and the Family"
"Body Language"
"Do It Yourself Again: Self-Help"
"Devices for the Stroke Patient"
"Facts about Strokes"
"Strokes: A Guide for the Family"
"Stroke: Why Do They Behave That Way?"

Organizations

ALS Society of America, 12011 San Vicente Blvd., Suite 350, Box 49001, Los Angeles, CA 90049

American Parkinson's Disease Association, Inc., 147 E. 50 Street, Suite 103, New York, NY 10022

Committee To Combat Huntington's Disease, 250 W. 57 Street, Suite 2016, New York, NY 10019

Epilepsy Foundation of America, 1828 L Street, N.W., Suite 406, Washington, D.C. 20036

Institute of Rehabilitation Medicine, 400 E. 34 Street, New York, NY 10016

Muscular Dystrophy Association of America, Inc., 1790 Broadway, New York, NY 10019

Muscular Dystrophy Association, Inc., 810 Seventh Avenue, New York, NY 10019

Myasthenia Gravis Foundation, Inc., New York Academy of Medicine Building, 2 E. 103 Street, New York, NY 10029

Myasthenia Gravis Foundation, 15 E. 26 Street, New York, NY 10010

National ALS Foundation, Inc., 185 Madison Avenue, New York, NY 10016

National Council for Homemaker-Home Health Aide Services, Inc., 1740 Broadway, New York, NY 10019

National Easter Seal Society for Crippled Children and Adults, 2023 W. Ogden Avenue, Chicago, IL 60612

National Huntington's Disease Association, 1441 Broadway, Suite 501, New York, NY 10018

National Institute of Neurological Disease and Stroke, National Institutes of Health, Bethesda, MD 20014

National Multiple Sclerosis Society, 257 Park Avenue South, New York, NY 10010

National Paraplegia Foundation, 33 N. Michigan Avenue, Chicago, IL 60601

National Parkinson Foundation, 1501 N.W. Ninth Avenue, Miami, FL 31316

National Safety Council, 425 N. Michigan Avenue, Chicago, IL 60611

Office of Vocational Rehabilitation, U.S. Department of Health, Education and Welfare, Washington, D.C. 20402

Parkinson's Disease Foundation, Inc., William Black Medical Research Building, Columbia Presbyterian Medical Center, 640 W. 168 Street, New York, NY 10032

Rehabilitation Services Administration, Department of Health, Education and Welfare, 330 C Street S.W., Washington, D.C. 20201

United Cerebral Palsy Associations, Inc., 66 E. 34 Street, New York, NY 10016

United Parkinson Foundation, 220 S. State Street, Chicago, IL 60604

Musculoskeletal

Books

Adams, J. C.: *Outline of Fractures*, Churchill Livingstone, Edinburgh, 1978.

——— *Outline of Orthopaedics*, 8th ed., Churchill Livingstone, Edinburgh, 1976.

Aladjem, H.: *The Sun is My Enemy*, Prentice-Hall, Inc., Englewood Cliffs, N.J., 1972.

Aston, J. N.: *A Short Textbook of Orthopaedics and Traumatology*, 2d ed., J. B. Lippincott Company, Philadelphia, 1976.

Baldonado, A. F., and D. A. Stahl: *Cancer Nursing: A Holistic Multidisciplinary Approach*, Medical Examination Publishing Co., Inc., Garden City, N.Y., 1978.

Bates, B.: *A Guide to Physical Examination*, 2d ed., J. B. Lippincott Company, Philadelphia, 1979.

Blau, S. P. and D. Schultz: *Lupus, the Body Against Itself*, Doubleday & Company, Inc., Garden City, N.Y., 1977.

Blauvelt, C. T., and F. R. T. Nelson: *A Manual of Orthopaedic Terminology*, The C. V. Mosby Company, St. Louis, 1977.

Buck, B., and A. D. Lee: *Amputation: Two Views*, The Nursing Clinics of North America, W. B. Saunders Company, Philadelphia, 1976.

Burnside, K. R., et al.: *Health Assessment in Clinical Practice*, Prentice-Hall, Inc., Englewood Cliffs, N.J., 1980.

Caillet, R.: *Soft Tissue Pain and Disability*, F. A. Davis Company, Philadelphia, 1977.

Christensen, J. B., and I. R. Telford: *Synopsis of Gross Anatomy*, 3d ed., Harper & Row, Publishers, Incorporated, New York, 1978.

Cyriax, J.: *Textbook of Orthopaedic Medicine*, vol. 1: *Diagnosis of Soft Tissue Lesions*, Baillière, Tindall, London, 1978.

Farrell, J.: *Illustrated Guide to Orthopaedic Nursing*, J. B. Lippincott Company, Philadelphia, 1977.

Friedman, L. W.: *The Psychological Rehabilitation of the Amputee*, Charles C Thomas, Publisher, Springfield, Ill., 1978.

Fries, J. F.: *Arthritis: A Comprehensive Guide*, Addison-Wesley Publishing Company, Inc., Reading, Mass., 1979.

Hartman, T. J.: *Fracture Management: A Practical Approach*, Lea & Febiger, Philadelphia, 1978.

Hilt, N. E., et al.: *Manual of Orthopedics*, The C. V. Mosby Company, St. Louis, 1980.

Hollinshead, W. H.: *Functional Anatomy of the Limbs and Back*, W. B. Saunders Company, Philadelphia, 1976.

Implementing Patient Education in the Hospital, American Hospital Association, Chicago, 1979.

Lewis, R. C.: *Handbook of Traction, Casting and Splinting Techniques*, J. B. Lippincott Company, Philadelphia, 1977.

Malasanos, L., et al.: *Health Assessment*, The C. V. Mosby Company, St. Louis, 1977.

Melvin, J. L.: *Rheumatic Disease: Occupational Therapy and Rehabilitation*, F. A. Davis Company, Philadelphia, 1980.

Polley, H. F., and G. G. Hander: *Rheumatologic Interviewing and Physical Examination of the Joints*, 2d ed., W. B. Saunders Company, Philadelphia, 1978.

Ramamurti, R. P.: *Orthopaedics in Primary Care*, The Williams & Wilkins Company, Baltimore, 1979.

Rowe, J. W., and L. Dyer: *Care of the Orthopaedic Patient*, Blackwell Scientific Publications, Ltd., Oxford, 1977.

Self Help Manual for Patients with Arthritis, prepared by the Arthritis Health Professions Section of the Arthritis Foundation and published by the Foundation, Atlanta, 1980.

Turek, S. L.: *Orthopaedics—Principles and Their Application*, J. B. Lippincott Company, Philadelphia, 1977.

Zvaifler, J. N., and C. A. Robinson: *Rheumatoid Arthritis*, Disease-a-Month Yearbook, Medical Publishers, Inc., Chicago, 1974.

Periodicals

Armstrong, L., and R. Patterson: "Arthroscopy: A New Approach to Knee Surgery That Affects Patient Care," *RN*, **35:**39 (January 1978).

"Arthritis—A Two-Part Report," *Consumer Reports* (June and July 1979).

Bassett, C. L.: "Current Concepts of Bone Formation," *J Bone Joint Surg* [*Am*], **44A:**1217 (1962).

Bear, E. D., et al.: "Taking a Health History," *Am J Nurs*, **77:**1190–1193 (July 1977).

Bowden, S.: "New Surgery for Arthritic Hands," *Nursing,* **6:**46 (August 1976).
Brown-Skeers, V.: "How the Nurse Practitioner Manages the Rheumatoid Arthritis Patient," *Nursing,* **9:**26 (June 1979).
Chamberlain, M. A.: "Aids and Equipment for the Arthritic," *Practitioner,* **224:**65–71 (1980).
Craven, R. F., and T. D. Curry: "When the Diagnosis is Raynaud's," *Am J Nurs,* **81:**1007–1009 (May 1981).
Deyerle, W. M., and S. A. Grossland: "Broken Legs Are To Be Walked on," *Am J Nurs,* **77:**31 (December 1977).
Eggland, E. T.: "How To Take a Meaningful History," *Nursing '77,* **22:**30 (July 1977).
Ehrlich, G.: "Arthritis Management—Treating Rheumatoid Arthritis with Behavioral and Clinical Strategy," *Nurs Digest,* **4:**24 (Winter 1976).
Figley, B. A., et al.: "Human Sexuality: A Comprehensive Approach to Sexual Health in Rheumatic Disease," *Topics Clin Nurs,* **1:**69 (January 1980).
Gallagher, L. L.: "When Your Patient Has a Shoulder Arthroplasty: Here's How To Help," *Nursing,* **10:**46–49 (July 1980).
Gever, L. N.: "Reducing the Side Effects of Steroid Therapy," *Nursing,* **10:**59 (September 1980).
Good, A. B.: "Reiter's Disease," *Postgrad Med,* **61:**153, 1977.
Hudak, C.: "A Pyramidal Treatment Plan for the Patient with Arthritis," *Nurse Pract,* **2:**19 (May–June 1977).
Irby, R.: "Diagnostic Tests That Identify Connective Tissue Diseases," *Consultant,* **18:**157 (October 1978).
Janul, L. C.: "Polymyositis-Dermatomyositis: A Perplexing Disorder," *Am J Nurs,* **77:**1184 (1977).
Koffler, D.: "The Immunology of Rheumatoid Diseases," *Clin Symp,* **31:**2–36 (1979).
———: "Systemic Lupus Erythematosus," *Scientific American,* **243:**94–102 (August 1980).
———: "The Management of Gout," *Hosp Pract,* **14:**75 (1979).
Mignogna, S. L.: "Specialized Needs of the Immobilized Patient," *Nursing Care,* **11**(1):26–35 (January 1978).
Millard, L.: "Low Back Pain: Guide to Evaluation," *Hosp Med* **14:**79–90 (September 1978).
Moore, T. M., M. H. Myers, and J. P. Harvery: "Collateral Ligament Laxity of the Knee," *J Bone Joint Surg,* **58A**(5):594–598 (July 1976).
Nowotny, M. L.: "If Your Patient's Joints Hurt, The Reason May Be Osteoarthritis," *Nursing,* **10:**39–41 (September 1980).
Nute, L. F., et al.: "Nursing Care of Patient Undergoing a Total Hip Arthroplasty," *ONA,* **3:**43–54 (February 1976).
Rand, P. H.: "Evaluation of Patient Education Programs," *Phys Ther,* **58:**851 (1978).
Rickel, L.: "Emotional Support for the Multiple Myeloma Patient," *Nursing,* **6**(4):76–80 (April 1976).
Shealy, C. N.: "Holistic Management of Chronic Pain," *Topics Clin Nurs,* **2:**1–8 (April 1980).
Shivock, C.: "Total Knee Replacement Arthroplasty," *ONA J,* **4:**179 (July 1977).
Simkin, P. A.: "Management of Gout," *Ann Intern Med,* **90:**812 (1979).
Simpson, A.: "Arthritis: A Joint Approach," *Nurs Mirror,* **152:**28–29 (1981).
Spruck, M.: "Gold Therapy for Rheumatoid Arthritis," *Am J Nurs,* **79:**1246–1248 (July 1979).
Swanson, A. B.: "Reconstructive Surgery in the Arthritic Hand and Foot," *Clin Symp,* **31:**2–32 (1979).
Taylor, J. F.: "Osteomyelitis: The Acute Form," *Nurs Times,* **72:**486–488 (Apr. 1, 1976).
———: Osteomyelitis: The Chronic Form," *Nurs Times,* **72**:535–537 (Apr. 8, 1976).
Templeton, C. G., et al.: "Weight Control: A Group Approach for Arthritis Clients," *J Nutr Educ,* **10:** 33–35 (January/March 1978).
Tobeason, S. J.: "The Arthritis Patient Comes to Surgery," *AORN J,* **32**(4):608–613 (October 1980).
"Total Joint Arthroplasty Symposium, Part I," *Mayo Clin Proc,* **54:**491–550 (August 1979).
"Total Joint Arthroplasty Symposium, Part II," *Mayo Clin Proc,* **54:**557–612 (September 1979).
Viellion, G.: "Nursing Care of a Patient in Traction," *Am J Nurs,* **79:**1771–1798 (October 1979).
Waterson, M.: "Exercises To Help Manage Your Rheumatoid Arthritis," *Nursing,* **9:**32 (1979).
Watts, R. J.: "Impact of Chronic Illness on Sexual Health," *Issues Ment Health Nurs,* **2:**67–83 (December 1979).
Webb, K. J.: "Early Assessment of Orthopaedic Injuries," *Am J Nurs,* **74:**1048–1053 (June 1974).
White, J. F.: "Rheumatology Nursing: A Specialty You Can Tailor to Your Talents," *Nursing,* **9:**108 (October 1979).
———and G. L. Ziegler: "Patient Management of Systemic Lupus Erythematosus (SLE)," *Crit Care Update,* **8:**5–15 (August 1980).
Zeitlin, D. J.: "Psychological Issues in the Management of Rheumatoid Arthritis," *Psychosomatics,* **18:**7 (1977).

Organizations

American Orthotics and Prosthetics Association, 1440 N Street N.W., Washington, D.C. 20005
The Arthritis Foundation, 1212 Avenue of the Americas, New York, NY 10036
National Institute of Arthritis, Metabolism and Digestive Disease, National Institutes of Health, Bethesda, MD 20014
Veterans' Administration Prosthetic Center, Veterans' Administration, 252 Seventh Avenue, New York, NY 10001

Pamphlets

Dubois, E. L.: "Information for Patients with Lupus Erythematosus," American Lupus Society, Torrance, Calif.
Epstein, W. V., and G. Clewley: "Living with SLE," Milberry Union Bookstore, San Francisco.
Feinberg, J.: "Principles of Joint Protection and Work Simplification," Indiana University Medical Center, Indianapolis.
Haviland, N., et al.: "A Workbook for Consumers with Rheumatoid Arthritis," American Occupational Therapy Association, Rockville, Md.
"Lupus and You: A Guide for Patients," St. Louis Park Medical Center Research Foundation, Minneapolis, Minn.
"Rheumatoid Arthritis: Patient Education Workbook," Multipurpose Arthritis Center, University of Alabama, Birmingham.
"Self-Help Devices for Arthritic Patients," Institute of Rehabilitation Medicine of New York University Medical Center, published by Merck, Sharp & Dohme.

Section 11

Problems in Special Situations

Chapter 58

NURSING ROLE

Medical and Traumatic Emergencies

Barbara J. Lockwood

Learning Objectives

1. Differentiate between medical and traumatic emergencies.
2. Describe the purpose of an emergency medical service system.
3. Explain the role of history taking in an emergency situation.
4. Identify the sequential components of a head-to-toe assessment appropriate in an emergency situation.
5. Explain the emergency care of victims with sudden obstructed airway, near drowning, heat and cold exposure, burns, and various kinds of poisoning.
6. Differentiate between blunt, penetrating, contrecoup, and crushing trauma.
7. Describe the emergency care for eye and facial injuries, intraabdominal injuries, extremity injuries, and head and spinal cord injuries.
8. Compare the emergency treatment for pneumothorax, flail chest, and pericardial tamponade.
9. Describe the legal responsibilities of a nurse in emergency care situations.

The definition of an *emergency* is determined by the client. While most medical personnel consider emergencies to be life-threatening events, the public now considers an emergency to be an illness or injury for which the client requires or desires the immediate attention of a physician.[1] This chapter discusses only life-threatening emergencies. For clarity, emergencies are divided into two groups: medical emergencies and traumatic emergencies. *Medical emergencies* are defined as all acute physiologic crises not directly caused by a traumatic impact to the body and generally not requiring surgical intervention. *Traumatic emergencies* are all physiologic crises which are directly caused by impact to the body and generally require surgical intervention.

OVERVIEW OF EMERGENCY CARE

Care of the emergency victim has evolved over the last 20 years into a specialized branch of medicine and nursing. Educational programs specific to emergency care in medical and nursing schools are becoming more common. Paraprofessionals, such as emergency medical technicians (EMT) and paramedics (EMT-P), are now trained to deliver qualified prehospital care. Sophisticated transportation systems, some using small planes and helicopters, have been developed. Many of these programs utilize nurses to deliver prehospital care[2] (Fig. 58-1).

This chapter was reviewed by Ann Dumas, R.N., B.S., CCRN, formerly Staff Nurse, Emergency Room, University of New Mexico Hospital, Albuquerque, New Mexico; Student, School of Law, University of New Mexico, Albuquerque, New Mexico.

Emergency Medical Service System

Emergency care is the responsibility of the community as well as the medical facilities providing the service. The community's commitment to decreasing morbidity and mortality has stimulated rapid growth in emergency care. The *emergency medical service (EMS) system* was developed to integrate all elements required in the delivery of quality emergency care. The nine features of an effective EMS system include:[3]

1. Communication system
2. Transportation system
3. Effective prehospital care delivered by qualified personnel
4. Designated emergency care facilities with 24-hour coverage by qualified physicians and nurses
5. Medical facilities with adequate ancillary departments (blood bank, radiology, 24-hour operating room availability, etc.)
6. Disaster preparedness (e.g., civil defense plans)
7. Emergency psychiatric services
8. Educational programs to train and provide continuing education to all those providing emergency care
9. Public information campaign to ensure public understanding of how to enter the EMS system when an emergency arises (e.g., distribution of emergency phone numbers)

All individuals and communities who either deliver or

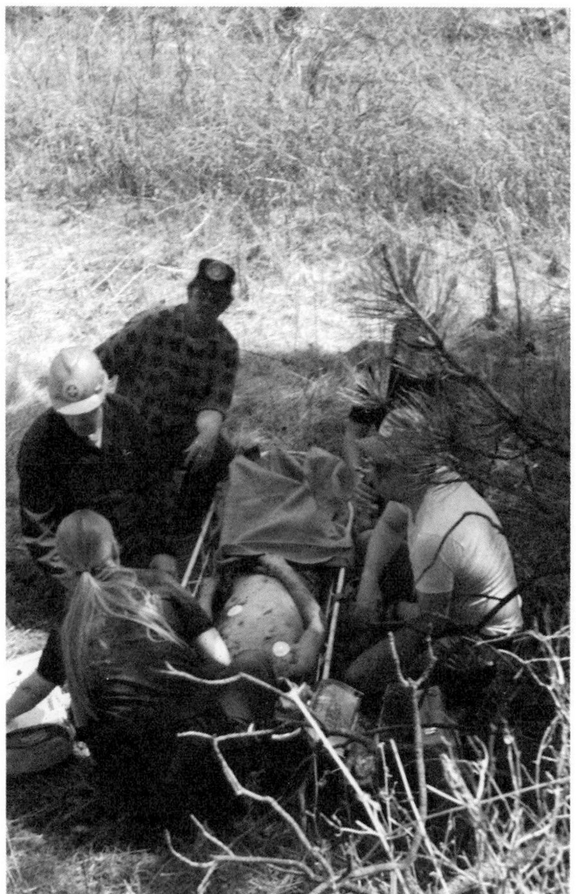

Figure 58-1 Rescue workers and a flight nurse give emergency care to the victim of a fall. *(Photo by Dan Turner.)*

receive emergency care are affected by how well the EMS system works.

Emergency Nursing

The integrated nature of the EMS system has affected the roles that personnel assume while delivering emergency care. There is a great deal of overlap between medical and nursing roles. The degree of intervention depends more on training than on title or job classification. Since there is no clear-cut distinction between medical and nursing roles, all medical and nursing interventions are discussed together in this chapter.

Emergency nursing is one of the most challenging specialties in the field of health care. This specialty requires the nurse, whether in the hospital emergency department or at the emergency site, to use a sound knowledge base, clinical skills, and the nursing process. The principles of crisis intervention as well as the actual use of emergency skills are important to the victim and family in the emotion-laden, stressful environment of an emergency situation. Rapid assessment, history taking, appropriate intervention, and emotional support for the family and victim take place in a very short time period.

The emergency nurse must also take part in health promotion by teaching clients about accident prevention and basic emergency care in the home. Public awareness can greatly reduce the number of accidents as well as the morbidity and mortality in emergencies which go untreated prior to the victim's arrival at an emergency care facility. The emergency nurse needs to be aware of clients who continually return to the hospital with injuries. They may be accident-prone or the victims of battering. Health care teaching specific to each emergency is described in this chapter.

ASSESSMENT OF THE EMERGENCY VICTIM

Recognition of a life-threatening illness or injury is one of the most important aspects of emergency care. A differential diagnosis (medical) is not as important as recognizing dangerous clinical manifestations and initiating action to reverse or avert a crisis. Therefore initial contact with the victim requires a brief, accurate history and a rapid, thorough assessment.

History Taking

The history of the accident or illness is important because it can provide clues to the cause of the crisis and may verify what the assessment reveals. The client may be unable to give a history, but family, friends, and witnesses can frequently give accurate information if the right questions are asked. The history should include the following:

1. What is the chief complaint? What caused the person to seek attention?
2. How long ago did the accident occur? How long ago did the client become ill?
3. Where did the accident occur? Where did the client become ill?
4. Describe the accident or illness. How did it happen?
5. What has happened since the onset of the crisis?
   - **a.** Has the client been moved?
   - **b.** Has emergency care been started at the scene of the illness or accident?
   - **c.** What are the client's subjective complaints?

   d. Witnesses' (if any) descriptions of the client's behavior since the onset
6. Health care history
   a. Allergies
   b. Current medications client is taking
   c. Chronic or recent health problems

Interview Technique

Obtaining an accurate history in an emergency situation is dependent on the nurse's interviewing technique. She must avoid using medical jargon and leading the client. "Does the pain in your chest radiate down your left arm?" is a poor question because it leads the client. A better question is: "Is your pain only in your chest?" The nurse must remain nonjudgmental toward the historian or risk losing important information. "Listen" to the nonverbal communication, because it is as important to a complete history as are the verbal responses to questions. People who are emotionally distraught by a crisis may not give accurate information. There are also situations in which the historian wishes to protect himself or someone else. For example, a woman who stabs her husband may be unwilling to discuss the situation. The nurse needs to verify confusing and conflicting information with other family members and/or witnesses.[4]

Assessment Process

Because emergencies require rapid intervention, the physical assessment process must begin as the history is being taken. The initial assessment takes in the victim as a whole and the environment, including interpersonal interactions. People who seek help for a physical complaint are in a state of crisis. Entry into the EMS system is often an intimidating, frightening experience. People do not have the opportunity to prepare for coping with an emergency in the same way they prepare for an anticipated hospitalization. Besides the fear of what is happening to them, they must place themselves under the care of total strangers. There is little time to develop a relationship between the client and family and the nurse. The entire range of crisis behaviors, some seemingly inappropriate, are seen by EMS personnel. The nurse must realize that the suspicious behavior that may be exhibited by client and family is not directed at her but rather is a normal behavior under the circumstances. People need to know what the nurse is doing for them. It is the responsibility of the emergency personnel to maintain open communication throughout the history and assessment period.

Certain behaviors should alert the EMS nurse to potential problems. Inconsistent histories given by several family members may signal a problem such as wife abuse. The client who curses and verbally abuses the nurse may be severely hypoxic, intoxicated, or have a serious head injury. As the assessment proceeds the nurse must continue to observe behaviors and interactions along with physical signs.

Continued behavioral assessment is the first principle of a thorough assessment. Other principles of assessment are:

1. Make the assessment quickly.
2. Conduct the assessment systematically.
3. Compare your assessment findings with the history.
4. *Listen* for client complaints, labored breathing, breath sounds, heart sounds, and bowel sounds.
5. *Look* at skin color and body movement and for the presence of blood.
6. *Feel* for deformities and areas that elicit pain.
7. *Smell* for breath odors, such as alcohol, and gasoline on clothes.

A systematic head-to-toe assessment of the emergency victim starts with the ABCs (Table 58-1): establish that the client has a patent *airway,* is *breathing,* and has *circulation* as evidenced by heart sounds and pulses. (Refer to Chap. 28 for the management of cardiac arrest.) Next determine whether the client has any external bleeding. If this is present, stop the bleeding by exerting pressure directly over the bleeding site. If bleeding continues, pressure may be applied on major arteries proximal to the injury (Fig. 58-2). This may require the assistance of another person. If the airway is open, a pulse is present, and there is no obvious bleeding, the immediate fear of a life-threatening situation is decreased.

Examination of the body begins with the head and neck. The client's level of consciousness is assessed. If consciousness is decreased, the cause must be sought. The history may include epilepsy with grand mal seizures. An alcohol smell on the breath may explain the diminished level of consciousness, or a large depression over the right temporal area may be palpable. The pupil size and reaction to light are recorded. The head is palpated for depressions, hematoma, and areas of softness as well as for pain. Neck examination includes palpation and visualization of the trachea to ensure that it is in the midline and not deviated to the left or right; a deviated trachea may signal a life-threatening tension pneumothorax. Pain in the cervical spine area may signify fracture of a cervical vertebra.

The physical assessment continues with the chest, spine, abdomen, and pelvis, and lastly the

Table 58-1
Head-to-Toe Assessment of Emergency Victims

Airway

Breathing

Circulation

Head and neck
- Level of consciousness—cause for decrease
- Pupil size and reaction to light
- Examine eyes, ears, nose, and mouth
  - Bleeding
  - Foreign body
  - Drainage
  - Pain
  - Cyanosis
- Examine head:
  - Lacerations
  - Depressions
  - Contusions
  - Pain
- Examine neck:
  - Stiffness
  - Pain in cervical vertebrae
  - Midline trachea
  - Distended neck veins
  - Bleeding
  - Ability to swallow

Chest
- Symmetry of chest wall, anterior and posterior
- Motion: equal movement with respiration
- External signs of injury or illness:
  - Petechiae
  - Signs of external injury
  - Bleeding
  - Cyanosis
  - Pain
  - Respiratory distress
  - Breath sounds
  - Pain or deformity of vertebrae

Abdomen and pelvis
- Symmetry of external abdominal wall and bony structures
- External signs of injury or illness
- Pain—localizing or rebound
- Bowel sounds
- Rigidity or distension of abdomen

Extremities
- Signs of external injury
- Pain
- Movement—arms and legs
- Sensation in each limb

Peripheral pulses
- Present
- Quality

Adapted from W. Phipps, *Medical-Surgical Nursing: Concepts and Clinical Practice,* The C. V. Mosby Company, St. Louis, 1978, p. 421.

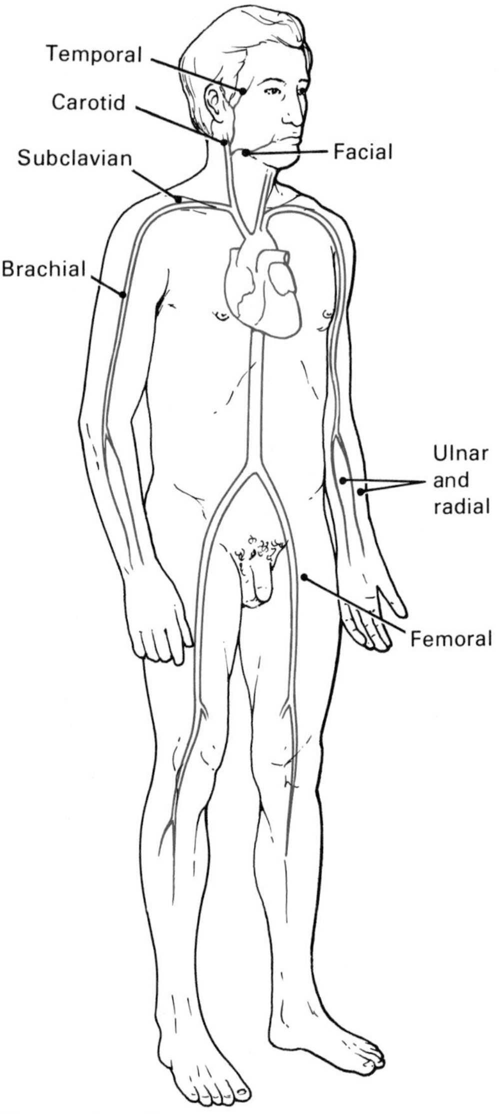

Figure 58-2 Pressure points for control of hemorrhage.

extremities. Each region is checked for symmetry, motion, external signs of illness or injury (open wounds, hematomas, altered skin color, rashes) and palpated for deformities and pain. Regardless of the victim's chief complaint, a thorough head-to-toe assessment and an accurate history are critical in an emergency situation.

CRISIS INTERVENTION

Crisis intervention techniques can be well utilized by the emergency nurse to help clients and families cope with the threat of an emergency. The client experiences crisis because he has lost security and control over his life. The client's reaction to the crisis will partially depend on preestablished coping patterns. An emergency may compound a preexisting crisis, e.g., a death in the family may have occurred recently. Therefore nurses should use the following crisis intervention techniques:[5]

1. Present oneself to the client as calm, empathetic, hopeful, and willing to assume responsibility.
2. Focus on release of emotion.
3. Foster mature behavior.
4. Explore impact of the emergency with the client.
5. Explore unsatisfied needs.
6. Give the client summary and feedback.
7. Structure planning with emphasis on the client (family) taking charge by selecting appropriate alternatives.
8. Review future possibilities of stress, ways to resolve problems, and sources of help.

The type of emergency and the client's and family's ability to deal with their needs and feelings will determine which intervention techniques are needed.

MEDICAL EMERGENCIES

The nursing role in the management of many types of emergencies has been discussed in earlier chapters. Acute respiratory failure (Chap. 22), anaphylactic shock (Chap. 10), rape (Chap. 46), myocardial infarction (Chaps. 27 and 28), diabetic ketoacidosis and insulin reaction (Chap. 41), and head and spinal cord injuries (Chaps. 53 and 54) are all seen relatively often by the emergency nurse.

This section will focus on prehospital care for the medical emergency victim. As stated previously, medical emergencies include all physiologic crises which are not directly caused by an impact to the body. This section also includes acute situational crises such as drowning and poisoning. The emergency management of these victims generally does not require surgical intervention.

Sudden Obstructed Airway

Sudden obstructed airway is caused by the aspiration of foreign material into the trachea, resulting in inadequate respiration. This phenomenon has been called the "cafe coronary" because it frequently occurs in restaurant patrons who aspirate a large piece of meat or other whole food and is often mistaken for a myocardial infarction. The victims are rarely seen in the emergency room with the obstruction still in place. If the obstruction is still in place upon arrival at the emergency room, the client will be in cardiopulmonary arrest.

The signs of acute respiratory distress progress as the victim is unable to clear the airway. Immediately following aspiration of foreign material the following danger signs will signal the need to intervene: ineffective or absent cough, high-pitched, crowing noises on inhalation, clutching the throat (universal distress signal), inability to speak, cyanotic skin and/or lips.[6] If the obstruction is not removed the victim will become unconscious from hypoxia and rapidly develop cardiopulmonary arrest.

The American Heart Association has developed appropriate protocols to treat this emergency.[7] All basic life support classes teach a technique to remove the obstruction. The sequence for the conscious victim is:

1. Confirm that airway is completely obstructed or breathing is ineffective (ask victim if able to speak).
2. Deliver four back blows (between the shoulder blades, with the heel of the hand).
3. Deliver four manual thrusts (chest thrust or abdominal thrust).
4. Repeat back blows and manual thrusts until they are effective or until victim becomes unconscious.

Figure 58-3 depicts the correct position of both the conscious victim and the rescuer for the back blows and the manual thrusts.

If the victim is unconscious, additional steps are indicated to clear the airway. After delivering the back blows and manual thrusts, the victim's head is turned to the side and the mouth is "swept" with the fingers to remove any loosened object. The rescuer then attempts to ventilate the victim with mouth-to-mouth resuscitation (Fig. 58-4). The four maneuvers continue until the obstruction is cleared or the victim is transferred to an emergency medical facility. The nurse is responsible for teaching the client that sudden airway obstruction can be prevented by proper chewing and avoiding excessive laughter and talking while chewing. In addition, excessive intake of alcohol depresses the gag reflex and should be discouraged.

Cricothyroidotomy

If attempts at ventilation and removal of the foreign body are not successful and equipment is not

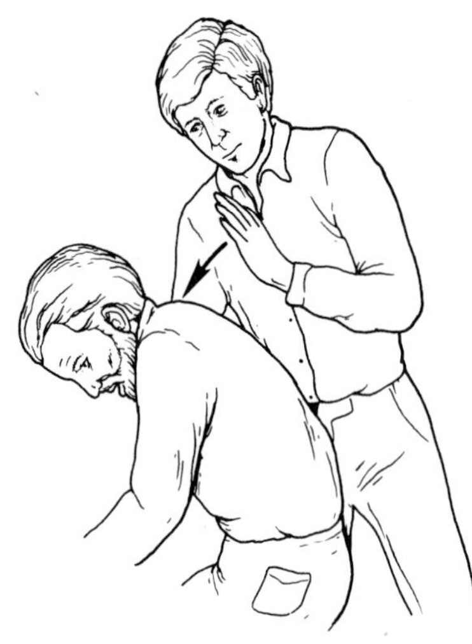

4 Back blows

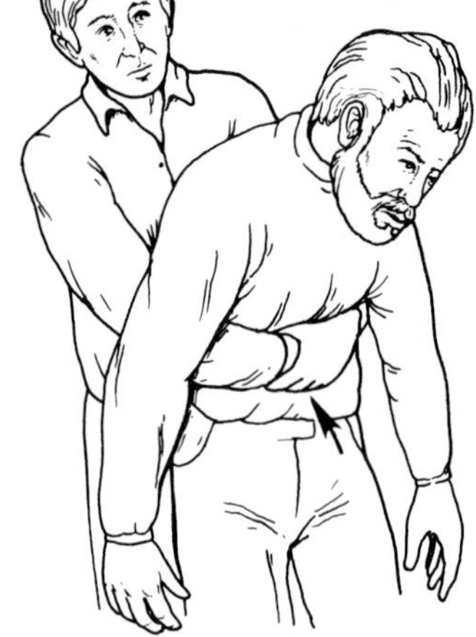

4 Abdominal thrusts

Figure 58-3 Clearing the obstructed airway of the conscious victim, using four back blows and four chest thrusts or abdominal thrusts. *(Reproduced by permission of the American Heart Association.)*

available for endotracheal intubation or tracheostomy, a cricothyroidotomy (cricothyroid puncture) may be performed. This procedure provides a temporary airway by puncturing the cricothyroid membrane with a large (10-gauge) polyethylene needle or scalpel (Fig. 58-5). This method maintains an airway until more definitive therapy can be instituted. Cricothyroidotomy may also be used in other conditions causing acute airway obstruction (e.g., laryngeal edema from anaphylactic shock).

Near Drowning

Near drowning is a common medical emergency which compromises the respiratory system and can lead to cardiac arrest. Drowning, the fourth most common cause of accidental death, may occur in fresh or salt water.[8] Persons have recovered from near drowning after being submerged for as long as 25 minutes. Therapy is vigorous and is directed at correcting hypoxia and severe acid-base and fluid imbalances and supporting basic physiologic functions.

Most drowning victims aspirate water but some do not, because of laryngeal spasm. Prognosis is better for the latter, because fluid imbalance and acid-base disturbances are less severe. Table 58-2 describes the significant clinical differences between clients who have aspirated salt water versus fresh water. While the amount of water aspirated may be small, the osmotic gradient of the fluid causes fluid imbalances in the body. Fresh water, being hypotonic, is rapidly absorbed into the circulatory system. Salt water, being hypertonic, draws fluid from the circulation into the alveoli.[9] Additional fluid is frequently swallowed by the near-drowning victim. Large amounts of fresh water are rapidly absorbed via the gastrointestinal system, causing hypervolemia.

The nursing role in caring for the near-drowning victim includes observing for signs of hypoxia, pulmonary edema, and gastric distension. Other measures are monitoring urine output, central venous pressures, body temperature, and level of consciousness. Hypoxia can be reversed by giving mouth-to-mouth resuscitation, suctioning the oral pharynx, and inserting an endotracheal tube and mechanically ventilating the client with 100% oxygen. If pulmonary edema is present or if alveoli are collapsing, mechanical ventilation using positive end-expiratory pressure (PEEP) may be required to improve gas exchange across the alveolar-capillary membrane. PEEP is discussed in Chap. 21. Efforts to mechanically drain water from the lungs are fruitless and delay appropriate treatment.[10]

Near-drowning victims may become profoundly acidotic secondary to hypoxia. Metabolic acidosis, hypoxia, and severe hypothermia may also be present and may result in ventricular fibrillation.[11] Arterial blood gases are routinely measured to monitor oxygen and carbon dioxide levels and acid-base imbalances. Hyperventilation (to correct respiratory acidosis) and intravenous sodium bicarbonate (to correct metabolic acidosis) therapy are begun early. Hypothermia can

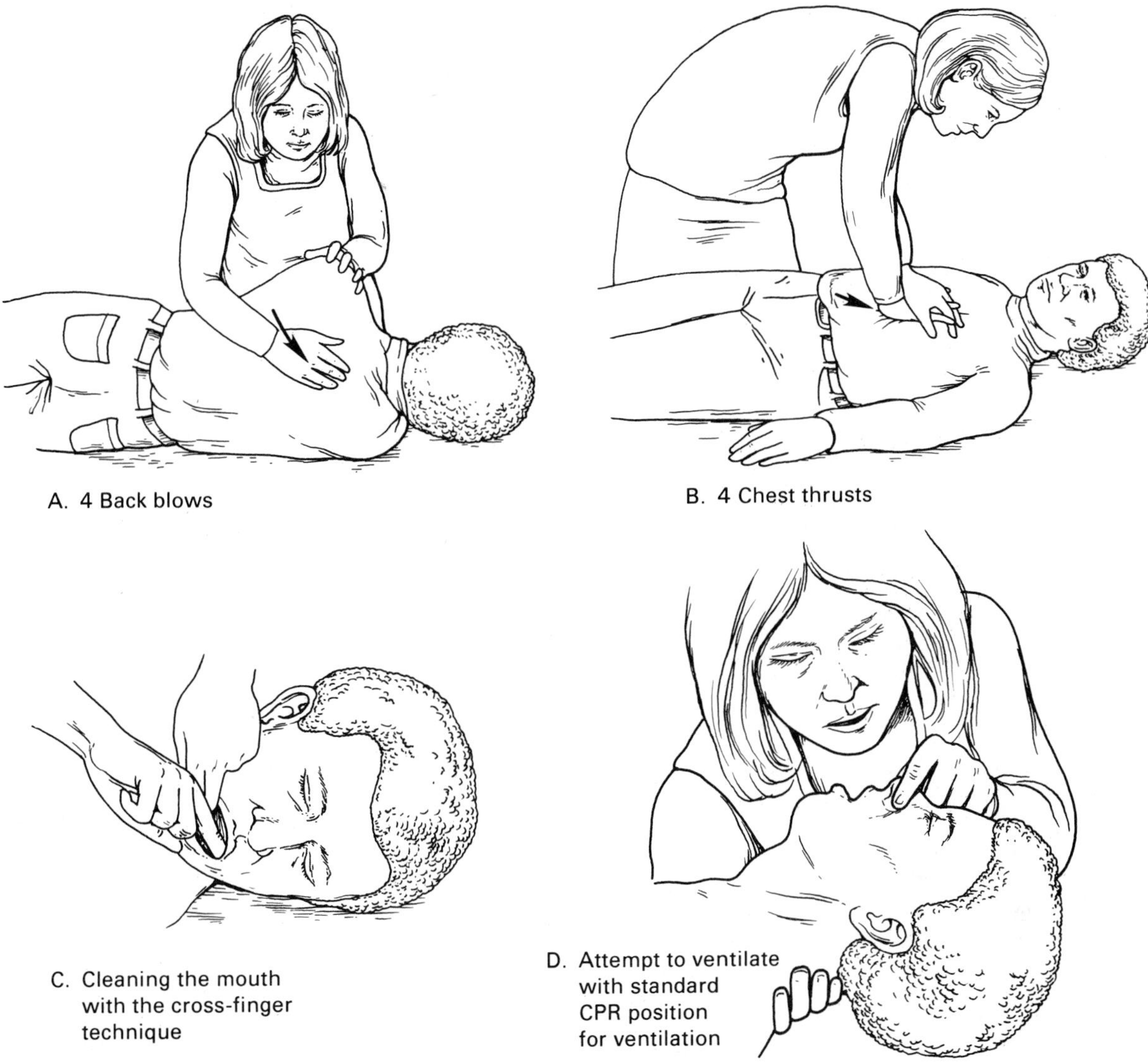

A. 4 Back blows
B. 4 Chest thrusts
C. Cleaning the mouth with the cross-finger technique
D. Attempt to ventilate with standard CPR position for ventilation

Figure 58-4 Clearing the obstructed airway of the unconscious victim, using four back blows and four chest thrusts or abdominal thrusts, and clearing the mouth with the cross-finger technique. *(Reproduced by permission of the American Heart Association.)*

prevent the return to a normal pH, so hypothermic clients should be warmed as rapidly as possible. Use of a mechanical hypothermia blanket is the most effective method.

After ventilation is started and fluid therapy to correct acid-base imbalances is begun, a nasogastric tube, indwelling catheter, and central venous pressure line are inserted. The nasogastric tube decompresses the stomach to remove swallowed water and prevent the aspiration of vomitus and debris. Urine output is monitored by the use of an indwelling catheter. Diuretic therapy is often instituted to bring the fluid imbalance under control and correct pulmonary edema. Central venous pressure readings reflect the severity of fluid overload and indicate the effectiveness of diuretic therapy. The level of consciousness is carefully monitored by the use of a neurological check sheet. Deterioration in neurological status may indicate cerebral edema, increased hypoxia, or profound acidosis. Near-drowning victims may also have a head injury,

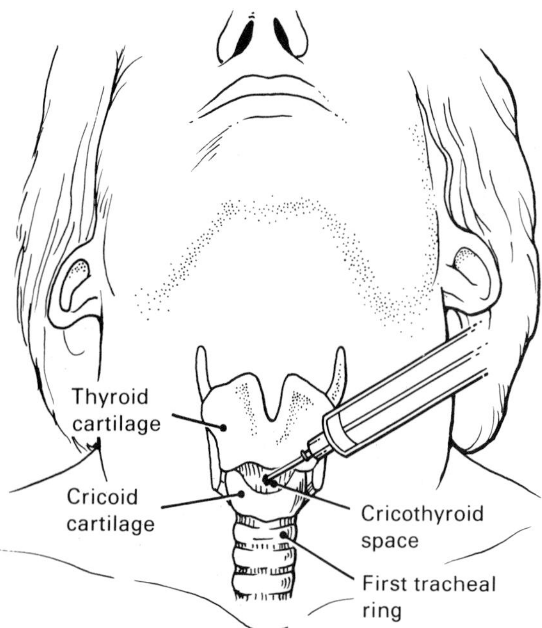

Figure 58-5 Cricothyroid puncture is performed by inserting a large-gauge needle into the cricothyroid space. This procedure provides a temporary airway in acute airway obstruction.

which would cause prolonged alteration in level of consciousness when all other monitored parameters are returning to normal.

Thermal Emergencies

Thermal emergencies encompass all conditions caused by extremes in temperatures. These emergencies include heat cramps, heat exhaustion, heat stroke, burns (thermal, electrical, and chemical), cold exposure, and frostbite. If left untreated, these conditions can progress to loss of limb or life.

Heat cramps, heat exhaustion, and heat stroke

Table 58-3 describes the clinical manifestations and management of three common emergencies that occur in hot weather. Heat cramps and heat exhaustion are common following profuse sweating in hot weather. They are due to excessive loss of sodium. Heat stroke occurs when the body receives more heat externally than it can dissipate. All three heat emergencies are frequently seen in persons engaged in sports.

People with chronic renal, pulmonary, and cardiac illnesses are more likely to develop problems in hot weather. Increased environmental temperature accompanied by profuse diaphoresis raises the body temperature rapidly. When this occurs the body's oxygen requirement is increased. The respiratory rate increases to meet this demand. The heart rate also increases to meet tissue demands for a higher oxygen level. These physiologic responses to heat continue to raise the body temperature. Clients with diseased cardiac or pulmonary systems cannot tolerate the increased demand forced on them. Regardless of the body's effort to compensate, it cannot generate increased oxygen levels.

Certain drugs known to be phototoxic enhance the problems caused by sun and excessive heat. These drugs include phenothiazines, thiazides, antihistamines, tolbutamide (Orinase), and chlorpropamide (Diabinese).[12]

When obtaining the history, the nurse in the emergency room should note whether a client has cardiac, respiratory, or renal disease or is taking any phototoxic drugs. Following appropriate treatment, client teaching must be aimed at preventing recurrence of the emergency. The client on phototoxic drugs should be warned that these drugs make one very susceptible to heat emergencies.

Burns

The management of burns is one of the most serious long-term problems in health care today (Chap. 13). Initial management of the burn victim is critical. First the burning agent must be removed. Flames should be extinguished and smoldering clothing remove. Also remove all jewelry, as it conducts heat and may cause constriction problems. If the burns are caused by chemicals, the involved area must be flushed with copious amounts of water. Once the burning has stopped, the victim should be covered with a clean sheet or any available clean covering to prevent dirt from entering the wounds. Butters and oils should never be applied to new burns; oils trap heat and can cause deep burns long after the burning agent is removed.

Because massive amounts of fluid are lost through burned skin or into interstitial spaces, hypovolemic shock may develop quickly, and the fluid volume must be replaced as quickly as possible. A central venous pressure (CVP) line and indwelling catheter are inserted immediately to monitor fluid volume. Arterial blood gases and carbon monoxide levels are evaluated. If inhalation burns are suspected, intubation is carried out immediately, before local edema makes the procedure more difficult.

Smoke inhalation can result in carbon monoxide (CO) poisoning, chemical injury to the lungs, and

Table 58-2
Significant Clinical Differences between Aspiration of Salt and Fresh Water

Clinical Parameter	Salt Water	Fresh Water
Hypoxia	Increased hypoxia, fluid in alveoli	Alveolar collapse due to altered surfactant, atelectasis, uneven ventilation
Blood volume	Hypertonic fluid draws water into alveoli Hypovolemia Increased blood osmolarity and viscosity	Hypotonic water absorbed into circulation rapidly Transient hypervolemia Decreased blood osmolarity and viscosity Elevated CVP
Serum electrolytes	Hyperkalemia from severe acidosis and hypoxia Clinical picture complicated by large amounts of salt water	Hyperkalemia from severe acidosis and hypoxia
Hemoglobin	No difference	Hemolysis results in drop in hemoglobin
Central venous pressure	Initial rise in CVP, followed by rapid drop to zero (consistent with hypovolemic shock)	Continual rise of CVP
Neurological effects	Lethargy, drowsiness, coma due to electrolyte imbalance	Cerebral edema due to hypervolemia resulting in decreased level of consciousness
Urinary system	Acute renal failure due to tubular necrosis caused by hypoxia and hypotension	Acute renal failure due to hemolysis and hypotension

Adapted from William L. Orris, "Aquatic Medical Emergencies," in Carmen G. Warner (ed.), *Emergency Care,* 2d ed., The C. V. Mosby Company, St. Louis, 1978.

upper airway obstruction from laryngeal edema. Burned nasal hairs, soot in the sputum, and hoarseness are symptoms of smoke inhalation. Management requires administration of 100% oxygen until carbon monoxide levels decrease and respiratory distress is alleviated.

Certain burns are more serious than they initially appear. Burns of the hands, feet, and genitalia and circumferential burns are indications for hospital admission. Electrical burns may present with small entrance wounds and extensive injured tissue hidden below.

Because burns are such devastating injuries, the emergency nurse is obligated to educate the public. Correction of conditions such as frayed electrical cords and malfunctioning appliances will reduce the likelihood of electric shock and burns. Fire prevention measures in the home and out of doors also will reduce the incidence of these tragic accidents.

Cold exposure–hypothermia

Hypothermia has been briefly discussed in the section on near drowning. Persons who engage in winter sports or become lost in wilderness areas where night temperatures are low are also susceptible to hypothermia. Other groups at risk are alcoholics, street people, and the elderly. Alcohol causes peripheral vasodilatation, making one more susceptible to the cold. Street people may not be able to cope with sudden drops in temperature. The elderly may reduce their heating facilities to cope with rising energy costs.

Hypothermia occurs when the heat produced by the body is less than the amount of body heat lost into the environment. Heat is lost as radiant energy from the body in large amounts through the head and thorax and through respiration. As heat is lost, the peripheral vascular system constricts in an attempt to conserve heat. If the clothing is wet, evaporation speeds heat loss. Wind also speeds heat loss by

Table 58-3
Heat Cramps, Heat Exhaustion, Heat Stroke: Clinical Manifestations and Management

Thermal Emergency	Clinical Manifestations	Management
Heat cramps	Severe pain and cramps in lower extremity muscles and abdomen, faintness, dizziness, weakness	Increase sodium chloride intake: oral tablets, intravenous infusion
Heat exhaustion	Pale skin, profuse sweating, nausea and vomiting, rapid weak pulse, lowered blood pressure; dilated pupils may be present; transient loss of consciousness	Place client in cooler environment: loosen clothing; apply cold compresses; elevate legs above heart level
Heat stroke	Elevated temperature (up to 41°C [106°F]), reddish flush to skin, hot and dry skin, initial elevation of blood pressure, bounding pulse, rapid and irregular respirations, agitation, coma	Reduce body temperature: ice bath, hypothermia blanket, chlorpromazine or diazepam to reduce shivering; elevate head of bed. Hospitalize! Oxygen, intravenous fluid replacement, supportive care

Adapted from Hugh E. Stephenson, Jr., "Heat Emergencies," in Hugh E. Stephenson and Robert S. Kimpton (eds.), *Immediate Care of the Acutely Ill and Injured*, 2d ed., The C. V. Mosby Company, St. Louis, 1978, pp. 117–120.

lowering the environmental temperature, increasing the heat requirement. The body produces heat largely via caloric intake. As cold temperatures persist, shivering and movement are the body's only mechanisms to produce heat. However, these mechanisms also speed heat loss.

If left untreated, hypothermia can be fatal. Clinical manifestations of progressively worsening hypothermia include uncontrollable shivering, slow, slurred speech, amnesia, loss of muscle coordination, drowsiness, and coma. Unconsciousness generally occurs when the core body temperature is approximately 29°C (84°F).[13] Wet clothing, wind, and alcohol in the system (producing vasodilatation) increase the severity of and susceptibility to hypothermia.

Treatment of hypothermia is aimed at warming the victim rapidly. The first step is to move him to a warm, dry environment as quickly as possible. Wet clothing must be removed. Several ways to speed warming are the use of (1) warmed fluids by mouth if the victim is conscious, (2) warmed intravenous fluids, (3) warmed oxygen mist, and (4) a hypothermia blanket set to warm.

Following the emergency, the nurse should teach the client how to avoid future problems. People should never travel to high elevations or venture out into cold temperatures unless they are prepared with extra dry, warm clothing, high-sugar foods for extra calories, and a plan for survival should an accident occur.

Frostbite

Frostbite occurs in the same situations which produce hypothermia. When a portion of the body is exposed to freezing temperatures for a prolonged period, vasospasm occurs and circulation ceases. The manifestations range from numbness and total anesthesia of the affected extremities to evidence of necrotic tissue. Emergency management requires moderately rapid rewarming of the affected part, as by submersion of the extremity in a water bath at approximately 43°C (110°F). Massage should never be used, since this may increase tissue damage. All clothes which constrict the frozen extremity should be removed. Any blisters should be left intact. The victim should not be allowed to smoke cigarettes because of their vasoconstricting effect. Gentle exercise to increase blood flow should be encouraged. Efforts should be made to promote normal blood circulation until definitive care can begin.[14] If the victim is left untreated, frostbite may result in amputation of the affected part.

Poisonings

Poisonings may be accidental or purposeful, as in the case of suicide attempts. It is important that the nurse be nonjudgmental during the initial interview with the client; the accuracy of the history may be dependent on her ability to remain neutral. This is especially true when inteviewing people who have attempted suicide or parents who have carelessly left poisonous agents easily available to children. Only 50 percent of all poison histories are accurate.[15] The history should include the type of poisoning present, how much toxin the victim was exposed to, the length of time since the exposure occurred, symptoms appearing since the poisoning, and past medical history (including allergies and present medications being taken by the victim). If contact is made with the victim prior to arrival in the emergency room, he should be instructed to bring the poison container to the hospital.

Poisonings may be of the surface or topical type (organophosphate pesticide) or may involve inhalation (carbon monoxide), ingestion (pills or food), or injection (insect and snake bites).

Surface toxins

Surface toxins must be washed from the victim with copious amounts of water as soon as possible. Special attention must be given to those body areas which serve as pockets collecting the toxin, such as the ears and the navel.

Inhaled toxins

Inhaled toxins are difficult to treat and may result in chemical pneumonitis. Appropriate treatment includes removing the victim from the toxin source, keeping him quiet, administering oxygen, and observing for respiratory distress.

Ingested toxins

Ingested toxins are common and may range from an overdose of medication to food poisoning. Some toxins require immediate induction of vomiting, while others contraindicate this. Generally, inducing vomiting is contraindicated in the following circumstances: (1) ingestion of strong bases or acids, (2) absence of gag reflex, (3) unconsciousness, and (4) seizures. If none of these conditions exists, vomiting should be induced even if the ingestion occurred several hours earlier. Vomiting can be induced by giving the adult victim 30 mL syrup of ipecac by mouth, followed by 6 to 8 ounces of oral fluid. The dose may be repeated once if necessary.[16] All gastric contents should be saved for laboratory analysis. Another method of removing the toxin is insertion of an Ewald (large nasogastric or orogastric) tube into the client's stomach and lavage with at least 3 L saline.

Treatment of the poison victim is directed at removing the toxin from the body, supporting the body systems until the crisis is past, and giving an antidote if the poison is known and if there is a specific antidote to it. Frequently the specific poison which caused the crisis is not known. Supportive care must be given whether or not an antidote is available. It is important to remember that the so-called universal antidote (a mixture of burnt toast, magnesium oxide, and tannic acid) has no place in poison management; it is a waste of precious time to give this worthless mixture.[17] Table 58-4 describes some common poisons with their specific antidotes.

Table 58-4
Specific Antidotes for Some Common Poisons

Poison	Antidote
Carbon Monoxide	Oxygen
Cyanide	Cyanide kit: amyl nitrite, sodium nitrite, sodium thiosulfate
Organophosphate insecticides: parathion, malathion	Atropine, 2-PAM (pralidoxime)
Diphenhydramine (Benadryl), atropine, potato leaves, tricyclic antidepressants	Physostigmine
Phenothiazines	Diphenhydramine (Benadryl)
Narcotic ingestion	Naloxone (Narcan)

Adapted from Barry Rumack, John B. Sullivan, Jr., and Robert G. Peterson, *Management of Acute Poisoning and Overdose,* The Rocky Mountain Poison Center, Denver, Colo., 1980, pp. 16–21.

Since many ingested poisons can be reabsorbed in the lower gastrointestinal tract, an alert victim may become comatose and critically ill at a later time. Cathartics and activated charcoal are used to decrease the possibility of gastrointestinal reabsorption. Activated charcoal is given orally or through an Ewald tube and then removed from the gastric tract by vomiting or aspiration of stomach contents via the tube. It has no known contraindications and can absorb a number of poisons from the GI tract. Cathartics are used to decrease toxicity by moving poisons through the gastrointestinal system rapidly and thereby reducing absorption. Magnesium-containing cathartics are contraindicated in renal failure, as are oil-based cathartics in pesticide poisonings. Magnesium sulfate (adult dose 15 to 30 g) is a commonly used cathartic.[18]

Food poisoning is also a type of poison ingestion. Frequently a large number of people become ill following the ingestion of the same contaminated food. This can help speed identification of the toxic agent. Food poisoning may be caused by chemicals in the food or by bacterial toxins. Chemical food poisons include antimony (from gray-enameled utensils), cadmium (caused by acid liquids in cadmium-plated containers), sodium cyanide (cockroach poison), and zinc (caused by cooking or storing acid foods in galvanized iron utensils). These poisons cause gastrointestinal symptoms which develop within a few minutes to 2 hours. Bacterial sources of food poisoning include *Clostridium botulinum* (found in improperly canned vegetables and preserved meat and fish), *Salmonella* (caused by contamination of food by rat feces, the housefly, and human carriers) and *Staphylococcus* (in milk, mayonnaise, and cream contaminated by infected humans). Treatment of food poisoning is supportive and symptomatic. Botulism is the most severe form and causes respiratory paralysis and death if untreated (Chap. 53). Salmonella and staphylococcus poisoning cause severe gastrointestinal distress (nausea, vomiting, and diarrhea).[19] For more detailed discussion of food poisoning, refer to Chap. 32.

Injected toxins

Insect Bites Insect bites, especially from bees, yellow jackets, hornets, and wasps, can cause an anaphylactic reaction in a hypersensitive individual. (Treatment of anaphylactic reaction is discussed in Chap. 10.) The stinger of the insect is often left in the skin after the bite and continues to release venom. The stinger should be removed by a scraping motion with a fingernail, knife, or needle (tweezers may cause more venom to be released by squeezing the stinger).

Local treatment of bites consists of applying ice and sodium bicarbonate (baking soda) or a weak ammonia solution to the bite site to counteract the acid in the insect venom. Persons known to be allergic to insects should carry emergency insect kits that contain epinephrine.

Snakebite Poisonous snakes in the United States include rattlesnakes, ground rattlers, copperheads, moccasins, and coral snakes. It is important to become familiar with the types and identifying characteristics of poisonous snakes in the region of the country in which one lives.

Local reactions to snakebite are intense burning pain and rapidly developing edema, sometimes accompanied by bleeding. Generalized toxic reactions from snake venom include nausea and vomiting, dizziness, tachycardia, GI bleeding, and respiratory problems. Sloughing of the tissue may occur around the area of the bite.

The treatment of snakebite is somewhat controversial. Some general principles of emergency care include the following:

1. Identify the snake and/or bring it to emergency room for identification.
2. Apply tourniquet above the level of the bite. It should be applied tight enough to minimize lymphatic and venous return without constricting arterial flow.
3. Wash, incise, and apply suction to bite area. The incision should be approximately 0.6 cm long and 0.3 cm deep. Suction is applied by suction cups or the mouth. These procedures are useful only if done within 20 minutes of the bite.
4. Do *not* apply ice to the bite area.
5. Administer appropriate antivenin serum by intravenous infusion. Because antivenin is made from horse serum, the client should be skin-tested for possible hypersensitivity reactions prior to administration.

Nurse's role in education

The nurse must be aware of the responsibility of educating the public to the dangers of poisonous substances in the hope of preventing these types of emergencies. Initial treatment measures should be taught to the public, since early treatment can save lives. Parents should know what poisons they routinely keep in their homes and how to store them properly out of the reach of small children. All homes should have syrup of ipecac available to induce emesis early following acute poisoning. People who work around dangerous substances should be taught how to decontaminate one another should an accident occur. Everyone should have the telephone number of the local poison control center. These centers give poison treatment information over the telephone that is specifically focused on prehospital care.

TRAUMATIC EMERGENCIES

Traumatic emergencies include all physiologic crises which are directly caused by impact to the body and generally require surgical intervention. Traumatic injuries may affect only one system (e.g., a fractured humerus) or many systems (multiple trauma).

Trauma is the leading killer of young adults.[20] Not only does trauma kill but it leaves countless numbers of people permanently disabled. The rehabilitation of these victims alone costs huge sums. It is for these reasons that so much attention has been focused on the care of the trauma victim.

Nursing interventions in all the possible combinations of trauma are beyond the scope of this chapter. Broad concepts are presented, with emphasis on the principles of trauma care. Specific injuries are mentioned because they are common causes of trauma and illustrate the principles of care.

While many people envision the accident scene as a large auto collision with tremendous activity, many accidents also occur in out-of-the-way places. Regardless of the site or the injuries, the principles of trauma management must always be followed:

1. Obtain a rapid, accurate history.
2. Make a rapid, thorough head-to-toe assessment (Table 58-1).
3. Stop all external bleeding by applying direct pressure and/or pressure at major arteries proximal to the injury (Fig. 58-2).
4. Treat shock. Most multiple trauma victims die of blood loss. The other injuries can wait if bleeding is stopped and fluid volume replaced. Medical antishock trousers may be used (Fig. 58-6).
5. Do not move the client until the proper immobilization equipment is present. Never assume that there is no spinal injury.
6. Transport the client quickly to the *nearest facility* able to treat the victim.
7. Constantly reassess the victim's condition and treat symptoms as they occur; e.g., oxygen for cyanosis.
8. Always expect the worst.

Traumatic Injuries

Traumatic injuries fall into four major categories: (1) blunt trauma, (2) penetrating trauma, (3) contrecoup trauma (acceleration-deceleration), (4) crushing trauma. *Blunt trauma* occurs when the body impacts on a blunt object such as a steering wheel. The external injury may appear minor, but the impact may cause severe, life-threatening internal injuries such as a ruptured spleen. *Penetrating trauma* occurs when a foreign body impales or passes through the body tissues (e.g., gunshot wounds and stabbings). *Contrecoup trauma,* like blunt trauma, is caused by the impact of parts of the body against other objects. This type of injury differs from blunt trauma primarily in the velocity of the impact. Internal organs are rapidly forced back and forth within the bony structures which surround them, so that internal injury is sustained not only on the side of the impact but also on the opposite side where the organ hit bony structure. If the velocity of impact is great enough, organs and blood vessels can literally be torn from their point of origin. Many head injuries are caused by contrecoup trauma. *Crushing trauma* may vary in severity from a crushed finger to a crushed chest. Table 58-5 describes some common traumatic injuries as they relate to the above categories of trauma and the mechanism of injury.

Facial and Ocular Injuries

Traumatic injuries to the face are often accompanied by injury to the eye. Table 58-6 describes some common facial and ocular injuries, their associated clinical manifestations, and the recommended emergency management. Facial injuries may be immediately life-threatening because of bleeding into the posterior oral pharynx. A patent airway must be maintained to prevent asphyxiation.

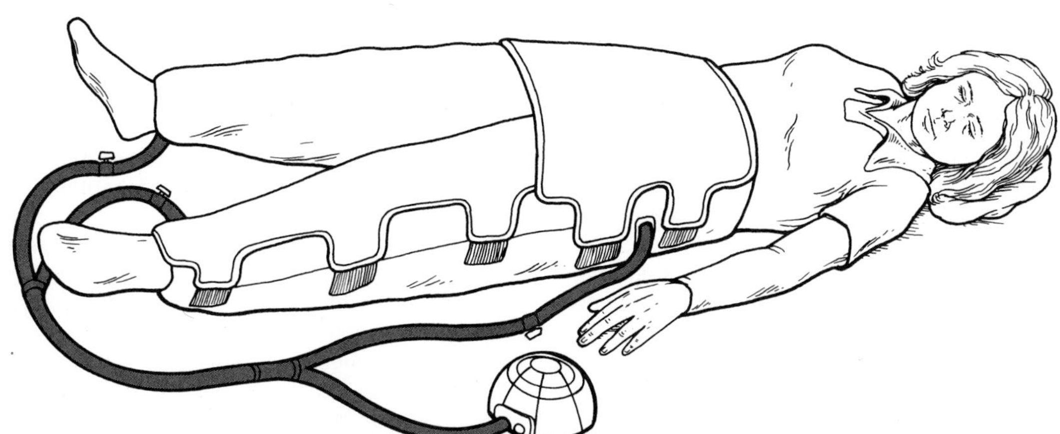

Figure 58-6 Medical antishock trousers (MAST) counteract internal bleeding and hypovolemia by developing a pressure of up to 104 mmHg around the legs and abdomen in order to slow or stop arterial bleeding; force blood from the lower body to the heart, brain, and other vital organs in the upper body; and prevent blood from circulating to the lower extremities. Circulation in the feet should be assessed frequently. MAST should be removed only if a physician is present, IV fluids are available, and surgical facilities are ready if needed.

Table 58-5
Common Traumatic Injuries Related to the Mechanism of Injury

Mechanism of Injury	Related Common Injury
Blunt trauma	
Blunt steering-wheel injury to chest	Rib fractures, flail chest, pneumothorax, hemopneumothorax, cardiac contusion, pulmonary contusion, pericardial tamponade, great vessel tears
Shoulder-harness seat belt injury	Fractured clavicle, dislocated shoulder, rib fractures, pulmonary contusion, pericardial contusion or tamponade
Lap seat belt injury	Fractured bladder, lower abdominal injuries, fractured pelvis, sciatic nerve damage, great vessel tears, fractured liver, lacerated or ruptured spleen
Penetrating trauma	
Gunshot or stab wound to chest	Open pneumothorax, hemopneumothorax, pericardial tamponade, esophageal damage, tracheal tear, great vessel tears
Gunshot or stab wound to abdomen	Liver, spleen, stomach, bladder, pancreas, small intestine, and large intestine damage, renal damage, great vessel tears
Contrecoup trauma	
Blunt-object contact with right side of head	Associated left-sided cerebral contusion
Crush injury	
Heavy equipment crushing thorax	Pneumothorax and hemopneumothorax, flail chest, great vessel tears and rupture, decreased blood return to heart with decreased cardiac output

Facial fractures near the eye can cause secondary eye injury. This is particularly true of orbital bone fractures. Ocular injuries may cause permanent loss of the eye or loss of vision if left untreated. All eye injuries require a visual acuity test to assess the limitation of vision. If the victim is unable to view an eye chart, hold up several fingers to establish his ability to see. Victims will usually tell you if the image is blurred. The majority of eye injuries are from foreign bodies. Never remove an impaling object from the eye! Cover the eye and calm the victim until qualified help and special equipment are available.

Chemical burns to the eyes require prompt action. Flush the eyes immediately with copious amounts of saline for at least 20 minutes. This may be done by using IV solution tubing as a tiny hose. Even small amounts of chemical left in the eye can cause further damage. If the victim says a solution got in his eye, assume that it is potentially damaging and proceed appropriately.

Thoracic Injuries

Thoracic injuries range from simple rib fractures to life-threatening tears of the aorta, vena cava, and other major vessels. The most common thoracic emergencies are described in Table 58-7. This table does not include major vessel tears because these victims require immediate fluid replacement and surgery; there is little the nurse can do except assist in getting the client to surgery as rapidly as possible.

Pneumothorax

Pneumothorax should be suspected following any blunt trauma to the chest wall. It can be caused by penetration of the lung by a fractured rib or by rupture of an alveolar bleb in the client with chronic obstructive lung disease. Pneumothorax associated with trauma may be accompanied by hemothorax—a condition called *hemopneumothorax.* The hemothorax may be minor, or the victim may lose his entire blood volume into the thoracic cavity.

A pneumothorax may be open or closed. *Closed pneumothorax* has no associated external wound; *open pneumothorax* includes an open chest wound. This type of chest wound is caused by a penetrating injury of the chest wall such as a stabbing or gunshot wound and is often referred to as a *sucking chest wound.* An open pneumothorax should be covered with a vented dressing. This allows air to escape from the vent and decreases the likelihood of tension pneumothorax developing. (A *vented* dressing is one secured on three sides, with the fourth side left untaped.) If the object which caused the open chest wound is still in place, do not remove it until a physician is present! An object piercing tissues should be secured with tape and dressings so it does not move inside the victim.

Table 58-6
Common Ocular and Facial Injuries: Clinical Manifestations and Emergency Management

Injury	Clinical Manifestations	Emergency Management
	Eye Injuries	
Chemical		
Acid, base	History, pain, loss of vision	Immediate irrigation of affected eyes with large amounts of water for 20 min. If chemical base, irrigation required for longer period of time. Instillation of topical anesthetic may be necessary to decrease pain.
Blunt ocular trauma		
Blowout orbital fracture	Limitation of eye movement, diplopia, anesthesia of cheek; swelling around eye may or may not be present	Ice to reduce swelling; surgical intervention.
Blunt trauma to eye	Avulsion of eye contents; hyphema (blood visible in anterior chamber); loss of vision	Protect eye with loose, nonocclusive dressing.
Penetrating trauma to eye and foreign bodies	Subjective sensation of having something in the eye; pain	Protect eye with loose dressing. Wait for definitive treatment by a physician.
	Facial Injuries	
Fractures		
Frontal bone	Rapid edema may mask underlying fractures	Secure airway. Remove foreign material, blood, etc. Suction. Tracheostomy may be necessary. Control hemorrhage with pressure packing. Definitive fixation of fractures by a physician.
Periorbital	May have frontal sinus involvement (see Eye Injuries)	
Nasal	Nasal bones displaced; epistaxis	
Zygomatic arch	Depression of zygomatic arch	
Maxilla	Segmental motion of maxilla	
Mandible	Dental fractures, bleeding, limited motion of mandible	

Tension pneumothorax will kill the victim within minutes if left untreated. Large amounts of air trapped in the pleural cavity not only collapse the lung on the side of the injury but displace the heart and major blood vessels to the other side of the chest and collapse the opposite lung. The normal negative pressure inside the chest is lost, and intrathoracic pressure starts to rise. This interferes with the normal return of blood to the heart and ultimately decreases cardiac output. Cardiopulmonary collapse and death result. It is for this reason that nurses and paramedics are now being trained to insert large-bore needles and chest tubes into the chest wall to release the trapped air.

Flail chest

Flail chest is a condition in which several adjacent ribs are fractured in two or more places. This causes a portion of the chest wall to lose its continuity with the rest of the rib cage and move in the opposite direction from the rest of the thorax (Fig. 58-7). The loss of chest wall integrity causes a loss of normal intrathoracic negative pressure, and cardiopulmonary collapse and death may result if the victim is left untreated. On inspiration the intact chest wall expands while the flail section sinks into the chest. When the intact chest wall relaxes on expiration, the flail section bulges outward. This is called *paradoxical respiration.* If the flail chest is severe, air ceases to move in and out of the trachea and moves from side to side within the chest. This condition is fatal, since no ventilation takes place.

Nurses and paramedics have been taught the skill of intubation and mechanical ventilation because it is the only way to ensure stabilization of the chest wall and ventilation. Definitive treatment of the flail chest requires internal stabilization by the use of mechanical ventilation with positive end-expiratory pressure (PEEP)(see Chap. 21).

Table 58-7
Thoracic Injuries: Clinical Manifestations and Emergency Management

Injury	Definition	Clinical Manifestation	Emergency Management
Pneumothorax	Collection of air between chest wall and lung	Dyspnea, pain, decreased movement of involved chest wall, diminished breath sounds on injured side	Insertion of large-bore needle with attached one-way valve to release air from pleural cavity; chest tube insertion to underwater seal or one-way valve.
Hemothorax	Collection of blood between chest wall and lung; usually occurs with pneumothorax	Same as above	Insertion of chest tube and aspiration of pleural cavity. Treat hypovolemic shock if present.
Tension pneumothorax	Same as pneumothorax, but no air can escape during expiration; rapid increase of air in pleural cavity causes shifting of intrathoracic organs and increased intrathoracic pressure	Cyanosis, air hunger, violent agitation, trachea deviated to side opposite injury, subcutaneous emphysema	Insertion of chest tube or large-bore needle to relieve air pressure in thorax. Treat hypoxia.
Flail chest	Two or more adjacent ribs fractured in two or more places, causing loss of stability of chest wall	Paradoxical movement of chest wall, respiratory distress, cyanosis; may occur in conjunction with any of three injuries above	Internal stabilization of chest wall by intubation and mechanical ventilation with PEEP. Oxygen therapy. Sedation.
Cardiac tamponade	Rapid collection of blood in pericardial sac from laceration of blood vessels; prevents heart from pumping blood because pericardium is inelastic	Muffled and distant heart sounds, falling or absent blood pressure or pulses, steadily increasing central venous pressure. Neck veins may be distended	CPR if no pulses present. Immediate aspiration of blood from pericardium with needle and syringe by physician. Surgery to repair torn vessel.

Pericardial tamponade

Pericardial tamponade may be caused by blunt trauma or by a penetrating wound (Table 58-7). If left untreated, it is fatal. Since the pericardiocentesis is a highly sophisticated skill, it has not been routinely taught to nurses. If pulses are absent, cardiac massage should be started until the pericardial sac can be aspirated (Cardiac tamponade is discussed in Chap. 29.)

Intraabdominal Injuries

Intraabdominal injuries may be caused by either blunt or penetrating trauma. As already indicated, an object piercing tissues should never be removed until a physician is present; the impaling object tends to decrease bleeding by direct pressure on the site, and once it is removed the bleeding may increase. Common injuries of the abdomen include lacerated liver, ruptured spleen, pancreatic trauma, mesenteric artery tears, diaphragmatic rupture, urinary bladder rupture, great vessel tears, renal injury, and stomach or intestinal rupture. All these injuries may result in massive blood loss and hypovolemic shock. Surgery must be carried out as early as possible to repair the damaged organs and stop the bleeding. Common sequelae to intraabdominal trauma are peritonitis and massive infection, particularly when the bowel is perforated.

Clinical manifestations of abdominal trauma are (1) guarding and splinting of the abdominal wall; (2) a hard, distended abdomen; (3) decreased or absent bowel sounds; (4) bruising over the abdomen; (5) pain; (6) pain over the scapula caused by irritation of the phrenic nerve by free blood in the abdomen; and (7) signs of hypovolemic shock. Intraabdominal injuries are often associated with low rib fractures, fractured femur, fractured pelvis, and thoracic injury. If any of these injuries are present, the victim should be observed for abdominal trauma.

Paracentesis is an important diagnostic tool in the evaluation of abdominal trauma. The two methods used are four-quadrant tap and peritoneal lavage. The four-quadrant tap uses a spinal needle attached to a saline-filled syringe. This procedure involves inserting the needle (a sterile one each time) into all four quadrants of the abdomen and gently aspirating. A positive finding is aspirated nonclotted blood.

The second procedure is the diagnostic peritone-

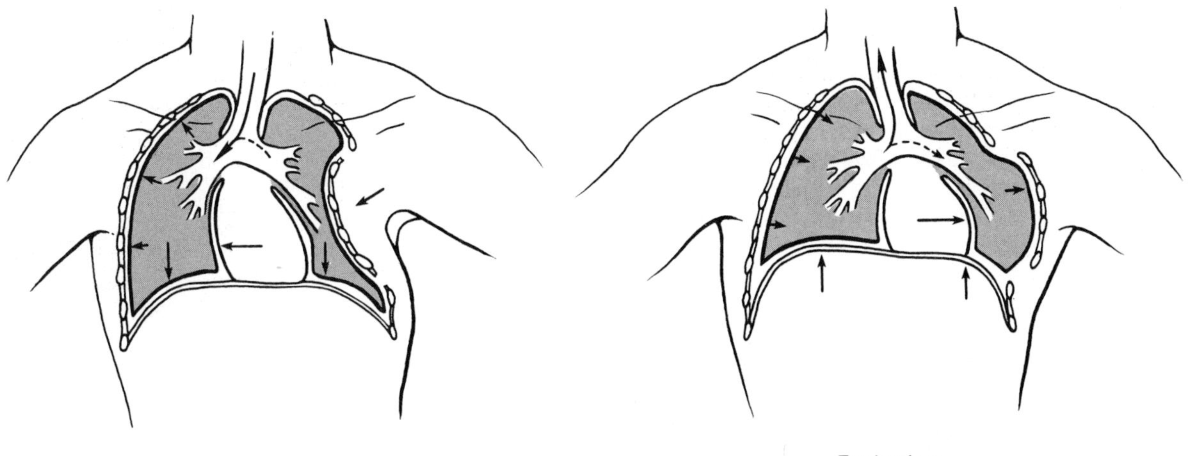

Figure 58-7 Flail chest produces paradoxical respiration. On inspiration the flail section sinks in with the mediastinal shift to the uninjured side. On expiration the flail section bulges outward with the mediastinal shift to the injured side.

al lavage. In this procedure the abdomen below the umbilicus is locally anesthetized and a large angiocatheter or peritoneal dialysis catheter is inserted into the abdomen. A syringe is attached to the catheter, saline is infused, and fluid is aspirated. The fluid is observed for gross abnormalities, especially blood, and is sent to the laboratory for microscopic evaluation. Positive findings include any of the following:

RBC>100,000 per cubic millimeter
High amylase level
Presence of bacteria
Presence of bile

If the results are positive, surgery is indicated immediately. If the results are negative, continued observation of the client is warranted.

Emergency care of the victim of intraabdominal trauma focuses on fluid replacement and prevention of hypovolemic shock. Intravenous lines are started and volume expanders or blood are given if the victim is hypotensive. A nasogastric tube is inserted to decompress the stomach and prevent the aspiration of vomitus. No pain medication is given, because analgesics can mask the progression of clinical manifestations.

Extremity Injuries and Fractures

Extremity injuries and fractures cause a large number of people to seek emergency care. Injury to the extremities may involve bone, muscle, and blood vessels. Emergency care focuses on maintaining or restoring circulation to the extremity, properly immobilizing it, and decreasing the discomfort of the victim. Fractured and crushed extremities should be immobilized before the victim is moved. This decreases the pain and guards against further injury to the limb. Extremities are never manipulated or moved from their original position unless pulses are absent distal to the injury. When this occurs, traction must be applied to the affected limb until pulses are palpable. This is done by stabilizing the limb above the injury, supporting the limb with both hands, and gently (never forcibly) pulling its distal end. This technique requires at least two people. All open wounds should be covered with dressings and overt bleeding stopped with direct pressure. If there is any doubt about the status of the limb, it is better to splint and immobilize it prior to moving the victim than to risk causing further damage.

Head and Spinal Cord Injury

Head and spinal cord injuries frequently occur together, especially following diving accidents and falls. Emergency care of these victims is often complicated by the presence of other injuries. Head-injured victims usually present with elevated blood pressure and a slow pulse. If the victim has a rapid pulse and low blood pressure, he is probably also injured internally. Shock is always treated first, because the head injury will not cause death as rapidly as hemorrhage. Other signs of cranial injury are decreased level of consciousness, aberrant pupillary reaction to light, and hyperventilation or other respiratory alteration.

Spinal cord injury, especially injury of the cervical spine, is often associated with cranial injury. All victims of multiple trauma should be treated as if they have a spinal injury. They should be kept immobile, with the head left in the position it was found. Back boards and scoop stretchers are used to immobilize the spine and facilitate moving the victim to medical help. The head should be immobilized with sandbags. Many victims of vertebral fractures have been left paralyzed because a "helpful" onlooker moved them and caused the spinal cord to be severed. Movement and sensation should be assessed in all four extremities prior to moving the victim to a hospital. This will establish a baseline of functioning before edema develops in the spinal cord.

TRIAGE

Triage (sorting) is a method of managing emergency or disaster situations so that the greatest numbers of lives are saved. A triage system identifies and categorizes the victims so that the most critically injured (the most life-threatening injuries) are treated first. The process involves constant reassessment of the casualties as the situation changes.

Using triage principles high priority is given to cardiac arrest, hemorrhage, respiratory insufficiency, and altered level of consciousness. Intermediate priority is given to closed fractures and minor burns. A low priority is given to ambulatory victims with minor tissue injuries or with dazed affect and no apparent physical injuries.

The case study that accompanies Fig. 58-8 offers a basis for applying the principles of triage and emergency management.

LEGAL IMPLICATIONS OF EMERGENCY CARE*

Good Samaritan Laws

Most states have enacted Good Samaritan laws which release a person administering emergency care from civil liability. These laws do not apply if the emergency care provider acts in a grossly negligent manner or gives the care with the expectation of being paid. In determining negligence, the nurse would be held to the *reasonable person standard,* which is defined as performing those actions which would be taken by a reasonable nurse in a similar situation. The key is to do the best the nurse can do under the circumstances.

Once a nurse begins providing care, that care should be continued until another health care provider (e.g., the EMT) assumes the responsibility for care. Some states have included continuity of care in their statutes, requiring provision of continuing care to an accident victim. If the nurse has any doubts about the quality of care provided by another health care provider, it would be advisable to continue care during the

*This section was written by Virgil H. Lewis, R.N., B.S.N., M.A., J.D.

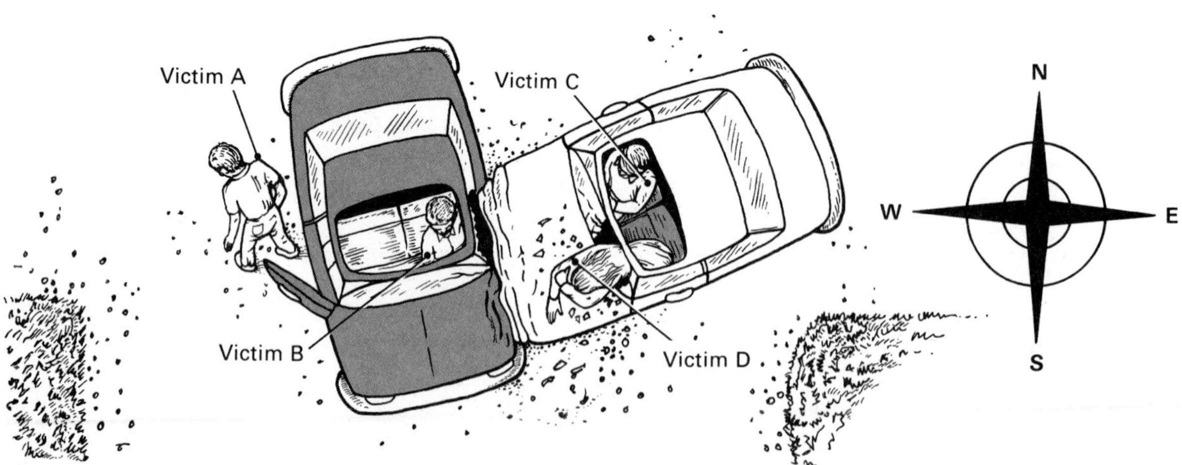

Figure 58-8 Multiple trauma situation resulting from traffic accident. (See case study for explanation of events.)

transportation of the accident victim to an emergency medical facility.

Vermont is the only state which has passed legislation requiring a person to give aid during an emergency. Failure to assist an accident victim, if such an act would not endanger the rescuer, is punishable by a fine of $100. Other states rely on the Good Samaritan laws to encourage emergency care. Health professionals should know the statutes regarding such care in their state.

Emergency Room Care

The emergency room nurse is frequently confronted with medicolegal decisions, especially when there has been criminally caused injury or death. Hospitals should have procedures detailing the *preservation of evidence,* including clothes, specimens, and statements of the client. Statements made by the client immediately following an accident or criminal activity are often admissible in court as an exception to the "hearsay rule." If an autopsy is planned after a death, all clothing should be left intact and blood, wounds, and bullet fragments left untouched.

Complete *documentation* of the client's chief complaint, clinical manifestations, treatment given, and results of treatment is essential. Documentation ensures continuity of care as well as a written record that can be used as legal evidence. The hospital should have a policy of recording every action taken for the client during emergency care at the time the action is taken.

Emergency situations often involve obtaining *informed consent* from the client. It is the physician's responsibility to explain the nature and risks of the procedure. However, the nurse may be delegated the responsibility for getting the consent signed or witnessing the signing. If consent cannot be obtained because of the client's condition, emergency care may be performed under an implied consent doctrine. Once the client regains the capability to make decisions, consent must be obtained for additional procedures.

An important factor in decreasing malpractice suits arising from emergency room situations is establishing rapport with the client and family. It is important to establish meaningful contact in a seemingly depersonalized environment. When the client and family are at a high stress level, otherwise insignificant comments or gestures may easily be misconstrued. The highest level of professionalism should be practiced by all nursing staff. Malpractice litigation has often resulted from the anger and suspicions of clients even when no negligence has occurred.

Case Study / **Multiple Trauma Situation**

Vehicle 1 was traveling south at a speed of 40 mph. The driver did not yield for the red light and was hit by vehicle 2 which was traveling west at 45 mph. By the time the police arrive at the scene, a crowd has gathered with many angry motorists honking their horns because traffic is blocked in four directions.

There are four victims of the accident. Victim A is walking around aimlessly and appears dazed. He has a small hematoma above his right eye with no other apparent injuries. He denies loss of consciousness and is oriented.

Victim B is still in the car. She is conscious but pinned in the car by the dashboard and door. She complains of pain in her left arm and leg with limited movement. She has an open wound on her left leg, and there is a noticeable amount of blood on the floor of the car.

Victim C is unconscious and sprawled over the hood of the car, having been thrown through the windshield. He has multiple lacerations over his face. He has a depression over the left frontal bone and profuse bleeding from the mouth and nose. His eyes are swollen shut. He is still breathing, with a palpable, weak pulse of 60.

Victim D is unconscious and has no apparent injuries. He is still sitting in the car and with his seat belt strapped. However, he is not breathing, is cyanotic, and has a weak, thready pulse. The rescuers removed his lower denture plate but could not find his upper plate. They are unable to breath into his lungs.

Discussion Questions

1. What injuries might you suspect victims A and B have?
2. What precautions should be taken in removing victim B from the car?
3. What is the significance of victim C not wearing a seat belt?
4. What are possible causes of unconsciousness in victim C? What injuries might he have?
5. What probably caused the obstructed airway in victim D? Explain the steps to clear an obstructed airway.
6. Apply the principles of triage in this situation.

REVIEW QUESTIONS

The number of the question corresponds to the same-numbered objective at the beginning of the chapter.

1. A differentiating feature between medical and traumatic emergencies is that
   a. medical emergencies are not as life-threatening as traumatic emergencies
   b. medical emergencies are situational and not physiologic crises
   c. traumatic emergencies are caused by a direct impact to the body
   d. traumatic emergencies always require surgical intervention

2. Which of the following is *not* part of an EMS system?
   a. public information campaign
   b. transportation system
   c. disaster preparedness
   d. rehabilitative care facility

3. An important principle of history taking in emergency situations is to
   a. obtain history after giving emergency care
   b. record history before giving care
   c. verify history with family members or friends
   d. ask leading questions to facilitate the process

4. Which of the following should be done before making an assessment of an emergency victim?
   a. make sure client is breathing
   b. obtain verbal permission to give care
   c. obtain written permission to give care
   d. leave emergency scene to summon help

5. A person who has overdosed on aspirin is brought unconscious to the emergency room. Initial treatment would be to
   a. wait for an antidote
   b. give the universal antidote
   c. give syrup of ipecac
   d. aspirate stomach with Ewald tube

6. Which of the following is considered a blunt injury?
   a. crushing injury of chest
   b. impact with steering wheel
   c. gunshot wound
   d. contrecoup trauma

7. The primary purpose of peritoneal lavage is to
   a. dialyze off toxic substances
   b. remove ascitic fluid
   c. remove foreign particles
   d. assess for internal bleeding

8. Definitive treatment of a flail chest would include
   a. cricothyroid puncture
   b. chest tube insertion
   c. oxygen administration
   d. intubation and mechanical ventilation

9. Which of the following emergency measures would be considered negligence on the part of the nurse?
   a. discarding bloody, torn clothes of a rape victim
   b. witnessing the signing of a consent form
   c. initiating CPR at an accident site
   d. discontinuation of care when the EMT arrives

REFERENCES

1. James D. Mills, "Introduction: Overview of Field of Emergency Medicine," in A. L. Jenkins and J. H. van de Leuv (eds.), *Emergency Department Organization and Management,* 2d ed., The C. V. Mosby Company, St. Louis, 1978.
2. Barbara Lockwood, "New Horizons: Flight Nursing," in C. Hudak et al. (eds.), *Critical Care Nursing,* 2d ed., J. B. Lippincott Company, Philadelphia, 1977, pp. 5–18.
3. Stephen P. Murphy, "Elements of an Emergency Medical Care System," in Carmen G. Warner (ed.), *Emergency Care: Assessment and Intervention,* 2d ed., The C. V. Mosby Company, St. Louis, 1978, pp. 1–12.
4. Jeanie Barry, "Emergency Assessment," in J. Barry, *Emergency Nursing,* McGraw-Hill Book Company, New York, 1978, pp. 165–166.
5. Thomas N. Rusk and Barbara J. Edwards, "Psychiatric Emergencies," in Carmen G. Warner (ed.), *Emergency Care: Assessment and Intervention,* 2d ed., The C. V. Mosby Company, St. Louis, pp. 151–157.
6. American Heart Association, *Cardiopulmonary Resuscitation: Airway Obstructions,* 1978, p. 53. Reprinted with permission of the American Heart Association.
7. Ibid., pp. 54 and 55.
8. Hugh E. Stephenson, Jr., and Robert S. Kimpton (eds.), *Immediate Care of the Acutely Ill and Injured,* 2d ed., The C. V. Mosby Company, St. Louis, 1978, p. 75.
9. William Orris, "Aquatic Medical Emergencies," in Carmen G. Warner (ed.), *Emergency Care: Assessment and Intervention,* 2d ed., The C. V. Mosby Company, St. Louis, 1978, p. 289.
10. Stephenson, op. cit., pp. 75–78.
11. Ibid., p. 76.
12. Ibid., p. 117–120.
13. Orris, op. cit., p. 295.
14. Stephenson, op. cit., p. 123.
15. Barry H. Rumack, John B. Sullivan, Jr., and Robert G. Peterson, *Management of Acute Poisoning and Overdose,* The Rocky Mountain Poison Center, Denver, Colo., 1980, p. 1.
16. Ibid., pp. 9, 22.
17. Ibid., p. 12.
18. Ibid., pp. 12–13.
19. Georgia B. Nolph, "Poisonings," in Hugh E. Stephenson, Jr., and Robert S. Kimpton (eds.), *Immediate Care of the Acutely Ill and Injured,* 2d ed., The C. V. Mosby Company, St. Louis, 1978, p. 175.
20. Lewis M. Flint, Jr., "Trauma: Today's Challenge for Critical Care," *Heart Lung,* **7**(2):247 (March–April 1978).

Chapter 59

NURSING ROLE

Radiation Accidents

Anita Ann Wagner Garman
Delores C. Lesher
Audrey S. Bomberger

Learning Objectives

1. Describe the properties and characteristics of different types of ionizing radiation.
2. Identify the major sources of ionizing radiation.
3. Describe the acute and chronic physiologic and psychological effects of radiation on human beings.
4. Determine the role of nursing in the hospital planning and preparation for radiation accidents.
5. Explain the nursing management of clients who have been exposed to radiation.

A *radiation accident* is an unforeseen occurrence, either actual or suspected, which involves exposure of or contamination on or within human beings and/or the environment by ionizing radiation.[1] With the increased use of radiation in nuclear medicine and industry and as a source of nuclear power, the potential for radiation accidents has increased. Thus far, the safety record for radiation is very good. The number of radiation accidents is low and seldom involves more than one to three persons. In the United States fewer than eight persons have been irradiated under accidental circumstances and have died as a result of the exposure.

In March 1979, radiation was accidentally released into the atmosphere from a nuclear power plant at Three Mile Island, Pennsylvania. No one received a dose of radiation beyond the recommended safety levels.[2] However, there was an overreaction to the potential danger at Three Mile Island by the news media as well as the population in the surrounding community and across the nation. This reaction indicates the confusion, frustration, fear, and moral dilemmas which result from dissemination of insufficient information as well as erroneous reports regarding the crisis and its implications. Another contributing factor to the overreaction was the absence of well-rehearsed contingency plans for radiation accidents.

This chapter gives a glossary of the terms used in nuclear science (Table 59-1) and discusses several aspects of radiation, including a historical review of radiation research, some basic facts regarding its nature and source, and the biological effects of exposure. In addition, the nursing implications of radiation exposure are presented.

This chapter was reviewed by Major Charles E. Day III, Chief, Health Physics, USA Environmental Health Agency, Aberdeen Proving Grounds, Maryland, and by Colonel Thomas Lew Pitchford, U.S. Army, Academy of Health Sciences, Ft. Sam Houston, San Antonio, Texas.

Table 59-1

Glossary of Terms Used in Nuclear Science

Accelerator Device designed to impart high kinetic energy to charged particles (electrons, protons) by imparting high velocities to them.

Atom Smallest amount of an element which has the chemical properties of that element. An atom consists of a central nucleus carrying a positive electrical charge around which electrons move in orbits. All atoms of the same atomic number (i.e., same number of protons) are atoms of the same element, regardless of the number of neutrons present.

Atomic energy Term sometimes used to denote nuclear energy.

Atomic mass Actual mass of an individual atom including protons, neutrons, and electrons.

Atomic number Number which is equal to number of protons in the nucleus. It is also equal to the number of orbital electrons.

Cobalt 60 Radioactive isotope which is an important source of gamma radiation used in industry, research, and cancer therapy. It is usually made by neutron irradiation in a reactor.

Contamination Presence of radioactivity in a material or place where it is undesirable.

Decay (radioactive) Spontaneous nuclear transformation in which particles of gamma radiation are emitted or x-radiation is emitted. When a radioactive atom disintegrates it is said to decay.

Decontamination Removal or reduction of radioactive contamination.

Electron Negatively charged particle.

Gamma radiation High-energy electromagnetic radiation which is similar to x-rays or visible light. Gamma rays are emitted in the process of nuclear transition.

Half-life Time necessary for half of a large sample of decaying particles (such as radioactive nuclei) to decay to half its original value, that is, for half the atoms present to disintegrate.

Table 59-1 (Continued)

Ionization Any process by which an atom, molecule, or ion gains or loses electrons.

Ionizing radiation Any electromagnetic or particulate radiation capable of producing ions by interaction with matter. Knocks electrons from atoms during its passage and thereby leaves ions in its path.

Irradiation Exposure of materials to radiation.

Isotopes Atoms whose nuclei have the same atomic number but different mass numbers.

Mass number Number equal to the number of neutrons plus protons in a nucleus. For most atoms it is fairly close to the atomic mass. For example, lead 208 has 82 protons and 126 neutrons. Its mass number is 208. Its atomic mass is 208.0422 atomic mass units.

Neutron Elementary particle with no electric charge located in a nucleus. Outside a nucleus the neutron is radioactive. The number of neutrons in an atom of a given element can vary, resulting in nuclei that have the same atomic number but different mass numbers. These variants are called *isotopes* of the element.

Nuclear fission Splitting of a heavy nucleus into two or more parts, usually accompanied by the emission of neutrons and gamma rays. Although fission can occur spontaneously, it is usually caused by a neutron hitting the nucleus.

Nuclear fusion Reaction between two light nuclei resulting in the production of at least one nuclear species heavier than either initial nucleus.

Nuclear reaction A process in which a particle hits a nucleus, often forming a compound nucleus which can decay by giving off the same particle with the same or less energy or by giving off another particle. The resultant or product nucleus is sometimes radioactive.

Nuclear reactor Device in which a self-sustaining nuclear-fission chain reaction can be maintained and controlled.

Nuclide Almost a synonym for nucleus. Nuclides are distinguished from one another by the number of neutrons and protons.

Radiation Electromagnetic waves such as light or particulate rays such as alpha, beta, and gamma rays.

Radioactivity Spontaneous decay of radioactive nuclides by the emission of alpha, beta, or gamma rays. It is possible to make radioactive nuclides using nuclear reactions. Some naturally occurring radioactive elements also exist (e.g., uranium).

Rem (roentgen equivalent man) Unit or dose of ionizing radiation which gives the same biological effect as that from 1 roentgen of x-radiation or gamma radiation. For gamma or beta rays 1 rem is approximately equal to 1 rad.

Roentgen Unit of ionizing radiation.

X-rays Electromagnetic waves similar to light but of much shorter wavelength.

HISTORICAL REVIEW OF RADIATION AND RADIOACTIVITY

Radiation has been present in our world since the beginning of time. The most familiar source of radiation is the sun, a good example of a radiation emitter. However, it was not until the late 1800s that significant advances began to be made in observing and describing radiation and radioactivity. In 1895 Roentgen identified penetrating radiations which he called *x-rays.* Shortly thereafter Becquerel discovered that uranium emitted radiation. In the early 1900s the work of Planck and Einstein showed that there were many types of radiation including heat, visible light, ultraviolet light, and radio waves. In addition to displaying properties associated with continuous waves, these types of radiation also displayed properties associated with discrete bundles of electromagnetic energy, or *photons.* Most such photons arise from vibrations of electrons in matter and differ only in their energies. (Any beam of photons can be referred to as *electromagnetic radiation.*)

In 1911 Rutherford conceptualized the atom as being composed of a tiny central core, the nucleus. It contained all the positive charge and essentially all the mass of the atom. Surrounding the nucleus was a nearly empty region containing the light, negatively charged electrons which balance the positive charges of the nucleus (Fig. 59-1). In 1919 Rutherford found that energetic protons were released when the nitrogen nucleus was bombarded by alpha particles.

In 1932 Chadwick's identification of the neutron triggered a rapid succession of major developments in nuclear research[3] (Table 59-2). Extensive radiation technology concerned with the production of energetic radiations for research, medicine, and industry was also developed.

NATURE OF RADIOACTIVITY

One reason radioactivity is surrounded by such a mysterious aura is that while it is all about us it cannot be seen, heard, smelled, or felt. Since it cannot be detected by our body senses, we tend to ignore or not acknowledge its presence in our lives. Radiation is surrounded with a mystique and a fear which is heightened by the memory of atomic warfare. Much of the mystique can be overcome by understanding what radiation is, where it originates and how it affects our bodies.

Structure of Matter

Matter is composed of compounds (e.g., water and salt) made up from various elements such as

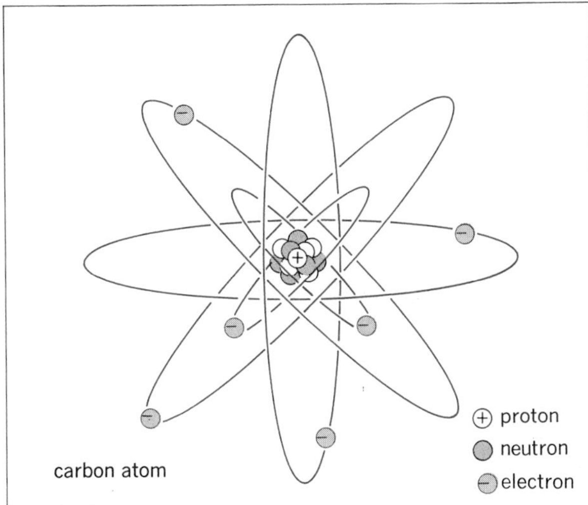

Figure 59-1 Schematic view of an atom. *(From A. J. Vander, J. H. Sherman, and D. S. Luciano, Human Physiology: The Mechanisms of Body Function, 3d ed., McGraw-Hill Book Company, New York, 1980.)*

hydrogen, oxygen, sodium, and chlorine. An *element* is the smallest unit of matter retaining chemical characteristics specific to that unit. Elements are composed of atoms, which in turn are composed of particles called *neutrons, protons,* and *electrons.* The presently accepted model of the atom postulates the existence of a relatively heavy central core, or *nucleus,* which is composed of two kinds of particles: protons (positive charge) and neutrons (neutral charge). The nucleus has a series of surrounding orbitals or energy levels containing very small negatively charged particles, the electrons (Fig. 59-1). The charges of the proton and electron constitute the fundamental units of electrical charge.

The number of protons in the nucleus of an atom determine the *atomic number (Z),* which is also equal to the number of electrons in a neutral atom. Electrons determine the chemical properties of the atom. The *mass number (A)* is equal to the total number of protons and neutrons in the nucleus. Helium has an atomic number of 2 and a mass number of 4 (composed of two neutrons and two protons).

The term *nuclide* refers to the species of atom which displays the same mass number and number of protons. The term *isotope* refers to the species of atom which displays a different mass number but the same atomic number. Consequently, isotopes constitute different nuclides of the same element, for example cobalt 59 ($A=59$, $Z=27$) and cobalt 60 ($A=60$, $Z=27$). Nuclides and isotopes can be categorized as stable or unstable. An example of a stable isotope would be cobalt 59, which does not change its nuclear state or emit radiation spontaneously. In contrast, cobalt 60 is an unstable isotope, because its nuclear state changes spontaneously and it emits radiation.

Table 59-2
Developments in Nuclear Science and Technology

1934 Enrico Fermi split the atom while bombarding uranium with neutrons.
1939 Discovery of enormous amounts of energy released from fission of uranium.
1942 Development of first self-sustaining fission reaction in a nuclear reactor by Enrico Fermi and colleagues.
1945 Explosion of nuclear-fission devices developed under the direction of J. Robert Oppenheimer. First nuclear detonation at Trinity Site, New Mexico. Nuclear detonations at Hiroshima and Nagasaki, Japan.
1952 Production of thermonuclear explosions.
1954 Commissioning of first nuclear-powered submarine, the Nautilus.
1960s Development of commercial nuclear power plants.

Nature of Radiation

Radiation is the emission of radiant energy in the form of waves or particles. *Ionization* is the transfer of energy from radiation to matter, including living cells. The principal way *ionizing radiation* transfers energy in cells is by the removal of orbital electrons from neutral atoms of the cell. This removal of orbital electrons makes the atom a positive ion altering biochemical molecules—an alteration that can lead to cellular dysfunction, damage, or death. If enough cells are altered by ionizing radiation, a tissue effect may be manifested. Ionizing radiation is made up of energetic particles and electromagnetic radiation from both naturally occurring and artificially produced nuclear reactions.

Types of ionizing radiation

Alpha, beta, and gamma are three common types of ionizing radiation (Fig. 59-2).

Alpha (α) *rays* (also called *alpha particles*) are heavy, slow-moving particles identical to the helium nucleus ($^{4}_{2}He$). Alpha radiation travels only a few centimeters in air and has low penetrative ability, usually being stopped by a sheet of paper or by the skin. The potential hazard of alpha-emitting materials is the possibility of their being inhaled or ingested. Alpha particles are generally emitted during radioactive decay only by elements of high atomic number (82 or higher) and are usually accompanied by one or more of the other types of radiation.

Beta (β) *radiation* (also called *beta particles*) consists of fast-moving, lightweight particles which are identical to an atom's electron and carry a single

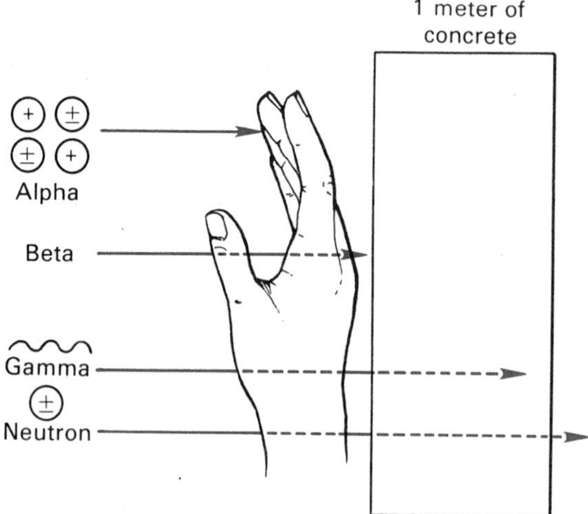

Figure 59-2 Relative penetrative ability of four types of ionizing radiation.

negative charge. Beta rays travel further in air and are more penetrating than alpha rays. Some beta radiation can penetrate through the skin a few millimeters into living tissues. Most beta radiation can be stopped by 0.1 inch or less of aluminum, but the most energetic can penetrate up to 0.3 inch of aluminum.

Gamma (γ) *radiation* is almost always accompanied by one or more of the other types of radiation, i.e., alpha or beta particles. It can be very energetic and is highly penetrating. Gamma radiation displays both wave and particle properties, as do x-rays and visible light. Because of its penetrative ability, considerable amounts of shielding such as concrete or lead may be required for protection from certain gamma-radiation sources. Radioactive iodine (^{131}I) used in medicine is an example of an emitter of both gamma and beta rays.

A fourth type of radiation is *neutron radiation.* Neutrons are used to cause fission and split atoms in nuclear reactors. Neutrons outside of a nucleus are radioactive. Neutron radiation is more penetrating than other particle radiations because the neutrons have no electrical charge and therefore are not attracted or repelled by other charged particles.

Units of measurement

Radiation is measured in various units. *Dose* refers to the amount of ionizing radiation energy absorbed per unit mass of irradiated material at a specific location such as a part of the human body. Absorbed doses of radiation are expressed in a unit called the *rad.* When dealing with biological matter, it becomes important to try to relate dose-specific observable biological effects to equivalent amounts of absorbed radiation. Thus rads are multiplied by various correcting factors to obtain a unit dose equivalent called the *rem.* For most radiation situations, especially those commonly found in a hospital, the rad and the rem are numerically equal. The *millirad* (mrad) or the *millirem* (mrem) are the normal units or measures utilized when specifying permissible doses. *Dose rate* is the amount of ionizing radiation received per unit of time and is usually expressed in rads or millirads per hour.

Over 100 rads of external, penetrating radiation must be absorbed during a short period of time over a substantial portion of the body before most people will show significant clinical manifestations. However, intense radiation to a small portion of the body will cause a local reaction. Intense x-radiation or beta radiation to the skin may cause reddening and ulceration.

SOURCES OF RADIATION

Natural Sources

Radiation sources can be classified as natural or artificial. Natural radiation is present everywhere and varies in amount with geographical location. Although the amount of natural radiation is relatively low, it is measurable and cannot be considered negligible. In the United States the dose range from natural radiation accumulated per year varies from 80 to 500 mrem, with the average dose being about 100 to 120 mrem.

Everyone is exposed to a certain amount of natural radiation which can be classified as cosmic, terrestrial, and internal. High-energy cosmic radiation comes from the sun and stars. The amount of cosmic radiation absorbed by humans can be calculated by adding 1 mrem per year for every foot of elevation one lives above sea level to the average dose of 40 mrem per yer (Fig. 59-3). (Cosmic radiation at sea level is 40 mrem per year.)

Terrestrial sources such as rocks, soil, and water are also types of natural radiation. Natural radioactive elements such as uranium and thorium are widely distributed in soil and rocks. It is therefore understandable that the type of home a person lives in will affect the amount of radiation received from earthen-type building materials. Internal sources of natural radiation include radioactive potassium and carbon.

Artificial Sources

The second source of radiation is the artificial, or synthetic. This source of radiation has a wide variety of

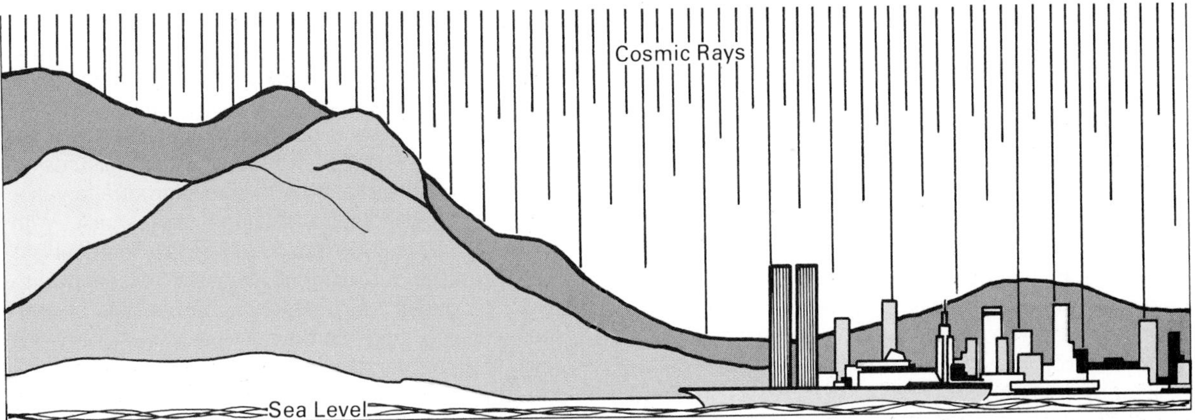

Figure 59-3 Natural radiation from cosmic rays. Cosmic radiation at sea level is 40 mrem per year. For every foot of elevation above sea level, 1 mrem per year should be added to find the total amount of cosmic radiation absorbed by each person.

applications, including medicine, industry, research, and warfare. All these uses constitute potential sources of radiation accidents or excessive radiation exposure.

Medical uses include diagnostic as well as therapeutic procedures. Diagnostic procedures using x-rays and radioactive isotopes are common. X-rays are used to diagnose a wide variety of disorders including dental problems, fractures, and tumors. Radioisotopes are used in procedures related to brain, liver, thyroid, and renal scans. Therapeutic procedures primarily involve the treatment of persons with cancer. Radiation therapy for cancer clients is discussed in Chap. 11.

An important industrial type of synthetic radiation is the use of nuclear power for the production of energy. The first nuclear power plants were built in the 1960s. Synthetic radiation is used in agriculture (gamma radiation increases the shelf life of various vegetables), in the oil industry (radioactive needles can sense the profile of the earth layers), and in many other areas for production and testing of various materials.

The use of radiation in *research* is important in many disciplines including physics and chemistry. Radiocarbon dating with the isotope carbon 14 has been used for many years.

Utilization of synthetic radiation is for the most part constructive. Its use for warfare is destructive and is one reason for people's fear of radiation. Another area of concern and possible fear is the disposal of nuclear wastes from both nuclear weapon testing and power plants.

EFFECTS OF RADIATION EXPOSURE ON THE HUMAN BODY

Somatic Effects

The somatic or bodily effect of ionizing radiation is cellular damage. This damage may manifest itself clinically as acute radiation syndrome or in a more chronic form such as cancer.

Cellular effects

Our knowledge of the effect of radiation upon the living cell is limited by our understanding of the nature of the cell. While a detailed discussion of cellular effects is beyond the scope of this text, it is important to understand that the transfer of radiation energy to a cell alters or disrupts the molecular structure of the cell, most notably the structure of DNA. When the molecules affected are essential for the normal functioning of the cell, the cell suffers injury or dies. The more cells affected, the greater the impact on the organism.

Dose, dose rate, and cell sensitivity are major variables in determining the cellular response to ionizing radiation. Very high doses can be tolerated if received in small increments and distributed over a long period of time. This tolerence is due to the repair and regenerative processes of the body. Cellular sensitivity to radiation is influenced by cell metabolic activity, rate of division, and stage of differentiation. This explains in part why certain organs of the body are more sensitive than others to ionizing radiation (Table 11-14). The most radiosensitive, in order, are (1) testes, (2) hematopoietic system, (3) gastrointestinal tract, and (4) skin. Because the physiologic effects of ionizing radiation take place at the cellular level, they usually manifest themselves after a latent period of days or weeks. However, after high doses of radiation the response is seen within hours after exposure.

Acute radiation syndrome

The acute radiation syndrome (Table 59-3) is the response of the body to extremely high doses of radiation. Many types of tissues having varying sensitivities to radiation are involved when the whole body is irradiated. The clinical manifestations are determined by the types and amount of tissues(s) involved as well as the type of radiation received, the dose, and the dose rate. It is the damage to the most sensitive and vital tissues such as the hematopoietic system that decides the outcome for the organism.

The prognosis and treatment of radiation injury depend upon the clinical picture presented. Survival is almost impossible after a single exposure of a large portion of the body to penetrating gamma radiation of 1000 to 5000 rads. The clinical course is one of erythema of the face and body within minutes of exposure, followed later by hypotension due to vasodilatation, disorientation, seizures, and shock. With doses of 1000 to 5000 rads, death results in about 3 to 7 days and is due primarily to gastrointestinal damage. The gastrointestinal syndrome consists of nausea, vomiting, and diarrhea with a loss of epithelial cells, fluid, and electrolytes. With doses of 5000 rads or more, death results in a matter of hours from damage to the central nervous and cardiovascular systems.

With whole-body radiation in doses between 200 and 1000 rads, survival depends primarily on the

Table 59-3
Acute Radiation Syndrome*

Phase and Parameter	Dose Ranges: Subclinical Range 0–100 rads	Sublethal Range: 100–200 rads	Sublethal Range: 200–600 rads	Sublethal Range: 600–1000 rads	Lethal Range 1000–5000+ rads
Initial (prodromal) phase					
Incidence of nausea and vomiting	None	5–50%	50–100%	75–100%	100%
Time of onset	—	Approx. 3–6 h	Approx. 2–4 h	Approx. 1–2 h	Less than 1 h
Duration	—	Less than 24 h	Less than 24 h	Less than 48 h	Less than 48 h
Latent phase†					
Duration	—	More than 2 weeks	Approx. 7–15 days	None to approx. 7 days	None
Secondary phase					
Organ system responsible	None	None	Hematopoietic		Gastrointestinal; cardiovascular; central nervous
Clinical manifestations	None	Moderate leukopenia	Severe leukopenia; infection; hemorrhage; more than 300 rads: erythema, epilation		Erythema of face and body, nausea and vomiting; diarrhea, imbalance of fluid and electrolytes. Hypotension, disorientation, seizures, shock
Time of onset after exposure	—	2 weeks or more	Several days to 2 weeks; epilation within 2–3 weeks		Erythema within minutes, other symptoms within hours to 3 days
Critical period after exposure	—	None	4–6 weeks		1–48 h up to 14 days

*Single high-dose-rate exposure of whole body.
†Latent phase is a period of apparent well-being between the initial phase and secondary phase. Fatigue may be present.

ability of the cells of the hematopoietic system to regenerate spontaneously. It is this system which presents the major medical problem. The clinical manifestations of acute radiation syndrome at these levels usually begin within 1 to 6 hours of exposure with nausea and vomiting and occasionally diarrhea. Within 3 to 4 days a sense of fatigue is experienced which lasts months, with gradual improvement. Infection and hemorrhage occur within 4 to 6 days after the initial phase has subsided. With doses over 300 rads, erythema is present and epilation (hair loss) may take place 2 to 3 weeks after exposure. The hematopoietic syndrome is manifested by an initial increase in granulocytes 2 to 4 days after exposure, followed by a decline and a decrease of lymphocytes which reaches a minimum just below 1000/μL within 1 to 4 days after exposure.

An exposure of the whole body to 100 to 200 rads results in a moderate biological response. In this instance survival is probable. A prolonged depression of the formed elements of the blood may not occur. For exposures of less than 100 rads, symptoms are almost entirely lacking and survival is expected.

Latent effects

It has long been established that radiation is a carcinogenic (cancer-inducing) agent. Radiation has been implicated as one of the causes of leukemia, skin carcinoma, and osteosarcoma as well as lung and thyroid carcinomas. At low doses of radiation, the predominant effect is cell damage. Since the cells are still able to replicate, the result may be tumor formation and development of genetic diseases. At higher radiation doses, the cells are either killed or become sterile, resulting in impaired function due to a decrease in the number of cells in a given organ. The functional derangements vary in severity according to the amount of the affected organ that is destroyed. As cell death or sterilization approaches 100 percent, the likelihood of tumor formation or genetic effects decreases to zero.

The amount of time which passes between radiation exposure and the appearance of a radiation-associated problem is called the *latent period*. In contrast to the latent phase associated with the acute radiation syndrome, this period can range from 1 to 30 years before tumor formation and functional or developmental abnormalities occur, depending upon the organs involved and the amount of radiation absorbed. The period of increased risk will continue for some time after exposure; after this time, the likelihood of developing an abnormality decreases.

The amount of radiation that is necessary to induce the various cancers remains controversial.[4] The fact remains that the incidence of radiation-induced cancer appears to have decreased.[5] This can be partially explained by (1) the decreased misuse of radiation as a panacea for illnesses of all types and (2) the implementation of strict regulations regarding use along with a lowering of maximum permissible doses to occupationally exposed personnel and the general population.

Genetic Effects

Since controlled studies of the effects of radiation on human mutation rates are not feasible, investigations have been limited to other mammals and insects, with results extrapolated to humans.[6,7] Considerable caution must be exercised in such extrapolation to human genetics. Laboratory experiments have revealed that radiation is a mutagenic agent. Without exception the biological effects produced by radiation are identical to mutations which occur naturally. Consequently, they are not distinguishable from naturally occurring abnormalities on an individual basis. Furthermore, animal experiments have shown that mutations produced by radiation are recessive and may not be manifested for many generations. This latter finding may explain why a mutagenic effect was not observed in the first-generation offspring of the Hiroshima and Nagasaki survivors.[8]

Although postwar Hiroshima and Nagasaki provided a population of irradiated humans for study, it must be remembered that the magnitude of exposure was not controlled and could only be estimated. In addition, by genetic standards the exposed population was small. Consequently, the genetic effects on humans from ionizing radiation remain largely unclear at present. However, when there is concern about genetic abnormalities, all future babies must be *assumed* to be at some risk (albeit very small) from the moment of significant irradiation of the ovaries or testicles of their parents.

Psychological Effects

Ionizing radiation also has a psychological effect on humans. The psychological consequences of an unanticipated radiation exposure are even more difficult to quantify than the physiologic effects. The physical damage (although it may not be observable) may create psychological reactions; and there are psychological problems which do not directly result from actual physical injury but which complicate treatment. For example, the injury can intensify previously existing emotional problems. In general, the pretrauma behavior is the best predictor of behavioral reactions to stress.

For those who do not have a technical background in the physical sciences, radiation may hold a nuclear mystique. One author describes this mystique as being based on three perceptions:[9]

1. Radiation is emitted from strange, esoterically named substances.
2. Radiation requires a high level of technology for production.
3. Radiation is associated with immense power and capacity for destruction.

People with these perceptions may overreact to an injury involving radiation and thereby complicate their treatment and recovery.

Too often, irradiated persons, in addition to having to cope with their own emotions, are placed in the position of having to provide emotional support to family, friends, and even hospital staff, because the latter have incorrect perceptions of radiation. They may display a negative or avoidance reaction toward the irradiated person, fearing that they will be contaminated or in some way harmed by the radiation. If this negative reaction is displayed by others, the irradiated person may never be given the kind of psychological support he would probably receive if he had other injuries or illnesses.

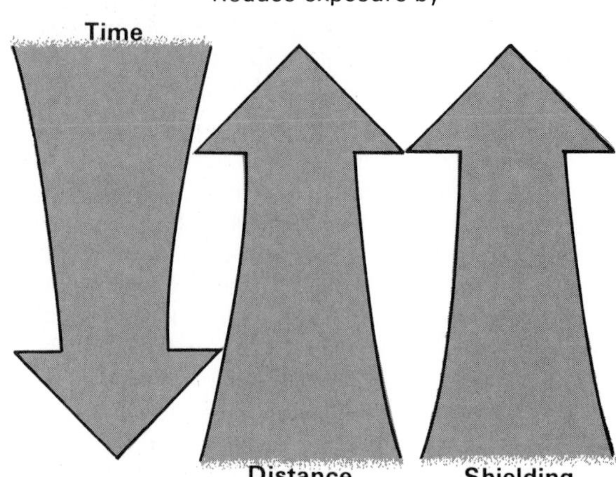

Figure 59-4 Exposure to ionizing radiation can be reduced by decreasing the time spent near the source, increasing the distance from the source, or increasing the amount of shielding between the source and the object irradiated.

NURSING ROLE IN RADIATION ACCIDENTS

Health Promotion and Maintenance

While nuclear reactor plants tend to command the focus of attention regarding radiation, more concern and caution should be extended to low-dose, long-term radiation. This applies to situations such as caring for or assisting clients during x-ray or fluoroscopic procedures, especially when portable equipment is being utilized. It also applies to the use of radiation therapy in the treatment of clients with cancer (Chap. 11). Such exposure to radiation by health care personnel and their clients can be greatly reduced if simple precautions based on the following principles of time, distance, and shielding are practiced (Fig. 59-4):

Time—The longer one remains in the vicinity of the radiation source, the more radiation one receives. Therefore it is essential to carry out the necessary procedures and then move away from the source. Since radiation is emitted at varying rates depending upon the source, it is important to know the dose rate and to plan accordingly the amount of time to be spent near the source. The amount of radiation absorbed is given by the equation: dose rate × time = dose.

Distance—The farther one is from the source of radiation, the less radiation will be absorbed. In administering care to a radioactive client, it is often helpful to the staff to mark on the floor distances from the client and the amount of time that can be safely spent at each distance. For example, 1 minute can be spent next to the bed, 5 minutes 3 feet away, etc. The radiation protection officer is the one who determines the distances and the times.

Shielding—Various materials such as lead, other heavy metals, iron, or concrete are used as shields. They vary in their effectiveness according to their thickness and the type of radiation involved. In general, increasing the amount of shielding decreases the amount of exposure.

Time, distance, and shielding are also discussed in Chap. 11. In addition to being alert to radiation hazards within the hospital setting, nurses should be aware of actual or potential radiation hazards within their community. For example, it is important for planning purposes to know the most likely sources of radiation accident within the community and the likely number of resulting casualties. A good resource person for this type of planning is the health physicist. This is a person with recognized technical and/or professional qualifications in the protection of human beings and their environment from the harmful effects of radiation.[10]

The International Commission for Radiation Protection (ICRP) and the National Council for Radiation Protection (NCRP) have established guidelines and recommendations for acceptable levels of radiation exposure. While these vary according to individual categories, they have all been set at levels at which biological effects are not detectable. People are divided into two categories, radiation workers and the general public. Radiation workers are those who, in the course of their work, incur a relatively high likelihood of exposure to ionizing radiation. The maximum permissible occupational dose for a radiation worker is 5 rem in any one year.[11] This radiation exposure is minimal, particularly when safety precautions are taken. Few radiation workers receive even one-tenth of the permissible values; consequently detectable effects of radiation are not observed in radiation workers except in cases of radiation accident.

A film badge should be worn by all those who work with radiation or clients who are radioactive. The photographic film is darkened by nuclear radiation. Thus the radiation exposure of the wearer can be checked by inspecting the film and comparing it with known standards. Film badges are also discussed in Chap. 11.

The second category includes the general public, for whom the maximum permissible dose of radiation is 0.5 rem per year. Radiation exposure to a fetus should not exceed 0.5 rem during the entire gestation period of the mother.[12] For women who are not radiation workers, the NCRP-recommended exposure of a 0.5-rem-per-year dose limit is sufficiently low to keep them within acceptable levels during pregnancy. However, women of childbearing age who are radiation workers should be considered potentially pregnant, and their assigned duties should reflect this consideration.

Acute Intervention

Nurses who work with clients receiving some type of radiation therapy, nurses working in emergency rooms likely to receive radiation accident victims, and occupational health nurses employed at nuclear reactor sites should all be familiar with the following general nursing considerations and guidelines.[13]

There should be standing orders or standard operating procedures (SOP) specifying the procedures to be followed upon receipt of an irradiated person. These should state in sequence the procedures to be performed and the persons to be notified, such as the physician, radiation protection officer (health physicist), hospital administrator, etc. The standing orders should also include where and how to obtain a survey meter and protective clothing (if applicable) and the procedures and designated area for initial treatment and decontamination.

An assessment should be made of the nature of the accident, the type and amount of radiation exposure or radioactive contamination involved, and the body areas that may have been irradiated or contaminated. If possible, this information should be obtained before the client arrives from someone at the scene of the accident or from the client.

Exposures to radiation can take place in two forms, external and internal, and they may occur simultaneously. *External* radiation involves a source of radiation entirely outside the body. The radiation strikes a person and, depending upon its physical characteristics, deposits energy as it passes through the body much as an x-ray does. Energy will be absorbed, but the exposed person does not become radioactive and thus presents no radiation hazard to other personnel. Alternatively, radioactive contamination may be deposited on the skin. This material may enter the body through wounds, inhalation, or ingestion, producing what is known as *internal radiation,* or *internal radioactive contamination.* Since decontamination may have been initiated at the site of the accident, it is important to assess how much decontamination remains to be done. The removal of the client's outer garments will remove the greater part of the surface contamination in most cases.

Upon arrival at the facility, the client should be checked with a survey meter for contamination. This should be done as the stretcher is removed from the ambulance and before it enters the hospital.

If the client is seriously injured, emergency lifesaving assistance should be given immediately. This takes precedence over decontamination. Unfortunately, there have been incidents when first aid such as stopping hemorrhage was given belatedly because the personnel in attendance were afraid of being contaminated themselves.

If contamination is present or suspected, precautions should be taken to prevent or minimize its spread by removing contaminated clothing from the client, isolating the client from others, and ensuring that personnel in direct contact with the client wear protective clothing. Instruction should also be given to ambulance personnel on how to decontaminate themselves and the ambulance. Someone with expertise in decontamination should supervise to ensure compliance with instructions.

The contaminated client and any wounds should be handled as one would handle a surgical procedure. Gown, gloves, cap, and mask should be worn by personnel because these items serve as protective clothing.

If external contamination is suspected, the following should be saved: clothing, bedding from ambulance (if applicable), blood, urine, feces, vomitus, and all metal objects such as jewelry, belt buckles, and dental plates. Everything should be labeled with name, body location, time, and date. All items should be saved in plastic bags which are taped, closed, and placed in an appropriately covered container clearly marked "Radioactive—Do Not Discard."

If the client is radioactive, the length of time that attendants may spend in caring for the client should be limited by the exposure they may receive. If the radiation dose rate is sufficiently high, time, distance, and shielding precautions should be in operation. The staff should be rotated if treatment procedures will require much time. Only the personnel necessary to perform the treatment should be near the client, and protective clothing should be worn. The radiation protection officer should inform personnel whether it is necessary for personnel to wear film badges or pocket dosimeters to determine or monitor the amount of exposure.

Calm efficiency will have a soothing effect on the client. There should be no suggestion of reluctance or avoidance in rendering care on the part of the nurse (or others). With proper precautions there is less health risk to staff with a radioactively contaminated client than with a client with an infectious disease. Much of the care rendered by the nurse will be supportive in nature, particularly when high doses of radiation are involved.

Chronic Management

Earlier in the chapter, potential latent or chronic effects of ionizing radiation were discussed. Since there are many carcinogens, it is not always possible to determine the cause of cancer.

The ongoing nursing management of the client depends on the primary clinical picture. If anemia and infection are the main problems, they are treated accordingly (see Chap. 24).

Irradiated clients may need long-term psychological rehabilitation, depending upon the severity of their reaction to the radiation injury. The nurse's therapeutic approach to the client will be determined by his need, not by the fact that he was once irradiated. The initial response by nursing staff is extremely important and may have a significant effect upon the client's immediate response as well as his future need for psychological help.

REVIEW QUESTIONS

The number of the question corresponds to the same-numbered objective at the beginning of the chapter.

1. Which of the following types of ionizing radiation has low penetrative ability but is most hazardous to humans if the radiation emitter is inhaled or ingested?
   a. alpha
   b. beta
   c. gamma
   d. neutron

2. In the United States the natural background dose accumulated per year varies from
   a. 10 to 50 mrem
   b. 80 to 500 mrem
   c. 10 to 50 rem
   d. 80 to 500 rem

3. Ionizing radiation damages tissue most commonly by
   a. passing through the tissue without being absorbed
   b. decreasing the kinetic or heat energy of the molecules
   c. transferring its energy by ejecting or dislodging the cellular electrons
   d. transferring its energy by ejecting or dislodging the cellular protons

4. In planning care for the client with internal radiation the nurse should know that all the following afford some protection from ionizing radiation *except*
   a. shielding
   b. dosimeters
   c. distance
   d. time

5. In decontaminating a client with external contamination or suspected internal contamination, which of the following would be saved and labeled "Radioactive—Do Not Discard"?
   a. blood, urine, feces, and vomitus
   b. shoes, outer garments, and underwear
   c. metal jewelry, belt buckles, and dental plates
   d. all the above

REFERENCES

1. E. L. Saenger, *Perspectives on Radiation Accidents,* Hospital preparation for the Management of Radiation Accidents Seminar sponsored by the University of Cincinnati Medical Center, Sept. 29 and 30, 1980.
2. L. Battista et al., *Population Dose and Health Impact on the Accident at Three Mile Island Nuclear Station,* U.S. Government Printing Office, Washington, D.C., May 10, 1979.
3. J. Shapiro, *Radiation Protection,* Harvard University Press, Cambridge, Mass. 1972.
4. L. S. Taylor, "Some Nonscientific Influences on Radiation Protection Standards and Practice: The 1980 Sievert Lecture," *Health Phys,* **39**:851–874 (1980).
5. E. Travis, *Primer of Medical Radiobiology,* Year Book Medical Publishers, Inc., Chicago, 1975.
6. A. G. Searle, *Genetic Effects of Neutrons in Mammals and Their Implications for Risk Assessment in Man: Biological and Environmental Effects of Low-Level Radiation,* vol. 2, International Atomic Energy Agency, Vienna, 1976, pp. 461–471.
7. P. B. Selby, "Radiation-Induced Dominant Skeletal Mutations in Mice: Mutation Rate, Characteristics, and Usefulness in Estimating Genetic Hazard to Humans from

Radiation," The Sixth International Congress of Radiation Research, Tokyo, 1979, pp. 537–544.
8. Travis, loc. cit.
9. S. M. Bunin, *Psychological Aspects of Acute Radiation Accidents: Handling Radiation Accidents,* International Atomic Energy Agency, Vienna, 1969.
10. J. G. Kereiakes, "The Health Physicist," Hospital preparation for the Management of Radiation Accidents Seminar sponsored by the University of Cincinnati Medical Center, Sept. 29 and 30, 1980.
11. *Radiation Protection for Medical and Allied Health Care Workers,* National Council on Radiation Protection and Measurements, Report No. 48, Washington, D.C., 1976.
12. Ibid.
13. *Nurses—Emergency Handling of Radiation Accident Cases,* U.S. Atomic Energy Commission, 1969.

Chapter 60

NURSING ROLE IN MANAGEMENT

Addictive Behavior

Karen H. May McArdle
Patsy L. Orth Duphorne

Learning Objectives

1. Identify general theories of causation of addictive behaviors.
2. Differentiate between physiological and psychological dependence.
3. Describe the addictive cycle.
4. Describe common features of addictive behaviors.
5. Describe the incidence and at-risk population for specific addictive behaviors.
6. Describe the clinical manifestations and complications of smoking, obesity, caffeinism, and alcoholism.
7. Classify abused drugs according to type, street name, route of administration, effects, and complications.
8. Describe the assessment and medical and nursing management of drug overdose and alcohol withdrawal syndrome.
9. Identify potentially dangerous interactions between alcohol and other chemical substances.
10. Describe nursing management for the alcoholic client undergoing surgery.
11. Describe the general nursing role in assessment and management of addictive behaviors.
12. Identify treatment programs available to clients with addictive behaviors.
13. Describe common problems in the process of recovery from an addiction.

Any substance capable of inducing physiological or psychological dependency is a candidate for use in addictive behavior. Because this behavior may fall short of physiological addiction yet be harmful to the individual, the term *substance abuse* has been adopted as a substitute for *addiction*. It more accurately suggests the common situation and suggests the wide range of substances involved. Besides the well-known drugs of addiction, the list of substances implicated in substance abuse includes glue, nicotine, caffeine, and even food.

The nurse may encounter the substance abuser anywhere—in the emergency room, the hospital ward, the place of employment, the school, the family, or social settings. The substance abuser could be the skid-row vagrant but is more likely to be a coworker, neighbor, family member, or client.

This chapter focuses on five kinds of substance abuse: smoking, obesity, caffeinism, drug abuse, and alcohol abuse. It presents causes, common aspects, and physiological and psychological consequences of abuse. Treatment approaches are described, and the role of the nurse in the assessment and management of the client in an acute care setting is discussed.

CAUSES OF ADDICTIVE BEHAVIOR

Nearly everyone uses sustances susceptible to abuse on occasion. Why do some develop addictive behavior and others do not? The answer is complex and not completely known. Etiological theories may be grouped into four general models: medical, psychodynamic, social-learning, and sociocultural. These models are presented in their pure form. In actual situations, there is much overlap of causes for a specific addictive behavior.

The *medical model* emphasizes the disease concept and looks at physiological problems either as genetic predispositions or as physical changes caused by addiction. Problems may be caused by differences in metabolic rates, lack of certain enzymes in the breakdown of substances such as alcohol, dietary deficiencies such as deficiency of the vitamin B complex, hormonal reactions to stress, brain damage, and unusual responses of the nervous system to substances. In addition, genetic predisposition or genetic transmission is associated with alcoholism and obesity. Intensive biochemical studies are under way to identify receptors and transmitters in the brain for opiates and to clarify the role of endorphins (morphinelike substances produced by the body) in addiction.[1]

The *psychodynamic model* focuses on interpersonal or intrapersonal needs and problems which underlie the symptoms of addiction. A connection with a personality disorder or neurosis is sought. A description of the "addictive personality" (a myth not supported by research) often includes low self-esteem, poor communication skills, and inadequate relationships with others.

The *social-learning model* focuses on early learning of potentially addictive behaviors through modeling by parents and the belief that this behavior relieves

This chapter was reviewed by Sandra J. Ciske, Treatment Director, Northwest Treatment Center for Alcoholism, Seattle, Washington.

tension. The addictive behavior is strongly reinforced in an attempt to prevent withdrawal symptoms. It is also reinforced socially and emotionally because it may help the substance abuser cope with his environment.

The *sociocultural model* looks at the cultural influences on behaviors, including the rituals, practices, or taboos which may limit or enhance such behaviors. Additional influences include society's moral, ethical, or legal responses (deterrents) to addiction.

COMMON ASPECTS OF ADDICTIVE BEHAVIORS

All addictive behaviors have certain common features or themes as shown in Table 60-1. These themes may be present in the initiation or maintenance of addictive behaviors; they may not all be present in every individual, or they may be found in varying degrees. Because of the serious implications these themes have for assessment and nursing management, it is essential that they be assessed with each person suspected of addiction.

HEALTH PROMOTION AND MAINTENANCE

Health professionals have frequent opportunities to encourage and support the development of positive and healthy patterns of behavior to cope with frustration and stress. Some approaches that the health professional may use to aid the client are:

1. Helping people find ways to express feelings either through direct expression verbally or indirectly through physical exercise
2. Introducing relaxation techniques
3. Providing factual information about the physical and emotional risks associated with addictive behaviors
4. Describing observations of problematic behaviors to increase awareness
5. Speaking out publicly against known health hazards such as smoking and alcohol and drug abuse
6. Modeling healthy patterns of coping rather than negative, addictive behaviors
7. Supporting the efforts of others to change addictive behaviors

TERMS USED TO DESCRIBE ADDICTIVE BEHAVIORS

Physiological Dependence

Addiction is a process of physiological dependence which is characterized by the two primary components of tolerance and withdrawal syndrome. The first component, *tolerance*, develops with repeated use. It refers to the need to continually increase the amount of a substance used to obtain the desired

Table 60-1
Common Features of Addictive Behaviors

Biophysical Dimension	Psychological Dimension	Sociocultural Dimension	Environmental Dimension
At risk for chronic or terminal illnesses	Self-destructiveness	Family dysfunction (behavioral disorders in other family members)	Increased risk taking (inattention, accident-proneness)
Physical changes due to substance abuse	Denial	Alienation or isolation from family and friends	Inappropriate response to life crises (accidents, trauma, hospitalization, moves, or job changes)
Tolerance	Projection	Modeling influence or peer pressure for substance use	Reliance on environment for structure and support
Withdrawal symptoms	Manipulation	Poor social skills (particularly among adolescents)	External responsiveness (allowing outside cues to control consumption or use)
Relapse, or the abstinence violation effect (occuring when user attempts to stop the substance)	Compulsive behavior		
	Impulsive behavior		
	Low frustration tolerance		
	Stress reduction (initial decrease in tension, but with long-term abuse and increased tension)		
	Distortion of reality		
	Depression		
	Helplessness		
	Poor body image or low self-esteem		
	Craving (emotional response to felt need or desire for substance following decreased use or abstinence)		
	Loss of control (not being able to stop once a substance is used)		

effect. For example, if two beers produce a "high" initially, later it may take six and finally twelve or fifteen to produce the same effect. However, tolerance by itself does not indicate addiction. Furthermore, tolerance develops more rapidly with some substances such as heroin, than with others such as alcohol. Tolerance usually decreases with heavy substance abuse over a period of time because of a slowing of metabolism secondary to liver damage.

The second component of addiction is the *withdrawal syndrome*, a predictable pattern of response when the regular use of a chemical is discontinued, interrupted, or decreased without substitution. For example, when regular heavy use of alcohol is suddenly stopped, it is predictable that anxiety, tremors, nausea, and other symptoms will follow.

Psychological Dependence

Psychological dependence refers to the subjective need for a chemical or object. In other words, a person thinks he needs the substance. It has also been termed *habituation*. It is a primary motivator in addiction, as it is a strong reinforcer of continued substance use. Psychological dependence may occur without physiological dependence for certain substances such as marijuana and nicotine (Table 60-2). If the dependence is only psychological, there will be no physiological symptoms upon withdrawal.

ADDICTIVE CYCLE

The addictive cycle is an unhealthy response pattern learned in order to deal with stress or anxiety or fulfill an unsatisfied need (Fig. 60-1). Such needs may include hunger, sex, security, belonging, self-confidence, elevation of mood, or a change in behavior. The addictive response pattern is a means to avoid problem solving. In the development of this cycle, psychological dependence develops prior to physiological dependence. The dependence is reinforced through continued use when a problem, need, or stressful situation arises. This pattern of coping is generalized to a wide variety of situations and its original intent is lost. The fulfillment of the need helps the person maintain a distance from the problem. In many cases the action of the substance frees the abuser from responsibility for personal behavior. This cycle may be continuous or interrupted, stopping and starting as numerous attempts are made to regain control over use of the abused substance. During these interruptions, withdrawal symptoms may occur. Depending upon the substance and the severity of the withdrawal syndrome, the abuser may require hospitalization. However, the cycle is usually continued to avoid the unpleasant and sometimes fatal effects of withdrawal.

ADDICTIVE BEHAVIORS

Smoking (Tobacco Abuse)

Incidence

Smoking is the most common form of drug abuse in our society. It has a much greater potential for the development of dependence than alcohol. The trends in smoking have varied over the past 10 years, but the

Table 60-2
Dependency in Substance Abuse

Drug Class or Type	Tolerance	Psychological Dependence	Physiological Dependence
Stimulants			
Caffeine	Yes	Yes	No
Nicotine	Yes	Yes	No
Amphetamines	Yes	Yes	No
Cocaine	No	Yes	No
Depressants			
Heroin	Yes	Yes	Yes (rapid)
Codeine	Yes	Yes	Yes
Morphine	Yes	Yes	Yes
Methadone	Yes	Yes	Yes
Barbiturates	Yes	Yes	Yes
Alcohol	Yes	Yes	Yes
Hallucinogens			
Marijuana	No	Yes	No
LSD	Mild	Yes	No
PCP	?	?	?

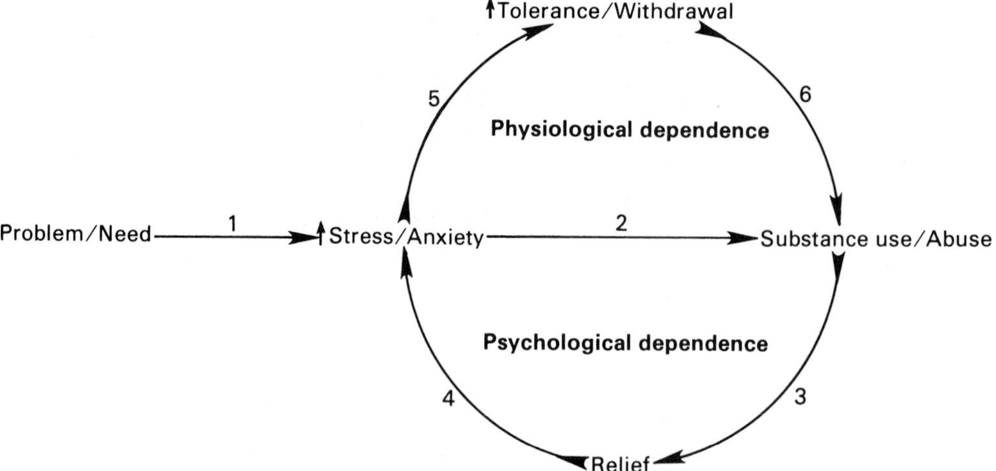

Figure 60-1 The addictive cycle. *Step 1*: The problem or need arouses stress or anxiety and is dealt with through substance use. *Steps 2 to 4*: The cycle of substance use, relief, and recurring stress or anxiety is repeated until psychological dependence is established. Interrupting the cycle brings about anxiety but not physical symptoms. *Steps 5 to 6*: Physiological dependence usually follows psychological dependence. Increased tolerance is a sign of physical adaptation. Withdrawal symptoms then follow abstinence.

percentage of smokers appears to be decreasing. The percentage of women smokers has not decreased as much as that of males, however, and the greatest increase in smoking is among teenage girls.[2] In 1977 about 53 million Americans smoked. More than 30 million Americans have quit smoking.[3] It has been estimated that a person's life is shortened 14 minutes for each cigarette smoked.[4]

Both smokers and nonsmokers are at risk from the effects of smoking on their health. Pipe and cigar smokers usually puff and do not inhale, hence are considered to be at lower risk for developing health problems than cigarette smokers. Occupations involving smoke or dust increase the risk of illness and early death in a person who also smokes. Children who are most likely to smoke include those whose parents, siblings, or friends smoke.

Effects of use

Smoking is a stimulant that fulfills a need unique to the individual. It is the response to stress and tension which is important in both the initiation and the continuation of this behavior. Tobacco contains more than 100 known chemical compounds, including at least 15 known carcinogens and a number of hydrocarbons or solvents which may cause death.[5] Two of the most damaging substances are nicotine and carbon monoxide.

Nicotine is such a potent drug that the nicotine removed from one cigar, if injected intravenously, would be a fatal dose![6] Nicotine is absorbed through the lungs in smoking, through the buccal mucosa in chewing, and through the nasal mucosa in snuffing. When taken by these routes, nicotine initially bypasses the liver and goes directly to the brain and other parts of the body. The clinical manifestations of smoking are listed in Table 60-3.

All tobacco smoke contains *carbon monoxide*. When the smoke is inhaled, the carbon monoxide combines with blood hemoglobin and prevents the hemoglobin from carrying oxygen. This decreased oxygenation of blood may explain the smoker's shortness of breath during exertion.

Smoking has adverse effects on a developing fetus. It has been observed that fetal breathing move-

Table 60-3
Clinical Manifestations of Smoking (Nicotine Related)*

Raised arousal level
Decreased attention to extraneous stimuli
Fine tremor (nicotine tremor)
Shortness of breath
Decreased appetite
Antidiuretic effect
Decreased aggressiveness
Sedation (with large doses)

*Found in varying degrees in nicotine users.

ments are reduced when the mother smokes. The birth weights of babies of mothers who smoke tend to be lower than average. In mothers who smoke, a 200 to 300 percent increase in prematurity and twice as many aborted and stillborn babies have been noted, compared to mothers who do not smoke.[7] These infants are also more susceptible to bronchitis and pneumonia during the first 2 years of life.[8]

Smoking is an addictive behavior. Tolerance develops rather quickly, as indicated by the need to increase the number of cigarettes smoked daily. When tobacco is suddenly withdrawn from a regular user, subjective and objective symptoms appear which include craving, irritability, depression, drop in pulse rate and blood pressure, constipation, sleep disturbance, and changes in the EEG.

Complications

A major concern in smoking involves accidental death due to fires from careless habits, especially smoking in bed. Smoking predisposes to respiratory disease (especially chronic obstructive pulmonary disease), cardiovascular disease, and increased incidence of cancer of the mouth, throat, and lungs. The incidence of cancer of the mouth, throat, larynx, and stomach is higher for cigar and pipe smokers. There also appears to be an association between smoking and the development of peptic ulcers and cirrhosis of the liver. Women over 35 who smoke and take birth control pills have an increased risk of hemorrhage, especially cerebral hemorrhage.

Obesity

Incidence

Obesity may be described as the condition of being 15 percent or more over the ideal body weight based on height and frame.[9] Obesity generally occurs when more calories are taken in than are utilized by the body for energy. Physiological causes of obesity are the exception rather than the rule. Approximately 20 to 40 percent of the American population is overweight.[10] Being overweight does not necessarily mean being overnourished. Obese persons may be malnourished, especially when the greater part of their caloric intake is obtained from carbohydrates.

Etiology

The tendency for obesity to occur in families may reflect metabolic or genetic predispositions as well as learned behaviors and rituals surrounding eating. The behaviors affecting eating are usually learned early by the child. Modeling practices of parents or significant others make lasting impressions. Eating patterns may be influenced by one's culture, ethnic background, or religion. Peer influences, age group, and lifestyle also prescribe certain eating practices and patterns. The child learns quickly that good children eat everything. They may also be rewarded by sweets. The child may also learn that certain foods, particularly sweets, help the hurt go away. The adult transfers this behavior to current situations by, for instance, enjoying a piece of chocolate cake after getting a traffic ticket.

Appetite and Hunger *Hunger* is a physical sensation resulting from contractions of an empty stomach. *Appetite*, a psychophysiological phenomenon, is the desire or craving for food and is not dependent upon an empty stomach. Major reward centers are found in areas within the hypothalamus in the brain and appetite is concerned with the hypothalamus. When certain areas of the brain are stimulated, extreme hunger and food-searching behavior result. The hypothalamus also contains a satiation center. When this center is stimulated, hunger is resolved and eating stops. If the satiation center is damaged, a tremendous appetite results from the loss of control. Since the appetite is not satisfied, gross obesity results.

Eating causes biochemical changes in the reward center of the brain. Because of these changes, overeating and dieting become more complex issues than merely satisfying hunger.

Types of obesity

The two basic types of obesity are juvenile and adult onset. In *juvenile obesity* there are a greater number of adipose cells than normal and some enlargement of these cells. A generalized distribution of fat is observed over the entire body. *Adult onset obesity* begins during the adult years or during pregnancy and is characterized by a normal number of cells, enlargement of these cells, and a central distribution of fat. This type of obesity is often caused by metabolic disorders and can be a predisposing factor in hypertension.

Diagnosis of the type of obesity is based on history of onset, metabolic findings, and observation of the distribution of fat. During weight loss the cell size may decrease but the number of cells does not change, so it is more difficult for the juvenile-onset obese person to lose weight and maintain the weight loss.[11]

Complications

The obese client is a greater surgical risk because of potential postoperative complications such as infection, pulmonary disorders, abdominal distension, and phlebitis. Obesity increases the risk for cerebrovascular disease and coronary heart disease. Pulmonary and cardiac failure may be associated with massive obesity, and there may be aggravation of some diseases such as degenerative joint disease, angina pectoris, hypertension, and adult-onset diabetes. There may also be an increased risk for certain types of cancer, including cancer of the colon and gallbladder.

Starvation diets predispose to hyperuricemia, electrolyte depletion, and ketosis. Compulsive dieting or use of stimulants such as amphetamines may lead to anorexia nervosa, so a diet should be undertaken with medical supervision.

Weight loss

Weight loss is dependent on a number of factors. One of these factors is body image—the more positive the body image during and after weight loss, the more successful it will be. The ability to respond to internal cues (hunger) rather than external cues is essential for tuning in to one's own body. The amount of activity or energy exerted may help or hinder this process, although increased exercise seems to be most effective for adult-onset obesity.[12] Support systems such as the family members' response to the obese person's dieting and weight loss are important in predicting success. The individual's motivation for making changes in his own behavior is also very important.

Maintenance of weight loss can be more difficult than the weight loss itself unless permanent behavior modifications have been made. Reexposure to stressors often precipitates the old eating patterns and weight gain.

Caffeinism (Caffeine Abuse)

Incidence

Approximately 80 percent of adults and 30 percent of youths (12 to 17 years old) use coffee. Adults and youths were found to have similar rates (60 percent) for the consumption of tea.[13] One cup of coffee contains approximately 100 to 150 mg caffeine, which is considered a therapeutic dose. The content of caffeine in tea varies according to how it is brewed and the use of additives such as milk or sugar. A cup of tea averages 60 to 75 mg caffeine and a glass of cola 40 to 60 mg caffeine.

Caffeine is a xanthine derivative which occurs naturally in a number of plants such as coffee beans, tea leaves, cocoa, and cola nuts. It is also found in medications such as Excedrin, Vanquish, Anacin, Bromo Seltzer, and cold preparations.[14]

Effects of use

Caffeine is one of the most widely used stimulant drugs in the world. It is readily available in the form of coffee, tea, and cola drinks. Caffeine is absorbed by the gastrointestinal tract and rapidly distributed throughout the body. Peak blood plasma levels occur within 30 minutes after ingestion. Caffeine crosses the placenta and is also secreted in the milk of lactating females. High doses of caffeine stimulate the respiratory center and may be useful in reversing respiratory depression in cases of drug overdose.

The clinical manifestations of caffeine use are listed in Table 60-4. Some of the physiological actions help to explain caffeine's effectiveness in increasing work output and prolonging the time one can perform physically exhausting work.

Caffeine interferes with sleep by increasing sleep onset time, decreasing dreaming (REM) sleep, and decreasing deep sleep time. Coffee taken in the evening is more likely to have adverse effects on light users than on regular or heavy users (5 to 6 cups or more per day). Coffee taken in the morning by regular or heavy users is required to avoid morning tiredness and irritability.

Caffeine is considered to be an addicting substance, although the question of tolerance is still being debated. The most common and best substantiated withdrawal symptom is headache. It occurs about 18 hours after abstinence begins and can be relieved by caffeine use. Other effects of withdrawal include irritability, sleepiness, and feelings of decreased contentment, alertness, and energy.

Complications

Caffeine is contraindicated in patients with glaucoma because it can significantly raise the intraocular pressure when the glaucoma is unregulated, resulting in a caffeine-induced headache.

Table 60-4

Clinical Manifestations of Caffeinism*

Increased alertness and thinking
Increased respirations
Relaxation of smooth visceral muscles
Decreased peristalsis
Possible interference with REM and deep sleep
Increased speed of motor tasks
Increased myocardial contractions
Diuresis
Jitteriness
Nervousness
GI upset

*Found in varying degrees in caffeine users.

Toxic effects of caffeine include ringing in the ears, flashes of light, insomnia, increased sensibility, tachycardia, arrhythmias, and hypotension. In heavy coffee drinkers, blood lipid level may be increased, which may lead to increased incidence of angina and myocardial infarction. Habitual users are reported to have slightly higher blood pressure, increased basal metabolic rates, and increased blood glucose levels. In high doses, caffeine influences behavior patterns and may precipitate anxiety states.

Drug Abuse

Billions of dollars are spent each year for legal and illegal drugs that are used to alter mood, thinking, awareness, and consciousness. Addictive behaviors related to drug abuse primarily represent either illicit use or misuse of prescribed chemical substances. Those who practice illicit use are frequently associated with a drug culture which uses its own jargon and supports drug-seeking behaviors (Table 60-5). Misuse of prescribed medications, particularly amphetamines and tranquilizers, has become a major problem in our society.

The substances discussed in this section are classified as (1) stimulants, (2) depressants, and (3) hallucinogens according to their primary effect in altering mind or body functions (Table 60-6).

Stimulants

Drugs classified as stimulants are listed in Table 60-5.

Incidence of Problem About 8 billion amphetamines are manufactured legally each year. Stimulant drugs account for 5.4 percent of all prescriptions, or nearly 13 million prescriptions. The highest incidence of stimulant use is in the 18- to 25-year-old category.[15]

Effects of Use Stimulants are often taken to elevate the mood, increase alertness, and decrease appetite. The use of stimulant drugs for weight control has greatly decreased because of the adverse effects

Table 60-5
Addictive Substances

Substance	Street Names	Administration
	Stimulants	
Cocaine	Cake, snow, big, candy, girl, charlie, corinne, gold dust, coke, bernice, flake, stardust	Sniffed, injected, oral
Amphetamine (Benzedrine)	Uppers, bennies, splash, peaches, hearts, roses	Oral, injected
Dextroamphetamine (Dexedrine)	Dexies, oranges, copilots, Christmas trees	Oral, injected
Biphetamine (Benzedrine & Dexedrine combination)	Footballs	Oral, injected
Methamphetamine (Methedrine)	Crystal, meth, speed	Oral, injected
Cigarettes (nicotine)	Fags, coffin nails	Smoked, sniffed, chewed
Caffeine		Oral
	Depressants (Downers)	
Amobarbital (Amytal)	Goof balls, fool pills, downs, blue heavens, blue devils	Oral, injected
Amobarbital & secobarbital (Tuinal)	Tooies, rainbows, Christmas trees, double trouble	Oral, injected
Pentobarbital (Nembutal)	Yellow jackets, dolls, goof balls, nimbies	Oral, injected
Phenobarbital (Luminal)	Purple Hearts, pink lady, phennies	Oral, injected
Secobarbital (Seconal)	Reds, red birds, red devils, seccy	Oral, injected
Glutethimide (Doriden)	Cibas	Oral, injected

Table 60-5 (Continued)

Substance	Street Names	Administration
Marijuana (leaves of the *Cannabis sativa* plant) THC, hashish (resin of the cannabis plant)	Pot, grass, hemp, reefer, tea, weed, gage, Mary Jane, Acapulco gold, Panama red, hash	Oral, sniffed, smoked ("tokes"—inhalations)
Heroin	H, horse, smack, scag, stuff, Harry Scat, junk	Sniffed, smoked, intravenous injection (called *mainlining*), subcutaneous injection (called *skin popping*)
Codeine	Schoolboy, junk	Oral
Morphine	M, white stuff, monkey morf	Oral, injected
Methadone	Dolly, dolls	Oral, injected
Alcohol, ethanol, ethyl alcohol	Booze, juice	Oral
	Hallucinogens	
LSD	Acid, trips, big D, sugar cubes, 25, instant Zen	Oral, injected
Psilocybin	Magic mushrooms	Oral
DMT, *N,N*-dimethyltryptamine	AMT, businessman's high, businessman's trip or lunch	Injected, smoked
Morning glory seeds	Pearly gates, flying saucers, heavenly blue	Oral
Mescaline (peyote)	Mesc, white light, blue caps, pink wedge, big chief, cactus, button tops	Oral, injected
4-Methyl-25-dimethoxy-methylphenethylamine	STP, DOM	Oral
Ketamine hydrochloride	Green, 1980 supergrass (when used with marijuana, it is called K, jet, superacid, purple mauve, special LA coke, super C)	Smoked, injected
Methyl-3, 4-methylenedioxyamphetamine	MDA, love drug	Oral
Phencyclidine (Sernyl)	PCP, hog, elephant tranquilizer, horse tranks, angel dust (when sprinkled on leaves such as mint or parsley, it is known as crystal joints, superweed, angel hair, CJ, or KJ)	Snorted, smoked, oral
Solvents such as airplane glue, automobile paint, gasoline, paint thinners		Sniffed

of the drugs. Also, it is now recognized that after about 2 weeks of taking these drugs, their anorectic property becomes ineffective.

The major effects of stimulants are presented in Table 60-6. *Amphetamines*, originally used in the treatment of narcolepsy, are one type of stimulant (Fig. 60-2). They cross the blood-brain barrier rapidly and produce wakefulness, hyperactivity, anorexia initially, diaphoresis, some increase in metabolic rates, hypertension, and peripheral vascular constriction. The amphetamine user may become febrile, restless, irritable, and acutely psychotic.

With frequent or heavy use, amphetamine psychosis often develops. As a result of this paranoid state, the abuser may become violent and destructive. The person admitted to the hospital in this paranoid state is potentially dangerous to himself and others. He will generally require hospitalization until the symptoms clear, in 48 to 72 hours.

Fatigue and depression are common upon withdrawal of amphetamines. Grand mal seizures may occur when amphetamines are suddenly discontinued. Fatal overdose results in convulsions and coma prior to death.

Cocaine, another type of stimulant, mimics the effects of amphetamines. It is the most expensive stimulant on the illegal drug market. It is rapidly absorbed across all mucous membranes and can be taken intravenously as well as sniffed. It produces tremendous euphoria. When it is taken intravenously, the effect has been described as a whole-body orgasm.

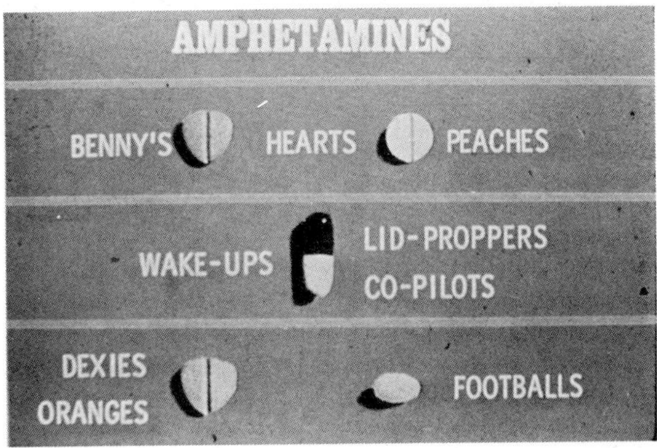

Figure 60-2 Amphetamines are known by various street names.

When cocaine is taken intravenously, a brief but intense vasoconstriction occurs. Collapse and scarring of the veins at the injection site may occur. When the drug is sniffed the severe vasoconstriction that occurs may damage the nasal septum and mucosa.

Table 60-6
Effects of Drugs by Major Classification

Classification	Physiological Effects	Psychological Effects
Stimulants	Stimulation of central nervous system Vasoconstriction Rapid development of tolerance Increased pulse and blood pressure Diaphoresis	Mood elevation Paranoia Increased alertness Hyperactivity
Depressants	Depression of central nervous system Hypotension Slowed heart beat and respiration Increased reaction time Analgesia or anesthesia	Tranquility Drowsiness Confusion
Hallucinogens	Increased pulse, blood pressure, and respirations Increased salivation Dilated pupils Probable inhibition of some neurotransmitters Rapid production of tolerance for psychedelic response	Distortion of senses and perceptions Flashbacks Behavior changes Auditory and visual hallucinations

Because of stricter controls and more limited use of amphetamines, a new class of drugs called *legal stimulants* is gaining popularity. These look-alike drugs are similar in appearance to pharmaceutically prepared drugs, and many contain numbers and markings. They also have similar street names such as "pink hearts" and "black beauties." The chemical ingredients are basically caffeine or ephedrine or combinations of these two drugs with phenylpropanolamine or diphenhydramine. All these drugs are central nervous system stimulants. They are sold in capsule or tablet forms without prescriptions (Fig. 60-3).

Complications There are serious complications with the use of stimulants. Marked weight loss may occur, primarily from decreased food intake rather than increased metabolism. Scarring and collapse of veins occur with the intravenous use of cocaine. Damage to the nasal septum and mucosa occurs when cocaine is sniffed. Myocardial failure and cerebrovascular accidents are potential adverse effects from the use of stimulants. Several fatalities have been associated with the use of legal stimulants.

Depressants

Drugs classified as depressants are listed in Table 60-5.

Incidence of Problem In 1977, 8.5 million Americans took prescription sleeping pills at least once; of those, 2.1 million took the drug every night for 2 months or more.[16]

The popularity of sedatives and hypnotics has decreased, because they have been found to provide only short-term therapeutic effectiveness and have a high abuse potential. Their use has frequently resulted in overdose or suicide.

Effects of Use Depressants act primarily on the central nervous system (Table 60-6). They depress cardiac and respiratory function. They are largely detoxified in the liver and are excreted in the urine. The therapeutic functions of the depressant category of substances are to relieve anxiety (sedative), to induce sleep (hypnotic), and to provide analgesia or anesthesia.

Common terms for most depressant drugs are tranquilizers, sleeping pills, and pain pills. The tranquilizer category of drugs is such a large field of study that it is not included in this chapter. The reader is referred to psychiatric nursing texts and psychopharmacology texts for information concerning such drugs as chlorpromazine (Thorazine), chlordiazepoxide (Lib-

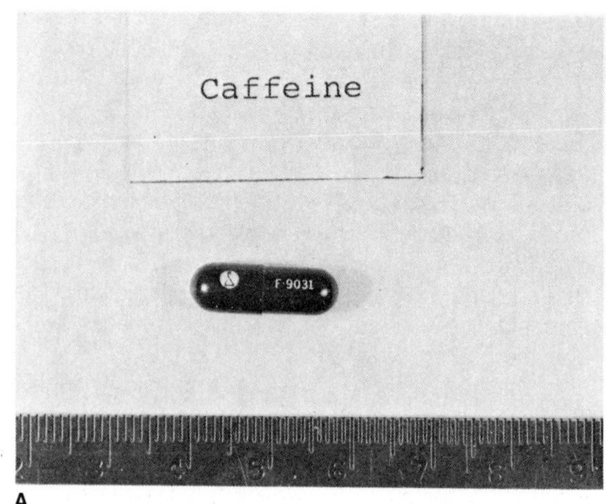

A

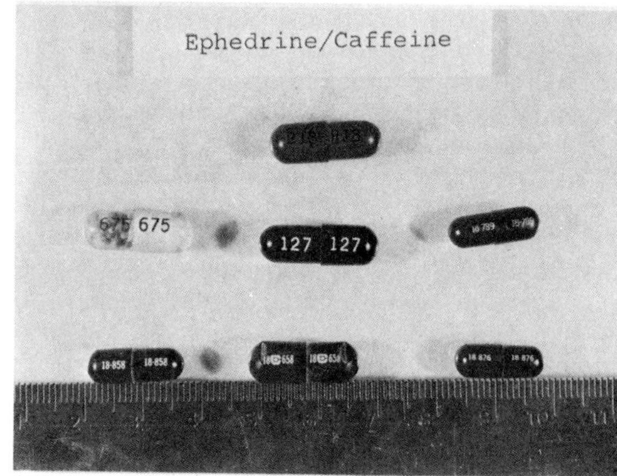

B

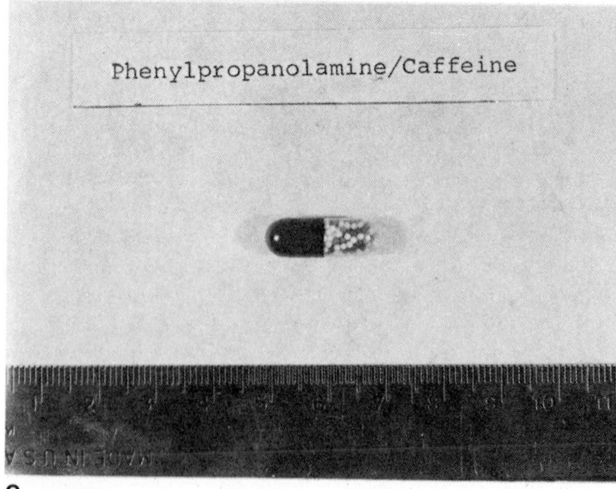

C

Figure 60-3 A new class of legal stimulants is gaining in popularity (Scales in centimeters.)

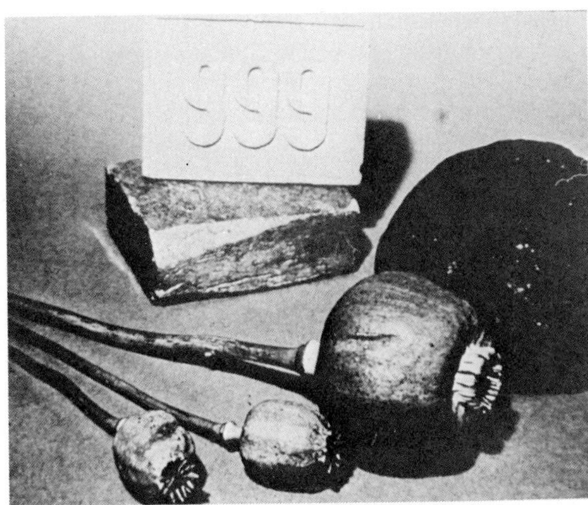

Figure 60-4 Opium is obtained as a milky exudate from the unripened capsule of the opium poppy (left), prepared as gum opium (right). The most active constituent is morphine, seen as a block of morphine base in the background.

rium), and diazepam (Valium). Diazepam is probably the most abused prescription drug in our society.

Morphine and codeine are pure derivatives of opium (Fig. 60-4). Narcotics such as methadone and meperidine (Demerol) are synthetically produced. Heroin, which is prepared from morphine, is a severe respiratory depressant and has no legal use. All narcotics have a high potential for addiction and abuse. The primary therapeutic purpose of narcotics is analgesia. Tolerance develops quickly when narcotics are used to seek a "high." Accidental overdose is most likely to occur following a period of hospitalization when the user has no access to narcotics. When narcotics are taken irregularly for pain relief, tolerance builds up slowly and addiction is uncommon.

Methadone (Dolophine, Amidon, Adanon), also known as "dollies" and "10-8-20," is a federally controlled substance. It acts to block the action of heroin, particularly the euphoric high, and it decreases the craving for heroin. Methadone is long-acting, effective orally and inexpensive and generally has few side effects. It has been widely used in maintenance programs to help clients withdraw from heroin and other narcotics. Urine checks may be made periodically to evaluate a client's compliance with the program. Because of the development of physical dependency with methadone and its potential for illicit use, alternative drugs are being studied for use in withdrawal programs. Buprenorphine is a drug which is nonaddictive, causes few withdrawal symptoms, and is less likely to cause respiratory depression than methadone. The use of this drug is currently under investigation.

Opiate antagonists are used therapeutically to counteract the respiratory depression associated with narcotic overdose. These drugs include levallorphan tartrate (Lorfan), and naloxone hydrochloride (Narcan). When one of these is given intravenously, it can reverse respiratory depression in minutes. In the presence of narcotic addiction, opiate antagonists precipitate rapid withdrawal symptoms. These drugs also have diagnostic value; if the respiratory depression is not caused by narcotics, the drugs are generally ineffective.

Barbiturates are prescribed primarily for their sedative or hypnotic action (Fig. 60-5). Generally speaking, the more rapidly a barbiturate acts, the greater its potential for misuse and abuse; the longer a barbiturate acts, the greater its potential for chronic poisoning and accidental overdose.

Legal downers have become prominent on the market to replace barbiturates. These are "look-alike" drugs similar to legal stimulants, which encourages users to think and feel as if they were taking the real thing. Many times they are used in conjunction with legal stimulants to bring the user "back down." A serious medical crisis may be potentiated by the use of these drugs.

Complications Complications with the use of depressant drugs include overdose and pulmonary edema. These problems sometimes occur within minutes after the dose is taken. Pulmonary edema may be due to respiratory and cardiovascular depression or to allergic reaction to the drug or to the elements with which the drug may be mixed (cut). If the drug is

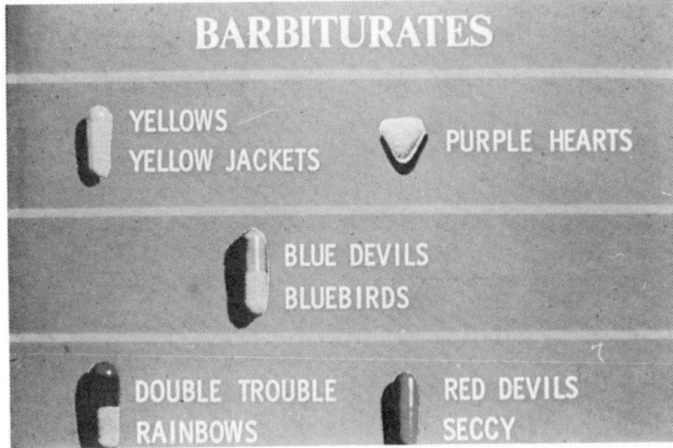

Figure 60-5 Barbiturates are sold under various street names.

injected, the complications may include local abscesses, endocarditis, tetanus, thrombophlebitis, hepatitis, and peripheral vascular disease. Narcotics pass the placental barrier and may create withdrawal problems for the newborn within a few hours after birth. Adverse effects of depressants include fever of 39 to 40°C lasting 24 to 48 hours. Cardiac arrhythmias often occur from the quinine used to cut the narcotic.

Hallucinogens

Drugs classified as hallucinogens are listed in Table 60-5.

Incidence of Problem Since hallucinogens are not legal or prescribed drugs, there are no data from which to determine incidence of their abuse. It is estimated that there are about 45 million marijuana smokers in the United States, and this number is continually increasing.

Effects of Use The hallucinogens are rapidly absorbed from the gastrointestinal tract and mucous membranes. They are detoxified by the liver. Acting as sympathomimetic drugs, they can increase blood pressure, pulse, temperature, and salivation and cause dilated pupils (Table 60-6).

Psychological effects include distortion of the senses and visual and auditory hallucinations. Hallucinogen users may experience a phenomenon called *synesthesia*. This is a subjective experience in which the user may hear light, see sound, and experience other distortions. Tolerance to psychedelic effects occurs rapidly with repeated use.

Flashbacks may occur up to 18 months after the last drug use. Flashbacks are the periodic return of drug-related imagery and feelings in the absence of drug use. They seem to occur more frequently with multiple use and in those with preexisting psychiatric disorders. Flashbacks may be precipitated by unusual stress or falling asleep. A *bad trip* is an acute anxiety and panic reaction which may be experienced by naive users immediately following drug use.

No deaths have been attributed directly to the use of hallucinogens other than solvents (glue, paint). Death can occur indirectly, however, from drug-induced causes such as driving with distorted senses, jumping off high places believing one can fly, or engaging in other such dangerous behavior.

During the first 3 to 5 hours following the usual dose, there is a generalized self-awareness of effects such as shifts in bodily sensations and perceptions. During the next 4 to 5 hours, a period of self-centeredness and ideas of reference occurs. (The term *ideas of reference* indicates a faulty type of thinking in which external events or incidents are referred to oneself.) By 12 to 24 hours after hallucinogen use, there may be some letdown and fatigue.

Marijuana is the most widely used illicit drug. Marijuana is derived from the leaves and flowers of the hemp plant, *Cannabis sativa* (Fig. 60-6). The major psychoactive component is delta-9-THC (tetrahydrocannabinol), which is responsible for 95 percent of the drug effect. Although marijuana may be either smoked or taken orally, it is usually smoked, as a smaller amount is needed in smoking to produce the desired effect. In the process of smoking, one-half to three-fourths of the THC may be lost. Special smoking holders or pipes are employed to recover more of the THC.

Marijuana has similarities to the stimulants, sedatives, analgesics, and psychomimetics. The subjective effects are largely dependent upon the personality and expectations of the user and the social setting. Sense perceptions may be increased in scope and intensity, and imagery becomes stronger. Time-space perception is changed and the passage of time is overestimated. Impairment of immediate memory is a common phenomenon with marijuana use.

The most consistent physiological effects of marijuana are an increase in heart rate, bronchodilatation, and reddening of the conjunctivae. The effects usually occur whithin minutes after smoking and persist for 3 to 4 hours. Following these immediate and short-term responses, it takes approximately 5 to 8 days for one-half of the THC in a single marijuana cigarette to clear out of one's system. When marijuana is taken orally, effects occur in about 30 to 60 minutes and persist for 5 to 7 hours.

Research studies indicate that marijuana may

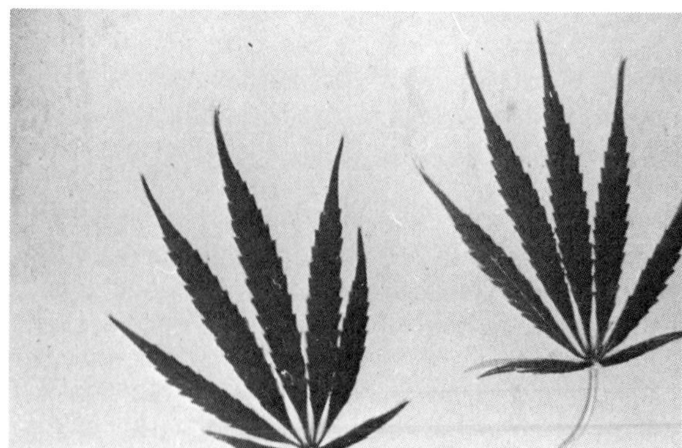

Figure 60-6 Marijuana leaves. Cannabis, or hemp plant, exists as both male and female plants. The female plant's leaves and flowers produce the psychoactive principle, primarily THC, as a sticky resin.

have injurious effects on the reproductive tract, the lungs, cellular metabolism, and the brain. The cannabinoids found in marijuana have an attraction for organs with high fat content and therefore collect in the brain, testes, and ovaries. Marijuana is considered more harmful to the lungs than tobacco. It may also suppress the immune system, specifically the T lymphocytes. This alteration may lead to a proliferation of bacteria and an inability to fight off infection. Marijuana is thought to have a greater carcinogenic potential than tobacco because of the release of irritating chemicals such as carbon monoxide, formaldehyde, and nitrogen in the lungs.[17,18]

Glue sniffing and inhaling the vapors of other solvents to produce a hallucinogenic experience is a deadly game. Spray paint has rapidly become the leading substance abused in this category, surpassing toluene-based glues and gasolines. Inhalants are generally classified as depressants with an initial excitement phase similar to that of alcohol. The physiological effects of inhaled solvents are generally those of an acute brain syndrome. There may be irritation of the eyes, double vision, dizziness, ringing in the ears, slurred speech, dilated pupils, pain in the head, neck, and chest, drowsiness, fever blisters, nausea, vomiting and diarrhea, and unsteady gait. Seizures, convulsions, coma, and death may ultimately result. The psychological effects are similar to alcohol intoxication and include transient euphoria, giddiness, confusion, bizzare behavior, and visual hallucinations.

Complications With high doses of marijuana, the user may be subject to postural hypotension. Bronchitis and asthma may occur with chronic heavy smoking of marijuana. Conjunctival vascular congestion, elevated blood sugar, urinary frequency, and occasional nausea, vomiting, or diarrhea may also result. Symptoms of withdrawal from marijuana may include anxiety, sleeplessness, sweating, lack of appetite, nausea, and general malaise. Cannabis psychosis may result from chronic heavy use. Heavy marijuana use eventually leads to apathy and general deterioration in all aspects of living.[19]

The inhalation of various solvents may cause problems of severe liver, lung, kidney, and central nervous system damage due to direct toxicity of the agents. In chronic users, irritation of nasal and oral mucous membranes may occur. Bone marrow suppression, macrocytic or aplastic anemia, cerebral edema, and hepatic necrosis may also result.

Inhalants may sensitize the heart to circulating epinephrine. This may result in fatal arrhythmias leading to ventricular fibrillation and death. Accidental death may also occur as a result of suffocation when the user is breathing the fumes, the oxygen supply is cut off, or the bag over the face becomes fixed.

Acute management of drug overdose

Assessment Nursing assessment of the overdose client includes continual observation of physical, psychological, and behavioral symptoms. The depressant category of drugs (sedative-hypnotics, narcotics, and solvents) presents the greatest threat to life. Clinical manifestations of overdose may include aggression, agitation, ataxia, depression, disorientation, fever, hallucinations, hypotension, needle tracks, pinpoint pupils (with narcotics), dilated pupils (with sedative-hypnotics), respiratory depression, slurred speech, coma, and convulsions. The nurse's sense of smell may provide clues if solvents have been inhaled.

Diagnostic Studies Blood samples may be tested for drugs. A positive drug test is usually repeated in 12 hours. A urinalysis may be performed to detect the presence of barbiturates, alcohol, narcotics, hallucinogens, and amphetamines. Methadone may not be detected in the urine.

Fluid intake should be restricted before the client gives the urine sample; otherwise a false negative may result. The nurse must be certain that the sample to be tested is from the client and that nothing has been added to it. To avoid decomposition the sample should be taken to the laboratory immediately or kept under refrigeration until analyzed.

Medical Management Medical management is aimed at maintaining the cardiac and respiratory systems and clearing the body of chemicals. General medical management is summarized in Table 60-7.

Nursing Management Aggressive nursing management is important for the drug overdose client (Table 60-8). The immediate goals of nursing management are to maintain the airway and to protect the

Table 60-7

Medical Management of Drug Overdose

1. Treatment of respiratory depression with
   a. opiate antagonists: levallorphan tartate (Lorfan) 0.5 mg IV or naloxone hydrochloride (Narcan) 0.4 mg IV
   b. suctioning
   c. tracheostomy
   d. assisted ventilation
2. Gastric lavage
3. Forced diuresis with thiazides and mannitol
4. Peritoneal dialysis or hemodialysis
5. Restraints if necessary

Table 60-8
Nursing Care Plan for the Client with Drug Overdose

Client Problem	Expected Outcome	Nursing Intervention
Acute toxicity (poisoning)	No evidence of abused substances in body	Assist with gastric lavage, forced diuresis with diuretics, or peritoneal dialysis. Monitor intake and output.
Respiratory depression	Respiratory rate 14–20/min	Maintain patent airway. Monitor respirations. Suction as needed. Administer opiate antagonists as ordered.
Cardiovascular depression	Blood pressure above 100/60. Pulse rate above 60/min	Monitor blood pressure and pulse q 30 min. Stimulate client by talking, touching, etc. Assist with CPR if arrest occurs.
Cardiovascular stimulation	Blood pressure below 150/90. Pulse below 100/min	Monitor blood pressure, pulse, and temperature q 30 min. Give treatments or medications as ordered. Provide quiet environment.
Inadequate intake and output	Fluid intake of 3000–5000 mL/day. Urinary output of 900 mL/day	Monitor intake and output. Observe for manifestations of fluid overload. Maintain intravenous infusion at ordered rate. Ensure patent urinary drainage from bladder. Report urine output <30mL/h.
Increased anxiety (aggression/agitation, withdrawal/depression, suicide thoughts)	Ability to cope with mild to moderate levels of anxiety. No destructive or self-destructive behaviors or thoughts. Ability to interact and communicate needs appropriately	Provide support and reassurance. Be alert to changes in feelings and behavior. Assess degree of depression, intention of suicide, and refer for psychiatric help if high degree. Stay with client. Decrease external stimulation. Communicate in simple, calm manner.
Confusion, disorientation, delusions (paranoid), hallucinations	Clear, alert mental status. Orientation to reality. No delusions or hallucinations	Orient to place, time, and person with each contact. Explain all treatments and procedures in simple direct manner. Keep environment clear and visible with adequate lighting. Do not reinforce ideas by agreeing or disagreeing.
Ataxia or convulsions	No injuries due to falls, no convulsions	Provide bed rails and tongue blade. Apply restraints if necessary. Assist in ambulating.

client from injury. A patent airway is essential if other lifesaving measures are to be of value. Overdose clients may present in an agitated state. Care is needed to protect them from injuring themselves or others.

Vital signs, level of consciousness, and pupillary reflexes should be checked as often as every 10 to 15 minutes until stable, then every 30 minutes, and finally every 4 hours. Siderails should be raised on the bed. Intake and output should be measured accurately.

If the client is comatose, he should be turned frequently. Meticulous skin care should be carried out. Artificial tear solutions or eye patches are used to prevent corneal damage. Nursing care of the unconscious client is discussed in Chap. 52.

Extremely agitated, delusional, or hallucinating clients need a quiet, nonstimulating environment. These clients should not be left alone, as they are extremely frightened, and isolation may increase behavioral symptoms. The nurse must frequently orient the overdosed client—*where* he is, *who* the nurse is, and *what* is happening. The nursing approach should be calm, nonthreatening, and supportive.

Since the overdose may have been a suicide attempt, the client should be observed carefully for further attempts. A psychological assessment to determine the degree of hopelessness, helplessness, and depression is important. A specific suicide assessment questioning motive, plans, and means may be appropriate.

Alcohol Abuse (Alcoholism)

Alcohol is a frequently abused and easily acquired substance. Its misuse affects jobs, family, and health. Alcoholism presents two major problems. First, the effects of chronic alcoholism and withdrawal present serious physiological and psychological problems. Second, the interactions of alcohol with other substances can produce undesirable results (see the section on Interactions of Alcohol and Other Substances).

Incidence

Alcoholism is a major public health problem. Four out of five persons in the United States use alcoholic drinks. Of those who consume alcohol, about one in ten is an alcoholic. Twenty-five billion dollars is spent each year on alcohol-related illnesses, lost time on the job, and property damage resulting from intoxication.[20] The National Council on Alcoholism has compiled a number of risk factors for becoming an alcoholic.[21]

Effects of use

Alcohol is a depressant drug. Its effect on the central nervous system is directly proportional to the blood alcohol level. Alcohol requires no digestion. Approximately 20 percent of alcohol is absorbed unchanged from the stomach and about 80 percent is absorbed from the small intestine. The absorption rate of alcohol can be altered in various ways. When taken on a full stomach, alcohol is absorbed more slowly because protein and fats retain the alcohol in the stomach. Plain water mixed with alcohol slows absorption by diluting its concentration. Soda water increases the rate of absorption because the CO_2 it contains causes rapid movement of alcohol from the stomach to the small intestine. The rate of absorption is increased by strong emotions. When large amounts are ingested, 10 to 15 percent may be eliminated unchanged by the kidneys, lungs, and skin.

Once absorbed into the bloodstream, alcohol goes almost immediately to the liver for metabolism The first step in oxidation occurs when the enzyme *alcohol dehydrogenase* breaks down the alcohol to form acetaldehyde and H_2O (Fig. 60-7). The rate of oxidation established during this step averages 15 g (1 ounce) of alcohol per hour. The second step occurs when the enzyme *acetaldehyde dehydrogenase* converts acetaldehyde and H_2O into acetic acid. The familiar hangover is thought to be produced by the cumulative effect of acetaldehyde. If this enzyme is inhibited by Antabuse or genetic differences, as in some Japanese and native Americans, a lowered tolerance or an Antabuse reaction occurs. The symptoms of this reaction are flushing, decreased blood pressure, tachycardia, diaphoresis, headache, and difficulty breathing. The final step of metabolism occurs when acetic acid breaks down into CO_2 and H_2O. The energy produced by this process amounts to about 7 calories per gram (Fig. 60-8). Fructose or fruit juice may speed up metabolism and may be useful in treating acute intoxication.

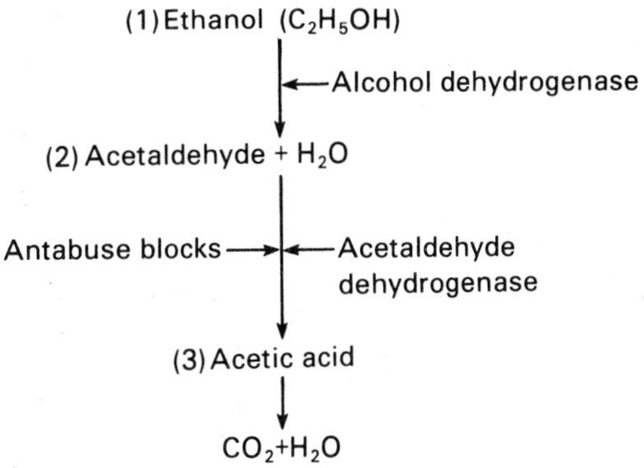

Since alcohol is evenly distributed in the body by the bloodstream, the *blood alcohol level* (BAL) can be correlated with the psychophysiological effects on the body. Alcohol is measurable within 15 to 20 minutes after ingestion and reaches a peak in 60 to 90 minutes. Usually no measurable alcohol is present by 12 to 24 hours after the last drink. The BAL is affected by the amount consumed, the rate of drinking, one's body weight, the concentration of the drink, and the

(1) Ethanol (C_2H_5OH)
↓ ← Alcohol dehydrogenase
(2) Acetaldehyde + H_2O
Antabuse blocks → ↓ ← Acetaldehyde dehydrogenase
(3) Acetic acid
↓
$CO_2 + H_2O$

Figure 60-7 Metabolism of alcohol.

Table 60-9
Risk Factors Related to Alcoholism

History of alcoholism in family
History of total abstinence
Broken or disrupted home
Last or near last child in large family
Female relatives with history of recurrent depression
Heavy smoking
Cultural groups:
- Irish
- Scandinavian
- Native American
- Eskimo

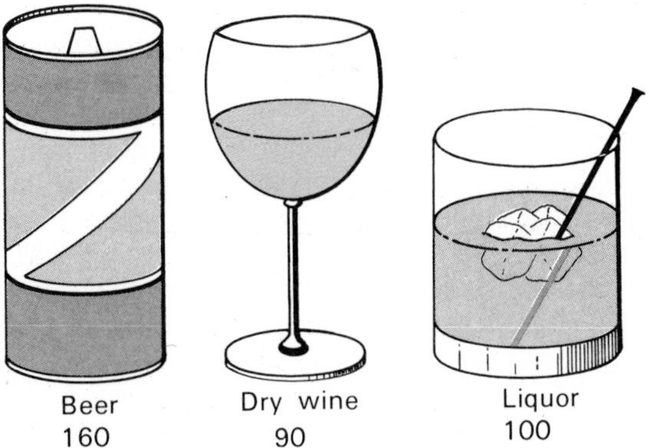

Figure 60-8 Approximate caloric content of various alcoholic drinks.

Table 60-10

Correlation of Basal Alcohol Level (BAL) and Psychophysiological Effects

BAL, mg%*	Psychophysiological Effect
20	Light and moderate drinkers begin to feel some effects. Approximate BAL reached after one drink.
40	Most people begin to feel relaxed.
60	Judgment mildly impaired. People less able to make rational decisions about their capabilities (e.g., to drive).
80	Definite impairment of muscle coordination and driving skills. Legally drunk in some states.
100	Clear deterioration of reaction time and control. Legally drunk in most states.
120	Vomiting unless this level reached slowly.
150	Balance and movement impaired. Equivalent of $\frac{1}{2}$ pint of whiskey circulating in bloodstream.
300	Many people lose consciousness.
400	Most people lose consciousness and some die.
450	Breathing stops; eventual death.

*Basal alcohol level is generally recorded in milligrams of alcohol per 100 mL blood, or milligrams percent (mg%). BAL is determined by how much alcohol is consumed, how fast it is consumed, and individual's weight.

Adapted from William R. Miller and Ricardo F. Munoz, *How to Control Your Drinking,* Prentice-Hall, Inc., Englewood Cliffs, N.J., 1976, p. 11.

menstrual cycle. Generally, the larger the person the more alcohol he can tolerate, unless most of his size is due to fat. The BAL has a fairly predictable correlation with psychophysiological phenomena in the person who has not developed a tolerance for alcohol (Table 60-10).

Alcohol inhibits the antidiuretic hormone (ADH) responsible for retaining body fluids, and it increases blood sugar for about an hour after ingestion. It has an anesthetic effect on minor aches and pains. Alcohol is a gastric irritant because it stimulates the secretion of hydrochloric acid. It decreases inhibitions and enhances mood. The drinker may become happy, hostile, violent, or quite social and amorous. It slows motor reactions and hence increases reaction time. It may cause tunnel vision or double vision in higher doses. Alcohol in low doses tends to increase sexual arousal; with high doses of alcohol, sexual arousal is decreased.

Alcohol also decreases critical thinking and judgment, leading to risk taking and decreased concentration. A major effect is on memory. *Blackout*, or the inability to recall events or actions occurring while intoxicated, is an early warning sign of alcoholism. Jellinek has identified four stages of alcoholism;[22] these are shown in Table 60-11.

Complications

Chronic alcoholism shortens a person's life by about 12 years. Alcohol accelerates the aging process. Chronic use by a pregnant woman may produce the *fetal alchohol syndrome* which includes mental retardation and physical and developmental disabilities in the baby. Neurological damage may result in conditions such as Korsakoff's psychosis, alcoholic pellagra, and Wernicke's syndrome. Cardiac disor-

Table 60-11

Jellinek's Phases of Alcohol Addiction

Phase I—Prealcoholic phase
Sign: Increase in tolerance
Behaviors: Occasional, then constant, relief drinking

Phase II—Prodromal phase
Sign: Ushered in by first blackout
Behaviors: Guilt, sneaking and gulping drinks, alibi system

Phase III—Crucial phase
Sign: Addiction, loss of control
Behaviors: Rationalization, social withdrawal, neglect of food, grandiose and aggressive behavior, morning drinks

Phase IV—Chronic phase
Sign: First bender, decrease in tolerance
Behaviors: Obsession with drinking, physical and moral deterioration, impaired thinking, indefinable anxieties, collapse of alibi system

Note: All symptoms do not necessarily occur in all alcoholics, nor do they always occur in the same sequence. It may take from 5 to 20 years for the male to move from heavy drinking to the chronic phase, often a briefer period for female.

ders include cardiomyopathy, angina pectoris, myocardial infarction, and atrial fibrillation or *holiday heart syndrome* (high alcohol consumption associated with weekend or holiday drinking without heart disease). Pancreatitis, cancer of the esophagus, Mallory-Weiss syndrome (tear at the junction of the stomach and esophagus), esophageal varices, and cirrhosis are also found.

Other adverse reactions include pathological intoxication and withdrawal syndrome. *Pathologic intoxication* is characterized by sudden rage or a psychotic type of reaction to small amounts of alcohol. The *withdrawal syndrome* consists of three phases—the shakes, acute hallucinosis, and delirium tremens.

The alcoholic surgical client

Preoperative Nursing Care Identification of the alcoholic client in the preoperative period is important. The nurse needs to be alert to cues such as alcohol on the breath or increasing agitation. Many alcoholics are undiagnosed at the time of admission for surgery. In addition, the alcoholic is often debilitated and may require health promotion measures prior to surgery. Unless the surgery is a true emergency, the client should not be operated on during the withdrawal phase. Since withdrawal symptoms or delirium tremens (DTs) usually do not begin until 12 to 48 hours after the last drink, surgical procedures should be delayed 48 to 72 hours, if possible. If a known alcoholic requires emergency surgery, intravenous alcohol may be given until the critical phase of the postoperative period is past.

Drug-alcohol interactions pose a potential hazard to the client. Depending upon the drug used and upon the physical state of the client, he may require much more or much less of a drug to produce the desired therapeutic effect. Preoperative medication doses need to be adjusted accordingly. The anesthesiologist needs to be informed if the client is a known or suspected alcoholic.

The client who is tolerant of alcohol may also be tolerant of other medications, including anesthetics. The usual dosage of sedative or anesthetic may not be adequate, and the client may be taken into surgery wide awake and alert.

The acutely intoxicated client may easily be oversedated because sedative drugs act additively with alcohol. Phenothiazines should be used cautiously because of their tendency to produce hypotension. Chloral hydrate inhibits the oxidation of ethyl alcohol, and this can result in central nervous system depression.

Another danger to the alcoholic surgical client is multichemical use. Often the client who abuses alcohol also abuses other drugs. It is not uncommon to find significant concentrations of sedatives in the blood of the alcoholic. To add more medication to the client's system which already contains two types of depressants can be risky. This is why a complete drug history on admission can be helpful in preventing the problem. However, the substance abuser is often reluctant to admit use of an addictive substance.

Postoperative Nursing Care The alcoholic client takes longer to become fully responsive in the immediate postoperative period if alcohol is circulating in his system. Because many alcoholics are also heavy smokers, they are particularly susceptible to severe respiratory complications, especially acute bacterial pneumonia. Early ambulation and deep breathing are of prime importance postoperatively to prevent pulmonary complications. Chronic emphysema and bronchitis are not uncommon in the alcoholic.

Temperature should be carefully monitored during the postoperative course. Elevations may occur from a variety of causes including gram-negative septicemia, pneumonia (bacterial or aspiration), active cirrhosis, or hepatitis.

The alcoholic is generally more susceptible to infections because of a poor nutritional state and the inability of the cirrhotic liver to fight against infection. The immune response and mobilization of leukocytes to the area of injury is also depressed in the alcoholic.

Management of acute withdrawal from alcohol

Assessment The detoxification process, or drying out, is initiated when alcohol intake is stopped or drastically reduced. Acute detoxification without drugs generally will last about 2 to 3 days. Drugs such as chlordiazepoxide (Librium) and diazepam (Valium) potentiate the effect of alcohol, slow metabolism, and increase the length of the withdrawal period. If the client is addicted to these drugs, the withdrawal period will be lengthened.

The nursing assessment of the alcoholic client experiencing severe withdrawal symptoms includes observing clinical manifestations of three stages. The first stage is the *shakes*. This stage is characterized by a period of tremulousness and occurs about 5 to 35 hours after the last drink. In addition to tremors, acute anxiety, anorexia, nausea and vomiting, insomnia, and increased pulse and blood pressure may be noted.

The next stage is called *acute hallucinosis*. This stage is characterized by altered sensory perception. Hallucinosis may become the primary source of discomfort for the client and may signal impending delirium tremens. In this stage the person may also continue to experience the manifestations of the first stage.

The third stage is known as *delirium tremens* (DTs). Manifestations of this stage include disorientation to time, place, and person, increased psychomotor activity and agitation, hallucinations, delusions, and fear. Physiologically there are increases in blood pressure, pulse, and respirations and fever accompanied by diaphoresis. Seizures, or *rum fits*, generally of the grand mal type, may be seen within the first 48 hours or later if other depressants are interacting with alcohol. Delirium tremens occur from 24 to 72 hours after the last drink and is life-threatening, with mortality rates ranging from 5 to 30 percent.[23]

Complications associated with withdrawal include aspiration pneumonia, peripheral vascular collapse, infection, myocardial infarction, and traumatic injuries such as burns, lacerations, or fractures. Because of the potential medical problems inherent in withdrawal, medical personnel are primarily concerned with management of acute withdrawal. Clients may be referred to outpatient facilities for help with the long-term effects and behavioral changes of alcoholism.

Diagnostic Studies Blood alcohol level (BAL), as previously discussed, is important in diagnosis. It provides an indication of the amount of alcohol consumed. A person with a fairly high BAL (150 mg/mL, or 150 mg%) and few observable symptoms is probably quite tolerant of the effects of alcohol and may be a potential alcoholic.

Two other means of measuring alcohol concentration are the *Breathalyzer* and a *urinalysis*. Usually 5 to 10 percent of the alcohol is excreted through breathing and in the urine; samples of each therefore show proportionate alcohol concentration. An *intoximeter* (Breathalyzer) is used for monitoring the use of alcohol in treatment programs (Fig. 60-9). Urine samples may also be utilized for this purpose. Law enforcement officials may use these indicators to identify persons who are driving while intoxicated (DWI). A BAL greater than 100 mg% is the usual legal guideline for intoxication.

Another diagnosic indicator is the Michigan Alcoholism Screening Test (MAST), which provides a quick screening tool for potential alcoholics and serves as a predictor of treatment outcome. The short form of the MAST is given in Table 60-12.

Direct interviewing of the client and his family or friends is valuable to obtain a psychosocial history. This will assist the nurse in identifying drinking patterns or behavior clues such as job losses, absences from school, falling grades, divorce or separation, or behavior problems of children. A complete physical

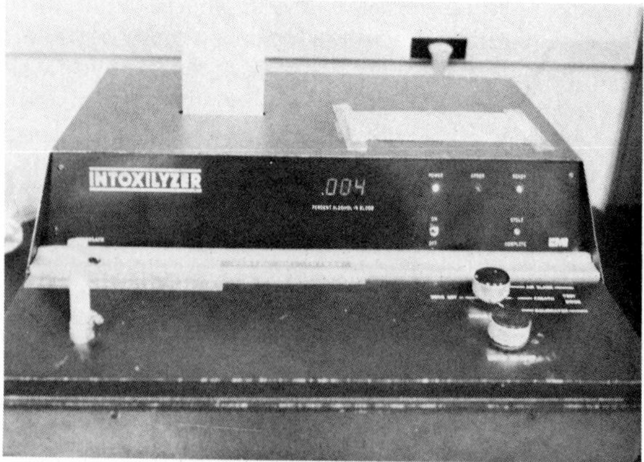

Figure 60-9 The Breathalyzer or intoximeter can obtain an indirect measurement of blood alcohol level.

assessment including a health history may reveal physical manifestations of alcohol abuse.

Medical Management Medical management is aimed at preventing withdrawal from becoming physiologically overwhelming and bringing the body systems back into equilibrium. Some general medical approaches are outlined in Table 60-13.

Nursing Management The nursing role in client care during alcohol withdrawal is primarily to provide rest and prevent injury (Table 60-14). A quiet, nonstimulating environment is essential. As external stimuli increase, the risk of alcoholic hallucinosis and seizures also increase. The nurse has a vital role in helping the client maintain contact with reality and talking him down from agitated states by providing support and reassurance. Psychological assessment includes attention to the presence and degree of depression as well as the response of friends, family, or support systems to the alcoholic client. Suicide attempts may be a sequel to a drinking bout.

Safety measures include maintaining bed rest if the client is unsteady. Bed rails may be necessary and restraints may be needed if there is no one to stay with the client. An open airway must be maintained. Close observation for signs of respiratory depression are important. If the client is stuporous or in a coma, positioning on the side will help prevent aspiration. During the night, a light should be left on in the room. A light that is not too bright will help reduce confusion by avoiding shadows and unclear objects in the environment. A light helps maintain a sense of reality orientation. The nurse should explain all treatments in a simple, direct manner. The client may need to be assisted with personal hygiene and skin care.

Table 60-12
Short Michigan Alcoholism Screening Test

1. Do you feel you are a normal drinker? (A normal drinker is a person who drinks less than or as much as most other people.) (No)*	Yes_____	No_____
2. Does your wife, husband, a parent or other near relative ever worry or complain about your drinking? (Yes)	Yes_____	No_____
3. Do you ever feel guilty about your drinking? (Yes)	Yes_____	No_____
4. Do friends and relatives think you are a normal drinker? (One who drinks less than or no more than most other people.) (No)	Yes_____	No_____
5. Are you able to stop drinking when you want to? (No)	Yes_____	No_____
6. Have you ever attended a meeting of Alcoholics Anonymous? (For your personal concerns about your own drinking.) (Yes)	Yes_____	No_____
7. Has drinking ever created problems between you and your wife, husband, a parent or other near relative? (Yes)	Yes_____	No_____
8. Have you ever gotten into trouble at work because of drinking? (Yes)	Yes_____	No_____
9. Have you ever neglected your obligations, your family, or your work for two or more days in a row because you were drinking? (Yes)	Yes_____	No_____
10. Have you ever gone to anyone for help about your drinking? (Yes)	Yes_____	No_____
11. Have you ever been in a hospital because of your drinking? (Yes)	Yes_____	No_____
12. Have you ever been arrested for drunken driving, driving while intoxicated, or driving under the influence of alcoholic beverages? (Yes)	Yes_____	No_____
13. Have you ever been arrested, even for a few hours, because of other drunken behavior? (Yes)	Yes_____	No_____

*Alcoholism-indicating responses appear in parentheses.
Scoring: 0–1, Nonalcoholic; 2, possibly alcoholic; 3 or more, alcoholic.
Melvin Selzer, Amiram Vinokur, and Louis van Roojen, "A Self-Administered Short Alcoholism Screening Test (SMAST)," *J. Stud. Alcohol,* **36**(1):86 (1975).

Vital signs should be monitored every 1 to 4 hours, depending upon the severity of the client's condition. Adequate nutrition is best maintained by giving small, frequent feedings. Intake and output should be monitored to assess overhydration or dehydration. Fruit juices and Gatorade are useful in speeding up metabolism and replenishing lost fluids.

When the benzodiazepine class of drugs (chlordiazepoxide, diazepam) are used in withdrawal, the nurse should be aware that gradual decreases in these drugs are necessary to prevent a second withdrawal syndrome. These drugs are best absorbed from the oral route and should be given orally whenever possible. Smokers generally require more of these drugs than nonsmokers to achieve the desired response.

Interactions of alcohol and other substances

The combined use of alcohol and drugs has skyrocketed within the past 30 years. Research findings now indicate that these practices can increase serious physiological effects and lead to changes in behavior. Psychoactive substances such as marijuana and cocaine are commonly combined with alcohol. The most frequently combined drugs are minor tranquilizers and alcohol. This combination can

Table 60-13

Medical and Pharmacological Management of Alcohol Withdrawal

1. Benzodiazepines as chlordiazepoxide (Librium) 50 mg IM or PO q 4–6 h for agitation
2. Tranquilizers as chlorpromazine (Thorazine) 25 mg IM or 100 mg PO for nausea and vomiting
3. Hypnotics as flurazepam (Dalmane) 30 mg h.s. prn
4. Anticonvulsants as diphenylhydantoin (Dilantin) 100 mg PO t.i.d. or magnesium sulfate 1 g IM and repeat in 6 h for seizure control
5. Vitamin regimen as multivitamins, B complex, and vitamin C
6. Fluids as tolerated but do not force fluids
7. Catheterize prn
8. Restraints prn

be fatal. The combination of alcohol and other drugs is the second most frequent cause of drug-related medical crises.[24]

Alcohol may interact with a drug in one of four ways (Table 60-15):

1. The combination may be *antagonistic* (the effect of either substances is blocked or decreased). A substance which is known to produce this effect with alcohol is disulfiram (Antabuse). In some cases, stimulants such as caffeine may have a weak antagonistic effect.
2. The interaction may cause an *additive* effect (the effect of the combination is equal to the effects of the two substances added together). Substances in this category include antihypertensives, antihistamines, and marijuana.
3. Another type of interaction, called the *synergistic* effect, is also termed *potentiating* or *supraadditive*. A synergistic effect occurs when two drugs taken together have a combined effect greater than if their individual effects were simply added together. This group is the most hazardous, as the effect is usually not anticipated. Substances which are known to produce this effect with alcohol include anticonvulsants, some antidepressants, anesthetics, ethanol analogs (chloral hydrate, paraldehyde), opiate derivatives, barbiturates, and major and minor tranquilizers. The combination of tobacco and alcohol has a synergistic effect that increases 15 times the risk of cancer of the neck and esophagus.
4. Another type of interaction is *cross tolerance* or *reverse synergism*, in which a sensitivity is developed to other drugs so that it takes a greater amount of a drug to obtain the same effect. This effect is found when alcohol is combined with depressants, opiates, anticonvulsants, and anesthetics.

Table 60-14

Nursing Care Plan for the Client in Alcohol Withdrawal

Client Problem	Expected Outcome	Nursing Intervention
Shakes*	No falls or injuries. No shaking, no restless or unnecessary motions	Monitor vital signs 1–2 h. Provide safety bed rails. Assist with walking and personal hygiene as needed. Provide support and reassurance. Administer benzodiazepines, tranquilizers, hypnotics, vitamins, and anticonvulsants as outlined in Table 60-13.
Acute hallucinosis	No hallucinations. Contact with reality	Stay with client. Provide quiet, nonstimulating environment. Keep room well lighted. Continue interventions as described under Shakes.
Delirium tremens	Minimal shaking and motor activity. No injuries or delusions. Orientation to time, place, and person. No seizure activity	Assess and monitor signs and symptoms at least q 30 min. Provide safety measures such as bed rails and assistance with walking and eating. Orient to environment with each contact. Employ calm, matter-of-fact approach. Explain procedures and what is expected of client. Do not reinforce fears by agreeing or disagreeing. Use tongue blade and prevent injury during seizures. Use restraints as needed.
Depression and suicidal thoughts	No depression. No evidence of suicidal thoughts or self-destructive behaviors	Assist client with expression of thoughts and feelings, especially anger, guilt. Assess degree of depression, intention of suicide. Make referral if probably suicidal.

*During the stage of shakes, anorexia, nausea and vomiting, and increased pulse and blood pressure are also seen. The specific nursing care of these problems is discussed in other chapters.

Table 60-15
Alcohol-Drug Interactions

Alcohol Combined with	Type of Interaction	Alcohol Combined with	Type of Interaction
Barbiturates	Synergistic	Ethanol analogs Chloral hydrate Paraldehyde	Synergistic
Minor tranquilizers Meprobamate (Equanil, Miltown) Benzodiazepines Diazepam (Valium) Chlordiazepoxide (Librium)	Synergistic	Narcotics Morphine and opiates Hydromorphone (Dilaudid) Meperidine (Demerol) Propoxyphene (Darvon)	Synergistic
Major tranquilizers Chlorpromazine (Thorazine) Thioridazine (Mellaril) Reserpine (Serpasil)	Synergistic	Marijuana	Additive
Antidepressants MAO inhibitors Isocarboxazid (Marplan) Nialamide (Niamid) Phenelzine (Nardil) Tricyclics Imipramine (Tofranil) Desipramine (Norpramin, Pertoran) Nortriptyline (Aventyl) Amitriptyline (Elavil)	Synergistic/antagonistic	Antialcohols Disulfiram (Antabuse) Calcium carbimide (Temposil)	Antagonistic
		Hypoglycemics Tolbutamide (Orinase) Tolazamide (Tolinase) Chlorpropamide (Diabinese) Acetohexamide (Dymelor)	Antagonistic
		Antibiotics Chloramphenicol, isoniazid (INH) griseofulvin, metronidazol (Flagyl)	Antagonistic
Stimulants Caffeine (coffee, tea, cola) Amphetamines Methylphenidate (Ritalin)	Antagonistic/synergistic	Antianginals Nitroglycerin	Additive
Anticonvulsants Diphenylhydantoin (Dilantin)	Synergistic	Analgesics Aspirin	Additive
Antihistamines	Additive/(?)synergistic	Antihypertensives Reserpine (Serpasil) Methyldopa (Aldomet) Hydralazine (Apresoline) Guanethidine (Ismelin)	Additive
Anesthetics Ether Chloroform	Synergistic	Nicotine	Synergistic

Compiled from FDA Drug Bulletin, *Alcohol-Drug Interactions,* June 1979, and Ernest P. Noble (ed.), *Third Special Report to the U.S. Congress on Alcohol and Health from the Secretary of Health, Education and Welfare,* June 1978. Generic names for drugs used, with trade names in parentheses. The listing of drugs in each category is not all-inclusive. Individual alcohol-drug interactions may vary according to amount of each drug used, physical condition of user, stage of addiction, and possible genetic differences.

ASSESSMENT OF ADDICTIVE BEHAVIORS

Problems in Identification of Addictive Clients

It is not an easy task to identify the addicted person in the emergency room or on the hospital unit. It is rare for people to seek treatment for an addiction; instead, they present with feigned or real symptoms to obtain certain drugs or chemicals. In the early stages of addiction, the abuser is often not aware that there is a problem, so he does not seek help. If an addiction problem is becoming apparent, the usual reaction is denial. The person may say "I only drink beer, not alcohol," or "Marijuana is safer than being an alcoholic," or "My parents are overreacting." It requires patience, persistence, and skill to deal with a client who denies he has a problem.

Addicted clients are skilled at moving the focus of attention away from themselves. They are adept at discouraging questions that require direct answers. They fear exposure if they are involved in the use of illicit drugs. The substance abuser does not want to jeopardize any chances of obtaining the addictive substance. He is unwilling to give up the temporary good feeling associated with the substance abuse.

These clients are able to *confabulate* (to fill in the

gaps of their story), and rather than give truthful answers they give the answer they think the nurse wants to hear. Attempts to manipulate and play on the sympathetic feelings of others are common. They may play one staff member against another and by this means become the "victim" so that the nurse will "rescue" them. The importance of effective staff communication cannot be overemphasized when working with addictive clients.

The substance abuser has a good alibi system and rationalizes or blames others for his behavior. Such comments as "My job is so stressful, I have to have a few drinks to calm down," or "My home life is so bad that I need my junk to make living there bearable" are examples.

Careful investigation and assessment of complaints can help to screen out malingering. This same type of assessment may be helpful in determining what specific substance is being abused.

Clues in Identification

There are clues to alert the nurse to the possibility that a client may be a substance abuser (Table 60-16). These clues may be in the client's physical appearance, mental status, or history. In the course of recounting the history, the client may mention changes in lifestyle, family or marital conflict, problems with maintaining employment, or legal entanglements. His mental status should be assessed and inquiry made about psychiatric admissions. Features of physical appearance such as poor grooming or body odor are important clues.

Nursing Role in Assessment

Once the possibility of addictive behavior has been perceived, the nurse should focus the interview on the client's habits related to smoking, drinking, eating, and drug use. Amounts or doses consumed

Table 60-16
Clues to Types of Drug Abuse

Depressants	Stimulants	Hallucinogens
	Mental Status	
With barbiturates and alcohol, mild to severe organic brain syndrome with recent and remote memory loss; cognitive faculties reduced With narcotics, cognitive faculties intact; may present as immature, withdrawn, and detached Alcoholic may be rude, arrogant, or belligerent Frequent requests for pain pills or sleeping pills Passive personality	Mood swings Uninhibited behavior Ethical deterioration with long-term use of cocaine Hypervigilant Suspicious or paranoid	Cognitive faculties intact Possible evidence of primary thought disorders Hallucinations Confusion, anxiety, or panic
	Physical Appearance and Condition	
Constricted pupils in narcotic use Skin sallow or blemished with acne; red and puffy face and hoarseness of voice in alcoholic Scratches, bruises, or other signs of injury in alcohol or barbiturate user Needle or track marks in narcotics user Gingivitis and caries Slurred speech Clumsy, slow-moving, ataxic Odor of alcohol Decreased vital signs	Dilated pupils Cold and clammy skin in habitual cocaine users Needle marks or coke burns Gingivitis and caries Jerky, rapid, startled movements Aggressiveness Increased temperature, pulse, and respirations	Reddened conjunctivae in marijuana users Hazardous behavior

daily or weekly, duration of the habit, and general health status should be noted. Specific information related to recent changes in health status such as cough, weight gain or loss, infections, or chronic problems should be obtained. It may be useful to validate this information with other family members or friends, since the client may tend to underestimate or disregard the significance of these behaviors.

If the client admits to an addictive behavior, further information is needed. Using an open and nonjudgmental style, the nurse should ask the client his reasons for starting the behavior, reasons for continuing it, and what behavior controls have been tried. It is also important to know what motivates the client to seek help and what sources of support are available. A careful initial assessment provides a data base upon which a realistic treatment program can be built.

GENERAL NURSING MANAGEMENT OF ADDICTIVE BEHAVIORS

The nurse can assume an important role in the treatment plan for an addicted client, by validating addictive behaviors and motivating clients to change them. Several approaches are useful to achieve change. First, caring confrontation allows the nurse to enlist the client's help in treatment by sharing her observations and impressions in an open and nonjudgmental manner with the client. Initially these observations may be met with firm denial. By consistently focusing on the specific effects of these behaviors for that client, the nurse may get across the message of caring and concern.

An educational approach to addiction is important. This increases the client's awareness of the addictive cycle and teaches the effects of substance use on the body and mind, interactions of substances, and treatment alternatives. The nurse can encourage a realistic but hopeful attitude by providing support and guidance in the change process. Attitude is expressed nonverbally as well as verbally. Frequently it is the nurse's nonverbal attitude which is a barrier to an effective working relationship with the client. It is important to examine one's attitude, both verbal and nonverbal, toward addictive behavior and addictive clients. Sometimes events or persons in one's own background may trigger ineffective emotional responses to these clients.

The nurse can teach the client to use simple relaxation techniques or substitute positive behaviors such as hobbies, jogging, or meditation. It is important to recognize that addictive behaviors are resistant to change. Stopping the substance use (abstinence) does not meet the emotional need or replace the peer group pressure often associated with addictive behavior.

TREATMENT ALTERNATIVES

In order to start treatment it is important to consider the client's physical and emotional condition, past history, and available resources. The client needs to know that there are various approaches for each addictive behavior. One approach may be more effective for some persons than for others. It is important to reinforce the message that if one treatment is not effective, another may be more helpful. The selection of treatment is the decision of the client and his family. This decision needs to be made when the client is ready and committed to change.

The type and outcome of treatment are closely tied to the client's motivation and reasons for initiating and maintaining the addictive behavior. Treatment goals reflect a focus on one of the four models discussed in the earlier section, Causes of Addictive Behavior.

Medical Model

The medical model emphasizes the treatment of the disease or the effects of the addictive behavior. During the detoxification process, persons with severe symptoms may be hospitalized and supported with drugs like diazepam or chlordiazepoxide to prevent the development of complication. Upon discharge the client may be given an antagonist such as Antabuse or methadone to deter the use of alcohol or heroin. Tranquilizers such as diazepam may be given to the client to use at home. The client will generally be referred to a community resource or outpatient treatment facility for support or follow-up.

The process of weight loss may be viewed as similar to alcoholic or drug detoxification. Hospitalization may be used for bypass surgery, jaw wiring, or fasting in weight-reduction programs (Chap. 33). Dieters may be given amphetamines, hormones, diuretics, or a variety of low-calorie diets and exercise programs.

In the medical model, withdrawal from the substance and abstinence are only part of the addictive cycle. This may be only the beginning of a lifestyle change dealing with associated social, occupational, and family problems. A possible problem in the medical model is alleviating one addiction while substituting another negative addiction. For example, the use of diazepam to assist in the withdrawal from alcohol may result in a new addiction to the diazepam. In addition, the combination of this drug with alcohol has a synergistic effect and may also cause cross tolerance.

Psychodynamic Model

The psychodynamic model focuses treatment on the person's underlying needs and problems. A variety of psychotherapeutic approaches may be employed by a trained therapist (nurse, psychiatrist, social worker, psychologist), including one-on-one therapy, group therapy, or family therapy. These approaches may be found in an inpatient treatment facility, on special units for alcoholics or drug abusers, or on the general medical unit. Outpatient treatment facilities also provide counselors for individual and group therapy. These methods are also used for family therapy. Some therapeutic community programs such as Odyssey House which have this focus include a structured living setting for treating the dependency, sense of futility, and other emotional problems of the drug addict. The aim of Odyssey House is to return clients to community life.[25]

In general, group therapy and family therapy are useful because the social-reference group plays a major role in the motivation and maintenance of behavior. *Group therapy* provides the opportunity for members of the group to find support and caring among other members with similar problems. It allows the members to share feelings of frustration, anger, and hurt. Group therapy helps members going through change to learn new coping and interactional skills. Groups have been found to be more effective than one-on-one therapy as less denial, manipulation, and projection usually occur in relating to the therapist.

During the past decade *family therapy* has gained support. The family of the alcoholic is usually very disrupted by alcoholic behavior. The family members need help in learning how to cope more effectively with the alcoholic as well as how to function as a family unit. Families are highly influential in assisting the abuser to stop or change his behavior and need to be included in the treatment process whenever possible.

Problems in the psychodynamic model chiefly arise from the refusal of clients or families to get involved unless participation is made mandatory through the legal system. The expense and the length of time needed for these programs may also be barriers. It is important to remember that looking *only* at the underlying problems may not stop or change the addictive behavior.

Social-Learning Model

The social-learning model focuses on the learning of new behaviors to replace addictive patterns of behavior. Approaches associated with this model include educational information-giving classes in school, community groups, and behavioral therapy. School programs are aimed at prevention and providing information about the use or abuse of substances in primary and secondary schools and colleges. Community self-help groups are therapeutic in supporting changes in behavior, identifying causes or "triggers" of patterns of abuse, and providing specific advice or plans to reach goals. Examples of these groups are Weight Watchers, Take Off Pounds Sensibly (TOPS), Overeaters Anonymous, Synanon, Alcoholics Anonymous (AA), Alanon, Alateen, and Women for Sobriety.

Behavioral therapy or *behavior modification* is based on principles of learning. It involves conditioning procedures that may either reinforce desired behaviors or extinguish undesirable behaviors or both. There are a wide variety of techniques which not only decrease or remove the addictive behavior but also support healthy alternative behaviors. Behavioral therapy aims at modifying or changing behavior and includes self-help programs, aversion therapy, biofeedback, desensitization, conditioning, hypnosis, positive imagery, and behavioral-alternatives training. *Self-help programs* and books are popular and effective for assisting some highly motivated people to change behavior. Most self-help programs teach techniques for self-management which include self-monitoring, relaxation, assertiveness, dealing with uncomfortable feelings, and developing a more positive self-concept. Programs and clinics for controlling drinking, losing weight, and quitting smoking are based on these techniques. "I Quit Smoking" kits and smoking clinics are available in many communities.

Aversion therapy is frequently used in the treatment of addictive behavior. It attempts to "turn off" the behavior through associating it with painful or unpleasant responses. It may take the form of chemical agents of aversion such as Antabuse, electrically produced aversion as seen in some biofeedback programs, or verbally produced aversion to prevent overeating. *Conditioning* may also be used; the consequences of the behavior are either reinforced or punished with certain conditions added. For example, if the obese woman loses 10 pounds in a month, she may buy a new dress.

Hypnosis is used in a number of clinics to decrease the desire for the addictive behavior. It implants the association of a behavior such as smoking with unpleasant responses such as nausea or vomiting. *Positive imagery* may be employed in obesity to provide mental suggestions for behavioral changes in eating. *Environmental management* is effective in treating obesity. Changes such as setting regular mealtimes, eating at the table, and making fruits and vegetables available for snacks could be made to reinforce positive eating behaviors.

The drawback with the use of the social-learning model is that most persons lack the motivation to consistently follow a program long enough to develop new behaviors.

Sociocultural Model

The sociocultural model of treatment emphasizes the legal or economic consequences of the behavior. Persons arrested for driving while intoxicated may be required to attend groups such as AA, driving school, individual counseling sessions, or occupational alcoholism programs. Laws providing for involuntary commitment of the alcoholic to a treatment program are in effect in many states.

Many treatment programs combine approaches from all of these models. It is important to consider personal characteristics, type of addiction, motivation for treatment, current medical and mental status, and resources. Only then can an individualized treatment program be designed. Combined treatment programs working with both alcoholics and drug addicts have been effective for some clients.

ROAD TO RECOVERY

Detoxification is the first step in breaking the addictive cycle. This is usually considered the initial treatment stage, although some persons may go through this period without medical supervision. Detoxification may be successfully and safely accomplished within a relatively short time. The next step, *maintenance* of this stage, may take the form of abstinence or controlled use, depending on the client's treatment goal and substance abuse. This correlates with the dieter's maintenance of the desired weight. Treatment, which may involve a variety of forms as discussed in the previous section, is essential to a successful outcome. The client must master a new lifestyle that utilizes other avenues of stress relief and pleasure. At this step it is important for him to have supportive resources and professional help.

Preventing readdiction is a continous challenge that does not end when a goal has been maintained for a specific period of time. *Relapse* within the first 3 months after treatment is a common occurrence with all addictive behaviors. Studies show that two-thirds of those addicted to alcohol, smoking, or heroin relapse within 3 months (Fig. 60-10).

Two theories may explain why relapse occurs. The first theory postulates an *abstinence violation effect*, which occurs when the drinker takes one drink, feels guilty, and reasons that he might as well continue drinking.[26] A conditioning response may occur in abstinent narcotic addicts who see friends using drugs or who experience other stimuli associated with drug-seeking behavior which cause cravings.[27] The second theory is based on *abstinence phobia*, an anxiety reaction noted in overreaction to withdrawal and to becoming substance-free. This reaction reflects the client's feelings of inadequacy and lack of skills in being normal and facing his real self.[28] This reaction even occurs in persons losing weight, who may have a difficult time dealing with the reactions of others to their new self.

In preventing relapse, it is important for the nurse to help the client anticipate those times when it may be most difficult to maintain his goal, such as holidays, birthdays, anniversaries, and times of personal loss or illness. It is essential for the client and nurse to work out several plans which are realistic and acceptable for use during periods of stress or craving. The nurse needs to encourage the client to seek help during particularly stressful periods in order to prevent relapse before readdiction occurs. The nurse should provide the client with a list of available community resources.

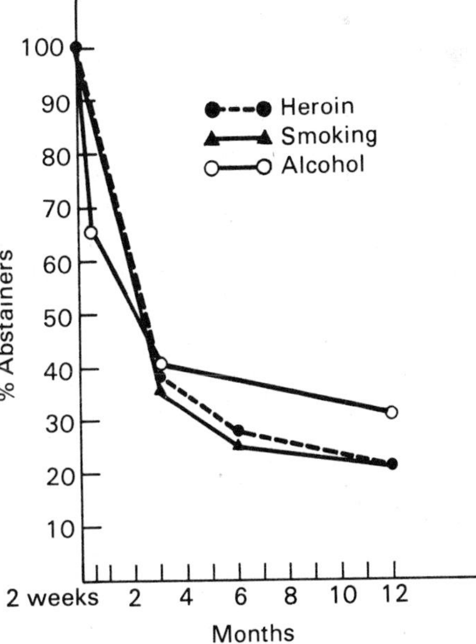

Figure 60-10 Relapse rate over time for heroin, tobacco smoking, and alcohol use. [*From W. A. Hunt et al., Relapse Rates in Addiction Programs, J. Clin Psychol,* **27:***455 (1971).*]

Case Study / Addictive Behaviors

Bill, 37 years old, and Mary, 35 years old, have been married for 15 years. Their marriage has been stormy the last 4 years, with frequent brief periods of separation. They have two children: Willie is 10 years old and Janet is 15.

Bill smokes about two packs of cigarettes per day. He currently works as a stock clerk in a local department store. He has had frequent changes in employment in the past 6 years because of absenteeism. He drinks daily and he becomes angry when any mention of his drinking habits and behavior are mentioned. His childhood religious upbringing frowned on alcohol use. He does not attend church now.

Mary has had a weight problem most of her life. However, she had managed to keep her weight controlled until the past 6 years. She is trying to be a good wife and mother in an attempt to keep the family together. She has had some part-time employment and currently is working evening hours in a donut shop. She has just signed up to attend meetings of a Weight Watchers group, since her previous diet attempts have failed.

Willie is in the fifth grade and is doing average work for his age. He has no particular interests or hobbies and spends most of his time at home watching TV. He tries to be helpful to his mother. He is generally very quiet and withdrawn when his father is at home.

Janet is a freshman in high school. She was kept back in seventh grade because of failing grades, and since that time she has managed to just get by in most of her classes. She spends a great deal of time away from home in the company of her friends. She drinks alcohol with her friends on occasional weekends, smokes marijuana about 3 times a week, and usually attends parties every weekend where she has tried uppers, downers, and hallucinogens. She has not been involved with the police.

Discussion Questions

1. In what ways does the father's alcohol addiction influence the family?
2. What are the possible connections between the parents' childhood and their currect situation?
3. Who in the family exhibits the most normal social behavior?
4. Make a prediction describing the life situation of each family member 10 years from now without any intervention.
5. What type of defense does Bill use regarding his drinking behavior?
6. What are some possible causes for Mary's failure to diet successfully?
7. What are some possible referral resources for each family member?
8. What are some potential physical and emotional problems for each family member?
9. If you were a relative or friend of this family, what would you advise each person to do?

REVIEW QUESTIONS

The number of the question corresponds to the same-numbered objective at the beginning of the chapter.

1. The social-learning model of addiction causation focuses on
   a. underlying interpersonal needs
   b. cultural influences
   c. parental modeling of behaviors
   d. genetic transmission

2. Withdrawal symptoms are characteristic of
   a. psychological dependence
   b. physiological dependence
   c. abstinence violation effect
   d. loss of control

3. What happens when a substance is stopped after psychological dependence has been established?
   a. increased anxiety with no physical symptoms
   b. decreased tolerance
   c. increased tolerance
   d. increased anxiety with withdrawal symptoms

4. Which of the following is *not* a common characteristic of addictive behaviors?
   a. being at risk for chronic or terminal illnesses
   b. responding to external rather than internal cues
   c. having a high frustration tolerance
   d. exhibiting self-destructiveness

5. Which of the following is *not* considered a risk factor for becoming alcoholic?
   a. history of abstinence
   b. heavy smoking
   c. stable home
   d. near youngest in age in large family

6. Physiological complications of smoking may include
   a. cancer of the mouth and throat, lung disease
   b. adult-onset diabetes, hyperuricemia, anorexia
   c. myocardial infarction, hypertension, anxiety attacks
   d. synesthesia, hypotension, anemias

7. Which group of effects would most probably be observed with the use of depressants?
   a. rapid tolerance, vasoconstriction, increased pulse, paranoia
   b. synesthesia, flashbacks, sympathomimetic and anticholinergic effects
   c. confusion, drowsiness, tranquility, hypotension
   d. suicidal thoughts, hallucinations, withdrawal, blank stare

8. During alcohol withdrawal a quiet, nonstimulating environment is primarily important to
   a. decrease the client's loud, aggressive behavior
   b. decrease the risk of alcoholic hallucinosis and seizures
   c. prevent depression and suicide thoughts
   d. promote secondary withdrawal

9. The most hazardous group of alcohol-drug interactions is the group which produces
   a. cross tolerance
   b. antagonistic effects
   c. additive effects
   d. synergistic effects

10. During surgery, it is important to remember that the alcoholic will generally
   a. need less anesthesia initially
   b. need more anesthesia initially
   c. experience withdrawal symptoms 72 to 96 hours after the last drink
   d. experience hypertensive episodes

11. It is often difficult for the nurse to identify the source of drug addiction because
   a. many substances produce similar effects
   b. most addicts will not talk to her
   c. brain damage takes away primary symptoms
   d. all addicts act the same

12. Treatment approaches associated with the social-learning model include
   a. self-help programs, aversion therapy, environmental management, hypnosis
   b. involuntary commitment, mandatory attendance at meetings of groups, occupational programs for abuse
   c. one-on-one therapy, group therapy, family therapy
   d. detoxification, treatment of medical problems

13. The most common problem during the recovery process is
   a. infection or physical injury
   b. depression or suicide thoughts
   c. positive addiction
   d. relapse

REFERENCES

1. A. Goldstein, "Recent Advances in Basic Research Relevant to Drug Abuse," in Robert L. Dupont, Avram Goldstein, and John O'Donnell (eds.), *Handbook on Drug Abuse*, National Institute on Drug Abuse, January 1979, p. 443.
2. American Lung Association, *Women Are Kicking the Cigarette Habit*, January 1978.
3. National Cancer Institute, "Progress Report on a Nation Kicking the Habit," *The Smoking Digest,* U.S. Public Health Service, October 1977.
4. K. L. Melmon and H. F. Morrelli, *Clinical Pharmacology*, 2d ed., The Macmillan Company, New York, 1978, p. 1020.
5. K. L. Jones et al., *Drugs: Substance Abuse*, 2d ed., Canfield Press, San Francisco, 1975, pp. 69–70.
6. R. J. Gibbins et al., *Research Advances in Alcohol and Drug Problems*, John Wiley & Sons, Inc., New York, 1976, p. 26.
7. O. S. Ray, *Drugs, Society and Human Behavior*, The C. V. Mosby Company, St. Louis, 1972, p. 105.
8. G. Burckhardt, "WHO Expert Committee on Smoking Gives Serious Warning," *Int J Health Educ,* **21**(4): 228 (1978).
9. R. McLain and F. W. Widlak, "Patients' Self-Concept and Weight Reduction: Use of Covert Sensitization," *Issues in Ment Health Nurs,* **2**(2):2 (December 1979).
10. G. MacGovern, *Diet Related to Killer Diseases; II, Obesity*, U.S. Government Printing Office, Washington, D.C., 1977, pp. 1–3.
11. K. L. Mahan, "A Sensible Approach to the Obese Patient," *Nurs Clin North Am,* **14**(2): 233–234 (June 1979).
12. Ibid., p. 239.
13. H. I. Abelson et al., *National Survey on Drug Abuse*; Vol. 1: *Main Findings*, National Institute on Drug Abuse, 1977, p. 99.
14. C. S. Farkas, "Caffeine Intake and Potential Effect on Health of a Segment of Northern Canadian Indigenous People," *In J Addict,* **14**(1): 32 (1979).
15. Ray, op. cit., p. 169.
16. "Update on Sedative Hypnosis," *FDA Drug Bull*, August 1979, pp. 16–17.
17. Joan D. Rittenhouse (ed.), *Consequences of Alcohol and Marijuana Use*, National Institute on Drug Abuse Pub. No. (ADM) 80-920 (1979).
18. Peggy Mann, "Marijuana Alert: 1. Brain and Sex Damage," *Reader's Digest*, December 1979, pp 139–144.
19. Walter X. Lehmann, "Marijuana Alert: 2. Enemy of Youth," *Reader's Digest*, December 1979, pp. 144–146.
20. Ray, op. cit., p. 13.
21. Criteria Committee, National Council on Alcoholism, "Criteria for the Diagnosis of Alcoholism," *Am J Psychiatry,* **129**(2): 133-134 (August 1972).
22. E. M. Jellinek, "Phases of Alcohol Addiction," *Q J Stud Alcohol,* **13**:677 (December 1952).
23. P. K. Burkhalter, *Nursing Care of the Alcoholic and Drug Abuser*, McGraw-Hill Book Company, New York, 1975, p. 30.
24. E. P. Noble (ed.), *Third Special Report to the U.S. Congress on Alcohol and Health* from the Secretary of Health, Education and Welfare, June 1978.
25. J. Densen-Gerber, *The Odyssey House Story*, Doubleday & Company, Inc., Garden City, N.Y. 1973.
26. G. A. Marlatt, "A Cognitive-Behavioral Model of the Relapse Process," in Norman A. Krasnegor (ed.), *Behavioral Analysis and Treatment of Substance Abuse*, National Institute on Drug Abuse Research Monograph, June 1979, p. 196.
27. N. M. Valentine and Roger E. Meyer, "Narcotic Antagonists: Treatment Tool for Addiction," *Nurs Clin North Am,* **11**:545 (September 1976).
28. S. M. Hall, "The Abstinence Phobia," in N.S. Krasnegor (ed.), *Behavioral Analysis and Treatment of Substance Abuse*, National Institute on Drug Abuse Research Monograph, June 1979, pp. 61, 64.

BIBLIOGRAPHY FOR SECTION 11

Trauma and Emergencies

Davis, M. D., et al.: "Diagnosis and Management of Blunt Abdominal Trauma," *Ann Surg,* **183**(6):672–678 (1976).

Drury, L. R.: "Evacuation and Early Care of the Trauma Patient," *Heart Lung,* **7**(2):249–252 (March–April 1978).

Fitzgerald, M. D.: "Burn Management," *Crit Care Quarterly,* **1**(3) (December, 1978).

Geelhoed, G. W.: "Blunt and Penetrating Chest Trauma," *Family Practice,* **17**(2):100–106 (Feb. 1978).

Gilroy, A., et al.: "Initial Assessment of the Multiply Injured Patient," *Nurs Clin North Am,* **13**(2):177–190 (June 1978).

Hutchinson, R.: "What to Do—and What to Worry About—When Treating Stings and Bites," *Nursing 77,* **7**:69–71 (June 1977).

Sproul, C. W., et al. (eds.): *Emergency Care: Assessment and Intervention,"* The C. V. Mosby Company, St. Louis, 1974.

Willis, J. C., et al.: "Prehospital Care-Nursing Perspective," *Heart Lung,* **7**(2):253–256 (March–April 1978).

Wingert, W. A., and Wainschel, J.: "A Quick Handbook on Snakebites," *Med. Times,* **105**:68–75 (April 1977).

Radiation Accidents

Kuntz, E.: "Ready to Evacuate Area?" *Modern Healthcare,* 14–16 (May 1979).

Mettler, F. A.: "Emergency Management of Radiation Accidents," *College Emergency Physicians,* **7**:8 (August 1978).

Norwood, W. D.: *Health Protection of Radiation Workers,* Charles C Thomas, Publisher, Springfield, Ill. 1975.

Addictive Behavior

Books

Abel, E. L.: *The Scientific Study of Marijuana,* Nelson-Hall Publishers, Chicago, 1976.

Cahn, Sidney: *The Treatment of Alcoholics,* Oxford University Press, New York, 1970).

Chafetz, Morris E., et al.: *Frontiers of Alcoholism,* Science Press, New York, 1970).

Davidson, Sharon: The Assessment of Alcoholism, in Sharon V. Davidson (issue ed.), *Family and Community Health, Alcoholism and Health,* **2**(1):1–32, (May 1979.)

Estes, Nada J., and M. Edith Heinemann: *Alcoholism: Development, Consequences, and Interventions,* The C. V. Mosby Company, St. Louis, 1977.

Gibbins, Robert J., et al.: *Research Advances in Alcohol and Drug Problems,* vol. III, John Wiley & Sons, Inc., New York 1976.

Hofman, F. G.: *A hanbook on Drug and Alcohol Abuse: The Bio-Medical Aspects,* Oxford University Press, New York 1975.

Lowenfels, Albert B.: *The Alcoholic Patient in Surgery,* The Williams & Wilkins Company, Baltimore, 1971.

McNichol, Ronald W.: *The Treatment of Delerium Tremens and Related States,* Charles C Thomas, Publisher, Springfield, Ill., 1970.

Miller, William R. (ed.): *The Addictive Behaviors: Treatment of Alcoholism, Drug Abuse, Smoking and Obesity,* Pergamon Press, New York, 1980.

Miller, William R.: Problem Drinking and Substance Abuse: Behavioral Perspectives, in Norman A. Krasnegor (ed.), *Behavioral Analysis and Treatment of Substance Abuse,* NIDA Research Monograph 25, Government Printing Office, Washington, D.C., 1975, pp. 158–177.

Nahas, G. G.: *Keep Off the Grass,* Pergamon Press, New York, 1979.

Periodicals

Aldoory, Shirley: "The Chemical Curtain: Polydrug Abuse Among Women," *Alcohol Health and Research World,* 28–36 (Winter 1978).

Barnes, Gordon E.: "Solvent Abuse: A Review," *The International Journal of the Addictions,* 1–26 (1979).

Bernstein, Leonard: "Medical Hazards of Aerosols," *Post-Graduate Medicine,* **52**:67 (Dec. 1972).

Betts, Virginia T.: "Psychotherapeutic Intervention with the Addict-Client," *Nurs Clin North Am,* **11**:551–558 (September 1976).

Clements, J. Eugene, and Richard Simpson: "Environmental and Behavioral Aspects of Glue Sniffing in a Population of Emotionally Disturbed Adolescents," *The International Journal of the Addictions,* 129–134 (1978).

Cohen, S.: "Glue Sniffing," *JAMA,* **231**(6):653–654 (February 1975).

Cotroneo, Margaret, and Barbara R. Krasner: "Addiction, Alienation and Parenting," *Nurs Clin North Am,* **11**:517–525 (September 1976).

Doyle, N. C.: "Marijuana and the Lungs," *Am Lung Assoc Bull,* **65**:2–7 (November 1979).

DuPont, R. L.: "Just What Can You Tell Your Patient About Marijuana?" *Resident Staff Physician,* **23**:103–104 (1980).

———: "Marijuana Smoking-A National Epidemic," *Am Lung Assoc Bull,* **66**:2–7 (September 1980).

Huber, G. L.: "Marijuana, THC, and Pulmonary Antibacterial Defenses," *Med Resident,* **77**:403–410 (1980).

Iveson, I.: "Cannabis Sativa. Behind the Smoke Screen," *Nurs Mirror,* **150**:30–31 (1980).

Korman, Maurice, Frank Trimboli, and Ira Semler: "A Comparative Evaluation of 162 Inhalant Users," *Addictive Behaviors,* **5**:143–152 (1980).

Korobkin, Rowena, Arthur K. Asbury, Austin S. Summer, and Sart D. Nielsen: "Glue Sniffing Neuropathy," *Arch Neurol,* **5**:158–161 (1975).

Massengale, O., H. Glaser, R. LeLievre, J. Dodds, and M. Klock: "Physical and Psychologic Factors in Glue Sniffing," *New Eng J Med,* **269**:1340–1344 (1963).

Mitcheson, M.: "Government Health Warning for Cannabis?" *Midwife,* **15**:142–143 (April 1979).

Reed, Susan W.: Assessing the Patient with an Alcohol Problem, *Nurs Clin North Am,* **11**(3):483–491 (1976).

Rottenberg, R.: "Answering Questions About Marijuana," *Nurs Mirror,* **150**:112–113 (May 30, 1980).

Silberberg, N. E., and M. D. Silberberg: "Glue Sniffing in Children: A Position Paper," *J Drug Education,* **4**(3) (Fall 1974).

Vourakis, Christine, and Gerald Gennett: Angel Dust—Not Heaven Sent, *Am J Nurs,* **79**:649 (1979).

Wyse, George: "Deliberate Inhalation of Volatile Hydrocarbons," *Can Med Assoc J,* **106**:71–73 (January 6, 1973).

Organizations

Al-Anon, Family Group Headquarters, P. O. Box 182, Madison Square Station, New York, NY 10010

Alcoholics Anonymous World Services, Inc., Box 459 Grand Station Station, New York, NY 10011

Department of Health, Education & Welfare, Food and Drug Administration, Rockville, MD 20857

National Council on Alcoholism, 133 East 62 Street, New York, NY 10024

National Clearing House for Drug Abuse Information, 5600 Fishers Lane, Rockville, MD 20856

National Drug Abuse Foundation, 6500 Randall Place, Falls Church, VA 22044,

Take Off Pounds Sensibly—TOPS, International Headquarters, 4575 South 5 Street, Milwaukee, WI 53207

Weight Watchers International, 800 Community Drive, Manhasset, NY 11030

Appendix A

Laboratory Values

Diane Germain

The tables in this appendix list some of the most common tests, their normal values, and possible etiologies of abnormal values. Laboratory values may vary with different techniques and/or different laboratories. Possible etiologies are presented in alphabetic order. Abbreviations appearing in the tables are defined as follows:

<= less than
>= greater than
g= gram
L= liter
mEq= milliequivalent
mL= milliliter
dL= deciliter
mmHg= millimeter of mercury
fL= fentoliter
mm= millimeter
mg= milligram
ng= nanogram (one billionth of a gram)
pg= picogram (one trillionth of a gram)
μg= microgram (one millionth of a gram)
μU= microunit
μL= microliter
IU= international unit
mOsm= milliosmoles
U= unit

This appendix was reviewed by Barbara Fricke, M.S. (ASCP); Patricia Olson, M.T. (ASCP) SC; Cecilia Dail, M.T. (ASCP); and Penelope Allen, M.T. (ASCP)—faculty, Medical Technology Program, University of New Mexico, Albuquerque, New Mexico.

Table 1
Chemistries (Serum, Plasma, Whole Blood)

		Possible Etiology	
Test	**Normal Value**	**Higher**	**Lower**
Acetone	0.3–2.0 mg/dL	Diabetic acidosis High fat diet Low carbohydrate diet Starvation	
Albumin	3.5–5.0 g/dL	Dehydration	Chronic liver disease Malabsorption Malnutrition Nephrotic syndrome
Aldolase	1.0–7.5 U/L	Skeletal muscle disease	Renal disease
Alpha-amino acid nitrogen	3.5–7.0 mg/dL	Infectious hepatitis Poisoning from carbon tetrachloride, arsenic, chloroform	Bacterial pneumonia Insulin administration
Alpha-1-antitrypsin	200–400 mg/dL	Acute and chronic inflammation Arthritis Stress syndrome	Chronic lung disease (early onset) Malnutrition Nephrotic syndrome
Alpha-1-fetoprotein	<25 ng/mL	Cancer of testes and ovaries Carcinoma of liver	

Table 1 (Continued)

		Possible Etiology	
Test	**Normal Value**	**Higher**	**Lower**
Alpha-hydroxybutyric dehydrogenase (α-HBD)	0–140 μU/mL	Hemolytic anemia Leukemia Malignant melanomas Muscular dystrophy Myocardial infarction Nephrotic syndrome	
Ammonia	30–70 μg/dL	Severe liver disease	
Amylase	60–160 Somogyi units/dL	Acute and chronic pancreatitis Mumps (salivary gland disease) Perforated ulcers	Acute alcoholism Cirrhosis of liver Extensive destruction of pancreas
Antinuclear antibody (ANA) (*Note*: This test is often considered a serology test.)	Negative or titer <1:10	Chronic hepatitis Rheumatoid arthritis Scleroderma Systemic lupus erythematosus	
Anti-DNA antibody test (*Note:* This test is often considered a serology test.)	≤20%	(Same as antinuclear antibody)	
Ascorbic acid	0.4–2.0 mg/dL	Excessive ingestion of vitamin C	Connective tissue disorders Hepatic disease Renal disease Rheumatic fever Vitamin C deficiency
Bicarbonate	20–30 mEq/L	Compensated respiratory acidosis Metabolic alkalosis	Compensated respiratory alkalosis Metabolic acidosis
Bilirubin	Total: 0.2–1.3 mg/dL Indirect: 0.1–1.0 mg/dL Direct: 0.1–0.3 mg/dL	Biliary obstruction Impaired liver function Hemolytic anemia Pernicious anemia Prolonged fasting	
Blood gases			
pH: Arterial Venous	7.35–7.45 7.35–7.45	Acidosis	Alkalosis
PCO_2: Arterial Venous	35–45 mmHg 42–52 mmHg	Compensated metabolic alkalosis Respiratory acidosis	Compensated metabolic acidosis Respiratory alkalosis
PO_2: Arterial Venous (*Note*: Since arterial blood gases are influenced by altitude, the value for PO_2 decreases as altitude increases. The lower value here is normal for an altitude of 1 mile.)	75–100 mmHg* 30–50 mmHg	Administration of high concentration of O_2	Chronic lung disease Decreased cardiac output
Blood urea nitrogen	See urea nitrogen		

Table 1 (Continued)

Test	Normal Value	Possible Etiology: Higher	Possible Etiology: Lower
C-reactive protein (CRP) (*Note:* This test is often considered a serology test.)	Negative	Acute infections Any inflammatory condition Widespread malignancy	
Calcium	9–11 mg/dL (4.5–5.5 mEq/L)	Acute osteoporosis Hyperparathyroidism Vitamin D intoxication	Acute pancreatitis Hypoparathyroidism Liver disease Malabsorption syndrome Renal failure Vitamin D deficiency
Carbon dioxide (CO_2 content)	20–30 mEq/L	(same as bicarbonate)	
Carcinoembryonic antigen (CEA) (*Note:* This test is often considered a serology test.)	≤2.5 ng/mL	Carcinoma of liver Carcinoma of pancreas Chronic cigarette smokers Inflammatory bowel disease Other cancers	
Carotene	50–200 µg/dL	Cystic fibrosis Hypothyroidism Pancreatic insufficiency	Dietary deficiency Malabsorption disorders
Chloride	95–105 mEq/L	Cardiac decompensation Metabolic acidosis Respiratory alkalosis Steroid therapy Uremia	Addison's disease Diarrhea Metabolic alkalosis Respiratory acidosis Vomiting
Cholesterol	150–270 mg/dL (varies with age)	Biliary obstruction Hypothyroidism Idiopathic hypercholesterolemia Renal disease	Anemia Extensive liver disease Hyperthyroidism Malnutrition Steroid therapy
Cholesterol, HDL (high-density lipoproteins)	Male: >55 mg/dL Female: >45 mg/dL		
Cholinesterase (RBC)	0.65–1.00 U	Exercise	Acute infections Insecticide intoxication Liver disease Muscular dystrophy
Pseudocholinesterase (plasma)	4–10 U/L		
Complement components			
C1q	14–20 mg/dL		Acute glomerulonephritis Lupus erythematosus Vasculitis associated with rheumatoid arthritis
C4	20–40 mg/dL		
C3	120–167 mg/dL		
Coomb's			
Direct	Negative	Acquired hemolytic anemia Anti-RH antibodies in pregnant women Blood incompatibilities Presence of irregular antibody in serum Transfusion reaction	
Indirect (*Note*: These tests are often considered serology tests.)	Negative		
Copper	80–150 µg/dL	Cirrhosis Female on contraceptives	Wilson's disease

Table 1 (Continued)

		Possible Etiology	
Test	**Normal Value**	**Higher**	**Lower**
Cortisol	8 A.M.: 5–25 μg/dL 8 P.M.: <10 μg/dL	Cushing's syndrome Pancreatitis Stress	Adrenal insufficiency Panhypopituitary states
Creatine	0.2–1.0 mg/dL	Active rheumatoid arthritis Biliary obstruction Hyperthyroidism Renal disorders Severe muscle disease	Diabetes mellitus
Creatine phosphokinase (CPK) Creatine kinase (CK)	Male: 5–55 U/L Female: 5–35 U/L	Hypothyroidism Musculoskeletal injury or disease Myocardial infarction Severe myocarditis	
Creatinine	0.5–1.5 mg/dL	Severe renal disease	
Fluorescent treponemal antibody (FTA) (*Note*: This test is often considered a serology test.)	Negative	Syphilis	
Folic acid (folate)	3–25 ng/mL		Alcoholism Hemolytic anemia Madequate diet Malabsorption syndrome Megaloblastic anemia
Glucose, fasting	70–120 mg/dL	Acute stress Cerebral lesions Cushing's disease Diabetes mellitus Hyperthyroidism Pancreatic insufficiency	Addison's disease Hepatic disease Hypothyroidism Insulin overdosage Pancreatic tumor Pituitary hypofunction Postgastrectomy dumping syndrome
Glucose tolerance (GTT), fasting	70–120 mg/dL	Diabetes mellitus	Hyperinsulinism
30 min	30–60 mg/dL above fasting		
60 min	20–50 mg/dL above fasting		
120 min	5–15 mg/dL above fasting		
180 min	Fasting level or lower		
Haptoglobin	70–200 mg/dL	Infectious and inflammatory processes	Hemolytic anemia
Hepatitis B surface antigen (HB_s Ag) (*Note*: This test is often considered a serology test.)	Negative	Hepatitis A	

Table 1 (Continued)

Test	Normal Value	Possible Etiology: Higher	Possible Etiology: Lower
Immunoglobulin			
IgA	100–400 mg/dL	Cirrhosis Rheumatoid arthritis	Hereditary telangiectasia Malabsorption syndromes
IgD	0–40 mg/dL	Chronic infection	
IgE	<1 mg/dL	Anaphylactic shock Atopic disease (allergies)	
IgG	650–1800 mg/dL	Hepatitis Rheumatoid arthritis Scleroderma	
IgM (*Note*: These tests are often considered serology tests.)	40–250 mg/dL	Biliary cirrhosis Hepatitis Rheumatoid arthritis	Hepatoma
Insulin	4–24 μU/mL	Acromegaly Adenoma of islet cells Untreated mild cases of Type II diabetes	Diabetes mellitus
Iron, total	50–150 μg/dL	Excessive RBC destruction	Iron-deficiency anemia
Iron-binding capacity	250–410 μg/dL	Iron-deficient state Oral contraceptives Polycythemia	Cancer Chronic infections Pernicious anemia Uremia
Ketone bodies	Negative	Marked ketonuria	
Lactic acid	5–20 mg/dL	Acidosis Congestive heart failure Shock	
Lactic dehydrogenase (LDH)	95–200 U/L 80–120 U (Wacker)	Congestive heart failure Hemolytic disorders Hepatitis Metastatic cancer of liver Myocardial infarction Pernicious anemia Pulmonary embolus Skeletal muscle damage	
Lactic dehydrogenase isoenzymes			
LDH_1	10–25%	Myocardial infarction Pernicious anemia Pulmonary embolus Sickle-cell crisis	
LDH_2	25–40%	Myocardial infarction Pulmonary embolus Sickle-cell crisis	
LDH_3	15–25%	Malignant lymphoma Pulmonary embolus	
LDH_4	0–10%	Lupus erythematosus Pulmonary infarction	
LDH_5	0–5%	Congestive heart failure Hepatitis Pulmonary embolus and infarction Skeletal muscle damage	

Table 1 (Continued)

Test	Normal Value	Possible Etiology: Higher	Possible Etiology: Lower
Lipase	0.2–1.5 U/mL	Acute pancreatitis Hepatic disorders Perforated peptic ulcer	
Magnesium	1.5–2.5 mEq/L	Addison's disease Hypothyroidism Renal failure	Chronic alcoholism Hyperparathyroidism Hyperthyroidism Hypoparathyroidism Severe malabsorption
Monospot or Monotest (*Note*: These tests are often considered serology tests.)	Negative	Infectious mononucleosis	
Osmolality	285–295 milliosmoles (mOsm/kg)	Chronic renal disease Diabetes mellitus	Addison's disease Diuretic therapy
Oxygen saturation (arterial)	95–98%	Polycythemia	Anemia Cardiac decompensation Respiratory disorders
pH	See blood gases		
Pepsinogen	350–750 U/mL		Achlorhydria Pernicious anemia
Phenylalanine	0–2 mg/dL	Phenylketonuria	
Phosphatase, acid	0–11 IU/mL 1–4 U (King-Armstrong)	Advanced Paget's disease Cancer of prostate Hyperparathyroidism	
Phosphatase, alkaline	5–13 U (King-Armstrong)	Bone diseases Marked hyperparathyroidism Obstruction of biliary system Rickets	Excessive vitamin D ingestion Hypothyroidism Milk-alkali syndrome
Phosphorus, inorganic	2.8–4.5 mg/dL	Healing fractures Hypoparathyroidism Renal disease Vitamin D intoxication	Diabetes mellitus Hyperparathyroidism Vitamin D deficiency
Potassium	3.5–5.5 mEq/L	Addison's disease Diabetic ketosis Massive tissue destruction Renal failure	Cushing's syndrome Diarrhea (severe) Diuretic therapy Gastrointestinal fistula Pyloric obstruction Starvation Vomiting
Proteins			
Total Albumin Globulin	6.0–8.0 g/dL 3.5–5.0 g/dL 2–3.5 g/dL	Burns Cirrhosis (globulin fraction) Dehydration	Congenital agammaglobulinemia Liver disease Malabsorption
Albumin/globulin ratio	1.5:1–2.5:1	Multiple myeloma (globulin fraction) Shock Vomiting	Malnutrition Nephrotic syndrome Proteinuria Renal disease Severe burns

Table 1 (Continued)

Test	Normal Value	Possible Etiology: Higher	Possible Etiology: Lower
Pyruvic acid	0.3–0.9 mg/dL	Acute phase of some infections Diabetes Thiamine deficiency	
Renin			
Supine	1.4–2.9 ng/mL/h	Renal hypertension	Increased salt intake Primary aldosteronism
Upright	0.4–4.5 ng/mL/h		
Rheumatoid factor (RA factor) (*Note*: This test is often considered a serology test.)	Negative or titer <1:20	Rheumatoid arthritis Sjögren's syndrome Systemic lupus erythematosus	
RPR (*Note*: These tests are often considered serology tests.)	Nonreactive	Syphilis	
Sodium	135–145 mEq/L	Dehydration Impaired renal function Primary aldosteronism Steroid therapy	Addison's disease Diabetic ketoacidosis Diuretic therapy Excessive loss from GI tract Excessive perspiration Water intoxication
Testosterone			
Male	400–120 ng/dL	Polycystic ovary Virilizing tumors	Hypofunction of testes
Female	30–150 ng/dL		
T_4 (thyroxine)	5–12 μg/dL	Hyperthyroidism Thyroiditis	Cretinism Hypothyroidism Myxedema
T_3 uptake	25–35%	Hyperthyroidism Metastatic neoplasms	Hypothyroidism Pregnancy
T_3	110–230 ng/dL	Hyperthyroidism	
Thyroid-stimulating hormone (TSH)	1.9–5.4 μU/mL	Myxedema Primary hypothyroidism	Secondary hypothyroidism
Transaminases			
Serum glutamic-oxaloacetic (SGOT), or aspartate amimotransferase (AST);	15–45 U/L	Liver disease Myocardial infarction Pulmonary infarction Acute hepatitis Liver disease Shock	
Serum glutamic-pyruvic (SGPT), or alanine aminotransferase (ALT)	5–36 U/L		
Triglycerides	40–150 mg/dL	Diabetes mellitus Hyperlipidemia Hypothyroidism Liver disease	Malnutrition
Urea nitrogen (BUN)	10–30 mg/dL	Increased protein catabolism (fever, stress) Renal disease Urinary tract infection	Malnutrition Severe liver damage

Table 1 (Continued)

Test	Normal Value	Possible Etiology	
		Higher	**Lower**
Uric acid	Female: 2.5–5.5 mg/dL Male: 4.5–6.5 mg/dL	Eclampsia Gout Gross tissue destruction High protein weight reduction diet Leukemia Renal failure	Administration of uricosuric drugs
Vitamin A	15–60 μg/dL	Excess ingestion of vitamin A	Vitamin A deficiency
Vitamin B_{12}	200–1000 pg/mL	Myeloid leukemia	Extreme vegetarianism Malabsorption syndrome Pernicious anemia Total or partial gastrectomy
Zinc	50–150 μg/dL		Alcoholic cirrhosis

Table 2
Hematology

Test	Normal Value	Possible Etiology	
		Higher	**Lower**
	Coagulation Tests		
Bleeding time (IVY)	1–6 min	Defective platelet function Thrombocytopenia von Willebrand disease	
Partial thromboplastin (PTT)	60–70 s	Deficiency of factor VIII, IX, and X, XI, XII (hemophilia, liver disease)	
Activated partial thromboplastin time (APTT)	33–45 s	Heparin therapy	
Prothrombim time (Protime, PT)	12–15 s	Anticoagulant therapy Deficiency of factor I, II, V, VII, and X Inadequate vitamin K in diet Liver disease	
Fibrinogen	200–400 mg/dL	Burns (after 1st 36 h) Inflammatory disease	Burns (during 1st 36 h) DIC Severe liver disease
Fibrinolysin (whole blood clot lysis)	None in 24 h	Acute DIC Massive hemorrhage Primary fibrinolysis	
Erythrocyte count*	Male: 4.5–6.0 million/μL (mm^3) Female: 4.0–5.0 million/μL (mm^3)	Dehydration High altitudes Polycythemia vera Severe diarrhea	Anemia Leukemia Posthemorrhage

Table 2 (Continued)

Test	Normal Value	Possible Etiology: Higher	Possible Etiology: Lower
		Erythrocyte Indices	
Mean corpuscular volume (MCV)	82–98 cubic microns (μ^3)	Macrocytic anemia	Microcytic anemia
Mean corpuscular hemoglobin (MCH)	27–31 pg per cell	Macrocytic anemia	Microcytic anemia
Mean corpuscular hemoglobin concentration (MCHC)	32–36%	Spherocytosis	Hypochromic anemia
Erythrocyte sedimentation rate (ESR)	Male: <15 mm/h Female: <20 mm/h	*Moderate Increase:* Acute hepatitis Myocardial infarction Rheumatoid arthritis *Marked Increase:* Acute and severe bacterial infections Malignancies Pelvic inflammatory disease	Malaria Severe liver disease Sickle-cell anemia
Hematocrit*	Male: 40–54% Female: 38–47%	Dehydration High altitudes Polycythemia	Anemia Hemorrhage Overhydration
Hemoglobin*	Male: 13.5–18.0 g/dL Female: 12.0–16.0 g/dL	COPD High altitudes Polycythemia	Anemia Hemorrhage
Platelet count* (thrombocytes)	150,000–400,000/μL (mm³)	Acute infections Chronic granulocytic leukemia Chronic pancreatitis Cirrhosis Collagen disorders Polycythemia Post splenectomy	Acute leukemia Disseminated intravascular coagulation Thrombocytopenic purpura
Reticulocyte count	0.5–1.5% of RBC	Hemolytic anemias Metastatic carcinoma in bone marrow Polycythemia vera	Hypoliferative anemia Macrocytic anemia Microcytic anemia
White blood* cell count	5–10,000/μL (mm³)	Inflammatory and infectious processes	Aplastic anemia Side effects of chemotherapy and irradiation
Differential: 1. Segmented neutrophils	40–60%	Bacterial infections Collagen diseases Hodgkin's disease	Aplastic anemia Viral infections
2. Band neutrophils	0–3%	Acute infections	
3. Lymphocytes	20–40%	Chronic infections Lymphocytic leukemia Mononucleosis Viral infections	Adrenocortical steroid therapy Hodgkin's disease Whole body irradiation

Table 2 (Continued)

Test	Normal Value	Possible Etiology	
		Higher	Lower
4. Monocytes	4–8%	Chronic inflammatory disorders Malaria Monocytic leukemia	
5. Eosinophils	2–4%	Allergic reactions Eosinophilic and granulocytic leukemia Parasitic disorders	Steroid therapy
6. Basophils	0–1%	Acute severe infections Myeloproliferative diseases	Anaphylactic reaction
Sickle-cell preparation	Negative	Sickle cell	
Lupus erythematosus (LE preparation)	No LE cells seen	Lupus erythematosus Rheumatoid arthritis	

*Components of complete blood count (CBC).

Table 3
Urine Chemistry

Test	Specimen	Normal Value	Possible Etiology	
			Higher	Lower
Acetone	Random	Negative	Diabetes mellitus High-fat, low carbohydrate diets Starvation states	
Aldosterone	24 h	2–26 μg/day	*Primary Aldosteronism:* Adrenocortical tumors *Secondary Aldosteronism:* Cardiac failure Cirrhosis Large dose of ACTH Salt depletion	ACTH deficiency Addison's disease Corticosteroid therapy
Amylase	24 h	1000–5000 Somogyi U/day	Acute pancreatitis	
Bence Jones protein	Random	Negative	Multiple myeloma	
Bilirubin	Random	Negative	Hepatitis	
Calcium	24 h	100–250 mg/day	Bone tumor Hyperparathyroidism Milk-alkali syndrome	Hypoparathyroidism Malabsorption of calcium and vitamin D

Table 3 (Continued)

Test	Specimen	Normal Value	Possible Etiology: Higher	Possible Etiology: Lower
Catecholamines Epinephrine Norepinephrine	24 h	<20 μg/day <100 μg/day	Pheochromocytoma Progressive muscular dystrophy	
Chlorides	24 h	110–250 mEq/day	Addison's disease	Burns Excess perspiration Kidney Menstruation
Copper	24 h	<30 μg/day	Cirrhosis Wilson's disease	
Coproporphyrin	24 h	50–200 μg/day	Lead poisoning Oral contraceptive use Poliomyelitis	
Creatine	24 h	<100 mg/day	Carcinoma of liver Endocrine diseases (hyperthyroidism, diabetes, Addison's disease) Infections, burns Muscular dystrophy Skeletal muscle atrophy	Hypothyroidism
Creatinine	24 h	0.8–2.0 g/day	Anemia Leukemia Muscular atrophy *Salmonella*	Renal disease
Creatinine clearance	24 h	85–135 mL/minute		Renal disease
Estrogens	24 h	Female ovulation peak: 28–100 μg/day Luteal peak: 22–105 μg/day Menses: 4–25 μg/day Pregnancy: Up to 45,000 μg/day Menopausal female: 1.4–19.6 μg/day Male: 5–18 μg/day	Gonadal or adrenal tumor	Agenesis of ovaries Endocrine disturbance Ovarian dysfunction
Glucose	Random	Negative	Diabetes mellitus Low renal threshold for glucose resorption Physiological stress Pituitary disorders	
Hemoglobin	Random	Negative	Extensive burns Glomerulonephritis Hemolytic anemias Hemolytic transfusion reaction	
17-Hydroxy-corticosteroids	24 h	Male: 3.5–12 mg/day Female: 3–10 mg/day	Adrenal cancer Cushing's syndrome	Addison's disease Hypofunction of anterior pituitary

Table 3 (Continued)

Test	Specimen	Normal Value	Possible Etiology: Higher	Possible Etiology: Lower
5-Hydroxy-indoleacetic acid (5-HIAA)		2–9 mg/day	Malignant carcinoid syndrome	
17-Ketosteroids	24 h	Male: 10–22 mg/day Female: 6–16 mg/day	Autonomous tumor of adrenals Cushing's syndrome Adrenal hyperplasia Interstitial cell tumor of testes Hyperpituitarism Severe stress	Adrenal cortical insufficiency Diabetes mellitus Hypogonadism Hypopituitarism
Lead	24 h	<100 μg/day	Lead poisoning	
Metanephrine	24 h	<1.3 mg/day	Pheochromocytoma	
Myoglobin	Random	Negative	Crushing injuries Electric shock Extreme physical exertion	
pH	Random	4.0–8.0	Chronic renal failure Compensatory phase of alkalosis Salicylate intoxication Vegetable diet	Compensatory phase of acidosis Dehydration Emphysema
Phenylpyruvic acid	Random	Negative	Phenylketonuria	
Phosphorus, inorganic	24 h	0.9–1.3 g/day	Fever Hypoparathyroidism Nervous exhaustion Rickets TB	Acute infections Nephritis
Porphobilinogen	Random	Negative	Acute intermittent porphyria Liver disorders	
Protein	Random	Negative	Congestive heart failure Nephritis Nephrosis Physiologic stress	
Protein (quantitative)	24 h	<150 mg/day	Cardiac failure Inflammatory processes of urinary tract Nephritis Nephrosis Toxemia of pregnancy	
Sodium	24 h	40–250 mEq/day	Acute tubular necrosis	Hyponatremia
Specific gravity	Random	1.003–1.030	Albuminuria Dehydration Glycosuria	Diabetes insipidus
Titratable acidity	24 h	20–50 mEq/day	Metabolic acidosis	Metabolic alkalosis
Uric acid	24 h	250–750 mg/day	Gout Leukemia	Nephritis
Urobilinogen	24 h	0.5–4.0 mg/day	Hemolytic disease Hepatic parenchymal cell damage Liver disease	Complete obstruction of bile duct
Uroporphyrins	Random	Negative	Porphyria	

Table 4
Miscellaneous Values

	Normal	Possible Etiology: Higher	Possible Etiology: Lower
		Gastric Analysis	
Free hydrochloric acid	0–30 mEq/L	Hypermotility of the stomach	Pernicious anemia
Total acidity	15–45 mEq/L	Gastric and duodenal ulcers	Gastric carcinoma
Combined acidity	10–15 mEq/L	Zollinger-Ellison syndrome	Severe gastritis
		Feces	
Color			
Brown	Various colors depending on diet		
Clay	Biliary obstruction or presence of barium sulfate		
Tarry	If more than 100 mL of blood in GI tract		
Red	Blood in large intestine		
Black	Blood in upper gastrointestinal tract or iron medication		
Fecal fat	<6 g/day	Chronic pancreatic disease Obstruction of common bile duct Malabsorption syndrome	
Urobilinogen	30–220 mg/100 g of stool	Hemolytic anemias	Complete biliary obstruction
Mucus	Negative	Mucous colitis Spastic constipation	
Pus	Negative	Chronic bacillary dysentery Chronic ulcerative colitis Localized abscesses	
Blood*	Negative	Anal fissures Hemorrhoids Malignant tumor Peptic ulcer Ulcerative colitis	
		Cerebrospinal Fluid	
Pressure	60–150 mmH_2O	Hemorrhage Intracranial tumor Meningitis	Head injury Spinal tumor Subdural hematoma
Blood	Negative	Intracranial hemorrhage	
Cell count	WBC: 0–8 cells/μL RBC: None	Inflammation or infections of the CNS	
Chloride	100–130 mEq/L	Uremia	Bacterial infections of CNS (meningitis, encephalitis)
Glucose	45–75 mg/dL	Diabetes mellitus Viral infections of CNS	Bacterial infections and TB of the CNS
Protein			
Lumbar	15–45 mg/dL	Guillain-Barré syndrome Poliomyelitis Traumatic tap	
Cisternal	15–25 mg/dL	Syphilis of CNS	
Ventricular	5–15 mg/dL	Acute meningitis Brain tumor Chronic infections Multiple sclerosis	

*Ingestion of meat may produce false positive results. Client may be placed on a meat-free diet for 3 days prior to test.

Table 5
Toxicology of Common Drugs

Barbiturates		**Therapeutic level**	**Toxic level**
	Short-acting	1–5 mg/dL	>5 mg/dL
	Intermediate-acting	5–14 mg/dL	>30 mg/dL
	Long-acting	15–35 mg/dL	>40 mg/dL
Carbon monoxide (carboxyhemoglobin)	Normal findings		
	Urban nonsmokers	<5% saturation of hemoglobin	
	Suburban nonsmokers	<1.5% saturation of hemoglobin	
	Rural nonsmokers	0.5–2.0% saturation of hemoglobin	
	Smokers	1.5–5.0% saturation of hemoglobin	
	Heavy smokers	5–9% saturation of hemoglobin	
	(Symptoms present with >20% saturation)		
Diazepam (Valium)	Therapeutic level 0.05–0.25 mg/dL Toxic level 0.5 mg/dL Lethal 2 mg/dL		
Digitalis preparations		**Therapeutic level**	**Toxic level**
	Digoxin	1–2 ng/mL	>3 ng/mL
	Digitoxin	14–30 ng/mL	>30 ng/mL
Dilantin	Therapeutic level 10–30 ng/mL		
Ethanol	**Basal alcohol level**	**Effect**	
	20 mg% (20 mg/dL)	Light drinkers begin to feel relaxed.	
	40 mg% (40 mg/dL)	Most people begin to feel relaxed.	
	80 mg% (80 mg/dL)	Impairment of muscle coordination and driving skills. Legally drunk in some states.	
	100 mg% (100 mg/dL)	Deterioration of reaction time and control. Legally drunk in most states.	
	120 mg% (120 mg/dL)	Vomiting occurs unless this level is reached slowly.	
	150 mg% (150 mg/dL)	Balance and movement are impaired. Equivalent of $\frac{1}{2}$ pint whiskey circulating in bloodstream.	
	300 mg% (300 mg/dL)	Most people lose consciousness.	
	400 mg% 400 mg/dL)	Most people lose consciousness and some *die*.	
	450 mg% (450 mg/dL)	Breathing stops.	
Methanol	>20 mg/dL—may be fatal		
Salicylates	Therapeutic level 15–25 mg/dL Toxic level 30 mg/dL Lethal level >60 mg/dL		

Appendix B

Diet Therapies

Virginia M. Hunter
Donna J. Rodriguez

This appendix was reviewed by Elizabeth Anne Linnehan, R.D., Assistant Professor of Nutrition, Nursing Department, Molloy College, Rockville Center, New York, and Elizabeth G. Meyer, R.N., M.S.N., Assistant Professor, Northern Virginia Community College, La Plata, Maryland.

Table 1
High Calorie, High Protein Diet

	Traditional U.S.	Spanish-American	Black
Breakfast	Large orange juice 1 toast with butter or jelly Cream of Wheat with 2 T skim milk powder 2 poached eggs	Large apple juice Flour tortilla with butter Atole with 2 T skim milk powder 2 fried eggs	½ grapefruit Biscuits and gravy Grits with 2 T margarine Omelet with 2 eggs
	High protein milk (2 T skim milk powder added)	High protein milk	High protein milk
Lunch	Cheeseburger on bun with double meat patty, lettuce, tomato French fried potatoes	2 burritos with extra cheese, meat Lettuce and tomato salad with dressing Biscochitos	Split pea soup with ham hocks Grilled cheese sandwich Watermelon wedge
	High protein milkshake	High protein milk	High protein milk
Dinner	Spaghetti with 4 oz meat sauce, parmesan cheese Green beans with 2 T margarine Bread with butter Tapioca pudding	2 tamales with red chili sauce Spanish rice Peas with 2 T butter Custard	4 oz fried chicken Sweet potato Mustard greens with 2 T butter Biscuit Vanilla ice cream
	High protein milk	High protein milk	High protein milk
Snack	Fruit yogurt	Cottage cheese with fruit	½ sandwich with peanut butter Banana

Table 2
Low-Sodium (2 g) Diet

General principles

1. Cook without salt.
2. Do not use table salt.
3. Avoid foods listed in Table 12, High-Sodium Foods.
4. Limit milk to 2 c per day.

Sample Menu Plan for Low-Sodium (2 g) Diet

	Traditional U.S.	Spanish-American	Black
Breakfast	1 c milk $\frac{3}{4}$ c Puffed Wheat Sugar Toast Margarine Scrambled egg Coffee	$\frac{1}{2}$ c milk $\frac{1}{2}$ c Cream of Wheat Sugar Tortilla Fried egg Coffee	$\frac{1}{2}$ c milk $\frac{1}{2}$ c grits Boiled egg 2 t butter 1 biscuit made with low sodium baking powder Coffee
Lunch	$\frac{1}{2}$ c chicken salad sandwich with 1 t mayonnaise Fresh fruit 1 c milk Iced tea	$\frac{1}{2}$ c beans, pinto $\frac{1}{2}$ c chili with meat Tossed salad with oil and vinegar Tortilla $\frac{1}{2}$ c gelatin dessert Coffee	2 oz fried fish Creamed carrots Roll and butter Canned fruit Soda
Dinner	3 oz roast beef 1 baked potato 2 t sour cream 2 t margarine $\frac{1}{2}$ c green beans 1 dinner roll $\frac{1}{2}$ c sherbet Coffee	3 oz fried steak $\frac{1}{2}$ c fried potatoes $\frac{1}{2}$ c zucchini or corn 1 c chocolate pudding Bread and butter or margarine Coffee	3 oz pork chop $\frac{1}{2}$ c boiled potatoes $\frac{1}{2}$ c greens cooked without salt pork 1 c ice cream Sugar cookies Coffee

The above diet is designed for a 2-g sodium restriction. To limit the sodium intake further:

1000 mg Na:	Restrict milk to 1 c Use salt-free butter and vegetables
500 mg Na:	Restrict milk to 1 c Meat limited to 4 oz Use salt-free butter, bread, vegetables, and starches

Table 3

Comparison of Low-Fat Diet with Low Cholesterol, Low Saturated Fat Diet

Diet Principles (Low Fat)

1. Visible fat (e.g., butter, cream, margarine, salad dressing, cooking oil) is restricted to 1 t per meal.
2. Only lean meats, skim milk, and no more than 7 eggs per week are used.
3. Foods high in fat content (e.g., avocados, fat meat, olives, nuts) are avoided.
4. Foods are not prepared with added fat for cooking.

Diet Principles (Low Cholesterol, Low Saturated Fat)

1. The fat content of the diet is modified to increase the ratio of polyunsaturated fatty acids to saturated fatty acids.
2. Organ meats and shellfish are restricted because they are high in cholesterol although low in total fat.
3. Only 3 whole eggs per week are used because egg yolk is high in cholesterol. Egg white may be used as desired.
4. Vegetable oils are used in cooking and food preparation. Coconut, olive palm, and peanut oils are not allowed because of their high content of saturated fats.
5. If weight reduction is desired, calorie level should be specified.

	Traditional U.S.		Spanish-American		Black	
	Low Fat	**Low Cholesterol, Low Saturated Fat**	**Low Fat**	**Low Cholesterol, Low Saturated Fat**	**Low Fat**	**Low Cholesterol, Low Saturated Fat**
Breakfast	$\frac{1}{2}$ c orange juice $\frac{3}{4}$ c dry cereal 1 poached egg 1 slice toast with 1 t margarine or butter 1 c skim milk Coffee with sugar	$\frac{1}{2}$ c orange juice $\frac{3}{4}$ c dry cereal Low cholesterol egg 1 slice toast with 1 t special vegetable oil margarine 1 c skim milk Coffee with sugar	1 banana $\frac{1}{2}$ c oatmeal 1 hard-boiled egg 1 flour tortilla 1 skim milk Coffee with 1 t cream	1 banana $\frac{1}{2}$ c oatmeal 1 corn tortilla with 1 t special vegetable oil margarine 1 c skim milk Coffee with sugar	$\frac{1}{4}$ cantaloupe $\frac{1}{2}$ c corn meal mush 1 scrambled egg 1 slice toast with 1 t butter or margarine 1 c skim milk Coffee with sugar	$\frac{1}{4}$ cantaloupe $\frac{1}{2}$ c corn meal mush 1 slice toast with 1 t special vegetable oil margarine 1 c skim milk Coffee with sugar
Lunch	2 oz baked chicken Mashed potato Tossed salad with vinegar, lemon juice Bread with 1 t margarine or butter Angel food cake Iced tea with sugar and lemon	Baked chicken (skinless) Mashed potato with 1 t special vegetable oil margarine Tossed salad with vinegar, vegetable oil margarine Angel food cake Iced tea with sugar and lemon	2 oz lean hamburger Hamburger bun Lettuce, tomato, pickle 1 t mayonnaise Sherbet Carbonated beverage	$\frac{3}{4}$ c dry cottage cheese with peach slices Saltine crackers Cucumber and tomato slices 1 t special vegetable oil Sherbet Carbonated beverage	2 oz baked fish Baked potato Zucchini Bread with 1 t butter or margarine Gelatin dessert Lemonade	Fried fish (scale fish only; cooked with allowed oils) Fried potatoes (cooked with allowed oils) Zucchini Cornbread (made with allowed oils) Gelatin dessert Lemonade
Dinner	2 oz lean roast beef Rice Green beans Dinner roll with 1 t butter or margarine Canned peach 1 c skim milk	Lean roast beef Rice with 1 t special vegetable oil margarine Green beans Dinner roll with 1 t special vegetable oil margarine Canned peach 1 c skim milk	Green chili stew (made with 2 oz lean beef cubes, potato slices, tomato, chili) 1 flour tortilla Pudding (made from skim milk and egg whites) Fruit punch	Green chili stew (made with lean beef cubes, potato slices, tomato, chili) 1 corn tortilla with 1 t special vegetable oil margarine Pudding (made from skim milk and egg whites) Fruit punch	2 oz lean pork chop Corn on the cob Okra Bread with 1 t margarine or butter Watermelon slice Buttermilk	Breaded lean pork chop Corn on the cob with 1 t special vegetable oil margarine Okra Biscuit (made with allowed oils) Watermelon slice Buttermilk

Table 4
1200-Calorie Weight Reduction Diet

	Exchanges	Traditional U.S.	Spanish-American	Black
Breakfast	1 meat	1 scrambled egg	1 hard-boiled egg	1 oz ham
	2 bread	1 slice toast ¾ c dry cereal (unsweetened)	1 flour tortilla ½ c Cream of Wheat	2 griddle cakes/diet syrup
	1 fruit	½ small banana	½ c orange juice	⅓ c pineapple juice
	1 fat	1 t margarine 1 sausage link*	1 slice bacon	1 t margarine
	1 dairy	1 c low-fat milk	1 c whole milk	1 c whole milk
	Beverage	Coffee	Coffee	Coffee
Lunch	2 meat	1 slice bologna 1 slice cheese	Cheese enchiladas (made with 2 oz cheese, 2 corn tortillas, chili sauce)	2 oz baked breaded pork chop
	2 bread	2 slices bread		1 corn muffin
	Vegetable	Lettuce, pickles	Tomato wedges	Spinach
	1 fruit	Fresh grapes (12)	2 canned peach halves (packed in water)	Fresh orange
	Beverage	Diet soda	Artificially sweetened lemonade	Unsweetened iced tea
Dinner	2 meat	2 oz roast beef	Chili con carne (made with ½ c ground beef, ½ c pinto beans and chili powder)	2 oz baked chicken
	1 bread	Baked potato (with 1 t margarine*)		Corn on the cob
	Vegetable	Cooked carrots	Tossed salad	Okra
	1 fruit	¾ c strawberries	Fresh apple	Fruit cocktail (packed in water)
	1 milk	1 c low-fat milk	1 cup low-fat milk	1 cup low-fat milk

*1 extra fat exchange allowed for each cup of 2% lowfat milk; 2 extra fat exchanges allowed for each cup of skim milk.

Table 5
Post-Gastrectomy (Dumping Syndrome)

Purpose To slow the rapid passage of food into the intestine; to control symptoms of the dumping syndrome (dizziness, sense of fullness, diarrhea, tachycardia) which sometimes occur following a partial or total gastrectomy.

Diet Principles

1. Meals are divided into six small feedings to avoid overloading intestines at mealtimes.
2. Fluids should not be taken with meals, but at least 30–45 minutes before or after meals. This will help prevent distension or feeling of fullness.
3. Concentrated sweets (honey, sugar, jelly, jam, candies, sweet pastries, sweetened fruit) are avoided because they sometimes cause dizziness, diarrhea, and sense of fullness.
4. Protein and fats are increased to promote rebuilding of body tissues and meet energy needs. Meat, cheese, eggs, and milk products are specific foods to increase in the diet.
5. Amount of time these restrictions should be followed vary from client to client. Your health care provider will decide the proper amount of time for you to remain on this prescribed diet according to your condition and progress.

	Traditional U.S.	Spanish-American	Black
Breakfast	1 poached egg 1 slice toast 2 sausage Margarine	1 fried egg 1 corn tortilla 2 slices bacon Margarine	1 oz ham 2 biscuits with 2 t gravy ½ c buttermilk

Table 5 (Continued)

	Traditional U.S.	Spanish-American	Black
10:00 snack	$\frac{3}{4}$ c dry cereal $\frac{1}{2}$ c milk $\frac{1}{2}$ fresh banana Sugar substitute*	$\frac{1}{2}$ c atole $\frac{1}{2}$ c milk 2 unsweetened canned peach halves Sugar substitute*	$\frac{1}{2}$ c grits with 2 T margarine added $\frac{1}{4}$ cantaloupe
Lunch	Grilled cheese sandwich with 2 oz cheese, lettuce 2 unsweetened pear halves	1 burrito with 1 oz meat, 1 oz cheese, $\frac{1}{2}$ c pinto beans, 1 flour tortilla $\frac{1}{2}$ diet gelatin dessert with fruit cocktail added	2 oz fried fish $\frac{1}{2}$ c buttered rice $\frac{1}{2}$ c mustard greens 1 fresh apple
2:00 snack	$\frac{1}{2}$ c plain yogurt 2 graham crackers	$\frac{1}{2}$ c cottage cheese 5 soda crackers	2 t peanut butter 1 slice bread
Dinner	2 oz tomato meatloaf $\frac{1}{2}$ c mashed potatoes with gravy $\frac{1}{2}$ c buttered green beans $\frac{1}{2}$ c unsweetened applesauce	2 tamales $\frac{1}{2}$ c buttered corn 1 fresh orange	2 oz fried pork chop $\frac{1}{2}$ c black-eyed peas $\frac{1}{2}$ c buttered carrots 1 fresh plum
8:00 snack	$\frac{1}{2}$ sandwich with 1 slice bread, 1 oz roast beef, lettuce, mayonnaise	1 corn tortilla with 1 oz melted cheese and green chili	$\frac{1}{2}$ sandwich with 1 slice bread, 1 slice salami, lettuce, mayonnaise

*If allowed by health care provider.

Table 6

High Fiber Diet

Purpose To increase bulk in the daily diet. The bulk provided in the high fiber diet helps to stimulate the intestinal tract and mobilize its contents. This diet is useful for relief of constipation and for clients with diverticulosis.

The following foods are recommended for increasing bulk in the diet.

Food Groups	Food Recommended (High Fiber)
Breads	Whole wheat and whole grain breads, crackers
Cereals	Bran-type cereals such as bran flakes, 100% bran, shredded wheat, oatmeal
Cereal products and flours	Wheat germ, wild rice, buckwheat, cornmeal, millet, rice, bran, whole wheat
Fruits	Fresh fruits with skins: apples, figs, apricots, pears, plums, peaches, berries. Dried fruits: apricots, figs, pears, prunes, dates, currants, raisins
Vegetables	Raw vegetables such as cauliflower, carrots, celery, lettuce, spinach, tomatoes, radishes, mushrooms, cabbage
Meat alternates	Legumes, nuts, seeds
Desserts and sweets	Bran muffins (plain or with dried fruit added) or cookies, oatmeal cookies with raisins
Miscellaneous	Nuts, popcorn

Table 6 (Continued)

Sample Meal Pattern		
Breakfast	**Lunch**	**Dinner**
$\frac{1}{2}$ fresh grapefruit $\frac{1}{2}$ c All-Bran Scrambled egg Whole wheat toast Butter or jam Milk Coffee	Roast beef sandwich on 2 slices whole wheat bread, lettuce, tomato Tossed salad Fresh apple Milk Coffee	Fried chicken Baked potato Peas Coleslaw Whole wheat bread Oatmeal cookies Milk Coffee

Table 7

Low Residue (Fiber) Diet

The low residue diet provides food low in fiber, which will result in a small amount of fecal material in the lower intestinal tract.

Foods	Foods Included	Foods Excluded
Beverages	Carbonated drinks, coffee, tea, cocoa, strained fruit juices	Alcohol, fruit juices with pulp
Bread	White bread, rolls, rusk, melba toast, crackers	Bread and crackers containing whole grain flour or bran, any hot breads such as biscuits, muffins, waffles, or pancakes
Cereals	Cooked refined or strained cereals: Cream of Wheat, Cream of Rice, farina, grits, dry cereals without bran, noodles, spaghetti, and macaroni	Whole grain cereals. Cereals containing bran, nuts, and raisins. Shredded Wheat
Meat	Lean, tender ground beef, lamb, pork, veal or fish, broiled, stewed or baked; canned tuna or salmon; shellfish; crisp bacon, chicken or turkey without skin, liver, cream style peanut butter	Fried, smoked, pickled, or cured meats, highly seasoned ham, fried fish, luncheon meats
Egg	All but fried	Fried or uncooked eggs
Cheese	Milk, cheese (American, cheddar), cottage cheese	All other cheese
Milk	Limit to 1–2 c (if tolerated) including that used in cooking. Plain yogurt	Fruit yogurt
Fats	Butter, margarine, cream, oil, crisp bacon, mayonnaise, plain gravy	Any other. Rich or spiced gravies
Soup	Cream and vegetable soups made from foods allowed and with milk allowed, bouillion, broth, may add strained vegetable juices	Cream and vegetable soups made with foods not allowed (peas and dried beans)
Vegetables	Tender carrots, beets, or asparagus. Strained vegetables, potatoes without skins, vegetable juices	Raw vegetables, all vegetables not strained, dried beans, peas, and legumes
Fruit	Strained fruit juices, ripe bananas, applesauce, pears, peaches, peeled apricots, Napoleon cherries	Raw fruits, fruits with skins, seeds

Table 7 (Continued)

Foods	Foods Included	Foods Excluded
Desserts	Plain desserts (custards and puddings, plain ice cream from milk allowance), sherbert, plain gelatin desserts, angel food cake, sponge cake, plain butter cake, plain cookies	Nuts, coconut, raisins, rich desserts (pies, rich cakes, cobblers)
Condiments	Allspice, cinnamon, mace, paprika, salt, ground thyme, sugar, vinegar, lemon juice	All others

For a more restricted residue diet, milk should be eliminated.

Table 8
Low Protein Diet for Hepatic Failure

General principles

1. Limit protein to 20 g per day at onset of severe hepatic failure.
2. Protein must be from high biological value protein sources.
3. Diet must be high in calories.
4. Fat limited only to prevent early satiety.
5. Increase protein in diet by 10-g increments as tolerated without causing signs/symptoms of hepatic encephalopathy.
6. Sodium is also usually restricted as well as fluid when edema and ascites are present.

	Traditional U.S.	Spanish-American	Black
Breakfast	$\frac{1}{2}$ c grape juice with 2 T Polycose powder* French toast made with low protein bread, 1 egg—serve with salt-free butter and syrup $\frac{1}{4}$ c milk	$\frac{1}{4}$ c cranberry juice with 2 T Polycose powder Low protein toast with 3 salt-free butters and 2 t jelly 1 egg omelet with 3 salt-free butters $\frac{1}{4}$ c milk	$\frac{1}{4}$ c prune juice with 2 T Polycose powder Low protein toast with 3 salt-free butters 1 egg fried in 3 salt-free butters $\frac{1}{4}$ c milk
Snack	Jelly beans	Hard candy	Sugar mints
Lunch	$\frac{1}{4}$ c half and half $\frac{1}{2}$ c Cream of Wheat with 3 salt-free butters Small tossed salad with 3 T oil and vinegar‡ Applesauce with whipped topping or Lipomul† Peas with 3 salt-free butters	$\frac{1}{4}$ c half and half $\frac{1}{2}$ c cornmeal cereal (atole) with 3 salt-free butters Small guacamole salad Gelatin with whipped topping or Lipomul Corn with 3 salt-free butters	$\frac{1}{4}$ c half and half $\frac{1}{2}$ c grits with 3 salt-free butters Cucumbers in sour cream Peaches with whipped topping or Lipomul Sweet potatoes with brown sugar and 3 salt-free butters
Snack	Low protein cookies	Low protein bread cubes with whipped cream and strawberries	Popsicles made with Polycose
Dinner	$\frac{1}{2}$ baked potato 3 salt-free butters $\frac{1}{4}$ c sour cream $\frac{1}{2}$ c green beans with 3 salt-free butters Low protein toast with 3 salt-free butters and 2 t jelly $\frac{1}{4}$ c milk	$\frac{1}{2}$ c fried potatoes with 1 melted salt-free butter $\frac{1}{2}$ c zucchini with 3 salt-free butters Low protein toast with 3 salt-free butters and 2 t marmalade $\frac{1}{4}$ c milk	$\frac{1}{2}$ c mashed potatoes $\frac{1}{2}$ c fried okra Low protein toast with 3 salt-free butters and 2 t jam $\frac{1}{4}$ c milk

*Polycose is a brand name product made by Ross Laboratories.
†Lipomul is a fat emulsion made by Upjohn.
‡One must keep in mind the possibility of esophageal varices and avoid crisp foods if they are present.

Table 9

Low Protein Diet for Renal Failure

Diet allowance

40 g Protein
2 g Sodium
40 mEq Potassium
1500 mL Fluid

	Exchanges	Traditional U.S.	Spanish-American	Black
Breakfast	1 fruit	60 mL grape juice	60 mL apple juice	Applesauce
	1 bread	Toast or corn flakes	Tortilla	Grits
	1 meat	Scrambled egg	Fried egg	Poached egg
	3 fat	2 margarine or butter 30 mL cream Jelly	2 butter 30 mL cream Jam	2 butter 30 mL cream Jam
	Beverage	250 mL decaffeinated coffee	250 mL decaffeinated coffee	250 mL decaffeinated coffee
	Dairy	120 mL milk	120 mL milk	120 mL milk
Lunch	1 meat 2 bread	Salt-free tuna $\frac{1}{4}$ c 2 slices bread	2 enchiladas (using $\frac{1}{4}$ c ground beef, 2 corn tortillas, and shredded lettuce)	Fried chicken leg Cornbread $\frac{1}{2}$ c rice
	Vegetable	Lettuce and cucumber	Chili sauce	Zucchini
	Fruit	Canned plums	Canned pears	Canned peaches
	2 fat	2 T salt-free mayonnaise	2 T oil for cooking	1 butter 1 T oil for cooking
		Hard candy	Jelly beans	Hard candy
	Beverage	250 mL carbonated beverage	250 mL carbonated beverage	250 mL carbonated beverage
Dinner	1 meat	1 oz fried fresh fish	1 oz chicken	1 oz pork
	1 bread	$\frac{1}{2}$ c mashed potatoes (using presoaked potatoes)	1 salt-free corn or flour tortilla to make chicken taco	Salt-free corn on the cob
	Vegatable	Salt-free green peas	Tossed salad	Salt-free green beans
	Fruit	Fruit cocktail	Canned pineapple	Grapes
	3 fat	30 mL cream 1 T oil for cooking 1 butter	30 mL cream Salt-free dressing 2 T	30 mL cream 2 butter
	Beverage	250 mL fruit punch 250 mL decaffeinated coffee	250 mL fruit punch 250 mL decaffeinated coffee	250 mL fruit punch 250 mL decaffeinated coffee
Snack		120 mL gelatin dessert with whipped topping	180 mL Popsicle	Butterballs
		140 mL carbonated beverage*	80 mL carbonated beverage	320 mL carbonated beverage

*Coke is an acceptable beverage.

Table 10
Menu Plan for 1800-Calorie Diabetic Diet

	Exchanges	Traditional U.S.	Exchanges	Spanish-American	Exchanges	Black
Breakfast	$\frac{1}{2}$ milk 2 bread 1 meat 1 fat 1 fruit	$\frac{1}{2}$ c low-fat milk 1 slice toast $\frac{3}{4}$ c corn flakes Scrambled egg 1 margarine (+ $\frac{1}{2}$ from low-fat milk) $\frac{1}{2}$ c orange juice Coffee	$\frac{1}{2}$ milk 2 bread 1 meat 1 fat 1 fruit	$\frac{1}{2}$ c whole milk $\frac{1}{2}$ c atole 1 6″ tortilla Fried egg 1 butter $\frac{1}{2}$ c grapefruit juice Coffee	$\frac{1}{2}$ milk 2 bread 1 meat 1 fat 1 fruit	$\frac{1}{2}$ c buttermilk 1 cup grits Poached egg 1 butter (+ 1 from buttermilk) $\frac{1}{3}$ c apple juice Coffee
Lunch	$\frac{1}{2}$ milk 2 breads 3 meat 2 fat 1 fruit 1 vegetable	$\frac{1}{2}$ c low-fat milk 2 halves of a hamburger bun 3 oz hamburger 2 tablespoons French dressing Small apple Tossed salad Diet soda	3 bread 3 meat 1 fat 1 fruit 1 vegetable	$\frac{1}{2}$ c potatoes $\frac{1}{4}$ c beans $1\frac{1}{2}$ corn tortillas 1 oz cheese $\frac{1}{2}$ c ground beef 1 t oil for frying $\frac{1}{2}$ c pineapple (drain syrup) Lettuce and tomatoes Fruit-flavored diet drink	3 bread 3 meat 1 fat 1 fruit 1 vegetable	1 c rice 1 2″ square cornbread 3 oz fried chicken 1 t oil for frying $\frac{1}{2}$ c peaches (drain syrup) $\frac{1}{2}$ c zucchini Unsweetened iced tea
Snack	1 fruit	Small orange	1 fruit	2 small apricots	1 fruit	1 c watermelon
Dinner	$\frac{1}{2}$ milk 2 bread 3 meat 1 vegetable 1 fruit	$\frac{1}{2}$ c low-fat milk $\frac{1}{2}$ c mashed potatoes 1 small dinner roll 3 oz chicken $\frac{1}{2}$ c green beans $\frac{1}{2}$ c fruit cocktail (drain syrup) Coffee	3 bread 3 meat 1 vegetable 1 fruit	1 6″ tortilla Green chili stew made with 1 c potatoes, 3 oz stew meat, tomatoes and green chili $\frac{1}{2}$ c pears (drain syrup) Coffee	3 bread 3 meat 1 vegetable 1 fruit	1 c fried potatoes 1 2″ biscuit 3 oz pork chop Stewed tomatoes $\frac{1}{2}$ c applesauce Coffee
Snack	$\frac{1}{2}$ milk 1 bread 1 meat 1 fat	$\frac{1}{2}$ c low-fat milk 4 crackers 1 oz cheese 1 margarine	2 bread 1 meat 1 fat	Sandwich—2 slices bread 1 slice lunchmeat 1 pat butter	2 bread 1 meat 1 fat	Sandwich—2 slices bread 2 T peanut butter 1 pat butter

Table 11
High Potassium Foods

Fruits

Apricots
Apricot nectar
Avocado
Banana
Cantaloupe
Currants, fresh
Dates
Dried fruit
Figs, fresh, dried
Elderberries, raw
Grapefruit
Grapefruit juice
Honeydew melon
Nectarine
Orange, fresh
Orange juice
Papaya, fresh
Peach, fresh
Pear, fresh
Pineapple, fresh
Pineapple juice
Pomegranate
Prunes, fresh, dried
Prune juice
Raisins
Tangerine

Vegetables

Artichokes
Broccoli
Dried beans, lima, pinto, red,
White, cooked, mung, soy
Dried peas, split
Leafy greens—collard, spinach
Swiss chard, turnip
Mushrooms, fresh, cooked
Parsnips
Potato, sweet or white
Pumpkin
Rhubarb
Rutabagas
Squash, winter
Tomatoes
Tomato juice
V-8 juice
Yams

Miscellaneous

Bran cereals and breads, wheat germ
Brown sugar, molasses
Chocolate, cocoa
Nuts and seeds

Table 12
High-Sodium Foods

Beverages	Mineral water, club soda Dutch processed cocoa
Breads	Saltines, baking powder biscuits, muffins, Bisquick, pretzels, salted snack crackers and chips Quick breads such as cornbread, nut bread, etc. Pancakes, waffles, including mixes
Cereals	Instant cooked cereal Processed bran type cereals Commercial Granola
Dairy	Commercial buttermilk Regular cheese
Desserts	Commercial baked products Baked products and puddings made from mixes
Fats	Bacon fat; salted nuts or seeds Commercial dips (sour cream type, etc.) Regular salad dressings and mayonnaise
Juices	Tomato juice, V-8 juice, Clamato, bloody mary mixes
Meat	Smoked or cured products—bacon, ham, sausage, salt pork, hot dogs, lunch meat, corned or chipped beef, organ meats, shellfish, sardines, herring, anchovies, caviar, kosher meats, canned tuna fish and salmon, mackerel
Potato or substitute	Salted potato chips, salted french fries, instant potatoes, rice, or noodle mixes
Seasonings	Salt, excessive amounts of baking powder, baking soda Celery, onion, and garlic salt and other seasoned salt and peppers. Meat tenderizers, Ac'Cent, msg, worcestershire, soy sauce, mustard, catsup, horseradish, chili sauce, tomato sauce, barbeque sauce, steak sauce
Soup	Commercial soups, bouillon cubes, or powdered dehydrated soups
Vegetables	Sauerkraut, tomato juice, V-8 juice, vegetables in creamed or seasoned sauces. Frozen vegetables processed with salt or sodium
Miscellaneous	Olives, pickles, salted popcorn, commercially prepared entrees (frozen or canned, e.g., pot pies, TV dinners, etc.) Mexican, Italian, Oriental dishes as ordinarily prepared

Table 13
Vegetarian Protein Sources

Combinations of vegetable and grain proteins in the correct proportions and/or nonmeat proteins such as milk, cheese, etc. can provide complete proteins (all 8 essential amino acids).

Some complementary protein sources are:

$\frac{1}{4}$ c beans + $\frac{2}{3}$ c rice
$1\frac{1}{2}$ T soybeans + $\frac{3}{4}$ c rice
$\frac{1}{3}$ c sesame seeds + 1 c rice
$\frac{3}{4}$ c rice + 1 c skim milk *or* 5 T dry nonfat milk
$\frac{3}{4}$ c rice + $1\frac{1}{4}$ oz cheese
$2\frac{1}{2}$ T beans + $\frac{3}{4}$ c bulgur
$\frac{2}{3}$ c whole wheat flour + $2\frac{1}{2}$ T soy flour
$\frac{1}{4}$ c beans + 1 c cornmeal *or* 6 corn tortillas
$2\frac{1}{2}$ T whole wheat flour + $\frac{2}{3}$ c dry milk + 1 c cornmeal
$\frac{1}{3}$ c beans + 1 oz cheese
$\frac{1}{4}$ c peanuts + $\frac{1}{3}$ c sunflower seeds

All the above are raw ingredients. Each combination provides the same amount of protein available in a 3-oz steak.

Table 14
Low Cost Protein Supplements

(Each supplies approximately 7 g of protein, equal to 1 oz of meat)

Food	Amount
Brewer's yeast	$2\frac{1}{3}$ T
Cheese	1-in cube
Cottage cheese	$\frac{1}{4}$ c
Egg	1
Milk, whole, low-fat, skim	$\frac{7}{8}$ c
Peanut butter	2 T
Pinto beans	$\frac{1}{4}$ c
Poultry	1 oz
Soybeans (cooked)	1 c + 2 T
Split peas, lentils (cooked)	7 T (or $\frac{1}{2}$ c)

Appendix C

Answer Key to Review Questions

CHAPTER 1

1. a
2. d
3. b
4. d
5. a
6. a
7. c

CHAPTER 2

1. a
2. c
3. d
4. b
5. d
6. b
7. a
8. b

CHAPTER 3

1. b
2. b
3. b
4. d
5. a
6. d

CHAPTER 4

1. b
2. d
3. c
4. d
5. c
6. d
7. d

CHAPTER 5

1. b
2. d
3. c
4. b
5. c
6. a
7. c
8. d

CHAPTER 6

1. b
2. b
3. c
4. a
5. a
6. c
7. a
8. d

CHAPTER 7

1. b
2. a
3. c
4. b
5. d
6. a
7. a
8. d
9. d

CHAPTER 8

1. b
2. b
3. b
4. a
5. c

CHAPTER 9

1. a
2. c
3. b
4. c
5. d
6. b
7. d
8. a
9. c
10. b

CHAPTER 10

1. d
2. d
3. b
4. a
5. c
6. d
7. c
8. b
9. a
10. d
11. c
12. c

CHAPTER 11

1. d
2. a
3. c
4. a
5. c
6. b
7. d
8. d
9. d
10. b
11. d
12. a
13. d
14. a
15. c

CHAPTER 12

1. c
2. b
3. b
4. b
5. a
6. c
7. d
8. d
9. a

CHAPTER 13

1. c
2. a
3. c
4. b
5. c
6. c
7. a
8. b
9. b

CHAPTER 14

1. b
2. d
3. a
4. a
5. b
6. c

CHAPTER 15

1. c
2. a
3. c
4. b
5. b
6. b
7. d
8. a

9. b
10. d

CHAPTER 16

1. a
2. c
3. c
4. a
5. a
6. a
7. b
8. d

CHAPTER 17

1. b
2. a
3. d
4. a
5. d
6. c
7. b
8. b
9. c
10. c

CHAPTER 18

1. c
2. b
3. b
4. a
5. c
6. d
7. a
8. c
9. d
10. d

CHAPTER 19

1. b
2. b
3. c
4. c
5. b
6. d
7. a
8. d

CHAPTER 20

1. c
2. a
3. c
4. d
5. c
6. a
7. b
8. a
9. a
10. d
11. d
12. c
13. a

CHAPTER 21

1. a
2. b
3. b
4. d
5. c
6. b

CHAPTER 22

1. d
2. a
3. b
4. b
5. a
6. c
7. d

CHAPTER 23

1. c
2. a
3. b
4. c
5. c
6. a
7. d

CHAPTER 24

1. c
2. d
3. b
4. d
5. c
6. c
7. d
8. a
9. b
10. d
11. c
12. d
13. c
14. b
15. c
16. c

CHAPTER 25

1. c
2. b
3. a
4. d
5. c
6. a
7. b
8. a
9. c
10. d

CHAPTER 26

1. a
2. c
3. b
4. a
5. a
6. d
7. a
8. c
9. b
10. a
11. b
12. b
13. c
14. b

CHAPTER 27

1. b
2. d
3. b
4. a
5. c
6. d
7. c
8. d
9. c
10. b
11. a
12. b

CHAPTER 28

1. a
2. c
3. d
4. c
5. d
6. a
7. b
8. a
9. d
10. b
11. c

CHAPTER 29

1. a
2. a
3. b
4. c
5. c
6. d
7. d

CHAPTER 30

1. a
2. d
3. c
4. a
5. b
6. a
7. b
8. c
9. c
10. d

CHAPTER 31

1. d
2. a

3. a
4. c
5. b
6. d
7. a
8. a

CHAPTER 32

1. a
2. a
3. d
4. b
5. a
6. a
7. d
8. b
9. b
10. c
11. a

CHAPTER 33

1. b
2. d
3. c
4. a
5. c
6. c
7. a
8. a
9. d
10. b
11. c

CHAPTER 34

1. b
2. c
3. a
4. c
5. a
6. d
7. a
8. d
9. b
10. a
11. a
12. a
13. a
14. a
15. d

CHAPTER 35

1. b
2. d
3. b
4. c
5. b
6. a
7. c
8. d
9. c
10. a
11. d

CHAPTER 36

1. b
2. c
3. b
4. d
5. c
6. c
7. b

CHAPTER 37

1. b
2. b
3. c
4. c
5. b
6. b
7. a
8. a
9. d
10. d
11. c
12. c

CHAPTER 38

1. b
2. b
3. d
4. c
5. b
6. b
7. c
8. c
9. b
10. c
11. c

CHAPTER 39

1. d
2. c
3. c
4. a
5. c
6. d
7. b

CHAPTER 40

1. b
2. c
3. d
4. c
5. a
6. a
7. b
8. a

CHAPTER 41

1. b
2. a
3. b
4. b
5. d
6. c
7. c
8. d
9. c

CHAPTER 42

1. a
2. d
3. a
4. d
5. b
6. d
7. c
8. d
9. a

CHAPTER 43

1. c
2. d
3. b
4. a
5. b
6. e
7. c

CHAPTER 44

1. d
2. a
3. a
4. d
5. c
6. b
7. c

CHAPTER 45

1. a
2. d
3. d
4. c
5. b
6. b

CHAPTER 46

1. c
2. c
3. d
4. b
5. b
6. c
7. a
8. d
9. b
10. c
11. d
12. d
13. b
14. a
15. d

CHAPTER 47

1. d
2. b

3. d
4. d

CHAPTER 48

1. c
2. a
3. d
4. b
5. d
6. d
7. a
8. c
9. b
10. d

CHAPTER 49

1. b
2. c
3. d

CHAPTER 50

1. d
2. c
3. b
4. a
5. d
6. c
7. a
8. a
9. c

CHAPTER 51

1. c
2. c
3. b
4. a
5. d
6. d
7. b

CHAPTER 52

1. a
2. b
3. b
4. c
5. b
6. b
7. a
8. a
9. a
10. b

CHAPTER 53

1. c
2. d
3. b
4. c
5. a
6. a
7. b
8. c

CHAPTER 54

1. d
2. b
3. c
4. d
5. a
6. c
7. d
8. a
9. c
10. d
11. d
12. a
13. b

CHAPTER 55

1. b
2. c
3. c
4. b
5. c
6. c
7. c

CHAPTER 56

1. a
2. d
3. c
4. d
5. d
6. a
7. c
8. c
9. a
10. b
11. a
12. d
13. c
14. b

CHAPTER 57

1. c
2. b
3. c
4. b
5. d
6. a
7. d
8. b

CHAPTER 58

1. c
2. d
3. c
4. a
5. d
6. b
7. d
8. d
9. a

CHAPTER 59

1. a
2. b
3. c
4. b
5. d

CHAPTER 60

1. c
2. b
3. a
4. c
5. c
6. a
7. c
8. b
9. d
10. b
11. a
12. a
13. d

INDEX

INDEX